OXFORD MEDICAL PUBLICATIONS

OXFORD TEXTBOOK OF SURGERY

EDITORS

PETER J. MORRIS

Nuffield Professor of Surgery and Chairman
Nuffield Department of Surgery
Oxford Radcliffe Hospital
The John Radcliffe
Oxford

RONALD A. MALT

Professor of Surgery
Harvard Medical School
Surgical Chief
Liver, Biliary, and Pancreas Center
Massachusetts General Hospital

OXFORD TEXTBOOK OF SURGERY

Edited by

PETER J. MORRIS AND RONALD A. MALT

VOLUME 1

New York Oxford Tokyo
OXFORD UNIVERSITY PRESS
1994

Oxford University Press, Walton Street, Oxford OX2 6DP

Oxford New York
Athens Auckland Bangkok Bombay
Calcutta Cape Town Dar es Salamm Delhi
Florence Hong Kong Istanbul Karachi
Kuala Lumpur Madras Madrid Melbourne
Mexico City Nairobi Paris Singapore
Taipei Tokyo Toronto
and associated companies in
Berlin Ibadan

Oxford is a trade mark of Oxford University Press

Published in the United States
by Oxford University Press Inc., New York

A catalogue record for this book is available from the British Library

Library of Congress Cataloging in Publication Data
(cataloging Data available)
ISBN 0 19 261800 8 (Two Volume Set)
ISBN 0 19 262603 5 (Vol 1)
ISBN 0 19 262604 3 (Vol 2)
(Available as a two volume set only)

Typeset by Create Publishing Services Ltd, Bath
Printed in Hong Kong

Preface

The Oxford Textbook of Surgery aims to present a picture of surgery in its totality. To achieve this it has brought together the experience of surgical practice from two major clinical schools on opposite sides of the Atlantic, namely the Oxford University Clinical School and the Massachusetts General Hospital Clinical School of the Harvard Medical School, for most of the contributors are on the staff of one or the other or have worked in one or other institution in the past. In some instances former visiting Professors have been brought into play but the vast majority of contributors can claim some allegiance to one or other institution. We have found, not surprisingly perhaps, that, with one or two notable exceptions, such as, for example, in the approach to cancer of the prostate, the practice of surgery in the United Kingdom and the United States does not differ remarkably. Each subject has been covered by an expert in the field writing from his or her own wisdom and experience, but remembereing past needs and difficulties during training days.

In this book we have approached surgery from a practical point of view and have attempted to cover most aspects of general surgery (an entity less easily defined nowadays) as well as giving an overview of the various specialist branches of surgery ranging from orthopaedics and neurosurgery through cardiothoracic surgery to plastic surgery. To achieve detailed coverage of every aspect of surgery in one textbook is obviously impossible, but our aims were to produce a book which could be used as a source of reference by general surgeons, either trained or in training, both in the Western world and in developing countries, and equally to provide a ready source of reference for surgeons in specialist branches of surgery, such as neurosurgery and orthopaedic surgery. We hope that with this approach general surgeons will not only get a feeling for current practice in their own areas of interest but will also be able to obtain sufficient information about problems presenting in their patients that involve, or might involve, another speciality. Similarly the specialist surgeon can also find sufficient material in the Textbook concerning some problem in general surgery or another specialist branch of surgery to be able to reassure a patient or to use for teaching purposes. We feel strongly that there is still a major need for a comprehensive textbook of surgery in this age of increasing specialization. Our approach should also prove invaluable to the medical undergraduate as well as to the surgeon practising in developing countries, where the general surgeon remains truly a generalist.

We have endeavoured to make the text become alive and attractive by the widespread use of colour for illustrations and tables, a major innovation for a textbook of surgery. This aim has certainly been achieved in our opinion by our publishers, Oxford University Press. Our thanks are due to their staff.

We are grateful to all our contributors who have been most patient during the gestation of the book. We especially wish to thank Mr Steve Westaby and Dr John Baldwin who organized the cardiac surgery section, Mr Chris Adams who planned the neurosurgery section, Dr Steve Dretler for the urology section, and Dr Michael Ehrlich of Brown University (formerly MGH) who, with his department, dealt with the whole of the orthopaedic section.

We hope that you will find this book an attractive and readily approachable treatise on surgery in its entirety, whether you be practising, training, or studying in the Western world or indeed in a developing country with limited resources.

Peter J. Morris
Oxford

Ronald A. Malt
Boston

Volume 1 Contents

Volume 2 Contents

Contributors

WILLIAM M. ABBOTT
Professor of Surgery, Harvard Medical School; Chief of Vascular Surgery, Massachusetts General Hospital, Boston, USA

C. B. T. ADAMS
Senior Consultant Neurosurgeon, Radcliffe Infirmary, Oxford; Lecturer in Neurosurgery, University of Oxford

N. SCOTT ADZICK
Associate Professor of Surgery and Pediatrics, University of California, San Francisco, USA

EDWARD AKELMAN
Chief, Division of Hand, Upper Extremity, and Microvascular Surgery, Brown University Medical School, Rhode Island Hospital, Providence, USA

MARK S. ALLEN
Consultant in General Thoracic Surgery, Mayo Clinic; Assistant Professor of Surgery, Mayo Medical School, Rochester, Minnesota, USA

ALEX F. ALTHAUSEN
Associate Professor of Surgery, Harvard Medical School; Urologist, Massachusetts General Hospital, Boston, USA

PHILIP C. AMREIN
Assistant Professor of Medicine, Harvard Medical School, Boston, Massachusetts, USA

J. P. ANTHONY
Senior Registrar, Obstetrics and Gynaecology, Oxford Radcliffe Maternity Hospital

NICHOLAS ARCHER
Consultant Paediatric Cardiologist, Oxford Radcliffe Hospital

BRUNO ARENA
Visiting Fellow in Gynecologic Oncology, Women's & Infants' Hospital, Brown University, Providence, Rhode Island, USA

HUGH AUCHINCLOSS
Associate Visiting Surgeon, Massachusetts General Hospital and Associate Professor of Surgery, Harvard Medical School, Boston, USA

ROBERT J. BAIGRIE
Clinical Lecturer, Nuffield Department of Surgery, University of Oxford Clinical Medical School, Oxford Radcliffe Hospital

MICHAEL T. BAILIN
Instructor in Anesthesia, Harvard Medical School; Assistant Anesthetist, Massachusetts General Hospital, Boston, USA

JOHN C. BALDWIN
Professor and Chief, Cardiothoracic Surgery, Yale University, New Haven, Connecticut, USA

DAVID H. BARLOW
Nuffield Professor of Obstetrics and Gynaecology, University of Oxford, Oxford Radcliffe Hospital

HUGH BARR
Consultant Gastrointestinal Surgeon, Gloucestershire Royal Hospital; Hunterian Professor, Royal College of Surgeons of England

BARBARA BASSIL
Instructor in Surgery, Harvard Medical School; Associate in Urology, Massachusetts General Hospital, Boston, USA

GLENN E. BEHRINGER
Honorary Surgeon, Massachusetts General Hospital, Boston, USA

MALCOLM K. BENSON
Consultant Physician, Osler Chest Unit, Oxford Radcliffe Hospital

DAVID L. BERGER
Resident in Surgery, Massachusetts General Hospital; Clinical Fellow in Surgery, Harvard Medical School, Boston, USA

ALAN R. BERRY
Consultant Surgeon, Northampton General Hospital, Northampton, UK

KENNETH I. BICKERSTAFF
Consultant Surgeon, Princess Royal Hospital, Telford, Shropshire, UK

LUCA M. BIGATELLO
Instructor in Anesthesia, Harvard Medical School, Massachusetts General Hospital, Boston, USA

PETER C. BLOCK
Associate Director, St Vincent Heart Institute, Portland, Oregon, USA

LAWRENCE F. BORGES
Associate Visiting Neurosurgeon, Massachusetts General Hospital, Boston, USA

WILLIAM D. BOYD
Senior Registrar, Obstetrics and Gynaecology, Oxford Radcliffe Hospital

MELBOURNE D. BOYNTON
Assistant Professor of Orthopedic Surgery, Medical College of Wisconsin, Milwaukee, USA

ALLAN R. BRASIER
Associate Professor of Internal Medicine, University of Texas Medical Branch, Galveston, USA

DAVID C. BREWSTER
Associate Clinical Professor of Surgery, Massachusetts General Hospital and Harvard Medical School, Boston, USA

JULIAN BRITTON
Consultant Surgeon, Oxford Radcliffe Hospital

CHERYL J. BUNKER
Assistant Physician, Massachusetts General Hospital; Instructor in Medicine, Harvard Medical School, Boston, USA

WALTER J. BURDETTE
Adj. Professor, University of Houston; Chief, Thoracic and Cardiovascular Surgery, Park Plaza Hospital, Houston, Texas, USA

KEVIN G. BURNAND
Professor of Vascular Surgery, United Medical and Dental Schools of Guy's and St Thomas's Hospitals, St Thomas's Campus, St Thomas's Hospital, London

MICHAEL J. CALLAM
Consultant Surgeon, Bedford General Hospital, UK

RICHARD P. CAMBRIA
Associate Professor of Surgery, Harvard Medical School; Associate Visiting Surgeon, Massachusetts General Hospital, Boston, USA

W. BRUCE CAMPBELL
Consultant Vascular and General Surgeon, Royal Devon and Exeter Hospital, Exeter, UK

JAMES CARMICHAEL
CRC Professor of Clinical Oncology, University of Nottingham, UK

LEN E. S. CARRIE
Consultant Anaesthetist, Nuffield Department of Anaesthetics, Oxford Radcliffe Hospital

DAVID C. CARTER
Regius Professor of Clinical Surgery, Edinburgh University Medical School, Edinburgh, UK

JANE E. CARTER
Yale University School of Medicine, New Haven, Connecticut, USA

PAUL H. CHAPMAN
Chief of Pediatric Neurosurgery, Massachusetts General Hospital, Boston, USA

R. W. CHAPMAN
Consultant Gastroenterologist, Oxford Radcliffe Hospital

F. MARK CHARNOCK
Consultant Obstetrician and Gynaecologist, Oxford Radcliffe Maternity Hospital

MACK L. CHENEY
Assistant Professor of Orolaryngology, Harvard Medical School; Director, Facial Plastic and Reconstructive Surgery, Massachusetts Eye and Ear Infirmary, Boston, USA

GEORGE W. CHERRY
Principal Clinical Scientific Officer, Department of Dermatology, Oxford Radcliffe Hospital

T. K. CHOI
Queen Mary Hospital, Hong Kong

S. C. SYDNEY CHUNG
Senior Lecturer in Surgery, Prince of Wales Hospital, The Chinese University, Hong Kong

P. JANE CLARKE
Consultant Surgeon, Oxford Radcliffe Hospital

CAROL A. COBB
Part-time Senior Registrar, Gastroenterology Unit, Oxford Radcliffe Hospital

RICHARD COBB
Consultant Surgery, Birmingham Heartlands Hospital, Birmingham, UK

JEAN-MARIE COLLARD
Oesophageal Surgeon, St Luc Academic Hospital, Louvain Medical School, Brussels, Belgium

JACK COLLIN
Consultant Surgeon, Oxford Radcliffe Hospital; Reader in Surgery, University of Oxford

R. E. CONDON
Ausman Foundation Professor and Chairman of the Department of Surgery, The Medical College of Wisconsin, Milwaukee, USA

ALASDAIR K. T. CONN
Chief of Emergency Services, Massachusetts General Hospital, Boston, USA

BAIRBRE L. CONNOLLY
Colin McStay Research Fellow, Children's Research Centre, Our Lady's Hospital for Sick Children, Crumlin, Dublin, Ireland

DAVID J. CONTI
Associate Professor of Surgery, Albany Medical College; Director, Section of Transplantation, Albany Medical Center Hospital, New York, USA

MARTIN T. CORBALLY
Consultant Paediatric and Transplant Surgeon, Our Lady's Hospital for Sick Children, Crumlin, Dublin, Ireland

A. BENEDICT COSIMI
Professor of Surgery, Harvard Medical School; Chief, Transplantation Unit, Massachusetts General Hospital, Boston, USA

JAMES L. COX
Evarts A. Graham Professor of Surgery, Washington University Medical School, St Louis, Missouri, USA

DAVID CRANSTON
Consultant Urological Surgeon, Oxford Radcliffe Hospital

THOMAS G. CROPLEY
Assistant Professor, Division of Dermatology, Department of Medicine, University of Massachusetts Medical Center, Worcester, USA

ROBERT M. CROWELL
Director, Brain Aneurysm/AVM Center, Massachusetts General Hospital, Boston, USA

ALEKSANDAR CURCIN
Assistant Professor of Orthopedics, University of Maryland School of Medicine, Baltimore, USA

A. S. DAAR
Professor and Chairman, Department of Surgery, College of Medicine, Sultan Qaboos University, Muscat, Sultanate of Oman

WILLARD M. DAGGETT
Professor of Surgery, Harvard Medical School; Visiting Surgeon, Massachusetts General Hospital, Boston, USA

M. J. DAVIES
Professor of Cardiovascular Pathology, St George's Hospital Medical School, University of London, UK

THOMAS C. B. DEHN
Consultant Surgeon, Royal Berkshire Hospital, Reading, Berkshire, UK

FRANCIS L. DELMONICO
Associate Professor of Surgery, Harvard Medical School; Director, Renal Transplantation, Massachusetts General Hospital, Boston, USA

ZAREH DEMIRJIAN
Massachusetts General Hospital, Boston, USA

RONALD W. DESKIN
Associate Professor of Otolaryngology and Pediatrics, University of Texas Medical Branch, Galveston, USA

JULES L. DIENSTAG
Associate Professor of Medicine, Harvard Medical School and Physician, Massachusetts, General Hospital, Boston, USA

RICHARD DOLL
Emeritus Professor of Medicine, University of Oxford

PATRICIA K. DONAHOE
Marshall K. Bartlett Professor of Surgery, Harvard Medical School and Chief of Pediatric Surgical Services, Massachusetts General Hospital, Boston, USA

DANIEL P. DOODY
Assistant Professor of Surgery, Harvard Medical School and Associate Visiting Surgeon, Massachusetts General Hospital, Boston, USA

STEPHEN P. DRETLER
Director, Kidney Stone Center, Massachusetts General Hospital, Boston, USA

NICHOLAS DUDLEY
Consultant Surgeon, Oxford Radcliffe Hospital

BRUCE C. DUNPHY
Director and Chief, Division of Gynaecology, Foothills Hospital, Calgary, Alberta, Canada

JOHN D. EDWARDS
Chief, Vascular Surgery; Assistant Professor of Surgery, Creighton University School of Medicine, Omaha, Nebraska, USA

THOMAS K. EGGLIN
Assistant Professor of Radiology, Yale University of Medicine, New Haven, Massachusetts, USA

MICHAEL G. EHRLICH
Professor and Chairman, Brown University School of Medicine; Surgeon-in-Chief, Department of Orthopedics, Rhode Island Hospital, Providence, USA

C. C. ENTWISTLE
Medical Director, Regional Blood Transfusion Centre, Oxford

RICHARD L. FABIAN
Director of Head and Neck Surgery, Massachusetts General Hospital and Massachusetts Eye and Ear Infirmary; Associate Professor in Otolaryngology, Harvard Medical School, Boston, USA

PAUL D. FADALE
Assistant Clinical Professor; Chief, Division of Sports Medicine, Brown University Medical School, Rhode Island Hospital, Providence, USA

CHARLES M. FERGUSON
Associate Visiting Surgeon, Massachusetts General Hospital: Assistant Professor of Surgery, Harvard Medical School, Boston, USA

T. BRUCE FERGUSON
Associate Professor of Surgery, Division of Cardiothoracic Surgery, Washington University, St Louis Missouri, USA

CARLOS FERNÁNDEZ-DEL CASTILLO
Instructor in Surgery, Massachusetts General Hospital and Harvard Medical School, Boston, USA

PIERRE FOËX
Nuffield Professor of Anaesthetics, University of Oxford

MANSON FOK
Senior Lecturer in Surgery, The University of Hong Kong, Queen Mary Hospital, Hong Kong

ROBERT G. FORMAN
Senior Lecturer and Consultant in Obstetrics and Gynaecology, United Medical and Dental Schools of Guy's and St Thomas's Hospitals, Guy's Hospital, London

HAMISH McA. FOSTER
Director, Special Surgical Unit, John Hunter Hospital, Newcastle, Australia

ALLEN FOSTER
Medical Director, Christoffer Bindenmission; Senior Lecturer, Institute of Ophthalmology, London

KENNETH L. FRANCO
Assistant Professor of Surgery, Yale University of Medicine, New Haven, Connecticut, USA

PATRICIA M. FRANKLIN
Senior Transplant Nurse Practitioner, Oxford Transplant Centre, Oxford Radcliffe Hospital

DAVID P. FRANKLIN
Vascular Surgeon, Director of Vascular Laboratory, Geisinger Medical Center, Danville; Clinical Assistant Professor of Surgery, Jefferson Medical College, Thomas Jefferson University, Philadelphia, Pennsylvania, USA

MARVIN P. FRIED
Associate Professor of Otology and Laryngology, Harvard Medical School; Chief, Division of Otolaryngology, Beth Israel Hospital and Brigham & Women's Hospital, Boston, Massachusetts, USA

ELLEN M. FRIEDMAN
Associate Professor of Otolaryngology, Head and Neck Surgery and Communicative Sciences and Pediatrics, Baylor College of Medicine; Chief of Service, Pediatric Otolaryngology, Texas Children's Hospital, Houston, USA

DAVID M. FRIM
Clinical Fellow in Surgery, Harvard Medical School, and Senior Resident in Neurosurgery, Massachusetts General Hospital, Boston, USA

JOHN A. FROEHLICH
Clinical Assistant Professor, Adult Reconstructive Surgery/ Sports Medicine, Brown University School of Medicine, Rhode Island Hospital, Providence, USA

HENNING A. GAISSERT
Fellow in Cardiothoracic Surgery, Washington University, St Louis, Missouri, USA

WALTER H. GAJEWSKI
Assistant Professor, Brown University School of Medicine, Women and Infants Hospital, Providence, Rhode Island, USA

WILLIAM J. GALLAGHER
Combined Medical Staff, Everett, Washington State, USA

G. GREGORY GALLICO, III
Associate Professor of Surgery, Harvard Medical School; Surgeon, Massachusetts General Hospital, Boston, USA

CHRISTOPHER S. GARRARD
Consultant and Clinical Lecturer in Intensive Care, Oxford Radcliffe Hospital

MARK C. GEBHARDT
Associate Professor of Orthopedic Surgery, Harvard Medical School, Massachusetts General Hospital and Children's Hospital, Boston, USA

PAUL L. F. GIANGRANDE
Consultant Haematologist, Oxford Haemophilia Centre, Oxford

MICHAEL D. G. GILLMER
Consultant Obstetrician and Gynaecologist, Oxford Radcliffe Hospital

STEPHEN GOLDING
Lecturer in Radiology, University of Oxford and Consultant in Charge, Computed Tomography Unit, Oxford Radcliffe Hospital

ANDREW C. GORDON
Clinical and Research Fellow in Paediatric and Neonatal Surgery, Oxford Radcliffe Hospital

MALCOLM H. GOUGH
Honorary Consultant Surgeon, Oxford Radcliffe Hospital

C. O. GRANAI
Associate Professor/Director of Gynecologic Oncology, Brown University/Women & Infants Hospital, Providence, Rhode Island, USA

CHRISTOPHER S. GRANT
Associate Professor of Surgery, College of Medicine, Sultan Qaboos University, Muscat, Sultanate of Oman

DEREK W. R. GRAY
Reader in Surgery and Consultant Surgeon, Oxford Radcliffe Hospital

CATHERINE R. GREBENIK
Consultant Anaesthetist, Oxford Radcliffe Hospital

ANDREW GREEN
Assistant Professor of Orthopedic Surgery, Brown University and Rhode Island Hospital, Providence, USA

MICHAEL J. GREENALL
Consultant General Surgeon and Surgical Oncologist, Oxford Radcliffe Hospital

BRIAN GRIBBIN
Consultant Cardiologist, Oxford Radcliffe Hospital

D. MERVYN GRIFFITHS
Consultant and Senior Lecturer in Neonatal and Paediatric Surgery, Wessex Regional Centre for Paediatric Surgery, Southampton General Hospital, Southampton, UK

HERMES C. GRILLO
Chief of Thoracic Surgery, Massachusetts General Hospital: Professor of Surgery, Harvard Medical School, Boston, USA

EDWARD J. GUINEY
Professor of Paediatric Research, University College Dublin; Consultant Paediatric Surgeon, Our Lady's Hospital for Sick Children, Temple Street Children's Hospital, and National Children's Hospital, Dublin, Ireland

PETER B. H'DOUBLER
Consultant Surgeon, Saint Joseph's Hospital, Atlanta, Georgia, USA

DAVID I. HAMILTON
Professor of Cardiac Surgery, University of Edinburgh, UK

GEORGE HAMILTON
Consultant Vascular Surgeon, Royal Free Hospital and School of Medicine, London

GRAEME L. HAMMOND
Professor of Surgery, Yale University School of Medicine, New Haven, Connecticut, USA

DAMIAN C. HANBURY
Clinical Lecturer in Urology and Transplantation, Oxford Radcliffe Hospital

LINDA J. HANDS
Clinical Reader and Consultant Surgeon, University of Oxford, Oxford Radcliffe Hospital

WOLFGANG HARRINGER
Research Fellow in Surgery, Massachusetts General Hospital and Harvard Medical School, Boston, USA

MICHAEL R. HARRISON
Professor of Surgery and Pediatrics; Director, Fetal Treatment Center, University of California, San Francisco, USA

W. HARDY HENDREN
Chief of Surgery at Children's Hospital, Boston; Robert E. Gross Professor of Surgery, Harvard Medical School, Boston, Massachusetts, USA

PATRICIA L. HIBBERD
Assistant Professor of Medicine, Harvard Medical School; Assistant in Medicine, Massachusetts General Hospital, Boston, USA

ROBERT S. D. HIGGINS
Surgical Director, Thoracic Organ Transplants, Division of Cardiothoracic Surgery, Henry Ford Hospital, Detroit, Michigan, USA

GEORGE T. HODAKOWSKI
Research Fellow in Surgery, Massachusetts General Hospital and Harvard Medical School, Boston, USA

HERBERT C. HOOVER
Associate Professor of Surgery, Harvard Medical School, Boston, Massachusetts, USA

BRIAN HOWDEN
Professional Officer, Monash University, Department of Surgery, Monash Medical Centre, Melbourne, Australia

MARGARET N. A. HUGHES
Clinical Scientist, Department of Dermatology, Oxford Radcliffe Hospital, Oxford

MICHAEL J. HULSTYN
Assistant Professor of Orthopedic Surgery, Brown University School of Medicine, Rhode Island Hospital, Providence, USA

IMTIAZ HUSAIN
Associate Professor of Urology, College of Medicine, King Saud University, Riyadh, Saudi Arabia

KEITH B. ISAACSON
Assistant Professor in Reproductive Biology, Obstetrics, and Gynecology, Harvard Medical School; Assistant in Gynecology, Massachusetts General Hospital, Boston, USA

PAULA JABLONSKI
Senior Lecturer, Monash University, Department of Surgery, Monash Medical Centre, Melbourne, Australia

MARSHALL L. JACOBS
Associate Cardiothoracic Surgeon, The Children's Hospital of Philadelphia; Associate Professor of Surgery, University of Pennsylvania, Philadelphia, USA

D. P. JEWELL
Consultant Physician, Oxford Radcliffe Hospital; Clinical Lecturer, University of Oxford

GORDON J. JOHNSON
Rothes Professor of Preventive Ophthalmology, International Centre for Eye Health, Institute of Ophthalmology, London

RICHARD P. JUNIPER
Consultant Oral and Maxillofacial Surgeon, Oxford Radcliffe Hospital

DAVID A. KEITH
Associate Professor of Oral and Maxillofacial Surgery, Harvard School of Dental Medicine, Massachusetts General Hospital, Boston, USA

RICHARD KERR
Clinical Reader and Consultant Neurosurgeon, Radcliffe Infirmary, Oxford

M. G. W. KETTLEWELL
Consultant Surgeon, Oxford Radcliffe Hospital; Fellow, Green College, Oxford

SAMUEL H. KIM
Pediatric Surgeon, Massachusetts General Hospital and Associate Clinical Professor of Surgery, Harvard Medical School, Boston, USA

WALTER W. K. KING
Reader in Surgery; Chief, Head and Neck Unit, Department of Surgery, Prince of Wales Hospital, The Chinese University of Hong Kong

ANDREW N. KINGSNORTH
Senior Lecturer in Surgery, Royal Liverpool University Hospital, Liverpool, UK

KIMBERLEY SAUNDERS KIRKWOOD
Assistant in Surgery, Massachusetts General Hospital, Boston, USA

WOLFRAM TRUDO KNOEFEL
Fellow in Surgery, Massachusetts General Hospital and Harvard Medical School, Boston, USA

DANIEL B. KOPANS
Director of Breast Imaging, Massachusetts General Hospital; Associate Professor of Radiology, Harvard Medical School, Boston, USA

JOHN G. KRAL
Professor of Surgery, Kings County Hospital, State University of New York, Brooklyn, USA

HILLEL LAKS
Professor and Chief, Cardiothoracic Surgery, UCLA School of Medicine, Los Angeles, California, USA

PETER M. LAMONT
Clinical Reader in Surgery, Oxford University and Consultant Surgeon, Oxford Radcliffe Hospital

GLENN M. LaMURAGLIA
Assistant Professor of Surgery, Harvard Medical School, Massachusetts General Hospital, Boston, USA

JOHN G. G. LEDINGHAM
Professor of Clinical Medicine and May Reader, University of Oxford Medical School, Oxford

KING-TEH LEE
Associate Professor of Surgery, Kaohsiung Medical College Hospital, Taiwan, Republic of China

GEORGE V. LETSOU
Assistant Professor of Surgery (Cardiothoracic), Yale University, New Haven, Connecticut, USA

ARTHUR K. C. LI
Professor and Chairman, Department of Surgery, Prince of Wales Hospital, The Chinese University, Hong Kong

RICHARD S. LIMBIRD
Assistant Clinical Professor, Brown University Hospitals, Providence, Rhode Island, USA

DAVID R. M. LINDSELL
Consultant Radiologist, Oxford Radcliffe Hospital

J. M. LITTLE
Professor of Surgery, Westmead Hospital, NSW, Australia

T. J. LITTLEWOOD
Department of Haematology, Oxford Radcliffe Hospital

MICHAEL T. LONGAKER
Chief Resident in Surgery, UCSF Medical School, San Francisco, California, USA

CAROL A. LORENTE
Instructor in Oral and Maxillofacial Surgery, Harvard School of Dental Medicine; Clinical Associate in Oral and Maxillofacial Surgery, Massachusetts General Hospital, Boston, USA

JAMES W. LUCARINI
Instructor in Otolaryngology, Harvard Medical School, Boston, Massachusetts, USA

PHILLIP R. LUCAS
Surgeon-in-Charge, Division of Spine Surgery, Rhode Island Hospital, Brown University School of Medicine, Providence, USA

H. KIM LYERLY
Assistant Professor of Surgery and Pathology and Member of the Cancer Center, Department of Surgery, Duke University Medical Center, Durham, North Carolina, USA

OLUWATOPE A. MABOGUNJE
Senior Consultant in Surgery, Sultan Qaboos University Hospital, Muscat, Sultanate of Oman

I. Z. MACKENZIE
Reader in Obstetrics and Gynaecology, Nuffield Department of Obstetrics and Gynaecology, University of Oxford, Oxford Radcliffe Hospital

RONALD A. MALT
Professor of Surgery, Harvard Medical School, Massachusetts General Hospital, Boston, USA

PANKAJ S. MANKAD
Royal Hospital for Sick Children and Royal Infirmary, Edinburgh, UK

HENRY J. MANKIN
Chief of Orthopedic Service, Massachusetts General Hospital; Edith M. Ashley Professor of Orthopedics, Harvard Medical School, Boston, USA

MICHAEL N. MARGOLIES
Visiting Surgeon, Massachusetts General Hospital; Associate Professor of Surgery, Harvard Medical School, Boston, USA

CHRISTOPHER G. MARKS
Consultant Surgeon and Director of Surgery, Royal Surrey County Hospital, Guildford, Surrey, UK

VERNON C. MARSHALL
Professor and Chairman, Monash University Department of Surgery; Chairman, Division of Surgery, Monash Medical Centre, Melbourne, Australia.

ROBERT L. MARTUZA
Professor and Chairman, Department of Neurosurgery, Georgetown University Medical Center, Washington, DC, USA

DOUGLAS MATHISEN
Associate Professor of Surgery, Harvard Medical School, Boston; Associate Surgeon, Massachusetts General Hospital, Boston, USA

GEORGE M. MATOOK
Captain, United States Air Force, Department of Orthopedic Surgery, USAF Hospital, Tinker Air Force Base, Oklahoma City, USA

CHARLES J. McCABE
Associate Chief, Emergency Services, Massachusetts General Hospital; Assistant Professor of Surgery, Harvard Medical School, Boston, USA

FRANCIS J. McGOVERN
Clinical Instructor, Harvard Medical School; Assistant in Urology, Massachusetts General Hospital, Boston, USA

MICHAEL J. McKENNA
Assistant Professor, Harvard Medical School/Massachusetts Eye and Ear Infirmary, Boston, USA

HENRY McQUAY
Clinical Reader in Pain Relief, Oxford Radcliffe Hospital

D. L. McWHINNIE
Surgical Tutor, University of Oxford, Oxford Radcliffe Hospital

BRYAN F. MEYERS
Clinical and Research Fellow in Surgery, Massachusetts General Hospital, Harvard Medical School, Boston, USA

JONATHAN MICHAELS
Clinical Lecturer, Nuffield Department of Surgery, Oxford Radcliffe Hospital

LUC A. MICHEL
Chief of General Surgery, University Hospital of Mont-Godinne, Yvoir, Belgium

HAMISH R. MICHIE
Clinical Lecturer in Surgery, Oxford Radcliffe Hospital

ANDREW MITCHELL
Consultant Surgeon, Milton Keynes Hospital, Buckinghamshire, UK

ASHBY C. MONCURE
Associate Clinical Professor of Surgery, Harvard Medical School; Visiting Surgeon, Massachusetts General Hospital, Boston, USA

M. JOCELYN MORRIS
Associate Specialist in Chest Diseases, Oxford Radcliffe Hospital

PETER J. MORRIS
Professor of Surgery, University of Oxford, Oxford Radcliffe Hospital

NEIL MORTENSEN
Consultant Surgeon, Department of Colorectal Surgery, Oxford Radcliffe Hospital

JOHN T. B. MOYLE
Consultant Anaesthetist, Milton Keynes Hospital, Buckinghamshire, UK

JOHN A. MURIE
Consultant Vascular Surgeon, The Royal Infirmary, Edinburgh, UK

NAOFUMI NAGASUE
Associate Professor of Surgery, Shimane Medical University, Izumo, Japan

BARRY N. NOCKS
Assistant Professor of Surgery, Harvard Medical School; Associate Urologist, Massachusetts General Hospital; Director of Urology, Spaulding Rehabilitation Hospital, Boston, USA

DANIEL J. NOLAN
Consultant Radiologist, Oxford Radcliffe Hospital

TIM O'BRIEN
Research Fellow in Urology, Oxford Radcliffe Hospital

ROBERT G. OJEMANN
Professor of Surgery, Harvard Medical School; Visiting Neurosurgeon, Massachusetts General Hospital, Boston, USA

TERENCE O'KELLY
Wellcome Research Fellow, University Department of Pharmacology and Department of Surgery, Oxford

CHRISTOPHER S. OGILVY
Assistant Professor of Surgery, Harvard Medical School; Assistant Visiting Neurosurgeon, Massachusetts General Hospital, Boston, USA

RANDY W. OPPENHEIMER
Attending Physician, Scripps Memorial Hospital, San Diego, California, USA

PAOLO ORTU
Research Fellow in Surgery, Massachusetts General Hospital, Harvard Medical School, Boston, USA

INGEGERD ÖSTMAN-SMITH
Consultant Paediatric Cardiologist, Oxford Radcliffe Hospital

LESLIE W. OTTINGER
Visiting Surgeon, Massachusetts General Hospital, Boston, USA

RICHARD D. PAGE
Senior Registrar in Cardiothoracic Surgery, The Cardiothoracic Centre, Liverpool, UK

A. P. PANDEY
Professor of Urology, Christian Medical College Hospital, Vellore, India

NICHOLAS PAPANICOLAOU
Associate Professor of Radiology, Harvard Medical School; Head, Division of Genitourinary Radiology, Massachusetts General Hospital, Boston USA

ANDREW J. PARRY
Senior Registrar in Cardiothoracic Surgery, Papworth Hospital, Cambridge, UK

DINAH V. PARUMS
Clinical Tutor in Pathology, Nuffield Department of Pathology, Oxford Radcliffe Hospital

MARK S. PASTERNACK
Chief, Pediatric Infectious Disease Unit, Massachusetts General Hospital; Associate Professor of Pediatrics, Harvard Medical School, Boston, USA

ARUN PAUSAWASDI
Professor of Surgery, Faculty of Medicine, Siriraj Hospital, Mahidol University, Bangkok, Thailand

A. PENNATHUR
Massachusetts General Hospital, Boston, USA

LESTER C. PERMUT
Assistant Professor of Surgery, UCLA School of Medicine, Los Angeles, California, USA

CRAIG A. PETERS
Assistant Professor of Surgery, Harvard Medical School; Assistant in Surgery (Urology), Children's Hospital, Boston, Massachusetts, USA

RAVI PILLAI
Consultant Cardiothoracic Surgeon, Oxford Radcliffe Hospital: Clinical Lecturer, University of Oxford

CHARLES E. POLETTI
Neurosurgeon, Hartford Hospital, Connecticut, USA

BRUCE A. J. PONDER
CRC Professor of Human Cancer Genetics, University of Cambridge, UK

MICHAEL D. POOLE
Director, Oxford Craniofacial Unit, Radcliffe Infirmary, Oxford

FRANCESCO PUMA
Massachusetts General Hospital, Boston, USA

GEORGE K. RADDA
British Heart Foundation Professor of Molecular Cardiology, MRC Magnetic Resonance Spectroscopy Unit, Oxford Radcliffe Hospital

N. RANGABASHYAM
Professor of Surgery, Rajah Muthaiah Medical College, Annamalai University, Annamalai Nagar, South India

PETER J. RATCLIFFE
University Lecturer and Consultant Physician, Renal Unit, Oxford Radcliffe Hospital

DAVID W. RATTNER
Assistant Professor of Surgery, Harvard Medical School, Massachusetts General Hospital, Boston, USA

STEVEN D. RAUCH
Assistant Professor of Otolaryngology, Harvard Medical School, The Massachusetts Eye and Ear Infirmary, Boston, USA

JUSTIN A. ROAKE
Consultant Surgeon, Nuffield Department of Surgery, Oxford Radcliffe Hospital

GRANT V. RODKEY
Visiting Surgeon, Massachusetts General Hospital; Associate Clinical Professor of Surgery, Harvard Medical School, Boston, USA

JERROLD ROSENBERG
Assistant Professor of Rehabilitation Medicine, Brown University Medical School, Providence, Rhode Island, USA

FRED ROSEWARNE
Assistant Director, Department of Anaesthetics, Royal Melbourne Hospital, Victoria, Australia

ROBERT H. RUBIN
Chief of Transplantation Infectious Disease and Director of the Clinical Investigation Program, Massachusetts General Hospital; Associate Professor of Medicine, Harvard Medical School, Boston, USA

PAUL S. RUSSELL
John Homans Professor of Surgery, Harvard Medical School; Visiting Surgeon and Former Chief of the Transplantation Unit, Massachusetts General Hospital, Boston, USA

ROBB H. RUTLEDGE
Clinical Professor, Department of Surgery, University of Texas, Southwestern Medical Center, Fort Worth, USA

DANIEL P. RYAN
Instructor in Pediatric Surgery, Harvard Medical School, Boston, Massachusetts, USA

DAVID C. SABISTON
James B. Duke Professor of Surgery; Chairman, Department of Surgery, Duke University Medical Center, Durham, North Carolina, USA

SALAH D. SALMAN
Lecturer, Harvard Medical School; Director of the General Otolaryngology Service; Director of the Sinus Center, Massachusetts Eye and Ear Infirmary, Boston, USA

JUAN A. SANCHEZ
Assistant Professor of Clinical Surgery, University of Miami School of Medicine, Florida, USA

ADRIAN SAVAGE
Senior Registrar, Oxford Radcliffe Hospital

J. GORDON SCANNELL
Clinical Professor of Surgery, Emeritus, Harvard Medical School; Senior Surgeon, Massachusetts General Hospital, Boston, USA

ISAAC SCHIFF
Joe Vincent Meigs Professor of Gynecology, Harvard Medical School; Chief, Vincent Memorial Obstetrics and Gynecology Service, Massachusetts General Hospital, Boston, USA

DAVID SCOTT
Clinical Associate Professor, Monash University; Head, Transplantation Surgery, Monash Medical Centre, Melbourne, Australia

JOHN W. SEAR
Clinical Reader in Anaesthetics, Nuffield Department of Anaesthetics, University of Oxford

JOHN D. SEIGNE
Assistant in Urology, Massachusetts General Hospital; Instructor in Surgery, Harvard Medical School, Boston, USA

STEWART SELL
Professor of Pathology, Medical School, University of Texas at Houston, USA

JONATHAN S. T. SHAM
Senior Lecturer in Radiation Oncology, University of Hong Kong, Queen Mary Hospital, Hong Kong

ROBERT C. SHAMBERGER
Associate Professor of Surgery, Harvard Medical School and Senior Associate in Surgery, Children's Hospital, Boston, Massachusetts, USA

J. SHAPIRO
Instructor in Otology and Laryngology, Harvard Medical School, Boston, Massachusetts, USA

PAI-CHING SHEEN
Professor of Surgery, Kaohsiung Medical College Hospital, Taiwan, Republic of China

PAUL C. SHELLITO
Assistant Professor of Surgery, Harvard Medical School; Associate Visiting Surgeon, Massachusetts General Hospital, Boston, USA

BASIL J. SHEPSTONE
University Lecturer in Radiology, University of Oxford, Radcliffe Infirmary, Oxford

BRADFORD J. SHINGLETON
Ophthalmic Consultants of Boston, Massachusetts, USA

DANIEL SHOSKES
Fellow in Renal Transplantation, Department of Urology, Cleveland Clinical Foundation, Cleveland, Ohio, USA

MICHAEL E. SINCLAIR
Consultant Anaesthetist and Clinical Lecturer, Nuffield Department of Anaesthesia, Oxford Radcliffe Hospital

ARTHUR J. SOBER
Associate Professor of Dermatology, Harvard Medical School; Associate Chief of Dermatology, Massachusetts General Hospital, Boston, USA

PATRICIA M. SOLGA
Assistant Professor of Orthopedic Surgery, Brown University School of Medicine, Providence, Rhode Island, USA

R. G. SOUTER
Consultant Surgeon, Milton Keynes General Hospital, Buckinghamshire, UK

GAVIN P. SPICKETT
Consultant and Senior Lecturer in Clinical Immunology, Newcastle General Hospital and University of Newcastle upon Tyne, UK

DAVID D. STARK
Massachusetts General Hospital, Boston, USA

GORDON M. STIRRAT
Professor of Obstetrics and Gynaecology, University of Bristol, UK

ROBERT M. STRAUSS
Massachusetts General Hospital, Boston, USA

NICHOLAS S. A. STUART
ICRF Clinical Research Fellow, Oxford Radcliffe Hospital

JOHN G. N. STUDLEY
Consultant Surgeon, James Paget Hospital, Great Yarmouth, Norfolk, UK

HERMAN SUIT
Andres Sorrino Professor of Radiation Oncology, Harvard Medical School; Chief of Radiation Oncology, Massachusetts General Hospital, Boston, USA

THOROLF SUNDT III
Massachusetts General Hospital, Boston, USA

OWEN S. SURMAN
Associate Professor of Psychiatry, Harvard Medical School; Psychiatrist, Massachusetts General Hospital, Boston, USA

MORTON N. SWARTZ
Professor of Medicine, Harvard Medical School and Massachusetts General Hospital, Boston, USA

BROOKE SWEARINGEN
Assistant Professor, Harvard Medical School, and Assistant Visiting Neurosurgeon, Massachusetts General Hospital, Boston, USA

P. K. H. TAM
Reader in Paediatric Surgery, University of Oxford, Oxford Radcliffe Hospital

AKIHIRO TANIMOTO
Massachusetts General Hospital, Boston, USA

HECTOR M. TARRAZA
Assistant Professor of Gynecologic Surgery, University of Vermont Medical School, Portland, USA

PETER J. TEDDY
Consultant Neurosurgeon, Department of Neurological Surgery, Radcliffe Infirmary, Oxford

W. HAMISH THOMSON
Consultant General Surgeon, Gloucestershire Royal Hospital, Gloucester, UK

DAVID J. TIBBS
Honorary Consulting Surgeon, Oxford Radcliffe Hospital

RONALD G. TOMPKINS
Chief of the Burn and Trauma Services, Massachusetts General Hospital; Chief of Staff, Shriners Burns Institute, Harvard Medical School, Boston, USA

PETER G. TRAFTON
Associate Professor of Orthopedic Surgery, Brown University Medical School, Providence, Rhode Island, USA

B. TROTMAN-DICKENSON
Research Fellow in Radiology, Royal Brompton National Heart and Lung Hospital, London

GLENN A. TUNG
Instructor in Radiology, Harvard Medical School; Assistant in Radiology, Massachusetts, General Hospital, Boston, USA

WILLIAM TURNER
Assistant, Department of Urology, Inselspital, University of Berne, Switzerland

ROBERT G. TWYCROSS
Macmillan Clinical Reader in Palliative Medicine, University of Oxford; Consultant Physician, Sir Michael Sobell House, Oxford Radcliffe Hospital

MUNEYASU URANO
Professor of Radiation Medicine, University of Kentucky Medical Center, Lexington, USA

GUS J. VLAHAKES
Associate Visiting Surgeon, Massachusetts General Hospital and Harvard Medical School, Boston, USA

JOHN C. WAIN
Assistant Professor of Surgery, Harvard Medical School, Boston, Massachusetts, USA

TIMOTHY C. WANG
Assistant in Medicine, Massachusetts General Hospital; Instructor in Medicine, Harvard Medical School, Boston, USA

CHARLES WARLOW
Professor of Medical Neurology, Department of Clinical Neurosciences, University of Edinburgh, UK

ANDREW L. WARSHAW
Harold and Ellen Danser Professor of Surgery, Harvard Medical School; Chief of General Surgery and Associate Chief of Surgical Services, Massachusetts General Hospital, Boston, USA

DAVID J. WEATHERALL
Regius Professor of Medicine, University of Oxford

EDWARD W. WEBSTER
Professor of Radiology (Physics), Harvard Medical School; Chief, Division of Radiological Sciences, Department of Radiology, Massachusetts General Hospital, Boston, USA

WILLIAM I. WEI
Professor of Otorhinolaryngology, University of Hong Kong, Queen Mary Hospital, Hong Kong

ARNOLD-PETER C. WEISS
Assistant Professor of Orthopedics, Brown University School of Medicine and Rhode Island Hospital, Providence, USA

MARK C. WEISSLER
Associate Professor of Otolaryngology–Head and Neck Surgery, University of North Carolina, Chapel Hill, USA

CLAUDE E. WELCH
Senior Surgeon, Massachusetts General Hospital; Clinical Professor of Surgery Emeritus, Harvard Medical School, Boston, USA

JOHN P. WELCH
Attending Surgeon, Hartford Hospital, Hartford, Connecticut; Professor of Clinical Surgery, University of Connecticut School of Medicine, Farmington, Connecticut; Assistant Professor of Surgery, Dartmouth Medical School, Hanover, New Hampshire, USA

STEPEHN WESTABY
Cardiac and Thoracic Surgeon, Oxford Heart Centre

RICHARD I. WHYTE
Assistant Professor, Section of Thoracic Surgery, University of Michigan, Ann Arbor, USA

JOSEPH W. WILKES
Instructor in Oral and Maxillofacial Surgery, Harvard School of Dental Medicine, Boston, Massachusetts, USA

ANDREW R. WILKINSON
Reader in Paediatrics and Perinatal Medicine, University of Oxford; Consultant Paediatrician, Oxford Radcliffe Hospital; Fellow, All Souls College, Oxford

CHRISTOPHER G. WILLETT
Assistant Professor in Radiation Oncology, Harvard Medical School; Associate Radiation Oncologist, Massachusetts General Hospital, Boston, USA

ROBIN C. N. WILLIAMSON
Professor and Director of Surgery, Royal Postgraduate Medical School, Hammersmith Hospital, London

ROGER S. WILSON
Chairman, Department of Anesthesiology and Critical Care Medicine, Memorial Sloan-Kettering Cancer Centre; Professor of Anesthesiology, Cornell University Medical College, New York, USA

CHRISTOPHER G. WINEARLS
Consultant Nephrologist, Renal Unit, Oxford Radcliffe Hospital

DIETMAR H. WITTMANN
Associate Professor of Surgery, Section of Trauma and Emergency Surgery, Medical College of Wisconsin, Milwaukee, USA

JOHN WONG
Professor of Surgery, The University of Hong Kong, Queen Mary Hospital, Hong Kong

WILLIAM C. WOOD
Joseph Brown Whitead Professor and Chairman, Department of Surgery, Emory University, Atlanta, Georgia, USA

CAMERON D. WRIGHT
Assistant Professor of Surgery, Harvard Medical School, Massachusetts General Hospital, Boston, USA

MICHAEL J. YAREMCHUK
Associate Professor of Surgery, Harvard Medical School; Associate Surgeon, Massachusetts General Hospital, Boston, USA

DAVID T. ZELT
Resident in Vascular Surgery, Massachusetts General Hospital, Harvard Medical School, Boston, USA

NICHOLAS T. ZERVAS
Higgins Professor of Neurosurgery, Harvard Medical School and Chief, Neurosurgical Service, Massachusetts General Hospital, Boston, USA

Dose schedules are being continually revised and new side-effects recognized. Oxford University Press makes no representation, express or implied, that the drug dosages in this book are correct. For these reasons the reader is strongly urged to consult the drug company's printed instructions before administering any of the drugs recommended in this book.

Wound healing 1

1 Wound healing

GEORGE W. CHERRY, MARGARET A. HUGHES, ANDREW N. KINGSNORTH, AND FRANK W. ARNOLD

INTRODUCTION

'Nowhere is the gap between basic research and clinical application more glaring than in the biology of wound healing'

Earl A. Peacock Jr (1983)

Modern advances in molecular biological research techniques have increased the gap between our understanding of the mechanisms of wound healing and the clinical application of this knowledge, as pointed out by Peacock in 1983. A number of factors besides the expansion of new knowledge have contributed to this distance, although probably the most important is that, in healthy individuals, tissue repair after acute injury is thought to occur at a maximum rate and is not really impaired unless adversely affected by localized or systemic conditions (Table 1).

Table 1 Local and systemic factors that adversely affect wound healing

Local	Systemic
Impaired blood supply	Arterial disease
Bacterial and fungal infection	Venous hypertension
Foreign body reactions	General malnutrition
Complications following radiotherapy	Diabetes mellitus
Excessive use of topical corticosteroids	Marfan's syndrome
	Whole body irradiation
	Immunosuppressant drugs and corticosteroids
	Vitamin A and C deficiencies
	Anticoagulants
	Obesity

Recent clinical studies, designed to demonstrate increased healing of acute wounds with therapeutic agents resulting from advances in basic research, such as growth factors and, in particular, epidermal growth factor, have yielded conflicting results. In addition, the clinical significance of improving the healing of acute donor site skin graft wounds by 1 or 2 days is debatable.

However, with regard to chronic wounds there has been a major improvement, over the past decade, in decreasing the gap between basic wound healing research and clinical application. An augmentation in the healing rate of these wounds would not only be beneficial to the patients but also to health care budgets. Chronic leg ulceration alone in the United Kingdom has been estimated to cost £300 million to £600 million per annum—similar to the cost of tobacco-related diseases.

There has been a renewed interest in recent years into the pathophysiology of venous ulcers, resulting in knowledge of the role of leakage of fibrinogen and other blood substances across the capillaries due to chronic venous hypertension (Fig. 1). These pathological changes have been shown to be accompanied by an impairment of the microcirculation in patients with venous leg ulcers. Similar microcirculation impairment has been seen in patients with type I insulin-dependent diabetes, in which healing also is defective.

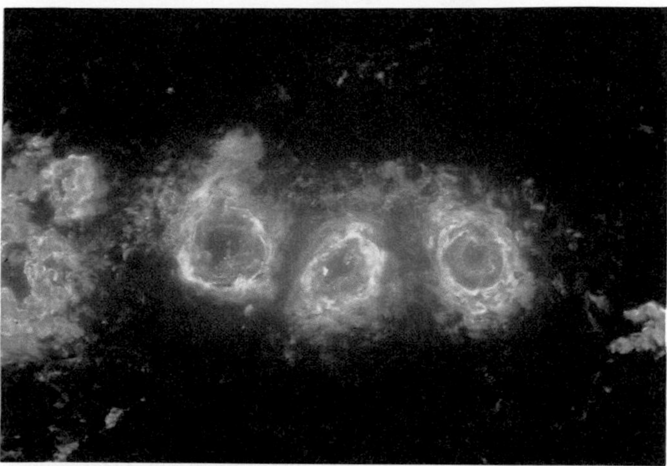

Fig. 1 Immunohistological section of a biopsy from the centre of a venous ulcer stained with antifibrin monoclonal antibody, demonstrating pericapillary fibrin staining (green fluorescence).

Another example where basic research has finally been utilized clinically is that of the practice of maintaining a moist wound environment under occlusive dressings to enhance healing. An increase in healing compared to wounds left exposed to air was demonstrated in animal studies in 1962 and a year later in humans. Because of the improved healing of skin wounds that occurs with occlusive dressings, the latter are now used as controls in experimental and clinical studies to test the efficacy of growth factors and other healing promoters (Fig. 2).

There is a lack of standardized clinical definitions to describe the status of both acute and chronic wounds. This can be a problem in the dissemination of the results of clinical wound healing studies. In order to overcome this problem in chronic wounds, Knighton has established a classification of non-healing wounds, based on up to 20 clinical and wound status parameters, to generate what is termed a wound severity index (Table 2). His

Table 2 Chronic wounds severity score (Knighton *et al.* 1986)

Wound diagnosis	Score*
Venous ulcers	30.0 ± 13.9
Arterial insufficiency	24.2 ± 7.8
Diabetes	22.1 ± 13.0

*Based on Knighton's wound severity index.

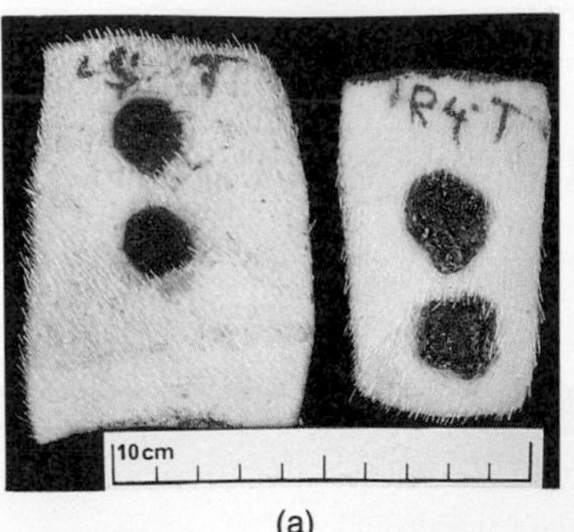

(a)

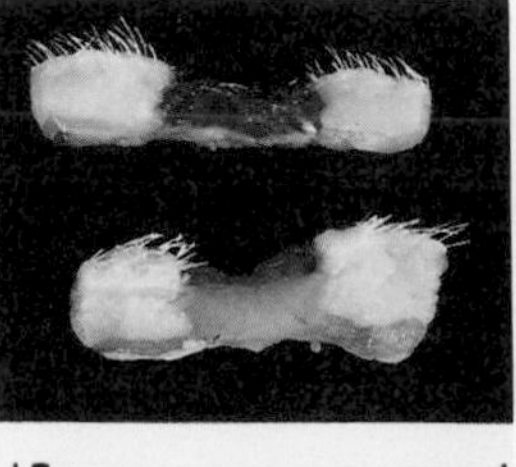

(b)

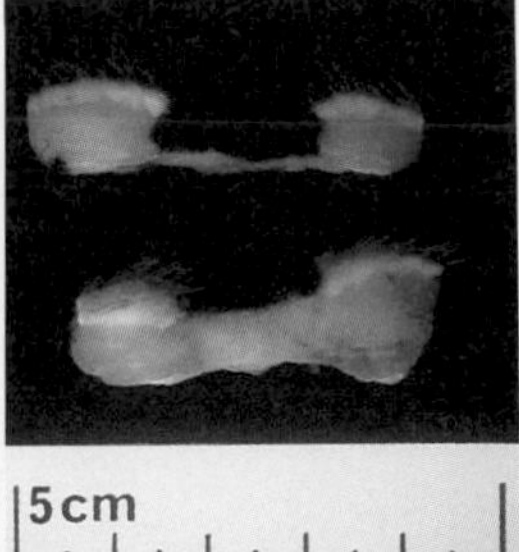

(c)

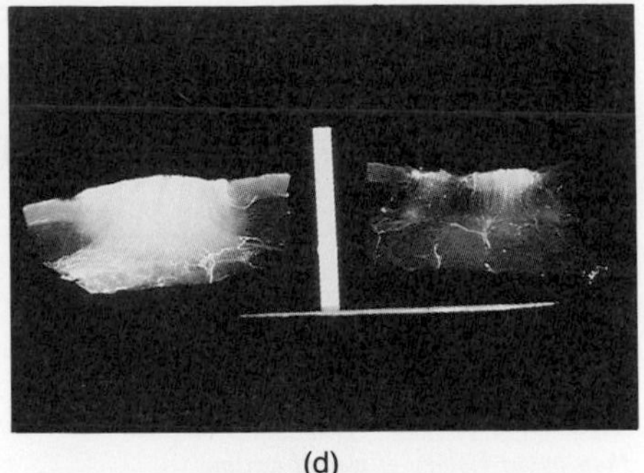

(d)

Fig. 2 (a) Seven-day-old full-thickness wounds, initially 2 cm in diameter, made on the left and right flanks of a pig. Wounds on the left side were treated with an occlusive hydrocolloid dressing (DuoDerm/Granuflex) and the wounds on the right were treated with a non-occlusive dressing. The wounds treated with the hydrocolloid dressing have marked improved healing without scab formation. (b) Cross-sections of same wounds (top = non-occlusive dressing). (c) Intravenous fluorescein dye was given prior to removal of the tissue to demonstrate the blood supply of wounds. The top wound exposed to the air with the non-occlusive dressing has little or no perfusion compared to the lower wound, which was treated with the hydrocolloid dressing and exhibits an excellent blood supply. (d) Microangiograms of similarly treated wounds, demonstrating increased morphological blood supply in the left wound which was treated with the hydrocolloid dressing.

assessment of wounds includes a number of variables ranging from the size, depth, extent of undermining, bone exposure, arterial blood supply, and duration of the lesion.

To a number of patients the most important perception of healing is not necessarily acceleration of healing, but the appearance of the resultant scar. For the burn patient, in addition to the cosmesis of the scar, the functional recovery of the injured tissue is of great importance. This goal has been accomplished for a number of years by using pressure garments to manage excess scar tissue formation in these patients. Over the past decade, research workers in Australia, the British Isles, and the United States have shown that covering hypertrophic scars with a silastic gel sheet results in both clinical and elastometrical improvement of the scars, without exerting pressure. The mode of action of this therapy in preventing hypertrophic scar formation is still not known, but studies by Quinn and colleagues have ruled out any pressure effect, temperature alteration, oxygen tension change, or occlusion as a factor.

Thus it appears that the gap between basic research and clinical utilization in wound healing is narrowing, particularly in the treatment of chronic wounds. This is evident in the amount of research that is being carried out currently on wound dressings and healing promoting agents, such as growth factors. The aim of this chapter is to review the basic science of wound healing, as well as to illustrate how this research is affecting the clinical management of wounds.

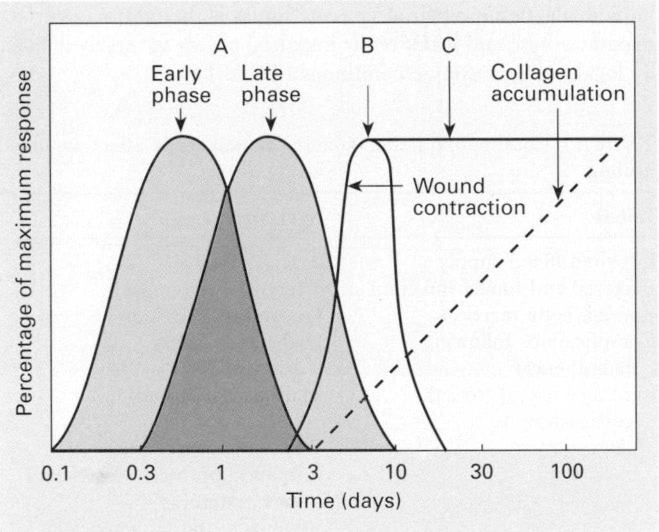

Fig. 3 Phases of wound repair. (A) Early phase of inflammation—accumulation of neutrophils; late phase of inflammation—accumulation of macrophages; (B) repair phase—formation of granulation tissue; (C) scar formation and maturation.

HEALING PHASES

In order to describe the complex cascade of events that follows injury, it is convenient to look at this process as a number of overlapping phases: inflammation, formation of granulation tissue with angiogenesis, and scar formation (extracellular matrix remodelling) (Figs. 3 and 4).

Injury to tissue leads to loss of structural integrity, instigating the coagulation cascade to prevent localized haemorrhage. In skin, mucosa, and gut especially, injury is also complicated by the invasion of micro-organisms. These events play an important role in initiating the defence and repair mechanisms by sealing off severed vessels and transferring blood constituents, circulating cells, and bioactive substances to the site of the wound (Fig. 5). This transferral and the ensuing defence processes constitute the early aspect of wound healing, commonly referred to as the inflammatory phase.

It has been stated by Peacock and others that the inflammatory reaction in soft tissue, which begins literally seconds after injury, is the same whether caused by a surgeon's sterile blade or by invading bacteria after a street injury. Qualitatively, inflammation is the same, but it is likely to be more prolonged in the latter case. More specifically, the mechanism of leucocyte adhesion to the vascular wall after injury followed by diapedesis, a major part of the inflammatory response, is essentially the same in all wounds whether resulting from surgery or trauma.

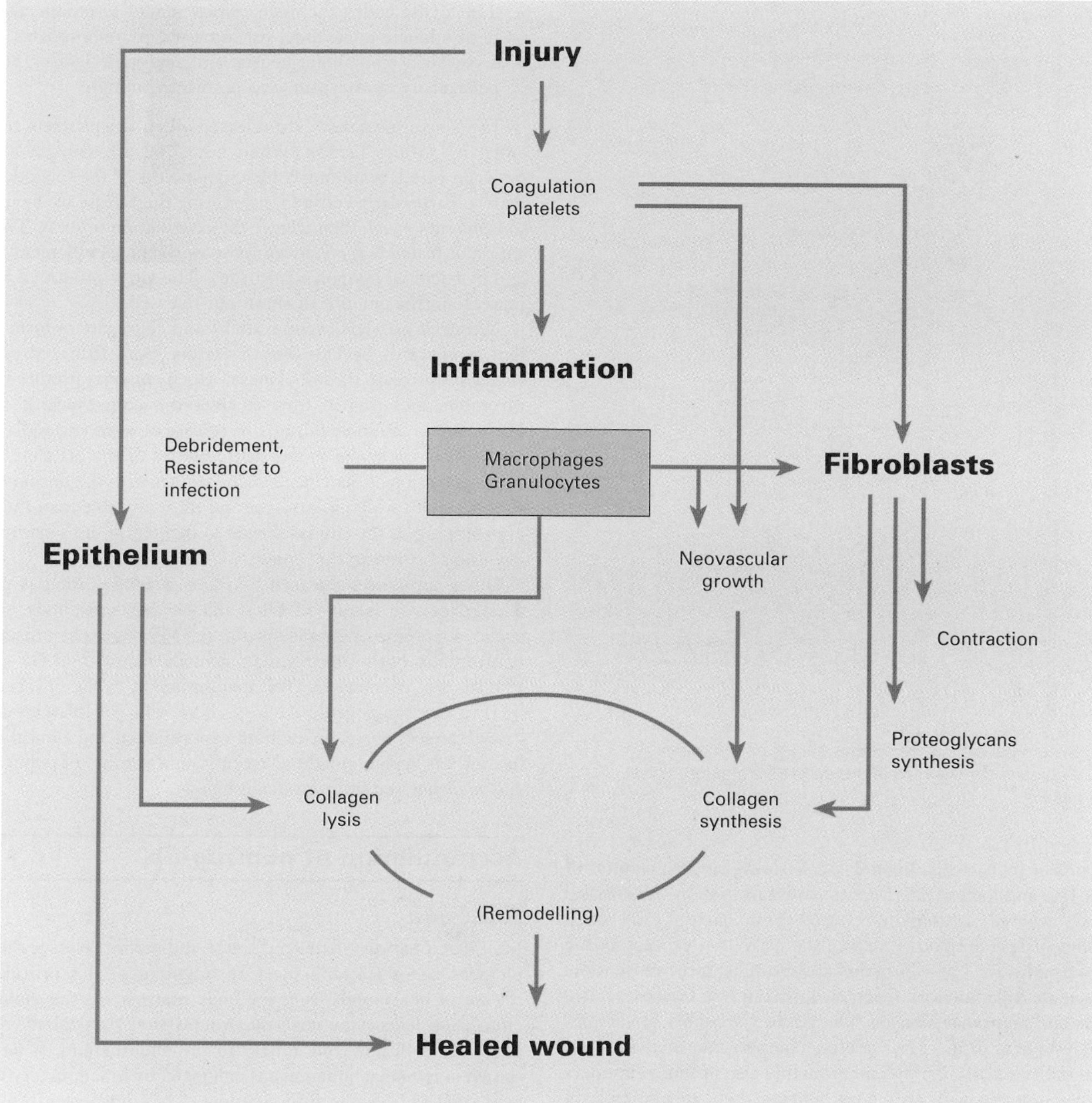

Fig. 4 A general flow diagram of wound healing. Note the central role played by inflammation.

Sequence in inflammation

The inflammatory phase is triggered by two classes of mediators (soluble signal factors): those controlling vessel permeability and those attracting or trapping cells. The clinical signs of inflammation are caused by changes in blood vessels—with dilatation leading to erythema, and endothelial cell separation allowing plasma extravasation, producing localized swelling. There are overlapping stages but, in general, the order of arrival at the wound site from an intravascular space is thought to occur in the following sequence: plasma with soluble components and cellular constituents, first platelets, then neutrophils, followed by monocytes and lymphocytes. The migration of epithelial cells to resurface the injured tissue begins during this phase, mediated by the above events.

Alterations in microvascular permeability after injury allow both fluid and plasma components to pass to the tissue. Vasoactive amines and peptides (including histamine from mast cells, serotonin from platelets, and bradykinin from neutrophils) cause the reversible opening of junctions between endothelial cells and allow the passage of neutrophils and monocytes.

Hageman factor (factor XII), a plasma glycoprotein, is activated by adsorption on to fibrillar collagen, leading to the generation of bradykinin and initiation of the complement cascade. The complement system is composed of 20 interacting soluble proteins in the serum and extracellular fluid, which can be activated by IgM and IgG antibodies bound to antigens on the surface of micro-

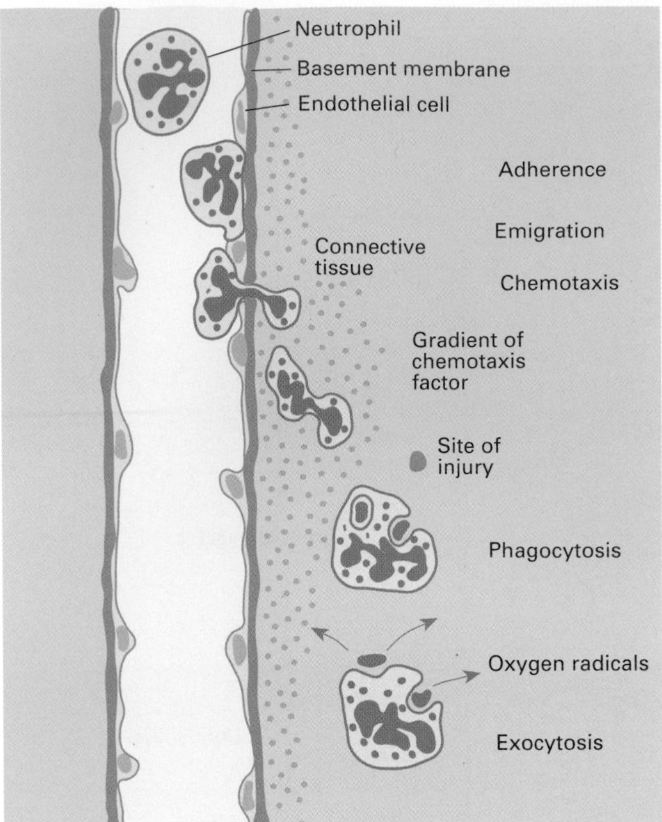

Fig. 5 Scheme depicting the various stages of neutrophil accumulation and participation in the early inflammatory phase of wound healing.

organisms or by bacterial lipopolysaccharides. Large quantities of IgM or IgG antibodies lead to complement fixation by the classical pathway, whereas endotoxin released from bacteria and small quantities of IgG antibody enhance the activation process by the alternate pathway. These proteins are the substances responsible for the acute inflammatory reaction. IgM can lyse Gram-negative bacteria and neutralize viruses. The C5 to C9 factors of complement combine to form a large protein complex that mediates lysis of bacterial cell walls. Complement factors also opsonize invaders (coat their antigen with antibody), making them recognizable to phagocytic cells. The factor C5a is also chemotactic, attracting polymorphonuclear cells, neutrophils, to the site. The complement component C3b binds to specific receptor proteins on phagocytic cells and to microbial cell walls and enhances the ability of the phagocytes to bind, ingest, and destroy micro-organisms.

Platelets

The earliest circulating cell or cell fragment detected in the injury site is the platelet. Platelets contain three types of organelles involved in haemostasis and initiation of the inflammatory phase.

1. α-Granules, which contain adhesive glycoproteins such as fibrinogen, von Willebrand factor, fibronectin, thrombospondin, and also growth factors—platelet-derived growth factor (PDGF), transforming growth factors α and β (TGF-α and TGF-β), and platelet factor 4.
2. The 'dense body', the main storage site of serotonin, also contains adenine nucleotide, calcium, and pyrophosphates.
3. Lysosomes, containing neutral and acid hydrolysases, elastase, collagenase, antitrypsin, and α_2 macroglobulin.

The above substances are released when the platelets are activated by various factors. When injury occurs, contact is made between platelets and insoluble components of the subendothelial matrix, particularly collagen, promoting the release of the α-granule contents which then trigger the coagulation process. The activation of platelets is enhanced by some of the complement factors and by bacterial lipopolysaccharides. The latter produce a 50-fold increase in the amount of serotonin released.

Activated platelets become sticky and aggregate to form a plug that temporarily occludes small vessels. Both damaged platelets and tissues release thrombokinase, which converts prothrombin to thrombin, and this in turn ensures the conversion of soluble fibrinogen to insoluble fibrin. The release of serotonin and adenine nucleotides contained in the dense bodies of the platelets induce the aggregation of platelets, which interact with the fibrin network to form a clot which is stronger and more durable than the initial platelet plug. If the clot is allowed to dehydrate, it transforms to a dry eschar covering the wound.

Other substances released by the α-granules, such as platelet derived growth factor (PDGF), and by the dense body, such as cyclic adenosine monophosphate (cAMP) are chemotactic for neutrophils; both transforming growth factor-β (TGF-β) and PDGF are chemotactic for macrophages, while TGF-α and TGF-β are angiogenic factors. The role of platelet-derived growth factors in enhancing both experimental and clinical wound healing has been highlighted recently in a number of publications, and is elaborated in more detail below.

Accumulation of neutrophils

Adhesion

Interaction between damaged tissue and serum releases the complement factor C3, and the C3e fragment of this provokes the release of neutrophils from the bone marrow. At the same time, circulating leucocytes near the wound site, particularly neutrophils, cease to flow and adhere to the endothelium. It has been shown *in vitro* that adherence is enhanced by inflammatory mediators, such as C5a (the fifth component of complement), platelet-activating factor, and leukotriene. There is a very fast initial response, with onset of adherence as early as 30 s after injury and with a maximum response at 2 min.

The binding of leucocytes to endothelium results from the interaction of complementary receptors in both cell types. Their expression is enhanced by cytokines and bacterial lipopolysaccharide. Physical factors, such as haemodynamic shear stress, also influence adherence. This first stage of adherence is critical. While there is some evidence that some wounds can heal without the presence of neutrophils, patients with leucocyte adhesion deficiency, lacking an essential glycoprotein, are unable to mobilize neutrophils or monocytes, and exhibit decreased pus formation and impaired wound healing.

Diapedesis

Vasopermeability factors act on actin microfilaments inside the endothelial cells and effect the reversible opening of junctions so that neutrophils are able to pass between the endothelial cells to the extravascular space. It is suggested that the secretion of elastase and other enymes by the neutrophils enables them to degrade elastin and components of the endothelial basement membrane.

Migration

Molecules released by platelets following disruption of the blood vessels, e.g. kallikrein (an enzyme that leads to the formation of vasodilating peptides) and fibrinopeptides, diffuse to the site of the wound and set up a concentration gradient of chemotactic factors which attract the neutrophils that have traversed the endothelium through the extracellular space to the injury site.

Phagocytosis

At the site the neutrophils form the first line of defence against the invading micro-organisms. The neutrophils phagocytose bacteria, then kill the ingested cells by the production of microbiocidal substances—oxygen metabolites such as hydroxyl radicals, hydrogen peroxide, and the superoxide ion. Release of some of these substances to the outside of the cell may also lead to tissue damage and prolong the inflammatory phase. Some bacteria may be killed by non-oxidative mechanisms, but these are not defined *in vivo*. If bacterial contamination is low, the density of neutrophils declines, but if numbers of micro-organisms persist, the bacterial lipopolysacharides continue to promote the arrival of further neutrophils. The neutrophils are unable to regenerate their enzymes and so themselves decay after phagocytosis.

Accumulation of macrophages

The macrophage is indispensable in the degradation of injured tissue debris and in the reparative phase of wound healing (Fig. 6). If the macrophages are inhibited, wound healing is radically impaired.

Normal tissues contain very few macrophages, but, in response to chemotactic factors released after injury, circulating monocytes are attracted to the site of injury several hours after the first neutrophils arrive. Endothelial cells in wounded tissue also play a role in this process, and have been shown to regulate the preferential adhesion of monocytes and lymphocytes to endothelium.

At the injury site, monocytes differentiate into macrophages. One of the signals promoting this differentiation is the binding of fibronectin to surface receptors on monocytes, which induces the activation of the receptors for phagocytosis. Macrophages develop functional complement receptors and undertake similar operations to the neutrophils. However, further interactions with the interferons, and subsequently with bacterial or viral products, induce further differentiation into a fully activated phenotype. Interferons enhance endocytosis and phagocytosis and modulate the surface receptor functions of newly migrated macrophages. Ingestion of bacteria by endocytosis triggers the primary oxygenase which converts molecular oxygen to the superoxide, which then reacts to produce hydrogen peroxide and hydroxyl

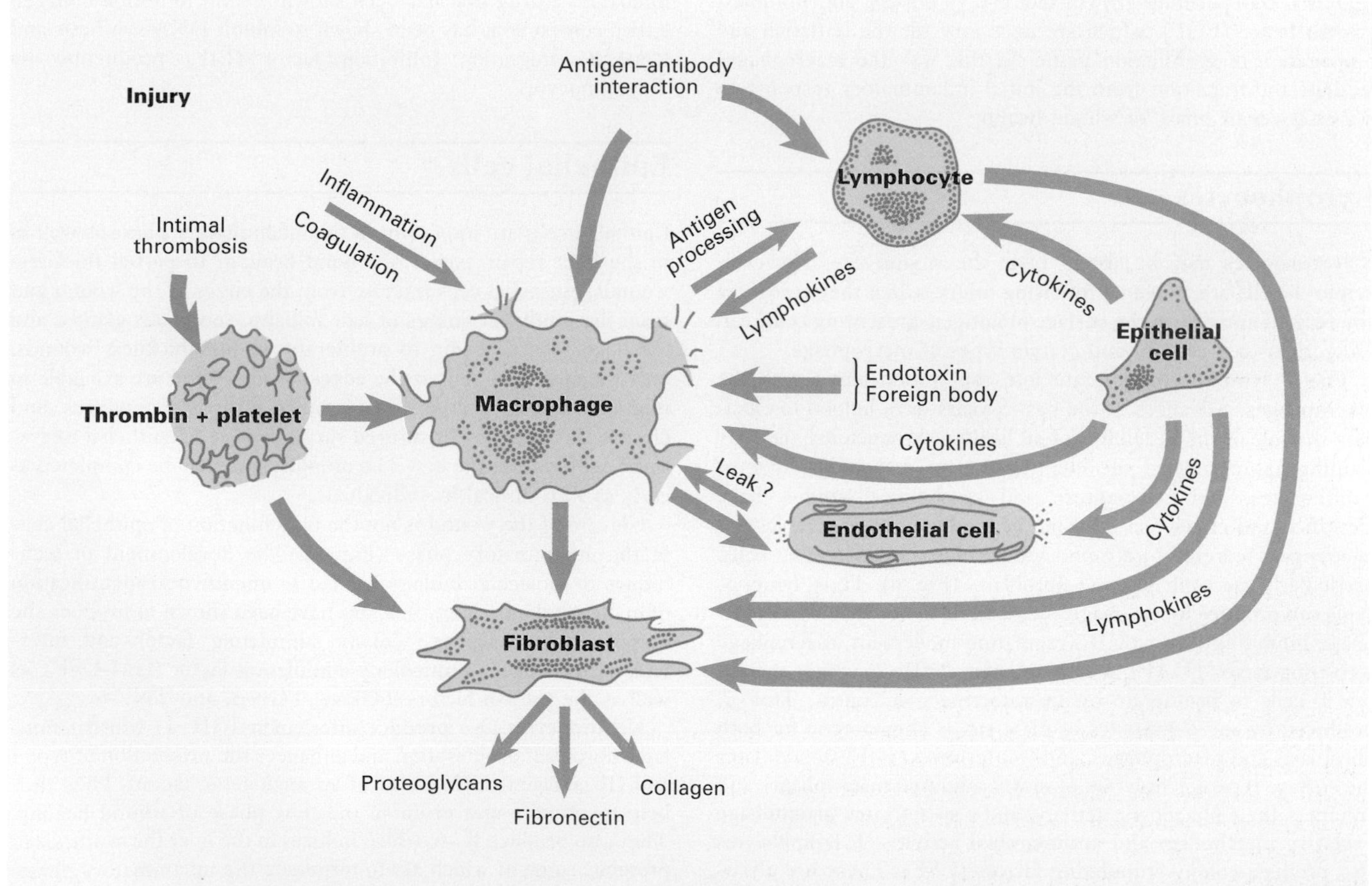

Fig. 6 Cellular biology of wound healing. Note the central role played by the macrophage.

radicals required for microbiocidal activity. Oxygen is essential. If the partial pressure of oxygen falls below 30 mmHg, macrophages are inactivated; their phagocytosing potential is reduced. The relationship between oxygen pressure and healing has been shown to be linear, explaining the beneficial role of oxygen pressure in repair.

The activated macrophage is the major effector cell for degrading and removing damaged connective tissue components, collagen, elastin, and proteoglycans. Initial degradation takes place extracellularly—up to several millimetres from the macrophage. Collagen and other fragments are then ingested and degraded by the cathepsin enzymes and other peptides. In contrast to neutrophils, macrophages can continue to synthesize the necessary enzymes, thus persisting for a longer time. They also phagocytose the decaying neutrophils.

Apart from their role in debridement, macrophages secrete chemotactic factors which bring additional inflammatory cells to the wound site. Macrophages also produce prostaglandins, which are strongly vasodilatory and affect the permeability properties of microvessels. The macrophages act after the amines and kinins, and are produced on demand, prolonging the inflammatory phase. Prostaglandins also augment the adenyl cyclase activity in T lymphocytes, which accelerates the mitosis of other cells.

The angiogenesis stimulated in the early phase of wound healing has been shown to be related to the presence of macrophages. Increased levels of lactate production, up to 15-fold, have been found in wounded tissue, and have caused macrophages to produce and release angiogenic substances. The macrophages also produce growth factors, such as platelet-derived growth factor (PDGF), transforming-growth factor-β (TGF-β), and fibroblast growth factor (FGF), which are necessary for the initiation and propagation of granulation tissue. In this way the macrophages mediate the transition from the initial inflammatory response to the early repair phase of wound healing.

Lymphocytes

B lymphocytes may be absent from the wound site. However, helper T cells are activated following injury, when they recognize any foreign antigen on the surface of antigen-presenting cells, e.g. Langerhans cell in skin, and certain types of macrophage.

The T lymphocytes migrate into the wound along with the macrophages. Advances in the past 5 years have helped to elucidate the role of the T cell in wound healing. Monoclonal antibody staining has permitted the identification of sets and subsets of lymphocytes, and cell culture and biochemical studies have identified and characterized some of the lymphokines, molecular messengers secreted by lymphocytes, which influence other cells, particularly macrophages and fibroblasts (Fig. 6). Thus, lymphocytes can produce macrophage chemotactic factor (MCF), macrophage inhibiting factor (MIF) regulating movement, macrophage activating factor (MAF), and interleukin-2 (IL-2) which enables the T cells to proliferate by an autocrine mechanism. TGF-β, produced by the α-granules of platelets, is chemotactic for both fibroblasts and macrophages, and γ-interferon (γ-IFN) modulates the surface receptor function of newly migrated macrophages and enhances their phagocytic activity, and also activates macrophage oxidative metabolism and antimicrobial activity. T lymphocytes also produce colony stimulating factors (CSF). These are glycoproteins that act on neutrophils and macrophages through specific receptors which have recently been identified—granulocyte-CSF, macrophage-CSF, granulocyte/macrophage-CSF, and interleukin-3 (IL-3).

The colony stimulating factors are very potent, being effective at very low concentrations (pg/ml). They are involved in the stimulation of proliferation, and of the commitment of the monocyte to differentiation and maturation. They stimulate the function of phagocytosis, and the production by macrophages of substances such as prostaglandins, tumour necrosis factor (TNF), γ-IFN, and further colony stimulating factors. As quantities are very small, it is not known whether all cells are able to produce colony stimulating factors. They are induced *in vivo* by the presence of micro-organisms. Colony stimulating factors are currently in clinical use for the treatment of neutropenia, both congenital and induced by cancer therapy. It has been suggested that there could be a prophylactic role for them in abdominal and genitourinary surgery, where infections are common.

Macrophages and lymphocytes have been shown to be present from day 1 in wounds, although lymphocytes are fewer in number than macrophages. In a study on human wounds by Martin and colleagues, macrophages peaked between 3 and 6 days and lymphocytes between 8 and 14 days. Thus they persist into the early repair phase of wound healing. Both macrophages and lymphocytes disappear from mature wounds by an unknown mechanism, but in abnormal scars both persist long afterwards. In hypertrophic scars, macrophages and lymphocyte levels have been found to be very high 4 to 5 months after wounding, and lymphocytes were still present at 40 per cent of the high level after 2 years. It has been suggested that control of lymphocytes might be a useful approach to control of scarring. It is of interest that minoxidil, a drug that has been shown *in vitro* to inhibit collagen lattice contraction, has been shown to inhibit DNA synthesis and leucocyte migration inhibition factor (LIF) production by T lymphocytes.

Epithelial cells

Epithelial cells are important in the inflammatory phase as well as in the later repair aspect of wound healing. In partial thickness wounds, epithelial cells migrate from the edges of the wound and from the epithelial linings of hair follicles, sebaceous glands, and sweat glands and begin to proliferate. In full thickness wounds, only the epithelial cells at the edges of the wound are available to migrate, because of the destruction of dermal appendages, and closure takes longer. In sutured surgical wounds epithelial migration begins within the first 24 h of injury and may be completed as early as 72 h in healthy individuals.

Closure of the wound is not the only function of epithelial cells in the inflammatory phase (Fig. 4). The development of techniques in molecular biology has led to unequivocal identification of many cytokines. Keratinocytes have been shown to produce the granulocyte/macrophage colony stimulating factor and interleukin-3 (IL-3) or multicolony stimulating factor (GM-CSF), as well as the growth factors TGF-α, TGF-β, and TNF-α.

Keratinocytes also produce interleukin-1 (IL-1) which stimulates fibroblast proliferation and enhances the production of type I and III collagen mRNA and of an angiogenic factor. Thus they help to prepare and promote the next phase of wound healing. They also produce IL-6, which induces in the liver the synthesis of proteins, some of which act to terminate the inflammatory phase.

By definition, chronic ulcers have a deficit in epithelialization. This could arise through reduced cell proliferation, or excess cell loss. Early studies of mitotic frequency at the edge of superficial ulcers failed to show any difference between those which healed expeditiously with treatment and those which did not. It is therefore probable that the surface extracellular matrix of such wounds governs the process of wound closure by forming an environment which may be either permissive of, or prohibitive for, epithelial cell adhesion and migration. The nature of these interactions remains relatively unexplored.

FORMATION OF GRANULATION TISSUE

Various chemotactic, growth, and activating factors produced in the inflammatory phase are concerned in the initiation and development of granulation tissue which lasts from about day 4 to day 21 after wounding. Granulation tissue comprises a loose matrix of fibrin, fibronectin, collagen, and glycosaminoglycans, particularly hyaluronic acid, containing macrophages, fibroblasts, and ingrowing blood vessels. In deep wounds, granulation tissue serves as a scaffold for new tissue ingrowth. In incisional wounds during this phase the wound begins to gain tensile strength, although it is during this early period that wound dehiscence and evisceration most frequently occur.

Fibroblasts

In the initial phase after wounding, fibroblasts migrate into the wound site 24 h after injury. During this phase of healing (4 to 21 days) the fibroblasts are activated and undergo a burst of proliferative and synthetic activity, initially producing high amounts of fibronectin, and then synthesizing the other protein components of the extracellular matrix, including collagen and elastin, and glycosaminoglycans. The fibroblasts align themselves along the wound axis and form cell to cell links, which contribute to the contraction of the wound.

There has been much discussion about the type and origin of fibroblasts that appear in the wound. These fibroblasts have characteristics in between those of normal resting fibroblasts and smooth muscle cells. This altered phenotype, which has been called the 'myofibroblast' is more mobile and more contractile than the inactivated fibroblast, and disappears on the completion of wound healing. Early distinctions between fibroblasts and myofibroblasts were based on ultrastructural criteria, but immunochemical analyses have, more recently, led to identification of subspecies of myofibroblasts based on permutations of expression of vimentin, desmin, and a smooth muscle actin. It has now been shown that smooth muscle cells in culture can reversibly modulate from contractile to synthetic cells, i.e. the reverse of the myofibroblast development, and this may reflect changes occurring *in vivo*. In addition, it has been demonstrated that smooth muscle genes can be switched on transiently in certain circumstances by other non-muscle cells, including macrophages and some epithelial cells. It is still not known what controls the change in phenotype.

Complex factors influence the behaviour of the fibroblasts in the formation of granulation tissue. Migration is promoted by TGF-β (produced by platelets and keratinocytes). Proliferation is promoted by thrombin, by serotonin (produced by platelets), by interleukin-1 (IL-1) produced by keratinocytes, by fibroblast growth factor from macrophages, and by epidermal growth factor. Synthetic activity is promoted by IL-1 and factor XIII for collagen, and by thrombin, epidermal growth factor, and TGF-β for fibronectin, while lysyloxidase activity is augmented by serotonin. Some remodelling of the extracellular matrix may take place at this stage. Degradative activity, which is also necessary for remodelling, is enabled by the promotion of collagenase synthesis by prostaglandin E_2.

Angiogenesis

Research into factors influencing angiogenesis has been directed at means of inhibiting new vessel growth in regard to tumour metastasis or, in the case of wound repair, means of stimulating angiogenesis to enhance healing.

Hypoxia following injury, if not so severe as to lead to tissue death associated with ischaemia, acts as a major stimulus for angiogenesis, which is required for restoration of blood flow. Along with fibroblast proliferation, neovascularization is a common feature of granulation tissue in the early phase of healing. One stimulus for new vessel growth is fibroblast growth factor, while other angiogenic factors, such as those secreted by macrophages and other cells, also contribute to the neovascularization. The growth of vessels in surgical wounds starts from capillary loops a few days after surgery, and vascularization may be complete in 6 to 7 days. In burns, development is later and may be complete in 12 to 16 days. The secondary wound (reopened and resutured) revascularizes at a significantly faster rate than a control wound which has not been reopened and resutured (Fig. 7 (a, b)). This aspect of the importance of angiogenesis in wound healing has been observed in other types of wounds where differences in regional vascularity and healing are directly related.

The endothelial migration seen in granulation tissue is supported by the increased fibronectin in this tissue. Mitotic activity leads to the formation of capillary buds which sprout from blood vessels adjacent to the wound and extend into the wound space. There is a gradual establishment of flow. Endothelial cell proliferation is stimulated by a low wound $P\text{O}_2$ in the early stages, but growth of vessels is later enhanced by a high wound $P\text{O}_2$ which is also essential for the synthesis of collagen necessary for the complete formation of the vessels. The pattern of vascular growth is probably the same in the healing of skin, muscle, and intestinal wounds. In fractured bones, vessel growth can be stimulated by repeated muscle contraction which increases bone blood flow, while vascularization is reduced by immobilization.

Modulation of angiogenesis is currently a very active area of research; inhibition of vessel growth in tumours and its promotion in wounds are both appealing therapeutic strategies. Progress has been hampered by difficulty in quantifying the dynamic process of neovascularization without interfering with it. Laser-Doppler flow measurements have been found to correlate with vessel counts in experimental wounds, and may offer a non-invasive and repeatable method. However, conventional laser-doppler techniques show large variations between readings even at adjacent points. Recently, a scanning laser-doppler device has been developed, which overcomes this difficulty and which allows the imaging of blood flow in surface wounds. It has been used to study the evolution of blood flow over time in experimental and clinical wounds.

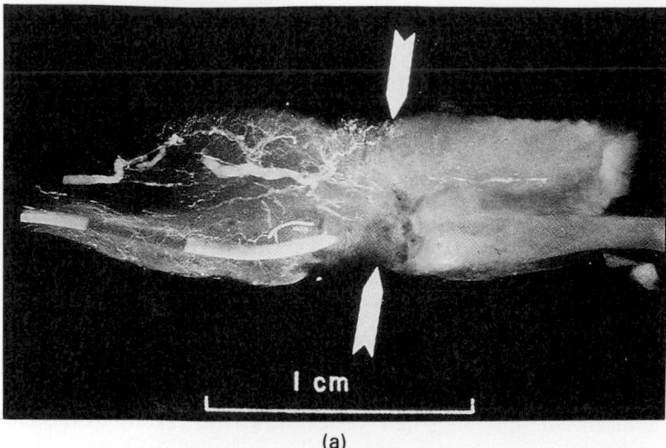

(a)

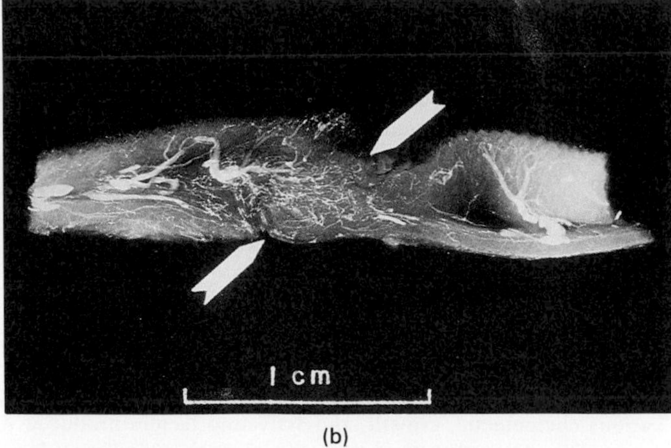

(b)

Fig. 7 (a) Microangiogram of a cross-section of a primary wound perfused from the left side. A small amount of dye is seen in the distal pedicle, but no vessel can be seen crossing the wound at 5 days. (b) Five-day-old secondary wound. Note the excellent filling of all the vessels and perfusion of small vessels which have grown across the wound.

Contraction

Wound closure by contraction, the inward movement of the edges of the injured tissue, is a normal part of the healing process. However, in some wounds, such as full thickness freeze injury, contraction does not occur. Wound contraction begins between days 8 and 10 after injury (Fig. 3). It is controlled both by the fibroblasts and by the extracellular matrix, and is due to the fibroblasts applying tension to the surrounding tissue matrix. *In vivo* it has been demonstrated that with contraction there is constant centrifugal tension. The rate of contraction has been shown to be constant for animals of a particular species or strain, and independent of the shape of wounds. However, there is marked interspecies variation. Contraction makes a much greater contribution to closure of full thickness wounds in rats than in man, which adds to the difficulty of extrapolating from experimental studies to the clinical situation.

COLLAGEN—MATRIX FORMATION AND REMODELLING

Collagen synthesis plays an important role in the early stages of healing and the formation of the granulation matrix. Production of collagen remains a major process in wound repair for several weeks after wound closure, and the collagen continues to undergo remodelling for 2 years or more until the injured tissue is finally restored.

Collagen is the major component by weight of the extracellular matrix of the skin, accounting for about 60 to 80 per cent of the dry weight of the tissue. There are known to be at least 13 different genetically distinct collagen types (Table 3), six of which occur in human skin.

Extracellular matrix

The extracellular matrix of tissues is composed of various polysaccharides and proteins and their complexes. These are secreted by cells *in situ* and different amounts and types are assembled to form diversely organized structures related to the functions of the particular tissue. The matrix not only serves as a support, but has a role influencing the behaviour of the cells in contact with it, affecting their development, migration, proliferation, shape, and metabolism, all of which are important with regard to wound healing.

Table 3 Collagen types (modified from Uitto 1989)

Collagen type	Chain composition	Tissue distribution
I	$[\alpha1(I)]_2\alpha2(I)$	Ubiquitous in most connective tissues, including skin, bones, tendons, ligaments, etc.
III	$[\alpha1(III)]_3$	Skin, blood vessels, predominant in fetal tissues and in early wounds
IV	$[\alpha1(IV)]_2\alpha2(IV)$	Basement membranes, anchoring plaques
V	$[\alpha1(V)]_2\alpha2(V)$ $[\alpha1(V)]_3$	Ubiquitous
VI	$\alpha1(VI)\alpha2(VI)\alpha3(VI)$	Extracellular microfibrils
VII	$[\alpha1(VII)]_3$	Skin, fetal membranes

The polysaccharides are glycosaminoglycans—long, unbranched chains of disaccharide repeating units. They fold with wide curvature in a random fashion and absorb large amounts of water, filling much of the extracellular space. Proteoglycans are formed by the combination of a number of glycosaminoglycan chains with a protein, and may contain up to 95 per cent (w/w) carbohydrate. Glycoproteins, on the other hand, are composed of short, branched oligosaccharide chains, containing from 1 to 60 per cent carbohydrate. The proteins of the extracellular matrix are principally structural proteins such as collagen and elastin, and adhesion proteins such as fibronectin and laminin.

All collagen molecules are composed of three polypeptide α-chains, with a left-handed triple-helix configuration. The chains have about 1000 amino acids and have a distinctive amino acid composition of 33 per cent glycine and 20 per cent of the imino acids, proline and hydroxyproline, with a particular repeating trimeric sequence of glycine–X–Y, where either X or Y is often proline.

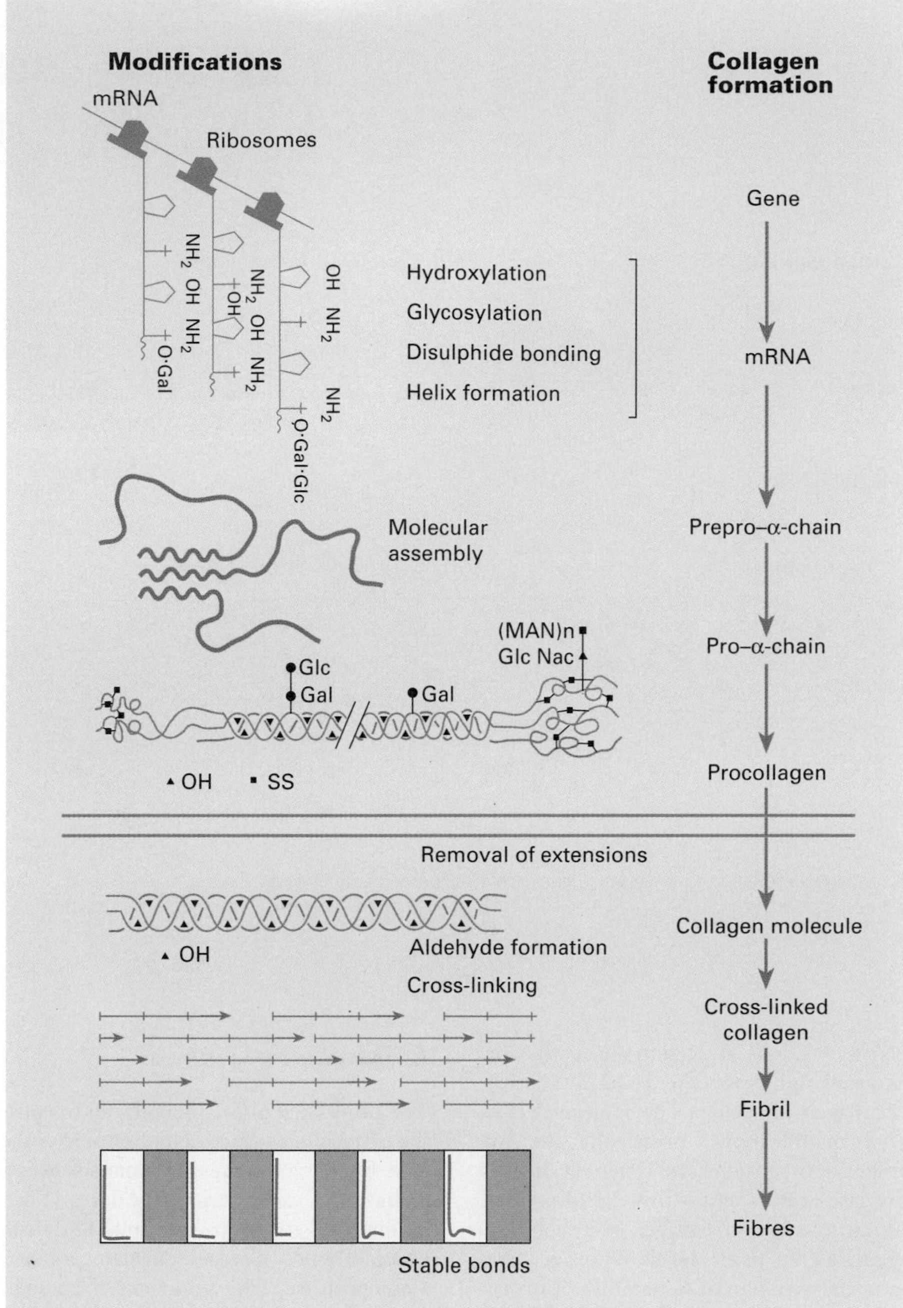

Fig. 8 Collagen biosynthesis: intracellular and extracellular stages, the double line represents the cell membrane; GLc, glucose; Gal, galactose; GlcNac, *N*-acetylglucosamine; SS, disulphide.

Synthesis of collagen

The synthesis of collagen involves a progression in the combination of amino acids to form chains which associate to form molecules, and then association to form fibrils which aggregate into fibres or bundles. Fibroblasts are the major cell type to synthesize collagen. The first stages of synthesis take place intracellularly, to produce procollagen molecules which undergo activation stages in the extracellular space (Fig. 8).

Intracellular synthesis

In the nucleus the genes are activated and there is translation of mRNAs, specific for single polypeptide chains. The mRNAs pass into the cytoplasm and are translated on the ribosomes of the endoplasmic reticulum, the three polypeptide chains being synthesized simultaneously (Fig. 8). The three α-chains may be identical (as in type III collagen), or a hybrid molecule consisting of two identical chains and a different third chain (as in type I), or three different chains (as in type VI). The molecule is a triple-chain molecule by the time it is detached from the ribosomes. The

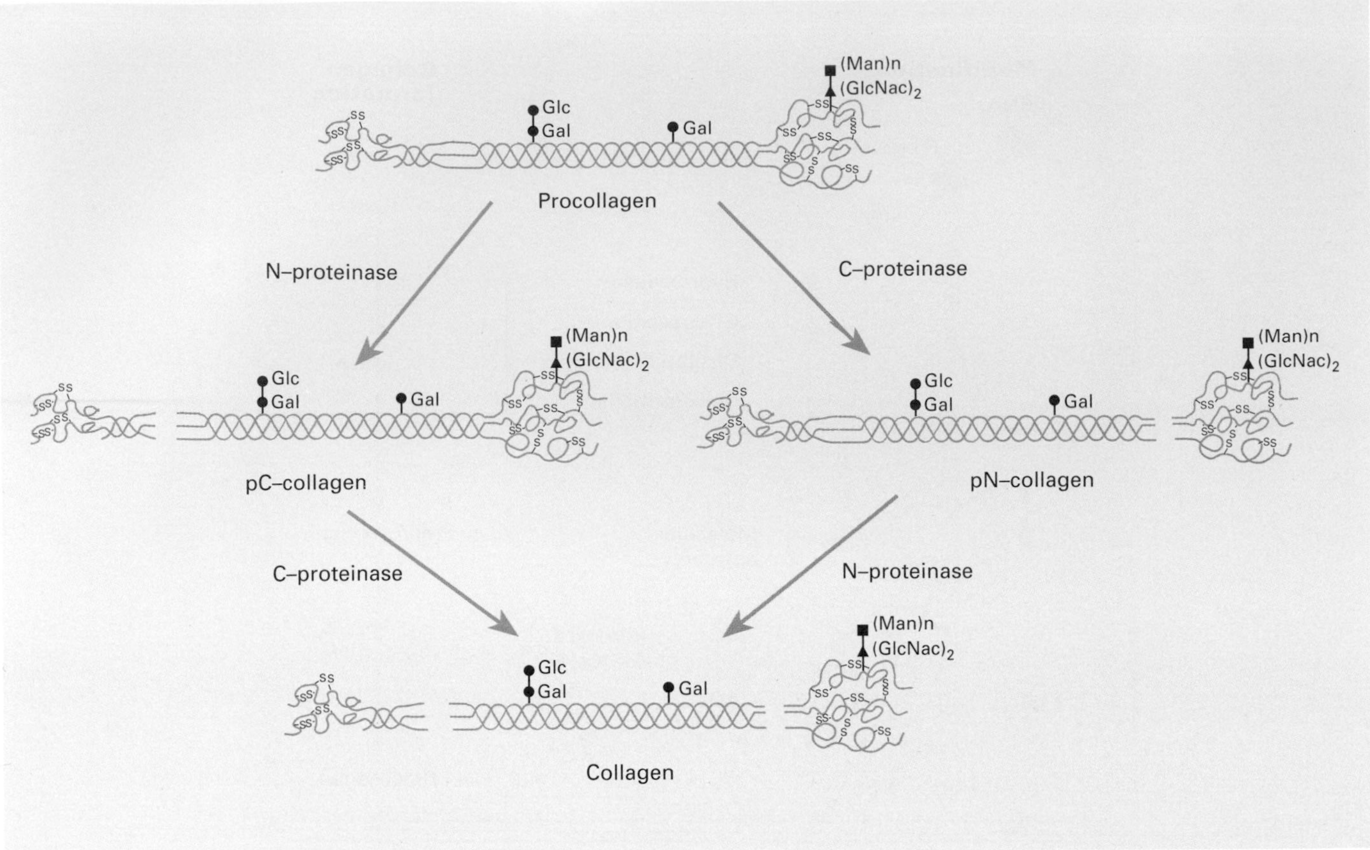

Fig. 9 Cleavage of the procollagen molecule to collagen. There is no obligatory sequence.

small, regularly spaced glycine residues situated in the central area of the chains allow them to pack tightly together to form the triple helix. This is the preprocollagen molecule. The molecules then undergo post-translational modifications, principally the hydroxylation of a large number of the proline and lysine residues by the enzymes lysyl hydroxylase and 3- and 4-prolyl hydroxylase. Hydroxylation is a rate-limiting step for collagen secretion, and appears to be tightly regulated by tissue levels of oxygen and lactate. The non-enzymatic glycosylation of some of the hydroxylysine residues also takes place at this stage. The hydroxy groups of hydroxyproline residues form interchain hydrogen bonds, which contribute to the stabilization of the triple-stranded helix. The 4-hydroxyproline moieties stabilize the collagen triple helix at physiological temperature (if not hydroxylated it unwinds above 24 °C). The hydroxylysine-saccharide units are also factors in the proper subunit alignment and the subsequent assembly of fibres. This precursor procollagen molecule has extension non-helical peptides of 15 to 20 amino acids in non-collagenous sequences at both ends of the chains. These propeptides contain both intra- and intermolecular disulphide bonds, giving a globular form and probably serving as the starting point for the rapid triple-helix formation. They also prevent intracellular formation of large collagen fibres. These post-translational modifications result in the formation of the procollagen molecule, which is then transported to the Golgi apparatus, enclosed in vesicles, and taken via the microtubules to the cell surface.

Extracellular synthesis

The processing of the procollagen to collagen fibres takes place in the extracellular space. The first step is the activation of the molecule by the cleavage of amino- and carboxy-peptide ends by amino- and carboxyl-propeptidases (Fig. 9). Lack of, or defects in, one of these enzymes results in defective fibres, e.g. type VII Ehlers–Danlos disease, dermatosporaxis in calves lacking the aminoprotease. The sequence of charge and hydrophilic amino acids in the collagen molecule is such that it allows self-assembly of collagen into fibrils *in vitro*, possibly because the helical portions allow electrostatic interaction with adjacent collagen molecules, but the *in-vivo* process is considered to be more complex. The ε-amino group of certain lysine and hydroxylysine residues is converted to aldehyde by the extracellular enzyme lysyl oxidase. The aldehydes react to form covalent bonds between the short, non-helical end of the collagen molecules, thus cementing the overlaps. The polymerization of many molecules in a staggered arrangement gives rise to the typical periodicity of 60 nm seen in electron microsope sections (Fig. 10) and this arrangement maximizes the tensile strength of the structure. At this stage type III fibrils have diameters of 40 to 60 nm and type I 100 to 500 nm. The size of the collagen fibrils may depend on the order of cleavage of the non-helical domains, cleavage of the carboxy-terminal first resulting in thin fibrils and of the amino-terminal first leading to thick fibrils.

The build-up of the propeptides released in the transformation

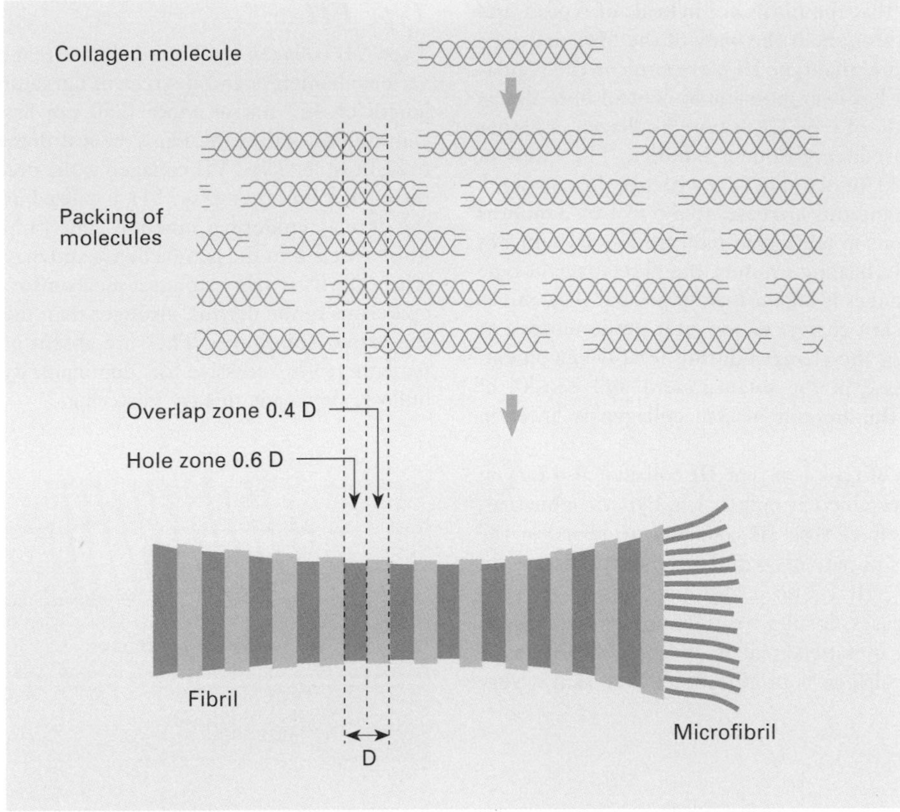

Fig. 10 Staggered packing of collagen molecules to form fibrils.

of procollagen to collagen inhibits collagen synthesis and thus provides a feedback for switching off the process of synthesis. The failure of this feedback system may be a contributory factor in excessive scarring.

Cross-links

The aggregates of collagen molecules formed in the extracellular space then undergo cross-linking. The extent and types of cross-links, or ratios of types, vary from tissue to tissue, with age, and in disease. In skin, the collagen produced after injury is initially stabilized by cross-links derived from hydroxyallysine. In normal wound healing this changes to cross-links derived from the modified amino acid allysine, but this change does not occur in hypertrophic scars. With time, these cross-links change to 'mature', more stable cross-links, which have not been completely characterized.

In skin the major mature cross-link may be hydroxyaldohistidine. In most other connective tissues a hydroxypyridinium cross-link is predominant. The greater the number of cross-links, the stiffer a tissue will be, although stiffness may also be influenced by the type of cross-link. In normal bone, for example, the hydroxypyridinium cross-link occurs with a frequency of 0.24 moles per mole of collagen.

Abnormal numbers or types of cross-links can lead to malformation of tissue. The hydroxypyridinium cross-link prevalent in bone also occurs in hypertrophic scars, but is not found in normal skin or in normal mature scar tissue. Increased hydroxylation of lysine residues can occur in hyperglycaemic states, and affects the types of cross-links as well as the number. In one study of diabetic patients, the numbers of five different types of cross-link were shown to increase between three- and six-fold. Clinical assessment of hand contracture was associated with an increased number of cross-links, which was also correlated with the duration of diabetes and with skin changes.

The organization of the collagen in tissues is also influenced by the kinds and amounts of non-collagenous macromolecules that the cells secrete along with the collagen. In addition, the fibroblasts have a mechanical role in the assembly, crawling over the collagen, pulling and compacting it. The final architecture of the collagen network is related to its function. Thus collagen fibres in the papillary dermis are aligned in thin bundles almost perpendicular to the basement membrane and they hold up the dermal papillae. Some of the fibres glide into the loops of the anchoring fibrils attached to the basement membrane. In the reticular dermis the thick, undulating bundles are nearly parallel to the epidermal plane, and are connected by interlacing fibres, allowing the tissue to resist stress in all directions. In the hypodermis interlacing collagen fibres surround the adipocytes.

Types of collagen

At one time it was suggested that there might be different phenotypes of fibroblast, each synthesizing a particular type of collagen, but it has been shown that at least types I, III, and VI can be all synthesized by the same cells.

Types I and III

Types I and III, the interstitial collagens, are the major types of collagen in skin, the rod-shaped molecules providing its tensile strength. It is suggested that the fibrils are hybrids of types I and III, with type I present throughout the body of the fibril and type III round the periphery, and that type III plays a role in the regulation of fibril diameter. It has been possible to control fibre size *in vitro* by changing the ratio of type III to type I collagen, a higher proportion of type III producing thinner bundles. The ratios of type I to type III in normal human skin vary with age. In a 15-week fetus the ratio is 0.8 to 1 and this increases to 3.6 to 1 by 3 months after birth. Determinations in adult skin indicate I to III ratios of between 3.5 and 6 to 1. In healing wounds, the percentage of type III collagen in the early stages is higher than in normal skin, and as healing progresses there is a change to a greater predominance of type I collagen, mirroring the changes during fetal development. There is a linear decrease in the total amount and density of collagen with age, and the amount of skin collagen is lower in females than males.

Ratios of the amounts of type I to type III collagen also vary in disease, having been determined as only 2 : 1 in hypertrophic scar, but 19 : 1 in keloid. Levels of type III collagen are raised in the nodules and contractures of patients with Dupuytren's disease. In diabetic patients the type III:I ratio is also high, and finger contraction occurs in some cases. Insulin treatment causes expression of type III collagen in the mesangial matrix. In Ehlers–Danlos type IV disease, no type III collagen is produced, and the skin is very thin.

Type IV

Type IV collagen is a major component of the basement membrane in the dermal–epidermal junction to which basal keratinocytes attach preferentially. It is also produced by endothelial cells and forms an essential element of the microvascular wall. The triple-helix conformation is interrupted by non-collagenous segments lacking the Gly–X–Y repeat sequence. The procollagen molecules are not cleaved after secretion, they retain their propeptides and therefore their globular regions. The carboxy-terminal globular domains of pairs of molecules associate 'head to head', and further lateral associations between amino terminals, stabilized by disulphide bonds, allow the formation of a sheet-like polygonal mesh. The higher carbohydrate content, with disaccharides of glucose and galactose attached to the hydroxylysine residues, also contributes to the formation of the mesh. Several layers of such sheets are eventually joined together by covalent bonds, making it more flexible than types I and III.

Type V

Type V collagen is ubiquitous and interfaces between the cell surface and the surrounding matrix. It has a chain length similar to that of the interstitial collagens, but an amino acid content more like that of the basement membrane collagens. It does not contain any disulphide bonds.

Type VI

Improved techniques have shown type VI collagen to be more abundant in skin and other tissues than was previously thought. In cultured fibroblasts the ratio of amounts of I : VI mRNA was 3 : 1, indicating that type VI could be more abundant than type III, and the expression in cultured cells reflected that in skin sections. Type VI collagen is a heterotrimer, composed of three different α-chains, which have unusually large globular domains at the ends of the polypeptides. It has a high cysteine content and is highly disulphide bonded. The chain length is short.

Type VII

Type VII collagen is a homopolymer that aggregates in bundles of various diameters and degrees of curvature. It has a longer chain length of 467 nm or more (750 nm has been measured). Discontinuities within the triple-helical domain allow the molecules to be flexible. Type VII collagen is the predominant component of the anchoring fibrils (Fig. 11), localized in the sub-basal lamina of the dermal–epidermal junction. The carboxylate terminals of the fibrils insert into the lamina densa and may extend into the dermis. These fibrils are the strongest mechanism for the adherence of the epidermis to the dermis, stronger than the attachment effected by the hemidesmosomes. They are absent or reduced in the skin of patients with recessive or dominant dystrophic epidermolysis bullosa; this leads to easy blistering.

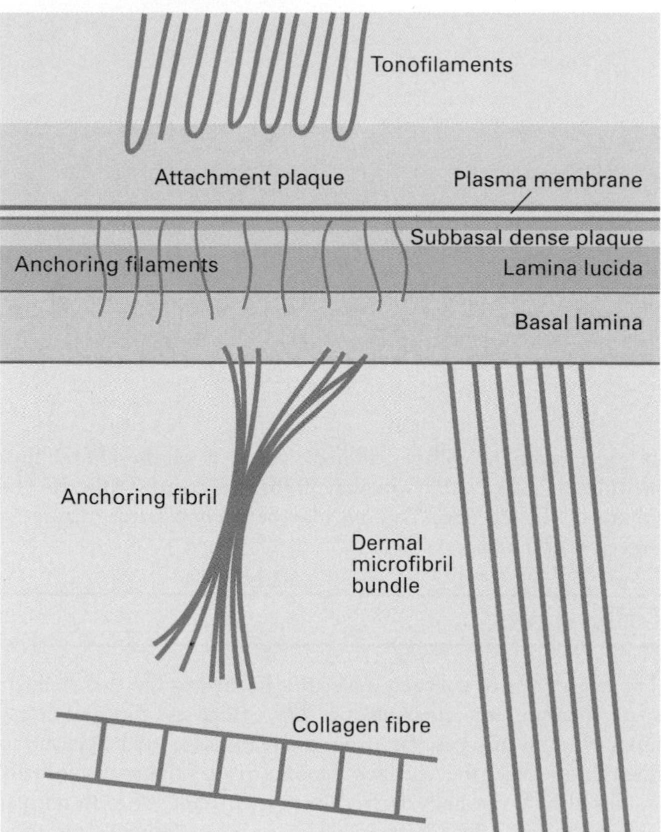

Fig. 11 Epidermal–dermal junction in the region of a hemidesmosome.

Collagenolysis

In the extracellular space, procollagenase is transformed to collagenase which cleaves the helical portion of the collagen molecule, causing the fragments to unwind. The single-stranded polypeptides are then susceptible to degradation by extracellular proteinases and peptidases, or undergo endocytosis and are degraded by intracellular enzymes. Some procollagen may be retained and degraded in the cell rather than secreted. There is some evidence for this, but the mechanisms are not understood. Mature collagen may also be absorbed by phagocytosis. Mature banded collagen found in vacuoles in the cytoplasm of fibroblasts must have come from the extracellular space, because it is only there that such collagen is formed. If it were from the intracellular synthetic pathway, it would be in the form of procollagen. The peak levels of collagen phagocytic activity have been shown to correspond with the period when a change of configuration and fibre orientation was occurring.

There is a relationship between the stability of the collagen triple helix and the degree of intracellular degradation of collagen. Underhydroxylated collagen is non-helical at 37 °C and its secretion rate is only one-tenth that of fully hydroxylated collagen. Non-helical collagen is degraded in the lysosomes. Degradation produces free hydroxyproline, which is a measure of collagen degradation because proline hydroxylation occurs after translation.

In health, the synthesis and degradation of collagen is finely regulated to maintain the optimal level of collagen. Imbalance is associated with disease states, such as scleroderma, as well as alterations in wound healing. In scleroderma, *in-vitro* studies indicate that collagen accumulation is due to enhanced synthesis rather than any other process. On the other hand, excessive collagen degradation is responsible for the imbalance in recessive dystrophic epidermolysis bullosa. Skin from friction blisters in these patients produced high concentrations of collagenase in organ culture, and a radioimmunoassay study found that this reflected the *in-vivo* pathology, the concentration of collagenase being ten-fold that in normal skin. Increased collagenolysis may occur with more normal levels of collagenase if the collagen is abnormal, e.g. collagen synthesized under hyperglycaemic conditions is more susceptible to degradation. Imbalance may also be due to defective regulation of cellular growth, leading to low collagen levels, as in focal dermal hypoplasia. Lesions show the absence of dermal connective tissue, the epidermis apposing on to fat tissue, separated by a thin layer of reticulate fibres. Measurement of the proliferative capacity of fibroblasts from adjacent skin in culture indicated a population doubling time twice as long as normal and a saturation density only one-fifth that of controls. The rate of collagen synthesis was normal.

The failure of regulation also causes a problem in the formation of keloids, when the synthesis and breakdown are both stimulated, but the former to a greater extent, thus leading to imbalance and overgrowth. The remodelling of scar tissue also requires the degradation and synthesis of collagen.

Collagen and wound healing

In the adult, the normal repair of wounds occurs by the formation of granulation tissue and its organization to a scar. Scar is a dynamic, metabolically active tissue. Precise regulation of collagen metabolism during the repair process is exerted by cytokines (see below) and by the interactions of the extracellular matrix with fibroblasts. *In vitro*, fibroblasts in contact with collagen fibrils in a three-dimensional lattice show decreased production of types I and III collagen, but enhanced gene expression and activation of collagenase. Experimental studies on collagen deposition in wounds show some variation between species and some differences that may be due to the particular experimental techniques. Some studies in mice showed little collagen in the granulation tissue after 1 week, but another study in rats showed the presence of some collagen from day 1. Recent work on rat wounds indicated that type III collagen was synthesized within 10 h after injury. Collagen synthesis is maximal between 14 and 21 days, although increased collagen deposition may be provoked to occur earlier by electric stimulation. After 21 days the rate of synthesis and the volume density of collagen in the wound return to the normal level. However, the tensile strength of the tissue continues to increase for a considerable time, up to 60 days or even 1 year. Wound tensile strength is a physical measurement which reflects the degree of intermolecular cross-linking, rather than collagen biosynthesis. Its increase is due to the formation of further cross-links and a change to more stable forms which lead to reorientation of the direction of the bundles. Breaking of the tissue occurs by disruption of the connection between fibres in the bundles and by slipping of molecules one over the other in the fibre. Between 3 weeks and 2 months after the injury, cellularity decreases, as does fibroblast cytoplasm volume.

Fetal wound healing

In contrast to the healing by scar formation in the adult, the healing of fetal wounds up to the early third trimester of gestation proceeds without scar formation. Collagen is deposited more quickly in the fetal wound than in the adult, but is rapidly organized and is not excessive. It is thought that this might be due to glycosaminoglycans, which are also deposited. The nature and ratios of the glycosaminoglycans, which affect the cross-linking of collagen fibrils and the migration of fibroblasts, vary in different stages of wound healing. Hyaluronic acid, in particular, the content of which is high in the fetal wound matrix and which is found wherever there is tissue regeneration or repair, has been shown *in vitro* to facilitate the movement of fibroblasts. While hyaluronic acid is present only in the early stages in adult wounds, it is present throughout the process in fetal healing and the wound is closed by mesenchymal ingrowth on to the hyaluronate-enriched matrix. An *in-vitro* study of the activity of a hyaluronic acid stimulating factor in sheep detected levels ten-fold higher in the fetal serum than in the serum of normal adults. In animal models there is variation in the open-wound healing response in the fetus of different species—wounds in sheep contracting, while those in the rabbit and monkey heal without contraction, as in the human.

The relevance of reduced scar formation in fetal wound healing and the potential application to clinical healing has been highlighted in recent work by Ferguson and colleagues. These workers have stated that fetal wound healing is characterized by a reduced growth factor profile and have demonstrated that neutralizing TGF-β activity by antibodies results in decreased wound scarring in adult rats. While this method is not applicable in the clinic, it clearly demonstrates that the modulation of scarring may be an attainable goal.

Wound remodelling—pharmacological control

One of the problems with scar tissue is that it tends to remain somewhat weaker and more brittle than previously unwounded tissue. A second problem is that it tends to contract abnormally. A third problem in certain people is that of overhealing, leading to

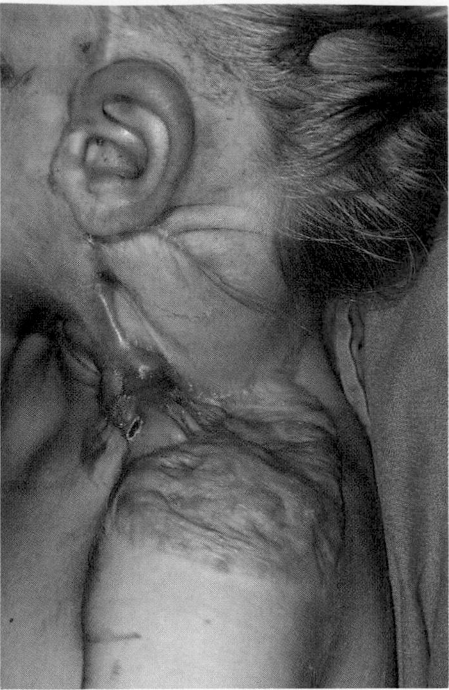

Fig. 12 Hypertrophic scar on a young child.

hypertrophic scars or keloids (Figs. 12 and 13). Some clinical differences between keloids and hypertrophic scars are listed in Table 4. While some researchers consider that there is spontaneous regression of hypertrophic scars eventually, others maintain that many such scars persist indefinitely. Biochemical

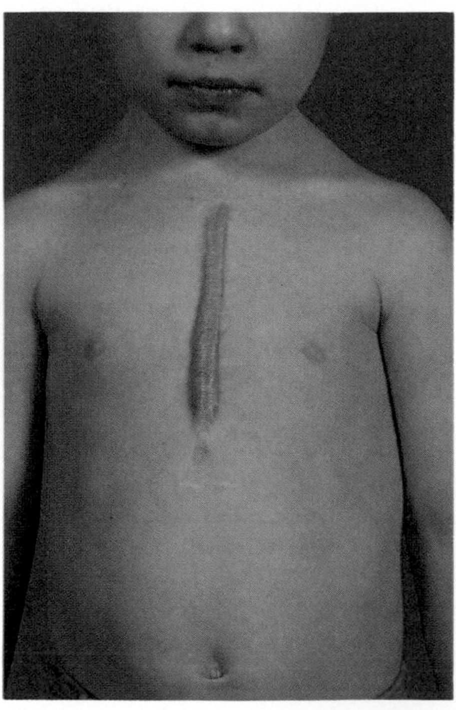

Fig. 13 Keloid scar.

Table 4 Hypertrophic scars and keloids (from Brody 1981)

Hypertrophic scars	Keloids
Develop soon after surgery	May not begin for many months
Usually subside with time (maturation)	Rarely subside with time
Limited boundary	Overgrow their boundaries
Size commensurate with injury	Minor injury may produce large lesion
Occur with motion (compression)	Independent of motion
Usually occur across flexor surfaces (joints, abdomen, etc.)	Areas of high predilection (ear-lobes, presternal skin), rarely across joints
Improve with appropriate surgery	Often worsened by surgery

differences between hypertrophic scar, keloid, and normal skin have also been characterized. Keloids have a greatly increased proportion of type I to type III collagen compared with normal skin, whereas in hypertrophic scars the ratio is lower than normal. Glycosaminoglycan contents are also abnormal in hypertrophic scars. One study determined the level of hyaluronic acid in hypertrophic scar to be less than half that of normal skin, while the level of chondroitin 4-sulphate was six times higher, as was also the case in granulation tissue. Either the chondroitin sulphate continues to be formed in the hypertrophic scar or it is not removed.

One reason for the imperfect characteristics of scar tissue is that the newly formed collagen pattern in a wound is abnormal, and that rapid intermolecular cross-linking while fibres are being formed leads to their being irreversibly fixed. The use of scanning electron microscopy to study collagen morphology led to the hypothesis that if the cross-linking could be temporarily delayed or slowed, a more nearly physiological collagen pattern would have time to develop.

Attempts to delay or inhibit the cross-linking of collagen have met with some success, e.g. β-aminoproprionitrile and other nitriles inhibit lysyl oxidase, the enzyme that deaminates the lysyl ε-amino group to aldehyde, an early step in the formation of intermolecular cross-links. D-Penicillamine reacts with aldehyde groups and so blocks cross-linking of newly formed collagen, but it may also make existing cross-links more labile. Improvement has also been effected using corticosteroids which inhibit fibroblast migration and proliferation and collagen synthesis. Compression has also been of benefit in some cases.

As described in the introduction, silastic gel is being used in the treatment of abnormal scars and is now licensed for use in the United States. γ-Interferon, which suppresses collagen synthesis *in vitro* and in animal models *in vivo*, leads to improvement in keloids in a small group of patients. An *in-vitro* study has shown that calcium antagonists reduce extracellular matrix component synthesis in a connective tissue equivalent. Cryosurgical treatment has also led to considerable improvement in one group of 45 patients. Increased understanding of the regulation of scarring has led to the suggestion that the inhibition of helper T cells by cyclosporin or compounds with similar properties should be investigated. A further approach to the control of different phases of wound healing, including hypertrophic scar and keloid formation, is that of influencing cell–matrix adhesion by using monoclonal antibodies or synthetic peptides.

Experimental wound-healing models

A wound is a very complex biological system and detailed studies of repair processes and the factors that influence them require both *in-vivo* and *in-vitro* models. An *in-vitro* model is more of a closed system, allowing the isolation of a tissue and investigation of modulation without the complication of other factors. While *in-vitro* models are only partial, and cannot be extrapolated directly, they do allow perceptions which may be valid *in vivo*.

One *in-vitro* model that has proved useful is the hydrated collagen lattice. An acidic type I collagen solution polymerizes *in vitro* when raised to physiological pH and ionic strength, forming a three-dimensional gel. If fibroblasts are incorporated into the polymerizing solution, they organize and align collagen fibrils and compact them, causing the lattice to contract. Such a lattice provides a simple model for connective tissue, and has been used as an *in-vitro* model for connective tissue contraction and scar contracture in wound healing. The degree and speed of contraction of the lattice are related to the cell density, to the concentration of collagen and of serum, and also to the type of cell involved, and to the presence of drugs or other factors. This model has been used recently by the authors to investigate the effect of different concentrations of minoxidil on the contraction of type I collagen lattices. In these studies minoxidil was found to inhibit the contraction of lattices in a dose-dependent manner (Fig. 14). Inhibition was evident in 24 h and was reversible to an extent depending on the length of time of exposure to the particular minoxidil dose. Washing out the minoxidil after 2 days for a dose of 4 mmol (800 μg/ml) or after 6 days for 2 mmol, led to the resumption of contraction (Fig. 15). Visualization of cells with MTT (3-(4,5-dimethylthiazol–2-yl)-2,5-diphenyltetrazolium bromide), which is metabolized to a blue formazan by the mitochondria of living cells, showed that the inhibition during the first 48 h was not due to fibroblast death. However, prolonged exposure beyond the 2 or 6 days, respectively, led to cellular death. Resumption of contraction with exchange to normal medium coincided with the return of rounded cells to an elongate morphology and to proliferation (Fig. 16). A lower dose of 0.5 mmol slowed contraction but did not affect morphology (as observed in the light microscope) nor cell proliferation.

The finding that minoxidil inhibits lattice contraction as well as fibroblast proliferation *in vitro*, and that the inhibition of contraction is reversible, supports the suggestion that it might be of therapeutic significance in cases of fibrotic disease and excessive scar formation.

Another study of the collagen lattice model showed the contraction of type III collagen lattices to be faster and to a greater degree than type I hydrated collagen lattices with identical numbers of cells. This could well be correlated with the high type III:I ratios in patients with Dupuytren's contraction and diabetics, certain of whom suffer hand contracture. In another *in-vitro* study using hydrated collagen lattices, fibroblasts from patients with Dupuytren's disease showed a consistently higher contractility than normal skin fibroblasts.

REGULATION OF WOUND HEALING BY PEPTIDE GROWTH FACTORS

Growth factors are messenger peptides secreted from a number of cell types integral to the repair mechanism. In general, growth factors are mitogens and chemoattractants. They show a remarkable specificity for cell types, acting selectively to induce cells into the wound environment in an orderly sequence, beginning with neutrophils, followed by macrophages, fibroblasts, and endothelial cells. As previously stated, the functions of these cells in wound healing include removal of cellular debris, leading to the formation of granulation tissue and its replacement with collagen and, subsequently, mature scar tissue. Growth factors are also released from blood on coagulation and subsequently are contributed by macrophages and probably by fibroblasts.

To date, the following growth factors have been shown to play a pivotal role in wound healing:

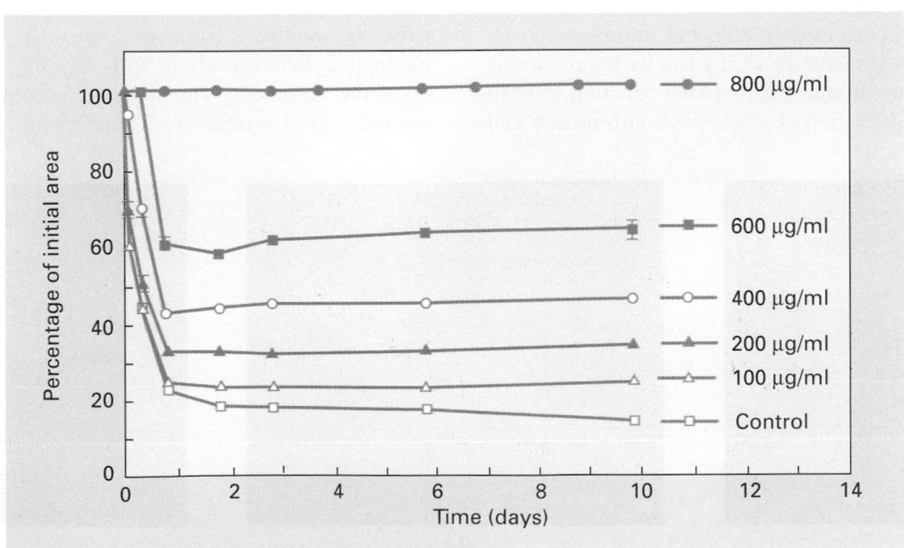

Fig. 14 Effect of minoxidil on lattice contraction by human skin fibroblasts, 74-year-old, third passage. Collagen concentration = 0.9 mg/ml, cell density = 6.7 × 10^4 cells/ml. Each point is a mean (± SEM) of three lattices.

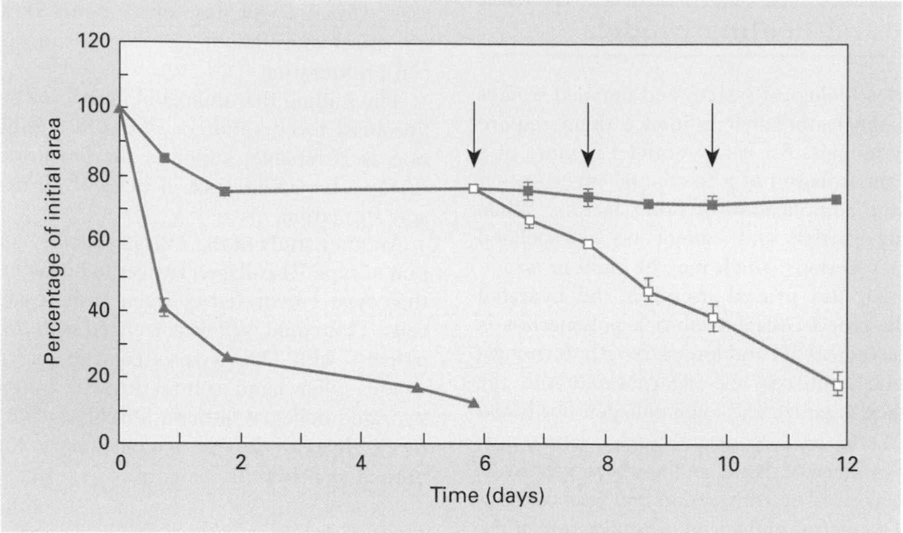

Fig. 15 Reversibility of the inhibition of contraction by minoxidil, 400 μg/ml, human foreskin fibroblasts, fourth passage. Collagen concentration = 0.65 mg/ml, cell density = 6.7 × 10^4 cells/ml. Control (▲); minoxidil 400 μg/ml (■); minoxidil removed (□); exchange of medium (↓). Each point is a mean (± SEM) of four lattices except for the minoxidil treatment up to day 6, which is a mean of eight lattices.

1. Transforming growth factor beta (TGF-β) is a potent stimulator of the synthesis of matrix proteins, such as collagen and fibronectin, and of glycosaminoglycans. It is present in high concentration in blood platelets and is released instantaneously into the wound at the site of injury. Multiple forms of TGF-β and the TGF-β receptor exist; these may generate a complex and diverse range of interacting signals on matrix, mesenchyme, and endothelial cells, some of which are inhibitory and some of which are stimulatory.
2. Platelet-derived growth factor (PDGF) has a more restricted target-cell specificity in comparison with other growth factors, but it is a major serum mitogen, also released from the α-granules of platelets, inducing fibroblast proliferation, matrix production, and maturation of connective tissue. Its particular attributes are effects on cell surface (cytoskeleton) motility, mainly directed at smooth muscle cells and fibroblasts.
3. Basic fibroblast growth factor (b-FGF) has its main stimulatory effect on the growth and differentiated function of fibroblasts and on the proliferation of vascular smooth muscle cells and endothelial cells. Therefore it has a major function as an 'angiogenesis peptide'.
4. Epidermal growth factor (EGF) and its homologue, transforming growth factor alpha (TGF-α), generally stimulate cell proliferation by binding to the EGF receptor in a variety of tissue types. They are also released from α granules of platelets.

Numerous other growth factors and cytokines have been proved to be, or are likely to be present in wounds. These include insulin-like growth factor (IGF), platelet derived endothelial cell growth factor (PDECGF), vascular endothelial growth factor (VEGF), heparin binding epidermal growth factor (HB-EGF), and granulocyte monocyte colony stimulating factor (GMCSF). Their role(s) are still uncertain. The situation is further confused by the fact that many growth factors, notably TGF-β, PDGF, and IGF exist as multiple 'isoforms'. Growth factor activity is also modulated by association with binding proteins, and depends upon the availability and type of receptor(s) present. Thus, for example, IGF1 is transferred from blood and local sites of produc-

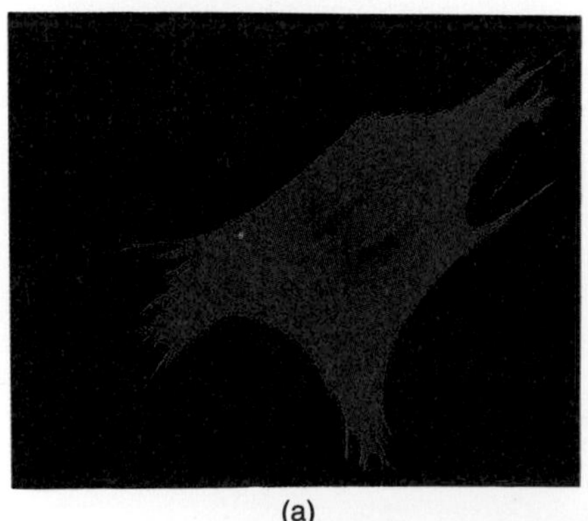
(a)

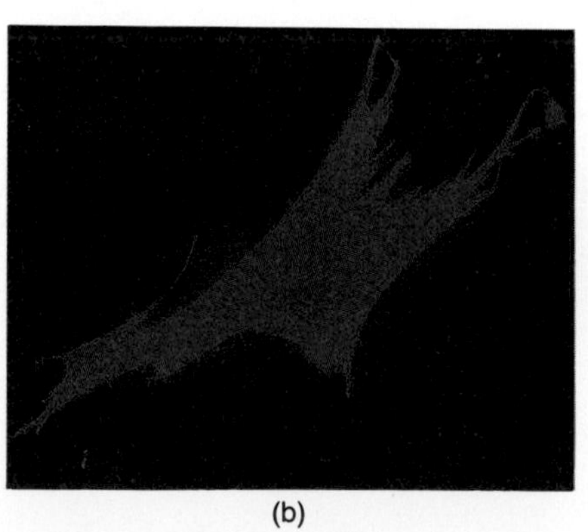
(b)

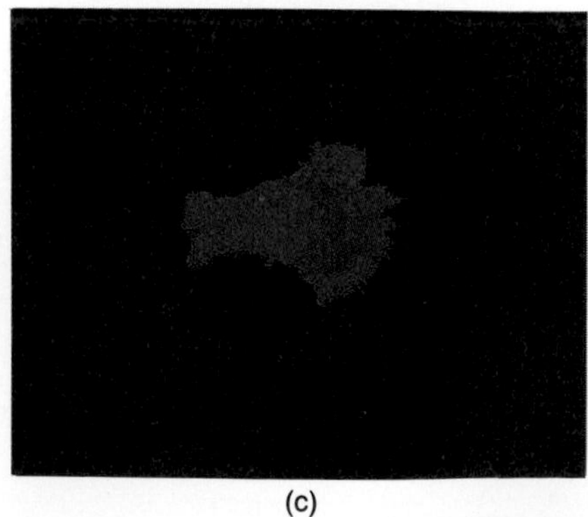
(c)

Fig. 16 Morphology of normal human skin fibroblasts in a monolayer, demonstrating actin fibres stained with rhodamine-phalloidin (× 400). (a) Control; (b) minoxidil, 100 μg/ml—little change in morphology, reflecting minor inhibition seen in gel contraction with this dose; (c) minoxidil 800 μg/ml—marked alteration in structure correlating with complete inhibition of gel contraction at this dose, but reversible up to 2 days.

tion to its cellular targets via a sequence of binding proteins, whose affinities are modulated by the pH of the wound environment. Alterations in the levels of binding proteins, and elevations of IGF antagonists have been found in situations associated with defective repair, including diabetes, malnutrition, uraemia, and jaundice.

The function of growth factor receptors and of post-receptor signalling pathways is also important. *In vitro*, high levels of several growth factors have been shown to reduce (down-regulate) expression of the relevant receptor at the cell surface. As a result, increasing levels of growth factor are ultimately associated with decreased cellular responses.

The pattern of growth factor expression in human wounds is being described by the techniques of immunoassay of wound fluid and of immunohistochemistry of biopsies. Unfortunately, these methods recognize antigenic determinants on the growth factor molecules, not their biological activity. Thus, for example, chronic venous ulcers have been found by Ferguson and colleagues to contain high levels of growth factors, including FGF, PDGF, and TGF-β, predominantly distributed in the fibrin cuffs around the blood vessels. It is not known whether these growth factors are biologically active, and if so whether they are sequestered or able to diffuse, or whether the appropriate receptors are expressed on adjacent wound cells.

The early response to injury

Thrombin, formed from the clotting cascade, stimulates the release of growth factors from α-granules of platelets. TGF-β, PDGF, and EGF are released locally and are chemotactic for both macrophages and fibroblasts. Macrophages play a critical role in subsequent events because they secrete a large repertoire of peptides involved in wound-healing mechanisms. These peptides include TGF-β, PDGF, b-FGF, EGF, TGF-α, and tumour necrosis factor (TNF). Phenotypic changes occur in macrophages as the wound matures, as evidenced by variation in their abilities to secrete peptides under basal or stimulated conditions. This modification in synthetic activity presumably leads to differential production of matrix, collagen, or ground substance at a particular time in the maturation of the wound. In addition, growth factors such as b-FGF have a strong influence on cellular movement within the wound, stimulating chemotaxis followed by synthetic activity when cells are positioned to deliver their products. PDGF may be a multifunctional 'first signal' peptide at the site of injury, being the first messenger stimulating fibroblast proliferation.

Role of the extracellular matrix

Extracellular matrix proteins provide a spatial organization that strongly influences the proliferation, differentiation, shape, and migration of cells. Growth factors modify the extracellular matrix and, by so doing, modify cell-surface matrix receptors and cellular receptors which, in turn, affect synthetic activity and the ultimate speed of wound repair. In the resting state, the matrix acts as a reservoir for inactive growth factors which are liberated or solubilized at the time of injury and are then free to transduce intracellular signals for replication and matrix synthesis. Experimentally, it can be shown that the action of TGF-β depends on the type of substratum in which it is acting, since in a non-retracting fibrin lattice, which restricts TGF-β mobility, matrix and collagen synthesis is impaired. In fact, TGF-β itself influences stromal formation because it regulates the splicing pattern of the ground-substance molecule fibronectin–mRNA precursor in granulation tissue.

Two latent proenzymes (metalloproteinases) have an important influence on extracellular matrix structure and function. These metalloproteinases are synthesized by fibroblasts and are characterized as collagenases (which degrade interstitial collagens) and stromalysin, (which degrades basement membrane proteins, including type IV collagen). Angiogenesis can only take place once the surrounding basement membrane has been degraded, allowing angiogenic cells to migrate and proliferate in the wound. Furthermore, the proteolytic activity of these metalloproteinases is regulated by endogenous tissue inhibitors of metalloproteinases. b-FGF has been shown to be a regulator of collagenase synthesis, thus affecting tissue remodelling during angiogenesis. *In vitro*, TGF-β increases the production of tissue inhibitors of metalloproteinases.

Cell culture studies

Using simple chemotactic assays, TGF-β and PDGF can be shown to influence movement of monocytes at physiological concentrations. b-FGF, TGF-β, and PDGF are chemotactic for fibroblasts. b-FGF is mitogenic and chemotactic for endothelial cells *in vitro*, reaffirming its critical role in angiogenesis and granulation tissue formation. In culture, many peptide growth factors are both mitogenic to fibroblasts and also increase their synthetic activity in a differential manner. In respect of synthetic activity, TGF-β appears to be the most active, stimulating the transcription of mRNA for both procollagen and matrix proteins, and increasing the production of these proteins in a number of cell lines *in vitro*. However, it is likely that many of the actions observed *in vitro* are not strictly analogous to the compartmentalization of function within the wound microenvironment.

Wound chambers

The implantation of a subcutaneous wound chamber represents an experimental form of injury that allows the examination of the organization of granulation tissue, excluding the process of re-epithelialization. A specific number of parameters such as cellularity, collagen content, DNA content, and matrix protein synthesis are used to assess this healing process. After a few days, wound fluid from such implanted chambers contains EGF/TGF-α, TGF-β, and PDGF-like activity. Activated monocytes from wound chambers have increased transcript numbers of the mRNA species TGF-α, TGF-β, and PDGF.

Subcutaneous implantation of a polyvinyl alcohol sponge provokes an inflammatory reaction within the interstices of the sponge, which accelerates accumulation of cellular elements. Small quantities of EGF incorporated into pellets embedded within the sponge, or injected daily into the sponge in an albumin carrier, increase cellularity, nucleic acid content, collagen, and glycosaminoglycan content in the granulation tissue. The synthetic effects are dose-dependent, and the observed accumulation of hydroxyproline is increased significantly by as little as 1 µg/day EGF.

In the wire mesh-type Hunt–Schilling wound chamber implanted subcutaneously in rats, exogenous TGF-β as a single injection soon after implantation increases the deposition of collagen. TNF has no effect on its own, although it inhibits the effects of TGF-β while not influencing those of PDGF. These experiments demonstrate the importance of the interaction between peptides within a wound.

A cylindrical chamber produced from polytetrafluoroethylene (PTFE) allows granulation tissue to grow along the lumen. Cellularity can be increased two- to six-fold by a single injection into the chamber lumen of small concentrations (100–400 μg) of PDGF, TGF-β, and b-FGF in a collagen gel. The half-life of iodinated peptides within the gel is in the region of 20 h and the most potent peptide is TGF-β.

Hunt and colleagues are using miniaturized porous chambers in human studies. Subcutaneous implantation can be performed under local anaesthesia, and is only slightly more traumatic than the insertion of an intravenous cannula. These 'human wound models' have been used to investigate the effects of tissue hypoxia, underperfusion during and after surgery, and parenteral nutrition before operation, and on rates of collagen synthesis. Eventually, they may be applied to determine variations in intrinsic healing potential, to predict wound failure and dissect its mechanisms, and to select patients for experimental treatments.

Animal studies

The first clue to the involvement of growth factors in wound healing became apparent from experiments using topical application of EGF to a standardized back wound in mice. Enhanced wound closure was observed both in control and sialectomized animals receiving EGF, indicating that the local delivery of wound-healing factors accelerated healing. EGF incorporated into multilamellar liposomes to prolong release, but not when given as a single dose, doubles tensile strength in skin wounds of rats at 7 days after wounding. A single dose of 2 μg TGF-β in a collagen vehicle increases tensile strength by 51 per cent at 9 days, whereas PDGF in saline does not produce any significant effect on breaking strength. The acceleration of the healing process is accompanied by increased infiltration into the wound of mononuclear cells and fibroblasts and by collagen deposition. The beneficial effects of collagen as a vehicle for peptide growth factors in these models is demonstrated by the fact that 2 μg of PDGF in a collagen suspension doubles the strength of wounds at 5 days, an effect which is still apparent at 40 days. Histological analysis of the wounds treated with these growth factors demonstrated an *in-vivo* chemotactic response of macrophages and fibroblasts and an increase in type I collagen. With both TGF-β and PDGF a dose–response curve is apparent. Wounds treated with both peptides demonstrate an augmented cellular infiltrate and, in the case of PDGF, increased staining with a monoclonal antibody procollagen type I. Recombinant b-FGF 400 μg, infiltrated into healing incisional wounds on the third day post-wounding, increased breaking strength assessed on days 5, 6, and 7 by 39 per cent. However, this peptide had no effect on wound collagen content, although histological examination showed better organization and maturation in b-FGF treated wounds. Effects are presumably due to earlier accumulation of fibroblasts and/or collagen cross-linking. Local TNF increases wound disruption strength by one-half in incisional wounds in mice in a narrow dose range (50–500 μg). Outside this range, its effect on wound strength appears to be inhibitory and associated with a dense inflammatory infiltrate.

The depth of wounding has an important bearing on whether its repair can be accelerated by exogenous application of peptide growth factors. For instance, in full-thickness skin incisions in pigs treated twice daily with EGF for 14 days, no benefit was observed in treated animals. However, in partial-thickness dermal wounds, EGF and TGF-β increased epithelialization, cellularity, and thickness of the dermis, presumably through generation of epithelium from dermal appendages. In an excisional skin model, increased staining for collagen matrix protein mRNA after treatment with exogenous TGF-β has been found. The staining for TGF-β mRNA itself was also increased, indicating that TGF-β was autostimulatory, accounting, at least in part, for the persistent effects of single doses of this peptide.

Healing deficits

Uncontaminated surgical wounds in healthy patients heal by primary intent simply with the support of wound sutures. It is unlikely that, in this situation, growth factors will be a useful adjunct. The greatest therapeutic benefit of these peptides is likely to be derived in situations where impaired healing results in increased morbidity or mortality for patients. In animals, a wound-healing deficit can be defined artificially and the impairment in healing can be successfully ameliorated by growth factors.

However, impaired acute healing in animal models bears an indeterminate relationship to the common human problems of chronic wound healing failure. In essence, it has not yet proved possible to create good analogues of venous, arteripathic, or decubitus ulcers, if only because laboratory animals do not live long enough to achieve the tissue changes seen in some of these conditions in man.

Steroids

The wound-healing deficit induced by the use of corticosteroids is well documented. In steroid-sensitive animals, treatment causes a prolonged monocytopenia, preventing macrophage migration into the wound and thus diminishing this essential element of the wound-healing cascade. The *in-vitro* effects of steroid treatment are to depress fibroblast proliferation and inhibit procollagen and matrix protein synthesis. A single local application of TGF-β (10–40 pmol/wound) in a collagen suspension in the rat reverses a 50 per cent wound-healing deficit resulting from methylprednisolone treatment. PDGF in the same model fails to reverse the wound-healing deficit, but does increase fibroblast numbers in the wound. However, these fibroblasts lack enhanced expression of procollagen type I. Wound macrophages remain absent from both PDGF and TGF-β treated wounds. In steroid-treated pigs, local applications of exogenous TGF-β reverse the depression of matrix protein synthesis, procollagen mRNA, and TGF-β mRNA. In methylprednisolone-treated rats, daily injection of 5 μg EGF in an albumin carrier into a polyvinyl alcohol sponge restores collagen and matrix protein levels to normal.

Irradiation

Local irradiation impairs wound healing by depleting dermal fibroblasts and decreasing the proliferative potential of endothelium, whereas total body irradiation depresses bone marrow-derived elements, virtually eliminating wound macrophages. A single application of 2 to 10 μg of PDGF in a collagen vehicle partially reverses the surface irradiation wound-healing deficit in the skin of rats 7 days after creation of the wound. PDGF does not reverse the wound-healing deficit seen with total body irradiation. These studies support the hypothesis that PDGF requires the presence of activated wound macrophages for activity *in vivo*.

Cytotoxics

Cytotoxic treatment decreases circulating white cells and impairs the formation of granulation tissue in a wound chamber. Adriamycin treatment reduces the level of TGF-β and PDGF-like activity in aliquots of wound fluid removed from wound chambers. Injection of TGF-β into the wound chamber returns granulation tissue formation to a normal level. Incisional wound healing is impaired by Adriamycin treatment, and the strength of wounds can be returned to normal by a single intra-incisional application of 2 μg of TGF-β or 50 mg TNF in a collagen vehicle.

Diabetes

Neovascularization is impaired in wound healing in diabetics. In implanted Hunt–Schilling wound chambers in diabetic rats, PDGF restores granulation tissue formation and angiogenesis to normal. The influx of connective tissue cells, DNA synthesis, and collagen deposition are increased, effects that are augmented by the addition of insulin to PDGF. In diabetic mice, 0.5 μg b-FGF applied locally to an open wound once a day increases granulation tissue thickness, infiltrated cells, capillary number, and tissue strength of full-thickness punch biopsy wounds. Moreover, in diabetic rats, the wound-healing deficit is improved in a differential manner by b-FGF and TGF-β: collagen synthesis in polyvinyl alcohol sponges increases 136 per cent at day 9 by a single application of 2 μg TGF-β but tensile strength is unaltered, whereas b-FGF suppresses collagen synthesis and increases cellularity. EGF induces a selective increase in the synthesis of type I collagen, whereas insulin returns collagen activity to normal and causes temporary inhibition of proteolytic activity directed primarily at type I collagen.

Non-cutaneous tissue

The maturation of intestinal wounds differs from the maturation of skin wounds, and is mainly reflected in the rate of accumulation of collagen. Fibroblasts are present in low numbers in intestinal submucosa and collagen is generated by smooth muscle cells. TGF-β augments collagen production in smooth muscle cells by 100 per cent and non-collagen proteins by 40 per cent *in vitro*. EGF has no effect on collagen synthesis in smooth muscle, indicating that modulation of wound repair in intestine differs from that in skin. The gain in strength of intestinal wounds is far more rapid than in skin whether assessed by measurement of anastomotic bursting strength or breaking strength of linear enterotomy wounds. Continuous intraperitoneal delivery of 0.5 μg EGF/kg.day increases by 20 per cent the tensile strength of linear enterotomy wounds in stomach, ileum, and colon at 5 days. This is accompanied by an increase in cellularity. In the rabbit stomach, topical application of TGF-β (0.1–2 μg per wound) to partial thickness (excluding mucosa) longitudinal wounds, accelerates wound breaking strength by 4 days. PDGF (10 μg/wound) does not enhance gastric wound strength but increases cellular influx 2.9-fold, whereas TGF-β does not affect cellularity.

Human studies

Clinical trials are awaiting a clear definition of the efficacy of individual growth factors. In anticipation of clinical application of growth factors, the United States Food and Drug Administration has discussed guidelines to be adopted prior to phase 1 clinical studies. The first clinical trials with EGF were negative, possibly due to lack of purity before recombinant DNA techniques were available. Daily application of 5 μg EGF to suction blisters on the anterior abdominal wall failed to improve healing, nor did local EGF affect epithelial healing after penetrating keratoplasty. Alternative reasons for this negative effect have been investigated in the alkali-burned cornea of rats, showing the effect to be due to a lack of adherence of regenerated epithelium to underlying stroma. EGF has no effect on endothelial cell or stromal cell regeneration, and hence there is no adherence of epithelium to underlying stroma due to the absence of a basement membrane. Further developments will have to address such problems and it is likely that a wound-healing cocktail will contain a number of peptides to stimulate various elements of the wound-healing cascade. A clinical trial using skin-graft donor sites has demonstrated that 10 μg EGF/ml applied in an antibiotic cream at each wound dressing reduces the length of time to healing by 1.5 days.

As mentioned previously, platelets contain numerous growth factors, which can be released by incubation with thrombin. Knighton has reported that topical application of autologous platelet lysate may accelerate the healing of chronic wounds. These findings remain to be confirmed by further studies.

A large number of phase I and II clinical trials of single growth factors are in now progress. Most are being carried out in chronic venous, decubitus, or neuropathic-diabetic ulcers (Table 5). Some encouraging preliminary results have been reported for diabetic and decubitus ulcers.

Table 5 Early trials of exogenous growth factors in human wounds (as of April 1993)

Agent	Venous ulcer	Decubitus ulcer	Diabetic ulcer	Donor site
EGF	−	0	−	+*
PDGF	0	+	+	0
FGF	−	+	0	−
TGF-β	0	+	0	0

+, beneficial compared with control.
−, no benefit compared to control.
0, not reported.
* This study in burns patients has been contradicted by an equivalent one in normal volunteers.

WOUND DRESSINGS

'A material which, when applied to the surface of a wound, provides and maintains an environment in which healing can take place at the maximum rate.'

Thomas (1986)

Wound dressings have been utilized since the beginning of time, and some of the dressings used today in plugging and concealing wounds, such as lint and cotton wool, would not seem out of place to practitioners of medicine in early civilizations. In the classification of wound-healing products, these dressings have been referred to as passive. New dressings, such as polymeric films, polymeric foams, particulate and fibrous polymers, hydrogels, and hydrocolloids, have been classified as interactive dressings, providing a microenvironment which is conducive to healing. One of the hydrocolloid dressings (DuoDerm/Granuflex), to which a considerable amount of clinical and experimental research has been devoted, provides a wound-healing environment that, in addition to improving healing, also stimulates angiogenesis (Figs.

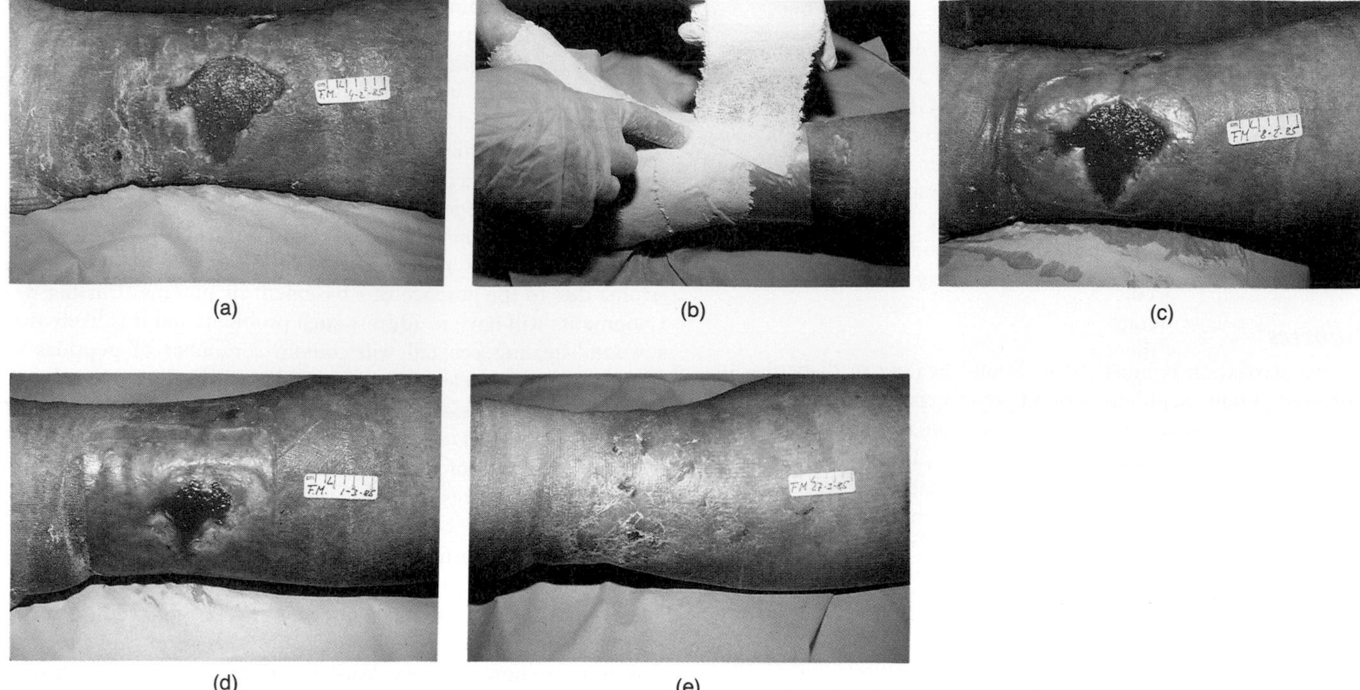

Fig. 17 (a) Venous ulcer before treatment with hydrocolloid dressing under a zinc paste bandage and outer compression bandage. (b) Paste bandage being applied over a hydrocolloid dressing. (c) Four days after treatment with hydrocolloid dressing. Note the increased granulation tissue compared to (a). (d) A marked decrease in the size of the ulcer 4 weeks after using hydrocolloid dressing. (e) Ulcer completely healed.

17, 18). The third part of this classification is that of active products which actively stimulate healing beyond that of the normal biological maximum.

Occlusive dressings and wound infection

One of the worries that clinicians have in using some of the new occlusive dressings in the treatment of chronic wounds is that, because of their impermeability to oxygen, this will lead to an environment that will increase wound infection. A recent review of more than 103 published papers, comparing the clinical infection rate between conventional and occlusive dressings, found a clinical infection rate of 2.08 per cent with wounds treated with occlusion compared to 5.37 per cent with conventional dressings. One of the reasons for this finding might be the ability of some occlusive hydrocolloid dressings to increase wound angiogenesis and local blood supply, thus providing an environment not conducive to bacterial growth (Figs. 2 and 17(c)).

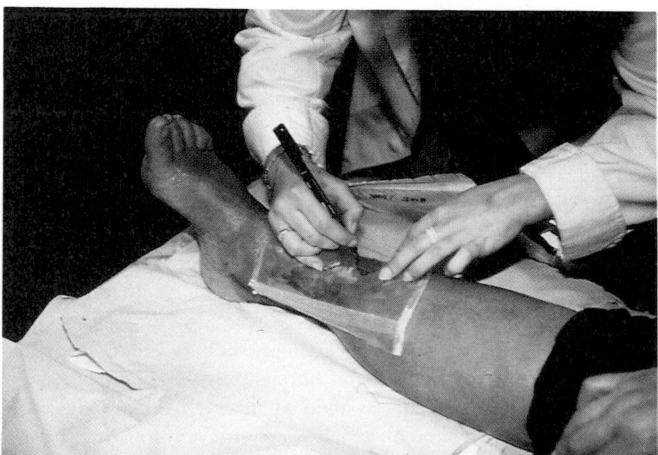

Fig. 18 Photographs are useful in assessing the healing of chronic ulcers, to measure wound area changes with treatment, but similar assessments can be made by tracing ulcer size using plastic films.

Cultured autografts and allografts

Biological wound coverage other than by conventional skin-grafting techniques has gained prominence with the use of cultured epidermal autografts and allografts. The latter grafts, although initially thought not to be rejected by the host, have since been shown to be replaced rapidly by host keratinocytes, thus acting as a temporary wound coverage but significantly stimulating the healing process.

In the future, dressings that deliver specific growth factors, pharmacological agents to stimulate healing, or serve as transducers to provide physical forces to the wound (such as electrical stimulation, ultrasound, or other stimuli) will be available to manage chronic wounds. These are being evaluated currently in a number of clinical and experimental studies.

THE FUTURE

At the time of writing, the explosive increase in our understanding of tissue repair and its defects is just beginning to be translated into practical strategies. This burst in wound healing knowledge is reflected in the newly established Wound Healing organizations in the United States and Europe 'The Wound Healing Society' for the former and the 'European Tissue Repair Society'.

It is important to define realistic clinical objectives. In acute wound healing, the major problems are wound failure (including anastomotic leakage, hernia recurrence, and some types of fracture non-union) and over-healing in its many guises (adhesions, strictures, contractures, and hypertrophic and keloid scarring). Although technical errors are a major and preventable cause in some cases, intrinsic defects in wound healing potential are also important. Human wound healing models as described in this chapter may help to predict repair failure and permit the selection of patients for new therapies.

In chronic wounds the main aims will be to induce healing in patients where this was previously impossible, to accelerate it, and to prevent recurrence.

Several important developments will be required to realize the promise of growth factors and other new agents. Local pharmacology of wounds is in its infancy; new delivery systems will be required to apply these agents precisely to the site and at the time they are needed. The plethora of new agents will mandate careful investigation to determine which ones are optimal for which clinical situation. Finally, the design of clinical trials, including ethical issues, recruitment criteria, and choice of endpoints, remains a serious problem. Successful resolution of these issues promises finally to close the gap between basic research and clinical application.

FURTHER READING

Abatangelo G, Davidson JM, eds. *Cutaneous development, aging and repair.* Padova: Liviana Press, 1989.

Ahn ST, Monafo WW, Mustoe TA. Topical silicone gel: a new treatment for hypertrophic scars. *Surgery* 1989; **106**: 781–7.

Arnold F, West DC. Angiogenesis in wound healing. *Pharmacol Ther* 1991; **52**: 407–22.

Brody GS. Hypertrophic scar contracture. *Plast Reconstr Surg* 1981; **67**: 673–84.

Brown GL, *et al.* Enhancement of wound healing by topical treatment with epidermal growth factor. *N Engl J Med* 1989; **321**: 76–9.

Clark RAF, Henson PM, eds. *The molecular and cellular biology of wound repair.* New York: Plenum Press, 1988.

Dineen P, ed. *The surgical wound.* Philadelphia: Lea and Febiger, 1981.

Ehrlich HP, Buttle DJ, Bernanke DH. Physiological variables affecting collagen lattice contraction by human dermal fibroblasts. *Exp Molec Pathol* 1989; **50**: 220–9.

Folkman J, Klagsburn M. Angiogenic factors. *Science* 1987; **235**: 442–7.

Hendriks T, Mastboom WJB. Healing of experimental intestinal anastomoses: Parameters for repair. *Dis Colon Rect* 1990; **33**: 891–901.

Hinman C, Maibach H, Winer G. The effect of air exposure and occlusion on experimental human skin wounds. *Nature* 1963; **200**: 377–9.

Hudlickà O, Tyler KR. *Angiogenesis: the growth of the vascular system.* London: Academic Press, 1986: 123–7.

Hunt TK, ed. *Wound healing and wound infection: theory and surgical practice.* New York: Appletone Century-Crofts, 1980.

Hutchinson JJ, Lawrence JC. Wound infection under occlusive dressings. *J Surg Infec* 1991; **17**: 63–94.

Janssen H, Rooman R, Robertson JIS, eds. *Wound healing.* Petersfield: Wrightson Biomedical, 1991.

Kingsnorth AN, Vowles R, Nash JRG. Epidermal growth factor increases tensile strength in intestinal wounds in pigs. *Br J Surg* 1990; **77**: 409–12.

Knighton DR, Fietel VD, Austin L, Ciresi KF, Butler EL. Classification and treatment of chronic nonhealing wounds. *Ann Surg* 1986; **204**: 322–30.

Krasner D, ed. *Chronic wound care.* King of Prussia; Pennsylvania: Health Management Publications, 1990.

Ksander GA, Sawamura SJ, Ogawa Y, Sundsmo J, McPherson JM. The effect of platelet releasate on wound healing in animal models. *J Am Acad Dermatol* 1990; **22**: 781–91.

Lydon MJ, *et al.* Dissolution of wound coagulum and promotion of granulation tissue under DuoDERM™. *WOUNDS* 1989; **1**: 95–106.

McGaw WT, Ten Cate AR. A role for collagen phagocytosis by fibroblasts in scar remodelling: An ultrastructural stereologic study. *J Invest Dermatol* 1983; **81**: 375–8.

McGee GS, *et al.* Recombinant basic fibroblast growth factor accelerates wound healing. *J Surg Res* 1988; **45**: 145–53.

McGrath MH, Simon RH. Wound geometry and the kinetics of wound contraction. *Plast Reconstr Surg* 1983; **72**: 66–73.

Marks RM, Barton SP, Edwards C, eds. *The physical nature of the skin.* Lancaster, England: MTP Press, 1988.

Martin CW, Muir IFK. The role of lymphocytes in wound healing. *Br J Plast Surg* 1990; **43**: 655–62.

Myers MB, Cherry GW. Rate of revascularisation in primary and disrupted wounds. *Surg Gynecol Obstet* 1971; **132**: 1005–8.

Nanney LB. Epidermal and dermal effects of epidermal growth factor during wound repair. *J Invest Dermatol* 1990; **94**: 624–9.

Pasyk KA, Thomas SV, Hassett CA, Cherry GW, Faller R. Regional differences in capillary density of the normal human dermis. *Plast Reconstr Surg* 1989; **83**: 939–47.

Peters RM, Peacock EE, Benfield JR, eds. *The scientific management of surgical patients.* Boston: Little Brown & Co, 1983: 27–63.

Phillips T, Dover J. Leg ulcers. *J Am Acad Dermatol* 1991; **25**: 965–87.

Pricolo VE, Caldwell MD, Mastrofrancesco B, Mills CD. Modulatory activities of wound fluid on fibroblast proliferation and collagen synthesis. *J Surg Res* 1990; **48**: 534–8.

Quinn KJ, Evans JH, Courtney JM, Gaylor JDS, Reid WH. Non pressure treatment of hypertrophic scars. *Burns* 1985; **12**: 102–8.

Rayman G, Williams SA, Spencere PD, Smaje LH, Wise PH, Tooke JE. Impaired microvascular hyperaemic response to minor trauma in type I diabetes. *Br Med J* 1986; **292**: 1295–8.

Rothe M, Falanga V. Growth factors: their biology and promise in dermatologic disease and tissue repair. *Arch Dermatol* 1988; **125**: 1390–8.

Rowsell AR. The intra-uterine healing of foetal muscle wounds: Experimental study in the rat. *Br J Plast Surg* 1984; **37**: 635–42.

Russell RCG, ed. *Recent Advances in Surgery 11.* Edinburgh: Churchill Livingstone, 1982.

Ryan TJ, ed. *Beyond occlusion: dermatology proceedings*, Int. Congress and Symposium Series, No. 137, Paris. London: Royal Society of Medicine, 1988.

Shah M, Foreman DM, Ferguson MWJ. Control of scarring in adult wounds by neutralizing antibody to transforming growth factor β. *Lancet* 1992; **339**: 213–14.

Singh G, Foster CS. Epidermal growth factor in alkali-burned corneal epithelial wound healing. *Am J Ophthalmol* 1987; **103**: 802–7.

Steenfos HH, Hunt TK, Scheuenstuhl BS, Goodson WH. Selective effects of tumour necrosis factor-alpha on wound healing in rats. *Surgery* 1989; **106**: 171–6.

Thomas S. The role of foam dressings in wound management, In: Turner TD, Schmidt RJ, and Harding KG, eds. *Advances in Wound Management.* Chichester: John Wiley & Sons, 1986.

Tsuboi R, Rifkin DB. Recombinant basic fibroblast growth factor stimulates wound healing in healing-impaired db/db mice. *J Exp Med* 1990; **172**: 245–51.

Uitto J, Olsen PR, Fazio MJ. Extracellular matrix of the skin: 50 years of progress. *J Invest Dermatol* 1989; **92**: 61s–77s.

Uitto J, Perejda AJ, eds. *Connective tissue disease: molecular pathology of the extracellular matrix.* New York: Marcel Dekker, 1987.

Zouboulis CC, Orfanos CE. Cryosurgical treatment of hypertrophic scars and keloids. *Core J in Dermatol* 1991: 11–12.

Surgical infections and AIDS 2

2.1 Surgical infections

R. E. CONDON AND DIETMAR H. WITTMANN

DEFINITION

Surgical infections are those best treated by operative intervention or those that follow surgical procedures and occur in the operative wound or at a distant site. Surgical infections may be classified as primary infections occurring spontaneously, those following tissue injuries, or those following planned surgical trauma such as an operation.

PHYSIOLOGY

The unique feature of all surgical infections is tissue necrosis. In post-traumatic surgical infection tissue necrosis is induced by mechanical or other physical trauma, while in primary or spontaneous surgical infection tissue necrosis is induced by the pathophysiological process. Inflammation is the response to tissue necrosis, leading to the events visible at the surface which were well described by Celsus and refined by Galen as rubor (redness), tumor (swelling), calor (heat), dolor (pain), and functio laesa (loss of function). These symptoms describe the effects of the host responses which, when controlled and properly regulated, result in elimination of necrotic material and prepare the way for tissue repair. The same mechanisms of inflammation are employed to eliminate invading micro-organisms.

Inflammation is characterized by increased blood flow, increased vascular permeability, recruitment of cells that phagocytose microbes and damaged tissue, secretion of preformed mediators, generation of additional mediator compounds, and the local or regional accumulation of these biochemically active compounds and inflammatory cells. The magnitude of the inflammatory response and of its symptoms is dependent on the burden of tissue injury and on the number and pathogenicity of the invading micro-organisms. If toxins or other bacterial products continuously destroy tissue, or exceed the capability of the host to confine the challenge to body integrity, the inflammatory process will continue and may then result in multisystem malfunction.

The sequence of events occurring early in the inflammation process is the result of activation of inter-relating systems that provide considerable duplication of biological effects. For example, the peptides of the clotting, kinin, and complement systems may each produce vasodilation. Duplication maintains the integrity of the response even in the face of dysfunction of one component part; it also provides the basis for additive and even deleterious effects recognized clinically as autoaggressive multisystem organ failure.

Local phase of infection

Surgical infections take a relatively uniform course once initiated. First, there is local inflammation following the initial tissue injury. Macrophages may not be capable, however, of phagocytosing all the dead cells and detritus, and remaining necrotic tissue is an excellent nutrient medium for bacterial growth. Bacteria, in turn, release toxins that destroy additional tissue and thus fuel the infectious challenge. Bacteria may invade surrounding tissue slowly or rapidly, depending on their production of specific toxins (spreading factors). The host, in turn, answers with further inflammation in an attempt to confine the infection. If successful, dead tissue, foreign bodies, and micro-organisms are destroyed and removed, and a scar is formed.

If the extent of tissue injury and number of bacteria exceed the capability of the host to terminate an infection locally, an abscess may form (Fig. 1). During the early phases of inflammation there is exudation of plasma, and thus fibrin, through widened spaces between endothelial cells and through open injured vessels. As the infection progresses, this inflammatory process spreads centrifugally from the initial focus of infection, with macrophages and fibrin deposition attempting to confine the infection faster than bacterial toxins can destroy the tissue. The progress of the infection is eventually stopped through the formation of a pyogenic membrane, inside which dying phagocytes and bacteria release toxins that liquefy the abscess contents. The resulting high osmolarity attracts water, increasing the pressure inside the abscess capsule, while oxygen and nutrients diffuse poorly through the

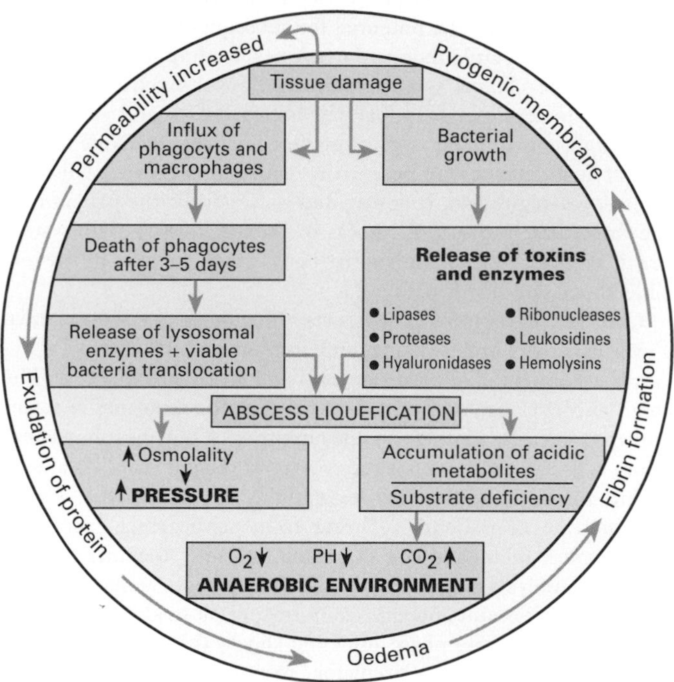

Fig. 1 Pathophysiological events in an abscess. The pyogenic membrane forms as the result of events of early inflammation. Proteases and other enzymes are released from phagocytes and bacteria, leading to liquefication of the contents of the abscess cavity. The increased osmolality leads to attraction of water, increasing the pressure within the abscess. The environment is basically anaerobic with accumulation of acidic metabolites and an oxygen deficit. In this environment many antibiotics are not effective.

abscess capsule, promoting anaerobic glycolysis. An abscess is therefore characterized by high pressure, low pH, and low oxygen tension, and represents an ideal environment for the multiplication of anaerobic bacteria. It is poorly permeated by antibiotics. This is particularly true of aminoglycosides, which are inactive at the pH commonly found in an abscess. The best treatment of an abscess is drainage: local host defences are so intensely concentrated around the abscess capsule that additional antibiotic therapy, except for the period immediately before and during drainage, is rarely indicated.

Systemic phase of infection

If local circumscription of infection is not possible, either by removing the bacteria or by abscess formation, micro-organisms eventually invade the bloodstream and may reach distant organs. The presence of bacteria in the bloodstream (bacteraemia) transiently occurs in healthy individuals. In patients, bacteria often will be found on the intravascular portion of catheters. Non-toxin producing, mostly non-multiplying bacteria can sometimes be isolated by blood culture, but these cause no or only mild systemic symptoms: bacteraemia may, however, progress to systemic disease, especially in immunocompromised and postoperative patients. If the condition is persistent and associated with multiplication of bacteria in the bloodstream, and with the death of large numbers of bacteria as a consequence of host defence mechanisms, then a serious state of infection termed sepsis or septicaemia ensues. Septicaemia is characterized not only by invasion and multiplication in the bloodstream of large numbers of bacteria but also by the potential for subsequent sudden overload of the host with endotoxin and cytokines, leading to septic shock. Sepsis is the clinical symptomatic state resulting from the host response to septicaemia. Liberated bacterial exo- and endotoxins are deleterious to many organ functions; equally, cytokine mediators of host defences are potentially damaging if there is failure of their down-regulation. It not treated successfully, the patient may die immediately of septic shock, or later following multisystem organ failure: 1 ng endotoxin/kg body weight results in irreversible shock and death within 2 h.

Clinically, symptoms of sepsis resemble those of endotoxaemia. Fever usually is high, spiking, and accompanied by chills. Tachycardia accompanies or precedes fever and is proportional to it. The total leucocyte count may not be particularly abnormal in sepsis and may even be low due to consumption of polymorphonuclear white cells. The differential count is more reliable: there is always a shift to the left. Petechial lesions may be seen in the skin or conjunctivae of patients suffering from septicaemia caused by streptococci, meningococci, or pseudomonads. Anaemia secondary to haemolysis may appear rapidly when septicaemia is due to staphylococci, pseudomonads, coliforms, or clostridia. During the initial hyperdynamic phase of septic shock, the peripheral vasodilation is explained by a circulatory response which aims to compensate for the inability of cells to use oxygen. The last stage of septic shock is hypodynamic due to exhaustion. Shock is common in septicaemia caused by Gram-negative organisms, but occurs relatively less often with Gram-positive infection. Metastatic abscesses, especially of the bone, brain, or spleen, are not unusual after an episode of septicaemia: any injured tissue is easily infected during septicaemia. Diagnosis is aided by a high index of suspicion.

Thermolabile exotoxins are released by living bacteria, particularly Gram-positive organisms, while thermostabile endotoxins are released by all bacteria after death. Endotoxins are complex moieties of high molecular weight consisting of phospholipids, polysaccharides, and proteins derived from the outer cell wall, particularly of Gram-negative rods such as *Escherichia coli*. Clinically measurable effects of endotoxin include fever, consumptive coagulopathy, increased vagotonus, hyperglycaemia followed by hypoglycaemia, leucopenia or leucocytosis, increased levels of plasma lipids, release of hepatic enzymes, thrombocytopenia, and reduced serum iron concentration.

Low doses of endotoxin primarily affect the reticuloendothelial system. Animal studies have shown a marked reduction of clearance of particulates such as colloidal carbon during endotoxaemia. Mediators such as collagenases, pyrogenic prostaglandins, and coagulation factors are released from macrophages, and after 7 days antibodies against endotoxin are produced. Endotoxins act directly on the hypothalamic temperature regulation centre to cause fever, reinforcing the activity of pyrogenic substances released from dying neutrophilic granulocytes. Erythropoiesis is shifted from the bone marrow to the spleen, resulting in leucopenia followed by leucocytosis after 2 to 6 h. In small doses, endotoxins increase phagocytic activity and bacterial killing. Thrombocytopenia, accompanied by thrombocyte aggregation and lysis, results in the release of ADP, vasoactive amines, histamine, serotonin, and platelet factor III, which in turn may lead to consumptive coagulopathy. In the extrinsic coagulation system, endotoxins cause release of a tissue factor derived from macrophages, as well as platelet factors and thromboplastins. In the intrinsic system, factor XII (Hageman factor) is activated, leading to disseminated intravascular coagulation.

Endotoxin has a profound effect on metabolism. Initially, it induces hyperglycaemia, which is followed after several hours by hypoglycaemia. Hyperlipidaemia results from altered metabolism of free fatty aids, cholesterol, phospholipids, and triglycerides. Protein synthesis by the liver is stimulated; lactate dehydrogenase transaminases and phosphokinases are released, increasing the serum concentration of these enzymes. Release of adrenocorticotrophic hormone, cortisone, and growth hormone is increased; thyrotropin and luteinizing hormone are not affected. Plasma iron and total iron binding capacity are reduced. A vagotonic effect results in loss of thirst and appetite, stomach emptying is delayed, and diarrhoea may occur.

DIAGNOSIS

History and physical examination

The early accurate diagnosis of surgical infections is essential: delayed treatment can result in overwhelming sepsis and multisystem organ failure. The history and physical examination are the surgeon's most important diagnostic tools. The classical signs of tumor, rubor, calor, dolor and functio laesa are indicative of localized surgical infections. Clinical symptoms of systemic sepsis include disturbed sensorium, tachypnoea, tachycardia, hypotension, fever, oliguria, and high output heart failure. In postoperative patients, the sudden appearance of tachypnoea and hypotension suggests Gram-negative septicaemia. The condition has a potential mortality rate of 30 to 50 per cent, but early diagnosis and treatment markedly improves the chance of survival.

The entire body must be examined; all dressings should be

removed. Inspection and palpation of an area of suspicion might reveal the first three of the classical signs of infection. Removal of an intravenous cannula dressing may reveal purulent drainage or thrombophlebitis. Rectal examination may show tenderness and induration as signs of a developing pelvic abscess. Auscultation of the chest may reveal the presence of pneumonia before it is evident on a chest radiograph.

The patient should be examined for clues to the source of infection such as pain or redness in the surgical wound or at an intravenous infusion site, or purulent sputum, cough, pleuritic pain, rales, or dullness in the chest, diarrhoea, dysuria, or flank pain. Pain in the shoulder and an immobile diaphragm suggest a subphrenic abscess. A pelvic or prostatic mass on rectal examination may indicate an abscess, and headache or nuchal rigidity may indicate a central nervous system infection.

Haematology, urinalysis, and radiology

Most bacterial infections produce an increase in the leucocyte count and a shift to the left in the differential count, or a relative lymphopenia. This increase in the proportion of the more immature forms of polymorphonuclear leucocytes may signal infection before a rise in the total leucocyte count is evident. The differential count may also reveal lymphocytosis in viral infections, monocytosis in tuberculosis, eosinophilia in parasitic infections or hypersensitivity reactions (drug allergy), and toxic granulation of leucocytes in acute bacterial infection. A leukaemoid response (a total white count over 25 000 cells/mm^3), may be seen in septicaemia, pneumococcal pneumonia, liver abscess or cholangitis, suppurative pancreatitis, necrotic bowel, or retroperitoneal phlegmon. Leucopenia is a sign of overwhelming bacterial infection and carries a bad prognosis. Viral infection, typhoid perforation of the bowel, or tuberculosis may also present with leucopenia. Anaemia may be associated with infection caused by bacteria, such as *Clostridium perfringens*, group A streptococci, or coagulase-positive staphylococci, which produce haemolytic enzymes.

Routine chest films may reveal generalized or focal atelectasis, or may indicate intra-abdominal infection through signs of gastrointestinal leakage or free air identified under one of the diaphragms. In the investigation of patients with suspected intra-abdominal infection, flat, upright, and decubitus films may reveal a localized air–fluid level, suggesting an intra-abdominal abscess, or a spreading air bubble pattern suggestive of infection with a gas-producing organism. Specialized radiological procedures are often helpful in confirming the diagnosis of intra-abdominal abscess. These studies include ultrasonography and computerized tomography (CT); the choice of technique depends primarily on the expertise of the local radiologist. Although a gallium scan may be helpful in special circumstances, this examination is subject to appreciable error and is difficult to interpret in a patient who has had a recent operation.

Bacteriology

Observation of exudates and secretions such as wound drainage, urine, and sputum for odour, colour, and consistency may be useful in diagnosing. Grape-like odours occur with pseudomonal infections, urea-like odours with Proteus infections, and faeculent odours with anaerobic organisms such as Bacteroides, fusobacteria, clostridia, and peptostreptococci. A Gram stain offers the earliest clue to the cause of an infection, particularly when a specific monobacterial infection is suspected. If multiple infecting organisms are present the Gram stain usually shows a variety of pathogenic bacteria. Notes should be taken of the numbers of polymorphonuclear leucocytes on the slide (few, many, loaded) and whether organisms can be seen inside them. Acid-fast and fungus stains can be used if such infections are likely. Pathogens recovered most frequently from the exogenous and endogenous flora are shown in Fig. 2. Bacteria often responsible for intra-abdominal infections are listed in Table 1.

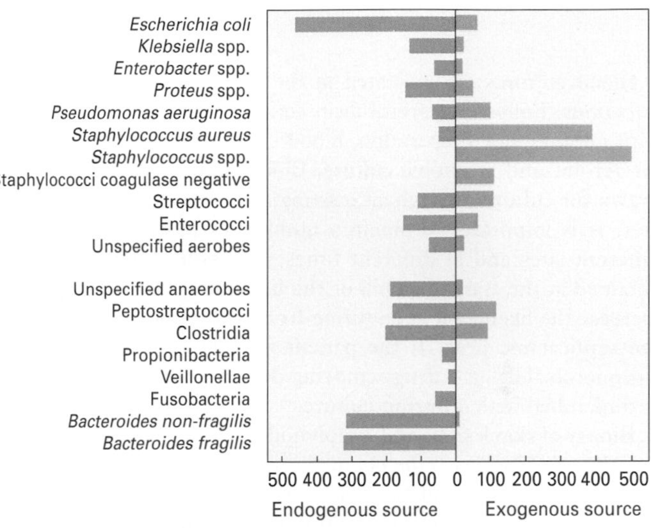

Fig. 2 Bacteria isolated from surgical infections, contrasting those stemming from an exogenous (bone and joint) and an endogenous (intra-abdominal) source. Data for exogenous bacteria from Wittmann DH. Wertigkeit der Antibiotika bei posttraumatischen Knocheninfektionen (evaluation of antibiotics in bone infections). In: Cotta H., Braun A., eds. *Knochen-und Gelenkinfektionen (bone infections)*. Berlin: Springer-Verlag, 1988. Data for endogenous bacteria taken from Howard R. Microbes and their pathogenicity. In: Simmons, RL, Howard R J. eds. *Surgical Infectious Disease*. Norwalk, CT: Appleton Century Crofts, 1986: 11–28.

Technique of obtaining the specimen

Purulent material from the deepest aspect of the wound should be aspirated into a syringe and any air evacuated. Pus is the best medium in which to preserve bacteria for transport to the laboratory. The capped syringe is sent for aerobic and anaerobic culture and for determinations of antibiotic sensitivity. Alternatively, a moist swab can be used to obtain bacteria from a site of suspected infection. Ideally, anaerobic specimens should be transported immediately in a CO_2-filled tube and plated within 1 h of sampling; fastidious organisms may otherwise die, resulting in a false-negative culture result. If the specimen is held overnight, it should be placed in an anaerobic sterile vial or tube; under no circumstances should an anaerobic specimen be refrigerated. Generally speaking, *Escherichia coli* (aerobe) and *Bacteroides fragilis* (anaerobe) are the usual causes of wound infection following gastrointestinal or gynaecological operations, while staphylococci are the usual causative organisms when intra-abdominal viscera have not been resected or opened.

Table 1 Pathogens isolated from 900 patients with intra-abdominal infections

Aerobic bacteria		Obligate anaerobic bacteria	
E. coli	51%	Bacteroides, unspecified	72%
Enterococci	17%		
Proteus species	16%	Fusobacteria	7%
Klebsiella species	14%	Veillonella	2%
Enterobacter species	6%	Propionibacteria	5%
Pseudomonas species	7%	Clostridia	23%
Streptococci	12%	Peptostreptococci	21%
Staphylococci	5%		
Other	8%	Other	21%

Data from Wittmann DH. *Intra-abdominal Infection: Pathophysiology and Treatment*. New York: Marcel Dekker, 1991.

Blood cultures are indicated in the investigation of all serious infections. Following careful disinfection of the venipuncture site with an iodophor preparation, blood samples should be obtained for aerobic and anaerobic culture. Blood should not ordinarily be drawn for culture through an existing intravenous needle or catheter. It is important to obtain a number of blood cultures from different sites and at different times; if possible, they should be obtained at the start of a chill or the beginning of a fever spike to increase the likelihood of culturing from a specimen drawn during the septicaemic peak. If the patient is receiving treatment with antimicrobial drugs a drug removing device is helpful in obviating antimicrobial action during culture.

Biopsy of skin lesions and lymph nodes may be helpful, although lymph node biopsies in the inguinal region should be avoided. If no nodes are palpable and the diagnosis is obscure, a blind scalene node biopsy may sometimes be productive. Specimens should be sent for routine bacteriological, acid-fast bacillus, and fungal cultures, as well as for histological examination. Skin tests, except for tuberculosis, have limited use: serological tests are more reliable then skin tests for the diagnosis of fungal disease.

While culture and sensitivity tests are essential, the latter results need to be interpreted appropriately since the tests are not always reproducible and must be viewed with caution. Sensitivity reports are an oversimplification of the complex foundations on which antimicrobial chemotherapy is based and are usually based on disc diffusion tests, which are highly sensitive to small technical and environmental changes. They may not correlate with the actual minimal inhibitory or bactericidal concentration of an antibiotic or with the concentration of antibiotic achieved at the site of infection. Routine disc sensitivity tests are generally of little value to the clinician. The minimal inhibitory concentration or the minimal bactericidal or fungicidal concentration is more useful clinically.

THERAPY OF SURGICAL INFECTIONS

All wounds whether made at the operating table or resulting from trauma, provide an environment for bacterial growth. Infections can be minimized if wound management follows the principles below.

1. Tissue should be handled gently, and operative trauma kept at a minimum.
2. Further contamination should be minimized by use of aseptic techniques.
3. Devitalized tissue, debris, and traumatic foreign bodies should be removed.
4. Complete haemostasis should be achieved.
5. Blood supply is essential for healing and should not be impaired.
6. Formation of dead space should be avoided during closure.
7. The wound should be closed with layer-to-layer approximation without tension.
8. Operative time should be kept to a minimum to reduce the numbers of bacteria entering the wound.
9. The wound may be irrigated with liberal amounts of sterile saline Ringer's lactate solution prior to closure.

Resistance of the host to infection is intimately involved with the magnitude of trauma and the early inflammatory response. Three primary factors interact in infection: the extent of tissue injury, the inoculum (quantity) and toxic products (quality) of infecting micro-organisms, and the host defence capacity. Meticulous, atraumatic technique is important: the extent of tissue injury is crucial in the development of subsequent bacterial infection. Debridement is important to reduce the amount of necrotic material, allowing phagocytes to concentrate on invading micro-organisms. If the initial wound is contused and fringed with loose tissue, scalpel excision of the wound edges often leaves less traumatized issue. Any fresh wound almost invariably becomes contaminated as long as it is exposed to the environment. In this context, the operating room is not sterile, and bacteria can be isolated from the wound exudate of even primarily healing wounds. Bacteria require 6 to 8 h to multiply to a concentration which is virulent and which is accompanied by invasion of adjacent tissues. During this time debridement of necrotic tissue and primary wound closure carries little risk of infection. However, infections frequently complicate healing of wounds if primary closure is completed later than 6 to 8 h after injury.

General principles of therapy

Non-localized infections (cellulitis, lymphangitis) should be treated with antibiotics, preferably penicillin G in high doses, as well as local heat, rest, immobilization, and elevation. Local moist heat relieves pain and increases blood and lymph flow: it is best applied by intermittent moist compresses, which hastens localization. Prolonged application of heat encourages oedema and satellite infection. Surgical incision and drainage are not usually indicated.

In a localized infection (abscess, infection of a closed space), the most important therapeutic modality is the operative reduction or elimination of invading and multiplying bacteria and the removal by drainage of factors promoting bacterial growth. Antimicrobial therapy is effective only in conjunction with operative reduction of the bacterial inoculum. Incision and drainage is thus indicated whenever infection is localized or occurs in a closed space. Fluctuance of most superficial abscesses signals the appropriate time for drainage. When in doubt, needle aspiration may be diagnostic, especially in deeper infections. The incision must be large, placed in the most dependent area of the abscess, and kept open to prevent skin closure before the deepest site of infection is controlled. Superficial wound abscesses should be packed lightly with gauze after drainage, while deeper abscesses are kept open by sump drains or tubes.

Antibiotic therapy

The goal of antibiotic therapy is to achieve a concentration of antibiotic in the infected tissue that exceeds the minimum inhibitory concentration for at least three-quarters of the time between successive doses. Drug pharmacokinetics vary considerably with patient age and disease. Antibiotics are usually given in insufficient doses, particularly at the onset of treatment, if only manufacturers' recommendations and disc sensitivity data are used to determine the dose and dosing interval. Clinically appropriate doses are recorded in a review by the authors (Condon and Wittmann 1992) which should be consulted for further information. Suggestions about initial empiric therapy for surgical infections originating from various sources are recorded in Table 2.

Systemic antibiotics are not usually indicated for the treatment of uncomplicated wound abscess which can be drained through an incision which does not open new tissue planes or expose new tissue to contamination by the contents of the abscess. Since overlying tissues must be opened to drain deep abscesses, antibiotics should be administered during the period immediately before and during incision and drainage. A longer period of therapy with parenteral antibiotics is indicated in immunocompromised patients, or when there is evidence of septicaemia (systemic toxicity, high fever), or progression of infection despite adequate drainage. If infection persists the first question to be asked, before systemic antibiotics are given, is whether incision and drainage has been adequate, and whether there may be another unrecognized and undrained surgical infection.

Antimicrobial treatment should be specific: that is, directed against the causative pathogens based on either the clinical diagnosis or a specific bacteriological diagnosis. When the bacteriological diagnosis is uncertain, empirical or calculated antibiotic therapy should be targeted at the most likely pathogens and the following points should be considered.

1. The spectrum of pathogens known to be typical.
2. The pathogenicity, synergism, and antagonism exhibited by bacteria in various mixed infections.
3. The concentration of antibiotic which can be achieved at the site of infection.
4. The side-effects of antimicrobials.
5. The negative interaction of antibiotics with host defence mechanisms.
6. The results of well controlled clinical studies of unselected patients.

Antibiotics that reliably kill bacteria should be given preference, such as penicillin for infections by group A streptococci or clostridia and cefotaxime against *E. coli* and Klebsiella.

Risk factors

Several factors increase the risk of a patient acquiring infection (Table 3). These risk factors may be related to the patient's capability to defend against an infectious threat, the infectious challenge itself, as represented by the number and pathogenicity of bacteria, the extent of associated injury, and environmental factors such as the hospital bacterial flora. The surgeon should be alert to these factors and tailor therapeutic or preventive strategies to the specific circumstances. For example, antibiotic prophylaxis is usually not indicated before a clean or aseptic operative procedure, but may very well be useful in an insulin-dependent diabetic. The dilemma for the surgeon is to decide when bacteriological contamination of an open ulcer, for example, becomes a clinically significant risk or is associated with tissue-penetrating disease.

Improper preoperative management is an organizational problem and can increase the postoperative infection rate. Common errors include failure to give a preoperative bath with antiseptic soaps or solutions, and shaving of the operative site the night before operation. Shaving is probably not indicated in most patients; when practised, it should be limited to the immediate preoperative period.

Table 2 Initial empiric therapy for surgical infections

Bacteria on Gram stain	Source	Initial calculated antibiotic therapy
In chains Gram + cocci	Soft tissue	Penicillin G (high dose; 10 million U 8-hourly)
In clusters Gram + cocci	Soft tissue	Penicillin G (high dose; 10 million U 8-hourly) Clindamycin or methicillin
Gram − rods	Abdomen	Cefotaxime
	Pulmonary	Ceftriaxone
	Biliary tract	Cefazolin
Gram + rods	Soft tissue	Penicillin G
Mixed G+ and G−	Intra-abdominal abscess	Cefotaxime + metronidazole, or ampicillin-sulbactam
	Multiple injuries, especially extremities	Cefotaxime + clindamycin

Table 3 Risk factors for infection

Patient related
Malnutrition
Immune compromise
Obesity
Renal insufficiency
Pulmonary dysfunction
Cardiovascular disease
Endocrine and metabolic disorders
Injury related
Location
Extent
Environment related
Contamination
Superinfection
Hygiene
Long-term ICU stay

Long-term ICU treatment

Changes in the microbial flora of the skin, respiratory tract, and gastrointestinal tract are seen in the most seriously ill patients, regardless of the underlying disease. Resistant Gram-negative organisms, staphylococci, and fungi usually colonize such patients shortly after admission to the hospital. Factors increasing the incidence of colonization are antibiotic administration, use of inhalation therapy equipment, immunosuppressive or irradiation therapy, and depressed neurological status. Administration of multiple potent antimicrobials disturbs the patient's microbial ecological system since not only pathogenic but also symbiotic bacteria are eliminated. For example, therapy with imipenem often leads to elimination of too many bacteria, and, in the susceptible patient, allows superinfection with fungi or other resistant bacteria which are normally of low pathogenicity. These situations should be avoided by discontinuing antimicrobials at the earliest possibility or changing early to a narrow spectrum regimen directed only at pathogenically important micro-organisms.

Scoring severity of infection

Many scoring systems have been developed to assess the severity of disease. The Surgical Infection Society currently proposes the use of the APACHE-II system to compare treatment regimens. The APACHE score consists of an Acute Physiology Score and a Chronic Health Evaluation (Fig. 3). There are disease-specific weighting factors to calculate mortality. For patients with intra-abdominal infection, a score of 21 correlates with a mortality risk of 50 per cent (Fig. 4).

SKIN AND SOFT TISSUE INFECTIONS

Infections with a single organism usually follow minor trauma, and are limited to the skin and subcutaneous tissues. However, even minuscule lesions may become life threatening; examples are streptococcal erysipelas, cellulitis, phlegmon or lymphangitis, clostridial infections including gas gangrene, tetanus, and some staphylococcal infections.

Primary infections

Group A streptococci may cause cellulitis and erysipelas: once inoculated beneath the skin, the defensive barriers are easily breached by the toxins released by streptococci; in addition the lymphatic system is frequently involved. Clinically, there is oedema with reddening of the skin (Fig. 5). Penicillin G is the treatment of choice since it kills all group A streptococci, a remarkable property that has not changed since the introduction of this drug more than 45 years ago. Before the discovery of penicillin, invasive group A streptococcal infection had a mortality rate of 90 per cent. Anaerobic streptococci (peptostreptococci) are part of the normal flora of the mouth and gastrointestinal tract. In contrast to other streptococcal wound infections, these organisms produce a thin, brown discharge, often with crepitation in the infected tissue (anaerobic cellulitis). Treatment consists of wide incision and drainage, and administration of 10 million units (6 g) of penicillin G 6-hourly. Cephalosporins, clindamycin, chloramphenicol, and metronidazole are second choice agents against anaerobic cocci.

Folliculitis, furunculosis, and carbuncle

These infections are usually due to *Staphylococcus aureus*, although in patients receiving antibiotics, Gram-negative bacteria and Candida may be the cause. Folliculitis originates within one hair follicle; furunculosis represents infection of several hair follicles in a circumscribed area; a carbuncle (boil) is a confluent infection involving multiple contiguous follicles in which the infection is limited to the subcutaneous tissue by thick overlying skin and dense subcutaneous fascia. Carbuncles usually are found on the back of the neck and torso. Warm skin compresses and good local hygiene are usually sufficient therapy for folliculitis and most cases of furunculosis. Carbuncles require incisions for drainage and treatment with antistaphylococcal penicillins, erythromycin or clindamycin.

Hydradenitis suppurativa

This infection of apocrine sweat glands is usually seen in young adults and is due to staphylococci or anaerobes (especially peptostreptococci). Often, only complete excision of the infected tissue down to deep fascia, with subsequent grafting or delayed closure, is curative.

Bite wounds

Human bite wounds are contaminated with a combination of aerobic non-haemolytic streptococci, anaerobic streptococci, *B. melaninogenicus*, spirochaetes, and staphylococci. The original wound must be treated by debridement, thorough irrigation, and immobilization. Systemic antibiotics, usually penicillin, must be administered. If the infection becomes established, radical debridement of the infected area is imperative and must be accompanied by antibiotic therapy.

Infections of dog and cat bite wounds are caused by *Pasteurella multocida* in 25 to 50 per cent of cases; otherwise, the spectrum of bacteria is the same as that seen in human bite wounds. The antibiotics of choice are high dose penicillin G, amoxicillin/clavulanic acid or oral cefuroxime.

* Begining: Date .... Time .... Ending: Date .... Time	**APACHE-II**	Patient study number	Patient initial

	RAW VALUES MIN	RAW VALUES MAX	+4	+3	+2	+1	0	+1	+2	+3	+4
* Temerature (rectal)			≥ 41°	39°–40.9°		38.5°–38.9°	36°–38.4°	34°–35.9°	32°–33.9°	30°–31.9°	≤ 29.9°
Blood pressure S/D											
$\frac{2\times \text{diastolic} + \text{systolic}}{3}$ = mean			≥160	130–159	110–129		70–109		50–69		≤49
Heart rate			≥180	140–179	110–139		70–109		55–69	40–59	≤39
Respiratory rate			≥50	35–49		25–34	12–24	10–11	6–9		≤5
(a) if FiO_2 ≥50 then use A-aDO2 (A-aDO2 = FiO_2 (713) - $PaCO_2$–PaO_2) * FiO_2	a. A-aDO2 ___		≥500	350–499	200–349		<200				
(b) If FiO_2 <50 then record only PaO_2 PaO_2 .... $PaCO_2$	b. PaO2 ___						>70	61–70		55–60	<55
Arterial pH			≥7.7	7.6–7.69		7.5–7.59	7.33–7.49		7.25–7.32	7.15–7.24	<7.5
or serum CO_2 Record only if no ABGs			≥52	41–51.9		32–40.9	22–31.9		18–21.9	15–17.9	<15
Serum sodium			≥180	160–179	155–159	150–154	130–149		120–129	111–119	≤110
Serum potassium			≥7	6–6.9	5.5–5.9		3.5–5.4	3–3.4	2.5–2.9		<2.5
Serum creatinine			≥3.5	2–3.4	1.5–1.9		0.6–1.4			<0.6	
Haematocrit			≥60	50–59.9	46–49.9		30–45.9		20–29.9		<20
White blood count			≥40		20–39.9	15–19.9	3–14.9		1–2.9		<1
Acute physiology score (APS)											

* GLASGOW COMA SCALE	AGE	CHRONIC HEATH EVALUATION	APACHE-II SCORE
Circle appropriate responses Eyes open: 4-spontaneously 3-to verbal stimuli 2-to painful stimuli 1-no response Motor response: 6-to verbal command 5-localizes to pain 4-withdraws to pain 3-decorticate 2-decerebrate 1-no response Verbal- non-intubated 5-oriented and converses 4-disoriented and talks 3-inappropriate words 2-incomprehensive sounds 1-no response Verbal - intubated 5-seems able to talk 3-questionable ability to talk 1-generally unresponsive Neurological points 15 - GCS = ...	Age Points ≤44 0 45-54 2 55-64 3 65-74 5 ≥75 6 Age points	Any one of the following chronic conditions Liver - Cirrhosis with PHT or encephalopathy Cardiovascular - Class IV angina or at rest or with minimal self care activities Pulmonary - Chronic hypoxaemia or hypercapnoea or polycythaemia of PHT > 40 mm Hg Kidney - Chronic peritoneal or haemodialysis Immune - Immunocompromised host Non-operative or emergency postoperative patient +5 Chronic health points	APS points .... Neurologic points .... Age points .... Chronic health points .... Total APACHE-II ....

Fig. 3 Form to record data utilized to determine the APACHE-II score.

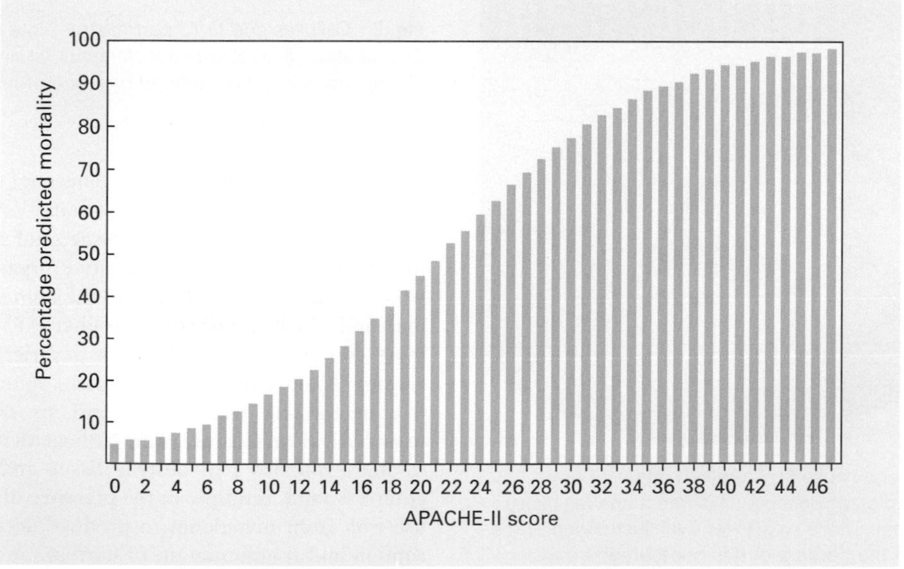

Fig. 4 Correlation of APACHE-II score and mortality risk in intra-abdominal infection. Data from Nyström PO, *et al. World Journal of Surgery*, 1990; **14**: 148–58.

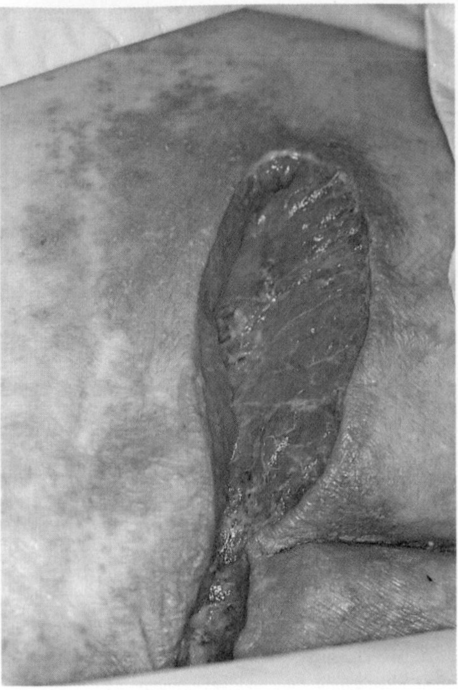

Fig. 5 Secondary wound erysipelas due to haemolytic *Streptococcus pyogenes*. A superficial wound infection had previously been treated by drainage and packing with resulting granulation of the subcutaneous tissues. Nonetheless, and reflecting the invasive capacities of streptococci, this infection began 4 days after opening of the wound. The infection responded to oral penicillin.

Synergistic gangrene

Chronic progressive bacterial gangrene is caused by the synergistic action of microaerophilic non-haemolytic streptococci, and aerobic haemolytic staphylococci (Fig. 6). The incubation period is 7 to 14 days. Cellulitis is followed by gangrenous ulceration that is progressive unless treated. Radical excision of the ulcerated lesion and its gangrenous borders is imperative, along with administration of large system doses of penicillin. Burrowing ulcers are caused by a combination of microaerophilic streptococci and staphylococci (Meleney's ulcer). Such lesions have a characteristic metallic sheen, cause necrosis of large areas of skin, and may produce sinus tracts in the underlying tissue. These should be incised, drained, and treated with high doses of penicillin (10 million units every 6 h).

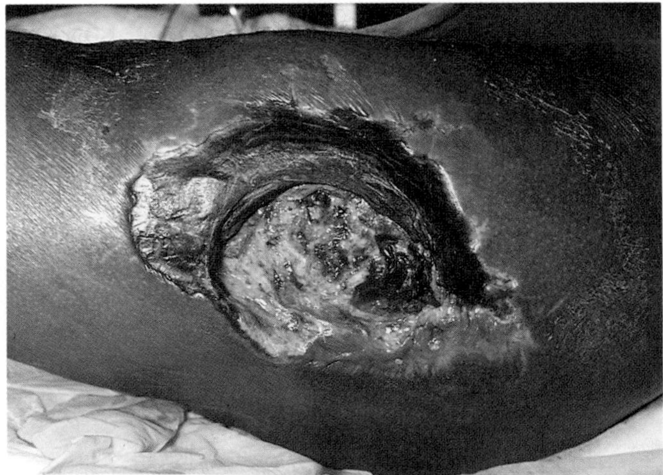

Fig. 6 Synergistic gangrene caused by a mixed infection by anaerobic streptococci and staphylococci. This infection was caused by self-injection with heroin. There was extensive destruction of the deep tissues extending to the borders of this photograph.

Non-clostridial gangrenous cellulitis caused by *B. melaninogenicus* and anaerobic streptococci is typified by a progressive gangrenous infection of the skin and adjacent areolar and fascial tissues. Prompt incision and drainage, and administration of large doses of penicillin are necessary. Supportive treatment is imperative, since toxaemia with dehydration, fever, and prostration rapidly develops.

Clostridial cellulitis is a serosanguineous, crepitant, septic process of subcutaneous, retroperitoneal, or other areolar tissue, caused principally by *C. perfringens* (also known as *C. welchii*). It differs from gas gangrene in that the infection does not involve muscle (Fig. 7), but spreads rapidly via fascial planes. Extensive gangrene results from vascular thrombosis. Systemic effects are moderate if the infection is treated promptly with early surgical debridement and penicillin therapy.

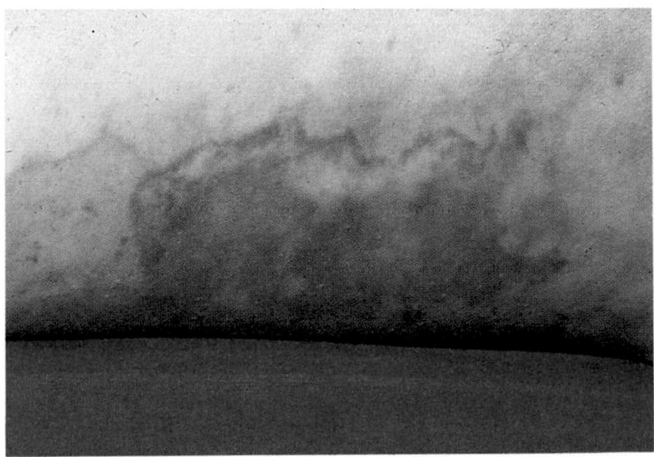

Fig. 7 Cellulitis due to *C. perfringens*. Note the ecchymotic discoloration of involved subcutaneous fat and the advancing border of cutaneous infection defined by a line of erythema.

Clostridial myonecrosis (gas gangrene) is an anaerobic infection of muscle characterized by profound toxaemia, extensive local oedema, massive necrosis of tissue, and a variable degree of gas production (Fig. 8). The causative organisms are the clostridia which abound in soil, dust, and the alimentary tract of most animals and which are usually saprophytic. *C. perfringens*, which is the most common cause, produces a variety of potent toxins, including hyaluronidase, collagenase, four different haemolysins, five necrotizing lecithinases, and six other necrotizing lethal toxins. All clostridia owe their pathogenicity to elaboration of such soluble exotoxins that destroy tissue and blood cells. Clostridia enter a wound, multiply in the presence of devitalized muscle, and use iron from myoglobin to produce necrotizing exotoxins. Disruption and fragmentation of normal muscle cells and capillaries

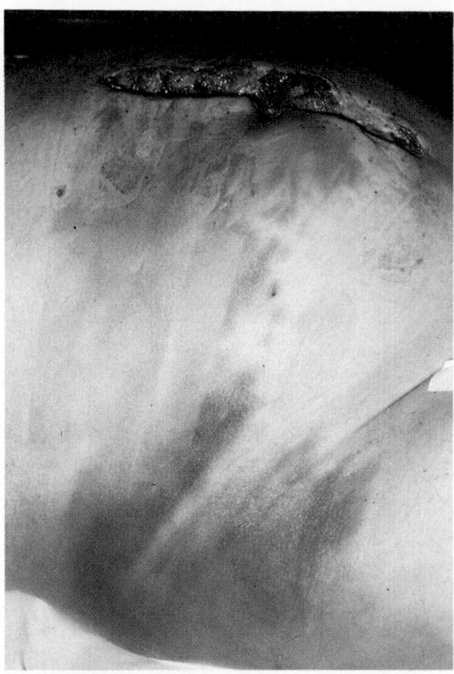

Fig. 8 Myonecrosis due to *C. perfringens*. Note the bronzing of skin. This infection spread to this state in only 24 h following an operation for pelvic infection.

result in further necrosis, haemorrhage, and oedema. There is no fibrin formation or polymorphonuclear leucocytic reaction. The affected muscles are at first red and friable, but progress to a purplish black, stringy, pulpy mass. The presence of gas is variable. The affected area swells and discharges a brownish, malodorous fluid. The overlying skin initially shows blotchy ecchymoses (marbling), then blackens, and finally sloughs.

The diagnosis of gas gangrene is based on typical clinical findings, as well as on the presence of large Gram-positive rods in the wound fluid. Delay in diagnosis, even for just a few hours, greatly increases the mortality. Immediate removal of involved muscle groups is necessary: amputation is indicated if the remaining viable muscles are insufficient for useful function. High intravenous doses of penicillin and whole blood are given preoperatively and postoperatively. Multiple treatments with hyperbaric oxygen (oxygen at 3.03 kPa) may reduce the amount of debridement necessary and lower the mortality, but muscle resection should not be delayed in anticipation of hyperbaric therapy. Untreated gas gangrene is always fatal; the fatality rate in treated patients ranges from 25 to 40 per cent.

Tetanus

This is caused by a spore-forming obligate anaerobe, *Clostridium tetani*, found in the faeces of humans and animals and capable of prolonged survival in soil. Two exotoxins are produced: tetanospasmin, a neurotoxin, and tetanolysin, a haemolysin. Dead muscle and clotted blood provides an ideal culture medium for germination of tetanus spores, and compound fractures with devitalization of muscle are very susceptible to such infection, as are small puncture wounds harbouring a clot deep in the tissues. Locally produced tetanolysin contributes to optimal growth conditions through its lecithinase, gelatinase, esterase, and lipase activities. Tetanospasmin, the neurotoxin responsible for the clinical features of the disease, does not act peripherally or locally but is carried to and acts on the central nervous system. In order to neutralize blood-borne toxin, antitoxin must be present before tetanospasmin becomes fixed by nerve cells. Antitoxin given when symptoms are apparent only limits further intoxication of nerve cells and cannot reverse developing symptoms.

There is considerable variability in progression of the disease from onset. There may be a prodromal period of headache, stiff jaw muscles, restlessness, yawning, risus sardonicus, and wound pain, typically beginning 1 to 2 weeks after trauma but occasionally as early as 1 day or as late as 2 months after injury. The active stage follows in 12 to 24 h, with trismus, facial distortion, opisthotonos, pain, clonic spasms, and seizures. Acute asphyxia is a major hazard and may result from either spasm of the respiratory muscles or aspiration. The shorter the incubation period, the poorer the prognosis.

Human immune globulin, 3000 units intramuscularly, should be given immediately to neutralize circulating toxins. An additional 1000 units are injected into and immediately proximal to the wound, followed by wide debridement. Five hundred units of intramuscular immune globulin may be given daily subsequently. If symptoms persist for longer than 2 weeks, the large initial doses of immune globulin may be repeated. An airway must be established; tracheostomy will be needed in every patient with more than prodromal symptoms and should be performed before the situation becomes urgent. Respirator support and oxygenation may be needed. Muscle spasms may be controlled with intravenous midazolam or diazepam, or with intramuscular meprobamate or chlorpromazine. If spasms persist, curare or another muscle blocker should be given. Additional sedation is usually not needed if muscle relaxant therapy has been adequate, but is best achieved with intramuscular barbiturates if required. The patient should be placed in a quiet room, with environmental stimulation kept at a minimum to avoid triggering seizures. Intravenous thiopental (Pentothal) may be needed to control seizures. High doses of penicillin G (5–10 million units) will establish a sufficient antibacterial tissue concentration. With appropriate early care, 75 per cent of patients survive with no neurological impairment.

Principles for tetanus prophylaxis

Tetanus is absolutely preventable by prior active immunization. Effective active immunization (not associated with a fresh wound) is accomplished by injection of 0.5 ml fluid or adsorbed toxoid, repeated after 2 and 20 months.

Immediate meticulous surgical care of the fresh wound is of prime importance. Removal of devitalized tissue, blood clots, and foreign bodies, obliteration of dead space, and prevention of tissue ischaemia in the wound are the objectives of initial treatment. If the wound is grossly contaminated, penicillin should be administered. Wounds which are seen late or are grossly contaminated should be left unsutured after debridement, protected by a sterile dressing for 3 to 5 days, and closed by delayed primary suture if the tissues appear clean and healthy. Active and passive immunization should be accomplished with 0.5 ml tetanus toxoid and tetanus immune globulin, 250 to 1000 units, as outlined in Table 4. Patients not previously immunized should receive injections of 0.5 ml fluid or adsorbed toxoid, repeated after 2, 6, and 20 months.

Table 4 Tetanus prophylaxis in wound management*

History of tetanus toxoid doses	Clean, minor wound		All other wounds	
	Toxoid†	Immune globulin	Toxoid†	Immune globulin
Less than 3 or unknown	Yes	No	Yes	Yes
Three or more‡	Yes if ⩾ 10 years since last booster	No	Yes if ⩾ 5 years since last booster	No

* Modified from *Mortality and Morbidity Weekly Reports*, August 8, 1991.

† For children less than 7 years, DTP is preferred (DT if pertussis vaccine is contraindicated). For older children and adults, combined diphtheria-tetanus (DT) is preferred to tetanus toxoid alone.

‡ If only fluid toxoid has been used, a dose of adsorbed toxoid should be used in all cases.

Infections of the hand

The most common hand infections are paronychia, pulp infection, and subcutaneous abscesses, including felon and bacterial tenosynovitis. The therapeutic goal is to restore full hand function. Elevation, immobilization in the position of function, and heat in the form of hot wet packs changed every 2 to 4 h are helpful. Hot soaks may be used for 20 min every 4 h. Ten million units of penicillin 6-hourly are effective in severe infections. Abscesses and other local collections of pus should be drained promptly; generally the volar aspect is incised. Important principles of managing hand infections are summarized in Table 5.

Breast abscess

Anaerobic and staphylococcal infections of the breast occur in two forms: puerperal (postpartum) and spontaneous (non-puerperal). A puerperal breast abscess is usually caused by staphylococci; non-puerperal breast abscesses (Fig. 9) may also be due to anaerobes, usually *Peptostreptococcus magnus* (Table 6). Excision of the involved duct through a periareolar incision is indicated for persisting or recurring non-puerperal breast abscess.

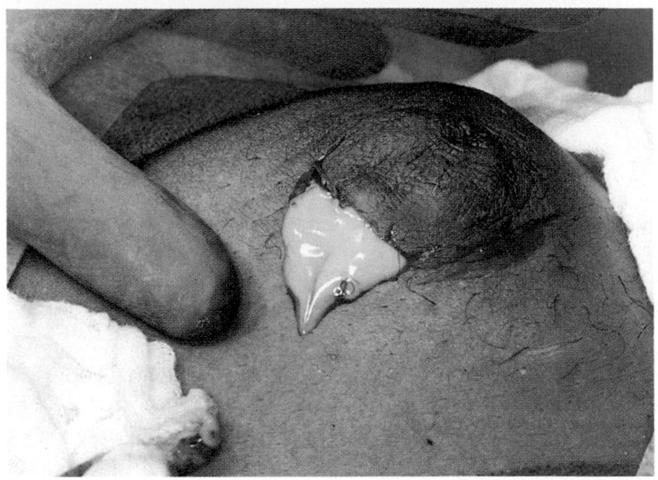

Fig. 9 Non-puerperal breast abscess. The pus was viscid and creamy yellow. The culture grew *Bacteroides ureolyticus*, two strains of Peptostreptococcus and an ampicillin-sensitive *E. coli*. Despite the clinical appearance of the pus, no staphylocci were present. This case illustrates the necessity to document infections by culture.

Pilonidal disease

A subcutaneous area located in the intergluteal cleft over the sacrum becomes infected when ingrown hair leads to formation of a foreign body sinus and triggers growth of mixed bacterial species, often with a predominance of anaerobes. Initial lesions are treated by unroofing, leaving the deep epithelialized wall of the sinus track intact, accompanied by epilation of surrounding skin

Table 5 Principles of management of hand infections

Establish the diagnosis before initiating therapy
Obtain a culture and give a tetanus booster or vaccination
Establish adequate anaesthesia; use a tourniquet whenever possible
Do not inject local anaesthetic into infected tissue
Incise/excise and drain mature lesins avoiding incisions in '*no-man's land*' overlying the distal palm and proximal phalanges
Elevate the extremity
Immobilize the extremity with a dorsal plaster splint
Apply wet dressings to the wound and change them frequently
Use antibiotics in high doses
Do not close puncture or human bite wounds
Do not close wounds which have been in contact with dishwater or other contaminated fluids, or in which contamination with sand or dirt has occurred
Do not drain a felon with a puncture type incision; equally, do not incise every painful digit

Table 6 Bacteria recovered in non-puerperal breast infection

Genus	No. of organisms
Aerobes	
Staphylococcus*	24
Streptococcus	4
Bacillus	2
Corynebacterium	1
Escherichia	1
Proteus	1
Pseudomonas	2
Anaerobes	
Actinomyces	3
Clostridium	2
Fusobacterium	1
Mitsuokella	1
Bacteroides*	8
Lactobacillus	3
Eubacterium	3
Propionibacterium*	16
Peptostreptococcus*	34
Veillonella	2

*Predominant genera.

From Walker A, Edmiston CE, Krepel CJ, Condon RE. *Archives of Surgery*, 1988; **123**: 908–11, with permission.

and allowing secondary healing. No additional antibiotic therapy is required, although wide excision and healing by secondary intention may be required if infection is recurrent or persistent.

Perianal abscess

Anaerobic infections of the perianal soft tissue originate from anal ducts and glands and present as localized subcuticular or subcutaneous foci immediately adjacent to the pigmented epithelium of the anal verge and canal. They do not burrow into deeper tissues, but must be clearly differentiated from perirectal and deeper abscesses by digital rectal examination. If tenderness precludes adequate investigation a thorough examination can be completed under anaesthesia. Before fluctuance occurs, antibiotic therapy for 2 to 3 days together with twice-daily sitz baths will often resolve the infection. If a fluctuant collection is present, perianal incision allows drainage; antibiotics are discontinued but sitz baths should continue until all inflammation has resolved.

Perirectal abscess

Burrowing, intersphincteric, ischiorectal, and supralevator abscesses originate in the rectal crypts and glands at the upper end of the anal canal. Goodsall's rule is incorrect; burrowing abscesses may originate at any point of the anorectal circumference. Typically, the abscess burrows directly radially from the infected gland or crypt of origin to present on the perianal skin at a slight distance from the anal verge. Burrowing may also occur in the subcutaneous tissues around the anus to form a more or less complete 'horseshoe abscess'. Alternatively, the infection may burrow between the anal sphincters or through the sphincters into the ischiorectal space, from which it may extend superiorly into the supralevator space, before dissecting subcutaneously to perianal skin. All forms of perirectal abscess are potentially more dangerous than a simple perianal abscess, and the two infections should not be confused. Examination under anaesthesia (regional block or general) is essential to make an accurate diagnosis. Drainage through a wide perianal incision is the treatment of choice. *Bacteroides* species, clostridia, and peptostreptococci predominate as causative organisms; the most common causative aerobe is *Proteus mirabilis*. The drainage wound should be packed open, packs changed frequently, and sitz baths taken twice daily. Additional antibiotic therapy after completion of drainage is not necessary in patients with normal immunological function.

THORACIC INFECTION

Lung infection may follow chest trauma which includes pulmonary contusion or rib fractures. Pulmonary infections may be caused by a variety of micro-organisms: aspiration following major trauma is a common cause of bronchopneumonia, usually caused by oral anaerobes. Treatment consists of a broad spectrum cephalosporin, such as cefotaxime, in combination with clindamycin.

Pleural empyema may follow haemothorax as well as pneumonia or other pulmonary infection, and is usually due to the same organisms as those which caused the lung infection. It may also follow elective thoracotomy. Empyema always requires closed tube drainage. If the lung does not completely expand, open pleural debridement (decortication is a misnomer) is essential. Antimicrobial therapy is directed against causative bacteria which may include anaerobes. Pulmonary infections, particularly those which follow aspiration of oral or gastric fluids, may progress to intrapulmonary abscess. Obligate oral anaerobes are often involved, but these may be difficult to isolate in routine culture. Percutaneous needle aspiration is often helpful for diagnosis. Antibiotic therapy should include anaerobic coverage with metronidazole, and open drainage may be required.

Infections of the heart

Surgical infections of the heart include endocarditis and pericarditis. Tuberculous pericarditis may require pericardiectomy, and endocarditis due to enterococci, *Streptococcus viridans*, pneumococci, and other bacteria also may require operative treatment. Subacute bacterial endocarditis is usually caused by streptococci of the viridans group (70 per cent of cases), *Enterococcus faecalis*, or group D streptococci. All streptococci are sensitive to parenteral penicillin at a dose of 6 million units (3.6 g) every 24 h for 4 weeks. The penicillin sensitivity of *Enterococcus faecalis* is variable; ampicillin is the best treatment for infections with this organism. Enterococci are generally resistant to cephalosporins and aminoglycosides.

ABDOMINAL INFECTION

Peritoneal infection

Contamination of the abdominal cavity may follow penetrating abdominal trauma or blunt trauma associated with intestinal rupture. Such patients usually undergo early operation, and intra-abdominal infection does not occur; unless operated on within 24 h of traumatic perforation, an intra-abdominal infection is likely. Secondary peritonitis may follow a variety of pathological conditions, including peptic ulcer perforation, pancreatitis, gallbladder perforation, bowel ischaemia due to strangulation or vascular compromise, small or large bowel perforation, genitourinary infection, and perforation of an intra-abdominal abscess. The source of infection must be controlled by closure or exteriorization, and the abdominal cavity must be cleansed of bacteria, toxins, and adjuvants such as bile, mucus, barium, blood, and necrotic tissue. Additional further influx of bacteria or adjuvants must be prevented. Multiple planned relaparotomies (staged abdominal repair) may be required for advanced cases with an APACHE-II score of 14 or greater.

Biliary infections

These are almost always associated with calculous disease. The infection progresses from acute cholecystitis to cholangitis or empyema of the gallbladder and, occasionally, to internal fistula formation; alternatively, the acute infection may settle into repetitive episodes of chronic cholecystitis. Uncomplicated gallstones are associated with bacteribilia (culture-positive bile) in 30 to 50 per cent of cases. The most important and frequently recovered pathogenic bacteria are *E. coli*, klebsiellae, and clostridia. Treatment consists of cholecystectomy and drainage of the bile duct system, following which infection usually resolves with antibiotic therapy. In immunocompromised patients broad-spectrum penicillins and third-generation cephalosporins are indicated.

Liver abscess

This may be due to amoebae, salmonellae, or to a mixed bacterial population, and usually follows appendicitis, bacterial or other forms of colitis, or biliary tract infection. Echinococcal cysts occasionally become secondarily infected. Obligate anaerobes are found in over 50 per cent of liver abscesses. Percutaneous drainage is needed if the abscess has developed a rind or wall within the liver. Specific antibiotic treatment will cure the infection, provided that the underlying condition is eliminated.

Pancreatitis and pancreatic abscess

Pancreatitis begins as a chemical inflammation, but more than half of the fatalities are due to infection. Pancreatic abscesses develop within the necrotic pancreatic tissue and require drainage; planned multiple laparotomies have been advocated for severe cases. Antibiotic therapy includes a third-generation cephalosporin combined with metronidazole; imipenem or sulbactam/ampicillin are good alternatives.

Appendicitis

Appendectomy (Fig. 10) is required. Antibiotics given prior to surgery are effective mainly for prophylaxis of infection in the incisional wound, and in uncomplicated appendicitis need not be continued following completion of the operation. Continued administration of antibiotics is indicated when the disease has progressed to gangrene, perforation, abscess, or diffuse peritonitis. Abscesses may be drained percutaneously with the help of ultrasound or CT, or open drainage by laparotomy may be established. Obligate anaerobes are always present. *E. coli* may cause lethal sepsis. In severe cases of diffuse peritonitis, a third-generation cephalosporin must be combined with metronidazole for therapy; ampicillin/sulbactam also has been successful.

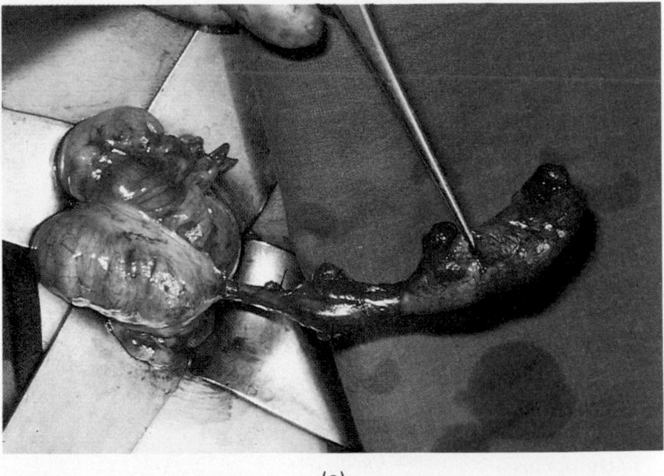

(a)

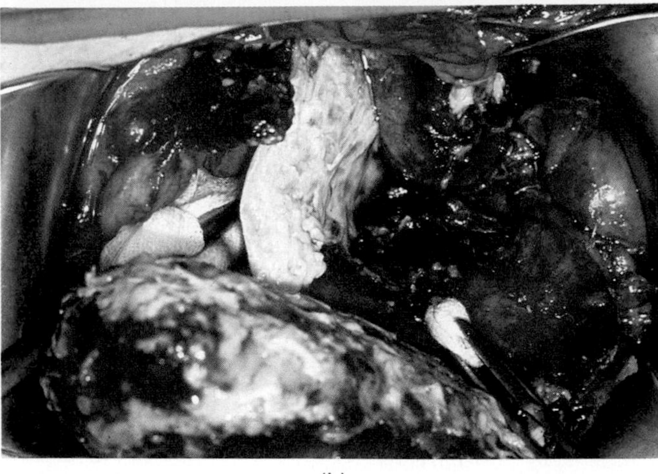

(b)

Fig. 10 The range of infection associated with appendicitis is broad. (a) Illustrates a case of simple, catarrhal appendicitis treated by early operation. (b) Illustrates a case of neglected, perforated appendicitis with formation of a complex lower abdominal abscess associated with necrosis of adjacent tissues.

Diverticulitis

More than half of patients over 50 years of age in the Western world have colonic diverticula, but only a minority develop symptoms. Diverticulitis may occur at any time and is usually treated with bowel rest and antibiotics. The disease is due to anaerobic organisms; 500 mg metronidazole every 12 h is the treatment of choice. If septicaemia develops, a third-generation cephalosporin may be included. Other drug combinations active against *B. fragilis* and *E. coli* may be used. Perforation of a diverticulum results in either diffuse peritonitis or a peridiverticular abscess (Fig. 11). The abscess itself may secondarily perforate and cause diffuse peritonitis; laparotomy and resection of the diseased colon segment is the treatment of choice. Primary anastomosis has been successful in selected cases; if this is not appropriate or possible,

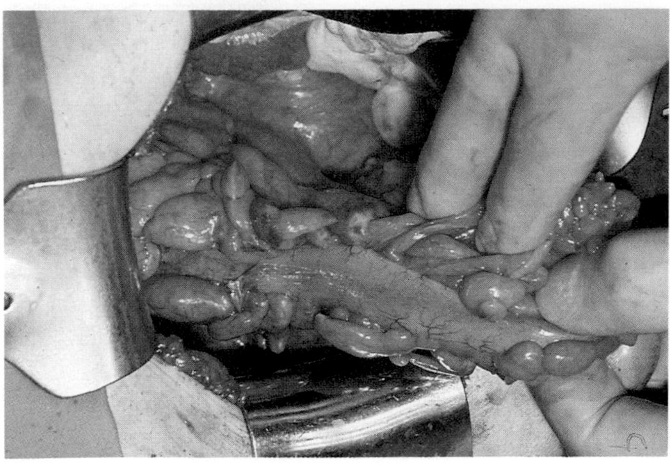

Fig. 11 A contained diverticular abscess originating in a diverticulum of the sigmoid colon.

an end-colostomy and mucus fistula may be performed, but Hartmann's procedure should be avoided if possible. Later restoration of bowel continuity entails some further risks of mortality and morbidity, but the magnitude of such risks is generally exaggerated in reports in the literature.

FEMALE GENITAL TRACT INFECTION

Infections of this region are mostly non-surgical (in the sense that operative drainage or debridement of tissue is not usually necessary to control the infection), and the mainstay of therapy is the administration of appropriate antibiotics. Sexually transmitted infections are diagnosed by the presence of specific micro-organisms in cultures of cervical exudate. Pelvic inflammatory disease is usually due to gonococci, while endometritis, adnexitis, and myometritis are caused by mixed infection with aerobic and anaerobic intestinal bacteria. These infections are treated with antibiotics; transvaginal drainage is needed in some cases. Occasionally, a persisting tubal abscess may need resection.

GENITOURINARY TRACT INFECTION

The most common form of urinary tract infection involves only the urinary bladder, occurs primarily in women due to the relatively short length of the urethra, and is caused by coliform organisms. Such infections usually respond readily to increased fluid intake and administration of an oral penicillin or cephalosporin, although recurrence is common. Urinary bladder infection is also common following the placement of a Foley catheter. Although closed urinary drainage systems delay the onset of bladder infection, infection always occurs eventually if the catheter remains in place, the route of infection being through the urethra external to the catheter. Such infections are usually caused by coliform bacteria. Antibiotics should not ordinarily be used to treat this form of urinary bladder infection unless the catheter can be removed; the continued presence of the catheter assures continuing infection and administration of antibiotics only results in emergence of resistant organisms. Acidifying bladder washes are partially effective in controlling bladder infection in this situation.

If the ureteropelvic junction is incompetent, backwash of infected bladder urine into the ureter and renal pelvis may result in acute pyelitis, accompanied by septicaemia and even septic shock. Chronic pyelonephritis is usually haematogenous in origin and may result in a nephric or perinephric abscess which may rupture and cause peritonitis. Drainage is required and antibiotic treatment should be specific and should include a drug active against anaerobes such as metronidazole.

BONE AND JOINT INFECTION

Post-traumatic ostitis

This is seen primarily in unstable fractures in which moving fragments continuously produce friction and necrotic tissue; unless the fracture is stabilized, the infection cannot be controlled. Staphylococci are the predominant causative micro-organisms but *P. aeruginosa* is isolated in 10 per cent of cases. Obligate anaerobes are present in more than 10 per cent of the cases, but are usually missed by routine culture techniques, and Gram-negative facultative anaerobes may become a problem. Following operative stabilization of the fracture, specific intravenous antimicrobial therapy should be continued for 4 weeks. The bone concentration of the chosen antibiotic should be greater than its minimum inhibitory concentration for the infecting bacteria.

Osteomyelitis

In adults, antimicrobial therapy should be specific for the infecting organism and should achieve a bone concentration above its minimum inhibitory concentration. A swab is insufficient as a bacteriological specimen; open biopsy to obtain a piece of infected tissue for culture and determination of antibiotic sensitivity is preferred. Haematogenous osteomyelitis in adults (usually immunocompromised individuals) may require operative drainage and sequestrectomy. Haematogenous osteomyelitis in children can be treated successfully if parenteral antibiotics are administered early in the disease, but if a large subperiostal abscess or a sequestra forms, operative management is required. Osteomyelitis of the spine may present as a groin abscess and is usually seen in immunocompromised patients: staphylococci, mycobacteria, and salmonellae are the most common causative micro-organisms. Specific antimicrobial therapy is mandatory and bone biopsy may be required to provide adequate samples for culture and sensitivity studies. The chosen antibiotic needs to reach bone concentrations above their minimum inhibitory concentration for the pathogen involved.

CENTRAL NERVOUS SYSTEM INFECTION

Subdural empyema accounts for 10 to 32 per cent of intracranial suppurations. Acute frontal sinusitis and mastoid infections are the most common antecedent cause, but infected subdural collections occur in 2 per cent of patients following meningitis and are most commonly caused by Gram-positive cocci. Early drainage is essential to prevent a further increase of intracranial pressure (neurosurgical emergency).

Metastatic and primary brain abscess may follow meningitis, or may be due to haematogenous or direct spread from mastoiditis or nasal sinus infection. Anaerobic bacteria and *Staphylococcus aureus* are most commonly found in these conditions. Prompt incision and drainage is required.

POSTOPERATIVE INFECTIONS

Wound infection

Any purulent discharge from a closed surgical incision (not just from around a suture) with inflammation of the surrounding tissue, with or without a positive culture, should be considered as a wound infection. A rare case of sterile fat necrosis will be included, but this is better than overlooking a true infection. Superficial (suprafascial) wound infection in the early postoperative period is diagnosed on clinical findings, as well as on the results of a Gram stain of needle-aspirated material. The earliest sign of such infections is induration, accompanied by erythema and increasing pain: excessive wound pain is a commonly overlooked sign, particularly in patients with wound infections caused by Gram-negative organisms. Immediate therapy consists of reopening the wound and evacuating the pus; antibiotics are not usually required.

Deep wound infections involving fascia and muscle are more serious, and are usually accompanied by infection in one of the main body cavities or in bone or a joint. They usually occur as the result of a technical error. Drainage, control of any source of continuing infection, and antibiotic therapy are indicated.

Necrotizing fascitis

This is a serious mixed infection due to a haemolytic streptococci or staphylococci and peptostreptococci, and associated with excessive collagenase production, leading to dissolution of connective tissue. The infection involves the epifascial tissues of an operative wound, laceration, abrasion, or puncture. It may be immediately fulminant or may remain dormant for 6 or more days before beginning to spread rapidly. Subcutaneous and fascial necrosis accompanies extensive undermining of the skin, resulting in gangrene. Treatment is excision of the entire area of fascia affected, administration of large doses of penicillin (12–30 million units/day), and appropriate systemic support.

Postoperative peritonitis

Fifteen to 30 per cent of all intra-abdominal infections occur following an operation. The diagnosis is usually delayed. The most common cause is a technical error compromising the vascular supply to an anastomosis, resulting in necrosis and leakage of intestinal contents into the peritoneal cavity. Iatrogenic perforation of a hollow viscus is another cause. An intra-abdominal haematoma may become secondarily infected, resulting in an abscess. Treatment is operative, as in other forms of secondary peritonitis, although non-operative drainage with ultrasound or CT guidance is a valid option for an abscess not associated with an anastomosis (Fig. 12). Antimicrobial therapy is more difficult due to the possible selection of resistant bacteria by preoperative antibiotic therapy. Antibiotics administered should not only cover the specific bacteria isolated, but should also be effective against possible pathogens from the facultative and obligate anaerobic bowel flora; usually a third-generation cephalosporin plus metronidazole is sufficient. Other options are imipenem or ampicillin-sulbactam. If a resistant Pseudomonas, Enterobacter, or Serratia presents problems for treatment, the synergism seen between aminoglycosides and β-lactam antibiotics should be exploited. Enterococci rarely cause a problem and need not be treated specifically when otherwise adequate aerobic and anaerobic antibiotic coverage is provided.

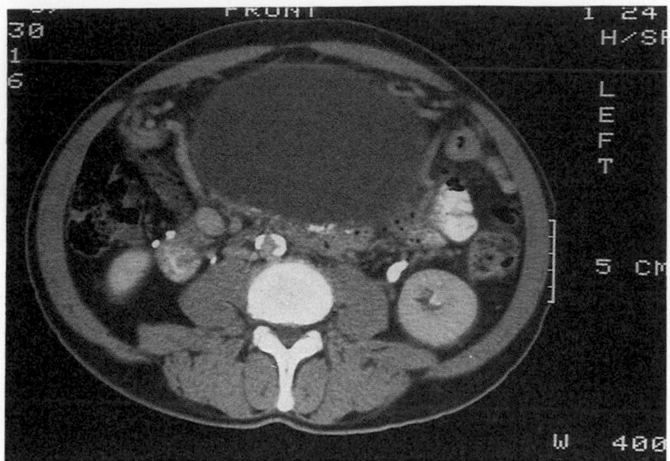

Fig. 12 A large intra-abdominal abscess demonstrated by computed tomography and easily drained percutaneously.

Pulmonary infections

These are common following thoracic and upper abdominal operations. Pain and the supine posture interfere with adequate diaphragmatic and chest wall respiration resulting in atelectasis, and subsequent bronchopneumonia or lobar pneumonia. Treatment of mild cases involves physical therapy and adequate analgesia to allow for full expansion of the lungs. If antimicrobial therapy is likely to be required for suspected pneumonia, transtracheal aspiration should be used to obtain a specimen for culture before therapy is started. If indicated, infected secretions can be removed by bronchoscopy, and a reliable specimen can be obtained for Gram stain, culture, and determination of antibiotic sensitivity. A variety of micro-organisms, such as streptococci, pneumococci, staphylococci, meningococci, gram-negative anaerobes, and fungi may be isolated. The result of the Gram stain will help in choosing the initial antibiotic for calculated therapy. Aspiration pneumonia is usually due to anaerobic oral bacteria. If gastric juice is also aspirated, a severe infection may result (Mendelson syndrome) which has a high mortality risk. Pleural empyema may develop following thoracic or abdominothoracic operations, or following postoperative pneumonia. The contribution of anaerobic organisms is usually underestimated. Tube thoracostomy drainage and rethoracotomy are treatment options. Initial antimicrobial therapy should be based on the result of a Gram stain and should also include a drug such as metronidazole or clindamycin, active against anaerobes.

Mediastinitis

This carries a high mortality and is most commonly seen following oesophageal resection. Treatment consists of adequate operative drainage and administration of antimicrobials fully active against endotoxin-producing Gram-negative bacteria and obligate anaerobes; a third-generation cephalosporin, combined with metronidazole will cover most pathogenic bacteria. Imipenem may be required. Interpretation of bacteriological results is difficult since antibiotics will usually have been given before a proper specimen can be obtained during the operative drainage procedure. The gaps in bacterial coverage of antibiotics previously given should influence the current choice of antibiotic. Sternum infection is seen following median sternotomy and most commonly is due to staphylococci. If antibiotic treatment is not initially successful, the sternum must be reopened to allow for drainage.

Urinary tract infection

A Foley catheter, if required, should be connected to a closed drainage system and should be removed as soon as possible. Specimens of urine should be sent for culture and sensitivity testing every 5 days, and at the time of catheter removal. Suprapubic urinary bladder catheterization is preferable for long-term bladder drainage since the risk of infection is considerably reduced. A colony count of 10^6/ml bacteria in fresh urine is highly suggestive of active infection. Dysuria is not always present. Hemorrhagic cystitis is usually caused by *E. coli*. If the infecting organism is unknown, a Gram stain will help in selecting an appropriate antibiotic.

Line infection/intravenous catheters

One-third of intravenous catheters become colonized with bacteria within 2 days of placement. Bacteraemia will occur in 1 per cent of patients with an intravenous catheter in place for longer than 48 h, and the risk of septicaemia increases to 5 per cent with increasing duration of catheterization. An intravenous catheter should always be removed and cultured whenever bacteraemia is suspected. Intra-arterial catheters may also be the site of sepsis and should be similarly handled.

Infections of vascular prostheses are most commonly due to staphylococci. Treatment may require removal of the artificial vascular graft. Antimicrobial wound treatment without graft removal succeeds in selected situations.

ANTIBIOTIC PROPHYLAXIS

The scientific basis for the use of prophylactic antibiotics in surgery was laid by Miles and Burke in the late 1950s when they were able to show that infections could be prevented only when antimicrobials were given prior to or at the time of the infectious challenge. Antibiotics given 3 h following a challenge with infectious bacteria were ineffective in preventing infection. A surgical incision exposes normally sterile tissues to a non-sterile environment; some contamination occurs with any operation. Bacteria may start multiplying before effective host defences are established, and if initially present in a concentration exceeding 100 000 organisms/g tissue, may exceed the host defence capacity. Host defences also recognize damaged and dead tissue, which are eliminated by the same humoral and cellular mechanisms as those used to defeat invading bacteria. Thus, there is a need for gentle operative technique to minimize the volume of damaged tissue and for adherence to principles of aseptic surgery to reduce the level of bacterial contamination.

Following closure of the wound, its environment is sealed by local intravascular coagulation and the events of early inflammation which initiate wound healing: this may explain why postoperative administration of antibiotics is ineffective in preventing wound infection. Antibiotics administered preoperatively diffuse into the peripheral compartment, in this case the wound fluid; since the wound is saturated with antimicrobials at the time it becomes contaminated, potentially invading bacteria are inhibited from multiplying and many are killed.

For years the basic principles concerning appropriate timing in administering antibiotics for prophylaxis were not accepted. Although a controlled trial demonstrating the efficacy of antibiotic prophylaxis in potentially contaminated operations was reported by Bernard and Cole, other reports produced conflicting conclusions. Nearly 10 years after the description of the decisive or vulnerable period by Burke, the data from a controlled clinical trial proving that antibiotics were effective only when given in the immediate preoperative period were reported and widely accepted by surgeons. Doubts about the efficacy of antibiotic prophylaxis persisted well into the 1970s, but during the last two decades many excellent studies have been published, so that today antibiotic prophylaxis is an established practice and the principles for optimal preventive antibiotic administration are widely accepted.

The principles of antibiotic prophylaxis are:

1. Use an antibiotic with efficacy against the bacteria likely to contaminate the wound as demonstrated in a controlled clinical trial.
2. Use full doses of the chosen antibiotic.
3. Administer the antibiotics preoperatively at a time such that effective tissue concentrations will have been achieved when intraoperative contamination occurs.
4. If the operation is prolonged beyond 3 or 4 h, give another dose. Otherwise, single dose prophylaxis is effective in most clinical situations.
5. Employ antibiotic prophylaxis whenever the risk of wound infection is increased.

Single dose prophylaxis

The first prospective controlled trial which investigated the proper postoperative duration of antibiotic prophylaxis was performed by Strachan and colleagues in 1977. A single preoperative dose of cefazolin was compared with a regimen of cefazolin given for a period of 5 days after operation. The infection rate following a single dose of antibiotic was 3 per cent; that following multiple postoperative dosing was 5 per cent. Although there was no statistically significant difference between these figures, the slight numerical difference in favour of the single dose seen in this study was also found in many subsequent studies which tested the same hypothesis for various indications. The most prudent and conservative interpretation of the results of all of these studies is that, at the very least, single dose prophylaxis is as effective as multiple dosing, and is preferable because it is less likely to alter antibiotic resistance patterns of bacteria in a hospital. It is astonishing in the presence of this evidence (Table 7) that multiple dose prophylaxis still is used today in many institutions.

Table 7 Single dose prophylaxis versus multiple dose prophylaxis; results of prospective randomized trials in colon operations

Number of studies	27
Single dose	
Operations performed	510
Infections seen	22
Infection rate (%)	4.3
Multiple dosing	
Operations performed	493
Wound infections seen	34
Infection rate (%)	6.9

Table 8 Critical values for duration of operation*. If the duration of operation exceeds T hours (T is the 75th percentile of duration for each specific procedure) the risk of infection in increased.

T(hours)	Typical operations
1	Appendectomy, limb amputation, caesarian section
2	Hernia repair, cholecystectomy, exploratory laparotomy, open reduction of fracture, hysterectomy, ventricular shunt, mastectomy
3	Thoracotomy (all), gastric, small bowel, colon operations (all), spinal fusion, joint prosthesis, nephrectomy, vascular surgery (all)
4	Hepatobiliary–pancreatic operations (all), prostatectomy, head and neck surgery, craniotomy
5	Cardiac surgery (all)
7	Organ transplantation

Data from Culver DH, *et al. American Journal of Medicine*, 1991; **91**(Suppl. 3B): 152S–157S.

The risk of infection

The risk of developing a wound infection has traditionally been determined by stratifying operations into classes: clean, clean-contaminated, contaminated, and dirty, based on the relative degree of intraoperative bacterial contamination. This scheme ignores other important factors, such as the functional state of host defences and the amount of tissue trauma engendered by the operation, which also help to determine the risk of developing a wound infection. Regression analysis of outcome in a very large number of surgical patients has indicated that the factors controlling the risk of developing a wound infection are: heavy bacterial contamination as reflected in an operation classed as contaminated or dirty; impaired host defences as reflected in an ASA score of 3 or higher; and long duration of operation. The critical time is procedure-specific (Table 8).

Any patient exhibiting one or more of these risk factors should be given antibiotic prophylaxis. In addition, prophylaxis should be administered whenever a prosthesis is to be inserted during the operation.

Specific recommendations

In the discussion of selected specific clinical circumstances, we have used the results of published controlled studies which fulfil most of these following criteria: prospective conduct of the study, definition of entrance criteria and drop-out conditions, consideration of risk factors, unbiased randomization, double-blind assessment of clinical and bacteriological outcome, and appropriate statistical analysis.

Colorectal operations

The risk of wound infection following colorectal operations without prophylaxis is of the order of 40 per cent. A single dose of parenteral antibiotics or effective oral antibiotic bowel preparation can reduce the incidence of postoperative infection to less than 10 per cent. The two essential steps in effective prophylaxis for an elective colon operation are thorough mechanical cleansing of the bowel, preferably by polyethylene glycol purgation, and oral administration of antibiotics: neomycin and erythromycin base are effective. Parenteral antibiotics alone are less reliable in this situation. Since the risk associated with administering a single parenteral dose of a β-lactam antibiotic is minimal, we now employ combined oral and systemic prophylaxis (Table 9). The use of parenteral antibiotics alone is not recommended in an elective surgery situation, but is the only regimen available for emergency operations.

Table 9 Preparation for elective colorectal operation

Preoperative day
1. Oral polyethylene glycol–electrolyte solution (Colyte, Golytely) orally, 4 litres over 2 h, beginning at 10:00 a.m.
2. If chronic constipation or extensive diverticulosis exists, double the purgation volume and start 2–3 h earlier
3. If the patient cannot swallow the required volume in the required time, pass a nasogastric tube and into duodenum administer purgation by lavage, removing the tube when complete
4. Clear liquid diet only on this day
5. Neomycin, 1 g together orally at 1 p.m., 2 p.m., and 10 p.m.
6. Nothing by mouth after midnight

Operation day
1. Evacuate the rectum completely into a commode before transport to the operating suite
2. Administer ampicillin-sulbactam, 2 g IV (other parenteral antibiotics of equivalent spectrum may be used instead)
3. Commence operation at 8:00 a.m.
4. If the operation is scheduled later in the day, adjust the oral neomycin–erythromycin dosing schedule appropriately so that the operation starts 19–20 h after the first dose.

Appendectomy

Antibiotic prophylaxis for patients undergoing surgery for acute appendicitis includes a treatment aspect for the intra-abdominal infection, as well as a prophylaxis aspect as regards infection of the abdominal wound. Antibiotics are of questionable therapeutic value in simple acute appendicitis, but are certainly therapeutic when perforated appendicitis and peritonitis are present. For all other circumstances, single dose prophylaxis is justified. The high risk of wound infection following perforation justifies leaving the subcutaneous wound open.

The best results are obtained with antibiotics active against aerobic as well as anaerobic bacteria. In studies in which an aminoglycoside or a cephalosporin was used in combination with either clindamycin or metronidazole, only seven of 261 patients (2.7 per cent) developed a wound infection. The best current regimen seems to be metronidazole combined with cefazolin.

Gastroduodenal operations

The incidence of postoperative wound infections following stomach operations correlates directly with the number of bacteria within the stomach which, in turn, correlates with the acidity of the stomach and the underlying pathology. The 'acid barrier' which effectively kills swallowed bacteria in normal individuals may be altered by H_2-receptor antagonists given during the 12 h before operation. All groups of antibiotics have been studied as prophylaxis for gastroduodenal operations. First-generation cephalosporins are as effective as any other group of β-lactam drugs and are as effective as aminoglycosides.

Recommended prophylaxis for gastroduodenal operations involves interdicting use of acid secretion blocking or neutralizing agents for 1 or 2 days preoperatively, including when ordered as part of the anaesthetic premedication, and administration of 2 g of cefazolin on induction of anaesthesia.

Biliary tract operations

Although the normal biliary tree rarely harbours any bacteria, in the presence of disease the biliary tract should be viewed as bacterially contaminated. The number of bacteria is influenced by a variety of factors, primarily the presence of biliary stones or a stricture (Table 10). The risk of infection following an operation for biliary disease without antibiotic cover is about 16 per cent. Numerous clinical trials have employed a variety of antibiotic regimens in biliary operations (Table 11).

Single dose antibiotic prophylaxis is appropriate in bile tract surgery. Although enterococci are frequently recovered from bile, their presence can be ignored in choosing an antibiotic for prophylaxis when cholecystectomy is being performed for calculous disease. The agent of choice remains 2 g of cefazolin given about 30 to 45 min prior to the operation. Second choice agents may be cefuroxime, cefamandole, sulphamethoxazole-trimethoprim, or cefotaxime. The use of ceftriaxone is not recommended because of its long half-life. Cholangitis (fever, chills, jaundice) involves a more faeculent spectrum of bacteria, including the regular presence of anaerobes. In this circumstance, ampicillin-sulbactam, 2 g, is preferred.

Table 10 Bacteria isolated from biliary tract*

	No of isolates	Percentage distribution
AEROBES	1183	95
E. coli	434	35
Klebsiella	154	12
Enterobacter	45	4
Proteus	99	8
Pseudomonas	19	2
Other Gram-negative bacteria	36	3
Streptococci	162	13
Enterococci	159	13
Staphylocci	75	6
Obligate anaerobes	65	5
B. fragilis	9	1
Peptostreptococci	20	2
Clostridia	29	2
Other anaerobes	1	
All bacteria	1248	100

*Data from Condon RE, Wittmann DH. The use of antibiotics in general surgery. In: Wells, SA, ed. *Current Problems in Surgery*. Chicago: Mosby Year Book, 1991.

Vascular operations

The risk of infection is increased by the clinical setting in which most vascular reconstructions are performed: electively for arterial insufficiency, implying some degree of tissue ischaemia, or as an emergency for trauma. The frequent need for insertion of a prosthesis for bypass or repair further disables host defence mechanisms and increases the risk of infection. Overall, the risk of infection following vascular surgery is of the order of 4 per cent.

Table 11 Antibiotic prophylaxis in biliary operations*

Prophylactic agent(s)	No. of trials	No. of patients	Infected No.	Infected Rate (%)
Cefotetan	1	90	13	14
Mezlocillin	2	359	24	7
Cefamandole	5	431	24	6
Gentamicin	2	202	11	5
Cefazolin	7	494	26	5
Cefonocid	2	99	4	4
Cefoxitin	2	92	3	3
Cefuroxime	5	353	10	3
Piperacillin	1	50	1	2
Cefotaxime	2	87	0	0

*Data from Condon RE, Wittmann DH. The use of antibiotics in general surgery. In: Wells SA, ed. *Current Problems in Surgery*. Chicago: Mosby Year Book, 1991.

Table 12 Vascular operations and antibiotics used as prophylactic agents*

Prophylactic agent(s)	No. of trials	No. of patients	Infected No.	Infected Rate (%)
Cephaloridine	1	27	6	22
Cephradine	2	75	0	0
Cefazolin	1	225	2	1
Cefotaxime	1	134	4	3
Oxacillin	1	168	4	2
Cephalothin	1	232	2	1

* Data from Condon RE, Wittmann DH. The use of antibiotics in general surgery. In: Wells SA, ed. *Current Problems in Surgery*. Chicago: Mosby Year Book, 1991.

The bacteria of concern are *S. aureus*, *E. coli* and other enteric Gram-negative rods, which are the cause of early postoperative infections, and the *S. epidermidis* group of organisms which cause indolent late graft infections. A few controlled clinical trials have been reported (Table 12), but recent increases in resistance among staphylococci, especially *S. epidermidis*, mandate care in the choice of antibiotic for prophylaxis.

Recommended prophylaxis is cefazolin administered at induction of anaesthesia, as long as two-thirds or more of *S. epidermidis* group isolates in the hospital are sensitive to this antibiotic. If *S. epidermidis* resistance is a problem, ampicillin-sulbactam or sulphamethoxazole-trimethoprim are currently effective alternatives. If methicillin-resistant staphylococci are a problem, vancomycin (for the staphylococci) plus cefotaxime or aztreonam (for the coliforms) should be effective.

FURTHER READING

Bernard HR, Cole WR. The prophylaxis of surgical infection: the effect of prophylactic antimicrobial drugs on the incidence of infection following potentially contaminated operations. *Surgery* 1964; **50**: 161–8.

Bohnen JMA, Solomkin JS, Dellinger EP, Bjornson HS, Page CP. Guidelines for clinical care: anti-infective agents for intraabdominal infection: A surgical infection policy statement. *Arch Surg*, in press.

Burke JF. The effective period of preventive antibiotic action in experimental incisions and dermal lesions. *Surgery* 1961; **50**: 161–8.

Condon RE, Wittmann DH. The use of antibiotics in general surgery. In Samuel A. Wells, ed. *Current Problems in Surgery*. Chicago: Mosby Year Book, 1991.

Condon RE, Wittmann DH. The use of antibiotics in surgery. *Curr Probl Surg* 1992; in press.

Culver DH, *et al.* Surgical wound infection rates by wound class, operative procedure, and patient risk index. *Am J Med* 1991; **91** (Suppl 3B): 152S–157S.

Finald M, McGowan JE, Jr. Nosocomial infections in surgical patients. Observations on effects of prophylactic antibiotics. *Arch Surg* 1976; **111**: 143–5.

Friedrich PL. Zur bacteriellen Aetiologie und zur Behandlung der diffusen Peritonitis. *Arch Klin Chir* 1902; **68**: 524.

Kanus WA, Draper EA, Wagner DP, Zimmerman JE. APACHE II: A severity of disease classification system. *Crit Care Med* 1985; **13**: 818.

Karl RC., Mertz JJ, Veith FC, Dineen P. Prophylactic antimicrobial drugs in surgery. *N Engl J Med* 1966; **275**: 305–308.

Miles AA, Miles EM, Burke J. The value and duration of defense reactions of the skin to primary lodgment of bacteria. *Br J Exp Path* 1957; **38**: 79–96.

National Nosocomial Infections Surveillance (NNIS) System. Nosocomial infection rates for interhospital comparison: limitations and possible solutions. *Infect Control Hosp Epidemiol* 1991; **12**: L609–21.

Nyström PO, *et al.* Proposed definitions for diagnosis, severity scoring, stratification, and outcome for trials on intraabdominal infection. *World J Surg* 1990; **14**: 148–58.

Polk HD, Jr, Lopez-Mayor JF. Postoperative wound infection: a postoperative study of determinant factors and prevention. *Surgery* 1969; **66**: 97–103.

Seabrook GR. Pathobiology of graft infections. *Sem Vasc Surg* 1990; **3**: 81–8.

Strachan CJ, *et al.* Prophylactic use of cefazolin against sepsis after cholecystectomy. *Br Med J.* 1977; **1**: 1254–6.

Wittmann DH. *Intra-abdominal Infection: Pathophysiology and Treatment.* New York: Marcel-Dekker, 1991.

Wittmann DH, Bergstein JM, Frantzides CT. Calculated empiric antimicrobial therapy for mixed type surgical infectious disease. *Infection* 1991; **19**: in press.

2.2 The surgical management of acquired immune deficiency disease

WALTER J. BURDETTE

INTRODUCTION

Acquired immune deficiency syndrome (AIDS) has attracted widespread attention and fear because of its uniform fatality, its association with a controversial lifestyle, and its continued rapid increase in incidence. The groups in which the disease was originally prevalent included homosexuals, users of intravenous drugs, and recipients of blood carrying the virus. Now they also include heterosexuals and children of infected mothers. Racial and geographic disparity still exists. In the United States, the annual rates per 100 000 population vary from 0.1 in South Dakota to 40.6 in New York state, 47.7 in Puerto Rico, and 71.2 in New York City.

The geographic rankings in descending numbers of AIDS cases reported are the United States, Uganda, Zaire, Brazil, France, Malawi, Tanzania, Italy, Kenya, and Spain. So far the disease has yielded only to improvement in palliation.

Most cases of AIDS are treated by medical specialists, but many diagnostic and therapeutic problems require surgical participation. Experience with surgical management of AIDS has now been sufficiently extensive to provide some general guidelines for appropriate approaches to problems with a given set of clinical findings. In addition to the responsibilities associated with surgical treatment, the surgeon has the duty to protect personnel and himself from the dangers of infection prevalent in an environment where medical personnel are exposed to infected blood and body fluids and the danger of injury with a contaminated instrument.

HIV AND AIDS

Acquired immune deficiency syndrome was first diagnosed in 1981, but subsequent retrospective studies have documented cases earlier than this. The search for the cause of the clinical syndrome resulted in the isolation of a virus from tissue by Montagnier *et al.* in 1983 which he called lymphadenopathy-associated virus (LAV). In 1984 Gallo *et al.* cultured a virus from AIDS patients and identified it as HTLV-III. The official name given at that time to the AIDS virus was HTLV-III/LAV, and this may be encountered in the early literature. However, the International Committee for Taxonomy of Viruses changed the name to human immunodeficiency virus (HIV), and the structure of this retrovirus is now known. Following invasion of a cell by this virus, viral RNA is converted to DNA by reverse transcriptase, which is integrated into the host genome, and undergoes replication. When this phenomenon occurs in helper/inducer CD4 lymphocytes, for which the virus has a predilection as the CD4 molecule acts as a receptor for the virus, they are destroyed as the newly produced viral particles are released. The cellular immune response of the host is impaired, leading to increased susceptibility to infections and to uncommon tumours in immunocompetent individuals. Patients infected with HIV virus do not show clinical symptoms when immunosuppression is not severe; they are said to be affected with AIDS-related complex (ARC) which later progresses to the clinical syndrome of AIDS. Viral infection can be screened by using an enzyme-linked-immunosorbent assay, but diagnosis of an individual case requires the Western blot test. Immunity is not conferred by infection with this virus.

DIAGNOSIS OF AIDS

When laboratory evidence of infection with HIV is present, a diagnosis of AIDS may be made with even a presumption of the following complicating diseases: Kaposi's sarcoma, infection with *Pneumocystis carinii*, cerebral lymphoma, non-Hodgkin's lymphoma, pneumonia, disseminated mycobacterial infection, cytomegalovirus retinitis, or toxoplasmosis of the brain (Figs. 1–11). In the absence of a positive test for HIV infection, the diagnosis of AIDS may be made when there is definitive diagnosis of candidiasis of the oesophagus or tracheobronchial tree, non-Hodgkin's lymphoma, HIV encephalopathy, Kaposi's sarcoma, *Pneumocystis carinii* pneumonia, extrapulmonary cryptococcosis, extrapulmonary *Mycobacterium avium* or *M. kansasii* infection, prolonged cryptosporidiosis, cerebral toxoplasmosis, herpes simplex infection lasting longer than 1 month, progressive multifocal leucoencephalopathy, pulmonary lymphoid hyperplasia or pneumonia in a young child, or a T4 helper/inducer lymphocyte count below $400/mm^3$.

OPERATIVE MANAGEMENT

Major operations are not often indicated in AIDS patients. However, biopsy, endoscopy of alimentary tract and bronchi, closed thoracotomy with thoracic drainage, and provision of vascular access are frequently required. In the early stages of the disease these patients can be treated as any other patient with symptoms, signs, and laboratory results indicating that operative management is required. Later the risk is increased and the usual clinical signs of disease may be lost. Patients with AIDS may require both elective and emergency abdominal operations, but there is a five-fold higher mortality rate following emergency rather than elective procedures. The most frequent abdominal emergencies are intestinal obstruction (including volvulus), gastrointestinal haemorrhage, perforation, and peritonitis. Elective procedures are usually those carried out for diagnosis in the presence of a mass or pain, splenectomy, operation to relieve partial or intermittent bowel obstruction, cholecystectomy for the treatment of Salmonella sepsis, and cytomegalovirus infections. Wound healing is not usually a problem following abdominal operations. Fortunately, more than twice as many operations are performed electively rather than as emergency procedures. When patients are operated on in an emergency, especially late in the disease, it may be advisable to use retention sutures and not to close the skin primarily. In reality, it is necessary to return to the measures used before the advent of antibiotic medications for management of surgical complications. The variety of procedures performed in any given facility varies widely. For example, those in descending order in one group of cases with AIDS were biopsy, including cerebral stereotactic localization with biopsy or culture, endoscopy, abdominal procedure, thoracic procedure, rectal operation, and insertion of sinus windows. The use of a vena cava filter when thrombophlebitis first occurs is advocated by some clinicians.

INFECTIONS IN AIDS

Many infections in patients with AIDS are similar to those found in other types of immune suppression, such as those associated with measures used to prolong survival of grafts and following chemotherapy. The clinical conditions occurring most often are those normally combated by helper (CD4) T cells and related cell-mediated immune responses. Infecting organisms which are normally damaged or eliminated by antibody-mediated and non-specific immune mechanisms do not constitute the same problem as such potentially lethal organisms as *Pneumocystis carinii*, Toxoplasma, and Cryptococcus. Abdominal symptoms encountered are usually the result of infections with cytomegalovirus, mycobacteria, or *Salmonella typhimurium*.

Infections with cytomegalovirus may result in perforation and bleeding; in the case of cytomegalovirus enterocolitis, the appearance of the mucosal surface may be somewhat deceptive and confused with ulcerative colitis. When operation is required on such

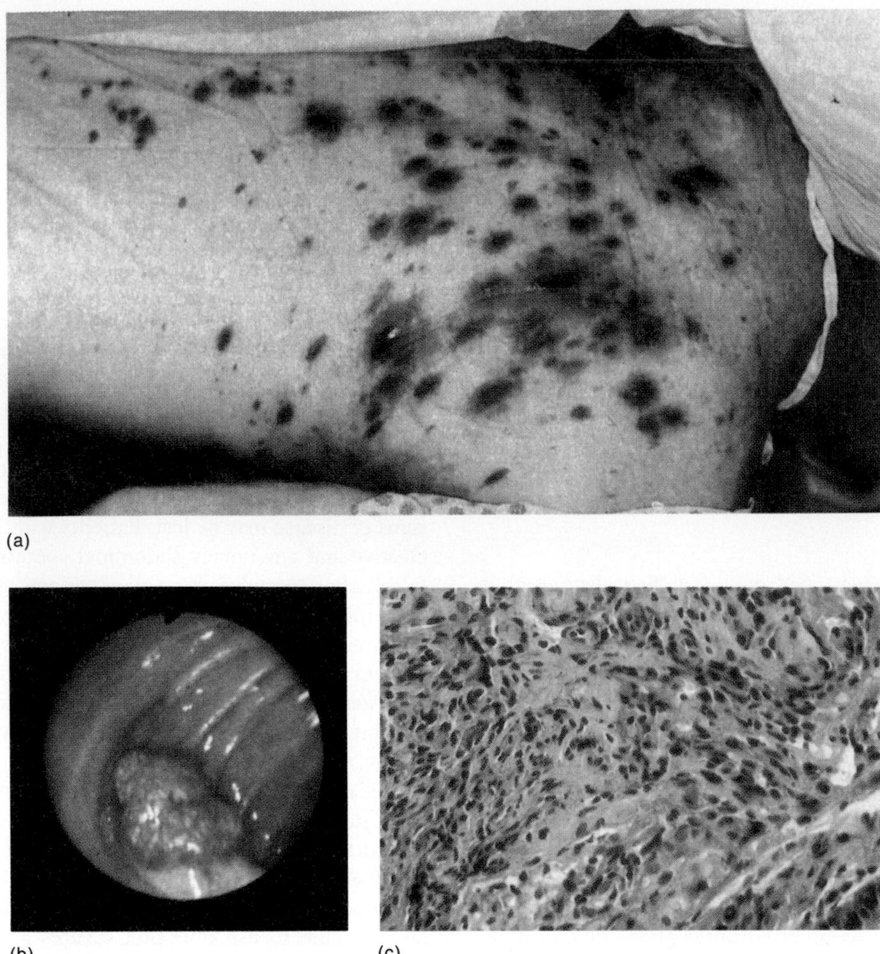

(a) (b) (c)

Fig. 1(a) Kaposi's sarcoma of the skin in a patient with AIDS. (b) Endoscopic appearance of Kaposi's sarcoma of the duodenum in a patient with AIDS. (c) Microscopic appearance of Kaposi's sarcoma of the stomach in a patient with AIDS.

bowel it is best not to reanastomose the gut since localized disease may not be apparent grossly on inspection of the mucosa. An enterostomy should be used instead. Retention sutures and allowing the skin to close by second intention should also be considered.

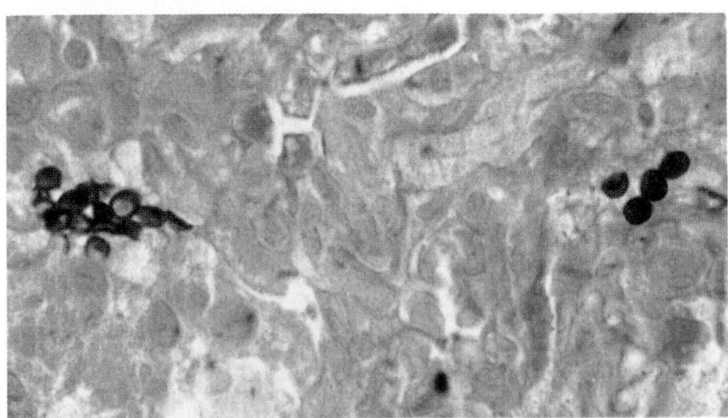

Fig. 2 Pulmonary infection with *Pneumocystis carinii* in a patient with AIDS.

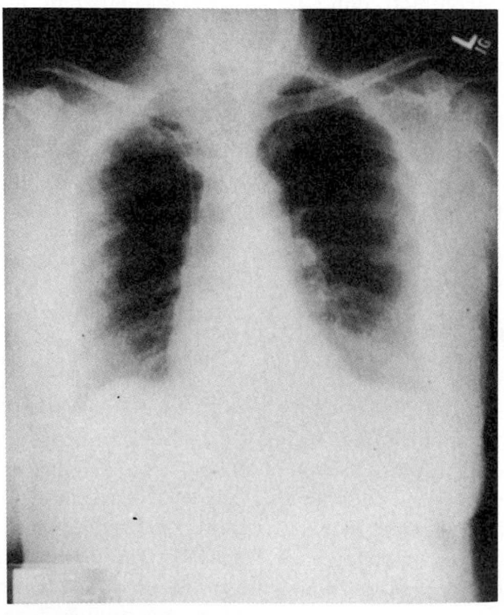

Fig. 3 Radiographic appearance of lungs infected with *Pneumocystis carinii* in a patient with AIDS.

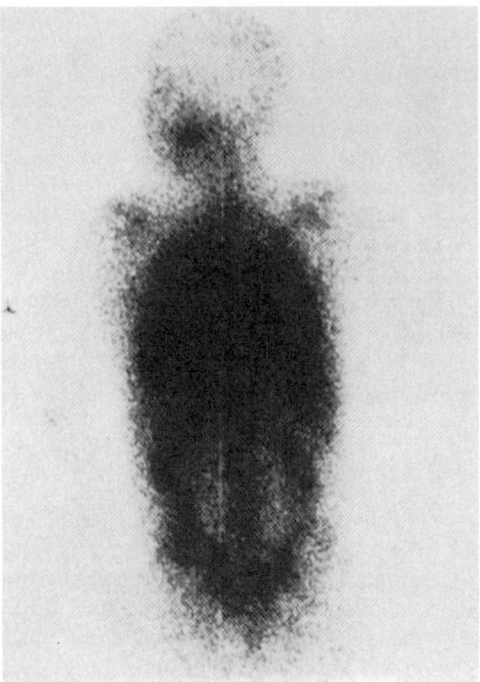

Fig. 4 Corresponding gallium scan of the same patient in Fig. 3 illustrating the more sensitive detection of the infection with *Pneumocystis carinii*.

Mycobacterium avium intracellulare is one of the most frequent of the unusual infecting organisms encountered. In the case of lymphadenopathy and other manifestations of infections with *M. avium*, diagnosis by means other than biopsy of retroperitoneal nodes can be successful in most cases and should be attempted before an operative approach is undertaken. Diagnosis may be obtained from needle biopsies of liver and bone marrow and from blood cultures. Abscess of the spleen in patients with mycobacterial infection may necessitate splenectomy which may also be indicated for treatment of thrombocytopenia. Infections with *Mycobacterium tuberculosis* and *M. kansasii* also occur in AIDS patients, but not as often as *M. avium* infections. Other abscesses, infection of the liver, and generalized peritonitis also may be the result of infection with mycobacteria. The presence of intra-abdominal infection may necessitate ileocolic resection, drainage of abscesses, and exploratory operation.

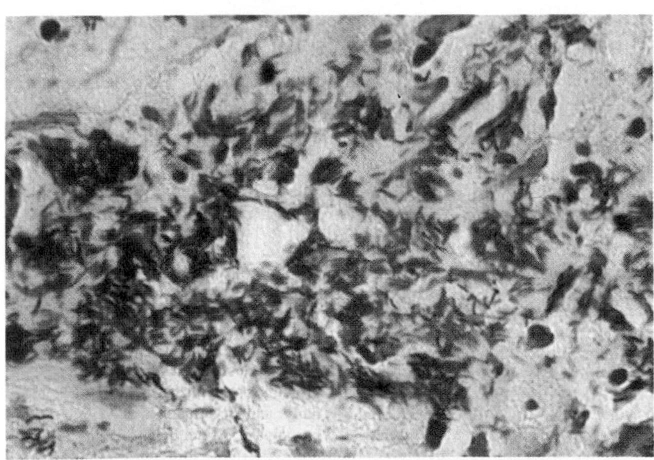

Fig. 5 The microscopic appearance of myriads of *Mycobacterium avium* in a patient with AIDS.

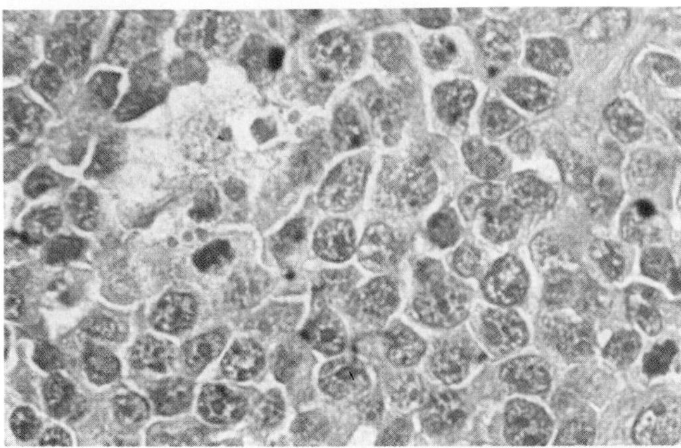

Fig. 6 Burkitt's lymphoma of the liver in a patient with AIDS.

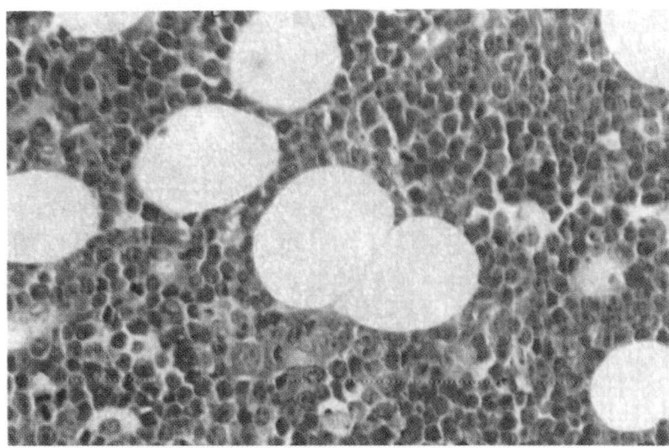

Fig. 7 Large-cell lymphoma in AIDS.

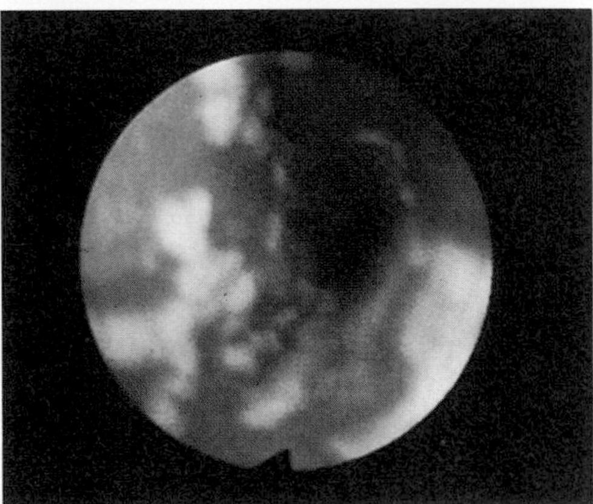

Fig. 8 Endoscopic view of cytomegalovirus infection causing ulcers of the colon in AIDS.

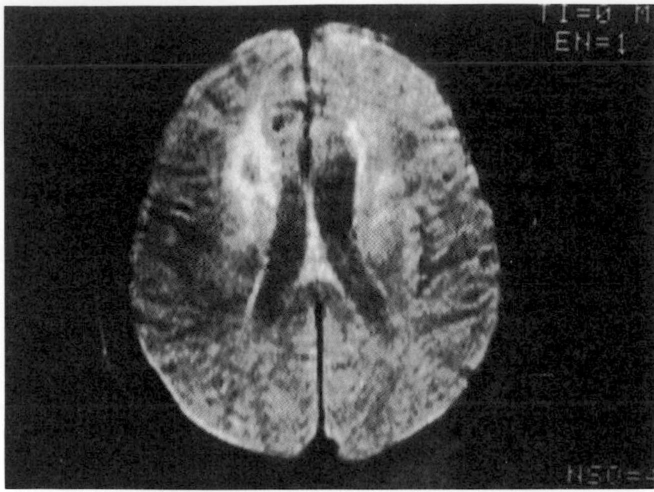

Fig. 9 Computerized cerebral tomogram showing the appearance of leucoencephalopathy in a patient with AIDS.

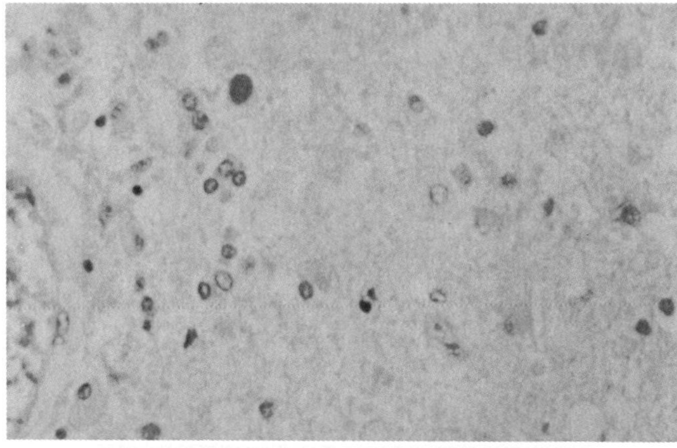

Fig. 10 Microscopic appearance of viral inclusions in the brain of a patient with AIDS.

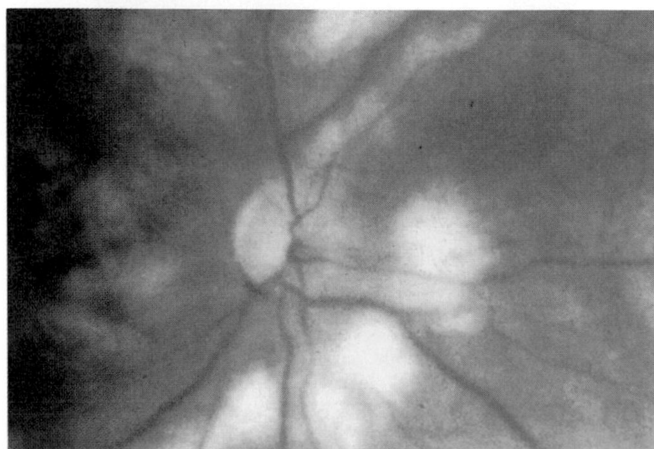

Fig. 11 Cytomegalovirus retinitis in a patient with AIDS.

Salmonella typhimurium infection may require vigorous antimicrobial therapy, and cholecystectomy may be necessary to control sepsis, particularly when gallstones are present. This organism can weaken the arterial wall, and may produce pseudoaneurysms of aorta, iliac, or femoral arteries requiring repair.

The types of infection encountered in patients with AIDS varies, depending on location and facility. For example, in one series infecting agents encountered were Candida, Pneumocystis, cytomegalovirus, Mycobacteria, herpes, hepatitis viruses, Cryptosporidium, Staphylococcus, Histoplasma, organisms causing blastomycosis and lues, and Legionella. Others not found in this study but occurring elsewhere fairly frequently include Aspergillus, Listeria, Mucor, Nocardia, Strongyloides, Toxoplasma, Salmonella, and Zygomycetes.

TUMOURS IN AIDS

The two types of tumours encountered most frequently in AIDS patients and whose complications may require surgery are non-Hodgkin's lymphomas and Kaposi's sarcoma. Other tumors such as melanoma, astrocytoma, and basal and squamous cell carcinoma may also be found. Although first described as cutaneous nodules in the lower extremities of elderly Mediterranean males, Kaposi's sarcoma can be disseminated in AIDS patients, involving any organ, including the skin, gastrointestinal tract, liver, and lungs. When present in the alimentary tract the prognosis is poor; diagnostic endoscopic biopsy may or may not give positive results because of the location of the tumour in the submucosa. The presence of Kaposi's sarcoma in the gut can lead to dysphagia, abdominal pain, haemorrhage which can be massive, perforation, a syndrome similar to toxic megacolon and ulcerative ileocolitis, malabsorption syndrome, and bowel obstruction. Non-Hodgkin's lymphoma, a high grade B-cell lymphoma, can cause gastrointestinal bleeding, obstruction, perforation, and may present as an abdominal mass. Resection of the tumours or bypassing them usually yields the desired result. Radiation and chemotherapy possibly may accelerate a fatal outcome because of the resulting increase in immunosuppression.

PULMONARY PROBLEMS IN AIDS

Neoplasms and infections of the lung occur frequently in AIDS patients; life-threatening pneumonia affects approximately two-thirds of patients with the disease. Bronchoscopic biopsy and lavage have been a successful means for diagnosing diffuse lesions, but are less so with focal disease. Pneumocystis, cytomegalovirus, fungi, and atypical mycobacteria are the most common aetiological agents. When endoscopic biopsy or washings are not appropriate or successful in making a diagnosis of Kaposi's sarcoma or lymphoma, an open lung biopsy may be necessary. In patients with pneumothorax, closure of the pulmonary defect may be indicated when closed thoracotomy and thoracic drainage tube(s) fail, but caution must be exercised in adopting this option. Removal of a tumour of the lung early in the disease has been undertaken successfully without complications, and the opportunity should not be missed because of the fear of a fatal outcome at that time. Haemoptysis from an aspergilloma can be sufficiently severe to require thoracotomy with resection since bronchial artery embolization and intracavitary amphotericin have not been very successful treatments. Bronchial lavage and biopsy has reduced the number of thoracotomies necessary for diagnosing the nature of pulmonary infections and, at times, tumours. However, pneumothorax is not an uncommon complication of a vigorous approach to pulmonary biopsy via the bronchoscope. Closed thoracotomy and insertion of one or two thoracic tubes for closed drainage is then necessary. A balloon catheter may be useful for clearing the lumen of an obstructed thoracic drainage tube. Although the use of bronchoscopy for diagnosing infections in adults has almost superseded open lung biopsy, this is not necessarily the case in infants and children. Creation of a pericardial window for drainage can be done through a subxiphoid approach perhaps even by video-assisted thoracoscopy. The wisdom of placing a patient on a respirator is often debatable, although there may be sufficient recovery to discontinue this management early in the course of AIDS. Tracheostomy is almost never indicated because of the danger of overwhelming infection and difficulty in containing the contamination.

OTHER COMPLICATIONS OF AIDS

Neurological complications of AIDS includes the presence of intracerebral masses, encephalitis, meningitis, myelitis, radiculitis, and progressive multifocal leucoencephalopathy. Symptoms, including progressive dementia, are present in 40 per cent of patients. Infections with papovavirus, Varicella-zoster virus, cytomegalovirus, and herpes simplex, and non-viral infections such as cryptococcosis and tuberculosis can occur. Stereotactic localization, biopsy, and culture of accessible sites may be indicated occasionally.

Oral lesions may include candidiasis and hairy leucoplakia. Kaposi's sarcoma and mycobacterial infections can be localized in the upper alimentary tract, and both infections and tumours may lead to bleeding, ulceration, and obstruction that can be life threatening. Cervical lymphadenopathy may be troublesome, but biopsy does not often alter clinical management. Maxillary sinus infections may require drainage.

Infections of the soft tissues usually are caused by multiple aerobic and anaerobic organisms. Bacteria other than Clostridia also produce gas in these lesions, and pentamidine ulcers may be quite troublesome to treat. Proctocolitis is the most common problem for AIDS patients in some locations. Because of depressed immune responsiveness, operations in anal and rectal areas must not be undertaken except in unusual circumstances. A minor procedure may result in an overwhelming cellulitis and may require a colostomy.

THERAPEUTIC AGENTS USEFUL IN AIDS

Much research is in progress to develop drugs effective against HIV itself and against the infections that occur in AIDS patients. Of the former zidovudine (AZT) is widely used as a treatment of AIDS and is moderately effective, while those that are used currently to treat *Pneumocystis carinii* infections are pentamidine isothionate, dapsone, co-trimoxazole, and zidovudine. Others such as clindamycin and primaquine show some promise. Alone and in combination, a battery of drugs is required to produce any therapeutic response to infections with *Mycobacterium avium*. Those used most frequently are aminoglycosides, ciprofloxacin, clofazimine, ethambutal, imipenem, isoniazid, and the rifamycins. Gancyclovir is used for retinal and gastrointestinal damage resulting from infections with cytomegalovirus. Foscarnet will be licensed soon. Initially amphotericin B was the only drug at all effective for infections with *Cryptococcus neoformans*; itraconazole and fluconazole also show some promise. Pyrimethamine and sulphadiazine are used for treating *Toxoplasma gondii* infection. The extensive and prolonged damage that herpes simplex viruses 1 and 2 can produce in AIDS patients responds to acyclovir, provided that the infecting strains are not resistant. Chemotherapy and/or irradiation for the tumours that appear in AIDS patients follows the same protocols as for patients with the same tumours who do not have AIDS. Unfortunately treatment is limited by toxic effects, some of which are similar to those caused by HIV. The spectrum of drugs and manner of combining and administering them both to treat infections and tumours in AIDS, is rapidly changing, resulting in improved palliation, but no cures are available at present.

PROTECTION OF HEALTH-CARE WORKERS FROM HIV

The chief sources of HIV infection in health-care workers have been blood and tissues, semen, vaginal secretions, or other body fluids containing blood. Pleural, peritoneal, pericardial, amniotic, synovial, and cerebrospinal fluids are also potential sources of infectious virus. Contact with oral or other mucous membranes and skin lesions of patients, droplets that are airborne, and laboratory specimens containing the virus should also be avoided. There is no evidence that the virus occurs as an aerosol from the lungs.

Routes of transmission to the surgeon and other health-care workers are via mucous membranes, transcutaneously after prolonged contact or when dermatitis or other conditions have destroyed the normal dermal barrier, and percutaneously by injuries from sharp instruments contaminated with infected blood. The risk of transfer of infectious virus by a needle puncture has been calculated as 0.4 per cent. The transfer of virus to health-care workers has occurred most frequently during manual handling and loading of needles, hand-to-hand transfer of sharp instruments, during lengthy procedures associated with blood loss, emergencies, management of trauma, and obstetric, gynaecological, orthopaedic, vascular, and cardiothoracic procedures.

Preventive measures include the identification of patients with AIDS and ARC. (When precautions are universal in suspected groups, this is not mandatory.) No surgeon or member of an operating team should participate if he or she has defects in skin and/or immune barriers. Operating gowns should prevent passage of fluids completely or an effective apron should be worn in addition to an ordinary gown. Helmet head covering and protective eye wear should also be used. Needles should be handled with instruments only, and there should be no hand-to-hand passing of sharp instruments. The use of staples and cutting cautery should be considered when feasible. During emergencies on the ward and in the emergency room and intensive care units the improper use and disposal of large-bore needles is a known source of transfer of HIV to health-care workers. The urgency of the moment should not cause the usual precautions to be abandoned. Double gloving is advisable in the operating room, and gloves should always be used when dressing wounds or examining orifices and when handling contaminated materials. Gloves should be discarded in an appropriate container immediately after use.

After a procedure has been completed and gloves removed, the hands must be washed thoroughly. If there has been contamination of broken skin or injury with sharp instrument or needle the area should be cleansed thoroughly but application of caustic material to the site is not recommended. Evidence for the effectiveness of immediate initiation of therapy with the antiretroviral agent, zidovudine (AZT), which inhibits the production of provirus, is incomplete. The person affected should be tested for HIV antibody at the time and periodically over the following 6 months, and should refrain from transmitting blood, semen, and milk or donating an organ to others for at least 12 weeks.

The usual measures for sterilizing instruments and customary cleaning of the operating room are adequate. Cleaners should wear protective gloves, gown, helmet head covering and eye wear or shield. Discarded needles should not be bent or replaced in an individual container. Both needles and disposable blades should be discarded in a puncture-proof, sealed container. A reliable system of transfer of specimens either to the laboratory or to a site of disposal should be adopted so that no specimen or other item contaminated with infected body fluids, blood, or tissue is lost or arrives in the laboratory without the nature of the material being known to the receptionist. When ventilation of the patient is necessary, disposable equipment should be available and mouth-to-mouth resuscitation should never be attempted.

Much has been published about the rights of the patient with AIDS for treatment and the rights of health-care personnel when managing their treatment. Knowledge of the methods of transmission and the dangers of infection with HIV virus and adoption of the precautions suggested while caring for these patients should reduce the danger of contracting AIDS sufficiently to remove most objections about risks of exposure and provide adequate numbers of personnel willing to provide the therapy required.

SUMMARY

The surgeon has a role to play in the clinical management and diagnosis of the protean manifestations of AIDS. Familiarity with its unusual features is required to ensure appropriate and effective management of complications requiring attention in a manner that avoids risk to the surgical team.

A wide range of unusual infections with clinical manifestations and the appearance of non-Hodgkin's lymphomas and Kaposi's sarcoma at multiple sites in patients with AIDS are problems encountered with increasing frequency by the surgeon. To make diagnosis and management more difficult, warning clinical signs often are effaced late in the disease because of deranged immune responses.

Biopsy, endoscopy, procedures to provide vascular access, and closed thoracotomy drainage are frequently required in the management of AIDS.

Exploration of the abdomen for relief of obstruction, drainage of abscesses, biopsy and resection of tumours, splenectomy, cholecystectomy, appendectomy, and colostomy and ileostomy may be required in the care of patients with AIDS. Emergency abdominal procedures have a much poorer prognosis than elective operations and often require deviation from usual modes of treatment. Anal and perineal procedures should not be undertaken except in exceptional circumstances. Tracheostomy is almost never advisable. Thoracotomy can be performed successfully in selected patients. Intubation requires careful evaluation of indications before initiating the use of a respirator in selected cases.

Operations should not be undertaken by those with defective dermal and immune barriers. Appropriate protective gowns, eye wear, and double gloves should always be used when any procedure is done at any location, and no manual handling of needles or hand-to-hand passage of sharp instruments is permissible. Exposure to the AIDS virus requires immediate cleansing of the site and subsequent testing for HIV, but the usefulness of immediate administration of zidovudine or other therapy is unknown.

FURTHER READING

Bell DM, Shapiro CN, Holmberg SD. HIV and the surgical team. *Bull Am Coll Surg* 1990; **75**: 7–15.

Burdette W.J. The role of the surgeon in the management of AIDS. *Surg Rounds* 1988; **11**: 22–37.

Centers for Disease control. HIV/AIDS Surveillance. *US Dept Health Human Serv Rep* 1992; **October**: 1–18.

Centers for Disease Control. Recommendations for preventing transmission of infection with human T-lymphotropic virus type III/lymphadenopathy-associated virus during invasive procedures. *MMWR* 1986; **35**: 21–3.

Dupont JR, Bonavita JA, DiGiovanni RJ, Spector HB, Nelson SC Acquired immunodeficiency syndrome and mycotic abdominal aortic aneurysms: a new challenge? Report of a case. *J Vasc Surg* 1989; **10**: 254–7.

Kaiser LR, Hiatt JR. Surgical considerations in the management of the immunocompromised patient. *Crit Care Clin* 1988; **4**: 193–208.

Kleinhaus S, Weinberg G, Sheran M, Boley SJ. The management of surgery in infants and children with the acquired immune deficiency syndrome. *J Pediatr Surg* 1985; **20**: 497–8.

Lipsett P, Allo MD. AIDS and the surgeon. *Surg Clin N Am* 1988; **68**: 73–88.

Mathew A, Raviglione MC, Niranjan U, Sabatini MT, Distenfeld A. Splenectomy in patients with AIDS. *Am J Hematol* 1989; **32**: 184–9.

Myer A. A. The surgical management of AIDS and HIV-infected patients. *Adv Surg* 1989; **22**: 57–73.

Miller JI. The thoracic surgical spectrum of acquired immune deficiency syndrome. *J Thoracic Cardiovasc Surg* 1989; **92**: 977–80.

Mills J, Massur H. AIDS-related infections. *Sci Am* 1990; **263**: 50–7.

Velley JF, Lefevre P, Curtet M, Couraud L. 2 cases of pulmonary excision in patients with acquired immunodeficiency syndrome. What is the role of surgery in AIDS? *Ann Chir* 1989; **43**: 143–6.

Wilson SE, *et al.* Acquired immune deficiency syndrome (AIDS). Indications for abdominal surgery, pathology, and outcome. *Ann Surg* 1989; **210**: 428–33.

Anaesthesia and the operating room 3

3.1 Anaesthesia for surgeons

JOHN W. SEAR AND FRED ROSEWARNE

INTRODUCTION

Contemporary surgical practice has developed in parallel with advances in the preoperative assessment and perioperative management of patients with increasingly complex underlying medical problems. In this chapter, we will consider some of these medical problems as well as briefly discussing current anaesthetic practice and postoperative care.

PREOPERATIVE ASSESSMENT

The assessment of the patient with coexisting medical disease is covered in detail elsewhere.

Cardiovascular system

Ischaemic heart disease

Clinical history includes determination of the presence of angina (either on exercise or at rest) and whether the patient has suffered known myocardial infarction in the past. Evaluation of exercise tolerance may be important in a patient with angina who is undergoing major surgery and who may be subjected to stress factors such as large fluid shifts or aortic cross clamping. The resting ECG is often normal in patients with ischaemic heart disease, but may show evidence of previous infarction (presence of Q waves, T wave inversion, or persistent ST segment elevation suggesting a ventricular aneurysm). This is significant, as the myocardial tissue will often be contracting either hypo- or akinetically, and the poor contractility be further depressed by the effects of most volatile anaesthetic agents (see below). Further tests to evaluate left ventricular function include either multiple gated acquisition (MUGA) or thallium scanning, and the predictive value of these in the preoperative assessment of the patient undergoing major vascular surgery is discussed elsewhere (Chapter 5.2).

In patients with known clinical or ECG evidence of previous myocardial infarction, the risk of reinfarction is increased by the combined effects of anaesthesia and surgery in the early post-infarct period. However, the risk falls to that seen in comparable patients not undergoing surgery by 6 months, and hence, elective surgery should be postponed for this period of time.

Care should be taken to maintain optimum drug therapy in the patient with ischaemic heart disease, who may be receiving β-adrenoceptor blocking drugs, calcium channel blockers, nitrates, or diuretics. Since abrupt cessation of therapy may worsen pre-existing angina, all medication should be continued up to the time that preoperative drugs are given. Patients with angina at rest may require additional perioperative medication, including transdermal or intravenously administered nitrates.

Postoperatively, the effects of abdominal surgery may decrease the gastrointestinal absorption of orally administered drugs, and medication must be provided by other routes, such as intravenous infusions, sublinguinal or intranasal calcium channel antagonists, and sustained release preparations of nitrates and β-adrenoceptor antagonists.

Laboratory testing must include assessment of plasma electrolytes and haemoglobin, the electrocardiogram, and chest radiograph. Other tests may be indicated by the presence of coexisting or predisposing factors, such as diabetes mellitus or hypertension.

Hypertension

A similar strategy is useful in the assessment of patients with hypertension, in whom adequacy of medication and the presence or absence of the end-organ manifestations of hypertension (hypertensive heart disease with left ventricular hypertrophy and myocardial ischaemia, hypertensive nephropathy and retinopathy, cerebrovascular disease manifest as strokes or transient ischaemic episodes) should be evaluated. Current drugs used in the treatment of hypertension include β-adrenoceptor and calcium channel blockers, angiotensin converting enzyme inhibitors and other vasodilators. As in the patient with myocardial ischaemia, abrupt cessation of treatment may lead to rebound of symptoms and severe hypertensive episodes; this is especially important in hypertensive patients treated with the α_2- agonist, clonidine. Drug treatment may be withheld if the patient exhibits preoperative orthostatic hypotension, if there is inadequate time available for optimization of drug therapy or there is an urgent need for the surgery to proceed.

The surgeon (and anaesthetist) is often faced with an untreated hypertensive patient presenting for elective surgery, and it is therefore important to have a strategy in deciding whether surgery is cancelled or allowed to proceed. Based on the WHO definition of hypertension (systolic pressure above 160 mmHg or diastolic pressure above 95 mmHg), we can recognize four groups of patients: those with diastolic pressure less than 110 mmHg but more than 95 mmHg on at least three occasions following admission; those with diastolic pressure above 110 mmHg but less than 120 mmHg on at least three occasions following admission; those with diastolic pressure over 120 mmHg on at least three occasions following admission and those in whom diastolic pressures are normal, but systolic pressures are elevated (often 200–250 mmHg).

There is little evidence of increased cardiovascular risk associated with anaesthesia in the first group of patients, and the anaesthetist is safe to proceed in the absence of end-organ damage. Other recent approaches to the management of mild hypertension include the prescribing of a single dose of a β-adrenoceptor blocking drug as part of premedication, or the administration of preoperative clonidine.

In patients with a diastolic blood pressure of 110 to 120 mmHg, but no evidence of end-organ disease, there is a need to balance the urgency of the surgery against the potential risks associated with anaesthesia. These patients should be carefully monitored before, during and after surgery, and active management of blood

We are grateful to Dr J. W. Mackenzie for his contribution to the section on postoperative pain relief.

pressure should be undertaken. If end-organ disease is present the operation should be cancelled, and appropriate treatment instituted.

Anaesthetists and physicians agree that individuals with a diastolic pressure of over 120 mmHg should have their elective surgery postponed, while appropriate measures are taken to control the blood pressure. Although patients with a systolic arterial pressure of above 160 mmHg are defined as hypertensive, they are usually suffering not from hypertension but from arteriosclerosis. Whether any reduction in the perfusion pressure may lead to organ underperfusion, with resulting ischaemia and dysfunction of the heart, kidneys or brain, is debated.

When treatment prior to surgery is thought to be appropriate, the operation should be postponed for 4 to 6 weeks to allow optimization of therapy and resetting of the autoregulatory mechanisms of the body. Uncontrolled hypertension and tachycardia in the postoperative period require active and aggressive treatment: both increased blood pressure and tachycardia may cause an imbalance of coronary supply and demand, with the development of myocardial ischaemia.

Congestive cardiac failure

General and regional anaesthesia are both contraindicated in the presence of acute heart failure. The combination of congestive cardiac failure with general anaesthesia will result in cardiac muscle depression and pronounced hypokinesia; regional techniques such as extradural and intrathecal blocks may lead to decreased systemic vascular resistance, with significant decreases in blood pressure because of venous pooling. The reduction in systemic vascular resistance may also lead to an increased cardiac output.

Whatever anaesthetic approach is used, intraoperative inotropic support with drugs such as dopamine, dobutamine or dopexamine may be required. Any significant increase in systemic vascular resistance caused by these agents may, however, lead to further reductions in stroke volume.

Clinical and radiological evidence of left ventricular failure in patients with ischaemic heart disease is linked with a poor clinical prognosis. Patients with congestive cardiac failure should undergo plasma urea and electrolyte monitoring before surgery. Patients receiving cardiac glycosides, and presenting with arrhythmias may have digitalis toxicity: digitalis levels should be checked.

The anaesthetist may be asked to provide sedation or analgesia for patients with chronic congestive cardiac failure undergoing endoscopic procedures such as cystoscopy and colonoscopy. Unfortunately, these procedures are frequently performed in areas with poor lighting, with reduced assistance for the anaesthetist and little monitoring equipment. If these procedures cannot be undertaken under light sedation with supplemental oxygen therapy, a full relaxant general anaesthetic with rapid sequence induction will need to be performed. Patients undergoing gastroscopy for acute indications often have significant quantities of blood in their stomachs, and are at risk of aspiration. Optimal monitoring should be available for these highly unstable patients.

Valvular heart disease

Mitral valve disease

The natural history of mitral valve disease is one of progressive impairment of myocardial function over a long period of time. Important factors in preoperative assessment are a history of, or the presence of left ventricular failure and atrial fibrillation, which carries the risk of systemic embolism to the brain or legs. With time, changes occur in left atrial function leading to increases in pulmonary vascular pressures, with reduced pulmonary compliance and increased work of respiration.

Anaesthetists should be aware of the importance of avoiding bradycardia, which, in the presence of relatively fixed stroke volume, will decrease cardiac output, and increase tachycardia; hence, decrease will diastolic filling time and further increase left atrial pressure, and hypovolaemia.

Aortic valve disease

The natural history of aortic valve disease is shorter, in terms of symptomatology, than that of mitral valve disease. There is progressive hypertrophy of the left ventricular muscle, leading to left ventricular failure. The main symptoms are angina, syncope (Stokes–Adams attacks), and dyspnoea of effort; as left ventricular failure develops, orthopnoea, paroxysmal nocturnal dyspnoea, and congestive cardiac failure become apparent.

Anaesthesia in these patients should therefore avoid reductions in systemic vascular resistance. In aortic stenosis, this decreases coronary perfusion and may lead to falls in cardiac output. Conversely, any increase in systemic vascular resistance in patients with aortic regurgitation will further reduce forward blood flow. Bradycardia which, again, will lead to decreased cardiac output because of the relatively fixed stroke volume, should also be avoided, as should tachycardias, arrhythmias, and myocardial depression, which may occur with the use of volatile anaesthetic agents.

Patients with valvular heart disease present several important problems to the surgeon and the anaesthetist. Appropriate antibiotic prophylaxis against bacterial endocarditis should be provided. Drugs of choice include ampicillin or amoxycillin (or erythromycin in the penicillin-sensitive patient). These should be given prior to induction of anaesthesia, laryngoscopy and intubation to ensure peak drug concentrations at the time of any instrumentation of the oral cavity. Gentamicin should be added in patients scheduled for gastrointestinal or genitourinary surgery and instrumentation. The use of anticoagulants needs to be controlled in patients with prosthetic valves, and in those with atrial fibrillation and a history of systemic emboli (see later). The relatively fixed cardiac output means that techniques and procedures involving significant fluid shifts are especially hazardous.

Arrhythmias

A number of arrhythmias may be detected on ECG monitoring undertaken as part of the preoperative assessment of the elective general surgical patient.

If atrial fibrillation is present the ventricular rate should be controlled to about 100 beats/min or less, and there should be a ventriculo-radial deficit of less than 20 beats. Atrial flutter should be treated prior to surgery, with digoxin or amiodarone, or by cardioversion. Ventricular tachycardias and ventricular ectopics which are either multifocal or are occurring more frequently than 1 in 5 beats should be treated preoperatively. The anaesthetist and surgeon must consider the need for preoperative insertion of a temporary (or permanent) pacing wire in patients with any type of heart block. A permanent artificial cardiac pacemaker should be inserted when the patient has complete (third degree) heart block, the sick sinus syndrome or symptomatic bradycardia (rate less than 35 beats/min). Temporary pacing should be instituted for patients with any symptomatic heart block, Mobitz type II block, or right bundle branch block and left axis deviation on the ECG, indicative of bifascicular block involving the left anterior fascicle of the left bundle, and sick sinus syndrome.

Respiratory system

All general anaesthetic agents are respiratory depressants, both in terms of the responses to hypoxia and to hypercapnia. In addition, anaesthetized patients who are breathing spontaneously show loss of the intercostal component of ventilation. During anaesthesia, both spontaneous ventilation and intermittent positive pressure ventilation result in a reduction in functional residual capacity of approximately 400 ml. This may be compounded by a similar reduction occurring on adopting the supine posture, as well as by the effects of obesity, upper abdominal surgery and crystalloid infusion. Thus, the functional residual capacity decreases towards the closing volume (that volume at which there is significant basal airway closure). The closing volume also increases markedly with age, obesity, smoking, and crystalloid infusion, with the result that airway closure occurs during anaesthesia and surgery, increasing the alveolar–arterial $P\text{O}_2$ difference.

Anaesthesia is also associated with a redistribution of ventilation away from dependent lung areas, while there is little change in perfusion. This mismatching of ventilation and perfusion results in a 'true shunt' developing. Matching of perfusion to ventilation requires an intact pulmonary vascular response to hypercarbia, acidosis and hypoxia (hypoxic pulmonary vasoconstriction). Most volatile anaesthetic agents inhibit the hypoxic pulmonary vasoconstriction reflex, while it is preserved with the intravenous agents. During general anaesthesia there is, therefore, a need to increase the inspired oxygen concentration to maintain a normal arterial $P\text{aO}_2$.

Physiological dead space is also increased (by up to 50 per cent) during intermittent positive pressure ventilation as a result of ventilation of underperfused or non-perfused alveoli. Thus, this will increase the $P\text{aCO}_2$ and so compound the effect of general anaesthetics as respiratory depressants.

These physiological changes which occur during anaesthesia and surgery also allow several groups of patients who are at risk of developing postoperative pulmonary complications to be identified. In cigarette smokers, hypersecretion of mucus and an increased closing volume will predispose to basal air trapping, leading to possible atelectasis and pneumonia. Obesity is associated with a decreased total pulmonary compliance, with an increased work of breathing, leading to early postoperative respiratory fatigue, in addition to changes in lung volume. This is particularly important in patients undergoing upper abdominal or thoracic surgery. Malnourished patients have a poor energy reserve, again predisposing to respiratory fatigue, while in the elderly lung volumes and altered sensitivity to anaesthetic agents and to opioids is increased. Patients with pre-existing lung disease are an obvious high-risk group. All of the above risk factors are further complicated by surgical problems which may influence postoperative lung function. These include surgery lasting more than 4 h; type of surgical incision; transverse incisions are associated with less disturbance of pulmonary function than midline incisions; and bowel distension, which decreases pulmonary function, particularly if an upper abdominal incision is used.

Clinical features of lung disease, relevant to preoperative assessment

Symptoms which must be assessed include dyspnoea, cough, sputum production, haemoptysis, chest pain, and wheeze. Factors contributing to these symptoms include a history of smoking or occupational exposure to dust, and associated cardiovascular pathology (ischaemic heart disease, cardiac failure, hypertension, cor pulmonale).

Examination should concentrate on evidence of obstructive airway disease, evidence of poor respiratory expansion, including kyphoscoliosis and neuromuscular weakness due to myasthenia gravis or a myopathy, evidence of increased work of breathing manifested by increased respiratory and heart rates, tracheal tug, use of accessory muscles and intercostal indrawing, nature and quantity of sputum, evidence of an active chest infection, and evidence of respiratory failure or right heart failure with cor pulmonale, both of which are poor prognostic indicators in patients requiring elective general surgery.

Chronic obstructive airway disease

Excessive mucus secretion is coupled with a variable degree of airway obstruction due to both bronchial oedema and retained secretions. In some patients, the disease progresses to hypoxia, hypercapnia and right ventricular failure. These patients show a loss of ventilatory sensitivity to CO_2, and depend on their hypoxic ventilatory drive. Other patients develop emphysema associated with lung overdistension, alveolar parenchymal destruction, loss of elastic pulmonary compliance, and airway obstruction. These patients have an increased physiological dead space, and hyperventilate to maintain normocapnia.

For both groups, assessment should address normal exercise tolerance, previous response to surgery and response to bronchodilator therapy. Excessive sputum should be removed by physiotherapy and postural drainage, and infection should be treated with antibiotics.

The presence of a reversible element to the obstructive airways disease, which may be sensitive to bronchodilator drugs, should be assessed, and preoperative blood gases analysed in those patients who may require ventilatory support in the immediate postoperative period.

Preoperative investigations include spirometry and measurement of arterial blood gases (see Section 3.4). The ratio between the forced expiratory volume in 1 second (FEV_1) and forced vital capacity (FVC) should be above 0.7; and the FEV_1 should be more than 1 litre. Patients with an FEV_1/FVC of less than 0.5; and an FEV_1 less than 1 litre have an increased risk of postoperative morbidity. However, recent studies have shown that patients with FEV_1 values between 0.3 and 1 litre need have little extra morbidity. The best preoperative predictors of the need for postoperative ventilation are preoperative $P\text{aO}_2$ and presence of dyspnoea at rest.

Asthma

Preoperative assessment should elicit the frequency and severity of asthma attacks, factors provoking attacks, drug history, and whether the patient has ever required ventilatory support. Elective surgery should not be undertaken unless the asthma is well controlled, with peak flow values above 250 to 300 l/min, and minimal or no diurnal 'dips' in peak flow. In patients with a marked seasonal fluctuation in symptoms, it is better not to undertake elective surgery during the poor season. For the severe asthmatic with intractable airway obstruction, especially those already on inhaled steroid therapy, a short course of systemic steroids (prednisolone 40–80 mg/day, reducing) may be useful. Where feasible, regional anaesthetic techniques should be employed. Where this is not possible general anaesthesia may be undertaken using a minimal intervention regimen or 'balanced anaesthesia. In the first approach spontaneous ventilation is supplemented, where appropriate, by regional anaesthetic techniques. Opioid analgesia and sedation are kept to a minimum. The aims are to avoid stimulating an irritable tracheobronchial tree and to minimize respiratory depression. Alternatively, asthmatics are managed using standard 'balanced anaesthesia' with a few modifications. The patient receives preoperative physiotherapy and inhaled salbutamol prior to going to theatre. The induction dose is higher than usual to avoid irritation of the trachea during intubation. Histamine releasing drugs such as *d*-tubocurarine, atracurium, and morphine are avoided.

Chronic infections

Bronchiectasis is characterized by the overproduction of purulent sputum from disorganized and dilated bronchi. Causes in the older adult population include whooping cough, measles or tuberculosis. There may be some degree of airway obstruction, often poorly responsive to bronchodilator therapy. Patients should be admitted at least 3 days prior to surgery for postural drainage, physiotherapy, and treatment with antibiotics. Where appropriate regional anaesthesia is safest; if it is not possible patients should be intubated to allow for controlled ventilation and clearance of secretions. Endobronchial anaesthesia may prevent soiling of non-infected lung by the infected side. Postoperative care is important, and the recent introduction of the mini-tracheostomy tube has assisted the clearance of secretions in these patients where effective coughing is limited by pain from the operative site.

General anaesthesia is not contraindicated in younger children with cystic fibrosis, but care should be given to timing, such that surgery is undertaken at the optimum time of the child's well being. Early discharge prevents or reduces the risk of pulmonary colonization by hospital-acquired organisms.

Influence of intercurrent therapy on anaesthesia and surgery

Steroid therapy

The normal response of the adrenal cortex to stress and trauma (including surgery and anaesthesia) is described elsewhere. In the patient receiving either steroid or adrenocorticotrophin therapy for the treatment of systemic diseases, failure to supplement the normal daily dose of enteral steroids may result in acute adrenocortical insufficiency. Preoperative stimulation tests will identify those patients unable to mount a response due to exogenous steroid suppression of native adrenocortical synthesis. In these individuals, maintenance therapy must be supplemented with additional doses of hydrocortisone. Regimens which have been advocated include 100 mg IV at induction of anaesthesia, followed by 100 mg every 6 hours for 3 days, and 25 mg IV hydrocortisone at induction, followed by 100 mg every 24 h. Alternatively, the normal daily steroid dose of all patients can be supplemented with hydrocortisone, the dose depending on the nature of the surgery. For minor procedures, a single dose of 100 mg IV hydrocortisone at induction is the sole supplement: an additional 100 mg 12 h later is advisable in those undergoing major surgery.

Serum urea and electrolytes levels and blood glucose should be monitored before surgery, and fluid balance should be carefully checked. Adrenal insufficiency in the postsurgical patient may be manifest as true collapse, or as malaise, lethargy, muscle weakness, and postural hypotension. Treatment should be by fluid infusion of colloid and crystalloid. These patients are often resistant to inotropes and large doses of steroids may be necessary.

Other medical problems

Diabetes

Between 2 and 2.5 per cent of the population are known to be diabetic and there may be an equal number of undiagnosed diabetic patients. Diabetics affects about one in six patients over the age of 65 years, and one in four over the age of 85 years.

The perioperative mortality of diabetic patients varies between 4 and 13 per cent; most deaths result from the diseases associated with diabetes, including atherosclerosis, nephropathy, hypertension and ischaemic heart disease, and infection. In addition, a high proportion of patients suffer from autonomic and peripheral neuropathies, which may lead to postural hypotension or sudden cardiac arrest. Myopathy with muscle weakness may result in excessive increases in the plasma potassium concentration following the administration of suxamethonium. It has been estimated that 63 per cent of diabetic patients have symptoms or signs of cardiovascular disease, 44 per cent have peripheral vascular disease, and 24 per cent suffer from cerebrovascular disease.

Hyperglycaemia may result from a deficiency of insulin, insulin resistance and accelerated hepatic glucose production due to increased glucagon (non-insulin-dependent diabetes mellitus , type II), or from a lack of insulin (insulin-dependent diabetes mellitus,—type I). Ninety per cent of diabetic patients have type I disease: they are often obese and have normal or elevated plasma insulin levels. These patients are not prone to ketosis, but they may develop non-ketotic hyperosmolar coma. The insulin-dependent patient often has an abrupt onset of polyuria, polydipsia, weight loss, and fatigue.

The diagnosis of diabetes is made on the basis of a fasting venous blood glucose level above 140 mg/dl (7.8 mmol/1), and an abnormal glucose tolerance test: blood glucose concentration in excess of 200 mg/dl (11.0 mmol/1) 2 h after ingestion of 75 g of glucose.

Treatment of diabetes

Patients maintained by dietary treatment alone require no special medication before surgery, although some patients may need insulin therapy at least transiently during the postoperative period.

The oral hypoglycaemic agents in common usage are the sulphonylureas and biguanides. The former group (tolbutamide, chlorpropamide, glibenclamide, and glipizide) enhance insulin secretion by the pancreas, probably by increasing cyclic AMP levels in the β-cells. The pharmacological characteristics of these drugs are shown in Table 1. Because of the longer duration of action of chlorpropamide, the drug should ideally be stopped 24 to 36 h before surgery. The side effects of sulphonylurea therapy include hypoglycaemia, cholestatic jaundice, rashes, agranulocytosis, goitre, and inappropriate ADH secretion.

The mechanism of action of the biguanides, such as phenformin and metformin, is ill defined, but they appear to increase peripheral extrasplanchnic glucose utilization by a shift from oxidative to anaerobic metabolism. As such, they have been associated with the development of lactic acidosis.

Insulin has a number of different physiological effects. As well as its major effect of increasing peripheral uptake and utilization of glucose, and reducing glycogenolysis, it also decreases gluconeogenesis, increases formation of protein from amino acids, and increases synthesis of glycogen. Present day insulin preparations may be derived from bovine or porcine, or human sources; the former may be allergenic, leading to the development of tolerance.

Table 1 Oral hypoglycaemic agents. Normal daily dosages, duration of effect, elimination half-life, protein binding, and main site of metabolism for commonly used orally hypoglycaemic agents

	Dose/day (mg)	Duration (h)	Half-life (h)	Protein binding	Main site of metabolism
Tolbutamide	500–1000	6–10	4–10	96	Hepatic
Chlorpropamide	100–500	20–60	24–42	95	Renal (hepatic)
Glipizide	5–40	6–12	3–7	95	Hepatic
Glibenclamide	2.5–30	10–15	10–16	99	Hepatic

Insulin preparations vary in their times to onset, peak and duration of action; as well as in their origin. Short-acting preparations are soluble, while the longer acting insulins are formulated either as a zinc suspension, or as a suspension with protamine sulphate (isophanes) (Table 2).

Preoperative management

The signs and symptoms of diabetes should be assessed as should any associated pathology which may be present. Laboratory tests should include a full electrolyte, urea, and creatinine screen, blood count with white cell differential, chest radiograph, and ECG (Table 3). Many patients will be receiving other coincidental therapy, which should be optimized before surgery (e.g. β-adrenoceptor blocking drugs, calcium channel inhibitors, angiotensin converting enzyme inhibitors, other antihypertensive agents, digitalis).

Plasma and whole body potassium levels may be decreased in patients with uncontrolled diabetes, and additional supplementation needs to be given before surgery. Diabetic autonomic neuropathy is manifest in its earliest stage as a lack of variation of the cardiac rate, with a tendency to higher than average resting heart rates. Other features include postural hypotension, and intraoperative episodes of bradycardia and hypotension occurring unexpectedly without apparent precipitating causes. A cardiac autonomic neuropathy is present in between 20 and 40 per cent of all diabetics and is associated with a poor prognosis.

Effect of anaesthetic agents on blood glucose level

Plasma glucose concentrations are generally unaffected by anaesthesia, but rise during surgery, the extent of the increase depending upon the applied surgical stimulus. Extradural anaesthesia reduces the glycaemic response. Ether is the only volatile anaesthetic agent which has a significant effect in increasing the plasma glucose concentration, although thiopentone may also have an effect on the plasma glucose concentration by action on hepatic phosphorylase. Hyperglycaemia is the result of a synergistic interaction between three hormones: adrenaline, glucagon, and insulin. Adrenaline increases plasma glucose concentration by inhibiting insulin secretion, stimulating hepatic glycogenolysis, and reducing tissue sensitivity to insulin. Glucagon acts primarily to increase glucose production, but also increases glucose utilization. Increased plasma cortisol enhances the duration of the additive effects of adrenaline and glucagon.

Perioperative management

Although the major hazard in the diabetic patient is hypoglycaemia, it is now recognized that acute hyperglycaemia during surgery may result in altered host defence mechanisms, extracellular dehydration and electrolyte imbalance, intracellular dehydration, and impaired wound healing. The blood glucose level is best maintained in the range 4 to 8 mmol/1, with 6 mmol/1 being optimal. There is now much evidence linking chronic hyper-

Table 2 Insulin preparations. Types of insulin preparation used in man, with indication of their times to onset of effect, time of peak effect, and duration of effect

	Source	Onset (h)	Peak (h)	Duration (h)
Short acting*				
Soluble and neutral	B	0.25	2–5	5–8
Human Actrapid	H hp	0.5	2–5	8
Humulin S	H hp	0.5	1–3	7
Intermediate acting				
Semilente	B hp	1–2	3–8	10–20
Isophane	B,P,H	2–3	6–14	18–28
Humulin I	H hp	1	2–8	20
Mixtard	P hp	1	2–8	24
Long acting				
Human Monotard	H hp	2	7–15	22
Ultralente and PZI	4–5	12–24	24–36	
Biphasic				
Suspension: RAPITARD P hp				
Isophane:				
MIXTARD P hp				
HUMAN MIXTARD H				
HUMULIN M1 to M4 H hp				

B = bovine; H = human; P = porcine; hp = highly purified.

* Intravenously administered soluble or human insulins have a short half-life (5 to 10 min), and a duration of effect less than 30 min. These properties may be useful in the acute management of perioperative hyperglycaemia.

Table 3 Aspects of the management of the surgical diabetic patient

Optimization of blood glucose control
Patients treated by diet alone
Patients on oral hypoglycaemic drugs
Patients maintained on insulin
Assessment of other pathology present
Cardiovascular system
Renal
Retinopathy
Neuropathies: peripheral and autonomic
Infections: local or systemic

glycaemia with the end-organ pathology responsible for the long-term complications of diabetes.

Elective surgery in non-insulin-dependent diabetics

Most non-insulin-dependent diabetics secrete sufficient endogenous insulin to carry them through minor surgery (that not involving penetration of a body cavity or transection of a major limb bone) and do not need transient insulin therapy provided that glucose-containing solutions are withheld. When major surgery is undertaken exogenous insulin will usually be needed to prevent the development of ketosis. In all patients, oral hypoglycaemic agents should be discontinued before surgery and recommenced whenever possible the next day.

Elective surgery in the insulin-dependent patient

Various management regimens for the insulin-dependent patient have been suggested. These include a 'laissez-faire' minimal intervention approach, the 'split-normal-dose' regimen where the patient receives 25 to 50 per cent of the usual morning dose of insulin plus 5 per cent dextrose solution at a rate between 100 and 200 ml/h, regular administration of low-dose IV insulin or an infusion of insulin with the simultaneous infusion of 5 per cent dextrose (with adjustment of the rates of infusion of the insulin and/or glucose based on frequent blood glucose estimates), and an intensive glucose–insulin–potassium regimen. When monitoring these methods of diabetic control, blood glucose determinations are preferable to urine glucose analysis, since anaesthesia and surgery change the renal threshold to glucose excretion. An alternative approach is the administration of a long-acting insulin preparation the evening before surgery to achieve basal normoglycaemia, followed by IV insulin alone in doses (based on weight, height and blood glucose level) sufficient to maintain the peroperative plasma glucose level at between 4 and 8 mmol/1.

Fluid replacement should be given as normal saline solution (0.154 M). Higher blood glucose levels (and therefore higher insulin requirements) are found in patients receiving either 5 per cent dextrose or Hartmann's solution (Ringer's lactate) the latter being an important gluconeogenic precursor, especially in starved or catabolic patients.

Postoperative management

Various regimens of postoperative management have been described. Those based on sliding scales of urinary glucose level are no longer applicable because of the ready availability of blood glucose reflectance meters. Sliding scale doses of insulin given subcutaneously every 4 to 6 h based on plasma glucose concentrations, although preventing the extremes of hyper- and hypoglycaemia, often cause considerable fluctuations in diabetic control. Continuous infusion of insulin at a fixed rate (1–2 units/h) does not seem to improve glucose control over subcutaneous insulin administration, nor over the glucose—potassium—insulin regimen. A recently described bedside algorithm for postoperative diabetic care has been based on infusion of dextrose saline (100 ml/h) and potassium, and a separate infusion of insulin at a rate varying according to 2-hourly blood glucose estimations. This regimen aims to maintain the plasma glucose level between 6.7 and 10.0 mmol/1, with an insulin infusion rate varying between 0.5 and 5.0 U/h. There is, therefore, no standard procedure: each patient must be treated as an individual and the blood glucose titrated to the range 4.3 and 6.6 mmol/l during surgery and the postoperative period. There are few data to suggest that any of the above regimens for optimal intraoperative control is better than the others.

Chronic renal failure

Renal function may be impaired as a result of parenchymous disease, or as a result of ageing. Patients with impaired renal function present a number of clinical problems of importance to the anaesthetist and surgeon.

Acid–base and electrolyte imbalance

Patients with chronic renal failure are unable to excrete acid metabolites. This results in metabolic acidosis, low plasma bicarbonate, hyponatraemia, hyperchloraemia, and hyperkalaemia. Hyperphosphataemia is associated with low serum calcium concentrations. Although the uraemic patient can tolerate mild to moderate degrees of hyperkalaemia, most authorities suggest that serum potassium levels of greater than 5.5 mmol/1 to 6.0 mmol/1 should be reduced prior to anaesthesia and surgery. This is of importance as a number of intraoperative factors may further increase the plasma potassium, including spontaneous ventilation, hypoventilation, repeated administration of suxamethonium, and the administration of stored blood. Methods of reducing high serum potassium concentrations include haemodialysis and haemofiltration, glucose–insulin therapy, administration of bicarbonate, hyperventilation, and calcium resonium enema (30–60 g).

Anaemia

Patients with chronic renal failure may present with a normochromic, normocytic anaemia of complex aetiology. Causes include decreased red cell production as a consequence of reduced erythropoietin synthesis and release, bone-marrow depression by uraemia, decreased red cell life-span, repeated blood losses during haemodialysis, and aluminium toxicity. Other factors include deficiency of iron, folate, and vitamins B_6 and B_{12}. These problems are now less prominent with the use of biosynthetic erythropoietin, which increases haemoglobin concentrations towards normal values.

Hypertension and ischaemic heart disease

These conditions affect 60 to 70 per cent of patients with chronic renal failure. Patients requiring treatment for hypertension (other than adequate haemodialysis) often show refractory hypertension, necessitating large doses of combination antihypertensive drugs (β-adrenoceptor blocking drugs, calcium channel antagonists, vasodilators, and angiotension converting enzyme inhibitors). Anaesthetic agents may interact with each of these, resulting in exaggerated hypotensive or bradycardic responses. In addition, these patients show exaggerated pressor responses to laryngoscopy and tracheal intubation, and to surgical stimulation. Medication must, therefore, be optimized before any elective surgery is undertaken. Patients with chronic renal failure (especially those on haemodialysis) are also liable to suffer from accelerated atherosclerosis, uraemic cardiomyopathy, and pericarditis.

Coagulation

Uraemic patients may present with bleeding problems, due to platelet dysfunction and thrombocytopenia, as well as decreased levels of platelet factor III which reduces platelet adhesiveness. Any preoperative abnormalities of coagulation (seen as a prolonged bleeding time, but unaltered prothrombin time or partial thromboplastin time) should be treated by platelet transfusion, cryoprecipitate or infusions of deamino-D-arginine vasopressin.

Central venous system

Uraemia initially manifests as malaise, fatigue, and reduced mental ability; patients may later progress to myoclonus and fitting, coma and death. Peripheral neuropathies are common in the lower limbs, and these may involve the autonomic nervous system, leading to postural hypotension.

Gastrointestinal tract

Common gastrointestinal symptoms in patients with uraemia are anorexia, nausea and vomiting, gastrointestinal haemorrhage, diarrhoea, and hiccups. Chronic renal failure patients also show a delayed gastric emptying time, as well as increased volume and acidity of the gastric contents. Preoperative use of antacids and histamine H_2-receptor antagonists is indicated.

Protection of veins, shunts, and fistulae

All functioning shunts and fistulae must be protected during anaesthesia and surgery, with the sphygmomanometer cuff placed on the contralateral arm. Non-invasive blood pressure monitor cuffs must not be placed on the arm containing fistulae or shunts. The present generation of non-invasive blood pressure monitors has reduced the indications for intra-arterial blood pressure monitoring, but damage to future vascular access sites by arterial cannulation is unlikely with the new Teflon cannulae, especially for short-term intraoperative monitoring.

Venous access should be restricted (if at all possible) to distal sites on the dorsum of the hand, with preservation of all forearm and antecubital fossa veins. Central venous cannulation (useful as a guide to maintaining intraoperative normovolaemia) is best achieved via the subclavian or internal jugular routes.

Anaesthesia for general surgery in patients with chronic renal failure

Uraemic patients may show unusual drug responses due to intercurrent therapy, reduced plasma protein binding of intravenous drugs, and low plasma pseudocholinesterase activity. Electrolyte imbalance may affect the successful reversal of competitive neuromuscular blockade.

All intercurrent therapy should be continued up to the morning of surgery, and a history of peptic ulceration or discomfort, or symptoms of hiatus hernia or gastric reflux should be treated with antacids and/or H_2-receptor antagonist drugs. Rapid sequence induction is more commonly used in patients with renal impairment because of the increased incidence of delayed gastric emptying shown by these patients. Care should be exercised with the use of central acting antiemetic drugs (phenothiazines, butyrophenones) as they can result in prolonged sedation and extrapyramidal side-effects in the patient with chronic renal failure. The introduction of routine preoperative haemofiltration or dialysis has improved greatly the medical status of surgical patients with chronic renal failure. Preoperative laboratory investigations should therefore include estimation of plasma electrolytes and creatinine, haemoglobin and haematocrit, platelets, and a clotting screen. In the diabetic patient with renal failure, preoperative monitoring of the blood glucose is imperative.

Premedication should be carefully chosen; the orally administered short-acting benzodiazepines (temazepam) offer suitable anxiolysis and mild sedation. Intramuscular opioid premedication is best avoided because of the propensity towards bleeding and the increased sensitivity of the uraemic patient to drugs of the morphine series.

Anaesthesia is best induced with either the combination hypnotic–opioid (using sleep doses of etomidate or thiopentone) or, in patients undergoing major abdominal or body-cavity surgery and in whom there is a history of recent myocardial infarction or poor left ventricular function, moderate to high doses of fentanyl or sufentanil followed by monitoring in the intensive care unit. Both regimens will attenuate the haemodynamic responses to induction, laryngoscopy and intubation, and surgical stress. Diisopropylphenol (propofol) should be used with care in these patients because of the marked hypotension which can occur due to peripheral vasodilation.

Neuromuscular blockade is best achieved with incremental doses of agents which rely minimally on the kidney for their elimination (vecuronium, atracurium, or mivacurium), and with careful monitoring of the extent of neuromuscular blockade. Similarly, doses of analgesic drugs should be titrated against effect. Since active metabolites of pethidine and morphine accumulate in patients with chronic renal failure, the intraoperative use of drugs of the anilino-piperidine group (fentanyl, alfentanil, sufentanil) is preferred. Enflurane is generally avoided because of the tendency for fluoride ion to accumulate during longer cases, although the clinical significance of this is debated for routine surgery.

Liver disease and anaesthesia

The four main functions of the liver are metabolism of glucose, amino acids, fatty acids, and cholesterol; production of bile, which is involved in absorption of drugs and fat from the intestines; detoxification of drugs and waste products; and synthesis of proteins (including albumin, clotting factors, and transport proteins). Each of these aspects may influence the safe conduct of anaesthesia.

Drug metabolism

The liver is the principal organ of drug metabolism, and changes in liver blood flow, hepatocellular function, and both the plasma protein concentration and the extent of drug binding will all affect drug pharmacokinetics. In addition, drugs administered during anaesthesia or in the perioperative period may affect hepatic function, either by alterating liver blood flow or through direct cellular effects. Halothane, for example, has been shown to exacerbate liver dysfunction, whereas isoflurane does not alter function in the cirrhotic liver. Patients with cirrhosis show a variable degree of alteration in drug metabolism; drugs undergoing phase 1 metabolism (oxidation, reduction, hydroxylation) have a greater impairment in clearance than drugs metabolized through conjugation reactions.

Preoperative assessment

This should include evaluation of the patient's general condition, the presence of jaundice, the state of nutrition and hydration, the presence of encephalopathy, and evidence of clotting disorders. Liver disease may also affect cardiorespiratory and renal function. Grading of the severity of liver disease can help predict outcome.

Cardiorespiratory status

Patients with cirrhosis may have reduced systemic vascular resistance, increased cardiac output, and both systemic and pulmonary shunting of blood. The last may result in hypoxia and may be associated with impaired hypoxic pulmonary vasoconstriction and hypoventilation. Analysis of arterial blood gases may show lowered tensions of O_2 and CO_2. Hepatomegaly and ascites cause an increase in the pulmonary closing volume, leading to basal atelectasis. There may be associated pleural effusions.

Renal status

There is a high incidence of postoperative renal failure in jaundiced patients undergoing abdominal surgery: one study reported an incidence of 17 per cent, with a mortality rate of 100 per cent. In addition, there is prognostic importance in the value of the preoperative creatinine; a value of 130 μmol/l is associated with a worse prognosis. Patients with cirrhosis are liable to develop the hepatorenal syndrome, the aetiology of which is complex. Measures to prevent its occurrence include maintenance of fluid and sodium balance, avoidance of nephrotoxins, and aggressive treatment of infection.

Haemostatic status

Decreased synthesis of clotting factors may lead to a haemorrhagic tendency during surgery and the postoperative period. Predisposing factors include a pre-existing coagulopathy, a dilutional coagulopathy due to rapid fluid replacement, an exaggerated fibrinolytic response, and the complicating metabolic problems of hypothermia, hypocalcaemia, and acidosis.

Patients with liver disease have reduced levels of clotting factors II VII, IX, and X, which may respond to the administration of vitamin K. Levels of factors V and XI are also often reduced, and this should be treated by the infusion of fresh frozen plasma. Similarly, platelet deficiency can be overcome by platelet infusions. Factor VIII levels often remain normal in severe liver disease, as it is synthesized by the reticuloendothelial system. A low level is usually indicative of disseminated intravascular coagulation.

Preoperative laboratory tests should include the thrombin time, activated partial thromboplastin time, prothrombin time, and platelet count. The history, clinical examination, and laboratory tests can together provide an indication of the degree of risk. Increased mortality is associated with serum albumin below 30 g/l, presence of infection, white blood cell count above 10000/ml, treatment with more than two antibiotics, serum bilirubin above 50 μmol/l, presence of ascites, malnutrition, and the need for emergency surgery. The administration of preoperative oral bile salts has been shown to reduce the incidence of both endotoxaemia and postoperative renal impairment in patients with obstructive jaundice. Other protective measures include the intraoperative administration of mannitol and dopamine.

Premedication

Intramuscular drugs should, in general, be avoided because of the pre-existing bleeding tendency, and even small doses of opiates may induce the development of acute liver failure. Hence most anaesthetists favour an oral short-acting benzodiazepine or no premedication. H_2-receptor antagonists may be prescribed if there is a risk of gastric ulceration, as may vitamin K.

General anaesthesia

The anaesthetic sequence currently used by most units treating significant numbers of patients with liver disease is thiopentone, atracurium, and isoflurane for maintenance, with ventilation to normocapnia. Isoflurane maintains hepatic oxygen supply better than other agents, while atracurium depends on breakdown by Hoffman degradation rather than by hepatic metabolism. Occasional patients show resistance to atracurium due to increased binding by raised levels of globulin. Although plasma cholinesterase levels may be deficient in patients with liver failure, there is no contraindication to the administration of suxamethonium when clinically indicated; however the duration of its effect may be prolonged. Analgesia is usually provided by incremental doses of fentanyl or sufentanil. Many anaesthetists do not use nitrous oxide during prolonged surgery because of the development of bowel distension through diffusion of nitrous oxide into the gut. Intraoperative fluids (normal saline, blood, 5 per cent dextrose) should aim to maintain normovolaemia, a haemoglobin above 10 g/dl and normoglycaemia (4–7 mmol/l). Mannitol may be necessary to maintain a urinary output of about 1 ml/kg.

Hepatic encephalopathy

This may develop due to primary acute hepatocellular dysfunction or as a complication of cirrhosis, where it may be precipitated acutely by excessive alcohol ingestion. The encephalopathy may be due to decreased synthesis of essential cerebral metabolites (other than glucose) or to the accumulation of gut-derived substances affecting neurological function. The latter theory is favoured, with ammonia, mercaptans, fatty acids, and octopamine being implicated. The benzodiazepine antagonist, flumazenil, has recently been shown to improve encephalopathy clinically and electrophysiologically in about 80 per cent of subjects.

Anaemia

The normal range of haemoglobin concentration is 13.5 to 17.5 g/dl in men, and 11.5 to 15.5 g/dl in women. Anaemic patients may be asymptomatic, although lassitude and decreased exercise tolerance are common features. The patient may be pale. If anaemia is moderate or severe, physical examination may reveal cardiomegaly and functional heart murmurs. In the perioperative patient, tissue oxygenation is dependent upon arterial oxygen content, capillary blood flow, and the position of the oxyhaemoglobin dissociation curve.

Oxygen content

This is determined from the partial pressure of oxygen and the percentage haemoglobin saturation according to the following equation:

$$\text{Content} = (\text{Hb} \times 1.34 \times Sa\text{o}_2) + (P\text{o}_2 \times 0.0225)$$

where Hb = haemoglobin content g/dl, $Sa\text{o}_2$ = oxygen saturation, $Pa\text{o}_2$ = partial pressure of oxygen, and 0.0225 = ml oxygen dissolved/100 ml blood/kPa oxygen tension.

In normal arterial blood, haemoglobin is almost fully saturated (96–98 per cent) in the patient breathing room air. In the patient with anaemia, the decreased oxygen content (due to the decreased amount of haemoglobin) can be partially offset by increasing the inspired oxygen concentration.

Capillary blood flow

This varies with cardiac output, systemic vascular resistance and blood viscosity: although capillary blood flow increases because of reduced viscosity, this is offset by the reduction in oxygen content of the blood. Hence any factor causing a further fall in oxygen delivery, such as blood loss or myocardial depression, will cause tissue hypoxia.

Oxyhaemoglobin dissociation curve

At rest, basal oxygen consumption is about 250 ml/min. This is achieved through extraction by the tissues of about 5 ml oxygen per 100 ml blood. Mixed venous saturation is approximately 75 per cent and the mixed venous PO_2 about 5.3 kPa. The oxyhaemoglobin dissociation curve will be shifted to the left by hypothermia, reduced 2,3-diphosphoglycerate levels, or alkalosis. This leads to further reduction of $P\bar{v}O_2$ at 75 per cent saturation, and impaired tissue oxygenation. A right-shift of the oxyhaemoglobin dissociation curve will allow oxygen to be released to the tissues from haemoglobin, but only at higher $PaCO_2$ levels.

Provided that cardiac output, and therefore tissue perfusion, remains unaltered, anaemia causes a reduction in both capillary and tissue PaO_2. In patients with chronic anaemia two important physiological compensatory mechanisms come into play: levels of 2,3-diphosphoglycerate in red cells are increased, shifting the oxyhaemoglobin dissociation curve to the right, and cardiac output is increased due to reduced blood viscosity, so effectively reducing peripheral vascular resistance and capillary dilatation in response to the reduced oxygen content of the blood.

Packed cell volume versus viscosity

The relationships between haemoglobin concentration, blood viscosity, and oxygen flux and the tissues are shown in Fig. 1.

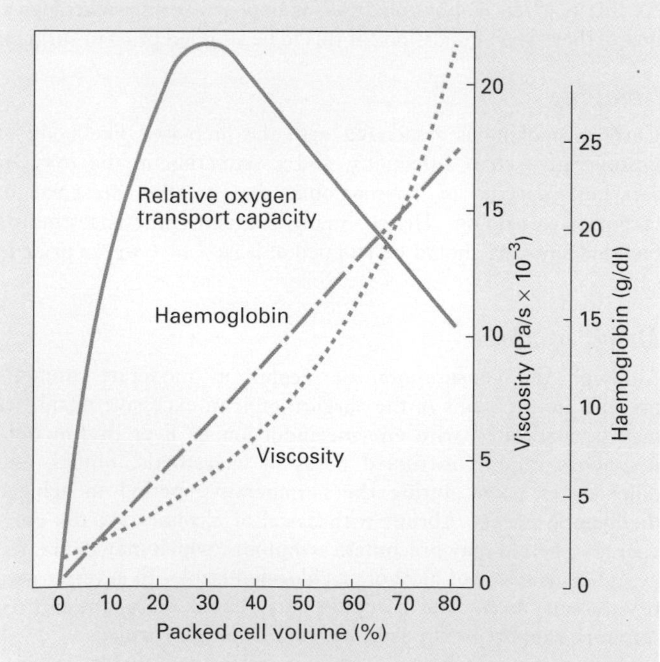

Fig. 1 The relationships between haemoglobin concentration, blood viscosity, and oxygen flux in the tissues.

Although arterial oxygen content increases linearly as packed cell volume increases, there is also an accompanying increase in viscosity, which reduces capillary blood flow. As shown in Fig. 1, there is an optimal packed cell volume at which the balance between viscosity and arterial oxygen content results in the maximum volume of oxygen being transported to the tissues in a given time. This optimum packed cell volume is about 30 per cent, and the haemoglobin concentration, 8 to 9 g/dl.

Effects of anaemia on anaesthesia and surgery

There is no substantial evidence to show that normovolaemic anaemia increases the morbidity associated with surgery although risks are increased in the presence of other factors which may impair tissue oxygenation, such as pre-existing lung disease or hypovolaemia. Similarly, there are insufficient data to suggest that anaemia is associated with poorer wound healing, and it has been suggested that healing of colonic anastomoses is optimal if the haemoglobin level is maintained in the range 10 to 12 g/dl.

Since inhaled anaesthetic agents have a reduced solubility (15–25 per cent) in anaemic blood, the concentration of anaesthetic in the blood will increase more rapidly than normal. Although this increases the rates of onset of and recovery from anaesthesia, there is also the risk of overdosage or toxicity. The depressant effect which these drugs have on the cardiovascular system may be exaggerated in the anaemic patient.

Respiratory alkalosis (due to excessive mechanical ventilation) and hypothermia shift the oxyhaemoglobin dissociation curve to the left, reducing tissue oxygen release, while intraoperative hypovolaemia (secondary to blood loss) may decrease cardiac output and cause splanchnic vasoconstriction. Blood lost during surgery must therefore be replaced promptly. Pain and shivering in the postoperative period increase systemic vascular resistance and result in tissue hypoxia. Thus, oxygen should be administered to the anaemic patient in the immediate postoperative period, and subsequently if pulmonary function is impaired. Attention must be paid to cardiovascular function, avoiding hypovolaemia by appropriate administration of crystalloid, colloid, or blood, and treating arrhythmias or reduced cardiac output promptly.

Sickle-cell diseases

These are caused by the inheritance of the sickle-cell gene, either alone or in combination with another haemoglobinopathy. The most common genotypes are homozygous sickle-cell disease (SS), sickle-cell trait (SA), sickle-cell haemoglobin C (SC), and sickle cell β-thalassaemia (Sβthal). Under conditions of reduced oxygen tension, sickle haemoglobin undergoes gelation, altering the malleability of the erythocyte, which assumes an elongated sickle shape. These misshapen cells cause sludging of the blood in the capillaries leading to an increased blood viscosity, thromboembolic episodes and cell haemolysis. To reduce the risk of sickling during surgery, elective operations should be performed only when the patient is not having a crisis, and is free from infection. Safe and simple general anaesthesia in these patients requires adequate oxygenation, ventilation to normocapnia, maintenance of the circulating volume, and good postoperative care. The induction of hyponatraemia may reduce the risk of sickling, as may deliberate raising of pH. In patients with severe sickle-cell disease scheduled for major surgery, preoperative transfusion to decrease the absolute percentage of HbS to less than 40 per cent reduces the risk of vaso-occlusion, as well as suppressing the bone marrow, thereby resulting in decreased production of sickle cells.

Preoperative assessment should include the prescribing of

adequate premedication, as anxiety may precipitate crises due to the associated vasoconstriction. The use of 50 per cent oxygen in nitrous oxide, supplemented by isoflurane, is the current technique of choice. Intraoperative monitoring should include oximetry and capnography (if available). The use of automated non-invasive blood pressure cuffs has been questioned because of a possible increase in problems due to stasis and sickling while a sphygmomanometer cuff is inflated. Postoperatively, arterial hypoxaemia is common, and this may be exacerbated by the depressant effects of postoperative analgesia. Oxygen should be given for 24 to 48 h after surgery. Local hypoxaemia and acidosis must be avoided, so tourniquets should not be applied for limb surgery, and major regional nerve blockade is contraindicated, as is intravenous regional anaesthesia.

Although sickle-cell trait (SA) patients are less at risk, adequate oxygenation is essential throughout the perioperative period.

Drug therapy and pre-existing conditions

Drug therapy

Tricyclic antidepressants

Severe arrhythmias, including ventricular ectopic beats, may occur in the spontaneously breathing patient receiving volatile inhalational agents, especially halothane. The incidence appears greatest in patients undergoing oral surgery.

Monoamine oxidase inhibitors

The intraoperative administration of vasopressor agents to patients receiving treatment with monoamine oxidase inhibitors may result in hypertensive crises. Monoamine oxidase inhibitors may also interact with opioids, resulting either in 'excitatory' signs (hypertension, hyperpyrexia, convulsions) or marked central nervous system depression (especially respiratory centre depression). After consultation with the patient's psychiatrist, monoamine oxidase inhibitors should, if possible, be discontinued at least 2 weeks prior to anaesthesia and surgery.

Lithium

This treatment for manic depression may potentiate the effects of both depolarizing and non-depolarizing muscle relaxants, and the drug is therefore best discontinued prior to anaesthesia, following discussion with the psychiatrist concerned.

Antiepileptic drugs

Surgery and anaesthesia may influence the disposition of these agents, resulting either in subtherapeutic drug concentrations, which increase the risk of seizures, or toxicity. Postoperatively, binding of phenytoin is reduced due to changes in the plasma concentrations of albumin, α_1-acid glycoprotein and free fatty acids. Drug binding and distribution may also be influenced by changes in acid–base status. Another important side-effect of chronic antiepileptic therapy (especially with phenobarbitone, phenytoin and carbamazepine) is hepatic microsomal enzyme induction: patients may require increased doses of both hypnotic and analgesic drugs for adequate anaesthesia and pain relief. Other enzyme-inducing agents include rifampicin, isoniazid, spironolactone, phenylbutazone, alcohol, cigarette smoking, and drugs such as the anabolic steroids.

Anticoagulant therapy

Warfarin is best discontinued 3 to 4 days preoperatively and replaced with an infusion of heparin (24 000 units per 24 h). Before induction anaesthesia, the International Normalized Ratio should be well below 1.5; any residual effect of warfarin should be reversed by vitamin K (phytomenadione) administration. Fresh frozen plasma or clotting factor concentrates may be administered to patients receiving warfarin who require emergency surgery.

Heparin treatment is usually discontinued just before surgery, the best time for stopping being at the time of oral premedication (the biological half life of the anticoagulant being dose-dependent, but ranging between 0.5 and 3 h). Postoperatively, when the patient is tolerating oral intake, warfarin treatment should be recommenced with an oral loading dose of 8 to 10 mg; the International Normalized Ratio should be checked at 48 h, and if it is greater than 2 to 2.5, heparin is discontinued.

For perioperative prophylaxis against deep venous thrombosis or pulmonary embolism, 5000 units of heparin should be given subcutaneously with premedication, and then continued 12-hourly for 3 days after surgery. The efficacy of this therapy is not usually monitored, but the risk of haemorrhagic episodes is increased in patients concurrently receiving antiplatelet therapy such as low-dose aspirin. Use of the new low molecular weight heparins is said to provide prophylaxis against thrombosis without the risk of haemorrhagic episodes. Additional prophylaxis may include elasticized or inflatable stockings and calf stimulators.

Oral contraceptives

The combination of surgery and oral contraception increases the incidence of postoperative deep venous thrombosis, and intake of the oral contraceptive pill should be discontinued at least 4 to 6 weeks before surgery. If emergency surgery is required in a woman currently using oral contraception, prophylaxis against deep venous thrombosis may take the form of low-dose heparin, intraoperative infusion of dextran 70, and elasticated stockings. In theory, this increased risk of deep venous thrombosis should not exist in patients taking the progesterone-only pill.

Hormone replacement therapy

As this is given in physiological (as opposed to pharmacological doses) there is no indication for this to be stopped prior to surgery.

Smoking

Chronic smoking is associated with the increased likelihood of postoperative chest infections, and a reduction in the oxygen-carrying capacity of haemoglobin due to the presence of carboxyhaemoglobin. Hence, many surgeons and anaesthetists feel that smoking should be stopped at least 3 to 4 weeks prior to surgery.

Drugs of abuse

Although the consumption of alcohol in moderate amounts presents no problems to the surgical patient, excessive quantities may be associated with enzyme induction or liver dysfunction. Alcoholics require increased doses of anaesthetic, opioid, and other drugs given during the perioperative period to achieve therapeutic effects. Abrupt withdrawal of alcohol over the perioperative period may precipitate symptoms, which may be treated by judicious doses of alcohol or chlormethiazole. In severe cases, seizures may occur which require intravenous diazepam and respiratory support before commencing chlormethiazole.

Other drugs of importance include marijuana, opioids, cocaine, and LSD. Again, withdrawal symptoms may occur perioperatively. The association of drug abuse with carriage of bloodborne infections such as hepatitis B or HIV should be considered, and appropriate precautions taken.

Inherited conditions

There are a number of genetic and familial conditions that influence anaesthetic practice, three of which are of major importance.

Plasma pseudocholinesterase deficiency

Deficiency of this enzyme, which is responsible for the metabolism of suxamethonium, procaine, 2-chloroprocaine, and tetracaine, may be either acquired or inherited. The latter may be expressed as both homozygous and heterozygous conditions, and causes variable degrees of prolongation of the duration of suxamethonium, causing apnoea, and the need for intermittent positive pressure ventilation. Delineation of the genotype in affected patients and if necessary, in their relatives, can be made by measuring the percentage enzyme inhibition caused by dibucaine (10^{-5} M) and fluoride. A silent gene, lacking enzyme activity, and other genetic variants exist (e.g. C_5).

Porphyria

This group of diseases is caused by inherited defects or acquired dysfunction of the enzymes responsible for haemopoiesis. Hepatic (acute intermittent) porphyria presents the most important problems to the anaesthetist and occurs about 1 in 100 000 live births in the United Kingdom, although higher rates occur in other countries (e.g. Sweden, southern Africa). The condition is due to a deficiency of uroporphyrinogen I synthase, which is diagnosed by an increased urinary concentration of aminolevulinic acid and porphyrobilinogen. Acute attacks may be precipitated by a number of anaesthetic-related drugs including barbiturates, flunitrazepam, the contraceptive pill, and prochlorperazine.

Preoperative examination of the patient should include careful assessment of the cardiovascular system for tachycardia and hypertension and of the central nervous system for neuritis, neuropathies (motor, sensory, and autonomic), and bulbar palsy. Regional anaesthesia is contraindicated as neurological complications may arise. Other forms of the disease which also have anaesthetic implications but which are less common include hereditary coproporphyria and porphyria cutanea tarda hereditaria. The same drugs may precipitate crises in these patients.

Malignant hyperpyrexia

This defect of muscle calcium transport is inherited as an autosomal dominant characteristic located on chromosome 19. The disease is characterized by heat production (> 1°C rise/h), muscle rigidity, excess lactate and CO_2 production, hypoxia, hyperkalaemia, respiratory and metabolic acidosis, and myoglobinuria. The incidence is about 1:200 000 surgical patients in the United Kingdom.

For the disease to be expressed, a genetically sensitive individual must be exposed to a trigger agent (inhalational agent, suxamethonium, and possibly nitrous oxide). A greater incidence of the condition is found among patients undergoing surgical correction of squints and hernia and minor orthopaedic procedures. Morbidity is high (24 per cent). Management of an attack involves intravenous administration of dantrolene, withdrawal of likely precipitating agents and supportive therapy, including control of hyperkalaemia and acidosis, surface and peritoneal cooling, and treatment of cardiac arrhythmias. Specific therapy with dantrolene sodium (1–10 mg/kg IV) has reduced the mortality, and the drug may also be used as prophylaxis in susceptible individuals. As the disease is genetically inherited, 'at-risk' individuals should be screened by the *in-vitro* examination of a muscle biopsy taken under local anaesthesia. Abnormal contracture following exposure to caffeine is the principal diagnostic test, combined with electron microscopy.

Preoperative laboratory testing

Preoperative laboratory testing of patients scheduled for elective surgery allows quantitation of an abnormality detected by history and physical examination, detection of significant abnormalities not revealed by history and examination, and offers medicolegal protection to medical staff.

There is general agreement that assessment of the severity of pre-existing disease is important. This allows the patient to be restored to optimum health before surgery, allows any support likely to be needed in the perioperative period to be predicted, and also assists in risk–benefit decisions. A detailed discussion of preoperative preparation of patients with the various commonly encountered diseases is outside the scope of this section.

'Screening' of asymptomatic patients in the belief that detection of abnormalities will improve perioperative course and outcome is of great significance. Until recently, minimal data have been available to support the assertions made. However, there has been increased evaluation of the benefits of preoperative laboratory testing of patients in the last decade. A retrospective study of patients undergoing inguinal herniorrhaphy or stripping of varicose veins, found only 63 abnormal results in 1972 tests, and in no instance was patient management influenced by these results. Similar results have been found by other workers and it is concluded that history and physical examination determine which tests are appropriate in all but a small minority of patients.

The use of a battery of tests to provide medicolegal protection has also been questioned. One review concluded that there was no benefit to patient management or cost–benefit from routine screening of asymptomatic patients. In addition, potential legal problems may be generated when false-positive results occur. Retrospective studies have shown that unexpected positive results in asymptomatic patients are generally ignored: for example, anaemia found on routine screening of children was ignored in 74 per cent of cases.

The tests recommended for asymptomatic patients undergoing routine surgery are shown in Table 4.

Premedication

Agents used for premedication form part of the anaesthetic technique, with the provision of analgesia or supplementation to volatile agent-nitrous oxide or hypnotic infusion-nitrous oxide anaesthetics. The primary indications for preoperative medication are anxiolysis, sedation especially in paediatric patients, analgesia, amnesia, vagolysis to reduce salivary secretions, and prophylaxis against postoperative nausea and vomiting and hence aspiration pneumonitis.

Anxiolysis

Most patients experience some anxiety prior to surgery and this is best allayed by the combination of careful and sensitive discussion of the issues of concern to the patient and the use of anti-anxiety drugs, the most common agents being the benzodiazepines (dia-

Table 4 Recommended screening tests for asymptomatic patients undergoing minor body-surface surgery

Age (years)	Male	Female
<40	–	Hb or Hct
40–59	ECG, urea, glucose	Hb/Hct, ECG, urea, glucose
>60	ECG, urea, glucose CXR, Hb/Hct	Hb/hct, ECG, urea, glucose, CXR

Hb = haemoglobin; Hct = haematocrit; ECG = electrocardiograph; CXR = chest radiograph.

zepam, lorazepam, or temazepam) and some of the opioids (morphine, pethidine, and papaveretum).

Sedation

This may also be achieved by administration of benzodiazepines or opioids. In children antihistamines such as trimeprazine (which can be given by the oral route) or rectal administration of ketamine or methohexitone can be used.

Amnesia

Many anaesthetists regard amnesia of the events leading up to anaesthesia and surgery as desirable, especially in the very young and in patients having repeated general anaesthetics. Amnesic drugs may also reduce the risk of awareness occurring during anaesthesia, allowing a lighter depth of anaesthesia to be maintained. The most effective amnesic agents are the benzodiazepines (especially lorazepam and midazolam). The anticholinergic agent, hyoscine, also exhibits amnestic properties.

Analgesia

The routine use of analgesic drugs as part of the premedication, except in patients experiencing severe acute or chronic preoperative pain has been criticized by some anaesthetists. However, the preoperative administration of analgesic drugs (both opioids and non-steroidal anti-inflammatory drugs) reduces the dose of induction agent and maintenance agents necessary for clinically adequate anaesthesia. In addition, the use of analgesia (either as part of the premedication, or intraoperatively) provides patient comfort in the initial postoperative period. The main disadvantages of all opioid drugs are their association with nausea and vomiting, and the risk of respiratory depression.

Antivagal actions

The response to many noxious stimuli is the development of a vagally medicated bradycardia. Intramuscularly administered anticholinergics have been shown to be ineffective in preventing these responses. Routine use of antisialogogues has major disadvantages: the patient suffers an unpleasant dry mouth during the preoperative period, and dry mucous membranes are sticky and easily damaged during laryngoscopy and intubation. Present use of these agents tends to be reserved for infants, and in those situations where a dry mouth is advantageous, (such as for intra-oral surgery). Hyoscine is the most potent of the antisialogogues available and has the additional advantage of producing amnesia and sedation. In the elderly, however, there is a significant incidence of perioperative confusional states.

Antiemetics

Drugs used for premedication may either reduce the emetic effects of the anaesthetic agents employed, or aid gastric emptying. The first group includes the antihistamines and butyrophenone drugs, as well as hyoscine; gastric emptying can be facilitated by administration of metoclopramide, and the gastrokinetic drug, cisapride. Additional effective medications include transdermal hyoscine, and the 5-hydroxytryptamine antagonist, ondansetron.

Agents to decrease gastric acidity are normally administered only to those patients either at risk of regurgitation of gastric contents into the pharynx with tracheal aspiration, such as the pregnant patient, those with a hiatus hernia or strong clinical history of gastric reflex, the obese, and those with clinical evidence of gastric stasis, or in those procedures associated with a high incidence of nausea and vomiting, such as laparoscopy. Such antacid therapy aims to reduce acid production, and to raise the gastric pH of residual contents to above 2.5. The first is achieved by administration of histamine H_2-receptor antagonists (cimetidine, ranitidine, famotidine, or nizatidine) or the hydrogen-pump antagonist omeprazole given over several hours pre-surgery; the second is by alkalis such as sodium citrate or magnesium trisilicate given orally 15 to 30 min prior to induction.

Antihistamine drugs such as the phenothiazines promazine, chlorpromazine, and promethazine may also offer protection against the drug-mediated release of endogenous histamine and other autocoids in the atopic individual. Their protection is usually incomplete, and co-administration of sodium cromoglycate and hydrocortisone may be of benefit in the highly sensitized patient.

Methods of premedicant drug administration

Although the most popular rates of administration are by the intramuscular (the traditional method) and oral routes, alternatives such as intravenous, rectal, and transdermal routes have specific indications.

Orally administered premedicants may be less effective than those administered parenterally. Gastric emptying and drug absorption will be influenced by pain, anxiety, opioids, and intra-abdominal pathology. However, the oral route is considered by many to be the route of choice for children, and it is the preferred route in patients with bleeding disorders (patients receiving anticoagulants, haemophiliacs, or those with other coagulation defects, and patients with liver and renal failure).

The timing of the premedication is of importance since maximum antisialogogue and antivagal effects need to be achieved before induction of anaesthesia: thus the majority of drugs are given 1 to 2 h preoperatively. For more rapid onset of anxiolysis, the short-acting benzodiazepine temazepam has been advocated, especially for use in day-care anaesthesia.

GENERAL ANAESTHETIC PHARMACOLOGY AND PRACTICE

Safe general anaesthesia depends upon the administration and maintenance of an 'adequate anaesthetic dose' without the accompanying development of unwanted or adverse side-effects; the monitoring, where possible, of the depth of anaesthesia by clinical signs (such as heart rate, blood pressure or autonomic responses), or a derivate of brain activity, such as EEG or evoked potentials, relating, where possible, the presence of clinically adequate anaesthesia with a defined plasma drug concentration; and the prompt recovery of normal brain activity through the use of drugs that undergo rapid elimination and have no residual depressive effects on the central nervous system or other systems.

Induction of anaesthesia

Unconsciousness may be induced by intravenous hypnotics alone or in combination with other agents (including opioids). Hypnotics (with the exception of ketamine) do not possess analgesic properties nor do they relax skeletal muscle. Although they are rarely used alone for the maintenance of anaesthesia, their use will reduce the requirement for other anaesthetic agents.

Thiopentone is still the archetypal hypnotic drug, providing a rapid, effective and safe onset of anaesthesia. Its non-hypnotic properties include cardiorespiratory depression, and, in large doses, prolonged recovery. Absolute contraindications are rare and include proven barbiturate allergy or a history of acute intermittent porphyria. Thiopentone should be used cautiously, with reduced dosage and careful titration of dose to effect in patients with respiratory obstruction or inadequate airway control before induction of anaesthesia, in severe cardiovascular collapse or shock, and in those with status asthmaticus, cardiovascular disease (ischaemic heart disease, hypertension, valvular heart disease), hypovolaemia, acute adrenocortical insufficiency, or uraemia.

Methohexitone and thiamylal have faster clearance rates than thiopentone, and both are broken down to inactive metabolites. The side-effects of methohexitone include pain on intravenous injection, a tendency to venous thrombophlebitis, and exaggerated involuntary movements, especially in the unpremedicated patient and patients with epilepsy.

Etomidate (a carboxylated imidazole) has the advantage of not inducing histamine release, and is therefore indicated for use in asthmatic and atopic patients. Induction of anaesthesia causes only minimal haemodynamic and respiratory changes. Pain on injection and myoclonic activity during induction have limited its use for routine surgery.

Ketamine is the only hypnotic agent possessing analgesic activities. In contrast to other agents, ketamine increases sympathetic autonomic activity, and is therefore useful for the rapid induction of anaesthesia in patients requiring high sympathetic activity for maintenance of cardiovascular function (e.g. in the presence of pericardial tamponade, and hypotension). Indications for the use of ketamine include: poor-risk surgical patients (e.g. those with poor myocardial function or hypovolaemia); debridement, application or removal of painful dressings and skin grafting in patients suffering from burns; short diagnostic or surgical procedures, including cardiac catheterization; and postoperative pain relief.

Propofol (di-isopropyl phenol) causes comparable cardiovascular and respiratory depression to thiopentone when used for induction of anaesthesia. Induction is often accompanied by pain on injection, especially when small veins are employed, with coughing and hiccoughing, and involuntary movements. It has a high clearance rate and can therefore be used for both induction and maintenance of anaesthesia, especially where prompt and complete recovery is important (e.g. day case surgery). The low incidence of nausea, vomiting, and headache is important for the ambulant patient. Because of its pharmacological effects, propofol should be used with care in patients with compromised cardiac function (ischaemic heart disease, hypertension) or hypovolaemia.

Midazolam, a water-soluble benzodiazepine, should be used to provide sedation, amnesia, and sleep—but not anaesthesia. It has a shorter duration of action than diazepam, but may cause unexpected ventilatory and cardiovascular depression, especially in patients with chronic obstructive pulmonary disease, hypotension associated with hypovolaemia, and in the elderly.

Maintenance of anaesthesia

Anaesthesia may be maintained by infusions of hypnotic agents, volatile agents, or opioids, alone or in combination.

Intravenous infusion anaesthesia

Use of intravenous infusions of anaesthetics has increased in popularity due to development of drugs with higher systemic clearance and metabolism to inactive metabolites, such as propofol or methohexitone. Some indications for the use of intravenous techniques include day-case anaesthesia, military or 'field' anaesthesia (where nitrous oxide is not available), and as a supplement to cardiopulmonary bypass or regional anaesthesia.

Volatile anaesthetic agents

More commonly, volatile or inhalational agents provide the basis of general anaesthesia. The differing physicochemical properties of the different volatile agents will affect their pharmacological effects. Thus, agents with low blood/gas solubilities (e.g. nitrous oxide, desflurane, and sevoflurane) will cause rapid onset and recovery of central nervous system effects. The oil/gas solubility provides one index of potency, defined in terms of the minimum alveolar concentration (MAC), which is the alveolar concentration preventing a response to a surgical incision in 50 per cent of subjects (Table 5).

Table 5 Minimal alveolar concentration values (indices of potency of inhalational anaesthetics).

Agent	MAC
Nitrous oxide	105–110
Halothane	0.75
Enflurane	1.68
Isoflurane	1.15
Desflurane	6–6.2
Sevoflurane	1.71

MAC = minimum alveolar concentration (concentration of anaesthetic in oxygen required to inhibit response to the initial surgical stimulus in 50 per cent of subjects, i.e. ED_{50}).

Nitrous oxide is a weak anaesthetic agent (minimum alveolar concentration 105–110 per cent), which cannot alone suppress the somatic, autonomic, or haemodynamic responses to noxious stimuli during clinical use. However addition of nitrous oxide at inspired concentrations of 60 to 70 per cent significantly decreases the dose requirements of other more potent volatile agents (as well as those of the hypnotic and opioid drugs). Relative contraindications to the use of nitrous oxide include the need for high inspired oxygen concentrations (e.g. during bronchoscopy and upper airway surgery), and its high diffusibility into air-filled spaces so increasing their volume or pressure: this occurs in the presence of a pneumothorax, after pneumoencephalography, after tympanoplasty, in patients with grossly dilated bowel due to intestinal obstruction, and where air embolism may occur. Nitrous oxide should be avoided if possible during the first 4 weeks of pregnancy, because of its effects on organogenesis: the arguments concerning its effect on theatre pollution are covered in the section on medico-legal issues below.

Halothane, enflurane, and isoflurane are highly potent volatile agents, but have narrow margins of safety between their anaesthetic effects and cardiovascular depressive properties. They therefore have to be administered by calibrated vapourizers. All three separate components of the anaesthetic triad may be achieved with these agents; however the concentrations required to achieve appropriate anaesthetic depth may result in excessive hypotension through the combination of myocardial depression, vascular smooth muscle relaxation, and depression of the sympathetic nervous system. Thus, the inspired drug concentration tends to be regulated according to an adverse effect of the volatile agents—cardiovascular depression. This is most significant with enflurane, and may be exaggerated in the patients with hypovolaemia or congestive cardiac failure. Cardiovascular depression is less severe with halothane; other side-effects which may favour the choice of halothane as the volatile supplement include low pungency and laryngeal irritability, bronchodilation, and uterine muscular relaxation.

Isoflurane exhibits all of the favourable properties of the other two volatile agents, combined with a faster uptake and elimination, and minimal biotransformation, with its associated reduced risk of renal and hepatic toxicity. Although isoflurane produces vasodilation, this is accompanied by a reflex increase in sympathetic activity that either maintains or increases both heart rate and cardiac output. However hypotension may occur in patients with decreased sympathetic reserve, such as those receiving β-adrenoceptor blocking drugs.

In appropriate concentrations, all three agents are able to control the hyperdynamic responses to noxious stimulation during surgery. Dose requirements for volatile agents can be reduced by combination therapy with other centrally acting drugs (hypnotics, sedatives, and opioids), as well as achieving relaxation through use of myoneural blocking drugs. Other non-hypnotic effects of the volatile agents include possible alterations in myocardial blood flow distribution with development of ischaemia (the so-called coronary steal phenomenon) with isoflurane; increased cerebral blood flow and intracranial pressure (seen with both halothane and enflurane in clinical concentrations, but with isoflurane only at concentrations above 1.5 per cent); risk of seizures during enflurane anaesthesia, especially in presence of hypocarbia; hepatotoxicity (with halothane, enflurane, and possibly isoflurane); fluoride-induced nephrotoxicity due to enflurane biotransformation; malignant hyperpyrexia (may be triggered by all three agents), and impaired cellular-mediated immunity.

Opioids

Opioid drugs may be given for premedication, introperative supplementation, or postoperative analgesia. As premedicants, or as supplements during anaesthesia, small doses of morphine (0.03–0.5 mg/kg) or pethidine (meperidine) (0.5–1.0 mg/kg) reduce the dosage requirements of the inhaled and other intravenous agents. Provided that ventilation is maintained, the side-effects of these doses are relatively minor and easily controlled. The newer synthetic opioids (fentanyl, sufentanil, and alfentanil) were developed to provide greater potency but with fewer side effects and greater margins of safety. Because of their minimal effects on the heart and circulation, opioids are sometimes used alone to maintain anaesthesia in high-risk patients. However, the major disadvantage of these agents when used alone is their limited anaesthetic efficacy (resulting in liability to awareness, recall, and sympathetic autonomic responses to noxious stimuli). In addition, large doses of opioids cause respiratory depression, necessitating postoperative respiratory support.

Adverse effects of anaesthetic agents

The safety of contemporary anaesthesia has been well documented; however, adverse effects may occur with all anaesthetic agents. Adverse effects of the volatile agents have been previously described. The adverse effects encountered with intravenous agents may be divided into non-hypnotic side-effects and anaphylactic or anaphylactoid responses.

Non-hypnotic adverse effects of intravenous anaesthetic agents

Overdose may be absolute, due to acute excess administration, or to accumulation as a result of reduced elimination or metabolism, or relative, due to patient factors such as hypovolaemia, extremes of age, intercurrent disease (especially cardiac, renal, or hepatic impairment), and drug–drug interactions. Other problems may be due to bacterial contamination of the agent or the use of incompatible drug mixtures. For example, precipitation occurs if thiopentone and *d*-tubocurarine, or vecuronium are administered in the same syringe, or via the same intravenous cannula without flushing between drugs. Exaggerated pharmacological effects which may occur include excessive hypotension or bradycardia. These are seen following administration of large doses of the intravenous hypnotic agents and opioids, respectively. Idiosyncratic effects are not predictable from the pharmacology of the individual drug. Examples include porphyria, malignant hyperpyrexia, plasma pseudocholinesterase deficiency, glucose 6-phosphate dehydrogenase deficiency, and the genetic polymorphism of drug metabolism—fast and slow acetylators of hydralazine, slow and fast hydroxylators of desbrisoquin, or propranolol.

The incidence of these adverse drug responses is higher than that of the true allergic or immunological reactions.

Anaphylactoid and anaphylactic reactions

Mechanisms of anaphylaxis

Most drugs administered during anaesthesia are of low molecular weight (less than 1000 Da). Alone they are not capable of initiating an immune response with the production of specific antibodies. However, many drugs are able to combine *in vivo* with a carrier protein (hapten) to form an antigenic moiety. The extent of basophil and mast cell degranulation induced depends on the amount of drug injected, the affinity of the drug for the antibodies, and the amount of cell-bound antibodies produced.

Anaphylactic reactions

These depend upon classical antigen–antibody interactions that activate the complement cascade via the classical pathway. Complement activation results in mast cell disruption and the release of histamine and other autocoids which increase vascular permeability, and so allow the passage of phagocytes from extravascular sites to enter the bloodstream and break down the antigens.

Anaphylactoid reactions

These occur as a result of a direct pharmacological effect or some other non-immunological response by which the drug causes release of histamine. Some drugs, particularly those with basic properties (e.g. *d*-tubocurarine, suxamethonium, morphine, thiobarbiturates, and trimetaphan), cause direct competitive displacement of histamine (another basic molecule) from the mast cell. As will be discussed later, predisposing factors exist which may also play a role in the genesis of these anaphylactoid responses.

The main aetiologies of these anaphylactoid hypersensitivity reactions to drugs can be subdivided into activation of the alternative pathway of complement and direct pharmacological effects.

Alternative complement pathway

Unlike the classical pathway, preformed antibodies to a particular antigen are not necessary for alternative pathway activation. Hence prior exposure to the drug or endotoxin is not necessary.

Direct pharmacological effects of drugs

Although adverse drug reactions may involve activation of one or other of the complement pathways, the majority are better described as anaphylactoid in nature, and occur as a result of a dose-related direct effect of the drug upon mast cells and basophils. Such reactions may be manifest as either local cutaneous signs, or as more severe systemic signs and symptoms of histamine release. With drugs such as thiopentone and some of the neuromuscular blocking agents, a flush and weal reaction is often seen following their intravenous injection. The systemic features of the reactions are usually mild (hypotension, tachycardia), and without the other stigmata of histamine release. Why some of these cases (for which no immunological basis will be found on subsequent testing) progress to more generalized systemic symptoms is uncertain.

Factors predisposing to the development of allergic reactions include patient factors, possible pharmacological factors, and potential at-risk patient groups.

Patient factors

Adverse reactions are rarer in children than in adults, but there is probably no sex difference in incidence. The apparently higher incidence in gynaecological patients may be related to pregnancy.

There is a high incidence of adverse reactions on first or subsequent exposure to certain IV anaesthetics in the pregnant patient, which may be due to the choice of drugs used for short gynaecological procedures. The immune status of these patients is also altered, and this may play a role.

Hypersensitivity reactions to IV anaesthetic drugs are more common in atopic individuals and asthmatics. The increased incidence of hypersensitivity reactions to first exposure in the atopic individual is small compared with the higher incidence of hypersensitivity reactions seen in patients receiving repeat administration of the same anaesthetic agent. The impression among some anaesthetists that adverse reactions are more common in nervous, anxious patients is not supported by any data. Apart from patients with a history of previous anaphylaxis or a proven sensitivity to one or more drugs, there are no other predictors of at-risk groups.

Pharmacological factors

Many of the intravenous anaesthetic agents are poorly water soluble and hence glycols, macrogols, and non-ionic surfactants are added to increase their solubility. These solvents may trigger complement activation.

Clinical features of allergic reactions

There is considerable variation in the severity and magnitude of the clinical features among different reactors. Factors that influence the severity of the symptoms include the amount of drug injected, the reactivity of basophils and mast cells; the responsiveness of the bronchial and vascular smooth muscle, and the activity of the autonomic nervous system. Control of peripheral autonomic nervous system activity is also regulated by higher centres. Thus, the increased emotional activity of the asthmatic patient prior to anaesthesia and surgery may both enhance any existing symptomatology, and exaggerate any adverse response to IV drug administration.

Table 6 Symptoms and signs occurring during acute hypersensitivity reactions to intravenous anaesthetic agents

Cutaneous flushing or development of an overt rash
Pruritus
Cough
Tachycardia
Bronchospasm
Hypotension
Cardiac arrest

The various symptoms that may occur during adverse reactions are shown (Table 6). The maximum intensity of the symptoms often occurs rapidly, usually within 30 min of IV drug administration. All of the clinical features can be attributed to mast cell and basophil degranulation, and this knowledge has been used in some of the methods used for preoperative prophylaxis in patients with a history of drug allergy. The usual order of the main clinical symptoms is skin changes, hypotension with tachycardia, and bronchospasm with resulting arterial hypoxia.

Skin changes are characterized by the classic triple response described by Lewis. Erythema is caused by dilatation of capillaries over the face, arms, and mantle; weal formation arises from increased vascular permeability causing fluid transudation, and flares are presumably due to an axon reflex response. Hypotension and tachycardia result from the transudation of fluid from the vascular to extravascular spaces. Histamine also causes vascular smooth muscle dilatation, and hence the venous pooling of blood may occur. The accompanying tachycardia is probably not a baroreflex response, but rather the chronotropic effect of increased circulating catecholamine levels following their release by histamine from the adrenal medulla. Bronchospasm is the most life-threatening of the symptoms, and treatment must primarily be aimed at preventing severe arterial hypoxia.

Following the successful treatment of an allergic reaction, the causative agent must be identified wherever possible. The laboratory diagnosis depends on the results of a number of routine haematology tests, including measurement of haematocrit. Changes in platelet and white cell numbers may be small, but of significance. Disappearance of basophils (expressed as a percentage of the total leucocyte count) is indicative of a type I response. Serial measurements should be made of the plasma concentrations of total IgE antibodies and complement proteins (C2, C4, and breakdown products C3a, C3b and C1 esterase inhibitor) during the 72 h after an adverse reaction. Metabolism of both C3 and C4 is indicative of an immune reaction which does not involve IgE antibodies, while C3 conversion alone is an indicator of a specific non-immune mechanism. In contrast to atopic patients who have increased levels of IgE, some individuals (10–20per cent) have very low levels of this immunoglobulin. Such people appear to be prone to non-immune mediated clinical reactions, and may produce positive intradermal tests to drugs which have a high potential for inducing histamine release.

Other *in-vivo* and *in-vitro* diagnostic tests which may be useful for later assessment to establish the identity of the drug responsible for the reaction include intradermal skin testing, the IgE

Table 7 Management of allergic reactions

AIMS:
- Correct arterial hypoxaemia
- Restore intravascular fluid volume
- Inhibition of further release of chemical mediators

ROUTINE
- STOP ADMINISTRATION OF ANTIGEN
- AIRWAY
- ADDED INSPIRED OXYGEN
- ADRENALINE—either intravenously, intramuscularly or via the endotracheal tube (depending on the severity of the reaction). Dose 4–8 μg IV for hypotension; 0.5 ml of 1:1000 (0.5 mg) for cardiovascular collapse
- FLUIDS—both crystalloids and colloids, although the former may be ineffective in some cases
- BRONCHODILATORS—if there is bronchospasm, give aminophylline or adrenaline. If during anaesthesia, consider use of halothane, diethyl ether, ketamine, or isoflurane for relief of bronchoconstriction
- POSITIVE PRESSURE VENTILATION—especially in cases of pulmonary oedema
- INOTROPES—to support circulation. Adrenaline 2–4 μg/min; noradrenaline 2–4 μg/min; isoprenaline 0.5–1 μg/min
- ANTIARRHYTHMICS
- CONSIDER CEREBRAL RESUSCITATION—if prolonged period of cardiac arrest or low output, or arterial hypoxaemia. Useful drugs include mannitol, dexamethasone, frusemide, IPPV with mild hypocapnia
- CORRECT ACIDOSIS
- NO BENEFIT FROM STEROIDS IN ACUTE PHASE; but methylprednisolone may be helpful in cases thought to be complement-mediated
- NO AGENT AFFECTS GASTROINTESTINAL SYMPTOMS
- ISOPRENALINE increases dead space, and may increase arterial hypoxaemia
- ANTIHISTAMINES only useful in angioneurotic oedema

inhibition test, leucocyte histamine release test, basophil degranulation test, radio-allergosorbent test, and delineation of specific antibodies.

Treatment of allergic reactions to drugs

The management of severe histamine release reactions has been comprehensively reviewed. The aims of treatment must be to correct hypoxia, inhibit further release of chemical mediators, and restore the vascular fluid volume (preferably with colloids). When the combination of adrenaline and adequate volume does not produce improvement, then noradrenaline may be lifesaving. Table 7 lists a management approach to allergic reactions.

There is considerable controversy as to whether steroids should be given routinely. Cortisol does not inhibit the allergen–antibody interaction, nor the release of vasoactive amine from mast cells and basophils. Thus, steroids are probably only indicated for the treatment of severe bronchospasm. Other stimulant drugs, such as isoprenaline, should only be given cautiously in the presence of cardiac arrhythmias or hypovolaemia. Vasoconstrictors should also be used with care, as they can provoke acute pulmonary oedema when coupled with rapid fluid infusion. Anticholinergic drugs, such as atropine, may attenuate the release of histamine by decreasing the intracellular concentrations of the second messenger, guanosine monophosphate. However, only limited data from which to draw conclusions are available. In cases of severe or intractable bronchospasm, there is need for drugs other than aminophylline. These include glucocorticoids, adrenaline, isoprenaline, salbutamol, and even general anaesthetic agents with bronchodilator properties (diethyl ether, halothane, ketamine, and isoflurane). Persistent vasodilatation can be reversed by dopamine, dobutamine, ephedrine, or adrenaline, given by repeat bolus doses or infusion. There is no evidence of any acute value in the administration of H_1 and H_2-blocking drugs; however these drugs may have a role in prophylaxis.

Management of these patients after recovery should include counselling and an explanation of the significance of hypersensitivity, reassurance as to future anaesthesia, and registration of the patient with Medic Alert or similar organizations. In addition, a clear summary of the reaction should be placed in the patient's notes, and sent to the general practitioner.

Management of the patient who has previously suffered an allergic reaction

Although the occurrence of a first exposure reaction of any drug is unpredictable, steps can be taken to prevent hypersensitivity reactions occurring on subsequent exposures. These include use of local rather than general anaesthesia where possible, although hypersensitivity to the ester type of local anaesthetics has been reported. When general anaesthesia is essential, the use of adequate preoperative anxiolysis and premedication may reduce stress. Preoperative prophylaxis should be aimed at both reducing histamine release, and at blocking its systemic effects. Sodium cromoglycate stabilizes mast cells, and so prevents degranulation and histamine release, salbutamol prevents bronchospasm, and hydrocortisone antihistamines (H_1-receptor antagonists; e.g. chlorpheniramine or terfenadine and H_2-receptor antagonists e.g. cimetidine or ranitidine) may also be administered. The last two groups of drugs inhibit histamine release, but also compete at the receptors to attenuate the decreases in systemic vascular resistance.

Repeat exposure to any drug that the patient has received intravenously in the recent past should be avoided and inhalational agents rather than IV agents should be used whenever possible, although caution should be taken to avoid repeat exposures to halothane. Plasma expanders such as Haemacel and Dextran should not be used.

LOCAL ANAESTHETICS

These produce a transient and completely reversible blockade of nerve function, and hence an interruption of sensory perception. The first agent used in clinical practice was cocaine, described for ophthalmological surgery by Köhler in 1884. Procaine, the archetypal aminoester was synthesized in 1905, while the amide anaesthetic lignocaine (lidocaine) was introduced in 1943.

Local anaesthetics act by blocking sodium channels in the axon membrane and inhibiting sodium conductance, whilst having minimal effects on potassium currents. Other pharmacological actions relate to their interaction with calcium ions, perhaps by inhibiting the binding of calcium ions to phosphatidylserine.

The anaesthetics bind to a receptor site at the internal opening of the sodium channel, and some drugs such as benzocaine may actually penetrate the nerve membrane and cause conformational changes which lead to a decrease in the diameter of the sodium channel. Most of the local anaesthetic drugs have a pK_a value close to physiological pH, and will therefore exist in both ionized and unionized forms. Diffusion of drugs through the epineurium and nerve membrane can only occur in the unionized form, the fractions in the two forms being governed by the Henderson–Hasselbach relationship ($pH = pK_a + \log \text{ionized/unionized}$). Blockade of the sodium channels is therefore dependent upon the presence of the ionized form of the local anaesthetic. Following blockade of these channels, there is a decrease in the rate and degree of the depolarization phase of the action potential, with failure to achieve the threshold potential and therefore no development of a propagated action potential.

Structure–activity relationships of local anaesthetic agents

Two types of drug can be recognised clinically—esters, such as cocaine, procaine, chloroprocaine, and tetracaine, and amides which include prilocaine, lignocaine, mepivacaine, and bupivacaine. The ester drugs are readily broken down by hydrolyase enzymes (e.g. plasma cholinesterase), and hence tend to be shorter acting. The amide drugs are broken down in the liver. One of the metabolites of the ester local anaesthetic drugs is para-amino benzoic acid, which is capable of inducing allergic reactions in some patients. The pharmacological properties of the different local anaesthetic agents are related to their lipid solubility, protein binding and pK_a values (Table 8).

Table 8 Physicochemical properties of different local anaesthetic agents in current clinical use

	pK_a	Lipid solubility	Protein binding (%)
Esters			
Procaine	8.9	0.02	5.8
Chloroprocaine	8.7	0.14	–
Tetracaine	8.6	4.1	75.6
Amides			
Prilocaine	7.7	0.9	55
Lignocaine	7.7	2.9	64.3
Mepivacaine	7.6	0.8	77.5
Bupivacaine	8.1	27.5	96

Lipid solubility is the primary determinant of anaesthetic potency, while protein binding influences the duration of anaesthetic activity. Procaine and chloroprocaine are agents with low potency and short duration, lignocaine, mepivacaine, and prilocaine have intermediate effects, and tetracaine and bupivicaine have long duration of effect with high potency.

The duration of effect of a local anaesthetic agent can be prolonged by addition of a vasoconstrictor such as adrenaline which decreases the rate of vascular absorption of drug from the site of administration. As well as producing conduction blockade, local anaesthetics have other important adverse effects on the cardiovascular and central nervous systems, and the neuromuscular junction.

Most local anaesthetic agents readily cross the blood–brain barrier, initially causing excitation and then, at higher doses, central nervous system depression. There is good correlation between the plasma concentration of lignocaine and associated central nervous system toxicity. At pharmacological concentrations, local anaesthetic agents exert effects on cardiac and peripheral vascular smooth muscle to cause arterial dilation and myocardial depression. At toxic concentrations, the combined effects of peripheral vasodilation, depressed myocardial contractility and depression of the heart rate and myocardial conducting pathways may result in circulatory collapse and cardiac arrest. Some of the local anaesthetic agents, such as procaine, have a quinidine-like effect on the heart, increasing the refractory period, raising the threshold for stimulation and prolonging the conduction time. Local anaesthetic agents also affect transmission at the neuromuscular junction, and may potentiate the effects of both depolarizing and non-depolarizing muscle relaxants.

In addition to these three main adverse effects, IV or topically administered local anaesthetic agents also have the ability to suppress the haemodynamic responses to laryngoscopy and endotracheal intubation, as well as decreasing the minimum alveolar concentration, and hence dose maintenance requirements, for volatile anaesthetic agents.

Systemic toxicity of local anaesthetic agents

Accidental intravascular injection of an excessive amount of local anaesthetic into the epidural space can cause profound systemic effects. Toxicity is related to type of local anaesthetic agent and total dose administered, site of injection, rate of injection (intravascular injection), use of vasoconstrictors, and is increased in shock where relatively more of the cardiac output is directed to the heart and brain. Acidosis also increases toxicity.

The toxic effects which occur with lignocaine are directly related to the blood concentration as shown in Table 9.

In general, the cardiovascular system is more resistant to the effects of local anaesthetic drugs than is the central nervous system, the dose ratio being of the order of 3.5 to 6.7:1. However, this ratio is low for bupivacaine, and this has resulted in cases of

Table 9 Toxic effects associated with lignocaine

Lignocaine (mcg/ml)	Reaction
2–4	Antiarrhythmic Circumoral numbness Dizziness Irrational behaviour
6	Visual disturbances
8	Muscular weakness
10	Unconsciousness
20	Respiratory arrest
25	Cardiovascular depression

Table 10 Maximum doses and signs of toxicity for commonly used local anaesthetic agents

	Maximum dose (mg)		Important toxic side-effects
	Plain	With adrenaline	
Amethocaine	100	–	Cardiac depression, may cause asystole and ventricular fibrillation
Bupivacaine	175	250	Cardiotoxicity, drowsiness, convulsions
Cinchocaine	50	–	
Chloroprocaine	800	1000	Neurotoxicity Prolongation of effect of suxamethonium
Cocaine	200	–	Sympathetic stimulation, excitement, restlessness, headache, vomiting, myocardial depression, cardiac arrhythmias
Etidocaine	300	400	Less toxic than bupivacaine
Lignocaine	300	500	Convulsions, twitching, psychotic reactions
Mepivacaine	350	500	Less cardiotoxic than bupivacaine
Prilocaine	400	600	Methaemoglobinaemia
Procaine	500	700	CNS toxicity, may prolong the effect of suxamethonium, reduced procaine metabolism in patients with deficiency of pseudocholinesterase

Amide drugs (bupivacaine, cinchocaine, etidocaine, lignocaine, mepivacaine, prilocaine) have all been reported to precipitate malignant hyperpyrexia.

cardiovascular collapse following release of the tourniquet in patients given bupivacaine for intravenous regional analgesia, and following the use of 0.75 per cent bupivacaine in obstetric epidural practice. Cardiotoxicity appears to be related to the physicochemical characteristics of the local anaesthetic agents—namely high potency, high lipid solubility, and high plasma protein binding, and appears to be increased in the pregnant patient. The predisposition to ventricular arrhythmogenicity is due to the presence of butyl groups within the local anaesthetic side-chains (seen with bupivacaine but not with mepivacaine). Toxicity is influenced by acid–base status, hypercapnia, and acidosis reducing the threshold for convulsive activity and the threshold for cardiac depression. Other systemic effects, apart from the allergic reactions and those listed above, include development of methaemoglobinaemia, neurotoxicity, and initiation of episodes of malignant hyperpyrexia (see Table 10).

Systemic toxicity can be prevented by the establishment of venous access in all patients before the institution of regional anaesthesia, by the use of appropriate doses (Table 10), by checking for accidental intravenous administration, and by using vasoconstrictors (to reduce systemic absorption) whenever possible.

If systemic toxicity does occur, oxygen should be administered, with careful monitoring of cardiovascular effects, and convulsive or CNS excitatory activity should be treated with diazepam or midazolam. Facilities for intubation and ventilation as well as drugs for support of the circulation should be available at all times.

Allergic reactions to local anaesthetic agents

Allergic responses to local anaesthetic agents in current use are rare (constituting probably less than 1 per cent of all reactions to drugs). In most patients, other causes of drug reactions are responsible, e.g. systemic toxicity, simple fainting, or reactions to added adrenaline. The recommended maximum dosage of these agents is shown in Table 10.

The ester group of local anaesthetics is more liable to provoke adverse reactions as these drugs contain both a *p*-aminobenzoic acid group, and methyl- or propyl-paraben as the added preservative. The systemic effects of adrenaline are undoubtedly the cause of some of the reported adverse reactions to the local anaesthetics. Use of 1/800 000 adrenaline in dental anaesthesia is frequently accompanied by tachycardia, palpitation, and chest tightness, although angina is rare.

Hypersensitivity reactions to the amide anaesthetic agents are unusual, but allergy to lignocaine has been reported.

SPECIFIC ASPECTS OF ANAESTHESIA

The surgeon or anaesthetist may also be required to attend patients presenting with specific problems where an appreciation of the problems encountered by the anaesthetist are important.

Neuroanaesthesia

Physiology

Cerebral blood flow is maintained constant despite changes in perfusion pressure: this phenomenon is termed autoregulation and is also seen in the renal circulation. The normal cerebral blood flow is 44 ml/100 g tissue/min which equates to between 600 and 800 ml/min in an adult brain. Regional blood flow varies with grey matter receiving 80 ml/100 g/min and white matter 20 ml/100 g/min. Approximately 85 per cent of cerebral blood flow is supplied by the carotid circulation, and the remainder by the vertebral arteries. The cerebral oxygen consumption (measured as cerebral metabolic rate for oxygen, $CMRO_2$) is of prime importance in anaesthesia for neurosurgical patients, since blood flow to the brain is frequently impaired due to raised intracranial pressure. The normal $CMRO_2$ is about 3 ml/100 g tissue/min. Beyond certain limits, autoregulation of cerebral blood flow is lost and perfusion pressure determines cerebral blood flow. Autoregulation is maintained within a range of perfusion pressures of 60 to 150 mmHg. The mechanism of autoregulation is not fully understood, and several theories have been advanced. These include a direct response to distension from perfusion pressure (myogenic theory or Bayliss effect), metabolic theory (local metabolic vasodilator products control arteriolar smooth muscle diameter directly), and a prominent role for innervation of cerebral blood vessels, although the role of autonomic factors in controlling autoregulation is not clear.

Intracranial pressure

Factors influencing intracranial pressure include production of cerebrospinal fluid. This is produced by the choroid plexus at a rate of about 0.4 ml/min and is subsequently reabsorbed by the arachnoid villi. Other factors are cerebral blood flow, venous pressure—a raised venous pressure due to coughing or straining is reflected in a rise in intracranial pressure, and arterial CO_2. An elevated $Pa\text{CO}_2$ causes marked vasodilation. The time course of this effect has been disputed but ranges of 20 s to 5 to 8 min have been quoted. Cerebrovascular disease reduces but does not abolish CO_2 responsiveness of vessels. Oxygen availability also has an effect on intracranial pressure, which increases in response to a lowered arterial $P\text{O}_2$ at levels below about 40 mmHg. The combination of hypoxia and hypercarbia has a synergistic effect on cerebral blood flow. High oxygen concentrations have a mild vasoconstrictor effect which is more marked under hyperbaric conditions. Brain bulk changes affect intracranial pressure, and the effect is determined by the extent and the rate of change. Compliance curves can be plotted for intracranial pressure against intracranial volume and these show that within physiological limits, compensatory mechanisms maintain a relatively constant intracranial pressure. However, when compensatory mechanisms are exhausted, further increases in intracranial volume (blood clot, etc) produce greater increases in intracranial pressure.

Variations in perfusion

Normally, cerebral blood flow matches tissue perfusion needs; however areas of brain with localized damage, such as may occur near tumours, trauma, or infarcts, may receive blood flow in excess of their metabolic needs. This has been termed 'luxury perfusion syndrome' and is due to a localized loss of autoregulation. If carbon dioxide levels are raised, nearby intact autoregulated vessels will dilate causing a reduced blood flow through the areas of adjacent damaged non-autoregulating vessels, the 'intracerebral steal effect'. If, however, carbon dioxide levels are lowered, normal vessels vasoconstrict and hence blood flow increases to the damaged areas (inverse steal or Robin Hood syndrome).

Pathophysiology of space–occupying lesions

Trauma produces a large increase in brain bulk due to clot formation, localized oedema from damaged cells and cellular disruption. Gunshot wounds produce the greatest rise in intracranial pressure because of the effects of the velocity of the projectile. Intracerebral aneurysms in themselves rarely produce a large increase in intracranial pressure. However, an episode of bleeding is followed by a marked rise in pressure due to the clot formation and cerebral oedema associated with damage to neurones. Cerebral arteriovenous malformations may be functional space-occupying lesions even in the absence of haemorrhage. Tumours, abscesses, and hydrocephalus also affect intracranial pressure.

Compensatory mechanisms

The ability of compensatory mechanisms to act is dependent on the rate of rise of intracranial pressure as well as the integrity of the responses and the region involved. A slow growing meningioma in the posterior fossa may reach substantial size before causing problems due to raised intracranial pressure, whereas a rapidly expanding intracerebral haematoma may cause pressure related symptoms quickly.

Control of intracranial pressure

Osmotic diuretics produce a transient reduction in total body water, including that in the cerebrum. Mannitol is the principal agent currently employed, a dose of 1 to 1.5 g/kg being given IV over about 20 min. Mannitol may cause a rise in blood pressure if administered rapidly, and in the presence of blood–brain barrier damage it may leak out and cause fluid retention in these regions. For this reason, many anaesthetists prefer frusemide in doses of 20–40 mg IV, which produces a rapid diuresis without these potential adverse effects.

Hypoxia and hypercarbia have a synergistic effect, increasing cerebral vasodilation and hence intracerebral blood flow. Arterial oxygen tension should be maintained above 100 mmHg and $Pa\text{CO}_2$ should not exceed 40 mmHg (5.3 kPa). During anaesthesia, $Pa\text{CO}_2$ should be maintained in the range 25 to 30 mmHg (3.3–4 kPa). The elderly are less tolerant of prolonged hypocardia which has been shown to lead to postoperative memory impairment.

Cortisone, dexamethasone, and hydrocortisone have also been used to control intracranial pressure. The maximal effect is exerted on the oedema surrounding cerebral tumours. If steroids have been administered for a prolonged period of time, the risk of adrenal suppression becomes significant and gradual tapering off rather than abrupt cessation of therapy should occur.

Hypothermia is effective in reducing cerebral metabolic needs and hence provides protection against cerebral hypoxia. Technically it is very difficult to achieve: surface cooling methods are generally slow and cumbersome and the possibility of overshoot to below a core temperature of about 32°C leads to an increasing risk of ventricular irritability and difficult-to-treat ventricular arrhythmias occur. Cardiopulmonary bypass has been used intraoperatively but problems of haemostasis and technical difficulty have limited its adoption.

Lumbar drainage of cerebrospinal fluid may be used to increase exposure to the pituitary gland and to aneurysms which have not bled. Its use in patients with raised intracranial pressure is potentially hazardous due to the likelihood of herniation of the cerebellar tonsils through the foramen magnum, or 'coning'. In certain cases neurosurgeons may use an intraoperative ventricular tap to drain cerebrospinal fluid and thus assist exposure.

Anaesthetic aspects

Anaesthetic drugs affect intracranial pressure through their effects on cerebral vasodilatation and on the cerebral metabolic rate for oxygen. Some agents, such as methohexitone and enflurane, also have an effect on the seizure threshold. Postoperative somnolence or respiratory depression may cause significant problems following infusions of opiates and barbiturate. Anaesthetic doses of thiopentone reduce cerebral blood flow and $CMRO_2$. For this reason, thiopentone has been widely used in neuroanaesthesia. However, its infusion is associated with delayed recovery because of its partial metabolism to an active, more slowly cleared metabolite (pentobarbitone) and to a saturation of the hepatic metabolic pathways. Ketamine causes a dose-dependent rise in cerebral blood flow of 61 per cent; if 67 to 70 per cent nitrous oxide is administered as well, there are further increases in $CMRO_2$ (by up to 16 to 20 per cent). For these reasons, it is not used in neuroanaesthesia.

Of the volatile anaesthetic agents, halothane is a potent cerebral vasodilator and causes an increase in cerebral blood flow of about 13 per cent. Enflurane also increases cerebral blood flow, but of greater significance is its production of EEG abnormalities. For these reasons neither agent is used in neuroanaesthesia. Isoflurane at doses below 1 per cent has been shown to produce minimal change in cerebral blood flow or $CMRO_2$ and for these reasons it is widely used in neuroanaesthesia. In concentrations above 1 per cent, isoflurane increases the intracranial pressure in hydrocephalic patients, and then its use is not recommended until the brain has been surgically decompressed.

Anaesthesia for neurosurgical patients

The assessment of these patients may be very difficult due to the lack of co-operation accompanying confusion associated with raised intracranial pressure. The level of consciousness and whether this is stable or fluctuates should be noted. A history of early morning headaches, vomiting, or photophopia is indicative of raised intracranial pressure. If there is a significant impairment of conscious state, a history should be obtained from relatives, because of difficulties in eliciting drug allergies, medications, and previous anaesthetic problems from people with impaired levels of consciousness. Adequate physical examination is frequently difficult in patients who have significantly raised intracranial pressure because of lack of co-operation. A full neurological examination need not normally be performed by the anaesthetist.

Trauma patients should have a thorough examination to exclude possible sites of concealed blood loss or active bleeding: these may be very difficult to diagnose or treat once a craniotomy is proceeding. Assessment should also include likelihood of cervical spine damage, pneumothorax, or lung trauma, as these will have a marked bearing on intraoperative and postoperative management. The combination of significant head and chest injuries is usually an indication for postoperative respiratory support because of the importance of maintaining optimal oxygenation postoperatively and the difficulties of performing adequate chest physiotherapy in people with impaired consciousness. Patients with profound rises in intracranial pressure may manifest pulmonary oedema. The aetiology is uncertain but is believed to be mediated centrally via catecholamine release. Hypertension also frequently accompanies severe raised intracranial pressure.

Laboratory investigations should include serum urea and electrolytes, haemoglobin, and clotting studies. Patients over 40 years should also have chest radiographs and ECG performed.

A detailed account of the anaesthetic considerations in all neurosurgical conditions is not appropriate. However aspects relating to the more frequently encountered problems will be mentioned.

Management of trauma patients is influenced by the need to protect the patient's airway because of faciomaxillary damage and impaired conscious state, the need for respiratory support because of impaired respiratory drive or thoracic problems, management of acute blood loss from other sites, and the possibility of coexisting cervical spine injury.

Anaesthesia is usually induced on the operating table with monitoring equipment attached to the patient. All trauma patients should be assumed to have a full stomach and thus a rapid sequence induction technique is used. Cervical spine damage should usually be assumed unless it is actually excluded by imaging or, more rarely, by a good history of the injury sustained. Monitoring will be determined mainly by the other injuries sustained, but would normally include ECG, blood pressure, oximetry, and inspired oxygen content. A urinary catheter should be *in situ*. Maintenance of anaesthesia will vary with anaesthetist's preference and patient's condition; however use of agents causing cerebral vasodilation or increased cerebral metabolic rate, such as ketamine, halothane, or enflurane, are usually avoided.

Patients with severe multiple injuries or significant combined head and chest injuries usually require respiratory support in the intensive care unit. No hard and fast rules can be given regarding postoperative management, but the maintenance of optimal respiratory function is of paramount importance. The Pao_2 should be maintained above 100 mmHg (13.3 kPa) and the $Paco_2$ should be below 40mmHg (5.3 kPa). Antiepileptic medication is routinely given intraoperatively because of the risk of seizures.

Anaesthetic considerations for outpatient anaesthesia

Outpatient anaesthesia has progressed in both the United States and Europe from the performance of simple procedures under local anaesthesia to the total anaesthetic care of patients with complex medical problems. This allows costs per patient per operation and disruption of the patient's personal life to be reduced and also decreases the risk of exposure to hospital-acquired infections.

Preoperative evaluation and patient selection

Patients scheduled for outpatient surgery must be willing and able to comply with both preoperative and postoperative instructions. Although initial experiences in most day surgery units were limited to ASA group I and II patients (American Society of Anesthesiologists classification of stress), some units are now accepting medically stable ASA group III patients. The imposition of a rigid age range is illogical as there appears to be no age-related increase in recovery time or incidence of postoperative anaesthetic complications.

Careful selection of patients is of prime importance to the efficient running of a day surgical unit. A full history and physical examination are required before surgery and this can be conducted either by the surgeon in the outpatient clinic or by the anaesthetist. The latter may see patients either in a special pre-anaesthetic assessment clinic, or by prior arrangement in the day-care unit. Details of the patient's past medical and drug histories can be obtained readily by a simple questionnaire completed at the outpatient clinic. In many centres, this questionnaire alone is used as the major screening tool in deciding the suitability of the patient for day case anaesthesia and surgery.

Preoperative assessment should also include the facility for performing simple laboratory tests, depending on the patient's age, state of health and concurrent drug history. For young healthy outpatients undergoing body surface surgery, there is no evidence of the value of any routine laboratory tests for male patients, and only a haemoglobin estimation is worthwhile for females. Patients with controlled chronic diseases (hypertension, diabetes mellitus) will require additional laboratory screening (electrolytes, urea or creatinine, blood sugar) as appropriate.

There is considerable disagreement between the United States and Great Britain over the length of surgery that can be performed on an outpatient basis. In the United Kingdom, much surgery is limited to less than 30 min duration, while in the United States, operations lasting 2 to 3 h are successfully conducted in many outpatient facilities. Studies have shown no correlation between anaesthetic time and recovery (or discharge) time.

One of the major causes of 'surgical' readmissions following out-patient surgery is inadequate pain relief; hence the adequate provision of pain relief is of paramount importance. Although injection of long-acting local anaesthetic drugs (bupivacaine, mepivacaine) at the site of incision may help to decrease postoperative analgesic requirements, pain can be controlled in many patients with conventional oral analgesic drugs such as codeine, paracetamol, mefenamic acid, and dextropropoxyphene. The recent introduction of the non-steroidal anti-inflammatory agents diclofenac and ketorolac, with their 'morphine sparing effects' has led to a major reconsideration of the methods of providing analgesia for the outpatient.

Premedication

The use of premedication in the outpatient setting has been the subject of much debate and interest: although it has been stated (without supporting data) that premedication prolongs the recovery period, appropriate premedication (e.g. rapid and short-acting analgesic drugs) may decrease recovery times as a result of their ability to reduce anaesthetic requirements. Furthermore, premedication with analgesic or sedative drugs does not appear to increase the percentage of outpatients at risk of developing aspiration pneumonitis. However, excess administration of centrally acting sedative and analgesic drugs has been shown to impair motor co-ordination and psychomotor performance for up to 5 to 12 h.

Because outpatients may have a greater residual gastric volume than inpatients at the time of induction of anaesthesia, many authorities have recommended the routine administration of oral antacids, with or without gastrokinetic agents, before outpatient surgery. Unfortunately, colloid antacid suspensions can produce serious pulmonary sequelae if aspirated, and the reliability and efficacy of a single dose (30 ml) of sodium citrate has been questioned. Moreover, the use of oral antacids will *per se* increase the residual gastric volume. Histamine H_2-receptor antagonists and the gastrokinetic agents metoclopramide and cisapride are of greater efficacy.

Since prolonged fasting does not guarantee complete gastric emptying, there is further controversy over the length of the period of fasting before outpatient surgery, especially as there is good evidence that preoperative hunger and thirst contribute significantly to preoperative anxiety. Furthermore, prolonged fasting may result in the patient arriving in the anaesthetic room with a plasma glucose concentration of less than 4 mmol/l. Ingestion of 150 ml of water as late as 2 h prior to surgery has been reported to decrease significantly the severity of thirst without increasing the gastric volume in fasted outpatients.

Postoperative nausea and vomiting is a common problem after general anaesthesia, and can delay discharge as well as leading to unexpected hospital admissions from outpatient facilities. Factors alleged to increase the incidence of nausea and vomiting include body habitus, type of surgery (laparoscopy, orchidopexy, strabismus surgery, therapeutic terminations of pregnancy), assisted ventilation using a face mask (with the resultant passage of air into the stomach) and poor choice of anaesthetic agents (e.g. combinations involving all or some of fentanyl, etomidate, nitrous oxide, isoflurane). Droperidol (5–75 μg/kg IV) has been found to be an effective prophylactic antiemetic in both children and adults undergoing treatment as outpatients. Other authors favour the combination of low dose droperidol (0.5–1.0 mg IV) and metoclopramide. Other promising treatments include transdermal hyoscine, and the newer drugs domperidone and ondansetron.

Anaesthesia

The ideal outpatient anaesthetic agent should provide rapid and smooth onset of hypnosis, intraoperative amnesia and analgesia, good surgical conditions, and a short recovery period with minimal or no complications. There are no good criteria for excluding endotracheal intubation as part of any outpatient anaesthetic technique, although the introduction of the largyneal mask has reduced the need for endotracheal intubations where neuromuscular relaxation is not required. Of greatest importance to the efficient and safe conduct of outpatient anaesthesia and surgery is the seniority of the operators. The outpatient facility is not the remit of either junior anaesthetists or surgeons in training; cases should be managed by senior personnel experienced in the types of anaesthesia and surgery best suited to the patients.

POSTOPERATIVE PAIN RELIEF

There is an increased awareness of deficiencies in the traditional management of peroperative pain. In recent years there has been rapid expansion of knowledge of both the mechanisms of pain and alternative approaches to pain control. One of the major problems in pain management has always been the objective assessment of pain and the problems related to observer bias by medical and nursing staff. By defining pain as 'what the patient says hurts', we can remove this bias. The inadequacy of the traditional intramuscular opioid regimen is generally acknowledged and the incidence of inadequate pain relief by this method varies between 25 and 70 per cent.

A patient's analgesic requirements may be affected by surgical factors such as site of surgery and type of incision, anaesthetic factors, including type of anaesthesia and incidence of vomiting, patient factors, including age and sex, concurrent drug therapy, and psychological factors, such as cultural background, past experience, the understanding of pain, fear, and anxiety, and the ability of the patient to cope. Past bad experiences can affect later treatment of pain.

Physiological effects of pain

Pain and its inadequate control may affect many body systems, resulting in morbidity. Decreased O_2 and increased CO_2 due to diaphragmatic splinting and impaired intercostal muscle function will cause a decreased tidal volume and decreased functional residual volume. This may lead to sputum retention, atelectasis, decreased cough and infection. Sympathetic stimulation causes tachycardia and hypertension which can lead to myocardial ischaemia, increased peripheral resistance, and increased O_2 consumption. Reduced mobility because of pain may increase the incidence of deep vein and pulmonary thromboembolism. Increased gastric statis and reduced intestinal motility increase the incidence of postoperative vomiting. Other problems include urinary retention, restlessness, anxiety, increased postoperative confusion and impaired sleeping, and endocrine effects including increases in cortisol, catecholamines, aldosterones, and ADH. This results in sodium and water retention, and the anti-insulin effects of those hormones worsen diabetic control.

Opioid receptors

Opioid receptors were first identified in 1973, and the endogenous opioids were isolated in 1975. The enkephalins, endorphins, and other endogenous peptides are released in response to pain. Five receptor sub-types have been identified: mu, delta, kappa, sigma, and epsilon (Table 11).

Side-effects of opioids are generally dose-dependent. Respiratory effects include respiratory depression, impaired CO_2 response, and suppressed cough reflex.

Table 11 Different pharmacological properties attributable to the various types of opioid receptor

	Opioid receptors		
Effect	μ	κ	σ
Analgesia	Supraspinal and spinal	Supraspinal	–
Respiration	Depressed	Depressed	Increased
Mood	Euphoria	Sedation or dysphoria	Dysphoria
Pupil size	Miosis	Miosis	Mydriasis
Morphine withdrawal	Suppressed	?Suppressed	Not suppressed

Effects on the central nervous system include sedation, euphoria, miosis, nausea and vomiting, and muscle rigidity after high doses of opiates.

Other side effects include myocardial depression (dose-dependent), reduced myocardial oxygen consumption, vasodilation due to direct histamine release, bradycardia, delayed gastric emptying and gastrointestinal motility, and some opiates may cause spasm of the spincter of Oddi. Retention of urine and itching may also occur. Potency varies between opiates, but the maximal effect is similar.

Approaches to pain management (Table 12)

The so-called multimodal approach to pain relief employs combinations of different agents and techniques to control postoperative pain. The pre-emptive use of analgesics allows doses of opioids to be reduced: once pain is established, pain relief requires higher total doses, with the associated increase in incidence of undesirable effects such as sedation and respiratory depression. Combining opioids with local anaesthetic agents and prostaglandin synthetase inhibitors (non-steroidal anti-inflammatory drugs) further reduces total opioid dosage and increases the safety margin. The role of anxiety in postoperative pain and the importance of reducing anxiety by explanation and reassurance should be appreciated and incorporated in overall pain management.

Table 12 Different therapeutic approaches available for the management of acute postoperative pain

OPIOIDS
- Intramuscular (as required)
- Oral opioids
- Intravenous infusion
- Patient controlled analgesia (PCA)*
- Epidural opiates bolus or via syringe pump*

LOCAL ANAESTHETIC AGENTS
- Nerve blocks
- Interpleural catheter*
- Plexus blocks
- Indwelling epidural catheter*

NSAIDs*

COMBINATION TECHNIQUES
- Epidural opioids and local anaesthetic agents*
- NSAIDs and opioids*

* Newer techniques—the efficacy remains to be established in all patient groups.

Intramuscular opioids, as required

With this regimen, a fixed, prescribed dose of opioid is given as required. There are many problems with this system. Failure may occur because of pharmacokinetic factors, such as variability in absorption, distribution, metabolism, and excretion. Plasma concentrations of morphine are a poor reflection of the drug concentration in the central nervous system. Pharmacodynamic factors may also result in failure of pain relief: the 'minimum effective analgesic concentration' shows a four- to five-fold variability in surgical patients undergoing the same operation. Administration factors also play a role. The delay between the patient perceiving pain and nursing staff being able to administer opiate means that there is frequently a significant painful period between doses. The interpatient variability in dose requirement is not appreciated and patients with higher dose requirements are inadequately treated.

Oral opioids

These can be given as solutions or tablets, or as sustained-release suppositories (e.g. morphine sulphate, sustained release tablets, MST)). However, the vomiting and delayed gastric emptying which follows some surgery means that drugs are poorly absorbed and have variable efficacy. In addition, some opioids undergo extensive first pass or presystemic metabolism in the walls of the intestine and the liver before entering the circulation; this reduces their bioavailability. The effective dose is less than the administered dose.

Intravenous infusions

One of the disadvantages of intramuscular or intravenous bolus dosing is the constantly changing plasma drug concentration, causing either toxic effects or subtherapeutic ineffective concentrations over a period of time.

A drug infused at a constant rate takes five half-lives to reach steady state. For morphine, which has a $T_{1/2}$ of 1.5 to 4 h, 20 h may be needed to reach a stable analgesic level. A loading dose is needed, yet this is often forgotten when altering infusion rates. Problems arise when a plateau is established which is too high or low compared with the therapeutic window. Drug or metabolites may accumulate, particularly when rates are not reduced with reducing requirements. Requirements reduce markedly after 24 to 48 h and at night during sleep, allowing for reduction of infusion rates.

Respiratory depression and hypoxia are a significant complication with all opioid administration techniques, but these are especially seen with constant rate intravenous infusions, and hence careful respiratory monitoring is mandatory. Because the rate of increase of the plasma opioid concentration is slow, the infusion allowed may not provide total analgesia, so necessitating 'intravenous bolus top-up doses.

Patient controlled analgesia

This modification of intravenous infusion techniques uses a computerized syringe pump to deliver bolus doses whenever the patient presses a button. A lockout period ensures that the full effect of the dose is achieved before patient can deliver more drug. Advantages include reduction in swings in blood concentration and reduced side-effects, removal of observer bias or judgement of analgesic requirements and tailoring drug requirements to changing analgesic needs. Some studies have also suggested a reduced total requirement.

Local anaesthetic blocks

The most commonly used local anaesthetic agents are lignocaine, prilocaine, and bupivacaine. The duration of effect varies, but most blocks will provide 2 to 4 h of analgesia; occasionally the effect will last for 8 to 12 h. The advantages of this technique are that profound analgesia can be produced without opioid side-effects and without respiratory depression. However, although local blocks can block wound pain, tissue-related pain is not relieved. In addition, toxic side-effects of local anaesthetics limit the volume of agent which can be used and there is a risk of damage to adjacent structures or tissues, including intravenous or intra-arterial injection, pneumothorax, haemorrhage, infection, and permanent nerve damage.

Techniques for the administration of local anaesthetic blocks include wound infiltration, nerve blocks, epidural blocks, paravertebral blockade, and intrapleural blockade. The role of the last is still to be evaluated. The advantage of the last two techniques is that, unlike epidural blockade, there is no effect on limb or bladder innervation, and no sympathetic blockade.

Oral non-opioid drugs

These may be classified into the peripheral acting, non-steroidal anti-inflammatory drugs and centrally acting drugs such as paracetamol and nefopam. Paracetamol (acetaminophen) has analgesic and antipyretic effects, but no anti-inflammatory activity. High doses can cause hepato- and nephrotoxicity. Non-steroidal anti-inflammatory drugs all act by inhibition of prostaglandin synthase. However, their potency as inhibitors of this enzyme does not parallel their therapeutic efficacy; other factors are involved. Since they are weak acids, they accumulate in the parietal cells of the stomach and inhibit local prostaglandins that are responsible for a protective role in the mucosa. This action is possibly responsible for the high incidence of gastric irritation, although newer drugs have a lesser effect on the stomach.

Newer drugs which may have a role in postoperative pain relief are diclofenac, piroxicam, and ketoralac. They have several important properties: when used as adjuvants to conventional therapy; they have been shown to exhibit a 'morphine-sparing' effect; in conjunction with opioids, they may lessen the incidence of opioid-induced side-effects; and they can be given orally, rectally or intramuscularly. These drugs are the current first-line treatment for mild to moderate pain, and especially for bone pain. First choice drugs are the propionic acid derivatives (ibuprofen and ketoprofen, or naproxen); other drugs include salicyclates (where the adverse effects may be reduced by taking the drug with food) or benoylate; while third choice are drugs such as indomethacin, sulindac, and folmetin.

Mixed opioid agonist–antagonists, and partial agonist drugs

These have been advocated as suitable analgesic agents for postoperative pain relief without the side-effects of pure opioid agonists. The archetypal mixed agonist–antagonist was nalorphine, which acts as an antagonist at low doses. In higher doses, it has mild agonist properties. The partial agonists act at the κ and δ receptors as well as the μ receptors. Examples include buprenorphine and butorphanol.

Epidural opiates and local anaesthetic agents

The epidural space is bounded by the ligamentatum flavum and dura. By placing a catheter in this space, continuous administration of epidural opiates is possible. More lipid soluble opiates tend to remain at the dermatome segments of administration, whereas morphine (water soluble) may spread via the cerebrospinal fluid to the brain-stem. Delayed respiratory depression, including apnoea, has been documented up to 18 to 24 h after morphine administration. This is less of a problem with lipid soluble drugs.

Advantages of the epidural route over conventional intravenous techniques include superior analgesia, improved lung function, less sedation, and improved mobility, as well as earlier hospital discharge. Disadvantages include pruritus, nausea, vomiting, and urinary retention with opiates.

Local anaesthetics such as bupivacaine cause sympathetic blockade which may lead to hypotension, and reduced concentrations are used to minimize this complication. Combinations of local anaesthetic and narcotic are synergistic at the spinal cord level and are being used increasingly. Other complications include epidural haematoma, neurological sequelae at time of catheter insertion or removal and, rarely, infection.

Many authors believe that spinal opioids are highly effective, and that they may produce superior analgesia to parenterally administered drugs. Compared with local anaesthetic agents given extradurally or intrathecally, opioids do not cause hypotension. However, the advantages are not seen in all patients. There may be incomplete analgesia (unblocked segments), and there is patient variability in dose–response relationships. In addition, techniques are time-consuming, technically demanding and must be carried out with full aseptic precautions, and there is a high incidence of nausea and vomiting, pruritus, and urinary retention. Respiratory depression may occur, and this may be delayed for several hours after drug administration, especially with morphine.

PERIOPERATIVE FLUID BALANCE

The body's fluid balance can be considered in terms of the quantity of fluid—the circulating blood volume and its distribution, and the quality of that fluid, as characterized by plasma or serum osmolality, sodium and potassium concentrations and pH (Table 13).

The distribution of the circulating blood volume will not be covered here, except to emphasize its important role in the maintenance of normal cardiac output.

Abnormalities of fluid balance during surgery and the perioperative period

The homeostatic control of reabsorption and excretion of water and salts by the kidney is achieved through a number of different hormones and mechanisms, several of which are influenced by the stress responses to anaesthesia and surgery.

Water excretion is impaired during the perioperative period, as a result of increased secretion of ADH or AVP. Sodium excretion is also reduced, while excretion of potassium and nitrogen is increased, as a result of the increased levels of corticosteroids (glucocorticoids and mineralocorticoids) that are present in the body during this period. The increased release of ADH, which may persist for up to 72 h postoperatively, is due both to osmotic and non-osmotic factors. The latter pathways include stimulation of arterial baroreceptors through hypotension, stimulation of left atrial receptors by intermittent positive pressure ventilation, pain, the emotion or anxiety associated with surgery, hypoglycaemia, and β-adrenoceptor stimulation. Although morphine was generally believed to stimulate ADH release, this has subsequently

Table 13 Water, sodium, and potassium balance in the body

	Water	Na^+	K^+
Total body content	0.64 l/kg	57 (mmol/l)	47 (mmol/l) (men) 40 mmol/l (women)
Distribution (%)			
Intracellular	67	5–10	96
Extracellular	33	50	4
Bone		40–45	
Exchangeable amount (%)		60–70 (40 mmol/kg)	c.95
Daily normal intake	1750 ml	100–250 mmol	50–100 mmol
80% from food and drink			
20% from intermediary metabolism			
During fasting (i.e. postoperatively) 1–2 ml/kg.h			
Regulation:	Serum osmolality and ADH ANF	95% renal: glomerular filtration rate Aldosterone ANF ?Prostaglandins ?Kallikrein	Filtration Reabsorption Secretion

Replacement crystalloid fluids
Physiological saline (0.9% NaCl) = Na^+ 150 mmol/l.
Dextrose (5%) = 200 cal/l; no electrolytes.
Dextrose (4%)/0.18% NaCl = Na^+ 30 mmol/l.
Compound sodium lactate = Na^+ 131, K^+ 5, Ca^{2+}2, Cl^- 111, lactate 29 mmol/l.

been shown to be incorrect. In fact, opioids alone inhibit ADH release by increasing the osmoregulatory threshold to secretion. However, significant increases do occur due to surgical stimulation.

Sodium retention occurs as a result of stress factors accompanying anaesthesia and surgery. There is an increase in plasma aldosterone release from the adrenal glomerular cells, as well as an alteration in renal haemodynamics with redistribution of renal blood flow away from the tubular regions. The third factor is the so-called 'third space effect'—secretion of fluid in spaces such as the bowel in patients undergoing prolonged abdominal surgery, pleural fluid, and peritoneal fluid (ascites).

All of the volatile anaesthetic agents so far investigated, including ether, cyclopropane, isoflurane, enflurane, and halothane, cause a decrease in urinary volume and an associated increase in urinary osmolality. The decrease in urinary volume is brought about by a decrease in renal blood flow and a secondary decrease in glomerular filtration rate. This reduction in urinary volume influences the quantity of perioperative fluid required by the patient.

Most of the factors so far described promote salt and water retention. For over 30 years, there has been conjecture over the presence of a 'natriuretic factor'. This has now been isolated from cardiac atrial tissue and is a peptide that induces a diuresis, natriuresis, and moderate kaliuresis (atrial natriuretic factor, or atriopeptin). The peptide is synthesized as a 151 amino-acid sequence (pre-pro-atrial natriuretic factor), is stored within atrial myocytes as a 126 amino-acid pro-hormone (pro-atrial natriuretic factor or atriopeptigen), and is then cleaved to provide an active 28 amino-acid peptide. It has a short circulating half-life (about 3 min), and is metabolized in the kidney, as well as at other sites. Physiologically increased concentrations of atrial natriuretic factor are found after intravascular volume expansion which leads to atrial stretching, and after high sodium diets. Levels are also increased in cardiac disease, and in volume overloaded patients with chronic renal failure.

Atrial natriuretic factor increases the glomerular filtration rate without altering total renal blood flow. It causes vasoconstriction of the efferent glomerular vessels, inhibits angiotensin II, antagonizes the effects of noradrenaline, and blocks renin release, and hence aldosterone secretion. Data are conflicting on the effects of anaesthesia and surgery on atrial natriuretic factor levels in man. Fentanyl-isoflurane anaesthesia was associated with no increase in atrial natriuretic factor in patients undergoing infrarenal aortic clamping or carotid artery surgery, but there were increases following thoracic aortic clamping. Levels of atrial natriuretic factor seen during cardiac surgery for coronary artery grafting or valve replacement were higher than were seen in healthy controls. This increase in atrial natriuretic factor during bypass may act as the stimulus to promote the postsurgical diuresis that occurs despite the high circulating levels of ADH, glucocorticoids, and mineralocorticoids.

Other hormones which promote intrarenal vasodilatation and salt excretion include the prostaglandins (PGD_2, PGE_2, and PGI_2), and the kinins (bradykinin and kallidin) which enhance the effects of the prostaglandins, and modulate the renin–angiotensin system.

Other perioperative hormonal changes influencing fluid balance include increases in levels of growth hormone and prolactin in response to the stress and trauma of surgery. Both of these hormones may lead to salt and water retention. There are conflicting data on the effects of surgery on oestrogen levels in the perioperative period, but increased oestrogen levels would lead to salt and water retention.

Perioperative fluid requirements

Perioperative fluid requirements depend on the length and complexity of the surgery. Requirements for routine surgical practice in the United Kingdom and the rest of Europe would be approximately 7 ml/kg of normal saline or 5 ml/kg of an isotonic solution containing sodium and potassium, such as Hartmann's solution (Ringer's sodium lactate). The anaesthetist should be aware of the risk of fluid overload, particularly in patients with cardiac or renal disease.

About 30 ml/kg of water is required over the first 24 h after surgery to achieve a fluid balance comparable with preoperative conditions. Sodium (1–2 mmol/kg) and potassium (1 mmol/kg) are also required. Measured extra losses, such as those due to blood loss or third-space effects, must also be replaced.

The hypovolaemic patient presents postoperatively with low blood pressure, low central venous pressure, low cardiac output and, probably, low pulmonary capillary wedge pressure. A number of therapeutic manoeuvres are available for the management of these low-perfusion conditions.

PERIOPERATIVE COMPLICATIONS

Intraoperative complications

Since 1980, numerous studies have been published concerning critical incidents during anaesthesia. A critical incident is defined as some event which either contributed directly to an adverse outcome or which, if not rectified, would have caused an adverse outcome. Critical incident analysis was developed during the Second World War during the training of aircrew and has been widely adopted in anaesthesia in the various quality assurance programmes run at local and national levels. Resulting from this analysis, priority areas in education can be established to improve patient outcome from anaesthesia. Unfortunately, problems relating to the adequacy of checking of equipment before use continue to cause significant problems.

Aspiration of gastric contents

This is a major cause of anaesthetic morbidity. The traditional fasting period prior to surgery has become increasingly questioned in recent years. It may be harmful to deprive children of fluids for this amount of time, and more recent recommendations involve feeding with clear fluid to within 2 h of surgery. If emergency surgery is required waiting 4 h does not guarantee that gastric emptying will occur: following trauma, gastric emptying effectively ceases and hence delay of the surgery does not decrease the risks of aspiration. Most anaesthetists would now elect to induce anaesthesia as early as practicable and then use Sellick's manoeuvre (cricoid pressure) combined with a rapid sequence induction to reduce the incidence of aspiration. If aspiration occurs, prompt airway suctioning and the maintenance of adequate oxygenation are the cornerstones of therapy. Cricoid pressure should be applied to reduce the chance of further aspiration. The patient may need to be placed in the lateral position and oxygen saturation should be monitored. The urgency of surgery and the extent of inhalation should be considered when deciding whether to proceed or to defer surgery. If saturation remains satisfactory postoperatively in the recovery room, no further treatment is necessary. Inadequate or falling saturation is an indication for monitoring in a high dependency area. The role of steroids is debated and the use of prophylactic antibiotics is no longer encouraged.

Faulty delivery of anaesthetic gases

Problems with the delivery of anaesthetic gases may rapidly lead to hypoxic brain damage unless prompt diagnosis and correction are instituted. The routine use of oxygen analysers and capnography with appropriately set alarms allows the early detection and correction of the majority of these faults before physiological changes ensue. Oximetry is a relatively late and non-specific detector of failure of gas delivery. There are numerous potential causes of a failure of gas delivery and removal, and these are outlined in Table 14. It should be noted that all of these problems have been reported.

Table 14 Causes of failure of gas delivery

Gas supply system
- Cylinders: exhausted, contaminated, wrong cylinder connected
- Pipelines: misconnections or damage during building repairs.

Anaesthetic machine
- Rotameter damage and backbar leaks
- Inadvertent delivery of high concentrations of CO_2
- Inadvertent delivery of volatile agent when vaporizer assumed to be off

Breathing circuit problems
- Disconnection, obstruction, and leaks in the circuit
- Carbon dioxide accumulation due to inadequate minute ventilation, faults with CO_2 absorber units, or exhausted soda lime

Endotracheal tube problems
- Failed intubation resulting in hypoxia or aspiration
- Undetected oesophageal intubation
- Traumatic intubation
- Kinking and obstruction of the endotracheal tube (mimics asthma)
- Endotracheal tube cuff herniation
- Bronchospasm: mainly due to light anaesthesia or irritation of the carina by the endotracheal tube. Less often, asthma or aspiration may cause bronchospasm
- Wrong choice of endotracheal tube leading to intraoperative problems

Transurethral resection of the prostate syndrome

Absorption of irrigation fluid following transurethral resection of the prostate may lead to neurological and cardiovascular changes. The incidence of this complication has been estimated to be as high as 3.9 per cent. Water has been replaced by glycine as an irrigant because of problems due to water toxicity. Glycine, however, may also be absorbed into the circulation, causing dilutional hyponatraemia, hyperammonaemia, and fluid overload. This causes neurological and circulatory changes. Neurological symptoms include apprehension, disorientation, nausea and vomiting, visual disturbances, and coma or seizures. Symptoms occur between 15 min after surgery has commenced up to several hours after surgery has ended. Cardiovascular changes include bradycardia, raised central venous pressure, hypertension, angina, and ECG changes.

Several factors affect the onset of the TURP syndrome including hydrostatic pressure of the irrigant, the experience of the surgeon (which affects the number of venous sinuses opened), duration of surgery, peripheral venous pressure, and the type of fluid used for irrigation. The clinical effects of hyponatraemia relate to both the speed of onset and the extent of the fall in serum sodium. A gradual fall is better tolerated neurologically than is an abrupt fall. As glycine is metabolized to other amino acids, ammonia is produced, and this contributes to the development of

Table 15 Effect of alterations of body chemistry during transurethral resection of prostate on level of consciousness; the relationship between serum sodium and neurological state

Na^+ (mmol/l)	Neurological state
<120	Restless, confused, mild disorientation
<115	Nausea, drowsy
<100	Seizures, coma

Normal range 134–143 mmol/l.

neurological sequelae, in combination with hyponatremia (Table 15). In addition, elevated serum glycine levels (above 4000 µmol/l) have been associated with visual disturbances.

Diagnosis is generally made clinically, and hence spinal anaesthesia has become the most popular technique for this operation. This allows assessment of the patient's mental state to be made throughout the operation. In addition, co-existing respiratory disease is common in this group and spinal anaesthesia is well tolerated by such patients. Following clinical diagnosis, the surgeon should be informed whilst electrolytes and osmolarity are checked.

The osmolal gap (the difference between measured and calculated osmolalities) is increased in the TURP syndrome, due to the presence of an osmotically active particle (glycine) which contributes to measured osmolality but which is not included in the equation for estimation of osmolality.

$$\text{Osmolality} = 2 \times [\text{Na}] + \text{glucose} + \text{urea (all in mmol/l)}$$

Mildly symptomatic patients experience nausea, vomiting, confusion, and visual disturbances and have a serum sodium above 120 mmol/l. Treatment involves cessation of surgery, reassurance, administration of a diuretic, and ophthalmic consultation if visual disturbances occur. In severe cases, involving loss of consciousness, other causes of loss of consciousness should be excluded (Table 16).

Table 16 Causes of delayed return of responsiveness following surgery

Raised intracranial pressure
Occurs in patients with undetected space-occupying lesions who are subjected to significant fluid shifts such as those accompanying major blood loss (e.g. during gastrointestinal haemorrhage or vascular surgery, during TURP, or associated with surgery for major trauma)
Drugs
Atypical response to sedation—benzodiazepines, premedication, hyoscine
Hypercarbia
Secondary to oversedation
Metabolic
Diabetes, hypothyroidism
Psychiatric

Management involves assessment and support of the airway and ventilation in those with impaired conscious state. The degree of hyponatremia should be assessed: a serum sodium level below 120 mmol/l is life-threatening. The optimal rate of correction of hyponatraemia is controversial. While it is claimed that rapid correction of chronic hyponatraemia may lead to demyelination, the significance of this in acute hyponatraemia is uncertain. Hypertonic saline should be administered slowly until the serum sodium exceeds 120 mmol/l. Many use frusemide in addition to reduce fluid overload. Patients with renal failure may need dialysis to correct abnormalities.

Patient care

The anaesthetized patient has lost his normal protective reflexes and is therefore vulnerable to a variety of traumatic problems including slips or falls during patient transfer or if sides are absent, pressure sores, corneal ulcers, diathermy burns, electrocution, and peripheral nerve palsies. Urinary bladder distension causes increased sympathetic drive and pain, tachycardia, or occasional arrhythmias in the recovery room.

Air embolism

This may occur when veins at a level above the heart are held distended by bone rather than collapsing due to atmospheric pressure. Situations predisposing to this include neurosurgical procedures performed in the sitting position and prone laminectomies, and it may also occur during total hip replacement during reaming of the femur. Rarely, gases may be injected into the circulation directly, for example during laparoscopy (carbon dioxide embolism). The features of air embolism depend on several factors, including volume of gas involved, speed of gas entrainment and presence of a patent foramen ovale where gas may reach the left side of the heart, causing symptoms in coronary and cerebral circulations.

Human error

Many factors have been shown to affect vigilance levels of anaesthetic personnel. The ergonomics of the anaesthetic machine have been increasingly examined in recent years. The original Boyle's machine has evolved into a complex piece of equipment with numerous modifications that comply with increased demand for safety features. On newer machines dials and controls have been regrouped into a tidier and more easily visualized unit. There has also been the need to produce a machine which is easy to clean following the increased number of 'dirty cases' currently being undertaken. The placement of monitors on the anaesthetic machine and the machine's placement with respect to the patient affect the ease and frequency of observations made by the anaesthetist.

Postoperative complications

When complications occur in the recovery room or in the perioperative period the importance of consultation with the anaesthetist who gave the anaesthetic cannot be over-emphasized. The anaesthetist may be able to suggest other causes for the problem, and may wish to see the patient to discuss these problems further.

Respiratory

Postoperative respiratory depression is most commonly due to opiates used for pain relief. However, other causes may include over-sedation, recurarization, or the development of pulmonary oedema. Consultation with the anaesthetist is important. When respiratory depression is severe, immediate respiratory support is necessary, using an Ambu bag or similar device.

Atelectasis may occur when inadequately treated pain limits chest movement, and pre-existing disease may increase the severity. Optimal analgesia and intensive physiotherapy are needed. Occasionally, bronchoscopy may be required to remove sputum.

Cardiovascular system

Cardiac failure occurs when reduced myocardial contractility is unable to cope with the additional stress of fluid shifts and drug-induced depression of myocardial contractility. Clinical manifestations range from dyspnoea, which may mimic asthma in mild cases to frank pulmonary oedema with frothy sputum. Management involves optimization of oxygenation, posture, and diuretics and in severe cases intermittent positive pressure ventilation may be required. The ECG should be reviewed as ischaemia or arrhythmias will worsen cardiac output.

Postoperative hypertension may be due to pain, or to the withdrawal of preoperative antihypertensive medication. Optimal pain relief should be ensured before further antihypertensive medication is given. Initially, drugs should be given intravenously to reduce delays and to ensure that reliable blood levels are achieved.

Hypotension is most commonly due to inadequate fluid replacement. Drain tubes should be checked for correct function and concealed blood loss should be excluded. Following spinal or epidural anaesthesia, especially in patients whose operations were performed in the lithotomy position, fluid shifts can occur because of the loss of sympathetic tone. In the absence of demonstrable fluid problems, ischaemia, arrhythmia, and drug-induced myocardial depression should be excluded. Uncommon causes of postoperative hypotension include relative cortisol deficiency in steroid-dependent patients and subclinical hypothyroidism.

Atrial fibrillation is the most common arrhythmia arising postoperatively. Patients previously maintained on digitalis may suffer arrhythmias following cessation of therapy or due to poor absorption in the presence of abdominal conditions. Following ECG confirmation of the arrhythmia, specific therapy should be commenced. Rapid atrial fibrillation with haemodynamic instability may require intravenous verapamil or in very severe cases, DC countershock. Pre-existing disease, pain, poorly controlled hypotension, intraoperative events, and suboptimal oxygenation, especially in combination with hypertension or tachycardia, may lead to ischaemic events in the perioperative period.

Nervous system

Confusion is common in the perioperative period, especially in the elderly. Diagnosis is frequently difficult and management is often suboptimal. Diagnosis is frequently made by exclusion of possible causes and in many cases no obvious cause for the acute brain syndrome is ever discovered (Table 17).

Table 17 Causes of postoperative confusion in the general surgical patient

Hypoxia—This must be excluded before attempting to sedate the patient
Alcohol withdrawal
Pain, particularly in patients who are still drowsy
Drugs of addiction. Especially in emergency cases, illicit use may have preceded the accident which necessitated the operation
Pre-existing psychological or psychiatric conditions are frequently overlooked
Sensory isolation especially in elderly patients or patients in intensive care where loss of the 'night-day' cycle frequently leads to confusion
Drugs
Benzodiazepines: (especially in elderly patients)
Ketamine: emergence delirium can occur, especially in bright, noisy surroundings
Butyrophenones (droperidol)
Scopolamine premedication in 'elderly' patients

Relatively inexperienced house staff often have to manage patients with acute postoperative confusional states. Hypoxia must be excluded, either by oximetry or blood gas estimation. Review of the anaesthetic chart or recovery room notes will often reveal a likely cause; however, in the majority of cases no cause is ever ascertained. Management involves reassurance of the patient and staff, combined with measures to prevent damage to suture lines, intravenous equipment and wound drains. Sedation should be used cautiously if at all.

The anaesthetized patient is vulnerable to nerve injury because of the loss of protective reflexes. Nerves especially vulnerable are the ulnar nerve at the elbow, the lateral popliteal nerve during lithotomy, the brachial plexus (lower nerves during abduction, and upper plexus in the Trendelenburg postion) and the supraorbital nerve.

If nerve damage following surgery is suspected, early anaesthetic consultation is recommended, followed by neurological referral.

Miscellaneous

Urinary retention

This is a frequent complaint especially in patients confined to bed following surgery. Inability to pass urine may be related to fluid deficiency, pain, or difficulties managing bottles and bedpans, especially in noisy or crowded wards.

Catheter-related problems, and postoperative urinary tract infections, although not relevant to the anaesthetic management, need careful follow-up.

The development of incontinence following spinal or epidural anaesthesia needs immediate follow-up by the anaesthetist in consultation with a neurologist.

Jaundice

Postoperative jaundice is an uncommon problem. Full clinical and biochemical assessment is important. Halothane hepatitis is a rare postoperative event and its diagnosis is generally made by exclusion. Many cases of 'halothane hepatitis' have turned out to be infection with cytomegalovirus or other viruses. Jaundice may also rarely occur following enflurane anaesthesia. Up to 1987 six cases had been reported; thus the incidence of jaundice is significantly lower than that following halothane anaesthesia and the mortality in established cases is also lower. Death occurred in 21 per cent of enflurane hepatitis cases compared with 50 per cent of halothane cases.

Suxamethonium apnoea (see above)

Management in the operating theatre should be supportive until other metabolic pathways eliminate the suxamethonium. Sedation should be administered to reduce unpleasant recollections of awakening whilst paralysed.

Vomiting

This is one of the most common and distressing postoperative complications. The incidence of vomiting ranges from 10 to 50 per cent depending on the type of surgery. Many factors contribute to the incidence of vomiting, including use of opiates, type of surgery (gynaecological surgery has a very high incidence), gastrointestinal distension (due to ileus), and early ambulation.

Dental damage

The anaesthetist should be notified immediately, to allow early dental consultation. Crowned, capped, and carious teeth are especially vulnerable to damage during anaesthesia and surgery. Damage may be caused at intubation, by oral airways, or during suctioning of the patient.

Rashes

Skin rashes may be caused by reaction to anaesthetic agents, antibiotics, adhesive dressings, or skin prep solution. Management is generally conservative, but well demarcated lesions related to areas of adhesive or skin preparation require follow-up to prevent recurrence in future operations.

Sore throat

The incidence of sore throat following endotracheal intubation varies between 2 and 70 per cent of cases. Predisposing factors are the use of red-rubber endotracheal tubes, cigarette smoking, difficult or traumatic intubation, prolonged intubation, and prior laryngeal pathology. Conflicting results have been found with 'high volume-low pressure' cuff designs used for short-term intubation. The management of postintubation sore throat is conservative; reassurance is usually all that is required.

Muscle pains

The development of muscle pains is common in fit, ambulant, muscular young subjects given suxamethonium to facilitate endotracheal intubation. The pain may be quite severe and resembles that caused by unaccustomed exercise. Management involves notification of the anaesthetist concerned, reassurance of the patient, and non-opioid analgesics.

HAZARDS TO OPERATING ROOM STAFF

Pollution from anaesthetic agents

During the 1970s and 1980s there was substantial interest in the possible deleterious effects of chronic exposure of operating room personnel to trace concentrations of volatile anaesthetic agents. Possible problems included increased abortion rate amongst female staff, decreased fertility rates, and effects on concentration and performance, as well as possible immunological effects. As a result of this concern, scavenging of anaesthetic agents has become widespread practice throughout the world.

Over the last decade, there has been debate over the real implications of these observations as a survey of practising hospital female doctors aged less than 40 years has failed to support these findings. The results to date reveal no significant correlation between miscarriage rates or incidence of congenital anomalies and hours spent in operating suites or the doctor's medical specialty. However, during the 1980s scavenging has been almost universally adopted in an attempt to alleviate any problems; in many countries it is mandatory. The belief that adoption of such scavenging measures has eliminated the problem has been disputed by recent evidence suggesting exposure levels are frequently quite high. Reasons include faulty scavenging, high gas flow techniques with frequent periods when the mask is not applied to the face, and the practice of leaving the gas flow running between cases.

Further legislation in the United Kingdom has been enacted as the Control of Substances Hazardous to Health (COSHH) regulations. These were adopted in 1990, and require assessments of the level of pollution in theatre environment to be made.

Scavenging

This may be active, when applied suction extracts the gases vented from the anaesthetic machine, or passive when the gases pass along large diameter tubing and are released into the atmosphere. Problems have occurred with both types of system. The application of suction directly to the lungs causing failure of ventilation of the patient can occur, or obstruction of tubing can lead to barotrauma. Currently, only active scavenging may be installed in new anaesthetic installations in the United Kingdom.

Circle absorber systems

These may be employed in place of the traditional 'T-piece' apparatus used in the United Kingdom. They lead to a reduction in fresh gas flows of at least 50 per cent, so resulting in lower volumes of waste gases for removal as well as reduced volatile agent costs.

Low flow and closed circuit techniques

These can be used to reduce flows further, but they require higher levels of monitoring and have not achieved widespread acceptance.

Regional (local anaesthetic) techniques

These reduce pollution but are not always practicable.

Total intravenous anaesthesia

This eliminates pollution but currently available agents are expensive, and the techniques are not suited to all cases (see earlier).

Improvements in practice

Improvements in practice such as turning flows off between cases, or not moving masks from the face during cases, further reduce pollution.

Improvements to theatre ventilation

Improvements to theatre ventilation, including non-recycling of theatre air, lead to lower pollutant levels but are very costly.

The wider issue of environmental pollution by anaesthetic agents is less clear. However, it has been stated that the contribution by anaesthetic agents to ozone layer depletion is minimal, that the effects of nitrous oxide on the greenhouse effect are complex, and that the overall effect of anaesthetic agents on global pollution is minimal.

Fires and explosions in the operating environment

The risks of fires and explosions have declined since the decline in use of explosive volatile anaesthetic agents. Whilst these older agents had great merits, the proliferation of electrical devices in the operating suite has greatly increased the risks involved with their use.

The principal problems in contemporary practice are listed below.

Diathermy in the presence of pooled alcoholic skin preps

This hazard continues to occur and has been commented on detrimentally by the various Colleges and Defence Unions.

Laser surgery

This is of especial concern when surgery involves the upper airway and oesophagus. A variety of ingenious devices have appeared in an attempt to minimize the risk of ignition of the endotracheal tube (for example some anaesthetists have wrapped foil or foil-tape around conventional PVC or rubber endotracheal tubes). Cases have been reported in which the foil has unwrapped and ignition has nonetheless still occurred. A variety of purpose-built endotracheal tubes have appeared including those where aluminium powder is deposited on the surface to dissipate the generated heat, and those with saline filled cuffs and metal spirals embedded in the wall of the tube. In all cases the goal is to reduce the chance of ignition from a casual contact with the laser beam. Recently a fire occurring with one of these tubes has been reported. The ultimate problem relates to the enhanced flammability of plastics in the presence of high concentrations of oxygen or nitrous oxide. Interest and research have therefore centred on the use of total intravenous anaesthetic techniques (employing infusions of propofol or methohexitone), low inspired oxygen concentrations, and avoiding the use of nitrous oxide.

Fires due to electrical faults

All faulty mains voltage equipment must be discarded or sent for repair. Problems have occurred with surgical headlights, heating blankets, and junction boxes.

Uncommon causes of fires and explosions

These include diathermy into gas-containing viscera (during bowel surgery) or diathermy in a nitrous oxide inflated abdomen during laparoscopy; anaesthetic machine mishaps due to oil and grease contamination of pipelines resulting in explosions when exposed to high oxygen concentrations; and trailing ends of fibreoptic light sources left on paper drapes.

Electrical safety

This is discussed in Chapter 3.3.

Acquired immune deficiency syndrome (AIDS)

There are 25 to 100 carriers of HIV for each person with the clinical picture of AIDS. A recent estimate suggested that, on average, each anaesthetist is likely to encounter three HIV carriers in a year of clinical practice. Infection with HIV leads to inevitable damage to the immune system followed by the development of tumours or opportunistic infections. It is now generally accepted that most carriers will develop AIDS within 8 years of exposure and that death will usually occur within a year.

The HIV virus contains RNA and the enzyme 'reverse transcriptase' which generates DNA from RNA. The virally generated DNA becomes incorporated into the host's DNA, and subsequently codes for the production and release of virus particles which infect other host cells. It is this combination with host DNA which makes effective treatment and vaccination difficult at the present time.

Prevention remains the only therapeutic 'option' available. The public have been exposed to an extensive advertising campaign which has produced only a small change in social behaviour. Estimates on seroconversion following a single needlestick injury vary widely, but a figure of 1 per cent has been quoted. The delay between inoculation and seroconversion can be long, and the risks of seroconversion following mucous membrane contact (such as produced by the 'aerosol' of blood and bone fragments produced during orthopaedic surgery) have not been estimated. There are clear implications for anaesthetic and surgical practice regarding the precautions to be taken for all patients (irrespective of their HIV status) as well as presently unanswered questions regarding staff testing for HIV, routine patient testing for HIV status, and the exposure of trainees to patients known to have AIDS.

MEDICOLEGAL ASPECTS OF ANAESTHETIC AND SURGICAL PRACTICE

Informed consent

There is general agreement that, in the United Kingdom, the attitude of the public is considerably less legalistic than in North America. However, for consent to be legally valid, the doctor should provide sufficient details and information about proposals for treatment to enable the patient to form a proper decision as to his or her choices.

It is not necessary under English law to explain every possible complication of the proposed procedure, and the degree of explanation may well vary between individuals, having regard to factors such as education, cultural background, pre-existing anxiety, and urgency of surgery, as well as physical status. The term 'informed consent' has different meanings in different contexts. Similarly, the use of 'blanket' consent forms affords very little protection. Although legally consent does not require written documentation, it is to be recommended as the long intervals existing between incident and litigation may leave both parties unable accurately to recall what was said. A record that the consent was given after an adequate discussion of the potential risks and benefits is of greater value. Clinical judgement is required regarding the provision of an adequate explanation on the one hand, and needless discouragement of a patient from undergoing necessary surgery on the other. In emergency situations, the opportunity for detailed discussion is curtailed, and it is recommended that associated non-urgent procedures be deferred until the patient can give adequate consent.

Awareness

It has been estimated that 0.5 per cent of patients undergoing balanced anaesthesia involving relaxants may recall intraoperative events. Of these, 10 per cent may experience pain or remember paralysis. In many cases the anaesthetist is not notified of this complication and the opportunity to discuss the circumstances leading to the awareness was lost. Of those patients pursuing litigation, in many cases the lack of a sympathetic acceptance of the legitimacy of the complaint and explanation of why it may have occurred has contributed to the seeking of legal redress.

When awareness has occurred the anaesthetist should be informed at the earliest opportunity so as to allow discussion whilst the patient is still in hospital. Advice from the Medical Defence Union recommends that the patient should be reassured that their experience was genuine, and that in the absence of faulty equipment or anaesthetic technique, their experience was a sequel to the use of balanced anaesthetic techniques where the volatile agent concentration is minimized to avoid potentially toxic effects.

Dreams may occur either during anaesthesia or at any time in the perioperative period. They do not usually involve the operation but may be very distressing. Awareness can usually be prevented by careful checking of the anaesthetic machine to detect for disconnections or faulty apparatus, and by intraoperative vigilance. However, awareness may be difficult to avoid under some circumstances (e.g. in the patient undergoing caesarian section, or the critically ill patient receiving general anaesthesia under life-threatening circumstances), and this highlights the importance of meticulous record keeping. Whether patients should be told before the operation of the risk of awareness has not been resolved; however, most would currently argue against this as routine practice.

Perioperative deaths

Ever since the first cases of death associated with anaesthesia, both surgeons and anaesthetists have either formally or informally audited their complications. At present in the United Kingdom, it is the responsibility of the anaesthetist to report to the coroner (or his equivalent in Scotland and Northern Ireland) cases where either death has occurred within 24 h of surgery, or where it has occurred later but the patient has failed to recover complete consciousness after the operation. Similar mechanisms exist for reporting perioperative mortality in the United States and many other countries in the Western world. However, until recently, there were few data available to allow determination of the incidence of perioperative mortality in different patient groups.

In 1982, Lunn and Mushin published the results of their study on deaths occurring within 6 days of anaesthesia. This was a voluntary study encompassing five regions in the United Kingdom. Their conclusions were that 0.6 per cent of patients die within 6 days of surgery and that in only 1 in 10 000 cases was anaesthesia solely responsible for death.

In 1987, the Confidential Enquiry into Perioperative Deaths (CEPOD) was published. This study spanned 30 days after surgery and involved three regions in the United Kingdom; it excluded certain patient groups (e.g. cardiac surgery patients, children and neonates, obstetrics patients). The last group is audited in the United Kingdom by the Triennial Confidential Enquiry into Maternal Mortality. Only three deaths were judged solely due to anaesthesia, giving a rate of 1 in 185 000. The main conclusions made were: the need for the availability of proper recovery facilities; the provision and utilization of essential monitoring; and the adequate supervision of trainees. Of particular importance is the consultation between surgeon and anaesthetist regarding emergency cases, and those patients suffering from intercurrent illness. Too frequently, there is inadequate notification to allow optimization in management of those patients suffering from multisystem illness.

Anaesthetic agent toxicity – halothane hepatitis

The toxicity of volatile anaesthetic agents has been known since the introduction of diethyl ether and chloroform. Concern over modern agents led to the National Halothane Survey in the United States by Bunker in 1969. It was found that the incidence of hepatic toxicity following halothane was no greater than that after the earlier agents. Further studies highlighted the problem of 'unexplained hepatitis following halothane'.

The quoted incidence for 'halothane-associated hepatitis' varies between 1:2500 and 1:36 000 exposures, and is substantially lower in children at between 1:82 000 to 1:200 000. Halothane does not function as a classical liver toxin; there is no dose-dependent degree of liver damage, nor a recognized mechanism of action, nor are its effects consistent in different species. Investigations have centred on the various metabolic pathways halothane may follow under different circumstances. Halothane may undergo reductive or oxidative metabolism with production of trifluoroacetic acid, and inorganic chloride, bromide, and fluoride. The diagnosis of halothane hepatitis is one of exclusion, as there is no pathognomonic test available. The recommended interval between halothane anaesthetics recommended by the Committee on Safety of Medicines is 3 months (although the logic of this may be questioned in the light of an assumed immune aetiology in at least some cases). It is also recommended that halothane is contraindicated if undefined fever and jaundice have developed after halothane anaesthesia. Cirrhosis, chronic hepatitis, and liver tumours were not seen as contraindications.

Toxicity after enflurane and isoflurane may also occur, but is rarer than after halothane.

3.2 Surgical diathermy

JOHN T. B. MOYLE

The word diathermy means through heating. Surgical diathermy is a technique that allows bleeding from small blood vessels to be arrested without the need for mechanical clips or sutures and enables tissues to be cut without the use of a knife, with sealing of small blood vessels at the same time. It is carried out by the application of heat to small areas of tissue in a highly controlled way. In microsurgery the heat may be applied with a needle which has been preheated in a flame (for example in ophthalmic surgery, or by applying a piece of resistance wire through which an electric current is passed (as in cautery of the nasal septum). However the heat is usually generated by passing a radiofrequency electric current through the tissues themselves.

Animal tissue is a conductor of electricity but has a considerable resistivity. Resistivity is the intrinsic property of a material to resist the passage of electricity: the higher the resistivity, the poorer a conductor and vice versa. When an electric current is passed through a poor conductor energy is lost in the form of heat and the temperature of the material increases. The amount of heat produced depends upon the current (amperes) and the resistance of the tissue (ohms). The heating power developed may be expressed as

$$W = RI^2$$

(where W = power (W), R = resistance (Ω), and I = current). One watt of power is converted into 1 J/s heat. Surgical diathermy uses 30 to 400 watts of power, depending upon the degree of heating required.

Under normal circumstances, passing the required amount of current through the body, either as direct current or at conventional mains frequency (50 Hz in the United Kingdom and Europe, 60 Hz in North America) would cause severe muscle spasm, intense pain, and fatal cardiac arrhythmias. However as frequency is increased, more current may be passed through the body with fewer of these effects, allowing the use of higher currents and, therefore, higher temperatures (Fig. 1). For this reason, surgical diathermy uses radiofrequency currents in the range 0.5 to 1.5 MHz.

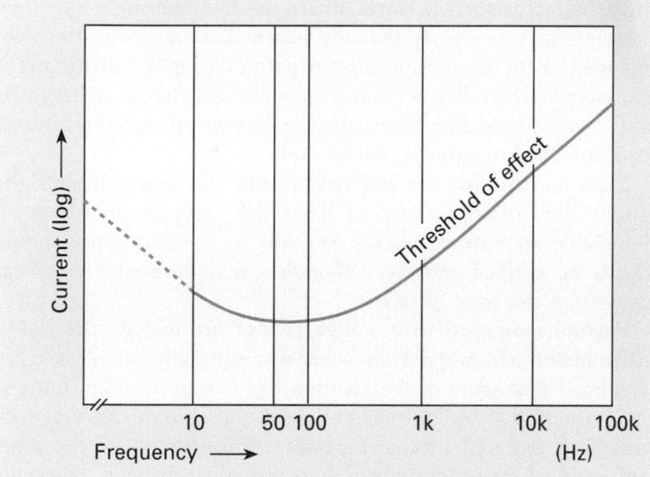

Fig. 1 Variation of the threshold of pathophysiological effects of electric current with frequency.

Application of radiofrequency current across living tissue would cause heating of the whole volume. It is therefore necessary to limit the amount of tissue heated to avoid damaging the surrounding mass. This goal is achieved ensuring a high current density in the volume of tissue that requires diathermy and a very low current density in all other tissues. The same heating effect will occur along all of the current pathway but the temperature will only rise significantly where the current density is high. Where there is a low current density the rise in temperature will be totally dissipated by the large volume of surrounding tissues. An understanding of the concept of current density is vital to the safe use of radiofrequency surgical diathermy.

There are two ways of delivering a high current density to a localized area: monopolar and bipolar diathermy. With the monopolar technique the current is passed through a large volume of tissue (Fig. 2) from an 'indifferent' or 'plate' electrode of comparatively large surface area which is in good electrical contact with a large area of the body. The current then passes through an active electrode of very small contact surface, which is under the control of the surgeon. A very low current density is therefore passed

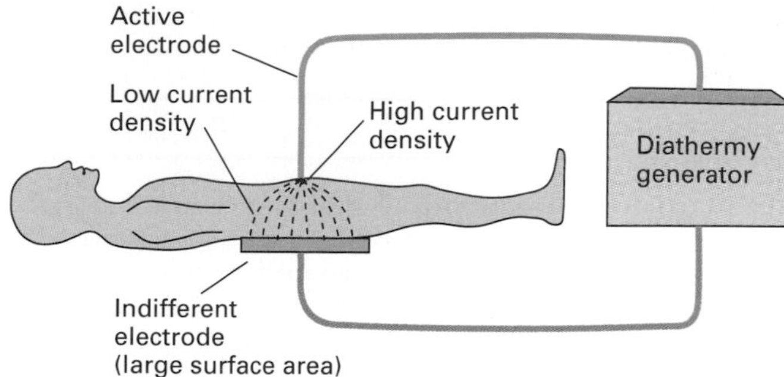

Fig. 2 Two-dimensional representation of monopolar diathermy.

through most of the body, but at the point of contact between the active electrode and the tissues the current density is very high, and therefore has a large heating effect.

Bipolar surgical diathermy involves the current being passed between two point electrodes, in the form of insulated forceps limbs placed immediately adjacent to the tissue to be heated (Fig. 3). A very high current density, and hence a high heating effect, is produced over a very small volume of tissue, with virtually no heat generated elsewhere in the body. Bipolar diathermy can only be used with relatively low currents and is only suitable for the coagulation of small blood vessels. Its greatest application is in microsurgery, especially of the hand, and in neurosurgery.

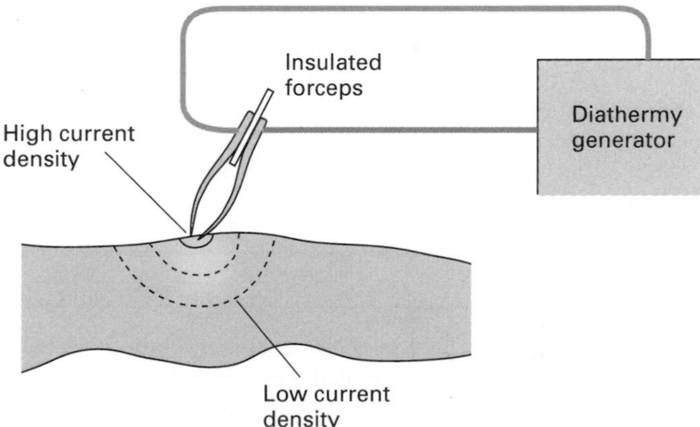

Fig. 3 Two-dimensional representation of bipolar diathermy.

GENERATORS

Radiofrequency surgical diathermy generators are basically continuous wave radio transmitters without antennae. The earliest types consisted of a spark-gap and a tuned circuit supplied with electricity. Production of an arc across the gap caused the circuit to oscillate at its resonant frequency for as long as current was supplied to it. With the advent of vacuum valves (radio tubes) the quality of the diathermy current improved and it became more controllable. Such valves are expensive and large, requiring power supplies for their filaments as well as high tension for the output current, and are less reliable than the semiconductors which have superseded them.

Modern diathermy generators employ high-power, high-frequency transistors which provide an output equivalent to that available from valve generators. Although the main part of the generator is a high-powered radiofrequency oscillator, semiconductor electronics and microprocessors are used to control the oscillator, monitor its performance, and to monitor safety, especially in regard to the connection of the indifferent electrode.

Waveform

The waveforms of the radiofrequency currents used in surgical diathermy have been chosen empirically. Tissue to be cut has to be heated very rapidly, but only in close proximity to the tip of the electrode. Cutting is achieved by striking an arc between the tip and the tissue, thus charring it: a continuous sinuosoidal waveform of high power is the most effective. Coagulation requires less heat applied over a slightly greater volume of tissue: this is best achieved by repetitive short bursts of a few cycles of the current. There are some applications, such as transurethral prostatectomy, where a combination of these two waveforms may be blended to achieve more widespread coagulation during cutting.

Many manufacturers produce machines which generate complex waveforms for special situations but their advantages are hard to prove.

Endoscopic diathermy

Radiofrequency diathermy is most commonly used to coagulate small blood vessels, using appropriate forceps, and to cut tissues, using a fine pointed electrode. Both of these procedures may be carried out endoscopically using appropriate insulated electrodes. The most frequent applications for such techniques are the treatment or removal of bladder tumours and hypertrophic prostate tissue. This requires distension of the bladder with a non-conductive fluid, such as a glycine solution, and the use of a blended current.

Appropriate electrodes may also be used via a fibreoptic gastroduodenoscope or a laparoscope.

Dangers

Skin damage is probably the most common surgical problem associated with radiofrequency diathermy. It is caused either by coagulation of blood vessels close to the skin, or by inadvertent contact between a skin edge and a conducting instrument while treating deeper tissues.

Knowledge of the principle of current density obviates the disaster of inadvertent coagulation of pedicles. The classical cause of this problem is the use of monopolar diathermy on the testicle whilst it is supported in the surgeon's hand. The current density is then very high in the spermatic cord, which has a small cross-sectional area and is the sole current pathway between the rest of the body and the testis. Whenever monopolar diathermy is used in this situation, the testicle should remain in contact with the main bulk of the body with, if possible a saline-soaked swab to improve conduction. This disaster can be totally avoided by the use of bipolar diathermy.

Increased current density is also the cause of skin burns caused by poor contact between the indifferent 'plate' electrode and the skin. This, and also faults in the indifferent electrode lead, may cause skin burns at other sites as the current attempts to find other pathways to complete the circuit. The generator should have self-diagnosis systems for lead faults, the indifferent electrode must be carefully applied, and the patient's skin must be protected from contact with any other conductive material which may form an alternative current pathway.

There is an enormous variety of internal and external electronic cardiac pacemakers and one must assume that they may all be inhibited or even damaged by radiofrequency diathermy, unless the manufacturer's data states otherwise. If diathermy is vital then it is necessary to ensure that the pacemaker and its lead are not included in the maximum current pathway: bipolar diathermy is the safer method. There is also an increased risk of arrhythmias and even intracardiac burns due to leakage of current through leads attached to external pacemakers.

Explosion and fire are still risks during diathermy, despite the almost total disappearance of flammable anaesthetic agents. If flammable anaesthetic agents are still in use diathermy should ideally be avoided entirely, although it may be used if it is kept away from the zone of risk.

Factors associated with a high risk of fire include the use of inflammable skin preparation solutions, especially when there is a likelihood that some of the solution has flowed into skin folds or the perineal area and not been allowed to evaporate. Several such fires have required extensive plastic reconstruction of the groin and perineal area. The atmosphere around a patient, especially under the surgical drapes, during general anaesthesia has an increased concentration of oxygen. Because nitrous oxide supports combustion as well as, if not better than, oxygen, special care must be taken when diathermy is used in the oral cavity, where the concentration of oxygen/nitrous oxide is always elevated. Methane in obstructed bowel may detonate if struck by a diathermy spark, especially if mannitol has been used as a bowel evacuant.

3.3 Electrical safety in anaesthesia and surgery

JOHN T. B. MOYLE

The subject of electrical safety in the operating theatre and elsewhere in health-care facilities, is of the utmost importance for the following reasons:

(1) electronic equipment is now ubiquitous in health care;
(2) in no other sphere of life is the deliberate ohmic connection of electronic equipment to living tissue entertained; and
(3) the sick patient is more susceptible to the unwanted effects of electrical energy than is the healthy person.

HARMFUL EFFECTS OF CURRENT ELECTRICITY

There are a number of ways by which an electric current passing through living tissue may cause damage. With an understanding of these mechanisms, electrical safety enters the realm of common sense.

Table 1 Approximate resistivity of body tissues at 50 Hz (derived from Geddes and Baker 1967)

Material	Resistivity (ohm/cm)
Blood	150
Urine	30
Skeletal muscle	300
Cardiac muscle	750
Lung	1275
Fat	3000
Liver	800
Nerve tissue	500
Bone	500–6000

Risk of electrical damage may occur whenever the body, or part of it, becomes part of an electrical circuit. The amount and variety of morbidity and mortality depend upon the magnitude of the current, the time for which it passes through the body, and, to a certain extent, the frequency of the applied current.

From Ohm's law, $I = E/Z$ where I is the current in amperes, E = the potential difference in volts across Z, which is the resistance (or impedance with alternating current (a.c.)). The current passing through the body therefore depends not only upon the magnitude of the applied voltage but also upon the electrical resistance of the body; the lower the resistance, the higher the current. If the skin was perfectly dry, the skin resistance alone would be between 100 000 ohm and 300 000 ohm. However, water and, especially, perspiration reduce this resistance dramatically, such that the average resistance may be assumed to be between 50 ohms and 10 000 ohm when assessing electrical risk. Table 1 shows the approximate resistivity of body tissues at 50 Hz.

The morbidity of excessive currents passing through the living body may be due to one or more of the following:

(1) electrical energy being converted into heat which will cause damage proportional to the product of time and current; this may even progress to charring (a process made use of in radio frequency surgical diathermy);
(2) hypoxaemic damage due to respiratory muscle spasm, or temporary cardiac arrhythmia; permanent cardiac damage may also ensue;
(3) chemical burns at contact points due to electrolysis—this type of morbidity only occurs when there is a direct current (d.c.) component to the electric current.

Death from electrocution may occur due to asphyxia caused by the respiratory muscle spasm, respiratory arrest due to CNS dysfunction, or because of cardiac asystole or arrhythmia.

Damage to any particular part of the body is dependent upon current density or current per unit cross-sectional area of the current pathway. This concept is illustrated in Fig. 1.

Table 2 shows the effects of increasing current at 50 or 60 Hz through the human trunk. These values vary greatly under different conditions, the most obvious of which is the route that the current takes through the body—the most dangerous of which is that which passes through the axis of the heart. Other factors causing variation include sex, body weight, and state of health of the area of contact, and the frequency (see Chapter 3.2), the waveform, and the duration of the electric shock.

Figure 2 shows the relationship between time/current and the probability of the pathological effect.

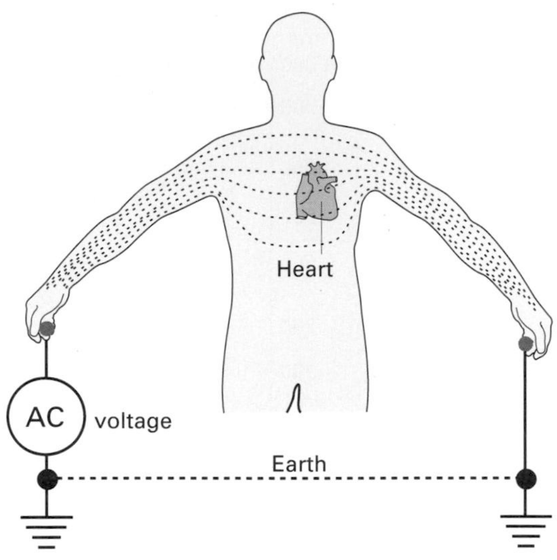

Fig. 1 Current density

Table 2 The effects of electric current at 50 Hz or 60 Hz through the human trunk

Threshold of perception	1 mA
Pain	5 mA
'Let-go' current, severe pain, and muscle spasm	15 mA
Respiratory muscle spasm	50 mA
Ventricular fibrillation	80–100 mA
Sustained myocardial contraction	>1000 mA

Microshock

The concept of microshock is important in anaesthesia, intensive care, and thoracic surgery. If electrical contact is made internally, especially on or close to the heart, very low currents, as low as 10 μA, may initiate arrhythmias. The resistance of skin contact is eliminated and the current density at the interface between the contact and the heart is very high (see Fig. 3). Microshock may occur during thoracic surgery, but the risk is much more common when conductive saline is used as the fluid in a cardiac catheter, pulmonary artery catheter, or a central venous pressure catheter, as leakage current may pass through a pressure transducer.

PROTECTION AGAINST ELECTRICAL INJURIES AND ELECTROCUTION

The philosophy of electrical safety in medicine has a different bias from that in the domestic or industrial situation. The reasons for this are:

1. Only in the medical environment is direct electrical connection with the body necessary (surgical diathermy, electrocardiogram, electromyogram, electroencephalogram, etc.);
2. Any protective cut-out system must be sensitive enough to protect against currents above preset, but very low, values due to fault conditions, passing through the body. Such sensitive devices are very likely to trip-out in non-fault conditions; this would also be dangerous to life, in the case of ventilators, dialysis machines, and extracorporeal circulation pumps.

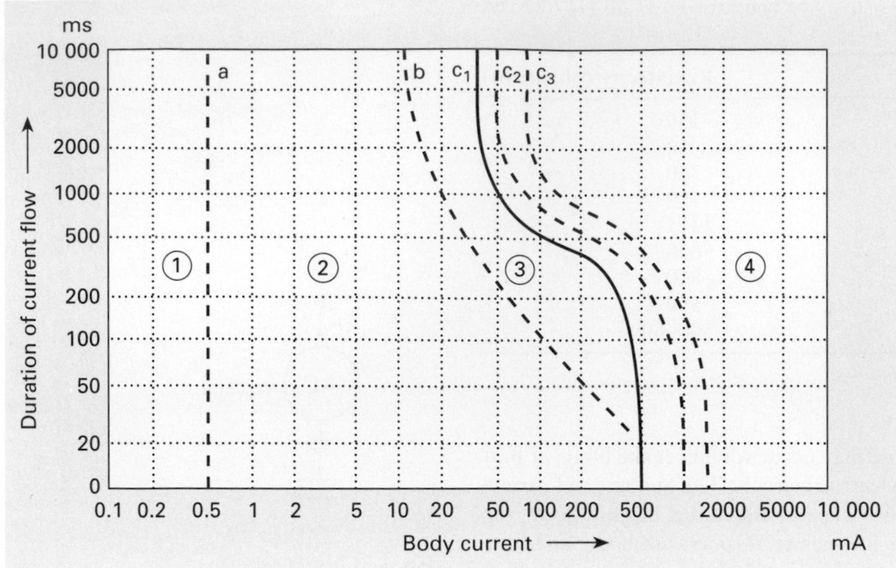

Fig. 2 Time/current zones of effects of AC currents (15 Hz to 100 Hz) on persons. The point 500 mA/100 ms corresponds to a fibrillation probability of the order of 0.14 per cent. (Reproduced with permission from IEC 1984, who retain the copyright.)

Zones	Physiological effects
Zone 1	Usually no reaction effects
Zone 2	Usually no harmful physiological effects
Zone 3	Usually no organic damage to be expected. Likelihood of muscular contractions and difficulty in breathing, reversible disturbances of formation and conduction of impulses in the heart, including atrial fibrillation and transient cardiac arrest without ventricular fibrillation increasing with current magnitude and time
Zone 4	In addition to the effects of Zone 3, probability of ventricular fibrillation increasing up to about 5% (curve C_1) up to about 50% (curve C_2), and above 50% beyond curve C_3. Increasing with magnitude and time, pathophysiological effects such as cardiac arrest, breathing arrest and heavy burns may occur

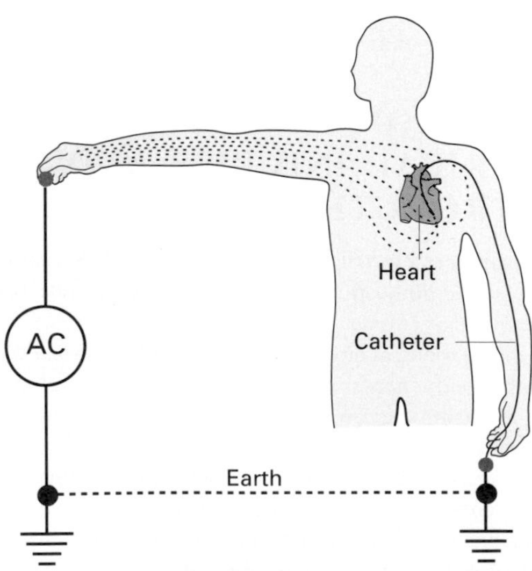

Fig. 3 The concept of microshock.

3. Protective cut-outs would have to be built into each piece of electronic apparatus and designed in such a way that a fault condition occurring in one piece of equipment did not cause the power supply of other life-supporting equipment to be tripped-out.

Electrical safety in the domestic and industrial environment and for the doctor's surgery (office), where single items of diagnostic apparatus which are not life supporting and conventional office equipment are used, is nowadays provided by a device called an earth leakage circuit breaker (ELCB). The principle of the ELCB is shown in Fig. 4. The live and neutral conductors are passed through a ferrite ring, thus forming the single turn primary of a transformer. The secondary winding consists of many turns of fine-gauge wire, which are connected to a solenoid. Under normal conditions, with no fault in the apparatus supplied through the ELCB, the current in the neutral conductor is equal and opposite in polarity to that in the live conductor, and therefore there is no change in the magnetic field and no current is induced to energize the solenoid.

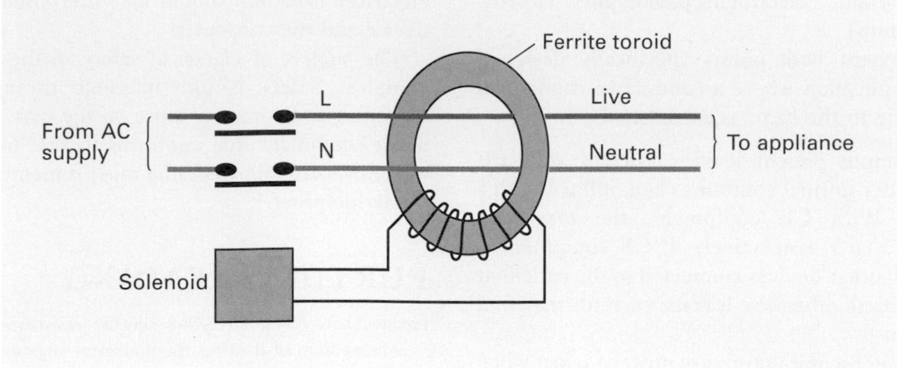

Fig. 4 Principle of the earth leakage circuit breaker (ELCB).

If a fault occurs such that electrical leakage current passes out of the system, say, through a human body, then there will be an imbalance of current between the live and neutral conductors and a voltage will be induced to energize the solenoid. Energization of the solenoid mechanically disconnects the live and neutral conductors from the apparatus. The ELCB has to be manually reset after the fault condition has been rectified. ELCBs are normally arranged to supply more than one socket outlet, which means that a single fault may disconnect the supply from a number of pieces of equipment.

PREVENTION OF GROSS ELECTROCUTION IN THE OPERATING THEATRE

The ELCB is unsuitable for use in the operating theatre and intensive care unit for the following reasons.

1 Permissible levels of electric current that may be allowed to pass through the sick, and so electrically susceptible, patient are much lower than those permissible in the fit and healthy person.
2 If an ELCB is designed to be extra-sensitive, it is always more prone to erroneous cut-outs.
3 An electrical current may be deliberately allowed to pass through the patient and may not all return to the equipment in use, but may find an alternative pathway. This may be at extremely low levels in monitoring equipment, but at increasing levels through (muscle or nerve) stimulators, to appreciable values with surgical diathermy.

Because of these problems, the idea in medical electronics is to use ever more rigorous design safety criteria, and by patient–circuit isolation rather than the use of ELCBs.

All equipment that may come into contact with a patient should have been designed and manufactured to comply with the relevant national and international standards. International agreement about safe design is published by the International Electrotechnical Commission (IEC) in the Standard IEC 601 (= BS 5724). This standard is published as IEC 601 Part 1, which contains all the general requirements for all equipment. There are an increasing number of Part 2s being published, which contain particular requirements for each type of equipment.

The main protection against electrocution in the operating theatre and elsewhere in the health-care facility is insulation, which minimizes the leakage current that may pass through the human body. Insulation, which also refers to the protective housing of equipment, must be designed so that possible leakage currents do not exceed levels set out in Standard IEC 601 even if the earth connection is inadequate. Earth conductors at mains supply outlets should be tested regularly, and the external cables of equipment should also be inspected carefully on a regular basis. These tests should be carried out by qualified engineering staff. However, electrical safety is also the responsibility of the users of the equipment.

1. Avoid portable distribution boards whenever possible.
2. Use ceiling-mounted pendant supplies whenever possible, as they are less likely to be damaged than those on the floor and are unlikely to become wet. Keep water and electricity apart.
3. Avoid the use of long mains supply cables, and avoid damage to cables by knotting, equipment wheels, etc.
4. Notify engineering staff of any visible damage to equipment or cables.
5. Make sure that regular maintenance records are kept and are available for inspection by the user.

One area where a potential risk of electric shock or burns is not common sense, except to an engineer, is when high frequency currents are in use, for example with radio frequency surgical diathermy. In normal use, insulation between two conductors or a single conductor and the body may be entirely adequate for d.c. or 50 Hz. However, this insulation may become the dielectric of a capacitor formed between the body and a 'conductor' at high frequency. (The resistance or impedance of a capacitor decreases as frequency increases.) Thus, at high frequencies, high currents may pass along unexpected routes, causing electrocution or burns. Burns may even occur between the body and metalwork that is not intentionally a conductor but is earthed. Burns due to this mechanism have occurred via the metalwork of operating tables and through the transducers of pulse oximeters (modern pulse oximeter transducers are isolated so that an earth pathway at high frequency cannot occur).

PREVENTION OF MICROSHOCK

Conventional safety measures may not protect the 'electrically susceptible' patient sufficiently. IEC 601 classifies the extra requirements in the design of equipment where there is risk of microshock.

Category BF Equipment having an applied part with intentional connection to the patient (e.g. electrocardiogram, electroencephalogram, electromyogram).

Category CF Equipment with points specifically designed for application where a conductive connection directly to the heart is established.

In general, the maximum patient leakage current with BF equipment is 100 μA under normal conditions and 500 μA with a single fault condition. With CF equipment, the maximum currents are 10 μA and 50 μA, respectively. If CF equipment is connected to a patient, all other devices connected to the patient at that time should be CF rated, otherwise leakage currents may find other routes to the heart.

In this day and age of microcomputers, care must be taken when computing equipment is connected in any way to monitoring apparatus, as most computing equipment is not protected to the same high specification as medical equipment and the safety standard of such monitoring equipment is immediately lowered, by definition, to that of the computing equipment. Some form of electrical isolation should be interposed between the medical device and the computer.

The subject of electrical safety in the health-care situation is complex. Safety is only possible through good maintenance, vigilance, and common sense on the part of the user, and by only using equipment that conforms to IEC 601. However well these guidelines are followed, one must remember that nothing is absolutely foolproof.

FURTHER READING

Geddes LA, Baker LE. The specific resistance of biological material—A compendium of data for the biological engineer and physiologist. *Med Bio Engineer* 1967; 5: 271–93.

IEC 479-1 *Effects of passing current through the human body*. Geneva: International Electrotechnical Commission, 1984.

IEC 601-1 *Safety of medical electrical equipment, Part 1: General requirements*. Geneva: International Electrotechnical Commission, 1979.

Martin TL. *Malice in Blunderland*. New York: McGraw Hill, 1973; 5.

3.4 Interpretation of lung function tests in the surgical patient

M. JOCELYN MORRIS

In patients scheduled to undergo surgery, lung function tests are often performed to detect those whose lung function is so poor that the risks of general anaesthesia are unacceptable; those whose lung function is moderately impaired such that any further deterioration due to postoperative pulmonary complications will put them immediately at risk and those with pulmonary disease who may benefit from energetic implementation of respiratory therapy such as effective bronchodilatation, physiotherapy, and prophylactic steroid therapy, prior to surgery.

With modern anaesthetic techniques there are virtually no patients who cannot be adequately ventilated and oxygenated during anaesthesia. The problems arise in the postoperative period, when hypoventilation is common and other pulmonary complications such as sputum retention, chest infection, and pulmonary emboli may supervene or cardiac output may be reduced. The particular vulnerability of chest patients to these complications arises from their mechanical inability to increase ventilation, from the marked decrease in oxygen content of the blood caused when small decreases of arterial $P\text{a}O_2$ occur in patients who are already hypoxaemic, and in some diseases from reduced sensitivity to rising $P\text{a}CO_2$, which normally causes ventilation to increase.

History is important in pinpointing those patients who need to undergo lung function tests prior to surgery: the most important warning symptom is shortness of breath. Past history of lung disease may be relevant, including recurrent chest infections which may indicate those likely to suffer from sputum retention and postoperative chest infection.

Investigations of lung function can be divided into tests which assess lung mechanics, those which assess gas transfer, and those which assess control of breathing.

LUNG MECHANICS

The best test for assessing lung mechanics is expiratory spirometry which, when correctly performed, gives very reproducible results. The equipment for this test is inexpensive and is portable. The main disadvantage is that it depends on the co-operation and maximum voluntary effort of the patient and these are assumed in the interpretation of the results. The elements required for the successful performance of the manoeuvre are maximum inspiration and complete and maximally forced expiration. Several attempts at this manoeuvre may be required, with repeated instructions, encouragement, and demonstrations of the sort of breath needed, before success is achieved. A normal expiratory spirogram is shown in Fig. 1(a). Predicted normal values for forced expired volume in the first second (FEV_1) and for forced vital capacity (FVC) (the total volume expired) depend on age, sex, height, and race, while the ratio of FEV_1/FVC is related to age. The measured values should be related to those predicted for a particular patient (Table 1). There is a wide range of normal values, the standard deviation for FEV_1 and FVC being 0.5 litres. An initial test may miss a diagnosis of mild disease since the subject may have to lose up to 2 l from his expired volume before falling out of the range into which 95 per cent of normal subjects fit. Since there is a large reserve of respiratory function, failure to detect mild disease is not a serious problem in surgical patients.

The results of this test allow lung function to be classed as normal, obstructive disease, or restrictive disease. If the volumes are not normal, distinction between obstructive and restrictive disease can be made from the FEV_1/FVC ratio: if this ratio is reduced there is an obstructive problem, (Fig. 1(b)). Predicted

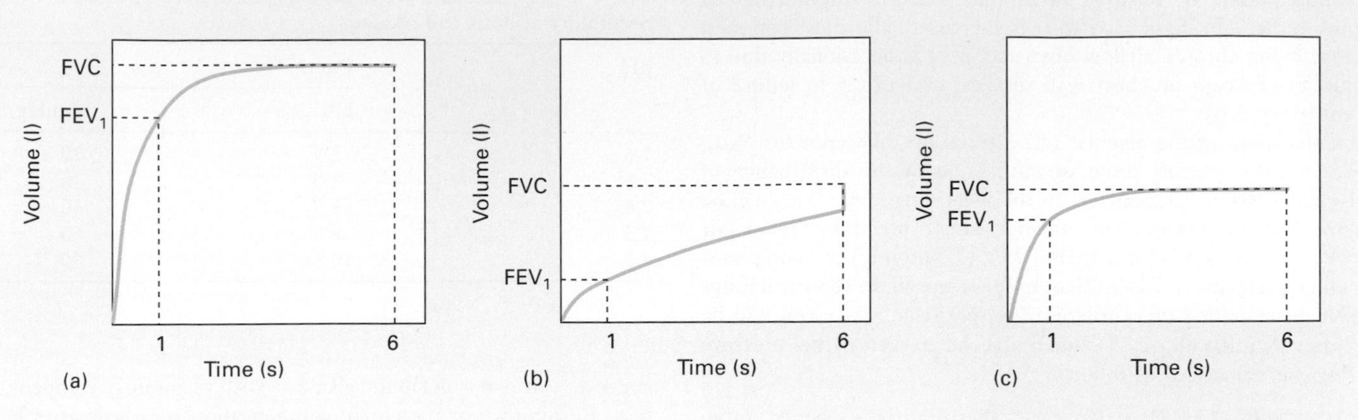

Fig. 1 Typical spirograms demonstrating (a) normal, (b) obstructive, (c) restrictive patterns of lung function.

Table 1 Rough guide to the severity of disturbance in lung mechanics

	Obstructive FEV_1 (percentage predicted)	Restrictive FVC (percentage predicted)
Mild	50–80	50–80
Moderate	35–50	35—50
Severe	< 35	< 35

FEV_1/FVC ratio is 83 per cent at age 20 to 25, and 67 per cent at age 70 years.

Diseases associated with airflow obstruction in the intrathoracic airways include smoking-induced chronic airflow obstruction (emphysema, chronic bronchitis), asthma, bronchiectasis, and, in infants, bronchiolitis. Central intrathoracic airways are narrowed in carcinoma of trachea, tracheomalacia, extrinsic compression, carcinoma of the larynx, vocal cord paralysis, epiglottitis, croup, large tonsils, and when there is an inhaled foreign body. In obstructive lung disease maximal expiratory flow rates are reduced, and these are reflected in a reduced FEV_1/FVC ratio. It is useful to obtain a measurement of slow vital capacity, that is maximum inspiration to total lung capacity followed by complete gentle expiration. In patients with obstructive disease this slow vital capacity (VC) may be considerably greater than the fast (maximally forced) expired volume (FVC). It this is so the ratio FEV_1/VC will be lower than FEV_1/FVC emphasizing that the problem is predominately one of airflow obstruction.

In restrictive lung disease the volumes are reduced but the FEV_1/FVC is ratio is normal, indicating that the airways do not offer abnormal resistance to flow (Fig. 1(c)). The element of the test which is poorly performed is the maximal inspiration—patients with restrictive disease are limited as to the size of the breath they can take in. Cause of inspiratory restriction include weakness of inspiratory muscles, rigid chest wall (ankylosing spondylitis, scoliosis), pleural disease, stiff lungs (alveolitis, fibrosis, congestion), and exclusion of part of the lung from the manoeuvre (collapse, consolidation, previous resection).

These tests of lung mechanics indirectly evaluate dyspnoea and work of breathing and give a measure of respiratory reserve, limitations of which may become important postoperatively when additional lung pathology may be present. Assessment of lung mechanics is often not possible before emergency surgery, in seriously ill patients, or in the early postoperative period, because of the maximal breaths required. More sophisticated lung function tests should be performed in the lung function laboratory in patients in whom the results of spirometry indicate severe disease and who are well enough to attend. Hyperinflation, the hallmark of airflow obstruction, can be assessed by the measurement of the static lung volumes, total lung capacity (TLC), functional residual capacity (FRC), and residual volume (RV) by helium dilution or whole body plethysmography. Direct measurements of airway resistance can be made: both the degree of hyperinflation and the increase in airways resistance parallel the decrease in maximum expiratory flow rates in airflow obstruction, and so can be roughly predicted from the simpler maximum effort tests. Peak flow (maximum expiratory flow) will be reduced in both obstructive and restrictive disease and this does not, therefore, distinguish between these two diagnoses.

GAS TRANSFER

Measurements of gas transfer are, on the whole, tests of ventilation perfusion (V/Q) matching. V/Q mismatching tends to be severe in patients with significant mechanical problems and major reduction of spirometric lung volumes. Of the tests available to assess gas transfer from alveolus to pulmonary capillary and vice versa, the best is measurement of arterial blood gases. Three items of information are obtained—arterial partial pressure of oxygen ($Pa{O_2}$), partial pressure of carbon dioxide ($Pa{CO_2}$) and the pH. These can be analysed both separately and together to build up a picture of lung function.

If, in a patient breathing air at sea level, the $Pa{O_2}$ is below the value predicted from the patient's age, hypoxaemia is present.

Predicted $Pa{O_2}$ (kPa) = 0.133 (104 − 0.24 age), SD 1.05
Predicted $Pa{O_2}$ (mmHg) = 104 − 0.24 age, SD 7.9

For example, predicted $Pa{O_2}$ is 13.2 kPa (99 mmHg) at age 20 and 11.6 kPa (87 mmHg) at age 70 years. A diagnosis of respiratory failure is made when the $Pa{O_2}$ is 8 kPa (60 mmHg) or below. Respiratory failure is divided into classes. In type 1, $Pa{CO_2}$ is normal or reduced (normal range 4.6–6.0 kPa, 35–45 mmHg). This is typically seen in pulmonary embolism, 'shock' lung, asthma, pulmonary fibrosis, pneumonia, and the emphysematous 'pink puffer'. In Type 2, $Paco_2$ is increased, the most common cause being chronic airflow obstruction; it is occasionally due to muscle weakness or chest wall disease, and rarely to failure of ventilatory drive.

Calculation of the alveolar (A) arterial (a) difference for Pao_2, $P(A - a)o_2$, enables some quantification of the disturbance of alveolar–arterial gas transfer. In the ideal lung $P(A - a)o_2$ will be zero, but in practice in normal lungs breathing room air $P(A-a)o_2$ should be less than 1 kPa (7.5 mmHg) in young subjects and less than 2.7 kPa (20 mmHg) at age 60. In abnormal lungs with mismatching of ventilation and perfusion $P(A-a)o_2$ will be greater than the above. Assumed alveolar oxygen partial pressure (PAo_2) is calculated as follows:

$PAo_2 = PIo_2 - Paco_2/R$ (R = respiratory exchange ratio, assumed to be 0.8)

PIo_2 = inspired oxygen concentration/100 × (barometric pressure − water vapour pressure)
Therefore when breathing air

$P(A-a)o_2 = 20 - Paco_2/0.8) - Pao_2$ (kPa)
$(P(A-a)o_2 = (150 - Paco_2/0.8) - Pao_2$ (mmHg)

When added oxygen is being inspired, even in normal lungs, $P(A-a)o_2$ widens, so comparisons between sequential measurements become difficult if different concentrations of oxygen are being given. Usually hypoxaemia is associated with an increased $P(A-a)o_2$, but if there is global underventilation, for example, due to oversedation, $Paco_2$ and $PAco_2$ may rise sufficiently such that PAo_2, and therefore Pao_2 falls. In this situation the calculated $P(A-a)o_2$ is normal, despite the presence of hypoxaemia. This indicates that the problem is one of underventilation of normal lungs. More usually, in the type 2 respiratory failure of chronic airflow obstruction one finds hypoxaemia, hypercapnia, and an increased $P(A-a)o_2$, indicative of the V/Q mismatching seen in abnormal lungs.

A reduced $Paco_2$ indicates hyperventilation, while an increased $Paco_2$ is indicative of hypoventilation. When ventilation perfusion mismatching is present there is a disparity between the ventilation required to achieve normal Pao_2 and normal $Paco_2$. Because of the linear CO_2 dissociation curve overventilation of one part of the lung (areas with high V/Q), can compensate for underventilation of another part (low V/Q regions). For oxygen, which has a sigmoid dissociation curve, this does not occur (Fig. 2). Breathing hard and increasing the Pao_2 in blood coming from the more normal areas of lung does not increase significantly the oxygen content (saturation) of this blood and therefore of the mixed pulmonary venous blood. This difference between the behaviour of carbon dioxide and oxygen results in type 1 respiratory failure.

The pH indicates whether an acidaemia or alkalaemia is present, while the $Paco_2$ indicates the respiratory contribution to the disturbance of acid–base state. The relationship between pH and $Paco_2$ indicates whether compensation has occurred (Table 2). For example if the $Paco_2$ is low,the patient is hyperventilating and there is a respiratory alkalosis. The pH will indicate whether this is acute and uncompensated (pH $>$ 7.4) or more chronic and compensated (pH near 7.4). It takes several hours for compensation of plasma bicarbonate by renal adjustment to begin, and days to complete. A useful working rule is that compensation does not bring the pH quite back to normal. A slightly acid pH with an elevated $Paco_2$ suggests a primary respiratory acidosis with metabolic compensation. A slightly alkaline pH with an elevated $Paco_2$ suggests a primary metabolic alkalosis with respiratory compensation. Respiratory or metabolic compensation for alkalosis is less complete and less predictable than that for acidosis. Respiratory compensation for a primary metabolic disorder occurs quite quickly, so the presence of compensation is not useful in determining how long the acid–base disorder has existed. Acute change in blood gases and pH superimposed on chronic changes are more difficult to interpret unless the results of serial measurements of blood gases are available.

Table 2 Approximate predictions of pH in uncompensated respiratory acidosis and alkalosis

pH	$Paco_2$	
	kPa	mmHg
7.6	2.5	20
7.5	4.0	30
7.4	5.5	40
7.3	8.0	60
7.2	10.5	80

Other tests of gas transfer include measurement of oxygen saturation by ear or finger pulse oximetry. This is a valuable non-invasive test for screening or for obtaining serial or continuous measurements. From the shape of the oxygen dissociation curve (Fig. 2) it can be seen, however, that this test will not detect early deterioration in gas exchange well. The Pao_2 may have fallen considerably before the oxygen saturation falls measurably, and saturation may then fall precipitously with only a further small decrease in Pao_2. Transcutaneous O_2 and CO_2 electrodes are not yet sufficiently robust in performance for routine use outside the intensive care unit. In the patient able to attend the lung function laboratory before surgery, measurement of transfer of carbon monoxide is a useful non-invasive screening test, particularly in the assessment of patients with pulmonary fibrosis, in whom CO transfer may be reduced when the lung volumes are still normal.

Acute changes in both lung mechanics and gas transfer are less

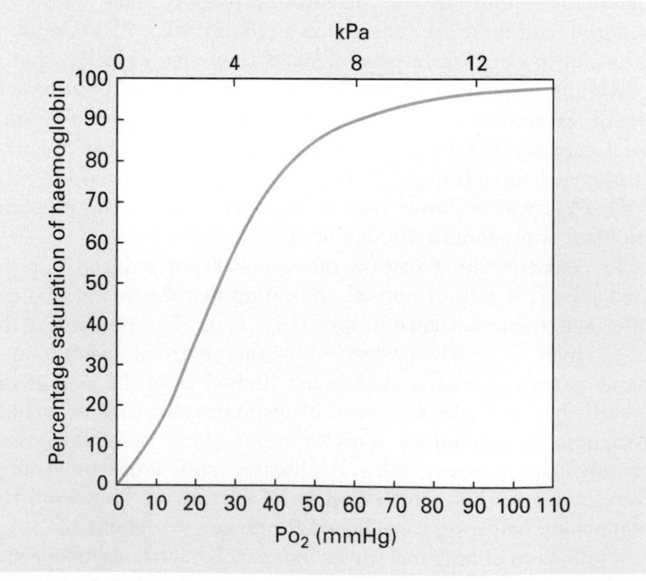

Fig. 2 Haemoglobin oxygen dissociation curve.

well tolerated by the patient than are chronic, slowly developing changes.

CONTROL OF BREATHING

Minute ventilation is normally controlled so that $Pa\text{O}_2$ and $Pa\text{CO}_2$ remain constant, despite varying metabolic demand for uptake of oxygen and excretion of carbon dioxide. Ventilation is driven by the rhythmic output from the brain-stem respiratory centre, the output of which is modulated by a falling $Pa\text{O}_2$ and increasing $Pa\text{CO}_2$ and cerebrospinal fluid acidity, and by reflexes arising from airways, alveoli, and chest wall. Formal assessment of control of breathing is not usually made before surgery, though if the preoperative $Pa\text{CO}_2$ is high it indicates either that control mechanisms have failed to increase ventilatory drive or that the mechanical problems are so great that ventilation cannot be increased despite increased drive. Opiates may depress respiratory drive postoperatively, but the benefits of early mobilization, coughing, and chest physiotherapy which are allowed by adequate pain relief are thought to outweigh this depressive effect. In patients with chronic airflow obstruction, the hypoxic drive to ventilation is important; oxygen must initially be given at low concentrations and its effect on $Pa\text{CO}_2$ monitored. It can be seen from Fig. 2 that in any patient with $Pa\text{O}_2$ near the knee of this curve a small decrease in $Pa\text{O}_2$ postoperatively due to hypoventilation may cause a sharp drop in oxygen saturation and oxygen carrying capacity.

Ideally perhaps, all patients should undergo expiratory spirometry and pulse oximetry before major surgery; however, a careful history of dyspnoea and recurrent chest infections will usually indicate those in whom preoperative lung function assessment is mandatory.

FURTHER READING

Gibson GJ. *Clinical Tests of Lung Function*. London: Macmillan Press (New York: Raven Press), 1984.

3.5 Blood transfusions and blood substitutes in surgical practice

C. C. ENTWISTLE

GENERAL PRINCIPLES

Blood lost due to surgery or trauma does not necessarily require replacement by transfusion. Circulating fluid is readily replaced from extravascular reserves, protein is regenerated in days and, in an otherwise healthy person, red cells are replaced over the next few days or weeks.

Transfusions may be warranted where blood loss is considerable, and especially if it is rapid, when further blood loss or imminent major surgery is likely, if the patient is suffering from symptomatic anaemia or if absorption of haematinics is impaired.

Blood to be transfused comes from donations, each bag from a single donor, and despite rigorous screening, each carries a small risk. Every recipient therefore requires individual assessment, and should only be transfused where the balance of risks is in favour of transfusion being performed.

PATIENT NEEDS

A minimum preoperative haemoglobin level of 100 g/l is no longer regarded as essential since many patients with lower haemoglobin levels tolerate surgery and seem to recover just as well.

Operative blood loss should be measured if at all possible. The patient initially requires restoration of blood volume. For small losses (under 20–25 per cent blood volume) simple fluids such as saline solution are adequate, safe, and inexpensive replacements, even though their renal excretion is rapid. Greater losses (up to 30–35 per cent blood volume) are better countered by infusion of colloid plasma substitutes such as solutions of modified starch, gelatin, or dextrans. All are widely available commercially, are much less expensive than plasma-derived equivalents, and are ready for use at ambient temperatures for any patient regardless of blood group, (though samples for blood grouping and compatibility tests should be taken before some dextrans are given). Because these products have molecular weights of 30 to 70 kDa they remain in the circulation to maintain plasma oncotic pressure for much longer than simple electrolyte solutions. They are only slowly metabolized or excreted over a period of about 2 days and are excellent stop gap agents for use while red cell products are awaited. They have no procoagulant activity.

When losses involve about 50 per cent of blood volume (or less in the elderly or patients with respiratory insufficiency), and especially if this loss is rapid, effective replacement of oxygen carrying capacity, as well as volume replacement, is vital. Blood, commonly now supplied as red cell concentrates, is necessary. Replacement of plasma proteins and coagulation factors is rarely indicated when blood loss is less than about one blood volume, even though there is little of either in red cell products. Extravascular fluids provide a large protein reservoir and coagulation usually remains unaffected even when levels of clotting factors are only one-third of normal: these factors are regenerated within hours except in patients with pre-existing liver disease.

Patients suffering massive blood loss need to be provided with sufficient appropriate products, which may include fresh frozen plasma and cryoprecipitates: platelet concentrates are required to counter platelet depletion from haemodilution and to correct for any functional impairment of circulating platelets.

MECHANICS OF PROVIDING BLOOD

Patient and sample identification

Clinicians contemplating transfusion should have a working knowledge of transfusion medicine, and be familiar with local facilities and practices. Blood request forms are legal documents; they must give unambiguous patient identification (date of birth is very useful), and state clearly what is required and by when. A brief prior visit to the local blood bank can promote good future communication. Blood samples for grouping, antibody screening, and compatibility testing (cross-matching) must be adequately labelled, and this is best done as the sample is taken. Mistakes in identification and in mislabelling of samples are among the most common causes of fatal transfusion reactions.

Grouping, antibody screening, and crossmatching

Blood groups are determined by antigens on cells, and can be shown as an agglutination reaction induced by reference antisera (Fig. 1). Such tests are performed either manually, on slides or in tubes or microwell systems, or by automated methods. Antibody screening involves testing the patient's serum for the presence of any rhesus, Kell, or other minor blood group antibodies which cause agglutination of a well-characterized panel of cells.

Compatibility testing consists of excluding *in vitro* antibody activity against donor cells, which if given, would provoke a transfusion reaction.

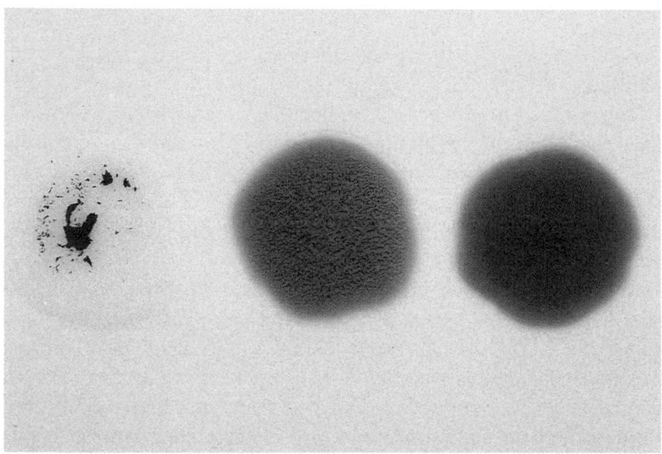

Fig. 1 Agglutination reactions in red cell typing. Strong positive (left), weak positive (centre), negative (right).

This is performed by adding serum in a 2 : 1 ratio to 3 per cent donor cells suspended either in low-ionic strength saline or normal saline; the mixture is then incubated at 37°C for 15 min (low ionic strength saline) or 45 min (normal saline), following which it is examined for agglutination, or even haemolysis, which indicate incompatibility. No single procedure detects all clinically important antibodies, but as a minimum, the indirect antiglobulin test should always be performed if possible. In this, an antiglobulin reagent (of animal or monoclonal origin) is added to cells which have been incubated as above; any cells coated with patient's antibody will then agglutinate, again indicating incompatibility. Recommended technical details are published elsewhere.

Anticipated requirements

The possible need for blood should always be anticipated. One or 2 per cent of patients carry atypical blood group antibodies, present either naturally or as a consequence of previous pregnancy, transfusion, or transplantation, and provision of compatible blood for these patients can sometimes prove difficult. For patients likely to require a transfusion a clotted blood sample should be grouped, screened for atypical antibodies and, where appropriate, special blood obtained and full compatibility tests done. At least a day's notice should be allowed for routine requests to be assimilated into the busy laboratory workload.

In emergencies, time may only allow shortened cross-matching, and even unmatched blood may have to be provided within 5 to 10 min. Unmatched blood can be of the same ABO group as the patient, or of Group O since Group O cells will not react with either anti-A or anti-B antibodies (Table 1); it must also be rhesus D negative if the recipient is a female of potentially child-bearing age. If Group O blood is given to patients of Group A, B, or AB, concentrated cells are preferable since the donor plasma and its anti-A and anti-B antibodies are largely removed (although even if given they would be rapidly diluted in the recipient's circulation and most would cause little if any clinically significant problem). These measures may be life-saving but errors are more likely to be made, patient antibodies to other groups may be missed, and transfusion reactions are more common. Whatever blood is given, it should never be ABO incompatible, for example, A Group to a Group O patient, since immediate, severe, and sometimes fatal intravascular haemolysis can follow, depending on the strength of that patient's antibodies. Incompatibility involving other blood

Table 1 Distribution of the most important blood groups in the United Kingdom

System	Groups of red cells	Per cent in population	Antibodies present in serum
ABO	O	47	Anti-A, anti-B
	A	42	Anti-B
	B	8	Anti-A
	AB	3	Neither
RHESUS	D positive	85	Normally no antibodies
	D negative	15	1–2 per cent if previous transfusion, pregnancy, or transplant
KELL	K positive	9	
	K negative	91	
Other systems			As for rhesus and Kell, but sometimes naturally-occurring antibodies also present

Major differences from these figures occur in other populations e.g. Group B over 20 per cent in the Middle East, Indian subcontinent, and many Afro-Caribbean countries; rhesus D negative is almost unknown in the Far East.

group systems (e.g. rhesus, Kell, Duffy) leads to reticuloendothelial sequestration of mistransfused cells rather than to immediate lysis, and is a much less severe clinical result.

Maximum surgical blood ordering schedules

To make the best use of the group and screen system, both to minimize hazards to patients from avoidable urgent blood requests and wastage of laboratory resources on blood not then used, blood banks are increasingly being encouraged through active clinical audit to use maximum surgical blood ordering schedules. Under these schedules, compatibility tests are only performed based upon ongoing review of previous blood usage by given surgeons for essentially similar clinical situations.

PRODUCTS AVAILABLE

Homologous blood

Almost all transfusion services are based upon blood collected from healthy unpaid volunteer donors. Because of national demands for self-sufficiency in blood and plasma-derived products, notably factor VIII for haemophilics, the use of whole blood is rapidly giving way to red cell preparations, supplied either as concentrates or as suspensions in optimal additive solutions, the plasma being removed for fractionation. Red cells in optimal additive solutions have excellent viability and the suspension viscosity is comparable to that of whole blood.

Whole blood may still be preferable for paediatric patients and blood transfused into babies should have been stored for less than 7 days and also be known to be cytomegalovirus antibody negative. There is no convincing evidence that 'donor fresh' blood has any magic haemostatic properties; perioperative haemorrhagic states, exclusive of surgical causes, are often attributable to platelet deficiency or malfunction and should be corrected appropriately. In some countries, though not in the United Kingdom, so-called 'directed' blood donations are used, usually from close family members, especially parents for their own children. Although such donations are better than no blood, they offer little advantage over conventional supplies and indeed may not always be quite as safe.

Autologous blood

A patient's own blood can be collected and reinfused, thus eliminating some of the hazards of homologous transfusions. A preoperative deposit of up to about four donations (450 ml blood each) can be made by basically healthy patients within the 5 weeks prior to planned (e.g. orthopaedic) surgery. Patients as young as 8 to those over 80 can predonate blood, provided that the necessary local facilities are available. Case selection should minimize the taking of blood unlikely to be needed. Where 'cross-over' of untransfused units into the routine blood bank is practised the patient-donor and blood must satisfy safety standards for homologous donations.

Intraoperative haemodilution is another means of providing autologous blood. Two units of blood are drawn in the anaesthetic room and replaced with crystalloid solution or plasma substitute: that fresh and platelet-rich blood is then immediately available if needed. The patient's blood viscosity is also lowered, which aids tissue perfusion and oxygenation—this is particularly valuable in vascular surgery.

Peroperative salvage may also be practised: shed blood is collected, and the red cells are washed and filtered ready for reinfusion, usually within minutes. Peroperative salvage is most cost-effective where substantial blood loss is predicted.

Some other blood products

Platelet concentrates

These are made from individual donations but are rarely needed in routine surgery. In patients suffering major blood loss, and particularly during cardiac surgery with prolonged bypass, in those with renal failure, and those taking aspirin or other antiplatelet drugs, circulating platelets may be deficient in number (under $100 \times 10^9/l$), function, or both, making active platelet support essential. Patients with haematological disorders may need prophylactic platelet transfusion as well as replacement, for example to cover insertion of a Hickman line, splenectomy, and of course for intercurrent surgery. In all these situations a haematologist should be consulted and reasonable notice given to obtain appropriate products.

Fresh frozen plasma

This is essentially normal plasma containing citrate anticoagulant and its use is indicated when massive blood loss (over one blood volume) occurs, or when there is mixed coagulation impairment, for instance due to warfarin overdose, liver disease, or as part of disseminated intravascular coagulation. The last occasionally complicates prostatic or chest surgery and some obstetric situations. Fresh frozen plasma should then be given (1 litre initially) to supplement other transfusions. In such cases, haematological advice should be sought. Fresh frozen plasma should not be used as a volume expander; safer products are available.

Cryoprecipitates

These concentrates, which include factor VIII, fibrinogen, von Willebrand factor and some other factors are also made from individual donations. While most cryoprecipitates are given to patients with haemophilia A (see below), or von Willebrand's disease, they can provide a source of fibrinogen in patients with disseminated intravascular coagulation, and act as a substrate for 'fibrin glue', activated by thrombin for sealing large raw surfaces (pleura, liver etc.), for patients undergoing vascular surgery, and many other applications.

Clotting factor concentrates

These are best provided purified from plasma pools and subjected to viral inactivation to prevent transmission of HIV, etc. These concentrates and cryoprecipitates are critical in the proper management of surgery in haemophilics, but should always be given in collaboration with the local haemophilia service to ensure that adequate and correct treatment is given and monitored.

TRANSFUSION COMPLICATIONS

Immediate

Sites of vascular access may become inflamed, thrombose, or become dislodged; if so, resiting is indicated.

Over-transfusion, particularly in the elderly, can be avoided by accurate fluid balance control. Overhydration is treated by judicious use of diuretics and digoxin and reduced fluid input.

Allergic reactions, predominately cutaneous, are commonly attributed to unidentified foreign proteins in donor blood. These reactions are usually uncomfortable for the patient rather than serious, although severe anaphylactic reactions can occur. Treatment with antihistamines and intravenous hydrocortisone is usually effective.

Non-haemolytic febrile transfusion reactions are common. Some are associated with patient alloimmunization to HLA, platelet (HPA), or granulocyte-specific antigens following previous pregnancy, transfusion, or transplantation. These reactions are rarely serious and resolve either spontaneously after discontinuation of the offending unit, or with administration of antipyretics and symptomatic measures. In-line microaggregate, or the more effective though expensive white cell removal filters, reduce the incidence and severity of non-haemolytic febrile transfusion reactions in patients who react repeatedly.

Haemolytic reactions due to red cell incompatibility are similar to non-haemolytic febrile transfusions reactions, with the addition of rigors and perhaps loin pain and collapse. Such reactions should be exceedingly rare provided there have been no clerical or laboratory errors. Treatment is as for non-haemolytic reactions but the possible occurrence of intravascular lysis and complement activation make critical observation of renal function essential; dialysis may be necessary.

Delayed

Poorly sustained haemoglobin level (overt or occult bleeding excluded) may be due to elimination of transfused blood near the end of its shelf-life or accelerated destruction due to an anamnestic antibody response after previous pregnancy or transfusion; mild jaundice with elevated unconjugated serum bilirubin can occur.

An immunosuppressive 'transfusion effect' may follow transfusions of homologous blood. This results in depression of humoral and cellular immune responses which persists for many months. Renal graft survival may be improved but metastatic spread of certain tumours (particularly colorectal) may be potentiated and susceptibility to wound and other postoperative infections is increased.

Transmitted infections are the most serious complication. Despite routine virological donor screening, about one donation in every million carries low levels of hepatitis B virus or is HIV positive, despite a negative antibody test (especially in the early 'window' stages of infection). Hepatitis C virus is present in up to 1 in 500 of some donor populations, is readily transmissible through transfusion, and accounts for almost all cases of non-A, non-B hepatitis. Up to one-half of the recipients become chronic carriers and later develop chronic hepatitis, and perhaps cirrhosis and even hepatoma. Routine screening of donors for hepatitis C virus antibodies should reduce the incidence of these complications.

Cytomegalovirus is ubiquitous, although more endemic in some populations than others. While cytomegalovirus causes little more than a brief glandular fever-like illness for most patients and is a recognized cause of a similar postcardiotomy syndrome, it can cause serious morbidity and mortality in premature babies and immunosuppressed patients such as transplant recipients. Depending on local populations and facilities, blood negative for cytomegalovirus antibody can be provided or alternatively, virus-carrying white blood cells can be largely filtered out.

Rarely blood and its products can become contaminated with bacteria; some Gram-negative organisms proliferate even during storage at 4°C. Transfusion of such blood very rapidly leads to severe, often irreversible, endotoxin shock.

SUMMARY

Transfusions form an integral part of overall patient care, demanding definition of specific needs and complementary treatment. While careful surgical technique will minimize blood loss, particular aspects must be addressed, such as large raw areas, prolonged bypass, pre-existing coagulation problems, and platelet deficiency. Supplementary measures may be helpful, including use of fibrinolytic inhibitors during surgery and haematinics afterwards. Knowledge of the blood products given and monitoring of progress are essential to ensure anticipated effects are achieved and that adverse complications are expeditiously treated. Patients undoubtedly benefit from transfusion, but like any other prescribed medication, this must only be given when justified.

FURTHER READING

Auck TF, Carey P. Autologous transfusion practice—international forum. *Vox Sang*, 1990; **58**: 234–53.

Blumberg N, Heal JM, Murphy P, Agarwal MM, Chuang C. Association between transfusion of whole blood and recurrence of cancer. *Br Med J*, 1986; **293**: 530–3.

British Committee for Standards in Haematology Blood Transfusion Task Force. Guidelines for autologous transfusion. *Clin Lab Haematol*, 1988; **10**: 193–201.

British Committee for Standards in Haematology Blood Transfusion Task Force. Guidelines for implementation of a maximum surgical blood ordering schedule. *Clin Lab Haematol*, 1990; **12**: 321–7.

British Society for Haematology and British Blood Transfusion Society. Guidelines for compatibility testing in hospital blood banks. *Clin Lab Haematol*, 1987: **9**: 333–41.

Dienstag JL. Non A non B hepatitis I. Recognition, epidemiology and clinical features. *Gastroenterology*, 1983; **85**: 439–62.

Friedman BA. An analysis of surgical blood usage in United States Hospitals with application to maximum surgical blood ordering schedule. *Transfusion*, 1979; **19**: 268–78.

Gilbert GL, Hayes K, Hudson IL, James J. Prevention of transfusion-acquired cytomegalovirus infection in infants by blood filtration to remove leucocytes. *Lancet*, 1989; i: 1228–31.

Goldfinger D. Controversies in transfusion medicine: directed donations (pro). *Transfusion*, 1989; **29**: 70–4.

Hogman CF, Rosen I, Andreen M, Akerblom O, Hellsing. Haemotherapy with red cell concentrates and a new red cell storage system. *Lancet*, 1983; **i**: 269–72.

Page PL. Controversies in transfusion medicine: directed donations (con). *Transfusion* 1989; **29**: 65–70.

Simpson MB. Platelet transfusion in selected clinical situation. In: *Platelets*. American Association of Blood Banks, 1988: 129–65.

Sirchia G, Wenz B, Rebulla P, Parravicini A, Carnelli V, Bertolini F. Removal of white cells from red cells by transfusion through a new filter. *Transfusion*, 1990; **30**: 30–3.

Care of the critically-ill patient

4

4 Critical care of the surgical patient

CHRISTOPHER S. GARRARD

INTRODUCTION

The critical care unit has become an integral and essential part of a modern acute hospital, providing an environment for the observation and treatment of the severely ill patient. Many large hospitals are able to support separate medical, surgical, neurosurgical, and respiratory units, while in smaller institutions, a single multidisciplinary unit serves the needs of several specialties.

Critical care demands many clinical skills that are not always obtained during the course of basic medical or surgical training. Specific training, is therefore, widely acknowledged to be essential for those embarking on a career in critical care, regardless of their primary specialty. The critical care clinician must be able to sustain the physiological equilibrium of the patient by pharmacological and mechanical means. This requires constant surveillance of the patient, anticipation of adverse events and aggressive intervention when necessary (proactive management). Meticulous attention to detail of each organ system is essential and yet the patient must always be considered as a physical and psychological whole. Time is of the essence; when intervention is planned, it should be undertaken quickly and without delay.

A major component of critical care is counselling and support for the relatives and friends of the patient. Time must be set aside to explain the reasons for, and the consequences of, investigations and therapy. This responsibility cannot be delegated to the junior surgical or nursing staff but should be undertaken by the most senior member of the surgical team. Not only is this an essential part of the surgeon's responsibility to the patient, but it also minimizes errors in communication and the risk of litigation.

As with other aspects of health care delivery, the nurse fulfils the key role in the provision of critical care. The intense and unremitting nature of critical care practice places severe burdens upon nurses, and the clinician must provide a team approach to support nursing staff. A 'one to one' nurse to patient ratio is highly desirable and is probably the most important factor in ensuring quality of care.

The following chapter deals with several critical care topics, classified according to the major organ systems.

4.1 Cardiovascular aspects

CHRISTOPHER S. GARRARD

CARDIOPULMONARY RESUSCITATION

Cardiac arrest may complicate the clinical course of both medical and surgical patients and the provision of prompt and efficient cardiopulmonary resuscitation is a basic skill required by all critical care personnel. The critical care unit provides an ideal environment for successful cardiopulmonary resuscitation following cardiac arrest. The rate of survival after cardiac arrest is higher in the critical care unit than in other areas of the hospital because the event is usually witnessed, the rhythm is usually ventricular fibrillation, and all the necessary personnel and equipment are immediately available. Outlook is poorest when cardiac arrest complicates renal failure, respiratory failure, or other metabolic disorders, including sepsis. Prodromal events such as hypoxaemia, arrhythmias, and electrolyte disturbances should be detected before circulatory failure occurs, and prompt intervention may prevent cardiac arrest.

Whenever possible the cause of cardiac arrest should be ascertained. It may be rapidly apparent that the serum potassium had been rising during the proceeding hours or that there had been a prodromal arrhythmia. In the postoperative cardiac surgical patient, electromechanical dissociation due to haemopericardium must always be considered. Such information and the clinical background may influence significantly the approach to resuscitation. Because the critical care unit patient is invariably undergoing ECG monitoring, ventricular fibrillation is usually recognized and treated immediately. Even in the highly advantageous environment of the critical care unit, however, a disciplined approach to basic cardiopulmonary resuscitation procedure still needs to be followed.

The conduct of cardiopulmonary resuscitation

A resuscitation team leader should supervise the resuscitation. Ideally, this individual should have little active role in resuscitation procedures but should direct the treatment priorities, coordinate the participants, and assess the effectiveness of resuscitation. One team member should maintain cardiac massage while another provides ventilatory support. Another member should establish medication access, preferably by a central venous route, if not previously established, while another records interventions and medications administered.

The ABC (Airway, Breathing, Circulation) order of assessment and resuscitation should be followed. In many cases the patient will already be intubated; if not, the airway must be secured (oral airway will suffice) and ventilation provided initially by face mask and Ambu bag (self-inflating ventilation bag). Two hands are required to produce an adequate seal with an anaesthetic face mask, and another individual should provide ventilation. If the patient is already on a mechanical ventilator, 'bagging' the patient with 100 per cent O_2 will permit better synchronization with cardiac massage: slow inflations of the lungs sufficient to cause visible expansion of the chest wall are required. A major arterial pulse, such as the carotid, should be checked since a malfunctioning arterial line may not accurately reflect cardiac output.

Controversy still surrounds the use of the precordial (chest) thump. When a defibrillator is immediately to hand and when the patient is already monitored it probably has little role in the resuscitation procedure.

Circulation support

The ratio of cardiac compressions to each ventilated breath should be 5:1, with a compression rate of 60 to 80 per minute. Whatever cardiac compression rates are achieved, they must not interfere with effective ventilation. Recent clinical trials have not confirmed the superiority of simultaneous compression-ventilation cardiopulmonary resuscitation, as was suggested by animal studies. No more than 10 s should be permitted for any manoeuvre that demands temporary cessation of chest compression.

Assessment of the efficacy of cardiopulmonary resuscitation is difficult. An intra-arterial pressure trace is an ideal indicator of cardiac output but is not always available. End-tidal CO_2 greater than 2 kPa (15 mmHg) has recently been shown to indicate efficient resuscitation and favourable outcome, while an end-tidal CO_2 less than 1.5 kPa (10 mmHg) predicts a poor outcome. Administration of bicarbonate during resuscitation will tend to raise end-tidal CO_2, misleading the clinician into believing resuscitation is more effective than it really is.

All medications should be administered by a central venous cannula or by the transtracheal route: the latter is particularly suitable for the administration of adrenaline (double dose).

Definitive measures

The measures that need to be applied depend upon the underlying cause of cardiac arrest. The most common arrhythmia is ventricular fibrillation which should be treated with immediate defibrillation. If defibrillation at 200 J produces no response, this should be repeated. If there is still no response, defibrillation at 360 J should be performed. If this is also unsuccessful, defibrillation at 360 J should be repeated after intravenous administration of 1 mg adrenaline (epinephrine) and then lignocaine (100 mg intravenously).

If this is still unsuccessful, alternative paddle positions (anteroposterior) or another antiarrhythmic drug should be tried. In refractory cases attempts should be made at electrical placing by either external or internal electrodes.

Cardiopulmonary resuscitation should be attempted for up to 2 min after each drug, and should not be interrupted for more than 10 s, except for defibrillation. Differentiating 'coarse' from 'fine' fibrillation has been thought to predict response to defibrillation. However, the standard approach outlined above should still be adhered to. Recent work in animal models has shown that the frequency characteristics of the pattern of ventricular fibrillation are determined by the duration of fibrillation. Such a tool, may in the future, serve to predict outcome. Once an effective cardiac output is achieved, a continuous infusion of adrenaline (epinephrine) in doses of 1 to 10 mg/h can be given to support the myocardium and circulation. In the young patient with an otherwise good prognosis, supramaximal doses may be administered. Other inotropes and pressors can be used with equal effect. Arterial blood gases and electrolytes should be monitored, and a chest radiograph obtained.

Adrenaline has largely replaced lignocaine (lidocaine) as the first pharmacological agent to be administered in cardiac arrest patients. Adrenaline, and possibly noradrenaline (norepinephrine), may increase cerebral perfusion during basic life support, although they probably do not enhance the efficacy of defibrillation. Lignocaine is effective in the treatment of ventricular tachycardia and in ventricular fibrillation prophylaxis. However, evidence to support its use in cardiopulmonary resuscitation is lacking and lignocaine may actually render the heart more refractory to electrical defibrillation.

Administration of sodium bicarbonate is no longer recommended, except where efficient ventilation can be maintained during prolonged resuscitation. After prolonged resuscitation it may be reasonable to consider administering 50 mmol of sodium bicarbonate (50 ml of 8.4 per cent) if there is persistent metabolic acidosis. Unfortunately, the buffering effect of bicarbonate results in the generation of carbon dioxide which readily diffuses into the intracellular compartment and may therefore worsen intracellular acidosis. The best way of controlling the acidosis observed during cardiopulmonary resuscitation is to establish effective ventilation and ensure an adequate circulation. Other alkalinizing agents, such as the combination of sodium carbonate and bicarbonate (Carbicarb®), although not widely available, may offer an alternative method of correcting severe acidosis.

There is no limit to the number of defibrillations which can be attempted, assuming that the cardiac rhythm diagnosis is correct. Changing both paddle positions and the defibrillator itself should be considered, together with administration of other antiarrhythmic drugs such as bretilium.

Electromechanical dissociation

Electromechanical dissociation is the presence of QRS complexes without apparent ventricular contractions, as evidenced by a palpable pulse or arterial pressure waves. Caution should always be exercised when using an arterial line to obtain an index of cardiac contractility, since such a device may give false information. If in doubt, the carotid or femoral pulse should be checked. Electromechanical dissociation is managed in the same way as any cardiac arrest situation except that intravenous adrenaline (1 mg) should be administered immediately.

It is essential to exclude and correct hypovolaemia, which may be disguised by pressor administration or may form part of sepsis syndrome. Pneumothorax/haemothorax should be considered in all trauma victims, while cardiac tamponade may complicate postoperative cardiac cases. Pulmonary embolism must always be considered in the postoperative patient.

Treatable electromechanical dissociation must be managed aggressively. In many cases cardiac arrest is unheralded but in retrospect it may be apparent that physiological changes were present, indicative of events such as cardiac tamponade or pneumothorax. Acute and severe blood loss will eventually result in electromechanical dissociation: volume resuscitation requires insertion of several large bore cannulae for the transfusion of blood and blood products. In patients likely to survive, emergency thoracotomy, internal cardiac massage, and cross-clamping of the descending aorta may all be required before an effective cardiac output can be achieved.

Any patient maintained on intermittent positive pressure ventilation who manifests increasing airway pressures may be developing a pneumothorax. There may be insufficient time to obtain a chest radiograph, and tube thoracostomy (possibly bilateral) may have to be performed immediately. Tamponade may develop following cardiac surgery, and the clinician must be alert to the implications of a falling cardiac output and oliguria in the face of a rising central venous pressure. The decision to reopen a sternotomy wound is never made lightly, but prompt intervention may be the only way of saving the patient who is developing tamponade. Cardiac massage in this situation is probably ineffectual at best and at worst may disrupt coronary artery vein grafts.

If hyperkalaemia or hypocalcaemia is suspected, or if calcium antagonists have recently been administered, calcium chloride (10 ml of 10 per cent) should be administered.

Asystole

Asystole has grave prognostic implications, since treatment is much less effective than is the case for ventricular fibrillation. It is critical that errors in identifying asystole are excluded. Faulty equipment or very fine ventricular fibrillation may lead to the incorrect assumption that asystole is present. If any doubt exists the patient should be treated as for ventricular fibrillation.

Adrenaline, 1 mg followed by atropine 2 mg, should be administered through a central venous line. Isoprenaline (isoproterenol) may be administered if these first two agents fail to re-establish ventricular fibrillation or another rhythm. As with refractory ventricular fibrillation, persistent asystole may respond to either external or internal electrical pacing. There are few, if any, indications for the intracardiac administration of medication: the risk of myocardial damage is high and the benefits questionable.

Cerebral resuscitation

A final indicator of the success or failure of cardiopulmonary resuscitation is the subsequent level of cerebral function. Many of the factors determining the development of neurological sequelae are self-evident, such as the duration of circulatory standstill. Other factors, such as the rapidity with which circulatory and metabolic homeostasis can be achieved, also have a significant bearing on neurological outcome. Aspects of cerebral resuscitation are considered further elsewhere.

CIRCULATORY FAILURE

Circulatory failure not due to cardiac arrest can be divided broadly into hypovolaemic, cardiogenic, and distributive types. Because of the hypotension and tachycardia associated with these forms of circulatory failure they are often referred to as shock syndromes. The causes of these three types of circulatory failure are summarized in Table 1.

Hypovolaemic circulatory failure

The clinical response to intravascular volume depletion varies considerably, depending upon the rapidity of depletion and the peripheral vasoconstrictor responses. The classic clinical picture includes orthostatic hypotension, tachycardia, pallor, tachypnoea, cold vasoconstricted peripheries, oliguria, and mental obtundation. Minor volume depletion may be unmasked by the inadvertent

Table 1 Classification of the circulatory failure syndromes

I. Hypovolaemic circulatory failure
  Haemorrhage
    External and internal
    Crush injury
  Severe burns
  Acute electrolyte depletion
    Upper and lower gastrointestinal losses
    Addison's disease
    Diabetes mellitus and insipidus
II. Cardiogenic circulatory failure
  Disorders of contractility
    Ischaemic heart disease
    Hypoxaemia
    Cardiomyopathies
    Sepsis syndrome
    Drug induced
  Disorders of pump mechanics
    Valvular disorders
    Cardiac tamponade
    Constrictive pericarditis
  Disorders of afterload
    Systemic hypertensive
    Coarctation of aorta
    Pulmonary hypertension
    Pulmonary embolism
  Disorders of rhythm
    Tachy- and bradyarrhythmias
III. Distributive circulatory failure
    Sepsis syndrome
    Post-traumatic
    Anaphylactic
    Neurogenic
    Endocrinological

administration of a vasodilator such as glyceryl trinitrate or the commencement of positive pressure ventilation. Prolonged periods of hypovolaemic shock result in permanent tissue injury developing either during the period of hypoperfusion or during subsequent reperfusion).

Management and monitoring

Clinical evaluation of the degree of hypovolaemia precedes any attempts to establish invasive monitoring. The blood pressure, degree of orthostasis, tachycardia, sweating, and peripheral vasoconstriction, together with signs of end-organ hypoperfusion such as neurological obtundation and cardiac arrhythmias will impress on the clinician the urgency of therapy. A simple clinical classification of the degree of hypovolaemia is shown in Table 2 and provides a guide to the blood volume deficit. Transfusion must be commenced via large bore (14 gauge), peripheral intravenous cannuli before time-consuming attempts to establish central venous pressure and arterial lines are made.

Venous access is of prime importance. Small peripheral venous and triple lumen central lines are generally inadequate for rapid, large volume transfusions. Several large peripheral lines combined with a large bore (8 or 8.5 Fr) central line will usually suffice. If a peripheral cut down is required, the insertion of the cut end of a sterile giving set (without the connector) directly into a vein ensures rapid transfusion.

The patient should be placed in the 'feet up–head down posture', and given oxygen supplementation. *In extremis*, with profound hypotension and a cardiac arrest situation developing, adrenaline (epinephrine) in 1 mg boluses should be considered. In trauma patients, whose injuries may be associated with uncontrollable blood loss, no rate or volume of transfusion will save the patient's life unless emergency surgery is undertaken.

An arterial and central venous pressure monitoring line greatly facilitates assessment of resuscitation. Correction of blood pressure, resolution of tachycardia, and an increase in central venous pressure (approaching 10–12 mmHg, relative to the right atrium) indicate satisfactory volume expansion; warming of the skin, absence of orthostatic hypotension, urine production of 0.5 to 1 ml/kg.h, and resolution of metabolic acidosis indicate re-establishment of organ perfusion.

Transfusion fluids

When undertaking fluid resuscitation the clinician must first address the issue of what fluid and how much? Although there is controversy regarding the selection of crystalloid versus colloid, some rationalization can be applied on a case by case basis. The supporters of crystalloid fluids point out that hypovolaemia affects both the intravascular and interstitial spaces and that crystalloids are distributed readily to both spaces in a ratio of 1:3. The proponents of colloidal solutions emphasize the urgency of expanding the intravascular space to defend the circulation. Some agents, such as the hydroxyethyl starches, produce a volume expansion greater than the transfused volume due to their osmotic properties. Obviously, patients with slowly developing hypovolaemia secondary to long-standing gastroenterological losses, and who may be haemoconcentrated will benefit from balanced electrolyte replenishment. The massively bleeding trauma patient could be initially and briefly supported with any fluid. Very soon, however, haemodilution effects and coagulation defects will mandate blood and blood product replacement. Clearly, it is the volume and speed of replacement that determines outcome more than the initial selection of the type of fluid.

When massive transfusion is required, blood should always be warmed and replacement of clotting factors considered on a continual basis. The difficulty of achieving a balance between undertransfusion and overtransfusion should not be underestimated,

Table 2 Classification of severity of hypovolaemia

	Class 1	Class 2	Class 3	Class 4
Heart rate (beats/min)	<100	>100	>120	>140
Blood pressure	Normal	Normal	Decreased	Decreased
Pulse pressure	N or increased	Decreased	Decreased	Decreased
Capillary refill	Normal	Delayed	Delayed	Very delayed
Blood loss (l)	Up to 0.75	0.75–1.5	1.5–2.0	2.0 plus
Blood loss (%)	Up to 15	15–30	30–40	>40

even with all appropriate monitoring facilities. Remember that prolonged hypoperfusion carries the risk of organ tissue damage, while fluid overload, although not well tolerated in the elderly, can be reversed with diuretics or haemofiltration.

Cardiogenic circulatory failure

The initial clinical evaluation of cardiogenic failure should determine the nature of the failure (systolic versus diastolic), the underlying cause and the severity of the problem. A full clinical history and physical examination should be performed to detect ischaemic heart disease, hypertension, alcoholism, viral syndrome, valvular heart disease, or congenital heart disease. A 12-lead ECG should be obtained to identify acute myocardial infarction, left ventricular hypertrophy, heart block, or arrhythmias. Chest radiography is required for the assessment of heart size and pulmonary vascular markings, and pleural effusion.

If the patient is suffering from acute pulmonary oedema or cardiogenic shock, treatment should begin immediately. If there is less urgency an echocardiogram provides information about the size, thickness, and performance of the heart. The Doppler mode provides unique, non-invasive assessment of valvular function and allows for detection of intracardiac shunts.

The treatment of cardiogenic failure is based upon the manipulation of myocardial contractility, cardiac preload and afterload. This is achieved by the administration of inotropes, fluids, diuretics, and vasodilators, alone or in combination. The success or failure of therapy should be measured against clear therapeutic endpoints, such as a doubling of cardiac output, or a 25 per cent fall in pulmonary artery wedge pressure. The electrocardiogram, systemic arterial pressure, cardiac output, and pulmonary artery wedge pressure should be carefully monitored throughout the period of therapy. An arterial cannula is essential for monitoring patients receiving vasodilator or inotropic therapy, particularly when the blood pressure is labile. Flow-directed pulmonary artery catheters are most useful when there is uncertainty regarding left ventricular filling pressure or cardiac output.

Myocardial preload

Preload is best represented by the ventricular end-diastolic volume although clinically it is more convenient to use ventricular end-diastolic pressure. The end-diastolic pressure is, in turn, approximated by the atrial pressures; right atrial pressure for the right ventricle and pulmonary artery wedge pressure for the left ventricle. Increases in preload are associated with increases in both the extent and velocity of muscle fibre shortening, which combine to produce an increase in stroke volume. Heart failure is characterized by a limited increase in left ventricular stroke work for a given rise in left ventricular end-diastolic pressure (Fig. 1).

The relationship between end-diastolic pressure stroke and volume is non-linear, and in the failing heart contractility is less responsive to increases in end-diastolic pressure. Nevertheless, alterations in preload are important determinants of cardiac performance in both normal and failing hearts. The response of heart muscle to changes in preload produces a functional reserve capable of improving cardiac output. A simple method of confirming the relationship of ventricular end-diastolic volume and ventricular end-diastolic pressure involves the use of a rapid fluid challenge. A significant and persistent rise in end-diastolic pressure following fluid challenge without an increase in cardiac output suggests that further fluid loading may be ill advised. Conversely, improved systemic arterial pressure and urine output without much change in end-diastolic pressure suggests that further fluid loading may be beneficial. A summary of factors that alter preload is shown in Table 3.

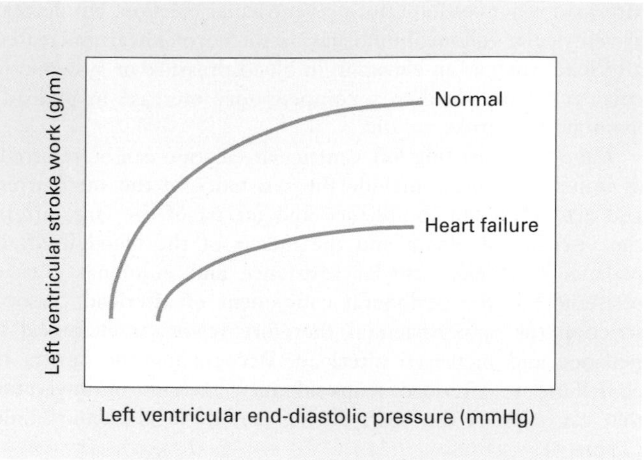

Fig. 1 Ventricular performance curves for normal subjects and patients with congestive heart failure. The failing heart is less responsive to increases in preload than the normal heart.

Central venous pressure

Any attempts to modulate preload require continuous and accurate measurement of central venous pressure and pulmonary artery wedge pressure. Central venous pressure should be transduced and displayed on the bedside monitor: it is difficult to estimate this with confidence using water manometry. Pressure should be measured at the peak of the 'a' wave (if in sinus rhythm) and at end-expiration. Electronic 'mean' venous pressures may overestimate central venous pressure in mechanically ventilated patients and underestimate pressure in those breathing spontaneously. Since the venous pressure is such a critical parameter it should be measured by the clinical attendant at the time and not taken from the previously documented clinical record.

Myocardial afterload

Afterload reflects the stress distributed within the ventricular wall during ventricular ejection and is determined by impedance factors opposing ventricular ejection and by ventricular wall tension. Wall tension in turn is determined by the La Place relationship between ventricular cavity radius and pressure. Thus,

Table 3 Factors that modulate preload

Factors that increase preload
Venoconstriction
Transfusion
'Head down' position
Factors that decrease preload
Venodilation
Hypovolaemia
Raised intrathoracic pressure
Positive pressure ventilation
Tension pneumothorax
Cardiac tamponade
Loss of atrial 'pump'

afterload is not constant during ventricular ejection, but decreases as ventricular volume diminishes. In the normal heart, increases in afterload, such as an elevation in blood pressure or systemic vascular resistance, lead to a compensatory increase in preload to maintain the stroke volume.

The forces resisting left ventricular ejection can be referred to as impedance: these include the resistance of the small arteries and arterioles, the compliance and inertia of the large arteries, the viscosity of blood, and the inertia of the blood itself. Impedance (systemic vascular resistance and pulmonary vascular resistance) is the peripheral component of afterload. Vasoconstriction (or polycythaemia) therefore results in increased impedance and increased afterload. Recognizing the factors that contribute to afterload helps identify avenues of intervention that can support the heart during periods of circulatory failure (Table 4).

Table 4 Factors that modulate afterload

Factors that increase afterload
Increased aortic impedance
Arteriolar constriction
Dilatation of ventricular cavity
Factors that decrease afterload
Decreased aortic impedance
Arteriolar dilatation
Reduction in ventricular cavity radius

Although few therapeutic situations require an increase in afterload, one such situation arises during conditions of isolated right ventricular failure, as might occur following myocardial infarction. Left ventricular preload is low because of impaired right ventricular output. Any factor reducing left ventricular afterload, such as volume depletion, vasodilators, or epidural anaesthetics, may preferentially reduce right heart coronary perfusion by reducing systolic pressure. Right ventricular function then becomes further impaired. If right ventricular dilatation then occurs the displacement of the interventricular septum further reduces left ventricular ejection. Left ventricular function will not improve until left ventricular afterload is increased by the administration of a systemic vasoconstrictor to improve right ventricular coronary blood flow.

Therapeutic benefit is more commonly derived by reducing afterload in cardiac failure. This is usually achieved by the administration of vasodilators to reduce impedance. Such drugs may have difference effects on arterial resistance, arterial compliance, and left ventricular volume. The greatest benefit will be seen in hypertensive patients, but significant effect can still be obtained in normotensive patients with heart failure in whom systolic arterial pressure exceeds 90 mmHg. Several agents are available, including sodium nitroprusside, glyceryl trinitrate, hydralazine, and the angiotensin converting enzyme inhibitors. In addition to the use of pharmacological agents, aortic impedance can be minimized by avoiding polycythaemia and maintaining a haemoglobin concentration of between 9 and 11 g/dl. The intra-aortic counterpulsation balloon pump is also effective in reducing aortic impedance and has the advantage of maintaining coronary filling pressure.

Therapeutic manipulation of preload and afterload

Sodium nitroprusside

Nitroprusside is a vasodilator that acts directly on both arteriolar and venous smooth muscle. At least part of its action may be related to inhibition of platelet aggregation and thromboxane A_2 synthesis, together with it synergism with prostacyclin. It exerts its effects directly on vascular smooth muscle rather than through a receptor system and, by reducing systemic vascular resistance, it reduces myocardial oxygen consumption and improves myocardial function. Nitroprusside has been shown to be a direct dilator of vessels within the substance of the myocardium resulting in increased coronary blood flow and markedly decreasing coronary vascular resistance. Venodilation causes some reduction in preload by increasing the capacity of the venous bed. This in turn may be useful in decreasing pulmonary congestion. A theoretical concern regarding the use of nitroprusside in patients with myocardial ischaemia is that the drug might cause preferential shunting of flow into non-ischaemic areas (the coronary steal phenomenon).

Nitroprusside dilates the cerebral circulation as well as other vascular beds. This is potentially dangerous in patients with preexisting intracranial hypertension, and may indicate a need for intracranial pressure monitoring. Nitroprusside does not impair normal cerebral autoregulation.

Pulmonary circulation

Nitroprusside dilates the pulmonary circulation. By blocking hypoxic vasoconstriction it may reduce arterial oxygenation in 10 to 20 per cent of patients due to increased pulmonary venous admixture.

Metabolism

Nitroprusside is an iron co-ordination complex which is metabolized in the blood to cyanide and then to thiocyanate (via rhodanese) and excreted in the urine. The thiocyanate metabolite itself has a mild hypotensive effect which is dose dependent and does not appear to plateau. Hypotension is generally reversed within 5 to 10 min of stopping infusion of the drug.

Indications

Nitroprusside is indicated in the treatment of congestive heart failure, in acute myocardial infarction, aortic insufficiency, acute mitral insufficiency due to papillary muscle dysfunction, or ischaemic ventricular septal defect. It should be avoided in patients with mitral or aortic stenosis. Nitroprusside is particularly appropriate therapy for hypertensive patients with acute myocardial infarction and persistent chest pain or left ventricular failure, and for normotensive patients with severe pump failure. The drug should be avoided in hypotensive patients, although it can be successfully used in conjunction with inotropic agents or intra-aortic balloon counterpulsation. Pulmonary artery catheter monitoring is generally required. Nitroprusside is particularly suitable for the treatment of hypertensive crises. In view of this propensity to induce excessive hypotension, an arterial line is generally considered to be an essential prerequisite of nitroprusside therapy. Almost all hypertensive patients will respond, although nitroprusside resistance has been described in patients with severe hypertension and renal failure. An additive hypotensive effect is seen with other drugs and it is generally wise to institute other antihypertensive therapy as soon as the blood pressure is controlled.

Dose

Generally, only modest doses of nitroprusside are needed: an initial infusion of 10 to 15 μg/min can be increased by 10 μg/min every 5 to 15 min. Most patients with heart failure show a positive response to 70 to 140 μg/min (1–2 μg/kg.min). In patients with pulmonary oedema accompanying congestive heart failure, nitroprusside is also started at a dose of 10 to 15 μg/min, but the dose is more rapidly increased (20 μg/min increments every 3–5 min) in order rapidly to reduce filling pressure and relieve symptoms. During infusion, the pulmonary artery wedge pressure should not be allowed to fall below 15 mmHg and the mean arterial pressure should be maintained at 70 mmHg (diastolic BP >50 mmHg). Initial doses of 0.5 to 1 μg/kg.min are generally effective in the treatment of hypertensive crises.

Response to therapy

A positive response to nitroprusside infusion consists of either a drop in the pulmonary artery wedge pressure or an increase in cardiac output (or both). A decrease of 20 to 50 per cent in pulmonary artery wedge pressure and an increase in cardiac output of 20 to 40 per cent are considered positive responses. If blood pressure falls without an improvement in cardiac output or a decrease in pulmonary artery wedge pressure, nitroprusside should be discontinued or an inotrope added.

The dose required to produce a given hypotensive effect in patients with hypertensive crisis is variable, but the maximum recommended dose is about 8 μg/kg.min. Since the drug deteriorates in the light, the administration set should be opaque or covered in aluminium foil. Once diluted nitroprusside remains stable for about 24 h under such conditions. Longer term medications can be substituted once blood pressure control is obtained with nitroprusside.

Toxicity

Since nitroprusside is metabolized to thiocyanate, excessive amounts administered over long periods to patients with severely compromised renal function can result in the accumulation of thiocyanate. Side-effects include nausea, vomiting, hiccups, mental confusion, and psychotic behaviour. The clinical manifestations of thiocyanate toxicity are lactic acidosis, confusion, hyper-reflexia, convulsions, tinnitus, and blurred vision. Infusion rates below 3 μg/kg.min for less than 72 h are not usually associated with toxicity. Monitoring blood thiocyanate levels may be necessary in patients requiring infusions for longer than 2 to 3 days: thiocyanate levels below 10 mg/dl are considered satisfactory.

Glycerine trinitrate (GTN, TNG, nitroglycerine)

Nitrates cause direct relaxation of vascular smooth muscle. Their predominant effect is on the capacitance vessels (veins), although arterioles are also dilated at higher doses. Nitrates may act on smooth muscle by releasing prostacyclin from vessel endothelial cells. Both glycerine trinitrate and nitroprusside exert a similar effect on preload with nitroprusside causing a greater decrease in afterload.

Glycerine trinitrate has an antianginal effect, although there is controversy over the mechanism of action. Several studies suggest that its major effect is due to systemic venodilation, which reduces preload and ventricular size, and in turn decreases left ventricular end-diastolic pressure, intramyocardial wall tension, and myocardial oxygen consumption. The drug may also decrease ischaemia by promoting epicardial and collateral coronary blood flow. Within the usual dose range, glycerine trinitrate has minimal effects on arteriolar tone: blood pressure and cardiac output are rarely affected unless preload is markedly reduced or unless significant myocardial hypoxia is relieved. In the higher dose range, glycerine trinitrate acts in a similar fashion to nitroprusside, causing a fall in systemic vascular resistance, increasing cardiac output, and decreasing blood pressure.

Metabolism

Glycerine trinitrate is widely distributed in the body and is rapidly metabolized to dinitrates and mononitrates, with a half-life of approximately 4 min.

Indications

Because glycerine trinitrate has little direct effect on blood pressure but has a profound effect on pulmonary artery wedge pressure, it may be preferable to nitroprusside in patients without hypertension who have heart failure and pulmonary oedema. The intravenous dosage is highly variable but can be started at 10 μg/min and adjusted every 5 to 10 min until the desired haemodynamic response (drop in pulmonary artery wedge pressure) is achieved. The dose which is usually effective in patients with heart failure is 30 to 100 μg/min. If no benefit is derived at a dose of 400 to 500 μg/min, other pharmacological options should be considered. High doses of glycerine trinitrate over several days are well tolerated. Continuous infusion is titrated to produce relief of chest pain or reversal of ischaemic ECG changes. It is essential that left ventricular filling pressure is adequate, otherwise significant hypotension may ensue. Occasionally, a precipitous fall in blood pressure in response to glycerine trinitrate administration may be the first indication that a particular patient is intravascularly depleted.

Toxicity

Side-effects include headache, sinus tachycardia, and hypotension. Rare complications include methaemoglobinaemia, paradoxical hypertension with bradycardia, and exacerbation of hypoxaemia.

Diuretics

Short-acting loop diuretics are considered an essential component of the treatment of acute heart failure. Frusemide (furosemide) in doses of 10 to 100 mg should be administered intravenously to patients with increased preload. Extremely large doses of frusemide (250–4000 mg/day) have been recommended in patients with reduced renal function but are unlikely to produce a meaningful diuresis: the addition of 2.5 to 5 mg of oral metolazone to frusemide is preferred. Intravenous bumetanide, a potent and short-acting loop diuretic, in doses of 0.5 to 2 mg, may be effective in patients resistant to frusemide.

Although the optimal response to diuretic therapy is a reduction in left ventricular filling pressure and increased urine output, the response of left ventricular pump function to diuretics is variable. Loop diuretics are of great value in patients with decompensated heart failure and should be used as needed to control pulmonary congestion. In the absence of a significant and sustained diuresis in patients with renal failure short-term reliance on venodilators may buy time while alternative means such as haemofiltration are established.

Myocardial contractility

The terms contractility and myocardial performance should not be confused: they are not synonymous. Myocardial performance is the sum total of preload, afterload, contractility, and heart rate, and is usually measured as cardiac output, while contractility is only one component of myocardial performance. Contractility is the final determinant of cardiac output and can be defined as the force of ejection, independent of afterload or preload. Contractility is not fixed but variable: it improves with adrenergic stimulation and increased coronary blood flow, and worsens due to the action of pharmacological and physiological depressants (barbiturates, general anaesthesia), metabolic abnormalities (hypothyroidism, sepsis), and loss of ventricular substance (myocardial infarction). Some of the factors that influence contractility are listed in Table 5.

Table 5 Factors that influence myocardial contractility

Factors that increase contractility
Sympathetic stimulation
Endogenous catecholamines
Exogenous catecholamines and inotropes
Increased myocardial oxygen delivery
Factors that decrease contractility
Myocardial hypoxia
Myocardial ischaemia
Metabolic depressants
Pharmacological depressants

The direct measurement of contractility is technically difficult since most techniques, such as ejection fraction, may be influenced by the relative state of preload or afterload at the time the measurement is made. However, it is conceptually important because it can be increased by a number of inotropic agents commonly used to treat circulatory failure. The most reliable and commonly used inotropic agents include dopamine, dobutamine, adrenaline (epinephrine), noradrenaline (norepinephrine), isoprenaline (isoproterenol), and glucagon.

Therapeutic manipulation of contractility

Dopamine

Dopamine is the immediate precursor of noradrenaline in the catecholamine synthetic pathway. It has both α- and β-adrenergic effects but differs from other catecholamines by producing vasodilation in renal, mesenteric, coronary, and intracerebral arterial vascular beds. This dopaminergic effect is not blocked by β-blockers. Since dopamine acts on a variety of receptors, and each receptor has a different dose–response relationship in different patients, a wide range of haemodynamic effects may be elicited under different conditions. Dopamine exerts β_1-adrenergic activity, mainly by releasing noradrenaline from myocardial storage sites. It also increases contractility and heart rate by its direct action on β-adrenergic receptors, effects which are blocked by β-blockers. α-Adrenergic effects causing vasoconstriction occur at high doses. In addition to its direct effect on α-adrenergic receptors, dopamine may also cause contraction of vascular smooth muscle by acting on a serotonin or tryptamine-sensitive receptor.

Cardiovascular effects

Low doses (0.5–2 μg/kg.min) may cause minimal increase in cardiac output contactility. Its major effect is an increase in renal blood flow and urine output due to stimulation of dopaminergic receptors. The renovascular effect is probably the most commonly exploited property of dopamine, but it may be lost at infusion rates greater than 5 μg/kg.min, when there is an increase in cardiac contractility. At even higher doses (>10 μg/kg.min) the α-adrenergic effects increase. Pulmonary artery and pulmonary artery wedge pressure may increase at high doses of dopamine. In addition, dopamine may increase intrapulmonary shunt fraction, resulting in a fall in oxygenation.

Dopamine selectivity increases renal and mesenteric blood flow by its action on dopaminergic receptors, but some of the renal effects of dopamine may be due to the inhibition of aldosterone secretion resulting in a natriuresis and increased urine output.

Dose

Intravenous administration of dopamine results in near steady-state levels in 5 min. The half-life of intravenously administered dopamine is approximately 1 min: it is metabolized by both catechol-*O*-methyl transferase and monoamine oxidase enzyme systems, and is ineffective when given orally. Dopamine is inactivated by bicarbonate and other alkaline solutions. The initial dose depends on specific aims of therapy: for the promotion of renal or splanchnic blood flow doses of 1.5 to 2.5 μg/kg.min are generally adequate, while a vasopressor effect is only achieved at doses greater than 5 μg/kg.min. Most patients show a pressor response to dopamine infusion at doses below 20 μg/kg.min, although some may require infusion rates in excess of 50 μg/kg.min. At these levels there are significant vasoconstrictor effects.

Toxicity

Arrhythmias are generally associated with administration of high doses of dopamine or the presence of myocardial ischaemia, metabolic acidosis, or hypoxaemia. Dopamine may increase myocardial conduction and precipitate a rapid ventricular response in patients with atrial fibrillation.

Peripheral gangrene may be seen in patients with profound shock treated for a prolonged period with large doses of dopamine. Hypotension may occur secondary to vasodilation in certain patients receiving low doses of dopamine: a specific vasopressor should be administered until an adequate blood pressure is obtained. Other side-effects include nausea, vomiting, angina pectoris, and, occasionally, hyperglycaemia. Tissue necrosis due to local extravasation is a serious complication and for this reason dopamine should be routinely administered via a central vein. If peripheral extravasation does occur, the area should be infiltrated locally with 10 ml of normal saline containing 5 to 10 mg of phentolamine.

Interactions with other drugs

Dopamine is metabolized by the monoamine oxidase system. and its effects are therefore greatly potentiated in patients receiving monoamine oxidase inhibitors. These effects may persist several weeks after cessation of such inhibitors. Phenothiazines, haloperidol, and tricyclic antidepressants have mild α-adrenergic blocking actions which may reduce the peripheral vasoconstricting effects of dopamine. Propanolol and other β-blocking agents blunt the cardiac stimulation produced by dopamine.

Dobutamine (DBT)

Dobutamine is a synthetic catecholamine that was the product of a systematic attempt to design a pure β_1-adrenergic agent. Dobutamine is structurally related to isoprenaline (isoproterenol) and acts directly on β_1-adrenergic receptors in the myocardium. Unlike dopamine, dobutamine does not enhance noradrenaline release from nerve endings, nor does it act on dopamine receptors. Its action is therefore not potentiated by monoamine oxidase inhibitors. The predominant β_1-receptor action increases myocardial contractility, and it has less effect on heart rate than does dopamine. Dobutamine has relatively weak β_2- and α-receptor activity, with peripheral vasodilation predominating. It has a short half-life (<2.5 min) in patients with heart failure: this becomes important if it is necessary to reverse an adverse effect such as ventricular tachycardia. There are no biologically active metabolites of dobutamine.

Cardiovascular effects

At low to moderate dose levels, dobutamine increases myocardial contractility, causes peripheral vasodilation, and augments renal blood flow. Some increase in heart rate can be expected. In addition, a decrease in pulmonary artery wedge pressure often accompanies the improved cardiac output.

Pulmonary effects

Dobutamine increases cardiac output and by doing so increases intrapulmonary venous admixture. Relief of pulmonary venous congestion brought about by a reduction in pulmonary artery wedge pressure improves pulmonary compliance and reduces the work of breathing.

Metabolism

Dobutamine is metabolized by catechol-*O*-methyl transferase and glucuronide transformation in the liver, most of the drug being eliminated unchanged by the kidneys and biliary tract. Its elimination follows first-order kinetics.

Dose

Positive inotropic effects occur with doses as low as 0.5 µg/kg.min, although the usual initial dose is 2 to 2.5 µg/kg.min. Therapeutic effects of the drug usually plateau at 15 to 20 µg/kg.min. Dobutamine is useful in the treatment of cardiogenic and septic shock if the associated hypotension is not severe. If hypotension is a problem, noradrenaline (norepinephrine) or high doses of dopamine may need to be added.

Toxicity

Cardiac arrhythmias are the most frequent toxic side-effect, but these are less common than with dopamine or isoproterenol. Hypotension may occur, especially if preload is inadequate. Tolerance may be observed after prolonged continuous infusion, an effect that is related to down-regulation of β-receptors. Dobutamine is contraindicated in patients with obstructive cardiomyopathy since it may increase cardiac outflow obstruction. The ventricular response in atrial fibrillation may be increased.

Noradrenaline (norepinephrine)

Noradrenaline is the neurotransmitter of postganglionic sympathetic nerves and is released from the adrenal medulla. In the heart, it is synthesized and stored in granules in myocardial adrenergic nerve endings. It is a β_1-agonist and has minimal effects on β_2-receptors. α-Adrenergic receptor effects result in marked peripheral vasoconstriction and increased left ventricular afterload.

Cardiovascular effects

Cardiovascular effects are not apparent with doses below 2.5 µg/min, but above that, noradrenaline increases systolic pressure proportionately more than diastolic pressure. This results in a significant increase in systemic vascular resistance and mean arterial pressure. Heart rate may be slowed by a baroreceptor reflex and cardiac output remains unchanged or slightly reduced. Noradrenaline is a potent venoconstrictor, and increases venous return by decreasing vascular capacitance. Noradrenaline increases afterload, preload, and contractility and can greatly increase myocardial work and oxygen demand. Coronary blood flow may be increased through an increase in the filling pressure gradient between the mean arterial pressure and the left ventricular end-diastolic filling pressure. Right ventricular perfusion may be greatly enhanced since the majority of right-sided coronary flow occurs during systole.

Pulmonary effects

Noradrenaline may be a respiratory stimulant through its action on the carotid bodies. It has little effect on bronchial smooth muscle, but it will increase pulmonary vascular resistance: this is potentially disadvantageous in patients with underlying pulmonary hypertension.

Other vascular effects

Physiologically, noradrenaline is a potent vasoconstrictor of the renal artery bed. This effect can be ameliorated to some degree by concurrent administration of low dose dopamine. Noradrenaline produces vasoconstriction in the liver and splanchnic beds, resulting in decreased flow. However, in patients with distributive (septic) shock noradrenaline may increase renal blood flow and enhance urine production by increasing perfusion.

Noradrenaline does not vasoconstrict vessels supplying the brain, although α_2-adrenergic receptors are present on these vessels. The powerful pressor effects of noradrenaline may maintain cerebral perfusion during periods of circulatory collapse; indeed, noradrenaline may be as effective as adrenaline in supporting the circulation during cardiac arrest.

Metabolism

Noradrenaline is enzymatically degraded in the liver and kidneys. There is also reuptake at β-adrenergic and non-neuronal receptor sites.

Dose

The pressor effects of noradrenaline may be beneficial in distributive (septic) shock, where there is systemic vasodilation and peripheral hypoperfusion as evidenced by low systemic vascular resistance and lactic acidosis. Noradrenaline will support myocardial and cerebral perfusion effectively while cardiac output and oxygen delivery is carefully monitored. Although there are theoretical limits to the dose that can be safely administered, the dose can be progressively increased to achieve the desired effect. It is essential to exclude volume depletion before resorting to pressor therapy. Following calcium-channel blocker overdose, intravenous calcium and noradrenaline may quickly restore vascular tone.

Toxicity

Systemic vasoconstriction resulting in organ ischaemia, especially of the dermal, renal, and mesenteric vascular beds, may produce irreversible injury. These effects must be weighed against the potential benefits. Palpitations, angina, headaches, hyperglycaemia, and hypocalcaemia may follow noradrenaline administration.

Adrenaline (epinephrine)

Adrenaline is a naturally occurring catecholamine with α-, β_1-, and β_2-adrenergic activity. For circulatory support it may be infused in doses of between 0.01 and 0.2 µg/kg.min. Although the oxygen supply to oxygen demand ratio may be adversely affected, adrenaline may improve peripheral perfusion. It is particularly, useful in the treatment of distributive circulatory failure, such as the sepsis syndrome and anaphylactic reactions. Although the same effects can be achieved by combinations of agents with predominantly α-adrenergic effects (noradrenaline) and β-adrenergic effects (dobutamine), adrenaline still has a place in the current management of circulatory failure.

Isoprenaline

Isoprenaline (isoproterenol) has both β_1- and β_2-adrenergic activity, and produces peripheral vasodilation and an increase in myocardial contractility and heart rate. The tachycardia and reduced coronary perfusion pressure results in a much reduced oxygen supply to oxygen demand ratio. It is therefore not the drug of choice for use in patients with myocardial failure, but it may have application in severe bradycardias not associated with myocardial ischaemia.

Glucagon

Glucagon is a pancreatic polypeptide that has inotropic and chronotropic effects which are not dependent on β-receptor responsiveness. By directly stimulating adenylcyclase it increases intracellular AMP concentration. Although not a first-line drug for use in circulatory failure, it may be effective when other inotropes have failed.

Phosphodiesterase inhibitors

Milrinone and enoximone are powerful phosphodiesterase inhibitors which may be beneficial in patients with severe heart failure who are unresponsive to dobutamine or dopamine. These agents have combined inotropic and vasodilator properties and are effective even in the presence of β-receptor down-regulation.

The selection of inotropes and vasodilators in cardiac failure

Dobutamine and dopamine have very different haemodynamic profiles and should not be considered to be interchangeable. Because dopamine causes substantial peripheral vasoconstriction and can increase pulmonary capillary wedge pressure, it should be used cautiously in patients with acute heart failure who have increased peripheral vascular resistance and elevated wedge pressures. Dobutamine may be preferable to dopamine for the treatment of acute congestive heart failure, while nitroprusside is preferable when the systolic pressure is above 90 mmHg. Combinations of all three drugs are commonly used. A logical regimen in a patient with severe congestive heart failure would be nitroprusside and dobutamine with infusion of low (renovascular) doses of dopamine. Recently introduced inotropic agents such as the β-adrenergic agonists amrinone and dopexamine and the phosphodiesterase inhibitors milrinone and enoximone combine inotropic and vasodilator properties (afterload reduction) and theoretically reduce the risk of increasing myocardial work.

The effects of inotropes, vasodilators, and diuretics on myocardial performance are well represented by the plot of left ventricular stroke work index and pulmonary artery wedge pressure. In the failing heart there is greatly reduced myocardial performance for a given preload. As shown in Fig. 2, the depressed curve of heart failure can be shifted toward normal by inotropic drugs, or vasodilator drugs.

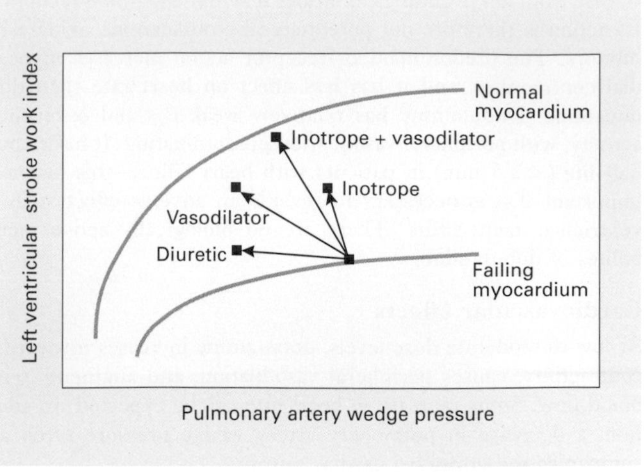

Fig. 2 The effects of inotrope, vasodilator, and diuretic upon the relationship of left ventricular performance and pulmonary artery wedge pressure.

These effects may be complementary when the drugs are infused together. Note that diuretics usually reduce filling pressure without augmenting output. An inotrope such as dobutamine may not only increase contractility but may also reduce pulmonary artery wedge pressure, while dopamine may increase pulmonary artery wedge pressure, especially at high doses.

Ultimately, oral inotropes and vasoactive agents will be needed to replace acute systemic therapy. Several effective oral agents, including diuretics, cardiac glycosides (digoxin), nitrates, hydralazine hydrochloride, and the angiotensin converting enzyme inhibitors, are available for the treatment of stable or compensated congestive failure. Of these the combination of diuretics and angiotensin converting enzyme inhibitors has had the most impact on morbidity. Patients should be supervised while a low dose of an oral agent (such as captopril 6.25 mg, or enalapril maleate 2.5 mg) is administered and the intravenous drug is gradually discontinued. Cautious dose increases are needed in order to avoid hypotension, especially if the patient is volume depleted. If the first dose of an angiotensin converting enzyme inhibitor is tolerated, doses should be increased until a maintenance dose is achieved. Since angiotensin converting enzyme inhibition tends to increase serum potassium levels, potassium supplementation should be very cautious and serum levels need to be monitored. Angiotensin converting enzyme inhibitors may also cause acute renal failure, particularly in patients with chronic azotaemia and renal artery stenosis, making it important to monitor serum creatinine and blood urea nitrogen levels.

Disturbances in heart rate

Heart rate is an important determinant of cardiac output. Since cardiac output is determined by the product of heart rate and stroke volume, cardiac output for a given stroke volume will increase as heart rate increases. As heart rate falls, the diastolic filling interval lengthens, stroke volume increases, and cardiac output is protected. However, at very low heart rates (approaching 40 beats/min) there is insufficient stroke volume reserve to compensate for the fall in rate and blood pressure may fall. The presence of an effective atrial pump helps to prime the ventricle and, in slow supraventricular and idioventricular rhythms, bradycardia is less well tolerated. In the clinical setting it is therefore essential to determine whether bradycardias are associated with circulatory failure. If blood pressure is maintained, continued observation may be all that is required; if hypotension develops, active intervention is required. Sinus bradycardia usually responds to atropine (0.6 mg) but other rhythms may need administration of isoprenaline (isoproterenol) or electrical pacing. In the severely ill ventilated patient, who often has multiple organ system failure, sinus bradycardias may accompany tracheal suctioning, even in the absence of hypoxaemia or metabolic disturbances. Pretreatment with atropine will generally prevent these episodes. Alternatively suctioning can be performed through an airtight port attached to the swivel connector of the endotracheal tube. The explanation for such episodes is unclear but they must represent the unopposed activity of the vagal system.

The effect of tachycardia on cardiac output depends on the underlying contractile state of the myocardium, and when contractility is impaired cardiac output may fall. In this situation, cardiac output can be increased by an increase in heart rate up to approximately 110 beats/min. In the presence of heart disease, heart rates greater than 160 beats/min are badly tolerated, while in patients with healthy myocardia heart rates of up to 180 beats/min are associated with an intrinsic increase in contractility that accompanies the tachycardia. In patients with ischaemic heart disease increased heart rate seriously raises myocardial oxygen consumption. Some prosthetic cardiac valves function poorly at high cardiac rates due to the inertia of the valve mechanism and attempts should be made to keep heart rates below 120 beats/min.

Sinus tachycardia is usually a physiological response to a specific event or series of events, which may include endotoxaemia, fever, or hypovolaemia. Until the underlying cause is remedied the tachycardia will remain. Attempts to slow sinus tachycardia with myocardial depressant agents, such as β-adrenergic blockers, is not recommended.

Arrhythmias

Arrhythmias developing in patients in the intensive care unit are commonly the result of metabolic disturbances, hypovolaemia, increased afterload, or hypoxaemia. A concerted effort must be made to identify and correct these disturbances before resorting to treatment with antiarrhythmic agents. Indeed, resistance to these agents can be expected until the underlying abnormalities are corrected. Thereafter, the urgency with which arrhythmia needs to be corrected is determined by the severity of the haemodynamic disruption. Obviously, the onset of shock may necessitate emergency electrical cardioversion, while arrhythmias in the absence of haemodynamic disturbance can be managed with appropriate antiarrhythmic drugs or elective electrical cardioversion. As a general rule, ventricular arrhythmias produce greater haemodynamic disturbance than supraventricular rhythms. A summary of treatment regiments for both supraventricular and ventricular arrhythmias is shown in Fig. 3.

Distributive circulatory failure

The treatment of distributive circulatory failure provides one of the most challenging aspects of critical care. Although there are several causes of distributive circulatory failure, including anaphylaxis and neurogenic shock, it is the sepsis syndrome that accounts for most cases. The pathophysiology and principles of management of the sepsis syndrome provides a model that can be applied to most forms of distributive circulatory failure irrespective of cause.

Sepsis syndrome

The sepsis syndrome, and associated multiple organ system failure, is the most common cause of death in critical care patients. It represents the host response to endotoxaemia caused by a wide range of micro-organisms. Sepsis syndrome is characterized by low peripheral vascular resistance which, in the presence of normal cardiac function, is coupled with increased cardiac output (high output failure) and low filling pressures. However, cardiac function, along with the function of other organ systems, may be greatly impaired. Those patients who do not generate high cardiac outputs in the face of a septic insult generally have a poor prognosis.

Definition

The definition of the sepsis syndrome is based upon the demonstration of signs of infection, shock, and evidence of organ system dysfunction as described in Table 6.

Table 6 Clinical features of the sepsis syndrome

Evidence of fever and shock
1. Fever $>$ 38°C or hypothermia $\leqslant$ 36.6°C core temperature
2. Tachycardia $\geqslant$ 90 beats/minute
3. Tachypnoea $\geqslant$ 20 breaths/minute or requiring mechanical ventilation
4. Hypotension, systolic blood pressure $\leqslant$ 90 mmHg or $\geqslant$ 40 mmHg fall in systolic pressure, with adequate fluid filling
5. Evidence for localized focus of infection

Together with other clinical evidence of toxicity or end-organ failure
1. Metabolic acidosis, pH $\leqslant$ 7.3 corrected for $P\text{CO}_2$ changes, or a base deficit $\geqslant$ 5
2. Arterial hypoxaemia with $P\text{O}_2 \leqslant$ 10 kPa
3. $P\text{aO}_2$: $F\text{IO}_2$ ratio $\geqslant$ 33 ($P\text{aO}_2$ in kPa) or 250 ($P\text{aO}_2$ in mmHg)
4. Increased plasma lactate
5. Oliguria $\leqslant$ 0.5 ml/kg.h for 1 h
6. Coagulation defect with prothrombin time 1.5 times control or PTT 1.2 times control
7. Thrombocytopenia $\leqslant$ 100 000 or more than 50% fall within 24 h
8. Acute deterioration in mental status
9. Any other sign of organ system failure (see Table 7)

Pathogenesis and pathophysiology

Sepsis syndrome is the pathophysiological responses to systemic infection or endotoxaemia. The clinical syndrome can be produced by a wide range of organisms including Gram-positive and Gram-negative bacteria, protozoa, viruses, and fungi. In a significant proportion of cases an infective organism is never isolated. Although endotoxaemia is not consistently present in early sepsis, it is usually present in late, severe sepsis syndrome with multiple organ system failure and is associated with a poor prognosis. Systemic endotoxaemia may also result from translocation of endotoxin and bacteria from the intestinal lumen into the circulation and may explain the development of sepsis syndrome in trauma and burn patients (Fig. 4).

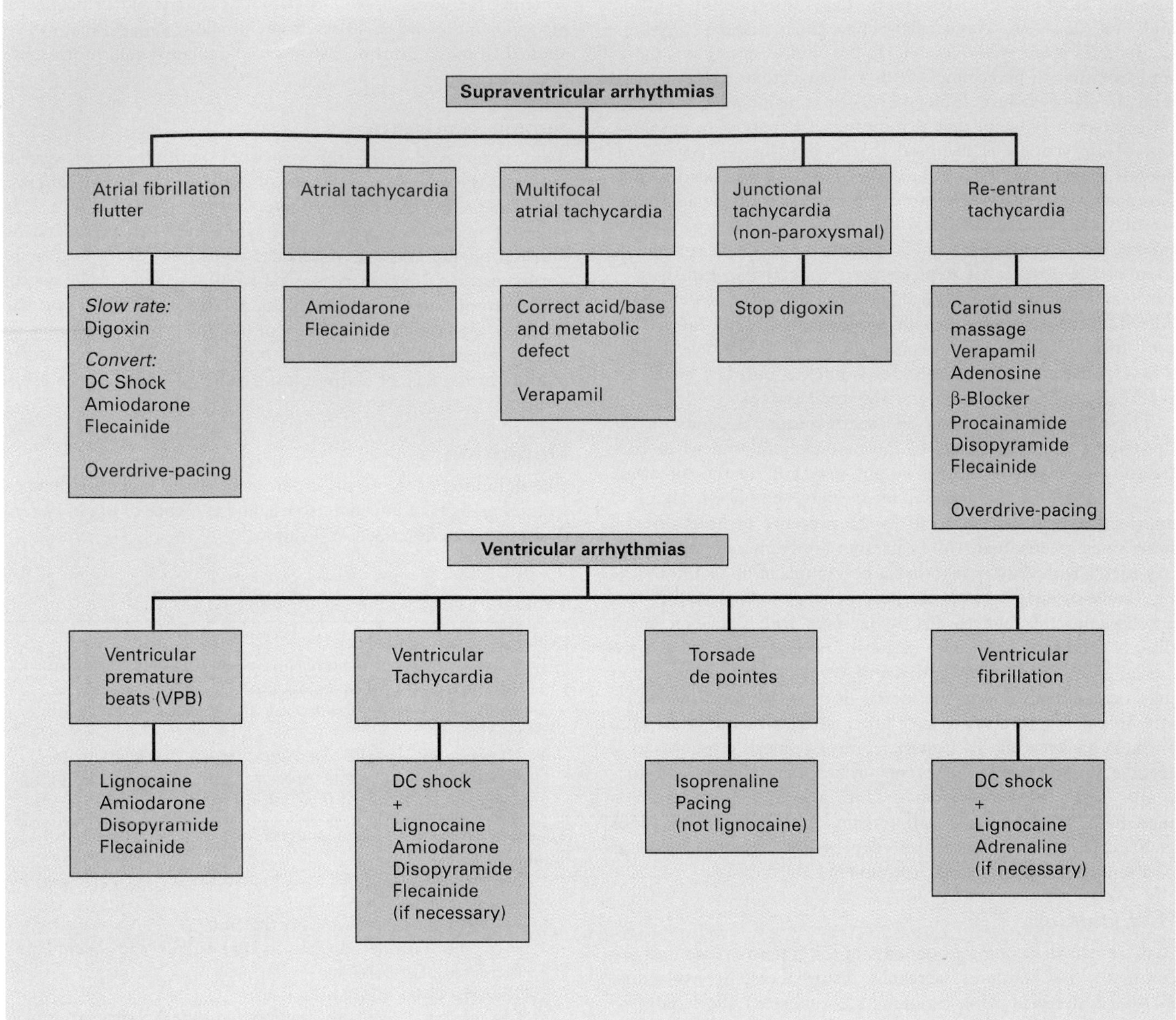

Fig. 3 Algorithms for the treatment of supraventricular and ventricular arrhythmias.

Spillover of endotoxin into the circulation is known to occur in patients with inflammatory bowel disease such as Crohn's disease and in those with obstructive jaundice. Bile salts may have a beneficial effect by binding endotoxin, and therefore their absence may predispose towards endotoxaemia. The presence of circulating micro-organisms and endotoxins appears to trigger an immunological and inflammatory cascade with complement activation and the release of a number of host-derived mediators, including tumour necrosis factor, interleukins, and myocardial depressant factor. These mediators are probably responsible for the systemic vasodilation, hypotension, and multiple organ system failure which are often seen.

The presence of multiple organ system failure is usually only too apparent to the clinician, although formal diagnostic criteria can be defined and are summarized in Table 7. Not surprisingly, the greater the number of organ systems involved the worse the prognosis.

Upper gastrointestinal tract colonization

Colonization of the upper gastrointestinal tract, particularly with Gram-negative organisms, may be a significant aetiologic factor in sepsis. It may also play a role in the perpetuation of the sepsis syndrome. Colonization of the stomach and upper small bowel in the critically ill patient provides a major source of endogenous infecting organisms. Colonization of the upper gastrointestinal tract is promoted by parenteral administration of antibiotics which are excreted in saliva, bile, and intestinal mucus, and which suppress the endogenous intestinal anaerobic flora. Other factors that promote colonization are listed in Table 8. Gastrointestinal tract colonization provides a reservoir of pathogens that not only increase the enteric endotoxin pool but also increase the risk of nosocomial lung infection developing following the aspiration of gastrointestinal contents.

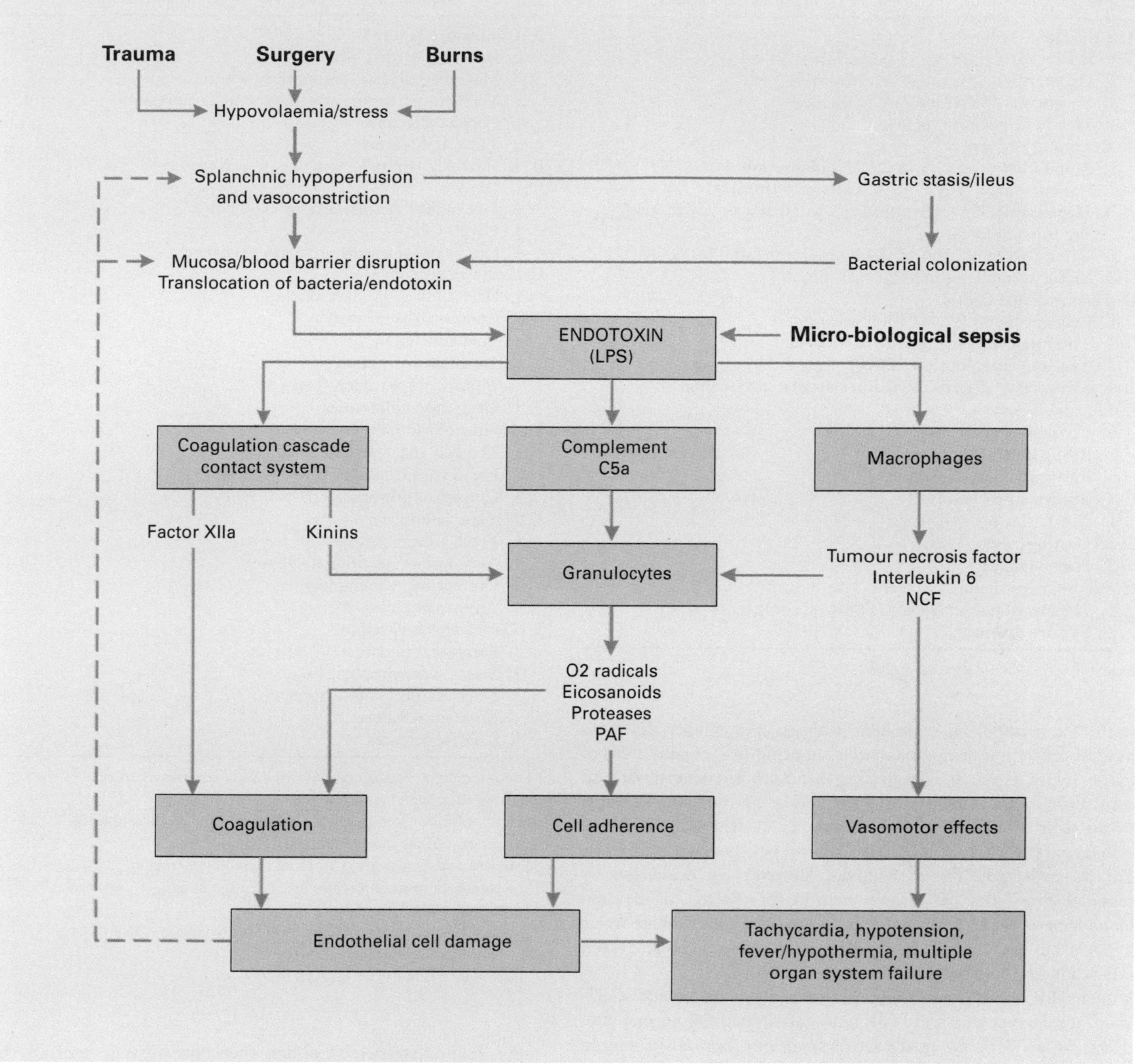

Fig. 4 Possible interactions leading to the sepsis syndrome.

Selective decontamination of the digestive tract

Selective decontamination of the digestive tract with orally administered non-absorbable antimicrobial agents has been recommended as a method of reducing the colonization of the upper gastrointestinal tract in the critically ill patient. This reduces nosocomial lung infections, although there has not been a consistent reduction in mortality. The procedure appears to be well tolerated and resistant strains of colonizing micro-organisms do not commonly develop. Selective decontamination may, therefore, be recommended in patients with severe multiple injuries and in those in whom persistent endotoxaemia is suspected.

Several 'recipes' have been proposed, including the combination of oral polymyxin, amphotericin, and gentamicin with a systemic β-lactam such as ceftazidime. This combination is administered as a paste for the oral cavity and as a mixture to pass through the digestive tract. Polymyxin is particularly effective in reducing faecal endotoxin levels.

Oxygen transport considerations in the sepsis syndrome

Sepsis syndrome is characterized by defective oxygen utilization in the face of a high cardiac output. The reduced oxygen consumption may be associated with raised blood lactate levels, suggesting

Table 7 Criteria for the presence of organ system failure

A. Circulatory failure
 1. Bradycardia (rate ⩽ 50 beats/min)
 2. Hypotension (Mean BP ⩽ 50 mmHg
 3. Ventricular tachycardia or fibrillation
 4. Metabolic acidosis (pH ⩽ 7.2)
B. Respiratory failure
 1. Respiratory rate ⩽ 5 or ⩾ 40 breaths/min
 2. Hypercapnoea ($Pa\text{CO}_2$ ⩾ 6.7 kPa or 50 mmHg)
 3. Hypoxaemia ([A-a]$P\text{O}_2$ gradient ⩾ 50 kPa or 350 mmHg)
C. Acute renal failure
 1. Urine output ⩽ 400 ml/24 h or ⩽ 150 ml/8 h
 2. Rising serum creatinine ⩾ 150 mmol/l
D. Haematologic failure
 1. Leucopenia (WBC ⩽ 1000 cells/mm^3)
 2. Thrombocytopenia (platelets ⩽ 20 000/mm^3)
 3. Anaemia (haemocrit ⩽ 20%)
 4. Evidence of disseminated intravascular coagulation
E. Hepatic failure
 1. Coagulation defect (INR ⩾ 2.0)
 2. Rising hepatic enzymes
 3. Rising alkaline phosphatase
F. Gastrointestinal failure
 1. Ileus
 2. Gastroparesis
 3. Haemorrhage
G. Neurological failure
 1. Depressed consciousness (Glasgow coma score ⩽ 6)
 2. Seizure disorder

INR = international normalized ratio.

anaerobic metabolism consistent with an intracellular defect in oxygen utilization or microvascular shunting that creates areas of tissue hypoxaemia. It is probable that both elements exist and contribute to the impaired oxygen uptake by the tissues. When tissue hypoxia becomes more severe, as evidenced by a fall in venous oxygen saturation ($S\text{vO}_2$) below 60 per cent hyperlactaemia can be expected. Tissue hypoxia, however, as evidenced by reduced $S\text{vO}_2$, may be present even in the absence of elevated blood lactate levels. A normal or high $S\text{vO}_2$ does not exclude tissue hypoxia but merely reflects the degree of reduced tissue oxygen utilization and high output state.

In health, oxygen consumption is largely independent of delivery until oxygen delivery falls below about half the normal rate, that is, below 7 ml/kg. In the sepsis syndrome, not only is oxygen consumption reduced, but there appears to be delivery dependent oxygen consumption at all levels of delivery. This claim has been challenged on the grounds that the formulae for calculating oxygen consumption and delivery, using the Fick principle, both contain the common elements of cardiac output and the oxygen content of arterial blood, and that they are therefore inevitably correlated. Indeed, when oxygen uptake is derived from analysis of exhaled gases, no such delivery dependence of oxygen consumption is found. Irrespective of how this controversy is resolved, the underlying principles of using combinations of inotropes and vasopressors to optimize cardiac output and oxygen delivery still pertain, although it remains to be conclusively demonstrated that such methods improve survival.

Table 8 Factors associated with upper gastrointestinal tract colonization

1. Parenteral antibiotics
2. Suppression of gastric acid secretion
3. Gastroparesis and ileus
4. Level of invasive instrumentation
5. Absence of enteral feeding
6. Extremes of age

Table 9 Management overview of organ system support

A. Circulatory failure*
 1. Optimize cardiac preload
 2. Maximize cardiac contractility with inotropes
 3. Maintain perfusion pressures with vasopressors
 4. Correct anaemia
 5. Treat arrhythmias
B. Respiratory failure*
 1. Oxygen
 2. Mechanical ventilation
 3. PEEP/CPAP
 4. Extra- and intracorporeal gas exchange
C. Acute renal failure
 1. Haemofiltration/haemodialysis or:
 2. Conservative measures
  Fluid restriction
  Potassium restriction
  Appropriate nitrogen intake
 3. Drug dose adjustment
D. Haematologic failure
 1. Red cell and platelet transfusion
 2. Fresh frozen plasma (INR < 1.5)
 3. Correct antithrombin III deficiency
E. Hepatic failure
 1. Fresh frozen plasma
 2. Appropriate nutritional support
 3. Correct hypoalbuminaemia
 4. Adjust drug dosage
F. Gastrointestinal failure
 1. Parenteral nutrition
 2. Stress ulcer prophylaxis
 3. Selective decontamination
G. Neurological failure
 1. Control seizures

*Optimization of circulatory and respiratory parameters to achieve the following therapeutic goals:
 Increased mean blood pressure to 75 per cent premorbid levels
 Increased cardiac index above 4.5 l/min.m^2
 Increased oxygen delivery to more than 600 ml/min.m^2
 Increased oxygen consumption to 170 ml/min.m^2
This should lead to:
 Reduced blood lactate and correction of metabolic acidosis
 Urine output more than 0.5 ml/kg.h
 INR = international normalized ratio.

Management of the sepsis syndrome

Management is aimed at organ system support, the suppression or amelioration of the toxic effects of the septic process, and, most important, the identification and eradication of the septic focus. Some forms of organ system support, such as mechanical ventilation and haemofiltration, are readily achievable, while the support of the brain, circulation, and gastrointestinal tract has to be approached indirectly by trying to attain supranormal levels of oxygen delivery (Table 9).

In addition to organ system support, specific interventions aim at the eradication of the septic focus or at inhibiting the inflammatory cascade. Appropriate antibiotics must be selected, but these will eventually prove ineffective unless surgical drainage of large foci of infection is undertaken.

Identification and eradication of the septic focus

An aggressive approach to clinical, radiographic, sonographic, and microbiological surveillance is required if the focus of infection is to be identified and eradicated. The investigations should be directed along the lines suggested by a thorough understanding of the clinical problems. Recognizing the limitations of non-invasive investigations should encourage early diagnostic laparotomy. The clinical features of intra-abdominal sepsis may be difficult to elucidate in the sedated patient receiving potent analgesics.

Immunotherapy

Many attempts have been made to interrupt the inflammatory cascade of sepsis. Corticosteroids appear to be ineffective, as do specific inhibitors of leukotriene and prostenoid production. With the advent of improved assays for endotoxin it has been shown that endotoxaemia predicts impending sepsis in the febrile patient and correlates with clinical events and the development of lactic acidosis. Recent experience with administration of antibody against the lipopolysaccharide component of endotoxin in patients with Gram-negative sepsis has shown a significant reduction in overall mortality, particularly in those presenting with shock. Such immunotherapy against endotoxins and cytokines may, in time, become the standard for specific intervention in sepsis.

PHYSIOLOGICAL MEASUREMENT IN CIRCULATORY FAILURE

Flow-directed pulmonary artery catheter

The flow-directed pulmonary artery catheter is a multilumen tube used for the catheterization of the right-sided circulation. It incorporates a balloon, of about 1.5 ml capacity, at the tip: this facilitates the passage of the catheter into the pulmonary artery as well as allowing the determination of left-sided filling pressures. A thermistor at the tip enables the determination of cardiac output by the thermodilution technique. Newer catheters include the capacity for sequential atrioventricular pacing as well as fibreoptics for continuous monitoring of mixed venous oxygen saturation. Most recently, a pulmonary artery catheter has been introduced which incorporates a rapid response thermistor facilitating the estimation of right ventricular ejection fraction and, therefore, right ventricular end-diastolic volume.

At the proximal, hub end of flow-directed pulmonary artery catheter there are several ports and connections; a distal and proximal port, a balloon inflation port, a thermistor connection, and, in some, a fibreoptic connection.

There has been much controversy regarding the risk/benefit of the pulmonary artery catheter in both coronary care and intensive care, fuelled partially by the lack of published prospective trials. It is therefore incumbent on each clinician to determine the true need for its insertion. Indications for pulmonary artery catheterization are constantly evolving; however, current indications are summarized in Table 10.

Table 10 Indications for pulmonary artery catheter insertion

1. Refractory hypotension
2. Cardiogenic circulatory failure
3. Cardiovascular monitoring during PEEP
4. Acute right ventricular myocardial infarct
5. Assessment of cardiac valvular and septal defects
6. Assessment of therapy in severe chronic congestive heart failure
7. Electrophysiology studies and cardiac pacing
8. Preoperative staging of high-risk patients

The utility of data derived from pulmonary artery catheterization rests upon the fact that there are limits to the reliability and accuracy of clinical methods of determining pulmonary artery pressure, pulmonary vascular resistance, left atrial pressure, peripheral vascular resistance, and cardiac output. Several studies have revealed that even when radiographic and clinical criteria are critically evaluated the presence or absence of left ventricular failure cannot always be reliably predicted. Another test of the utility of pulmonary artery catherization is whether or not meaningful alterations in therapy result from the information derived from the flotation catheter. It has been estimated that in between one- and two-thirds of patients investigated by this means therapeutic alterations are made as a result of the information obtained.

Given the large amount of potentially valuable information obtainable from the catheter, it would be tempting to use it in most critically ill patients. However, the incidence of serious complications is high enough to mitigate against its routine use. Some of the complications related to the pulmonary artery catheter are listed in Table 11.

Table 11 Some complications associated with the use of pulmonary artery catheters

1. Overwedging with pulmonary infarction
2. Arrhythmias
3. Air embolus
4. Endocarditis
5. Sepsis
6. Thrombocytopenia
7. Catheter knotting
8. Pneumothorax
9. Tricuspid valve avulsion
10. Pulmonary artery branch rupture and haemorrhage

The overall incidence of complications is difficult to assess. However, many of the serious complications can be avoided by adhering to standard procedures. Checking the chest radiograph following insertion of the catheter should detect pneumothorax and over-distal placement of the catheter tip (overwedging). Furthermore by ensuring that the pulmonary artery pressure trace returns after each deflation of the balloon, lung infarction should be prevented. By adopting strict aseptic insertion techniques, using a plastic sheath around the external portion of the catheter, and by removing the catheter within 72 h the risk of sepsis and endocarditis is reduced.

Insertion of the flow-directed pulmonary artery catheter

Correct and skilful insertion technique cannot be learnt from a textbook but requires careful instruction by an experienced clinician. However, a few recommendations and comments can be made at this juncture. Full aseptic technique requires the wearing of surgical gown, cap, mask, and gloves, and preparation of as much of the equipment as possible before touching the patient.

This includes attaching three-way taps, flushing all channels with heparinized saline, checking the integrity of the balloon, and completing *in-vitro* calibration of the pulmonary artery catheter oximeter (if used). The use of the internal jugular route, particularly the right internal jugular, facilitates placement. Prior insertion of a pulmonary artery catheter sheath (8–8.5 Fr) makes later replacement with either another pulmonary artery catheter or a triple lumen catheter very much more convenient. As the catheter is introduced its natural curvature should be maintained such that it will be directed through the tricuspid valve and up into the right ventricular outflow tract (with the balloon inflated). The catheter should be advanced slowly, about 2 cm every 2 s, watching its distal port pressure trace. As each heart chamber is entered (right atrial and right ventricle), the pressure should be noted. Once in the pulmonary artery the catheter should be advanced until it wedges, the pulmonary artery wedge pressure (or pulmonary artery occlusion pressure) being monitored. When the balloon is deflated the pulmonary artery trace should reappear. Subsequent inflation of the balloon should initially continue to give a pulmonary artery trace: as the catheter uncoils and advances, it will again wedge. This should be the ideal catheter position. A portable chest radiograph will confirm the catheter position. Right atrial and pulmonary artery wedge pressures should be recorded at the top of the 'a' wave at end-expiration.

Measurement of pressures

Right atrial waveform, pulmonary artery systolic, diastolic, and mean pressures, and pulmonary artery wedge waveform should be measured. In the spontaneously breathing patient, the pulmonary artery wedge pressure reflects left atrial pressure. The relationship of pulmonary artery wedge pressure to left ventricular end-diastolic pressure is more complex however. Pulmonary artery wedge pressure provides an accurate indication of left ventricular end-diastolic pressure, provided that the latter is low and there is no mitral valve disease. At high left ventricular end-diastolic pressures (30–35 mmHg), the pulmonary artery wedge pressure is usually 5 to 10 mmHg lower. The pulmonary artery diastolic pressure is generally 1 to 2 mmHg greater than the pulmonary artery wedge and can be used as a crude index of left atrial pressure, again assuming that there is no mitral valve or pulmonary disease. The pulmonary artery wedge pressure is not usually higher than the pulmonary artery diastolic pressure and should never be greater than the mean pulmonary artery pressure. When this occurs (assuming no mitral regurgitation) the discrepancy is usually caused by overwedging of the catheter or by improper measurement of the pulmonary diastolic pressure.

Measurement of cardiac output

This generally requires the averaging of three reasonably close, sequential measurements. Ideally, ice-cooled saline (at 9°C) should be injected at the same point during the respiratory cycle, at end-expiration. This may be difficult to achieve and in practice it is probably satisfactory to adopt random injection timing and derive an average value for cardiac output. Cardiac index is obtained by dividing the cardiac output by the body surface area: the normal range is 2.8 to 3.6 $l/min.m^2$.

Mixed venous saturation

Blood sampling from the pulmonary artery allows the determination of venous oxygen saturation (Svo_2), venous oxygen tension (Pvo_2), and venous oxygen content (Cvo_2). This is obtained through the distal port of the catheter when it is in position in the pulmonary outflow tract. It is important that the specimen is aspirated slowly (3 ml/min) to avoid obtaining an arterialized specimen. The laboratory determination of Svo_2 is most accurately performed using an oximeter and should not be derived from the Pvo_2. Pulmonary artery catheters incorporating direct continuous oximetry provide a unique facility to monitor Svo_2.

Derived haemodynamic parameters

Haemodynamic parameters can be derived using various formulae and a hand-held calculator or microcomputer, or can be calculated directly by newer generations of cardiac output computers or physiological monitors. The variables needed to calculate derived values are listed in Table 12. These derived haemodynamic parameters can be classified in two major categories, pump performance, and oxygen transport and utilization, and are shown in Table 13.

Table 12 Additional variables required to calculate derived haemodynamic indices

1. Blood pressure—systolic, diastolic, and mean. Most modern physiological monitoring systems provide accurate mean values. Failing this, the mean value can be calculated as: MAP = diastolic BP + 1/3 (systolic BP − diastolic BP)
2. Body surface area (BSA) from appropriate nomogram
3. Heart rate
4. Haemoglobin concentration
5. Arterial blood gases at a defined Fio_2 and barometric pressure (P_B)

Data reflecting pump performance

Cardiac index (cardiac output divided by body surface area) and stroke index (cardiac index divided by heart rate) relate cardiac output to the patient's body surface area. Systemic vascular resistance and pulmonary vascular resistance represent the peripheral component of afterload (that is, impedance). Their derived calculation is based on a rearrangement of Poiseuille's law (the hydraulic resistance equation):

$$R = \frac{P_i - P_o}{Q}$$

where R = resistance, P_i = pressure at inflow, P_o = pressure at outflow, Q = blood flow.

From this:

$$\text{SVR} = \frac{(\text{MAP} - \text{CVP})80}{\text{CO}} \text{ dyne/s.cm}^5$$

and

$$\text{PVR} = \frac{(\text{PA} - \text{PAWP})80}{\text{CO}} \text{ dyne/s.cm}^5$$

where MAP = mean (systemic) arterial pressure, CVP = central venous pressure, SVR = systemic vascular resistance, CO = cardiac output, PA = mean pulmonary arterial pressure, PAWP = pulmonary artery wedge pressure, and PVR = pulmonary vascular resistance.

Systemic vascular resistance is increased in low flow states, such as cardiogenic and hypovolaemic shock, secondary to endogenous or exogenous vasoconstrictors, and in systemic hypertension. It is decreased in states associated with high cardiac output, including trauma, sepsis, burns, liver disease, and anaemia, and in Addison's disease.

Table 13 Categories of haemodynamic parameters derived from pulmonary artery catheter data

1. Data reflecting pump performance
   (a) Cardiac index (CI = CO/BSA)
   (b) Stroke volume (SV = CO/HR)
   (c) Stroke index (SI = CI/HR)
   (d) Systemic vascular resistance (SVR)
   (e) Pulmonary vascular resistance (PVR)
   (f) Left ventricular stroke work index (LVSWI)
   (g) Right ventricular stroke work index (RVSWI)
2. Data reflecting oxygen transport and utilization
   (a) Oxygen content—arterial ($Ca{O_2}$), venous ($Cv{O_2}$) and pulmonary capillary ($Cc{O_2}$)
   (b) Arteriovenous oxygen content difference (a-$vD{O_2}$)
   (c) Oxygen consumption ($\dot{V}{O_2}$) or oxygen uptake
   (d) Oxygen delivery ($D{O_2}$) or oxygen transport or oxygen availability
   (e) Oxygen extraction ratio or oxygen utilization ratio ($\dot{V}{O_2}/D{O_2}$)
   (f) Alveolar–arterial oxygen difference (A–$aD{O_2}$)
   (g) Shunt fraction ($\dot{Q}s/\dot{Q}t$) or venous admixture ($\dot{Q}va/\dot{Q}t$)

Pulmonary vascular resistance tends to be elevated in heart failure, pulmonary embolus, chronic obstructive pulmonary disease, adult respiratory distress syndrome, and mitral valve disease and decreased in vasodilated states and in hypovolaemia.

Left and right ventricular stroke work indices are derived parameters reflecting cardiac contractility. They are measures of the external work of the ventricle during each contraction and are represented as:

$$\text{LVSWI} = \text{SI} \times \text{MAP} \times 13.6$$

and

$$\text{RVSWI} = \text{SI} \times \text{PA} \times 13.6$$

where MAP = mean (systemic) arterial pressure, PA = mean pulmonary arterial pressure, and SI = stroke index (CI/HR).

The left ventricular stroke work index is elevated in some types of hypertension, aortic stenosis, and stress states (trauma, burns, and sepsis), and decreased in hypovolaemic, cardiogenic, and late septic shock. The right ventricular stroke work index is usually elevated in patients with pulmonary hypertension and valvular heart disease and decreased in hypovolaemic and cardiogenic shock. Identical stroke work indices can be obtained by doubling the stroke index and halving the pressure (volume work) or by halving the stroke index and doubling the pressure (pressure work). However, myocardial oxygen consumption is considerably greater when the heart is performing pressure work than when it is performing volume work. The extent of myocardial oxygen demand can be approximated using the rate–pressure product (heart rate × systolic blood pressure). Values above 12 000 are indicative of significantly increased myocardial work and increased myocardial oxygen demands.

Data reflecting oxygen transport and utilization

Oxygen delivery

Oxygen delivery is the amount of oxygen leaving the heart to be delivered to the tissues in ml/min (normal range 640–1200 ml/min) or, expressed as an index based on body surface area, the oxygen delivery index (normal range 500–720 ml/min.m^2) Oxygen delivery indicates the integrity of the interactions between the cardiac pump, the oxygenating function of the lungs, and the carrying capacity of red blood cells. It does not provide an index of what the tissues do with the oxygen once it is delivered (oxygen uptake or extraction). Oxygen delivery is calculated from the product of cardiac output and the oxygen content of the blood ($Ca{O_2}$ ml/dl of blood).

$$\text{Oxygen delivery} = \text{cardiac output} \times Ca{O_2} \times 10\ \text{ml/min}$$
$$\text{Oxygen delivery index} = \text{cardiac index} \times Ca{O_2} \times 10\ \text{ml/min.m}^2.$$

Oxygen consumption index

Oxygen consumption is the amount of oxygen (in ml) consumed by the body's tissues per minute. Normal values range from 190 to 250 ml/min and the oxygen consumption index (corrected for body surface area) ranges from 100 to 160 ml/min.m^2. These variables are calculated as:

$$\text{Oxygen consumption} = \text{CO} \times (Ca{O_2} - Cv{O_2}) \times 10\ \text{ml/min.m}^2$$
$$\text{Oxygen consumption index} = \text{CI} \times (Ca{O_2} - Cv{O_2}) \times 10\ \text{ml/min.m}^2$$

In normal subjects, resting oxygen consumption is broadly unchanged over a wide range of values of oxygen, the oxygen extraction ratio varying to maintain a stable consumption. The normal physiological response to a fall in oxygen delivery is to increase oxygen extraction. Oxygen uptake, derived from analysis of inspired and expired respiratory gases, during steady state conditions will produce values equivalent to oxygen consumption.

Arteriovenous oxygen content difference

The arteriovenous oxygen content difference is calculated as the difference between arterial and mixed venous oxygen content ($Ca{O_2} - Cv{O_2}$). It is increased in conditions of increased oxygen extraction (decreased cardiac output, anaemia, and increased oxygen consumption) and may be decreased in high cardiac output states, in states associated with significant atrioventricular shunting, and with conditions in which impaired oxygen utilization occurs (sepsis). The oxygen extraction ratio is calculated as the arteriovenous oxygen content difference divided by the arterial oxygen content ($Ca{O_2} - Cv{O_2}$) and reflects the fraction of delivered oxygen that is consumed: the normal range is 22 to 30 per cent. It varies in a similar way to the arteriovenous oxygen content difference.

The utility of oxygen transport measurement

A characteristic feature of cardiogenic shock is arterial hypoxaemia which, in association with the reduced cardiac output, causes profound falls in oxygen delivery and a subsequent rise in blood lactate. The administration of oxygen may improve haemodynamic parameters and produce a fall in lactate concentrations. The reduced oxygen delivery and hyperlactataemia are associated with an increase in oxygen extraction ratio and a marked reduction in venous oxygen saturation. The profound fall in venous oxygen saturation is of particular importance if the overall mixed venous saturation is less than 50 per cent, indicating that some tissues are significantly hypoxaemic. This results in anaerobic metabolism and increased lactic acid production. The treatment of cardiogenic circulatory failure should therefore be aimed at increasing cardiac output and at increasing venous oxygen saturation. The outcome of cardiogenic shock following acute myocardial infarction is considerably better in those patients whose cardiac index is greater than 2.2 l/min.m^2. Attempts should therefore be made to achieve cardiac indices greater than this using a combination of preload optimization, inotropes, and vasodilators, and then to maximize oxygen on-loading by supplemental oxygen and if necessary intubation and mechanical ventilation.

Alveolar–arterial oxygen gradient (A-aDO_2)

The alveolar-arterial oxygen gradient (A-aDO_2) is a relatively sensitive but non-specific index of cardiopulmonary function. Gradients are normal when hypoxaemia is secondary to high altitude or alveolar hypoventilation (<2.6–3.3 kPa or 20–25 mmHg). In the presence of a normal cardiac output, the gradient provides a rough index of venous admixture and has the added advantage that a mixed venous blood sample is not required for its determination. However, it does require the $F\text{io}_2$ to be accurately known. Determination of the gradient may offer predictive information—very high gradients are associated with severe cardiopulmonary disease—as well as offering a means to monitor therapy. It is calculated as:

$$\text{A-aDO}_2 = P\text{Ao}_2 - P\text{ao}_2$$
$$P\text{Ao}_2 = (P\text{B} - 47)\,(F\text{io}_2) - (1.25 \times P\text{aCo}_2)$$

where $P\text{Ao}_2$ = partial pressure of oxygen in alveolar air.

Shunt fraction (Qs/Qt) and venous admixture (Qva/Qt)

The shunt fraction (Qs/Qt) measures the fraction of total blood flow that is not oxygenated during its passage through the lungs, and is calculated when the $F\text{io}_2$ = 100 per cent. When it is calculated at an $F\text{io}_2$ of below 100 per cent, it is more correctly referred to as the venous admixture (Qva/Qt). Pulmonary conditions which cause shunting, such as pneumonia, atelectasis, and secretions, have primary effects on the shunt fraction. In patients who have diseased lungs, changes in shunt may simply reflect changes in pulmonary blood flow rather than changes in the intrinsic disease process. The effect of blood flow on shunt depends to some degree whether the lungs are normal, diffusely diseased, or have lobar or regional abnormalities. Venous admixture or shunt varies directly with cardiac output in patients with normal or diffusely abnormal lung (the higher the cardiac output, the greater the shunt) and inversely with cardiac output in patients with unilateral lung abnormalities. The resultant effect of cardiac output and shunt on the $P\text{ao}_2$ is complex and depends on whether the alteration in pulmonary shunt predominates over the change in mixed venous blood oxygen content.

The shunt equation is a mathematical derivation, partly based on the Fick equation. The derivation of the shunt equation involves making certain physiological assumptions which are in part theoretical. Since oxygen consumption represents the product of blood flow cardiac output times the atroventricular oxygen content difference ($C\text{ao}_2 - C\text{vo}_2$), the Fick equation, can be expressed as:

$$V\text{o}_2 = Q\text{t} \times (C\text{ao}_2 - C\text{vo}_2)$$

The shunt equation is expressed as the ratio of oxygen content differences between pulmonary capillary blood ($C\text{co}_2$), an assumed quantity based on the knowledge of the partial pressure of oxygen in the alveolus $P\text{Ao}_2$ and the oxygen content of arterial and mixed venous blood respectively. It is represented as:

$$\frac{Q_s}{Q_t} = \frac{(C\text{co}_2 - C\text{ao}_2)}{(C\text{co}_2 - C\text{vo}_2}$$

In order to calculate the shunt fraction one must carry out the following steps.

1. Obtain mixed venous blood through the distal line of the pulmonary artery catheter together with a direct pulmonary venous saturation if a fibreoptic pulmonary artery catheter has been used.
2. Measure arterial blood gases.
3. Calculate $C\text{ao}_2$ = (haemoglobin × 1.34 × $S\text{ao}_2$) + ($P\text{ao}_2$ × 0.022)
4. Calculate $C\text{vo}_2$ = (haemoglobin × 1.34 × $S\text{vo}_2$) + ($P\text{vo}_2$ × 0.022)
5. Calculate $P\text{Ao}_2 = (P\text{B} - 47)F\text{io}_2 - (P\text{aCo}_2 \times 1.25)$
6. Calculate $C\text{co}_2$ using $P\text{Ao}_2$ from step 5, i.e. $C\text{co}_2$ = (haemoglobin × 1.34 × $S\text{co}_2$) + ($P\text{Ao}_2$ × 0.022) (assume $S\text{co}_2$ = 100 per cent, a reasonable assumption providing the patient is on supplemental oxygen).

(N.B. The oxygen solubility factor is quoted as 0.022 ml/kPa, the equivalent factor for mmHg is 0.003.)

The normal shunt fraction is less than 10 per cent. Shunts below 10 per cent are rarely seen in patients receiving positive pressure ventilation. Calculated true shunts greater than 30 per cent are considered incompatible with prolonged spontaneous ventilation. Below 20 per cent the weaning process should be considered if the cardiac status is good.

LACTIC ACIDOSIS

Lactic acidosis is a pathological state characterized by persistent elevation of the serum lactate concentration together with significant acidaemia. Lactic acidosis should always be suspected in a patient with metabolic acidosis and an increased anion gap which cannot be explained by uraemia or ketonaemia. The onset of clinical manifestations may resemble diabetic ketoacidosis, with sudden malaise, weakness, anorexia, nausea, and vomiting. An early sign of lactic acidosis is hyperpnoea or abdominal pain. In contrast to diabetic ketoacidosis, there is no polyuria, polydipsia, or acetone odour, and the fluid deficit is usually less marked.

Lactic acidosis may occur during anaerobic conditions when oxidative metabolism via the Krebs' cycle or gluconeogenesis is prevented. It may be associated with impaired end-organ function, such as liver or kidney disease, which greatly decreases the metabolic capacity for lactate. Lactate is metabolized either via oxidative metabolism (Krebs' cycle) to CO_2 and H_2O, or by gluconeogenesis to glucose. Both of these pathways depend on intact aerobic metabolism and need intact mitochondrial function, a favourable redox state, and adequate ATP. Gluconeogenesis from lactate occurs in the liver and kidneys and provide a continuous supply of glucose that would be otherwise wasted to tissues.

Increased lactate levels can exist without acidosis as is seen when lactate production exceeds metabolic capacity, even with intact oxidation metabolism, and good end-organ function. When this occurs (for example in hyperventilation and stress), pyruvate is converted to lactate. However, the elevation in lactate is generally modest (5 mmol/l) and acidosis, as noted above, is usually absent.

Types of lactic acidosis

Type A lactic acidosis is associated with poor tissue perfusion and hypoxaemia and is the most common type. The initial hydrolysis of a relatively large amount of ATP would initially release more H^+ than lactate.

Type B lactic acidosis not associated with a decreased oxygen supply and lactic acidosis is due to increased glycolysis or decreased gluconeogenesis. Hydrogen ion and lactate production tend to be equimolar. Type B lactic acidosis has been subdivided into three subtypes: type B_1 is associated with disorders such as diabetes mellitus, renal and hepatic disease, infection, and leukaemia; type B_2 is due to drugs, chemicals, and toxins such as phenformin, ethanol, and methanol; type B_3 covers congenital forms of lactic acidosis such as Von Gierke's disease.

Normal lactate levels are 0.5 to 1.6 mmol/l for arterial blood and 0.5 to 2 mmol/l for venous blood. It is essential that a tourniquet is not applied during venesection. Most patients with lactic acidosis have an anion gap that averages 22 to 27 mmol/l. The increase in the anion gap is usually greater than the decrease in HCO_3^-, in contrast to diabetic ketoacidosis, in which the increase in the anion gap is identical to the decrease in HCO_3^-.

Clinical examples

Tissue hypoxia

Lactic acidosis is usually associated with tissue hypoxia, being common when cardiac output is greatly impaired but rare in patients with uncomplicated anaemia or hypoxaemia. As cardiac output decreases to 30 per cent of normal the major compensatory mechanism of increased oxygen extraction is insufficient to prevent tissue hypoxaemia. In the presence of arterial hypoxaemia and even severe anaemia, in tripling of cardiac output and a tripling of oxygen extraction results in a ninefold increase in oxygen delivery and ensures adequate oxygen delivery. Chronic lactic acidosis may develop in patients with severe congestive heart failure, and tissue hypoxia may exist in the presence of high cardiac output if blood distribution is disturbed, as occurs in the sepsis syndrome. The resolution of such a lactic acidosis is then considered a marker of efficacy of therapy provided liver function is unimpaired.

Seizures

Lactic acidosis may accompany grand mal seizures and is generally self-limiting. Specific treatment of the acidosis is unnecessary, although resolution of lactic acidosis may be slower in patients with pre-existing liver disease.

Diabetes mellitus

Lactic acidosis used to be observed in patients with diabetes mellitus following phenformin administration; it is now rare since this side-effect was recognized. Lactic acidosis occasionally develops in patients with diabetic ketoacidosis and extreme volume depletion. It may also be evident in liver disease: basal lactate metabolism is generally normal in cirrhotics but the reserve is much decreased. Rising lactate levels in acute fulminant hepatitis are associated with a poor prognosis.

Hypoglycaemia

Lactic acidosis in association with hypoglycaemia is generally confined to infants and children, but has been noted occasionally in adults with either hepatic or renal disease.

Malignancy

Lactic acid levels are occasionally increased in patients with acute leukaemia, lymphomas, and intra-abdominal neoplasms. It has been attributed to the over-production of lactate by the tumour and appears to be related to the tumour burden.

Asthmatics

Twenty per cent of asthmatics admitted to hospital may exhibit excess lactate production from the respiratory muscles, with some contribution from lactate under-utilization due to hypoperfusion of skeletal muscle and liver. The presence of lactic acidosis correlates with a peak expiratory flow rate of 60 l/min or less and might suggest that respiratory fatigue is imminent and that the patient may require ventilatory assistance.

Drugs

Several drugs or toxins including, phenformin, salicylates, ethylene glycol, and methanol may be associated with lactic acidosis.

Treatment

Type A lactic acidosis

Therapy is directed at correcting or alleviating the underlying cause: this might include the administration of blood, fluids, and drugs to correct circulatory failure by optimizing myocardial performance. The underlying principle should be to maintain adequate levels of oxygen delivery. Mortality is high (>75 per cent) in patients with persistent lactic acidosis despite appropriate measures.

Type B lactic acidosis

No specific form of current therapy has been shown to reduce the mortality rate associated with Type B lactic acidosis. Administration of sodium bicarbonate has been recommended to maintain the arterial pH above 7.2: below this there is myocardial depression and reduced cardiac output, while at a pH below 7.0, utilization of lactate by the liver is impaired. The dose of bicarbonate required can be estimated by multiplying the desired increase in HCO_3^-, in mmol, by 50 per cent of the patient's body weight in kg. However, bicarbonate stimulates glycolysis whilst depressing other oxidative reactions and therefore enhances lactate production. This increase in lactate production may contribute to the mortality associated with lactic acidosis. In diabetic ketoacidosis, bicarbonate delays the fall in blood lactate and total ketone bodies, even though it improves the pH. The relative risks and benefits of correcting a metabolic acidosis with bicarbonate are more thoroughly considered below.

Haemodialysis and peritoneal dialysis do not correct the cause of lactic acidosis but do restore the buffer pool. Dialysis and haemofiltration may supplement bicarbonate therapy by making space for additional fluid volume to be administered. Haemodialysis and haemofiltration fluids generally use lactate or acetate as the buffer. The buffering effect depends upon conversion to bicarbonate which may be impaired in patients with severe lactic acidosis or liver disease. In such circumstances a bicarbonate buffer may be preferable, with the above limitations being acknowledged.

ALKALI THERAPY OF METABOLIC ACIDOSIS

Severe metabolic acidosis due to diabetic ketoacidosis, sepsis syndrome or renal failure is a common clinical problem in the critical care unit. Arguments have been voiced both for and against the use of specific alkalinizing agents to correct the acidosis rapidly in an attempt to avoid the complications of the acidotic state. Severe acidosis has several serious and life threatening effects, including circulatory failure due to reduce myocardial contractility, increased systemic and pulmonary vascular resistance, and enhanced arrhythmogenesis. In addition, end-organ receptor sensitivity to inotropes and pressors may be diminished, reducing the efficacy of these agents. Unfortunately, controlled studies of the effects of correction of metabolic acidosis with bicarbonate have failed to demonstrate improved haemodynamics. Additionally, and depending upon the alkalinizing agent selected, certain risks are associated with alkali therapy (Table 14).

Table 14 Unwanted effects of alkali therapy

1. Sudden electrolyte shifts to and from the intracellular space (particularly calcium and potassium)
2. Increased osmolarity with concentrated alkali
3. Shift in oxyhaemoglobin dissociation curve reducing peripheral tissue oxygen off-loading
4. Increased intracellular acidosis due to diffusion of CO_2 into cells (generated from bicarbonate)
5. Risk of cardiac arrest with pH > 7.55

The convenience of arterial blood gas measurement, reflecting extracellular pH, has unfortunately diverted attention away from the need to correct intracellular acidosis. In addition, when tissue perfusion is poor, as occurs during cardiopulmonary resuscitation, arterial alkalaemia can coexist with venous and intracellular acidosis.

Sodium bicarbonate

Several bicarbonate solutions are available, some of which include salts of weak acids such as citrate (Shohl's solution) or lactate (lactated Ringer's solution) and require the metabolism of these precursors to bicarbonate (Table 15).

Table 15 Bicarbonate preparations

Preparations	Bicarbonate content
5% bicarbonate solution	595 mmol/l
8.4% bicarbonate solution	1000 mmol/l
Shohl's solution	100 mmol/l
Lactated Ringer's solution	28 mmol/l

Hypertonic solutions are theoretically of advantage when hyponatraemia is present or in patients with circulatory overload. Isotonic solutions may be used when there is a risk of producing a hyperosmolar state or when volume expansion is desired. It is not unusual for patients with severe acidosis to require more than 200 mmol of bicarbonate per hour: such resistance to bicarbonate therapy usually denotes ongoing acid production, as might occur in a lactic acidosis secondary to sepsis. When bicarbonate neutralizes hydrogen ion CO_2 and H_2O are produced according to the formula

$$H^+ + HCO_3^- \rightarrow H_2CO_3 \rightarrow H_2O + CO_2$$

In the presence of an adequate circulation and alveolar ventilation the excess CO_2 is quickly eliminated by the lungs and pH restored to normal. In patients with circulatory collapse or ventilatory failure, CO_2 accumulates in the blood and, although the buffering capacity by bicarbonate is enhanced the effect upon pH is less than expected. Cell membranes are readily permeable to CO_2 (unlike bicarbonate and hydrogen ions), and intracellular pH may paradoxically fall following the administration of bicarbonate. This paradoxical response is of particular importance with regard to cerebral and cardiac function, resulting in raised intracranial pressure and refractory heart failure, respectively.

Hyperosmolality and hypernatraemia may be serious side-effects of sodium bicarbonate therapy, with each milliequivalent of bicarbonate providing twice the osmolar load. Severe and prolonged hypernatraemia can be associated with serious neurological sequelae including death.

Salt solutions of weak acids, such as acetate and lactate, can be used to improve base deficit indirectly. These act as bicarbonate precursors and are effective because of the subsequent generation of bicarbonate. The onset of effect is clearly slower than the equivalent doses of bicarbonate. Solutions which depend on hepatic metabolism to bicarbonate for their efficiency (e.g. lactated Ringer's, Shohl's solution) should be used with caution in patients with severe liver disease. Acetate is also contraindicated in diabetic ketoacidosis, when acetyl-CoA is already present in excess.

Tris-hydroxymethylaminomethane (THAM)

Tris-hydroxymethylaminomethane is an aminoalcohol which has an osmolality similar to that of plasma. A 0.3 M solution is a more powerful buffer than bicarbonate and produces a lower osmolar and sodium load than bicarbonate in equivalent doses. THAM should be infused slowly at rates not exceeding 2 mmol/min, to avoid an excessively rapid fall in arterial $P\text{CO}_2$. After the infusion of 40 to 50 mmol, arterial blood gases can be repeated to assess benefit and determine whether further administration is required.

The buffering activity of THAM differs from bicarbonate in several important respects. By buffering carbonic acid, bicarbonate is generated and CO_2 is removed from plasma. By reducing extracellular and intracellular CO_2, intracellular pH rises, unlike the situation following bicarbonate administration, which may exaggerate intracellular acidosis. The non-ionized fraction of THAM also diffuses directly into the intracellular space and acts as a buffer within the cell. THAM appears to have a positive inotropic and antiarrhythmic effect by correcting myocardial acidosis. Hypoventilation may occur following its administration due to the reduced CO_2 and resetting of chemoreceptor responsiveness, in which case mechanical ventilation may be required. Other, adverse effects of THAM are shown in Table 16.

Table 16 Disadvantages of tris-hydroxymethylaminomethane

1. Central venous administration required due to alkaline pH
2. Accumulates in renal failure
3. Increased glycogen oxidation may cause hypoglycaemia
4. May induce hypoventilation

Experimental evidence suggests that intraneuronal acidosis following head injury can be harmful and that THAM can correct intracerebral acidosis, reduce oedema, and improve the energy state of brain tissue. Preliminary results of a clinical trial of this therapy in severely head injured and comatose patients showed slightly improved survival.

Sodium carbonate

Sodium carbonate acts as a hydrogen ion acceptor and a bicarbonate precursor. Carbonate preferentially buffers hydrogen ions, producing bicarbonate as follows:

$$CO_3^- + CO_2 + H_2O \rightarrow 2HCO_3^- \text{ (uptake of } CO_2\text{)}$$
$$H^+ + HCO_3^- \rightarrow H_2CO_3 \text{ (uptake of } H^+\text{)}$$

and

$$CO_3^{2-} + H^+ \rightarrow HCO_3^- \text{ (uptake of } H^+\text{)}$$

As with THAM sodium carbonate produces a fall in extracellular and intracellular CO_2, and therefore reduces intracellular pH. However, it exerts no direct intracellular buffering due to its highly ionized state.

A combination of sodium carbonate and sodium bicarbonate (Carbicarb®), has the attraction of bicarbonate (rapid activity without the need for metabolism to an active form) and the ability of carbonate to act as a CO_2 acceptor. Generally, a lower dose of Carbicarb is required compared to bicarbonate. In hypoxic lactic acidosis induced in animal models, Carbicarb proved superior to bicarbonate in correcting pH, reducing lactate levels, and protecting against hypotension.

Sodium dichloroacetate

Dichloroacetate has been shown to improve acidosis and support the circulation in some cases where bicarbonate therapy has failed. Dichloroacetate stimulates phosphodehydrogenase activity, increasing pyruvate oxidation, which in turn generates bicarbonate and reduces blood lactate levels. By this mechanism it is also able to reduce brain lactate more rapidly than is the case without therapy. Although dichloroacetate decreases the morbidity and mortality of experimentally induced lactic acidosis in dogs, it has yet to be shown to improve survival rates significantly in patients. There appear to be no major short-term complications from dichloroacetate therapy but chronic use carries a risk of drowsiness, paralysis, and polyneuropathy.

FURTHER READING

Cardiac arrest and circulatory failure

American Heart Association. Standards and guidance for cardiopulmonary resuscitation (CPR) and emergency cardiac care (ECC). *JAMA*, 1986; **255**: 2905–89.

Braunwald E. On the difference between the heart's output and its contractile state. *Circulation*, 1971; **43**: 171–74.

Berkowitz C, *et al.* Comparative responses of dobutamine and nitroprusside in patients with chronic low output cardiac failure. *Circulation*, 1977; **56**: 918–24.

Callahan M, Barton C. Prediction of outcome of cardiopulmonary resuscitation from end-tidal carbon dioxide concentration. *Crit Care Med*, 1990; **18**: 358–62.

Chatterjee K. Vasodilator therapy for heart failure. In: Cohn JN, ed. *Drug treatment of heart failure*. New York: York, 1983; 151–78.

Gaasch WH, Apstein CS, Levine HJ. Diastolic properties of the left ventricle. In: Levine HJ, Gaasch WH, eds. *The ventricle: basic and clinical aspects*. Boston: Martinus Nijhoff, 1985: 143–70.

Goldberg LI. Cardiovascular and renal actions of dopamine: potential clinical applications. *Pharmacol Rev*, 1972; **24**: 1–29.

Krischer JK, Fine EG, Weifeldt ML, Guerci AD. Comparison of prehospital conventional and simultaneous compression–ventilation cardiopulmonary resuscitation. *Crit Care Med*, 1989; **17**: 1263–69.

Royal College of Physicians. Resuscitation from cardiopulmonary arrest. Training and organisation. *J R Coll Phys*, 1987; **21**: 1–8.

Wilson JR, Reichek N, Dunkman WB, Goldberg S. Effect of diuresis on the performance of the failing left ventricle in man. *Am J Med*, 1981; **70**: 234–9.

Oxygen uptake, sepsis syndrome and multiple organ system failure

Alverdy JC, Aoys E, Moss GS. Total parenteral nutrition promotes bacterial translocation from the gut. *Surgery*, 1988; **104**: 185–90.

Duff JH, *et al.* Defective oxygen consumption in septic shock. *Surg Gynecol Obstet*, 1969; **128**: 1051–60.

Edwards JD, *et al.* Use of survivors' cardiorespiratory values as therapeutic goals in septic shock. *Crit Care Med*, 1989; **17**: 1098–103.

Ledingham IMcA, Alcock SR, Eastaway AT, McDonald JC, McKay IC, Ramsay G. Triple régime of selective decontamination of the digestive tract, systemic cefotaxime and microbiological surveillance for prevention of acquired infection in intensive care. *Lancet*, 1988; i: 785–90.

Matushak GM, Rinaldo JE. Organ interactions in the adult respiratory distress syndrome during sepsis. *Chest*, 1988; **94**: 400–6.

McArdle AH, Palmerson C, Brown RA, Brown HC, Williams HB. Early enteral feeding of patients with major burns: prevention of catabolism. *Ann Plastic Surg*, 1984; **13**: 396–401.

Parker MM, *et al.* Profound but reversible myocardial depression in patients with septic shock. *Ann Intern Med*, 1984; **100**: 483–90.

Ramsay G. Endotoxaemia in multiple organ failure: a secondary role for SDD. In: van Saene HKF, Stoutenbeek CP, Lawin P, Ledingham IMcA, eds. *Infection control by selective decontamination*. Berlin: Springer Verlag, 1989: 135–42.

Ravin HA, Rowley D, Jenkins C, Fine J. On the absorption of bacterial endotoxin from the gastrointestinal tract of the normal and shocked animal. *J Exp Med*, 1960; **112**: 783–90.

Rush BF, *et al.* Endotoxaemia and bacteraemia during haemorrhagic shock. *Ann Surg* 1988; **207**: 549–54.

Shibutani K, Komatsu T, Kubal K. Critical level of oxygen delivery in anaesthetized man. *Crit Care Med*, 1983; **11**: 640–3.

Shoemaker WC, Appel PL, Kram HB. Prospective trail of supranormal values of survivors as therapeutic goals in high risk surgical patients. *Chest*, 1988; **94**: 1176–218.

Shoemaker WC, Appel PL, Kram HB, Waxman K, Tai-Shion L. Prospective trial of supranormal values of survivors as therapeutic goals in high-risk surgical patients. *Chest*, 1988; **94**: 1176–86.

Stoutenbeek CP, van Saene HKF, Miranda DR, Zandstra DF. The effect of selective decontamination of the digestive tract on colonisation and infection rate in multiple trauma patients. *Intensive Care Med*, 1984; **10**: 185–92.

Wilmore DW, *et al.* The gut: a central organ after surgical stress. *Surgery*, 1988; **104**: 917–23.

Wellman W, Fink TC, Benner F, Schmidt FW. Endotoxaemia in active Crohn's disease. Treatment with whole gut irrigation and 5-aminosalicylic acid. *Gut*, 1986; **27**: 814–20.

Zieglar TR, *et al.* Increased intestinal permeability associated with infection in burn patients. *Arch Surg*, 1988; **123**: 1313–19.

Pulmonary artery catheter

Baele PL, McMichan JC, Marsh HM, Sill JC, Southorn PA. Continuous monitoring of mixed venous oxygen saturation in critically ill patients. *Anesth Analg*, 1982; **61**: 513–17.

Boyd KD, Thomas SJ, Gold J, Boyd AD. A prospective study of complications of pulmonary artery catheterizations in 500 consecutive patients. *Chest*, 1983; **84**: 245–9.

Forrester JS, Diamond GA, Swan HJC. Correlative classification of clinical and hemodynamic function after acute myocardial function. *Am J Cardiol*, 1977; **39**: 137–45.

Groeneveld ABJ, Thijs LG. Pulmonary artery catheterization in septic shock. *Clin Intensive Care*, 1990; **1**: 111–15.

Guyton AC, Lindsey AW. Effect of elevated left atrial pressure and decreased plasma protein concentration on the development of pulmonary edema. *Circ Res*, 1959; **7**: 649–57.

Lategola M, Rahn H. A self guiding catheter for cardiac and pulmonary arterial catheterization and occlusion. *Proc Soc Exp Biol Med*, 1953; **84**: 667–8.

Pinilla JC, Ross DF, Martin T, Crumb H. Study of the incidence of intravascular catheter infections and associated septicaemia in critically ill patients. *Crit Care Med*, 1983; **11**: 21–5.

Robin ED. The cult of the Swan-Ganz catheter: Overuse and abuse of pulmonary flow catheters. *Ann Intern Med*, 1985; **103**: 445–9.

Shah KB, Rao TK, Langhlin S, El-Etr A. A review of pulmonary artery catheterization in 6,245 patients. *Anesthesiology*, 1984; **61**: 271–5.

Stevenson LW, Perloff JK. The limited reliability of physical signs for estimating hemodynamics in chronic heart failure. *JAMA*, 1989; **261**: 884–8.

Swan HJC, Ganz W, Forrester J, Marcus H, Diamond G, Chonette D. Catheterization of the heart in man with use of a flow-directed balloon tipped catheter. *N Engl J Med*, 1970; **283**: 447–51.

Vincent J-L, Thirion M, Brimioulle S, Lejeune P, Kahn RJ. Thermodilution measurement of right ventricular ejection fraction with a modified pulmonary artery catheter. *Intensive Care Med*, 1986; **12**: 33–8.

Lactic acidosis and alkali therapy

Bersin RM, Arieff AI. Improved hemodynamic function during hypoxia with Carbicarb, a new agent for the management of acidosis. *Circulation*, 1988; **77**: 227–33.

Effron MB, Guarnieri T, Frederkisen JW, Greene HL, Weisfeldt ML. Effects of tris (hydroxymethyl) aminomethane on ischemic myocardium. *Am J Physiol*, 1978; **235**: H167–74.

Jaffe AS. New and old paradoxes. Acidosis and cardiopulmonary resuscitation. *Circulation*, 1989; **80**: 1079–83.

Kruse JA, Haupt, MT, Puri VK, Carlson, RW. Lactate levels as predictors of the relationship between oxygen delivery and consumption in ARDS. *Chest*, 1990; **98**: 959–62.

Rosner MJ, Elias KG, Coley I. Prospective, randomized trial of THAM therapy in severe brain injury: preliminary results. In Hoff JT, Betz AL, eds. *Intracranial Pressure VII*. Berlin: Springer, 1989: 611–15.

Shapiro JI. Functional and metabolic responses of isolated hearts to acidosis: effects of sodium bicarbonate and Carbicarb. *Am J Physiol*, 1990; **258**: H1835–9.

Stacpoole PW. Lactic acidosis: the case against bicarbonate therapy. *Ann Intern Med*, 1986; **105**: 276–9.

Stacpoole PW, Lorenz, AC, Thomas RG, Harman EM. Dichloroacetate in the treatment of lactic acidosis. *Ann Intern Med*, 1988; **108**: 58–63.

von Gazmuri RJPM, Weil MH, Rackow, EC. Cardiac effects of carbon dioxide-consuming and carbon dioxide-generating buffers during cardiopulmonary resuscitation. *J Am Coll Cardiol*, 1990; **15**: 482–90.

Weil MH, Ruiz CE, Michaels S, Rackow EC. Acid base determinants of survival after cardiopulmonary resuscitation. *Crit Care Med*, 1985; **13**: 888–92.

4.2 Renal aspects

CHRISTOPHER S. GARRARD

OLIGURIA

An appreciation of the significance of oliguria, and its early recognition is essential if steps are to be taken to preserve renal function in the critically ill patient. The minimum effective urine volume is determined by the obligate solute load which has to be excreted each day. In healthy individuals, about 800 mmol can be eliminated in as little as 650 ml of urine. Even in those taking a high carbohydrate, low sodium, low nitrogen diet, any degree of renal impairment greatly increases the minimum obligate urine volume. As a rough guide, a urine requirement of 1 ml/kg.h provides adequate solute clearance. At 0.5 ml/kg.h (840 ml for a 70-kg patient) azotaemia will only be avoided if renal function is normal. Urinary tract catheterization is often necessary, but is invasive. Having accepted the potential complications associated with urinary catheters it is all the more important to monitor urine volumes constantly and to take appropriate action if necessary. Table 1 outlines a simple approach to the evaluation and treatment of oliguria. Complete anuria should always, of course, prompt consideration of a blocked urinary catheter.

Relying on only a limited number of the criteria listed in Table 1 may lead to an erroneous conclusion regarding the volume status of the patient. Several other pitfalls may mislead the unwary. In the patient with sepsis, oedema (extravascular fluid) may coexist with marked intravascular hypovolaemia, indicated by a low central venous pressure and positive response to a fluid challenge. Conversely, the central venous pressure and pulmonary artery wedge pressure can easily be overestimated in patients on positive pressure ventilation if measurements are not made at end expiration.

There can be no substitute for personally measuring the venous pressure and, in doing so, confirming the calibration and zeroing of the equipment. Over-reliance upon fluid balance records, even when accurately maintained, can mislead since the compliance of the major capacitance vessels can change.

Several urinary measurements may help to distinguish potentially reversible prerenal azotaemia from established intrinsic renal failure: these include sodium concentration (U_{Na}), osmolality (U_{osm}), urine to plasma urea nitrogen ratio, urine to plasma creatinine ratio (U_{cr}/P_{cr}, fractional excretion of sodium (FE_{Na}), and renal failure index (RFI). Table 2 shows the differences between these indices for prerenal and renal azotaemia.

Table 1 Evaluation of oliguria in the critically ill

Prompted by:
Urine volume <0.25 ml/kg.h for 2 h (e.g. <10 ml)
or
Urine volume <0.5 ml/kg.h for 4 h (e.g. <30 ml)

What is the evidence to suggest volume depletion?
1. Clinical evaluation
    - Jugular venous filling
    - Skin turgor
    - Oedema
    - Hypotension
    - Tachycardia
    - Thirst
2. Fluid balance over preceding 24, 48, 72 h
3. Central venous pressure/pulmonary artery wedge pressure
4. Urinary Na^+, fractional Na^+, excretion
5. Response to rapid fluid challenge
    - In terms of urine volume
    - In terms of central venous pressure/pulmonary artery wedge pressure

Table 2 Comparison of prerenal azotaemia and acute renal failure

Index	Prerenal azotaemia	Acute renal failure
U_{osm}	High U_{osm}	Isosthenuria
U_{Na}	<20 mmol/l	>40 mmol/l
FE_{Na}	$<1\%$	$>1\%$
U_{cr}/P_{cr}	$>20{:}1$	$<15{:}1$
Urine sediment	Normal	Cellular casts

See text for abbreviations.

Calculation of fractional excretion of sodium (FE_{Na})

Filtered and excreted sodium can be calculated as follows:

$$FE_{Na} = \frac{\text{urine Na}}{\text{filtered Na}} \times 100(\%)$$

If urine sodium = urine volume × U_{Na} and filtered sodium = GFR × P_{Na}, then

$$FE_{Na} = \frac{U_{Na}V}{\text{GFR} \times P_{Na}} \times 100(\%)$$

$$FE_{Na} = \frac{U_{Na}V}{(UcrV/Pcr) \times P_{Na}} \times 100(\%)$$

$$FE_{Na} = \left(\frac{U_{Na}}{P_{Na}}\right) \times \left(\frac{P_{cr}}{U_{cr}}\right) \times 100(\%)$$

where GFR is the glomerular filtration rate (ml), P_{Na} is the plasma sodium concentration (mmol/l), U_{Na} is the urine sodium concentration (mmol/l), P_{cr} is the plasma creatinine concentration (mmol/l), U_{cr} is the urine creatinine concentration (mmol/l), and V is the urine flow rate (ml/min).

Since creatinine is essentially not reabsorbed or secreted, the urinary concentration of creatinine is a function of water reabsorption. Sodium, however, is actively reabsorbed by the tubules, such that the final U_{Na} depends upon sodium reabsorption as well as the amount of water reabsorbed by the tubules. The renal failure index (RFI) offers no advantages over the FE_{Na} but may be calculated thus:

$$\text{RFI} = U_{Na} \times \frac{P_{Cr}}{U_{Cr}}$$

Application of fractional excretion of sodium (FE_{Na})

In the oliguric patient, a FE_{Na} below 1 per cent is consistent with prerenal azotaemia. A FE_{Na} of less than 0.4 per cent is even more specific. Conversely, an FE_{Na} of greater than 1 per cent may be consistent with renal damage, although a FE_{Na} greater than 3 per cent is much more indicative of intrinsic renal disease. Values between 1 per cent and 3 per cent are therefore less conclusive. A low FE_{Na} may, under certain circumstances, be an unreliable guide since patients with intrinsic renal failure occasionally have a FE_{Na} of 1 per cent. Conversely, there are hypovolaemic conditions in which the FE_{Na} can be paradoxically high (Table 3).

Table 3 Limits of reliability of FE_{Na} values

Causes of FE_{Na} less than 1 per cent in patients with intrinsic renal failure
- (a) Non-oliguric acute renal failure
- (b) Early acute glomerulonephritis (without tubular damage)
- (c) Renal failure associated with severe renal vasoconstriction
    - Hepatorenal syndrome
    - Sepsis syndrome
    - Non-steroidal anti-inflammatory drugs
    - Renal vasculitides
    - Radiocontrast-induced acute renal failure
    - Myoglobinuria and haemoglobinuria
- (d) Renal hypoperfusion
    - ACE inhibitor
    - Renal artery stenosis
    - Normovolaemic burns patient
    - Renal transplant rejection
    - Cyclosporin nephrotoxicity

Cause of a FE_{Na} greater than 1 per cent in the hypovolaemic patient
- (a) Chronic renal disease
- (b) Diuretic use within 12 to 24 h of testing FE_{Na}
    - Thiazides
    - Frusemide
    - Osmotic diuretics
    - Glycosuria
- (c) Metabolic alkalosis with alkaline urine (pH $<$ 7.0)
- (d) Addison's disease

The increase in the urine sodium produced by diuretics persists much longer following ingestion of thiazides than after frusemide, ethacrynic acid, or the osmotic diuretics. By 24 h after the last dose of diuretic, FE_{Na} can again be adopted as an indicator of prerenal azotaemia.

There are rare situations where the sodium cation is an unreliable indicator of the nature of renal dysfunction. This is the case when there is sodium wasting such as occurs in the patient with a metabolic alkalosis due to the loss of upper gastrointestinal tract secretions. In such a situation, a urinary chloride level of less than 20 mmol/1 (or FE_{Cl} less than 1 per cent) is indicative of volume depletion.

Management of prerenal azotaemia

Once the clinician is reasonably confident that the observed oliguria is due to volume depletion the obvious response is to administer fluid, the nature of which is dictated by the degree of urgency, electrolyte status and the haemoglobin concentration of the patient. Colloidal solutions expand the intravascular space rapidly, while electrolyte solutions are distributed across intra- and extracellular compartments. Blood is preferred when the patient is anaemic. If fluid is infused rapidly (500 ml in 30 min) the response to volume expansion is similar regardless of the type of fluid. The haemodynamic and renal response to a fluid bolus will often resolve any doubts as to the intravascular volume status of the patient. Fluid resuscitation should be performed quickly and under the personal supervision of the clinician. It is insufficient simply to increase the infusion rates of existing fluids and re-evaluate the patient 6 to 12 h later.

The administration of dopamine in so called 'renovascular' doses (about 2.5 µg/kg.min) may reverse the renal vasoconstriction that is a feature of the volume depleted state. Provided that sufficient fluid resuscitation has been undertaken, renovascular dopamine may promote a diuresis. Whether this approach can prevent the onset of vasomotor nephropathy remains to bc conclusively proven.

Vasoconstrictor agents have often been considered likely to contribute to renal vasoconstriction and have therefore been contraindicated in prerenal azotaemic states. Contrary to this opinion, recent experience in sepsis has suggested that pressor agents such as noradrenaline, by increasing systemic blood pressure, may encourage a diuresis more effectively than inotropes such as dobutamine that have peripheral vasodilator properties.

In the patient with sepsis syndrome or primary cardiac failure the insertion of a pulmonary artery catheter to optimize preload, combined with the use of inotropes or pressors, may be necessary to ensure the preservation of renal function.

ACUTE RENAL FAILURE

Overall mortality from acute renal failure remains in excess of 50 per cent, although there has been an indication of improved survival in recent years. Less than 10 per cent of patients with uncomplicated acute renal failure die, but in those with multiple organ system failure the mortality rate from acute renal failure rises to above 70 per cent, and may approach 100 per cent when four organ systems fail. Renal failure therefore represents a serious complication in the critically ill patient.

Once renal failure is established, additional renal insult must be avoided and consideration paid to the reduction in fluid and drug elimination. Acute renal failure may be grouped into four broad categories: ischaemic injury, nephrotoxicity, glomerular disorders, and vascular disorders (Table 4).

Table 4 Some causes of acute renal failure in intensive care

Vasomotor nephropathy (acute tubular necrosis)
Sepsis syndrome
Severe polytrauma
Massive haemorrhage
Transfusion reaction
Myoglobinuria
Pancreatitis
Dehydration
Gastrointestinal losses
Ileus
Nephrotoxic agents associated with renal failure
Antibiotics (e.g. aminoglycosides, penicillin)
Radiographic contrast media
Heavy metals
Anaesthetic agents
Organic solvents
Insecticides
Disease of glomeruli and small vessels
Acute glomerulonephritis
Systemic lupus erythematosus
Polyarteritis nodosa
Henoch–Schönlein purpura
Wegener's granulomatosis
Goodpasture's syndrome
Serum sickness
Malignant hypertension
Haemolytic-uraemic syndrome
Drug-induced vasculitis
Abruptio placentae
Disease of large renal vessels
Renal arterial thrombosis, emboli, or stenosis
Bilateral renal vein thrombosis

Although more than 80 per cent of renal failure in the critical care unit patient will be due to vasomotor nephropathy (acute tubular necrosis) the clinician must remain alert to the possibility of other aetiologies. It may be necessary to rule out an obstructive uropathy or an active glomerulitis. Although intravenous urography with nephrotomograms will define renal size and detect caliceal and ureteric dilation of obstruction, the renal ultrasonogram visualizes the kidney without the risk of exacerbating renal failure, particularly in the diabetic patient. Retrograde urography may still be necessary to identify accurately the level of obstruction and facilitate the placement of stents. Occasionally, renal biopsy may be indicated when the aetiology is obscure and the urine sediment is consistent with a glomerulopathy.

Treatment

The most immediate clinical problem for the patient who has recently developed renal failure is the maintenance of an appropriate intravascular volume in the face of a large obligate fluid input due to drug administration and total parenteral nutrition. By concentrating the nutrients, reducing drug diluent volumes, and using syringe pumps instead of volumetric pumps, fluid overload van be minimized. Hyperkalaemia can be temporarily controlled by the use of glucose and insulin infusion (1 unit soluble insulin to each 2 g of glucose) or ion exchange resins. Although high levels of urea and related metabolites are well tolerated in the ambulant or stable patient with renal failure, an early and aggressive approach to renal support with haemofiltration or haemodialysis is preferable in the patient with multiple organ system failure. Thus, the threshold for embarking upon haemofiltration or haemodialysis should be much lower in the critically ill than in the uncomplicated renal failure patient. Instead of waiting for volume overload, bleeding, uraemic pericarditis, hyperkalaemia, or acidosis, renal replacement therapy should be started early to maintain metabolic state as near normal as possible. Such use of renal replacement therapy is associated with an improved outcome, and the overall approach to patient management is greatly simplified once haemofiltration is established. Fluid balance is readily achieved and, provided adequate caloric intake is available, nitrogen intake does not need to be restricted. Full profile amino acid solutions are probably as effective as the special solutions of essential and branch chain amino acids. Energy requirements should be met using a balance of carbohydrate and lipid to deliver 45 to 50 kcal/kg.day. Where renal function is impaired for longer than 2 to 3 weeks some consideration has to be given to supplementation with vitamins and other essential elements such as zinc.

Recovery from a reversible renal pathology such as vasomotor nephritis is typically heralded by a polyuric phase followed by a plateau in serum creatinine lasting a few days, before creatinine levels consistently fall.

Renal replacement therapy

Renal replacement therapy can take the form of peritoneal dialysis, intermittent haemodialysis, continuous ultrafiltration, continuous haemofiltration, or continuous haemodiafiltration. Continuous arteriovenous or venovenous haemofiltration provide relatively simple and effective renal replacement therapy which is particularly well suited to the critical care patient. Although haemodialysis removes certain solutes, such as potassium, more efficiently, haemofiltration causes less haemodynamic disturbance and facilitates the regulation of fluid balance.

Peritoneal dialysis is suitable for patients with acute renal failure who have not had abdominal surgery and are not excessively catabolic. However, peritoneal dialysis has been largely superseded by haemofiltration, although it may still be preferred in patients suspected of carrying hepatitis B virus or HIV, or in very young children.

Indications for renal replacement therapy

The need for renal replacement therapy must be evaluated in each individual patient. Although there are threshold values for hyperkalaemia (>6.0 mmol/l), blood urea (>40 mmol/l), or severe acidosis (pH < 7.2) which would justify renal replacement therapy, the overall clinical status, including the need to make room for drugs and nutrition, all need to be considered. The aim of renal replacement therapy is to remove uraemic toxins and maintain electrolyte, acid/base and fluid balance.

In the patient with uncomplicated renal failure, maintaining the plasma urea below 30 mmol/l would generally be considered acceptable. In the critically ill patient lower target values approaching 20 mmol/l are preferred.

Continuous haemofiltration

Continuous haemofiltration is achieved by passing heparinized blood at flow rates of between 100 and 200 ml/min through a highly permeable haemofilter. The modern high-flux, biocompatible haemofilters, made from polyamide, polyacrylonitrile, or polysulphone, have negligible effects on platelets, neutrophils, or complement.

Plasma water passes through the haemofilter membrane and is drained into a collecting system (Fig. 1). Blood cells and proteins are not filtered through the membrane and are returned to the patient. The haemofiltrate contains all of the water soluble components of plasma and thus enough urea and creatinine are removed to control the patient's biochemistry. At haemofilter blood flows of 200 ml/min, about 1 litre of filtrate will be produced each hour. Since the clearance of creatinine and urea by the membrane is close to 100 per cent, a filtration rate of 1 l/h (24 l/day) results in a clearance of about 17 ml/min, which is adequate for all but the most catabolic patient. Since the plasma concentration of potassium is very low, only about 100 mmol can be removed each day. Haemofiltration is therefore not the most efficient treatment for hyperkalaemia although any correction of metabolic acidosis lessens the risks associated with an elevated serum potassium.

Haemofiltration modes

Several techniques are available to the clinician depending upon the availability of local expertise and the needs of the patient. The simplest mode is spontaneous continuous ultrafiltration which requires arterial and venous access such as that provided by a Scribner shunt (Fig. 1(a)). Filtered volume is not replaced and relief from fluid overload can be achieved quickly.

The volume of filtrate removed by the haemofilter can be replaced by a suitable haemofiltration replacement fluid which contains a lactate buffer. The replacement fluid may be infused through the return (venous) blood line or proximal to the haemofilter (predilution). The latter technique improves blood flow through the filter and increases haemofiltration efficiency. The reinfusion of a suitable haemofiltration fluid converts spontaneous continuous ultrafiltration to continuous arteriovenous haemofiltration (Fig. 1(b)). The filtration rate is regulated by a gate clamp on the filtrate outflow tubing. Tightening of this clamp reduces the filtration rate as does raising the level of collection bag.

A feature of these two techniques is that as the blood pressure falls in response to fluid withdrawal, the rate of blood flow and therefore filtration is reduced. The absence of a blood pump further adds to the safety and simplicity of this technique.

An alternative to continuous arteriovenous haemofiltration is continuous venovenous haemofiltration (Fig. 1(c)), which requires the insertion, by the Seldinger technique, of a double lumen venous catheter in the jugular, subclavian, or femoral vein. Infection of these catheters is a potential hazard and they should not be used for any other purpose. All access sites, whether arteriovenous or venovenous, should always be kept uncovered and in direct view of the attending nurse so that disconnections are immediately apparent. Pumped continuous venovenous haemofiltration can maintain clearances approaching 17 ml/min but requires close monitoring and safety alarms. The relative efficiency of this tech-

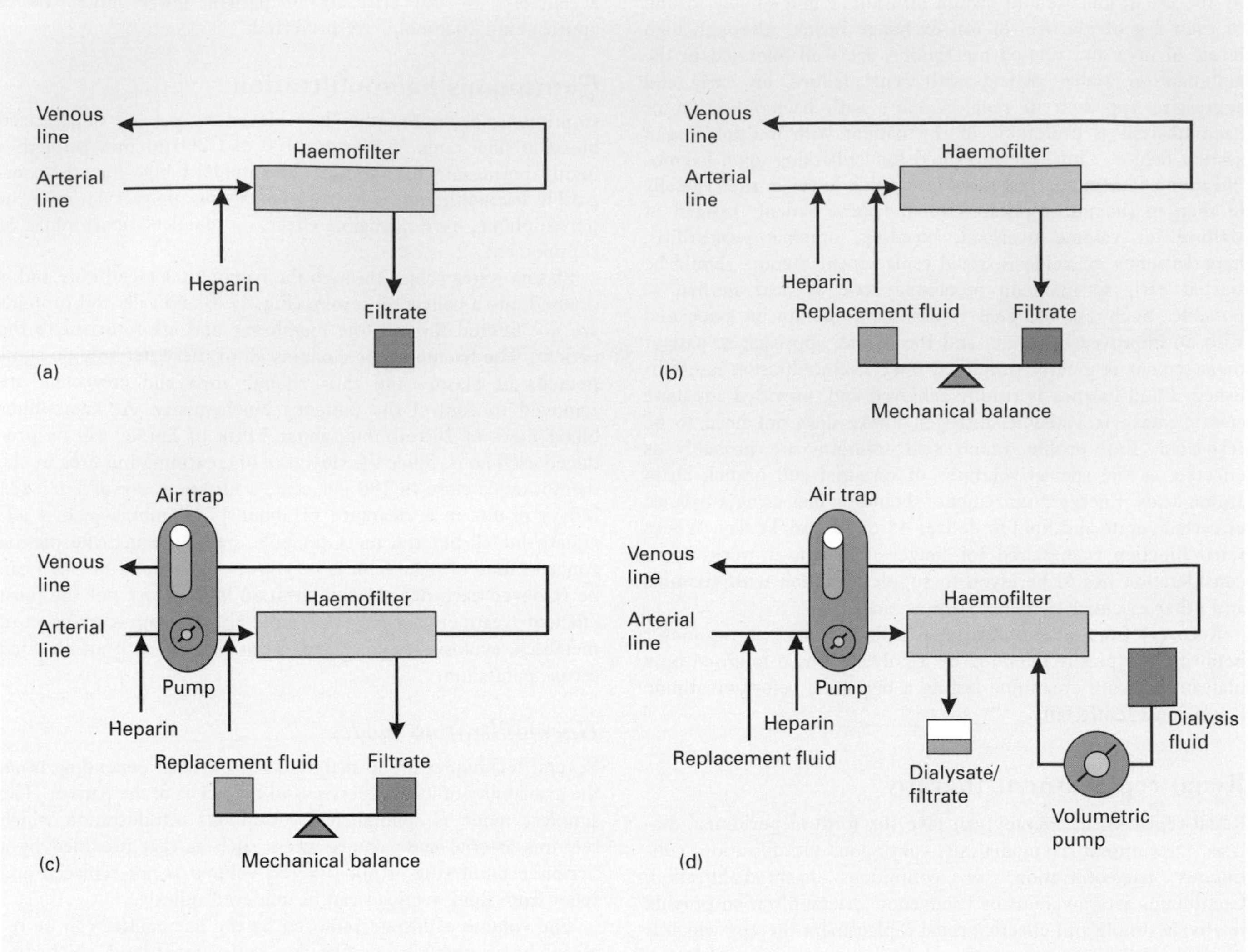

Fig. 1 (a) Schematic of an extracorporeal circuit for spontaneous, continuous ultrafiltration. (b) Schematic of an extracorporeal circuit for continuous arteriovenous haemofiltration (CAVH). (c) Schematic of an extracorporeal circuit for continuous venovenous haemofiltration (CVVH). (d) Schematic of an extracorporeal circuit for continuous venovenous haemodiafiltration (CVVHD).

nique and ease of vascular access make it suitable for routine intensive care renal replacement.

Continuous arteriovenous or venovenous haemodiafiltration (Fig. 1(d)) offers yet another alternative. Haemofiltration replacement fluid is pumped by a volumetric infusion pump in a countercurrent direction, to the filtrate side of the haemofilter membrane. Dialysate fluid flow rates of only 1 to 2 l/h are required to obtain clearance rates that are over twice that of haemofiltration alone.

Haemofiltration protocol

The entire extracorporeal circuit must be thoroughly flushed through with 1 to 2 l of heparinized saline (5 units of heparin/ml) to exclude all air from the system. This is a simple procedure for continuous arteriovenous haemofiltration but rather more involved with continuous venovenous haemofiltration or haemodiafiltration, which require blood pumps. Suitably trained nurses or specialists in intensive care can undertake all aspects of haemofiltration if specialized renal unit personnel are unavailable. Some recommend administration of 5000 units of heparin to the patient, but this is generally not necessary. Maintenance of fluid balance is achieved by either adding replacement fluid intermittently each hour or by using a mechanical or microprocessor controlled balance which will ensure a preset fluid balance (such as zero, − 500 ml, − 1000 ml). With the mechanical balance system, fluid balance goals can be changed at the end of each 4-l cycle if necessary. Microprocessor controlled balances allows continuous adjustment of fluid balance. Gradual slowing of filtration rate, as evidence by a lengthening of the cycle time usually indicates impending failure of the filter due to blood clots.

Anticoagulation

Continuous infusion of 500 to 1000 units of heparin per hour into the haemofilter input blood line will generally prevent clotting within the extracorporeal circuit. Since there is significant filtration of the heparin, this produces very little systemic anticoagulation: the dose of heparin represents a compromise between the need to prevent the haemofilter clotting and the avoidance of systemic effects. In patients at great risk from bleeding the use of low molecular weight heparin or prostacyclin should be considered. In the uraemic patient, the extracorporeal circuit can often be maintained without any anticoagulant for some days. The viability of haemofilter circuits is difficult to predict even with heparin. Some remain functioning for 5 or 6 days while other repeatedly fail after 24 h.

Effects on acidosis and temperature

Most haemofiltration replacement fluids contain lactate as a buffer. Conversion to bicarbonate is impaired in patients with renal and hepatic disease and correction of the metabolic acidosis may be therefore be slower than expected. If necessary, non-buffered replacement fluid can be used and bicarbonate infused separately to correct the acidosis. In contrast, a marked metabolic alkalosis may be precipitated by lactate buffer, particularly if the patient is small and the filtration rates high.

Hypothermia (temperature $<35°C$) can develop with high replacement fluid flow rates unless the fluid is warmed with a blood warmer. Even with warmed fluid, the fever associated with sepsis may be abated, suggesting that circulating cytokines are actively removed by the filtration process.

Drug therapy and nutrition

There are few data regarding the clearance of commonly used non-protein bound drugs, including antibiotics. Efficient veno-venous haemofiltration provides the equivalent of a creatinine clearance of almost 20 ml, a value that is often quoted in drug package inserts as a guide for drug dosage. Wherever possible drug levels should be monitored. Once haemofiltration is established dietary nitrogen restriction is no longer necessary and standard parenteral and enteral nutrition preparations can be used.

ANION AND OSMOLAL GAPS

Anion gap

The anion gap can be a useful guide in resolving biochemical disturbances in the critically ill patient. The anion gap is calculated by sum of the concentrations of the principal anions, chloride and bicarbonate, subtracted from the sodium concentration i.e. $[Na^+] - ([Cl^-] + [HCO_3^-])$. The normal value is in the range 7 to 18 mmol/l. Low values are seen in a variety of conditions, including hypoalbuminaemia, bromide or iodide toxicity, and myeloma. However, the changes are sufficiently small as to render the recognition of low anion gaps to be of little clinical use. In contrast, a raised anion gap, due to excess of anions other than chloride and bicarbonate, may be of clinical value. These anions include lactate, citrate, and acetate, present usually as the sodium salts, but may also be inorganic or organic acids. When this is the case the increased anion gap is associated with a metabolic acidosis (Table 5). Not all metabolic acidosis is associated with a raised anion gap, however. When acidosis is caused by the primary loss of bicarbonate or the gain of hydrochloric acid, there are no foreign anions present and the sodium ions are balanced by appropriate though abnormal amounts of chloride or bicarbonate (Table 6).

Table 5 High anion gap metabolic acidosis

1. Renal failure
2. Lactic acidosis
3. Ketoacidosis
   - β-Hydroxybutyric acid
   - Acetoacetic acid
4. Intoxication:
   - Salicylate
   - Methanol
   - Ethylene glycol
   - Paraldehyde
   - Sulphur
5. Non-ketotic hyperglycaemia
6. Rhabdomyolysis

In high anion gap acidosis, the fall in bicarbonate approximates the rise in anion gap. In mixed acid–base disorders the change in anion gap may be more or less than that expected from the change in bicarbonate: an oversimplistic approach to the application of anion gap theory may therefore mislead the clinician. Any consensus of opinion reached by the use of anion gap analysis must pass the test of being consistent with the overall clinical picture.

Osmolal gap

The osmolal gap is the difference between the measured and the calculated osmolality.

$$\text{Calculated osmolality} = ([Na^+] \times 2.0) + [\text{urea}] + [\text{glucose}] + [\text{potassium}]$$

The factor of 2.0 applied to the sodium concentration (in mmol/l) allows for the osmolal contribution of the anions that balance sodium cations. Estimates of osmolal gap produce values of 0 ± 6 mosmol/l. The clinical utility of the osmolal gap rests upon identifying patients with toxins, drugs or certain plasma constituents present in excessive amounts in their serum. Ethanol, methanol, and ethylene glycol are common toxins associated with

Table 6 Normal anion gap metabolic acidosis

1. Loss of bicarbonate
   - (a) Gastrointestinal
     - Diarrhoea
     - Pancreatic fistula
     - Ileostomy
     - Ureter—bowel diversion
   - (b) Renal tract
     - Renal tubular acidosis
     - Acetazolamide therapy
     - Post-hyperventilation
2. Dilutional
   - Rapid saline infusion
3. Administration of hydrochloride donors
   - (a) Ammonium chloride
   - (b) Arginine hydrochloride
   - (c) Lysine hydrochloride
   - (d) Hydrochloric acid

a raised osmolal gap. The osmolal gap will be raised in patients receiving a mannitol for the treatment of raised intracranial pressure and the size of the gap parallels the plasma mannitol concentration.

As with the anion gap, the osmolal gap may help elucidate the underlying cause of certain electrolyte disturbances. However, neither are a substitute for a careful and systematic clinical evaluation of the patient.

FURTHER READING

Cameron JS. Acute renal failure in the intensive care unit today. *Intensive Care Med*, 1986; 12: 64–70.

Emmett M, Narins RG. Clinical use of the anion gap. *Medicine*, 1977; **56**: 38–54.

Gennari FJ. Serum osmolality uses and limitations. *N. Engl J Med*, 1984; **310**: 102–5.

Golper TA, Pulliman J, Bennett WM. Removal of therapeutic drugs by continuous arteriovenous haemofiltration. *Arch Intern Med*, 1985; **145**: 1651–2.

Henderson LW, Colton CK, Ford CA. Kinetics of haemodiafiltration: II. Clinical characterisation of a new blood cleansing modality. *J Lab Clin Med*, 1975; **85**: 372–91.

Kramer P, Wigger W, Rieger J, Mathaei D, Scheler F. Arteriovenous haemofiltration: a new and simple method for treatment of overhydrated patients resistant to diuretics. *Klin Wochenschr*, 1977; **55**: 1121–2.

Rainford D, Sweny P, eds. *Acute renal failure*. London: Farrand Press, 1990.

Smithline N, Gardner KD Jnr. Gaps anionic and osmolal. *JAMA*, 1976; **236**: 1594.

Steiner RW. Interpreting the fractional excretion of sodium. *Am J Med*, 1984; **77**: 699–702.

Stevens PE, Riley B, Davies SP, Gower PE, Brown EA, Kox W. Continuous arteriovenous haemodialysis in critically ill patients. *Lancet* 1988; ii: 150–2.

Zarich S, Fang LST, Diamond JR: Fractional excretion of sodium: exceptions to its diagnostic value. *Arch Intern Med*, 1985; **145**: 108–12.

4.3 Respiratory aspects

CHRISTOPHER S. GARRARD

ACUTE LUNG INJURY AND ADULT RESPIRATORY DISTRESS SYNDROME

Acute lung injury has a wide range of causes and a broad spectrum of severity. In its mildest form the only evidence for lung dysfunction may be an increase in the alveolar–arterial oxygen gradient (A-a)Do_2, without clinical signs of lung congestion, radiographic changes or reduction in lung compliance. The more severe forms of acute lung injury are generally referred to as the adult respiratory distress syndrome. The most common conditions associated with the development of this syndrome are listed in Table 1.

The severity of the disease process depends upon the nature, severity, and duration of the insult to the lungs. Adult respiratory distress syndrome associated with aspiration, fat embolism, pancreatitis, or sepsis may be more severe than the lung injury associated with a brief episode of hypovolaemic shock or mismatched blood transfusion. In view of the heterogeneity of disease a simple scoring system, such as that shown in Table 2, should be used to quantify the severity of acute lung injury.

The incidence of adult respiratory distress syndrome is uncertain, but it may effect 5 to 10 per cent of patients at risk. Clearly, the criteria by which the condition defined will be reflected in the incidence, morbidity, and mortality reported in any particular series. The observation that mortality has changed little over the past two decades may indeed reflect a trend towards a stricter definition. It is evident that patients do not usually die of hypoxaemia but from the complex disturbances that result from multiple organ system failure. The management of patients with adult respiratory distress syndrome is therefore aimed at many facets of organ system support.

Recognition of moderate to severe adult respiratory distress syndrome is not difficult. The patient has acute respiratory distress, requires an increasing $F\text{io}_2$ (greater than 0.5) to maintain a $P\text{ao}_2$ of more than 7.0 kPa (50 mmHg) and usually has extensive lung infiltrates on the chest radiograph. With mechanical ventil-

Table 1 Conditions associated with adult respiratory distress syndrome

1. Circulating factors
    - Sepsis syndrome
    - Shock syndromes of any cause
    - Severe polytrauma
    - Pancreatitis
    - Blood transfusion
    - Postcardiopulmonary bypass
    - Neurogenic pulmonary oedema
    - Drugs
        - Heroin
        - Paraquat
        - Aspirin
        - Protamine
        - Heparin
2. Pneumonia
    - Bacterial
    - Viral
    - Legionella
    - Protozoa
3. Lung contusion
    - Trauma
4. Aspiration injury
    - Gastric juice
    - Smoke
    - Chemicals
    - Drowning
5. Embolization
    - Amniotic fluid
    - Fat embolism

Table 2 Adult respiratory distress syndrome lung injury score

		Value
1. Chest radiographs score		
No alveolar consolidation		0
Aleolar consolidation confined to 1 quadrant		1
Aleolar consolidation confined to 2 quadrants		2
Aleolar consolidation confined to 3 quadrants		3
Aleolar consolidation in all 4 quadrants		4
2. Hypoxaemia score ($Pa\text{O}_2$ in mmHg/unity for kPa/unity, divide by 7.5)		
$Pa\text{O}_2/F\text{I}\text{O}_2$	>300	0
$Pa\text{O}_2/F\text{I}\text{O}_2$	225–299	1
$Pa\text{O}_2/F\text{I}\text{O}_2$	175–224	2
$Pa\text{O}_2/F\text{I}\text{O}_2$	100–174	3
$Pa\text{O}_2/F\text{I}\text{O}_2$	<100	4
3. PEEP score (when ventilated)		
PEEP	$\leqslant$5 cmH_2O	0
PEEP	6–8 cmH_2O	1
PEEP	9–11 cmH_2O	2
PEEP	12–14 cmH_2O	3
PEEP	$\geqslant$15 cmH_2O	4
4. Respiratory system compliance score (when available)		
Compliance	$\geqslant$80 ml/cmH_2O	0
Compliance	60–79 ml/cmH_2O	1
Compliance	40–59 ml/cmH_2O	2
Compliance	20–39 ml/cmH_2O	3
Compliance	$\leqslant$19 ml/cmH_2O	4

The final value is obtained by dividing the aggregate sum by the number of components that were used.

No lung injury (score = 0)
Mild to moderate lung injury (score = 0.1–2.5)
Severe lung injury (score >2.5)

Reproduced from Murray JF, Matthay MA, Luce JM, Flick MR. An expanded definition of the adult respiratory distress syndrome. *Am Rev Resp Dis*, 1988; **138**: 720–723, with permission.

ation, the lungs are stiff and require high inflation pressures. Calculated effective, static, and dynamic compliance (C_{dyn} and C_{stat}) are low usually being less than 20 ml/cmH_2O (30 ml/mmHg). Cardiogenic pulmonary oedema should be excluded by measurement of the pulmonary artery wedge pressure (<18 mmHg). The Murray lung injury score will usually be more than 2.5. Calculated venous admixture reveals a shunt fraction between 30 and 50 per cent.

There is no specific therapy at present for acute lung injury, except to suppress or remove the injurious agent, avoid aggravating the condition, and supporting the patient until lung function recovers. Adult respiratory distress syndrome may require prolonged periods of mechanical ventilation and can be associated with a mortality of more than 50 per cent. Above all, the clinician must anticipate its development, with the aid of an awareness of the precipitating causes (Table 1). A proactive approach to the management of these underlying disease processes may help prevent or ameliorate progression to respiratory failure.

Pathogenesis

The pathogenesis of adult respiratory distress syndrome is complex, being the product of several processes such as complement activation, neutrophil accumulation, platelet aggravation, and mediator release. In patients with trauma and sepsis, endotoxaemia is responsible for initiating complement activation and other components of the immune–inflammatory cascade. Complement activation causes leucocyte sequestration in pulmonary capillaries which, in turn, injures endothelial cells through the release of toxic superoxide radicals, arachidonic acid metabolites, cytokines, and proteases.

Unfortunately, monitoring complement activation appears to have little value in predicting the development or the clinical course of adult respiratory distress syndrome. It is also clear that the condition can still develop in the most severely neutropenic patients. Bronchoalveolar lavage studies have detected the presence of neutrophils, proteolytic enzymes, chemotactic factors, antiproteases, and cytokines in lung washings. Activation of the clotting system may further aggravate the pathophysiological disturbances by causing intravascular coagulation and platelet aggregation within the pulmonary vascular bed. Furthermore, the platelet and fibrin aggregates release vasoactive substances, such as serotonin, histamine, and prostaglandins that, in combination with fibrinogen degradation products, damage the endothelium and pulmonary microvasculature.

Complicating the picture further is the possibility that supportive measures such as oxygen and positive pressure ventilation may themselves promote or prolong lung injury.

Pathology

Adult respiratory distress syndrome is characterized by diffuse alveolar epithelial and endothelial damage. In the early stages, the alveolar interstitium becomes infiltrated with inflammatory cells and the alveoli spaces filled with proteinaceous and haemorrhagic fluid. Hyaline membrane formation and capillary microembolism are common features. Leakage of plasma through damaged pulmonary endothelium results in interstitial and alveolar oedema and may alter the properties of surfactant. Alveolar type I cells are replaced by cuboidal microvillous Type II cells, disturbing alveolar wall architecture and exacerbating the effects of pulmonary capillary injury. There may be progression to pulmonary fibrosis with obliteration of the pulmonary alveolar and microvasculature architecture. Despite the extensive pathological changes that may be found on biopsy, good physiological recovery is possible.

Pathophysiology

The pathological changes result in reduced functional residual capacity, increased venous admixture (shunt), reduced lung compliance, and refractory hypoxaemia. The role played by abnormal surfactant in the pathophysiology of adult respiratory distress syndrome is unclear, but its severity seems to be related to the proportion of the abnormal surfactant. Bronchoalveolar lavage fluid obtained from patients with adult respiratory distress syndrome contains aggregated and inactive surfactant. Unlike the experience with respiratory distress in the neonate, surfactant replacement in the adult condition has produced inconsistent results.

Management of adult respiratory distress syndrome

The aim of respiratory support is to achieve adequate oxygen on-loading at the lungs without impeding cardiac output. To help maintain oxygen delivery in the haemoglobin concentration should be maintained above 11 g/100 ml of blood. Oxygen, intermittent positive pressure ventilation and positive end-expiratory pressure form the basis of respiratory support in adult respiratory distress syndrome. Although constant positive airway pressure can be delivered by a tight-fitting anaesthetic face mask in the spontaneously breathing patient, endotracheal intubation is generally required. The endotracheal tube should be of the high volume/low pressure cuffed variety and the cuff inflated to a pressure not exceeding 30 cmH_2O.

The ventilator selected to support the patient should have the facility to deliver the basic modes of ventilation, control mechanical ventilation, assist control, synchronized intermittent mandatory ventilation, and pressure support. The best mode of ventilation is not known but selection should be based upon whichever achieves ventilation goals for the lowest peak and mean airway pressure.

Oxygen

Most patients will require a $F\text{io}_2$ of more than 0.6 to achieve an acceptable $P\text{ao}_2$ (one that satisfies the oxygen delivery requirements of the patient). For example a patient on 100 per cent oxygen and 20 cmH_2O positive end-expiratory pressure, with a haemoglobin concentration of 12 g/100 ml and a $P\text{ao}_2$ of 7.0 kPa (53 mmHg) might appear dangerously hypoxaemic. Yet this low $P\text{ao}_2$ may satisfy oxygen requirements provided the cardiac output is adequate. Oxygen extraction by the tissues drives the mixed venous oxygen content to lower than normal values. The clinician must therefore be alert to evidence of tissue hypoxaemia, such as metabolic acidosis, mental obtundation, or cardiac arrhythmias. If such evidence is not present it may be reasonable to assume that oxygen delivery is adequate. If doubt exists about the adequacy of oxygen delivery, a flow directed pulmonary artery catheter can be inserted to measure cardiac output and mixed venous saturation and to calculate oxygen delivery.

Positive end-expiratory pressure

This recruits lung units partly to restore the reduced functional residual capacity to normal. Positive end-expiratory pressure of 5 to 20 cmH_2O (0.5–2.0 kPa) is added in increments of 5 cmH_2O until an acceptable $P\text{ao}_2$ is reached. Current practice encourages the use of the lowest pressure that will meet oxygenation goals. 'Best' or 'optimal' positive end-expiratory pressure is the pressure that maximizes oxygen delivery, with the lowest $F\text{io}_2$, lowest venous admixture, and highest effective compliance. Concern over barotrauma has led to a more conservative approach to the use of positive end-expiratory pressure in recent years.

Ventilation settings of the mechanical ventilator may be as crucial as the level of positive end-expiratory pressure with regard to causing barotrauma. Conventional high tidal volume settings of 10 to 12 ml/kg may be inappropriate in the patient with adult respiratory distress syndrome and non-compliant lungs. Increasing the ventilation rate and reducing the tidal volume will reduce peak airway pressures at the cost of higher VD/VT and higher mean airway pressure. A deliberate policy of 'permissive hypercapnia', allowing the $P\text{co}_2$ to rise to between 7 and 9 kPa, can be achieved by reducing both the tidal volumes and ventilator rate. This results in lower mean and peak airway pressures. The attendant respiratory acidosis is usually well tolerated and ultimately compensated for.

A feature of the patient with adult respiratory distress syndrome is the extensive gravity dependent lung collapse that is best visualized by CT scan. To a large degree this is a consequence of nursing the patient for prolonged periods in the supine position. Sitting the patient as upright as possible minimizes the volume of dependent lung. In the persistently hypoxic patient, significant improvement in oxygenation may be obtained by rolling the patient into a prone position every 6 to 8 h.

Non-conventional forms of ventilation such as high frequency ventilation have potential advantages in supporting patients with adult respiratory distress syndrome. In randomized studies peak airway pressures are lower but mean airway pressure and mortality are unchanged. Inverted I:E ratio ventilation (inspiration to expiration ratio) has been claimed to reduce the positive end-expiratory pressure level for a given $P\text{ao}_2$. However, the mean airway pressures are inevitably raised by such techniques.

Extracorporeal membrane oxygenation for respiratory failure was abandoned over a decade ago following controlled, randomized investigation. With the availability of improved oxygenators there has been renewed interest in combining extracorporeal partial CO_2 removal and low frequency conventional ventilation. Whether this approach offers significant advantages over permissive hypercapnia techniques remains to be seen. Both techniques are aimed at reducing the deleterious effect of positive pressure upon the alveolar epithelium and may therefore hasten recovery from adult respiratory distress syndrome.

Intravenous gas exchange devices (IVOX®) have been developed that may offer the safest alternative to conventional ventilation and gas exchange techniques. These devices will require extensive evaluation before they replace or supplement conventional ventilation techniques.

Circulatory support

Fluid administration should be regulated to ensure adequate cardiac output without aggravating the pulmonary oedema. Measurement of pulmonary capillary wedge pressure using a flow directed pulmonary artery catheter may provide a more reliable assessment of the filling status of the patient than measurement of central venous pressure. The information provided by measures of cardiac output and derived indices of vascular resistance rationalizes the use of inotropes, pressors, and afterload reduction. Pulmonary hypertension is not an uncommon feature of adult respiratory distress syndrome, and although attempts to reduce the pulmonary arterial pressures have not reduced mortality, significant increases in oxygen delivery can be obtained with agents such as prostacyclin. Despite an increase in venous admixture with prostacyclin, the increases in cardiac output and mixed venous saturation produce enhanced oxygen delivery and improved $P\text{ao}_2$.

There is no strong evidence to favour colloidal over crystalloid replacement fluid. The volume of fluid is more critical: the type of fluid should be selected to ensure electrolyte equilibrium and defend plasma colloid osmotic pressure. Diuretics should be used to reduce intravascular volume as needed. If the patient becomes oliguric, early haemofiltration will be needed to maintain fluid balance. Nutritional support in the form of enteral feeding or total parenteral nutrition can be started early in the course of adult respiratory distress syndrome.

Specific treatments to inhibit mediator cascades are largely experimental. Multicentre randomized studies have failed to show significant benefit from corticosteroids, non-steroidal anti-inflammatory agents, or vasodilator prostaglandins. Anecdotal reports of high dose steroids (40–60 mg prednisone/day) in 'chronic' respiratory distress suggest some benefit in terms of oxygenation and lung compliance. However, the use of steroids in the acute phase afforded no benefit in multicentre, controlled studies.

Antiendotoxin monoclonal antibodies significantly reduce mortality in septic shock and may therefore prevent or moderate adult respiratory distress syndrome in this group of patients. As yet, this hypothesis and others aimed at alternative components of the immunoinflammatory cascade have not been formally tested.

Outcome

Provided that multiple organ system support can be maintained, a positive attitude towards final recovery is justified. Even after periods of mechanical ventilation, a high $F\text{io}_2$ and positive end-expiratory pressure for up to 3 to 4 months a good functional outcome is possible. Biopsy proven pulmonary fibrosis does not inevitably mean that there is fixed, irreversible pathology. A mortality rate of over 50 to 60 per cent is generally quoted for the last decade, although most recent reports have shown a fall in mortality to about 20 per cent. Pulmonary function testing 1 year following recovery may show a reduction in vital capacity with a mild obstructive defect. In many patients the only abnormality may be a reduction in carbon monoxide transfer.

MECHANICAL VENTILATION

The provision of efficient and safe mechanical ventilation is a skill that must be mastered by all physicians practising critical care. The basic principles still pertain despite the introduction of complex and sophisticated mechanical ventilators and the overabundance of studies claiming superiority of certain techniques over others. The application of common sense and sound physiological doctrine will serve better than devotion to an attractive technical innovation.

Indications for intubation and mechanical ventilation

Although mechanical ventilation is not to be undertaken lightly since it is associated with much morbidity and some mortality, failure to intervene promptly can have catastrophic consequences for the patient. The indications for mechanical ventilation fall into two broad categories: inadequate alveolar ventilation with increasing $P\text{co}_2$, and inadequate gas exchange with increasing alveolar–arterial oxygen gradient and arterial hypoxaemia. Guidelines for mechanical ventilation in acute respiratory failure are shown in Table 3. The physician must always exercise clinical judgement in the interpretation of these guidelines and anticipate problems before they arise. For example, one of the simplest criteria for mechanical ventilation is a respiratory rate of 35 breaths per minute or more. If a patient with a respiratory rate of 30 breaths per minute is clearly becoming fatigued an early elective intubation is preferred to an emergency procedure an hour or so later. Similarly, a progressive fall in vital capacity in a patient with myasthenia gravis receiving full medication may indicate a need for ventilatory support, although the critical value of less than 15 ml/kg is not broached.

Table 3 Guidelines for introduction of mechanical ventilation

A. *General indications in acute respiratory failure (after Pontoppidan et al.)*

1. Inadequate ventilation
   Indicated by:
   (a) Apnoea, upper airway obstruction, unprotected airway
   (b) Respiratory rate > 35 breaths/min (normal range 10–20)
   (c) Vital capacity < 15 ml/kg (normal range 65–75)
   (d) Tidal volume < 5 ml/kg (normal range 5–7)
   (e) Negative inspiratory force < 25 cmH_2O (normal range 75–100)
   (f) $P\text{aco}_2$ > 8 kPa (60 mmHg) (normal range 4.7–6.3 kPa (35–47 mmHg)
   (g) V_D/V_T ratio > 0.6 (normal range < 0.3)
2. Inadequate gas exchange oxygenation
   Indicated by:
   (a) $P\text{ao}_2$ < 8 kPa, (60 mmHg) on $F\text{io}_2$ > 0.6
   (b) Alveolar-arterial oxygen gradient (A-a)Do_2 on $F\text{io}_2$ 1.0 > 47 kPa (350 mmHg) (normal range 3.3–8.7 kPa (25–65 mmHg)

B. *Specific indications, with or without previous respiratory pathology*

3. Chronic obstructive lung disease
   (a) Failure of conservative measures
   (b) Inability to co-operate with care
   (c) Decreased consciousness
   (d) Cardiac instability
   (e) Apnoea
   (f) Severe respiratory acidosis
   (g) Acute management of nocturnal obstructive hypoventilation.
4. Chronic restrictive lung disease
   (a) Severe hypoxaemia
   (b) Fatigue and impending exhaustion.
5. Severe acute asthma
   (a) Failure of conservative measures
   (b) Obtundation
   (c) Cardiac instability
   (d) Increasing $P\text{aco}_2$
   (e) Fatigue and impending exhaustion.
6. Head trauma
   Unconscious, unprotected airway, cerebral oedema, apnoea, or global hypoventilation.
7. Chest trauma
   Flail chest with hypoventilation and hypoxaemia
   Pulmonary contusion with hypoxaemia
8. Neuromuscular weakness
   Apnoea or progressive hypoventilation (see above)
   Airway protection, nocturnal hypoventilation/hypoxaemia
   Organophosphate poisoning
9. Other neurological disorders
   Status epilepticus, tetanus, high cervical spine injury
10. Upper airway protection
    Loss of consciousness, neck and oropharyngeal trauma, epiglottitis, acute neuromuscular event
11. Drug overdose
    Apnoea, hypoventilation, airway protection, seizures

Selection of airway access

Endotracheal intubation will be the preferred technique in most cases. Orotracheal intubation is particularly suited to emergency intubation while nasotracheal intubation requires a little extra time. A coagulation defect or thrombocytopenia makes nasotracheal intubation inadvisable due to risk of serious haemorrhage. Whatever technique is selected, intubation should be performed in a safe and expeditious manner by the most experienced clinician available: this will usually be an anaesthetist or trained specialist in intensive care. Neuromuscular relaxant drugs should only be used to facilitate intubation by experienced personnel. Complications of endotracheal intubation are due to occlusion or displacement of the tube, and airway trauma. The appropriate endotracheal tube size for most adult males is 8 to 9 mm internal diameter; and for women, 7 to 8 mm. For children, a rough calculation using the child's age in years divided by 4, plus 4.0 will provide the tube internal diameter in mm. These smaller tubes are generally uncuffed.

It is essential that the endotracheal tube be securely anchored and the cuff inflation pressure restricted to less than 30 cmH_2O. The latter can be achieved by always using high volume, low pressure cuffed tubes and allowing a small cuff leak during each ventilator cycle (minimal leak technique). Alternatively, cuff inflation pressures can be measured periodically using an anaeroid manometer and adjusted accordingly. Contrary to popular belief, higher cuff pressures do not improve airway protection against aspiration but only serve to damage the tracheal mucosa and risk later stenosis.

Tracheostomy

Tracheostomy should replace endotracheal intubation for specific indications and not merely after the elapse of a predefined time interval. Using modern endotracheal tubes and techniques, endotracheal intubation can be tolerated without permanent harm to the airway for months if necessary. It has been shown that most mucosal damage is caused in the first week of intubation with little additional change thereafter.

However, much can be gained by the judicious selection of patients for tracheostomy either as the preferred primary route for airway access or as a replacement for endotracheal intubation. The common indications for replacement include the need for chronic or permanent ventilation, to help weaning after previously failed attempts at extubation, to facilitate oral nutrition, or the presence of upper airway complications of endotracheal intubation. Indications for primary tracheostomy are considered elsewhere.

The same principles of cuff pressure management apply to tracheostomy tubes as to endotracheal tubes. Tracheostomy is associated with fewer but more serious complications than endotracheal intubation. These include tube displacement, pneumothorax, severe haemorrhage, and wound infection.

Minitracheostomy

Minitracheostomy tubes are 3.5- to 4.0-mm diameter, cuffless tubes inserted percutaneously through the cricothyroid membrane, usually under local anaesthesia. A Seldinger technique for introduction of the minitracheostomy tube offers an alternative to the direct trochar method. Minitracheostomy allows suctioning lung secretions without the need for formal endotracheal intubation or tracheostomy.

Cricothyroidotomy

A cricothyroidotomy may be preferred in life-threatening, upper airway obstructions where endotracheal intubation is not feasible and there is insufficient time to perform tracheostomy. Performed under local anaesthesia, a full sized tracheostomy tube can be inserted (6–8 mm internal diameter) to facilitate mechanical ventilation. In emergency conditions, temporary oxygenation (30 min) can be aided by the intermittent insufflation of 100 per cent oxygen at 50 PSI (15 l/min) via a 14-gauge cannula inserted through the cricothyroid membrane. Interruption of oxygen flow is regulated by a simple Y piece adaptor.

Features and applications of a mechanical ventilator

Most adult patients are supported on volume/time cycled, pressure limited ventilators (volume ventilator or flow generator). The volume/time cycled ventilators deliver preset tidal volumes regardless of changes in lung compliance or impedance. The price paid for this desirable characteristic is that the inflation pressures must rise to overcome the mechanical load. To protect the patient against inadvertently high pressures, a pressure limit must be set. When this limit is reached the ventilator terminates inspiration regardless of the volume delivered and triggers an alarm.

Neonates and infants may be satisfactorily ventilated using time cycled, pressure limited devices (pressure ventilator or pressure generator). The pressure limited paediatric ventilator offers simplicity and reliable ventilation although the delivered tidal volume is difficult to measure. In the premature neonate these are not serious limitations and pressure limited ventilation is the preferred technique.

Specifically designed, compact, lightweight ventilators, driven by cylinder oxygen and using fluid logic circuits are available for transporting ventilator dependent patients. They are pressure generators and can be used for both adults and children. By entraining air, a choice of either 60 per cent or 100 per cent oxygen is available.

Drive mechanisms

All ventilators possess a drive mechanism that propels the air/oxygen gas mixture into the patient. Some deliver the gas to the patient directly (single circuit) or indirectly through a dual circuit. There are several types of drive mechanisms that determine the flexibility, the available ventilation modes, and the ability to deliver preprescribed tidal volume in the face of abnormal lung mechanics.

Schematics of a simple positive pressure ventilator and ventilator circuit during inspiratory and expiratory phases are shown in Figs. 1 and 2.

Control and monitoring mechanisms

The control mechanism that cycles the ventilator from inspiration to expiration may be electromechanical, or electronic (using microprocessor technology). Modern mechanical ventilators tend to fall into the latter category and offer a degree of sophistication that has greatly improved the safety and efficiency of mechanical ventilation.

Depending upon the indications for ventilation, the clinician must select the mode of ventilation, choose the ventilation parameters, and adjust the ventilator alarms. The most commonly available ventilator modes include control mechanical ventilation, assist control (triggered ventilation), intermittent mandatory ventilation (IMV or SIMV), and pressure support, although some others are used.

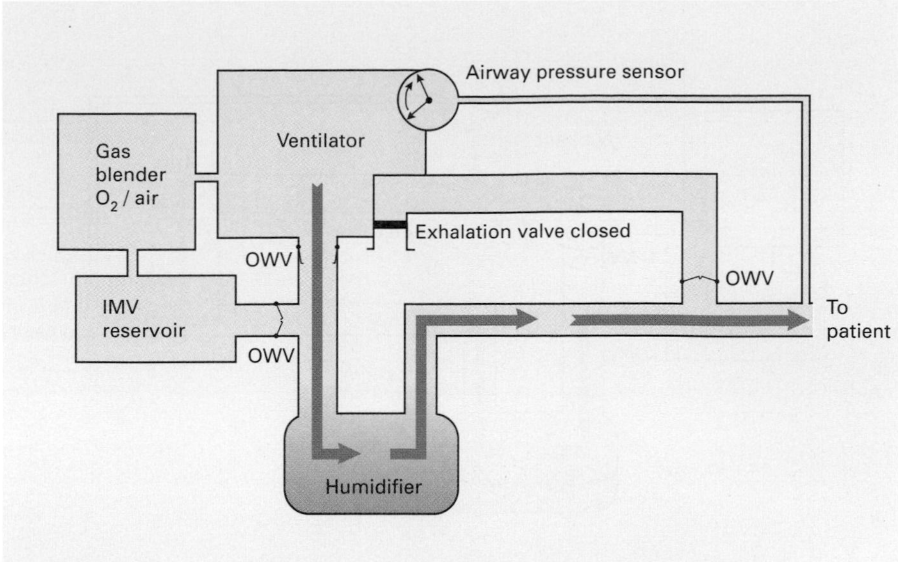

Fig. 1 Schematic of ventilator circuit during positive pressure inflation of the lungs. The direction of gas flow is indicated by the broad arrows. One-way valves (OWV) assure unidirectional flow and the expiratory valve ensures lung inflation.

Control mechanical ventilation

This provides time and volume cycled, pressure limited breaths at preset rates, but does not allow the patient to breathe spontaneously. This mode is suitable for the paralysed or heavily sedated patient.

Assist control or triggered ventilation

This synchronizes the ventilator to the patient's own respiratory rhythm, delivering a volume preset, pressure limited tidal volume. A trigger sensitivity must be selected (usually −0.5 to −2.0 cmH_2O) by which the patient can initiate volume preset breaths above the set rates. Patients have a tendency to hyperventilate on assist control. As a safety requirement, a high respiratory rate alarm is needed and a 'back up' ventilation rate must be set in the event of apnoea. Assist control is better tolerated than control mechanical ventilation and the patient requires less sedation.

Intermittent mandatory ventilation

This was originally devised for weaning but is now widely adopted as a maintenance mode (see Fig. 3). It provides the opportunity

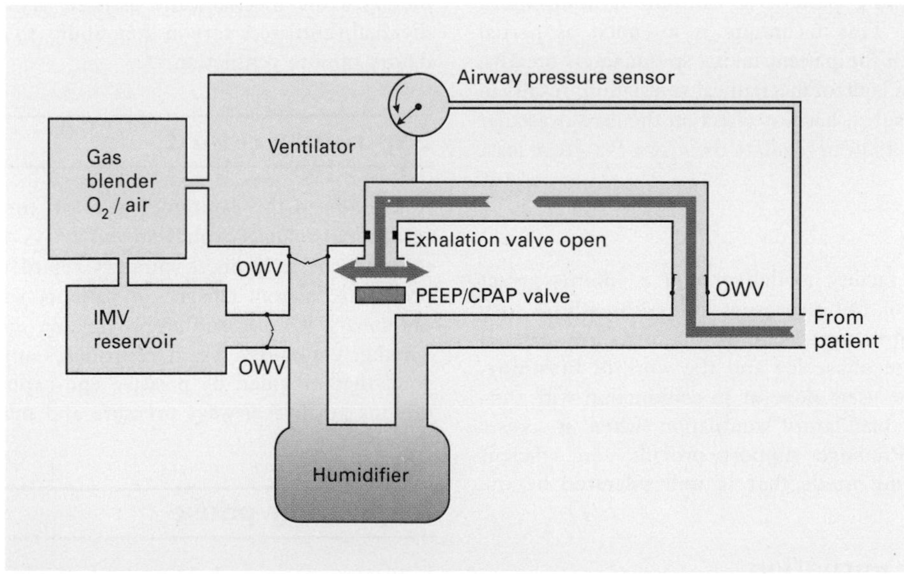

Fig. 2 Schematic of ventilator circuit during exhalation. Expiratory valve is opened permitting passive exhalation. The direction of gas flow is indicated by the broad arrows. PEEP/CPAP valve partially occludes expiratory flow to produce desired PEEP/CPAP level.

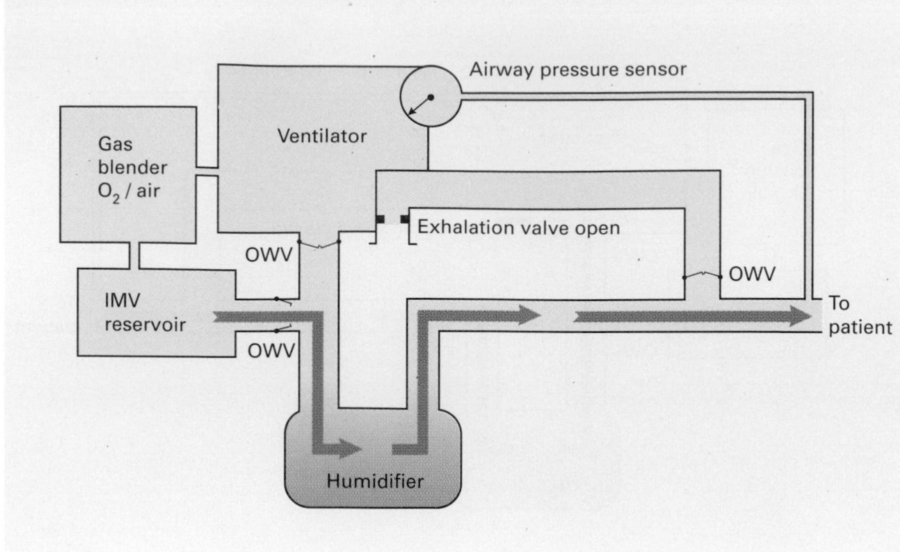

Fig. 3 Schematic of ventilator circuit during spontaneous inspiration in intermittent mandatory ventilation (IMV) mode. The IMV reservoir can consist of a distensible anaesthetic bag which is constantly filled from the air/oxygen blender and results in a continuous gas flow around the ventilator circuit (continuous flow IMV). Alternatively, access to a reservoir of gas mixture at ambient pressure can be triggered by the patients own inspiratory effort (demand valve IMV). The direction of gas flow is indicated by the broad arrows. Positive pressure cycled breaths are triggered by the patient's own ventilatory effort but only up to the set mandatory rate (synchronized IMV).

for the patient to breathe spontaneously and supplement the positive pressure minute ventilation. In the standard intermittent mandatory ventilation mode there is a theoretical risk of stacking a ventilator breath on top of a spontaneous breath. However, this does not appear to be a significant problem and an appropriately set pressure limit should prevent this causing inadvertent overinflation of the lungs. More modern ventilators use the triggering or assist facility to synchronize the machine breaths with the patient's own spontaneous breathing pattern (synchronized intermittent mandatory ventilation). This technique is intended as partial ventilation support. With the patient taking spontaneous breaths, it is better tolerated than control mechanical ventilation, results in lower mean airway pressures, has less effect on the cardiovascular system, and allows the patient to regulate their own $P\text{CO}_2$ to at least some degree.

Pressure support

This uses a triggering facility to deliver, not a volume preset breath as in assist control, but a pressure limited breath (as with paediatric pressure ventilation). The inspiratory flow rate is usually high to minimize phase lag and the work of breathing. Pressure support may be used alone or in conjunction with synchronized intermittent mandatory ventilation when it assists spontaneous breaths. Pressure support provides an efficient maintenance and weaning mode that is well tolerated by the patient.

Other modes of ventilation

Pressure release, high frequency and inverse I:E ratio ventilation have their proponents. Evidence to indicate significant superiority of these modes over conventional methods of ventilation is not convincing. High frequency ventilation in its several forms has been recommended for use following reconstructive laryngeal, tracheal, or bronchial surgery or for patients with bronchopleural or bronchocutaneous fistulae. Even these applications may not offer much advantage, if any, over conventional modes. Mandatory minute ventilation is an innovative mode whereby the combined spontaneous and mechanical ventilation must reach a minimum preset level. As the patient's spontaneous ventilation increases the mechanically assisted breaths become fewer. Individual ventilators vary in their ability to achieve successful mandatory minute ventilation.

Expiratory retard

Restriction of the expiratory gas flow through a flow-dependent resistance prolongs expiration and delays the airway pressure drop to atmospheric levels. Expiratory retard was claimed to prevent premature airway closure in patients with chronic obstructive pulmonary disease and improve lung emptying. It is doubtful whether expiratory retard contributes any additional benefit beyond that provided by positive end-expiratory pressure or continuous positive airways pressure and may increase the work of breathing.

Inspiratory pause

Inspiratory pause or hold prolongs the inspiratory phase and delays the onset of expiration. As such it is thought to increase oxygenation by improved ventilation distribution and reduced V/Q mismatch. Like positive end-expiratory pressure and continuous positive airways pressure, it increases mean airway pressure, and may have cardiovascular effects. It is doubtful whether inspiratory pause contributes significantly to patient management.

Sighs

Before the advent of high tidal volume ventilation and positive end-expiratory pressures and continuous positive airways pressure, sighs were added to the ventilation protocol to prevent progressive atelectasis. Each sigh was delivered 2 to 6 times per hour and was equivalent to about twice the conventional tidal volume. The risks of barotrauma probably outweigh the theoretical benefits.

Ventilator parameters

Once a ventilation mode has been selected (at least temporarily), ventilatory parameters must be set before attaching the patient to the ventilator. The ventilator parameters include:

1. Tidal volume;
2. Ventilation rate;
3. Inspiratory/expiratory (I:E) ratio;
4. Flow waveform;
5. FiO_2 (0.21 to 1.0);
6. Pressure limit;
7. Positive end-expiratory pressure/continuous positive airway pressure (0 to 20 cmH_2O).

Tidal volume

The delivered, inspiratory tidal volume may be set at 10 to 12 ml/kg body weight. This should be reduced if the patient has restrictive lung disease or has undergone lobectomy or pneumonectomy. Using respiratory rates of more than 10 breaths per minute with such tidal volumes will provide full ventilatory support. If the patient is breathing spontaneously, an intermittent mandatory ventilation mode will be preferred at rates between 4 to 8 breaths per minute. If assist control or pressure support is chosen the respiratory rate will be the patient's spontaneous rate.

I:E ratio, inspiratory flow rate

The rate of inspiratory to expiratory time (I:E ratio) will generally range from 1:2 to 1:4. This provides sufficient time for full passive exhalation. In patients with obstructive lung disease failing to allow adequate time for exhalation results in hyperinflation (auto- or intrinsic positive end-expiration pressure). The higher the set respiratory rate the shorter expiration becomes and the I:E ratio falls. This may lead to the paradoxical situation in the patient with chronic obstructive pulmonary disease where the PCO_2 rises as the ventilator rate is increased.

The I:E ratio can be adjusted in several ways depending upon the make of ventilator. In some, a ratio can be selected directly, while in others, the inspiratory flow rate determines the duration of inspiration. An acceptable range for inspiratory flow rates is between 30 and 60 l/min (0.5–1.0 l/s).

Inspiratory waveforms

Many volume and time cycled (flow generator) ventilators allow the choice of several waveforms. Although there is little evidence to favour one over the other, a square waveform delivers the tidal volume in the least time and with higher peak pressures. A decelerating flow pattern results in lower peak pressures, longer inspiratory intervals, and lower I:E ratios.

Inspired oxygen concentration (FiO_2)

This should be constantly adjusted to provide adequate arterial oxygenation without hyperoxia. Too high a FiO_2 is frequently the cause of failure to wean patients with chronic obstructive pulmonary disease from a mechanical ventilator.

Pressure limit

Setting a pressure limit about 10 cmH_2O above the peak pressure reached during each ventilator cycle protects the patients against inadvertently high pressures experienced during coughing or straining. Hitting the pressure limit terminates inspiration and sounds an alarm.

Positive end-expiratory pressure/continuous positive airways pressure

Maintaining airway pressure above barometric pressure in a spontaneously breathing patient is called constant positive airway pressure. The same pressure applied to a patient on intermittent positive pressure ventilation is called positive end-expiratory pressure. This technique is used to correct lung volume (FRC) in conditions characterized by reduced lung volume such as adult respiratory distress syndrome or cardiogenic pulmonary oedema. It may also be of benefit in patients with flail chest segments since it acts to splint the chest wall.

Positive end-expiratory pressure/continuous positive airways pressure is achieved by the inclusion of a resistance at the expiratory end of the breathing circuit. Ideally this resistance should be as close to a threshold resistor as possible, such as an underwater column. In practice most of the valves produce some flow-dependent retardation of expiration that increases the work of breathing in a spontaneously breathing patient.

Bypassing the oropharynx by an endotracheal tube is known to cause a fall in FRC in both adults and children. The application of low levels of continuous positive airways pressure (3–5 cmH_2O) reverses this effect and has therefore been suggested as part of routine management of the intubated patient ('physiological continuous positive airways pressure'). The usual indication for positive end-expiratory pressure is the presence of refractory hypoxaemia due to acute lung injury. Starting at 5 cmH_2O the pressures are increased progressively until satisfactory oxygenation is achieved for a FiO_2 ideally less than 0.6. It is rarely necessary to exceed levels of 20 cmH_2O. Assessment of the effects of such treatment can be made in several ways by calculating the venous admixture or shunt fraction, oxygen delivery or effect static compliance of the lungs. Clearly, following the PaO_2 alone takes no account of the effects of positive pressure upon cardiac output. Continuous measurement of mixed venous SaO_2 with a suitable flow directed pulmonary artery catheter is a particularly good method of evaluating the response to a change in airway pressure.

Ventilator monitors and alarms

The ventilation monitors and alarms that must be set and maintained include:

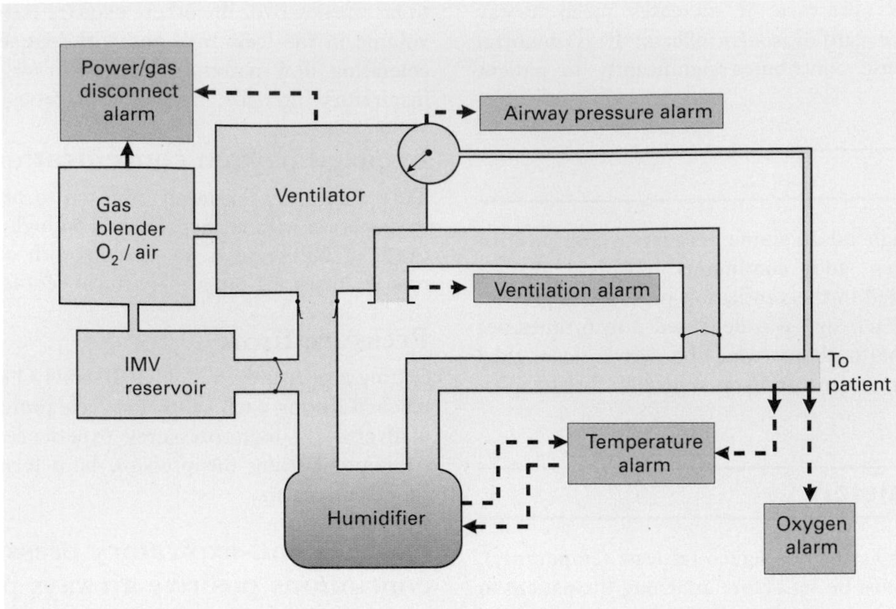

Fig. 4 Schematic of ventilator circuit showing minimum alarm/monitoring facilities on a mechanical ventilator. The pressure alarm monitors inflation pressures (peak and mean) and also detects patient disconnection which results in the circuit pressure falling to and remaining at zero. Ventilation alarms monitor the expiratory tidal volume and minute ventilation providing confirmation that the ventilation objectives are being met. The ventilation alarms will also detect disconnection or apnoea. The temperature of inhaled gases is monitored within the humidifier and at the patient's mouth. Excessively high temperature causes an alarm and automatically down regulates the humidifier heater.

1. Exhaled tidal volume, exhaled minute ventilation;
2. Airway pressure/disconnect;
3. Peak and mean airway pressures;
4. $F\text{IO}_2$;
5. Inhaled gas temperature.

Exhaled volume and minute ventilation

The ability to measure exhaled tidal volume and minute ventilation is a great asset and aid in evaluating the efficiency of ventilation. By setting low limit alarms the safety of mechanical ventilation is greatly enhanced and supplements the airway pressure/disconnect alarm (Fig. 1(d)).

Airway pressures

Careful monitoring of peak and mean airway pressures is essential in the patient supported with a flow generating (volume/time cycled) ventilator. A step increase in peak pressure may indicate a change in lung compliance, airway resistance, displacement of the endotracheal tube into a main bronchus, or even a pneumothorax. The pressure alarm should therefore be set 5 to 10 cmH_2O above the normal peak pressure (Fig. 4).

Inspired oxygen concentration

An oxygen sensor just proximal to the endotracheal tube ensures that any sudden fall in $F\text{IO}_2$ is detected immediately and before the patient can desaturate.

Gas temperature

Strict control of the temperature of the inhaled gases is essential to avoid thermal injury and to ensure effective humidification of inspired gases. Modern humidifiers are usually of the 'wick' variety that efficiently humidify high gas flows. Heat/moisture exchangers placed between the ventilator circuit Y-piece and the endotracheal tube provide an alternative method of humidification particularly for short-term ventilation. Inspired gas should leave the humidifier at about 40°C and reach the endotracheal tube at close to 37°C (Fig. 4). A low voltage heating element can be incorporated into the inspiratory limb of the circuit to reduce gas cooling and water condensation.

Clinical monitoring of mechanical ventilation

An essential aspect of monitoring is regular clinical examination of the patient, and inspection of the ventilator and ventilator circuit. Expansion of the chest should be symmetrical with each ventilator cycled breath (control mechanical ventilation, intermittent mandatory ventilation), assisted breath (assist control or pressure support), or unassisted spontaneous breath (intermittent mandatory ventilation). Auscultation should confirm air entry and detect any added sounds. The patient should be sat up or rolled side to side to allow inspection of the whole of the chest. The endotracheal tube should be secure and as comfortable as possible for the patient. The endotracheal cuff pressure should be checked (<30 mmHg) or a small leak should be audible with a stethoscope on the side of the neck. The ventilator circuit should feel warm but be free of significant amounts of condensed water. The humidifier temperature and water level should be checked.

The pulse oximeter has contributed significantly to the monitoring and safety of patients on mechanical ventilation. Not only does it provide a continuous measurement of oxygenation but also reduces the need for arterial blood gas sampling.

Much can be appreciated from watching the ventilator pressure gauge with each cycle. In addition to evaluating peak inspiratory pressure the clinician will be able to judge whether the patient is 'fighting' the ventilator. Comparing inspiratory and expiratory tidal volumes may indicate a leak in the circuit, either at circuit connections or at the endotracheal tube cuff. When peak pressures are high, the internal compliance of the ventilator and circuit (about 2 to 2.5 ml/cmH_2O) may account for much of the volume loss. A rough assessment of the compliance of the lung can be made by following the peak inflation pressures. However, it is preferable to calculate effective static and dynamic compliance in the following way.

Effective dynamic compliance

$$C_{dyn} = \frac{V_T\text{exh} - ([P_{peak} - \text{PEEP}] \times 2.0)}{P_{peak} - \text{PEEP}}$$

Effective static compliance

$$C_{stat} = \frac{V_T\text{exh} - ([P_{pause} - \text{PEEP}] \times 2.0)}{P_{pause} - \text{PEEP}}$$

where C_{dyn} = effective dynamic compliance (ml/cmH_2O), C_{stat} = effective static compliance (ml/cmH_2O), $V_T$exh = exhaled tidal volume (ml), P_{peak} = peak airway pressure (cmH_2O), P_{pause} = inspiratory pause pressure (cmH_2O), PEEP = positive end expiratory pressure (cmH_2O), and the figure 2.0 represents the internal compliance (ml/cm H_2O) of the ventilator and circuit. The product $P_{peak} \times 2.0$ indicates the volume of gas contained within the ventilator circuit that does not enter the patients lungs but is measured as exhaled V_T.

The effective dynamic compliance is always less than the effective static compliance by about 10 ml/cmH_2O. Greater differences indicate airways obstruction is contributing to the peak airway pressure. Normal values for effective dynamic compliance range between 50 and 80 ml/cmH_2O depending upon the size of the patient. Dynamic compliance will fall with both bronchoconstriction or lung restriction as in adult respiratory distress syndrome. Static compliance is relatively unaffected by bronchoconstriction. In severe adult respiratory distress syndrome, static compliance may fall to as low as 10 to 20 ml/cm H_2O from the normal range (60 to 90 ml/cmH_2O).

Specific strategies in ventilator management

Restrictive lung disease

Patients with restrictive lung diseases such as sarcoidosis or fibrosing alveolitis should be ventilated with small tidal volumes of between 5 and 8 ml/kg at rates of 15 to 20 breaths per minute. Oxygen need not be restricted in the manner recommended for patients with chronic obstructive pulmonary disease.

Chronic obstructive pulmonary disease

Although most patients with acute on chronic respiratory failure can be managed successfully without mechanical ventilation, a small proportion fail to respond to conservative measures and require ventilatory assistance. In many cases, the need for mechanical ventilation is the direct result of injudicious oxygen therapy. Low rate synchronized intermittent mandatory ventilation (6–8 breaths per minute) or low pressure levels of pressure support are ideal for such patients with acute on chronic respiratory failure. The $P\text{a}CO_2$ should be reduced very slowly towards but not to normal levels. The $F\text{i}O_2$ rarely needs to be higher than 0.35. High ventilator rates (> 14 per minute) are associated with high values of V_D/V_T (>0.5). Paradoxically, as the ventilator rates are increased in an attempt to increase minute ventilation, the $P\text{a}CO_2$ may rise. To avoid intrinsic or autopositive end-expiratory pressure the I:E ratio should be maintained at 1:2 or higher. Weaning can begin as soon as the precipitating cause of respiratory failure has been corrected. Weaning will be unsuccessful if there is any underlying metabolic alkalosis or if the patient receives sedative or analgesic agents. The $P\text{a}CO_2$ can be allowed to rise slowly to above normal levels provided sufficient time is given for the blood pH to correct and the $F\text{i}O_2$ kept below 0.35. Carbon dioxide production can be minimized by providing balanced nutrition with calories being provided by both lipid and carbohydrate.

Asthma

Probably less than 1 per cent of acute severe asthma attacks require mechanical ventilation. However, it is apparent that some patients suffer cardiac arrest and die each year because intubation and mechanical ventilation was not performed in time. Hypercarbia alone is generally insufficient indication for ventilation but a combination of a rising $P\text{a}CO_2$, fatigue, failure of conservative measures, or arrhythmias does call for elective intubation and mechanical ventilation.

Since asthma has a prevalence of between 4 and 8 per cent in the United Kingdom and the United States, it is not uncommon for a postoperative patient on a mechanical ventilator to develop bronchospasm. Asthmatic patients are difficult to ventilate and usually require high inflation pressures. Hypoxaemia may persist despite the addition of high concentrations of oxygen and is the result of mucus plugging of the airways. A philosophy of 'permissive hypercapnia' or 'controlled hypoventilation' should be adopted with the $P\text{a}CO_2$ remaining at elevated levels (7–8 kPa, 50–70 mmHg). Lower tidal volumes and respiratory rates are therefore possible. Lower inspiratory flow rates result in lower peak pressures and reduced risk of barotrauma. Deaths in ventilated asthmatic patients are usually the result of barotrauma, hypotension in volume depleted patients, arrhythmias, or lung infection.

Maximal bronchodilator therapy, including corticosteroids, is continued throughout the period of mechanical ventilation supplemented if necessary with inhalational anaesthetics such as isoflurane or the intravenous anaesthetic ketamine. Both of these agents are potent bronchodilators. Rehydration and adequate humidification of inspired gases will usually mobilize secretions and mucous plugs; if not, bronchoalveolar lavage may be indicated.

The use of extracorporeal membrane oxygenation and CO_2 removal has been reported in acute asthma. These must be considered exceptional cases and such techniques cannot be generally recommended.

Bronchopleural/bronchocutaneous fistulae

Although bronchopleural and bronchocutaneous fistulae can occur after trauma or lung infection, many arise during the postoperative period following lobectomy or pneumonectomy. It is generally appreciated that early weaning and extubation is preferred in these patients. Occasionally, postoperative complications necessitate a longer period of ventilation when there is significant risk of dehiscence of the bronchial stump. To reduce the risk of this, low tidal volume, high respiratory rate ventilation should be adopted to minimize inflation pressures. High frequency ventilation would appear to be ideally suited to the prevention of bronchopleural fistula, although evidence to prove superiority over conventional ventilation is lacking.

The development of bronchopleural fistula is heralded by clinical deterioration, reduced chest wall movement on the affected side, tracheal deviation, and a sudden increase in inflation pressures. Emergency tube thoracostomy must be performed converting the bronchopleural fistula into a bronchocutaneous fistula. Compensation for the loss of tidal volume through the fistula is easily made by adjusting the ventilator but if the leak is large, endobronchial intubation may be necessary. Bronchopleural and bronchocutaneous fistulae are unlikely to close until the patient is weaned from the ventilator.

Weaning

More than 80 per cent of patients who are ventilated postoperatively can be weaned simply by clinically evaluating their spontaneous ventilation on a 'T-piece' or similar circuit. The remainder require a progressive reduction in ventilatory support until measurement of ventilation parameters can be made. These parameters include the negative inspiratory force and vital capacity. A negative inspiratory force greater than $-25\ \text{cmH}_2\text{O}$ or a vital capacity greater than 10 ml/kg usually indicates sufficient ventilatory reserve for spontaneous ventilation. These parameters cannot be applied to patients with severe chronic obstructive pulmonary disease, in whom blood gases have to be followed with each reduction in ventilation support. Failure to wean a patient successfully should prompt the questions addressed in Table 4.

Intermittent mandating ventilation or pressure support modes are very suitable for a gradual weaning process. Assist-control can also be used to wean patients by progressively reducing the tidal volume.

Table 4 Questions to ask when weaning is difficult

1. Is the endotracheal tube of optimal size? Small endotracheal tubes of <7 mm internal diameter have a high resistance.
2. Has the patient been seated upright to aid lung mechanics?
3. Is there evidence of airway obstruction that would improve with bronchodilator or steroid therapy?
4. Are there respiratory depressant drugs being administered?
5. Is there evidence of occult neuromuscular disease? Exclude interactions with aminoglycosides.
6. Is there evidence of hypothyroidism, hypophosphataemia, or hypomagnesaemia?
7. Is there a metabolic alkalosis? If so this should be corrected with potassium chloride and volume as appropriate.
8. Is there evidence of malnourishment on history or simple laboratory test such as serum albumin.
9. Is tracheostomy indicated?
10. In patients with chronic obstructive pulmonary disease, are the target blood gases similar to the premorbid values?
11. Is there evidence of diaphragmatic dysfunction due to phrenic nerve injury?

Complications of mechanical ventilation

Several complications of mechanical ventilation can be attributed to the local effects of the endotracheal tube upon the airway. These include airway obstruction due to endotracheal tube displacement and pressure necrosis leading to vocal cord injury and subglottic stenosis. The risk of nosocomial pneumonia is increased in the intubated patient.

Other complications are the direct consequence of positive pressure ventilation. Haemodynamic effects such as reduced cardiac output, reduced renal perfusion, and salt and water retention are primarily the result of mechanical, neuroreflex, and humoral factors.

Interstitial lung damage may occur due to positive pressure ventilation and this has prompted renewed interest in extracorporeal systems for the management of patients with acute respiratory distress syndrome. However, the greatest concern relates to the risk of pneumothorax, pneumomediastinum, pneumopericarium, or subcutaneous emphysema. Pneumothorax is the most feared complication because it is associated with rapid deterioration unless dealt with quickly. Tube thoracostomy is mandatory since progression to a tension pneumothorax is very likely. Prophylactic thoracostomy tubes are not recommended, even in the presence of pneumomediastinum. Sudden clinical deterioration associated with a rise in inflation pressures and absence of breath sounds should raise the question of pneumothorax. Emergency decompression with a 14-gauge cannula may produce temporary relief and may have a diagnostic role, but tube thoracostomy should be performed without delay and without radiographic confirmation if necessary. Blunt dissection through the parietal pleura with forceps and digital exploration of the pleural space prior to insertion of the thoracostomy tube is essential if lung damage is to be avoided. Thoracostomy tubes with rigid metal stylets must not be used under any circumstances.

FURTHER READING

Ashbaugh DG, Bigelow DB, Petty TL, Levine BE. Acute respiratory distress syndrome in adults. *Lancet*, 1967; **ii**: 319–23.

Barnes PK. Principles of lung ventilators and humidification. In: Scurr, C. Feldman S, eds. *Scientific Foundations of Anaesthesia*. London: William Heinemann, 1982:533–43.

Bernard GR, *et al.* High dose corticosteroids in patients with the adult respiratory distress syndrome. *N Engl J Med*, 1987; **317**: 1545–70.

Cameron PD, Oh TE. Newer modes of mechanical ventilatory support. *Anaesthesia Intensive Care*, 1986; **14**: 258–66.

Danek SJ, Lynch JP, Weg JG, Dantzker DR. The dependence of oxygen uptake on oxygen delivery in the adult respiratory distress syndrome. *Am Rev Resp Dis*, 1980; **122**: 387–95.

Downs JB, Block AJ, Vennum KB. Intermittent mandatory ventilation in the treatment of patients with chronic obstructive pulmonary disease. *Anesth Analg*, 1974; **53**: 437–43.

Downs JB, Kelin EF, Desautels D, Modell JH, Kirby RR. IMV: A new approach to weaning patients from mechanical ventilators. *Chest*, 1973; **64**: 331–5.

Downs JB, Olsen GN. Pulmonary function following adult respiratory distress syndrome. *Chest*, 1974; **65**: 92–3.

Duchateau J, *et al.* Complement activation in patients risk of developing the adult respiratory distress syndrome. *Am Rev Resp Dis*, 1984; **130**: 1058–64.

Elliott CG, Morris AH, Cengiz M. Pulmonary function and exercise gas exchange in survivors of adult respiratory distress syndrome. *Am Rev Resp Dis*, 1981; **123**: 455–92.

Fairley HB. Critique of intermittent mandatory ventilation. In: Kirby R, Graybar GB, eds, *Intermittent mandatory ventilation*. Boston: Little, Brown and Co., 1980: 79–90.

Fowler, AA, *et al.* Adult respiratory distress syndrome: risk with common predispositions. *Ann Intern Med*, 1983; **98**: 593–7.

Gattinoni L, *et al.* Treatment of acute respiratory failure with low frequency positive-pressure ventilation and extracorporeal removal of CO_2. *Lancet* 1980; **ii**: 292–4.

Gotloib L, Barzilay E. The impact of using the artificial kidney as an artificial endocrine lung upon severe septic ARDS. *Intensive Crit Care Digest*, 1986; **5**: 3–5.

Hammerschmidt DE, Weaver LJ, Hudson LD, Craddock PR, Jacob HS. Association of complement activation and elevant plasma-C5a with adult respiratory distress syndrome: pathophysiological relevance and possible prognostic value. *Lancet*, 1980 **i**: 947–9.

Haynes JB, Hyers TM, Giclas PC, Franks JJ, Petty TL. Elevated fibrinogen degradation products in adult respiratory distress syndrome. *Am Rev Resp Dis*, 1980; **122**: 841–7.

Heenan TJ, Downs JB, Douglas ME, Ruiz BC, Jumper L. Intermittent mandatory ventilation. Is synchronization important? *Chest*, 1980; **77**: 598–602.

Hickling KG. Extracorporeal CO_2 removal in severe adult respiratory distress syndrome. *Anaesthesia Intensive Care*, 1986; **14**: 45–53.

Hickling KG, Henderson, SJ, Jackson R. Low mortality associated with low volume pressure limited ventilation with permissive hypercapnia in severe adult respiratory distress syndrome. *Intensive Care Med*, 1990; **16**: 372–7.

Hurst JM, Branson RD, Davis KJ, Barrette RR, Adams, KS. Comparison of conventional mechanical ventilation and high-frequency ventilation. A prospective, randomized trial in patients with respiratory failure. *Ann Surg*, 1990; **211**: 486–91.

Kariman K, Burns SR. Regulation of tissue oxygen extraction is disturbed in adult respiratory distress syndrome. *Am Rev Resp Dis*, 1985; **132**: 109–114.

Kirby RR, *et al.* High level PEEP in acute respiratory insufficiency. *Chest*, 1975; **67**: 156–63.

Kumar A, *et al.* Continuous positive-pressure ventilation in acute respiratory failure. *N Engl J Med*, 1970; **283**: 1430–6.

Mohsenifar Z, Tashkin DP, Goldbach P, Campisi DJ. Relationship between O_2 delivery and O_2 consumption in the adult respiratory distress syndrome. *Chest*, 1983; **84**: 267–71.

Montgomery AB, Stager MA, Carrico J, Hudson LD. Causes of mortality in patients with the adult respiratory distress syndrome. *Am Rev Resp Dis*, 1985; **132**: 485–9.

Murray JF, Matthay MA, Luce JM, Flick MR. An expanded definition of the adult respiratory distress syndrome. *Am Rev Resp Dis*, 1988; **138**: 720–3.

National Heart Lung and Blood Institute, Division of Lung Diseases. *Extracorporeal support for respiratory insufficiency*. Bethesda, MD:National Institutes for Health, 1979; 243–5.

Ognibene FP, *et al.* Adult respiratory distress syndrome in patients with severe neutropenia. *N Engl J Med* 1986; **315**: 547–51.

Pepe PE, Hudson LD, Carrico CJ. Early application of positive end expiratory pressure in patients at risk for the adult respiratory distress syndrome. *N Engl J Med*, 1984; **311**: 281–6.

Pepe PE, *et al.* Clinical predictors of adult respiratory distress syndrome. *Am J Surg*, 1982: **144**: 124–30.

Petty TL, Ashbaugh DG. The adult respiratory distress syndrome: clinical features, factors influencing prognosis and principles of management. *Chest*, 1971; **130**: 66–71.

Petty TL, Silvers GW, Paul GW, Stanford RE. Abnormalities in lung elastic properties and surfactant function in adult respiratory distress syndrome. *Chest* 1979; **75**: 571–4.

Pontoppidan H, Geffin B, Lowenstein E. Acute respiratory failure in the adult. *N Engl J Med*, 1972; **287**: 690–9.

Qvist J, Pontoppidan H, Wilson RS, Lowenstein E, Laver MB. Haemodynamic responses to mechanical ventilation with PEEP: the effect of hypervolaemia. *Anesthesiology*, 1975; **42**: 45–55.

Rinaldo JE. Mediation of ARDS by leukocytes. Clinical evidence and implications for therapy. *Chest*, 1986; **89**: 590–3.

Rinaldo JE, Petty TL. Indicators of risk, course, and prognosis in adult respiratory distress syndrome (ARDS). *Am Rev Resp Dis*, 1986; **133**: 343–4.

Rinaldo JE, Rogers RM. Adult respiratory distress syndrome. *N Engl J Med*, 1986: **315**: 578–80.

Rocker GM, Wiseman MS, Pearson D, Shale DJ. Diagnostic criteria for adult respiratory distress syndrome: time for reappraisal. *Lancet* 1989; **i**: 120–3.

Rotman HH, Lavelle TF, Dimcheff DG. Vendenbelt RJ, Weg JG. Long term physiological consequences of the adult respiratory distress syndrome. *Chest*, 1977; **72**: 190–2.

Saldeen T. The microembolism syndrome. *Microvasc Res*, 1976; **11**: 227–59.

Simpson DL, Goodman M, Spector SL, Petty TL. Long term follow-up and bronchial reactivity resting in survivors of the adult respiratory distress syndrome. *Am Rev Resp Dis*, 1978; **117**: 449–54.

Smith RA, Desautels DA, Kirby RR. Mechanical ventilators. In: Kirby RR, Smith RA, Desautels DA, eds. *Mechanical Ventilation*. New York: Churchill Livingstone, 1985; 327–474.

Tate RM, Repine JE. Neutrophils and the adult respiratory distress syndrome. *Am Rev Resp Dis*, 1983; **128**: 522–9.

Weigel JA, Norcross JF, Borman KR, Sayder WH. Early steroid therapy for respiratory failure. *Arch Surg*, 1985; **120**: 536–40.

Weiland JE, *et al.* Lung neutrophils in the adult respiratory distress syndrome. Clinical and pathophysiological significance. *Am Rev Resp Dis*, 1986; **133**: 218–25.

Weinberg P, *et al.* Biologically active products of complement and acute lung injury in patients with the sepsis syndrome. *Am Rev Resp Dis* 1984; **130**: 791–6.

Wood LH, Prewitt RM. Cardiovascular management in acute hypoxemic respiratory failure. *Am J Cardiol* 1981; **47**: 963–72.

4.4 Infection in the critical care unit

CHRISTOPHER S. GARRARD

NOSOCOMIAL INFECTION IN THE CRITICAL CARE UNIT PATIENT

Incidence

Nosocomial infection is one which develops at least 48 h after admission to hospital. It affects about 15 to 40 per cent of critical care unit patients, and contributes to approximately 75 per cent of late deaths in such units. The terms colonization, infection, and sepsis are often used interchangeably, but should be used only within the limits of the following definitions. Colonization is defined microbiologically as the presence of a potentially pathogenic organism on two or more consecutive occasions. In contrast, infection is the presence of many pathogenic organisms, with leucocytes and the clinical signs of inflammation. Sepsis is a syndrome comprising the clinical signs of infection (fever and leucocytosis) and organ system failure. An infecting organism may or may not be identified. Wider aspects of the sepsis syndrome are considered in more detail elsewhere.

Predisposing factors

The incidence of nosocomial infection is dependent upon the length of stay in the critical care unit, the number of invasive procedures or degree of intervention, the nature of the underlying illness, and mode of presentation. These factors are to some extent interdependent: the longer a patient remains in the critical care unit the more interventions and procedures are likely to be performed.

The impact of the underlying illness and the type of patient can be judged by examining the different rates of infection in medical and surgical intensive care units. Burns and general surgical critical care units have infection rates of about 30 per cent, compared with less than 15 per cent in general medical units. Coronary care units have rates of infection of 5 per cent, which is similar to that of the general wards.

The performance of invasive procedures has a great effect upon the incidence of nosocomial infection. Endotracheal intubation and mechanical ventilation carries a 20 to 60 per cent incidence of pneumonia, while up to 30 per cent of patients with a urinary catheter develop urinary tract infections. Up to 15 per cent of infections are line-related, and strict rules regarding the insertion and management of arterial and venous catheters need to be rigorously enforced. Generally speaking, no vascular lines other than tunnelled feeding catheters and those required for haemodialysis or haemofiltration should remain in place for more than 5 days. Factors associated with an increased incidence of vascular catheter infections include the infusion of hypertonic solutions, frequent disconnection of infusion lines, and the length of time the catheter remains *in situ*. Peripheral intravenous lines usually need to be changed more frequently because of local non-bacterial inflammation. The incidence of wound-related infection depends upon the type of surgery performed but accounts for about 15 per cent of critical care infections.

The longer a patient remains in the critical care unit the higher the incidence of infection: after 24 h about 10 per cent of patients become infected, while more than 90 per cent can be infected after 2 weeks.

Infection control

The keys to infection control include the adoption of preventative measures, the early recognition of infection, and the application of disciplined antibiotic policies. The Centres for Disease Control Guidelines (1985) address the important issues of hand washing, disinfection, and isolation procedures, together with strict control of antibiotic therapy and prophylaxis. These measures are aimed at the elimination of environmental organisms and prevention of cross-infection. Their impact has not been as great as might have been expected, consistent with the recognition that the patient's own endogenous bacterial flora serves as the source of most nosocomial infection.

Identification of organisms

Rigorous surveillance techniques must be applied to identify the organisms responsible for the infection. Specimens must be carefully preserved and transported rapidly to the laboratory: loss of a microbiological specimen through carelessness may adversely affect morbidity or even mortality. Table 1 lists the bacteria most commonly identified in nosocomial infections. Although there is considerable variation from unit to unit the common pathogens generally include *E. coli, Staph. aureus, P. aeruginosa*, and enterococci.

Table 1 Bacterial flora commonly associated with nosocomial infection

Organism	Percentage
Coliforms	20
S. aureus	10
P. aeruginosa	10
Enterococcus spp.	10
Klebsiella spp., *Enterobacter* spp., *S. epidermidis*, *Proteus* spp., *Candida* spp., and others	50

The usual sites sampled in the microbiological survey of a potentially infected or septic patient are shown in Table 2. Clearly, surveillance should be directed primarily at the site suggested by the clinical picture. However, much time may be saved by applying a broad approach and simultaneously sampling all potential sites of infection.

NOSOCOMIAL PNEUMONIA

Nosocomial pneumonia occurs 0.5 to 1 per cent of hospital patients. A high proportion of these cases are seen in critical care

Table 2 Antimicrobial surveillance in the septic patient

1. Wounds and discharge sites
2. Lung and airways
   (a) Tracheal aspirate
   (b) Blind bronchial lavage
   (c) Bronchoscopic lavage
3. Urine
4. Blood
   (a) Two sites
   (b) Fresh venepuncture
   (c) Skin preparation with alcohol
5. Invasive line tips
6. CSF
7. Others, needle aspirates

units where the incidence of nosocomial pneumonia may reach 5 to 25 per cent. Such pneumonias may be responsible for up to a quarter of critical care deaths. Several factors predispose towards nosocomial pneumonia in critical care patients: some of these are summarized in Table 3.

Most reports of nosocomial pneumonia in the critical care patient have used purely clinical criteria to establish the diagnosis. Conventional criteria include fever, leucocytosis, purulent sputum, and the appearance of new or progressive infiltrates on chest radiographs. While these criteria are probably satisfactory for general hospital patients they are not specific enough for use in the critically ill. The onset of fever and leucocytosis may be the result of a variety of infectious or even non-infectious pathologies. Since colonization of endotracheal tubes with oropharyngeal bacteria is inevitable within a few hours of intubation, simple endotracheal aspirates may not reliably reflect lung colonization.

Table 3 Factors predisposing towards nosocomial pneumonia in critical care patients

1. Advanced age
2. Obesity
3. Cigarette smoking
4. Low Glasgow coma score
5. Diabetes mellitus
6. Malignant disease
7. Oropharyngeal colonization with Gram-negative organisms
8. Gastric colonization increased in ileus and reduced gastric acidity
9. Chronic heart, lung, or renal disease.
10. Endotracheal intubation

A more specific approach to the diagnosis of pneumonia in critical care patients is the adoption of microbiological surveillance based on quantitative cultures of material obtained by a protected specimen brush and bronchoalveolar lavage. A clinically significant infection is suggested by the presence of more than 10^3 colony forming units (c.f.u.) in 1 ml of lavage fluid, or in the 1 ml of saline in which the protected specimen brush has been agitated. Prospective studies of nosocomial pneumonia diagnosed by protected specimen brushing show the incidence increases from less than 10 per cent at 10 days to more than 25 per cent at 30 days. Critical care patients with pneumonia have a mortality rate about twice that of patients without pneumonia. Bronchoalveolar lavage offers the potential advantage that Gram staining of a centrifuge deposit of the fluid obtained may provide an early indication of pneumonia: if more than 25 per cent of white cells in the centrifuge deposit contain intracellular organisms it is highly likely that the patient has pneumonia. Recent studies have shown that blind bronchial lavage with an undirected catheter is almost as sensitive and specific as fibreoptically guided bronchoalveolar lavage.

Measures to reduce the risk of nosocomial pneumonia

Bacteria enter the lungs by several portals: from contamination of the inspired air by infected equipment, by aspiration of oropharyngeal secretions, or as blood-borne infection. Significant improvement has been achieved in the avoidance of infection from contaminated ventilator circuits and humidification systems. Changing ventilator circuits every day is associated with a higher incidence of nosocomial lung infection than when the circuits are changed every 2 to 3 days; leaving the ventilator circuits unchanged for the entire duration of the patient's admission does not appear to add to the risk of pneumonia. If a humidifier is used in the ventilator circuit, a closed system which maintains the level of sterile water within the humidifier is preferable to intermittent topping up. Sheathed suction catheter systems allow a single catheter to be used for 24 h without repeated disconnection of the ventilator circuit from the endotracheal tube. Suctioning can be continued without interruption of either intermittent positive pressure ventilation or continuous positive airways pressure. Although lung infection rates are no lower than those associated with conventional suction catheters there are benefits from reducing the risk of contamination of nursing staff and cross-infection. Humidification can also be achieved using heat/moisture exchangers that also serve as microbiological filters and may reduce the rate of airway contamination.

Stress ulcer prophylaxis

Antacids and H_2-blockers increase gastric pH and may encourage bacterial colonization of the gastric secretions. Aspiration of gastric fluid is likely to be associated with a higher risk of nosocomial lung infection. The possible adverse effects of H_2-blockers and their questionable efficacy make routine prescription of these agents difficult to justify. Effective stress ulcer prophylaxis can be achieved by instilling sucralfate, a cytoprotective agent that does not increase gastric pH, into the stomach. It has been suggested that introducing small volumes of enteral feed (30 ml every 2 h), even in the presence of an ileus, achieves the same results. Patients receiving enteral nutrition do not need stress ulcer prophylaxis.

Selective digestive tract decontamination

In view of the potential role of oropharyngeal and gastric secretions in the development of nosocomial pneumonia it is logical to reduce the rate of colonization of these secretions. Combinations of non-absorbable topical antibiotics such as polymyxin, tobramycin, and amphotericin with a short course of a systemic broad-spectrum antibiotic significantly reduce lung infection rates. Surprisingly, selective digestive tract decontamination has little impact upon mortality, except possibly in trauma patients. Development of microbial resistance does not as yet appear to be a complication of this procedure although anecdotal experience suggests it might encourage the spread of methicillin resistant staphylococci.

The translocation of micro-organisms and endotoxin from the bowel lumen directly into the circulation has been linked with the development and persistence of the sepsis syndrome; this has been cited as a reason for inhibiting or eliminating intestinal colonization. Although routine selective digestive tract decontamination cannot yet be recommended, its use in selected patients might still be considered.

Other measures

Nasojejunal feeding tubes have advantages over the more widely used nasogastric tubes for enteral nutrition since they facilitate such feeding even in the presence of gastric paresis and are associated with a lower risk of aspiration of gastric contents.

The heavily sedated or obtunded patient should be moved regularly from side to side to discourage the development of dependent lung collapse. At other times the patient should be sat upright to reduce the risk of aspiration.

Management

All ventilated, critical care patients who are considered to have nosocomial pneumonia on clinical grounds should undergo fibreoptic bronchoscopy for bronchoalveolar lavage or protected specimen brushing. As an alternative, lavage can be performed through a non-directed catheter passed as far into a lobar bronchus as possible. If possible, cytopathological examination of the centrifuge sediment from bronchoalveolar lavage fluid should be performed. If more than 25 per cent of white cells contain organisms, empirical therapy should be commenced, based on the results of Gram staining. The range of bacteria isolated by protected specimen brushing in two studies of nosocomial pneumonia is shown in Table 4.

Any empirical antibiotic regimen for patients with nosocomial pneumonia must provide broad-spectrum cover and minimize the risk of allowing multiresistant organisms to develop. A combination of an aminoglycoside and an antipseudomonal β-lactam largely satisfies these requirements, and has the additional benefit of antimicrobial synergy. These attributes are particularly desirable for treating *Pseudomonas aeruginosa* infections, which carry a high mortality rate. If a staphylococcal infection is indicated on Gram stain, then antistaphylococcal antibiotics should be included in the regimen. Therapy should be modified or discontinued if less than 10^3 c.f.u./ml are isolated from quantitative cultures obtained by protected specimen brushing. The duration of antibiotic treatment necessary to eradicate the infecting organism has not been determined: depending upon the clinical response, antibiotics can usually be stopped after 5 to 7 days. Anaerobic or staphylococcal lung infections may require up to 4 weeks therapy.

Table 4 Lung bacteria identified by protected specimen brush in patients with nosocomial pneumonia

	Fagon *et al.* (1989)	Torres *et al.* (1989)
	(52 patients) No. (%)	(20 patients) No. (%)
Gram-negative bacteria		
P. aeruginosa	16 (31)	7 (35)
Acinetobacter spp.	8 (15)	6 (30)
Proteus spp.	8 (15)	—
B. catarrhalis	5 (10)	—
Haemophilus spp.	5 (10)	—
E. coli	4 (8)	3 (15)
Klebsiella spp.	2 (4)	3 (15)
Enterobacter spp.	1 (2)	1 (5)
Miscellaneous	1 (2)	1 (5)
Legionella spp.	1 (2)	2 (10)
Gram-positive bacteria		
S. aureus	17 (33)	5 (25)
S. pneumoniae	3 (6)	1 (5)
Other streptococci	8 (15)	4 (20)
Corynebacteriae spp.	4 (8)	
S. epidermidis	1 (5)	
Anaerobes	1 (2)	1 (5)
Polymicrobial flora	21 (40)	10 (50)

N.B. Several polymicrobial cultures obtained.

INFECTION IN THE IMMUNOCOMPROMISED HOST

The most common causes of immunocompromise are malignancy, chemotherapy, corticosteroid treatment, immunosuppressive treatment after transplantation, and acquired immune deficiency syndrome (AIDS). Immunocompromise can take the form of failure of phagocytosis, defective cell-mediated immunity, defective antibody-mediated immunity, and splenectomy. Opportunistic infections can usually be managed outside the critical care unit unless respiratory or renal failure intervenes. Some degree of deficiency of both cellular and antibody-mediate immune response is observed in trauma and burns patients, and this may increase their susceptibility to infection.

Failure of phagocytosis

A reduction in the number or function of neutrophils, monocytes, or macrophages increases susceptibility to infection. Pyogenic abscesses or osteomyelitis caused by *Staph. aureus*, Enterobacteriaceae, *Serratia marcesens*, and fungi are common. Failure of macrophage function may result from their impaired migration to the infection site (as in diabetes mellitus) or from a failure of opsonization, which requires the interaction of antibody and complement on the surface of the micro-organism. Deficiency of systemic antibodies or complement, whether congenital or acquired, will therefore result in impaired phagocytosis.

Complement deficiency

Congenital deficiencies of complement components 6, 7 or 8 are associated with recurrent systemic infections by *Neisseria meningitidis* and *N. gonorrhoea*. Deficiency of the early components C2 or C3, although rare, may predispose to recurrent viral and bacterial infections. Acquired complement deficiency, which may occur in immune complex disease such as systemic lupus erythematosus (SLE) and some subtypes of glomerulonephritis, will encourage the progression of a localized infection to systemic sepsis. In an acute exacerbation of SLE, low complement levels are often used as a marker of disease activity. Thus, low complement levels might lead to the conclusion that conditions such as lung infiltrates or encephalopathy are due to the primary disease process and not to infection. Clearly this may not be appropriate.

Granulocytopenia

Granulocytopenia is one of the most common causes of immunocompromise in critical care patients. Patients with fewer than 1000 granulocytes/mm^3, including immature precursors, are considered to be granulocytopenic and are at increased risk of infection. Severely granulocytopenic patients with white cell counts less of than 500/mm^3 are at particular risk. Leucocyte transfusions are not effective in correcting this immune defect, but there may be a place for the use of recombinant granulocyte/monocyte colony stimulating factor (GMCSF).

Cellular immunodeficiency

Congenital forms of cell-mediated immunodeficiency such as Di George syndrome or Wiskott-Aldrich syndrome are rare, and most cases are due to an acquired defect in the number of function of T lymphocytes. Impaired cell-mediated immunity can be demonstrated by an absence of delayed hypersensitivity to Candida, mumps- or tuberculin (PPD) antigens. The T-lymphocyte count (CD3$^+$ and CD4$^+$) may also be reduced.

The causes of acquired cell-mediated immunodeficiency include lymphoproliferative diseases such as Hodgkin's lymphoma, steroid and immunosuppressive therapy, sarcoidosis, and acquired immunodeficiency syndrome (AIDS). Some impairment of cell-mediated immunity is also found in patients undergoing chronic haemodialysis.

Cell-mediated immunity stems from the interaction of effector T cells with antigen presenting monocytes and macrophages. The presentation of surface antigen (from the pathogen) by presenting cells, to the effector lymphoctes, is an essential prerequisite to the cell-mediated immune mechanism. As even pathogens that reside intracellularly are accessible to the presenting phagocytes, and therefore to the effector lymphoctes, cell-mediated immunity is particularly effective against a wide range of intracellular organisms, some of which are listed in Table 5. Susceptibility to infection with non-intracellular organisms, such as fungi is also found in cell-mediated immunodeficiency.

Defective humoral immunity

Defective humoral or antibody-mediated immunity results from deficient B lymphocyte maturation or differentiation. The subsequent failure of plasma cells to produce immunoglobulin results in antibody deficiency. Defective antibody-mediated immunity can be demonstrated in the laboratory by assay of IgM, IgG and IgA and their subclasses. Blood B-cell count may be low and the *in-vivo* antibody response to Pneumococcus polysaccharide or tetanus toxoid may be impaired. Antibody deficiency occurs in chronic lymphocytic leukaemia, multiple myeloma, and in congenital or acquired hypogammaglobulinaemia. Occasionally a thymoma may underlie an acquired hypogammaglobulinaemia. The usual pathogens are *Haemophilus influenzae*, Pneumococcus, *Pseudomonas aeruginosa*, and *Neisseria meningitidis*.

Treatment of defective antibody-mediated immunity relies upon appropriate use of antibiotics supplemented by immunoglobulin infusion in doses of 200 to 500 mg/kg. Immunoglobulin administration may need to be repeated each month.

Splenectomy

Splenectomy may result from trauma, staging of Hodgkin's disease, or as part of the treatment of hereditary spherocytosis or idiopathic thrombocytopenic purpura. Patients with sickle cell disease may be functionally asplenic.

Pathogens affecting these patients are the encapsulated bacteria such as Pneumococcus, *H. influenzae*, and Meningococcus. Splenectomized patients, especially children, may develop a fulminant septicaemia that is rapidly fatal unless immediately treated (post-splenectomy syndrome). Prophylactic pneumococcal and H. *influenzae* vaccination is indicated before surgery is undertaken in these patients.

Sites of infection and organisms

The granulocytopenic patient usually experiences infection of the lungs, skin, alimentary tract, oropharynx, and oesophagus. The urinary tract and liver are less commonly involved. Common pathogens include *Pseudomonas aeruginosa, Klebsiella pneumoniae, Escherichia coli, Staphylococcus aureus, Candida albicans*, and *Aspergillus* spp. Patients with cell-mediated immunodeficiency experience infections in similar sites but with a slightly different spectrum (Table 5). Nocardial infection may be especially common in cardiac transplant patients: the lung is the most common site of infection, and bronchoalveolar lavage or transbronchial biopsy is usually required for diagnosis. Treatment is with sulphisoxazole (6–12 g/day) or trimethoprim/sulphamethoxazole.

Table 5 Infections associated with cell-mediated immunodeficiency

1. Bacteria
   - *Salmonella* spp.
   - *Listeria moncytogenes*
   - *Nocardia* spp.
   - *Legionella pneumophila*
2. Mycobacteria
   - *M. tuberculosis*
   - *M. avium-intracellulare*
3. Fungi
   - *Candida* spp.
   - *Aspergillus* spp.
   - *Mucor* spp.
   - *Cryptococcus* spp.
4. Protozoa
   - *Pneumocystis carinii*
   - *Toxoplasma gondii*
   - Cryptosporidia
5. Viruses
   - Cytomegalovirus
   - Herpes zoster
   - Herpes simplex
   - Epstein-Barr
6. Parasites
   - *Strongyloides stercoralis*

Prevention of infection

Since many infections are caused by the patient's own endogenous bacteria attempts have been made to reduce infection using isolation procedures and special environmental units: results have been disappointing. Selective decontamination of the oropharynx and upper gastrointestinal tract using non-absorbable antibiotics have failed to increase long-term survival. In contrast, antifungal prophylaxis using ketoconazole has been effective in reducing the incidence of oesophageal candidiasis. As with the immunocompetent patient, the risk of infection is related to the level and number of interventions: invasive procedures should therefore be limited to essential diagnostic investigations. Stool softeners should be administered to prevent bacterial translocation and anorectal abrasion.

Microbiological surveillance

Careful physical examination of the patient is an essential prerequisite to locating and identifying an infection. The oropharynx, ears, and sinuses should be checked daily. Fundoscopic eye examination may reveal fungal infection. Culture samples should be obtained from the sites listed in Table 2, with the addition of oropharyngeal and stool specimens.

The appearance of new infiltrates on chest radiographs indicates an opportunistic pneumonia until proven otherwise. Although sputum should be stained (Gram and special stains) and cultured, fibreoptic bronchoscopy for bronchoalveolar lavage, brushing, and transbronchial biopsy may be required. Occasionally open lung biopsy is needed to establish a diagnosis.

Antibiotics treatment

The use of antimicrobial prophylaxis suffers from the major disadvantage that bacterial resistance almost always develops. Confirmed or even suspected infection requires immediate and effective treatment: the source or type of infection may not be identified despite careful physical examination and microbiological surveillance and empirical antibiotic therapy may have to be started based on clinical probability. The selected antibiotics need to be effective against Gram-negative and Gram-positive bacteria such as *E. coli*, *Pseudomonas* spp., *S. aureus*, and *S. epidermidis*. A combination of a third-generation cephalosporin or penicillin derivative such as piperacillin with an aminoglycoside (gentamicin, netilmicin) and a penicillinase-resistant penicillin such as nafcillin or oxacillin would eliminate most of the likely organisms.

Aminoglycoside resistance may occur, particularly to gentamicin, and may explain a lack of response to treatment. Antibiotic treatment should generally be continued until cultures become negative and signs of infection resolve.

Fungal infection

Persistent fever in the face of apparently adequate antibiotic therapy should always raise the question of fungal infection. Systemic fungal infections are difficult to diagnose and carry a high mortality rate. Simultaneous colonization of the skin and other sites such as the oropharynx, oesophagus, and urinary tract makes systemic infection more likely but not inevitable. Blood cultures for fungi can be negative in up to 50 per cent of patients with systemic fungaemia and, unfortunately, serological tests cannot differentiate clearly between colonization and systemic infection. The addition of amphotericin B to the treatment regimen should be seriously considered in cases of suspected candidiasis, despite the risks of nephrotoxicity. A less toxic antifungal agent such as fluconazole might be considered as an alternative, particularly for the treatment of Candida infections. Other fungi such as Aspergillus and Mucor should be considered, especially if in patients presenting with a lung infection. Bronchoscopy, bronchoalveolar lavage, and transbronchial biopsy are usually needed to establish the diagnosis of invasive aspergillosis or mucormycosis: treatment is with amphotericin B. Cryptococcal infections usually present with meningitis, pneumonitis, or disseminated infection. Examination of cerebrospinal fluid (Gram stain or India ink preparation with latex agglutination tests for cryptococcal antigen) may confirm the diagnosis. Any skin lesions should be scraped and Gram stained. Transbronchial biopsy is required in the case of suspected cryptococcal pneumonitis. Cryptococcus infection should be treated with amphotericin B and flucytosine.

Pneumocystis carinii

This protozoan is a common cause of pneumonia in the immunosuppressed patient. Patients present with breathlessness, tachypnoea, cough, and hypoxia, and physical examination reveals scattered crackles on auscultation, although chest findings can be minimal. The chest radiographic appearances are non-specific and may take the form of diffuse bilateral interstitial or lobar infiltrates. The infection is generally fatal if not treated. The treatment of choice for *P. carinii* is trimethoprim (20 mg/kg) and sulphamethoxazole (100 mg/kg), given four times a day for up to 14 days. Failure of clinical response within 3 to 6 days or the development of side-effects such thrombocytopenia may require therapy to be changed to pentamidine isothionate, 4 mg/kg per day. Side-effects such as neutropenia, azotaemia, and cardiotoxicity may be avoided by administering pentamidine as an aerosol. Corticosteroids can be added to reduce the interstitial inflammatory response and have improved survival in AIDS patients with Pneumocystis pneumonia.

Toxoplasma gondii

Toxoplasma gondii disseminates widely through multiple organ systems, with death usually resulting from encephalitis or myocarditis. Serological tests for Toxoplasma are not reliable, the diagnosis being best established by identifying the organism in cerebrospinal fluid. Treatment is with a combination of sulphadiazine and pyrimethamine.

Viral infections

Of the viral infection that must be considered herpes simplex, herpes zoster, and cytomegalovirus are commonly encountered in transplant recipients. If infection with these agents is confirmed immunosuppressive therapy generally needs to be discontinued and specific antiviral agents administered. Gancyclovir is effective against cytomegalovirus, and acyclovir is effective against herpes simplex and herpes zoster. Both agents are associated with bone marrow suppression and nephrotoxicity.

ANTIBIOTIC THERAPY IN INTENSIVE CARE

The major issues that must be addressed when prescribing antibiotics are listed below.

1. Does the nature and severity of infection justify the use of antibiotics?

2. Are antibiotics being used as prophylaxis, specific therapy for an identified organism, or as empiric therapy?
3. What are the appropriate dosage regimens and is combination therapy required?
4. What are the criteria for discontinuing treatment? What is considered to represent a 'course' of treatment?

Of these, the first and last questions are the most important and the most difficult to answer: whether to start treatment with antibiotics, and when to stop. The selection of an antibiotic for use in critical care patients should be based on a sound appreciation of the clinical presentation and the microbiological laboratory findings. The patient with fever, leucocytosis, and a site of infection does not necessarily require treatment with antibiotics: inappropriate or unnecessary antibiotic therapy being associated with increased mortality. Conversely, it is not unusual to begin empirical therapy in a patient who is critically ill before an organism or a site of infection can be identified. If possible, empirical therapy is selected according to the nature or suspected site of infection. For example an aspiration pneumonia will require a different antimicrobial agent or combination of agents than would be selected for intra-abdominal sepsis. After commencing antibiotics, the clinical response to therapy and results of bacterial stains and cultures will determine whether treatment should continue, cease, or be modified. The ideal length of antibiotic treatment has not been determined, but 5 days would generally be adequate for most infections. Beyond this time the possibility of development of resistant microbial strains increases.

β-Lactams

The β-lactams, which include the penicillins, cephalosporins, carbapenems, and monobactams (see Table 5), have found wide application in critical care. These antibiotics bind to specific penicillin-binding receptor proteins on the cytoplasmic surface of the bacterial cell wall, the inner membrane, releasing autolysins that disrupt the cell wall structure as the organism replicates.

β-Lactam resistance has evolved by alteration of the penicillin-binding protein receptors, by alteration of the pores that allow egress of the antibiotic through the cell wall, or by production of β-lactamase, a bacterial enzyme which causes hydrolytic destruction of the β-lactam ring with subsequent loss of antibacterial activity. β-Lactamase may be produced by the organism either continuously or after exposure to a β-lactam agent. The development of organisms resistant to multiple antimicrobial agents is a significant problem in the intensive care unit.

Penicillins

Pneumococcal or meningococcal meningitis, streptococcal endocarditis, and anaerobic lung abscesses (but not those caused by *Bacillus fragilis*) may be treated with penicillin G. To maintain minimal inhibitory serum concentrations, 1- or 2-hourly dosing may be necessary in meningitis. The penicillins often cause rashes, anaphylaxis, haemolytic anaemia, potassium-losing nephropathy, and pseudomembranous colitis. In patients with renal failure high serum concentrations of penicillins may induce seizures.

Broad-spectrum penicillins

Ampicillin and amoxicillin have an extended range of activity to include Gram-negative bacteria such as *Escherichia coli*, *H. influenzae*, *Proteus mirabilis*, *Salmonella* spp., and *Shigella* spp. Combination of these penicillins with an aminoglycoside for serious enterococcal infections reduces the emergence of resistance.

Penicillinase-resistant penicillins

Resistance to nafcillin and oxacillin seriously restricts the use of these agents in the treatment of staphylococcal infections in the critical care unit. These antistaphylococcal penicillins are indicated primarily when organisms can be reasonably predicted to be sensitive: when resistance is a possibility, an alternative agent such as vancomycin should be prescribed. The addition of an aminoglycoside enhances the efficacy of the penicillins, particularly in serious infections such as endocarditis or osteomyelitis.

α-Carboxy penicillins

Carbenicillin and ticarcillin, are antipseudomonal penicillins effective not only against *Pseudomonas aeruginosa*, but also against most Enterobacteriaceae, penicillin-sensitive Gram-positive organisms, and several anaerobes. These are generally unsuitable for empirical therapy because of their unpredictable activity against *Klebsiella pneumoniae* and enterococci. Like methicillin, the antipseudomonal penicillins may induce a potassium-losing nephropathy if used in high doses.

Ureidopenicillins

Piperacillin, mezlocillin, and azlocillin are extended spectrum penicillins. Azlocillin is effective against *Pseudomonas aeruginosa*, but less predictable in its activity against other Gram-negative bacilli. Mezlocillin and piperacillin are effective against all the organisms sensitive to carbenicillin and ticarcillin, but also very active against Klebsiella, enterococci, Serratia, and Citrobacter.

The half-life of ureidopenicillins is about 1.3 h and the recommended dose for critically ill patients is 3 to 4 g every 4 h. Resistance to the ureidopenicillins frequently emerges when it is used as empirical monotherapy and ideally they should be combined with an aminoglycoside such as gentamicin or netilmicin.

Cephalosporins

Due to their broad spectrum of activity, the cephalosporins are among the most frequently prescribed parenteral antibiotics for the critically ill. Because of their relative safety, these agents have been used extensively for surgical prophylaxis as well as treatment regimens.

Cephalosporins have been classified in terms of generations to denote similarities in chemical structure and chronology of release. However, it is probably better to consider the cephalosporins in terms of their potency and spectrum of activity. For example, first-generation cephalosporins are less active against aerobic Gram-negative bacilli than second-generation cephalosporins, while the third-generation agents are effective against a wide spectrum of organisms including Gram-negative bacilli. In addition, first-generation cephalosporins are generally more effective against Gram-positive cocci than are third-generation agents. Thus, first-generation cephalosporins are usually prescribed for staphylococcal or non-enterococcal streptococcal infections in patients with penicillin allergy without anaphylaxis.

All of the cephalosporins are relatively ineffective against enterococci or methicillin-resistant staphylococcal infections. Cross-sensitivity with penicillin allergy may be observed, taking the form of rash, anaphylaxis, neutropenia, drug fever, and pseudomembranous colitis. Occasionally there may be elevation of hepatic enzyme levels and haematological disturbances such as thrombocytopenia, leucopenia, or anaemia.

Cefotaxime, ceftriaxone, and ceftizoxime show similar spectra of activity in ill patients. However, they are relatively ineffective against *Pseudomonas aeruginosa*, methicillin-resistant staphylococci, and enterococci. Due to its ability to penetrate the blood–brain barrier, cefotaxime has been widely used in the treatment of Gram-negative bacillary meningitis. Ceftazidime has the benefit of being effective against *Pseudomonas aeruginosa* infections.

Carbapenems

Imipenem is a broad spectrum carbapenem combined with the dehydropeptidase inhibitor, cilastatin, which inhibits its enzymatic breakdown. Imipenem's activity against aerobic Gram-negative bacilli, including *Pseudomonas aeruginosa*, is comparable with that of aminoglycosides. It activity against *Staphylococcus aureus* and streptococci is similar to that of nafcillin.

Resistant strains of *Pseudomonas aeruginosa* have developed following imipenem therapy, and *Pseudomonas cepacia*, *Pseudomonas maltophilia*, and *Enterococcus faecium* are also resistant to imipenem.

The broad spectrum of imipenem makes this agent highly suitable for empirical therapy for the critically ill, especially when used in combination with an aminoglycoside and metronidazole. Seizures have been reported after the administration of large doses of imipenem or in patients with renal failure.

Monobactams

Aztreonam, is a monobactam antimicrobial, with a somewhat narrower spectrum of activity than other β-lactams. It has an antimicrobial spectrum similar to the aminoglycosides: although effective against *Pseudomonas aeruginosa*, combination with an aminoglycoside for pseudomonal infections may inhibit the development of resistant strains (Table 6).

β-Lactamase inhibitors

Several derivatives of the natural penicillins have broad spectra of activity. By combining these penicillins with β-lactamase inhibitors the activity spectrum can be broadened further to create a major class of antibiotics. The addition of the β-lactamase inhibitor clavulanic acid greatly enhances the activity of ticarcillin or amoxicillin, and broadens its spectrum of activity against anaerobes, *Staphylococcus aureus*, and aerobic Gram-negative organisms.

Aminoglycosides

Aminoglycosides, alone or combined with other antibiotics, remain an essential part of therapy for life-threatening Gram-negative infections. Variations in drug distribution mandate close monitoring of serum concentrations to achieve the therapeutic effect without toxicity.

The parenteral aminoglycosides most commonly used in the treatment of serious systemic infections include gentamicin, netilmicin, amikacin and tobramycin. The *in-vitro* antimicrobial activities of these aminoglycosides are similar, in terms of their activity, against Gram-negative organisms such as *Pseudomonas aeruginosa*.

The combination of an aminoglycoside with a β-lactam or with a monobactam antibiotic has been shown to enhance the *in-vitro* susceptibility of Gram-negative bacilli, especially *Pseudomonas aeruginosa*. Enterococci are generally resistant to penicillin, ampicillin, or vancomycin alone, but these drugs do exhibit synergy with the aminoglycosides. Gentamicin exhibits more synergy than streptomycin, tobramycin, or amikacin.

The plasma half-life and distribution, are similar for most aminoglycosides. The pharmacokinetics change in the critically ill patient with sepsis, heart failure, renal failure, or hepatic disease, and similar changes occur following surgery and during pregnancy. These factors tend to increase the volume of distribution so that loading and maintenance doses of the aminoglycosides have to be increased. Aminoglycosides are distributed throughout the extracellular fluid compartment, but because penetration of the blood–brain barrier is minimal, levels within the cerebrospinal fluid and brain tissue are poor. The aminoglycosides are excreted largely unchanged by glomerular filtration. The distribution and elimination of aminoglycosides are also influenced by the weight, age, and the state of hydration of the patient.

Gentamicin, netilmicin, and tobramycin require a loading dose of between 2 and 3 mg/kg followed by maintenance doses of 1.5 to 2.0 mg/kg. For amikacin, the loading dose is 10 to 12 mg/kg, followed by doses of 8 mg/kg. The loading dose and subsequent doses of these aminoglycosides are infused intravenously over 30 min. Maintenance doses are required every three to four half-lives: in the presence of normal renal function this would be every 8 to 12 h. In the anuric patient doses may need to be repeated only once every 24 h or even less frequently.

Although monitoring of aminoglycoside levels is laborious and expensive, combination therapy represents the best way of achieving an antimicrobial effect without encouraging the development of resistant strains. Plasma levels should be measured after the third or fourth dose, and then daily, before and 30 min after each dose.

Side-effects associated with aminoglycoside use include nephrotoxicity, ototoxicity, and accentuation of neuromuscular blockade. Aminoglycoside nephrotoxicity usually becomes evident within 5 to 7 days of commencing therapy: increased serum creatinine values are an indicator of established nephrotoxicity. Predicting nephrotoxicity is difficult but the presence of factors such as volume depletion and previous aminoglycoside treatment probably increase the risk. Factors associated with nephrotoxicity are trough concentrations greater than 2 μg/ml, the cumulative dose, and treatment courses longer than 2 to 3 weeks. Some degree of renal impairment may be observed in up to 25 per cent of patients receiving aminoglycoside therapy. However, the true nephrotoxic risk is difficult to assess since aminoglycosides tend to be used in patients already at risk of renal failure from their underlying illnesses. Indeed, concern over nephrotoxicity may divert attention away from otoxicity the implications of which are just as serious in terms of disability.

Quinolones

The fluoroquinolones represent a unique group of antibiotics. Recently available examples, such as ciprofloxacin, have a much broader spectrum of activity than the earlier quinolones, with

Table 6 Common antibiotics and their use in the critical care unit

Antibiotic	Organisms and applications
Penicillins	
Penicillin G	*Streptococcus* spp., Neisseria spp., *E. coli*, *Proteus mirabilis*, *Salmonella* spp., *Shigella* spp., most anaerobes (except *B. fragilis*).
Broad-spectrum penicillins	
Ampicillin	As for penicillin G except anaerobes; *H. influenzae* usually sensitive.
Penicillinase-resistant penicillins	
Methicillin, nafcillin, oxacillin	*Staph. aureus*, streptococci, and sensitive strains of *Staph. epidermidis*
Carbenicillin, ticarcillin	*Pseudomonas aeruginosa*, Enterobacteriaceae, non-penicillinase-producing Gram-positive cocci, *H. influenzae*, some *Bacteroides* spp.
Ureidopenicillins	
Mezlocillin	As for carbenicillin, plus *Enterococcus* spp., *Klebsiella* spp., *Serratia* spp., *Citrobacter* spp., and *Bacteroides* spp.
Piperacillin	As for mezlocillin, but also very active against *Pseudomonas aeruginosa*
Cephalosporins	
First-generation	
Cefazolin, cephalothin, cephradine	*Escherichia coli*, Klebsiella, *Proteus* spp., methicillin-sensitive *Staphylococcus aureus*, *Staphylococcus epidermidis*, streptococci, prophylaxis for clean surgery
Second-generation	
Cefamandole	As for cefazolin, plus *Haemophilus influenzae*, and some *Proteus* spp.
Cefuroxime	As for cefamandole, plus *Neisseria* spp. CNS application due to good blood–brain barrier penetration.
Cefoxitin	As for cefazolin, plus indole-positive *Proteus* spp. and *Bacteroides fragilis*; prophylaxis for surgery when *B. fragilis* may be present (e.g. gastrointestinal, genitourinary)
Third-generation	
Cefotaxime	As for cefamandole, but greater efficacy against Gram-negative bacilli, including *H. influenzae*, *Enterobacter* spp., and *Serratia* spp. Penetrates blood-brain barrier well and therefore used in Gram-negative bacillary meningitis in adults.
Ceftizoxime	As for cefotaxime plus anaerobes but except *B. fragilis*.
Ceftriaxone	As for cefotaxime but once daily dosage
Cefotetan	Similar to cefotaxime for Gram-negative bacteria, with some anaerobic activity
Ceftazidime	As for cefotaxime for Gram-negative bacteria; *Pseudomonas aeruginosa*, but with poor Gram-positive coverage
Carbapenems	
Imipenem/cilastatin	*Strep. pneumoniae*, Enterobacteriaceae, *Steph. aureus*, *Listeria* spp., *H. influenzae*, *Neisseria* spp., *P. aeruginosa*, *E. coli*, anaerobes including *B. fragilis*
Monobactams	
Aztreonam	Enterobacteriaceae, *E. coli*, *Proteus mirabillis*, *Klebsiella* spp., *H. influenzae*
β-Lactamase inhibitors	
Clavulanic acid	Combined with ticarcillin, enhanced activity against *B. fragilis* and *Pseudomonas aeruginosa*, *Staph. aureus*, and aerobic Gram-negative organisms
Sulbactam	Combined with ampicillin enhanced activity against *Bacteroides* spp., *Staph. aureus*, and aerobic Gram-negative organisms
Aminoglycosides	
Gentamicin	Enterobacteriaceae, *Klebsiella* spp., *Serratia* spp., *Pseudomonas aeruginosa*
Amikacin	As for gentamicin, but maybe effective against gentamicin-resistant enterobacteriaceae, and *Pseudomonas* spp.
Netilmicin	As for gentamicin but may be effective against gentamicin-resistant enterococcus and *Pseudomonas* spp.
Tobramycin	Similar to gentamicin but with enhanced activity against *Pseudomonas aeruginosa*
Streptomycin	Tuberculosis (combination therapy) tularaemia
Antianaerobic agents	
Metronidazole	Anaerobes, including *B. fragilis*, *Clostridium* spp., *Trichomonas* spp.
Clindamycin	*Bacteroides* spp., including *B. fragilis*, other anaerobes, *Streptococcus* spp., some activity against *Staphylococcus aureus*
Fluoroquinolones	
Ciprofloxacin	Wide spectrum including Gram-negative bacilli and *Staph. aureus*. Ineffective against *B. fragilis*
Others	
Erythromycin	*Mycoplasma pneumoniae*, *Legionella* spp., *Bordetella pertussis*, *Corynebacterium* spp., *H. influenzae*
Tetracycline	*Mycoplasma pneumoniae*, *Brucella* spp., non-chloera Vibrio, *Bacteroides* spp., *Rickettsia rickettsii*
Vancomycin	Methicillin-resistant staphylococcus, *Streptococcus faecalis*, *Clostridium difficile*
Trimethoprim/ sulphamethoxazole	*Pneumocystis carinii*, *Pseudomonas* spp., (except *Pseudomonas aeruginosa*), Nocardia
Chloramphenicol	*Haemophilus influenzae*, Neisseria, *Salmonella typhi*, *Brucella* spp., Gram-positive cocci, *Rickettsia* spp., *Clostridium* spp., *B. fragilis*

significant activity against Gram-negative bacilli and *Staphylococcus aureus*. Approximately 50 per cent of methicillin-resistant strains of *Staphylococcus aureus* are sensitive to ciprofloxacin, although it has limited activity against *Bacillus fragilis* and aerobic streptococci.

Tissue penetration is excellent with both oral and systemic ciprofloxacin, and fluid and tissue concentrations may exceed serum levels, except in bronchial secretions, cerebrospinal fluid, and saliva. A potential draw back of the fluoroquinolones may be the ease with which resistant strains develop. Like the β-lactams, combination therapy with aminoglycosides may be necessary in the critically ill patient.

Antianaerobic antibiotics

A wide range of antibiotics, including clindamycin, metronidazole, chloramphenicol, the extended spectrum penicillins cefoxitin, imipenem, and piperacillin are effective in treating anaerobic infections. The third-generation cephalosporins such as cefotetan, moxalactam, and ceftizoxime and more effective against *Bacteroides* spp. than the earlier generations of cephalosporins.

In view of the relative safety of metronidazole the inclusion of this agent in combination therapy is usually justified, especially if lower intestinal pathogens are a potential threat.

Clindamycin is the agent that is most often associated with the development of pseudomembranous colitis although several other antibiotics, including the cephalosporins, may also be implicated. Metronidazole therapy has been associated with neutropenia, polyneuropathy, and convulsions.

Other agents

Several antibiotics that have specific applications can be identified. These include erythromycin, tetracycline, vancomycin, trimethoprim/sulphamethoxazole, and the antituberculous agents. In addition specific antiviral and antifungal drugs are being used in critically ill patients with increasing frequency.

Erythromycin is the drug of choice for the treatment of Legionella infection, which should be considered in patients with pneumonia, renal impairment, gastrointestinal symptoms, or neurological abnormalities. Erythromycin therapy should be started intravenously at 1 g, 6-hourly. Erythromycin offers significant activity against other community-acquired infections, such as pneumococcal and mycoplasmal pneumonia.

Tetracycline remains the drug of choice for patients with Rocky Mountain spotted fever, brucellosis, or non-cholera Vibrio infections. The maximum adult daily dose of this agent is 2 g.

Vancomycin is usually effective against serious methicillin-resistant staphylococcal infections. It is also suitable for patients who have a history of anaphylactic reaction to penicillin. Vancomycin may be infused over at least 1 h at a dose of 1 g, repeated 8-h to 12-hourly in patients with normal renal function. In critically ill patients with suspected staphylococcal infection, vancomycin can be started before specific identification and sensitivities are available. Flucloxacillin/methicillin can be introduced later when sensitivities are known. As with the aminoglycosides peak and trough serum concentrations must be closely monitored for dose adjustment after 48 h: dose requirements are much reduced in the presence of renal failure.

Trimethoprim/sulphamethoxazole is most often used in the treatment of *Pneumocystis carinii* pneumonia. Pentamidine given either parenterally or by nebulization is an alternative therapy, particularly in AIDS patients. Trimethoprim/sulphamethoxazole has been recommended for use in the management of severe Nocardia infections, which characteristically respond to treatment with sulphonamides.

FURTHER READING

Barsa M, Imipenem. First of a new class of beta-lactam antibiotics. *Ann Intern Med*, 1985; **103**: 552–60.

Brown AE. Neutropenia, fever and infection. *Am J Med*, 1984; **76**: 421–5.

Centres for Disease Control. CDC definitions for nosocomial infections. *Am Rev Resp Dis*, 1988; **139**: 1058–9.

Chandrasekar PH, Kruse JA, Mathews MF. Nosocomial infection among patients in different types of intensive care units at a city hospital. *Crit Care Med*, 1986; **14**: 508–10.

Chastre JY, *et al.* Diagnosis of nosocomial bacterial pneumonia in intubated patients undergoing ventilation: comparison of the usefulness of bronchoalveolar lavage and the protected specimen brush. *Am J Med*, 1988; **85**: 499–506.

Chastre J, *et al.* Quantification of BAL cells containing intracellular bacteria rapidly identifies ventilated patients with nosocomial pneumonia. *Chest*, 1989; **95**: 190S–2S.

Craven DE, *et al.* Nosocomial infection and fatality in medical and surgical intensive care unit patients. *Arch Intern Med*, 1988; **148**: 1161–8.

Daschner F. Nosocomial infections in the intensive care unit. *Intensive Care Med*, 1985; **11**: 284–7.

Donowitz GR, Mandell GL. Beta-lactam antibiotics. *N Engl J Med*, 1988; **318**: 419–426, 490–499.

Dreyfuss D, *et al.* Prospective study of nosocomial pneumonia and of patient and circuit colonization during mechanical ventilation with circuit changes every 48 hours versus no change. *Am Rev Resp Dis*, 1991; **143**: 738–43.

Duma RJ. Aztreonam, the first monobactam. *Ann Intern Med*, 1987; **106**: 766–7.

Fagon JY, *et al.* Detection of nosocomial lung infection in ventilated patients. *Am Rev Resp Dis*, 1988; **138**: 1210–6.

Fagon JY, *et al.* Nosocomial pneumonia in patients receiving continuous mechanical ventilation. *Am Rev Resp Dis*, 1989; **139**: 877–84.

Gerding DN. *et al. Clostridium difficile*-associated diarrhea and colitis in adults: a prospective case controlled epidemiologic study. *Arch Intern Med*, 1986; **146**: 95–100.

Johnanson WG, Sedenfeld JJ, Gomez P, De Los Santos R, Coalson JJ. Bacteriologic diagnosis of nosocomial pneumonia following prolonged mechanical ventilation. *Am Rev Resp Dis*, 1988; **137**: 259–64.

Johanson WG, Pierce AK, Sanford JP, Thomas GD. Nosocomial respiratory infections with Gram-negative bacilli. The significance of colonization of the respiratory tract. *Ann Intern Med*, 1972; **77**: 701–6.

Joshi JH, Schimpff SC. Infections in the compromised host. In: Mandell GL, Douglas RG, Jr, Bennett JE, eds. *Principles and Practice of Infectious Diseases.* New York: John Wiley and Sons, Inc, 1985: 1644–9.

Leu HS, Kaiser DL, Mori M, Woolson RF, Wenzel RP. Hospital acquired pneumonia. Attributable mortality and morbidity. *Am J Epidemiol*, 1989; **129**: 1258–67.

McA Ledingham I, *et al.* Triple regimen of selective decontamination of the digestive tract, systemic cefotaxime, and microbiological surveillance for prevention of acquired infection in intensive care. *Lancet*, 1988; **i**: 785–90.

Neu HC. The emergence of bacterial resistance and its influence on empiric therapy. *Rev Infect Dis*, 1983; **5**: 59–520.

Schimpff SC. Acquired immunodeficiency syndrome. In: Moossa AR, Robson MC, Schimpff SC. eds. *Comprehensive Textbook of Oncology*. Baltimore: Williams and Wilkins, 1986: 605–14.

Smith C R, *et al.* Cefotaxime compared with nafcillin plus tobramycin for serious bacterial infections: a randomized, double blind trial. *Ann Intern Med*, 1985; **101**: 469–77.

Stoutenbeck CP, *et al.* The effect of selective decontamination of the digestive tract on colonization and the infection rate in multiple trauma patients. *Intensive Care Med*, 1984; **10**: 185–92.

The choice of antimicrobial drugs. *Med Lett Drugs Ther*, 1988; **30**: 33–40.

Torres A, *et al.* Diagnostic value of quantitative cultures of bronchoalveolar lavage and telescoping plugged catheters in mechanically ventilated patients with bacterial pneumonia. *Am Rev Resp Dis*, 1989; **140**: 306–10.

Torres A, *et al.* Incidence, risk, and prognosis factors of nosocomial pneumonia in mechanically ventilated patients. *Am Rev Resp Dis*, 1990; **142**: 523–8.

4.5 Critical care management of the trauma patient

CHRISTOPHER S. GARRARD

INTRODUCTION

Death following trauma has a trimodal distribution: the first peak of fatality occurs within seconds or minute of injury; the second peak occurs during the next few minutes to hours following injury and includes the so-called 'golden hour' which affords the clinician the best opportunity to safeguard the patient's life; the third peak occurs after several days and is a consequence of sepsis and multiple organ system failure. Clearly, the deaths occurring in the second and third periods may be influenced by the critical care clinician. A systematic approach to improving survival during the first hour has been the aim of the Advanced Trauma Life Support courses developed and sponsored by the American College of Surgeons. The basic philosophy of these courses carries through to intensive care management of trauma. Intensive care is generally required for patients requiring high levels of observation or organ system support such as mechanical ventilation. Retrospectively, the Injury Severity Score (ISS) correlates with the need for organ system support such as mechanical ventilation: patients requiring admission to a critical care unit usually have scores above 20. The aim of trauma critical care is to resuscitate and sustain the trauma victim while avoiding secondary complications.

Intensive care management can be considered in three phases. An acute resuscitative phase, an intermediate or consolidating phase and a late phase associated with secondary complications.

PHASE 1. ACUTE RESUSCITATION PHASE

This phase begins as soon as the patient is transferred to intensive care from the emergency room, trauma unit or referring hospital. While it is the responsibility of the referring physician to ensure that such transfers are conducted safely with the patient as stable as possible, the receiving physician should participate in defining standards of care prior to initiating transfer. Most urgent investigations will have already been performed but others may still be required after admission to the intensive care unit. During the first few minutes on the intensive care unit the patient will be rapidly reassessed by the receiving physician. Simultaneously the transferring physician provides a brief, verbal review of prehospital history and subsequent management.

The following initial evaluation plan is based upon the *Advanced Trauma Life Support Instructor Manual* (American College of Surgeons Committee on Trauma 1988)

Assess the airway and cervical spine

If the patient is not intubated, the airway should be checked. In intubated patients, patency of the airway, the position of the endotracheal tube, and cuff pressure of the tube should be ascertained.

Any difficulty or complications associated with intubation should be known, and the endotracheal tube should be examined to determine whether size and length are appropriate. If there are any causes for concern over the position or function of the endotracheal tube it should be changed. Procedures, including endotracheal intubation, can only be performed while control of the cervical spine is maintained.

The cervical spine must be stabilized until a cervical spine fracture can be excluded. All cervical spine films should be reviewed personally: the cervical spine should be assumed to be unstable until proven otherwise. The patient may be received in the critical care unit on a full spinal board, with stiff neck collar with sandbag support. This should be retained until the cervical spine can be cleared or a suitable replacement instituted.

Assess breathing

If chest movement and air entry are not adequate and symmetrical, the reason should be determined. Signs of cyanosis should also be looked for.

The position of the endotracheal tube should be confirmed to exclude endobronchial intubation, and pneumothorax or haemothorax that could have developed since the initial evaluation should be excluded. If chest drains are already *in situ* they should be functioning normally; if not, there may be a need for a new thoracostomy tube.

If the patient is mechanically ventilated, any change in inflation pressures since initial assessment should be recorded. A sudden rise in peak inflation pressure may suggest pneumothorax, haemothorax or airway obstruction. The latter may take the form of a local obstruction due to kinked endotracheal tube, mucus or a foreign body, or generalized obstruction with wheezing, consistent with asthma.

All trauma patients must receive supplemental oxygen, and this should continue until any possible causes of hypoxaemia have been excluded. Pulse oximetry is an ideal way of monitoring oxygenation. Unless there are reasons to suspect chronic obstructive pulmonary disease the concentration of oxygen need not be restricted.

There is good evidence that oxygen uptake is increased during the immediate post-traumatic period, resulting in reduced mixed venous saturation. Supplemental oxygen, mechanical ventilation and inotropic support may therefore be required to ensure adequate oxygen delivery. It is essential that inotropic support is not confused with the need for adequate volume replacement.

Assess circulation and bleeding

Monitoring of vital signs, pulse, skin capillary refill, and blood pressure will determine whether there is continued blood loss: multiple fractures can be responsible for effective blood losses of over 40 per cent of total blood volume, and intra-abdominal bleeding should also be considered. Peritoneal lavage or abdominal CT may be performed if this was not carried out in the emergency room.

The total transfused volume of fluid should be determined, including crystalloid, colloid, and blood products. The availability of type-specific or cross-matched blood and quantity should be determined.

All patients suffering major trauma should have good venous access established during initial resuscitation, with at least two 14-gauge venous catheters. A single lumen central line may provide a satisfactory portal for drug administration and central venous pressure monitoring but is inadequate for aggressive volume resuscitation.

Assess neurological disability

Is the patient alert? Does the patient respond to verbal commands or is the patient unconscious? This simplified ATLS neurological score (alert, responds to voice, responds to pain, unresponsive; AVPU) should be repeated to detect any change since admission and then replaced by the Glasgow Coma Score. Any change in pupil size and reactivity since admission should be recorded.

Assess total body surface

The patient should be examined from top to toe, and any further injuries identified. Results should be correlated with earlier findings.

The entire surface of the patient must be inspected on admission to the critical care unit, especially the head and back. The history of the trauma event and the resulting injuries should be reviewed carefully. Could there be any other injuries that have not been excluded?

Formal internal fixation and stabilization of fractures will often be undertaken during the first 24 h to facilitate nursing care and reduce the risk of fat embolus.

Anticipation of events related directly to the original injury and unrelated complications is the key to good management. Table 1 lists some of these events in order to their probable chronology.

Table 1 Time of onset of trauma associated complications

Event	Time after injury
Cardiac rupture	<1 h
Diaphragmatic tear	<1 h
Aortic rupture	<1 h
Pneumothorax	<1 h
Haemothorax	<1 h → 6 h
Pneumomediastinum	<1 h → 6 h
Splenic rupture	<1 h → 6 h
Oesophageal rupture	6 h → 1 day
Small bowel perforation	6 h → 1 day
Lung contusion	0 h → 2 days
Cerebral oedema	6 h → 4 days
Fat embolism	6 h → 4 days
Delayed splenic rupture	1 → 4 days
Pancreatitis	1 → 4 days
Bronchial tear	<1 h → 7 days
Respiratory failure	<1 h → 7 days +
Cardiac contusion	1 h → 7 days
Renal failure	1 → 10 days
Nosocomial infection/sepsis	2 → 10 days

Neuroendocrine responses to trauma

During the 24 h following injury, changes in neurological and endocrine activity have a significant effect on the clinical course. Activation of the sympathetic nervous system defends the circulation against hypovolaemia by venous and arteriolar vasoconstriction and by increasing the rate and force of myocardial contraction. Metabolically there is glycogenolysis, fat mobilization, and reduced insulin secretion. Decreased blood volume leads to decreased perfusion of the kidney and increased renin secretion, which in turn activates angiotensin II and stimulates aldosterone release. Consequently, the circulation is further protected by vasoconstriction and salt and water retention. In response to pain, nausea, or any reduction in left atrial filling pressure, ADH secretion is also promoted, increasing the resorption of water from the distal renal tubules and collecting ducts. The adrenocortical response to severe trauma consists of an increase in ACTH from the anterior pituitary. Cortisol levels increase three- or four-fold unless there is adrenal insufficiency.

PHASE 2. INTERMEDIATE CONSOLIDATING PHASE

After the first 24 h most direct effects of injury will have declared themselves and will have been treated. Patients are typically haemodynamically stable, may have some degree of gas exchange impairment (due to lung contusion) and a proportion will require mechanical ventilation. If intubation is indicated in patients who have suffered crush injury, burns, or spinal cord injury, the use of depolarizing muscle relaxants should be avoided in view of the risk of sudden hyperkalaemia. Gastric paresis and a full stomach may be present 24 h after trauma and represent a significant hazard during intubation. Analgesia should be maintained to keep the patient comfortable and sedation should be used judiciously, particularly following head injury. Renal function is usually unimpaired at this stage unless there has been outflow obstruction or renal damage due to crush injury and myoglobinuria. Nutritional support is commenced, preferably as enteral feeding, but as total parenteral nutrition if necessary. If enteral feeding is not possible stress ulcer prophylaxis is required, preferably with a cytoprotective agent such as sucralfate.

Selective digestive tract decontamination has been recommended to reduce the rate of upper gastrointestinal tract colonization by Gram-negative organisms. Despite its rather marginal benefits in routine use, trauma patients may benefit most from such treatment. The focus of critical care management in the intermediate consolidating phase is to avoid iatrogenic complications and limit the risk of subsequent nosocomial infection.

PHASE 3. LATE PHASE WITH SECONDARY COMPLICATIONS

Secondary complications begin to appear towards the end of the first week of admission, but may occur within 48 h.

Infection

Hospital-acquired infection by endogenous bacteria is a continual threat, to the patient. The incidence of nosocomial infection increases with increasing severity of injury, the number and level of invasive clinical procedures, and the length of admission. After 10 days of critical care admission very few patients escape some form of hospital-acquired infection. The systemic signs of infection, fever, and leucocytosis may herald the appearance of the sepsis syndrome with organ system failure, although leucocytosis may be absent in the severely injured patient. In many patients the type of injury will suggest the source of infection, while in ventilated patients nosocomial pneumonia must always be considered. The stress of trauma and gastrointestinal tract colonization with Gram-negative organisms may result in bacterial or endotoxin translocation across the intestinal wall into the circulation, precipitating the sepsis syndrome.

Respiratory failure

The respiratory system is commonly involved with differing degrees of respiratory impairment. The most severe examples are manifest as the adult respiratory distress syndrome, which requires a prolonged period of mechanical ventilation. Adult respiratory distress syndrome following trauma may result from lung contusion, fat embolism, massive blood transfusion, aspiration of gastric contents, or in association with the sepsis syndrome. Lung contusion and, by the same token, myocardial contusion, must be suspected in any patient with fractured ribs, sternal fracture, or anterior flail segment. Ventilator management is directed at maintaining adequate arterial oxygenation without circulatory embarrassment, oxygen toxicity, or barotrauma.

Fat embolism syndrome

In its classical form, fat embolism syndrome presents with dyspnoea, skin petechiae, hypoxaemia, thrombocytopenia, falling haemoglobin, and fat globules in the urine. It is most common in patients with extensive and multiple fractures, occurring in up to 5 per cent of patients with combined pelvic and femoral fractures. Fat droplets may activate platelet aggregation with resultant consumption coagulopathy. Fat lodging in the lung is converted by lipase to free fatty acid that causes acute lung injury. Petechial haemorrhages over the torso, axillae, and conjunctivae probably result from a combination of thrombocytopenia and circulating fatty acids. Treatment is supportive and includes vasopressors, inotropes, and mechanical ventilation. There is some evidence to suggest that treatment with high-dose corticosteroids may reduce platelet aggregation. Other agents such as aspirin and heparin carry a significant risk of haemorrhage and are not recommended.

Renal failure

In the oliguric patient prerenal azotaemia and obstructive uropathy must be excluded before attributing renal failure to vasomotor nephropathy (acute tubular necrosis). Haemofiltration or haemodialysis should be commenced once reversible renal impairment has been excluded.

Cardiovascular failure

Most cardiovascular problems relate to the initial acute resuscitative phase. However, during the late phase the effects of myocardial contusion and sepsis syndrome may be associated with impaired myocardial contractility and hypotension. Appropriate use of inotropes and vasoactive agents may be required to support the circulation. Late hypovolaemia resulting from secondary haemorrhage or delayed rupture of the spleen should always be considered.

FURTHER READING

American College of Surgeons Committee on Trauma. *Advanced Trauma Life Support Instructor Manual*. Chicago: ACS, 1988.

Chandrasekar, PH, Kruse JA, Mathews MF. Nosocomial infection among patients in different types of intensive care units at a city hospital. *Crit Care Med*, 1986; **14**: 508–10.

Cournard A, *et al.* Studies of the circulation in clinical shock. *Surgery*, 1943; **13**: 964–95.

Cowan BN, Burns HJG, Boyle P, Ledingham I. McA. The relative prognostic value of lactate and haemodynamic measurements in early shock. *Anaesthesia*, 1984; **39**: 750–5.

Craven DE, *et al.* Nosocomial infection ad fatality in medical and surgical care unit patients. *Arch Intern Med* 1988; **148**: 1161–8.

Edwards JD. Oxygen transport following major trauma. In: Vincent, J. L. (ed. *Update in Intensive Care and Emergency Medicine*. Berlin: Springer Verlag, 1988; **5**: 25–31.

Shoemaker WC, *et al.* Pathogenesis of respiratory failure (ARDS) after haemorrhage and trauma. *Crit Care Med*, 1980; **8**: 504–12.

Stoutenbeck CP, *et al.* The effect of selective decontamination of the digestive tract on colonization and the infection rate in multiple trauma patients. *Intensive Care Med*, 1984; **10**: 185–92.

4.6 Central nervous system aspects

CHRISTOPHER S. GARRARD

THE TREATMENT OF BRAIN INJURY

Preventative of brain injury (cerebral protection) is only possible in certain circumstances such as in patients undergoing cardiopulmonary bypass. Hypothermia and the barbiturates are particularly effective for this. Therapy commenced during a cerebral insult may be referred to as cerebral preservation while cerebral resuscitation describes any therapy begun after brain injury. Cerebral preservation occurs in the cold water drowning victim who makes a good neurological recovery despite a prolonged period beneath the water.

MECHANISMS OF BRAIN INJURY

Several processes interact at cellular level to determine the viability of brain tissue following injury. Each of these processes can be altered or ameliorated by brain-orientated intensive care. The rapid re-establishment of cerebral blood flow is of critical importance: brain oxygen stores are depleted in about 10 s and brain glucose and ATP stores are depleted 5 min following circulatory arrest. Some cerebral neurones are able to tolerate normothermic ischaemia for somewhat longer periods and the most extreme form of cellular damage, autolysis of brain tissue, begins after 1 to 2 h of no blood flow.

After circulatory arrest of more than 5 min, reperfusion and reoxygenation may cause irreversible brain damage, in the same way that other organ systems may be damaged. However, the widely held belief that a normothermic circulatory arrest lasting longer than 5 min is incompatible with recovery of normal brain function is not always correct. Several studies in animal models have shown good cerebral recovery after periods of circulatory arrest of more than 15 min and there have been reports of humans recovering after arrest times of up to 15 min.

The degree of brain injury, regardless of the nature of the insult, depends first upon the severity and duration of the injury and second, upon the speed and efficiency of resuscitation. To this should be added a third factor, the early application of brain-orientated intensive care.

BRAIN-ORIENTATED INTENSIVE CARE

Brain-orientated intensive care is broadly based and comprises several modalities (Table 1). All organ systems must be actively supported and function restored as quickly as possible. The period immediately following cardiopulmonary resuscitation for circulatory arrest may be characterized by persistent metabolic acidosis and impaired cardiac contractility: the myocardium may need to be supported with inotropes and gas exchange maintained by mechanical ventilation until any acidosis resolves. Bicarbonate infusion is best avoided since alkalinizing agents may worsen cerebral and myocardial intracellular acidosis.

The systemic blood pressure should be supported with vasopressors if autoregulatory mechanisms are impaired. Cardiac arrhythmias must be rigorously controlled. Biochemical abnormalities such as hyperglycaemia should be corrected. If sodium bicarbonate has been used injudiciously during resuscitation, serum osmolality may be significantly increased: the use of mannitol as an osmotic diuretic could further exaggerate the hyperosmolar state and serial measurements of serum osmolality may need to be made. Hyperglycaemia should be controlled with insulin if necessary since preischaemic hyperglycaemia has been shown to worsen the outcome of both global and focal cerebral ischaemia.

The management of blood pressure in patients with brain injury and raised intracranial pressure is controversial. Hypotension

Table 1 Some modalities of cerebral intensive care

1. Restoration of the circulation by regulation of:
    - Cardiac contractility/rhythm
        - Inotropes
        - Pacing
        - Mechanical support
    - Vascular tone
        - Vasopressors
        - Hypotensive agents
    - Intravascular filling
        - Central venous pressure/pulmonary arterial wedge pressure monitoring
        - Transfusion
2. Prevent agitation or restlessness
    - Sedatives
        - Benzodiazepines
        - Barbiturates
        - Propofol
    - Neuromuscular relaxants
        - Non-depolarizing
3. Prevent or treat seizures
    - Benzodiazepines
    - Barbiturates
    - Phenytoin
    - Valproate
4. Ventilator support
    - Moderate hyperventilation
    - Normoxia
5. Regulation of intracranial pressure
    - Hyperventilation
    - Mannitol
    - Loop diuretic
    - Sedation
6. Maintain normothermia
    - Suppress hyperthermia
    - Hypothermia?
7. Moderate haemodilution
8. Specific pharmacologic agents
    - Barbiturates
    - Calcium-channel blockers
    - Free radical scavengers

carries the risk of global hypoperfusion, while hypertension, although maintaining perfusion pressure, encourages the development of cerebral oedema. Common sense dictates a strategy aimed at avoiding extremes of blood pressure, with target systolic blood pressures between 100 and 160 mmHg. To this end, direct intra-arterial blood pressure monitoring is preferred to non-invasive methods. Theoretically, vasodilators such as hydralazine, nitroprusside, and nitroglycerin should be avoided since they could cause stealing of blood flow away from the brain. In practice, however, agents such as nitroprusside and nitroglycerin are very effective in reducing blood pressure.

Hyperthermia unrelated to infection may be observed in the early phases following head injury or brain ischaemia. Active efforts to lower the temperature should be made with antipyretic (acetaminophen) and cooling. Small intravenous doses of chlorpromazine (2.5 mg for adults) may be effective when other measures fail. It is well recognized that hypothermia at the time of cerebral injury protects the brain against anoxic insult.

Cerebral oedema and the reduction in cerebral perfusion brought about by raised intracranial pressure is a particular problem in trauma and encephalitis. Almost 80 per cent of patients with severe head injury have some degree of elevation in intracranial pressure; 50 per cent of deaths are directly attributable to raised intracranial pressure. It has also been estimated that up to one-third of deaths due to head injury may occur without any such increase. Cerebral oedema following circulatory arrest is less commonly associated with increased intracranial pressure. The normal pressure, of less than 15 mmHg at rest, with wide swings according to body activity and position, is determined by the relationship of the intracranial and intraspinal volume to the restricted rigid skull vault and the more compliant spinal subarachnoid space. The volume compartments within the skull are the brain, the cerebrospinal fluid, and the intravascular blood. Cerebrospinal fluid and blood are displaced as brain tissue swells. The relationship between intracranial pressure and increases in volume is not linear, but is roughly exponential. At high pressures (>25 mmHg) a small increase in volume causes a steep rise in pressure, but little damage is caused until cerebral blood flow becomes restricted. An intracranial pressure which is sustained at above 50 mmHg results in greatly reduced cerebral perfusion and is usually fatal.

Considerable controversy exists regarding the effects on outcome of monitoring intracranial pressure. Evidence to show that such monitoring significantly improves survival following head trauma is less than convincing, but neurological deterioration often appears to follow episodes of raised intracranial pressure, and patients with persistently raised intracranial pressure generally have a poor outcome. If attempts to lower intracranial pressure are to be made at all, measurement would seem logical: the clinician can then titrate therapy to achieve an acceptable cerebral perfusion pressure (mean arterial pressure minus mean intracranial pressure) of greater than the critical level of 40 mmHg. Perfusion pressures in the range 60 to 80 mmHg are ideal, but are not always attainable.

Clinical signs are poor indicators of intracranial pressure: temporal lobe lesions may be associated with third nerve signs at a lower pressure than lesions elsewhere and diffuse bilateral cerebral lesions cause pupillary enlargement only when pressure is considerably greater than 25 mmHg. Sixth nerve palsy is commonly described but is not a reliable indicator of raised intracranial pressure.

Currently available techniques for the measurement of intracranial pressure use either a hollow subarachnoid screw (Richmond bolt), ventricular catheter, or miniature strain gauges. Intraventricular catheters probably carry a higher risk of infection but also provide a more reliable measurement.

A recent innovation, infrared transmission cerebral spectroscopy, may provide a convenient and non-invasive method of evaluating the state of oxygenation of the brain by measuring the haemoglobin saturation of predominantly mixed venous cerebral blood. Whether this technique will provide clinically useful information remains to be seen but initial evaluations appear encouraging.

Mechanical hyperventilation to reduce the $P\text{CO}_2$ to below 3.5 kPa (<30 mmHg) will rapidly lower intracranial pressure by causing cerebral vasoconstriction. These effects are seen within minutes, but are dissipated within 1 to 2 h. Further reduction in intracranial pressure requires a further increase in the level of hyperventilation and reducing the level of ventilation may result in an increase in pressure unless the underling pathology has been reversed. An excessive reduction in $P\text{CO}_2$ or elevation in arterial pH may reduce cerebral perfusion and oxygen offloading and may therefore be counter productive. Hyperoxia should probably be avoided. Hyperventilation necessitates higher mean airway pressures and the ventilator should be regulated to produce the highest alveolar ventilation for the lowest inflation pressures. This can often be attained using an assisted mode such as volume assist or pressure assist in a non-paralysed patient. If the patient is intolerant of this approach and becomes agitated, full sedation and, if necessary, neuromuscular relaxation will allow the patient to be maintained on SIMV (synchronized intermittent mandatory ventilation) or a control mode of ventilation. Although hyperventilation is an established mode of treatment of raised intracranial pressure, there are no clinical trials proving its efficacy, and one recent study has suggested poorer long-term outcome (3–6 months) in patients hyperventilated following head injury. In experimental models of brain injury, hyperventilation neither reduces brain lactate nor improves the energy state (phosphocreatine: inorganic phosphate ratio) of the brain.

Hyperosmolar therapy with mannitol and frusemide (furosemide) is widely recommended for production of a sustained reduction in intracranial pressure. Mannitol can be administered as a single bolus dose of 0.5 to 1 g/kg body weight, or repeated as an infusion of 0.25 to 0.5 g/kg. This induces an osmotic gradient that reduces intracranial pressure for 3 to 4 h in most patients. Side-effects, due to systemic dehydration and intravascular volume depletion, including the precipitation of a non-ketotic hyperosmolar state in diabetics, may be seen with mannitol. Frusemide (furosemide) complements the action of mannitol, but may be less effective when used alone.

Barbiturate administration following acute cerebral injury may have several beneficial effects. Control of agitation and restlessness by sedative agents minimizes intracranial pressure changes, and seizures should be prevented. Barbiturates may also possess specific cerebral protective properties, although this is contentious and offers an avenue for further investigation. Clinical studies in humans have produced conflicting results, but some cerebral protection appears to have accrued from the use of barbiturates in patients with Reye's syndrome. There are sound reasons why barbiturates should protect the brain following injury (Table 2).

Of the barbiturates available, thiopentone (pentothal) is an excellent sedative agent and anticonvulsant. With prolonged use it

Table 2 Potential cerebral protective effects of barbiturates

1. Decrease cerebral oedema
2. Reduce the cerebral metabolic rate
3. Reduce intracranial pressure
4. Decrease free fatty acid formation
5. Scavenge free radicals
6. Silence EEG activity
7. Reduce brain infarct size in focal ischaemia
8. Increase tolerance to carotid occlusion

is distributed widely throughout the body and its effects are then slow to clear. Until properly conducted clinical studies can convincingly show a specific cerebral protective effect of barbiturates, justification for their use will be limited to the sedative and anticonvulsant effects.

The calcium-channel blockers, particularly nimodipine, improve survival following subarachnoid haemorrhage by reversing cerebral vasospasm. They probably act by reducing the intracellular release and accumulation of free ionized calcium and inhibition of mitochondrial activity, which occurs during ischaemia and reperfusion. Studies in animals and in man have examined the potential protective effect of calcium-channel blockers in a much wider range of cerebral injury with some indication of a beneficial response following cardiac arrest. Despite a degree of cerebral selectivity, the use of calcium-channel blockers may be limited by adverse effects such as systemic hypotension.

Free radicals are short-lived highly reactive compounds that are released during the reperfusion of ischaemic neuronal issue and initiate sustained lipid peroxidation. Free radical scavengers such as superoxide dismutase, desferrioxamine, thiopentone, vitamin E, vitamin C, glutathione, chlorpromazine, mannitol, and some dextrans have been used in an attempt to reduce the effects of reperfusion injury of several organs including the brain. Preliminary studies have shown no protective effect of desferrioxamine and a calcium-channel blocker in a dog ischaemic brain model, although desferrioxamine alone appeared to reduce cerebral damage following shorter periods of cerebral ischaemia. The use of free radical scavengers cannot yet be recommended, however rational their application may seem.

Corticosteroids have no beneficial effect in cerebral oedema associated with head injury, and their effects following cardiac arrest have not been adequately explored. Their use in brain-orientated intensive care, other than to reduce high intracranial pressure associated with brain metastases, cannot be recommended.

The interaction of certain drugs with γ-aminobutyric acid receptors may have some application in cerebral protection. Drugs such as diazepam (benzodiazepine receptor agonist), baclofen (γ-aminobutyric acid B agonist), valproic acid (γ-aminobutyric acid transaminase inhibitor), and pentobarbital (an effector of γ-aminobutyric acid A receptors) require further evaluation as protective agents.

THE PATIENT IN COMA

Coma is a state of depressed level of consciousness and should be distinguished from the abnormal content of consciousness that results in confusion, delirium, or psychosis. The drowsy patient (level) may also be confused (content), although the converse may not be true. The level of consciousness should always be quantified in terms of some standard such as the Glasgow Coma Score (Table 3). By accurately recording coma scores, small changes in conscious level can be recognized and if necessary, acted upon. Most patients admitted to intensive care in coma will have a score of less than 6.

Table 3 Glasgow Coma Score

	Points
Eye opening (maximum 4 points)	
Spontaneous	4
To speech	3
To pain	2
None	1
Verbal response (maximum 5 points)	
Orientated	5
Confused conversation	4
Inappropriate words	3
Incomprehensible sounds	2
None	1
Best motor response (maximum 6 points)	
Obeys commands	6
Localizes to pain	5
Withdraws to pain	4
Abnormal flexion	3
Extensor response	2
None	1

Highest score = 15, lowest = 3.

The level of consciousness emanates from the reticular activating system and the cerebral hemispheres. Transient loss of consciousness (concussion) after head trauma has been attributed to rotation of the hemispheres about the midbrain/diencephalic junction. Ultrastructural changes occur in the brain neurones, even with very transient loss of consciousness after trauma. Prolonged loss of consciousness (coma), whether or not related to trauma, is usually associated with lesions in either both hemispheres, one hemisphere with compression of the upper brainstem, or in the brain-stem reticular activating system. When coma is due to injury to the reticular activating system, other signs of brain-stem dysfunction such as pupillary, caloric, and oculomotor signs are usually apparent.

The predominant causes of coma vary from centre to centre: drug intoxication and head injury may be more common in the inner city while metabolic disease such as diabetic coma, cerebrovascular events, and mass lesions may predominate in other hospitals. A careful clinical history and physical examination are therefore paramount in determining the underlying cause of coma. A list of common causes of coma is shown in Table 4.

Diagnosis

Diagnostic dilemmas often arise when coma is due to drugs or metabolic causes, when physical signs may be consistent with both cerebellar and brain-stem lesions, depending upon the severity of the metabolic disturbance. However, pupil size and reactivity are usually well preserved despite severe obtundation.

Patients with severe myasthenia gravis, Guillain-Barré syndrome, or basilar artery thrombosis may appear to be in coma although they may be receptive. The so called 'locked-in' syndrome due to cranial nerve and limb paralysis may be extremely

Table 4 Some common causes of coma

Primary CNS causes
1. Vascular
    - Haemorrhage
    - Infarction
    - Vasculitis
2. Trauma
    - Direct neuronal damage
    - Secondary haemorrhage
    - Secondary ischaemia/hypoxia
    - Cerebral oedema
3. Infection
    - Encephalitis
    - Meningitis
    - Abscess
4. Postictal
5. Malignancy
    - Primary mass
    - Metastases
    - Oedema

Secondary CNS causes
1. Drugs
    - Alcohol
    - Sedatives
    - Narcotics
2. Metabolic
    - Glucose metabolism-hyper/hypoglycaemia
    - Osmolar disturbances
    - Endocrine disorders–pituitary, adrenal, thyroid
    - Electrolyte disturbances
    - Hypoxia/hypercarbia
    - Hepatic encephalopathy
    - Uraemic encephalopathy
    - Extreme hypo/hyperthermia
3. Circulatory failure
    - Cerebral hypoperfusion
        - Sepsis syndrome
        - Heart failure
        - Hypovolaemic shock

difficult to distinguish from coma: the clinical significance of this becomes only too apparent when considering patients as potential organ donors.

Computerized tomography (CT) of the head may define anatomical abnormalities and confirm a clinical diagnosis. Although the CT scan is generally a safe procedure and is available to most critically ill patients it should not be used indiscriminantly, bearing in mind the risks associated with transporting the patient to the radiography department. Conversely, changes in coma score may mean that repeated scans are necessary to determine the requirement for surgical intervention.

The pupillary reflex must be assessed with care and attention: a cursory evaluation with a poor light source is clearly inadequate. Contraction of only 1 mm is sufficient to indicate pupillary responsiveness. Unequal pupils may be found following the instillation of mydriatics or direct trauma to the eye.

The presence of full and conjugate eye movements indicates an intact pons and midbrain. Normally, turning the head from side to side will cause the eyes initially to move conjugately in the opposite direction followed quickly by eye movement in the direction of head movement. The presence of 'doll's eyes', which remain fixed in relation to the head, indicates brain-stem damage and should be confirmed by caloric testing. Abducted (outward looking) eyes are common in stuporous or drowsy patients and should not be interpreted as a bad prognostic sign. As coma deepens the eyes may become fixed in the primary position.

Limb movement affords the most reliable method of detecting asymmetric neurological function. Movements of a limb away from the body (i.e. pushing away) indicate an intact corticospinal pathway and this type of purposeful limb should always be distinguished from flexion, extension, or pronation. The triple flexion response of the hip, knee, and ankle joints in response to tactile stimuli is not necessarily purposeful since it is integrated at the level of the spinal cord.

Management

Protection of the airway takes precedence over all other aspects of management. Failure to protect the airway and control the cervical spine in a comatose patient with head injury must be considered to be serious omissions. Positioning of the patient in the semiprone or Fowler's position may be adequate in the drowsy patient with an intact gag reflex but as consciousness fades, endotracheal intubation may be required. The technique of intubation should combine speed, safety, and avoidance of factors that may increase intracranial pressure.

Prognosis

Predicting the outcome of coma, regardless of the underlying cause, is a difficult task. Apart from unequivocal brain death there are no clinical signs that confidently predict outcome. Young patients may have many early clinical signs consistent with poor outlook and yet may make a full recovery. Assessment of prognosis based on neurological findings should be interpreted broadly, and in conjunction with the patient's age and prior medical condition. The clinician's approach to management should also incorporate a consideration of the patient's premorbid wishes, if these are known.

Prognostication in cases of head injury is usually more accurate than in non-traumatic coma, for which there are many aetiologies. While more than 90 per cent of patients in whom pupillary or oculomotor reflexes are absent in the first 6 h following injury will die, 4 per cent may still make a significant recovery: this proportion is large enough to make the clinician hesitate to abandon support in the first 24 h. Some favourable and unfavourable signs of recovery in the comatose head injury patient are summarized in Table 5. Such signs can be cautiously applied to patients with coma due to other causes, but with less confidence.

Somatosensory evoked potentials may offer useful information, particularly in children. Absence of cortical responses with preserved lower level brain potentials appears to be a reliable indicator of poor outlook in anoxic coma and following head injury.

In practice, an expectant policy allowing time for the development of convincing signs, full evaluation, and neurological consultation to take place seems to be the most acceptable. In those patients in whom the outlook is grave, family and relatives can come to terms with reality. A period of 48 to 72 h may be needed initially. The primary physician should indicate clearly the management policy to nursing staff and house staff, particularly after

Table 5 Predictive signs of outcome in head injury patients

Favourable signs of recovery in first 72 h
Early wakening
Verbal response
Intact caloric response
Fending off external stimuli
Normal muscle tone
Unfavourable signs in the first 24 h
Absent spontaneous eye opening
Absent spontaneous eye movement
Absent pupillary response
Absent corneal reflex
Absent caloric response
Absent deep tendon reflexes
Absent muscle tone

full and frank discussion with the nearest relatives. In some cases, extubation may be possible and more conservative management plans adopted.

BRAIN DEATH

The accurate and reliable determination of brain death has become an essential part of clinical practice in the critical care unit. Brain-dead patients need to be identified so that either unnecessary life support can be discontinued or so that transplantation organ donation can be considered and organized. It is unnecessary to establish the diagnosis of brain death, unless organ transplantation or the cessation of life support measures is deemed appropriate.

The criteria used acknowledge the fact that independent, self-sustaining life is not possible in patients with brain-stem death. It is also inevitable that within a short period of time (usually hours, but at most 2 or 3 days) circulatory collapse and cardiac arrest will occur which will be unresponsive to any medical measures.

Before undertaking brain death testing in the comatose patient several preconditions must be satisfied. First, a definitive cause for coma must be established. Second the patient requires mechanical ventilation and third, enough time must have elapsed from the onset of coma to determine that the brain injury is irreversible. This time interval will vary according to the cause of the brain injury. For example, following head trauma or a major intracranial haemorrhage 6 to 12 h may be sufficient time to be sure that recovery is not possible. In the case of hypoxic brain injury secondary to cardiac or respiratory arrest 24 to 48 h may be needed. If any doubt exists as to possible effects of drugs, periods extending up to 7 days may need to be considered. The elimination of drugs and duration of activity is extremely variable. Some agents, such as nortriptyline, diazepam, methadone, and phenobarbitone have prolonged plasma half-lives of between 10 and 150 h and may therefore have very extended activity.

Brain death criteria

The tests of brain-stem function include many of the cranial nerve reflexes and the activity of the respiratory centre. Pupillary reaction to light depends upon the integrity of the optic nerve, the midbrain, and, the oculomotor nerve (III). The corneal reflexes are dependent on the afferent trigeminal (V) and the facial nerve (VIII).

Dysfunction of both cerebral hemispheres disinhibits the brain-stem reflex mechanisms for conjugate eye movements. Normally, turning the head from side to side elicits easy or 'loose' conjugate eye movements in the oppositive direction. Brain-stem dysfunction cause one or both eyes to fail to move fully and conjugately. Abducens nerve (VI) palsy indicates pontine dysfunction or diffuse increase in intracranial pressure. Oculomotor nerve (III) palsy with absence of full adduction of one eye also indicates midbrain pathology. The pattern of spontaneous respiration may become periodic when both hemispheres are affected, and irregular or absent when the inferior pons and medulla are involved.

Established hospital guidelines for the diagnosis of brain death should be rigorously adhered to. The completion of a standard form to be made part of the patient's record is generally desired. Table 6 lists many of the most widely accepted brain death criteria.

Table 6 Criteria for the diagnosis of brain death

Preconditions
1. Patient is in coma, receiving mechanical ventilation
2. Definitive diagnosis of the cause of coma
3. Enough time elapsed to ensure irreversibility
4. Two doctors perform the tests independently (the doctors should be of senior rank and clearly identified)

Exclusion criteria
1. The patient cannot be hypothermic ($< 35°C$)
2. There must be no residual effects of sedative, anaesthetic, or neuromuscular relaxant drugs
3. Other metabolic or endocrine disease such as hypothyroidism, polyneuropathy, or myasthenia gravis must be excluded

Signs
1. Unreactive pupils to bright light
2. Absent corneal reflexes
3. Absent vestibulo-ocular reflexes
   No cold caloric responses (exclude ear wax)
   'Doll's eyes'
4. Absent purposeful movement
5. Absent motor response to pain stimulation
6. Absent decorticate or decerebrate posturing
7. Absent respiratory effect during formal apnoea test

A formal document must be signed, dated, and the time of completion of testing recorded. If brain death is confirmed this recorded time becomes the legal time of death.

Specific criteria for the diagnosis of brain death may vary in minor details depending on local or national recommendations. These variations may include the requirement for two sets of observations, about 24 h apart, and an EEG showing electrocerebral silence. An advantage of performing two tests lies not in improved accuracy, but provides time for the co-ordination of transplant teams. Some protocols require the radiographic demonstration of absent cerebral blood flow.

The conduct of the apnoea test may also vary from centre to centre but relies on achieving an indisputable CO_2 stimulus to respiration in the absence of respiratory depressants such as sedatives, narcotics, neuromuscular relaxants, or hypoxia. The patient should be monitored with continuous ECG and pulse oximetry if available. Mechanical ventilation should be adjusted to stabilize the $P\text{CO}_2$ at a normal high level. The patient should then be preoxygenated with 100 per cent O_2 for about 10 min. The ventilator can then be disconnected at the endotracheal tube and a catheter passed down the endotracheal tube to facilitate insufflation of oxygen at 1 to 2 min. The patient is carefully observed to detect any respiratory movement of the chest or abdomen. Arterial oxygen saturation can be accurately monitored with a pulse oximeter. After 5 to 10 min blood gases can again be sampled. The patient is then temporarily supported with the ventilator until the blood gases confirm a high CO_2 stimulus (6.5 kPa, 50 mmHg) and the absence of hypoxia. In practice $P\text{CO}_2$ values between 8 and 10 kPa can be achieved by this protocol. If no respiratory effort has been detected and other signs of brain-stem dysfunction have been demonstrated the patient may be considered brain dead.

It is the responsibility of the doctor performing the tests of brain death to explain the implications of such tests to relatives before the tests are completed. It is essential that the relatives are aware that survival is not possible in the presence of positive brain death criteria.

FURTHER READING

Abramson NS. *et al.* Randomized clinical study of thiopental loading in comatose survivors of cardiac arrest. *N Engl J Med*, 1986; **314**: 397–403.

Ames A III, Nesbett FB. Pathophysiology of ischemic cell death. I. Time of onset of irreversible damage; importance of the different components of the ischemic insult. *Stroke*, 1983; **14**: 219–23.

Bircher N, Safari P. Cerebral preservation during cardiopulmonary resuscitation. *Crit Care Med*, 1985; **13**: 185–90.

Bruce DA, Gennarelli T, Langfitt T. Resuscitation from coma due to head injury, 1978; *Crit Care Med*, **6**: 254–8.

Cooper P. *et al.* Dexamethasone and severe head injury. A prospective, double blind study. *J Neurosurg*, 1979; **51**: 307–10.

Farber JL, Chien KR, Mittnacht S. The pathogenesis of irreversible cell injury in ischemia. *Am J Physiol*, 1981; **102**: 271–81.

Fleischer JE, *et al.* Failure of deferoxamine, an iron chelator, to improve neurologic outcome following complete cerebral ischemia in dogs. *Stoke*, 1987; **18**: 124–7.

Gudeman S, Miller J, Becker D. Failure of high-dose steroid therapy to influence intracranial pressure in patients with severe head injury. *J Neurosurg*, 1979; **51**: 301–6.

Jennet B, *et al.* Predicting outcome in individual patients after severe head injury. *Neurosurgery*, 1979; **4**: 283–8.

Kirsch JR, Helfaer MA, Koehler RC, Traystman RJ. Brain ischaemia and reperfusion injury. In Bihari D, Holiday JW, eds. *Update in Intensive Care and Emergency Medicine*. Berlin: Springer-Verlag, 1989; 66–84.

Lim KH. *et al.* Prevention of reperfusion injury of the ischemic spinal cord: use of recombinant superoxide dismutase. *Ann Thoracic Surg*, 1986; **42**: 282–6.

Lind B, Snyder J, Safer P. Total brain ischemia in dogs: cerebral physiological and metabolic changes after 15 minutes of circulatory arrest. *Resuscitation*, 1975; **4**: 97–101.

Marshall LF, *et al.* Pentobarbital therapy for intracranial hypertension in metabolic coma. Reye's syndrome. *Crit Care Med*, 1978; **6**: 1–6.

McCormick PW, *et al.* Noninvasive cerebral optical cerebral spectroscopy for monitoring cerebral oxygen delivery and haemodynamics. *Crit Care Med*, 1991; **19**: 89–97.

Michael R, *et al.* Mechanisms by which epinephrine augments cerebral and myocardial perfusion during cardiopulmonary resuscitation in dogs. *Circulation*, 1984; **69**: 822–35.

Pallis C. *ABC of brain stem death.* Torquay: British Medical Journal/Devonshire Press, 1983.

Plum F, Posner J. *The Diagnosis of Stupor and Coma.* Philadelphia: Davis, 1980.

President's Commission for the Study of Ethical Problems in Medicine and Biomedical and Behavioral Research. *Defining Death. Medical, Legal and Ethical Issues in the Determination of Death.* Washington: US Government Printing Office, 1981.

Rockoff M, Marshall L, Shapiro H. High-dose barbiturate in therapy humans: A clinical study of 60 patients. *Ann Neurol*, 1979; **6**: 194–8.

Safar P, Bircher N. Cardiopulmonary cerebral resuscitation. *An Introduction to Resuscitation Medicine*. World Federation of Societies of Anaesthesiologists. 3rd edn. London: Balliere Tindall, 1986.

Safar P, Grenvik A, Abramson NS, Burcher N, eds. Reversibility of clinical death: symposium on resuscitation research. *Crit Care Med*, 1988, **16**: 919–1086.

Schanne FAX, *et al.* Calcium dependence of toxic cell death: A final common pathway. *Science*, 1979; **206**: 700–3.

Shapiro HM. Postcardiac arrest therapy. Calcium entry blockade and brain resuscitation. *Anesthesiology*, 1985; **62**: 384–7.

Shiu GK, Nemoto EM. Barbiturate attenuation of brain free fatty acid liberation during global ischemia. *Neurochemistry*, 1981; **37**: 1448–56.

Smith DS, Rehncrona S, Siesjo BK. Barbiturates as protective agents in brain ischemia and as free radical scavengers *in vitro*. *Acta Physiol Scand*, 1980; **42**: 129–34.

Steen PA, *et al.* Cerebral blood flow and neurologic outcome when nimodipine is given after complete cerebral ischaemia in the dog. *J Cerebral Blood Flow Metab*, 1984; **4**: 82–7.

Todd MM, Chadwick HS, Shapiro HM, Dunlop BS, Marshall LF, Dueck R. The neurologic effects of thiopental therapy following experimental cardiac arrest in cats. *Anesthesiology*, 1982; **57**: 76–86.

Wei EP, *et al.* Effects of oxygen Radical on cerebral arterioles. *Am J Physiol*, 1985; **248**: H157–H162.

4.7 Gastrointestinal aspects

CHRISTOPHER S. GARRARD

HEPATIC DYSFUNCTION

Varying degrees of hepatic dysfunction, with a variety of causes, are seen in the surgical patient admitted to the critical care unit. There is usually evidence of cholestasis, hepatocellular injury, or a combination of both. Cholestasis is associated with elevation of serum alkaline phosphatase levels and conjugated bilirubin, while hepatocellular damage results in enzyme elevation and increased prothrombin time. Extrahepatic cholestasis should be excluded by ultrasonography of the gallbladder and biliary tree.

The most common causes of hepatic dysfunction in the critical care unit include:

(1) total parenteral nutrition
(2) hepatic hypoperfusion
(3) drug induced causes
(4) hepatitis

Total parenteral nutrition

Elevation of the liver enzymes (aspartate aminotransferase), alkaline phosphatase, and serum bilirubin, is often seen 2 to 6 days after the start of intravenous nutrition. Ultrasonography may be required to exclude extrahepatic obstruction. The underlying aetiology is unclear, but histologically examination shows elements of fatty infiltration as well as periportal inflammation and intrahepatic cholestasis. Secondary bacterial colonization of the biliary tract may also play a role. Biochemical abnormalities can be quite marked, but the clinical course is generally benign. Transition to enteral feeding is associated with resolution of the biochemical and pathological abnormalities.

Hepatic hypoperfusion

Hypoperfusion of the liver due to sepsis syndrome, cardiogenic shock, haemorrhagic shock, burns, or trauma can result in mild to severe hepatic dysfunction, depending upon the severity and prolongation of the ischaemic insult. Elements of intrahepatic cholestasis may be present in patients with sepsis syndrome, although the major liver injury is probably a consequence of hypoperfusion associated with endotoxaemia.

Drug-induced liver disease

A wide range of drugs may be associated with intrahepatic cholestasis, hepatitis, or even massive necrosis. These include erythromycin, chlorpromazine, tolbutamide, and the anabolic steroids (cholestatic) isoniazid, methyldopa, nitrofurantoin (hepatitis-like), carbon tetrachloride, and acetominophen (massive necrosis).

Hepatitis

A, B, or non-A, non-B hepatitis should be considered in any patient developing jaundice and the biochemical features of hepatitis. Serological screening and blood precautions should be undertaken.

ACUTE HEPATIC FAILURE

Hepatic failure that develops acutely over a period of several days or weeks without pre-existing liver disease is referred to as fulminant hepatic failure. It is due to sudden, massive necrosis of hepatocytes, and is followed rapidly by the onset of encephalopathy. In the critical care unit, the likely cause is either viral hepatitis or an overdose of acetaminophen (paracetamol).

Aetiology

Viral hepatitis accounts for up to 70 per cent of cases of acute hepatic failure. The most common causative agent is hepatitis B virus, reported to be responsible for 25 to 75 per cent of cases of viral hepatitis. Hepatitis A is somewhat less common, while non-A, non-B hepatitis accounts for about 30 per cent of cases. Non-A, non-B hepatitis usually follows a slightly slower, but still progressive, course and carries a high mortality—more than 80 per cent. Hepatitis C (non-A, non-B hepatitis group) is often found in association with hepatitis B and is now recognized as major cause of chronic progressive liver disease. The association of hepatitis D (delta agent) with hepatitis B is a serious finding and is usually followed by a rapid deterioration in liver function.

Drug reactions and overdose with acetaminophen (paracetamol) account for about 20 per cent of cases of acute liver failure. Other drugs, such as non-steroidal anti-inflammatory agents and antidepressants, are associated with lesser degrees of liver dysfunction but can cause acute liver failure. Halothane anaesthesia is often proposed as a cause of drug-induced hepatic failure, but increased awareness of this and the avoidance of repeated halothane anaesthesia have greatly reduced this problem. Drug overdose explains about 10 per cent of cases of acute hepatic failure, the most common agents being acetaminophen and ferrous sulphate.

Fulminant hepatic failure is a common feature of *Amanita phalloides* poisoning: ingestion of 50 g of the mushroom is frequently fatal. Other toxins, such as carbon tetrachloride, methylbromide, chloroform, and xylene may occasionally produce acute hepatic failure. Rare causes of fulminant hepatic failure include profound hypovolaemic shock, Budd–Chiari syndrome, fatty liver of pregnancy, Reye's syndrome, Wilson's disease, and hyperthermia.

Clinical features

Jaundice and fetor hepaticus may often be apparent, while other characteristic signs of liver dysfunction, such as spider naevi, ascites, and liver palms, are generally absent. The serum levels of bilirubin and transaminases are usually elevated, although some patients progress to coma before bilirubin levels become significantly elevated.

Hepatic encephalopathy is usually attributed to neurotoxic materials such as ammonia and mercaptans, derived from the metabolism of nitrogenous compounds in the bowel. These compounds enter the systemic circulation having bypassed the liver through anatomic or functional shunts. Entry of aromatic amino acids into the central nervous system may also account for neurological disturbances. The severity of hepatic encephalopathy can be classified into the four stages shown in Table 1.

Table 1 Classification and mortality of hepatic encephalopathy

Stage I :	subtle personality changes, with inappropriate behaviour; normal EEG, <30% mortality
Stage II :	more confusion, drowsiness, metabolic flap; EEG becomes abnormal, 30% mortality
Stage III:	stupor (but rousable) and incoherent speech, 50% mortality
Stage IV:	Coma (no verbal response), >80% mortality

Most patients with stage IV coma have intracranial pressures raised to more than 30 mmHg. Factors that may precipitate or be associated with hepatic encephalopathy include the administration of sedative or hepatotoxic drugs, bleeding into the gastrointestinal tract, increased dietary protein, and diuretic-induced hypokalaemic alkalosis.

Haemorrhagic manifestations result from decreased synthesis of clotting factors II, V, VII, IX, and X, disseminated intravascular coagulation, and splenic sequestration of platelets. Active bleeding from varices, gastritis, and peptic ulcers further deplete clotting factors, and these should be managed aggressively by replenishing clotting factors with fresh frozen plasma and undertaking surgical or endoscopic intervention if necessary.

Renal failure may complicate hepatic failure for several reasons.

Gastrointestinal haemorrhage or overuse of diuretics may result in prerenal azotaemia. Severe or prolonged hypotension, sometimes in association with use of nephrotoxic drugs, may result in vasomotor nephritis (acute tubular necrosis). A serious complication of hepatic failure is the hepatorenal syndrome, a poorly understood condition that results in functional renal failure without clear histopathological lesions in the kidneys: normal renal function returns only if the liver function recovers.

Nosocomial infection occurs in up to 30 per cent of patients and is a common cause of death. There may be a qualitative defect in immune defences due to impaired reticuloendothelial cell clearance, and abnormal leucocyte migration and complement-dependent opsonization.

The adult respiratory distress syndrome is common in patients with end-stage liver failure and is almost uniformly fatal. Impaired clearance of vasoactive substances by the hepatic reticuloendothelial system may contribute to the development of acute lung injury.

Spontaneous bacterial peritonitis should always be suspected in the patient with ascites: this may occur in the absence of peritonism, leucocytosis, or fever. A diagnostic abdominal paracentesis is essential.

Hypoglycaemia may develop because of reduce hepatic glycogen reserves and decreased gluconeogenesis.

Treatment

The treatment of hepatic encephalopathy includes reducing the gastrointestinal protein load by restricting dietary protein intake, preventing gastrointestinal bleeding, and encouraging intestinal emptying with agents such as lactulose. In stage I and II encephalopathy, protein intake should be restricted to less than 40 g per day, and this should be further reduced to less than 20 g per day in patients with stages III and IV encephalopathy. Caloric intake, preferably as dextrose, should be maintained in excess of 2000 calories per day. Patients with liver damage may be lipid intolerant, and the presence of lipaemic serum requires a reduction of lipid intake. Increased levels of aromatic amino acids (tryptophan, tyrosine, and phenylalanine) may result in decreased synthesis of normal neurotransmitters and, therefore, enhanced synthesis of false neurotransmitters. Such false transmitters may contribute to encephalopathy, although this process might be reversed by the administration of branched-chain amino acids. Neomycin, 0.5 to 1 g administered orally every 6 h, suppresses ammonia production by colonic bacteria. The addition of lactulose, initially in doses of 50 ml orally every 2 h, acts as an osmotic laxative and decreases ammonia absorption from the intestinal lumen by increasing gut intraluminal acidity.

If there is evidence of cerebral oedema, mannitol may be given. There is no evidence that corticosteroids such as dexamethasone have any beneficial effect upon cerebral oedema in this setting or upon the underlying hepatic failure.

Fluid and electrolyte balance requires continuous and meticulous attention. Patients with hepatic failure are generally intolerant of sodium loads and hypokalaemia is poorly tolerated. Volume depletion must be avoided to minimize the risk of vasomotor nephropathy and central venous pressure monitoring is almost obligatory. Target central venous pressures of 8 to 12 mmHg will generally ensure adequate preload. Lower pressures, especially in patients receiving assisted ventilation, carry the risk of volume depletion. If oliguria develops the differential diagnosis includes prerenal azotaemia and the hepatorenal syndrome. Both conditions are associated with a low fractional excretion of sodium (FE_{Na}) so that exclusion of volume depletion is critical to clinical management.

Haemodialysis or haemofiltration should be performed in patients with renal failure if recovery is expected or liver transplantation envisaged. It may be difficult to distinguish between hepatorenal syndrome and vasomotor nephropathy. If doubt exists over the precise cause of renal failure an active approach to management with haemofiltration is indicated.

Use of all types of sedation should be minimized as far as possible. If the use of sedatives cannot be avoided, continuous infusion of a short acting benzodiazepine such as midazolam is acceptable, provided the infusion is discontinued intermittently to reassess the need for sedation. Coexistent renal failure further reduces the clearance of a wide range of medication and lactate.

Coagulopathy is assessed by daily monitoring of the prothombin time. Although there may be little response to the administration of vitamin K, this should be given empirically in doses of 10 mg intravenously daily for 3 days. Vitamin K stores may be severely depleted in the presence of liver necrosis, and supplementation ensures that vitamin K is available if there is any hepatocellular regeneration.

Fresh frozen plasma should be given to patients with severe bleeding or as prophylaxis before an invasive procedure. A target prothrombin time of less than one and a half times control is required for most surgical procedures. Clotting factor concentrates should be avoided since they may precipitate disseminated intravascular coagulation; this is otherwise uncommon unless there is associated sepsis. The most common site of bleeding is the gastrointestinal tract. Bleeding from sites other than surgical wounds, is somewhat infrequent.

Hypoglycaemia should be expected in all patients with fulminant hepatic failure. In the encephalopathic patient the symptoms of hypoglycaemia may not be apparent and hypoglycaemia will only be detected by regular monitoring of blood sugar levels. Dextrose should be administered intravenously as intermittent boluses, or as a continuous infusion if necessary. Administration of glucagon is inappropriate in patients with depleted glycogen stores.

Death secondary to acute hepatic failure usually results from cerebral oedema, sepsis, or haemorrhage. Mortality is related to the stage of encephalopathy (Table 1). Those patients who survive fulminant hepatic failure have a high probability of complete recovery as the liver regenerates over the following 3 to 4 months.

HEPATORENAL SYNDROME

The hepatorenal syndrome refers to renal failure of unknown aetiology which occurs in a fully hydrated patient with severe, often progressive, liver disease. Urine biochemistry is characteristic and renal histopathology is unremarkable. The pathogenesis of the hepatorenal syndrome appears to involve intense intrarenal vasoconstriction and alteration in renal cortical blood flow, possibly due to an imbalance of prostaglandins and thromboxane. Less than 5 per cent of patients with the hepatorenal syndrome survive unless they undergo successful orthotopic liver transplantation. Renal failure is reversed after liver transplantation suggesting that it is due to circulating or systemic factors. Excessive use of diuretics, sepsis, abdominal paracentesis, and gastrointestinal haemorrhage are associated with an increased risk of the hepatorenal syndrome.

Clinical presentation

Typically, patients who develop the hepatorenal syndrome have signs of advanced liver disease, such as icterus, ascites, palmar erythema, spider angiomata, and hepatic encephalopathy. Laboratory findings confirm hepatic failure, with elevated serum levels of bilirubin, liver enzymes, and ammonia. The impaired synthetic function of the liver usually results in hypoalbuminaemia and prolongation of the prothrombin time. Hyponatraemia, hypokalaemia, and alkalosis are common accompaniments. Hyponatraemia results from proximal tubular reabsorption of sodium and water with non-osmotic release of vasopressin. The first sign of hepatorenal syndrome is usually oliguria. The major differential diagnoses include prerenal azotaemia and vasomotor nephropathy (acute tubular necrosis). The patient with hepatorenal syndrome appears well hydrated and volume depletion can usually be excluded. The fractional excretion of sodium (FE_{Na}) is less than 1 per cent and the urinary sodium less than 10 to 15 mmol/l, in contrast to vasomotor nephropathy, which characteristically has a high urinary sodium content—over 30 mmol/l. If prerenal azotaemia is suspected a cautious fluid challenge consisting of about 250 ml of crystalloid or colloid infused over 30 min can be tried. If doubt remains regarding the volume status of the patient, a flow directed pulmonary artery catheter should be inserted for accurate assessment of left heart filling pressures. The urine sediment should be examined carefully. The presence of cellular casts suggests vasomotor nephropathy rather than hepatorenal syndrome. Obstructive uropathy should be excluded by renal ultrasound or if necessary, retrograde pyelography.

Treatment

When treating any patient with advanced liver disease, it is essential to avoid factors that precipitate the hepatorenal syndrome. Adequate nutrition must be maintained and electrolyte abnormalities corrected. Diuretics should be used judiciously and ascites drained only for specific indications. Any intercurrent infection must be treated aggressively. The use of certain drugs, such as the non-steroidal anti-inflammatory agents, angiotensin-converting enzyme inhibitors, and tetracyclines should be avoided and aminoglycosides should not be used unless this is unavoidable.

There is currently no specific treatment for the hepatorenal syndrome: therapy is directed at supporting the underlying liver disease. Haemodialysis and haemofiltration may control the metabolic disturbances of renal failure but the outcome is determined by the degree of liver impairment. A summary of these supportive measures is shown in Table 2.

Pharmacological agents that have been used in an attempt to reverse the hepatorenal syndrome include dopamine, isoproterenol (isoprenaline), phenoxybenzamine, phentolamine, aminophylline, mannitol, metaraminol, epinephrine (adrenaline), papaverine, and prostaglandin A1. All have been without effect in double-blind studies. Recovery of renal function has occurred following peritoneojugular (LaVeen) and portacaval shunting procedures. Orthotopic liver transplantation appears to offer the best hope for reversal of the hepatorenal syndrome but is only available for a relatively small group of suitable patients.

Table 2 Supportive measures in the hepatorenal syndrome

Fluid and electrolytes
Exclude volume depletion, insert central venous pressure or pulmonary artery catheter
Optimize fluid balance
Water restriction
Sodium restriction
Administer dDAVP
Correct hypokolaemia
Haematology/coagulation
Blood
Fresh frozen plasma
Vitamin K
Encephalopathy
Restrict protein intake
Ensure adequate carbohydrate
Gastrointestinal tract emptying
Branch-chain amino acids
Infection
Antibiotics
Reduce endotoxaemia
Support circulation
Ascites
Diuretics
Paracentesis
Colloid infusion
Peritoneal/venous shunting
Portosystemic shunting
Nutrition and bed rest

Ascites

Abdominal ascites is a common feature of the patient with the hepatorenal syndrome. The common indications for reduction of ascites include abdominal pain, intravascular coagulation and renal vein compression, gastro-oesophageal reflux (with erosion of varices), and restriction of ventilation by diaphragm splinting. Simple measures such as bed rest and salt restriction are essential preliminary measures. Spironolactone or amiloride, combined if necessary with a loop diuretic, can then be added. In a proportion of patients direct drainage of ascitic fluid is required. The aim is to drain sufficient fluid to alleviate symptoms without inducing the hepatorenal syndrome. Infusion of colloid should accompany the paracentesis to ensure that the patient does not become volume depleted. Paracentesis is occasionally followed by a brisk diuresis, particularly if the renal veins have been compressed by the ascitic fluid.

ACUTE PANCREATITIS

Mild acute pancreatitis has a mortality of less than 3 per cent and rarely requires critical care management. Ten per cent of patients with pancreatitis have severe disease, however, accompanied by multiple organ system failure. Although early reports of severe acute pancreatitis were associated with a mortality of up to 75 per cent more recent mortality figures have fallen towards 20 per cent. Most cases of pancreatitis are the result of either alcohol abuse or cholelithiasis. Other causes of pancreatitis are listed in Table 3.

Table 3 Causes of acute pancreatitis

Frequent (80–90%)
- Alcoholism
- Cholelithiasis
- Idiopathic (10%)

Occasional (10–15%)
- Postoperative pancreatitis
- Trauma
- Penetrating peptic ulcer
- Drugs (thiazides, sulphonamides, azathioprine)
- Virus (mumps, infectious mononucleosis)
- Hypercalcaemia
- Hyperlipidaemia
- Ampullary obstruction

Rare (less than 3%)
- Connective tissue disease
- Oestrogens
- Hypothermia
- Malnutrition
- Afferent loop syndrome
- Translumbar aortography

Clinical presentation

Acute pancreatitis should be considered in any patient presenting with abdominal pain, nausea, and vomiting. Other common clinical signs and symptoms of acute pancreatitis are shown in Table 4. Abdominal pain is invariably present and radiates to the back in 50 per cent of patients. Acute haemorrhagic pancreatitis often presents dramatically with shock, confusion, coma, oliguria, and abdominal ecchymoses.

Table 4 Clinical presentation of acute pancreatitis

Signs and symptoms	Percentage of cases
Abdominal pain	90
Nausea or vomiting	70
Fever	70
Abdominal distension/ascites	60
Shock	20
Dyspnoea	20
Icterus	20
Confusion/coma	10
Cullen's or Gray-Turner's sign	<5
Subcutaneous fat necrosis	<2

Laboratory confirmation usually rests on the detection of elevated levels of serum or urinary amylase. Elevated serum amylase also may be found in patients with intestinal obstruction, bowel perforation or infarction, pregnancy, renal failure, major burns, and carcinomas of the lung, oesophagus, or ovary. Isoenzyme analysis may help differentiate pancreatic and salivary sources of amylase.

Treatment

The treatment of severe acute pancreatitis can follow either of two philosophies. The first involves the surgical removal of necrotic material to reduce the risk of organ system failure and secondary infection. The second adopts a conservative approach delaying surgery until indicated for complications such as haemorrhage or infection.

Regardless of the management philosophy, the critical care treatment during the acute, toxaemic phase is directed at the management of primary pancreatic failure (diabetes mellitus), hypovolaemia secondary to fluid sequestration, and multiple organ system failure. Analgesia can be achieved using agents such as pethidine or a synthetic opiate (alfentanil). Morphine probably should be avoided in view of a propensity to cause spasm of the sphincter of Oddi.

Late complications result from local, intra-abdominal, and systemic infection and often progress to the sepsis syndrome. This late phase has a significant effect on the final mortality from acute pancreatitis and requires all the resources of the critical care unit.

Hyperglycaemia and ketoacidosis require volume replacement, continuous insulin infusion according to blood sugar levels (2–8 units/h is generally adequate), provision of intravenous dextrose, and correction of electrolyte imbalance. Metabolic acidosis can also result from lactic acidosis and, occasionally, from renal failure.

Hypocalcaemia occurs in about 25 per cent of patients, usually within the first week of the illness. Hypocalcaemia is associated with hypoalbuminaemia, calcification of areas of intra-abdominal fat necrosis, and parathyroid dysfunction.

Treatment is supportive, there being no specific, effective therapeutic agent available. Drugs such as somatostatin, glucagon, cimetidine, aprotinin (trasylol), and anticholinergics do not appear to be effective. Peritoneal lavage is favoured by some, as is open drainage of the pancreatic bed following pancreatectomy. Much more extensive and controlled evaluation of these forms of treatment is required.

Multiple organ system involvement in pancreatitis

Any of the major organ systems can be involved in patients with acute pancreatitis. Organ system failure in pancreatitis is one of the most common indications for critical care unit admission. Since organ system failure is responsible for most of the deaths associated with pancreatitis, prevention, or at least early recognition, is paramount.

Cardiovascular system

The electrocardiogram may show prolongation of the ST interval and non-specific T-wave changes. Tachyarrhythmias can develop and are probably related to the metabolic abnormalities of pancreatitis or coexistent alcoholic cardiomyopathy. Hypotension may result from bradykinin release and abdominal fluid sequestration. The intravascular fluid deficit can be large, requiring several litres for replacement, and central venous pressure monitoring is generally required. The nature of the replacement fluid is probably less critical than the volume. Fluid resuscitation should continue until a central venous pressure of about 10 mmHg can be achieved and satisfactory urine output of 0.5 to 1.0 ml/kg.min is maintained.

Respiratory system

More than half of all patients with pancreatitis will have chest radiographic changes such as patchy infiltrates, collapse, or pleural effusion. Pleural effusions of an exudative type occur in up to 15 per cent of patients, the left hemithorax being most commonly involved. Arterial hypoxaemia is evident in up to 75 per cent of patients: this usually responds to supplemental oxygen but about 20 per cent of patients require endotracheal intubation and positive pressure ventilation.

Host defence

Leucocytosis, fever, and complement activation are features of acute pancreatitis. As with all intensive care patients, nosocomial infection is increasingly likely after the second week of admission. However, use of antibiotics should be reserved for patients with clear signs of infection of sepsis. Prophylactic antibiotics are not recommended.

Gastrointestinal system

Gastric erosions and ileus are common accompaniments of acute pancreatitis. Prophylaxis against stress associated gastric erosions and total parenteral nutrition should be provided for the mechanically ventilated patient. Ulcer prophylaxis can be provided by cytoprotective agents (sulcralfate), antacids, or H_2 blockers. The last increase gastric pH, and may increase the risk of nosocomial pneumonia.

Haematologic system and coagulation

Anaemia may result from pancreatic or gastric bleeding. Patients with alcoholic cirrhosis and oesophageal varices are at further risk of gastrointestinal haemorrhage. Prolongation of prothrombin time may occur due to coexistent liver failure or disseminated intravascular coagulation: replacement of clotting factors with fresh frozen plasma is indicated, particularly if there is active bleeding. Platelet transfusion also may be required if there is bleeding in the presence of a platelet count of less than 50 000/mm^3.

Renal system

Prerenal azotaemia and vasomotor nephropathy will occur unless rigorous fluid resuscitation is undertaken. Any fall in hourly urine volumes to below 0.5 ml/min.kg should prompt an immediate evaluation of the volume status of the patient using all measures available. In established renal failure haemofiltration provides a convenient means of controlling the fluid balance, electrolyte balance, and azotaemia. Only rarely is haemodialysis is required.

Central nervous system

Agitation, confusion, and even seizures may occur, possibly due to breakdown of cerebral lipid fractions.

FURTHER READING

Boyer TD. Major sequelae of cirrhosis. In: Wyngaarden JB, Smith JH, Jr, eds. *Cecil Textbook of Medicine*. 18th edn. Philadelphia: WB Saunders. 1988; 847–52.

Epstein M, Perez G, Oster JR. Management of renal complications of liver disease. *J Intensive Care Med*, 1988; 3: 71–86.

Ettien JT, Webster PD. The management of acute pancreatitis. *Adv Intern Med*, 1980; **25**: 169–98.

Fraser CL, Arieff AI. Hepatic encephalopathy. *N Engl J Med*, 1985; **313**: 685–873.

Gordon DG, Tedesco FJ. Recognising systemic manifestations of acute pancratitis. *J Crit Illness*, 1987; **2**: 77–83.

Imrie CW. The management of severe acute pancreatitis. *Clinics Crit Care Med*, 1987; **11**: 93–107.

Jensen DM. Portal-systemic encephalopathy and hepatic coma. *Med Clin NAm*, 1988; **70**: 1081–92.

Mayer DA, *et al.* Controlled trial of peritoneal lavage for the treatment of severe acute pancreatitis. *N Engl J Med*, 1985; **312**: 399–404.

O'Grady JG, *et al.* Coagulopathy of fulminant hepatic failure. *Semin Liver Dis*, 1986; **6**: 159–63.

Payne JA. Causes and complications of fulminant hepatic failure. *J Intensive Care Med*, 1986; **1**: 216–23.

Ranson JHC. Etiologic and prognostic factors in human acute pancreatitis: a review. *Am J Gastroenterol*, 1982; **77**: 633–8.

Rattner DW, Warshaw AL. Surgical intervention in acute pancreatitis. *Crit Care Med*, 1988; **16**: 89–95.

Scharschmidt BF. Acute and chronic hepatic failure and hepatic transplantation. In: Wyngaarden JB, Smith JH, Jr, eds. *Cecil Textbook of Medicine* 18th edn. Philadelphia: WB Saunders, 1988.

Sweny P. The hepatorenal syndrome. In: Rainford D, Sweny P, eds. *Acute Renal Failure*. London: Farrand Press, 1990: 83–112.

Williams R, Gimson A. Management of acute liver failure. *Clin Gastroenterol*, 1985; **14**: 93–104.

4.8 The role of cytokines in bacterial sepsis

HAMISH R. MICHIE

INTRODUCTION

Humoral and cell-mediated immune responses represent a highly specific and sophisticated defence mechanism against invading pathogens associated with minimal injury to host tissue. Unfortunately a considerable time must generally elapse following infection before these specific responses are evoked (in the absence of previous exposure or vaccination). Antigen-specific immune responses are usually preceded by a non-specific acute inflammatory response of varying degree. Host responses to inflammation are often similar whether evoked by Gram-positive or Gram-negative bacteria, viruses, parasites, or even in 'sterile' circumstances such as in acute pancreatitis or severe burns. In certain clinical situations the inflammatory response may aid survival but, as shown in Fig. 1, a penalty must always be paid in terms of host autoinjury. Sometimes the inflammatory response is itself the lethal event, the invading micro-organisms otherwise being quite harmless.

The concept of host autoinjury as the principal cause of death in many infections was given strong support when James D. Watson (of DNA double helix fame) demonstrated that a single mutation in a certain strain of mouse (C3H HEJ) was associated with virtu-

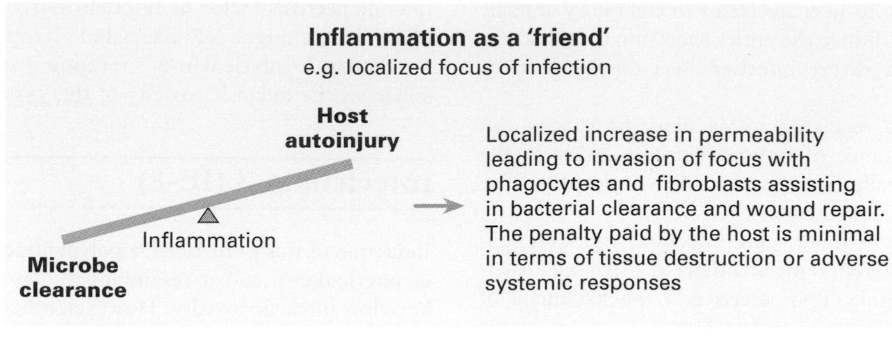

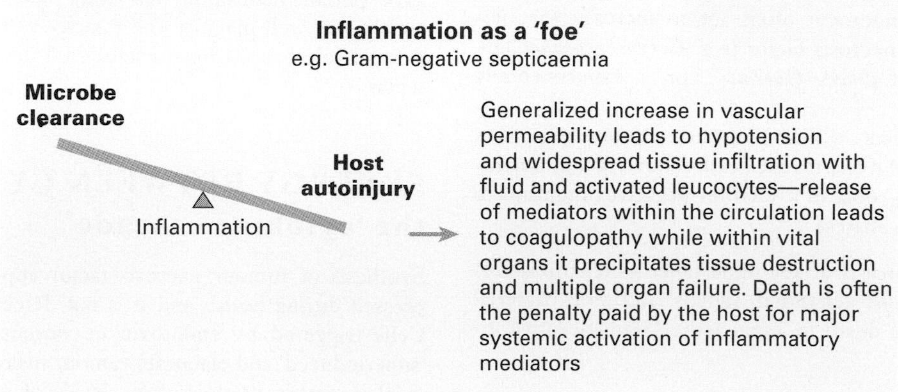

Inflammation as a 'foe'
e.g. Gram-negative septicaemia
Microbe
clearance
Host
autoinjury
Inflammation
Generalized increase in vascular permeability leads to hypotension and widespread tissue infiltration with fluid and activated leucocytes—release of mediators within the circulation leads to coagulopathy while within vital organs it precipitates tissue destruction and multiple organ failure. Death is often the penalty paid by the host for major systemic activation of inflammatory mediators

Fig. 1 Acute inflammation largely confined to a septic focus is an intrinsic component of the healing mechanism. Intravascular activation of the same mechanism causes the entire body to behave like a massive wound, with intravascular mediator activation, capillary leak, and often lethal consequences.

ally complete protection against the effects of an otherwise lethal injection of live Gram-negative bacteria or their associated endotoxins. By transplanting cells between 'sensitive' and 'resistant' strains it could be shown that the lethality of endotoxin was due to proteins synthesized by reticuloendothelial cells. This, and other research, enhanced the growing belief that the key to enhancing survival following severe sepsis did not lie with better antibiotics but with therapies that prevented induction of the inflammatory response to a lethal degree. Against this was the concern that blunting the inflammatory response might itself render the host succeptible to lethal secondary infection.

A major breakthrough in the understanding of sepsis has occurred in the last decade with the revolution in molecular biology. Techniques have been developed to characterize and assay the mediators that are evoked following severe inflammation which cause host autoinjury and death. These mediators are collectively refered to as cytokines.

CHARACTERISTICS OF CYTOKINES

Although there is no universally accepted definition, to be considered a cytokine a molecule must show the following features.

1. It must be a protein or polypeptide.
2. It must be a mediator of a component of inflammation.
3. It must be evoked as part of the immune response to an antigen (although micro-organisms acting through different receptors may be far more potent inducers than antigen-generated stimuli).
4. It must have no intrinsic chemical or enzymatic activity.
5. It must bind to specific protein receptors on target cells.
6. It must alter the behaviour of the target cell.

Cytokines may be regarded as the hormones of disease and like true hormones the target cell may be the cell of origin (autocrine action), an adjacent cell (paracrine action), or a distant cell (endocrine action). Cytokines are biologically active in concentrations a thousandfold less than true hormones. They also exist in multiple forms. Finally their biological effects long outlive their appearance in the circulation. These considerations explain why it has been so difficult to monitor cytokine activity during human critical illness.

A large number of cytokines (>30) have now been characterized. The bulk of available evidence suggests that the following cytokines are most important in the mediation of lethal sepsis: (1) tumour necrosis factor; (2) interleukin-1; (3) interleukin-6; (4) interleukin-8. Although these cytokines were originally believed to be principally the products of monocytes/macrophages it is now clear that they are synthesized to a significant extent by other cells including neutrophils, lymphocytes, endothelial cells, and glial cells in the central nervous system. The following is a brief description of the key inflammatory cytokines.

Tumour necrosis factor (TNFα, cachectin)

Tumour necrosis factor is synthesized as a 25-kDa precursor and processed to produce a 17-kDa product which is actively secreted into the circulation. A large amount of evidence supports a key role for this cytokine in critical illness.

1. Administration of tumour necrosis factor to laboratory animals or cancer patients will induce the entire spectrum of host alterations associated with severe infection in a dose-dependent manner.
2. In human volunteers receiving intravenous *Escherichia coli* endotoxin, the appearance of tumour necrosis factor in the circulation is temporally and quantitatively related to the clinical response to endotoxaemia.
3. In patients with overwhelming acute infection, e.g. meningococcal septicaemia or cerebral malaria there is a striking association between circulating TNF levels and the likelihood of death.
4. Agents which sensitize human beings or animals to the adverse effects of endotoxin often act to increase the biosynthesis of tumour necrosis factor (e.g. *Corynebacterium parvum*, *Bacillus Calmette-Guerin*, or experimentally D-galactosamine).
5. Monoclonal antibodies which neutralize tumour necrosis factor have been shown to prevent death following administration of a lethal (LD_{100}) dose of live Gram-negative organisms to animals, including primates).

The last piece of evidence is of key importance as it emphasizes the point that it is host-generated signals and not bacterial poisons *per se* that cause death in lethal acute Gram-negative infection.

Interleukin-1 (IL-1)

Interleukin-1 exists in α and β forms of which the latter is considered the more important mediator of sepsis. It is a 33-kDa polypeptide that has little structural similarity to tumour necrosis factor and acts through an independent receptor. Unlike tumour necrosis factor it has no leader sequence that allows its secretion by cells so that it remains cell bound and therefore extremely difficult to detect during sespis. Detectable levels of interleukin-1β may reflect lysis of the cell of origin rather than active secretion.

Administration of interleukin-1β to animals and human beings will replicate virtually all the responses seen in acute infection. It appears to be about 100 times less potent than tumour necrosis factor and has never been shown to be intrinsically lethal to any animal. It magnifies greatly the biological effects of tumour necrosis factor (by a factor of about 100) and it is currently believed that much of the lethality of acute infection is attributable to tumour necrosis factor and interleukin-1β acting synergistically. Furthermore tumour necrosis factor stimulates interleukin-1β production and agents which block the interleukin-1β receptor also prevent death in primates receiving an LD_{100} dose of *Escherichia coli* endotoxin.

Interleukin-6 (IL-6)

Interleukin-6 is a 26-kDa polypeptide produced principally by monocytes or endothelial cells which have been activated by tumour necrosis factor or interleukin-1β. Monoclonal antibodies against interleukin-6 have also been shown to provide protection in animals against lethal Gram-negative infection. Interleukin-6, when administered as a sole agent appears to be of low toxicity, the only significant host response being a marked increase in hepatic acute-phase protein synthesis. Recent evidence suggests that tumour necrosis factor or interleukin-1β increase the expression of GP 130, a target cell-associated glycoprotein that binds to the interleukin-6/interleukin-6 receptor complex and greatly enhances the intrinsic toxicity of this cytokine.

Interleukin-8 (IL-8)

Induction of this 6- to 10-kDa polypeptide appears to parallel that of interleukin-6 and it resembles the latter in that it appears to have low intrinsic toxicity. However, when it is present in association with tumour necrosis factor or interleukin-1β it appears to have potent neutrophil activating and chemotactic properties which may well magnify the toxicity of the other cytokines. No definite role has yet been established for this cytokine in human sepsis.

SYNERGY BETWEEN CYTOKINES—the 'cytokine cascade'

Synthesis of tumour necrosis factor appears to be strongly repressed during health and it is not detectable in the circulation. Cells triggered by endotoxin or various other stimuli become 'superinduced' and elaborate tumour necrosis factor as their principal secretory product. Low levels of endotoxaemia appear to trigger tumour necrosis factor without significant circulating interleukin-1β and in this cytokine milieu, fever and neurohormonal and acute-phase protein alterations occur but without lethal responses such as hypotension or coagulopathy. These lethal responses occur if tumour necrosis factor levels become high enough for significant secondary synthesis of interleukin-1β or the other synergizing cytokines to occur. These observations may explain why monoclonal antibodies against any of the key cytokines, when given prophylactically, will prevent death following lethal bacterial challenge in animals.

Individual variations in cytokine production

It is well recognized that individuals differ greatly in their systemic response to a infected focus. For example, 20 per cent of individuals with established acute appendicitis show no fever, tachycardia, anorexia, or neutrophil leucocytosis. The remainder exhibit these changes to a varying extent. Even established peritonitis may be associated with minimal signs of systemic toxicity in some individuals while others rapidly progress to septic shock and death. Recent evidence suggests that this individual variation may be related to differences between individuals in the magnitude of the cytokine response following a standard stimulus. It has been shown that a variation of over one hundredfold exists between individuals in terms of monocyte-secreted tumour necrosis factor following a standard dose of endotoxin both *in vitro* and *in vivo*. The endotoxin-resistant mouse (C3H HEJ) has a defect on chromosome 4 that prevents synthesis of tumour necrosis factor. It appears that there are comparable human beings who secrete very little tumour necrosis factor after endotoxin stimulation ('low responders'). It has recently been shown that responder status is closely related to haplotype on the Class 2 histocompatibility complex (i.e. tissue type). Tissue typing may be a method which can be used in the future to identify, prospectively, individuals at high risk of death if sepsis ensues (e.g. following major gastrointestinal surgery).

Mechanisms of cytokine mortality in severe sepsis

The induction of the cytokine cascade represents an inappropriately severe host response to an inflammatory stimulus and leads to death through the following mechanisms.

1. Hypothermia;
2. Coagulopathy;
3. Visceral hypoperfusion and reperfusion injury;
4. Lactate acidosis and acidaemia;
5. Myocardial depression;
6. Peripheral vasodilation;
7. The capillary leak syndrome which is believed to induce profound hypotension and multiple organ failure.

All of these alterations may be induced by tumour necrosis factor or interleukin-1β but they do not act directly. Figure 2 illustrates the principal efferent mechanisms by which cytokines exert their lethal effects.

Blocking the cytokine cascade

This field is still in its infancy and only a small fraction of the potential agents that may be of value have been tested in infected human beings. In severe surgical sepsis (e.g. pancreatic abscess or acute gastrointestinal anastomosis disruption) mortality is still 'sticking' at 50 to 70 per cent and there is little prospect that better antibiotics or haemodynamic support will alter this. There is good reason, however, to believe that modification of the cytokine cascade might reduce mortality. Figure 2 illustrates the theoretical ways in which this could be done. The advantages and disadvantages of each approach will be considered briefly.

Inhibiting endotoxin-induced generation of cytokines

Blockade of endotoxin is an attractive concept because the toxic moiety of the molecule (lipid A) is common to all Gram-negative strains. Furthermore endotoxin is not a fundamental component of the immune system and therefore inhibiting endotoxin should not cause immunosuppression in any way. A human monoclonal antibody against lipid A has recently been evaluated in Phase 3 clinical trials and has been shown to reduce mortality following Gram-negative bacteraemia by 39 per cent. This represents a major advance in the therapy of Gram-negative infection but the use of this agent is complicated by the following considerations: (1) it is expensive; (2) there is no ideal way to predict whether shock is caused by a Gram-negative organism while there is still a therapeutic window and probably only 40 per cent of individuals receiving this agent will, in retrospect be candidates to benefit from it; (3) it is ineffective against septic shock induced by non-Gram-negative pathogens. Other methods which have been proposed for modifying cytokine production following endotoxaemia include:

1. Blocking the effects of endotoxin on its target cell. The mechanism whereby endotoxin triggers the target cell to secrete cytokines has recently been clarified. Firstly the lipid A component of endotoxin binds to the LPS binding protein (LBP). The endotoxin/LBP complex then binds to the CD14 receptor of target cells which acts as the signal triggering cytokine synthesis. It is possible that anti-CD14 antibodies may render target cells resistant to endotoxin but this has not been investigated therapeutically. Additionally, the azurophilic granules of neutrophils contain an endogenous inhibitor of the LPS binding protein called bactericidal permeability-increasing protein (BPI). Levels of bactericidal permeability-increasing protein appear to be deficient in severe sepsis and it can be shown that exogenously administered bactericidal permeability-increasing protein significantly protect animals from the lethal effects of endotoxin. The clinical evaluation of bactericidal permeability-increasing protein is about to commence.
2. Blocking the intracellular signal generated by the interaction between endotoxin, its binding protein, and the CD14 receptor. Unfortunately this secondary signal has not yet been identified but its characterization might allow therapies that rendered the individual temporarily resistant to the effects of endotoxin.
3. Blockade of cytokine synthesis. Glucocorticoids are potent inhibitors of tumour necrosis factor synthesis but only if given prophylactically. It appears that these agents stimulate inhibitors that impede the signals stimulating cytokine synthesis but are powerless to arrest activation once it is in progress. Current clinical evidence does not favour a role for these agents in most instances of severe sepsis.

Monoclonal antibodies against cytokines

This is an extremely promising approach as unlike antiendotoxin antibodies these agents might be more generally applicable in severe inflammatory states rather than just those initiated by endotoxin. Clinical trials have now commenced with antitumour necrosis factor and anti-interleukin-1 antibodies and results should soon be available. Experimentally they are most effective when given prophylactically and concerns have been expressed as to their potential role in established sepsis. Against this animal models of lethal endotoxaemia are not really representative of typical human sepsis and septic shock and there is a small body of evidence suggesting that antitumour necrosis factor antibodies significantly attenuate hypotension associated with septic shock, although it has not yet been shown that they diminish mortality.

Inhibitors of cytokine receptors

Concerns have been raised about the inherent immunogenicity of anticytokine antibodies and the use of natural or synthetic inhibitors of cytokine function may circumvent this problem. Approaches undergoing or about to undergo clinical evaluation include:

1. Use of a naturally occuring interleukin-1 receptor antagonist. Animals or human beings exposed to endotoxin elaborate a 23- to 25-kDa peptide that competes with interleukin-1 for occupancy of its receptor but has no agonist properties. This moiety is termed the interleukin-1 receptor antagonist (IL-1 ra). It prevents death in otherwise lethal endotoxaemia. It has also been tested in Phase II studies in patients with various types of sepsis (Gram-negative, Gram-positive, and fungal) and was found to reduce mortality significantly (from 45 to 16 per cent). If this finding is confirmed in double-blind clinical trials it will represent a major advance in the therapy for severe sepsis.
2. Use of soluble tumour necrosis factor receptors. Soluble

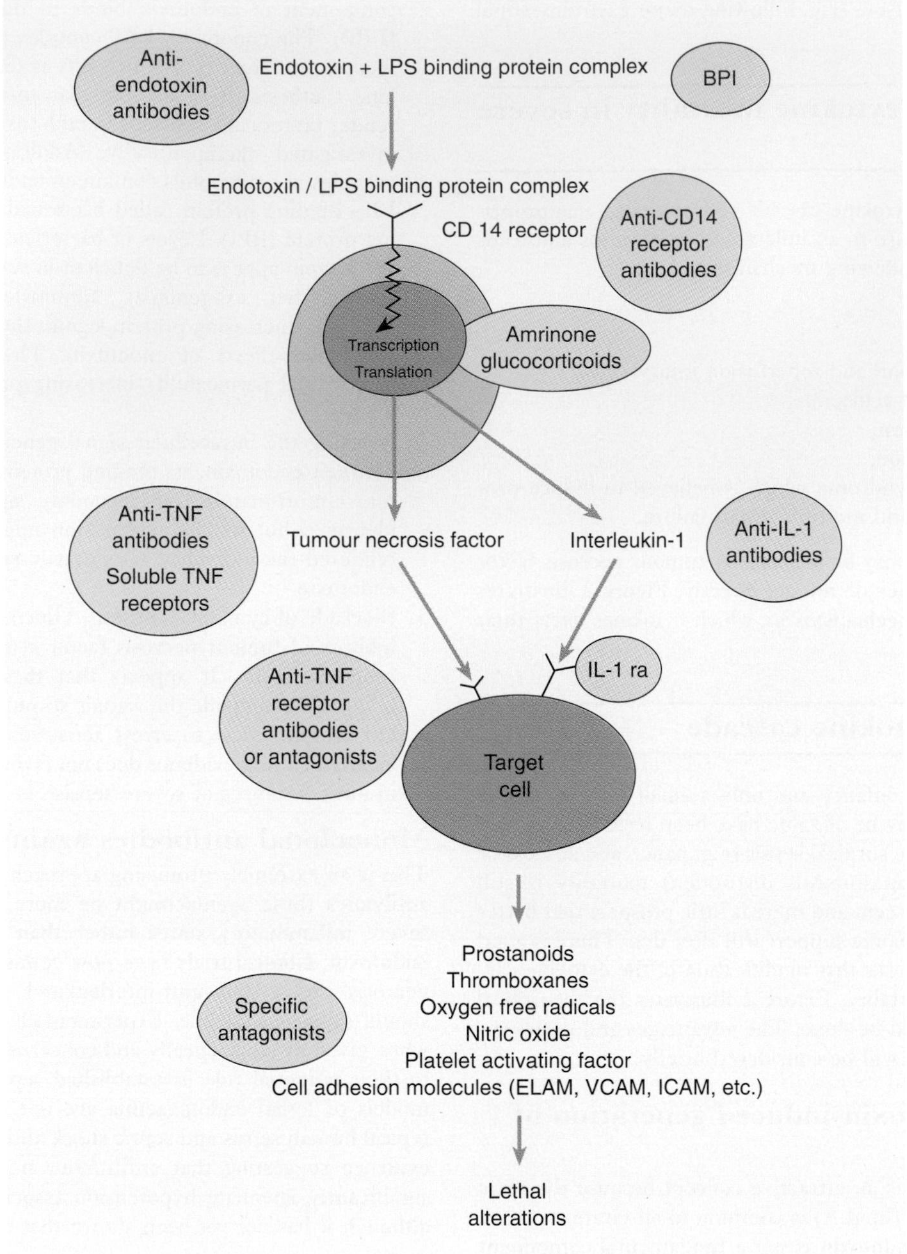

Fig. 2 Host autoinjury occurs through a pathway that has recently been elucidated. The relative contributions of the various mediators remain to be clarified. Potential antagonists of this pathway are shown in bold circles.

tumour necrosis factor receptors are detectable in the bloodstream during health and become elevated during severe sepsis. Again the shedding of receptors into the bloodstream may represent a beneficial host response to limit cytokine activity and this protective mechanism may become overwhelmed in severe sepsis. Gram-negative septic shock in the baboon may be attenuated by use of large amounts of soluble tumour necrosis factor receptors administered exogenously. Attempts are being made to conjugate soluble tumour necrosis factor receptor fragments to an antibody to increase their half-life in the circulation.

Although anticytokine therapy is in its infancy it is clear that following severe inflammatory or infective episodes the host not only releases large amounts of potentially lethal cytokines but also releases potential antidotes to these cytokines such as soluble receptors and endogenous antagonists. Lethal effects of cytokines are probably seen when these antidotes are exhausted, leading to unopposed synergistic cytokine activity. The current interpretation is that both interleukin-1 and tumour necrosis factor orchestrate the deleterious effects of infection and that blocking the activity of either one of these cytokines prevents the full consequences of the disease.

IMMUNOTHERAPY AGAINST SURGICAL SEPSIS

As stated earlier septic shock and multiple organ failure have a multifactorial aetiology but surgical patients are particularly at risk.

CYTOKINES IN CHRONIC SEPSIS

The major thrust of cytokine research has been involved with attenuating the host response to acute infection. It is becoming apparent that cytokines such as tumour necrosis factor and interleukin-1 may also mediate chronic events in sepsis including immunosuppression, accelerated proteolysis, and generalized cachexia and anorexia. At present the data are confusing and controversial and different but similar models reveal conflicting results. If cytokines are of importance as mediators of cachexia it is probable that they act in concert with other mediators such as stress hormones and by altering neurohormonal set-points within the hypothalamus and elsewhere within the central nervous system.

FURTHER READING

Beutler B. Cytokines in shock 1992. In: Lamy M, Thijs LG, eds. *Update in Intensive Care and Emergency Medicine*. Berlin: Springer-Verlag, 1993: 51–67.

Dinarello CA. Blocking cytokines in infectious disease. In: Lamy M, Thijs LG, eds. *Update in Intensive Care and Emergency Medicine*. Berlin: Springer-Verlag, 1993: 362–76.

Dinarello CA, Wolff SM. Mechanisms of disease—the role of interleukin-1 in disease. *N Engl J Med* 1993; **328**: 106–13.

Lowry SF, van Zee KJ, Moldawer LL. Strategies for modulation of tissue cytokine responses to sepsis. In: Lamy M, Thijs LG, eds. *Update in Intensive Care and Emergency Medicine*. Berlin: Springer-Verlag, 1993: 345–61.

Michie HR, *et al.* Detection of circulating tumor necrosis factor following endotoxin administration. *N Engl J Med* 1988; **318**: 1481–6.

Ohlsson K, *et al.* Interleukin-1 receptor antagonist reduces mortality from endotoxin shock. *Nature* 1990; **348**: 550–2.

Ziegler EJ, *et al.* Treatment of Gram-negative bacteremia and shock with human antiserum to a mutant *Escherichia coli*. *N Engl J Med* 1982; **307**: 1225–30.

Ziegler EJ, *et al.* Treatment of Gram-negative bacteremia and septic shock with HA–1A human monoclonal antibody against endotoxin. *N Engl J Med* 1991; **324**: 429–36.

5 Medical problems in the surgical patient

5.1 Respiratory problems

LUCA M. BIGATELLO AND ROGER S. WILSON

INTRODUCTION

Pulmonary complications are a major source of morbidity in surgical patients, second only to cardiovascular events as a cause of perioperative death. The overall incidence of pulmonary complications following all types of surgery is approximately 5 per cent. Several risk factors have been associated with a higher rate of pulmonary complications, including age, male gender, emergency surgery, American Society of Anesthesiology physical status classification, and the length of the surgical procedure.

While these conditions contribute to an overall increase of perioperative complications, two additional factors specifically predispose to the development of pulmonary complications: pre-existing respiratory disease and surgery of the chest or upper abdomen. Clinically important atelectasis, bronchospasm, retained secretions, and infectious complications may develop in 20 to 70 per cent of patients with pre-existing respiratory disease. This, in the most severe cases, can result in acute respiratory failure and the need for prolonged mechanical ventilation. Death from pulmonary complications occurs in 7 per cent of surgical patients with moderate to severe chronic lung disease. A recent prospective study confirmed that pulmonary complications occur in 33 per cent of patients with mild to moderate chronic lung disease who undergo upper abdominal surgery.

Evaluation for surgery must consider the effects of anaesthesia and surgery on respiratory function. In addition, special consideration has to be given to patients who are at high risk for perioperative pulmonary complications and to those who are scheduled to undergo lung surgery. Finally, optimization of their clinical status should be performed preoperatively, in an attempt to minimize morbidity.

EFFECT OF SURGERY AND ANAESTHESIA ON RESPIRATORY FUNCTION

Pulmonary function is altered in several ways during and after surgery. Important aspects include the breathing pattern, lung volumes, gas exchange, and defence mechanisms. These changes occur to some degree in every surgical patient, but have a greater impact in those with pre-existing respiratory disease.

Ventilation

Under normal circumstances, spontaneous minute ventilation (tidal volume × respiratory rate) increases in response to elevated arterial carbon dioxide tension and to a reduction of the arterial oxygen tension. Most drugs used during anaesthesia impair this normal ventilatory response to hypercapnia and hypoxaemia. Opioids can produce profound respiratory depression. Even small doses of morphine sulphate (for example, 7.5 mg subcutaneously) can blunt the ventilatory response to hypercapnia and hypoxia, and all the currently available opioid agonists seem to exert a similar effect at equipotent analgesic doses. The inhalational anaesthetics halothane, enflurane, and isoflurane also depress respiratory drive. Ventilatory response to hypoxaemia is virtually abolished at inspired concentrations of halothane as low as 0.1 to 0.2 per cent, which are likely to be present still during early recovery from general anaesthesia (Fig. 1.). The potent inhalational agents decrease spontaneous minute ventilation, producing a decrease in tidal volume and resultant rapid, shallow breathing. This pattern increases the ratio of dead space to tidal volume (V_D/V_T), leading to CO_2 retention, and may facilitate the development of alveolar collapse and atelectasis.

Lung volumes

Changes in static lung volumes occur during surgery and anaesthesia. In 1933 Beecher reported a decrease in vital capacity of approximately 45 per cent and in functional residual capacity of approximately 20 per cent after laparotomy. These changes persisted from 1 to 2 weeks postoperatively. Subsequent studies confirmed and extended this original observation. The following characteristics have been established: functional residual capacity is reduced during general anaesthesia by about 20 per cent below the value measured in the awake, supine position. This change occurs early in the course of the surgical procedure, appears not to be influenced by use of muscle relaxants, and is more pronounced in the elderly. Upper abdominal incisions and thoracotomy are associated with the largest decrease in lung volumes postoperatively, followed by lower abdominal surgery; peripheral procedures do not cause persistent changes. The cause of the reduction in lung volumes was elucidated in 1974 by Froese and Bryan. Using lateral chest radiograms they found that the diaphragm ascended into the chest by about 2 cm during anaesthesia with or without paralysis, and this change accorded roughly with the decrease in functional residual capacity (Fig. 2).

Breathing at low lung volumes may affect gas exchange. A 20 per cent reduction in functional residual capacity added to an equivalent decrease secondary to assumption of the supine position brings the resting lung volume (the functional residual capacity) quite close to residual volume. This circumstance may favour the development of atelectasis in the dependent zones of the lung following induction of general anaesthesia. Resistance to airflow also increases at lower lung volumes. Airway resistance is inversely proportional to the fourth power of the radius of the airway. At a reduced functional residual capacity, small decreases in volume result in a marked increase in resistance, which may cause hyperinflation and air-trapping in patients with asthma or chronic obstructive pulmonary disease.

Gas exchange

Uncomplicated general anaesthesia produces abnormalities in gas exchange that may become clinically significant in patients with pre-existing respiratory disease. Adequate gas exchange is dependent upon homogeneous matching of ventilation and perfusion

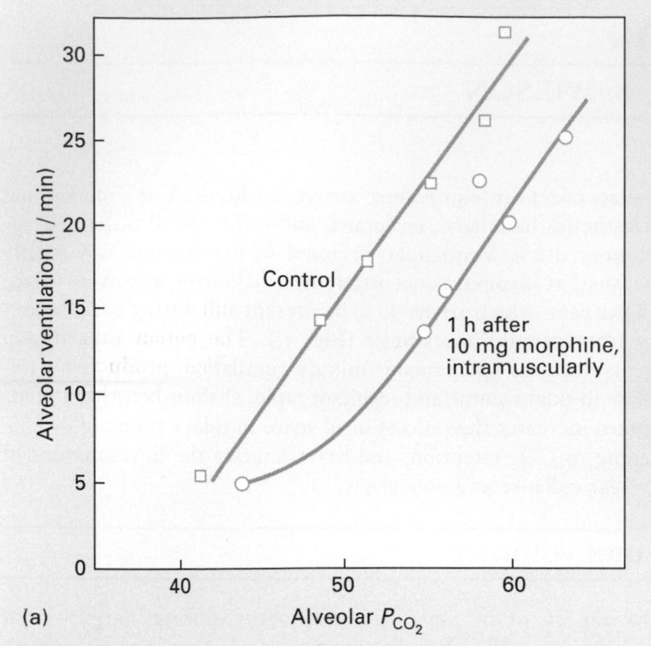

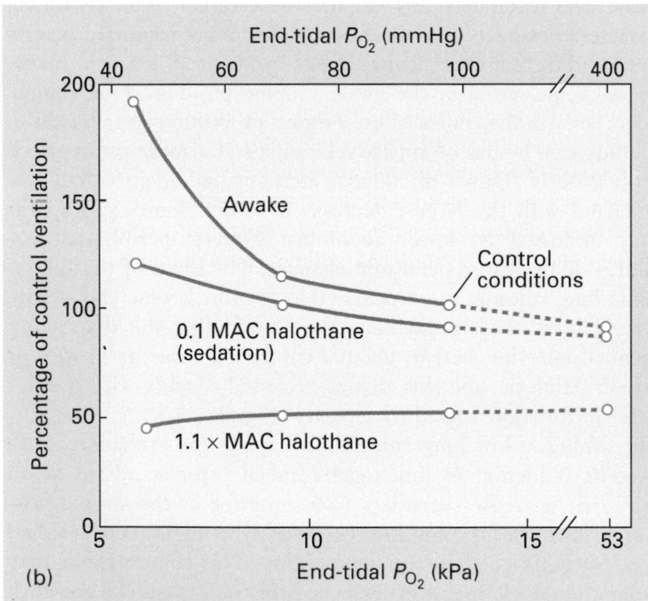

Fig. 1 (a) Effect of opioids on the ventilatory response to hypercapnia: alveolar $P\text{CO}_2$ is plotted against minute ventilation before and 1 h after administration of morphine sulphate, 10 mg IM. (b) Effect of halothane anaesthesia on ventilatory response to hypoxia. MAC is the minimal alveolar concentration required for anaesthesia.

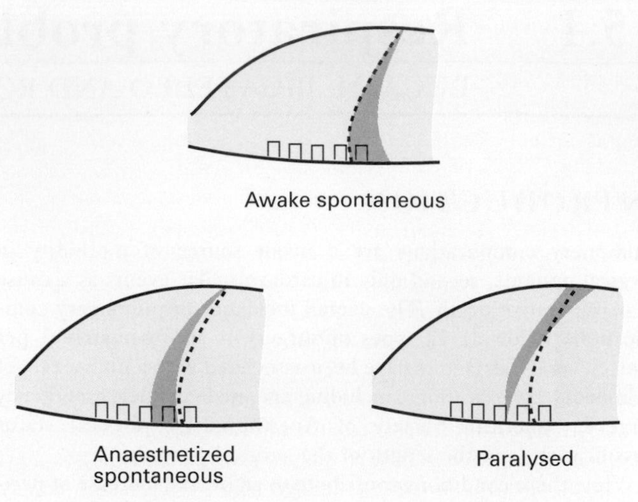

Fig. 2 Diagrammatic comparison of the position of the diaphragm in the awake and anaesthetized patient. The broken line is the end-expiratory position of the diaphragm in the awake, supine state. The shaded area indicates the respiratory excursions of the diaphragm.

at the alveolar level. Inspired gas delivered to lung regions that have no pulmonary capillary blood flow cannot take part in gas exchange and, conversely, pulmonary blood flow distributed to regions without ventilation cannot be oxygenated. The term ventilation/perfusion ratio (V/Q) is commonly used to refer to this relationship. Considering the lung as a whole, typical resting values may be 4 l/min for alveolar ventilation and 5 l/min for pulmonary blood flow. Thus, the overall V/Q ratio would be 0.8, which happens to be close to the normal ratio between CO_2 production and O_2 consumption (respiratory quotient). In fact, ventilation and perfusion are not uniformly distributed and may range all the way from unventilated to unperfused alveoli, with infinite gradation in between.

A simplified approach to V/Q physiology is shown in Fig. 3. The ventilated but unperfused alveoli comprise the dead space, the perfused but unventilated alveoli the shunt, and gas exchange is confined to the 'ideal' alveoli. In clinical practice, arterial hypoxaemia is frequently the result of low V/Q ratios rather than of a true shunt and is more correctly referred to as venous admixture. Usually, an increased dead space may be offset by increasing minute ventilation. An abnormal venous admixture up to about 30 per cent may be corrected with higher inspired oxygen concentrations.

In the awake individual with normal lungs, the amount of inefficient ventilation causing venous admixture is minimal, resulting in an alveolar/arterial $P\text{O}_2$ gradient of about 10 mmHg. During uncomplicated general anaesthesia the alveolar/arterial $P\text{O}_2$ gradient may increase to 30 to 50 mmHg. The increase is secondary to the reduction in lung volumes and its effects on the development of atelectasis with alveolar and/or airway closure and resultant V/Q mismatch. Furthermore, inhalational anaesthetics may impair gas exchange by inhibiting the physiological mechanism of hypoxic pulmonary vasoconstriction that tends to divert pulmonary blood flow away from areas of low ventilation to regions of increased ventilation, preserving the V/Q relationship and arterial oxygenation.

Elimination of CO_2 is also affected during general anaesthesia, as a result of changes in the ratio of dead space to tidal volume (V_D/V_T). Changes in V_D/V_T as they occur during general anaesthesia are shown diagrammatically in Fig. 4. The anatomical

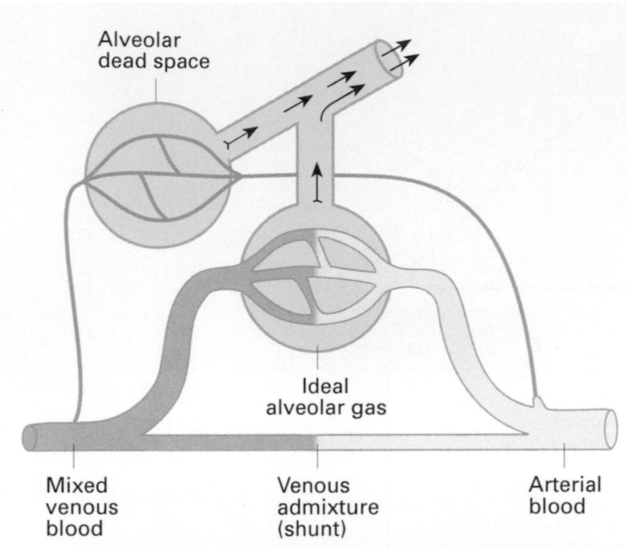

Fig. 3 Diagrammatic representation of the efficiency of gas exchange in the lung, considered as a three-compartment model. Gas exchange occurs only in the 'ideal' alveoli. The alveolar dead space consists of alveolar units which are ventilated but not perfused. The venous admixture is the result of pulmonary blood flow through alveoli which are not ventilated. In the real situation, infinite gradations of ventilation and perfusion occur.

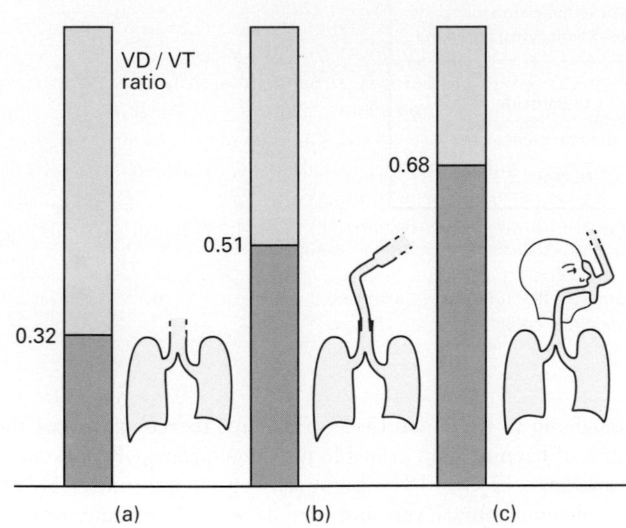

Fig. 4 Changes in dead space as a fraction of tidal volume during general anaesthesia. (a) From the carina downwards; (b) including the endotracheal tube and connectors; and (c) including the face-mask and connectors.

dead space ($(V_D/V_T)_a$; oral cavity, pharynx, and conducting airways) measures about 30 per cent of the tidal volume in spontaneously breathing individuals. During general anaesthesia, the $(V_D/V_T)_a$ also includes that segment of the anaesthetic circuit in which the gas flow is bidirectional (endotracheal tube or face-mask and tubing distal to the 'Y-piece' connector). When the trachea is intubated, the $(V_D/V_T)_a$ is slightly decreased because the upper airway is bypassed. When anaesthesia is administered by face-mask, on the other hand, the volume of the mask adds further dead space, and the $(V_D/V_T)_a$ increases to approximately 40 per cent.

The term 'physiological dead space', $(V_D/V_T)_{phys}$, defines areas of the lung parenchyma beyond the conducting airways where gas exchange does not occur. In the awake individual with normal lungs, no significant $(V_D/V_T)_{phys}$ is detectable. During general anaesthesia, the $(V_D/V_T)_{phys}$ increases to approximately 30 per cent of the tidal volume. Thus, a seemingly adequate minute ventilation of 5 to 6 l may result in an alveolar ventilation as low as 2 to 3 l per minute, which could cause CO_2 retention.

Studies carried out with the aid of the multiple inert gas washout technique allow summarization of the effects of anaesthesia on gas exchange as follows.

1. The alveolar/arterial Po_2 gradient is increased during anaesthesia, and this change is markedly affected by age.
2. The decrease in Po_2 is secondary to an increased distribution of flow to areas of decreased ventilation, most commonly the dependent areas.
3. The increase in V_D/V_T seems to be secondary to increased distribution of ventilation to areas of lesser perfusion.
4. The major differences are between the awake and anaesthetized state; paralysis and controlled ventilation do not greatly alter overall gas exchange.

Host defences

Inspired air is normally warmed and humidified in the nasopharynx. This process facilitates the clearance of airway secretions by optimizing ciliary function. Anaesthetic gases are essentially dry as they leave the standard anaesthesia machine; dryness tends to damage the respiratory epithelium. Endotracheal intubation exacerbates this problem by bypassing the upper airway. The cough mechanism is depressed during general anaesthesia as well as during spinal anaesthesia. The combination of these factors predisposes to inflammation of the respiratory mucosa and to retained secretions, which may favour alveolar collapse, bronchospasm, and infection.

Normal function of the immune system in humans is altered in the immediate postoperative period. Unfortunately, clinical testing in this area is confronted with the difficulty of separating the effects of multiple intraoperative factors that may impact on immunity. It appears that many of the immune changes seen in surgical patients are primarily the result of the surgical trauma and of endocrine responses, rather than of the anaesthetic exposure itself. *In-vitro* studies suggest that anaesthetic agents may have a direct effect on granulocyte and monocyte function and on the release of immunological mediators. The clinical significance of these observations, however, is not defined at the present time. A synopsis of the possible effects of anaesthetic agents on different components of the immune response is shown in Fig. 5.

CLINICAL EVALUATION OF THE PATIENT WITH PULMONARY DISEASE

Identification of patients at increased risk for perioperative respiratory complications is important since optimization of their clinical status can decrease morbidity. During clinical evaluation,

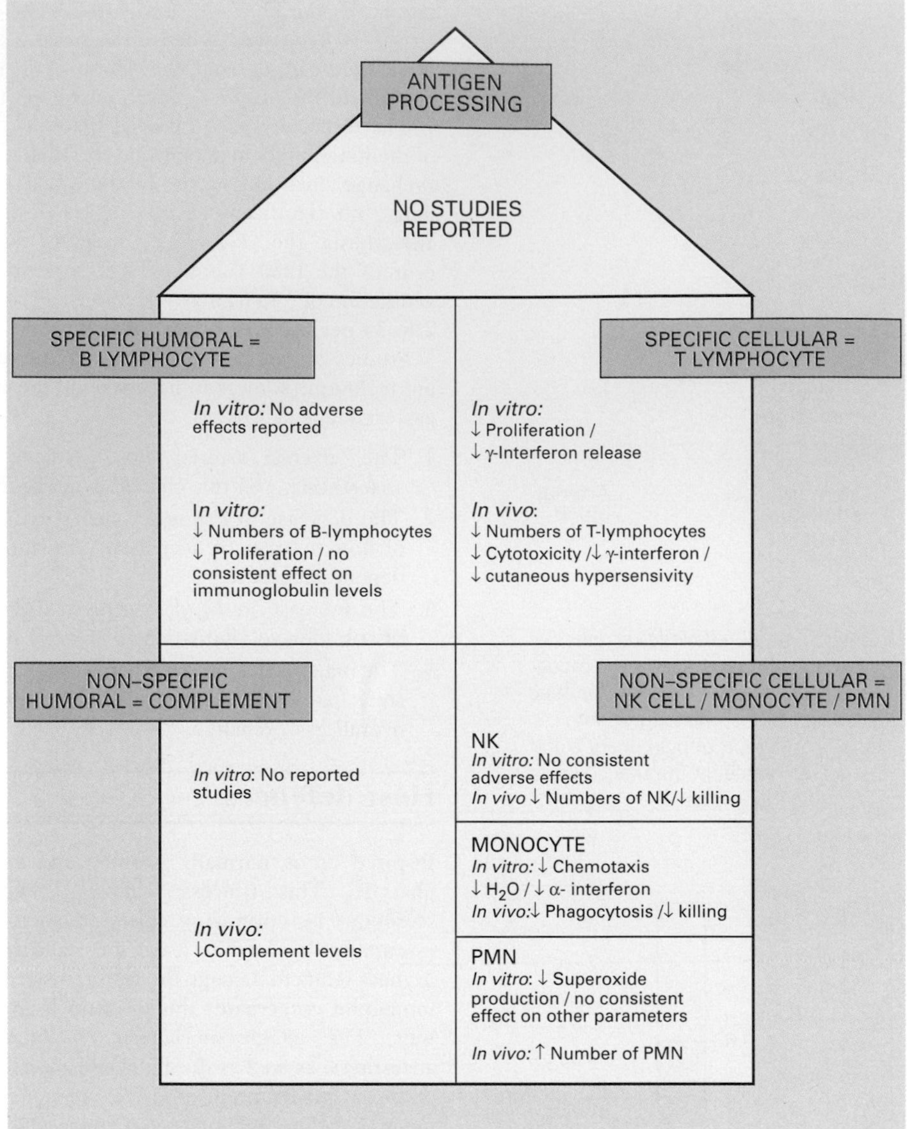

Fig. 5 Effects of anaesthetic agents (primarily halothane) on the function of immune components. NK–natural killer cell, PMN—polymorphonuclear cells.

one should give emphasis to the current respiratory status of the patient, to coexisting cardiovascular disease, to a prior history of treatment for pulmonary disease, to occupational exposures, and to the use of medications such as bronchodilators or corticosteroids. Among the risk factors possibly associated with an increased rate of perioperative pulmonary complications, the following have been reported consistently.

Cigarette smoking

This is associated with an increased perioperative mortality because of the effects of smoking on both the cardiovascular and respiratory systems. A history of tobacco use is a sensitive predictor of lung disease and of postoperative respiratory complications: compared with non-smokers, cigarette-smokers have a two- to threefold greater incidence of perioperative pulmonary complications. Smoking also increases the concentration of carboxyhaemoglobin in the blood (3–15 per cent), thereby reducing the amount of haemoglobin available for oxygen transport. Cessation of smoking 12 to 18 h preoperatively significantly lowers carboxyhaemoglobin levels and may decrease heart rate, arterial blood pressure, and catecholamine levels. The impact of smoking cessation on the incidence of perioperative pulmonary complications, however, is not detectable unless smoking is discontinued for more than 8 weeks before surgery. This conclusion is in agreement with the observed improvement in respiratory symptoms and lung volumes that occurs over a period of months following the cessation of smoking.

Obesity

Obesity reduces total lung volume and functional residual capacity, thus predisposing to hypoxaemia and atelectasis. Lower pre- and postoperative arterial oxygen saturation was found, compared with non-obese controls, in patients undergoing jejunoileal bypass for morbid obesity. The scanty data available from studies with a precise definition of obesity suggest that postoperative hypoxaemia and atelectasis are common in obese patients, but that the risk of severe respiratory morbidity is in general not increased.

Asthma

A major concern when managing patients with bronchial asthma is the potential for exacerbation of bronchospasm secondary to stimulation of the airways. Severe bronchospasm may occur during endotracheal intubation, often as a result of 'light anaesthesia', bronchial secretions, and surgical manipulation of the viscera or the airway. Early studies suggested an increased risk of perioperative respiratory complications in patients with bronchial asthma when compared to non-asthmatics. However, even steroid-dependent asthmatic patients were shown to tolerate major surgery if proper perioperative care was given. Anaesthetic considerations in asthmatic patients include the use of volatile agents, which induce a direct bronchodilator effect independent of adrenergic stimulation. Ketamine exhibits bronchodilator properties. Opioids effectively blunt airway reflexes; synthetic opioids, such as fentanyl, do not induce histamine release and may decrease airway irritability during intubation and extubation of the trachea. When possible, regional anaesthesia or general anaesthesia administered by face-mask may be a valuable alternative to endotracheal intubation.

Chronic obstructive pulmonary disease

Patients with chronic obstructive pulmonary disease have been identified as a group at increased risk for perioperative respiratory complications, as opposed to those with restrictive disease in whom expiratory flow rate and cough mechanism are preserved. Many critical values of pulmonary function have been associated with an increased incidence of postoperative pulmonary complications. A summary of abnormal values of pulmonary function tests associated with increased perioperative respiratory complications is reported in Table 1. Although it is clear that patients with chronic obstructive pulmonary disease are at higher risk than is the normal population, no one best test or combination of tests has emerged as a predictor of morbidity. In fact, other studies fail to show a reproducible correlation between abnormal values of pulmonary junction tests and the rate of pulmonary complications. Thus, the predictive value of abnormal pulmonary function tests as indictors of surgical risk in patients with chronic obstructive pulmonary disease seems to be generic. Given that abnormal pulmonary function tests are usually associated with symptoms, they might be no more specific than the information gathered during a careful history and physical examination.

Table 1 Pulmonary function tests criteria suggesting increased risk of postoperative respiratory morbidity

	Abdominal surgery	Thoracic surgery
FVC	<70% predicted	<70% predicted
	<75% predicted	<2 l
FEV_1	<70% predicted	<2 l
	<2 l	<800 ml*
FEV_1/FVC	<65% predicted	<50% predicted
FEF	<50% predicted	
MEFR	<200 l/min	<200 l/min
MVV	<50% predicted	<50% predicted
$Paco_2$	>45 mmHg	>45mmHg
MPAP		>30 mmHg
$\dot{V}o_2$		>1 l/m

FVC, forced vital capacity; FEV_1, forced expiratory volume in 1 s; FEF, forced expiratory flow between 25 and 75 per cent of FVC; MEFR, mid-expiratory flow rate; MVV, maximum voluntary ventilation; $Paco_2$, arterial carbon dioxide tension; MPAP, mean pulmonary artery pressure; $\dot{V}o_2$, oxygen consumption; *, predicted post-resection FEV_1.

Preoperative considerations for pulmonary resection

Virtually all patients with bronchogenic carcinoma of the lung have chronic obstructive pulmonary disease. While surgical therapy offers the best prospect of long-term survival, removal of lung tissue may reduce postoperative function, predisposing to long-term mechanical ventilatory support and possible death. When evaluating patients for lung surgery one should be able to predict postoperative function. The most frequently used method to predict lung function following lung resection is pulmonary scintigraphy. Ventilation scans with xenon-133, perfusion scans with technetium microaggregate, or combined $\dot{V}/\dot{Q}$ scans are equally effective in predicting postoperative forced vital capacity and forced expiratory volumes in 1s (FEV_1). The selective function of the segment to be resected can be evaluated, and the predicted postoperative FEV_1 calculated. A predicted post-excision $FEV_1 \leqslant 800$ to 1000 ml is generally considered of poor prognostic value.

Post-resection disability is related not only to limitations in ventilation but also to alterations in pulmonary blood flow and pressure; thus, criteria that stratify patients according to their ability to exercise have been studied. Measurement of maximum oxygen consumption, pulmonary artery pressures, and calculated pulmonary vascular resistances during bicycle ergometer testing have been advocated as possible criteria that could identify operative candidates who would otherwise not be considered for thoracotomy based on the results of pulmonary function tests. The predictive value of exercise testing needs confirmation in larger studies.

Optimization of pulmonary function

The efficacy of preoperative prophylactic measures in decreasing pulmonary complications has been clearly substantiated. Patients with abnormal pulmonary function tests who underwent a preoperative regimen of bronchodilators and physiotherapy had a postoperative rate of pulmonary complications of 21 per cent, as opposed to a 60 per cent incidence in patients with similar pulmonary function tests who did not receive preventive treatment.

Preoperative evaluation would be of limited value unless prophylactic measures are instituted in those patients identified as being at increased risk. High-risk categories of patients include those with chronic obstructive pulmonary disease as indicated by abnormal pulmonary function tests (particularly when scheduled for thoracic or upper abdominal surgery), smokers, and patients with acute respiratory infections or active bronchospasm. General measures that may be beneficial include the cessation of smoking, hydration, humidification of inspired gases, antibiotic treatment of infections, and treatment of associated cardiovascular and metabolic disease. More specifically, respiratory function may be improved over a short period of time before surgery by means of a programme of chest physical therapy and pharmacological treatment.

Chest physical therapy

This includes breathing and coughing exercises, postural drainage, ambulation, and the use of mechanical aids to lung expansion. Physiotherapeutic treatment should be planned and carried out by specialized personnel in order to ensure maximal patient compliance. Preoperative education is likely to be more effective than attempting to teach principles of physiotherapy in the presence of postoperative pain and medications.

Several kinds of mechanical aids to physiotherapy are available. Intermittent positive pressure breathing (IPPB), popular in the 1960s and 1970s, is not always well tolerated and may transiently decrease pulmonary compliance. Forced expiratory exercise by means of blow bottles and similar devices is no longer recommended because of the potential for hyperinflation and air-trapping. Currently, manoeuvres designed to increase the functional residual capacity, such as incentive spirometry and continuous positive airway pressure by face-mask, are used more frequently. Preoperative IPPB, incentive spirometry, and deep-breathing exercises seems to be equally effective in reducing the incidence of pulmonary complications following upper abdominal surgery, as compared with no respiratory treatment. However, the use of IPPB is frequently associated with unpleasant side-effects such as bloating and abdominal distension.

Pharmacological therapy

Table 2 summarizes the characteristics of the most common agents used preoperatively in patients with pulmonary disease. Fluidification of bronchial secretions and resolution of bronchospasm are the main goals of this treatment. Bronchodilator therapy should be aggressively pursued even in those patients with chronic obstructive pulmonary disease who do not seem to respond to a single administration during pulmonary function testing: some of these patients will benefit from repeated treatments over the course of few days. End-points of preoperative pharmacological treatment should be the resolution of acute symptoms such as bronchospasm and dyspnoea, and improvement in the patient's level of activity, as well as in the ability to expectorate and perform physiotherapeutic manoeuvres. Repeating a set of pulmonary function tests may offer an objective documentation of the effects of treatment.

NON-INVASIVE RESPIRATORY MONITORING

Non-invasive respiratory monitoring is now available almost routinely in the operating room and in the intensive care unit.

Pulse oximetry

Pulse oximetry provides continuous measurement of arterial oxygen saturation by spectrophotometry. Oxygenated and

Table 2 Pharmacological agents in the preoperative treatment of patients at risk for pulmonary complications

Agent	Mechanism	Route	Side-effects	Comments
Mucolytics				
Acetylcysteine*	Cleavage of disulphide bonds of mucoproteins	Nebulized	Bronchospasm	Concomitant nebulization of bronchodilator may prevent bronchospasm
Normal saline	Fluidification of mucus	Nebulized	Bronchospasm	As above
Bronchodilators				
Cromolyn sodium	Prevents degranulation of mast cells	PO Nebulized	Headache, diarrhoea	Effective only for prophylaxis, should be continued perioperatively
Sympathomimetics Isoproterenol Adrenaline	Increased intracellular cyclic AMP through stimulation of adenylate cyclase; bronchial smooth muscle relaxation	IV SC Nebulized	Tachycardia, arrhythmias, hypertension	Haemodynamic effects limit their clinical use; very low dose (0.25–0.5 mg/min) of adrenaline is often devoid of haemodynamic effects
Albuterol Terbutaline Metaproterenol	Selective stimulation of β_2-adrenergic receptors	Nebulized	Tachycardia	Fewer haemodynamic effects than non-selective agents; dose can be titrated to side-effects, which are short lived
Anticholinergics Atropine Glycopyrrolate Ipratropium	Bronchial smooth muscle relaxation (large airways)	Inhaled nebulized (IV)	Tachycardia, drying of secretions	Minimal haemodynamic effects with glycopyrrolate and ipratropium; may be effective as adjunctive therapy
Methylxanthines Aminophylline Theophylline	Phosphodiesterase inhibition, adenosine block, catecholamine release, diaphragmatic contractility	PO IV	Nausea, vomiting, tachycardia, supraventricular arrhythmias, seizures	Weak bronchodilators, poorly understood mechanism, serious toxicity, long half-life; not ideal for acute bronchospasm
Corticosteroids	Decrease inflammation of the respiratory mucosa	PO IV Inhaled	Immunosuppression, poor wound healing, salt retention, hypertension, suppression of endogenous steroidogenesis	Very effective in exacerbations of bronchospasm; delayed onset; rapid taper minimizes side-effects

PO, by mouth; IV, intravenous; SC, subcutaneous. *Randomized trials show no evidence of efficacy for acetylcysteine in the common applications.

reduced haemoglobin have different spectra of light absorption: the relative concentration of oxygenated haemoglobin (expressed as percentage saturation) in arterial blood is derived by a microprocessor from the ratio of absorption of two different wavelengths specific for the two forms of haemoglobin. The sensing unit of the pulse oximeter (oxysensor) can be applied to areas of the body (fingertips, toes, earlobes, nose, tongue) where a light beam is shone through and recorded by an emitting and a receiving diode. Adequate arterial blood flow is necessary in order to provide an adequate signal: motion, vasoconstriction, hypothermia, and very low blood pressure interfere with the detection of the signal. The intraoperative use of continuous oximetry identifies episodes of arterial oxygen desaturation earlier and more frequently than does clinical observation. Postoperatively, pulse oximetry is widely employed during immediate recovery from general anaesthesia and in the intensive care unit. Continuous monitoring of arterial oxygen saturation in these settings may reveal episodes of hypoxaemia that could otherwise go undetected. During weaning from mechanical ventilation, recording of arterial oxygen saturation may allow for changes in ventilatory parameters with less frequent arterial blood sampling.

Capnometry

This provides measurement of end-tidal CO_2 and display of exhaled CO_2 waveforms (capnography). The most commonly used capnometers continuously withdraw a small (150 ml/min) sample of gas distally to the 'Y-piece' connector of the breathing circuit. Modifications to face-masks, nasal airways, and nasal cannulas have been designed to facilitate capnography in the awake patient, enabling the capnograph to serve as an apnoea monitor. The CO_2 tension recorded at end-expiration (end-tidal CO_2) reflects the $P\text{CO}_2$ in the alveolar gas, which in normal circumstances is slightly lower (2–4 mmHg) than the arterial $P\text{CO}_2$. A higher arterial to end-tidal $P\text{CO}_2$ gradient reflects an increase in V_D/V_T. A sudden fall in the end-tidal $P\text{CO}_2$ may be due to an acute decrease in cardiac output, to pulmonary embolism or to air embolism. Useful applications of capnometry in the operating room include: detection of accidental oesophageal intubation by absence of a CO_2 waveform, inadequate ventilation, disconnection of a component of the breathing system, CO_2 rebreathing from an exhausted CO_2 absorber or a malfunctioning valve. Capnometry may allow early detection of air embolism during sitting craniotomy, spinal fusion or hip surgery, by a sudden decrease of end-tidal CO_2 secondary to a decreased cardiac output or to sampling of gas lower in CO_2, which diffuses into the alveoli from the pulmonary capillaries. Capnography may be useful in the intensive care unit in mechanically ventilated patients, where the adequacy of ventilation in response to physiological or mechanical changes may be assessed immediately.

ANAESTHETIC TECHNIQUE

No evidence exists that the type of anaesthetic technique affects the outcome of patients with chronic respiratory disease. Potential advantages of a regional anaesthetic (spinal, epidural, extremity blocks) are avoidance of the reduction in respiratory volumes and consequent alterations in gas exchanges associated with general anaesthesia, as well as the potential benefit of not intubating the trachea. On the other hand, a regional anaesthetic may weaken the function of respiratory muscles and blunt the proprioceptive reflexes from the diaphragm, causing hypoventilation; oversedation of an awake patient may also lead to hypoventilation, particularly in the elderly. Few studies have looked at the outcome of patients with respiratory disease in respect to the use of regional versus general anaesthesia, and the results of these are contradictory: although two large studies report better outcomes following spinal or epidural anaesthesia, the finding was not reproduced when comparable groups of patients were studied. Not surprisingly a universally applicable answer is not available. When suitable, extremity blocks (brachial, lumbosacral, ankle block) are intuitively a safe alternative, since they do not interfere with respiratory mechanics. Spinal or epidural anaesthesia may be very effective in a co-operative patient for procedures of the lower extremities or lower abdomen, while they may turn out an unwise choice in an elderly patients with dyspnoea at rest, scheduled for long and traumatizing surgery. Most instances are not so clear-cut, and the decision must ultimately be made by an experienced anaesthesiologist. The statement often forwarded, that a patient with severe chronic obstructive pulmonary disease 'needs a spinal' because he or she 'may never be extubated' is inappropriate.

Another approach now commonly employed for thoracic and upper abdominal surgery utilizes epidural analgesia in combination with 'light' general endotracheal anaesthesia. A mixture of a narcotic analgesic and local anaesthetic (for example, fentanyl 10 μg/ml in bupivacaine 0.075–0.125 per cent at 3–6 ml/h) is infused into the epidural space via a catheter inserted into the thoracic or lumbar spine, while general anaesthesia is maintained with nitrous oxide in oxygen and, if necessary, supplemented with a low concentration of a volatile agent. The epidural infusion can be continued beyond the surgery for analgesia. The adjunct of epidural analgesia greatly reduces the amount of general anaesthetic, facilitates extubation, and provides excellent pain relief postoperatively without significant ventilatory depression. The possible impact of this combined technique on the development of postoperative pulmonary complications has been assessed in several studies. While a few studies indicate a beneficial effect when compared to general anaesthesia alone, others found no difference; none, however, found higher rates of complication in the epidural groups. These studies are difficult to compare because of the different definitions of pulmonary complications, and the lack of uniformity with anaesthetic techniques used. However, the satisfaction of patients was uniformly superior when epidural analgesia was continued postoperatively, compared with intermittent intramuscular injection of opioids.

POSTOPERATIVE RESPIRATORY FAILURE

Many of the mechanisms that affect respiratory function during anaesthesia and surgery persist for a variable period of time postoperatively. In most instances, pulmonary complications may be viewed as a continuation of physiological derangements initiated on the operating table. Characteristically, postoperative patients breath rapidly, with shallow tidal volumes; vital capacity is reduced for several days postoperatively. Prolonged immobilization, tight bandages, splinting from incisional pain, and diaphragmatic dysfunction, all contribute to the persistence of low lung volumes.

The most important changes occur after thoracic and upper abdominal surgery. However, any type of surgery, when associated with immobilization, malnutrition, advanced age, and a decreased respiratory reserve, may create grounds for pulmonary complications. Patients with long-standing respiratory failure are particularly vulnerable in the perioperative period: pulmonary or systemic complications may easily result in acute respiratory failure requiring mechanical ventilation.

Causes of inability to sustain spontaneous ventilation at the end of surgery include excessive administration of volatile anaesthetics, narcotic analgesics, or muscle relaxants; prolonged and traumatizing procedures with large fluid requirement; and intraoperative complications such as lung collapse, pneumothorax, pulmonary oedema. In these circumstances, treatment of the intercurrent complication is generally sufficient to allow rapid recovery of respiratory function. Inability of sustaining adequate spontaneous ventilation later in the postoperative course is most frequent in patients with severe chronic obstructive pulmonary disease. Frequent causes of acute respiratory failure at this time are: pneumonia, tracheobronchitis, aspiration pneumonitis and cardiac failure. Pneumonia impairs gas exchange and decreases lung compliance: excessive bronchial secretions increase airway resistance and worsen bronchospasm. Patients with limited respiratory reserve tolerate poorly the consequent increased work of breathing and will require prolonged mechanical ventilation.

GUIDELINES FOR MANAGEMENT OF POSTOPERATIVE RESPIRATORY FAILURE

Hypoxaemia

Hypoxaemia may initially be treated with enriched inspired oxygen concentrations provided by a non-rebreathing face-mask, high-flow oxygen delivery systems, or by continuous positive airway pressure delivered by mask. Adjustable positive pressure ventilation triggered by the patient's inspiratory effort can also be delivered mechanically without the use of an eudotracheal tube. These systems may be effective in the short-term management of acute respiratory failure secondary to exacerbations of chronic pulmonary disease or to congestive heart failure. No data are available, however, in surgical patients. The potential for gastric distention associated with positive airway pressure without endotracheal intubation suggests the need for cautious use of these techniques in patients recovering from gastrointestinal surgery.

Endotracheal intubation

Ultimately, the surgical patient with acute respiratory failure may require endotracheal intubation and mechanical ventilation to avoid exhaustion, acidosis, and hypoxaemia. Intubation should be carried out by an experienced physician. Oral intubation under direct laryngoscopy is generally the easier route, and the one of choice in unstable patients when rapid re-establishment of the airway is mandatory. Nasal intubation is better tolerated during prolonged mechanical ventilation; the endotracheal tube is more effectively secured and accidental extubation less likely. Potential drawbacks include the possibility of mucosal damage and bleeding, which can make subsequent laryngoscopy very difficult, the limited internal diameter and length of the endotracheal tube, and the possibility of subsequent sinusitis. Naso-tracheal intubation should be avoided in patients with coagulopathies, and in those with major fractures of the facial bones or of the base of the skull. Table 3 summarizes issues concerning the oral and nasal approaches to intubation.

Nutrition

Patients with acute or chronic respiratory failure are often chronically ill and malnourished, and the added stress of surgery and infection further depletes their metabolic reserves. When tolerated, enteral nutrition may be used instead of total parenteral nutrition. This route seems to be more physiological, preserves the function of the intestinal mucosal barrier, and avoids the possible complications related to the use of parenteral nutrition, including morbidity resulting from venous access.

Table 3 Nasal versus oral intubation

	Nasal intubation	Oral intubation
Advantages	May be carried out without laryngoscopy when visualization or neck motion is limited	More easily carried out by inexperienced personnel
	Easily secured in place	Large-bore and shorter-length tubes can be utilized
	Improved patient comfort	
	Easier oral access and care	
Disadvantages	Choanal size limits diameter of the tube	Easily dislodged
	Occasional difficulty in suctioning	May be occluded if precautions are not taken to prevent the patient from biting on the tube
	Relative contraindications	May be poorly tolerated by some patients
	Risk of epistaxis in patients with coagulopathy	
	Obstruction of paranasal sinuses; long-term use may be associated with bacteraemia secondary to sinusitis	

Table 4 Guidelines for postoperative analgesia in adult intubated patients

	Agent and dose	Comments
Continuous IV infusion of opioids	Morphine sulphate: 5 mg/h, up to 20–30 mg/h; fentanyl, 50–100 mg/h	Little or no haemodynamic effects (mild bradycardia) respiratory depression; tachyphylaxis; mild sedative effect; no amnesic effect
Patient-controlled analgesia	For example, morphine sulphate, 1–2 mg boluses at lockout intervals of 10 min	Little or no haemodynamic effects (mild bradycardia) respiratory depression; tachyphylaxis; mild sedative effect; no amnesic effect
Continuous epidural infusion	Preservative-free morphine: 0.25–1 mg/h; fentanyl: 3–10 μg/ml in 0.1% bupivacaine, at 5–10 ml/h	Special training for nursing personnel necessary; delayed (up to 24 h) respiratory depression with morphine
Intercostal nerve blockade	0.5% bupivacaine with adrenaline 1:200 000, 4–5 ml per level	Repeated (every 4–8 h) blocks required; potential for pneumothorax intravascular injection, infection
Non-steroidal anti-inflammatory	Indomethacin: 25–50 mg PO or PR	Often effective for pain from thoracotomy and chest tubes
Non-steroidal anti-inflammatory	Ketorolac: 15–60 mg IM	Analgesic effect possibly as potent as IM morphine; potential for coagulopathy

IV, intravenous; PO, by mouth; PR, by way of the rectum; IM, intramuscular.

Physical therapy

As outlined earlier, a programme of physical therapy, including postural drainage, deep-breathing exercises, and early mobilization should be undertaken by specialized personnel. Getting the patient out of bed is a most effective lung expansion manoeuvre, which may generate a 10 to 20 per cent increase in functional residual capacity. Ambulation with the help of a nurse and a respiratory therapist is possible in co-operative intubated patients.

Analgesia and sedation

Adequate analgesia is essential postoperatively since pain can result in tachycardia and hypertension and limit respiratory and general activity. Intermittent intramuscular injections do not allow reliable pain control. In patients in the intensive care unit, where respiratory function can be closely monitored, opioids should be given intravenously.

In recent years, neuroaxial administration of opioids has become common practice in many surgical intensive care units. Preservative-free morphine injected intrathecally (1 mg or less) or epidurally (2–4 mg), can give excellent analgesia for 24 to 36 h. The epidural route is more frequently used, since it carries less risk of postdural puncture headache and infection, and thus is safer when prolonged drug delivery is desirable. Continuous epidural infusion through an indwelling catheter allows the use of short-acting, highly lipid-soluble opioids, such as fentanyl, thereby limiting the potential for ventilatory depression. Since opioids and local anaesthetics block different nociceptors in the spinal cord, mixtures of the two can be used to improve analgesia and minimize side-effects.

Self-administered analgesia (patient-controlled analgesia) allows standard drugs such as morphine or meperidine to be given from bedside devices operated directly by the patient. These devices typically employ infusion pumps with safety limits on infusion rates. Patient-controlled analgesia provides more stable blood levels of opioids when compared to intermittent *pro re nata* administration, and consequently better pain control with smaller overall amounts of the drug.

Regional nerve blocks may also be considered: multiple intercostal nerves blockaded with a local anaesthetic (for example, 0.5 per cent bupivacaine with adrenaline 1:200000) provide 4 to 8 h of analgesia following thoracotomies and subcostal and flank incisions. Non-steroidal anti-inflammatory agents may be an effective alternative or adjunct to opioids; ketorolac is a new non-steroidal anti-inflammatory agent with analgesic properties comparable to morphine but with no detectable respiratory depression.

Guidelines for postoperative analgesia for the mechanically ventilated patient are summarized in Table 4.

Sedation and adequate sleep is also an important aspect of the care of these patients; the practice of withdrawing or minimizing sedation in intubated patients to facilitate weaning is, in many cases, inappropriate. Benzodiazepines and neuroleptic agents are frequently used for sedation. In patients requiring large doses of sedatives because of excessive agitation, a continuous infusion may be appropriate. Midazolam (a short acting benzodiazepine) or propofol (an ultra-short-acting potent hypnotic) administered in continuous infusion can provide satisfactory sedation without untoward haemodynamic and respiratory effects; recovery after discontinuation of the infusion was almost immediate in the majority of patients.

Respiratory measures

The extent of acute lung disease is a major determinant of the patient's ability to sustain spontaneous ventilation: extubation will not be possible while major parenchymal damage from pneumonia or trauma persists, causing hypoxaemia, increased dead space, and impaired lung compliance. Appropriate antibiotic therapy must be guided by serial cultures. Fluid balance should be evaluated daily, and diuretic therapy administered when clinical evidence of fluid retention develops. Bronchospasm mandates aggressive treatment, as outlined earlier; factors capable of precipitating bronchospasm include pulmonary oedema, direct stimulation of the airways, pain, agitation, and (although probably not commonly) β-blockade therapy. Chest physical therapy should be accompanied by adequate analgesia. Excessive amounts of bronchial secretions may hinder extubation: treatment of tracheobronchitis with antibiotics, inhalation of mucolytics, and chest physical therapy enhance the patient's ability of clearing secretions.

Breathing through a narrow, long tube increases the patient's work and may limit weaning. A major increase in resistance occurs in adults if endotracheal tubes below size 7.0 (internal diameter in mm) are used, in conjunction with an increase in minute ventilation. Above this size, resistance does not increase appreciably, and the discomfort and risk of changing the tube is not justified in most patients.

The timing of an elective tracheostomy is not defined. Airway damage by the endotracheal tube has become less common since the introduction of high-volume, low-pressure cuffs. It is generally accepted that patients can be safely ventilated through an oro- or nasotracheal tube for 7 to 14 days. Elective tracheostomy has a low incidence of complications and is often unexpectedly welcomed by the patient, who appreciates the lower resistance to breathing and the better comfort as compared with an oro- or nasotracheal tube. Modifications of the tracheostomy tube allow the patient to talk when he is not mechanically ventilated (fenestrated tracheostomy) and during positive pressure ventilation ('talking' tracheostomy).

MODES OF MECHANICAL VENTILATION

Modern ventilators for use with patients in intensive care units are capable of delivering different modes of ventilation, allowing greater versatility in the choice of the modality that seems most appropriate for each patient. Regardless of the mode selected, the first decisions to be made when starting a patient on ventilatory support are about tidal volume, respiratory rate, and inspired oxygen concentration. Tidal volumes 50 to 80 per cent larger than spontaneous are often necessary to compensate for the circuit compressible volume and the increased physiological dead space, $(V_D/V_T)_{phys}$. Since ventilator circuits include humidifiers and long, large-bore corrugated tubing, a considerable percentage of the tidal volume is compressed in the system and never reaches the patient. Most systems have compressible volume loss factors of 3 to 5 ml/cmH_2O airway pressure. Thus, with a peak airway pressure of 50 cmH_2O, 150 to 250 ml of volume is lost. $(V_D/V_T)_{phys}$ may increase because of dilation of the airways and decreased cardiac output during positive pressure ventilation, and because of the lung disease itself.

Slow respiratory rates and large tidal volumes are generally employed in patients with chronic obstructive pulmonary disease, in whom a short expiratory time impairs CO_2 elimination and favours air-trapping. Rapid rates may be employed safely in patients with restrictive disease.

The duration of inspiration may be controlled in three different ways, depending upon the design of the ventilator. In volume-cycled modes, such as continuous mandatory ventilation, intermittent mandatory ventilation, and assist/controlled ventilation, inspiration terminates when the preset volume is delivered. In the absence of a leak, this method guarantees the tidal volume, independent of changes in compliance and resistance. In pressure-cycled modes, such as pressure-limited ventilation, inspiration terminates when a preset mouth pressure is reached. In this mode, pressure but not volume has to be dialled to determine tidal volume, which, consequently, is not guaranteed and is affected by changes in respiratory compliance and resistance. In time-cycled ventilators, inspiration terminates after a preset time, and tidal volume depends on the inspiratory flow rate; these ventilators are still used in the operating room, but are not practical for prolonged ventilation in the intensive care unit.

Inspired oxygen concentration ($F\text{IO}_2$) is generally regulated to the lowest possible level to maintain adequate arterial oxygen tension (60 to 80 mmHg) in order to avoid oxygen toxicity. The 'safe' level of $F\text{IO}_2$ in humans is not known: oxygen toxicity is directly related to $F\text{IO}_2$ and to the length of exposure. Inspired concentrations of O_2 below 50 per cent should be safe even for prolonged periods of time. Arterial oxygenation may be improved, and $F\text{IO}_2$ decreased, by applying positive end-expiratory pressure.

Positive end-expiratory pressure (PEEP) improves oxygenation in patients with acute respiratory failure by increasing functional residual capacity, by redistributing oedema fluid to the interstitial compartment, and possibly by decreasing cardiac output and shunting. Although there is a progressive increase in arterial P_{O_2} with an increase in functional residual capacity, increasing levels of positive end-expiratory pressure are associated with the potential for hyperinflation, increased intrathoracic pressure, decreased preload and increased afterload to the right ventricle, shifting of the intraventricular septum with decreased filling of the left ventricle, and barotrauma. Since benefits and complications of PEEP must be balanced, there is no agreement on what is the optimal level.

We will illustrate the salient features of a few among the most common modalities of mechanical ventilation, emphasizing that none has been proved to be universally superior and that the choice is dictated by the characteristics of each individual patient, the time course of the respiratory failure, and the preference of experienced physicians.

Controlled mandatory ventilation

This implies that the machine is fully sustaining the task of breathing. Controlled mandatory ventilation necessitates suppression of the patient's spontaneous efforts, accomplished either with overventilation or with heavy sedation and occasionally with paralysis. This mode is reserved for patients with absent respiratory drive or with the most severe degrees of failure and is obviously not ideal during the process of withdrawal of mechanical support.

Intermittent mandatory ventilation

This allows spontaneous breathing complemented by a variable input from the ventilator. The amount of ventilation provided can be progressively reduced as the patient's clinical condition improves. Intermittent mandatory ventilation is a simple and effective mode of weaning. A potential problem of this method is the inability of some patients to couple their spontaneous activity with the mechanical breaths. In the synchronized modification of intermittent mandatory ventilation the patient's breath inhibits the mechanical cycle, which is delivered only after a preset pause.

Assist/controlled ventilation

This allows the patient to initiate every breath spontaneously; the machine responds to the negative pressure exerted by the patient's inspiratory effort by delivering a preset tidal volume. By progressively decreasing the size of the assisted breath, the patient is allowed more work until the input from the ventilator becomes negligible. Although very appealing in principle, assist/controlled ventilation has several drawbacks. The less than perfect design of many 'demand valves' may cause either an excessive work to trigger the mechanical breath or, on the other hand, the delivery of breaths in response to stimuli such as coughing or moving, which may cause periods of distinct discomfort to the patient. Also, since the size of the assisted breath is the only variable that can be set, this does not always match the patient's pattern of breathing: when the patients peak-inspiratory flow is higher than the one supported by the ventilator the mechanical breath may reach the patient while exhalation has started, causing discomfort and increased work of breathing.

Inspiratory pressure support ventilation

This is a relatively new mode of assist ventilation. A preset amount of pressure is delivered in response to the patient's inspiratory effort; the tidal breath is delivered at an inspiratory flow (80–100 l/min) which is always higher than the patient's, thus avoiding dysynchrony. The only preset parameter is the inspiratory pressure; the patient controls the entire breathing cycle, receiving a smooth assistance from the ventilator. Potential advantages of this method are a more physiological pattern of breathing, decreased work of breathing, and slower respiratory rate, as compared with intermittent mandatory ventilation, and the potential for less barotrauma. The success of inspiratory pressure support ventilation is also due to the much improved overall design of the ventilators that can supply it; these ventilators, however, are also extremely expensive, and they should be reserved for the few patients who might really benefit from advanced modes of ventilatory support.

Discontinuation of mechanical ventilation

Once the patient who has been subjected to prolonged mechanical ventilation finally gets close to being separated from the machine, some objective criteria to predict the success of extubation, are appropriate. Bedside measurements of respiratory system mechanics are easily obtainable: suggested values include a forced vital capacity approaching 1 litre, a tidal volume of 300 to 400 ml, a negative inspiratory force lower than 40 cmH_2O, and a respiratory rate lower than 30 breaths/min.

Common sense should warn against predetermined criteria: if they are too strict, few patients will fail, but many others will be subjected to unnecessarily prolonged mechanical support. If liberal criteria are chosen, many patients inevitably fail. The answer is that no index or combination of variables can be an accurate predictor. Only the daily observation of the patient's progress, coupled with the observation of many previous states and with continuous learning about the underlying pathophysiology can improve the success rate in the treatment of respiratory failure.

FURTHER READING

Aitkenhead AR, Pepperman ML, Willatts SM, *et al.* Comparison of propofol and midazolam for sedation in critically ill patients. *Lancet* 1989; 704–8.

Appelberg M, Gordon L, Fatti LP. Preoperative pulmonary evaluation of surgical patients using the vitalograph. *Br J Surg* 1974; **61**: 57–9.

Beecher HK. Effect of laparotomy on lung volume: demonstration of a new type of pulmonary collapse. *J. Clin Invest* 1933; **12**: 651.

Bersten A, *et al.* Treatment of severe cardiogenic pulmonary edema with continuous positive airway pressure delivered by face-mask. *N Engl J Med* 1991; **325**: 1825–30.

Brochard L, *et al.* Reversal of acute exacerbations of chronic obstructive lung disease by inspiratory assistance with a face-mask. *N Engl J Med* 1990; **323**: 1523–30.

Celli BR, Rodriguez KS, Snider GL. A controlled trial of intermittent positive pressure breathing, incentive spirometry and deep breathing exercises in preventing pulmonary complications after abdominal surgery. *Am Rev Respir Dis* 1984; **130**: 12–15.

Froese AB, Bryan AC. Effects of anesthesia and paralysis on diaphragmatic mechanics in man. *Anesthesiologgy* 1974; **41**: 242–55.

Gaensler EA. Analysis of ventilatory defects by timed capacity measurements. *Am Rev Tuberc* 1951; **65**: 256.

Gracey DR, Divertie MB, Didier EP. Preoperative pulmonary preparation of patients with chronic obstructive pulmonary disease. *Chest* 1979; **76**: 123–9.

Keagy BA, *et al.* Elective pulmonary lobectomy: factors associated with morbidity and operative mortality. *Ann Thorac Surg* 1985; **40**: 349–52.

Latimer RG, *et al.* Ventilatory patterns and pulmonary complications after upper abdominal surgery determined by preoperative and postoperative computerized spirometry and blood gas analysis. *Am J Surg* 1971; **122**: 622–32.

Oh SH, Patterson R. Surgery in corticosteroid-dependent asthmatics. *J Allergy Clin Immunol* 1974; **53**: 345–51.

Pedersen T, Eliasen K, Henriksen H. A prospective study of risk factors and cardiopulmonary complications associated with anesthesia and surgery: risk indicators of pulmonary morbidity. *Acta Anesthes Scand* 1990; **34**: 144–55.

Pontoppidan H. Mechanical aids to lung expansion in non-intubated patients. *Am Rev Respir Dis* 1980; **122**: 109–19.

Stein M, Cassara EL. Preoperative pulmonary evaluation and therapy for surgical patients. *JAMA* 1970; **211**: 787–90.

Tarhan S, *et al.* Risk of anesthesia and surgery in patients with chronic bronchitis and chronic obstructive pulmonary disease. *Surgery* 1973; **74**: 720–6.

Tisi GM. Preoperative evaluation of pulmonary function. *Am Rev Respir Dis* 1979; **119**: 293–346.

Vaughan RW, Engelhart RC, Wise L. Postoperative hypoxemia in obese patients. *Ann Surg* 1974; **180**: 877–82.

Veterans Affairs TPN cooperative study group. Perioperative total parenteral nutrition in surgical patients. *N Engl J Med* 1991; **325**: 525–32.

Warner MA, Divertie MB, Tinker JH. Preoperative cessation of smoking and pulmonary complications in coronary artery bypass patients. *Anesthesiology* 1984; **60**: 380–3.

5.2 Cardiological problems

PIERRE FOËX

Anaesthesia and surgery carry increased risks in patients suffering from cardiovascular disease. This problem is accentuated in the elderly. Ischaemic heart disease, chronic lower respiratory tract infection, and cardiac failure are the disorders which are most commonly associated with postoperative deaths. Over the last decade, better preoperative assessment and the introduction of more sophisticated monitoring have increased the safety of surgery in patients with cardiovascular disease, as it has become possible for the anaesthetist to detect changes in the circulation before life-threatening complications occur. Nevertheless, myocardial infarction, progressive myocardial ischaemia, dysrhythmias, congestive cardiac failure and cerebrovascular accidents continue to occur relatively frequently, reflecting the trend to undertake invasive surgical procedures even in the severely ill patient. Relatively silent cardiac diseases are often initially diagnosed when a patient is admitted for surgery. Medical history, clinical examination, interpretation of the electrocardiogram, chest radiographs, and renal function tests form the basis of the preoperative evaluation. The need for this assessment to be supplemented by echocardiography, radionuclide cardiac imaging, cardiac catheterization, and angiography is, however, increasing. Objective data are required to enable decisions to be made about the overall surgical and anaesthetic strategy, including the extent of cardiovascular monitoring and the need for postoperative management in a high dependency or intensive care unit, as the most conscientious clinical assessment often fails to detect serious physiological abnormalitics which should be remedied before anaesthesia and surgery. This requires familiarity with cardiovascular drugs which may modify haemodynamic responses to stresses.

CARDIOVASCULAR DISEASES

Coronary artery disease

Ischaemic heart disease is the most common cause of death in developed countries, accounting for 30 per cent of all deaths in men, and 25 per cent of deaths in women. Its incidence increases markedly with age and its presence is a major threat to surgical patients.

Recent infarction

The risk of perioperative myocardial infarction is increased 30- to 300-fold in patients who have suffered a previous infarction; when surgery takes place within 3 months of the infarction the risk of reinfarction may be as high as 25 per cent. However, the delay between myocardial infarction and surgery is only one factor which needs to be taken into consideration. The type of surgical procedure is also important: reinfarction is more likely to occur after abdominal, thoracic, and prolonged surgery than after body surface surgery. The quality of the patient's ventricular function is paramount, as an ejection fraction of less than 40 per cent increases the risk of perioperative cardiac morbidity and mortality dramatically. Indeed, the presence of left ventricular failure at any time after myocardial infarction has been shown to be the most significant factor associated with mortality after emergency surgery for appendicitis or hip fracture. Persistence of angina after infarction is also an ominous sign, as it indicates the presence of compromised myocardium.

The inevitability of high morbidity and mortality rates associated with anaesthesia and surgery after a recent myocardial infarction has recently been questioned. Extended monitoring of ECG, arterial, central venous, and pulmonary capillary wedge pressure, combined with aggressive management of cardiovascular abnormalities during the perioperative period, may reduce the risk of reinfarction to about 5 per cent. To keep variations of heart rate, arterial pressure and pulmonary wedge pressure within very narrow limits, however, patients must be admitted to an intensive care unit for a relatively long period. It remains safer, in most circumstances, to delay elective surgery for at least 3 months after myocardial infarction.

Angina

Angina is a well recognized risk factor for perioperative morbidity and mortality, but there are subsets of patients in whom the risks are particularly high. Unstable angina is associated with risks comparable to those of recent myocardial infarction. Unless surgery can be considered life-saving, patients should be made stable before any other procedure is undertaken. Disabling angina increases the risk of perioperative ischaemia, while mild angina is a threat mostly for patients with preoperative ST–T segment abnormalities.

Silent ischaemia

Over the last decade it has become obvious that many patients suffer from silent myocardial ischaemia, which can be detected by exercise testing or ambulatory ECG monitoring.

There are three types of silent myocardial ischaemia. Type 1 is observed in patients without any symptoms and occurs in about 2.5 per cent of the male population aged between 39 and 59 years, about 40 per cent of whom will develop symptomatic coronary artery disease. Type 2 occurs in about 16 per cent of patients who have suffered myocardial infarction, and Type 3 occurs in patients suffering from angina. In these patients 75 per cent of all episodes of ischaemia are silent, and only 25 per cent are painful.

The absence of pain may be a reflection of less severe ischaemia, a smaller affected area, or a different distribution of impairment of coronary blood flow. However, it is more likely that patients with silent ischaemia have a higher pain threshold, related to higher levels of plasma endorphins.

Silent ischaemia has been reported in 20 to 90 per cent of patients presenting for coronary artery surgery or vascular surgery, and is known to increase the risk of postoperative complications. This may be due to the association between silent ischaemia and poor left ventricular function.

Coronary artery bypass grafts

The risk of perioperative infarction after successful coronary artery revascularization is low, and both morbidity and mortality are close to those of patients without heart disease. Thus, coronary revascularization is often advocated before major surgery is undertaken in patients with coronary heart disease. The low incidence of cardiovascular complications may be somewhat misleading, however, since the morbidity and mortality associated with the coronary revascularization itself should be taken into account; this makes the place of coronary revascularization prior to major surgery controversial. When it is indicated in its own right, for example, in patients with unstable angina, correctable disabling angina, or triple vessel disease, coronary revascularization should be performed first. When the indications are less clear cut, it is probably advisable only before surgery which is likely to be associated with major haemodynamic instability, such as major vascular surgery. In some patients, coronary bypass surgery improves cardiac function, probably because some areas of the left ventricle are still viable, if not functional. The concept of 'hibernating' myocardium explains this situation: myocardium with very poor blood supply may cease to contract, yet receives enough blood to maintain cell viability. Reperfusion restores mechanical activity and cardiac function. In patients with pre-existing ventricular dysfunction this does not always occur after coronary graft procedures and left ventricular function may remain severely compromised.

Causes of ischaemia

Autoregulation of the coronary circulation is impaired in the face of coronary artery disease and the balance between oxygen demand and supply is easily compromised, leading to regional myocardial ischaemia. The major causes of ischaemia are: tachycardia, during which oxygen demand is increased while oxygen supply is impaired because of the shorter duration of diastole; hypotension, during which coronary perfusion pressure is reduced (as coronary blood flow through narrowed vessels is directly proportional to the perfusion pressure) so that the reduction in perfusion may be greater than the reduction in oxygen demands; hypertension, which increases oxygen demand, in the face of an insufficient coronary flow reserve; and left ventricular overfilling, which increases wall tension and oxygen demand, while compromising coronary blood flow because of the augmented tissue pressure. These cardiovascular abnormalities are responsible for perioperative myocardial ischaemia and infarction.

Abnormalities of left ventricular wall motion are frequently detected in patients suffering from coronary artery disease. Non-invasive diagnostic methods relying on radionuclides (radionuclide cineangiography, perfusion scans), and ultrasound (echocardiography) are of proven value and should be used systematically in the preoperative assessment of patients with significant coronary artery disease. Where substantial abnormalities of wall function are present, or if left ventricular aneurysms are discovered, the negative inotropy of most anaesthetic agents is likely to cause severe depression of global cardiac function.

It is becoming increasingly obvious that clinical assessment of left ventricular function is difficult, especially in patients whose activity is limited by peripheral vascular disease or other disabilities. Radionuclide studies show that severe dysfunction is frequently present in patients who appear essentially asymptomatic: about one-third of patients presenting for major vascular surgery have ejection fractions below 50 per cent.

Arterial hypertension

It is convenient to consider that systolic pressure above 160 mmHg, and diastolic pressure above 90 mmHg define arterial hypertension. Hypertension is present in between 10 and 20 per cent of the adult population and carries the risk of serious cardiovascular complications such as stroke, ischaemic heart disease, peripheral vascular disease, and renal dysfunction.

Clinical examination may reveal an enlarged heart and signs of left ventricular failure. The chest radiograph and electrocardiogram may confirm left ventricular hypertrophy. Signs of previous myocardial infarction, myocardial ischaemia, and disorders of intraventricular conduction are often noted. The cerebral complications of hypertension include transient ischaemic attacks and major cerebrovascular accidents. Renal complications may be shown by proteinuria, and elevated serum creatinine and urea. Inspection of the retina may show diminished vessel calibre, nipping, and flame-shaped haemorrhages. Approximately 90 per cent of hypertensive patients suffer from essential hypertension; only 10 per cent have secondary hypertension. Some causes of secondary hypertension are listed in Table 1, and it is a possibility that must be kept in mind.

Table 1 Causes of secondary hypertension

1. Renal diseases
   - (a) Unilateral renal disorders
     - Renal artery stenosis
     - Obstructive nephropathy
     - Pyelonephritis
   - (b) Bilateral renal disorders
     - Glomerulonephritis
     - Interstitial nephritis
     - Pyelonephritis
     - Polycystic disease
     - Collagen vascular disease
     - Obstructive uropathy
2. Adrenal disorders
   - Primary aldosteronism
   - Cushing's syndrome
   - Phaeochromocytoma
3. Drug-associated
   - Oral contraceptives
   - Corticosteroids
   - Sympathomimetics
4. Other causes
   - Coarctation of the aorta
   - Pre-eclampsia
   - Raised intracranial pressure
   - Tetanus

Hypertension is associated with a high incidence of perioperative hypertensive crises, dysrhythmias and myocardial ischaemia, and increases the risk of reinfarction.

While maintenance of the antihypertensive drug regimen is essential in order to ensure cardiovascular stability and prevent rebound hypertension, the need to initiate antihypertensive therapy before anaesthesia and surgery in untreated patients is more controversial. As postponement of surgery may cause considerable inconvenience to patients and disrupt operative programmes, it is essential to identify patients in whom the risks of anaesthesia and surgery will be significantly improved by treatment of their hypertension. This may be done in considering the severity of the hypertensive heart disease (Table 2).

Table 2 Classification of severity of hypertension

Diastolic pressure	Category
<90 mmHg	Normal
90–104 mmHg	Mild hypertension
105–115 mmHg	Moderate hypertension
>115 mmHg	Severe hypertension

The presence of mild hypertension increases the risks of anaesthesia and surgery but there is no evidence that treatment reduces this risk. Moderate hypertension poses a more substantial threat, especially in the presence of target organ disease, such as significant coronary, cerebrovascular, or renal disease; treatment of hypertension prior to elective surgery is then recommended. In severe arterial hypertension optimal treatment before elective surgery is essential as the incidence of dysrhythmias and/or myocardial ischaemia is far higher in untreated than in treated patients. A major cause for concern is the possibility of very large increases in arterial pressure accompanied by tachycardia and increases in the pulmonary wedge pressure at the time of endotracheal intubation, extubation, and during the recovery period. The increase in pulmonary wedge pressure may represent both failure of the left ventricle to eject and reduced ventricular compliance. Hypertensive crises may result in strokes, myocardial infarction, pulmonary oedema, or life-threatening dysrhythmias. Treatment of hypertension blunts these responses, especially when it includes β-adrenoceptor blockers.

If treatment of hypertension is indicated, it should be continued for several weeks before surgery since 'cosmetic' reductions in blood pressure will be obtained very quickly, but improvement of the underlying vascular hyper-reactivity will occur gradually over weeks and not days.

Regional anaesthesia is often considered a safe alternative to general anaesthesia in untreated hypertensive patients. This is not true: lumbar epidural anaesthesia has been shown to cause greater reductions in systolic and diastolic arterial pressure in untreated than in treated hypertensive patients.

Hypertension and left ventricular hypertrophy

As left ventricular hypertrophy reduces ventricular compliance, excessive volume loading may cause pulmonary oedema, while reduced filling may result in a dramatic reduction in cardiac output. Moreover, in patients with left ventricular hypertrophy marked discrepancies may exist between right and left ventricular filling pressures. Monitoring the pulmonary capillary wedge pressure may therefore be essential for safe perioperative management after major surgery.

Hypertension in the elderly

Isolated systolic hypertension is due predominantly to the loss of elasticity of the aorta and its major branches. The high pressure increases myocardial oxygen consumption and may cause myocardial ischaemia. However, the treatment of isolated systolic hypertension may be associated with subjective complaints and objective deterioration of cardiac, cerebral, or renal function; in addition titration of blood pressure is often difficult. Treatment of purely systolic hypertension in the elderly is probably not justified before surgery, but adequate cardiovascular monitoring is essential to enable excessive hypo- or hypertension to be detected and treated immediately.

When both systolic and diastolic pressures are elevated, the risk of cardiovascular complications are increased in the elderly as well as in younger patients. Antihypertensive treatment reduces the risk of complications but it is important to achieve the reduction gradually in order for cerebral autoregulation to return to normal limits.

Heart failure

Incipient right or left ventricular failure, indicated by the presence of a third heart sound or distended jugular veins, increases the relative risk of complications by 2 to 10 times. Overt ventricular failure must be treated before any surgical procedure is undertaken in order to reduce the risk of postoperative pulmonary oedema, and invasive monitoring may be necessary to maintain optimal ventricular filling throughout the perioperative period.

Low ejection fractions are associated with increased risks of anaesthesia and surgery. The author's personal views regarding major surgical procedures are as follows: when the ejection fraction is greater than 50 per cent, cardiac function is likely to be adequate and the risks are acceptable in the absence of other risk factors, such as reversible myocardial ischaemia and impaired pulmonary or renal functions. When the ejection fraction is between 40 and 50 per cent, the risks are increased, and the presence of additional risk factors should prompt reconsideration of the type of surgery, with a view to performing the most limited operation possible. Postoperative care in an intensive care or high dependency unit is necessary. When the ejection fraction is between 30 and 40 per cent, whether or not additional risk factors are present, management must be carefully considered. Surgery may be postponed to allow optimal medical treatment; alternatively, less extensive procedures may have to be selected; surgery may be delayed until the balance of risk is increasingly in favour of surgery rather than abstention, or surgery may be cancelled altogether. Again, intensive care management after major surgery is essential. Ejection fractions less than 30 per cent are usually observed in patients who have intermittent left ventricular failure. Recent episodes of left ventricular failure may require admission of the patient to an intensive care unit prior to surgery so that full monitoring may be implemented and treatment optimized with intravenous drugs ahead of major procedures if, and only if, surgery is deemed essential.

Valvular disease

The incidence of rheumatic fever has fallen in the Western world, but many elderly patients still suffer from rheumatic heart disease; others suffer from degenerative valvular disease and the prevalence of valvular disease in people over the age of 65 may be as high as 4 per cent.

Aortic stenosis is now the most common valvular lesion; it leads to the development of a pressure gradient between the left ventricle and the aorta. Left ventricular hypertrophy develops as a result of increased stroke work; hypertrophy is accompanied by an increase in diastolic stiffness and an increase in end-diastolic pressure. Raised ventricular pressure and increased muscle mass augment myocardial oxygen consumption, but myocardial blood flow is impaired due to the reduction in aortic diastolic pressure. During the perioperative period, close attention must be paid to changes in heart rate and arterial pressure. Increases in heart rate are poorly tolerated because they reduce the duration of diastole and thus decrease coronary blood flow. Similarly, interventions which reduce systemic vascular resistance decrease both the coronary perfusion pressure and coronary blood flow and may precipitate myocardial ischaemia (Table 3).

Aortic regurgitation causes an increase in left ventricular stroke volume with a corresponding increase in left ventricular cavity size. In moderately severe aortic regurgitation, the stroke volume may be double the normal value. End-diastolic pressure in the aorta is low. Forward flow is facilitated by a relatively low vascular resistance, while regurgitant flow is increased by peripheral vasoconstriction, or by the prolonged diastole associated with bradycardia.

Mitral stenosis impedes left ventricular filling. Flow through the narrowed mitral valve depends on the left atrial pressure, which determines early diastolic flow, and the contribution of atrial systole, which determines late diastolic flow. As duration of diastole is an important determinant of ventricular filling, tachycardia is poorly tolerated. Atrial fibrillation further compromises ventricular filling, especially when the ventricular rate is fast. In patients with mitral stenosis, the main benefit of digitalis therapy is to maintain heart rate below 80 per minute. In many patients, mean left atrial pressure is greater than 15 mmHg. Factors which facilitate overfilling of the atria will rapidly lead to pulmonary oedema.

Mitral regurgitation results in dilatation of both left atrium and left ventricle. The regurgitant flow causes high pressure in the atrium during systole, but there is no obstruction to diastolic forward flow except in combined stenosis and regurgitation. Any increase in systemic vascular resistance will limit left ventricular forward ejection and exaggerate retrograde flow into the atrium.

Cardiomyopathies

Hypertrophic obstructive cardiomyopathy is characterized by massive ventricular hypertrophy associated with failure of the ventricles to relax adequately. Systolic function is maintained and rapid ejection often causes pressure gradients within the cavity of the ventricle. Interventions that increase the inotropic state of the myocardium worsen left ventricular function, while this is improved by drugs that reduce contractility, hence the beneficial effects of β-adrenoceptor blockers and calcium antagonists.

Dilated cardiomyopathy implies marked dilatation and impaired contractile performance. The ejection fraction is usually extremely low. Previous viral myocarditis and excessive alcohol consumption are the main predisposing factors.

Cerebrovascular disease

Cerebrovascular disease is responsible for death in 9 per cent of men and 15 per cent of women in the United Kingdom. The symptoms and signs of previous cerebrovascular accidents are easily detected when they have resulted in a significant functional deficit. However, transient disturbances of cerebral function should not be overlooked as they may indicate the presence of atherosclerotic lesions of the cerebral vasculature. Particular attention should be paid to reduced carotid artery pulsation and to carotid artery bruits, as carotid artery stenosis may be responsible for transient ischaemic attacks. The question of carotid angiography and carotid endarterectomy may have to be considered, as hypotensive episodes during any type of surgery may precipitate a stroke in patients with significant carotid artery stenosis. The prognosis of postoperative stroke is poor, with a mortality of about 50 per cent. If carotid disease is asymptomatic, prophylactic carotid endarterectomy is probably not indicated.

Carotid artery disease may be considered a marker for coronary disease, as the mortality associated with carotid artery surgery is predominantly due to myocardial infarction.

A high proportion of patients suffer from both cerebrovascular and hypertensive disease. Their management is difficult because their blood pressure can be very labile during anaesthesia and postoperatively. The incidence of neurological deficit is greater in patients who develop hypertension after surgery and neurological deficits are much more likely to occur in untreated or poorly controlled hypertensive patients. Hypertensive crises can cause intracerebral haemorrhages. Gradual control of blood pressure is necessary in order for cerebral autoregulation to return to near normal.

Peripheral vascular disease

Between one-third and two-thirds of patients undergoing peripheral vascular surgery suffer from coronary heart disease, and the

Table 3 Adverse haemodynamic interventions in valvular diseases

Type of lesion	Event	Mechanism	Effect
Mitral stenosis	Bradycardia Tachycardia Atrial fibrillation	Fixed stroke volume Reduced filling time Loss of atrial contribution to ventricular filling	Reduced cardiac output
Mitral regurgitation	Peripheral vasoconstriction	Increased regurgitant flow	Decreased forward flow
Aortic stenosis	Bradycardia	Fixed stroke volume	Reduced cardiac output
	Tachycardia Peripheral vasodilatation vasodilatation	Reduced diastolic time Reduced coronary perfusion pressure	Reduced coronary flow
Aortic regurgitation	Bradycardia	Increased regurgitant flow	Reduced cardiac output
	Peripheral vasoconstriction	Increased regurgitant flow	

morbidity and mortality associated with anaesthesia and surgery are higher in such patients than in those undergoing non-vascular surgery. Clinical evaluation is often inadequate because of physical inactivity, and objective assessment of cardiac function and myocardial perfusion is invaluable, especially in patients presenting for surgery of the abdominal aorta and other intra-abdominal vessels. About one-third of these patients have low cardiac output and ejection fraction less than 50 per cent.

The high incidence of complications following surgery of the abdominal aorta is a reflection of major haemodynamic disturbances. Cross-clamping of the aorta causes a sudden, large increase in left ventricular afterload. In patients with compromised left ventricular function, the pulmonary wedge pressure increases, reflecting acute left ventricular dilatation associated with acute myocardial ischaemia. Myocardial ischaemia is particularly common when cross-clamping is applied above the renal arteries or the coeliac axis. Administration of vasodilators may be required to prevent or treat myocardial ischaemia during aortic cross-clamping. Removal of the clamps has three effects: firstly, vascular resistance is abruptly reduced; secondly, the sudden return of acidic blood to the heart causes cardiac depression; thirdly, the circulating volume is reduced because vasodilatation has developed in the lower limbs. Adequate volume loading before the gradual removal of cross-clamps is essential.

It is often assumed that surgery of limb vessels is relatively well tolerated because it does not cause major haemodynamic instability. While peripheral vascular surgery is better tolerated than aortic surgery, cardiovascular complications and mortality are still more frequent than in non-vascular surgery, reflecting the association with hypertensive and coronary disease. Indeed, in elderly patients vascular surgery for limb salvage carries a mortality rate of up to 16 per cent.

Dysrhythmias and heart blocks

Any rhythm other than sinus rhythm is associated with a significant increase in the risk of cardiac complications because preoperative dysrhythmias reflect the underlying heart disease.

Dysrhythmias

Atrial dysrhythmias may precede the development of atrial tachycardia and atrial fibrillation. The loss of correctly timed atrial contraction reduces the ventricular filling, particularly when the ventricular rate is fast. In patients with atrial fibrillation or atrial flutter sinus rhythm should be restored if possible, or the ventricular rate controlled, prior to surgery. Fluid load may be poorly tolerated and, for major surgery, patients with atrial fibrillation may benefit from perioperative monitoring of the pulmonary capillary wedge pressure.

Ventricular ectopic activity is often associated with organic heart disease or digitalis toxicity. Premature ventricular beats frequently occur in patients with ventricular wall dysfunction and poor ejection fraction. Cardiac function may worsen: many anaesthetic agents depress cardiac performance, and alter the electrophysiology of the myocardium either by a direct effect on the conduction tissue or by enhancing the arrhythmogenic activity of adrenaline.

Heart blocks

Heart blocks (Fig. 1) usually have an organic cause and may be accentuated by vagal stimulation, digitalis, β-adrenoceptor antagonists, and calcium antagonists. Anaesthesia may precipitate the development of complete heart block in patients with a wide range of atrioventricular or intraventricular conduction disorders by several mechanisms. Some anaesthetic agents, particularly the halogenated inhalational anaesthetics, decrease atrioventricular conduction. Secondly, anaesthesia often causes dysrhythmias, and premature beats are known to facilitate the development of post-ectopic heart block. Thirdly, alterations of serum potassium concentration may occur: acute hypokalaemia may be caused by respiratory alkalosis (hypocapnic intermittent positive pressure ventilation), while acute hyperkalaemia may follow the rapid infusion of large quantities of stored blood. These changes exacerbate dysrhythmias and compromise conduction, and insertion of a temporary pacemaker is often necessary before elective or

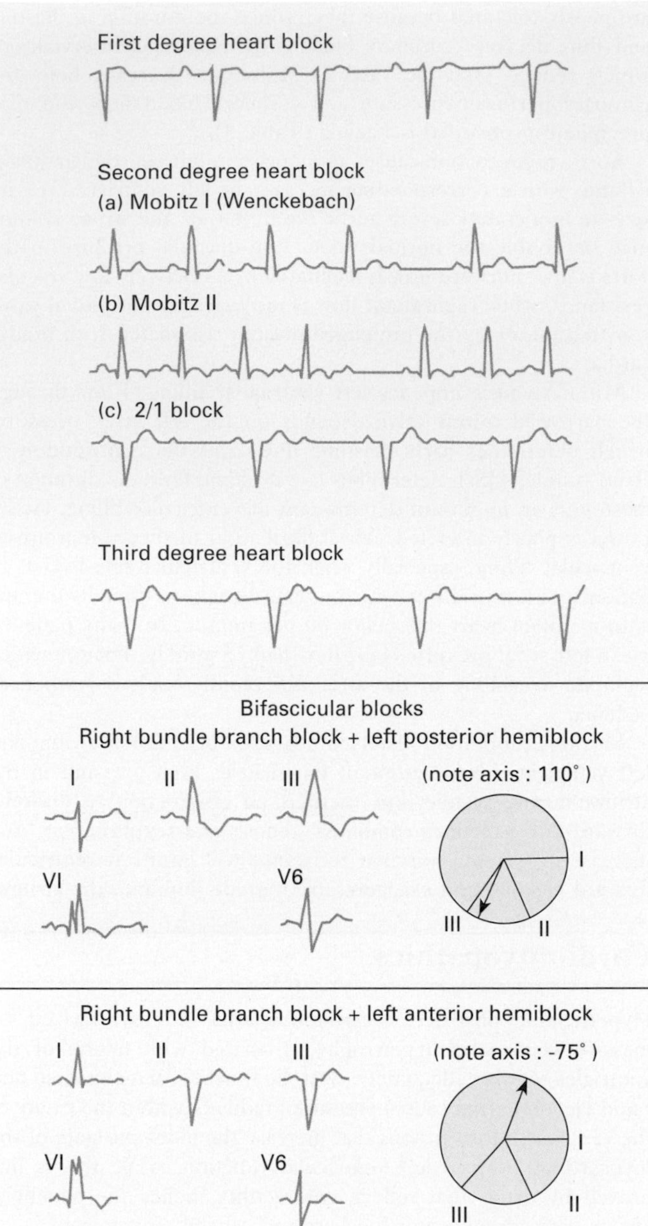

Fig. 1 Typical examples of heart blocks.

Table 4 Indications for temporary pace-makers

Symptomatic first degree heart block
Symptomatic second degree Mobitz I heart block
Second degree Mobitz II heart block
Third degree heart block
Symptomatic bifascicular block
Left bundle branch block and first degree heart block
Sick sinus syndrome
Slow rates unresponsive to drugs

emergency surgery, even though permanent pacing may not be necessary (Table 4).

Insertion of a temporary pacemaker is not usually recommended in asymptomatic patients with uncomplicated first degree heart block. Such patients do, however, occasionally develop profound bradycardia accompanied by hypotension while under general anaesthesia. Temporary pacing should be considered when this type of block is unresponsive to atropine, and must also be considered when first degree heart block is accompanied by bundle branch block. In Mobitz type I (Wenckebach) block, temporary pacing is necessary only when the patient is symptomatic. However, temporary (or permanent) pacing is necessary in Mobitz type II second degree heart block and in third degree heart block.

The question of whether temporary pacing is required in patients with a bifascicular block is unsettled. Bifascicular blocks can be identified relatively easily: right bundle branch block with left axial deviation of greater than −75° is associated with left anterior hemiblock; right bundle branch block with right axial deviation greater than 110° is associated with left posterior hemiblock. Whenever patients with bifasicular blocks have experienced symptoms which can be attributed to transient complete heart block, temporary pacing is necessary. In totally asymptomatic patients, the risk of anaesthesia facilitating the development of complete heart block is probably very small. Complete left bundle branch block accompanied by first degree heart block is also an indication for temporary pacing.

The sick sinus syndrome represents a group of disturbances of impulse formation in the sinoatrial node which can easily lead to severe arrhythmias, including cardiac arrest during anaesthesia and surgery. The diagnosis should be suspected if there are periodic episodes of slow sinus rate alternating with tachycardia. Establishment of temporary pacing before anaesthesia and surgery is recommended since bradycardia may result from treatment of tachycardia, and this is usually refractory to drug therapy.

Regional anaesthesia is not safe in patients with conduction disorders: absorption of lignocaine injected into the extradural space may cause sinus bradycardia and induce heart blocks, especially in patients with bundle branch block. The same criteria for insertion of a temporary pacemaker should be applied before regional anaesthesia and before general anaesthesia.

Patients with permanent pacemakers

Most pacemakers are implanted prophylactically for atrioventricular blocks or sick sinus syndrome, and they have recently been implanted for the control of recurrent tachydysrhythmias. Over the past 30 years the complexity of pacemakers has increased and they are now classified by the chamber paced, activity sensed, mode of response, and type of programmability. Prior to anaesthesia and surgery it is essential to establish the type of pacemaker, the risk of programmes being lost during diathermy, and the means of inducing a fixed rate, which may be necessary during the procedure, particularly when electrocautery is used.

The risk of interference by electrocautery is minimized by placing the indifferent diathermy plate well away from the pacemaker, and limiting the duration of electrocautery to 1-s bursts at intervals of at least 10 s.

Global assessment of risk

Several authors have tried to determine which clinical preoperative factors contribute to the development of cardiac complications in patients undergoing major non-cardiac surgery. The index of cardiac risk in non-cardiac surgery developed by Goldman and his colleagues was based on the relationship between postoperative complications and preoperative assessment data in just over 1000 patients. Using discriminant analysis to identify the factors that contributed significantly to the cardiac risks of anaesthesia and surgery, they produced an index which was able to predict the prognosis in over 80 per cent of cases (Table 5). When applied to a selected population of patients undergoing surgery for abdominal aortic aneurysm this index tended to underestimate the risk of complications. This is not surprising in view of the marked cardiovascular disturbances which occur during major vascular surgery.

Another index, developed by Detsky and colleagues takes coronary artery disease into account more fully, considering not only recent myocardial infarction (within 6 months) but also older infarcts and severe angina (Table 6). Patients with a low score

Table 5 Multifactorial index of cardiac risk (After Goldman *et al.* 1977 and Goldman 1987)

(a)

Risk factor	No. of points
S_3 gallop; increased venous jugular pressure	11
Previous myocardial infarction (less than 6 months)	10
Premature ventricular ectopics (more than 5 per min)	7
Atrial dysrhythmias, rhythm other than sinus	7
Age greater than 70 years	5
Emergency operation	4
Severe aortic stenosis	3
Poor general condition	3
Intraperitoneal or intrathoracic operation	3

(b)

	Unselected non-cardiac surgery	Abdominal aortic surgery
Class I 0–5 points	1%	7%
Class II 6–12 points	7%	11%
Class III 13–25 points	14%	38%
Class IV > 26 points	78%	No patient operated on

Sources: Goldman *et al.* (1977), Jeffrey *et al.* (1983)

Table 6 Cardiac risk index (after Detsky *et al.* 1986)

Coronary heart disease	
Myocardial infarction within 6 months	10
Myocardial infarction more than 6 months	5
Angina Class 4 (Canadian Cardiovascular Society)	20
Angina Class 3 (Canadian Cardiovascular Society)	20
Unstable angina within 3 months	10
Cardiogenic pulmonary oedema	
Within 1 week	10
Ever	5
Valvular disease	
Suspected critical aortic stenosis	20
Dysrhythmias	
Any rhythm other than sinus rhythm	5
More than 5 premature ventricular beats/min at any time prior to surgery.	5
Poor general status	
Age over 70	5
Emergency operation	10

(0–5) have below average risk, while higher scores predict an above average risk of cardiovascular complications.

Global indices of risk are useful but have their limitations, as the severity of heart disease is often underestimated by pure clinical assessment. More detailed preoperative assessment, including functional evaluation of ventricular function, is becoming an integral part of indices of risk in patients undergoing major surgery.

FURTHER INVESTIGATIONS

Chest radiograph

Although the cost-effectiveness of the routine chest radiograph has been questioned, it provides important information in patients with heart disease. Diagnostic alterations of the cardiac shadow, such as prominent left atrium or marked left ventricular hypertrophy, may be observed in valvular heart disease. Cardiomegaly (heart shadow >50 per cent of the diameter of the thorax) in patients with coronary artery disease is usually associated with a low ejection fraction, and substantial enlargement of the left ventricle in hypertensive heart disease is associated with poor diastolic ventricular function. Pulmonary congestion and presence of pleural effusion may also indicate impaired cardiac function.

Electrocardiography

Although the resting electrocardiogram is normal in 25 to 50 per cent of patients with coronary heart disease, the ECG remains a very important preoperative test in these patients. Characteristic patterns associated with ischaemia, injury, and infarction are easy to recognize (Fig. 2). When Q waves extend to a large area on the precordial leads, left ventricular function is likely to be substantially reduced. Abnormalities of the ST segment or T wave suggestive of myocardial ischaemia are associated with a three-fold increase in perioperative ischaemia. Patients with coronary artery disease who are admitted for elective surgery following previous investigations should undergo repeat ECG: totally silent myocardial infarction often occurs within the days preceding admission. Overlooking a very recent infarction is a most serious hazard.

Characteristic patterns of ventricular or atrial hypertrophy are seen in valvular heart disease, and in severe arterial hypertension (Fig. 2).

Holter monitoring

Continuous ambulatory ECG recording is of considerable value in the diagnosis of dysrhythmias. Short episodes of tachyarrhythmias, including ventricular tachycardia, may indicate that the dysrhythmia is potentially life-threatening and may warrant drug therapy prior to anaesthesia and surgery. Similarly, in the presence of conduction disorders, continuous ECG monitoring may reveal episodes of complete heart block demonstrating the severity of what may otherwise be considered a relatively benign conduction disorder.

Over the past 5 years the use of continuous ambulatory monitoring has revealed that many episodes of myocardial ischaemia are completely silent. Such silent ischaemia accounts for 75 per cent of ischaemic episodes in patients with stable angina and 90 per cent of episodes of ischaemia in those presenting for coronary artery bypass grafting. As silent ischaemia is an adverse factor in both stable and unstable angina, 24-h ECG monitoring is likely to become an important preoperative test in patients with coronary heart disease presenting for surgery.

Exercise electrocardiography

Exercise electrocardiography has a high specificity in the prediction of coronary disease and gives an indication of the coronary reserve. Exercise-induced ischaemia usually occurs in territory supplied by coronary arteries that are moderately or severely obstructed, or which develop vasospasm during exercise. There is a good correlation between poor exercise tolerance and perioperative cardiac complications in patients undergoing vascular surgery.

Echocardiography

M-mode echocardiography represents a one-dimensional view of the heart plotted against time, while two-dimensional echocardiography enables evaluation of an entire sector of single-dimensional beams. The latter makes it possible to obtain estimates of muscle mass, ejection fraction, velocity of fibre shortening, and end-diastolic and end-systolic volumes. Segmental wall motion abnormalities due to myocardial ischaemia can be described qualitatively and quantitatively. Images in multiple planes are necessary to obtain accurate estimations of ejection fraction and volumes.

Both the extent of left ventricular hypertrophy and the degree of diastolic dysfunction can be determined in patients with arterial hypertension. After myocardial infarction the size of ventricular aneurysms can be assessed, as can papillary muscle abnormalities and the presence of mural thrombi. In valvular heart disease the anatomy of the valves can be examined. Other conditions such as pericardial effusion, presence of clots after cardiac surgery, and atrial myxoma can be detected.

Advances in Doppler technology have made it possible to measure flow across the heart valves; forward and regurgitant flows can be estimated, and pressure gradients across stenoses may be calculated. Such measurements correlate well with direct measurements obtained at cardiac catheterization.

The introduction of transoesophageal echocardiography (the transducer being attached to the distal end of a gastroscope) has

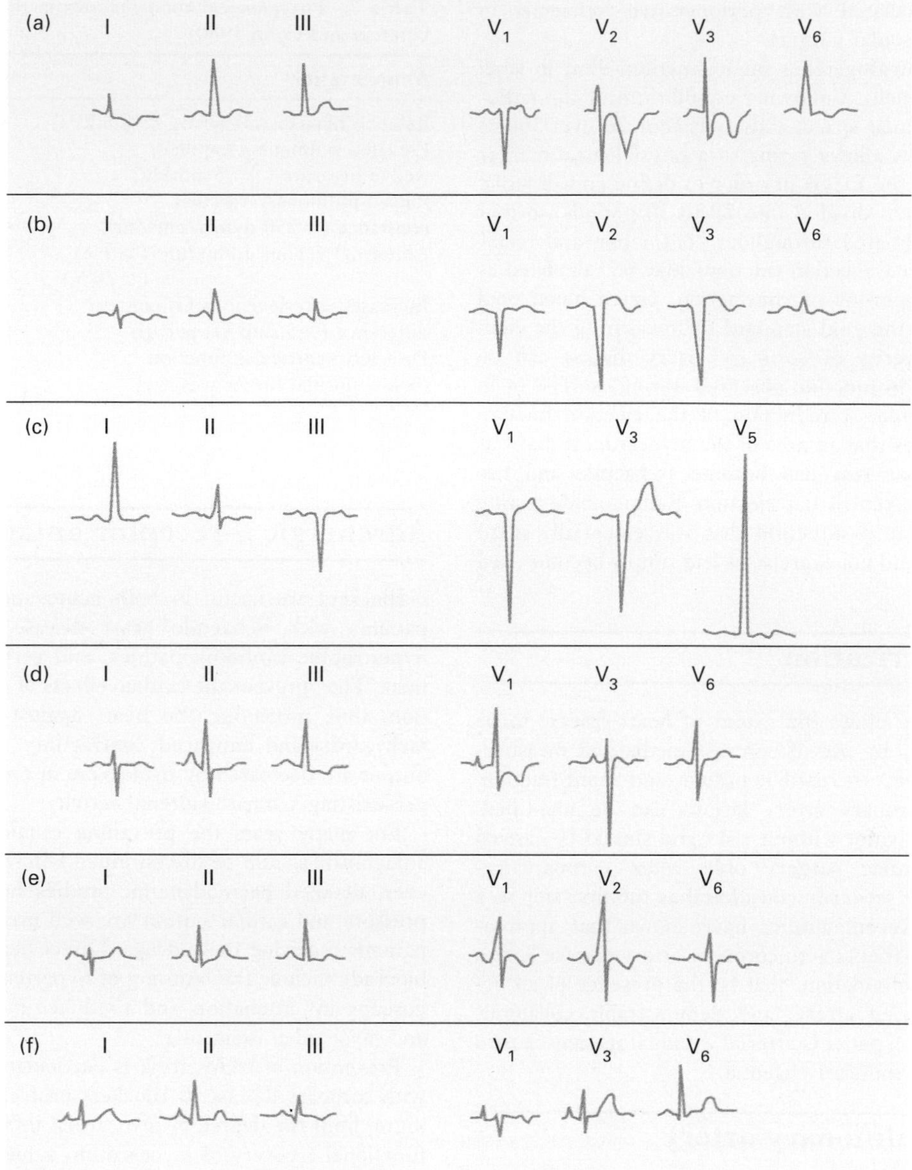

Fig. 2 Typical ECG patterns of myocardial ischaemia (a), myocardial infarction (b), left ventricular hypertrophy (c), right ventricular hypertrophy (d), left atrial hypertrophy (e), and right atrial hypertrophy (f).

made it possible to obtain high quality images during anaesthesia and surgery. In awake patients, high quality images of dissection of the thoracic aorta, prosthetic valve dysfunction, intracardiac thrombi, cardiac and paracardiac masses, and acute mitral regurgitation can be obtained. This technique is particularly useful when standard echocardiography is inconclusive because of chest trauma.

Nuclear imaging

Scintillation cameras detect γ-rays emitted by radiopharmaceuticals. Multicrystal cameras (dynamic studies) and single probe detectors (ejection fraction, cardiac output, pulmonary transit time) extend the range of studies.

Myocardial imaging is used extensively to determine the presence and size of myocardial infarction and the presence of areas of poor perfusion. Hot-spot imaging relies on the avidity of infarcted segments for technetium–99m pyrophosphate. Uptake is detectable as early as 12 to 16 h following infarction, while the maximum abnormality is seen at 48 to 72 h. Cold-spot imaging relies on the uptake of thallium (^{201}Tl) being proportional to regional myocardial blood flow: areas of ischaemia, infarction, or decreased perfusion appear as cold spots. Perfusion scans may be entirely normal at rest, even in the presence of significant coronary stenoses; heterogeneity of thallium uptake may become obvious during metabolic stress or infusion of a coronary vasodilator such as dipyridamole. Repeat imaging at rest 3 to 4 h later may show that some perfusion defects have disappeared. Reversible defects indicate transient myocardial ischaemia without infarction, and their presence is associated with perioperative ischaemia in patients undergoing vascular surgery.

Gated blood pool imaging relies on technetium-99m to label serum albumin or red cells. Following equilibrium of the radionuclide in the intravascular space, activity is counted over 300 to 500 cardiac cycles. This allows gating to a physiological marker (usually the R wave of the ECG) in order to define end-diastole. The cardiac cycle is then divided into 20 to 30 periods, so that dimensions can be estimated throughout contraction and relaxation. Global and regional ejection fractions may be calculated as well as extent and synchrony of contraction. Gated blood pool imaging is regarded as the gold standard for measuring the ejection fraction. The severity of coronary artery disease can be gauged by the changes in function observed during exercise or in response to dipyridamole. A reduction of the ejection fraction during exercise indicates that an area of the myocardium that was functioning normally at rest has become ischaemic and has stopped contributing to ventricular ejection. Radionuclide testing often reveals ventricular dysfunction that was essentially silent because the patients could not exercise or had simply become used to their disability.

Cardiac catheterization

Cardiac catheterization allows the extent of heart disease to be delineated anatomically by use of contrast media and measurement of intracardiac pressure, cardiac output, and shunt fraction. The exact site of coronary artery lesions can be identified. Coronary angiography is not without risks and should be carried out prior to non-cardiac surgery only when coronary revascularization is being seriously considered as the first step in a staged management. Recent studies have shown that approximately 25 per cent of patients with coronary artery disease have a 'steal prone' coronary circulation, that is, the presence of an occluded artery, a stenosed artery, and demonstrable collaterals between the two. In such patients arterial vasodilators may cause a steal phenomenon and induce ischaemia.

Preoperative pulmonary artery catheterization

The insertion of a balloon-tipped pulmonary artery catheter allows left and right ventricular filling pressures, cardiac output, and mixed venous oxygen saturation to be measured and oxygen consumption and physiological shunt to be calculated. There is a high incidence of unrecognized cardiorespiratory abnormalities, particularly in the elderly (Table 7), and identification and accurate estimation of functional defects makes it possible to postpone surgery in order to initiate further treatment, to modify the operation itself, or to cancel surgery altogether if the risks are unacceptable.

CARDIOVASCULAR MEDICATION

The preoperative assessment of patients with cardiovascular disease cannot be complete without considering their long-term cardiovascular medication. Adrenergic β-adrenoceptor blockers, calcium antagonists, angiotensin converting enzyme inhibitors, nitrates, and cardiac glycosides are commonly used and may interact with drugs given during anaesthesia or during recovery from surgery.

Table 7 Physiological abnormalities in the elderly (after Del Guercio and Cohn 1980)

Abnormality	Percentage of patients
Relative hypoxaemia ($Pa\text{O}_2$ < 8.8 kPa)	44
Elevated pulmonary capillary wedge pressure (>7.5 mmHg)	46
Raised pulmonary vascular resistance (>250 dyn/s/cm^5/m^2)	46
Abnormal venous admixture (>9%)	82
(>20%)	22
Increased arteriovenous O_2 content difference (>5.2 ml O_2 per dl)	23
Poor left ventricular function (below normal function curve)	22

Adrenergic β-receptor antagonists

β-Blockers are useful in both acute and long-term therapy of patients with ischaemic heart disease, arterial hypertension, hypertrophic cardiomyopathies, and certain forms of dysrhythmias. They prevent the cardiac effects of β-adrenoceptor stimulation, thus protecting the heart against the adverse effects of tachycardia and enhanced contractility. Heart rate and cardiac output are decreased by β-blockers in proportion to the patient's pre-existing sympathoadrenal activity.

For many years the prevailing opinion was that β-receptor antagonists should be discontinued before elective surgery. However, detailed haemodynamic studies have shown that arterial pressure and cardiac output are well maintained in hypertensive patients receiving these drugs. Direct benefits of β-adrenoceptor blockade include the blunting of hypertensive responses to laryngoscopy and intubation, and a reduced incidence of dysrhythmias and myocardial ischaemia.

Prevention of tachycardia is particularly important in patients with coronary disease. β-Blockers protect the ischaemic myocardium, limit the degree of myocardial infarction, and improve the functional recovery of myocardium subjected to short periods of ischaemia. Maintenance of such therapy throughout the perioperative period is therefore strongly recommended. However, β-blockade also modifies some of the responses of the circulation and if hypovolaemia occurs the adrenergic stimulation which is normally responsible for tachycardia will be substantially blunted. Reliance on tachycardia as an indicator of the severity of hypovolaemia may therefore cause unnecessary delays in fluid replacement in these patients.

Calcium antagonists

Calcium antagonists are used extensively in the management of supraventricular dysrhythmias, angina, and arterial hypertension. As calcium ions play a crucial role in the electrical activity of the heart and the excitation–contraction coupling of cardiac and vascular smooth muscle, calcium antagonists can be expected to cause marked alterations in the cardiovascular system. The selective inhibition of transmembrane and intracellular Ca^{2+} fluxes is responsible for the depression of sinus node activity and atrioventricular node conduction, the negative inotropy, and the vasodilatation that attend the administration of calcium antagonists.

Verapamil causes myocardial depression and decreases sinus node and atrioventricular node activity. It is effective in slowing the atrial rate in sinus tachycardia and is most effective in terminating re-entrant paroxysmal supraventricular tachycardias. It slows the ventricular rate in atrial fibrillation and atrial flutter. Verapamil is also used in the management of coronary heart disease, as it decreases myocardial oxygen consumption and may cause coronary vasodilatation.

Nifedipine is predominantly a vasodilator and is ineffective in the management of supraventricular arrhythmias mediated by reflex sympathetic overactivity. Nifedipine has become a very important drug in the management of arterial hypertension, angina, and coronary spasm.

The effects of diltiazem are intermediate between those of verapamil and those of nifedipine. It is used mostly in the management of ischaemic heart disease, though it is also effective in the management of supraventricular dysrhythmias.

New calcium antagonists, such as nicardipine and nimodipine, have recently been introduced: like nifedipine, they are nitrendipine derivatives. Nicardipine is used in the treatment of angina and hypertension, while nimodipine is used mostly to prevent or treat cerebral vasospasm.

The reflex-mediated adrenergic responses to calcium antagonists are suppressed by the addition of β-blockers, and the possibility of adverse interactions between β-blockers and calcium antagonists must be recognized, particularly when they are administered intravenously.

Halogenated anaesthetics reduce calcium fluxes in cardiac cells and may potentiate the negative inotropy and chronotropy of the calcium antagonists. This in no way indicates that calcium antagonists should be discontinued before elective surgery, but monitoring must be sufficiently detailed for early warning signs of adverse effects to be detected immediately.

Calcium antagonists offer little or no protection against perioperative myocardial ischaemia. In this respect they appear to be much less effective than β-blockers, probably due to their inability to protect the heart against the effect of sympathetic overactivity. They do not prevent increases in heart rate.

Angiotensin converting enzyme inhibitors

Angiotensin converting enzyme inhibitors cause peripheral vasodilatation and, in patients with normal renal circulation, increase renal plasma flow, decrease renal vascular resistance, and have little effect on glomerular filtration. However, in patients with renal artery stenosis, these drugs may precipitate renal failure, as the reduction of vascular resistance in the efferent arteriole reduces the glomerular filtration pressure.

Angiotensin converting enzyme inhibitors are becoming increasingly important in the management of congestive heart failure because they increase cardiac output and exercise tolerance; they also prolong survival. They are also effective in controlling blood pressure in hypertensive patients. Unlike other vasodilators, they do not cause sodium retention because the renin–angiotensin–aldosterone system is blocked.

Converting enzyme inhibitors may minimize the pressor responses to intubation and surgical stimulation without causing exaggerated reductions in blood pressure in response to induction or maintenance of anaesthesia.

Nitrates

Nitrates cause venodilatation and, to a lesser extent, arteriolar vasodilatation: these combined effects decrease left ventricular wall tension and myocardial oxygen consumption. Glyceryl trinitrate causes a reflex tachycardia which may counteract this beneficial effect, unless a β_1-adrenoceptor antagonist is also administered. Glyceryl trinitrate redistributes coronary blood flow to the subendocardium by increasing collateral coronary blood flow. It is effective in the treatment of unstable angina, coronary artery spasm (Prinzmetal's variant angina) and in acute myocardial infarction as a means of limiting infarct size.

Cardiac glycosides

The cardiac glycosides inhibit transport of sodium and potassium ions across cell membranes by inhibiting the Na^+, K^+-ATPase. One major effect is the release of sequestered calcium ions from the mitochondria of the failing heart, thus enhancing calcium availability in the sarcoplasmic reticulum and improving contractile force. This advantage is counteracted by a marked increase in systemic vascular resistance. Thus, in acute care units, the combination of vasodilators and inotropes such as dopamine or dobutamine is used routinely instead of cardiac glycosides.

Digitalis preparations increase central vagal activity, delaying the atrioventricular conduction time, an effect well suited to the treatment of atrial fibrillation, atrial flutter, and occasionally the termination of supraventricular tachycardia in the Wolff–Parkinson–White syndrome.

Cardiac glycosides may accumulate in patients with poor renal function, and toxic blood concentrations may be achieved following administration of conventional doses. This tendency may be enhanced following anaesthesia and surgery because of the alterations in renal function associated with the stress response to surgery. Digitalis toxicity may be precipitated during anaesthesia because respiratory alkalosis exacerbates the effects of hypokalaemia, especially in patients taking diuretics. Nevertheless, the use of digoxin to maintain normal heart rate (55–70 beats/min) in patients with atrial fibrillation has the advantage over all the other antiarrhythmics of having positive rather than negative inotropic effects. This may be important in patients with poor left ventricular function.

Preoperative administration of digitalis has been advocated to minimize the effect of potent anaesthetic agents on the heart, and to minimize the incidence of perioperative tachyarrhythmias. However, the risk of intraoperative dysrhythmias is increased. Laver and Lowenstein have advocated the following guidelines: acute digitalization is justified in the patient with preoperative heart failure; digitalis is best continued until the evening before operation in patients with chronic atrial fibrillation if the ventricular rate is in excess of 80 beats/min; preoperative digitalization may be considered for reducing the incidence of supraventricular dysrhythmias in patients undergoing abdominal or intrathoracic operations in whom a previous myocardial infarction is associated with abnormal left ventricular function; preoperative digitalization should be discouraged if it is intended solely to counteract the cardiac depression of anaesthesia.

CONCLUSION

Rigorous preoperative assessment is essential in order to identify patients in whom the cardiac risks of anaesthesia and surgery are particularly high. Cardiologists and radiologists are frequently called upon to establish the nature and severity of cardiac disorders and to perform objective tests of cardiac function, as unrecognized poor cardiac function is associated with excessive morbidity and mortality. Sound management rests on communication between surgical and anaesthetic teams in order to define the safest strategy for the perioperative period. Collaboration with cardiologists is essential in order to ensure the best therapy of cardiovascular abnormalities, both pre- and postoperatively.

FURTHER READING

Al Wathiqui M H, Farber N, Pelc L, Gross GJ, Brooks HL, Warltier DC. Improvement in functional recovery of stunned myocardium by long-term pretreatment with oral propranolol. *Am Heart J*, 1989; **117**: 791–8.

Barnes RW. Asymptomatic carotid disease in patients undergoing major cardiovascular operations: can prophylactic endarterectomy be justified? *Ann Thoracic Surg* 1986; **42**: S36–S40.

Brunner HR, Gavras H, Waeber B, Textor SC, Turini GA, Wauters JP. Clinical use of an orally acting converting enzyme inhibitor, captopril. *Hypertension* 1980; **2**: 558–66.

Carliner N, *et al.* Routine preoperative exercise testing in patients undergoing major non-cardiac surgery. *Am J Cardiol* 1985; **56**: 51–8.

Chung F, *et al.* Calcium channel blockade does not offer adequate protection from perioperative myocardial ischemia. *Anesthesiology* 1988; **69**: 343–7.

Clements FM, de Bruijn NP. Perioperative evaluation of regional wall motion by transoesophageal two-dimensional echocardiography. *Anesth Analg* 1987; **66**: 249–61.

Cohn PF. Silent myocardial ischemia: classification, prevalence, and prognosis. *Am J Med* 1985; **79** (Suppl 3A): 2–6.

Coriat P, Harari A, Ducardonet A, Targot JP, Viars P. Risk of advanced heart block during extradural anaesthesia in patients with right bundle branch block and left anterior hemiblock. *Br J Anaesth* 1981; **53**: 545–7.

Cutler BS, Leppo JA. Dipyridamole thallium 201 scintigraphy to detect coronary artery disease before abdominal aortic surgery. *J Vasc Surg* 1987; **5**: 91–100.

Dagnino J, Prys-Roberts C. Strategy for patients with hypertensive heart disease *Clin Anaesthesiol* 1989; **3**: 261–89.

Deanfield JE, Selwyn AP, Chierchia S, Maseri A, Ribiero P. Myocardial ischaemia during daily life in patients with stable angina: its relation to symptoms and heart rate changes. *Lancet* 1983; **ii** 753–8.

Del Guercio LRM, Cohn JD. Monitoring operative risk in the elderly. *JAMA* 1980; **243**: 1350–5.

Detsky AS, Abrams HB, Forbath N, Scott JG, Hilliard JR. Cardiac assessment for patients undergoing non-cardiac surgery. *Arch Intern Med* 1986; **146**: 2131–4.

Dirksen A, Kjoller E. Cardiac predictors of death after non-cardiac surgery evaluated by intention to treat, *Br Med J* 1988; **297**: 1011–3.

Foëx P. Pharmacology of cardiovascular drugs. *Clin Anaesthesiol* 1989; **3**: 131–61.

Foster ED, Davis KB, Carpenter JA, Abele S, Fray D. Risk of noncardiac operation in patients with defined coronary disease: The coronary artery surgery study (CASS) registry experience. *Ann Thoracic Surg* 1986; **41**: 42–50.

Gifford RW Jr. Myths about hypertension in the elderly. *Med Clin N Am* 1987; **71**: 1003–11.

Goldman L. Multifactorial index of cardiac risk in non-cardiac surgery: ten-year status report. *J Cardiothorac Anesth* 1987; **1**: 237–44.

Goldman L. Assessment of the patient with known or suspected ischaemic heart disease for non-cardiac surgery. *Br J Anaesth* 1988; **61**: 38–43.

Goldman L, *et al.* Multifactorial index of cardiac risk in noncardiac surgical procedures. *N Engl J Med* 1977; **297**: 845–50.

Haagensen R, Steen PA. Perioperative myocardial infarction. *Br J Anaesth* 1988; **61**: 24–37.

Hertzer NR, *et al.* Coronary artery disease in peripheral vascular patients. A classification of 1000 coronary angiograms and results of surgical management. *Ann Surg* 1984; **199**: 223–33.

Jeffrey CC, Kunsman, J Cullen, DJ, Brewster, DC. A prospective evaluation of cardiac risk index. *Anesthesiology* 1983; **58**: 462–4.

Knight AA, *et al.* Perioperative myocardial ischemia: importance of the preoperative ischemic pattern. *Anesthesiology* 1988; **68**: 681–8.

Laver MB, Lowenstein E. Anesthesia and the patient with heart disease. In: Johnson RA, Haber E, Austen WG, eds. *The practice of cardiology*. Boston; Little Brown and Company, 1980: 1090–1109.

Leppo J Plaja J, Gionet M, Tumolo J, Pasakos JA, Cutler BS. Non-invasive evaluation of cardiac risk before elective vascular surgery. *J Am Coll Cardiol* 1987; **9**: 269–76.

Morise AP, *et al.* The prediction of cardiac risk in patients undergoing vascular surgery. *Am J Med Sci* 1987; **293**: 150–8.

Prys-Roberts C, Meloche R, Foëx P. Studies of anaesthesia in relation to hypertension. I. Cardiovascular responses of treated and untreated patients. *Br J Anaesth* 1971; **43**: 122–137.

Raby KE, *et al.* Correlation between preoperative ischemia and major cardiac events after peripheral vascular surgery. *N Engl J Med* 1989; **321**: 1296–300.

Rao TLK, Jacobs KH, El-Etr AA. Reinfarction following anesthesia in patients with myocardial infarction. *Anesthesiology* 1983; **59**: 499–505.

Sorensen MB, Engell HC. Preoperative haemodynamic evaluation of patients submitted for major surgery. *Acta Anaesth Scand* 1978; **22**: 391–9.

Steen PA, Tinker JH, Tarhan S. Myocardial reinfarction after anesthesia and surgery. *JAMA* 1978; **239**: 2566–70.

Zaidan JR. Pacemakers. *Anesthesiology* 1984; **60**: 319–34.

5.3 Renal problems

CHRISTOPHER G. WINEARLS AND PETER J. RATCLIFFE

Surgeons and nephrologists share the management of patients with chronic renal failure, acute renal failure, and structural disease of the urinary tract. The presence of pre-existing chronic renal disease requires modifications to the management of patients undergoing surgery and this is discussed first. Acute renal failure is a dreaded complication of surgery: although dialysis and haemofiltration allow many patients to survive with recovery, the mortality rate remains high. Prevention and management of acute renal failure will be discussed in the second part of this section.

SURGERY IN PATIENTS WITH CHRONIC RENAL DISEASE

As the safety of surgery increases and the indications for particular procedures widen, surgery is being undertaken in a greater number of older patients and in those with pre-existing illnesses. Surgeons will therefore be operating on patients with pre-existing chronic renal impairment, for conditions unrelated to their renal failure, and performing procedures related to the provision of and complications of renal treatment (e.g. vascular access operations, parathyroid surgery, renal transplantation).

Preoperative assessment

Modification of pre- and postoperative management will depend on the severity of renal failure, which is best assessed by measurement of the glomerular filtration rate. This can easily be measured by the urinary creatinine clearance before elective surgery is undertaken, but in more urgent situations this opportunity may not arise. In this circumstance, the serum creatinine is the best guide to renal function, but reference to age, sex, and body mass (which determine muscle mass and creatinine production rate) is essential in relating serum creatinine level to the adequacy of renal function. An estimate of the glomerular filtration rate (GFR) is provided by the formula:

$$\text{GFR (ml/min)} = \frac{(140 - \text{age in years}) \times \text{weight in kg} \times S}{0.82 \times \text{serum creatinine } (\mu\text{mol/l})}$$

For males, $S = 1$; females, $S = 0.85$.

A value of serum creatinine at the upper limit of the 'normal range' (150 μmol/l) would reflect a creatinine clearance of 75 ml/min in a young male weighing 80 kg, but only 18 ml/min in an elderly female weighing 40 kg. Clearly, the implications of a further decline of 5 to 10 ml/min, which might easily arise during apparently uncomplicated surgery, will be quite different in the two patients.

The preoperative examination should include particular attention to the state of hydration: patients with renal disease have a limited capacity to regulate their salt and water excretion and are therefore particularly liable to imbalances in either direction. Clinical signs may, however, be more difficult to interpret. Tachycardia may be obscured by β-blockade and an acute reduction in systemic blood pressure may have simply brought a previously high blood pressure into the normal range. Useful signs of severe intravascular depletion are cool extremities, peripheral cyanosis, and a postural fall in blood pressure: in very sick patients this may be manifest simply by sitting the patient with their legs over the side of the bed. The jugular venous pressure will be low unless there is coincident myocardial or pericardial disease. Severe overhydration will usually be manifest, as in patients with normal renal function, by a raised jugular venous pressure, and signs of peripheral or pulmonary oedema. Pulmonary oedema is particularly serious, since in those with severe renal failure even large doses of diuretics may not be effective. In such patients, and in any maintenance dialysis patient with pulmonary oedema, emergency dialysis or haemofiltration will be required. In young patients with good cardiovascular function, overhydration is less easily detected and may be manifest as resistant hypertension without significant oedema.

Attention should be directed to the detection and assessment of cardiovascular disease, since severe coronary and hypertensive heart disease is common in patients with renal disease. Coronary disease may be present in young adults, particularly those with renal failure from diabetic glomerulosclerosis in whom myocardial infarction is sometimes painless. Hypertension is associated with all forms of renal disease, although the prevalence varies and increases with the severity of renal failure. About 80 per cent of patients with end-stage renal disease require antihypertensive treatment. The pathogenesis is poorly understood, but in severe renal failure, sodium retention is an important factor. When this is controlled by dialysis, the number of patients requiring antihypertensive treatment can be reduced to about 20 per cent.

Antihypertensive treatment should be maintained during surgery, unless intercurrent illness has produced severe hypotension. This is particularly important with drugs such as clonidine or β-blockers, the abrupt withdrawal of which may cause rebound phenomena. Hypertension is associated with increased anaesthetic risk and since there is evidence that treatment, particularly with β-blockers, reduces the incidence of arrhythmias and myocardial ischaemia under anaesthesia, elective surgery is usually deferred when elevated blood pressure is found unexpectedly in the preoperative assessment. It is important, however, to be sure that unexpectedly raised blood pressure in patients with closely monitored renal disease is not simply a manifestation of anxiety. In dialysis patients, unexpected hypertension may be due to fluid overload, which will require removal by dialysis. It is again important to be sure of this diagnosis since removal of excessive fluid by dialysis prior to surgery will increase the risk of dangerous intraoperative hypotension.

When assessing patients on maintenance dialysis much can be learnt from the dialysis records. For instance, in patients with limited cardiac reserve, fluid losses and vasodilation during haemodialysis may provide sudden and severe hypotension, a problem which may also be manifest during anaesthesia. Records of such problems during haemodialysis may forewarn the surgeon and anaesthetist. In addition, dialysis records should indicate pre- and postdialysis weights and blood pressures, which will be of importance in assessing preoperative fluid balance.

Clinical examination and history should usually be supplemented by simple investigations which include a full blood count, measurement of serum creatinine and electrolytes, electrocardiogram, and a chest radiograph. A full blood count will be important in assessing the need for pre- or perioperative transfusions (see below). In acutely ill patients comparison with previous values may indicate serious blood or other fluid loss.

The use of serum creatinine in the estimation of renal function has been described. This is a less satisfactory guide to the adequacy of dialysis since the characteristics of dialysis membranes differ from those of the glomerular filter. For instance, in patients maintained by continuous ambulatory peritoneal dialysis a serum creatinine level above 1200 μmol/l can often be tolerated well, while such levels in a haemodialysis patient would usually indicate inadequate dialysis. Of much greater importance is measurement of the serum potassium: the risk of cardiotoxicity is very high when this rises above 7 mmol/l, and the level which is acceptable preoperatively will depend on whether the patient has renal function or is dialysis dependent, and on the type of surgery planned. For instance, minor surgery in patients with moderate chronic renal failure could proceed if the serum potassium is less than 6 mmol/l whereas in the dialysis patient undergoing major surgery a preoperative serum potassium of less than 4.5 mmol/l should be the aim.

The electrocardiogram may reveal the presence of hypertensive or ischaemic heart disease: the detection of acute ischaemia and arrhythmias is particularly important. The chest radiograph will show the cardiac diameter. A sudden increase in diameter reflects serious overhydration, but may also indicate acute pericardial or myocardial disease. Pulmonary oedema requires prompt treatment.

Analysis of arterial gases will be helpful in selected patients. In the presence of severe anaemia, arterial hypoxaemia is difficult to detect clinically and is also more serious. Patients with acute surgical pathology and severe renal disease will often have an important metabolic acidosis with respiratory compensation. In this situation, sudden and often inadvertent changes in respiration, consequent on sedation, anaesthesia, or analgesia, may cause large changes in arterial pH and consequently the plasma potassium.

Anaesthesia and analgesia

Modifications of anaesthetic technique and drug prescription will depend on the severity of renal failure, the presence or absence of disease in other organs, and the type of surgery. In the main these issues are dealt with elsewhere, but certain simple principles should be understood by all involved in the care of the patient.

The use of forearm veins for intravenous infusions may damage potential sites for vascular access, and this is a very serious consideration in any patient who is, or may become dependent on dialysis for life support. It is particularly important to avoid damage to the cephalic venous system. Intravenous infusions should be sited in veins outside the forearm or on the ulnar side of the hand.

Premedication

Delayed gastric emptying is common in patients with serious renal disease, particularly when renal disease complicates diabetes and severe autonomic neuropathy is present. Premedication with agents such as metoclopramide may be helpful in reducing the risk of gastric aspiration. Most renal patients are all too aware of the increased risk they face during intercurrent illness and anxiolytic drugs such as benzadiazepines will often be helpful. These may be given orally as increased bleeding times in haemodialysis patients are a relative contraindication to intramuscular agents. Opiate analgesia should be used with care (see below).

Monitoring

If substantial fluid loss is expected, particularly in patients with known cardiovascular instability, central venous pressure should be monitored. Blood pressure is best monitored using an automated sphygmomanometer: intra-arterial monitoring is rarely required, but if it is considered essential, the dorsalis pedis artery is the site of first choice in order to avoid damage to vessels which may be required later for creation of vascular access. Where anaemia and cardiorespiratory disease coexist, the use of pulse oximetry to ensure maintenance of optimal blood oxygenation will be helpful.

Induction of general anaesthesia

Anaesthesia may result in sudden hypotension requiring resuscitation with intravenous fluid or even pressor agents. Care must be taken to avoid overhydration, particularly in haemodialysis patients in whom preservation of renal function is not an issue, and excess fluid will require dialysis or haemofiltration for removal. The risk of hypotension is also present during spinal and epidural analgesia, and in these circumstances it may be even more difficult to control. Even in patients without renal disease, renal blood flow is usually reduced and autoregulation is impaired under surgical anaesthesia. A variety of renal vasoconstrictor mechanisms contribute to this, including activation of the sympathetic nervous system and the renin-angiotensin system. An important defence is provided by the vasodilatory action of renal prostaglandins (I_2 and E_2). In patients with significant renal disease this mechanism assumes greater importance and prostaglandin synthetase inhibitors should not be used in the perioperative period.

Postoperatively

The most serious, and potentially fatal immediate postoperative complication is respiratory depression. With the use of modern muscle relaxants such as atracurium, which are rapidly cleared by mechanisms independent of renal function, the problem of recurarization due to the action of muscle relaxants outlasting their antagonist should not, in theory, occur. Nevertheless, respiratory depression, and even respiratory arrest is a very important, and rather unpredictable risk after major surgery in patients with severe renal failure. Prolonged and excessive action of sedative and analgesic drugs, and impaired gas exchange arising from undiagnosed pulmonary oedema, may contribute.

The action of most opiate analgesics is prolonged in renal failure. This is particularly striking in the case of morphine and probably arises from retention of active metabolites such as morphine 6-glucuronide. Potentially fatal respiratory depression may also unpredictably complicate the use of relatively modest doses of supposedly milder agents such as dihydrocodeine and dextropropoxyphene. Probably the most predictable agent is pethidine, although retention of the pethidine metabolite, norpethidine, has been reported to account for symptoms of neuromuscular excitability. Facilities for the continuous observation of these patients in the first 2 h after surgery are therefore essential.

Fluid and electrolyte balance

Patients with chronic renal failure but otherwise good health generally maintain sodium and water balance until the glomerular filtration rate is reduced very severely (below approximately 10 ml/min). This is achieved by a corresponding large increase in the proportion of the filtered sodium and water which is excreted. Similarly, to produce a given change in excretion of sodium and water at low glomerular filtration rate requires a magnification of the tubular response: for instance, a response which is effected by kidneys with a glomerular filtration rate of 120 ml/min from a change in fractional excretion of sodium from 0.5 to 3 per cent, will require a change from 5 to 30 per cent, if the filtration rate is only 12 ml/min. It is therefore not surprising that one of the earliest effects of chronic renal disease is a limitation in the power of the kidney to compensate for changes in sodium and water intake.

In healthy individuals with a normal solute intake, water excretion can be varied from approximately 20 ml to 1500 ml/h; in renal disease this range is reduced in both directions. The reduction in capacity for water excretion will, in most cases, be very much greater than the reduction in glomerular filtration rate, since during surgery other factors such as non-osmotic ADH release impair water excretion. Many patients with severe renal disease will be at risk of water intoxication from commonly prescribed postoperative regimens which include 2 to 3 litres of 5 per cent dextrose/day. Since the precise limitations of renal compensation are difficult to predict, the problem can only be avoided by strict attention to fluid balance, corroborated by daily weighing of the patient.

In some surgical situations, such as the relief of urinary obstruction, and after renal transplantation, massive diuresis and natriuresis may be encountered. In these patients, it may be necessary to adjust the rate of intravenous replacement on an hourly basis, and also to adjust the sodium concentration of the replacement fluid regularly in the light of urinary sodium concentration.

In dialysis patients without residual renal function, great care is required to maintain fluid and electrolyte balance. Patients should be dialysed prior to surgery, but because of increased arrhythmias and haemodynamic instability immediately after dialysis, where possible, an interval of a few hours should be allowed before induction of anaesthesia. Avoidance of hyperkalaemia is of paramount importance, and can sometimes be difficult, even in patients with only mild renal disease. In general, as with sodium and water, although potassium balance is maintained in chronic renal disease, capacity for excretion is severely limited. This may be particularly serious in diabetic patients, who are liable to develop hyporeninaemic hypoaldosteronism which further reduces potassium excretion. In patients with significant renal disease, potassium supplements and potassium-sparing diuretic agents should only be used when serum potassium is low or declining.

In dialysis patients serum potassium should be measured before dialysis is terminated and should be reduced below 4.5 mmol/l. In dialysis patients known to have difficulty in maintaining potassium balance, provision for increased preoperative dialysis should be made and a calcium resonium enema should be given prior to surgery.

Anaemia and bleeding

Patients with severe renal failure are almost invariably anaemic, but severe anaemia in patients presenting for surgery should be less frequent now that recombinant erythropoietin is available. Anaemia is usually well tolerated, except in patients with coexisting ischaemic heart disease, and major surgery, such as for renal transplantation, is feasible in many patients with haemoglobin levels as low as approximately 6 g/dl. Nevertheless, a higher preoperative haemoglobin level, in the range 8 to 10 g/dl, will provide a greater safety margin in the event of haemorrhage and itself reduces the bleeding time. Blood should be cross-matched for any procedure during which a brisk haemorrhage is possible and, if the surgical indication is not immediate, consideration should be given to preoperative transfusion, particularly in patients with cardiac disease. Patients with renal failure have a bleeding diathesis, which is in part a consequence of abnormal platelet function. Such patients are liable to ooze from incisions and particularly careful attention to surgical haemostasis is required. Medically the problem can be limited by ensuring that the patients are well dialysed, transfused to haemoglobin levels of 8 to 10 g/dl preoperatively, and that heparin used during dialysis has been cleared or reversed. The administration of platelets is not effective but there are measures that can be applied in patients who are at particular risk of bleeding or who continue to ooze after surgery. Cryoprecipitate produces a temporary improvement in bleeding time. The synthetic vasopression analogue 1-deamino 8-D-arginine vasopression (0.3 μg/kg IV) is effective for about 48 h. Conjugated oestrogens provide an improvement in bleeding time which lasts up to 14 days.

Drug prescription

Special care must be taken with the use of all drugs, not only because their elimination may be slowed and their bioavailability altered in patients with renal failure, but also because they may directly or indirectly reduce residual renal function. Before prescribing it is prudent to ask whether these considerations apply and, if they do, whether prescription is essential, whether there is an alternative drug, and whether the dose needs to be modified. A list of commonly used drugs that may adversely affect renal function is given in Table 1.

Table 1 Drugs which may aggravate renal failure

Drug	Mechanism
Antimicrobials	
Aminoglycosides	
Amphotericin B	Tubular damage
Pentamidine	
ACE inhibitors	Reduce GFR
Corticosteroids	Catabolism
Cyclosporin	Reduce GFR
Cytotoxics	Hyperuricaemia
Diuretics	Hypovolaemia
NSAIDs	Reduce GFR
Tetracyclines	Catabolism
Vitamin D analogues	Hypercalcaemia

Because the elimination of many drugs is dependent on renal function, the dose and frequency of administration must be changed in patients with renal failure (Table 2). In a patient receiving maintenance dialysis the mode of dialysis also has an

Table 2 Drugs to be prescribed with special care in renal failure

Class	Comment
Antimicrobial	
Aminoglycosides	Reduce dose, ototoxic
Acyclovir	Reduce dose
Cephalosporins	Reduce dose
Co-trimoxazole	Reduce dose
Ethambutol	Reduce dose or avoid, retinal toxicity
Ganciclovir	Reduce dose
Nitrofurantoin	Avoid, neuropathy
Penicillins	Avoid very high doses, fits
Vancomycin	Reduce dose, ototoxic
Anaesthetic drugs	
Pancuronium	Avoid, prolonged paralysis
Gallamine	Avoid, prolonged paralysis
Opiates	Reduce dose, prolonged effect
Gastrointestinal	
Metoclopramide	Be aware of extrapyramidal effects
H_2-antagonists	Reduce dose
Magnesium salts	Monitor magnesium concentration
Cardiac	
Digoxin	Reduce dose and frequency
β-Blockers	May need to reduce dose
Spironolactone, amiloride	Avoid, hyperkalaemia
ACE inhibitors	Monitor creatinine and K^+
Clofibrate	Avoid, muscle injury
Oral hypoglycaemics	
Chlorpropamide	Avoid, hypoglycaemia
Tolbutamide	Reduce dose
Biguanides	Avoid, lactic acidosis

important effect: for example, haemodialysis removes gentamicin from the circulation very rapidly so that it should be administered at the end of dialysis, following which high levels will persist in the plasma until the next treatment. In contrast peritoneal dialysis will remove gentamicin continuously at a low rate.

ACUTE RENAL FAILURE AS A COMPLICATION OF SURGERY

Definition

Acute renal failure following surgery may be defined operationally as 'a reduction in renal function sufficient to cause clinical problems' to distinguish it from the very much more common occurrence of acute renal functional impairment, often recognized simply by a rise in the plasma creatinine concentration. A reduction in excretory capacity may occur on a background of pre-existing chronic renal functional impairment, when it is referred to as 'acute on chronic renal failure'. In this situation a relatively minor reduction in renal function can cause clinically important problems.

Incidence

The annual incidence of severe acute renal failure requiring dialysis is 30 to 60/million population/year, but less than half of these cases have a surgical cause. In addition, five to ten times as many patients develop transient renal impairment, which can be managed without recourse to dialysis, but which requires careful attention to water and electrolyte balance.

In Oxford, between 1988 and 1990, 190 patients with acute renal failure were referred for renal support and of these 39 per cent had a surgical cause (Table 3). This compares with the 32-year experience of the General Infirmary at Leeds where 1347 patients were treated between 1956 and 1988. In 638 (47.4 per cent) of these the acute renal failure arose from surgical conditions (Table 4). These figures are typical of Western civilian practice, except that in the United States of America trauma is a more common cause of surgical acute renal failure than in the United Kingdom.

Table 3 Surgical acute renal failure, Oxford Renal Unit 1989–1990

Surgery	*n*	Percentage of surgical cases	Percentage of total cases
Cardiac	16	22	8
Abdominal	18	24	9
Urological	14	19	7
Vascular	18	24	9
Trauma	8	11	4
Total	74	100	39

Survey of acute renal failure in Oxford in a 24-month period during which a total of 190 patients required haemodialysis or haemofiltration for acute renal failure.

Table 4 Acute renal failure—surgical causes. General Infirmary at Leeds 1956–1988

	n	Deaths	Actuarial 1-year survival (%)
General surgery	445	253	40.5
Cardiovascular	81	49	37.5
Trauma	94	43	52.2
Burns	17	14	17.6
Urinary obstruction	116	72	32.7
Renal stones	18	8	54.3
Retroperitoneal fibrosis	10	5	44.4
Bladder tumour	49	36	20.0
Malignancy	52	38	23.2
Pancreatitis	24	17	29.2
Surgical sepsis	126	88	29.3
All surgery	638	359	41.2

Prospective audit of surgical practice has defined circumstances associated with a particularly high risk of acute renal failure. There is, for example, a 20 per cent incidence of acute renal failure following abdominal aortic aneurysm rupture compared to only 3 per cent following elective repair. About 10 per cent of patients undergoing hepatobiliary surgery develop renal impairment but only 3 per cent require renal support. Two other high risk situations are acute pancreatitis and extensive burns: about 20 per cent of patients with greater than 15 per cent burns and 4 per cent of those with acute pancreatitis develop acute renal failure, and in both circumstances the mortality rate is high.

Aetiology and classification

The causes of acute renal failure are generally classified according to whether they act at prerenal, renal or postrenal sites (Table 5).

Prerenal failure arises in an otherwise healthy kidney as a simple consequence of hypoperfusion. The low perfusion pressure may be confined to the kidney, as with bilateral renal artery stenoses (Fig. 1) or stenosis of the artery to a single functioning kidney, but hypoperfusion is more often systemic and in surgical practice most commonly arises from hypovolaemia or sepsis.

Table 5 Aetiology of acute renal failure in surgical practice

1. Hypoperfusion (prerenal)	Shock
	Hypovolaemia
	Cardiogenic
	Septic
	Renal arterial disease
	Aortic dissection
	Embolism
2. Renal injury (renal)	Acute tubular necrosis (following 1)
	Toxic
	Drugs
	Myoglobin
	Haemoglobin
	Glomerulonephritis
	Associated sepsis
	Interstitial nephritis
	Antibiotics
3. Obstruction (postrenal)	Bilateral ureteric
	Retroperitoneal fibrosis
	Lymphoma
	Malignancy bladder
	Cervix
	Unilateral ureteric
	stones
	papilla
	tumour
	Bladder outflow
	Prostatic hyperplasia or carcinoma
	Urethral stricture

Postrenal causes are those of obstruction to urine flow. For obstruction to cause acute renal failure it must either be bilateral or affect a single functioning kidney. Bilateral ureteric obstruction is most often caused by retroperitoneal fibrosis, retroperitoneal lymphoma (Fig. 2), or malignant disease invading the base of the bladder. Bladder outflow obstruction is usually a result of prostatic disease or urethral stricture. Renal stones and sloughed papillae cause acute on chronic renal failure when they obstruct the only or better functioning of two kidneys.

Renal causes

Acute renal failure arising from intrinsic damage to the kidney is commonly due to 'acute tubular necrosis'. Definition is difficult since the pathogenesis in man is poorly understood, but this form of renal disease is generally associated with a severe haemodynamic disturbance or nephrotoxic exposure; acute renal failure is presumed to arise from tubular damage. The term 'necrosis' is widely used but inaccurate, since frank necrosis of tubular cells is not usually striking when tissue is examined histologically.

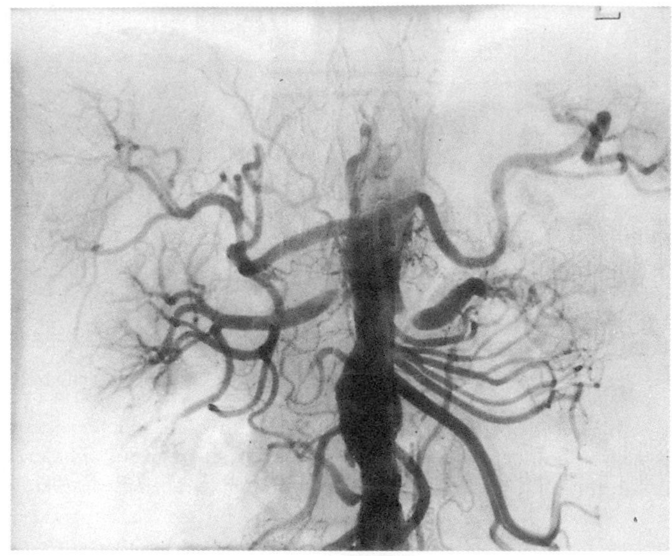

Fig. 1 Aortogram showing bilateral renal artery stenosis. This patient developed acute renal failure following coronary artery bypass grafting. (By courtesy of Dr E.W.L. Fletcher.)

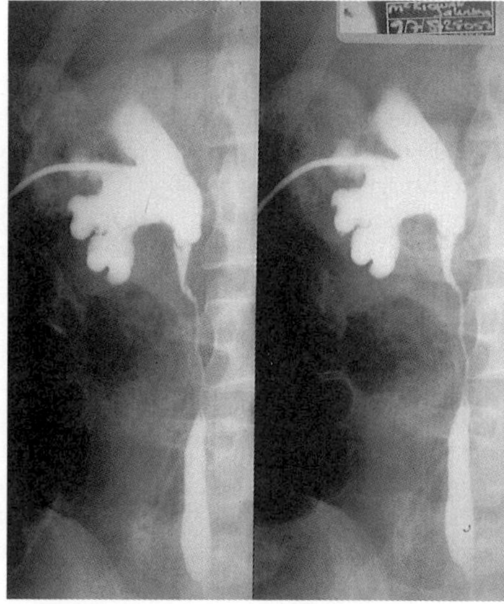

Fig. 2 Antegrade pyelogram in a patient with lymphoma and retroperitoneal lymph nodes, showing dilated renal calices.

In most clinical settings, the risk of acute tubular necrosis is rather unpredictable: a particular reduction of systemic blood pressure, or loss of intravascular volume cannot be precisely related to the risk of acute renal failure. Following exposure to potential nephrotoxins such as aminoglycoside antibiotics, haem proteins and radiographic contrast media, the risk of acute renal failure is usually low, not clearly dose dependent, and more obviously related to the coincidence of other potentially damaging influences. Many of the agents commonly listed as causing acute tubular necrosis might therefore more accurately be termed risk factors. Risk will also depend on the patient's underlying condition (Table 6): those with conditions such as heart failure, chronic liver disease, obstructive jaundice, chronic hypertension, or diabetes, in

Table 6 Conditions predisposing to the development of acute renal failure

Congestive heart failure
Chronic hypertension
Chronic liver disease
Obstructive jaundice
Systemic sepsis
Exposure to aminoglycosides, radiocontrast media
Renovascular disease
Chemotherapy for malignant disease
Multiple myeloma
Diabetes mellitus

which there are pre-existing abnormalities of renal haemodynamics will be at greater risk from a particular insult. The type of surgery is also important: operations or conditions associated with sepsis or severe tissue injury (for instance after trauma, burns, or major vascular occlusion) are associated with an increased risk of acute tubular necrosis.

Patients with acute renal failure caused by glomerular or interstitial disease usually present to physicians but may be referred to urologists when the striking symptoms are of haematuria or renal pain.

Pathophysiology

Since the kidney has a high resting blood flow, a low arterial–venous oxygen difference, and good autoregulatory capability it is not immediately clear why it should be susceptible to hypoperfusion injury. Regional disparities in oxygenation are well recognized and may leave certain regions at risk despite high overall blood flow, or renal perfusion may suffer an unusually severe reduction in certain forms of haemodynamic shock. The risk of renal injury is strongly dependent on the type of shock, being high in septicaemic shock and low in simple haemorrhagic shock (e.g. following gastrointestinal haemorrhage). The most severe threat to renal perfusion probably arises from multiple interactions such as activation of vasoconstrictor mechanisms, including the sympathetic nervous system and renin angiotensin system, loss of compensatory vasodilation such as by inhibition of prostaglandin production, and vascular injury itself, which may complicate septicaemia and endotoxaemia.

For some risk factors, a direct nephrotoxic action is clear. These include exposure to heavy metals such as *cis*-platinum, organic solvents, polyene antibiotics, amphotericin B, and prolonged administration of aminoglycoside antibiotics. Other precipitating factors such as myoglobin, haemoglobin,and radiographic contrast media have a clear association with acute renal failure, but renal injury is by no means invariable, and the mechanism of damage is not yet adequately explained.

Several mechanisms have been proposed to explain the near complete loss of renal function associated with acute tubular necrosis (Table 7). Tubular injury may prevent function directly, either by luminal blockage or by permitting back leakage of filtrate; or filtration itself may be reduced, either primarily, or secondary to feedback signals arising from impaired tubular transport or raised luminal pressures. Since these mechanisms may all operate at different times or may coincide and interact, it has been impossible to obtain a simple unifying explanation, even for the relatively simple animal models of acute renal failure.

Table 7 Mechanisms of excretory failure in acute tubular necrosis

Glomerular (either primary or via feedback from tubular signals)
Reduced perfusion
Reduce ultrafiltration coefficient (probably arising from reduced capillary surface area)
Tubular
Backleakage of filtrate across damaged epithelium
Obstruction by intraluminal debris or compression of the tubules by swollen cells.

The most immediate consequence of an abrupt loss of renal function is, of course, retention of the waste products of metabolism. The rate of accumulation is dependent not only on the severity of renal failure but on the rate of production. Increased catabolism is observed postoperatively and is particularly severe in patients with sepsis, burns, or trauma. Acute renal failure in this setting is marked by particularly rapid rises in urea, creatinine, urate, phosphate, acidaemia, and most importantly potassium. Massive muscle injury, which is not always traumatic, and may for instance complicate sepsis, ischaemia, prolonged coma, unusually strenuous exercise, or alcoholic intoxication, will lead to the particularly rapid onset of dangerous hyperkalaemia, hypocalcaemia, and hyperphosphataemia.

Management

Diagnosis

Acute renal failure is usually detected by a rise in the plasma creatinine or urea concentrations, or as a fall in urine output. Normal urine output alone can be falsely reassuring since many patients with acute renal failure are not oliguric; it is essential to monitor urea and creatinine in any patient at risk of developing postoperative renal failure.

Essential early diagnostic steps are the exclusion of urinary obstruction, the exclusion or treatment of prerenal failure, and the detection of pre-existing chronic renal disease. In each case assessment of the clinical history is vital. Urethral obstruction should be excluded immediately by palpation of the bladder.

Exclusion of obstruction

The risk of ureteral obstruction depends on the underlying pathology, being increased following pelvic or retroperitonal surgery for malignant pathologies, or in the presence of a single kidney. It may lead to renal pain or to the classical pattern of alternating polyuria and oliguria. Ultrasound examination is the key investigation and will detect almost all cases, with occasional failures when the investigation is performed early after acute obstruction or when the urinary system is encased with malignant tissue.

Recognition and correction of prerenal failure

The possibility of prerenal failure should be apparent from clinical examination. Although systemic blood pressure will not always be low in a supine patient there will generally be evidence of impaired circulation, such as cool extremities and postural hypotension. If external fluid losses are not apparent, the possibility of fluid sequestration, sepsis, or cardiac dysfunction must be considered. The diagnosis of prerenal failure is made by restoration of renal function when the haemodynamic problem is corrected.

The type of replacement fluid (blood, colloid, or crystalloid) should ideally reflect what has been lost. In circumstances where this is not clinically apparent or where blood is not available immediately, circulatory resuscitation should be commenced with isotonic crystalloid or colloid solutions. Controversy still surrounds the arguments for and against crystalloid or colloid solutions and in most circumstances either is acceptable. Colloid solutions are more expensive and have the potential to cause anaphylactoid reactions, but they are confined, at least partially, to the vascular compartment for a short period of time and can increase plasma oncotic pressure. Although the action on Starling forces may be slight and short-lived it may be significant in patients with coincident lung or cardiac disease who are on the verge of developing pulmonary oedema. Our practice is to use isotonic crystalloid solution in most circumstances and reserve the use of colloid solutions for resuscitation of shocked patients and those in whom intravascular depletion is combined with interstitial oedema. Colloid solutions are either albumin-containing preparations such as plasma protein fraction or carbohydrate polymer solutions such as Haemacel. Because of rapid availability and freedom from vasodilatory effects sometimes seen with plasma protein fraction, Haemacel is very suitable while blood becomes available, and up to 1500 ml may be infused. Some concern has been raised by the reporting of acute renal failure apparently occurring as a consequence of dextran infusions. The risk is small and may not be present with all carbohydrate polymers, but it is wise to use plasma protein fraction if large volumes of colloid replacement are to be given.

The aim of correcting the deficit as precisely and rapidly as possible is best achieved by administering fluid rapidly, but in relatively small aliquots: about 250 to 500 ml should be administered over approximately 30 min, and central venous pressure should be measured accurately after each aliquot of fluid. As vascular capacitance is filled this will remain low, but it will rise rapidly once repletion is achieved, and 250 ml aliquots of fluid are appropriate once any shift has been discerned. In some situations, such as severe haemorrhage, venoconstriction will be important. This will relax as volume replacement proceeds and may lead to a further fall in central venous pressure, which requires differentiation from continued fluid loss. If renal function does not immediately improve great care must be taken to avoid overhydration. Once volume replacement is achieved it is common to give an intravenous dose of either mannitol (10–20 g) or frusemide (40–80 mg) to promote a diuresis. This manoeuvre is justified on several grounds. First it provides reassuring evidence that renal perfusion has been re-established somewhat sooner than might otherwise be the case. Secondly, these agents might actually reduce the risk of acute tubular necrosis (see below). If in a volume-replete patient these manoeuvres do not induce a diuresis of at least 40 ml in the following hour then 'acute tubular necrosis' has probably become established.

Much is made of the importance of urinary electrolyte measurements in the assessment of the oliguric patient. Classically, in prerenal failure, tubular function should be intact and is reflected by a urine specific gravity of above 1.030 and an osmolality greater than 400 mosmol/kg H_2O, a urine to plasma urea ratio above 7, and a fractional excretion of sodium of less than 1 per cent. The distinction is often blurred by diuretic therapy and pre-existing renal disease, and is not a great help in management. The overriding concern is to achieve prompt and precise correction of the haemodynamic problem, something which will often require a period of continuous bedside medical attendance.

Recognition of pre-existing chronic renal failure

The possibility or pre-existing renal failure should have been excluded in the preoperative assessment but if not may be suspected from a history of renal disease or hypertension, unexplained anaemia, or if reduced kidney size is demonstrated by ultrasonography. If these exclusions are made, renal failure develops postoperatively in a situation of recognized risk, and the urine deposit is not very cellular, a presumptive diagnosis of acute tubular necrosis can be made. In other situations, for instance if renal failure is found on admission, diagnostic assessment of the full range of renal diseases will be required. History should involve careful enquiry about drug or toxin exposure. Examination should include a search for cutaneous signs of vasculitis and microscopic examination of fresh urine looking for red cells, red cell casts, white cells, and bacteria.

Immediate management and indications for urgent dialysis

Renal failure is often recognized rather late, presenting the clinician with the need to treat dangerous hyperkalaemia immediately and assess the need for urgent dialysis. The risk from hyperkalaemia is of sudden arrhythmic death; early electrocardiographic abnormalities are increased 'T' wave amplitude, while later, ominous changes are broadening of the QRS complex, and flattening and eventual disappearance of the P wave. Eventually, the electrocardiogram comes to resemble a sine wave and cardiac standstill follows. Treatment is required urgently if the serum potassium is above 8 mmol or there are electrocardiographic changes (Fig. 3).

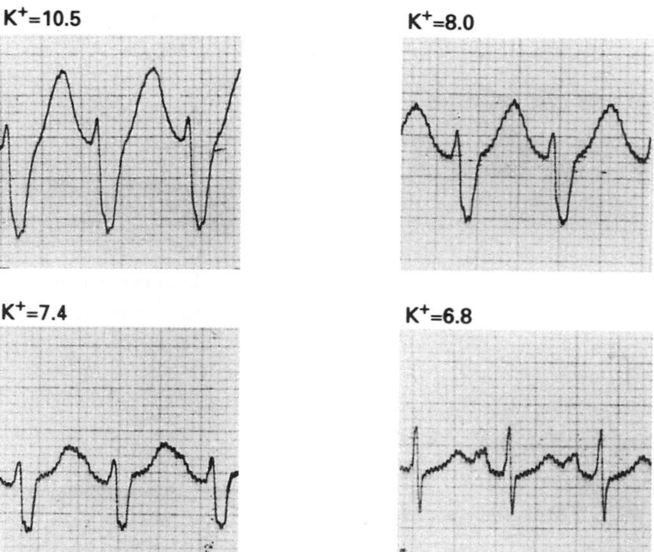

Fig. 3 Electrocardiogram demonstrating the features of severe hyperkalaemia.

The immediate management is intravenous administration of calcium. Calcium gluconate (10 ml of 10 per cent) should be given over 1 to 2 min and repeated until the electrocardiogram improves. Additional measures should be undertaken to reduce the serum potassium. In patients without serious fluid overload, hypertonic sodium bicarbonate (4.2 per cent) may be given intravenously in a dose of 50 mmol (100 ml). Entry of potassium into cells is promoted by correction of acidosis and also by the hypertonic sodium. Serum potassium may also be reduced acutely by insulin, which promotes cellular entry by stimulation of Na, K-ATPase. To prevent hypoglycaemia, glucose is given concurrently, a typical regimen being 50 g glucose intravenously with 15 units soluble insulin. Monitoring is required to detect hypoglycaemia in unconscious patients and if this cannot be provided (e.g. during a transfer) it is safer, in non-diabetic patients, to omit insulin and rely on the endogenous insulin response to glucose infusion. Following control of hyperkalaemia by these measures, provision for urgent dialysis should be made unless renal function has been restored.

Fluid overload manifesting as pulmonary oedema is also an immediate indication for ultrafiltration using a dialysis machine, haemofiltration, or peritoneal dialysis (see below). A marked metabolic acidosis should be treated with sodium bicarbonate only if there is hyperkalaemia or cardiogenic shock. This will have only temporary benefit and is not a substitute for dialysis or measures to improve tissue perfusion.

Prophylaxis and attempts at reversal

Since many treatments when applied before the insult are effective in ameliorating or preventing acute renal failure in experimental models, it might be expected that prophylactic measures would be important in surgery. However, since many of the measures, such as use of vasodilators, may exacerbate hypotension they are difficult or dangerous to apply in clinical practice. Prophylactic administration of dopamine, mannitol, or frusemide, coupled with intravenous fluid sufficient to maintain or even expand the plasma volume, will almost certainly reduce the incidence of acute renal failure after high-risk procedures such as aortic surgery and surgery in jaundiced patients. Of these measures, the most important is maintenance of blood volume. The use of prophylactic mannitol is also established practice in aortic surgery, a suitable regimen consisting of infusion of 10 g as a hypertonic 20 per cent solution after induction of anaesthesia followed by infusion at a rate of 10 g/h during the procedure.

In patients with established acute tubular necrosis such measures can usually increase the urine output moderately, but there is no evidence that they lessen the severity or duration of renal failure or that they improve survival. However, when renal failure is first detected it is difficult to know whether any reversible element exists. In this situation it is usual to attempt to improve renal perfusion and urine flow by the intravenous administration of dopamine (1–2 µg/kg.min) and frusemide (5–10 mg/min) for 1 to 2 h. Whilst there is no certain evidence of efficacy, there is little short-term risk associated with these procedures.

General measures (Table 8)

Apart from the control of fluid and electrolyte balance a number of measures have become part of the routine management of patients with acute renal failure and are based on common sense, and knowledge of the causes of death and morbidity, rather than on the results of rigorous clinical trials.

The first is the prevention and prompt treatment of infection. To avoid nosocomial infection the number of intravascular catheters should be kept to a minimum and there should be a low threshold for changing these. Bladder catheters should either be removed or connected to a closed drainage system. Samples should be examined frequently for bacteria and Candida. Fever should be promptly investigated. Antibiotic treatment will often be required before microbiological identification of the pathogen is available. The usual sites of sepsis are surgical wounds, the abdominal cavity, the lungs, central venous catheters, and the urinary tract. Surgeons should have a low threshold for re-exploring the abdomen in patients who have developed renal failure following abdominal surgery or penetrating injury since in these seriously ill patients clinical signs and imaging are too insensitive to detect residual sepsis.

Table 8 General measures in the management of acute renal failure

1. Avoid and treat infection
    - Remove unnecessary lines and catheters
    - Regular surveillance cultures
    - Use narrow spectrum antibiotics
    - Regular search for deep sepsis
    - Good mouth, wound, vascular access care
2. H_2-antagonists to prevent stress ulceration
3. Nutritional support
    - Enteral if possible
    - Parenteral through tunnelled line
    - Provide for hypercatabolism
4. Maintain haemoglobin > 10g/dl
5. Prescribe prudently
    - Avoid certain drugs
    - Modify dose and interval

The second general measure is the maintenance of adequate nutrition. This is more difficult in patients with renal failure, but with attention to fluid balance it is usually possible to provide both sufficient calories and sufficient nitrogen. The nutritional requirements will depend on the degree of catabolism. Depending on the method of renal replacement being used, adjustments in the potassium, phosphate, and sodium concentrations of parental nutrition solutions will be required. Gastro-intestinal haemorrhage was a common cause of death but is seldom fatal today, perhaps because anticoagulation is minimized and the prescription of H_2-receptor antagonists or cytoprotective agents is routine. Most patients with surgical acute renal failure have received broad-spectrum antibiotics and therefore are at risk of developing *Clostridium difficile* toxin-related colitis. Stools should be tested regularly for the toxin, and prompt treatment with oral metronidazole or vancomycin should be instituted.

Finally it should again be emphasized that the metabolism and excretion of many drugs is altered in renal failure. Each prescription should be checked to determine whether dose modifications are required (see Table 2).

Renal replacement techniques

Peritoneal dialysis

Peritoneal dialysis via a rigid catheter inserted percutaneously or by surgical implantation of a soft catheter is still widely used for the treatment of acute renal failure as it is inexpensive and can be instituted without recourse to specialized equipment. Continuous peritoneal dialysis has three possible advantages over haemodialysis: a lower risk of exacerbating bleeding because heparinization is not required, less cardiovascular instability, and a lower risk of disequilibration. In practice these problems can be minimized or overcome with modern haemodialysis techniques. Peritoneal dialysis requires an intact peritoneum, a watertight abdomen, and a safely inserted dialysis catheter. It also needs a significant amount of nursing supervision. Other potential problems include difficulties in maintaining dialysate flow, peritoneal infection, protein losses, limited efficacy in hypercatabolic patients and, when a rigid catheter is used, immobilization of the patient. The choice of peritoneal dialysis is often made for practical reasons such as lack of haemodialysis equipment, but it is the treatment of choice in infants. It should not be used in hypercatabolic patients or those with any past or recent intra-abdominal pathology, because adhesions make catheter placement hazardous.

Intermittent haemodialysis

Intermittent haemodialysis is the orthodox treatment for acute renal failure and it is the most practical way to treat mobile patients. Access to the vascular system is either via catheters placed in central veins or by the use of an arteriovenous shunt. Treatment should be started before complications make it urgent. The first dialysis treatment is generally short, lasting 2 to 3 h. Depending on whether the patient is severely catabolic, subsequent treatments will need to be undertaken daily or on alternate days, aiming to keep the pretreatment blood urea below 33 mmol/l and to avoid fluid overload. In patients with an unstable cardiovascular system bicarbonate-buffered dialysate is used in preference to acetate. The dialysis treatment is used as an opportunity to administer blood transfusions, allowing the extra fluid to be removed by ultrafiltration.

The risk of bleeding can be minimized if low doses of heparin are used, and if necessary this can be reversed at the end of dialysis by the administration of protamine sulphate. There is some evidence to suggest that the use of low molecular weight heparin reduces the risk of bleeding, and this is used in some units for patients requiring dialysis in the early postoperative period. Heparin requirements can be further reduced by the use of prostacyclin to inhibit platelet function. The drug is short-lived and is given as an infusion immediately before, and during, the dialysis treatment. In most regimens prostacyclin does not replace heparin, but is used in combination with a reduced dose. The disadvantages are expense and hypotension. If a patient is actively bleeding when dialysis is required, dialysis can even be performed without heparin, provided the lines have been primed with heparin-containing saline and the blood flow is maintained over 200 ml/min.

The particular limitation of intermittent haemodialysis is the need to establish fluid balance for a 24- to 48-h period during a 3- to 4-h treatment. Thus to control fluid balance ultrafiltration has to be rapid, risking hypotension, cardiac ischaemia, and arrhythmias. Haemodialysis treatment also needs to be frequent to avoid rapid and large changes in the concentrations of plasma urea and other molecules which may generate transcellular osmotic gradients leading to 'disequilibration'; a syndrome which probably arises from the rapid entry of water into the brain cells and which leads to coma and fits. Another disadvantage of haemodialysis is the sequestration of white cells which occurs in the lungs as a result of complement activation at the dialysis membrane. Although this sequestration is short-lived it can aggravate hypoxia.

Continuous treatments

These limitations of intermittent haemodialysis stimulated the development of the continuous treatments, which are particularly applicable to the immobilized patient with multiple system failure being managed in the intensive care or high dependency unit. The advantages of these forms of treatment are that they can be used in patients with low systolic blood pressures and provide continuous metabolic control and fluid balance with very little perturbation to the cardiovascular system. This means that there are no constraints on the administration of parenteral nutrition, blood products, and drugs. A disadvantage is the need for continuous heparinization, but with low doses and removal by the filter this should not lead to dangerous systemic anticoagulation. The treatments can only be safely used if the patient has continuous bedside nursing supervision, is immobile, and is unlikely to dislodge the catheters. The use of these catheters is not without its problems. Arterial catheters can cause limb ischaemia in patients with pre-existing peripheral vascular disease, and damage to the vessel wall can lead to thrombosis, aneurysm formation, and leakage of blood into the retroperitoneal space.

There are a number of forms of continuous renal replacement treatment. The simplest is continuous arteriovenous or venovenous haemofiltration, with continuous replacement of the filtrate with fluid which has the electrolyte composition of plasma but which is buffered with lactate rather than bicarbonate (Fig. 3). Using either a Quinton-Scribner shunt, or femoral vascular catheters, a circuit containing a low pressure filter is established. This allows production of ultrafiltration that can be varied from 2 to 3 l/day to 24 l/day by altering the pressure across the filter and the blood flow. Venovenous circuits require a blood pump: since this introduces the risk of potentially fatal air embolism a venous air trap detector and automatic safety switch is mandatory. Low volume haemofiltration (6 l/day) controls fluid balance and substitutes partially for dialysis but needs to be supplemented by haemodialysis treatments, which can be shorter and less frequent. High volume haemofiltration (in excess of 15 ml/min) makes haemodialysis unnecessary but fluid imbalance can occur very rapidly and scrupulous monitoring is needed. This can be achieved by computerized pumped haemofiltration fluid replacement or by using a simple gravity feed device controlled by a balance system (see Fig. 4) which returns fluid in direct proportion to that removed.

Another variation is continuous arteriovenous haemodialysis. The circuit is the same as that for continuous arteriovenous haemofiltration, but a low resistance dialysis filter is used. The blood flow is kept low (less than 100 ml/min) and the negative pressure across the membrane is adjusted to control ultrafiltration. The additional component is the slow pumping of dialysis fluid, countercurrent through the dialysate compartment of the filter. Full equilibration in the dialyser is necessary to provide optimal clearance of nitrogenous waste products (15–20 ml/min). The effluent from the filter consists of dialysate and ultrafiltrate. Since most of the membranes used have a high ultrafiltration capacity, scrupulous attendance to fluid balance on an hourly basis, or by a continuous replacement system is again required.

Prognosis

The survival of patients with acute renal failure following surgery depends largely on the underlying disease. The majority of deaths occur in the first week of acute renal failure, and are due to cardiorespiratory or multisystem failure. Sepsis, gastrointestinal haemorrhage, pancreatitis, liver failure, and cerebral damage also contribute to mortality. Overall survival has almost certainly improved over the three decades since dialysis was introduced, although this has not always been easy to demonstrate. In the Leeds series survival improved from 38.4 per cent in patients treated between 1956 and 1959 to 47.4 per cent in the 1980 to 1988 cohort. This improvement was confined to the older patient group (over 45 years), probably because improvements in postoperative care,

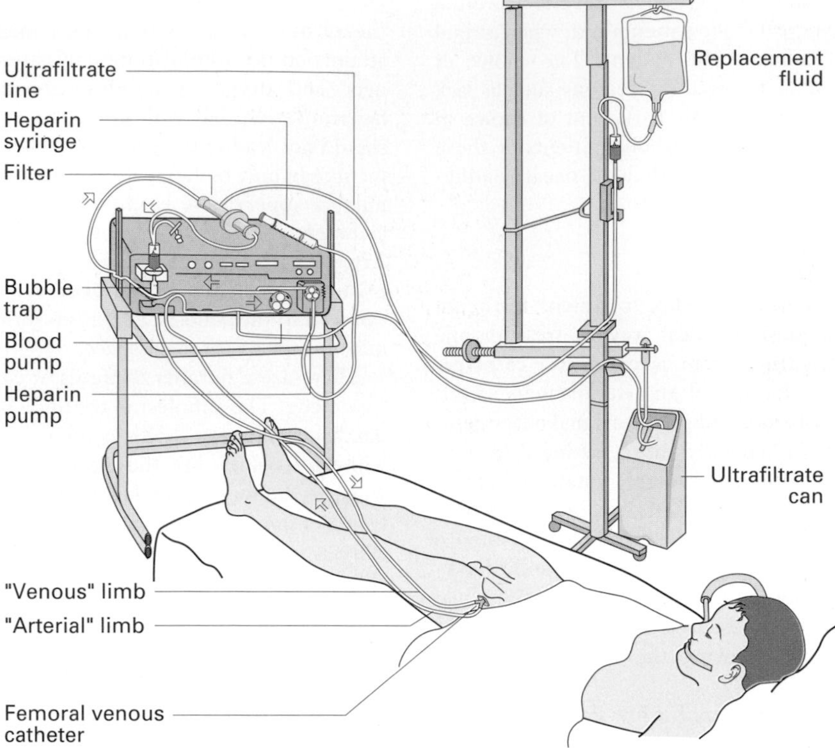

Fig. 4 Diagram of a patient undergoing pumped venovenous haemofiltration for acute renal failure using a gravity feed balance system for infusion of replacement fluid.

Table 9 Patients with a poor prognosis

1. Superadded adult respiratory distress syndrome
2. Prolonged requirement for inotropic support
3. Unresolved sepsis
4. Jaundice developing during acute renal failure
5. Underlying premorbid organ dysfunction
    - Cardiac failure
    - Chronic liver disease
    - Haematological malignancy

antibiotics, parental nutrition, and renal support systems have been balanced by the risks of performing more complex surgery in older and less healthy patients.

Treatment for acute renal failure is usually undertaken in the hope that if the patient survives the kidneys will recover. This is not always the case. Persistent renal failure is sometimes seen after severe shock, where the pathology is usually cortical necrosis. Chronicity is also more likely in the elderly and in those with pre-existing renal impairment. When acute renal failure occurs in certain settings or is associated with particular complications the prognosis is particularly poor (Table 9). There is, however, no proven method of establishing that the prognosis of a patient with acute renal failure is hopeless, so that decisions to discontinue renal support in severely ill patients must be made individually.

FURTHER READING

Badr K, Ischikawa I. Prerenal failure. A deleterious shift from renal compensation to decompensation. *N Engl J Med* 1988; **319**: 623–9.

Bennett WM, Blythe WB. Use of drugs in renal failure. In: Schrier RW, Gottschalk CW, eds. *Disease of the Kidney*. 4th edn. Boston: Little Brown and Company, 1988: 3437–506.

Berisa F, *et al*. Prognostic factors in acute renal failure following aortic aneurysm surgery. *Q J Med* 1990; **76**: 689–98.

Berns AS. Nephrotoxicity of contrast media. *Kidney Int* 1989; **36**: 730–40.

Better OS, Stein JH. Early management of shock and prophylaxis of acute renal failure in traumatic rhabdomyolysis. *N Engl J Med* 1990; **322**: 825–9.

Bihari DJ, Neild GH, eds. *Acute Renal Failure in the Intensive Therapy Unit*. Berlin: Springer Verlag, 1990.

Frost L, Pedersen RS, Ostgaard SE, Hansen HE. Prognosis in acute pancreatitis complicated by acute renal failure requiring dialysis. *Scand J Urol Nephrol* 1990; **24**: 257–60.

Graybar GB, Work J, Barber WH. Anesthetic considerations for the dialysis patient. *Semin Dialysis* 1989; **2**: 108–16.

Holt SDH. The management of acute renal failure: surgical aspects of sepsis. In Rainford D, Sweny P, eds. *Acute Renal Failure*. London: Farrand Press, 1990; 221–34.

Kjellstrand CM, Jacobson S, Lins LE. Acute renal failure In: Maher JF, ed. *Replacement of Renal Function by Dialysis*. 3rd Edition. Dordrecht: Kluwer Academic Publishers, 1988; 616–49.

Myers BD, Moran SM. Hemodynamically mediated acute renal failure. *NEngl J Med*, 1986; **341**: 97–105.

Turney HJ, Marshall DH, Brownjohn AM, Ellis CM, Parsons FM. The evolution of acute renal failure. 1956–1988. *Q J Med* 1990; **74**: 83–104.

Wait RB, Kahna KD. Renal failure complicating obstructive jaundice. *Am J Surg*, 1989; **157**: 256–63.

5.4 Hepatic problems

CAROL A. COBB AND R. W. CHAPMAN

INTRODUCTION

Postoperative liver dysfunction is a common problem. Although the incidence after elective abdominal surgery is less than 1 per cent, much higher rates occur after major surgery, multiple trauma, and prolonged intervention. The majority of cases are mild, transient, and resolve spontaneously, but occasionally the liver injury may be severe and result in fulminant liver failure and/or chronic liver disease. There are many aetiological factors, and in any one patient the pathogenesis is often multifactorial (Fig. 1).

In this section the clinical presentation, investigation, diagnosis, treatment, and prevention of hepatic problems in the surgical patient are discussed. Patients with normal preoperative liver function are considered separately from those with preexisting liver disease. Primary liver diseases, details of hepatobiliary surgery, liver transplantation, and surgical treatment of portal hypertension and ascites are dealt with elsewhere.

THE SURGICAL PATIENT WITH NORMAL PREOPERATIVE LIVER FUNCTION

Introduction

Postoperative hepatic dysfunction in surgical patients with normal liver function can be classified into three groups: those due to (1) overproduction of bilirubin; (2) hepatocellular dysfunction; and (3) extrahepatic biliary obstruction (see Table 1).

Table 1 Causes of hepatic dysfunction in the surgical patient with normal preoperative liver function

Overproduction of bilirubin
haemolytic anaemias
blood transfusion
resorption of blood
sepsis
Gilbert syndrome
Hepatocellular dysfunction
Hepatic
ischaemia-induced hepatitis
post-transfusion hepatitis
coincident viral hepatitis
drugs
total parenteral nutrition
fasting
obesity
diabetes mellitus
Cholestatic
ischaemia-induced cholestasis
sepsis
drugs
total parenteral nutrition
Extrahepatic biliary obstruction
bile duct injury
common bile duct stones
postoperative pancreatitis
acalculous cholecystitis

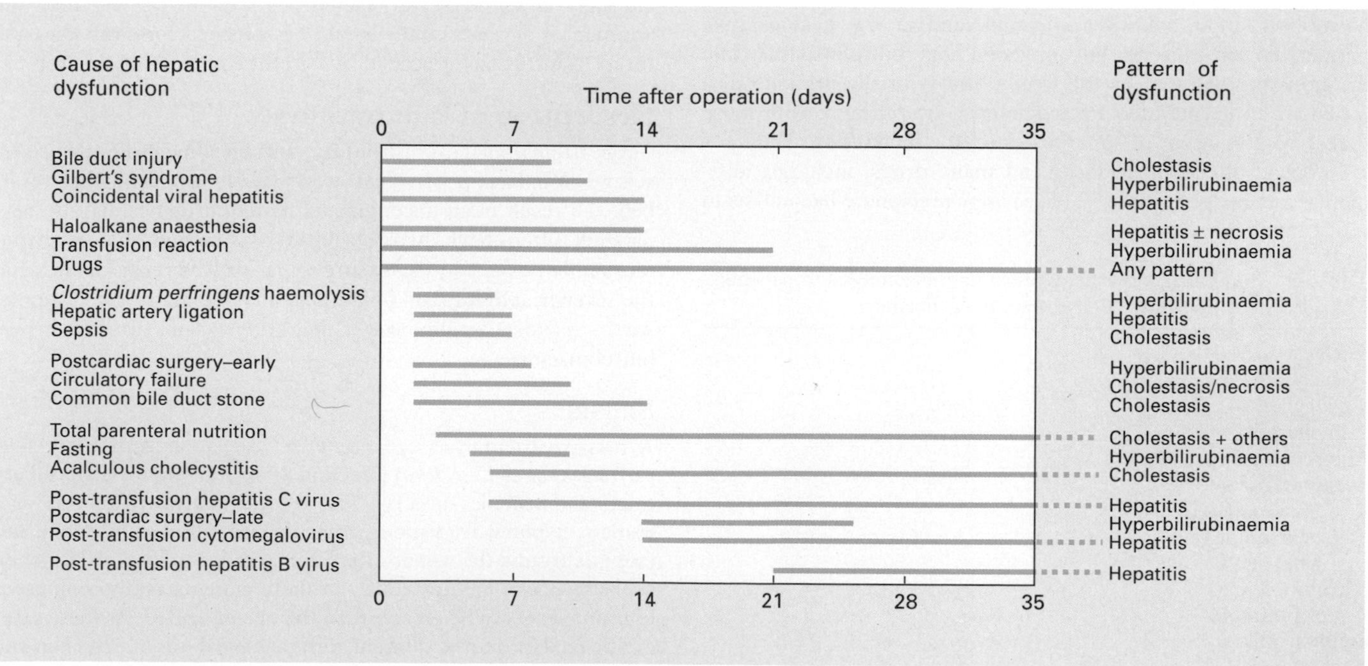

Fig. 1 Onset of hepatic dysfunction in relation to cause and pattern.

Overproduction of bilirubin

In a healthy individual the liver conjugates up to 500 μmol of bilirubin per day as a result of the breakdown of red blood cells. The liver is capable of handling several times this quantity without the occurrence of hyperbilirubinaemia and only if haemolysis is severe or occurs in conjunction with hepatocellular insufficiency does jaundice develop. Unconjugated bilirubin comprising 90 per cent of the total is suggestive of haemolysis. When the level of unconjugated bilirubin is excessively high there appears to be a concomitant rise in the conjugated fraction. The cause of significant haemolysis may be haemolytic anaemia, blood transfusion, resorption of haematomata, sepsis, or open-heart surgery.

Haemolytic anaemias

Congenital and acquired haemolytic anaemias can be associated with postoperative jaundice (see Table 2).

Table 2 Haemolytic conditions associated with postoperative liver dysfunction

Sickle-cell disease
Hereditary spherocytosis
Glucose 6–phosphate dehydrogenase deficiency
Pyruvate kinase deficiency
Non-immune acquired haemolytic anaemias

In surgical patients with sickle-cell disease there are increased risks as acute haemolysis and severe pain can be precipitated by infection, dehydration, acidosis, and hypoxia. In the postoperative period the earliest signs of infection must be treated promptly, especially as these patients have splenic hypofunction and are susceptible to bacterial infection. Patients from the African continent, parts of Asia, the Arabian peninsula, and southern Europe should be screened for sickle-cell disease.

Patients with hereditary spherocytosis may also experience a haemolytic crisis following infection, and in the postoperative period this can cause an unconjugated hyperbilirubinaemia. The diagnosis is suggested by the family history or the presence of a raised mean corpuscular haemoglobin concentration, with more than 1 to 2 per cent of spherocytes on the blood film.

Surgery, infection, acidosis, and many drugs, including antibiotics and analgesics (see Table 3), may precipitate haemolysis in patients with glucose 6-phosphate dehydrogenase deficiency. At least 10 million people worldwide have this red cell enzyme deficiency, and thus patients from the Mediterranean, South East Asia, the Middle East, and West Africa should be screened preoperatively. The cresyl blue decoloration test or the methaemoglobin reduction test can be used in screening, and the diagnosis made by enzyme assay.

Table 3 Some drugs that may precipitate haemolysis in patients with glucose 6-phosphate dehydrogenase deficiency

Analgesic
acetanilide
salicylates
phenacetin
Antimicrobial
antimalarials
primaquine
pentaquine
pamaquine
Nitrofurans
nitrofurantoin
Sulphonamides
Nalidixic acid
Antihelminthics

Pyruvate kinase deficiency is another red cell enzymopathy in which infection can precipitate haemolysis. Patients should be aware of their diagnosis but macrocytosis and an abnormal enzyme assay will confirm the diagnosis.

Causes of non-immune acquired haemolytic anaemia include disseminated intravascular coagulation, vasculitis, pneumococcal, meningococcal, and Gram-negative sepsis, *Clostridium perfringens* (was *C. welchii*) infection, burns, drowning, and some drugs. These are covered in other parts of this section.

Blood transfusion

Immediate and delayed haemolytic reactions may occur following blood transfusion. Within 24 h of the transfusion of one unit of stored blood at least 10 per cent undergoes haemolysis. Transfusion of two units of blood should not result in an increase in the serum bilirubin. If transfusion is rapid, massive, or occurs in a patient with impaired liver function, the capacity of the liver to conjugate bilirubin may be exceeded. Jaundice in this situation occurs 10 to 12 h after transfusion. Incompatibility of transfused blood may result in a severe immediate haemolytic reaction, which may occur if there are antibodies to the donated blood in the recipient's plasma. Jaundice appears at 12 h after commencing transfusion, peaks at between 24 and 36 h, and lasts for a total of 4 or 5 days.

Delayed haemolytic transfusion reactions are seen between 3 days and 3 weeks post-transfusion, with the peak reaction being at around 7 to 10 days. They are due to a secondary immune response, and in the majority of cases there has been sensitization to red cell antigens through past transfusion or pregnancy. This response is often to Rhesus and Kidd antigens, and is seen clinically as extravascular haemolysis with fever, jaundice, and anaemia. A serum sample should be screened for antibodies and future transfusions preceded by careful compatibility testing.

Resorption of haematomata

Large haematomata, crush injury, and bleeding from major vessels result in large pools of extravascular blood which, when resorbed, can result in an unconjugated hyperbilirubinaemia. As these patients often have hepatocellular dysfunction due to hypotension, hypoxia, and major surgery, as well as renal impairment, the severity and duration of jaundice may be marked. In a similar way, massive pulmonary infarction can cause hyperbilirubinaemia.

Sepsis

A massive haemolysis can occur in association with *Clostridium perfringens* (was *C. welchii*) infection 24 to 72 h after gastric, biliary tract, and colonic surgery. The typical clinical picture is of a restless, hypotensive patient, an acute rise in serum bilirubin, and crepitus around the wound site. Several causes of liver dysfunction probably occur simultaneously in these patients as the conjugated bilirubin level can be greater than the unconjugated. As these cases can be fatal, prompt treatment with massive doses of penicillin and hyperbaric oxygen are imperative. Meningococcal, pneumococcal, and Gram-negative sepsis can cause haemolysis through disseminated intravascular coagulation and secondary microangiopathic haemolysis. As sepsis can also cause intrahepatic cholestasis, a combination of the two factors may cause marked jaundice.

Open-heart surgery

Early and late rises in bilirubin are seen after open-heart surgery. Early onset jaundice may be seen in up to 23 per cent of such patients and the main contributing factors are hypoxia, severity of right-heart failure preoperatively, and number of units of blood transfused. Although it has been suggested that cardiopulmonary bypass and prosthetic valves cause haemolysis, these are probably not significant contributors to the increased bilirubin. Late jaundice due to an autoimmune haemolytic anaemia has been reported where anaemia and jaundice, exacerbated by repeat transfusion, occur a few weeks after surgery. The presence of antiglobulin antibodies confirms the diagnosis; steroids are the treatment of choice.

Gilbert syndrome

Gilbert syndrome is low-grade chronic hyperbilirubinaemia found in 3 to 7 per cent of the population, with a male to female ratio of 2–7 : 1. It presents in the second or third decade as a raised level of unconjugated bilirubin. The serum bilirubin does not exceed 100 μmol/l and is usually less than 50 μmol/l. Liver function tests, routine haematology tests, and liver biopsy are normal. Haemolysis and acquired liver disease should be excluded and the diagnostic tests are: a two- to threefold increase in bilirubin induced by a 48-h fast and resolved by resumption of a normal diet; normal postprandial serum bile acids and reduced bilirubin UDP-glucuronyl transferase activity in a liver biopsy. The syndrome is probably inherited in an autosomal dominant fashion with variable penetrance.

The reduced bilirubin UDP-glucuronyl transferase activity is associated with reduced hepatic clearance of bilirubin and this, in combination with a possible mild compensated haemolytic state, is thought to cause the hyperbilirubinaemia. The main precipitating factor seems to be fasting, and it is primarily lipid withdrawal that is to blame. In the postoperative period, a raised bilirubin level may be noted particularly during episodes of vomiting, especially in pregnancy and febrile illnesses. Gilbert syndrome must be considered in the differential diagnosis of hepatic dysfunction in such patients.

Circulatory failure

Circulatory failure/surgical shock

Circulatory failure contributes to hepatic dysfunction in many surgical situations, although it is rarely the sole cause of the liver abnormality. Major trauma, burns, sepsis, massive blood loss, and surgery can be precipitants of ‘shock’, and these factors often occur together. In particular, gastrointestinal blood loss and septicaemia increase the risk of liver dysfunction when associated with hypotension. Cholestasis is the most common pattern of injury following hypotension, and this is a benign complication with a good prognosis. Prolonged hypotension, which is often associated with increased right atrial pressure, results in an ischaemic hepatitis, for example in open-heart surgery. There is an initial striking elevation of serum transaminases, up to 200 times the normal level, a marked decrease in prothrombin time, and a typically delayed bilirubin rise. These dramatic changes are seen within hours of surgery, and where no severe liver damage has occurred they revert rapidly to normal with restoration of liver blood flow and oxygenation. However, massive centrilobular hepatic necrosis can occur, and the ischaemic hepatitis can progress to fulminant hepatic failure, which has a high mortality rate. The clinical manifestation of hypoxic liver cell necrosis inevitably postdates the hypoxic event, and other causes, especially a viral hepatitis, must be considered.

Massive haemorrhage in combination with massive transfusion (for example, more than 20 units of blood) puts the liver particularly at risk of liver damage, should the patient survive. Major trauma patients are particularly at risk of this form of liver damage as well as that due to direct liver injury. In one study, 2 per cent of patients with major trauma and shock developed significant jaundice.

Patients with major burns form another group in which circulatory failure is an important factor in the aetiology of the associated hepatic dysfunction. Haemolysis often adds to the bilirubin load on the liver.

Hepatic artery ligation

The normal liver usually tolerates hepatic artery ligation without significant sequelae unless the flow of portal-vein blood is inadequate because of vascular stricture and sepsis. Minimal derangement of bilirubin and alkaline phosphatase levels occur, and moderate increases in the transaminase levels in the first week may be the only consequence. Hepatic arterial collateral vessels develop very rapidly and this, in combination with the portal circulation, reduces the ischaemic insult. Extensive mobilization of the liver can involve division of the ligamentum and triangular ligament and if this precedes hepatic artery ligation, massive liver necrosis may result. If infarction occurs, the amounts of bilirubin and transaminases rise rapidly to high levels.

Post-transfusion hepatitis

Post-transfusion hepatitis is the single most important complication of blood-product transfusion.

The first case of post-transfusion hepatitis was reported in 1885 after a patient received human serum. In the early 1980s the incidence of post-transfusion hepatitis in Europe and the United States was between 2 and 20 per cent. In 1991 it was suggested that the incidence in Italy may have fallen to around 5 per cent. The change in blood donor selection, surrogate testing for non-A, non-B post-transfusion hepatitis (with alanine aminotransferase and anti-HBc (antibody to hepatitis B core antigen) testing), and the modification of transfusion practice (less homologous and more autologous transfusions) have reduced the incidence. With an increase in the sensitivity and specificity of diagnosing hepatitis C virus (HCV) carriage in the future, the low risk of developing post-transfusion viral hepatitis will become extremely low. The viruses known to cause post-transfusion hepatitis are listed in Table 4.

Hepatitis B virus (HBV)

The estimated number of carriers of HBV worldwide is 120 million, and in the United States of America there are at least 900 000 carriers. Transmission of HBV by blood transfusion has been reduced dramatically by the screening of donor blood, although

Table 4 Infective agents that can cause post-transfusion hepatitis

Hepatitis B virus (HBV)
Hepatitis C virus (HCV)
Hepatitis D virus (HDV)
Human immunodeficiency virus (HIV)
Cytomegalovirus (CMV)
Epstein–Barr virus (EBV)
Parenterally acquired non-A, non-B, non-C virus(es)

today parenterally acquired HBV infection can still occur in transfused patients because genetic mutations in the virus result in falsely negative screening tests.

The clinical picture of acute HBV infection is very variable, from asymptomatic to fulminant hepatic failure. A fulminant fatal post-transfusion illness is seen in the elderly. Recovery without sequelae is the rule, but 5 to 10 per cent of infants and children with acute HBV infection develop chronic infection, as do 90 per cent of neonates. The mortality of hepatitis B infection is 1 to 3 per cent, and treatment with α-interferon is available for selected patients with chronic HBV infection. However, post-exposure prophylaxis by administration of hepatitis B immunoglobulin and HBV vaccine is also available.

Prevention of post-transfusion hepatitis B is mainly through the screening of donated blood. Donor education, voluntary and not commercial donations, and attempts to discourage donors at risk of carrying transmissible diseases are other important measures. A combination of alanine aminotransferase and antihepatitis B core (anti-HBc) antibody assays have been used since 1986 to exclude many donors at risk of hepatitis C and human immunodeficiency virus infection as well as HBV infection. More recently, more specific tests have become available.

Hepatitis B surface antigen (HBsAg) was used to screen those infected with HBV, but more recently it has been shown that HBV variants exist due to mutations in the genome. Such mutations can result in the HBsAg test being negative and post-transfusion hepatitis B infection, including fulminant disease, has occurred. Screening for anti-HBc positivity should prevent this.

Hepatitis C virus (HCV)

Hepatitis C virus is an RNA virus with homology to the flaviviruses and is the most common cause of post-transfusion hepatitis, accounting for up to 95 per cent of cases. Both plasma and cell products are infective. The infection rate of transfused patients is 7 to 10 per cent. The estimated prevalence of HCV infection among volunteer blood donors around the world varies from 0.2 to 1.7 per cent. For example, in New York it is 0.9 to 1.4 per cent; in western Europe, 0.7 per cent; in Japan, 1.5 per cent; and in Hungary, 1.7 per cent.

The incubation period is 5 to 12 weeks, although after transfusions of a particularly large volume of infected blood this may be shortened to between 1 and 4 weeks. Clinically, the disease is mild with only a moderate elevation of transaminase levels. Rarely, a fulminant hepatitis may occur which has a high mortality. Levels of bilirubin and the transaminases may rise for a second, or even third, time in the first few months of the infection. Diagnosis is mainly by exclusion as seroconversion may take up to 6 months or more. Tests for antibodies to HCV are widely available but the false positive rate is high. Repeat assays using different varieties of antibody, or the immunoblot technique as opposed to the enzyme-linked immunosorbent assay (ELISA), improve the specificity. The polymerase chain reaction (PCR) method will identify viral RNA in the serum and is the most accurate technique, but at the present time it is expensive and not widely available. Histologically, there are lymphoid follicles in the portal tracts, showing mild chronic inflammation bordering on chronic active hepatitis. There may be parenchymal inflammation and focal necrosis, as well as some fatty change. Chronic infection is also clinically mild and occurs in 85 per cent of patients or more. At least 41 per cent of patients develop chronic active hepatitis and 20 per cent develop cirrhosis. HCV also greatly increases the risk of development of hepatocellular carcinoma, four times more so than HBV. The time interval between infection and end-stage liver disease may be in the order of 25 years. Treatment of HCV-infected patients with α-interferon has been proved to be effective, but the optimum timing of treatment in such a protracted disease process is still unclear.

Prevention was initially through donor education, exclusion of high-risk individuals as donors, and surrogate testing using serum aspartate transaminase levels and anti-HBc tests. Since September 1991 blood donors in the United Kingdom have been screened for HCV infection by methods involving the use of antibodies to viral components. Any positive blood is rejected despite the high false positive rate.

Hepatitis D virus (HDV)

Hepatitis D virus only infects individuals already infected with HBV. The incubation period is 30 to 50 days and chronic infection is the most common outcome. Diagnosis is made by finding serum IgM anti-delta. Acceleration towards cirrhosis may occur when HBV-infected patients then acquire HDV infection. Prevention of post-transfusion HDV infection is the same as for HBV.

Human immunodeficiency virus (HIV)

Human immunodeficiency virus, when acquired by transfusion, can cause a hepatic illness very similar to hepatitis B or C. The antibody appears between 1 and 2 months after exposure. The risk became apparent in 1982 to 1983 and was highest with unheated, non-pasteurized pooled plasma products (e.g. factor VIII). Appropriate treatment and screening of all donors now exists and should prevent infection in this way. Through aggressive donor education the incidence of HIV positivity among donors in the United Kingdom is 1 in 50 000.

Cytomegalovirus (CMV)

Cytomegalovirus transmission commonly occurs after transfusion but infection is usually subclinical and benign. A glandular fever-like illness is typical at 2 weeks to 3 months after exposure. Clinically, fever, splenomegaly, jaundice, raised aminotransferase levels, and atypical lymphocytes may occur. However, massive hepatic necrosis and granulomatous hepatitis have been reported. Immunocompromised patients are at most risk and may also develop a fatal pneumonitis or disseminated infection. Virus can be cultured from saliva or urine and IgM antibody to CMV can be detected in the serum. In the United Kingdom, 50 to 60 per cent of the population is anti-CMV antibody positive. Only a few of these are infective but there is no readily available test for infectivity.

Epstein–Barr virus (EBV)

The EBV causes infectious mononucleosis or glandular fever and can be transmitted parenterally. Clinically there is fever, right upper quadrant pain, with or without pharyngitis, and lymphadenopathy. Hyperbilirubinaemia occurs in about 50 per cent, transaminases are raised to 20 times the normal level in up to 80 per cent, and one-third of patients have a raised alkaline phosphatase. The Paul–Bunnell or monospot test is usually positive and the diagnosis is made by finding a raised IgM anti-EBV capsid antibody. The sinusoids and portal tracts are infiltrated with large mononuclear cells. The histology may be similar to that for hepatitis A, B, or C. Fatal acute hepatic necrosis is rare and chronic hepatitis and cirrhosis do not occur. As infection with this virus is common, and infectivity cannot be specifically tested for, screening is not performed.

Coincidental viral hepatitis

Patients incubating a hepatitic virus may come to surgery and anaesthesia. Postoperative deterioration in liver function frequently occurs and a mortality rate of 31 per cent in 36 such patients has been reported. Those patients who died had viral or alcoholic hepatitis. Thus viral serology should be part of the investigation of a patient with hepatitic liver dysfunction occurring early after surgery.

Drugs

Many drugs used in the peri- and postoperative period have been associated with liver dysfunction. Almost every naturally occurring liver disease affecting man can be mimicked by the toxic effect of drugs on the liver. Drugs can affect bilirubin metabolism at any stage, causing hyperbilirubinaemia. The drug or its metabolite can be hepatotoxic or can precipitate a hypersensitivity reaction. Hepatocellular dysfunction may be due to cellular necrosis or intrahepatic cholestasis. Factors that increase the risk of drug-induced hepatic injury include liver disease, increasing age, female sex, and genetic polymorphism.

The list of potentially hepatotoxic agents is large and ever increasing. Some of the drugs used in the perioperative period are listed in Table 5. The general anaesthetic drugs are discussed separately. Alternative causes of liver dysfunction should be sought but there are often several potential candidates. A hepatitic picture must lead to exclusion of a viral aetiology, and the differentiation of intrahepatic and extrahepatic cholestasis is important. Liver biopsy will only rarely give a diagnosis. Diagnostic challenge is not recommended, as a severe reaction can occur and the mortality from drug hepatitis with jaundice is approximately 10 per cent.

General anaesthetic drugs

Halothane, a haloalkane, was first introduced in 1956. Within 4 years there had been several reports of postoperative liver necrosis ascribed to halothane usage. The National Halothane Study gave the incidence of fatal hepatic necrosis as 1 in 35 000. Two subsequent, again retrospective, studies gave an incidence of between 1/6000 and 1/20 000.

Halothane hepatitis is associated with a 75 per cent incidence of multiple exposures, particularly where subsequent exposure is within 3 months. Female and obese patients are more at risk, and enzyme induction by other drugs further increases this risk. Liver injury occurs 1 to 15 days after exposure, and jaundice appears on approximately the seventh day, but may be later if liver injury follows the first exposure to halothane. There is fever, eosinophilia (in 8–32 per cent), arthralgia, and a non-specific skin rash. The transaminase levels are grossly elevated, for example 500–2000 IU/l, whereas the alkaline phosphatase level is often less than twice the normal level.

Histologically, the main feature is centrilobular necrosis, varying from multifocal spotty necrosis to massive necrosis. Ballooning degeneration of hepatocytes, inflammatory infiltrate, stromal fibrosis, fatty change, and occasionally granulomatous aggregates are also seen. Distinction from a viral hepatitis may be difficult.

Two types of halothane-induced hepatotoxicity are thought to exist: a mild subclinical form occurring in up to 20 per cent of patients exposed (abnormal liver function tests are the only manifestation) and a second, rare, fulminant form, due to severe necrosis which may be fatal. Five factors have been postulated in the pathogenesis of halothane hepatotoxicity: toxic products of metabolism, hypersensitivity, regional hepatic hypoxia, genetic predisposition, and altered hepatocellular calcium homeostasis.

Enflurane hepatitis has been proposed in 30 to 50 reports and, although these remain a subject of contention, the liver injury reported is similar to that induced by halothane.

Isoflurane has also been reported to cause liver damage. Whereas halothane undergoes 30 per cent biotransformation, with enflurane it is only 2 per cent and with isoflurane 1 per cent. Metabolic transformation is probably the key to haloalkane liver injury and the difference in the degree of biotransformation may explain the much lower incidence in the last two agents. Desflurane is the newest and most promising agent but is still being studied.

Total parenteral nutrition

Since its advent in the 1960s, parenteral nutritional support has become safer, more reliable, and progressively more efficient. However, complications still occur and hepatobiliary abnormalities are the second most common problem, after catheter sepsis, which result in cessation of parenteral feeding. There are a number of different patterns of liver dysfunction that have been attributed to total parenteral nutrition, but the patients in whom these problems occur have several other concomitant risk factors for hepatic disease and it is often impossible to blame any one of these. The clinical picture, hepatobiliary dysfunction, liver histology, pathogenesis, and management of hepatic problems associated with total parenteral nutrition can usefully be discussed by comparing adults and infants.

Total parenteral nutrition in adults

Whereas the main hepatic problem in infants on total parenteral nutrition is cholestasis, in adults it is hepatocellular damage. In adults the presentation of liver injury is less severe and can be divided into abnormalities occurring during short-term therapy and those occurring during longer-term total parenteral nutrition. Fatty liver, intrahepatic cholestasis, and non-specific triaditis are features of short-term treatment, and steatonecrosis and chronic liver disease are seen with long-term feeding. When dextrose was the primary source of non-protein calories, quite dramatic rises in transaminase levels occurred. As the formulation of total parenteral nutrition has changed, so have the abnormalities seen. Since the introduction of lipid emulsions as an additional source of calories, abnormalities in liver function tests have become less frequent, a late and slow rise in alkaline phosphatase and bilirubin is the most frequent finding. These changes are most notable when

Table 5 Some hepatotoxic drugs used in surgical patients

Drug	Effect
Analgesics	
Acetaminophen (paracetamol)	Acute hepatitis
Dextropropoxyphene	Cholestasis
Anti-inflammatory agents	
Benoxaprofen	Cholestasis
Diclofenac	Acute or cholestatic hepatitis
Ibuprofen	Acute or cholestatic hepatitis
Indomethacin	Acute hepatitis
Phenylbutazone	Acute or cholestatic hepatitis: granulomata
Sulindac	Acute or cholestatic hepatitis
Antibacterials and antifungals	
p-Aminosalicyclic acid	Acute hepatitis
Augmentin®	Cholestasis
Chloramphenicol	Acute hepatitis
Erythromycin estolate	Cholestasis
Ethionamide	Acute hepatitis
Flucloxacillin	Cholestasis
Fucidic acid	Cholestasis
Griseofluvin	Cholestasis
Isoniazid	Acute hepatitis: chronic active hepatitis
Ketoconazole	Acute or cholestatic hepatitis
Nitrofurantoin	Acute hepatitis: chronic active hepatitis
Penicillin	Acute or cholestatic hepatitis: granulomata
Pyrazinamide	Acute hepatitis
Rifampicin	Cholestasis: unconj. hyperbilirubinaemia
Tetracycline	Steatosis: (pancreatitis)
Antimetabolites	
Azathioprine	Acute hepatitis: cholestasis: peliosis: veno-occlusive disease
Bleomycin	Steatosis
Busulphan	Cholestasis
Chlorambucil	Acute hepatitis
Cyclosporine	Cholestasis
Fluorodeoxyuridine	Sclerosing cholangitis
6-Mercaptopurine	Acute hepatitis: cholestasis
Methotrexate	Chronic hepatitis: cirrhosis
Thioguanine	Acute hepatitis: veno-occlusive disease
Cardiovascular drugs	
Amiodarone	Alcoholic hepatitis-like cirrhosis
Diltiazem	Granulomata
Methyldopa	Acute hepatitis: chronic active hepatitis
Nifedipine	Cholestasis
Perhexilene	Alcoholic hepatitis-like cirrhosis
Procainamide	Cholestasis
Quinidine	Acute hepatitis: granulomata
General anaesthetic agents	
Enflurane	Acute hepatitis
Fluroxene	Acute hepatitis
Halothane	Acute hepatitis
Isoflurane	Acute hepatitis
Methoxyflurane	Acute hepatitis
Trichloroethylene	Acute hepatitis
Hypoglycaemic agents	
Chlorpropamide	Cholestasis
Glibenclamide	Cholestasis
Tolbutamide	Cholestasis
Psychotropic agents	
Phenothiazines	Cholestasis
Miscellaneous drugs	
Oral contraceptive drugs	Cholestasis: Budd–Chiari syndrome
Carbamazepine	Cholestasis
Corticosteroids	Steatosis

excessive amounts of fat (e.g. more than 3 g/kg body weight) are given.

Short-term total parenteral nutrition

Fatty change is the most benign hepatic lesion seen within the first 14 days of total parenteral nutrition, and is often paralleled by a rise in the transaminase levels. Periportal fat infiltration is the first change, but this may progress to pan- or centrilobular infiltration. The rise in transaminase levels that usually accompanies these changes most commonly resolves spontaneously, even when total parenteral nutrition is continued. The lipid is mainly triglyceride, and the likely cause of its accumulation is increased hepatic synthesis combined with impaired export of triglyceride. Dextrose- and glucose-based feeds are clearly associated with fatty liver. Most total parenteral nutrition formulations should now contain lipid emulsions, and this has been shown to decrease the incidence of steatosis. Excess lipid will result in fat accumulation, but this is seen within the Kupffer cells and hepatic lysosomes. Essential fatty acid deficiency can result in a fatty liver and tryptophan degradation products have also been implicated. Primary systemic deficiency of carnitine also results in a fatty liver. Low systemic and hepatic carnitine levels have been found in patients on long-term total parenteral nutrition, with sepsis, and in stress states. Whether the inclusion of carnitine, a non-essential amino acid, in total parenteral nutrition would prevent or reverse the fatty change is not known. Malnutrition itself can produce a fatty liver, as can starvation and sepsis. Increased tissue release and increased hepatic uptake of free fatty acids, combined with increased synthesis of triglyceride, result in the fatty change.

Intrahepatic cholestasis occurs after more than 2 weeks of treatment, at a time when the transaminase levels are returning to normal and the bilirubin and alkaline phosphatase levels are starting to rise. The histological changes that accompany this cholestatic picture are bile-duct proliferation, canalicular bile plugging, centrilobular cholestasis, bile pigment within hepatocytes, and a periportal infiltration with granulocytes and lymphocytes. In the majority of cases the cholestasis resolves on discontinuation of feeding. Reduction in the dose of lipid infused will reduce the levels of bilirubin and alkaline phosphatase. In one study, cholestasis was reported in 14 of 27 patients on total parenteral nutrition, and it was suggested that cholestasis in these patients predisposes them to cholelithiasis. Patients on total parenteral nutrition for more than 6 weeks were also shown to develop biliary sludging, as shown by ultrasound scanning. Normal feeding for 4 weeks returned the bile to normal. Progressive liver disease has not been seen in adults receiving total parenteral nutrition for up to 6 months.

The pathogenesis of the cholestasis remains unclear, but several factors have been implicated. The underlying condition and nutritional status of the patient, as well as the infection and treatment (including transfusion, surgery, and drugs), may also play a role. Various amino acids and toxins have been blamed. Deficiency of taurine may be a factor in as much as taurine is involved in the metabolism of bile acids and may prevent the accumulation of lithocholic acid. This secondary bile acid has been found in excess in patients with both inflammatory bowel disease and cholestasis associated with total parenteral nutrition, and has been implicated as a hepatotoxin. Metabolic products of tryptophan have been suggested as toxins. Lipid emulsion in doses above 3 g/kg.day have been shown to cause intrahepatic cholestasis; however, a further study giving 3.5 g/kg.day of fat was not accompanied by cholestasis. Decreased hepatic biliary flow due to reduced neural and hormonal stimulation from a rested bowel may contribute to this pattern of cholestasis. Bacterial overgrowth secondary to stasis or intestinal surgery and portal endotoxaemia are possible additional factors in these patients.

Non-specific triaditis occurs in patients with inflammatory bowel disease receiving total parenteral nutrition; this relatively minor change is accompanied by very marked derangement of liver function tests. This group of patients may have liver abnormalities that predate the total parenteral nutrition, and these may have been exacerbated by the parenteral nutrition.

Long-term total parenteral nutrition

Chronic progressive liver disease in adults on total parenteral nutrition is rare but has been demonstrated in patients receiving treatment for more than 6 or even 12 months. Such long-term total parenteral nutrition is given to patients who often require multiple transfusions and hepatotoxic drugs, and in whom the underlying disease is chronic, complicated, and may have involved extensive and repeated surgery. Again, it is impossible to isolate total parenteral nutrition as the only factor causing liver problems. Three studies give an incidence for progressive liver disease of between 5 and 15 per cent. The changes seen in short-term total parenteral nutrition were also seen in many of these patients, and beyond 6 months' therapy a cholestatic picture of liver function was the common finding. Histologically the common changes seen in these studies were cholestasis, hepatocyte necrosis, an alcoholic hepatitis-like picture, steatonecrosis, and early cirrhosis. The pathogenesis could involve any or all of the factors mentioned under shorter-term total parenteral nutrition, as the limited number of cases makes studies difficult. Total parenteral nutrition is the only source of nutrition in these patients, and juggling with the constituents of the feed formula and cyclical feeding are often the only therapeutic options. The prognosis may be poor in patients with short-bowel syndrome.

Total parenteral nutrition in infants

Nutritional support of premature infants is now the most common use of total parenteral nutrition in paediatric medicine, and liver dysfunction has been noted in this group of patients throughout the development of this therapy. Children with chronic and/or extensive gastrointestinal disease make up the majority of the remainder. Infants receiving total parenteral nutrition are at risk of five types of hepatobiliary disease: fatty change, intrahepatic cholestasis, biliary sludging, gallstones, and acute acalculous cholecystitis.

Early in the course of total parenteral nutrition a liver biopsy may demonstrate mild fatty change and hydropic swelling of hepatocytes. These changes are not precursors of cholestatic disease, they occur infrequently and are reversible on stopping the total parenteral nutrition. In animal and human studies the data suggest that excess carbohydrate is to blame. However, deficiency of essential fatty acids may be another cause.

The first reported case of cholestasis related to total parenteral nutrition was in a premature infant in 1971. Most premature infants are at risk of heart failure, sepsis, necrotizing enterocolitis, and treatment with blood transfusion and multiple drugs. All of these may cause hepatobiliary problems and thus it is difficult to ascribe hepatic complications to total parenteral nutrition alone. The incidence of cholestasis increases with duration of total parenteral nutrition and also with decreasing gestational age and birth weight. In 1979 it was found that cholestasis occurred in 23 per cent of infants with respiratory problems receiving total parenteral nutrition. If treatment was for more than 60 days, the incidence rose to 60 per cent and to 90 per cent after 80 days. Duration of therapy is often a function of the gestational age, as is birth weight, and these are therefore not independent variables. Immature hepatic function may be the primary factor in the liver disease seen in infants.

Monitoring of premature infants on total parenteral nutrition is important and the commonly used 'liver function tests' are not useful. A rise in unconjugated bilirubin occurs late in the course of cholestatic disease in these patients and total bilirubin is commonly raised in premature infants with no liver disease. Alkaline phosphatase is unhelpful as there is a preponderance of the bone isoenzyme in infants, and this isoenzyme is also affected by the child's nutritional status. Transaminase levels can also be unreliable as the levels do not correlate with the degree of cholestasis associated with total parenteral nutrition. γ-Glutamyl transpeptidase is the most sensitive test, but lacks specificity. Serum bile salt levels have also been found to be good indicators of cholestasis, but there is a normal developmental delay in bile salt metabolism, giving rise to elevated levels. A combination of γ-glutamyl transpeptidase and serum bile salts may be a more specific test. Ultrasound scanning and endoscopic retrograde cholangiopancreatography (ERCP) will help to exclude extrahepatic cholestasis and it may also be necessary to perform a liver biopsy. Although the liver histology may be non-specific, a biopsy can identify other causes of cholestasis, such as cytomegalovirus hepatitis or extrahepatic obstruction. It can also indicate the urgency of cessation of the total parenteral nutrition and the prognosis of the liver pathology. Cholestasis early in treatment with total parenteral nutrition is seen as bile pigment in the hepatocytes, bile plugs in canaliculi, pseudorosette formation, and a varying degree of triaditis, with or without eosinophils. Cholestasis with longer-term total parenteral nutrition may show portal and lobular fibrosis, expansion of the portal tracts with portal ductular proliferation, and bile plugs in the interlobular ducts. Patients with intrahepatic cholestasis in whom total parenteral nutrition is continued may develop micronodular cirrhosis. The clinical cholestasis that reverses on stopping the total parenteral nutrition is accompanied by reversal of most of the histological findings. Some portal fibrosis may persist and where cirrhosis occurs the prognosis is poor, liver failure being the most common cause of death in these patients.

The pathogenesis of this cholestasis is still unclear, but there are many candidates. As has been stressed previously, it is often difficult to separate several risk factors for hepatic injury in the population of patients on total parenteral nutrition. Sepsis, transfusion, drug therapy (including anaesthesia), and the underlying disorder may all contribute. In premature infants there is, in addition, immature hepatic function: there is decreased hepatic uptake of bile salts, bile salt synthesis is reduced, ileal uptake of bile salts is inefficient, and the ability to detoxify lithocholic acid is impaired. These factors may make the premature infant particularly susceptible to hepatic injury. Hepatotoxins of various types have been suggested and most of the contents of total parenteral nutrition have been implicated.

Biliary sludging is seen in children and adults on long-term total parenteral nutrition and in 1983 it was shown that up to 100 per cent of adults receiving more than 6 weeks' total parenteral nutrition develop 'sludge'. This thick bile may be responsible for varying degrees of extrahepatic cholestasis, and liver histology may show bile plugging of interlobular ducts. Two infants have been described with refractory cholestasis that improved after surgical disimpaction of biliary sludge. Thus, an infant with cholestasis during total parenteral nutrition should also be investigated for an extrahepatic cause, with ultrasound scanning, computerized tomographic scanning, ERCP, possibly liver biopsy, and biliary decompression if necessary.

Gallstones can occur in infants and adults on total parenteral nutrition. In 1990 a study reported that, over a 3-year period, five of seven infants with choledocholithiasis were premature and had sepsis and/or were receiving total parenteral nutrition. Even in infants, ERCP is an effective therapeutic approach. Biliary sludging, cholelithiasis, and acalculous cholecystitis associated with total parenteral nutrition are more thoroughly discussed in relation to adults (see above).

Management of hepatic complications of total parenteral nutrition

The majority of abnormalities are minimal and self-limiting and may require no therapy. The only effective means of reversing cholestasis in these patients is to replace total parenteral nutrition with oral feeding. Infants, in particular, may be dependent on parenteral feeding, and in such patients there are several important factors to consider. Liver disease due to drugs or infection should be excluded as well as any extrahepatic obstruction. The latter may need urgent correction. If hepatic dysfunction persists and no other cause is found, the carbohydrate content of the feed should be adjusted. The Harris and Benedict equation is used to predict the patient's carbohydrate need, but this is not accurate and does not account for the 'stress state' (for example nutritional state, tissue damage, infection) of the patient. Glucose utilization has been shown to be maximal at around 5 to 6 mg of dextrose/kg.min, and this is probably the maximum dose above which lipogenesis occurs. Overfeeding should also be excluded and corrected. Any calorie input lost in reducing the dextrose delivered is replaced by protein or fat. Fat should supply approximately 30 per cent of the required calories but the total quantity should not exceed 3 g of fat/kg.day. In feed formulations that do not contain fat, an essential fatty acid deficiency may be the cause of the liver dysfunction, and a lipid emulsion should be introduced. Four per cent of the daily non-protein calories supplied by linoleic acid will correct this deficit. As discussed above, there are several amino acids that, when added to the feed formulation, may help to prevent the hepatic problems. If the quantity and source of calories is appropriate, then 'cyclic' nutrition can be tried. This involves giving all total parenteral nutrition over a 10- to 12-h period, with no calories given during the remainder of the 24 hours. This has been shown to prevent or reverse the liver disease. In patients with increasing cholestasis, in whom total parenteral nutrition cannot be stopped, copper, manganese, and aluminium should be withheld as they are normally excreted in the bile and may accumulate in the liver and basal ganglia, causing permanent damage.

Fasting

Mild hyperbilirubinaemia can be precipitated by fasting and is due mainly to an unconjugated bilirubin rise. The majority of patients showing this effect are probably those with Gilbert syndrome. Fatty change is also seen, particularly in acute weight loss or starvation. This is related to the increase in serum fatty acids and increased fatty acid turnover precipitated by decreased availability of glucose, a rise in glucagon levels, and increased sympathetic nervous activity. Obese subjects who lose weight rapidly may show a transient elevation of serum liver enzymes.

Obesity

Fatty change in the liver is seen in up to 50 per cent of obese subjects, with occasional periportal inflammation and fibrosis. Steatonecrosis and cirrhosis have been reported but this may be due to coexistent diabetes mellitus or alcoholic liver disease. Fifty per cent of obese patients can be shown to be glucose intolerant, and this and excess dietary fat and carbohydrate in relation to protein intake may be involved in the aetiology of steatosis. The fatty infiltration is perivenular and diffuse. Liver function tests may be abnormal and reflect more severe histological change. The changes are, in general, benign and non-progressive, and can be reversed by weight loss.

Diabetes mellitus

Diabetic patients also show fatty change in the liver; the majority are non-insulin-dependent diabetics who are also overweight. Steatosis is very rare in juvenile-onset insulin-dependent patients. Symptoms are rare, an enlarged, slightly tender liver may be found on examination, and liver function tests may be slightly deranged in about 20 per cent of diabetics, but do not correlate with histology. The fatty change is centrilobular and diffuse. Weight loss and good diabetic control will resolve these abnormalities.

Steatonecrosis may also occur and this is seen in the non-insulin-dependent group. It has been suggested that the incidence of cirrhosis among diabetics is twice that of the general population. This suggestion is unproven and may originate in the number of cirrhotic patients with glucose intolerance that have wrongly been classified as primary diabetics.

Emergency biliary surgery in diabetic patients has a higher than expected mortality. This is due in part to the disruption of glucose control caused by surgery, the increased risk of infection due to leucocyte dysfunction, and poorer wound healing.

Sepsis

Sepsis can produce a deep jaundice, which may be cholestatic and occurs 2 to 4 days after the onset of bacteraemia. In 1969 a study showed an incidence of jaundice of 0.6 per cent in 1140 patients with bacteraemia; however, hepatic dysfunction was shown in 1979 to have little effect on survival when compared with the primary infection. Pneumonia, Gram-negative bacteraemia, intra-abdominal abscess, and pyelonephritis can all cause a raised bilirubin. Gram-negative infection in infants frequently causes cholestasis. Endotoxins may be the main culprit as they have been shown to inhibit bile secretion, although cytokines have been implicated more recently. As in most cases of hepatic dysfunction discussed here, sepsis is rarely the only factor that can be implicated and thus the aetiology may be multifactorial. Biochemically and histologically, the changes are very similar to those observed with circulatory failure, with a moderate rise in conjugated bilirubin, aminotransferases, and alkaline phosphatase levels. However, an increase in the unconjugated bilirubin level also occurs, giving a rise in total bilirubin out of keeping with the increase in liver enzymes. Hepatic histological changes include biliary stasis, fatty change, and periportal inflammation. Extrahepatic biliary obstruction must be excluded. Pneumococcal, meningococcal, and Gram-negative sepsis may cause haemolysis by disseminated intravascular coagulation or a secondary microangiopathic haemolysis, and in these conditions the rise in unconjugated bilirubin will be prominent.

Benign postoperative intrahepatic cholestasis

'Benign postoperative intrahepatic cholestasis' is unlikely to be a specific entity. It occurs in situations where blood loss is a prominent problem and is probably due to a combination of hypotension and multiple blood transfusions. Caroli in 1950 was the first to describe the occurrence of postoperative cholestatic jaundice. Benign postoperative intrahepatic cholestasis has been included in all lists of causes of postoperative jaundice since about this time. The aetiology of postoperative cholestasis is discussed within this section, and the majority of cases given this label in the past now have a definable cause.

Extrahepatic obstruction

Bile-duct injury

Bile-duct injury can follow cholecystectomy, common bile duct exploration, or any upper abdominal operation. If unrecognized at operation, jaundice, biliary fistula, or biliary peritonitis will occur in the early postoperative period. Prompt surgical repair helps to prevent permanent liver damage.

Common bile-duct stones

Retained common bile-duct stones after cholecystectomy and/or exploration of the common bile duct are uncommon. In the majority of cases, ERCP will both diagnose and treat this problem by sphincterotomy. Reoperation is required if ERCP fails or is not available. Some practitioners advocate visualization and, if necessary, clearance of the bile duct at ERCP prior to cholecystectomy. Occasionally, blood may collect in the common bile duct and cause obstruction.

Postoperative pancreatitis

Acute postoperative pancreatitis is uncommon and the cause is unknown. Thirty per cent of patients may be jaundiced, and oedema of the head of the pancreas is thought to result in some degree of obstruction and a low-grade hyperbilirubinaemia.

Acalculous cholecystitis

Acute non-calculous cholecystitis can occur after major trauma, burns, surgery that does not involve the upper abdomen, and in patients receiving long-term total parenteral nutrition, especially infants. It accounts for about 1 per cent of all cases of cholecystitis. A Japanese series of acalculous cholecystitis after gastrectomy demonstrated an incidence of 0.64 per cent. The aetiology is unknown, but it has been suggested that biliary stasis is important.

Postoperative cholecystitis occurs most commonly in the fifth to seventh decade, but in patients with trauma or burns this form of cholecystitis is seen most frequently in the second to fourth decade. The sex ratio is also different in these two groups; females predominate in the former, males in the latter. The postoperative form tends to follow a major surgical procedure. This form of cholecystitis can occur up to 1 month after the operation. Right upper quadrant pain and tenderness is usually accompanied by nausea, vomiting, and fever. The observed bilirubin rise is variable but may be up to 85 μmol/l; levels of transaminases and alkaline phosphatase are only mildly raised. Ultrasound may show enlargement of the gallbladder and, by definition, no gallstones are seen. ERCP is often necessary to exclude other causes of obstruction, although surgery should not be delayed in these already seriously ill patients. Histologically, the gallbladder shows vascular dilatation, congestion, and oedema in all layers, without fibrosis. Abscesses of varying size may be seen in the gallbladder wall and the mucosal surface is necrotic and ulcerated. Perforation is frequent.

Acalculous cholecystitis occurs in patients receiving total parenteral nutrition for more than 3 months with an incidence of 4 per cent.

The level of mortality has been given as between 33 and 75 per cent. However, this may pertain only to major trauma patients and reflects the already much increased mortality in this group.

THE SURGICAL PATIENT WITH PRE-EXISTING LIVER DISEASE

Introduction

Patients with liver disease may require surgery as a consequence of the disease or for unrelated problems. Any surgery involving the liver itself, the biliary system, or the blood vessels associated with the liver has the potential to cause hepatocellular dysfunction, bleeding problems, nutritional difficulties, and infection. Where there is impaired liver function in such patients the problems discussed in this section become doubly important.

Anaesthesia and surgery in a patient with pre-existing liver disease have the potential to cause deterioration in liver function and even acute liver failure. Peri- and postoperative haemorrhage and postoperative infection are the other major complications. Factors that should be considered in these patients are the nature of the liver disease, the preoperative assessment of the liver disease, fluid balance, renal function, drug metabolism and adverse effects, nutrition, maintenance of liver blood flow, and prevention of complications.

Preoperative management

The nature and severity of the liver disease should be confirmed before surgery whenever possible, as there are specific risk factors related to the underlying liver pathology.

In patients with known liver disease, assessment of hepatic function is important preoperatively. Standard liver tests (aspartate aminotransferase, alanine aminotransferase, alkaline phosphatase, γ-glutamyl transferase) do not give a good guide to hepatic function. Serum bilirubin in cirrhotic patients can be used as a predictor of dysfunction. Serum albumin and liver-dependent clotting factor measurement will assess the synthetic capacity of the liver. The indocyanine green clearance test can also be used to assess function and hepatic blood flow. As haemorrhage and infection are important complications in these patients, platelet count, haemoglobin level, white blood-cell count and differential, blood grouping, and cross-matching of sufficient fresh blood is essential. Serum urea estimation is often unreliable in assessing renal function in liver disease, as hepatic dysfunction causes a low urea. Electrocardiogram, chest radiograph, and screening for any infection are also mandatory. Further specific tests may be required and are mentioned below as appropriate.

Improvement of the preoperative status of patients with liver disease can significantly decrease their operative morbidity and mortality. Specific attention should be given to:

(1) correction of coagulopathy to normal by administering vitamin K and fresh frozen plasma;
(2) improving the nutritional status;
(3) treatment of renal impairment;
(4) treatment of infection;
(5) control of ascites.

The nutritional status of patients with liver disease is discussed separately below.

Patients positive for hepatitis B virus (HBV) or C virus (HCV)

The HBV- or HCV-positive patient that comes to surgery is at risk of postoperative deterioration in liver function and is also a risk to all staff involved in his or her care. Hepatitis B surface antigen assay is a good screening test but anti-HBc positivity is more reliable in atypical cases (see above). Anti-HCV antibody can be detected and if specific testing for HCV infection by PCR is not freely available, positivity should be confirmed by alternative antibody assay techniques. Both HBV and HCV infection are associated with periods of mild, or even subclinical, liver disease, and both can result in chronic liver disease and cirrhosis. Liver function and associated complications of chronic liver disease must therefore be identified prior to surgery.

Acute hepatitis

Surgery should be avoided if possible in acute hepatitis as acute liver failure may be precipitated, liver function is unpredictable, and the specific cause may not yet be identified (for example, viral serological tests may not become positive until some weeks after the acute illness). One study reported a 61 per cent morbidity and 31 per cent mortality following surgery in patients with undiagnosed acute liver disease. The deaths from hepatic failure occurred in those patients with viral or alcoholic hepatitis.

Obstructive jaundice

Patients with obstructive jaundice are at risk of postoperative renal failure, haemorrhage, and deterioration in liver function. It has been shown that patients with liver disease and hyperbilirubinaemia have abnormal renal structure and function, abnormal circulatory haemostasis, and deterioration in the gastrointestinal barrier to infection, and all these contribute to the postoperative risk of renal failure. Increased levels of unconjugated and conjugated bilirubin and bile salts damage the middle segment of the proximal convoluted tubule, producing changes very similar to those caused by anoxia. Decreased creatinine clearance occurs preoperatively in 30 per cent of patients with obstructive jaundice, and this is seen particularly in patients with coincident sepsis. This is due to decreased renal blood flow, which is more marked in the cortex and results in impaired ability of the kidney to concentrate urine, as well as susceptibility to sodium and water depletion. The cause may be decreased sensitivity to catecholamines. Patients with obstructive jaundice have lowered peripheral vascular resistance, renal salt wasting, some loss of left ventricular function, and pooling of blood in the splanchnic bed. Thus, a small volume of blood loss can result in a marked fall in arterial blood pressure, which will obviously exacerbate any renal failure. Endotoxins have been found in the circulation of 50 to 70 per cent of patients with obstructive jaundice, and these toxins also cause defects in renal structure and function. In particular, they increase renal vascular resistance, cause endothelial swelling, fibrin deposition, and low-grade disseminated intravascular coagulation. Bile salts disrupt endotoxins in the gut lumen but in obstructive jaundice this is prevented and endotoxins readily reach the portal circulation. Hyperbilirubinaemia, bile salt retention in the liver, and the endotoxins impair the reticuloendothelial phagocytotic function of the Kupffer cell system and endotoxins enter the general circulation. Table 6 lists the parameters that help identify the patient at risk of postoperative renal failure.

Table 6 Parameters that identify the patient particularly at risk of renal failure

Age (>60 years)
Haematocrit < 30%
White blood-cell count > 10 000/mm^3
Albumin < 30 g/l
Hyperbilirubinaemia
Raised alkaline phosphatase
Raised serum creatinine
Weight loss
Malignant disease

The principles of preoperative treatment of these patients include the treatment of sepsis, avoidance of nephrotoxic drugs, treatment of renal impairment, and the correction of hypovolaemia, hypoalbuminaemia, hyponatraemia, and anaemia. Preoperative renal failure will require correction of fluid balance, administration of antibiotics, and dialysis if necessary.

Chronic liver disease and cirrhosis

Chronic liver disease can be associated with adequate liver function where there is no hyperbilirubinaemia, hypoalbuminaemia, or coagulopathy. If infection and renal impairment are also excluded, specific preoperative treatment may not be necessary. Perioperatively, particular consideration of fluid balance, ventilation, liver blood flow, and drug metabolism is important. There is still a risk of liver decompensation, haemorrhage, and infection postoperatively. Peri- and postoperative management are discussed below.

Cirrhosis may be associated with well-compensated liver function, assessed as above. However, surgery in cirrhotic patients has a high mortality, reported to be 80 per cent in patients with advanced cirrhosis undergoing cholecystectomy. Child's classification is a useful guide to the preoperative assessment of risk in these patients, which is made more accurate by the addition of the prothrombin time (see Table 7). Prothrombin time, serum albumin, and the presence of infection (white blood-cell count >10 000/mm^3) are regarded as the most useful indicators of risk. The risk is further increased when these patients undergo gastrointestinal surgery and is highest following hepatobiliary surgery.

Cirrhosis is also associated with renal abnormality. The latter is accompanied by proteinuria and haematuria. Renal failure may occur in 50 to 75 per cent of cirrhotics. It may be prerenal, due to

Table 7 Child Pugh risk assessment

	Group A	Group B	Group C
Serum bilirubin (g/l)	<40	40–50	>50
Serum albumin (g/l)	>35	28–35	<28
Ascites	None	Mild	Moderate–severe
Encephalopathy	Absent	Grade I–II	Grade III–IV
Prothrombin time (prolonged from control)	Normal	<2.5 s	>2.5 s
Surgical risk	Good	Moderate	Poor
Mortality (%)	3–10	10–30	50–80

acute tubular necrosis, or it may have no obvious cause, when it may be labelled the hepatorenal syndrome. Preoperatively these patients should be assessed daily for weight change, ascites, oedema, and pyrexia. The sodium balance must be estimated; urine volumes, urine and serum osmolarity, serum creatinine, urea, sodium, potassium, and albumin must be checked; and haemoglobin, haematocrit, and liver function must be tested. Deranged coagulation will require daily vitamin K injections, but where hepatocellular function is poor these may not correct the abnormalities and fresh frozen plasma will be needed to cover any invasive tests or bleeding episodes as well as perioperatively.

Infection, hypoalbuminaemia, and ascites should be treated. The last should be treated by nutritional support (see below) along with paracentesis and albumin infusion. Urinary catheterization and a central venous catheter are essential but, again, infection must be avoided.

Nutritional status in patients with liver disease

Perioperative malnutrition increases the morbidity and mortality of any operation. In the patient with liver disease, malnutrition will compound the already significant risk of complications. Obstructive jaundice results in malabsorption of fat and steatorrhoea. If obstruction is prolonged, malnutrition will develop. Inevitably, chronic parenchymal liver disease is associated with protein–calorie malnutrition. Glucose intolerance is seen in 50 to 80 per cent of cirrhotics, deficiencies of vitamins A, C, and E, folic acid, and zinc result, and there is a deficiency of branched-chain amino acids. These, and the nature of the liver disease, result in compromised immune defence, and postoperative infection and wound dehiscence are common problems.

Malnutrition can be identified from a history of weight loss, the patient's height to weight index, body composition, protein turnover, serum albumin, urinary urea, and the immune status, as well as a number of other detailed tests.

Nutritional support can be given as oral supplements, enteral or parenteral feeding. Oral feeding is obviously the most efficient, cheap, and safe, when it is appropriate. Enteral feeding is well tolerated in obstructive jaundice. Special formula feeds are available for patients with chronic liver disease. They contain a high proportion of branched-chain amino acids which may be deficient and which also help reduce protein catabolism, another factor in the malnutrition in these patients. When such patients require surgery, parenteral feeding is often the only method available. Extensive investigation and preparation often dictates periods of starvation preoperatively and may also be a factor delaying surgery. Parenteral feeding regimens need to be tailored to the patient. If there is no glucose intolerance, glucose solutions can be the major source of calories; but if sugar intolerance exists, fat and protein content must be increased. Lipid emulsions seem to be well tolerated by patients with liver disease. Insulin resistance may be a problem, particularly in patients with infection. In patients with well-preserved liver function, and no past or presenting encephalopathy, standard formulations are acceptable. If there is a risk of encephalopathy, or if it already exists, a mix containing less phenylalanine, tyrosine, tryptophan, and methionine, and more arginine and branched-chain amino acids is recommended. Vitamins A, D, E, K, and C, folic acid, zinc, and copper must be regularly supplemented.

The maximum benefit to be gained from preoperative parenteral feeding comes from 10 to 14 days of therapy. The aim should be to correct the amino acid profile, reach a positive nitrogen balance, and scrupulously avoid infection. Renal failure is often a further problem, volume and electrolytes must be carefully monitored, and the formula may need to be adjusted further. If the patient is requiring haemodialysis or haemoperfusion, this will assist the control of fluid balance. In obstructive jaundice, if there is no hepatocellular dysfunction, standard supplemented oral, enteral, and parenteral feeding regimens can be used. Obstructive jaundice should not be left untreated any longer than necessary (see above).

Monitoring is vital and should consist of at least 8-hourly tests of blood sugar; daily weight, urea, creatinine, and electrolyte measurements; biweekly determinations of calcium, phosphate, liver function, and albumin; and weekly measurement of zinc and magnesium levels and culture of blood, urine, and any other drained fluid. The duration of feeding should be reviewed constantly.

Intraoperative management

The principal intraoperative concern is anaesthetic technique. Basic principles pertain to patients with liver disease, but protein binding, metabolism, and liver blood flow are particularly important considerations. An experienced anaesthetist should be employed where liver disease and hepatobiliary surgery are combined. In patients with well-compensated liver disease, standard drugs may be appropriate. The premedication may be affected by albumin levels, and the response to opiate drugs at this time may be helpful in assessing the dose requirements postoperatively. Narcotic analgesics and the benzodiazepines may have very prolonged action in patients with hepatocellular dysfunction.

During surgery there are several specific problems. Periods of hypotension or hypoxia will compromise liver function and precipitate renal failure more readily than in other patients. There may be derangement of blood coagulation. Rapid or large-volume transfusions of blood products may be required. Hepatobiliary disease and renal impairment will modify most drug pharmacokinetics and dynamics.

Of the haloalkanes, isoflurane is the best agent to use in these patients (see above); however, inhalation agents should be avoided. It should also be noted that prolonged use of nitrous oxide may cause additional liver damage. Liver blood flow, hepatocellular dysfunction, and plasma protein concentration are the factors affecting anaesthetic drug kinetics and dynamics intraoperatively. All anaesthetic techniques cause a reduction in hepatic blood flow, as do hyperventilation, increased sympathetic tone, and surgical manipulation of the liver and abdominal viscera. Good liver perfusion is also important for the clearance of endotoxins and lactate, and metabolic acidosis is another potential problem. A fall in liver blood flow will reduce the clearance of drugs and enzyme activity intraoperatively and the potential for a postoperative deterioration in liver function will be increased.

Control of ventilation must also be precise, as hypoxia, acidosis, and hyperventilation can all affect liver and renal function adversely, both intra- and postoperatively. Central venous catheterization, a urinary bladder catheter, and an arterial line are mandatory. In patients with cirrhosis and renal impairment, sodium-containing fluids should be used judiciously. Fresh blood and fresh frozen plasma must be readily available, and in long operations electrolytes, blood sugar, and coagulation will need to be monitored regularly.

The importance of avoiding infection during all anaesthetic and surgical techniques cannot be stressed too often.

Postoperative management

The immediate postoperative concern is whether to reverse the anaesthetic or whether ventilatory support should be continued in an intensive care unit. Reasons to continue ventilation in these patients include:

(1) the persistent effect of anaesthetic and/or neuromuscular blocking agents—in obstructive jaundice, neuromuscular blocking drugs will have prolonged action;
(2) massive intraoperative blood loss and transfusion;
(3) anticipation of further bleeding;
(4) any episode of cardiac arrest during the operation;
(5) significant preoperative lung disease;
(6) failure to maintain adequate arterial oxygenation;
(7) Post-sternotomy, cardiopulmonary, or left-heart bypass.

Regular assessment of liver function in the postoperative period will allow the early identification of deterioration. All the factors discussed in the first part of the section pertain to these patients also.

Central venous catheters should be left in place to monitor fluid balance, especially in relation to risk of bleeding and renal failure. Haematological monitoring must include daily coagulation testing and the prompt correction of abnormalities. Intravenous vitamin K should be given daily.

Constant vigilance against infection is mandatory in postoperative patients with liver disease. All catheters and drainage systems must be watched and handled by experienced staff. Blood, urine, and drained fluids must be monitored regularly for infection. Cirrhotic patients are particularly prone to chest infection, and chest physiotherapy should be rigorous in these patients. Consideration of peritoneal infection is important, as this can be an occult cause of deteriorating liver function. Biochemical monitoring should be routine as renal function is at risk. When haemorrhage, hypotension, and infection coexist, small volumes of concentrated urine, with a urine to plasma osmolarity ratio greater than 1.05, indicate potential renal failure. This is reversible if recognized and treated promptly. Established renal failure can be oliguric or high output.

Upper abdominal, subcostal, and sternotomy incisions are associated with severe postoperative pain, which is made worse by prolonged procedures. Patients with liver disease often require these operative procedures, and thus pain relief is particularly important. Septicaemia and coagulation abnormalities may limit the administration of analgesia by epidural methods. Doses of other intravenous or inhalational analgesics should be low initially, and they must be monitored carefully. The duration of action of benzodiazepines and narcotic analgesics can be very prolonged in patients with hepatocellular disease.

FURTHER READING

The surgical patient with normal preoperative liver function

Barbara JA, Contreras M. Non-A, non-B hepatitis and the anti-HCV assay. *Vox Sang* 1991; **60**(1): 1–7.

Clark RJS, Doggart JR, Lavery T. Changes in liver function after different types of surgery. *Br J Anaesth* 1976; **48**: 119–22.

Du Priest R, Khaneja S, Cowley A. Acute cholecystitis complicating trauma. *Ann Surg* 1979; **189**: 84–6.

Flint LM Jr, Polk HC Jr. Selective hepatic artery ligation: limitations and failures. *J Trauma* 1979; **19**: 319–21.

McIntyre N, Benhamou J-P, Bircher J, Rizzetto M, Rodes J, eds. *Oxford textbook of clinical hepatology*. Oxford: University Press, 1991.

Nunes G, Blaisdell FW, Margaretten W. Mechanism of hepatic dysfunction following shock and trauma. *Arch Surg* 1970; **100**: 546–56.

Powell-Jackson P, Greenway B, Williams R. Adverse effect of exploratory laparotomy in patients with unsuspected liver disease. *Br J Surg* 1982; **69**: 449–51.

Ray DC, Drummond GB. Halothane hepatitis, *Br J Anaesth* 1991; **67**: 84–99.

Saidi F, Donaldson GA. Acute pancreatitis following distal gastrectomy for benign ulcer. *Am J Surg* 1963; **105**: 87–96.

Sirchia G, *et al.* Prospective evaluation of post-transfusion hepatitis. *Transfusion* 1991; **31**: 299–302.

Takahushi T, Yamamura T, Utsunomiya J. Pathogenesis of acute cholecystitis after gastrectomy. *Br J Surg* 1990; **77**: 536–9.

Utili R, Abernathy CO, Zimmerman HJ. Endotoxin effect on the liver. *Life Sci* 1977; **20**: 553–68.

Zimmermann HJ. Even isoflurane (editorial). *Hepatology* 1991; **13**(6): 1251–3.

Zimmerman HJ, Fang M, Utili R, Seeff LB, Hoofnagle J. Jaundice due to bacterial infection. *Gastroenterology* 1979; **77**: 362.

Total parenteral nutrition

Allardyce DB. Cholestasis caused by lipid emulsion. *Surg Gynecol Obstet* 1982; **154**: 641–3.

Beale EF, Nelson RM, Bucciarelli RL, Donnelly WH, Eitzman DV. Intrahepatic cholestasis associated with parenteral nutrition in premature infants. *Paediatrics* 1979; **64**: 342–7.

Bowyer BA, Fleming CR, Ludwig J, Petz J, McGill DB. Does long-term parenteral nutrition in adult patients cause chronic liver disease? *J Parenteral Enterol Nutr* 1985; **9**: 11–17.

Craig RM, Neumann T, Jeejeebhoy KN, Yokoo H. Severe hepatocellular reaction resembling alcoholic hepatitis and cirrhosis after massive small bowel resection and prolonged total parenteral nutrition. *Gastroenterology* 1980; **79**: 131–3.

Fisher RL. Hepatobiliary abnormalities associated with total parenteral nutrition. *Gastro Clin N Am* 1989; **18**(3): 645–66.

Fouin-Fortunet H, Le Quernec L, Erlinger S, Lerebours E, Colin R. Hepatic alterations during total parenteral nutrition in patients with inflammatory bowel disease: a possible consequence of lithocholate toxicity. *Gastroenterology* 1982; **82**: 932–7.

Grant JP. *Effects of cyclic vs. continuous TPN in hospitalized patients*. American Gastroenterology Association Postgraduate Course. Nutrition in Gastroenterology. 1987.

Grant JP, *et al.* Serum hepatic enzyme and bilirubin elevation during parenteral nutrition. *Surg Gynecol Obstet* 1977; **145**: 573–80.

Jeejeebhoy KN, Anderson GH, Nakhooda AF, Greenberg GR, Sanderson I, Marliss EB. Metabolic studies in total parenteral nutrition with lipid in man. Comparison with glucose. *J Clin Invest* 1976; **57**: 125–36.

Jonas A, Yahav J, Fradkin A, Kessler A. Choledocholithiasis in infants: Diagnostic and therapeutic problems. *J Pediatr Gastroenterol Nutr* 1990; **11**(4): 513–17.

Messing B, De Oliveira FJ, Galian A, Bennier JJ. Cholestase au coeurs de la nutrition parenterale totale; mise an evidence de facteurs favorisants; association à une lithiase vesiculare. *Gastroenterol Clin Biol* 1982; **6**: 740–7.

Rabeneck L, Freeman H, Owen D. Death due to TPN-related liver failure. *Gastroenterology* 1984; **86**: 1215–19.

The surgical patient with pre-existing liver disease

Aranha GB, Sontag SJ, Greenle HB. Cholecystectomy in cirrhotic patients; a formidable operation. *Am J Surg* 1982; **143**: 55–60.

Garrison RN, Cryer HM, Howard DA, Polk HC. Clarification of risk factors for abdominal operations in patients with hepatic cirrhosis. *Ann Surg* 1984; **199**: 648–54.

Gelman SI. Disturbances in hepatic blood flow during anaesthesia and surgery. *Arch Surg* 1976; **111**: 881–3.

Greenway B, Williams R. Adverse effect of exploratory laparotomy in patients with unsuspected liver disease. *Br J Surg* 1982; **69**: 449–51.

O'Keefe SJ, El-Zayadi AR, Carraher T, Davis M, Williams R. Malnutrition and immune competence in patients with liver disease. *Lancet* 1980; **ii**: 615–17.

Silk DBA. Parenteral nutrition in patients with liver disease. *J Hepatol* 1988; **7**: 269–77.

5.5 Haematological problems

PAUL L. F. GIANGRANDE AND T. J. LITTLEWOOD

INTRODUCTION

Bleeding in association with surgery is a common problem encountered by surgeons and of referral to haematologists. An understanding of the mechanism of blood coagulation is important in order to understand the basis of disorders of haemostasis and the common laboratory tests.

BLOOD COAGULATION

The fundamental step in blood coagulation is the formation of insoluble fibrin strands. The cleavage of small polypeptide chains from the soluble parent fibrinogen molecule is sufficient to achieve this transformation. However, this is only the last step in a series of enzymatic reactions that take place during coagulation (Fig. 1). The coagulation cascade is initiated in two ways. The extrinsic arm is activated when tissue factor forms a complex with factor VII. The resultant complex activates factor X directly, which has a central role in both pathways. Factor X may also be activated through the intrinsic pathway, when negatively-charged subendothelial collagen is exposed and activates factors XII and XI. Factor X forms a complex with calcium and factor V. This complex cleaves prothrombin to produce thrombin, which in turn cleaves fibrinopeptides A and B from soluble fibrinogen to yield insoluble fibrin strands.

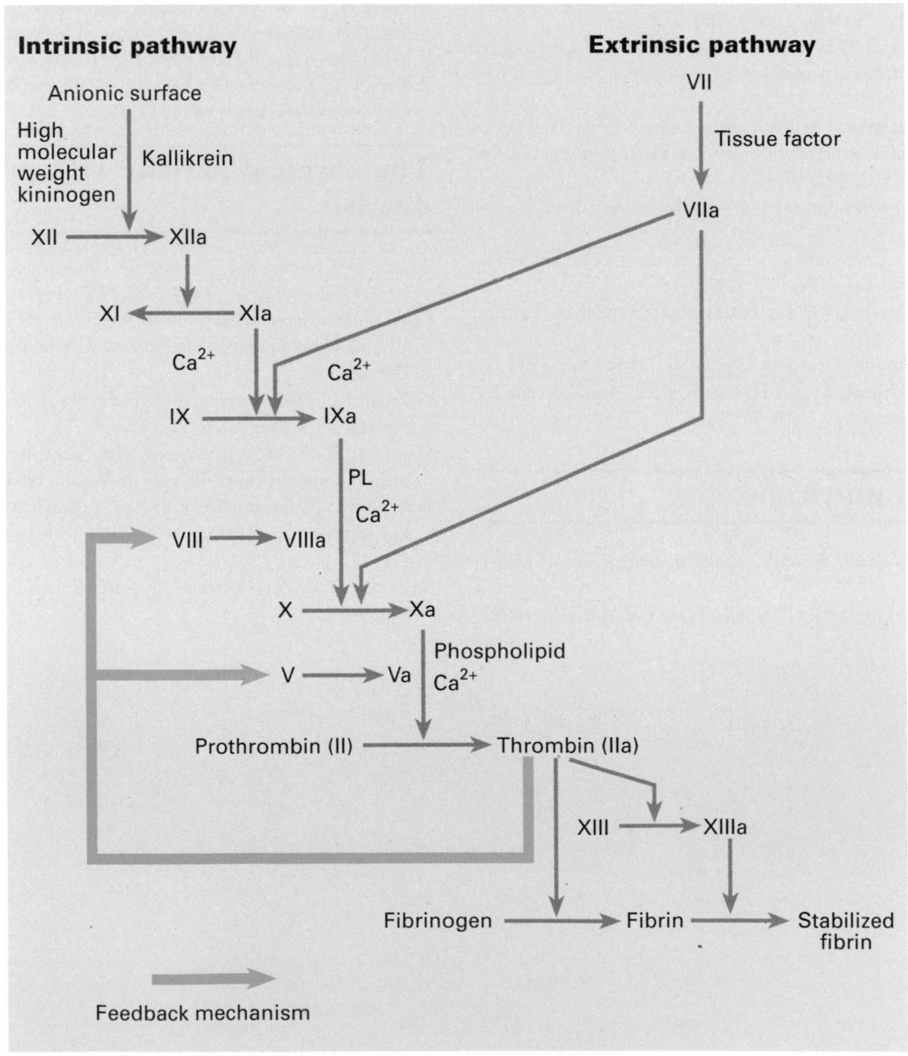

Fig. 1 Blood coagulation pathway.

The basic tests included in a clotting screen are the prothrombin time and the kaolin cephalin clotting time: the former tests the extrinsic pathway, and the latter tests the intrinsic pathway (see below).

There are naturally occurring anticoagulants. The most important of these are antithrombin III, protein C, and protein S. Deficiency of these factors may result in a thrombotic tendency (see below).

Platelets are essential for normal haemostasis. They are particularly important in the formation of the primary response to vascular injury, when activated platelets coalesce to form a platelet plug in the transected vessel.

Laboratory tests of haemostasis

Coagulation tests are carried out on blood anticoagulated with sodium citrate. In contrast to other laboratory samples, it is very important that the correct volume of blood is collected in the appropriate tube. Tests must be carried out on fresh samples as coagulation factors are labile, and if there is undue delay in sending a specimen to the laboratory there will be spurious prolongation of the clotting times. Contamination with heparin (e.g. from indwelling cannulae) will also result in spurious results. It is not possible to state normal ranges which are universally applicable for most clotting tests, as individual laboratories are likely to use slightly different techniques and reagents. Individual laboratories will issue their own normal ranges.

Prothrombin time (PT)

Brain extract (rich in tissue factor) and calcium are added to the test plasma, and the time taken for a clot to develop is measured. The prothrombin time is a test of the function of the extrinsic pathway, and is sensitive to isolated or combined deficiencies of factors II, V, VII, X, and fibrinogen.

Prothrombin time ratio

The results of a prothrombin time are usually expressed as a ratio, comparing the result obtained on the patient test plasma to that obtained on a normal plasma sample

$$\text{prothrombin time ratio} = \frac{\text{PT (s) of test sample}}{\text{PT of normal sample}}$$

The normal prothrombin time ratio should be close to 1.0. The International Normalized Ratio (INR) is for practical purposes the same as the prothrombin time ratio.

Kaolin cephalin clotting time

Kaolin, phospholipid, and calcium are added to the test plasma, and the time taken for a clot to appear is measured. Kaolin activates factor XII, just like collagen. The kaolin cephalin clotting time thus tests function of the intrinsic pathway, and is sensitive to isolated or combined deficiencies of factors XII, XI, X, IX, VIII, V, II, or fibrinogen.

Thrombin time

Thrombin is added to patient plasma, and the time taken for a clot to develop is measured. The thrombin time is prolonged when the fibrinogen level is low, or in the presence of inhibitors of thrombin (e.g. heparin).

Platelet count

Normal range is 150 to 400×10^9/l. Significant bleeding may occur when the count falls below 80×10^9/l. Abnormal bleeding may occasionally occur if platelet function is abnormal, even when the platelet count is normal or even increased (e.g. myelodysplasia, polycythaemia).

Bleeding time

The bleeding time is a simple test of platelet function. A sphygmomanometer cuff is inflated to 40 mmHg around the upper arm. A 5-mm incision is made with a special blade. The incision is wiped with blotting paper every 30 s, and the bleeding time is taken as the time when blood stops oozing. The normal bleeding time is less than 9 min. The bleeding time will be prolonged in association with thrombocytopenia and disorders associated with defective platelet function (e.g. von Willebrand's disease, some cases of myeloproliferative disease).

ACQUIRED DISORDERS OF COAGULATION

Acquired disorders of haemostasis are encountered much more frequently than congenital defects. In order to exclude the possibility of a congenital disorder of coagulation (for which specific therapy may be available) it is important to try to establish from a personal history whether there have been spontaneous haemorrhagic problems (e.g. epistaxis, haemarthrosis, gastrointestinal bleeding) in the past or bleeding after previous surgery (e.g. tonsillectomy, appendicectomy) or dental extractions. The family history should also be elicited. Symptoms of congenital disorders of haemostasis usually appear early in life. However, it should be borne in mind that mild forms of congenital disorders such as haemophilia may only become evident after surgery or major trauma. Acquired disorders of haemostasis may present in a number of ways, ranging from sudden life-threatening bleeding after surgery or childbirth at one end of the spectrum to minor purpura or an increased bruising tendency at the other.

When unexpected bleeding is encountered during surgery, the following possibilities should be considered:

Disseminated intravascular coagulation

Pathogenesis

In most circumstances, initiation of coagulation is a local phenomenon and this is an appropriate reaction to local vascular injury which has resulted in bleeding, e.g. at the site of a surgical incision. Disseminated intravascular coagulation (DIC) is a consequence of explosive activation of the coagulation cascade throughout the vascular tree. Paradoxically, this results in a bleeding tendency and symptoms related to vascular occlusion are relatively rare. This is because the initial thrombus formed in response to the triggering of disseminated intravascular coagulation undergoes very rapid lysis. If the initial trigger persists, further cycles of coagulation and instantaneous lysis rapidly result in the depletion of coagulation factors, including fibrinogen, and consumption of platelets.

The principal causes of disseminated intravascular coagulation that are encountered in clinical practice are listed in Table 1.

Most cases of disseminated intravascular coagulation are triggered by septicaemia. Gram-negative organisms are often implicated. Malignant disease is also an important cause, particularly

Table 1 Principal causes of disseminated intravascular coagulation in clinical practice

Severe infections (e.g. septicaemia)
Malignant disease (metastatic carcinoma, leukaemia)
Shock
Severe burns
ABO incompatible transfusion
Obstetric disorders
Eclampsia
Abruptio placentae
Amniotic fluid embolism
Retained dead fetus
Intravascular haemolysis (e.g. infusion of hypotonic saline, systemic absorption of hypotonic fluids after prostatectomy)

when there are multiple metastases. Carcinoma of the lung, pancreas, stomach, and prostate are particularly associated with this complication. Promyelocytic leukaemia is also frequently complicated by disseminated intravascular coagulation.

Clinical features

In overt cases, there is widespread bruising with extensive purpura. There may be persistent oozing of blood from surgical wounds and venepuncture sites. Bleeding from mucosal surfaces (e.g. epistaxis) is common. Occasionally, there are signs of vascular occlusion in the distal limbs.

Laboratory features

In fulminant cases of disseminated intravascular coagulation the blood is incoagulable. Both the kaolin cephalin clotting time and prothrombin time are markedly prolonged, but will be corrected by the addition of normal plasma to the patient's plasma. The thrombin time is also prolonged, reflecting depletion of fibrinogen. The fibrinogen level is usually below 1.0 g/l (normal range 2–4 g/l). Levels of fibrin degradation tests in the blood will be very high, reflecting hyperfibrinolysis. The platelet count is usually reduced, and may be less than 50×10^9/l in severe cases. Examination of the blood film typically reveals the presence of fragmented erythrocytes.

Treatment of disseminated intravascular coagulation

It is important to identify the underlying cause (see Table 2). Treatment of the underlying condition removes the stimulus for further consumption of coagulation factors.

Fresh frozen plasma should be infused, as this is a good source of coagulation factors, including fibrinogen. As a rough guideline, three to four packs will be required initially. Cryoprecipitate is a very good source of fibrinogen, and has the advantage of being more concentrated so that volume overload may be avoided. If available, cryoprecipitate should be given as well as fresh frozen plasma. Platelet concentrates should also be transfused: 10 to 12 packs should suffice as initial therapy. There is no convincing evidence that administration of antithrombin III concentrates is beneficial. It is important not to overlook the fact that patients often need blood in addition to plasma products. Maintenance of circulating blood volume and an adequate haemoglobin level are important objectives, as tissue hypoxia will only exacerbate disseminated intravascular coagulation.

Contrary to what might be imagined, administration of inhibitors of fibrinolysis (e.g. tranexamic acid) are of no value in the treatment of disseminated intravascular coagulation. The use of such agents may precipitate overt thrombosis. In the past low doses of heparin were administered in cases of disseminated intravascular coagulation, in an attempt to break the vicious cycle of initial thrombosis and subsequent lysis. Such therapy is no longer widely advocated, and it is usually possible to control the activation process by judicious use of blood products and treatment of the underlying cause.

Table 2 Recommendations on reversal of oral anticoagulant therapy

A. *Life-threatening haemorrhage*:
Immediately give 5 mg vitamin K_1 by slow intravenous infusion and a concentrate of factor II, IX, X, with factor VII concentrate (if available). The dose of concentrate should be calculated based on 50 i.u. factor IX/kg body weight

If no concentrate is available fresh frozen plasma should be infused (about 1 l for an adult) but this may not be as effective

B. *Less severe haemorrhage such as haematuria and epistaxis*:
Withhold warfarin for 1 or more days and consider giving vitamin K_1 0.5–2.0 mg intravenously

C. *INR of greater than 4.5 without haemorrhage*:
Withdraw warfarin for 1 or 2 days and then review

D. *Unexpected bleeding at therapeutic levels*:
Investigate possibility of underlying cause such as unsuspected renal or alimentary tract disease

Liver disease

Haemostatic abnormalities in liver disease

The liver is the principal site of synthesis of coagulation factors. Both acute and chronic liver diseases are thus frequently associated with haemostatic abnormalities. Thrombocytopenia of moderate severity ($50–100 \times 10^9$/l) is a frequent finding in patients with chronic liver disease. Another factor which contributes to the bleeding tendency of chronic liver disease is increased fibrinolytic activity, associated with a decreased plasma level of naturally occurring α_2-antiplasmin.

The most frequent haemorrhagic problems are oesophageal and gastrointestinal haemorrhage, as well as bleeding from biopsy sites and during and after surgery. Bleeding into soft tissues is only rarely encountered.

The most common laboratory findings are a marked reduction in the plasma levels of all coagulation factors except factor VIII. Both the prothrombin time and kaolin cephalin clotting time are prolonged.

Therapy

Vitamin K should be administered when it is suspected that the haemorrhagic disorder is due, at least in part, to deficiency of the vitamin (see below). Fresh frozen plasma contains all of the coagulation factors and inhibitors present in blood and is suitable for the correction of the multiple abnormalities associated with liver disease. Usually two to three bags of fresh frozen plasma should suffice to correct the haemostatic defect.

Platelet concentrates are usually of little use in patients with liver disease and thrombocytopenia, as the infused platelets are rapidly sequestered in the liver and spleen. Desmopressin (DDAVP) at a dose of 0.3 μg/kg can be used to shorten the bleeding time before invasive procedures such as biopsy or laparoscopy.

Inhibitors of fibrinolysis, such as tranexamic acid, may be useful in the management of upper gastrointestinal bleeding.

Chronic renal failure

Patients with chronic renal failure often have a bleeding tendency, due in part to poor platelet function. This may be corrected by dialysis. Those with nephrotic syndrome, by contrast, may develop thrombotic complications such as renal vein thrombosis and deep venous thrombosis. The most frequent haemorrhagic manifestations observed in uraemic patients, whether on chronic haemodialysis or not, are usually from mucosal surfaces (gastrointestinal bleeding, epistaxis, menorrhagia). Retroperitoneal haemorrhage, bleeding into the pericardial and pleural spaces, and intracranial haemorrhage may develop occasionally. Patients do not usually bleed after surgical procedures, but renal biopsies are sometimes complicated by the formation of an intrarenal haematoma.

Prolongation of the bleeding time, associated with a normal or only slightly reduced platelet count and normal coagulation tests are the usual findings in uraemia. There is an inverse relationship between the haematocrit and the bleeding time in renal failure. Haemodialysis or transfusion of platelet concentrates may produce transient shortening of the bleeding time. The infusion of eight to ten bags of cryoprecipitate in uraemic patients is usually followed by shortening or even return to normal of the bleeding time. DDAVP (desmopressin) at a dose of 0.3–0.4 μg/kg usually restores the bleeding time to normal in uraemic subjects 1 h after intravenous infusion. Transfusion of red cell concentrates in order to correct anaemia and maintain the haematocrit above 0.30 also shortens the bleeding time. Administration of erythropoietin has a similar effect.

Vitamin K deficiency

Vitamin K is necessary for the synthesis of coagulation factors II (prothrombin), VII, IX, and X. Vitamin K is fat soluble and is absorbed effectively only in the presence of bile salts. Some vitamin K is also synthesized by colonic bacteria. Little vitamin K is stored in the body and in certain conditions symptoms of deficiency may become evident within a few weeks.

Deficiency of vitamin K is associated with prolongation of both the prothrombin time and the partial thromboplastin time. The thrombin time and plasma fibrinogen concentration are normal, which helps in the exclusion of disseminated intravascular coagulation, and the platelet count is normal. Typical haemorrhagic manifestations are easy bruising, and bleeding from sites of injury or from the gums or gastrointestinal tract.

Debilitated patients undergoing surgery are particularly vulnerable, as dietary deficiency may be compounded by the administration of broad-spectrum antibiotics which kill off gut bacteria that synthesize the vitamin. Vitamin K will not be effectively absorbed from the gastrointestinal tract when there is obstruction of the bile duct. Malabsorption of vitamin K may also occur in a number of other conditions, e.g. coeliac disease, intestinal fistulae. Vitamin K deficiency as a consequence of partial biliary tree obstruction may contribute to the development of impaired haemostasis in chronic hepatic disorders such as cirrhosis. An injection of vitamin K may shorten an abnormally long prothrombin time in such cases.

Anticoagulants

Obviously, the consumption of anticoagulants will result in a bleeding tendency! Where unexpected bleeding occurs during or after surgery, consideration should be given to the possibility that the patient is on anticoagulant therapy. This problem may arise when urgent surgery is carried out, without full medical details of the patient being available (e.g. the patient is unconscious).

Where the possibility is suspected, further details may be sought from others involved in the medical care of the patient. Patients taking oral anticoagulants usually carry a medical advisory card. The diagnosis may be confirmed by the finding of a significantly prolonged prothrombin time. The kaolin cephalin clotting time is often only slightly prolonged, and the thrombin time is normal. The platelet count will also be normal.

Warfarin and its congeners are competitive inhibitors of vitamin K. Measures which have been recommended to reverse anticoagulant therapy are shown in Table 2.

Bleeding after cardiopulmonary bypass may be due to the presence of heparin (see below). Contamination with heparin of blood samples drawn from venous cannulae for clotting studies is a very common cause of spurious laboratory results. This may lead to further time-consuming tests and delays in surgery before it can be confirmed that the patient does not have a disorder of haemostasis. Blood for clotting studies should be drawn from a peripheral vein if venous cannulae are flushed with heparin. Inadvertent full heparinization of patients prior to surgery has been reported. In these cases, full-strength heparin was used to flush indwelling venous cannulae, rather than the specific dilute preparations. The use of low-dose subcutaneous heparin does not significantly alter laboratory tests of haemostasis and does not result in a generalized bleeding tendency during surgery.

Administration of streptokinase as thrombolytic therapy (e.g. for myocardial infarction) within 10 days or so after surgery or other invasive procedure such as biopsy may be hazardous as serious bleeding may ensue.

Massive blood transfusion

Blood collected in citrate phosphate dextrose with added adenine (CPDA1) has a shelf life of 35 days at 4°C. However, levels of all the coagulation factors decline during storage. Platelets in stored blood also rapidly lose their viability.

For these reasons, haemorrhagic problems may develop when a patient's blood is replaced by large quantities of stored blood within a short period of time. Microvascular bleeding is a typical manifestation of the impaired haemostasis. Examples include bleeding from mucous membranes, oozing from catheter sites which persists after application of pressure, continuous oozing from surgical wounds, and generalized petechiae. Impaired haemostasis is, of course, only one of several important problems encountered in patients receiving a massive blood transfusion. These include hypocalcaemia due to citrate overload, hyperkalaemia, and hypothermia.

When there is no underlying medical complication, replacement of up to one blood volume (8–10 units of blood in an adult) is not likely to be associated with significant haemostatic problems. Laboratory tests of coagulation may help to identify patients who need additional blood components to improve haemostasis when larger volumes of blood are transfused. A platelet count of less than 50×10^9/l, prothrombin time ratio of 1.8 or more, and a plasma fibrinogen level of 0.5 g/l or less are strongly associated with microvascular bleeding. Platelet support may be required once the patient has received 15 or more units of blood. Fresh frozen plasma is a source of coagulation factors, including fibrinogen.

Cardiopulmonary bypass

Excessive bleeding in association with cardiopulmonary bypass surgery is often a problem. Several factors contribute.

Thrombocytopenia is often present during cardiopulmonary bypass. There is also impairment of platelet function, associated with prolongation of the bleeding time. Platelet dysfunction is related to contact with the synthetic surface of the oxygenator, and probably the induced hypothermia. Many patients with coronary artery disease may be taking aspirin. Patients taking aspirin before cardiopulmonary bypass surgery are at risk of excessive blood loss during the procedure. It is therefore recommended that aspirin be discontinued at least 5 days before cardiopulmonary bypass. Despite abnormalities in platelet number and function, there is no evidence that routine perioperative transfusion of platelet concentrates is necessary.

Cardiopulmonary bypass is associated with a drop in the plasma levels of most coagulation factors, which is primarily attributable to haemodilution. As with platelet concentrates, it is not necessary routinely to transfuse fresh frozen plasma during cardiopulmonary bypass.

Heparin is routinely administered in order to prevent extracorporeal clotting in the oxygenator. Protamine sulphate is administered at the end of surgery in order to neutralize remaining heparin. In gross excess protamine itself acts as an anticoagulant. Following initial adequate heparin neutralization, the reappearance of active heparin in the bloodstream may occur 2 to 6 h later. This rebound effect is caused by the delayed return of sequestered extravascular heparin which occurs when peripheral perfusion improves. Thrombocytopenia may complicate heparin therapy in about 5 per cent of patients receiving the drug. The onset of thrombocytopenia is typically between 6 and 12 days after exposure to the drug. This is due to the development of an antibody which induces platelet activation. The possibility of heparin-induced thrombocytopenia should always be considered in the differential diagnosis when thrombocytopenia develops after cardiopulmonary bypass. Platelet concentrates should only be transfused if there are bleeding complications as arterial thrombosis has been reported after transfusion of platelets.

The administration of aprotinin, an inhibitor of plasmin, significantly reduces intraoperative and postoperative blood loss associated with cardiopulmonary bypass. The requirement for blood transfusion is reduced, and the actual operating time may be shortened.

CONGENITAL DISORDERS OF COAGULATION

Haemophilia

Haemophilia is the most common congenital disorder of coagulation and affects 1 in 10 000 males. Haemophilia A is caused by a deficiency of factor VIII in the circulating blood. In its severe form (less than 2 per cent of the normal factor VIII) it is characterized by recurrent joint bleeds, intramuscular bleeding, and excessive bruising after trauma. Recurrent bleeds may result in crippling arthritis. Haemophilia B (Christmas disease) is a clinically identical disorder caused by deficiency of factor IX. Both conditions show X-linked inheritance, but in one-third of cases of haemophilia there is no preceding family history as the condition results from a new mutation. Female carriers invariably have a high enough factor level to protect them from spontaneous haemorrhagic complications, although treatment with coagulation factor concentrate may be required before surgery.

Inhibitory antibodies

Some 6 per cent of patients with haemophilia A and 1 per cent of those with haemophilia B develop inhibitory IgG antibodies directed against the infused factor. Management of patients with high titre antibodies can be difficult. A satisfactory clinical response may often be obtained by increasing the dose of human factor VIII administered, although the antibody titre may be subsequently boosted. Porcine factor VIII may be effective where the antibody titre against human factor VIII is very high.

The patient's plasma must be screened for the presence of inhibitory antibodies prior to surgery. Elective, non-urgent surgery is not advisable if a patient is known to have inhibitory antibodies.

Liver disease in haemophilia

Chronic liver disease is a problem in many haemophiliacs. This is usually due to persistent infection with hepatitis B or C. All patients who are likely to receive coagulation factor concentrates should be vaccinated against hepatitis B. Documentation of abnormal hepatic function is of practical importance to the surgeon for a number of reasons.

1. In established liver disease, the synthesis of a number of coagulation factors is disturbed. Fresh plasma may be required in addition to factor concentrate to ensure haemostasis.
2. The dosage of certain drugs may need to be modified.
3. There is a potential risk to staff of infection through needlestick injuries.

Liver transplantation has been carried out in a small number of haemophiliacs with serious liver disease, and this has the added bonus of curing haemophilia as both factor VIII and factor IX are synthesized by hepatocytes. Of course, this radical treatment cannot be routinely applied to haemophiliacs!

HIV infection and AIDS

Approximately one-third of haemophiliacs in the United Kingdom were infected with the human immunodeficiency virus (HIV) between the years 1979 and 1985. The extent to which haemophiliacs in various countries were infected with HIV is very variable. Infection with HIV is associated with a progressive decline in the number of CD4+ T lymphocytes in the blood. Cellular immunity is compromised and patients may eventually develop opportunistic infections. Thrombocytopenia is seen in approximately 10 per cent of patients infected with HIV. Thrombocytopenia is clearly particularly dangerous in haemophiliacs who already have a bleeding tendency. Zidovudine therapy usually raises the platelet count considerably.

There is no evidence that surgery accelerates progression to AIDS by promoting the decline in the number of CD4+ T lymphocytes. Many surgeons are concerned about the possibility of transmission of HIV (see also Chapter 2.2). However, the risk of infection to health care workers through body fluids or inoculation is much less than that associated with hepatitis B. A prospective study of needlestick injuries among health care staff and involving patients known to be infected with HIV has demonstrated a risk of infection of around 0.3 per cent. The vast majority of such injuries are associated with the resheathing of needles: this should be avoided, and all used needles should be discarded in a suitable container immediately after use. Needlestick injuries amongst surgeons due to suture needles appear to be less dangerous than injuries associated with hollow needles used for venepuncture. The prophylactic administration of zidovudine after a needlestick injury does not guarantee protection against infection, and the drug has a number of toxic effects. The risk of transmission through blood or other bodily fluids coming into contact with intact skin is negligible.

Practical management of a patient with haemophilia scheduled for surgery

Wherever possible, elective surgery should be carried out in a centre experienced in the management of haemophilia. All registered patients should carry a medical card which states the precise diagnosis, factor level, inhibitor status and blood group. The HIV status of a patient will not be stated on the card. It must be remembered that female carriers of haemophilia A or B may themselves also have low levels of factor VIII or IX respectively, and may require treatment prior to surgery or dental work.

Patients scheduled for elective surgery should be admitted 1 or 2 days beforehand for blood tests (Table 3). Patients with severe haemophilia are likely to need infusions of concentrate for at least 7 to 10 days after any type of surgery. They will often need, therefore, to stay in hospital for a longer period than other patients and this must be planned for accordingly. It is all too common to see patients scheduled for discharge 2 days after 'minor' surgery. There is no such thing as 'minor' surgery for haemophiliacs.

Table 3 Preoperative check list

1. Check supplies of concentrate are adequate for treatment period
2. Is any other surgical work scheduled?
3. Blood tests for:
   Baseline factor level
   Inhibitory antibody screen
   Hepatitis HBsAg status
   Antihepatitis B antibody (anti-HBs) status
   Antihepatitis C antibody (anti-HCV) status
   Anti-HIV status
   Liver function tests (including prothrombin time)
   Full blood count
   Group and save plasma or cross-match as appropriate

All patients receiving coagulation factor concentrates (even high-purity ones) should be vaccinated against hepatitis B. If some time has elapsed since completion of the course of vaccination, immune status should be checked and the antibody level (anti-HBs) checked. Surgeons dealing with haemophiliacs should certainly be vaccinated against hepatitis B. No vaccine is as yet available against hepatitis C.

In some countries where concentrate is not readily available, some units have achieved considerable savings by good co-ordination of activities. If a patient is scheduled to have surgery and will be in hospital and having concentrate for some days thereafter, other procedures can be carried out at the same time (e.g. dental work, excision of skin lesions, vasectomy etc.).

On the day of surgery, concentrate should be infused within 1 h before surgery: a dose of 50 i.u./kg of factor VIII or 75 i.u./kg of factor IX should suffice to boost the plasma level to well within the normal range. Pre- and postinfusion plasma levels of factor should be checked in the laboratory to confirm that a suitable level has been achieved for surgery. After surgery, twice-daily bolus infusions of factor VIII will be required for at least 5 days. Further daily doses may be required for a further 5 days or so, until soft tissue healing is achieved. Factor IX has a longer half-life, and only one infusion a day is necessary. Analgesics must not be given by intramuscular injection, and aspirin is contraindicated.

To minimize the risk of bleeding from wounds, it is sensible to change dressings after infusion of a dose of concentrate. Similarly, physiotherapy is best scheduled immediately after infusion. Intramuscular injections (e.g. premedication prior to surgery, postoperative analgesia) must not be given, as a large intramuscular haematoma is likely to develop.

Deep venous thrombosis is not a problem in patients with haemophilia A, and prophylaxis (e.g. heparin, low-dose warfarin) is not necessary, even in orthopaedic surgery. Such treatment may also interfere with laboratory monitoring of plasma factor levels after infusion of concentrate. Thrombosis has been reported in patients receiving prothrombin-complex concentrates, and high-purity factor IX concentrates are to be recommended for patients with haemophilia B undergoing surgery.

Other congenital disorders of coagulation

Very occasionally, patients with isolated congenital deficiencies of other coagulation factors may be encountered. Deficiencies of fibrinogen, factor V, factor X, factor VII, factor XI, or XIII may be associated with a serious bleeding tendency. Similar practical guidelines to those set out above apply. Specific plasma-derived concentrates of most of these coagulation factors are available commercially.

INVESTIGATION OF THE PATIENT WITH A BLEEDING TENDENCY

It is not necessary to perform tests of haemostasis on all patients scheduled for elective surgery. However, if a history of a possible bleeding tendency emerges during outpatient investigation, patients should certainly be referred for investigation prior to surgery.

Basic tests of coagulation include the prothrombin time, kaolin cephalin clotting time, and the platelet count. Where the platelet count is normal (or even elevated) a bleeding time should be measured to exclude the possibility of congenital or acquired defects of platelet function. It is important to try to distinguish between congenital disorders on the basis of the personal and family history. Table 4 is intended only as a guideline to how the screening test may help in the diagnosis of specific defects.

Where bleeding is encountered during surgery and there is no obvious source of haemorrhage, a prothrombin time, kaolin cephalin clotting time, and platelet count should be requested in the first instance. The administration of two to three units of fresh

Table 4 Laboratory investigation of a patient with a bleeding tendency

Disorder	Prothrombin time	Kaolin cephalin clotting time	Thrombin time	Platelets	Bleeding time	Notes
Heparin	N	↑↑	↑↑	N	N	Reptilase time normal
Diffuse intravascular coagulation	↑↑	↑↑	↑↑	↓	↑	Fibrin degradation tests elevated Erythrocyte fragments on blood film
Liver disease	↑	↑	N or ↑	N or ↓	N or ↑	Transaminases
Functional platelet defect	N	N	N	N	↑(↑)	
Vitamin K deficiency	↑↑	↑	N	N	N	Echis carinatus time normal Similar findings with warfarin
Haemophilia	N	↑↑	N	N	N	Confirm with specific factor assay
von Willebrand's disease	N	↑↑	N	N	↑(↑)	Confirm with specific factor assay

N – Normal
↑ – increased
↓ – decreased

frozen plasma is a useful practical measure until the cause is identified. Platelet concentrates should be given if the platelet count is below $50 \times 10^9/l$.

THROMBOPHILIA

The term thrombophilia is used to describe familial or acquired disorders of the haemostatic mechanism which predispose to thrombosis. Inherited deficiencies of antithrombin III, protein C, and protein S are important causes of a thrombotic tendency. Antithrombin III inactivates factors IX, X, XI, and thrombin. Protein C and its cofactor protein S are vitamin K-dependent proteins which inactivate factors V and VIII. Such patients are particularly vulnerable to the development of deep venous thrombosis and/or pulmonary embolism after surgery if adequate precautions are not taken.

At present, the great majority of thrombotic episodes remain unexplained in that no underlying disorder may be identified. Occasionally, acquired blood disorders associated with a definite thrombotic tendency may be diagnosed after an episode of thrombosis. These include thrombocytosis secondary to myeloproliferative disease, polycythaemia, and the lupus anticoagulant. The development of a lupus anticoagulant is associated with prolongation of the kaolin cephalin clotting time and, in about a quarter of cases, prolongation of the prothrombin time. The former is not corrected by the addition of normal plasma to the patient's own plasma. There may be thrombocytopenia. Despite these findings, the patient is paradoxically at risk of thrombosis and there is no undue risk of haemorrhage (even in association with surgery). Although originally described in association with systemic lupus erythematosus, it is important to appreciate that the great majority of cases arise in people who have no evidence of the disorder and who are perfectly well.

Consideration should be given to investigating patients encountered in clinical practice who have thrombosis at an unusually early age, or in an unusual site (e.g. mesenteric vein thrombosis), or where there is a suggestion of a familial tendency to thrombosis. Laboratory testing for thrombophilia is difficult once a patient is anticoagulated, as heparin reduces the plasma level of antithrombin III whilst warfarin boosts the plasma level of antithrombin III but lowers the level of proteins C and S. Investigation is best deferred until the patient has been off anticoagulants for at least 2 months.

Management of individuals with thrombophilia

By no means all patients with documented thrombophilia will experience spontaneous thrombosis during their lifetime. Studies suggest that approximately half of such patients will experience spontaneous thrombosis. Where deficiency of antithrombin III, protein C, protein S, or lupus anticoagulant are identified in patients without a history of thrombosis, it is not usual practice to initiate long-term prophylactic warfarin therapy as this treatment itself is not without risks. However, such patients should certainly receive some form of prophylaxis to cover surgery and pregnancy. Standard low-dose subcutaneous heparin therapy is perfectly satisfactory for general surgery. Higher doses of heparin or low-intensity anticoagulation with warfarin are advisable to cover major orthopaedic procedures. Affected women should not take oestrogen-containing oral contraceptives or hormone replacement therapy after the menopause. Plasma-derived concentrates of antithrombin III are available and may be given in addition to subcutaneous heparin to cover surgical procedures. Concentrates of protein C and S are not yet available.

An episode of thrombosis in a person with documented thrombophilia should be treated with heparin and warfarin in the standard fashion. Patients with antithrombin III deficiency may require more heparin than usual in order to achieve an adequately prolonged kaolin cephalin clotting time. Consideration should be given to long-term oral anticoagulation following an episode of thrombosis, if there are no contraindications.

HAEMOGLOBINOPATHIES

Sickle-cell disease

Subjects with sickle haemoglobin (HbS) are found throughout tropical Africa, scattered in countries bordering the Mediterranean, in the Middle East and India. With the ease of world travel there can be no surgeon who can assume that a patient with sickle-cell disease requiring surgery will not come under his or her care.

Operating on a patient with sickle-cell disease significantly increases the risk to the patient of sickle-related complications. These may vary in severity from a painful limb crisis to life threatening neurological or respiratory crises but the risk may be minimized by appropriate perioperative care.

Dehydration, anoxia, hypothermia, and hypotension must be avoided. Local or regional anaesthesia may be preferable to general anaesthesia but limb tourniquets must not be used in order to avoid local tissue anoxia. For very minor surgery of short duration the above precautions may be adequate. For more major surgery the level of HbS should be reduced by blood transfusion. The most effective, albeit complicated, method is to exchange transfuse the patient preoperatively with the aim being to reduce the percentage of HbS from a predicted starting point of approximately 90 per cent to below 20 per cent. Once this is achieved the HbS percentage is maintained below 20 per cent by regular transfusions of red cells until the patient is mobilized and active postoperatively.

If an initial exchange transfusion is not carried out transfusion of red cells should be given with care to avoid unduly raising the blood viscosity.

If emergency surgery is necessary in an unprepared patient an exchange transfusion to lower the HbS as far as possible is the best measure if time and the patient's condition allow. Otherwise, adherence to the general measures described above should be performed. Wound and pulmonary infections in the postoperative period should be rigorously sought and treated.

Finally, patients with sickle-cell disease may have minor cardiac and renal impairment but this will be rarely severe enough, at least in younger patients, to occasion any alarm peroperatively.

Sickle-cell trait

The risk for patients with sickle-cell trait undergoing surgery is not much greater than for normal individuals. However, the simple precautions of avoiding dehydration, anoxia etc. should be followed. Preoperative blood transfusion is not needed.

Thalassaemia

Patients with thalassaemia trait can undergo surgery without any special precautions whatsoever. In contrast, patients with β-thalassaemia major or anaemic patients with thalassaemia intermedia (a hotch-potch of thalassaemic disorders of a severity somewhere between thalassaemia major and thalassaemia trait) should be transfused up to a normal haemoglobin preoperatively. There is no need for exchange transfusion in this group.

The optimal routine treatment for patients with β-thalassaemia is regular blood transfusion to maintain a normal haemoglobin level. Those patients who have not simultaneously undergone a rigorous iron chelating programme may become iron overloaded and the clinical consequences of this, especially the risk of impaired cardiac function, will be of importance to the surgeon and anaesthetist in a patient needing surgery. There have recently been some encouraging reports of improvement in cardiac function in iron overloaded patients after aggressive high-dose therapy with desferrioxamine. Therapeutic benefit may take many months to achieve but is worthwhile if time allows.

Splenectomy is a common operation in thalassaemic patients. The increased risk of infection after splenectomy is well described. Briefly, patients should receive Pneumovax preoperatively and then penicillin by mouth for a minimum of 2 years postoperatively. In addition, an interesting thrombotic problem has been identified in some patients after splenectomy. Persistent thrombocytosis after splenectomy occurs predictably in patients where anaemia persists. The thrombocytosis may be associated with life threatening thromboembolic complications and this phenomenon has been well documented in patients with HbH disease. HbH disease occurs where there is a failure of three of the four α globin genes to form α globin chains with the clinical phenotype that of thalassaemia intermedia. A number of reports cite persistent thrombocytosis in these patients after splenectomy and the subsequent development of thrombophlebitis and thromboembolism.

In patients with a persistent thrombocytosis ($>500 \times 10^9$/l) after splenectomy it is wise to use life-long aspirin postoperatively and treat with warfarin those patients who develop signs of superficial thrombophlebitis or other thrombotic events despite the aspirin.

MYELOPROLIFERATIVE DISORDERS

Among these disorders are included chronic myeloid leukaemia, primary proliferative polycythaemia (formerly known as polycythaemia rubra vera), essential thrombocythaemia, and myelofibrosis. In each of these disorders the platelet count may be significantly raised (often greater than 1000×10^9/l) and in the perioperative period this may greatly enhance a thrombotic tendency. In addition, patients with polycythaemia will have a high haemoglobin associated with an increase in red cell mass which will further enhance the risk of thrombosis. The situation may be further complicated by an increased haemorrhagic tendency due to abnormal platelet function in each of the above disorders giving rise to the situation where a single patient is simultaneously at increased risk of thrombosis and bleeding.

Wherever possible surgery in such patients should be planned and appropriate treatment given to the patient to render the blood counts normal or near normal preoperatively. Once this is achieved it is good practice to give antithrombotic prophylaxis peroperatively. Preoperative coagulation tests should include, in addition to the platelet count, a bleeding time, prothrombin time, and activated partial thromboplastin time. Patients with a prolonged bleeding time, with the implication of impaired platelet function, should have platelets available to be transfused in the operative and postoperative period as necessary.

Patients with uncontrolled myeloproliferative disorders who are admitted with acute surgical problems requiring emergency surgery are at significant risk of thrombotic and haemorrhagic complications. Patients with polycythaemia may be venesected down to a normal haemoglobin relatively quickly (isovolumetric replacement of red cells by colloid is recommended) but a high platelet count cannot be quickly corrected. Perioperative anticoagulation is essential to reduce the risk of thrombosis. Bleeding perioperatively can be managed as above with platelet transfusions and fresh frozen plasma if there is prolongation of the prothrombin or activated partial thromboplastin time.

Perhaps the single most commonly performed operation in myeloproliferative disorders is splenectomy. The indications for this operation are beyond the scope of this section (see Chapter 37). A number of reports of splenectomy in the management of myeloproliferative disorders have been published. Mortality rates vary from 4 to 28 per cent and complication rates from 47 to 56 per cent. The major reported causes of morbidity were haemorrhage despite apparently appropriate precautions, followed by infection and thrombosis. Infections in one series occurred in 21 of 96 patients after splenectomy with the respiratory system, wound, and subphrenic space being the affected sites. The high mortality and morbidity rates for splenectomy in patients with myeloproliferative disorders compare unfavourably with the relatively trouble free course seen in patients undergoing splenectomy for autoimmune disorders such as idiopathic thrombocytopenic purpura, and autoimmune haemolytic anaemia (see later).

LYMPHOPROLIFERATIVE DISORDERS

The indications for splenectomy in patients with lymphoproliferative disorders are lessening. Fewer staging laparotomies and splenectomies in patients with Hodgkin's disease are performed nowadays compared with 10 to 20 years ago and splenomegaly with hypersplenism due to tumour infiltration in patients with lymphoma can often be successfully treated by chemotherapy.

Nevertheless there remains a steady trickle of patients, often elderly and with massively enlarged spleens, who require surgery either for local symptoms induced by the splenomegaly, hypersplenism, or both (see also Chapter 37). Thrombocytopenia is the most common haemostatic abnormality and platelet transfusions may be needed perioperatively. Infection and bleeding are the most common complications but the postoperative risks are substantially less in patients with lymphoproliferative disorders compared with myeloproliferative disorders.

MYELODYSPLASIA

Myelodysplasia is a clonal disorder of bone marrow resulting in the production of morphologically and functionally abnormal red cells, white cells, and platelets. Infection and bleeding are common complications. The median survival is between 2 and 3 years from diagnosis and approximately one-third of patients will develop acute myeloid leukaemia in the terminal stages of their illness. In the early stages a typical patient may be noted to be mildly anaemic (often with a raised mean cell volume), leucopenic, and thrombocytopenic, or any combination of these.

From a surgical point of view the major risks are of haemorrhage and infection. Even if the platelet count is normal it is likely that functionally the platelets will be abnormal and a preoperative bleeding time should be checked. As with the myeloproliferative disorders platelets for transfusion should be available perioperatively and close attention given to prompt treatment of postoperative infection.

AUTOIMMUNE DISORDERS

Idiopathic thrombocytopenic purpura

Splenectomy is a standard form of treatment in patients with idiopathic thrombocytopenic purpura who have failed to achieve a sustained response to primary drug therapy. In childhood idiopathic thrombocytopenic purpura up to 80 per cent of patients will remit spontaneously or after treatment with prednisolone and/or intravenous immunoglobulin (IV IgG). In contrast, first-line therapy results in sustained complete remission in only around 25 per cent of adults with this disorder.

Up to 90 per cent of patients with idiopathic thrombocytopenic purpura who have failed to respond to prednisolone, or who relapse after the withdrawal of prednisolone, will obtain a rapid rise in platelet count after treatment with intravenous immunoglobulin; unfortunately the response is usually shortlived. However, maintenance therapy with intravenous immunoglobulin may achieve long-term remission in 40 to 50 per cent of patients.

The expense of maintenance intravenous immunoglobulin means that splenectomy is the most common treatment option in patients who have failed to achieve a sustained response with prednisolone.

Improvement in the platelet count preoperatively can be achieved with prednisolone in those patients who have previously shown a response to this drug, or with intravenous immunoglobulin which improves the platelet count in up to 90 per cent of patients with idiopathic thrombocytopenic purpura.

The risk of adrenal suppression in patients treated with prednisolone for weeks or months preoperatively would necessitate increasing doses of steroid perioperatively. Also patients treated with prednisolone have an increased risk of perioperative infection. Intravenous immunoglobulin does not carry these risks and its use preoperatively may enhance the response to splenectomy. In preparing a patient for surgery intravenous immunoglobulin is the treatment of choice where the means and facilities allow it to be given. A typical dose is 0.4 g/kg body weight/day for 5 days. Platelet transfusion perioperatively should rarely be required nowadays.

Splenectomy will return the platelet count to normal, or substantially improve it, in around 60 to 70 per cent of patients. Only a small number (about 10 per cent) will be left with continuing haemorrhagic problems.

AUTOIMMINE HAEMOLYTIC ANAEMIA

Splenectomy is the treatment of choice for the patients with autoimmune haemolytic anaemia who fail to respond to treatment with prednisolone. Splenectomy is effective in more than 50 per cent of cases. In contrast to patients with idiopathic thrombocytopenic purpura intravenous immunoglobulin has little or no place in the management of patients with autoimmune haemolyic anaemia. There are no specific precautions to be taken preoperatively. Severe anaemia can be corrected by blood transfusion although the half-life of the transfused red cells will be markedly shortened by immune destruction.

Postoperatively a transient increase in platelet count (often to $>1000\times10^9/l$) is common and perioperative antithrombotic prophylaxis should be given.

FURTHER READING

Bickerstaff KI, Morris PJ. Splenectomy for massive splenomegaly. *Br J Surg* 1987; **74**: 346–49.

Blood Transfusion Task Force, British Committee for Standardization in Haematology. Guidelines for transfusion for massive blood loss. *Clin Lab Haematol* 1988; **10**: 265–73.

Bloom AL, Forbes D, Thomas DP, Tuddenham EGD, eds. *Thrombosis and haemostasis*. 3rd edn. Edinburgh: Churchill Livingstone, 1993.
British Committee for Standards in Haematology. Guidelines for the use of fresh frozen plasma *Transfusion Med* 1992; **2**: 57–63.
Cohen AR, Mizanin J, Schwartz E. Rapid removal of excessive iron with daily dose intravenous chelation therapy. *J Pediatr* 1989; **115**: 151–5.
Dacie JV. *The Haemolytic Anaemias*, Vol. 2. Edinburgh: Churchill Livingstone—Longman Group UK Ltd, 1988.
Danforth DN, Fraker DL. Splenectomy for the massively enlarged spleen. *American Surgeon* 1991; **52**: 108–13.
Duthie RB, Rizza CRC, Giangrande PLF, Dodd C. *Management of musculoskeletal problems in haemophilia*. Oxford: University Press, 1993.
Gill PG, Souter RG, Morris PJ. Splenectomy for hypersplenism in malignant lymphomas *Br J Surg* 1981; **1**: 29–33.
Hirsch J, Dacie JV. Persistent post-splenectomy thrombocytosis and thrombo-embolism. A consequence of continuing anaemia. *Br J Haematol* 1966; **12**: 44–53.
Jacobs P, Wood L, Dent DM. Splenectomy in the chronic myeloproliferative syndromes. *S Afr Med J* 1992; **81**: 499–503.
Mitchell A, Morris PJ. Surgery of the spleen. *Clinics in Haematol* 1983; **12**: 565–90.
Morris PJ, Cooper IA, Madigan JP. Splenectomy for hypersplenism in malignant lymphoma. *Lancet* 1975, **ii**: 250–2.
Poller L, Thomson JM, eds. *Thrombosis and its management*. Edinburgh: Churchill Livingstone, 1993.
Rizza CRC, Lowe GDO, eds. *Haemophilia and its management*. London: Balliere Tindall, 1994.
Woodman RC, Harker LA. Bleeding complications associated with cardiopulmonary bypass. *Blood* 1990; **76**: 1680–97.

5.6 Psychological care

OWEN S. SURMAN

FEAR OF SURGERY

Two types of fear commonly encountered in the surgical patient are fear of bodily injury and fear of death, typically fear of not awakening from anaesthesia (narcosis anxiety). Other common sources of apprehension are fear of pain, fear of cancer being discovered at operation, fear of intraoperative wakefulness, and fears of non-specific factors common to the hospital experience such as separation from job and family. Studies of patients undergoing orthopaedic and gynaecological surgery have demonstrated that high levels of anxiety precede hospital admission and persist for several days following operative intervention.

ORIGIN OF PREOPERATIVE ANXIETY

Past trauma

The surgical experience recalls early life stress. For some, parental separation at a time of childhood surgery, or unpleasant exposure to a mask for anaesthesia induction may trigger abnormal fear of surgery in adulthood. Those with a traumatic past are especially vulnerable.

Identification

Emotional adaptation to surgery may differ, according to expectations derived from the surgical experience of relatives. Patients encountering a similar disease process may observe, share, and compare outcomes in a way that modifies the impact of events: visits from recipients of organ transplants improve the hopes and coping skills of patients awaiting a suitable organ.

Expectation

Surgery is often a source of hope and improved identity, as in the case of cosmetic procedures and transplantation. In other instances, however, surgery may represent a substantial loss. The burden of mastectomy or colostomy has inspired the formation of successful self-help groups. Although there is an implicit gain for the patient whose life is maintained by removal of cancer or whose proximal limb is saved by amputation of a gangrenous distal part, the subjective or symbolic meaning of operative intervention is also of significance to recovery. Emotional outcome is particularly influenced by the patient's knowledge and orientation to perioperative events, particularly the realistic appraisal of what can be expected. Two factors that increase perioperative anxiety are unpredictability and underestimation of pain and risk.

PREOPERATIVE PSYCHOLOGICAL EVALUATION

Patients with psychopathological states require identification and specialized medical management.

Personality disorder

The different types of personality disorder have in common a basic problem with trust and a pattern of failed or strained relationships. Problems with medical compliance may occur as well as strain in the doctor–patient relationship. The patient may discharge him or herself. Costly litigation, or even personal injury to the caregiver or a colleague, may follow from the perceived injustice of a malcontent. Some patients who are unlikely to benefit from surgery may seek an operation or a series of operations in a neurotic attempt to gain attention.

In addition to identifying personality pathology, it is important to recognize normal variations in coping style, particularly individual tendencies toward anxiety and in locus of control. Some attribute the outcome of events to external factors beyond control, while others perceive events to be under greater personal influence. Some patients may adopt an avoidance or denial approach to the threat of surgery, while others may exaggerate risks. More stress is encountered among the young, among those with an 'excess of recent life events' and among those with medical conditions that are relatively demanding. Good outcomes are more likely for those with an active and energetic orientation.

Affective disorder

The depressed patient may be irritable, agitated, or quietly withdrawn. Postoperative mobilization is a challenge and impaired nutrition undermines the process of surgical repair. Treatment of depression requires supportive psychotherapy, psychopharmacological intervention, and social support. When depression is secondary to surgically correctable physical impairment, successful operative intervention is most often followed by improvement in mood and well being. For example, hysterectomy is often preceded by psychiatric morbidity, which decreases after the operation.

Anxiety disorder

Anxiety may result from misconceptions about surgery, from anniversary reaction to past trauma, or from the impact of new learning or increased physical impairment on established coping skills. Those who deny their disease are especially likely to react anxiously to detailed preoperative information. Isolated phobias, such as needle phobias, claustrophobia, or pathological dread of anaesthesia are occasionally encountered, as are generalized anxiety states and multiple phobias with panic attacks.

Treatment of anxiety begins with preoperative teaching and formation of a therapeutic alliance. Some patients may derive considerable support from contact with others who have successfully completed a similar operative procedure. Such peer group support has been useful in a variety of surgical settings. Those who are unresponsive to these measures or who have chronic anxiety disorders often benefit from psychotherapy and treatment with anxiolytic agents.

Cognitive impairment

Impaired cognition in patients requiring surgery is most frequently of metabolic origin and is associated with increased risk of postoperative delirium. Functionally psychotic, demented or retarded patients must be recognized, however. The Mini-Mental State test is an excellent screening tool for delirium and dementia but has a high rate of false-positive results among those with less than 9 years of education and among people aged 60 or more.

Alcoholism

Alcoholic patients are often exquisitely sensitive to rejection and given to pathological denial. Preoperative recognition of the potential for delirium tremens and of the higher risk of postoperative delirium is important in patients with a history of alcoholism. Postoperative delirium may occur in the form of delirium tremens, as a manifestation of alcohol withdrawal, or, delirium may occur *de novo* in an otherwise recovered alcoholic with established sobriety.

INFORMED CONSENT

Three aspects of the informed consent process can be valuable tools in establishing a good doctor–patient relationship.

Bonding

Along with a statement of risks and benefits, the consent process is a declaration of clinical goals. A factual, caring presentation marks the beginning of a collaborative bond for patient and surgeon.

Teaching

Patients must be informed of discomfort associated with the procedure and about availability of pain relief. The need for intravenous therapy, indwelling catheter, drains, and endotracheal tube should be discussed, as well as the customary length of the operation and the anticipated time for recuperation in hospital and following discharge. The surgeon must provide information about necessary postoperative care including medication, diet, activity restriction, and medical visits. The patient should know of complications, including psychological difficulties, commonly associated with the procedure, and the risk of dying. Information should be addressed in a candid but constructive fashion. A visit to areas of the hospital dedicated to postoperative care can be beneficial, as is the opportunity for contact with other patients who have had similar surgery.

Observing

The informed consent process allows the surgeon an opportunity to observe the patient's mental status. Preoccupation with excessive detail may be evidence of anxiety or paranoia. Failed comprehension may signal encephalopathy, internal distraction, or deficient intellect. Dress and deportment are a statement of self worth as well as personal management and socioeconomic status. A despondent, tearful, or lethargic manner signals depression. Attempts by the patient at good-natured evasion of a proper alcohol and drug history may be a clue to pathological denial. An ingratiating attitude coupled with criticism of former physicians is typical of paranoid individuals. Adjustment problems or evidence of greater psychopathology should be followed by formal psychiatric consultation and by social service intervention when there is a need for additional perioperative support.

INNOVATIVE SURGERY

The pace of medical science has made some former experimental procedures routine. New experiments with the artificial heart and transplantation of multiple organs have aroused the interest of ethicists and health policy planners. The economics of current health care has put a spotlight on quality of life aspects for all such interventions.

Patient selection

The selection process for emerging surgical technology is based on capacity to benefit from the procedure, degree of present need, and time of initial presentation. The need to establish a priority list among patients is a source of stress for physicians; this intensifies as patients die while waiting for treatment. Since patients with a specific medical handicap or psychosocial impairment may have differing levels of limitation, suitability for costly new procedures, such as heart transplantation, is best determined on an individual basis to avoid discrimination. Factors such as older age and prior alcoholism may not be valid reasons for excluding people who otherwise appear to have a good chance of recovery and long life.

REDUCTION OF PREOPERATIVE STRESS

Education and support

Emphasis should be on individual concerns. Patients need to know that pain is normal and that early postoperative mobilization is healthy. The surgeon should review past difficulty with specific analgesic drugs, anaesthetic agents, or other medications essential to the operation. Patients should be encouraged to request pain medication as needed and they should be reassured about fears of addiction.

Disfigurement is a frequent source of worry but may be couched in understatement such as 'Will I be able to wear a bikini?' Other common worries concern sexual function, future childbearing capacity, return to active life-styles, and loss of privacy. Some may wish to maintain access to aspects of their work. Dietary considerations, visiting arrangements, health care directives, and financial issues should be discussed. A preoperative visit with a medical social worker, or dietitian may be helpful. Patients with histories of lengthy medical problems, such as those with juvenile onset diabetes, often have firm opinions about their medical needs. When they do, preoperative discussion with the nursing staff is beneficial since it helps to accommodate to specific needs. It is equally important to shape expectations and to encourage patients to modify their life-styles. Timely referral to a smoking cessation programme or substance abuse clinic may make a profound difference to postoperative outcome.

Specialized intervention

A preoperative visit by the anaesthetist has benefits compared to sedation alone. In a study of patients undergoing abdominal surgery, those who were taught about the normality of postoperative pain and encouraged to request analgesics when needed had greater postoperative comfort and used far fewer narcotics than those receiving no information about pain control. Subsequent studies have employed preoperative interventions such as support, teaching, hypnosis, and relaxation training, and have looked at varying measures of postoperative outcome. Although methodological problems exist, such as lack of 'blind' controls, these studies document a major reduction of time in hospital. For example, in one study the hospital stay of elderly patients undergoing repair of a fractured femur was 12 days shorter in those who received additional care by a psychiatrist compared with a similar group treated a year earlier without psychiatric support.

Patients undergoing surgical procedures benefit from information that fosters healthy expectations and from behavioural or cognitive techniques that provide effective coping strategies and an enhanced sense of control. The challenge is to refine these interventions in a manner that allows for differences in individual coping style, variation in operative requirements, and nature of the relationship between the patient and members of the surgical team.

Some researchers have attempted to modify the risk of postoperative delirium. Supportive preoperative visits by a psychiatrist were shown in two studies to reduce the incidence of delirium following cardiac surgery. In a third study, preoperative psychiatric support combined with autohypnosis training failed to produce a statistically significant reduction in postcardiotomy delirium relative to controls with routine care. However, the number of patients who became delirious was insufficient to provide a conclusive result. In a more recent study 64 cardiac surgery patients informed by a nurse investigator of the possibility for unusual postoperative experiences were better able to cope with changes in cognition or perception.

Preoperative participation of a psychiatrist may be especially helpful in high risk procedures and when there is a critical demand for patient self-monitoring and compliance. Whenever the surgeon suspects significant psychopathology, or when there is a prior history of postoperative psychiatric difficulty or past medical non-compliance, a psychiatrist should be consulted.

PREOPERATIVE MANAGEMENT OF PSYCHIATRIC DISORDERS

Personality disorder

When a personality problem is identified, collaboration among primary physician, psychiatrist, and surgeon is necessary. Consistency is essential. The marginally adaptive patient should be enlisted in a specific care plan with a minimum of ambiguity. Good communication among caregivers helps with the demanding dependency of such patients and the emotions they may arouse. Paranoid and obsessive individuals manage best when one member of the team is designated as doctor in charge. The designated physician is ideally one who can relate to the patient and who can expend the time for repeated questions and detailed review of the care plan. At times one can advantageously enlist an interested family member who is a reassuring influence.

Major depressive disorder

If the patient is depressed, psychiatric help should be requested. It is often advisable to postpone the operation and to treat the depressive disorder. However, if a surgically correctable condition is strongly contributory to the mood disorder, there is little benefit in delay. In other instances the surgery may be urgent or the mood disorder intractable. Appropriate antidepressant medication should be given through the first preoperative day, and resumed postoperatively as soon as the patient can safely take sips by mouth. There are isolated reports of adverse interaction between tricyclics and anaesthetic agents, but the morbidity of recurrent depression carries a greater risk. Because combined use of halothane and tricyclic antidepressants may increase catecholamine levels, sympathomimetic agents should be used with caution in such situations.

Since antidepressants are metabolized in the liver, careful dosing and measurement of serum levels of the drug are required in patients with abnormal liver function. Imipramine is available for parenteral administration. Fluoxetine should be used with attention to its long half-life and with knowledge that it may increase levels of some other drugs. In all instances the anaesthetist and surgeon should be informed of medication requirements. Although there has been some controversy about preoperative use of monoamine oxidase inhibitors, they can be administered safely. Numerous patients have successfully undergone surgery and reported their prior monoamine oxidase inhibitor treatment after the operation.

Monoamine oxidase inhibitors interfere with the breakdown of central nervous system depressants. Potentially fatal adverse reactions are known to occur with meperidine, atropine, or other anticholinergic agents and with barbiturates. However morphine, oxycodone, and codeine can be used postoperatively for analgesia. Because monoamine oxidase inhibitors increase the level of catecholamines in peripheral nerve endings and potentiate the effect of sympathomimetic agents, hypertensive crisis may result from the use of pressors and the diet must be low in tyramine (which is especially high in aged cheese). Hypertensive crisis may also occur when monoamine oxidase inhibitors are combined with other classes of antidepressants such as tricyclics, serotonin uptake inhibitors (e.g. fluoxetine), or bupropion.

Anxiety disorder

Anxiety may be acute in onset and related to fear of surgery, or it may represent a chronic emotional disorder or personality trait. Some patients may not acknowledge distress, or may do so with difficulty because of social custom or personality style. It is best to ask the patient about special concerns. Some patients dread specific types of intervention, such as endotracheal tube placement. Since the average patient knows little about anatomy, much can be learned by eliciting misconceptions. It is helpful to know how patients have coped with prior surgery and with other stressful events. In a recent study of 1420 patients undergoing surgery at University of Iowa Hospital and Clinics, the best predictor of postoperative psychological distress was found to be preoperative psychological distress.

Anxiety may be increased by an over-zealous account of the planned procedure. However, an excessively paternal approach is insufficient to allow for the education and discussion necessary for the patient to make a judgement about the procedure and postoperative outcome.

Minor tranquillizers in the benzodiazepine class are a useful adjunct to psychological support. Shorter acting agents (for example alprazolam, lorazepam, oxazepam) are preferable for use in elderly and debilitated patients. Oxazepam and diphenhydramine are most easily metabolized in the liver and are the anxiolytic and sedative hypnotic agents of choice in patients with impaired hepatic function. The prescribing physician should be aware of the half-life and the potency of psychotropic agents and of the patient's past psychopharmacological history. Patients with debilitating anxiety should be referred for psychiatric assessment.

Panic disorder

Panic disorder, with or without agoraphobia, responds effectively to alprazolam, imipramine, or monoamine oxidase inhibitors. Ideally, monoamine oxidase inhibitors are best avoided or gradually discontinued 2 weeks prior to the operation. However, they can be continued when there is insufficient time for withdrawal, when anxiety symptoms are severe, or if alternative agents have proved ineffectual. Although imipramine has a slower onset of response than does alprazolam, it can be effectively instituted when surgery is elective, and it is available for parenteral administration. Sudden cessation following chronic administration of anxiolytics is often associated with rebound anxiety as well as by withdrawal symptoms. When oral medication cannot be administered a parenterally administered benzodiazepine can be used to provide sedation. Intravenous lorazepam and oral alprazolam are equipotential for the treatment of generalized anxiety. Lorazepam is also available for sublingual administration.

Phobic disorder

For patients with simple phobias a combination of behaviour therapy and anxiolytic agents can be helpful.

Hex or predilection to death

Hackett and Weisman give the example of a farmer whose certainty of postoperative fatality presaged his cardiovascular death 3 days after subtotal gastrectomy. These patients are noteworthy for the absence of anxiety or depression. When such a conviction is evident surgery is best avoided, if possible.

Functional psychosis

Psychotic patients often accommodate satisfactorily to the structure of a busy surgical service. Actively suicidal individuals require continuous close supervision by special duty nurses. Antipsychotic agents should be administered in full dose throughout the pre- and postoperative period. Aliphatic substituted phenothiazines (e.g. chlorpromazine,) are more likely to be associated with hypotension than the high potency neuroleptics (e.g. haloperidol). Patients should be managed in a simple direct manner aided, where possible, by supportive family members. The patient should be sheltered from stressful interpersonal relations. Competency should be established or appropriate guardianship arranged in consultation with hospital legal advisers.

Preoperative encephalopathy

Organic central nervous system disorders should be addressed with an appropriate search for underlying metabolic, infectious, and neurological causes. An unexpected rise in serum ammonia is sometimes evident in patients in whom other liver function tests are relatively mildly impaired. Treatment depends on the cause. Standard techniques should be employed, with reference to clock, calendar, availability of special personal effects, and gentle review of the daily routine. Excessive sedation should be avoided. Supportive nursing techniques and family visits often reduce agitation; low doses of haloperidol are also helpful. Caution is necessary when drugs are administered to patients with hepatic dysfunction. Diphenhydramine is a gentle treatment for insomnia. Benzodiazepines may cause confusion in the elderly, but some do benefit from low doses of short-acting agents.

Postoperative encephalopathy

Supportive care should be coupled with a search for specific aetiology. Anaesthetic agents or intolerance to specific analgesic agents or their metabolites (normeperidine delirium is an example) should be suspect as well as idiosyncratic reaction or toxicity to other medication. Depression of central nervous system function may be evidence of postoperative cardiopulmonary or infectious complication or of endocrinopathy. Postoperative delirium requires energetic treatment when agitation, mood lability, hallucinations, and delusions pose a threat to medical management. When delirium occurs in the intensive care unit, pharmacological intervention may include intravenous morphine, haloperidol, or lorazepam. A psychiatric consultant should visit daily, when possible, until the patient's sensorium is clear. Return of normal consciousness may be associated with feelings of shame or guilt among patients who retain memory for delusional material or perceptual aberrations. It is therefore wise to 'debrief' patients as cognition returns to baseline and to explain events in a supportive fashion. Patients are comforted to know that delirium does not represent a weakness of character or spirit but is rather a product of understandable biological events and environmental stress.

Although delirium was once a frequent complication of cardiovascular surgery, its incidence following coronary artery bypass grafting and cardiotomy has declined with improvement in surgical technology. The risk of delirium is increased with increasing age and lessened tolerance to decreased perfusion pressure, severity of physical illness, history of myocardial infarction, preoperative organic brain syndrome, duration of extracorporeal circulation, sustained mean arterial pressure under 50 mmHg during bypass, and postoperative hypotension requiring pressure pressors or an intra-aortic balloon pump. In a study of 23 patients undergoing aortic valve replacement, a previously unreported association was found between low preoperative cholesterol level, which was attributed to a probable catabolic state, and to postoperative psychopathology.

Steroid-induced psychosis following organ transplantation has become less frequent. Cyclosporin encephalopathy has been most frequent among liver transplant recipients and is characteristically associated with other signs of toxicity such as tremor, impaired renal function, and elevated blood pressure.

Delirium may occur secondary to alcohol withdrawal in current drinkers or in the recovered alcoholic in the absence of recent alcohol abuse. Another cause of delirium is acute sensory deprivation. Complex partial seizures should also be considered in the differential diagnosis.

Alcoholism

The one reported drink per night may be from a bottomless glass. Preoperative detoxification is best whenever possible; however, prevention of withdrawal is a primary goal. Supplemental nutritional support should be instituted and full doses of chlordiazepoxide should be administered every 4 to 6 h in patients suspected of alcoholic withdrawal. Intravenous alcohol is an alternative. Patients with addictive disorders may provoke an angry response from otherwise caring physicians. Participation of a psychiatric consultant is desirable.

Recovered alcoholics may feel vulnerable and are often apprehensive about a stress-related relapse. Patients who are attending Alcoholics Anonymous may be especially vigilant about perioperative medications and the potential euphoriant effects of narcotic analgesics. When psychotropic agents are advisable, pain should be taken to point out the medical indication. Some hospitals sponsor weekly Alcoholics Anonymous meetings. Supportive visits from 'safe' companions may reduce perioperative stress.

Drug-addicted patients

Treatment is similar to that of the alcoholic patient. Barbiturate requirements for patients addicted to depressants are established with a test dose of phenobarbital. Narcotic addicts who require surgery should not undergo drug withdrawal until after the operation. Pain relieving medication should be given in addition to that required for daily maintenance. After surgery, drug withdrawal can be approached in a standard method.

Pain intolerance

Inadequate analgesia is the most likely cause of persistent postoperative pain. Tolerance may occur among those receiving frequent daily analgesics over a period of weeks, but addiction is rare. Depression, anxiety, and tolerance to opioids increase postoperative analgesic needs and should be considered whenever pain persists in the absence of postoperative complications. Antidepressants of traditional narcotic adjuvants can be highly beneficial. Psychiatric consultants who are familiar with relaxation techniques and hypnosis can often provide symptom relief.

AWARENESS DURING OPERATIONS

Blacher reported six patients in whom postoperative symptoms of irritability, preoccupation with death, and nightmares were associated with expressed doubts about their sanity. All had experienced wakefulness at some point during their operation, unknown to the anaesthesiologist, and all benefited once a link was established between that event and their postoperative anxiety. One study reported a 1 per cent incidence of awareness among 490 patients undergoing various operative procedures who were interviewed by the same anaesthesiologist in each of the first three postoperative days. Studies of awareness, memory, and hearing among patients who were apparently unconscious under anaesthesia have led to surgeons being cautioned to avoid making disparaging or frightening remarks.

FURTHER READING

Aberg T, *et al.* Adverse effects on the brain in cardiac operations as assessed by biochemical psychometric and readiologic methods. *J Thorac Cardiovasc Surg* 1984; **87**: 99–105.

Abram HS, Gil BF. Prediction of post-operative psychiatric complications. *N Engl J Med* 1961; **265**: 1163.

Anthony JC, *et al.* Limits of the 'Mini-Mental State' as a screening test for demential and delirium among hospital patients. *Psychol Med* 1982; **12**: 397–408.

Blacher RS. On awakening paralyzed during surgery. *JAMA* 1975; **234**: 67–8.

Craven JL, Bright J, Dear CL. Psychiatric psychosocial and rehabilitative aspects of lung transplantation. *Clin Chest Med* 1990; **11**: 247–57.

Dubin WR, Field AL, Gastfriend DR. Postcardiotomy delirium: a critical review. *J Thorac Cardiovasc Surg* 1979; **77**: 586–99.

Egbert LD, Battit GE, Welch GE, Bartlett MK. Reduction of postoperative pain by encouragement and instruction of the patient. *N Engl J Med*, 1964; **270**: 825.

Engvall WR. Awareness during anesthesia. *Semin Anesth* 1988; **7**: 55–61.

Gath D, Cooper P, Day A. Hysterectomy and psychiatric disorder: I. Levels of psychiatric morbidity before and after hysterectomy. *Br J Psychiat* 1982; **140**: 335–50.

Jarvik ME. Drugs used in the treatment of psychiatric disorders. In: Goodman LS, Gilman A, eds. *The Pharmacological Basis of Therapeutics.* 3rd edn. London: Collier-Macmillan, 1969: 191–8.

Johnston M. Anxiety in surgical patients. *Psychol Med* 1980; **10**: 145–52.

Johnston M. Pre-operative existential status and post-operative recovery. In: Wise TN, ed. Advances in psychosomatic medicine. Guggenheim, FG ed. *Psychological Aspects of Surgery*. Basle: Karger, 1986; 1–20.

Layne OJ, Yudofsky SC. Postoperative psychosis in cardiotomy patients: the role of organic and psychiatric factors. *N Engl J Med* 1971; **284**: 518.

Levitan SJ, Kornfeld DK. Clinical and cost benefits of liaison psychiatry. *Am J Psychiatr* 1981; **138**: 790–3.

Lundberg SG, Guggenheim FG. Sequelae of limb amputation. In: Wise TN, ed. Advances in psychosomatic medicine. Guggenheim FG, ed. *Psychological Aspects of Surgery*. Basle: Karger, 1986; 199–210.

Lazarus HR, Hagens TH. Prevention of psychosis following open heart surgery. *Am J Psychiatr* 1968; **124**: 1190.

Marks RM, Sachar EJ. Under-treatment of medical inpatients with narcotic analgesics. *Ann Intern Med* 1973; **78**: 173.

Meninger KA. Polysurgery and polysurgical addiction. *Psychoanal Q* 1934; **3**: 173.

Merrikin KJ, Overcast TD. Patient selection for heart transplantation: When is a discriminating choice discrimination? *J Health Politics, Policy Law* 1985; **10**: 7–32.

Mumford E, Schlesinger HJ, Glass GV. The effects of psychological intervention on recovery from surgery and heart attacks: an analysis of the literature. *Am J Public Health* 1982; **72**: 144–51.

Naber D, Bullinger M. Neuroendocrine and psychological variables relating to postoperative psychosis after open-heart surgery. *Psychoneuroendocrinology* 1985; **10**: 315–24.

O'Hara MW, *et al.* Psychological consequences of surgery. *Psychosom Med* 1989; **51**: 356–70.

Owen JF, Hutelmyer CM. The effect of preoperative intervention on delirium in cardiac surgical patients. *Nursing Res* 1982; **31**: 60–2.

Ray C. The surgical patient: psychological stress and coping resources. In: Biver JR, ed. *Social Psychology and Behavioral Medicine.* New York: John Wiley & Sons, 1982.

Surman OS. Post noxious desensitization: some clinical notes on the combined use of hypnosis and systematic desensitization. *Am J Clin Hypnosis* 1979; **22**: 54–60.

Surman OS. Psychiatric aspects of organ transplantation. *Am J Psychiatry* 1989; **146**: 972–81.

Surman OS, Purtilo R. Organ transplants for ugly ducklings: II Allocation of scarce resources to unusual recipients. *Psychosomatics* 1992; **33**: 203–12.

Surman OS, Hackett TP, Silverman EL, Behrendt DM. Efficacy of psychotherapy for patients undergoing cardiac surgery. *Arch Gen Psychiatry* 1974; **30**: 830.

Weisman AD, Hackett TP. Psychosis after eye surgery: establishment of specific doctor-patient relationship in prevention and treatment of black patch delirium. *N Engl J Med* 1958; **258**: 1284.

Weisman AD, Hackett TP. Predilection to death. Death and dying as a psychiatric problem. *Psychosom Med.* 1961; **23**: 232–56.

Wilson SI, Vaughan RW, Stephen CR. Awareness, dreams and hallucinations associated with general anesthesia. *Anesth Analg Curr Res* 1975; **54**: 606–17.

Imaging in surgical practice 6

6.1 Conventional radiology

BASIL J. SHEPSTONE

Even though it is over a century since the discovery of X-rays by Wilhelm Roentgen on 8 November 1885 and in spite of the major advances in imaging techniques which are presented in subsequent sections, plain radiographs still command an important place in surgical practice. As the value of plain radiography will be illustrated extensively in specialist chapters, this section will concentrate mainly on the chest radiograph and plain films of the urinary tract.

THE CHEST

The posteroanterior chest radiograph is still the mainstay of the standard medical examination. In hospital practice a routine film on admission will provide a baseline for later comparison, following surgery, when infection, oedema, or collapse might supervene. The lateral projection is no longer carried out routinely, but may be necessary to localize a lesion anatomically (for interventional purposes) or to obtain a view of a structure not seen on the posteroanterior view, for example the right-ventricular border, the left-atrial border, the oblique fissure, the posterior costophrenic angle, or the spine. It is also useful for the differential diagnosis of mediastinal masses.

The key to successful diagnosis of the chest radiograph is its systematic examination, which must include the soft-tissue shadows (breast, muscles, cutaneous tissues), the diaphragmatic and subdiaphragmatic areas (of great importance to the surgeon), the bony cage (ribs, clavicles, scapulae, spine, proximal humeri), the lung fields, the heart, and mediastinum. Whenever possible, bilateral and symmetrical structures must be carefully compared.

Although it is the duty of the radiographer to produce a technically perfect product, it is still imperative that the film reader checks that this is achieved. For example, positioning must be exact with both left and right costophrenic angles and apices within the film area. The scapulae must not overlap the bony cage. Penetration, as tested by the thoracic vertebrae just being visible through the heart shadow, must be assessed. Underpenetration may produce a useless white film, whereas an overpenetrated film, although looking very black, can be salvaged by the use of a bright light. Rotation with respect to the cassette, which can cause discrepancies in the appearance of the left and right lung fields, must be checked by making sure that the angles made by the clavicle with the vertical are the same on each side. Finally, the degree of inspiration must be checked by counting the number of ribs, preferably on the right side, that appear above the right hemidiaphragm. Ten posterior ribs are the norm. If more than this number can be counted and there is also flatness of the hemidiaphragms, with a decrease in the number and size of the lung markings, chronic obstructive disease may be present.

The routine view is, of course, taken in the posteroanterior position (which refers to the direction of the beam) so that the anteriorly-situated heart can be as close to the film as possible (Fig. 1). This enables an accurate estimation of the so-called cardiothoracic ratio to be made (the ratio of the width of the cardiac shadow at its widest point to the diameter of the thorax at its widest point). The normal cardiothoracic ratio is less than 50 per cent.

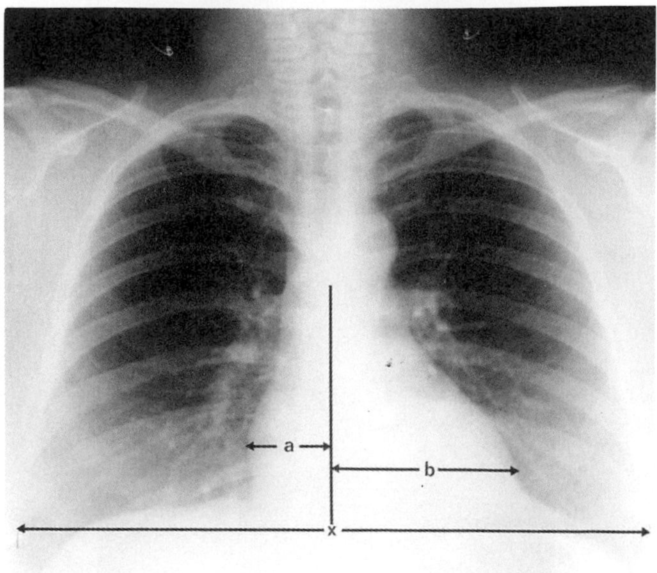

Fig. 1 A normal posteroanterior chest radiograph showing how to calculate the cardiothoracic ratio (equal to $(a+b)/x$) and which should normally be less than 0.5.

Tumours of the lung and mediastinum

The routine chest radiograph is still the first investigation of choice in the diagnosis of bronchial carcinoma (Fig. 2). Either the primary tumour or one of its secondary effects or complications may be seen, or both. Among the latter is identification of metastases to the mediastinum or elsewhere.

The primary tumour may present as an opaque nodule, but tumours are not the only cause of pulmonary nodules and the differential diagnoses include abscesses or granulomata, infarctions, haematomas, focal collagen disease, retention cysts, sequestrated segments, arteriovenous malformations, and hamartomas. Also, the lesion may be pleural based, when encysted pleural effusions and fibromata are possible. Finally, the lesion may not lie within the pulmonary parenchyma itself, but on the surface of the body e.g. a large wart or mole (Fig. 3).

Malignant tumours may be primary or secondary carcinomas, but may also be lymphomas or plasmacytomas.

A bronchial carcinoma often blocks the bronchus from which it arises and in this case leads to absorption collapse of the affected segments or lobes (Fig. 4). Superimposed infection then also usually occurs. Unless there is another good reason for the collapse in an adult (e.g. bronchiectasis with inspissated pus, asthma with mucoid impaction, or inhaled foreign body) bronchial carcinoma must always be suspected. Cavitating lesions may be due either to tumours or abscesses, although an area of infarction can also break down (Fig. 5).

A hilar mass may represent metastases to the mediastinal lymph

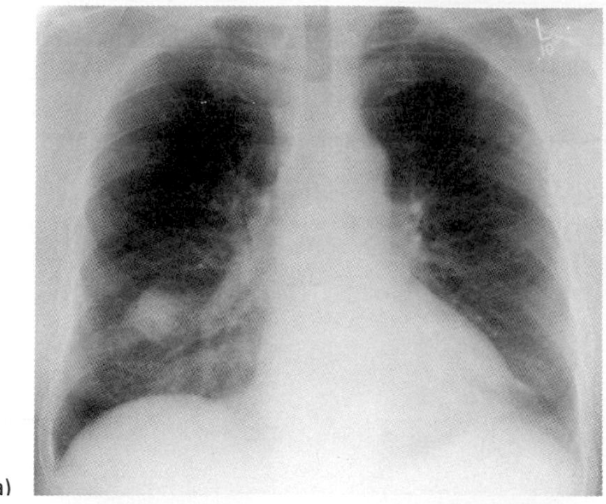

(a)

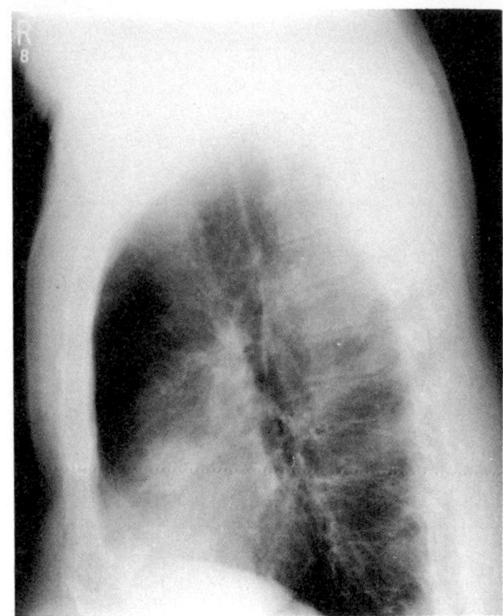

(b)

Fig. 2 Primary bronchial carcinoma presenting as a solitary nodule in the right lung (by courtesy of Dr Fergus Gleason).

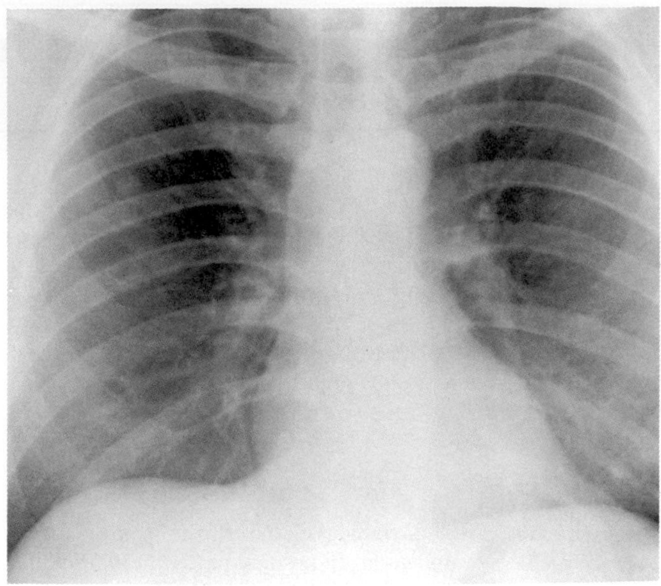

Fig. 3 A skin wart appearing as a solitary nodule in the right upper zone of an otherwise normal chest radiograph.

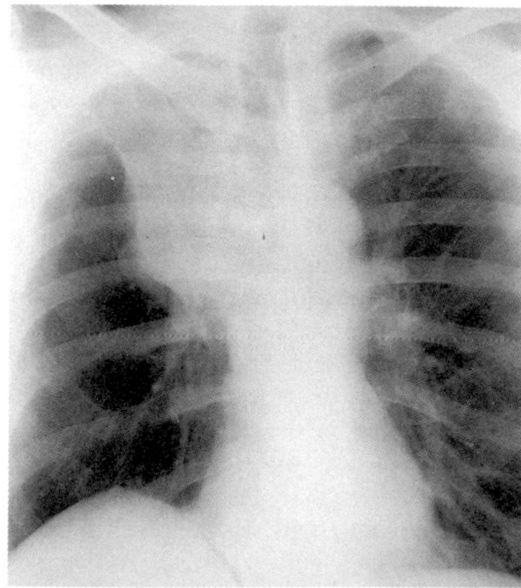

Fig. 4 Collapse of the right upper lobe due to a bronchial carcinoma, with elevation of the horizontal fissure and the right hilum.

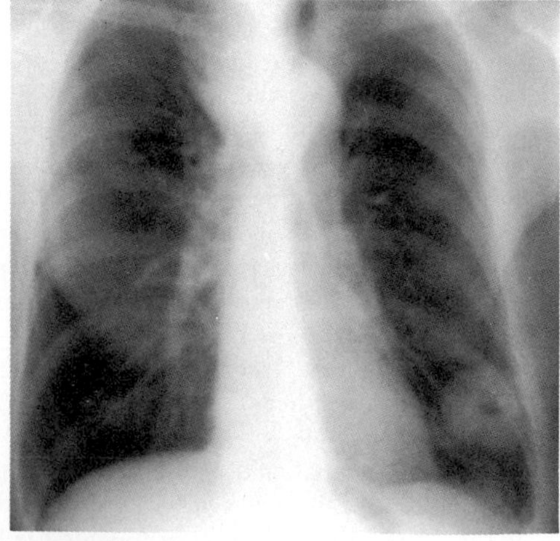

Fig. 5 A cavitating tumour at the left base.

nodes (Fig. 6) and a pleural effusion may also arise as a result of a malignant tumour (Fig. 7), although infection and infarction can also cause unilateral effusions. Failure of major organ systems like the heart, kidneys, and liver are also common causes of effusions, but these are usually bilateral. A hilar carcinoma or metastases to the mediastinal nodes can involve the phrenic nerve, with subsequent elevation and paresis of a hemidiaphragm (Fig. 8).

In an apical or so-called 'Pancoast' tumour there is often lysis of the adjacent ribs. Metastases to bone in general may present as lytic or sclerotic lesions, depending on the aggressiveness of the tumour. Alternatively, they may present with pathological fractures.

The lungs are a common site for haematogenous metastases, where they often produce multiple round nodules of different sizes (Fig. 9) (as opposed to granulomatous disease, where the nodules are usually small and of similar size (Fig. 10)). Alternatively, lymphatic spread may show a reticular, almost fibrous-looking appearance, often with septal lines and is referred to as lymphangitis carcinomatosa (Fig. 11).

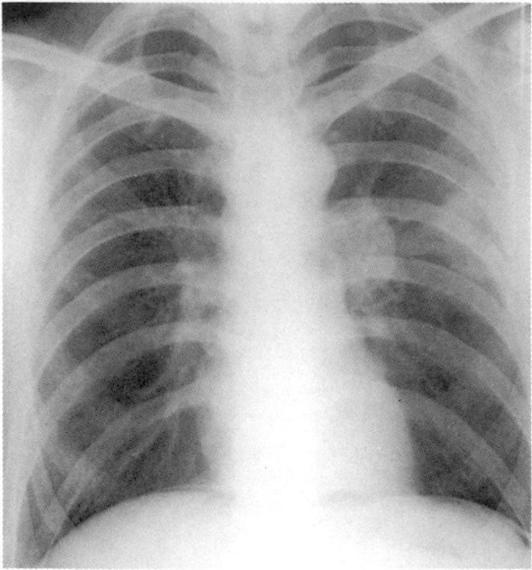

Fig. 6 An enlarged left hilar node due to an associated bronchial carcinoma appearing as an amorphous cavitating lesion.

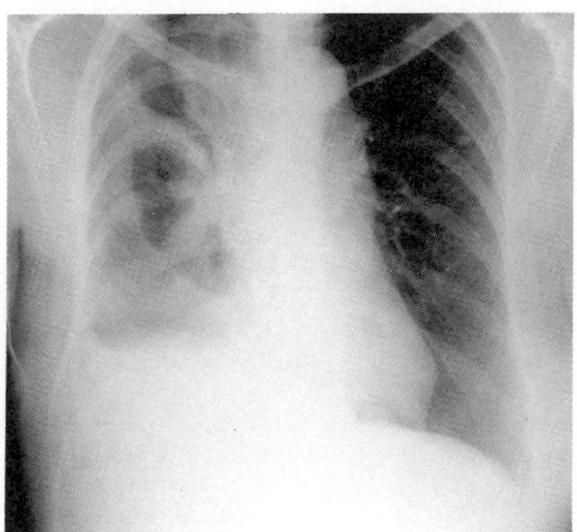

Fig. 7 A right malignant pleural effusion in a woman who has undergone right mastectomy.

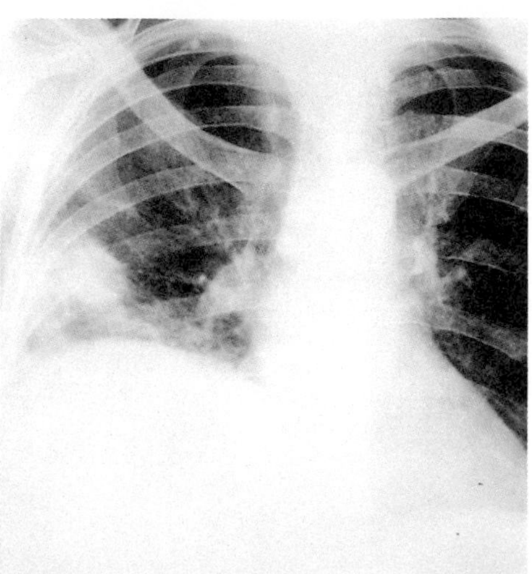

Fig. 8 A raised right hemidiaphragm due to phrenic-nerve paralysis in a patient with carcinoma of the right lung.

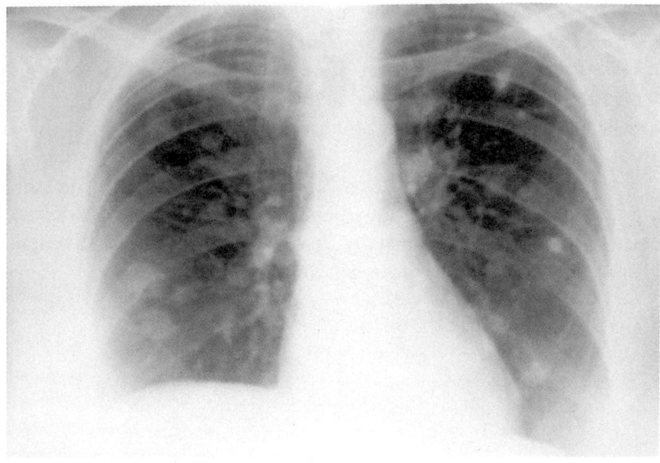

Fig. 9 Pulmonary metastases in a patient with a primary renal carcinoma.

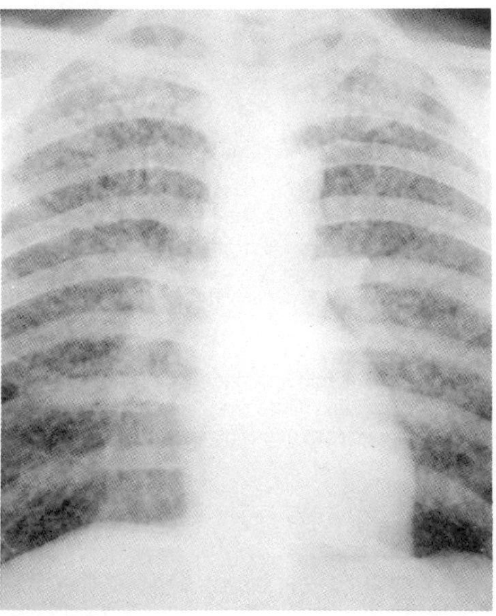

Fig. 10 Miliary tuberculosis.

Lymphoma usually affects the mediastinum. Hodgkin's disease, which is the most common of the lymphomas, normally affects the paratracheal glands, leading to local enlargement and generalized widening of the superior mediastinum (Fig. 12). Leukaemia and sarcoidosis can, however, lead to similar appearances, although sarcoidosis classically enlarges the hilar glands.

Infections of the lungs

These usually present as diffuse, water-dense opacities (Fig. 13). Lobar pneumonia is now not often seen, but when it is, the opacity usually outlines an entire lobe. If resolution is incomplete, fibrosis may appear and bronchiectasis may be seen as a late sequel. The more common bronchopneumonia gives similar densities, but they are usually more patchy and are seen mainly in the lower lobes. Pneumonitis gives a similar picture, with the opacities usually confined to one segment of a lobe.

The very common acute or chronic bronchitis may show nothing on chest radiography because bronchi are air-filled structures superimposed on an air-filled background and thus comply with the rules of radiology that a structure or an area of pathology can be seen only if its radiographic density is different from that of an adjacent tissue.

In bronchiectasis, however, the bronchi do become thick enough to be seen and so may be seen as end-on ring shadows or else small cystic areas, usually at the bases (Fig. 14). Bronchography is necessary before resection is considered.

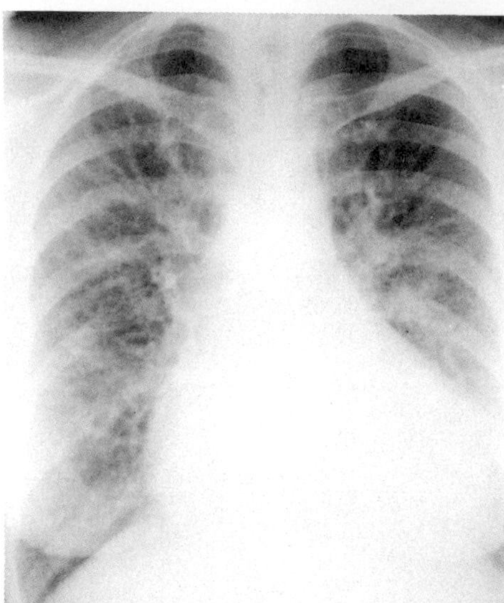

Fig. 11 Lymphangitis carcinomatosa in a patient with a primary carcinoma of the pancreas. (Note the septal lines, which are not pathognomonic of interstitial pulmonary oedema. They are also seen in the pneumoconioses.)

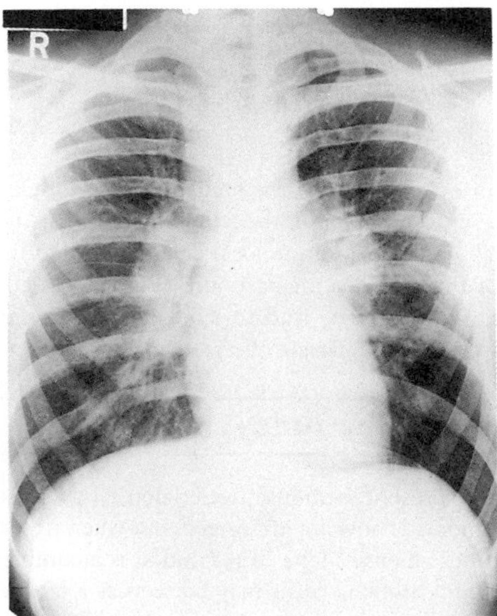

Fig. 12 Bilateral enlargement of the hilar nodes and the right paratracheal nodes in a patient with leukaemia. These appearances are also encountered in lymphoma and sarcoidosis.

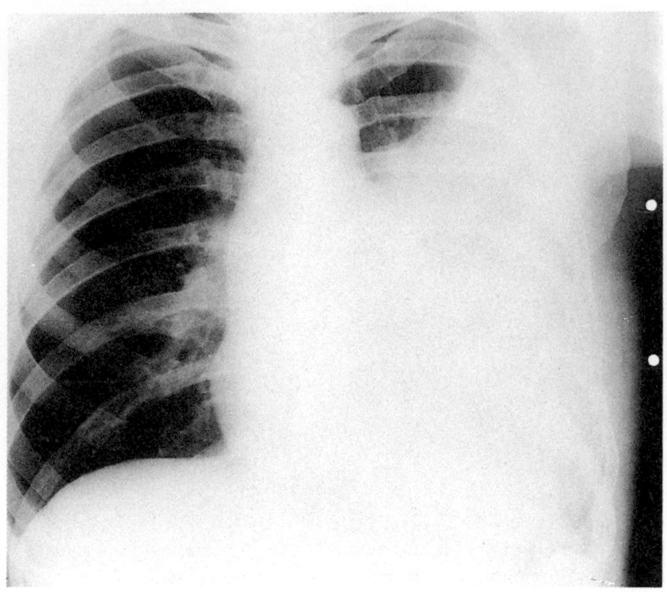

Fig. 13 Widespread left-sided pneumoniac consolidation.

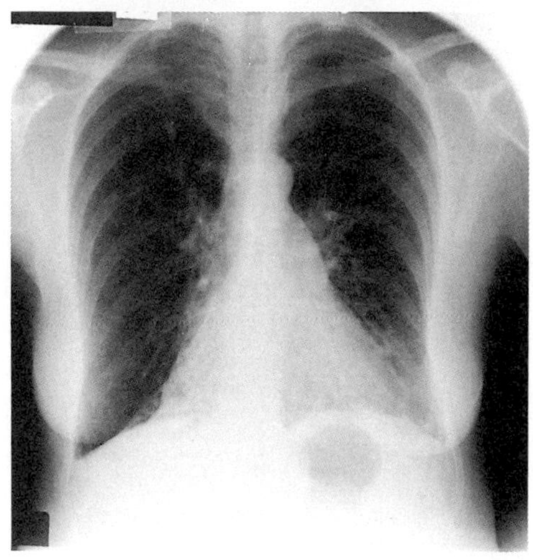

Fig. 14 Lower-zone bronchiectasis (with collapse of both right middle and lower lobes due to inspissated pus).

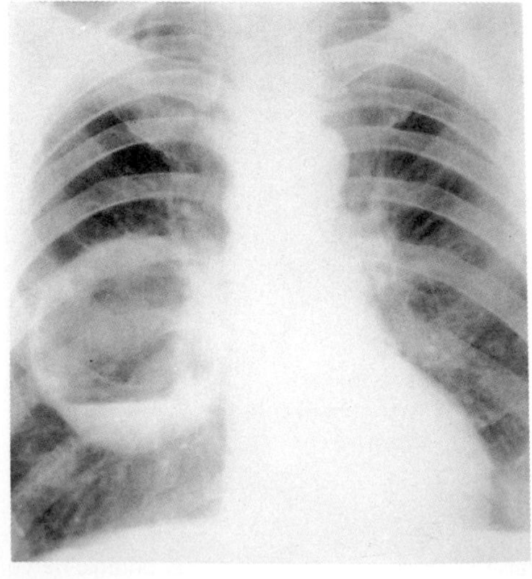

Fig. 15 A large pyogenic cavitating abscess in the right lung.

Infected areas, especially those distal to an occluded bronchus, may break down to form local abscesses with fluid levels (Fig. 15).

The characteristic radiographic appearance of tuberculosis in children is an area of water density with enlarged hilar glands in the affected side. It is important to remember that tuberculosis is the only infection which can enlarge hilar lymph nodes enough to make them visible on the routine chest radiograph. Alternatively the disease can present with a miliary pattern, consisting of multiple small round opacities of similar size throughout the chest (Fig. 10). In adult infections, the disease has a tendency to spread to the posterior segment of the upper lobe and appear as an apical lesion which can cavitate. A mycetoma may later appear in the cavity (Fig. 16).

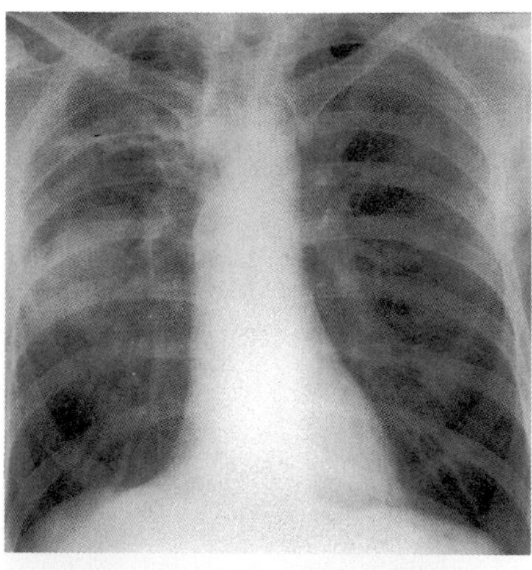

(a)

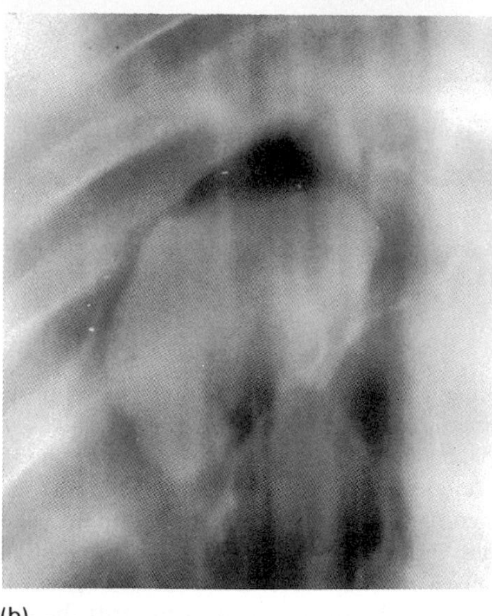

(b)

Fig. 16 An aspergilloma in an old tuberculous cavity at the apex of the right lower lobe.

In patients who are immunosuppressed for any reason, but especially as a result of AIDS, unusual opportunistic infections may occur, for example those from *Pneumocystis carinii* or cytomegalovirus (Fig. 17).

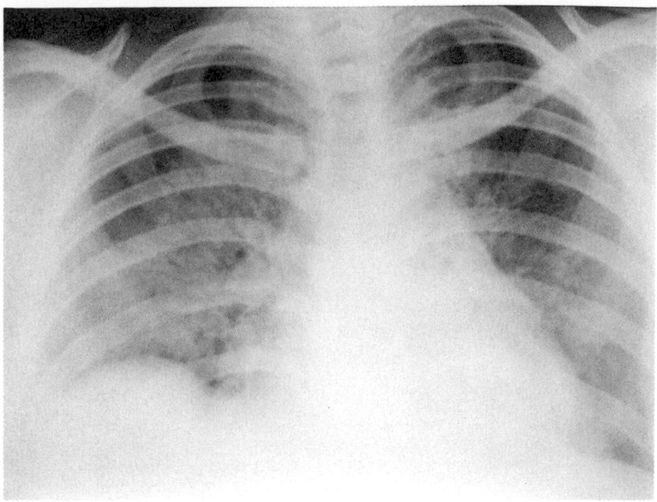

Fig. 17 *Pneumocystis carinii* infection in a patient with AIDS.

Obstructive airways disease

Obstructive airways disease includes the various types of emphysema and asthma and presents radiologically as elongated, translucent lung fields with flattened diaphragms, prominent hilar shadows, and a decrease in the number and size of the lung markings. In emphysema, bullae may occur. These are translucent areas where the alveolar walls have broken down and appear as black areas which are devoid of lung markings and are delineated by fine, curvilinear markings (Fig. 18).

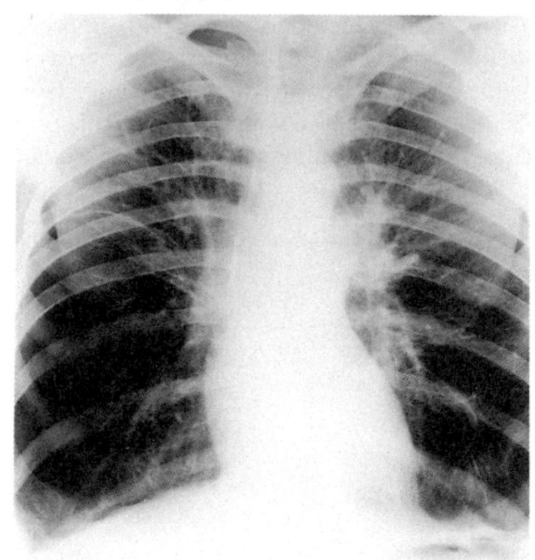

Fig. 18 An elderly man with bullous emphysema.

Sarcoidosis

Like tuberculosis, this disease is characterized by non-caseating granulomatous lesions which can affect the lungs, skin, eyes, and even bone. In the lungs, the disease classically presents with symmetrical, bilateral hilar, and paratracheal gland enlargement

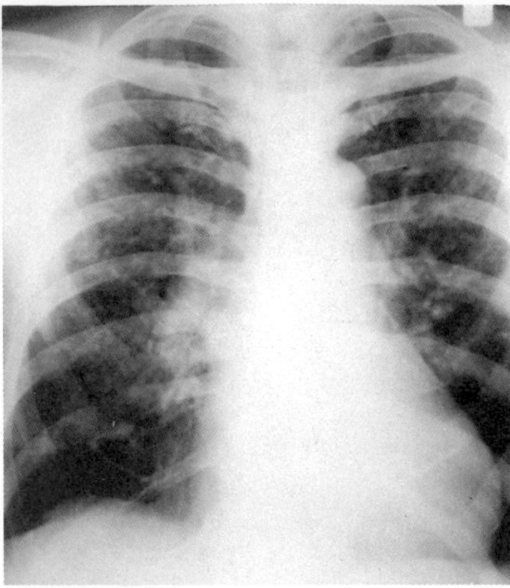

Fig. 19 The nodular-reticular pattern characteristic of sarcoidosis (some hilar lymphadenopathy is still visible).

(Fig. 12). If the disease progresses, the lung fields may demonstrate a nodular-reticular pattern, (Fig. 19) which proceeds to fibrosis and emphysema.

The pneumoconioses

This is a collective name for a group of conditions usually arising in workers from industrial enterprises such as mining where foreign substances are inhaled. These include silica, iron, tin, talc, asbestos, and beryllium. Silicosis is perhaps the most common of the pneumoconioses. In the early stages there is a widespread small-nodular pattern, which once again may proceed to fibrosis and bullous emphysema. In silicosis the fibrotic areas often occur bilaterally and symmetrically in the upper lung fields and are 'geometric' in shape—so-called conglomerate masses characteristic of the entity known as pulmonary massive fibrosis (Fig. 20).

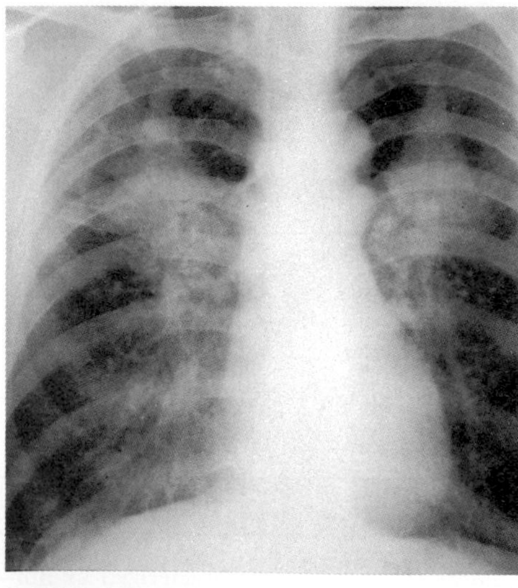

Fig. 20 A retired coal miner with progressive massive fibrosis due to silicosis. The symmetrical rhomboid opacities in the upper zones are called 'conglomerate masses'.

The pleura

Pleural tumours are rare, but the malignant pleural tumour mesothelioma occurs in workers with asbestos. Such workers may also develop pleural or diaphragmatic calcification and are prone to develop asbestosis *per se*, which gives a characteristically diffuse reticular pattern to the lung fields.

Pleural effusions may be free or encysted (Fig. 7 and 21 respectively). When free, they manifest as basal opacities which initially fill the costophrenic angles and then rise up the hemithorax towards the axilla, usually with a meniscus. They may be seen following infections like pneumonia or tuberculosis, infarctions, or malignancy. They are also seen as complications of cardiac failure, hypoproteinaemic states (like hepatic failure), and renal failure (the 'uraemic lung'). Empyema, or pus in the pleural space, which was common in tuberculosis, is now rarely seen as a post-pneunomic complication.

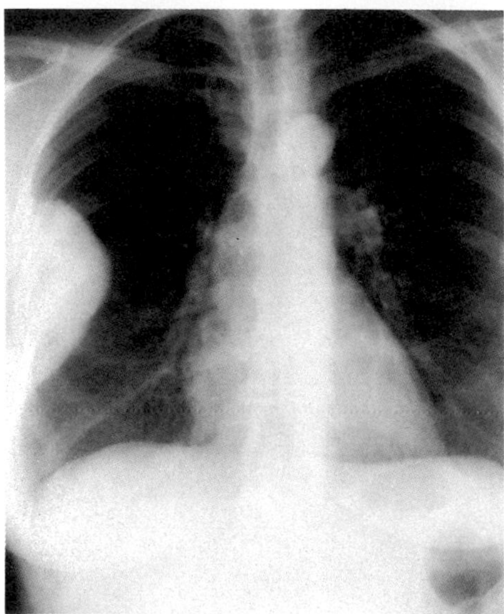

Fig. 21 An encysted pleural effusion in the right midzone following an infection.

Spontaneous pneumothorax is common in young people and, although sometimes ascribed to the rupture of a bulla, its aetiology is usually unknown (Fig. 22).

Pneumothorax may also be due to trauma and is often associated with rib fractures. Tension pneumothorax occurs when air continues to enter the space, but cannot escape because the tear in the pleura acts like a one-way valve. It is therefore essential to observe any shift in the mediastinal structures towards the opposite side and, if so, to equilibrate the pressures immediately.

The heart

The posteroanterior chest radiograph can yield information about the cardiac diameter, enlargement of individual chambers, and the state of the pulmonary vasculature. The cardiothoracic ratio has already been considered.

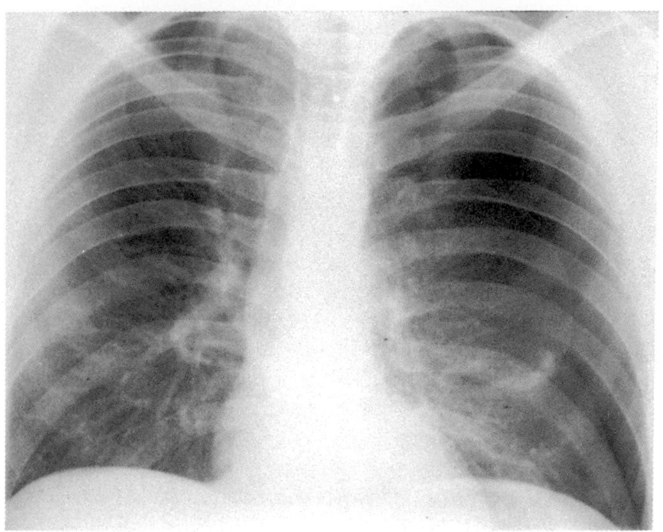

Fig. 22 A left-sided pneumothorax in a young man with some shift of the mediastinum to the right.

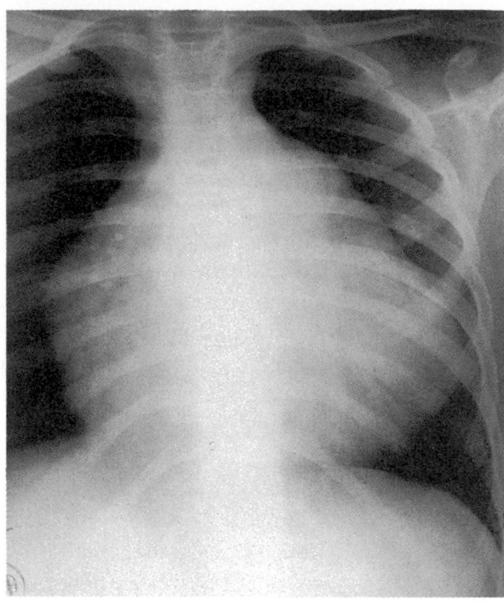

Fig. 23 A child with Fallot's tetralogy showing the misnamed 'boot-shaped' heart and oligaemic lung fields.

In the posteroanterior view the right heart border is formed by the right atrium with the superior vena cava entering it from above. On the left side three protuberances may be seen. The top one is the aortic knuckle, the next one the pulmonary outflow tract (opposite the left main pulmonary artery which constitutes the left hilum—normal lymph nodes and bronchi are invisible), and the lower one is the border of the left ventricle. The left atrium lies behind the heart, but occasionally the prominent auricular appendage of an enlarged left atrium will form a further protuberance between the pulmonary outflow tract and the left ventricular border. On the lateral view, the right ventricle forms the anterior border and the left atrium most of the posterior border, where it is a close relation of the invisible oesophagus.

The diagnosis of left-ventricular enlargement is made on the posteroanterior view when its border moves outwards and the apex downwards. Right-ventricular enlargement is diagnosed on the lateral view by noting that the anterior border has risen up higher behind the sternum. On the posteroanterior view, it manifests as a lateral shift of both the left and right heart borders, but with the apex tilted upwards (forming the imaginatively-named 'boot-shaped heart') (Fig. 23). In biventricular enlargement the left and right borders are also displaced laterally, but the apex stays in its normal horizontal plane. The right-ventricular component is again observed on the lateral view, where left-ventricular enlargement shifts the lower posterior border too little for detection.

Isolated right atrial enlargement is very rare, but would shift the right-hand border laterally. Left atrial enlargement, arising mainly from mitral-valve disease, forms a double shadow behind the heart as the enlarged chamber penetrates posteriorly and towards the right, surrounded by air-filled lung which provides the contrast. It will also splay the carina, resulting in a left main bronchus pointing laterally rather than downwards towards the left costophrenic angle. The proof of an enlarged left atrium is obtained from looking at a lateral chest after the patient has swallowed some barium. The enlarged left atrium will then indent the contrast-filled oesophagus as it curves round the posterior border of the heart towards the hiatus (Fig. 24).

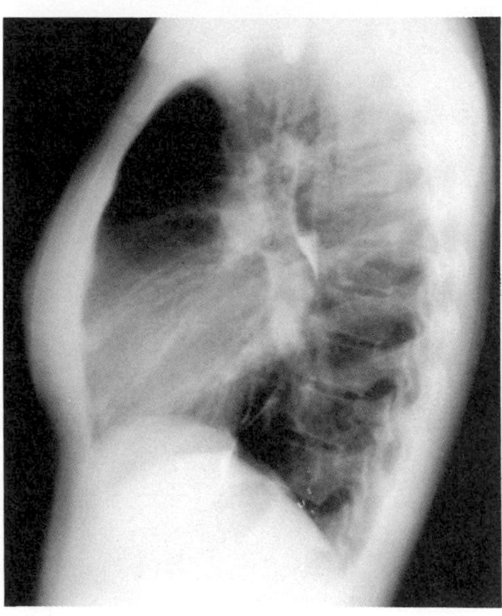

Fig. 24 Lateral chest with barium showing indentation of the barium column in a patient with a large left atrium due to mitral stenosis.

Pulmonary appearances in heart disease

The appearance of the lungs provides major clues to the diagnosis of heart disease. Normally the lower-zone vessels are more prominent and larger than the upper-zone vessels and the outer rim of the chest is usually free of lung markings. Because of the disposition of the left and right pulmonary arteries and bronchi, the left hilum is slightly higher than the right and as they emerge from the hila, the main right and left pulmonary arteries have a largely vertical configuration. The pulmonary veins, on the other hand, return to the left atrium, which is about 5 cm below the hila. The veins returning from the upper zones therefore run vertically, whereas those draining the lower zones run horizontally. It is, thus, not possible to differentiate between arteries and veins in the upper half of the lung fields, whereas in the lower half, arteries are vertically disposed and veins horizontally.

In pulmonary venous hypertension (the chief causes of which are mitral-valve disease and left-ventricular failure) both the vertical upper-zone and the horizontal lower-zone veins become larger. The latter are seen coming in right from the periphery, an area where there are normally no markings. As the pressure rises, pulmonary oedema will occur, which first fills the interstitial and then the alveolar spaces. The lower zones become hazy and vessel differentiation is lost. This and true upper-zone venous enlargement contribute to the characteristic 'upper-lobe diversion', when the upper-lobe vessels appear larger and more prominent than the lower-lobe vessels. Interstitial oedema may appear as septal lines in the costophrenic angles, but these are short-lived as water, accumulating on each side, soon obliterates these distended interlobular lymphatics. A much more certain sign is peribronchial oedema or 'cuffing' when the normally-invisible end-on bronchi become visible as black holes because of the surrounding fluid—a variant of the so-called 'air bronchogram' (Fig. 25). There may be pleural effusions to a greater or lesser degree, or if no treatment is offered, full-blown perihilar alveolar oedema which presents as widespread cotton-wool-like opacities in the central areas (Fig. 26).

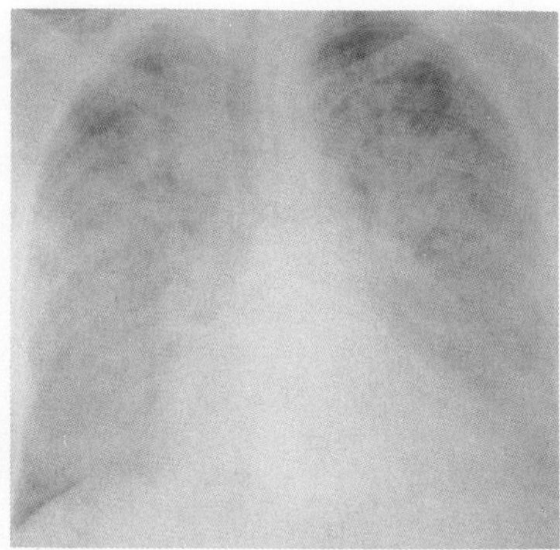

Fig. 26 Florid alveolar pulmonary oedema, in this case due to congestive cardiac failure, but which is not pathognomonic of this condition as it can occur wherever there is alveolar damage.

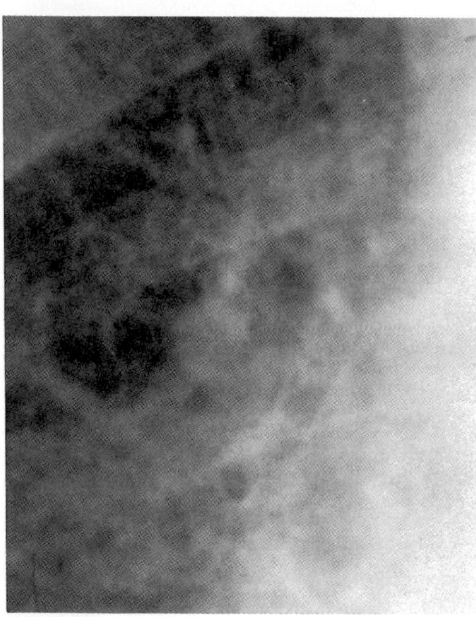

Fig. 25 Detail of a chest radiograph of a patient with pulmonary oedema to demonstrate 'peribronchial cuffing'—a variant of the 'air-bronchogram' sign.

In pure pulmonary arterial hypertension, which arises when there is either increased pulmonary blood-flow (e.g. anaemia, thyrotoxicosis, left-to-right shunts) or peripheral arterial close-down (e.g. primary pulmonary arterial hypertension, pulmonary emboli, chronic obstructive lung disease) there is so-called pulmonary plethora with an enlarged pulmonary outflow tract, left and right main pulmonary arteries, and the rest of the vertically-disposed arterial tree (Fig. 27). Obviously it may also arise from pulmonary venous hypertension and the two varieties often occur together, usually in left-heart failure.

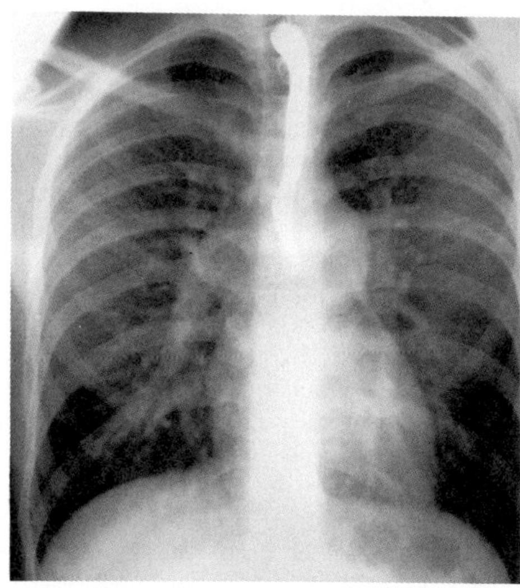

Fig. 27 A patient with pulmonary arterial hypertension due to left-to-right shunt. Note the large pulmonary outflow tract.

Decreased-pulmonary flow (pulmonary oligaemia) is seen in obstruction in the pulmonary outflow tract at or below the pulmonary valves. The classical example is Fallot's tetratology (Fig. 23).

Pericardial perfusions and cardiac calcifications

These are traditionally classified under the headings inflammatory, non-inflammatory, and malignant, and in fact the causes are very similar to those producing pleural effusions.

The common inflammatory causes are suppurative, viral, tuberculotic, and rheumatic. Non-inflammatory causes include heart-failure, uraemia, and myocardial infarction. The effusion could also be due to blood in the pericardial sac from trauma or from a ruptured aortic or left-ventricular aneurysm.

Constrictive pericarditis may be a sequel to viral or tuberculous pericarditis and is sometimes seen after haemorrhage into the pericardium or in one or two of the collagen diseases. Subsequent fibrosis of the pericardium may lead to cardiac tamponade and right-heart failure. About half of the cases lead to calcification (Fig. 28).

Cardiac calcification may also be seen in the mitral and aortic valves, the coronary arteries, and in the left atrium, where it occurs as mural thrombus (Fig. 29).

Mediastinal opacities

A lateral view is mandatory for the differential diagnosis of mediastinal opacities, the usual approach being to separate those occurring in the anterior, middle, and posterior compartments.

Anterior compartment

The normal structures in this compartment are the thymus, retrosternal lymph nodes, the ascending aorta and, occasionally, a retrosternal extension of the thyroid.

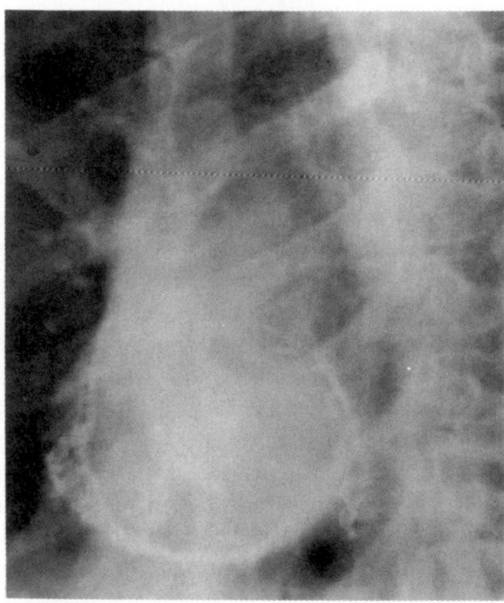

Fig. 28 An old oblique chest film showing a calcified pericardium due to tuberculosis.

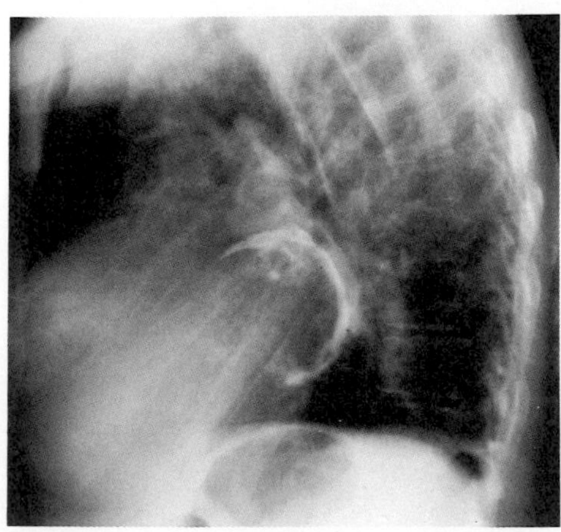

Fig. 29 Calcified left-atrial thrombus.

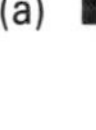

(a)

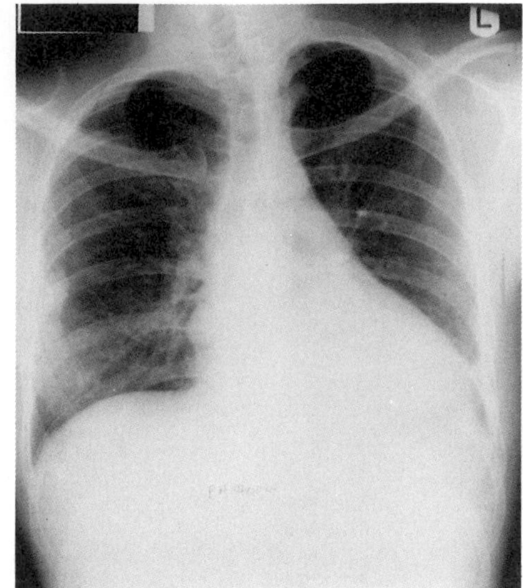

(b)

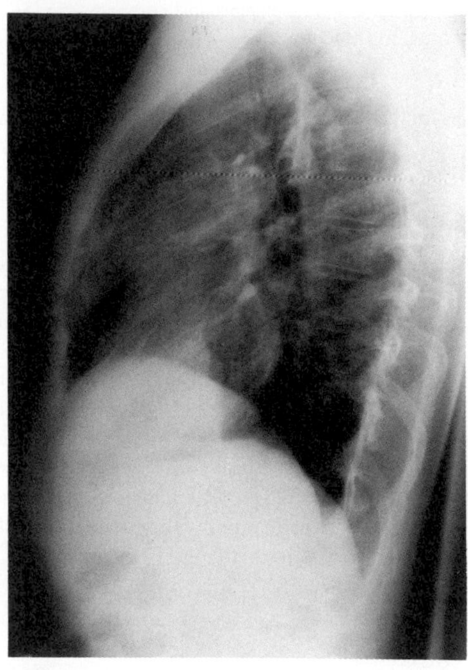

Fig. 30 Posteroanterior (a) and lateral (b) chest film of a patient with myasthenia gravis who was found to have a thymoma occupying the anterior translucent space (by courtesy of Dr Fergus Gleeson).

Opacities occurring in this compartment may therefore be due to thymomas (Fig. 30), enlarged lymph nodes, aneurysm of the ascending aorta, or retrosternal goitre (Fig. 31). Other possibilities are dermoid tumours, pericardiocoelomic cysts, parathyroid adenomas, and hernia of Morgagni.

Middle compartment

Middle-mediastinal structures include the aortic arch and its branches, the pulmonary artery, the inferior and superior venae cavae, and the heart.

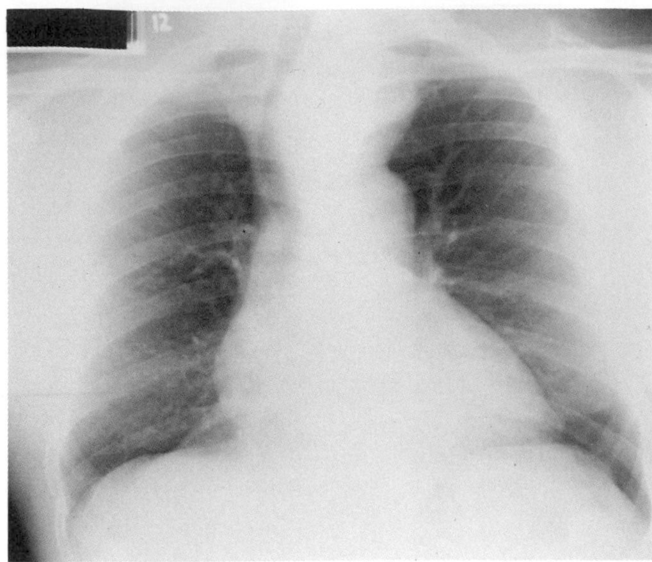

Fig. 31 Posteroanterior chest radiograph of a patient with a retrosternal goitre which is displacing and compressing (a fundamental sign) the trachea.

Anomalies may be due to a big left atrium, aortic aneurysm, bronchial cyst, enlarged hilar lymph nodes (due to lymphoma, leukaemia, sarcoidosis, tuberculosis, or metastases).

Posterior compartment

Structures normally occurring in this compartment are the trachea and bronchi, oesophagus, descending aorta, lymph nodes, vagi, spine, and nerves emerging through the intervertebral foramina.

Abnormalities include tumours of neurogenic origin (neurofibroma, ganglioneuroma, neuroblastoma, myelocele, and meningomyelocele), paravertebral abscess, aneurysm of the descending aorta, sequestrated lung segments, reduplication cysts of the oesophagus, loculated pleural effusions, corrective-tissue tumours, Zenker's diverticulum, and oesophageal lesions (achalasia (Fig. 32), hiatus hernia (Fig. 33), leiomyoma, and sub- or epiphrenic diverticula).

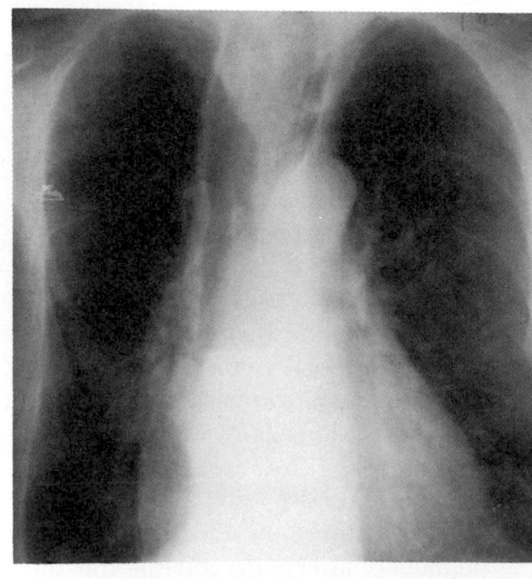

Fig. 32 Achalasia of the oesophagus with a fluid level.

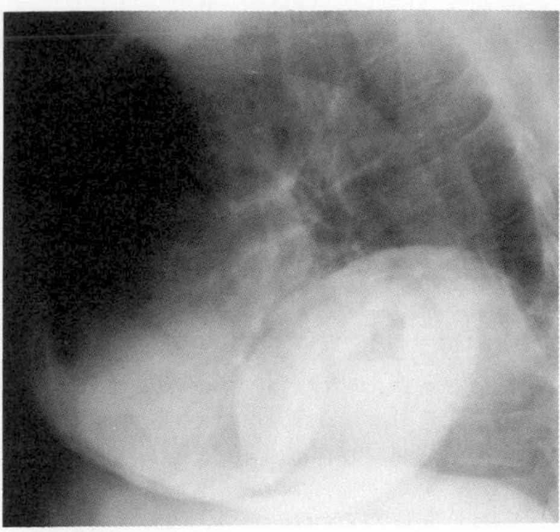

Fig. 33 Lateral chest of an obese woman with a large hiatus hernia occupying most of the posterior mediastinum.

The postoperative chest

After general surgery, poor respiratory effort and retained secretions lead to local collapse, often referred to as 'plate atelectasis', which usually appears as horizontal lines in the lower zones. Pleural effusions are also common, but both of these entities resolve soon after surgery. General anaesthesia may lead to aspiration pneumonia or even to the full-blown adult respiratory distress syndrome. The radiographic appearances of this syndrome are indistinguishable from pulmonary oedema due to cardiac failure, fluid overload, or any form of alveolar damage. Pulmonary emboli may lead to an oligaemic area of lung with vessel cut-off, but it is usually diagnosed on pulmonary perfusion–ventilation scintigraphy. When the resulting infarction becomes established it manifests as a water-dense wedge which may cavitate.

A subphrenic collection of pus, blood, or fluid can lead to eleva-

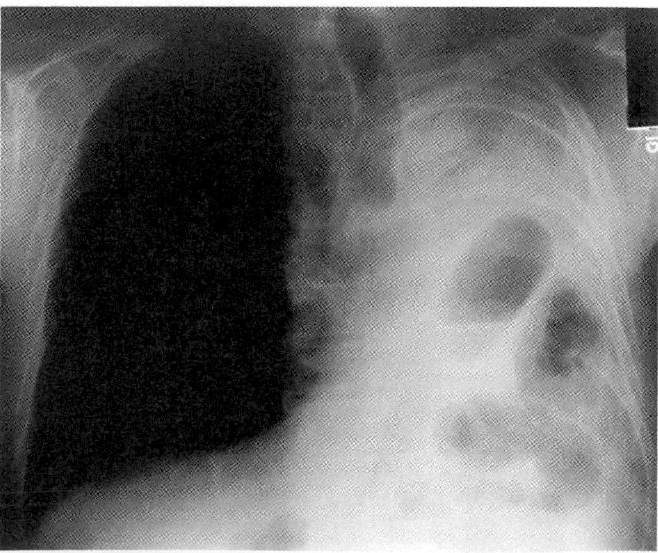

Fig. 34 Chest radiograph of a man who has undergone a left upper lobectomy.

tion of the hemidiaphragm and an associated 'sympathetic' pleural effusion. Air under the diaphragm is common after abdominal surgery, but it may arise from an anaerobic infection or perforation of a viscus. Occasionally it may arise from the lung or via the vagina in women.

The hallmark of a thoracotomy is a resected 4th, 5th, or 6th rib. Partial regeneration of the rib can take place. After a lobectomy or a sublobectomy resection, the remaining lung should expand to fill the volume previously occupied by the resected segment. This will be accompanied by appropriate shift of landmarks. However, in spite of drainage, pleural effusions, empyema and haemothorax can occur and it is not uncommon to see a mixture of expanded lung and organizing fluid densities (Fig. 34). Poor closure of a bronchus can lead to bronchopleural fistula and early surgical emphysema in the soft tissues is a common occurrence. After pneumonectomy there is a combination of hyperinflation of the remaining lung with consequent shift of the mediastinum towards the side of the operation and the accumulation of fluid in the pneumonectomy space. Any chest operation can lead to phrenic nerve damage and elevated hemidiaphragm, but the nerve is often crushed deliberately to reduce the size of the treated hemithorax.

Open-heart surgery is done via a sternal split, radiographic evidence for which is the presence of wire sternal sutures. A widened mediastinum and associated pleural effusions are common and air may enter any of the pleura, pericardium, or peritoneum. Sudden widening of the mediastium may indicate haemorrhage or an aortic dissection. The postpericardotomy syndrome is characterized by pain, fever, and pleurisy and the cardiac outline is enlarged by a pericardial effusion visible with echocardiography.

THE GENITOURINARY TRACT

Plain abdominal radiographs are essential before embarking upon contrast studies of the kidneys. As the perinephric fat is translucent, the kidneys are often visible lateral and parallel to the psoas lines, opposite T12, L1, and L2 and with the left kidney about 1.5 cm higher than the right. As the perirenal fat line persists after nephrectomy, the evidence for this operation is a resected rib and not an absent renal outline.

Even on plain film it may be possible to recognize an enlarged or shrunken kidney. The latter could be due to chronic pyelonephritis, chronic glomerulonephritis, or renal ischaemia, whereas enlargement may be due to hydronephrosis, a tumour, or simply to compensatory hypertrophy. Bilaterally enlarged kidneys may be due to polycystic disease or to bilateral hydronephrosis. Kidneys are also enlarged in acute situations such as acute pyelonephritis.

Calcification in the renal area is very common and usually due to renal calculi, the majority of which are opaque (Fig. 35). Diffuse calcification of the parenchyma, known as nephrocalcinosis, is uncommon, but may be seen in tuberculosis, hyperparathyroidism, renal-tubular acidosis, medullary sponge kidney, and in milk-alkali syndrome (Fig. 36). Renal cysts and tumours are occasionally identified by calcification in adjacent involved kidney.

Renal stones can travel down the ureters and appear in the bladder or urethra (Fig. 37). Encrustations on papillary bladder tumours may be visible on the plain film (Fig. 38), as can the florid calcification in the walls of the bladder and ureter in schistosomiasis.

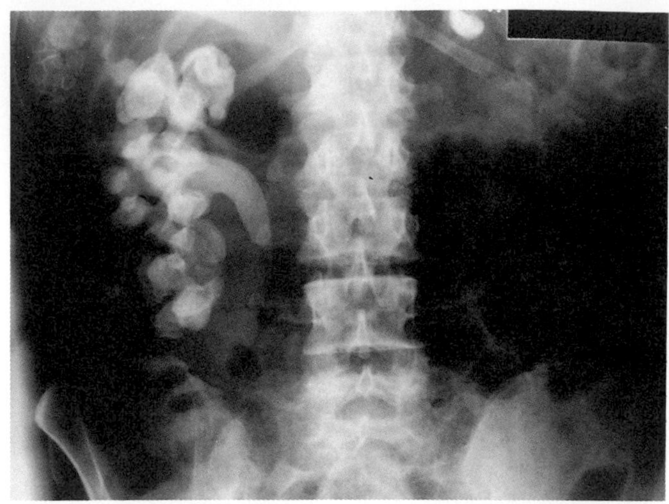

Fig. 35 A large staghorn calculus in the right kidney.

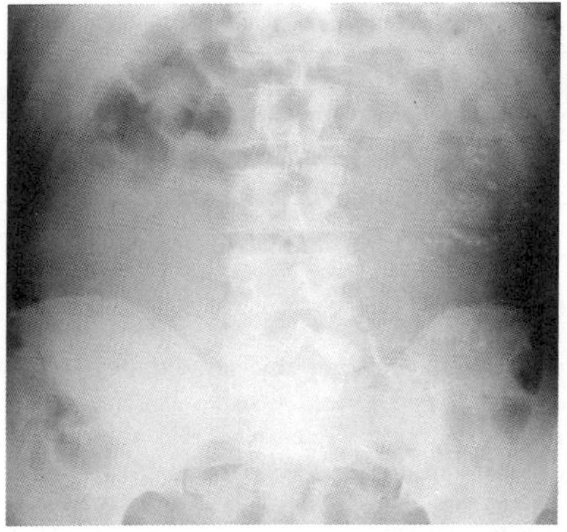

Fig. 36 Nephrocalcinosis in a patient with hyperparathyroidism.

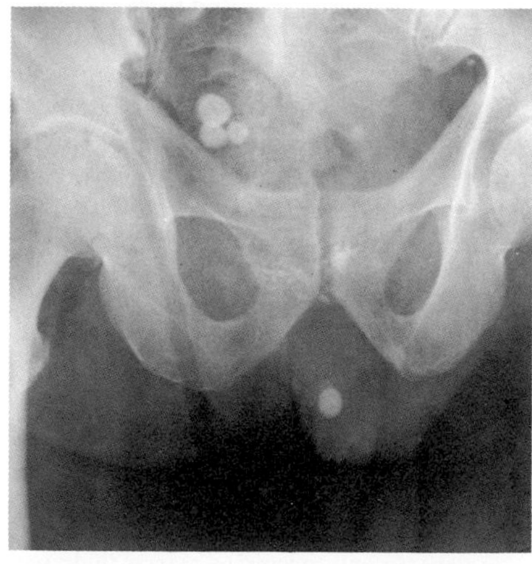

Fig. 37 A patient with calculi in a vesical diverticulum and in the urethra. He also has a calculus in a calcified prostate.

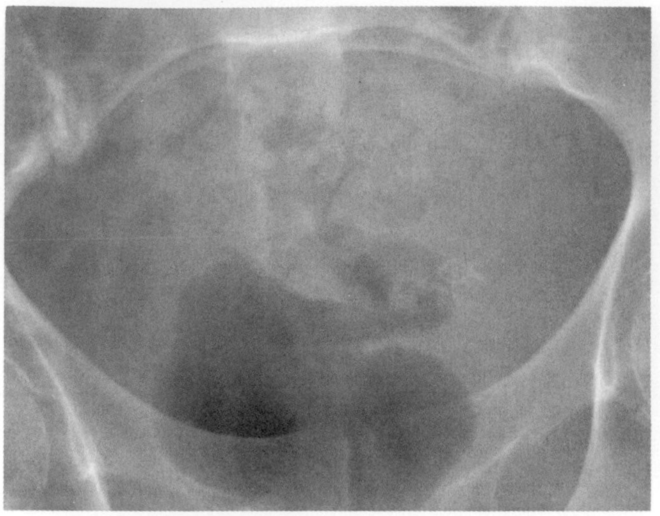

Fig. 38 Plain film of the pelvic outlet showing amorphous calcific deposits on a papillary transitional-cell tumour in the bladder.

Adrenals

The adrenals are nowadays usually investigated by ultrasound, CT, or radionuclide techniques. In areas where tuberculosis is common, this involves the adrenals leading to Addison's disease and calcification in the adrenal areas on the plain film. This could also arise from haemorrhage into the adrenal in infancy and theoretically in certain tumours, notably neuroblastoma.

FURTHER READING

Davidson AJ, ed. *Radiology of the Kidney*. Philadelphia: WB Saunders Co, 1985.

Fraser RG, Pare JAP. *Diagnosis of Diseases of the Chest*. 2nd edn. Philadelphia: WB Saunders Co, 1977–1979.

Grainger RG. Allison DJ, eds. *Diagnostic Radiology. An Anglo-American Textbook of Imaging*. Vols 1, 2, and 3. Edinburgh: Churchill Livingstone, 1986.

Sutton D. *Textbook of Radiology and Imaging*. 4th edn. Edinburgh: Churchill Livingstone, 1987.

Sutton D, Young JWR, eds. *A Short Textbook of Clinical Imaging*. London: Springer-Verlag, 1990.

6.2 Computed tomography

STEPHEN GOLDING

INTRODUCTION

In the two decades since computed tomography (CT) was introduced by Sir Godfrey Hounsfield it has become established as a powerful diagnostic tool and one that is relevant to many branches of surgery. Used appropriately, CT is capable of making a major impact on management decisions.

The technology of CT is outside the scope of this chapter and the interested reader is referred to Hounsfield (1973) or to Pullan (1979). In essence, the scanner rotates an X-ray tube around the patient in an arc and the emergent radiation beam is measured by photoelectric detectors. A computer is used to display the measurements as an image representing a cross-sectional 'slice' of the patient, based on the density of tissues to X-rays and their 'attenuation value' (Fig. 1). The image can be thought of as a cross-sectional radiograph but unlike radiography there is no superimposition of structures and the detector/computer system makes the technique very sensitive. The principal advantages of CT over conventional techniques stem from this fact.

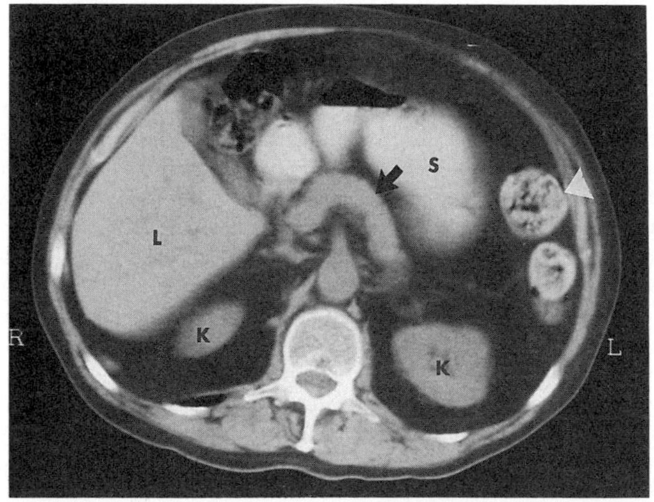

Fig. 1 Normal CT section of the upper abdomen, showing the liver (L), the kidneys (K), and the pancreas (arrow). Note that the organs are identified because the intervening fat has a lower attenuation value than other soft tissues. Oral contrast medium has been given and outlines the stomach (S) and descending colon (arrowhead).

THE TECHNIQUE

Preparation

From the patient's point of view CT examination is simple. In the majority of examinations all the patient has to do is lie on the couch while the machine makes the readings (Fig. 2). Preparation is minimal; some departments prefer to starve their patients for a few hours beforehand if intravenous contrast media are to be given.

Patients undergoing examination of the abdomen and pelvis are required to drink a dilute contrast medium in order to opacify the bowel and distinguish this from local structures with similar attenuation values (Fig. 1). This contrast medium is also administered rectally for examinations of the pelvic viscera. Examination for gynaecological indications requires a full bladder and the use of a vaginal tampon as an anatomical marker.

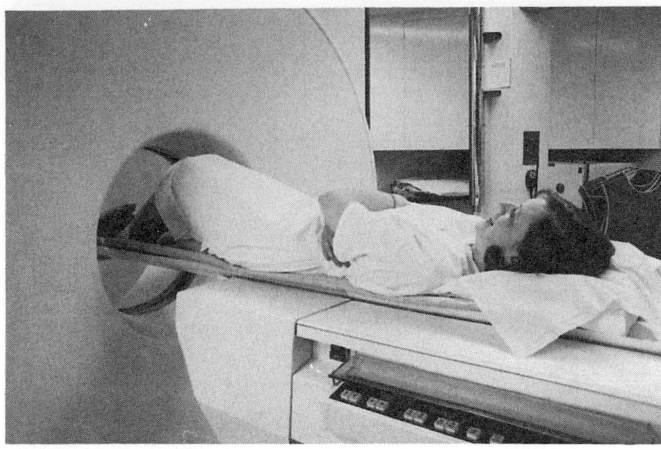

Fig. 2 The usual examination position for patients undergoing CT. Greater comfort is provided by using the support behind the knees.

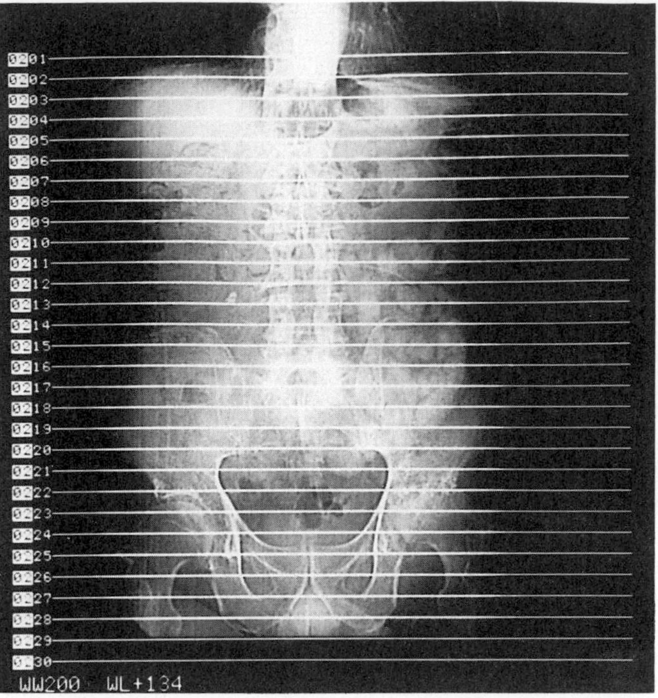

Fig. 3 Digital radiograph obtained at the start of the examination, showing the area to be examined. This examination records thirty sections, taken from the dome of the diaphragm to the pelvic floor.

Barium retained in the colon after previous gastrointestinal radiology produces artefacts on CT and barium studies should be deferred if CT is required. Large metal prostheses such as hip transplants may cause sufficient interference to prevent successful imaging around them. Metal clips used for haemostasis or for marking the margins of tumours also produce significant artefacts.

Sedation is only rarely required for patients undergoing CT. Premedication may be useful for those in pain so that they are able to lie still. General anaesthesia is required if involuntary or uncontrollable movement may be a problem, particularly in children, although many infants can be examined satisfactorily after a feed or under sedation.

Examination technique

Examination is usually carried out with the patient supine, although specialized indications may require specific positions. Exposures typically last a few seconds, and suspended respiration is required when the chest or abdomen are being examined; a diagnostic examination may not be possible if the patient has difficulty holding their breath, as respiratory movement may cause artefact. Other areas can be studied during quiet respiration. Where exposures of the abdomen last longer than 5 s an antiperistaltic agent (e.g. hyoscine butylbromide, Buscopan, or glucagon) reduces movement artefact caused by peristalsis.

Most CT machines can produce a digital radiograph of the examination area (Fig. 3) at the start of the examination. This allows the examination to be planned accurately and also provides a computerized record of the sections.

The examination produces sequential sections taken through the area of interest, the section thickness and inter-slice interval being determined by the size of the organ under investigation. Routine examinations of the chest, abdomen, or pelvis usually use sections 8- to 10-mm thick, whereas a specific examination of the adrenal glands may require 5-mm sections, and 2-mm sections may be needed to display the auditory ossicles. Axial sections are standard, although if the patient can be positioned appropriately in the gantry, sections can be obtained in coronal or other planes; this is required in only a minority of examinations.

The image

The CT section is a cross-sectional radiograph in which the tissues are displayed on a grey scale according to their attenuation value. Dense structures such as cortical bone appear light, whereas low density areas like air appear dark, as is the case with conventional radiographs. The attenuation of tissues on CT is displayed on a wider scale than can be shown effectively on one image, however. The display console therefore allows the image to be manipulated so that areas at different points on the attenuation scale can be examined. This allows discrimination of, for example, the fine detail of the lungs, at the lower end of the attenuation scale (Fig. 4).

The basic image data can also be manipulated in other ways. Measurements from a small area can be reprocessed to give a high resolution image; this is useful for demonstrating small structures such as the auditory ossicles or trabecular detail in bone (Fig. 5). Information from contiguous thin sections may be reformatted in different planes, or in three-dimensional perspective views, to provide a more anatomical display. Such images are helpful in communicating the orientation of lesions but rarely add further diagnostic information.

Enhancement

Enhancement refers to the commonly used technique of scanning following the intravenous administration of iodine-containing contrast medium. This increases the attenuation of areas which have a circulation, and allows their differentiation from avascular structures such as abscesses, cysts and devascularized tissue.

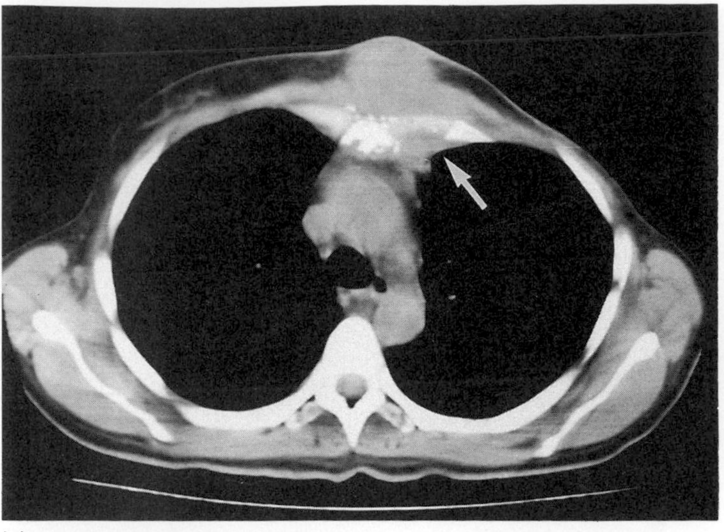

(a)

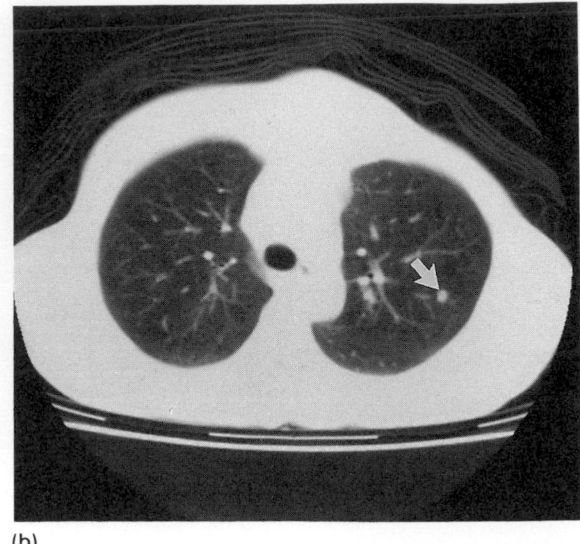

(b)

Fig. 4 (a) CT section at the level of the arch of the aorta, displayed at window levels and widths appropriate to soft tissue. The section shows a large soft tissue mass arising in the anterior chest wall, with erosion of the sternum and extension into the mediastinum (arrow). This was due to recurrent carcinoma of the breast. Such images are useful to plan treatment fields for radiotherapy. (b) The same section displayed on lower window levels, showing the structure of the lungs. A small pulmonary metastasis is seen in the left lung (arrow), and was not detected on chest radiographs.

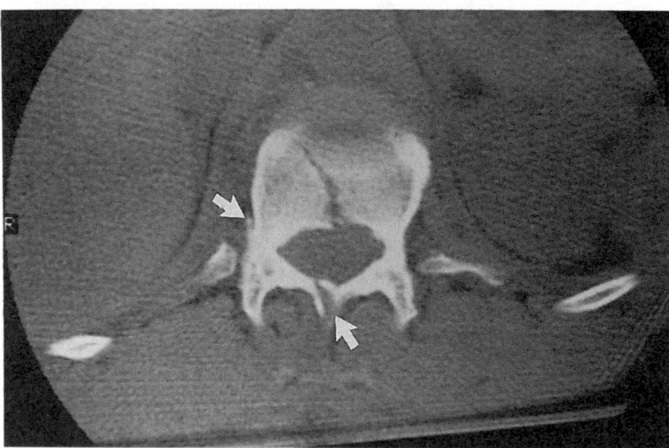

Fig. 5 High resolution CT image obtained in a patient with rotational injury at the thoracolumbar junction. There is a sagittal fracture of the vertebra body. Note that high resolution display also reveals fractures of the neural arch and base of the right pedicle (arrows).

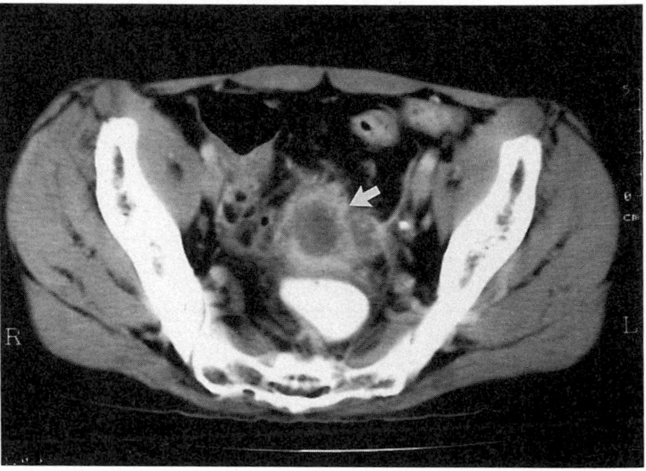

Fig. 6 CT section of the pelvis in a patient with a diverticular abscess. Intravenous contrast medium has been given and outlines granulation tissue around the abscess cavity (arrow). This facilitates identification of inflammatory fluid collections.

However it is commonly used to aid diagnosis by increasing the contrast between normal and abnormal tissues, hence the term 'enhancement'. This technique is routine in the examination of the liver, kidney and brain, and in the investigation of abdominal sepsis or trauma (Fig. 6).

Specialized techniques

As circulating blood increases in attenuation after enhancement, examination of blood vessels can be made by taking sections soon after injection, usually during the first or second circulation of the injection bolus. This may be used to distinguish tortuous vessels from other pathology and also to demonstrate vascular disease such as aortic aneurysm or dissection (Fig. 7). Examination during direct injection of local veins or through an arterial catheter (CT arteriography) is also recommended in specific indications, although the standard technique suffices for most vascular studies. Many CT machines allow rapidly repeated exposures to be made at one level following an intravascular bolus of contrast medium, with the resulting alteration plotted by the computer against time. This technique, 'dynamic CT', produces an accurate measurement of tissue perfusion but is little used in practice, although it is a useful research tool. Combined with incremental table movement, dynamic CT gives an overview of an organ in one phase of perfusion. This is sometimes used in examination of vessels and in a detailed search for small space-occupying lesions in the liver.

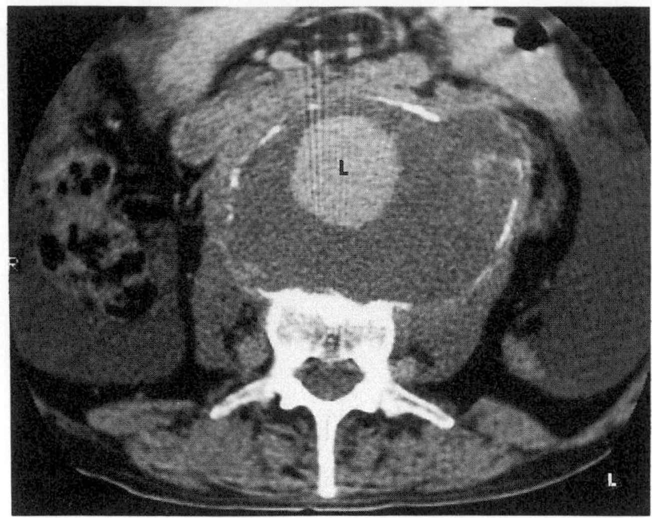

Fig. 7 High resolution CT section of the abdomen in a patient with a large aortic aneurysm. The aortic wall is partly calcified. Contrast medium outlines the patent lumen (L) within extensive mural thrombus. Note that the aneurysm has eroded the vertebral body posteriorly and that on the left side there has been partial rupture of the wall.

The cross-sectional display produced by CT has also been applied to other contrast procedures in radiology in order to obtain more information. Examples include examination after intrathecal or intra-articular injection (CT myelography and CT arthrography, respectively). In both cases cross-sectional definition is used to produce images of areas which are difficult to assess by the corresponding conventional technique.

The precise tissue map of CT images has been used successfully to direct treatment beams in radiotherapy and it is now common for radiotherapy to be planned on the basis of CT images, using specially constructed computer hardware.

Advantages and disadvantages of CT

The principal advantage of CT is that it provides a clear, accurate display of tissues without superimposition of structures. Disease processes may be detected at an earlier stage than is possible with other techniques, and lesions may be detected in areas which are difficult to assess with conventional imaging. The technique is not limited to specific organs: since all of the tissues in a body section are displayed it can be used to search for disease sites.

The clinical advantages of CT are well illustrated by its role in neurosurgery, one of its first areas of application. The technique offered for the first time the ability to image cerebral anatomy and pathology directly. Invasive and indirect tests such as arteriography and encephalography were largely replaced, and more accurate diagnosis became possible.

Although CT is effective in disease detection and localization, characterization of lesions is more difficult, since many have similar attenuation characteristics. For example, it may not be possible to distinguish fibrotic masses from benign or malignant neoplasms on the basis of their CT appearance alone. Biopsy is therefore usually required for definitive diagnosis.

The other main disadvantages of CT are the high capital cost of the equipment and the fact that it employs ionizing radiation. The absorbed radiation dose from CT varies according to examination technique, but it is generally similar to that encountered with other major radiological procedures such as angiography or barium enema. CT is therefore used with care around radiosensitive structures such as the eye, or in children and young people, and only for over-riding indications in pregnant women.

Relationship to other techniques

In the abdomen, pelvis, and musculoskeletal soft tissues, ultrasound offers an alternative to CT as a sectional imaging technique. The relative strengths of the two are too complicated to discuss in detail here, but in general, if a good quality image is obtained by ultrasound, the two techniques are usually comparable in application. However, the results of ultrasound, unlike CT, are limited by the presence of bowel gas and bone, and if these prevent good images being obtained, CT is more reliable. Ultrasound is also attenuated by fat, making the technique more suitable for slim patients, whereas a moderate amount of body fat improves image quality in CT. Ultrasound is of limited use in the chest.

The technique which most resembles CT is magnetic resonance imaging (MRI). Like CT, MRI is a cross-sectional technique, but unlike CT, examination in any plane is possible. MRI has the advantage of not employing radiation, and it discriminates between soft tissues to a degree unequalled by any other technique. However MRI is expensive and of limited availability. Movement artefact is a problem in studying the abdomen, because scan times are long and there is, as yet, no generally available contrast medium to label the bowel, as there is in CT. Little signal is obtained from lung and MRI does not compare with CT in this area.

THE INDICATIONS

It is the golden rule of investigational medicine that no patient is examined unless the results influence clinical management. This is particularly true of CT: examinations should always be tailored to the clinical problem. However, when used appropriately, CT has proved to be a powerful factor in clinical management decisions in a wide range of applications. All surgical specialities are major users of CT services. Table 1 lists the clinical indications for which CT is currently recommended; these are divided according to clinical subspeciality although there is some overlap.

In recent years the indications for CT have had to be reassessed in the light of growing experience in MRI and its availability. MRI has become an established investigational tool in the neurosciences and in orthopaedics, and to a lesser extent in gynaecology (Table 1). For technical reasons MRI is unlikely ever to be applicable to the diagnosis of conditions affecting the lungs or cortical bone. Haemorrhage can produce confusing appearances on MRI and CT therefore remains the technique of choice in patients who have suffered trauma.

The main advantages of CT in clinical practice stem not only from its accuracy in detecting disease but also from the fact that a convincing normal examination virtually excludes the presence of lesions of any size. When an abdominal mass is suspected, for example, CT is the most accurate technique for demonstrating disease and indicating its organ of origin (Fig. 8), but is also more reliable than ultrasound in excluding disease when there is none present. The technique can therefore be used to select patients

Table 1 Applications of computed tomography in surgery

1. General surgery
   - Detection and localization of palpable abdominal masses, or neoplasms of solid intra-abdominal organs
   - Detection of intra-abdominal abscesses
   - Diagnosis and preoperative assessment of aortic aneurysm and dissection*
   - Diagnosis of focal liver disease and obstructive jaundice (if ultrasound unhelpful)*
   - Staging of neoplasms of the liver, pancreas, kidney, lymphatic system
   - Evaluation of complications of pancreatitis
   - Evaluation of trauma to the chest, abdomen, and pelvis
2. Orthopaedic surgery
   - Diagnosis and preoperative evaluation of discovertebral disease*
   - Diagnosis and staging of musculoskeletal neoplasms*
   - Evaluation of major skeletal trauma
   - Detection and evaluation of congenital and degenerative joint disease*
   - Assessment of osteomyelitis prior to evacuation*
   - Diagnosis of avascular necrosis of bone and joints*
3. Neurosurgery
   - Detection and localization of all structural disease of the brain*
   - Diagnosis and preoperative evaluation of structural lesions of the spinal cord*
   - Monitoring treatment response and detecting relapse of neoplasms of brain and spinal cord*
   - Diagnosis and evaluation of cerebral trauma
   - Diagnosis of sensorineural deafness and blindness
4. Urology
   - Differential diagnosis of renal masses (where other techniques fail)
   - Preoperative staging of carcinoma of the kidney, prostate, and bladder*
   - Staging, monitoring treatment and surveillance of testicular tumours
   - Evaluation of renal trauma
   - Investigation of ureteric obstruction (where other techniques fail)
   - Diagnosis and preoperative evaluation of retroperitoneal fibrosis
   - Evaluation of structural complications of renal transplants*
   - Detection of the undescended testicle*
5. ENT surgery and ophthalmology
   - Diagnosis of conductive hearing loss
   - Diagnosis and staging of neoplasms of the larynx, pharynx, sinuses, salivary glands, and oral cavity*
   - Evaluation of severe facial trauma
   - Preoperative assessment for endoscopic sinus procedures
   - Investigation of unilateral exophthalmos
   - Evaluation of lesions of the optic globe*
6. Thoracic surgery
   - Localization, differential diagnosis and preoperative evaluation of mediastinal masses
   - Staging carcinoma of the bronchus and of the oesophagus*
   - Diagnosis and preoperative evaluation of aortic aneurysm and dissection*
   - Evaluation of severe chest trauma
   - Staging prior to resection of solitary pulmonary metastases
7. Gynaecology
   - Staging advanced neoplasms of the cervix, uterus, and ovary
   - Treatment monitoring and detection of relapse of advanced neoplasms
   - Pelvimetry*
8. Plastic surgery
   - Preoperative planning for reconstructive surgery, especially of the face
   - Staging cutaneous neoplasms before radical resection

The asterisks indicate where MRI, if available, may replace CT.

who require surgical intervention. Similar observations apply to patients with suspected intra-abdominal abscesses (Fig. 6), in whom lesions close to the bowel are difficult to detect by ultrasound; CT more reliably confirms or excludes a focal collection. CT is also a reliable technique for excluding significant damage to intra-abdominal organs in patients who have suffered abdominal trauma (Fig. 9). In all three instances the exclusion of disease has a major effect on the clinical management of the patient.

The ability of CT to delineate masses accurately has produced a major advance in the management of malignant disease. In addition to the diagnostic role outlined above, the technique is recommended for assessing the local extent of the majority of solid tumours and distinguishes reliably between patients with resectable disease and those in whom an attempted resection is pointless (Fig. 8). In addition, CT is used to detect malignant lymph node enlargement in the chest, abdomen, and pelvis (but cannot,

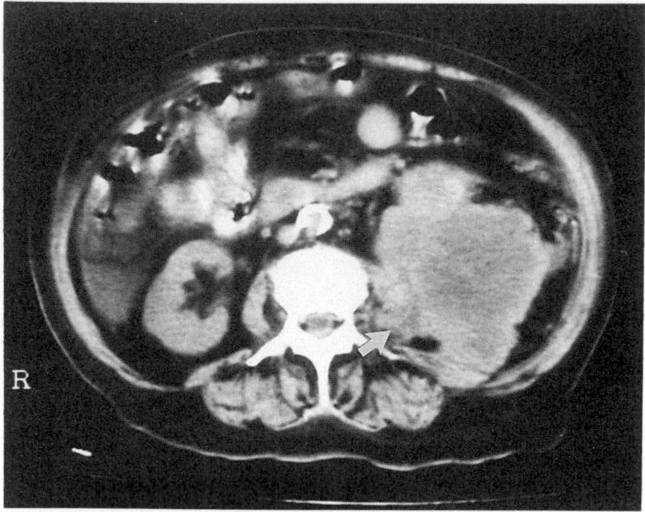

(a)

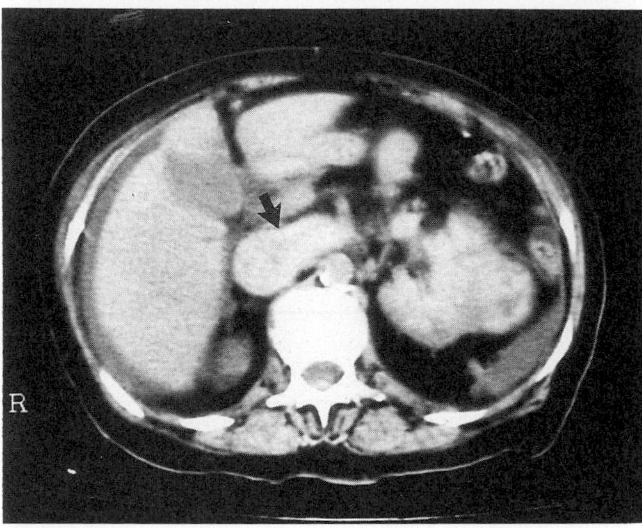

(b)

Fig. 8 (a) CT section of the abdomen in a patient who presented with an abdominal mass due to carcinoma of the left kidney. Examination was obtained for tumour staging. The left kidney is replaced by an inhomogeneous mass which has obliterated the fat plane posterior to the kidney and infiltrated the left psoas muscle (arrow), indicating that the tumour is unresectable. (b) A section slightly higher shows tumour expanding the left renal vein and entering the inferior vena cava (arrow). Assessment of the renal vein is an essential component of tumour staging by CT.

unlike lymphography, demonstrate small tumour deposits in nodes of normal size) and has become the technique of choice for demonstrating metastases to the brain, lungs (Fig. 4), liver, and adrenal glands. Disease staging protocols based on CT results have now been defined for the majority of malignant tumours, with the aim of excluding disease spread and therefore identifying those patients suitable for radical treatment.

The combined cross-sectional display of bone and soft tissue has made CT an important technique in orthopaedics, allowing the assessment of stability of spinal fractures, demonstrating the

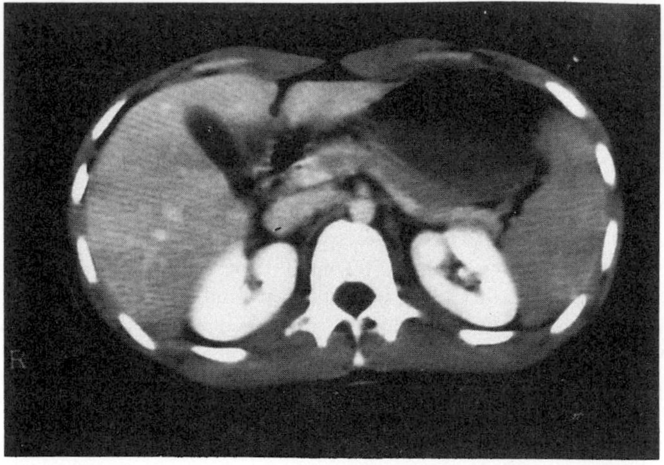

Fig. 9 CT section of the upper abdomen in a patient involved in a road traffic accident. There was extensive laceration to the right side of the trunk. The demonstration by CT of normal anatomy in the body wall and normally enhancing hepatic parenchyma deep to this excludes significant intra-abdominal damage despite extensive right abdominal tenderness and guarding.

disposition of fracture fragments prior to surgical fixation (Fig. 5), and planning corrective surgery in joint disease.

CT-guided interventional techniques

A wide range of percutaneous therapeutic procedures are now performed under CT control. The principal advantage of the technique is that it permits the operator to site an instrument with confidence and safety, even in relatively inaccessible areas of the body. The most common technique is CT-guided biopsy (Fig. 10): aspiration for diagnostic cytology or cutting needle biopsy for histological diagnosis can be undertaken in virtually any area of the body. CT-guided drainage can also be used in the

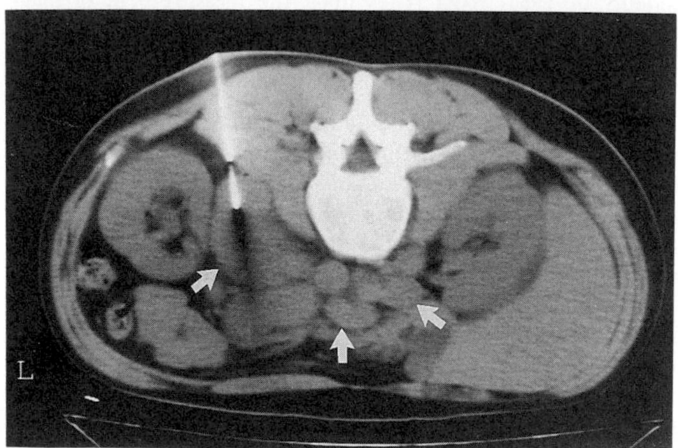

Fig. 10 CT guided biopsy. The patient presented with abdominal pain and fever. CT showed extensive retroperitoneal lymphadenopathy (arrows). CT guidance was used to site a Trucut needle in the lymph node mass, providing a histological diagnosis of non-Hodgkin's lymphoma.

treatment of most deep-seated abscesses and other pathological fluid collections. Guided neurolysis, tumour lysis by alcohol injection, and laser therapy are also possible.

CONCLUSION

Although the capital and running costs of CT are high, the technique is undoubtedly cost effective. It can be used to achieve an early diagnosis in patients who would otherwise need to undergo a large number of alternative investigations, and it can be performed on an outpatient basis, reducing costs for inpatient investigation. Moreover, the diagnostic and therapeutic applications of CT frequently replace exploratory laparotomy, or other major surgical procedures. Maximization of these cost benefits is heavily dependent on good patient selection, and calls for close liaison between the surgeon and the radiologist.

In the future the clinical role of CT will need to be reassessed as MRI develops, particularly in examination of the abdomen, where further development of MRI is to be expected. For the present, CT is the mainstay of cross-sectional imaging.

FURTHER READING

Genant HK. Symposium on computed tomography. *Orth Clin N Am* 1985; **16**: 357–89.

Golding SJ. Computed tomography and tumour staging. *Curr Imaging* 1990; **2**: 2–8.

Golding SJ, Husband JE. CT-Guided interventional techniques. *Interventional Radiol* 1990; **5**: 101–23.

Hounsfield GN. Computerised transverse axial scanning. *Br J Radiol* 1973; **46**: 1016–22.

Moore AT, Dixon AK, Wheeler T. Cost-benefit evaluation of computed tomography. *Health Trends* 1987; **19**:8–12.

Muller PR, Simeone JF. Intraabdominal abscess: diagnosis by sonography and computed tomography. *Radiol Clin N Am* 1983; **21**: 425–43.

Pullan BR. The scientific basis of computerised tomography. In: Lodge T, Steiner R, eds. *Recent Advances in Radiology* No. 6. Edinburgh: Churchill Livingstone, 1979; 1–15.

Williams MP, Scott IHK, Dixon AK. Computer tomography in 101 patients with a palpable abdominal mass. *Clin Radiol* 1984; **35**: 293–6.

Wing VW, Federle MP, Morris JA, Jeffrey RB, Bluth R. The clinical impact of CT for blunt abdominal trauma. *Am J Roentgenol* 1985; **145**: 1191–4.

Wittenberg J, Fineberg HV, Ferrucci JT. *et al.* Clinical efficacy of computed body tomography. *Am J Roentegenol* 1980; **134**: 1111–20.

6.3 Magnetic resonance imaging

AKIHIRO TANIMOTO AND DAVID D. STARK

INTRODUCTION

Introduction to MRI

The use of magnetic resonance imaging (MRI) has been rapidly expanding since it was introduced as a new clinical imaging modality in 1981. MRI relies upon the measurement of magnetization in tissues and it can distinguish tissue structures with far better contrast resolution than other imaging techniques. In contrast to computerized tomography (CT), MRI can provide images in arbitrary planes, including sagittal, coronal, and even oblique directions. CT displays only X-ray beam attenuation coefficients, while MRI uses four biophysiochemical parameters to produce images: resonant frequency, proton density, relaxation times (T_1 and T_2), and motion. Scanning methods in MRI are called 'pulse sequences'. Images are often classified as 'T_1 weighted', 'T_2 weighted' or 'proton density weighted', terms which refer to the source of the signal difference or relative brightness as displayed on the image.

There are few hazards or contraindications to MRI. The strong magnetic fields used in MRI may cause suppression of cardiac pacemakers due to induced current, or motion of intracranial aneurysmal clips. Clips on coronary arteries and other organs rarely migrate, however, because the torque in the field strength is 1.5 tesla or less. Modern types of heart valves and stainless steel orthopaedic implants which do not exhibit ferromagnetism are also unaffected by MRI.

Physical basis of nuclear magnetic resonance

A proton (nucleus of hydrogen) can be compared with a tiny elementary magnet. In a natural environment, the magnetic moments m of individual protons in the body are pointed in random directions. It follows that their sum, or macroscopic magnetization, M, is zero. If placed in a constant magnetic field B_0, many of the tiny elementary magnets spontaneously undergo a transient orientation in the direction of the field. Therefore, a small magnetization vector M_z appears parallel to B_0. The nuclear magnetic resonance phenomenon can be observed when protons absorb radiowaves at a specific frequency (the Larmor frequency). On a macroscopic scale, the magnetization vector M will be rotated away from its M_z equilibrium position parallel to B_0. The angle between M and B_0 will become greater as the applied radiowave has a longer duration or greater power. In MRI, a transmitted radiowave that shifts vector M perpendicular to B_0 (transverse or XY plane) is called a 90° pulse. As vector M is then parallel to the XY plane (M+M_{xy}), the value of longitudinal magnetization M_z is zero. Resonance occurs when the magnetization rotating in the transverse plane emits radiowaves that can be detected by the imaging system.

When the radiowave excitation pulse ceases, total magnetization M slowly returns to its equilibrium state. This phenomenon is called 'relaxation'. Once the 90° pulse has been terminated, M_{xy} decays and M_z grows. This return of longitudinal magnetization (M_z) is characterized by the relaxation time T_1. T_1 values vary among tissues according to the mobility of the hydrogen (proton)-

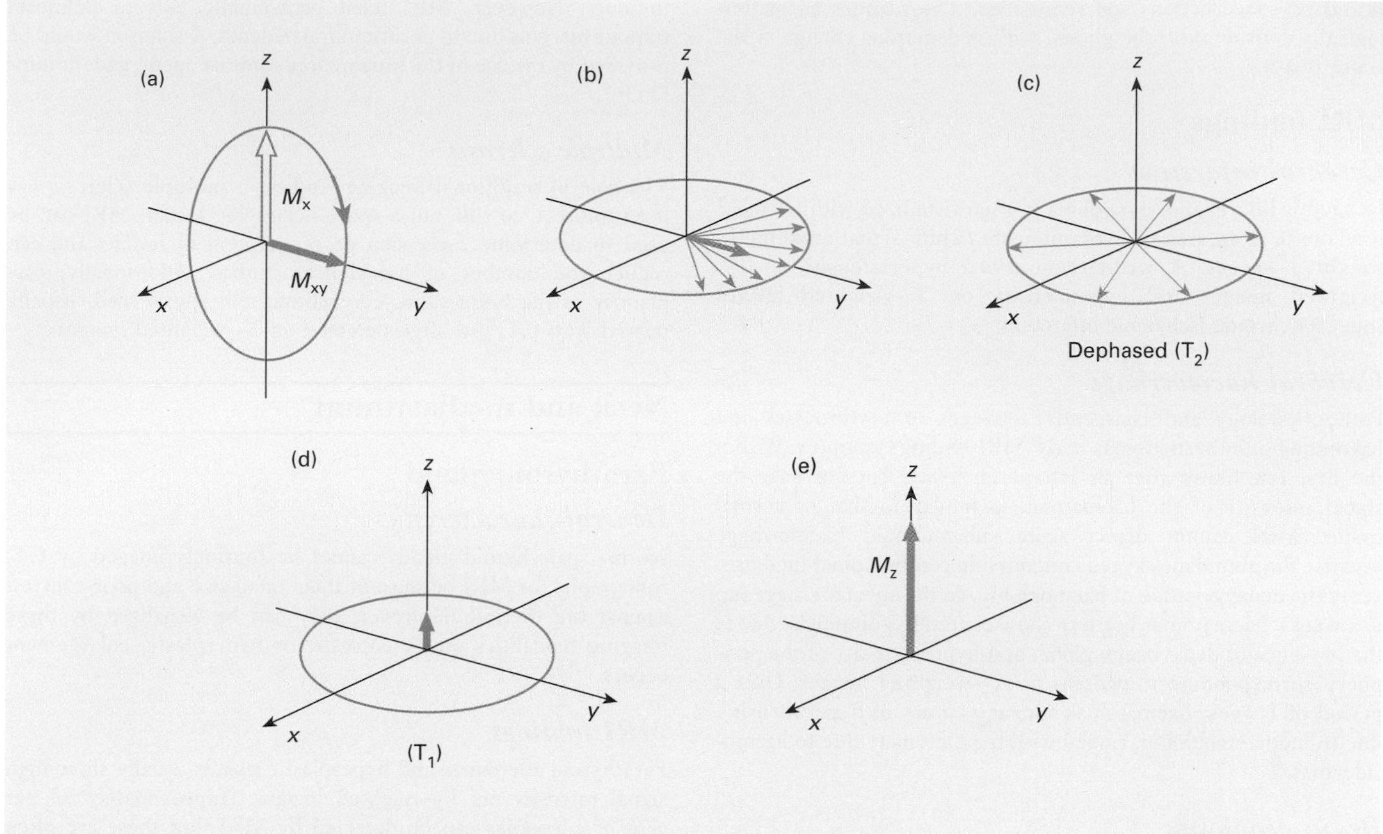

Fig. 1 Behaviours of macroscopic magnetization after 90° pulse.
(a) By 90° pulse, the longitudinal magnetization M_z is rotated to the xy plane (M_{xy}). (b), (c) M_{xy} (transverse magnetization) begins to dephase as a function of T_2. (d), (e) During the dephasing, the magnetization returns to the equilibrium state as a function of T_1. An electric current forming MR images is induced in an antenna by the variation of the magnetic field caused by inphase rotation of protons in the transverse plane (M_{xy}).

containing molecules. Water molecules (such as cerebrospinal fluid) have a very long T_1, while lipid molecules (such as fat tissues) have a very short T_1.

The 90° pulse that shifts equilibrium magnetization from M_z to M_{xy} also places the nuclear magnetic moment 'in phase', which means that they are moving in exact alignment. However, transverse magnetization is progressively dephased (protons lose alignment) soon after the pulse ceases. This phenomenon, known as transverse relaxation, is characterized by the relaxation time T_2 (Fig. 1).

Nuclear magnetic resonance in biological tissues is measured by detecting transverse magnetization M_{xy} before it relaxes (dephases). An electric current is induced in an antenna by the variation of the magnetic field caused by in-phase rotation of protons in the transverse plane (M_{xy}). This electrical signal (the MR signal) represents the magnetic characteristics of each tissue. The amplitude and timing of various signals is mathematically converted to represent the number of protons present in a tissue (proton density) or the relaxation time (T_1 and T_2).

CLINICAL APPLICATIONS

Brain

General characteristics

Numerous studies in this field have been documented since MRI was first introduced to the clinical environment. MRI promises to be a unique tool, providing high quality images of the brain with few motion artefacts.

Cerebral infarction

Cerebral infarction refers to a sudden and focal neurological deficit with an associated ischaemic abnormality in a localized region of the brain due to thrombosis. The hypoxia that occurs with ischaemia initially leads to an increase in the intracellular water content; tissue necrosis results if the ischaemia is persistent.

Cerebral haemorrhage

Intracranial haemorrhage can appear as various pathophysiological states, including intraparenchymal haemorrhage, intratumoural haemorrhage, haemorrhagic infarction, subarachnoid haemorrhage, epidural or subdural haemorrhage, and vascular malformations.

Brain neoplasms

Precisely defining the extent of the tumour and grading the malignancy are the most important goals of any imaging study because of the implications for patient management and evaluation of treatment. So many classifications of brain tumours have been provided that a knowledge of general neuropathological features is essential for analysing magnetic resonance images.

Multiple sclerosis

The clinical course of multiple sclerosis is usually described as a relentless stepwise progression of neurological dysfunction, manifested by exacerbations and remissions. The plaques are pathologically considered to be gliosis, with oedematous change in the acute phase.

MRI findings

Cerebral infarction

Ischaemic infarct and/or oedema is often visualized within 6 to 12 h of onset as an area of hyperintensity (white signal area) on T_2 weighted images. A well-circumscribed hyperintensity on T_2-weighted images and hypointensity on T_1-weighted images suggests chronic ischaemic infarction.

Cerebral haemorrhage

Pathophysiology and consecutive changes of erythrocytes and haemoglobin in haematomas make MRI findings complex. Within the first few hours after an intraparenchymal haemorrhage the signal intensity of the haematoma is similar to that of normal tissue. MRI cannot depict acute subarachnoid haemorrhage because the abundant oxygen contained in cerebrospinal fluid prevents the deoxygenation of haemoglobin. In the subacute stage (up to a week), haematomas begin to show central hypointensity due to the presence of deoxyhaemoglobin and hyperintensity of the periphery corresponding to oedema on T_2-weighted images. Over a period of 1 week, haematomas appear as areas of hyperintensity, due to methaemoglobin, ringed with hypointensity due to haemosiderin.

Brain neoplasms

Because the tumour may contain cysts, calcification, haemorrhage, and necrosis, a single signal pattern is not found. Peritumoural oedema increases relaxation times and makes it difficult to detect the tumour margin. Tumours often extend beyond the rims apparent on CT scans, and similar difficulties may reasonably be expected when MRI is employed.

Multiple sclerosis

The characteristic MRI findings consist of multiple, usually small, lesions with prolonged relaxation times, most commonly located in the periventricular region. The T_2-weighted spin echo technique is currently the best method for detecting multiple sclerosis: this is positive in between 80 and 100 per cent of patients with definite multiple sclerosis by established clinical criteria.

Advantages of MRI over other methods

Cerebral infarction

The advantages of MRI over CT are apparent when delineating small infarcts in the brain-stem and cerebellum and lacunar infarcts in the basal ganglia. MRI can detect hyperacute ischaemic changes in the brain by 6 h after onset, while CT is usually useful in detecting them after 24 h.

Cerebral haemorrhage

MRI is less useful for detecting acute (within 1 day) cerebral haemorrhage. However, it gives a dynamic window through which a variety of haemorrhagic conditions may be observed.

Brain neoplasms

Multiplanar capabilities and a reduction in artefacts from the skull can demonstrate relationships between brain tumours and the skull better than CT, particularly in patients with infratentorial tumours. However, MRI itself occasionally fails to delineate tumour margins due to peritumoural oedema. A solution would be provided by the use of the intravenous contrast agent, gadolinium-DTPA.

Multiple sclerosis

The role of traditional imaging studies in multiple sclerosis has been indirect, to rule out a space-occupying lesion. MRI can be used to determine regression or progression of lesions and can reduce the number of paraclinical studies. Additionally, tiny plaques in the brain-stem, cerebellum, and spinal cord, usually missed with CT, are often detected on T_2-weighted images.

Neck and mediastinum

Parathyroid gland

General characteristics

Normal parathyroid glands cannot be routinely imaged by CT, sonography, or MRI because of their small size and poor contrast against the thyroid. However, they can be visualized by these imaging modalities once neoplastic or hyperplastic enlargement occurs.

MRI findings

Parathyroid adenomas and hyperplastic glands usually show high signal intensity on T_2-weighted images. Approximately 75 per cent of adenomas can be detected by MRI, but these are often indistinguishable from posterior thyroid adenomas.

Advantages of MRI over other methods

MRI may be particularly valuable in patients with recurrent or persistent hyperparathyroidism following surgical exploration performed without preoperative localization of the tumours, since it is free of artefacts due to surgical clips or postoperative fibrous tissue. However, sonography is preferred as the first modality as it is a sensitive and inexpensive method, capable of detecting 80 per cent of parathyroid tumours.

Mediastinum

General characteristics

Enlarged mediastinal lymph nodes are the most common mass lesions, accounting for 25 per cent of all mediastinal diseases. Thymomas, teratomas, neurogenic tumours, and bronchogenic and pericardial cysts are also common.

MRI findings

Mediastinal lymph nodes are easily visible on T_1-weighted images, standing out clearly against hyperintense mediastinal fat. Mediastinal tumours such as thymoma, germ cell tumours, and neurogenic tumours usually have similar signal intensities to those of lymph nodes. Cystic lesions containing serous fluid can be distinguished from complicated cysts and solid lesions by their long relaxation times.

Advantages of MRI over other methods

MRI may be more efficient than CT for the detection of hilar adenopathy: the condition can be distinguished from pulmonary vessels and bronchi without the need for intravenous contrast because of the superb contrast afforded by the lack of a signal from flowing blood. However, accurate discrimination between cancer and inflammation is still impossible by MRI: size criteria analogous to those used in CT (> 1 cm) are used to identify abnormal nodes. MRI cannot provide tissue-specific diagnosis of mediastinal tumours on the basis of signal intensity, but can indicate spatial relationships between tumours and adjacent structures by its multiplanar capabilities.

Abdomen

Liver

General characteristics

Among the wide spectrum of hepatic diseases, detection, characterization, and staging (if malignant) of liver tumours currently command the greatest interest in clinical imaging. MRI has been remarkably advanced and employed in the diagnosis of focal hepatic diseases over recent years, and its efficacy has been described by many investigators.

MRI findings

Metastatic liver tumours

Hepatic metastases often show well-defined margins and homogeneous internal morphology, with hypoechoic T_1-weighted images and slightly hyperechoic T_2-weighted images compared to normal liver parenchyma. Primary and metastatic liver tumours of different histology can be distinguished from each other: MRI commonly demonstrates specific morphological features that suggest the correct tissue diagnosis (Fig. 2).

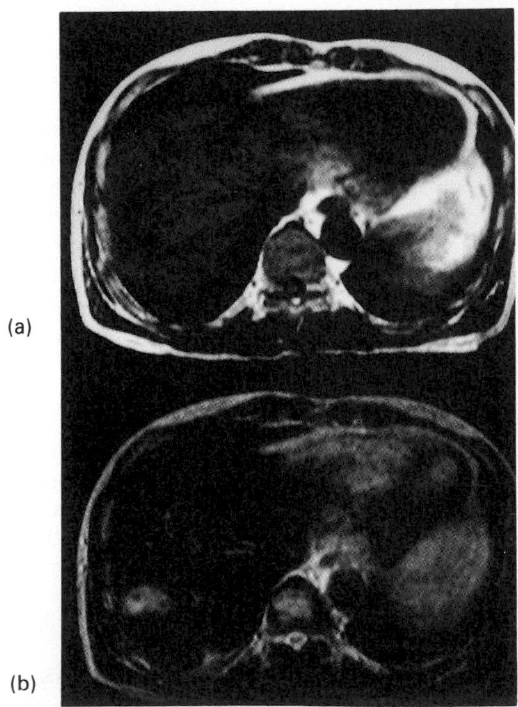

Fig. 2 Liver metastasis from colonic cancer. (a) T_1-weighted image shows a low intensity mass in the right lobe. (b) T_2-weighted image shows a high intensity mass.

Hepatic cell carcinoma

Hepatomas usually show signal intensities similar to those of metastases. However, about 10 per cent of hepatomas display a bright signal on T_1-weighted intensities because of steatosis; this is very rare in metastases. T_2-weighted images are more reliable for the detection of hepatomas than are T_1-weighted images: using the latter method, 40 to 50 per cent appear as a low intensity capsule, considered to be fibrous tissue.

Haemangioma

Cavernous haemangiomas essentially comprise a blood lake. They typically produce well-defined low signal lesions on T_1-weighted images and extremely high intensity signals with T_2 weighting (Fig. 3). The specificity of MRI in detecting haemangiomas more than 2 cm in diameter is over 90 per cent.

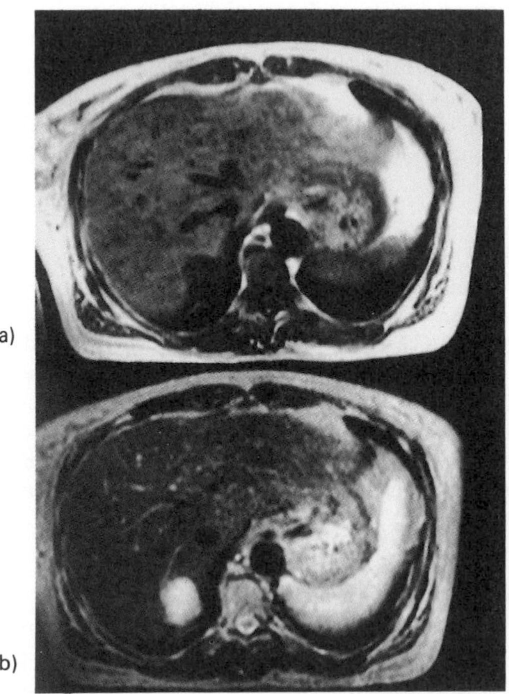

Fig. 3 Liver haemangioma. (a) T_1-weighted image shows a clearly-margined low intensity mass in the right lobe. (b) On T_2-weighted image, a mass shows a very high signal intensity.

Focal nodular hyperplasia

Focal nodular hypoplasia usually shows similar signal intensity to normal liver parenchyma on T_1-weighted images and slightly higher intensity on T_2-weighted images, with compression of hepatic vascular structures. MRI may demonstrate the characteristic stellate scar of focal nodular hyperplasia, which is not generally encountered in hepatic adenomas, but its differentiation from other hepatic tumours is often difficult.

Liver cirrhosis

Cirrhosis usually produces non-specific signal intensities from the liver and can be diagnosed by its morphological features, such as enlargement of the left and caudate lobe, irregularity of liver surface, enlarged portal veins, or prominent collateral veins and splenomegaly, which can also be seen on CT. Regenerating nodules in cirrhotic liver sometimes show high signal intensity in T_1-weighted images due to steatosis, which is indistinguishable from hepatomas with fatty metamorphosis.

Fatty liver

Focal fatty liver infiltration often shows regional high intensity on T_1-weighted images, mimicking hepatomas with fatty metamorphosis, but may be clinically diagnosed by its isointensity on T_2-weighted images.

Advantages of MRI over other methods

The diagnostic performance of MRI varies substantially, depending on the instruments used, use of pulse sequences and other techniques, lesion size, and tumour histology. In general, T_2-weighted images can show significant differences in the internal structures of hepatic tumours and provide unambiguous tissue contrast betwen lesions and normal hepatic parenchyma, while T_1-weighted images show the anomaly in a similar way to CT. Many CT criteria can be directly applied to T_1-weighted images. Failure to obtain good T_2-weighted images is the most common reason for failure to reach a diagnosis. At present, MRI is not always superior to other modalities, but it is an important adjuvant.

Metastases

One study showed MRI to have a sensitivity of 64 per cent in the detection of individual metastatic liver tumours, compared with 51 per cent for CT ($p<0.0001$). The sensitivity for identifying individual patients with liver metastases was 82 per cent, compared with 80 per cent for CT (non-significant). The specificity of MRI in patients without hepatic metastases was 99 per cent, versus 94 per cent for CT ($p<0.05$). In planning resection of liver metastases, MRI has the advantage over CT because of its superior specificity.

Hepatic cell carcinoma

MRI can detect 85 per cent of tumours smaller than 2 cm and 100 per cent of those larger than 2 cm (an average of 97 per cent, compared with 98 per cent for CT). MRI can be almost equivalent to CT in the detection of primary tumours, but often demonstrates secondary nodules missed on CT. MRI is sometimes valuable, therefore, in staging hepatomas when planning surgical approaches for resection, avoiding exploration in patients with unresectable disease. However, total image diagnosis including CT, sonography, and selective angiography is still imperative to assess daughter nodules accurately. Tumour thrombi up to the second branches of the portal system can be usually visually by MRI, but it is difficult to demonstrate portal invasion.

Haemangiomas

MRI (especially T_2-weighted imaging) is superior to other imaging modalities in diagnosing and delineating cavernous haemangionas from other malignant tumours. Small (< 1 cm) haemangiomas can be demonstrated reliably on T_2-weighted images when sufficient anatomical resolution is achieved. CT usually requires both precontrast and contrast scans to diagnose haemangiomas and sometimes fails to demonstrate small lesions. MRI can prevent patients from requiring a second examination such as sonography or selective angiography after CT.

Biliary tract

General characteristics

Cholelithiasis often accompanies inflammatory processes and malignancies in the biliary system. Diagnostic imaging allows the cause of obstructive jaundice to be determined and enables malignancies to be staged.

MRI findings

T_2 weighted MRI shows as a signal void (dark signal) surrounded by high intensity bile. Thickening of the gallbladder wall and a dilated biliary system are routinely demonstrated.

Advantages of MRI over other methods

MRI does not seem to have any advantages over CT or sonography. Stone disease accounts for a considerable proportion of biliary pathology and represents a physical limitation for MRI as crystalline structures produce no signal. In addition, the poor spatial resolution of MRI is a disadvantage for the study of small biliary structures such as the common bile duct. The applications of MRI are, therefore, limited; they include detection of hepatic metastases from gallbladder cancers and cholangiocarcinomas, but not diagnosis of primary lesions.

Pancreas

General characteristics

The pancreas is an important target for surgeons because of the high mortality rate associated with pancreatic neoplasms. Detecting pancreatic cancer, determining the stage, and differentiating it from pancreatitis are undoubtably the major goals in imaging of the pancreas.

MRI findings

Pancreatic carcinomas

Pancreatic carcinomas larger than 2 cm produce focal mass lesions that are detectable by MRI using morphological criteria analogous to CT. These are associated with the appearance of the tumour and with indirect signs of biliary obstruction and invasion to the neighbouring structures. The contrast between tumour and pancreas derived from longer T_1 and T_2 of the tumour may clearly delineate the boundary of the tumour, but the invasion to adjacent tissues is often ambiguous because of the relatively poor spatial resolution of MRI.

Pancreatitis

The characteristics of pancreatitis on MRI are similar to those described with CT. Observed signs include alterations in the pancreatic volume, abnormal colour, dilatation of the pancreatic duct, fluid collections or pseudocysts, and peripancreatic infiltration. However, small pancreatic calcifications are often undetectable on MRI because they do not generate a signal, while the high sensitivity of CT in detecting small calcifications is well known.

Advantages of MRI over other methods

CT is apparently superior to MRI for detecting and staging pancreatic tumours. Motion-induced ghost artefacts from surrounding fat and gastrointestinal tract are major problems that produce poor quality magnetic resonance images. MRI does not allow a definitive diagnosis between cancer and pancreatitis. The major advantage of MRI in staging pancreatic carcinomas is its sensitivity for detection of hepatic metastases.

Gastrointestinal tract

General characteristics

Neoplasms of the gastrointestinal tracts are common, and while advances in barium studies and endoscopic procedures allow accurate diagnosis, assessment of invasion beyond the gut wall or of metastasis to other organs is essential to enable therapy to be planned.

MRI findings

MRI has not been used in the diagnosis of gastrointestinal tract tumours due to its poor spatial resolution, motion artefacts, and poor contrasts between tumours and the bowel wall. However, extension of oesophageal and rectal carcinomas into adjacent structures can be detected with relative success due to fewer motion artefacts and the high contrast of surrounding fat tissue. In other parts of the gastrointestinal tract, MRI usually illustrates only large masses fixed to other abdominal structures.

Advantages of MRI over other methods

MRI can be equal or superior to CT in staging of rectal cancers since high quality pelvic images can be obtained. The multiplanar capabilities of MRI allow studies to be performed in the sagittal plane to delineate rectal anatomy. With current resolution, MRI is unlikely to be able to distinguish mucosal tumours from those invading muscle. However, MRI can reliably detect invasive tumours beyond the bowel wall; this is useful in assisting the planning of surgical excision. Sagittal and coronal images can clearly delineate the relationship between the tumour and the rectal sphincter, allowing planning of a sphincter-saving operation. MRI may be equal or superior to CT in detecting pelvic lymphadenopathy and is more specific in identifying the normal patient, but the criteria for lymphadenopathy depends upon the size of nodes: the borderline for enlarged nodes has been reported as ranging from 12 mm to 20 mm.

Kidney

General characteristics

The detection of renal masses has been dramatically improved by the advance of imaging modalities. At present, the major application of MRI to the kidneys include staging of kidney cell carcinomas and characterization of retroperitoneal masses.

MRI findings

Renal cell carcinomas

The detection of renal cell carcinoma using MRI is sometimes difficult, particularly when lesions are smaller than 2 cm, because its signal intensities are similar to those of renal parenchyma. There is no morphologically specific finding in this disease (Fig. 4).

Angiomyolipoma

The appearance of angiomyolipoma on MRI depends upon the fatty component of the tumour, as with CT. It becomes impossible to differentiate renal angiomyolipoma from renal cell carcinoma if the fat component is poorly contained.

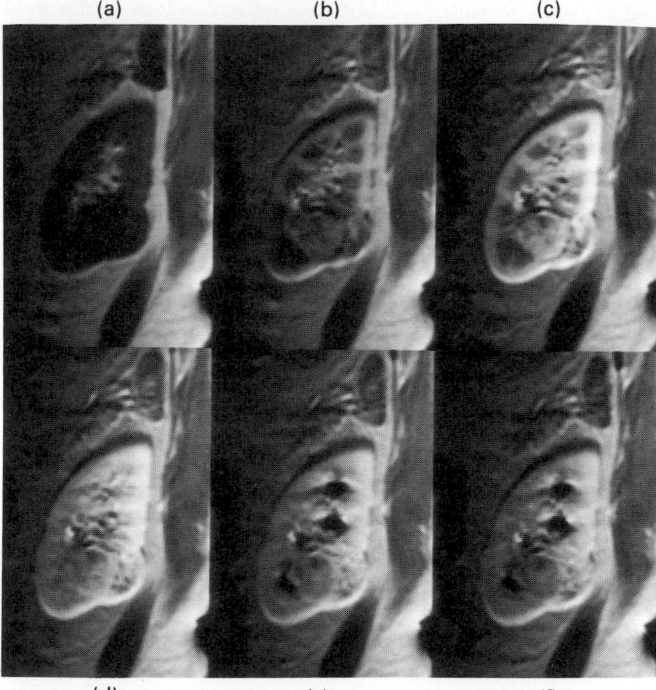

Fig. 4 Left renal cell carcinoma (sagittal view). (a) T_1-weighted image shows an isointensity mass in the lower pole of the left kidney. The contour of the tumour is not apparent. (b)–(f) After the bolus injection of gadolinium-DTPA, the contour of hypervascular tumour is clearly demonstrated.

Haemorrhagic cysts

Haemorrhagic cysts occasionally mimic solid tumours on CT. They produce a very high intensity signal on both T_1- and T_2-weighted images and can be delineated from tumours.

Stones

Renal stones are not usually detected, except for staghorn calculi, which show a signal void.

Advantages of MRI over other methods

MRI has similar results to contrast-enhanced CT in the staging of renal cell carcinoma, with an overall accuracy of 91 per cent. Evaluation of vascular extension and invasion of adjacent organs are two areas in which CT is less reliable than multiplanar resonance. Studies in coronal and sagittal planes allow more accurate differentiation of polar renal masses, adrenal masses, retroperitoneal tumours, or tumours of liver origin, which are notoriously poorly delineated in transverse planes on CT. Multiplanar studies are also useful for evaluating the extent of intravenous tumour thrombus. There are no specific signal characteristics that allow one to differentiate between malignant and inflammatory retroperitoneal lymph nodes using MRI.

MRI has not been extensively applied to the evaluation of renal pelvic tumours (transitional cell carcinomas) since intravenous urography and antegrade/retrograde pyelography have high diagnostic accuracy.

Intravenous contrast agents such as gadolinium-DTPA can be

used in MRI, as with CT. MRI has no advantages in this field because CT and sonography are apparently better able to detect renal mass lesions than MRI.

Adrenal gland

General characteristics

Non-invasive evaluation of adrenal gland morphology has been facilitated by the advance of CT, which has good spatial resolution. Adrenal tumours are divided into functioning and non-functioning; the former can be diagnosed by hormonal assays, but the latter have to be differentiated from metastases.

MRI findings

There are no tissue- or hormone-specific findings which allow differentiation between adenomas, carcinomas, and metastases. The diagnosis is usually established on the basis of morphological appearance, as with CT, rather than signal intensities.

Advantages of MRI over other methods

The advantages of MRI in this field lie in its multiplanar capabilities that allow adrenal tumours to be differentiated from tumours of adjacent structures. There appears to be an overlap of approximately 25 per cent in the signal characteristics of malignant (metastatic) and benign adrenal tumours. Needle aspiration biopsy is still imperative to characterize tissue reliably.

Pelvis

Uterus

General characteristics

Cervical carcinoma, endometrial carcinoma, and uterine myoma are common disorders requiring surgical treatment. While gynaecological examinations can provide some information about tumour staging, imaging is essential for the accurate diagnosis of uterine cancers.

MRI findings

T_2-weighted images provide superior contrast resolution of the zonal anatomy of the uterine body and the boundary between the uterus and cervix, the isthmus and the vagina. Delineation of these structures allows the depth of myometrial invasion and vaginal invasion of uterine neoplasms to be determined: tumours appear as high intensity lesions in low intensity muscular structures. T_2-weighting is also sensitive in demonstrating as low intensity masses uterine leiomyomas as small as 0.5 cm, and can determine the site of origin as submucosal, intramural, or subserosal.

Advantages of MRI over other methods

The advantages of MRI over CT in this field are multiplanar capability and the superior contrast resolution obtained with T_2-weighted images. MRI has been reported to be able to demonstrate Stage II lesions in cervical cancers and Stage I, II, and III lesions in endometrial cancers, but it cannot detect Stage 0 lesions of either. T_2-weighted imaging in the sagittal plane may be useful in detecting rectal or vesical invasion; however CT is the most accurate method for staging advanced cervical cancers. MRI is as accurate as CT in demonstrating lymph node involvement but benign and malignant adenopathy cannot be separated.

Another potential of MRI is the capability of imaging obstetric patients, since it avoids any prenatal exposure to radiation.

Ovary

General characteristics

Ovarian neoplasms are currently classified according to a WHO scheme based on histogenesis: epithelial origin, stromal origin, and germ cell origin. Up to 10 per cent of neoplasms are metastases from other sites. Preoperative imaging affects only the type of operative approach, since all patients with malignant ovarian tumours should undergo laparotomy. In patients with benign tumours, imaging may be used for follow-up, but laparotomy is eventually needed to rule out malignancy.

MRI findings

Benign cystic ovarian tumours typically appear as low intensity on T_1-weighted images and high intensity on T_2 weighting, but often contain haemorrhage and protein-rich fluid, causing a high intensity T_1-weighted image. Some kinds of ovarian tumours, for example, ovarian fibroma, show characteristic low intensity on T_2-weighted images but most ovarian tumours show non-specific findings that do not allow differentiation of benign from malignant.

Advantages of MRI over other methods

MRI has not been sufficiently evaluated in the diagnosis and staging of ovarian tumours. Its multiplanar capabilities may be of value in detecting the spread of malignant tumours to adjacent organs, but MRI has not been proved to be more useful than CT or sonography in differentiating between benign and malignant tumours. MRI and CT are equally effective in the detection of pelvic and retroperitoneal lymphadenopathy, and MRI can also be used to characterize some specific ovarian tumours, such as fibroma, polycystic ovary, and endometrial cyst. Dermoid cysts, the most common benign ovarian tumours, are better characterized on CT than by MRI.

Bladder

General characteristics

Bladder tumours are classified histologically as transitional cell carcinoma (most common), adenocarcinoma (from urachal remnants), squamous cell carcinoma, sarcoma, and others. Since most superficial tumours are treated by endoscopic resection, imaging should be performed, particularly to stage bladder tumours which have extended beyond the muscular layer of the wall and to assess metastases.

MRI findings

T_1-weighted images and PDWI can usually delineate tumours from urine and perivesical fat, while T_2 weighting allows differentiation of tumour from adjacent normal bladder wall. Disruption of the low intensity line of the bladder wall on T_2-weighted images correlates with invasion beyond the deep muscular layer.

Advantages of MRI over other methods

Reported accuracies of MRI in staging bladder tumours range from 73 to 85 per cent, which is similar to or slightly better than CT (59–88 per cent). MRI is unreliable in predicting the depth of bladder wall invasion, especially in delineating invasiveness of superficial tumours (less than Stage B2) from invasive tumours (more than Stage B2).

Prostate

General characteristics

Prostatic cancer is the second most common cancer in men. Although digital rectal examination is still recommended as the best screening technique for the detection of potentially curable tumours, transrectal sonography and MRI have been recently introduced as complementary techniques.

MRI findings

MRI demonstrates the zonal anatomy of the prostate, allowing characterization of prostatic nodules and of prostatic cancers. T_2-weighted imaging allows the prostate to be divided into a hyperintense peripheral zone and a hypointense central and transitional zone. Prostatic carcinoma develops predominantly (about 70 per cent of cases) in the peripheral zone, although benign prostatic hyperplasia predominantly (95 per cent of cases) affects the transitional zone. Prostatic nodules arising from the peripheral zone are, therefore, likely to be malignant.

Advantages of MRI over other methods

MRI can provide excellent tissue contrast in the prostate, but the shape and signal intensity of prostatic carcinoma are non-specific and mimic benign prostatic hyperplasia unless extracapsular extension or metastases are obvious. The accuracy of MRI in differentiating stages A and B (confined to the prostate) from Stage C and D (extracapsular extension or metastases) has been reported to range from 52 to 89 per cent.

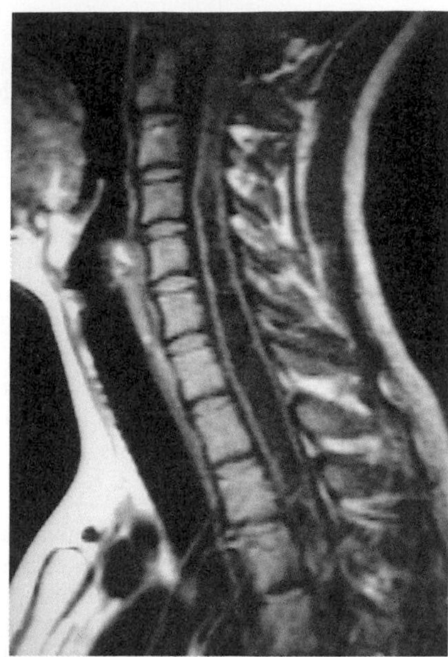

Fig. 5 Syringomyelia (sagittal view). T_1-weighted image shows a longitudinal low intensity within the spinal cord.

Orthopaedics

Spine

General characteristics

Disease of the spine can be divided into three categories: intramedullary (intraspinal cord) lesions, intradural extramedullary lesions, and extradural lesions, including intervertebral disc diseases.

MRI findings

Intramedullary lesions

Syringomyelia and hydromyelia appear as low intensity images with T_1 weighting and as high intensity lesions spreading longitudinally within the spinal cord with T_2 weighting (Fig. 5). In patients with Arnold–Chiari malformation, MRI which includes the posterior fossa of the skull can show the cerebellar tonsils and vermis projecting into the upper cervical spinal canal. Intramedullary plaques of multiple sclerosis may appear as high intensity on T_2-weighted images, but are not visible on T_1-weighted images.

Intramedullary spinal tumours (ependynomas and astrocytomas) have no reliable characteristic magnetic resonance feature, but appear as lesions with prolonged T_1 and T_2. Spinal arteriovenous malformation may be sometimes demonstrated as a high intensity lesion with a spotty signal void, consistent with abnormal large vessels detectable on T_2-weighted images.

Intradural extramedullary lesions

Paravertebral extension of the dumb-bell shape intradural extramedullary tumours (neurofibroma, neurinoma, etc.) are usually well demonstrated on T_2-weighted images but poorly differentiated with T_1 weighting from contiguous muscle (Fig. 6). Spinal meningiomas show similar signal intensities to neural tissues on both T_1- and T_2-weighted images.

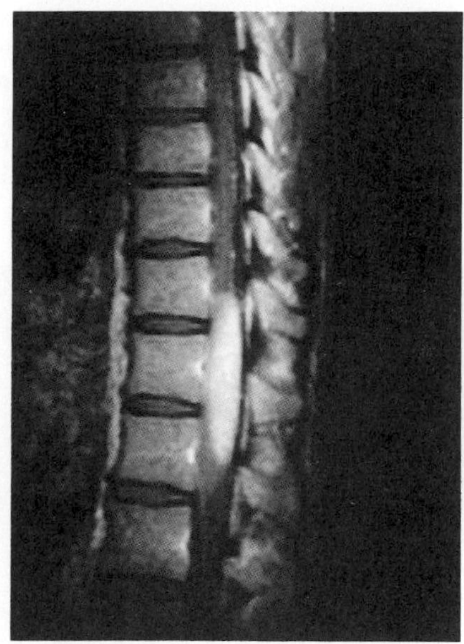

Fig. 6 Neurinoma (sagittal view). T_1-weighted image after the injection of gadiolinium-DTPA shows high intensity mass within the spinal canal.

Extradural lesions

Degenerative discs usually produce lower signal intensities than normal on T_2-weighted images. Protruded or extruded fragmented discs are easily visible on T_1-weighted and PD weighted images. Involvement of the spine by metastatic tumours is demonstrated as low intensity vertebrae on T_1-weighted imaging.

Advantages of MRI over other methods

For the investigation of almost all conditions of the spine, MRI is an alternative to contrast myelography and is complementary to radiographs and CT scans. Sagittal scans of the spine and oblique scans along disc spaces are particularly helpful.

Intramedullary lesions

Syringomyelia and hydromyelia can be demonstrated in their superior and inferior extents in most cases (about 90 per cent). CT-myelography is the most effective way in confirming syringomyelia when results of MRI are equivocal. MRI is the only method capable of demonstrating intramedullary plaques of mutiple sclerosis. A survey examination of the brain in patients with suspected spinal lesions of multiple sclerosis may demonstrate lesions compatible with this diagnosis.

Intradural extramedullary lesions

Intradural extramedullary tumours can be demonstrated on MRI as well as on CT, but secondary erosivė changes of the subarticular canal are less precisely visualized than with CT. Calcification is frequently difficult or impossible to detect on MRI. The intravenous contrast agent gadolinium-DTPA may be valuable, particularly in detection and estimation of extent of tumours.

Extradural lesions

Degenerative disc diseases (spondylosis, disc herniation, and canal stenosis) are widely applicable to investigation by MRI. There is 83 per cent agreement between the results of preoperative MRI and surgical findings in patients with degenerative disc diseases, a rate equivalent to that of CT–myelography. T_2-weighted imaging in the sagittal plane is useful in the survey of degenerative discs, which show lower signal intensities than normal (Fig. 7). Sagittal T_1-weighted imaging allows simultaneous visualization of multiple metastatic tumours affecting the vertebrae; this is impossible with CT.

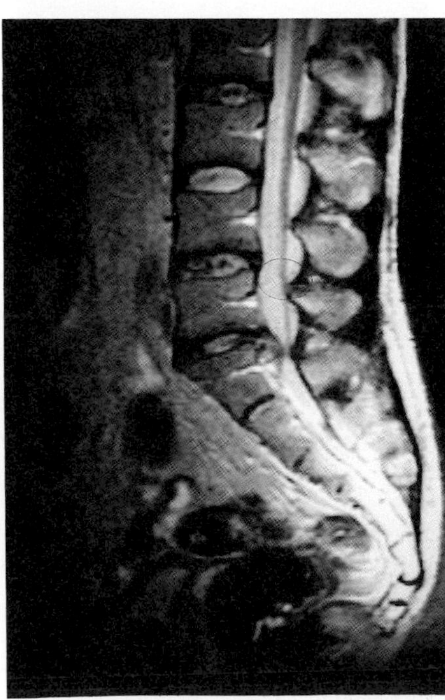

Fig. 7 Lumbar disc herniation (sagittal view). T_2-weighted image shows the extrusion and caudal migration of L5–S1 intervertebral disc compressing the spinal cord.

MRI findings complementary to plain radiographs in the assessment of vertebral disorders, such as atlantoaxial subluxation, spondylosis, spondylolisthesis, and tethered cord syndrome (myelomeningocele with dysgenesis of the spina and lipoma).

Knee joint

General characteristics

Injuries of the knee joint, such as meniscal tears, ligament injuries and fractures, arthritis, and neoplasms are routinely encountered. Plain films, CT, and arthrography are used for diagnosis. The use of MRI in the assessment of knee joint diseases is increasing because of its capability to be used in multiple image planes and fewer problems with motion artefacts.

MRI findings

Excellent visualization of menisci and ligaments can be achieved by coronal and sagittal MRI. For example, meniscal tears show disruption of low intensity meniscus in high intensity intra-articular fat or fluid on T_2-weighted images.

Advantages of MRI over other methods

MRI may be helpful in evaluating patients with minor knee injuries and may reduce the need for arthrography and arthroscopy. Meniscal tears that are difficult to detect on arthroscopy can be demonstrated, along with surrounding fluid or blood. Images along the longitudinal direction of the femur, tibia, and fibula are useful to show the extent of marrow involvement in patients with bone tumours.

Glenohumeral joint (Fig. 8)

General characteristics

The most common clinical indications for MRI are pain or restricted range of motion in the shoulder, patients referred with suspected rotator cuff tears or impingement, defects in the glenolabrum, infections, and neoplasms.

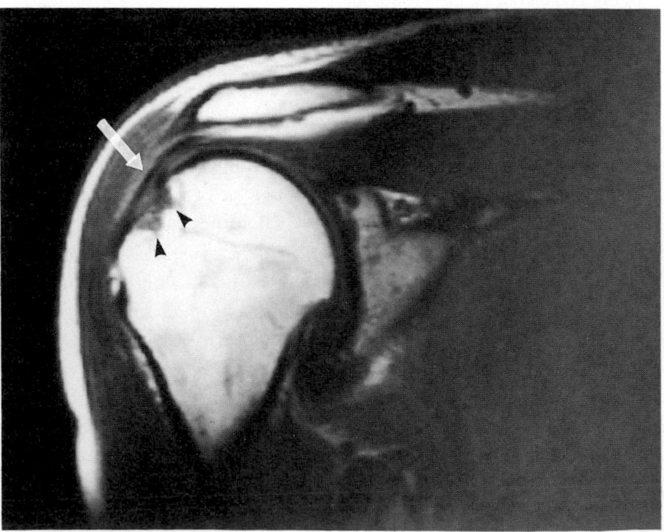

Fig. 8 Injury of supraspinous tendon of the right shoulder (coronal view). T_1-weighted image shows the slight swelling of the tendon (arrow) and associated detachment of humeral head (arrowhead).

MRI findings

Sagittal T_2-weighted imaging is well suited for evaluating rotator cuff disease. Tendinitis and fluid collections show as high intensity lesions, often associated with the cuff tear. Disruption of the labrum, the main cause of recurrent anterior dislocation, are seen as linear high intensity lesions on T_2-weighted imaging.

Advantages of MRI over other methods

Routine radiography, radionuclide studies, CT, and sonography have been important techniques for evaluating the glenohumeral joint, but arthrography has been essential when surgical treatment is considered. MRI may reduce the indications for arthrography by its excellent soft tissue contrast and multiplanar capability.

Hip joint

General characteristics

Although there are numerous causes of hip pain, MRI has progressed most rapidly in evaluating patients with suspected avascular necrosis of the femoral head because of its high sensitivity and specificity.

MRI findings

Early in the course of avascular necrosis, an inhomogeneous loss of signal intensity can be seen on T_1-weighted images. A low intensity line of demarcation may also be evident at the margin of the necrotic zone during the early phase, when radiographs are typically normal.

Advantages of MRI over other methods

MRI permits early detection of avascular necrosis of the hip.

FURTHER READING

Bernardino ME, Steiberg HV, Pearson TC. Comparison of MRI and angiography in the determination of shunt patency for portal hypertension. *Radiology* 1986; **158**: 57–61.

Berquist TH, *et al.* Magnetic resonance imaging of the chest: a diagnostic comparison with computed tomography and hilar tomography. *Magnetic Resonance Imaging* 1984; **2**: 315–27.

Berquist TH. Shoulder and arm. In: Berquist TH, ed. *MRI of the Musculoskeletal System*, 2nd edn. New York: Raven Press, 1990: 313–56.

Biondetti PR, Lee JKT, Ling D, Catalona WJ. Clinical stage B prostate carcinoma: staging with MR imaging. *Radiology* 1987; **162**: 325–9.

Bradley WG Jr, Crooks LE, Newton TH. Physical principles of NMR. In: Newton TH, Potts DG, eds. *Modern Neuroradiology*, Vol. 2. San Francisco: Clavadel, 1983: 15–61.

Brant-Zawadzki M, *et al.* Primary intracranial tumour imaging: a comparison of magnetic resonance and CT. *Radiology* 1984; **150**: 435–40.

Brant-Zawadzki M, *et al.* Basic principles of magnetic resonance imaging in cerebral ischaemia and initial clinical experience. *Neuroradiology* 1985; **27**: 517–20.

Butch RJ, *et al.* Staging rectal carcinoma by MR and CT. *Am J Roentgenol* 1986; **146**: 1155–60.

Butch RJ, Stark DD, Malt RA. Magnetic resonance imaging of focal hepatic nodular hyperplasia. *J Comput Assist Tomogr* 1986; **10**: 874–7.

Buy J-N, *et al.* MR imaging of bladder carcinoma: correlation with pathologic findings. *Radiology* 1988; **169**: 695–700.

Bydder GM, *et al.* Enhancement of cervical intraspinal tumors in MR imaging with Gd-DTPA. *J Comput Assist Tomogr* 1985; **9**: 847–51.

Choyke PL, Kressel HY, Pollack HM, Arger PM, Axel L, Mamourian AC. Focal renal masses: magnetic resonance imaging. *Radiology* 1984; **152**: 471–7.

Dooms GC, Hricak, H, Crooks LE, Higgins CB. Magnetic resonance imaging of the lymph nodes: comparison with CT. *Radiology* 1984; **153**: 719–28.

Dooms GC, *et al.* Cholangiocarcinoma imaging by MR. *Radiology* 1986; **159**: 89–94.

Ebara M, *et al.* Diagnosis of small hepatocellular carcinoma: correlation of MR imaging and tumor histologic studies. *Radiology* 1986; **159**: 371–7.

Ferruci JT Jr. MR imaging of the liver. *Am J Roentgenol* 1986; **147**: 1103–16.

Gallimore G, Harms SE. Knee injuries: high-resolution MR imaging. *Radiology* 1986; **160**: 457–61.

Gamsu G, *et al.* Magnetic resonance imaging of benign mediastinal masses. *Radiology* 1984; **151**: 709–13.

Glazer GM, *et al.* Evaluation of focal hepatic masses: a comparative study of MRI and CT. *Gastrointest Radiol* 1986; **11**: 263–8.

Gomori JM, *et al.* Intracranial haematomas: imaging by high field MR. *Radiology* 1985: 87–92.

Grossman RI. Haemorrhage. In: Stark DD, Bradley WG Jr, eds. *Syllabus: a Categorical Course in Diagnostic Imaging—MR Imaging*. Radiological Society of North America 1988: 189–95.

Hricak H, *et al.* Uterine leiomyoma: correlation of MR, histopathologic findings and symptoms. *Radiology* 1986; **158**: 385–91.

Hricak H, Thoeni RF, Carrol PR, Demas BE, Marotti M, Tanagho EA. Detection and staging of renal neoplasms: a reassessment of MR imaging. *Radiology* 1988; **166**: 643–9.

Idy-Perenti I, Bittoun J. Physical basis. In: Vanel D, McNamara MT, eds. *MRI of the Body*. Paris: Springer-Verlag, 1989: 1–29.

Kerlin P, *et al.* Hepatic adenoma and focal nodular hyperplasia: clinical, pathologic and radiologic features. *Gastroentrology* 1983; **84**: 994–1002.

Lee BCP, Deck MDF. Sellar and juxtasellar lesion detection with MR. *Radiology* 1985; **151**: 143–7.

Lee JKT, *et al.* Magnetic resonance imaging of abdominal and pelvic lymphadenopathy. *Radiology* 1984; **153**: 181–8.

Lee BCP, *et al.* MR imaging of syringomyelia and hydromyelia. *Am J Neuroradiol* 1985; **6**: 221–8.

Li KC, *et al.* Distinction of cavernous hemangioma from hepatic metastases with MRI. *Radiology* 1988; **169**: 409–15.

Mitchell DG, Rao VM, Dalinka MK. Femoral head avascular necrosis: correlation of MR imaging, radiographic staging, radionuclide imaging and clinical findings. *Radiology* 1987; **162**: 715.

Modic MT, *et al.* Imaging of degenerative disc disease. *Radiology* 1988; **168**: 177–86.

Mueller NL, Gamsu G, Webb WR. Pulmonary nodules: detection using magnetic resonance and computed tomography. *Radiology* 1985; **155**: 687–90.

Nelson RC, Chezmar JL, Sugarbaker PH, Bernardino ME. Hepatic tumors: comparison of CT during arterial portography, delayed CT, and MRI imaging for preoperative evaluation. *Radiology* 1989; **172**: 27–34.

Peck WW, Dillon WP, Norman D, Newton TH, Wilson CB. High-resolution MR imaging of pituitary adenomas at 1.5 T: experience with Cushing disease. *Am J Roentgenol* 1989; **152**: 145–51.

Renig JW, *et al.* Adrenal masses differentiated by MR. *Radiology* 1986; **158**: 81–4.

Rummeny E, *et al.* MR imaging of liver neoplasms. *Am J Roentgenol* 1989; **152**: 493–9.

Schiebler ML, *et al.* Prostatic carcinoma and benign prostatic hyperplasia: correlation of high-resolution MR and histopathologic findings. *Radiology* 1989; **172**: 131–7.

Sipponen JT, Sepponen RE, Sivula A. Nuclear magnetic resonance (NMR) imaging of intracerebral haemorrhage in the acute and resolving phases. *J Comput Assist Tomogr* 1983; **7**: 959.

Stark DD, Moss AA, Goldberg HI, Davis PL, Federle MP. Magnetic resonance and CT of the normal and diseased pancreas: a comparative study. *Radiology* 1984; **150**: 153–62.

Stark DD, *et al.* Detection of hepatic metastases by magnetic resonance: analysis of pulse sequence performance. *Radiology* 1986; **159**: 365–70.

Stark DD, Wittenberg J, Butch RJ, Ferrucci JT Jr. MR detection of hepatic metastases: a randomized controlled comparison with CT. *Radiology* 1987; **165**: 339–406.

Stark DD, *et al.* Magnetic resonance imaging and spectroscopy of hepatic iron overload. *Radiology* 1985; **154**: 137–42.

Stark DD, *et al.* Magnetic resonance imaging of the neck. II. Pathologic findings. *Radiology* 1983; **150**: 455–61.

Stark DD, Clark OH, Moss AA. Magnetic resonance imaging of the thyroid, thymus and parathyroid glands. *Surgery* 1984; **96**: 1083–90.

Stark DD, Moss AA, Goldberg HI. Nuclear magnetic resonance of the liver, spleen and pancreas. *Cardiovasc Interventional Radiol* 1986; **8**: 329–341.

Stark DD, *et al.* Magnetic resonance imaging of the neck. I. Normal anatomy. *Radiology* 1983; **150**: 447–54.

Stark DD, Goldberg HI, Moss AA, Bass NM. Chronic liver disease: evaluation by magnetic resonance. *Radiology* 1984; **150**: 149–51.

Steiner E, *et al.* Imaging of pancreatic neoplasms: comparison of MR and CT. *Am J Roentgenol* 1989; **152**: 487–91.

Sze G, *et al.* Gadolinium-DTPA in the evaluation of intradural extramedullary spinal disease. *Am J Neuroradiol* 1988; **9**: 153–63.

Webb WR, *et al.* Evaluation of magnetic resonance imaging of the normal and abnormal pulmonary hila. *Radiology* 1984; **152**: 89–94.

Wehrli FW. Principles of magnetic resonance. In: Stark DD, Bradley WG Jr, eds. *Magnetic resonance Imaging*. St Louis: Mosby, 1988: 3–23.

Winkler ML, Hricak H, Higgins CB. MR imaging of diffusely infiltrating gastric carcinoma. *J Comput Assist Tomogr* 1987; **11**: 337–9.

6.4 Gastrointestinal radiology

DANIEL J. NOLAN

ROLE OF PLAIN ABDOMINAL RADIOGRAPHS IN DIAGNOSIS OF THE ACUTE ABDOMEN

Plain radiographs are the initial imaging procedure performed in most patients who present with suspected acute disorders of the gastrointestinal tract. Radiographs of the abdomen and chest can provide essential diagnostic information.

Examination technique

A supine view of the abdomen and an upright view of the chest are the basic views considered essential in most patients. The upright chest radiograph is an important part of the examination: pain from pleural or lung disorders may present initially with abdominal pain and this is the most reliable view for showing free intraperitoneal air. Decubitus and upright views of the abdomen are also occasionally helpful. It may be necessary to proceed to contrast studies, ultrasound, or computed tomography (CT) if plain radiographs are unhelpful or inconclusive.

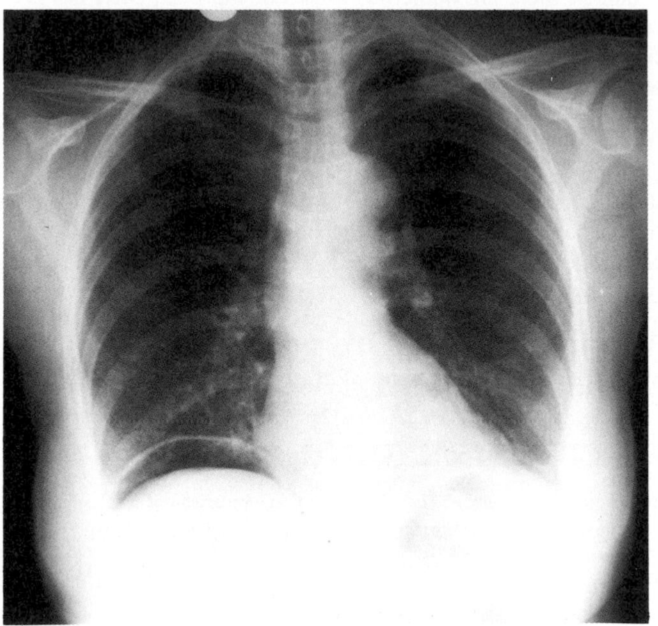

Fig. 1 Pneumoperitoneum—chest radiograph. A collection of air is noted between the liver and right hemidiaphragm.

Pneumoperitoneum

Spontaneous pneumoperitoneum normally indicates that a duodenal or gastric ulcer has perforated, or that the colon has perforated due to diverticulitis, acute colitis, carcinoma, or trauma. Perforation of the small intestine is uncommon. Free intraperitoneal air is demonstrated in 60 to 90 per cent of plain radiographs performed in patients with pneumoperitoneum, depending on how carefully the examination is performed. The upright posteroanterior chest and left lateral decubitus (right side up) abdominal radiographs are the best views for demonstrating the presence of pneumoperitoneum.

With good radiographic technique as little as 1 ml of intraperitoneal air can be detected. A small amount of free intraperitoneal air is demonstrated as a sickle-shaped collection of air between the liver and the diaphragm on the chest view (Fig. 1) and between the liver and the abdominal wall on the left lateral decubitus view. Larger collections of air may outline the liver. When a relatively large amount of free intraperitoneal air is present characteristic signs may be seen on the supine radiograph. These include gas outlining the outer wall of the intestine (Rigler's signs), a triangular collection of gas between intestinal loops, and gas outlining the gallbladder, the lower border of the liver, lesser sac, and the falciform ligament (Fig. 2). The characteristic 'football sign' is seen most frequently in infants, when a large amount of gas outlines the lateral limits of the peritoneal cavity.

Small intestinal obstruction

Causes of small intestinal obstruction include adhesions, bands and hernias, inflammatory lesions such as appendix abscess, diverticulitis, Crohn's disease, and neoplasms.

Small intestinal obstruction can be diagnosed on plain abdominal radiographs in 60 to 70 per cent of patients, and the supine

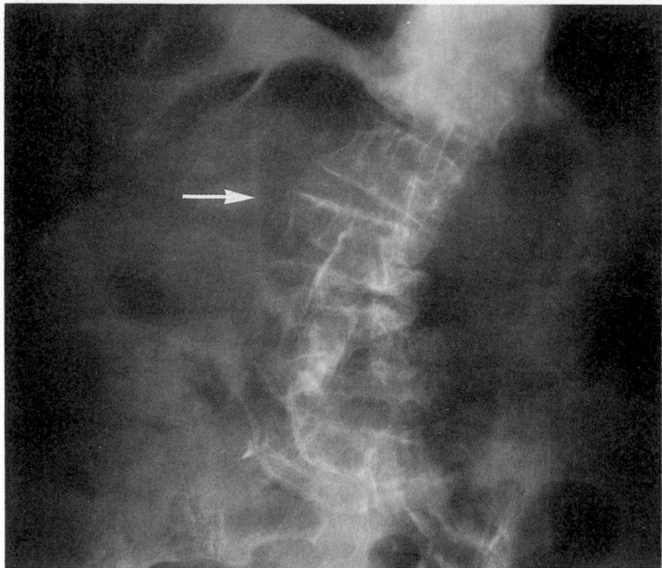

Fig. 2 Pneumoperitoneum. Free intraperitoneal gas is seen outlining the falciform ligament (arrow) on a supine view of the abdomen.

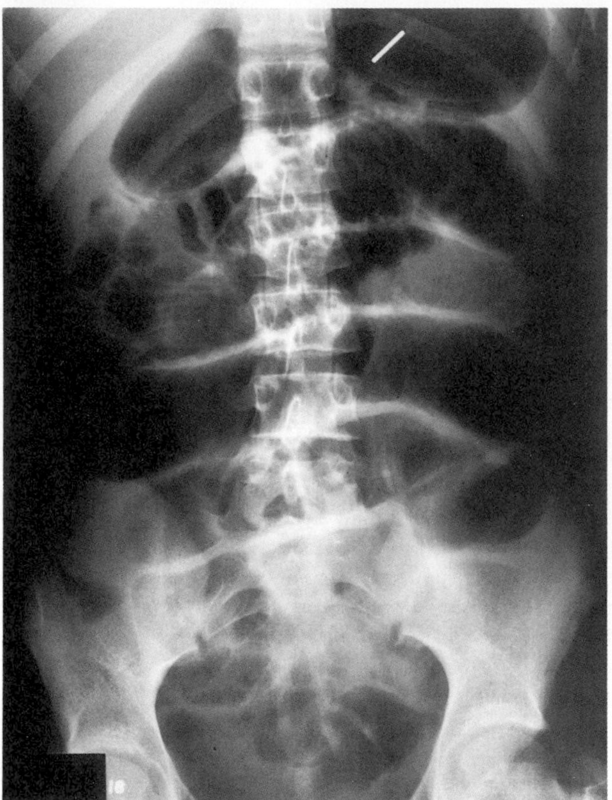

Fig. 3 Small intestinal obstruction. Dilated gas-filled loops of small intestine are seen in the centre of the abdomen. Very little gas is present in the colon. Note the nasogastric tube in the stomach.

abdominal view is the most reliable for making the diagnosis. Typical features are gas-distended loops of jejunum and ileum arranged in transverse loops across the central portion of the abdomen (Fig. 3). Little or no gas is seen in the colon in most

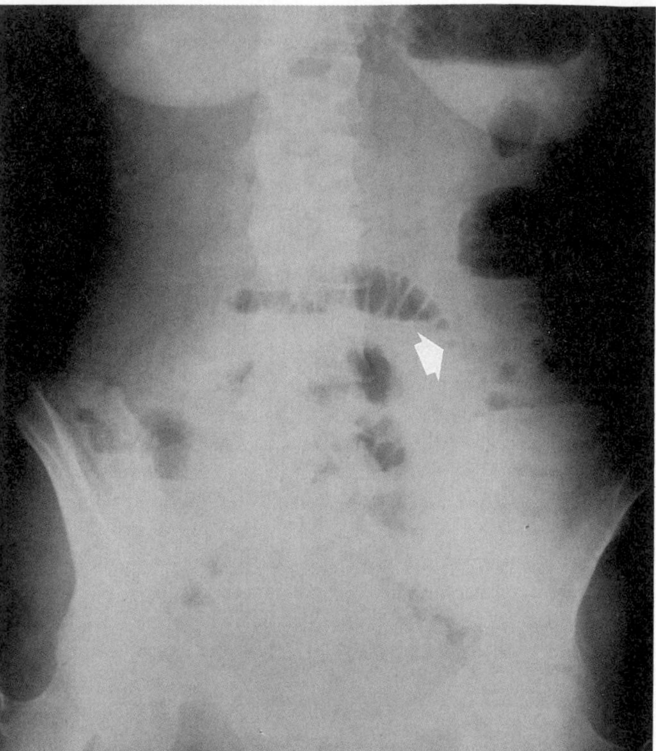

Fig. 4 Small intestinal obstruction. An upright view of the abdomen shows the typical 'string of beads', sign (arrow).

patients with obstruction of the small intestine, but a moderate or normal amount of colonic gas may be present if the lumen of the small intestine is not completely occluded. If the obstructed loops are fluid-filled they are more difficult to identify, but an upright view in such patients shows the classical 'string of beads' sign due to multiple small collections of gas above the fluid (Fig. 4). This is a diagnostic sign of small intestinal obstruction even in the absence of gas-distended loops of intestine.

Plain abdominal radiographs may have a normal appearance in patients with small intestinal obstruction, due to vomiting in cases of high obstruction or because of the intermittent nature of the obstruction.

Closed-loop obstruction occurs when a single loop of intestine is obstructed at two points, one proximal and one distal. Gas and/or fluid may be seen in a round or oval-shaped loop that remains constant in position on different views.

The characteristic appearances of gallstone ileus, caused by impaction of a gallstone in the small intestine, include evidence of intestinal obstruction, visualization of the obstruction calculus, and, in about one-third of cases, air in the biliary tree.

Large intestinal obstruction

The plain radiographic appearance of obstruction of the large intestine will depend on whether or not the ileocaecal valve is competent. When the valve is competent there is usually considerable dilatation of the colon as far as the obstruction, including marked caecal dilatation, usually with no dilatation of the small intestine. The ileocaecal valve is incompetent in most patients and dilatation of the colon and the small intestine is seen, with the caecum only showing slight dilatation. Fluid-filled distension of the proximal colon is seen when the obstructive lesion is proximal to the splenic flexure.

The site of transition between dilated gas- or fluid-filled colon and collapsed empty colon normally identifies the site of the obstructing lesion. If there is any doubt about the diagnosis an instant single-contrast barium or water-soluble contrast enema, performed with the contrast medium passing as far as the dilated colonic segments, confirms the presence or absence of obstruction. When obstruction is confirmed the cause is frequently identified. Caecal volvulus should be suspected when a haustrated and disproportionately enlarged air-filled viscus is seen anywhere in the abdomen; the caecum is usually absent from the right iliac fossa and distended small intestine is seen to the right of the dilated caecum. Sigmoid volvulus can frequently also be diagnosed on plain abdominal radiographs: the characteristic appearance is that of a grossly enlarged, gas-filled sigmoid colon arising from the pelvis and deviating to the left or right flank. The apex of the loop is positioned high in the abdomen and may lie under and elevate the diaphragm. Three dense curved lines, representing the walls of the enlarged loop, converge towards the stenosis over the left part of the sacrum (Fig. 5).

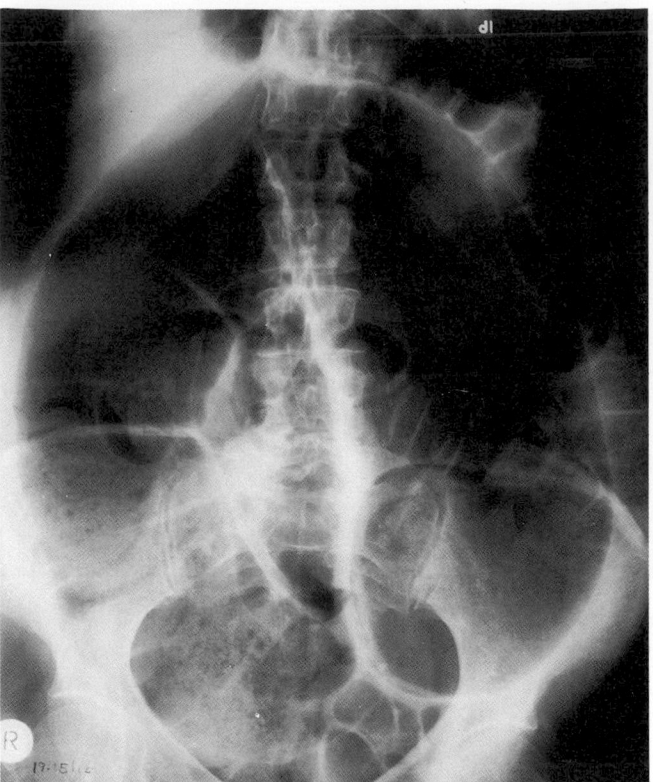

Fig. 5 Sigmoid volvulus. The sigmoid colon is grossly distended with gas and the walls of the enlarged loop converge over the left part of the sacrum. The ascending colon and transverse colon are loaded with faeces and are normal in size. Note Paget's disease involving the left hemipelvis.

Acute colitis

The supine view of the abdomen frequently yields important diagnostic information in acute ulcerative colitis. When air is present in the colon the mucosal edge and haustral pattern give an indication of the severity of the inflammation. In the segments where there is faecal residue active mucosal disease is unlikely. Patients with toxic megacolon, a potentially lethal complication of ulcerative colitis, show dilatation of the transverse colon (exceeding 5.5 cm in width). Other signs of toxic megacolon include loss of the normal haustral pattern, an irregular contour to the colonic wall, and numerous, broad-based rounded inflammatory polyps (pseudopolyps) projecting into the lumen of the dilated segment (Fig. 6). Perforation is a serious complication of toxic megacolon.

Mesenteric infarction

Acute mesenteric ischaemia and infarction may occur when emboli arising in the heart following atrial fibrillation, myocardial infarction, a left atrial myxoma, or deep venous thrombosis via a patent foramen ovale lodge in the superior mesenteric artery. Other causes of mesenteric infarction include cardiogenic shock and penetrating or blunt trauma to the abdomen. Plain abdominal radiographs show distended loops of small intestine shortly after the onset of symptoms; the number and size of the distended loops increase later. Specific radiological signs may develop, including thickening and oedema of the valvulae conniventes, thickening of the intestinal wall, air in the intestinal wall (Fig. 7), and air in the intrahepatic portal veins.

Paralytic ileus

Paralytic (adynamic) ileus is one of the more common forms of intestinal obstruction and usually occurs throughout the gastrointestinal tract, although occasionally involving only one segment. It is a risk that is present for 3 to 4 days after an abdominal operation. Other causes of paralytic ileus include intestinal ischaemia, sepsis, intraperitoneal inflammation such as acute appendicitis, cholecystitis, pancreatitis, retroperitoneal haematoma, fracture of the spine, ureteric colic, thoracic lesions such as basal pneumonia, rib fractures, or myocardial infarction.

Dilated loops of small and large intestine with air–fluid levels are frequently seen on plain abdominal radiographs. It may be impossible to distinguish adynamic ileus from obstruction and a contrast study may be required to establish the correct diagnosis. When there is localized inflammation, such as in appendicitis, cholecystitis, or pancreatitis, the ileus may develop in one or two adjacent loops of small intestine called 'sentinel loops'.

CONTRAST STUDIES OF THE GASTROINTESTINAL TRACT

Barium-enhanced examination of the upper gastrointestinal tract is used to evaluate the oesophagus, stomach, and duodenum. The double-contrast barium examination, which is now used routinely in the great majority of centres, is quick and easy to perform and takes about 10 to 15 min.

High-density barium is used to coat the mucosal surfaces and a gas-producing agent is used to distend the stomach and duodenum. An intravenous injection of hyoscine butylbromide

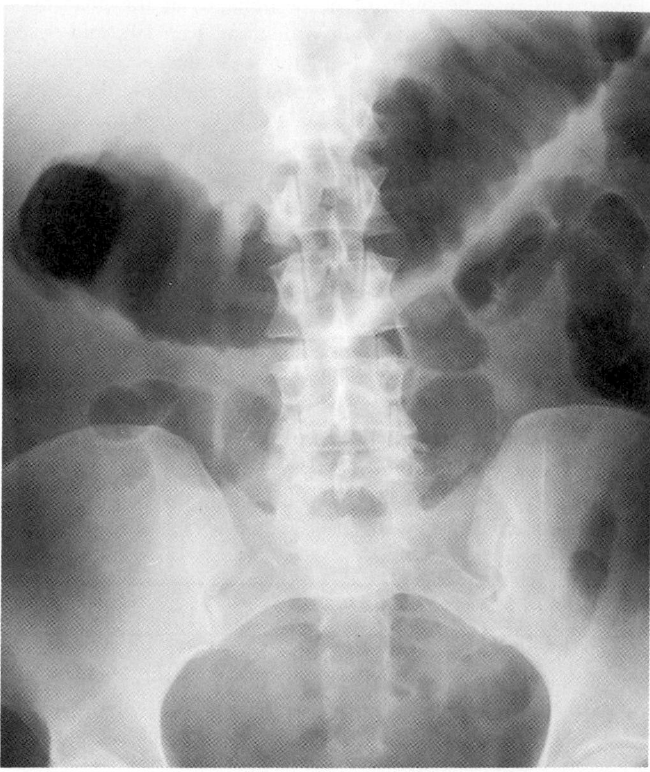

Fig. 6 Toxic megacolon in ulcerative colitis. The transverse colon is dilated, there is loss of the normal haustral pattern, and multiple broad-based inflammatory polyps are present in the dilated segment. An increased amount of gas is noted in the small intestine.

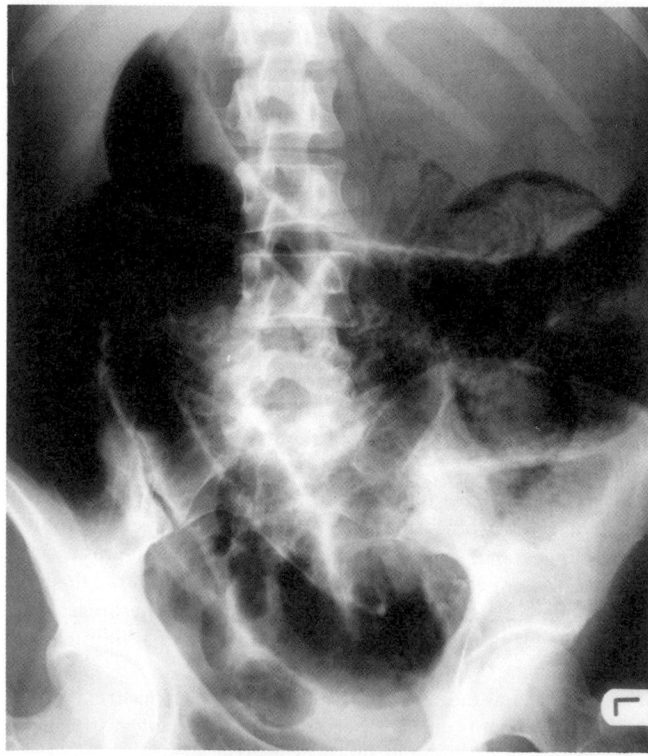

Fig. 7 Intestinal infarction. The small intestine is dilated and there is extensive gas in the wall of the intestine.

(Buscopan) or glucagon is given to relax smooth muscle. Double-contrast views of the oesophagus are obtained when the barium is swallowed quickly, so that the swallowed air distends the oesophagus enabling mucosal views to be obtained.

Oesophagus

The oesophagus extends from the cricopharyngeus to the gastro-oesophageal junctions. Dysphagia (difficulty in swallowing) is a distressing symptom caused by narrowing of the lumen of the oesophagus. Causative factors include carcinoma of the oesophagus, carcinoma of the fundus of the stomach invading the lower oesophagus, benign strictures, extrinsic neoplasms compressing the oesophagus, and oesophageal webs. A food bolus may impact in the oesophagus during severe oesophageal spasm.

Carcinoma of the oesophagus appears on barium studies as an irregular stricture with mucosal destruction and shouldering of the margins, as an infiltrating constricting lesion, or as an irregular polypoid mass (Fig. 8).

When carcinoma of the fundus invades the lower oesophagus the primary tumour may be obvious as a large mass in the fundus. In other cases a carcinoma is seen at the oesophagogastric junction with little indication of whether the neoplasm originates in the lower oesophagus or fundus of the stomach.

The oesophagus may be compressed by enlarged neoplastic mediastinal lymph glands or primary carcinoma of the bronchus. Carcinoma of the bronchus occasionally invades the oesophagus, resulting in an oesophagobronchial fistula that can be identified on a barium swallow.

Most benign strictures result from gastro-oesophageal reflux and are usually located in the lower oesophagus just above the oesophagogastric junction. There may be an associated hiatal hernia. Such strictures usually appear as smooth segments of narrowing, although there may be some irregularity of the mucosa without mucosal destruction (Fig. 9). It may be impossible to distinguish a benign oesophageal stricture from primary carcinoma.

Prolonged nasogastric intubation may result in the development of oesophageal strictures, and the accidental ingestion of corrosive acids or alkalis can also result in severe damage to the oesophagus with subsequent stricture formation. Certain medication in tablet form, including tetracycline, quinidine, and potassium chloride, may lodge in the oesophagus at the level of the aortic arch, causing oesophagitis and occasionally strictures.

Hiatus hernias, classified as sliding and rolling, are seen as herniations of stomach through the diaphragmatic hiatus into the thorax. Sliding hiatal hernias are by far the more common type and are present when both the oesophagogastric junction and stomach herniate into the thorax. While only a small amount of stomach may herniate in some patients, in others the whole stomach is affected. Hiatal hernias are reducible when they move in and out of the thorax and non-reducible when part of the stomach remains fixed in the thorax. The rolling type of hiatal hernia, also known as para-oesophageal hernia is seen when the oesophagogastric junction remains in its normal position below the diaphragm, the stomach herniating into the thorax beside the normally positioned lower oesophagus.

Oesophageal webs are seen as shelf-like defects in the cervical oesophagus extending from the anterior wall in a posterior direction. Some webs are circumferential and allow a jet of barium to pass through the centre.

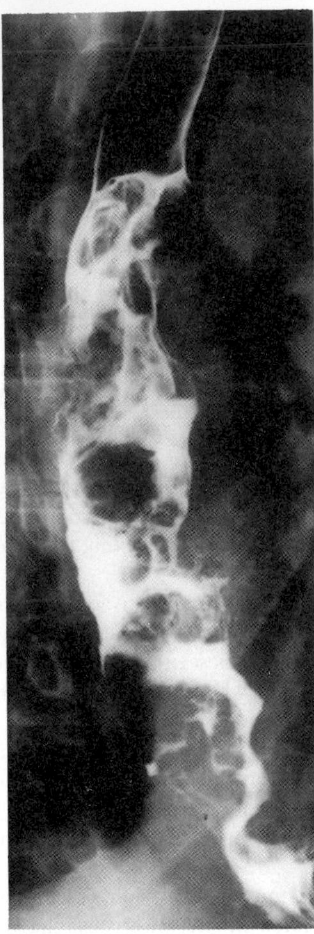

Fig. 8 Carcinoma of the oesophagus. An extensive irregular polypoid mass is seen involving the lower half of the oesophagus.

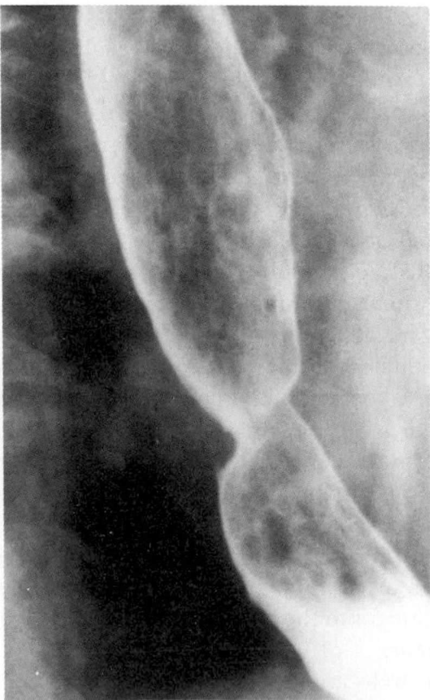

Fig. 9 Benign oesophageal stricture. A short segment of smooth narrowing is noted in the lower oesophagus.

Diverticula may be seen in the oesophagus at the pharyngo-oesophageal junction (Zenker's diverticulum; Fig. 10), mid-oesophagus, or at the distal end of the oesophagus (epiphrenic diverticulum). Most mid-oesophageal and epiphrenic diverticula are asymptomatic. Zenker's diverticula may be small and difficult to recognize or can be large, compressing the adjacent oesophagus and soft tissues. The formation of Zenker's diverticulum is often related to gastroesophageal reflux and as a result there is an association between benign oesophageal strictures and Zenker's diverticula. For this reason, a barium swallow should always be performed in patients who present with dysphagia before proceeding to endoscopy, which can result in perforation of the diverticulum, with serious consequences.

Oesophageal varices represent dilated venous collaterals, and usually result from portal venous hypertension. They are seen on barium examination as serpiginous or oval filling defects, mostly in the lower oesophagus and extending upwards to involve the middle third of the oesophagus (Fig. 11). Obstruction to the superior vena cava may result in upper oesophageal varices.

Stomach

The most frequently encountered disorders of the stomach are ulceration and carcinoma. Gastric ulcers are seen as small or large, round or oval collections of barium with a surrounding zone of radiolucency due to oedema. Folds frequently radiate from the edge of the ulcer crater. The most frequent sites of gastric ulceration are the lesser curve and the posterior wall of the stomach (Fig. 12). So-called 'sump ulcers' may develop on the greater curve aspect of the gastric antrum and lower body of the stomach in patients taking analgesic medications (Fig. 13), commonly in the elderly. They develop because of the combined effect of gravity and the corrosive action of the drugs. Occasionally these sump ulcers penetrate through the gastric wall and result in the formation of a gastrocolic fistula.

Erosions are mostly present in the antrum and appear as small collections of barium with surrounding oedema, often located on gastric mucosal folds.

Carcinoma of the stomach is seen as an ulcerating, polypoid, or infiltrating lesion. Ulcerating carcinomas, sometimes called malignant ulcers, show thickening or distortion of the folds at the edge of the crater and fusion or amputation of the folds by an area of induration at the ulcer edge. Malignant ulcers are often shallow with a nodular or uneven pattern in the base of the crater and have ill-defined or irregular outlines. If malignancy is suspected an adequate number of endoscopic biopsies should be obtained at the earliest opportunity.

Polypoid carcinomas appear as irregular polypoid filling defects in the stomach (Fig. 14). Infiltrating carcinomas characteristically produce marked narrowing of the lumen of the stomach and when they involve the whole stomach, show the characteristic 'linitis plastica' appearance (Fig. 15); however, mucosal biopsies obtained at endoscopy from areas of linitis plastica often fail to show evidence of malignancy. Metastatic carcinoma of the breast may infiltrate the wall of the stomach and also result in a 'linitus plastica' appearance.

The clinical and radiological features of primary gastric lymphoma, which accounts for 2.5 per cent of malignant gastric neoplasms, frequently resemble those of gastric lesions, particularly carcinoma. Since the prognosis of primary gastric lymphoma is much better than that of carcinoma, accurate diagnosis is impor-

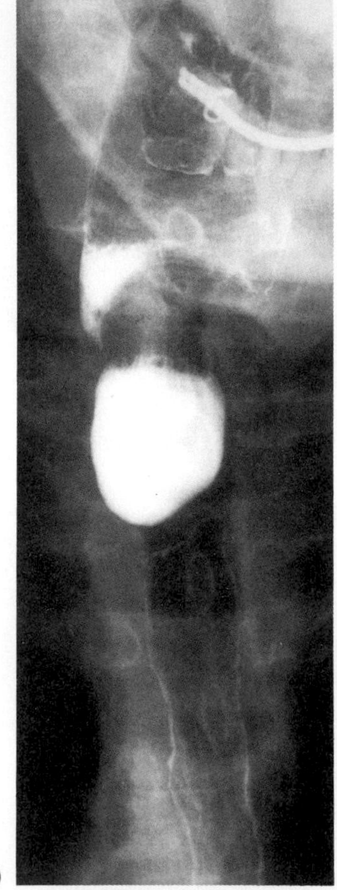
(a)

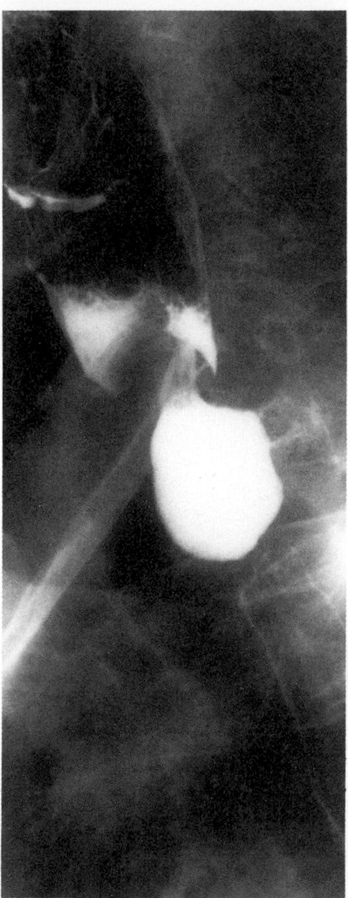
(b)

Fig. 10 Zenker's diverticulum (a,b). Anteroposterior and lateral views of the upper oesophagus show a moderate sized Zenker's diverticulum.

tant. Characteristic radiological features include a mass that may be partially effaced by the barium, gross hypertrophy of the mucosal folds that become more effaced as the stomach is distended (Fig. 16), and one or more large gastric ulcers seen in association with mucosal hypertrophy. Narrowing and rigidity of the gastric antrum may be seen, sometimes extending across the pylorus into the duodenum. Duodenal ulceration is occasionally found in association with a gastric mass.

Duodenum

Benign peptic ulceration is common and is the most frequently encountered disorder in the duodenum. The barium examination is an accurate technique for detecting and demonstrating duodenal ulcers, provided a good double-contrast examination technique is used. Ulcer craters in the duodenum appear as single or multiple sharply defined, constant collections of barium, sometimes with a surrounding zone of oedema or with folds radiating from the crater. Most ulcers have a diameter of less than 1 cm (Fig. 17). Some patients may have considerable deformity of the duodenal cap due to previous ulceration, making it difficult to detect an active ulcer crater. The degree of deformity varies considerably and, when marked, can result in duodenal stenosis.

A number of malignant neoplasms may involve the duodenum. Primary neoplasms of the duodenum are uncommon, and can be classified into carcinoma of the papilla of Vater and true carcinoma of the duodenum. Carcinoma of the papilla of Vater appears as an enlarged papilla with irregular borders, sometimes with ulceration. Non-papillary carcinomas of the duodenum are adenocarcinomas and are seen as ulcerative, polypoid or annular lesions, similar to the appearances of carcinomas in other parts of the gastrointestinal tract. Lymphomas and sarcomas of the duodenum are sometimes encountered.

The duodenum may be invaded by malignant neoplasms from adjacent organs or may be the site of metastic deposits. Carcinoma of the head of the pancreas frequently involves the duodenal loop, causing widening, a double contour, irregularity of the inner border, or stricture formation. The reversed '3' sign of Frostberg is a characteristic but infrequent finding. Carcinoma of the body or tail of the pancreas may invade the distal duodenum. The duodenum may also be invaded by malignant neoplasms in adjacent organs such as the colon, right kidney, and gallbladder. The duodenum may be the site of metastatic deposits from malignancies elsewhere, particularly malignant melanoma.

The duodenum is affected by Crohn's disease in about 4 per cent of patients who have the disease elsewhere in the small intestine or colon. The appearances are similar to those in the more distal parts of the small intestine. Crohn's disease may cause tubular narrowing of the gastric antrum and proximal duodenum in continuity, resulting in the 'pseudo post-Billroth I' appearance.

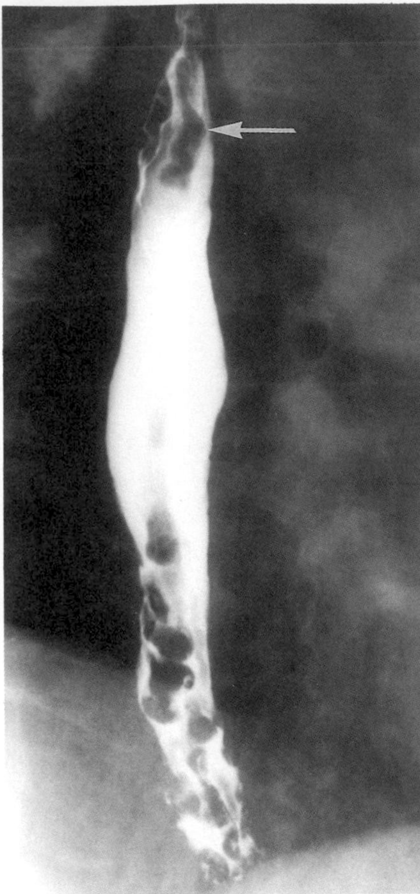

Fig. 11 Oesophageal varices. Multiple oval filling defects are seen in the lower oesophagus. A serpiginous filling defect can also be identified in the mid-oesophagus (arrow).

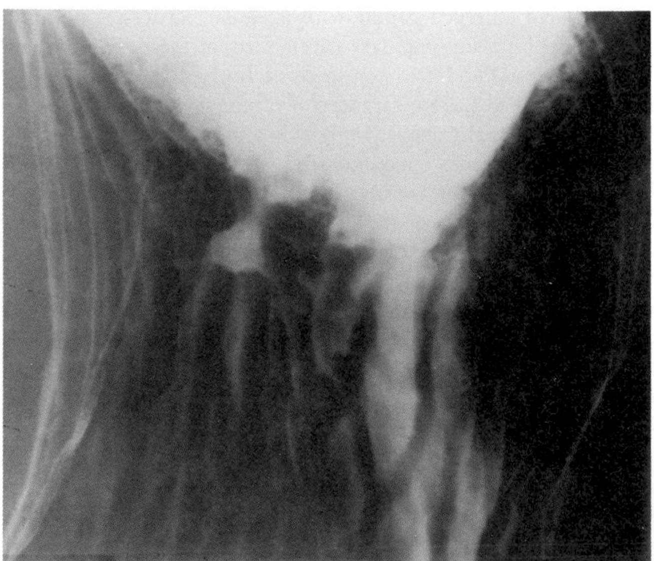

Fig. 12 Gastric ulcer. A small ulcer crater is seen on the posterior wall of the body of the stomach with folds radiating from the edge of the crater.

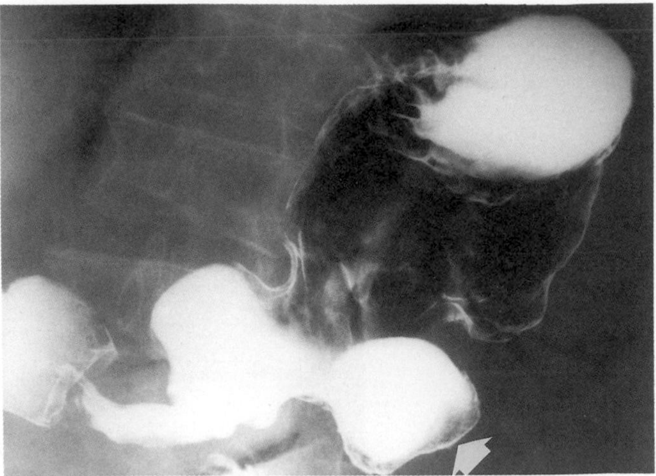

Fig. 13 Gastric ulcer. A large 'sump ulcer' (arrow) is seen arising from the greater curve aspect of the lower body of the stomach.

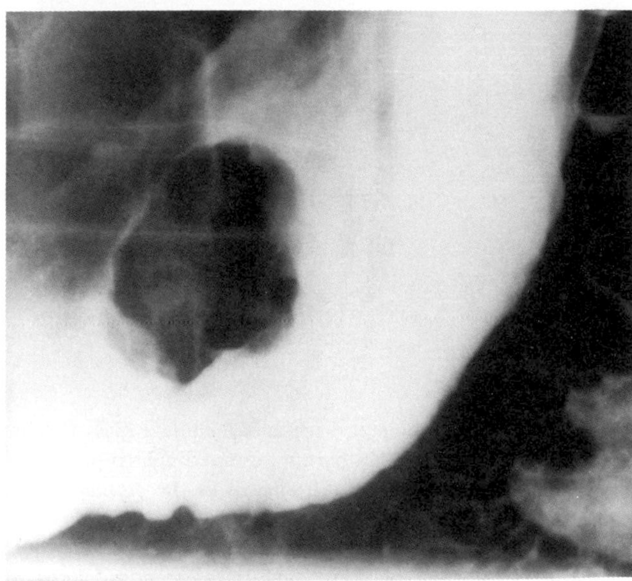

Fig. 14 Carcinoma of the stomach. An irregular polypoid mass is seen in the mid-body of the stomach. Most polypoid carcinomas are larger than this when first detected.

Intramural duodenal haematoma can result from blunt abdominal trauma, anticoagulant therapy, or blood dyscrasia. On barium studies an intramural haematoma is seen as a concentric obstructive lesion in the second or third part of the duodenum, sometimes giving a 'coiled spring' appearance.

Duodenal diverticula are seen fairly frequently on barium examination and these have little clinical significance in the majority of patients.

Small intestine

Barium studies play an important role in the investigation of patients with known or suspected disorders of the small intestine.

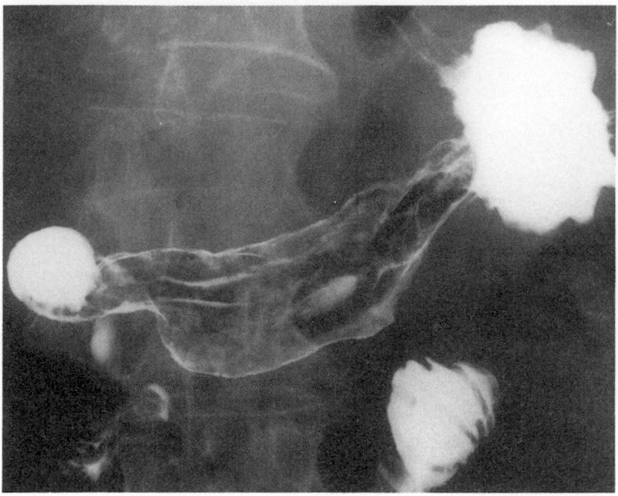

Fig. 15 Infiltrating carcinoma. An extensive infiltrating carcinoma has resulted in contraction of the stomach with irregularity of muscosal folds—the typical 'linitis plastica' appearance.

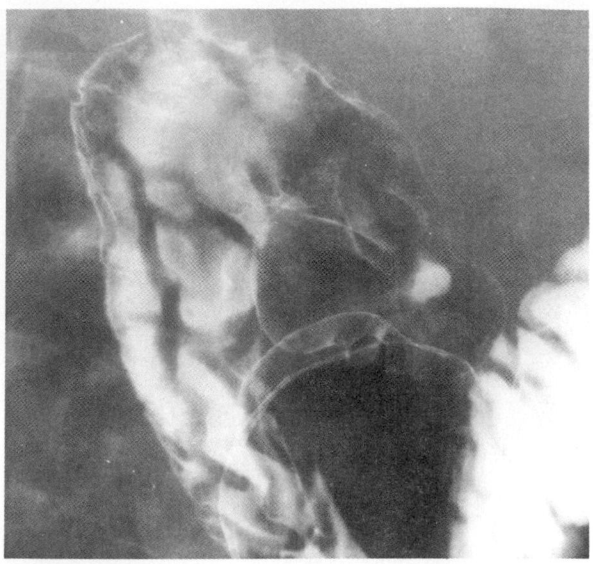

Fig. 17 Duodenal ulceration. A moderate sized collection of barium is seen outlining a duodenal ulcer crater. There is slight deformity of the deuodenal cap and a number of folds radiate from the oedematous edge of the ulcer.

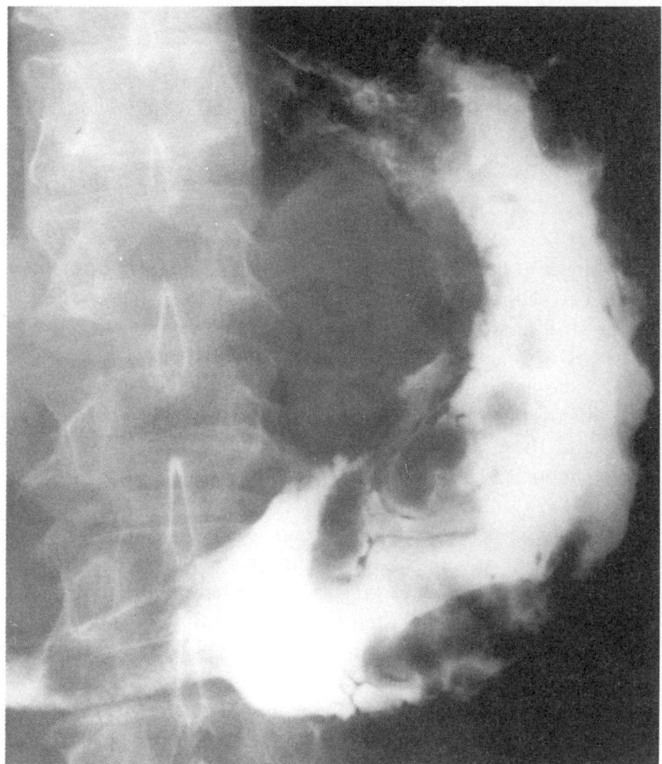

Fig. 16 Gastric lymphoma. There is marked hypertrophy of the mucosal folds in the fundus and body of the stomach.

There is continuing debate as to which of the several available techniques should be used for routine examination of the small intestine. The barium follow-through and small bowel enema (enteroclysis) are used most frequently. The barium follow-through is a well established technique and is the preferred method of many radiologists, but the small bowel enema is being increasingly adopted in many centres. The barium follow-through is normally performed after the barium examination of the oesophagus, stomach, or duodenum by taking films when the barium passes into the small intestine. The small bowel enema is performed by passing a special radio-opaque nasogastric tube so that its tip lies in the distal duodenum or proximal jejunum and infusing dilute barium to outline the small intestine. A double-contrast technique using barium and an aqueous solution of methylcellulose is used in some centres. The small bowel enema is superior to the follow-through as the loops of jejunum and ileum are distended during the examination, making it easier to detect any abnormalities that may be present. The terminal ileum is frequently shown when barium refluxes through the ileocaecal valve during barium enema examinations.

Disorders that are disclosed as morphological changes in the small intestine on barium examination include Crohn's disease, neoplasms, chronic radiation enteritis, Meckel's diverticulum, jejunal diverticulosis, tuberculosis, and ischaemia.

Crohn's disease is characterized by a variety of radiological signs. Ulceration is common and is seen as fissure ulcers, discrete mucosal ulcers, longitudinal ulcers, sinuses, and fistulae (Fig. 18). Single or multiple strictures are a frequent finding: tight strictures cause obstruction and result in dilatation of the more proximal intestine. Other signs of Crohn's disease including thickening of the valvulae conniventes, cobblestoning, asymmetrical lesions, skip lesions, and a mass in the right iliac fossa displacing adjacent loops of intestine.

Primary neoplasms of the small intestine are uncommon. Carcinoid tumours, located mostly in the distal ileum, may give a variety of radiological appearances. Characteristically, a carcinoid tumour appears as an intraluminal filling defect, but it may also be seen as a localized stricture or as a mass in the right iliac fossa causing distortion of a number of adjacent ileal segments. Primary carcinoma of the small intestine is nearly always located in the jejunum and has a radiological appearance similar to that of

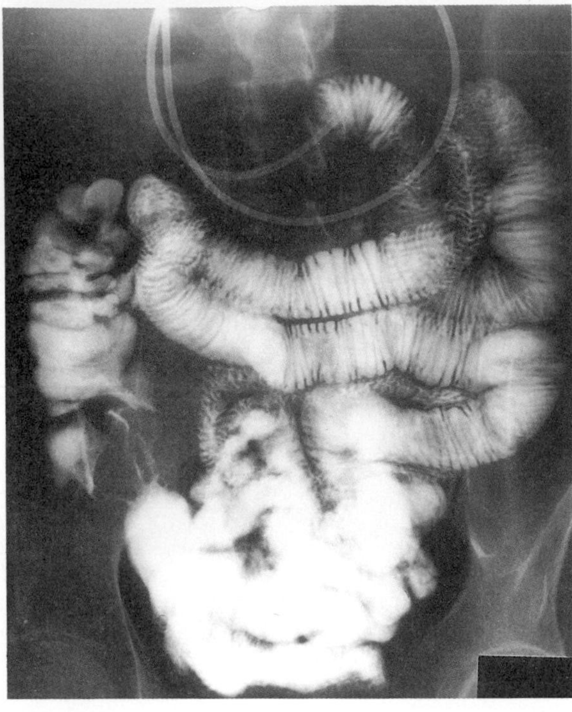

(a)

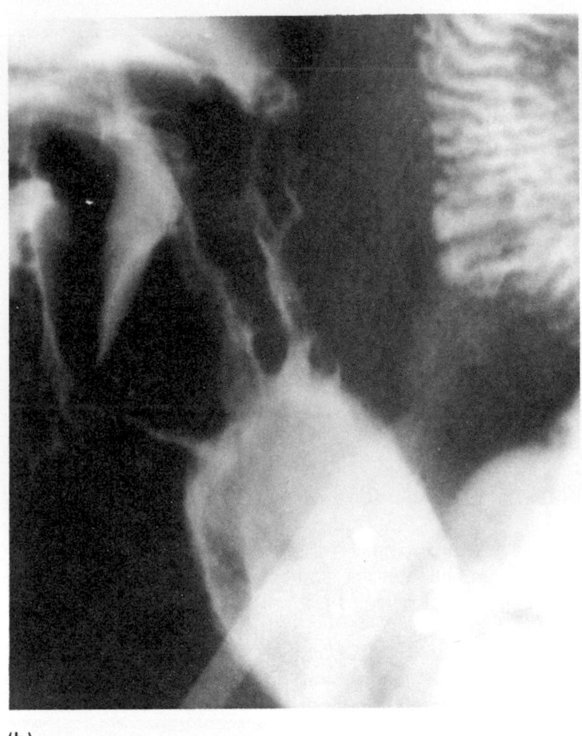

(b)

Fig. 18 Ileal Crohn's disease (a,b). The distal ileum is grossly abnormal with the lumen of the terminal ileum replaced by a number of ileocaecal fistulae. There is slight dilatation of the intestine proximal to the fistulae. The patient presented with abdominal pain, weight loss, and diarrhoea. On physical examination a mass was palpated in the right iliac fossa

carcinoma of the colon. Lymphomas, which are multiple in 40 per cent of patients, are mostly seen in the ileum, although they may be located anywhere in the small intestine. Ulceration and cavitation is a frequent finding in lymphomas. Leiomyomas and leiomyosarcomas may be seen as either round intraluminal filling defects, or as cavitating masses related to the small intestine.

Chronic radiation enteritis develops in a small number of patients following radiotherapy to the abdomen and pelvis. The radiological changes include thickening of the valvulae conniventes, single or multiple stenoses, adhesions, sinuses, and fistulae. Meckel's diverticulum is seen as a solitary pouch arising from the antemesenteric border of the ileum.

Barium examination in patients with small intestinal obstruction shows the site of obstruction as an abrupt transition from distended or dilated small intestine to collapsed distal loops. Causes of obstruction that may be identified include neoplasms, Crohn's stricture, adhesions, or internal herniae. Other disorders of the small intestine that may be demonstrated on barium examination include jejunal diverticulosis, tuberculosis, and ischaemia.

Colon

The barium enema remains a widely used technique for the detection of carcinomas and adenomas in the colon, the diagnosis and evaluation of diverticular disease and its complications, and for assessing the extent and severity of inflammatory bowel disease. The double-contrast barium technique is the method of choice in most centres, although a single-contrast examination is performed in patients with suspected colonic obstruction. Water-soluble contrast studies are performed mostly to examine the anastomosis in patients who have undergone recent sigmoid resection.

Digital examination of the rectum and sigmoidoscopy are the initial diagnostic procedures in the investigation of colonic disorders, and these should always be performed before a barium enema is requested. If a rectal biopsy is performed, an interval of at least 7 days should be allowed before a barium enema is performed to avoid the risk of perforation.

A clean colon, a satisfactory barium suspension, the use of a smooth muscle relaxant, and good examination technique are necessary to obtain consistently good results. The colon is cleansed by using a combination of cathartics, low residue diet, and increased fluid intake on the day before the examination. A cleansing enema may be required on the morning of the examination. The examination is performed by infusing barium into the colon and replacing much of the barium with air to give a double-contrast effect before taking the radiographs. Hyoscine butylbromide or glucagon is given intravenously to produce smooth muscle relaxation.

Most carcinoma of the colon has reached a fairly advanced stage by the time the patient presents with clinical symptoms. Carcinoma is shown as a constricting lesion with mucosal destruction, a narrow irregular lumen and shouldered margins, and a sharp transition between the neoplasm and adjacent normal colon. In some cases the carcinoma is seen as an irregular intraluminal polypoid filling defect (Fig. 19); other carcinomas appear as asymmetrical infiltrating lesions with mucosal destruction.

Occasionally the carcinoma is shown as a large ulcerating mass. Multiple primary carcinomas are seen in the colon at the time of presentation in 3 to 5 per cent of patients.

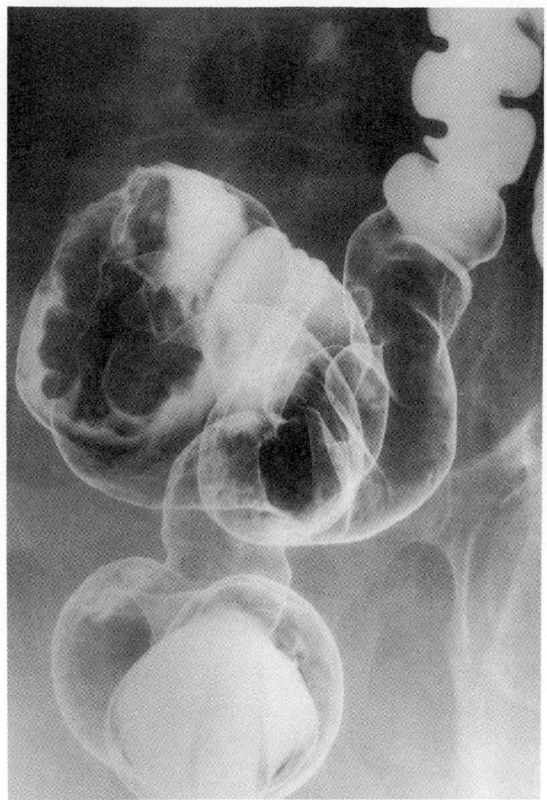

Fig. 19 Carcinoma of the colon. A large irregular polypoid filling defect is shown in the distal sigmoid colon on barium enema examination.

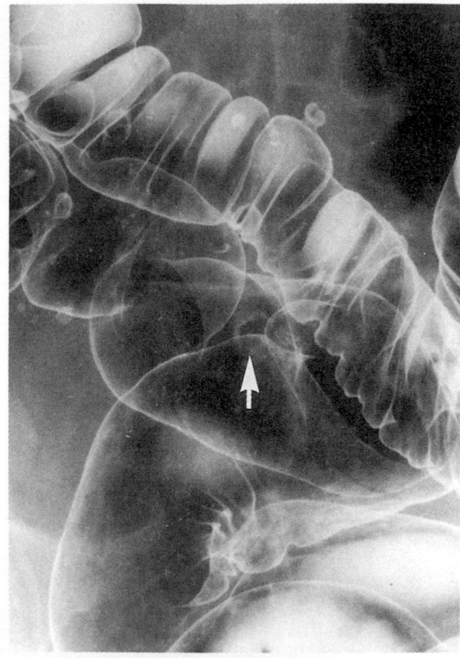

Fig. 20 Adenomatous polyp. Barium enema shows a small, sharply defined, irregular filling defect in the mid-sigmoid colon (arrow). A number of diverticula can also be identified.

Since strong evidence suggests that adenomas are the precursors of the great majority of colorectal carcinomas, the detection and removal of adenomas in the colon and rectum is important. Adenomas are shown as either sessile (Fig. 20) or pedunculated small filling defects, usually less than 1 cm in diameter. Villus adenomas may be larger and have a frond-like appearance.

Flexible sigmoidoscopy, and colonoscopy are now widely available for examining the colon. The relative roles of barium studies, flexible sigmoidoscopy and colonoscopy have not been established. A small number of centres now perform flexible sigmoidoscopy before barium enemas. The majority of polyps and carcinomas develop in the sigmoid colon and investigation by combined flexible sigmoidoscopy and barium enema improves the detection rate, particularly in patients with diverticular disease, in whom small carcinomas and polyps may be obscured by the diverticula.

Ulcerative colitis, Crohn's colitis, and ischaemic colitis account for the great majority of patients with inflammatory bowel disease who are assessed with barium studies. The diagnosis of ulcerative colitis should be firmly established on the basis of a rectal biopsy taken at sigmoidoscopy. The double-contrast barium enema is an excellent technique for demonstrating the extent and severity of inflammation and the presence or absence of an associated carcinoma (Fig. 21). Mucosal ulceration may be mild, moderate or severe and will extend in a proximal direction from the rectum in continuity to involve part or all the colon with associated loss of the normal haustral pattern. Patients with chronic ulcerative colitis show narrowing of the lumen and shortening of the colon.

The typical features of Crohn's colitis are inflammation, often in the form of aphthous ulcers, strictures, asymmetrical lesions, skip lesions, and predominant involvement of the right side of the colon. The distal sigmoid colon and rectum are nearly always spared, although perianal sinuses and fistulae (Fig. 22) are a recognized feature. Ischaemic colitis characteristically shows oedematous changes in the splenic flexure that either return to normal in about 4 to 6 weeks, or result in stricture formation.

Diverticular disease is a frequent finding in middle-aged and older patients. Diverticula appear as single or multiple small outpouchings, most frequently in the sigmoid colon, although they may be present in any part of the colon. Acute inflammation (diverticulitis) complicates diverticular disease in a small minority of patients. A paracolic abscess may be shown on barium enema as displacement and narrowing of the intestinal lumen with an altered mucosal pattern. Unlike carcinoma of the colon, the mucosal pattern in the narrowed segment is intact, although it may be distorted, and there is no shouldering of the margins. In some cases it may be impossible to distinguish a paracolic inflammatory mass from carcinoma. A soft tissue mass, gas lucency, air–fluid level, or barium in an extraluminal cavity may be seen in diverticulitis. The characteristic drape sign is occasionally seen, and is caused by bending of adjacent empty diverticula towards the abscess. Paracolic abscess may result in colonic or sometimes small intestinal obstruction. Fistulae may be identified as tracks of contrast medium passing from the colon to adjacent viscera. The more common fistulae are colovesical and coloenteric, fistulae to

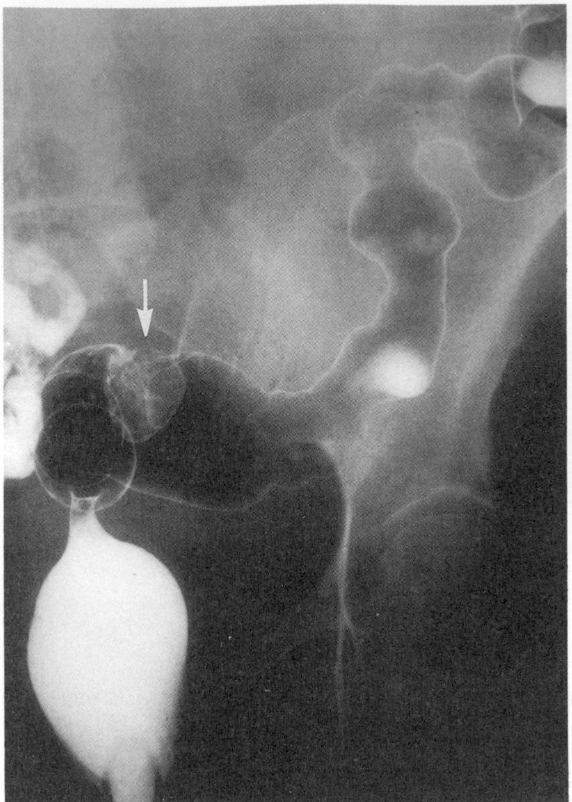

Fig. 21 Ulcerative colitis and carcinoma. The sigmoid colon is shortened and shows minimal mucosal ulceration, consistent with mild active inflammation in chronic ulcerative colitis. A polypoid carcinoma is also seen in the distal sigmoid colon (arrow).

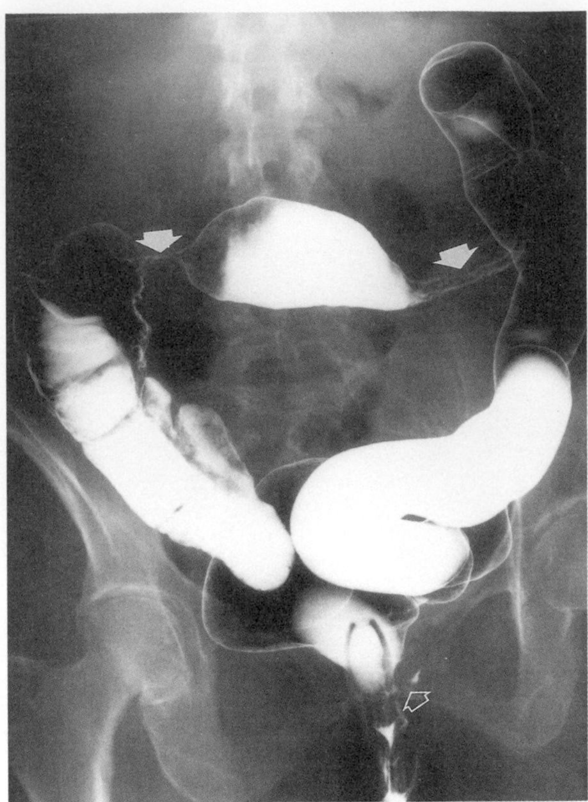

Fig. 22 Crohn's colitis. There is quite marked shortening of the proximal colon and two tight strictures can be identified in the transverse colon (arrows). Note also the perianal sinus track (open arrow).

the skin, genital tract, ureter, stomach, hip, perineum, and soft tissues of the thigh being less common. Longitudinal paracolic fistulae appear as a track of barium running parallel to the colon in the paracolic tissues.

COMPUTED TOMOGRAPHY (CT) (see also Section 6.2)

Computed tomography (CT) is only occasionally used as the initial investigation when disorders of the hollow organs of the digestive system are suspected. CT can, however, provide useful further information about neoplasms and other conditions that involve the gastrointestinal tract.

Initial optimism that CT would be a reliable method for staging oesophageal carcinoma prior to surgery has not been confirmed. It is sensitive in detecting liver metastases and invasion of the tracheobronchial tree but is unreliable for assessing mediastinal soft tissue extension, aortic invasion, and coeliac axis lymph node involvement. Endoscopic ultrasound is proving to be a more accurate technique for staging oesophageal carcinoma, since the depth of infiltration can be accurately assessed and lymph node metastases can be detected. However, endoscopic ultrasound has the disadvantage that an expensive dedicated endoscope is required.

CT has a limited role in evaluating the stomach: it is most useful for the preoperative staging of gastric carcinoma and for helping to confirm the diagnosis of linitis plastica. The characteristic appearances of gastric varices on CT can be helpful when the diagnosis is difficult on barium studies. The role of CT in visualizing the duodenum is mostly limited to showing changes in adjacent organs such as the pancreas that also involve the duodenum.

CT also has a limited role in the investigation of the small intestine, although in certain patients with Crohn's disease CT is useful for investigating abdominal masses, and in particular for demonstrating abscesses and fistulae. An abscess appears as a fluid collection in the mesentery or retroperitoneum bordered by a thick contrast-enhancing wall. Gas within the fluid in the form of scattered bubbles or air–fluid levels is diagnostic. The extraintestinal extent of lymphomas and other intestinal neoplasms can be defined by CT. Dilated fluid-filled loops of obstructed intestine show characteristic appearances on CT and this can be an important finding when obstruction is not suspected.

In the colon CT is important in evaluating patients who have undergone surgical resection for carcinoma. In the immediate postoperative period surgical complications can be diagnosed. It is also a sensitive method for detecting local and distant recurrent neoplasm. CT is being used increasingly in the initial evaluation of suspected acute diverticulitis. Sigmoid diverticulitis is seen on CT as localized thickening of the colonic wall in association with inflammatory changes in the pericolic fat or an adjacent abscess. Fistulae, distant abscesses, intestinal or ureteric obstruction, and peritonitis are complications that can be identified on CT.

ANGIOGRAPHY

The main indication for performing gastrointestinal angiography is in the diagnosis and treatment of gastrointestinal bleeding. If endoscopy fails to identify the origin of an acute bleeding episode, selective catheterization of the coeliac axis, superior mesenteric artery, and inferior mesenteric artery is normally performed. Angiography is successful in locating the bleeding site in up to 90 per cent of patients who continue to bleed during the investigation. Embolization may be undertaken during angiography in patients who are unsuitable for surgery. Single vessels such as the left gastric, gastroduodenal, and gastroepiploic arteries can be embolized because of the rich collateral circulation in the upper gastrointestinal tract.

Diagnostic angiography plays an important role in the location of bleeding from the small intestine, which is beyond the reach of endoscopy. Some patients will present with acute bleeding, while others have a long history of obscure bleeding with negative endoscopy and barium studies. Superselective arteriography may be required to pinpoint the site of bleeding in the small intestine accurately. If a lesion demonstrated by angiography in the small intestine is likely to be difficult or impossible to identify at surgery, intraoperative angiography is indicated. The catheter is left in the superselected branch vessel supplying the lesion during the subsequent operation. The anatomical location of the abnormality is then confirmed by an intraoperative angiogram of the individual loops. A modification of the technique involves injecting a small amount of methylene blue through the superselectively placed catheter.

Angiodysplasia, which is usually located in the caecum and ascending colon, can cause obscure gastrointestinal bleeding. It cannot be identified on barium studies but it may be recognized by an experienced endoscopist. Angiography is an excellent technique for diagnosing this condition.

FURTHER READING

Allison DJ, Hemingway AP, Cunningham DA. Angiography in gastrointestinal bleeding. *Lancet*, 1982; **2**: 30–3.

Allison DJ, Hemingway AP. In: Nolan DJ, ed. *Radiological atlas of gastrointestinal disease*. Chichester: John Wiley, 1983: 281–309.

Anderson JR, Mills JOM. Caecal volvulus: a frequently missed diagnosis? *Clin Radiol*, 1984; **35**: 65–9.

Athanasoulis CA, *et al*. Intraoperative localisation of small bowel bleeding sites with combined use of angiographic methods and methylene blue injection. *Surgery*, 1980; **87**: 77–84.

Balthazar EJ. Colon. In: Megibow AJ, Balthazar EJ, eds. *Computed tomography of the gastrointestinal tract*. St Louis: Mosby, 1986: 279–385.

Balthazar EJ, Megibow AJ, Naidich DP, LeFleur RS. Computed tomographic recognition of gastric varices. *Am J Roentgenol*, 1984; **142**: 1121–5.

Banfield WJ, Hurwitz AL. Esophageal stricture associated with nasogastric intubation. *Arch Intern Med*, 1974; **134**: 1083–6.

Bartram CI. Radiology in the current assessment of ulcerative colitis. *Gastrointest Radiol*, 1977; **1**: 383–92.

Cho KC. Computed tomography in colonic diverticulitis. In: Herlinger H, Megibow AJ, eds. *Advances in gastrointestinal radiology*. St Louis: Mosby, 1991: 85–99.

Day EA, Marks C. Gallstone ileus. Review of the literature and presentation of thirty-four new cases. *Am J Surg*, 1975; **129**: 552–8.

Dehn TCB, Nolan DJ. The role of the small bowel enema in the early postoperative obstruction. *Gastrointest Radiol*, 1989; **14**: 15–21.

Dixon PD, Nolan DJ. The diagnosis of Meckel's diverticulum: a continuing challenge. *Clin Radiol*, 1987; **38**: 615–19.

Field S. The acute abdomen—the plain radiograph. In: Grainger RG, Allison DJ, eds. *Diagnostic radiology: an Anglo-American textbook of organ imaging*. Edinburgh: Churchill Livingstone, 1986: 719–742.

Field S, Guy PJ, Upsdell SM, Scourfield AE. The erect abdominal radiograph in the acute abdomen: should its routine use be abandoned?. *Br Med J*, 1985; **290**: 1934–6.

Frostick SP, Collin J, Daar AS, Kettlewell M, Nolan DJ. Non traumatic intra-mural haematoma: an unusual cause of duodenal obstruction. *Br J Surg*, 1984; **71**: 313–14.

Gough IR. Strangulating adhesive small bowel obstruction with normal radiographs. *Br J Surg*, 1978; **65**: 431–4.

Gourtsoyiannis NC, Nolan DJ. Lymphoma of the small intestine: radiological appearances. *Clin Radiol*, 1988; **39**: 639–45.

Greenall MJ, Levine AW, Nolan DJ. Complications of diverticular disease: a review of the barium enema findings. *Gastrointest Radiol*, 1983; **8**: 353–8.

Hodges PC, Miller RE. Intestinal obstruction. *Am J Roentgenol*, 1955; **74**: 1015–25.

Jeffree MA, Barter SJ, Hemingway AP, Nolan DJ. Primary carcinoid tumours of the ileum: the radiological appearances. *Clin Radiol*, 1984; **35**: 451–5.

Love L. Large bowel obstruction. *Semin Roentgenol*, 1973; **8**: 299–322.

Marshak RH, Lindner AE, Maklansky D. Diverticulosis and diverticulitis of the colon. *Mt Sinai J Med*, 1979; **46**: 261–76.

Mellins HZ, Rigler LG. The roentgen findings in strangulating obstructions of the small intestine. *Am J Roentgenol*, 1954; **71**: 404–15.

Mendelson RM, Nolan DJ. The radiological features of chronic radiation enteritis. *Clin Radiol*, 1985; **36**: 141–8.

Miller RE. The technical approach to the acute abdomen. *Semin Roentgenol*, 1973; **8**: 267–79.

Miller RE. The radiological evaluation of intraperitoneal gas (pneumoperitoneum). *CRC Crit Rev Diagn Imaging*, 1973; **4**: 61–85.

Miller RE, Nelson SW. The roentgenologic demonstration of tiny amounts of free intraperitoneal gas: experimental and clinical studies. *Am J Roentgenol*, 1971; **112**: 574–85.

Miller RE, Becker GJ, Slabaugh RD. Detection of pneumoperitoneum: optimum body position and respiratory phase. *Am J Roentgenol*, 1980; **135**: 487–90.

Nadrowski L. Ileus. In: Nelson RL, Nyhus LM, eds. *Surgery of the small intestine*. Norwalk, Connecticut: Appleton & Lange, 1987: 295–305.

Nolan DJ, Gourtsoyiannis NC. Crohn's disease of the small intestine: review of 100 consecutive patients examined with a barium infusion technique. *Clin Radiol*, 1980; **31**: 597–603.

Nolan DJ, Cadman PJ. The small bowel enema made easy. *Clin Radiol*, 1987; **38**: 295–301.

Papadopoulos VD, Nolan DJ. Carcinoma of the small intestine. *Clin Radiol*, 1985; **36**: 409–13.

Privett JTJ, Davies ER, Roylance JR. The radiological features of gastric lymphoma. *Clin Radiol*, 1977; **28**: 457–63.

Quint LE, Glazer GM, Orringer MB, Gross BH. Esophageal carcinoma: CT findings. *Radiology*, 1985; **155**: 171–5.

Scott JR, Miller WT, Urso M, Stadalnik RC. Acute mesenteric infarction. *Am J Roentgenol*, 1971; **113**: 269–79.

Takemoto T, Ito T, Aibe T, Okito K. Endoscopic ultrasonography in the diagnosis of oesophageal carcinoma, with particular regard to staging it for operability. *Endoscopy*, 1986; 18: 22–5.

Teplick JG, Teplick SK, Ominsky S, Haskin M. Esophagitis caused by oral medication. *Radiology*, 1980; **134**: 23–5.

Welborn JK, Ponka JL, Rebuck JW. Lymphoma of the stomach. *Arch Surg*, 1965; **90**: 480–7.

Young WS, Englebrecht HE, Stoker A. Plain film analysis of sigmoid volvulus. *Clin Radiol*, 1978; **29**: 553–60.

6.5 Ultrasound imaging

DAVID R. M. LINDSELL

The applications of ultrasound in surgical practice are widespread (Table 1). The great majority of examinations are performed either in obstetric patients or are undertaken to study the abdomen. It is not within the scope of this chapter to consider in detail obstetric ultrasound. The ability to obtain images of the fetus and placenta without the use of ionizing radiation has greatly enhanced obstetric practice, and in the United Kingdom most pregnancies will be scanned at some stage during their course. It is possible to assess accurately gestational age, placental position, and the presence of many different fetal anomalies as well as assessing different parameters in the growth-retarded fetus.

Table 1 The applications of ultrasound in surgical practice

Obstetrics
Abdomen
Infant brain
Eye
Thyroid and parathyroid
Salivary glands
Breast
Heart
Pleura
Joints and soft tissues
Scrotum
Vascular system
Trauma
Interventional procedures

The use of non-ionizing radiation makes ultrasound safe; it is also relatively inexpensive and can be performed at the patient's bedside. A number of different organs can be viewed at the same examination and in a short space of time. Ultrasound is therefore widely practised by surgeons, cardiologists, and neonatologists as well as radiologists.

Ultrasound has limitations, in that the interpretation of images obtained is dependent on the skill of the operator and image quality is degraded by obesity and by the presence of bowel gas.

THE ABDOMINAL MASS

Patients with a palpable or suspected abdominal mass are investigated in a variety of ways. If there is a strong clinical suspicion that the mass originates in the colon, for example, then a barium enema examination may be requested as the initial examination. Since it is unusual for the organ of origin of a mass to be known, patients are frequently referred initially for examination by either ultrasound or computed tomography (CT). Both CT and ultrasound have a positive predictive value of between 95 per cent and 100 per cent in determining the presence or absence of an abdominal mass, and the predicted organ of origin of a mass is correct in 90 per cent of patients examined with either technique. CT is slightly more sensitive in its ability to define the exact nature of a mass. Since there is little to choose between the two techniques, the ease, lower cost, and lack of exposure to ionizing radiation, make ultrasound the method of choice.

THE HEPATOBILIARY SYSTEM

Ultrasound examination of the right hypochondrium includes a detailed assessment of liver texture, the bile ducts, gallbladder, and right kidney.

Gallbladder

Ultrasound has replaced the oral cholecystogram for the detection of gallstones, not so much because of its greater sensitivity but rather because it enables examination of other structures at the same time. There is little difference in the sensitivity of the two examinations in the detection of gallbladder pathology. It is not possible to state the actual sensitivity, since a negative examination by either technique is often the end point and thus false negative diagnoses are only rarely detected.

In acute cholecystitis the gallbladder is distended and thick-walled, and stones will usually be seen (Fig. 1). Pericholecystic inflammatory change may also be visible. As it is possible to localize the position of the gallbladder precisely, direct pressure on this area by the transducer will elicit a positive ultrasound Murphy's sign.

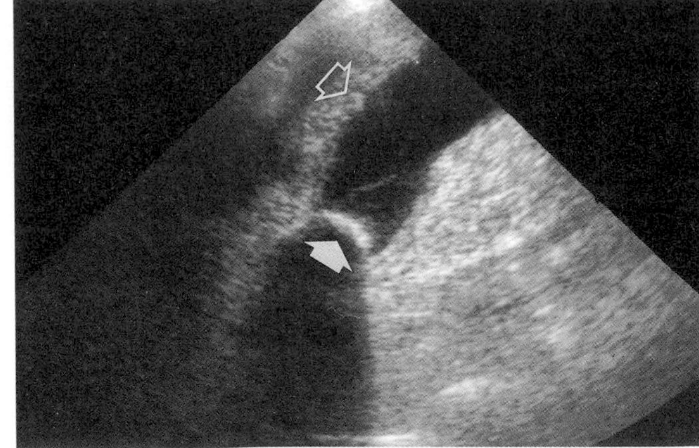

Fig. 1 An acutely inflamed thick walled gallbladder (open arrow) with a large stone (closed arrow) impacted in Hartmann's pouch.

Bile ducts

The ability of ultrasound to detect bile duct dilatation, in the intrahepatic bile duct especially, approaches 100 per cent and it is the primary investigation in patients with suspected obstruction

(Fig. 2). If biliary dilatation is detected, the level of obstruction needs to be defined: this is possible in 95 per cent of cases, while the cause of the obstruction can be determined in 85 per cent of patients. The sensitivity varies depending on the obstructing lesion (Table 2). Direct visualization of tumours of the ampulla of Vater is rare, as is the precise diagnosis of sclerosing cholangitis.

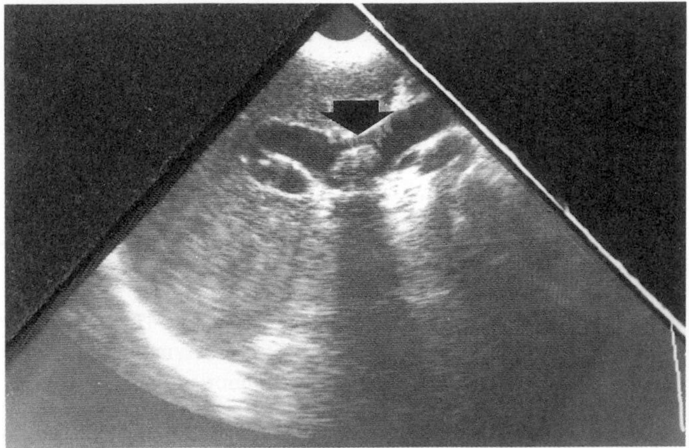

Fig. 2 A large stone (arrow) within a dilated common bile duct.

Table 2 Sensitivity of ultrasound in defining the cause of biliary obstruction

	Sensitivity(%)
Pancreatic masses	97
Choledocholithiasis	82
Cholangiocarcinoma	96
Chronic pancreatitis	67

Once the diagnosis of biliary obstruction has been made it may be appropriate to perform a CT scan if ultrasound has failed to demonstrate the cause of obstruction or if surgery is contemplated.

Liver

Although ultrasound has a major role in investigating diffuse hepatocellular disease, in surgical practice it is most commonly used to determine the presence of focal liver lesions (Fig. 3). It is able to differentiate between solid and cystic lesions, and if there is any doubt about the nature of a mass guided aspiration can be performed to determine whether the lesion is a benign or malignant tumour or whether it is an abscess or cyst. The use of ultrasound at the time of surgery, with a sterile transducer applied directly to the liver, has led to a reappraisal of the sensitivity of preoperative investigations in the detection of liver tumours. Intraoperative ultrasound is currently the most sensitive method of detecting liver tumours: 40 per cent of the lesions detected by this method are not palpable at surgery. Preoperative assessment with either ultrasound or conventional CT has a sensitivity of 60 to 70 per cent in the detection of liver tumours. In some centres magnetic resonance imaging is preferred as it has the ability to differentiate between benign capillary haemangiomas and metastases.

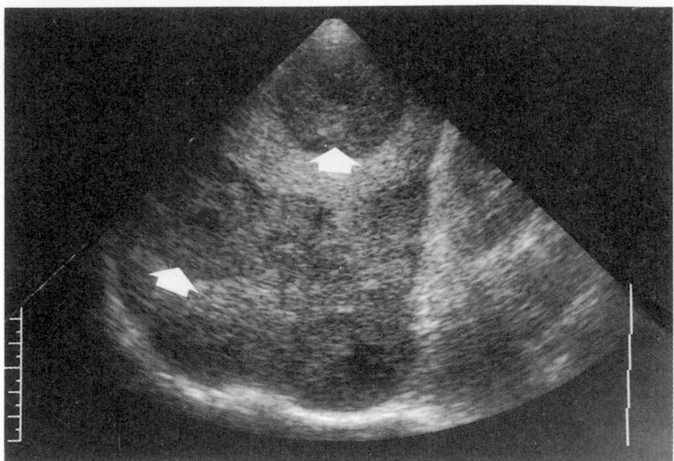

Fig. 3 Focal areas (arrows) of reduced echogenicity within the liver due to metastases.

PANCREAS

Ultrasound fails to produce a good image of part or all of the pancreas in 25 per cent of patients, due to the presence of overlying bowel gas. In the majority of patients in whom the pancreas is clearly seen detection of abnormalities is sensitive. If the pancreas is poorly visualized and if surgery is contemplated, or in acute pancreatitis, CT should also be performed.

Pancreatic tumours

Focal masses of altered echogenicity are usually due to adenocarcinoma. Occasionally guided percutaneous biopsy is required to allow differentiation of such masses from focal areas of pancreatitis or rare benign tumours. Endocrine tumours of the pancreas are often small and difficult to detect preoperatively by any technique: intraoperative ultrasound visualizes these with a sensitivity approaching 100 per cent.

Acute pancreatitis

During an acute attack of pancreatitis the coexisting ileus may obscure the pancreas. CT is the preferred investigation, particularly as this allows an assessment of pancreatic necrosis. Ultrasound can be used to evaluate the gallbladder and biliary tree and to monitor pancreatic fluid collections.

Chronic pancreatitis

A combination of endoscopic retrograde pancreatography and ultrasound is the most sensitive method for detecting chronic pancreatitis. In a few patients CT will provide additional information. There is, however, poor correlation between the findings on any imaging study and the degree of pancreatic dysfunction other than in patients with the most severe disease.

RENAL TRACT

Ultrasound reliably demonstrates the shape, size, and echogenicity of the kidneys and the nature of mass lesions. It will also demonstrate renal tract dilatation. The normal non-dilated ureter is not visualized. The bladder and prostate are well seen with both transabdominal and transrectal ultrasound. Ultrasound is therefore the primary imaging modality in renal failure, urinary tract infection, and in the assessment of bladder outflow obstruction.

Renal tract obstruction

Ultrasound is a highly sensitive means for the detection of renal tract dilatation. While dilatation usually indicates obstruction this is not always so, and obstruction in its early phases does not always produce dilatation. Ultrasound provides no functional information and the level of obstruction may be difficult to discern. For these reasons it will often need to be followed by urography, antegrade pyelography, or renal scintigraphy. Urinary tract calcification, especially in the ureters, may not always be detected by ultrasound and a plain abdominal radiograph should usually accompany any ultrasound examination of the renal tract. Patients with symptoms suggestive of ureteric calculi should undergo urography rather than ultrasound examination.

Renal tract tumours

Ultrasound is more sensitive and more specific than urography in the detection of renal mass lesions other than tumours of the renal pelvis, which are also more reliably diagnosed by CT. Ultrasound may be used to determine whether mass lesions detected by urography are cystic or solid (Fig. 4). Tumours of the ureter are poorly detected by ultrasound unless they are causing hydronephrosis. Tumours of the bladder are better detected by transabdominal ultrasound than urography, their respective sensitivities being 77 per cent and 61 per cent, respectively. The combination of transabdominal and transrectal ultrasound increases the sensitivity to 95 per cent.

The initial investigation in patients with haematuria is usually urography. If cystoscopy is not to be performed then the urogram should be accompanied by an ultrasound scan. If ultrasound is used as the first investigation there is a risk that urothelial tumours of the renal pelvis and ureter will be missed. These tumours are however very much less common than renal cell carcinoma and bladder tumours.

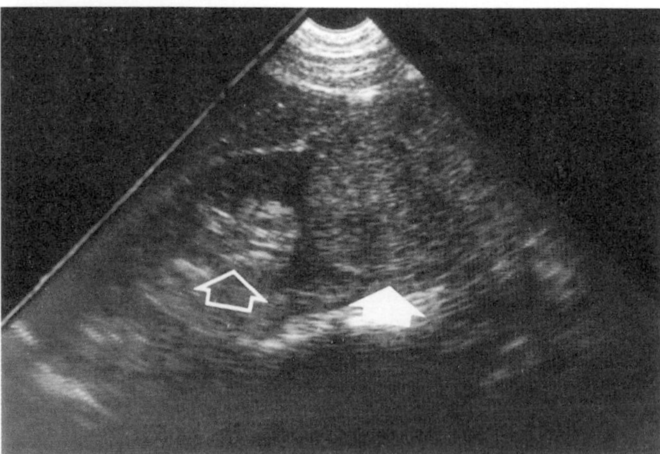

Fig. 4 A solid renal cell carcinoma (closed arrow) arising from the lower pole of the kidney (open arrow).

Prostate

Transabdominal ultrasound permits a two-dimensional volumetric assessment of the degree of intravesical enlargement of the prostate, as well as assessment of residual urine volume. It is therefore preferred to urography in patients with bladder outflow obstruction. Transrectal ultrasound gives improved resolution of images of the prostate itself, allowing breaches of the capsule and adjacent lymph node involvement by tumours to be detected.

ULTRASOUND IN GYNAECOLOGY

The uterus and ovaries may be visualized by both transabdominal and transvaginal scanning. Transvaginal ultrasound has the advantage that the transducer is nearer the midline pelvic structures and may therefore be of a higher frequency, which improves the resolution of the image. This method of scanning is preferred in the early detection of pregnancy and in the assessment of abortion and ectopic pregnancy. The higher frequency limits the depth of penetration of the ultrasound wave and more laterally situated pelvic masses are often better assessed by transabdominal scanning.

Pelvic masses

The role of ultrasound in the assessment of a pelvic mass is to determine the nature and size of the mass as well as its organ of origin. Ultrasound reliably differentiates between solid and cystic lesions in the pelvis. In general terms most ovarian lesions are cystic and most uterine lesions are solid; there is some overlap, however, and the organ of origin is then inferred by visualizing either the normal ovaries or the normal uterus and excluding these as the cause for the mass. A very large mass may obscure normal structures, making the organ of origin more difficult to predict. Features suggestive of malignancy in ovarian lesions are a multiloculated appearance and the presence of solid elements within the mass (Fig. 5). Ultrasound is of limited value in the evaluation of malignancy of the uterine body or cervix although uterine fibroids are well visualized. Ultrasound will also permit differentiation between masses of gynaecological origin and other pelvic masses, such as bowel lesions.

Recently much attention has been given to the possibility of using ultrasound to screen for ovarian cancer. Using transabdominal ultrasound imaging, the odds that a positive result on screening indicates the presence of a primary ovarian cancer are 1 in 67. The sensitivity can be improved by using transvaginal colour flow Doppler ultrasound, which reduces the number of false positive results. Colour flow Doppler ultrasound machines cost two to three times as much as conventional ultrasound equipment, however.

Acute pelvic pain

In young women it can be difficult to differentiate between appendicitis, pelvic inflammatory disease, and complications of ovarian cysts. In this clinical setting ultrasound is of value if a positive diagnosis of one of these causes for the pain can be made.

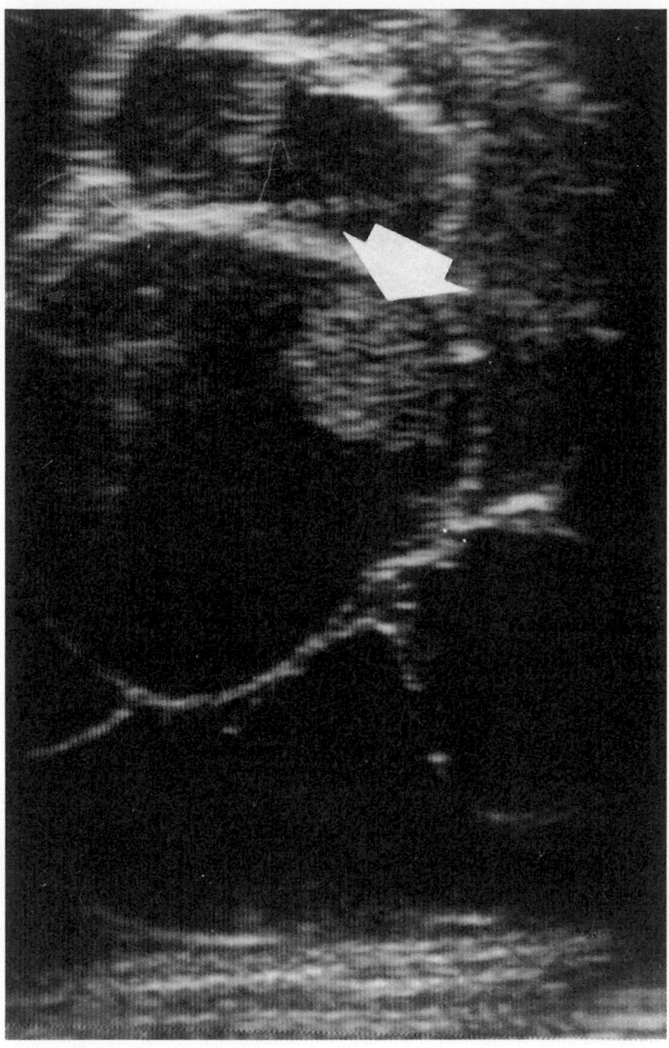

Fig. 5 A multiloculated cystic ovarian tumour containing one small area of solid tissue (arrow).

Ectopic pregnancy

The advent of transvaginal ultrasound has increased the likelihood of making a positive diagnosis of ectopic pregnancy. It also permits the earlier diagnosis of an intrauterine pregnancy, which effectively eliminates the diagnosis of ectopic pregnancy as the two only very rarely coexist. Some form of pelvic abnormality will be seen in three-quarters of patients with an ectopic pregnancy, although the ectopic gestation sac and embryo will be seen in only 40 per cent. As 25 per cent of patients with ectopic pregnancy will have a virtually normal scan it is imperative that the scan is always performed in conjunction with an accurate measurement of human chorionic gonadotrophin.

Infertility

Not only does ultrasound allow an assessment of the morphology of the pelvic organs but it also permits monitoring of cyclical ovarian and endometrial changes. For the purposes of *in-vitro* fertilization, transvaginal ultrasound allows accurate needle aspiration of ovarian follicles to harvest ova.

THE GASTROINTESTINAL TRACT

With the exception of the diagnosis of pyloric stenosis in infancy, ultrasound does not have a primary role in the investigation of the gastrointestinal tract. However tumours of the gastrointestinal tract will often be obvious on ultrasound, although it may be difficult to differentiate these from inflammatory masses such as diverticular masses. Bowel wall thickening and stricture formation is also often apparent in conditions such as Crohn's disease. Ultrasound has a sensitivity of more than 80 per cent and a specificity of 95 per cent in the diagnosis of acute appendicitis without perforation and it has been advocated that it should be used routinely in an attempt to reduce the negative appendicectomy rate. The sensitivity is much lower in patients with perforated appendices, although it has been argued that this does not matter as the need for surgery will be obvious. This fact, and the fact that ultrasound will not detect up to 20 per cent of cases of acute appendicitis, means that it should be used judiciously. It should probably be confined to patients with equivocal clinical findings and young women, in whom it will exclude a gynaecological cause for the pain. Surgeons should be aware of the high specificity of a positive diagnosis but must equally be aware that a negative result must be treated with caution.

ENDOSCOPIC AND INTRALUMINAL ULTRASOUND

Much of the recent development in ultrasound has related to the technological advances that now permit the incorporation of ultrasound transducers into endoscopes and the development of intraluminal transducers. Using transducers attached to upper gastrointestinal tract endoscopes it is now possible to obtain images of the oesophagus and heart with a transducer within the oesophagus and to visualize the pancreas, duodenum, and common bile duct with a transducer in the stomach or duodenum. If the endoscope is able to pass through an oesophageal tumour, ultrasound is more sensitive than CT for local staging. It is able to define extension through the layers of the oesophagus, extension to adjacent organs, and spread to local lymph nodes. If the tumour cannot be passed then CT is superior for the detection of mediastinal extension.

Ultrasound examination of the rectum and colon can be performed using either a rectal transducer or a transducer incorporated into a colonoscope. Correlation of the ultrasound results with histological analysis of the resected specimen according to the 1987 TNM classification gives overall accuracy rates of 81 per cent for rectal tumours and 93 per cent for colonic tumours. Some problems have been found with T2 tumours, which may be accompanied by peritumoural inflammation and abscess formation. The possibility of false positive diagnosis of lymph node metastasis is a problem.

Distant metastases within the abdomen can only be detected by abdominal ultrasound or CT.

ABDOMINAL ABSCESSES

Ultrasound, CT, and nuclear medicine techniques may be used to detect intra-abdominal abscesses. No technique is capable of specifically determining whether an identified fluid collection is infected or not, and percutaneous aspiration of the fluid should always be performed. Many comparative studies of the sensitivity of the three techniques have been performed: those for ultrasound range from 60 to 100 per cent, for CT from 78 to 100 per cent, and for nuclear medicine techniques 75 to 100 per cent. Abscesses in the suphrenic spaces, the right upper quadrant, perirenal areas, and the midline of the pelvis are well seen with ultrasound. CT has the advantage of not being affected by open wounds, dressings, and bowel gas, unlike ultrasound, and CT is better able to image the mesentery and retroperitoneum. Ultrasound should be used initially to look for an abscess. If this is inconclusive then CT will overcome most of the problems that make the ultrasound scan unsatisfactory. Nuclear medicine techniques using either gallium-67 or labelled white cell scanning should be reserved for those patients in whom intra-abdominal sepsis is strongly suspected but in who a definitive diagnosis cannot be reached by the other two techniques.

INTERVENTIONAL ULTRASOUND

Percutaneous fluid drainage and biopsy procedures can be guided by conventional fluoroscopic screening, CT, or ultrasound. The method chosen will be influenced by the site within the abdomen and the individual preference of the operator. Masses or abscesses within the retroperitoneum, mesentery, or pelvis are often better approached using computed tomography as this provides better visualization of, and therefore avoidance of, the bowel. Superficial lesions, lesions in the liver, and collections in the suphrenic spaces can usually be approached with ease using ultrasound.

The ability to drain abscesses percutaneously has totally changed the management of such patients. Surgery with its greater morbidity, mortality, and cost can often be avoided, or at least deferred until the patient's general condition improves. Success rates of 75 to 85 per cent for percutaneous abscess drainage procedures are common.

Percutaneous biopsy may be performed using either a fine needle to obtain specimens for cytological examination or using larger needles for histological specimens. If accurate cytology is available then fine needle aspiration biopsy is preferred because of its lower complication rate. Large surveys of the complication rate of fine needle biopsy in Europe and the United States reveal mortality rates between 0.006 and 0.031 per cent and rates of tumour seeding along the needle tract of between 0.003 and 0.009 per cent. Most deaths have been due to haemorrhage following liver biopsy or, less commonly, pancreatitis after pancreatic biopsy.

Many other procedures including nephrostomy, biliary drainage, and percutaneous pancreatography can be performed using ultrasound guidance.

OTHER APPLICATIONS OF ULTRASOUND IN SURGERY

Thyroid and parathyroid

The ability to differentiate between cystic and solid areas allows assessment of focal or diffuse thyroid enlargement. Most lesions within the thyroid are palpable, and the availability of fine needle aspiration biopsy for cytology means that there is often no value in imaging thyroid nodules, particularly as ultrasound cannot reliably separate benign from malignant lesions.

Ultrasound will frequently detect enlargement of the parathyroid glands if they are in a conventional site but it is unable to detect hyperplasia of the glands. In the search for a parathyroid adenoma it should therefore be the first investigation (Fig. 6). In rare instances ultrasound can be used to guide aspiration of impalpable thyroid and parathyroid lesions. Occasionally ablation of a parathyroid adenoma by ultrasound guided alcohol injection has been performed in patients unfit for surgery. Any mass in the neck or region of the salivary glands can be evaluated with ultrasound and its nature and organ of origin characterized.

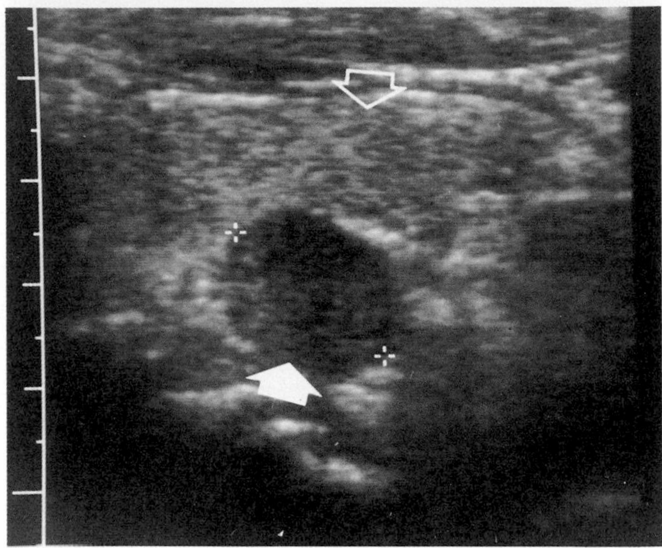

Fig. 6 A parathyroid adenoma (closed arrow) situated posteriorly to the thyroid (open arrow).

Male genital tract

Ultrasound is highly sensitive in the detection of non-palpable testicular tumours and may therefore be used to exclude the presence of a tumour in patients with non-specific scrotal symptomatology. Tumour echo patterns vary and classification of tumour type is not possible (Fig. 7). Some benign testicular conditions such as orchitis may mimic tumours. If a tumour is detected then abdominal ultrasound should be performed to detect lymph node metastases, although actual staging is performed using CT.

Epididymo-orchitis may produce characteristic thickening of the epididymis which may aid in its differentiation from testicular torsion. Ultrasound imaging of the testis is unreliable in diagnosing torsion, and radionuclide imaging is currently the investigation of choice, with a reported sensitivity of 90 per cent. Continuous wave Doppler stethoscopes and conventional duplex Doppler ultrasound have given unreliable results. Recent studies using colour flow Doppler ultrasound report sensitivities of 86 and 100 per cent and specificity of 100 per cent in the detection of testicular torsion, and this may well be the method of the future.

Trauma to the testis, such as testicular rupture and testicular and paratesticular haematoma are well demonstrated.

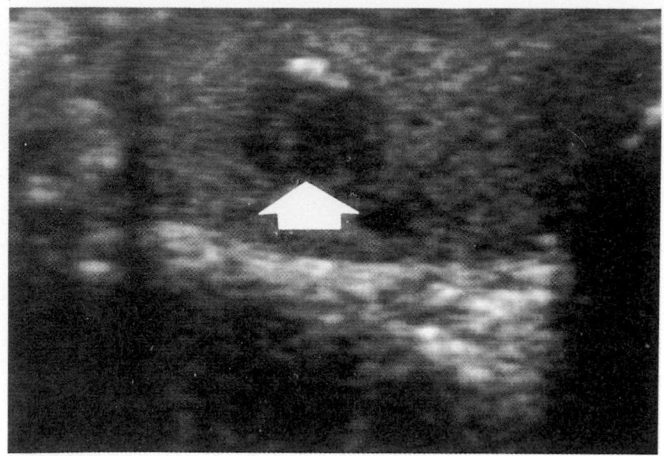

Fig. 7 A small impalpable testicular tumour (arrow) containing a small area of calcification.

The value of duplex ultrasound in the investigation of penile erectile dysfunction is currently being assessed. Initial studies suggest that this may be a valuable technique as it is possible to assess peak systolic velocity in the cavernosal arteries as well as diminished flow in diastole as indicators of the adequacy of the veno-occlusive mechanism.

Breast

Although there are those who support the use of ultrasound as a primary imaging technique, it is most often used to clarify the cystic or solid nature of a mass detected on X-ray mammography or in breasts that appear particularly dense on mammography. Ultrasound should be used initially in the assessment of inflammatory breast disease as abscesses can be localized, and percutaneous drainage can be performed. It may also be used to evaluate breast masses in young patients.

Musculoskeletal system

One of the earliest applications of ultrasound in the evaluation of musculoskeletal system, and still one of the most commonly performed examinations, is the examination of painful hips, particularly in children. This is an extremely simple and accurate technique for detecting fluid within the joint and, if appropriate, for guiding joint aspiration.

Dynamic examination of the hip in infancy using ultrasound allows detection of congenital dislocation at a time when the femoral head is not ossified and is therefore not visible on the plain radiograph. Other applications of ultrasound to the musculoskeletal system are the detection of non-radio-opaque foreign bodies, the evaluation of rotator cuff and Achilles' tendon injuries and the assessment of soft tissue masses and haematomas.

Vascular system (see also Chapter 7)

Duplex ultrasound imaging of the extracranial carotid arteries is now widely performed in patients who have experienced a transient ischaemic attack. It may be used to determine which patients go on to angiography and possible surgery. In experienced hands ultrasound has a 92 to 95 per cent accuracy as compared with conventional arteriography in the analysis of extracranial carotid artery disease. If the duplex examination demonstrates a completely normal vessel in a patient with a classical transient ischaemic attack or stroke the cause is unlikely to lie in the extracranial carotid artery. Duplex ultrasound may be used to evaluate the arterial and venous systems of the arms and legs, and in many centres it has replaced venography for the diagnosis of lower limb venous thrombosis. Thrombosis in the popliteal, femoral, and proximal external iliac veins is readily confirmed or excluded, although thrombosis confined to the deep veins of the calf is less easy to demonstrate. Venography is therefore preferred if anticoagulation is to be used for thrombosis confined to the deep calf veins.

The intra-abdominal vasculature, particularly the hepatic and portal venous systems and the renal vasculature, may be readily evaluated with duplex and colour flow Doppler ultrasound. The altered dynamics of the portal venous system in portal hypertension and obstruction to the hepatic veins are all well demonstrated. Doppler evaluation in possible renovascular hypertension has been disappointing but the assessment of the renal venous system and the characterization of renal perfusion in renal transplants is more promising. Not only does duplex ultrasound of the transplanted kidney give an indication of rejection but it will also detect obstruction of the kidney and the presence of perirenal fluid collections such as lymphoceles and urinomas.

With very few exceptions ultrasound demonstrates the presence or absence of abdominal aortic aneurysms and can be used for subsequent monitoring of their size. It is less reliable than angiography and computed tomography in establishing the relationship to the renal arteries and less reliable than computed tomography in detecting a leaking aneurysm.

FURTHER READING

General

Bourne T, Campbell S, Steer C, Whitehead MI, Collins WP. Transvaginal colour flow imaging: a possible new screening technique for ovarian cancer. *Br Med J*, 1989; **299**: 1367–70.

Campbell S, Bhan V, Whitehead MI, Collins WP. Transabdominal ultrasound screening for early ovarian cancer. *Br Med J*, 1989; 299: 1363–7.

Cooperberg PL, Gibney RG. Imaging of the gallbladder. *Radiology*, 1987; **163**: 605–13.

Ferrucci JT. Liver tumour imaging: current concepts. *Am J Roentgenol*, 1990; **155**: 473–84.

Freeny PC. Radiology of the pancreas: two decades of progress in imaging and intervention. *Am J Roentgenol*, 1988; **150**: 975–81.

Lindsell DRM. Ultrasound imaging of pancreas and biliary tract. *Lancet*, 1990; **335**: 390–3.

Puylaert JBCM, *et al.* A prospective study of ultrasonography in the diagnosis of appendicitis. *N Engl J Med*, 1987; **317**: 666–9.

Spencer J, Lindsell D, Mastorakou I. Ultrasonography compared with intravenous urography in the investigation of adults with haematuria. *Br Med J*, 1990; **301**: 1074–6.

Thorsen MK, *et al.* Diagnosis of ectopic pregnancy: endovaginal vs transabdominal sonography. *Am J Roentgenol*, 1990; **155**: 307–10.

Webb JA. Ultrasonography in the diagnosis of renal obstruction. *Br Med J*, 1990; **301**: 944–6.

Specific

1. Hepatobiliary, pancreatic, and gastrointestinal ultrasound.

Kurtz AB, Goldberg BB. Gastrointestinal ultrasonography. *Clinics in diagnostic ultrasound 23.* New York: Churchill, Livingstone, 1988.

2. Genitourinary ultrasound.
Hricak H. Genitourinary ultrasound: *Clinics in Diagnostic Ultrasound 18*. New York: Churchill Livingstone, 1986.
3. Gynaecological ultrasound.
Steel WB, Cochrane WJ. Gynecologic ultrasound: *Clinics in Diagnostic Ultrasound 15*. New York: Churchill Livingstone, 1984.
4. Endoscopic and intraoperative ultrasound.
Rifkin MD. Intraoperative and endoscopic ultrasonography: *Clinics in Diagnostic Ultrasound 22*. New York: Churchill Livingstone, 1987.
5. Vascular and Doppler ultrasound.
Taylor KJW, Strandness DE. Duplex Doppler ultrasound: *Clinics in Diagnostic Ultrasound 26*. New York: Churchill Livingstone, 1990.

6.6 Imaging in children

DAVID R. M. LINDSELL

TECHNIQUES

The development of techniques such as ultrasound, computed tomography (CT), radionuclide scintigraphy and magnetic resonance imaging has greatly enhanced our diagnostic capabilities in children. Many conditions still require conventional radiographic examinations and contrast studies to make a diagnosis. The chosen imaging modality will be the one that provides most diagnostic information in the shortest time while minimizing the discomfort and radiation dose to the child. In this latter respect ultrasound and magnetic resonance imaging have the advantage that they do not use ionizing radiation.

Contrast studies of the gastrointestinal tract are usually performed with barium, but when aspiration or intestinal perforation are likely to be present the newer low osmolarity water-soluble contrast media are safer. The use of Gastrografin® is rarely indicated, except possibly in the treatment of meconium ileus. Many congenital abnormalities, such as diaphragmatic hernia, duodenal atresia, omphalocele, and congenital hydronephrosis can be diagnosed antenatally by ultrasound, and the obstetrician and paediatric surgeon forewarned. If appropriate the mother can then be transferred prior to delivery to a paediatric surgical unit. It is beyond the scope of this section to consider antenatal diagnosis and paediatric surgical conditions occurring outside the abdomen.

GASTROINTESTINAL OBSTRUCTION IN THE NEWBORN AND YOUNG INFANT

Oesophageal atresia and tracheo-oesophageal fistula

The diagnosis of oesophageal atresia is usually suspected clinically and can be confirmed on a chest radiograph, which will show a soft catheter passed into the oesophagus coiling back on itself. Further confirmation can be obtained by injecting a small quantity of air down this catheter: this will distend the proximal oesophageal pouch. Contrast medium should not be injected as this may lead to aspiration.

A tracheo-oesophageal fistula is present in 85 per cent of infants with oesophageal atresia, and an abdominal radiograph will show gas within the intestine: the abdomen is gasless in those without a fistula. Tracheo-oesophageal fistula can occur in isolation: contrast studies of the oesophagus may be necessary to demonstrate the fistula, which often runs upwards from the oesophagus to the trachea in the lower part of the neck.

Imaging studies are also necessary to demonstrate coexisting abnormalities, which are present in about 50 per cent of patients. These include vertebral and renal abnormalities, duodenal and anal atresia, and congenital heart disease.

Hypertrophic pyloric stenosis

Since ultrasound uses non-ionizing radiation, it has now replaced barium studies in the diagnosis of pyloric stenosis in the small percentage of babies in whom the clinical diagnosis is in doubt. The interpretation of ultrasound is operator-dependent, and if such expertise is not available a barium study should be performed.

Ultrasound clearly demonstrates the hypertrophied muscle, and the length and thickness of the pyloric muscle can be measured to confirm the diagnosis (Fig. 1(a)).

Barium studies demonstrate a narrow elongated pyloric canal with indentations on the gastric antrum and duodenal bulb from the thickened muscle (Fig. 1(b)).

Duodenal obstruction

Duodenal obstruction may arise from a number of causes (Table 1); the radiographic appearances depend on whether or not the obstruction is complete. If it is complete, as in duodenal atresia, the classical 'double bubble' appearance of air and fluid in the distended stomach and proximal duodenum is seen (Fig. 2). If the baby has recently vomited or if a nasogastric tube has been passed the abdomen may appear almost gasless. In this situation the obstruction can be seen if 15 to 20 ml of air are injected through the nasogastric tube. Plain radiographs may be virtually normal in patients with partial obstruction, and contrast studies may be necessary to demonstrate abnormalities such as a duodenal web or bowel malrotation.

Malrotation of the intestine

During the embryonic period the duodenojejunal loop rotates 270° around the superior mesenteric artery axis in an anticlockwise direction. The caecocolic loop, which initially lies inferiorly to the superior mesenteric artery, also rotates 270° in an anticlockwise direction. Finally the caecum and ascending colon become fixed to

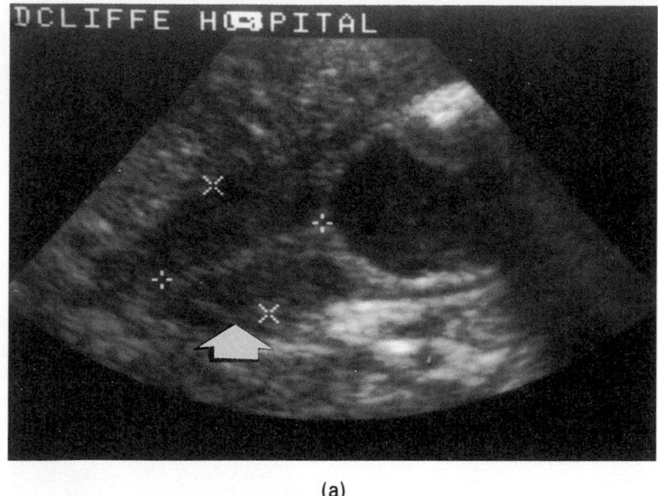

(a)

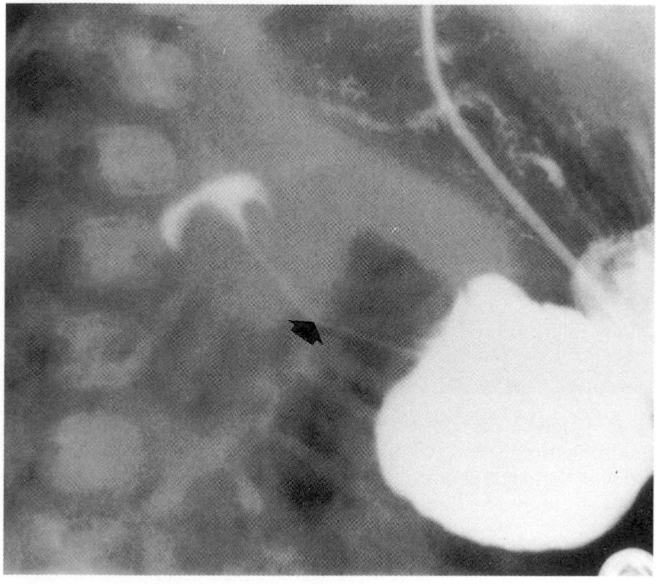

(b)

Fig. 1 (a) and (b) Ultrasound demonstrating the hypertrophied muscle (white arrow) and barium meal demonstration of the elongated narrowed pyloric canal (black arrow) of hypertrophic pyloric stenosis.

Table 1 Causes of duodenal obstruction

Duodenal atresia or stenosis
Duodenal obstruction associated with malrotation
Annular pancreas
Duodenal web
Preduodenal portal vein
Duodenal duplication cyst
Extrinsic compression by adjacent masses

the posterior peritoneum. If this process is interrupted at any point then malrotation or non-rotation results.

Intestinal obstruction, with the possibility of vascular compromise, is due to either an associated volvulus or extrinsic compression from peritoneal Ladd's bands. Abdominal radiographs may either suggest duodenal or small bowel obstruction. The

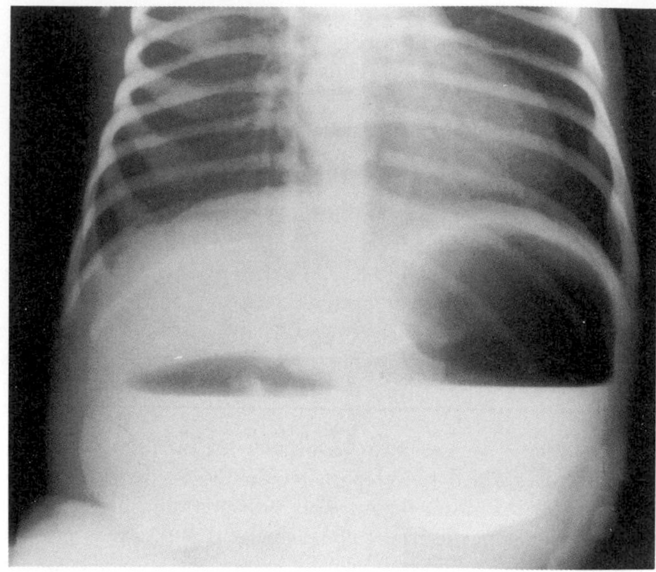

Fig. 2 'Double bubble' appearance of two fluid levels in the dilated stomach and proximal duodenum of duodenal obstruction.

diagnosis of malrotation is made by an upper gastrointestinal tract contrast study. This demonstrates the duodenojejunal flexure and ligament of Treitz to be in an abnormally low position or in the right side of the abdomen rather than in their normal position, which is in the left side of the abdomen on a level with the duodenal bulb. Although the position of the caecum is also abnormal, its position is variable in the neonate, and contrast studies of the upper rather than the lower gastrointestinal tract are therefore more reliable.

If a volvulus is present then the affected segment of bowel will appear twisted, whereas Ladd's bands give an extrinsic impression on the bowel outline. Rarely, malrotation presents less acutely, with cyclical abdominal pain and vomiting or malabsorption.

SMALL BOWEL OBSTRUCTION

The main causes of small bowel obstruction are listed in Table 2.

Table 2 Causes of small bowel obstruction

Small bowel atresia or stenosis
Meconium ileus
Hernia (internal or external)
Volvulus (usually associated with malrotation)
Duplication cyst
Intussusception
Intestinal aganglionosis
Inspissated milk curd syndrome

Abdominal radiographs show dilated loops of small bowel with air–fluid levels on erect and decubitus views. It can be difficult to differentiate between small and large bowel obstruction in young infants, because the normal differentiating features of valvulae conniventes of the small bowel and haustrae of the colon are not apparent in this age group. The anatomical position of the dilated loops of bowel may be helpful but it may be necessary to perform a contrast study of the colon simply to define the level of obstruction. It is also important to differentiate between an ileus and obstruction. Infants often develop ileus secondary to septicaemia and metabolic disturbances.

Occasionally a 'bubbly' appearance is present in the right side of the abdomen; this is due to meconium mixed with air and may be seen in meconium ileus, ileal atresia, or Hirschsprung's disease. If perforation occurs during the intrauterine period the spilt meconium produces a sterile peritonitis, with the formation of peritoneal calcification or, less often, rim calcification in a 'meconium pseudocyst'. Ascites may be present.

Meconium ileus

This condition, seen almost exclusively in babies with cystic fibrosis, causes small bowel obstruction due to thick tenacious meconium in the distal ileum. This prevents the normal bowel contents from entering the colon, which, as a result, is often a 'microcolon'. Ileal atresia is usually associated with a colon of normal calibre, as it is frequently caused by a vascular accident late on in fetal life.

The abdominal radiograph shows dilated small bowel loops, but is often remarkable for the lack of fluid levels due to the very sticky meconium within the bowel. Fifty per cent of babies with meconium ileus have other abnormalities, such as intestinal atresia or volvulus, and this should be suspected if many fluid levels are present on the radiograph.

The diagnosis of meconium ileus is confirmed by a water-soluble contrast study of the large bowel with reflux of contrast into the distal ileum. This will demonstrate 'balls' of inspissated meconium in the terminal ileum (Fig. 3).

Some success has been reported in the non-operative treatment of meconium ileus. Hyperosmolar water-soluble contrast material is refluxed amongst the impacted meconium and may relieve the obstruction both through its lubricating effect and the fact that it pulls fluid into the bowel lumen. Reported success rates for this procedure vary but a rate of 50 per cent can be achieved. The procedure is, however, only appropriate in uncomplicated cases, which account for less than half the total number. The baby has to be very closely monitored as the hyperosmolar effect of the contrast media may lead to considerable fluid and electrolyte imbalance.

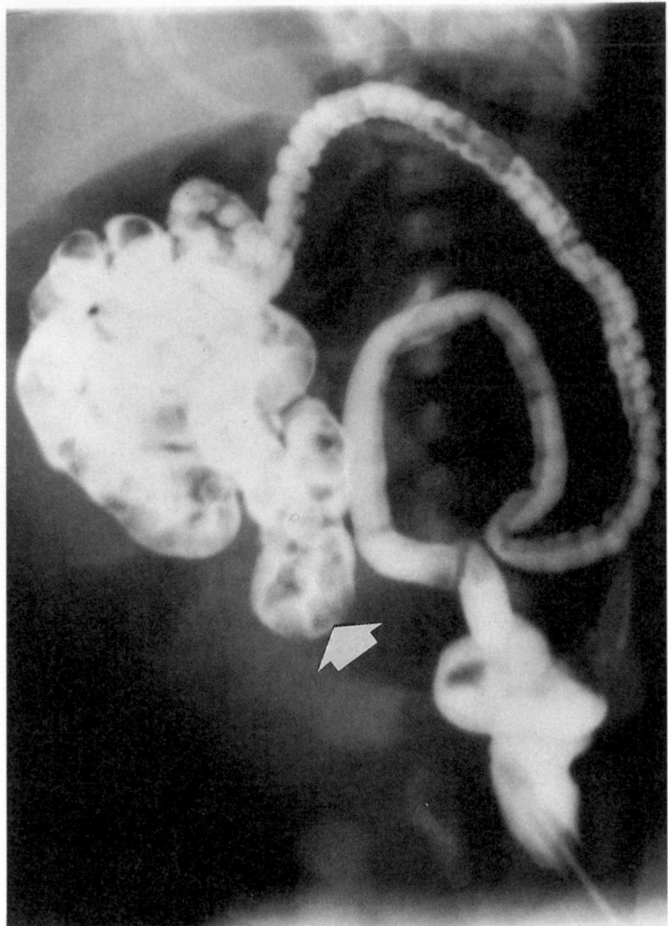

Fig. 3 Large bowel contrast study demonstrating the 'microcolon' of meconium ileus and reflux of contrast around meconium 'balls' (arrow) in the distal ileum.

Intussusception

In infants over the age of 3 months the most common causes of small bowel obstruction are intussusception and obstructed herniae. The appearance of intussusception on plain radiographs vary from a virtually normal radiograph to a picture of marked small bowel obstruction. A soft tissue mass of the intussusception itself will be visible in about one-half of the patients, or there will be an absence of the normal colonic gas pattern in the right side of the abdomen (Fig. 4). The diagnosis can be confirmed by either ultrasound or contrast examination of the colon.

Once the diagnosis has been confirmed a decision has to be taken whether to attempt non-operative reduction with either barium or gas or whether to proceed directly to surgery. This requires close co-operation between the surgeon and the radiologist. The surgeon must carefully assess the child: signs of peritonitis and bowel ischaemia are contraindications to non-operative reduction, as is radiographic evidence of perforation.

Non-operative treatment has for many years relied on hydrostatic pressure from a barium or water-soluble contrast enema to reduce the intussusception. Recently there has been renewed interest in the use of gas, with suggestions that better rates of reduction can be achieved; in addition, the procedure is cleaner and quicker. Reported series suggest a successful reduction rate using barium of between 50 and 80 per cent, whereas most studies using gas report rather better figures of 75 to 95 per cent. Factors which suggest that the procedure is less likely to be successful are a history of longer than 24 h, the presence of small bowel obstruction, and an intussusception in the distal colon. The incidence of perforation of the bowel during non-operative reduction is between 0.4 and 1.2 per cent. If gas is being used then perforation may lead to respiratory embarrassment due to gross pneumoperitoneum. The spillage of barium and faecal material into the peritoneum was thought to be associated with a very high morbidity: recent studies suggest that an immediate laparotomy reduces the long term sequelae to a minimum. The rate of recurrence of the intussusception following non-operative reduction is similar to that following surgery (4–10 per cent).

LARGE BOWEL OBSTRUCTION

The causes of large bowel obstruction are listed in Table 3. As previously discussed the differentiation between large and small

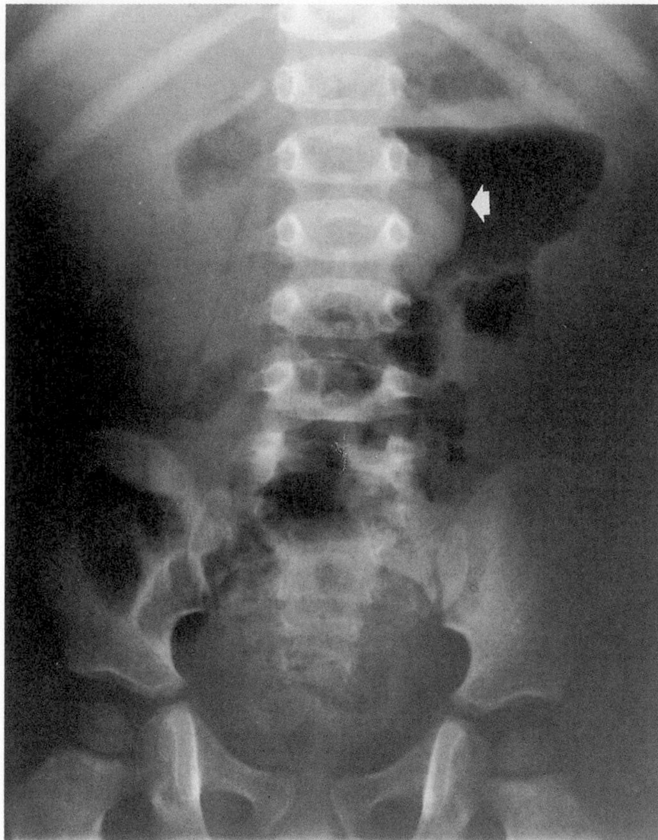

Fig. 4 Plain radiography showing the soft tissue mass (arrow) of an intussusception.

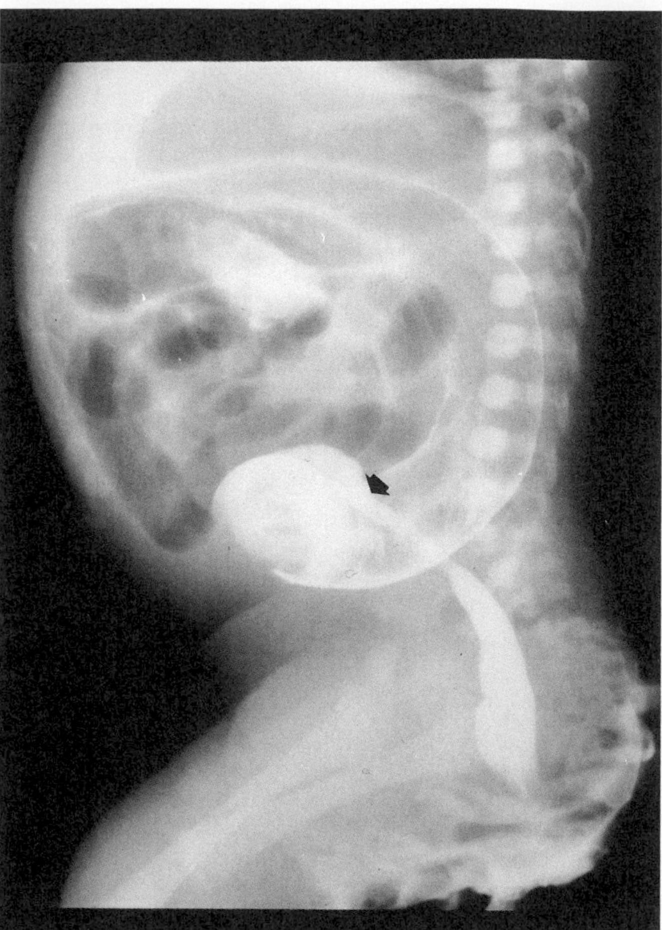

Fig. 5 Large bowel contrast study in Hirschsprung's disease demonstrating the transition zone (arrow) between distended but normally innervated proximal colon and the collapsed abnormally innervated distal colon and rectum.

Table 3 Causes of large bowel obstruction

Hirschsprung's disease
Anorectal atresia or stenosis
Meconium plug syndrome
Colonic atresia or stenosis
Extrinsic compression by cysts or tumours

bowel obstruction may be difficult using plain radiographs alone. It may be necessary to perform a contrast study of the colon to define the level of obstruction as well as to differentiate obstruction from ileus.

Hirschsprung's disease

The majority of infants with Hirschsprung's disease present with large bowel obstruction in the first week of life. The remainder usually present in the first 3 years with constipation. The definitive diagnosis is made by rectal biopsy. Plain abdominal radiographs suggest a distal large bowel obstruction or, in the rare instance of total aganglionosis of the colon, small bowel obstruction. Contrast studies using low osmolality water-soluble contrast will define a transition zone in 70 per cent of affected infants (Fig. 5). This transition zone demarcates the proximal normally innervated and dilated bowel from the distal abnormally innervated bowel which is of normal or reduced calibre.

Meconium plug syndrome

This condition occurs most commonly in premature infants and infants of diabetic mothers. The colon is normally innervated but plain radiographs suggest large bowel obstruction. Contrast studies demonstrate plugs of meconium obstructing the distal colon. The condition is probably due to functional immaturity of the colon and is self limiting. The act of performing a contrast study will dislodge the meconium.

Anorectal anomalies

These include ectopic anus, imperforate anus, rectal atresia, and anal or rectal stenosis. In these conditions, imaging defines the relationship of the atretic segment to the levator ani pelvic sling and the integrity of sphincters and their nerve supply. Both CT and magnetic resonance imaging can be used for this purpose. Fistulae can be demonstrated by contrast studies of the bladder, urethra, and vagina, and associated malformations such as renal ectopia, hydronephrosis, spinal and cardiac anomalies, and oesophageal or duodenal atresia can also be visualized.

Prior to complex imaging of the pelvic musculature and renal and gastrointestinal tracts, plain radiographs will show a degree of large bowel obstruction. Spinal abnormalities will also be apparent and if a fistula is present gas may be visible within the bladder (Fig. 6). A 'cross table' radiograph, with the baby prone and with its pelvis raised, is sometimes used to assess the distance between the most distal loop of bowel containing gas and the perineum. This may be misleading as the bowel proximal to the atresia may be plugged by meconium and not visible on the radiograph. This film should be delayed until the baby is about a day old to allow gas to reach the distal bowel.

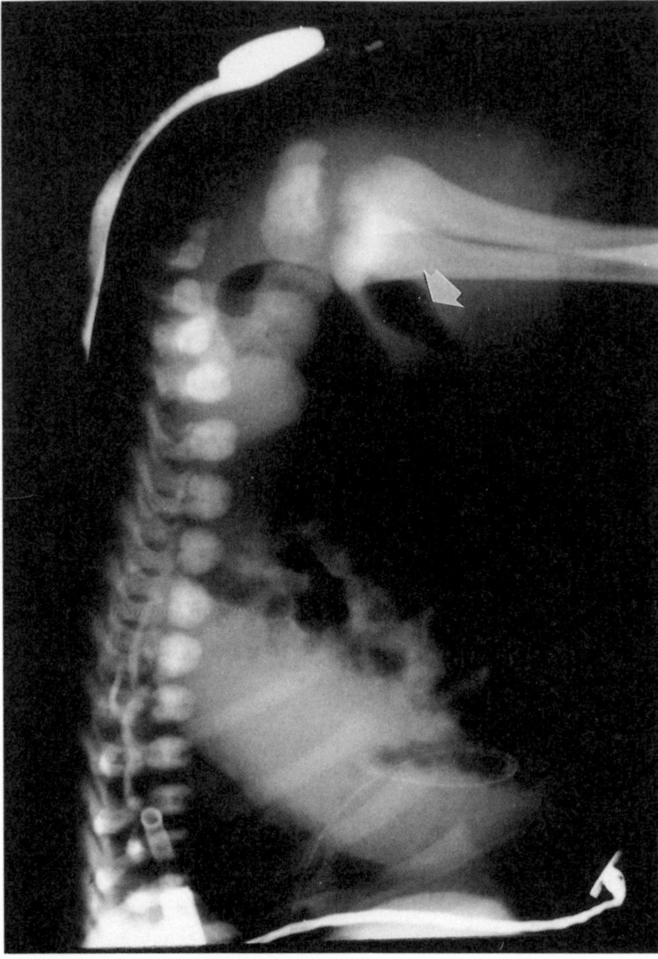

Fig. 6 'Lateral invertogram' in baby with imperforate anus demonstrating air within the bladder (arrow) due to a fistula from the bowel.

NECROTIZING ENTEROCOLITIS

The diagnosis of necrotizing enterocolitis is both a clinical and radiological one, as radiographic abnormalities may not always be apparent. Radiographic abnormalities include intestinal ileus and distension, and bowel wall thickening. Intramural gas leads to lucencies in the bowel wall which may be linear, circular, or 'bubbly' (Fig. 7). Air may pass from the bowel wall into the mesenteric venous system and become apparent in the portal vein. If perforation occurs, free air will be visible in the peritoneal cavity and abscesses may form. Free air is best seen on decubitus radiographs but the first signs, including visualization of both sides of the bowel wall, the falciform ligament, and umbilical artery remnants, may be detected on a supine film. Long term sequelae are stricture formation and, rarely, enterocolonic fistulae. These can be demonstrated by contrast studies of the bowel.

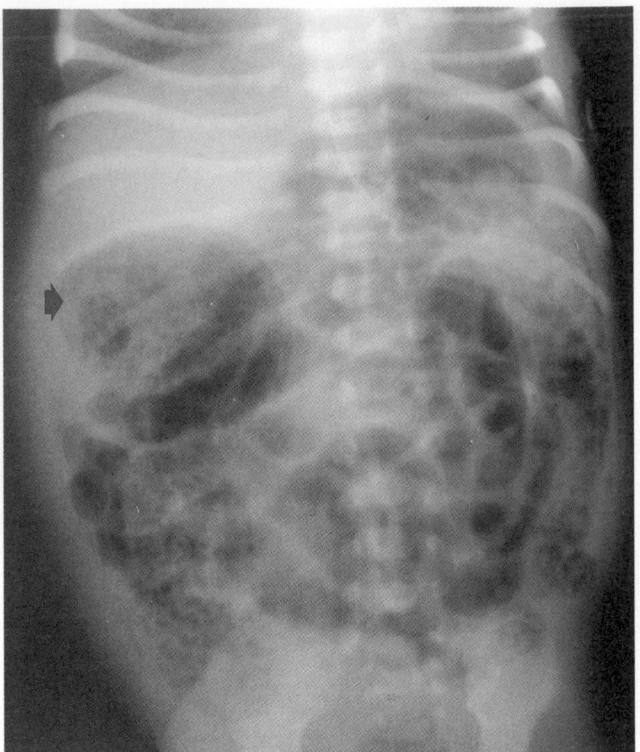

Fig. 7 Intramural air (arrow) in a severe case of necrotizing enterocolitis.

ABDOMINAL MASSES

In the immediate neonatal period most abdominal masses are renal in origin, due either to cystic disease or to hydronephrosis. Other masses occurring at birth are omental, mesenteric or duplication cysts, choledochal cysts, ovarian cysts, and adrenal haemorrhage. Tumours such as Wilms' tumour and neuroblastoma are more common around the age of 2 or 3 years; liver tumours, which are much less common, can occur at any age. The role of imaging is primarily to define the organ of origin of the mass, to define its nature and, if the mass is a tumour, whether there is evidence of spread. Ultrasound is the initial investigation of choice. This may be supplemented by CT or magnetic resonance imaging where appropriate.

Hydronephrosis

Hydronephrosis may be due to obstruction, vesicoureteric reflux or the prune belly syndrome. Obstruction most commonly occurs at the pelviureteric junction. Ultrasound determines whether hydronephrosis is present, whether it is unilateral or bilateral, whether the ureters are dilated, and whether the bladder and posterior urethra are normal. It gives no information about function, however: the intravenous urogram provides some information about function, but this is best assessed by radionuclide diuretic renography using technetium-99m either labelled to diethylene-triamine-penta-acetate (DTPA) or mercaptoacetyltriglycine (MAG 3) renography.

Renal cystic disease

There are many forms of renal cystic disease in infancy. The most common cause of an abdominal mass is multicystic dysplastic kidney, which must be differentiated from gross hydronephrosis as renal cysts and dilated calices can be confused. Multicystic dysplastic kidney is usually unilateral, and a number of non-communicating cysts of varying size are seen. An anomaly of the contralateral kidney, such as pelviureteric obstruction, is occasionally seen. A technetium-99m labelled dimercaptosuccinic acid (DMSA) scintigram will demonstrate a non-functioning kidney. A micturating cystourethrogram should also be performed to assess whether vesicoureteric reflux is occurring on the contralateral side. Infantile polycystic kidney disease is almost invariably bilateral. The ultrasound appearances of large highly echogenic kidneys are characteristic, although the actual cysts are usually small and therefore not seen.

Wilms' tumour

Wilms' tumour is the most common urinary tract tumour of childhood, and together with neuroblastoma, it is the most common solid organ tumour outside the central nervous system. Initial imaging with ultrasound or urography demonstrates an intrarenal solid mass which may expand within the kidney or protrude from the surface (Fig. 8). Areas of cystic necrosis may be present. Calcification is seen in about 5 per cent of patients on plain radiographs and in 10 per cent of those examined with CT. Chest radiography, ultrasound, and CT are used for tumour staging. Close attention is paid to the presence of pulmonary or hepatic metastases, lymph node involvement, and involvement of the contralateral kidney, which occurs in 5 per cent of cases.

Neuroblastoma

Neuroblastoma arises in the adrenal glands or anywhere in the sympathetic chain. The imaging protocol depends on the site of origin: about 70 per cent of these tumours occur within the abdomen and half of these originate in the adrenal gland. Within the abdomen, ultrasound demonstrates a solid extrarenal mass which may displace the kidney. Calcification is seen in 50 per cent of plain radiographs and in up to 80 per cent of CT studies. CT is also used to assess local spread, including spread into the spinal canal, and metastatic disease. Scintigraphy is required to detect skeletal metastases. Iodine-131 or iodine-123-*m*-iodobenzylguanidine (MIBG) may be used to detect the primary tumour and any metastases, as well as monitoring response to therapy. The role of magnetic resonance imaging in both neuroblastoma and Wilms' tumour is still being evaluated.

IMAGING IN URINARY TRACT INFECTION

Imaging studies in children with urinary tract infection allow the early detection of conditions such as hydronephrosis and vesico-

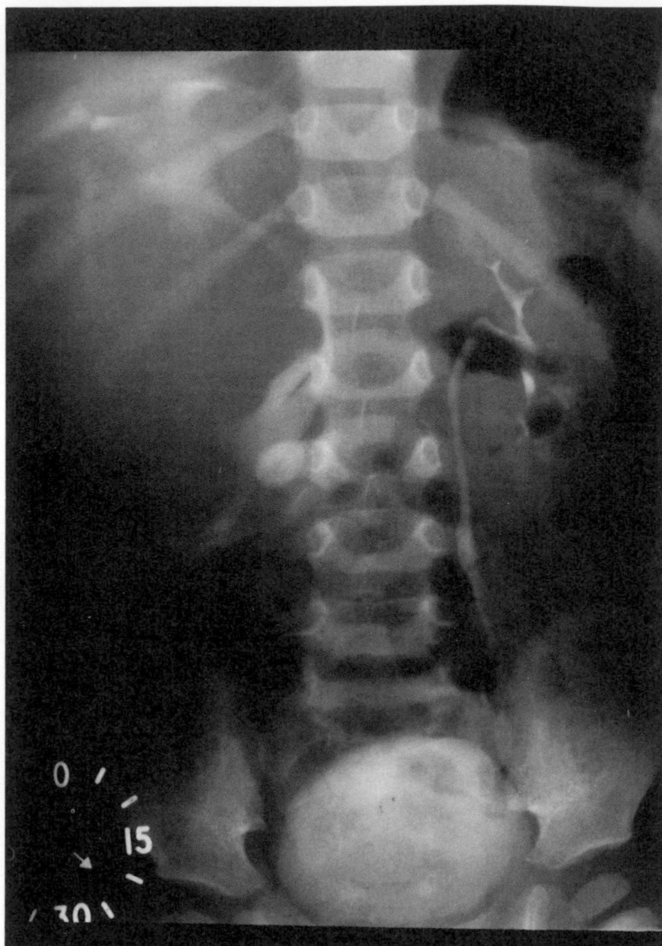

Fig. 8 Classical urogram of a Wilms' tumour showing a large intrarenal mass lesion.

ureteric reflux, which may lead to irreversible renal damage. If damage has occurred, the severity can be assessed.

As previously stated, hydronephrosis can be evaluated by ultrasound, intravenous urography, and renal scintigraphy. Vesicoureteric reflux is assessed by a micturating cystourethrogram (Fig. 9). This may also demonstrate urethral abnormalities such as posterior urethral valves, ectopic ureters, and ureteroceles. Less commonly, reflex can be demonstrated by direct or indirect radionuclide cystography.

Renal scarring is best demonstrated by technetium-99m labelled dimercaptosuccinic acid (DMSA) scintigraphy (Fig. 10). This also permits quantification of split renal function. Ultrasound is unreliable in the detection of mild or even moderate degrees of renal scarring.

In the young infant (under 1 year of age) an ultrasound scan to detect hydronephrosis and a micturating cystourethrogram to detect reflux are performed. Between the age of 1 and 5 years there is debate as to the most appropriate investigations. One approach is to perform an ultrasound scan and a DMSA scintigram initially, followed by a cystogram if either show scarring or a dilated urinary tract, suggestive of reflux. After the age of 5 years an ultrasound scan and a plain abdominal radiograph, to detect renal calcification and spinal anomalies, are probably all that is required. In all age groups, if an abnormality is detected, then the appropriate

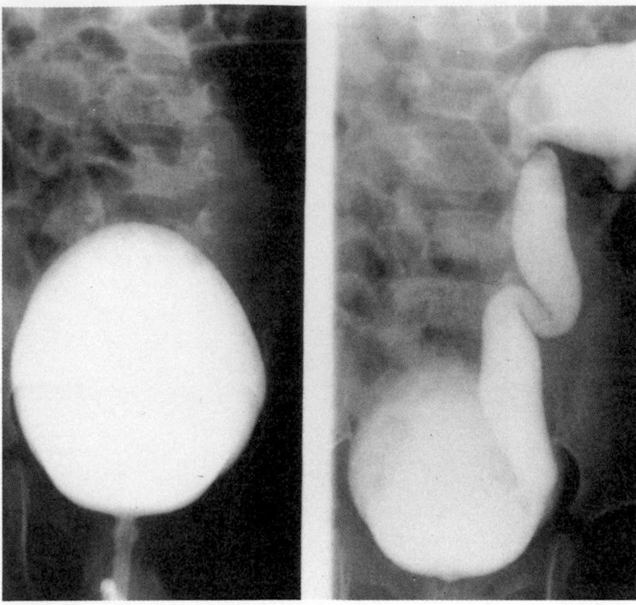

Fig. 9 Micturating cystourethrogram demonstrating vesicoureteric reflux.

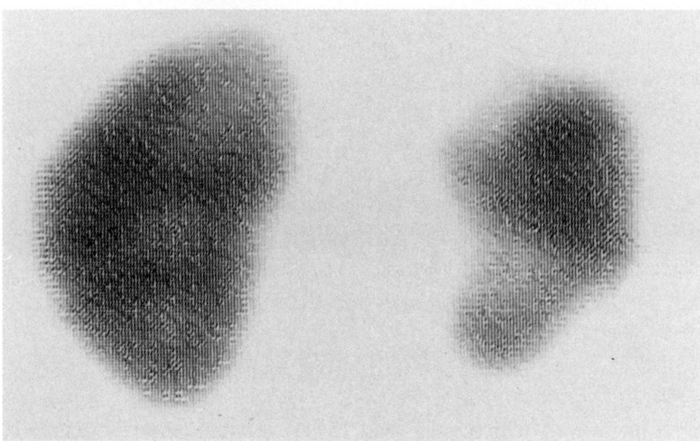

Fig. 10 Technetium-99m DMSA scintigraphy demonstrating renal scarring. Split junction: left = 64 per cent, right = 36 per cent.

imaging protocol will be followed depending on whether obstruction, reflux, or scarring are suspected.

BILIARY ATRESIA

The diagnosis of biliary atresia must be made quickly so that surgery can be performed in the first 2 months of life. Ultrasound is performed initially to exclude other causes of biliary obstruction such as choledochal cyst, although the two may coexist. The gallbladder is not usually visualized in patients with biliary atresia, but examination of the liver is otherwise normal. Following ultrasound examination biliary excretion is assessed using either [^{123}I]- bromosulphthalein or [^{99}Tc^{m}] iminodiacetic acid compounds. Reported sensitivity in differentiating atresia from hepatitis varies between 85 and 100 per cent. The final diagnosis and differentiation may depend on liver biopsy and operative cholangiography.

MECKEL'S DIVERTICULUM

This may occasionally be detected on plain radiographs as a fluid filled or air filled mass containing debris, or a calcified enterolith may be seen. Contrast studies of the small intestine may fill the diverticulum but the standard method of detection relies on technetium scintigraphy. Provided that the diverticulum contains ectopic gastric mucosa then the scintigram should be positive.

FURTHER READING

Aaronson IA, Cremin BJ. Cysts of the kidney. In: *Clinical Paediatric Uroradiology*. Edinburgh: Churchill Livingstone, 1984: 76–99.

Aaronson IA, Cremin BJ. Tumours of the urinary tract. In: *Clinical Paediatric Uroradiology*. Edinburgh: Churchill Livingstone, 1984: 307–34.

Bell RS, Graham CB, Stevenson JK. Roentgenologic and clinical manifestations of neonatal necrotising enterocolitis. *Am J Roentgenol*, 1971; **112**: 123–34.

Berdon WE, Slovis TL, Campbell JB, Baker DH, Haller JO. Neonatal small left colon syndrome: its relationship to aganglionosis and meconium plug syndrome. *Radiology*, 1977; **125**: 457–62.

Bisset GS, Kirks DR. Intussusception in infants and children: diagnosis and therapy. *Radiology*, 1988; **168**: 141–5.

Boechat MI, Kangarloo H. MR Imaging of the abdomen in children. *Am J Roentgenol*, 1989; **152**: 1245–50.

Boechat MI, *et al.* Primary liver tumours in children: comparison of CT and MR imaging. *Radiology*, 1988; **169**: 727–32.

Bower RJ, Sieber WK, Kiesewetter WB. Alimentary tract duplications in children. *Ann Surg*, 1978; **188**: 669–74.

Carty H, Pilling, DW, Majury C. Iodine-123 BSP scanning in neonatal jaundice. *Ann Radiol*, 1986; **29**: 647–50.

David R, *et al.* The many faces of neuroblastoma. *Radiographics*, 1989; **9**: 859–82.

Gans SL. Classification of ano-rectal anomalies: a critical analysis. *J Pediatr Surg*, 1970; **5**: 511–13.

Gu L, *et al.* Intussusception reduction in children by rectal insufflation of air. *Am J Roentgenol*, 1988; **150**: 1345–8.

Hibi S, Todo S, Imashuku S, Miyazaki T. Iodine-131 meta-iodobenzylguanidine scintigraphy in patients with neuroblastoma. *Pediatr Radiol*, 1987; **17**: 308–13.

Hope JW, Borns PF, Berg PK. Roentgenologic manifestations of Hirschsprung's disease in infancy. *Am J Roentgenol*, 1965; **95**: 217–29.

Houston CS, Wittenborg MH. Roentgen evaluation of anomalies of rotation and fixation of the bowel in children. *Radiology*, 1965; **84**: 1–17.

Kluth D. Atlas of oesophageal atresia. *J Pediatr Surg*, 1976; **11**: 901–19.

Kohda E, Fujioka M, Ikawa H, Yokoyama J. Congenital anorectal anomaly: CT evaluation. *Radiology*, 1985; **157**: 349–52.

Leonidas JC, Berdon WE, Baker DH, Santulli TV. Meconium ileus and its complications, a reappraisal of plain film roentgen diagnostic criteria. *Am J Roentgenol*, 1970; **108**: 598–609.

Martin GI, Kutner FR, Moser L. Diagnosis of Meckel's diverticulum by radio isotope scanning. *Pediatrics*, 1976; **57**: 11–12.

Nussbaum AR, Sanders RS, Hartman DS, Dudgeon DL, Parmley TH. Neonatal ovarian cysts: sonographic–pathologic correlation. *Radiology*, 1988; **168**: 817–21.

Rescorla FJ, Grosfeld JL, West KJ, Vane DW. Changing patterns of treatment and survival in neonates with meconium ileus. *Arch Surg*, 1989; **124**: 837–40.

Ros PR, Olmsted WW, Moser RP, Dachman AH, Hjermstad BH, Sobin LH. Mesenteric and omental cysts: histologic classification with imaging correlation. *Radiology*, 1987; **164**: 327–32.

Rosenfield NS, *et al.* Hirschsprung disease: accuracy of the barium enema examination. *Radiology*, 1984; **150**: 393–400.

Sato Y, *et al.* Congenital anorectal anomalies: MR Imaging. *Radiology*, 1988; **168**: 157–62.

Snyder WH, Chaffin L. Malrotation of the intestine. In: Mustard WT, Ravitch MM, Snyder WH, Welch KJ, Benson CD, eds. *Pediatric Surgery*. Chicago: Year Book Publishers, 1969: 808–17.

Westra SJ, de Groot CJ, Smits NJ, Staalman CR. Hypertrophic pyloric stenosis: Use of the pyloric volume measurement in early US diagnosis. *Radiology*, 1989; **172**: 615–19.

Working group of the research unit, Royal College of Physicians. Guidelines for the management of acute urinary tract infection in childhood. *J R Coll Phys*, 1991; **25**: 36–42.

6.7 Nuclear medicine techniques

BASIL J. SHEPSTONE

BASIC CONCEPTS

Nuclear medicine uses the properties of radioactive and stable nuclides to diagnose morphological and/or physiological disorders and to provide therapy using unsealed radioactive sources.

One great advantage that nuclear imaging techniques have over other imaging modalities is that they represent function rather than morphology. Another is that, although ionizing radiation is used, adverse reactions are rare. A third advantage is that many of the techniques demonstrate exquisite sensitivity in detecting disease, but this is accompanied by the great disadvantage that radionuclide studies are seldom specific; that is, although certain notable exceptions occur, pathognomonic appearances are rare.

It is well known that radioactive substances can emit α- or β-particles, or else γ-rays. α-Particles are emitted only by the naturally occurring radionuclides, such as radium, which are no longer used in medicine. β-Particles, because of their short path length before they are absorbed, are useful for therapy but useless for diagnosis as they cannot emerge from the body. This leaves only γ-rays which, like X-rays, can pass out of the body and be detected externally.

The currently used unit of radioactivity is the becquerel (Bq), which is the Système International unit and equal to one disintegration per second. As this unit is a very small amount, the commonly used multiple is the megabequerel (MBq), where 1 MBq = 10^6 disintegrations per second. The older unit, the curie (Ci) = 3.7×10^{10} disintegrations per second, so 1 millicurie (mCi) = 37 MBq.

RADIOPHARMACEUTICALS

The basic radiopharmaceutical is a γ-emitting radionuclide attached to a compound which is specially tailored to target a particular organ system or physiological process. The quantities used are generally small and so the radiopharmaceuticals neither disturb the process under investigation nor provoke hypersensitivity reactions.

The most popular radionuclide used currently is called technetium-99m (where 99 is the mass number and m means 'metastable'; it can also be written $^{99}Tc^{m}$). Like all metastable radionuclides, technetium-99m has the triple advantages of being a pure γ-emitter, having a short half-life, and being readily available from a longer-lived generator containing its parent radionuclide. In fact it is now used so widely that γ-ray detectors are specifically designed to function optimally at the γ-ray energy of technetium-99m.

Technetium-99m originates from the generator as the pertechnetate, $^{99}Tc^{m}O_4$, but it can, for example, be attached to human serum albumin macroaggregates which blockade the pulmonary capillaries and can be used to detect pulmonary emboli. It can be linked to phosphates or phosphonates which undergo chemiabsorption on to bone crystal in order to image bone. Reticuloendothelial uptake in liver, spleen, and bone marrow is effected by linking it to sulphur or tin colloid, which is phagocytosed. In the form of the pertechnetate it can be taken up by active ion transport into gastric mucosa, thyroid, and salivary glands. Hepatocyte and biliary-tract imaging uses the active cellular transport and excretion of $^{99}Tc^{m}$-labelled substituted carbamoyliminodiacetic acid. It can also be chelated with, say, dimercaptosuccinic acid, which will be taken up by the renal cortical cells to produce renal images. Chelated to diphenyltriaminepenta-acetic acid it can measure the glomerular filtration rate. The most exciting recent compound linked to technetium-99m is hydroxymethylpropylamine oxime ('Ceretec', 'Exametazime': Amersham), which crosses the blood–brain barrier and can be used, say, to investigate neuropsychiatric disorders such as Alzheimer's dementia and schizophrenia.

Other radionuclides are, of course, also used in nuclear medicine. Examples are thallium-201 (^{201}Tl) chloride for myocardial imaging, and gallium-67 (^{67}Ga) citrate for the detection of tumours and infective/inflammatory foci. Indium-111 (^{111}In) has been used to label white cells (to detect infection) or monoclonal antibodies (to detect targets as diverse as tumours or areas of endometriosis). Iodine-123 (^{123}I) has replaced one of the original radionuclides used in nuclear medicine, iodine-131 (^{131}I), in the diagnosis of thyroid disorders.

All of the above radionuclides are called single-photon emitters as they emit single γ-ray photons. However, there is also a class of so-called positron-emitting radionuclides, that emit two photons, a positive electron (or positron), and a conventional negative electron in coincidence at an angle of 180° to each other. These charged subatomic species cannot exist as such for any length of time and are annihilated by their opposite number, yielding two high-energy γ-rays. Among the positron-emitting radionuclides are important biological atoms, such as oxygen-15 (^{15}O), nitrogen-13 (^{13}N), carbon-11 (^{11}C), and fluorine-18 (^{18}F), which can be incorporated into a variety of tracers. Fluorine-18, for example, has been incorporated into fluorodeoxyglucose and has revolutionized neurophysiology and neuropathology.

Unfortunately, these potentially most useful radiopharmaceuticals are produced in cyclotrons and have extremely short half-lives (of the order of a few minutes). Therefore the necessary in-house facilities needed to produce these include the cyclotron, on-line radiochemical processing, purification, and sterilization, and a positron camera—an exorbitantly expensive facility.

It is the ability of radiopharmaceuticals to act as indicators of physiological processes which separates nuclear medicine from most other imaging processes, such as computed tomography and ultrasound, which are largely conveyors of morphological information. However, exceptions exist. The intravenous urogram, for example, is a functional as well as a morphological study.

MAPPING THE DISTRIBUTION OF RADIOPHARMACEUTICALS

The distribution within the body of single-photon-emitting radionuclides (γ-emitters) is mapped by means of a scintillation, or gamma, camera (Fig. 1). A modern camera can either accumulate flat ('planar') images or rotate around the body to reconstruct, via the computer, tomographic images in the transverse, sagittal, or coronal planes.

The basic component of such cameras is a thallium-activated sodium iodide crystal, which can convert γ-rays into light photons. The latter are then converted into electrons and subsequently aggregated into amplified filtered pulses. The pulses, suitably distributed spatially, can then produce maps of the distribution of radioactivity on either X-ray or polaroid film, or on to light-sensitive paper. Otherwise, pulses may be stored in the memory banks of a computer for later manipulation.

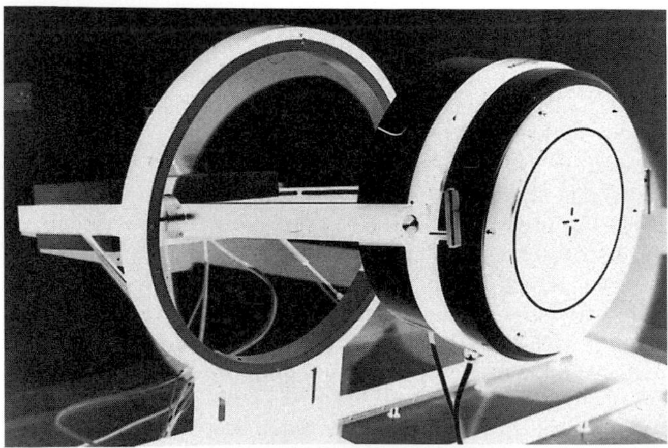

Fig. 1 A modern gamma-camera.

In order to screen out unwanted γ-rays, both from the patient and from other sources of radiation in the imaging suite or from background radiation, collimators are used. These usually consist of a lead slab penetrated by many small holes, and acting like a sieve, keeping out γ-rays from any direction except those from the organ of interest. Further sorting of unwanted energies is done electronically.

The data can therefore be in either digital or analogue form, but the two are interconvertable. So-called 'regions of interest' can, for example, be drawn around areas of physiological interest (such as the renal cortex, the left ventricle, the oesophagus) and count-rate changes within these regions can be derived as activity–time curves. In this way, for example, renograms can be produced to demonstrate the passage of a radiopharmaceutical such as $^{99}Tc^{m}$-diphenyltriaminepenta-acetic acid through the kidney.

Positron detectors detect the pair of γ-rays resulting from the positron–electron annihilation; in order to do this they are placed on either side of the source, usually in a ring formation, and only register a count if both detectors detect photons in coincidence. Image-control techniques are then used to reconstruct the cross-sectional image. Single-photon-emission tomography uses the rotating gamma-camera to detect photons from multiple angles (180° or 360°) around the patient and an associated computer to reconstruct multiple slices. Technetium–99m and iodine–123 are the common radionuclides used for single-photon-emission tomography, and the principal organs of interest are the brain and the myocardium.

IMAGING DISEASE PROCESSES

The skeleton

Bone blood flow and bone turnover are the major factors determining the uptake of radiopharmaceuticals into bone. In the resting state, about one-third of the maximum potential blood flow through bone is excluded by sympathetic tone, and so processes that alter this tone also affect bone blood flow. Chemiabsorption on to recently deposited or exposed bone crystal is the principal method of radiopharmaceutical uptake.

Normal bone will therefore be active ('warm' rather than 'hot'), with the larger bones, such as the pelvis, and the joints predominating. Diseased areas show up as photon-abundant or 'hot' areas due to increased blood flow, bone turnover, or loss of sympathetic tone. However, a purely lytic area, such as an osteoclastoma or an infarct, can be photon-deficient ('cold'), and extraosseous uptake of bone-seeking radionuclides is well described, for example in paretic states, neuropathies, areas of necrosis, and infarction.

$^{99}Tc^{m}$ complexed organic and inorganic phosphate compounds are the major bone-seeking tracers, to which hydroxyl groups are often added to improve crystal binding. The currently favoured compounds are the diphosphonates. The skeleton takes up about 60 per cent of the injected dose, the rest being excreted through the kidneys and, at the same time, providing renal scintigrams, which are crude assessments of renal function. Skeletal scintigraphy is usually done in three phases, detecting flow, equilibrium uptake, and the so-called late crystal phases.

As with most radionuclide studies, skeletal scintigraphy is exquisitely sensitive (10^{14} times as sensitive as plain skeletal radiography), but non-specific. Its main use in modern nuclear medicine is the detection of metastases and, nowadays, requests for skeletal scintigraphy constitute nearly half of the routine workload of most general nuclear medicine departments (Fig. 2).

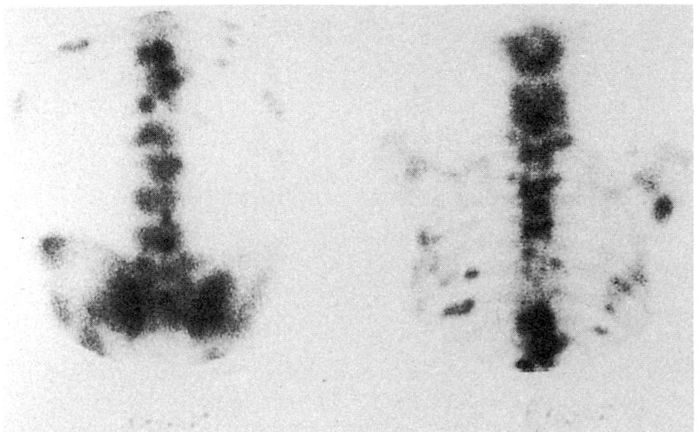

Fig. 2 Part of a skeletal scintigram obtained using ^{99}Tc^{m}-HMDP. The very black areas are foci of increased uptake due to increased flow to, and osteoblast stimulation around, skeletal metastases from a primary breast cancer.

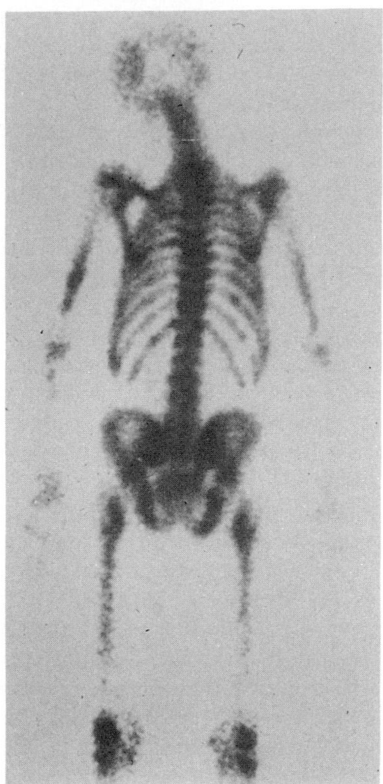

Fig. 3 A skeletal scintigram using ^{99}Tc^{m}-HMDP, showing generalized increased bone uptake of tracer, but with no sign of renal uptake. This constitutes the 'superscan' resulting from diffuse metastatic spread from a bronchial carcinoma.

Some 20 to 30 per cent of bone metastases are seen on skeletal scintigraphy, but not on radiographs. However, in about 5 per cent of cases or less, the reverse is true and it is possible that processes infiltrating the bone marrow, such as myeloma and leukaemia, will be missed on skeletal scintigraphy.

A variant of the appearance of metastatic disease in the skeleton is the so-called 'superscan', when the whole skeleton shows relatively uniform high uptake with little in the way of discrete foci. It might even be reported as normal until it is noted that no renal images are present—an indication of the fact that nearly all the dose has been taken up by rapidly metabolizing bone and very little is left to excrete through the kidneys (Fig. 3). However, this pattern may also be seen in metabolic bone disease.

Benign bone tumours show varying degrees of uptake. That in an osteoid osteoma may be almost pathognomonic with a central, very hot nidus, surrounded by an oval of slightly lesser intensity (Fig. 4). Most other bone neoplasia show varying degrees of uptake and are usually investigated by plain radiography, computed tomography (CT), or magnetic resonance imaging (MRI). However, multifocality can be demonstrated easily on scintigraphy.

As far as trauma is concerned, 80 per cent of all fractures show increased uptake by 24 h, and nearly all are visible by 3 days. Injury often removes the sympathetic drive, resulting in generally increased, but diffuse, uptake—a situation called the reflex sympathetic dystrophy syndrome. Failure to see increased flow at a fracture site a few weeks after injury suggests a lack of bone union. On skeletal radiography, rib fractures usually present as focal areas of increased uptake arranged in a vertical line, as opposed to metastases, which are randomly located. In many parts of the skeleton, such as wrist, ankle, face, and base of skull, fractures not seen on conventional radiology may be detected easily on scintigraphy. This includes stress fractures of the tibia.

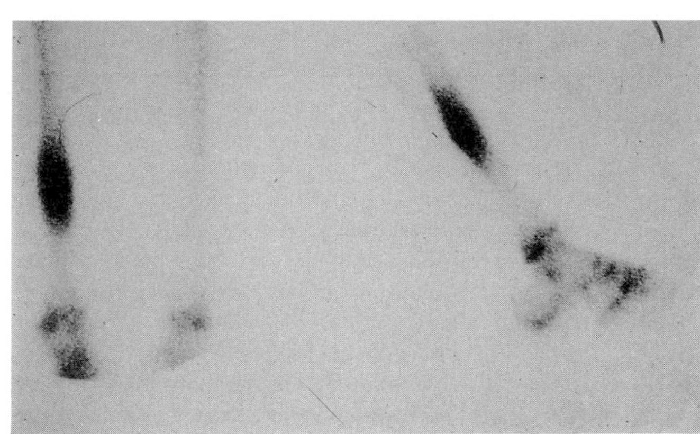

Fig. 4 A skeletal scintigram using ^{99}Tc^{m}-HMDP, showing the characteristic high uptake in an osteoid osteoma, with its oval configuration and very 'hot' nidus.

Avascular necrosis of the femoral head or the scaphoid may be detected as areas of photon deficiency during both the flow and crystal phases. In the case of hip fractures, account must be taken of the fact that a photon-deficient head can be due to tamponade of the artery by surrounding oedema. To distinguish between necrosis and oedema, a bone-marrow scintigram using ^{99}Tc^{m}-sulphur or

^{99}Tc^{m}-tin colloid, which is phagocytosed by the marrow reticuloendothelial cells, will demonstrate whether the marrow has survived or not. The marrow will survive in generalized oedema, but not in avascular necrosis.

Skeletal scintigraphy can detect osteomyelitis both on the flow study, which demonstrates increased blood flow to the affected area, and on the delayed study due to bone turnover. Radiographic changes may not occur before 1 to 2 weeks. The technique is also useful in distinguishing between osteomyelitis and cellulitis, as the latter produces only increased flow, while osteomyelitis shows both increased flow and increased bone turnover. Bone injured in any way can produce misleading images as reactive bone shows a high affinity for radionuclides for up to 9 months after a fracture.

The problem is at its most frustrating in the case of a prosthetic hip replacement, which can become loose or infected, or both. The problems may be solved by using an infection-seeking agent such as gallium-67 citrate or ^{111}In-labelled white cells, but the problem may be extremely difficult to resolve.

Radionuclides, such as technetium-99m methylene diphosphonate (HMDP) can also be used to investigate metabolic bone disease, such as Paget's disease, renal osteodystrophy, primary hyperparathyroidism, osteoporosis, and a number of other rarer conditions. These can be detected, quantified, and followed-up easily, using serial scintigraphy or bone absorptiometry.

The skeletal scintigraphic agents, notably technetium-99m pyrophosphate, are often taken up in soft tissue. The best known is uptake in areas of myocardial or cerebral infarction or ischaemia, while this uptake is also quite common in necrotic tumours and a host of other situations, including scar tissue in the lungs of patients in chronic renal failure.

Skeletal scintigraphy can also be used for the detection and follow-up of joint disease, such as rheumatoid arthritis, where there is a strong correlation with clinical symptoms.

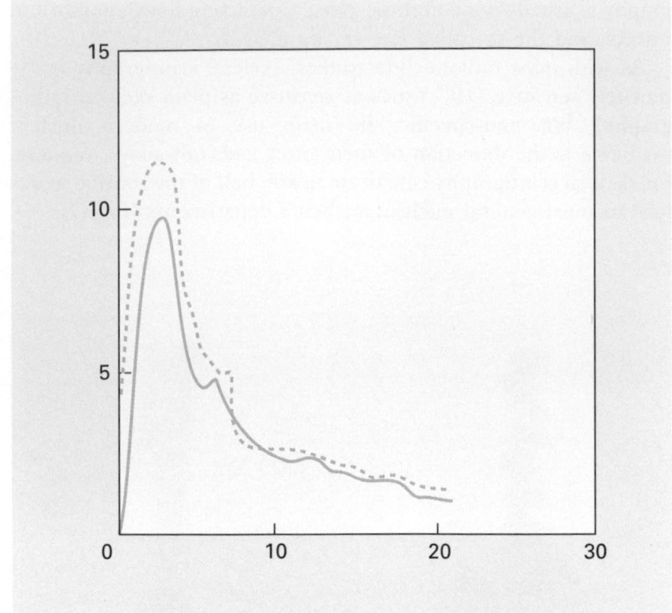

Fig. 5 Normal gamma-camera renogram of left (solid curve) and right (dotted curve) kidneys using ^{99}Tc^{m}–mercaptoacetyltriglycine. Each curve shows a rising vascular phase, a sharp handling peak of good amplitude, and a rapidly descending excretory phase; *Y*-axis, percentage of injected dose; *X*-axis, time in minutes after injection.

The urogenital tract

Kidney

Reasonable renal images may be obtained using ^{99}Tc^{m}-dimercaptosuccinic acid, and this should be used in patients allergic to iodine-containing contrast media and so unable to undergo intravenous urography. All renal masses show up as photon-deficient areas. A renal column of Bertin, which may appear as a mass on urography, shows photon-abundance on scintigraphy. However, the principal use of the technique is for the detection of renal scarring, especially in children, which is notoriously difficult or impossible to detect with intravenous contrast. By measuring the uptake of labelled dimercaptosuccinate by each kidney, an assessment of relative renal function can be made, and renal scintigraphy has also been found to be sensitive in the detection of renal trauma.

A second useful tracer technique for investigating the kidneys is renography. This is usually performed with ^{99}Tc^{m}-diphenyltriaminepenta-acetic acid or ^{99}Tc^{m}-mercaptoacetyltriglycine. The normal renogram is a computer-generated activity–time curve depicting the passage of radionuclide through the kidney, and is obtained by defining a 'region of interest' over the kidneys. The normal renogram is shown in Fig. 5. Its analysis is complex, utilizing so-called deconvolutional analysis and deriving transit times, but it seems to be just as useful it if is interpreted simply. The rising part of the curve (Phase I, or 'vascular phase') is a function of radionuclide reaching the kidney; the peak (Phase II, or 'handling phase') is related to the efficiency of parenchymal function, while the descending part of the curve (Phase III, or 'excretory phase') shows the rate of washout of tracer from the renal area. Much of the activity 'seen' by the gamma-camera will be background activity, and ideally this should be subtracted from the renal curves.

In parenchymal failure there is a normal vascular phase, but the handling peak is of poor count rate and broadened. One of the most difficult diagnoses to make without invasive contrast angiography is that of renovascular hypertension. However, renography following the administration of angiotensin-converting enzyme inhibitors is now reported to increase the accuracy of the test. An example of its use is given in Fig.6.

In obstructive situations one might expect a renogram similar to that shown in Fig. 7(a), where the vascular and handling phases are normal, but the excretory phase fails to descend normally and may even continue to rise. However, a similar curve is obtained when there is hydronephrosis without current obstruction. In this instance the administered tracer simply pours into the dilated pelvicaliceal system. The curve will eventually descend, but not within the 30 min or so normally assigned to a renogram study. There is, however, a very simple way of distinguishing between this 'floppy-bag' scenario and true obstruction, and that is to perform a diuretic-provocation renogram. There will be prompt clearance of tracer from the pelvis in the cases of non-obstructive hydronephrosis, as shown in Fig. 7(b).

Radionuclide methods for detecting vesicoureteric reflux can be direct or indirect and are excellent for follow-up studies as the radiation dose to the patient is much lower than for voiding cystourethrography. The direct test is similar to its radiographic counterpart in that technetium-99m is instilled into the bladder via a catheter and images are recorded as the patient voids

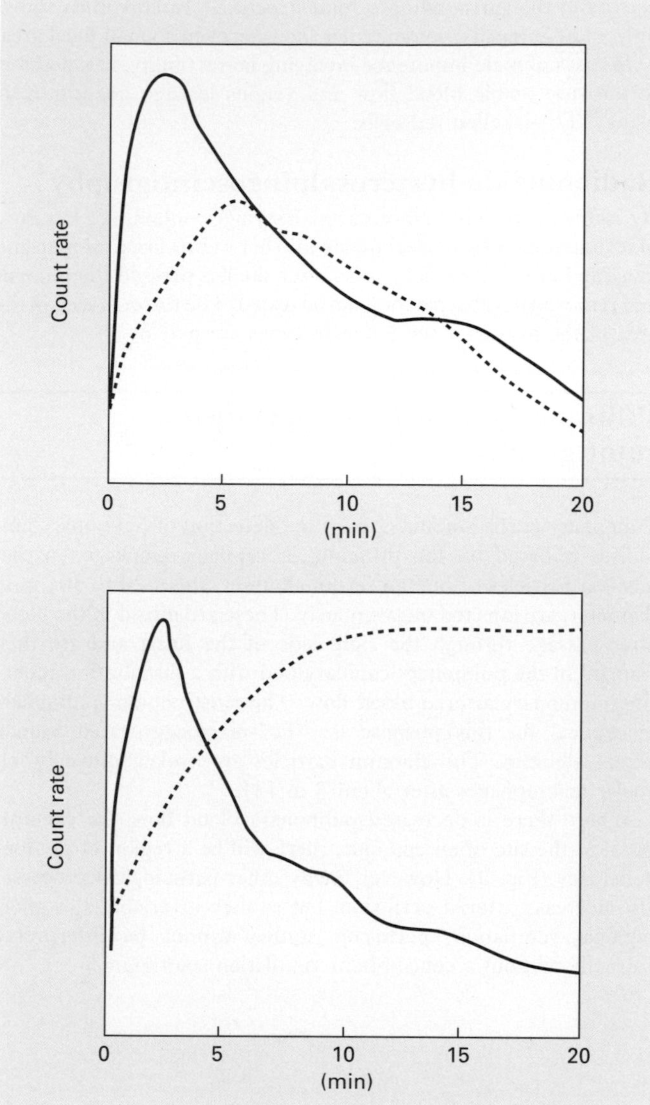

Fig. 6 Above: iodine-123 orthohippurate renogram in a hypertensive man with right-sided renal artery stenosis prior to angioplasty. Abnormal right side (dotted line) and normal left (continuous line). Below: during the administration of an angiotensin-converting enzyme inhibitor (captopril) the left renogram is unchanged, but the right side has altered dramatically.

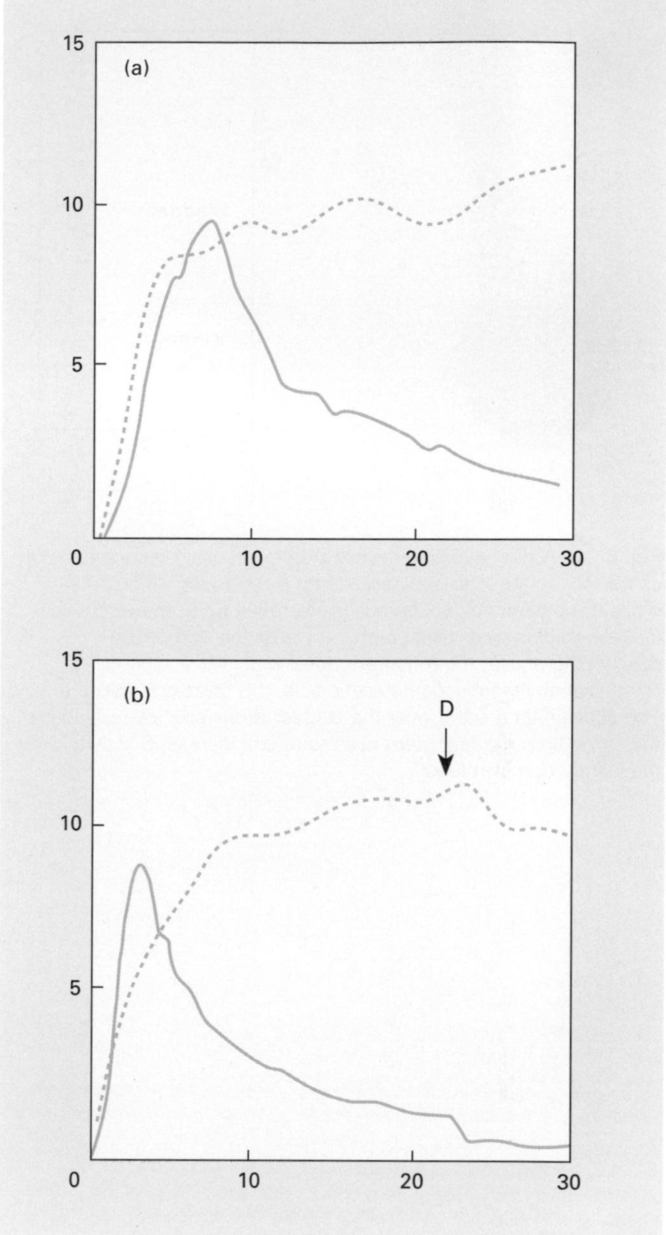

Fig. 7 (a) Renogram, showing obstructive pattern on right side; (b) gamma-camera renogram with diuretic provocation, showing a normal left renogram, but the right renogram shows little response to diuretic (D). Graphical conventions as in Fig. 5 (the normal renograms).

(Fig. 8(a)). The indirect study can be done as part of a conventional renogram, with the patient being asked to void near the end of the excretory phase. If reflux is present, the curve will show a sharp rise, as shown in Fig. 8(b).

Serial renograms can be very useful in monitoring renal grafts after transplantation. Apart from being able sometimes to detect early rejection 1 to 2 days before biochemical abnormalities become obvious, the method is useful for detecting acute tubular necrosis (where the renogram steadily rises), renal vessels, ureteral obstruction, thrombosis, and extravasation. $^{99}Tc^{m}$-sulphur colloid is also useful in identifying graft rejection, as macrophages accumulating in the failing transplant take up this agent to the same extent as the liver and spleen.

Kidneys with active pyelonephritis take up gallium-67 citrate for much longer (about 72 h) than normal kidneys (24 h).

Any of the above studies may be coupled with measurements of total glomerular filtration rate and effective renal plasma flow using ^{51}Cr-ethylenediaminetetraacetic acid clearance and iodine-123 orthohippurate or $^{99}Tc^{m}$-mercaptoacetyltriglycine, respectively.

Testicular imaging and penile blood flow

Radionuclide methods can also be used to investigate acute testicular pain, which can be due to torsion or acute epididymitis. In the former, a cut-off in the flow of the testicular artery is accompanied by decreased vascularity of the testes and increased

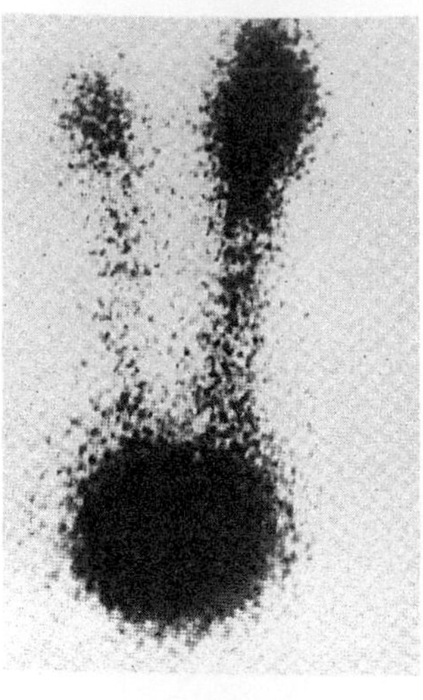

(a)

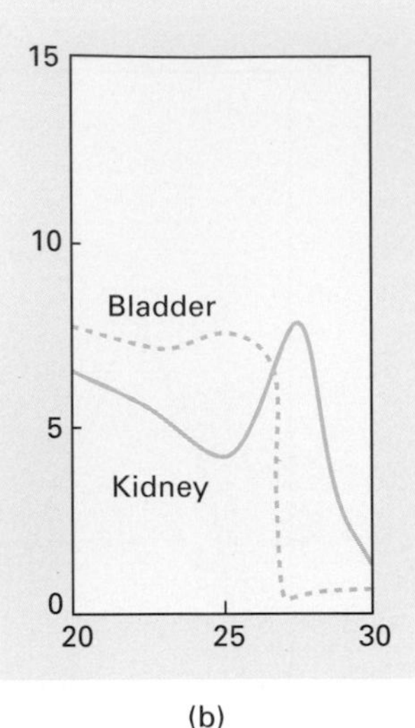

(b)

Fig. 8 (a) A direct voiding cystoureterogram using technetium-99m as pertechnetate in saline instilled into the bladder via a catheter while the patient voids. There is gross reflux up both ureters. (b) Indirect voiding cystoscintigraphy. towards the end of the descending phase of a renogram done with ^{99}Tc^{m}-diphenyltriaminopenta-acetic acid, this child was asked to void. The activity–time curve over the bladder drops precipitously, but at the same time the renogram rises to reflect increased activity over the kidney due to reflux.

activity of the surrounding scrotal structures. Epididymitis shows only a low-intensity, semicircular focus or even a small focal area.

In cases of male impotence involving inerectibility, it is possible to measure penile blood flow and venous leakage quantitatively using ^{99}Tc^{m}-labelled red cells.

Radionuclide hysterosalpingoscintigraphy

By asking the patient to insert a small syringe containing a low dose of technetium–99m pertechnetate into her vagina like a tampon and imaging her pelvis an hour or so after she has pressed the plunger and removed it, tubal patency can be tested. The tracer is seen in the area of the ovaries if the fallopian tubes are patent.

Pulmonary ventilation–perfusion scintigraphy

Pulmonary perfusion imaging for the detection of pulmonary embolism is based on the principle of capillary blockage, in that labelled particles of human serum albumin, about 20 to 50 μm in diameter, are injected intravenously. These are mixed in the blood after passage through the right side of the heart and are then trapped in the pulmonary capillary bed with a distribution reflecting pulmonary arterial blood flow. The most popular radiopharmaceutical for this purpose is ^{99}Tc^{m}-macroaggregated human serum albumin. The albumin particles are broken down by alveolar macrophages after about 3 to 12 h.

Where there is decreased pulmonary blood flow, for example distal to the site of an embolus, there will be a region of photon-deficiency (Fig. 9). However, many other pathological processes also decrease arterial perfusion, but as they invariably also affect regional ventilation, perfusion studies cannot be interpreted correctly without a concomitant ventilation scintigram.

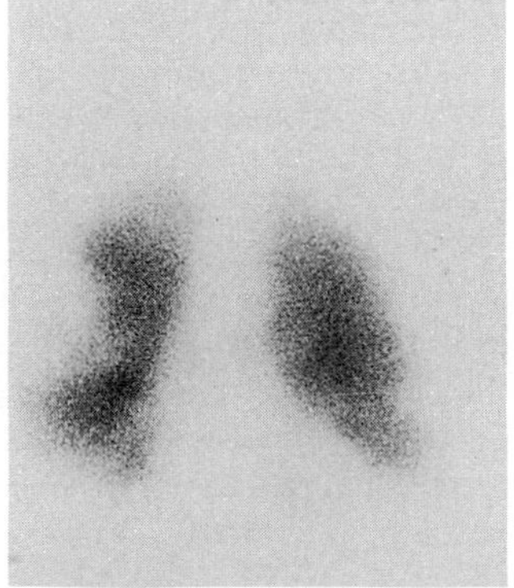

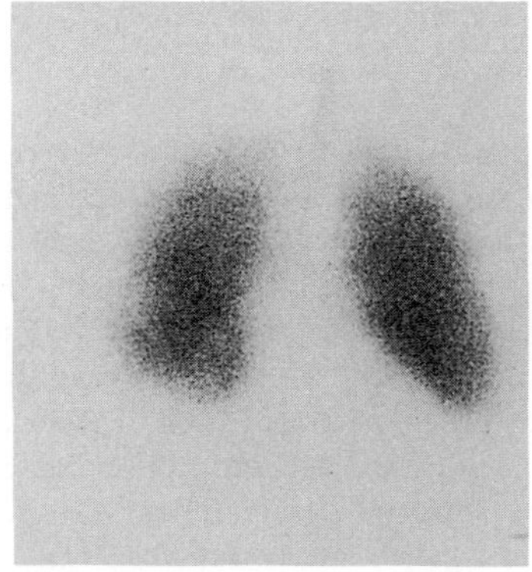

Fig. 9 Perfusion–ventilation scintigrams using ^{99}Tc^{m}-macroaggregated albumin and ^{81}Kr^{m} gas, respectively. The labelled macroaggregates stick in the pulmonary capillary bed. The pair of scintigrams show an unmatched perfusion defect typical of a pulmonary embolus in the right mid-zone.

Ventilation scintigraphy can be documented using inert gases such as xenon-133 (^{133}Xe) or krypton-81m (^{81}Kr^{m}), or as an aerosol such as ^{99}Tc^{m}-diphenyltriaminepenta-acetic acid delivered through a nebulizer. A more recent agent is technetium-99m pseudogas, which is an ultrafine, mainly monodispersed aerosol. It is generated when a spray of technetium-99m pertechnetate solution is ethanol is burnt. Krypton-81 gas is the safest and most popular agent, and it simply inhaled in oxygen by the patient standing in front of, or lying under, the gamma-camera. It is derived from a rubidium-81 (^{81}Rb) generator.

The sensitivity of pulmonary perfusion imaging approaches 100 per cent in detecting emboli in a given patient but, when compared with pulmonary angiography, both tests miss some emboli and the specificity is low. The following is a simplistic guide to interpretation using perfusion and ventilation scintigraphy and the contemporaneous chest radiograph.

1. Normal: if pulmonary perfusion is normal, then it can be assumed that both ventilation scintigraphy and the chest radiograph will be normal.
2. Unmatched perfusion defect(s): here abnormal perfusion with a photon-deficient defect occurs with normal ventilation and a chest radiograph which is either normal or shows oligaemia and vessel cut-off in the affected area. This is diagnostic of early reversible pulmonary embolus.
3. Matched perfusion defect(s), where perfusion defect(s) correspond exactly with the ventilation defect(s). In this instance the patient will either have known obstructive airways disease (e.g. emphysema or asthma), the hypoxia causing vessel close-down and so a perfusion defect, or else he will have opacities on the chest radiograph corresponding to the matched defect(s). The diagnosis is then that of the opacities, such as neoplasia, collapse, infection, oedema, effusion, fibrosis, haemorrhage and, of course, established infarction. Therefore a matched defect may mean that a patient has had an embolus, albeit a little late for early anticoagulation.

The above schema is, in fact, very difficult to operate in practice, due to on-going controversy as to what constitutes a significant perfusion defect. The result is that opinions are usually given as probabilities. In the case of normal perfusion, there need be no further evaluation for pulmonary embolism. Where there is clinical suspicion of emboli, but with a low probability of embolism on scintigraphy, no further evaluation is needed and also no treatment unless there is radiographic evidence of deep venous thromboses. If the probability of emboli is high, anticoagulation is imperative, but angiography is unnecessary. In the intermediate probability range,management depends on whether the clinical suspicion of pulmonary embolism is high or low. If it is high, either venography or angiography is necessary, and anticoagulation is necessary if either are positive. However, if the clinical suspicion is low, further angiography or venography is unnecessary and the appearances are usually due to a different disease.

Liver and biliary system

The liver–spleen scintigram, using ^{99}Tc^{m}-sulphur or ^{99}Tc^{m}-tin colloid, was once one of the most frequently used procedures in nuclear medicine. Its decline has not been due to a lack of accuracy, but to the ability of ultrasound and cross-sectional imaging techniques, such as CT and MRI, to characterize lesions and their surrounds much more effectively.

However, one existing technique worth describing is that of hepatic arterial perfusion scintigraphy, which is used for the mapping of hepatic metastases and involves the delivery of ^{99}Tc^{m}-macroaggregated albumin (as described above for use in pulmonary perfusion scintigraphy) through a catheter inserted into the common hepatic artery, just distal to the origin of the gastroduodenal artery. The technique is derived from that used to deliver chemotherapeutic agents. In this way the hepatic arterial perfusion scintigraphy technique 'locks in' the pattern of chemotherapy delivery for later imaging. This ensures chemotherapy delivery to the entire liver tumour burden and identifies inadvertent delivery to the gut or to the systemic circulation via arteriovenous shunting.

The use of ^{99}Tc^{m}-labelled red blood cells has become valuable for the characterization of known liver masses. The method relies on the fact that most cavernous haemangiomas have decreased perfusion, but increased blood-pool activity. This state of affairs is mimicked only by the rare angiosarcoma. The combined use of this radiopharmaceutical and single-photon-emission tomography can detect haemangiomas as small as 1 cm diameter. Advances in single-photon-emission tomography technology, such as high-resolution and dynamic single-photon-emission tomography, have improved this figure to less than 1 cm.

The standard liver-spleen scintigram, which relies on the uptake of ^{99}Tc^{m}-labelled colloid by the reticuloendothelial cells of the spleen and their counterpart, the Kupffer cells in the liver, still serves as a quick and easy procedure for the establishment of hepatosplenomegaly and is highly sensitive in assessing diffuse liver disease. The patterns in alcoholic liver disease (small liver, left-lobe hypertrophy, shift of colloid uptake to an enlarged spleen) and in isolated hepatic venous obstruction (Budd–Chiari syndrome with its 'hot' caudate lobe) are particularly well recognized.

In general, the combined use of ^{99}Tc^{m}-sulphur colloid imaging, gallium-67 citrate imaging, hepatobiliary imaging (see below) and radiolabelled red cell imaging allow the histological characterization of mass lesions, not yet realized by CT and MRI. Such a combination of methods is very useful in the characterization of focal nodular hyperplasia, hepatic adenoma, focal fatty replacement, cavernous haemangioma, hepatocellular carcinoma, and macroregenerating nodules.

The introduction of ^{99}Tc^{m}-labelled substituted carbamoyliminodiacetic acid compounds has permitted a non-invasive method of investigating hepatobiliary disorders. These so-called bifunctional agents are extracted from the blood by the hepatocyts and are concentrated in bile. In this way one obtains an estimate of hepatocyte function and an image of the biliary excretion pathway. A great advantage of the method is that it can be used when bilirubin levels are as high as 30 mg per cent.

The technique should be the first choice in the diagnosis of acute cholecystitis, where the cystic duct is obstructed. A normal study demonstrates, in temporal sequence over about an hour, the liver, common bile duct, gallbladder, duodenum, and jejenum. If the gallbladder is not seen within 30 min of the intravenous injection of the ^{99}Tc^{m}-labelled compound, acute cholecystitis is present (always provided the patient has a gallbladder!) (Fig. 10). Concomitant ultrasound is useful when thickening of the gallbladder wall, a pericholecystic collection, or a stone in the cystic duct can be found. A similar technique can be used in jaundiced neonates to distinguish between biliary atresia and neonatal hepatitis. In general, however, jaundice is always investigated by ultrasound in the first instance.

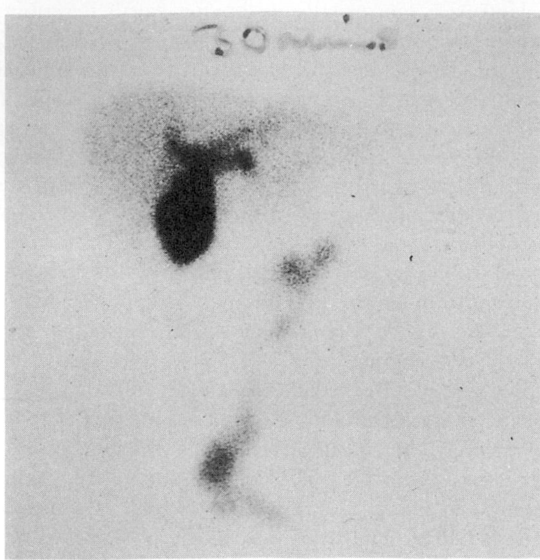

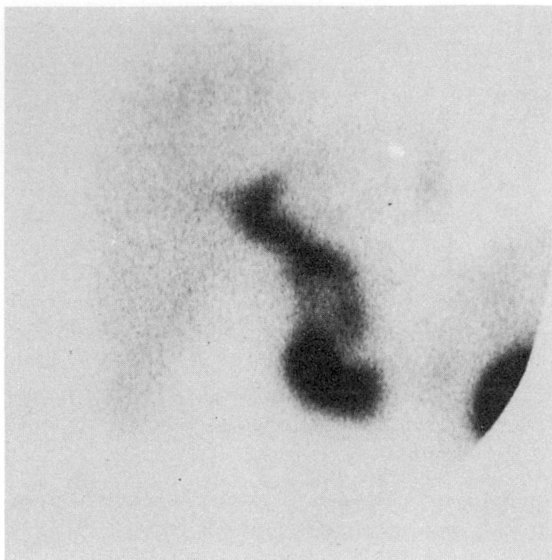

Fig. 10 Cholecystoscintigraphy using $^{99}Tc^{m}$-labelled substituted carbamoyliminodiacetic acid in a normal subject 30 min after injection (left) and in a patient with acute cholecystitis (right) 60 min postinjection. The gallbladder is clearly visible early in the study in the normal situation, but not even after 1 h in cholecystitis.

The role of the technique in chronic cholecystitis is limited, but in the postoperative patient it is useful in assessing biliary leaks, functional patency of the biliary system and for detecting cystic-duct remnants. It is also the only reliable way of demonstrating enterogastric reflux quantitatively under physiological conditions.

The spleen, bone marrow and lymphatic system

As stated above, $^{99}Tc^{m}$-labelled sulphur, tin, or antimony trisulphide colloid, which is trapped by the reticuloendothelial cells, can be used to image the liver, spleen, bone marrow, and lymphatic system.

The spleen may be imaged without concomitant hepatic activity by injecting autologous red cells, denatured by keeping them in a water-bath at 40°C for about 1 h and labelled with technetium-99m. The technique is usually reserved for searching for splenuniculi.

The distribution of bone marrow (or at least its reticuloendothelial elements, which usually coincide with the haematopoietic elements) varies with age as the functioning marrow withdraws from the extremities into regions said to be 'covered by an Edwardian bathing costume'. Any deviation from this pattern, say in myelofibrosis (marked decrease in marrow elements) or in the chronic haemolytic anaemias (extension of the marrow space), can be detected easily. The method is also useful for monitoring bone-marrow transplants and for deciding on optimal sites for marrow aspiration.

Injections of $^{99}Tc^{m}$-antimony trisulphide between the webs of the toes will enable the extent and integrity of the lower limb lymphatics to be evaluated. This technique may therefore be used to assess patients with Milroy's disease. Similar techniques can be used to evaluate lymphoedema in the arms and to plot the position of the internal mammary chain prior to chest wall irradiation for appropriate medially situated breast cancers.

Gastrointestinal tract

The liver and hepatobiliary systems have already been discussed. The salivary glands can be imaged following intravenous injection of technetium-99m as the pertechnetate, when the normal parotid and submaxillary glands become visible. Sublingual glands are too small to be seen. The activity can be discharged with a sialogogue. There is no uptake from, or discharge into, the four glands in true xerostomia or Sjögren's syndrome, whereas these are normal in cases of psychological origin. The method may also be helpful in the diagnosis of Warthin's tumour (papillary cystadenoma lymphomatosa) where there is no uptake or excretion of tracer.

Structural disease of the oesophagus is correctly investigated using endoscopy and barium meal, but the investigation of oesophageal function may be performed using radionuclides. The principal indications are either gastro-oesophageal pain, dysphagia, or one of the neuromuscular disorders. The two principal radionuclide tests for the investigation of these conditions are the measurement of oesophageal transit time and the physiological oesophageal reflux test. Reflux in babies can be determined by adding $^{99}Tc^m$-sulphur colloid or $^{99}Tc^m$-diphenyltriaminepenta-acetic acid and by taking late images over the chest to look for aspiration of tracer.

Abnormalities of gastric emptying are common after surgery for peptic ulceration, and include dumping syndrome, diarrhoea and gastric stasis. Early dumping is due to rapid gastric emptying associated with a fall in plasma volume. Late dumping is due to reactive hypoglycaemia resulting from rapid emptying. Gastric emptying-studies using liquid and solid meals labelled with $^{99}Tc^m$-, ^{111}In-, or $^{113}I^m$-diphenyltriaminepenta-acetic acid can assess such problems. They are not indicated in all postoperative patients, but dumping or stasis must be confirmed before any further surgery is contemplated.

In acute gastrointestinal haemorrhage, the site of bleeding is usually localized by angiogram studies. However, radionuclide angiography is more sensitive for the detection of such bleeding, and can be a valuable guide to selective abdominal arteriography. The two tracers commonly used for this purpose are $^{99}Tc^m$-labelled sulphur colloid or red cells. Labelled red cells are better than colloid for detecting intermittent bleeding or bleeding near the liver and spleen. They can also be used for serial imaging over 24 h as the labelled cells continue to circulate. One disadvantage of the technique is that target:non-target ratios are low due to the high circulating background of labelled cells (Fig. 11). Another is that blood leaking into the bowel may be displaced both distally and proximally and this may result in the false identification of the bleeding site. Finally, free pertechnetate can concentrate in gastric or colonic secretions. Radionuclide angiography using this method is reported to detect bleeding rates of 0.1 ml/min, which compares favourably with a rate of only 0.5 ml/min for contrast angiography.

The rationale for the use of radiocolloid for the detection of bleeding is that intravascular colloid is cleared rapidly by the hepatic and splenic phagocytes, leaving visible any colloid extravasating from a bleeding site. This method is useful in detecting active lower gastrointestinal tract bleeding and in monitoring the efficacy of therapy. The use of colloid yields a higher target:non-target ratio than that of labelled red cells as the background is rapidly cleared of activity. A disadvantage is that bleeding sites near the liver or spleen are difficult to detect.

Rectal bleeding in children may be due to bleeding from ectopic gastric mucosa in a Meckel's diverticulum. Gastric mucosa will take up pertechnetate with an accuracy of between 85 and 95 per cent in children.

The thyroid and parathyroid

Thyroid gland

It is well known that the thyroid traps inorganic plasma iodide, which is later organified to form the thyroid hormones tri-iodothyronine (T_3) and thyroxine (T_4). Iodine uptake studies using iodine-131 as sodium iodide were among the very first procedures in nuclear medicine to be carried out in the clinical situation, shortly after this fission product of uranium-235 became available after the Second World War. Today, the radionuclide of choice is the much safer iodine-123, with iodine-131 used mainly for therapy of toxic nodules, as a result of its high output of β-particles.

A number of functional thyroid studies can be performed using iodine-123; namely, uptake tests to distinguish between hypo-, eu-, and hyperthyroidism; thyroid stimulating hormone (TSH) or thyrotropin releasing hormone (TRH) stimulation and repression tests to distinguish between disorders of the thyroid–pituitary–hypothalamic axis and the gland itself; and the perchlorate wash-out test to evaluate whether organification of iodide is normal.

Functional morphology can be assessed using iodine-123 or technetium-99m as pertechnetate (which is trapped, but obviously

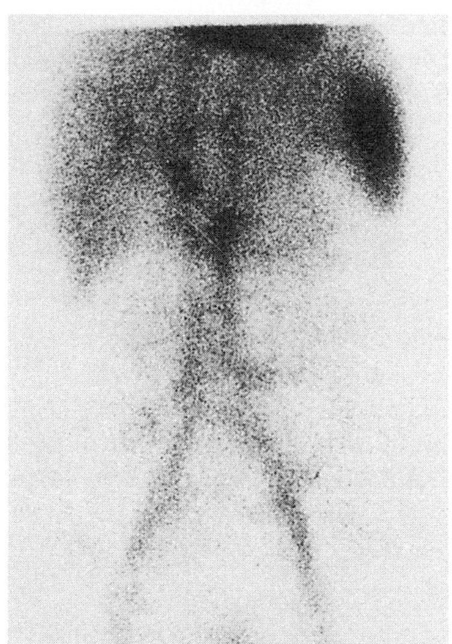

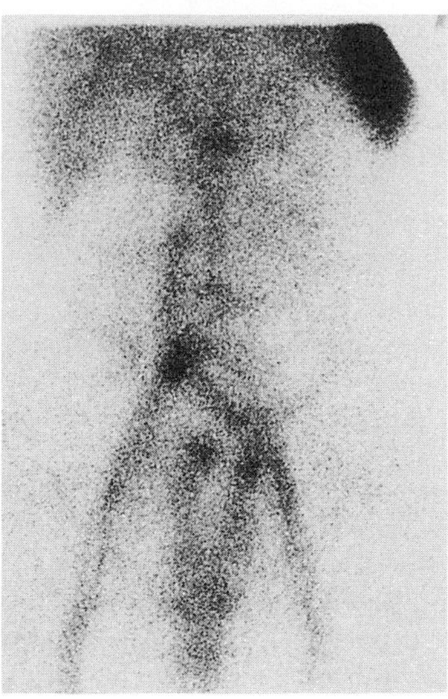

Fig. 11 A search for lower gastrointestinal bleeding using $^{99}Tc^m$-labelled red cells. There is gradual accumulation of tracer in the distal sigmoid colon and rectum, but the background of circulating labelled red cells can make discrimination difficult. Left, early; right, late.

not organified by the thyroid). Ectopic thyroid tissue, which may occur in the neck anywhere from the back of the tongue to behind the sternum, may be mapped. Thyroglossal cysts are usually detected clinically, but scintigraphy is employed to ensure that such clinically detected masses do not contain thyroid tissue. Even the normal thyroid image may show anatomical deviations, with one lobe larger than the other or, rarely, just a solitary dominant lobe. Pyramidal lobes are also seen from time to time. One should also never underestimate the amount of regrowth of thyroid tissue that can take place after partial, or even so-called complete, thyroidectomy.

Abnormal thyroid images can demonstrate focal or diffuse tracer uptake, and such uptake can, in turn, be photon-abundant ('hot') or photon-deficient ('cold'). The division of thyroid nodules into hot or cold is important, as 15 to 20 per cent of cold nodules may be malignant, whereas hot nodules are nearly always benign and usually toxic. Unfortunately, there is no way of distinguishing further between the various causes of cold nodules (benign adenomas, carcinomas, metastases, cysts, haematomas, focal thyroiditis, abscesses, or combinations of these) using radionuclide methods, but ultrasound can, of course, distinguish between cystic and solid lesions, and the advent of fine-needle aspiration has, in any case, enabled a preoperative diagnosis of thyroid nodules to be made. The rarer medullary carcinoma of the thyroid, which produces hypercalcitonaemia, may be detected with technetium-99m in its pentavalent state coupled to dimercaptosuccinic acid.

Toxic goitres include the hyperplastic, hyperfunctioning gland of Graves' disease. As opposed to this diffuse variety of goitre, one gets the uninodular or multinodular toxic goitre, in which the overactive areas suppress normal tissue—the so-called 'hot nodule'. While acute suppurative thyroiditis is rare, subacute thyroiditis is a painful, but self-limiting problem, which is probably of viral origin. It produces generalized decreased uptake. Hashimoto's thyroiditis is, by contrast, chronic and painless, and is probably due to lymphocytic infiltration causing an organification defect. Early images in this condition show an enlarged gland with normal or enhanced trapping, but later images show poor, uneven uptake.

In cases of hypothyroidism one may not even have sufficient counts to produce an image, but such a 'non-image' can provide diagnostic information which is just as useful as in any other, more dramatic, imaging situation. Euthyroid goitres simply show enlargement with normal uptake.

Parathyroid glands

It is estimated that a surgeon seeking the source of excess parathormone will find the source on exploration most of the time, but is less than 75 per cent successful on re-exploration, and in this instance nearly all available imaging techniques have to be employed.

The thallium-201/technetium-99m pertechnetate subtraction technique is arguably the most useful imaging test. Thallium-201 is a potassium analogue and, besides its well-known property of being taken up in the mycardium, is also localized in parathyroid adenomas and a variety of other neoplasias. Normal parathyroid glands are not visible. The problem is that thallium-201 chloride is also taken up by a normal thyroid and so one has to subtract electronically a thyroid image taken after an injection of pertechnetate from one taken previously after an injection of thallium-201 in the same position. The technique is more complex than this simple description would lead one to believe, but it is claimed that about 80 per cent of parathyroid adenomas can be localized by this method. It is not useful in secondary hyperparathyroidism.

Adrenals

Adrenal medulla

Neoplasia derived from the neural crest, so called apudomas, may be imaged using the noradrenaline and guanethidine analogue. ^{131}I- or ^{123}I-labelled *m*-iodobenzylguanidine, which is taken up at sites of catecholamine storage granules. This has proved to be useful in localizing benign and malignant phaeochromocytomas, paragangliomas, neuroblastomas, carcinoid and medullary carcinomas, and has also been used therapeutically in these conditions.

Adrenal cortex

When used with appropriate suppressive manoeuvres, such as the administration of dexamethasone, uptake of the cholesterol analogue, ^{131}I- or ^{75}Se-labelled norcholesterol, can supply evidence of adrenocortical hyperfunction. Adrenal cortical imaging is particularly appropriate to the localization of resectable neoplasia, or in the identification of a suspected adrenal remnant following surgery. Symmetrically increased uptake denotes adrenocorticotropic hormone (ACTH)-dependent hyperplasia, while asymmetrical uptake indicates ACTH-independent hypercorticalism. A unilateral image usually represents a neoplasm, commonly an adenoma. Adrenal carcinoma may destroy normal adrenal tissue with the resultant absence of an image.

The method is particularly useful in distinguishing between ACTH-induced adrenal hyperplasia and primary adrenal tumours that produce hypercorticalism. Results are only slightly less reliable in detecting Conn's tumours, producing hyperaldosteronism. The technique can also be used to distinguish between adrenal and ovarian causes of hirsutism.

Cardiovascular system

Modern techniques in nuclear medicine provide valuable information about cardiac structure, pathology, perfusion, and function. Four principal radionuclide techniques are available:

(1) radionuclide ventriculoscintigraphy and the evaluation of ventricular function;
(2) radionuclide or 'first-pass' angioscintigraphy;
(3) myocardial perfusion scintigraphy;
(4) infarct-avid scintigraphy.

Radionuclide ventriculoscintigraphy

The cardiac blood pool may be imaged using ^{99}Tc^{m}-labelled red cells. Images of the ventricles (usually the left) in systole and diastole are obtained by gating the gamma-camera to the patient's electrocardiographical signal (notably the R wave) and summing counts obtained over many cardiac cycles.

The most important functional parameter of the left (or right) ventricle that can be calculated is the ejection fraction which is identified as:

$$\text{Ejection fraction} = \frac{\text{end diastolic counts} - \text{end systolic counts}}{\text{end diastolic counts}}.$$

In spite of the slight errors inherent in the method, the left-ventricular ejection fraction is a sensitive indicator of dysfunction. The value is normally greater than 50 per cent. Patients who have had recent infarction show ejection fraction decreases that correlate well with the volume of infarcted tissue, and so the parameter can serve as a guide to prognosis. It is, similarly, an excellent indicator of therapeutic effectiveness and can be assessed at rest or during exercise.

The method can also be used to generate contours of the ventricular blood pool in end-diastole and end-systole, which can be manipulated to assess wall-motion abnormalities such as hypokinesia, akinesia, and dyskinesia. This can also be accomplished by producing phase and amplitude maps from Fourier analysis of the activity–time curves of the summed counts over several cardiac cycles. Right-ventricular scintigraphy is also possible, but less accurate as there is no one view of the heart (compared with the left anterior oblique view of the left ventricle) on which the right ventricle is completely circumscribed.

Estimates of regurgitant fractions, in patients with aortic and mitral valve disease, and ventricular volumes can also be derived from radionuclide ventriculography and the method can be useful in the timing of valve-replacement surgery.

Radionuclide angiography

This is also known as 'first-pass' angioscintigraphy and documents an injection of technetium-99m as pertechnetate or labelled autologous red cells as it passes through the superior vena cava, the right atrium and ventricle, the lungs, the left atrium and ventricle and, finally, the aorta. There must be no chamber dilatation, delay in transit, or recirculation (Fig. 12). The method can be used to detect any gross anatomical aberration in patients with congenital heart disease, such as right-to-left shunts. By computer analysis of activity-time curves over the lungs, left-to-right shunts can actually be quantified down to shunts as small as 10 per cent. In this way, the closing of shunts can be detected and the degree of success of corrective surgery can be observed.

First-pass scintigraphy can also be used for screening large, obstructed vascular lesions in the superior vena cava or the aorta, and it is occasionally helpful in the detection of peripheral vascular obstruction.

Myocardial perfusion scintigraphy

Myocardial cells treat thallium-201 chloride in the same way as they do potassium and so regional myocardial uptake of thallium-201 reflects intact myocardial perfusion to viable myocardium. Regions of ischaemia, acute infarction, or scarring appear as focal decreased uptake, and to distinguish among these it is essential to derive images after stress and then later at rest. An ischaemic area will 'fill in', whereas a scar will not.

Myocardial perfusion imaging can be used to differentiate ischaemic from idiopathic cardiomyopathy, to evaluate collateral coronary vessels or angioplasty, and to assess coronary bypass grafts.

There has been much interest recently in the replacement of thallium-201 by the more favourable $^{99}Tc^{m}$-labelled isonitriles, such as $^{99}Tc^{m}$-sestamibi.

Infarct-avid scintigraphy

This method, which can be used to detect both myocardial and cerebral infarcts between 12 h and 10 days after the event, depends on the property of ischaemic, infarcted, or necrotic tissue to take up certain bone-seeking tracers, such as technetium-99m pyrophosphate. A more recent advance embracing the same principle is the use of ^{111}In-labelled Fab fragments of antimyosin, which will bind to areas of myosin released in acute infarction.

Thrombus detection

While contrast venography provides the gold standard for detecting deep-vein thrombosis in the lower limb, it is not without its contraindications. ^{125}I-fibrinogen could detect clots in the calf only on direct counting and could not be imaged. $^{99}Tc^{m}$-fibrinogen could produce a scintigram but has been withdrawn from the market, probably because of the risk of HIV contamination. More recently, ^{111}In-platelets have been used for the detection of emboli, thrombi, and atherosclerotic lesions, with varying degrees of success.

The central nervous system

Magnetic resonance imaging is now unquestionably the modality of choice in delineating cerebral lesions. Conventional cerebral scintigraphy using tracers such as technetium-99m, as pertechnetate or glucoheptonate, which only pass through the blood–brain barrier when a lesion is present, is rare nowadays but may still be useful in detecting early cerebral infections and in the differential diagnosis of cerebral infarction.

Cerebral radionuclide angiography may, however, still be a very useful rapid and non-invasive way of investigating the cerebral circulation. Any vascular lesion, such as an arteriovenous malformation, meningioma, or glioma, will be seen as a focal area of increased activity, while photodeficient areas are seen in cerebrovascular accidents, subdural haematomas, and in massive carotid occlusions. A characteristic sequence in patients who have recently had strokes is the so-called 'flip-flop' phenomenon, where there is diminished perfusion on the side of the brain involved during the arterial phase, but which changes to increased activity during the later venous phase (Fig. 13). Jugular reflux, which occurs in the superior mediastinal syndrome, also produces a characteristic diagnostic picture.

Emission-computed tomographic imaging of the brain

Unfortunately, this very important branch of nuclear medicine has, as yet, little part to play in neurosurgery, but it is of undoubted importance in the investigation of neuropsychiatric disorders, such as the dementias, schizophrenias, the epilepsies, and even the depressive illnesses—none of which has hitherto been amenable to radiological diagnosis. Of all of these conditions, the epilepsies are arguably of the greatest interest to the neurosurgeon because it is possible to resect the sources of seizure disorders if they can be identified anatomically (Fig. 14). Epileptogenic foci show areas of decreased perfusion and metabolism interictally, but become areas of hyperperfusion during a seizure.

The principal agents used for these studies are ^{18}F-deoxyglucose and oxygen-15 in positron-emission tomography studies and $^{99}Tc^{m}$-hydroxymethylpropylamine oxime in single-photon-emission tomography studies. The last agent can also be used as an aid in the diagnosis of cerebral death.

Any isotope can be used in the evaluation of ventriculovenous shunt patency and ^{111}In-diphenyltriaminepenta-acetic acid cistinography can assist in the diagnosis of normal-pressure hydrocephalus.

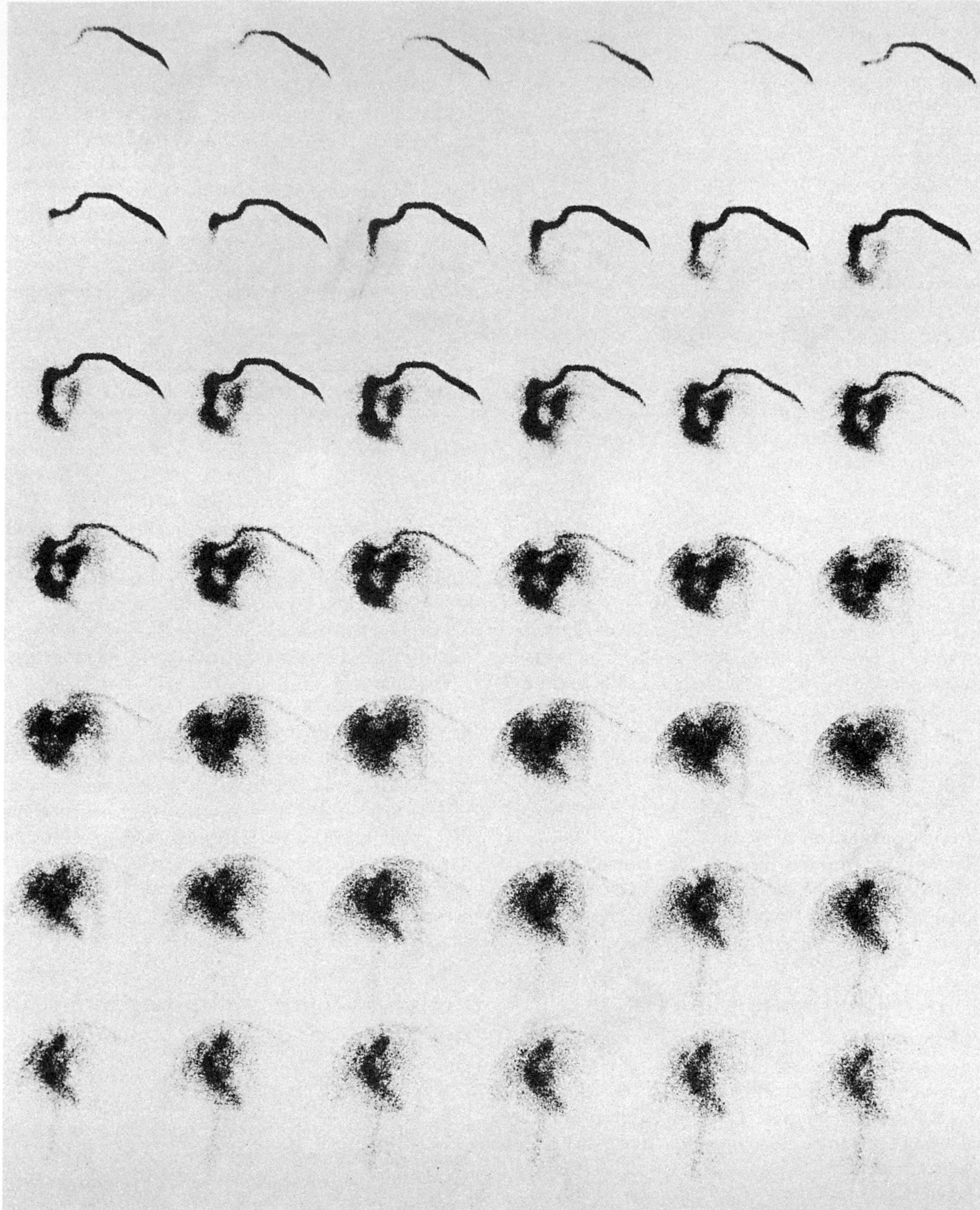

Fig. 12 A first-pass cardiac study using $^{99}Tc^{m}$-labelled red cells. The tracer enters the heart by way of the superior vena cava and the right atrium and ventricle, thence via the pulmonary outflow tract to the lungs. The left atrium and ventricle and the aorta are then seen before mixing takes place.

Dacrocystoscintigraphy

In the investigations for epiphora, patency of the nasolacrimal ducts may be investigated under physiological conditions by instilling a drop of normal saline containing a few bequerels of technetium-99m as pertechnetate into each conjunctival sac, and documenting the progress of the tracer through the canals into the nose (Fig. 15).

Tumour imaging

Many of the methods used for detecting benign and primary and secondary malignant tumours have already been discussed, but it is also necessary to describe radionuclide methods specifically designed to image tumours in general. These include mainly gallium-67 citrate scintigraphy and the use of labelled monoclonal antibodies against tumour-associated antigens.

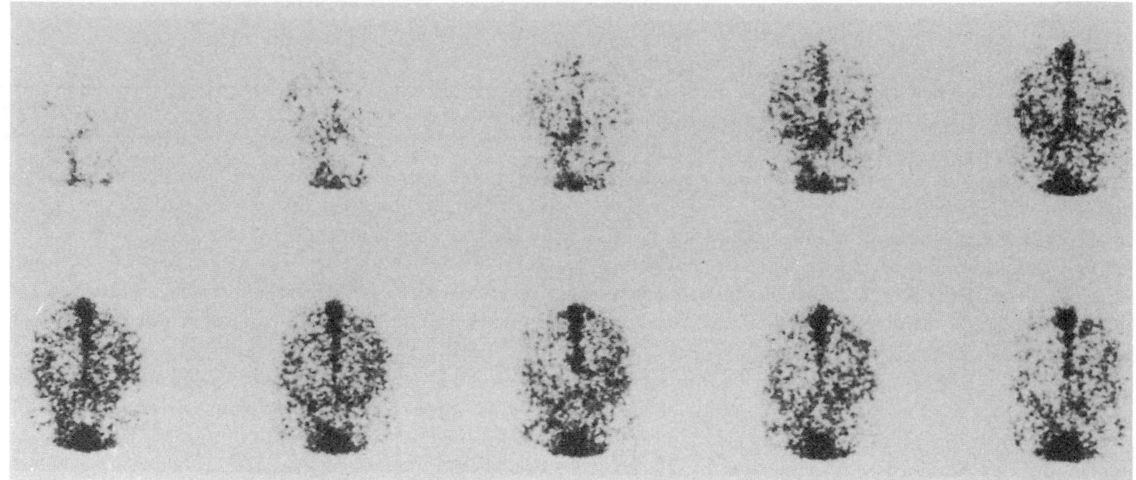

Fig. 13 Radionuclide angiogram using technetium-99m as pertechnetate. The delayed appearance of the tracer in the left hemisphere (reader's right) is due to cerebrovascular disease in the left carotid and/or the left middle cerebral artery. During the later venous phase, activity in the right hemisphere decreases, to reveal the relatively increased flow in the left hemisphere—the so-called 'flip-flop' phenomenon.

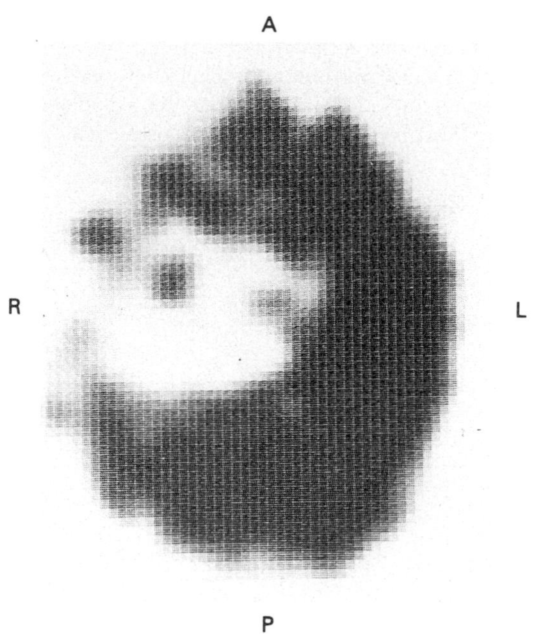

Fig. 14 A section through the brain of an 8-year-old girl with partial seizure disorder, showing a photon-deficient area in the right frontal zone.

Gallium-67 citrate was initially a bone-seeking agent and it was being used for this purpose in a patient with Hodgkin's disease when its propensity to seek out lymphomatous nodes was realized. It is, however, also taken up by a number of normal tissues, such as lymphoid tissue (notably Waldeyer's ring), lacrimal glands, liver, spleen, breasts, genitalia, and faeces, making the observation of any abnormal gallium-67 uptake difficult.

Nevertheless it is useful for detecting the extent of intrathoracic lymphoma, with a sensitivity of 75 to 80 per cent and it can detect primary bronchial carcinoma with a sensitivity of 80 to 85 per cent. However, it was soon found to be an infection/inflammation-seeking agent as well, and so it lacks specificity. Also, it does not concentrate as well in adenocarcinomas as in other types. If primary lung cancer concentrates gallium-67 citrate, detection of its spread to mediastinal nodes has a sensitivity approaching 100 per cent, compared to mediastinoscopy. However, specificity is much lower, at 53 to 60 per cent.

With the advent of polyclonal antibodies against tumour-

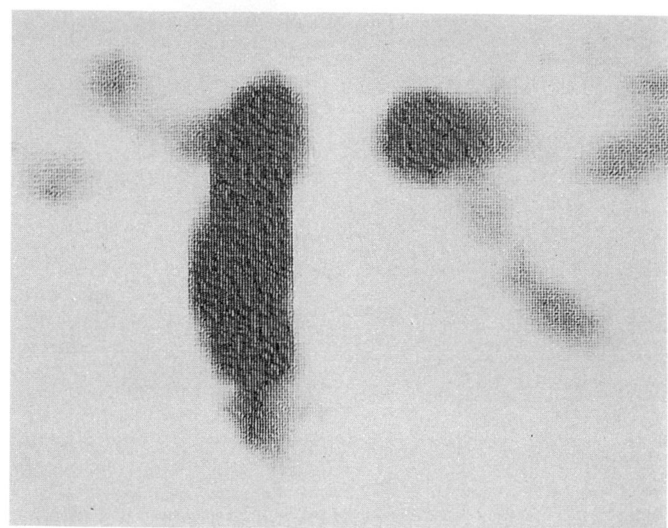

Fig. 15 Dacrocystoscintigraphy, showing normal rapid flow of tracer from the conjunctiva through the lacrimal canal on the right, but hold-up on the left.

associated antigens, followed closely by the now ubiquitous monoclonal antibodies, hopes of finding tumour-specific radiopharmaceuticals were rekindled, as were hopes of using them at high activities for therapy. Antibodies can be labelled with specific radionuclides (iodine-123), indium-111, and even technetium-99m as pertechnetate) and provide at least the potential for the specific delivery of radionuclides to a particular cancer for detection and treatment.

Polyclonal antibodies are mixtures of antibodies having affinity for the tumour as well as, unfortunately, cross-reactive affinities towards other tissues. One of the first and best of these to be tried was carcinoembryonic antigen. Monoclonal antibodies, produced by hybridoma technology are, on the other hand, directed against relatively specific antigenic determinants in the neoplastic cell, and so are less eager to react with normal cells. However, this lack of cross-reactivity is not absolute, and much effort is being expended in producing antibody fragments, such as the $F(ab)_2$ fragments, which have little or no cross-reactivity with normal tissue.

Preliminary results in cancers with well-characterized antibodies to specific tumour-associated antigens have been encouraging, for example in malignant melanoma (Fig. 16), ovarian cancer, and cutaneous T-cell lymphoma. In these instances success is probably due to the fact that the antigen–antibody reaction probably occurs on the cell surface.

Therapeutic studies show some promise, but at the present time both diagnostic and therapeutic applications have not lived up to their initial theoretical promise. Exciting new developments are taking place in tumour receptor imaging. For example, radioligands which bind oestrogen and somatostatin receptors in breast carcinoma have been used to image these tumours and their secondaries and to monitor, for example, the efficacy of tamoxifen, which can be seen to make oestrogen-positive tumours (about 65 per cent of the total) disappear.

Infection/inflammation-seeking tracers

Intra-abdominal infection and inflammation are major surgical problems, to which all imaging modalities (but particularly ultrasound) can contribute. As far as radionuclide imaging is concerned, the best-known agents for seeking out inflammatory or infective foci have been gallium-67 citrate and $^{99}Tc^{m}$-labelled colloids, but these have been superseded by radiolabelled white cells (either pure polymorphonuclear leucocytes or mixed white cells) labelled *in vitro* with indium-11 chelates or $^{99}Tc^{m}$-hydroxymethylpropylamine oxime. More recently, microcolloids, monoclonal antibodies, and immunoglobulins have been introduced.

Gallium-67 citrate has been used for some time and has a particular reputation for seeking chronic infection. It is simple to use and requires no special preparation, but—as stated above—it targets so many normal structures that there are few areas where the target:non-target ratio is high enough to engender analytical confidence. It is also difficult to image technically as it has three so-called photopeaks which make gamma-camera tuning difficult. This makes its sensitivity for assessing intra-abdominal sepsis rather low (about 60 per cent). Its specificity is also low because it is a tumour seeker, and sequential studies over 3 days have to be carried out to enhance accuracy.

On the other hand, it is now a simple matter to label leucocytes with either indium-111 oxime, indium-111 tropolone, or technetium-99m hydroxymethylpropylamine oxime (the same sub-

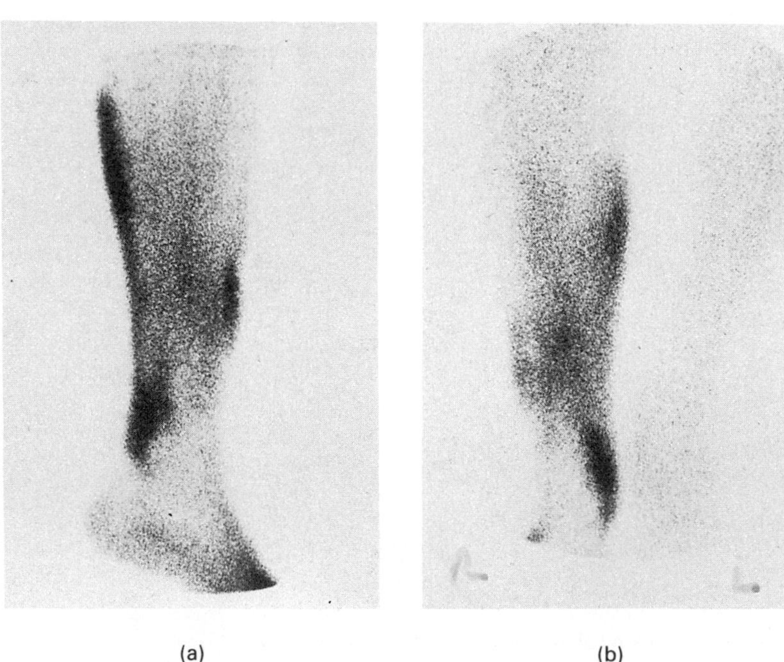

(a) (b)

Fig. 16 Scintigrams from a subject with suspected metastatic melanoma on whom immunoscintigraphy was performed using $^{99}Tc^{m}$-labelled monoclonal antibodies to the high molecular weight melanoma-associated antigen. There were no palpable lesions in the areas of increased uptake. (a) Lateral view of right leg; (b) anterior view of both legs.

stance as is used for cerebral perfusion and tumour imaging). Indium is transported by blood constituents as if it was iron, and so it is effectively trapped by iron-binding proteins in the plasma and on the surface of all blood cells. Therefore, in order to label white cells, the plasma has to be removed first (from about 60 ml of whole blood), followed by the red cells and platelets. Finally, if it has been decided to label only granulocytes, these have to be separated off from the other white cells. The appropriate white cells are incubated with indium-11 oxime or tropolone and re-suspended in platelet-poor plasma for re-injection into the patient. It would appear that pure granulocytes are not significantly superior for the detection of acute soft-tissue infections so, as their preparation requires an extra stage, it seems just as effective to label mixed white cells.

There is, as expected, normal leucocyte uptake in the haematopoietic areas of the bone marrow, liver, and spleen, but no renal or bowel activity as in the case of gallium-67 citrate. This method therefore provides a larger clear background in which to identify sepsis. Focal areas close to the liver and spleen may be imaged by using $^{99}Tc^{m}$-sulphur colloid to outline the liver and spleen and then subtracting these areas electronically from the overall image.

When the inflammatory response due to intra-abdominal sepsis is marked, early imaging at 4 h after re-injection of the labelled leucocytes can be obtained (Fig. 17). However, with less acute responses, uptake is slower and may be seen only at 24 h. Delayed imaging can distinguish between abscess and exudate in Crohn's disease and ulcerative colitis. The labelled exudate moves distally, whereas the activity over an abscess obviously remains static. Leucocyte abundance in the bowel is always pathological.

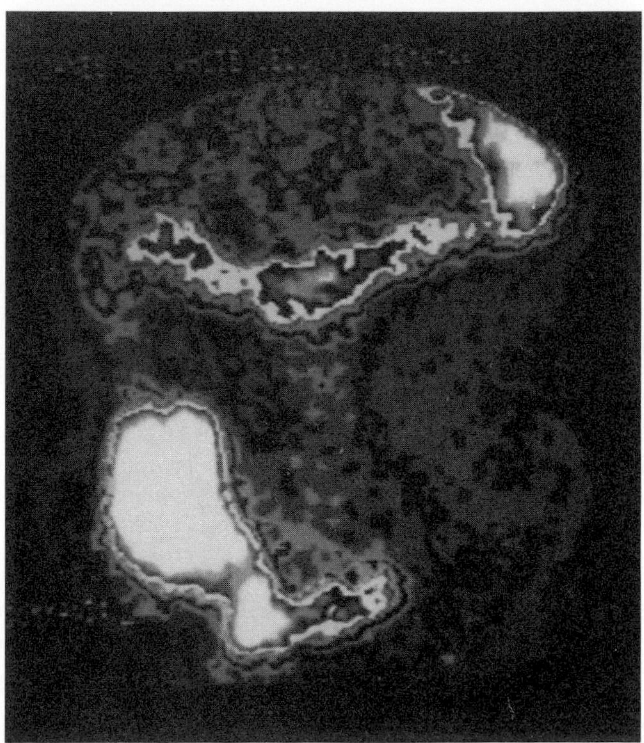

Fig. 17 An early labelled leucocyte study using indium-111 tropolone on a patient with Crohn's disease of the large bowel with a large abscess in the right iliac fossa. This was still visible 24 h later, whereas the rest of the uptake, presumably in exudate, has been passed.

The sensitivity of indium-111 tropolone-labelled mixed white cells is 100 per cent in detecting acute soft-tissue infections, but drops to 85 per cent in mixed infections. The specificity is about 92 per cent, with false-positive results due to uptake in inflammatory conditions such as acute pancreatitis and inflammatory bowel disease, necrotic tumours, dissolving haematomas, and in patients on non-steroidal anti-inflammatory agents. Swallowed saliva may also produce misleading appearances. The more recent techniques using white cells labelled with $^{99}Tc^{m}$-hydroxymethylpropylamine oxime and $^{99}Tc^{m}$-human immunoglobulin have yet to be widely evaluated.

When intra-abdominal infection is suspected and localizing signs are present, or if scintigraphy is negative or inconclusive, then ultrasound or computed tomography must be used. If not, leucocyte scintigraphy should otherwise be the investigation of choice, with a negative study virtually excluding infection. However, a positive study is seldom sufficient to allow surgical drainage without further help from ultrasound or computed tomography.

NUCLEAR PATHOLOGY

The non-imaging branch of nuclear medicine is often referred to as nuclear pathology. Although not strictly the province of the surgeon, some of the tests under this heading could be useful in clinical or research situations.

Paramount among these tests is the ability to estimate accurately almost infinitesimal amounts of certain hormones, enzymes, and drugs in the blood using competitive binding assays, especially those using so-called radioimmunoassay techniques involving radioactive tracers, particularly iodine–125.

The assessment of a number of physiological parameters involves the use of radionuclides. These include measurements of body composition (especially blood and plasma volumes), circulation and blood flow, tumour turnover, and metabolism.

SAFETY OF NUCLEAR MEDICINE STUDIES

The universally adopted policy in radiation protection is to keep radiation doses as low as reasonably achievable (the ALARA principle), and so it is important that the clinician considers that the potential gain for the patient in using a radioactive test will exceed potential risks. Non-essential, repetitive examinations and the use of radionuclides with large β-irradiation components must be discouraged. All ionizing radiation investigations on pregnant women are to be avoided unless the clinical benefit far outweighs the risk. In addition, it is essential to use sensitive detection equipment, good handling techniques, and highly trained personnel. If technetium–99m is used as the basis of most studies in nuclear medicine, absorbed doses will be of the same order as those incurred in conventional radiography and often far less.

FURTHER READING

Adazraki NP, Mishkin FS. eds. *Fundamentals of nuclear medicine.* 2nd edn. New York: The Society of Nuclear Medicine, 1988.

Maisey MN, Britton KE, Gilday DL, eds. *Clinical nuclear medicine.* London: Chapman and Hall Medical, 1991.

Mistry R. *Manual of nuclear medicine procedures.* London: Chapman and Hall, 1988. (A detailed how-to-do-it recipe book.)

6.8 Nuclear magnetic resonance spectroscopy

GEORGE K. RADDA

Nuclear magnetic resonance (NMR) is a means by which the magnetic properties of certain atomic nuclei can be observed. These nuclei are 'polarized' when placed in a uniform magnetic field and can then be studied through their interaction with low energy radiowaves. The signals (often referred to as resonances) collected from the sample have frequencies that depend on the applied magnetic field and are characteristic of the different nuclei; for example, hydrogen (^{1}H) produces a different signal from phosphorus (^{31}P). In magnetic resonance imaging (MRI) the signals from the hydrogen atoms contained in tissue water and fat are spatially encoded by the use of magnetic field gradients, and are reconstructed to produce the anatomical images that have such widespread practical clinical applications. For each type of nucleus, the precise frequency of the resonance is also governed by the way in which the electrons surround the nucleus; that is, the chemical properties of a molecule containing that particular atom. We can therefore identify and quantitatively measure specific molecules in a sample. The data are collected in the form of high resolution NMR spectra, which record the frequency dependence of the resonances. The term NMR spectroscopy is still widely used in the scientific community but in the clinical context it is most commonly referred to as magnetic resonance spectroscopy (MRS).

MRS is used to study aspects of the biochemistry of selected regions of the human body by detecting and quantitatively measuring specific metabolites. For example, using phosphorus (^{31}P), MRS signals from adenosine triphosphate, adenosine diphosphate, phosphocreatine, and inorganic phosphate are observable (Fig. 1). In addition, the inorganic phosphate resonance gives a direct measurement of intracellular cytoplasmic pH. These parameters can be used to evaluate the relationship between energy supply and demand in tissues and organs, often referred to as 'energy metabolism'.

Applications of MRS in surgery must still be largely considered as research. Knowledge of alterations in the cellular metabolism of diseased tissue not only increases our understanding of the disease but may be of clinical benefit. For example, a quantitative and objective measure of tissue ischaemia, when clinical examination and routine tests are equivocal, would help in deciding when tissue damage is irrevocable and may, therefore, indicate when reconstructive surgery is futile. Many diseases have been studied by MRS.

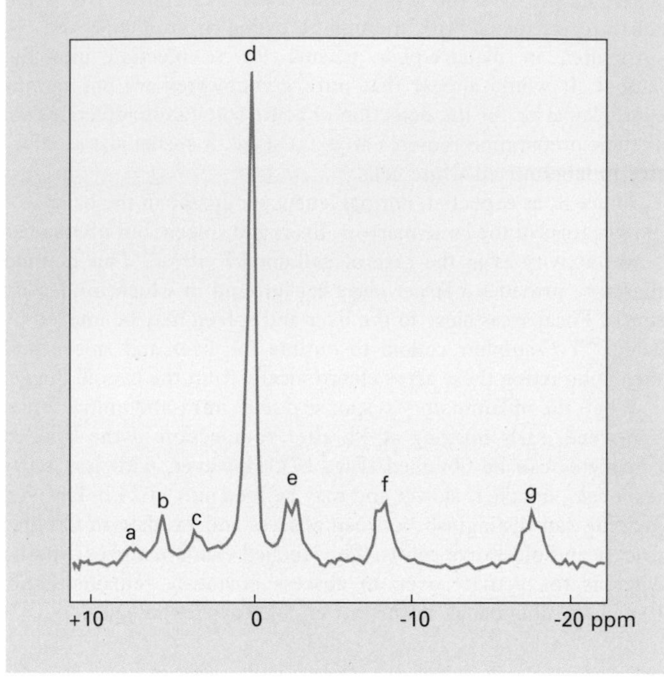

Fig. 1 ^{31}P NMR spectrum of human gastrocnemius muscle: a, phosphomonoesters (including sugar phosphates); b, inorganic phosphate; c, phosphodiesters; d, phosphocreatine; e, γ-ATP; f, d-ATP; g, β-ATP.

PERIPHERAL VASCULAR DISEASE AND TISSUE BIOCHEMISTRY

When patients with advanced peripheral vascular disease causing rest pain are studied by ^{31}P MRS, the foot muscle (extensor digitorum brevis) shows marked abnormalities in phosphate-containing metabolites, the most consistent being relatively high levels of inorganic phosphate and low phosphocreatine concentrations. The changes are usually rapidly reversed by surgical restoration of blood supply. MRS measurements on this muscle provide a sensitive index of disease and a means of quantifying ischaemia. They relate more closely to the patient's symptoms than do conventional measurements of ankle pressure. In conditions that produce pain similar to that caused by vascular disease, such as arthritis of the spine, MRS clearly defines the condition causing the pain.

Patients with intermittent claudication suffer from pain and cramp in their calf muscle during exercise because blood flow is limited. Changes in calf muscle metabolism during rest and during and after exercise (plantar flexion) have shown that patients with claudication use up more muscle phosphocreatine than do control subjects. At the same time, the muscle cells of patients become more acid due to lactate production, indicating impaired oxygen supply. The rate of metabolic recovery after exercise is slower in patients with claudication, and this appears to provide the most sensitive index for objectively assessing the severity of the disease. The measurements are relatively simple, provided that the expensive instrumentation is available, can be repeated easily and, in principle could be used as part of the routine clinical evaluation prior to surgical treatment (Fig. 2).

MRS IN TRANSPLANTATION SURGERY

The metabolic viability of isolated, cold-preserved organs can be conveniently examined by ^{31}P MRS and this has provided the basis of much work on kidney and heart preservation in animal models.

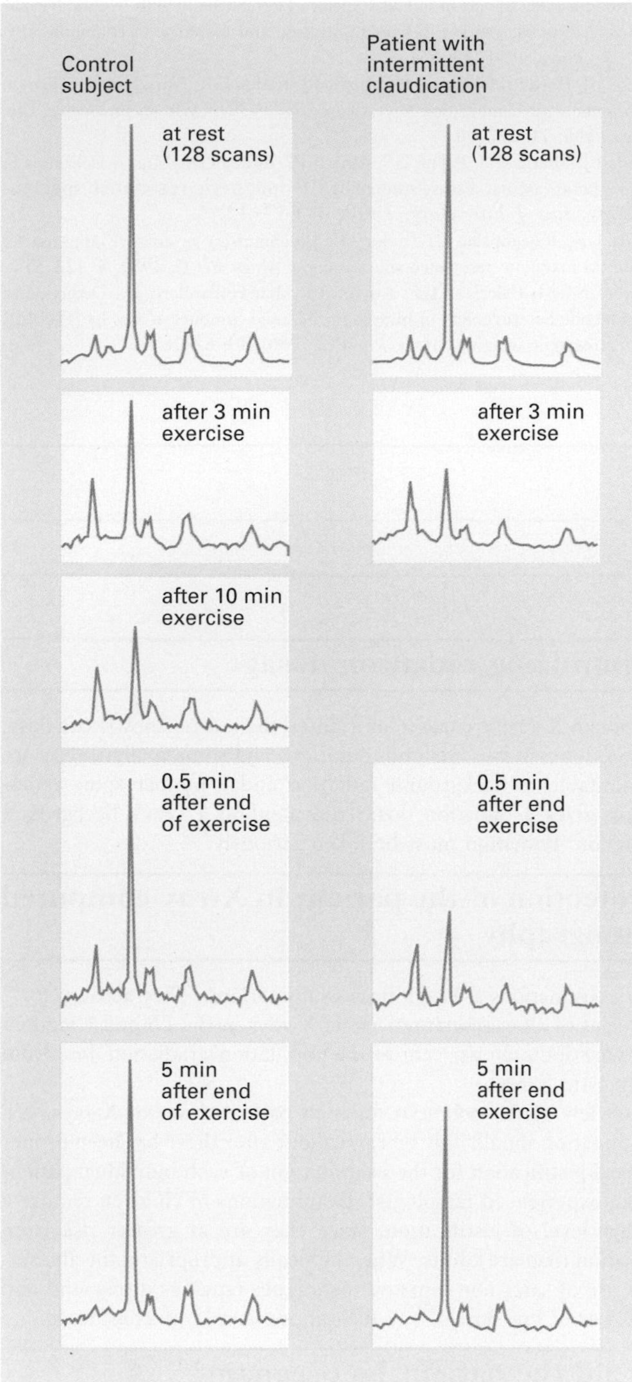

Fig. 2 Calf muscle spectra obtained before, during, and after exercise.)

Several groups have examined the energy state of isolated human kidneys during cold ischaemia, prior to transplantation, and have shown that while the signal from adenosine triphosphate gradually decreases with time, that due to inorganic phosphate increases. Intracellular acidification is dependent on the nature of the preservation medium used. Initial function of the kidney after transplantation appears to reflect the adenosine triphosphate content of the preserved organ. While the method has not been explored further, largely because organ preservation is not a major problem in renal transplantation as practised today, it is likely that similar investigations in cardiac transplantation may be more helpful.

Preliminary reports on the MRS examination of transplanted human hearts indicate that phosphocreatine adenosine triphosphate ratio *in vivo* decreases during rejection. Such measurement may provide an alternative and non-invasive approach for the early detection of rejection. If these studies are confirmed, the need for regular cardiac biopsies could be eliminated.

CANCER

One of the most obvious applications of MRS is to investigate the nature of solid tumours and their response to therapy. From the point of view of surgery, methods for determining tumour type, grading, and potential response to chemotherapy are important in clinical management. ^{31}P MRS has provided much new information about tumours, particularly in the brain: the bioenergetic characteristics of menangiomas for example, are significantly different from those of gliomas. However, because of the large diversity of metabolic patterns in human tumours, the greatest application of ^{31}P MRS may not be in characterizing tumour respiratory activity in general terms, but in identifying the intrinsic biochemical characteristics of tumour due to its particular environment and physiological state. This may help clinical decisions in specific cases. In a more general sense it appears that there are some characteristic changes in the spectroscopic signals associated with phospholipid metabolism and structures. In particular it has been suggested that the levels of the metabolites phosphoethanolamine and phosphocholine may reflect cellular growth and proliferation in some complex way. Nevertheless, up until now no clear relationships between tumour grades and metabolism have been observed.

In some recent empirical studies, proton (^{1}H) spectroscopy has been used to correlate tumour grade with spectral patterns. In ^{1}H spectroscopy of the brain the main signals are from choline-containing compounds, creatine and phosphocreatine and *N*-acetyl aspartate. High lactate concentrations are observed in some tumours. It remains to be established whether any of these signals could be used for tumour grading or for distinguishing between malignant and benign tumours.

Once an unequivocal diagnosis of cancer is made, pathological and clinical staging will determine decisions about appropriate treatment. No single system of staging is applicable to all cancers but several non-invasive staging procedures are routinely used. Hepatic spread is not uncommonly the initial manifestation of cancer elsewhere, yet diagnosis of hepatic metastases is often difficult in patients without advanced disease. The sensitivity of CT scanning and ultrasound for diagnosing diffuse liver involvement is poor.

Some recent studies have shown that hepatic spread of lymphoma produces biochemical changes that can be detected by ^{31}P MRS of the liver: elevated phosphomonoester levels (likely to be from phosphoethanolamine) have been found in patients with hepatic infiltration. This increase in the phosphomonoester signal approximately relates to clinical stage and in several patients there was some indication that the spectroscopic measurement was more sensitive to infiltration than conventional techniques. In addition, the monoester signal appears to provide a useful marker of the response of lymphoma cells to chemotherapy and of recurrent progressive disease.

Although MRI gives direct anatomical guidance to the surgeon, MRS has unique contributions to make in patient management and therapeutic decision making prior to surgery.

FURTHER READING

Cadoux-Hudson TA, Blackledge MJ, Rajagopalan B, Taylor DJ, Radda GK. Human primary brain tumour metabolism *in vivo*: a phosphorus magnetic resonance spectroscopy study. *Br J Cancer* 1989; **60**: 430–6.

den Hollander JA, *et al.* Potentials of quantitative image-localized human ^{31}P nuclear magnetic resonance spectroscopy in the clinical evaluation of intracranial tumors. *Magn Res Q*, 1989; **5**: 152–68.

Dixon RM, Angus PW, Rajagopalan B, Radda GK. Abnormal phosphomonoester signals in ^{31}P MR spectra from patients with hepatic lymphoma. A possible marker of liver infiltration and response to chemotherapy. *Br J Cancer*, 1991; **63**: 953–8.

Hands LJ, Bore PJ, Galloway G, Morris PJ, Radda GK. Muscle metabolism in patients with claudication investigated by P-31 NMR spectroscopy. *Clin Sci*, 1986; **71**: 283–90.

Hands LJ, Sharif MH, Payne GS, Morris PJ, Radda GK. Muscle ischaemia in peripheral vascular disease studied by ^{31}P-magnetic resonance spectroscopy. *Eur J Vasc Surg*, 1990; **4**: 637–42.

Radda GK, Rajagopalan B, Taylor DJ. Biochemistry *in vivo*: an appraisal of clinical magnetic resonance spectroscopy. *Magn Res Q*, 1989; **5**: 122–51.

Segebarth CM, Baleriaux DF, Luyten PR, den Hollandere JA. Detection of metabolic heterogeneity of human intracranial tumours *in vivo* by ^{1}H NMR spectroscopic imaging. *Magn Res Med*, 1990; **13**: 62–76.

6.9 Imaging guidelines

DAVID LINDSELL

INTRODUCTION

With the development of multiple imaging techniques such as ultrasound, computed tomography, magnetic resonance imaging, and photon emission tomography in addition to conventional radiography, contrast radiography and vascular radiology it is important that clinicians have guidance on the appropriateness and merits of these techniques. A useful test is one whose result—positive or negative—will alter patient management; many requests for imaging do not. Each unnecessary test increases costs, may add to patient irradiation, blocks the service, lowers standards, and harms morale. Other than for medicolegal reasons the chief causes of wasteful use of tests are:

1. *Imaging when results are unlikely to affect patient management* because the anticipated 'positive' finding is usually irrelevant (e.g. degenerative spinal disease) or because a positive finding is so unlikely.
2. *Examining too often*, i.e. before the disease could have progressed or resolved or before the results will influence treatment.
3. *Imaging when it has already been done*, e.g. at another hospital, in outpatient or accident and emergency clinics.
4. *Failing to explain the purpose of the examination*, so that the wrong films are taken or an essential view is omitted.
5. *Doing the wrong study*; imaging techniques change all the time.

A guideline is 'not a rigid constraint on clinical practice, but a concept of good practice against which the needs of the individual patient can be considered'. So while there have to be good reasons for ignoring guidelines they should not be regarded as absolute rules. No set of guidelines will command universal support and any problems should be discussed with your own radiologists. The guidelines discussed here reflect the practice in the United Kingdom. They have been adapted for local needs and surgical practice from the second edition of the Royal College of Radiologists' (UK) Guidelines. Copies of the Royal College of Radiologists Guidelines can be obtained from the Royal College of Radiologists, 38 Portland Place, London, W1N 3DG, UK. They may vary from one hospital to another and from one country to another. They may need to be adapted to suit local circumstances.

Minimizing radiation dosage

Although X-rays are taken for granted there is no known safe dose. Some 'spontaneous' genetic mutations and some malignancies are attributable to background radiation and a lumbar spine radiograph gives a radiation dose equivalent to a year's background radiation. Radiation must be taken seriously.

Protection of the patient in X-ray computed tomography

CT examinations are high dose examinations. They account for 2 per cent of all examinations using X-rays in the United Kingdom but contribute 20 per cent of the population's radiation dose from diagnostic X-rays.

In view of the potential for high patient doses of X-rays, CT examination should only be carried out after there has been proper clinical justification for the examination of each individual patient by an experienced radiologist. Examinations of children require a higher level of justification, since they are at greater risk from radiation than are adults. When clinically appropriate, the alternative use of safer non-ionizing techniques (such as ultrasound and MRI) or of low dose X-ray techniques should be considered.

Could the patient be pregnant?

Irradiation of any area between the diaphragm and the knees should be avoided in pregnancy unless there are over-riding clinical considerations. If the patient is, or might be, pregnant the department of radiology must be informed.

Using the guidelines

In general these guidelines only deal with areas of difficulty or controversy. Straightforward indications for examinations are not discussed, nor are the indications for examinations where the requests are routinely evaluated by a radiologist, e.g. CT, MRI, or arteriograms.

The sections are laid out by systems with further sections for accident and emergency, trauma, paediatrics, ultrasound, mammography, and nuclear medicine. There are three columns. The first gives the clinical situation which may be the basis for requesting an examination. The next column is the guideline on whether or not the investigation is appropriate, and the third provides explanatory comments. The guidelines used are:

1 *Indicated.* This guideline is used to indicate the most appropriate investigation for that clinical situation, and may differ from the examination requested.
2 *Six-week rule.* These are situations in which experience shows that the clinical problem usually resolves with time and we therefore suggest deferring the study for 6 or 8 weeks and only performing it if the symptoms are still a problem. Acute back or neck pain are common examples.
3 *Not indicated routinely.* This emphasizes that while no guidelines are absolute the request will only be carried out if a clinician gives strong arguments for it. An example would be a patient with backache in whom there were findings to suggest disease other than degenerative disease.
4 *Not indicated.* Examinations in this category are those where the supposed rationale for the test is untenable. A cervical spine radiograph may be requested in patients with suspected vertebrobasilar insufficiency 'to show degenerative changes'. In fact all patients in this age group have degenerative changes and it is impossible to know whether or not those changes affect the vertebral arteries.
5 *Specialist clinicians only.* These are studies that will only be performed for consultants who have relevant clinical expertise to evaluate the clinical findings and act on the imaging results.
6 *Limited examination.* Here the study is confined, as explained above, usually to a single view intended to show any major abnormality, e.g. lateral skull for epilepsy in the absence of localizing signs.

CHEST

Clinical situation	Guideline	Comment
Preoperative	Not indicated routinely	Exceptions before cardiopulmonary surgery, in suspected malignancy or tuberculosis. Note that many patients with cardio-respiratory disease have a recent film available.
Chest wall pain (as opposed to pleuritic pain)	Six-week rule	Conditions such as Tietze's disease do not show on radiography. Main purpose is reassurance.
Chest trauma Mild	Not indicated routinely	Showing a rib fracture does not alter management. A posteroanterior film only is taken (see accident and emergency section)
Moderate/severe	Indicated (see accident and emergency section)	
Upper respiratory tract infection	Not indicated	
Pneumonia Adults (follow-up)	Indicated	To confirm clearing in middle-aged and elderly: pointless to re-examine at less than 7 to 10-day intervals as clearing can be slow
Children (follow-up)	See paediatric section	

Notes

1. Chest radiographs account for 33 per cent of all examinations.
2. Less than two out of ten chest radiographs show an abnormality.
3. The average radiation dose from a chest radiograph examination is 0.02 mSv. The average dose from a CT scan of the chest is 400 times that of a chest radiograph.

FACIAL BONES AND SKULL RADIOGRAPHS

Clinical situation	Guideline	Comment
Headaches	Not indicated	Neither skull, sinus, or neck radiographs are useful in the absence of focal signs or symptoms
Sinusitis	Not indicated routinely: specialist request	Thickened mucosa is non-specific and may occur in asymptomatic subjects. Refractory cases need ENT opinion.
Temporomandibular joints	Specialists only	Performed for faciomaxillary surgeons or rheumatologists. Findings nearly always negative because the symptoms arise in the meniscus of the joint.
Orbits? metallic foreign body (prior to MRI)	Indicated	Only if clear history of eye injury whilst using metallic materials.
Middle and inner ear symptoms including vertigo	Specialist only	Evaluation of these symptoms and signs need ENT, neurosurgical, or neurological expertise.

FACIAL BONES AND SKULL RADIOGRAPHS (*cont.*)

Clinical situation	Guideline	Comment
Visual disturbances	Not indicated	Plain films are rarely positive and negative findings may be misleading. May need CT or MRI.

Notes

1. The average radiation dose from a skull radiograph examination is 0.1 mSv (five times that of a chest radiograph). A CT scan of the head gives a radiation dose about 20 times as great.
2. Radiation can damage the lens of the eye.

CERVICAL SPINE

Clinical situation	Guideline	Comment
Acute neck pain	Six-week rule	1. Usually due to disc/ligamentous changes undetectable on radiography.
Chronic neck pain	Not indicated routinely	Degenerative changes begin in early middle age regardless of symptoms. Examination only indicated for neurological signs or suspicion of non-degenerative disease.
Torticollis without trauma	Not indicated	Deformity is due to spasm: no significant bone changes are seen. Sometimes indicated in children.
Headache	Not indicated	No value.
Suspected vertebrobasilar disease	Not indicated	Degenerative disease is universal in middle age and there is no way of telling if the vertebral arteries are affected.

THORACIC SPINE

Clinical situation	Guideline	Comment
Pain without trauma	Six-week rule	Degenerative changes are invariable from middle age. Examination rarely useful in the absence of neurological signs or evidence of metastases or infection.

LUMBAR SPINE

Clinical situation	Guideline	Comment
Acute pain without trauma	Six-week rule	Most such patients recover: radiograph seldom show relevant findings. Older patients with possible osteoporosis are an exception.
Chronic back pain with no clinical evidence of infection or neoplasm	Not indicated routinely	Degenerative changes are universal and non-specific from middle age. Main value in younger patients (e.g. with spondylolisthesis or ankylosing spondylitis) or in patients over 60 for osteoporotic changes.
? Disc prolapse	Not indicated routinely	Plain film changes are rarely specific. Demonstration of a disc prolapse requires MRI, radiculography, or CT. 'Normal' radiographs may be falsely reassuring. Most patients with major disc prolapse have normal radiographs. Indicated for persistent, progressive, unremitting pain, or neurological signs.
Prephysiotherapy	Not indicated routinely	
? Spina bifida occulta (sacral dimple) with no clinical signs or symptoms	Not indicated	About 10 per cent of individuals have minor lumbosacral anomalies.

Notes

1. In the absence of neurological signs lumbar spine radiographs reveal significant disease (e.g. malignancy, ankylosing spondylitis) in about 1 per cent of patients presenting with acute back pain outside hospital.
2. The average radiation dose from three views of the lumbar spine is 2.4 mSv (120 times that of a chest radiography examination).

PELVIS AND HIPS

(Combined lumbar spine and pelvis examination is not appropriate: the sacroiliac joints are shown on lumbar spine views and there must be specific reasons for requesting both examinations.)

Clinical situation	Guideline	Comment
Hip pain—full movement	Not indicated routinely	Many middle-aged patients have short-lived 'twinges'. Only if symptoms and signs are persistent with well advanced osteoarthritic changes will hip replacement be contemplated.
Hip pain—limited movement	Six-week rule	

COCCYX

Clinical situation	Guideline	Comment
Coccydynia/injury to coccyx	Not indicated	Neither condition has radiographic findings which influence management.

KNEES

Clinical situation	Guideline	Comment
Knee pains without locking or restricted movement	Not indicated routinely	Most symptoms are from soft tissues. Osteoarthritic changes are common from late middle-age. Radiographs should be taken at the time of an orthopaedic or rheumatological consultation after full clinical examination.
Knee pains with locking or restricted movement	Indicated	Many films are normal but radiography is necessary to exclude opaque loose bodies.
? Osgood–Schlatter's disease	Not indicated	Apophyseal irregularity is non-specific: the key radiographic finding is soft tissue swelling so radiographs add nothing to clinical examination.

ANKLES AND FEET

Clinical situation	Guideline	Comment
Feet—hallux valgus	Orthopaedic surgeons only	Main value in assessment prior to surgery.
Plantar fasciitis? calcaneal spur	Not indicated	Plantar spurs are common incidental findings. The pain is from plantar fascial 'inflammation' seldom seen on radiography. Scintigraphy is more sensitive.

SKELETAL SURVEY

Clinical situation	Guideline	Comment
? Metastatic disease	Not indicated routinely	Skeletal scintigram preferred. Selected views to evaluate 'hot spots' on radionuclide scans.
? Myelomatosis	Indicated	Skeletal scintigram may not show myeloma changes
? Renal bone disease	Indicated	

MULTIPLE JOINT SURVEY

Clinical situation	Guideline	Comment
? Inflammatory joint disease	Not indicated	Concentrate on symptomatic joints. Scintigraphy will identify active joints. Exception—take radiographs of feet when symptomatic hands are radiologically normal.

PLAIN ABDOMEN

Clinical situation	Guideline	Comment
Acute abdominal pain	Indicated	Supine abdomen for gas pattern and erect chest film for subphrenic gas and for lung changes ± ultrasound.

PLAIN ABDOMEN (*cont.*)

Clinical situation	Guideline	Comment
Intestinal obstruction	Supine examination indicated. Erect examination rarely indicated	Careful evaluation of the supine view is usually enough. Occasionally an erect view is required to clarify the supine film or if a senior clinician has a strong suspicion of obstruction, but only after inspection of the supine film first.
Suspected biliary disease, pancreatitis	Not indicated	Request ultrasound
Aortic aneurysm	Not indicated	Ultrasound indicated
Non-specific abdominal pain, urinary retention, acute urinary tract infection, haematemesis and melaena, acute peptic ulceration, appendicitis	Not indicated	No useful information. Ultrasound may be helpful in some situations, e.g. urinary tract conditions and appendicitis.
Palpable mass	Not indicated	Request ultrasound. If doubtful discuss with radiologist about possible CT.
Renal size assessment	Not indicated	Ultrasound is the examination of choice.
? Renal (ureteric) colic or pain with haematuria	Normally as part of emergency IVU	See under IVU.
Constipation	Specialist request only	Senior gastroenterologists and geriatricians for distribution of faecal shadowing. Many normal adults are constipated: it is impossible to assess significance of radiological signs.
Lost intrauterine contraceptive device (IUCD)	Not indicated	Ultrasound indicated. If not seen on ultrasound then radiography may be indicated.

Notes

1. The average radiation dose from a plain abdominal radiograph is 1.5 mSv (75 times that of a chest radiograph) and from an abdominal CT examination 8.0 mSv (400 times that of a chest radiograph).

BARIUM EXAMINATION OF OESOPHAGUS

Clinical situation	Guideline	Comment
Dysphagia	Indicated	Distinguish between true dysphagia with food sticking at a particular level and vague discomfort not related to swallowing or eating.
Globus syndrome	Indicated	Usually due to cricopharyngeus overaction, often secondary to reflux. May require cine or video swallowing for its demonstration.
Chest pain ? hiatal hernia/reflux	Not indicated routinely	Reflux and oesophagitis are best diagnosed clinically or by pH monitoring. Barium studies are of limited value. 1. Reflux/hiatal hernias are common and may be present when chest pain has other causes. 2. Reflux is variable: failure to show it does not exclude it. Endoscopy is advisable if reflux symptoms do not respond to therapy.

BARIUM EXAMINATIONS OF STOMACH AND DUODENUM

Clinical situation	Guideline	Comment
Duodenal ulcer (follow-up)	Not indicated	Ulcer scarring makes it hard to assess activity: clinical history (or endoscopy) is better.
Dyspepsia	Not indicated routinely, particularly for those under 45	Non-ulcer causes of dyspepsia are reflux (+/− oesophagitis), dysmotility (diffuse discomfort with nausea early and distension late in the day), aerophagy, ulcer-like dyspepsia (may need

BARIUM EXAMINATIONS OF STOMACH AND DUODENUM *(cont.)*

Clinical situation	Guideline	Comment
		endoscopy during an attack). Features suggesting non-ulcer dyspepsia include steady weight, patient remaining well, but known to be 'a worrier'. Features pointing to early investigation are: age over 40, weight loss, anaemia, woken by pain, pain radiating to back, periodicity, smoking, taking non-steroidal anti-inflammatory drugs, history of ulcer, vomiting, localized pain.
Gastric ulcer (follow-up)	Endoscopy preferred	Premalignant potential of gastric ulcers requires confirmation of healing.
Gastrointestinal bleeding	Not indicated	Endoscopy preferred.
Pancreatic/biliary disease	Not indicated	Ultrasound, endoscopy, CT preferred.
Upper gastrointestinal tract resection/ operation, recent	Indicated (water soluble contrast study)	To assess integrity of anastomoses and satisfactory transit to small bowel.
Old	Not indicated	Endoscopy is more sensitive routinely for possible ulceration. Barium studies may be useful in assessing gastric remnant emptying and anatomy/motility of small bowel.

Notes

1. The average radiation dose from a barium meal is 5.0 mSv (250 times that of a chest radiograph).

BARIUM EXAMINATION OF SMALL BOWEL

Clinical situation	Guideline	Comment
Intestinal blood loss (chronic or recurrent)	Indicated	After upper tract endoscopy and barium enema or colonoscopy.
Malabsorption	Not indicated routinely	Indicated for jejunal diverticulosis or if intestinal biopsy is normal or if complications (e.g. lymphoma) are suspected.
Small bowel disease suspected, e.g. Crohn's disease	Indicated	
Small bowel obstruction Acute	Only indicated after discussion with radiologist	Small bowel series may provide more precise information on cause and site of obstruction.
Small bowel obstruction Chronic or recurrent	Indicated	Small bowel barium enema the examination of choice.

BARIUM EXAMINATION OF LARGE BOWEL

Many patients with bowel symptoms have irritable bowel syndrome (IBS) and may be managed by a trial of non-proprietary medicines. In others symptoms originate in the distal colon. All patients should have prior sigmoidoscopy which may rule out the need for barium studies. All patients should undergo rectal examination to ensure that they are suitable for intubation and to rule out a rectal carcinoma.

Double contrast barium enema (DCBE) is a useful study only if the bowel is properly prepared. If this is not possible it is a waste of time.

Clinical situation	Guideline	Comment
Inflammatory bowel disease or tumour suggested by abdominal pain, rectal bleeding, change in bowel habit	Indicated	Defer for 7 days if biopsy has been undertaken.
Large bowel obstruction (acute)	Indicated after consultation	Single contrast study to define narrowed area only.
Ulcerative colitis Acute exacerbation	Not indicated routinely	Plain film studies are usually sufficient for evaluation. Suspected toxic megacolon is an

BARIUM EXAMINATION OF LARGE BOWEL (*cont.*)

Clinical situation	Guideline	Comment
		absolute contraindication. For less severe cases an 'instant' enema without preparation may be discussed with the radiologist.
Chronic long-term follow-up	Not indicated routinely	Frequency of follow-up studies requires radiological/gastro-enterological consultation. Colonoscopy may be preferred.

Notes

1. The average radiation dose of a barium enema is 9.0 mSv (450 times that of a chest radiograph).

BILARY TRACT EXAMINATION

Clinical situation	Guideline	Comment
Gallstones/ cholecystitis suspected	Ultrasound indicated	Cholecystography is only indicated if good views are not obtained with ultrasound. Plain films only show about 20 per cent of stones. Ultrasound allows examination of other related organs—liver, right kidney, pancreas.
Jaundice	Ultrasound indicated	Ultrasound is very sensitive for bile-duct calibre, gallstones, many types of liver disease. Discuss further investigation with radiologist.

INTRAVENOUS UROGRAPHY

Clinical situation	Guideline	Comment
Haematuria	Indicated	Useful survey of urinary tract particularly for collecting system lesions. If normal discuss with urologist and radiologist. Ultrasound more sensitive for bladder lesions. Cystoscopy also needed.
Hypertension without evidence of urinary disease	Not indicated	IVU is insensitive for renal artery stenosis. Hypertension in younger adults and not responding to medication may require digital angiography or radionuclide imaging.
Urinary retention and symptoms of bladder outflow obstruction	Not indicated	Ultrasound preferred. Allows evaluation of upper tract and bladder emptying. Best carried out in conjunction with urine flow measurement Some symptoms attributed to prostatic enlargement have other causes, e.g. bladder instability and may not improve with prostatectomy.
? Renal mass.	Not indicated	See abdominal mass. Ultrasound preferred +/− CT
Renal (ureteric) colic	Indicated—limited examination only	Findings highly specific for obstruction but disappear rapidly when pain ceases. Delayed films (up to 24 h) may be necessary to show site of obstruction. If acute pain has subsided a plain film and ultrasound are appropriate as follow-up studies.

Notes

1. The average radiation dose from an IVU is 4.6 mSv (230 times that of a chest radiograph).

IVU/MICTURATING CYSTOGRAM

Clinical situation	Guideline	Comment
Urinary tract infection, recurrent in young women	Rarely indicated	Most cases relate to onset of sexual activity. Indications for investigation (ultrasound and plain film) are: breakthrough on treatment, presence of unusual organisms, previous urinary tract disease. In diabetics or in renal failure ultrasound is preferable because of risk of contrast damage and/or poor concentration. Micturating cystogram is rarely useful.
Urinary tract infection—other adults	IVU rarely indicated. Ultrasound and plain abdominal radiograph preferred.	IVU indicated for sterile pyuria, recurrent infection associated with ureteric pain, possible papillary necrosis.
Enuresis	Not indicated	See also under paediatric imaging.

MULTIPLE IMAGING STUDIES

Clinical situation	Guideline	Comment
Metastatic adenocarcinoma ? source e.g. barium meal, barium enema, IVU, etc.	Rarely indicated Specialist request only	Demonstration of primary source very rarely affects clinical management. Current exceptions are breast, ovary, thyroid.

VENOGRAPHY

Clinical situation	Guideline	Comment
Suspected deep venous thrombosis	Indicated but ...	Ultrasound preferred for demonstration of thrombus in popliteal and femoral vein. Therefore, if thrombus confined to veins in calf is unimportant or if

VENOGRAPHY (*cont.*)

Clinical situation	Guideline	Comment
		clinical examination suggests thrombus above knee request ultrasound.
Suspected deep venous thrombosis during pregnancy	Limited venogram indicated after ultrasound	Ultrasound should be performed first to assess the popliteal, femoral, and external iliac veins. If this is normal then a limited venogram to assess the veins in the calf to midthigh can be performed.

ACCIDENT AND EMERGENCY AND TRAUMA IMAGING

Skull

The key clinical questions in head injury are:

1 Is there evidence of brain injury?
2 Is there evidence of intracranial haemorrhage or raised intracranial pressure?
3 Is there a skull fracture? If so, is it depressed?
4 Are other systems/areas involved?

CT can answer questions 1 and 2, skull radiographs cannot.
The key management questions are:

1 Does the patient need admission for observation?
2 Is CT scan and/or neurosurgical opinion required?

These questions underlie appropriate policies.
Note that if a decision is made to admit for observation, skull radiography becomes unnecessary unless a depressed fracture is suspected.

Facial bones

Clinical situation	Guideline	Comment
Nasal trauma	Not indicated	Management of the bruised nose will depend on local arrangements: usually a follow-up visit to ENT will determine the need for radiographs.
Eye Trauma Radio-opaque missile injury	Indicated if history suggestive of penetrating injury	History important as signs are often minimal. Films with eyes up and eyes down. CT or ultrasound may also be used.

Facial bones (*cont.*)

Clinical situation	Guideline	Comment
Middle third injury	Indicated but patient co-operation essential	May be advisable to delay until patient's condition has improved. Discuss with oral surgeon.
Mandible injury	Indicated but not for non-traumatic dislocation	Orthopantomography and anteroposterior mandible preferred.
Temporomandibular joint(s)	ENT/oral surgeons only	

Cervical spine/neck

Clinical situation	Guideline	Comment
Fully conscious minor head injury without neck pain or facial trauma	Not indicated	
Unconscious head injury/unconscious patient	Indicated	Cervical spine radiographs can be difficult to evaluate and need careful inspection. 1. Should show C7/T1. Up to one-third of fractures occur here. 2. Should show odontoid peg; not always possible at time of initial study. 3. May need 'swimmers' view, obliques, tomography, CT. Discuss with radiologist.
Neck injury with pain	Indicated	As above. Flexion/extension views not usually indicated in acute trauma. Discuss with senior radiology or orthopaedic staff.
Neck pain without injury	Not indicated routinely	Radiography only if there are neurological symptoms/signs.
Pharyngeal/upper oesophageal foreign body	Soft tissues of neck if foreign body radio-opaque	Differentiation from calcified cartilage can be difficult. May proceed to laryngoscopy, endoscopy, barium swallow. See abdomen for foreign body below neck level.

Dorsal and lumbar spine

Clinical situation	Guideline	Comment
Trauma	Indicated	
Acute back pain (no trauma)	Six-week rule, unless metastatic disease or infection suspected	Refer if there are neurological signs
Chronic back pain	Not indicated	Refer to outpatients department or back to general practitioner.

Pelvis and sacrum

Clinical situation	Guideline	Comment
Trauma to coccyx	Not indicated	Does not affect management.
Major trauma patient or fall with inability to bear weight	Indicated	Physical examination may be unreliable.

Limbs

Clinical situation	Guideline	Comment
Ankle injury	Not indicated routinely	Indicated if bony tenderness.
Injury—foot and ankle	Rarely indicated together	Clinicians must choose which film they want.
Soft tissue foreign body 1. Metal, glass, painted wood	Indicated	All glass, except that of light bulbs, is opaque; some paint is opaque. Two normally penetrated (i.e. not soft tissue) views needed.
2. Plastic, wood	Not indicated	These are not usually opaque.

Special points in major trauma

Clinical situation	Guideline	Comment
Major trauma	*Earlier guidelines apply but whenever there is major trauma:*	

Special points in major trauma (*cont.*)

Clinical situation	Guideline	Comment
	1. Lateral cervical spine.	Must see C7/T1
	+ 2. Chest film	Beware pitfalls of supine chest radiographs.
	+ 3. Pelvis	Clinical examination not sufficient.
	Other considerations: Abdomen	Plain film not useful. Ultrasound/ diagnostic peritoneal lavage/CT useful if in doubt.
	Urinary tract	Remember deceleration injury to renal arteries ?One film IVU. Beware bladder/urethral injury ?urethrogram/ cystogram. If CT with contrast performed then IVU not needed.

Chest radiography

Clinical situation	Guideline	Comment
Chest trauma Mild	Not indicated routinely	
Moderate/severe	Indicated	A posteroanterior film is taken for pneumothorax, fluid, lung contusion, or aortic trauma.
Stab injury	Indicated	
? Sternal fracture	Lateral sternum preferred	

Abdomen

Clinical situation	Guideline	Comment
? Obstruction	Supine view indicated Erect view rarely indicated	Careful evaluation of the supine film is usually enough. Fluid levels are non-specific and may be misleading.

Abdomen (*cont.*)

Clinical situation	Guideline	Comment
? Perforation	Supine indicated Erect posteroanterior chest view indicated	Chest film is more sensitive in detecting small amounts of free gas. Lateral decubitus abdominal film indicated if patient cannot sit or stand.
Blunt or stab injury	Supine indicated Erect posteroanterior chest indicated	Ultrasound valuable for detecting haematomas and injury to some organs, e.g. spleen.
Swallowed foreign body	Abdomen view rarely indicated but lateral chest view indicated	Most swallowed foreign bodies pass from the stomach but: 1. When lodged in the oesophagus even coins can cause symptomless erosion. Many oesophageal foreign bodies will only be seen on a lateral chest film: dentures vary in radio-opacity. 2. Leakage of mercury salts from swallowed batteries is dangerous. Therefore, all cases must have a lateral chest film and then: (i) an abdominal film if endoscopic removal/operation is proposed; (ii) an abdominal film if foreign body is a swallowed battery. (iii) an abdominal film if lateral chest film is clear and there is doubt if a foreign body has been swallowed at all. In units with a metal detector, its use is preferable.

Urinary tract imaging

Clinical situation	Guideline	Comment
Renal (ureteric) colic—two-film IVU	Indicated	The diagnostic urographic signs are often only present during pain. It may not be appropriate to examine if pain has subsided. The presence/absence of obstruction is clear on the 20-min film. If the site of the stone is not obvious, films for up to 24 h may be needed.
Possible renal trauma/IVU/ultra-sound/CT/ angiography	Indicated but with radiological/ urological consultation: choices are affected by local policies	Renal tract may need investigation where renal trauma is suspected, e.g. after loin injury, stab wound, etc. +/− haematuria. Renal parenchymal injury, perirenal blood/fluid, and renal perfusion can be shown but management is usually conservative so the most important issue is the normality of the other kidney; a single film IVU is usually enough. In major abdominal trauma especially after deceleration injury, renal artery damage may be overlooked. Here, too, a one-film IVU is helpful if CT is not performed.
Pelvic injury/ urethral bleeding	Urethrogram indicated	To show urethral integrity, leak, rupture, +/− cystogram if urethra is normal and there is suspicion of bladder leak.

IMAGING IN CHILDREN

It is important to minimize radiation dose in children especially in those with long-term problems

Chest radiography

Clinical situation	Guideline	Comment
Acute chest infection	Not indicated routinely	Many infections only involve the bronchi. If signs/symptoms suggest lung infection, a radiograph will show/rule out parenchymal involvement or collapse. With simple consolidation follow-up is not required after good response to treatment. If there is collapse and/or failure of treatment, follow-up is essential.
? Inhaled foreign body	Indicated	Inspiratory/ expiratory films are required for evidence of air trapping. Chest screening or high kV views may be needed in very young children. History of inhalation is often not clear. Bronchoscopy should be performed if in doubt.
Sudden unexplained wheeze	Indicated	May be due to inhaled foreign body.
Preoperative chest radiograph	Not indicated	As for adults.

Plain abdomen

Clinical situation	Guideline	Comment
Non-specific abdominal pain	Paediatrician, paediatric surgeon, gastroenterologist only	Careful clinical history and examination needed, with ultrasound for specific problems: these should be discussed with radiologists.
? Constipation	Not indicated	
? Intestinal obstruction in neonates	Indicated	Discuss first with radiologist.

Plain abdomen (*cont.*)

Clinical situation	Guideline	Comment
? Intussusception (plain film)	Indicated (supine and erect views to include diaphragms)	Expert ultrasonography is preferable +/− air or barium enema. Erect abdomen or chest film if clinical suspicion of perforation.
Swallowed foreign bodies	Rarely indicated (except for mercury batteries)	See comments in accident and emergency section.
Trauma to abdomen	Not indicated routinely	Ultrasound or CT are more specific, particularly in spleen/liver/kidney trauma. Horizontal beam film may show signs of perforation.
? Intestinal obstruction	See adult section	

Barium studies

Clinical situation	Guideline	Comment
Recurrent vomiting	Paediatrician, paediatric surgeons, gastroenterologist only	This symptom covers a wide spectrum from obstruction in the neonatal period to those children who reflux or posset and children with migraine. Most infants can be managed by careful clinical evaluation and a plain abdominal film.
? Necrotizing enterocolitis	Paediatrician/ paediatric surgeons only	Dangerous in the acute phase: may be needed after recovery to rule out possible stricture formation. Use water-soluble contrast.
Rectal bleeding	Paediatrician, paediatric surgeons, gastroenterologist only	If Meckel's diverticulum is a possibility do isotope scan first. Colonoscopy may be preferable to barium enema.
Possible intussusception	Indicated but . . .	Contraindicated in the presence of free gas or with peritonism or shock. Needs surgical/ radiological consultation. Where appropriate expertise is available ultrasonic diagnosis and pneumatic reduction may be better than barium enema.

Urinary tract

Clinical situation	Guideline	Comment
Enuresis—IVU or micturating cystogram	Not indicated	Investigation is only required for daytime frequency/urgency/ wetting; then urodynamic study may be undertaken to confirm/rule out bladder instability or neuropathy. Micturating cystogram may show ectopic ureter. Cystoscopy may be needed to detect an ectopic ureter.
Continuous wetting	Limited IVU indicated	To exclude duplex system with ectopic ureter.
Urinary tract infection—IVU.	Rarely indicated	Imaging options are under continual review and appropriate choices need familiarity with the field. Currently plain film, ultrasound, DMSA scan, and micturating cystogram are commonly utilized. Discuss with radiologist.
Hypertension	Paediatricians only	Renal tract and renovascular disease are relatively common in hypertensive children. Subtle scars may only be evident on DMSA.

Urinary tract (*cont.*)

Clinical situation	Guideline	Comment
		Further investigation should be discussed with radiologist.
Renal (ureteric) colic	Indicated	See accident and emergency section.
? Obstruction (e.g. chronic renal pain)	Indicated	Ultrasound the first investigation.

Skull and sinus radiography

Clinical situation	Guideline	Comment
Head injury	Not indicated routinely	See accident and emergency section. Same indications apply as in adults.
? Sinusitis	ENT surgeons and paediatricians only	Sinuses are poorly developed before 6–9 years and sinus radiographs are of little clinical value. Muscosal thickening can be a normal finding in the sinuses of children.
Mouth breathing—postnasal space for ? adenoid enlargement	ENT surgeons and paediatricians only	Adenoid hypertrophy is normal in children. Radiographs are only useful if operation is contemplated.

The spine

Clinical situation	Guideline	Comment
Back or neck pain	Indicated	Back pain is uncommon in children without a cause. Follow-up needed if infection is suspected. Skeletal scintigraphy is indicated if there is bone pain and plain films are normal.
? Spina bifida occulta (or for enuresis)	Not indicated	Spina bifida occulta is common and not in itself significant. Neurological signs would require evaluation.

Limbs and joints

Clinical situation	Guideline	Comment
? Non-accidental injury	Indicated for affected area Skeletal survey for senior clinicians only	Careful clinical and radiological examination essential. Skeletal survey requires radiological involvement to ensure adequate quality. Skeletal scintigram is sensitive for occult injury.
Limb injury—opposite side for comparison	Not indicated routinely	The one possible exception is the opposite elbow when there is a strong clinical evidence of elbow fracture with no radiological evidence and no available radiologist.

OBSTETRIC ULTRASOUND

Clinical situation	Guideline	Comment
Early pregnancy bleeding/ viability	Indicated	Ultrasound will confirm pregnancy location (i.e. intra- versus extrauterine). viability, and gestational age.
Suspected ectopic pregnancy	Indicated	A sensitive pregnancy test should also always be performed. The presence of an empty uterine cavity on ultrasound in a patient with symptoms of an ectopic pregnancy and a positive pregnancy test is highly suspicious of this diagnosis.
Placental localization Antepartum haemorrhage Placenta praevia	Indicated	The identification of a low lying placenta is a common finding on scanning before 20 weeks and in the absence of bleeding is not an indication for repeat scanning. Identification of a retroplacental

OBSTETRIC ULTRASOUND (*cont.*)

Clinical situation	Guideline	Comment
		haemorrhage is extremely difficult and ultrasound cannot exclude the diagnosis of abruptio placenta.

PELVIMETRY

Ideally MRI should be used to obtain pelvimetry measurements, when indicated, in both pregnant and non-pregnant women. If MRI is not available then low dose conventional radiography or CT techniques should be used.

NON-OBSTETRIC ULTRASOUND

Clinical situation	Guideline	Comment
Abdominal ultrasound		
Suspected gallstones or cholecystitis	Indicated	If gallbladder is not well seen, oral cholecystogram with upright screening films may be used. Biliary radionuclide scan may be added for acute gallbladder symptoms.
Suspected liver metastases	Indicated (with reservations)	Contrast enhanced CT is more sensitive. MRI is used for possible capillary haemangiomas.
Abnormal liver function tests	Not indicated routinely	Little value when the cause is obvious, e.g. alcoholism, but with unexplained abnormality, it is useful for liver size and to rule out focal abnormalities, e.g. metastases and biliary obstruction.
Jaundice or liver function tests with obstructive pattern	Indicated (with exceptions)	Shows dilated ducts in patients with obstruction (except in some cases of sclerosing cholangitis). Not needed with clear-cut hepatitis/ drug-induced jaundice.
Pancreatitis	Indicated	Pancreas often appears normal: purpose is to show gallstones and monitor presence/absence of pseudocysts. CT is more sensitive especially for pancreatic calcification and necrosis.
Suspected pancreatic tumour	Indicated (with reservations)	Useful in slim patients. In obese patients, or if ultrasound is negative/equivocal, use CT or MRI.
? Abdominal aortic aneurysm	Indicated	Useful in diagnosis and follow-up. For suspected leak or dissection CT is preferable, but should not delay urgent surgery.
Suspected abdominal sepsis	Indicated	Shows subphrenic/ subhepatic spaces and pelvis well, but is less useful in midabdomen. If negative and clinical suspicion is high, use CT. With abdominal wounds and enterostomies it may be appropriate to use CT directly.
Suspected lymph node enlargement	Not indicated routinely	CT is more sensitive and specific.
Suspected acute appendicitis	Not routinely indicated	Clinical history/examination pre-eminent but in skilled hands appendiceal disease may be shown. Also used for suspected pelvic/adnexal disease.
Pelvic ultrasound		
Suspected pelvic mass	Indicated	
Pelvic pain	Occasionally indicated	In absence of clinical findings, ultrasound rarely gives diagnostic information.
Suspected pelvic inflammatory disease	Indicated	Negative result does not rule out infection.

NON-OBSTETRIC ULTRASOUND (*cont.*)

Clinical situation	Guideline	Comment
Urinary tract ultrasound		
Renal failure	Indicated	A normal scan does not always exclude obstruction.
Suspected renal colic	Not indicated	IVU is more sensitive during pain. Ultrasound + plain abdominal film may be used in cases with severe contrast allergy.
Haematuria	Indicated	See IVU section.
Urinary tract infection		
In children	Indicated	See section on children.
In adults	Not indicated routinely	Low yield investigation; main use, with plain film, for recurrent or breakthrough infections.
Suspected renal mass	Indicated	For primary diagnosis: CT is preferable for staging and for assessment of complex/cystic masses.
Prostatic enlargement	Indicated	For upper tracts and bladder pre- and postvoiding preferably with flow rates.
Hypercalcaemia or hyperpara-thyroidism	Indicated	Primary investigations to visualize parathyroid adenoma and nephrocalcinosis.
Suspected prostatic malignancy	Not indicated routinely except to assess upper tracts	Transrectal ultrasound +/− biopsy after clinical examination and prostate-specific antigen levels.
Suspected scrotal mass and/or pain	Indicated	
Suspected testicular torsion	Not indicated routinely	Torsion is a clinical diagnosis; colour flow Doppler is useful to diagnose inflammatory conditions.

NON-OBSTETRIC ULTRASOUND (*cont.*)

Clinical situation	Guideline	Comment
Vascular ultrasound		
Suspected deep vein thrombosis	Indicated, if there is clinicoradio-logical agreement	More sensitive with colour flow Doppler, insensitive for calf vein thrombi.
Peripheral limb arterial disease	Indicated	Depends on local expertise and equipment.
Transient ischaemic attacks thought to be arising in carotid territory	Indicated	Not useful as a screening method for asymptomatic bruits.

RADIONUCLIDE IMAGING (SCINTIGRAPHY)

It is important to understand that many of these investigations are best used in conjunction with other imaging techniques: this is emphasized by the use of the terms 'firstline', 'secondline', and 'complementary' for their categories. CLINICIANS SHOULD INDICATE THE FUNCTION BEING INVESTIGATED, BECAUSE THIS WILL DETERMINE WHICH ISOTOPE IS USED.

Clinical situation	Guideline	Comment
Skeletal system (bone scan)		
Known primary tumour; ? bone metastases	Firstline	A radionuclide scan assesses the whole skeleton, and is more sensitive than plain radiography.
Myelomatosis	Not routinely indicated	Bone scans fail to show myeloma changes in about 50 per cent of patients but may be useful in staging and follow-up where the scan is positive.
Bone pain	Secondline	Increased activity on a bone scan is non-specific, but may be demonstrated in the presence of normal radiographs.
Trauma	Secondline	Bone scan is useful for detection of undisplaced fractures (e.g. femoral neck) and stress fractures, where plain films may be normal or equivocal.

NON-OBSTETRIC ULTRASOUND (*cont.*)

Clinical situation	Guideline	Comment
Non-accidental injury	Specialist request only	Selected plain radiographs to evaluate hot spots. Good for occult, sometimes multiple injuries.
Osteomyelitis	Secondline (firstline in children)	Bone scan is sensitive in early detection of osteomyelitis. Radiographs can be normal in first 2 to 3 weeks. Labelled white cell scan will distinguish infection from other lesions. May be difficult to interpret in metaphyses of children.
Painful prosthesis	Secondline	Radiographs first. A normal bone scan excludes significant complications. May need labelled white cell scan to distinguish loosening from infection.
Gastrointestinal system		
Acute gastrointestinal bleeding	Secondline following endoscopy	Labelled red cell or colloid scan. Barium precludes the use of radionuclides or angiography, and therefore should be deferred in the acute situation. Radionuclide studies are more sensitive than angiography and can detect bleeding rates as low as 0.1 ml/min.
? Meckel's diverticulum	Firstline	Pertechnetate scan. Detects ectopic gastric mucosa.
Inflammatory bowel disease	Complementary to endoscopy and barium studies	Labelled white cell scan. White cell study assesses activity and extent of disease. Seek advice of radiologist.
Acute cholecystitis	Complementary to ultrasound	Biliary radionuclide scan shows cystic duct obstruction in acute cholecystitis. Seek advice.

RADIONUCLIDE IMAGING (*cont.*)

Clinical situation	Guideline	Comment
? Postoperative biliary leak	Firstline with ultrasound	Biliary radionuclide scan will show an active leak.
Biliary atresia	Firstline	Biliary radionuclide scan. Biliary atresia excluded by demonstration of activity within bowel.
Metastatic or primary tumour of liver/spleen	Not indicated	Use ultrasound and/or CT, MRI.
Liver/spleen trauma	Not indicated	Ultrasound and/or CT is superior.
? Haemangioma of the liver	Not indicated routinely	Use MRI or, if not available, CT.
Respiratory system (V/Q scan)		
Suspected pulmonary embolism	Firstline	Interpreted together with current radiograph. Equivocal cases may need pulmonary angiography if available.
Cardiovascular system		
Chest pain	Secondline after stress ECG	Thallium/isonitrile myocardial perfusion study. Detects presence, location, and extent of myocardial ischaemia. In patients unable to exercise, pharmacological stress (dipyridamole, dobutamine) can be used.
Evaluation of ventricular function	Firstline to quantify ventricular function	Can assess prognosis in patients after acute myocardial infarction.
Infection/inflammation		
Pyrexia of unknown origin	Secondline after ultrasound or CT	Labelled white cell or gallium scan. White cell scan is better in cases of postoperative sepsis. Gallium will accumulate at sites of tumour (e.g. lymphoma) and infection. Seek advice. Gallium gives a high radiation dose.

RADIONUCLIDE IMAGING (*cont.*)

Clinical situation	Guideline	Comment
Renal system		
Hypertensive young adult, without renal disease: ? renal artery stenosis	Complementary to ultrasound	Ultrasound to assess relative renal sizes. Renogram will detect 'functional' stenosis and will exclude significant unilateral renal artery stenosis. May require digital angiography. IVU is insensitive.
Dilated pelvicaliceal system? Pelvi-ureteric junction obstruction	Secondline after ultrasound	Determines presence or absence of obstruction and divided renal function.
Acute renal failure	Complementary to ultrasound	Ultrasound will detect an obstructive cause. Renogram assesses perfusion and function of kidneys and obstruction to outflow.
Failing renal transplant	Complementary to Doppler ultrasound	May differentiate acute rejection from acute tubular necrosis. Choice of investigation depends on local arrangements.
Urinary tract infection (paediatric)	Firstline with ultrasound	DMSA scan and/or micturating cystogram. Exact mode of investigation depends on local practice. DMSA is more sensitive than ultrasound in detecting scarring.
? Renal space-occupying lesion	Not routinely indicated	DMSA scan. Ultrasound and/or CT recommended. Main use in suspected pseudotumour.
? Vesicoureteric reflux	Indicated	Alternative to contrast cystogram.
Endocrine system		
Evaluation of thyroid nodules or thyrotoxicosis	Secondline after biopsy or ultrasound	Differentiation of Graves' disease from toxic nodular goitre. To determine functional status of nodules.

RADIONUCLIDE IMAGING (*cont.*)

Clinical situation	Guideline	Comment
? Ectopic thyroid tissue (e.g. lingual thyroid)	Firstline	CT and/or ultrasound may also be used to assess retrosternal extension.
Hypercalcaemia/ hyperpara-thyroidism	Secondline to ultrasound, MRI	Parathyroid subtraction scan. Preoperative location of parathyroid adenoma. Vein sampling may also be helpful. Seek advice.
Adrenal medullary tumour	Firstline with CT/ultrasound	MIBG scan. Location of phaeochromo-cytoma.
Adrenal cortical tumours. Conn's, Cushing's syndromes	Secondline after CT/ultrasound	Selenocholesterol scan. Differentiation of unilateral adenoma from bilateral hyperplasia.

MAMMOGRAPHY

Mammography is indicated for the diagnosis, preoperative assessment, and management of breast cancer.

Clinical indications for mammography

Where there is clinical suspicion of breast cancer, e.g. a suspicious lump, residual lump following aspiration of a cyst, or a single duct discharge, then referral to a breast clinic/breast surgeon is advisable PRIOR TO ANY RADIOLOGICAL INVESTIGATION.

Mammography is unlikely to influence the management of:

1. Breast pain and/or tenderness in the absence of other clinical signs;
2. Generalized breast lumpiness;
3. Long-standing nipple inversion;
4. Symptoms related to the contraceptive pill.

Mammography should not be requested:

1. As a routine prior to or during hormone replacement therapy;
2. In the management of cyclical mastalgia without clinical signs;
3. As the firstline investigation in women under 35 unless there is a STRONG clinical suspicion of breast cancer. The sensitivity of mammography in detecting malignancy is reduced in the young glandular breast and cancer is uncommon in this age group.

Breast ultrasound

The radiologist may decide that ultrasound is a more appropriate method of investigation to solve the clinical problem. Ultrasound is not suitable for screening at any age.

Remember that although mammography is the best method of detecting early breast cancer, it is not 100 per cent sensitive. A negative mammogram does not exclude breast cancer. All imaging results must be considered in the context of the clinical findings.

Mammography in high risk groups

Routine mammography may be justified at any age in women who are at high risk of developing premenopausal breast cancer. This includes those with histological risk factors from previous surgery and first-degree relatives of those who have had premenopausal breast cancer. Mammography should be supervised by a breast clinic or specialist.

Mammography in women with a family history of breast cancer

Local policies and availability vary and general guidelines are not appropriate. Many departments and screening units offer a service only through prior referral to a breast clinic or specialist.

Women with a mother or sister who developed breast cancer before menopause, or in whom two or more close relatives (mother, sister, aunt, grandmother) developed breast cancer, are at higher risk. Appropriate counselling and a personal plan for mammography may be required. If the family history is of post-menopausal breast cancer, referral to the clinic or specialist may be delayed until the age of 35. Where the family history is of premenopausal cancer, referral at an age 10 years younger than the first-degree relative who developed breast cancer may be advisable.

A single first-degree relative who develops postmenopausal breast cancer confers only a slight increased risk to others and routine mammography is not usually indicated in women under the age of 50.

Population screening programme in asymptomatic women in the United Kingdom

Age 50–64	Indicated—mortality reduction proven. All women registered with a general practitioner invited every 3 years
Age 65 and over	Not indicated routinely—women can self-refer to screening programme centres, but are not invited automatically
Under 50	Not indicated—mortality reduction not yet proven. United Kingdom national trial in progress.

The arteries 7

7.1 The pathobiology of atherosclerosis

DINAH V. PARUMS

INTRODUCTION

Cardiovascular disease remains the chief cause of death in the United States and Western Europe, and atherosclerosis, the principal cause of myocardial and cerebral infarction, accounts for the majority of these deaths.

One of the problems in the study of the nature of human atherosclerosis lies in the lack of unanimity about the definition of the histopathological structure of the lesion. The name 'atheroma' was commonly used by the Greek writers to describe the yellow, intimal plaques or nodules containing 'gruel-like' material. 'Arteriosclerosis' was introduced in 1829 by Lobstein as a generic term for all diseases of the artery in which there is thickening of the vessel wall with induration (Table 1). Arteriosclerosis remains the acceptable collective term for what is known popularly as hardening of the arteries. The term 'atherosclerosis' was introduced by Marchand in 1904. The World Health Organization gives the definition of atherosclerosis as 'a variable combination of changes of the intima of arteries consisting of focal accumulations of lipid, complex carbohydrates, blood and blood products, fibrous deposits and calcium deposits associated with medial changes.'

Table 1 Types and location of arteriosclerotic lesions

Name	Predominant initial lesion	Arterial size
Atherosclerosis	Intima (inner media)	Large and medium
Mönckeberg's	Media	Large and medium
Arteriolosclerosis	Intima/media	Arterioles
Mucoid (cystic) medial necrosis	Media	Large
Endarteritis	Intima	Small
Polyarteritis	Intima, media, and adventitia	Medium and small
Infectious arteritis	Adventitia/media	Large and medium
Giant cell arteritis	Media	Medium and small
Takayasu's arteritis	Intima and media	Large and medium

NORMAL ARTERIAL ANATOMY

Arteries are compliant, distensible structures with a flat internal surface. They consist of three layers; the intima, the media, and the adventitia.

At birth, the intima consists of a single layer of endothelial cells which rests on the basement membrane and is separated from the media by the internal elastic lamina. The media consists of interconnected smooth muscle cells which, in muscular arteries, are separated from the adventitia by the external elastic lamina. Large elastic arteries such as the aorta possess a media which contains numerous parallel elastin fibres. Vasa vasorum, found in the adventitia of larger arteries, provide oxygenation and nutrition to the outer layers of the artery.

Normal arterial physiology is shown in Table 2.

Table 2 Normal arterial physiology

Endothelial cell function
1. Permeability barrier
2. Non-thrombogenic and antithrombogenic (Factor VIII—von Willebrand factor, cyclo-oxygenase, prostacyclin, heparan sulphate)
3. Metabolism of vasoactive substances (endothelium derived relaxing factor (EDRF)—now known to be nitric oxide, angiotensin converting enzyme (ACE))
4. Production of growth factors and growth inhibitors (e.g. interleukin-1 (IL-1))
5. Connective tissue production
6. Oxidation of low density lipoprotein (LDL)

Smooth muscle cell function
1. Contractility
2. Connective tissue production
3. Lipid metabolism (LDL, cholesterol, prostaglandin)
4. Proliferation is induced by platelet derived growth factor, monocyte derived growth factor, endothelial cell derived growth factor, LDL, and prostacyclin

NORMAL LIPID PHYSIOLOGY

Lipoproteins

Triglycerides and other lipids are insoluble in plasma and are therefore transported as lipoproteins, aggregates of variable size, lipid, and protein content. These lipoproteins are usually classified by their density on ultracentrifugation, the lipoprotein with the lowest density and the greatest triglyceride content having the highest flotation number (Table 3).

Table 3 Major classes of lipid and their associated proteins

Associated apoprotein	Lipid	Function of protein moiety
AI, AII	HDL	Activation of transferase
B	VLDL, LDL	Triglyceride transport Binds to LDL receptor, with uptake into cells
CI, CII, CIII	VLDL, HDL	Activate and inhibit lipoprotein lipase
D	HDL	
E	VLDL, HDL, IDL	Control of clearance of VLDL, chylomicron remnants

High density lipoprotein (HDL), very low density lipoprotein (VLDL), low density lipoprotein (LDL), and intermediate density lipoprotein (IDL) are classified by their ultracentrifugation properties

Apoproteins

Apoproteins are the lipid-free protein components of the plasma lipoproteins. They play a role in receptor recognition and enzyme regulation and maintain the structural integrity of the lipoprotein particles.

Apoproteins are divided into classes A, B, C, D, and E, and are further divided into subclasses (Table 3). Apoprotein A is the major protein in high-density lipoprotein. Apoprotein A1 binds phospholipid and activates lecithin cholesterol transferase.

Apoprotein B accounts for 90 per cent of the protein of low-density lipoproteins and is a major protein of chylomicrons and very-low-density lipoproteins. Apoprotein B has a role in the transport of triglycerides.

Apoprotein CII activates the lipoprotein lipase of adipose tissue, while apoprotein E is involved with recognition of the remnant particle by the liver.

The absorption of dietary fat

Dietary fat accounts for between 30 and 50 per cent of the energy intake of many people. In the small intestine, partial hydrolysis of fats occurs due to the action of lipases, and in the presence of bile salts, cholic and chenodeoxycholic acids, and some phospholipid, micelles are formed, followed by absorption of non-esterified fatty acids and monoglycerides in the duodenum and proximal jejunum.

Monoglycerides are re-esterified in the mucosal cells to form triglycerides. Dietary cholesterol esters are hydrolysed by pancreatic enzymes and cholesterol is absorbed in the small intestine where it combines with triglycerides, phospholipids, and specific apolipoproteins in the mucosal cells. The combination leads to the formation of triglyceride-rich chylomicrons which are secreted into the lymphatic circulation. Here, changes in cholesterol, phospholipid, and apoproteins occur, including the loss of apoprotein AII and uptake of apoproteins C and E.

Although triglycerides, phospholipids, and cholesterol have important functions in the body and are vital components of cell structure, raised levels of these lipids in the circulation are associated with an increased incidence of ischaemic heart disease.

Fat transport

Very-low-density lipoprotein is synthesized in the liver and is the form in which endogenously synthesized triglycerides are transported. Triglyceride is gradually removed from the chylomicrons and very-low-density lipoprotein by the action of lipoprotein lipase. This enzyme is present in adipose tissue and in capillaries at tall sites. Its activity is stimulated by apoprotein CII and also by insulin. Glycerides and non-esterified fatty acids which are released from chylomicrons are taken up by muscle, where they provide the main energy source for aerobic metabolism. Excess is stored as triglyceride in adipose tissue.

As triglycerides are removed, the remnant particle becomes smaller; some of the more water soluble components on the surface, such as phospholipid, unesterified cholesterol, and apoprotein C become redundant and transfer to high-density lipoprotein. The remaining chylomicron remnant is intermediate-density lipoprotein, some of which is metabolized by the liver and some of which is probably metabolized in the tissues to low-density lipoprotein.

Low-density lipoprotein is the main cholesterol carrier in the plasma, and is removed from the circulation at a much slower rate than that of many other particles. Low-density lipoprotein is bound to cells by high affinity receptors. When it enters the cell it is degraded in lysosomes to liberate cholesterol: dietary cholesterol inhibits the activity of enzymes responsible for endogenous cholesterol synthesis. The number of cell receptors is regulated by intracellular cholesterol levels.

High-density lipoproteins form the other group of lipoproteins in the circulation; these are mainly synthesized in the liver and intestinal mucosa. Phospholipids and cholesterol are transferred to high-density lipoproteins, where cholesterol esters are formed by the action of lecithin cholesterol acyl transferase.

THE FUNCTION OF LIPIDS

Triglycerides

These are derived from animal and plant dietary sources and account for up to 95 per cent of the lipids in adipose tissue. They are a source of energy during periods of starvation. During periods of adequate feeding, triglycerides can be synthesized in the body and stored.

Phospholipids

Phospholipids are fundamental components of cell membranes.

Cholesterol

Dietary cholesterol is derived mainly from dairy products and eggs: diets high in saturated fat are generally high in cholesterol. The average intake in people eating Western diets is 300 to 500 mg per day, but it may be as high as 1000 mg.

Cholesterol is also synthesized in the body and is excreted in bile salts and bile as free cholesterol.

Cholesterol is an important component of cell membranes and is particularly involved in the regulation of membrane fluidity and stability. It is transported round the body as a component of lipoproteins and is also an important precursor of steroid hormones and bile acids.

No other blood constituent varies so much between or within populations as plasma cholesterol level, with a range of 100 to 275 mg/dl (2.6 –7.1 mmol/1).

HYPERLIPIDAEMIA

A high level of circulating lipoproteins usually results from an increase in their synthesis due to a diet high in saturated fat and/or a genetically determined reduction in their removal from the circulation. Depending on the type of particles this causes an increase in the concentration of cholesterol and/or triglycerides in the plasma. Table 4 is one classification of familial hyperlipidaemia, based on the World Health Organization (Frederickson) classification. Familial hyperlipidaemia is one of the most common inherited conditions, affecting at least 1 in every 500 people in the United Kingdom. In some populations, such as Lebanese and Afrikaaners, the incidence is much higher. It is inherited in an autosomal dominant manner.

Conditions which may cause secondary hyperlipidaemia include diabetes mellitus, hypothyroidism, excessive alcohol intake, obesity, nephrotic syndrome, pregnancy, biliary obstruction, myeloma, and intake of drugs such as thiazide, steroids, β-blockers, and oral contraceptives.

Table 4 Typical lipoprotein patterns in hyperlipidaemia

Type	Chylomicrons	VLDL	LDL	HDL
I	High	Normal or low	Normal or low	Normal or low
IIA	Normal	Normal	High	Normal
IIB	Normal	Raised	High	Normal
III	Normal	VLDL/LDL raised and abnormal in composition		
IV	Normal	Raised	Normal	Normal
V	Normal	Raised	Normal	Normal

EPIDEMIOLOGY OF ATHEROSCLEROSIS

Incidence

Atherosclerosis and its complications are the leading cause of morbidity and mortality in the Western world, accounting for more than 50 per cent of all deaths. Over 80 per cent of these deaths are due to arteriosclerosis and hypertension combined.

Prevalence

Atherosclerosis shows a prevalence of nearly 100 per cent in adults. The severity of the disease varies from mild to severe when comparisons are made between groups, individuals, and even within individuals. In general, atherosclerosis increases with age, but it is not thought to be an intrinsic biological ageing process as most mammalian species age without spontaneously developing atherosclerosis.

Males are affected more frequently than females, but the differences tend to diminish with increasing age: the ratio of affected males to females is 6:1 at ages 35 to 44, but 2:1 in the 65 to 74 age group.

Heredity

Heredity influences the severity of atherosclerosis directly by affecting arterial wall structure and function and indirectly through such factors as hypertension, hyperlipidaemia, diabetes, and obesity.

Risk factors

Epidemiological studies (such as the Framingham study) show that certain habits, diseases, and lifestyles are more important than others and offer different degrees of risk (Table 5). It must be realized that advanced atherosclerosis and its clinical complications are uniquely human conditions. It is not possible to follow the progression of atherosclerosis within an individual, and epidemiology has to rely on the assessment of clinical consequences of atherosclerosis, such as myocardial infarction, as they apply to populations. Although these risk factors may be important in the development of these clinical complications; they do not necessarily *per se* reflect what is going on at the level of the intimal lesion in a single individual.

Table 5 Risk factors for atherosclerosis

High risk factors
- Smoking
- Hypetension
- Hyperlipidaemia (raised LDL)
- High fat diets

Other probable risk factors
- Diabetes mellitus (hyperglycaemia)
- Elevated blood uric acid (gout)
- Hypothyroidism
- Renal disease
- Familial history of premature atherosclerosis

Factors having an uncertain role
- Sedentary life
- Obesity
- Anxiety

The degree of atherosclerosis may potentially be decreased by:
- Low fat diets
- Exercise
- High levels of high density lipoprotein (HDL)

PATHOLOGY

Types of lesions

The lesions seen in atherosclerosis consist of fatty streaks, fibrous plaques, and complicated or advanced plaques.

Fatty streaks are yellow, flat lesions arising between the intima and internal elastic lamina, consisting of macrophages containing cholesterol and cholesterol esters derived from plasma. Although they occur at all ages, fatty streaks are most commonly seen in the aorta of children. These lesions can regress, and there is still debate as to whether they progress to advanced plaques.

Fibrous plaques are grey-white, elevated lesions consisting of subendothelial proliferations of smooth muscle cells, collagen, and variable amounts of extracellular lipid (Fig. 1). They appear

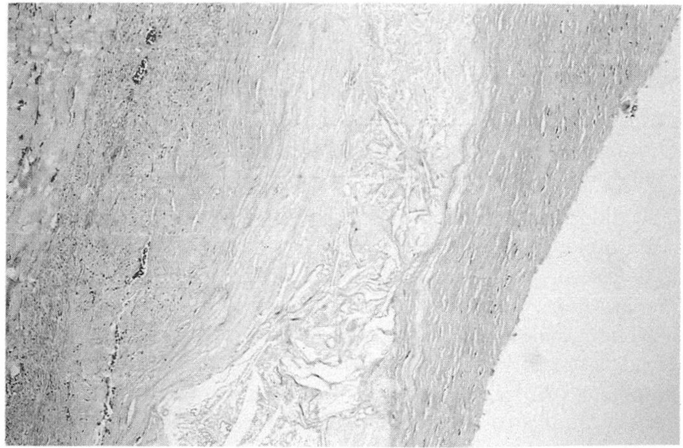

Fig. 1 This light micrograph shows a fibrous atheromatous plaque. Note the cholesterol clefts which are left behind as soluble lipids are removed during tissue processing. There are some cells within the atheroma, but these are sparse (haematoxylin and eosin).

in the second and third decades of life at bifurcation points in arteries and the aorta.

Complicated/advanced plaques are pale yellow-grey or white raised lesions of varying size affecting the intima and inner media. They give rise to local complications (Fig. 2) and are clinically the most important type of lesion.

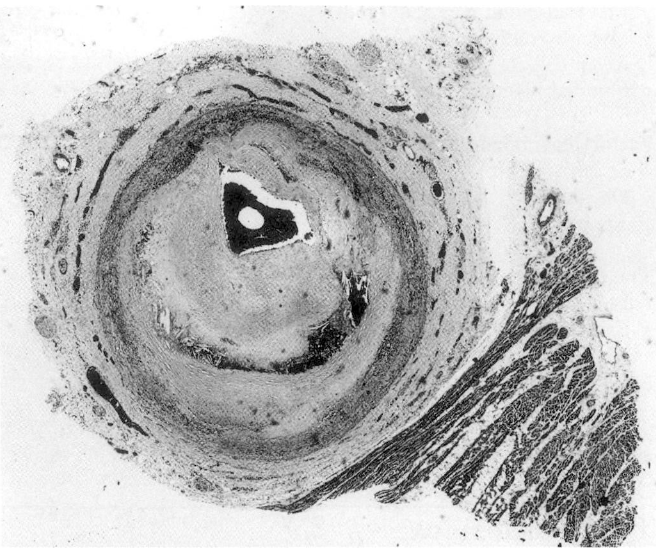

Fig. 2 This low power light micrograph shows a coronary artery which is almost completely occluded with atheroma and organized thrombus. In addition, the plaque has fissured, resulting in haemorrhage. The coronary artery media is thinned and there is a mild adventitial chronic inflammatory cell infiltrate.

The local sequelae of the advanced plaque give rise to the clinical complications of atherosclerosis, most commonly ischaemia and infarction.

The local complications of advanced atherosclerosis include stenosis of the arterial or aortic lumen, plaque ulceration and fissuring (with or without atheroemboli), thrombosis (with or without thromboemboli), calcification, haemorrhage into the plaque, aneurysm formation (with or without thrombosis and thromboemboli), and chronic inflammation (chronic periaortitis) see Section 7.2 (Fig. 2.)

Patterns of lesion distribution

The abdominal aorta is affected more often than the thoracic aorta. Atherosclerosis is particularly seen around ostia of branch vessels. It is rare in pulmonary arteries, except in the presence of pulmonary hypertension.

Major anatomical patterns include involvement of coronary arteries, the terminal abdominal aorta and its branches, the innominate, carotid, and subclavian arteries and their branches, and visceral branches of the abdominal aorta including the renal arteries.

Although these patterns of distribution are fairly characteristic, clinical experience suggests that there is some selectivity in their occurrence in different categories of patients. Some patients, for example, are prone to cerebrovascular disease with little or no evidence of disease at other sites. It is unclear which factors are most important in determining anatomic patterns of involvement.

Pathogenesis of atherosclerosis

Multiple theories of atherogenesis have been proposed (Table 6). Perhaps the earliest and best known theories were those elaborated in 1844 by Carl von Rokitansky (the thrombogenic theory) and in 1835 by Rudolph Virchow (the lipid inhibition theory). Virchow also believed that atheroma was a chronic inflammatory process involving the intima. While it is now evident that platelets, fibrin, lipids and mononuclear cells do play a part in atherogenesis, the key question is, how? Many theories of atherogenesis still abound; it is likely that multiple factors which affect the status of the arterial wall and the composition and dynamics of the blood are involved.

Table 6 Theories of atherogenesis

Theory	Main element
Haemodynamic	Endothelial cell injury
Encrustation (Rokitansky)	Thrombosis
Lipid imbibition (Virchow)	Cholesterol-LDL-macrophage
Response to injury (Ross)	Vessel wall and platelets
Neoplastic (Benditt)	Smooth muscle cells
Viral (Benditt)	Endothelial/smooth muscle cells
LDL uptake (Brown and Goldstein)	Cholesterol-LDL-macrophages

In the past decade, the cellular nature of atherosclerosis has been realized and more clearly understood. Many immunological and molecular biology studies have been performed on experimentally induced lesions in animal models but an increasing amount of research is being undertaken in man. We are only just beginning to understand how hypercholesterolaemia and hypertension might lead to the development of atherosclerosis.

It is now clear that the principal changes that take place in the artery wall during atherogenesis occur largely within the intima of medium and large arteries. The key factors include the entry of cells and non-cellular substances, including lipids (principally low-density lipoproteins), from the plasma.

Role of the arterial wall

Intimal injury and smooth muscle cell proliferation

Injury to the intima causes proliferation of smooth muscle cells and myofibroblasts (cells with phenotypic characteristics of both smooth muscle cells and fibroblasts) within the intima. Proliferation can be seen in experimental animal models and in man as part of an age-related phenomenon, known as diffuse intimal thickening. Cultured smooth muscle cells *in vitro* are capable of synthesizing extracellular matrix components such as collagen, elastin, and mucopolysaccharides. Smooth muscle cells can also metabolize lipoproteins and accumulate cholesterol esters.

Reponse to injury theory

Mechanical, chemical, or immunological damage to the endothelium, results in entry of plasma constituents such as lipoproteins and fibrinogen, together with cellular elements including platelets, monocytes, and lymphocytes. Platelet-derived growth factor can induce smooth muscle cell proliferation, forming a plaque which then progresses due to lipid infiltration and modification, further proliferation of monocytes, platelets and lymphocytes, and smooth muscle cell proliferation and collagen production and degradation.

Monoclonal theory

Cells in atheromatous plaques of black females were observed by Benditt and coworkers to be monotypic for the A or B isoenzyme of glucose 6-phosphate dehydrogenase. This was interpreted as evidence that atherosclerosis represents a neoplastic intimal lesion. There is, however, a recognized tendency to monotypism in other benign, non-neoplastic proliferative lesions, such as scar tissue.

Viral theory

Herpes virus particles and viral DNA can be detected in early atherosclerotic lesions in humans. How this relates to atherogenesis is still unclear.

Role of lipids

Dietary evidence

This remains a surprisingly controversial area. Dietary fat intake is probably important, since human populations consuming typical diets high in saturated fats and cholesterol have high mean serum cholesterol levels and have high mortality rates from coronary artery disease.

Recent studies performed on large numbers of hypercholesterolaemic individuals who have been treated with drugs that reduce plasma cholesterol levels have shown that decreasing cholesterol levels over time decreases the incidence of the clinical sequelae of atherosclerosis. As a result, guidelines for the reduction of serum cholesterol levels have been drawn up. Plasma cholesterol levels below 200 mg/dl are acceptable; levels between 200 and 240 mg/dl should be treated by diet; levels above 240 mg/dl should be treated by diet together with cholesterol lowing agents such as 3-hydroxy–3-methylglutaryl coenzyme A reductase and bile acid sequestrants.

Hyperlipidaemia

Patients with genetically determined hyperlipoproteinaemia (Table 4) and marked hypercholesterolaemia due to nephrotic syndrome, diabetes mellitus, and untreated myxoedema, have severe atherosclerosis. However, the correlation between the severity of atherosclerosis and cholesterol levels within an individual is imperfect: the state of circulating lipids, rather than the level, may be of importance.

Low-density lipoprotein

Low-density lipoprotein is the main carrier of plasma cholesterol to the tissues of the body. Studies on patients with familial hypercholesterolaemia have shown that hepatocytes, fibroblasts, and smooth muscle cells carry high affinity receptors for plasma low-density lipoprotein, which are down-regulated when this lipoprotein is plentiful. Patients with familial hypercholesterolaemia have defective receptors.

Low-density lipoprotein can be modified by malonation and oxidation, principally by macrophages or exogenous agents. Macrophages, endothelial cells, and smooth muscle cells also contain non-saturable, 'scavenger receptors' or 'modified low-density lipoprotein receptors' which are not down-regulated and which preferentially take up modified low-density lipoprotein.

High levels of circulating high-density lipoprotein appear to be protective, even in individuals with raised cholesterol levels.

Oxidized lipids

Ceroid is the name given to the insoluble yellowish pigment present in mammalian tissues, especially in the presence of vitamin E deficiency. It is regularly seen in association with human atherosclerotic plaques and can be regarded as the hallmark of the advanced lesion. It is insoluble in lipid solvents and is therefore recognizable in routinely processed tissue sections by lipid stains such as Oil Red O (Fig. 3). It is thought to consist of polymerized products of oxidized lipoproteins, predominantly low-density lipoproteins, within macrophages.

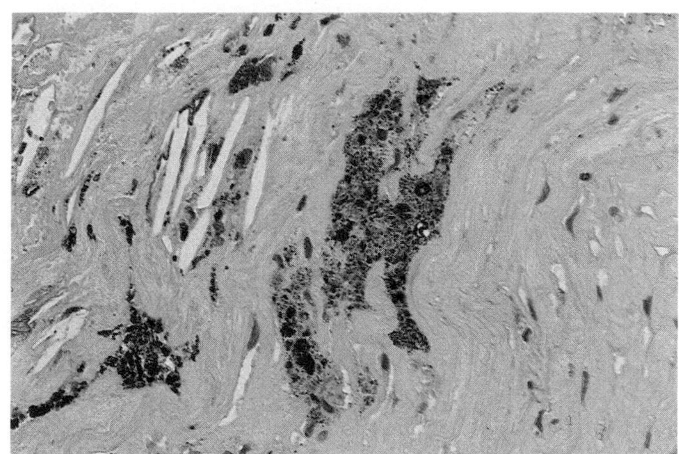

Fig. 3 This light micrograph shows ceroid rings and granules, both within macrophages and extracellularly in the base of the atheromatous plaque. This section has been stained with Oil Red O which, in this routinely processed tissue section, stains insoluble lipid.

Oxidized lipids are toxic and immunogenic: they can act as chemoattractants for leucocytes and induce cell proliferation. Their effects could account for the progression and some of the complications of atherosclerosis.

Experimental/animal models

Lesions resembling atherosclerosis can be induced in experimental animals by a combination of high lipid diets and intimal injury.

Role of cells in atherosclerosis

Endothelial cells

The endothelium is able to modify and transport lipoproteins, to form vasoactive substances, to participate in leucocyte adherence, to produce growth factors, and to participate in procoagulant and anticoagulant activity.

Injury to endothelial cells or exposure to cytokines can induce endothelial cells to express genes for mitogens such as platelet-derived growth factor and interleukin-1. This may be of importance in the progression from early to advanced atherosclerotic plaques. Endothelial cells express class II major histocompatibility antigens and are involved in antigen presentation; this may be of importance in immunologically induced endothelial damage and in recruitment of lymphocytes into the lesion.

In advanced plaques, the endothelium no longer remains, but new vessel formation is seen at the base of the plaque. The endothelial cells at these sites may perform similar functions.

Smooth muscle cells

Smooth muscle cells are the principal source of collagen in the fibrous plaque; they can take up and modify lipoprotein and they are an important source of platelet-derived growth factor. Smooth muscle cells are present in diffuse intimal thickening and their numbers are increase in larger lesions.

Macrophages/monocytes—the macrophage hypothesis

Foam cells, which are present in fatty streaks and at the edges of most advanced plaques, are macrophages (Fig. 4) and macrophages are found in the necrotic base of the advanced atherosclerotic plaque.

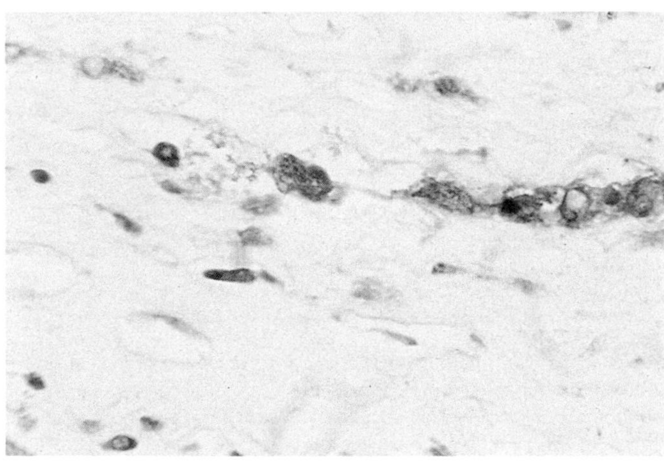

Fig. 4 This light micrograph shows a section of a human atherosclerotic plaque stained immunohistochemically with a monoclonal antibody which recognizes human monocyte/macrophages (stained brown).

In terms of the development of the clinical complications of atherosclerosis, the most important roles of the macrophage include their interactions with lipoproteins—secretion of monokines which recruit and modulate the behaviour of other cells (platelet-derived growth factor, fibroblast growth factor, transforming growth factor α and β, colony-stimulating factor-1, tumour necrosis factor, and interleukin-1), release of enzymes; release of oxygen radicals, and their ability to modify lipoprotein, rendering it toxic, immunogenic, and more amenable to the scavenger receptor pathway.

Platelets

Platelets produce growth factors and mitogens, the best known being platelet-derived growth factor, an endothelium-derived growth factor-like substance, and transforming growth factor-β. Platelets play an important role in thrombosis and in the coagulation process: they may be sources of mitogens during the development of early atherosclerotic lesions, when mural thrombus forms at sites of endothelial damage. In advanced plaques, lesions may progress at sites of fissuring due to secondary thrombosis, which may, in turn lead to smooth muscle cell proliferation and collagen deposition.

Lymphocytes

T lymphocytes, but not B lymphocytes, are present within early and advanced atherosclerotic plaques, but the reason for their presence remains unclear: it may imply that immunological phenomena are involved in atherogenesis or in the progression of atherosclerosis. These lymphocytes are activated and strongly express major histocompatibility class II antigens.

Both T and B lymphocytes are seen in the adventitia in chronic periaortitis (see Section 7.2), when the atheroma thins the media.

Role of haemodynamic factors

The location of fibrous plaques at bifurcation points and branch points can be best explained by consideration of increased haemodynamic forces at these sites. There is a direct relation between hypertension and atherosclerosis in systemic arteries. Atherosclerosis is only seen in the pulmonary arteries in association with pulmonary hypertension.

Role of thrombogenic factors

Mural thrombi may become organized to the endothelium and resemble fibrous plaques. Fibrin and platelets are associated with developing plaques, and thrombosis may be important in their extension. Intraplaque haemorrhage and fissuring exposes collagen, which is highly thrombogenic.

Do theories of atherogenesis explain clinical risk factors?

Hyperlipidaemia

Low-density lipoprotein is the source of lipid in early atherosclerotic plaques and of the large amounts of cholesterol in advanced plaques. Individuals with Type II or Type IV hyperlipoproteinaemia (Table 4) have more atherosclerosis. These individuals have high circulating levels of low-density lipoprotein without necessarily having a raised serum cholesterol.

Cigarette smoking

Cigarette smoking is the factor with the strongest epidemiological association with the incidence and severity of atherosclerosis. A series of glycoproteins derived from tobacco has been associated with an immune response within the vessel wall. Increased serum concentrations of carbon monoxide in smokers are also thought to be injurious to the endothelium.

Hypertension

Hypertension acts synergistically with other risk factors for atherosclerosis. Altered haemodynamic properties of blood flow, causing endothelial injury, and humoral mediators of blood pressure, such as renin and angiotensin may be involved. The specific mechanisms by which hypertension increases the severity of atherosclerosis, however, still remain unclear.

Diabetes mellitus

Many diabetic individuals are hypercholesterolaemic. The mechanisms underlying the increased severity of atherosclerosis seen in those who have normal cholesterol levels are unknown. Some diabetics have decreased levels of high-density lipoprotein and are often hypertensive. Specific factors in the arterial wall or present in the plasma of diabetics may account for these observations remain unidentified.

Regression of atherosclerosis

Although fatty streaks experimentally induced in animals are reversible, there is still controversy over whether advanced atherosclerotic lesions in humans can regress. Some studies have shown that angiographically demonstrable lesions in hypercholesterolaemic patients, become smaller with a combination of diet and cholesterol-lowering drugs.

A possible mechanism by which regression may occur is by lipid-laden intimal macrophages re-emerging into the blood, although there is no evidence that this occurs in man.

FURTHER READING

Ball M, Mann J. *Lipids and Heart Disease: a Practical Approach*. Oxford: University Press, 1988.

Benditt EP, Benditt JM. Evidence for a monoclonal origin of human atherosclerotic plaques. *Proc Natl Acad Sci USA*, 1973; **70**: 1753–56.

Brown MS, Goldstein JL. A receptor-mediated pathway for cholesterol homeostasis. *Science*, 1986; **232**: 34–47.

Mitchinson MJ, Ball RY. Macrophages and atherogenesis. *Lancet*, 1987; **ii**: 146–9.

Parums DV. Inflammatory mediators and atherosclerosis. *Biochem Soc Trans*, 1990; **18**: 1069–72.

Ross R. The pathogenesis of atherosclerosis—an update. *N Engl J Med*, 1986; **314**: 488–500.

Woolf N. *The Pathology of Atherosclerosis*. London: Butterworth, 1982.

7.2 Chronic periaortitis

DINAH V. PARUMS

INTRODUCTION

In 1890, in the first volume of *Archives of Surgery*, Hutchinson commented that, in elderly patients, arteries are liable to a spreading inflammation which glues the artery to its sheath. He noted that inflammation was the hallmark of atheroma, differentiating it from senile change or fatty degeneration.

Chronic inflammation in the aortic adventitia is commonly seen in association with advanced atherosclerosis when the aortic media is thinned (Fig. 1). This condition is known as chronic periaortitis. Chronic periaortitis is most common, and most severe, at sites where atherosclerosis is also most severe (see Section 7.1), notably in the lower abdominal aorta.

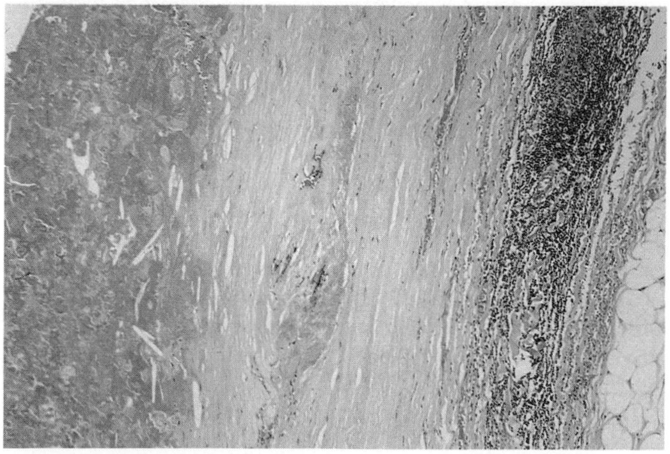

Fig. 1 A low power light micrograph of a section from an atherosclerotic abdominal aortic aneurysm taken during elective repair. Note the advanced atherosclerosis (left) with thinning and disruption of the aortic media and a dense inflammatory infiltrate in the aortic adventitia (right) (haematoxylin and eosin).

The inflammatory cells consist of lymphocytes and plasma cells (Fig. 2). The degree of inflammation varies: it is usually minimal, or subclinical, and is only noted on histological examination. Occasionally, the inflammation is severe enough to be visible macroscopically or on computed tomography (CT) scan. At this stage it is likely to produce clinical effects. Clinical chronic periaortitis can be seen in dilated or undilated aortas.

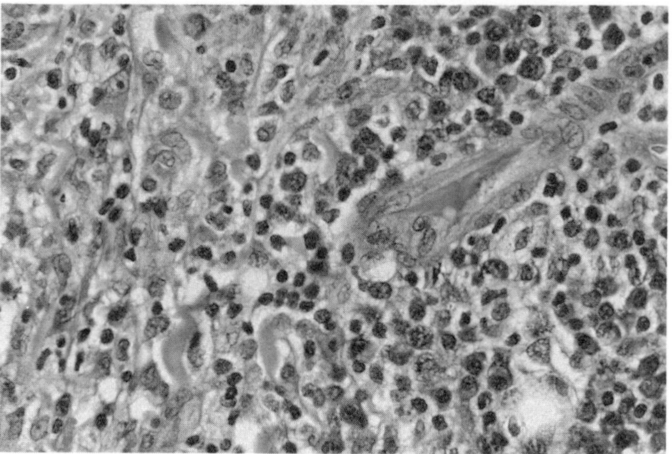

Fig. 2 This light micrograph shows chronic inflammatory cells, lymphocytes, plasma cells, and macrophages, seen here clustered around the vasa vasorum in the adventitia (haematoxylin and eosin).

'IDIOPATHIC RETROPERITONEAL FIBROSIS'

'Idiopathic retroperitoneal fibrosis' was first described by Albarran in 1905 but is best known by the name of Ormond who described it in 1948. It is typically a disease of middle-aged to elderly males who develop chronic inflammation and fibrosis around the lower abdominal aorta (see Section 7.1). This inflammatory process tends to drag neighbouring hollow structures towards the midline. The disease usually presents as a urological problem with obstruction of one or both ureters, often resulting in hydronephrosis.

The periaortic distribution of the idiopathic retroperitoneal fibrosin first emerged from necropsy studies (Fig. 3) and has been confirmed by CT (Fig. 4). The presentation is associated with a raised erythrocyte sedimentation rate and there is often a dramatic response to steroids. Histopathological examination reveals advanced aortic atherosclerosis with medial disruption and adventitial infiltrates of lymphocytes and plasma cells. The degree of atherosclerosis is not always appreciated as the fibrous tissue alone is often submitted for histological examination following surgical mobilization of the ureters.

A similar chronic inflammatory process around the thoracic aorta occurs much less commonly. This is known as idiopathic mediastinal fibrosis. The histopathological findings in these two conditions are identical, and they may occur in contiguity through the diaphragm.

Retroperitoneal fibrosis has been associated with the use of methysergide, an indole derivative with a strong structural similarity to serotonin which is used in the treatment of migraine. Its mechanism of action is uncertain but in the context of idiopathic retroperitoneal fibrosis it is suggested that the vessel wall is damaged by vasospasm provoked by the drug simulating the peripheral effects of serotonin. Idiopathic retroperitoneal fibrosis in patients treated with methysergide is often accompanied by fibrosis at other sites.

The rapidity with which patients with ureteric obstruction respond to corticosteroid treatment supports the view that the ureter is not blocked by fibrosis but rather by oedema and inflammation. This is confirmed histologically, although it is not known whether this oedema and inflammation obstructs the ureter directly or indirectly, by interfering with nerves or blood supply. Despite the value of steroid therapy, almost all surgeons still regard ureterolysis as the first line of management.

The term idiopathic retroperitoneal fibrosis is misleading: the disease is not idiopathic, but secondary to atherosclerosis; it is not retroperitoneal, but periaortic. The term is also misleading because it allows the incorporation of eccentric causes of fibrosis in the retroperitoneum, such as malignant neoplasm, endometriosis and diverticulitis (Table 1) into the category of what is a periaortic disease.

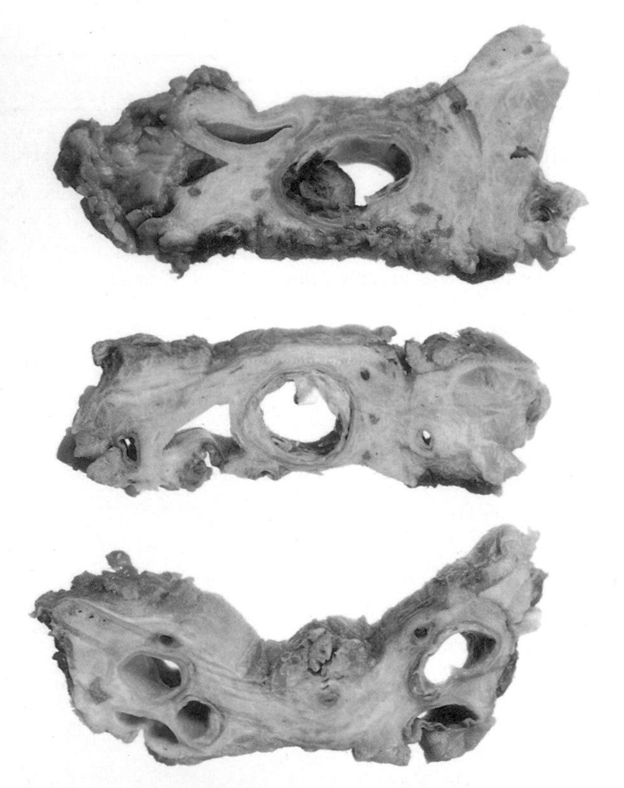

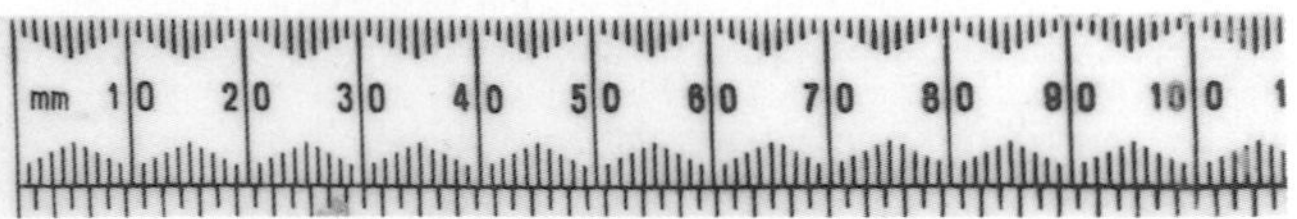

Fig. 3 The macroscopic appearance of the abdominal aorta, removed at necropsy and sectioned transversely down its length from a case of 'idiopathic retroperitoneal fibrosis'. The top section shows the area of maximal periaortic thickening (25 mm) just below the renal artery origin where the aortic diameter is 24 mm maximally. The middle section is at the aortic bifurcation and the bottom section shows the inflammation and fibrosis around the internal and external iliac vessels. The ureters are encased in fibrous tissue and the inferior vena cava is also involved.

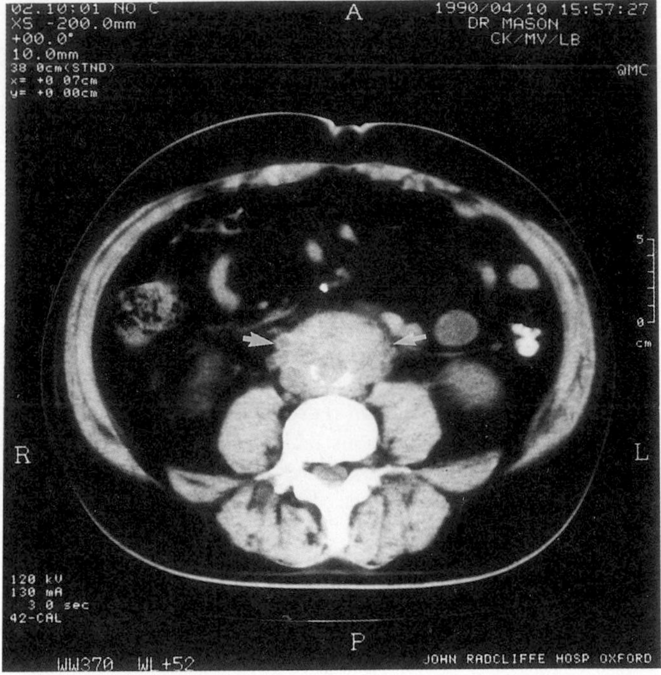

Fig. 4 An abdominal CT scan from a case of idiopathic retroperitoneal fibrosis which shows a dense, periaortic mass, 25 mm in thickness. The aorta is 24 mm in diameter. There is an associated right hydronephrosis due to obstruction of the right ureter by the inflammatory process.

Table 1 Causes of retroperitoneal fibrosis

Non-malignant
Diverticulitis
Endometriosis
Infection
Postirradiation
Crohn's disease
Inflammatory pseudotumour
Idiopathic retractile (sclerosing) mesenteritis
Intra-abdominal (mesenteric) desmoid
Fibromatoses of infancy and childhood
Paraganglioma
Gardner's syndrome
Drugs—methysergide, hydralazine, ergotamine
Malignant
Sarcoma
Lymphoma
Myeloma
Metastatic carcinoma

'INFLAMMATORY ANEURYSM'

Occasionally, the surgeon sees an abdominal aortic aneurysm encased in fibrous tissue that extends into the retroperitoneum (Figs. 5 and 6). These so-called 'inflammatory aneurysms' of the aorta have a reported incidence of 2.5 to 10 per cent of all aortic aneurysms.

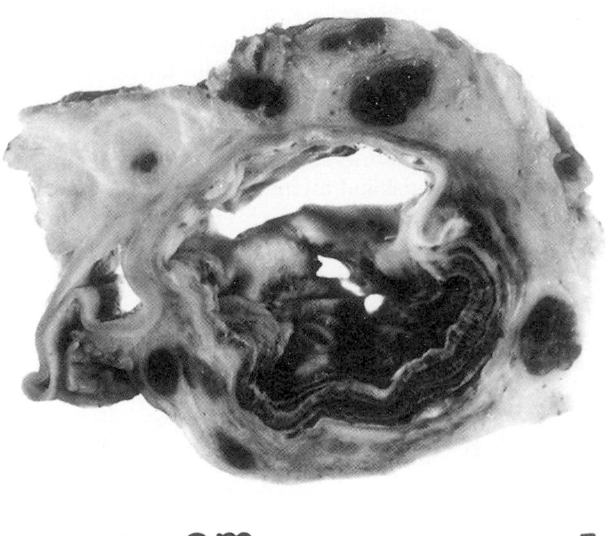

Fig. 5 The macroscopic appearance of the abdominal aorta, removed at necropsy and sectioned transversely down its length from a case of inflammatory aneurysm. This section shows the area of maximal periaortic thickening (18 mm) just below the renal artery origin where the aortic diameter is 48 mm maximally.

Inflammation of the aorta ('aortitis') has been recognized as an entity since the late sixteenth century when aortic aneurysm was known to be associated with syphilis. From the fifteenth century until the beginning of this century, syphilis was widespread in many countries and was probably the most common cause of aortitis. Today, there are numerous rare causes of aortitis which can lead to aneurysm formation (Table 2).

Abdominal aortic aneurysms are most commonly associated with advanced atherosclerosis. The aneurysm is secondary to thinning of the aortic media, probably due to the atherosclerosis. For some time, surgeons and pathologists have tended to classify these abdominal aortic aneurysms as either 'atherosclerotic' or 'inflammatory'. Recent large reviews from the Mayo Clinic in the

Table 2 Causes of aortitis resulting in aneurysm formation

Infectious
Syphilis
Bacterial, e.g. Staphylococcus, Pseudomonas, Pneumococcus, Salmonella, *E. coli*
Tuberculosis
Fungi
Non-infectious
Giant cell aortitis
Idiopathic aortitis (Takayasu's)
Polyarteritis nodosa
Rheumatoid arthritis
Rheumatic fever
Ankylosing spondylitis
Relapsing polychondritis
Behçet's disease
Infantile polyarteritis or Kawasaki disease
Systemic lupus erythematosus
Sarcoidosis
Cardiac myxoma embolus
Church–Strauss syndrome
Wegener's granulomatosis

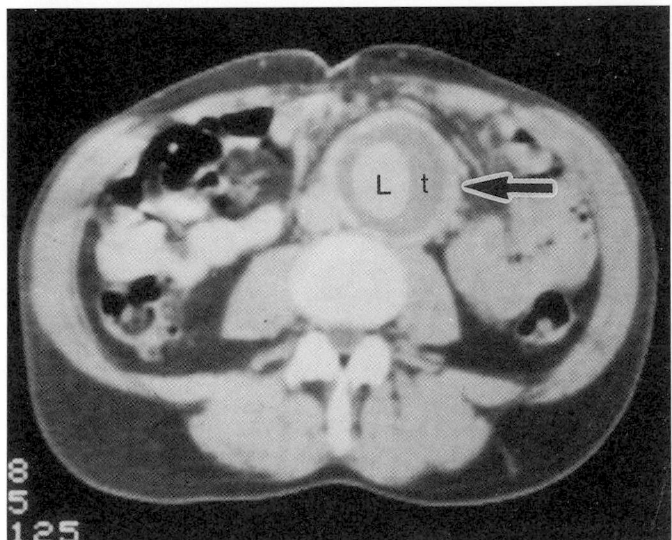

Fig. 6 A contrast enhanced abdominal CT scan from a case of inflammatory aneurysm which shows a dense, periaortic mass 8 mm in thickness (arrow). The aorta is 55 mm in diameter. The lumen (L) is opacified but not the thrombus (T) within the sac. Note the relation of the inflammatory tissue peripheral to the flecks of calcium present in the right lateral portion of the aortic wall.

United States and from Cambridge and Oxford in the United Kingdom have confirmed that all atherosclerotic abdominal aortic aneurysms are inflamed, but to a varying degree. The factors that determine the degree of chronic inflammation associated with atherosclerosis at this site remain unknown.

To add to the confusion, the term perianeurysmal retroperitoneal fibrosis has been used to describe the condition in which ureteric blockage has occurred as a result of fibrosis around atherosclerotic aneurysms of the abdominal aorta. The inflammatory infiltrate is the same as that seen in both idiopathic retroperitoneal fibrosis and inflammatory aneurysms, there is a raised erythrocyte sedimentation rate, and the disease responds to treatment with corticosteroids. Ureteral disease may occur in up to 23 per cent of patients with inflammatory aneurysms. The term inflammatory aneurysm is, therefore, misleading, since it perpetuates the image of aneurysm secondary to an inflammatory process. While this may be the mechanism underlying mycotic aneurysm, which is very rare, both medial thinning, giving rise to aneurysmal dilatation, and adventitial inflammation are sequelae of atherosclerosis (see Section 7.1).

CHRONIC PERIARTERITIS

Inflammation and fibrosis are frequently seen around coronary arteries in association with advanced atherosclerotic plaques. In this situation, the triad of atherosclerosis, medial thinning, and adventitial inflammation is termed chronic periarteritis.

CHRONIC PERIAORTITIS: A LOCAL COMPLICATION OF ATHEROSCLEROSIS

The unifying concept of chronic periaortitis as a local complication of atherosclerosis brings together the conditions previously termed idiopathic retroperitoneal fibrosis, inflammatory aneurysm, and perianeurysmal retroperitoneal fibrosis as part of a spectrum of the same disease, having in common advanced atherosclerosis, medial thinning, and adventitial chronic inflammation.

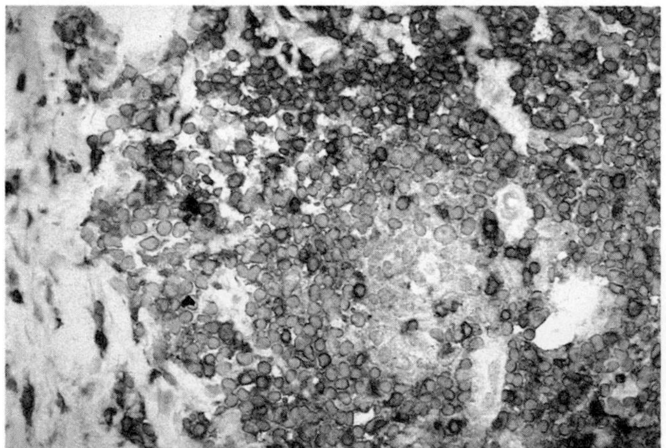

Fig. 7 Double immunohistochemical labelling of T lymphocytes by antibody CD3 (brown) and B-lymphocytes by antibody 4KB 128 (red) in the aortic adventitia in chronic periaortitis.

The histopathological findings—including characterization of the inflammatory cell populations (Fig. 7), clinical presentation and CT appearances of idiopathic retroperitoneal fibrosis, and inflammatory aneurysms show no important differences except that in the latter, the aortic diameter is increased. The factors which determine why some atherosclerotic aortas dilate and others do not are unknown, but hereditary defects in aortic collagen and elastin may play a role (see Section 7.1).

Inflammation is more likely to be a consequence of the atheroma than a cause, since inflammation is not seen in the adventitia of normal arteries and aortas, or in atherosclerotic plaques. In these cases, the media is intact. Immunoglobulin-secreting plasma cells occur in the aortic adventitial infiltrate in chronic periaortitis; this has been interpreted as evidence that chronic periaortitis is due to an autoimmune reaction to a component of the atherosclerotic plaque, likely to be a component of oxidized lipid or ceroid (see Section 7.1). Immunoglobulin, predominantly IgG, is associated with ceroid in plaques in patients with severe chronic periaortitis. Furthermore, antibodies to oxidized low-density lipoprotein and ceroid are detectable in patients with severe chronic periaortitis.

Computed tomography (CT) has an established role in the preoperative diagnosis of chronic periaortitis, by demonstrating the periaortic mass. Shrinkage of the periaortic mass does occur in response to steroid therapy of idiopathic retroperitoneal fibrosis. The mass in chronic periaortitis probably shrinks as part of its natural history. The variable proportion of cells and fibrous tissue seen histologically in chronic periaortitis suggests that in its early stages the tissue is highly cellular and contains immature fibroblasts; later it evolves into predominantly fibrous tissue, contracting as it does so. Contraction would account for the 'dragging' of mobile structures, such as the ureters, medially towards the aorta.

Finally, the core of textbook chronic periaortitis, or rather idiopathic retroperitoneal fibrosis and inflammatory aneurysm, is surrounded by a substantial and mysterious fringe of clinical associations which are ill-defined and which vary in both their severity and characteristics, examples being pulmonary hyalinizing granuloma, lymphomatoid granulomatosis, Reidel's thyroiditis, and sclerosing cholangitis. Studies of idiopathic retroperitoneal fibroses and inflammatory aneurysms have not confirmed these associations.

FURTHER READING

Albarran J. Rétention renale par periureterité; liberation externe de l'uretere. *Assoc France Urol*, 1905; **9**: 511–7.

Baker LRI, *et al.* Idiopathic retroperitoneal fibrosis; a retrospective analysis of sixty cases. *J. Urol*, 1988; **60**: 497–503.

Hutchinson J. On the diseases of the arteries. *Arch Surg* 1890; **1**: 84–6.

Mitchinson MJ. Chronic periaortitis and periarteritis. *Histopathology*, 1984; **8**: 589–600.

Ormond JK. Bilateral ureteral obstruction due to envelopment and compression by an inflammatory retroperitoneal process. *J Urol*, 1948; **59**: 1072–9.

Parums DV. The spectrum of chronic periaortitis. *Histopathology*, 1990; **16**: 423–31.

Pennell RC. *et al.* Inflammatory abdominal aortic aneurysms: a thirty year review. *J Vasc Surg*, 1985; **2**: 859–69.

7.3 The pathobiology of vasculitis

DINAH V. PARUMS

INTRODUCTION

Vasculitis can be defined as inflammation of vessel walls accompanied by a demonstrable structural change. The inflammation may be acute or chronic and the structural change may be accompanied by necrosis, often termed fibrinoid necrosis, or by fibrosis. The terms vasculitis, arteritis, and angiitis are used synonymously.

Inflammation and necrosis of vessels may be produced by infections with micro-organisms, by many chemical and physical agents, and by hypersensitivity phenomena. The pathological and clinical effects are widely variable depending upon the size and type of the vessels involved, their number and distribution, the chronicity of the lesions, and the presence of complications. The variable distribution throughout the body of vessels affected produces a highly variable and often bizarre clinical picture; circulation of vital organs (brain, heart, kidneys) may be affected. Acute forms of the disease may run a rapid course with all the lesions at the same stage of development; chronic forms show a more prolonged course with lesions in various stages of development and periods of remissions and exacerbations.

Complications include thrombosis, rupture of vessels with haemorrhage, vascular occlusion, and aneurysm formation (see Table 2 in Section 7.2).

CLASSIFICATION OF VASCULITIS

Few other diseases cause as much diagnostic and clinical controversy as the vasculitides and there is still no single, universally accepted classification system. This is largely because the pathogenesis of many of the vasculitic syndromes remains poorly understood, but also because of their varied clinical presentation and because their clinical and pathological features frequently overlap (see Section 7.9.3).

An aetiological classification of vasculitis

A classification system is only of value if it aids diagnosis and thus allows the most appropriate clinical management to be carried out. A clinicopathological classification based on the size of the affected vessel is given in Table 1. Although the most rational and memorable form of classification is one based on aetiology, in most instances the aetiology is unclear or unknown.

Table 1 Clinicopathological classification of vasculitis

I Infectious
II Non-infectious

1. Involving large, medium and small vessels
   - (a) Idiopathic (Takayasu's arteritis)
   - (b) Giant cell arteritis and aortitis
   - (c) Vasculitis and aortitis of rheumatic disease
2. Involving medium-sized and small vessels
   - (a) Thromboangiitis obliterans
   - (b) Polyarteritis (polyarteritis nodosa, Kawasaki disease)
   - (c) Granulomatosis vasculitis (Wegener's, Church–Strauss, sarcoid)
   - (d) Vasculitis of collagen vascular disease (rheumatic fever, rheumatoid arthritis, systemic lupus erythematosus, Behçet's disease, systemic sclerosis, Sjögren's)
3. Involving small blood vessels
   Serum sickness, Henoch-Schönlein purpura, drug-induced, malignancy-associated, mixed cryoglobulinaemia, hypocomplementaemia, inflammatory bowel disease, primary biliary cirrhosis, Goodpasture's syndrome, transplant vasculitis.

Infectious

Infectious vasculitis is the only form of the condition which is completely understood. Small, medium-sized, and large vessels may be infected by pyogenic bacteria, mycobacteria, fungi, Rickettsia, viruses, protozoa, or spirochaetes (*Treponema pallidum*). With regard to the last, syphilis deserves special mention.

Syphilis

Syphilitic disease of the large arteries is rare, since it occurs in the tertiary stage of the disease, which is now seldom left untreated for the long periods required for this to occur. Syphilitic aortitis has four main manifestations: syphilitic aortitis, syphilitic aneurysm, aortic insufficiency, and syphilitic coronary ostial stenosis. In syphilitic aortis the inflammatory process actively disrupts and destroys the lamellar units which make up the aortic media, resulting in replacement fibrosis. The inflammation is most prominent at the vasa vasorum which are surrounded by chronic inflammation featuring abundant plasma cells. These vessels may undergo endarteritis obliterans. Although these appearances are seen mainly in the ascending aorta and the arch, the descending aorta may also be affected. The intima may show the classical 'tree bark' appearance of intimal thickening.

Non-infectious

Hypersensitivity

A number of conditions characterized by inflammation and segmental necrosis of small vessels are attributed to immunologically mediated injury and are grouped under the generic term 'necrotizing vasculitis'. Necrotic regions often contain considerable amounts of fibrin (fibrinoid necrosis) (Fig. 1).

Immune complexes have been implicated in the pathogenesis of various forms of vasculitis in humans. In some patients, these immune complexes have been shown to contain hepatitis B virus, hepatitis A virus, cytomegalovirus, HTLV–1, HTLV–3, or parvovirus.

The model for these forms of vasculitis is that seen in experimentally induced serum sickness (the Arthus reaction). Immune complexes may also lodge in the glomerular basement membranes, producing an acute necrotizing glomerulonephritis.

Acute (hypersensitivity (leucocytoclastic) vasculitis)

Patients may have a history of short duration (weeks) of hypersensitivity to drugs or foreign proteins. Small veins, arteries, and

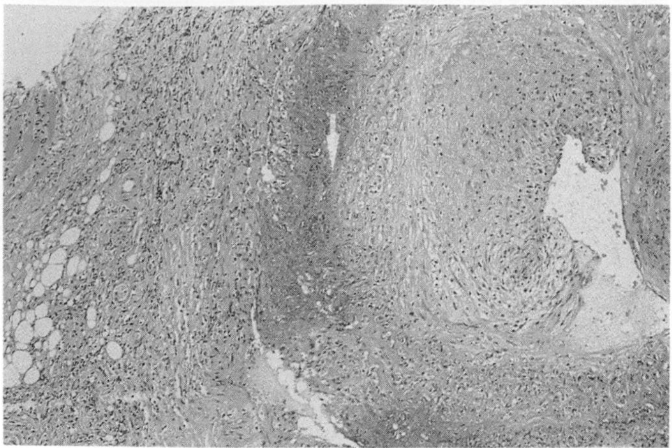

Fig. 1 This light micrograph shows the appearances of the necrotizing vasculitis of polyarteritis nodosa. Note the mixed acute and chronic inflammatory cell infiltrate and fibrinoid necrosis of the vessel wall (haematoxylin and eosin).

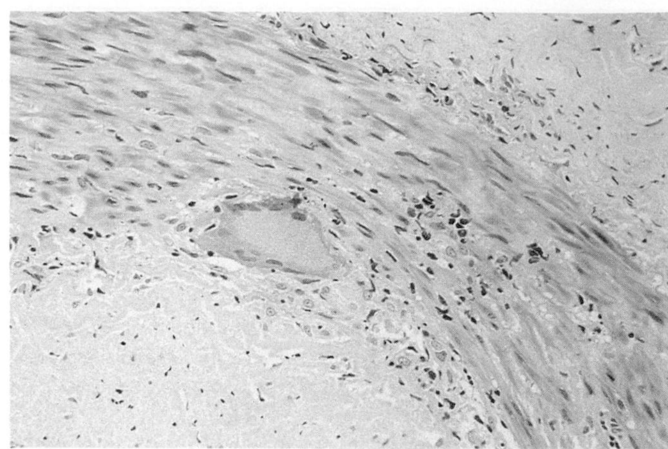

Fig. 2 This light micrograph shows giant cell or temporal arteritis. Note the giant cell granuloma formation associated with destruction of elastin (haematoxylin and eosin).

capillaries are affected. Lesions may be self-limited and regress, may cause death, or may progress to become chronic. Renal glomeruli may be affected, particularly in some distinct syndromes such as Henoch–Schönlein purpura, vasculitis associated with malignancy, and essential mixed cryoglobulinaemia. There is clinical, histological, and probably aetiological overlap between hypersensitivity vasculitis and the vasculitis seen in some of the collagen vascular diseases.

Chronic—polyarteritis nodosa and the polyarteritis group

Although these lesions may be produced experimentally by repeated exposure to an antigen, in man a specific antigen is rarely isolated. Hypertension is often present but no causal relation has been established. The natural history is one of months or years of remission, exacerbation, and eventual death: 60 per cent of patients die within 1 year.

Lesions at various stages may be seen, even within the same vessel. The more common form, polyarteritis nodosa, affects both arteries and veins, mainly in the kidneys, skin, heart, liver, gastrointestinal tract, pancreas, skeletal muscle, peripheral nervous system, and central nervous system, but not in the lungs. It is a disease which affects mainly young adults, with a female to male ratio of 3 : 1.

Kawasaki disease (mucocutaneous lymph node syndrome) is a form of polyarteritis which occurs in infancy and childhood, classically in children under 5 years, and most commonly in those under 1 year of age. The child presents with a fever, rash, and oedema of the palms and soles; desquamation of the fingertips may be present. There is also an acute, non-suppurative swelling of the cervical lymph nodes. Death, which occurs in less than 1 per cent of patients, is due to myocardial infarction following involvement of the coronary arteries. This disease is likely to be an infantile form of polyarteritis nodosa.

Erythema nodosum is a vasculitis of the skin and subcutaneous tissue, usually in the lower extremities, which occurs in association with many disorders that exhibit hypersensitivity phenomena, including sarcoidosis and inflammatory bowel disease.

Granulomatous

Among the conditions which may be termed 'granulomatous vasculitis' are included Wegener's granulomatosis, lymphomatoid granulomatosis, Churg–Strauss syndrome, necrotizing sarcoidal vasculitis, and bronchocentric granulomatosis. Because these usually present with symptoms and signs in the respiratory tract they have been termed by some as 'pulmonary angiitis and granulomatosis': this term is now out of date. Lymphomatoid granulomatosis, which was thought to be similar in many ways to Wegener's granulomatosis, is now known to be a T-cell lymphoma.

Autoantibodies to neutrophil cytoplasmic components including antineutrophil cytoplasmic antibody are associated with Wegener's granulomatosis and have been detected throughout the spectrum of vasculitis, excluding giant cell arteritis. In addition to providing evidence for an autoimmune aetiology for vasculitis, such serological findings may form the basis of new classification systems (see Section 7.9.3).

Giant cell arteritis (temporal arteritis; cranial arteritis) presents with focal granulomatous inflammation of medium and small arteries (especially cranial vessels) of the elderly. This inflammation is localized to and destroys elastin fibres (Fig. 2), and probably represents an autoimmune reaction to components of elastin. There is a female to male ratio of 3:1. Patients present with headache, throbbing temporal pain and tenderness, or with fever and malaise. The disease usually follows a benign course over 6 to 12 months, but blindness and death may occur. There is a dramatic response to steroids. Giant cell aortitis which may affect the thoracic or abdominal aorta and which may be associated with dissecting aneurysm formation is present in 10 per cent of patients.

Wegener's granulomatosis is an acute, necrotizing granulomatous disease of the arteries, veins, and adjacent tissues of the upper respiratory tract. It may be associated with focal or diffuse glomerulonephritis. There is a dramatic response to cyclophosphamide.

Churg–Strauss syndrome is a multisystem vasculitis which involves pulmonary and splenic vessels and is associated with bronchial asthma and eosinophilia. The vascular lesions resemble polyarteritis nodosa histologically.

Takayasu's arteritis (pulseless disease) presents as a clinical syndrome of ocular disturbance, and marked weakness of pulse in the upper extremities, related to fibrous thickening of the aortic arch with narrowing or obliteration of the origins of the great vessels. It may also affect the origin of large vessels in the abdominal aorta, e.g. renal arteries. It is predominantly seen in young women (female to male ratio of 9 : 1), with an average age of onset of 30 years. Aneurysms, haemorrhage, and thrombosis are common.

Thromboangiitis obliterans (Buerger's disease) is characterized by segmental, thrombosing, obliterative acute and chronic inflammation of arteries and veins, usually of the legs, leading to gangrene. It is almost exclusively seen in young male cigarette smokers.

Vasculitis of collagen vascular disease

The collagen vascular diseases include arthritis, myositis, carditis, and vasculitis. There is considerable overlap between the hypersensitivity and granulomatous categories of vasculitis in these conditions.

Rheumatoid arteritis occurs in a small number of men with rheumatoid arthritis affecting the spine (rheumatoid spondylitis). This is a true panarteritis, with necrosis and fibrosis of the media, obliteration of vasa vasorum, and intimal thickening. Between 25 and 30 per cent of patients have an aortitis, which may feature giant cells.

Behçet's syndrome, originally described as the triple symptom complex of recurrent oral and genital ulcers and relapsing iritis, is now recognized as a systemic disease which may involve any organ. The disease is most prevalent in patients from the Mediterranean, the Middle East, and Japan (prevalence 1 in 10 000). It is seen more commonly in men in the third decade of life. The vascular lesions consist of thrombophlebitis, arterial thrombosis, and aneurysm formation.

Endocarditis, myocarditis, pericarditis, valvular heart disease, atherosclerosis, and hypertensive heart disease are all seen in systemic lupus erythematosus. Lupus vasculitis causes a polyarteritis type of necrotizing vasculitis in small and medium-sized systemic, cerebral, and pulmonary vessels. It may also affect large vessels, including the aorta, producing a variety of lesions including a giant cell granulomatous aortitis.

The classic vascular lesion of scleroderma is seen most commonly in the kidney where it resembles the lesion seen in malignant hypertension.

Dermatomyositis is a multisystem disease characterized by vascular inflammation affecting primarily the skin and muscle. It is part of a continuum that includes polymyositis (in which the skin is spared).

Relapsing polychondritis is a systemic disease characterized by recurrent inflammation and destruction of cartilaginous structures of the ears, nose, trachea, larynx, and joints. Systemic vasculitis occurs, which shows histological similarity to polyarteritis nodosa.

Sjögren's syndrome is a chronic lymphoproliferative disorder. Small vessel, hypersensitivity vasculitis, either lymphocytic or leucocytoclastic, occurs in 10 to 15 per cent of patients.

FURTHER READING

Fauci AS, Haynes BF, Katz P. The spectrum of vasculitis. *Ann Intern Med* 1978; **9**: 660–78.

Lei JT. Systemic and isolated vasculitis. A rational approach to classification and diagnosis. In: Rosen PP, Fechner RE, eds. *Pathology Annual.* Norwalk, Connecticut: Appleton and Lange, 1989 (part 1); **24**: 25–114.

7.4 The non-invasive vascular diagnostic laboratory

JOHN D. EDWARDS AND WILLIAM M. ABBOTT

The concept of a clinical diagnostic vascular laboratory was first formulated two decades ago. Technological advances made in the 1960s allowed methods originally developed for research to be applied to the non-invasive evaluation of blood flow and blood pressure in clinical settings. The earliest such techniques involved indirect methods for evaluating cerebrovascular and peripheral vascular insufficiency. Rapid developments in the technology over the following 20 years have produced both indirect and direct methods of evaluation which provide both anatomical and physiological descriptions of vascular pathology. This chapter reviews the current technology and methods used in the diagnostic vascular laboratory and their various applications in the clinical evaluation and treatment of cerebrovascular and peripheral vascular disease.

The authors thank Victoria A. Hennessy for providing the illustrations used in this section.

CAROTID DISEASE

Indications for non-invasive carotid testing

Stroke represents the third leading cause of death in the United States today. Since extracranial carotid atherosclerotic disease is one of the major causes of stroke, its diagnosis and treatment is an important issue. Patients at risk for stroke include those who have suffered prior stroke or transient ischaemic attacks, and perhaps those with asymptomatic carotid bruits. Non-invasive studies should be performed on all such high-risk patients to identify those who might benefit from medical treatment or carotid endarterectomy. The studies can also be used to monitor the natural progression of carotid disease in patients with mild to moderate carotid stenosis in whom initial surgical therapy is not indicated, and to rule out postoperative restenosis in patients who have undergone carotid endarterectomy. Most vascular surgeons advocate studies 1, 3, and 12 months after surgery, and annually thereafter.

Non-invasive studies of carotid vascular function fall into the two main categories of direct and indirect tests: direct methods enable the carotid bifurcation itself to be examined while the indirect methods assess the effects of carotid stenosis on the distal circulation (such as ophthalmic artery pressure). Twenty years ago the only non-invasive tests available were indirect methods. In the past 10 years rapid progress in the development of Doppler and pulsed echo ultrasound technology has increased the use of direct methods. Several specialists have suggested that duplex scanning may be the only non-invasive test needed in the evaluation of carotid atherosclerotic disease. This approach, however, fails to take into account the valuable information regarding cerebral collateral flow that the indirect tests provide. Thus many laboratories use indirect tests such as ocular pneumoplethysmography as adjuncts to direct Doppler methods (Table 1).

Table 1 Tests

Direct tests	Indirect tests
Continuous wave Doppler	Periorbital Doppler
Duplex ultrasound	Ocular pneumoplethysmography
Triplex ultrasound	
Transcranial Doppler	

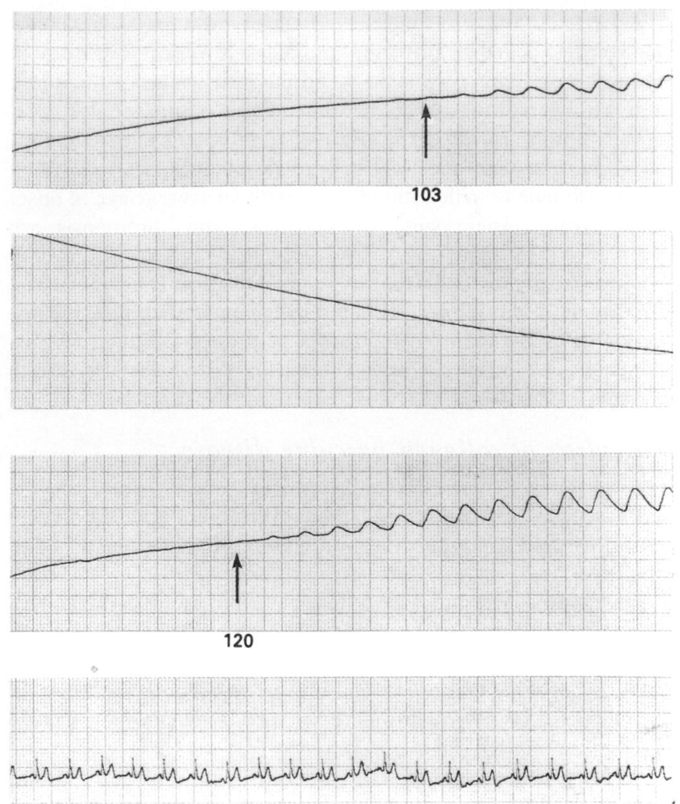

Fig. 1 Ocular pneumoplethysmography. Abnormal study in patient with severe right interal carotid artery stenosis. Upper tracing shows the reduced ocular pressure on the side of the stenosis.

OCULAR PNEUMOPLETHYSMOGRAPHY

Ocular pneumoplethysmography was initially designed as a non-invasive method for the determination of carotid stump pressure when applied in conjunction with common carotid test compression. The test then became popular as a non-invasive method of identifying haemodynamically significant carotid stenoses.

This technique uses suction ophthalmodynamometry for indirect measurement of the ophthalmic artery pressure. Small suction-cups applied to the sclera of each eye are capable of detecting arterial pulsations. The application of 300 mmHg suction pressure (500 mmHg in hypertensive patients) to the eye cups by an electric vacuum pump distorts the globe and increases the intraocular pressure. When the intraocular pressure increases above the ophthalmic artery pressure the arterial pulsations in the eye are abolished. The suction is then automatically reduced over a period of 30 s, while continuous strip chart recordings of the suction and the pulsations in the eye are made (Fig. 1). The systolic ophthalmic artery pressure in each eye is determined as the point at which pulsations first reappear. The pressure values recorded on the strip chart are actually measurements of the amount of suction: these values are converted to intraocular pressures using an analogue method.

The presence of haemodynamically significant carotid stenosis is indicated by differences in the ophthalmic artery pressures between the two eyes, the ratio of the ophthalmic artery to the brachial artery pressure, and the pulse amplitude. The test is considered abnormal if there is a difference of 5 mmHg or more between the two eyes; a difference of 1 to 4 mmHg and a ratio of less than 0.66 between the pressure in the ophthalmic artery and that in the brachial artery, a ratio of less than 0.60 between the pressure in the ophthalmic and brachial arteries; or a difference in amplitude of the first pulse of at least 2 mm (this last criterion is applied only to hypertensive patients, in whom the suction pressure does not obliterate the pulse). The accuracy with which haemodynamically significant carotid stenosis can be identified using these criteria is approximately 93 per cent. Ocular pneumoplethysmography is particularly valuable in patients in whom it is difficult to use direct tests; these include those with a densely calcified or highly tortuous carotid, those in whom the vessel has a high bifurcation, and immediately following carotid endarterectomy when the surgical incision prevents application of the Doppler probe. The study should not be performed in patients with glaucoma, lens implant, recent trauma, or those taking coumadin.

One of the most valuable applications of ocular pneumoplethysmography is as an adjunct to carotid duplex studies, to provide information regarding the status of the collateral cerebral circulation. The exact risk of stroke following a carotid arterial occlusion is difficult to predict and largely depends on the presence or absence of collateral flow, which may be extracranial, extracranial–intracranial, or intracranial. Extracranial collaterals may exist between the external carotid and subclavian or vertebral arteries; extracranial–intracranial collateral flow may occur between branches of the facial artery and the ophthalmic artery; intracranial collateral flow may involve the leptomeningeal vessels or the circle of Willis.

The adequacy of these collaterals can be assessed with ocular pneumoplethysmography since the ophthalmic artery pressure is a

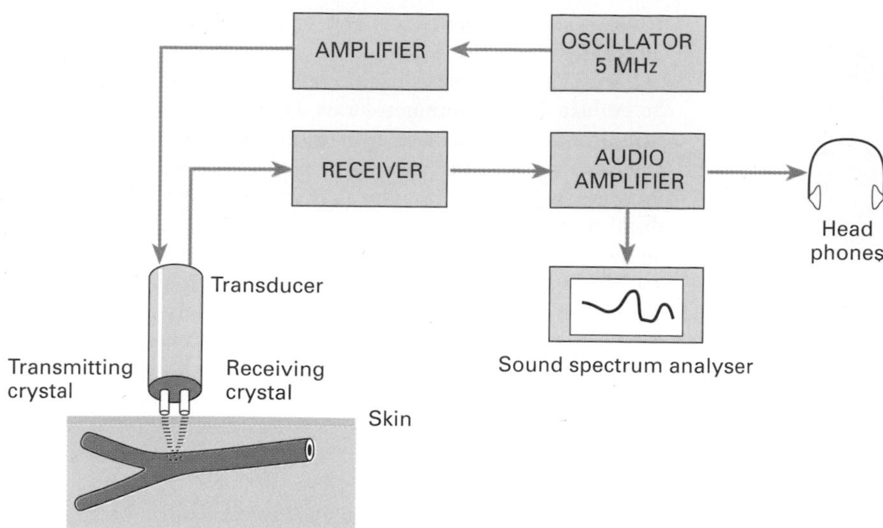

Fig. 2 Schematic of continuous wave Doppler study. In continuous wave Doppler the transmission and reception of the Doppler signal is continuous. The signal is processed for either audible or spectral analysis.

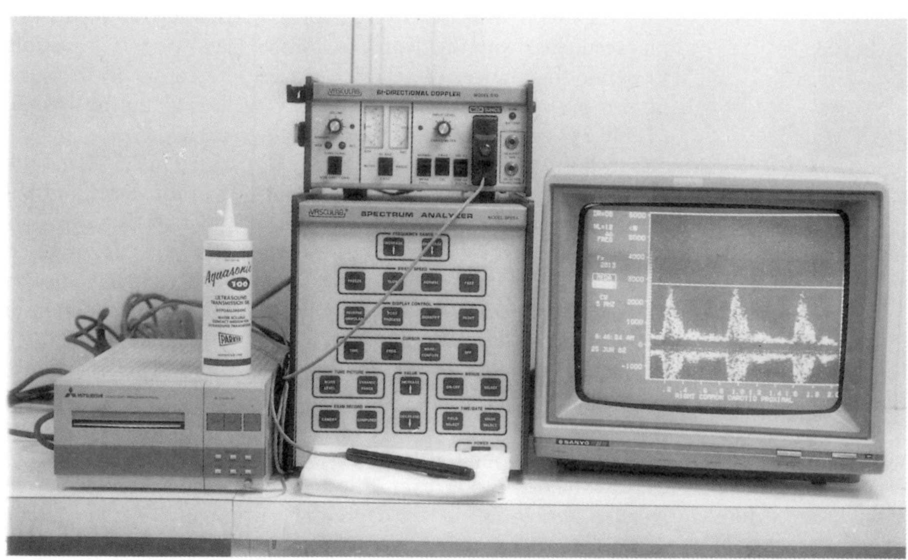

Fig. 3 Continuous wave Doppler equipment used for carotid examination. Left, fast Fourier transform spectrum analyser and 5-MHz probe. Right, spectral analysis of carotid artery displayed on video monitor.

reflection of both ipsilateral carotid flow and any collateral flow. Several studies have shown an increased risk of stroke in patients with abnormal results of ocular pneumoplethysmography compared to patients with carotid stenosis but a normal test. The combination of ocular pneumoplethysmography and ipsilateral common carotid artery compression provides a measure of the collateral ophthalmic artery pressure. Patients in whom this is less than 60 mmHg are at high risk for stroke should the carotid stenosis progress to occlusion. This test must be performed with extreme caution since the pressure applied to the common carotid artery could cause embolic stroke.

DIRECT STUDIES

Direct methods examine the carotid artery itself. The Doppler shift principle is used to identify abnormal velocities and flow patterns within the carotid artery, and B mode ultrasonography is used to identify the presence and characteristics of atherosclerotic plaque at the carotid bifurcation. Two types of ultrasonic Doppler velocity metering systems are currently popular: continuous-wave Doppler and range-gated pulsed Doppler.

Continuous-wave Doppler

Continuous-wave Doppler examination of the carotid artery is performed using a hand-held Doppler probe which contains two piezoelectric crystals, one for continuous transmission (usually at a frequency of 5 MHz) and the other for reception (Fig. 2). The probe is 'coupled' to the skin with an acoustic gel and held at an angle of 45 to 60° to the skin overlying the region of the common carotid artery in the area medial to the sternocleidomastoid muscle. The probe is advanced distally along the artery, guided by the audible signal and by the spectral frequency display on a video monitor (Fig. 3). The internal and external carotid arteries have unique Doppler shift frequency patterns: the internal carotid has high flow (and thus elevated frequency) in diastole due to the low resistance of the cerebral circulation. The external carotid, on the other hand, has low or almost no flow (Doppler shift frequency approaches 0 kHz) during diastole due to the normally high resistance of the external carotid system (Fig. 4). Because the continuous mode of transmission does not provide any spatial resolution, these unique Doppler patterns identify which artery is being

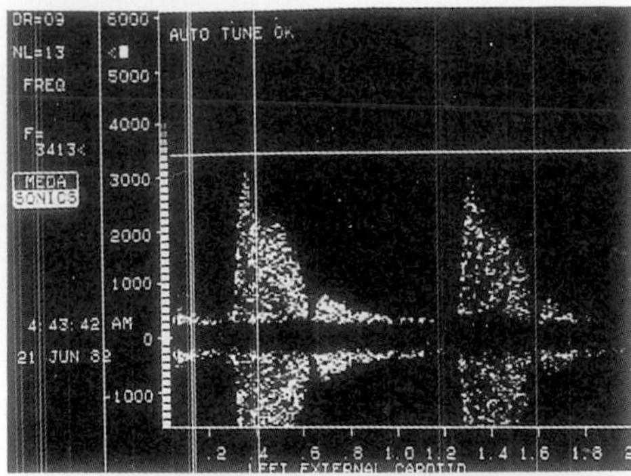

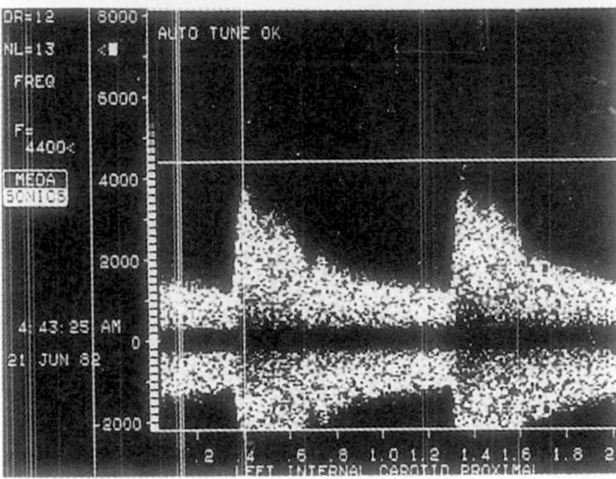

Fig. 4 Normal continuous wave Doppler spectrum from: left, external carotid; right, internal carotid. The internal carotid artery is identified by the high diastolic flow (and thus high frequency shift) during diastole due to low resistance of cerebral circulation.

examined. Pathological alterations in flow, such as increased distal internal carotid resistance due to disease, are a source of potential confusion when making this identification.

The audible Doppler signal provides a great deal of information regarding the presence of abnormal flow, but this is very subjective and does not result in a permanent record of the study. More sophisticated methods for analysis of the Doppler shift frequency data have therefore been developed: the most commonly used involves real-time sound spectrum analysis using fast Fourier transform to produce a graphic display of the Doppler spectrum obtained from insonation of the carotid artery. In the display, Doppler shift frequency (which corresponds to blood flow velocity) appears on the vertical axis and time is on the horizontal axis; the amplitude of any specific frequency is indicated by a continuous grey scale. The intensity of the grey scale reflects the number of red blood cells travelling at the velocity which produces that particular Doppler shift frequency. The vertical axis in the spectral display can be expressed as frequency (kHz) or as velocity (cm/s). If a continuous-wave Doppler probe transmitting at 5 mHz is directed at an incident angle of 60° to the carotid artery, a Doppler shift frequency of 1 kHz equals a blood flow velocity of 30 cm/s.

Carotid artery stenosis has two effects on blood flow which can be evaluated with continuous-wave Doppler and spectral analysis: turbulent flow and an increase in the flow velocity. As the degree of stenosis increases, the velocity of flow in the narrowed segment increases, as does the Doppler shift frequency. Flows immediately distal to the stenosis becomes increasingly turbulent, resulting in an increase in the range of frequencies represented in the spectral waveform (special broadening). The continuous nature of the ultrasound transmission used in the continuous-wave technique means that the entire cross-section of the carotid artery is insonated. Since normal blood flow is laminar, with blood travelling along the arterial wall flowing at a slower speed than that in the central portion of the artery, there is a certain amount of 'spectral broadening' in an entirely normal vessel, which makes spectral broadening more difficult to discern.

A variety of quantitative analytical methods may be applied to the frequency spectrum data in order to define more precisely the severity of disease in the carotid artery. One popular and fairly simple method of such analysis involves correlating the peak Doppler frequency with the degree of luminal narrowing. It is possible to define four ranges of severity of carotid stenosis on the basis of the peak Doppler shift frequency occurring during systole (Table 2).

The normal systolic peak frequency (f_{max}) is 0.5 to 2.5 kHz at the origin of the internal carotid and 2 to 3 kHz in the distal internal carotid artery. The lower f_{max} in the carotid bulb is due to its greater diameter. Frequencies of less than 5 kHz are usually seen in mild disease, while f_{max} in the 5- to 8-kHz range indicates moderate disease and represents a 30 to 50 per cent reduction in the diameter of the carotid lumen. When f_{max} is in the range 8 to 12 the stenosis is in the severe range, with a 50 to 70 per cent reduction in diameter. A peak frequency greater than 12 kHz places the lesion in the category of critical stenosis with a reduction of 70 per cent in diameter and 90 per cent in lumen area (Fig. 5). Such a critical stenosis produces a drop in pressure and flow across the stenosis, due to the severe degree of narrowing.

Another parameter frequently used to assess the spectral analysis is the carotid index which is a ratio of the peak systolic frequency in the internal carotid artery to that in the common carotid artery. The f_{max} and the carotid index correlates with the residual lumen diameter of the carotid artery: f_{max} 7.5 and a carotid index above 3.8 are indicative of a residual lumen of less than 2 mm. An f_{max} above 14 kHz and a carotid index of more than 7 almost always indicates a residual lumen diameter of less than 1 mm.

When the severity of a carotid stenosis progresses such that the cross-sectional area of the artery is reduced by more than 90 per cent, or a residual lumen diameter less than 1 mm (preocclusive range), the blood flow may approach zero as the stenosis approaches occlusion. This may result in a falsely low or absent

Table 2 Peak frequency ranges

Frequency range	Percentage diameter reduction (%)	Percentage area reduction (%)
<5 kHz	<29	<50
5 Khz < peak frequency < 8 kHz	>29–<50	>50–<75
8 Khz < peak frequency < 12 kHz	>50–<75	>75–<90
<12 kHz	>75	>90

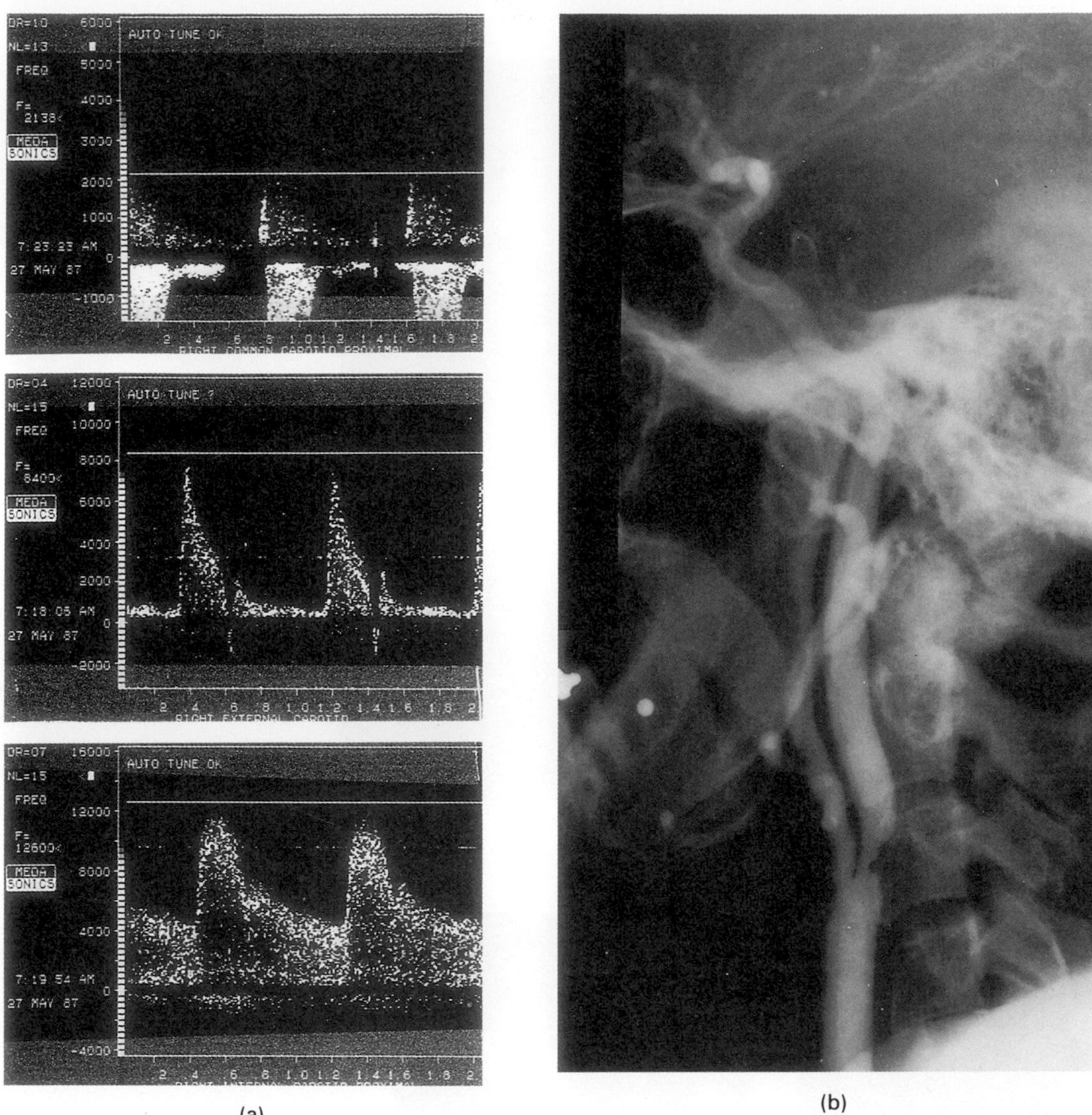

(a) (b)

Fig. 5 (a) Continuous wave Doppler spectral analysis revealing a 'critical stenosis' with peak systolic frequency shift of 12 kHz indicating a diameter reduction greater than 70 per cent. (b) Carotid arteriogram of patient in (a).

Doppler shift and a misdiagnosis of no stenosis or an incorrect diagnosis of occlusion, respectively. This potential for error must be kept in mind since either misdiagnosis would lead to surgery not being considered, leaving the patient at high risk for stroke (Fig. 6(a,b)).

A true carotid occlusion is indicated by the absence of a Doppler shift in the internal carotid artery, a decrease in peak velocity, and decreased or absent diastolic flow component in the common carotid artery (i.e. an increased pulsatility). The waveforms obtained from the common carotid artery are also asymmetrical, compared to those of the contralateral carotid artery, and the blood flow in the contralateral normal carotid may be elevated (Fig. 7(a,b).

Continuous-waver Doppler is a very effective and efficient method of direct non-invasive assessment of the carotid artery. However its lack of spatial resolution may result in occasional diagnostic errors. It may be difficult to ascertain the angle of incidence between the probe and the flow velocity vector in the carotid artery, which can produce errors in the Doppler shift frequency, especially when insonating very tortuous vessels. If the zone of high flow velocity is restricted to a small area in the artery it may be impossible to locate with the continuous-wave sound beam. Other sources of error include anatomical variations, insonating the wrong branch vessel, and the presence of venous flow. Some of these problems may be solved by visualizing the carotid bifurcation with B-mode ultrasound and using pulsed Doppler to allow more precise insonation of the vessel for velocity measurements.

Duplex scanning

Duplex scanning has become the most common non-invasive method in the examination of the carotid arteries. This technique combines the imaging capability of B-mode ultrasound and the velocimetric capabilities of range-gated (pulsed) Doppler in a

(a)

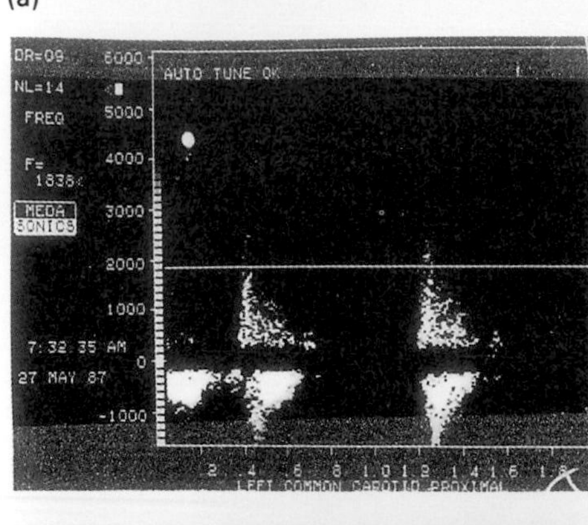

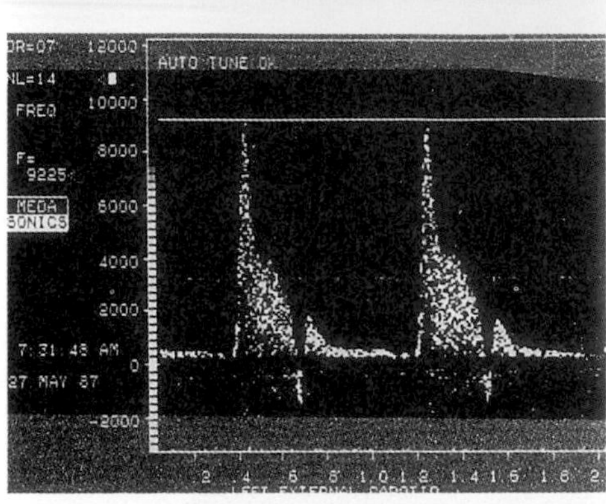

(b)

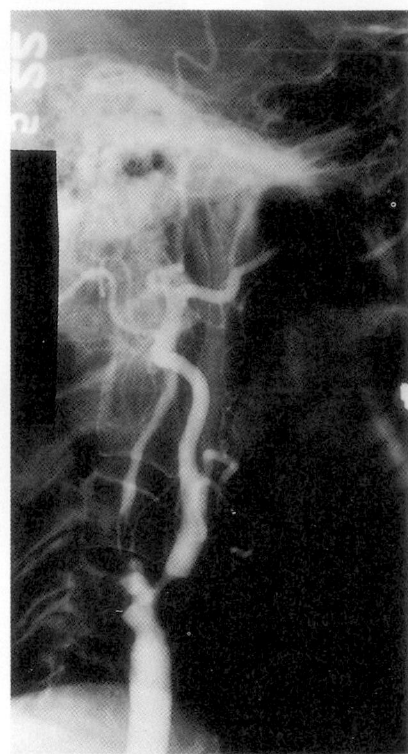

Fig. 6 (a) Continuous wave Doppler study of the carotid artery seen in (b). The study suggested an occlusion of the internal carotid artery. Left, absence of diastolic flow in the common carotid artery. Right, high peak frequency shift in the external carotid artery. No Doppler shift frequency could be discerned in the internal carotid artery. (b) Carotid arteriogram reveals classic 'string sign' confirming a minimal residual patent lumen in the internal carotid artery. The extremely low flow through the lesion could not be identified by Doppler, resulting in false positive diagnosis of carotid occlusion.

(a)

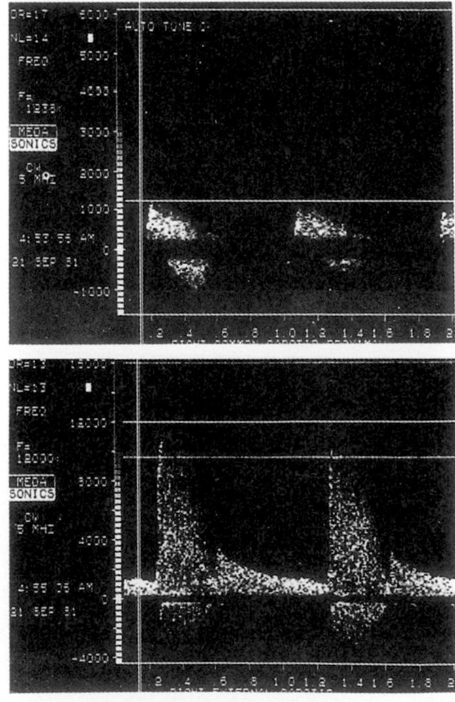

(b)

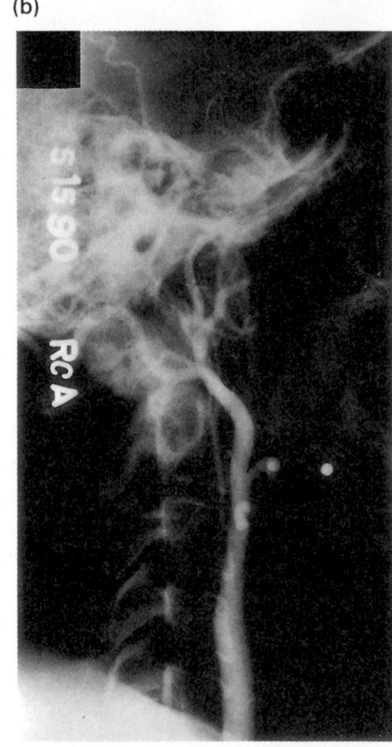

Fig. 7 (a) Continuous wave Doppler spectral pattern of internal carotid artery occlusion. Left, low peak systolic velocity in the common carotid artery. Right, high peak velocity in external carotid artery. No Doppler frequency shift found in the internal carotid artery. (b) Carotid arteriogram of patient in (a). Arteriogram confirmed occlusion of the internal carotid artery.

single instrument. B-mode ultrasound produces a standard two-dimensional image of the carotid artery, using the sound wave reflection that occurs between tissues of different acoustic densities (Fig. 8). This image provides a 'map' which may be used to direct the insonation of the vessel. The pulsed Doppler probe consists of a single crystal which serves both transmitting and receiving functions. By varying the time between emission and reception of the ultrasound signals, flow at different depths within the tissue can be investigated. The site which is actually studied for the Doppler shift effect has a small volume ($1\times1\times2$ mm).

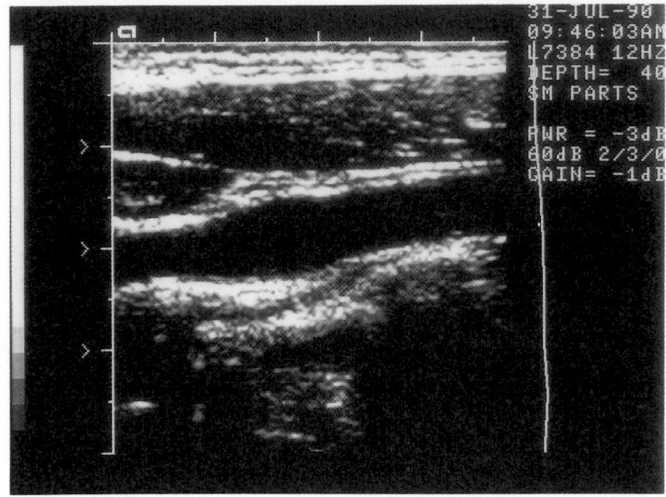

Fig. 8 Duplex scan. Longitudinal B-mode image of carotid artery.

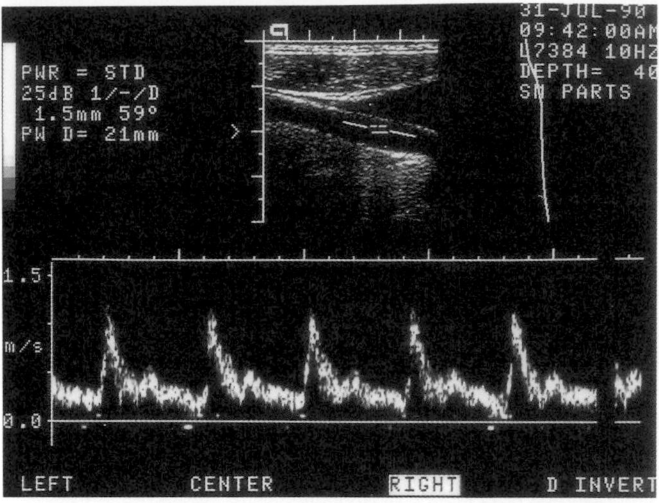

Fig. 9 Carotid duplex scan. Above: B-mode image. The oblique line in the image represents the angle of incidence of the Doppler beam. The cursor (gate) within the lumen of the artery is the sample volume of the pulsed Doppler. Below: pulsed Doppler spectral analysis.

Unlike continuous-wave Doppler, which provides a spectral array that represents the entire cross-section of the artery, pulsed (or range-gated) Doppler studies therefore provide a spectral pattern obtained from a small sample volume (gate) within the artery.

Rapid technological advances over the last decade have produced a wide variety of duplex scanners with different computer software capabilities and different transducer head designs. The transducers may be mechanical sector scanners or electrical linear or phased array transducers. The most versatile arrangement uses separate transducers for imaging and for Doppler examination, allowing the acquisition of the range-gated Doppler signal to be interpolated among the pulse-echo imaging signals. This provides continuous Doppler and real-time imaging without interruption of either modality.

The duplex scan is performed by placing the transducer on the neck overlying the region of the carotid bifurcation. A real-time B-mode image of the carotid artery is displayed on the monitor screen. The position of the Doppler sample volume (gate) is then adjusted by reference to a line that appears on the B-mode image indicating the angle of incidence between the Doppler beam and the carotid. The actual location of the gate is indicated on the monitor as a small rectangle. The scanner is equipped with a printer that can provide a hard copy of both the B-mode image and the Doppler spectral waveform (obtained by fast Fourier transform) on the same print. Depending upon the computer software package of the scanner, the Doppler signal analysis may include maximum and mean frequency waveforms, computed pulsatility index, and other analyses of the waveform. The spectral waveform is displayed on the same format as that described for continuous-wave Doppler. The grey scale which indicates frequency amplitudes may be in black and white or may be colour coded (Fig. 9).

Since the pulse method provides Doppler shift frequency data from a small volume within the artery, as opposed to the entire diameter of the vessel sampled by continuous-wave Doppler, the range of frequencies displayed in a normal artery is less when using the gated technique. Pulsed Doppler is thus more sensitive for detecting turbulent flow distal to a stenosis. The spectral broadening produced by the turbulent flow appears as a filling in of the spectral window on the waveform (Fig. 10).

The degree of carotid stenosis is assessed mainly on the basis of the spectral analysis, particularly with respect to peak systolic frequency, spectral broadening, end-diastolic frequency, and contour of the waveform. The vertical axis of the spectral plot may be expressed as either frequency or velocity. Various authors have described categories of severity of disease based on quantitation of the velocity or frequency shifts (Table 3).

Duplex scanning eliminates some of the difficulties inherent in continuous-wave Doppler examination by providing an image of the vessel which allows precise insonation of the vessel. However there are several potential sources of error that may affect duplex velocimetry. Low cardiac output or an innominate or proximal common carotid stenosis may decrease flow velocities, thus causing an underestimation of existing bifurcation disease. As with continuous-wave Doppler, if the stenosis is so severe that

Table 3 Pulsed Doppler criteria for carotid stenosis

Percentage stenosis	Peak systolic velocity (cm/s)	Peak diastolic velocity (cm/s)	Spectral broadening (bandwidth cm/s)
0	<110	<40	<30
1–39	<110	<40	<40
40–59	<130	40	<40
60–79	>130	>40	>40
80–99	>250	>100	>80

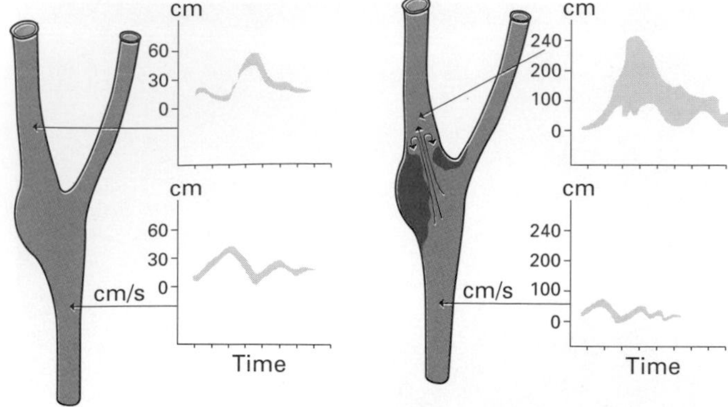

Fig. 10 Schematic illustration of 'spectral broadening'. Left, normal 'systolic window' represented as clear area under the peak frequency envelope. Right, carotid stenosis produces turbulent flow with resultant broad range of frequency shifts which fills in the systolic window on the spectral display.

there is minimal flow, the area of flow may be missed when positioning the gate, leading to a misdiagnosis of carotid occlusion. Despite these limitations, duplex scanning represents a powerful method of direct testing.

Colour flow duplex imaging

Standard duplex imaging provides Doppler shift data from single small volumes (1×1×2 mm) within the vessel lumen. Thus unless multiple samples are acquired sequentially (a very tedious task) a great deal of information about the flow within the vessel lumen, especially in the region of the carotid bifurcation, will be missed. By modifying the Doppler transducer, replacing the single gate receiver with a linear array multigate, simultaneous velocity measurements can be made across the entire diameter of the vessel. The velocity data is then colour coded and a real-time two-dimensional colour flow image is displayed superimposed on the B-mode image.

The 'Triplex' colour coding system assigns red and blue colours to flow velocity vectors of opposite direction (conventionally, the technician usually assigns red to flow in the arterial direction and blue to flow in the venous direction). Variations in Doppler frequency shift are indicated by changes in colour intensity: lighter shades of each colour represent higher flow velocities and maximum velocities appear white.

Triplex examination can provide definition of both normal and abnormal flow patterns in the region of the carotid bifurcation. The usual laminar flow pattern is disrupted at the normal carotid bifurcation, where a zone of boundary layer separation exists along the outer wall opposite the flow divider. In this region normal flow is in the reverse direction and appears as an area of blue on the Triplex scan (Fig. 11). In mild or moderate atherosclerotic disease the plaque will not produce haemodynamically significant stenosis but it will eliminate the normal contour of the bulb, eliminating the normal zone of boundary layer separation. Mild to moderate lesions will cause loss of this area of blue colour at the bifurcation. Haemodynamically significant stenosis will produce stream flow changes with high velocity (white) in the jet and turbulent flow (mixture of colours) just distal to the stenosis (Fig. 12).

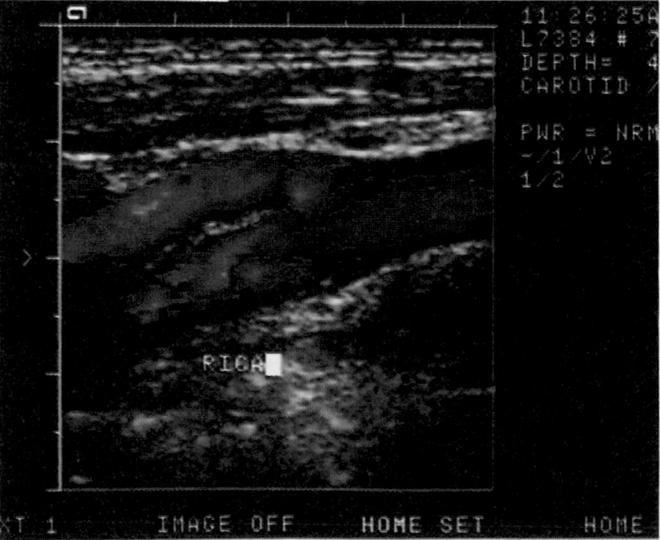

Fig. 11 Triplex scan of normal carotid bifurcation. The blue area indicates the normal zone of flow separation seen in the carotid bulb.

Transcranial Doppler

The direct studies discussed above provide excellent identification and quantification of extracranial carotid disease, but they do not provide direct information about the actual physiological effects of the carotid stenosis on cerebral perfusion because they fail to measure collateral cerebral blood flow. This is a critical issue, since collateral flow may provide adequate ipsilateral hemispheric perfusion in the presence of a 'critical' or haemodynamically significant carotid stenosis, while such a stenosis will have profound detrimental effects in the absence of adequate collateral flow. Direct studies are often supplemented with ocular pneumoplethysmography or supraorbital Doppler studies in an attempt to define collateral flow.

Transcranial Doppler was developed as a method for investigating intracerebral flow directly. A 2-MHz Doppler signal is used to insonate the vessels in the circle of Willis (Fig. 13) and its branches. Four different 'acoustic windows'—transtemporal, transorbital, suboccipital, and submandibular—are available for insonation of the intracranial vessels (Fig. 14). The transtemporal approach provides access to the anterior cerebral artery including the anterior communicating artery, as well as the posterior cerebral artery and the posterior communicating artery.

Changes in direction and velocity of flow in the various intracranial vessels can verify the presence of significant extracranial disease and can identify the presence of collateral flow. Decreased velocity of flow in the ipsilateral middle cerebral artery confirms the critical nature of the carotid stenosis. Increased velocity and reversal of flow in the contralateral anterior cerebral artery indicates the presence of collateral flow from the contralateral carotid via a patent anterior communicating artery.

The importance of transcranial Doppler as a clinical tool will undoubtedly increase as more experience is gained with the technique and as correlations between haemodynamic findings and clinical outcome are verified.

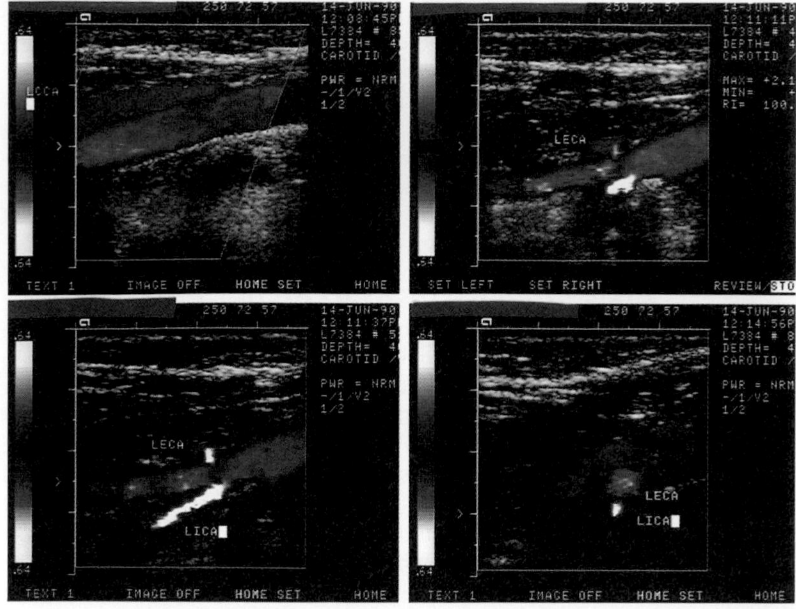

Fig. 12 Triplex study of severe stenosis of the internal carotid artery. The high velocity flow through the stenosis is represented by the white area in the lumen of the internal carotid artery.

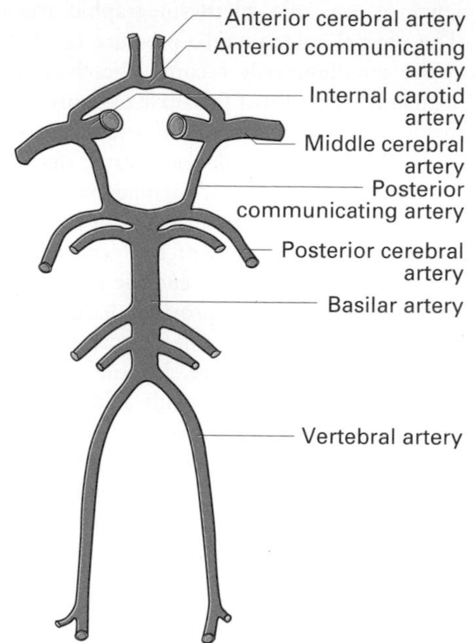

Fig. 13 Anatomy of the circle of Willis.

Applications of non-invasive carotid studies

Non-invasive testing of carotid function provides a safe, convenient, and reliable method for screening patients at risk for stroke, enabling identification of those who might benefit from therapeutic intervention. Patients at risk for stroke include those with a history of transient ischaemic attacks, amaurosis fugax, vertebrobasilar insufficiency, prior stroke, and asymptomatic carotid bruits. Transient ischaemic attacks affecting the carotid distribution may present as hemiparaesthaesia, hemiparesis, and/or speech difficulty. Amaurosis fugax presents as transient loss of vision in one eye. The patient often describes this transient monocular blindness as 'a shade being pulled down over the eye'. Vertebrobasilar insufficiency is usually characterized by dizziness, bilateral eye symptoms, ataxia, facial numbness, or bilateral extremity weakness or paraesthesiae.

Such symptoms are due to cerebral ischaemia, which may have a variety of possible aetiologies. These include cardiac arrythmias, cardiac thromboembolism, intracranial atherosclerotic disease, and carotid bifurcation disease. There is approximately a 50 per cent chance of the symptoms being due to carotid bifurcation disease, and patients suffering from transient ischaemic attacks have a 5.3 to 8.6 per cent risk of suffering a stroke per year; this is reduced to less than 1 per cent per year following uncomplicated carotid endarterectomy. Symptomatic patients should therefore undergo non-invasive carotid testing; identification of a significant lesion, on the appropriate side for the symptoms should prompt consideration of carotid endarterectomy.

Patients with asymptomatic carotid bruits may also be at increased risk for stroke: some studies have suggested that carotid stenoses of greater than 80 per cent carry a 12 per cent risk of stroke. If the results of non-invasive tests suggest the presence of such a lesion, consideration might be given to prophylactic carotid endarterectomy, although this is a controversial issue.

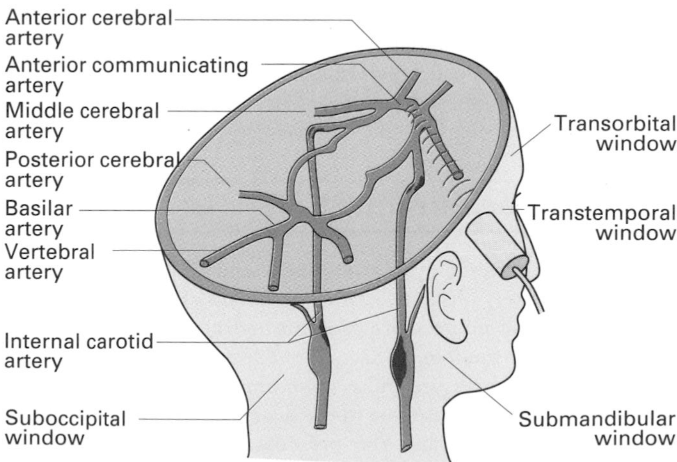

Fig. 14 Acoustic windows available for transcranial Doppler.

Until recently, non-invasive studies were used to identify patients with significant extracranial carotid disease; carotid arteriography would then be used to assess the patient for carotid surgery. The non-invasive diagnostic technology has advanced to the stage where redefinition of the indications for preoperative angiography is probably appropriate. In selected patients, such as those with lateralizing hemispheric symptoms and severe haemodynamically significant carotid disease, identified by non-invasive testing, it may be appropriate to proceed to carotid endartectomy without angiographic studies.

LOWER EXTREMITY ARTERIAL DISEASE

Indications for non-invasive vascular testing

A wide spectrum of clinical presentation is seen in patients with peripheral vascular occlusive disease, who may present with intermittent claudication, which may be mild or debilitating, ischaemic rest pain, ischaemic tissue loss, or gangrene. The diagnosis of peripheral vascular occlusive disease as the cause of the symptoms in these patients is often confounded by the presence of associated diseases such as neurological disorders, spinal stenosis (pseudoclaudication) and orthopaedic or rheumatological problems, and diabetes with its associated peripheral neuropathy and neuropathic, non-ischaemic pressure ulcers. Even when an obvious vascular aetiology exists, it is often difficult to determine the exact location of the most significant vascular lesion in the arterial tree. The mere radiological demonstration of a vascular lesion does not confirm its importance: it is the haemodynamic effect on the circulation that is important and this must be confirmed prior to considering any therapeutic intervention. A number of non-invasive studies allow analysis of the haemodynamic significance of any existing vascular pathology. These studies are often helpful in predicting the potential for healing of foot lesions or amputation sites and allow ischaemic and neuropathic foot pain to be differentiated. Haemodynamic studies also provide useful information when the results of peripheral vascular reconstructions or percutaneous angioplasty procedures are being evaluated, and in the detection of failing grafts. The tests also provide a means of assessing and following the progression of any vascular disease which does not require surgical intervention at the time of the patient's initial presentation.

Despite the large variety of studies available three basic parameters are analysed in the study of peripheral vascular disease: pressure, volume change, and flow velocity.

Pressure measurement

In the normal arterial system the large and distributing arteries produce relatively little resistance to blood flow and there is, therefore, almost no pressure gradient between the aorta and the small arteries of the foot. In fact, as the pressure pulse is propagated distally the pressure pulse wave amplitude and the systolic pressure actually increase due to the decreasing compliance of the distal arterial vessels and the presence of reflected waves. In patients with atherosclerotic peripheral vascular occlusive disease the arterial luminal narrowing which occurs at the sites of atherosclerotic plaque formation produces an increased resistance to flow and a resultant pressure drop across the stenoses. The measurement of distal lower extremity blood pressure therefore provides a method for detecting haemodynamically significant arterial occlusive disease. Since a critical stenosis will produce a pressure gradient across the lesion even before there is any reduction in total flow to the lower extremity, pressure measurement provides a very sensitive method for assessing the presence of physiologically significant arterial disease.

Ankle pressure measurement

Measuring the systolic arterial pressure at the ankle is a simple means by which any haemodynamically significant arterial lesion from the level of the aorta to the tibial arteries can be identified. The technique involves the placement of a blood pressure cuff around the calf at the level of the ankle. Since Korotkoff sounds are not audible with a stethoscope at this site the pulse is identified with either a continuous-wave Doppler sensor applied over the dorsalis pedis or posterior tibial artery or with a strain gauge plethysmograph or photoplethysmograph applied to the toe. The cuff is inflated well above the systolic arterial pressure and then slowly deflated: the ankle systolic pressure is recorded when the Doppler signal or pulsatile plethysmographic tracing is first identified. The normal ankle systolic pressure is 10 to 20 mmHg greater than the simultaneously recorded brachial systolic blood pressure. Calculating the ratio of the ankle pressure to the brachial pressure provides a convenient index of arterial disease.

The normal ankle: brachial index is greater than 1.0; a value below 0.92 indicates the presence of haemodynamically significant arterial disease. The degree of abnormality of the ankle: brachial index correlates with the location of the occlusive disease, the severity of the stenosis or occlusion, and the number of lesions in the arterial tree. In general, more proximal lesions have a greater effect on the index while higher values are associated with more distal (infrapopliteal) arterial disease. Multilevel disease, the so-called tandem lesion, is associated with a lower ankle: brachial index (Fig.15). The severity of the patient's symptoms correlates well with the ankle: brachial index, which decreases as the physiological effect of the arterial disease increases. Patients with claudication have a higher ankle: brachial index (0.6–0.8) than those with rest pain (0.26–0.35), while those with ischaemic ulcers have an ankle: brachial index between 0 and 0.25.

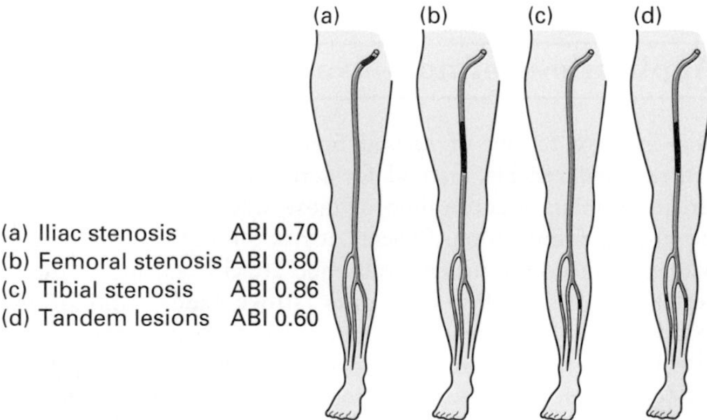

Fig. 15 In general, proximal occlusive lesions have the greatest effect on ankle: brachial indices.

Determination of the ankle:brachial index is a simple and reproducible test and is therefore a valuable diagnostic and prognostic tool which may be used to monitor the natural progression of arterial disease in a patient not yet requiring therapeutic intervention. It is also useful in assessing the results of peripheral bypass surgery. Several potential sources of error with this study must be recognized. Repeated determinations of ankle systolic pressures, made on the same day in the same patient, may vary by as much as 14 mmHg. Therefore a change in the ankle:brachial index of more than 0.15 is required before it is safe to conclude that a haemodynamically significant change has occurred. While an abnormal ankle:brachial index indicates the existence of arterial disease, it does not accurately locate the level of the lesion. In a significant proportion of patients with peripheral vascular occlusive disease, and especially in diabetic patients, medial calcification within the wall of the arteries (Monckeberg's sclerosis) produces incompressible vessels. In this instance the cuff pressure required to occlude flow in the underlying artery is greater than the blood pressure because additional pressure is required to collapse the calcified arterial wall. Falsely elevated ankle pressures and ankle:brachial indices are obtained, which underestimate the severity of the arterial occlusive disease. The ankle: brachial index may also underestimate the severity of lesions which produce no pressure gradient at rest but which produce a drop in pressure with the increased flow rates associated with exercise. The addition of other methods of measurement of pressure in the lower extremity increases the diagnostic accuracy of the study and provides further information concerning the severity and location of the arterial disease.

Post-exercise ankle:brachial index

The sensitivity of the ankle:brachial index in diagnosing mild to moderate stenotic disease may be increased by measuring the ankle pressure after exercising the patient. The principle involved is the physiological correlate of Ohm's Law: as the flow across a stenotic lesion increases, the pressure drop across that lesion also increases. Exercise, for example, on a treadmill, causes the peripheral resistance vessels distal to the stenotic lesion to dilate, resulting in an increased flow to the lower limb across the stenosis. The increased pressure drop that occurs with the increased flow can mean that a subcritical lesion at rest becomes haemodynamically significant on exercise.

This test is performed by measuring the ankle:brachial index at rest and again after the patient has exercised on a treadmill for 5 min (or until the patient is forced to stop due to claudication). The patient then resumes the supine position and the quality of the femoral, popliteal, and pedal pulses are immediately reassessed and ankle and brachial pressures are remeasured. Patients with arterial disease will always show a drop in the ankle pressure after exercise, the degree of which correlates with the functional significance of the disease. Multilevel arterial diseases will cause large pressure drops and proximal lesions have a greater impact than distal lesions (an iliac stenosis will produce a greater fall in the post-exercise ankle:brachial index than will a distal superficial femoral artery lesion). This occurs because of the larger muscle mass supplied by the more proximal vessel and the resultant greater diversion of blood flow.

'Reactive hyperaemia' may be used as an alternative to exercise to increase the rate of flow across a stenotic segment. This technique involves placing a pneumatic cuff on the thigh and inflating the cuff above systolic pressure for between 3 and 7 min. The temporary ischaemia produces distal vasodilatation; releasing the cuff causes a period of hyperaemic flow. The decrease in pressure that occurs with reactive hyperaemic flow across a stenosis correlates well with that seen following exercise. However, exercise testing is usually the preferred technique since it allows actual observation of the level of activity required to induce claudication and provides the vascular surgeon with a more objective measure of the patient's disability.

Segmental pressure measurement

Determination of segmental pressure provides greater definition of the atherosclerotic disease process by locating the level at which haemodynamically significant lesions exist. Segmental lower extremity pressures are measured most accurately by applying pneumatic cuffs around the high thigh, low thigh (just above the knee), around the calf just below the knee, and at the ankle. The segmental systolic pressures are then measured in the same manner as that described above.

The normal upper thigh pressure is 30 to 40 mmHg higher than the brachial pressure: this is actually an artefact of the size discrepancy between the thigh and the cuff. The pressure in the cuff is not completely transmitted to the underlying arteries and thus the measured systolic pressure is overestimated. If this apparent elevation in the thigh pressure is not detected then a haemodynamically significant iliac artery lesion or a proximal superficial femoral artery stenosis combined with a profunda stenosis probably exists.

Pressure gradients between any two levels do not normally exceed 20 mmHg, and gradients greater than 30 mmHg between any two segments indicate arterial disease in the intervening arterial segment. If a patient's low thigh pressure is 150 mmHg and the below-knee pressure measurement is 80 mmHg, for example, a popliteal arterial occlusion is probably present.

The technique of indirect non-invasive pressure measurement, by necessity, requires a blood pressure cuff placed at the level being studied and a pulse sensing device (Doppler flowmeter or photoplethysmograph) placed distally. This arrangement creates potential sources of error in interpreting segmental pressure data since segments of arterial disease may lie between the cuff and the sensing device. A proximal superficial femoral artery occlusion, for example, may falsely lower the high thigh pressure measurement, leading to a misdiagnosis of iliac arterial disease. If the cuff thigh size mismatch is excessive (as occurs in patients with large thighs) the apparently elevated high thigh pressure measurement may result in failure to diagnose a significant iliac artery lesion. Accurate assessment of patients with multisegment disease may also be difficult.

A salient component of the preoperative evaluation of the patient with peripheral arterial occlusive disease is the identification of the relative importance of proximal (aortoiliac) or so-called 'inflow' and distal (femoropopliteal or tibial) or so-called 'outflow' arterial stenoses. A critical assessment of the haemodynamic significance of lesions at the various levels is essential to enable the appropriate level for vascular bypass to be decided. The various lower extremity pressure measurements are very useful in this critical assessment. However, the potential artefacts inherent in the pressure measurements may lead to incorrect conclusions regarding the relative importance of lesions at various levels. Non-invasive arterial flow studies have therefore been developed which may be used along with the pressure measurement data in both diagnosing the presence of arterial occlusive disease and determining the relative importance of lesions present at various levels in the arterial tree. Despite all the advances in lower ex-

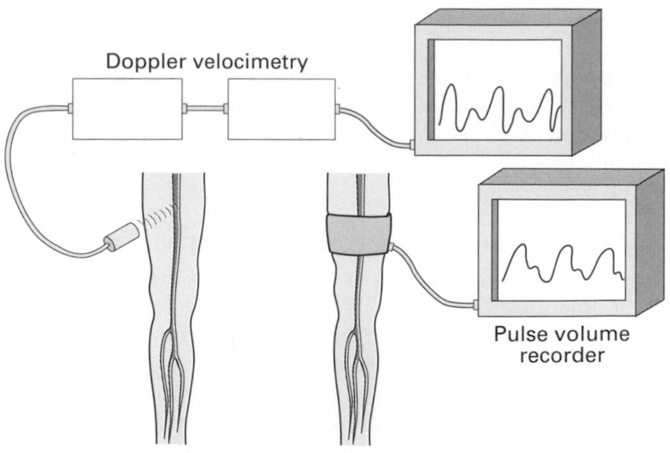

Fig. 16 Both Doppler velocimetry and plethysmography may be used to produce 'pulse waveforms' which are used to assess severity of lower extremity arterial disease.

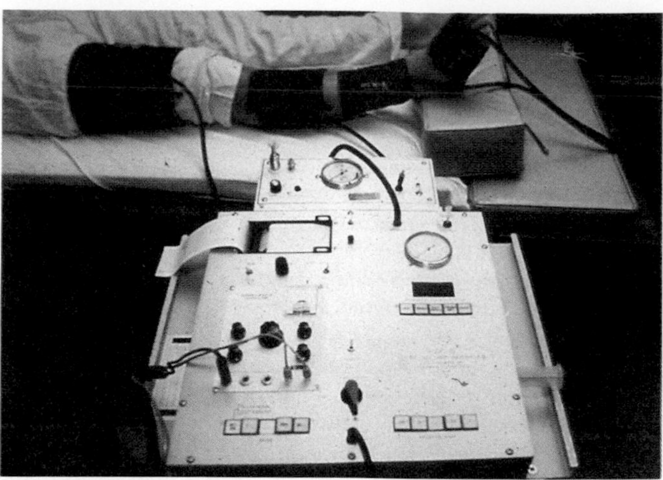

Fig. 17 Standard technique for performing segmental plethysmography. Note the difference in size of pneumatic cuffs placed at the various levels on the lower extremity.

tremity flow and pressure studies accurate assessment of iliac level disease is often elusive. A variety of indices such as the pulsatility index, damping factors, and inverse damping factors have been developed in an effort to bring better definition to the study of iliac disease. However, they add little to the information contained from the analysis of segmental pressures and flow waveform, discussed below.

Two parameters are available for non-invasive measurement of 'arterial flow': these are segmental volume change (plethysmography) and flow velocity (Doppler velocimetry). The data from studies of either of these parameters may be recorded and presented in waveform fashion. Analysis of the waveform 'pulse contours' provides valuable information which can be used in a collaborative fashion with segmental pressure studies critically to assess lower extremity arterial disease (Fig. 16).

Segmental pulse volume plethysmography

Plethysmography is the measurement of volume change. A variety of plethysmographs (e.g. mercury strain gauge, impedance and photoplethysmographs) are available, but the most convenient and commonly used device is an air-filled plethysmograph known as the pulse volume recorder. During cardiac systole the part of the limb being examined expands due to arterial inflow; during diastole the venous outflow exceeds arterial inflow and the limb contracts. The pulse volume recorder uses a pneumatic cuff as the segmental volume sensor and measures these changes in volume. Appropriately sized cuffs are placed on the proximal thigh, calf, and ankle (transmetatarsal and digital cuffs may also be used) (Fig. 17). The cuff at the site to be tested is inflated with air to a low pressure of 65 mmHg, bringing the volume sensing cuff into close approximation with the leg. The volume changes in the segment of the leg beneath the cuff produce changes in the air pressure within the cuff bladder; these are then converted to an analogue recording using a pressure transducer. The wave contour obtained closely resembles the waveform of the arterial pulse pressure (Fig. 18).

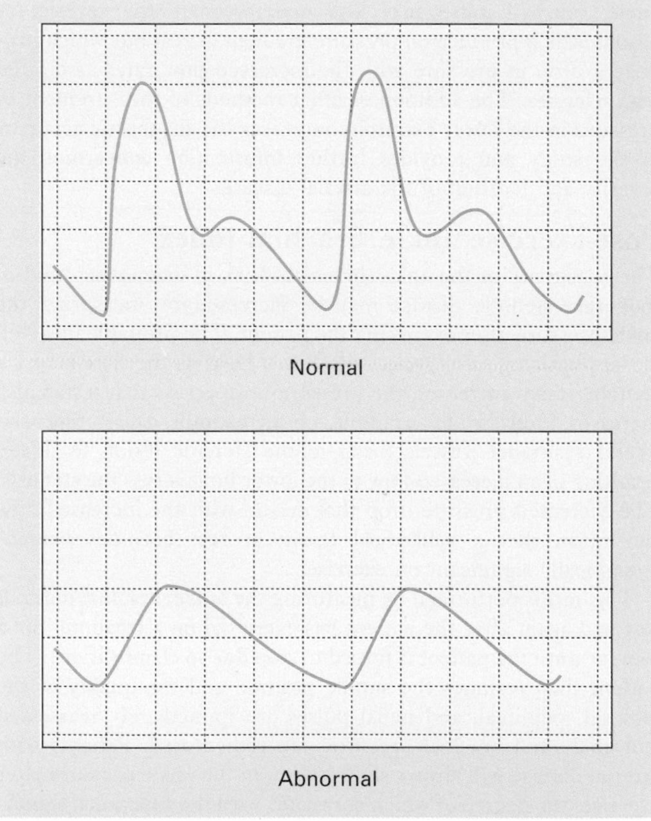

Fig. 18 Normal and abnormal pulse volume recordings. See text for description of the characteristics of normal and abnormal pulse volume recorder waveforms.

The contour obtained from pulse volume recording in a normal limb contains four important components: a steep slope in the anacrotic limb, a sharp systolic peak, bowing of the catacrotic limb towards the baseline, and a dicrotic notch. The last represents flow reversal and is due to the normal resistance present in the distal peripheral vascular bed. The presence of a dicrotic notch essentially rules out any haemodynamically significant arterial disease proximal to the pulse volume recorder cuff.

Contour changes that indicate the existence of arterial disease proximal to the cuff include loss of the dicrotic notch, decrease in the rate of rise in the anacrotic limb, rounding and delay in the systolic peak, bowing of the catacrotic limb away from the baseline, and decreased rate of fall in the catacrotic limb. The extent of the pulse wave contour abnormality correlates with the severity of the proximal arterial occlusive disease.

Quantitative as well as qualitative analysis of the pulse volume recorder waveform provides valuable information regarding the severity of the arterial disease proximal to the cuff. Waveform amplitudes are affected by a variety of factors other than arterial occlusive disease, including cardiac output, blood pressure, vasomotor tone, blood volume, muscularity of the limb, and position of the limb. Despite these other variables, progressively worse occlusive disease usually correlates with smaller pulse amplitudes. Five categories have been defined which classify the severity of the occlusive disease based on quantitative and qualitative analysis of the pulse volume recorder waveform (Table 4).

Analysis of the entire profile of segmental pulse volume recorder tracings from the thigh, calf, and ankle levels provides important information regarding the location and severity of occlusive disease. The different patterns resulting when haemodynamically significant disease occurs at different levels are useful in determining the location of physiologically significant disease (Fig. 19).

In the normal lower extremity the amplitude of the calf pulse wave seen on segmental pulse volume recording is larger than the thigh pulse wave. The phenomenon, which has been termed 'augmentation', is actually an artefact which results from the smaller size of the calf cuff compared to the thigh cuff: volume change produces a relatively greater pressure change in the smaller cuff than in the larger cuff (Fig. 20). The absence of the calf augmentation phenomenon indicates the presence of superficial femoral artery occlusive disease (Figs. 21, 22).

Table 4 Pulse volume recorder categories

	Chart deflection (mm)	
Category	**Thigh and ankle**	**Calf**
1	>15*	>20*
2	>15†	>20†
3	5–15	5–20
4	<5	<5
5	Flat	Flat

* With dicrotic notch.
† Without dicrotic notch.

In the presence of isolated iliac artery disease with an open distal system the pulse contours at all the levels on the affected side will be abnormal, but calf augmentation will still exist (Fig. 23). In the presence of occlusion of the superficial femoral artery and stenosis of the profunda femoral artery, segmental wave contours may lead to a false diagnosis of iliac artery disease: analysis of pulse volume recordings made at thigh level after exercise will usually allow differentiation between the two conditions. If an iliac lesion exists the post-exercise thigh pulse contour will deteriorate further, while a normal artery and diseased superficial femoral artery will produce no significant change in the contour after exercise. The degree of accuracy with which severity and location of arterial lesions can be assessed is greatly increased when analysis of pulse volume recordings is combined with segmental pressure studies.

Doppler velocimetry and Duplex scanning

Haemodynamically significant arterial stenosis produces changes in the arterial flow velocity and in the velocity pulse wave contour and disrupts laminar flow, creating turbulence. Each of these effects can be studied and the severity of the lesion estimated by Doppler examination. The same Doppler technology and methods used in the assessment of carotid disease may be applied to the study of lower extremity arterial disease. Unlike pressure measurements and plethysmography, which are indirect studies, Doppler studies provide direct information about the arterial disease.

Continuous-wave Doppler

A 'pencil' probe is most commonly used (Fig. 24), and is placed directly over the vessel to be insonated, maintaining a 45 to 60° angle of incidence to the vessel. To examine the common femoral artery the probe is positioned at or above the inguinal ligament to avoid inadvertent insonation of the superficial femoral or

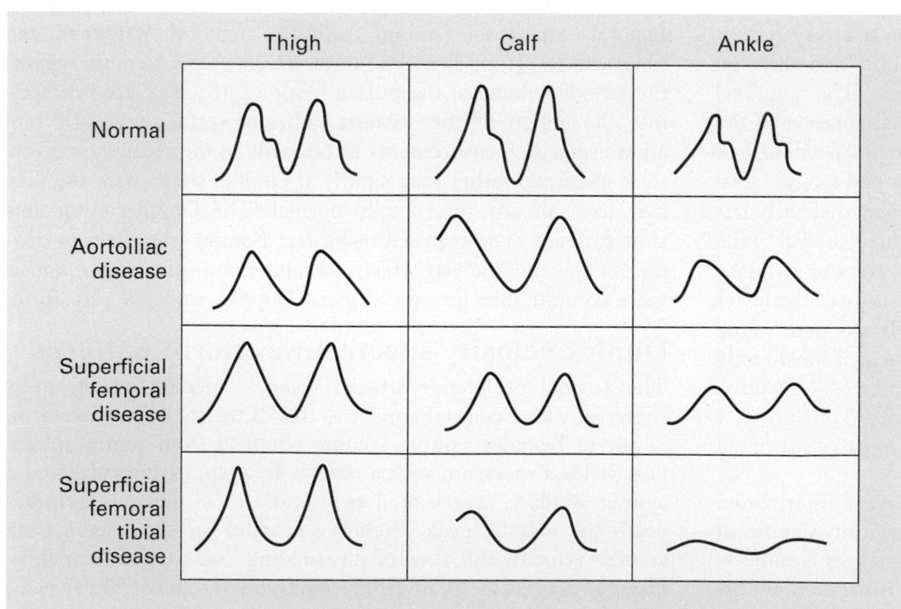

Fig. 19 Pulse volume recorder pattern recognition is useful in determining the distribution of lower arterial disease.

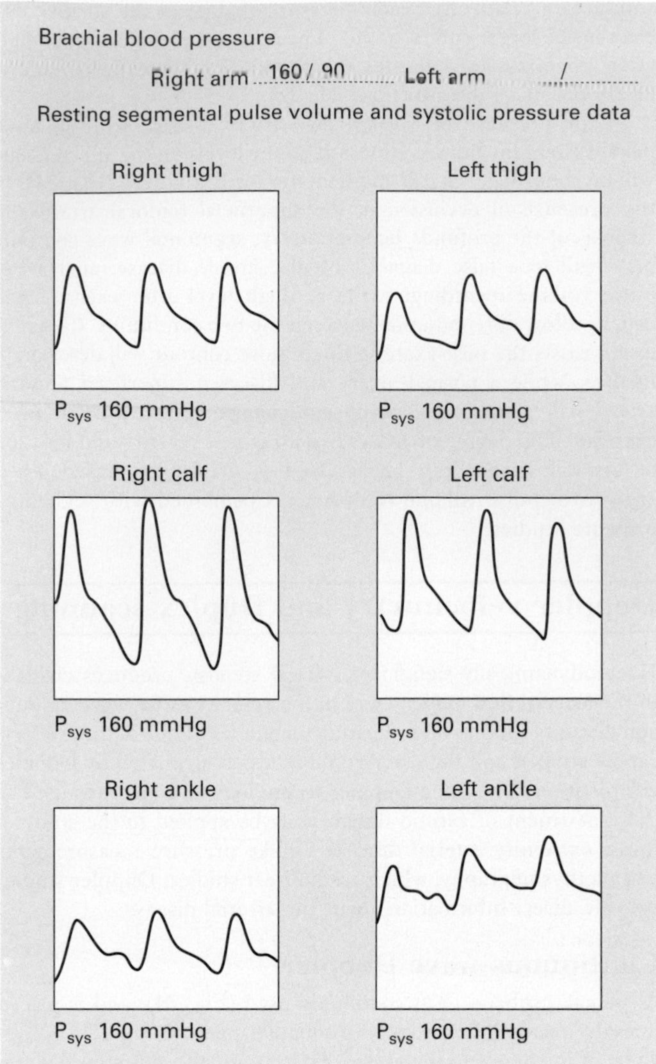

Fig. 20 Normal lower extremity segmental pulse volume recording. Note the presence of 'augmentation' at the calf level.

profunda femoral artery. The superficial femoral artery is best approached with the probe in a medial position and directed between the quadriceps and adductor muscles. The popliteal artery is located with gentle flexion and external rotation of the leg. The posterior tibial artery is insonated in its position just behind the medial malleolus. The dorsalis pedis and lateral tarsal (terminal branch of the peroneal) arteries are located slightly lateral to the extensor hallucis longus tendon and anteromedial to the lateral malleolus, respectively. Although these are the standard positions examined during the routine Doppler study of the lower extremities, arteries may be insonated at virtually any point along their course in the leg. This provides a versatile tool for directly examining arterial stenoses anywhere in the lower extremity. Where the arteries lie in a superficial location, a 10-MHz probe is used; arteries in deeper positions (e.g. peroneal) must be examined with a 5-MHz probe.

The audible Doppler signal provides important information which may suggest the presence of a haemodynamically significant stenosis. However, this type of Doppler signal analysis is subjective, and it provides no hard copy of the results. Most continuous-wave Doppler instruments used for peripheral arterial studies are equipped with zero-crossing frequency to voltage converters which produce a velocity analogue waveform which is recorded on a strip chart. The contour of the analogue waveform closely resembles that of the arterial pressure pulse (Fig. 25). However, this method may produce errors since the voltage output is proportional to the root mean square frequency rather than to the mean Doppler shift frequency, resulting in overestimation of low velocities and underestimation of high velocities. Despite these limitations, the analogue waveform provides excellent qualitative information about the arterial flow.

The normal analogue waveform is triphasic, with a rapid increase in velocity in early systole, followed by a rapid fall in velocity with reversal of flow in early diastole. In late diastole, there is a smaller forward flow component (Fig. 25(a)).

Arterial stenoses proximal to the segment being insonated will produce changes in the contour of the analogue waveform which correlate with the haemodynamic significance of the lesion. The earliest sign of a proximal stenosis is loss of the diastolic flow reversal, resulting in a biphasic waveform. As the severity of the stenosis increases, the slopes of the upstroke and downstroke decrease and the peak becomes rounded rather than peaked. Progressive dampening of the waveform results in a low amplitude monophasic waveform seen in patients with severe stenoses (Fig. 25(b–g)). Analysis of both the segmental analogue waveforms and pressures will usually provide sufficient data to enable haemodynamically significant arterial diseases to be diagnosed and will often allow accurate assessment of the location of the disease (Fig. 26).

Duplex scanning

Doppler velocimetry measurements can be made with far greater accuracy and precision when combined with duplex scanning technology. This greater definition is achieved at the price of greater technical complexity and longer time required to perform the study. Lower extremity arterial duplex scanning is performed by longitudinal imaging of the femoral, popliteal, and tibial arteries using real-time B-mode ultrasound. At the infrapopliteal level, the technical ease of the study is increased if triplex (colour duplex) capability is available: the colour technology reduces the acquisition time needed to locate the tibial vessels. Doppler flow velocity measurements are then obtained from the iliac, common femoral, superficial femoral, profunda femoral, popliteal, and tibial arteries. If the B-mode image visualizes any stenotic regions the sample volume of the pulsed Doppler may be placed directly into the region of the stenosis. This powerful diagnostic tool allows velocity measurements to be made in the areas most likely to be abnormal rather than simply at random sites where the flow may have already returned to normal. The Doppler frequency shift data are then analysed using fast Fourier transform to produce a spectral analysis which contains more information and is more accurate than the zero-crossed Doppler analogue waveform.

Duplex velocity spectral waveform patterns

The normal peripheral arterial velocity spectral waveform is triphasic, with a contour similar to that of the analogue waveform. A pulsed Doppler sample volume obtained from centre stream flow yields a spectrum with a narrow frequency bandwidth and a systolic window, represented as a clear area in the waveform beneath the systolic peak. Stenoses produce an increase in peak systolic velocity and spectral broadening due to turbulent flow. Haemodynamically significant lesions (stenosis above 50 per cent) cause loss of diastolic reversed flow and an increase in diastolic

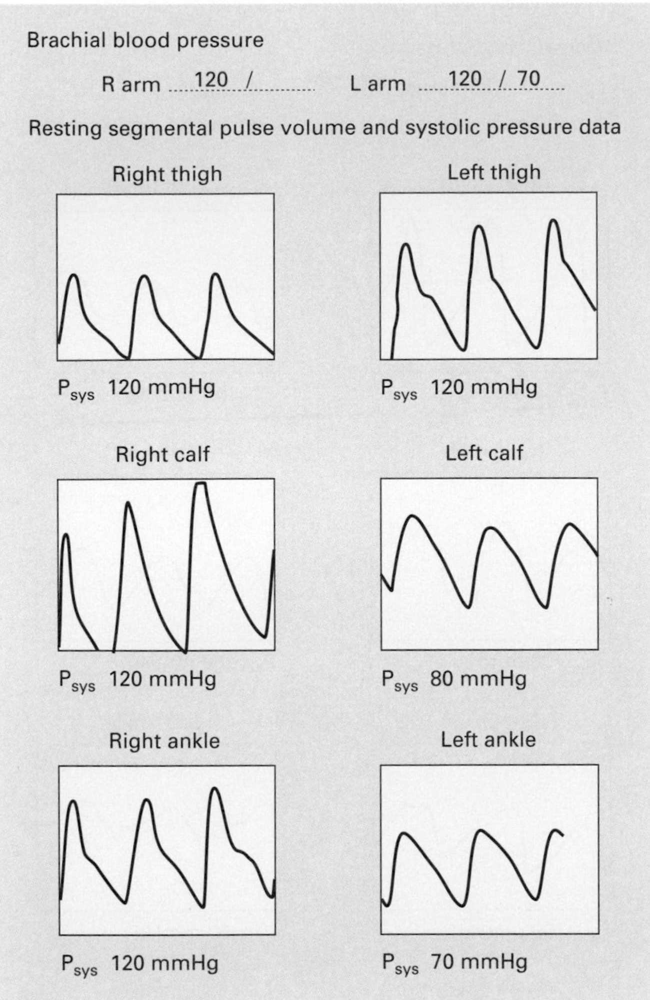

(a)

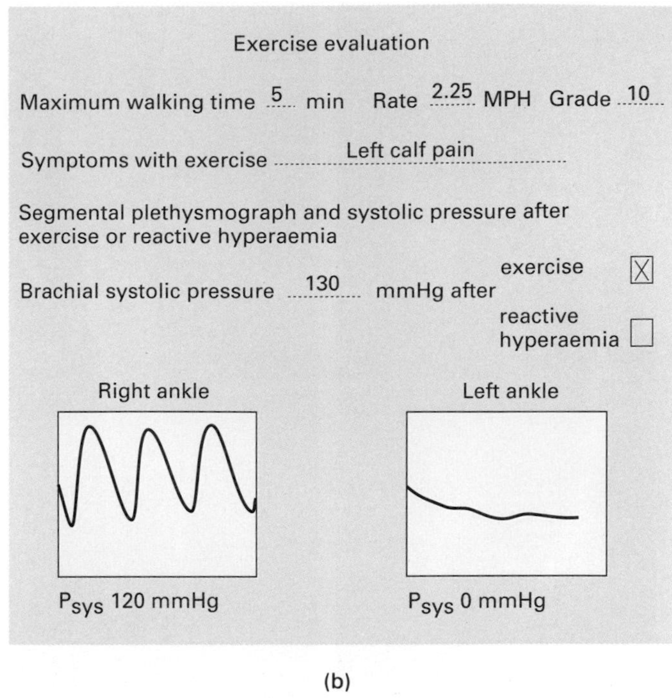

(b)

Fig. 21 Lower extremity pulse volume recording with post-exercise ankle pulse volume recording. The absence of normal calf augmentation on the left suggests a left superficial femoral artery occlusion. (a) At rest.(b) After exercise.

Table 5 Categories of stenosis

Category (percentage diameter reduction)	Spectral characteristics	Clinical interpretation
0 (normal)	Triphasic No spectral broadening Clear systolic window	Normal
1–19	Peak systolic velocity and waveform normal Spectral broadening present	Mild disease
20–49	30–50% increase in peak systolic velocity Marked spectral broadening	Moderate disease
50–99	50–100% increase in peak systolic velocity Loss of diastolic flow reversal Increase in peak diastolic velocity Extensive spectral broadening Monophasic waveform	Haemodynamically significant
100	No flow detected	Occlusion

forward flow. Analysis of waveform contour, peak systolic velocity, presence of diastolic reverse flow, peak diastolic forward flow, and spectral broadening allows arterial stenoses to be classified into five categories: normal, less than 20 per cent diameter reduction, 20 to 49 per cent diameter reduction, 50 to 99 per cent diameter reduction, and occlusion (Table 5).

A normal waveform is triphasic with a clear systolic window. When a minimal stenosis is present (less than 20 per cent diameter reduction) the waveform contour and peak systolic velocity are unaltered, but mild spectral broadening is seen. Stenoses in the moderate range (20 to 49 per cent) cause a 30 to 50 per cent increase in the peak systolic velocity and more marked spectral

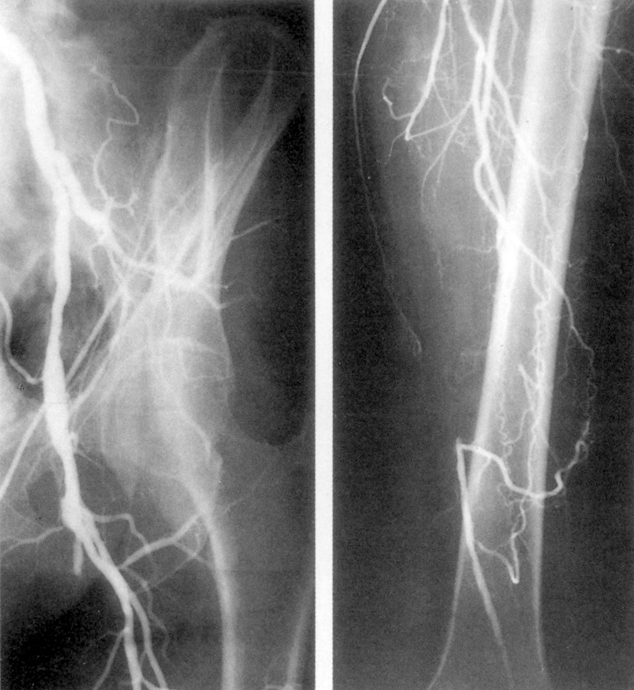

Fig. 22 Arteriogram of the patient in Fig. 21. The arteriogram confirms the occlusion in the superficial femoral artery. The post-exercise study reveals the typical deterioration in waveform and pressure that occurs distal to a haemodynamically significant lesion.

broadening, with filling in of the systolic window. The reverse flow component is usually still present. When severe arterial narrowing occurs (diameter reduction of 50 to 99 per cent) the lesion becomes haemodynamically significant. The pressure drop across the lesion results in reduced peripheral resistance, with resultant loss of the reversed flow component, and the peak diastolic forward flow is elevated. The waveform contour becomes monotonic and there is often a more than 100 per cent increase in peak systolic flow velocity (Fig. 27(a–d)).

TRANSCUTANEOUS OXYGEN TENSION MEASUREMENT

The studies reviewed in this chapter all provide haemodynamic evidence of the degree of arterial insufficiency that exists in a patient with peripheral vascular occlusive disease. Transcutaneous oximetry can provide valuable metabolic data which may be used to supplement the haemodynamic data provided by the other non-invasive tests. Transcutaneous oxygen tension provides information about the metabolic state of the tissue being studied and a measure of the adequacy of the arterial oxygen supply to the tissues.

Measurement of transcutaneous oxygen tension involves the placement of an oxygen-sensing electrode on the skin. The device used contains a small heating unit which warms the skin to a temperature conducive to efficient oxygen diffusion. The quantity of oxygen available for diffusion to the skin is a function of the arterial flow to the area and the amount of oxygen extracted from the blood to meet the metabolic requirements of the tissues. When arterial occlusive disease is severe the tissue perfusion becomes marginal and capillary oxygen perfusion decreases as the proportion of oxygen extraction must increase to meet the metabolic demands of the tissue.

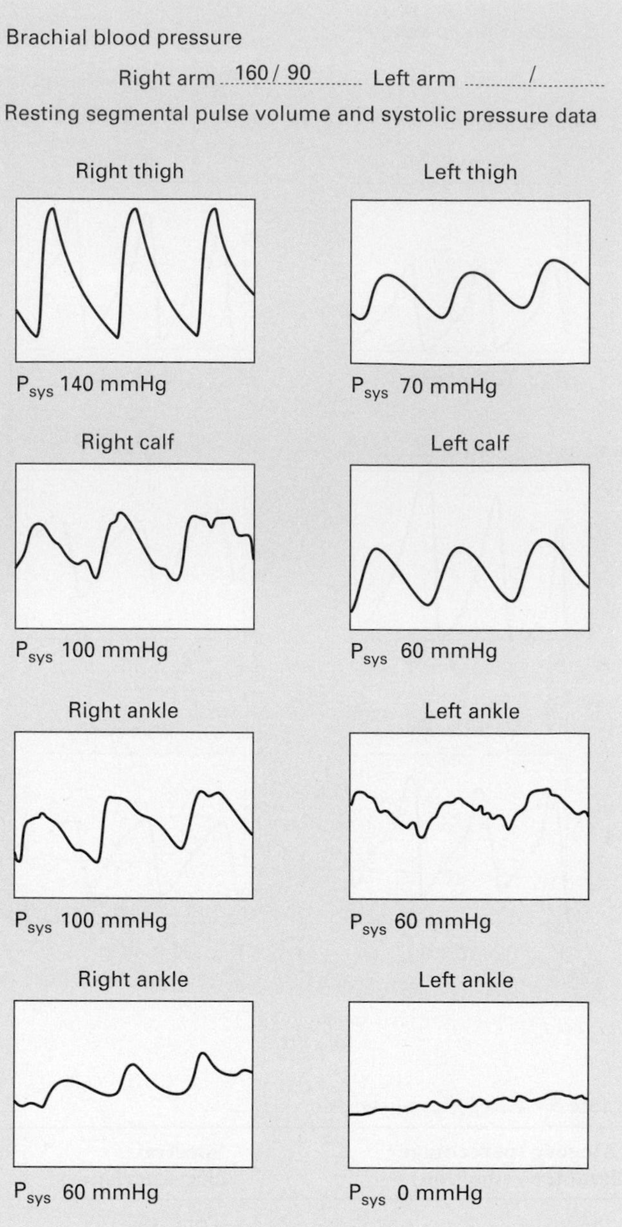

Fig. 23 Pulse volume recording of patient with isolated left iliac artery occlusion and right superficial femoral artery occlusion. Note the more severe post-exercise deterioration (lower tracing) on the side with the more proximal lesion (the left iliac lesion).

Transcutaneous oxygen tension is usually measured at the dorsum of the foot, medial aspect of the calf, and the thigh, with a reference electrode placed in the infraclavicular region. Comparing the value obtained at the lower extremity to that at the chest yields an index which can be compared to a normal value with regard to the patient's age, cardiac output, and arterial oxygen tension, as well as other factors. The normal value is approximately 60 mmHg, but this may decrease by 5 to 6 mmHg in a normal lower extremity. The normal transcutaneous oxygen tension index is 0.9.

Measurements of transcutaneous oxygen tension are not affected by mild or moderate arterial insufficiency; however severe

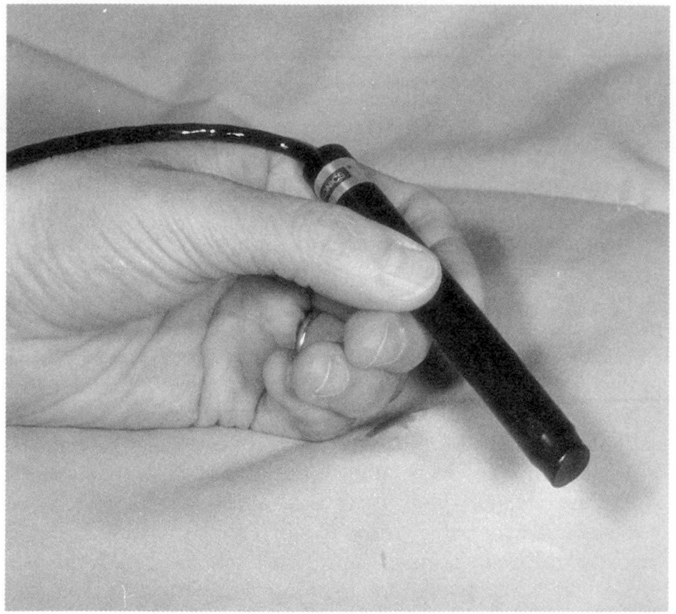

Fig. 24 Standard continuous wave Doppler probe.

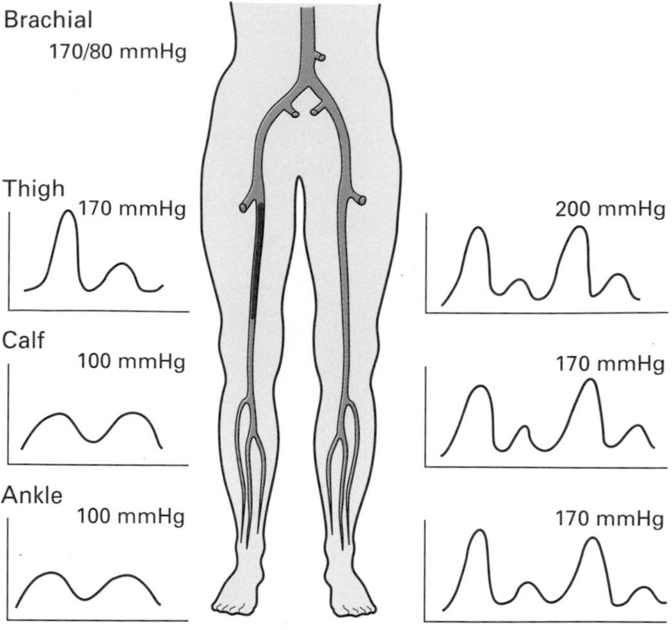

Fig. 26 Complementary analysis of segmental pressures and analogue Doppler or pulse volume recording waveforms increases the accuracy of the studies in diagnosing and locating the level of haemodynamically significant disease. In this example there is a superficial femoral artery occlusion.

peripheral vascular occlusive disease will produce significant changes in the oxygen tension measured at the foot. The study is therefore, often valuable in assessing a patient's risk for limb or tissue loss or in differentiating ischaemic rest pain from neuropathic pain: values of less than 20 mmHg, measured at the foot, are usually obtained in patients with rest pain, ischaemic ulcers, or gangrene.

APPLICATIONS OF THE NON-INVASIVE VASCULAR LABORATORY STUDIES

Intermittent claudication

Exertion-related lower extremity pain may be due to arterial disease, neurological disorders (pseudoclaudication), and orthopaedic or rheumatological problems. Segmental pressures and pulse volume recordings or Doppler velocity waveforms will differentiate vascular from other aetiologies. If ankle pressures greater than 50 mmHg and pulse volume recording categories of 2 or 3 (Table 4) are found, vascular claudication is unlikely. If the ankle pressure is less than 50 mmHg and the pulse volume recording category is 4 or 5, a vascular aetiology is likely. Exercise studies are very important in determining the cause of exertional leg pain: changes in the distal pressure and pulse volume or Doppler waveforms often confirm the diagnosis (Fig. 24).

Less than 5 to 8 per cent of claudicants will progress to the situation where limb loss is inevitable. However, severe claudication can be incapacitating, and the non-invasive studies are often used to supplement the history and physical examination in deciding whether surgical intervention is required.

Rest pain

In patients who present with foot pain at rest, the primary function of the vascular study is to differentiate neuropathic from ischaemic

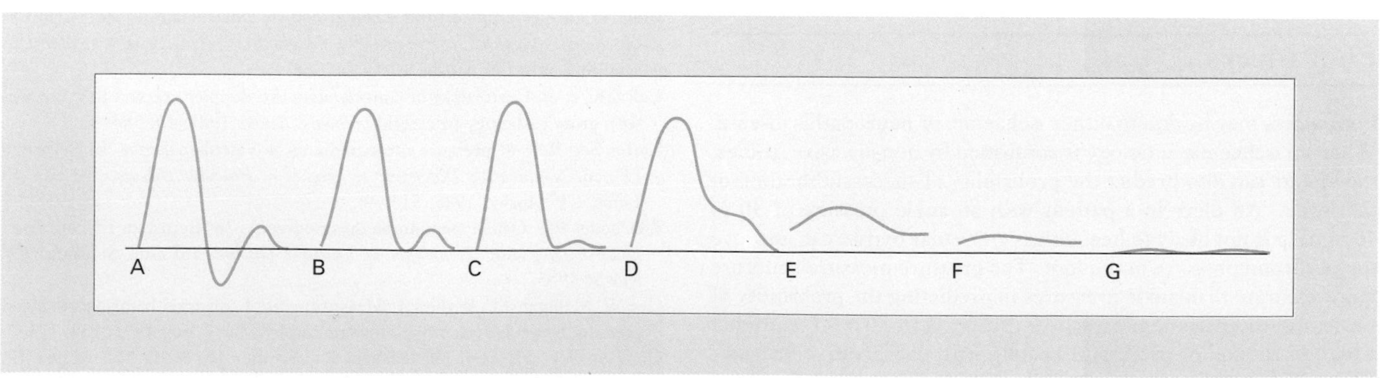

Fig. 25 Doppler velocity analogue waveforms. The waveform becomes increasingly abnormal with more severe arterial occlusive disease.

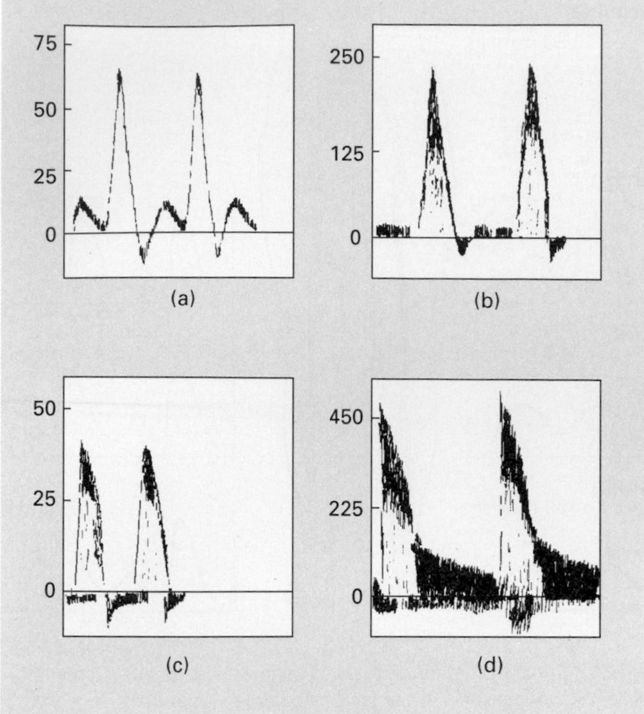

Fig. 27 Pulsed Doppler spectral analysis. (a) Normal artery. (b) Twenty per cent stenosis. (c) Twenty to 49 per cent stenosis. (d) More than 50 per cent stenosis.

foot pain: this is often difficult in diabetic patients. The pertinent studies include measurement of ankle and toe pressures and analysis of pulse volume recordings or Doppler waveforms, as well as measurement of transcutaneous oxygen tension. Ankle pressures less than 35 mmHg (less than 55 mmHg in diabetics) and pulse volume recording categories of 4 or 5 essentially confirm the diagnosis of ischaemic rest pain. If the ankle pressure is greater than 55 mmHg (greater than 80 mmHg in diabetic patients) and pulse volume recordings are in categories 1 to 3, ischaemic pain is unlikely. In diabetics with non-compressible vessels, the pulse volume or Doppler waveforms are more useful than the actual pressures, which may be deceptively high. Measurement of transcutaneous oxygen tension is also valuable in the assessment of the diabetic since non-compressibility of vessels has no effect on this measurement. If ischaemic pain is confirmed, the patient is at high risk for ischaemic tissue (limb) loss and should be evaluated for vascular bypass procedure.

Foot ulcers

Foot ulcers may be due to either ischaemic or neuropathic disease. When an ischaemic aetiology is confirmed by non-invasive studies, the results can also predict the probability of successful healing of the lesion. An ulcer in a patient with an ankle pressure of 30 to 40 mmHg is not likely to heal unless a vascular bypass can improve the perfusion pressure in the foot. Toe pressure measurements are more accurate than ankle pressures in predicting the probability of successful ulcer healing: pressures greater than 30 mmHg predict a high likelihood of successful healing with conservative management. Toe pressures less than this predict the need for revascularization to effect successful healing of the lesion.

Graft surveillance after distal bypass

Distal bypass grafts may fail for a variety of reasons, including retained venous valves, arteriovenous fistulae, anastomotic intimal hyperplasia, and progression of atherosclerosis in the graft or native arteries. Technical errors, myointimal hyperplasia, and progression of atherosclerotic disease cause graft failure by reducing graft blood flow below the thrombotic threshold velocity, below which thrombosis of the graft occurs. Postoperative surveillance allows the failing graft to be identified before occlusion occurs. Indirect physiological measurements such as ankle: brachial index segmental pulse volume recording or Doppler velocity analogue waveforms are probably not sensitive enough to detect reliably the failing but patent graft. Duplex scanning provides a very critical tool for such graft surveillance, providing both B-mode imaging, which defines anatomic complications of the graft (i.e. retained valves or intimal hyperplasia), and Doppler velocimetric data, which may identify a low flow state before thrombosis actually occurs. A low flow state exists when the peak systolic flow velocity is less than 45 cm/s or when a drop in velocity of greater than 30 cm/s occurs between serial measurements in the same graft. An abnormal B-mode scan or velocity measurement should prompt investigation with an arteriogram to assess the graft for possible revision.

FURTHER READING

Aaslid R, Markwalder TM, Nornes H. Noninvasive transcranial doppler ultrasound recording of flow velocity in basal cerebral arteries. *J Neurosurg* 1982; **57**: 769.

Baker JD, Dix D. Variability of doppler ankle pressures with arterial occlusive disease: an elevation of ankle index and brachial-ankle gradient. *Surgery* 1983; **89**: 134.

Baker JD, Barker WF, Machledeer HI. Evaluation of extracranial cerebrovascular disease with ocular pneumoplethysmography. *Am J Surg* 1978; **136**: 206–8.

Baker WH. *et al.* Diagnosis of peripheral occlusive disease: comparison of clinical evaluation and noninvasive vascular laboratory. *Arch Surg.* 1989; **11**: 1308–10.

Beach KW, Phillips DJ. Doppler instrumentation for the evaluation of arterial and venous disease. In Jaffe CC, ed. *Vascular and Doppler Ultrasound.* New York: Churchill Livingstone, 1984: 11–49.

Berkowitz HD, *et al.* Value of routine vascular laboratory studies to identify vein graft stenosis. *Surgery* 1981; **90**: 971–9.

Bernstein NM, Beloev ZG, Norris JW. The limitations of diagnosis of carotid occlusion by doppler ultrasound. *Ann Surg* 1988; **207**: 315–7.

Blackshear WM, *et al.* Detection of carotid occlusive disease by ultrasound imaging and pulsed doppler spectrum analysis. *Surgery* 1979; **86**: 698–706.

Brandyk DF. Monitoring after distal arterial reconstruction. In Bernstein EF, ed. *Recent Advances in Noninvasive Diagnostic Techniques in Vascular Disease.* St Louis: CV Mosby 1990: 247–58

Call GK, *et al.* Correlation of continuous-wave doppler spectral flow analysis with gross pathology in carotid stenosis. *Stroke* 1988; **19**: 584–8.

Carter SA. Role of pressure measurements in vascular disease. In Bernstein EF, ed. *Noninvasive Diagnostic techniques in Vascular Disease.* 3rd edn. St Louis: CV Mosby, 1985: 513–44.

Eikelboom BC. Ocular pneumoplethysmography. In: Bernstein EF, ed. *Noninvasive Diagnostic Techniques in Vascular Disease.* 3rd edn. St Louis: CV Mosby 1985.

Gee W, Mehigan JT, Wylie EJ. Measurement of collateral hemispheric blood pressure by ocular pneumoplethysmography. *Am J Surg* 1975; **130**: 121–7.

Goodson WF, Flanigan DP, Bishara Ra, Schuler JF, Kikta MJ, Meyer JP. Can carotid duplex scanning supplant arteriography in patients with facial carotid territory symptoms? *J Vasc Surg* 1987; **5**: 551–7.

Hausser CJ, Shoemaker WC. Use of a transcutaneous Po_2 regional perfusion index to quantify tissue perfusion in peripheral vascular disease. *Ann Surg* 1983; **197**: 337–43.

Harward TR, Bernstein EF, Fronek A. Continuous-wave versus range-gated pulsed doppler power frequency spectrum analysis in the detection of carotid arterial occlusive disease. *Ann Surg* 1986; **204**: 32–7.

Kameyaama M, Okinaka S. Collateral circulation of the brain with special reverence of atherosclerosis of the major cervical and cerebral arteries. *Neurology* 1963; **13**: 270–86.

Kempczinski RF. Segmental volume plethysmography in the diagnosis of lower extremity arterial occlusive disease. *J Cardiovasc Surg* 1982; **23**: 125–9.

Kempczinski RF. Segmental volume plethysmography: the pulse volume recorder. In Kempczinski RF, Yao JST, eds. *Practical Noninvasive Vascular Diagnosis*, 2nd edn. Chicago: Year Book Medical Publishers, 1987: 142–53.

Kohler TR *et al.* Duplex scanning for aortoiliac and femoropopliteal disease: a prospective study. *Circulation* 1987; **76**: 1074–80.

Leopold PW. *et al.* Duplex ultrasound: its role in the noninvasive follow-up of the *in situ* saphenous vein bypass. *J Vasc Technol* 1987; **11**: 183.

Megerman J, Abbott WA. Transcutaneous oxygen tension determination. In Kempczinski RF, Yao JST, eds. *Practical Noninvasive Diagnosis*. 2nd edn. Chicago: Year Book Medical Publishers 1987: 210–29.

Minh-Chau L, *et al.* Decreased graft flow velocity is a reliable predictor of impending failure of reversed vein grafts. *J Vasc Technol* 1988; **12**: 133.

Moll FL, Eikelboom BC, Vermeulen FE, VanLier JJ, Schulte BP. Dynamics of collateral circulation in progressive asymptomatic carotid disease. *J Vasc Surg* 1986; **3**: 470–4.

Moneta GL, Taylor DC, Strandness E. Noninvasive assessment of cerebrovascular disease. *Ann Vasc Surg* 1986; **1**: 489–501.

Moneta GL, *et al.* Operative versus nonoperative management of asymptomatic high grade internal carotid artery stenosis: improved results with endarterectomy. *Stroke* 1987; **18**: 1005.

Neumyer MM, Thiele BL. Evaluation of lower extremity occlusive disease with doppler ultrasound. In Taylor KJW, Burns PN, Well PNT, eds. *Clinical Applications of Doppler Ultrasound*. New York: Raven Press. 1988; 317–37.

Oh PIT, Provan JL, Amelie FM. The predictability of the success of arterial reconstruction by means of transcutaneous oxygen tension measurements. *J Vasc Surg* 1987; **5**: 356–62.

Otis SM, Ringelstein EB. Principles and applications of transcranial doppler sonography. In Bernstein EF, ed. *Recent Advances in Noninvasive Diagnostic Techniques in Vascular Disease*. St Louis: CV Mosby, 1990: 59–79.

Ramsey DE, Manke DA, Sumner DS. Toe blood pressure—a valuable adjunct to ankle pressure measurement for assessing peripheral arterial disease. *J Cardiovasc Surg* 1983; **24**: 43–8.

Spencer M. Continuous-wave doppler imaging of the carotid bifurcation. In Bernstein EF, ed. *Noninvasive Diagnostic Techniques in Vascular Disease*. 3rd edn. St Louis: CV Mosby 1985: 367–9.

Strandness DE, Jr. The Seattle data. In Bernstein EF, ed. *Recent Advances in Noninvasive Diagnostic Techniques in Vascular Disease*. St. Louis: CV Mosby 1990: 129–34.

Sumner DS. Noninvasive assessment of peripheral arterial occlusive disease. In Rutherford RB, ed. *Vascular Surgery*. Eastbourne: WC Saunders 1989; 61–111.

Sumner DS. Noninvasive assessment of peripheral arterial occlusive disease. In Rutherford RB, ed. *Vascular Surgery*. Eastbourne: WB Saunders 1989: 61–3.

Sumner DW, Strandness DE, Jr. Hemodynamic studies before and after extended bypass grafts to the tibial and peroneal arteries. *Surgery* 1978; **84**: 348.

Turnipseed WD, Acker CW. Postoperative surveillance. An effective means of detecting correctable lesions that threaten graft patency. *Arch Surg* 1985; **120**: 324–8.

Wells PNT. Instrumentation including color flow mapping. In Taylor KJ, Burns PN, Wells PNT, eds. *Clinical Applications of Doppler Ultrasound*. Raven Press 1987: 26–45.

Wieber DO, Whisnant JP. In Warlow C, Morris PJ, eds. *Transient Ischemic Attacks*. New York: Marcel Dekker, 1982; Ch. 1: 1–19.

Yao JST. Noninvasive techniques of measuring lower limb arterial pressures. In Bernstein EF, ed. *Noninvasive Diagnostic Techniques in Vascular Disease*. 3rd edn. St Louis: CV Mosby 1985: 83–90.

Zierler RE. Color-flow doppler imaging: normal and abnormal carotid studies. In Bernstein EF, ed. *Recent Advances in Noninvasive Diagnostic Techniques in Vascular Disease*. St Louis: CV Mosby, 1985: 37–41.

Zierler RE, Strandness DE, Jr. Duplex scanning for diagnosis of aortoiliac and lower extremity disease. *J Vasc Technol* 1987; **11**: 99–102.

7.5 Vascular prostheses

DAVID T. ZELT AND WILLIAM M. ABBOTT

INTRODUCTION

Dacron, and to a lesser extent Teflon, has become the major synthetic grafting material. Unlike nylon, Ivalon, and Vinyon-N which lose their tensile strength after implantation, Dacron and Teflon remain essentially unchanged even after long periods. Teflon is generally less reactive than Dacron. Poor reactivity may be a more or a less desirable property since it is associated with less tissue reaction, less incorporation of tissue into the graft, and less fibroblastic invasion.

Grafts may be fabricated as either a woven or knitted yarn. They can also be manufactured with a velour surface. Braided yarns have fallen from use as they tend to be quite bulky and difficult to handle; fabric prostheses are now made from multifilament yarn. In woven grafts, the threads are interlaced in a simple over-and-under pattern whereas a knitted fabric is made with threads that are looped to form a continuous interlocking chain. In general, the woven fabrics are less porous and stiffer than the knitted fabrics.

Velour is a variant of the Dacron fabric prosthesis developed in the later 1960s. The velour surface has loops of yarn extending upward at right angles to the fabric surface, giving the surface a velvety, plush texture. The velour finish can be made on the external, internal, or both surfaces of the graft. The velour configuration may possibly be important in providing a ‘trellis’ for the graft healing process.

An alternative to the fabric protheses is expanded Teflon or polytetrafluoroethylene which unlike the Dacron prostheses, is not a textile graft. Expanded polytetrafluoroethylene is a fluorocarbon polymer manufactured by forcibly expanding Teflon through a heating and stretching process. The result is a material consisting of solid nodes with interconnecting small fibrils. The length of the fibril determines the pore size which has been standardized to approximately 30 μm. Fluorine atoms in Teflon impart a highly electronegative surface charge to the graft, making it hydrophobic: this property is claimed to play a role in resistance to thrombosis. Early clinical experience with the expanded polytetrafluoroethylene graft was disappointing: aneurysm dilation developed in a number of grafts. The graft has since been reinforced by either a thin skin of polytetrafluoroethylene, thickened walls, or application of an external support coil.

An alternative to the fabric or polymeric vascular graft is the use of biological materials as a conduit. Bovine heterografts were the first biological graft developed for human implantation. These grafts stemmed from the work of Rosenberg who in 1956 described a process using the enzyme ficin that resulted in the production of pure collagen tube which was then tanned. The tanning process stabilizes the collagen tube by chemically cross-linking the collagen fibrils with dialdehyde starch. The chemically modified heterografts were prone to aneurysmal degeneration and, like the homografts, they were abandoned. The bovine heterograft was, however, a prototype for another tanned prosthesis: the human umbilical cord vein allograft stabilized with glutaraldehyde.

Early clinical experience with the human umbilical cord vein gave disappointing results. The grafts underwent degenerative changes early, with subsequent thrombosis and aneurysmal dilation. Although a glutaraldehyde stabilized and external Dacron mesh reinforced human umbilical vein was used for a while, degradation occurs within about 5 years.

SELECTION OF ARTERIAL GRAFTS

No single graft is suitable for every clinical situation. The choice of arterial substitute depends upon the diameter of the native vessel being replaced or bypassed, the anatomical location, whether a joint is being crossed, the presence of infection, the length of graft needed, and whether or not an autogenous substitute is an option.

Aortic grafts

The size of the vessel to be bypassed is obviously important in selecting the best graft. Since no autograft is of sufficient size to replace the aorta, prosthetic grafts are always necessary. Dacron grafts in either a woven or knitted configuration are the primary substitute, although polytetrafluoroethylene grafts are also available for aortic grafting. Knitted grafts are more pliable, softer, and easier to sew then are woven grafts. They are, however are more porous than woven grafts and must be rigorously preclotted before use to seal the interstices of the graft. During most operations employing porous, knitted grafts, 50 to 60 ml of blood is withdrawn from a convenient vessel prior to administration of systemic heparin and used to flush the prosthesis repeatedly until the interstices fail to pass blood. Knitted grafts impregnated with collagen do not need preclotting and are now available.

The choice of grafts for aortic replacement is arbitrary; all have good and fairly equivalent long-term patency. Special characteristics of each, however, makes one variety more favourable under certain circumstances. At the Massachusetts General Hospital and at Oxford Dacron grafts are the primary choice for aortic reconstruction, although expanded polytetrafluoroethylene is occasionally used, but usually in the smallest diameters. A knitted Dacron graft is ideal for elective aortic surgery because of its handling characteristics. However, with recent improvements in weaving technology, more woven grafts have been used in these institutions. In other circumstances, especially when blood loss is critical, such as with thoracic aortic surgery and ruptured aortic aneurysms, a woven Dacron graft is clearly the better choice.

Results have been good when using Dacron for arterial replacement of the aortofemoral system because of their high flow rate. Five-year patency rates approach 90 per cent for aortobifemoral bypass. By 10 years the patency rates fall to approximately 70 per cent. In a long-term study of nearly 1000 patients who underwent bypass for aortoiliac occlusive disease, Crawford *et al.* reported 10, 15, and 20-year patency rates of 79 per cent, 70 per cent, and 56 per cent respectively.

Extra-anatomic grafts

So-called extra-anatomic bypass grafting for aortoiliac disease gained popularity for the treatment of high risk patients who were considered to be unsuitable candidates for a major intra-abdominal operation. The two most common types of extra-anatomic bypass grafting are the axillofemoral and the femorofemoral bypasses. Both Dacron and expanded polytetrafluoroethylene have been used with similar success and patency rates. Patency rates after axillofemoral bypass range from 40 to 90 per cent at 5 years; the major determinant of patency is the status of the peripheral run-off. Femorofemoral bypass has patency rates comparable to those of aortofemoral grafting: 79, 68, and 60 per cent at 5, 10, and 15 years. At the Massachusetts General Hospital the femorofemoral bypass graft is used not only for the high risk patient, but also for the management of unilateral iliac occlusion in young patients, especially men, since avoiding para-aortic dissection eliminates the risk of sexual dysfunction. On the other hand, axillofemoral grafting is rarely used except in patients with aortic graft infection.

Infrainguinal grafts

The choice of grafting material for infrainguinal repairs is less straightforward than it is with aortic surgery. The material and the construction of the graft play a major role in determining the long-term patency. The anatomic location of the distal anastomosis and the status of the distal run-off are very important elements to consider when deciding which graft to use.

Undoubtedly the best patency and limb salvage rates are found when autogenous saphenous vein is used. In at least 20 per cent of patients, however, the saphenous vein is of inadequate length or calibre, or has been surgically removed for coronary artery bypass grafting or management of varicose veins. In general, veins less than 3 mm in diameter are inadequate for use as bypass conduits, and an alternative must be chosen. Other autogenous conduits such as the short saphenous veins, contralateral greater saphenous vein, or arm veins can be used. If these are also inadequate or unaccessible, a prosthetic graft must be used.

Currently expanded polytetrafluoroethylene and human umbilical vein grafts are the two prostheses more frequently used. In certain cases a composite or segmental graft can be used to allow more distal grafting when the vein is of insufficient length: such grafts make use of available vein as the distal segment of the bypass. The composite graft is joined to a more proximal segment of prosthetic graft, thereby producing a suitable length of conduit for distal revascularization. We do not often use a true composite graft for femoropopliteal grafting because currently available prothetic grafts perform as well or better. When mixed graft materials are used, it is usually as a sequential graft with the distal anastomosis to two or more segments.

Textile prostheses such as Dacron have markedly inferior patency rates in bypass to the popliteal artery compared to saphenous vein; 5-year patency results for bypass in the femoropopliteal position for saphenous vein and Dacron are 72 and 20 per cent respectively. Because of consistently poor results, Dacron grafts are no longer used for this type of procedure.

Without doubt expanded polytetrafluoroethylene has become the most commonly used synthetic conduit for infrainguinal reconstruction. Many papers have been published in recent years describing use of this material for distal reconstruction, but clearly defined indications for its use are lacking.

In a recent 6-year, prospective, multicentre, randomized comparison of autogenous saphenous vein and expanded polytetrafluoroethylene, Veith *et al.* demonstrated autologous saphenous vein to be superior for femoropopliteal bypasses, particularly when they cross the knee. By 4 years in the above-knee position, the differences between vein and expanded polytetrafluoroethylene were statistically significant, with saphenous vein showing a patency rate of 68 per cent, compared with 38 per cent for synthetic grafts. In the below-knee position, saphenous vein was also superior, with patency rates of 76 per cent and 54 per cent respectively. In the tibioperoneal location, saphenous vein grafts showed patency rate of 49 per cent, compared to 12 per cent for expanded polytetrafluoroethylene. The study failed to support the routine preferential use of expanded polytetrafluoroethylene grafts for either femoropopliteal or more distal bypasses. Flinn *et al.* reported an improved patency rate of 37 per cent when expanded polytetrafluoroethylene grafts were placed into the tibioperoneal location with the administration of postoperative warfarin.

Despite the many studies reporting significantly better patency and limb salvage rates following femoropopliteal bypass with saphenous vein some authors prefer expanded polytetrafluoroethylene, especially when placed above the knee. We use such synthetic grafts instead of vein only under specific circumstances and only in the above-knee position. Expanded polytetrafluoroethylene is rarely taken to the below-knee popliteal artery and virtually never to the tibial vessels. We favour an above-knee expanded polytetrafluoroethylene when operative time is important, in unstable or high-risk patients or in those requiring a femoropopliteal bypass in addition to a more extensive proximal inflow procedure such as an aortobifemoral bypass. Angiographic evidence of good run-off must be present to satisfy predictions of patency of the graft. Less than two-vessel run-off and the presence of diabetes reduces the 2-year patency of polytetrafluoroethylene grafts from 70 to 30 per cent.

Using expanded polytetrafluoroethylene to save the saphenous vein in case future coronary artery bypass grafting is necessary is unwarranted. Natural history and retrospective studies have shown that only a small percentage of patients who present with symptoms of peripheral vascular disease actually ever require coronary artery bypass grafting at a later time.

The difference in the patency rates of synthetic material and autogenous saphenous vein anastomosed to below-knee vessels may be partly due to the length of graft needed to reach the below-knee arteries, the technical difficulties in anastomosing the graft to a small artery, and to the difference in the elastic properties of the prosthesis and the host artery. Interposing a cuff of vein between an expanded polytetrafluoroethylene prosthesis and the artery produces patency rates of 91 per cent and 72 per cent for femoropopliteal and femorotibial grafts, respectively. This cuff of vein may decrease the compliance mismatch between host artery and prosthetic graft, but it is still not apparent whether it will improve long-term patency or reduce the development of neointimal hyperplasia. Decreased juxta-anastomotic neo-intimal hyperplasia is present in vein cuffed grafts in dogs. We have had only limited experience with the technique, since we so rarely use prostheses in these patients.

The glutaraldehyde-treated human umbilical vein is the most commonly used alternative to polytetrafluoroethylene for infrainguinal grafting. A comparison of these two materials found no differences for above-knee anastomoses. However, patency rates and limb salvage were better for human umbilical vein in below-knee anastomoses and in poor run-off situations. Other studies have also found that below-knee human umbilical vein grafts tend to have slightly better patency than expanded polytetrafluoroethylene, but human umbilical vein has the disadvantage of being technically difficult to handle. One study reported a 42 per cent dilation rate and a 57 per cent rate of aneurysm formation in patients with human umbilical vein grafts implanted for more than 2 years. Because of the appreciable incidence of thrombosis and aneurysmal degeneration we have not implanted an umbilical graft for several years.

AETIOLOGY OF GRAFT FAILURE

Graft failure is a major problem facing the vascular surgeon: patients are often more symptomatic after graft failure than they were before the bypass procedure. In a retrospective review of the outcome of failed femoropopliteal grafts, two-thirds of patients with failed grafts initially undertaken for claudication were no worse following graft occlusion. However, 24 per cent showed worsened ischaemia when the graft failed. A considerable number of patients were thereby converted to a limb-threatened status. Since all prosthetic grafts available are prone to complications, the vascular surgeon must understand the aetiologies of graft failure to enable him to reduce the risk of failure to a minimum.

Time period of graft failure

The causes of graft failure can best be divided into four time periods (Table 1). Acute graft failures (within 48 h) are usually secondary to technical errors in the creation of the anastomosis, a retained unlysed valve cusp, or placement of the graft at a site of poor inflow or outflow. Intraoperative angiography or angioscopy can provide detailed assessment of the anastomosis, and if an error such as an intimal flap or stenosis at the toe of the graft is recog-

Table 1 Aetiology of graft failure

Time period	Aetiology
0–24 to 48 h	Technical errors
0–2 months	Increased thomboreactivity
2–18 months	Intimal hyperplasia
>18 months	Progressive atherosclerosis

nized, the anastomosis can be repaired or revised. Reinspection of the preoperative angiogram must include assessment of the quality of the inflow vessels as well as the outflow. Areas of proximal stenosis revealed by angiography should be evaluated for haemodynamic significance by measuring intraluminal pressure gradients across the narrowed lumen. Significant blocks should be corrected before a more distal bypass procedure is performed. The blocks required proximal bypass or a balloon angioplasty.

Graft failure occurring between 2 days and 12 weeks after surgery is usually secondary to a heightened graft thromboreactivity. Thromboreactivity exists with all grafts or reconstructions but varies in intensity and duration and is governed by host factors (coagulability and blood flow), as well as by inherent properties of the graft (surface thrombogenicity and compliance). There may be a 'thrombotic threshold velocity' required to maintain graft patency and which reflects thromboreactivity. Velocities below a given level for any graft material will lead to thrombosis and closure of the graft.

Graft failure up to 18 months after operation is usually due to intimal hyperplastic lesions. Anastomotic intimal hyperplasia is commonly greater at the downstream or outflow anastomosis, and also occurs within the body of vein grafts. Its cause is unknown, but it is a very complex problem. Two major theories involve the response to injury hypothesis and the response of the vessel wall to new conditions of physical stress.

Graft failure after 18 months postoperatively is most often due to progression of atherosclerosis at or beyond the distal anastomosis. As discussed earlier the concept of distal progression of disease as a cause of late graft failure has been used by some as an argument in favour of using prosthetic material for femoropopliteal bypass, saving the saphenous vein for reconstruction of a more distal outflow vessel in those patient who develop further problems.

Structural failure

Structural failures are rare in modern day fabric prostheses. Some of the earlier grafts were flawed by friability, inability to hold sutures, and graft dilation; the knitted variety were more likely to fail. Complications associated with dilation include bleeding through graft interstices, fibre breakdown with resultant holes and tears, deposition of mural thrombus with possible graft occlusion or distal embolism, and development of anastomotic aneurysms. Almost all fabric prostheses dilate after implantation. An obligatory 15 to 20 per cent dilation occurs with knitted grafts, and this should not be viewed as a complication. In a small percentage of grafts, true aneurysmal dilation occurs. The risk of graft failure associated with dilation is unknown. In a study of 32 patients with knitted Dacron grafts to an average duration of 175 days no part of a graft dilated more than 94 per cent. Although woven grafts with interlocking yarns have little or no inherent stretch, knitted fabrics have much more stretch because of their looped structure. The loops straighten in the line of greatest stress, leading to dilation. Life-time followup of patients with these grafts is required. Advanced degeneration warrants replacement of the graft.

Anastomotic false aneurysm

An anastomotic false aneurysm results from a partial or complete separation of the prosthetic graft from the host artery. Although false aneurysms can occur at any site, they are most frequent at the common femoral artery, with a frequency rate of approximately 3 per cent. The aetiology of anastomotic false aneurysms is multifactorial. In the distant past, fragmentation of silk sutures was associated with many false aneurysms; now that non-absorbable, synthetic suture is used, suture failure is rarely a cause. In the majority of cases the sutures are intact, remaining attached to the graft with the tear occurring along the host artery. The cause of the tear may be due to atherosclerotic degenerative changes in the host artery wall. Endarterectomy at the site of the anastomosis weakens the anastomotic site and could be a predisposing factor leading to the formation of false aneurysms. Other contributing factors include a compliance mismatch between graft and host artery, infection, improper suturing technique, and tension on the suture line. Complications of false aneurysms include rupture, thrombosis, and embolism. In general, an anastomotic false aneurysm should be surgically repaired when diagnosed. In the elderly or high risk patient small false aneurysms (<2 cm) can be left untreated but require close monitoring. Any sign of expansion mandates repair.

Graft infection

Graft infection is one of the most devastating complications of arterial reconstruction. Although infection does not necessarily lead to graft thrombosis, it is a failure of the bypass procedure. The incidence ranges from 1 to 2 per cent for series reporting aortic prosthesis and up to 6 per cent for femoropopliteal grafts. Major morbidity and mortality is associated with the development of graft infection, and the entire infected graft must usually be removed to control the problem, followed by revascularization by an extra-anatomical route such as the obturator foramen.

OPTIMAL GRAFT DESIGN

The perfect graft material does not exist, although a number of characteristics have been suggested (Table 2). The graft must be available in a variety of sizes and lengths to accommodate aortic or distal tibial vessel bypasses. It should be easy to handle and suture. The graft must be non-fraying, pliable, and be able to conform to the artery to which it is being anastomosed. It should be durable, strong, and last the life expectancy of the patient without degeneration. The graft should be biocompatible, allowing healing with a non-thrombogenic surface; a graft that becomes completely lined with endothelium would be optimal. The prosthesis should match the viscoelastic properties of the host artery to which it is to be anastomosed. It should have a low associated infection rate, and a high, long-term patency rate. Unfortunately, no one arterial substitute, autogenous or prosthetic has all of these properties. An ideal graft however would have a perfect patency rate with no thrombotic occlusions, would not have pathological neo-intima, and would not develop infection, dilate, become aneurysmal, or otherwise breakdown and rupture.

Table 2 Characteristics of the ideal vascular prosthesis

1. Available in a variety of sizes and lengths
2. Ease of handling and suturability
3. Durable
4. Non-thrombogenic
5. Low infectivity
6. High patency rate
7. Viscoelastic properties similar to the host artery

Haemodynamic considerations

When replacing or bypassing an arterial segment with a vascular graft, one hopes that the graft will behave like the normal artery, providing non-turbulent, pulsatile flow. Unfortunately this is not always the case. A number of properties of the graft must be controlled in order to provide the most durable conduit, such as the diameter and the length in order to provide adequate flow to the distal arterial tree. Flow through a graft is best considered by the Poiseuille equation:

$$Q = \frac{(P_1 - P_2)r^4}{8nL}$$

where Q is the flow (cm^3 s), $P_1 - P_2$ represents the pressure gradient ($dynes/cm^2$) between two points separated by the distance L, r (cm) is the radius of the tube, and n the coefficient of viscosity of the fluid blood in poise (dyne s cm^2). Thus, graft diameter and length are the major determinants of resistance to steady flow.

Impedance is the equivalent to resistance in oscillating systems. Blood flowing through blood vessels is of course moved by pulsatile flow rather than by steady flow. As intraluminal pressure increases with systole, the arterial wall stretches and then returns to baseline during diastole. Thus, the distensibility or compliance of the vessel plays an additional important role in the impedance to pulsatile flow. Compliance is defined as the fractional change in diameter per unit change in pressure:

$$C = \frac{D}{DP}$$

The less compliant a vessel, the greater will be its impedance. Experimentally, compliant grafts are more likely to remain patent than stiff, non-compliant grafts. The consequences of a mismatch in viscoelastic properties (i.e. compliance) may therefore explain the inferior performance and decreased patency of small and medium sized grafts when a rigid graft is anastomosed to a compliant host vessel.

Biomaterial characteristics

It was hoped that prosthetic grafts would develop an endothelial lined surface with flow characteristics of the host artery. Initial observations in animals gave very encouraging results since implanted fabric prostheses 'healed' completely, with the production of a viable endothelial cell lined neointima. Prosthetic grafts in human beings do not develop such a neointimal lining; instead the grafts are lined by fibrin or a pseudointima. Subsequent clinical work has shown that man has a limited ability to organize the fibrin layer and that the ability to 'heal' the graft with an intimal lining is confined only to a small zone of pannus ingrowth adjacent to the ends of the graft.

Shortly after implantation, a 1 mm layer of fibrin forms on the inner surface of a fabric prosthesis. This layer is important in small diameter conduits and ultimately leads to occlusion of blood vessels less than 5 mm in diameter. The fibrin layer than becomes organized by ingrowth of fibroblasts arising from the bloodstream and most importantly, from ingrowth through the interstices of the graft wall. This organization is apparent within a few days after graft implantation and is completed within a few weeks. Capillaries traverse the graft interstices to nurture the neoinitimal lining.

Much work has gone into to determining the ideal porosity of textile grafts and to promote quicker healing and ingrowth on tissue into the prostheses. Porosity has been standardized in terms of the volume of filtered water passed per minute through 1 cm^2 of fabric at a water pressure equivalent to 120 mmHg. Grafts must be minimally porous at implantation to prevent massive haemorrhage but yet have maximum porosity for healing. Most knitted grafts have a porosity between 1200 and 1900 ml/cm^2.min. The tight woven grafts have porosity as low as 50 ml/cm^2.min. A newly developed velour graft acts a trellis for cellular ingrowth and leads to firm graft adherence to surrounding tissues.

FURTHER READING

Abbott WM, Bouchier-Hayes DJ. In: Dardik H, ed. *Graft Materials in Vascular Surgery*. Chicago: Year Book Medical Publishers, 1978: 59–78.

Abbott WM, *et al.* Effect of compliance mismatch in vascular graft patency. *J Vasc Surg* 1987; 5 376–82.

Birinyi LK, Douville EC, Lewis SA, Bjornson HS, Kempczinske RF Increased resistance to bacteremic graft infection after endothelial cell seeding. *J Vasc Surg* 1987; **5**: 193–7.

Brewster DC, Darling RC. Optimal methods of aortoiliac reconstruction. *Surgery* 1978; **84**: 739–48.

Brewster DC, LaSalle AJ, Robison JG, Strayhorn EC, Darling RC Factors affecting patency of femoropopliteal bypass grafts. *Surg Gynecol Obstet* 1983; **157**: 437–42.

Brewster DC, Lasalle AJ, Robison JG, Strayhorn EC, Darling RC Femoropopliteal graft failures. *Arch Surg* 1983; **118**: 1043–7.

Crawford ES, Bomberger RA, Glaeser DH, Salch SA, Russell WC Aortoiliac occlusive disease: Factors influencing survival and function following reconstructive operation over a twenty-five year period. *Surgery* 1981; **90**: 1055–67.

Dale WA. Arterial grafts: 1900–1978. In: Dardik H, ed. *Graft Materials in Vascular Surgery*. Chicago: Year Book Medical Publishers, 1978: 3–14.

Dardik H, *et al.* A decade of experience with the glutaraldehyde-tanned human umbilical cord vein graft for revascularization of the lower limb. *J Vasc Surg* 1988; **7**: 336–46.

Eickhoff JH, *et al.* Four years' results of a prospective, randomized clinical trial comparing polytetrafluoroethylene and modified human umbilical vein for below-knee femoropopliteal bypass. *J Vasc Surg* 1987; **6**: 506–11.

Flinn WR, *et al.* Improved long-term patency of infragenicular polytetrafluoroethylene grafts. *J Vasc Surg* 1988; **7**: 685–90.

Freischlag JA, Moore WS. Infection in prosthetic vascular grafts. In: Rutherford RB, ed. *Vascular Surgery*. 3rd edn Philadelphia: W. B. Saunders, 1989: 510–21.

Hasson JE, *et al.* Mural degeneration in the glutaraldehyde-tanned human umbilical vein graft: Incidence and implications. *J Vasc Surg* 1986; **4**: 243–50.

Houser LS Hashmi FH Jaeger VJ, Chawla SK, Brown L, Kemler RL. Should the greater saphenous vein be preserved in patients requiring arterial outflow reconstruction in the lower extremity? *Surgery* 1984; **95**: 467–72.

Julien S, *et al.* Biologic and Structural evaluation of 80 surgically excised HUV grafts. *Can J Surg* 1989; **32**: 101–7.

Lasalle AJ, *et al.* Femoropopliteal composite bypass grafts: current status. *Surgery* 1982; **92**: 36.

Leather RP, Shah DM, Karomody AM. Infrapopliteal arterial bypass for limb salvage: increased patency and utilization of the saphenous vein used '*in situ*'. *Surgery* 1981; **90**: 1000–8.

LoGerfo FW, Quist WC, Nowak MD, Cranshaw HM, Haudenschild CC. Downstream anastomotic hyperplasia: a mechanism of failure in Dacron arterial grafts. *Am Surg* 1983; **197**: 479–83.

Miller, A, *et al.* Routine intraoperative angioscopy in lower extremity revascularization. *Arch Surg* 1989; **124**: 604–8.

Nunn C, Carter MM, Donohue MT, Hudgins PC. Postoperative dilation of knitted Dacron aortic bifurcation grafts. *J Vasc Surg* 1990; **12**: 291–7.

Ottinger LW, Darling RC, Wirthlin LS, Linton RR. Failure of ultralightweight knitted Dacron grafts in arterial reconstruction. *Arch Surg* 1976; **111**: 145–9.

Ortenwall P, Wadenvik A, Risberg B. Reduced platelet deposition of seeded versus endothelial segments of expanded polytetrafluoroethylene. *J Vasc Surg* 1989; **10**: 374–80.

Ortenwall P, Wadenvik H, Kutti J, Risberg B. Endothelial cell seeding reduces thrombogenicity of Dacron grafts in humans. *J Vasc Surg* 1990; **11**: 403–10.

Prendiville EJ, Yeager A, O'Donnell TF, *et al.* Longterm results with the above-knee popliteal expanded polytetrafluoroethylene graft. *J Vasc Surg* 1990; **11**: 517–24.

Quinones-Baldrich WJ, Martin-Paredero V, Balier JD, Busuttil RW, Machleder HI, Moore WS. Polytetrafluoroethylene grafts as the first-choice arterial substitute in femoropopliteal revascularization. *Arch Surg* 1984; **119**: 1238–43.

Robison FG, Brewster DC, Abbott WM, Darling RC. Femoropopliteal and tibioperoneal artery reconstruction using human umbilical vein. *Arch Surg* 1983; **118**: 1039–42.

Rosenberg N. Physiologic factors in arterial grafting. In: Dardik H, ed. *Graft Materials in Vascular Surgery*. Chicago: Year Book Medical Publishers, 1978: 15–28.

Rutherford RB. High risk patient with aortoiliac disease. In: Brewster DC, ed. *Common Problems in Vascular Surgery*. Chicago: Year Book Medical Publishers, 1989: 150–6.

Rutherford RB, *et al.* Factors affecting the patency of infrainguinal bypass. *J Vasc Surg* 1988; 8 236–46.

Satiani B. False aneurysms following arterial reconstruction. *Surg Gynecol Obstet* 1981; **152**: 357–63.

Sauvage LR., Berger KE, Wood SJ, Yates SG, Smith JC, Mansfield PB. Interspecies healing of porous arterial prosthesis. *Arch Surg* 1974; **109**: 698–705.

Shue WB, *et al.* Prevention of vascular prosthetic infection with an antibiotic-bonded Dacron graft. *J Vasc Surg* 1988; **8**: 600–5.

Sterpette AV, Schultz RD, Feldhaus RJ, Pertz DJ. Seven year experience with polytetrafluoroethylene as above-knee femoropopliteal bypass graft. Is it worth while to preserve the autogenous saphenous vein? *J Vasc Surg* 1985; **2**: 907–12.

Suggs WD, Henriques HF, DePalma RG. Vein cuff interposition prevents juxta-anastomotic neointimal hyperplasia. *Ann Surg* 1988; **207**: 717–23.

Szilagyi DE, Elliott JR, Smith RF, Reddy DJ, McPharlin A. Thirty year survey of the reconstructive surgical treatment of aorto iliac occuluvive disease. *J Vasc Surg* 1986; **3**: 421–35.

Whittemore AD, Clowes AW, Couch NP, Mannick JA. Secondary femoropopliteal reconstruction. *Ann Surg* 1981; **193**: 35–42.

Veith FJ, *et al.* Six-year prospective multicenter randomized comparison of autologous saphenous vein and expanded polytetrafluoroethylene grafts in infrainguinal arterial reconstructions. *J Vasc Surg* 1986; **3**: 104–14.

7.6.1 Aortoiliac disease

JOHN D. EDWARDS AND DAVID C. BREWSTER

The infrarenal aorta and iliac arteries are among the most common sites of chronic atherosclerotic occlusive disease in patients with symptomatic arterial insufficiency of the lower extremities. Proper management of patients with aortoiliac disease requires an understanding of the various clinical presentations, the typical patterns of commonly associated infrainguinal arteriosclerotic disease, the incidence of coexistent cardiopulmonary disease, and the variety of surgical techniques available for therapeutic intervention. Proper patient selection, with careful history taking and physical examination, well accepted and standardized indications for surgery, appropriate preoperative testing and perioperative monitoring techniques, and use of appropriate procedures for each individual patient will usually result in a favourable clinical result with a low risk.

CLINICAL PRESENTATION

The initial manifestation of aortoiliac occlusive disease is intermittent claudication of the lower extremities, usually the buttock, hip, thigh, and calf muscle groups. The claudication is often more disabling than that associated with isolated femoropopliteal disease due to the larger number of muscle groups affected in more proximal occlusive disease. Some patients with aortoiliac disease, particularly those with disease affecting both inflow and outflow vessels, will present with claudicatory symptoms isolated to the calf. In addition to intermittent claudication, male patients with aortoiliac disease may present with the classic triad of diminished femoral pulses, lower extremity claudication, and impotence, known as the Leriche syndrome.

The symptoms experienced by an individual patient depend upon the distribution and severity of the occlusive process (Fig. 1). When disease is confined to the aortic bifurcation and the common iliac arteries (type 1 disease), limb-threatening ischaemia is rare and the symptoms are limited to claudication. Numerous

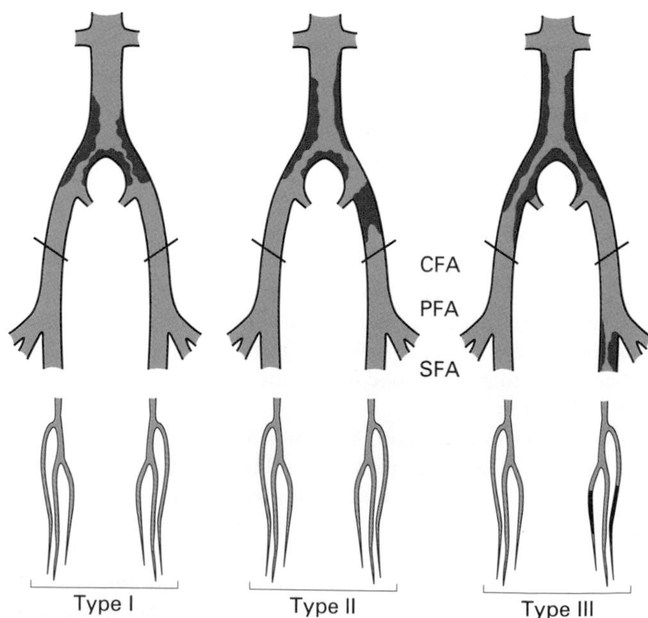

Fig. 1 Distribution of disease. Type I: disease localized to aortic bifurcation; type II: disease also involves external iliac arteries; type III: multilevel disease with infrainguinal arterial disease.

pathways of collateral circulation are often found in patients with type I disease, and these may result in only mild to moderate claudication, even when the aortoiliac segment is completely occluded. Haemodynamic compromise of the distal aortic segment may result in the recruitment of stem collaterals from the intercostal and lumbar arteries to anastomose with re-entry collaterals of the iliolumbar, gluteal, deep circumflex iliac, and epigastric arteries. Visceral collaterals involving the left colic branch of the superior mesenteric artery may reconstitute flow in the hypogastric artery via the marginal artery of Drummond and the haemorrhoidal plexus. Complete occlusions of the external iliac arteries may be compensated for by collateral flow through the gluteal branches of the hypogastric artery to the circumflex femoral branch of the profunda femoral artery ('cruciate anastomosis').

Type I disease is relatively infrequent (5–10 per cent) in patients with symptoms severe enough to warrant consideration for surgical revascularization. It is more common in younger patients in whom there is a lower incidence of associated coronary disease, hypertension, and diabetes. However, these patients often have abnormal lipid profiles (such as Frederickson Type IV hyperlipidemia). Type I disease is also unusual in that there is a high incidence of women with this disease pattern (nearly 50 per cent of patients).

The majority of patients with symptomatic aortoiliac occlusive disease will have a more widespread distribution of disease. Approximately 25 per cent of patients have extension of the disease process into the external iliac arteries (type II) and 65 per cent have the more widespread type III pattern of disease involving the aortoiliac segments and the infrainguinal arteries. Patients with Type III disease and the so-called 'tandem lesions' or combined segment disease present with more severe incapacitating claudication and may also develop limb-threatening ischaemia with rest pain and/or ischaemic ulcers and gangrene. The indication for revascularization in these patients is often limb salvage rather than claudication alone.

DIAGNOSIS

The clinical diagnosis of symptomatic aortoiliac disease is usually accurately established on the basis of a complete history and physical examination. Claudication occurring in the proximal muscle groups of the lower extremity, occurrence of the pain after walking a predictable distance, relief of the pain with only several minutes rest, and impotence in male patients is the classic description. Physical examination will often reveal auscultable bruits over the lower abdomen and the femoral regions. Femoral and distal pulses are usually diminished or absent and, in patients with more severe or type III disease, dependent rubor, elevation pallor and trophic skin changes may be seen in the feet and lower legs. However, claudication limited to the calf, the phenomenon of claudication despite normal distal pulses at rest, and pseudoclaudication may need to be considered in the differential diagnosis.

Some patients will present with symptoms of claudication limited to the calf despite the presence of haemodynamically significant inflow disease. This occurs most often in patients with multilevel (type III) disease, and it is important that they are recognized since inflow must be corrected to improve the symptoms. Physical examination will usually reveal diminished femoral pulses or bruits. Laboratory assessment of vascular patency, particularly good quality preoperative arteriography, sometimes including pressure measurements (see below), allows accurate assessment of the adequacy of aortoiliac inflow.

The presence of significant aortoiliac occlusive disease despite the normal pulses at rest is an important source of diagnostic confusion. This phenomenon is the physiological correlate of Ohm's Law: the stenosis of the aortoiliac segment may not be haemodynamically significant at the blood flow rates seen in the resting patient; with exercise, however, the rate of flow across the stenotic segment is increased, causing a greater drop in pressure across the stenosis. Pedal pulses that were present at rest may therefore vanish after 2 min on the treadmill, confirming the vascular aetiology of the symptoms. It is, therefore, important to include some form of post-exercise ankle pressure measurement in the evaluation of these patients.

Claudicatory symptoms must also be differentiated from non-vascular causes of lower extremity pain such as radicular pain caused by nerve root irritation from spinal stenosis (pseudoclaudication) or intervertebral disc herniation. These patients will often describe pain induced by simply standing as well as on walking, and this history will help distinguish these patients from claudicants. Patients with pseudoclaudication often need to sit or lie down in order to relieve the pain as opposed to simply stopping walking. A careful history may reveal the sciatic distribution of the pain, suggesting its true aetiology.

OPERATIVE INDICATIONS

It is generally agreed that limb-threatening ischaemia, clinically defined by the presence of untreated rest pain, ischaemic ulceration, or frank gangrene, will usually require major amputation; these signs and symptoms are, therefore, clear-cut indications for arterial reconstruction. In this patient population there are few contraindications to surgery, since revascularization by some means can usually be accomplished with morbidity and mortality rates equivalent to or lower than those associated with major amputations. Age is rarely, if ever, a contraindication. If direct aortoiliac reconstruction is deemed too great a risk, high-risk patients with multiple associated medical problems may be candidates for alternative techniques for lower extremity revascularization, such as extra-anatomical bypass, percutaneous transluminal angioplasty, atherectomy, or a combination of such procedures.

The need for surgical intervention must be dictated by the circumstances of each individual patient. Incapacitating claudication that prevents the patient from earning a living or that has a significant negative impact on the patient's desired lifestyle is generally considered an indication for surgery, provided that the patient is not at high risk for surgical complications, does not have a limited life expectancy secondary to associated medical problems, and has a generally favourable distribution of disease for correction. Patients with stable claudication will often experience significant improvement in their symptoms following conservative measures such as abstinence from smoking and pursuit of a daily exercise protocol, with weight reduction if appropriate. Surgical intervention should only be considered if these conservative treatments fail to improve the claudication.

An occasional but well recognized indication for aortoiliac arterial reconstruction is the phenomenon of atheroembolism (blue toe syndrome). The aortoiliac arteries are well-known as a source of emboli which may arise from the degeneration of unstable atherosclerotic plaque within this segment of the arterial tree. A clinical history of lower extremity arterial insufficiency is often lacking in these patients since the source of the atheroembolism may be a haemodynamically insignificant ulcerated or unstable plaque. Nevertheless, if the presentation is consistent with atheroembolism and if an aortogram reveals irregular, shaggy, or ulcerated atheromatous changes in the aortoiliac system (so-called 'degenerative aorta'), aortobifemoral bypass and exclusion of the native aortoiliac system may well be indicated to avoid further episodes of distal embolic events since, if left untreated, repeated episodes of microembolization may result in extensive tissue loss.

PREOPERATIVE EVALUATION

Preoperative evaluation of the patient with aortoiliac disease routinely includes assessment of the patient's cardiac, pulmonary, and renal function. Systemic atherosclerosis accounts for the fact that at least 40 per cent of patients requiring peripheral vascular reconstructive procedures have significant coronary artery disease. Myocardial infarction is the cause of more than 50 per cent of the perioperative deaths in patients undergoing peripheral vascular surgery, and the detection and management of coronary disease is, therefore, important. Traditional clinical cardiac risk assessment may be difficult in the patient awaiting peripheral vascular surgery who, due to claudication, leads a sedentary lifestyle: the absence of a cardiac history cannot safely be assumed to imply the absence of severe coronary disease. Unfortunately, most screening tests lack sensitivity and specificity for predicting postoperative cardiac complications, and the vascular surgeon often has to decide whether or not a patient requires preoperative cardiac catherization. Even coronary angiography may not allow anatomical findings to be related to the perioperative risk of a cardiac event.

Tests aimed at identifying the subset of patients truly at high risk of suffering perioperative cardiac ischaemic events due to coronary artery disease are being developed: dipyridamole thallium myocardial scintigraphy is sensitive in this respect. The dipyridamole thallium study identifies those patients who might require myocardial revascularization prior to aortic surgery or in whom an alternative to direct aortoiliac reconstruction might be advisable.

The high incidence of cigarette smoking and chronic obstructive airways disease in the atherosclerotic population places these patients at increased risk for pulmonary complications. Smoking, even in patients with no detectable lung disease, is associated with increased postoperative atelectasis and pneumonia: abstinence from smoking for 2 weeks prior to surgery is critical. In patients with clinical evidence of chronic obstructive airways disease, pulmonary function studies are often useful in directing and assessing preoperative preparation, which often includes chest physiotherapy, bronchodilators, and antibiotics. An FEV_1 of less than 800 ml and arterial blood gas tests revealing evidence of CO_2 retention identifies patients at high risk for pulmonary complications. Such complications may be avoided by combined thoracic epidural and general anaesthesia with immediate postoperative extubation and postoperative pain management using the epidural route.

Angiographic evaluation

If clinical evaluation indicates the need for revascularization and if the patient is a reasonable surgical candidate, angiography is the next stop in the evaluation. The angiogram should not be used as a diagnostic tool: clinical evaluation, history, and physical examination, often aided by non-invasive vascular laboratory testing, is usually sufficient to diagnose the problem and to determine the need for intervention. The angiogram is used to provide the anatomical details the vascular surgeon needs to select the appropriate operative approach. It may also be used to determine whether the atherosclerotic lesions may be amenable to some form of endovascular procedure such as percutaneous transluminal balloon angioplasty or atherectomy.

The arteriographic study should include the entire abdominal aorta as well as the infrainguinal runoff. Biplane aortograms will demonstrate any significant orificial lesions of the coeliac or superior mesenteric arteries which might alter the surgical approach. Oblique views of the pelvis are useful in identifying hypogastric arterial lesions as well as disease involving the origins of the profunda femoral arteries which might modify the distal anastomotic technique. Anatomical variations and/or occlusive lesions of the renal arteries should also be noted.

In patients with multilevel (type III) aortoiliac disease it may be difficult to ascertain the haemodynamic significance of the lesions at various levels, but this information is crucial since it determines whether an inflow, outflow, or combination procedure will be needed. Non-invasive laboratory testing such as Doppler analogue waveform analysis, segmental pulse volume recording, and pulsatility indices are often misleading: the presence of combined superficial femoral and profunda femoral disease may produce results that suggest the presence of proximal disease. Therefore, measurement of pull-back femoral pressures during the arteriogram can be extremely valuable in assessing the haemodynamic significance of iliac stenoses. A transfemoral retrograde catheter approach, usually undertaken at the time of diagnostic arteriography, allows measurement of intra-arterial pressures proximal to the level of disease and in the iliac or femoral vessels distal to the lesion (Fig. 2). A significant pressure gradient across the lesion is represented by a resting systolic pressure drop of more than 5 mmHg across the lesion or a fall in the femoral arterial pressure of more than 15 per cent in response to reactive hyperaemia, induced either pharmacologically (i.e. 30 mg papaverine) or with an occluding thigh cuff left in place for 3 to 5 min.

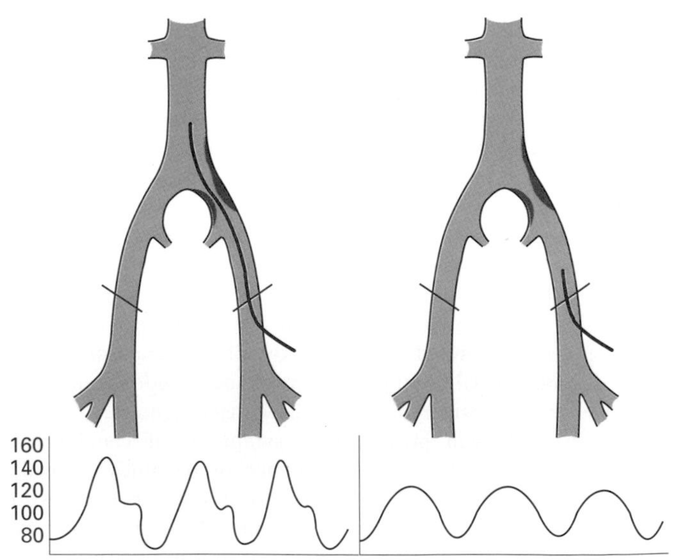

Fig. 2 Intra-arterial pressure measurement. Drop in systolic pressure of more than 5 mmHg across the iliac lesion or fall in femoral pressure more than 15 per cent with hyperaemic studies identifies a haemodynamically significant iliac stenosis.

SURGICAL TREATMENT OF AORTOILIAC DISEASE

Direct aortoiliac reconstruction with an aortobifemoral bypass using a prosthetic graft represents the most definitive and durable means of revascularization. In a small selected group of patients, direct aortoiliac endarterectomy may be appropriate. Extra-anatomical procedures or combination procedures using both endovascular techniques and extra-anatomical bypass, are applicable for patients considered to be too high a risk for direct repair. Proper selection of the relevant procedure depends upon critical analysis of three factors: the patient's general condition, the extent and the distribution of the atherosclerotic disease seen on the arteriogram, and the vascular surgeon's own experience and preference.

Aortoiliac endarterectomy

Aortoiliac endarterectomy may be used in those patients with truly localized (type I) disease. The advantages of this technique include the reduced risk of infection of the arterial reconstruction since no prosthetic material is used, a reduced incidence of wound complications since no groin incisions are needed, and establishment of antegrade inflow into the hypogastric arteries, potentially improving vasculogenic impotence in men more reliably than is the case with aortofemoral bypass. At present, these advantages over prosthetic grafting are rather minimal and the issue of improved potency is unproven. Careful patient selection is required for this approach. The atherosclerotic plaque should terminate at the common iliac bifurcation, allowing a satisfactory endpoint to the endarterectomy to be achieved without extending the arteriotomy more than 1 to 2 cm into the external iliac artery. The surgeon must verify that a secure endpoint has been achieved either with or without the use of tacking sutures.

Aortobifemoral bypass grafting

Aortofemoral bypass grafting is the preferred method of treatment of most patients with symptomatic aortoiliac disease. Initial graft patency rates approach 100 per cent, the 5-year patency rate exceeds 80 per cent, and the 10-year patency rate approaches 75 per cent. These excellent long-term results are due to several factors. First, use of aortofemoral bypass in preference to aorto-iliac bypass or extended aortoiliofemoral endarterectomies has eliminated the problem of graft failure due to the progression of disease or recurrent obliterative lesions in the external iliac artery segment. Secondly, prosthetic graft design and quality have steadily improved. Currently, a variety of reliable prosthetic grafts are available which have minimal tendencies to dilate or degenerate over time, and which have high long-term patencies in large vessel, high-flow situations. Such improved prosthetic grafts minimize the theoretical advantages of all autogenous reconstruction by means of aortobi-iliac endarterectomy. Avoidance of graft limb redundancy and matching the diameter of the graft limb to that of the femoral vessels are important factors in achieving a good result. Other important technical considerations involve the choice of methods for performing the proximal and distal vascular anastomoses.

Technical considerations in aortic grafting

Proximal anastomosis

Some controversy continues to exist regarding the advantages of end-to-end and end-to-side anastomosis of the graft to the proximal aorta, although most vascular surgeons prefer the end-to-end technique for several reasons. Theoretically, the end-to-end anastomosis is haemodynamically more sound: there is less turbulence, better flow characteristics and, unlike the end-to-side configuration, there is no chance of competitive flow in the native iliac arteries. The end-to-end technique also carries a lower risk of intraoperative distal embolic events, since the restoration of flow through the distal native aorta, where application of the distal clamp, in the end-to-side technique, may have loosened atherosclerotic debris or thrombus, is not required. The end-to-end technique also provides better visualization of the lumen of the proximal aorta, thus allowing any aortic thromboendarterectomy that might be needed in conjunction with the anastomosis to be performed. Finally, when using the end-to-end anastomosis, a short segment of the native aorta can be resected and the prosthetic graft thus allowed to lie in the aortic bed, where tissue coverage and reperitonealization can more adequately be obtained, thus potentially reducing the risk of a late aortoenteric fistula. (Fig. 3).

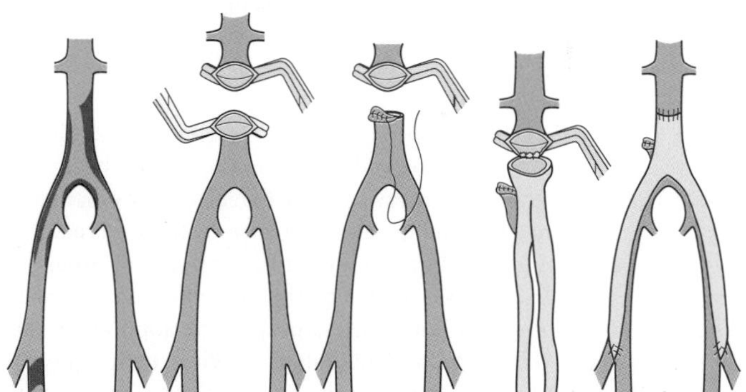

Fig. 3 Method of aortobifemoral bypass graft: end-to-end proximal aortic anastomosis.

There are, however, specific situations in which the end-to-side anastomotic configuration is preferred. These situations include patients in whom the distribution of atherosclerotic occlusive lesions would prevent retrograde perfusion of the hypogastric arteries and/or a patent inferior mesenteric artery, those with superior mesenteric and coeliac artery occlusive disease in whom prograde perfusion of the inferior mesenteric artery may be vital to intestinal viability, and those in whom aberrant or accessory renal arteries arise from the distal abdominal aorta (Fig. 4).

In patients in whom the atherosclerotic lesions have occluded the external iliac arteries bilaterally, transection of the proximal aorta, for purposes of performing end-to-end anastomosis, may devascularize the pelvis since no retrograde flow up the external iliac arteries from the level of the femoral anastomoses can occur. This potentially increases the risk of impotence, ischaemic colitis, buttock ischaemia, persistent hip claudication, and even paraplegia secondary to spinal cord ischaemia. Use of the end-to-side anastomosis in such circumstances allows continued native perfusion of the specific vessels in question while the graft bypasses the aortoiliac occlusive disease. The technical alternative to end-

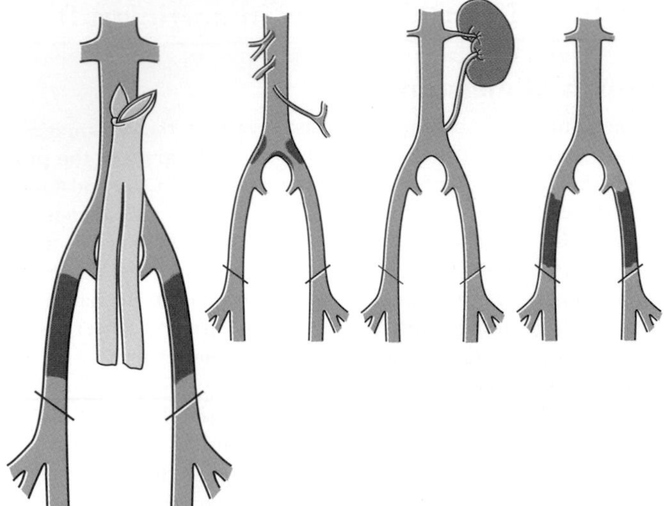

Fig. 4 Indications for end-to-side aortic anastomosis. End-to-side proximal anastomosis is indicated if the distribution of occlusive disease would cause an end-to-end anastomosis to jeopardize pelvic or visceral blood flow.

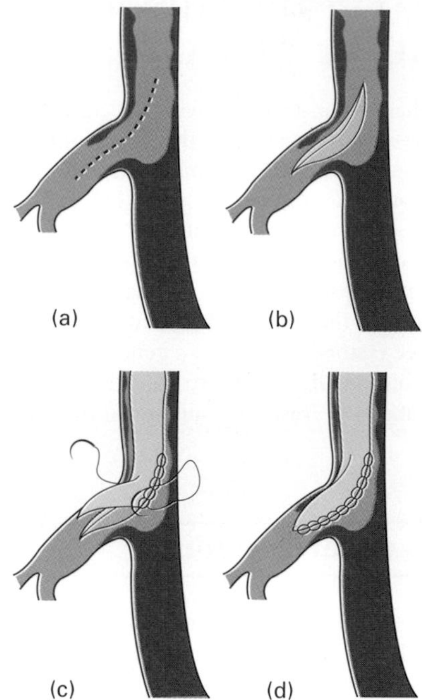

Fig. 5 Femoral profundaplasty. Graft patch profundaplasty should be used to ensure adequate outflow via profunda femoral artery.

to-side anastomosis in these cases would be reimplantation of, or side limb bypass grafts to, the inferior mesenteric, hypogastric, or renal arteries.

Distal anastomosis

When an aortic graft is inserted for the treatment of occlusive disease, the distal anastomosis should almost always be to the femoral artery. Extensive experience has revealed that creation of the distal anastomosis in the groin rather than to the external iliac artery avoids the increased graft failure rate seen due to progression of external iliac disease distal to the aortoiliac anastomosis. The use of prophylactic antibiotics, proper intraoperative skin preparation and draping, and meticulous surgical technique has avoided the increased graft infection rates that were feared with use of femoral level anastomoses.

Following completion of the proximal aortic anastomosis, the graft limbs are tunnelled to the groins retroperitoneally. In male patients surgical dissection in the region of the aortic bifurcation and the left common iliac artery is kept to a minimum to avoid injury to the autonomic nerve plexuses important for erectile and ejaculatory function. On the right side, the retroperitoneal tunnel is created directly anterior to the native iliac artery, placing the graft posterior to the ureter to avoid entrapment of the ureter by the limb of the graft. On the left, the tunnel is placed beneath the sigmoid mesocolon in a slightly lateral position to avoid nerve plexus injury. Again, care is taken to prevent ureteral entrapment. The distal anastomosis is then performed in an end-to-side fashion to the distal common femoral artery.

Profunda run-off

It is absolutely critical for graft limb patency for the distal anastomosis to allow adequate outflow, especially when the graft is placed in a patient with multilevel disease. Reconstruction for type III aortoiliac disease often involves placement of the distal anastomosis in a diseased common femoral artery in the setting of chronic occlusion of the superficial femoral artery and orificial stenosis of the profunda femoral artery. In such patients, ensuring adequate profunda outflow is the key to maintaining graft limb patency, and correction of any significant profunda stenosis is of paramount importance. If the profunda is free of orificial stenosis, measures 4 to 5 mm in diameter as determined by gentle graduated probe insertion, and has a length of 20 to 25 cm, outflow via the profunda alone is usually adequate to maintain graft patency.

The aortogram and run-off studies in patients with multilevel disease should include oblique views of the pelvis and groin to visualize the profunda orifice. One study reported a 59 per cent incidence of profunda stenosis in patients with lower extremity ischaemia in whom oblique views were obtained. If profunda stenosis is discovered during aortography or at surgery, there are several options which can be used to correct the stenosis. One standard technique involves extension of the femoral arteriotomy down the profunda, thus crossing the orificial stenosis (Fig. 5). The end of the graft limb is then fashioned with a long bevelled tip allowing the heel of the anastomosis to lie on the common femoral artery and the toe to lie down on the profunda. The anastomosis thus creates a graft patch profundaplasty. Some surgeons prefer to use autogenous tissue (endarterectomized superficial femoral artery or saphenous vein) to perform a separate profundaplasty. In this case, the prosthetic graft is anastomosed to the common femoral artery proximal to the patch profundaplasty.

Simultaneous distal grafting

The patient with type III aortoiliac (multilevel) disease often presents the therapeutic dilemma of whether an outflow procedure (e.g. femoropopliteal bypass) must be performed simultaneously with the aortobifemoral procedure. Eighty per cent of patients presenting with ischaemic rest pain will obtain adequate symptom relief following the inflow procedure alone if adequate profunda outflow is obtained. In patients who present with significant tissue loss in the foot, restoration of pulsatile flow in the foot may be required for successful healing, thus necessitating simultaneous distal grafting at the time of the inflow procedure. When claudication is the presenting symptom, reports suggest that 80 per cent of patients will experience improvement with the inflow procedure alone, although, in the author's experience, only 35 per cent of patients experience total relief of claudication.

Identification of patients likely to require synchronous distal bypass to obtain sufficient relief of ischaemic symptoms remains difficult. Preoperative non-invasive haemodynamic testing may provide useful data, although some investigators have found such studies unreliable. If unequivocally severe inflow disease in the aortoiliac segments is identified by absent or weak femoral pulses, severe lesions seen on angiography, or marked pressure gradients confirmed by intra-arterial femoral pressure measurements at the time of angiography, significant improvement may be expected with the inflow procedure alone. If clinical evaluation reveals only mild to moderate aortoiliac inflow, a small, diffusely diseased profunda femoris, poor profunda collateral development, or significant infrapopliteal disease, unfavourable results may be predicted from an inflow procedure alone.

In these situations intraoperative monitoring of calf or ankle peripheral vascular resistance (PVR) or ABI's may be used to assess the haemodynamic improvement following completion of the aortofemoral bypass, although improvement in the ankle PVR/ABI ratio may be delayed in the cold, vasoconstricted lower extremity. Good clinical acumen and surgical experience remain essential in deciding when to proceed with distal reconstruction. The use of intraoperative, adjunctive endovascular techniques such as transluminal balloon angioplasty, atherectomy, and laser/thermal angioplasty, to improve distal occlusive lesions following proximal graft insertion may result in more liberal use of synchronous distal revascularization if current studies reveal these procedures to be safe, reliable, and effective. At present, they are not commonly employed in these circumstances by the authors.

RESULTS OF DIRECT AORTOILIAC RECONSTRUCTION

Excellent early and late results of aortoiliofemoral reconstruction may be anticipated and may be achieved with highly acceptable patient morbidity and mortality rates. Numerous studies have reported 5-year patency rates of 85 to 90 per cent and 10-year rates of 75 per cent. Perioperative mortality rates of less than 3 per cent are commonplace in many centres. Patients with type III aortoiliac disease are most likely to have associated carotid and coronary arterial disease. Improved screening techniques and intensive perioperative monitoring associated with advances in anaesthetic management of these patients will result in still further improvements in perioperative complication rates.

ALTERNATIVES TO DIRECT AORTOILIAC RECONSTRUCTION

While direct reconstruction for aortoiliac occlusive disease using aortobifemoral bypass is the most definitive treatment, selected high-risk patients may not be suitable candidates for major surgery performed under general anaesthesia. A variety of 'extra-anatomical' bypass grafts, or a combination of endovascular techniques and extra-anatomical bypass grafts enable the vascular surgeon to achieve needed revascularization in such patients with reduced risk and acceptable patency rates.

The definition of the high-risk patient is a subjective process. Patients with a history of recent myocardial infarction, significant angina, a positive dipyridamole thallium study, and/or a left ventricular ejection fraction less than 35 per cent (per radionuclide ventriculography) are at high risk of suffering a perioperative myocardial event. Severe pulmonary disease also significantly increases the risks with associated general anaesthesia and major abdominal surgery: patients with severe dyspnoea, CO_2 retention, or FEV_1 of less than 800 ml/s fall into this category. Intensive intraoperative and postoperative monitoring techniques as well as improved anaesthetic techniques using combined general and thoracic epidural anaesthesia will often allow standard direct aorto-iliac reconstruction to be performed with acceptable risk, even in this high-risk category of patient. If the risk is deemed unacceptable, however, alternative bypass techniques can be offered.

EXTRA-ANATOMICAL BYPASS

Extra-anatomical bypass involves placement of a graft in an anatomical location remote from that of the artery which the graft bypasses. The most commonly employed extra-anatomical procedures include axillobifemoral, iliofemoral, and femorofemoral bypass. Such procedures may also be combined with various endovascular techniques in order to improve inflow to or outflow from the bypass graft. The procedure used depends upon the exact distribution of occlusive disease found on arteriographic studies.

Femorofemoral bypass graft

When the iliac occlusive disease is limited to the iliac system on one side, use of the contralateral patent iliac system as the source of inflow will allow use of a shorter prosthetic conduit with resultant improved long-term patency rates. The femorofemoral bypass graft may be used in this situation (Fig. 6). Failure of the graft due to progression of disease in the 'donor' iliac system is

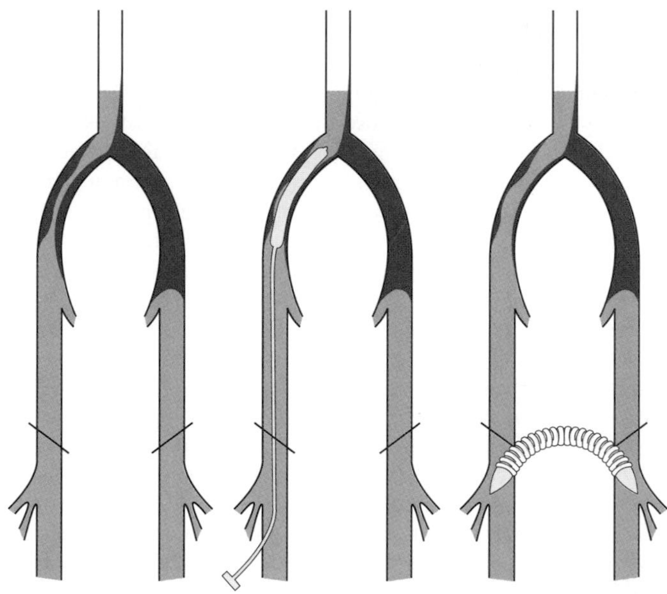

Fig. 6 Extra-anatomical bypass graft. Axillobifemoral bypass graft may be the procedure of choice in high-risk patients with aortic or bilateral iliac artery disease.

unusual: several authors have suggested that the increased flow through the donor iliac artery that occurs as a result of the femorofemoral bypass, may actually retard progression of atherosclerotic disease in the donor iliac system. Past concerns that the graft may create a 'steal', significantly reducing perfusion of the donor limb, are unfounded in the absence of any haemodynamically significant stenosis in the donor limb inflow. Severe outflow lesions on the donor side with occlusion or stenosis of the superficial femoral artery may result in a steal phenomenon, but this is not usually clinically significant.

The donor iliac artery must be evaluated with careful biplanar arteriography to establish clearly the absence of any haemodynamically significant inflow lesions. Physical examination and physiological testing are also important in assessing adequacy of the donor iliac system: non-invasive arterial testing may be very helpful in this assessment. The segmental pressures should disclose normal thigh pressures; pulse volume recordings at the thigh level should have an excellent contour, with brisk upstroke on the waveform, and femoral artery Doppler analogue waveforms should be triphasic. These non-invasive tests results suggest a patent iliofemoral system. When the superficial and profunda femoral arteries are diseased, these studies may falsely suggest disease at the iliac level: pull-back intra-arterial pressures obtained at the iliac and femoral levels will disclose the presence of any significant lesions. If arteriograms show an iliac stenosis that is apparently not haemodynamically significant, hyperaemic testing or pressure measurement obtained following administration of papaverine is necessary to be certain that the lesion will not become haemodynamically significant at the increased rates of flow that will occur after placement of the femorofemoral graft.

The status of outflow in the recipient limb is also a critical factor in determining the long-term patency of such grafts. One study showed that the patency rate of femorofemoral grafts was reduced from 92 per cent to 52 per cent if the superficial femoral artery in the recipient limb was occluded. The probability of salvaging the limb or of adequately relieving ischaemic symptoms by femorofemoral grafting is also reduced in the presence of significant outflow disease, even if the graft remains patent.

If the criteria above are applied when selecting patients for femorofemoral bypass the results are excellent and morbidity and mortality rates are low, even in high-risk patients. The procedure can be performed under epidural, spinal, or even local anaesthesia, completely avoiding any myocardial depressant effects of general anaesthesia and avoiding the need for mechanical ventilation in patients with severe pulmonary disease. The common femoral arteries are exposed through bilateral vertical groin incisions and the graft is placed in a subcutaneous, suprapubic tunnel from the donor to the recipient groin. A prosthetic graft of 8 mm in size is generally chosen. Many currently believe that externally reinforced polytetrafluoroethylene is the best available prosthesis for such application, since this is less likely to be occluded by external compression than are Dacron grafts. The conduit size should closely match that of the femoral arteries in order to prevent the deposition of laminated thrombus within the body of the graft that can occur when the graft is larger in diameter than the host vessels. The graft configuration which appears to provide the most optimal haemodynamics is a gentle 'C' configuration, in which the graft rises up through the suprapubic tunnel and then down again to the opposite femoral artery (Fig. 6).

Five-year cumulative femorofemoral graft patency rates of 75 to 80 per cent are common; these figures, combined with the simplicity of the procedure, and its low morbidity and mortality rates have led numerous authors to suggest the use of these grafts in low-risk as well as high-risk patients with unilateral iliac disease. In the sexually potent male patient, this approach has the additional advantage of avoiding the postoperative sexual dysfunction which may occur with direct reconstructions of the aorta. In general, however, good-risk patients are still best served by use of direct aortoiliac reconstruction.

AXILLOBIFEMORAL BYPASS GRAFT

High-risk patients with aortic or bilateral iliac artery occlusive disease who present with limb-threatening ischaemia are candidates for axillofemoral bypass as an alternative to either direct aortoiliac reconstruction or primary amputation (Fig. 7). In such patients the axillobifemoral bypass should be used in preference to the axillounifemoral graft, since the cumulative 5-year patency of the former is clearly superior. This improved patency rate has been attributed to the increased rates of flow in the axillary limb of the graft in the bilateral bypass.

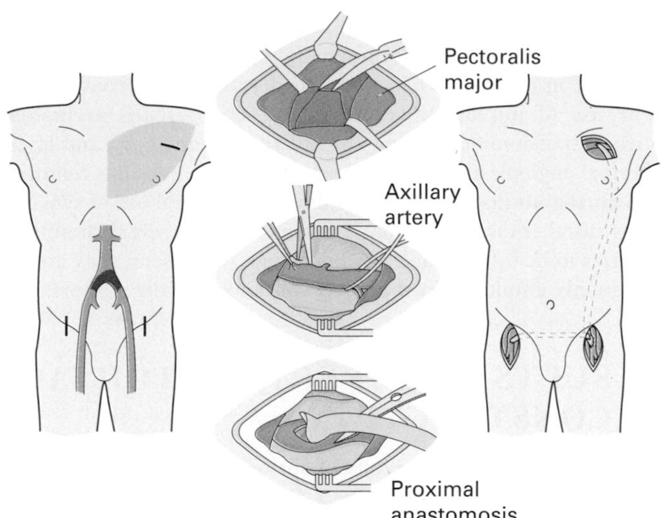

Fig. 7 Combined endovascular and extra-anatomical bypass procedure. Transluminal angioplasty of iliac artery stenosis provides 'inflow' for femorofemoral bypass of contralateral complete iliac artery occlusion. This combined technique allows use of a shorter prosthetic conduit than in axillofemoral bypass.

The axillary portion of the bypass graft is performed by exposing the first portion of the axillary artery using a skin incision placed beneath the clavicle. The pectoralis major muscle is divided in the tendinous portion near its insertion: this provides excellent exposure of the artery and also allows the bypass graft to lie at the appropriate angle as it emerges from the subclavicular fossa and enters the subcutaneous tunnel on the chest wall. Bilateral vertical groin incisions are used to expose the femoral arteries. The graft is then passed in subcutaneous tunnels from the subclavicular dissection to the ipsilateral groin and from that groin to the contralateral femoral artery (Fig. 7). This procedure usually requires general anaesthesia, at least during the blunt dissection of the subcutaneous tunnels: the subclavicular and femoral dissections may be performed under local anaesthesia. The prosthetic graft of choice is generally externally reinforced polytetrafluoroethylene, although some surgeons prefer Dacron grafts. The former will usually allow better results of graft thrombectomy if occlusion occurs. Prompt thrombectomy produces secondary patency rates of 60 to 70 per cent for occluded grafts. Although inferior to the long-term patency performance of aortobifemoral or femorofemoral grafts, axillobifemoral grafts offer a reasonable compromise in the high-risk individual. Paradoxically, the mortality rate of 5 to 10 per cent exceeds that of direct aortic grafting, although it must be remembered that such grafts are undertaken in patients in whom the risks associated with direct operation are almost certainly increased.

ENDOVASCULAR TECHNIQUES

Recent technological advances have produced a variety of endovascular techniques which, because of their decreased invasiveness, may be used alone or as an adjunct to surgical bypass techniques for treating aortoiliac occlusive disease in high-risk patients. These techniques include intra-arterial thrombolytic therapy for native occlusive lesions, transluminal balloon angioplasty, laser or thermal assisted balloon angioplasty, and atherectomy. Long-term follow-up of results of many of these techniques should be restricted to the high-risk patient felt to be unsuitable for standard aortobifemoral bypass. This does not apply, however, to balloon angioplasty for localized iliac disease, which has been evaluated for nearly a decade, and has been verified to be the procedure of choice for truly localized iliac stenotic lesions. Long-term patency and relief of ischaemic symptoms following percutaneous transluminal angioplasty for local iliac disease produces results equivalent to those of surgical treatment in patients with limited disease, and its advantages in terms of cost and morbidity are obvious. Iliac percutaneous transluminal angioplasty may also be employed as an adjunct to surgical revascularization, providing iliac inflow when distal surgical procedures are required. Transluminal balloon angioplasty may be used in these situations to provide inflow for femorofemoral bypass of a more extensive chronic atherosclerotic iliac occlusion on the contralateral side (Fig. 6). Adjunctive use of iliac percutaneous transluminal angioplasty in patients with bilateral iliac disease may also allow the use of shorter extra-anatomical bypass grafts, such as femorofemoral rather than axillofemoral grafts, and this may improve long-term patency rates. Long-term follow-up of patients treated using these combined techniques suggests that with appropriate patient selection (most importantly, those with fairly focal iliac disease), results equivalent or even superior to those achieved with standard arterial reconstruction can be achieved.

FURTHER READING

Bernhard VM, Ray LI, Militello JP. The role of angioplasty of the profunda femoris artery in revascularization of the ischemic limb. *Surg Gynecol Obstet* 1976; **142**: 840.

Boucher CA, Brewster DC, Darling RC, Okada RD, Strauss HW, Pohost GM. Determination of cardiac risk of dipyridamole-thallium imaging before peripheral vascular surgery. *N Engl J Med* 1985; **312**: 389

Brewster DC. Direct reconstruction for aortoiliac occlusive disease. In Rutherford RB, ed., *Vascular Surgery*. Philadelphia: WB Saunders Co., 1989; 667–691

Brewster DC, Darling RC. Optimal methods of aortoiliac reconstruction. *Surgery* 1978; **84**: 739.

Brewster DC, *et al.* Femoral artery pressure measurement during aortography. *Circulation* 1979; **60** (Suppl. 1): 120.

Brewster DC, *et al.* Aortofemoral graft for multilevel occlusive disease. Predictors of success and need for distal bypass. *Arch Surg* 1982; **111**: 1593.

Brewster DC, *et al.* Selection of patients for preoperative coronary angiography. Use of dipyridamole-stress thallium myocardial imaging. *J Vasc Surg* 1985; **2**: 504.

Brewster DC, Meier GH, Darling RC, Moncure AC, LaMuraglia GM, Abbott WM. Reoperation for aortofemoral graft limb occlusion. Optimal methods and long-term results. *J Vasc Surg* 1987; **5**: 305.

Brewster DC, *et al.* Long-term results of combined iliac balloon angioplasty and distal surgical revascularization. *Ann Surg* 1989; **210**: 324.

Brief DK, Brener FJ, Alpert J, Parsonnet V. Cross-over femoro-femoral grafts followed up five years or more. *Arch Surg* 1975; **110**: 1294.

Crawford ES, *et al.* Aortoiliac occlusive disease: Factors influencing survival and function following reconstructive operation over a twenty-five-year period. *Surgery* 1981; **90**: 1055.

Dalman RL, Taylor LM, Moneta GL, Yeager RA, Porter JM. Simultaneous arterial inflow procedures and femoral popliteal/tibial bypass procedures. *J Vasc Surg* 1991; **13**: 211.

Darling RC, *et al.* Aortoiliac reconstruction. *Surg Clin N Am* 1979; **59**: 565.

DeBakey ME, Lawrie GM, Glaeser DH. Patterns of atherosclerosis and their surgical significance. *Ann Surg* 1985; **210**: 115.

Flanigan DP, *et al.* Hemodynamic evaluation of the aortoiliac system based on pharmacologic vasodilatation. *Surgery* 1983; **93**.

Harris PL, Cave Bigley DJ, McSweeney L. Aortofemoral bypass and the role of concomitant femorodistal reconstruction. *Br J Surg* 1985; **72**: 317.

Hertzer NR, *et al.* Coronary artery disease in peripheral vascular patients. A classification of 1000 coronary angiograms and results of surgical management. *Ann Surg* 1984; **199**: 223.

Hertzer NR, *et al.* The risk of vascular surgery in a metropolitan community, with observations on surgeon experience and hospital size. *J Vasc Surg* 1984; **1**: 13.

Kalman PG, Hosang M, Johnston KW, Walker PM. The current role for femorofemoral bypass. *J Vasc Surg* 1987; **6**: 71.

Karayannacos PE, Yashon D, Vasko JS. Narrow lumbar spinal canal with 'vascular' syndromes. *Arch Surg* 1976; **111**: 803.

Lerich R, Moral A. The syndrome of thrombotic obliteration of the aortic bifurcation. *Ann Surg* 1948; **127**: 193.

LoGerfo FW, *et al.* A comparison of the late patency rates of axillobilateral femoral and axillounilateral femoral grafts. *Surgery* 1971; **81**: 33.

Malone JM, Moore WS, Golstone J. The natural history of bilateral aortofemoral bypass grafts for ischemia of the lower extremities. *Arch Surg* 1975; **110**: 1300.

Mannick JA, Williams LE, Nasbeth DC. The late results of axillofemoral grafts. *Surgery* 1970; **68**: 1038.

Peters RM. Identification, assessment and management of surgical patients with chronic respiratory disease. *Prob Gen Surg* 1984; **1**: 432.

Pierce GE, *et al.* Evaluation of end-to-side v. end-to-end proximal anastomosis in aortobifemoral bypass. *Arch Surg* 1983; **117**: 1580.

Picone AL, *et al.* Spinal cord ischemia following operations on the abdominal aorta. *J Vasc Surg* 1986; **3**: 94.

Piotrowski J, Pearce WH, Jones DN, Whitehouse T, Bell R, Pratt A, Rutherford RD. Aortobifemoral bypass. The operation of choice for unilateral iliac occlusion? *J Vasc Surg* 1988; **8**: 211.

Queral LA, *et al.* Pelvic hemodynamics after aortoiliac reconstruction. *Surgery* 1979; **86**: 799.

Royster RS, Lynn R, Mulcare RJ. Combined aortoiliac and femoropopliteal occlusive disease. *Surg Gynecol Obstet* 1976; **143**: 949.

Rutherford RB, *et al.* Serial hemodynamic assessment of aortobifemoral bypass. *J Vasc Surg* 1986; **4**: 428.

Rutherford RB, Patt A, Pearce WH. Extra-anatomic bypass: A closer view. *J Vasc Surg* 1987; **5**: 437.

Strandness DF. *Collateral Circulation in Clinical Surgery*. Philadelphia: WB Saunders Co., 1969.

Szilagyi DE, *et al.* A thirty-year survey of the reconstructive surgical treatment of aortoiliac occlusive disease. *J Vasc Surg* 1986; **3**: 421.

7.6.2 Femoral and distal arteries

JOHN A. MURIE AND MICHAEL J. CALLAM

INTRODUCTION

Obliterative atheromatous disease of the femoral and distal arteries does not exist in isolation but is part of a widespread vascular pathology; the cardiac, cerebral, and less commonly the mesenteric and renal circulations may be affected. Initial deposits of atheroma in the vessel wall are overlaid with hyaline collagenous material which projects into the arterial lumen. This plaque may ulcerate, leading to superimposed thrombosis which organizes and enlarges, further narrowing the vessel and causing turbulent flow. Turbulence accelerates the process leading to occlusion of the vessel.

The natural history of infrainguinal arterial disease is not a simple steady deterioration towards amputation; it is more often characterized either by stable intermittent claudication or even by symptomatic improvement as collateral channels enlarge. The risk of gangrene or pregangrene within a year of presentation is about 5 per cent, and about 2 per cent per annum thereafter. Of every 100 patients with claudication, approximately 40 will improve, 40 will remain unchanged, and 20 will require operation. However, the mortality rate of these patients is twice that of age and sex matched controls without peripheral vascular disease.

PRESENTATION AND CLASSIFICATION

The three cardinal features of peripheral lower limb ischaemia are intermittent claudication, rest pain, and gangrene, representing an increasing degree of severity of ischaemia. Intermittent claudication is a cramp caused by inadequate oxygenation of muscle. It is initiated by walking and relieved by rest; generally the calf muscles are most affected. Claudication distance remains roughly the same unless the underlying condition deteriorates, although the symptom is more pronounced on hurrying or going uphill.

Rest pain occurs when the blood supply is so poor that tissue perfusion is inadequate even at rest. The pain classically affects the toes or forefoot (the most distal part of the limb) although in severe cases it may involve the whole foot or calf. It is usually first noticed in bed, when the patient is horizontal, the beneficial effect of gravity is removed and the foot is warmed, thereby increasing metabolism. External stimuli are reduced at night and so pain may be appreciated more readily. Rest pain is helped by hanging the leg out of bed, standing, or even walking. As ischaemia progresses the pain becomes continuous, requiring opiate analgesia for its control. The third clinical feature is gangrene. This is the end stage of ischaemia when the circulation is so poor that necrosis ensues. It usually begins distally in the foot (Fig. 1).

In addition to the three cardinal features of ischaemia the concept of 'critical limb ischaemia' is useful in vascular surgery. This is defined as persistent rest pain requiring analgesia for more than 2 weeks, or ulceration, or gangrene of the foot, plus an ankle systolic pressure below 50 mmHg. In diabetics, owing to the unreliability of ankle pressure recording due to vascular calcification, the pressure criterion is replaced by absence of ankle pulses.

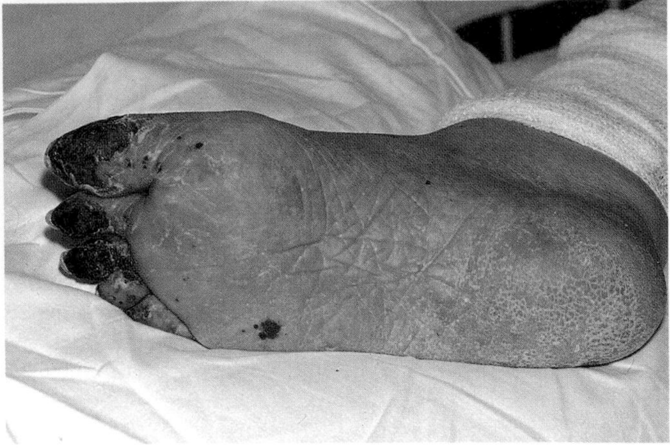

Fig. 1 Ischaemic gangrene affecting the toes of the foot.

ASSESSMENT

Assessment must establish the degree of ischaemia, whether it requires treatment and, if so, the most appropriate treatment. History and examination will usually identify the presence or absence of vascular disease and suggest its severity. Skin temperature, pallor on elevating the limb followed by dependent rubor, and the absence of pulses are particularly important features. The palpation of pulses should give the surgeon a rough idea of the site of arterial occlusion. More exact assessment requires a Doppler ultrasound probe and sphygmomanometer cuff to measure the highest opening systolic pressure of the three ankle arteries (Fig. 2). This is divided by the higher of the brachial systolic pressures to obtain an ankle/brachial pressure index, the normal value of which is greater than 1. Values of 0.6 to 0.9 are typical of claudication, 0.3 to 0.6 of rest pain, and below 0.3 of incipient or actual gangrene. In some individuals with apparently normal values at rest, occult disease may be uncovered if the ankle/brachial index falls after exercise.

The need for intervention is easy to assess in those with mild claudication or critical ischaemia. Between these extremes a balance must be struck between the risk to life and limb from any proposed procedure and the compromised lifestyle which may result from conservative management. This balance will be affected by the patient's social circumstances and by the results of further investigations to assess fitness for operation. Although simple palpation of pulses usually allows the approximate level of occlusion or stenosis to be recognized, if surgical or radiological

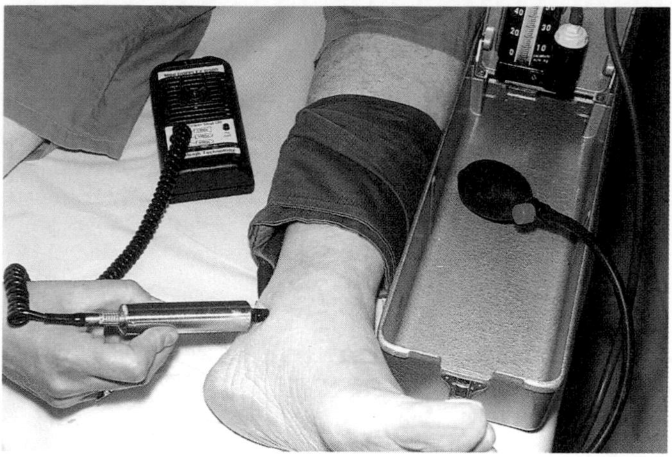

Fig. 2 Measurement of ankle/brachial index. The highest systolic pressure of the three ankle arteries is obtained using a hand held Doppler ultrasound probe. This is divided by the higher systolic pressure of the two brachial arteries.

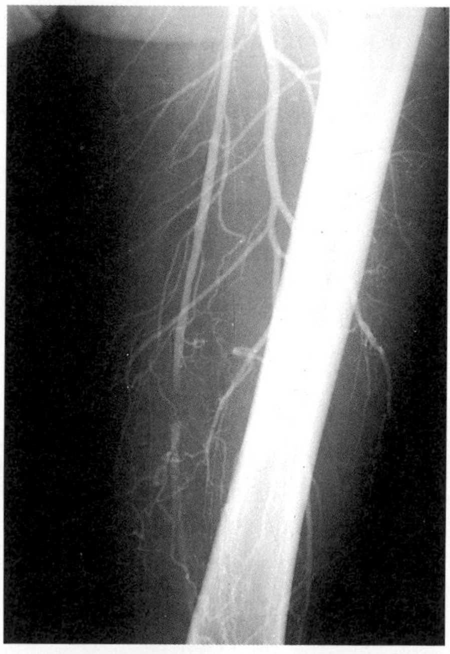

Fig. 3 Conventional angiogram showing classically sited occlusion in the distal superficial femoral artery.

intervention is intended some form of imaging is required to provide more detail: the standard imaging technique is angiography (Fig. 3). Radiographs are exposed after injection of radio-opaque contrast medium into the arterial tree through a fine catheter inserted via the femoral artery in the groin. Current techniques using non-ionic contrast media and narrow gauge catheters are safe, though invasive, and the angiogram remains the investigation of choice. Computerized (digital subtraction) angiography may be used as an adjunct to the basic conventional technique to highlight areas of special interest (Fig. 4). This modern method may also be employed on its own in some cases, using either an intra-arterial or an intravenous injection. The advantage of the former is that very

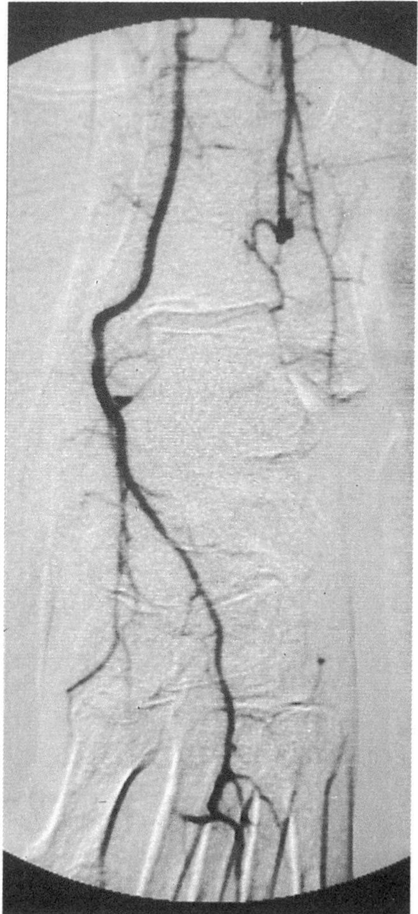

Fig. 4 Absence of complete pedal arch shown by intra-arterial digital subtraction angiography.

fine catheters may be used and small quantities of contrast media injected. The advantage of the latter is that the arterial tree does not have to be invaded at all. However the intravenous technique requires administration of a large volume of contrast agent, which debilitated patients may tolerate poorly. Furthermore, the image quality of intravenous digital subtraction angiography for the leg vessels is not particularly good.

It must be stressed that angiography should only be performed if intervention is intended. It allows an assessment of whether intervention is technically feasible and enables the most appropriate form of treatment to be chosen. The appearance of the aorta and iliac vessels is checked to confirm that there is no impairment of inflow to the leg. The sites of stenosis and occlusion in the leg arteries themselves are noted, and patency of the distal arteries (outflow) assessed. The usefulness of angiography in assessing patency of very distal arteries when an upstream occlusion is present has recently been questioned. The technique of pulse generated run-off may detect patent vessels at the ankle which have not been adequately demonstrated by angiography. A pneumatic cuff around the upper calf is mechanically inflated and deflated rapidly to generate a pseudopulse which is detected by a Doppler ultrasound probe over any patent ankle artery. In patients with critical ischaemia this may allow the possibility of a femorodistal bypass to be recognized in the presence of a negative angiogram.

Atheroma has a predilection for certain arterial sites and patterns of disease are recognizable: within the leg these common patterns are femoropopliteal disease and distal disease (Fig. 3). Nevertheless, atheroma is never entirely limited to one site, although relieving an obstruction at one site may result in a general relief of symptoms. The most common site of stenosis or occlusion in the femoropopliteal segment is the junction between the middle and distal thirds of the segment, where the superficial femoral artery exits through the adductor hiatus. Typically, an initial stenosis progresses to occlusion; this is followed by proximal propagation of thrombus to the origin of the superficial femoral artery; outflow from the common femoral is then solely into the profunda femoris artery. Although distal propagation of thrombus may occur, the popliteal artery usually stays patent because stasis here is prevented by inflow from the profunda femoris via the geniculate collaterals. There is, therefore, often a patent vessel which can accept the distal end of a bypass graft.

Distal obliterative disease which is not associated with proximal atheroma should raise the suspicion of another pathology, especially diabetes mellitus, arteritis, or previous embolic disease. However the most common distal disease is found in older patients and is accompanied by extensive proximal atheroma. Distal disease is not amenable to reconstructive surgery.

MEDICAL TREATMENT

Medical treatment may be indicated when the disease is not of sufficient severity to warrant operation (including angioplasty); when operation is impossible, inappropriate, or unsuccessful; or as an adjunct to operation. Several general measures are applicable to all patients whether or not they have surgery, for instance weight reduction in the obese, correction of anaemia or polycythaemia, treatment of hyperlipidaemia, and control of diabetes. The judicious treatment of heart failure and hypertension may also improve perfusion, but β-blocking drugs should be avoided as they may further compromise a diseased peripheral circulation.

Smoking is the most important correctable risk factor. Stopping smoking may be the only treatment that many patients require; claudication not infrequently improves spontaneously. Stopping smoking may not reduce atheroma that is already present, but continuation of smoking leads to an increased deposition and compromises the development of a collateral circulation. Smoking increases the risk of amputation and the incidence of graft occlusion after surgery.

Exercise is the other arm of effective conservation treatment: it may double the distance that can be walked before pain occurs in up to 80 per cent of patients. It has been suggested that selective exercise of those muscles which are most ischaemic produces the best results. Even rest pain may benefit from exercise, and it is prudent to recommend that patients exercise to the limit of comfort.

Apart from the above general measures, no other form of conservative treatment is widely accepted as likely to offer significant benefit in claudication or rest pain. A variety of drugs may occasionally offer a modest benefit; the most widely used are oxypentifylline (pentoxifylline) which alters red cell deformability so helping flow in the microcirculation, and naftidrofuryl which has an effect on ischaemic cell metabolism. More recently prostacyclin analogues have been used for their antithrombotic effect.

INDICATIONS FOR INTERVENTION

Subclinical disease

In a patient with unilateral symptoms it is not unusual to find angiographic evidence of early disease on the contralateral side. It is not yet known whether intervention for early asymptomatic disease confers benefit over a conservative policy and intervention in this group should occur only in the confines of a clinical trial addressing this question.

Intermittent claudication

Intermittent claudication represents the 'middle ground'. Any decision to intervene must take into account the possibility that spontaneous improvement may occur, especially if smoking is stopped and exercise adopted. Symptomatic improvement is especially likely within the first 6 months after onset of claudication. Consideration should be given to the degree to which the patient's lifestyle is affected and the hazard to life and limb that the proposed intervention might pose.

Rest pain and critical ischaemia

Rest pain or critical ischaemia despite appropriate medical management requires intervention if at all possible. Revascularization should generally be attempted if angiography and/or pulse generated run-off indicate that percutaneous transluminal angioplasty or reconstructive surgery is feasible. Nevertheless, in individual cases the chance of success may be recognizably slim and the decision to proceed will require fine judgement. There is a small group of patients, often unfit, who will benefit from primary amputation.

ALTERNATIVES TO SURGERY

Percutaneous transluminal angioplasty is a radiological technique in which a guidewire is introduced percutaneously through the common femoral artery to lie within a stenosis. A catheter with a

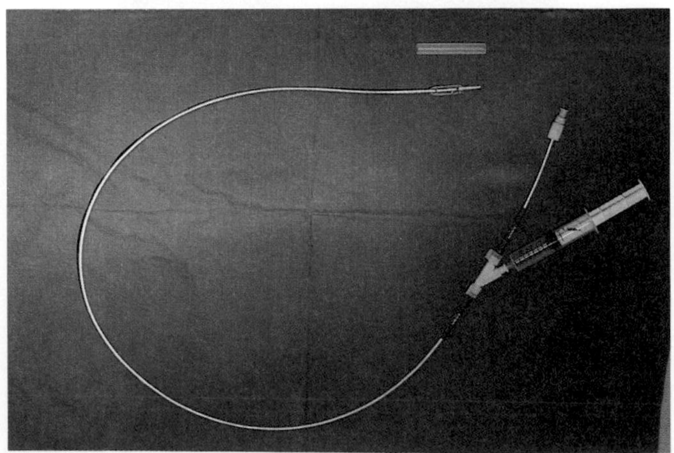

Fig. 5 Percutaneous transluminal angioplasty catheter.

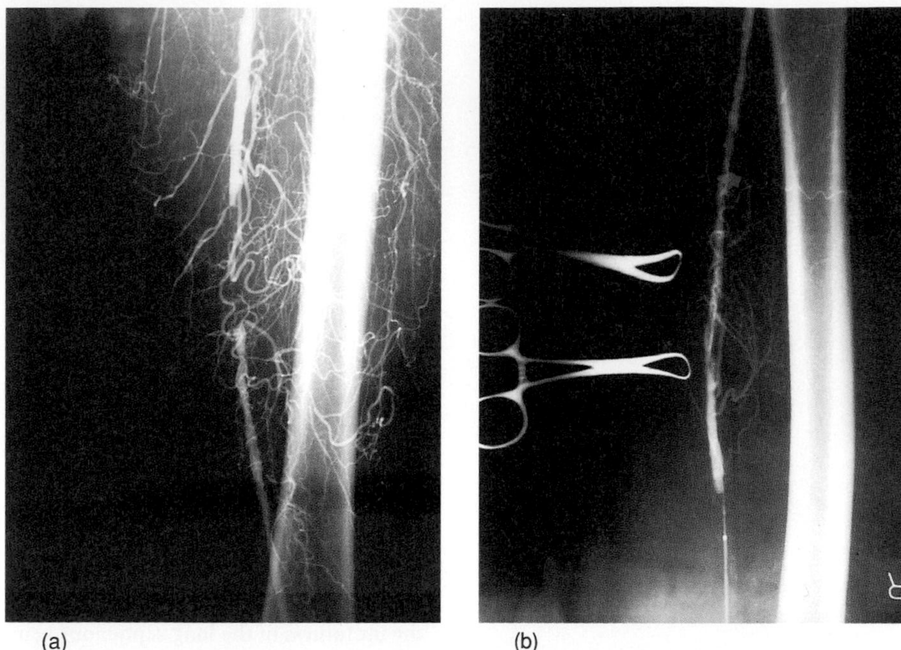

Fig. 6 (a) Angiogram showing superficial femoral artery occlusion. (b) Superficial femoral artery after percutaneous transluminal angioplasty. The previously occluded segment is marked by the two towel clips.

balloon at its end is introduced over the guidewire and the balloon is inflated within the narrowed segment (Fig. 5). Although introduced by Dotter and Judkins in 1964 for the treatment of atheromatous femoropopliteal disease, percutaneous transluminal angioplasty was made popular primarily by Gruntzig and his colleagues. Today the technique is regularly applied to the femoropopliteal segment and to many sites other than the leg (Fig. 6). It is carried out under local anaesthesia and is safe in experienced hands: the main complications of bleeding or thrombosis are unusual and can usually be remedied with surgical assistance. Percutaneous transluminal angioplasty is especially attractive for patients at the ends of the spectrum of disease severity, that is, those with minor claudication and for debilitated patients with severe ischaemia. Generally, occlusions up to 10 cm long are satisfactorily dealt with by this method.

It is sometimes impossible to push the guidewire and balloon catheter through an occlusion, especially if it is long. This may be overcome in some patients by burning through the occlusion using a laser (laser angioplasty). In general, the laser is not used to remove the bulk of atheroma but rather to allow proper placement of a guidewire and balloon catheter for conventional treatment. Laser angioplasty is a developing area and at this time is largely confined to specialist centres.

Mechanical atherectomy devices which may be introduced into the artery in a similar fashion to the angioplasty catheter are also available. The atherectomy catheter, however, has a cutting mechanism at its tip—a hollow core with side orifice and a sliding blade is a popular pattern, as is a high speed rotating cutter. These devices are used to cut through atheroma, retaining the resulting debris within their core for later removal. Their use is confined as yet to a few specialist centres.

The long-term results of laser angioplasty and atherectomy have yet to be assessed. They provide some hope for the use of minimally invasive procedures in the correction of arterial disease in the future and, if combined with a percutaneously inserted angioscope, may yet allow very sophisticated percutaneous arterial intervention.

When an acute occlusion occurs in a chronically atheromatous artery (usually the superficial femoral artery) it may cause limb threatening ischaemia for which emergency surgery used to be the only remedy. Today it is possible, in selected patients, to pass a long catheter percutaneously, via the common femoral artery, into the recent occlusion and to infuse a thrombolytic agent such as streptokinase or tissue plasminogen activator directly into the thrombus. If thrombolysis is successful the narrowed arterial segment may be improved by percutaneous transluminal angioplasty or selective operation.

OPERATIVE TECHNIQUES AND GRAFT MATERIALS

The choice of operation for patients with occlusive disease of the lower limb arteries depends on the site of the occlusion(s), the availability of a suitable graft, and the experience of the operator. Although a variety of local bypasses or patch angioplasties may occasionally be desirable, by far the most common procedure is a bypass from the common femoral artery to a distal vessel; this is usually the popliteal artery—either above or below knee level—but it may also be to the tibioperoneal trunk or to any of the three (crural) vessels of the lower leg. The modern technique differs little from that first described by Kunlin in 1948; a shunt is constructed in parallel with the occluded artery using end-to-side anastomoses both proximally and distally (Fig. 7). The rationale is to transport blood around an occluded segment while avoiding operative trauma to collaterals.

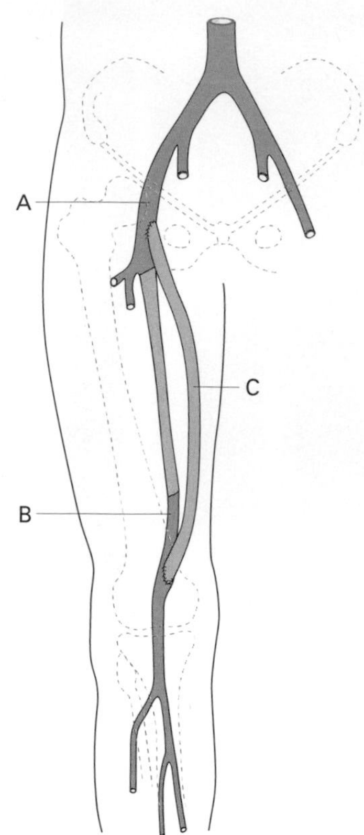

Fig. 7 Femoropopliteal bypass. A, common femoral artery; B, above knee popliteal artery; C, femoropopliteal bypass graft.

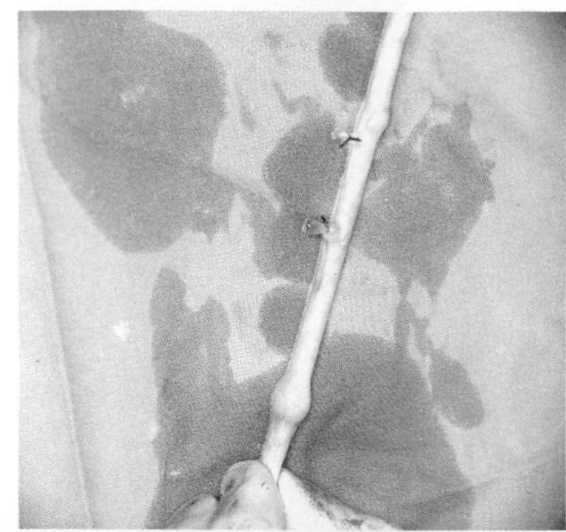

Fig. 8 Long saphenous vein excised, tributaries tied and dilated by saline injection to check for leaks before being used as a femoropopliteal bypass graft.

When available, the autogenous long saphenous vein is the best graft material for femorodistal bypass (Fig. 8). However, this vein may be too small in calibre, thrombosed, markedly varicose, or may have been removed surgically in the past. Also, its usable length may be too short for the proposed operation. The short saphenous, the cephalic, and the basilic veins may then be used, individually or in combination with themselves or with a limited length of long saphenous vein. It is common for the vein to be assessed visually at the time of operation, but it is possible to assess the usefulness of the long saphenous vein before surgery, either by duplex ultrasound scanning or by saphenography.

If the vein is inadequate it may be necessary to use a graft of synthetic material, the most popular of which is expanded polytetrafluoroethylene (PTFE) (Fig. 9). This inert substance has considerable resistance to thrombosis. Early patency rates for femoropopliteal bypass, both above and below knee, using such grafts are similar to those for autogenous vein (Fig. 10). Late patency rates are better when vein is used, especially at the below-knee site. Nevertheless, late graft occlusion is not always associated with limb loss, even when the original operation was undertaken for critical ischaemia, and limb salvage rates for vein and polytetrafluoroethylene femoropopliteal bypasses remain broadly similar.

An alternative to PTFE is glutaraldehyde-stabilized human umbilical vein supported by an external polyester mesh. This tanned graft is non-antigenic and resists biodegradation reasonably well. Patency rates compare favourably with those of PTFE but umbilical vein is expensive and aneurysmal degeneration of the graft has been described. Other less popular grafts are available,

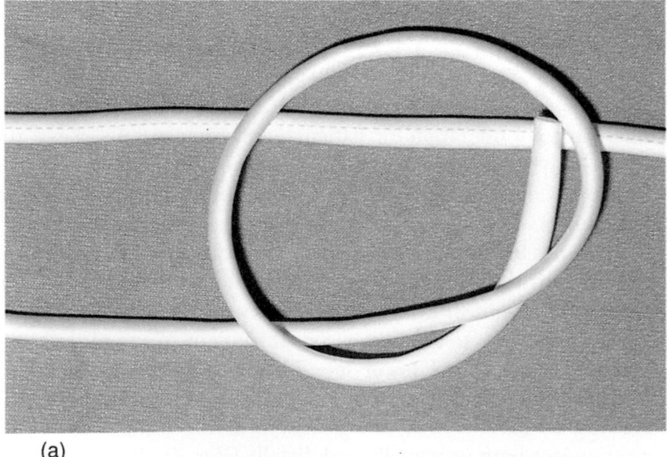

(a)

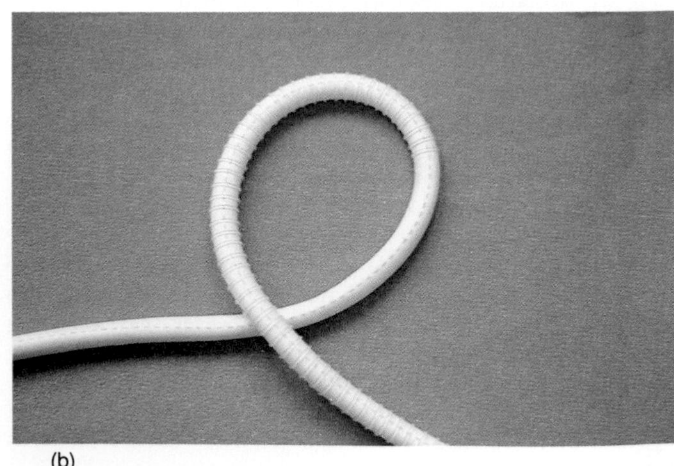

(b)

Fig. 9 (a) Polytetrafluoroethylene arterial prostheses. These are 6-mm diameter tubes, one of which has additional stiff external supporting rings (b).

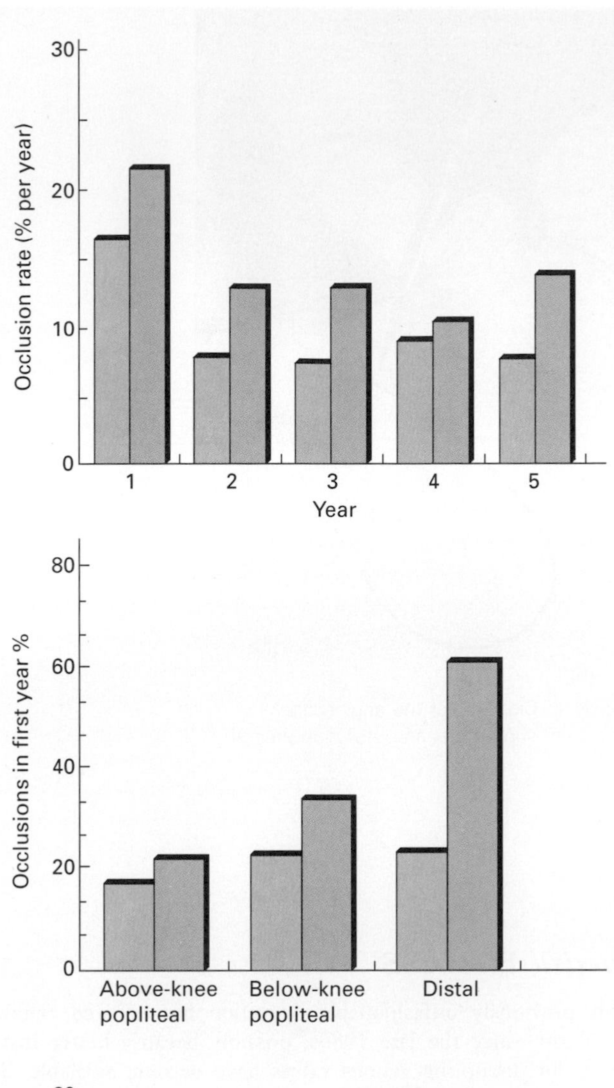

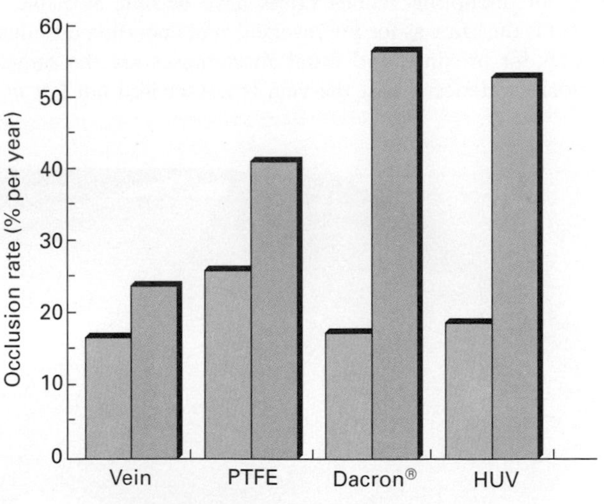

Fig. 10 (a) Occlusion rate for above-knee grafts for each year after surgery: ■ vein grafts, ■ mixed prosthetic grafts. (b) Occlusion rate in first year versus anastomotic site for vein and prosthetic grafts: ■ vein grafts, ■ prosthetic grafts. (c) Occlusion rate in first year for various graft materials in above and below knee situations: PTFE, polytetrafluoroethylene; HUV, human umbilical vein; ■, above knee; ■, below knee.

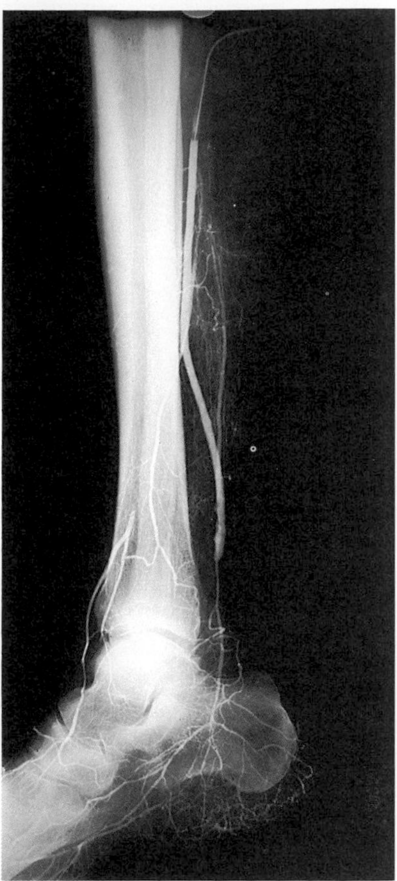

Fig. 11 Preoperative angiogram of femorocrural bypass, showing a good distal anastomosis with run off both distally and proximally into the posterior tibial artery.

such as those made from externally supported Dacron velour or ovine collagen.

When a graft of any type is inserted it is good practice to ensure at the end of the operation that the anastomoses, especially the distal one, are technically satisfactory and that flow through the graft is adequate to maintain patency. Several techniques are available. The electromagnetic flowmeter has been popular but it is difficult to achieve consistent results with this technique and peroperative Doppler ultrasonography is more satisfactory. To assess the integrity of an anastomosis the choice is between peroperative angiography (Fig. 11) which is cheap and readily available, and angioscopy which is now becoming increasingly popular in major vascular centres (Fig. 12). At the present time the authors' choice would be to use Doppler ultrasonography to assess the haemodynamics of the situation and angioscopy to assess the anastomoses. Nevertheless, if these techniques are not available it should not dissuade the surgeon from operating, especially in patients requiring limb salvage.

REVERSED AUTOGENOUS VEIN BYPASS

The most common reconstructive operation for occlusive disease below the inguinal ligament is a bypass from the common femoral to the popliteal artery, performed for occlusion of the superficial femoral artery. A bypass to the popliteal artery above the knee is

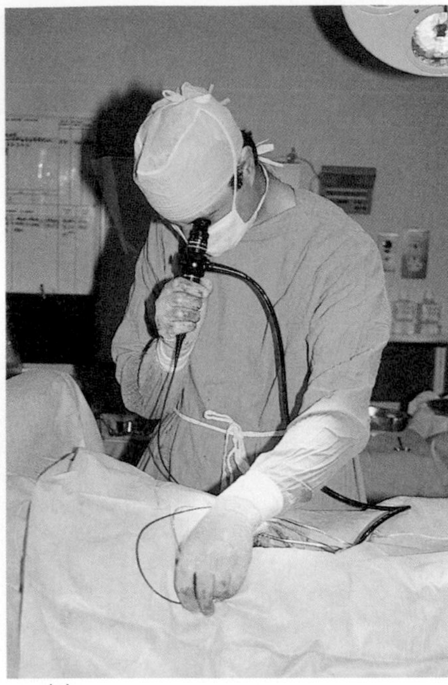

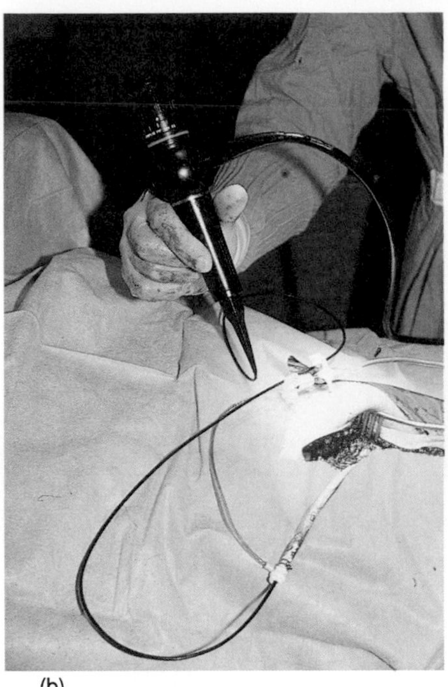

(a) (b)

Fig. 12 (a) Angioscopy to check the lower anastomosis. (b) Close-up of the angioscope passing through a valved introducer sheath. The instrument shown has an outer diameter of 2.2 mm.

the preferred option; if the above knee popliteal artery is very atheromatous or occluded then the below-knee vessel or even the crural vessels may be used.

Femoropopliteal bypass using reversed autogenous long saphenous vein is the archetypal operation. The popliteal artery is exposed via a medial incision and a satisfactory site for the lower anastomosis established. The femoral artery is exposed at the groin. A tunnel beneath sartorius is made between groin and suprageniculate politeal fossa, running orthotopically behind the knee if the infrageniculate site is to be reached. An adequate length of long saphenous vein is excised after tying and dividing its tributaries (Fig. 8) and heparin is administered to the patient. It is generally agreed that for use as a reversed femoropopliteal bypass graft, the vein must have a minimum diameter of at least 4 mm. The vein is checked for leaks and if satisfactory is reversed to deactivate the valves, and anastomosed in an end to side fashion to the arteries.

Either the proximal or the distal anastomosis may be made first, but the inexperienced surgeon should complete the distal anastomosis before the proximal as this allows the leg to be fully extended with the graft lying in the subsartorial tunnel after one anastomosis in such a way that the exact length of graft which is needed is easily recognized. On completion of both anastomoses the bypass may be checked by assessing the lower anastomosis, either by angiogram or angioscopy via an untied vein tributary which is tied after the check procedure. Adequacy of flow through the graft may be checked using an electromagnetic flow meter or Doppler ultrasonography. In general, there is no need to reverse the heparin at the end of the procedure, nor is there any need for external drains.

In-situ BYPASS

This previously unfashionable operation has enjoyed renewed popularity since the late 1980s, possibly because better instruments for disrupting venous valves have become available. The concept is the same as for the reversed vein operation inasmuch as the sites for proximal and distal anastomoses are the same; the essential difference is that the vein is not excised but left *in situ*.

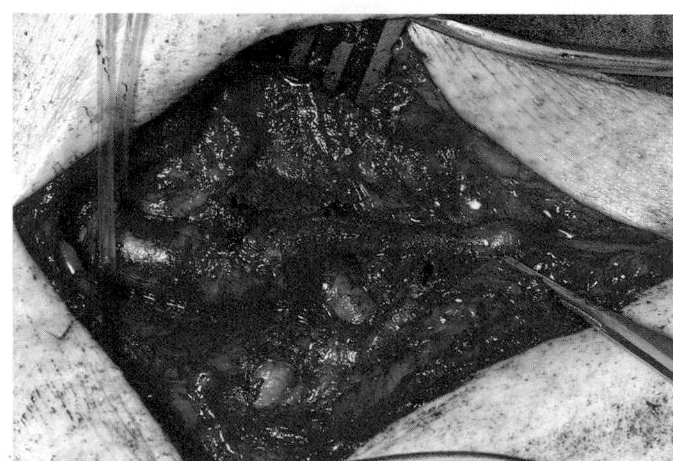

Fig. 13 *In-situ* femoropopliteal vein bypass. The long saphenous vein has been anastomosed end to side to the common femoral artery and the clamps released. The vein fills with arterial blood down to the first venous valve (at the tip of the forceps).

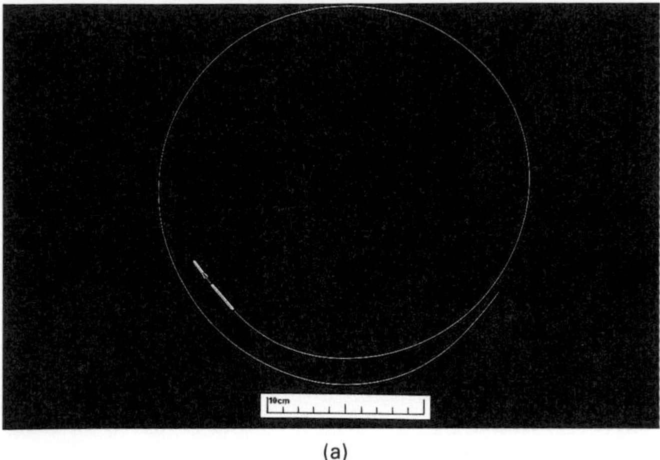

(a)

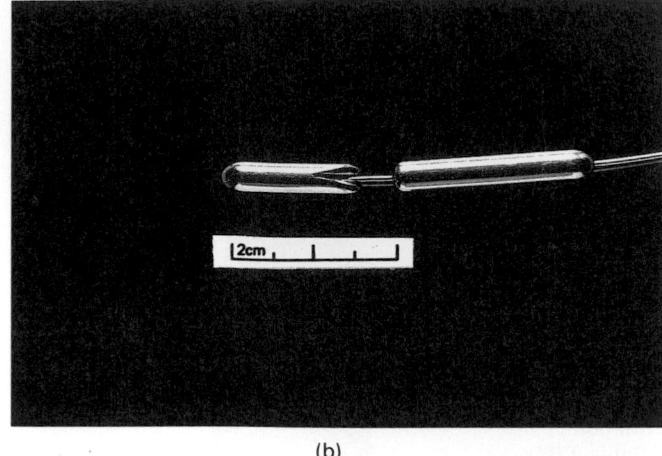

(b)

Fig. 14 (a) Hall valve cutter. (b) Close-up of head of valve cutter. The lower cylinder holds the vein open to allow the upper cylinder to disrupt the valves on traction.

The vein tributaries must all be recognized and tied off to prevent development of significant arteriovenous fistulae which compromise the graft blood flow distally, cause generalized oedema, and contribute to graft failure. The tributaries may be recognized by a variety of techniques from exposing the whole length of the vein for visual inspection (the authors' preference), to methods using Doppler ultrasonography, angiography, or angioscopy.

When using the vein *in situ* it is best to make the proximal anastomosis first and to declamp and allow the vein to fill with blood down to the first valve (Fig. 13). A valve cutter (valvulotome) is then introduced from the distal end of the vein up to the femoral anastomosis (Fig. 14). Withdrawing the valvulotome disrupts the valves and allows the blood to fill the graft as each set of valves is broken. Eventually the cutter is withdrawn followed by a spurt of pulsatile blood. The graft is then clamped and the lower anastomosis completed.

The major advantage of the *in-situ* technique, in addition to the fact that the vein and its blood supply is left largely undisturbed, is that the vein with the greater calibre in the groin is anastomosed to the large arteries, while the distal vein of smaller calibre is used in the anastomosis to smaller vessels further down the leg. It is therefore haemodynamically attractive and it is possible to achieve good results with a vein diameter of 3 mm or even less. Such grafts may be successful not only when anastomosed to the popliteal and proximal crural vessels, but even when the distal anastomosis is fashioned at ankle level. The technique, however, also has some technical disadvantages. Firstly, arteriovenous fistulae must be recognized and dealt with carefully. Secondly, the distal anastomosis may need to be made to a very small vessel and experience is required if this is to be successful. Such surgery is best done under magnification (×2.4 is adequate) and the result must be checked at completion by a peroperative angiogram or by angioscopy (if a thin enough scope is available).

FEMOPOPOPLITEAL BYPASS IN THE ABSENCE OF SUITABLE LONG SAPHENOUS VEIN

Autogenous ipsilateral long saphenous vein should be used for bypass from the common femoral artery to levels below the knee joint if possible. Some surgeons believe that the superiority of vein is such that if the long saphenous vein is compromised by severe varicosity, thrombosis, or small calibre, a search should be made for another vein source, such as the contralateral long saphenous, the short saphenous, cephalic, or brachial veins. These may be used in combination as a vein–vein composite graft. Many others believe that if the ipsilateral long saphenous vein is unavailable it is reasonable to use a manufactured alternative. The most commonly used are made from PTFE.

PTFE grafts come in a variety of calibres but 6 mm (occasionally 8 mm) is usually chosen for bypasses in the leg (Fig. 9). Some grafts are supported by external rings: these are an attractive adjunct, especially when the knee joint has to be crossed. The neointimal hyperplasia which occurs, especially at the distal anastomosis in PTFE grafts, has long been held to be the principle reason for their poorer patency (compared to vein) and it is likely that this tissue build-up is due to a compliance mismatch between the non-elastic graft and the expansile artery. The interposition of a piece of vein as a collar (Miller collar) between the PTFE and the artery has been suggested to be beneficial, but the results of meaningful trials of this promising method are still to be published.

OTHER OPERATIONS

In the presence of occlusive disease affecting the superficial femoral artery, the profunda femoris artery is the chief collateral channel between the iliac and popliteal arterial systems. In such circumstances, if the profunda is itself compromised, distal ischaemia is increased. Atheroma in the profunda shows a predilection for the area near its origin and reconstruction can be achieved by endarterectomy, by patch angioplasty (Fig. 15) or by a combination of both. Such surgery may be carried out in association with inflow reconstruction, such as an aortofemoral bypass in which a graft limb is extended beyond the common femoral artery into the profunda femoris. In general a femorodistal bypass, if feasible, will produce a better result than a profunda reconstruction alone.

Apart from the profunda femoris artery, the only other artery in the leg which is at all frequently managed by endarterectomy is the common femoral. Likewise, patch angioplasty is rarely used at

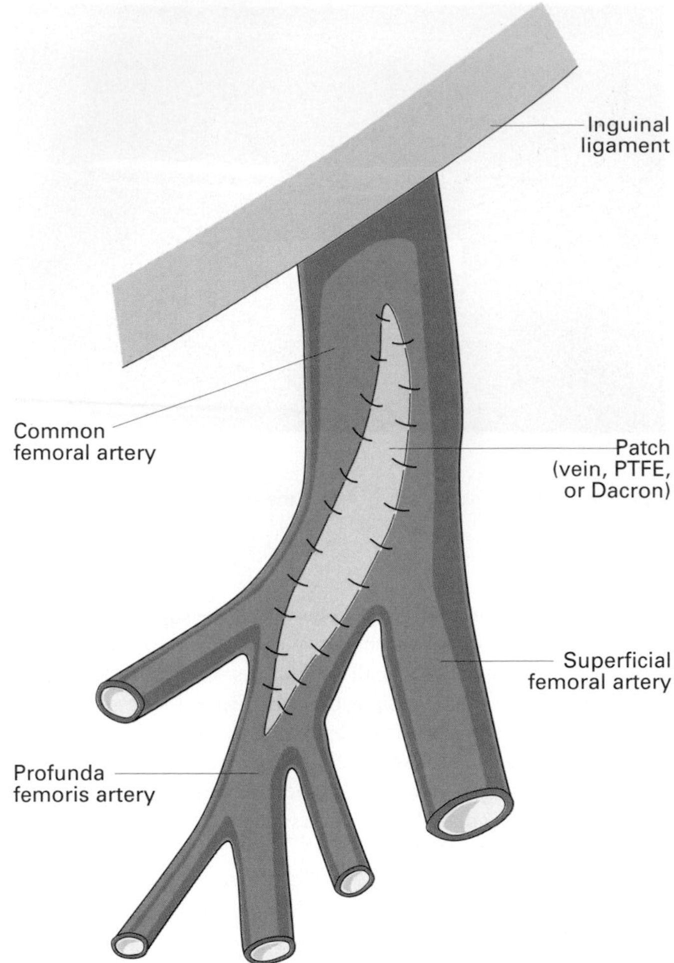

Fig. 15 Patch angioplasty of the origin of the profunda femoris artery (profundaplasty).

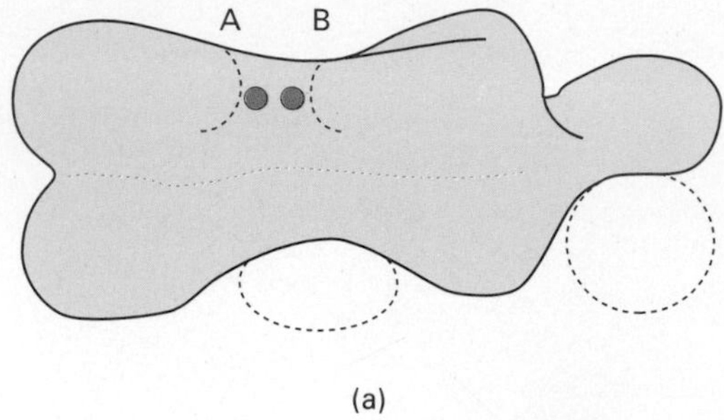

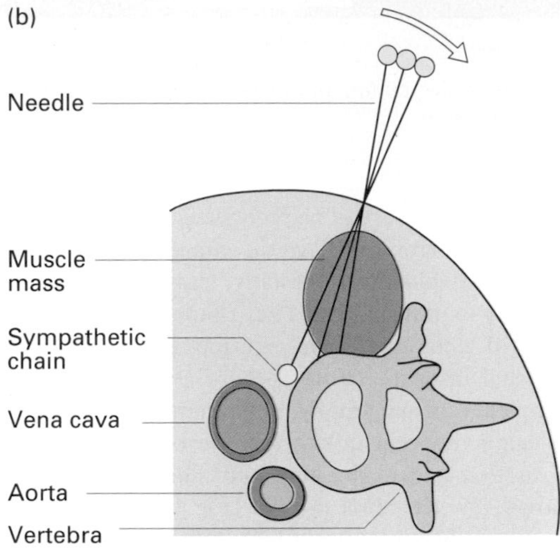

Fig. 16 Chemical sympathectomy. (a) Patient position. A, iliac crest; B, costal margin; ○ represents the two sites for injection. (b) Transverse view. Needles advanced to vertebral body then gradually swung until tangential to vertebral body at which point, after careful checking, injection may be made.

other native artery sites, although it has become fashionable for the relief of stenosis at graft–artery anastomoses and for the treatment of vein graft strictures.

LUMBAR SYMPATHECTOMY

The first lumbar sympathectomy was performed in 1924 and the operation has had variable popularity ever since. The advent of reconstructive surgery has put sympathectomy firmly in second place as a method of treatment of occlusive disease and at present its use can only be recommended as a last resort, for severe ischaemia when arterial bypass or reconstruction is not possible.

If either the collateral or the microcirculation is diseased, sympathectomy is unlikely to be of benefit. Its aim is to excise via a retroperitoneal route the sympathetic chain and ganglia from L4 to L2 (sometimes including L1), thereby increasing blood flow in the limb by decreasing vasomotor tone. The mechanism and effects of sympathectomy have been the subject of discussion for years, and they are complex; it is likely, however, that in suitable candidates skin capillary blood flow is increased. In contrast, the effect on skeletal muscle blood flow is controversial. Whatever the physiological effect, sympathectomy is extremely unlikely to benefit patients with claudication.

In the authors' experience, operative sympathectomy is only occasionally useful. Rather than submit patients to open surgery it may be more reasonable to perform a chemical sympathectomy by injecting 5 ml of 1:15 aqueous phenol at two separate sites along the lumbar sympathetic chain (Fig. 16). This requires only local anaesthetic and for many years was performed 'blind', although today the placement of needles should be monitored radiologically. In experienced hands a chemical sympathectomy is as effective as an operative procedure.

COMPLICATIONS

Early complications

Graft thrombosis

This may be due to inadequate inflow or, more likely, outflow which has not been recognized before surgery. It may also be due to a technically poor anastomosis, especially at the distal end of the graft. A balloon catheter thrombectomy is only likely to be successful in the long term if the underlying cause of the thrombosis is also corrected.

Haemorrhage

This is usually due to technical misadventure and the insertion of further sutures into an anastomosis may occasionally be needed. Very rarely it may herald an early anastomotic infection.

Lymph leak

This typically occurs from groin wounds, although wounds placed more distally in the leg are not immune. Most leaks stop spontaneously. Underlying grafts should be protected from the entry of external bacteria by administration of a broad spectrum antibiotic for the duration of leakage. Very rarely surgical closure of leaking lymph channels is necessary.

Oedema

This is not uncommon after bypass surgery in the leg and is often due to cell swelling and an increase in interstitial fluid in reperfused critically ischaemic limbs. Oedema may also be due to lymphatic hold-up, which may be expected to subside rapidly without active intervention. Finally, leg swelling may be due to relative immobility after surgery or to deep vein thrombosis.

Infection

Wound infection is uncommon and occurs most commonly in the groin wound. It is usually superficial. The underlying graft should be protected by administration of an appropriate antibiotic. If the anastomosis or graft becomes infected the material used for reconstruction will generally need to be removed and a new reconstruction, by an alternative clean route, attempted. This may be difficult to achieve.

Late complications

Thrombosis

This is the main cause of late graft failure and is generally due to progression of atheromatous disease,either proximally or distally. It may also be due to a cellular build-up at the anastomotic site of the graft (neointimal hyperplasia). Strictures may form in vein grafts and compromise flow, finally causing thrombosis. Such strictures are most common within the first year after graft insertion and should be recognized early by regular follow-up so that they may be repaired before thrombosis occurs. This requires either percutaneous transluminal angioplasty or a patch graft.

False or anastomotic aneurysm

When a leak occurs at an anastomosis the fluid may remain within the tissues and form a compartment contiguous with the artery/graft. Blood may flow freely in such a compartment and blood pressure will increase its size with time, forming a false aneurysm. An anastomotic aneurysm is a true aneurysm—it has an intimal lining—and reflects failing strength of the vessel wall at the site of anastomosis. Such aneurysms are more common after infection and may themselves be infected. They are also more common in patients with aneurysmal disease at other sites. Insertion of a graft which is too short, making it pull needlessly on its attached vessels, is a contributory factor in some cases.

Graft degeneration

A good quality autogenous saphenous vein of adequate calibre should rarely degenerate when used as an arterial conduit. Similarly, PTFE has been used in the leg for many years without major problems; this is probably true also for Dacron prostheses. The human umbilical vein graft may be prone to aneurysmal degeneration and other newer grafts—especially those of animal origin—must be regarded with caution at this time.

PREVENTION OF GRAFT OCCLUSION

Patients who have undergone angioplasty or reconstruction should be subjected to regular follow-up. Occlusion of grafts or angioplasty sites is common and most likely to occur within a year. Although early graft occlusion—within 30 days of insertion—is usually due to technical error and will occur before graft surveillance has started, intimal hyperplasia and fibrotic stricture may be identified in the medium term prior to occlusion. Patency may be prolonged and the life of a graft extended if problems can be identified and corrected by percutaneous transluminal angioplasty or surgery before occlusion; correction after occlusion has occurred is far less likely to be successful.

The form which surveillance should take has recently been widely discussed. Simple clinical review of symptoms and pulses will not give adequate warning of an impending occlusion. Serial assessment of the ankle/brachial pressure index is easy, non-invasive, and is an effective screening test; a decrease in the index of more than 0.15 suggests that a stenosis is developing. However, even this test will fail to identify graft stenosis before occlusion in some patients. Angiography, especially using digital subtraction techniques, has been suggested as the most effective form of screening, but is both invasive and expensive. Duplex ultrasonography is cheaper and gives an adequate non-invasive assessment of graft function. If the scan shows a suspicious area, particularly a graft segment where the velocity of flow is very high, angiography can be used to confirm the abnormality and allow planning of corrective treatment. The best follow-up at this time entails a duplex scan at 6 and 12 weeks after intervention and then at 3-month intervals to 1 year. The gain from follow-up beyond 1 year is likely to be limited.

Although graft surveillance is important it does not replace the traditional management of a vascular graft. This involves stopping the patient smoking, which significantly improves graft patency, correcting polycythaemia and hyperlipidaemia, and treating diabetes mellitus. Most surgeons do not routinely prescribe long-term antiplatelet or anticoagulant drugs as the evidence that they benefit graft patency is small. The exception perhaps is low dose aspirin (150 or 300 mg/day) for patients with fabricated grafts below the inguinal ligament.

FURTHER READING

Adar R, Critchfield GC, Eddy DM. A confidence profile analysis of the results of femoropopliteal percutaneous transluminal angioplasty in the treatment of lower extremity ischaemia. *J Vasc Surg* 1989; **10**: 57–67.

Ahn SS, *et al.* Removal of atheromatous lesions by angioscopically guided high-speed rotatory atherectomy. *J Vasc Surg* 1988; **7**: 292–300.

Beard JD, *et al.* Pulse generated run-off (PGR): a new method of assessing calf vessel patency. *Br J Surg* 1988; **75**: 361–3.

Beard JD, *et al.* Operative assessment of femorodistal grafts using a new Doppler flow meter. *Br J Surg* 1989; **76**: 925–8.

Beck AH, *et al.* Long term results of percutaneous transluminal angioplasty: a study of 4750 dilatations and local lyses. *Eur J Vasc Surg* 1989; 3: 245–52.

Becker GJ, Katzen BT, Drake MD. Non-coronary angioplasty. *Radiology* 1989; **170**: 921–40.

Bernstein EF, Fronek A. Current status of noninvasive tests in the diagnosis of peripheral arterial disease. *Surg Clin North Am* 1982; **62**: 473–87.

Berridge DC, *et al.* Tissue plasminogen activator in peripheral arterial thrombolysis. *Br J Surg* 1990; **77**: 179–82.

Bloor K. Natural history of arteriosclerosis of the lower extremities. *Ann R Coll Surg Engl* 1961; **28**: 36–8.

Brewster DC, *et al.* Femoropopliteal graft failures: clinical consequences and success of secondary reconstruction. *Arch Surg* 1983; **118**: 1043–7.

Clark, AM, *et al.* Anastomotic aneurysms of the femoral artery: aetiology and treatment. *Br J Surg* 1989; **76**: 1014–7.

Cotton LT, Cross FW. Lumbar sympathectomy for arterial disease. *Br J Surg* 1985; **72**: 678–83.

Dietrich EB, Timbadia E, Bahadir I. Application and limitations of laser assisted angioplasty. *Eur J Vasc Surg* 1989; **3**: 61–70.

Dormandy J. European consensus on critical limb ischaemia. *Lancet* 1989; **334**: 737–8.

Dormandy JA, Mahir MS. The natural history of peripheral atheromatous disease of legs. In: Greenhalgh RM, Jamieson CW, Nicolaides AN, eds. *Vascular Surgery: Issues in Current Practice*. New York: Grune & Stratton 1986: 3–17.

Dotter CT, Judkins MP. Transluminal treatment of arteriosclerotic obstruction. Description of a new technic and a preliminary report of its application. *Circulation* 1964; **30**: 654–70.

Dunlop MG, *et al.* Vacuum drainage of groin wounds after vascular surgery: a controlled trial. *Br J Surg* 1990; **77**: 562–3.

Ernst E. Peripheral vascular disease. *Br Med J* 1987; **299**: 873.

Ernst E, Matrai A. Intermittent claudication, exercise and blood rheology. *Circulation* 1987; **76**: 1110–4.

Green RM, Roedersheimer LR, DeWeese JA. Effects of aspirin and dipyridamole on expanded polytetrafluoroethylene graft patency. *Surgery* 1982; **92**: 1016–26.

Grigg MJ, Nicolaides AN, Wolfe JHN. Detection and grading of femorodistal graft stenoses: duplex velocity measurements compared with angiography. *J Vasc Surg* 1988; **8**: 661–6.

Gruntzig AR, Hopff H. Perkutane Rekanalisation chronischer arterieller Verschlusse mit einemneuen Dilatationskatheter. *Deutsch Med Wochenschr* 1974; **99**: 2502–5.

Haimovici H, Callow AD, De Palma RG, Ernst CB, Hollier LH, eds. *Vascular Surgery*. 3rd edn. Norwalk, Connecticut: Appleton and Large.

Harris PL, How TV, Jones DR. Prospectively randomised clinical trial to compare *in situ* and reversed saphenous vein grafts for femoropopliteal bypass. *Br J Surg* 1987; **74**: 252–5.

Hess H, Mietaschk A, Brucki R. Peripheral arterial occlusions: a six year experience with local low dose thrombolytic therapy. *Radiology* 1987; **163**: 753–8.

Hughson WG, *et al.* Intermittent claudication: factors determining outcome. *Br Med J* 1978; **i**: 1377–9.

Jelnes R, *et al.* Fate in intermittent claudication: outcome and risk factors. *Br Med J* 1986; **293**: 1137–40.

Juergens JL, Barker NW, Hines EA. Arteriosclerosis obliterans: a review of 520 cases with special reference to pathogenic factors and prognosis. *Circulation* 1960; **21**: 188–95.

Kakkasseril JS, *et al.* Efficacy of low dose streptokinase in acute arterial occlusion and graft thrombosis. *Arch Surg* 1985; **120**: 427–9.

Kannel WB, Shurtleff D. The Framingham study: cigarettes and the development of intermittent claudication. *Geriatrics* 1973; **28**: 61–8.

Kunlin J. Le traitemente de l'arterite obliterante par la greffe veineuse. *Arch Mal Coeur* 1949; **42**: 371.

Leopold PW, *et al.* Role of B-mode venous mapping in infrainguinal *in situ* vein—arterial bypasses. *Br J Surg* 1989; **76**: 305–7.

Michaels JA. Choice of material for above-knee femorodistal bypass graft. *Br J Surg* 1989; **76**: 7–14.

Miyata T, *et al.* A clinicopathological study of aneurysm formation of glutaraldehyde-tanned human umbilical vein grafts. *J Vasc Surg* 1989; **10**: 605–11.

Moody P, *et al.* Asymptomatic strictures in femoro-popliteal vein grafts. *Eur J Vasc Surg* 1989; **3**: 389–92.

Moody P, Gould DA, Harris PL. Vein graft surveillance improves patency in femoro-popliteal bypass. *Eur J Vasc Surg* 1990; **4**: 117–21.

Negus D, Irving JD, Friedgood A. Intra-arterial prostacyclin compared to Praxilene in the management of severe lower limb ischaemia: a double-blind trial. *J Cardiovasc Surg (Torino)* 1987; **28**: 196–9.

Pond GD, *et al.* Digital subtraction angiography of peripheral vascular bypass procedures. *Am J Roentgenol* 1982; **138**: 279–81.

Prevention of atherosclerotic complications with ketanserin trial group. Prevention of atherosclerotic complications: controlled trial of ketanserin. *Br Med J* 1989; **298**: 424–30.

Quick CRG, Cotton LT. The measured effect of stopping smoking on intermittent claudication. *Br J Surg* 1982; **69(suppl)**: 24–6.

Rutherford RB, ed. *Vascular Surgery*. 3rd edn. Philadelphia; W. B. Saunders: 1989.

Schubotz R, Muhlfellner O. The effect of pentoxifylline on erythrocyte deformability and on phosphatide fatty acid distribution in the erythrocyte membrane. *Curr Med Res Opin* 1977; **4**: 609–17.

Shaw SWJ, Johnson RH. The effect of naftidrofuryl on the metabolic response to exercise in man. *Acta Neurol Scand* 1975; **52**: 231–7.

Simpson JB, *et al.* Transluminal atherectomy for occlusive peripheral vascular disease. *Am J Cardiol* 1987; **61**: 97–101.

Skagseth E, Hall KV. *In situ* vein bypasses: experiences with the new vein valve strippers. *Scand J Thor Cardiovasc Surg* 1973; **7**: 53–8.

Strandness DE, Sumner DS. The relationship between calf blood flow and ankle blood pressure in patients with intermittent claudication. *Surgery* 1969; **65**: 763–6.

Thompson JF, *et al.* Intervention for graft stenosis: the role of surgery and transluminal angioplasty. *Br J Surg* 1989; **76**: 1017.

Towne JB. Role of fibrointimal hyperplasia in vein graft failure. *J Vasc Surg* 1989; **10**: 583–4.

Tyrrell MR, *et al.* Experimental evidence to support the use of interposition vein collars/patches in distal PTFE anastomosis. *Eur J Vasc Surg* 1990; **4**: 95–101.

Veith F, *et al.* Preoperative saphenous venography in arterial reconstructive surgery of the lower limb. *Surgery* 1979; **83**: 253–6.

Wiseman S, *et al.* The influence of smoking and plasma factors on prosthetic graft patency. *Eur J Vasc Surg* 1990; **4**: 57–61.

White GH, *et al.* Intraoperative video angioscopy compared with angiography during peripheral vascular operations. *J Vasc Surg* 1987; **6**: 488–95.

White RA, White GH. Laser angioplasty: development, current status, and future perspectives. *Sem Vasc Surg* 1989; **2**: 123–42.

Whittemore AD, *et al.* What is the proper role of polytetrafluoroethylene grafts in infrainguinal reconstruction. *J Vasc Surg* 1989; **10**: 299–305.

Wiseman S, *et al.* The influence of smoking and plasma factors on prosthetic graft patency. *Eur J Vasc Surg* 1990; **4**: 57–61.

Woelf KD, *et al.* Intraoperative assessment of *in situ* saphenous vein bypass grafts by vascular endoscopy. *Eur J Vasc Surg* 1988; **2**: 257–62.

Wolfe JHN, McPherson GAD. The failing femoro-distal graft. *Eur J Vasc Surg* 1987; **1**: 295–6.

7.6.3 Mesenteric arteries

LESLIE W. OTTINGER

Irrespective of the dominant systemic pattern of atherosclerotic disease, the mesenteric vessels are seldom spared. Autopsy studies show that even in middle age, more than 50 per cent stenosis is present in the coeliac axis and superior mesenteric arteries of about 6 per cent of subjects studied. The inferior mesenteric artery is similarly narrowed in twice as many. Most of these lesions, in fact, neither cause chronic symptoms nor lead to acute infarction. The circumstances under which they achieve clinical importance and the nature of these events is discussed in this section.

PATTERNS OF VISCERAL ISCHAEMIC INJURY

The major arteries that supply the intra-abdominal intestinal tract are the coeliac axis, the superior mesenteric artery, and the inferior mesenteric artery. The branches of each are interconnected by one or more peripheral arcades. There are also collateral points of junction between the three major vessels. For the coeliac axis and superior mesenteric artery these are the large pancreaticoduodenal arcades and small connections between the pancreatic and proximal jejunal vessels. One or two well-developed arcades similarly join the left branch of the middle colic artery and the superior branch of the inferior mesenteric artery. Proximal collateral inflow arises from the oesophageal and inferior phrenic arteries; distal inflow arises from branches of the hypogastric arteries.

Obliterative atheromatous disease in the mesenteric arteries is seldom diffuse. The initial and most severe lesions are almost invariably at their origins, the peripheral branches and collaterals being spared. The effectiveness of these collateral channels, especially when the superior mesenteric artery is occluded, is enhanced by gradual rather than sudden development of occlusion. Anatomical variations and prior occlusive disease also influence their role. Even complete occlusion of the origin of the inferior mesenteric artery is rarely significant except in limiting its effectiveness as a collateral source. An exception is ligation during operations of the aorta. The same statements apply to the coeliac axis. Here the exception is the coeliac compression syndrome, which is, in fact, a dubious clinical entity.

The spectrum of manifestations of mesenteric artery insufficiency extends from transient episodes of visceral pain to irreversible infarction. Three points along this spectrum are clinically important: intermittent insufficiency provoked by increased demand for perfusion during digestion; sustained insufficiency, a condition that invariably proceeds to actual ischaemic injury; and infarction, either partial or full thickness. Insufficiency and infarction are also common to the presentation of a superior mesenteric artery embolus. The challenge for successful management of obliterative atheromatous disease is to recognize occlusion during the early stages. The task is made difficult by the obscure nature of signs and symptoms prior to actual infarction.

INTESTINAL RESPONSE TO ISCHAEMIA

Despite the difficulty in directly measuring mesenteric blood flow in man, it is clear that there are marked increases during digestion, especially in the superior mesenteric artery. The classic presentation of intermittent ischaemia, provoked by a restriction of flow to such a degree that this increase in demand cannot be satisfied, is usually termed intestinal angina. Visceral pain, in fact, invariably accompanies small bowel ischaemia. When episodes are intermittent, however, its characteristics do not readily suggest the cause. It is aching in nature and poorly localized, being referred generally to the anterior abdomen. A useful clue in some patients is that it seems to be precipitated by meals.

A second clinical symptom of intermittent ischaemia is weight loss, usually the result of a decrease in intake rather than a loss of absorptive or digestive capacity. Even though many patients are not aware of a direct relationship between eating and pain, they progressively decrease their food intake in an effort to relieve advancing symptoms. An acute extensive ischaemic injury to the mucosa can affect absorptive capacity, but this is not generally a part of the chronic syndrome.

The third clinical manifestation of intermittent ischaemia which is even less specific, is disturbance in bowel function. Symptoms may include bloating, generalized abdominal discomfort, and a tendency toward diarrhoea or constipation.

Most patients with intestinal angina are elderly and have evidence of other obliterative atheromatous disease. An interesting physical sign is the presence of an epigastric bruit. In fact many do not have it, and most patients who do have a bruit do not have mesenteric vascular disease.

Some patients with abdominal angina are found to have multiple shallow antral gastric or post-bulbar duodenal ulcers. These are resistant to the usual therapy and are thought to reflect severe combined coeliac axis and superior mesenteric artery occlusive disease. Revascularization can allow healing.

Thrombosis of the origin of the coeliac axis or of the superior mesenteric artery is the end result of severe obliterative atheromatous lesions. It is often inconsequential, flow through the narrowed vessel origins having been restricted long enough for collateral channels to have become sufficient. This is not always the case; about one-half of the clinically significant cases of acute occlusion of the superior mesenteric artery have this aetiology. In other cases the coeliac axis or inferior mesenteric artery may represent a critical source for collateral flow in an extensively diseased system: their final occlusion may precipitate ischaemia and infarction. The site of infarction may be quite remote from the region directly supplied by the artery. Factors other than acute occlusion can also precipitate infarction in a patient with a severely compromised mesenteric circulation. These include central causes for hypotension and peripheral vasoconstriction, such as a cardiac arrhythmia or myocardial infarction, or any condition leading to hypovolaemia or shock. Hospital admission and angiographic studies may sometimes be such a factor. Nevertheless some patients with intestinal angina and no acute thrombotic lesion will have no apparent local or remote cause for infarction.

Sustained mesenteric insufficiency is characterized by persistent pain. If it is preceded by intestinal angina, the patient generally describes it as similar to that of intermittent episodes but more severe and unremitting. The majority of patients with symptomatic acute thrombosis will not have had prior mesenteric vascular symptoms: the duration of sustained insufficiency prior to infarction may vary from a few minutes to many days. The intensity of pain tends to wax and wane, and the actual severity of local ischaemia can be worsened by visceral artery spasm, bowel distension, and central factors that alter perfusion. Nevertheless, sustained mesenteric ischaemia almost always proceeds to frank infarction.

Early infarction involves only the mucosa and submucosa; sustained or profound ischaemia is associated with changes in the muscularis. The initial mucosal lesion is characterized by submucosal oedema and haemorrhage, followed by sloughing of the mucosa itself. This event releases blood into the lumen which may be detected in the gastric and rectal contents when infarction is extensive. Perforation of the bowel follows deep infarction, but may not occur for many hours.

The distribution of infarction caused by obliterative disease is variable, except when it is due to acute thrombosis of the superior mesenteric artery, when the distal small bowel and right colon are likely to be most severely affected. The infarct may also extend into areas dependent on this vessel for collateral supply, notably the left transverse and left colon. In other cases, the area of infarction may be in the distribution of the coeliac axis or patchy throughout the intestinal tract. Infarcts of the spleen, gallbladder, and liver are seen.

CLINICAL EVALUATION

Intermittent ischaemia with vague pain, weight loss, and fluctuating changes in bowel function is an obscure clinical entity. When ischaemic symptoms become continuous or infarction ensues the diagnosis is no longer elusive, but survival is by then unusual. It may be necessary to evaluate a large number of patients with a suggestive history to detect the few with intestinal angina. The demonstration of gastroduodenal ulcer disease, gallstones, or other unrelated conditions can delay the discovery of the actual cause of the symptoms.

A careful history centres on the characteristics of the pain and weight loss. Perhaps the most similar presentation is that of carcinoma of the pancreas, although bowel changes sometimes lead to an initial suspicion of colon disease. A recent history of peptic ulcer disease and findings of obliterative atheromatous disease in other systems, especially if premature, are helpful. In young women there is often a history of heavy cigarette smoking. Because of the infrequent occurrence of intestinal angina, the initial evaluation often centres on other diagnoses. It is important to persist until a correct diagnosis is established in any patient with abdominal pain and weight loss.

When available, flow Doppler studies may provide a useful direct measurement of mesenteric arterial flow. The critical examination is, however, the arteriogram. A lateral projection with supracoeliac injection into the aorta gives the most useful information about the patency of the origin of the coeliac axis and superior mesenteric artery. Selective injections are also of value but must be used with caution in symptomatic patients with severely compromised circulation, as they may precipitate infarction.

Only by correlation of the history and angiographic findings can the importance of vascular lesions be determined. Intermittent ischaemia is most often associated with extensive occlusive disease of at least two, and usually all three, major vessels. Continuous ischaemia is more frequently the result of acute occlusion of the superior mesenteric artery by thrombus or an embolus. Thromboses leading to infarction can occur in the absence of other severe mesenteric lesions. Continuous ischaemia may also represent the end-stage of extensive obliterative atheromatous disease, with or without acute thrombosis. It may also be the result of impending non-occlusive infarction, venous thrombosis, or even an aortic dissection. The aortic and mesenteric angiograms may sometimes suggest or support these diagnoses in the absence of lesions of major arteries.

MANAGEMENT

Intermittent ischaemia

The disability associated with intermittent ischaemia would be sufficient to merit correction in most patients; added to this is the risk of eventual infarction. No studies have predicted the magnitude of this risk, but it must be considered high in the severely symptomatic patient.

Treatment has centred on restoration of flow to the superior mesenteric artery and a number of surgical procedures that can accomplish this have been described. These include bypass grafts from the aorta or iliac artery, reimplantation of the superior mesenteric artery after resection of its diseased origin, thromboendarterectomy, either directly or through the open aorta, and side-to-side anastomosis of the main trunk or a branch to the aorta or iliac artery. If the aorta is severely narrowed or aneurysmal, resection and grafting may be indicated at the time of revascularization. The graft can then be used for the site of origin of a bypass or reimplantation. Of all these procedures, a graft from the supracoeliac aorta is perhaps the most uniformly feasible and satisfactory technique (Fig. 1(a)). Restoration of flow into the coeliac axis or one of its branches is not necessary for immediate success, but it may protect against future failure of the reconstruction because of progressive occlusive atheromatous disease. Angiodilatation provides a non-operative alternative to surgical reconstruction. The low risk in selected patients may justify the high recurrence rate.

Improvement of circulation immediately eliminates the pain of intermittent ischaemia. Recovery of normal gastrointestinal function may take months, and weight gain is slow, or non-existent in some patients.

Continuous ischaemia

Continuous ischaemia in patients with obliterative atheromatous disease precedes infarction, which is almost always fatal. Immediate diagnosis and intervention gives the only chance for survival. Prompt angiography can be useful, especially in patients with acute thrombosis of the superior mesenteric artery. Otherwise,

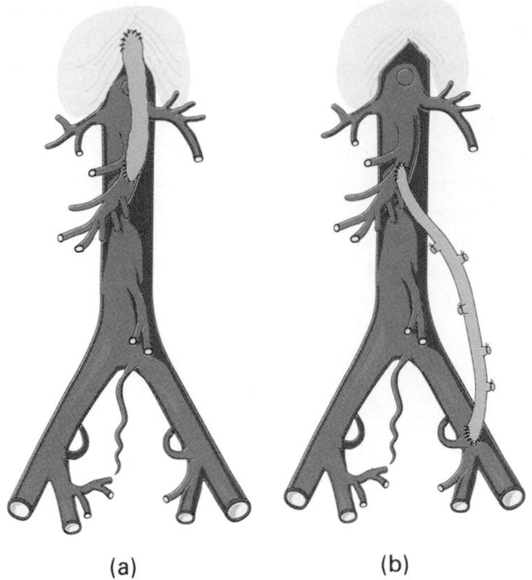

Fig. 1 (a) A bypass graft from the supracoeliac aorta to the superior mesenteric artery for revascularization in the management of intermittent mesenteric ischemia. (b) A bypass graft from the iliac to superior mesenteric artery, using a reversed segment of saphenous vein, in the management of acute thrombosis with infarction.

and in the presence of signs of advanced infarction or peritonitis, immediate laparotomy is the best choice.

In the early stages of threatened infarction the findings are subtle. The intestine does not show discoloration or haemorrhage but is grey, and there may be areas of spasm and hyperperistalsis. Faint collateral pulses can be palpated in some cases. The surgeon should be cautious about abandoning the diagnosis because there is no infarction: to do so always leads to later infarction. With these early findings, or if infarction is limited and other areas threatened, vascular reconstruction should be attempted. A good procedure is the construction of a bypass graft from the aorta or iliac artery to the superior mesenteric artery (Fig. 1(b)). A segment of saphenous vein may be superior in this circumstance. The superior mesenteric artery is exposed distal to the origin of the middle colic artery and opened to establish that no embolus is present. The arterotomy, if longitudinal, can be used for the distal anastomosis. The alternative of a thromboendarterectomy or a more complicated bypass seems less successful under these emergency conditions.

After restoration of circulation, the necessity for a bowel resection is assessed: a short period of observation should suffice. In patients with either very extensive obliterative disease or a marginal appearance of the intestine at completion of the operation, a second-look operation a few hours later has merit.

Infarction

Infarction, as a terminal event in obliterative atheromatous disease, has a dismal prognosis. Many patients are old and infirm and the infarction tends to be extensive. In an unselected series more than one-half of patients were moribund at the time of admission. In a few generally more fit patients with early diagnosis and limited infarction, arterial reconstruction with a resection, or even a resection alone, can succeed. The attempt is fruitless in the presence of extensive, advanced infarction with this underlying diagnosis.

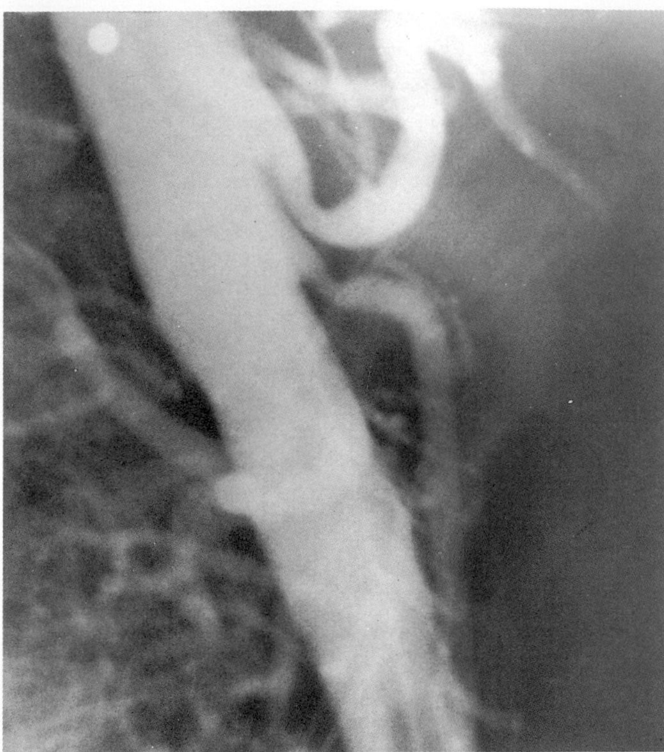

Fig. 2 Angiogram of the upper abdominal aorta in a 40-year-old patient with non-specific upper abdominal pain. Lateral view showing compression of both the coeliac axis and superior mesenteric artery by the median arcuate ligament.

Isolated coeliac artery disease

Pain relating to narrowing of the origin of the coeliac axis has been termed the coeliac axis compression syndrome. The lesion can be the result of compression of the artery by the median arcuate ligament when there is a relatively high origin of the artery or low termination of the ligament (Fig. 2). Fixed narrowing by fibroses or an obliterative atheromatous plaque is frequently found at surgical exploration.

Most patients are between 20 and 40 years old. Pain, which is quite non-specific, is felt in the upper anterior abdomen and may be precipitated by eating or exercise. The mechanism of pain is unknown, but there is no evidence that it is due to actual ischaemia. Asymptomatic compression of the coeliac axis is observed on many angiograms. Occlusion in the absence of advanced disease in the superior mesenteric artery is similarly inconsequential.

Surgical management is directed towards releasing the origin of the vessel and correcting any persistent narrowing. The placebo effect of these operations may well account for their unpredictable success and its variable duration. There is no associated risk of infarction and operations for isolated coeliac axis disease are rarely advisable.

FURTHER READING

Allende HD, Ona FV. Celiac artery and superior mesenteric artery insufficiency. Unusual cause of erosive gastroduodenitis. *Gastroenterology*, 1982; **82**: 763–6.

Beebe HG, MacFarlane S, Raker EJ. Supraceliac aortomesenteric bypass for intestinal ischemia. *J Vasc Surg*, 1987; **5**: 749–54.

Cherry RD, Jabbari M, Goresky CA, Herba M, Reich D, Blundell PE. Chronic mesenteric vascular insufficiency with gastric ulceration. *Gastroenterology*, 1986; **91**: 1548–52.

Colapinto RF, McLoughlin MJ, Weisbrod GL. The routine lateral aortogram and the celiac compression syndrome. *Radiology*, 1972; **103**: 557–61.

Croft RJ, Menon GP, Marston A. Does intestinal angina exist? A critical study of obstructed visceral arteries. *Br J Surg*, 1981; **68**: 316–18.

Cronstedt J. *et al.* Gastro-duodenal ulceration in abdominal angina. *Acta Chir Scand*, 1982; **148**: 687–92.

Dick AP, Graff R, Gregg DM, Peters N, Sarner M. An arteriographic study of mesenteric arterial disease. I. Large vessel changes. *Gut*, 1967; **8**: 206–20.

Evans WE. Long term evaluation of the celiac bond syndrome. *Surgery*, 1974; **76**: 867–71.

Marston A, Clarke JM, Garcia-Garcia J, Miller AL. Intestinal function and intestinal blood supply. *Gut*, 1985; **26**: 656–66.

Odurny A, Sniderman KW, Colapinto RF. Intestinal angina: percutaneous transluminal angioplasty of the celiac and superior mesenteric arteries. *Radiology*, 1988; **167**: 59–62.

Ottinger LW. The surgical management of acute occlusion of the superior mesenteric artery. *Ann Surg*, 1978; **188**: 721–31.

7.7.1 Abdominal aorta

JACK COLLIN

DEFINITION

An aneurysm is by definition an abnormal dilatation of an artery or vein, and the application of this general principle to the abdominal aorta has seldom presented any problems in routine clinical practice. The universal use of abdominal ultrasound as a basic diagnostic tool, and particularly the introduction of screening programmes for abdominal aortic aneurysms, has recently highlighted the need for a more precise definition to allow appropriate diagnosis of the many marginal aortic dilatations, or small aneurysms, which are now being discovered.

The diameter of the abdominal aorta, like other biological measurements, conforms to a normal population distribution curve. Median aortic diameter increases with age, is greater in men than in women, and is influenced by the race, weight, height, and prevalence of hypertension in the population studied. In men, after 60 years of age the shape of the curve becomes increasingly skewed to the right as the prevalence of abdominal aortic aneurysm increases. A definition of aneurysm based on deviation from the mean aortic diameter for a population will therefore be of limited value.

In some patients with an abdominal aortic aneurysm, dilatation may also involve the suprarenal or thoracic aorta, leading to a diagnosis of thoracoabdominal aortic aneurysm or generalized arterial ectasia, depending on the amount and extent of the dilatation. Any definition that relies solely on comparison of suspected aneurysm diameter with adjacent 'normal' aortic diameter will fail in the 5 per cent of patients whose aneurysms are not confined to the infrarenal aorta.

A modern definition of an aortic aneurysm takes into account the above facts and make due allowance for the inaccuracies of measurement inherent in even the most precise methods of diagnosis. The following definition is proposed: 'An aortic aneurysm is present when the maximum external diameter of the aorta either (1) is at least 4.0 cm; or (2) exceeds the diameter of the adjacent aorta by at least 0.5 cm.'

The imprecise but clinically useful term 'aortic ectasia' should be reserved for those cases where the aorta appears abnormally wide but is not aneurysmal by the above definition.

Table 1 Male to female ratio of incidence of death from ruptured abdominal aortic aneurysm (England and Wales, 1986)

Age (years)	M:F ratio
60–64	12.6
65–69	9.1
70–74	7.0
75–79	6.5
80 and over	4.0

EPIDEMIOLOGY

Aortic aneurysms are very rare before the age of 55 and are virtually confined to patients with Marfan's,. Ehlers–Danlos, or arteria magna syndromes. The common idiopathic abdominal aortic aneurysm is largely a disease of elderly men. Comparison of deaths from ruptured abdominal aortic aneurysm by age and sex reveal this to be 13 times more common in men than in women at age 60 to 65 years, but only four times more common in men than in women at over 80 years of age (Table 1). At age 85 almost three times as many women as men are still alive, so among the very elderly the numbers of men and women presenting with ruptured aneurysms is similar. The changing pattern of aneurysm presentation with age, combined with an increase in the number of elderly people in the populations of most wealthy nations, has led some surgeons to conclude erroneously that abdominal aortic aneurysm has increased in incidence disproportionately in women.

The annual risk of death from aortic aneurysm increases from 125 per 10^6 for men aged 55 to 59 years to 2728 per 10^6 at age 85+. At age 70 to 74 years, aortic aneurysms are responsible for 2.2 per cent of all deaths in men, and abdominal aortic aneurysms account for 77 per cent of these (Fig. 1). The disease is a particularly common cause of unexpected deaths, and more than 5 per cent of sudden deaths in men over 50 years of age investigated by autopsy are found to be due to ruptured abdominal aortic aneurysm.

In the past 30 years there has been a linear increase in the number of recorded deaths from aortic aneurysm in England and Wales. In part this can be explained by the progressive growth in

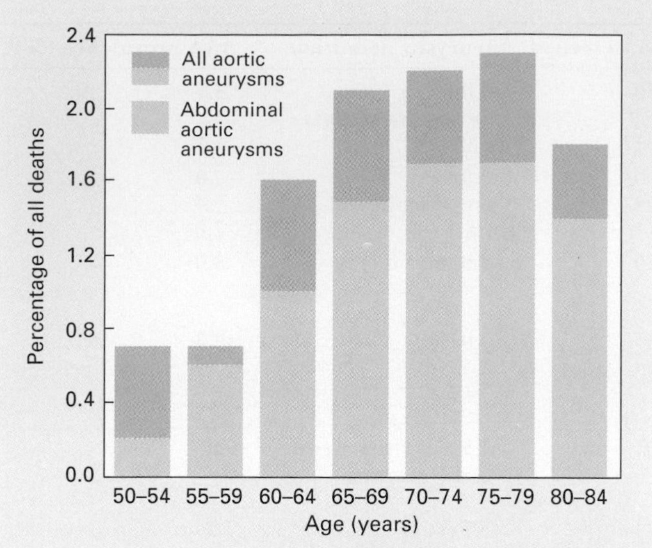

Fig. 1 Death from aortic aneurysm as a percentage of all deaths for men by age.

the number of elderly in the population, but age-specific death rates for aortic aneurysm have also increased over the age of 60. Some of the increase may be real, but much of the apparent change may be due to enhanced awareness of the disease, improved diagnosis, and altered referral patterns associated with the establishment of specialist vascular units. This issue is difficult to resolve because of the unreliability of national records of cause of death, which ultimately depend on the diagnostic acumen of the reporting doctor, seldom supported by autopsy evidence. In the United States a similar, but more rapid, increase in age-adjusted mortality for aortic aneurysm occurred between 1951 and 1968, but the number of recorded deaths then stabilized and, in Caucasian males, has declined at 2 per cent/annum since 1976, possibly as a consequence of the increasing impact of elective aneurysm surgery.

Reports from the early part of the century illustrate that there has been a qualitative as well as quantitative change in abdominal aortic aneurysm disease. Before the introduction of effective antisyphilitic therapy, the majority of aortic aneurysms were a manifestation of tertiary syphilis, and the mean age of presentation was consequently lower than at present. In developed countries, syphilitic aneurysms are now rare and idiopathic abdominal aortic aneurysms of the elderly represent the vast majority of cases seen.

There has been debate about the influence of racial factors on abdominal aortic aneurysms, with most studies focusing on comparison of black and white populations in the United States and South Africa. There is no doubt that the disease is seen less often in people of African descent than in Caucasians, but in both countries it is difficult to discover whether the differences simply reflect the lower life expectation and mean age of the black population and their poorer access to health care. The high prevalence of hypertension in these people gives theoretical grounds for suspecting that, age for age, abdominal aortic aneurysm might well be more common than in Caucasians. At present the evidence for racially determined differences in incidence must be regarded as suspect, and careful epidemiological studies will be required to resolve this issue.

Prevalence

The prevalence of any disease represents the total number of cases, both diagnosed and occult, present in the population at any given time, and should be distinguished from incidence, which is the number of new cases diagnosed over a specified period of time.

The majority of aortic aneurysms are asymptomatic and impalpable; consequently their prevalence in the community can be determined only by systematic screening. Although the results of many screening studies have been published, most are fundamentally flawed as measures of prevalence. The incidence of aortic aneurysm increases rapidly with age and is much higher in men than in women. Prevalence studies must therefore differentiate each 5- or 10-year age-group and men from women. Studies in patients with hypertension, atherosclerosis, or other diseases cannot produce prevalence data relevant to the whole population. Examination of all the data (Table 2) does, however, allow a number of conclusions to be drawn.

1. In men aged 65 to 74 the prevalence of abdominal aortic aneurysm of all sizes is around 5.5 per cent, and of diameter 4.0 cm or more is at least 2.0 per cent.
2. In patients with hypertension or atherosclerotic occlusive disease of the coronary, carotid, or limb arteries the prevalence of abdominal aortic aneurysm is 50 per cent higher than in the general population.

AETIOLOGY

The common abdominal aortic aneurysm of elderly men has been labelled as 'atherosclerotic'. This classification has little justification, has paralysed thinking, and needs to be re-examined. It is interesting to note that aneurysmal disease is encumbered by more than its fair share of unhelpful, or frankly misleading, descriptive terms, among which are atheromatous, mycotic, inflammatory, dissecting, and arteriovenous aneurysms. In the elderly the aorta, in common with every other artery, will have obvious features of atherosclerosis but this is not enough evidence to make credible a pathological diagnosis that does not fit with many known facts about the disease.

Tilson has compared patients with abdominal aortic aneurysms and those with occlusive aortoiliac disease. He found that the aneurysm patients were nine times more likely to be male; were, on average, 11 years older; and were much less likely to have had previous arterial surgery. Patients with occlusive disease were 16 times more likely to require reoperation after aortic surgery. In addition, aneurysm patients were, on average,more than 5 cm (2 inches) taller than patients with occlusive arterial disease, and had a significantly greater body surface area. In our own experience, aneurysms in patients who have associated occlusive arterial disease are generally smaller and may be less likely to rupture than in patients without severe atherosclerosis. This view is supported by the observation that mean growth rates for small aneurysms are 50 per cent faster when there is no obvious occlusive arterial disease.

Genetic predisposition

Surgeons have been aware for some years of the occasional occurrence of several cases of abdominal aortic aneurysm within families, but proof of the familial pattern of the disease has been

Table 2 Screening studies for abdominal aortic aneurysms

	City	Study group	No. screened	Aneurysm definition	AAA prevalence (%)
Healthy subjects	Oxford	Men 65–74 years	850	>4.0 cm or 5 mm > suprarenal aorta	5.7
	Chichester	Men and women 65–80 years	1312	⩾3.0 cm	5.8
Hypertensives	London	Men >50 years	200	⩾3.0 cm	7.0
	Birmingham	Men 65–85 years	94	5 mm > suprarenal	7.4
		Women 65–85 years	71	aorta	2.8
Atherosclerosis/ hypertension/ obesity	Portland	Men and woman >50 years attending cardiology clinic	120	⩾4.0 cm	5.0
	Vancouver	Men >55 years waist measure >101 cm hypertensive or atherosclerotic	45	⩾3.0 cm	13.3
	Minneapolis	Men 60–75 years with hypertension and/or coronary heart disease	201	>1.5 times suprarenal aortic diameter	9.0
	Nottingham	Men and women attending vascular clinic	104	>3.5 cm or 5 mm > suprarenal aorta	7.7

difficult to obtain because of the absence of symptoms and the advanced age of onset in most patients. Even carefully elicited family histories will often be unhelpful, since the majority of those with the aneurysm diathesis will die from other causes, and many who die from aneurysm rupture will have the wrong diagnosis recorded unless an autopsy is carried out. The problem is compounded by the absence of a common name for aortic aneurysm, which is consequently unfamiliar to the general public.

Recently, ultrasound screening studies have shown a prevalence of abdominal aortic aneurysm of 30 per cent in first-degree male relatives of patients with the disease. Because of the late age of onset, many of those with no evidence of an aneurysm at the time of screening could well develop the disease when they are older, so the lifetime prevalence in brothers and sons of aneurysm patients may be as high as 50 per cent. The search for the gene or genes responsible is hindered by the absence of three-generation families with confirmed aneurysm inheritance for genetic studies. It is likely that, with the rapid strides currently occurring in molecular biology, this problem will be solved in the next few years, using techniques such as paired sibling analysis.

Connective tissue degradation

Research efforts have concentrated on attempts to discover the mechanism of breakdown of collagen and elastin in the arterial wall of enlarging and ruptured abdominal aortic aneurysms. Several studies have shown the presence of proteolytic activity in tissue from aneurysmal aorta, but authentic collagenase has been shown to be present only when the aneurysm has ruptured. It is uncertain whether collagenolysis is the cause or a consequence of aneurysm rupture. Similar uncertainties surround the detection of elastase in the aortic wall and serum of aneurysm patients. The discriminant value of such analyses between patients with and without aneurysms has not always been confirmed, although recently a unique metalloprotease elastase has been found only in aneurysm patients. Recently, in one family in which aneurysms occurred in several members at an early age, it has been shown that the disease is linked to a genetically determined defect in type III collagen. It is possible that other genetic variations in type III collagen may account for some, if not all, cases of abdominal aortic aneurysm. Such a finding, although at present speculative, would mirror the situation in osteogenesis imperfecta where the disorder has been shown to be caused by a large number of different genetic variations in type I collagen.

Environmental potentiation

Abdominal aortic aneurysms have been shown to be associated with:

(1) male sex;
(2) advancing age;
(3) tobacco smoking;
(4) hypertension;
(5) chronic obstructive airways disease (irrespective of smoking history);
(6) occlusive arterial disease affecting coronary, carotid, and limb arteries.

In addition, aortic aneurysm is most common in Caucasians and those who are tall, but these are unlikely to be independent disease determinants and probably reflect racial differences in population–age structure and the relationship between height, longevity, and socioeconomic status.

The mechanisms by which environmental influences interact with underlying genetic predisposition to produce abdominal aortic aneurysm in an individual patient is at present uncertain, but the first three factors listed have by far the greatest importance. It is interesting that, in common with other diseases, the marked protective effect of female sex is progressively lost with advancing age, although even in the very elderly the risk of dying from aortic rupture is three times greater for men than for women.

NATURAL HISTORY

The great majority of abdominal aortic aneurysms are fusiform and are confined to the infrarenal segment. Small saccular aneu-

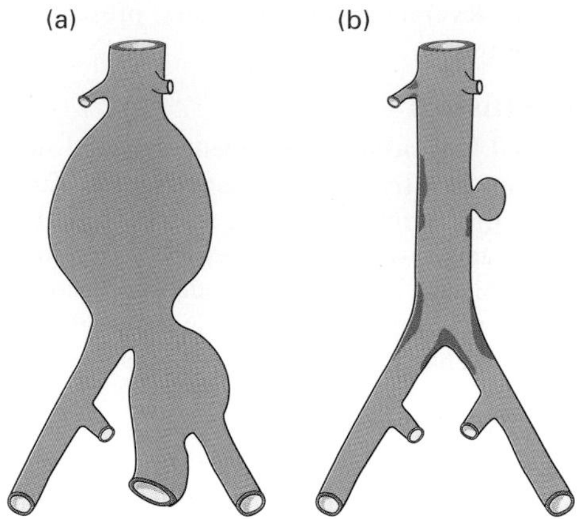

Fig. 2 (a) Large fusiform infrarenal abdominal aortic aneurysm continuous with aneurysms of the left common and internal iliac arteries. (b) A saccular aortic aneurysm associated with aortoiliac atheromatous occlusive arterial disease.

rysms are sometimes seen adjacent to atheromatous plaques in patients with predominant occlusive disease (Fig. 2), and rapidly growing infective 'mycotic' saccular aneurysms occasionally occur as a consequence of bacteraemia. Mycotic aneurysms are a local manifestation of systemic disease, require urgent medical and surgical treatment irrespective of size, and have a totally different natural history from that of the common idiopathic aortic aneurysms of the elderly discussed here.

The mean diameter of the infrarenal abdominal aorta increases with age in both men and women. An aortic aneurysm begins as a local accentuation of this normal ageing process. Physical laws predict that the rate of growth will increase with diameter, so once any local accentuation has started it can be expected to increase progressively with time. This explanation accounts for the three types of dilatation common seen, namely:

(1) a local aneurysm with normal adjacent arteries;
(2) generalized arterial ectasia;
(3) local dilatation within an ectatic arterial system.

Serial measurements have confirmed that growth rates increase as abdominal aortic aneurysms enlarge. The development of symptoms, risk of rupture, and clinical management of aortic aneurysms depend largely on their diameter, so it is convenient to discuss the natural history in relation to three somewhat arbitrary size ranges. It is important to remember, however, that the life-cycle of an individual aortic aneurysm is a continuous process from initial development to eventual rupture, the inevitability of which can be prevented only by elective surgery or prior death from some other disease. Looked at in this way, the description of an aortic aneurysm as a cancer of the artery is not quite so fanciful as it might seem.

Very small aneurysms (less than 4.0 cm diameter)

The prevalence of aneurysms less than 4.0 cm in diameter has become apparent only with the introduction of screening programmes for the disease. Two-thirds of all aneurysms detected by population screening are of this size, the reasons for which are interesting and help in understanding some important features of the disease.

1. The longest part of the life-cycle of any aneurysm will be when it is small, since incremental growth rates increase as the aneurysm enlarges.
2. Large aneurysms are more likely to be detected and present in routine clinical practice.
3. The larger an aneurysm becomes, the more likely it is to rupture and remove the patient beyond the benefits of screening.

Very small aortic aneurysms generally enlarge much more slowly than the large aneurysms which present in routine clinical practice, and median growth rates of 0.2 cm/annum are usual. Clinical and autopsy evidence indicates that even these very small aneurysms do sometimes rupture, but there are insufficient data for the risk to be quantified accurately. Several clinical follow-up studies have shown no cases of rupture occurring in such patients while the aneurysms remained very small, but ruptures did occur as the aneurysms grew.

Small aneurysms (4.0–5.9 cm diameter)

Autopsy studies of patients with an abdominal aortic aneurysm showed that more than one-third of aneurysms less than 6.0 cm in diameter had ruptured and caused death. Follow-up studies of patients with aneurysms less than 6.0 cm diameter managed conservatively have demonstrated a rupture rate of 6 per cent per annum over 3 years. Rupture rates tend to increase progressively with the length of follow-up as the aneurysms continue to expand. For aneurysms of 4.0 to 4.9 cm diameter the mean expansion rate is 0.5 cm/annum, increasing to 0.7 cm/annum for aneurysms of 5.0 to 5.9 cm diameter.

Large aneurysms (greater than 6.0 cm diameter)

Nowadays, patients with aneurysms of more than 6.0 cm diameter are invariably advised to have elective surgery. What we know of the natural history of large aneurysms comes from studies before operative treatment became possible in 1951 or from contemporary studies in patients too ill to undergo major surgery.

Studies from earlier in the twentieth century of clinical detection, and therefore presumably large and often symptomatic, abdominal aortic aneurysms report that most patients died within 3 years, and two-thirds of all deaths were from aneurysm rupture. Contemporary studies of patients with severe cardiac, respiratory, or other disease considered to make the risks of elective surgery unacceptably high show that aneurysm rupture accounts for half of all deaths.

CLINICAL PRESENTATION

The majority of abdominal aortic aneurysms are asymptomatic and are often discovered incidentally. The patient may notice a pulsatile epigastric mass for the first time typically while lying relaxed in bed or his bath. Large aneurysms in thin patients are readily detected on routine abdominal examination, but most are now discovered by ultrasonography or abdominal radiography performed to investigate unrelated symptoms. Urologists are a frequent source of referrals for many vascular surgeons, since prostatic hypertrophy and aortic aneurysm are both disorders of the elderly and detection of the aneurysm by abdominal palpation is easier during anaesthesia for prostatic resection. It is likely that much of the apparent increased incidence of abdominal aortic aneurysm over the past decade is attributable to general adoption of abdominal ultrasonography as the routine first-line investigation for abdominal symptoms.

In Britain, ruptured abdominal aortic aneurysm still accounts for around a third of all operations for the disease, but in the United States the figure for major vascular centres is currently between 5 and 20 per cent. Community studies have shown that 60 per cent of patients with ruptured abdominal aortic aneurysms do not reach hospital alive, while some of those who do are not operated upon. In Britain rupture of the abdominal aortic aneurysm is sadly still the way in which more than half of all cases present. In both the northern and southern hemispheres there is a seasonal variation in the incidence of aortic rupture, with more cases occurring in the winter months. The reason for this pattern is unknown, but may be related to the similar observed seasonal variation in mean blood pressure.

Symptoms and signs of aortic rupture

Typically, rupture of an abdominal aortic aneurysm produces the sudden unheralded onset of severe central abdominal and lumbar back pain. Some patients may have experienced dull back pain of lesser severity for hours or days before, due to acute aneurysm expansion immediately prior to rupture. The lumbar pain may be worse on one side, commonly the left, because of the direction in which the retroperitoneal haematoma spreads. There may be a variable degree of psoas spasm, and sometimes pain in the lower limb, due to compression of lumbar or sciatic nerve roots. Rupture of an internal iliac (hypogastric) artery aneurysm commonly produces maximal pain in the buttock and, rarely, blood may track with the sciatic nerve through the greater sciatic foramen to produce a gluteal haematoma.

Other early symptoms and signs depend on the volume of acute blood loss. Once the posterior peritoneum is breached, the patient will rapidly bleed to death into the peritoneal cavity, and most immediate deaths are due to intraperitoneal rupture. Survival after rupture depends on an intact posterior peritoneum, tissue tamponade, and early emergency surgery. When the connective tissue tamponade provided by the retroperitoneum is very effective, or the leak is small, only modest haemorrhage may occur, and these patients can survive long journeys to hospital and several days before exsanguinating haemorrhage occurs. The self-selection of such patients for transfer to distant tertiary referral centres may be partly responsible for the superior results of some units. In most cases, tamponade is less effective and arrests acute haemorrhage only when assisted by hypotension secondary to blood loss. These patients exhibit pallor, sweating, tachycardia, and anuria, and transfusion alone by raising the blood pressure will result in further haemorrhage. Immediate surgery to clamp the aorta above the site of rupture offers the only chance of survival.

Uncommon presentations

The great majority of abdominal aortic aneurysms will present as described above, but it is a common disease and any vascular surgeon will see several cases in his career, presenting in each of the following ways.

Aortic occlusion

Turbulent blood flow occurs in all aneurysms and slow transit of contrast medium is often seen on angiography. Turbulent flow contributes to the formation of the mural thrombus which is present in most aneurysms. Sometimes the thrombotic process is more extensive and the aorta may occlude. Occlusion usually does not involve the renal artery origins but is frequently accompanied by acute critical ischaemia of the lower limbs.

Distal embolization

Mural thrombus can become dislodged from within the aneurysm, perhaps as a consequence of direct abdominal trauma, and lodges as emboli in the arteries of the lower limb. One or two per cent of all emboli to the lower limb arise from this source.

Ureteric occlusion

Around 10 per cent of abdominal aortic aneurysms are of the 'inflammatory' type, with a variable degree of perianeurysmal fibrosis. One or both ureters can become encased in fibrous tissue and occluded, either by being drawn medially towards the aortic aneurysm or, more commonly, where they cross an 'inflammatory' common iliac aneurysm. The patient may present with hydronephrosis or anuria and renal failure.

Aortocaval fistula

This generally occurs in association with aortic rupture into the retroperitoneum, which consequently tends to dominate the clinical picture. In these circumstances the aortocaval fistula is usually only diagnosed peroperatively, when dramatic venous bleeding is seen on opening the aneurysm sac after aortic cross-clamping. Rarely, the aortic aneurysm may rupture only into the inferior vena cava and produce the characteristic clinical picture of venous engorgement and visible arterial pulsation in veins, accompanied by high-output cardiac failure.

Aortoenteric fistula

The majority of aortoenteric fistulae are seen as late complications of aortic surgery, and spontaneous fistulation into the gut from an aorta which has not been operated upon is extremely rare. Fistulae usually occur into the duodenum and present with haematemesis and melaena. The treatment of this condition is one of the most difficult in vascular surgical practice, since graft contamination and infection are inevitable.

Duodenal obstruction

The fourth part of the duodenum and duodenojejunal flexure is intimately adjacent to the abdominal aorta. A large infrarenal aortic aneurysm may therefore be a cause of external compression of the duodenum and high intestinal obstruction. The symptoms are those of duodenal distension with nausea and vomiting, which tends to be intermittent since the obstruction is incomplete.

MANAGEMENT

Symptomatic abdominal aortic aneurysms usually demand urgent or early treatment. The extent of preoperative investigation, assessment, and medical treatment may therefore need to be curtailed and the patient prepared for surgery as well as possible in the time available. The most immediate need for surgery arises in the patient with a ruptured aneurysm, and this is contrasted below with management of the asymptomatic patient. The management of other symptomatic presentations of the disease will fall somewhere between these two extremes, depending on how compelling the need for surgery.

Ruptured abdominal aortic aneurysm

The key fact to remember is that these patients are in the process of bleeding to death from the moment rupture occurs. More than half will die within the hour from haemorrhage into the peritoneal cavity, and it is unlikely that these patients could ever be saved. The majority of patients arriving at front-line hospitals will be suffering from some degree of circulatory collapse with hypotension. In this condition blood transfusion without arresting the haemorrhage is as futile as trying to fill a bucket with a hole in the bottom. The diagnosis should be made from the history and clinical examination. Investigations such as abdominal ultrasound or radiography are unnecessary, time consuming, and liable to cause fatal delay. The patient should be transferred immediately to the operating theatre, the only permissible investigation being the taking of a blood sample for cross-matching. In the operating theatre all preparations for the operation are carried out before the induction of anaesthesia, which should take place only when the surgeon is poised to make the abdominal incision. Anaesthesia is liable to induce severe hypotension as the vasoconstrictor tone which has been maintaining circulation to vital organs is abolished. At this stage transfusion is given to the extent necessary to sustain essential functions. Only when the aorta above the rupture has been controlled and securely clamped should full transfusion to restore normal blood pressure be given.

In a number of patients with ruptured abdominal aortic aneurysm the haemorrhage is so well contained by the surrounding connective tissue that there are no obvious clinical signs of blood loss. Such individuals can survive long journeys to tertiary referral centres and may live for several days before the connective tissue finally gives way and fatal haemorrhage occurs. These patients are liable to be misdiagnosed as suffering from other conditions, of which the most common are ureteric colic, pancreatitis, and sciatica. To establish the diagnosis, ultrasonography or computerized tomography may be required. Once the diagnosis is certain, operation is required with appropriate urgency since fatal haemorrhage can occur at any time. It is particularly tragic to see a patient who arrived at the hospital in good condition transferred to the operating theatre in a collapsed state after prolonged delay.

Asymptomatic abdominal aortic aneurysm

The only substantial reason for treating the patient with an asymptomatic abdominal aortic aneurysm is to prevent his premature death at some indeterminate future date from aneurysm rupture. At present the only treatment known to reduce this risk is elective surgical replacement of the aneurysmal aorta. A decision to recommend treatment must therefore be based on balancing the operative mortality and morbidity against the risk of aneurysm rupture. The limited information available on the natural history of abdominal aortic aneurysms shows a general relationship between aneurysm diameter and rupture risk. For abdominal aortic aneurysms of 4.0- to 5.9-cm diameter the risk of death from rupture is around 5 per cent/annum and for diameter above 6.0 cm is of the order of 15 per cent/annum. Since the disease is unlikely to produce any distressing symptoms unless the aneurysm ruptures, it seems unreasonable to ask a patient to accept an immediate operative mortality risk greater than the annual expectation of death from the untreated disease. It is essential therefore that every patient should be carefully investigated and the individual risks of surgery assessed so that an informed judgement can be made in each case.

'Inflammatory' abdominal aortic aneurysm

Inflammatory aneurysms comprise around 10 per cent of all abdominal aortic aneurysms encountered in clinical practice but since they are commonly symptomatic, this probably over-represents the prevalence of the inflammatory variant of aortic aneurysms in the entire population. The pathogenesis of this disorder is still the subject of debate, but the original suggestion that the inflammation is a response to leakage of blood from contained aortic rupture is no longer tenable. The macroscopic appearance at operation is of two types: (1) an angry hyperaemic periaortic inflammation, or (2) a chronic fibrotic icing-sugar aortic wall, but both types may be seen at different points on the same aneurysm. Histologically, the wall of all aortic aneurysms shows evidence of an inflammatory response and the difference between the macroscopically inflamed and non-inflamed aneurysm is quantitative rather than qualitative. The condition is best regarded as a chronic periaortitis and has much in common with idiopathic retroperitoneal fibrosis. Recent work by Parums and Mitchinson in Cambridge, England has advanced the theory that the periaortitis is an immune response to antigens, principally ceroid, leaking from atheromatous plaques into the aortic adventitia. It is unclear whether the liberation of lipoproteins from atherosclerotic plaques is simply a consequence of aortic dilatation or a contributory factor to aneurysm formation.

Inflammatory aneurysms may present with symptoms or signs suggestive of the diagnosis, or they may be discovered incidentally during investigation or at operation for an asymptomatic or ruptured abdominal aortic aneurysm. The belief that inflammatory aortic aneurysms are less likely to rupture is not supported by any evidence and should not weigh heavily in management decisions. Even the thickest aortic walls of inflammatory aneurysms tend to be thin posteriorly where they lie in contact with the vertebral bodies, and rupture at this point is not uncommon. The diagnosis of inflammatory abdominal aortic aneurysm should be suspected in patients presenting with a history of abdominal and back pain and who have a tender but unruptured aneurysm. An elevated erythrocyte sedimentation rate will be present in half of those with an inflammatory aneurysm, and the diagnosis can be confirmed by demonstrating a thickened aortic wall on computerized tomography (Fig. 3) or magnetic resonance imaging.

In some patients one or both ureters may be obstructed by the periaortitis or, more commonly where they cross an inflammatory iliac aneurysm. Rarely, such patients may first present with renal failure, and the diagnosis of inflammatory aortic aneurysm be made secondarily. Hydronephrosis due to ureteric obstruction is usually best treated before elective aortic surgery, either by ureteric stenting or nephrostomy.

The presence of a stent in the ureter has the additional advantage of providing a useful guide to identification at operation when the ureters are encased in dense fibrosis. In general, following replacement of the aortic aneurysm the ureteric obstruction will resolve and operative dissection of the ureters to free them from the periaortitis is seldom necessary.

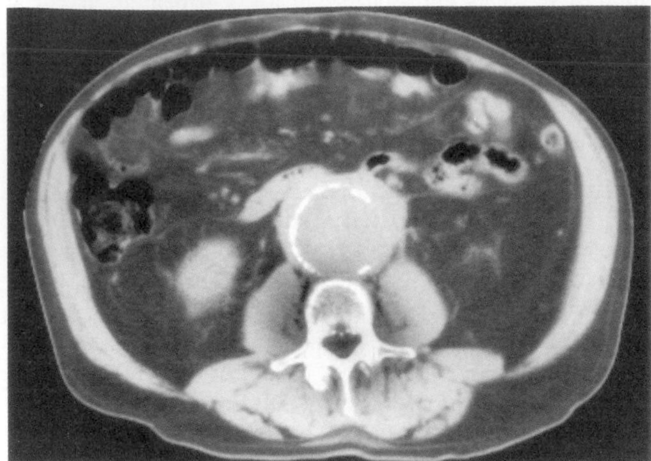

Fig. 3 CT scan of an inflammatory abdominal aortic aneurysm, showing the thick aortic wall.

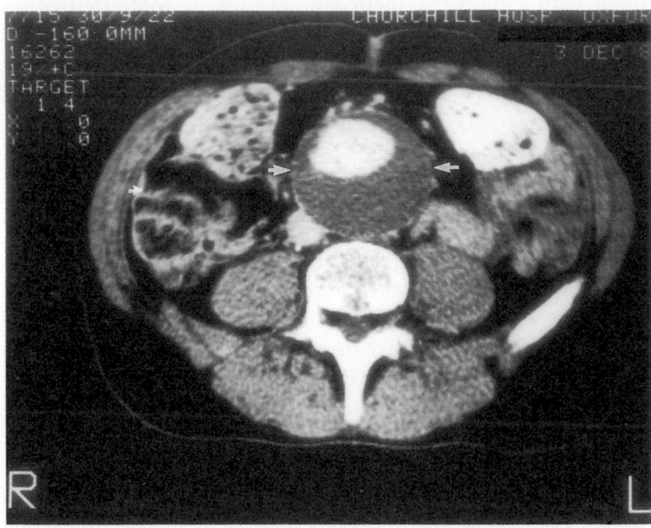

Fig. 4 CT scan of a large abdominal aortic aneurysm, showing mural thrombus.

Operative replacement of an inflammatory abdominal aortic aneurysm is difficult but can be satisfactorily performed in most patients by modification of a standard operative technique, since, fortunately, in the majority of instances the neck of the aneurysm is relatively free of periaortitis. Rarely, an elective operation may be too hazardous to continue when the aorta above the aneurysm is also inflamed. In such patients a case can be made for abandoning the procedure and treating for 3 months with systemic steroids to suppress the periaortitis before a further attempt at aneurysm replacement. 'He who fights and runs away lives to fight another day.'

Investigation of the aneurysm

The purpose of these investigations is to determine accurately the size and extent of the aneurysm, to note the thickness of the aneurysm wall and the presence of any localized saccular dilatation, and, finally, to assess the importance of coexistent occlusive or aneurysmal arterial disease elsewhere.

Ultrasonography of the abdominal aorta is the first-line investigation; its advantages are that it is cheap, freely available, accurate, reliable, and reproducible. Being non-invasive it can be repeated as often as required, either to confirm the original findings or to monitor growth of the aneurysm. Its main disadvantages are that it is observer-dependent and the permanent images produced can be difficult for anyone, other than the person who performed the scan, to interpret. Visualization of the suprarenal aorta and iliac arteries is often difficult and the study may be impossible in the grossly obese or when large amounts of bowel gas are present. It remains, however, the most useful investigation for measuring the diameter of an infrarenal aortic aneurysm.

Computerized tomography produces excellent permanent records of cross-sectional anatomy which are easy to interpret (Fig. 4). Its main uses are to discover the extent of any suprarenal aortic involvement and the thickness of the arterial wall, in order to detect 'inflammatory' aortic aneurysms. It can also be used to measure aortic diameter, but inaccuracies can occur if the section is not at right angles to the long axis of a tortuous aneurysmal aorta.

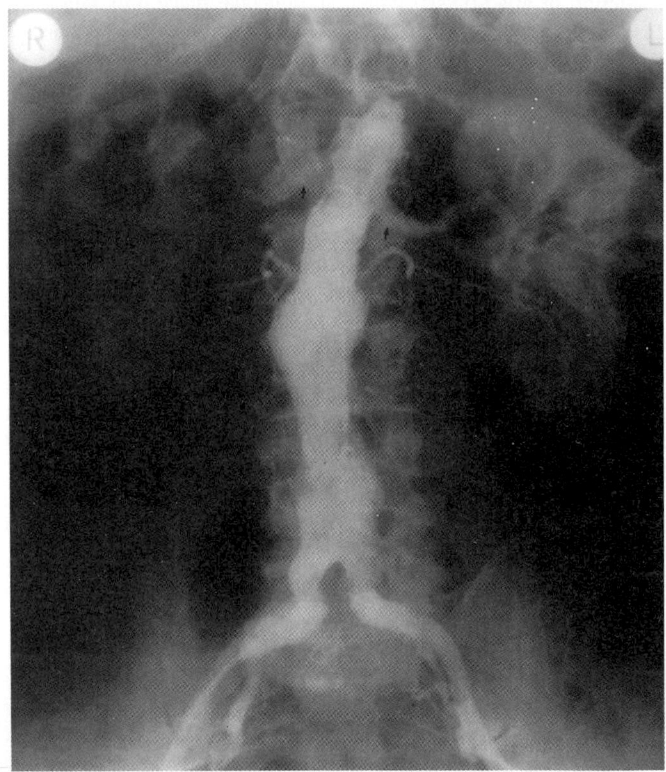

Fig. 5 Angiogram of an abdominal aortic aneurysm, showing the origin of renal arteries.

Magnetic resonance imaging (MRI) is available in some centres and the quality and definition of the images produced by the newer machines is now excellent. Since there is no radiation exposure it could well replace computerized tomography in many of its present uses.

Angiography (Fig. 5) is used mainly to discover the relationship of the renal arteries to the aneurysm and, by outlining the kidneys, may reveal relevant abnormalities, such as horseshoe or pelvic kidneys. When the aneurysm is large and blood flow turbulent or sluggish, it is sometimes difficult to obtain high-quality angiograms of the limb vessels from aortic injection of contrast, but this information can be of help in planning the extent of any arterial surgery required. The presence of iliac or femoral aneurysms or occlusive arterial disease in iliac, femoral, or more distal arteries of the limbs may be revealed.

Investigation of the patient

The purpose of these investigations is to discover how well the patient is likely to tolerate the trauma of a major arterial operation. Of particular importance are cardiac and respiratory function and the presence of carotid arterial or other coexistent disease.

Attention is paid in the history to symptoms of angina, breathlessness at rest or on exertion and previous myocardial infarction. All patients should have routine monitoring of their blood pressure and an electrocardiogram (ECG). Hypertension should be controlled and, if the history or ECG suggests possible abnormalities of myocardial function or blood supply, further investigations are essential. Echocardiography is useful for detecting abnormalities of valve or heart wall function, and the technique of multigated acquisition nuclear imaging allows a ventricular ejection fraction to be calculated at rest and after exercise. In some patients, coronary angiography will be indicated, and any coronary arterial disease discovered may need treatment by angioplasty or coronary artery bypass grafting before aortic surgery can be contemplated safely. Evidence of recent myocardial infarction is an important reason to recommend delaying elective surgery for all but the largest aneurysms, since the chances of further myocardial infarction and death are substantially increased by operation within 6 months of the infarct. Other relative contraindications to surgery are a low ventricular ejection fraction at rest or one which falls markedly on exercise, indicating inadequate blood supply to the myocardium.

Routine measures of respiratory function, such as peak expiratory flow and spirometry, are simple to perform as an extension of the normal clinical examination and should be a standard part of the assessment of all patients. More complex measurements of gas exchange are rarely necessary but, when required, the services of a respiratory function laboratory may prove helpful. Although poor lung function may be a contraindication to elective surgery, the presence of chronic obstructive airways disease is an important risk factor for aneurysm rupture. With the assistance of a chest physician, most patients can be improved to the point where the risks of elective surgery become acceptable.

The presence of carotid artery stenosis presents a more difficult problem to resolve, and debate still goes on about whether carotid endarterectomy should be performed before, during, or after aortic aneurysm surgery, or sometimes, indeed, whether it should be performed at all. Each case will need to be resolved on its merits, depending on the relative importance of the aortic aneurysm and carotid stenosis in the individual patient, but, in general, the patient with an asymptomatic internal carotid artery stenosis is not considered at risk of having a stroke during aortic surgery.

Because the majority of patients with an abdominal aortic aneurysm are old coexistent disease is common. Malignant disease discovered during investigation for the aneurysm presents a particular problem. It is difficult to be dogmatic about the treatment priority, but a rationale for therapy is outlined here. Generally, primary treatment for the cancer is given first, since delay is liable to reduce the chances of cure progressively while, on the other hand, provided rupture has not occurred, a large aneurysm is as easily replaced as a small aneurysm. If primary treatment of the cancer seems to have been successful, then the aortic aneurysm is replaced as soon as the patient has recovered from cancer surgery. If treatment of the cancer is definitely non-curative and life expectation is limited, aneurysm surgery is seldom advised, since in most patients death from aneurysm rupture will be a much better alternative than from carcinoma.

Operative mortality and morbidity

In the decade after the first replacement of an abdominal aortic aneurysm in 1951, operative mortality was high, at around 15 per cent. Over the past 30 years, as a result of surgical and anaesthetic refinements of technique and better pre- and postoperative management, elective operative mortality has been reduced to under 5 per cent in many vascular units and some centres are reporting less than 2 per cent. It would be a mistake to assume that the low mortality currently achieved in specialist units represents the common experience, and there is evidence that in many hospitals a figure of 10 per cent or more is still not unusual. Approximately 1 in 20 abdominal aortic aneurysms extends close to or above the origin of the renal arteries. Surgery in these cases may involve clamping the aorta above the renal arteries and sometimes their reimplantation. Operating on suprarenal aneurysms requires special skill and techniques, and inevitably is associated with greater hazard than the uncomplicated infrarenal aneurysm.

Elective aortic surgery remains a major operation and, even in the uncomplicated case, morbidity is considerable. Most patients can be discharged from hospital within 10 days of operation, but few will be restored to complete well-being in less than 2 months. Currently, there is debate about the long-term outlook for those who have undergone successful aortic aneurysm replacement. Some follow-up studies have shown a similar life expectation to that of the general population of the same age. This conclusion is disputed by others and seems to be inherently improbable given the known association of abdominal aortic aneurysm with a number of other diseases that impair life expectancy. There is no doubt, however, that the patient who survives surgical replacement of his aneurysm has a greater life expectation than one whose aneurysm is left untreated.

Operative technique

As with any operation, there are many variations in technique used by individual surgeons for routine operations, together with specific variations which may be employed to deal with special situations encountered. The standard techniques used by the author successfully over many years are described below and brief notes on useful or alternative techniques are appended after the main account.

Elective abdominal aortic aneurysm replacement

Preparation for the operation begins days or sometimes weeks before, to ensure that all the clinical information required is obtained and the patient is in the best state of health achievable at the time of operation. The main hazard peroperatively is sudden change in circulatory haemodynamics as a consequence of clamping and unclamping of the aorta, or blood loss. It is therefore essential that adequate monitoring of cardiac function and intravascular volume is in place before surgery begins.

The patient is placed supine on the operating table and the skin is prepared with antiseptic from the nipples to the knees—particular care must be made to ensure cleaning of the external genitalia. The operation field extends from the xiphisternum to mid-thighs, with the genitalia being securely excluded by towelling and the use of adherent skin drapes. A vertical midline abdominal incision is made from sternum to symphysis pubis and the peritoneal cavity opened. A complete inspection of all the intra-abdominal organs is made to exclude other pathology. The small intestine is retracted to the right and draped from the operative field, usually being retained within the abdomen, but in the obese better exposure is obtained if the intestine is exteriorized within a plastic 'gut' bag.

Minimal dissection of the retroperitoneum is employed to limit bleeding and it is unnecessary to mobilize adherent duodenum. The neck of the aneurysm is identified by palpation and the overlying peritoneum and fascia divided in the midline until the aorta is exposed. The inferior mesenteric vein is displaced to the left and seldom needs to be divided. Midline dissection continues until the left renal vein is identified, and fascial division is continued transversely at the lower border of the vein to free it and allow its retraction if required. Blunt dissection on both sides of the aorta in a strictly vertical plane continues until the vertebral body is encountered. Intravenous heparin is administered and the neck of the aorta clamped anteroposteriorly.

When the common iliac arteries are not aneurysmal, their dissection is easily accomplished by division of peritoneum and fascia over their anterior surfaces with blunt finger dissection down each side. The vessels are clamped anteroposteriorly. Common and internal iliac arteries may be aneurysmal and, in these circumstances, the external iliac arteries are clamped and back-bleeding from the internal iliac arteries controlled after the aortic aneurysm is opened.

The aortic aneurysm is inspected through the intact posterior peritoneum and the inferior mesenteric artery is oversewn with a transfixion suture at its origin. The posterior peritoneum and the aneurysm are then incised in the midline from the aneurysm neck to the aortic bifurcation, and the mural thrombus evacuated. At each end of the incision transverse scissor cuts are made so that half the circumference of the aorta is divided. Bleeding from lumbar vessels is controlled by direct pressure until permanently arrested by oversewing with transfixion sutures. At this stage the operative field should be bloodless and the ends of the aorta can be inspected and cleared of adherent thrombus.

In 80 per cent of cases a tube graft can be used, but where the iliac arteries are aneurysmal a bifurcated 'trouser' graft will be required. In the latter case it is preferable, and usually satisfactory, to anastomose each limb of the graft either to the termination of the common iliac artery or to the external iliac artery. It is desirable to retain circulation into at least one internal iliac artery to minimize the risk of gut or spinal cord ischaemia. The graft is stitched to the neck of the aneurysm, using an inlay technique and a monofilament prolene continuous suture. Exposure is improved by inserting a self-retaining rake retractor within the aneurysm sac. Three sutures are placed on each side of the midline of the aorta and graft posteriorly and the graft is 'parachuted' into place. The suture is continued on each side to the midline anteriorly, particular care being taken accurately to place the corner sutures in the lateral walls of the aorta. The anastomosis is tested for leaks at this stage, since subsequent haemorrhage from the posterior wall is more difficult to deal with.

The tube graft is cut to the appropriate length and the distal anastomosis made in exactly the same fashion. A vital step in the procedure is to ensure that no particulate material, atheroma, thrombus, or tissue remains inside the graft or iliac arteries proximal to the arterial clamps. Graft and proximal iliac arteries are therefore irrigated thoroughly with saline before the anastomosis is completed.

It is unnecessary to release the distal arterial clamps to achieve this end, and doing so may precipitate arterial thrombosis by exposing blood in the distal vessels to tissue thromboplastin from the operation site.

Five minutes before the anastomoses are completed the anaesthetist is warned that restoration of circulation to the legs is imminent so that circulatory volume can be appropriately and rapidly augmented when required. One distal clamp only is removed and the aortic clamp slowly released. This is a dangerous phase of the operation, and flow through the graft is titrated against the patient's blood pressure and heart filling pressure. Only when pressures are normal, with full restoration of blood flow to one limb, is the second distal clamp slowly released.

The operation is completed by meticulous haemostasis, and reversal of anticoagulation may be necessary to achieve this end.

Technical variations

Transverse incision

Many surgeons use a transverse, upper abdominal, dome-shaped incision for abdominal access. The abdominal wall muscles are cut in the line of the incision, which commences midway between the umbilicus and sternum and runs parallel to the costal margins. It is claimed that postoperative respiratory complications are reduced by this incision but it is more time consuming to make and close, bleeding is greater, and access to the iliac arteries is difficult.

Retroperitoneal approach

The patient is positioned corkscrewed on the operating table with the pelvis horizontal and the shoulders vertical. An incision is made from the tip of the left twelfth rib to the midline below the umbilicus. Abdominal wall muscles are cut in the line of the incision. The extraperitoneal plane is identified and the peritoneum retracted medially to expose the aorta. The left kidney may be retracted with the peritoneum or allowed to remain lying on the psoas muscle. Advocates of this approach point to the facility of the technique in obese patients and claim reduced postoperative morbidity. The disadvantage is that exposure of the right common iliac artery cannot readily be achieved.

The perirenal aneurysm neck

Aneurysms extending substantially above the origins of the renal arteries are discussed in the section on thoracoabdominal aortic aneurysms, but aneurysms with a neck at, or immediately above, the origin of the renal arteries can be dealt with by slight modification of the operative approach to the common infrarenal aortic aneurysm. The problem may be encountered unexpectedly at operation since, because of tortuousity of the aneurysmal aorta, many aneurysms appear on computerized tomographic scanning to extend above the renal arteries but experience shows that the majority prove at operation to be definitely infrarenal.

The aorta needs to be dissected and clamped above one or both renal arteries. To achieve this exposure the left renal vein must be freed from the aorta and retracted either superiorly or, occasionally, inferiorly. It will be necessary to divide either the left gonadal vein or sometimes the left adrenal vein to permit safe retraction, but division of the renal vein itself is rarely required. The anastomosis between graft and aorta is accomplished expeditiously with the renal arteries being incorporated within the proximal aorta as a single or double short tongue. After completion of the proximal anastomosis, the clamp is reapplied to the graft below the renal arteries and blood flow to the kidneys restored before attention is turned to the distal aortic anastomosis.

It is claimed that the retroperitoneal approach allows the perirenal aortic aneurysm to be dealt with as easily as the infrarenal aortic aneurysm and is part of the advocacy for general adoption of this approach.

Types of graft

In the early days of aortic surgery, aortic homografts were widely used but were abandoned because their use was inconvenient and they were prone to aneurysmal degeneration. They have been obsolete for 30 years and have only recently been reintroduced and advocated for use in the presence of established synthetic graft infection. Synthetic grafts in common use are of woven or knitted Dacron or polytetrafluoroethylene. Woven Dacron is stiffer and less permeable than the knitted material.

The problem of blood leaking at operation can be overcome by coating the knitted graft in various ways, but this adds to the cost disadvantage compared with the woven material. Polytetrafluoroethylene grafts are impermeable but suffer from two disadvantages. First, the aortic body of a trouser graft must be cut to the correct length with minimal tolerance if the legs are to lie at an acceptable angle. Secondly, polytetrafluoroethylene is prone to leak at stitch holes for a prolonged time, a problem which is increased when a large needle is used.

If a trouser graft is essential, anastomosis of the limbs to the iliac arteries is preferable, since this avoids additional incisions in the groins and consequently reduces the risk of contamination of the graft and graft infection.

The external iliac arteries invariably and mysteriously remain uninvolved by aneurysmal change, although they may become occluded by atherosclerosis.

Clear indications for aortofemoral grafting are the presence of large femoral artery aneurysms and external iliac artery stenosis or occlusion.

Ruptured abdominal aortic aneurysm replacement

Two-thirds of ruptured aneurysms leak either directly or secondarily into the peritoneal cavity within an hour or so and cause death from exsanguination. These patients usually die at home or on their way to hospital and thus do not come to surgery. Successful surgery is possible only because of temporary tamponade of the rupture by tissue pressure in the retroperitoneum, assisted by hypotension. These patients are on the brink of death and sustain fatal haemorrhage when the peritoneum ruptures, tissue tamponade fails, or the blood pressure is increased by injudicious transfusion before the rupture is secured. Most lives are saved by immediate transfer from emergency room to the operating theatre, but the operative mortality rate improves exponentially as the time between rupture and surgery increases by selecting for treatment only those with stable, contained rupture.

The patient is prepared for surgery while conscious on the operating table. Induction of anaesthesia should occur only when the surgeon is poised ready to make the incision. Blood pressure should be maintained at no more than 100 mm systolic until the aorta is controlled. This ideal may require rapid transfusion in order to maintain cerebral and myocardial perfusion on anaesthetic induction when compensatory vasomotor tone is suddenly relaxed. On opening the peritoneal cavity the posterior peritoneum is exposed by displacing the small intestine. The aorta above the aneurysm is identified by palpation and occluded by direct compression with the surgeon's left hand against the vertebral bodies. Only when the aorta has been securely occluded by compression should the posterior peritoneum over the upper part of the aneurysm be incised. The wall of the aneurysm should be exposed by sharp dissection with scissors through the haematoma and connective tissue, and only when the aortic adventitia is clearly identified is it permissible to use blunt finger dissection in the periadventitial plane to clear the neck of the aneurysm. Only when the neck of the aneurysm is securely occluded is it permissible to release the occlusion of aorta between fingers and vertebral bodies. The operation may then proceed as for an elective aortic aneurysm replacement.

Death from ruptured aneurysm is a direct consequence of blood loss. Patients will rarely survive if additional blood loss is caused by extensive, unnecessary, hasty, or careless dissection. Iatrogenic blood loss is most likely to occur from tearing of the left gonadal, left adrenal, or left renal vein by attempts to occlude the aorta by dissection of the aneurysm neck which is too hasty, too wide, and too high. Control of blood flow into the aneurysm must be achieved before any dissection is attempted.

High aneurysm rupture

When rupture of the aneurysm occurs close to the neck, it may prove difficult to dissect the neck clearly to allow initial aortic clamping at this level. In this situation the aortic neck can be identified from within the lumen of the aneurysm and a large Foley urethral catheter inserted. The balloon of the catheter is inflated in the aneurysm neck and tamponade of the aorta against the vertebral bodies is slowly released to confirm that the balloon is securely impacted. Careful external two-handed dissection of the neck of the aneurysm can then be performed and the balloon catheter replaced by an aortic clamp.

FURTHER READING

Collin J. Aortic aneurysm screening and management. In: Johnson CD, Taylor I, eds. *Recent advances in surgery*. Edinburgh: Churchill Livingstone, 1990.

Collin J, Araujo L, Walton J, Lindsell D. Oxford Screening Programme for abdominal aortic aneurysm in men aged 65–74 years. *Lancet*, 1988; **2**: 613–15.

Greenhalgh RM, Mannick JA. eds. *The cause and management of aneurysms*. Philadelphia: WB Saunders, 1990.

Parums DV, Mitchinson MJ. Serum antibodies to oxidised LDL and ceroid in chronic periaortitis. *J Pathol*, 1987; **151**: 57.

Pierce GE, guest ed. Abdominal aortic aneurysms. *Surg Clin N Am*, 1989; **69**: 4.

Tilson MD, A perspective of research in abdominal aortic aneurysm disease with a unifying hypothesis. In: Bergan JJ, Yao JST, eds. *Aortic Surgery*. Philadelphia: WB Saunders, 1989.

Veith FJ, ed. *Current critical problems in vascular surgery*. St. Louis: Quality Medical Publishing, 1989.

7.7.2 Femoral artery

RICHARD P. CAMBRIA

INTRODUCTION

Aneurysmal disease in the femoral triangle encompasses a spectrum of pathology; it includes both degenerative aneurysm in native vessels and the more commonly encountered false aneurysms. Whereas a true aneurysm is an abnormal dilatation involving all three layers of the vascular wall, a false aneurysm results from a rent in the integrity of either a native vessel or a previous vascular suture line, the 'wall' of the aneurysm being composed of surrounding scar and inflammatory tissue. The incidence, clinical importance, and management of these diverse lesions vary considerably.

CLASSIFICATION

Femoral artery aneurysms may be true aneurysms due to atherosclerotic degeneration of native vessels or false aneurysms that are either: (1) anastomotic aneurysms at the site of prior vascular reconstructions, or (2) false aneurysms, secondary to penetrating trauma or catheterization of the femoral artery (Table 1). Iatrogenic false aneurysm is the most commonly encountered lesion, in accordance with the ever increasing numbers and types of transarterial femoral catheterization procedures. An important complicating factor in the management of the false aneurysm is the presence or absence of infection. Infection can be the principal cause of the false aneurysm but an established femoral aneurysm of any type can be secondarily infected by haematogenous seeding. Acute necrotizing infection may be a cause of false aneurysm, particularly in intravenous drug abusers who use the femoral vessels as sites of vascular access.

Table 1 A classification of femoral artery aneurysm

True femoral artery aneurysms-atherosclerotic disease
False femoral artery aneurysms
1. Anastomotic aneurysms
2. Traumatic aneurysms (catheter injuries, penetrating wounds)

ATHEROSCLEROTIC FEMORAL ANEURYSM

While atherosclerotic femoral aneurysm is the second most common peripheral aneurysm (after popliteal artery aneurysm), it is, in fact, an uncommon clinical problem. Furthermore, atherosclerotic femoral aneurysms are generally detected in patients undergoing evaluation for aneurysmal disease elsewhere in the vascular tree. As is the case with the more commonly encountered popliteal aneurysm, atherosclerotic femoral aneurysm has a strong predilection for the male sex, is bilateral in over 70 per cent of the cases, and is seen in association with aortoiliac aneurysmal disease in 85 per cent of the patients. In the largest clinical series reported, only 3 per cent with aortic aneurysm had simultaneous femoral aneurysm.

Diagnostic uncertainty in femoral aneurysm disease generally involves the distinction between diffuse arteriomegaly and genuine aneurysm. In this regard, criteria similar to those developed for the definition of a popliteal aneurysm are appropriate. A femoral artery can be considered aneurysmal when its maximum diameter is 1.5 times or more that of the upstream normal external iliac artery. In addition to the physical examination, ultrasound evaluation combined with colour Doppler examination provides excellent resolution and a high degree of diagnostic accuracy. The demonstration of laminated thrombus within the aneurysm cavity is important in making the distinction between an ectatic artery and a true aneurysm. Ultrasound examination also allows an accurate measurement of size which may be important in determining whether aneurysm repair is indicated. As is the case in aneurysm disease in a variety of locations, angiography is not required for diagnosis, but it is essential in planning the technical details of operative repair.

Controversy exists as to the natural history and clinical importance of untreated femoral aneurysm. Much of the earlier literature simply reviewed operated cases, and an appreciation of the natural history was not available. Clearly, symptomatic aneurysms and those larger than 3 cm should be repaired. In one large series symptoms developed in less than 3 per cent of 40 patients followed without operation. We favour operations for all lesions larger than 3 cm, particularly if ultrasound examination demonstrates mural thrombus. These criteria are also applied to the patient with simultaneous aortic and femoral aneurysm; that is, the aortic graft may need to be carried to the femoral level if independent criteria for repair of the femoral aneurysm exists.

The technical aspects of operative repair relate to the extent of the aneurysm (Fig. 1). Femoral aneurysms have been classified as either Type I, terminating proximal to the common femoral artery bifurcation, or Type II, where the aneurysm involves the origin of the profunda femoris artery. Type I aneurysms are simply repaired with excision and interposition of a prosthetic conduit, as these arteries will generally be too large to repair with a vein graft. When the aneurysm extends into the femoral artery bifurcation, the details of the repair are somewhat more complex. Since these vessels tend to be large, a short segment of 12 × 6 mm Dacron bifurcation graft for separate anastomoses to the profunda and superficial femoral arteries is used. If concomitant femoral popliteal reconstruction is required to treat distal ischaemia, it will generally be necessary to carry out two separate reconstructions, with the femoral popliteal graft arising from the primary femoral artery reconstruction. The temptation simply to excise the anterior wall of the aneurysm, and close the defect with the proximal hood of a simultaneous femoropopliteal bypass graft should be avoided, as the remaining femoral artery may become aneurysmal.

FALSE ANEURYSM

Native vessel pseudoaneurysm

False aneurysm of the native femoral artery, secondary to percutaneous arterial catheterization, is a common problem for the

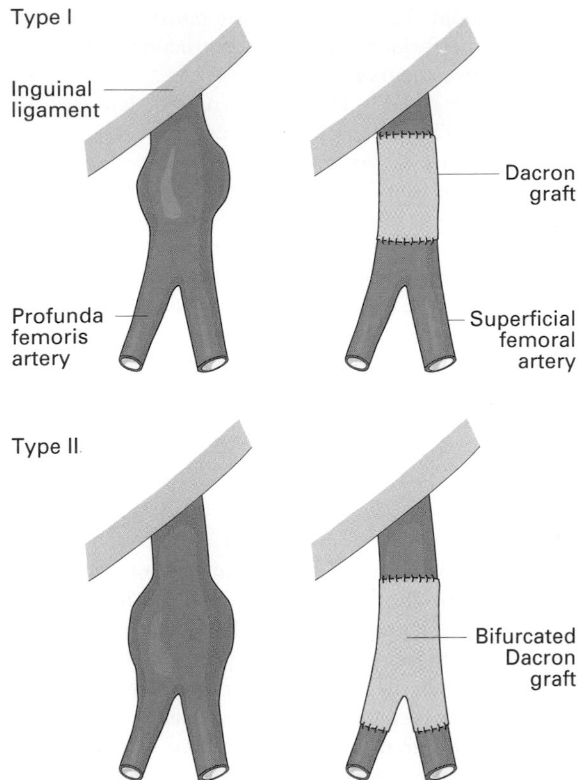

Fig. 1 Classification and repair of femoral artery aneurysms.

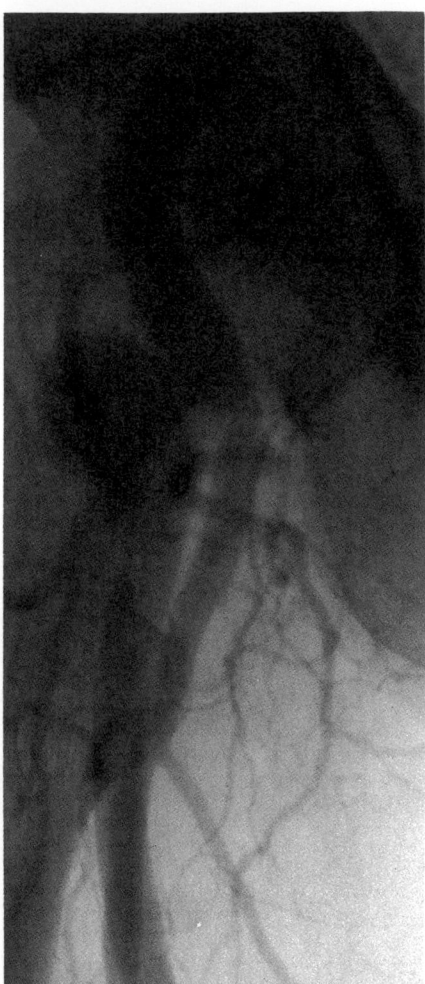

Fig. 2 Arteriogram demonstrating femoral artery false aneurysm.

vascular surgeon (Fig. 2). The incidence of this problem increases with the complexity and size of the catheters and sheaths introduced into the femoral artery: reported incidences for simple diagnostic cardiac catheterization are in the 0.5 per cent range, but this figure can increase to greater than 10 per cent after the percutaneous introduction of an intra-aortic counterpulsation balloon pump. Obviously, arterial complications of such procedures are not limited to false aneurysm formation and local thrombotic complications are even more common than false aneurysms. Traumatic femoral arteriovenous fistula formation can also occur, either in association with, or independent of, the false aneurysm. A characteristic systolic/diastolic murmur, audible with the stethoscope, is diagnostic of this condition.

While the diagnosis of femoral false aneurysm may be straightforward on the basis of a tender pulsatile mass, it may be difficult to distinguish a false aneurysm from an uncomplicated periarterial haematoma in the period immediately following the catheterization procedure. In such circumstances, a colour flow Doppler examination is simple, and accurate. A scan can frequently localize the origin of the false aneurysm, information that may be helpful in the planning of the operative repair. Despite the fact that indwelling sheaths may be left in the femoral artery for some period of time, infection in these lesions is distinctly uncommon.

Repair of native vessel femoral false aneurysm is generally indicated. Since the natural history of these lesions is to enlarge progressively, they can produce significant local pain and venous obstruction, and they are capable of thrombosis and distal embolization. Spontaneous thrombosis of false aneurysm occurs frequently. Patients after coronary artery balloon angioplasty were sequentially followed with colour Doppler scans and spontaneous obliteration was observed in small, otherwise undetected false aneurysms. We have observed this phenomenon in a few patients. It is also obvious that late appearance of progressively enlarging false aneurysms is seen in an active clinical practice. We routinely repair false aneurysms since such patients are generally referred with coexistent large haematomas or appreciable local pain. Affected patients are frequently undergoing investigation for acute cardiac problems, and repair under local anaesthesia is the preferred technique. Proximal control is obtained at the level of the inguinal ligament; distal control of the superficial and profunda femoris arteries is unusually not needed since control generally requires a fair amount of dissection in a patient under local anaesthesia. In addition, simply obtaining proximal control and then approaching the arterial defect directly through the aneurysm cavity simplifies the operation. Once the aneurysm cavity is entered, there is generally substantial back bleeding, even though the common femoral artery is clamped proximally. Bleeding can be controlled with a finger or cottenoid dissector, while the contents of the aneurysm cavity are evacuated and the anterior wall of the artery identified. Identification is a key technical manoeuvre, since failure to expose the arterial surface leads to placement of sutures in the extravascular tissues, and failure of the repair. Following the identification of the defect in the arterial wall, one or two monofilament sutures, placed parallel to the long axis of the artery will generally close the defect. Careful preoperative evaluation of the distal circulation is necessary to assess the possible requirement for distal catheter embolectomy, although embolectomy is rarely indicated. It is also critical to assess the adequacy of the distal circulation following repair. Repair is generally assessed by intraoperative pulse volume recordings. If these suggest a problem at the site of the repair, the surgeon must dissect the branches of the femoral artery, and reopen the femoral artery with the longitudinal arteriotomy. This usually occurs in the setting of a highly diseased femoral artery, and local repair with a vein patch angioplasty is required.

Infected femoral aneurysms present the surgeon with a difficult clinical problem, the goals of treatment being the eradication of intravascular sepsis and preservation of limb viability. Infected aneurysms in the femoral triangle occur in a variety of clinical settings, including infection of iatrogenic false aneurysm, usually secondary to bacterial contamination from indwelling catheters and sheaths, those occurring in intravenous drug abusers injecting themselves about the femoral triangle, and haematogenous inoculation of a true atherosclerotic aneurysm. Since true atherosclerotic aneurysms are uncommon, superinfection is rare. As stated above, despite the frequency of iatrogenic false aneurysm in a large hospital setting, secondary infection of these lesions is also rare.

The worst form of the disease is that found in intravenous drug abusers. Long-standing intravenous drug abuse combined with factors such as subsequent obliteration of available venous conduits, a proclivity for polymicrobial necrotizing infections, and the sociomedical stratum in which this problem is likely to be encountered, make this entity a challenging clinical problem; the dual goals of eradication of arterial sepsis and preservation of limb viability may not be feasible because of the nature of the infection. Infected femoral artery aneurysm in a drug abuser is generally associated with extensive arterial sepsis, frequently with the threat of rupture and bleeding through the overlying infected, and sometimes necrotic, skin. These patients frequently present themselves as a true vascular surgical emergency. The diagnosis may not be obvious, and appropriate blood cultures, careful physical examination for evidence of distal emboli, evaluation for concomitant infective endocarditis, and complete angiographic study to look for additional false aneurysms are indicated.

Clearly, the frequency with which the surgeon encounters this problem will be a function of the patient population he serves. Reddy and colleagues, in reporting the largest clinical series of infected femoral aneurysms in drug abusers, have outlined the principles of treatment in this particular clinical setting. These involve complete arterial excision back to healthy arterial wall, and closure of the transected artery with monofilament suture material, in addition to radical debridement of all surrounding necrotic and infected soft tissue. The obvious dilemma in this circumstance involves a decision about the need for, and technical aspects of, arterial reconstruction to maintain limb viability. Above-knee amputation is necessary in one-third of patients in whom arterial excision involves the common femoral artery bifurcation. If the sepsis is limited to the common femoral artery, such that the distal arterial closure can be completed above the femoral bifurcation, the surgeon can then anticipate continued limb viability by virtue of the circumflex femoral and profunda femoris collateral pathways. Thus, the wisdom of arterial reconstruction is tempered by the absolute need for immediate revascularization, and the nature of the patient. Reddy and colleagues advocate a selective approach to revascularization in the intravenous drug abuser and avoid insertion of prosthetic grafts because of the threat of late infection. Others have adopted a more aggressive policy towards limb preservation and performed routine reconstruction after excision of the infected false aneurysm.

The technical aspects of arterial reconstruction vary with the clinical setting. The bacteriology and extent of sepsis dictate the feasibility of either *in-situ* reconstruction or extra-anatomic reconstruction. One would not hesitate to place a vein patch repair or a saphenous vein interposition graft in a contaminated groin, but in the face of necrotizing arterial sepsis a vein patch would be doomed to fail, exposing the patient to the risk of early haemorrhage. The principles of treatment involve debridement of all infected arterial and soft tissues, placement of suture lines, whether arterial closures or anastomoses, in normal arterial tissue, and the interposition of healthy soft tissue coverage. Transposition of the proximal sartorius muscle over femoral arterial repairs in the groin is a simple, convenient, and effective means of providing soft tissue coverage.

Autogenous tissue should be used when placing a vascular reconstruction in a contaminated field. If necrotizing or frankly suppurative arterial sepsis is present, arterial excision and extra-anatomic reconstruction will be necessary. In this circumstance, preoperative arteriography is mandatory to plan the reconstruction. The obturator foramen bypass provides a convenient and effective means to circumvent arterial sepsis in the groin. Inflow for this bypass may be from either native iliac artery, aorta, or the ipsilateral limb of a previously placed aortofemoral bypass graft. Ideally, the extra-anatomic reconstruction is placed first, and groin exploration is accomplished following completion of the 'clean' procedure. A prosthetic conduit may be acceptable for an obturator foramen bypass, if the distal circulation is adequate to sustain its patency.

ANASTOMOTIC FEMORAL ANEURYSM

Anastomotic aneurysm occurs when either partial or total disruption of a suture line between a native vessel and vascular graft occurs, vascular integrity being maintained by a fibrous tissue capsule which constitutes the wall of the false aneurysm. Because of lack of tensile strength of this fibrous tissue capsule, the natural history of such an aneurysm is to continue to enlarge. In the femoral region, anastomotic aneurysm most commonly occurs at the site of the femoral anastomosis of an aortobifemoral bypass graft. Numerous clinical series have reported an incidence ranging from 2 to 8 per cent. In most reports, the femoral anastomotic aneurysm appears at a mean of 5 to 6 years after the initial operation, although this figure, as well as the overall reported incidence, varies with duration of follow-up. In the past, the aetiology of anastomotic aneurysm was attributed to the use of silk sutures, and poor quality control in the prosthesis itself. Since silk is a biological material, it is slowly absorbed with time.

Human beings never 'heal' a vascular prosthesis; integrity of the suture line is continuously dependent on the integrity of the sutures themselves. With the use of permanent, non-absorbable sutures, and improved prosthetic grafts, the aetiology of anastomotic aneurysm has gradually shifted to factors related to the host, rather than the implanted materials. Ongoing degeneration of a diseased arterial wall is the principal cause of development of anastomotic aneurysm in the modern era. However, a number of additional factors and early postoperative complications have been implicated as contributing to false aneurysm formation. These include graft infection, non-infectious postoperative wound complications, such as haematoma or seroma communicating with a fresh anastomosis, the need for local endarterectomy at the site of the femoral anastomosis, and inadequate suture bites on a thick, diseased femoral artery. In addition, since the femoral anastomosis is the most common site of an anastomotic aneurysm, physical factors relative to the distraction forces produced by joint motion and compliance mismatch between prosthesis and native artery contribute to false aneurysm formation.

The diagnosis of an anastomotic aneurysm is generally straightforward on the basis of physical examination and other confirmatory tests are not usually needed prior to complete angiography, which is necessary to plan the appropriate surgical therapy. A complete arteriographic study should be performed to search for additional false aneurysms at other suture lines, particularly at the proximal aortic suture line, since a subpopulation of patients afflicted with anastomotic aneurysm are subject to multiple aneurysms and multiple recurrences. As is the case with other false aneurysms, anastomotic aneurysms are likely to enlarge. They can cause symptoms of local compression and arterial ischaemia from embolism and *in-situ* thrombosis. In addition those located at aortic or iliac suture lines are capable of rupture. Thus, repair of all but the smallest false aneurysms is recommended.

The surgical management of anastomotic aneurysm initially relates to technical steps which are important in prevention of the problem. These have been alluded to above, and involve the use of permanent non-absorbable sutures, large suture bites on diseased femoral arteries, avoidance of excess tension, and careful attention to wound haemostasis and closure at the initial operation. Prophylactic antibiotics are used routinely.

Repair of femoral anastomotic aneurysm may be carried out under either general or regional anaesthesia. The old incision is reopened and proximal control of the graft is obtained above the aneurysm. Although dissection in a reoperated groin can be difficult, exploitation of the principles of traction and countertraction, and sharp dissection with a small scalpel blade, are very effective. There is no role for bypassing or avoiding the multiply operated groin simply because it may be difficult: bypassing does not prevent progressive enlargement of false aneurysms, and is likely to result in the sacrifice of the vital profunda femoris artery. Following control of the limb of the old graft and the native common femoral artery, the surgeon decides whether complete dissection of the distal vessels, for distal control, is appropriate. Since distal control may involve extended dissection with the possibility of injury to the profunda femoris artery, we prefer to open the aneurysm after proximal control is obtained and use intraluminal indwelling balloon catheters for distal control. Furthermore, if it subsequently becomes necessary to dissect out additional length of the profunda femoris artery, the balloon catheter serves as a stent of sorts. Initial distal control of the uninvolved profunda femoris artery, and then retrograde dissection to the area of the aneurysm, is neither necessary nor desirable. Following exposure and opening of the false aneurysm, it is important to instil heparinized saline solution into the now clamped limb of the aortofemoral graft, to prevent *in-situ* clot development during the period of clamping. At this point, a careful search for contributing factors to false aneurysm formation should be made. If any evidence of infection is present intraoperative Gram stains should be used to assess the necessity for extra-anatomic reconstruction. If only a portion of the old suture line is disrupted, the surgeon may be tempted to reclose this with additional interrupted sutures. This proclivity is to be avoided, as it increases the chance of a recurrence. Instead, the entire suture line should be taken down, and the native femoral artery trimmed back to healthy artery.

At this point, the surgeon must decide whether a new end-to-side type of reconstruction is feasible, or whether the new reconstruction should be in end-to-end fashion, thereby sacrificing retrograde flow in the native common femoral artery. The guiding principle should be a technically perfect reconstruction to undiseased distal artery, frequently carried out onto the profunda femoris artery in the manner of a profundaplasty. In such situations, the use of multiple interrupted sutures, at least at the toe and the heel of the reconstruction, is preferred. Reconstruction is generally accomplished with a new short segment of prosthetic graft, which is then simply sutured proximally to the amputated old prosthesis, in end-to-end fashion. Following completion of the reconstruction, adequacy of the distal circulation is ensured before leaving the operating room. Absolute haemostasis is obtained prior to wound closure.

FURTHER READING

Cambria RP, Tilson MD. Obturator foramen bypass grafts in groin sepsis. In: Ernst CB, Stanley JC, eds. *Current Therapy in Vascular Surgery*. Philadelphia: B. C. Decker, Inc. 1987: 224–30.

Cutler BS, Darling RC. Surgical management of arteriosclerotic femoral aneurysm. *Surgery* 1973; **74**: 764–8.

Graham LM, *et al.* Clinical significant of arteriosclerotic femoral artery aneurysm. *Arch Surg* 1980; **115**: 502–7.

Kresowik TF, *et al.* A prospective study of the incidence and natural history of femoral vascular complications after percutaneous coronary angioplasty. *J Vasc Surg* 1991; **13**: 328–36.

McCabe CJ, Moncure AC, Malt RA. Host artery weakness in the etiology of femoral anastomotic false aneurysm. *Surgery* 1984; **95**: 150–3.

Patel KR, Semel L, Clauss RH. Routine revascularization with resection of infected femoral pseudoaneurysms from drug abuse. *J Vasc Surg* 1988; **8**: 321–8.

Reddy, DJ, Smith RF, Elliott JP, Haddad GK, Wanek EA. Infected femoral artery false aneurysm in drug addicts: evolution of selective vascular reconstruction. *J Vasc Surg* 1986; **3**: 718–24.

Schellack J, Salam A, Abouzeid MA, Smith RB, Stewart MT, Perdue GD. Femoral anastomotic aneuryusm: a continuing challenge. *J Vasc Surg* 1987; **6**: 308–17.

Skillman JJ, Kim D, Baum DS. Vascular complications of percutaneous femoral cardiac interventions. Incidence and operative repair. *Arch Surg* 1988; **123**: 1207–12.

7.7.3 Popliteal artery

ASHBY C. MONCURE AND PETER B. H'DOUBLER

HISTORICAL PERSPECTIVES

Popliteal aneurysms hold an important place in the development of vascular surgery. Because of their accessibility to the examiner's hand and surgeon's scalpel, these were the first aneurysms to be diagnosed before death and to be treated surgically. In the fourth century, Antyllus used the technique of opening the sac after proximal and distal ligation in the popliteal fossa: infection and exsanguinating operative or postoperative haemorrhage were the usual results of this procedure. In the sixteenth century, Ambrose Paré stressed the importance of this operation and this remained the preferred surgical approach to this lesion until the eighteenth century. In 1785, John Hunter, the famous British surgeon, anatomist, physiologist, and pathologist, postulated that ligation of the non-dilated superficial femoral artery in the thigh would be a lesser and safer operation. The patient treated in this manner was a 45-year-old coachman whose symptoms were relieved until he died 15 months later of unrelated causes. The Hunterian ligation held a valuable place in the treatment of popliteal aneurysms for over a century.

Wright Post was the first American surgeon successfully to ligate a popliteal aneurysm in 1814. In 1902, Rudolph Matas of New Orleans began to use his technique of endoaneurysmorrhapy to repair popliteal aneurysms with good results. In the United Kingdom, Hogarth Pringle of Glasgow employed a saphenous vein graft to restore vascular continuity in the repair of a traumatic popliteal aneurysm. A patent graft was found at autopsy several years later. In 1916, 4 years after Pringle, Bertram Bernheim reported the first American experience with vein graft interposition.

AETIOLOGY

Popliteal aneurysms are the most common of peripheral arterial aneurysms and are often associated with other aneurysms, suggesting that there is a generalized pathogenetic mechanism. The two basic factors which contribute to aneurysmal formation are mechanical and mural. The first relates to the mechanical stresses transmitted to the arterial wall, and the latter to the strength and structure of the wall.

Most patients with popliteal aneurysms have arteriosclerosis. This degenerative process is associated with but not necessarily the cause of diffuse weakness of the elastin and collagen structural elements of the media which primarily confer strength on the vessel wall and may predispose a vessel to aneurysmal dilatation. The mechanical stresses which affect the popliteal artery include the systemic stress of hypertension. The artery above a bifurcation is more likely to become aneurysmal, possibly because of reflected pressure waves which cause arterial wall vibration and weaken the vessel wall. Aetiologic factors peculiar to the popliteal artery are the extrinsic stress on the artery from knee flexion and extension and the fixation of the vessel at the adductor hiatus. The presence of an arterial wall diffusely weakened by arteriosclerosis with the superimposition of some or all of these extrinsic and intrinsic mechanical stresses probably causes most popliteal aneurysms. The magnitude of the mechanical factors may determine whether a mild dilatation or a large aneurysm forms and the rate of its development.

Popliteal aneurysms are especially common in patients with arteriomegaly, a condition in which all the vessels show elongation, tortuosity, and diffuse dilatation, with evidence of arteriosclerotic narrowing. Multiple fusiform aneurysms, including those of the popliteal artery, are commonly associated with this condition.

Other less common causes of popliteal aneurysms include penetrating and blunt trauma, microbial arteritis caused by syphilis or other bacterial infection, and popliteal artery entrapment. In the last condition the artery is compressed by an aberrantly inserted gastrocnemius muscle and a post-stenotic aneurysm may develop. However, arteriosclerosis is the most common cause of aneurysm.

DIAGNOSIS

A popliteal artery aneurysm is suspected when a prominent expansile impulse can be felt in the popliteal space during physical examination of an asymptomatic patient. Further investigation of such a patient is necessary to confirm the presence of an aneurysm, document its size, and to determine whether mural thrombus is present within the aneurysm. Because of the high incidence of associated aneurysms a search for an occult abdominal aortic aneurysm, femoral aneurysm, and contralateral popliteal aneurysm is part of the evaluation of a patient with a suspected popliteal aneurysm.

The most common and least expensive diagnostic method is ultrasound: 'B' mode scanning, usually with the assistance of Doppler ultrasound, allows visualization of the vessel and is quick, accurate, and non-invasive. A popliteal artery dilated to greater than 2 cm diameter or a localized dilatation 1.5 to 2 times the size of the proximal vessel should be considered aneurysmal.

An arteriogram is not a good diagnostic test as it may miss an aneurysm when there is a normal calibre lumen within an aneurysm full of mural thrombus. It is however indicated in the planning of an operation as it defines the arterial anatomy and status of the distal runoff vessels (Fig. 1). Computerized tomography is a useful method of evaluating the popliteal space and provides detail about the arterial wall and intravascular contents, but is more expensive than ultrasound and should not be used for diagnosis. The most useful method of visualization of the popliteal artery is likely to be magnetic resonance imaging scanning, which shows excellent detail of the arterial wall and confirms the presence of mural thrombus. It may also obviate the need for arteriography in patients requiring surgical treatment, as the status of the adjacent arterial anatomy is clearly defined (Fig. 2).

The diagnosis of popliteal aneurysm is suggested by a variety of symptoms. Pain or swelling in the lower leg may be the result of pressure on nerves or venous return. Intermittent claudication, rest pain, or areas of skin necrosis can be the result of thromboemboli from the aneurysm. Rupture is a rare complication and

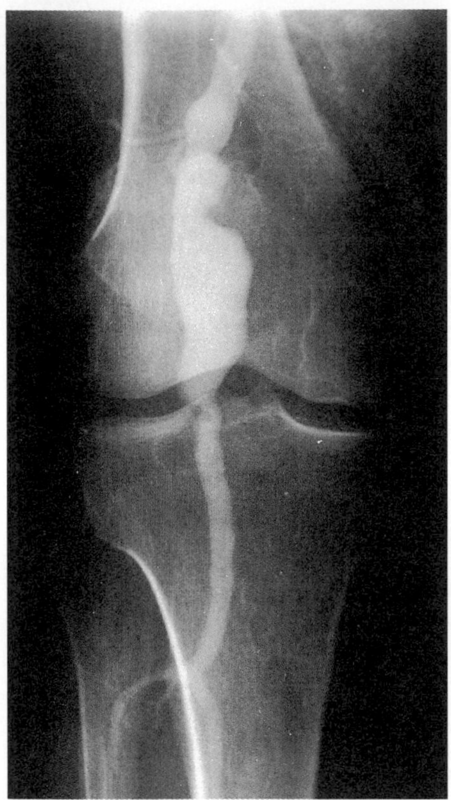

Fig. 1 Femoral contrast arteriogram demonstrating popliteal aneurysm just above the level of the knee joint.

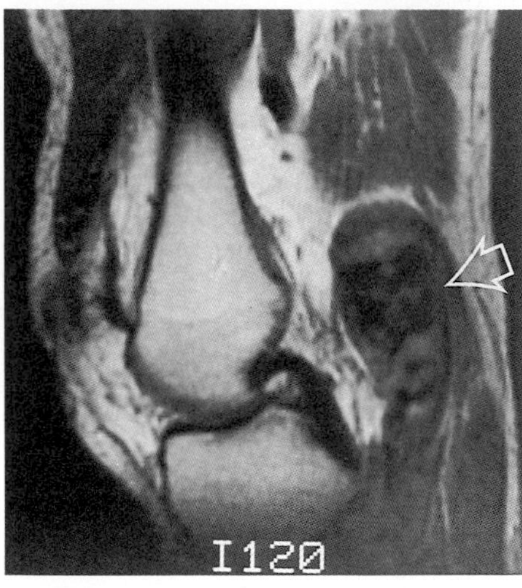

Fig. 2 Sagittal MRI of popliteal space shows large popliteal aneurysm with mural thrombus.

presents with sudden swelling and pain in the popliteal space, sometimes with signs of distal ischaemia. In a patient presenting with acute limb ischaemia, the diagnosis of popliteal aneurysm thrombosis should always be considered and is more likely if a prominent popliteal pulsation suggestive of a popliteal aneurysm is present on the unaffected side. It is important that this diagnosis is made as simple thromboembolectomy is unlikely to help such a patient.

CLINICAL BEHAVIOUR

Deposition of marginal laminar thrombus, a phenomenon common to most aneurysms, is responsible for the most frequent complications seen in this condition. Thrombotic and embolic complications are produced by dislodgement of the laminar thrombus within the aneurysm, with obstruction of the popliteal artery outflow tract and thrombosis of the aneurysm, or emboli may obliterate the distal tibial and peroneal arteries, producing severe ischaemia of the lower extremity. If the aneurysm is large, venous obstruction may be mechanically produced and lead to the formation of deep venous thrombosis. Neurological pain syndromes, particularly in the distribution of the sural nerve may also be produced by compression.

Occasionally, a popliteal aneurysm may rupture, but its containment within the popliteal space means that this complication is rarely life-threatening. It does, however, mandate urgent operation because of the severe pain produced and the threat of loss of the extremity secondary to distal arterial occlusion. Also rarely, a popliteal artery aneurysm may become infected as may other peripheral aneurysms.

MANAGEMENT

Linton described the natural history of popliteal aneurysms, reporting a 77 per cent limb loss and a 27 per cent mortality in 22 consecutive aneurysms encountered in 20 patients and treated conservatively. To avoid the high mortality and amputation rates experienced in this condition, operative management is recommended for all but very elderly, poor risk patients. This recommendation is reinforced by the finding of laminar thrombus present within the popliteal aneurysm upon examination by computed tomography or magnetic resonance imaging.

Operative management has the goal of preventing further complications of the aneurysm and restoration of adequate arterial perfusion to the extremity. This goal may be accompanied by bypass grafting of the popliteal aneurysm using autogenous saphenous vein with concomitant proximal and distal ligation of the aneurysm, by resection of the aneurysm with autogenous saphenous vein interposition grafting, or by resection of the aneurysm with end-to-end arterial anastomosis. Bypass grafting with proximal and distal ligation of the aneurysm has become the usual method of operatively managing the moderate sized popliteal aneurysm because of its simplicity of approach.

These techniques are best accomplished by operative exposure through the medial approach to the popliteal fossa, enabling harvest of greater saphenous vein and wide exposure of the arteries involved in the reconstruction through the same incision. This approach also provides the greatest flexibility to the surgeon, allowing more proximal and distal exposure to the arteries, if necessary, to accomplish the arterial reconstruction. Autogenous vein is greatly superior to prosthetic grafts in terms of long-term patency, and in the absence of an available saphenous vein arm veins should be sought for the reconstruction.

If the popliteal aneurysm is large and has produced symptoms attributable to compression of neighbouring veins or nerves the aneurysm should be resected or opened, and its branches ligated from within the aneurysm, prior to the arterial reconstruction. An aneurysm involving a short segment of popliteal artery may be best managed by resection and mobilization of the proximal and distal popliteal artery to allow end-to-end anastomosis without tension. An infected popliteal aneurysm must be resected and autogenous vein utilized in the reconstruction with an initial period of intravenous antibiotic treatment followed by oral antibiotic use indefinitely thereafter. Drug selection should be based initially on the results of Gram stain of the examined material and ultimately on the results of culture and antibiotic sensitivity testing.

Occasionally the clinical presentation may be that of acute arterial occlusion with inability to disobliterate the thrombus within the arterial tree distal to the aneurysm, using the usual method of Fogarty embolectomy catheters. In such circumstances, intraoperative use of urokinase, injected directly as a bolus in the non-perfused distal arterial tree (250 000 IU, reconstituted with 5 ml of sterile water for injection, further diluted with 50 ml 0.97 sodium chloride injection, USP), may be used to clear the distal arterial tree of thrombus, after which grafting around the popliteal aneurysm may be accomplished.

RESULTS OF TREATMENT

In general, the results of operative management of popliteal artery aneurysms are closely related to the status of the distal arterial tree and to the type of conduit employed. Patients undergoing successful revascularization have good early results. In the Massachusetts General Hospital series, patients with asymptomatic aneurysms treated operatively have uniformly good results (97.2 per cent) compared to those presenting with acute (70.7 per cent), or chronic symptoms (83.3 per cent). At 5-year follow up, 77.2 per cent of all saphenous vein grafts were patent, whereas only 29.5 per cent of Dacron prostheses remained patent.

FURTHER READING

Anton GE, Hertzer NR, Beven EG, O'Hara PJ, Krajewski LP. Surgical management of popliteal aneurysms. *J Vasc Surg* 1986; 3: 125–34.

Chitwood WR, Stocks LH, Wolfe WG. Popliteal artery aneurysms. *Arch Surg* 1978; **113**: 1078–82.

Edmunds LH, Darling RC, Linton RR. Surgical management of popliteal aneurysm. *Circulation* 1965: **32**: 517–23.

Evans WE, Vermillion BD. Popliteal aneurysm. In: Wilson SE, Veith FJ, Hoblon RW, Williams RA, eds. *Vascular surgery: principles and practice*. New York: McGraw-Hill, 1987: 501–3.

Linton RR. The arteriosclerotic popliteal aneurysm. *Surgery* 1949; **26**: 41–58.

MacGowan SW, Saif MF, Fitzsimons P, Bouchier-Hayes D. Ultrasound examination in the diagnosis of popliteal artery aneurysms. *Br J Surg* 1985; **72**: 528–9.

Reilly MK, Abbott WM, Darling RC. Aggressive surgical management of popliteal aneurysms. *Am J Surg* 1983; **145**: 498–502.

Rizzo RJ, Flinn WR, Yao JST, McCarthy WJ, Vogelzang RL, Pearch WH. Computed tomography for evaluation of arterial disease in the popliteal fossa. *J Vasc Surg* 1990; **11**: 112–19.

Weiner SN, Hoffman J, Bertstein RG, Koenigsbery M. The value of ultrasound in the diagnosis of popliteal aneurysm. *Angiology* 1983; **34**: 418–27.

Wychulis AR, Spittell JA, Wallace RB. Popliteal aneurysms. *Surgery* 1970; **68**: 942–52.

7.7.4 Carotid artery

JONATHAN MICHAELS AND PETER J. MORRIS

Aneurysms of the extracranial carotid artery are uncommon, the largest single reported series representing 37 of 8500 aneurysms treated at Baylor University over a 21-year period. They usually affect the common or internal carotid artery, rarely the external artery, and are bilateral in about 10 per cent of cases. True aneurysms are most commonly atherosclerotic, although mycotic and syphilitic aneurysms do occur, along with rarer degenerative and dysplastic conditions (Fig. 1). False aneurysms may occur following trauma and are seen increasing as a complication of previous carotid endarterectomy.

Most carotid aneurysms present as an asymptomatic, pulsatile neck swelling, or with transient or fixed neurological defects due to cerebral emboli. More rarely, they present with local pressure symptoms such as dysphagia or as an emergency following rupture. Examination usually demonstrates a pulsatile mass just below the angle of the jaw which may have a bruit and can sometimes be observed or palpated in the tonsillar fossa. They may, however, be sited anywhere from the root of the neck to the base of the skull.

The most common differential diagnosis of a pulsatile neck swelling is the more common and benign condition of a tortuous carotid artery (Fig. 2). This is usually seen in the root of the neck on the right and is asymptomatic. Other differential diagnoses should include masses overlying the carotid vessels with transmitted pulsation, particularly carotid body tumour, branchial cysts, and lymphadenopathy. Duplex ultrasonography is the first line of investigation: this is non-invasive, provides useful information about the size and extent of the aneurysm, and allows assessment of the contralateral carotid vessels. Angiography is usually required for accurate assessment of the anatomy (Fig. 3), with digital subtraction techniques providing enhanced images. CT or magnetic resonance techniques can provide excellent images showing the extent and situation of the aneurysm.

The natural history of untreated carotid aneurysms is not well documented, although small asymptomatic aneurysms may be treated conservatively, especially if the operative risks are high. Such treatment should include the use of antiplatelet agents such as aspirin to reduce the risk of cerebral emboli. The earliest reported surgical treatment was simple ligation of the carotid artery. This operation was first reported by Pare in 1552 for trauma and was carried out by Sir Astley Cooper in 1805 for a carotid aneurysm. His first attempt resulted in hemiplegia and early postoperative death but he successfully carried out the procedure on a similar case 3 years later.

Because of the risk of major stroke following carotid ligation the first choice for treatment is excision of the aneurysm with restora-

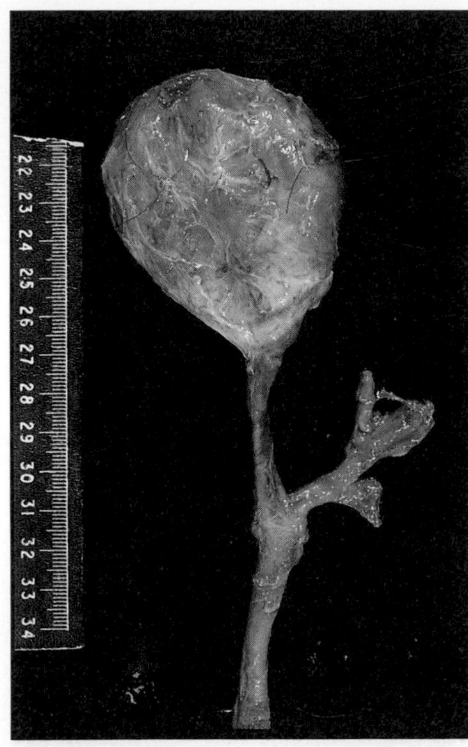

Fig. 1 Large aneurysm of the internal carotid artery found in a 45-year-old man who presented with a dense contralateral hemiparesis.

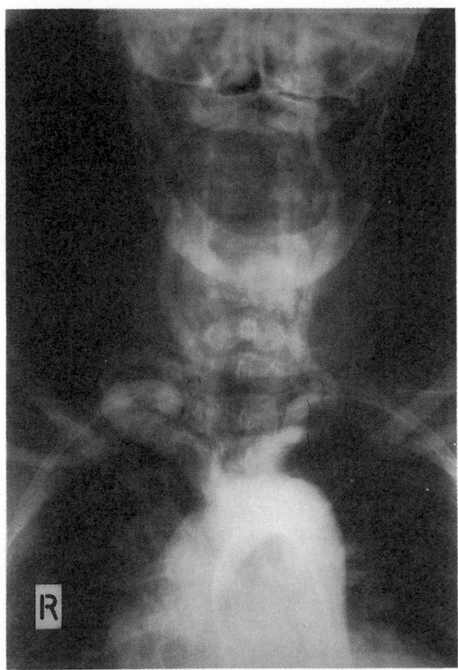

Fig. 2 Angiogram in a 70-year-old woman who presented with a pulsatile swelling in the root of the neck on the right showing a tortuous origin of the common carotid and subclavian artery.

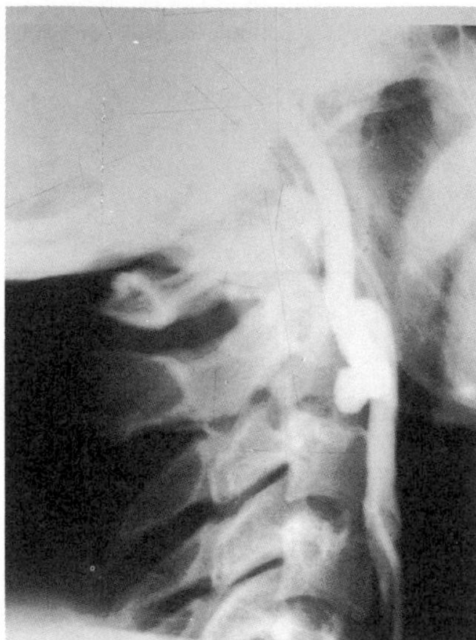

Fig. 3 Aneurysm which has occurred in a coiled redundant internal carotid artery.

tion of flow by direct anastomosis or graft. Primary anastomosis is frequently possible, as elongation of the artery often accompanies aneurysmal dilatation. Where this cannot be achieved the use of the external carotid artery, vein, or prosthetic graft is necessary. For false aneurysms the use of a patch angioplasty may be sufficient but the use of prosthetic materials should be avoided where possible, due to the implication of infection as a possible aetiological factor. The need for a peroperative shunt is controversial but it should be considered if there is a stump pressure of less than 55 mmHg or if there are EEG changes on applying clamps.

High aneurysms present the most difficult problem since surgical approaches require the removal of part of the mastoid bone or dislocation of the mandible. Where distal control would be difficult or dangerous, carotid occlusion may be the only alternative, but attempts should be made to improve upon the success of simple ligation. Graded occlusion may achieve this or one of a range of percutaneous techniques, such as inflatable, detachable occlusion balloons with concomitant extra-intracranial bypass if required.

FURTHER READING

Bergan JJ, Hoehn JG. Evanescent cervical pseudoaneurysms. *Ann Surg* 1965; **162**: 213–7.

Crandon IW, Teasdale E, Galbraith SL, Hadley DM. Carotid traumatic aneurysm treated by detachable balloon. *Br J Neurosurg* 1988; **2**: 507–11.

de Jong KP, Zondervan PE, van Urk H. Extracranial carotid artery aneurysms. *Eur J Vasc Surg* 1989; **3**: 557–62.

Goldstone J. Aneurysms of the extracranial carotid artery. In: Rutherford I, ed. *Vascular Surgery*. Philadelphia: WBS Saunders, 1984: 1279–87.

Hunt JL, Snyder WH. Late false aneurysms of the carotid artery: repair with extra-intracranial arterial bypass. *J Trauma* 1979; **19**: 198–200.

McCollum CH, Wheeler WG, Noon GP, DeBakey ME. Aneurysms of the extracranial carotid artery. *Am J Surg* 1979; **137**: 196–200.

Nicholson ML, Horrocks M. Leaking carotid artery aneurysm. *Eur J Vasc Surg* 1988; **2**: 197–8.

Raphael HA, Bernatz PE, Spittell JA, Ellis FH. Cervical carotid aneurysms: treatment by excision and restoration of arterial continuity. *Am J Surg* 1963; **105**: 771–8.

Sharma S, Rajani M, Mishra N, Sampathkumar A, Iyer KS. Extracranial carotid artery aneurysms following accidental injury: ten years experience. *Clin Radiol* 1991; **43**: 162–5.

Trippel OH, Haid SP, Kornmesser TW, Bergan JJ. Extracranial carotid aneurysms. In: Bergan JJ, Yao JST, eds. *Aneurysms: Diagnosis and Treatment*. New York: Grune and Stratton, 1982: 493–504.

7.7.5 Subclavian artery

JONATHAN MICHAELS

Aneurysms of the subclavian artery represent about 1 per cent of all peripheral arterial aneurysms. They fall into two distinct groups in terms of aetiology, presentation, and treatment: those of the intrathoracic and those of the extrathoracic portion of the subclavian artery. Those in the extrathoracic site are the more common, and about three-quarters of aneurysms at this site are related to thoracic outlet syndrome or to previous trauma (Figs. 1 and 2). The other major cause is atherosclerosis, which is responsible for the majority of intrathoracic aneurysms. Other, rarer causes include infection and degenerative conditions, and there have been a number of reports of aneurysms of an aberrant right subclavian artery. As would be expected the epidemiology parallels that of the underlying cause: atherosclerotic aneurysms occur in the elderly, while those associated with thoracic outlet syndrome are seen in young adults.

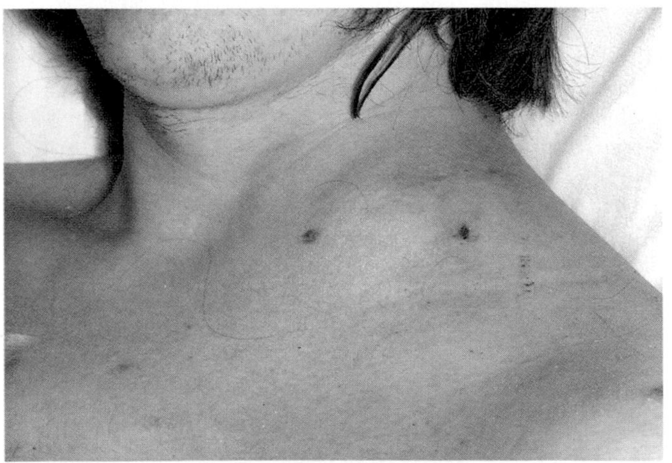

Fig. 1 Traumatic aneurysm of the left subclavian artery (by courtesy of Professor P. J. Morris).

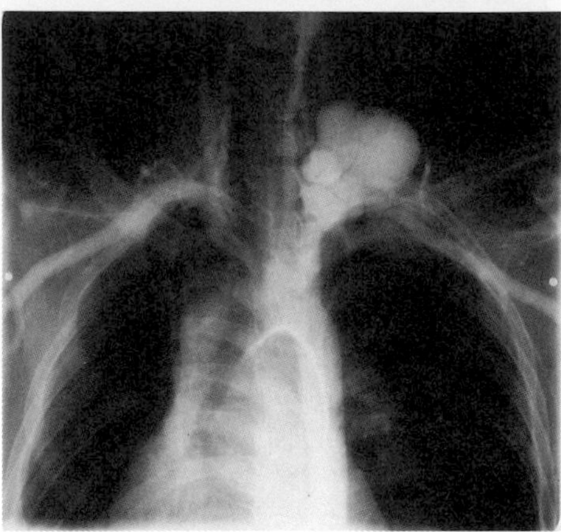

Fig. 2 Angiogram of patient in Fig. 1 showing a traumatic false aneurysm of left subclavian artery (by courtesy of Professor P. J. Morris).

Intrathoracic aneurysms present most often with an asymptomatic mediastinal shadow on a routine chest radiograph or with symptoms of local compression, and they must be differentiated from other mediastinal masses. Reported symptoms include chest and back pain, Horner's syndrome, venous congestion, and hoarseness. Symptoms due to distal embolization to the arm are an unusual presentation at this site but are seen in about two-thirds of patients with extrathoracic aneurysms. The emboli tend to be small, affecting digital vessels and leading to episodic symptoms, and may be confused with Raynaud's phenomenon. Whenever such symptoms are unilateral the possibility of a proximal arterial lesion should always be considered. Extrathoracic aneurysms are often associated with neurological symptoms of brachial plexus compression, although it may be difficult to determine the relative importance of the aneurysm and any associated thoracic outlet compression. Rupture of a subclavian aneurysm is a rare event but has been reported, as has acute ischaemia due to thrombosis.

Careful physical examination may reveal a pulsatile mass in the supraclavicular fossa, a bruit, or pulse deficits, and there may be evidence of associated thoracic outlet or upper mediastinal compression. Attention should also be directed to identifying coexisting aneurysms at other sites. Plain radiographs of the thoracic outlet and upper mediastinum may show the extent of the mass, a calcified arterial wall, or cervical ribs. Magnetic resonance imaging is also proving a useful investigation of the thoracic outlet, and is often able to detect fibrous bands causing obstruction. Conventional or digital subtraction angiography will demonstrate the arterial anatomy, extent of aneurysmal disease, and associated stenosis or thrombus, as well as showing occlusions of distal vessels if there have been previous emboli.

Because of the high risk of complications resulting in limb loss, elective surgical treatment is recommended for most subclavian aneurysms. Access to the intrathoracic subclavian artery is achieved through a lateral thoracotomy on the left or a median sternotomy for the right side. The extrathoracic subclavian vein can be approached through a supraclavicular incision after medial retraction of the phrenic nerve and division of the scalenus anterior. Additional exposure can be achieved by resection of the middle third of the clavicle or by dissection of the axillary artery below the clavicle. In cases of thoracic outlet syndrome it may also be necessary to resect a cervical rib or band, or the first rib if this is implicated.

The aim of the surgery is to exclude or remove the aneurysm with restoration of circulation. Direct arterial repair or patch angioplasty may be appropriate in some patients with false aneurysms. In most cases resection is possible, the arterial supply being maintained by either direct anastomosis or replacement with a venous or prosthesic graft. In difficult cases ligation may be less hazardous, the circulation being restored by extra-anatomical axilloaxillary or caroticosubclavian bypass.

FURTHER READING

Gordon RD, Garrett HE. Atheromatous and aneurysmal disease of the upper extremity. In: Rutherford I, ed. *Vascular Surgery*. Philadelphia: WB Saunders, 1984: 688–92.

Hobson RW, Israel MR, Lynch TG. Axillosubclavian arterial aneurysms. In: Bergan JJ, Yao JST, eds. *Aneurysms: Diagnosis and Treatment*. New York: Grune and Stratton, 1982: 435–47.

7.7.6 Visceral arteries

JACK COLLIN

INTRODUCTION

The visceral arteries comprise the coeliac, superior mesenteric, inferior mesenteric, and renal arteries together with all their branches. Aneurysms of these vessels are uncommon and in order of frequency rank below aneurysms of the abdominal and thoracic aorta, and those of the iliac, femoral, and popliteal arteries.

In common with other arterial aneurysms the majority are asymptomatic and since no easy non-invasive investigation can reliably detect their presence their true prevalence in the community is unknown. Any epidemiological data that exist are certainly suspect since they are obtained either from highly selected groups of patients undergoing angiography or computerized tomographic scanning or from autopsy studies in which small visceral aneurysms could easily be overlooked. No single vascular surgical unit has sufficient overall experience of visceral arterial aneurysms to allow useful analysis of the relative importance of different aetiologies or the indications for and results of various management options. Most accounts in the literature still comprise single case reports, small series, or larger analyses comprising collections of such cases from literature reviews. Any overview which attempts to give a didactic account of aetiology, presentation, and management of visceral artery aneurysms is therefore handicapped by the absence of a sound database and this fact should be borne in mind.

AETIOLOGY

In common with aneurysms of the aorta, the aetiology in the majority of cases is unknown, but the proximate cause is local failure of the connective tissue of the arterial wall to maintain the integrity of the vessel. Most patients are middle aged and, inevitably, atherosclerosis has been implicated, but in contradistinction to abdominal aortic aneurysms, a high proportion of cases occur in young people in their 30s and the majority of patients are women.

The single most interesting fact about this disease is that in developed countries ruptured visceral arterial aneurysm is now one of the major causes of maternal mortality. Between 1967 and 1982 there were 14 maternal deaths from this cause (10 splenic, three renal, and one hepatic artery aneurysm) in England and Wales, with most ruptures occurring in the last weeks of pregnancy. Similar observations in the United States have given rise to speculation by a number of authors that systemic and portal hypertension, increased cardiac output, and increased blood flow in some vessels, together with the hormonal and connective tissue changes in pregnancy may all be contributory factors.

A number of other aetiologies have been implicated with differing importance in various reports, including congenital malformations, trauma, arteritis, connective tissue disorders, and infection. Trauma, either accidental or iatrogenic during percutaneous biopsy, plays a major role in the causation of aneurysms within the liver or kidney but, fortunately, the majority are small and of no clinical significance (Fig. 1). Of the arteritides, Takayasu's disease is particularly important and can give rise to visceral aneurysm, with or without associated occlusive arterial disease.

In the past mycotic aneurysms were usually a consequence of bacterial endocarditis but more recently intravenous drug abuse and cardiac catheterization have contributed an increasing proportion of cases.

RELATIVE INCIDENCE OF INDIVIDUAL ANEURYSMS

Splenic aneurysms (Fig. 2) account for around two-thirds of all ruptured visceral artery aneurysms, with most of the remainder being ruptured renal, hepatic (Fig. 3), gastric, or superior mesenteric artery aneurysms (Fig. 4). Aneurysms of the inferior mesenteric artery are extremely rare, as are gastroduodenal and pancreaticoduodenal artery aneurysms.

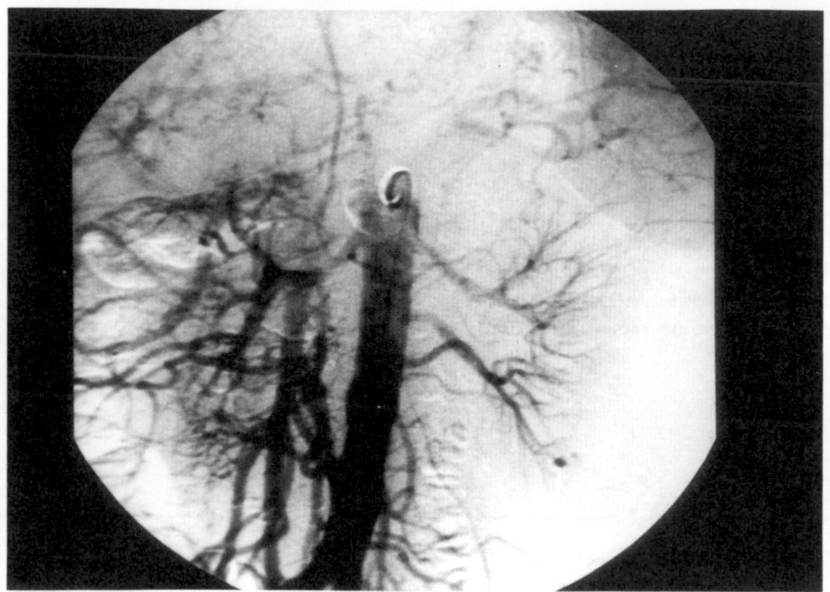

Fig. 1 Small renal artery aneurysm following renal biopsy.

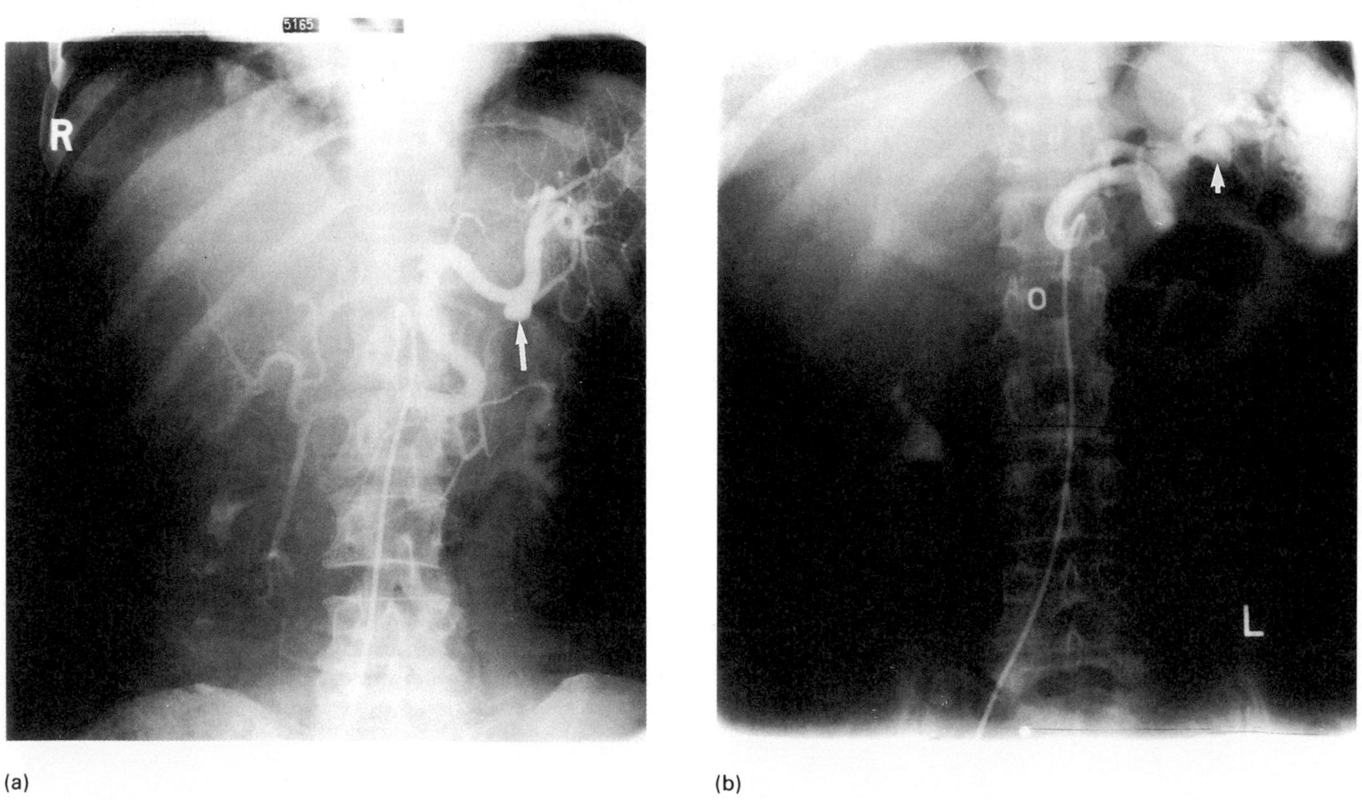

(a)

(b)

Fig. 2 (a) and (b) Splenic artery aneurysms.

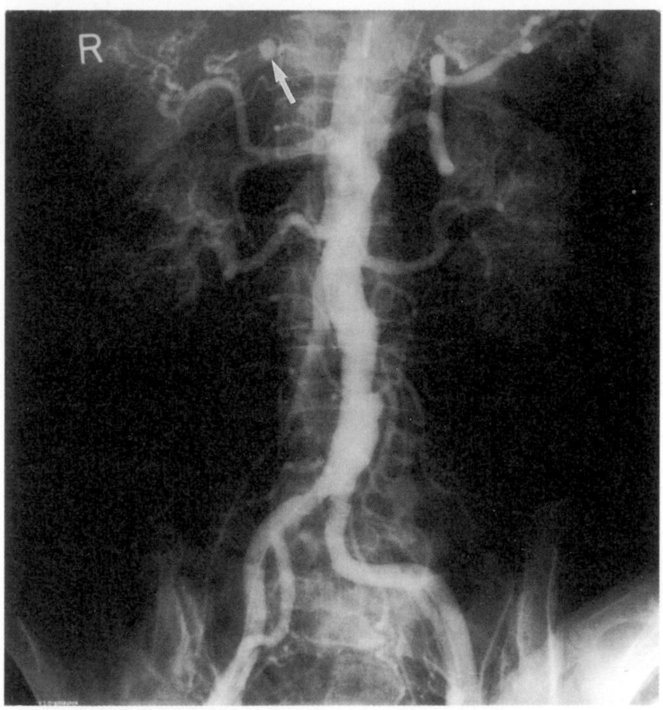

Fig. 3 Hepatic artery aneurysm.

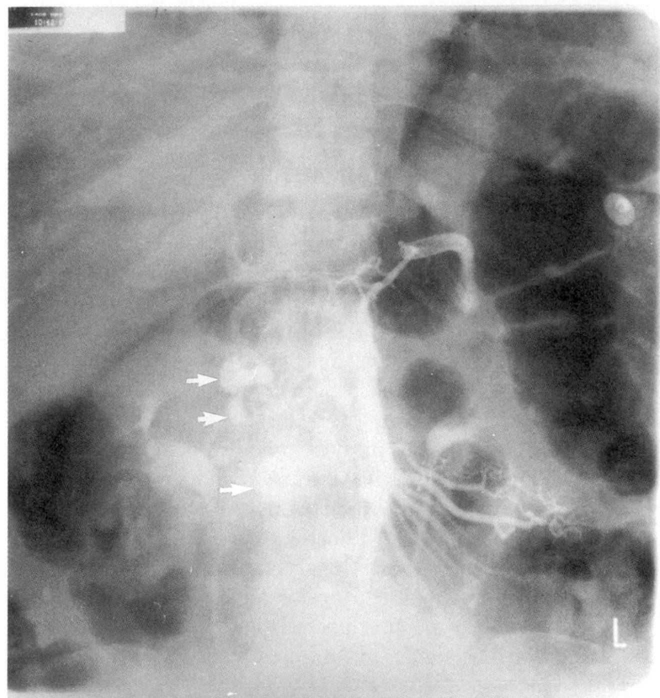

Fig. 4 Superior mesenteric artery aneurysm.

CLINICAL PRESENTATION

Most visceral artery aneurysms are asymptomatic or give rise to vague abdominal discomfort perhaps related to compression or stretching of adjacent nerves by aneurysm expansion. Occasionally hepatic, gastroduodenal, or pancreaticoduodenal aneurysms may produce bile duct compression and jaundice while splenic aneurysms may be associated with pancreatitis. Mesenteric aneurysms may produce gut ischaemia by releasing emboli from mural thrombus within the aneurysm. Apart from rupture, renal artery aneurysms are those most likely to give rise to major symptoms due to either hypertension or renal failure. This impression could well be flawed, however, since patients with hypertension or renal failure are more likely to undergo angiography and some aneurysms discovered will be incidental and insignificant findings.

The most dramatic symptoms occur when an aneurysm ruptures. Initially the rupture may be partially contained either by the adjacent connective tissue or, in the case of splenic, gastric, and hepatic artery aneurysms, within the lesser sac. In such circumstances the main symptoms are abdominal pain and a variable amount of circulatory collapse, depending on the volume of blood lost. Sooner or later the connective tissues which have partially contained the bleeding will give way with free rupture into the peritoneal cavity, and profound circulatory collapse.

Unusual presentations occur when a visceral aneurysm erodes into an adjacent structure, for example the hepatic artery into the common bile duct or a gastric, gastroduodenal, or pancreaticoduodenal artery into the foregut. The resultant haemobilia, haematemesis, and melaena are likely to be attributed preoperatively to other more common causes of upper gastrointestinal haemorrhage and even at operation the correct diagnosis may not be obvious.

DIAGNOSIS

The mainstay of precise anatomical diagnosis remains angiography with selective catheterization of the appropriate visceral artery. Angiograms will also display collateral circulation and allow planning of any operative procedure which may be necessary. Incidental diagnoses of visceral aneurysms will be made from abdominal radiographs if the aneurysm wall is calcified or from abdominal computerized tomograms. Computerized tomography may also give useful anatomical information or may be diagnostic in cases where a visceral aneurysm is suspected or presents as an abdominal mass.

The diagnosis of a ruptured visceral aneurysm is based on the clinical signs of circulatory collapse from blood loss together with evidence of intra-abdominal bleeding. The patient's condition will usually not permit time to be spent on confirming the diagnosis preoperatively, since emergency laparotomy to control the haemorrhage is mandatory.

MANAGEMENT

Management decisions are clear-cut and uncontroversial when a visceral artery aneurysm has ruptured: emergency surgery is lifesaving. There is considerable uncertainty about management of an intact aneurysm, particularly when it is asymptomatic, since not enough is known of the natural history of the disease for an informed recommendation to be made. When the aneurysm is very large or causes symptoms and is in an anatomical location which allows safe surgical exclusion, resection or arterial bypass to be performed, then surgery will usually be the sensible choice. An aneurysm discovered in early pregnancy or in a woman who plans to have children is also usually best treated by operation because of the risk of rupture during pregnancy.

The greatest uncertainty is caused by a small asymptomatic visceral artery aneurysm in an anatomical location where surgery is potentially difficult or dangerous. Many such aneurysms are best managed conservatively with regular monitoring of their size and the patient's condition. Others will lend themselves to treatment by interventional radiographic techniques, the scope of which continues to expand. Provided the aneurysmal artery can be cannulated the aneurysm can usually be satisfactorily occluded by the insertion of metal coils or inflatable detachable balloons.

Mycotic aneurysms of visceral arteries have the same sinister prognosis as they do elsewhere with a tendency to rapid enlargement and rupture. For this reason elective surgery is best undertaken as early as possible in conjunction with systemic antibiotic therapy to treat the underlying infection.

FURTHER READING

King TA, McDaniel MD, Flinn WR, Yao JST, Bergan JJ. Visceral artery aneurysms. In: Moore WS, ed. *Vascular surgery; a comprehensive review*. New York: Grune and Stratton 1983: 351–65.

Skudder PA. Visceral artery aneurysms. In: Persson AV, Skudder PA, eds. *Vascular Surgery*. New York: Marcel Dekker, 1987: 145–73.

7.7.7 Mycotic aneurysms

JOHN A. MURIE

INTRODUCTION

'Mycotic' is a term which was introduced in 1885 by Osler to describe aortic aneurysms caused by weakening of the arterial wall by infected emboli arising from bacterial endocarditis. This is now an uncommon cause of mycotic aneurysm and the term has come to be used to describe all infected aneurysms. Mycotic aneurysms may be 'true' (an arterial swelling lined by intima) or 'false' (an artery related swelling arising from a leak) and the point at which an infected artery or an infected anastomosis becomes a mycotic aneurysm is debatable, making an estimate of the incidence of the condition meaningless. In the mind of the vascular surgeon the term 'mycotic' is often associated with arteries, for, while infected venous aneurysms do occur and may even be described as mycotic, they are usually treated by simple excision and there is little risk of vascular insufficiency developing.

AETIOLOGY

Classification

The most useful classification is based on the putative status of the artery before infection and the source of infection. Arteries may be normal, atheromatous, aneurysmal, or may be associated with a prosthetic graft. The source of infection may be intravascular (septic emboli or bacteraemia) or extravascular (perivascular lymphatics, local abscess, trauma). Normal arteries are not thought to be affected by simple bacteraemia, while diseased arteries may be. An extravascular source of infection is often associated with more diffuse inflammation of the surrounding tissues than an intravascular source. This is especially so in cases of trauma where arterial disruption, haematoma and infection may eventually lead to a mycotic false aneurysm, the most common form of the condition, which is now frequently associated with the use of contaminated syringes by drug addicts.

Bacteriology

The type of organism recovered from a mycotic aneurysm depends on the source of infection and the location of the affected artery (Table 1). In the classical form of mycotic aneurysm due to infected emboli from bacterial endocarditis, Pneumococcus, Streptococcus, Haemophilus, and Enterococcus will usually be found. In non-endocarditic peripheral mycotic aneurysms Staphylococcus and Enterobacter are commonly present, but the list of other organisms isolated from such lesions is a lengthy one.

Salmonella is by far the most common infecting organism in mycotic aortic aneurysms. Nevertheless, numerous other bacterial species have been cultured from these lesions, including *Staphylococcus epidermidis* (of uncertain significance) and normal gut flora, the presence of which suggests that a bacteraemia arising from the gut may lead to organisms lodging in an already diseased aortic wall. A variety of other bacteria and fungi have been described in aortic lesions, including *Treponema pallidum* and *Mycobacterium tuberculosis*, which both have a prediliction for the aorta rather than other vessels.

Location

Forty per cent of mycotic aneurysms involve the femoral artery and 30 per cent affect the aorta; these two vessels are the most common sites of mycotic aneurysms. The most common cause is

Table 1 Bacteria grown from infected aneurysms

Aneurysm type	Bacteria
Peripheral (bacterial endocarditis associated)	Pneumococcus Streptococcus Enterococcus *Haemophilus influenzae*
Peripheral (other)	Staphylococcus Enterobacter Klebsiella Proteus *Escherichia coli* Pseudomonas Clostridium Bacteroides
Aortic	Salmonella Staphylococcus *Escherichia coli* Clostridium Bacteroides Streptococcus *Mycobacterium tuberculosis* *Treponema pallidum** Gonococcus*

*Where sexually transmitted diseases are not well controlled

trauma (in about 40 per cent of cases) followed by bacteraemia affecting an already diseased artery. It should be remembered, however, that virtually any artery can be the site of a mycotic aneurysm and that intravenous drug abuse and percutaneous catheterization procedures account for an increasing incidence of the problem in the brachial and femoral vessels. Other iatrogenic causes include aortic lesions in neonates monitored with umbilical catheters, and upper limb arterial lesions from infected needling of vessels or grafts in the vicinity of an arteriovenous fistula used for haemodialysis access. As a result the incidence of peripheral mycotic aneurysms is greater than that of aortic mycotic aneurysms.

CLINICAL

Presentation

This depends on many factors, not the least of which is the site of the aneurysm. The vast majority of peripheral aneurysms can be palpated, in contrast to most central aneurysms (Fig. 1). Typically, the patient has a fever, perhaps of 'unknown' origin and a history of bacterial endocarditis or operative or other trauma to the affected vessel. A mycotic aneurysm tends to enlarge rapidly and, if palpable, may appear as a tender, warm pulsatile mass with an overlying systolic murmur. Depending on the nature of the infective source, lesions may be multiple, and the natural history is of continued growth followed by rupture which, depending on the site and containment or otherwise by surrounding structures, may be rapidly fatal. A persistent fever of unrecognized origin is likely to be associated with slow and insidious aneurysmal growth, particularly if antibiotics have been administered at an early stage. Even if an aneurysm is recognized, the diagnosis may be elusive, especially if antibiotic therapy obscures the infective nature of the lesion.

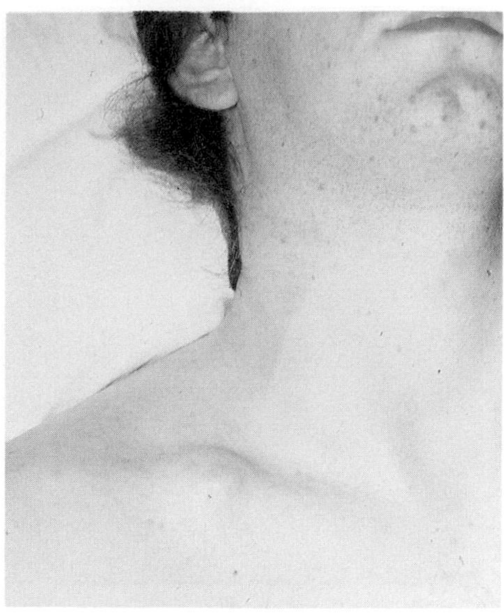

Fig. 1 An easily detectable peripheral (subclavian artery) mycotic aneurysm in a young man with bacterial endocarditis treated with antibiotics.

Diagnosis

There is usually a fever and the presence of petechiae is of great significance. Leucocytosis is very common unless antibiotics have been used. Blood cultures are useful in both diagnosis and management, and if venous samples fail to detect an organism, blood from an artery distal to the aneurysm should be tested.

Angiograms, although not in themselves diagnostic of infection, confirm the presence of an aneurysm and are essential for planned treatment. Non-calcified aneurysms in otherwise normal looking vessels should raise the question of a mycotic aetiology (Fig. 2). Ultrasonography, and particularly computed tomography, may be useful, particularly if fluid collections are visualized around prosthetic grafts: such a collection may be aspirated for bacteriological culture. Scanning using leucocytes labelled with a radioisotope of indium has proved useful in some centres.

TREATMENT

Prophylaxis with broad spectrum antibiotics such as cefuroxime is important in patients with a known septic focus and atheromatous occlusive disease or aneurysm or a vascular prosthesis. When confronted with an intact mycotic aneurysm, however, all infected tissue, including a thrombosed vascular prosthesis if present, must be excised. Open drainage may be both feasible and desirable in some cases. Alternatively, irrigation with antibiotic solution through a catheter may be used, along with systemic chemotherapy directed by appropriate culture.

Arteries should be ligated or oversewn, and anastomoses for bypass operations placed only in uninfected vessels using monofilament sutures. Ligation and excision of infected tissue without reconstruction is preferable, since any reconstruction is liable to further infection and this may lead to early catastrophic haemorrhage. If immediate reconstruction is deemed necessary to save life or limb it can often be performed away from the infected area, and it may even be done before excision of the infected lesion; for instance an axillofemoral bypass may be inserted before excising a mycotic

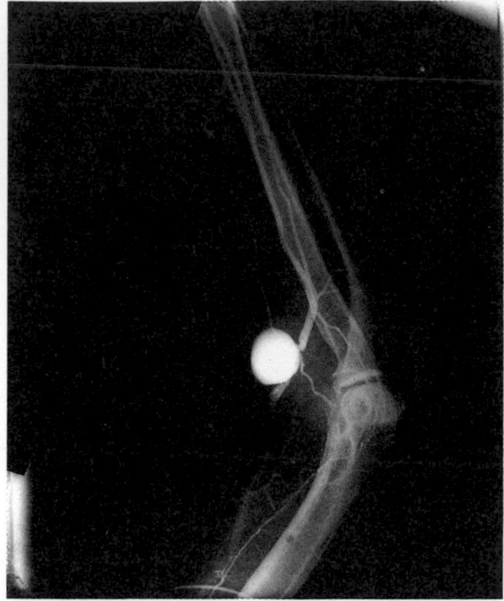

Fig. 2 Brachial artery mycotic aneurysm in an intravenous drug abuser. Note the normal appearance of the surrounding vessels.

abdominal aortic aneurysm. If reconstruction must be done at the same time and a graft must be placed near or in the area of excised infection, autogenous vein rather than grafts of foreign material should be used if at all possible. Even so, persisting infection with early anastomotic bleeding is a profound danger which may occur at any time from a few hours to several months after operation.

Although a mycotic aneurysm is a major operative challenge, conservative treatment is not appropriate. Antibiotic therapy alone will not prevent eventual rupture, and chemotherapy, guided by sensitivity reports from the bacteriology laboratory, is best used in conjunction with surgery. Antibiotics should be given systemically during the perioperative period and continued orally thereafter for several months.

RESULTS

So much depends on the location and aetiology of mycotic aneurysms that overall results are meaningless. Lesions arising from a bacterial endocarditis are generally treated successfully, with a 75 per cent early survival rate, while secondary infection of pre-existing, usually abdominal, aortic aneurysms has in the past been associated with a survival rate of only 10 to 20 per cent. Peripherally located lesions are generally associated with survival, although limb loss is not uncommon. In the future a better appreciation of the principles of treatment and the prolonged use of appropriate antibiotics may have a beneficial impact on this most difficult of vascular surgical problems.

FURTHER READING

Anderson CB, Butcher HR, Ballinger WF. Mycotic aneurysms. *Arch Surg* 1974; **109**: 712–17.

Baird RN. Mycotic aortic aneurysms. *Eur J Vasc Surg* 1989; **3**: 95–6.

Berridge DC, *et al.* ^{111}In-labelled leucocyte imaging in vascular graft infection. *Br J Surg* 1989; **76**: 41–4.

Brown SL, Busuttil RW, Baker JD, Machleder HI, Moore WS, Barker WF. Bacteriologic and surgical determinants of survival in patients with mycotic aneurysms. *J Vasc Surg* 1984; **1**: 541–7.

Dean RH, Meacham PW, Weaver FA, Waterhouse G, O'Neil JA. Mycotic embolism and embolomycotic aneurysm: neglected lessons of the part. *Ann Surg* 1986; **204**: 300–7.

Haimovici H. Peripheral arterial aneurysms. In: Haimovici H, Callow AD, DePalma RG, Ernst CB, Hollier LH, eds. *Vascular Surgery*, 3rd edn. East Norwalk, Connecticut: Appleton & Lange 1989: 670–4.

Ilgenfritz FW, Jordan FT. Microbiological monitoring of aortic aneurysm wall and contents during aneurysmectomy. *Arch Surg* 1988; **123**: 506–8.

McNamara MF, Finnegan MO, Bashi KR. Abdominal aortic aneurysms infected by *Escherichia coli. Surgery* 1985; **98**: 87–92.

Osler W. The Gulstonian lectures on malignant endocarditis. *Br Med J* 1885; **1**: 467–70.

Patel S, Johnston KW. Classification and management of mycotic aneurysms. *Surg Gynecol Obstet* 1977; **144**: 691–9.

Reddy DJ. Treatment of drug related infected false aneurysm of the femoral artery—is routine revascularization justified? *J Vasc Surg* 1988; **8**: 344–5.

Reddy DJ, Ernst CB. Infected aneurysms. In: Rutherford RB, ed. *Vascular surgery*, 3rd edn. Eastbourne: W. B. Saunders 1989: 983–96.

Infected femoral artery false aneurysms in drug addicts: evolution of selective vascular reconstruction. *J Vasc Surg* 1986; 3:718–24.

Sedwitz MM, Hye RJ, Stable BE. The changing epidemiology of pseudoaneurysm. Therapeutic implications. *Arch Surg* 1988; **123**: 473–6.

Taylor CM, Deitz DM, McConnell DR, Porter JM. Treatment of infected abdominal aneurysms by extraanatomic bypass, aneurysm excision, and drainage. *Am J Surg* 1988; **155**: 655–8.

Volgelzang RL, Sohaey R. Infected aortic aneurysms: CT appearance. *J Comput Assist Tomogr* 1988; **12**: 109–12.

Wilson SE, Van Wagenen P, Passaro E. Arterial infection. *Curr Probl Surg* 1978; **15**: 1–89.

7.8.1 Carotid artery

PETER J. MORRIS

INTRODUCTION

Atheromatous disease at the origin of the internal carotid artery is a significant cause of strokes. Its recognition as a cause of neurological symptoms is important, for it may be amenable to surgical correction by carotid endarterectomy. The usual indication for carotid endarterectomy is a transient ischaemic attack, although it may be performed in patients with an evolving stroke, a completed stroke, or an asymptomatic tight carotid artery stenosis. Transient stroke-like episodes, lasting minutes to hours, have been recognized for more than a century, but it was Chiari in 1905 who first described the association between thrombosis at the carotid bifurcation and distal embolism in the internal carotid artery, this association being further elaborated by Gunning and colleagues in Oxford.

The first carotid endarterectomy was performed by de Bakey in 1953, although several other carotid bifurcation reconstructions were performed during that decade. Over the next 30 years carotid endarterectomy became widely practised for both symptomatic and asymptomatic stenoses of the internal carotid artery. However, there were marked discrepancies in the operative rates in different parts of the world, there being, for example, 20 times more operations per million of population performed in North America compared to Great Britain in the 1980s. This difference reflected the controversy concerning the value of the operation in stroke prevention, remembering that the operation itself is associated with a significant risk of death and stroke. However, much of this controversy has now been resolved, at least in the management of the patient with transient ischaemic attacks. The interim results of two large multicentre trials in Europe and North America showed a marked beneficial effect of operation in preventing stroke in patients with transient ischaemic attacks and a tight (>70 per cent) stenosis of the internal carotid artery.

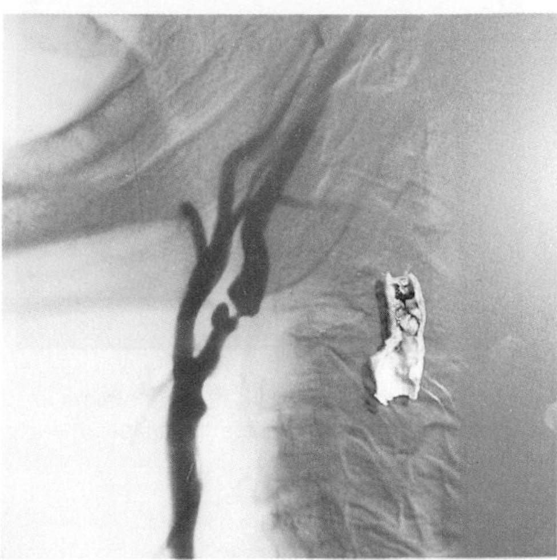

Fig. 1 Carotid angiogram showing a large atheromatous plaque at the origin of the internal carotid artery with a tight stenosis. The inset shows the endarterectomized specimen with thrombus within the lumen.

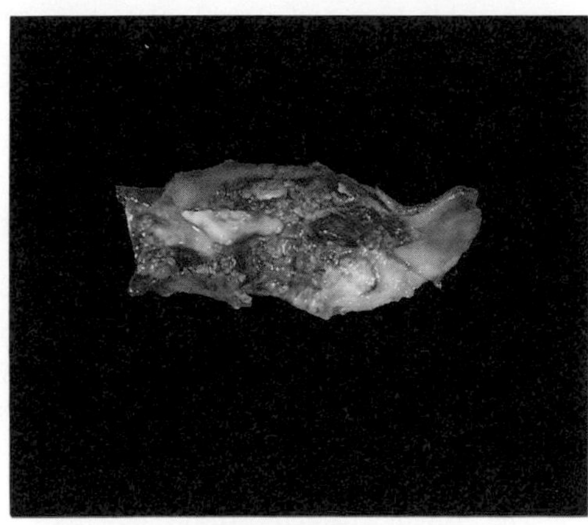

Fig. 2 An internal carotid endarterectomy specimen with thrombus within the lumen at the site of stenosis.

Pathophysiology of carotid distribution transient ischaemic attacks

Atheromatous plaques form at the carotid bifurcation, and especially in the carotid sinus. The lesion in the internal carotid artery is restricted in most instances to the origin of the artery and the carotid sinus, the artery distal to the lesion and the common carotid artery proximal to the lesion being relatively normal. The predilection for this area is undoubtedly due to the turbulence in flow created by the bifurcation and the dilated carotid sinus. The plaque may ulcerate, giving rise to thrombus formation in the bed of the ulcer or, if the plaque eventually produces a tight stenosis of the artery origin thrombus may form at the stenosed area of the plaque (Figs. 1 and 2). If thrombus is dislodged it will pass downstream, either to the retinal arteries via the ophthalmic artery or to the cerebrum via the middle cerebral artery, giving rise to a transient ischaemic attack, a complete stroke, amaurosis fugax, or a retinal infarct. An embolus from the same site in the plaque will tend to end up distally in the same place, for the bloodstream in the internal carotid artery is not random. Such patients suffer repeated attacks of amaurosis fugax, for example. Haemorrhage into an atheromatous plaque is also frequent and this can lead to sudden narrowing of the lumen as well as to ulceration. The latter may be associated with discharge of cholesterol crystals into the lumen which embolize distally, as well as thrombus formation in the bed of the ulcer. As the stenosis becomes more severe there is an increased risk of thrombosis and occlusion of the internal carotid artery, with a subsequent stroke, although occlusion does

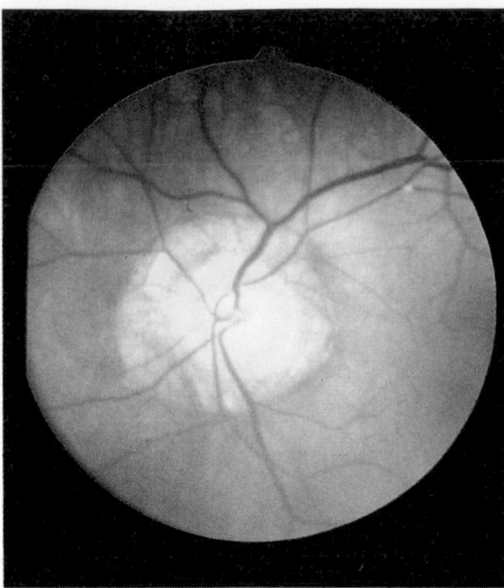

Fig. 3 Fundus of patient who had an episode of amaurosis fugax 24 h before showing a small refractile embolus peripherally (Hollenherst plaque).

not always result in a stroke. Alternatively, flow past the stenosis may become so poor as to produce transient ischaemic attacks on a purely haemodynamic basis. However, the bulk of carotid artery transient ischaemic attacks are embolic rather than haemodynamic. Such attacks in the carotid distribution may be due to emboli from proximal lesions located in sites other than the internal carotid artery, such as the heart. Three types of emboli can be detected in the retina (Fig. 3): white emboli of cardiac origin, causing segmental blockage and retinal infarcation, small white fibrin-platelet plugs which pass through the retinal circulation within minutes, and small refractile plaques (atheromatous debris).

CLINICAL PRESENTATION AND DIFFERENTIAL DIAGNOSIS

Symptoms of transient ischaemia in the carotid artery territory reflect its distribution to the eye and the anterior two-thirds of the brain. The most common symptoms are weakness, numbness, and clumsiness of the limbs, especially the arm, contralateral to the side of the lesion, or loss of vision on the side of the lesion (amaurosis fugax). The patient characteristically describes the loss of vision as being as if a blind had been pulled down (occasionally across) and as vision returns, usually in a few minutes, the blind retreats in the opposite direction. Dysphasia associated with a transient ischaemic attack is also common, especially if the left hemisphere is involved in a right-handed person. Amaurosis fugax usually lasts for only minutes while transient neurological defects last from minutes to hours.

Transient neurological deficits may be global rather than focal in nature and it is important to distinguish the two. Global symptoms include faintness, giddiness, vertigo, binocular visual loss, and syncope; these are due usually to a transient fall in blood pressure and hence cerebral perfusion. This seldom results in a focal deficit except where there is a tight carotid stenosis, as discussed earlier. The symptoms of vertebrobasilar ischaemia must also be recognized, but these are usually easily distinguished from transient ischaemic attacks in the carotid artery distribution (see Section 7.8.1).

Focal neurological deficits due to causes other than thromboembolism can present in a manner resembling a transient ischaemic attacks, but remembering that they exist will usually allow their exclusion (Table 1).

Table 1 Causes of transient focal neurological deficits not due to thromboembolism

Migraine	Hypoglycaemia
Focal epilepsy	Increased blood viscosity
Intracranial neoplasm	Polycythaemia, thrombocythaemia
Subdural haematoma	Sickle-cell disease
Intracranial aneurysm	Multiple sclerosis
Arteritis	Hysteria

Examination of the patient usually confirms that there is no residual neurological deficit. A bruit may be heard over the appropriate carotid bifurcation, but this is a relatively poor sign of an internal carotid artery stenosis, for an external carotid artery lesion may be the cause of a bruit. The absence of a bruit does not preclude a diagnosis of internal carotid artery disease as the cause of a transient ischaemic attack, as this is not uncommon in the presence of a very tight stenosis. Examination of the heart for evidence of valve disease as a possible source of emboli is also important. In patients who have had an attack of amaurosis fugax not long before being seen, examination of the fundi may be rewarding in that emboli may still be identified even though vision has recovered. If vision remains defective an embolus, usually refractile, can often be identified.

INVESTIGATION

There have been major changes in the investigation of carotid distribution transient ischaemic attacks in recent years. The gold standard has always been carotid angiography with the addition of CT scanning or magnetic resonance imaging (MRI) of the brain in recent years. However, the risk of a stroke being precipitated by angiography is between 1 and 4 per cent when this is performed for extracerebrovascular disease, and this has provided enormous impetus in recent years for the development of non-invasive methods of determining the presence of significant carotid artery disease. Oculoplethysmography and oculopneumoplethysmography have served this role for several years, at least in determining which patients should have angiography (see Section 7.4). However, the advent of the duplex scan, which combines real time B-mode scanning with Doppler sound spectral analysis, allows not only the carotid bifurcation to be imaged but also the degree of stenosis to be calculated. The addition of colour has further refined the technique: many vascular units perform a carotid endarterectomy on the basis of duplex scanning plus CT or MRI. In Oxford, for example, carotid endarterectomy is performed without angiography in 50 to 60 per cent of cases. Digital subtraction angiography has largely replaced conventional angiography but, in general, intra-arterial digital subtraction angiography is necessary to obtain satisfactory pictures, intravenous angiography having proved to be disappointing in that respect.

Transcranial Doppler analysis of blood velocity in the intracerebral arteries is a new approach to the evaluation of collateral cerebral blood flow, as is the development of probes for the duplex scanner which allow imaging of the intracerebral vessels. However, it is not yet possible to define their eventual role in diagnosis.

If there is any question of a cardiac focus for emboli an echocardiogram should be performed. Careful cardiac evaluation is always essential, however, for one-third of patients with carotid transient ischaemic attacks die of myocardial infarction within 5 years of undergoing carotid endarterectomy. Other investigations include all those that would be performed in any patient with atheromatous arterial disease, such as full blood count and blood lipid analysis.

MANAGEMENT OF CAROTID DISTRIBUTION TRANSIENT ISCHAEMIC ATTACKS

Once a diagnosis of a transient ischaemic attack in the carotid distribution has been made or even suspected then the patient should be given aspirin, 300 mg/day, and referred for evaluation by either a neurologist or vascular surgeon specializing in this area. Duplex scanning of the carotid arteries will usually enable a diagnosis of a carotid lesion to be established or excluded. A CT scan or MRI of the brain is advisable not only to exclude any other intracerebral lesion but also to show any existing areas of infarction. If a tight stenosis (>70 per cent) is present carotid endarterectomy is indicated, provided the patient's general health, in particular their cardiac status, is sound (Table 2). Age of itself is not a contraindication to carotid endarterectomy but the majority of patients will be between 65 and 75 years of age. If the stenosis is minimal, (0–29 per cent), surgery is not indicated: these patients have a worse outcome in terms of stroke than the non-surgical patients because of the perioperative mortality/stroke rate and the very low risk of a subsequent stroke associated with minimal lesions. These patients should be maintained on aspirin therapy. The appropriate treatment for moderate stenoses (30–70 per cent) is unclear at this time: both the North American and European trials are continuing to enter patients in this category. If not entered into trials carotid endarterectomy is probably best withheld at this time and the patients should be treated with aspirin. If transient ischaemic attacks continue to occur during treatment with aspirin, surgery or anticoagulation with warfarin or coumadin should be considered.

Table 2 The management of an internal carotid artery stenosis causing transient ischaemic attacks

Degree of stenosis	Management
70–99%	Carotid endarterectomy + aspirin + best medical management
30–69%	Aspirin + best management ? Carotid endarterectomy
0–29%	Aspirin + best medical management

Whatever the management, any hypertension should be well controlled and hyperlipidaemia treated by diet or, if severe, by cholesterol lowering agents. All patients are encouraged to stop smoking.

Table 3 Possible indications for carotid endarterectomy in the presence of a stenosis of the internal carotid artery

Transient ischaemic attack, including amaurosis fugax
Retinal infarction
Completed stroke
Evolving stroke
Asymptomatic internal carotid artery stenosis
Cerebral hypoperfusion

INDICATIONS FOR CAROTID ENDARTERECTOMY (Table 3)

Transient ischaemic attack

A transient ischaemic attack is defined as an acute loss of focal cerebral or ocular function with symptoms lasting less than 24 h and which, after adequate investigation is presumed to be due to embolic or thrombotic vascular disease. This definition not only includes transient neurological defects but also transient episodes of blindness (amaurosis fugax). The 24-h time period is arbitrary, but has been accepted for many years and indeed the majority of attacks last from minutes to hours. Those due to an atheromatous plaque at the origin of the internal carotid artery (Fig. 1), are by far the most common indication for carotid endarterectomy.

Retinal infarction

If an embolus lodges long enough in the retinal arteries, infarction of part or all of the retina may occur. This is regarded in the same light as amaurosis fugax with respect to indications for surgery.

Completed stroke

A patient whose neurological deficit lasts longer than 24 h but makes a full recovery or who is left with a permanent but stable neurological deficit and who has a stenosis of the internal carotid artery appropriate to the neurological signs is also a candidate for carotid endarterectomy, especially if a good recovery has been made.

Evolving stroke

This is a controversial indication. Early experience of carotid endarterectomy in this group of patients was accompanied by a high perioperative mortality (40–60 per cent) and the procedure was abandoned in this situation. However, cautious evaluation of the value of carotid endarterectomy in carefully selected patients with an evolving stroke or a fluctuating neurological deficit, where urgent investigations have confirmed the presence of an appropriate lesion, is now taking place in several centres.

Asymptomatic stenosis of the internal carotid artery

This is another controversial area. It has been an indication for carotid endarterectomy in a significant proportion of patients in the United States, but hardly at all in Great Britain. Retrospective and prospective studies of patients with a known asymptomatic stenosis of the internal carotid artery suggest that the risk of stroke in these patients is relatively low, and indeed less than the risk of myocardial infarction. Furthermore, when strokes do occur they are usually preceded by transient ischaemic attacks. The associated risk of death and stroke from the operation itself is, therefore, probably not outweighed by any benefit of subsequent stroke protection. If cardiac surgery is required, this is generally performed first, followed by the carotid surgery at a later date, rather than as a combined procedure, although again the indication for the carotid endarterectomy remains unresolved. There are a number of multicentre trials in progress comparing medical management plus carotid endarterectomy versus medical management alone in asymptomatic patients with a tight stenosis of the internal carotid artery, the first of which suggests, but not conclusively, that there may be a modest benefit of surgery. However, for the moment, until results of later trials are available, the controversy remains unresolved.

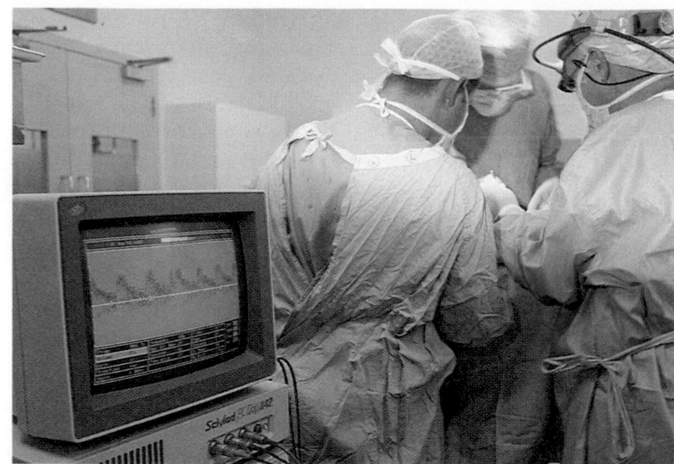

Fig. 4 Carotid endarterectomy in progress with continuous monitoring of middle cerebral artery velocity on the side of operation with transcranial Doppler.

Cerebral hypoperfusion

This is an extremely complicated clinical problem, in that there is no established method of determining whether a tight stenosis of the internal carotid artery, especially if bilateral, is responsible for transient neurological deficits by causing hypoperfusion rather than emboli. Certainly in some instances it must be, and the development of transcranial Doppler analysis and duplex scanning of the circle of Willis may in time allow patients with cerebral hypoperfusion, who would benefit from carotid endarterectomy, to be better defined. It is not likely to be a large number, based on the experience of the intracerebral–extracerebral reconstruction trial of several years ago.

CAROTID ENDARTERECTOMY

Timing of the operation

Once a firm diagnosis is established an elective operation can be planned as soon as possible. The risks of a stroke before surgery after the patient has started taking aspirin are relatively small and the risks of perioperative complications are reduced by taking the time for a careful evaluation of the patient and in particular his or her cardiac status.

Anaesthesia

Although some surgeons perform the operation under local anaesthetic, this is uncomfortable for the patient over the 1 to 2 h required (longer if a patch is used to close the arteriotomy) and most surgeons prefer a general anaesthetic. It is essential that blood pressure control is well established before the patient comes to surgery and it needs to be carefully monitored via an intra-arterial line throughout the procedure.

Monitoring of cerebral ischaemia

Where the operation is performed under local anaesthesia it is possible for the patient to report any neurological deficit, provided they have not required so much sedation as to lose their awareness of events. In patients under general anaesthetic, electroencephalography is valuable in units where the appropriate facilities exist (simple three-channel EEG monitoring is of no value). More recently monitoring of middle cerebral artery velocity on the side of the operation with transcranial Doppler is being widely adopted (Fig. 4). Whether this will prove an adequate measure of the maintenance of collateral flow remains to be seen.

Operation

The carotid bifurcation is exposed through an oblique incision along the anterior border of the sternomastoid (Fig. 5). Having exposed the carotid bifurcation, arterial pressures are measured in the common carotid artery proximal to the lesion and in the internal carotid artery distal to the lesion to establish the presence of a pressure gradient, and then the common carotid artery is clamped and the internal carotid pressure recorded. This is the stump pressure and is a measure of the collateral flow from the other side and the vertebrobasilar system via the circle of Willis. If the pressure is below 50 to 60 mmHg, surgeons who shunt selectively would consider that an indication for a shunt. Blood flow in the internal carotid artery may also be measured, using either an electromagnetic flow meter or more recently an ultrasound probe (OpDop). This provides a baseline for comparison with a similar measurement made after reconstruction.

The patient is then heparinized and clamps are applied to the common, internal, and external carotid arteries. An arteriotomy starting in the common carotid artery below the lesion is carried through the lesion into the internal carotid artery, distal to the disease (Fig. 6). If a shunt is to be used, it is inserted at this time. The two most widely used shunts are the Javid shunt and the Pruitt shunt (Fig. 7). The latter is more easily inserted and can be moved more easily out of the way during the endarterectomy (Fig. 8).

The endarterectomy requires identification of a plane between the plaque and the media: generally this lies somewhere between the outer one-third and inner two-thirds of the media. If the correct plane is identified the lesion comes away without difficulty.

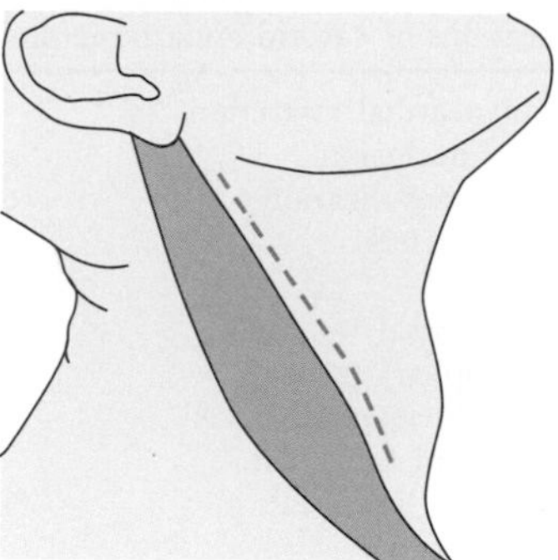

Fig. 5 Skin incision for carotid endarterectomy is made along the line of the anterior border of the sternomastoid.

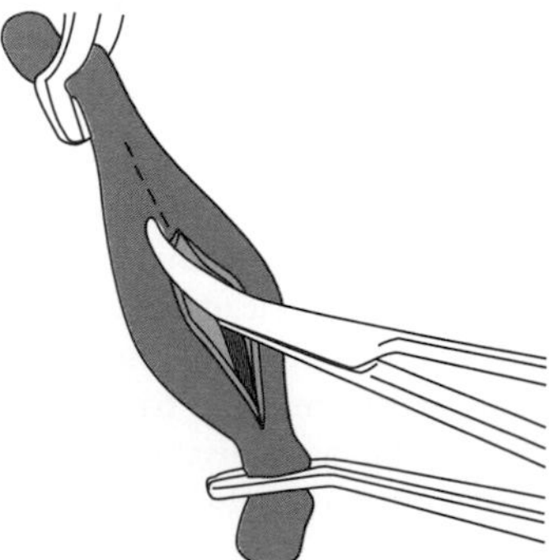

Fig. 6 Arteriotomy commencing in the common artery below the lesion in the internal carotid and carried up the artery through the plaque into the area distal to the lesion.

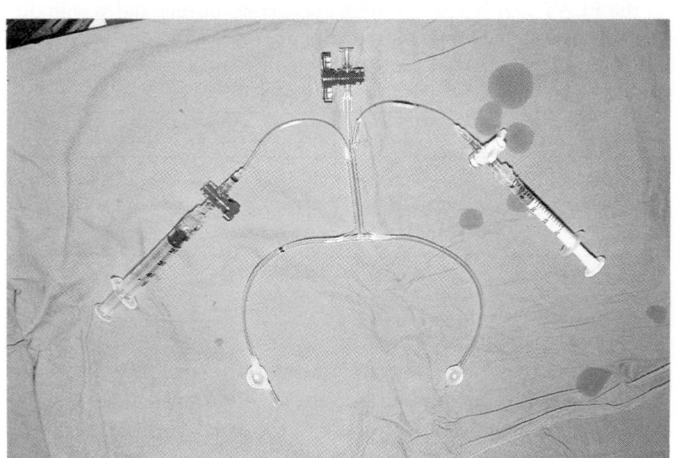

Fig. 7 Pruitt shunt with the balloons inflated.

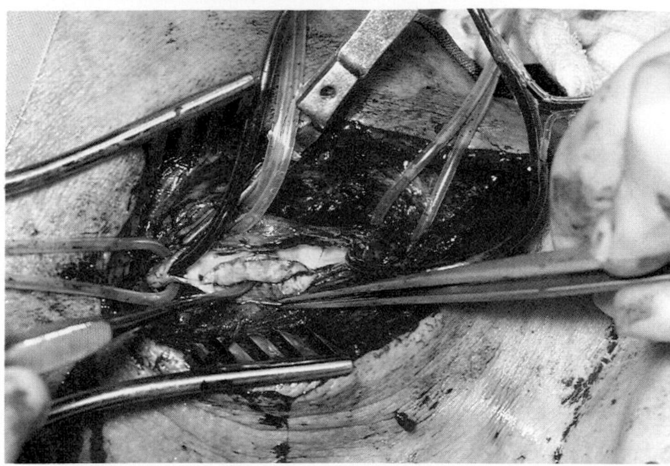

Fig. 8 Pruitt shunt in place while endarterectomy is proceeding.

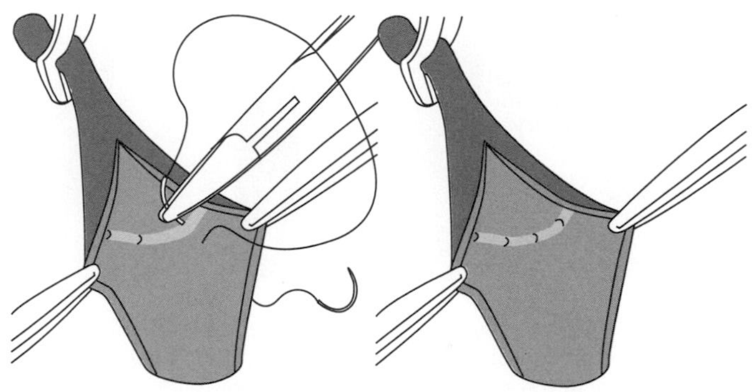

Fig. 9 Insertion of tacking sutures (7/0 Prolene) at distal flap to ensure that it is firmly adherent.

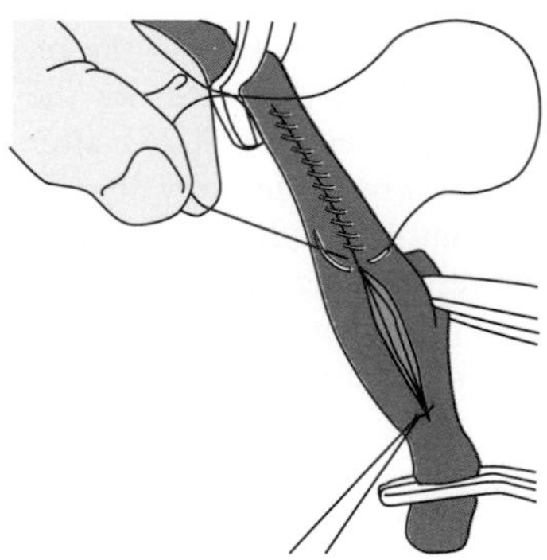

Fig. 10 Closure of arteriotomy with continuous 6/0 Prolene.

It is essential to obtain a tightly adherent distal flap in the internal carotid artery and if this is not the case it should be tacked down with some fine 7–0 prolene sutures (Fig. 9).

Having completed the endarterectomy the arteriotomy can be closed directly with a continuous prolene suture (Fig. 10) or with a vein (internal jugular vein or saphenous vein), polytetrafluoroethylene (Gore-Tex or Impra), or Dacron patch (Fig. 11). In recent years many vascular surgeons have routinely closed most arteriotomies with a patch, as the recognition of a relatively high incidence of recurrent stenoses, usually at the distal end of the endarterectomy has become apparent. Occasionally if the plaque is localized to the origin of the internal carotid artery and the external carotid is free of disease, the bifurcation can be reconstructed by suturing the posterior walls of these two arteries together and then suturing the anterior walls together; in effect this reconstructs a higher bifurcation, but widens the artery at the end of the endarterectomy (Fig. 12).

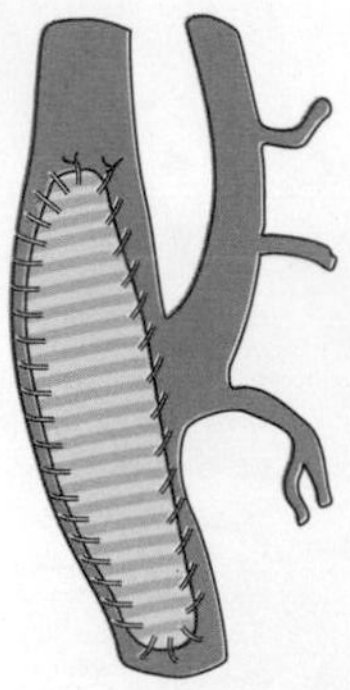

Fig. 11 Closure of arteriotomy with a knitted Dacron patch and 6/0 Prolene.

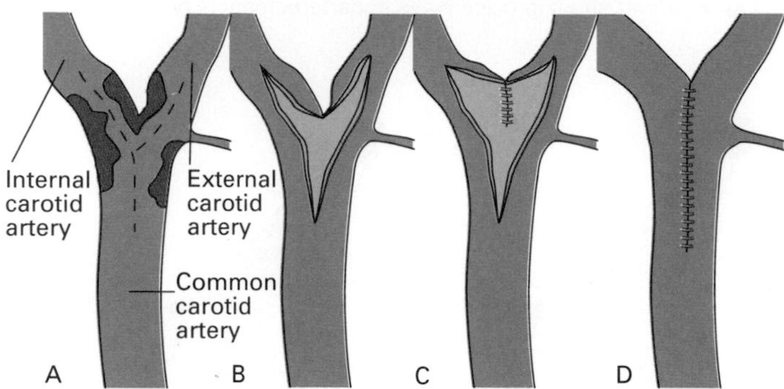

Fig. 12 Closure of arteriotomy using the external carotid artery such that the bifurcation is reconstructed at a higher level providing a wider artery at the site of the endarterectomy.

Postoperative monitoring

Following surgery the patient is kept in the recovery room until awake and then returned to the ward. As the vast majority of perioperative strokes occur in the first 24 h after operation neurological observations must be made every 30 min over the first 12 h and then every hour until 24 h. It is also important to maintain a stable blood pressure avoiding any periods of hypo- or hypertension. This should not generally be a problem if the patient has come to operation with well controlled blood pressure.

If any neurological deficit appears relevant to the side of operation, a rapid return to the operating room is indicated, with exploration of the neck and exposure of the carotid vessels. The endarterectomized site should be re-explored with removal of any thrombus; a careful inspection of the distal flap is mandatory. If thrombosis and occlusion of the internal carotid artery has occurred restoration of the cerebral flow may increase the likelihood of recovery or limit the extent of the neurological deficit. Although a CT scan of the brain and duplex scan of the operated side would be desirable, it is not practical to do this because of the loss in time in restoring flow in an occluded vessel that would result. Thrombus is found in less than 50 per cent of patients re-explored, and whether removing this will limit the evolving deficit is unknown. As any one surgeon's experience in this area is small it probably never will be, but it would instinctively seem an appropriate course to follow.

Table 4 Complications of carotid endarterectomy

Death – stroke or myocardial infarction
Stroke – thrombosis – occlusion
– embolization
– cerebral haemorrhage
Haematoma
Nerve pareses – hypoglossal
– glossopharyngeal
– facial 'marginal branch'
– recurrent laryngeal
– superior laryngeal
– accessory
Wound infection

Complications of carotid endarterectomy (Table 4)

The major complications of this procedure are death, either from stroke or a myocardial infarction, or a stroke. A stroke occurring during the operation or generally within the first 24 h of surgery may be transient or more severe, leading to a permanent disability. The combined perioperative mortality and stroke rate as defined in the European and North American trials (death or neurological deficit resulting in a permanent disability and occurring during and within 30 days of surgery) should be less than 5 per cent (Table 5). A neurological deficit may be due to thrombosis at the site of endarterectomy, with either occlusion or embolization, or an intracerebral haemorrhage.

Table 5 Combined mortality and disabling stroke rate (as defined in the ECST and NASCET trials) occurring during and within 30 days of carotid endarterectomy for tight stenosis (70–99 per cent) of the internal carotid artery in the two multicentre trials and in the author's personal experience for comparison.

Degree	Trial	No.	%
70–99%	North American trial (NASCET)	328	2.1
70–99%	European trial (ECST)	455	3.7
	Oxford (PJM)	305	2.5

As most patients are receiving aspirin significant haematomas are relatively common, but rarely need draining. Local nerve pareses are also not uncommon but are usually transient, recovering within weeks to months. Retraction is the usual cause of these local nerve pareses, which is often unavoidable, especially in the case of the hypoglossal nerve and a high carotid bifurcation. Retraction of the vagus may result in paresis of the superior or recurrent laryngeal nerve. In general the patient can be reassured that recovery will take place within a month or two.

Restenosis

The availability of duplex scanning after carotid endarterectomy has shown that the incidence of recurrent stenosis, commonly at the distal end of the endarterectomy, is much greater than hitherto believed, perhaps of the order of 15 to 30 per cent at 5 years. However, the development of symptoms related to the recurrent

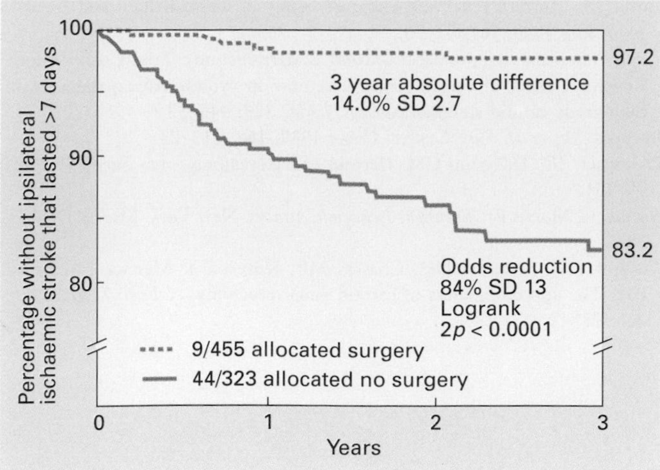

Fig. 13 Results of ECST showing survival free of any stroke that lasted more than 7 days in patients with 70 to 99 per cent stenosis allocated to surgical (n=455) or medical (n=323) treatment.

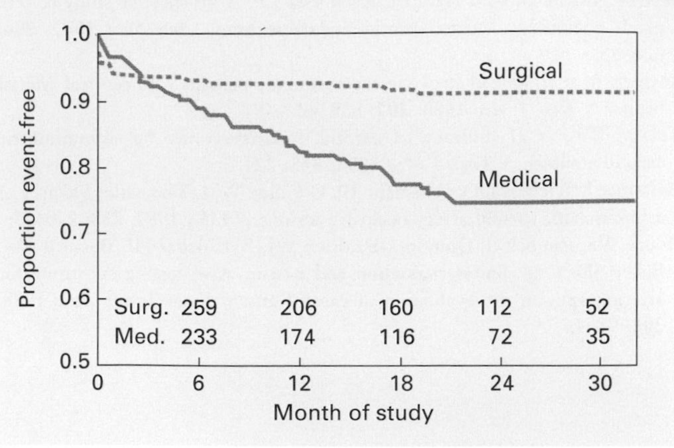

Fig. 14 Results of NASCET showing survival free of any ipsilateral stroke in patients with 70 to 99 per cent stenosis allocated to surgical (n=328) or medical (n=331) treatment.

stenosis is very uncommon. Restenosis may be due to myointimal hypertrophy or atheroma. In the absence of symptoms no treatment other than continued daily aspirin is necessary. The development of transient ischaemic attacks is an indication for reoperation. Whether the incidence of restenosis is less with patch closures is not known at this time.

PREVENTION OF STROKE

As carotid endarterectomy for stenosis of the internal carotid artery is an operation carried out in the expectation that it will prevent a subsequent stroke, it is perhaps surprising that it has taken nearly 30 years to establish that at least in the case of a tight symptomatic stenosis (>70 per cent) it does indeed do so. The simultaneous interim analyses of the European Carotid Surgery Trial (ECST) and the North American Symptomatic Carotid Endarterectomy Trial (NASCET) produced very similar results.

In the ECST 2518 patients who had had a carotid-territory non-disabling ischaemic stroke, transient ischaemic attacks, or retinal infarct and a stenotic lesion in the relevant internal carotid artery were randomized either to best medical management or best medical management plus carotid endarterectomy. All patients received antiplatelet therapy. For the 778 patients with a severe stenosis (70–99 per cent) the total risk of surgical death, surgical stroke, ipsilateral ischaemic stroke, or any other stroke was 12.3 per cent, compared to 21.9 per cent in the non-surgical group ($2p < 0.01$) (Fig. 13). In contrast, in the minimal stenosis group (0–29 per cent) there was little risk of ipsilateral ischaemic stroke in the non-surgical group so that any possible benefits of surgery were outweighed by the perioperative risks of surgery. It was not clear in the patients with a moderate stenosis (30–69 per cent) whether surgery was beneficial or not, and entry into the trial of such patients is continuing.

In the NASCET 659 patients with a severe stenosis (70–99 per cent) who had had a hemispheric or retinal transient ischaemic attack or a non-disabling stroke were randomized to best medical management or best medical management plus carotid endarterectomy. All patients received antiplatelet therapy. The cumulative risk of stroke at 2 years was 26 per cent in the non-surgical group but only 9 per cent in the surgical group ($p < 0.001$) (Fig. 14). In the moderate stenosis group (30–69 per cent), just as in ECST, there was no clear answer and entry to the trial is continuing. Patients with minimal stenoses were not entered into this trial.

Thus, these two trials convincingly demonstrate the beneficial effect of carotid endarterectomy in a patient with a tight symptomatic internal carotid artery. Furthermore the ECST shows that surgery is not indicated in patients with a symptomatic minimal stenosis. Studies of patients with a symptomatic moderate stenosis are continuing. It is not known whether the operation has a place in patients with a tight asymptomatic stenosis in reducing the risk of a subsequent stroke, but trials in progress at the present time should provide an answer to that question in due course.

FURTHER READING

Barnett HJM, Haines SJ. Carotid endarterectomy for asymptomatic carotid stenosis. *N Engl J Med* 1993; **328**: 276–8.

Chambers BR, Norris JW. Outcome in patients with asymptomatic neck bruits. *N Engl J Med* 1986; **315**: 860–5.

Chiari H. Uber des Verhalten des Teilungswinkels der Carotis communis bei der endarteritis chronica deformans. *Verl Dtsch Ges Pathol* 1905; **9**: 326–30.

DeBakey ME. Successful carotid endarterectomy for cerebrovascular insufficiency. *JAMA* 1975; **233**: 1083–5.

Eastcott HHG, Pickering GW, Robb CG. Reconstruction of internal carotid artery in a patient with intermittent attacks of hemiplegia. *Lancet* 1954; **ii**: 994–6.

European Carotid Surgery Trialist's Collaborative Group (1991). MRC European Carotid Surgery Trial: interim results for symptomatic patients with severe (70–99 per cent) or with mild (0–29 per cent) carotid stenosis. *Lancet* 1991; **337**: 1235–43.

Grotta JC. Current medical and surgical therapy for cerebrosvascular disease. *N Engl J Med* 1987; **317**: 1505–16.

Gunning AJ, Pickering GW, Robb-Smith AH, Ross Russell R. Mural thrombosis of the internal carotid artery and subsequent embolism. *Q J Med* 1964; **33**: 155–95.

Hankey GJ, Warlow CP, Sellar RJ. Cerebral angiographic risk in mild cerebrovascular disease. *Stroke* 1990; **21**: 209–22.

Hertzer NR, Bevin E, O'Hara PJ, Krajewski LP. A prospective study of vein patch angioplasty during carotid endarterectomy. *Ann Surg* 1987; **206**: 628–35.

Heyman A, *et al.* Risk of stroke in asymptomatic persons with cervical arterial bruits. *N Engl J Med* 1980; **302**: 838–42.

Hobson RW, *et al.* Efficacy of carotid endarterectomy for asymptomatic carotid stenosis. *N Engl J Med* 1993; **328**: 221–7.

Meissmer I, Wiebers DO, Whisnant JP, O'Fallon WM. The natural history of asymptomatic carotid artery occlusive lesions. *JAMA* 1987; **258**: 2704–7.

Moore WS, Ziomek S, Quinones-Baldrich WJ, Machleder HI, Busuttil RW, Baker JD. Can clinical evaluation and non-invasive testing substitute for arteriography in the evaluation of carotid artery disease? *Ann Surg* 1988; **208**: 91–4.

Murie JA, Morris PJ. Carotid endarterectomy in Great Britain and Ireland. *Br J Surg* 1986; **76**: 867–70.

North American Symptomatic Carotid Endarterectomy Trial Collaborators. Beneficial effect of carotid endarterectomy in symptomatic patients with high-grade carotid stenosis. *N Engl J Med* **325**: 445–53.

Sterpetti AV, *et al. Surg Gynecol Obstet* 1989; **168**: 217–23.

Thompson JE, Talkinton CM. Carotid endarterectomy. *Adv Surg* 1992; **26**: 99–131.

Warlow C, Morris PJ. *Transient Ischaemic Attacks.* New York: Marcel Dekker, 1982.

Winslow CM, Solomon DH, Chassin MR, Kosecoff J, Merrick NJ, Brook RH. The appropriateness of carotid endarterectomy. *N Engl J Med* 1988; **318**: 721–7.

7.8.2 Vertebrobasilar, subclavian, and innominate arteries

PETER J. MORRIS

INTRODUCTION

The vertebrobasilar arterial system supplies the brain-stem, occipital lobes, and medial aspects of the temporal lobes. Symptoms arising from ischaemia causing loss of function in one or more of these segments can produce a complex of symptoms (Table 1) which may be due to causes other than thromboembolism, especially when they occur in isolation. Because of the uncertainty of the diagnosis, surgery has played a far less prominent role in the management of vertebrobasilar transient ischaemic attacks than is the case for those in the carotid distribution. Nevertheless, epidemiological data from the Mayo Clinic in the 1970s suggested that the risk of stroke after a vertebrobasilar transient ischaemic attack was similar to that of patients with a similar attack in the carotid distribution. Thus identification of patients who might benefit from surgery is of considerable importance, although this has proved to be extremely difficult.

Table 1 Common symptoms of vertebrobasilar transient ischaemic attacks

Vertigo
Ataxia
Hemiparesis
Drop attacks
Sensory loss (unilateral or bilateral)
Diplopia
Binocular visual loss
Dysphagia
Dysarthria
Facial tingling or numbness (unilateral or bilateral)

PATHOPHYSIOLOGY

Obstruction of the origin of a single vertebral artery, usually by atheroma, should not result in distal ischaemia of the vertebrobasilar circulation if the contralateral vertebral artery is normal. In general, stenosis of the origins of both vertebral arteries is necessary to produce vertebrobasilar ischaemia; even then ischaemia may not occur if the internal carotid artery on each side is normal, along with a normal circle of Willis with intact posterior communicating arteries. However, there is often associated carotid bifurcation disease and intracerebral disease which, in association with disease of the origins of the vertebral arteries, can result in poor perfusion of the hindbrain. It should also be remembered that an intact so-called normal circle of Willis is found in only about 50 per cent of individuals.

In contrast to transient ischaemic attacks associated with stenoses of the internal carotid artery, those due to vertebrobasilar ischaemia are most often haemodynamic in origin. Whether it is also possible to produce temporary obstruction or kinking of the vertebral arteries in patients with cervical spondylosis by rotation of the neck is uncertain; although obstruction of a vertebral artery by osteophytes has been demonstrated, this should not result in symptoms unless there is associated disease in the contralateral vertebral artery.

A rather uncommon, but better defined, cause of vertebrobasilar ischaemia is the syndrome known as subclavian steal. In this condition there is a significant stenosis or even complete obstruction of the origin of the left subclavian artery, such that when the patient uses the left arm blood passing up the right vertebral artery passes into the left vertebral artery to feed the subclavian artery distal to the obstruction (Fig. 1).

In addition, stenosis or occlusion of the origin of the innominate

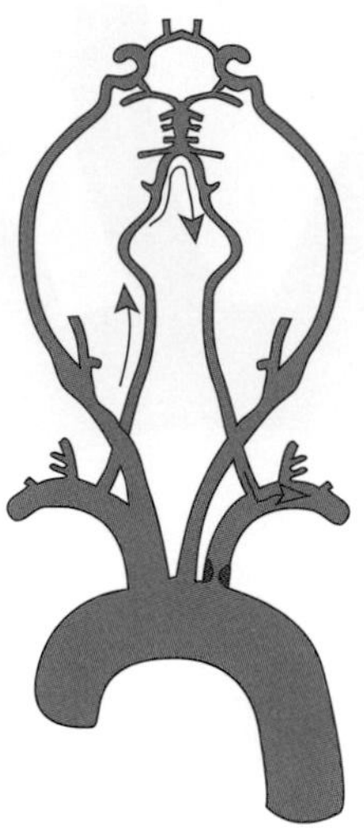

Fig. 1 Subclavian steal with a stenosis at the origin of the left subclavian artery and stealing of blood from the contralateral vertebral artery down the ipsilateral vertebral artery into the subclavian artery.

artery may be associated with steal down the right vertebral artery and internal carotid artery (innominate steal), causing symptoms associated with either vertebrobasilar ischaemia or carotid distribution ischaemia, or a combination of both.

CLINICAL PRESENTATION AND DIFFERENTIAL DIAGNOSIS

Vertebrobasilar transient ischaemic attacks are difficult to diagnose unless several symptoms occur together during an attack or in separate attacks. Vertigo is the most common symptom of vertebrobasilar ischaemia, but is more often due to other causes, such as disorders of the vestibule (it is important to establish that the patient is having true vertigo). Transient episodes of ataxia are also not uncommon. Other symptoms include diplopia, dysphagia, dysarthria, and drop attacks. The drop attacks are a striking phenomenon when the patient recalls just dropping to the ground without any prewarning symptoms, perhaps, but usually not, losing consciousness transiently, and then recovering immediately. Tingling and numbness of the face and mouth or, indeed, half the body may occur, as also may transient hemiparesis.

Visual loss is the second most frequent symptom after vertigo and is quite variable, ranging from reduced vision in one half field, perhaps accompanied by positive scotomata, to impairment of vision on both sides. Bilateral impairment of vision ranges from total blindness to a generalized mistiness of vision; positive or negative scotomata may occur as spots or moving lights which may be coloured.

The innominate steal or subclavian steal syndromes are classically produced by exercise of the arm on the appropriate side. Apart from bruits in the root of the neck these syndromes will be associated with a distinct pressure gradient between the arms on each side (at least 20 mmHg). However, it must be stressed that the presentation of patients with innominate or subclavian steal is not classical and the association of symptoms with a radiological finding is often difficult. A differential diagnosis of vertebrobasilar ischaemia includes the same causes as outlined in the differential diagnosis of carotid artery transient ischaemic attacks (Section 7.8.1).

INVESTIGATION

The investigation of patients with putative vertebrobasilar ischaemia is still based largely on angiography. An aortic arch study with selective viewing of both vertebral arteries and both carotid arteries, together with intracerebral views is required. The demonstration of stenoses at the origin of the vertebral artery does not necessarily confirm a diagnosis of vertebrobasilar ischaemia, and there is a lack of adequate functional tests of vertebrobasilar ischaemia. Duplex scanning of the vertebral arteries allows examination of the arteries in different positions of the neck. This, along with transcranial Doppler and duplex scanning of the circle of Willis, is likely to allow more precise definition of the relevance of extracerebral vascular disease, in particular vertebral disease, to symptoms compatible with a diagnosis of vertebrobasilar transient ischaemia.

Angiography remains an essential investigation for vertebrobasilar ischaemia, whatever the proposed cause might be. It demonstrates stenoses or occlusions of the origin of the left subclavian artery and the innominate artery, and also shows retrograde flow down the left vertebral in a subclavian steal syndrome (Fig. 2), and down the right carotid and vertebral in an innominate steal syndrome. Reverse flow can also be detected by duplex scanning the appropriate arteries in comparison with the contralateral side.

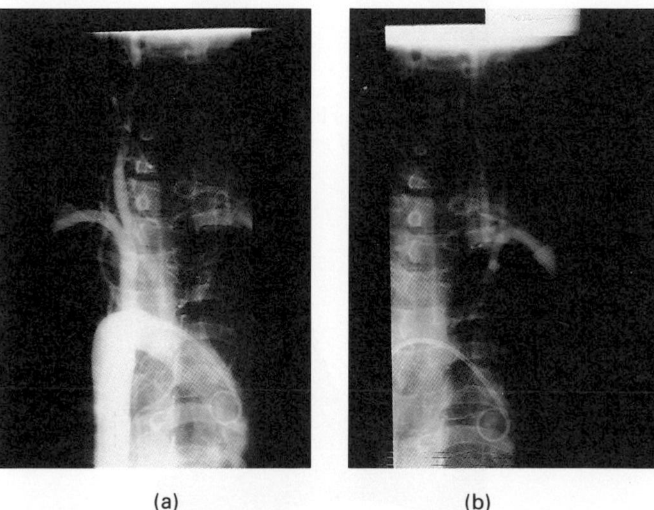

(a) (b)

Fig. 2 An angiogram in a patient with a subclavian steal showing obstruction of the origin of the left subclavian artery (a) and later films showing retrograde flow down the left vertebral artery into the subclavian artery distal to the obstruction (b).

INDICATIONS FOR SURGERY

In the presence of symptoms compatible with vertebrobasilar ischaemia, appropriate lesions demonstrable on angiography, such as bilateral vertebral artery stenoses, left subclavian artery stenosis with reverse flow down the left vertebral artery, or innominate artery stenosis with reverse flow down the common carotid and vertebral arteries on the right side, can be considered an indication for surgery. However, patients in whom a diagnosis can be reached of vertebrobasilar ischaemia due to a surgically correctable lesion are relatively few. The steal syndromes are the most clear-cut diagnoses, but even here the diagnosis often remains speculative and is only confirmed by a satisfactory outcome following surgical correction of the defect.

OPERATIONS

Vertebral artery

A stenosis of the origin of the vertebral artery may be approached directly and an endarterectomy performed at the origin or preferably through the subclavian artery (Fig. 3). Alternatively the vertebral artery can be divided distal to the lesion and reimplanted into the common carotid artery (Fig. 4). These procedures are performed through a transverse incision in the root of the neck, after division of the sternomastoid.

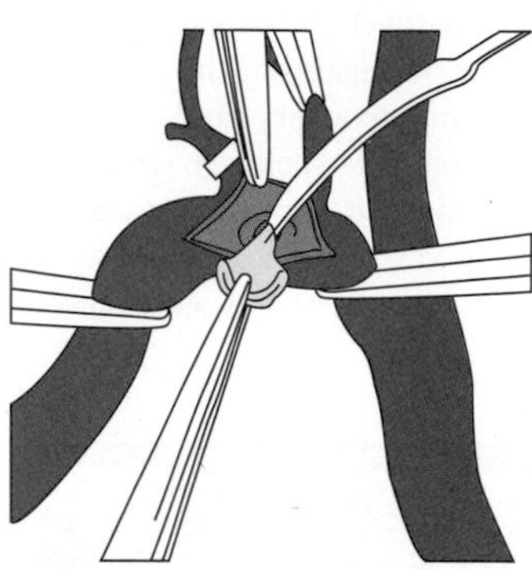

Fig. 3 The subclavian artery has been opened opposite the origin of the vertebral artery and a plug of atheroma extracted from the vertebral orifice.

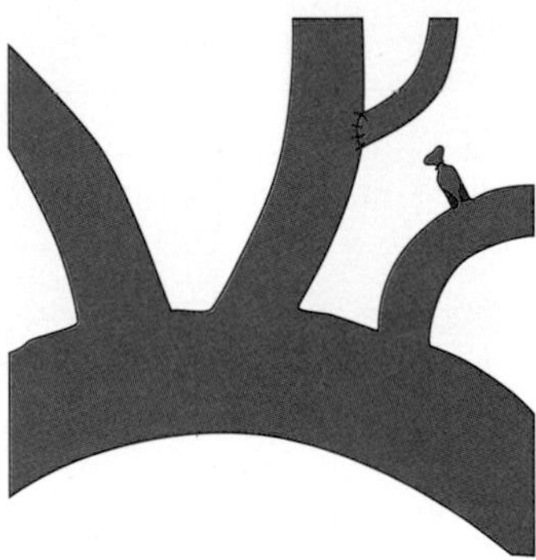

Fig. 4 The vertebral artery has been divided distal to the stenosis at its origin and reimplanted into the common carotid artery.

Subclavian steal

Although the original approach to a stenosis of the origin of the subclavian artery was via a left anterolateral thoracotomy with endarterectomy of the artery and closure with a patch, this is rarely performed today. The current operations of choice do not involve opening the chest. A graft, prosthetic or vein, is inserted end-to-side between the common carotid artery and the subclavian artery distal to the origin of the vertebral artery (Fig. 5). An approach which avoids clamping the common carotid artery involves running a graft, vein or prosthetic, from the axillary artery on the contralateral side subcutaneously just below the sternal notch to the axillary artery on the affected side (Fig. 6). Finally the subclavian artery may be divided proximal to the origin of the vertebral artery and anastomosed end-to-side to the common carotid artery (Fig. 7).

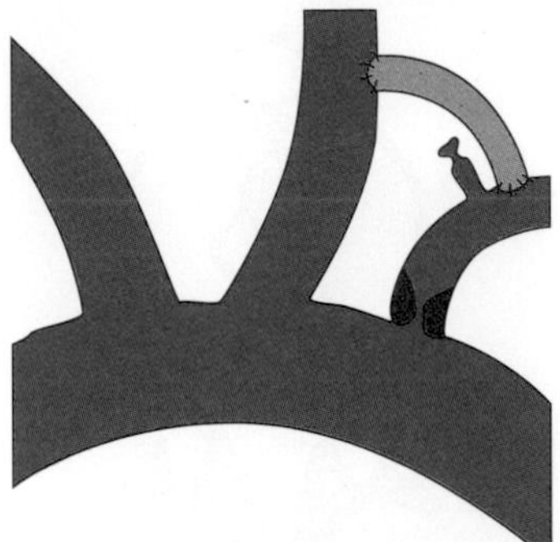

Fig. 5 Left carotid top left subclavian Dacron bypass graft.

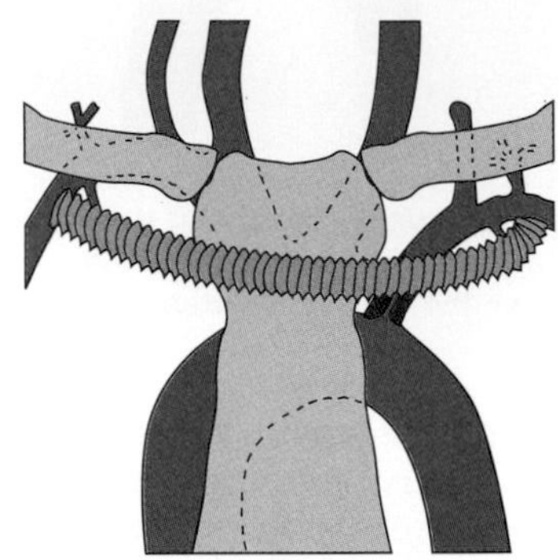

Fig. 6 Axilloaxillary graft, either saphenous vein or prosthetic, passes from between each axillary artery in front of the sternum.

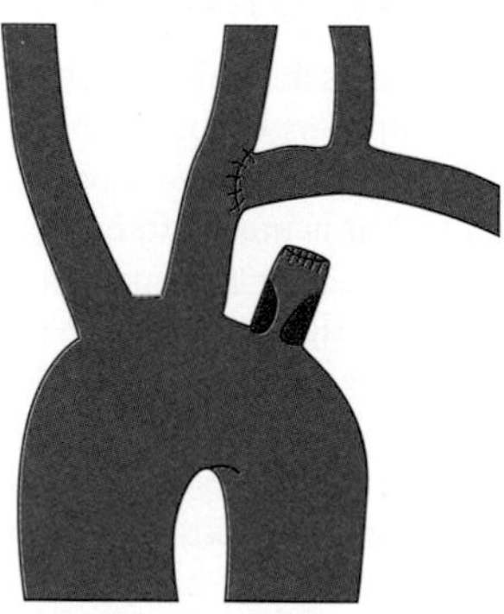

Fig. 7 The subclavian artery is divided in the root of the neck proximal to the origin of the vertebral artery and anastomosed end-to-side to the common carotid artery.

Innominate steal

Although it is possible to perform an endarterectomy directly on the origin of the innominate artery, the simplest approach is to run a Dacron graft off the arch of the aorta and anastomose it end-to-end to the distal innominate artery at its bifurcation (Fig. 8). The innominate artery and its origin from the arch of the aorta is best approached by a median sternotomy.

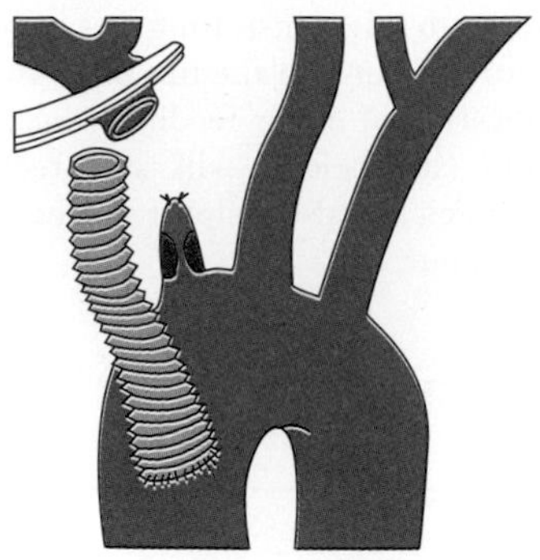

Fig. 8 The innominate artery is divided distal to the stenosis at its origin and a prosthetic graft (Gore-Tex or Dacron) run from the arch of the aorta to the distal innominate artery.

In the presence of complex disease, such as stenoses of the subclavian and innominate arteries, reconstruction can be satisfactorily performed with a bifurcated Dacron graft, the legs of the graft being anastomosed to the distal innominate artery and left subclavian artery distal to the stenosis but proximal to the vertebral artery.

RESULTS

Surgery for vertebrobasilar ischaemia, which now rarely involves opening the chest, can be performed with minimal morbidity. However, it is much more difficult to evaluate the efficacy of surgery in terms of relief of symptoms because of the varied nature of the symptom complex. Nevertheless with careful selection of patients, the outcome can be favourable. The outcome of surgery for innominate or subclavian artery steals in terms of symptom relief is much better in general than for vertebral artery surgery. If severe bilateral carotid stenoses are present in a patient with symptoms of vertebrobasilar ischaemia, the most appropriate procedure might well be a carotid endarterectomy.

FURTHER READING

Alpers BJ, Berry RG, Paddison RM. Anatomical studies of the circle of Willis in normal brain. *Arch Neurol Psychiatr* 1959; **81**: 409–18.

Cartlidge NEF, Whisnant JP, Elveback LR. Carotid and vertebro-basilar transient cerebral ischaemic attacks: a community study, Rochester, Minnesota. *Mayo Clinic Proc* 1977; **52**: 117–20.

Morris PJ. Surgery of vertebrobasilar disease. In: Warlow C, Morris PJ, eds. *Transient Ischaemic Attacks*. New York: Marcel Dekker 1982: 297–309.

7.8.3 Carotid body tumours

LINDA J. HANDS

Carotid body tumours arise from the chemoreceptor cells found at the carotid bifurcation. These are part of a widespread system of such cells which may give rise to tumours known as paragangliomas. Other examples of these are tumours of the vagal body or the glomus jugular and phaeochromocytomas. Patients can present at any age with a carotid body tumour but do so most commonly in the 5th and 6th decades. Although men were originally found to be more often affected, the sex ratio has recently reversed in favour of women.

PATHOLOGY

Carotid body tumours consist of epithelioid 'chief' cells arranged in clusters separated by trabeculae of well vascularized fibrous tissue. They have well-defined margins but lack a true capsule. Chemoreceptor cells are, in general, capable of secreting adrenaline and noradrenaline but carotid body tumours are virtually always non-secretory and therefore not associated with symptoms of hypertension. A histological diagnosis of malignancy is based on cellular atypia, mitosis, or local invasion but tends to be unreliable in predicting tumour behaviour. Most behave in a benign fashion; local invasion and lymph node metastases or haematogenous spread, especially to bone, are reported in less than 20 per cent of cases.

There appears to be a genetic susceptibility to these tumours and paragangliomas that arise in families are more likely to be bilateral or multiple. Carotid body tumours appear to be inherited on an autosomal dominant basis. Prolonged residence at high altitude is also associated with an increased incidence of carotid body tumours.

INCIDENCE

Paragangliomas are rare. Carotid body tumours occur most frequently but even they are uncommon, an incidence of 0.012 per cent of surgical specimens being reported at one hospital. Approximately 10 per cent of these patients have either bilateral or multifocal tumours of the chemoreceptor system. Ten per cent of patients have a genetic basis to their disease and in these the incidence of bilateral/multifocal tumours is approximately 30 per cent.

PRESENTING SYMPTOMS

The most common complaint is of a lump in the neck; this may have been present for a considerable time: one patient was reported to have presented after 47 years! The carotid bifurcation lies close to many important and sensitive structures (Fig. 1) and so expansion of the tumour may lead to cranial nerve paresis (VII, IX, X, XI, and XII) resulting in such symptoms as dysphagia, choking, or hoarseness. Symptoms are reported by approximately 10 per cent of patients.

DIAGNOSIS

It is vitally important to appreciate the possibility of a carotid body tumour in a patient who presents with a neck lump in the region of

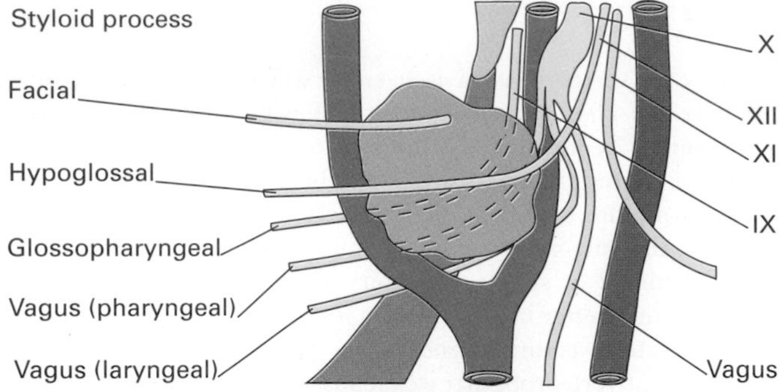

Fig. 1 Distribution of cranial nerves in relation to carotid body tumour. The cranial nerves are at greatest risk during dissection of the upper pole and the back of the tumour.

the carotid bifurcation. A misdiagnosis of lymph node enlargement followed by an attempt at excision biopsy can result in excessive blood loss and much embarrassment. Fine needle aspiration in the outpatient department may provide the answer, although this depends on the expertise of the local cytology department. Gray scale ultrasound imaging will confirm the relationship with the carotid bifurcation and should demonstrate splaying of the two branches by the tumour. Duplex scanning is probably more appropriate; it gives more precise identification of the vessels and the extent of their involvement. Angiography is usually performed if duplex or ultrasound examination suggests a carotid body tumour; it demonstrates splaying of the carotid bifurcation, a tumour blush, and often allows tumour feeding vessels to be identified (Fig. 2). In the future colour coded duplex scanning may be able to replace angiography by demonstrating not only the distortion of the carotid bifurcation but also the tumour vascularity. However, confident identification of major feeding vessels for embolization of large tumours (see below) will still require angiography. Enhanced CT images are also helpful in determining the upper level of a large tumour.

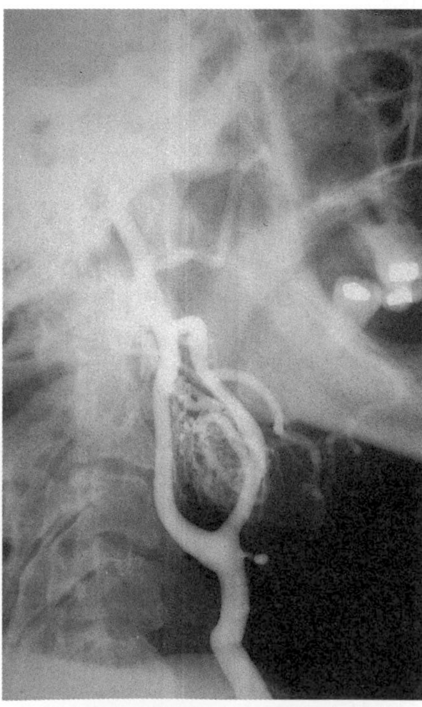

Fig. 2 Carotid angiogram showing the typical splaying of the carotid bifurcation by a carotid body tumour, and the origin of its blood supply from the external carotid artery.

TREATMENT

Conservative

If tumours are benign, their natural course is of slow enlargement with eventual compression of local structures resulting in symptoms such as nerve palsies. In the elderly patient without symptoms it may be appropriate to do nothing. However, it is much easier and safer to remove the tumour before extensive local invasion and so in most patients a surgical approach when the tumour is small is advocated. Untreated, 75 per cent asymptomatic patients eventually develop symptoms and 30 per cent will die from invasion of local structures or metastatic disease.

Surgical

Most patients in whom a diagnosis of carotid body tumour is made should undergo surgical excision.

Preoperative study

Embolization

These tumours are very vascular and if large, excision can result in excessive blood loss. In dealing with tumours greater than 3 cm in diameter it may be an advantage to shrink them preoperatively by embolization. It is essential that an experienced radiologist performs this manoeuvre. There are communications between the main feeding vessels of the tumour from the external carotid artery and the vertebral artery; embolization via the external carotid artery may result in brain embolization. Once the tumour has been successfully devascularized it is important that surgery is performed within the next 2 or 3 days or neovascularization occurs and the advantage is lost.

Direct and indirect pharyngoscopy/laryngoscopy

This is most important to assess cranial nerve involvement but is also useful to look for invasion of the pharynx by upward extension of the tumour, a rare occurrence.

CT scan/MRI

Either investigation is used to assess the extent of upward extension of the tumour and to determine any invasion of the skull base. Magnetic resonance imaging, especially with gadolinium enhancement, may provide some advantages over CT scanning: soft tissue contrast is probably better, an advantage when assessing the extent of invasion by a large tumour, and greater sensitivity allows detection of tumours down to 5 mm in diameter.

Crossmatch

There may be extensive blood loss during the surgery because of the vascular nature of the tumour and it is important that at least 4 units of blood are cross matched.

Operation

Anaesthesia

General anaesthesia should be used and nasal rather than oral intubation may be helpful to improve access to a tumour extending up under the mandible towards the base of the skull. Central venous pressure monitoring is mandatory and an arterial line is useful in view of the possibility of excessive blood loss

Surgeon

Experience with carotid artery surgery is important. It may be necessary to clamp the internal carotid artery, insert a shunt, and even to replace the artery with a length of saphenous vein. If the tumour is known to extend high in the neck the assistance of a craniofacial surgeon is often helpful.

Operative procedure

The side of the neck and lower jaw are prepared and draped. The groin should also be prepared in case a length of saphenous vein is required. An incision is made on the anterior border of sternomastoid and dissection extended deeply until the carotid arteries are exposed in their sheath. The common, internal, and external carotid arteries are each exposed and controlled beyond the tumour. Some surgeons advocate dividing the external carotid artery near its origin as soon as possible to reduce vascularity of the tumour and improve access (Fig. 3). Most would advocate at least clamping the artery at this point, although it is not often readily accessible. Heparin is not required prior to this manoeuvre.

The Connell technique in which a straight shunt is inserted via the common carotid artery into the internal carotid artery is another useful approach in that it excludes the external carotid artery from the circulation, thus effectively devascularizing the tumour. A straight Pruitt shunt is ideal for this purpose.

The tumour is dissected out along the white line which demarcates it from the adventitial tissue of the vessels. This dissection should start in the bifurcation and the tumour should be rolled upwards to get a clear view of the cranial nerves which run across the deep aspect of the upper part of the tumour. Good visualization is essential and haemostasis must be performed meticulously so that cranial nerves can be identified and preserved. However greatly they are involved it is usually possible to 'shell' the tumour off them. The only exception is the tumour diagnosed as a carotid body tumour which proves to be a vagal body tumour. This arises very close to the carotid bifurcation and can be easily mistaken for the former. The vagus nerve itself is involved and therefore has to be sacrificed. If a carotid body tumour extends well up in the neck, fracture of the styloid process will improve access. It may be necessary to dislocate forward the temporomandibular joint to gain access to its upper border. This is where preoperative CT scanning or MRI and peroperative assistance of a craniofacial surgeon become invaluable.

The Shamblin classification of carotid body tumours groups them according to the degree of invasion of the arterial wall. Those in Group 1 are easy to remove from the vessels, those in Group 2 require dissection in a subadventitial plane to remove them from the vessel, and in those in Group 3, the tumour encircles and invades the vessel to such an extent that it usually requires complete arterial excision and replacement, with a length of saphenous vein. A shunt may be used but it is often useful to have some means of cerebral monitoring such as ECG or transcranial Doppler to monitor distal flow during the procedure.

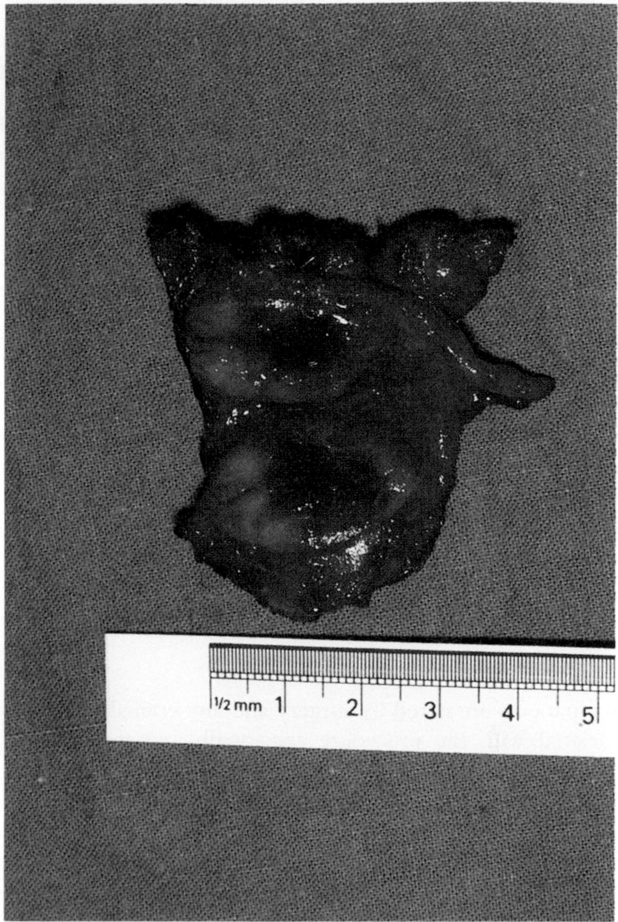

Fig. 3 The same carotid body tumour after resection. In this case the external carotid artery was ligated at its origin, divided, and removed with the tumour.

Approximately 50 per cent of carotid body tumours are in Shamblin Group 2 and 25 per cent in each of the other two groups.

Once the tumour is removed and adequate haemostasis achieved the wound should be closed over a vacuum drain which is left in for about 24 h or until significant discharge has ceased.

Postoperative care

The patient should be closely monitored postoperatively for central and peripheral neurological deficits (especially of cranial nerves IX, X, and XII, cervical sympathetic nerves, and the marginal mandibular branch of VII) and blood pressure well controlled, particularly if the internal carotid artery has been reconstructed. The incidence of cranial nerve defects associated with surgery has not declined over the years despite improvement in surgical technique (e.g. preoperative embolization to reduce bleeding preoperatively). Such problems are found particularly after removal of large tumours and are reported in 10 to 20 per cent of cases although most recover within a few weeks. Bilateral carotid body tumours should not be removed in the same operation. The incidence of nerve damage following surgery is sufficiently high to make bilateral recurrent laryngeal and hypoglossal nerve palsies a significant risk factor leading to respiratory and swallowing problems postoperatively. In patients who have had surgery to a previous carotid body tumour, resulting in cranial nerve palsy or carotid occlusion, the risks of operation on a contralateral tumour are considerable and radiotherapy (see below) may be preferable. Cerebrovascular accidents occur in less than 3 per cent of cases in most series.

Although the mortality of carotid body tumour removal used to be high (in 1950 it was reported at about 30 per cent) it now should be virtually zero because of innovations such as preoperative embolization, external carotid artery clamping, and well planned strategies for access high in the neck.

Radiotherapy

Radiotherapy has been promoted by some groups as a primary treatment. Few studies have compared this with surgery and none of these has been a randomized study. Most centres still recommend surgery, with radiotherapy used only for tumours too extensive to excise or as a backup treatment of those with recurrence. Radiotherapy as a primary treatment appears to slow progression of the disease but this is difficult to prove in a disease which naturally has a slow progression rate.

LONG-TERM OUTCOME

Most patients are cured by surgery and any cranial nerve palsies associated with the procedure are usually temporary although those caused by prolonged compression from the tumour itself are sometimes permanent. A few patients prove to have a malignant tumour, which may be diagnosed histologically, but this usually only comes to light when metastatic disease develops. If the tumour is known to be malignant because of local invasion or metastatic disease, local radiotherapy can be used to prevent local recurrence or to treat metastatic disease as it occurs. Most tumours are slow growing and survival for many years is possible even with established metastatic disease.

FURTHER READING

Hallett JW, Nora JD, Hollier LH, Cherry KJ, Pairolero PC. Trends in neurovascular complications of surgical management for carotid body and cervical paragangliomas: a fifty year experience with 153 tumours. *J Vasc Surg* 1988; **7**: 284–91.

La Muraglia EM, *et al.* The current surgical management of carotid body paragangliomas. *J Vasc Surg* 1992; **15**: 1038–44.

McPherson GA, Halliday AW, Mansfield AO. Carotid body tumours and other cervical paragangliomas: diagnosis and management in 25 patients. *Br J Surg* 1989; **76**: 33–6.

Vogl T, *et al.* Paragangliomas of the jugular bulb and carotid body: MR imaging with short sequences and GA-DTPA enhancement. *Am J Roentgenol* 1989; **153**: 583–7.

Williams MD, Phillips MJ, Nelson WR, Rainer WG. Carotid body tumour. *Arch Surg* 1992; **127**: 963–8.

7.9.1 Thoracic outlet obstruction

PETER J. MORRIS

INTRODUCTION

Obstruction of the subclavian artery or vein and pressure on the lower trunk of the brachial plexus may occur in the thoracic outlet due to a number of anatomical abnormalities, the best recognized being a cervical rib. The first successful removal of a cervical rib was undertaken by Coote in 1861. The clinical syndrome of thoracic outlet obstruction is a complex of clinical features, which may be either predominantly vascular or predominantly neurological. The syndrome has been given a number of descriptions over the years, each suggesting an aetiology, such as costoclavicular syndrome, scalenus anticus syndrome, and hyperabduction syndrome. However, the varied symptoms and signs in these patients are best grouped under the broad term thoracic outlet obstruction syndrome.

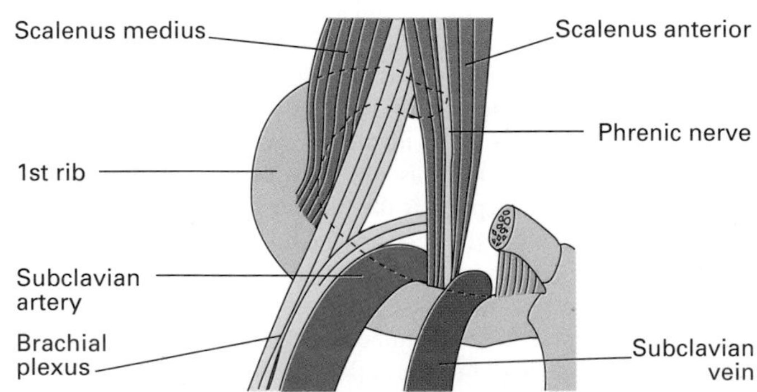

Fig. 1 The subclavian vein crosses the first rib in front of the insertion of scalenus anterior which separates it from the subclavian artery and the brachial plexus.

ANATOMY

The subclavian vein and artery cross the anterior half of the first rib, separated by the insertion of scalenus anterior into the scalene tubercle of the first rib (Fig. 1). The brachial plexus lies behind the vessels; the lower trunk of the plexus formed by the roots of C8 and T1 is the most inferior structure of the plexus and lies on the first rib. As these structures cross the first rib they lie behind and below the clavicle and the subclavius muscle attaching to the inferior aspect of the clavicle. After crossing the first rib the neurovascular bundle passes into the axilla below the coracoid process of the scapula with its attached pectoralis minor.

The most common cause of obstruction or pressure at the thoracic outlet is a cervical rib which passes beneath the brachial plexus and subclavian artery to attach to the scalene tubercle on the first rib. Not infrequently a cervical rib is incomplete but is replaced by a fibrous band which extends from the tip of the rib

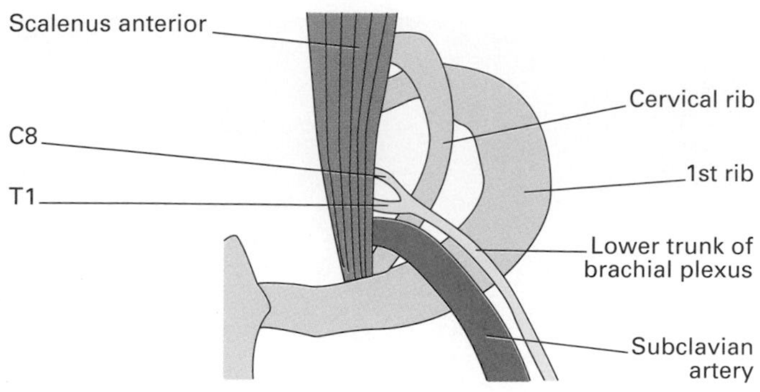

Fig. 2 A complete cervical rib attaching to the first rib at the scalene tubercle, with the subclavian artery elevated over it.

again to the scalene tubercle. The lower trunk of the brachial plexus may be stretched over a cervical rib or a fibrous band, as may the subclavian artery. This may also be squeezed in the angle between the scalenus anterior insertion and the cervical rib in certain positions (Fig. 2). Pressure on the brachial plexus and its lower trunk is sometimes due to a fibrous band lying along the medial border of scalenus medius as it passes to its insertion in the first rib. The insertion of scalenus anterior, which is quite fibrous, may sometimes be abnormal, with an extension running back along the first rib beneath the subclavian artery and obstructing it when the arm is in certain positions. The space between the clavicle and the first rib may be diminished in those with an old malaligned fracture of the clavicle or a hypertrophied subclavius muscle. This space also decreases as a result of poor posture: it is not uncommon for women to present with symptoms of thoracic outlet obstruction, either with or without a cervical rib, as they approach middle age.

The axillary vein may be obstructed as it crosses the first rib in front of scalenus anterior to become the subclavian vein if the space between the clavicle and first rib is decreased: this is usually associated with a large subclavius muscle or a fibrous anterior extension of the insertion of scalenus anterior.

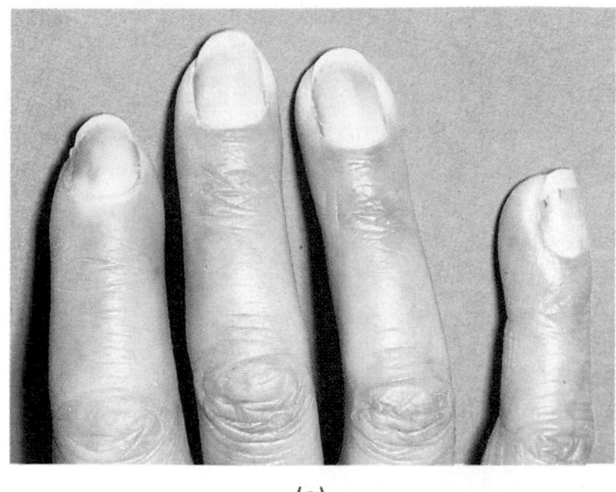

(a)

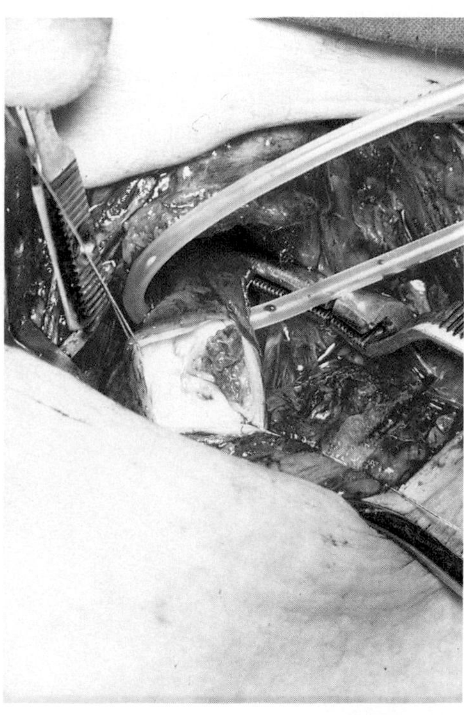

(b)

Fig. 3 A 62-year-old woman presented with (a) splinter haemorrhages in fingers (see nail of 5th finger) suggesting a proximal source of emboli. (b) She had a poststenotic aneurysm beyond a cervical rib compressing the artery which at operation was found to contain thrombus.

CLINICAL PRESENTATION

Patients present with any of a variety of symptoms and signs which may be predominantly vascular, predominantly neurological, or a combination of both. The majority of patients are women, usually between the ages of 20 and 40. Those with evidence of arterial obstruction may present with a history of Raynaud's phenomenon, nearly always unilateral, or of inability to use the arm on the involved side above the head for any period of time because of weakness in the arm and hand or pain and numbness in the fingers. On examination the subclavian artery may be prominent in the root of the neck when elevated by a cervical rib, which may indeed itself be palpable, and obliteration of the pulse can be readily achieved by a variety of manoeuvres, such as hyperabduction of the arm and bracing of the shoulders, which will be associated with pallor of the same hand. A bruit may be heard at rest or, more commonly, as the artery is compressed with one of the above manoeuvres. Occasionally older patients present with features of a subclavian aneurysm (which is really a post-stenotic dilation of the artery beyond an obstruction), giving rise to distal emboli from thrombus within the lumen of the aneurysm. Emboli from a subclavian aneurysm can produce distal signs ranging from splinter haemorrhages to gangrene of the finger tips (Fig. 3).

Patients with predominantly neurological symptoms often represent a difficult diagnostic group. Classically, pressure on the lower trunk of the brachial plexus results in paraesthesia of the ulnar aspect of the hand and forearm associated with certain posture, such as carrying a heavy basket or attempting to use the hand above the head. By the time of presentation there may be obvious weakness and wasting of the small muscles of the hand. There may be a tender point in the root of the neck over the plexus as it crosses a cervical rib. The patient often complains of pain with no appropriate segmental distribution in the shoulder, upper arm, or neck.

Finally many patients present with a combination of both vascular and neurological symptoms.

Venous obstruction at the thoracic outlet is an uncommon presentation, but this diagnosis should always be suspected in young people who present with an axillary vein thrombosis or intermittent swelling of the arm. They may participate in sports that can lead to hypertrophy of the subclavius muscle, such as surf board riding or butterfly swimming.

INVESTIGATIONS

A radiograph of the neck and upper chest will demonstrate cervical ribs (Fig. 4), but the absence of a rib does not exclude the diagnosis of thoracic outlet obstruction due to a fibrous remnant of an incomplete rib. A cervical rib, either complete or incomplete, will be visible on the radiograph, as will a prominent transverse process of the seventh cervical vertebra in the presence of a fibrous band. The presence of a cervical rib does not necessarily mean that this is the cause of the presenting symptoms. Cervical ribs are not uncommon and in most people do not give rise to problems.

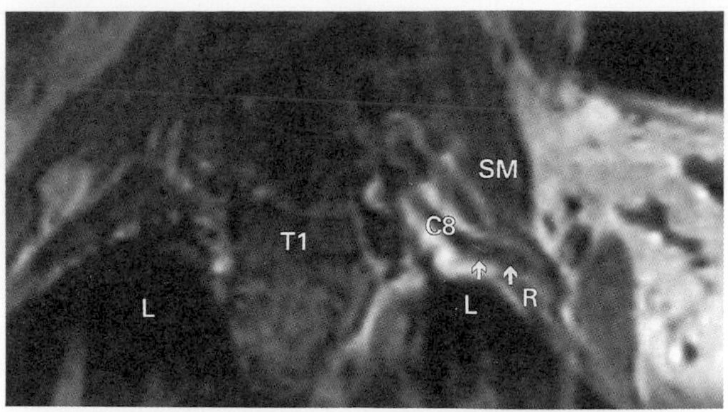

Fig. 5 MRI of thoracic outlet syndrome. A coronal T_1-weighted gradient recalled echo image through the apices of the lungs (L) and the body of the first thoracic vertebra (T1). The root of the C8 root (C8) is seen passing obliquely on scalenous medius muscle (SM). The C8 root is elevated (arrows) as it crosses the left first rib (R). (By courtesy of Dr N. Moore.)

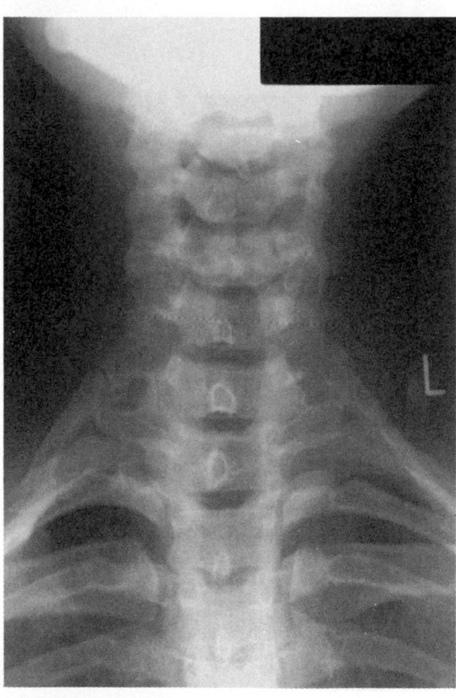

Fig. 4 A plain radiograph of the neck showing bilateral cervical ribs.

Magnetic resonance imaging (MRI) may be a useful addition to our diagnostic procedures, as it has the capacity to identify the brachial plexus and angulation of the lower trunk of the plexus over a fibrous band (Fig. 5). Our experience of MRI in the investigation of thoracic outlet obstruction in Oxford suggests that it is useful.

An arteriogram will demonstrate obstruction of the artery at the outlet with the arm abducted for example (Fig. 6), but this can be established clinically and does not need to be confirmed by angiography. The main indication for an arteriogram is to exclude the presence of thrombus within a possible subclavian aneurysm. However, the presence of both an aneurysm and intraluminal

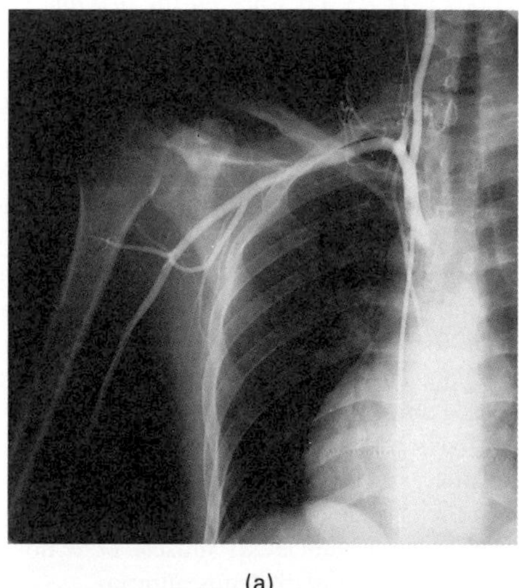

(a)

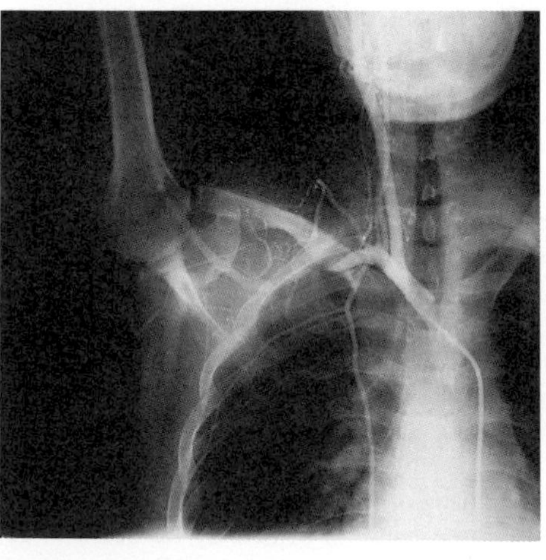

(b)

Fig. 6 (a) An arteriogram of the subclavian artery with the arm at the side, and (b) with the arm abducted showing complete obstruction of the artery at the thoracic outlet.

thrombus can be established by ultrasound, which further reduces the need for angiography.

A venogram will always be performed in a young patient presenting with a venous thrombosis and in the patient with intermittent swelling of the arm. A characteristic picture may be seen in the presence of obstruction, and sometimes a clinical diagnosis of axillary vein thrombosis will not be confirmed on venography, the clinical features being due to obstruction of the vein only at the thoracic outlet (Fig. 7).

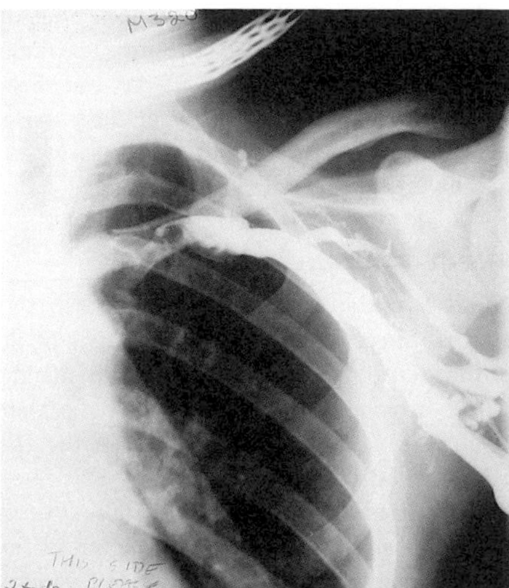

Fig. 7 A venogram in a patient with a diagnosis of subclavian vein thrombosis but in whom the vein was found to be patent at operation but obstructed at the thoracic outlet.

Neurophysiological studies are essential in establishing a neurological component to thoracic outlet obstruction and can provide a high degree of diagnostic accuracy in establishing the site of the problem at the brachial plexus level rather than at the level of the cervical spine or more distally.

In established 'classical' thoracic outlet syndrome there is a characteristic pattern of electrophysiological abnormality. The compound muscle action potential recorded from the thenar eminence is low, but median motor conduction velocity in the forearm and distal motor latency are normal. Preserved sensory nerve action potentials from the thumb, and index and third fingers, in the distribution of the C6 and C7 roots of the plexus, with normal conduction velocities across the wrist, serve to differentiate the condition from carpal tunnel syndrome. In contrast, the sensory nerve action potential from the fifth finger, in the C8 dermatome, is relatively reduced in amplitude or is absent. The hypothenar compound muscle action potential may also be reduced in amplitude, but less so than the response from abductor pollicis brevis. Normal motor and sensory conduction between the mid-arm and wrist exclude a peripheral ulnar nerve lesion.

Electromyography of the intrinsic hand muscles usually shows signs of chronic partial denervation consisting of scanty fibrillation potentials, prolonged polyphasic unstable motor unit action potentials which may have high amplitudes, and reduced density of the interference pattern. These findings are more prominent in the abductor pollicis brevis than in the first dorsal interosseous muscle, and in a few patients similar changes are seen in the forearm flexor compartment.

Other neurophysiological procedures which may be of help in diagnosis include measurement of F response (a late spinal response) latency, reflex latency measurement, recording of sensory nerve action potentials from the medial cutaneous nerve of the forearm, and cortical somatosensory responses following dermatomal stimulation. However, these tests are unlikely to be of value if the more characteristic changes are not observed. Measurement of proximal ulnar motor conduction velocity across the brachial plexus is now generally disregarded as a method of diagnosing the thoracic outlet syndrome. Typical findings in a patient with thoracic outlet compression due to a cervical rib are shown in Table 1.

Table 1 Results of electrophysiological studies in a patient with thoracic outlet compression due to a cervical rib

Motor conduction		
	Right median nerve	
		Abductor pollicis brevis inexcitable
	Right ulnar nerve	
		Abductor digiti minimi
		Compound muscle action potential 11 mV (normal)
		Conduction velocity (arm) 61 m/s (normal)
		F response latency 27.4 ms (normal)
Sensory conduction		
	Right thumb	
		Amplitude 37 μV (normal)
		Conduction velocity 58 m/s (normal)
	Right 3rd finger	
		Amplitude 27 μV (normal)
		Conduction velocity 58 m/s (normal)
	Right 5th finger	
		Amplitude 2 μV (low)
		Conduction velocity 53 m/s (normal)
Mixed nerve action potential		
	Right ulnar nerve wrist to mid-arm	
		Amplitude 8 μV (low)
		Conduction velocity 63 m/s (normal)
Electromyography		
	Right first dorsal interosseous	
		Fibrillation potentials, unstable polyphasic motor unit action potentials, reduced interference pattern
	Right flexor digitorum superficialis	
		Fibrillation potentials, unstable polyphasic motor unit action potentials, reduced interference pattern
	Right flexor carpi ulnaris	
		No abnormal spontaneous activity, normal motor unit action potential outline but high amplitude (10 mV). Normal interference pattern

DIFFERENTIAL DIAGNOSIS

The diagnosis of a vascular thoracic outlet obstruction is usually relatively straightforward, but may present problems in patients with bilateral Raynaud's phenomenon. However, symptoms due to thoracic outlet obstruction usually have an earlier onset in one hand. If the presenting feature is unilateral Raynaud's phenomenon, it is important to exclude an occupational cause such as the use of hand-held drills. It should also be remembered that arterial obstruction may occur proximal to the outlet, at the origin of the left subclavian or innominate arteries, and where this possibility exists an arch aortogram will be required.

The two major neurological diagnoses to be excluded are cervical spondylosis and carpal tunnel syndrome. MRI is the investigation of choice in the former, and neurophysiological studies the most useful investigation in the latter, but neither replaces a careful history and examination.

TREATMENT

Physiotherapy

Exercises designed to strengthen the muscles of the neck and shoulder girdle and the adoption of a more upright posture can relieve symptoms in many patients, especially women approaching middle age who often begin to droop across the shoulders, resulting in narrowing of the thoracic outlet. This should be the first approach in most patients unless they have florid symptoms of obstruction, definite neurological signs, or arterial changes, in which case it is better to proceed to surgery.

Surgery

The surgical approach to this condition depends on the cause. Cervical ribs, either complete or fibrous, should be excised. Additional bands in the scalenus medius are divided. If no obvious cause of compression is found, division of the scalenus anterior at its insertion (scalenotomy) has been widely practised in the past. However, definite evidence of vascular or neurological thoracic outlet obstruction in the absence of a cervical rib or fibrous band is now treated by excision of the first rib. If there is evidence of arterial damage such as a significant post-stenotic dilatation or an aneurysm of the subclavian artery, that section of the artery is excised and replaced with a short length of vein or a prosthetic graft such as polytetrafluoroethylene.

Surgical techniques

The techniques by which the above surgical procedures are performed are several and each has its protagonists. To some extent the technique should be dictated by the cause of the thoracic outlet obstruction.

Supraclavicular approach

With the patient in the prone position and a small sandbag behind the shoulders, a transverse incision is made above and parallel to the clavicle at the base of the anterior triangle. This is carried down through the platysma and the supraclavicular pad of fat to expose the scalenus anterior. The phrenic nerve crosses the anterior surface of the muscle from lateral to medial and should be carefully separated from the muscle and protected with a sling. Attention should be paid to the possible presence of an accessory phrenic nerve. The scalenus anterior muscle is then divided near its insertion, to expose the subclavian artery.

If a cervical rib or a fibrous remnant is present or any other fibrous band it will be obvious on palpation, and can be exposed by further dissection. The major advantage of the supraclavicular approach is that it allows the anatomy of the thoracic outlet to be fully visualized, together with any abnormality. A cervical rib is excised, being careful to take the rib back behind the plexus. This last part of the excision is usually best performed from the lateral aspect of the brachial plexus. A fibrous remnant of a cervical rib is divided and, depending on its length, an incomplete cervical rib is removed to ensure that the lower trunk of the brachial plexus is free of any potential pressure. Any other bands that are apparent, such as along the medial border of scalenus medius are also divided, especially in the absence of a cervical rib or fibrous remnant.

The supraclavicular approach is ideal for removal of a cervical rib or a fibrous remnant, and also allows inspection of the artery. If a segment of the artery has to be replaced the axillary artery can be exposed below the clavicle for distal control and placing of the distal anastomosis.

The subclavian vein is not seen through the supraclavicular approach and so it does not allow a possible venous obstruction to be defined; this is best achieved by the infraclavicular approach.

The first rib can be removed from above, but this procedure is less easy as exposure of the rib is often less than satisfactory. Removal of the first rib is best accomplished through the transaxillary approach or the infraclavicular approach.

Transaxillary approach

This is a popular method of resection of the first rib to relieve thoracic outlet compression. Some protagonists of this technique would argue that removal of the first rib and hence detachment of everything that attaches to it, such as the scalenus anterior, cervical rib, and fibrous bands, ensures that the thoracic outlet obstruction is relieved whatever the cause.

With the patient in a full lateral position, the upper arm is abducted to a right angle and forcibly retracted by an assistant. A transverse incision is then made on the medial aspect of the axilla, between the borders of pectoralis major anteriorly and the latissimus dorsi posteriorly, and deepened to expose the first rib. Care must be taken not to damage the nerve to the serratus anterior. The first rib is then excised after separating it from the attaching structures. The secret of good exposure is vigorous retraction of the arm, which usually requires assistants relieving one another at frequent intervals! This approach has the disadvantage that adequate access to the artery and vein is not possible.

Infraclavicular approach

The positioning of the patient is all important. The patient lies with a sandbag between the shoulder blades and a transverse incision is made beneath the clavicle from the coracoid process laterally towards the midline for some 5 cm. This incision is carried down to the pectoralis major, which is then divided with diathermy to expose the acromioclavicular fascia, incision of which allows the axillary vein and artery to be identified with the plexus behind the artery. The shoulder is then lifted forward, opening up the costoclavicular space and allowing the vein and artery to be retracted from the first rib, the anterior half of which is readily visualized. The rib is then excised as far forward as required and then back beyond the plexus. This approach is ideal for patients with venous or arterial obstruction, but has one disadvantage in that as excision of the rib proceeds posteriorly to take it back beyond the plexus, the view of the rib is sometimes poor.

Posterior approach

This is practised infrequently, for although it provides a good view of the neck and posterior part of a cervical rib or a first rib, the artery is not accessible, and it is a much more destructive approach than the others described. It is sometimes useful if a cervical sympathectomy needs to be performed in a patient who has had already undergone several neck explorations.

Table 2 Symptomatic outcome after removal of a cervical or first rib in 53 patients in Oxford presenting with thoracic outlet compression syndrome of a predominant vascular or neurological nature or a mixture of both

	Presentation	No.	Cured	Improved	Not improved
Cervical rib	Vascular	8	6	2	–
	Vascular/neurological	8	8	–	–
	Neurological	5	5	–	–
	Total	21	19	2	–
First rib	Vascular	17	8	8	1
	Vascular/neurological	7	6	–	1
	Neurological	5	3	–	2
	Total	29	17	8	4

Results

When an operation is performed for arterial obstruction, with a clearly established diagnosis the results are excellent (Table 2). If neurological compression at the thoracic outlet has been diagnosed without doubt, surgical relief of the obstruction will also produce a good outcome. If there is muscle wasting of the small muscles of the hand recovery will be slow; if this is long-standing it is unlikely to improve, although sensory symptoms and pain are relieved immediately. However, the diagnosis of neurological thoracic outlet compression is often far from clear, and in some instances surgery is performed almost as a diagnostic procedure, when both the patient and neurologist are desperate. Although some vascular surgeons feel that to be certain of relieving symptoms the first rib should always be removed even if a cervical rib is present, the Oxford experience does not support this concept (Table 2). Recurrence of symptoms usually occurs in the first 12 months but may occur later in a small number of patients due to fibrous scarring resulting in bands which produce pressure on the lower trunk of the plexus once again, or due to regrowth of a resected first rib, which may occur if the rib is removed subperiosteally. For this reason ribs should be removed with the periosteum.

FURTHER READING

Adson AW, Coffey JR. Cervical rib: a method of anterior approach for relief of symptoms by division of the scalenus anticus. *Ann Surg* 1927; **85**: 839–57.

Coote H. Exostosis of the left transverse process of the seventh cervical vertebra surrounded by blood vessels and nerves: successful removal. *Lancet* 1861; **i**: 360.

Davies AH, Walton J, Stuart E, Morris PJ. Surgical management of the thoracic outlet syndrome. *Br J Surg* 1991; **78**: 1193–5.

Eastcott HHG. Reconstruction of the subclavian artery for complications of cervical rib and thoracic outlet syndrome. *Lancet* 1962; **ii**: 1243–6.

Kieffer E. Arterial complications of the thoracic outlet syndrome. In: JJ Bergan, JST Yao, eds. *Evaluation and Treatment of Upper and Lower Extremity Disorders*. Orlando: Grune & Stratton, 1984: 249–75.

Lewis T, Pickering GW. Observations on maladies in which the blood supply to digits ceases intermittently or permanently, and upon bilateral gangrene of digits; observations relevant to so-called Raynaud's disease. *Clin Sci* 1934; **1**: 327–66.

Murphy JB. Case of cervical rib with symptoms resembling subclavian aneurysm. *Ann Surg* 1905; **41**: 399–406.

Murphy T. Brachial neuritis caused by pressure of 1st rib. *Aust Med J* 1910; **15**: 582–5.

Peet RM, *et al.* Thoracic outlet syndrome: evaluation of a therapeutic exercise programme. *Mayo Clin Proc* 1956; **31**: 281–7.

Roos DB. Transaxillary approach for 1st rib resection to relieve thoracic outlet syndrome. *Ann Surg* 1966; **163**: 354–8.

Roos DB. New concepts of thoracic outlet syndrome that explain etiology, symptoms, diagnosis and treatment. *Vasc Surg* 1979; **13**: 313–21.

Strange-Vognsen HH, *et al.* Resection of the first rib, following deep arm vein thrombolysis in patients with thoracic outlet syndrome. *J Cardiovasc Surg* 1989; **30**: 430–3.

Thompson JF, Webster JH. First rib resection for vascular complications of the thoracic outlet syndrome. *Br J Surg* 1990; **77**: 555–7.

Tilney P, Griffiths HTG, Edwards EA. Natural history of major venous thrombosis of the upper extremity. *Arch Surg* 1976; **101**: 792–6.

Vollmar J, Heyden B. Thoracic outlet syndrome with vascular complications. *J Cardiovasc Surg* 1979; **20**: 531–6.

7.9.2 Raynaud's syndrome

PETER M. LAMONT

INTRODUCTION

Maurice Raynaud first described a group of 25 patients with 'localasphyxia and symmetrical gangrene of the extremities' in 1862. He proposed that the observed changes were caused by vasospasm because most of the patients had palpable pulses at the wrist and patent large arteries were observed in those patients who underwent autopsy. Over the next 70 years it became apparent that this vasospastic condition could occur either in isolation or in association with other diseases, and so a distinction was made between Raynaud's disease (occurring in isolation) and Raynaud's phenomenon (secondary to an underlying disease). More recently this distinction has become less clear cut because some patients may develop collagen disorders several years after the onset of Raynaud's symptoms and patients with apparent primary Raynaud's disease may have low levels of autoantibodies present in their serum. For these reasons both primary and secondary Raynaud's conditions are now classified under the single banner of Raynaud's syndrome.

Raynaud's syndrome therefore describes the changes which result from intermittent vasospasm of the arterioles in the hands or feet; these classically occur following exposure to cold or as a result of emotional stimuli. The vasospasm resolves with warming, leading to the classical sequence of colour changes in the extremity from pallor to cyanosis to redness although, as with many classical descriptions of diseases, the full spectrum of colour changes is seldom seen in one individual patient. The syndrome may be primary, when no other condition can be identified after appropriate investigation, or it may be secondary to a wide variety of underlying disorders.

INCIDENCE

The majority of patients with Raynaud's syndrome are female, both because primary Raynaud's is classically described as a disease of young women and because many of the underlying disorders associated with secondary Raynaud's are more common in women. Of those who actually present with the syndrome, 70 to 90 per cent are female, although many individuals with mild to moderate cold sensitivity may not be disturbed by their symptoms enough to seek medical advice. Population surveys of Scandinavian women aged 18 to 60 years suggest an overall prevalence of Raynaud's syndrome of between 15 and 22 per cent in the general female population—a substantially higher number than is actually treated. Most of the women uncovered by such population surveys have primary Raynaud's syndrome and very few have associated collagen disorders. Secondary Raynaud's syndrome is much more common in patients who present to specialist units with an interest in the disorder. Only 30 per cent of patients presenting to specialist units have primary Raynaud's syndrome; the remainder have secondary Raynaud's syndrome, and one-half of these patients will have overt or suspected connective tissue diseases. This represents the single largest group of patients presenting to specialist units with Raynaud's syndrome. Such data confirm the clinical impression that secondary Raynaud's syndrome results in a greater severity of digital ischaemia than the primary form; patients with secondary Raynaud's syndrome are therefore more likely to present to a clinician for treatment.

PATHOGENESIS

Distinct colour changes in the hands or feet of Raynaud's patients in response to cold are the hallmark of the syndrome. Cold exposure produces profound pallor and numbness of the digits due to spasm of the digital arteries. The digital microvasculature dilates after a few minutes due to the accumulation of carbon dioxide and the products of hypoxic metabolism. As the vasospasm begins to relax a small amount of oxygenated blood enters these dilated vessels where it rapidly becomes desaturated and the pallor changes to cyanosis. As the digital vessels relax further, so normal blood flow is re-established and a reactive hyperaemia of the dilated microvasculature ensues as the cyanosis changes to rubor of the digits (Fig. 1).

Cold, emotional stimuli, or even cigarette smoking may induce an attack, and so severe is the vasospasm that its force overcomes the ability of the arterial blood pressure to keep the vessel walls apart, so that the digital arteries are completely closed during the attack (Fig. 2).

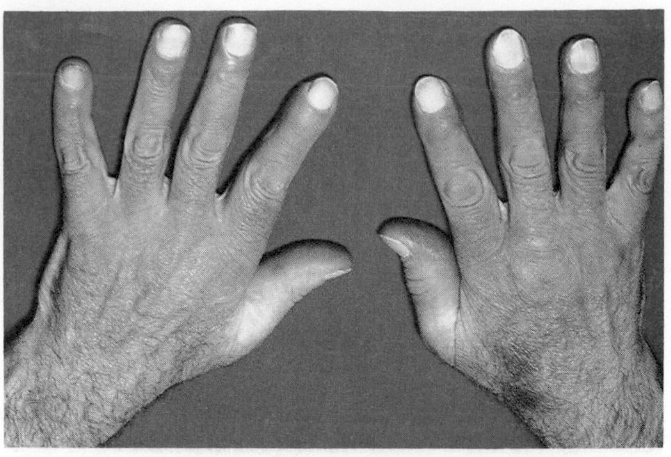

Fig. 1 The classical appearance of Raynaud's syndrome. The digits exhibit cyanosis changing to rubor as the hand rewarms during a Raynaud's attack.

The definitive picture of the pathogenesis of Raynaud's syndrome has yet to be described. The very number and variety of hypotheses put forward to explain the abnormal sensitivity to cold of the digital vessels attests to the presence of a continuing gap in our knowledge. Maurice Raynaud was the first to put forward his ideas on the pathogenesis of the digital vasospasm when he claimed that it was due to an 'enormous exaggeration of the excitomotor energy of the grey parts of the spinal cord which control the vasomotor innervation'. This eloquent description of sympathetic overactivity was challenged many years later by Sir Thomas Lewis, who published a series of papers on the subject in the 1930s. Lewis attributed the vasospasm to a local fault in the sensitivity of the digital arteries to cold stimuli and was able to induce attacks experimentally in the presence of an anaesthetized sympathetic supply. Conversely he was able to prevent an attack by keeping the hand warm when the rest of the body was cooled. Thus he concluded that, whatever the state of the sympathetic nervous outflow, provocation of a Raynaud's attack depended upon the local digital temperature. So persuasive were Lewis' experiments that the majority of subsequent work has concentrated on possible mechanisms of a local hypersensitivity to cold, and most workers have accepted that the central thermoregulatory system is normal in Raynaud's syndrome.

The normal vasospastic response to cold may be exaggerated if the digital vessel lumen is already narrowed by structural abnormalities. Microscopic abnormalities, ranging from slight intimal thickening through to frank intimal hyperplasia or even complete luminal obliteration, have been described in Raynaud's patients. The intimal thickening in most cases, however, is no worse than that in age-matched controls without Raynaud's syndrome and a purely structural abnormality seems an unlikely explanation for the excessive response to cold. Much attention has therefore turned to the functional aspects of vasoconstriction, with particular emphasis on sympathetic neurotransmission.

α-Adrenergic receptors sensitive to catecholamines in the digital vessel walls induce vasoconstriction in response to sympathetic stimulation. Sympathetic stimulation also induces the release of histamine, which is a vasodilator, from adjacent mast cells. Histamine H_2-receptors on the sympathetic nerve terminal in turn inhibit α-adrenergic neurotransmission. There is some evidence

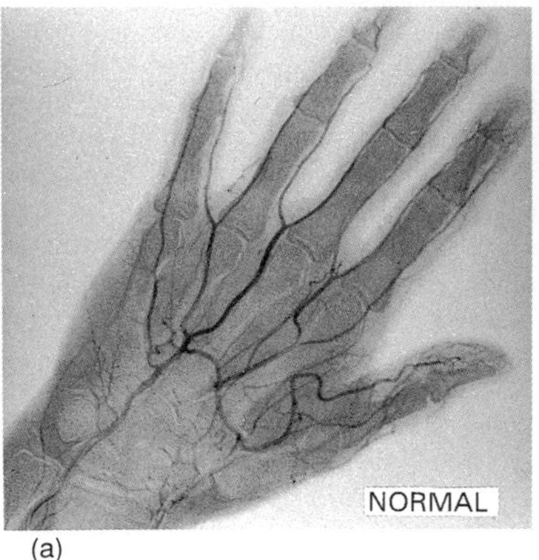

(a)

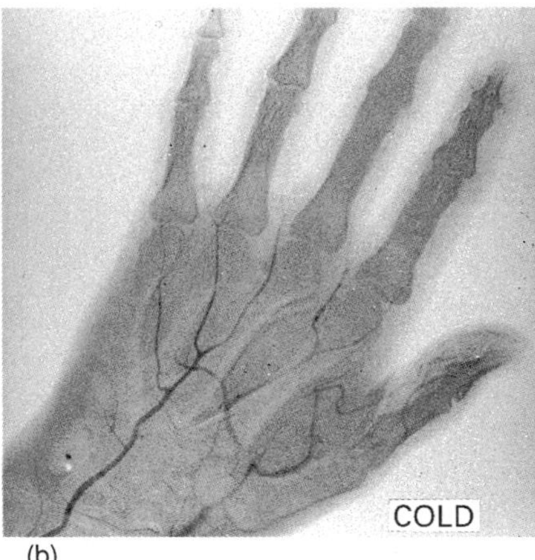

(b)

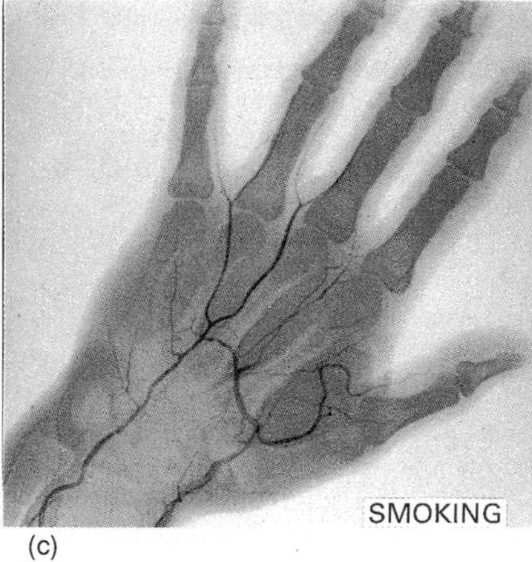

(c)

Fig. 2 The induction of digital vasospasm by cold and smoking. (a) The apparently normal angiogram of a 24-year-old female with primary Raynaud's syndrome. (b) Intense vasospasm prevents filling of the digital vessels after cold exposure in the same patient. (c) Cigarette smoking has the same vasospastic effect.

that this potential negative feedback control mechanism may be impaired in patients with Raynaud's syndrome. Under normal circumstances the digital vessels dilate rapidly when a cold stimulus sufficient to induce vasoconstriction is withdrawn. In Raynaud's patients this rapid postsympathetic vasodilation is delayed or absent and vasodilation occurs only when a warm stimulus is applied. While such an observation may be explained by excessive catecholamine release, by impaired catecholamine inactivation, by histamine depletion, or by mast cell dysfunction, none of these proposals has been clearly shown to underlie a Raynaud's attack. Catecholamine concentrations are certainly higher in the venous blood coming from the hand during a Raynaud's attack, but this phenomenon may be simply the result of a diminished blood flow.

The issue is complicated further by the observation that sympathetic stimulation normally has a similar effect on blood flow in the hand whether the hand is warm or cold. In Raynaud's patients the vasoconstrictor effect of sympathetic stimulation is significantly enhanced when the hand is cold compared to when it is warm. Cold itself may therefore sensitize or enhance local α-adrenergic receptor function in Raynaud's patients. While these data confirm the conclusions of Lewis that a local phenomenon underlies the onset of a Raynaud's attack, little progress has been made to date in establishing the underlying mechanism.

Several haemorheological phenomena have also been noted in the blood of Raynaud's patients. Both blood and plasma viscosity are increased and there is reduced red cell deformability, abnormal platelet adhesiveness, and reduced activity of the fibrinolytic system. It is difficult to interpret the relevance of these phenomena to the pathogenesis of Raynaud's syndrome.

At normal temperatures there is no significant difference in blood flow through the hands of normal individuals compared with Raynaud's sufferers, despite the increased viscosity in the latter group. As the hand is cooled the blood flow decreases more rapidly in Raynaud's syndrome than in normal controls and may cease altogether at 17 to 22°C, whereas there is still some flow in normal hands at these temperatures. The relative contribution of increased blood viscosity in Raynaud's patients to this cold sensitivity remains a matter for debate and it is not known whether viscosity is crucial to the pathogenesis of the syndrome or whether it is simply a secondary event.

Table 1 Disorders associated with Raynaud's syndrome

1. Connective tissue diseases
   - Scleroderma
   - Systemic lupus erythematosus
   - Dermatomyositis
   - Rheumatoid arthritis
   - Vasculitis
2. Occlusive arterial disease
   - Atherosclerosis
   - Thromboangiitis obliterans
   - Embolism
3. Trauma
   - Vibration injury
   - Cold injury
4. Neurovascular lesions
   - Thoracic outlet syndrome
   - Carpal tunnel syndrome
5. Miscellaneous
   - Ergotamine intoxication
   - Cryoglobulinaemia
   - Cold agglutinins

ASSOCIATED DISORDERS

A wide variety of other conditions may occur in association with Raynaud's syndrome (Table 1) and, in the case of the connective tissue disorders, the Raynaud's attacks may precede other features of the disease by several years. No single common thread has been identified among these disorders which may help to explain the pathogenesis of Raynaud's syndrome and not all of the patients with these disorders go on to develop Raynaud's syndrome. Patients who present with apparent primary Raynaud's syndrome may also exhibit abnormalities on immunological screening of their serum, although the significance of such findings is often uncertain.

Connective tissue disease

Secondary Raynaud's syndrome most commonly occurs in association with the connective tissue diseases. Between 40 and 80 per cent of patients with scleroderma will develop Raynaud's syndrome and the syndrome is often a presenting feature of scleroderma, although it may take several years after the onset of Raynaud's attacks before a definitive diagnosis is made. The incidence of Raynaud's syndrome is reported variously as 35 per cent in systemic lupus erythematosus, 22 per cent in dermatomyositis, and 11 per cent in rheumatoid arthritis. Many of these patients exhibit evidence of structural disease in the digital arteries on arteriography, with irregularity or obstruction of the lumen due to intimal proliferation. Such arteriographic changes are common in the connective tissue diseases and do not correlate with the presence or absence of Raynaud's attacks. Indeed many normal people over the age of 50 years have similar arteriographic findings and it is therefore difficult to implicate organic arterial obstruction on its own as a cause of the syndrome in patients with connective tissue disease.

Occlusive arterial disease

Raynaud's syndrome is seen in patients with arteriosclerotic disease in the limbs, particularly when the arteriosclerotic obstruction is sufficiently severe to reduce the digital blood pressure. When the digital blood pressure is low the normal vasospastic response to cold can more easily close off the vessel lumen against the reduced intravascular blood pressure. Thus although the sympathetic and local responses to cold are entirely normal and appropriate, the effects of cold-induced vasospasm are exaggerated and a Raynaud's attack ensues.

Thromboangiitis obliterans (Buerger's disease) is particularly associated with Raynaud's syndrome because, in addition to obstruction of the medium sized arteries of the forearm and calf, the digital vessels are commonly involved (Fig. 3). Such segmental involvement in the inflammatory thrombotic process results in a similar exaggeration of the normal vasospastic response to cold described above for arteriosclerosis because of the consequent reduction in digital blood pressure. Raynaud's attacks are the presenting feature of thromboangiitis obliterans in 12 to 25 per cent of patients and the disease itself may account for up to 12 per cent of the cases presenting to specialist units with Raynaud's syndrome. Thromboangiitis obliterans is particularly associated with smoking and remissions are often induced by abstinence from tobacco. Under these circumstances abnormalities of the digital pulses in the disease have sometimes been noted to disappear when the patient stops smoking, only to recur if the patient starts smoking again.

Trauma

Raynaud's syndrome is the classical occupational hazard of people who use vibrating tools such as chainsaws or pneumatic drills in their job. The attacks do not occur while the tool is being used, but later on when the hand is cooled. There may be a latent interval of several years between the regular use of a vibrating tool and the onset of the syndrome. The prolonged exposure to vibration may damage the endothelium lining the digital arteries and the subsequent subintimal fibrosis leads to widespread palmar and digital artery obstruction (Fig. 4). The suggestion that the vibration may have a direct effect on sympathetic nerve endings has not gained widespread support.

Cold injury may also induce Raynaud's syndrome and has also been noted as an occupational hazard, particularly in the frozen food processing industry. Chronic continued exposure to cold is

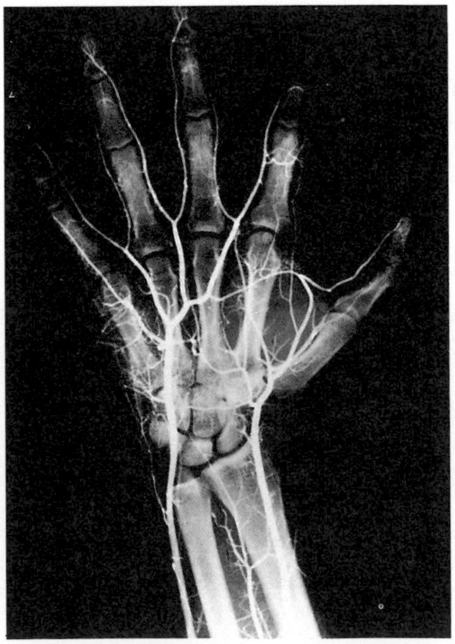

Fig. 3 Arteriogram of the hand of a male smoker with thromboangiitis obliterans. The proximal digital vessel on the radial aspect of the index finger is severely diseased. There is spasm of vessels in the third and fourth fingers and distal obliteration of vessels in the second and fifth fingers.

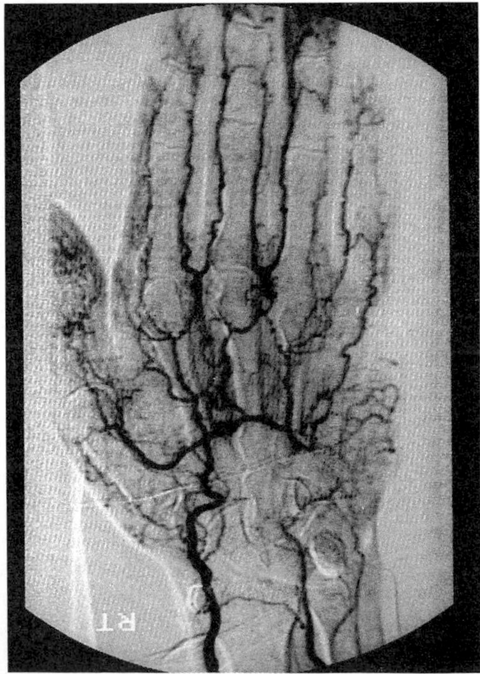

Fig. 4 Arteriogram of the hand of a man with a history of occupational exposure to high speed drills—the ulnar artery in the palm is obliterated and there is irregularity and occlusion of the digital arteries.

less important than rapid alternate cooling and warming of the hands such as occurs when workers handling frozen foods plunge their hands into warm water every few minutes to keep them warm. Alterations in working practices to avoid this alternate cooling and warming have substantially decreased the incidence of this particular occupational hazard.

Raynaud's syndrome may also be a long-term sequel in digits affected by frostbite.

Neurovascular lesions

Thoracic outlet syndrome may present with Raynaud's syndrome. It is unusual for both the neurological and vascular symptoms of thoracic outlet obstruction to coexist in the same patient and it is usually the vascular variety with subclavian artery stenosis, post-stenotic dilatation, and microembolization of the digital vessels which results in Raynaud's syndrome. Raynaud's syndrome may occur in patients with a coincident asymptomatic cervical rib and so it is important to demonstrate a definite vascular abnormality by angiography before attributing the Raynaud's syndrome to thoracic outlet obstruction.

Although carpal tunnel syndrome may be present in up to 15 per cent of patients with Raynaud's syndrome, nerve compression does not appear to contribute to the vasospasm, since division of the flexor retinaculum does not relieve the Raynaud's syndrome. A collagen disorder may underlie both conditions, so that they occur in association with each other without any specific cause and effect relationship.

Miscellaneous

Ergotamine is a potent vasoconstrictor used in the treatment of migraine. Prolonged use, especially in excessive dosages, may result in peripheral vasoconstriction manifesting as Raynaud's syndrome.

The presence of cold agglutinins or cryoglobulins in the blood produces hyperviscosity of the blood upon exposure to cold; blood flow in the digital arteries therefore virtually ceases in the digital vessels at low temperatures. Cold agglutinins adsorb on to red blood cells at temperatures between 24°C and 34°C and produce a reversible haemagglutination. The digital vessels are then plugged by masses of agglutinated red cells. Subsequent haemolysis of the agglutinated cells may produce haemoglobinuria and haemolytic anaemia.

Cryoglobulins in the blood obstruct the digital vessels by undergoing cold precipitation within them. The cryoglobulins may occur idiopathically but can also be secondary to a malignant reticulosis.

Changes in blood viscosity appear to be the primary mechanism for the obstruction to blood flow in these syndromes rather than any excessive response to sympathetic activity: the episodic digital ischaemia usually disappears if the cold agglutinins disappear.

DIAGNOSIS

The diagnosis of Raynaud's syndrome depends mainly upon the history of colour changes induced by cold exposure or occasionally by emotion. The involved extremity turns pale and numb when cold and makes a slow recovery when warmed, taking 15 to 45 min to pass through the stages of cyanosis and redness back to a normal colour. Pain in the digits is not a usual feature but may occur, particularly in the secondary varieties where there is digital vessel occlusion and a significant amount of ischaemic tissue damage, leading to ulceration and gangrene. This ischaemic damage may become so severe that the patient may require digital amputation despite the presence of a normal radial pulse (Fig. 5).

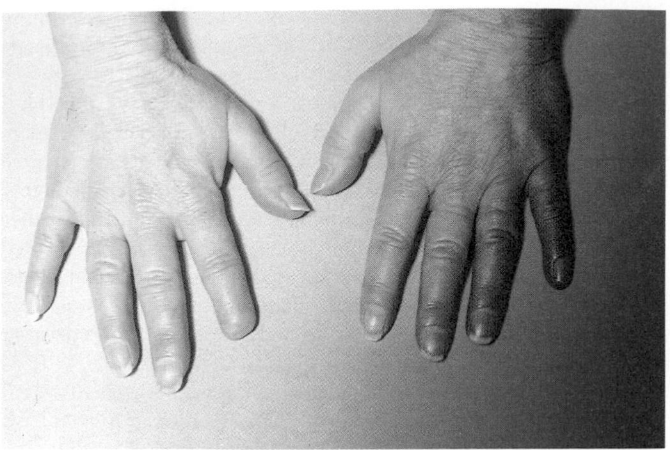

Fig. 5 Hands of a patient with scleroderma. The right index fingertip has been amputated for ischaemia and a Raynaud's attack is in progress in the left hand.

Such ischaemic tissue damage is extremely rare in the primary form of Raynaud's syndrome where the attacks are solely related to vasospasm and there is no obstructive element. Primary Raynaud's syndrome tends to occur in young women under 30 and is usually symmetrical, involving either the hands or the feet or both together. No associated disease is present and symptoms continue for 2 or more years without the development of any evident aetiology. Pain is unusual except when bacterial or fungal paronychia complicates the attacks.

Raynaud's attacks may be the presenting feature of a number of associated diseases, evidence for which should also be sought for in the history and examination. Patients with connective tissue disorders such as rheumatoid disease or systemic lupus erythematosus may complain of arthralgia and have stiff, painful and swollen joints. Patients with scleroderma may complain of dysphagia or diarrhoea and on examination may have a pinched face with a small tight mouth and inelastic skin. Telangiectasia may be present on the lips and hands and there may be missing digits where severe digital ischaemia has necessitated amputation.

Peripheral pulses should be felt for evidence of arteriosclerotic disease, and a history of heavy smoking may suggest the presence of thromboangiitis obliterans in a young male with Raynaud's symptoms. The presence of a subclavian bruit with Raynaud's syndrome in the ipsilateral hand suggests thoracic outlet obstruction, and there may also be differences in blood pressure between the two arms.

A careful history of drug use should be elicited, particularly if the patient takes migraine preparations containing ergotamine. The patient's occupational history is also important as they may have changed their job and only confess to cold exposure or the use of vibrating tools in a previous occupation on direct questioning.

The hands or feet themselves may look completely normal on examination, particularly in the warmth of the consulting room. The history of colour changes is usually sufficient to make the diagnosis, although the extremity can always be immersed in ice cold water for 30 s to induce an attack if confirmation is necessary. Special investigations are mainly directed at the detection of associated disorders: digital pressure and plethysmographic blood flow measurements are more useful as a research tool than for routine clinical use, and arteriography is not necessary in every patient with a clear history, although it can help to distinguish between purely vasospastic Raynaud's syndrome and that with an obstructive element in the digital vessels (Figs. 2 and 3). Arch arteriography is particularly useful when a more proximal arterial obstructive element is suspected, such as subclavian stenosis with thromboembolic obstruction of the digital vessels, as the proximal obstruction may be amenable to surgical correction.

Comprehensive investigation of the Raynaud's patient to rule out associated disorders should include radiography of the thoracic outlet to show the presence of a cervical rib; radiographs of the hands may show the joint disruption characteristic of rheumatoid arthritis or the subcutaneous calcinosis and sclerodactyly of scleroderma. Blood tests include a full blood count and an erythrocyte sedimentation rate, which may be elevated in connective tissue disorders. More specific screening tests include rheumatoid factor, antinuclear factor, anti-DNA antibody, serum protein electrophoresis, cryoglobulins, and cold agglutinin assays.

DIFFERENTIAL DIAGNOSIS

Acrocyanosis

Acrocyanosis is a separate vasospastic disorder of the hands or feet which occurs mainly in women and may be unilateral. The extremity feels cool, may be slightly oedematous, and has a constant blue discoloration which does not resolve in response to warmth (Fig. 6). Peripheral pulses are normal and ischaemic changes do not occur. The condition is due to cutaneous arteriolar vasospasm which is independent of temperature. The condition may respond to vasodilatory drugs used to treat Raynaud's syndrome and sympathectomy can produce good results if symptoms are severe.

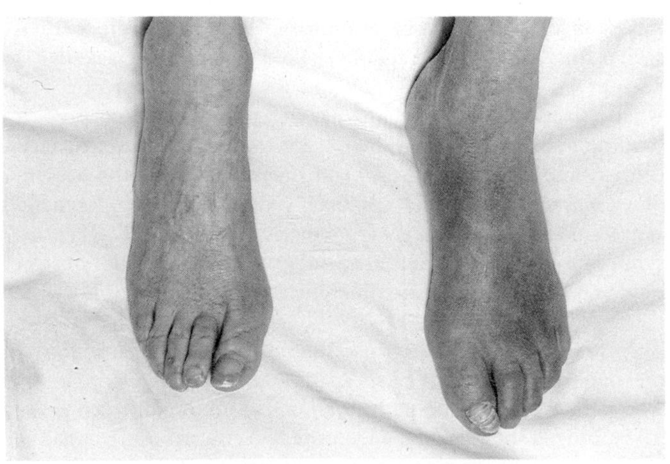

Fig. 6 Unilateral acrocyanosis in the right foot of an elderly woman. The reddish-blue discoloration was constant but otherwise asymptomatic and the foot pulses were intact.

Livido reticularis

Livido reticularis is also caused by cutaneous arteriolar vasospasm with secondary dilatation of associated capillaries and venules but the distribution is patchy and apparently random. There is patchy reddish-blue mottling of the lower legs and feet or occasionally of the arms and hands which persists irrespective of temperature, although it is often worse in the cold. The majority of cases occur in isolation but the disorder has been described in association with polyarteritis nodosa and systemic lupus erythematosus. No treatment is usually necessary other than reassurance and avoidance of cold.

TREATMENT OF RAYNAUD'S SYNDROME

General measures

No curative treatment is available for Raynaud's syndrome and the aim is therefore to palliate the symptoms by reducing the frequency and the severity of the attacks. Reassurance that the outlook is generally benign is important, especially in primary Raynaud's syndrome where progression to digital ischaemia and gangrene is extremely rare. The natural history of the syndrome includes long periods of remission, especially over the sùmmer months. The majority of patients can achieve a worthwhile response through the simple avoidance of cold and tobacco smoking. Smoking a cigarette may produce a fall in temperature of 2 to 3°C in the fingertips (Fig. 2) and smoking is absolutely contraindicated in patients with thromboangiitis obliterans, who should be advised that they run a very high risk of amputation if they continue to smoke. Techniques to keep the extremity warm range from advice to wear thick woollen gloves or socks in cold weather to the use of chemically activated handwarmers or electrically heated gloves, Perhaps less practical might be the advice to move to a warmer climate.

While the majority of patients can be managed satisfactorily with these conservative measures a few continue to have frequent or severe attacks or progress to digital ischaemia. For these patients the choice lies between drug therapy or sympathectomy.

Drug therapy

A variety of vasodilatory drugs with different modes of action are available and many have been advocated in the treatment of Raynaud's syndrome. Unfortunately the syndrome itself may remit spontaneously and there is also a strong placebo effect on the frequency and severity of attacks, so trials of drug therapy have to be very carefully controlled and the results interpreted with caution. A significant response to the drug is seen in many trials but only 30 to 60 per cent of the patients respond; in many cases the attacks continue and the drug response is only apparent as a reduction in the frequency or severity of the attacks without complete amelioration of the syndrome. Side-effects are common with these drugs and can be unpleasant. Some therapies are only effective when administered by the intravenous route, which requires hospital admission, and these have to be reserved for the most severely affected patients.

Despite these reservations a trial of the different drug therapies to see if one will induce a response is often worthwhile, because the only other alternative is surgery, the results of which are by no means guaranteed. As the outlook of the syndrome is generally benign, there is plenty of time to give drug therapy a reasonable trial, although the overall clinical impression is that marked improvements in symptoms are difficult to detect unless a strict diary of the frequency and severity of attacks is kept to allow comparisons before and after drug therapy to be made.

The best studied oral agents are nifedipine and thymoxamine and effective intravenous agents are iloprost and ketanserin.

Nifedipine

Nifedipine is a calcium channel blocking agent that interferes with the inward displacement of calcium ions through the slow channels of active cell membranes. In vascular smooth muscle cells the effect of this interference is a reduction in vascular tone with subsequent vasodilatation. Nifedipine is often used for the treatment of angina and hypertension and is the first choice of many clinicians for the treatment of Raynaud's syndrome. Side-effects are common and include headache, flushing, peripheral oedema, eye pain, and blurred vision.

Thymoxamine

Thymoxamine acts by competitive antagonism of α-adrenoreceptors and blocks vasoconstriction in the skin. There is a low incidence of side-effects with thymoxamine but only 25 to 30 per cent of patients may notice any subjective improvement in symptoms.

Iloprost

The prostanoids prostaglandin E_1 and prostacyclin are potent vasodilators and inhibit platelet aggregation; they are effective in severe Raynaud's syndrome but their rapid metabolism may limit their therapeutic potential. Iloprost is a more stable prostacyclin analogue, with a half-life 10 times longer than that of prostacyclin. Iloprost is administered as a 6-h intravenous infusion at a dose of 2 ng/kg.min on three consecutive days. The dose is reduced in 0.5 ng/kg.min increments if side-effects, which may include severe headache, dizziness, vomiting, and diarrhoea, occur. Studies in patients with severe secondary Raynaud's syndrome due to scleroderma report a 30 per cent reduction in the frequency of attacks and a 20 per cent reduction in their severity. Digital ischaemic lesions can heal after iloprost infusion but healing may not necessarily be significantly better than after placebo infusions. No orally effective prostanoid preparation is currently available and the severity of side-effects confines the use of intravenous preparations to hospital inpatients. Although the effects of iloprost on vasodilatation and platelet adhesion disappear almost as soon as the infusion is stopped, the clinical improvement may last for up to 6 weeks and repeated infusions may be given.

Ketanserin

Ketanserin is a serotonin receptor antagonist that antagonizes serotonin-induced vasoconstriction and platelet aggregation and inhibits the amplification by serotonin of vasoconstriction and platelet aggregation by other agents. Intravenous ketanserin improves finger blood flow and relieves ischaemic symptoms in severe secondary Raynaud's syndrome, but the effect is short-lived and wears off after the infusion is stopped. Oral ketanserin is also available and although it can improve finger blood flow, many studies have shown no subjective clinical improvement in Raynaud's symptoms over placebo.

Chemical sympathectomy

Reserpine is a rauwolfia alkaloid which depletes noradrenaline from sympathetic nerve terminals. Guanethidine has a similar effect and also prevents noradrenaline release from postganglionic neurones. Reserpine has been used orally to treat Raynaud's syndrome but the high incidence of side-effects associated with long-term use has made it an unpopular choice. Both reserpine and guanethidine may be administered intravenously into an affected extremity distal to a blood pressure cuff which is kept inflated above systolic pressure for 20 to 30 min during and after the injection. This so-called chemical sympathectomy does not produce lasting relief and is not effective in patients with advanced digital vessel obstruction, but may give short-term relief of severe symptoms in patients with predominantly vasospastic disease.

Surgical therapy

The mainstay of surgical treatment in Raynaud's syndrome is sympathectomy, although surgery may also be required when the syndrome is secondary to proximal vascular disease. In the latter cases it may be necessary to resect a cervical rib or band to relieve thoracic outlet compression, although first rib resection has also been advocated. Occasionally the subclavian stenosis and post-stenotic dilatation are so severe that local excision and vein graft replacement of the artery are required. The transaxillary approach to first rib resection is best avoided in this latter group of patients where the supraclavicular approach gives better proximal control of the artery.

Atherosclerotic disease in the brachial artery is rare but it is possible to bypass severely stenosed or occluded segments with a vein graft if the symptoms warrant it. The majority of patients with severely ischaemic digits due to Raynaud's syndrome have intact distal pulses and tolerate local amputation to control severe ischaemic pain or gangrene well. In many instances the middle or proximal phalanges can be preserved and primary closure of the amputation stump gives good healing. In severe cases digits may require amputation over a period of time as the disease progresses, particularly in patients with scleroderma. The more that can be preserved of each digit therefore, the better the long-term functional result.

Sympathectomy

The results of sympathectomy for Raynaud's syndrome are variable and there is considerable doubt over its long-term efficacy. Subjective clinical improvement is noted in 60 to 70 per cent of patients immediately after sympathectomy but 10 years later only 30 to 40 per cent of patients are still improved, which is not a statistically significant result compared to non-operated patients.

Good results from sympathectomy may be expected in patients with primary Raynaud's syndrome and in those patients whose secondary Raynaud's syndrome is due to embolic, traumatic, or atherosclerotic obstruction. Good results may also be obtained in patients with thromboangiitis obliterans but results have been uniformly poor in patients with connective tissue disorders. With the exception of the connective tissue disorders, where sympathectomy is usually best avoided, it is generally agreed that sympathectomy should be reserved for patients with recurrent ulceration of the fingertips or those who are severely incapacitated by vasospastic phenomena in spite of adequate medical management.

Lumbar sympathectomy may be performed either operatively or by percutaneous injection of phenol solution. An operative lumbar sympathectomy is performed through a small transverse muscle-splitting incision just above the level of the umbilicus and lateral to the rectus muscle. The sympathetic chain is approached retroperitoneally. Percutaneous sympathetic blockade is much more difficult in the cervical region and hand symptoms therefore require operative cervical sympathectomy. This operation is technically much easier through the transaxillary route than via the supraclavicular approach. Both approaches carry the risk of damage to the stellate ganglion resulting in a Horner's syndrome with ptosis, pupillary constriction, and facial flushing and dryness on the affected side. Resection of the second, third, and fourth thoracic ganglia appears in practice to produce effective sympathetic denervation of the arm and axilla without risking damage to the stellate ganglion. More recently cervical sympathectomy has been performed successfully endoscopically and this seems likely to become the routine approach to this procedure. Although abolished initially after sympathectomy, the vasomotor and sudomotor reflexes may return to the hand a year or more after surgery. Whether this return represents regeneration of nervous fibres or the gradual assumption of a greater role of residual sympathetic pathways is not known, but the phenomenon may account for the variable long-term results of sympathectomy in Raynaud's syndrome.

Summary of treatment

Most patients with Raynaud's syndrome can be managed with advice to stop smoking and to keep the extremity warm. Failure of these simple measures in patients without digital ischaemia is an indication for oral drug therapy with nifedipine or thymoxamine. The onset of digital ischaemia, especially in the connective tissue disorders, justifies a trial of intravenous iloprost therapy. Continued severe symptoms or ischaemia despite full medical treatment warrants consideration for sympathectomy. Local digital amputation may be the eventual outcome of severe ischaemic damage.

FURTHER READING

Cooke ED, Nicolaides AN. Raynaud's syndrome. *Br Med J* 1990; **300**: 553–5.

Lafferty K, Roberts VC, De Trafford JC, Cotton LT. On the nature of Raynaud's phenomenon: the role of histamine. *Lancet* 1983; **ii**: 313–14.

Lewis T. Experiments relating to the peripheral mechanisms involved in spasmodic arrest of the circulation in the fingers. A variety of Raynaud's disease. *Heart* 1929; **15**: 7–101.

Porter JM. Raynaud's syndrome and associated vasospastic conditions of the extremities. In: Rutherford RB, ed. *Vascular surgery*. Philadelphia: W. B. Saunders Company, 1984: 697–707.

Raynaud AGM. Nouvelles recherches sur la nature et la traitement de l'asphyxie locale des extrémités. *Arch Gen Med* 1874; **1**: 5.

Strandness DE, Sumner DS. Raynaud's disease and Raynaud's phenomenon. In: Strandness DE, Sumner DS, eds. *Haemodynamics for surgeons*. New York: Grune and Stratton, Inc., 1975: 543–81.

7.9.3 Vasculitis

GAVIN P. SPICKETT AND JOHN G. G. LEDINGHAM

INTRODUCTION

The term vasculitis embraces a wide variety of conditions in which inflammatory damage to blood vessels is a principal component. The clinical consequences of vasculitis depend on the size and nature of vessels involved, the organs they supply, and the nature of the underlying diagnosis. Most patients with vasculitides will present to physicians in the first instance, but patients with vasculitis affecting major arterial trunks may present to surgeons with, for instance, acute ischaemia of the limbs or abdominal organs. Wegener's granulomatosis is commonly first seen by ear, nose, and throat surgeons since it frequently affects the upper airways and eustachian tubes. Early recognition of a systemic vasculitis is important: most patients respond relatively favourably to medical treatment but have a poor prognosis if left untreated. The diagnosis is often difficult to prove, and in such cases delay in treatment can be particularly hazardous.

The vasculitides can be classified in a number of ways depending on clinical syndromes or histopathological features and size of vessels involved (see Section 7.3). None of these is yet very satisfactory and a retreat to the use of the simple term 'vasculitis' is increasingly favoured. It is important to recognize the considerable overlap which exists between the primary vasculitides, particularly with regard to the size of vessel affected. Table 1 lists the

Table 1 Classification of vasculitis

Primary	Secondary	Unclassified
Giant cell arteritis	Systemic lupus erythematosus	Buerger's disease
Takayasu's disease	Systemic sclerosis and variants	Behçet's disease
Wegener's granulomatosis	Rheumatoid arthritis	Kawasaki disease
Polyarteritis	Infection	
(a) Polyarteritis nodosa		
(b) Microscopic polyarteritis		
(c) Churg-Strauss variant		
Relapsing polychondritis	Cryoglobulinaemia	

Table 2 Presentation of systemic vasculitis to surgical specialities

	Symptoms	Diseases
General/vascular surgery	Peripheral ischaemia Gangrene	Takayasu's disease Buerger's disease Polyarteritis Systemic sclerosis
	Raynaud's phenomenon	Systemic sclerosis SLE Cryoglobulinaemia
	Abdominal pain Bowel perforation	Giant cell arteritis Polyarteritis Systemic sclerosis
	Pancreatitis	Polyarteritis
ENT surgery	Sinusitis/middle ear disease/deafness	Wegener's granulomatosis Cogan's syndrome
	Airway collapse	Polychondritis
	Stridor	Wegener's granulomatosis
Ophthalmological surgery	Iridocyclitis Uveitis Scleritis/episcleritis	Behçet's disease SLE Rheumatoid arthritis Wegener's granulomatosis
	Keratoconjunctivitis sicca	Sjögren's syndrome SLE Rheumatoid arthritis
	Retinal vasculitis Ischaemia	Giant cell arteritis Polyarteritis Behcet's disease
	Keratitis	Cogan's syndrome
Orthopaedic surgery	Arthralgia	Wegener's granulomatosis
	Arthritis	Polyarteritis Rheumatoid arthritis SLE

primary and secondary vasculitides. Primary vasculitides can be roughly subdivided by the size of the predominantly affected vessel and by the presence or absence of granulomata. Such a pathological classification as illustrated in Section 7.3 has little intrinsic merit and does not relate to the underlying triggering event.

MECHANISMS OF VASCULAR DAMAGE

The heterogeneous nature of the vasculitides indicates that there is no single explanation for the vascular damage; few primary vasculitic syndromes have a well understood cause. Epidemiological studies and circumstantial evidence suggest that Wegener's granulomatosis, microscopic polyarteritis, and Kawasaki disease may be triggered by infection, but the nature of the agent(s) is unknown. In the secondary vasculitides the mechanisms of vascular damage are related to the immunological products released as a result of the underlying disorder. The specificity of the disease processes for vessels of particular sizes has not been satisfactorily explained.

The inflammatory response involves non-specific phagocyte cells, macrophages, and neutrophils, which are attracted to areas of vascular damage by specific chemotactic factors. These may be released from the vascular endothelium itself, from adherent platelets, or by activation of the complement cascade. Complement is activated locally either by antigen and antibody (classical pathway) or by the damaged endothelium (alternative pathway). The natural amplification of complement activation means that deposition of a small quantity of immune complex rapidly leads to further complement breakdown, release of chemotactic factors, and cellular recruitment. The complement system is linked to the kinin system and the clotting cascade, both of which are activated, leading to increased vascular permeability and thrombus formation. As inflammation progresses, specific T lymphocytes may be recruited: these release lymphokines, further amplifying the cellu-

Table 3 Key investigations in system vasculitis

Investigation	*Giant cell arteritis*	*Takayasu's disease*	*Wegener's granulomatosis*	*Polyarteritis*	*SLE*	*Systemic sclerosis*	*Rheumatoid arthritis*	*Infection*	*Cryoglobulinaemia*	*Buerger's disease*	*Behçet's disease*	*Kawasaki disease*	*Relapsing polychondritis*
CRP[a]	+	−	+	+	+	−	+	+	−	−	+	+	+
ESR[b]	+	−	+	+	+	−	+	−	−	−	+	−	+
ANA[c]	−	−	−	−	+	+	+	−	+	−	−	−	−
ds-DNA[d]	−	−	−	−	+	−	−	−	−	−	−	−	−
ENA[e]	−	−	−	−	+	+	+	−	−	−	−	−	−
C3 + C4[f]	−	−	−	−	+	−	−	+	+	−	−	−	−
Cryoglobulins	−	−	−	−	+	−	+	+	+	−	−	−	−
Serum electrophoresis	−	−	−	−	+	−	+	−	+	−	−	−	−
Rheumatoid factor	−	−	−	−	−	−	+	−	+	−	−	−	−
c-ANCA[g]	−	−	+	+	−	−	−	−	−	−	−	+	−
p-ANCA[h]	−	−	−	+	−	−	−	−	−	−	−	−	−
Renal biopsy	−	−	+	+	+	+	−	−	+	−	−	−	−
Temporal artery biopsy	+	−	−	−	−	−	−	−	−	−	−	−	−
Angiography	+	+	−	+	−	−	−	−	−	+	−	−	−
Echocardiography	−	−	−	−	+	−	−	+	+	−	−	+	−

+, of value in diagnosis/monitoring; −, not helpful in diagnosis/monitoring.
[a]C-reactive protein. [b]Erythrocyte sedimentation rate. [c]Antinuclear antibody. [d]double stranded DNA. [e]Extractable nuclear antigens. [f]Third and fourth components of complement. [g]Classic antineutrophil cytoplasmic antibody. [h]Perinuclear antineutrophil cytoplasmic antibody.

lar response and promoting systemic effects, including the release of acute-phase proteins and fever. Vascular occlusion leads to local tissue infarction, which may be extensive when a major artery is involved. Healing of the vasculitic lesion may lead to local fibrosis.

The role of antibody in the vasculitis syndromes is poorly defined. Autoantibodies directed against various components of the cytoplasm of neutrophils and against endothelial cells have been described in primary vasculitis: although such antibodies may play a primary pathogenetic role in the disease, rather than being secondary markers of tissue damage, the evidence is far from conclusive. Antibody is more obviously involved in the pathogenesis of secondary vasculitis, as in cryoglobulinaemia and the connective tissue disorders.

INVESTIGATION OF POSSIBLE VASCULITIS

Presentations of vasculitis are protean: features which may lead to a surgical consultation are listed in Table 2. The diagnosis is often difficult to prove, and key investigations required to take a suspected diagnosis further are detailed in Table 3.

The inflammatory nature of the major vasculitides is manifest by an elevation in plasma levels of the acute-phase response proteins. C-reactive protein, which has a short half-life and rapid response time, is the most useful of these proteins for both diagnosis and monitoring therapy. For reasons that are unclear, certain closely related conditions such as systemic lupus erythematosus and systemic sclerosis tend to be associated with the production of very little C-reactive protein, while bacterial infection leads to substantial rises in the C-reactive protein levels. Infections masquerading as vasculitis and intercurrent infection in patients with established vasculitic illness may therefore make interpretation of high levels of C-reactive protein difficult. The erythrocyte sedimentation rate (ESR), an established marker of inflammation, is useful for diagnosis but of little value in monitoring therapy as it is largely dependent on the serum concentration of fibrinogen, which has a long half-life and a long response time. It is also affected by red cell morphology and the degree of anaemia. The ESR will nevertheless be raised in most vasculitides.

Serum immunoglobulins tend to be non-specifically elevated; monoclonal immunoglobulins (paraproteins) may be detected in Type II cryoglobulinaemia and also in Cogan's syndrome (ocular interstitial keratitis, often associated with various combinations of systemic vasculitis, aortitis, aortic valve disease, and musculoskeletal disease) and, less commonly, in the connective tissue disorders. A paraprotein can be identified rapidly by serum electrophoresis. Some abnormal immunoglobulin molecules (cryoglobulins) precipitate from the serum when it is cooled: if the peripheral skin temperature falls below this critical level *in vivo* precipitation may then damage cutaneous vessels. To identify a cryoglobulin, a sample must be taken at 37°C and transported at that temperature to the laboratory, where the clot is allowed to retract at the same temperature. The serum is then removed and then allowed to cool.

Complement levels are valuable indicators which can be used to monitor the activity of systemic lupus erythematosus; in addition,

Table 4 Autoantibodies associated with vasculitis

Antibody		Disease
Antinuclear antibody—homogeneous		SLE
speckled		SLE, Sjögren's syndrome, rheumatoid arthritis, mixed connective tissue disease, systemic sclerosis
nucleolar		systemic sclerosis, CREST syndrome
Anti-double-strand DNA		SLE
Anticentromere		Scleroderma, CREST
Anti-Ro	ENA[a]	SLE, Sjögren's syndrome
Anti-La	ENA[a]	('ANA-negative SLE')
Anti-Sm	ENA[a]	SLE
Anti-RNP	ENA[a]	SLE, mixed connective tissue disease
Anti-Scl 70	ENA[a]	Systemic sclerosis
Anticardiolipin Lupus anticoagulant		SLE, primary antiphospholipid syndrome
Antineutrophil cytoplasm (p-ANCA, c-ANCA)		Wegener's granulomatosis Polyarteritis

[a]ENA, extractable nuclear antigen.

levels are low in some types of cryoglobulinaemia. Both C3 and C4 are acute phase-proteins and their concentrations may be normal even when complement is being consumed; identification of C3 breakdown products may be helpful in demonstrating complement consumption.

Certain syndromes that are accompanied by vasculitis are characterized by the presence of autoantibodies which may be considered to be markers of the disease. This is mainly applicable to the connective tissue disorders (Table 4). In assessing the importance of these autoantibodies when making a diagnosis, it is important to recognize that, as the immune system ages, spontaneous production of raised levels of autoantibodies becomes more common: in middle-aged and elderly patients low levels are not necessarily indicative of disease. Autoantibody production may also occur transiently following infection, particularly with Epstein-Barr virus.

Rheumatoid factors are autoantibodies directed against the Fc region of human immunoglobulin. High levels are present in seropositive rheumatoid arthritis, and this is associated with the development of nodular and systemic disease. However, they are very poor specific indicators of rheumatoid arthritis since they are produced in response to other inflammatory stimuli and infections, and in the elderly. Their presence does not therefore indicate rheumatoid arthritis unless clinical features are also compatible with this diagnosis.

Antibodies to various neutrophil cytoplasmic antigens have been detected in the plasma of patients with vasculitis syndromes, particularly Wegener's granulomatosis, microscopic polyarteritis, and Churg–Strauss syndrome. In Wegener's granulomatosis and microscopic polyarteritis, the antibody which produces a coarse speckled staining of cytoplasm appears to be directed against a lysosomal serum protease (proteinase 3), whereas in necrotizing glomerulonephritis the perinuclear staining antibody probably recognizes myeloperoxidase, lactoferrin, or elastase in polymorphs. Although it has been suggested that these antibodies mediate tissue damage by activating neutrophils, this is as yet unproven. Rather stronger, but still inconclusive, evidence has been gathered to suggest that titres of cytoplasmic staining antibodies may confirm a suspected diagnosis of Wegener's granuloma, and may also be used to monitor progress and detect incipient relapse. These IgG antibodies have a half-life of some 3 weeks, so that when following response to treatment it is not useful to repeat assays at intervals of less than 4 to 6 weeks.

The high frequency of renal disease in vasculitis syndromes means that examination of the urine for protein and blood by stick testing, and careful microscopic examination for casts and red cells, is imperative. Plasma creatinine and urea measurements are crude but useful indices of glomerular filtration rate; when progressive renal disease is suspected, sequential measurements of 24-h urine protein and creatinine clearance should be performed. Renal biopsy may confirm vasculitis if an involved vessel is sampled, or if the histology is compatible with the renal manifestations of a systemic vasculitis illness. A negative biopsy of renal tissue, however, by no means excludes an arteritic illness.

Arteritis may be confirmed by biopsy of other tissues: those most commonly sampled include skin, muscle, temporal or occipital artery, sural nerve, epididymis, or liver; again it is essential to recognize the patchy distribution of vascular lesions and the need to examine the whole length of any biopsied vessel and to remember that negative findings do not exclude the diagnosis.

Imaging techniques have advanced substantially in the last 10 years. CT scanning or, better, magnetic resonance imaging, may allow accurate detection of vasculitic lesions in areas such as lungs and brain, which were previously difficult to investigate. Angiography has a major role in delineating the extent of vascular damage, particularly in patients with large vessel diseases such as Takayasu's disease and in polyarteritis nodosa, where the detection of characteristic aneurysms may be diagnostic. Echocardiography is the diagnostic test of choice in Kawasaki's disease and should be performed sequentially to monitor the size of the coronary artery aneurysms that are a characteristic feature of this illness.

VASCULITIS SYNDROMES

Giant cell arteritis

This condition, also known as temporal arteritis in view of its predilection for the temporal arteries, was first described in a hospital porter who was unable to tolerate his bowler hat because the pressure it exerted on the inflamed temporal vessels caused severe pain. This disease usually presents with severe headaches, accompanied by localized tenderness of the vessel in its course over the temple and scalp, and sometimes by fever and malaise. It is predominantly a disease of the elderly, particularly women, and is probably the most common form of vasculitis. It is not restricted to the temporal arteries but may involve other major vessels: in the scalp, occipital vessels are occasionally affected. Vasculitis of the facial artery may lead to severe jaw pain which is exacerbated by eating (jaw claudication), while vasculitis of the coronary arteries may cause myocardial ischaemia. Classically, vasculitis may affect the retinal artery, leading to sudden blindness. Vasculitis of arteries of the upper limb may lead to arm claudication, digital ischaemic lesions, and the need for a vascular surgical opinion.

Atypical presentations almost always cause diagnostic delay. There is usually tenderness over the inflamed artery if it can be palpated, C-reactive protein levels and the ESR are almost always raised, and there is usually a normochromic normocytic anaemia. Biopsy of an affected vessel shows characteristic giant cell granulomata, comprising mainly $CD4^+$ T lymphocytes, but a negative biopsy does not exclude the diagnosis. Angiography may be helpful when upper limb vessels are affected (Fig. 1).

The response to steroid therapy is rapid, but large doses (60–80 mg prednisolone/day) may be required. Immunosuppressive drugs such as cyclophosphamide (2 mg/kg.day) or azathioprine (2 mg/kg.day) have been used on occasions, but there is little evidence to suggest that the combination of prednisolone and these agents convey substantial advantages over prednisolone alone. The chief value of adding cyclophosphamide or azathioprine is in reducing the total dose of prednisolone needed to control chronic or unresponsive disease. Immediate therapy is mandatory, in view of the risk of visual impairment which occurs in up to 40 per cent of patients with temporal artery disease. The disease tends to regress in activity and may ultimately 'burn out', and steroids can usually be tailed off after some 1 to 2 years. The disease may relapse, however, and may persist for many years.

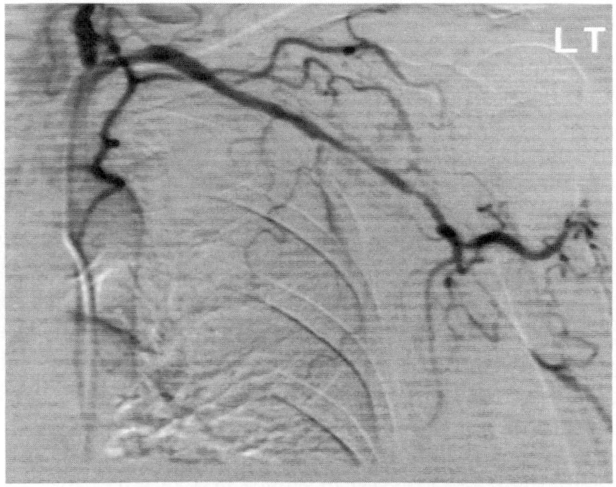

Fig. 1 Angiogram demonstrating the characteristic area of narrowing of the brachial artery in a woman who presented with symptoms of arm claudication and with ischaemic lesions of the fingers. (Kindly provided by Dr E.W.L. Fletcher.)

The aetiology is obscure: there is an association with polymyalgia rheumatica, and the two conditions may develop sequentially or even coexist in some patients. Polymyalgia rheumatica is a much milder illness, characterized by limb girdle stiffness, and it generally responds to lower doses of corticosteroids.

Takayasu's arteritis

Takayasu first described this disease following observations of retinal changes in a young Japanese woman in 1908. The disease is indeed predominantly one of young women, and although it was first described in Asian women and is still much more common in females, it is by no means racially restricted. It affects particularly the aortic arch and the large vessels of the branches arising from it, but it may extend to or affect only the descending thoracic and abdominal aorta and its primary branches. The pulmonary artery may also be involved.

The illness presents with a generalized inflammatory prodrome in around 70 per cent of patients, with fever, malaise, myalgia, and arthralgia. This is followed after a variable period by symptoms and signs of vascular occlusion including claudication of arms or legs, which commonly present to the vascular surgeon. Chest and back pain, breathlessness, and syncopal attacks may lead to medical consultation. The absence of peripheral pulses and the presence of bruits over affected vessels are characteristic. The renal artery is affected in over one-half of patients: hypertension is therefore common, and renal failure may be a late complication. Visual disturbance and ultimately blindness occurs in chronic cases. Death is usually due to congestive cardiac failure and/or myocardial infarction. The vessel most frequently affected is the subclavian artery (85 per cent).

The pathological features are those of a panarteritis, involving all layers of the elastic arteries. Secondary thrombosis and stenotic and aneurysmal lesions are common. Secondary atherosclerotic changes also occur in the damaged vessels.

There is usually evidence of an acute phase response with elevated levels of C-reactive protein and a rise in ESR, but there are no other specific markers. Duplex Doppler ultrasound will demonstrate reduced flow and arteriography will document the extent and nature of the lesions.

Medical treatment with 30 to 50 mg/day of prednisolone will reduce some of the inflammatory response, but it is uncertain whether the overall prognosis is affected. A few patients appear to have benefited from cyclophosphamide treatment, but studies of the effects of this drug are confused by the occurrence of spontaneous remission and sudden relapse. Surgical treatment involving appropriate vascular reconstruction is not contraindicated and may be successful in some cases, particularly when local inflammatory change has been damped down or abolished by corticosteroid or other immunosuppressive treatment.

Wegener's granulomatosis

Wegener's granulomatosis can be separated from other forms of arteritis by its characteristic clinical features, by its histopathology, and by its serological marker, the classical antineutrophil cytoplasmic antibody. None of these is, however, specific; even the histopathology is 'compatible with' rather than 'diagnostic of' the disease. Firm diagnosis, therefore, rests on the coincidence of typical clinical, histological, and serological features.

The pathology is that of a vasculitis affecting predominantly small arteries and veins, and is marked by a neutrophil and mononuclear cell infiltrate, accompanied by fibrinoid necrosis. Granulomata occur within these vessels and in the surrounding tissues and these have an abundance of multinucleate giant cells. The ESR and C-reactive protein levels are invariably raised in the acute phase. Serum immunoglobulin levels are also increased, while complement levels are invariably normal. Antineutrophil cytoplasmic antibodies, usually at high titre, are present in some 90 per cent of patients.

Most patients with Wegener's granulomatosis present with malaise, fever, and arthralgia; other features depend on the distribution and activity of the vascular lesions. The upper airways (nose, nasal sinuses, postnasal space, or eustachian tubes) are affected in 90 per cent of patients. These usually present to the ear, nose, and throat surgeon with chronic sinusitis, nasal discharge, usually with crusting and blood, nasal ulceration, and otitis media. Saddle nose deformity, due to erosion of nasal cartilage, is said to be a typical feature, but it occurs late in the disease.

Parenchymatous lesions in the lung may appear solid on chest radiographs, resembling neoplasms. Central necrosis may lead to fluid levels and the diagnosis of lung abscess or breaking down neoplasm. Infiltrative lesions are commonly misdiagnosed as tuberculosis. These manifestations present with cough, breathlessness, haemoptysis, and chest pain. Reduction of lung diffusing capacity is evidence of generalized interstitial disease, even in the absence of radiographically obvious lesions. Less commonly, submucosal granulomatous lesions sited in the sublaryngeal region may present with the features of extrathoracic obstruction, while localized airways obstruction is caused by lesions lower in the trachea or main bronchi. The clinical presentation of Wegener's granulomatosis affecting the kidney may vary from an abnormal microscopic deposit and modest proteinuria through to rapidly progressive glomerulonephritis, with or without nephrotic features. The disease may be confined to the upper airways, to the lungs, or to the kidney but, in many cases, lesions are found in all three sites. Ocular involvement has been documented with scleritis (Fig. 2), uveitis, and even scleromalacia perforans. When the upper nasal sinuses are affected, granulomata may spread to the retro-orbital space, causing proptosis or disorders of external ocular movement. Cutaneous evidence of vascular damage occurs in around 40 per cent of patients. The disease occurs predominantly in the middle-aged.

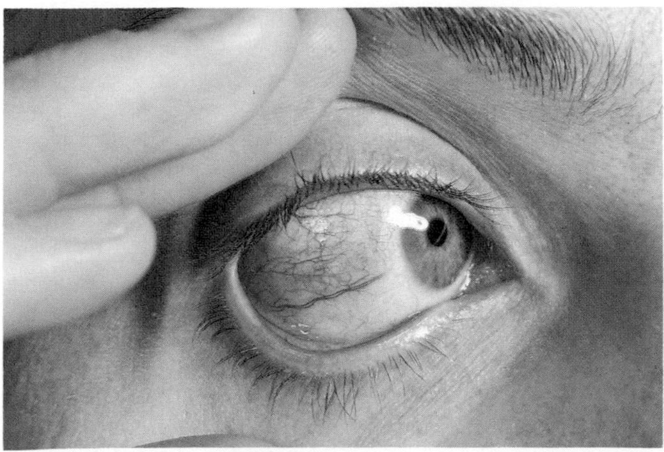

Fig. 2 Episcleritis in a patient with Wegener's granulomatosis.

The treatment of Wegener's granulomatosis is medical. In patients with life-threatening disease presenting with rapidly progressive glomerulonephritis and/or lung haemorrhage, pulsed methyl prednisolone (1 g daily for 3 days) and intravenous cyclophosphamide (2–2.5 mg/kg) can be effective, when followed by continued immunosuppression with prednisolone 30 to 40 mg/day and cyclophosphamide 2.5 mg/kg.day or azathioprine 2.5 mg/kg.day. When the presentation appears less immediately dangerous the same combination of high-dose steroids and cyclophosphamide or azathioprine can be used without the parenteral induction.

The disease appears to be suppressed by such treatment, rather than eradicated, though it may occasionally regress completely and not recur when treatment is withdrawn. More commonly there is a relapse sometimes after many years. Response to treatment is best monitored by a serial measurement of C-reactive protein and antineutrophil cytoplasmic antibody levels. There is laboratory and clinical evidence that relapse may be precipitated by intercurrent infection. The possibility that infusions of pooled immunoglobulin 0.5 g per kg per day for 4 days might be helpful as in idiopathic thrombocytopenic purpura is being explored in controlled clinical trials.

POLYARTERITIC SYNDROMES

Both microscopic polyarteritis (commonly) and polyarteritis nodosa (less often) may give rise to systemic manifestations, as in Wegener's granulomatosis, of malaise, fever up to 40°C (sometimes the only feature), myalgia, and weight loss. When the disease is confined to these manifestations diagnosis can be particularly difficult, even when it is suspected. Other presenting features, which are mostly medical, depend on the site and severity of the vasculitic process: some are more typical of the nodosa types, while others represent the microscopic categories of the condition. Surgical presentations are not uncommon.

Peripheral vascular disease may occur due to involvement of small vessels, which results in ischaemic lesions or frank gangrene of fingers or toes (Fig. 3). Ischaemic arteritic ulcers may occur particularly in the lower limbs, and there may be associated Raynaud's phenomenon. Embolic lesions or claudication may occur, as in giant cell arteritis, when vasa vasorum vasculitis results in stenosis or aneurysmal lesions of medium sized vessels.

Abdominal pain is a well-recognized presentation and probably results from vasculitis in the vessels of the splanchnic circulation. Symptoms are often rather vague and non-specific with ill-defined abdominal pain and occasionally modest diarrhoea or occult blood loss. An area of ischaemic gut or acute appendicitis of vascular origin may perforate, and mesenteric arterial vasculitis may result in a presentation of acute abdomen secondary to infarction of bowel or pancreas.

Renal manifestations present largely to physicians but infarction of the kidney (in polyarteritis nodosa) may result in loin pain, fever, vomiting, and blood and protein in the urine. This syndrome is often diagnosed as pyelonephritis, despite negative urine cultures, or of renal stone disease, despite the absence of firm evidence of a stone. The condition is rare and is best diagnosed by detection of the wedge-shaped infarcts by CT scanning of the

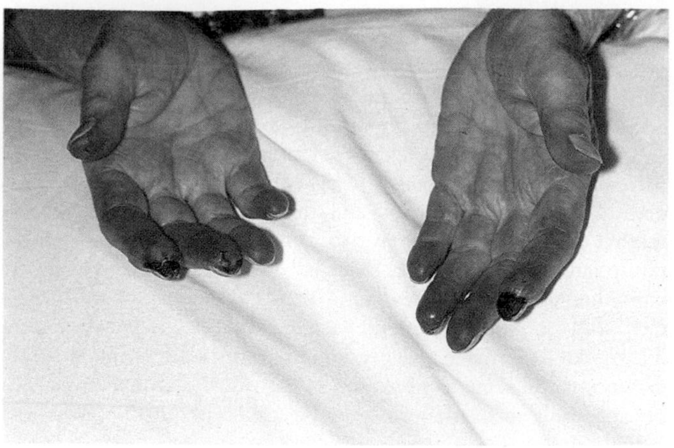

Fig. 3 The hands of a woman presenting with intractable digital ischaemia and who ultimately died of malignant hypertension as a result of systemic sclerosis involving the kidneys.

kidneys. Clinical vasculitis involving ureter, bladder, epididymis, and testis is rare but may result in haematuria or local pain and inflammation.

Obstructive uropathy due to retroperitoneal fibrosis may be quite commonly associated with a periaortitis (microscopic polyarteritis) surrounding the lower abdominal aorta. Vasculitis is sometimes evident from examination of biopsy material. CT scanning or magnetic resonance imaging in this situation shows soft tissue swelling as well as ureteric obstruction responsive to treatment with corticosteroids; mobilization of obstructed ureters into the peritoneum may be necessary.

The thoracic aorta, particularly the ascending arch, may be affected not only by giant cell arteritis and Takayasu's disease but also in relapsing polychondritis. In this rare condition, vasculitis surrounds tissues in which the glycosaminoglycan content is high. There may, therefore, be inflammation and vasculitis lesions over the cartilage of the ear, nose, trachea, larynx and, more rarely, the sclera and aortic collagen. As well as aortic aneurysm or dissection, perichondritis can result in collapse of tracheal tissue. Thoracic aortitis is not a common feature of microscopic or nodosa arteritis.

Although coronary arteries are probably rarely affected, this certainly occurs especially in giant cell arteritis. Vasculitis of the lung, particularly in Wegener's granulomatosis, may be misdiagnosed as a tumour and may present to a surgical team for biopsy or excision. In the Churg–Strauss variant, pulmonary infiltrates, asthma, and eosinophilia predominate and mononeuritis multiplex, which occurs in all forms of vasculitis, is perhaps especially common. Both forms of antineutrophil antibody have been found in this group of patients.

The eye is commonly affected by all vasculitis illnesses, presenting with episcleritis or scleritis more seriously, with vasculitis involving the retinal vessels or the optic nerve, diagnosed by ophthalmoscopy or fluorescein angiography. Anterior uveitis can also occur, but this is much less common. Cranial nerve lesions of the vasa nervorum may produce mononeuritis multiplex of the nerves supplying the external ocular muscles.

Diagnosis of these protean syndromes is often difficult. There are no absolutely diagnostic serological tests but the C-reactive protein level and ESR are almost always increased and a normochromic normocytic anaemia, together with polymorphonuclear leucocytosis, is common. Complement levels are normal or raised. Selective angiography is often valuable and may demonstrate characteristic small aneurysms, the structures which originally gave rise to the term 'nodosa'.

Polyarteritis nodosa is considered to be a 'immune complex disease' based on the link, in some parts of the world, with the presence of hepatitis B virus surface antigen. However, this is not a universal association and most patients in the Western world are not infected with this virus. The treatment is identical to that used in Wegener's granulomatosis, comprising high-dose corticosteroids and immunosuppression with cyclophosphamide or azathioprine. Again, the response to therapy is best monitored by review of clinical manifestations supported by regular review of haemoglobin, white cell count, C-reactive protein level, and ESR, although the latter is less sensitive.

Systemic sclerosis—scleroderma and CREST syndrome

Although in some patients manifestations of scleroderma are confined to the skin, there is often overlap with the more general organ involvement characteristic of systemic sclerosis. Not all clinicians would classify these disorders as vasculitic in origin, but they are associated with inflammatory cell infiltration and obstruction of small blood vessels with excessive collagen deposition. Again the many manifestations present very largely to physicians. Some particular features often lead to surgical consultations.

Raynaud's phenomenon is particularly common and may be the earliest feature of the disease. It may progress to ischaemic damage of fingers or toes, necrotic ulceration and ultimately the need for amputation. Other presentations which may be seen by the surgeon include dysphagia due to oesophageal disease; reflux oesophagitis may lead to stricture formation, and a barium swallow study shows the characteristic poor oesophageal motility. Less commonly, sclerosis of the small bowel may lead to disordered mobility, bacterial overgrowth, and malabsorption. Such patients may present with weight loss, nausea, vomiting, and diarrhoea. A small bowel enema shows characteristic local areas of dilatation and pseudodiverticula formation (Fig. 4). In advanced disease there may be complete loss of peristalsis, effectively intestinal obstruction, and some patients progress to a stage at which their survival is dependent on chronic parenteral nutrition. Perforation of the gut has been described and large bowel disease may also present with obstruction or infarction of the colon.

These syndromes rarely present any difficulty in diagnosis, which is usually obvious clinically. Serologically, they are characterized by a high level of antinuclear antibodies of speckled or nucleolar pattern and a specific autoantibody, Scl–70, which is found particularly in patients with systemic sclerosis. The anticentromere antibody is particularly associated with the CREST syndrome (C for Calcinosis circumscripta; R for Raynaud's; E for (o)esophageal disease; S for sclerodactyly; T for telangiectasia) an entity which, although often presenting as a discrete syndrome, also commonly overlaps with other manifestations of systemic sclerosis. No pharmacological agent is of any proven value in the treatment of systemic sclerosis. Management, therefore, revolves around the amelioration of symptoms and such immediate treatment as the particular clinical manifestations require. Sympathectomy or prostacyclin infusion may be of value, although limited in both time and effect, in the treatment of peripheral ischaemia.

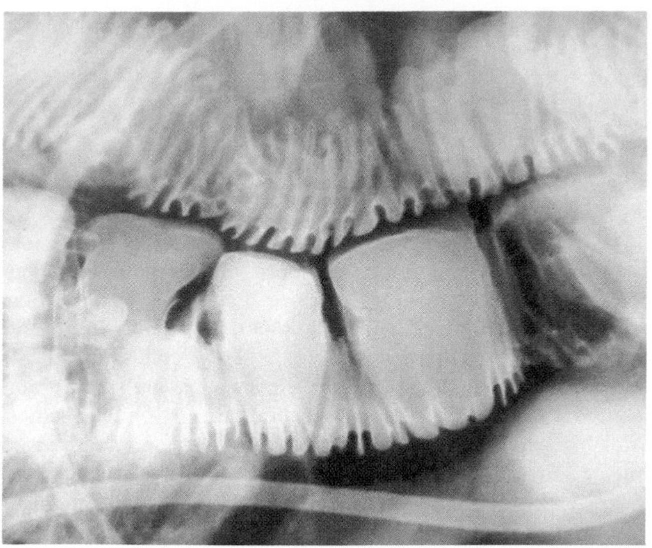

Fig. 4 Small bowel enema in a patient with systemic sclerosis showing dilatation and pseudodiverticular formation.

Broad spectrum antimicrobial (oxytetracycline) therapy is useful in controlling the gastrointestinal manifestations, which depend on overgrowth of bacteria. H_2-receptor antagonists or related agents may be helpful in the treatment of reflux oesophagitis and dysphagia, and pacemakers may be needed when disease affects the bundle of His and causes heart block. Total parenteral nutrition can be given if intestinal disease is sufficiently severe.

Systemic lupus erythematosus

The protean manifestations of this disorder almost always present to the physician, although Raynaud's phenomenon, with or without vasculitis of digital vessels of the upper or lower limbs, may be the only clinical feature in some women, who thus present to a surgical team. The diagnosis is suggested by the pattern of manifestations of the illness. Serological markers include a raised titre of antinuclear antibody, low concentrations of the third and fourth components of complement, increased binding of double-stranded DNA and/or the presence of anti-Ro, anti-La, and anti-SM antibodies. Elevated levels of antibodies to cardiolipin or antibodies interfering with clotting *in vitro*, the so-called 'lupus anticoagulant', are not infrequent findings. These phospholipid antibodies are mainly associated with otherwise unexplained venous or even arterial thrombosis, and perhaps with a history of recurrent abortion, possibly related to abnormal coagulation in the circulation of the pregnant uterus and resultant placental insufficiency.

Behçet's disease

Behçet's disease is a particularly poorly understood illness in which the pathology has a vasculitic component. It is classically characterized by recurrent orogenital ulceration, iridocyclitis with or without retinal vasculitis, and a number of cutaneous lesions. Although it may be more common in Japan and in the countries surrounding the Mediterranean, it is becoming increasingly recognized in the Caucasian population, most commonly in people in the third decade of life. There is a strong immunogenetic background to the disease: it is strongly associated with the HLA-B51 antigen in Turkey, Israel, France and the United Kingdom. HLA-DR7 in addition to B51 has been reported to be associated with retinal and neurological manifestations of the disease.

Histopathologically, affected tissues show a lymphomonocytic infiltration around affected epithelia and associated small blood vessels. The latter may be occluded by proliferation of endothelium and associated fibrinoid necrosis.

Mouth ulcers may be difficult to distinguish from those of lesser pathological significance. Ulcers in the genitalia may affect classically the labia, vagina, penis, and scrotum, and there may be an associated epididymo-orchitis. Skin manifestations include classical erythema nodosum as well as pustular lesions which are widely distributed but most common on the face and back. A characteristic feature is the development of pustular lesions at the sites of minor skin damage ('pathergy').

Among the most important manifestations presenting to surgeons will be those affecting the eye. Uveitis with or without hypopyon, iridocyclitis, retinal vascular lesions including infarction, optic atrophy, and choroidoretinitis are all dangerous complications and may lead to blindness. Neurological manifestations occur in up to 25 per cent of patients. Any part of the central nervous system may be affected, often in a series of episodes with focal neurological signs. If these arise in the hemispheres they may resemble stroke, but manifestations may also occur in the brain stem and cord. On occasion, the findings suggest inflammatory disease of the nervous system, meningitis, or encephalitis with pleocytosis of the cerebrospinal fluid.

Arthralgia and, on occasion, arthritis are commonly reported. Thrombophlebitis of superficial and deep veins may occur and more serious vascular complications include thrombosis, particularly of veins, sometimes such major vessels as the superior and inferior vena cava. Gastrointestinal manifestations are common and include diarrhoea, nausea, anorexia, and abdominal pain. On rare occasions ulceration of both colon and small bowel has been described, as have both malabsorption and pancreatitis. Aneurysmal changes in the aorta and its large branches may also occur. Pulmonary manifestations include shadows on chest radiographs, sometimes associated with haemoptysis and believed to be due to pulmonary vasculitis. Renal manifestations are very rare but both proteinuria and microscopic haematuria have been reported.

Treatment of mouth and genital ulcers with topical ointments or sprays containing both corticosteroids and tetracycline is often very effective, and uveitis may also respond to prednisolone eye drops. The more serious manifestations, particularly those of neurological or retinal disease, are best treated by a combination of corticosteroids and immunosuppressive agents, but the response is uncertain and often disappointing. There are also reports of apparently successful use of colchicine and of aspirin for thrombotic problems. High doses of prednisolone (up to 60 mg a day) appear to be necessary at the onset of serious complications; these are subsequently supplemented by azathioprine in a dose of 2 to 2.5 mg/kg.day. Cyclophosphamide has been used in the same dosage instead of azathioprine, but there is no convincing evidence that it is superior. Cyclosporin may have a particular role to play in the treatment of retinal manifestations, and thalidomide, although contraindicated in women of child-bearing age, has been reported to be beneficial in the treatment of skin and orogenital manifestations in occasional patients.

Kawasaki's disease

This is a systemic illness of children characterized in its onset by lymphadenopathy and mucosal ulceration, with vasculitis sometimes affecting the coronary arteries. The illness presents with fever, conjunctivitis, a skin rash, cervical lymphadenopathy, and oral ulceration. Desquamation of the skin may occur as a late feature. Although originally described in Japan, it occurs worldwide. The cause is likely to be infective, although no pathogen has been identified. The diagnosis is clinical, supported by a non-specific rise in the ESR and in C-reactive protein levels. Cardiac manifestations of the disease may be detected by electrocardiography (QT prolongation and ST segment changes with or without arrhythmias), and two-dimensional echocardiography or coronary angiography are mandatory to monitor the formation of coronary artery aneurysms and their progress. The pathology of coronary artery aneurysms is characterized by a panarteritis with fibrinoid necrosis and local aneurysm formation. Lymph node biopsy may show necrosis of the node with small vessel vasculitis and proliferation of immunoblasts.

In the acute phase of the disease, symptoms may be settled by high dose aspirin (30–50 mg/kg.day); corticosteroids are probably of no benefit and may even be harmful. Infusions of intravenous immunoglobulin at doses of 0.5 g/kg daily for 4 days are effective, but only if given within the first week of the onset of the disease.

Buerger's disease (thromboangiitis obliterans)

Whether or not this disorder exists as a specific entity is controversial, especially in the Western world. However it is a relatively common vascular condition in south-east Asia. The syndrome that suggests its diagnosis most commonly occurs in young men (male to female predominance 9 : 1) who are smokers. In the lower limb, ischaemic symptoms may produce clinical features ranging from claudication, sometimes felt in the arch of the foot, to ischaemic ulceration of the toes. Less commonly there may be Raynaud's phenomenon or claudication sometimes affecting the hand rather than musculature higher up the limb. Angiography reveals the presence of distal disease, such as obliteration of tibial and/or peroneal arteries in the leg. Histological examination of affected vessels does not reveal atheromatous change, but both arteries and neighbouring veins are characteristically infiltrated with neutrophils and small branches may have thrombosed. The only useful therapy is to persuade the patient to abandon smoking.

Lymphomatoid granulomatosis

This condition may be mistaken for Wegener's granulomatosis: the differentiation depends on the report of an experienced histopathologist. In both conditions there is granulomatous vasculitis in affected tissues, which are heavily infiltrated with atypical lymphocytes and plasma cells. Laboratory tests are unhelpful and the sedimentation rate is commonly normal. This disease which, in a significant but uncertain proportion of patients may proceed to malignant lymphoma, may respond well to immunosuppressive treatment with prednisolone and cyclophosphamide or azathioprine.

IMMUNOSUPPRESSIVE TREATMENT IN THE MANAGEMENT OF VASCULITIS

The mainstay of treatment for most primary inflammatory vasculitides is immunosuppression with high-dose prednisolone and either cyclophosphamide or azathioprine in a dose of 2 to 2.5 mg/kg.day. High dose methylprednisolone (500 mg to 1 g daily for 3 days) may be used in conjunction with intravenous cyclophosphamide (1 g/m^2) in patients with life-threatening complications, but the evidence demonstrating the superiority of this approach to high-dose oral therapy is uncertain. Both cyclophosphamide and azathioprine may cause a profound leucopenia and weekly blood counts are mandatory, at least in the initial stages of management. After high-dose and prolonged immunosuppression, administration of prophylactic septrin should be considered, since this is known to be useful in preventing Pneumocystis pneumonia in transplant recipients. Cyclophosphamide may also cause alopecia (reversible) and haemorrhagic cystitis, which may be prevented by the concomitant use of Mesna. Cyclophosphamide is also toxic to the gonads in both sexes, although the degree of toxicity is variable between individuals. Appropriate warnings must be given to patients, who should be offered the opportunity for sperm banking if a future family is to be considered. Long-term use of cytotoxic drugs, particularly chlorambucil and cyclosphosphamide, have been associated with an increased incidence of lymphoid malignancy later in life. Plasmapheresis, which has proven effective in myasthenia gravis, antiglomerular basement membrane disease, and in Guillain–Barré syndrome, has also been found useful by some groups, particularly when vasculitis affects the kidney.

FURTHER READING

Berstein RM. Humoral autoimmunity in systemic rheumatic disease. *J R Coll Phys*, 1990; **24**: 18–25.

Chajek T, Fainaru M. Behçet's disease: a report of 41 cases and a review of the literature. *Medicine*, 1975; **54**: 179–96.

Dahlberg PJ, Lockhart JM, Overholt EL. Diagnostic studies for systemic necrotizing vasculitis. *Arch Intern Med*, 1989; **149**: 161–5.

Fauci AS, Haynes BF, Katz PT, Wolff SM. Wegener's granulomatosis: prospective clinical and therapeutic experience with 85 patients for 21 years. *Ann Intern Med*, 1983; **98**: 76–85.

Hill GL, Moeliono J, Tumewu F, Bratacemadja, Tohandi A. The Buerger syndrome in Java. A description of the clinical syndrome and some aspects of its aetiology *Br J Surg*, 1973; **60**: 606–13.

Huston KA, Hunder GG, Lie JT, Kennedy RH, Elveback LR. Temporal arteritis: a 25 year epidemiologic, clinical and pathologic study. *Ann Intern Med* 1978; **85**: 162–7.

Levitt RY, Fauci AS. Polyangiitis overlap syndrome: classification and prospective clinical experience. *Am J Med*, 1986; **81**: 79–85.

McAdam LP, O'Hanlan MA, Bluestone R, Pearson CM. Relapsing polychondritis: prospective study of 23 patients and a review of the literature. *Medicine*, 1976; **55**: 193–215.

Ohta T, Shinoya S. Fate of the ischaemic limb in Buerger's disease. *Br J Surg*, 1988; **75**: 259–62.

Pisani RS, DeRemee RA. Clinical implications of the histopathological diagnosis of pulmonary lymphomatoid granulomatosis. *Mayo Clin Proc*, 1990; **65**: 151–63.

Raz I, Okon E, Chajek-Shaul T. Pulmonary manifestations of Behçet's syndrome. *Chest*, 1989; **95**: 585–9.

Rowley AH, Gonzalez-Crussi F, Shulman ST. Kawasaki syndrome. *Rev Infect Dis*, 1988; **10**: 1–15.

Savage COS, Winearls CG, Evans DD, Rees AJ, Lockwood CM. Microscopic polyarteritis: presentation, pathology and prognosis. *Q J Med*, 1985; **56**: 467–83.

Shelhammer JH, Volkman DJ, Parillo JE, Lawley TJ, Johnston MR, Fauci AS. Takayasu's arteritis and its therapy. *Ann Intern Med*, 1985; **103**: 121–6.

Specks U, Wheatley CL, McDonald TJ, Rohrbach MS, DeRemee RA. Anti-cytoplasmic autoantibodies in the diagnosis and follow-up of Wegener's granulomatosis. *Mayo Clin Proc*, 1989; **64**: 28–36.

Stanford MR, Graham K, Kasp E, Sanders MD, Dummonde DC. A longitudinal study of clinical and immunological findings in 52 patients with relapsing retinal vasculities. *Br J Ophthalmol*, 1988; **72**: 442–7.

Worrall JG, Snaith ML, Batchelor JR, Isenberg DA. SLE: a rheumatological view. Analysis of the clinical features, serology and immunogenetics of 100 SLE patients during longterm follow-up. *Q J Med*; 1990; **74**: 319–330.

Lancet leader: Cogan's syndrome. *Lancet*, 1991; **337**: 1011–12.

7.10 Renovascular disease

LINDA J. HANDS AND PETER J. MORRIS

RENOVASCULAR HYPERTENSION

Pathophysiology

In a classical experiment in 1934 Goldblatt and his colleagues showed that a clip partially occluding one renal artery of a dog caused hypertension. It has since been demonstrated that reduced renal perfusion stimulates renin release from the affected kidney. This in turn increases the conversion of angiotensinogen to angiotensin I. Angiotensin converting enzyme converts angiotensin I to angiotensin II and this sequence stimulates the release of aldosterone from the adrenal cortex (Fig. 1).

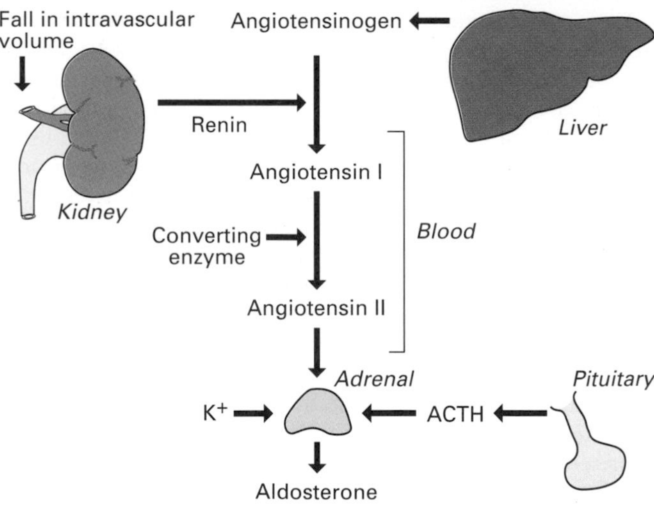

Fig. 1 The renin-angiotensin system.

In fact it is probably the vasoconstrictor action of angiotensin II which is responsible for the initial stages of hypertension. Salt and water retained under the influence of aldosterone are excreted by the other kidney. However, if there is only one kidney, or if the other kidney has been damaged by prolonged hypertension, the body is no longer able to excrete excess salt and water; hypertension is then due to increased intravascular volume. Thus, in the early stages of this disease the affected kidney secretes high levels of renin and renin production from the other kidney is suppressed. Later in the disease salt and water retention suppress renin production in both kidneys.

Causes of renal artery stenosis

In humans 70 per cent of renal artery stenoses are caused by atherosclerosis. Patients with this disease are usually elderly, often male, and frequently have other manifestations such as ischaemic heart disease and peripheral vascular disease.

The other major cause of renal artery stenosis, probably accounting for 20 per cent of cases, is fibromuscular dysplasia. There are three different forms of the disease, each affecting a particular layer of the arterial wall. The most common is medial dysplasia, characterized by hyperplasia of either the fibrous tissue or smooth muscle of the media (Fig. 2). Up to 70 per cent of cases of medial dysplasia are caused by medial fibroplasia, in which thickened fibromuscular ridges alternate with attenuated media so that the lumen is alternately stenosed and aneurysmal. This produces the so-called 'string of beads' sign on angiography (Fig. 3). Fibromuscular hyperplasia usually affects the distal two-thirds of the main renal artery and sometimes the primary branches. The

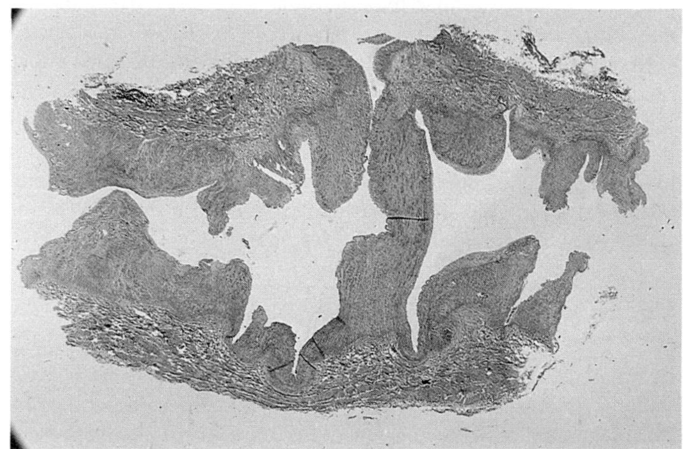

Fig. 2 Histology of the renal artery affected by fibromuscular dysplasia, showing medial proliferation in ridges.

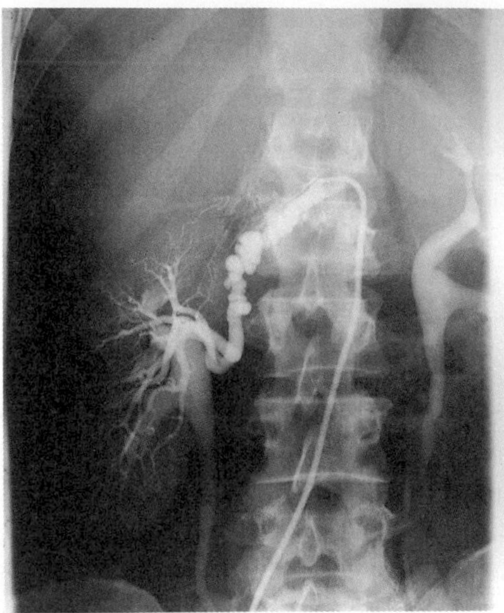

Fig. 3 Angiogram of a renal artery with fibromuscular dysplasia demonstrating the 'string of beads' sign.

entity occurs most often in young women. It commonly affects both renal arteries and occasionally the carotid and iliac arteries.

Other less common causes of renal artery stenosis include trauma, renal artery aneurysm (compressing the adjacent otherwise normal artery), arteriovenous fistulae (diverting blood from the kidney), neurofibromatosis, Takayasu's disease (an arteritis causing stenosis of arteries arising from the aorta and found mainly in young adults and children of Asian origin), and hypoplasia.

Renal artery stenosis and renovascular hypertension

Stenosis of an artery reduces blood flow appreciably only when the luminal diameter is reduced by 70 per cent. Even demonstration of such a stenosis of the renal artery on duplex scanning or arteriography in a hypertensive patient is not sufficient to warrant a diagnosis of renovascular hypertension. The renal artery disease may be an incidental manifestation of atherosclerosis in a patient with essential hypertension. Many nephrectomies and renal artery reconstructions were performed in patients with hypertension and renal artery stenosis before it was realized that fewer than half benefited from the procedure. The ultimate proof of renovascular hypertension is its cure by correction of the stenosis, but several tests have been developed that allow patients more likely to respond to such intervention to be selected.

Prevalence

In the general hypertensive population the prevalence of renovascular hypertension is only 1 to 5 per cent, but it is one of the few curable forms of hypertension. There are particular groups of individuals who are more likely to have renovascular hypertension and these need to be identified for further investigation. In addition, young adults with hypertension, although not necessarily more likely to have a renovascular cause, have a lot to gain by avoiding lifelong treatment if renovascular hypertension is discovered and corrected.

Patients with atherosclerosis often have renal artery stenosis. In patients unselected for hypertension who are undergoing angiography for peripheral vascular disease the prevalence of renal artery stenosis is about 30 per cent; 12 per cent of these have bilateral disease. In hypertensive patients with evidence of peripheral vascular disease the prevalence of renovascular hypertension, as opposed to merely renal artery stenosis, is about 14 per cent.

Patients with severe hypertension are more likely to have renovascular hypertension: the prevalence is 30 per cent in those with a diastolic pressure over 125 mmHg and up to 45 per cent in patients with accelerated hypertension and renal failure.

Age is another important factor. Thirty per cent of patients who develop a diastolic pressure greater than 105 mmHg after the age of 50 years have renovascular hypertension, and it is probably also more common in the elderly with renal failure. Over 70 per cent of older patients with a unilateral atrophic kidney have renal artery stenosis, and nearly 80 per cent of these have significant contralateral stenosis. Many have incipient or overt renal failure as a result, not necessarily accompanied by marked hypertension. At the other end of the scale, renal artery stenosis ranks with coarctation of the aorta as a major cause of hypertension in children.

The presence of a bruit, audible in the upper abdomen or flank, increases the likelihood of renal artery stenosis in any patient.

Progression of disease

This has only been studied in patients receiving medical treatment for their hypertension.

Repeated angiograms taken over 4 to 5 years show increasing stenosis in about 50 per cent of patients with atherosclerotic disease but in only 20 per cent of those with fibromuscular disease. Parallel changes in renal size and serum creatinine can also be detected. When the diameter of the renal artery is reduced by 75 per cent, between 12 and 40 per cent of those with atheromatous stenoses progress to complete occlusion within 1 year. Even at this stage the situation may not be irremedial. Sufficient renal tissue may be maintained by collateral vessels around the capsule and hilum to enable restoration of function if renal artery flow is reinstated (Fig. 4). One-third of patients with atheromatous disease present with bilateral renal artery stenosis; those with initially unilateral disease have a 40 per cent chance of contralateral renal artery stenosis developing within the next 4 years. Fibromuscular disease is even more likely to affect both renal arteries (60 per cent at presentation) although it is less likely to progress.

While one kidney is functioning normally, unaffected by either stenosis of its artery or hypertensive parenchymal damage, adequate excretion is maintained. However, if that kidney develops functional impairment the patient begins to slip into renal failure. Any kidney affected by renal artery stenosis tends to shrink, with loss of nephrons. This shrinkage can often be reversed by restoring blood supply, but once the kidney measures less than 8 cm in length function is unlikely to return. Thus intervention can be of benefit to patients with renal failure, provided it occurs before critical renal mass is lost. There is no correlation between renal function and blood pressure, either before or after treatment.

Acute pulmonary oedema occurs in up to 25 per cent of patients who have renal failure due to renal artery stenosis but it is reversed

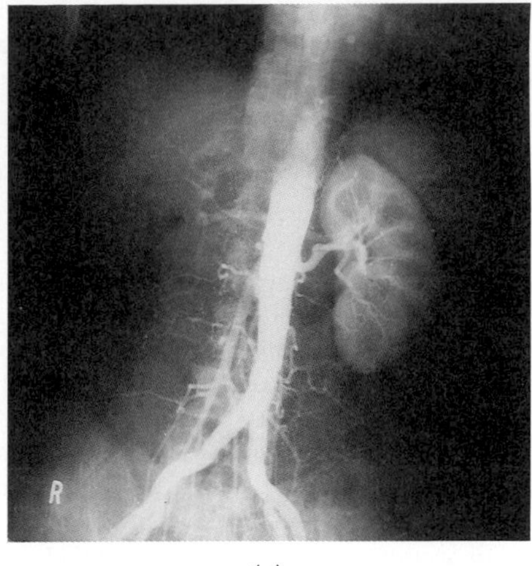

(a)

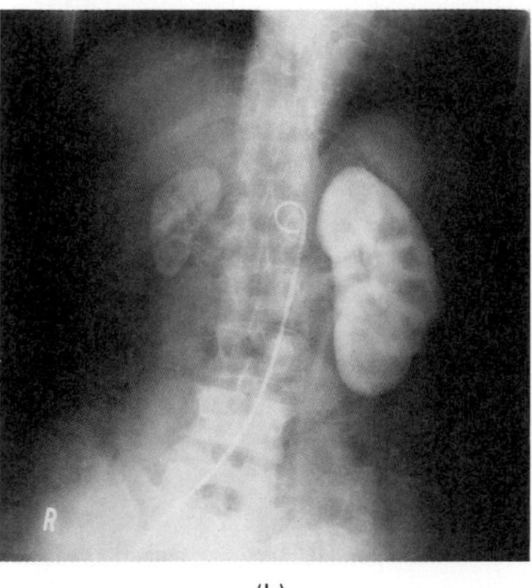

(b)

Fig. 4 Early (a) and late phase (b) of an angiogram showing late filling of the renal vessels via collaterals because of proximal renal artery occlusion.

by revascularization of the kidney. Renovascular disease must be excluded in any patients presenting with pulmonary oedema.

Diagnostic tests for renovascular hypertension

Demonstration of renal artery stenosis

Two initial requisites for the diagnosis of renovascular hypertension are hypertension and renal artery stenosis. Confirmation of the latter used to be left to the later stages of investigation because it required arteriography with its attendant risks. Two recent developments have changed that. Duplex ultrasonography is a non-invasive means of detecting renal artery stenosis both by visualization of the vessel and by measurement of the effect of stenosis on blood flow velocity and waveforms. In specialized centres prepared to devote time to each examination this test is both specific and sensitive. However many examinations are difficult to perform and interpret because of obesity or bowel gas: up to 50 per cent of examinations may have to be abandoned because of technical difficulties. The test also relies heavily on operator expertise. It is therefore unlikely to be useful as a screening test in its present form.

The other major advance is intravenous digital subtraction angiography. This technique requires injection of contrast medium into a vein rather than an artery, which considerably reduces associated morbidity. It relies on computer techniques to demonstrate the arteries when relatively low concentrations of contrast are present. There are several drawbacks to the method. A large amount of contrast has to be injected, which may further compromise renal function in patients with incipient or overt renal failure. Visualization of the vessels depends on cardiac output: output may be impaired in patients with ischaemic heart disease, and even in those with good cardiac output visualization of the renal arteries is often inadequate. Despite these reservations intravenous digital subtraction angiography is becoming a useful screening tool for renal artery stenosis in patients who have a high probability of renovascular hypertension on clinical grounds.

Renin levels

Once the diagnosis of renal artery stenosis in association with hypertension has been established, further investigations are required. The peripheral blood renin level is often elevated, but this is not always the case. Captopril, an angiotensin converting enzyme inhibitor, increases plasma renin levels in patients with renovascular hypertension and can be used to increase the accuracy of the test.

A more invasive test is measurement of renal vein renin by selective catheterization of each vessel via a femoral vein puncture. If unilateral disease is present the affected kidney should secrete high levels of renin and the contralateral kidney should have suppressed renin production. A ratio between the two kidneys of more than 1.5 has long been used as a highly specific (80–100 per cent) test for renovascular hypertension. Unfortunately the test lacks sensitivity: false negative rates of 20 to 50 per cent have been reported. Expressing the higher renin level as an increment relative to the inferior vena cava renin level is said to increase the sensitivity to 74 per cent. If the renal vein renin ratio is measured before and after administration of captopril, sensitivity of the test is increased, but at the expense of specificity.

Renin levels are influenced by fluid balance and by antihypertensive treatment. Ideally these tests should be performed when the patient has been off treatment for 2 to 3 weeks, with controlled sodium intake, and after 12 h of rest but it is often difficult to comply with such restrictions. Impaired renal function may also affect the test.

Isotope scanning

Radionuclide renal scanning is a less invasive means of assessing renal function. Labelled hippuran can be used to assess renal blood flow. However this alone offers no more than other measures of renal artery stenosis. A reduction in renal blood flow following exercise is said to predict a poor response to renal revascularization.

Labelled diethyltetraphenyl aminic acid is used more widely to provide a measure of glomerular filtration rate: in renal artery stenosis, uptake and excretion are delayed. Oral captopril administration produces a further fall in glomerular filtration rate in patients with renovascular hypertension, and makes this a relatively reliable test. Unfortunately most of these tests are only helpful in unilateral disease.

'The gold standard'

The 'gold standard' by which all these tests are assessed is the response of blood pressure to restoration of blood supply. There has been a suggestion that balloon dilatation of the renal artery at the time of intra-arterial angiography should be used as both test and treatment, in view of its low morbidity and mortality reported from certain centres. This approach is not in general use.

Angiography

Intra-arterial aortography is necessary prior to intervention to demonstrate the lesion accurately. Intravenous studies do not provide adequate resolution to plan treatment. A flush aortogram needs to be performed first so that any accessory renal arteries, which may be diseased, are detected and the origins of all the renal arteries adequately shown.

Treatment

Medical

The advent of powerful antihypertensive medications, such as β-blockers and, more recently, calcium channel blockers and angiotensin converting enzyme inhibitors, have brought blood pressure under satisfactory control in most patients. In patients with atheromatous disease the risks of any further intervention are increased because of their associated disease and age. If there is no evidence of renal failure and the blood pressure can be satisfactorily controlled by medication there is probably no justification for more aggressive intervention. However, a reduction in systemic pressure may reduce renal perfusion still further and lead to progressive renal failure. Renal function should be regularly monitored in these patients so that further intervention can be instituted before critical loss of renal substance. Angiotensin converting enzyme inhibitors can cause a reduction in glomerular filtration rate by removing the selective vasoconstrictive action of angiotensin II on the efferent arterioles and so precipitate renal failure. This is particularly likely to happen when there is a critical stenosis in a solitary kidney or bilateral disease.

Patients with fibromuscular hyperplasia are often diagnosed before or during middle age. The risks of intervention are lower and the outcome usually better than that in atherosclerotic patients. In addition, the advantage to the patient in terms of years free of treatment, or on reduced medication, are such that an attempt is usually made to restore blood supply.

Almost any child or young adult with hypertension due to renal artery stenosis should have the stenosis corrected; the results are good whatever the cause.

Percutaneous transluminal angioplasty

Percutaneous transluminal angioplasty of the renal artery is performed under angiographic screening. A guidewire is fed up to the renal artery from a femoral artery puncture site and then passed across the stenosis (or occasionally across an occlusion). Once in position a catheter bearing a balloon at its tip is slid over the guide wire. Inflation of the balloon disrupts plaque or stretches dysplastic vessel wall to remove the stenosis.

This technique works well in fibromuscular dysplasia: 50 per cent of patients are cured and maintain diastolic pressure below 90 mmHg without antihypertensive medication. Most of the remainder have improved blood pressure control, although they still require medication. Patients with atheromatous disease fare less well. The 'cure' rate is only about 20 per cent although a further 60 per cent are improved. Atheromatous disease of the renal artery is often an extension of aortic disease and limited to the renal artery ostium where it joins the aorta. In this situation satisfactory dilatation is usually unsuccessful because the balloon tends to bulge back into the aorta and only 25 per cent of patients have any long-term benefit.

Percutaneous transluminal angiography also has a place in the treatment of renal failure in this disease. Major centres are reporting a reduced or normal creatinine level in over 85 per cent of patients with renal failure due to either fibromuscular dysplasia or atherosclerosis.

Complications of percutaneous transluminal angiography probably arise in less than 10 per cent of cases, and range from a significant haematoma at the puncture site to renal artery thrombosis or dissection and segmental infarction of the kidney by distal embolization of fractured plaque or thrombus. Although facilities for emergency surgery used to be made available because of the potential risks of the procedure these risks are small; the chances of successful emergency surgical intervention are even smaller so this is probably no longer necessary. Restenosis occurs in fewer than 10 per cent of techically successful dilatations in patients with fibromuscular dysplasia but in at least 25 per cent of atheromatous lesions (15 per cent of non-ostial lesions). Mortality associated with the procedure ranges between 0 and 3 per cent but in most centres is less than 1 per cent.

Results vary slightly between different centres: those that have a more aggressive approach and use larger balloons tend to have better results without much increase in morbidity.

Surgery

Anaesthesia

Expert anaesthesia for renal artery surgery is critical. Application and removal of an aortic clamp causes large fluid shifts and imposes significant cardiac stress. Adequate monitoring with good intravenous access is essential. Minimal requirements are intra-arterial and central venous lines for measuring pressure, and many would also advocate a Swan-Ganz catheter.

Surgical access

There are several different surgical approaches to revascularization of the kidney. Exposure of the renal arteries may be transperitoneal or retroperitoneal, although the latter method is less suitable for the right renal artery. A combined approach may also be used in which the peritoneal cavity is opened via a transperitoneal incision and then the spleen, pancreas, splenic flexure of the colon and descending colon are mobilized and swung to the right to expose the aorta, the renal and superior mesenteric arteries, and the coeliac axis (Fig. 5).

Endarterectomy

Transaortic renal artery endarterectomy is often performed. The aorta is clamped and opened at the level of the renal arteries. A local endarterectomy of one or both vessels is performed, and can be extended to the aorta itself at this level if necessary (Fig. 6). This technique is particularly designed for the common situation when the renal artery disease is an extension of aortic plaque, narrowing only the ostium of the renal artery. It cannot be used if the disease is more distal in the vessel.

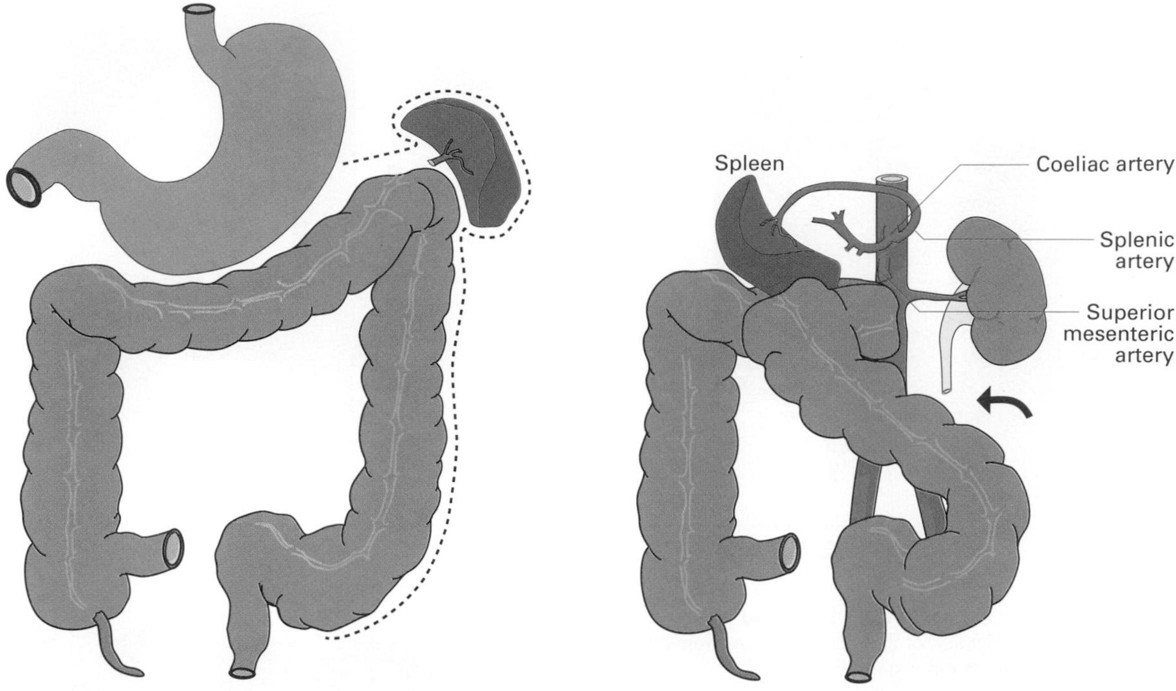

Fig. 5 The left colon, spleen, and pancreas are mobilized and swung to the right to expose the aorta, coeliac axis, and superior mesenteric and renal arteries.

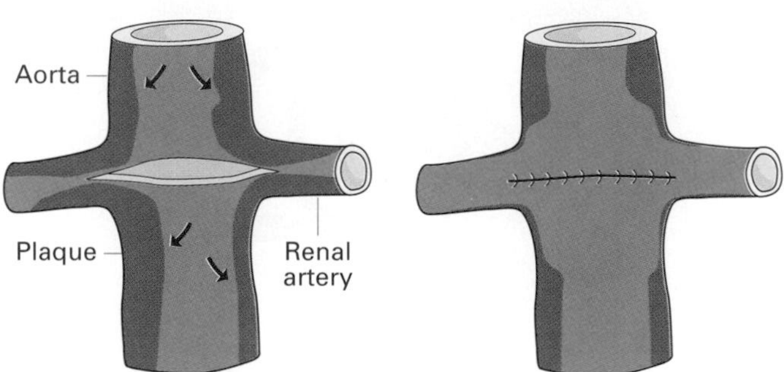

Fig. 6 Transaortic endarterectomy of the renal arteries.

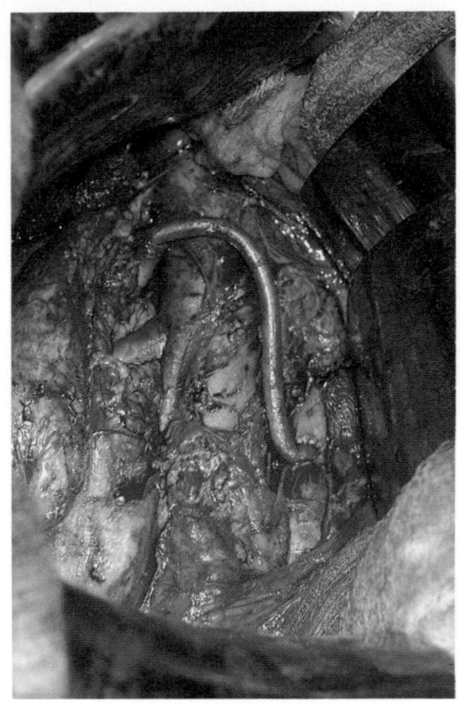

Fig. 7 Aortorenal bypass graft with saphenous vein.

Aortorenal bypass graft

The aorta is clamped, usually below the renal vessels to maintain flow in them as long as possible. A length of reversed saphenous vein is anastamosed to the aorta and then to the renal artery beyond the stenosis (Fig. 7). Graft of a synthetic material, such as polytetrafluoroethylene, may be used instead of vein.

Patients with atheromatous disease sometimes have occlusive aortoiliac disease or an abdominal aortic aneurysm which also requires treatment. In such cases it may be justifiable to replace the lower abdominal aorta with a graft at the same time. Patients with such extensive disease often have bilateral renal artery stenosis. Grafts can be run off the aortic graft to one or both renal arteries (Fig. 8).

Ilio- or viscerorenal reconstruction

Occasionally the aorta is so heavily calcified that aortorenal grafting would present serious technical problems. The iliac arteries may be relatively spared, especially on the anterior wall, and an iliorenal graft can be constructed using saphenous vein (Fig. 9). Failing this, or if there is reluctance to clamp the aorta in a high-risk patient, the visceral circulation can be used to donate blood to the kidney. The splenic artery, provided it is relatively free of atheroma, can be transected and anastamosed to the left renal

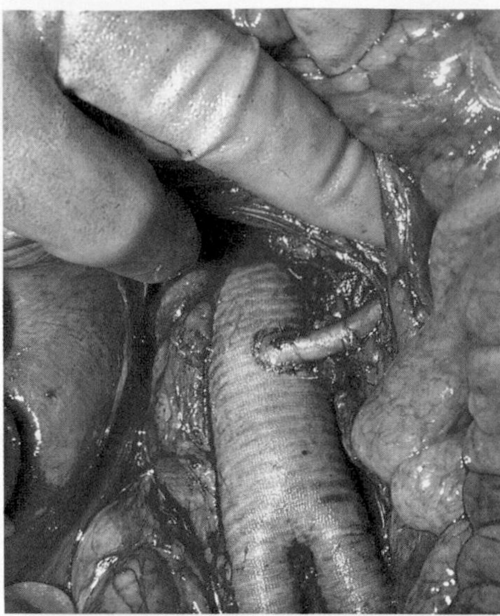

Fig. 8 Replacement of diseased aorta with a bifurcated Dacron graft, together with revascularization of the kidney with a saphenous vein graft from the aortic graft to the distal renal artery.

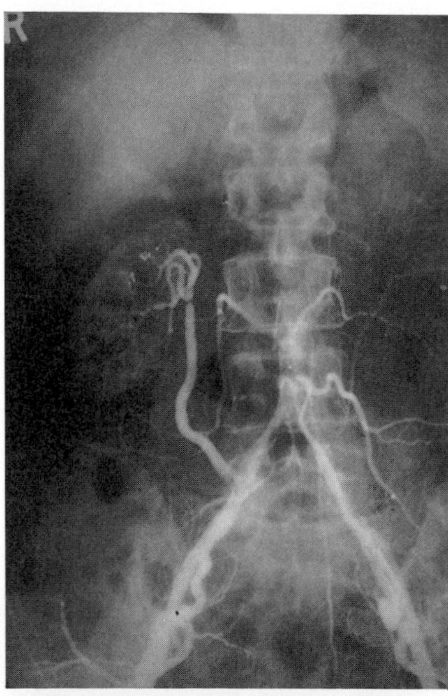

Fig. 9 Iliorenal saphenous vein bypass graft used when the aorta is heavily diseased and unsuitable as a site of graft anastomosis.

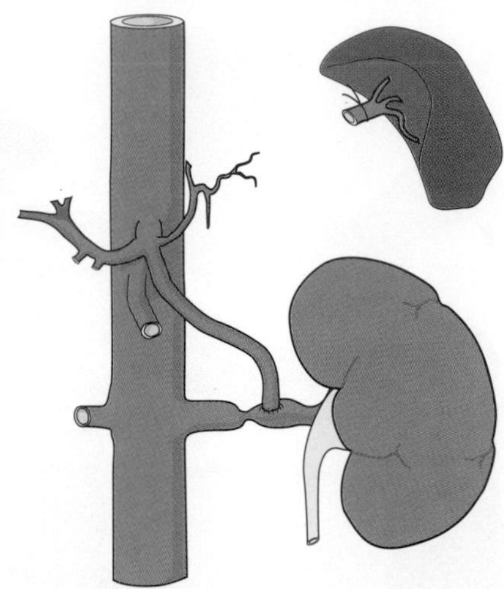

Fig. 10 Revascularization of the left kidney using the splenic artery.

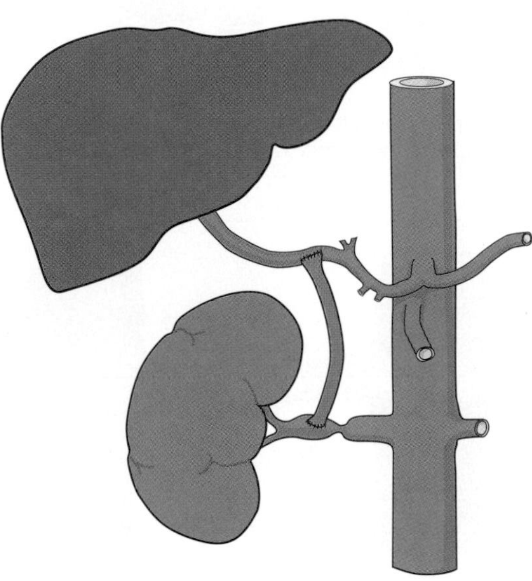

Fig. 11 Revascularization of the right kidney using a vein graft from the hepatic artery to the distal renal artery.

artery leaving the spleen *in situ* (Fig. 10). The hepatic artery can be used to supply the right kidney. A vein graft is usually taken from the side of the hepatic artery just beyond the gastro-duodenal artery and run down to the right renal artery (Fig. 11). Alternatively the gastroduodenal artery itself, the communication between the coelic axis and the superior mesenteric circulations, can be divided distally and anastamosed to the right renal artery if it is long enough. Reconstructions based on the visceral arteries should only be performed if significant coeliac axis disease (and in the case of gastroduodenal artery use, superior mesenteric artery stenosis) have been excluded on angiography.

Autotransplantation

In fibromuscular dyspasia particularly, there may be stenoses of smaller branches of the renal artery. Correction of these lesions requires microvascular techniques using vein graft; for this to be performed the kidney is usually removed from the body and perfused with cold fluid to protect aginst ischaemic damage. It is replaced as an autotransplant in the iliac fossa, anastomosing the artery and vein to the iliac vessels (Fig. 12).

Nephrectomy

Occasionally the kidney has shrunk too far for function to be saved by reperfusion, but it is still a source of renin, causing hypertension. In other cases it proves impossible safely to reperfuse the

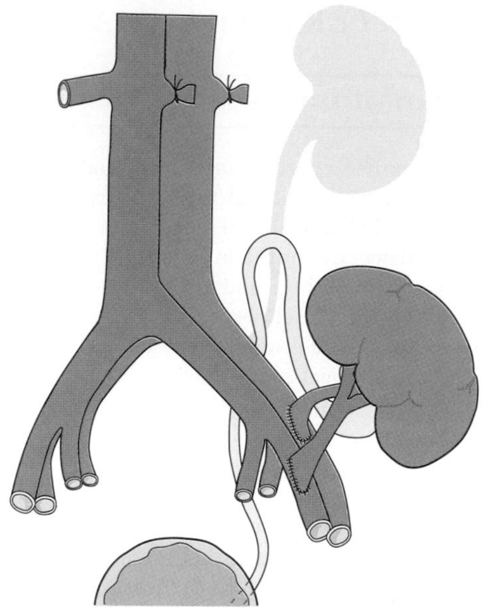

Fig. 12 Autotransplantation of the kidney.

kidney, either because of the extent of disease or the frailty of the patient, and the other kidney is functioning. In these circumstances nephrectomy may provide a simple and safe remedy for hypertension.

Results

The results of surgery in fibromuscular dysplasia of the renal artery are reasonably good. About 60 per cent of patients are 'cured' of their hypertension, 30 per cent have improved blood pressure control, and only 10 per cent fail to respond. Very few patients with fibromuscular dysplasia have renal failure but failure is usually also improved, or at least stabilized, by surgical intervention.

Patients with atheromatous disease respond rather less well. Less than 40 per cent are probably 'cured' of their hypertension, although slightly more are 'improved' and about 20 per cent fail to respond.

Renal failure occurs in about 15 per cent of patients with renovascular hypertension due to atheromatous disease compared with only about 2 per cent of those with fibromuscular dysplasia. Overall, approximately 50 per cent of patients with renal failure are improved, 40 per cent stabilized, and 10 per cent show further deterioration. These results are in the face of declining renal function prior to surgery and so stabilization of renal function is an improvement attributable to surgery. The benefits of surgery decline with increasing degrees of renal failure. Only 20 per cent of those with a serum creatinine greater than 180 μmol/l are improved, about 60 per cent stabilize, and 20 per cent fail to respond. Of those with a serum creatinine greater than 270 μmol/l about 30 per cent fail to respond, and the perioperative mortality rate, in one series, increased from 3 per cent to 13 per cent. Occasionally, patients with severe renal failure respond dramatically well to revascularization of the kidney. They tend to have bilateral renal artery occlusions and potentially functional renal tissue which has been maintained via collaterals. It is obviously important to be reasonably sure that such tissue exists before embarking on complicated, relatively high-risk surgery. The angiogram may show filling of the distal renal artery via collaterals (Fig. 4). Occasionally, but not always, a radioisotope scan demonstrates collateral blood flow reaching the kidney. Renal length on ultrasound is a fairly good guide: if less than 8 cm revascularization is unlikely to improve renal failure and may increase renovascular hypertension. Demonstration of viable glomeruli in a renal biopsy, taken either pre- or perioperatively, is also useful.

The mortality rate associated with renal artery surgery is low in patients with fibromuscular hypertension. In patients with atheromatous disease it is 3 to 10 per cent if surgery is confined to only one renal artery but this increases with extended surgery: aortic reconstruction with bilateral renal artery revascularization carries a perioperative mortality rate of up to 15 per cent. As might be expected the presence of significant atheromatous disease in the coronary and cerebral circulations increases mortality. It is probably also higher in those with renal failure.

A direct comparison between percutaneous transluminal arteriography and surgery in the treatment of renovascular hypertension cannot be made because the patient groups are dissimilar. The former is used mainly to treat young patients with fibromuscular dysplasia who are otherwise reasonably fit. It is not applicable to the patient with widespread atheroma affecting the aorta and extending into the renal arteries, who is also at much greater risk from surgery. The patients with fibromuscular dysplasia who come to surgery are those with complex branch lesions and those in whom percutaneous transluminal angioplasty has failed.

Overview of atheromatous renal artery disease

This disease encompasses a wide spectrum of patients. At one end is the man in his fifties with significant stenosis of one renal artery causing hypertension, with normal renal function, a slightly irregular aorta, mild asymptomatic peripheral vascular disease, and no evidence of significant heart disease. At the other extreme is the woman in her eighties with severe renal failure, hypertension, rest pain, and a history of several myocardial infarctions. In between are patients with any combination and severity of these problems.

If hypertension that can be controlled satisfactorily with medication is the main problem and the kidneys appear to be functioning adequately, no further intervention is required, provided renal function is monitored regularly. If hypertension is difficult to control or renal function starts to deteriorate and the lesion is a short stenosis or even occlusion, percutaneous transluminal angioplasty is indicated. However if the lesion is ostial, as it often is in these circumstances, this treatment may fail; if it succeeds the stenosis is likely to recur. In these circumstances many vascular surgeons would proceed directly to surgery.

In patients with more extensive atheromatous disease, who are usually older, both renal arteries and the aorta itself are involved. Thus the patient may have renal failure and lower limb ischaemia or an abdominal aortic aneurysm, both of which require treatment. However these patients also probably have significant myocardial ischaemia and will respond poorly to the stress of an aortic clamp; they also have cerebrovascular disease, which increases the risk of perioperative cerebrovascular accident. Hypertension may be controllable by medication, rest pain by analgesics, renal failure by dialysis, and the risks of aneurysm rupture can be ignored. However, this approach usually leads to a relatively poor quality of life. It is possible to replace the aorta and revascularize both kidneys, even in the elderly. Obviously the risks associated with such surgery depend on the patient's general health and the skill of the surgeon and anaesthetist. In major centres of such surgery the perioperative mortality has been reported as less than 6 per cent. Renal failure is improved or stabilized in all but 6 per cent, and hypertension improves in over 90 per cent. If the patient's health dictates it and the extent of associated disease allows, the kidneys may be reperfused via the visceral vessels to avoid the dangers of aortic clamping. Although surgical treatment of renovascular disease was previously restricted to the young and middle-aged, it is now being used in the treatment of the elderly, in whom medical treatment or percutaneous transluminal angiography prove unsatisfactory. The attendant risks to heart and brain can be reduced by careful monitoring, newer techniques, and even coronary artery bypass grafting or carotid endarterectomy prior to renal revascularization.

Overview of renovascular disease due to fibromuscular dysplasia

These patients are usually young, and have none of the stigmata of generalized vascular disease. They rarely develop renal failure, but they are at risk from cerebrovascular accidents or heart disease because of their hypertension: this must be detected and treated before the development of irreversible end-organ damage. Younger patients have a less satisfactory response to medical treatment, and surgical intervention is less hazardous. In general, fibromuscular renovascular hypertension responds well to either percutaneous transluminal angioplasty or surgical intervention, but the former is preferred since it is a relatively simple procedure with fewer associated risks. Most dysplastic lesions are amenable to percutaneous transluminal angioplasty, except for those in the smaller branches of the renal artery where the risks of dilatation are greater and the technical success rate diminishes. Surgery is usually only undertaken in patients in whom percutaneous transluminal angioplasty has failed or in whom the lesion is in the distal branches.

Children with renovascular hypertension

The most common cause of renovascular hypertension in children is fibromuscular dysplasia. Other causes include arteriovenous malformations, aneurysms, hypoplasia, Takayasu's disease, and neurofibromatosis. If the lesion is proximal it is occasionally possible to excise the affected artery and reanastamose the vessel to the aorta; however, a more complex procedure is usually required. Aortorenal bypass grafting is an option, but the use of saphenous vein in prepubertal children has led to aneurysmal dilatation or stricture formation in the graft at a later stage. This can be avoided by using autogenous artery, usually one of the internal iliac arteries. An alternative approach is to autotransplant the kidney. This approach is essential when microscopic bench repair of intrarenal abnormalities is required. Hypoplastic renal arteries are often associated with a low coarctation of the aorta, making this vessel unsuitable for bypass grafting. However the iliac arteries are usually spared, and either the kidney can be autotransplanted or an iliorenal graft constructed. Occasionally, especially in those patients with unilateral disease, the kidney is not worth salvaging and the only option is nephrectomy.

The results of surgery for renovascular hypertension in children are excellent, with a cure rate of 90 to 100 per cent.

RENAL ARTERY TRAUMA

Mechanism of injury

Deceleration in either a vertical or a horizontal direction imposes stretching and shearing forces on the renal artery because it joins the relatively mobile kidney to the fixed aorta. These forces cause intimal tears, particularly in the middle third of the artery, which may then lead to dissection and thrombosis of the vessel. Occasionally the entire vessel wall is disrupted and a perirenal haematoma forms. There is often remarkably little blood loss (and few concomitant physical signs) because of renal artery spasm. Blunt trauma to the kidney usually causes parenchymal damage, but it may disrupt the renal pedicle.

Complete occlusion or disruption of the main stem of the renal artery leads to renal infarction. Most of these injuries occur in young adult males with previously normal renal arteries. Development of cortical collateral vessels that might maintain viable renal tissue is usually poor. Thus in most of these patients there is a very narrow window of opportunity, probably within 1 to 2 h of injury and almost certainly within 6 h, in which to revascularize the kidney and recover function. There are reports in the literature of successful revascularization several days after injury, but these are relatively rare. Late revascularization is usually associated with development of renovascular hypertension and a need for nephrectomy. The patient may develop renovascular hypertension even if no attempt is made at revascularization, since ischaemic renal tissue survives, maintained by a partially occluded renal artery or cortical collaterals. The incidence of hypertension following trauma has been cited as between 10 and 50 per cent, but it is difficult to assess: not all cases of renal trauma are detected, and follow-up is incomplete on those that are detected. It develops between days and years after the injury and in up to 80 per cent of cases appears to be transient.

Symptoms and signs

Renal artery damage is often missed in the initial assessment since there are frequently few signs and often other injuries. It is more likely to be discovered at autopsy, during later urological assessment, or when the patient is evaluated for hypertension. At the initial presentation, patients may complain of unilateral flank pain, and occasionally of abdominal pain. Patients with severe disruption present with shock; those with lesser injuries have at least microscopic haematuria, some have loin tenderness and in a few a bruit can be heard in the upper abdomen or flank.

Investigations

Any trauma patient with even microscopic haematuria must undergo intravenous urography. This will demonstrate any abnormality in renal function and, very importantly, will confirm that the patient has another functioning kidney. Patients in whom the intravenous urogram is normal can be treated conservatively; if the examination shows no function on one side and the patient is haemodynamically unstable, immediate laparotomy is required to deal with the renal artery damage. If the patient is stable but has no function demonstrable in one kidney angiography or CT scan with contrast to demonstrate the arteries may be helpful as a prelude to reconstructive surgery, provided it does not delay intervention unduly.

A patient who presents with hypertension some time after trauma should undergo angiography to delineate any renal artery defect, in the same way as any other patient with renovascular hypertension.

Treatment

Most patients with renal trauma and normal renal function on intravenous urography can be managed conservatively. Those with severe disruption of the renal pedicle who present with profuse bleeding and absent renal function need emergency laparotomy. In these patients, extensive disruption often precludes reconstruction of the kidney, and nephrectomy is required.

The stable patient with absent renal function can either undergo surgery with a view to reconstruction or be treated conservatively. If more than 6 h have elapsed since the injury, reconstruction is unlikely to be successful and, unless both kidneys are non-functional, is probably not justified. The ischaemic kidney often shrivels and poses no further problem. If the other kidney is normal, renal function is maintained and relatively few patients develop troublesome renovascular hypertension. Laparotomy to remove an ischaemic kidney is unnecessary at this stage.

Reconstruction may be feasible if surgery is performed within 6 h of injury. Thrombectomy of the renal artery and excision of the affected segment with reanastomosis or vein interposition graft are usually required.

Patients known to have suffered trauma to the renal artery, especially those with non-functioning kidneys on intravenous urography should undergo regular blood pressure monitoring so that renovascular hypertension can be detected and treated before end-organ damage results.

RENAL ARTERY ANEURYSMS

Incidence

Renal artery aneurysms appear to be uncommon. Retrospective studies of postmortem reports put the prevalence at about 0.01 per cent; however many are small and intrarenal, and might not be detected on routine postmortem examination. Angiographic studies detect such aneurysms in up to 1 per cent of individuals (Fig. 13), although these are often selected for study on the basis of symptoms such as pain, haematuria, or hypertension, which might bias the findings. However, one prospective postmortem study found the prevalence to be 9.7 per cent in an apparently unselected series of individuals. Renal artery aneurysms occur with equal frequency in either sex and have been detected at all ages.

Pathology

The majority of these aneurysms are less than 1 cm in diameter and most are saccular. They occur with equal frequency in the main stem artery, in the primary branches, and in the peripheral branches. They are bilateral in up to 10 per cent of patients, and multiple aneurysms occur within one kidney in another 13 per cent. Many of these aneurysms occur at branch points, and as they sometimes occur in children they may be due to congenital weakness of the arterial wall at these points. They are rarely associated with atherosclerosis, despite the fact that about 20 per cent are calcified.

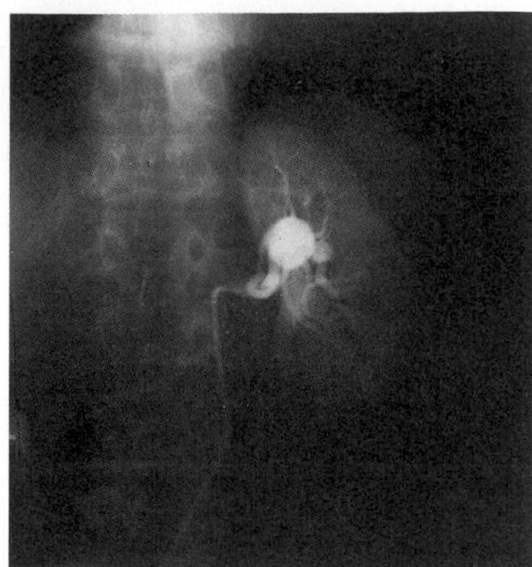

Fig. 13 Renal artery aneurysm (by courtesy of Dr E. W. Fletcher).

Fibromuscular dysplasia, and in particular the most common form, medial fibroplasia, is associated with microaneurysm formation in the main stem artery or its primary branches. However, these are usually considered separately from other renal artery aneurysms.

Consequences of renal artery aneurysms

The predominant risk is rupture. Rupture is most likely to occur during pregnancy, especially in the third trimester, but even then splenic artery aneurysm rupture is 4 to 5 times more common. It presents with abrupt onset of flank pain and hypotension and the mortality is high for both mother (56 per cent) and fetus (82 per cent). Few renal artery aneurysms which rupture in pregnancy are associated with medial hyperplasia, despite its occurrence mainly in young women. Prior to rupture they are usually asymptomatic, although a bruit may be audible.

Aneurysms may thrombose but, because they are saccular, rarely cause arterial occlusion. For the same reason they are unlikely to shed emboli into the distal renal vasculature. Occasionally they are associated with haematuria, presumably because of erosion into the renal pelvis.

Renal artery aneurysms have been associated with hypertension but are rarely the cause of it. Many of the patients in whom they are detected on angiography are investigated because of hypertension and the aneurysm is incidental: surgical treatment of the aneurysm does not usually cure the hypertension unless the aneurysm distorts and compresses the adjacent artery and causes a functional stenosis. Fibromuscular dysplasia may be associated with both hypertension and renal artery aneurysms but it is the stenotic component of the disease that is important in producing hypertension.

Treatment

An aneurysm detected in pregnancy should be repaired before the third trimester, despite the risks to the fetus. Females of child-bearing age should also have such an aneurysm repaired. The aneurysm can often be excised and the defect in the side of the artery closed with a vein patch. If the aneurysm is more extensive an aortorenal vein graft may be required. When multiple intrarenal aneurysms are present, *ex-vivo* reconstruction becomes necessary.

Unless a renal aneurysm is thought to be the cause of hypertension or troublesome haematuria from the renal artery, they rarely need treating in any other patients. Few patients with aneurysms experience problems, even over long periods of time.

RENAL ARTERIOVENOUS FISTULAE

Aetiology

Renal arteriovenous fistulae are uncommon. Approximately 30 per cent are congenital; nearly half of the acquired fistulae are secondary to renal biopsy and many follow renal surgery, such as nephrolithotomy or partial nephrectomy, or renal trauma. A few may arise from erosion of a renal artery aneurysm into an adjacent vein and they are sometimes seen in renal tumours. Fistulae occasionally develop in the renal pedicle following nephrectomy, probably due to mass ligature of the artery and vein. Fistula following renal biopsy seems particularly likely to occur if the patient is hypertensive prior to the procedure.

Pathology

Congenital arteriovenous fistulae are often large, complex, cirsoid malformations with multiple communications, and occupy much of the kidney (Fig. 14). Those which develop following biopsy are usually small and intrarenal (Fig. 15). Those associated with trauma may affect the intra- or extrarenal vessels and sometimes even the inferior vena cava.

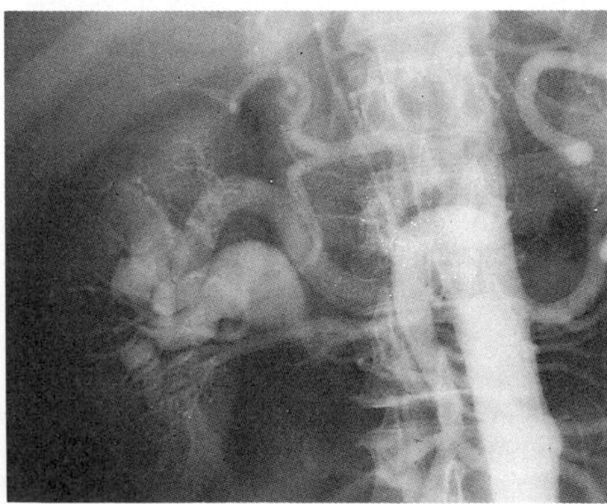

Fig. 14 Large arteriovenous fistula in hilum of kidney.

Small arteriovenous fistulae usually cause no problems. Larger fistulae are associated with two main problems. The first is due to the increased demands on cardiac output as blood is diverted through the low resistance fistula away from the general circulation. Systolic hypertension with a low diastolic pressure develops, and the patient may suffer high output cardiac failure. The second complication is the steal of blood from normal renal parenchyma to the fistula. Relative ischaemia of renal tissue stimulates renin production and leads to renovascular hypertension, so that diastolic pressure also rises. In a patient with pre-existing renal parenchymal disease, a fistula may also seriously compromise renal function. Rarely, an arteriovenous fistula ruptures to produce an intra- or extrarenal haematoma.

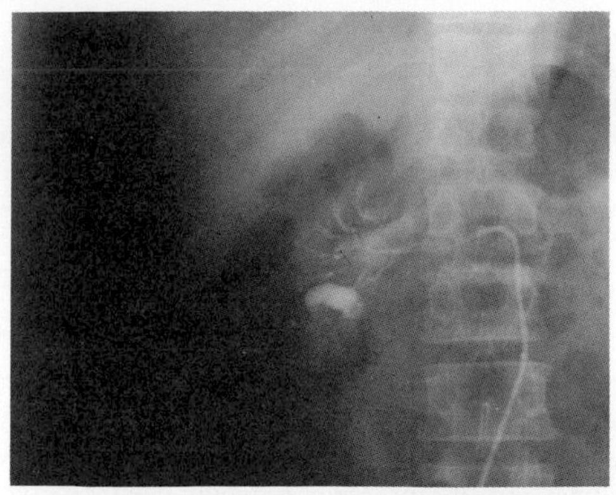

Fig. 15 Small arteriovenous fistula in the kidney following renal biopsy.

Symptoms and signs

About 60 per cent of patients have microscopic or macroscopic haematuria, but unless they have symptoms associated with heart failure or hypertension there are usually no significant problems in the history. On examination the only sign of the fistula itself is a continuous bruit audible in the upper abdomen or flank.

Investigations

An intravenous urogram may demonstrate reduced opacification of renal substance where blood has been diverted to the fistula, or distortion of the renal pelvis by an intrarenal fistula. In most cases, though, this investigation is of little help. Renal isotope scans may also demonstrate reduced perfusion but offer little more. The definitive investigation is the angiogram: this demonstrates the fistula, its feeding and draining vessels, and the extent of steal from the rest of the kidney.

Measurement of renal vein renin levels may not be helpful in the patient who has also developed renovascular hypertension, because the high flow of arterial blood through the renal vein dilutes renin washed out from the affected kidney.

Treatment

Most small intrarenal arteriovenous fistulae do not require treatment. The majority of those that develop following renal biopsy or trauma close spontaneously within 18 months.

Single intrarenal fistulae which cause problems can often be treated by embolization under radiographic control. Metal coils are usually placed in the segmental feeding vessel to promote thrombosis, often with temporary balloon catheter occlusion of the vessel proximal to this point to prevent the coils being carried through into the vein and systemic circulation.

Congenital arteriovenous fistulae are often too complex to treat by embolization and require surgery. This usually involves partial or complete nephrectomy because of the extent of renal disease.

Fistulae of the pedicle vessels are usually treated surgically. The fistula is excised and standard repair of the artery and vein performed, either by simple suture, vein patch, or interposition graft.

Hypertension associated with renal arteriovenous fistulae is improved or cured in 60 per cent of patients in whom the fistula is closed or the kidney removed. If the fistula is associated with trauma the response rate increases to 85 per cent.

FURTHER READING

Goldblatt H, Lynch J, Hanzai RF, Summerville WW. Studies on experimental hypertension–I, The production of persistent elevation of systolic pressure by means of renal ischaemia. *J Exp Med* 1934; **59**:347–79.

Jenkins AMc. Operations for renal ischaemia. In Bell PRP, Jamieson CW, Ruckley CV, eds. *Surgical Management of Vascular Disease*, 751–66.

Maldonado JE, Sheps SG, Bernatz PE, DeWeerd JH, Harrison EG. Renal arterio-venous fistula. *Am J Med* 1964; **37**:499–513.

Morris PJ. Renovascular hypertension: the indications for and the results of surgery. In: Bell PRP, Jamieson CW, Ruckley CV, eds. *Surgical Management of Vascular Disease*, 739–50.

Novick AC. Surgical correction of renovascular hypertension. *Surg Clin N Am* 1988; **68**:1007–25.

Peterson NE. Review article: traumatic bilateral renal infarction. *J Trauma* 1989: **29**:158–67.

Sos TA. Angioplasty for the treatment of azotaemia and renovascular hypertension in atherosclerotic renal artery disease. *Circulation* 1991; **83(suppl I)**:I1162–II166.

Tegtmeyer CJ, Bayne Selby J, Hartwell GD, Ayers C, Tegtmeyer V. Results and complications of angioplasty in fibromuscular disease. *Circulation* 1991; **83(suppl I)**:I155–I161.

Tham G, Ekelund L, Herrlin K, Lindstedt EL, Olin T, Bergentz S-E. Renal artery aneurysms. Natural history and progress. *Ann Surg* 1983; **197**:348–52.

van Bockel JH, van Schilfgaarde R, van Brummelen P, Terpstra JL. Renovascular hypertension. *Surg Gynecol Obstet* 1989; **169**:467–78.

7.11.1 Arterial emboli: limbs

W. BRUCE CAMPBELL

DEFFINITION AND AETIOLOGY

An embolus consists of undissolved material which is carried in the circulation and impacts in a blood vessel, usually blocking it. The most common source of arterial embolism is the left atrium in atrial fibrillation, accounting for two-thirds of all cases. Thrombus forms because of stasis in the enlarged and fibrillating atrium, and fragments detach to enter the arterial circulation (Fig. 1). Thrombi can also form on the damaged endocardium of the left ventricle after myocardial infarction, and arrhythmias cause these to detach and embolize. Other causes of emboli from the heart are shown in Table 1.

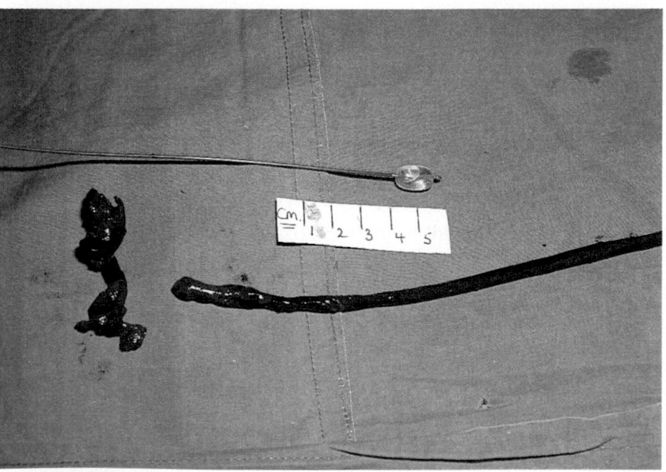

Fig. 1 To the left of the picture is embolic material from the left atrium, containing typical pale platelet thrombus. To the right lies a long length of propagated clot, extracted from the superficial femoral artery using the Fogarty embolectomy catheter shown above, with its balloon inflated.

Table 1 Sources of arterial emboli

The heart
Left atrium—atrial fibrillation
Left ventricle—after myocardial infarction
Mitral and aortic valves
Prosthetic
Rheumatic
Endocarditis
Uncommon causes
Congestive cardiac failure
Left ventricular aneurysm
Cardiomyopathy
Atrial myxoma
The arteries
Atheromatous embolism
Aorta ('shaggy aorta syndrome')
Stenosis in iliac or femoral arteries
Thrombus from aneurysms
Popliteal aneurysm
Aortic aneurysm
Others rarely
The veins
Rare—thrombus from deep veins passing through cardiac septal defect ('paradoxical embolism')
Tumour
Tumour invades artery and fragments detach
Foreign body
Examples
Detached fragment of arterial catheter
Bullet entering a major artery

Emboli can arise from the aorta and its branches (Figs. 2 and 3).

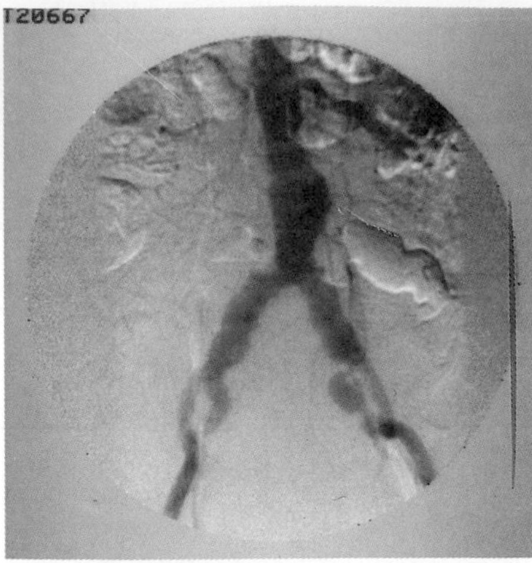

Fig. 2 Digital subtraction arteriogram of an ectatic and diseased aortoiliac system, which was the source of atheromatous emboli to both lower limbs. The patient was treated with an aortobifemoral graft.

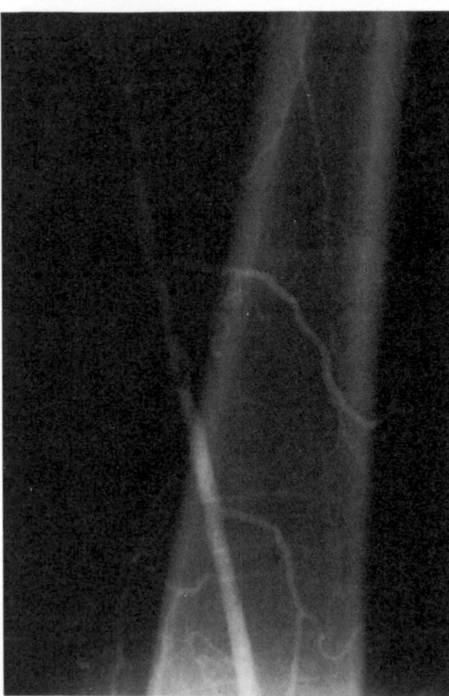

Fig. 3 Arteriogram showing a localized stenosis in the superficial femoral artery. The patient presented with signs of small emboli to the foot. A short segment of reversed saphenous vein was used to replace this segment of the artery.

Atheromatous plaques may rupture, allowing cholesterol debris to pass distally and block small arteries. Platelet thrombi forming on ulcerated atheromatous stenoses may also embolize. Thrombus forming in aneurysms due to abnormal patterns of blood flow can also form an embolism and this is a particular danger in the case of popliteal aneurysms. Table 1 lists the common sites of origin for arterial 'atheroemboli', and other rare causes of embolism. The clinical effects of small emboli are described later.

SITES AFFECTED BY EMBOLI

Emboli usually lodge at the bifurcations of arteries, because the diameter of each major branch is less than that of the main branching vessel.

Emboli to the limbs

In surgical practice most arterial emboli affect the limbs, the leg being affected six times more often than the arm (Table 2). Limb emboli are considered in detail below.

Table 2 Sites of occlusion of emboli to the limbs

Lower limb	
Aorta and iliac	26%
Femoral	45%
Popliteal	15%
Tibial	1%
Upper limb	
Subclavian	1%
Axillary	5%
Brachial	7%
	100%

From a series of 396 emboli (Panetta *et al.* 1986).

The brain and the eye

The brain is a frequent site of embolism, resulting in stroke. Small emboli passing up the internal carotid artery may also enter the retinal vessels, causing temporary or permanent blindness. If carotid atheroma is the source for recurrent emboli to the eye or brain then carotid endarterectomy may be required, although many patients are treated by antithrombotic drugs such as aspirin.

Mesenteric emboli

The superior mesenteric artery is usually affected, with clinical features of severe abdominal pain, sometimes vomiting or diarrhoea, and evidence of an embolic source (Table 1). Other features are a high white blood cell count and elevated serum amylase. A plain abdominal radiograph will show the absence of normal small bowel gas shadows centrally.

Urgent laparotomy is required and, if the bowel is still viable, embolectomy of the superior mesenteric artery can be performed. If there is doubt about bowel viability a 'second look' laparotomy should be performed 24 h later. In many cases the bowel is not viable and extensive resection is required. These patients require careful attention to replacement of fluid, electrolytes, and blood. If the whole small bowel has infarcted the patient will die.

PATHOPHYSIOLOGY

The effects of an embolus blocking a major limb artery depend on the level of the obstruction and on the capacity of collateral arteries to carry blood to the distal tissues. In the absence of good collateral flow there is stasis of blood in the arteries beyond the block and propagated clotting occurs (Fig. 1). Propagated clot also extends proximally to the next major branch. Reflex spasm of distal arteries is another effect of acute arterial occlusion. Clotting and spasm both make ischaemia worse.

Acute ischaemia due to an embolus causes hypoxia of the tissues and a failure to remove waste products; these are particularly damaging to muscle cells which have a rapid metabolic rate. Muscle death starts to occur after about 6 h. Initially ischaemia causes pain due to accumulation of metabolites, but as peripheral nerves become increasingly hypoxic paraesthesiae and eventually complete anaesthesia of the extremity occurs.

If the occlusion remains unresolved, venous thrombosis results from stagnation of blood flow: this is a late feature associated with a poor prognosis. 'Fixed staining' of the skin due to extravasation of blood into the tissues is another late sign (Fig. 4). Continued neglect results in gangrene.

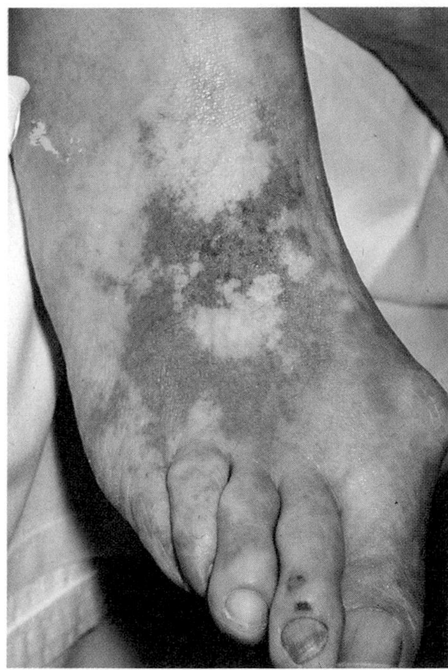

Fig. 4 Fixed staining of the skin. This is a late case of acute ischaemia and the foot could not be salvaged. Below knee amputation was done.

CLINICAL ASSESSMENT

Diagnosis of embolism causing acute ischaemia of a limb (Fig. 5)

The clinical features are best remembered as the 'six Ps'—pain, pallor, pulselessness, paraesthesiae, paralysis, and perishing cold. The onset of symptoms caused by an embolus is sudden, with pain and pallor occurring first. Colour change is variable and depends on the amount of collateral blood flow. If there are no established collaterals the extremity is white, sometimes with a bluish tinge. If some blood flow is maintained a pink colour remains, but capillary return is slower than normal. The more profound the ischaemia, the sooner paraesthesiae will be followed by anaesthesia. Loss of sensation is a serious sign and an indication for urgent treatment to restore blood flow. Paralysis is also a sign of advanced ischaemia.

Pulses distal to the occlusion are lost, while immediately proximal to the occlusion the pulse may be enhanced due to the high resistance caused by obstruction.

Acute ischaemia due to an embolus is a clinical diagnosis and special tests should not be necessary, but Doppler ultrasound investigation confirms absent or poor blood flow signals in the distal arteries, and the systolic pressure is unrecordable or low. An arteriogram is not necessary in the presence of an obvious embolic source (for example atrial fibrillation) and clear evidence of a sudden arterial occlusion, but angiography is worthwhile if there is any doubt about the diagnosis (Fig. 6).

Differential diagnosis

The main differential diagnosis is acute thrombosis occurring in arteries already narrowed by atherosclerosis (often called thrombosis *in situ* or acute-on-chronic ischaemia). The onset of ischaemia is often less sudden than in embolism and the degree of ischaemia is less profound, with preservation of a pink colour to the skin and intact sensation, due to established collateral arteries. There may be evidence of chronic arterial disease with a history of intermittent claudication, and absence of pulses with reduced systolic pressures in the contralateral limb. The absence of an obvious embolic source also supports a diagnosis of thrombosis rather than embolism. A generalized illness with hypotension or dehydration may be evident as a precipitating cause for acute thrombosis.

The distinction between embolism and thrombosis is not always easy, and in any doubtful case an arteriogram should be performed. If arteriography suggests thrombosis, then this can be treated by low dose infusion of a thrombolytic agent (for example streptokinase) through an arterial catheter. This method of treatment requires radiological facilities and expertise, and haematological monitoring of blood clotting during the infusion of the thrombolytic agent. When the thrombus has been lysed, transluminal angioplasty or bypass grafting may be indicated for repair of the underlying arterial stenoses.

Deep vein thrombosis is sometimes confused with arterial embolism, because it causes pain, reduced ability to move the limb, and colour change. This differential diagnosis should not be difficult: the limb with a venous thrombosis is swollen, sensation is not lost, and Doppler examination will confirm a normal arterial supply. Venous thrombosis occurring as a late sequel of arterial occlusion is accompanied by florid signs of neglected ischaemia.

TREATMENT

The first priority is relief of pain using strong analgesics such as morphine or pethidine (meperidine) given intramuscularly. An intravenous bolus of heparin should be given to reduce propagated clotting (5000–10 000 units). Continuous infusion of intravenous heparin is then commenced if any delay is anticipated in definitive treatment.

The ischaemic limb should never be actively warmed—this accelerates tissue damage. Measures to cool the limb are sometimes recommended but are generally impracticable. Another traditional recommendation is to nurse the patient with the limb dependent but any improvement from such a manoeuvre is likely

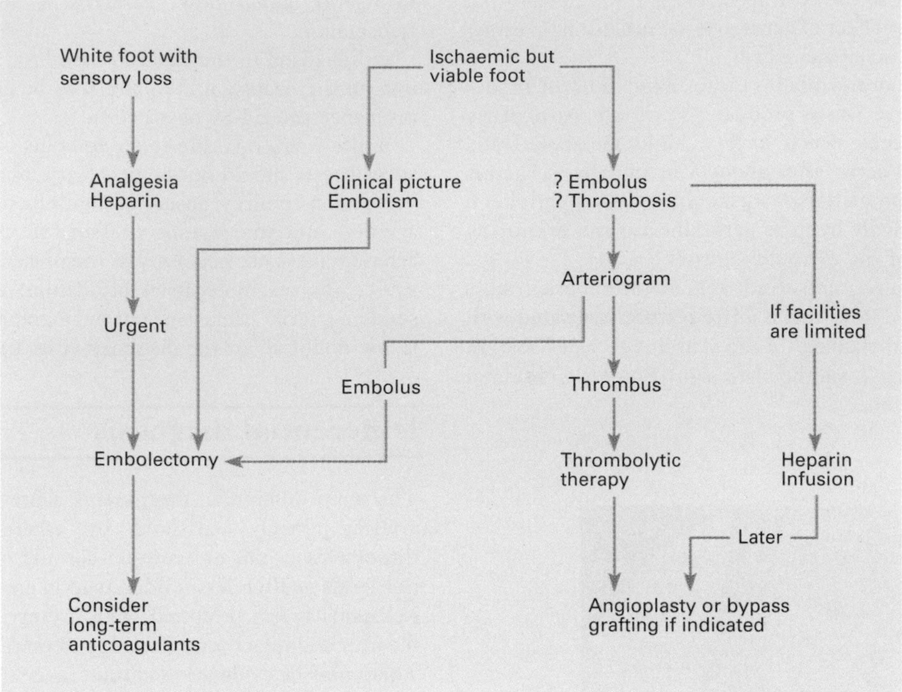

Fig. 5 Scheme for management of the acutely ischaemic limb.

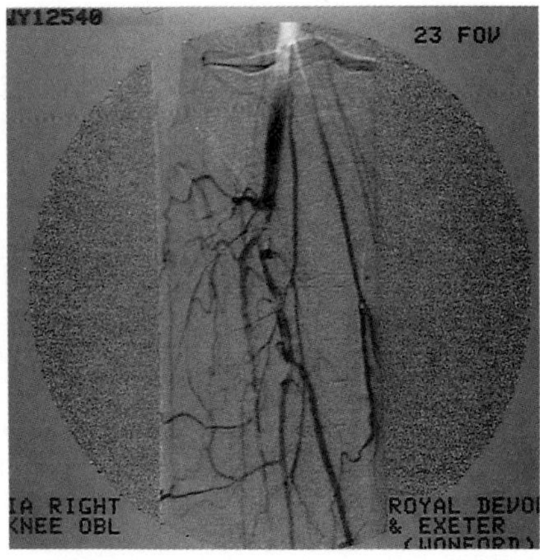

Fig. 6 Digital subtraction arteriogram showing embolic material at the bifurcation of the popliteal artery and in the tibioperoneal trunk.

to be marginal. Treatment for any acute medical condition, such as cardiac failure or arrhythmias, is commenced.

After these initial steps the aim should be emergency embolectomy as soon as possible to re-establish blood flow to the extremity. Embolectomy is usually performed under a local anaesthetic because most patients are elderly and unfit. The area to be anaesthetized should be marked and a dilute local anaesthetic, for example 0.5 per cent lignocaine (lidocaine), chosen so that a large volume can be used. It is helpful, but not essential, to have an anaesthetist in attendance to monitor the patient (ECG and blood gases) and to administer oxygen or sedation if this is required. An intravenous infusion should be set up before starting the operation.

Transfemoral embolectomy is the best initial approach for all lower limb emboli, while in the upper limb exposure of the brachial artery is required. For femoral embolectomy the incision should be vertical over the femoral artery, and should allow easy access up to the inguinal ligament. The common femoral artery is controlled with a sling as high as possible. Its bifurcation is exposed and slings are passed around the superficial and profunda femoris arteries, and also around any other branches.

In the upper limb it is easiest to approach the brachial artery through a longitudinal incision over the medial aspect of the upper arm, and this usually gives a satisfactory result. An approach through the antecubital fossa allows separate embolectomy of radial and ulnar arteries. This involves an S-shaped incision (medial above the elbow, curving across the antecubital fossa to the lateral aspect of the forearm). The bicipital aponeurosis is divided to reach the brachial bifurcation.

If the artery is non-pulsatile it is opened without any clamps in place. For simple embolectomy transverse incisions in arteries allow closure without the risk of narrowing the lumen. Longitudinal arteriotomy gives greater scope for reconstructive surgery but may require closure with a patch to avoid stenosis in narrow vessels.

A balloon embolectomy catheter of appropriate size is selected (Table 3) and the balloon is tested by inflating it with fluid (from a 1 ml or 2 ml syringe). The catheter is passed, proximally if it is necessary to remove clot and to ensure good inflow, and a proximal clamp is applied. After passing the catheter through an iliac clot into the aorta the contralateral limb must be checked at the end of the operation to ensure that embolic material has not been dislodged distally through the opposite iliac system.

The balloon catheter is passed distally and the clot withdrawn,

Table 3 Sizes of balloon embolectomy catheters at different sites

Site	Size of embolectomy catheter (French)
Iliac arteries (including aortic bifurcation)	5
Superficial femoral, popliteal, profunda	4
Tibial arteries	2 or 3
Brachial, ulnar, radial	3 or 4

These will vary depending on the calibre of the patient's arteries, but the sizes shown are a guide to those commonly used.

adjusting the balloon inflation pressure depending on the 'feel' of the catheter as it is withdrawn. Balloon catheters must be used gently, especially in vessels roughened by atheroma, to avoid intimal damage. The stilette should always be removed before passing the catheter. It should be possible to pass a catheter to the foot and passages are repeated until no further thrombus or clot is withdrawn. A balloon catheter should also be passed down the profunda femoris artery in the thigh. Distal flushing with about 100 ml heparinized saline (from 500 ml normal saline containing 5000 units heparin) is then performed through a soft catheter (for example a number 6 umbilical catheter) passed into the distal artery.

The patient should be warned to expect some discomfort during balloon withdrawal and also perhaps during flushing of the extremity with cold heparinized saline.

The arteriotomy is closed with a continuous non-absorbable suture (e.g. 0000 or 00000 polypropylene), checking inflow before final closure.

On releasing clamps the extremity should rapidly regain a pink colour with return of palpable pulses. If the result is unsatisfactory (the catheter fails to pass far enough or the foot is not improved) then an immediate arteriogram should be undertaken on the operating table with a proximal clamp in place to demonstrate the state of the distal vessels. The options thereafter are exposure of the popliteal artery for embolectomy or bypass surgery, or the use of thrombolytic agents. These are best performed by a surgeon with vascular expertise. If the expertise is not available and the foot is viable, then intravenous heparin therapy should be instituted.

If the material removed from the arteries is not typical thrombus it should be sent for histology to exclude a tumour embolus.

Swelling of the leg may occur after revascularization, and this can cause increased compartmental pressure leading to muscle necrosis if untreated. If there is any suspicion of raised intracompartmental pressure, a generous fasciotomy should be done. Compartment syndromes are more common after reconstruction for vascular trauma than after embolectomy.

Other methods of treating emboli

Embolectomy is the best treatment for arterial emboli. If in doubt about the management of an acutely ischaemic limb the artery should be explored with a view to an embolectomy. There is little to support the claim that embolectomy 'can do more harm than good', and an arteriogram can be performed at operation if embolectomy is not successful.

Thrombolytic therapy

Low dose intra-arterial streptokinase or urokinase can be effective in the treatment of embolism as for arterial thrombosis. This technique should only be used if the extremity is viable (sensation preserved). The infusion should be stopped after 48 h if there is no improvement, but if sequential radiographs show lysis then the infusion may be continued for up to 5 days. This method requires good radiological support.

Heparin therapy

Intravenous heparin alone can be used for the treatment of patients with acute limb ischaemia provided the limb is viable. This is safe management, especially when the facilities or expertise for vascular work are limited, or while awaiting a vascular opinion. Heparin minimizes propagated clotting and improvement may occur through natural clot lysis and the development of collaterals. The eventual state of the circulation to the limb is likely to be less good following heparin therapy alone than after successful embolectomy.

Percutaneous aspiration thromboembolectomy

This technique employs a specially designed catheter sheath system which can be used alone or in combination with thrombolytic drugs. The catheter is used to aspirate fragments of thrombus from the distal arteries and it is best suited to treating iatrogenic emboli resulting from intra-arterial catheterization or balloon angioplasty. This method is currently confined to specialist units.

Long-term anticoagulation after embolism

Administration of intravenous heparin in the immediate postoperative period reduces early recurrence of emboli. Thereafter, long-term anticoagulation is traditionally instituted (warfarin by daily oral administration) in the hope of preventing further emboli. Oral anticoagulants certainly should be used in patients in atrial fibrillation, but for patients with no obvious embolic source there is conflicting evidence of effect. Nevertheless, anticoagulation seems reasonable for all patients who will take warfarin reliably and from whom regular blood samples can be obtained for clotting studies. If haematological monitoring is difficult or if patients are unlikely to comply properly then the risk of haemorrhagic complications probably outweighs the benefits of long-term anticoagulation.

LATE PRESENTATION OF ARTERIAL EMBOLI

Patients with emboli may present many days after the acute event. Embolectomy may be successful even after a delay of a month but is rarely successful thereafter, because thrombus adheres to the vessel wall. Thrombolytic therapy may also be successful up to 1 month after impaction of an embolus.

Thrombolysis or intravenous heparin therapy are often used for these patients who present late but whose limbs have remained viable. If the obstruction is not relieved then arterial reconstruction can be performed at a later date if required.

THE MORTALITY AND MORBIDITY OF PERIPHERAL EMBOLI

Patients suffering embolism are often elderly and infirm, and up to 30 per cent die in the postoperative period. Factors associated with a higher mortality are increasing age, recent myocardial infarction, proximal (aortoiliac) occlusions, poor cardiac and pulmonary function, and pre-existing arterial disease.

Amputation is an uncommon sequel to embolism and is associated with delayed presentation. Limb loss following acute ischaemia is more commonly associated with thrombosis in diseased arteries than with emboli.

MICROEMBOLI

The small emboli that arise from arteriosclerotic arteries or aneurysms present either as isolated ischaemic digits (Fig. 7) or as ischaemic patches on an extremity. The main differential diagnoses are vasculitis and haematological disorders such as thrombocythaemia. 'Trash foot' is an important complication of grafting for aortic aneurysm and describes the passage of a shower of loose thrombus into the small vessels of the feet (Fig. 8).

Such small distal emboli are impossible to remove surgically. During aortic grafting prevention is the most important measure—gentle handling of the aneurysm, clamping the iliac arteries first, and flushing of blood both externally and, if possible, internally at the end of the procedure so that no thrombus or clots are allowed to pass into the limb arteries. When a localized arterial stenosis or aneurysm is identified as the cause for microembolism this should be dealt with appropriately—usually by bypass grafting (Figs. 2 and 3).

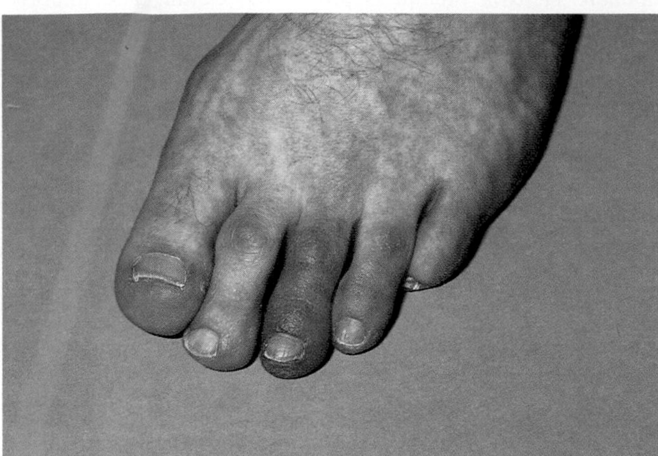

Fig. 7 An isolated ischaemic toe resulting from atheromatous embolism to the digital arteries.

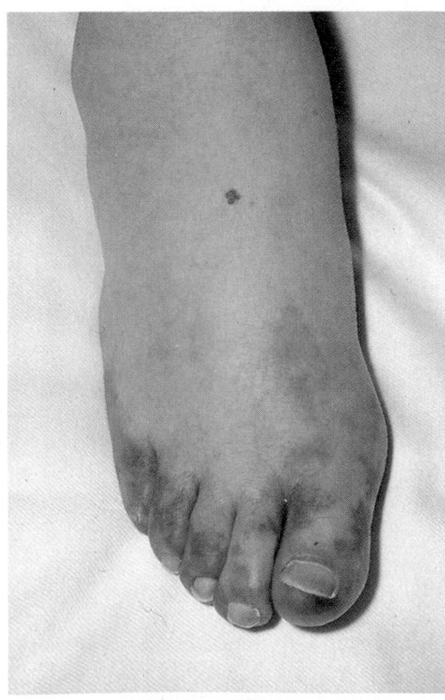

Fig. 8 'Trash foot'. A shower of embolic material has been carried to the small arteries of this foot during operation for aortic aneurysm.

FURTHER READING

Bergan JJ, Dean RH, Conn J, Yao JST. Revascularization in treatment of mesenteric infarction. *Ann Surg* 1975; **182**: 430–8.

Blaisdell FW, Steele M, Allen RE. Management of acute lower extremity arterial ischaemia due to embolism and thrombosis. *Surgery* 1978; **84**: 822–34.

Clason AE, Stonebridge PA, Duncan AJ, Nolan B, Jenkins AMcL, Ruckley CV. Morbidity and mortality in acute lower limb ischaemia: A 5-year review. *Eur J Vasc Surg* 1989; **3**: 339–43.

Clavien PA. Diagnosis and management of mesenteric infarction. *Br J Surg* 1990; **77**: 601–3.

Comerota AJ, White JV, Grosh JD. Intraoperative intra-arterial thrombolytic therapy for salvage of limbs in patients with distal arterial thrombosis. *Surg Gynecol Obstet* 1989; **169**: 283–9.

Connett MC, Murray DH, Wenneker WW. Peripheral arterial emboli. *Am J Surg* 1984; **148**: 14–9.

Dale WA. Differential management of acute peripheral arterial ischemia. *J Vasc Surg* 1984; **1**: 269–78.

Darling RC, Austen WG, Linton RR. Arterial embolism. *Surg Gynecol Obstet* 1967; **124**: 106–14.

Elliott JP, Hageman JH, Szilagyi DE, Ramakrishnan V, Bravo JJ, Smith RF. Arterial embolization: problems of source, multiplicity, recurrence, and delayed treatment. *Surgery* 1980; **88**: 833–45.

Field T, Littooy FN, Baker WH. Immediate and long-term outcome of acute arterial occlusion of the extremities. *Arch Surg* 1982; **117**: 1156–60.

Fogarty TJ, Cranley JJ, Krause RJ, Strasser ES, Hafner CD. A method for extraction of arterial emboli and thrombi. *Surg Gynecol Obstet* 1963; **116**: 241–4.

Galbraith K, Collin J, Morris PJ, Wood RFM. Recent experience with arterial embolism of the limbs in a vascular unit. *Ann R Coll Surg Engl* 1985; **67**: 30–3.

Green, RM, DeWeese JA, Rob CG. Arterial embolectomy before and after the Fogarty catheter. *Surgery* 1975; **77**: 24–33.

Hickey NC, Crowson MC, Simms MH. Emergency arterial reconstruction for acute ischaemia. *Br J Surg* 1990; **77**: 680–1.

Kazmier FJ. Shaggy aorta syndrome and disseminated atheromatous embolization. In: Bergan JJ, Yao JST, eds. *Aortic surgery*. Philadelphia: WB Saunders, 1989: 189–94.

Levin BH, Giordano JM. Delayed arterial embolectomy. *Surg Gynecol Obstet* 1982; **155**: 549–51.

Panetta T, Thompson JE, Talkington CM, Garrett WV, Smith BL. Arterial embolectomy: a 34-year experience with 400 cases. *Surg Clin N Am* 1986; **66**: 339–53.

Parent FN, Bernhard VM, Pabst TS, McIntyre KE, Hunter GC, Malone JM. Fibrinolytic treatment of residual thrombus after catheter embolectomy for severe lower limb ischemia. *J Vasc Surg* 1989; **9**: 153–60.

Petersen P, Godtfredsen J, Boysen G, Andersen ED, Andersen B. Placebo-controlled, randomised trial of warfarin and aspirin for prevention of thromboembolic complications in chronic atrial fibrillation. *Lancet* 1989; **i**: 175–9.

Scott DJA, Davies AH, Horrocks M. Risk factors in selected patients undergoing femoral embolectomy. *Ann R Coll Surg Engl* 1989; 71: 229–32.

Silvers LW, Royster TS, Mulcare RJ. Peripheral arterial emboli and factors in their recurrence rate. *Ann Surg* 1980; **192**: 232–6.

Tawes RL, *et al.* Arterial thromboembolism. A 20–year perspective. *Arch Surg* 1985; **120**: 595–9.

Turnipseed WD, Starck EE, McDermott JC, *et al.* Percutaneous aspiration thromboembolectomy (PAT): an alternative to surgical balloon techniques for clot retrieval. *J Vasc Surg* 1986; **3**: 437–41.

Walker WJ, Giddings AEB. A protocol for the safe treatment of acute lower limb ischaemia with intra-arterial streptokinase and surgery. *Br J Surg* 1988; **75**: 1189–92.

7.11.2 Arterial emboli: mesenteric arteries

LESLIE W. OTTINGER

Mesenteric ischaemia and infarction results from interruption of arterial or venous perfusion of all or part of the intestinal tract. The major causes are acute occlusion of the superior mesenteric artery, mesenteric venous thrombosis, and non-occlusive infarction. In general, the prognosis for survival is poor.

Acute superior mesenteric artery occlusion may be the result of either thrombosis or an embolus. Emboli account for about 20 per cent of all cases of acute ischaemia or infarction and about one-half of the cases of acute occlusion of the mesenteric artery. With early diagnosis and proper management, survival with preservation of most or all of the small intestine is readily achieved.

ANATOMICAL CONSIDERATIONS

Three vessels constitute the major arterial supply to the intra-abdominal intestine. These are the coeliac axis for the stomach and duodenum, the superior mesenteric artery for the jejunum, ileum, and right and transverse colon, and the inferior mesenteric artery for the left and sigmoid colon. It is unusual for an embolus to either the coeliac axis or the inferior mesenteric artery to produce infarction, because of the obtuse angle of the coeliac axis to the aorta, the small size of the inferior mesenteric artery, and the adequacy of collateral inflow to both. The superior mesenteric artery, in contrast, originates at an acute angle, is large and, at least when acute occlusion is proximal, seldom has the sufficient collateral flow to preserve viability of the entire area of intestine which it supplies. This artery is one of the most frequent sites of clinically apparent emboli to visceral vessels.

The first branches of the superior mesenteric artery are small, supplying the duodenum, pancreas, and proximal jejunum. The initial branch of any size is the middle colic artery. The superior mesenteric artery tapers rather rapidly distal to it, terminating in the arteries to the distal ileum. The usual sites at which an embolus lodges are at the origin of the middle colic artery, where it may or may not cause occlusion, and in the main trunk of the artery, within 5 cm distal to the origin of the middle colic artery. (Fig. 1). Occlusion at the origin of the superior mesenteric artery is almost invariably the result of thrombosis, not an embolus.

As with other peripheral emboli, most mesenteric emboli come from the heart. Common sources of emboli are atrial fibrillation, infarction of the ventricle with mural thrombus, and valvular excrescences. A few emboli come from the aortic wall itself, and some are iatrogenic, following aortic surgery or catheterization.

When occlusion of the superior mesenteric artery occurs gradually, collateral inflow from the other visceral vessels usually protects the intestine from ischaemic injury. When occlusion is acute, this collateral supply is not sufficient. Depending on the site at which an embolus lodges, the resulting ischaemic injury may extend from the proximal jejunum to the left transverse colon or, with a more peripheral site of occlusion, may involve only the ileum and right colon. Anatomical variation in collaterals and the presence of fragments of emboli peripherally mean that the ischaemic injury may be patchy and variable in its severity, especially in the early stages. However, the central area of supply, the ileum and caecum, usually sustains the most profound injury. A small embolus that enters a branch of the superior mesenteric artery may lead to a segmental infarct or to no ischaemic injury.

The mucosa is the only layer of the intestinal wall to have little resistance to ischaemic injury, becoming damaged rapidly by even relatively mild degrees of ischaemia. The first gross evidence of damage is submucosal oedema. This proceeds to haemorrhage and sloughing of the mucosa, with a small amount of intraluminal bleeding. If the deeper layers remain viable, or if arterial perfusion is restored, the mucosa regenerates: this may take several weeks, during which there is usually diarrhoea and sometimes a degree of malabsorption. In a few patients, the presence of deep ulcers leads to major haemorrhage from regenerating areas.

The initial response of the muscularis propria to ischaemia is spasm. Depending on the severity and duration of ischaemia, atony, infarction, and perforation can follow. Full thickness, irreversible infarction produces a characteristic foul-smelling bloody, peritoneal exudate. With restoration of arterial perfusion the viability of the outer layers may be preserved and chronic ulceration may lead to the development of strictures, which may take several weeks to become apparent.

Visceral pain is an invariable symptom of mesenteric ischaemia. Only in the obtunded or otherwise mentally impaired patient will it not suggest the diagnosis. In its absence, the diagnosis can be confidently excluded. Other symptoms and signs are less definite and depend on the extent, severity, and location of the ischaemic injury.

The course of ischaemic injury caused by an embolus is also variable. Short of removal of the embolus, the only factor likely to improve perfusion is remission of arterial spasm and the gradual enlargement of collateral vessels. Conversely, the ischaemic injury may be worsened by factors that further decrease perfusion, including hypoperfusion due to systemic hypotension and visceral artery spasm. Local factors, including oedema, haemorrhage, and distension, can also cause extension of the infarct. Although a superior mesenteric artery embolus can lead to immediate infarction and perforation within a few hours, this is not the usual course. Many patients will have symptoms for hours or even days before the development of irreversible infarction.

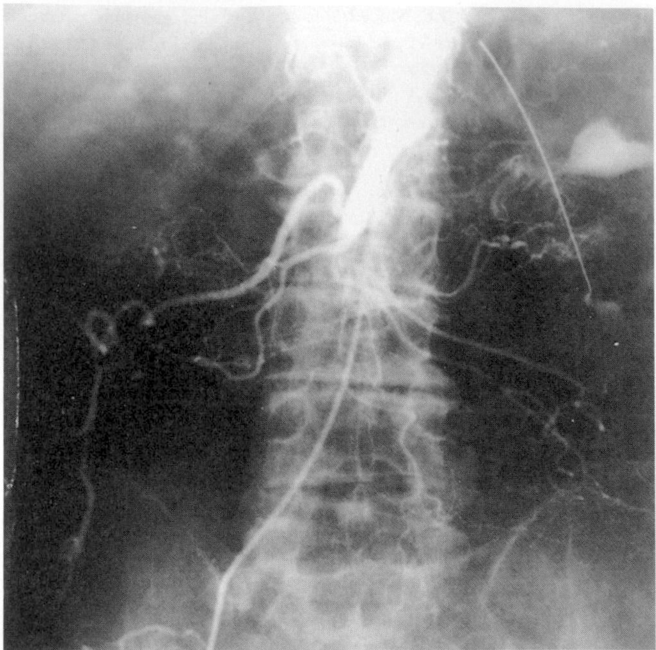

Fig. 1 (a) Selective superior mesenteric artery angiogram demonstrating occlusion of the artery by an embolus distal to the inferior pancreatoduodenal and middle colic arteries.

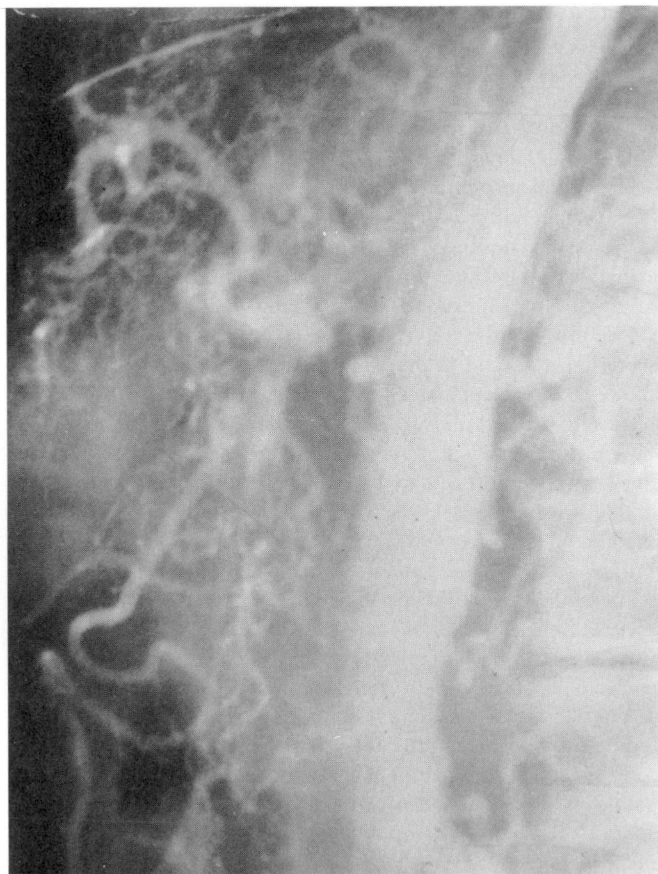

Fig. 1 (b) Lateral view in the same patient.

The collateral flow tends initially to lead to a gradient of severity of ischaemic injury, the peripheral areas being most spared. There is a tendency for areas of full thickness infarction to extend to include the marginal areas with the passage of hours. Eventually the initial patchy involvement will usually become an extended area of full thickness infarction.

CLINICAL PRESENTATION

Patients with mesenteric emboli almost always present with abdominal pain which tends to be steady and, being visceral in origin, poorly localized and referred generally to the mid-abdomen. Although traditionally thought to be sudden in onset and remarkably severe, this is not always true. There may be a vague onset and variable intensity, even with intermittent disappearance. Pain may have been present for several hours or even a few days.

The history may include vomiting, diarrhoea, or even tenesmus. Since signs of peritonitis are present only after perforation, there are initially no positive findings on physical examination. The gastric or rectal contents may contain gross or occult blood. At later stages, although the findings are non-specific, an intra-abdominal catastrophe is obvious, as is the need for laparotomy.

Diagnosis is most elusive during the early stages, when the chance for successful management is high. The decision to proceed with either angiography or laparotomy must be made on the basis of suspicion, not certainty. The diagnosis must be seriously entertained in any patient with unexplained abdominal pain, especially in those over 60 years old.

Laboratory tests are not so specific as to be useful in a positive way. Many patients, but not all, have a leucocytosis which may be extreme, counts exceeding 20 000/mm^3. The serum amylase is slightly elevated in 50 per cent of victims. Plain radiographs show no, or only non-specific, findings in most cases.

Arteriography is especially helpful in the patient with either a superior mesenteric artery embolus or thrombosis, but is less so in those with venous or non-occlusive infarction, though it may still yield useful indirect findings. The major application of arteriography is in the patient with a history suggesting an embolus, but without systemic or local findings to herald the later stages of infarction. In these patients, arteriography establishes the diagnosis, leading direct to an expeditious laparotomy. When the embolus is small and in a branch, arteriography may also eliminate the need for surgery, although this is quite an unusual site of embolism. As well as providing a certain diagnosis, the arteriogram provides the surgeon with useful information about the site of occlusion and patency of other visceral vessels.

Other radiographic studies, such as computer augmented tomography and indirect flow studies using a Doppler device show promise in helping to reach a diagnosis. They have not reached a level of development and application where they are generally useful or available.

MANAGEMENT

Even with the availability of angiographic therapeutic techniques, immediate laparotomy is the best approach for the management of the embolus and injured bowel. The ideal operation consists of an embolectomy followed by resection of any segment of non-viable bowel.

The surgeon must first confirm the diagnosis, then make an estimate of the extent and severity of ischaemic injury. In the early stages there may be no gross evidence of bowel injury, and there may even be faint peripheral pulses from collateral inflow. The diagnosis of superior mesenteric artery embolism should be abandoned only after the presence of a strong pulse in the main trunk is confirmed. In these early cases, an embolectomy can allow preservation of all of the intestine. Failure to perform an embolectomy invariably leads to infarction and a poor prognosis.

In the usual clinical setting, many patients have extensive infarction that is clearly irreversible. Experience and judgement are needed to decide whether a resection of most of the small bowel, with or without an embolectomy, should be performed. This decision should reflect the age and general condition of the patient and the amount of viable jejunum. Parenteral nutrition solutions have made a major contribution to management of patients with very extensive resections, and permanent home hyperalimentation is a measure to be considered. A successful outcome can be achieved in carefully selected patients with extensive infarction.

If the extent of injury is limited, decisions regarding resection or embolectomy must take into account the site of the embolus. Here, arteriography is helpful (Fig. 2). In a few cases, the embolus is in a peripheral vessel and perfusion to adjacent segments of bowel is normal: resection alone is all that is needed. A delayed reanastomosis may be selected for the colon. If the embolus is located centrally, even though the extent of the infarction is limited, resection alone is almost certain to fail. Further infarction can be anticipated, and an embolectomy is indicated.

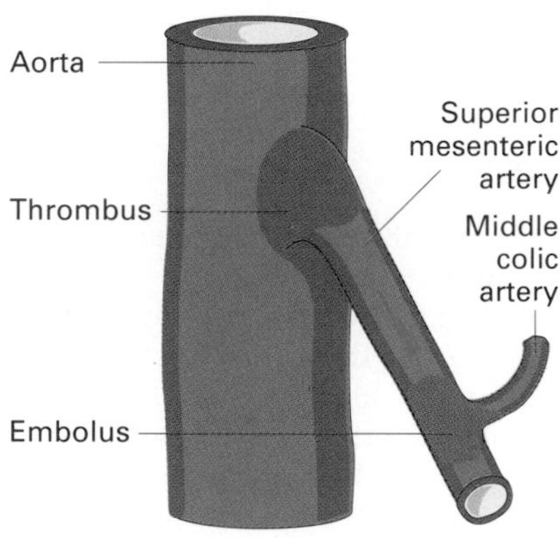

Fig. 2 The usual sites of occlusion with thrombosis and embolization in the superior mesenteric artery.

The technical demands for an embolectomy of the superior mesenteric artery are within the skills of the general surgeon. The approach to the vessel is at the base of the mesocolon, lifting the transverse colon in an anterior superior direction. The vein is usually to the right of the artery and most of its left branches pass posterior to it (Fig.3). The perivascular nerve plexus makes exposure somewhat more tedious than that for an extremity artery. This approach will lead to exposure just distal to the middle colic artery. A longitudinal arteriotomy is easier to close, especially in an atherosclerotic vessel, and can also serve as a site for bypass anastomosis if the diagnosis proves to be thrombosis at the origin of the superior mesenteric artery. In the presence of an embolus the pulse will be noted to end at or just beyond the middle colic artery. Embolectomy catheters can be used if the embolus is proximal to the arteriotomy and if there is distal propagation of thrombosis. The mesenteric vessels are fragile, and catheters should be used with care. The arteriotomy can usually be closed directly; eversion is neither necessary nor desirable. Rarely, a local endarterectomy or patch graft may be required.

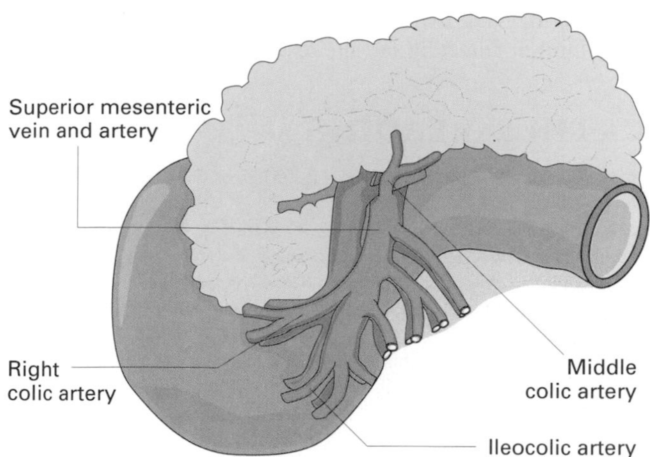

Fig. 3 The superior mesenteric vessels showing the relationship of the vein and its branches to the artery.

After mesenteric flow is restored, a period of observation is needed to determine which ischaemic segments of bowel are viable. Although fluorescein injections with observation under an ultraviolet light, and determination of pulsatile flow in the bowel wall by a Doppler device make objective assessment possible, these are usually unavailable, and the observation of an experienced surgeon carries the same degree of accuracy. If no doubt exists, non-viable segments should be resected. Depending on the apparent adequacy of arterial circulation, anastomosis may be performed, or stomas should be established.

When doubt continues after observation, clearly infarcted segments should be extirpated and a second-look operation scheduled. The second operation can be done at a convenient time, a few hours later, when there should be a clear demarcation of infarcted areas. The decision about reoperation should be made during the first operation, as the clinical course over the next few hours cannot serve as an indication that all is well. There is evidence that supports a policy of routine second-look operations after embolectomy.

Postoperative measures to prevent recurrence or extension of thrombus may be appropriate. These include the infusion of antispasm drugs, using angiographic techniques. More important is attention to the management of the cardiovascular system: hypovolaemia and peripheral vasospasm must be avoided. Anticoagulants prevent the formation of further emboli but must be used with caution for the first 24 h in the patients with a mesenteric artery suture line.

A number of specific postembolectomy complications can be described, all of which are relatively uncommon. Occlusion of the artery by thrombus or a new embolus will cause the original symptoms to recur and this is suggested in the patient who notes recurrence of pain. Early bleeding from the suture line follows anticoagulation; late bleeding usually means sepsis. Diarrhoea, often severe, is common, and parenteral nutrition can make an important contribution to survival. This subsides as the mucosal injury heals: persistence is indicative of extensive ulceration and stricture formation and a further resection will be needed. During the healing phase, mild bleeding is usual. Massive bleeding from deep ulcers may indicate the need for a resection. Angiography is often helpful in detecting the site of bleeding.

FURTHER READING

Boley SJ, Brandt SJ, Vieth FJ. Ischemic disorders of the intestine. *Curr Probl Surg*, 1978; **15**: 1–85.

Bulkley GB, Zuidema GD, Hamilton SR, O'Mara CS, Klacsmann PG, Horn SD. Intraoperative determination of small intestine motility following ischemic injury. *Ann Surg*, 1981; **193**: 628–37.

Clavian PA, Muller C, Harder F. Treatment of mesenteric infarction. *Br J Surg*, 1987; **74**: 500–3.

Gusberg R, Gump FE. Combined surgical and nutritional management of patients with acute mesenteric vascular occlusion. *Ann Surg*, 1974; 179: 358–61.

Jamieson WG. Acute intestinal ischemia. *Can J Surg*, 1988; **31**: 157–8.

Kaufman SL, Harrington DP, Sigelman SS. Superior mesenteric artery embolization: an angiographic emergency. *Radiology*, 1977; **124**: 625–30.

Ottinger LW. The surgical management of acute occlusion of the superior mesenteric artery. *Ann Surg*, 1978; **188**: 721–31.

Ottinger LW, Austen WG. A study of 136 patients with mesenteric infarction. *Surg Gynecol Obstet*, 1967; **124**: 251–61.

Shaw RS, Rutledge RH. Superior mesenteric embolectomy in the treatment of massive mesenteric infarction. *N Engl J Med* 1957; **257**: 595–8.

Sitses-Serri A, Mas X, Rouquita F, Figueres J, Saus F. Mesenteric infarction: an analysis of 83 patients with prognostic studies in 44 cases undergoing a massive small bowel resection. *Br J Surg*, 1988; **75**: 544–8.

Tomchik FS, Wittenberg J, Ottinger LW. The roentgenographic spectrum of bowel infarction. *Radiology*, 1970; **96**: 249–60.

Wilson C, Gupta R, Gilmour DG, Imrie CW. Acute superior mesenteric ischaemia. *Br J Surg*, 1987; **74**: 279–81.

7.12 Arterial and venous injuries

DAVID P. FRANKLIN AND RICHARD P. CAMBRIA

Trauma represents a major cause of death and morbidity in Western society, especially during the first four decades of life. Major vascular injuries are responsible for a substantial percentage of these deaths. Arterial and venous damage is seen in blunt and penetrating injuries involving both the extremities and body cavities. Direct vascular injuries are seen most frequently with penetrating trauma, especially in urban areas where civilian violence is increasing. The majority of vascular injuries that come to medical attention are in the extremities (Table 1.)

MECHANISMS OF INJURY

Penetrating injuries following stabbings or wounds caused by low-velocity bullets can result in lacerations, transections, or contusions of arteries and veins. False aneurysms can develop from arterial lacerations while arteriovenous fistulae can occur in combined arterial and venous injuries. High-velocity missiles cause severe vascular destruction along their paths. However, indirect injury also occurs by the missile's peripheral cavitational effect, with mural contusion, thrombosis, or delayed necrosis. Blunt trauma occurring with crushing injuries and fractures frequently results in arterial contusion, resulting in thrombosis or wall separation with subsequent false aneurysm formation. Arterial stretch injuries are often seen with shoulder girdle injuries and knee dislocations, causing intimal disruption with acute or delayed thrombosis due to intramural dissection. Rapid deceleration can result in arterial transection, as is seen especially in the thoracic aorta in victims of high-speed motor vehicle accidents.

DIAGNOSIS

Major haemorrhage with resultant hypotension is the hallmark of central, large vessel injury, while in the extremities distal ischaemia, expanding haematoma, or obvious arterial bleeding are essentially diagnostic of a vascular injury. Findings suggestive of a possible vascular injury include diminished distal pulses, proximity of the wound to a major vessel, or an adjacent nerve injury.

The presence of a distal pulse does not exclude an arterial injury: such pulses may well be present if collateral circulation is adequate, if intimal injury has not yet resulted in thrombosis, or if a side-branch injury has occurred, such as in damage to the deep femoral artery. Physical examination should always include auscultation in the region of injury: a bruit may indicate an intimal flap or a traumatic arteriovenous fistula formation. Haemorrhage or haematoma formation may be absent in traumatic arteriovenous fistulae because of blood flow into the low-pressure venous

Table 1 Location of vascular injuries

Site	Author	Year	Upper extremity	Lower extremity	Neck	Chest	Abdomen	Total
First World War	Makins	1922	367	648	176	–	11	1202
Second World War	DeBakey	1946	871	2471	34	–	49	2471
Korean War	Hughes	1958	109	304	14	–	7	304
Vietnam War	Rich	1970	416	840	76	4	354	1377
Los Angeles, California	Treiman	1966	67	86	14	10	56	233
Dallas, Texas	Perry	1971	213	141	65	14	75	508
Jackson, Mississippi	Hardy	1975	98	116	39	41	66	360
Houston, Texas	Mattox	1989	859	1102	694	1159	1946	5760

system. Diffuse swelling of an extremity can suggest venous injury, with secondary venous thrombosis or obstruction.

Arteriography is indicated when there is a need to establish a diagnosis or provide information critical to operative treatment. When the diagnosis is obvious, however, particularly in the extremities, direct exploration is frequently preferred: angiography adds little but prolongs the duration of ischaemia. Biplanar arteriography aids in the diagnosis of arterial injury by revealing the extent and location of injury. The presence of an intimal flap, arterial thrombosis, and formation of a false aneurysm or arteriovenous fistula can be confirmed with angiography. Arteriography should only be performed on haemodynamically stable patients. Unstable patients should proceed to the operating room, where intraoperative evaluation and arteriography can be performed as needed.

Penetrating trauma of the chest and abdomen usually requires immediate surgical exploration to confirm the diagnosis and allow prompt repair of the vascular injury. Vascular injuries of the body cavities due to blunt trauma, however, are frequently occult and, therefore, difficult to diagnose. The patient may initially be haemodynamically stable and the first signs of vascular injury may be delayed haemodynamic collapse. If a routine chest radiograph reveals mediastinal widening or haemothorax in the haemodynamically stable patient, aortography is mandatory to exclude injury of the descending thoracic aorta. CAT scanning in the haemodynamically stable patient frequently discloses retroperitoneal haemorrhage suggestive of injury to the aorta, inferior vena cava, or renal vasculature.

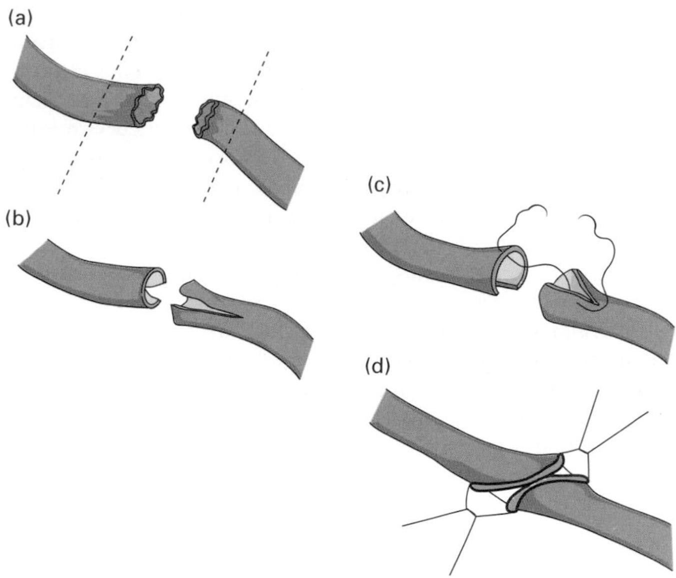

Fig. 1 Illustration of traumatic arterial transection repair by an end-to-end anastomosis. (a) Resection of injured arterial wall. Be certain that the artery is adequately mobilized to prevent excess tension on the anastomosis. (b) Spatulation of the divided artery. The spatulation is 180° apart on each side. (c) Approximate the 'toe' of the proximal end to the 'heel' of the distal end. (d) Sutures on each side allow stabilization and improve alignment during the repair.

PRINCIPLES OF SURGICAL REPAIR

While the management of different injuries is diverse, strategies share certain common principles of dealing with the injured vessel. These include achieving adequate surgical exposure for appropriate proximal and distal control, debridement or resection of the injured vessel, or both, so as to place suture lines in normal artery or vein, preference for autogenous rather than prosthetic conduits in contaminated surgical fields, and verification of the adequacy of the reconstruction.

First, proximal and distal control of the injury should be obtained. Blind clamping at the site of injury should be avoided, since it may cause further vessel or nervous injury. Appropriately placed incisions greatly aid in obtaining proximal control. The injured vessel should be inspected for thrombus before distal clamping and, if present, a thrombectomy should be performed with a Fogarty catheter.

Systemic anticoagulation during localized vascular repairs can aid in the prevention of thrombus formation. Systemic heparin is, however, generally not required for vascular repairs in the extremities, and it is often contraindicated in patients with major haemorrhage or associated multiple injuries, especially of the central nervous system. Regional heparin installation generally suffices when repairing an extremity injury.

Large vessel lacerations can frequently be repaired primarily using interrupted polypropylene sutures, which allow appropriate intima-to-intima reapproximation. Debridement of all areas of injured vessel wall is essential. In transected vessels, end-to-end anastomosis is required. Spatulation of the vessel ends in a cobra hood fashion (see Fig. 1) ensures adequate width of the vessel at the anastomosis. In mural contusion injuries, the vessels should be opened and inspected, and injured vessel wall segment resected. Repair can be performed with either a vein patch angioplasty or an end-to-end anastomosis.

Following debridement for extensive injury, excessive tension results in failure of an end-to-end repair, making interposition grafting necessary; autologous saphenous vein is the graft conduit of choice. Operative planning includes preparation of uninjured extremity for potential harvesting of a vein for use in the injured extremity as an arterial substitute. Removing a vein from an injured extremity adds to the risk of venous congestion from occult venous injury or delayed venous thrombosis. Some surgeons have advocated the use of polytetrafluorethylene (PTFE) prosthetic grafts in areas of minimal contamination, and in our view, it is the conduit of choice when a prosthetic graft must be placed in a contaminated field. Any graft type reconstruction must be provided with adequate soft tissue coverage. In areas of heavy contamination any graft is at risk for disruption, and arterial ligation with extra-anatomic reconstruction should be considered.

There has always been controversy over repair of venous injuries: advocates of repair say that improved limb blood flow favours patency of both arterial and venous reconstructions, as well as forestalling postphlebitic type sequelae. Those favouring simple ligation emphasize the likelihood of thrombosis in any graft placed in the venous circulation. We advocate a balanced approach: repair is appropriate if it can be simply accomplished, but complex reconstructions are avoided. Venous reconstruction needs strongly to be considered in patients with extensive soft tissue injury associated with the loss of important collateral venous drainage.

FALSE ANEURYSM (see Section 7.7.2)

A false aneurysm, or pseudoaneurysm, develops at a site of arterial injury where the adjacent non-vascular tissues contain the haemorrhage. Retraction and thrombosis are inhibited because the artery is not completely transected. Arterial flow is usually maintained at or beyond the level of injury. These events result in systemic arterial pressure at the site of injury and a resultant pulsating haematoma. Since the wall of the false aneurysm is not arterial wall, it does not contain elastic fibres; it will expand over time and in doing so may cause symptoms attributable to compression of adjacent structures; alternatively, contained rupture may occur. False aneurysms can also form following blunt trauma, such as with arterial contusion with necrosis of the arterial wall, or following penetrating trauma such as knife and bullet injuries.

Arteriography, cardiac catheterization, arterial blood pressure monitoring line placement, and arterial blood gas sampling can cause iatrogenic arterial injuries and false aneurysms. Few false aneurysms close spontaneously; their natural history is to enlarge and to produce local symptoms from compression, embolization, or haemorrhage. Surgical repair at the earliest convenience is advised.

ARTERIOVENOUS FISTULA

The traumatic arteriovenous fistula may develop when there is combined adjacent arterial and venous injury (Fig. 2). Arteriovenous fistulae may form acutely at the time of injury or may develop late following lysis of an intervening obstructing thrombus, or by rupture of a false aneurysm into an adjacent vein. Distal ischaemia is rare early in the formation of such a fistula; however as the fistula increases in size there is resultant dilation of the venous system with potential reversal of distal arterial flow and subsequent distal ischaemia. Large arteriovenous fistulae cause the proximal arteries to dilate to accommodate the tremendous blood flow.

Clinical manifestations of arteriovenous fistulae include venous hypertension with venous insufficiency, varicosities, swelling of the extremities, distal ischaemia, and the central cardiovascular complications of tachycardia, hypotension, and high-output heart failure. Repair of arteriovenous fistulae is best done early, before significant venous dilation and engorgement occurs. Interruption of the fistula and primary repair of the artery and vein are curative.

VASCULAR INJURIES OF THE EXTREMITIES

The majority of vascular injuries occur in the extremities, and vascular trauma occurs approximately twice as often in the lower extremities as in the upper limbs. The most difficult peripheral vascular injuries are located below the inguinal ligament, where improper treatment is more likely to result in amputation: an amputation rate of approximately 49 per cent was seen in the Second World War, when most arterial injuries were treated with arterial ligation. During the Vietnam war, where prompt arterial repair with improved techniques was often combined with concomitant venous repair, there were few amputations.

Penetrating trauma is the main cause of most vascular injuries. Such wounds are usually readily apparent, and peripheral arterial injuries are frequently suspected because of absent distal pulses and secondary ischaemia. Injury following blunt trauma may not be apparent until irreversible ischaemia has developed, particularly since actual thrombosis at the site of injury may be delayed.

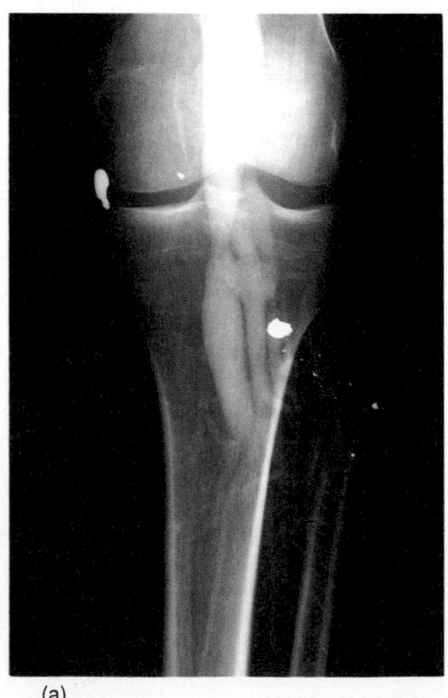

(a)

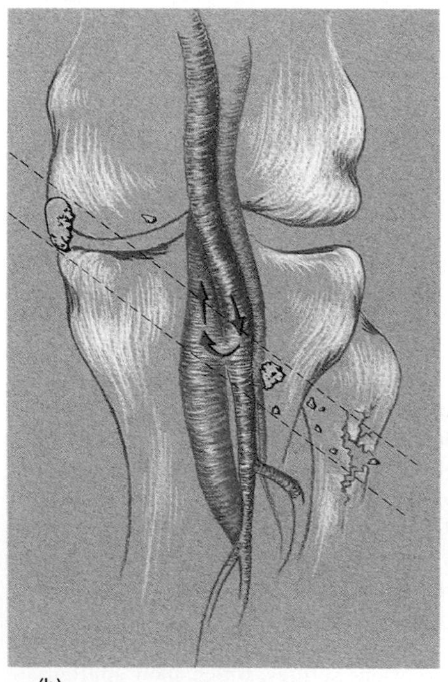

(b)

Fig. 2 Post-traumatic popliteal arteriovenous fistula. (a) Angiography shows an arteriovenous fistula in a patient with a small-calibre gunshot injury to the knee. (b) Gunshot injury to the knee. Notice the fragmentation of the bullet after striking the fibula. The largest missile fragment subsequently penetrates both popliteal artery and vein, with resultant arteriovenous fistula formation.

Table 2 The possibility of limb threatening ischaemia following arterial injury at various different sites.

High probability of severe ischaemia with occlusive injury
Popliteal artery
Common femoral artery
Both anterior tibial and posterior tibial arteries
Brachial artery proximal to profunda brachialis artery
Both radial and ulnar arteries
Moderate probability of significant ischaemia
Iliac artery
Superficial femoral artery
Subclavian artery
Axillary artery
Low probability of significant ischaemia
Brachial artery distal to profunda brachialis artery
Profunda femoris artery
Isolated tibial artery
Isolated radial or ulnar artery

Peripheral arterial injuries at certain levels are more prone to development of profound ischaemia and gangrene, while other sites of injury have a lower incidence of limb threatening ischaemia following injury or ligation (Table 2).

Injury of the axillary artery is usually due to penetrating trauma, although proximal humeral fractures, shoulder dislocations, and shoulder girdle stretch injuries are also associated with axillary artery injuries. Improper use of crutches can result in an aneurysm of the axillary artery. The brachial artery is most frequently injured as a result of penetrating trauma, and following brachial artery catheterization. The incidence of this catheterization complication approaches 1 per cent. Brachial artery injuries are occasionally seen in patients with posterior elbow dislocations and humeral fractures. Few patients with isolated axillary or brachial artery injury require amputation, but many patients will have ischaemic symptoms on exertion if arterial repair is not performed. Isolated radial or ulnar artery injuries are rarely associated with ischaemia or amputation. If primary arterial repair cannot be performed, ligation is well tolerated by the vast majority of patients with isolated radial or ulnar artery injury, but not both.

Injuries to the common femoral or superficial femoral arteries are often quite apparent because of loss of distal pulses and subsequent ischaemia, while injury to the profunda femoris artery may be difficult to diagnose because there are no signs of distal ischaemia. Local exploration or arteriography is frequently necessary to diagnose a profunda femoris injury, unless one detects an arteriovenous fistula or false aneurysm at the injury site. Patients with femoral shaft fractures and diminished distal circulation require arteriography to exclude superficial femoral artery injury. If they have rich collaterals, patients with superficial femoral artery injury may not experience profound ischaemia. Onset of ischaemia is frequently delayed because of thrombosis and loss of collateral flow secondary to stasis, traumatic swelling, or tourniquet use.

The popliteal region represents the greatest challenge in peripheral vascular trauma. Both penetrating and blunt trauma contribute to arterial and venous injuries in this area. Penetrating trauma, gunshot wounds more often than stab wounds, is clinically obvious in most cases. Blunt trauma is less obvious and is responsible for delay in treatment. Limited collaterals at the popliteal level, combined with injuries of the collateral arteries, often cause ischaemia resulting in eventual amputation. The amputation rate for popliteal arterial injuries in the civilian population is in excess of 30 per cent. As a result of the association of certain types of injuries with popliteal vascular injuries, an aggressive approach towards diagnosis and treatment is essential. All patients with knee injuries, whether blunt or penetrating, with an ischaemic appearing limb, should undergo urgent operation. Systemic heparin should be administered immediately, if no contraindication exists. Operative planning should give priority to revascularization if orthopaedic treatment will delay final revascularization more than 4 to 6 h from the time of original injury or ischaemia.

Following revascularization, arteriography is recommended to confirm patency of repair and distal outflow tract. Concomitant four-compartment fasciotomy should be routinely performed if extensive soft tissue injury exists or if ischaemia time is long. Venous repair is more critical at the popliteal level than at any other peripheral injury site and patency of one popliteal vein is desirable, especially when soft tissue injury is extensive. Venous thrombectomy may be required to open the venous system and venorrhaphy or interposition grafting may be required to correct the venous injury.

Arteriography should be performed in patients with knee injuries in which there is a significant incidence of popliteal arterial injury, even when there is no evidence of ischaemia. These injuries include penetrating trauma that traverses the popliteal fossa, knee dislocations, blunt knee trauma due to automobile bumpers, and fractures near the knee associated with resolution of ischaemia following fracture reduction. Orthopaedic tourniquets themselves can produce ischaemia and thrombosis. It is always important to evaluate prospectively the likelihood of a functional limb before embarking on complex reconstruction. Vascular salvage that results in major motor or sensory dysfunction in a limb may not be the ideal treatment, especially when the recovery time for associated orthopaedic and soft tissue injuries is considered. A paralysed extremity without sensory function is often best treated by early amputation rather than by extensive vascular, orthopaedic, and soft tissue reconstruction.

CAROTID AND VERTEBRAL ARTERY INJURIES

Vascular injury in the region of the neck is frequently suspected from a history of penetrating trauma, expanding haematoma, pulsatile bleeding, palpable thrill, audible bruit, or neurological deficit. Careful neurological evaluation is essential in all patients with cervical trauma. Patients with penetrating trauma and a diffusely abnormal lateralizing neurological examination frequently have extracranial cerebrovascular occlusion or embolization. More localized deficits can occur following cerebrovascular injury or direct injury to the brachial plexus, cervical plexus, or a cranial nerve. Patients suffering blunt trauma can have neurological deficits from closed head injuries or brachial plexus stretch injuries. Findings suggestive of carotid injury from blunt trauma include delayed onset of neurological symptoms due to delayed carotid thrombosis, transient ischaemic attacks due to emboli arising from a carotid intimal injury site, or Horner's syndrome due to carotid dissection. Angiography is appropriate for all patients with neurological deficits following cervical trauma. Patients who are haemodynamically stable and who have developed appreciable neurological deficit should have a preoperative CT scan of the brain.

Most vascular injuries in the neck are caused by penetrating trauma. To aid in evaluation of potential vascular injuries in the neck, one should determine the level of penetration before proceeding with exploration. Preoperative angiography is recommended for potential injuries to the proximal common carotid artery as well as the distal internal carotid artery at the base of the skull. Special preparations are frequently required for proximal and distal carotid artery injuries. Sternotomy is required for proximal control of common carotid injuries at its origin. Visualization of distal internal carotid artery injuries may require subluxation of the mandible, which requires preoperative placement of dental wires.

Operative exploration is warranted in all patients with neck injuries that penetrate the platysma, as well as all arterial injuries identified by angiography. In addition to preparing the neck region for surgery, the entire chest and a portion of the lower extremity, for saphenous vein harvesting, should be included in the operative field. The carotid bifurcation region is approached by an incision anterior to the sternocleidomastoid muscle. Carotid origin injuries require a median sternotomy. Proximal vertebral artery injuries are approached by a supraclavicular incision. With carotid injuries, proximal control is best achieved before identifying the site of arterial injury. Systemic anticoagulation is recommended unless contraindicated by other injuries. Limited injuries of the carotid system can often be repaired primarily. It is essential to resect all devitalized arterial wall. A temporary carotid shunt is used to reduce cerebral ischaemia time in severe injuries that require an end-to-end anastomosis, vein patch repair, or graft interposition. If graft interposition is planned, it is helpful to place the shunt through the graft prior to temporary shunt placement. Shunting is not required in repair of external carotid artery injury: arterial ligation is acceptable if simple repair is impossible. Ligation of the common or internal carotid artery should be avoided, if at all possible, because of the risk of stroke, except in patients with distal internal carotid artery injury at the base of the skull without adequate length of distal artery to allow repair and those with complete internal carotid occlusion with severe cerebral infarct. Patients with non-haemorrhagic stroke after carotid occlusion are likely to have conversion to a more severe haemorrhagic cerebral infarct if internal carotid circulation is restored. If carotid ligation is required, adjuvant heparin therapy may reduce the risk of thrombotic stroke.

The vertebral artery is less frequently injured, given its protected course in the transverse foramina of the cervical vertebrae. Since most vertebral arteries are paired and form a single basilar artery, vertebral ligation is acceptable in most cases. Preoperative angiography can help identify the location of vertebral artery injury and, equally important, the status of the contralateral vertebral artery. Primary repair of injuries to a single patent vertebral artery or a dominant vertebral artery should be carried out, if possible.

Venous injuries of the neck are best treated with primary repair or ligation; bilateral internal jugular venous ligations should be avoided, but extensive repairs with interposition grafts are rarely warranted. Special care is required when dealing with venous injuries to prevent air embolization at the site of injury. During venous ligation, one should protect the vagus nerve and other cranial nerves.

Postoperative care should include elevation of the head to reduce venous engorgement and swelling. Frequent neurological checks are essential to diagnose early postoperative complications at the site of repair. Prompt angiography, duplex scanning, or reoperation may be necessary to limit further neurological injury. Infusion of low molecular weight dextran, at a rate of 30 μl/h for 24 to 48 h following carotid artery repair helps prevent thromboembolic events.

THORACIC VASCULAR INJURIES

The most frequent sites of major injury in patients who have sustained blunt thoracic injuries are the proximal descending thoracic aorta and the proximal innominate artery. Both of these injuries are caused by high-speed motor vehicle accidents. Injury to the descending thoracic aorta occurs at the level of the ligamentum arteriosum, where the thoracic aorta is fixed in the posterior mediastinum. During the sudden deceleration which occurs in high-speed accidents the heart and aortic arch have continued forward momentum, resulting in a tear injury of the proximal, fixed, descending thoracic aorta. Innominate artery injury occurs most frequently from compression between the sternum and vertebral bodies, as well as from hyperextension of the neck. More severe injuries are usually fatal and never require medical attention.

Subclavian and intercostal vascular injuries can be associated with fractures of the clavicle or ribs.

The diagnosis of blunt thoracic vascular injuries is made from a combination of history, physical examination, and radiographic examinations as necessary. Pertinent points in the patient's history include motor vehicle accident at speeds greater than 70 km/h, sudden deceleration, driver of a vehicle, death of another victim in the accident, or loss of consciousness at the scene. Physical examination is frequently not very revealing until hypotension develops. Local findings include chest wall contusions, supraclavicular haematomas, clavicle or rib fractures, a systolic murmur, and diminished femoral or radial pulses. Chest radiographs are frequently abnormal in trauma victims, but suggestive findings of an aortic or great vessel injury include widened superior mediastinum, ill-defined or enlarged aortic arch shadow, apical pleural cap, left hemithorax, deviation of a nasogastric tube to the right with aortic injury or to the left with innominate artery injury, deviation of the trachea to the right or left mainstem bronchus inferiorly. Aortography is indicated in stable patients with these abnormalities, as well as in some patients with normal chest radiographs, but with an appropriate history suggestive of severe thoracic trauma. The unstable patient with an abnormal chest radiograph is often best served by immediate exploratory left thoracotomy.

Most thoracic injuries that reach medical attention involve entry wounds at the thoracic outlet or supraclavicular regions.

The approach and repair of thoracic vascular injury depends upon the location and type of injury. Injury to the descending thoracic aortic caused by deceleration is best approached by a left fourth intercostal space posterolateral thoracotomy. The aortic repair can be by primary end-to-end anastomosis or with an interposition Dacron graft. Adjuvant treatment recommended by some authors to reduce spinal cord ischaemia includes partial or complete cardiopulmonary bypass, or ascending aorta-to-descending aorta shunting, while others advocate a prompt clamp and repair technique.

The innominate vessels are approached by median sternotomy. Some penetrating injuries can be repaired primarily; however, extensive arterial injuries and deceleration injuries require the innominate artery to be resected and its origin to be oversewn at the aortic arch. Dacron graft placement from the right lateral side of the ascending aorta to the distal innominate artery is used in the reconstruction. Innominate venous injuries are best repaired primarily, when possible, but when this is not possible ligation is appropriate and is usually well tolerated.

The right subclavian vessels are approached by median sternotomy with right supraclavicular extension. In distal subclavian injuries, a supraclavicular approach, with or without clavicle resection, may be adequate. The proximal left subclavian artery can be controlled by a left third intercostal space anterolateral thoracotomy. For full visualization of the proximal left subclavian artery, a trap-door thoracotomy may be required through left third intercostal and left supraclavicular incisions, with an intervening partial median sternotomy. Subclavian venous repairs are often impractical because injuries are too extensive and multiple branches require venous ligation. Techniques of subclavian artery repair include end-to-end anastomosis and interposition grafting with Dacron or PTFE prostheses.

ABDOMINAL VASCULAR INJURIES

The major abdominal vasculature is largely protected from blunt injury because of its retroperitoneal location adjacent to the spinal column. Penetrating trauma, however, can cause vascular injury at any site. Major vascular injury with free intraperitoneal haemorrhage is frequently fatal or at best haemodynamically unstable, requiring immediately laparotomy for diagnosis and treatment. Haemorrhage arising within the retroperitoneum or mesentery may be contained, allowing stabilization and further evaluation.

An excretory urogram should be obtained in stable victims of penetrating trauma before exploratory laparotomy is undertaken. Failure to see one kidney is highly suggestive of a renal vascular injury. Computed tomography frequently reveals the presence or absence of a retroperitoneal haematoma. Patients with penetrating trauma should have exploration of retroperitoneal haematomas for possible aortic, caval, or renal vascular injuries. Arteriography is helpful in confirming renal artery injuries in patients with failure to visualize one kidney on urography.

Blunt abdominal trauma may produce avulsions of mesenteric arterial branches, of portal venous branches, or of renal vessels with resultant mesenteric, periportal, or retroperitoneal haematomas. Intimal injuries of visceral vessels due to blunt trauma may produce arterial thrombosis and subsequent ischaemia. Infrarenal abdominal aortic intimal injury from seat belt compression of an aorta during automobile accidents can result in aortic thrombosis and profound lower extremity ischaemia.

Pelvic fractures can be associated with large pelvic haematomas from cancellous bone disruptions, as well as vascular injuries. Arteriography is used to confirm hypogastric branch artery injuries. Arteriographic embolization is preferred to direct surgical ligation of the hypogastric arteries in patients with pelvic fractures and persistent haemorrhage.

A standard midline incision is appropriate for nearly all patients with abdominal vascular injuries. Extension into a left thoracoabdominal incision aids visualization of the proximal aorta. Appropriate exposure of the retroperitoneum depends on the vessels injured. Initial control of haemorrhage by packing the upper quadrants with laparotomy pads, as well as by evisceration of the small bowel, aids in the identification of the source of haemorrhage.

Suprarenal aortic injuries frequently require complete mobilization of the spleen, pancreas, stomach, and left colon to the right side of the abdomen to allow adequate exposure of the suprarenal aorta, coeliac axis, and the origin of the superior mesenteric artery. The infrarenal aorta and left renal vessels can be approached directly in the midline of the retroperitoneum just left of the root of the small bowel mesentery and below the transverse mesocolon. The inferior vena cava and right renal vessels are best seen by reflecting the right colon to the left and by extensive Kocher manoeuvre of the duodenum.

The iliac vessels are approached directly for proximal and distal control. The common iliac artery is best visualized at the aortic bifurcation in the midline of the retroperitoneum. The iliac veins are located posterior and to the right of the iliac arteries. In patients with extensive iliac venous injury, the common iliac artery may be divided over the site of venous injury. Following iliac venous repair or ligation, the common iliac artery can be reapproximated end-to-end. The distal external iliac arteries can be easily controlled just proximal to the inguinal ligament within the abdominal cavity. To avoid ureteral injury the retroperitoneum should be retracted and not divided in the region of the common iliac bifurcation.

Major arterial injuries in the abdomen can frequently be repaired by lateral arteriorrhaphy or end-to-end anastomosis. More extensive injuries to the aorta require patch aortoplasty with a PTFE patch or aortic replacement with a Dacron or a PTFE graft. When interposition grafting is required, the choice of vein, autologous artery, Dacron, or PTFE graft as a conduit, is determined by the size of the artery and amount of gastrointestinal contamination. PTFE is the prosthetic conduit of choice in contaminated surgical fields. If contamination is severe, arterial ligation and extra-anatomic reconstruction may be advisable. Injuries at the origin of a visceral artery frequently require revascularization grafting, such as an aortorenal or an aortosuperior mesenteric artery bypass. Coeliac and inferior mesenteric artery origin injuries can be ligated in most cases because of excellent collateralization from the superior mesenteric artery.

Venous injuries should be repaired if possible—most only require lateral venorrhaphy. To prevent tearing of these thin walled vessels vascular clamps should be avoided, and vessel loops or compression with sponge forceps should be used for temporary control. If repair of a venous injury is impracticable, ligation is acceptable. Ligation of the left renal vein should be as close to the inferior vena cava as is possible; venous drainage of the left kidney will proceed through the adrenal, gonadal, and lumbar veins. Injury to the right renal vein should be repaired, if at all possible, for the paucity of venous collateral branches may result in venous hypertension and renal dysfunction following right renal vein ligation.

Inferior vena cava injuries can frequently be repaired primarily using transient caval compression with sponge forceps or with partial-occlusion clamps. If complete occlusion is required to control caval haemorrhage, the surgeon should be aware of potentially major hypotension with caval clamping. Atriocaval shunting for suprarenal caval injuries as well as hepatic venous injuries has been described to maintain venous return during caval repair. Extensive caval injuries may require patch angioplasty or ligation. If the inferior vena cava repair results in a significant narrowing of the inferior vena cava, ligation is preferred to prevent the possibility of caval thrombosis and pulmonary embolism. Ligation of the iliac, hepatic, or portal veins as well as the inferior vena cava requires administration of additional fluid perioperatively. Following iliac or caval ligation, postoperative elevation of the lower extremities is recommended to reduce swelling. Concern over venostasis and potential deep venous thrombosis following major venous ligation warrants administration of subcutaneous heparin, 5000 units twice daily, in suitable patients.

FURTHER READING

Abbott WM, Darling RC. Axillary artery aneurysms secondary to crutch trauma. *Am J Surg* 1973; **125**: 515–20.

Accola KD, Feliciano DV, Mattox KL, Burch JM, Beall AC Jr, Jordon GL Jr. Management of injuries to the superior mesenteric artery. *J Trauma* 1986; **26**: 313–18.

Akins CW, Buckley MJ, Daggett W, McIlduff JB, Austen WG. Acute traumatic disruption of the thoracic aorta: a ten-year experience. *Ann Thoracic Surg* 1981; **31**: 305–9.

DeBakey ME, Simeone FA. Battle injuries of the arteries in World War II: an analysis of 2,471 cases. *Ann Surg* 1946; **123**: 534–79.

Fabian TC, Turkleson NL, Connelly TL, Stone HH. Injury to the popliteal artery. *Am J Surg* 1982; **143**: 225–8.

Feliciano DV. Approach to major abdominal vascular injury. *J Vasc Surg* 1988; **7**: 730–6.

Fisher DF Jr, Clagett GP, Parker JI, *et al.* Mandibular subluxation for high carotid exposure. *J Vasc Surg* 1984; **1**: 727–33.

Goldman MH, Kent S, Schaumburg E. Brachial artery injuries associated with posterior elbow dislocation. *Surg Gynecol Obstet* 1987; **164**: 95–7.

Graham JM, Feliciano DV, Mattox KL, Beall AC Jr. Innominate vascular injury. *J Trauma* 1982; **22**: 647–55.

Gregory RT, *et al.* The mangled extremity syndrome (M.E.S.): a severity grading system for multisystem injury of the extremity. *J Trauma* 1985; **25**: 1147–50.

Hardy JD, Raju S, Neely WA, Berry DW. Aortic and other arterial injuries *Ann Surg* 1975; **181**: 640–53.

Hewitt RL. Vascular injuries. In: Haimovici H, ed. *Vascular emergencies.* New York: Appleton-Century Croft, 1982: 261.

Hughes CW. Arterial repair during the Korean War. *Ann Surg* 1958; **147**: 555–61.

Makins GH. Injuries to the blood vessels. In: *Official history of the Great War Medical Service. Surgery of the War.* Vol. 2, London: His Majesty's Stationery Office. 1922: 170–296.

Mattox KL, Feliciano DC. Truncal vascular trauma: aorta, innominate vessels, vena cava, portal vein,and visceral arteries. In: Wilson SE, Veith J, Hobson RW II, Williams RA, eds. *Vascular surgery.* New York: McGraw-Hill,1987: 818–19.

Mattox KL, Holzman M, Pichard LR, Beall AC Jr, DeBakey ME. Clamp/repair a safe technique for treatment of blunt injury to the descending thoracic aorta. *Ann Thoracic Surg* 1985: **40**; 456–63.

Mattox KL, Feliciano DV, Burch J, Beall AC Jr., Jordan GL Jr, DeBakey ME. Five thousand seven hundred sixty cardiovascular injuries in 4,459 patients, epidemiologic evolution 1958–1987. *Ann Surg* 1989; **209**: 698–707.

McCollum CH, Mavor E. Brachial artery injury after cardiac catherization. *J Vasc Surg* 1986; **4**: 355–9.

Mullins RJ, Lucas CE, Ledgerwood AM. The natural history following venous ligation for civilian injuries. *J Trauma* 1980; **20**: 737–43.

O'Donnell TF Jr, Brewster DC, Darling RC, Veen H, Waltman AA. Arterial injuries associated with fractures and/or dislocations of the knee. *J Trauma* 1977; **17**: 775–84.

Orringer MD, Kirsch MM. Primary repair of acute traumatic aortic disruption. *Ann Thoracic Surg* 1983; **35**: 672–5.

Pasch AR, *et al.* Results of venous reconstruction after civilian vascular trauma. *Arch Surg* 1986; **121**: 607–11.

Pate JW. Traumatic rupture of the aorta: emergency operation. *Ann Thoracic Surg* 1985; **39**: 531–7.

Perry MO, Thal ER, Shires GT. Management of arterial injuries. *Ann Surg* 1971; **173**: 403–8.

Rich NM. Principles and indications of primary venous repair. *Surgery* 1982; **91**: 492–6.

Rich NM, Baugh JH, Hughes CW. Acute arterial injuries in Vietnam: 1000 cases. *J Trauma* 1970; **10**: 359–69.

Rovito PF. Atrial caval shunting in blunt hepatic vascular injury. *Ann Surg* 1987; **205**: 318–21.

Treiman RL, Doty D, Gaspar MR. Acute vascular trauma: a 15-year study. *Am J Surg* 1966; **111**: 469–73.

Trunkey DD, Lewis FR, eds. *Current therapy of trauma–2.* Toronto: BC Decker, 1986; xi.

Vaughan GD, Mattox KL, Feliciano DV, Beall AC Jr, DeBakey ME. Surgical experience with expanded polytetrafluorethylene (PTFE) as a replacement graft for traumatized vessels. *J Trauma* 1979; **19**: 403–8.

7.13 Percutaneous transluminal angioplasty and laser therapy

GLENN M. LaMURAGLIA AND THOMAS K. EGGLIN

ANGIOPLASTY

Angioplasty, the remodelling of an artery, traces its roots to the pioneering work of Dotter and Judkins in the early 1960s. They utilized a series of progressively larger coaxial catheters, passed across arterial obstructions to enlarge the lumen size. In the 1970s Gruentzig advanced the technique and broadened its application with the introduction of the non-elastomeric, polyvinylchloride angioplasty balloon mounted on a flexible, double-lumen catheter. Today, percutaneous transluminal angioplasty offers a safe and effective approach to the treatment of vascular stenoses in selected applications. The evolution of percutaneous transluminal angioplasty has continued with the development of new plastic materials for the construction of low-profile-high-pressure balloon catheters, hydrophilic coated guidewires, and improvement in digital imaging technology. While contemporary techniques continue to evolve, balloon angioplasty remains the mainstay of percutaneous transluminal therapy for atherosclerotic arterial stenoses. The contributions of novel techniques such as atherectomy, intravascular stenting, and laser angioplasty are still to be defined.

Mechanism of balloon angioplasty

Dotter and Judkins mistakenly believed that their coaxial technique resulted in remodelling and compression of atherosclerotic plaque. Instead, it is now known that plaque fracture, with or without localized dissection of the arterial media, is the major

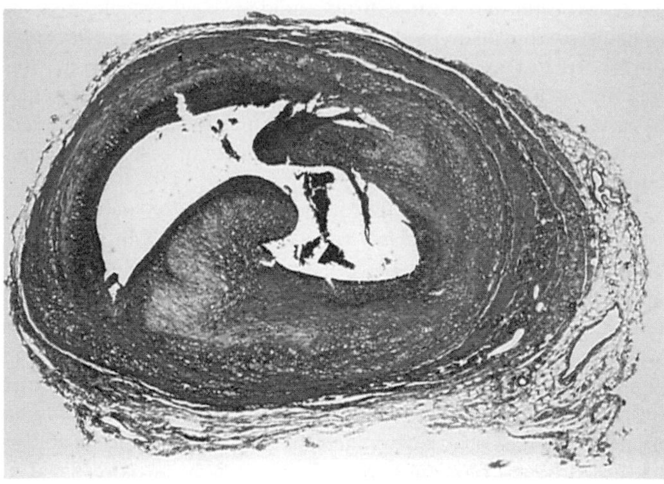

Fig. 1 Photomicrograph of the dissection of arterial plaque with balloon angioplasty. The cleft on the left demonstrates the dissection channel, while the right central portion demonstrates the original lumen. The specimen is of an artery 2 weeks after balloon angioplasty (magnification ×15).

mechanism of percutaneous transluminal angioplasty (Fig. 1); the result is demonstrated angiographically as clefts filled with contrast material. However, removal or distal embolization of plaque constituents is not a component of successful percutaneous transluminal angioplasty.

While overstretching to the point of adventitial rupture is obviously undesirable, lesser degrees of medial stretching represent an important part of the 'controlled' injury made with percutaneous transluminal angioplasty. Patients typically experience transient, localized discomfort related to balloon inflation, which is attributed to stretching of the media. Severe, unremitting pain is, instead, an unfavourable sign that should raise the suspicion of adventitial rupture or bleeding into adjacent tissues.

Indications

Peripheral

In the peripheral arterial system, percutaneous transluminal angioplasty can provide definitive therapy for claudication and limb-threatening ischaemia, or it may be used in combination with surgical procedures, such as iliac percutaneous transluminal angioplasty followed by femoropopliteal bypass. The ideal morphological indication for transluminal angioplasty is a single, short-segment stenosis in a medium to large vessel, such as an iliac (Fig. 2), femoral (Fig. 3), or popliteal artery. Other indications include multiple discrete short-segment stenoses or a short occlusion. Long-segment stenoses, long-segment occlusions, and stenoses in small (e.g. tibial) vessels may be treated by angioplasty, but with less immediate and long-term success.

The identification of appropriate targets for percutaneous transluminal angioplasty requires integration of the patient's clinical presentation, physical status, non-invasive vascular laboratory results, and, when possible, pressure gradients. Correlation of these data with the radiographic appearance of a lesion helps to determine whether intervention is warranted. Dilating stenoses without regard to the these factors, simply because a lesion is present and accessible, is inappropriate. Angioplasty is not entirely without risk, and the natural history of many lesions remains benign. In an attempt to avoid any ambiguity, many angiographers rely upon the demonstration of a significant intra-arterial pressure gradient (over 10 mmHg) before proceeding with angioplasty. For this reason, among others, appropriate haemodynamic monitors are an essential component of the angiography suite.

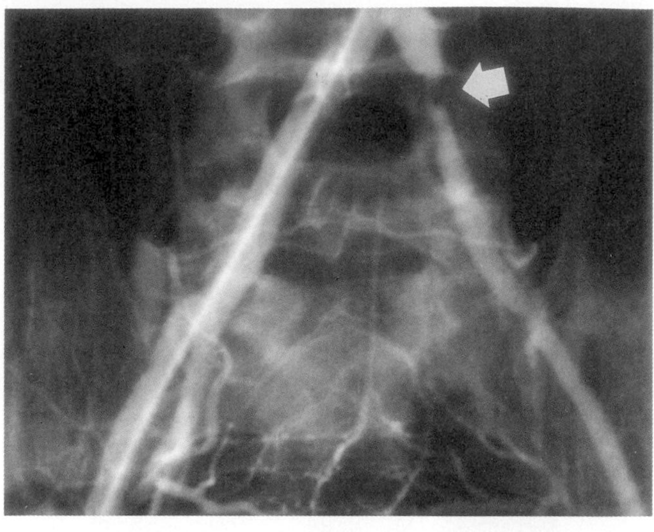

(a)

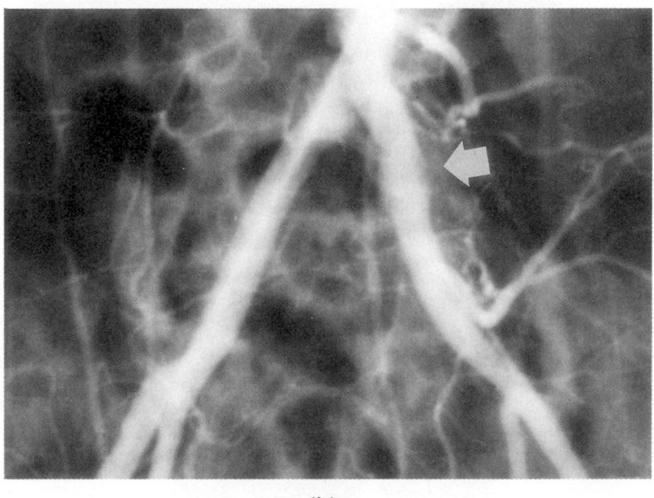

(b)

Fig. 2 (a) An angiogram of a localized severely stenotic common iliac artery. (b) The recanalized lumen of the same iliac artery after balloon dilatation.

Visceral

While the indications for peripheral angioplasty are well defined, the guidelines for visceral angioplasty are more ambiguous. For example, percutaneous transluminal renal angioplasty is most commonly performed to treat renovascular hypertension, but is also employed to preserve residual function in native or transplanted kidneys. An unsuccessful prior attempt at renal angioplasty does not affect the outcome of a subsequent surgical revascularization procedure as long as primary thrombosis of the renal artery is avoided.

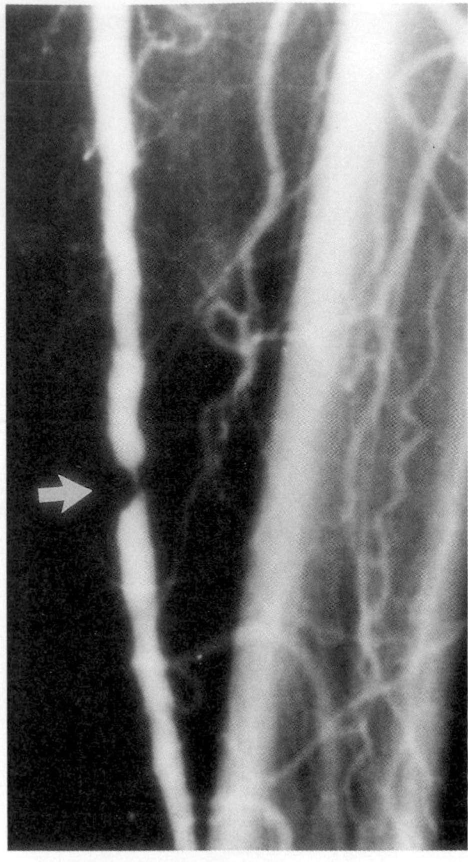

(a)

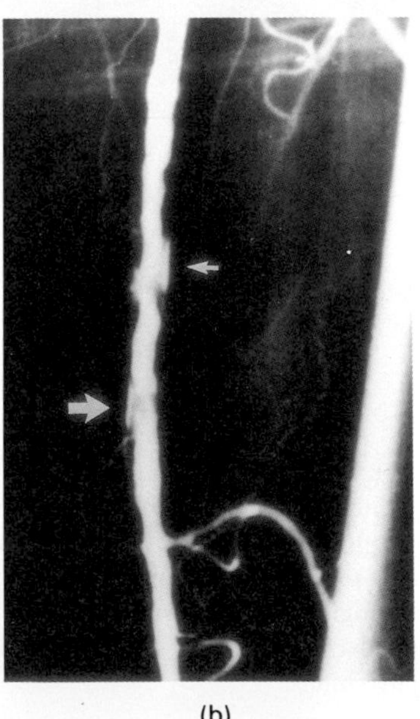

(b)

Fig. 3 A localized mid-superficial femoral artery stenosis (a) before and (b) after balloon angioplasty. The larger arrows demonstrate the lesion that had balloon angioplasty, the small arrow (b) demonstrates a dissection cleft noted as part of the procedure.

Since fewer than 5 per cent of patients with high blood pressure suffer from renovascular hypertension, it is frustrating and economically imprudent to screen large populations for that condition with standard arteriography. Suggestive signs and symptoms include hypertension with a bruit, sudden-onset, accelerated, or difficult to control hypertension, or onset of renal insufficiency during treatment with an angiotensin-converting enzyme inhibitor, such as captopril. Biochemical 'proof' of renovascular hypertension may be provided by asymmetric elevation of selective renal vein renin levels, with the assay being at least 1.5 times higher on the affected side.

The identification of appropriate targets for percutaneous transluminal renal angioplasty takes into account both the nature of the disease producing the renal artery stenosis (for example, atherosclerosis or fibromuscular dysplasia) (Fig. 4), and the location of the lesion in the renal artery. The distinction between these aetiologies is important since renal angioplasty is the treatment of choice for renovascular hypertension secondary to fibromuscular dysplasia, and since restenosis after angioplasty is more common in atheromatous renal artery stenosis than in fibromuscular dysplasia. Although fibromuscular lesions tend to be more distal in the main renal artery, or involve branch renal arteries, the atheromatous lesions are more likely to lie in the proximal renal artery. Proximal renal artery lesions may respond well to renal angioplasty (Fig. 5), but attempts at dilating stenoses that involve the origin of the renal artery are less likely to be successful (Fig. 6). Ostial stenoses are, in fact, often overhanging aortic plaques that are typically merely displaced by balloon inflation and, therefore, are impossible to fracture with a catheter in the renal artery.

Mesenteric ischaemia ('abdominal angina') manifests itself clinically as weight loss or postprandial abdominal pain, and is thought to be due to severe narrowing of at least two of the three arteries supplying the bowel. These abnormalities are best demonstrated using lateral or biplane aortography and, in several small

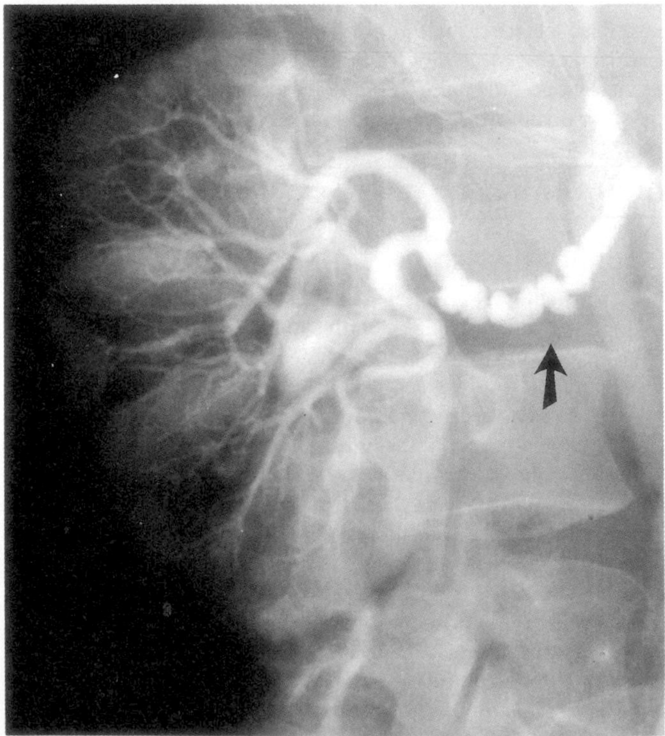

Fig. 4 An angiogram of fibromuscular dysplasia of a renal artery. The multiple lobulations in the artery (arrow) demonstrate the stenoses of the lesion.

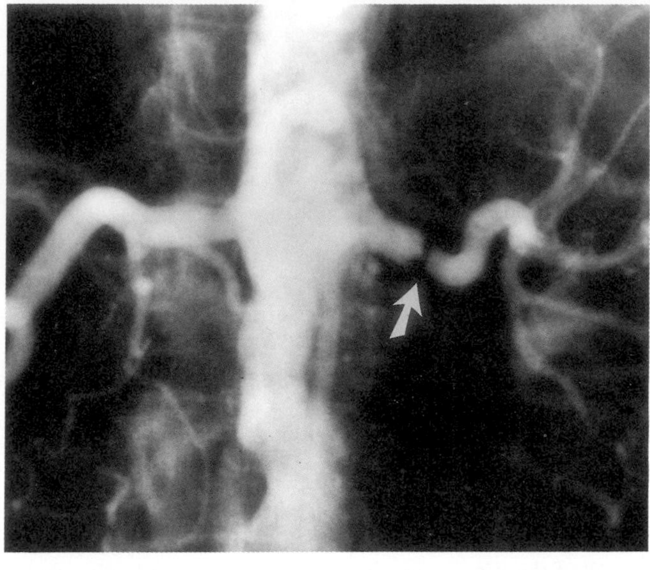

(a)

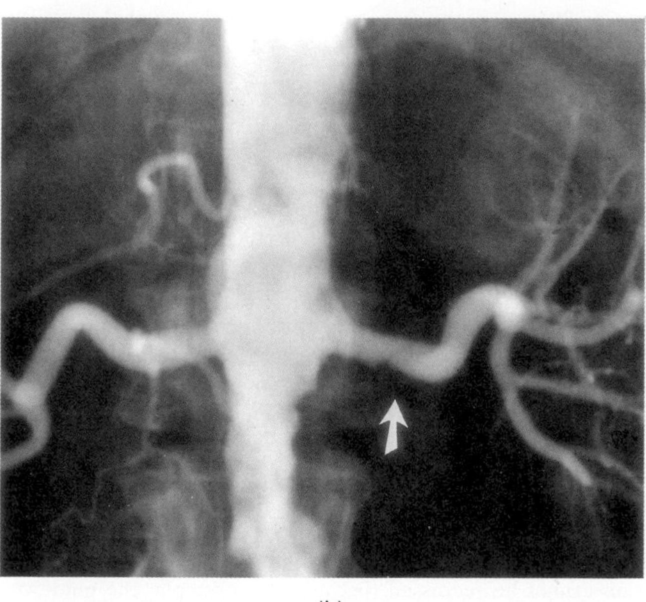

(b)

Fig. 5 An angiogram of a proximal renal artery stenosis (arrow) (a) before and (b) after balloon angioplasty. This atherosclerotic lesion is of the renal artery and not an aortic plaque.

series, angioplasty has enjoyed a high degree of success and almost no complications. Percutaneous transluminal angioplasty can be expected to be least effective in treating ostial lesions, which are the most commonly encountered, and the so-called median arcuate ligament syndrome.

Miscellaneous

Percutaneous transluminal angioplasty has also been employed to treat a number of disparate clinical problems, although none of the techniques is currently widely employed in clinical practice. For example, while lesions in the cervical portions of the carotid and vertebral arteries are accessible to the angiographer, fear of cerebral emboli has to date discouraged the widespread application of angioplasty at those sites. Lesions at the origin of the vertebral arteries account for approximately 40 per cent of all vertebrobasilar insufficiency, and at least 70 cases of vertebral percutaneous transluminal angioplasty have been reported, with varying results. Similarly, over 160 cases of carotid angioplasty for ischaemic cerebral symptoms have been described, but the data concerning complications and long-term follow-up are incomplete.

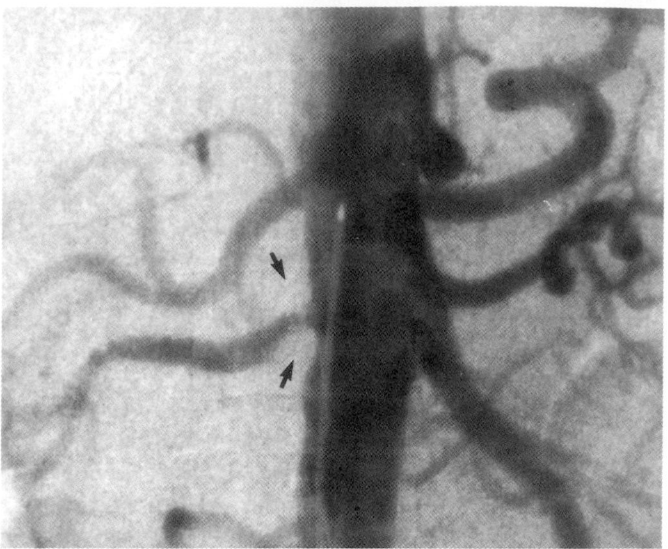

Fig. 6 Angiogram of renal artery origin stenosis, as demonstrated by the arrows. This lesion is primarily an aortic plaque, not a plaque of the renal artery. These lesions respond poorly to balloon angioplasty.

Technique

To define better a suspicious lesion seen on a diagnostic arteriogram, the radiologist can either obtain oblique views of the area or, as noted above, directly measure the change in intra-arterial pressure across the stenosis. After identifying a lesion to be dilated, the angioplasty may be performed at the conclusion of a diagnostic arteriogram or during a separate visit to the angiography suite. This decision is best made after considering the patient's ability to tolerate the additional time needed to dilate the stenosis and the amount of radiographic contrast that must be used to document the result.

Our approach to percutaneous transluminal angioplasty is based on a series of fundamental techniques, with minor modifications for specific anatomical sites (Fig. 7). The importance of experience cannot be overemphasized, especially in atypical or difficult cases, which require extensive deviation from these basic tools. Typically, this technique would involve the following steps:

(1) adequate definition of the haemodynamically significant lesion;
(2) navigation of the lesion with an appropriate guidewire;
(3) crossing the lesion with the selected angioplasty catheter;
(4) inflation of the balloon;

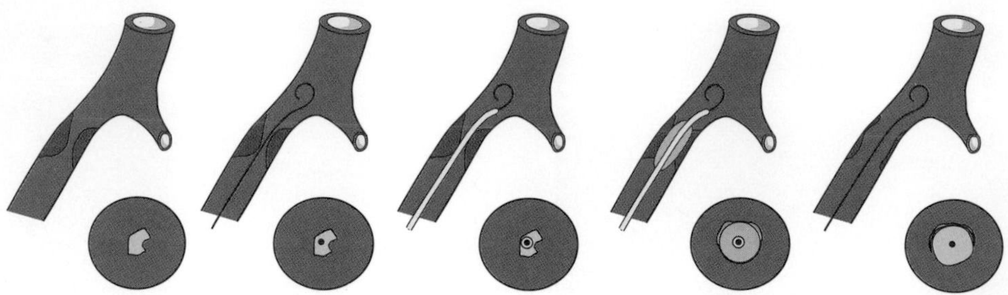

Fig. 7 The technique of balloon angioplasty including (a) identification of the lesion by angiogram; (b) passage of a guidewire across the lesion; (c) passage of balloon catheter across the lesion over the guidewire: (d) inflation of the balloon and performance of the balloon angioplasty; and (e) removal of the balloon catheter and repeat angiography while the guidewire is still in place. These schematics include a lateral and cross-section projection for each step described.

(5) repeat arteriography or manometry to demonstrate the effect of treatment;
(6) removal of the catheter and compression of the puncture site to achieve haemostasis.

Angioplasty catheters are described in terms of several variables: catheter shaft size (in the French scale; mm diameter/π), balloon outer diameter (in mm), and balloon length (in cm). For a particular case, the selected balloon has a diameter approximately equal to that of the 'normal' portions of the affected vessel and a length exceeding that of the lesion to be dilated. Employing the uncorrected dimensions (that is, not compensating for radiographic magnification) results in the use of balloons which are approximately 20 per cent larger than the native vessel, allowing for some over-distension, which is important in the mechanism of angioplasty. Typically employed balloon sizes range from 8 to 10 mm in the iliac arteries and about 6 mm in the superficial femoral artery. The size of the catheter shaft determines the size of the percutaneous arteriotomy and may affect the ability to traverse a particular lesion. Smaller catheters are often able to cross tighter stenoses, while larger catheters are stronger and may tolerate higher pressures. The development of so-called low-profile balloons, in essence larger balloons with a smaller cross-sectional diameter (due to tighter wrapping of the balloon and smaller catheter shaft size), has increased the number of lesions that can be successfully crossed and dilated.

The targeted lesion should be carefully crossed with an appropriate guidewire. To avoid the risk of intimal injury or extraluminal catheter passage after initial attempts at angioplasty, the wire should not be withdrawn across the stenosis until the conclusion of the procedure. Since balloon dilation requires transient arterial occlusion, intravenous heparin is administered prior to crossing the stenosis with a catheter, to minimize the risk of thrombosis. While not a risk in the iliac or superficial femoral arteries, spasm is a common complication of infrapopliteal or visceral angioplasty; intra-arterial nitroglycerine (50–200 mcg) is generally also administered at this time.

After advancing the catheter across the lesion, the balloon is inflated by hand under direct fluoroscopic visualization, using a 50 per cent mixture of low-strength contrast and saline in a 10 ml syringe and held in this position for 30 s. This method allows the angiographer to monitor the procedure for safety and often demonstrates the elimination of a 'waist' of stenotic plaque compressing the balloon as the lesion is dilated. While the routine use of a manometer is often unnecessary, it is helpful in avoiding balloon rupture. It is good practice to leave a set length of guide-wire extending beyond the catheter tip, in order to avoid traumatizing the wall of the vessel with that structure as the catheter contorts during balloon inflation. This precision becomes especially important when working near bifurcation points or smaller vessels. Follow-up radiographs or intra-arterial pressure measures can then be obtained in the same manner as for the original diagnostic study.

Femoropopliteal

In experienced hands, most above-knee stenoses are accessible by contralateral retrograde arterial puncture, obviating the need for a second arteriotomy after the diagnostic study. Arterial access for distal femoral and popliteal angioplasty may require antegrade puncture of the diseased vessel, which is technically more challenging than is the retrograde approach. Just as with retrograde access, the antegrade arteriotomy must be made below the level of the inguinal ligament, in order to permit adequate haemostasis with compression alone at the conclusion of the procedure. Retrograde popliteal artery puncture has been described as an alternative approach but is not widely applied. Technical success of percutaneous transluminal angioplasty is defined using the same criteria employed to measure the haemodynamic significance of the original lesion. In the procedure room, obliteration of a previously defined pressure gradient is the desired outcome. If the lesion cannot be recrossed (because, for example, the guidewire has been withdrawn or because adequate haemodynamic measurements cannot be obtained), the angiographer can rely upon improved postprocedure lower-extremity pulse-volume recordings. Repeat arteriography in the same plane as was used to demonstrate the original lesion can illustrate enlargement of the arterial lumen and contrast-filled clefts indicative of focal plaque fracture and medial dissection. If the angiographer is dissatisfied with the result, the dilation can be repeated using a balloon of larger diameter. The angiogram taken after percutaneous transluminal angioplasty is presently the best means of demonstrating the degree of medial dissection and the irregularity of the intima, and is, therefore, an important part of the postprocedure evaluation. Patients with extensive dissection and marked disruption of the intima are predisposed to arterial thrombosis and should be given the anticoagulant intravenous heparin, for 24 to 48 h after haemostasis is achieved.

Intimal injury with exposure of the media to the bloodstream is a necessary part of this technique, but is highly thrombogenic.

Therefore, aspirin is prescribed to inhibit platelet aggregation and clot formation at the treatment site. The effects of aspirin vary according to dose, and the dose that would be 'best' for most people has never been identified. Most physicians who perform percutaneous transluminal angioplasty prescribe either one baby aspirin (1.25 grain = 81.25 mg) or one adult aspirin per day. Some prescribe aspirin only around the time of the procedure while others prescribe it indefinitely.

Results

In general, the likelihood of technical success and long-term patency are directly related to the diameter of the vessel being dilated. In the iliac arteries (Table 1) initial success can be expected in over 90 per cent of cases, and most series report 5-year patency rates between 70 and 80 per cent. Few complete life-table analyses have been performed to assess the long-term patency of infrainguinal angioplasty procedures. Those available, while incomplete, suggest that approximately 80 per cent of femoropopliteal percutaneous transluminal angioplasty procedures are technically successful and that about two-thirds remain patent after 2 years of clinical follow-up (Table 2).

Table 1 Patency data from 2697 reported iliac percutaneous transluminal angioplasty procedures

	Mean (%)	Range (%)
Technical success	92	50–96
2-year patency	81	65–93
5-year patency	72	50–87

Adapted from Becker, Katzen, and Dake. *Radiology* 1989; **170**: 921–940.

Table 2 Patency data from 4304 reported femoropoliteal percutaneous transluminal angioplasty procedures

	Mean (%)	Range (%)
Technical success	81	70–93
2-year patency	67	43–79
5-year patency	67	54–73

Adapted from Becker, Katzen, and Dake. *Radiology*, 1989; **170**: 921–40.

The results of renal artery angioplasty remain more controversial. The indications for percutaneous transluminal renal angioplasty and reported rates of technical success vary widely amongst institutions, as do the definitions of technical success. A recent review of the largest percutaneous transluminal renal angioplasty series showed that renovascular hypertension may be cured in about one-quarter of patients, but that up to one-third of patients may derive no benefit. In both the short and long term, renal artery stenoses due to fibromuscular dysplasia respond more favourably to this technique than do those secondary to atherosclerosis (Table 3). For stenoses due to fibromuscular dysplasia, patency rates in excess of 90 per cent may be expected at 2 years, while fewer than 65 per cent of atherosclerotic lesions will remain patent after that interval.

Table 3 Outcome data after attempted angioplasty of 691 renal artery stenoses for treatment of hypertension

	Mean (%)	Range (%)
Atherosclerotic lesions		
Cured	19	9–29
Improved	52	29–75
Failed[a]	30	0–54
Fibromuscular lesions		
Cured	50	25–85
Improved	42	13–63
Failed[a]	9	0–25

[a] Excludes angioplasty failures. Adapted from Ramsay and Waller, *British Medical Journal*, 1990; **300**: 569–72.

Complications

As with diagnostic arteriography, the complications of percutaneous transluminal angioplasty may be divided into two groups: those due to direct arterial injury and those related to the administration of radiographic contrast (including acute renal failure and drug allergy). As a rule, the rate of complications is inversely related to vessel size and the experience of the operator. Approximately 2.5 per cent of patients who undergo angioplasty suffer a complication that requires surgery or other treatment. Entry-site trauma, including haematoma and pseudoaneurysm, occurs in 2 to 3 per cent of cases, while complications due to thromboemboli are identified after 4 to 5 per cent of angioplasty procedures. Arteriovenous fistula has been reported as a complication in less than 0.1 per cent of procedures; limb or organ loss and even death are described, but these are very uncommon complications of angioplasty.

LASER THERAPY

Although the ablation of atherosclerotic plaque by a laser was first described in 1962, the use of a laser for arterial recanalization is still experimental. Theoretical benefits offered by laser therapy include the ability to treat long-segment occlusion by debulking (instead of displacing atheromatous material as in balloon angioplasty), and the potential of treating the luminal surface to minimize myointimal proliferation. The introduction of laser systems initially generated intense scientific and proprietary enthusiasm on the part of investigators and manufacturers, but clinical experience with these devices has not met the exaggerated expectations. In the peripheral vascular system, laser recanalization is most frequently followed by balloon angioplasty, because the luminal diameter created is that of the probe (1–2 mm) which is insufficient to maintain flow. Lasers are, therefore, an adjunct to balloon angioplasty (Fig. 8). It is important to understand some fundamentals of laser energy delivery before summarizing clinical experiences.

Laser fundamentals

The word LASER is an acronym for light amplification by stimulated emission of radiation. Although several different laser systems have been used, major differences between them preclude their being compared to each other. Three fundamental charac-

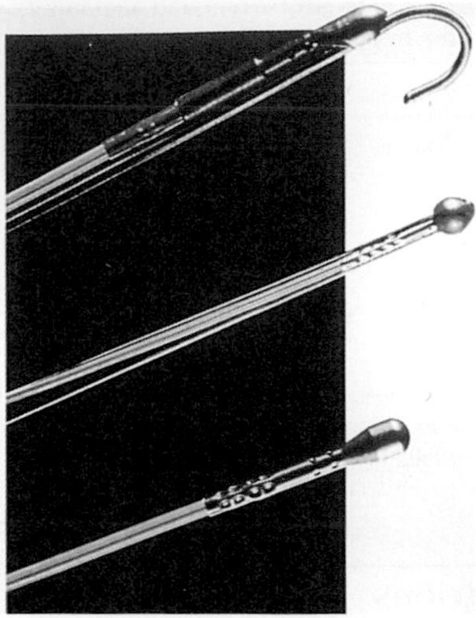

Fig. 8 Hot-tip probes produced by Trimedyne Corporation (Santa Anna, CA), demonstrating the metal cap placed on the distal portion of the fibreoptic device to convert the light energy into thermal energy.

teristics make each laser system unique; these are wavelength, pulse duration, and energy output.

The laser hardware consists of a resonator cavity that contains a translucent medium between a partial and totally reflecting mirror. The lasing medium, which gives the laser its name, is activated by an energy source, such as an electric current or a flashlamp. The specific molecules in the lasing medium are excited to their characteristic higher energy levels and, reaching a threshold, they produce a series of laser light emissions at specific wavelengths. The energy output at each wavelength is determined by the number of molecules at the corresponding energy level. The wavelength emitted is theoretically possible throughout the entire electromagnetic spectrum, ranging from X-rays through to microwaves.

Another laser parameter is the pulse duration or the amount of time that the laser emits light energy—from picoseconds (10^{-12} s) to continuous wave. The third important laser characteristic is energy, and the high concentration of coherent light energy produced provides lasers with many of their capabilities.

The laser radiation can interact in several different ways with the tissue by conversion of the light energy into other forms, which may or may not be desirable. There are essentially four different mechanisms of light energy conversion; they include luminescence, photothermal reaction, plasma formation, and photochemical reaction. The first three mechanisms have had applications in the therapy of atherosclerotic occlusive vascular disease.

Luminescence can be described as the emission of light energy from a molecule at specific longer wavelength(s), than the wavelength absorbed. The luminescence wavelength profile is usually a characteristic of the particular substance irradiated. It can be used for the identification of a particular tissue, as in the fluorescent discrimination between atherosclerotic plaque and normal arterial wall.

A photothermal reaction is the conversion of the light energy into heat energy. The effect on tissue depends on the method by which the energy is delivered, the amount delivered, the duration of the exposure, and the wavelength used. It is the mechanism employed for the ablation and recanalization of non-calcified atherosclerotic plaque, and the welding of blood vessels.

A plasma is a high-energy state resulting from a high-intensity, short-pulse duration ($<10^{-6}$ s) of laser light. Cavitation occurs, resulting in shock waves that disrupt tissue through a mechanical mechanism. It is through this mechanism that specific high-intensity laser systems can ablate calcified atheroma.

Laser targeting of tissue

Specific tissues can absorb different wavelengths of light because of their different biochemical composition. With the choice of a specific wavelength that is preferentially absorbed by the target tissue, selective tissue ablation can be performed. The energy of exposure and the duration of exposure are also important to avoid overriding this process or to permit diffusion of heat from the selected target to the adjoining non-targeted tissues. Two cardiovascular applications for this selective use of laser irradiation include the selective ablation of plaque and thrombus, the ablation of plaque having undergone clinical investigation. By choosing the appropriate wavelengths, one can target the yellow carotenoid chromophores in plaque, or the red haemoglobin chromophores in clot. In this fashion, one can irradiate the selected tissues at energies that ablate them, but which are below the thresholds of ablation of the surrounding normal or non-targeted tissues. This process can be expanded by the administration of exogenous chromophores that preferentially localize in the target tissue. Examples of this include the haematoporphyrin derivative, tetracycline, and carotenoids.

Clinical laser angioplasty: continuous wave

The initial clinical use and trials of laser therapy for the treatment of obliterative atherosclerotic disease utilized available commercial lasers, including the CO_2, neodymium:yttrium aluminium garnet (Nd:YAG), and Argon (Ar^+) lasers. Quartz fibres, commercially developed for the communications industry, improved the applicability of laser systems with wavelengths between 280 nm and 2.5 μm, because of their ability to transmit high-intensity radiation along their length without significant loss of energy. In these initial laser systems the energy was delivered in a continuous wave through the end of a cleaved fibre; it was difficult to control the irradiated energy during the ablation process. The elevated thermal effects, including tissue charring, unwanted coagulation, spasm, perforation, thrombosis, and subsequent development of aneurysms, limited the application of these systems. The development of the 'hot tip' was the first attempt at controlling the energy delivery of continuous-wave radiation by encasing the tip of the fibres with a metal jacket that was heated by the latter (Fig. 8). Although it improved the safety of laser recanalization of arteries, it has suffered several drawbacks. It is very user-dependent because it requires constant, rapid, to-and-fro motion, using a primarily mechanical means of recanalization; it causes vessel spasm and a large adjacent area of thermal injury; it is ineffectual against calcified plaque; and the devices advance along the mechanical path of least resistance—a problem with very eccentric plaques. Indeed, the primary mode of action of this device is probably mechanical and not related to any property of the laser energy. Clinical results have not been very promising in patients with clinically important atherosclerotic obstructive disease. Although the initial series claimed around a 90 per cent technical success rate and a 70 per cent 1-year patency, most of these lesions were short (<5 cm), superficial femoral obstructions in claudicators, and would probably respond in a similar fashion to conventional balloon angioplasty. When patients with critical ischaemia were treated, the results were significantly worse, with a less than 10 per cent 6-month clinical success rate.

Clinical laser angioplasty: pulsed laser

Although all clinical laser systems use thermal mechanisms of ablation, short-pulse laser ablation is much more efficient than is pure thermal vaporization because the former uses a microexplosive mechanism for the removal of tissue with the concomitant formation of microdebris (Fig. 9). Pulsed laser radiation is different from continuous-wave radiation because it delivers discrete quanta of irradiation at set time intervals of the order of picoseconds (10^{-12} s) to seconds. Although a chopped beam of continuous irradiation is technically considered a pulse, ablative pulsed laser irradiation has come to signify high-intensity light delivery; that is, a laser pulse that carries a significant amount of energy to ablate the irradiated tissue while being delivered in a short enough amount of time to cause minimal thermal effects to adjacent tissues. For most tissue this is adiabatic time-frame microseconds (10^{-6} s) to milliseconds (10^{-3} s). The type of tissue irradiated is therefore quite important, since mechanically weaker tissue will be more easily ablated at the same energy fluence than mechanically strong tissue. When pulses are of much shorter duration, one of the major problems that arises is that the intensity is too high to be able safely to couple the laser energy into a quartz fibre.

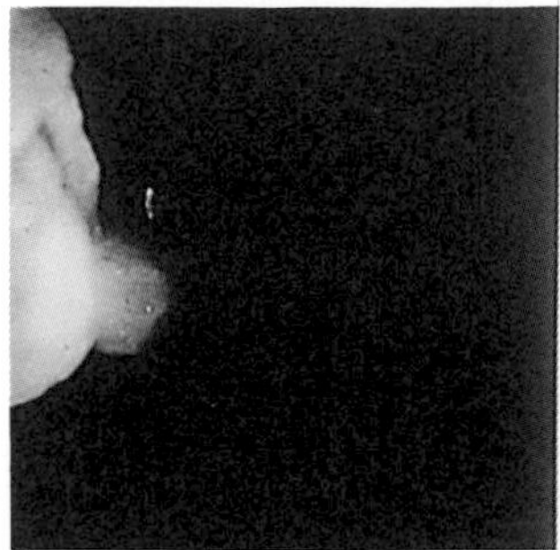
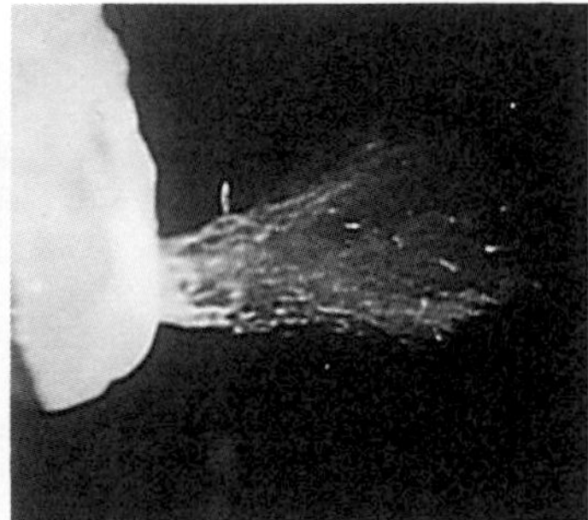

Fig. 9 These figures demonstrate 480 nm 1 μs pulse ablation of atherosclerotic plaque using high-speed flash photography. The microexplosive nature of ablation and the ensuing plume are evident at 15 μs and 150 μs after deposition of laser light. The microdebris can be seen ejecting from the atherosclerotic plaque (by courtesy of Martin R. Prince).

These considerations suggest that, depending on the application, the laser used, and the delivery system employed, there is an optimal laser pulse duration. However, it may be difficult to engineer the requisite power supply or to maintain activation of the lasing media for production of adequate laser output for specific pulse durations.

One other important factor in pulsed irradiation is the frequency of the pulses. If the laser pulse output is at a very high frequency, there may be accumulative thermal effect on the adjacent tissue that could make the system almost indistinguishable from continuous-wave laser irradiation. There are many variables that determine the optimal frequency. Despite the desire to obtain high efficiency by high pulse frequencies, power supply limitations usually keep the laser from a high delivery rate.

Pulsed lasers have not yet been used to a great extent in the treatment of atherosclerotic obstructive disease. There are three main systems: the 308 nm XeCl excimer, the pulse-dye, and the holmium:YAG (Ho:YAG), 2.1 μm laser. The infrared Ho:YAG laser is at a very early stage in its clinical application and there are only very scant data regarding its efficacy.

The pulse-dye laser used in Great Britain and in France is similar to the system used by the authors. Data concerning treatment of 'critical ischaemia' or severe disabling claudication demonstrate a 73 per cent acute clinical success rate and only a 10 per cent occlusion rate in the first 7-month follow-up. Data from use of the excimer laser are more extensive when used in peripheral arteries, but not all of the data are published. In one published series of 23 cases treated below the inguinal ligament, there was a 52 per cent success rate in recanalizing occluded arteries and an 80 per cent success rate in improving the luminal diameter in stenotic lesions. Of these cases, 47 per cent remained patent, with a mean follow-up to 10 months. These patients all had critical lower-extremity ischaemia (mean ankle/brachial index, 0.49), and all

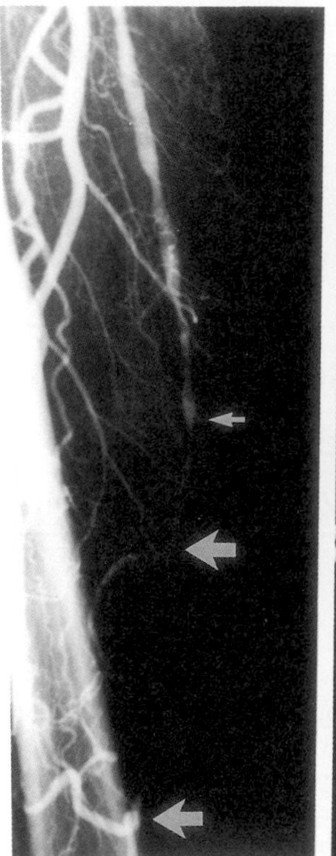
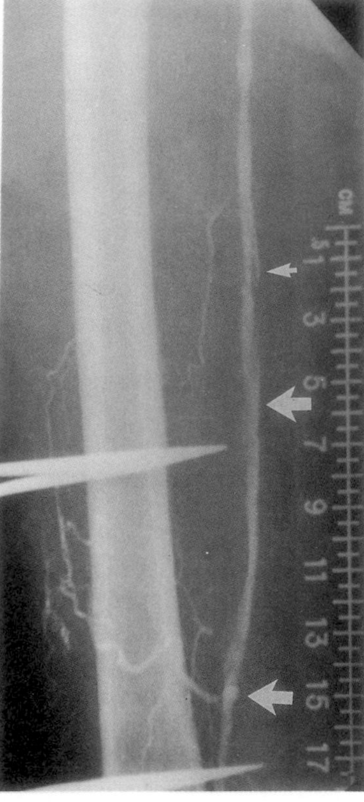

Fig. 10 Angiogram of a 10-cm occlusion before and after laser recanalization and balloon angioplasty. Of note, although the occluded segment was only 10 cm (large arrows), the stenotic segment was an additional 5 to 10 cm (small arrow), which required a balloon angioplasty and subsequent atherosclerotic plaque dissection. This phenomenon makes reporting of the length of the lesion or extent of disease difficult.

were treated with balloon angioplasty at the conclusion of the case. While these results are promising, it is still early to come to any conclusions about the effectiveness of these techniques.

The long-term patency of laser-treated atherosclerotic obstructive lesions is unknown. There are many theoretical and experimental advantages of pulsed systems over continuous-wave lasers, and most emerging new clinical laser systems for the treatment of obstructive atherosclerosis are of this type. However, there are several shortcomings (Fig. 10). At present most of these systems are limited to providing access for balloon angioplasty in total occlusions, and cannot provide the definitive therapy if used alone. Because they are relatively inefficient for tissue ablation, the inexperienced operator used them, mostly for mechanical advancement of the devices and not for ablation and removal of tissue. For this reason one may predict that the results of their use would be similar to those of balloon angioplasty.

FURTHER READING

Balloon angioplasty

Becker GJ, Katzen BT, Dake MD. *Noncoron Angiopl Radiol* 1989; **170**: 921–40.

Brewster DC, *et al.* Long-term results of combined iliac balloon angioplasty and distal surgical revascularization. *Ann Surg* 1989; **210**: 324–31.

Dotter CT, Judkins MP. Transluminal treatment of arteriosclerotic obstructions: description of a new technique and a preliminary report of its application. *Circulation* 1964; **30**: 654–70.

Gruentzig AR, Hopff M Perkutane rekanalisation chronischer arterieller verschlusse mit einem neuer dilatationskatheter: modification der Dottertechnik. *Deutsch Med Wochenschr* 1974; **99**: 2502–10.

Luscher TF, *et al.* Arterial fibromuscular dysplasia. *Mayo Clin Proc* 1987; **62**: 931–52.

Martin LG, Casarella WJ, Gaylord GM. Azotemia caused by renal artery stenosis: treatment by percutaneous angioplasty. *Am J Roentgenol* 1988; **150**: 839–44.

Ramsay LE, Waller PC. Blood pressure response to percutaneous transluminal angioplasty for renovascular hypertension: and overview of published series. *Br Med J* 1990; **300**: 569–72.

Schwarten, DE. Transluminal angioplasty of renal artery stenoses: 70 experiences. *Am J Roentgenol* 1980; **135**: 967–74.

Sniderman KW, Odurny A, Colapinto RF. Intestinal angina: percutaneous transluminal angioplasty of the celiac and superior mesenteric arteries. *Radiology* 1988; **167**: 59–62.

Laser

Decklebaum LI, Isner JM, Donaldson RF, Laiberte SM, Clarke RH, Salem DN. Use of pulsed energy delivery to minimize tissue injury resulting from carbon dioxide laser irradiation of cardiovascular tissues. *J Am Coll Cardiol* 1986; **7**: 898–908.

Litvak F, *et al.* Percutaneous excimer-laser and excimer-laser assisted balloon angioplasty of the lower extremity: Results of an initial clinical trial. *Radiology* 1989; **172**: 331–5.

McCarthy WJ, *et al.* Excimer laser-assisted femoral angioplasty: early results. *J Vasc Surg* 1991; **13**: 607–14.

Murray A, Mitchell DC, Grasty M, Wood RFM, Edwards DH, Basu R. Peripheral laser angioplasty with pulsed dye laser and ball tipped optical fibers. *Lancet* 1989: 1471–4.

Prince MR, LaMuraglia GM, Teng P, Deutsch TF, Anderson RR, Parrish JA. Selective ablation of calcified arterial plaque with laser induced plasmas. *IEEE J Quantum Electron* 1987; **QE-23**: 1783–6, 1987.

Wright JG, Belkin M, Greenfield AJ, Guben JK, Sanborn TA, Manzoian JO. Laser angioplasty for limb salvage: Observation on early results. *J Vasc Surg* 1989; **10**: 29–38.

7.14 Angioscopy in the treatment of peripheral vascular disease

DAVID T. ZELT, PAOLO ORTU, AND GLENN M. LaMURAGLIA

INTRODUCTION

Angioscopy, defined as the endoscopic visualization of the inner surfaces of blood vessels, has evolved from early attempts at endoscopic examination of intracardiac anatomy to its use in peripheral vascular surgery. Its importance became apparent in 1977 when Towne and Bernhard published their experience with a rigid arthroscope and choledochoscope during 91 vascular reconstructions. They concluded that the use of angioscopy during vascular reconstruction permitted a more precise repair. The use of these bulky rigid endoscopes did not, however, gain wide acceptance. In the 1980's 'ultrathin' and very flexible angioscopes that are easy to use were developed. These have provided unique information, different from that attained using conventional angiography.

THE EQUIPMENT

The basic components of the vascular endoscopy system are a fibreoptic imaging catheter containing illumination fibres, a high intensity light source, an irrigating system, and a video system with a camera and monitor.

Many larger imaging catheters or endoscopes (2.0–3.5 mm outer diameter) incorporate an irrigation channel into the catheter (Fig. 1). Some also have a working lumen for passage of microinstruments, a steering guidewire, or a laser fibre. A deflectable tip is available with some models for steerability.

The narrow or ultrathin angioscopes (0.8–1.7 mm outer diameter) can be used for intraoperative or percutaneous diagnosis and treatment of peripheral vascular and coronary artery disease. They are not actively steerable and are best used with a disposable coaxial catheter for irrigation.

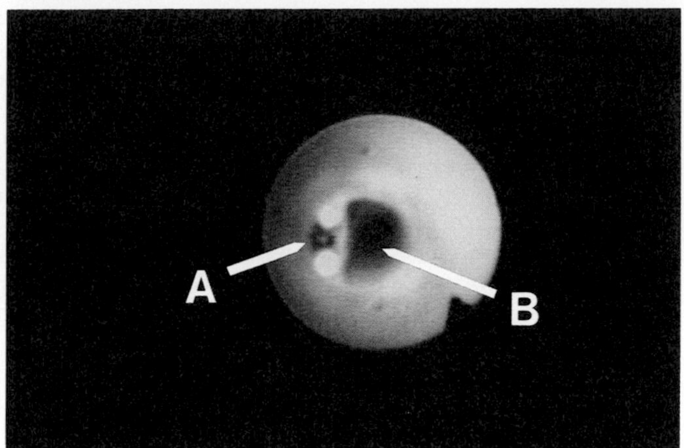

Fig. 1 Photograph of an angioscope within a vein as seen through a second angioscope. (a) Visual fibreoptic bundle and objective lens system with illumination fibres above and below. (b) Irrigation/working channel.

Pressurized heparin–saline (1 U/ml) is delivered through the irrigation channel or through another catheter to maintain a blood-free field for visual inspection. This solution can be delivered using a pressurized intravenous solution or through a commercially available foot controlled pump that regulates irrigation flow rates and can measure the volume of fluid administered. Excessive back bleeding can usually be controlled by increasing the irrigation fluid flow rate, but if this fails, control by external direct pressure, by an occluding balloon catheter, or by direct clamping of the artery may be necessary.

Although most angioscopes can be used with direct vision, indirect video imaging allows viewing by several people, video recording, and maintenance of a sterile field. Indirect video imaging employs a miniature camera mounted on to the angioscope catheter eyepiece. This provides a colour image 3 to 6 inches (8–15 cm) in diameter on a video monitor. A xenon light source of at least 300 W is generally used to provide illumination at the angioscope tip.

INDICATIONS

Diagnostic angioscopy

There are several important differences between arteriography and angioscopy. Conventional arteriography only provides a two-dimensional image of the arterial tree, which can be misleading without biplanar views. Although angiography does not provide information about the aetiology of the narrowed or obstructed segment, angioscopy can be used to differentiate between thrombotic and atheromatous elements of these lesions. Angioscopy is also an alternative to intraoperative arteriography for assessment of a graft and its anastomotic patency, but it cannot provide information about the distal run-off, as can arteriography.

Angioscopic criteria for the diagnosis of abnormal blood vessels include an oval or slit shaped cross-section, eccentric or concentric stenoses, inhomogeneous colour of the vessel wall, thrombotic deposits on the walls, ulceration, and slow restitution of blood flow after flushing of the lumen.

Findings at the time of the endoscopy may change the operative management: in one series this occurred in 14 per cent of patients examined. Revisions were necessary for misplaced sutures, redundant graft material, or atheromatous flaps not incorporated into the anastomosis causing partial obstruction of the lumen.

Angioscopy is becoming a valuable asset in the preparation of *in-situ* bypass grafts. Angioscopically directed localization and incision of the greater saphenous vein valves helps to ensure complete disruption of the valve cusps for an *in-situ* bypass (Fig. 2). The angioscope can also be used to identify venous side branches for ligation and to assess distal anastomotic patency. Venous injury by misplacement of the valvulotome into a side branch of a vein can be prevented by direct visualization. Angioscopy can also identify pathologically sclerotic vein segments and other venous abnormalities that could result in early graft failure.

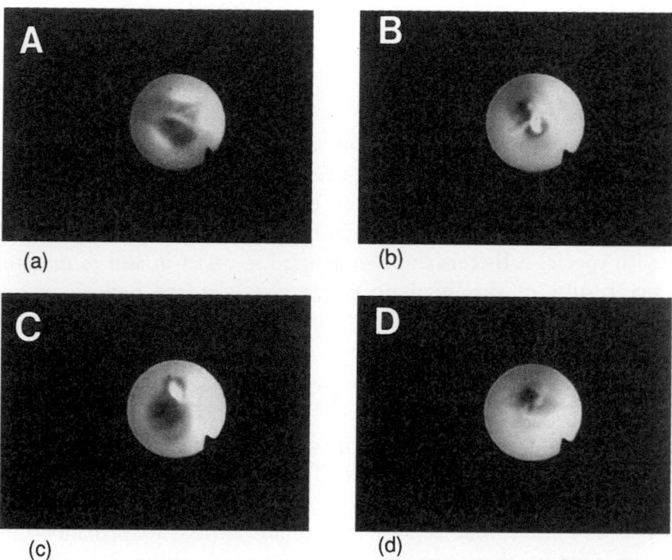

Fig. 2 Angioscopically guided valvulotomy. (a) Intact coapted vein cusps as seen from the angioscope; (b) a Mills valvulotome is guided under direct vision into one of the cusps; (c) after disruption of the first cusp, the valvulotome is positioned into the second cusp by 180° rotation of the valvulome; (d) completed valvulotomy with disrupted valve cusps.

Therapeutic angioscopy

Thromboembolectomy with the balloon catheter is generally performed as a blind procedure. As a result, the completeness of the thromboembolectomy is unknown, and intraoperative angiography is limited to the detection of a total occlusion or major thrombus. The addition of angioscopy to the procedure has several advantages over conventional thromboembolectomy including accurate detection, localization, and retrieval of the thrombus or embolus (Fig. 3). Angioscopy also facilitates the cannulation of bifurcating tributaries, such as the tibial vessels, with the balloon catheter. It is difficult to know the clinical impact of these procedures or the clinical significance of retained

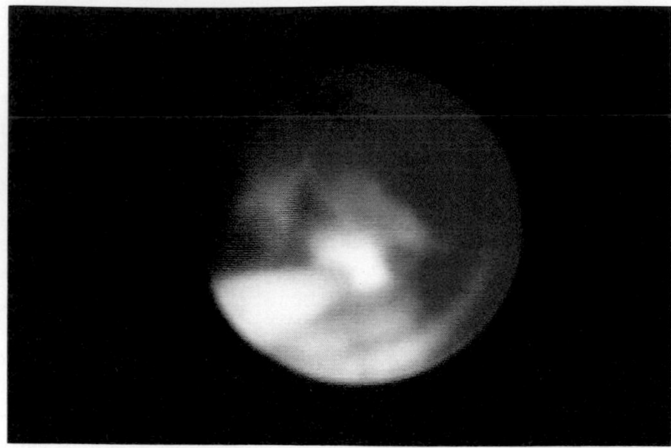

Fig. 3 Angioscopic visualization of retained thrombus in the limb of an aortofemoral bypass graft during thrombectomy. An inflated Fogarty balloon catheter is seen at the graft origin occluding arterial inflow for the procedure.

thrombus during thrombectomy since the 'blind' procedure has a relatively high success rate.

Angioscopically assisted intraluminal instrumentation has added a new dimension to the management of peripheral vascular disease. Angioscopes have been used to direct atherectomy and laser assisted angioplasty. Angioscopy performed percutaneously with special catheters can also be used to assist in and to monitor the results of thrombolytic therapy or standard balloon angioplasty.

PROBLEMS AND COMPLICATIONS

Despite the increasing popularity and use of angioscopy, few complications have been reported. The potential for injury to the vessel wall gives rise to most concern. After simulated angioscopic insertion into canine veins *in vivo*, minor intimal abnormalities are seen acutely; these are completely repaired within 2 weeks and veins which suffer subtotal loss of endothelium are replaced in 3 to 4 weeks.

Another complication secondary to any instrumentation of a blood vessel is arterial spasm. This problem may affect early patency and could increase the likelihood of vessel injury or perforation. Pretreatment with papaverine (0.5 mg/ml), especially useful in vein grafts, can be used to obviate the spasm.

Volume overload is a potential hazard which can arise if large volumes of irrigation fluid are used to keep a clear visual field. Fluid balances must be carefully monitored during angioscopy to avoid the development of pulmonary oedema, especially when a large irrigation catheter is used or when intra-arterial catheterization is needed, because larger volumes of irrigation may be required.

Magnification of intraluminal defects by the angioscopic optical system presents the vascular surgeon with the problem of interpreting their relevance. Towne and Bernhard reported a 29 per cent incidence of possibly important lesions identified by angioscopy. This incidence does not however, correlate with the early failure rate of vascular grafts. Clearly there is a definite learning curve to assess which lesions require correction or reconstruction and which may be ignored.

THE FUTURE

Angioscopy is becoming an important part of the vascular surgeons' armamentarium for both the diagnosis and treatment of peripheral vascular disease. By allowing the immediate detection and correction of technical errors and intravascular pathology its use may improve graft patency. For specific indications, angioscopy has also been shown to be an effective alternative to intraoperative angiography, but it is unlikely that angioscopy will replace angiography. As technological advancements improve angioscope systems and their use and indications widen, vascular surgeons will need to learn how best to use and interpret their findings. By carrying out routine angioscopy during arterial surgery, the vascular surgeon will be able rapidly to assess endovascular anatomy and thus potentially reduce graft failure rates and improve limb salvage.

FURTHER READING

Beck A, *et al.* Clinical application of percutaneous transluminal angioscopy. *Herz* 1988; **13**: 392–9.

Grundfest WS, *et al.* Introperative decisions based on angioscopy in peripheral vascular surgery. *Circulation* 1988; **78 (suppl I)**: 113–117.

LaMuraglia GM, *et al.* Angioscopically guided semi-closed technique for *in situ* bypass. *J Vasc Surg*, 1990; **12**: 601–4.

Miller A, *et al.* Routine intraoperative angioscopy in lower extremity revascularization. *Arch Surg* 1989; **124**: 604–8.

Towne JB, Bernhard VM. Vascular endoscopy: useful tool or interesting toy. *Surgery* 1977; **82**: 415–19.

White GH, White RA, eds. *Angioscopy: peripheral vascular and coronary applications.* Chicago: Year Book Medical Publishers, 1989.

White GH, White RA, Kopchok GE, Klein SR, Wilson, SE. Intraoperative video angioscopy compared with arteriography during peripheral vascular operations. *J Vasc Surg* 1987; **615**: 488–95.

White GH, White RA, Kopchok GE, Wilson SE. Angioscopic thrombolectomy: preliminary observations with a recent technique. *J Vasc Surg* 1988; 7: 318–25.

7.15 Thrombolytic therapy

GLENN M. LaMURAGLIA AND WILLIAM M. ABBOTT

Since heparin anticoagulation was found to have a beneficial effect in the treatment of thromboembolic disease there have been further efforts to improve the treatment of thrombotic disorders. Instead of using inhibitors of coagulation to shift the equilibrium of the clotting cascade, retarding the formation of thrombus with resulting slow absorption of clot, attempts were made to activate safely the endogenous serum fibrinolytic system. This goal can be achieved by the activation of the serum proteolytic precursor, plasminogen, to form plasmin (Fig. 1). In the presence of fibrin substrate, plasmin fragments fibrin and promotes active thrombus dissolution.

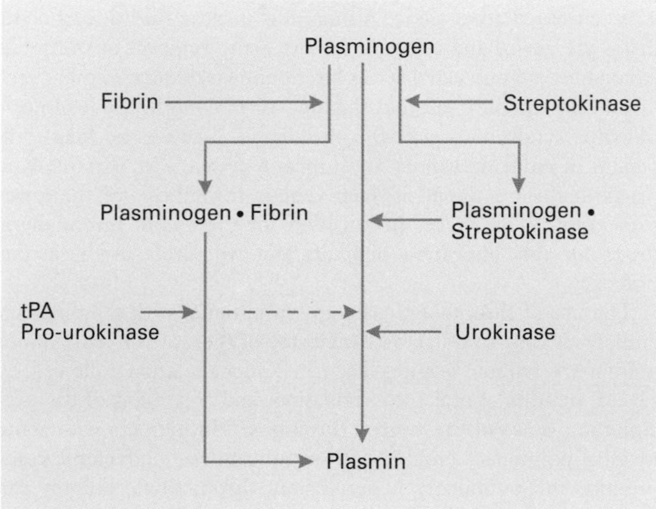

Fig. 1 The action of thrombolytic agents in the activation of plasminogen to plasmin.

THROMBOLYTIC AGENTS

Streptokinase

Streptokinase is a non-enzymatic polypeptide isolated from β-haemolytic streptococci and is the least expensive of the thrombolytic drugs. To initiate thrombolysis it must first combine with plasminogen in equal proportions to form an activated streptokinase–plasminogen complex that activates another plasminogen molecule to form plasmin. Sensitized individuals bear anti-streptococcal antibodies which inactivate streptokinase; the drug therefore has to be administered following a 100 000 to 250 000 IU loading dose. Intravenous doses of streptokinase average 100 000 IU/hour, while local intra-arterial administration usually requires 5000 to 10000 IU/hour. The half-life is short (23 min); however, the effects of plasmin activation may persist for longer.

Urokinase

Urokinase is an enzymatic two-chain polypeptide produced by endothelial and renal tubular cells. Originally isolated from urine, where it is found in a concentration of approximately 6 IU/ml, it is now obtained from tissue cultures of human kidney cells. Since urokinase is an endogenous human protein and is not antigenic, in contrast to streptokinase it does not cause allergic side-effects such as pyrexia, anaphylaxis, rash, and serum sickness. Since urokinase does not complex with antibodies or plasminogen present in the serum, its dose effects are more predictable than those of streptokinase. Intravenous administration is commonly started by a bolus of 4400 IU/kg followed by infusion of 4400 IU/kg.h. Local intra-arterial doses vary between 1000 and 6000 IU/min. Like streptokinase, the half-life of the drug is short (16 min).

Tissue plasminogen activator and pro-urokinase

To minimize the bleeding complications associated with the use of thrombolytic drugs, efforts have been undertaken to find plasminogen activators which are much more efficient in the presence of fibrin. This would mean that the activity of the thrombolytic drug could be limited to the thrombotic process, and little systemic fibrinolysis would occur. The benefits of the drug's clinical activity could thus be optimized, while haemorrhagic complications could be reduced.

Tissue plasminogen activator was the first 'clot specific' thrombolytic agent to be used clinically and is produced using recombinant genetic technology. This glycosylated protease is a poor activator of plasminogen to plasmin, except in the presence of fibrin, when this reaction is greatly enhanced, apparently due to specific molecular conformational changes noted *in vitro*. This results in the production of high concentrations of plasmin in thrombus. Despite high hopes of tissue plasminogen activator being a very specific drug for thrombus dissolution, initial clinical trials have been disappointing. In addition, plasma half-life of the drug is very short (approximately 5 min).

Pro-urokinase is an inactive precursor of urokinase which is converted to urokinase by plasmin. This activation is slow except in the presence of fibrin or its split products; it is therefore thought to have thrombus selectivity and, because of its rapid inactivation by thrombin, its use should theoretically be associated with fewer haemorrhagic complications. The half-life of pro-urokinase is 3 to 6 min, but clinical experience with it is limited.

CLINICAL USE

Indications

Thrombolytic therapy is indicated for the treatment of venous thrombosis, peripheral arterial occlusion, and myocardial infarction. The clinical aim of thrombolytic therapy is to achieve a faster and more thorough dissolution of thrombus than can be achieved by anticoagulation alone. Most clinicians agree that anticoagulation is primarily of use in preventing thrombus propagation, not in thrombolysis.

Several important factors need to be considered in patients prior to thrombolytic therapy. First, there must be unequivocal evidence that a thrombus is causing the clinically important vascular occlusion. Clot lysis is most successful when the thrombus is fresh or only a few days old. When occlusions are arterial, the ischaemia must not be severe enough to require emergency surgical intervention. There must be no contraindications to the use of the thrombolytic drug (Table 1): even with judicious use of these agents complications occur and these risks need to be weighed against the potential benefits of thrombolytic therapy.

Table 1 Contraindications to thrombolytic therapy

Absolute
Recent surgery (10 days)
Active bleeding
Stroke or intracranial disease (6 months)
Blood dyscrasia
Relative
Severe ischaemia
Recent trauma
Gastrointestinal bleeding/ulcers
Uncontrolled hypertension
Postpartum or pregnancy
Diabetic retinopathy
Atrial fibrillation
Aneurysmal disease

Cardiac indications

Thrombolytic drugs may be used to relieve acute coronary thrombosis during myocardial infarction. The clinical goal is for immediate clot lysis with reperfusion of the ischaemic cardiac muscle to limit the extent of infarction.

The optimal method by which this goal can be achieved is by the intravenous administration of thrombolytic drugs shortly after the onset of cardiac symptoms. Minimizing the delay between onset of symptoms and administration of the drug increases the likelihood of limiting the infarct: the thrombolytic drugs that hold the greatest appeal for this application are those with clot or fibrin 'selectivity'. Tissue plasminogen activator has found its widest application in patients with acute myocardial infarction: it should be given within 4 h of onset of coronary symptoms, as a loading dose (10 mg intravenously), followed by 50 mg/h for the next 2 h. Streptokinase has been shown to be as effective as tissue plasminogen activator in recent trials.

Thrombolytic drugs have also been administered very successfully via the intracoronary route at the time of acute cardiac catheterization. In the 70 to 80 per cent of patients in whom coronary flow is successfully re-established anticoagulation diminishes the risk of reocclusion while the stenotic lesion that precipitated the original thrombosis is treated.

Venous indications

Venous thrombosis or thromboembolism is a common and potentially life threatening problem. In cases of deep venous thrombosis, the objectives of therapy are inhibition of clot propagation and embolism and minimizing the venous injury precipitated by the thrombus, thus reducing the morbidity associated with venous insufficiency and the postphlebitic syndrome. The standard therapy of anticoagulants, bedrest, and elevation of the extremities effectively achieves the former objectives. It does not, however, minimize the venous inflammation, scarring, and valve injury with subsequent venous hypertension.

The effectiveness of thrombolytic drugs and anticoagulation in patients with deep venous thrombosis of the lower extremity has been compared in several studies. The pooled results indicate that thrombolytic therapy lyses 47 per cent of clots compared with 6 per cent lysis achieved with anticoagulation alone. The mode of acute treatment did not affect the incidence of pulmonary emboli. The incidence of bleeding complications was four times higher in patients treated with thrombolytic therapy than in those treated with anticoagulation alone. Although it is clear that thrombolytic drugs are useful and effective for the acute removal of thrombus from veins, no published series has demonstrated a clinical advantage of this therapy to avoid the long-term complications of postphlebitic syndrome years after the illness. There is no long-term benefit in reducing venous valve incompetence with thrombolytic drugs in the treatment of deep venous thrombosis of the lower extremities. This makes justification for the use of thrombolytic drugs for this indication difficult, and we rarely use it in our practice.

The use of thrombolytic therapy in patients with a pulmonary embolus is controversial. The mainstay of therapy for acute minor pulmonary emboli remains heparin anticoagulation followed by several months of oral anticoagulation, and treatment of the precipitating cause of the venous thrombosis. In patients with acute massive pulmonary emboli, with significant haemodynamic compromise and pulmonary hypertension, thrombolytic therapy can cause a more rapid improvement in haemodynamics and in the angiographic appearance of the emboli. There is no evidence that its use improves mortality rates, and at 7 days there were no differences in lung scans of patients treated with heparin alone and those treated with thrombolytic drugs. Again, bleeding complications are more common in patients treated with thrombolytic drugs. In our practice we use thrombolytic therapy in those few patients without contraindications who have symptomatic pulmonary emboli with dyspnoea and hypoxia, but not in patients with severe right heart failure, who should have surgical embolectomy. Most patients are therefore treated with heparin, followed by coumadin anticoagulation as clinically indicated.

Subclavian or axillary vein thrombosis is a specific type of venous thrombosis that can be successfully treated with thrombolytic therapy; its use in this setting is less controversial (Fig. 2). These thromboses can be precipitated by local intimal injury or effort thrombosis, thoracic outlet obstruction with venous compression, and by chronic indwelling venous catheters. Thrombolytic therapy has been used more frequently and with a higher degree of success in proximal upper extremity thrombosis for several reasons. Firstly, the clot is usually localized to the axillary–subclavian distribution, without distal extension down the arm veins. There is not usually a large number of venous tributaries present, in contrast to the situation when thrombus is present in

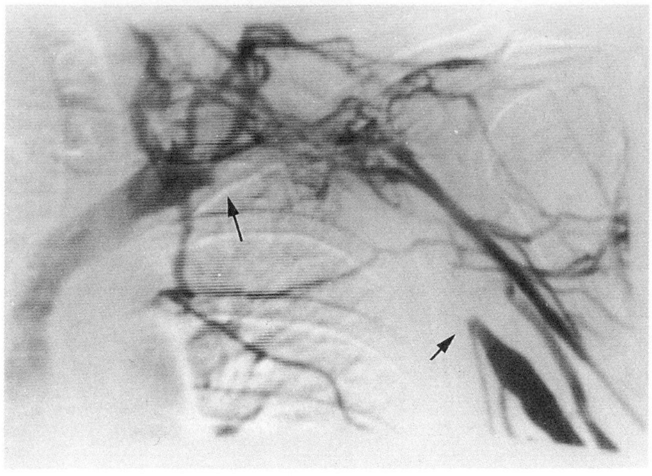

(a)

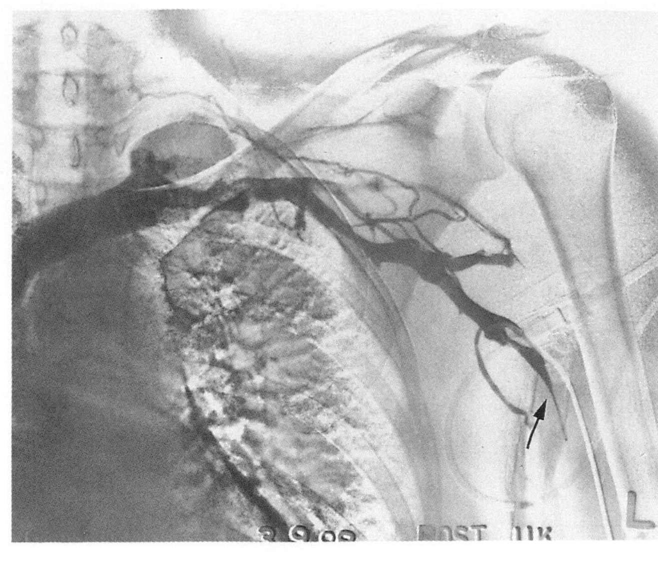

(b)

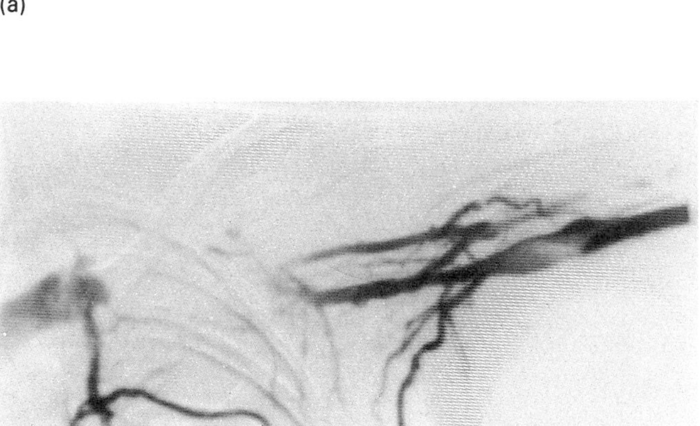

(c)

Fig. 2 Case demonstration of subclavian vein thrombolysis. (a) Thrombosed left axillary/subclavian vein (between arrows). (b) Recanalized axillary/subclavian vein through catheter injection (arrow). (c) Abduction venogram demonstrating thoracic outlet compression of vein.

the lower extremities. Another important factor is that catheters can readily be inserted into the axillary–subclavian venous thrombus, allowing the use of high dose local infusions that yield a higher lysis rate with a lower incidence of complications. Once recanalization of the vein has been established, the precipitating factor for the venous thrombosis can be ascertained and appropriately treated.

Arterial indications

The use of thrombolytic therapy in patients with an acute peripheral arterial thrombosis or embolus is controversial. It can, however, be very useful in the properly selected patient with an acute presentation, in whom ischaemic symptoms are not severe, where thrombus diffusely affects run-off, and when the risks for surgical intervention are high.

Before describing the criteria by which patients should be selected for arterial thrombolytic therapy, it is important to discuss its mode of administration. Historically, the drug was given intravenously to achieve a systemic thrombolytic state. Because the initial results were promising only for localized and acute artery occlusions, and were uniformly poor for thrombosed grafts, regimens of administration were altered to permit recovery of endogenous plasma levels of plasminogen. One of these protocols was 'burst' therapy, which called for a high dose intravenous administration of the thrombolytic drug for several hours followed by a recovery time of 12 to 24 h and a repeat of the cycle several times.

These intravenous methods have been largely replaced by intra-arterial infusion of the thrombolytic drug directly into the thrombus. Local injection of the drug into the thrombus can activate intra-clot, or local plasminogen, increasing the rapidity of lysis without totally depleting systemic concentrations of plasminogen. Lower doses of thrombolytic agents can also be used with this route of administration. Technical success can also be predicted during such local administration by the ability to pass a guidewire through the occlusion in question. After thrombolysis, sheaths are already in place for balloon angioplasty, if the lesion is suitable for such treatment (Fig. 3).

Although the technique by which thrombolytic therapy is administered is important, the aspect crucial to success is proper selection of patients. As well as recognizing an appropriate indication, it is important to determine that there are no contraindications to lytic therapy. Only patients who would otherwise be candidates for surgery because of their clinical presentations should be considered. This includes patients with an occluding thrombus precipitating a significant clinical end-organ ischaemia and a clinical presentation that would have a high likelihood of benefiting from its use (Table 2).

Recent arterial occlusions are clearly more responsive to thrombolytic therapy than well-organized, older clot. Therefore, a

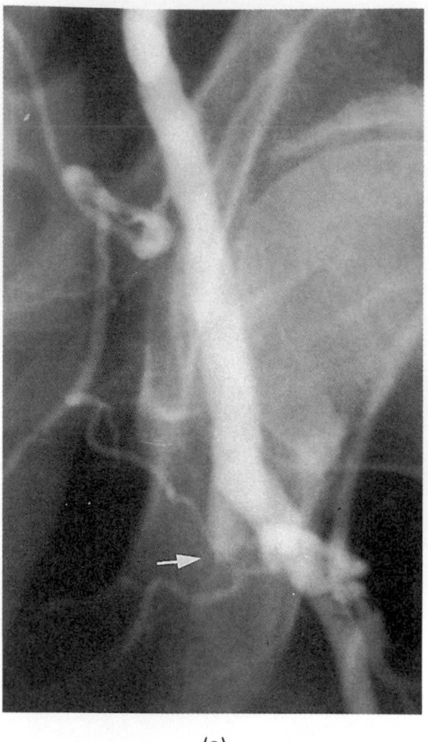

(a)

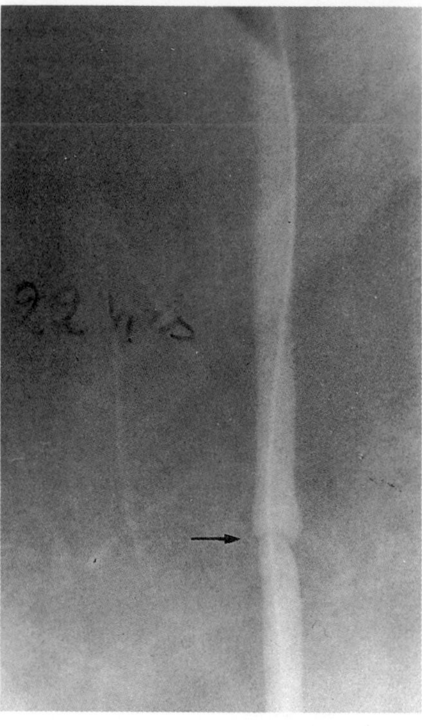

(b)

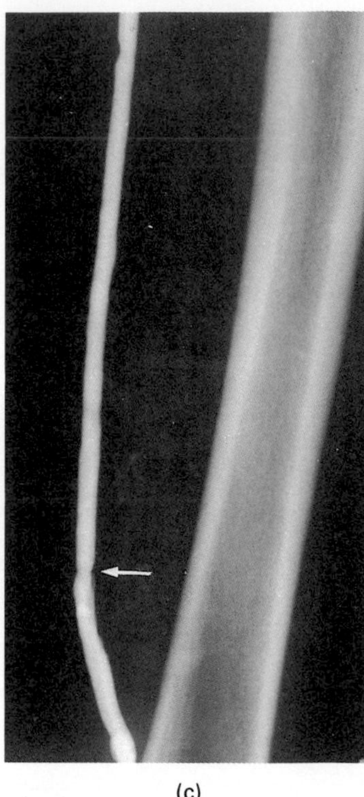

(c)

Fig. 3 Case demonstration of femoral–popliteal vein graft thrombolysis. (a) Left groin angiogram demonstrating proximal portion of the thrombosed vein graft (arrow). (b) After 22 h of thrombolytic therapy a vein graft stenosis is identified (arrow). (c) The vein graft after balloon angioplasty of the vein graft stenosis (arrow).

Table 2 Patients likely to benefit from intra-arterial thrombolytic therapy

Acute occlusions during balloon angioplasty or other interventional technique
Acute occlusion of native artery especially with loss of run-off (e.g. popliteal aneurysm)
Acute occlusion of vein bypass graft
Acute > chronic occlusion of prosthetic bypass graft
Patient with multiple vascular reoperations
Acute thrombosis in the setting of a prohibitive surgical risk

new thrombus that forms during an interventional technique or manipulation is the most likely to lyse. Acute occlusions of bypass grafts can be recanalized with thrombolytic therapy, followed by identification and treatment of the precipitating cause of the thrombosis: preoperative identification of the precipitating factor facilitates the subsequent procedure. Long-standing prosthetic bypass occlusions can be recanalized since they do not scar down as do thrombosed vein grafts but retain organized thrombus at either anastomosis with resorbed thrombus in their midportion. Thrombolytic therapy is often useful in acute arterial or graft occlusion in the presence of loss of outflow vessels (Fig. 4). Surgical thrombectomy of small or partially diseased arteries that have occluded as part of a graft or arterial thrombosis is often unsuccessful, and thrombolytic therapy can re-establish outflow before correction of the precipitating problem is attempted. In deciding whether to use thrombolytic therapy, other considerations include general surgical risk, complex anatomy, and scarring secondary to multiple operations.

Besides the usual contraindications to thrombolytic therapy there are specific contraindications for patients with arterial occlusions. Since implementation of the procedure and infusion to achieve clinical success can take up to 48 h, patients in whom end-organ viability is seriously threatened should not undergo thrombolytic therapy, but should immediately be taken to the operating room. Patients with early postoperative occlusion of a bypass graft should not be treated with thrombolytic therapy because of the high likelihood of substantial bleeding from the surgical site. An embolus in a surgically accessible vessel is not a good indication, especially when the added potential risk of further fragmenting an intracardiac thrombus and precipitating further emboli is considered. The presence of knitted Dacron grafts is considered a relative contraindication because of the reported incidence of bleeding through the graft wall if thrombolysis is performed before the graft is incorporated by the surrounding tissue (2–4 weeks).

Results of thrombolytic therapy for arterial or bypass occlusion varies with the technique, drug, and route of administration, but probably depend most of all on selection of patients. Experience from several units suggested that intravenous administration of thrombolytic therapy resulted in successful lysis in 38 per cent of 340 patients, with an incidence of major complications of 8 per cent. Intra-arterial administration of thrombolytic drugs does not change the complication rate (13 per cent), but more than doubles the success rate, to 78 per cent in 478 patients reviewed. These studies and their methods differed significantly and they include many early studies, performed when the technique was still evolving.

We exclusively use intra-arterial thrombolytic drugs for recan-

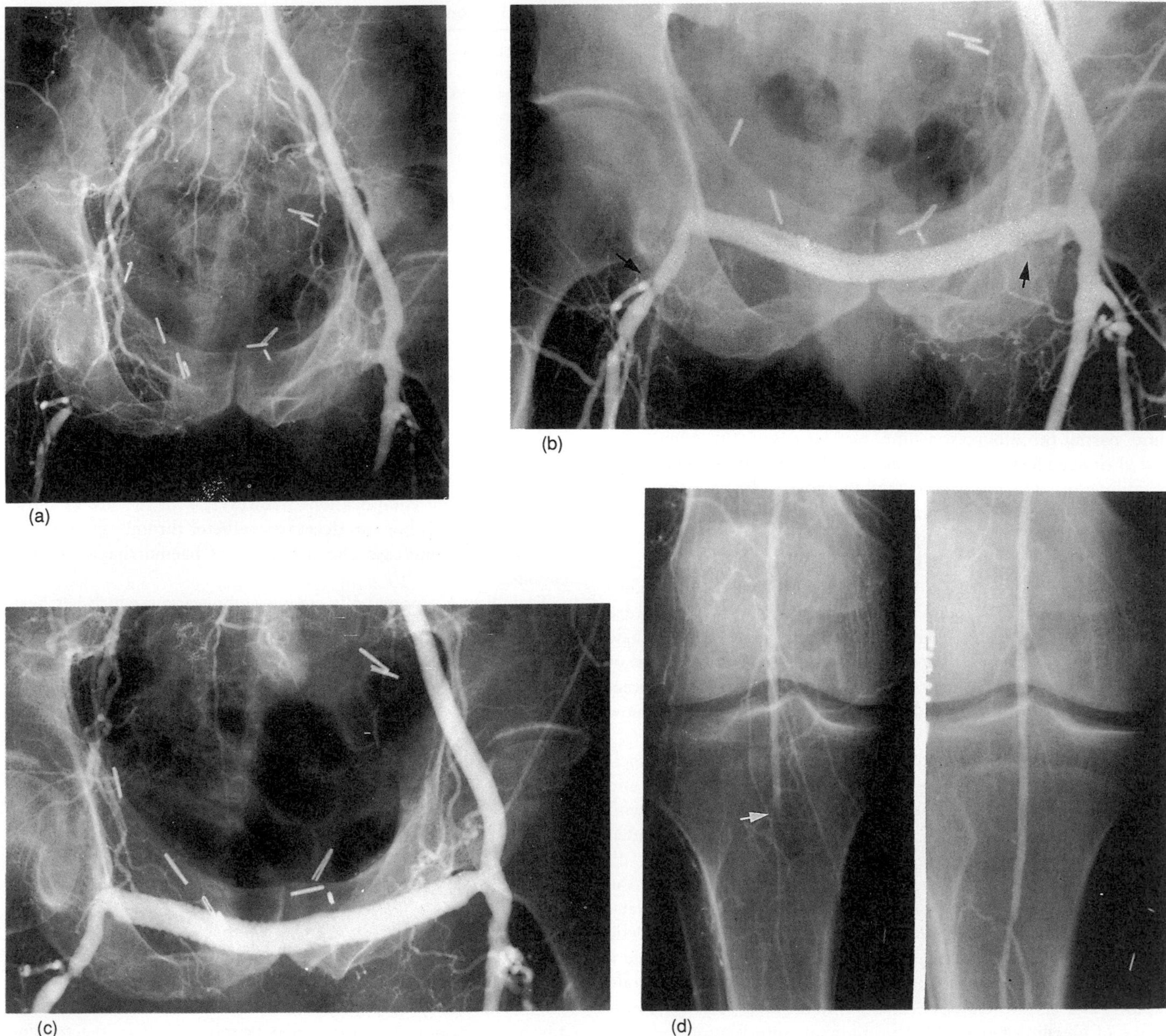

Fig. 4 Case demonstration of femoral–femoral prosthetic graft thrombolysis. (a) Thrombosed transpubic graft. (b) Partially recanalized transpubic graft with proximal thrombus (arrow) and right femoral stenosis (right arrow). (c) Totally recanalized graft after further thrombolysis. (d) Popliteal embolus (arrow) which occurred during thrombolysis, and was lysed after further drug administration.

alizing occluded peripheral arteries or bypass grafts. Attempts at recanalizing native arterial occlusions are undertaken in patients with recent onset of symptoms and minimal atherosclerotic disease in the adjacent vessels, suggesting focal disease. Attempts at intra-arterial thrombolysis are more frequently performed in patients with recent occlusions of infrainguinal bypass grafts. These distal reconstructions are more likely to benefit from thrombolysis which allows the precipitating cause of the thrombosis to be determined, distal run-off that may have been lost at the time of occlusion to be re-established, and balloon angioplasty for correction of the underlying problem to be used. Suprainguinal bypass grafts, such as thrombosed limbs of aortofemoral grafts, present a different problem. Invariably, the occlusion results from a problem with the distal anastomosis, revision of which can be performed at the time of surgical thrombectomy of the limb of the aortofemoral graft. Thrombolysis is therefore of little benefit in this setting.

Intraoperative indications

Intraoperative thrombolytic therapy has been used when residual thrombus has been identified on intraoperative arteriography or when there is evidence of distal run-off loss. The reported series are small and hard to interpret since they are anecdotal, with no control group. Success of thrombolytic therapy is also variably defined, from angiographic criteria to restoration of pedal pulses. Arterial flow in these patients was invariably restored after administration of the drug, and it is difficult to know how many of the 'thrombotic blockages' were thin thrombus films that would have opened in response to arterial pressure. Our indications for thrombolytic therapy are the angiographic presence of retained thrombus after thrombectomy or known loss of distal run-off. Reported success averages 69 per cent, with a 14 per cent incidence of bleeding complications, and an amputation rate of approximately 15 per cent. Both streptokinase and urokinase are effective, but we have used a regimen of two slow injections of 100 000 U of urokinase into the clamped distal circulation separated by 10 to 15 min.

MONITORING THROMBOLYTIC THERAPY

Before thrombolytic therapy is instituted, a standard haematological screen, including a complete blood count, prothrombin time, partial thromboplastin time, platelet count, thrombin time, and fibrinogen level should be performed to exclude an underlying coagulopathy. Once thrombolytic therapy is begun, haematological monitoring has two purposes: to ensure a lytic state, and to minimize haemorrhagic complications. To ensure a lytic state is necessary only if the procedure is unsuccessful. It is especially important if streptokinase is used, since high levels of antibodies can inactivate the drug and make the therapy ineffective. There are no good laboratory tests which can predict lysis or haemorrhagic problems. The thrombin time, which measures the clotting time of plasma after the administration of thrombin, is an indirect measure of the fibrinogen and fibrin split products: these can now be measured directly.

Some evidence suggests that low fibrinogen levels are associated with a higher incidence of haemorrhagic complications and that the patients who have serious problems are those with fibrinogen levels below 0.05 g/dl. It is therefore recommended that fibrinogen levels are checked and maintained above 0.05 g/dl, either by slowing the infusion of thrombolytic agent or by the administration of cryoprecipitate. Despite these published data, we have not used clinical laboratory testing during thrombolytic therapy other than a routine haematological screen to exclude a coagulopathy. The results of these tests are difficult to obtain rapidly, and careful clinical evaluation in an ICU setting for evidence of bleeding has resulted in minimal complications.

Complications of thrombolytic therapy

Some complications of thrombolytic therapy are common to all of the drugs, while others are specific to an individual drug (Table 3). Immunological reactions such as pyrexia, anaphylaxis, serum sickness, or a rash are limited to streptokinase because of its antigenic source: such complications are treated by stopping the infusion, with supportive care to treat the symptoms.

The most common complication is haemorrhage. Because bleeding is unpredictable, its potential occurrence is the major criterion for exclusion of patients from thrombolytic therapy. Bleeding can occur at the site of drug administration, from other puncture sites, or from areas of recent surgery as well as spontaneously in other anatomical areas. Treatment consists of stopping the infusion of the thrombolytic drug, treating the haemorrhagic area as warranted, and, if necessary, transfusing blood products to replenish coagulation factors. If bleeding is serious, cryoprecipitate, the only source of fibrinogen, must be replenished along with fresh frozen plasma. Administration of ε-aminocaprionic acid is not usually needed since the half-life of the thrombolytic agents is very short.

Table 3 Complications of thrombolytic therapy

Haemorrhage
Embolism
Pseudoaneurysm
Transgraft extravasation
Stroke
Compartment syndrome
Phlebitis
Myocardial infarction
Hepatic/splenic rupture
Loss of nails
Anaphylaxis, pyrexia, rash, or serum sickness (streptokinase only)

The administration of heparin during thrombolytic therapy to inhibit the formation of thrombus around catheters, or keep the thrombus from propagating has been said to increase the incidence of haemorrhagic complications. However, with the use of intra-arterial catheters, heparin decreases catheter thrombosis and does not appear to increase the incidence of haemorrhagic complications.

Embolism is a potentially serious complication, which has been inconsistently reported, but may have an incidence as high as 50 per cent. It can occur as a result of thrombus formation around the catheters used in intra-arterial infusion, the partial dissolution of thrombus and distal embolization in the same vessel, or as a washover from the thrombus into a more proximal vessel secondary to the breakup of clot and infusion into an occluded artery. These emboli may be clinically silent; however, they can temporarily produce worsening of ischaemia during the procedure. If emboli are identified, they are treated with continued thrombolytic therapy to the embolus, but if there is no clinical improvement surgical intervention may be required.

FUTURE TRENDS OF THROMBOLYTIC THERAPY

As thrombolytic therapy has been used for over two decades, advances continue. New drugs may be more selective in activating clot specific plasminogen without causing a systemic activation of the thrombolytic system. New and better delivery methods are being developed: coaxial systems that inject the drug at high speeds through many small side holes improve delivery of the drug and diminish the time of administration. New mechanical devices are being developed that work along with the thrombolytic drugs to break up the clot and remove it by suction. There are also pulsed laser systems that can selectively ablate thrombus, thereby enhancing the efficiency of the thrombolytic drug. Continued research will make thrombolytic therapy more widespread and safer in its applications for the treatment of thrombotic disorders.

FURTHER READING

Arneson H, Hoiseth A, Ly B. Streptokinase or heparin in the treatment of deep vein thrombosis: follow-up results of a prospective study. *Acta Med Scand* 1982; **211**: 65.

Belkin M, Belkin B, Bucknam CA, Straub JJ, Lowe R. Intra-arterial fibrolytic therapy: Efficacy of streptokinase vs urokinase. *Arch Surg* 1986; **121**: 769–73.

Bookstein JJ, Fellmeth B, Roberts A, Valji K, Davis G, Machado T. Pulsed-spray pharmacomechanical thrombolysis: preliminary clinical results. *Am J Roentgenol* 1989; **152**: 1097–100.

Durham JD, *et al.* Regional infusion of urokinase into occluded lower-extremity bypass grafts: long-term clinical results. *Radiology* 1989; **172**: 83–7.

Goldhaber SZ, *et al.* Randomised controlled trial of recombinant tissue plasminogen activator versus urokinase in the treatment of acute pulmonary embolism. *Lancet* 1988; **ii**: 293–8.

Gurewich V, Pannell R. A comparative study of the efficacy and specificity of tissue plasminogen activator and pro-urokinase: demonstration of synergism and of different thresholds of non-selectivity. *Thrombosis Res* 1986; **44**: 217–28.

LaMuraglia GM, Ortu P, Fillmore D, Obremski S, Athanasoulis C, Abbott WM. Selective laser photoablation enhances thrombolytic graft recanalization. *Surg Forum* 1990; **41**: 363–4.

Maizel AS, Bookstein JJ. Streptokinase, urokinase, and tissue plasminogen activator: pharmacokinetics, relative advantages, and methods for maximizing rates of consistency of lysis. *Cardiovasc Intervent Radiol* 1986; **9**: 236–44.

McNamara TO, Fischer JR. Thrombolysis of peripheral arterial and graft occlusions: improved results using high-dose urokinase. *Am J Roentgenol* 1985; **144**: 769–75.

Meissner AJ, *et al.* Hazards of thrombolytic therapy in deep vein thrombosis. *Br J Surg* 1987; **74**: 991–3.

Perrsson AV, *et al.* Burst therapy: a method of administering fibrinolytic agents. *Am J Surg* 1984; **147**: 531– .

Parent FN, Bernhard VM, Pabst TS, McIntyre KE, Hunter GC, Malone JM. Fibrinolytic treatment of residual thrombus after catheter embolectomy for severe lower limb ischemia. *J Vasc Surg* 1989; **9**: 153–60.

Rauwerda JA, Bakker FC, van den Broek TAA, Dwars BJ. Spontaneous subclavian vein thrombosis: a successful combined approach of local thrombolytic therapy followed by first-rib resection. *Surgery* 1988; **103**: 477–80.

Sharma GVRK, *et al.* Thrombolytic therapy. *N Engl J Med* 1982; **306**: 1268–76.

van Breda A, *et al.* Local thrombolysis in the treatment of arterial graft occlusions. *J Vasc Surg* 1984; **1**: 103–12.

Van De Werf F, *et al.* Coronary thrombolysis with tissue type plasminogen activator in patients with evolving infarction. *N Engl J Med* 1984; **310**: 609–13.

7.16 Vascular access and other techniques for dialysis and chemotherapy

DEREK W. R. GRAY

THE DEVELOPMENT OF VASCULAR ACCESS

Necessity is the mother of invention, and in the field of surgery vascular access is surely the best example of this truism, for a whole specialty has grown to meet the requirements of new fields such as dialysis and chemotherapy. The earliest vascular access was achieved by the introduction of intravenous glass cannulae in the early 1900s; these were replaced in the 1950s by plastic cannulae which allowed prolonged intravenous infusions. Attempts to extend the duration of infusion and to use more concentrated (and therefore irritant) solutions for intravenous feeding in the 1950s led to the development of central venous cannulation, made possible by the development of longer catheters and less thrombogenic plastics. This technology advanced in the 1970s with the introduction of Teflon and Silastic coated catheters, new tunnelling techniques, and the use of porous cuffs to anchor the catheters beneath the skin and perhaps provide a bacteria-proof seal. The central veins can now be used for long-term, high flow access sufficient for intravenous feeding, chemotherapy, and even haemodialysis, although their frequent use for haemodialysis is relatively recent.

The advent of haemodialysis, pioneered by Kolff in 1944, introduced a new requirement for repeated high volume blood flow both into and out of the circulation. Initially this was obtained by adapting the technique of intravenous cannulation to allow repeated catheterization of the femoral artery and vein, made safer by the introduction of the Seldinger guide wire technique. However, this approach rarely allowed dialysis for more than a few weeks. Permanent cannulation of arteries and veins always resulted in thrombosis, until the introduction of the Quinton–Scribner shunt using silastic tubing in association with Teflon coated vessel tips. The Quinton–Scribner shunt was the mainstay of haemodialysis for many years, but required relatively frequent revision and was prone to thrombosis and sepsis. A major advance was the realization that the formation of an artificial arteriovenous fistula resulted in massive enlargement of veins sufficient to allow repeated cannulation, and the Brescia–Cimino forearm fistula, first described in 1966, remains the mainstay of haemodialysis access today.

ANATOMICAL AND PHYSIOLOGICAL ASPECTS

Vascular access is only ever required to allow some form of medical treatment, and the surgery should be performed in such a way as to make the medical treatment as simple as possible. The first requirement of good access is prolonged patency or absence of thrombosis. The factors important in preventing thrombosis are the use of high flow vessels, non-thrombogenic materials and reduced blood clotting factors. The second requirement is minimal morbidity including a low rate of infection, and lack of disability caused by subsequent loss of the vessel.

For many patients these requirements are best met by using cannulae placed in large veins. Catheters inserted into the subclavian and internal jugular veins, with the catheter tip in the superior vena cava or right atrium, have high flow rates, and thrombosis of the vessel usually causes relatively little disability. Furthermore the good blood supply of the skin of the neck helps minimize infection. The leg veins and inferior vena cava have a slower flow and so thrombose more easily. Thrombosis often causes leg swelling or embolization and cannulae are at greater risk of infection.

In other patients a form of arteriovenous fistula is the best solution. Here the connection of the radial artery to the cephalic vein in the forearm is the preferred technique, giving high blood flow, low infection rate, and low thrombosis rate, with little morbidity if the vessels are lost. One arm is disabled during cannulation of the fistula, but this drawback is slight compared to the higher thrombosis and infection rate seen when leg vessels are used. Similar arguments apply to the use of cannulae (shunts) to connect arteries to veins.

PLANNED USE OF ACCESS SITES

It is now possible to keep patients in end-stage renal failure alive and well for many years, reliant on vascular access for regular therapy. The strengths and limitations of various forms of access in different patient groups have been learnt over the years, allowing the adoption of a flow diagram, which varies somewhat depending on the procedure planned and from unit to unit. A typical flow diagram for dialysis access is shown in Fig. 1. Forward planning is the key to good access surgery, allowing procedures to be performed on routine lists with sufficient time for fistulae to mature before use is required. The object of access surgery should be to avoid using all of the 'easy' access sites during the lifetime of the patient. Provision of a lifetime of access has been a particular problem for the young dialysis patient, but the recent success of renal transplant programs has meant that many patients can be relieved of the need to dialyse for large portions of their lives, and judicious planning of access is possible so as to maximize this benefit. Thus a patient who is likely to gain a rapid transplant should be given an early transplant rather than a fistula which is likely to thrombose if the transplant is successful. One of the most difficult messages to get across is the importance of preserving the cephalic veins, particularly because so often patients arrive via other services.

ACCESS FOR HAEMODIALYSIS

Anaesthesia

Patients with renal failure, both acute and chronic, are often a daunting prospect for a general anaesthetic when they first present. Fortunately local anaesthesia is adequate for most access procedures, although general anaesthesia is recommended for open internal jugular vein exposure in nervous patients. Administration of 1 per cent xylocaine with adrenaline is recommended to minimize oozing.

Preoperative preparation

It is important that patients are neither fluid overloaded nor dehydrated. There is a tendency to dehydrate recently dialysed patients, and it is best to have a drip running, dextran being a good choice because of its added anticoagulant properties. If a limb is to be used it should be shaved preoperatively, painted with betadine solution, and wrapped in cotton wool to keep it warm. A light premedication is often helpful to calm the nervous patient.

Postoperative management

The danger time for all forms of vascular access is during anaesthesia for another procedure, when dehydration, hypotension and inadvertent local pressure may result in thrombosis. Great care should be taken to avoid these risk factors. Patients with long-term indwelling cannulae must be scrupulous about covering the exit site and cannula ends with a sterile dressing, careful sterilization of the cannula prior to connection, and regular flushing of the cannula if not in use.

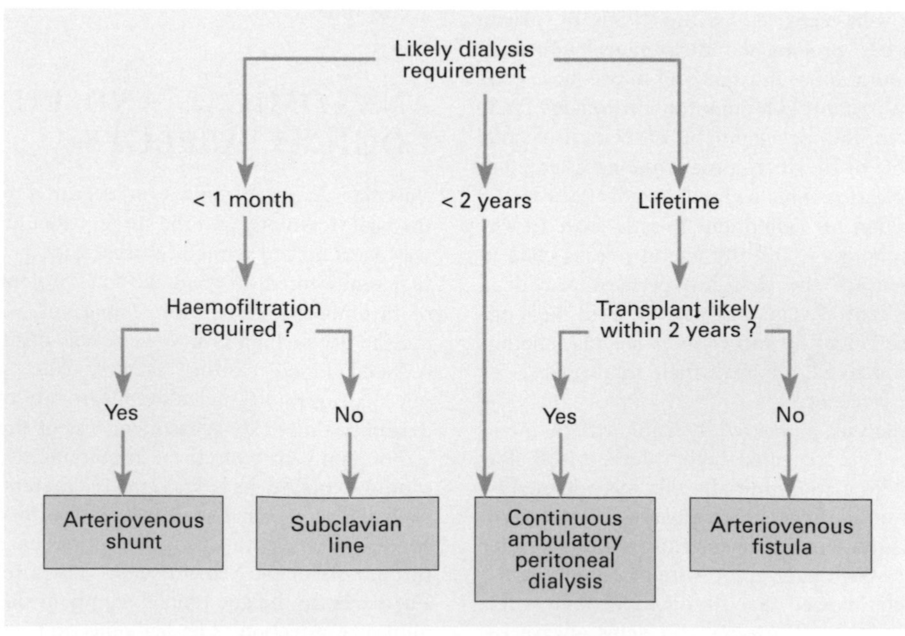

Fig. 1 Flow diagram to illustrate the options available for dialysis access for renal failure.

Techniques for acute access

Subclavian and jugular vein catheterization

The subclavian veins or internal jugular veins can be used to provide access for central venous monitoring, intravenous feeding or chemotherapy, when a single lumen catheter is usually adequate, or for haemodialysis, when a double lumen catheter is required (Fig. 2). In either case the catheter can usually be placed under local anaesthesia, with or without a short subcutaneous tunnel. The subclavian veins have the advantage of convenience, since neck lines tend to be obtrusive, but jugular line insertion is safer and also avoids the risk of later subclavian vein stenosis, which may create problems for forearm fistula formation. A number of commercial catheters are available. Most now use a smaller bore needle and syringe to locate the vein initially, followed by introduction of a flexible guide wire into the vein, withdrawal of the needle, and then advancement of the final catheter over the guide wire (Seldinger technique). There are several variations of techniques for the catheter insertion: those most commonly used are illustrated in Fig. 3 and described in Table 1.

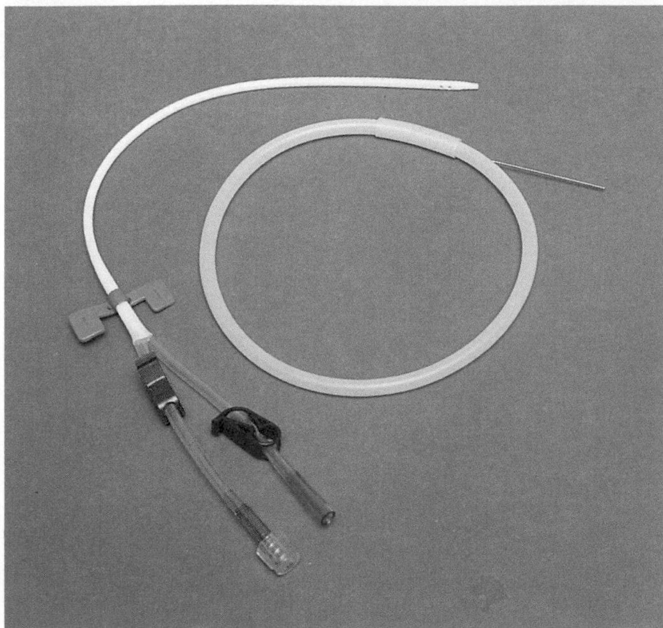

Fig. 2 Double lumen catheter with insertion guide wire. Note the clamps for temporary control of each lumen and caps for sealing between dialyses.

Removal of a catheter can usually be achieved by simple withdrawal, with local pressure to the puncture wound for 5 min.

Femoral vein catheterization

The femoral vein is now normally used only to provide access for single haemodialysis in the emergency situation and for venovenous haemofiltration. In this circumstance the femoral approach has the advantage over subclavian vein catheterization since the patient does not need to be placed head down (which can be difficult in fluid overloaded patients) and is more easily performed at the bedside, with less risk of complications, provided prolonged repeated dialysis is not attempted. The actual technique of cannulation is very similar to that employed for the subclavian vein, namely a Seldinger technique using a guide wire and double lumen catheter (Table 2). If arterial pressure is required

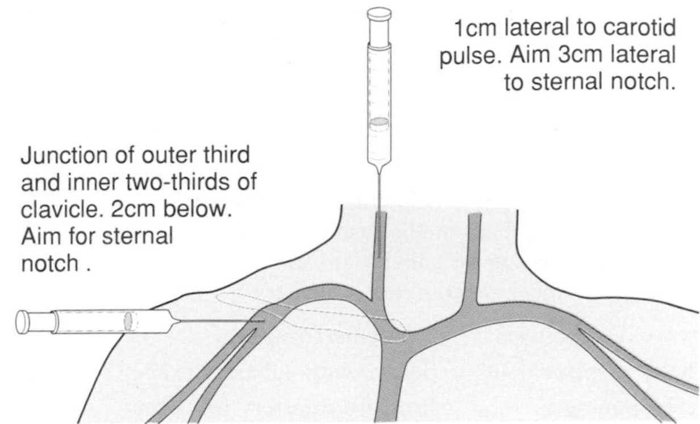

1cm lateral to carotid pulse. Aim 3cm lateral to sternal notch.
Junction of outer third and inner two-thirds of clavicle. 2cm below. Aim for sternal notch .

Fig. 3 Landmarks for subclavian and internal jugular line insertion.

Table 1 Internal jugular and subclavian vein catheterization

Positioning	
Head down	
Bolster between shoulders	
Points of technique	
Careful sterile field (operating theatre)	
Ensure good back flash of blood before inserting guide wire	
Ensure blood is venous (dark, non-pulsatile)	
Guide wire and catheter should slide in easily—never force (may cause a tear in a vital structure)	
Ensure catheter is filled with fluid and capped off	
Test flows with syringe	
Leave catheter capped with heparinized saline	
Check position by radiography	
Secure firmly (suture or adhesive drape)	
Common complications	*Prevention/treatment*
Arterial puncture	Check for and avoid prominent pulsation Withdraw needle Local pressure (3 min) Try different site
Air embolus	Head down. Catheter capped
Haemo/pneumothorax	Avoid excessive depth of penetration with needle Chest radiograph Chest drain if necessary
Sepsis	Sterile technique Antibiotic prophlaxis Use only for one purpose Catheter change with antibiotics
Thrombosis	Flush with heparinized saline regularly
Catheter embolus	Never withdraw catheter or guidewire through needle
Vessel erosion	Soft, round-ended catheter Change regularly
Arteriovenous fistulae	Avoid excessive penetration Fistulae require surgical exploration
Superior vena cava thrombosis	Avoid sepsis, prolonged cannulation

Table 2 Technique of femoral catheterization

Positioning	
Patient lying as flat as possible	
Legs at 30° with slight external rotation	
Points of technique	
Locate femoral pulse just below inguinal ligament	
Puncture vertically 1 cm medial using needle and syringe	
Insertion otherwise as for subclavian vein	
Radiograph to check position not necessary	
Common complications	*Prevention/treatment*
Catheter displacement	Secure with adhesive drape
Arterial puncture	Pressure to artery for 3 min
Retroperitoneal bleeding	Avoid puncture above inguinal ligament
Groin sepsis/thrombosis	Limit catheterization to under 7 days

for haemofiltration then the femoral artery can be cannulated using a similar technique.

The catheter can usually be removed by simple withdrawal followed by local pressure to the puncture site for 5 min. Prolonged bleeding may sometimes necessitate longer pressure. Occasionally a large haematoma or false aneurysm formation may require exploration.

Quinton–Scribner shunt

The Quinton–Scribner shunt was once the anchor of dialysis access, and can be used for both acute and long-term access, with the vessels of one limb lasting many years in some cases. Unfortunately, minor revisions are frequently required and in addition the device is inconvenient to dress and keep covered. However, the technique still has advantages for the patient with acute renal failure since it allows reliable access with less risk than subclavian puncture, particularly in patients with a bleeding tendency (as is often the case). In addition the arterial pressure can be used to 'drive' diafiltration systems. Either the radial artery/cephalic vein (Fig. 4) or posterior tibial artery/saphenous vein can be used, but

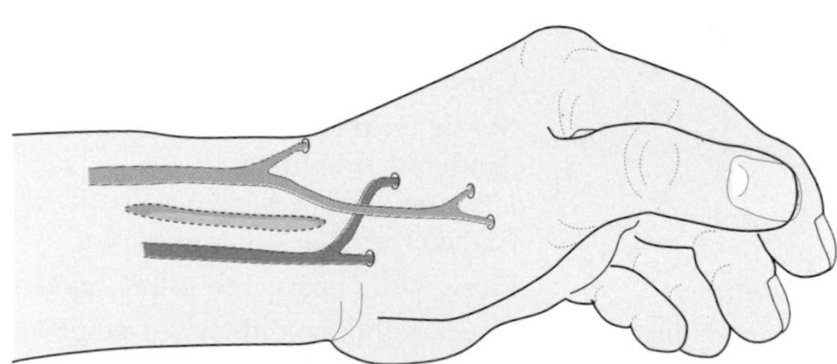

Fig. 4 Incision for exposure of cephalic vein and radial artery for either shunt insertion or fistula formation.

the forearm cannula is usually more practical once the patient is more mobile. This can also be converted to a fistula if needed later. Separate arterial and venous cannulae are placed which are joined together by a teflon connector when not dialysing (Figs. 5, 6 (a,b,c)). Local anaesthesia is usually adequate, and a so-called 'straight' silastic cannula is preferred (Fig. 5) since it allows simple thrombectomy using a short Fogarty-type embolectomy catheter. The largest possible Teflon vessel tip should be used to

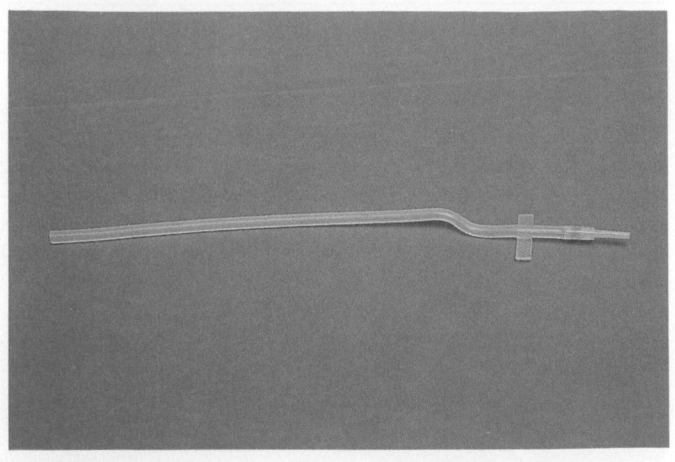

Fig. 5 A so-called 'straight' shunt cannula, which actually has a kink to allow easy passage through the skin. The side wings are intended to prevent rotation, but may erode through the skin if not placed deeply, and are removed by many surgeons prior to insertion. A teflon vessel tip is also shown.

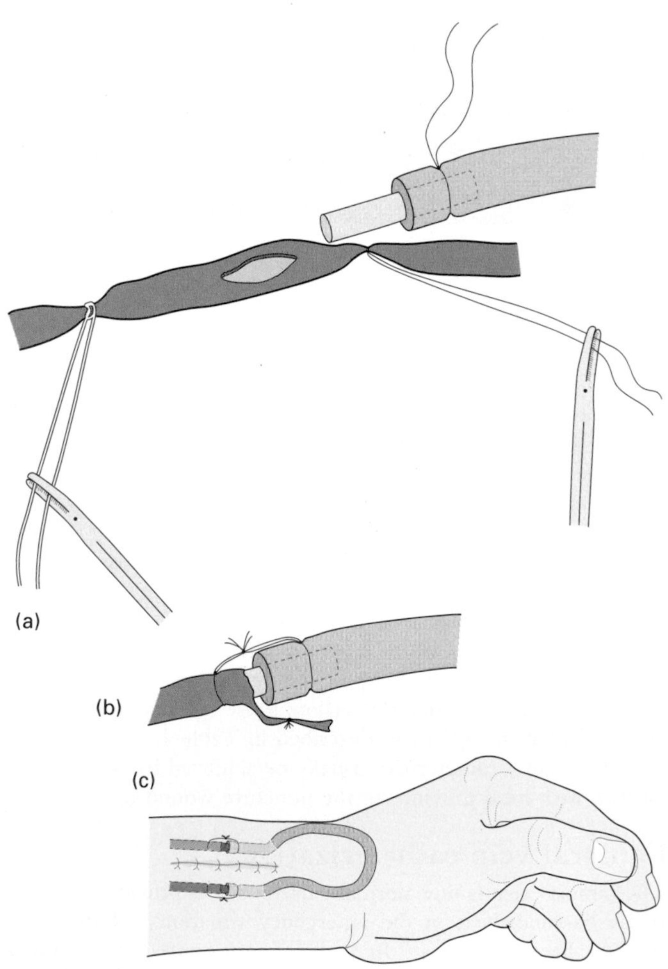

Fig. 6 (a) Insertion of cannula with vessel tip into vessel. (b) Cannula secured in vessel with silk ligatures. (c) Completed shunt with cannulae connected.

Table 3 Quinton–Scribner shunt insertion

Points of technique

1. Ensure other limb artery intact (dorsalis pedis or ulnar artery present by palpation or Doppler, Allen test)
2. Look for signs of subclavian vein stenosis/thrombosis (especially if previous subclavian catheter)
3. A single incision between the two vessels is best: avoid parallel incisions
4. Dissect cutaneous nerves away from the vein
5. Ensure vein is patent and accepts a good flow of heparinized saline
6. Dissect artery, ligating even the smallest branches
7. Cannulate and tunnel catheters ensuring no kinks or twists
8. Division of the distal vessel facilitates later removal

Common complications	*Prevention/treatment*
Thrombosis	Choose good vessels Ensure good hydration and blood pressure
Repeated thrombosis	Exclude technical error: Shunt angiogram Anticoagulation
Sepsis (usually caused by *Staphylococcus aureus*)	Prevent with prophylactic antibiotics and scrupulous asepsis Antibiotic treatment sometimes clears sepsis

cannulate the vessel (Table 3, Fig. 6 (a,b)). Another variety of cannula that has gained some popularity is the Buselmeier shunt, which has the advantage of keeping the shunt loop intact during dialysis, taking the flow to the machine off a side access port. In the event of clotting occurring in the dialyser the shunt will then keep working. The basic principles of insertion are similar.

Removal of cannulae may be required because of repeated thrombosis, sepsis that cannot be cleared, or when the shunt is no longer required. Provided clotting is normal and in the absence of sepsis the shunt can simply be clamped off for a period of at least 4 and preferably 7 days. Local anaesthetic is then infiltrated around the catheter tips and the cannulae removed by avulsion. In the presence of clotting disorders or sepsis it is wiser to remove the cannulae under direct vision and ligate the vessels with an absorbable ligature such as polyglycolic acid.

Techniques for long-term access

Arteriovenous fistulae

The connection of an artery to a vein results in steady widening of the vein and its tributaries, with increased rates of flow. Veins which were originally difficult to cannulate and unable to deliver the rate of flow sufficient for dialysis become ideally suited for repeated cannulation (Fig. 7). Once developed fully the fistula can remain patent indefinitely and provide permanent access. The ideal site, originally described by Brescia *et al.* is the radiocephalic fistula, but other sites are possible. Most fistulas can be formed under local anaesthesia, but maintenance of adequate hydration and a warm limb are particularly important for successful fistula formation. A recent innovation has been the use of a glyceryl trinitrate patch on the distal limb to encourage vasodilatation. For patients with a particular fear of needles, especially children, the use of EMLA (eutectic mixture of local anaesthetic) cream can allow painless cannulation.

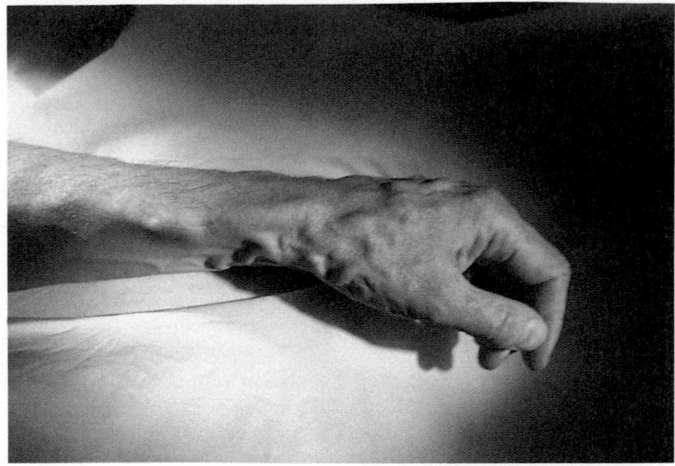

Fig. 7 Dilated veins after radiocephalic fistula formation.

For the creation of a radiocephalic fistula the incision and dissection should follow guidelines 1–5 (Table 3) outlined for shunt formation, although a slightly longer incision is needed (Fig. 4) and enough vessel should be dissected free to bring the two vessels side by side over approximately 2 cm without tension (Fig. 8 (a,b); Table 4). The cephalic vein is usually the best to use but occasionally other nearby tributaries will have suffered less trauma from previous infusions. Soft Silastic slings are used to control and approximate the vessels. The vessels are opened for a distance of 7 to 10 mm side by side, and the vein patency and size tested by injecting heparinized saline. The vessels are then anastomosed using continuous 6/0 or 7/0 Prolene suture, taking particular care not to narrow the lumen at the proximal end. A more precise anastomosis can be achieved using magnification loupes, but adequate anastomosis is possible without. Some surgeons prefer to tie

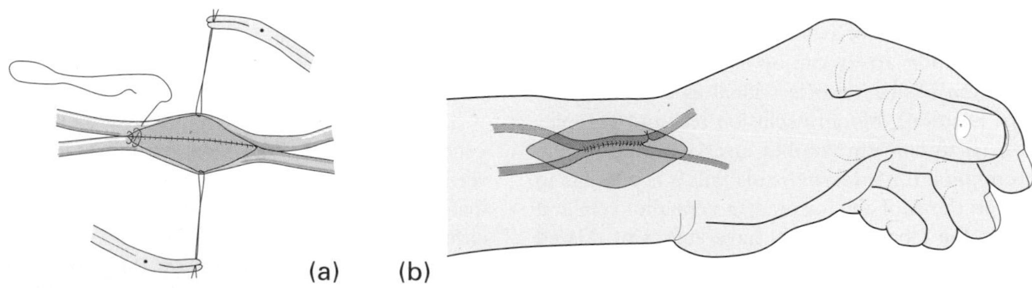

Fig. 8 (a) Anastomosis of artery to vein. (b) Completed radiocephalic fistula.

Table 4 Brescia–Cimino fistula formation

Common complications	Cause/prevention/treatment
Early thrombosis	Avoid unsuitable veins (too small or previously damaged by intravenous infusions) Check for technical error Correct dehydration Early thrombectomy
Haematoma	Carefully ligate all vessel tributaries
Failure to develop fully	Vein too small (<2 mm) or previously damaged by intravenous infusions
Early or late arm swelling	Subclavian vein stenosis/thrombosis Patients with previous subclavian catheterization should have a preoperative venogram
Distal venous hypertension (fistula thumb)	Tie off distal end of saphenous vein
Aneurysm formation (Fig. 9)	Avoid repeated needling in one place. May require reduction surgery
Late thrombosis	Poor needling technique causing perifistula haematoma. Evacuation or revision required
High venous pressures	Venous stenosis: angiogram Revision required
Heart failure	Only with high output fistula (20–50% of cardiac output): unusual with radial fistula. Reduce or reverse fistula
Distal ischaemia (steal)	Ligate distal artery or reverse fistula

off the distal vein or perform an end-to-side anastomosis in order to prevent the possibility of distal venous hypertension, but this is an uncommon complication that is relatively simple to deal with and leaving the distal vein initially may allow better run-off in the critical postoperative period. On releasing the slings a palpable thrill should be evident. The expected patency rate is variously reported at between 60 and 90 per cent at 1 year and 60 to 75 per cent at 5 years.

The general rule in fistula formation is that the non-dominant arm and the most distal site possible are used. It is possible to locate the radial artery distally in the anatomical snuffbox and at this point the artery lies close to the cephalic vein. However, the access for the anastomosis is more limited, making the procedure technically demanding, and should the cephalic vein prove to be unsuitable alternative veins are not available. If the radial artery is occluded or absent the ulnar artery can be used, together with a cephalic tributary or the basilic vein (less ideal as it tends to lie deep in an awkward position), but an occlusion test and Doppler studies should be used to confirm another arterial supply to the hand in case of thrombosis. If a forearm fistula fails it is possible to make a fistula between the cephalic (or median cephalic) vein and the brachial artery at the elbow, and still have sufficient dilated veins develop in the upper arm to allow satisfactory dialysis. In addition to the complications mentioned for radiocephalic fistula, the major complications of using this site are distal ischaemia due

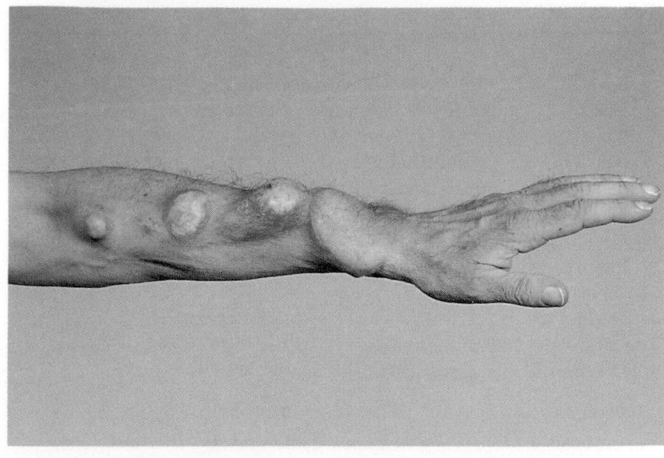

Fig. 9 Aneurysm formation in a radiocephalic fistula.

to stealing of blood and the development of cardiac failure due to massive fistula development. Both these complications can be minimized by limiting the diameter of the anastomosis to 6 mm.

In general a functioning fistula should not be closeed, even if a kidney transplant makes the fistula unnecessary, since it can never be certain that later dialysis will not be required. In fact many fistulae thrombose after successful transplantation. Indications for fistula closure include cosmetic appearance, extremely large flows leading to heart failure (see above) and, occasionally, sepsis and distal embolism. It is usually possible to dissect the fistula free, control the feeding vessels and take down the anastomosis. Often the artery can be reconstituted using fine Prolene suture, but the veins are best ligated.

Long-term central venous catheterization

Although a forearm fistula is the procedure of choice for long-term dialysis access it does have disadvantages (Table 4). The fistula cannot be used for dialysis for at least 4 weeks and often longer, since time is required for dilatation of the veins to occur. However, in some cases full development of the veins does not result, and thus a fistula may be a less attractive option in patients who present in renal failure and who require early dialysis. The waiting period can be covered by temporary dialysis via a subclavian line (see above), but the insecurity of this access makes most clinicians prefer inpatient treatment, and subclavian thrombosis and sepsis becomes more frequent with prolonged subclavian cannulation using temporary lines. In elderly patients with a limited life expectancy this waiting period may be a significant proportion of their remaining life. Some patients also have a horror of needles or have a phobia of needling themselves. Lastly, connection of an indwelling catheter is certainly less technically demanding than the insertion of two dialysis catheters into a fistula, and this may be an important factor in considering home dialysis in some patients.

The development of more efficient membranes has meant that venovenous dialysis can now be a long-term option, even though recirculation of 7 to 15 per cent of the blood may occur, and hence dialysis via a long-term central venous catheter represents another chronic access option (Table 5).

Although it is possible to use the subclavian vein, stenosis or occlusion is a common eventual outcome. The jugular veins are a better option, since loss of the external jugular veins or one inter-

Table 5 Complications of long-term central venous dialysis catheterization

Common complications	Cause/prevention/treatment
Catheter thrombosis	Frequent flushing
	Fill catheter with neat sodium heparin 5000 U/ml
	Slow low dose infusion of urokinase 10 000 units/h may clear partial blockages
	Use flexible guidewire to clear obstinate occlusions
Persistent occlusion	Change catheter over two guidewires (one each channel)
Intermediate occlusion of outflow	Reposition catheter tip in right atrium, short side away from atrial wall
Infection	Prophylactic antibiotics on insertion
	Use line only for dialysis
	Obsessional sterile connection technique
	Change catheter over guidewire using new tunnel and antibiotics
	Remove catheter
Superior vena cava thrombosis	Avoid positioning tip too high in superior vena cava
Atrial thrombin formation	Avoid positioning tip too low in atrium on tricuspid valve
	Both may respond to lytic therapy. Surgery occasionally required

nal jugular vein leads to no disability, and both internal jugular veins can be occluded with surprisingly little disability, provided there is a gap of some months between procedures.

The catheter must be robust and made of Silastic or other non-thrombogenic material with a cuff to allow tissue ingrowth; most have a double lumen with well designed caps and temporary occlusion clips (Fig. 10), although a single lumen (Francis) catheter based on an adapted peritoneal dialysis catheter, has also been used with success. Although the catheter can be placed in the external jugular vein of some patients, this vein is often too small and even if cannulation is successful malposition is common. The internal jugular vein is more certain to allow satisfactory cannulation. The internal jugular vein is approached at the lower end of sternomastoid, separating the sternal and clavicular heads (Fig. 11). Care must be taken in mobilizing the vein as small tributaries may be present, and avulsion may cause haemorrhage. The internal jugular vein must be carefully separated from the vagus behind and medial to it. The vein can be controlled by two double-looped slings and a purse-string suture of 4/0 Prolene inserted. The catheter is prefilled with saline, tunnelled to the wound, and the patient tipped head-down; the catheter is then inserted into the vein via an incision in the centre of the purse-string, which is then tied snugly around the catheter. A radiograph to check the position of the catheter should always be taken immediately and ideally the tip should be placed at the entrance to the right atrium. After closing the wound the patient should be nursed as upright as possible to minimize haematoma formation. Patency rates of 60 per cent at 2 years are claimed.

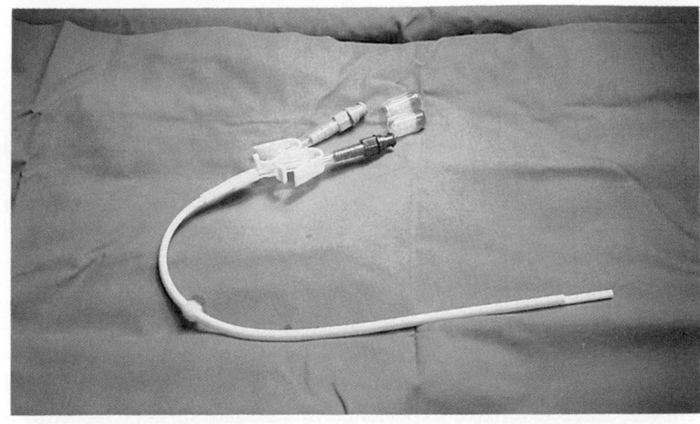

Fig. 10 Catheter for long-term venovenous dialysis. Note the dual lumen with staggered distal opening to minimize recirculation, temporary occlusion clamps, Dacron cuff, and caps for closure between dialyses.

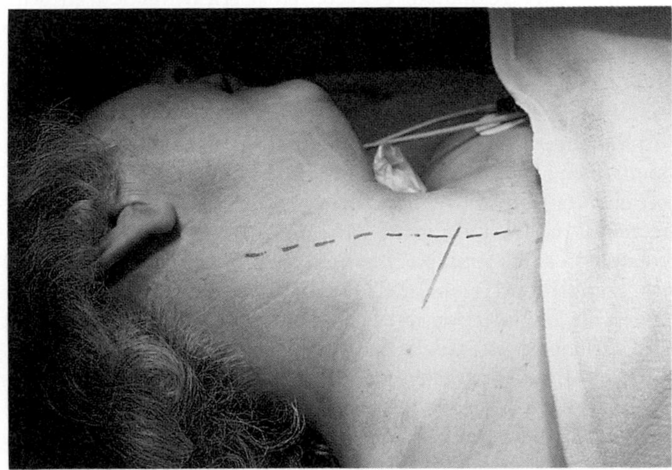

Fig. 11 Incision used for exposure of internal jugular vein. The anterior border of sternomastoid is marked by a dotted line.

Catheter removal is usually required for intractable thrombosis or sepsis (Table 5), and involves reopening of the original wound to free the Dacron cuff by sharp dissection. It is usually best to locate and divide the purse-string suture. The catheter is removed with the patient in the head-down position; bleeding can be controlled by a finger, whilst the track is closed with absorbable sutures.

Salvage procedures for patients with access problems

Expertise in the more complex access salvage techniques is not a skill that should be acquired easily, since it represents failure of the simpler procedures. Nevertheless, despite the greatest care, some patients eventually exhaust the simple access sites. This problem is most common in small women, where the vessels are naturally tiny, patients with vascular disease or Raynaud's phenomenon, diabetics, and patients with abnormal susceptibility to sepsis for some reason. A large number of ingenious techniques have been described for more complex access: only those that are commonly used will be described.

Venous transposition

A fistula may be functioning but unusable due to the deep-seated position or inaccessibility of the veins, for example the basilic vein. Mobilization of the vein to a more superficial position may prevent loss of an access site.

Interposition grafts

A vascular graft (either vein or prosthesis) inserted subcutaneously between a suitable artery and vein will allow repeated vascular access. Autologous saphenous vein is probably the conduit of choice, since extensive experience in vascular surgery has shown this to have a lower natural thrombogenicity and infection rate with repeated needling. However, saphenous vein is sufficiently strong to usually resist dilatation by persistent arterial pressure, a feature that is advantageous for vascular bypass grafts, but not ideal for access where needling of the graft is required. For this reason autogenous saphenous vein should only be used if a large vein is available. Patency rates of 70 per cent at 1 year and 65 per cent at 5 years are quoted. The alternative is a synthetic graft, with purpose-made Gore-Tex (using a tapered arterial end and loop reinforcement) probably being preferred over other synthetic grafts such as Dacron. Patency rates of 58 to 95 per cent at 1 year and 40 to 80 per cent at 2 years are claimed by various authors. Alternatives such as human umbilical vein, bovine artery, and human saphenous vein allografts have shown a higher complication rate from sepsis and aneurysm formation. An interesting technical modification is the addition of a connection port to the conduit to allow simple connection for dialysis without the need for cannulation (Haemasite). Two-year patency rates of 50 per cent with low infection rates are claimed for this prosthetic graft and thrombosis is easily cleared by opening the port.

In most patients the forearm and lower leg vessels have been used previously for either shunt or fistula formation, and the jugular veins may also have been used. The first requirement is location of a suitable artery and vein for anastomosis. In most patients a number of options are open: the radial artery may be patent, but since there are no suitable veins in the forearm a longitudinal graft needs to be run from the radial artery and connected to a cubital vein. In other patients the brachial artery and cubital veins are available and a forearm loop can be performed (Fig. 12). It is possible to cross the elbow joint to anastomose to the cephalic vein above the elbow, provided a reinforced graft is placed with the rings across the joint line. If these options are not possible a loop can be formed in the thigh, most simply by connecting the mobilized long saphenous vein as a loop anastomosed directly on to the common femoral artery. Other grafts are usable if anatomically possible: axillary artery to femoral vein and grafts between femoral vessels of opposite legs have been used. In these cases the basic technique is similar. The points of importance are listed in Table 6.

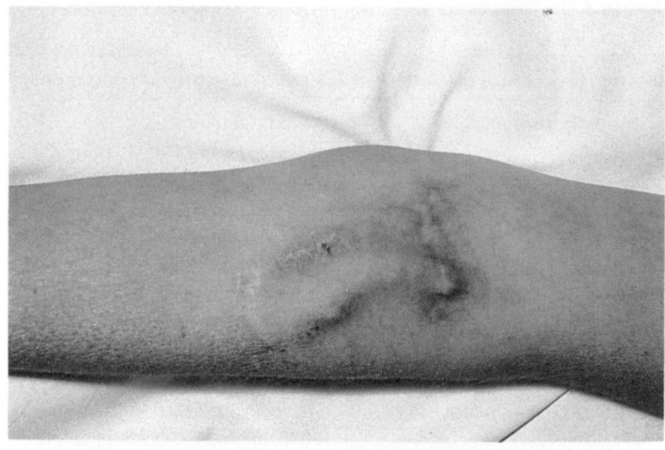

Fig. 12 Forearm saphenous vein loop between brachial artery and cephalic vein.

Table 6 Points of importance in formation of interposition grafts for dialysis access

Careful preoperative preparation, hydration, and anaesthesia
Prophylactic antibiotics
Choose widely patent, preferably untouched, vessels
Confirm proximal vessel patency preoperatively (radiology if necessary)
Use grafts at least 6 mm in diameter
Meticulous anastomosis technique avoiding vessel narrowing and intimal flaps
Careful tunnelling of grafts in the subcutaneous position (do not place too deeply—difficult to use)
Keep loops short and carefully avoid twists and kinks
Confirm rapid flow before closure
Early re-exploration of graft occlusions
On-table radiology if graft occludes
Late graft stenoses must be investigated by radiology and treated by percutaneous dilatation or early revision

Long-term haemodialysis access in children

Although the general principles outlined for adults also apply to children, the problems are increased by the small size of vessels available and the importance of psychological factors such as needle fear. Fortunately the introduction of EMLA cream allows the painless insertion of needles, making a fistula a far more attractive option than was previously the case. Since one must plan for a lifetime of renal replacement therapy decisions regarding the use of access sites are particularly important. General anaesthesia is recommended for all access-forming procedures.

Acute access for dialysis is a particular problem in children, since the subclavian veins are relatively difficult to cannulate percutaneously and tend to thrombose once cannulated. In neonates and many older children the best option may be peritoneal dialysis, which is discussed elsewhere. If this option is not available the best solution is usually to insert an internal jugular line under direct vision, using a cannula of as large a bore as can be inserted, with the tip of the cannula in the right atrium. The principles of insertion are similar to those described for adults. In many children the next option chosen would be early transplantation rather than fistula formation, in order to preserve the forearm site for future use.

In children in whom early transplantation is not an option the procedure of choice is again a radiocephalic fistula. Although the surgical principles are similar to the technique used in adults, experience of microsurgical techniques and special instruments are required.

VASCULAR ACCESS FOR TOTAL PARENTERAL NUTRITION

The requirements of access for parenteral nutrition differ from those of haemodialysis in that only a single line is required, and the flow rates needed are relatively small. However, the nutrients being delivered are highly irritant to vessels and it is thus not possible to use peripheral veins. The haemoglobin level of these patients is often near normal, as is platelet function, and so formation of an arteriovenous connection is contraindicated because of the likelihood of thrombosis, although this is a technique that has been used occasionally for total parenteral nutrition. The best solution is to use central venous cannulation, where the concentrated nutrients can be diluted rapidly enough to prevent vessel inflammation. The catheter used can be small bore, but must be made of non-irritant material such as silicone and in the case of permanent nutrition must be sufficiently robust for long-term use. Inclusion of a Dacron cuff is felt to be an advantage for prevention of track infection. A number of commercial catheters are now available (Fig. 13) and a major advance has been the recent development of totally implantable catheters with ports containing self-sealing membranes that allow intermittent cannulation (Fig. 14). The number of cannulations possible is still rather limited for the purposes of long-term total parenteral nutrition but it is certainly an option that is worth considering in children and for relatively short-term outpatient management, since the sepsis rate is low.

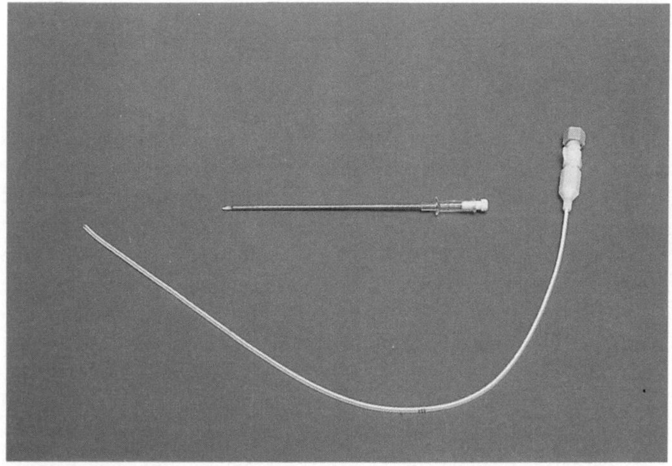

Fig. 13 Silastic catheter suitable for total parenteral nutrition, with needle for percutaneous insertion. The hub is detachable to allow removal of the needle and formation of a subcutaneous tunnel.

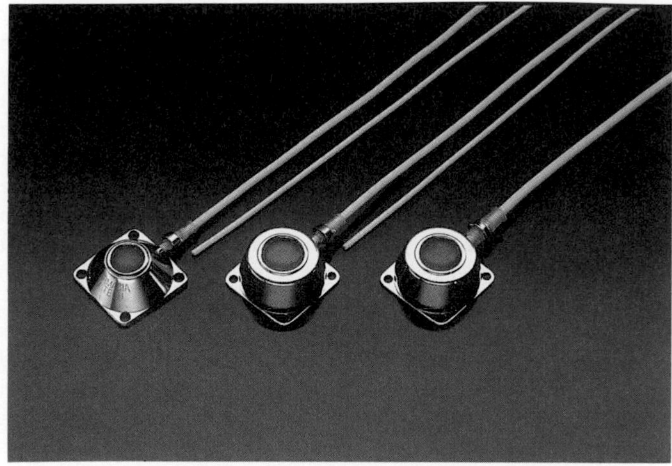

Fig. 14 Three varieties of implantable cannulae and ports for repeated access to venous, arterial, and peritoneal sites.

Access for short-term total parenteral nutrition

Percutaneous insertion of the catheter into the subclavian vein under local anaesthesia is the usual approach because the catheter can then be conveniently kept out of the way by strapping to the chest. The cannulation technique is similar to that described earlier for haemodialysis catheter insertion, but the proximal line should also be tunnelled out from the puncture site for a distance of about 5 cm. The complications include those noted for subclavian dialysis catheter placement, but sepsis is the most frequent problem. This usually arises from poor connection technique, particularly if the catheter is used for any purpose other than total parenteral nutrition; since many of these patients are in an intensive care unit the temptation to allow use of the line for blood sampling and drug delivery must be firmly avoided. Delivery of the daily requirement premixed in one bag also limits the number of bag changes and reduces the chance of infection.

Lines suspected of being infected may be cultured by taking blood from the line: a negative result is reliable, provided the patient has no antibiotics in the bloodstream at the time. Infected lines are best managed by removal and insertion of a fresh line on the other side, but occasionally infection can be cleared by changing the catheter over a guide wire, using a new subcutaneous tunnel, combined with intensive antibiotic treatment.

Access for long-term total parenteral nutrition

The catheters used for this purpose need to be considerably more robust and are consequentially larger. Insertion is often best undertaken by cannulation of the cephalic vein under local anaesthesia (Fig. 15), although percutaneous insertion into the jugular or subclavian vein is becoming possible even for cuffed catheters by the introduction of 'peel-away' insertion sheaths. The direction of the catheter is often incorrect at the first attempt when inserted by the cephalic vein route and radiographic screening

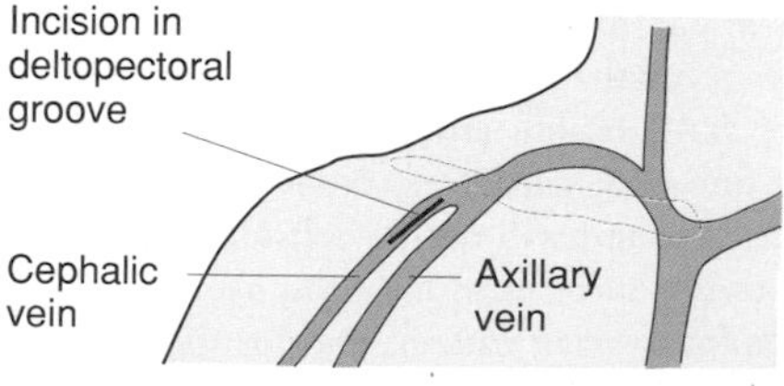

Fig. 15 Incision for cannulation of the cephalic vein.

should be undertaken during the procedure. Again the catheter should be tunnelled for at least 6 cm from the wound. Although the presence of a tunnel does not seem to influence the sepsis rate it is more convenient for the patient. The inclusion of a Dacron felt cuff is beneficial since the tissue ingrowth holds the catheter in place and may effectively seal the track to bacteria. The catheter tip must be smoothly rounded off and carefully positioned to lie free just at the entrance to the right atrium, since there have been descriptions of catheter perforation and thrombosis of the heart and great vessels. Sepsis is the main complication and attention to aseptic technique during bag changes must be meticulous.

Home total parenteral nutrition is mainly indicated in patients with short bowel syndrome. Meticulous training in catheter and bag changing technique is vital to prevent sepsis, which is the main complication. Suspected sepsis may be confirmed by finding bacterial counts at a ratio of greater than 5:1 in blood samples cultured from the catheter and a peripheral vein respectively. The most common causative organism is *Staphyloccus aureus*. Sepsis may be cleared by administration of urokinase and appropriate antibiotics via the catheter for 5 days. Occlusion may also occur due to lipid or calcium phosphate encrustation which may respond to local instillation of ethanol or 0.1 M hydrochloric acid respectively (into the catheter only and not systemically).

VASCULAR ACCESS FOR CHEMOTHERAPY

The treatment of a number of malignancies has been transformed by the advent of effective chemotherapeutic regimens, but the drugs used must be given intravenously at regular intervals, often for many weeks. Many of the therapeutic agents are highly irritant to peripheral veins and need to be delivered into high flow vessels. It has been suggested that constant infusion of chemotherapeutic agents may increase their efficacy and lower toxicity, but firm evidence for this point is lacking. Many chemotherapeutic drugs have toxic effects on the bone marrow and other organs and numerous blood samples need to be taken on a daily basis to monitor toxicity. Perhaps the most demanding example of intensive chemotherapy is that required for treatment of leukaemia, particularly when bone marrow transplantation is also required. There is, therefore, a need for reliable access to the central veins over a period of weeks to months and, in addition, a catheter that will allow both drug delivery and blood sampling at the same time is most useful. The most convenient catheter is a double lumen catheter of the Hickman variety (Fig. 16), which can be inserted under local anaesthesia into the cephalic or external jugular veins.

Patients suffering from leukaemia are often thrombocytopenic and neutropenic, and insertion of a line should only be attempted under full coagulation factor and platelet replacement with antibiotic prophylaxis. The line should normally be tunnelled to minimize infection, although in patients with absent platelets the tunnel may be kept very short.

A variety of alternative routes for delivery of drugs to allow treatment of apparently localized tumours have been described including the recanalized umbilical vein for hepatic perfusion, hepatic artery cannulation, and carotid artery and femoral artery perfusion via fine bore catheters. None has reached the status of accepted treatment and will not be considered further here. Some preliminary studies have examined the use of intraperitoneal delivery of drugs for ovarian cancer, and for this purpose a standard Tenckhoff catheter is ideal (see below).

Similar principles to those used in adults apply to insertion of

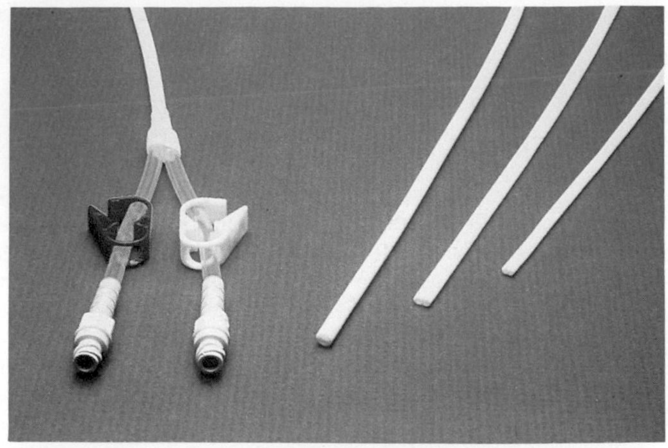

Fig. 16 Hickman-style catheter for medium- to long-term venous access. Three sizes of double lumen catheter are shown. Note the clamps for temporary control of each lumen.

lines for chemotherapy in children, but it is usually necessary to use the internal jugular vein for line insertion, although successful use of the long saphenous vein to cannulate the inferior vena cava has been described. General anaesthesia is normally required.

ACCESS FOR PERITONEAL DIALYSIS

The concept of using the peritoneum as a membrane for dialysis arose in the 1920s. It was initially employed to provide temporary renal replacement therapy, for example in cases where recovery of renal function was expected. The catheters used for this purpose were inserted using a 'blind' direct puncture technique with a trochar. Acute peritoneal dialysis catheters are still available (Trocath) but are probably used as much for diagnostic or therapeutic peritoneal lavage than for actual dialysis. The development that allowed long-term peritoneal dialysis was again the introduction of silastic non-irritant catheters, with the addition of cuffed tubes and use of a long subcutaneous tunnel. A variety of commercial catheter designs have been marketed, but the original Tenckhoff design is still the most popular and very effective, although the addition of a curl to the end of the catheter may help prevent displacement (Fig. 17). The requirements are for a catheter that allows rapid inflow and outflow of fluid, without leakage from the peritoneum and without allowing the introduction of agents which may cause sepsis. Complications of peritoneal dialysis catheter insertion are listed in Table 7.

Continuous ambulatory peritoneal dialysis has the advantage of being relatively cheap, simple to set up, and relatively easy to learn to run. The drawbacks are the relatively high readmission rate for complications, a tendency to obesity due to glucose absorption, and a short useful life, with approximately 50 per cent of catheters failing and requiring removal by 2 to 3 years. It is therefore not usually used for long-term dialysis of young, fit patients, but can be used as an option for patients where transplantation is expected within 2 years. It is also a favoured option for elderly patients, where survival is expected to be limited, and in diabetics and patients with other vasculopathies, where vessels suitable for haemodialysis may not be easily available. In addition, peritoneal dialysis using a smaller version of the Tenckhoff catheter is a good

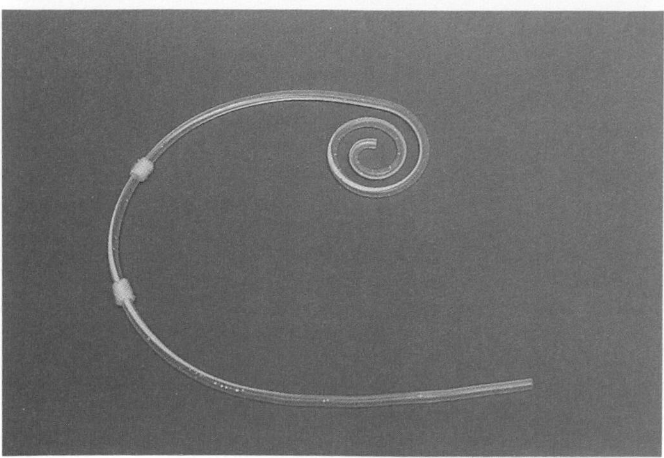

Fig. 17 Curled Silastic catheter for peritoneal dialysis with double cuff.

Table 7 Complications of peritoneal dialysis catheter insertion

Common complications	Cause/prevention/treatment
Leakage of fluid	Small peritoneal incision Careful insertion with snug ligatures Avoid usage (if possible) for 2 weeks (especially in the elderly)
Infection/peritonitis (usually caused by *Staphylococcus aureus*, especially in diabetics)	Good surgical technique Prophylactic antibiotics Meticulous connector sterility Regular antiseptic cleaning of exit site
Inadequate dialysis	
(i) catheter displacement	Carefully place catheter tip in pelvis Rectus tunnel fashioned pointing down Replacement under direct vision (± suture of tip)
(ii) obstruction by omentum	Carefully place catheter tip in pelvis Omentectomy
Bleeding/bowel perforation	Avoid forcible insertion Minor bleeding usually stops Direct vision placement in patients with adhesions (± adhesion lysis)
Groin or scrotal oedema	Usually due to an undetected hernia. Stop dialysis and repair hernia
External Dacron cuff erosion	Place cuff > 3 cm from skin exit Shave off cuff using scalpel

way of providing short- to medium-term dialysis for children, including neonates, and may provide sufficient time for successful transplantation to be performed. For chronic dialysis a double cuff catheter is not recommended as growth may cause puckering of the abdominal wall.

The catheter can be inserted by percutaneous puncture using a peritoneoscope, a technique that has firm advocates, but most surgeons prefer insertion by an open operative technique. Insertion under local anaesthesia is possible, but is only a comfortable procedure if no difficulties are encountered. General anaesthesia with relaxation is probably wiser in most patients. Prophylactic antibiotics are advisable. The catheter should be placed so that the subcutaneous tube and exit site is located either above or below the belt line, preferably on the opposite side to the side on which the patient normally sleeps (Fig. 18(a)). The peritoneum is best reached via the lower rectus sheath. A vertical or transverse incision can be used, opening the anterior rectus sheath. The rectus muscle can either be split or swept laterally to allow access to the posterior rectus sheath/transversalis fascia. A small incision in the peritoneum is then made, and a purse-string suture inserted. The catheter is then lubricated with sterile glycerine, loaded on to a blunt ended introducer and gently inserted along the anterior abdominal wall, over the bladder (and uterus in the female) and then slid down in front of the rectum. Some surgeons prefer to make a bigger peritoneal incision and insert the catheter under direct vision using sponge-holding forceps. A larger peritoneal incision also allows omentectomy to be performed safely, an addition that may reduce catheter failure due to occlusion by omentum. Omentectomy has been described as particularly important for peritoneal dialysis in children, although doubt has recently been cast on this dictum. The purse-string suture is then tied and stitched to the inner Tenckhoff Dacron cuff (Fig. 18(b)).

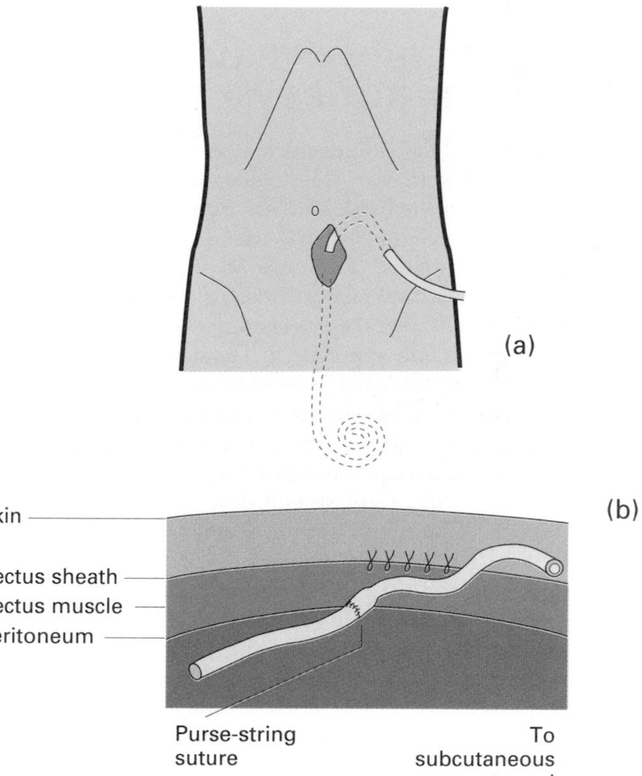

Fig. 18 (a) Incision and placement of peritoneal dialysis catheter. (b) Detail of peritoneal dialysis catheter insertion to show purse-string suture attaching catheter cuff to peritoneum and also the method of closure of the rectus sheath in order to keep the catheter pointing inferiorly.

The peritoneum can then be pulled up to allow an encircling ligature below the purse-string that helps prevent leakage of fluid from the stitch-holes. The catheter is then tunnelled to allow a gentle curve away from the peritoneum with the second cuff at least 3 cm from the skin exit. The rectus muscle and sheath should be closed snugly around the catheter so as to keep the catheter pointing into the pelvis (Fig. 18(b)), followed by the skin closure. On completion the catheter flow and absence of leakage should be tested by connection to a peritoneal dialysis bag and exchanging 1 l of saline rapidly.

The indications for catheter removal are repeated episodes of peritonitis, an infected catheter track unresponsive to antibiotics, loss of effective dialysis due to peritoneal thickening and return of renal function or a successful transplant rendering the catheter redundant. Removal can usually be accomplished under local anaesthesia. It is usually necessary to reopen the original insertion wound, freeing both the internal and external Dacron cuffs (where present) using sharp dissection. After removing the catheter the rectus sheath defect should be closed using a non-absorbable suture if there is no infection, to avoid later incisional hernia.

FURTHER READING

Bell PRF, Wood RFM. *Surgical aspects of haemodialysis.* 2nd edn. Edinburgh: Churchill Livingstone, 1983.

Bengmark S, ed. *The peritoneum and peritoneal access for dialysis.* London: Wright, 1989.

Brescia MJ, Cimino JE, Appel K, Hurwich BJ. Chronic hemodialysis using venipuncture and a surgically created arteriovenous fistula. *New Engl J Med* 1966; **275**: 1089–92.

Buselmeier TJ, Kjellstrand CM, Santiago EA, Simmons RL, Najarian JS. A new subcutaneous arteriovenous shunt. *Surgery* 1973; **73**: 512–20.

Kolff WJ, Berk HJ, Welle M, Van der Ley AJW, Van Dijk EC, Van Noordwijk J. The artificial kidney: a dialyser with a great area. *Acta Med Scand* 1944; **147**: 121–34.

Seldinger SI. Catheter replacement of the needle in percutaneous arteriography. *Acta Radiol* 1953; **39**: 369–76.

Sommer BG, Mitchell LH. *Vascular access for hemodialysis.* Chicago: Pluribus Press, 1989.

Tenckhoff H, Schechter H. A bacteriologically safe peritoneal access device. *Trans Am Soc Artif Org* 1968; **14**: 181–7.

Quinton W, Dillard D, Scribner BH. Cannulation of blood vessels for prolonged haemodialysis. *Trans Am Soc Artif Org* 1969; **15**: 104–13.

7.17 Limb amputation

DEREK W. R. GRAY

THE DEVELOPMENT OF AMPUTATION TECHNIQUES

For many centuries limb injuries have been common as a result of man's fascination with war. The outcome of even minor limb injuries inflicted on the battlefield was frequently fatal, in strong contrast to the minor importance accorded to such injuries in modern historical drama! The cause of these deaths was presumably sepsis from contaminated wounds containing devitalized tissue, but it was not until the last century that the important role of debridement was fully appreciated. The signs of increasing limb pain, swelling, and toxaemia were recognized as harbingers of death, and amputation the only cure. Despite the absence of aseptic technique, removal of the limb by incisions through healthy tissue with free drainage was often followed by recovery and healing. Although there are several descriptions of amputation dating back to Hippocrates the technique was popularized by Ambroise Paré around 1575 and was rapidly taken up by other military surgeons and then transferred to civilian practice. In the absence of true anaesthesia it was not possible to perform other than a guillotine type amputation and healing was always by secondary intention, although the later addition of a short flap by Yonge and Lowdham in 1679 made closure easier. To minimize the horrific experience surgeons became adept at rapid amputation, and apocryphal tales describe amputations performed in a few seconds, sometimes with the loss of the assistant's fingers.

The desire to replace an amputated limb with a prosthesis is as old as the procedure itself. There are many examples of false legs, mainly of wood, in ancient drawings and the use of a hook to replace the amputated forearm is also well known. The wooden peg-leg is common to many cultures and relied on the user kneeling on the weight-bearing surface. However there are also many examples of ingenious and complex artificial legs dating from the time of Pare.

The modern era of amputation surgery was heralded by the advent of anaesthesia and later by aseptic surgical techniques. It became possible to perform amputation using flaps fashioned to allow primary closure at a variety of levels. The huge number of amputees that followed the First World War provided a stimulus to the development of improved limb prosthetics, and many of the modern services originated at this time. Over the next few decades it was slowly appreciated that not all indications for amputation could be treated identically, and that patients presenting with infection or gangrene associated with loss of limb pulses had to be treated more cautiously in terms of amputation than patients undergoing amputation for trauma. Thus, Homans (1939) was voicing contemporary surgical opinion about the outcome of amputation in patients with vascular disease when he wrote 'amputations below the knee can almost never be expected to offer a healthy stump'. Fortunately, this view has been proven incorrect, but the technical demands of amputations performed for limb ischaemia are emphasized by this quotation.

INDICATIONS FOR AMPUTATION

As a consequence of increasing specialization in surgery, limb amputations are performed by different specialists, depending on the indications. Thus orthopaedic surgeons most often perform amputations for trauma, and vascular surgeons usually amputate for vascular disease. Although the techniques used for different indications are broadly similar there are some individual factors that must be considered.

Trauma

Since traumatic vascular injury is usually repairable, limb amputation is only indicated when there has been massive destruction of tissue, by either crush or blast injuries. The common causes are either motor accident or gunshot wounds in civilian practice. Ideally, the decision to amputate should be made immediately—a late amputation dictated by developing sepsis in an inadequately debrided limb represents a failure of management. Because the vascularity and health of the tissue proximal to the injury is usually good the amputation can be placed as distally as possible, within the limitation imposed by the need for excision of all devitalized tissue. Contamination with soil and dirt is common and in these cases the wound should be left open and closed secondarily after several days. Even if the early swelling of skin flaps prevents full closure by secondary suture, the basic health of the tissue will usually allow good healing by granulation and amputation at a higher level should be considered only if serious sepsis ensues.

Ischaemia

Amputation of the limb of a patient with rest pain, sepsis, or gangrene with the aim of primary wound healing is perhaps one of the greatest challenges to a surgeon. Several factors conspire against the healing process. Firstly the tissue at the line of incision has often only slightly better vascular perfusion than the critically ischaemic or frankly gangrenous tissue distally, and the lack of oxygen and nutrients delivered to this tissue means that the ability to form new vessels in granulation tissue and the metabolic processes involved in healing are greatly impaired, as is the ability to fight bacterial contamination. The lack of perfusion may be made worse by the frequent coexistence of poor cardiac function, respiratory disease and anaemia. Furthermore many patients have sepsis already within the limb and there may be considerable oedema as a result of this and other coexisting conditions such as heart failure. Many patients are diabetic, further reducing resistance to infection.

It therefore behoves the surgeon to pay attention to these factors and correct those that are correctable, wherever possible. Heart failure, anaemia, chest infection, and limb infection should all be treated, since this may make the crucial difference between success and failure. Unfortunately delay is not always humane or wise, since the toxaemia from an infected ischaemic leg may make factors such as heart failure worsen despite treatment until the limb is removed, and opiates required to treat severe rest pain may make a chest infection untreatable. The judgement to wait or proceed is often difficult and is probably best taken by the surgeon since other physicians may not appreciate the role of the ischaemic limb itself in dictating the general condition of the patient.

Malignancy

Amputation for a tumour affecting a limb is now a relatively rare occurrence, since most tumours can be controlled locally by a combination of radiotherapy and cytotoxic therapy, even if excision is not possible. When amputation becomes necessary it is always a planned procedure, usually in a limb with good vascularity without sepsis and the amputation is usually, therefore, technically quite straightforward. Psychological effects are likely to be the greatest problem in this group, since there is ample opportunity to brood on the forthcoming operation and the subsequent disability is compounded by the fear of recurrence of the tumour.

Congenital deformity

At one time amputation was considered the best option for a number of congenital deformities, on the basis that this gave superior cosmesis and would ultimately lead to better acceptance by society. However, it has now been realized that even patients with severely deformed limbs usually can obtain better function from the deformed limb, albeit with a number of prosthetic additions, than by amputating the limb and attempting to fit a conventional prosthesis. Furthermore, such patients are unlike normal limb amputees, in that they have never developed a body image of themselves with a full-size limb and do not adjust easily to a full-size prosthesis. A limb remnant represented by a single digit may be used to activate a control for a mechanized transport or prosthesis and should not be removed.

The only common exception to this rule is the deformity caused by congenital absence of the fibula, resulting in shortening of the lower leg. Conversion to a Symes amputation produces an end-bearing stump which may be fitted to a foot prosthesis that can result in remarkably normal function in young children.

Other indications for amputation

Amputation is rarely required for a limb that is severely deformed, useless, or painful from acquired disease. Examples of conditions that sometimes require amputation are neurological diseases leading to a painful flail limb and chronic osteomyelitis, where renal failure due to subsequent amyloidosis is a danger. These indications have become increasingly rare since the following points have been understood. Firstly, even a severely deformed limb can usually function better than a prosthesis. Secondly, a paralysed limb can still provide support following arthrodesis of appropriate joints or by the use of splints and gives better cosmesis. Thirdly, persistent severe pain of central neurological origin may make a limb useless but, unfortunately, removing the limb often does not result in relief since the pain persists in the 'phantom' limb.

THE CHOICE OF AMPUTATION SITE

The site of amputation is influenced by several factors. The overriding general principle is that the least mutilating procedure possible should always be chosen, a principle that is particularly important in the lower limb, where the retention of the knee joint results in much greater mobility after rehabilitation. However other factors are also important, the most obvious being the indication for amputation. In the case of amputation for malignancy the amputation must be performed at a site that is sufficiently proximal to ensure clearance of the malignant process and minimize the chances of recurrence. This usually means removing the limb at a level that includes the joint proximal to the lesion. In the case of amputation for trauma the amputation site should be as distal as possible, subject to the possibility of fitting a usable prosthesis. In the case of amputation for ischaemia the choice of amputation site is a balance between using as distal a site as is compatible with removing dead or near-dead tissue and a proximal site sufficient to ensure healing of the wound.

In the past the ease of fitting the limb for a prosthesis was also a factor. For instance, above or below knee prostheses were easier to fit and functioned better than through knee prostheses. However the steady advance in materials and design of prostheses has meant that this factor is less important than previously, although it is still difficult to get a good cosmetic result from a jointed prosthesis for long thigh amputations such as the Gritti-Stokes.

Clinical assessment

The most important requirement for successful amputation is skin healing, preferably by first intention. The skin that is to form the amputation flaps must at least be viable at the outset. Signs of demarcation, fixed staining, or anaesthesia of the flap skin are obvious contraindications to its use. The presence of excoriation, cellulitis, or frank ulceration are relative contraindications, although the likelihood that the phenomenon is entirely localized and that infection has been treated adequately must be considered. The tissues beneath the skin must also be healthy. The presence of deep tenderness and loss of function may signal necrosis of deep muscles or sepsis, which make an amputation unlikely to heal. The skin temperature is more a reflection of the ambient temperature, or the presence of sepsis or systemic illness and is not a reliable guide to subsequent healing. The absence of a pulse at the next most proximal palpation point has been said to be a contraindication to more distal amputation and vice versa, but this is certainly an unreliable sign. The decision about the level and type of amputation should also not be taken during the operation, since the degree of bleeding noted on incision of tissues at operation is a very poor guide to subsequent healing, being greatly affected by anaesthetic agents and transient hypotension.

The decision to undertake a more distal amputation is inevitably associated with a greater risk of failure to heal and the need for reamputation at a higher level. Furthermore, the exact magnitude of risk has been shown to vary considerably from centre to centre, and to make a rational decision it is necessary to know one's own results: a valuable contribution of continuous audit. The final decision should always take into account all of the factors influencing outcome including the physical and mental capacity of the patient to withstand a reamputation and whether the patient is likely to make use of the increased mobility that a joint saving amputation may give, to name just two.

Other assessment techniques

A variety of techniques for assessing the blood supply to the amputation flaps, including thermography, transcutaneous oxygen measurement, cutaneous perfusion measurement, xenon-133 clearance, Doppler ultrasound, and digital plethysmography have been described. There is no doubt that in the hands of enthusiasts these techniques can allow the correct choice of amputation site in a larger proportion of cases than is probably achieved by clinical judgement alone. However, all of the techniques require some degree of expertise in their performance and some are not readily available in many hospitals. No single technique has been shown to be sufficiently superior to the others to attain widespread acceptance, although transcutaneous oxygen measurement is probably the most valuable.

TECHNIQUES OF AMPUTATION

Anaesthesia and preparation

Although general anaesthesia is preferred by most centres it is possible to use local anaesthesia, nerve block, epidural, or spinal anaesthesia in appropriate situations. Some surgeons object to the use of techniques other than general anaesthesia on the grounds that the noise and motion associated with amputation is psychologically distressing to the patient, even in the absence of pain. However, the use of amnesic sedative agents during the procedure is highly effective and most patients remember nothing if such agents are used.

Local anaesthesia is only useful for digital amputation and has the potential disadvantage of causing local swelling of the tissues which may make closure less easy. There is also the theoretical (but in practice, remote) disadvantage of spreading infection. Local anaesthetic combined with adrenaline must never be used as this may further prejudice the blood supply.

Nerve block techniques have the advantage of avoiding the dangers of general anaesthesia and hypotension, but unfortunately tend to be unreliable, and conversion from nerve block to general anaesthesia in the middle of an amputation is distressing not only to the patient but also the theatre staff.

Epidural or spinal anaesthesia is usually very adequate for amputation of the lower limb, producing vasodilation as a by-product which certainly does no harm from the point of view of the procedure. A tourniquet should never be used for patients with vascular disease and is usually unnecessary even in patients with normal vessels. Broad spectrum antibiotics, such as penicillin, with activity against *Clostridium* spp. must always be given preoperatively.

After careful identification of the patient and the correct limb, the limb should be carefully painted with skin-prep prior to starting surgery, wrapping any gangrenous or infected portion in a plastic bag, sealed to the skin above by adherent non-porous tape. The incision lines for flap formation must always be marked out using a sterile marker.

Surgical technique

In modern surgical practice approximately 80 per cent of amputations are performed for ischaemia secondary to vascular disease. The life expectancy of this generally elderly group of patients is limited, mainly due to concomitant cardiovascular and cerebrovascular disease. Approximately 50 per cent of vascular amputees will die within 3 years. The main consideration in performing the amputation is to obtain stump healing. In non-vascular amputations, such as those for trauma or tumour, the patient is often young and a lifetime of prosthetic use must be anticipated. In these patients more advanced procedures to obtain maximal function may be indicated. Since the majority of surgeons perform lower limb amputations for ischaemia most of the techniques described below will be those recommended for this indication. Modifications and additional procedures applicable to amputation in non-ischaemic limbs will be considered as addenda to each technique. In those amputations indicated mainly for non-ischaemic disease, such as those in the upper limb, the reverse order will apply.

The amputation technique should be governed not only by the disease process and anatomical principles but also by the pros-

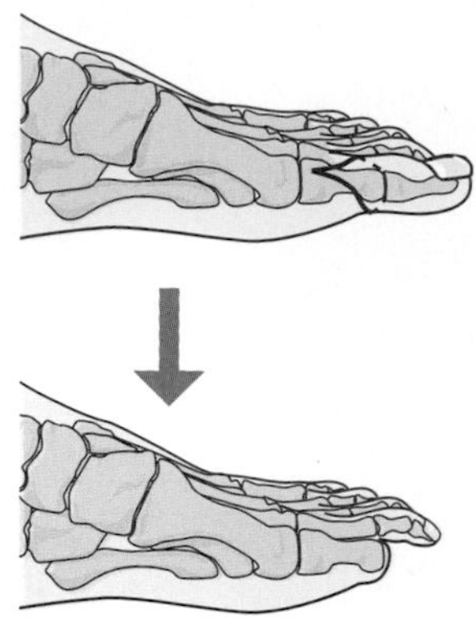

Fig. 1 'Racquet' incision for toe amputation.

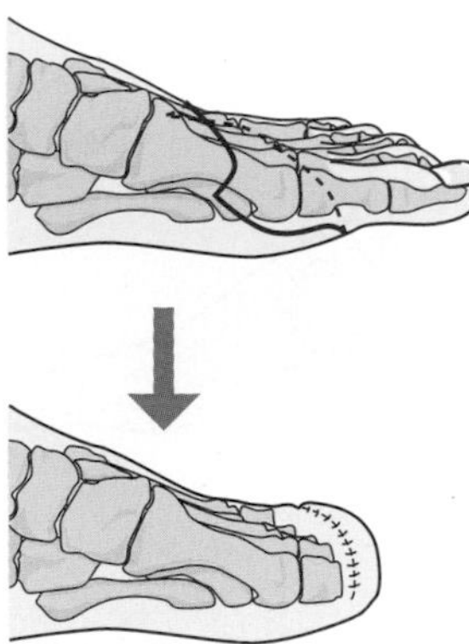

Fig. 2 Incision for transmetatarsal amputation, requiring a long viable flap of sole skin.

thesis available to replace the severed limb. A comment on the prosthesis available is therefore a necessary adjunct to the description of each amputation technique.

Lower limb amputations

Toe amputation

A 'racquet' shaped incision is recommended (Fig. 1). The tissues should be severed from the incision line directly down to the shaft of the phalanx and dissection of tissues should then continue proximally as close to the bone as possible, to avoid the possibility of damaging the digital vessels laterally and thus compromising the blood supply to the flaps and other digits. It is not usually wise to amputate just the distal phalanges for vascular disease and the dissection should continue up to the metacarpophalangeal joint, which is disarticulated to allow removal of the digit. The head of the metatarsal should then be removed by the careful use of nibbling forceps preventing further damage to the surrounding tissues. The bone should be nibbled back until the tissues can be seen to be falling in to cover approximately half of the cut end of the bone. Tendons should be pulled down with forceps, cleanly severed as short as possible, and allowed to retract. The incision should not be sutured closed but is best packed lightly with ribbon gauze, to limit bleeding, and allowed to heal by granulation. Prostheses are not usually required.

The usual indication for toe amputation in non-ischaemic limbs is for trauma. The wounds can be closed primarily provided that there is no danger of contamination. Amputation of distal phalanges may be contemplated for cosmetic reasons.

Transmetatarsal amputation

This amputation performed in an ischaemic limb allows surprisingly good function, despite the loss of the great toe, but is undoubtedly the amputation with the highest failure rate. The important requirement is an adequately vascularized flap of sole skin, allowing application of the technique shown in Fig. 2. It is uncommon to have an adequate vascular supply in the presence of gangrenous toes, and for this reason the amputation is not often performed for vascular disease. However the correct indications do occur sometimes in diabetic patients who have localized digital gangrene in the presence of foot pulses. If insufficient vascularized sole skin is available to ensure primary closure the amputation should not be performed as secondary closure often fails in patients with vascular disease. The dorsal transverse incision is first made over the metatarsals as shown (Fig. 2), incising through the dorsal tendons down to bone. The metatarsals are divided using a bone cutting forceps, or more satisfactorily, a power saw, and then the distal bones are elevated to allow careful dissection posteriorly close to the periostium and eventual separation and removal of the forefoot, leaving behind the sole, which should be kept as long as possible at this stage. Each metatarsal shaft should then be nibbled back for a distance of 1.5 cm using bone nibbling forceps to allow the tissues to fall in over the bone ends. The exposed tendons should then be removed from the sole flap by pulling down with forceps and then cleanly severing the tendon as short as possible. After ensuring haemostasis the flap is brought forward over the metatarsals and cut to the appropriate length to allow closure without tension, using deep interrupted absorbable sutures and an atraumatic skin closure (either steristrips or subcutaneous prolene inserted without instruments is preferred by the author).

In patients without ischaemic disease it is possible to leave the flaps open if gross contamination has occurred due to trauma, and use skin grafts later if full closure cannot be obtained.

A simple shoe filler is usually sufficient to provide a good functional result.

Transtarsal amputations (Chopart, Lisfranc)

Owing to the poor healing and inevitable equinus deformity caused by unopposed contraction of the ankle flexors these amputations are not recommended in either vascular or non-vascular patients.

Syme's operation

Syme's operation is the best amputation for patients with extensive non-ischaemic damage to the forefoot. The stump that is produced has the advantage of allowing considerable weight bearing, and thus allows considerable independence in the home without a prosthesis. It may suffice alone in areas where prostheses are not available. The defects of the procedure used to be difficulty in fitting a foot prosthesis because of lack of clearance from the ground, which has now been overcome, and poor cosmesis of the prosthesis in females, due to the thickness at the ankle: this is still a problem. There is a difference between the technique that can be used in children and in adults although the incisions used are similar (Fig. 3). In children the amputation uses the same heel flap to cover the end of the stump, but the amputation itself can consist

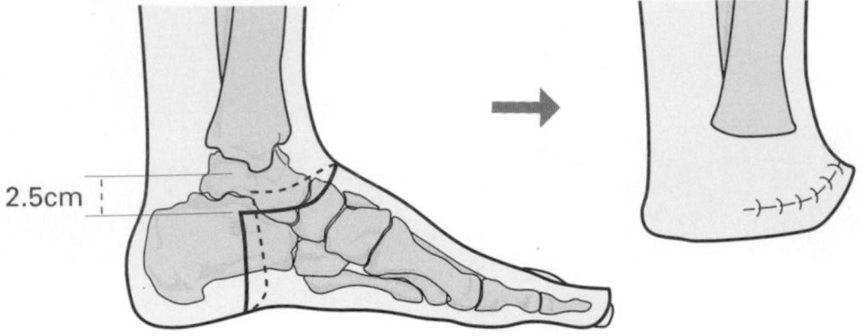

Fig. 3 Incision for Syme's amputation.

of simple disarticulation of the talus, followed by removal of the malleoli, leaving behind most of the joint surface. In adults the incision is made as shown in Fig. 3. The anterior incision is then deepened through the anterior tendons to allow disarticulation of the talus from the joint. The Achilles tendon is divided posteriorly and the talus and calcaneum are then dissected free from the heel by sharp dissection, staying close to the periosteum to avoid damage to vascular structures. The dissection is particularly difficult over the thin skin at the back of the heel, and there is a danger of 'buttonholing' the skin, which can again be avoided by staying close to the periostium. A variant operation described by Boyd is to leave a slice of the calcaneum attached to the heel skin, which can then be attached to the proximal cut bones in a similar manner to the Gritti-Stokes operation. This may lessen the trauma to the tissue but lengthens the stump.

Once the posterior flap has been dissected free the distal foot is removed, leaving the heel flap long at this stage. The exposed distal tibia and fibula are dissected free of adherent tissues staying on the periosteum. A transverse cut is then made approximately 1 cm above the ankle mortice. It is important that this cut is truly transverse, to prevent uneven pressure later when weight bearing. It is also important to leave some element of the malleolar prominence on each side, since this allows stabilization of the prosthesis and prevents rotation. After cutting tendons short and allowing them to retract and ensuring haemostasis the flap is brought over the cut end of the bone and trimmed to a suitable length without tension. The wound is closed by suturing the deep tissues of the heel pad to the deep fascia anteriorly with a suitable atraumatic skin suture.

Syme's amputation requires a relatively good blood supply to the heel pad and most patients that need to lose the foot from vascular disease do not have sufficiently good blood supply to allow this procedure. However, some diabetics with forefoot infection or gangrene may have normal ankle pulses and a Symes amputation can be successful.

Prostheses available are shown in Fig. 4.

Below-knee amputation

This is the most common amputation performed for vascular disease, and possibly the most demanding technically. Preserving the knee joint is of such major benefit in terms of rehabilitation that below knee amputation should usually be undertaken in all patients with non-reconstructible ischaemia distal to the calf, unless there are clear indications that the operation is certain to fail. Such contraindications would include necrosis of the potential posterior flap skin, or a patient who is certain not to benefit from the advantages of a below-knee prosthesis, for example where the knee has been arthrodesed. The operation described is a variant of the Burgess long posterior flap technique. A

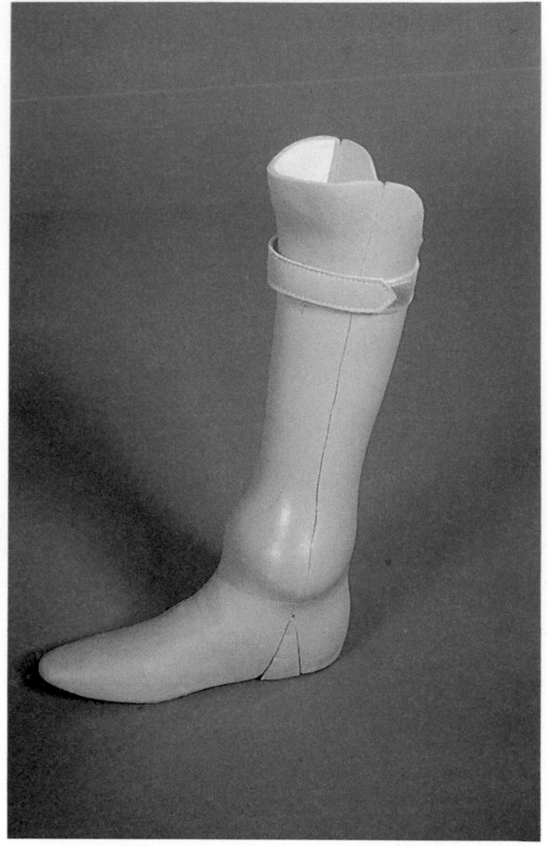

Fig. 4 Bivalved plastic prosthesis for Syme's amputation. Note the poor cosmetic result.

more complex technique, based on similar principles, is the skew-flap technique (see bibliography), which probably has similar healing rates but produces a more ideal conical stump.

The important principles of the technique are shown in Figs. 5 to 8. The stump should be as short as possible to maximize the chances of healing but long enough to allow optimal use of a below knee prosthesis: 9 cm from the knee joint line is ideal in thin legs, 11 cm in fat legs, and 7.5 cm can be regarded as the absolute minimum. A long posterior flap is used which should initially be kept as long as possible, and only trimmed prior to final suturing. The flap is based on half the circumference of the leg to maximize the blood supply from above. After outlining the flaps the skin incision is deepened through fascia, marking the tibia anteriorly to denote the later line of bone section. The muscle of the anterior and lateral compartments is divided to expose the fibula, ligating the anterior tibial vessels. The fibula is divided with a lateral bevel 1.5 cm proximal to the tibial line. The tibia is divided at the marked line with an anterior bevel and the lower leg removed by dissecting the posterior flap away from the bones. Bone dust should be washed away to prevent spur formation. Bleeding can be controlled by folding the flap forward and applying pressure. The bulk of the flap should be reduced by complete removal of the soleus muscle (Figs. 6, 7), which does not contribute to the blood supply of the flap. If the lateral portions of the gastrocnemius muscle bellies are particularly prominent these should also be trimmed to reduce 'dog-ears'. The posterior tibial and peroneal vessels are individually ligated whilst removing soleus. The flap is

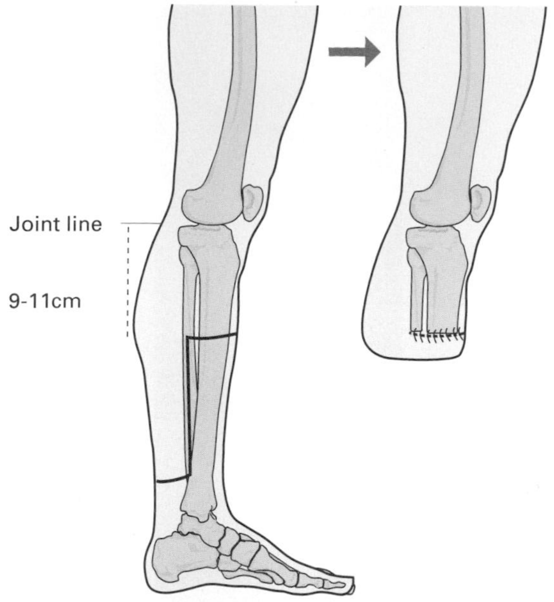

Fig. 5 Incision for below knee amputation. The posterior flap should be left as long as possible and only cut to an appropriate length prior to suturing.

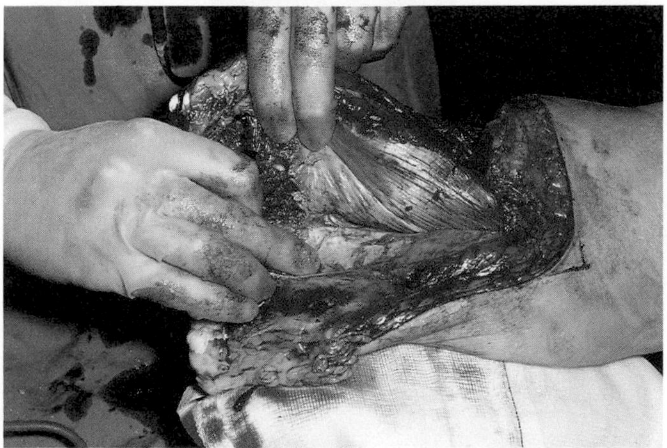

Fig. 6 Separation of the plane between soleus and gastrocnemius.

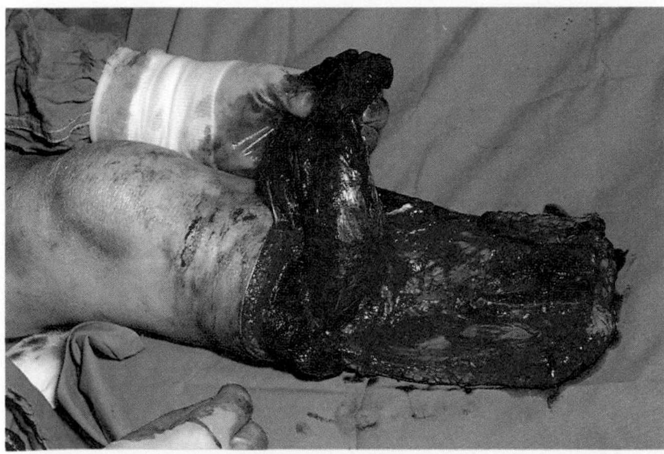

Fig. 7 Muscle bulk of soleus to be excised.

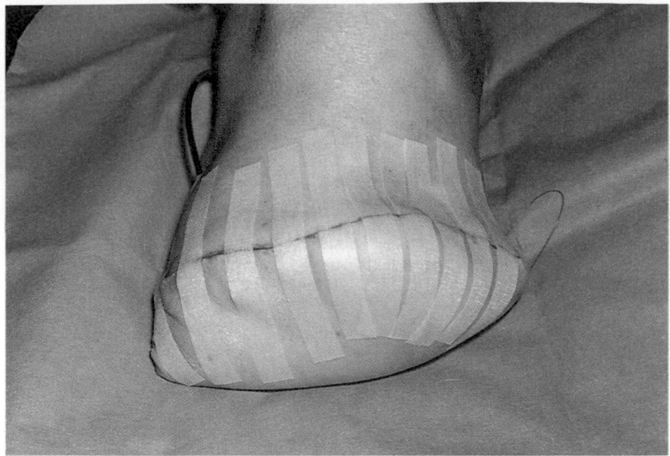

Fig. 8 Below-knee amputation before dressing.

then brought forward to the tibia, cut to a suitable length and sutured, deep fascia to periostium and deep fascia, over a vacuum drain. Skin closure should be performed with meticulous care of the skin. The author's preference is for subcuticular prolene inserted by hand needle, without the use of instruments, and covering steristrips (Fig. 8).

A longer stump may be of considerable benefit in young patients with non-ischaemic limbs: 15 cm is ideal. Short anterior or lateral flaps may be used to keep the scar away from the prosthetic bearing surfaces. More complex myodesis procedures may also allow better function. A fibula bone bridge can be inserted between the tibia and fibula to allow the Achilles tendon to be brought over and sutured to holes in the anterior tibia. The anterior and posterior tibial muscles can be sutured together over the interosseus membrane.

Most below-knee prostheses rely on a patellar tendon bearing socket with either strap or suction suspension (Figs. 9, 10). A variety of ankle joints with varying degrees of ankle and toe flexion are available.

Through-knee amputation (knee disarticulation)

In non-ischaemic limbs where the knee joint is non-functional or when the limb is damaged in such a way that a below-knee amputation is not possible this operation has several advantages: it is quick and easy to perform, using the lateral flaps shown in Fig. 11; the stump is end-bearing, has good leverage, and the bulbous bony shape can be used to suspend the prothesis. Modern polycentric knee prostheses have overcome many of the difficulties of limb-fitting and the cosmetic result is reasonable.

The flaps required to cover the bulbous end of the femur are of considerable length and use less-well vascularized lateral skin. Healing may thus be poor in patients with vascular disease. A below-knee amputation will heal as well and if the ischaemia is considered inadequate for a below-knee amputation a knee disarticulation is unlikely to heal either. This operation is not usually performed in patients with vascular disease, except where retention of the knee joint is contraindicated and a fast bloodless amputation is required.

Prostheses which are available tend to be rather bulky and of similar design to those used after Gritti-Stokes amputation with

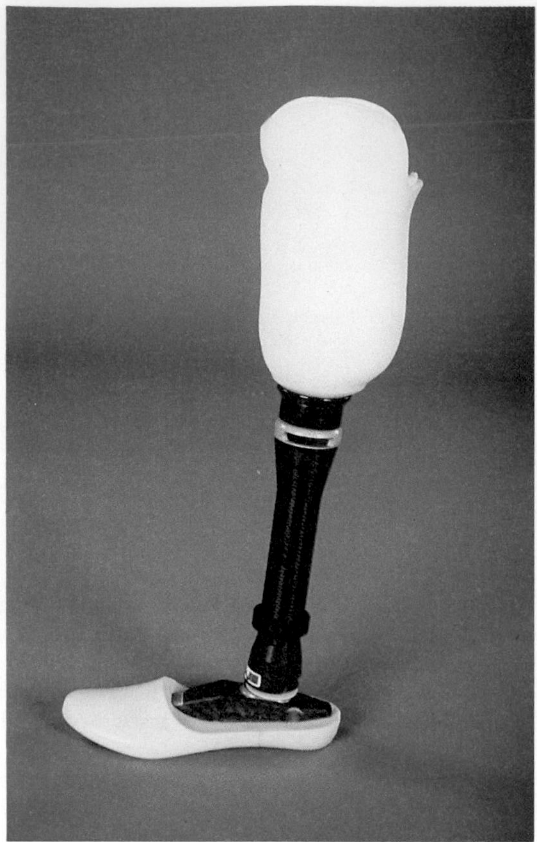

Fig. 9 Below-knee patella tendon bearing 'Endolite' prosthesis without cosmesis.

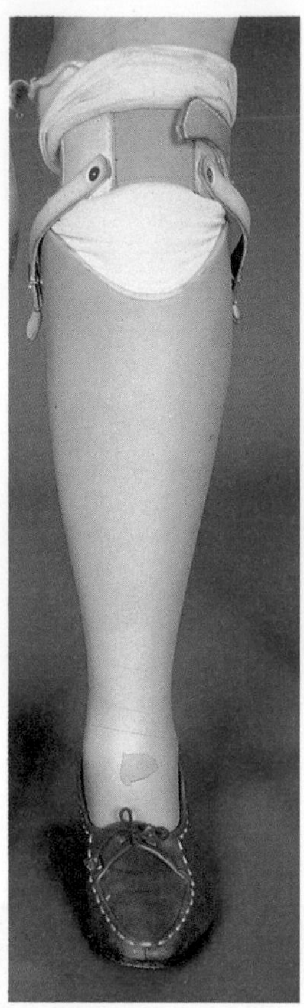

Fig. 10 Below-knee patella tendon bearing prosthesis with cosmesis and cuff suspension.

external joints (see Fig. 13). However the bulbous end can be used to allow suspension without a thigh corset and the socket can be end-bearing.

Gritti-Stokes amputation

The Gritti-Stokes amputation is a variety of through-knee amputation that has the advantage of using relatively well vascularized anterior skin, and so is useful for patients with or without vascular disease. The operation is useful for the few patients with ischaemic limbs who appear to have good perfusion below the knee but do not have the posterior flap of skin available to allow below-knee amputation (perhaps because of local infection or ulceration) and in those patients where retention of the knee joint is of no advantage. Gritti-Stokes amputation gives a long lever with partial end-bearing, although not as good as that obtained by knee disarticulation, and although the end is bulbous direct suspension of the prosthesis using the bulbous end is often not possible. Prostheses are good functionally but cosmetically inferior to those available for patients with above-knee amputation.

The basic points of the technique are shown in Fig. 12. The key point is the fixation of the patella remnant to the cut end of the femur. Some authorities recommend drilling the femur and using wire sutures for this purpose but the author has found that six strong absorbable sutures between the strong tissues at the periphery of the patella to the periosteum and surrounding tissues of the femur are adequate to ensure bony union. It is also helpful to make the cut through the femoral condyles proximal enough to

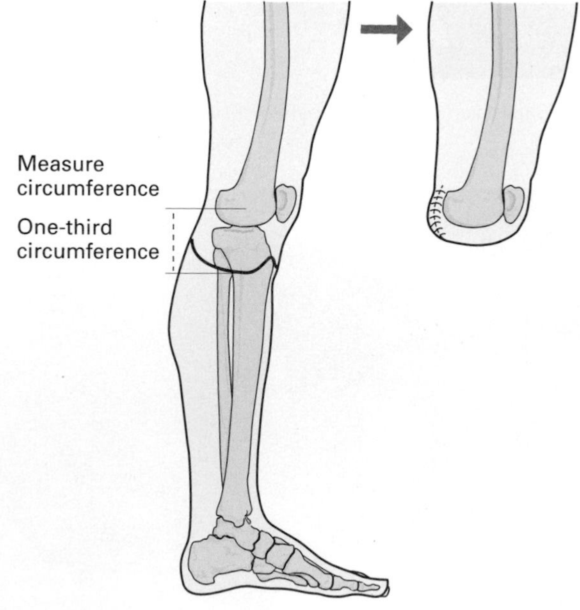

Fig. 11 Incision used for through knee-amputation (knee disarticulation) and final position.

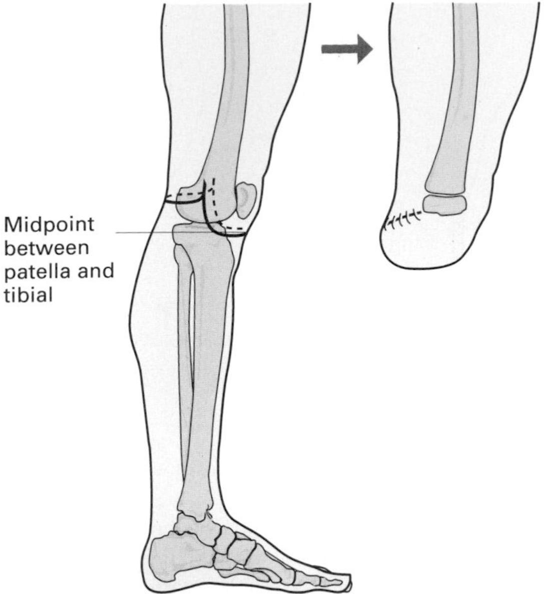

Fig. 12 Incision and principles of Gritti-Stokes amputation.

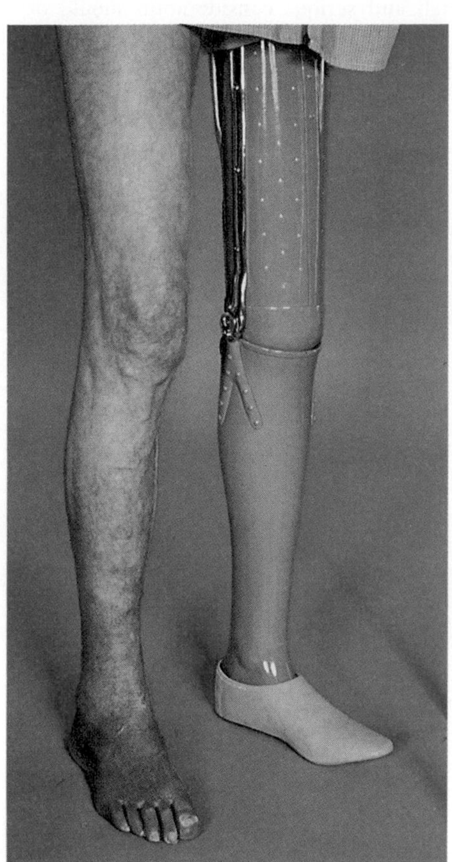

Fig. 13 Prosthesis for Gritti-Stokes amputation: an external knee joint must be used.

ensure there is relatively little tension and with a slight backward slope that encourages the patellar remnant to stay attached (Fig. 12).

Prostheses available are shown in Fig. 13.

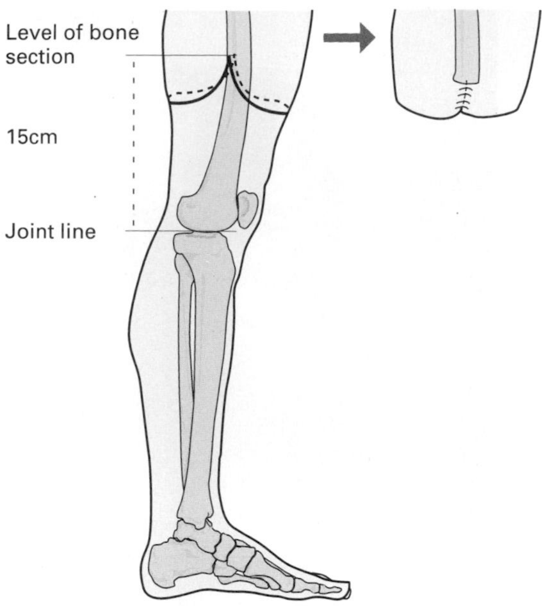

Fig. 14 Incision for above-knee amputation.

Above-knee amputation

The principles of the technique for patients with ischaemic limbs are shown in Fig. 14. Important points to note are that although a long femoral stump has advantages for leverage of a prosthesis this should not be at the expense of poor healing, as is often the case in excessively long stumps where the bone may be inadequately covered with soft tissues and the skin is stretched. In any case the site of division of the femur should not be more than 12 cm from the knee joint line to allow room for the knee mechanism in the prosthesis. The minimum length of stump that can be used to fit an above-knee prosthesis is 7.5 cm below the adductor muscle insertion. If the amputation must be shorter than this and it is hoped eventually to fit a prosthesis, a hip disarticulation should be performed, as this allows better fitting of modern prostheses and reduces weight.

The bone end should be rounded off and covered by suturing the deep fascia of the posterior flap, with its attached muscle, to the same structures anteriorly, enclosing a vacuum drain. The author prefers a subcuticular polypropylene suture with additional adhesive strips for closure.

Where amputation is performed in young patients with good vasculature the addition of more complex myodesis techniques to suture and overlap opposing groups of muscles using drill holes in the distal femur produces a stump that is a conical shape with better function. However these techniques do not work well in ischaemic limbs and may result in devitalization and failure of healing.

Prostheses available are shown in Figs. 15 and 16.

Hip disarticulation and hemipelvectomy

There is insufficient space to describe in detail the dissection required for these operations, which are usually performed in non-ischaemic patients, and the reader is directed to the references at the end of the chapter. The principle is to remove the required extent of the limb leaving a posterior flap with a layer of

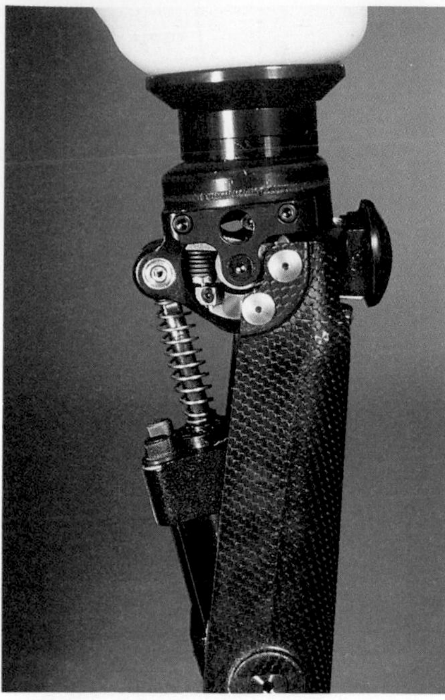

Fig. 15 Sophisticated knee joints are available to allow as near-normal gait as possible. Illustrated is a stabilized knee with pneumatic swing-phase control.

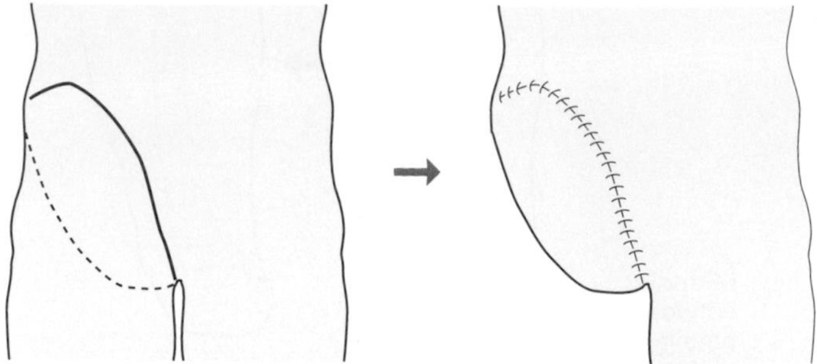

Fig. 17 Incision for hip disarticulation using a long posterior flap of skin and muscle to cover the defect.

viable muscle that can be used to cover and cushion the deep structures (Fig. 17).

Hip disarticulation and/or hemipelvectomy are rarely required for ischaemia, and when they are required infective gangrene is the usual cause. It is often not possible to produce the ideal flaps described for elective operations, and it is a question of using the best vascularized non-infected flap of skin available to cover the amputation site. Vascularized free flaps may be necessary. Mortality is high and serious consideration should be given in the elderly to non-intervention to allow death with dignity.

Prostheses available are shown in Fig. 18.

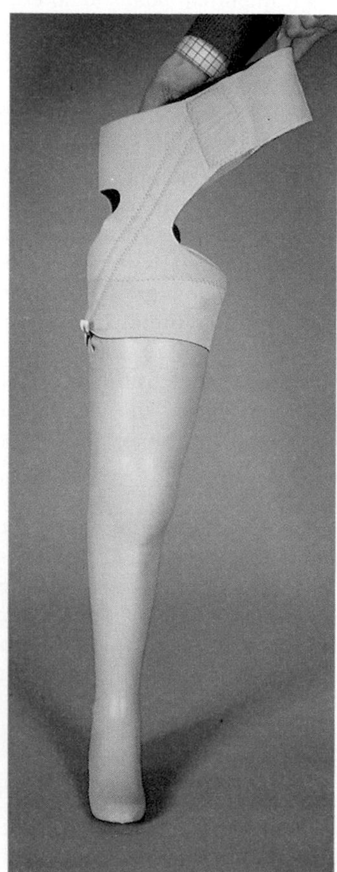

Fig. 16 Above-knee amputation prosthesis with cosmetic outer covering and soft neoprene suspension.

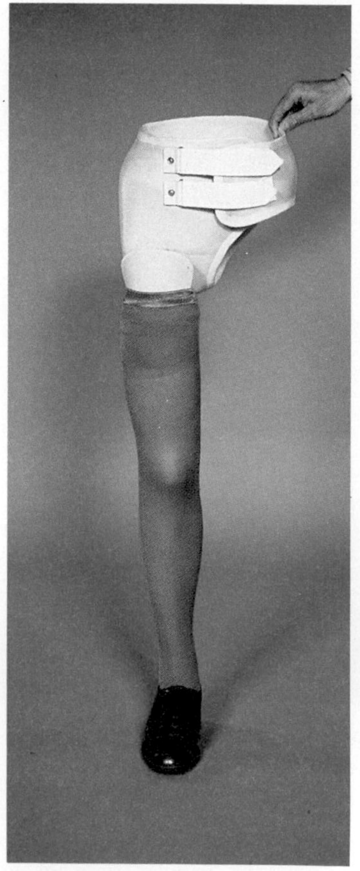

Fig. 18 Prosthesis for through-hip disarticulation. Note the anterior hinge joint.

Upper limb amputations

Finger and partial hand amputation

The usual indication is trauma and the general principle is to preserve as much viable tissue as possible, particularly preserving palmar surface skin and as much of the thumb as is practicable. Multiple injuries require specialist attention. Medial and lateral flaps should be used, which may be closed unless there has been gross contamination. If all the fingers and the palm of the hand are lost the wrist should be preserved since useful grip function can be obtained by use of an opposition plate.

Ischaemic fingers should be amputated as for ischaemic toes, (see above) leaving the wound open.

Cosmetic fingers are available but most patients choose to do without, since the prosthesis tends to get in the way.

Forearm amputation

The usual indication is for trauma. Equal length extensor and flexor flaps are fashioned as shown in Fig. 19, allowing bone section at around midforearm, if possible. Longer stumps than this have little advantage and tend to heal poorly. The minimum length that can work a forearm prosthesis is 5 cm below the biceps insertion. The extensor and flexor muscles are then sutured together under gentle tension over the bone ends, including the deep fascia with each bite.

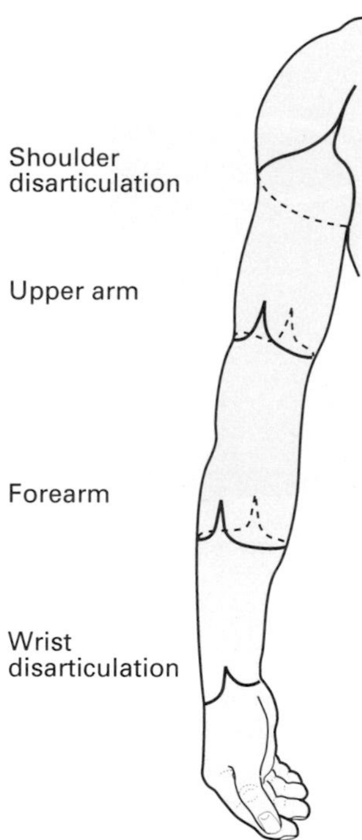

Fig. 19 Incisions used for amputations of the upper limb.

A variety of forearm prostheses are available (Figs. 20–22). Some use mechanical hands with the grip mechanism worked by a shoulder strap and cable (Fig. 20), or an electrically driven grip activated by muscle depolarization (Fig. 21). However, many patients find these cosmetic prostheses both heavy and functionally poor. The most functional prosthesis remains a split hook (Fig. 22) with special tools which can be fitted for specific tasks.

Elbow disarticulation

This amputation is not favoured, as fitting a useful prosthesis is difficult.

Above-elbow amputation

Equal length anterior and posterior flaps are used (Fig. 19). The bone should ideally be divided no closer than 9 cm above the medial epicondyle, to allow room for an elbow mechanism. The minimum length of humerus that allows an above-elbow prosthesis is 5 cm below the anterior axillary fold. However, provided that there are not over-riding reasons such as clearance of malignancy even a non-functional amputation across the humeral neck should be retained in preference to disarticulation, since it gives better cosmesis. The anterior muscle flap should be sutured over the bone end to the posterior muscle flap, with bites that include the deep fascia.

Although cosmetically acceptable prostheses are available, some with active grip using a shoulder activated cable (Fig. 23), the functional result is poor and these limbs are rarely used functionally if the patient has a normal contralateral arm.

Shoulder disarticulation and forequarter amputation

Virtually the only indication for these procedures is amputation for malignancy. There is insufficient space to discuss the details of the dissection required, but the incision for both is placed so as to allow a predominantly posterior flap to be brought forward to cover the amputation site, with an extension of the incision anterosuperiorly to allow access for proximal ligation of the limb vessels (Fig. 19). The operation results in considerable deformity which is difficult to disguise with prostheses that allow normal fit of clothing and retain function.

Although functional prostheses are available (see below) they are weighty and have poor function, so that many patients opt for a cosmetic shoulder filler only.

Auxiliary procedures for upper limp amputees

A number of complex operations have been described in the past to allow better function of arm prostheses. Most of these have now been abandoned and those that are still performed are usually not worth considering in a patient who has one normal arm. The formation of a skin-lined tunnel in the biceps muscle ('kineplastic tunnel') can sometimes be used to activate the terminal device of a forearm prosthesis. Patients that have lost both forearms can be given grip function by Krukenberg's operation, which separates the radius and ulna to act as separate jaws of a pincer. Although surprisingly good function can be obtained, the cosmetic penalties are considerable and are accepted by few patients.

Postoperative management

There are considerable differences in opinion on the dressing, bandaging, and prosthetic fitting of amputation stumps. It is the author's opinion that these differences stem from the experiences of different specialties dealing with either predominantly amputations performed for vascular disease or for non-vascular con-

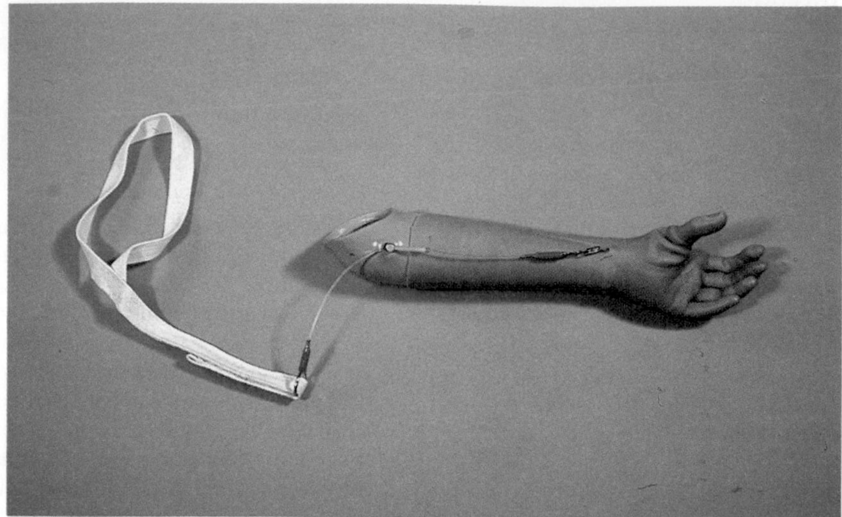

Fig. 20 Below-elbow amputation prosthesis with mechanical hand worked by a shoulder strap and cord.

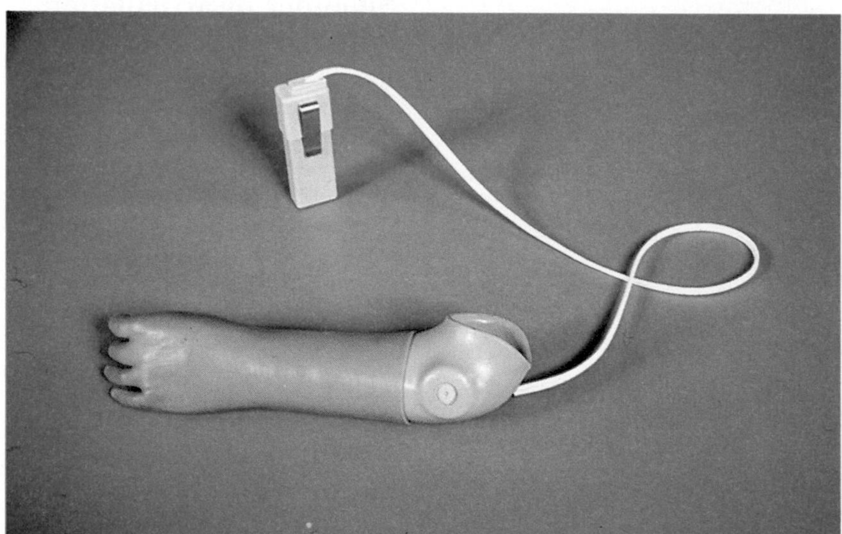

Fig. 21 Below-elbow prosthesis with electrically operated hand grip and myoelectric activator (child's).

ditions, and the management of these groups should probably be different.

Amputations for vascular disease should be dressed with a loose-fitting stump bandage, without compression. The bandage will tend to fall off unless supported by multiple longitudinal strips of adhesive tape, but compression may produce local necrosis of skin that is balanced on the edge of ischaemia, and a tourniquet effect, which is easily produced by inexpert bandaging, can be disastrous. Although the dressing is best left undisturbed if all is well, the stump must be viewed if there is any question of infection. The use of a plaster cast, suggested by some authors, is not recommended since it impedes the ease of access to the stump. Gentle active exercise should be encouraged by the physiotherapist, within the limits of pain. Some authorities recommend immediate fitting of a prosthesis and encourage rapid progression to walking within a few days. In the author's opinion this method may be possible in a centre with prosthetists able to attend at all times and the staff able to supervise walking properly, but for most hospitals such facilities are not available and this approach is potentially dangerous. The first goal is wound healing and the author recommends that the stump be left until primary healing of the wound is well under way, usually 2 weeks or more, before trying a few steps under supervision in a pneumatic pylon to regain bipedal balance. Subsequent progression to an adjustable training prosthesis encourages early learning of correct gait with moulding and shrinkage of the stump and the final prosthesis can often be fitted by 6 weeks.

Refinements such as preoperative physiotherapy and counsel-

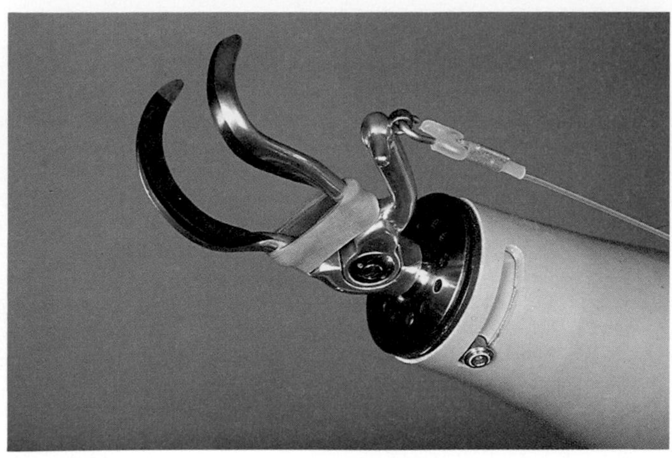

Fig. 22 Split hook prosthesis with wrist rotary action.

ling, postoperative compressive stump bandages, and plaster casts with fitted prostheses to allow immediate mobilization are applicable to young amputees, particularly those undergoing amputation for malignancy, and remarkable results can be obtained in this group.

Most patients, particularly the elderly, need to use a wheelchair some or all of the time around the house, and the home must be visited at an early stage to assess the modifications necessary for a wheelchair to be used before the patient returns.

Complications of amputation surgery

Early complications

Primary haemorrhage should be a rarity if blood vessels are ligated, but venous oozing is common and should be prevented from collecting and causing swelling and stump breakdown by insertion of a vacuum drain in all amputations. Infection is common, and is usually due to *Staphylococcus aureus* but other organisms such as *Clostridium* spp. may occur, particularly in ischaemic limbs. Strict aseptic technique, avoidance of excessive dressings and use of appropriate preventative antibiotics preoperatively and for at least 5 days postoperatively is recommended. Extensive infection despite these measures usually denotes inadequate blood supply and reamputation to a higher level is needed. Small areas of skin necrosis in the suture line may remain uninfected and subsequently heal, helped by wedge excision surgery if necessary, but extensive necrosis with pain should not be left until it becomes infected: early reamputation is a better option.

Late complications

Provided that skin healing is obtained most stumps can be fitted with a usable prosthesis and the site of the scar is usually immaterial. The exception is a scar that is adherent to a bony prominence since this will eventually ulcerate. Sometimes a thick skin graft or myoplastic flap can be swung in to cover the area, usually requiring the assistance of the plastic surgery department. Otherwise this problem may prevent satisfactory prosthesis use.

Some stumps with redundant tissue develop epidermoid cystic change at pressure points that often become infected. These can be excised, but unless the fundamental problem of chafing and maceration by the prosthesis is cured recurrence is inevitable. Terminal chronic oedema with verrucose hyperplasia occurs in stumps that are not supported sufficiently at the distal end (Fig. 24).

Stump neuromas, sometimes up to golfball size, are common, but unless they lie under a point of pressure and a trigger point is demonstrable they rarely need excision. Persistent stump or phantom pain is a problem in some patients. Sometimes ischaemia is the obvious cause but in others this is not the case. Phantom pain will usually lessen with time and techniques such as ultrasound therapy and transcutaneous electrical nerve stimulation may be helpful, combined at times with psychiatric support and antidepressive therapy.

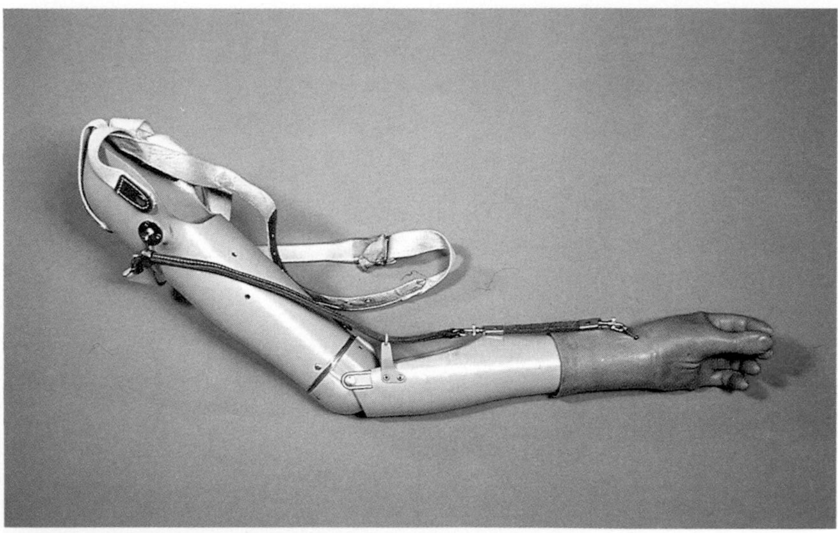

Fig. 23 Above-elbow prosthesis with mechanical hand and Bowden operating cable.

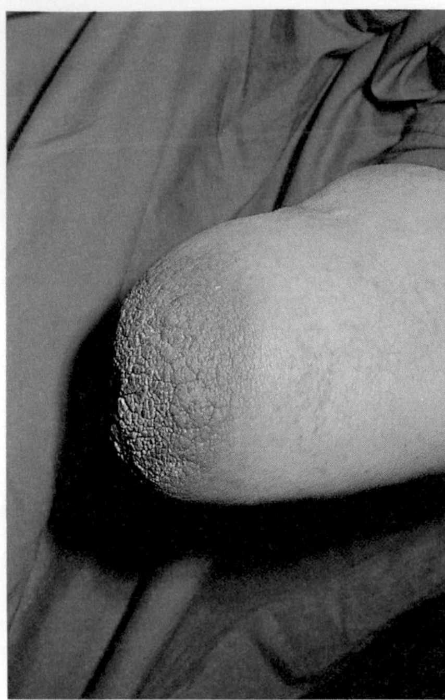

Fig. 24 Below-knee amputation stump with terminal verrucose hyperplasia due to inadequate distal support.

FURTHER READING

Burgess EM, Romano RL. The management of lower extremity amputees using immediate postsurgical prostheses. *Clin Orthop* 1968; **57**: 137–56.

Burgess EM, Romano RL, Zettl JH, Schrock RD. Amputations of the leg for peripheral vascular insufficiency. *J Bone Joint Surg* 1971; **53A**: 874–90.

Gray DWR, Ng R. Anatomical aspects of the blood supply to the skin of the posterior calf: technique of below-knee amputation. *Br J Surg* 1990; **77**: 662–4.

Greenhalgh RM, Jamieson CW, Nicolaides A, eds. *Limb salvage and amputation for vascular disease*. Philadelphia: Saunders, 1988.

Kostuik JP, Gillespie R, eds. *Amputation surgery and rehabilitation: the Toronto experience*. New York: Churchill Livingstone, 1981.

Moore WS, Malone JM, eds. *Lower extremity amputation*. Philadelphia: Saunders, 1989.

Murdoch G, Donovan RG, eds. *Amputation surgery and lower limb prosthetics*. Oxford: Blackwell Scientific, 1988.

Robinson KP, Hoile R, Coddington T. Skew flap myoplastic below-knee amputation: a preliminary report. *Br J Surg* 1982; **69**: 554–7.

Royal College of Surgeons. Report of a symposium on amputations and prosthetics held at the Royal College of Surgeons of England. *Ann R Coll Surg* 1967; **40**: 203–88.

Vitali M, Robinson KP, Andrews BG, Harris EE. *Amputations and prostheses*. 2nd edn. London: Balliere Tindall, 1986.

The veins 8

8.1 Venous disorders, vascular malformations, and chronic ulceration in the lower limbs

DAVID J. TIBBS

The veins of the lower limb must not be viewed as a series of inert venous conduits but rather as a complex pumping mechanism capable of returning venous blood to the heart against the force of gravity in the upright position. If active thrombosis is excluded, it is some form of failure in this mechanism that underlies nearly all venous disorders in the lower limb. The essentials of normal anatomy and physiology will be described first, especially those aspects that may undergo change and cause venous problems.

NORMAL ANATOMY AND PHYSIOLOGY

Essential properties of veins

Structure of the veins

Unlike arteries, the veins are specifically designed to allow flow in one direction only, towards the heart, and this is achieved by the presence of numerous valves arranged along their length (Fig. 1). Only in the common iliac veins, vena cava, the portal system, and in the cranial sinuses are these valves lacking. They form an essential part of the venous pumping mechanisms returning blood from the lower limbs against gravity and act to protect the peripheral tissues from back pressure set up by columns of blood when the patient is upright. Each valve is made up of two gossamer thin cusps which in spite of their delicate appearance are surprisingly strong (Fig. 2). The cusps are supported by the vein walls and their integrity as functioning valves depends on this support having sufficient strength to resist forces dilating the veins and tending to separate the cusps. The vein walls are thin but capable of considerable distension or contraction and these qualities are provided by circumferential rings of elastic tissue and smooth muscle. When the patient is upright and standing still, the veins are maximally distended and the diameter may be several times greater than in the horizontal limb at rest. The veins are very flexible; if the limb is elevated so that all blood leaves the veins, not only do they contract down to minimal size, but also collapse into a thin ribbon-like shape. Such a highly flexible, thin walled structure which collapses easily does not allow suction to be transmitted along its length and siphonage plays virtually no part in the movement of venous blood. It is incorrect to think of blood ever being sucked from one part of the venous system to another in the limbs.

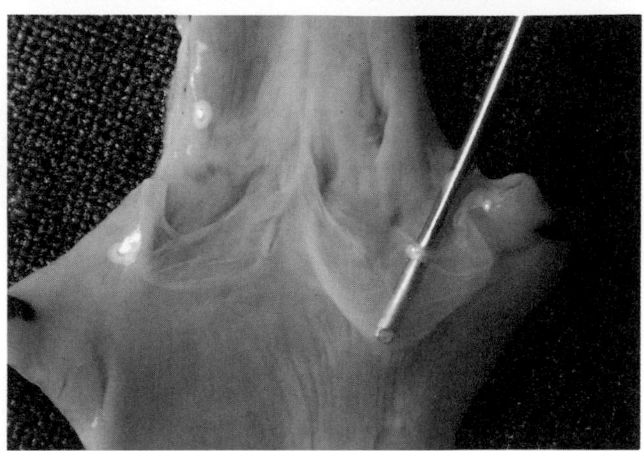

Fig. 2 A vein opened to show a pair of valve cusps. The probe lifts one cusp to display its delicate structure.

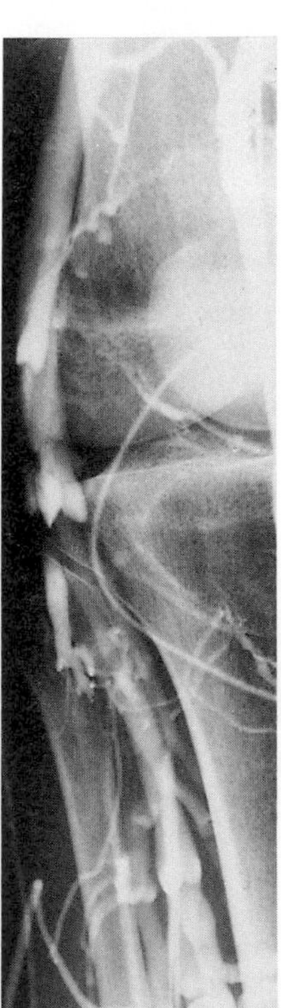

Fig. 1 Normal competent valves in a popliteal vein and its branches shown by phlebography. Such valves are essential for normal function in both superficial and deep veins.

As with arteries the interior of the veins is lined with endothelium, providing a non-thrombogenic surface, but in the case of veins, where slow flow and long periods of stasis might encourage thrombosis more easily than arteries, there is an enhanced protective mechanism providing prostacyclins to prevent aggregation of platelets, and actively forming fibrinolysins (plasmin) capable of dissolving thrombus and clot.

Arrangement of deep veins in the lower limbs

The deep veins lie beneath the deep fascia but do not all serve the same function, merely varying in size. They may be divided into two major categories.

The veins as conduits

The major veins in the limbs and the numerous branches joining them serve as conduits, taking blood back from the tissues towards the heart. These are the veins depicted in most anatomical diagrams starting as plantar veins running to tibial veins, through popliteal and superficial femoral veins to common femoral and iliac veins, and so into the inferior vena cava (Fig. 3). However, these veins make only a limited contribution to the active pumping of blood upwards against gravity which is so essential in the lower limbs and this function is largely dependent on the venous sinuses within muscle that act as highly efficient pumping chambers.

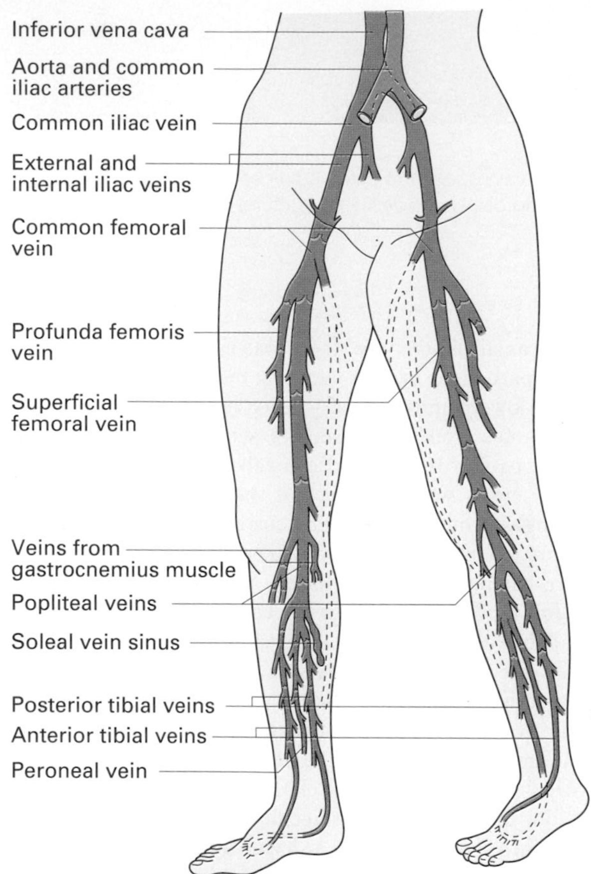

Fig. 3 The main venous conduits formed by the deep veins of the lower limbs; numerous branch veins join these.

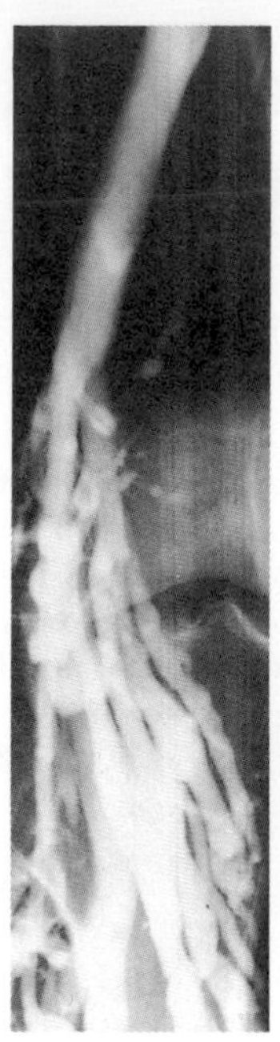

Fig. 4 Multiple venous sinuses within a gastrocnemius muscle. These are valved and act as pumping chambers for returning blood from muscle back to the heart against gravity. The soleus also has notably large venous sinuses but all muscles have similar provision for pumping although varying greatly in size, distribution, and number.

Veins as pumping chambers

The lower limbs have powerful muscles capable of great effort. During activity these require a copious flow of blood. Distributed throughout these muscles are numerous venous sinuses (Fig. 4). Their shape varies considerably in different muscles, some being long and thin (for example in the peroneal muscles) and others being broad and bulky, as found in the soleal and gastrocnemius muscles. The greater the effort required of the muscle, the larger the venous sinuses will be. Because the sinuses are surrounded by the muscle fibres they are strongly compressed when the muscle contracts and blood within them is driven out through connecting veins to join the main conduit veins (Fig. 5); the connecting veins

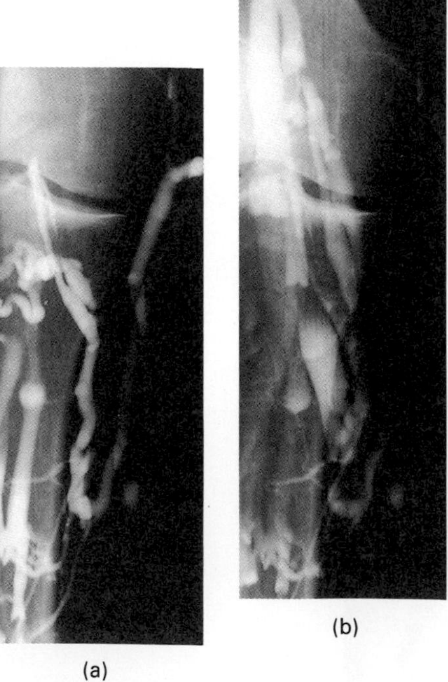

Fig. 5 Functional phlebograms demonstrating the pumping action of venous sinuses in gastrocnemius muscle. (a) During contraction, the sinuses are emptied. (b) After contraction, with muscle relaxed, the sinuses fall slack and allow easy refilling with blood ready to be expelled upwards with the next contraction.

are valved and situated at the heartward end of each sinus. Blood that has crossed the capillary beds of muscle passes through numerous small vessels into each sinus which fills to capacity from this source or until it is emptied by the next muscle contraction. In addition, veins communicating with superficial veins perforate the deep fascia and enter many sinuses near their distal ends (Fig. 6). The valves of these perforating veins allow flow inwards to the sinuses but prevent outward flow from them and, in this way,

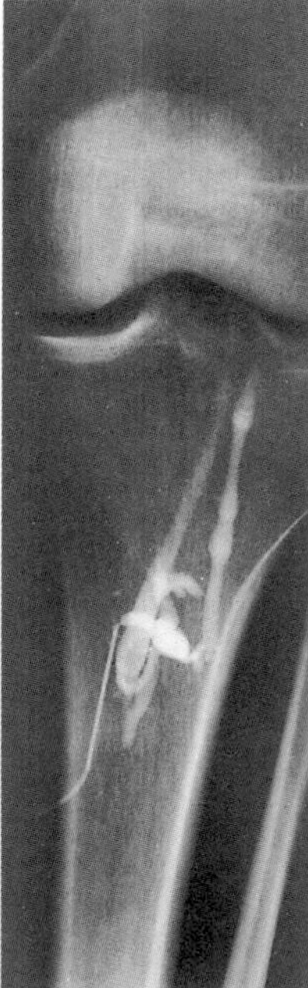
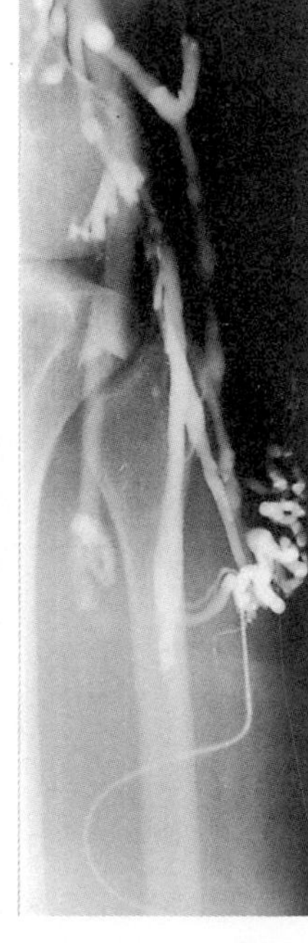
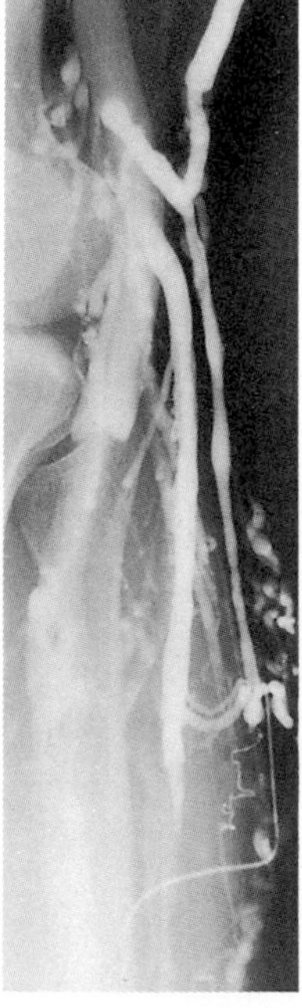

Fig. 6 Filling of a venous sinus in muscle from overlying superficial (varicose) veins. Phases of filling are viewed in two different rotations. A pair of perforating veins take flow directly from the superficial veins into a gastrocnemius sinus. Such inward flow is normal and often seen at all levels. A gastrocnemius sinus outlined in this fashion is easily mistaken for the neighbouring short saphenous vein, also shown here with an upward extension from it.

blood accumulated in superficial veins can enter the muscle sinuses when they are slack. Each sinus, together with the surrounding muscle fibres, forms an elegant and effective pumping chamber emptied at each contraction and propelling blood towards the heart. The valve arrangement in the conduit veins ensures that blood only moves in this direction and protects the sinus from unwanted reflux once contraction has ceased and the sinus is empty. Thus, the sinus can only fill from the intended sources, the muscular capillary beds, perforating veins, and interconnecting veins running between sinuses. All the muscles in the lower limbs, ranging from diminutive muscles, such as the plantar, to the massive muscles of the calf, contribute to this widespread pumping system which is often collectively termed the musculovenous pump. Sometimes this is referred to, for convenience, as the 'calf muscle pump': however, this implies that the muscles of the calf are the only ones that matter when, in fact, all muscle groups in the leg* and foot play an important part and are also implicated in any disorders that may arise.

* In this Section the term 'leg' is used in the anatomical sense, referring to the portion of lower limb below the knee.

Additional pumping mechanisms

Because of their valves, all veins are capable of contributing to venous return against gravity, in response to pressure by surrounding muscles or by any form of external pressure.

Changing the position of the limb from dependency to elevation will cause blood trapped between valves to empty proximally so that a form of pumping can be provided by repeatedly changing the position of the limb.

The underside of the foot provides a substantial pumping mechanism, partly because of the muscles within it, but perhaps even more so by the bodyweight compressing the underside of the foot against the ground at each footstep. The pool of blood in the capacious venous plexus under the foot is emptied upwards and, in the normal state, prevented from returning by valves in superficial and deep veins of the lower leg. Loss of effective valves here plays a significant part in venous disease.

Conclusion

Proper venous return from the lower limb depends upon an intricate pumping mechanism requiring numerous effective valves. Failure of the valves for any reason will reduce the effectiveness of venous return in the upright posture and may lead to an undesirable state of unrelieved venous pressure, or venous hypertension.

The superficial veins and perforating veins

Superficial veins

In addition to the deep vein systems of conduits and pumping chambers described above, there is a system of superficial veins lying outside the deep fascia subcutaneously. This commences as a network of fine veins mainly from the skin itself, that merge into branch veins running into two principal superficial veins, the long and the short saphenous veins (synonyms—greater or internal, and lesser or external). These, together with their branches, form two clearly identifiable systems but there is free interconnection between them. Figure 7 shows a typical arrangement of the superficial veins, including those branches commonly involved in venous disorders. There is much individual variation in the details and some of these variants will be discussed later. The long saphenous vein runs subcutaneously up the inner leg and thigh to the groin where it passes through the fossa ovalis to join the common femoral vein (Fig. 8). The short saphenous vein passes through the deep fascia somewhere between midcalf and knee and runs for a short distance beneath the fascia to end by joining the popliteal vein at a variable level but usually opposite the femoral condyles (Fig. 9); here it commonly gives off an upward extension (sometimes called the Giacomini vein) which may run deeply in continuity with the profunda femoris vein, or superficially curving round to join the long saphenous vein by its posteromedial branch in the upper thigh. Both saphenous systems have valves at intervals along their length and these valves become more numerous in the lower part of the leg, in keeping with the progressive increase in pressure to be resisted down the length of the limb when upright (Fig. 10).

The superficial veins, draining skin and subcutaneous tissues, play a major role in the regulation of body temperature. In hot conditions, greatly increased blood flow through the skin causes it to act as a radiator, aided by evaporation of sweat, very effectively losing body heat. The superficial veins dilate to remove the rapid

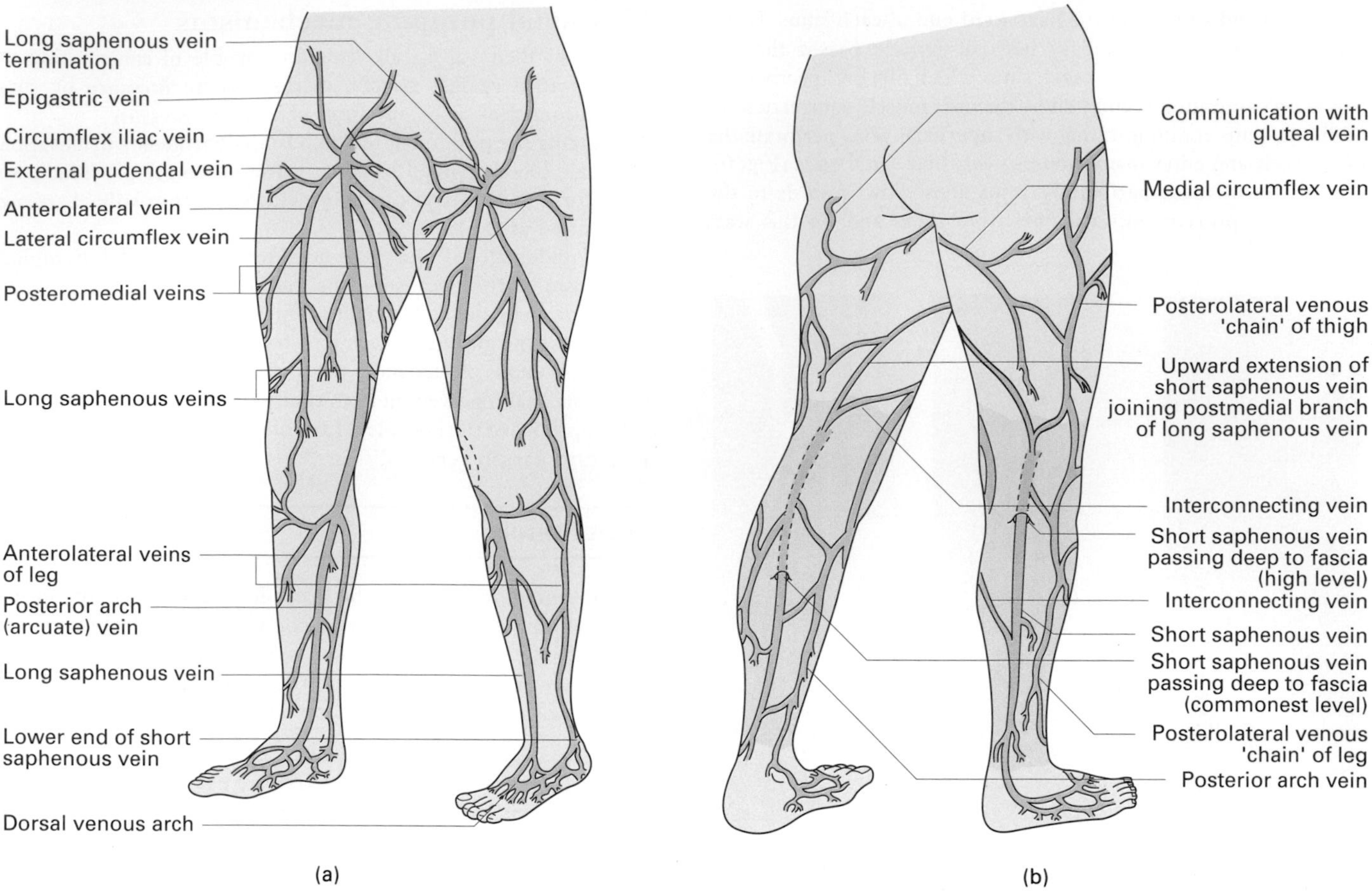

Fig. 7 The principal superficial veins are mainly arranged as the long and short saphenous systems. These empty into the deep veins via the saphenous terminations but also by numerous perforating veins. (a) Anterior aspect. (b) Posterior aspect.

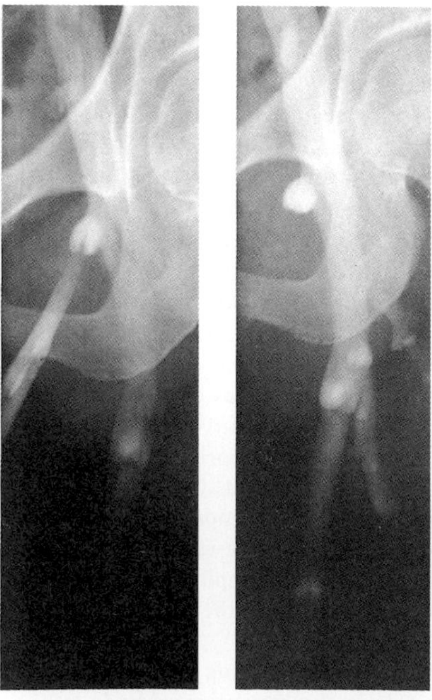

Fig. 8 A normal saphenous termination shown in two phases of filling at phlebography. Note the valve guarding its uppermost part and preventing reflux down it.

flow of blood and, in warm conditions or during exercise, these veins are maximally dilated, but in cold and inactive circumstances are constricted and inconspicuous. In venous disorders, enlarged or varicose veins will reflect these changes and in the very conditions in which patients wish to uncover their limbs the venous defects are most obvious.

Perforating veins

The saphenous veins empty blood at their terminations into popliteal and common femoral veins but they can also empty by numerous perforating veins running from the superficial veins through the deep fascia to join deep veins (Fig. 11). It has been estimated that there are over 60 such perforating veins distributed over all aspects of a lower limb. These perforators are often paired and many run directly into the deep conduit veins but, as previously said, others communicate with the venous sinuses in muscles (Fig. 6). Some perforators are more liable than others to be involved in venous disorders and have been given eponyms after the authority first drawing attention to them, but this is an oversimplification because other perforators, found extensively over the lower limbs, are, in fact, often implicated in venous disorders.

Most perforators are valved to allow only inward flow from superficial to deep veins but it is probable that the arrangement of fibres at the fascial apertures also plays a part in preventing outward flow when muscle contraction causes a sharp rise of pressure within the sinuses. Small perforators, less than 2 mm in diameter

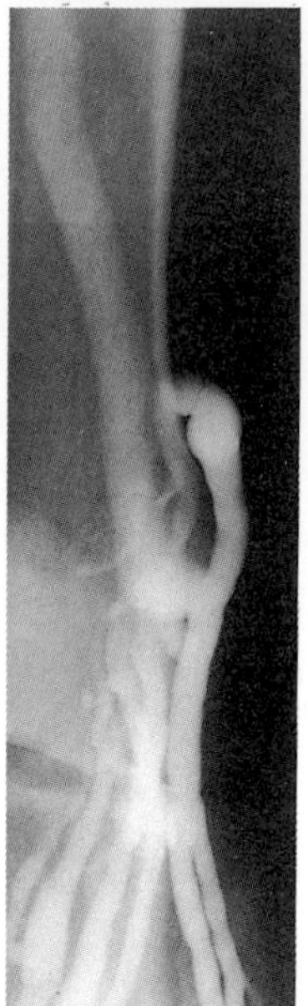
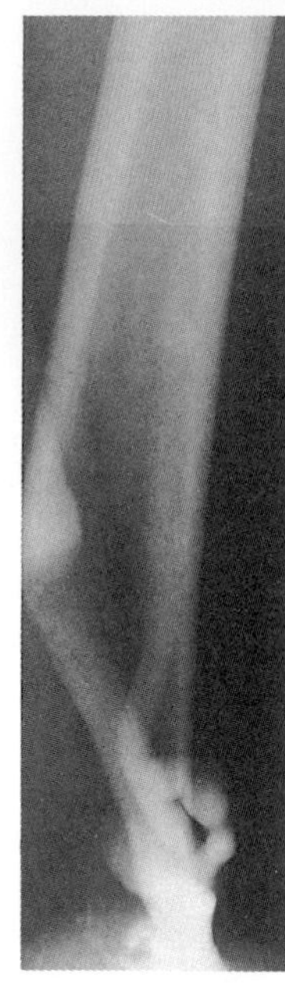
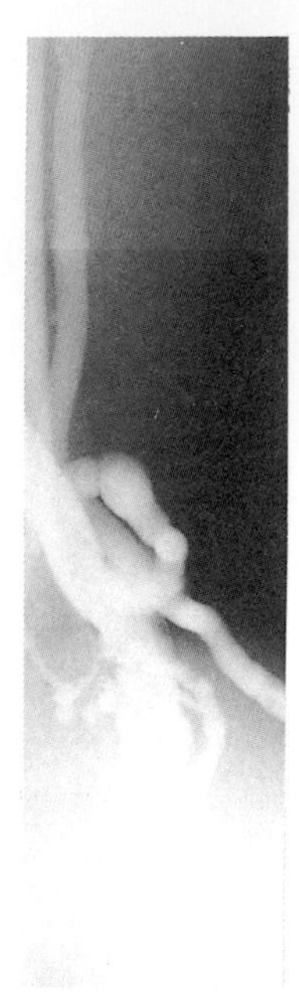

Fig. 9 A short saphenous termination shown in differing rotations at phlebography. In this example, the main junction with popliteal vein is at the most common level, opposite to the femoral condyles, and a substantial branch continues upwards (Giacomini vein) to join the profunda femoris vein. This upward extension commonly occurs and many variations are possible; for example, it may follow a superficial course to join the long saphenous vein posteromedially.

Inferior vena cava: No valves

Common iliac vein: No valves

External iliac and upper common femoral vein: Only 1 valve in 2 in 3 people, no valve in 1 in 3 people

Lower common femoral vein: No valves

Upper superficial and profunda femoris veins: 1 valve each in 1 in 3

Superficial femoral vein: 3 or 4 valves (variable)

Short saphenous vein: 1 upper valve, about 5 below

Tibial and peroneal veins: 8+ valves to ankle and numerous valves guarding muscular branches and sinuses

External iliac and upper common femoral veins: Valves absent on both sides in 1 in 10; absent on one side in 1 in 3: commonly absent in long saphenous incompetence and varicose veins

Long saphenous vein: 1 or 2 valves in first 4cm

Long saphenous vein of thigh: 5 valves (variable)

Knee joint

Long saphenous vein to ankle: 8+ valves

Valves in both superficial and deep veins more numerous below knee – in keeping with higher venous pressure and greater pumping requirements in more dependent parts

Fig. 10 Diagram indicating the distribution of valves usually present in superficial and deep veins.

tend not to be valved and presumably are responsible for equalization of pressure by outflow from deep to superficial veins.

When the limb is horizontal, superficial drainage is partly through the saphenous terminations and partly by the perforators to the deep veins. However, when upright, there is normally very little pumping action sending blood up the saphenous veins and the perforators play a major role in venous return from the superficial veins. When one stands still, the saphenous veins tend to fill steadily, but after muscular contraction, the resulting fall in deep venous pressure attracts flow from superficial to deep veins, through the perforators in the direction allowed by valves. Thus, in an upright and actively moving person most superficial drainage is by multiple perforators up the length of the limb rather than following each saphenous vein to its termination. When upright but motionless, both superficial and deep pressures remain equal, rising slowly in parallel fashion to maximal, and there is a slow drift of passive flow up both sets of veins; in this state, even a single movement causing muscle contraction to empty the deep veins will be immediately followed by flow from superficial veins, via perforators, into the deep veins. Because the saphenous veins and their branches have numerous valves the continuous column of blood in these veins becomes segmented between the valves as each part empties inwardly through its own group of perforators (Fig. 12). In this way, a continuous column of blood up a saphenous vein becomes a series of cascades between the valves.

Collateral flow

Reversed flow through perforators in a leg, that is to say outwardly from the deep veins, can often be demonstrated in apparently normal limbs when the popliteal vein is compressed so that surface veins are artificially caused to take on the role of collaterals. This phenomenon becomes a permanent feature in post-thrombotic deep vein obstruction where the perforators and superficial veins become part of a regular collateral system allowing continuous outflow, up the superficial veins, and past the underlying obstructed deep veins (Fig. 13). Such collateral veins may become greatly enlarged by forceful flow through them. In other circumstances, primary failure of the valve mechanism in a perforating vein may allow it to become the source of downflow in superficial veins with incompetent valves and this will be discussed presently. Occasionally, failure of perforator valves allows forceful ejection from intramuscular venous sinuses on contraction and causes enlarged, tortuous veins in the vicinity.

Creation of flow within veins

Only three forces create movement of venous blood in the limbs: arterial pressure across the capillary beds, the musculovenous pumps, and gravity.

1. In the arteries, pressure created at each heartbeat pumps the blood towards the peripheral capillary beds and is only slightly assisted or impeded by gravity, depending on the position of the limb. When standing upright and motionless, venous blood derived from peripheral capillary beds starts back towards the heart at a low pressure and slow delivery. This transcapillary flow leads to a slow build-up of pressure sufficient to give a drift of blood back to the heart. Eventually, this process causes a prolonged rise of capillary and venous pressure in foot and ankle region to 100 mmHg or more, which has undesirable consequences if maintained too long. This aspect will be discussed further.

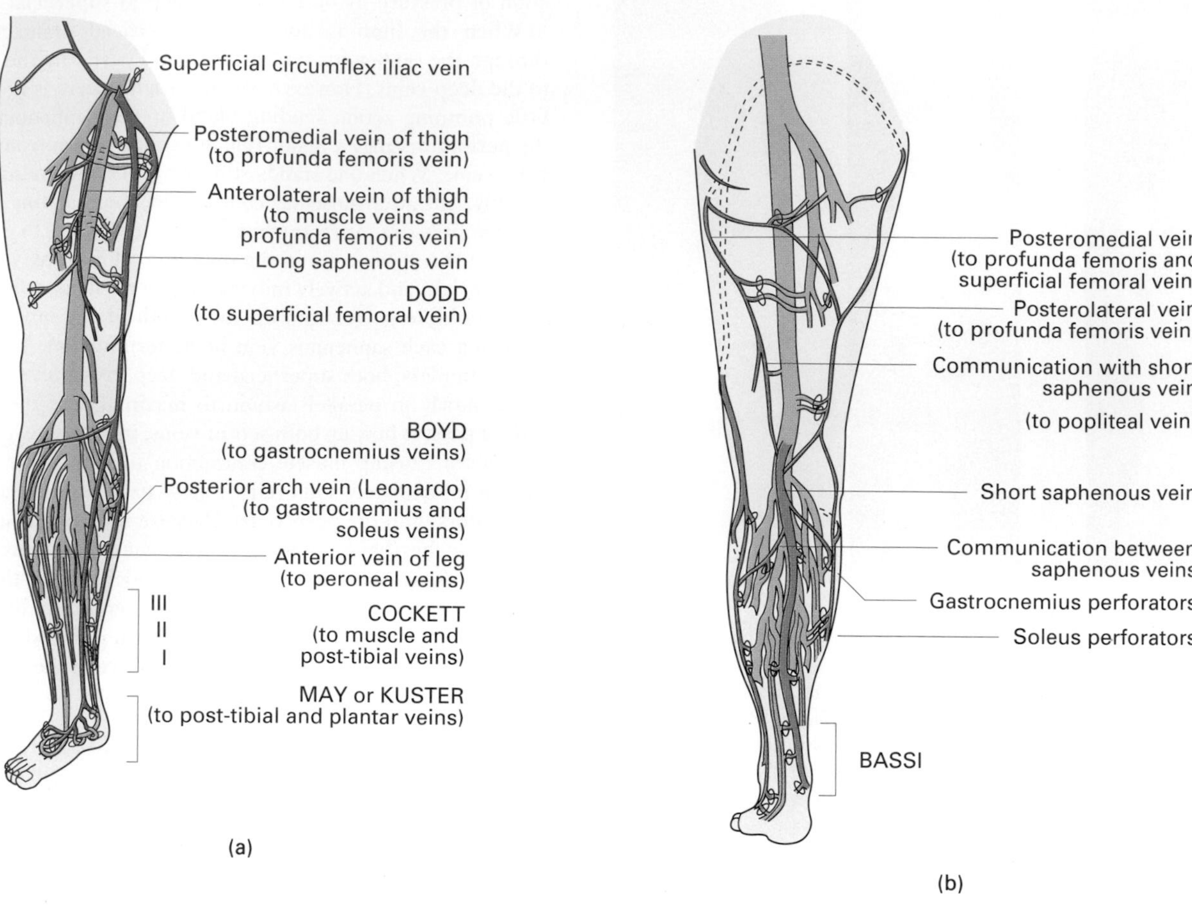

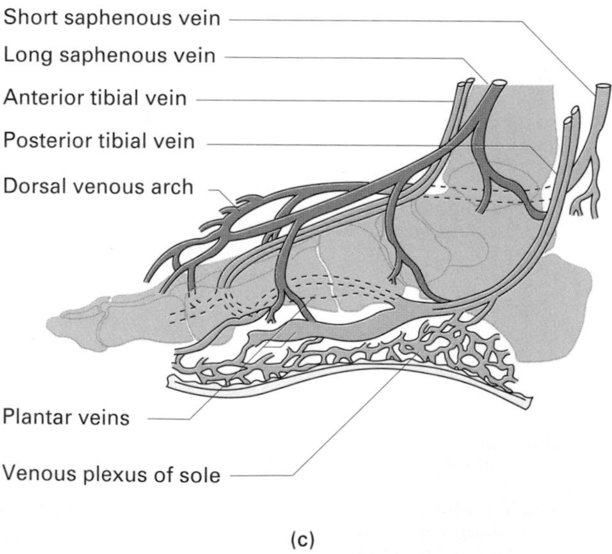

Fig. 11 Diagram of the principal perforator veins communicating between superficial and deep veins. Many have been given eponyms after authorities describing their importance in venous disorders. In addition to those shown here there are many more present at all levels, any of which may participate in venous problems. (a) Anterior aspect. (b) Posterior aspect. (c) The foot.

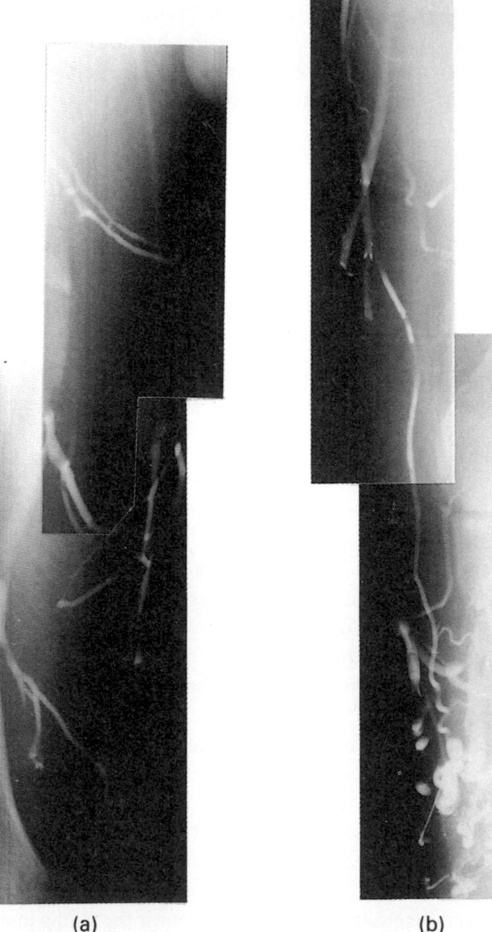

Fig. 12 Perforating veins in the thigh and their role in emptying the long saphenous vein in the upright position. Phlebograms from two limbs are shown. (a) Three sets of normal perforating veins have been outlined. The upper pair run posteriorly to join the profunda femoris; the lower ones run obliquely to the femoral vein in the mid and lower thigh. (b) Segmentation of blood into columns between valves in the thigh after repositioning the limb has partially emptied the saphenous vein.

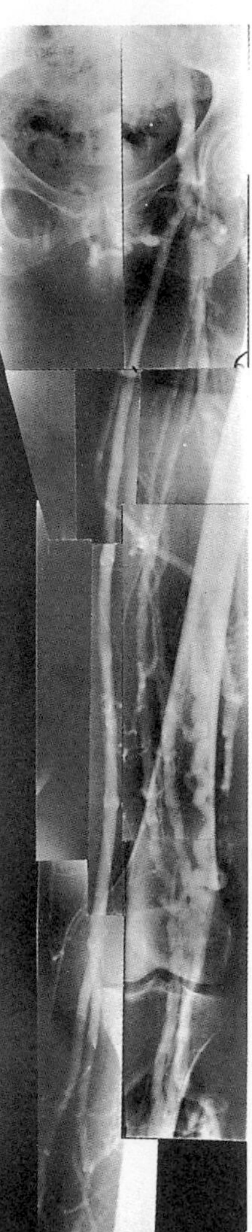

Fig. 13 Composite phlebogram of a limb with extensive obstruction of the deep veins following thrombosis some years previously. The long saphenous vein is shown acting as an important collateral channel past the deficient deep veins; although somewhat enlarged it is well valved and providing an excellent substitute. In the pubic region, branch veins are enlarged and tortuous by acting as collaterals across to the opposite side, compensating for left iliac vein occlusion.

2. By far the most powerful force creating venous return flow is the musculovenous pumping mechanism that can handle large volumes rapidly and generate a force well in excess of that required for venous return against gravity. Operation of the 'pump' (Fig. 14) is followed by a sharp fall in venous pressure in the lower part of the limb and, as will be seen later, extensive damage to this pumping system by thrombosis can seriously impair the well-being of the limb.
3. The third force causing venous flow is gravity itself. If the limb is elevated above the horizontal, flow towards the heart occurs by simple gravitational downflow without any need for assistance by transcapillary pressure or the musculovenous pump. Elevating the limb to promote venous flow is an important principle in the treatment of conditions where venous return is impeded for any reason. When the limb is in a dependent position, a normal set of valves in deep and superficial veins will, of course, prevent reflux of blood against the normal direction of venous flow. A failure of competence in the valves will, however, lead to retrograde flow down the limb when the patient first stands, or after an exercise movement has created slack veins in the lower part of the leg. In the superficial veins, this is the basis of the most common venous disorder of all, simple varicose veins.

Venous pressure changes within the lower limbs

When a person with normal veins rises from horizontal to upright position and the veins steadily fill by arterial inflow, the venous pressure in superficial and deep veins in the foot and ankle gradually rise over the next 30 to 60 s to that exerted by the column of blood from foot to heart level, about 100 mmHg, dependent upon overall height. This assumes that the subject stands still without movement because as soon as this occurs blood is pumped upwards and the pressure within them drops. A series of movements, such as walking, will empty the veins in the lower leg very effectively (Fig. 14) so that the pressure within them drops to around 20 mmHg and whilst movement continues it remains there (Fig. 15). On ceasing to walk and standing still the venous pressure again climbs steadily over the next minute to its previous

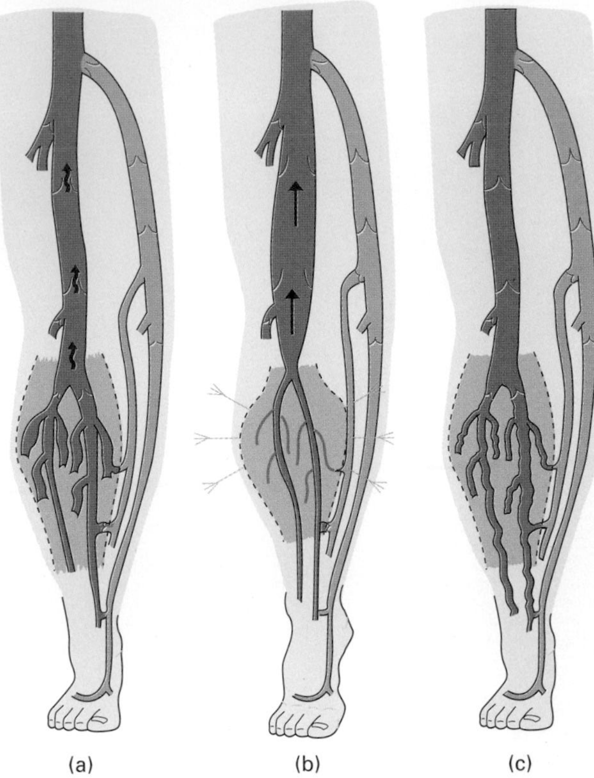

Fig. 14 Normal venous return against gravity in the upright position. (a) Standing still the veins fill to capacity in about 30 s. (b) With contraction of leg muscles the deep veins are compressed and empty upwards, the only direction permitted by valves. (c) With relaxation of muscle, the veins, protected from reflux by valves, are slack and refill slowly by arterial flow across capillary beds.

level but even a small single movement of the lower limb will cause a significant drop for many seconds. When capillary flow is greatly enhanced by muscular activity, each muscle contraction creates a corresponding increase in venous return and fall in the venous pressure. Without effective musculovenous pumping, removing the large flow of blood through contracting muscle, a most damaging rise in venous pressure occurs, giving severe venous hypertension. The characteristic changes and harmful effects caused by this will be discussed later but the causes for ineffective pumping are summarized in the next section.

DISORDERED VENOUS FUNCTION

Causes for failure in venous return and resulting venous hypertension

Venous insufficiency, a state of inadequate venous return in the upright position and accompanied by venous hypertension, may occur in the following circumstances.

1. The overwhelming of the pumping mechanism by massive downflow in superficial veins with deficient or defective valves, as often occurs in simple varicose veins.
2. Widespread impairment of the musculovenous pumping mechanism during active venous thrombosis, for example, acute deep vein thrombosis.
3. Obstruction or deformity in the main venous conduits as a consequence of venous thrombosis (post-thrombotic syndrome).
4. Loss of deep vein valve competence, or replacement of the deep veins by enlarged, valveless, collateral veins, as occurs in post-thrombotic states.
5. Inborn deficiency of deep vein valves or inherent weakness in the vein walls with consequent valve failure (valveless and weak vein syndromes).
6. Prolonged inactivity of the muscles with the limbs in a dependent position, as in paralysis or disease states inhibiting use of muscles. However, the blood flow through muscles will be correspondingly reduced and venous hypertension may not be too severe.

It should be noted that arteriovenous fistula, by direct arterial inflow to the venous side, can cause venous hypertension and the characteristic venotensive changes resulting from this (see later).

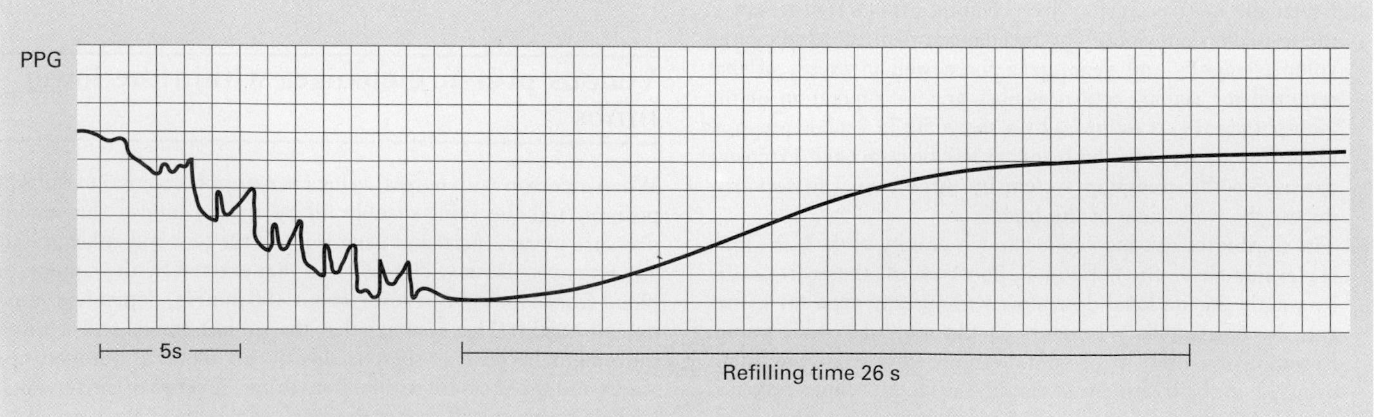

Fig. 15 A normal photoplethysmogram from the lower leg during and after five exercise movements in an upright position. This records the change in skin capillary filling, which in turn runs parallel with venous filling and venous pressure in that part of the limb. A substantial drop in filling accompanies exercise and recovers over the next 26 s. This recovery, or refilling, time is due to arterial inflow but will be unnaturally shortened if a venous disorder allowing reflux is present.

Signs of venous abnormality in the lower limb

There is much variation between individuals in the prominence of normal superficial veins when standing. Not only may the calibre of veins be very different between one person and another but the ease with which they are seen will differ greatly according to the depth of subcutaneous tissue and general skin texture. The superficial veins of a lean athletic person will appear large and easily seen but in the amply covered subject, perhaps with equally large veins, they will be far less obvious. Superficial veins may vary from one hour to the next in changing conditions of heat or cold. In women, the size of veins is greatly affected by the hormonal state; for example, there is obvious enlargement just before menstruation, and in pregnancy there is substantial prolonged enlargement which may be an important factor in the development of varicose veins. Other variations are related to vasomotor control; for instance, the tone of superficial veins in the lower part of the leg increases considerably on standing as part of a vasomotor reflex, adjusting veins to meet the increased pressure. For these reasons size alone is not a satisfactory indication of abnormality in a superficial vein unless the enlargement is gross. However, certain other changes may be present that allow immediate recognition of abnormality.

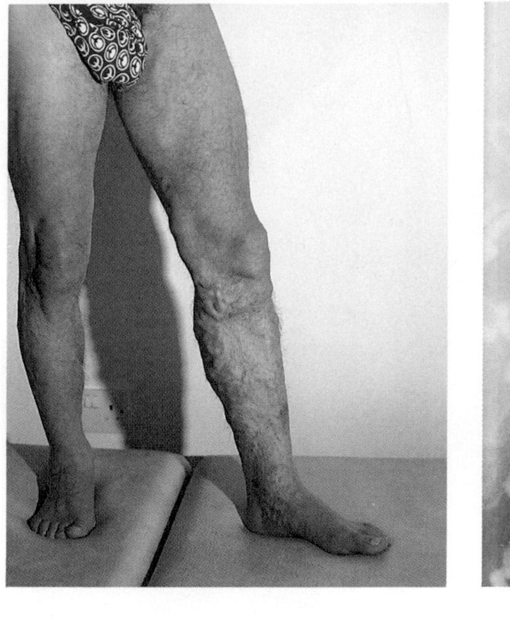

(a)

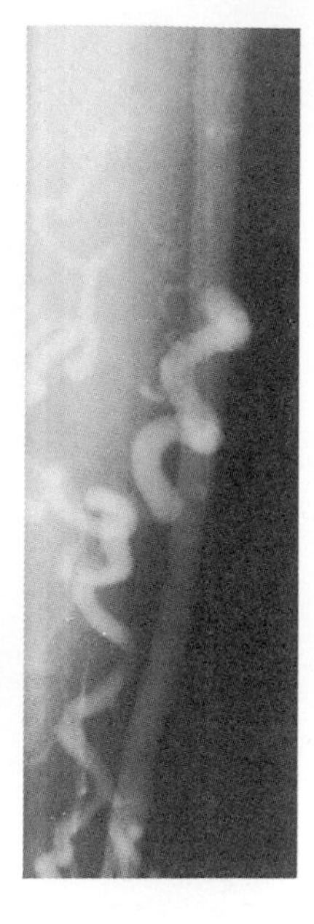

(b)

Fig. 16 Massive varicose veins arising from the long saphenous vein. (a) As seen clinically, running from lower thigh to the foot. (b) As seen on phlebography, a tortuous, enlarged posterior arcuate branch arising in the lower thigh. The long saphenous vein itself is enlarged but not tortuous.

Visible and palpable signs of venous abnormality

With patient standing

Tortuosity

This change in the veins has been recognized since antiquity and is the most significant visible sign of abnormality. The Latin 'varix' (pleural 'varices'), possibly derived from 'varus', meaning bent, specifically refers to tortuous dilatation of a vein. The word varicose is defined in medical dictionaries as describing veins that are tortuous, twisted, knotted, or lengthened. It may be seen in greatly varying forms, in small calibre veins running over a considerable distance, in a convoluted mass of enormously enlarged veins (Fig. 16), or, at the other extreme, a single bulge. This change is almost always associated, intermittently or continuously, with substantial flow in reverse direction to that natural for the vein. By far the most common example is seen in superficial vein incompetence where strong gravitational downflow occurs repeatedly in varicose veins, with progressive enlargement and increasing tortuosity in the affected veins. Conversely, high flow in a normal direction, at increased pressure, intermittently or continuously, will cause enlargement but seldom accompanied by tortuosity.

Saccules on the veins

A saphenous vein, as opposed to its branches, seldom becomes tortuous, perhaps because it is too robust, but often one or more saccules may be seen or palpated along its length (Fig. 17(a)). The term 'saphena varix' is given to a saccule which commonly develops close to the long saphenous termination (Fig. 17(b)). Usually a saccule is immediately below valve cusps (Fig. 17(c) and (d)) which are leaking heavily and the gross turbulence this causes on coughing gives rise to a characteristic, palpable thrill, readily confirmed by Doppler flowmetry and functional phlebography. It is possible that this turbulent jet of blood beneath the cusps creates a phenomenon similar to the post-stenotic dilatation in arteries described by Holman; occasionally a saccule arises within a cusp, but again this can be attributed to turbulence in malaligned cusps. However, this assumes that the initiating defect is the leaking valve but, alternatively, the primary fault could be weakening of the vein wall causing separation of the cusps and a resulting valvular incompetence, with the saccule as obvious evidence of structural failure in the wall. Perhaps it is most likely that both processes combine, each aggravating the other. However derived, the presence of a saccule is clear indication of an incompetent valve and, therefore, reversed flow down the vein when upright and exercising. Saccules are occasionally seen separately from valves but usually this dichotomy will be part of a more extensive process, with a grossly enlarged and sacculated vein due to generalized weakening of its walls.

Inky blue-black veins

Varicose veins commonly become adherent to overlying skin and may so stretch it that the dark blue venous blood shows through very clearly. This fragile covering will be vulnerable to minor trauma which may cause heavy haemorrhage.

Distended subdermal and intradermal venules

Extensive patterns of radiating venules are commonly seen around the ankle and on the foot (corona phlebectatica). These flares of veins (Fig. 18(a)) indicate venous congestion with increased venous pressure. They occur more readily in the weakened tissues of the elderly and are not necessarily the precursors of ulceration. These veins must be distinguished from small clusters of intradermal venules (thread or spider veins) seen on the thigh or upper leg increasingly as middle age approaches; these may signify under-

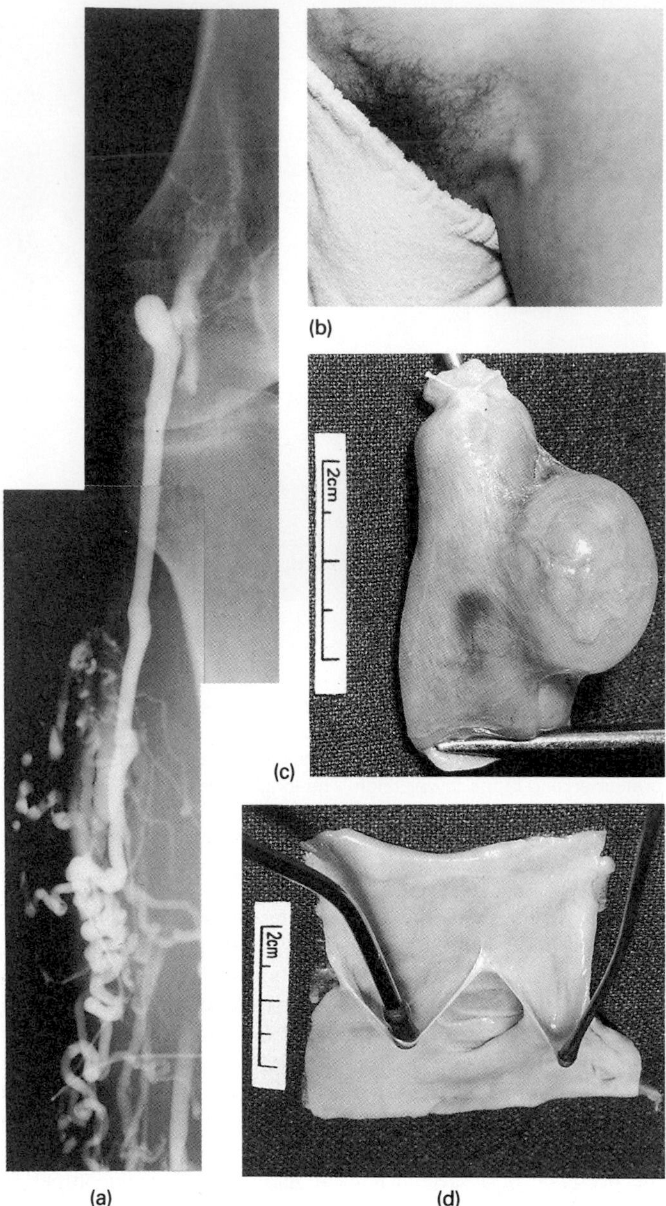

Fig. 17 Saphenous veins seldom show tortuosity but may develop a saccule below an incompetent valve. (a) A large saccule shown by phlebography on a short saphenous vein which is the source of extensive varicose veins. (b) Clinical appearance of a saphena varix, that is, a saccule arising immediately below the upper valve of the long saphenous vein in the groin. (c) A saphena varix distended with saline after surgical removal. (d) The same vein opened to display the mouth of the saccule immediately beneath the cusps.

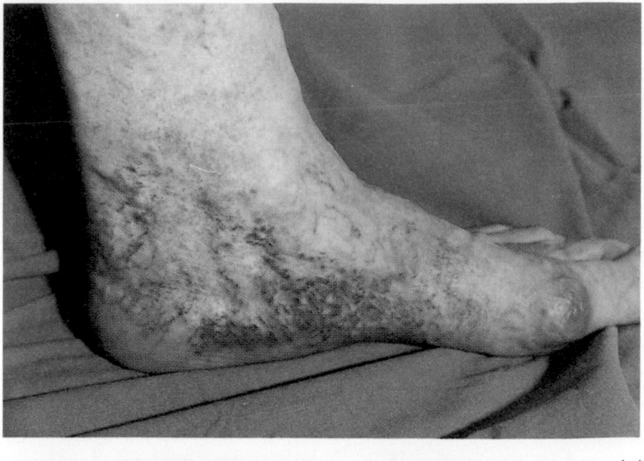

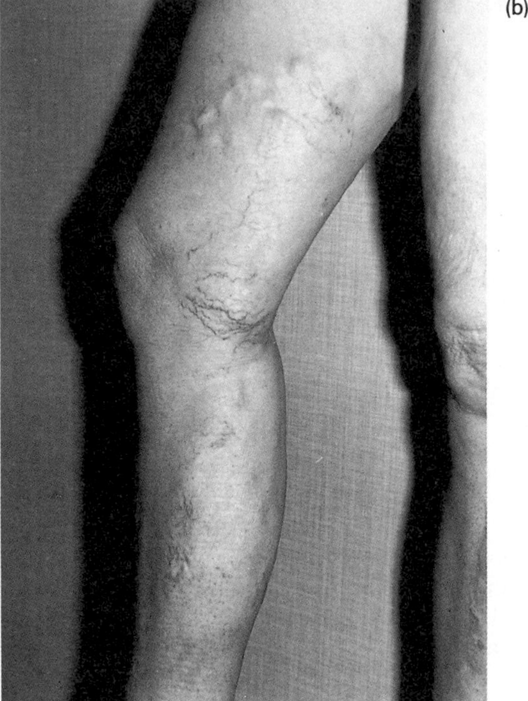

Fig. 18 Intradermal venules caused by venous stress. (a) A flare of grossly over-distended venules on the ankle and foot in long saphenous incompetence. Raised venous pressure from any cause may develop this, particularly in elderly people. (b) Venules behind the knee in a young woman overlying varicose veins running down the inner thigh and leg.

lying venous disorder (Fig. 18(b)) but often occur without any evidence of an abnormality.

Cough impulse

Varicose veins commonly give a palpable impulse when the patient coughs. This is because there is no functioning valve between the abdomen and the vein, and it confirms incompetence in the valves of deep and superficial veins leading down to this point. A high proportion of patients with incompetence in the long saphenous system lack any valves in the deep veins above the saphenous termination so that abdominal pressure is easily transmitted to varicosities in the limb.

Increased warmth in veins

Normally a superficial vein does not feel warm to the touch when compared with the neighbouring skin. Veins carrying a strong reversed flow of blood that has just emerged from a deep vein at true body temperature, as in simple varicose veins, often show obvious warmth to the touch, in comparison with skin alongside. This is valuable confirmation of the vein's abnormal state. Similarly, enlarged veins caused by arteriovenous fistula will feel warm to the touch.

With the patient lying

Hollows and grooves in the elevated limb

When the limb is elevated the veins will empty and the space occupied by large varicose veins becomes a hollow or a groove readily palpable or even visible. This is particularly marked when the surrounding tissues have become fibrotic in response to venous hypertension. Such hollows are often incorrectly diagnosed as fascial apertures enlarged by abnormal perforating veins. In fact, the hollow signifies no more than a large vein, but such a vein may have special significance, possibly related to surge from an underlying perforator.

The nature of varicose veins

Enlarged tortuous veins, that is to say, varicose veins, arise in three circumstances of unnatural flow.

1. *Simple (or primary) varicose veins.* These occur only in the superficial veins of the lower limbs and are by far the most common variety of varicose veins. Such veins have no competent valves and are subject to substantial gravitational downflow when the patient is upright and moving (see Fig. 30). This retrograde flow is in reverse to the natural direction allowed by valves and it is plausible to say that varicose veins are caused by the turbulent reversed flow beneath inadequate valves. Equally plausible, however, is to argue that veins with inherently weak walls expand in width and length so that valve cusps separate and allow reverse flow to occur. In this case, as with saphenous saccules discussed earlier, varicose veins could be the result of a vicious circle of weak walls and valve failure, causing turbulent, reversed flow expanding the walls still further. Certainly there are many studies by light and electron microscopy confirming degenerative changes in the wall structure in these circumstances but the question is whether this is a primary process or secondary to undue stress on the walls. This debate is unresolved and both circumstances may play a part, each aggravating the other. Whatever initiates the retrograde flow, it is a useful rule to regard tortuous veins as veins with intermittent or continuous reverse (retrograde) flow in them. Certainly this is true in commonplace, simple varicose veins, which are the expression of a dynamic phenomenon and not merely static distension.
2. *Secondary varicose veins.* Tortuosity is often seen in superficial veins carrying reversed flow as part of a collateral mechanism compensating for obstruction in a neighbouring deep vein. This is an acquired response and it seems that enforced reversed flow against the natural direction will cause enlargement and tortuosity in previously normal veins, for example, suprapubic veins acting as collaterals to iliac vein obstruction (see Fig. 58(d)), or in oesophageal varices in portal hypertension. By contrast, veins acting as collaterals but taking flow in their natural direction, enlarge but seldom show tortuosity, for example, in long saphenous branches overlying obstructed popliteal or femoral deep veins. The determining factor seems enforced reversed flow. (Note that clinical observation is often confused by the coexistence of deep vein obstruction and simple superficial vein incompetence in the same limb.)
3. *Arteriovenous fistula.* Tortuosity is often present in lesser veins in the vicinity of an arteriovenous fistula but the major veins leading from it enlarge without tortuosity.

Conclusion

Tortuosity (varicosity) in veins gives a strong indication of reversed flow in them and this may be due to either gravitational downflow in incompetent superficial veins (as in simple varicose veins) or enforced reversed flow. This occurs most commonly in collateral branch veins past deep vein obstruction but is also seen in veins near to arteriovenous fistula.

It is possible for both states to be present in the same limb.

Signs of venous hypertension (venotensive changes)

As explained above, venous hypertension of varying severity is a common consequence of venous disorder. Raised venous pressure will cause a corresponding increase in capillary pressure and, if sustained over long periods with inadequate relief, will cause characteristic changes in the skin and subcutaneous tissues. These are mainly the result of excess capillary transudation carrying with it protein molecules (Fig. 19) and leading to deposition of fibrin which forms a barrier to nutritional exchange between capillaries and the surrounding tissues. Other substances are also extravasated, including haemosiderin which eventually gives the characteristic brown skin pigmentation of venous hypertension. The venotensive changes listed below will take many months, or even years, to develop fully. They occur in varying combinations of severity and extent, and are to be found where the venous pressure is greatest. In this respect their position in the lower leg is gravitationally determined but an exception is seen with arteriovenous fistula where the high venous pressure is related to the arterial inflow in that vicinity. A number of conditions can cause venous hypertension, and the following changes may be seen in varying degree in any of them as a direct result of the raised venous pressure.

Venotensive changes

Swelling

This is mainly due to oedema which may be localized or found extensively over the limb, according to the nature of the venous abnormality causing it. The volume of overdistended veins can also make a significant contribution to the bulk of a limb, especially in foot and leg, when the patient is standing. It must be remembered that there are a number of other causes for oedema in a limb and these are summarized in Table 1 and Fig. 19. Inadequate lymphatic drainage causing oedema (see Chapter 9) can be an added component to venous disorders, particularly in congenital states.

Induration

A characteristic diffuse fibrosis develops in the subcutaneous tissues. This may vary from a slight thickening at an early stage, through to extensive areas of hard tissue in which the veins form large hollows and grooves evident when the leg is elevated. These changes may be accentuated by fat necrosis and chronic inflammatory changes. The terms 'lipodermatosclerosis' or 'liposclerosis' are often used to describe induration due to venous disorder.

Pigmentation

This is one of the most characteristic signs of venotension and is due to the accumulation of haemosiderin in the skin. It is often the earliest change to be seen and should immediately arouse

Table 1 Causes of oedema in lower limbs

Features	Diagnosis
Long-standing severe oedema of whole limb or moderate oedema up to knee level: unilaterally or bilaterally	
History of deep vein thrombosis Pigmentation Ulceration Enlarged superficial veins	Venous cause likely. Confirm with Doppler, phlethysmography, phlebography, ultrasonography
Brawny and non-pitting Peau d'orange. Crevices in skin	Lymphoedema. Photoplethysmography is normal. Radioactive uptake and gamma-camera can prove diagnosis. Lymphangiogram only if essential
Painful unilateral pitting oedema	
Painful Recent onset Acute process	May be due to one of the following: Deep vein thrombosis Superficial phlebitis Cellulitis; ?diabetes Lymphangiitis Injury Ischaemia (swelling due to hanging leg out of bed to relieve rest pain) Arteriovenous fistula of acute onset
Painless unilateral pitting oedema (but some discomfort when oedema is maximal):	
	May be due to one of the following: Venous causes: Superficial incompetence (varicosities) Deficiency or absence of deep vein valves Previous deep vein thrombosis (post-thrombotic limb) Subacute deep vein thrombosis Venous obstruction (tumour or cyst) Bilateral state with oedema suppressed on one side by ischaemia Early lymphoedema Combined states (e.g. lymphatic and venous disease both present) Arteriovenous fistula Tight bandaging in mid or upper limb Hysterical manifestation (*oedeme bleu* due to prolonged dependency or constricting band) Paralysed limb with prolonged dependency
Painless bilateral pitting oedema (but some discomfort when oedema maximal):	
	May be due to one or more of the following: Central cause, including heart failure, renal disease, liver disease, protein deficiency Malnutrition Unsuitable drug administration or undesirable response Excessive intravenous fluid and electrolyte therapy Obstruction to inferior vena cava or iliac veins by thrombosis, tumour, or ascites Overt or hidden malignancy Arteriovenous (aortovenacaval or iliac) fistula Symmetrical 'unilateral' state, that is, bilateral localized defects in lower limbs Ill-defined hormonal inbalance Prolonged dependency, e.g. air travel, habitual sleeping in chair, or paralysis Inborn or acquired (e.g. menopausal) tissue changes with increased capillary permeability

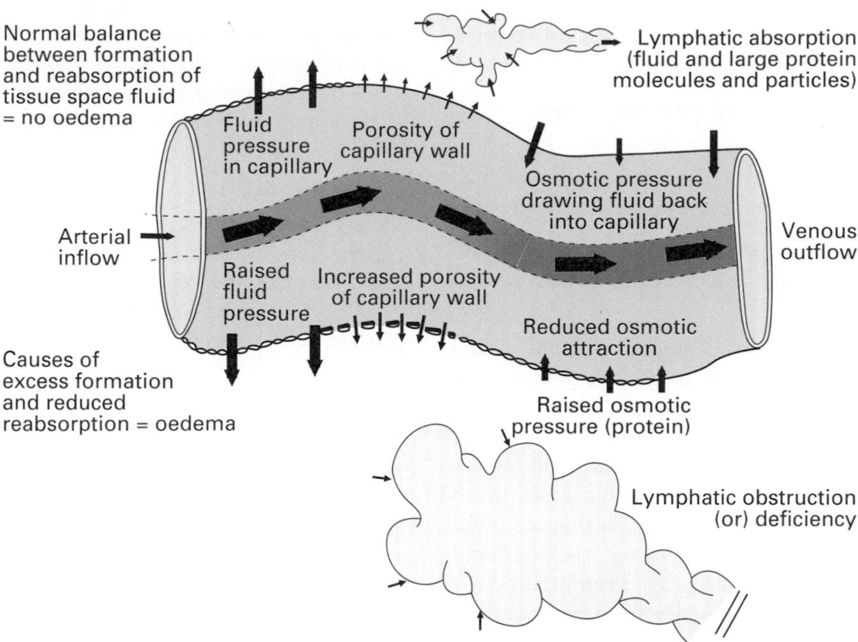

Fig. 19 Diagram of factors influencing formation and reabsorption of tissue fluid. The lymphatic system is responsible for removal of any large protein molecules that pass out of the capillaries and failure of this is a potent cause for oedema.

suspicion of a venous disorder. If accompanied by the other changes given here, it is diagnostic of venous hypertension (see Fig. 46(a) (iii)).

Ulceration

If venous hypertension and the changes it causes remain untreated, progressive deterioration in skin nutrition leads to small areas of tissue death which coalesce to form an ulcer. A venous ulcer will always be surrounded by pigmented skin and at least some induration (see Figs 47(a), 56(a), 57(g)) but there is great variation in severity and extent of these accompanying features; in long-standing ulcers the neighbouring skin may also show a characteristic white scarring known as 'atrophie blanche'. The changes given above are typical of venous ulceration and distinguish it from other forms of ulcer which often require completely different treatment. Correct diagnosis of the various ulcers that may be seen on the leg and foot is of considerable importance and is discussed later (see Ulcers of the leg).

Eczema and dermatitis

In venous hypertension the skin is particularly prone to eczema and is excessively vulnerable to any sensitizing agents or allergens applied to it. Pigmented areas are most affected, but often small patches of eczema can be seen overlying varicosities and clearly related to their distribution (see Fig. 46(a) (ii)). In these circumstances, pruritus will be a prominent symptom and scratching will damage the skin further. Once eczema has become established, it may appear on distant parts of the body as a more general sensitization. The appearance of eczema in the vicinity of varicose veins should always be a warning that progressive skin changes are likely. All too often eczema is aggravated by sensitization to medical products applied to the skin, or materials in the fabric of elastic stockings. Antibiotic creams are particular offenders in causing skin reactions.

Symptoms of venous disorder

When venotensive changes are not present

The symptoms accompanying abnormally enlarged or varicose veins without obvious venotensive changes are:

- Distress caused by unsightly and displeasing appearance;
- Aching in the vicinity of abnormal veins, particularly after prolonged standing;
- A feeling of heaviness towards the end of the day;
- In women, discomfort associated with varicose veins is most marked over a few days before menstruation. This is often described as aching, stinging, or burning and the veins become more prominent;
- Nocturnal cramps often appear related to varicose veins. This is particularly evident when the cramps occur only on the side affected by varicose veins. Moreover, attacks of cramp may cease following successful surgery to the veins. This association with varicosities is well established but ill understood; however, nocturnal cramp is a common condition in older people so that it is difficult to predict when elimination of varicosities will relieve it and no promise upon this should be given to patients before treatment. In the elderly, care must be taken to distinguish between simple cramp and ischaemic nocturnal rest pain; both are relieved by standing out of bed but in ischaemia the ankle pulses will be reduced or absent on palpation or Doppler flowmeter examination.

There is little relationship between the size of varicose veins and the discomforts complained of. Large, long-standing varicose veins may cause no admitted discomfort and, indeed, in these patients it may be difficult to persuade them to have treatment. Relatively small varicosities lying directly under the skin or intradermally, particularly if they have appeared recently, often seem to cause most discomfort, especially premenstrually in women.

Additional symptoms when venotensive changes are present

If venous disorder is accompanied by venotensive changes then one or more of the following symptoms is also likely to be present.

Pruritus This is commonly an early sign of venotensive skin change and repeated scratching by the patient may break the skin, possibly initiating an ulcer.

Increased discomfort The sense of general discomfort and heaviness or actual pain is increased. If an ulcer is present, this certainly causes discomfort, and often real pain if the ulcer is infected with *Staphyloccus aureus* or *Streptococcus viridans*. An ulcer will produce discharge varying from watery fluid through to frank pus and may be accompanied by unpleasant odour. Such manifestations cause the patient distress and a feeling of social insecurity, accentuated by the bandages or strong stockings used in treatment. Within a society venous ulcers are a significant cause for disability, often under-rated, and absence from work.

Venous claudication Extensive post-thrombotic venous obstruction in popliteal and femoral veins may so impede venous return that a few minutes of exercise cause considerable increase in venous pressure, well above the normal maximum. This is accompanied by a bursting sensation in the calf which quickly becomes unbearable and forces the patient to stop walking. (The term claudication, derived from the name of the Emperor Claudius, means 'limping'. It is most commonly used in connection with states of arterial insufficiency but is also used by neurologists for symptoms caused by compression of the cauda equina.) In venous claudication, the clinical features of venous obstruction will always be present and fully confirmed by the special investigations. Care must be taken to ensure that the claudication is not in fact due to arterial insufficiency coincidentally present with a venous disorder. In ischaemia, swelling of the foot can be due to the patient hanging the leg out of bed in order to relieve rest pain; this is not rare and, if the limb is elevated because it is misdiagnosed as a venous disorder, the severity of the condition is greatly aggravated and may lead to loss of the limb.

CLINICAL EXAMINATION AND SPECIAL INVESTIGATIONS

Clinical examination

The patient's complaint

It is important to have a clear statement by the patient of their complaint and the reason for dissatisfaction with their veins. Visible varicose veins tend to be blamed for any discomfort in the limb but this may have a very different origin and the symptoms must match the venous abnormality.

History

Certain aspects of medical history are important, particularly the likelihood of a previous deep vein thrombosis, so often long forgotten but yet a potent cause of venous disorder. In this respect, any history of 'white leg of pregnancy', major fractures of lower limbs or pelvis, prolonged immobilization in traction or plaster of Paris, or of major illness, should be enquired for. A family history and the age of first appearance of varicose veins may have a bearing upon prognosis and policy of management. Knowledge of previous treatment is essential as this will have fragmented anatomy of the superficial veins.

Examination

Unless stated otherwise, examination is carried out with the patient upright, that is to say in the position in which venous problems arise and venous defects are most evident. This is best done by asking the patient to stand on a strengthened couch or platform with appropriate handrails on the wall nearby.

Inspection

Careful inspection in good light is fundamental to observe the pattern of prominent veins and detect any skin changes of venous disorder (Fig. 20). The feet must be included in this and, if there is any hint of previous deep vein thrombosis, the pubes and lower abdomen must also be inspected. There is much to be learnt from the scars of any previous operations. If tortuous veins are present these must be traced along their full length and for this an oblique light throwing the veins into relief is most helpful. The following questions should be borne in mind.

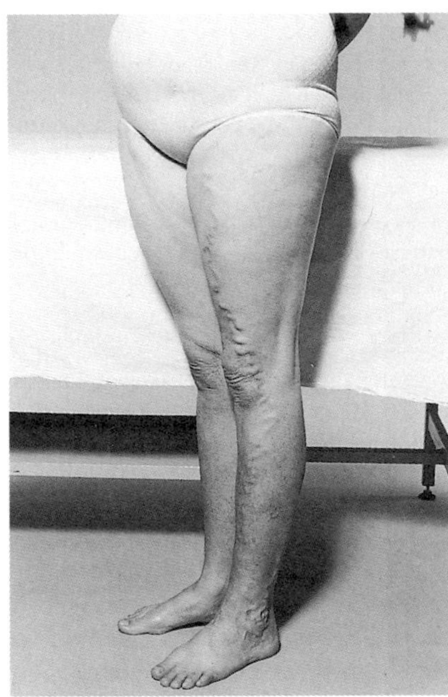

Fig. 20 Clinical examination. Careful inspection of all aspects of the limb and foot is essential. If there is any suggestion of previous deep vein thrombosis, the pubic region and lower abdomen must be included.

Do the veins fall within long or short saphenous distribution or is this uncertain; is another and unusual source possible?

Is visible evidence of venous hypertension present, particularly pigmentation, swelling, and ulceration?

Touch

Light touch, almost brushing the skin, is very helpful in detecting or locating veins. Consider the following questions.

> If there is apparent swelling, is there any pitting oedema?
> Are varicose veins 'hot' to touch, do they show a cough impulse?
> If there is an isolated bulge on the inner thigh, is there a thrill on coughing indicating an underlying jet of blood through a leaking valve?

Mapping out

This is a most important step, defining clearly the overall pattern of enlarged veins, including those that are not visible. The 'tap-wave' test is an essential skill in this respect.

Tap-wave test (percussion test of Chevrier)

In the standing patient with fully distended veins, a tap or sharp compression of a vein will send a corresponding wave of movement along its length, easily detected by light touch. Thus, one examining hand 'taps' on the vein in its lower part (so that valves do not dampen the effect) whilst fingers of the other hand locate the signal in its upper part (Fig. 21), moving progressively up the limb. In this way veins not detectable by any other clinical means are easily located and traced along their length. This procedure does not reveal much about function and is not reliable in assessing valve competence but it does swiftly map out the pattern of veins otherwise concealed from touch or sight, and this alone can turn speculative diagnosis to a probable one.

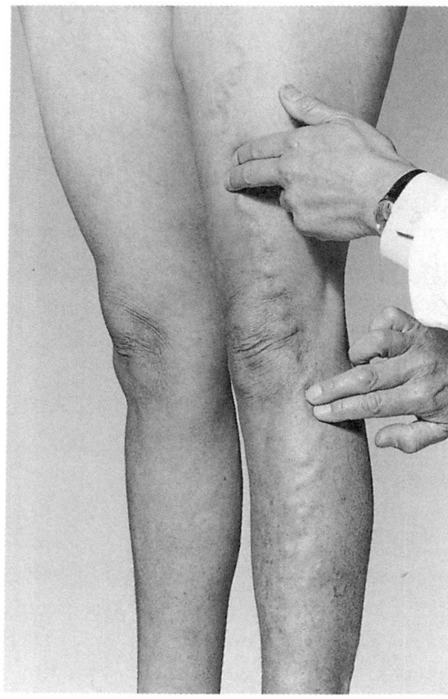

Fig. 21 Tap-wave test. With the veins fully distended by standing, the lower hand gives a tap or sharp compression on the vein to be traced. The distinctive percussion wave caused travels along the vein and is detectable by the upper hand even when the vein is not otherwise recognizable.

Examination with patient horizontal and the limb elevated

With the limb elevated to 45°, the veins will empty so that large subcutaneous veins become a gutter or a hollow. This can prove a valuable addition to 'mapping out', and in the detection of varicose veins concealed by subcutaneous fat the presence of a hollow helps in the recognition of early venous induration. It has already been pointed out that a hollow is seldom due to a fascial deficiency but is the site of a large varicosity and does not necessarily signify that an enlarged perforator underlies it.

Clinical tests

The features so far described give the observable changes that may be present in venous disorders. These give indirect evidence of abnormal function in veins but few are diagnostic of a specific state. Of the clinical tests, relying solely on the examiner's senses, only two are capable of giving a specific diagnosis. In both the following tests the use of an encircling rubber band to occlude superficial veins is avoided, partly because it may cause artefacts by constricting the deep veins, and also because it does not localize the superficial veins at fault.

The Trendelenburg type of test (selective occlusion test)

This test is based upon demonstration that temporary selective occlusion of one or more superficial veins by localized finger pressure will delay the filling of varicose veins when the patient first stands after the veins have been emptied by elevation of the limb (Fig. 22). It shows that the varicose veins fill by downflow in the vein selected for occlusion and, therefore, its valves must be incompetent. This is of great diagnostic value and accurately identifies simple (primary) varicose veins. When positive it is virtual proof of this, but no great reliance can be placed on a negative result in the exclusion of superficial vein incompetence, for example, when the likely pathway of incompetence has been misidentified (say, long saphenous), and the real source of incompetence is elsewhere (say, short saphenous) and has been overlooked. Other aspects of this test are considered later in the section discussing superficial vein incompetence, the state it is pre-eminent in recognizing.

Perthes' test

This type of test depends upon the change in the distended varicose veins of an upright patient exercising whilst a selected superficial vein is occluded to prevent downflow (Fig. 23). In the first stage it is shown that exercise by rising on the toes does not deflate the veins. Then, the main pathway of incompetence previously identified by selective Trendelenburg test, often a saphenous vein, is occluded by localized finger pressure and the patient is exercised as before. If the varicose veins become less prominent and softer to touch, it is clear that, when downflow in the superficial vein is prevented, exercise succeeds in emptying the varicose veins. This confirms that the deep vein pumping mechanism is functioning satisfactorily and the fault lies in the superficial vein under test which is capable of filling the varicosities as fast as they are emptied by the deep veins. A positive response gives meaningful confirmation of this; an uncertain or failed response raises suspicion of deep vein insufficiency but does not give acceptable

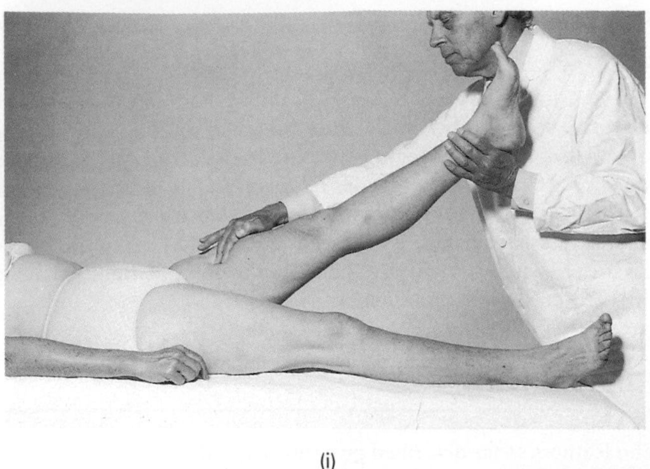

(i)

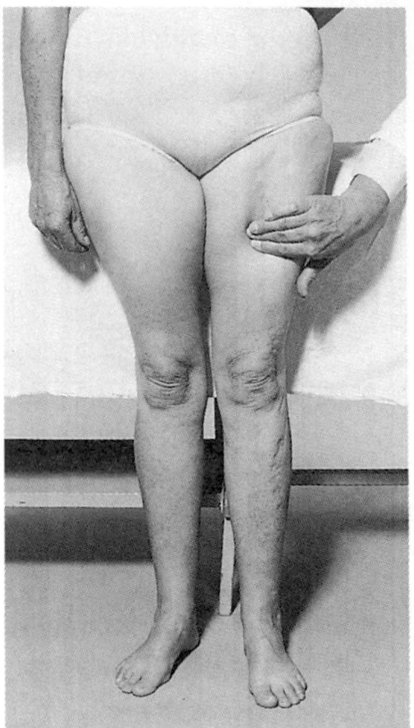

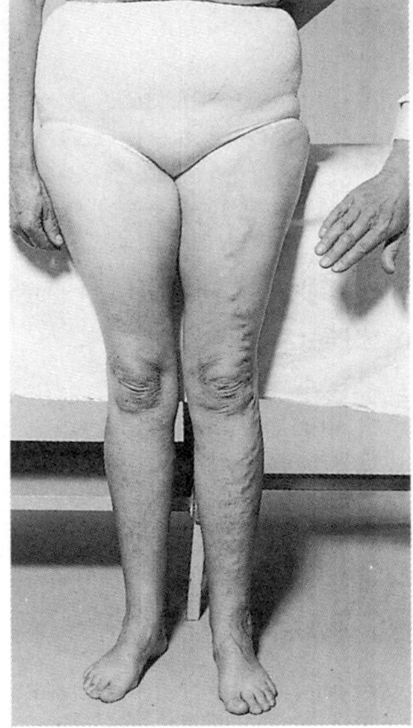

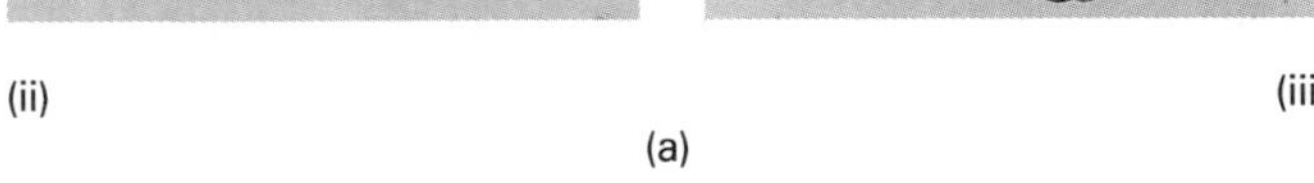

(ii) (iii)

(a)

Fig. 22 Selective occlusion (Trendelenburg) test.
(a) Long saphenous vein—anterolateral branch. (i) The veins are emptied by high elevation of the limb and the suspected pathway of incompetence is selectively occluded by compression with fingertips. (ii) With compression maintained, the patient stands and the varicose veins are observed. (At this stage, the patient may be exercised by rising on toes; absence of vein filling gives additional evidence that there is no significant perforator outflow.) (iii) After a short interval compression is removed. If the veins promptly fill only at this stage, incompetence in the valves of the vein under examination has been demonstrated and the test is considered positive.

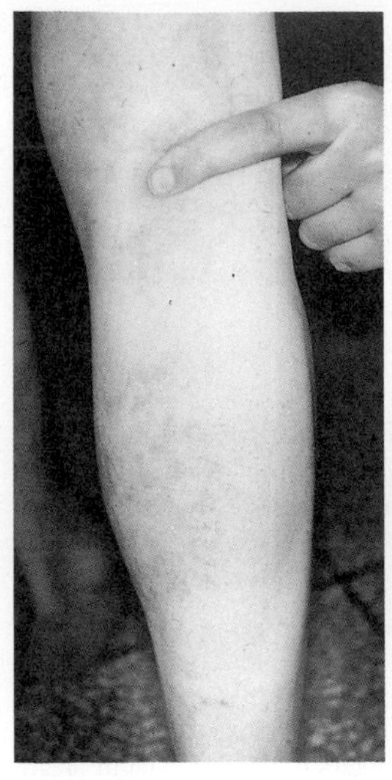

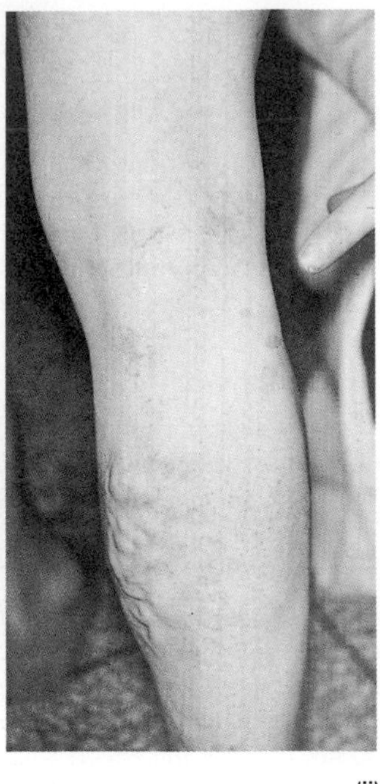

(i) (ii)

(b)

(b) Short saphenous vein. (i) Fingertip compression controls varicosities. (ii) The veins rapidly fill when compression is removed.

proof of this. This test is referred to again in the section on superficial vein incompetence.

With superficial vein incompetence these clinical tests can give a firm diagnosis, sufficient to act upon clinically. In other venous disorders reliance has to be placed on investigation with instruments measuring speed and direction of flow, pressure or volume change, or outlining of the veins and displaying their function by phlebography or ultrasonic imaging (ultrasonography).

Tests by electronic instruments and radiography

The basic defects that characterize venous disorder become apparent when exercising in an upright position and are readily detected by instruments and imaging techniques.

Demonstration of flow by ultrasound. The directional Doppler flowmeter and ultrasonography

Abnormal direction of flow

Flow in the direction that should be opposed by valves is abnormal and its presence indicates that the valves are incompetent or absent. A directional Doppler flowmeter (or more correctly, velocimeter) can detect this with great clarity. With this instrument a piezoelectric crystal in the probe emits a continuous ultrasound signal that is reflected back by red cells to a receiving crystal. According to the speed and direction of movement of the red cells, there is a Doppler shift in the phase of the signal which is recognized by the machine and made apparent audibly, by a needle gauge, by LED display, or by oscillograph; a permanent record is provided either by a chart recorder or by some form of computer printout. In order to facilitate the passage of ultrasound between probe and tissues a coupling gel is used on the skin. If a lightweight, flatheaded probe is used this can be held in the hand against skin without displacement when the patient moves (Fig. 24) and allows rapid repositioning of the probe so that several different sites may be examined in quick succession. The signal generated represents the speed of flow but not the volume;

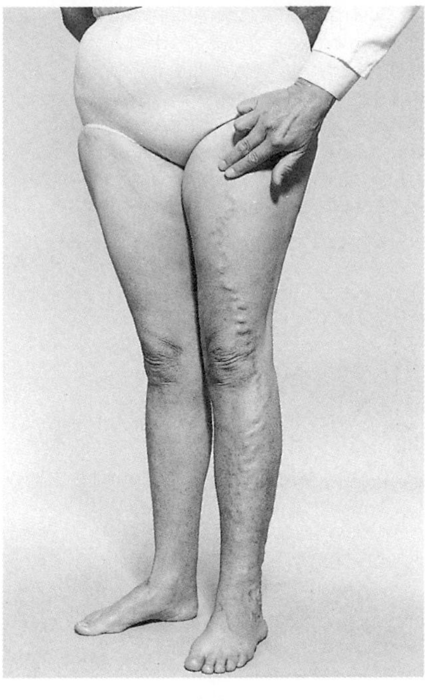
(a)

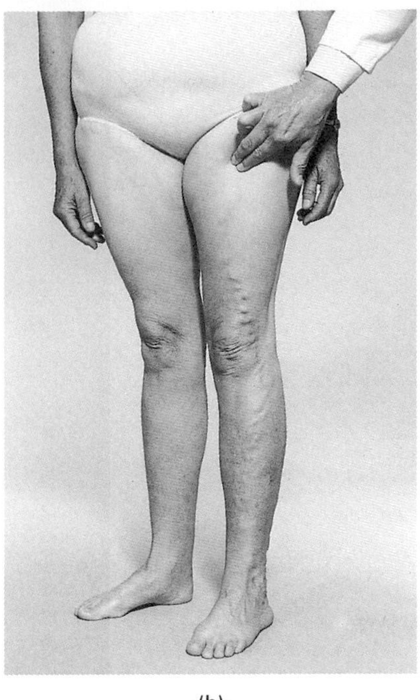
(b)

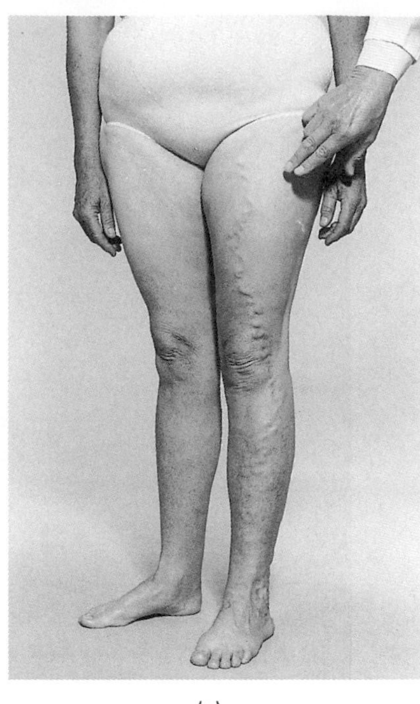
(c)

Fig. 23 Selective Perthes' test. (a) With the patient standing and the veins well filled, the suspected pathway of incompetence is compressed with fingertips and the patient asked to rise on toes three times. (b) With compression maintained, the veins are assessed. A positive response is shown if the veins have become visibly less prominent and have softened to touch. (c) On release of compression full prominence and firmness return promptly.

thus a high speed jet of blood leaking through valve cusps may cause a strong signal which can be misleading if more representative flow a short distance away is not sampled. However, such sharply localized, high velocity flow in itself confirms the presence of a leaking valve although it does not necessarily indicate the overall severity of incompetence. In tortuous veins, confused directional signals may be obtained due to the close proximity of conflicting flows or from uncertainty about the orientation, upwards or downwards, of the segment of tortuous vein under the probe. These difficulties can be resolved by asking the patient to cough in order to create a spurt of downward flow, or, by deliberately pressing the vein below the probe to cause a small peak of upward flow. The Doppler flowmeter is at its best over superficial veins such as a saphenous vein or its varicose branches. Much useful information can also be obtained from the deep veins, but here there may be uncertainty in distinguishing which deep vein is being picked up or, indeed, whether the signal is coming from an intervening superficial vein, for example, a short saphenous vein overlying the popliteal vein. The characteristic superficial vein flow patterns found in the various venous disorders are described later in this section. It is sufficient to say here that the directional Doppler flowmeter used in this way can give immediate positive confirmation of incompetence in superficial veins or give warning that deep vein problems may be present.

Pulsed beam ultrasonography provides a much more sophisticated demonstration by giving an image of veins and their valves on a display screen. It will show movement of these structures and also the direction and speed of blood flow within them. This is particularly valuable for detailed study of short lengths of deep veins and will be described further under Imaging techniques. Similarly, phlebography may be used to visualize the pattern of flow within superficial and deep veins.

Enhanced flow in the normal direction

Increased flow in superficial veins in the normal direction can be highly significant and occurs in two circumstances. It may occur when superficial veins, including saphenous veins, are acting as collaterals past occlusion in the underlying deep veins (see Figs. 13 and 57(b)). It will also be found in the veins above an arteriovenous fistula but here an added feature will be strongly pulsatile return flow in time with the heartbeats. This must be distinguished from the weak pulsation often noticed in fully distended veins, congested by a short period of standing without movement and due to transmission of pulsation from neighbouring arteries. It is most evident in venous disorders where valve incompetence causes rapid congestion within the limb; pulsation may also be found, and is easily seen, in cardiac failure with tricuspid valve incompetence.

Measurement and estimation of venous pressure in leg or foot

Failure in response of venous pressure to exercise

With exercise, in the upright position, the venous pressure within the limb normally falls, and when exercise ceases (Fig. 15) it takes at least 20 s before the original pressure is regained (restitution, refilling, or recovery time). In states of superficial or deep vein valvular incompetence the refilling time may be decisively shortened by reflux of venous blood down the limb and this is characteristic of conditions causing venous hypertension (Fig. 25). Measurements of venous pressure changes in response to exercise may be obtained by the following means.

By direct insertion of a needle or plastic cannula into a foot or ankle vein. The pressure is best measured by a calibrated

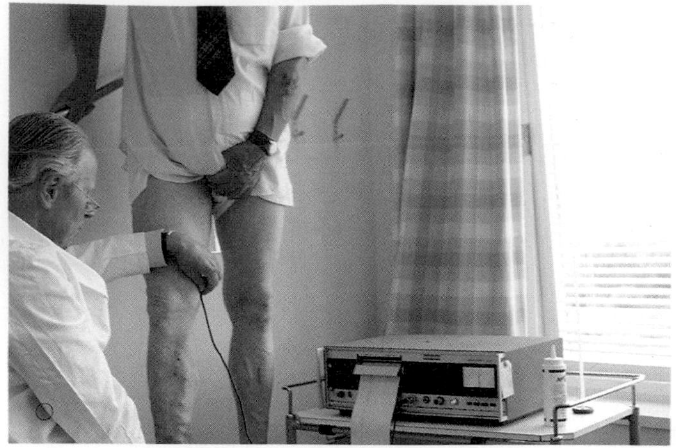

(a)

Fig. 24 Directional Doppler flowmetry (or, more correctly, velocimetry, because it is measuring velocity of flow) to the superficial veins is a simple but highly informative examination. (a) The probe is placed over the vein to be examined whilst the patient is standing and the response to coughing, calf compression, and exercise movements is given by audible and visible signals, and also by chart recorder. b) A chart recording of the responses in Doppler flow in an incompetent long saphenous vein; diagram of flow pattern.

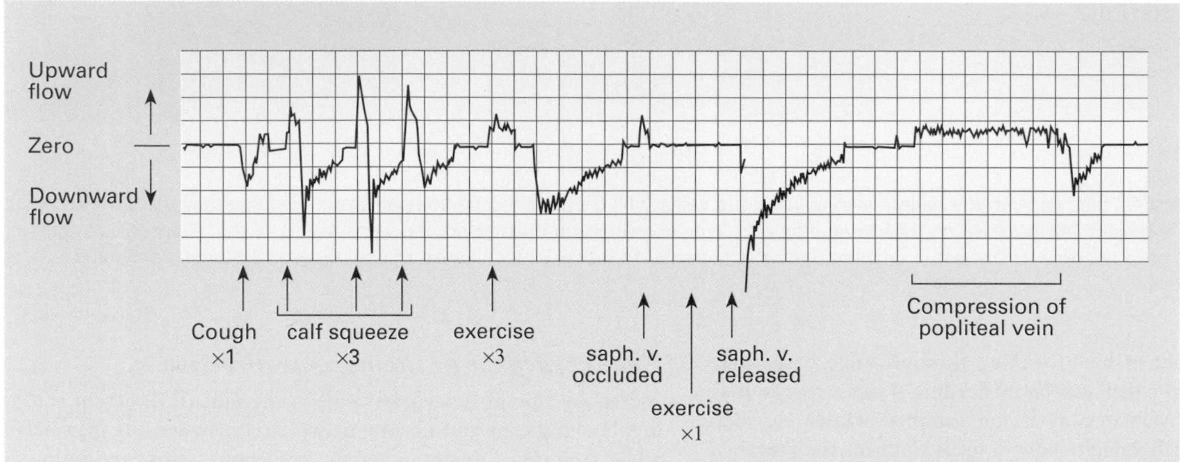

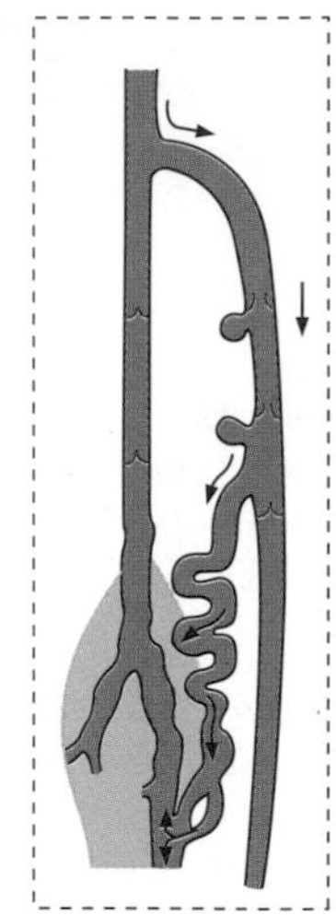

(b)

electronic transducer and the changes shown as a tracing on a chart recorder as they occur.

By indirect methods without the need to puncture a vein, and indicating the scale and rate of pressure changes rather than by giving accurate measurement. Photoplethysmography, described below, is a simple but effective way of doing this and in most circumstances can give a good estimation of valvular competence by gauging the recovery time.

Measurement of change in limb volume. Photoplethysmography

Failure in response of limb volume to exercise

The limb volume closely parallels the venous pressure so that when the patient is standing still it is maximal but after exercise, which has expelled blood from the limb, both venous pressure and limb volume will fall. The reduction in volume will indicate the amount of blood expelled by exercise; the time taken for the volume to return to its original value is a good indication of valve competence. With fully competent valves this will be at least 20 s, but when superficial or deep valve incompetence is present this will be shortened according to the severity of the condition. Various methods may be used for measuring and recording volume changes as they occur (plethysmography).

Fluid plethysmography The leg or foot is immersed in water within a fixed chamber and the amount of fluid displaced from this is measured. The weight of fluid may cause artefacts and the range of exercise possible for the patient is somewhat limited. Nevertheless, it is capable of giving reliable results.

Air plethysmography The leg is surrounded by an air-filled PVC chamber and the amount of air entering or leaving is measured to give changes in limb volume. It allows the patient more freedom of movement but must be carried out in conditions of stable temperature to prevent errors from thermal expansion or contraction of air within the container. In use, this proves to be a practical method, reliably indicating the speed and degree of volume change with exercise.

Electrical impedance plethysmography This method estimates the volume change within the limb by alteration in the electrical resistance which varies with the volume.

Strain gauge plethysmography The limb is encircled by a slender elastic tube containing mercury or similar electrically conducting fluid, the resistance of which will vary as the diameter of the elastic tube changes. Thus, when exercise reduces the volume, the elastic tube will shorten to give a broader diameter and the resistance will fall; as the volume is regained the tube is stretched and the resistance increases again. This method is simple to apply

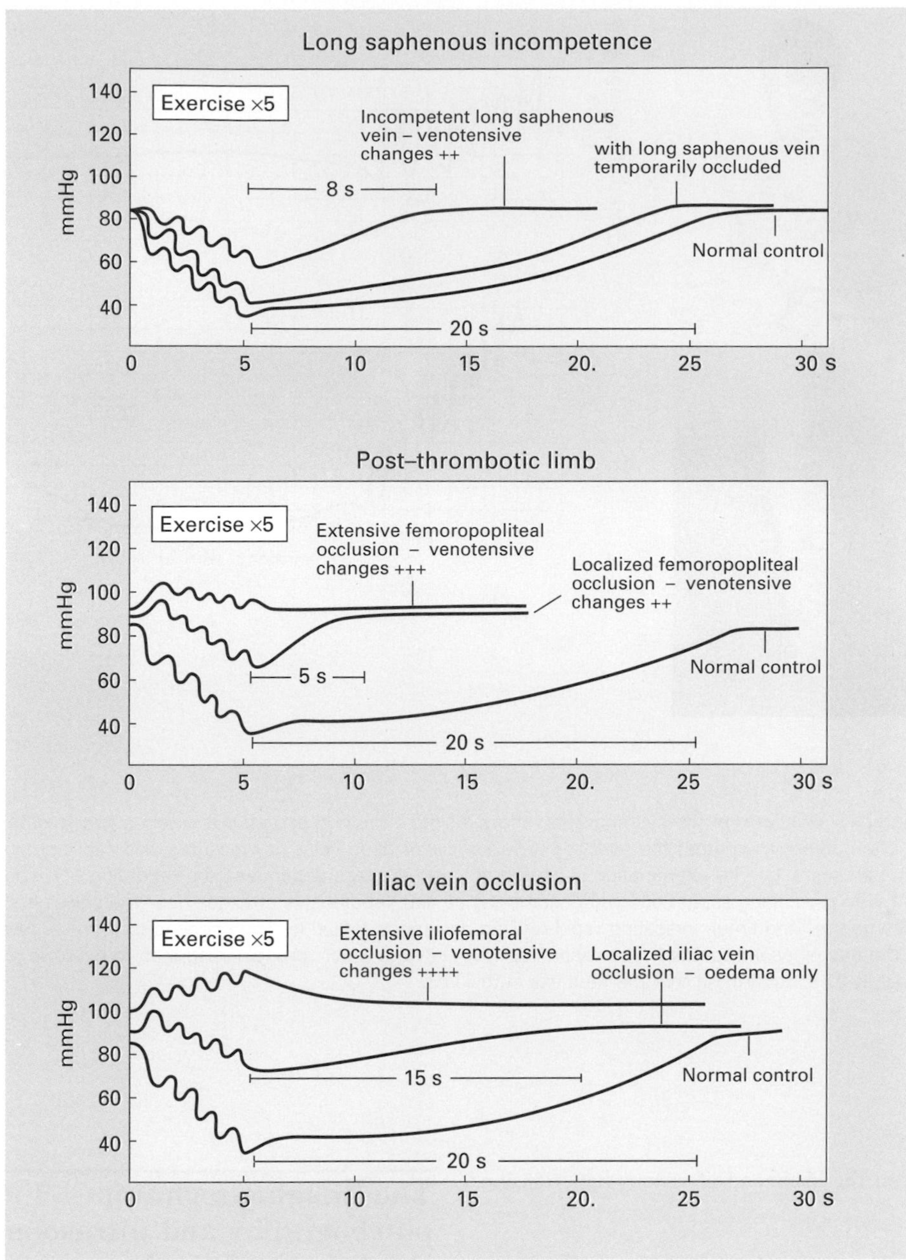

Fig. 25 Venous pressure changes in response to exercise and the refilling times in various venous disorders compared with the normal state.

and gives a good indication of the volume changes occurring in the limb. However, it is only sampling the changes at one or two levels and cannot measure the expelled volume; its main value is in gauging the recovery time.

Photoplethysmography This method (Fig. 26) photoelectrically estimates the number of red cells in the skin capillary bed underlying the transducer. A light emitting diode, which gives off no heat likely to cause artefacts, illuminates the capillary bed with infrared light. This is absorbed by haemoglobin in the red cells and the amount transmitted back to a photoelectric sensor will vary in accordance with the number of red cells underlying it. The signals are recorded as a line tracing on a chart recorder or computerized display. It has been shown that the degree of congestion of red cells in the skin capillaries bears a close relationship to the venous pressure in the limb and, thus, the signal from the photoplethysmograph closely parallels the venous pressure changes. It can certainly give a good estimation of the recovery time following exercise and this is its chief value. If two successive recordings are made, without changing the probe position or the instrument settings, comparison of the rate and extent of venous pressure change in different circumstances can be achieved, for example, in response to exercise with and without saphenous occlusion (see Fig. 34(c)). The method has certain vagaries but, with experience, can give a good portrayal of venous changes in the limb, taking only a few minutes and with no discomfort to the patient. It is a very practical method for assessing the effectiveness of musculovenous pumping, the overall

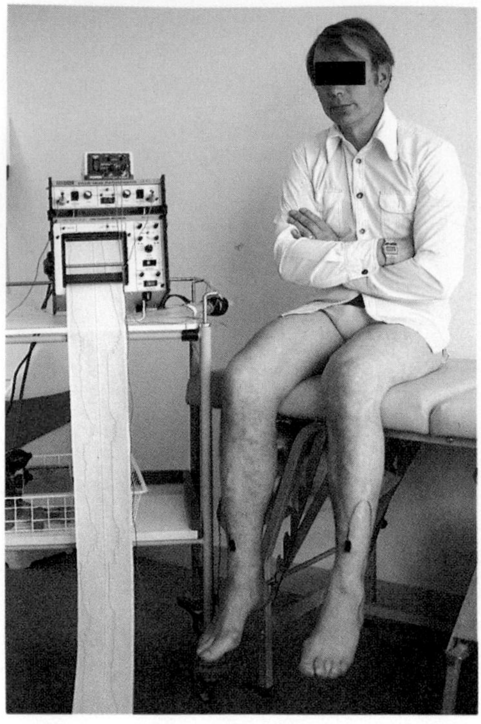

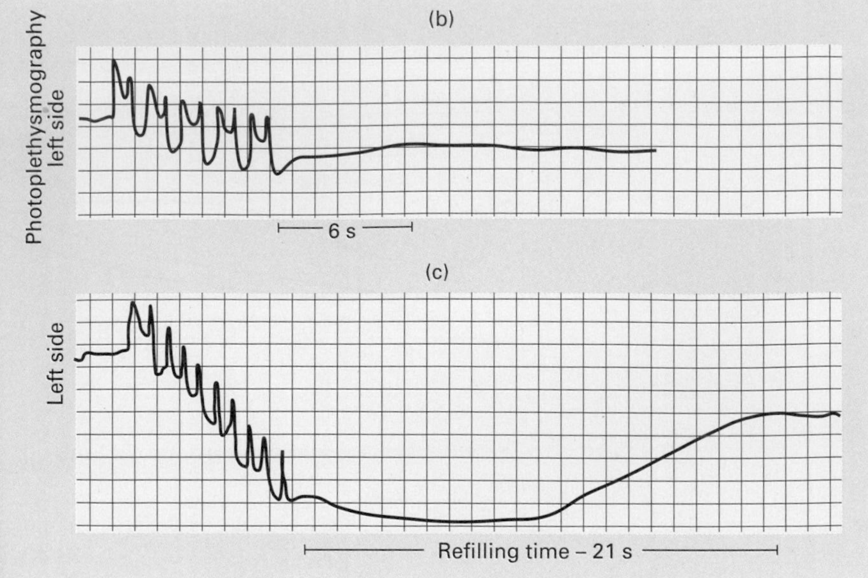

(a)

Fig. 26 Photoplethysmography. This form of plethysmography offers a simple method carried out within a few minutes and is able to confirm venous insufficiency and, often, to show whether the fault lies in superficial or deep veins. It measures skin capillary filling which is closely related to venous filling and pressure. (a) The examination is carried out with the legs dependent. (b) Recording of response to five exercise movements from a patient with gross long saphenous vein incompetence and venotensive changes near the ankle. A small fall is shown but this rises again in under 6 s (the refilling time), indicating rapid refilling by venous reflux. (c) The saphenous vein has been selectively occluded by fingertip pressure and the examination repeated. The recording now shows a much stronger response to exercise and prolongation of the refilling time to near normal at 21 s, confirming that the fault lies in this vein.

competence of valves, and the likelihood of venous hypertension being present.

Maximum venous outflow (MVO) Plethysmography, usually by strain gauge, may be used to measure the maximal speed at which venous blood can leave a limb and from this estimate any restriction in venous outflow. With the patient horizontal and the lower limbs elevated, a pneumatic cuff is used to cause venous congestion. The cuff is then abruptly released and, from the tracing on a chart recorder, reduction in volume (limb circumference if a strain gauge is used) over the first few seconds is expressed as a percentage of the total fall in volume. For example, in a normal limb 90 per cent of the total fall in volume will occur in the first 3 s (Fig. 27, left) but in ileofemoral obstruction with poor collaterals, perhaps only 45 per cent fall would occur in the same time (Fig. 27, right).

Although useful, estimation of maximal venous outflow does not give specific information and adds little to that gained from the other tests with instruments described above. However, it can help in excluding a venous cause in an oedematous limb, so that unnecessary phlebography is avoided but, overall, the information gained is greatly inferior to that from techniques visualizing veins.

The imaging techniques. Functional phlebography and ultrasonography by Duplex or colour flow scanning

If the special tests with instruments have not satisfactorily explained the nature of the venous disorder then a technique visualizing the veins can be used. This will not only display abnormal outline to the veins, such as occlusion or deformity, but will show if valves are defective or absent. In addition, abnormal patterns of superficial or deep venous flow, in response to exercise, can be demonstrated. The two main techniques are functional phlebography and ultrasonography.

Functional phlebography

Phlebography has been transformed over recent years by several factors, particularly the use of a non-irritating osmolar opaque medium, such as Iohexol, which causes no discomfort and does not precipitate phlebitis, the introduction of the image intensifier which allows prolonged viewing without exposing the patient to excessive radiation, and the realization that the patient must be examined in the position that causes venous problems (Fig. 28(a)

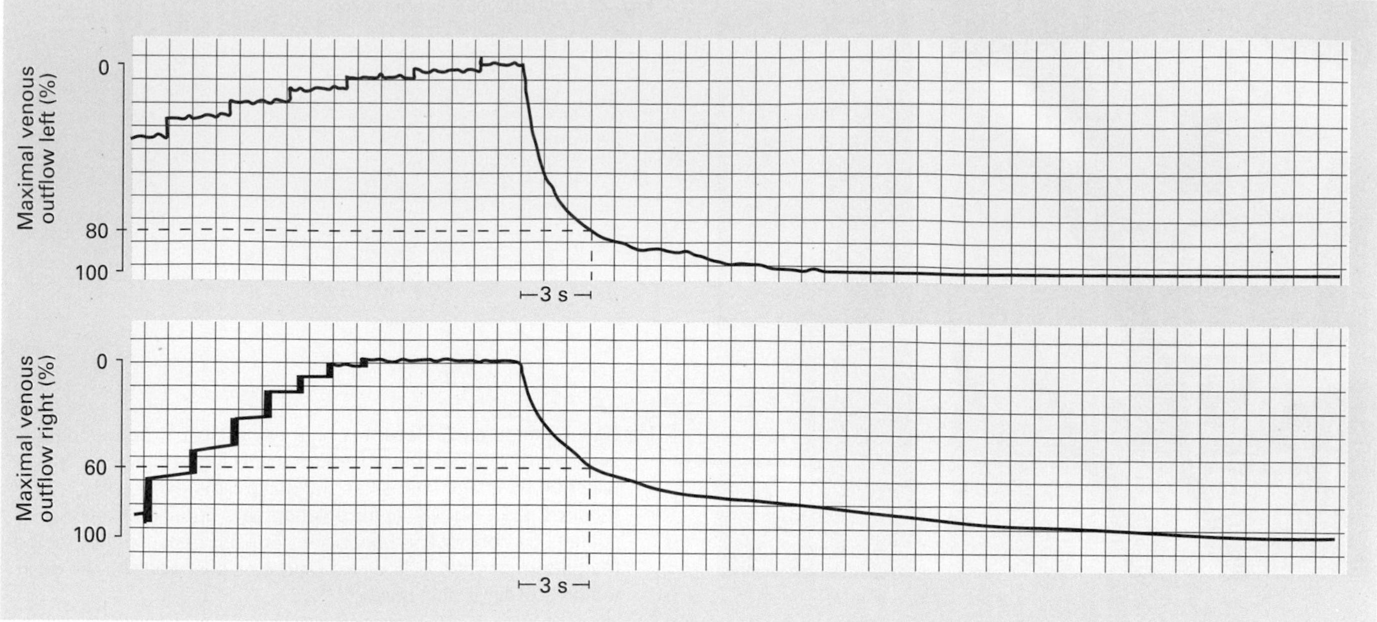

Fig. 27 Maximal venous outflow tracings from a patient with a history of a right deep vein thrombosis during pregnancy 20 years previously. The level of the recording is related to volume of the calf, and changes in this are due to variation in the amount of blood in veins. The initial rise shown is due to venous congestion caused by a pneumatic cuff on the thigh; the sharp fall is on release of the cuff and gives a measure of the rapidity with which venous blood can leave the limb. Left side: 80 per cent of the total fall occurs within the first 3 s. This is within the normal range. Right side: only 60 per cent of total fall occurs in the first 3 s, indicating restriction in venous outlet from the limb. Phlebography confirmed right iliac vein occlusion, but well compensated by pubic varicosities crossing to the opposite side.

(i)), that is to say, upright. With the exception of acute thrombosis in the deep veins, it is only when the patient is near upright and exercising intermittently that many features of venous disorder become apparent. The essence of functional phlebography is to study the functioning of the veins whilst they are working to return blood against gravity. This will allow valve function to be gauged and the causes for inadequate musculovenous pumping to be identified; occlusion or severe deformity in deep veins can be recognized, unnatural enlargement or tortuosity can be seen, and unusual flow patterns, for example collateral flow in superficial veins, are recognized. It is essential that the pattern of venous return should not be distorted by using such artefacts as constricting bands (Fig. 28(a) (ii)). The opportunity to witness events is very brief and is limited by the fact that only part of the limb can be viewed at one moment, the need to keep the amount of opaque medium within safe limits, and the rapidity with which the changes come and go with exercise.

It is not really possible for a radiologist to give comprehensive functional examination of a limb without knowing the likely nature of the problem that he should concentrate upon. It is essential that he should be well briefed by the surgeon or, even better, that the surgeon should be present, guiding the radiologist through the features to be looked for. For these reasons, functional phlebography is a skilled and rather specialized examination. It is important to record the rapidly changing events in some fashion for subsequent study and much can be learnt from this. Depending on the sophistication of apparatus, either multiple static films can be taken or the whole procedure recorded videographically. One problem is to know the relationship in depth of veins one to another and misinterpretation is all too easy without some method of clarification. The simplest way is to take two views of the limb in different rotations so that the relative shift in the veins gives an immediate understanding of their relationship. Before starting, various manoeuvres are rehearsed with the patient, such as exercise by rising up on the toes or rotating the limb inwards and outwards. Any movement by the patient causes immediate changes within the veins, dispersing the opacified blood and quickly creating a confused picture, and for this reason requests to exercise or rotate the limb must be carefully timed. Throughout the examination it must be remembered that only streams of opacified blood are seen and it is quite possible for a large vein to remain invisible because the opacified stream has chosen other channels; failure of a known vein to appear does not necessarily mean that it is occluded and different ways may have to be found to persuade opacified blood to enter it. Functional phlebography is not an easy method but it is immensely rewarding to those who familiarize themselves with it. It is not possible here to describe functional phlebography in detail, but some of the main manoeuvres will be outlined and examples of the results that can be obtained are given in the sections upon the various disorders. The method preferred by the Oxford Vascular Service is described here (Fig. 28(a) (iii)), but other centres have evolved their particular techniques for dynamic phlebography and obtain similar results.

Functional phlebography in the normal

If the patient is tilted foot down to 50° or more and contrast medium is introduced by needle into a superficial vein on the calf, it will be seen to drift down the superficial veins until checked by a valve and soon appear in the deep veins of the leg. This downward movement is because the specific gravity of the opaque medium is higher than that of blood. If injection is continued up to, say,

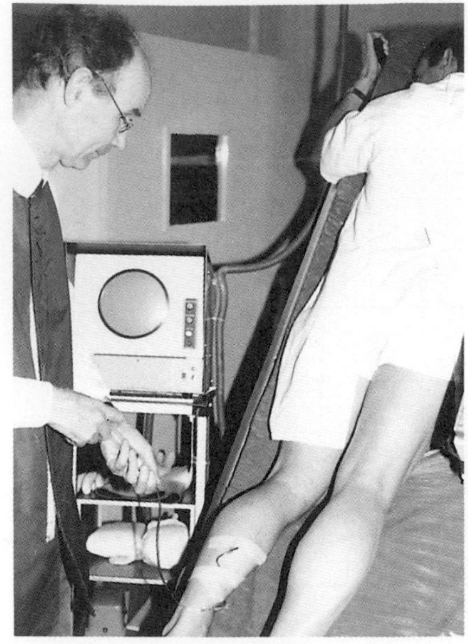

(i)

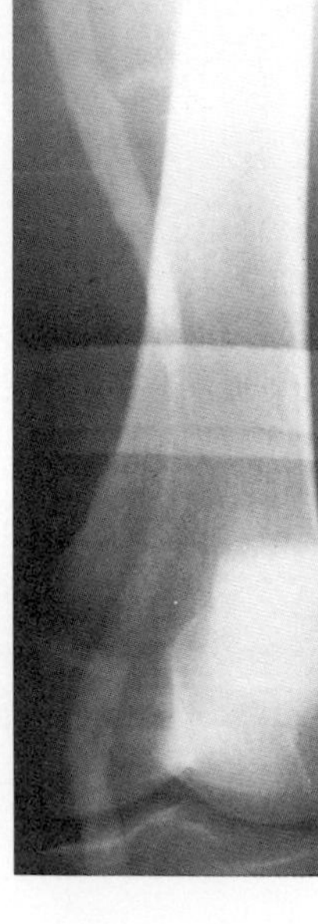

(ii)

Fig. 28 Functional phlebography.

(a) General features. (i) Patient is on a tilting table in near-upright position for most of the procedure. Outlining of the veins is watched by image intensifier and static films exposed as required. (See Fig. 48 (iii) for phlebograms obtained from this patient.) (ii) Constricting bands are not used because they distort the pattern of venous flow. (iii) Diagrams summarizing the main features of functional phlebology.

(iii)

		Superficial vein incompetence	Post-thrombotic syndrome	Valveless syndrome Inborn deficiency of valves deep and superficial
Needle into any convenient enlarged calf vein, small amount of contrast injected. Patient exercised (on toes) × 2	4 ml ex × 2	Flow down and into deep veins	Preferential flow up lower saphenous vein — accentuated by exercise ? move needle to foot vein	Contrast surges back and forth but appears in deep veins or leg via often large perforator(s)
Patient remains still whilst up to 150 ml injected	100-150 ml Passive filling	Outlines deep veins up to iliac veins (valves not shown)	Contrast travels upwards preferentially in lower saphenous vein and superficial veins Deep veins deformed or not outlined	Fills both deep and saphenous vein in parallel fashion
Patient exercised two or three times	Ex × 3	Spills over from upper deep vein to fall down saphenous vein	Blood pushed up superficial veins and collaterals Deep veins deformed or fail to fill	Blood in deep veins surges back and forth with each movement
Patient still. Table lowered to near horizontal until femoral vein shows distinct 'deflation' — but not emptied. Table then rapidly put to near vertical	Swill test	Valves shown as blood 'swills' back	Opacified blood rapidly cleared by fall-back. No valves seen in deformed veins	When returned to upright blood in deep vein falls down rapidly and contrast in upper thigh'disappears' Valves absent or defective
Patient still. Posture and table tilt varied to find optimal position to assist contrast 'up' superficial veins (varicography)	Upward trace	Further details of origin may be shown but unpredictable	Variably shows superficial and collateral veins	

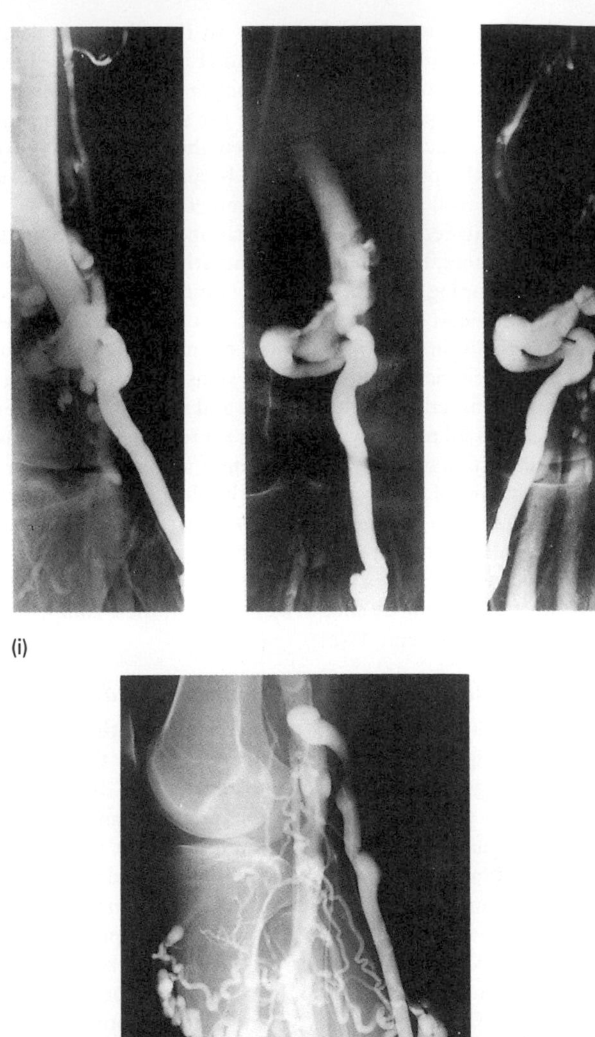

(c) Varicography. (i) When functional phlebography has been completed, varicography can be carried out to clarify anatomical details of superficial incompetence. In this illustration, a short saphenous termination is shown in three different rotations. Varicography usually requires a near-horizontal position to give an upward trace and this has the drawback of collapsing veins so that their size is misleading. It only gives outline and not function of the veins but this has already been ascertained by the preceding examination. (ii) Combination of functional and varicography techniques can give excellent demonstration of the venous disorder. In this example an enlarged, incompetent short saphenous vein gives rise to varicose veins that encircle the leg and join the long saphenous vein.

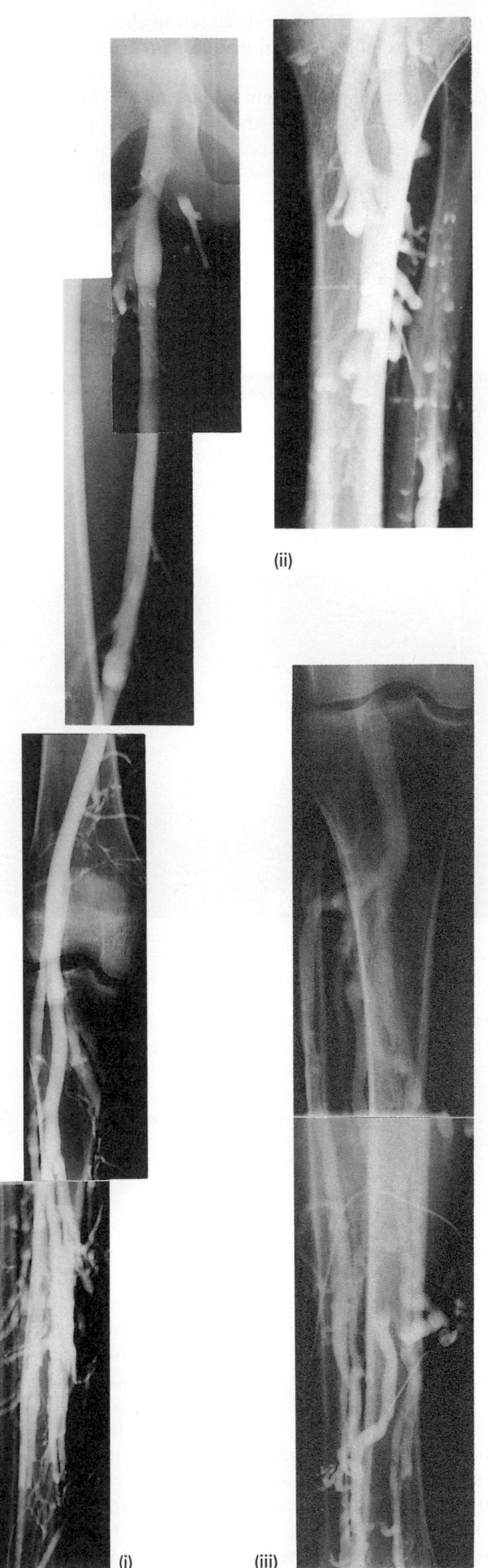

(b) Some basic manoeuvres (and see Fig. 48 (i–vi).) (i) Opaque medium, injected into calf veins whilst the patient remains still, fills the principal deep veins passively but valves are not well shown. (ii) The 'swill test' is used to display valves. The patient is tilted to near-horizontal and up again to empty partially and then refill the veins. It may require repeating to show different levels and in this illustration well valved tibial veins are shown. Since it disperses opacified blood it is best performed as the last stage in functional phlebography. (iii) In superficial incompetence opaque medium injected into calf varicosities will be swept down and into deep veins after an exercise movement (rising on toes), as shown here. If deep vein deformity or occlusion is present the medium is likely to be swept upwards, outlining superficial veins acting as collaterals (see Fig. 13).

100 ml, the deep veins will fill steadily so that they are clearly outlined up to the iliac veins and beyond (Fig. 28(b) (i)). Even a small exercise movement will cause rapid movement upwards in the deep veins with partial emptying of the superficial veins and segmentation of opacified blood between their valves. If movement continues the picture will quickly become confused and all opaque medium will soon leave the limb. During the phase of static filling, opacified blood enters tibial and peroneal veins by multiple perforators, but often it will similarly enter large venous sinuses, the pumping chambers, lying within muscles. This is a normal phenomenon but, for instance, if a single large gastrocnemius vein fills in this way it may be mistaken for a short saphenous vein. Static filling of the deep veins, as just described, is the first stage in functional phlebography and will test the ability of the deep veins to fill normally. Judicious exercise movements may be given during this stage and subsequently to study the patterns of flow. The valves of the deep veins can be shown by lowering the head of the table to near horizontal, so that the veins deflate slightly; the table is then rapidly returned to near vertical again (the swill test), which causes the valve cusps to fill and gives a clear impression of their number and, to some extent, their competence (see Figs. 1, 28(b)(ii), and 48(e)).

Functional phlebography in venous disorders

The procedure is carried out as described above, with the needle introduced through any convenient enlarged vein on the calf; this has the advantage that the direction of movement of the blood from these veins with slight exercise gives an important indication of function. When about 5 ml of medium has been injected the patient is asked to give a small exercise movement and the effect of this is watched on the screen. In simple incompetence of superficial veins the medium will sweep downwards and appear in deep veins (Fig. 28(b) (iii)); in occlusion or severe deformity of deep veins, the medium will be swept up the superficial vein as collateral flow (see Fig. 13). In other cases where perhaps both superficial and deep valves are incompetent heavy surge back and forth may be seen with exercise (Fig. 61(b)).

Other sites for injection may be used, including varicosities on the thigh. If the deep veins fail to fill and the opacified blood streams up superficial veins, as may happen in post-thrombotic syndrome, it may be necessary to reposition the needle to a foot vein to give maximum opportunity for outlining deep veins in the leg.

Varicography

Contrast medium injected moderately quickly, with the patient in only slightly head-up tilt, will tend to outline the vein in an 'upward' direction and, in effect, trace it to its 'origin'. In superficial incompetence this method is of value in showing the source of incompetence, for example, a short saphenous termination (Fig. 28(c) (i)) or a recurrent set of varicose veins of uncertain origin (see Figs. 53(a)(iii) and (b), (c), (d)). This method gives little information on function but it can be combined with information gained from functional phlebography to give comprehensive views of the veins at fault (Fig. 28(c) (ii)). However, the filling of veins by varicography is capricious and results can be misleading until experience is gained.

Ultrasonography (ultrasonic imaging)

Pulsed beam ultrasound scanning creates an image of tissue interfaces and moving blood on a video display unit. This can be used to portray a section through arteries and veins in any plane, from horizontal to vertical. The plane is chosen to show the structure under study to best advantage. In this way a portion of vein over some inches may be shown with its walls and valves clearly outlined and any movements by them demonstrated. The direction and speed of blood flow within the vessel at any point can be individually picked out by a Doppler flow facility and recorded separately (duplex); colour flow scanning (triplex) has the additional feature of displaying flow in a colour representing its direction of movement and showing the velocity by the intensity of the colour (Fig. 29). Thus, the vein walls and lumen can be outlined and flow studied, clot may be recognized by absence of flow and immobile vein walls, and the structure of valves and their competence can be scrutinized in detail. The anatomy of veins can be visualized preoperatively, for example, to demonstrate the level and manner of short saphenous termination; individual deep veins and their branches can be distinguished and flow patterns displayed, so that, for instance, incompetence in a gastrocnemius vein can be recognized (immediately apparent by colour flow) and the reflux within it estimated to assess its significance. This is possible because the diameter and speed of flow within any designated vessel can be measured and from this the volume of flow, either expelled upwards or refluxed downwards, can be calculated. In the popliteal vein this will indicate the effectiveness of the musculovenous pump below the knee or, conversely, the severity of reflux in the deep veins at that level.

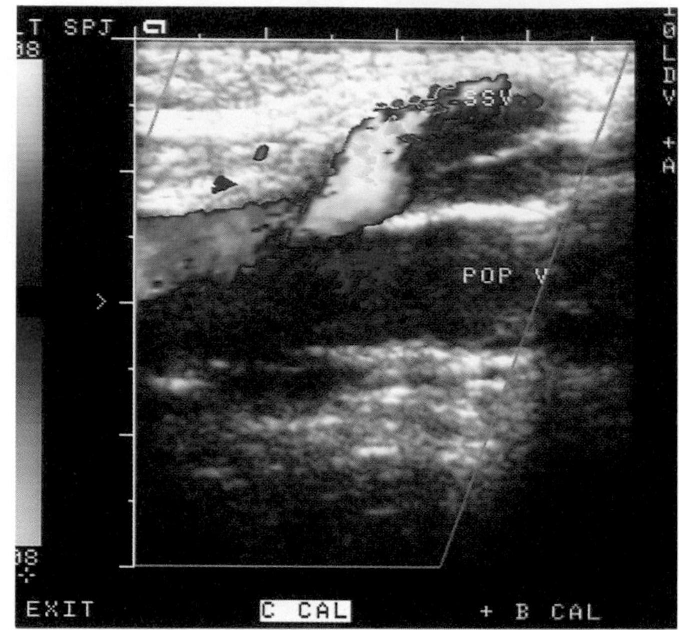

Fig. 29 Ultrasonographic colour flow imaging can give rapid display of veins, their valves, and direction and velocity of flow. In this illustration, the red colour outlines downward flow (away from heart) in the popliteal vein and into an incompetent short saphenous vein, the origin of varicose veins; upward flow (towards the heart) is represented in blue but this is minimal here because this phase has ceased with relaxation of calf muscle. This is an ideal way to examine, non-invasively, limited areas of special interest, such as the popliteal fossa.

The advantages of ultrasonography are that it is non-invasive and can be used for prolonged viewing with repeated cycles of exercise in a way not possible with phlebography and, moreover, the running costs are decidedly less. It is an excellent method for special study of localized areas of vein, both for research and in the practical management of some venous problems. It is already a practical alternative to phlebology for detecting acute thrombosis or in the display of specific structures, such as a short saphenous termination or a valve suspected of leaking. Its potential for future development is considerable and eventually it may displace phlebology for many purposes in the lower limb.

CLINICAL PATTERNS OF VENOUS DISORDER

Incompetence in superficial veins. Simple or primary varicose veins

In the upright position, each contraction of the muscles in a normal limb pumps blood upwards and it is prevented from returning by effective valves. The immediate reduction in the venous pressure and slackening of the deep veins in lower leg and foot caused by this gives opportunity for superficial veins to empty into the deep veins, ready to be pumped up with the next movement. Normally the valves in the superficial veins limit this inward flow so that only a short segment between each valve can empty through the corresponding perforating veins and disorderly widespread transfer of blood from superficial to deep veins is prevented. However, if there is extensive incompetence in the superficial valves, it is possible for blood to spill over from deep veins at high level, down the superficial veins and, finally, to enter the deep veins at low level every time these veins fall slack after muscle contraction (Fig. 30). This is the mechanism underlying the development of simple or primary varicose veins and is, by far, the most common venous disorder.

Such abnormal downflow is gravitationally determined. It only occurs when the patient is upright, or nearly so. In addition to muscular activity, it occurs as a single episode, when the patient rises from horizontal to vertical position, or when simple external pressure to calf or foot partially empties the deep veins. It will not occur with exercise unless there is a reasonably effective deep vein pumping mechanism. In this way, a retrograde circuit of flow is set up, spilling over from a deep vein somewhere above a musculovenous pumping mechanism, down incompetent superficial veins and through perforators to enter deep veins below the pumping mechanism. This may be any group of muscles in the leg or the foot itself, as described earlier. Endless repetition of this cycle of reversed flow causes the superficial veins to become enlarged and tortuous, that is to say, to become varicose veins. However, the main stem of the saphenous veins appears too robust to develop this change and it is the branch veins that do so. Varicose veins are the response to a dynamic process of strong reversed flow and not just by static distension.

A typical retrograde circuit (Fig. 31) is based on a superficial vein, often a long or short saphenous vein with defective or absent valves. The circuit has four components.

A source of outflow from deep to superficial veins at high level.

A pathway of incompetence running down the limb.

Re-entry points where superficial downflow joins the deep veins.

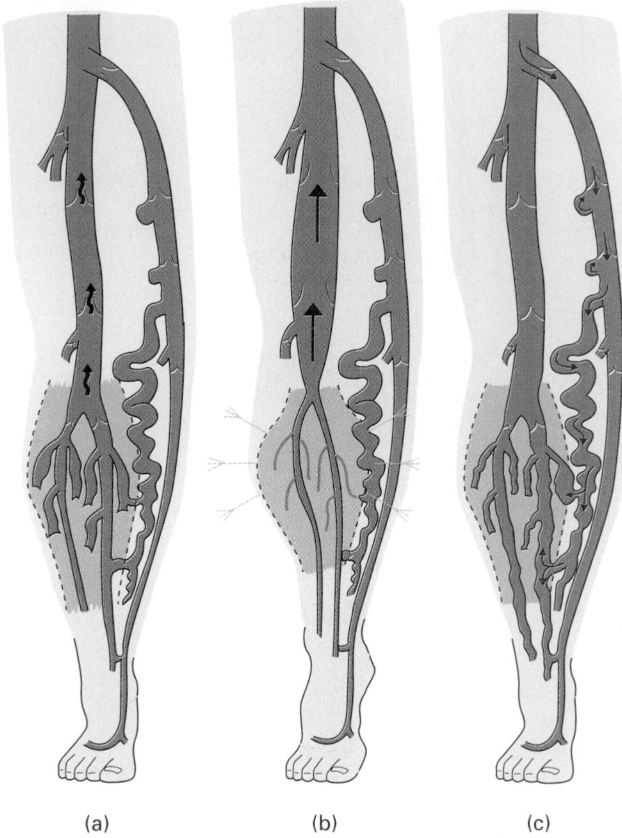

Fig. 30 The retrograde circuit of superficial vein incompetence in a standing patient. (a) Standing still. The veins are well filled with a slow upward drift in the main conduit veins. (b) On contraction of muscle. The leg veins are compressed and the blood driven upwards, emptying the deep veins. (c) On relaxation of muscle. The deep veins, protected from reflux by valves, are now slack. This allows a rush of blood down the pathway of incompetence (here the long saphenous vein and its varicosities), and via perforators into the deep veins so that they are filled prematurely from this unwanted source. This process is endlessly repeated in movements such as walking.

A return pathway provided by the deep veins and the musculovenous pumping mechanisms.

In a retrograde circuit based on an incompetent long or short saphenous vein, its upper end provides the source, its main stem and incompetent branches form the pathway of incompetence, and one or more perforating veins are the re-entry points (Figs. 32 and 33). The deep veins receiving this downflow may be principal conduits, such as the tibial veins, or the venous sinuses (pumping chambers) within any muscle group in the leg, or the veins of the foot (Fig. 33(b)). Although the source is usually the upper end of a saphenous vein, any communication between deep and superficial veins at high level may take on this role; not infrequently pelvic veins provide a source, especially during pregnancy, giving varicosities in vulva and upper thigh, and these may persist after childbirth (see Fig. 39). Less usual sources are particularly likely to occur when superficial vein anatomy has been fragmented by previous surgery, for example, after high saphenous ligation, a midthigh perforator may become the source of recurrence (Fig. 53(d) (iii)). There are numerous variations on this theme but

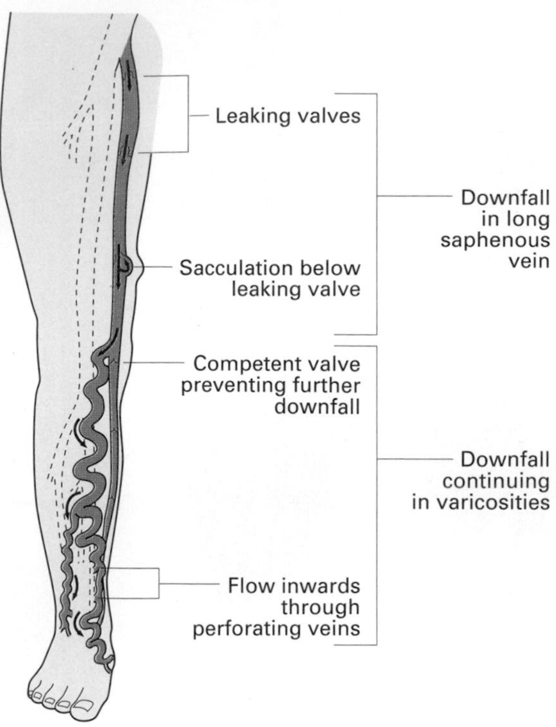

Fig. 31 The components of a typical retrograde circuit of superficial incompetence: a source (in this example, the saphenofemoral junction); a pathway of incompetence (long saphenous vein and varicosities); re-entry points to the deep veins (perforating veins); a return pathway up the deep veins (activated by the musculovenous pump). The other essential factor is gravity; the circuit's activity is maximal in the upright position but diminishes to extinction as the horizontal is approached.

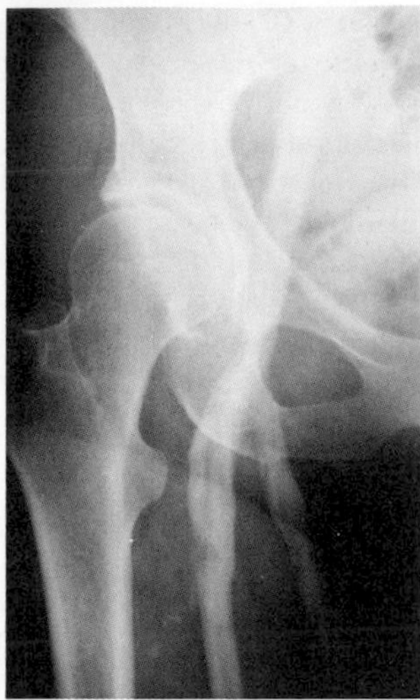

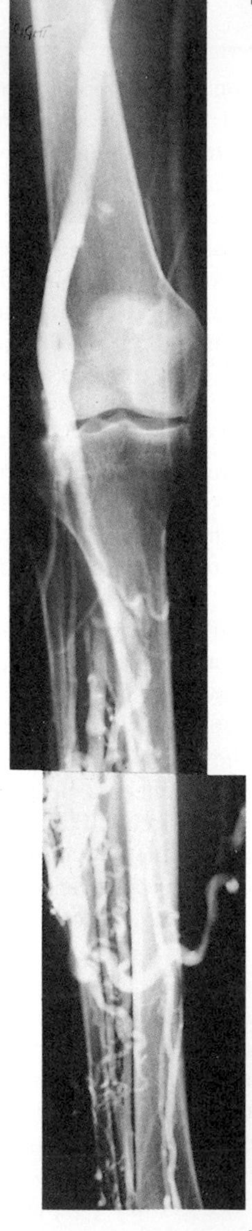

Fig. 32 Composite functional phlebogram of a retrograde circuit. Opaque medium injected into calf veins has entered the principal deep veins and, with exercise, it can be seen spilling over from the common femoral and down the long saphenous vein.

each has the same components, a higher level source, a pathway of incompetence, and re-entry point(s) provided by perforating veins at lower levels, including the foot. This state is usually curable by removal of the source and the pathway of incompetence, but enlarged re-entry points (one or more perforators) that allow backflow may also require closing off. An understanding of the retrograde circuit in superficial vein incompetence is essential in the good management of varicose veins and treatment will not be successful unless these components to the circuit are accurately recognized and effectively obliterated by sclerotherapy or removed by surgery. The more completely this is done, the more effective and permanent treatment will be. Several typical retrograde circuits of superficial vein incompetence are illustrated in Figs. 34, 35, 36, and 45.

Mixed patterns of superficial incompetence

These arise when there are two or more sources of incompetence causing the varicose veins, for example long and short saphenous vein incompetence both contributing to varicosities on the calf, or a pathway of incompetence that starts in long saphenous vein and then crosses over to join the short saphenous vein from which the varicose veins arise, or vice versa (Fig. 37).

Unusual or unexpected sources of superficial vein incompetence

It has already been mentioned that there are many possible unexpected sources of incompetent downflow in superficial veins, such

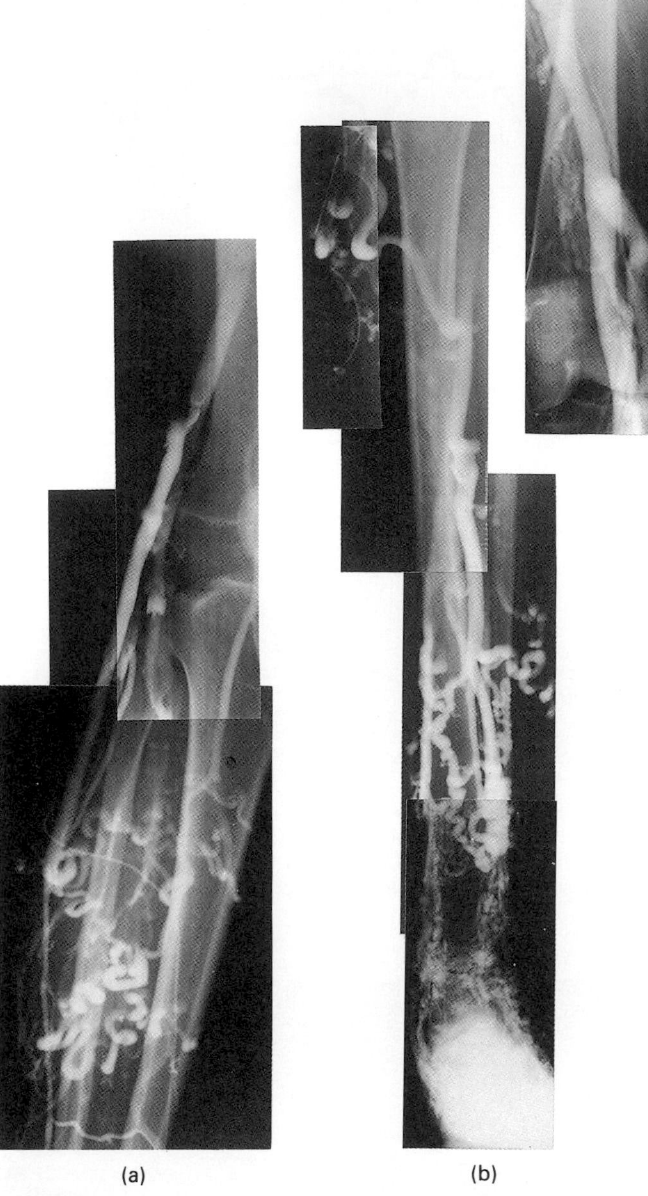

(a) (b)

Fig. 33 Short saphenous incompetence. (a) Composite pictures of short saphenous incompetence obtained by functional phlebography. (b) A retrograde circuit runs from a high level down to a low pressure area created by a venous pumping unit, and this includes the foot. Varicose veins, as part of the pathway of incompetence, often run to the underside of the foot, as shown in this composite phlebogram of short saphenous incompetence.

as the internal pudendal vein from the pelvic deep veins or when previous surgery has fragmented normal anatomy; moreover it is also possible for retrograde circuits of incompetence to arise in conjunction with other forms of venous disorder. Some examples of these less usual states are given below.

Unexpected sources

Varicosities from a long saphenous source may be visible in short saphenous territory or vice versa; one variant of this is a vein running upwards for a short distance before linking on to a branch of the other saphenous system and so giving rise to the apparent paradox of upward flow in a simple varicose vein (Fig. 38). With pregnancy, vulval varicosities arising via pudendal veins from the pelvic veins may appear and persist to provide an obscure source of superficial vein incompetence down thigh and leg (Fig. 39). In its most extreme form, this will be even more extensive, taking its source from massive incompetence in the ovarian veins and through the pelvic veins (Fig. 40(a) and (b)); it will be accompanied by severe premenstrual discomfort in the pelvis and in limb varicosities (pelvic congestion syndrome). This is exactly comparable with the equivalent state, in the male, of incompetence in a testicular vein leading to varicose veins at its lower end, but here outside the pelvis and showing as a varicocele in the scrotum; the venous return from this is to pelvic veins but it also has easy communication with veins in the upper thigh.

Intricate patterns

These patterns of incompetence follow an unexpected course, either by crossing over from one limb to the other or because flow passes from the source in an upward direction for an appreciable distance before cascading down the limb. An example of the former is long saphenous incompetence taking its origin via pubic varicosities crossing over from a surviving branches in a saphenous stump of the opposite side following inadequate surgery there (Fig. 41(a)). An example of paradoxical flow may be seen in an extension from the short saphenous vein running upwards to emerge on the inner aspect of midthigh and acting as the source of downflow in a long saphenous vein incompetent below this level (Fig. 41(b)); high ligation of the long saphenous vein will not cure this condition as the fault does not lie here.

Complex patterns

These occur when deep vein impairment and superficial vein incompetence coexist. Certainly, a saphenous vein acting as a collateral past deep vein occlusion is often oversized and incompetent but, as the predominant flow is continuous collateral upflow, confusion in diagnosis seldom arises. However, when the lower part of the limb has been spared thrombotic damage and is capable of effective pumping to produce an area of low venous pressure, it is possible for incompetent saphenous branches to spill down to the low pressure area and show the features of typical simple varicose veins. For example, if the femoral vein is occluded in midthigh, but there is no thrombotic damage to the deep veins below the knee, a saphenous vein acting as collateral may develop varicose side branches running down to the foot (Fig. 42(a) (i)). These veins may have no collateral function but become varicose by allowing flow down to the low pressure areas created in foot or lower leg by exercise. Similarly, in iliac vein occlusion, a typical long saphenous vein incompetence, with varicose veins, may develop in the limb beneath this, taking its source from the collateral flow passing from common femoral vein to uppermost saphenous branches and across the pubic region (Fig. 42(a) (ii)). A crossover variety of this sort occurs when an incompetent long saphenous vein of the opposite limb takes source from pubic collaterals that have crossed over to join its superficial epigastric and pudendal branches (Fig. 42(b) (i) and (ii)). It is important to recognize this since otherwise surgery to treat apparently simple saphenous incompetence may damage valuable collateral vessels.

Causation of incompetence of valves in superficial veins

The central feature of superficial vein incompetence is lack of effective valves in these veins. This may arise because there is an

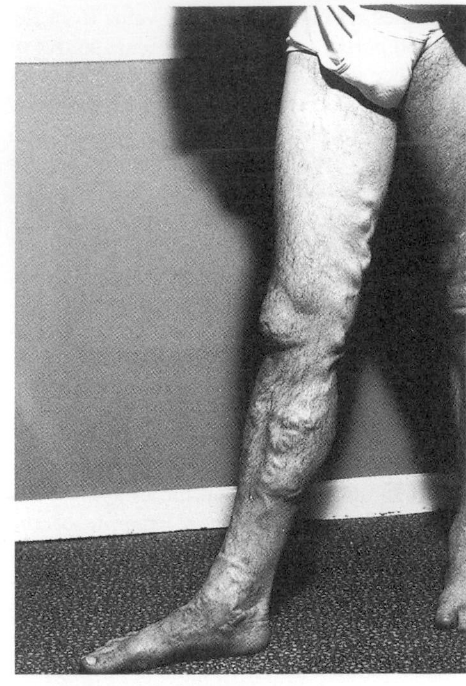

(a)

(a) A massive varicose vein arises from the long saphenous vein in the upper thigh (posteromedial branch in continuity with the arcuate vein) and runs down the length of the limb with branches continuing on to the foot. The presence of skin pigmentation indicates that downflow in the superficial veins is overwhelming the musculovenous pump sufficiently to cause venous hypertension. Selective (Trendelenburg) occlusion and Perthes' test were strongly positive.

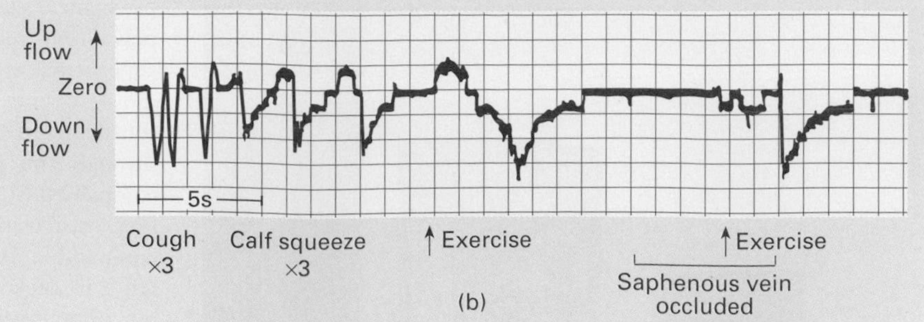

(b) Doppler flowmetry to long saphenous vein shows downflow after squeezing the calf and after exercise, but delayed when saphenous vein is occluded by finger pressure.

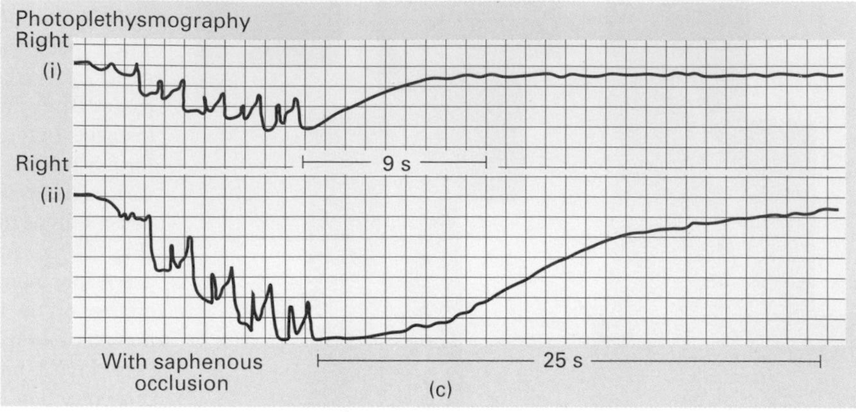

(c) (i) Photoplethysmogram showing refilling time of 9 s after five exercise movements. (ii) Photoplethysmogram repeated whilst the saphenous vein is occluded by finger pressure. The response is much stronger and the refilling time is now 25 s. These tests strongly indicate that surgery removing the long saphenous vein and varicosities should give a good result.

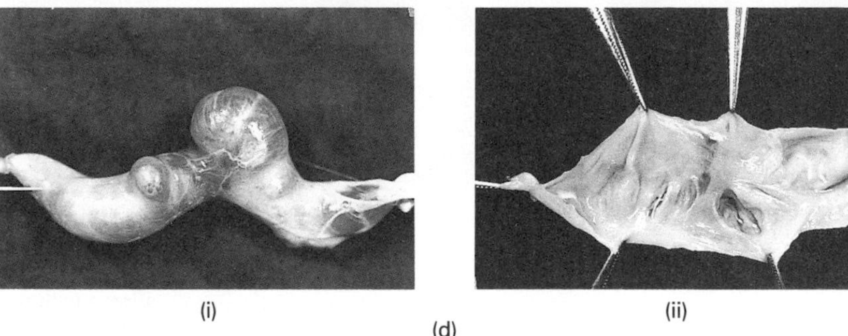

(i) (ii)

(d)

(d) Portion of the thigh varicosity after surgery. (i) Distended with saline to show sacculation in thinned and weakened walls. (ii) The vein opened to show its interior. Deep saccules are evident but no valves can be recognized. It is not known whether the weakened and expanded walls are a primary phenomenon or are secondary to the stress of turbulent downflow.

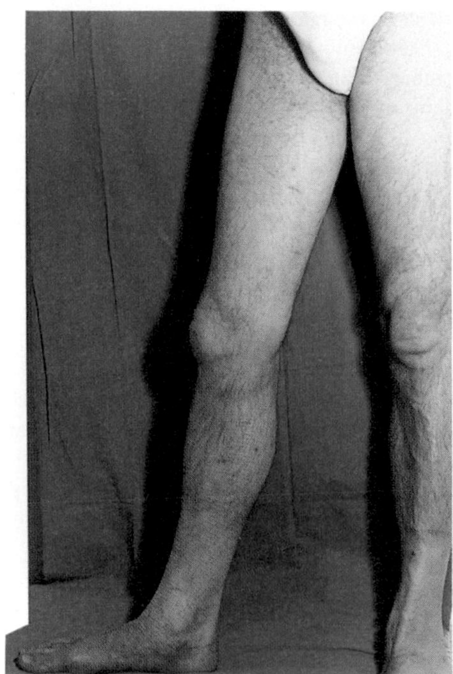

(e)

(e) Appearance 3 months after surgery. Discomfort has been relieved, there are no visible varicose veins, and pigmentation is much less. Photoplethysmography showed refilling in normal range at 25 s.

Fig. 34 Long saphenous incompetence. Clinical features and investigations.

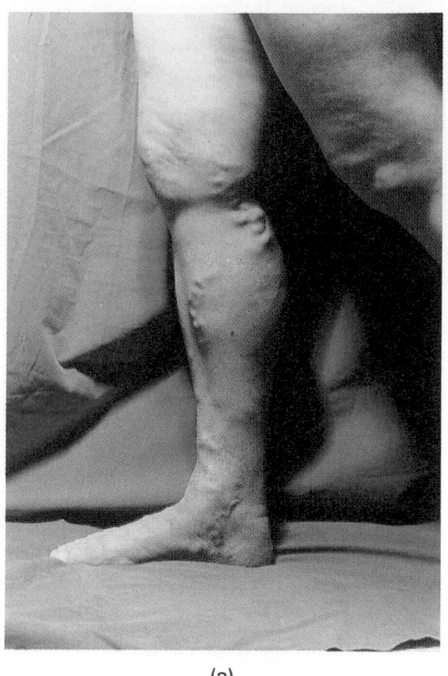
(a)

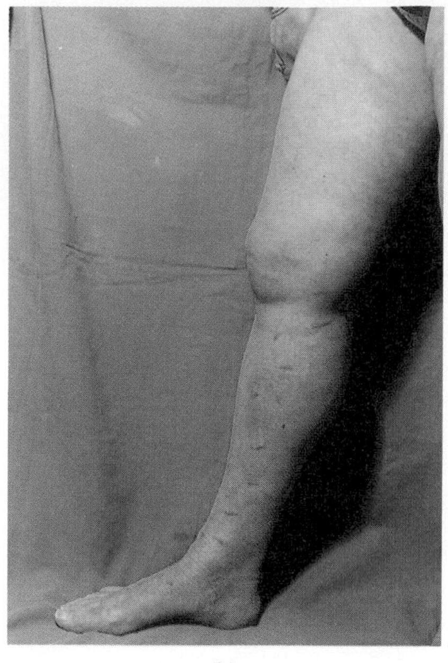
(b)

Fig. 35 Long saphenous incompetence; relief of symptoms with improved appearance and minimal scars. (a) Varicose veins, following two pregnancies, causing much discomfort, particularly around time of menstruation; large varicose veins can be seen running across the front of the ankle on to the foot. All tests and investigations were similar to the patient illustrated in Fig. 34. (b) Three months after surgery. Discomfort has gone and the patient is pleased with the appearance. Only small incisions closed with subcuticular stitches were used, or stab incisions and adhesive tape, in order to minimize scars.

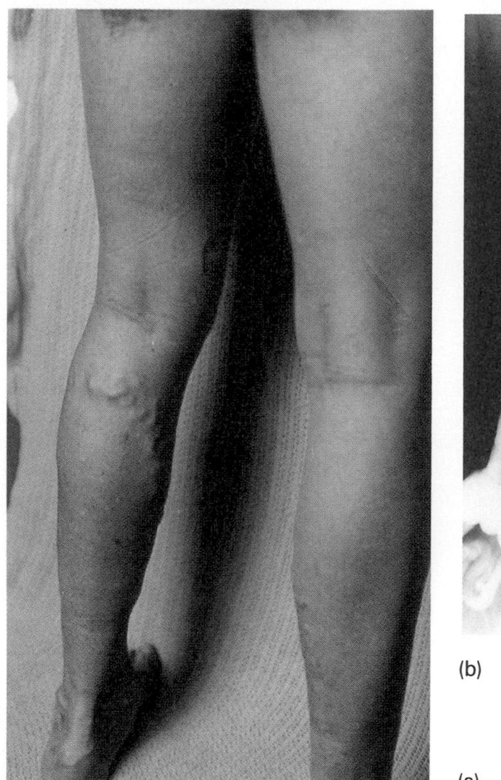
(a)

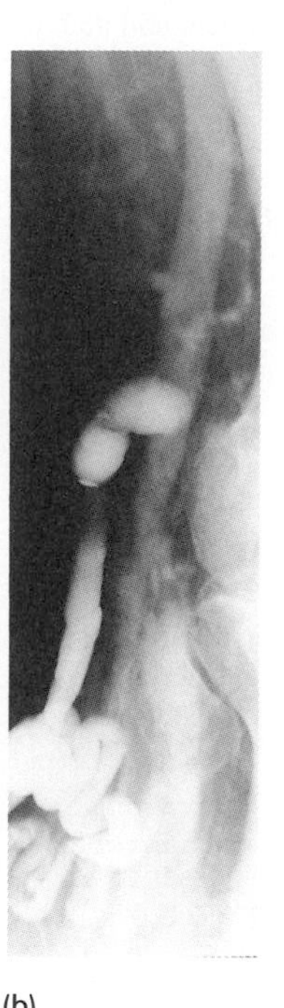
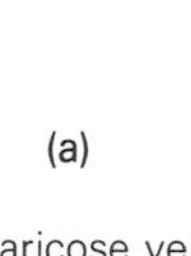
(b)

Fig. 36 Short saphenous incompetence and varicose veins in a young woman with a strong family history of vein problems. (a) Appearance of left limb. All clinical tests and special investigations confirmed short saphenous incompetence. (b) A phlebogram was obtained to show the level and manner of saphenous termination to guide the surgeon. This shows an enlarged saphenous vein terminating at the most common level and the varicose vein arising from it in upper calf.

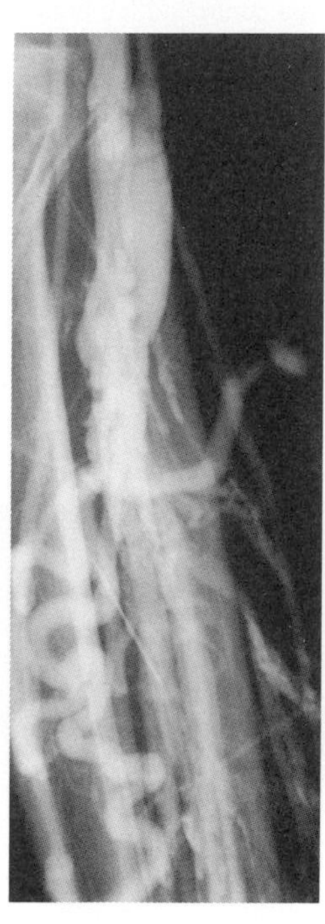

Fig. 37 Interconnection between the long and short saphenous systems. This is commonplace and the phlebogram here shows a varicose vein running obliquely from the short saphenous vein in the upper calf to join the long saphenous vein down which incompetent flow continued.

inborn weakness in the valve cusps or the vein wall, or there is a deficiency in the number of valves. Many patients give a family history suggesting an inherited defect and the fact that simple varicose veins not infrequently first appear at the age of 14 or 15 supports the belief that some form of inborn weakness is responsible in at least some patients. Some authorities believe that the fault is in the vein walls which allow valve cusps to separate and leak. This may certainly be true, but examples are seen where virtually no valves are present, or only vestigial ones, in the superficial veins concerned. It is likely that there are several different

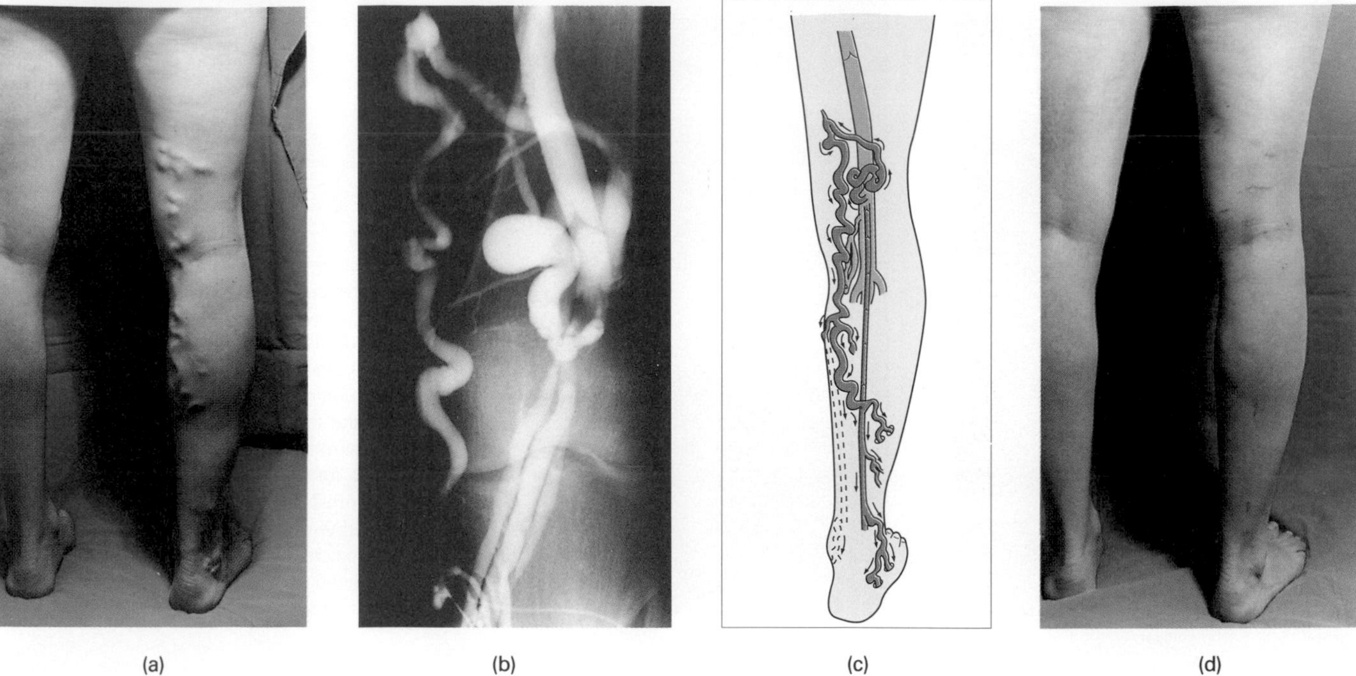

Fig. 38 Deceptive varicose veins. This varicose vein, in the mother of three children, had enlarged recently and caused discomfort. (a) On inspection, the vein shown here might be assumed to have an origin in the long saphenous vein but a selective occlusion test showed this was not so; however, pressure behind the knee controlled the entire varicose vein and its branches at the ankle. Doppler flowmetry confirmed that, after exercise, flow came up from the popliteal fossa and across to the uppermost visible point of the vein, and then down its length; this flow could be intercepted by finger pressure over the midpopliteal fossa. (b) Phlebography confirmed the origin of the varicosity as a tortuous vein arising from the short saphenous termination and winding upwards before descending posteromedially. (c) Diagram of the distribution of the vein shown by functional phlebography. In the lower leg it connects with both long and short saphenous veins as well as the deep veins by perforators. (d) With a good understanding of the unusual arrangement of this vein it was possible to remove it completely, with relief of symptoms and the improved appearance shown here.

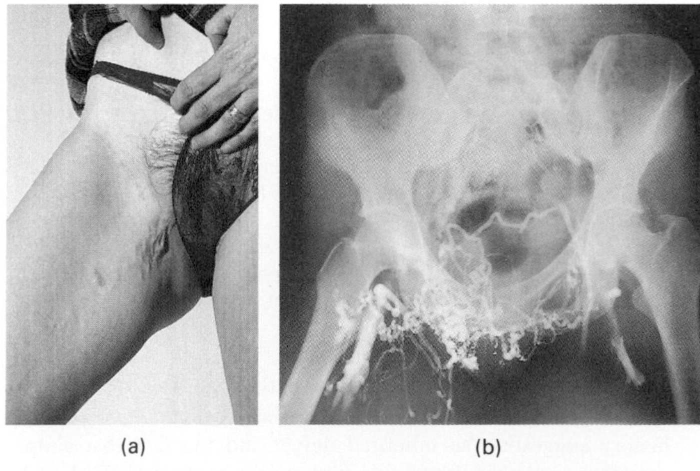

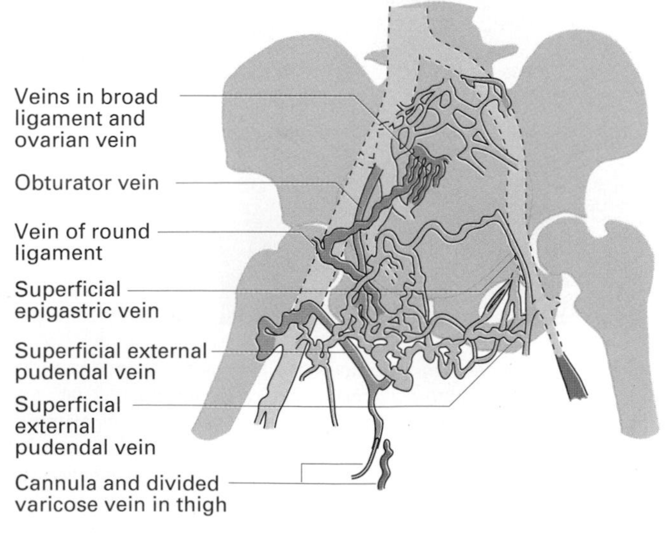

Fig. 39 Pelvic source of superficial incompetence. (a) A pudendal varicose vein taking its source from pelvic veins. The patient had developed large vulval varices during pregnancy but these subsided after childbirth leaving the vein shown here. (b) Phlebogram obtained through the pudendal varicosity during surgery. (c) Explanatory diagram of connections with pelvic veins. The internal pudendal vein, not identified here, is commonly implicated.

Fig. 41 Other patterns of incompetence.
(a) Intricate patterns of incompetence. (i) Crossover incompetence. Clinical appearance showing pubic varicosities, originating from the stump of a ligated long saphenous vein on the left side and providing the origin for substantial long saphenous incompetence, with venotensive changes, on the right side. (ii) Explanatory diagram.
(b) Paradoxical upflow. (i) These recurrent varicosities followed long saphenous surgery and appeared to have their source in midthigh. However, the varicose veins, and Doppler downflow in them, were controlled by pressure in the upper popliteal fossa, and from here Doppler upflow to the midthigh was detected after exercise and in unison with the pattern of downflow in the varicose veins. (ii) Composite phlebogram explaining this paradoxical flow. The varicosity originates from an upward extension of the short saphenous vein; there is also a lesser contribution from a long saphenous stump in the groin.

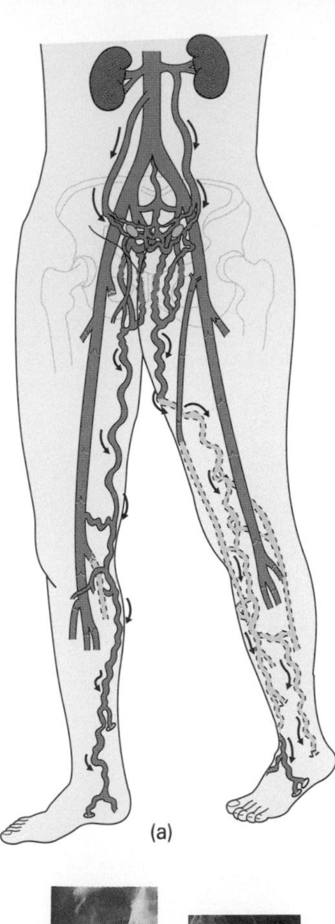

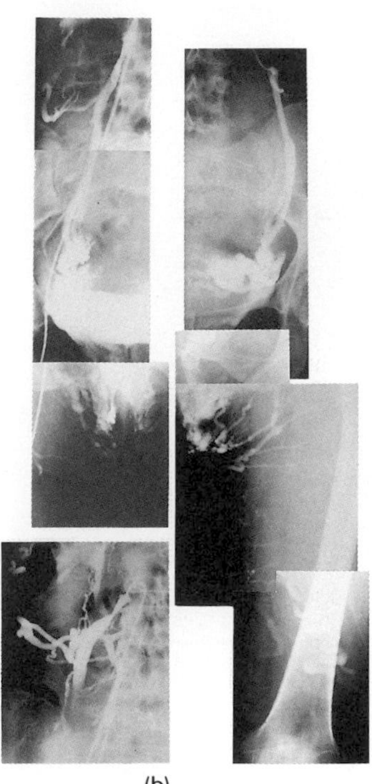

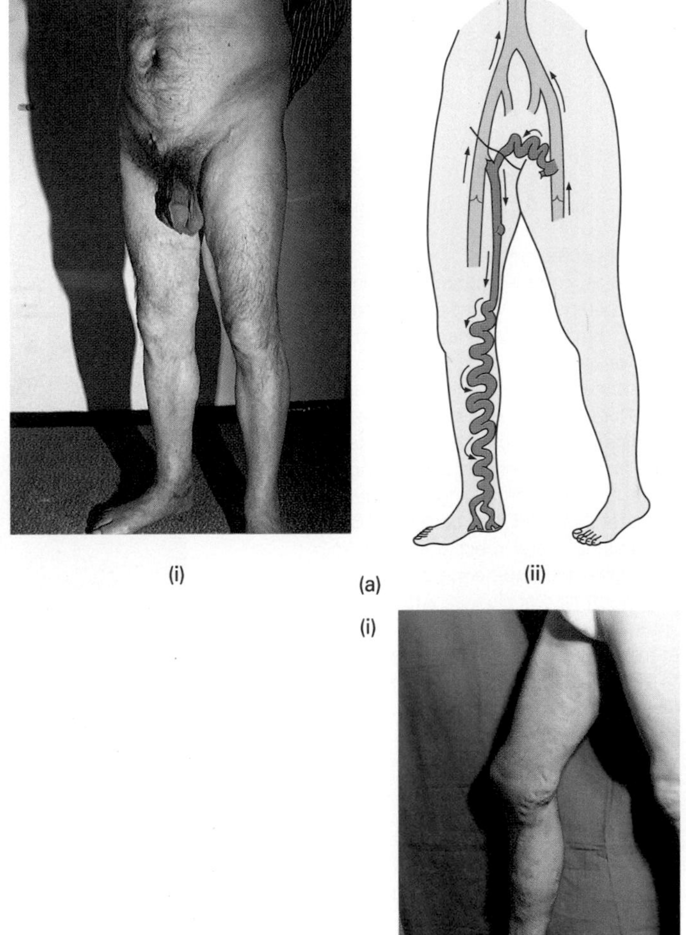

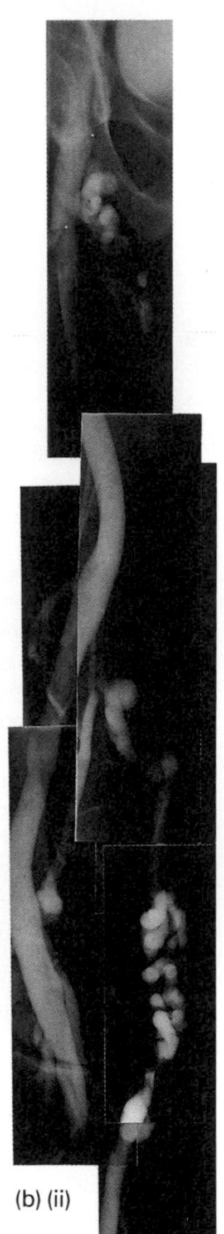

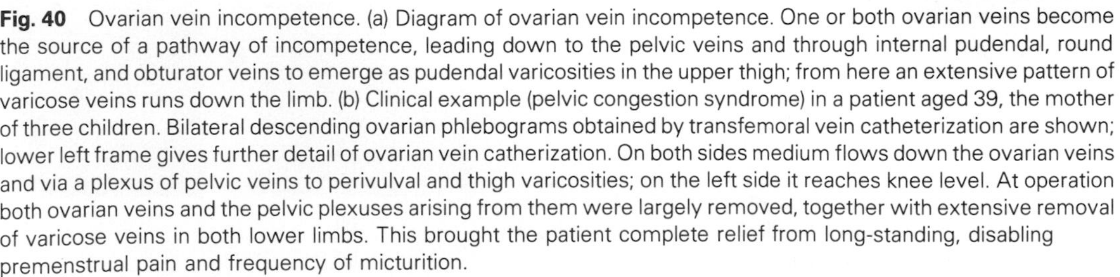

Fig. 40 Ovarian vein incompetence. (a) Diagram of ovarian vein incompetence. One or both ovarian veins become the source of a pathway of incompetence, leading down to the pelvic veins and through internal pudendal, round ligament, and obturator veins to emerge as pudendal varicosities in the upper thigh; from here an extensive pattern of varicose veins runs down the limb. (b) Clinical example (pelvic congestion syndrome) in a patient aged 39, the mother of three children. Bilateral descending ovarian phlebograms obtained by transfemoral vein catheterization are shown; lower left frame gives further detail of ovarian vein catherization. On both sides medium flows down the ovarian veins and via a plexus of pelvic veins to perivulval and thigh varicosities; on the left side it reaches knee level. At operation both ovarian veins and the pelvic plexuses arising from them were largely removed, together with extensive removal of varicose veins in both lower limbs. This brought the patient complete relief from long-standing, disabling premenstrual pain and frequency of micturition.

(ii)

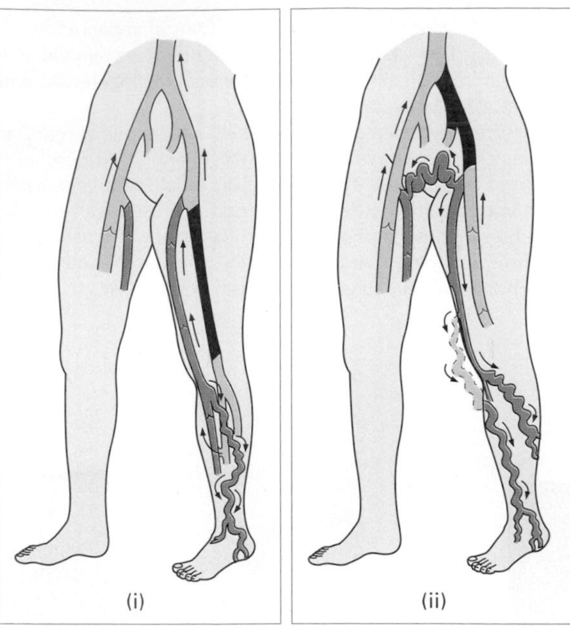

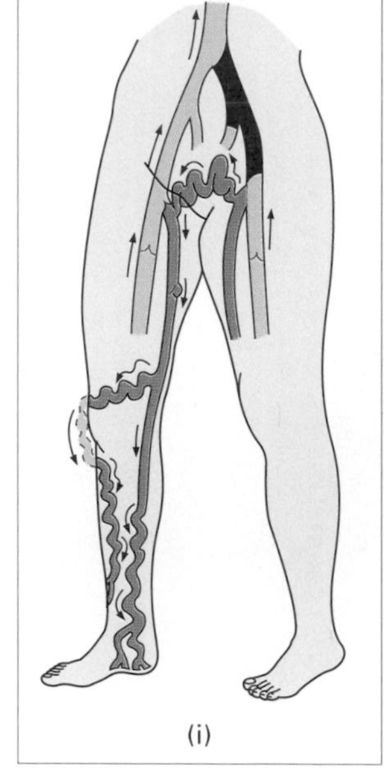

(a)

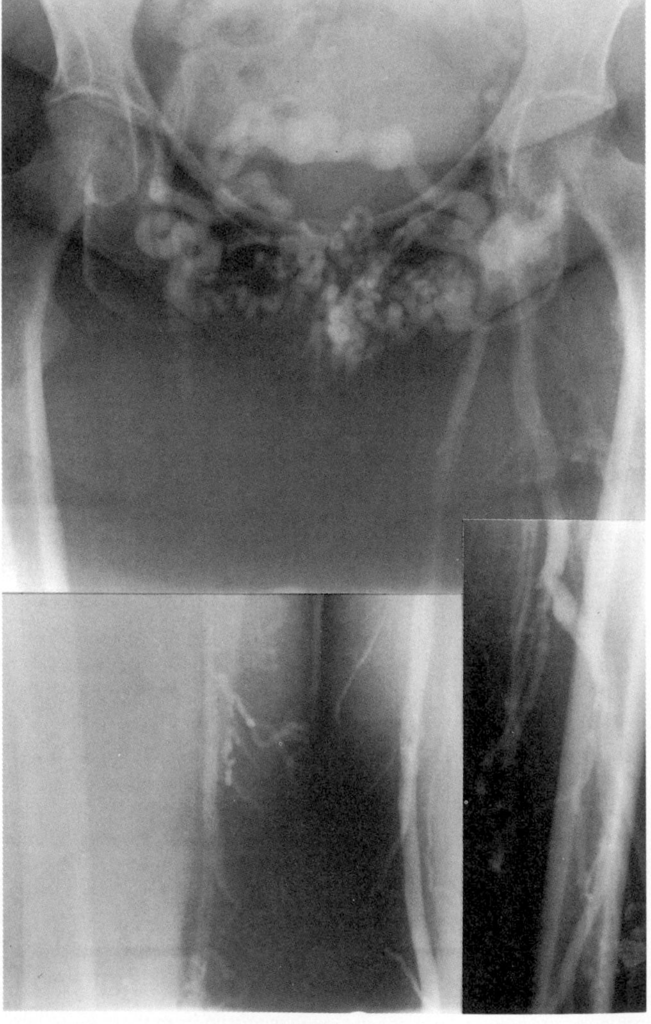

(ii)
(b)

Fig. 42 Complex patterns of incompetence.
(a) Diagrams of complex patterns, combining deep vein impairment with superficial vein incompetence. (i) Varicosities running down to the foot and originating from a long saphenous vein acting as collateral to an occluded femoropopliteal deep vein. (ii) Typical long saphenous incompetence and varicosities below left iliac vein occlusion. This is not uncommon and surgery may endanger pubic collateral veins originating from the saphenous termination.
(b) Crossover incompetence in iliac vein occlusion. (i) Long saphenous incompetence on right side arising from pubic varicosities acting as collaterals to left iliac occlusion. Surgery to right side could damage this collateral mechanism. (ii) An example of complex crossover incompetence shown by functional phlebography in left iliac occlusion. After three exercise movements, opaque medium injected into calf veins on the left side has travelled preferentially up the left long saphenous vein, across to the opposite side via pubic collateral varices, and down an incompetent right long saphenous vein, and is seen entering varices in the right thigh. Injection of medium was made at one site on the left leg only.

causes for valve failure, each leading to the same final result of incompetence and varicose veins. (See under Spectrum of valve deficiency.)

Aggravating factors

Many varicose veins first appear in pregnancy and although most will recede again, others will persist (Fig. 43). A likely mechanism is the dilating effect of oestrogen upon the vein walls, affecting their role in retaining valve cusps in good apposition and any uncovering any imperfections here. Apart from this, women are more prone to superficial vein incompetence than men in a ratio of about 2 : 1, again probably due to hormonal influence; this is supported by the fact that women's varicose veins are always more troublesome and prominent just before menstruation. Jobs involving prolonged standing have been shown to increase the likelihood of varicose veins and the incidence increases with age.

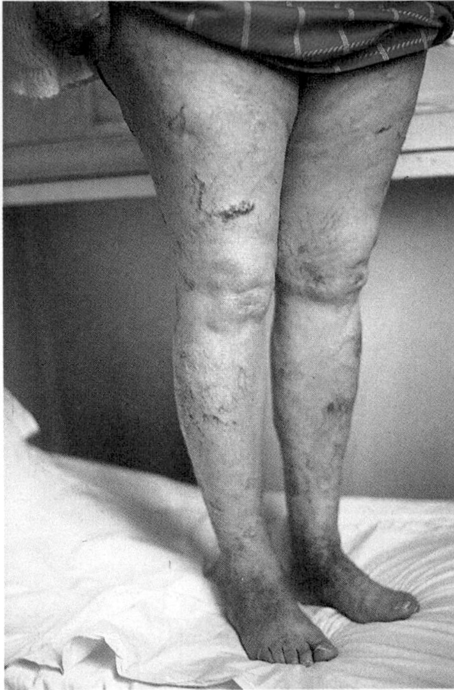

Fig. 43 Pregnancy can produce a widespread profusion of varicosities, including intradermal venules. These usually disappear when pregnancy is over but persisted in this patient.

Manifestations

Unsightly varicose veins are the most common expression of superficial vein incompetence and women are more likely to complain of this than men. Varying degrees of discomfort are attributed to the clearly visible defect and although this is usually correct, the possibility of another cause should not be overlooked. However, it is possible for the reverse to be true and for the patient to have heavy, uncomfortable legs, caused by substantial superficial vein incompetence but without any visible varicosities. This 'concealed' incompetence is not uncommon and is caused by a 'straight through' variety of saphenous incompetence which connects with perforators without any intervening varicosities (Fig. 44). Conversely, obvious varicose veins may seem unrelated to symptoms elsewhere in the limb, for example, the misleading pattern of varicosities found in the thigh when a large, clearly visible varicosity arises from the saphenous termination and 'bypasses' a competent valve in the uppermost long saphenous vein but then joins this vein in its incompetent lower part (Fig. 45).

The more severe forms of superficial vein incompetence, with or without varicosities, may overwhelm the pumping mechanism and give rise to venous hypertension. In mild cases this may cause an area of pigmentation, swelling, and slight induration near the ankle, perhaps with a tendency for eczema as shown in Fig. 46(a); in more severe cases venotensive changes will be more extensive and often include ulceration (Figs. 46(b), 47, and see Figs. 52, 63(a)), which is considered later in this Section. These changes are

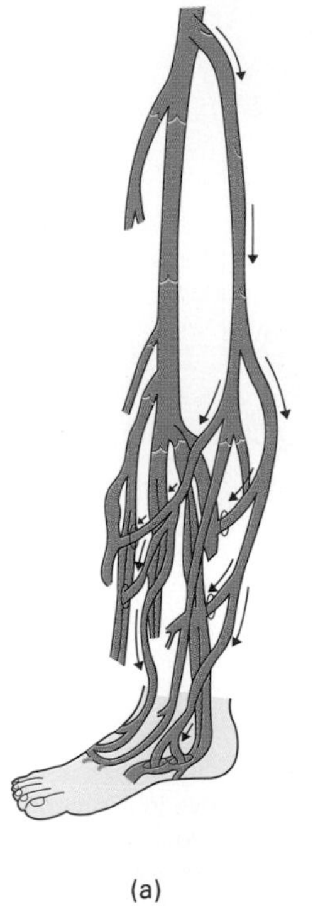

(a)

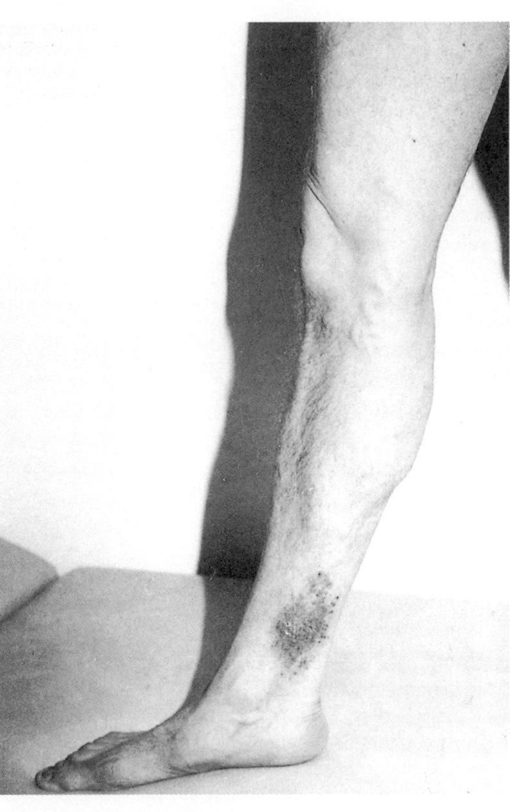

(b)

Fig. 44 Concealed superficial vein incompetence. Severe venotensive changes arising from superficial incompetence but not accompanied by obvious varicose veins. (a) Usually a pathway of incompetence includes visible varicose veins arising from a saphenous vein. However, it is possible for retrograde flow from a saphenous vein or posterior arch vein to enter perforating veins directly, without intervening varicose veins, and cause venotension in a relatively concealed fashion, as shown in this diagram. (b) Clinical example. This patient's only complaint was of an uncomfortable, itching, and discoloured patch above the ankle. Only one small varicose vein at knee level could be seen but, in fact, a massive incompetence in the long saphenous vein was present, detectable by tap-wave, and proved by Doppler flowmetry and photoplethysmography. Surgery to this vein relieved the symptoms and the skin changes subsided.

not specific to superficial vein incompetence (primary varicose veins) and it is important to remember that other venous conditions which create venous hypertension, such as deep vein impairment, can also be a potent cause but require different management.

Clinical examination and investigation

The general aspects of this have been considered in some detail earlier and will only be summarized here in relation to superficial vein incompetence. The history must always include enquiry for possible previous deep vein thrombosis with pregnancy, serious illness, or limb fractures. This will give warning that deep vein impairment is possible; it is then essential to examine the lower abdomen and pubic region for varicosities acting as collaterals past occluded iliac veins. The following procedure is appropriate and is carried out with the patient standing, the position in which venous problems become evident.

1. **Inspection** The general pattern of prominent veins and varicosities on all aspects of the limbs and on the lower abdomen is noted, together with any suggestion of saccules on the saphenous veins. The lower leg and foot are scrutinized for signs of venotension. If there is any possibility of diabetes the underside of the foot should be inspected to exclude neuropathic ulceration. General medical considerations should not be overlooked at this stage; because varicose veins are an obvious defect, symptoms are often wrongly attributed to them.

2. **Mapping out** The importance of commencing examination with a careful mapping out of the abnormal veins and other veins connecting with them cannot be overstated. This is done by inspection, palpation, and use of the tap-wave technique (see Fig. 21); the foot must be included and, if there is any suspicion of previous deep vein thrombosis, the lower abdomen and pubes. It may be combined with other observations on the varicosities, such as cough impulse and increased warmth; if there is a palpable saccule on a saphenous vein check for a thrill on coughing in keeping with a leaking valve here.

3. **Pathway of incompetence** The likely pathway of incompetence from which the varicosities arise should be selected, based on the findings at mapping out.

4. **Trendelenburg test** A selective Trendelenburg test, using fingers, not any form of tourniquet, should be applied to the suspected pathway of incompetence (see Fig. 22). This is the key test upon which diagnosis and decision for treatment depends. Perthes' test, exercising by rising on the toes with the pathway of incompetence occluded, is carried out as useful confirmation of the diagnosis (see Fig. 23).

In many cases the examination so far will have given clear evidence of the diagnosis and will have accurately identified the pathway of

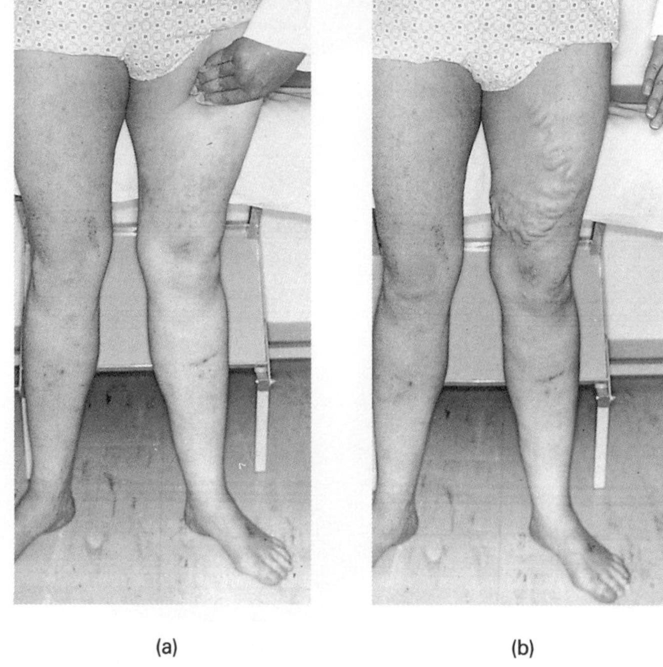

(a) (b)

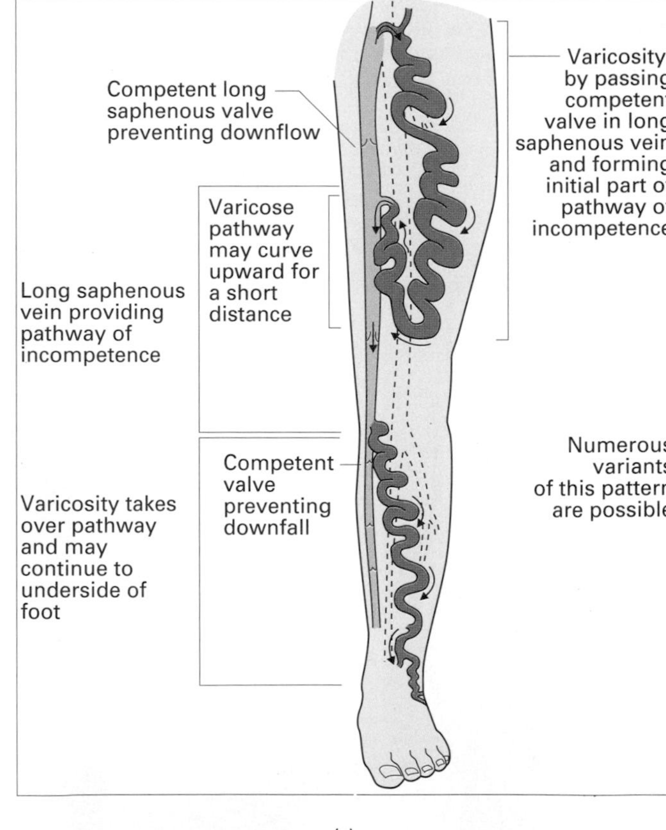

(c)

Fig. 45 Bypassing a valve in superficial incompetence. A functioning valve in a superficial vein is bypassed by a varicose vein which re-enters the incompetent portion of the vein below the valve. (a) Fingertip compression to the upper part of a thigh varicosity (anterolateral branch of saphenous vein) gives complete control, including varicose veins below the knee. (b) Release of compression causes immediate filling to varicose veins in thigh and leg. At surgery, syringe testing confirmed the presence of a functioning valve in the upper third of the saphenous vein but with gross incompetence below this level. (c) Explanatory diagram. This bypassing phenomenon occurs in many variants and is a common cause for confusion.

incompetence. However, sometimes the tests are inconclusive and, in any case, it is always useful to have further confirmation. This is easily and quickly provided by use of the directional Doppler flowmeter.

5. Directional Doppler flowmetry The probe is usually placed over the saphenous vein in the lower thigh or upper calf and the response to coughing, squeezing the calf, and rising on the toes noted (see Fig. 24). If the pathway of incompetence has been correctly identified, a burst of downflow should follow each exercise movement (Fig. 34(b)). If this does not occur, it is possible that the muscles so far exercised are not involved in the retrograde circuit and the effect of raising the foot clear of the ground, with knee straight, should be tried. If varicosities run to the foot this may produce a surprisingly vigorous response.

When downflow has been demonstrated, the test is repeated with the suspected pathway of incompetence occluded by finger pressure well above the probe to confirm that this eliminates the downflow (Fig. 34(b)). The Doppler flowmeter is also a valuable tool in mapping out and demonstrating interconnection between veins, for example, between varicose vein and saphenous vein, or long and short saphenous systems. This is done by placing the probe on one vein and giving sharp compression with the fingers to the other vein; if there is any connection the brief movement of blood this causes is easily transmitted to the vein under the probe.

6. Photoplethysmography If obvious venotensive skin changes are present, and especially if there is ulceration, further evidence will be needed to give positive confirmation of the cause as superficial vein incompetence. This may be elegantly provided by some form of plethysmography and a simple, practical way of carrying this out is by photoplethysmography (see Fig. 26). It can be used to demonstrate that an abnormally brief recovery time after exercise is restored to near normal when the suspected pathway of incompetence is selectively occluded by finger pressure (not a constricting band) (Fig. 34(c)). An unequivocal response can be accepted as sufficient evidence but if there are any remaining doubts, functional phlebography or ultrasonography may be advisable to exclude deep vein impairment.

7. Functional phlebography This should not be carried out as a routine in varicose vein cases but only when there are special features that require clarification. This method has already been discussed (Fig. 28) but the indications and findings in superficial vein incompetence are summarized here.

It gives positive identification of simple incompetence and demonstrates its source if other means have failed to do this.

It gives reassurance that the deep veins are normal and well valved or, conversely, that some form of deep vein impairment is present.

It assists the surgeon by displaying variable anatomy such as the termination of the short saphenous vein.

It identifies an unusual source of incompetence, such as the pelvic veins.

On phlebography the features of superficial vein incompetence causing varicose veins will be:

A demonstration of enlarged and tortuous veins arising from a pathway of incompetence such as a saphenous vein;

Downward flow in varicosities immediately following an exercise movement and entering the deep veins by perforators lower in the limb (Fig. 48(a)).

When the deep veins have been passively filled, not only will this confirm their normal outline but it also gives opportunity to demonstrate the source of incompetence. The patient is asked to make several exercise movements and the area of the suspected source is closely watched on the image intensifier. It is often possible to see spill-over from deep to superficial veins, with flow down the pathway of incompetence (Fig. 48(b), (c) and (d)), but the radiologist must be given clear guidance by the surgeon upon the probable source.

The swill test will give an overall impression of valves in the deep veins and will often give additional information about the source and pathway of incompetence (Fig. 48(e)).

In short saphenous and recurrent varicosities it may be easiest to locate the source by varicography, using the upward trace technique, as described earlier. The flow of medium will often follow the pathway of incompetence upwards and, via the source, into the deep veins (Fig. 48(f)). This upward flow is capricious and may be diverted before it reaches the objective but usually succeeds. The fact that the patient is near horizontal means that the veins are semicollapsed and this makes it more difficult to evaluate the importance of veins displayed.

8. Ultrasonography Ultrasonography by B mode duplex scanning or by colour flow imaging, previously described (see Fig. 29), is particularly useful in short saphenous incompetence where it can give positive confirmation of downflow in an incompetent vein and display the level of short saphenous termination. Similarly it can be used to display details of incompetence in a gastrocnemius vein causing perforator outflow in the calf, or in a groin recurrence.

Treatment of superficial vein incompetence and its manifestations

Varicose veins without accompanying venotensive changes

Here three levels of treatment may be recognized, cosmetic, alleviation of symptoms, and elimination of the underlying incompetent veins to give a lasting cure.

Cosmetic treatment

Lesser varicose veins can be disguised by appropriate make-up or the use of elastic support hose. Some patients will settle for these options but most will want the unsightly varicosities banished so that in summer the uncovered limb is blemish free. Sclerotherapy can accomplish this, often with lasting benefit, but in more gross varicose veins the best cosmetic result, and the most lasting, will be given by appropriate surgery, eliminating the source of incompetence without obvious scars, a skill the surgeon should be able to offer.

Relief of symptoms

Symptoms of heaviness and tiredness accompanying varicose veins can certainly be relieved by use of elastic support hose or elastic stockings (see Fig. 59(c)), combined with a policy of elevating the limb whenever possible (Fig. 49). However, this is not a cure and elastic support is often tedious to wear, particularly in hot weather. The most effective method will be the elimination of superficial vein incompetence by sclerotherapy or by surgery.

Elimination of the underlying cause

Treatment here will aim at a cure, that is to say complete elimination of the superficial incompetence which causes the unsightly

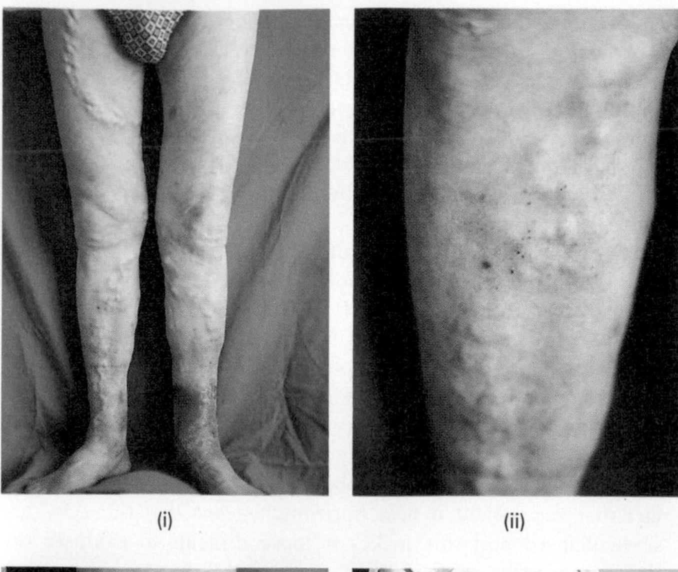

(i) (ii)

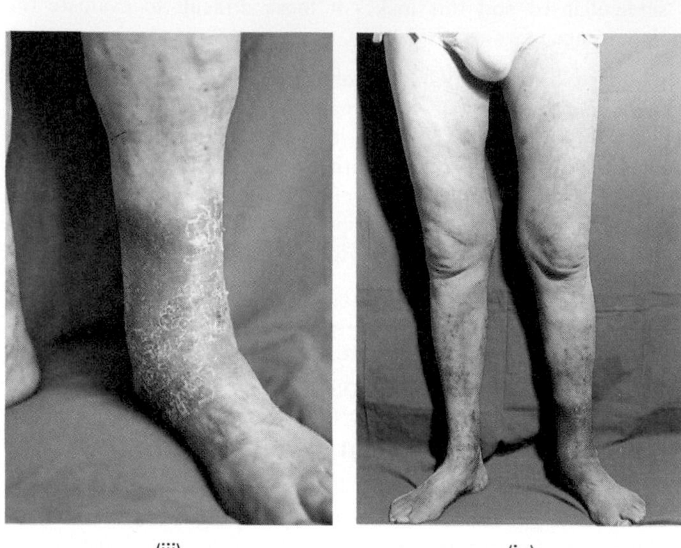

(iii) (iv)

Fig. 46 Consequences of venous hypertension (venotension) in superficial vein incompetence.

(a) Skin changes. (i) A patient with long-standing bilateral long saphenous incompetence. His main complaint was of discomfort and pruritus. (ii) Scratch marks over a varicose vein on the right shin confirm severe pruritus. (iii) Pronounced pigmentation and eczema at the left ankle are accompanied by induration and oedema. An area of eczema on the left inner thigh indicates a general skin sensitization. (iv) All tests confirmed simple incompetence in the superficial veins. Appropriate surgery completely relieved his symptoms and the improved state of the limbs 3 months later is shown here. (v) Preoperative recordings: *a* Doppler flowmetry (long saphenous veins). *b* and *c* Photoplethysmography on both sides. (vi) Postoperative photoplethysmography.

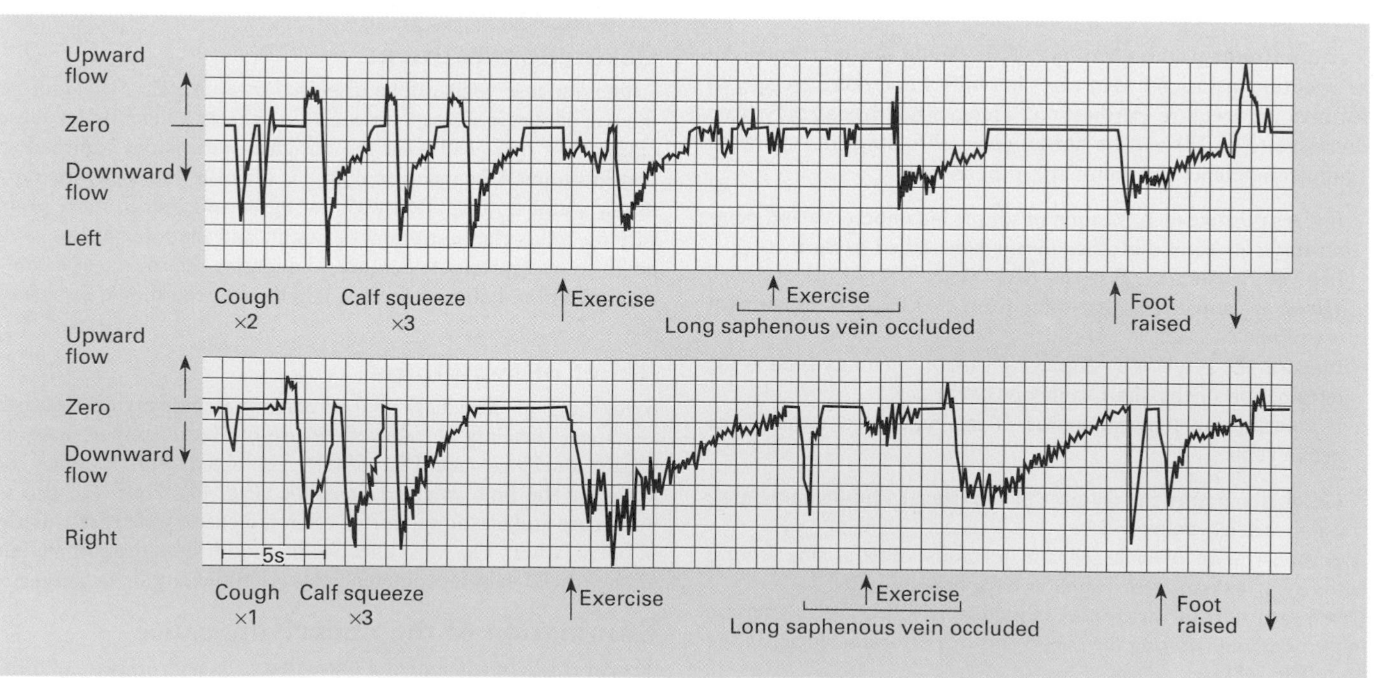

(v*a*)

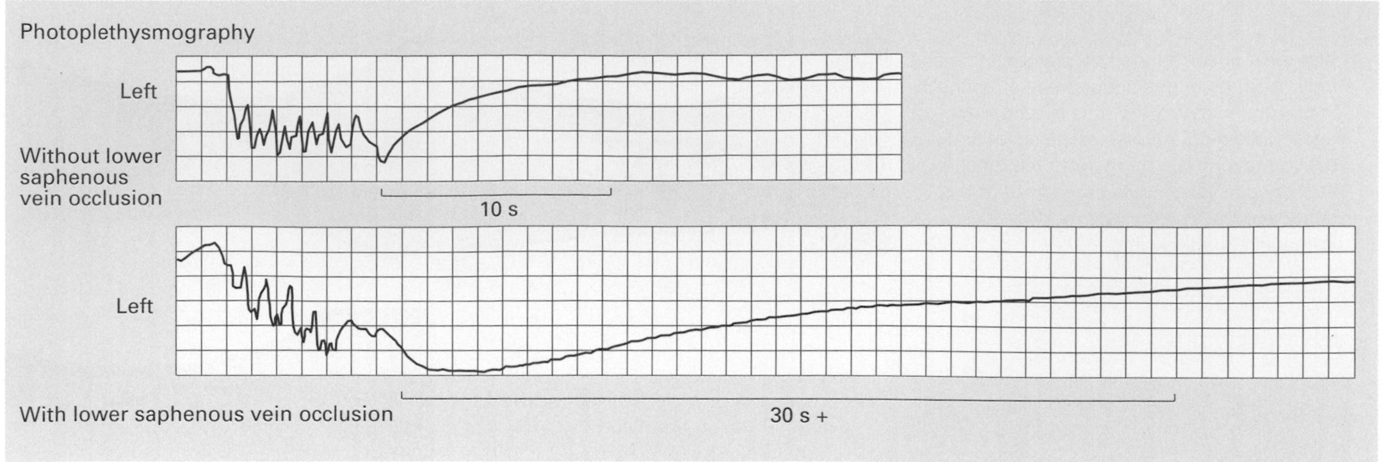

(v*b*)

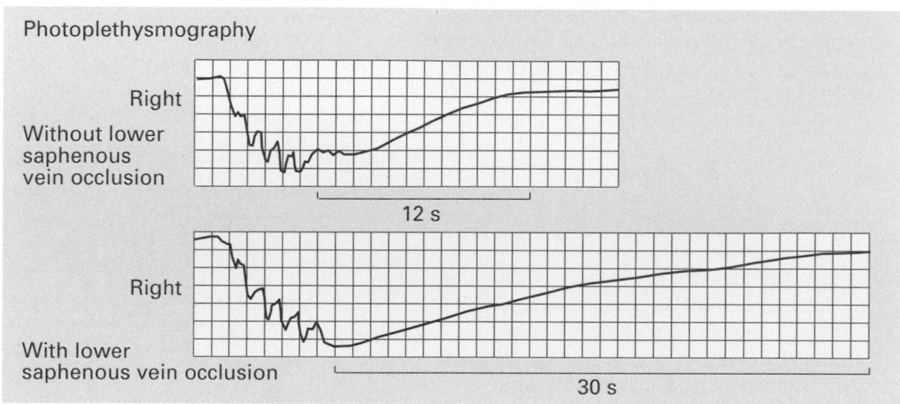

(v*c*)

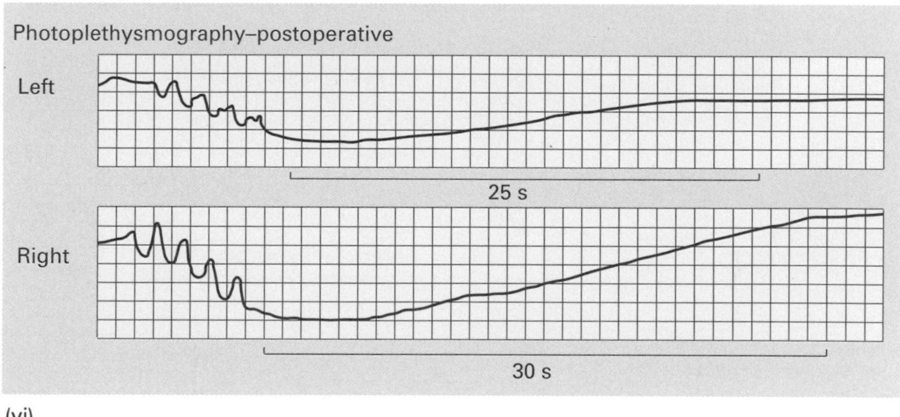

(vi)

(a)

(b)

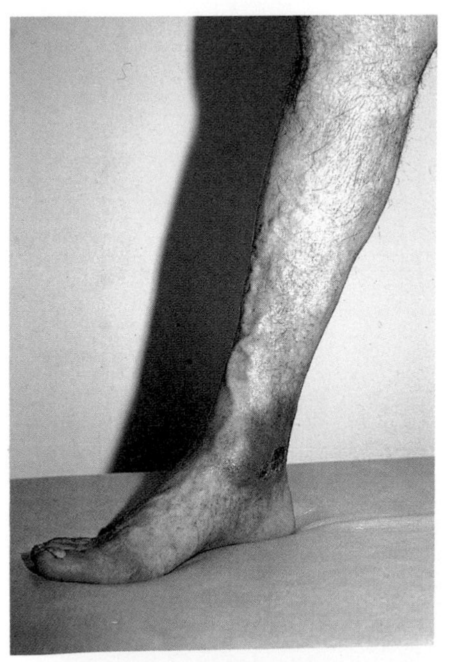

(b) Venotensive changes with a large varicose vein to the foot. This patient presented with venotensive pigmentation and a small painful ulcer near the ankle. A massive anterolateral tibial varicose vein originated from an incompetent long saphenous vein and ran on to the foot; Doppler flowmetry and photoplethysmography fully confirmed the diagnosis of venous hypertension from this cause. Surgery was advised but the patient would only accept sclerotherapy. This successfully obliterated the tibial varicosity with complete relief of symptoms and healing of the ulcer. The ulcer remained healed 1 year later.

(a) The ulcer is surrounded by pigmentation and induration. Its edges show areas of epithelial ingrowth indicating that it is in a healing phase following 10 days of elevation and active movements. Surgery to the long saphenous system was carried out at this stage and the patient was mobilized immediately afterwards.

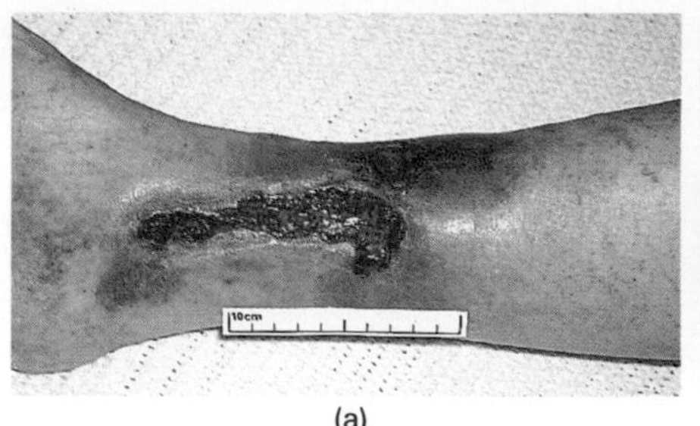

(a)

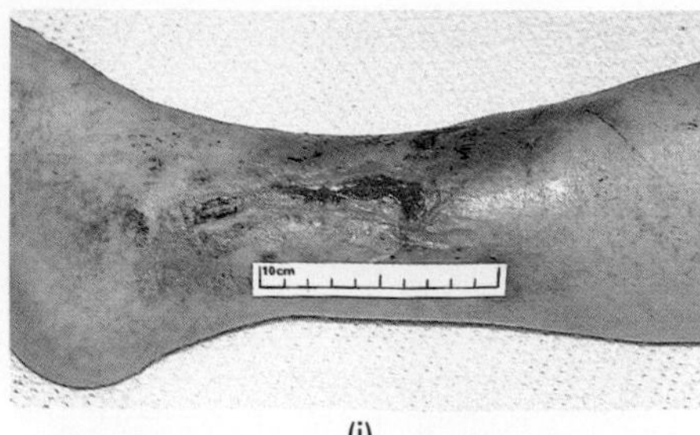

(i)

(ii)

(b)

(b) (i) The ulcer 1 month after surgery. It is healing well with active epithelial ingrowth. (ii) Two months after surgery, the ulcer has healed except for a crusted area in the upper part. At 3 months healing was complete.

Preoperative investigations.

(c) Doppler flow in the long saphenous whilst standing, showing downflow on coughing, after calf squeezing or exercise, but delayed during saphenous occlusion by finger pressure.

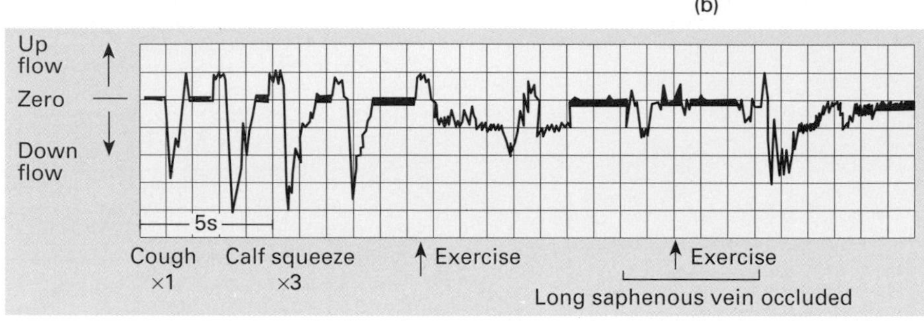

(c)

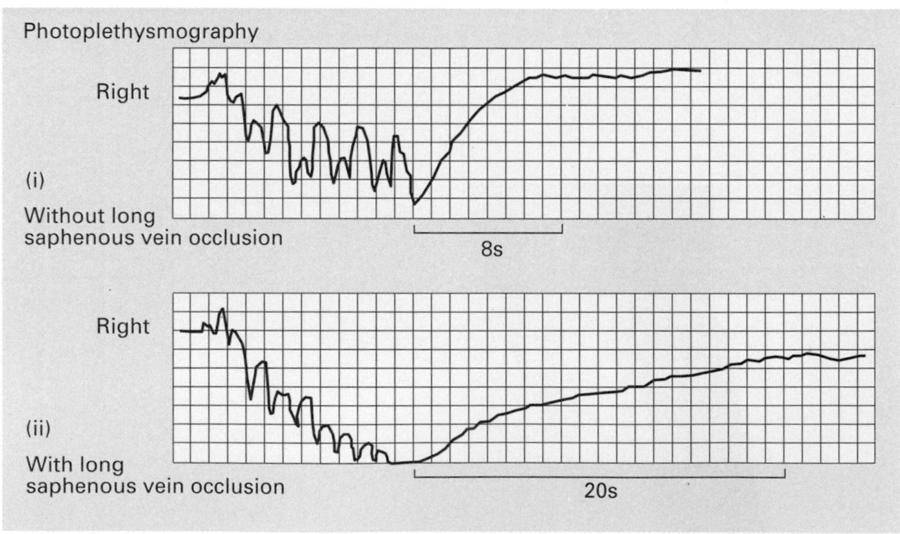

(d)

(d) (i) Photoplethysmography with refilling time of 8 s. (ii) Refilling time improved to over 20 s when the saphenous vein is occluded by finger pressure.

Fig. 47 Severe ulceration caused by long saphenous incompetence. It should be noted that severe ulceration such as this often develops because the musculovenous pumping mechanism is relatively weak and easily overwhelmed by superficial vein incompetence. Removing the factor of superficial incompetence makes it much easier to prevent ulceration but is not a complete cure because the weak musculovenous pump remains barely adequate. This was so in the patient illustrated who returned a year later, threatened with renewed ulceration because she had ceased taking any protective measures; with a policy of elevation whenever possible, and elastic support to the knee, the limb returned to good condition; the patient was urged to maintain these simple protective measures.

varicosities and symptoms from venous stress. The essentials are correct identification of the source and pathway of incompetence, and their obliteration by sclerotherapy or by surgery. Most failures in these aims are the result of inaccurate identification of the source or inadequate elimination of the pathway.

Compression sclerotherapy

With this method a suitable chemical, such as 3 per cent sodium tetradecylsulphate, is injected into the varicose veins, or the pathway of incompetence leading to them; this will destroy the endothelium and create a reaction within the veins that eventually seals them into a fibrous cord. To achieve this goal an 'empty vein–compression bandage' technique is used. The veins to be treated are identified whilst the patient is standing (Fig. 50(a) and (b)) and likely sites of injection marked with a felt-tipped pen. Injection into an artery is a grave hazard likely to cause extensive gangrene; this is most likely to happen in the vicinity of the ankle and this area should be avoided as far as possible. Although rare, measures to combat anaphylaxis must be at hand (adrenaline, hydrocortisone, antihistamine, intubation).

The patient is then repositioned sitting up on a couch with lower limbs horizontal (Fig. 50(c)), or with legs over the edge in moderate dependency to give slight distension of the veins. Needles, with syringes containing sclerosant attached, are inserted into selected veins and taped to the skin (Fig. 50(d)–(i)). The patient then lies flat, the limb is elevated to empty the veins, and the sclerosant is injected (Fig. 50(j)–(n)). In this way, a small quantity of sclerosant produces maximal effect without causing blood clot. While the limb is still in elevation, pressure pads are placed over the sites of injection and a firm bandage applied (Fig. 50(o)–(v)). This prevents blood from re-entering the veins when the patient stands and minimizes clot formation; it also presses the inner walls together to ensure that they will bond firmly with fibrous tissue. Provided that the veins are kept empty in this fashion little discomfort follows the procedure and obliteration of the vein is likely to be permanent (Fig. 50(w) and (x)). Compression is maintained for at least 3 weeks and the patient asked to exercise freely to discourage clotting spreading to the deep veins. Failure to apply effective compression will cause the injected veins to distend with clot so that they are painful (in fact, an induced superficial thrombophlebitis) and eventual recanalization of the vein is likely to occur; in a substantial vein, such as a saphenous vein, this will destroy any remaining valve function so that if the vein reopens it is a large conduit devoid of any restraint by valves and the recurrent state may be more severe than the original one. Although the method is very effective in small to medium calibre veins it does tend to give only temporary occlusion of the larger veins, particularly the saphenous vein itself, so that here recurrence not infrequently occurs after a year or two and further treatment is needed.

Sclerotherapy is seldom as complete as surgery in the obliteration of the incompetent veins and for this reason the patient will often be asked to attend at regular intervals so that further injections may be carried out to any returning varicosities. In this way, for a large set of veins, sclerotherapy tends to be a long-term policy of maintenance rather than the one-time cure intended with surgery. The use of compression bandaging, necessary with sclerotherapy, is undoubtedly tiresome and patients who have had treatment both by injection and by surgery often say that they preferred the surgical treatment. Sclerotherapy has its drawbacks, for example, a discoloration that may persist for many months afterwards, and although its exponents appear effortlessly to overcome these problems, it must not be regarded as an easy alternative to surgery with a requirement for little skill; quite the reverse is true. Injection into an artery, referred to above, is a potential disaster never to lose sight of; if, on sucking back, the needle produces any hint of arterial blood, by colour or pulsatile reflux, it should not be used but immediately repositioned elsewhere. Nevertheless, sclerotherapy is a most valuable method of treatment and in the case of lesser veins often can accomplish treatment scarcely possible for surgery. Perhaps the most reasonable view is to use surgery for the well defined patterns of saphenous incompetence, and use sclerotherapy to back this up when necessary or in the treatment of lesser varicosities. The combination of sclerotherapy with surgical treatment is discussed under Treatment of recurrent varicose veins.

Surgical treatment

The essential principle with surgery is that the source and the main pathway of incompetence are actually removed; in the case of a saphenous vein, this requires high ligation at its termination, flush with the deep vein, and stripping a substantial part of its length. Some typical procedures are illustrated in Figs. 51(a)–(p). If an incompetent saphenous vein is left in place, unstripped, it remains open as a valveless conduit running directly down to the low pressure areas beneath the musculovenous pumps, and is likely to form the basis of a new retrograde circuit of incompetence with renewed varicose veins (see under Recurrence below).

Surgical treatment should also remove the main varicosities through a series of small incisions (Fig. 51(m) and (n), otherwise these veins are liable to persist, much to the patient's disappointment, and will require final elimination by sclerotherapy. Moreover, these varicosities are the distal part of a pathway of incompetence and directly communicate with the low pressure areas so that they are constantly available to re-establish flow from higher levels; not only will they remain visible but they may progressively enlarge.

A further aspect that may require special attention is the site of inflow from incompetent superficial veins to the deep veins at low level, that is to say, the perforating veins. Usually, these are multiple points and it is not practical to identify and remove them surgically, nor is it necessary. However, in some cases one or two individual perforators have become enlarged and give heavy surge back and forth as the muscles contract and relax. When recognized, it is best to remove these veins, since otherwise they may form the source for a new pattern of varicosities running to the foot. However, the perforator must not be regarded as the main offender and its varying role in the venous disorders is considered later in this Section.

The best opportunity for surgical cure is at the first operation because recurrent veins based on a superficial vein anatomy fragmented by previous surgery are much more difficult to treat effectively. The first opportunity must not be wasted by inaccurate identification of the veins at fault or by inadequate surgery. Conscientious surgery for varicose veins is time consuming but very rewarding in terms of immediate comfort and lasting benefit to the patient.

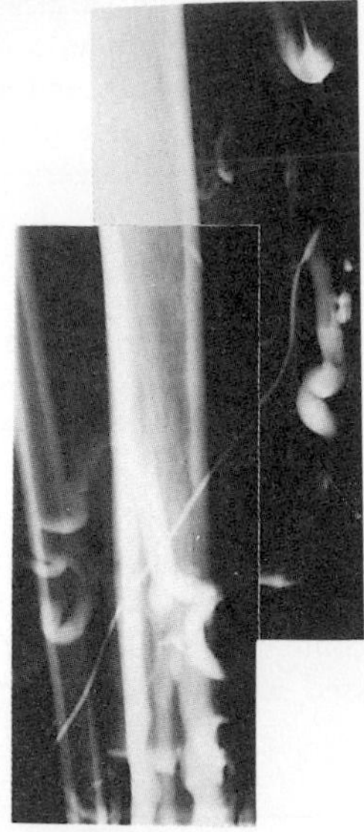

(a) Opaque medium (3 ml) has been injected into a varicose vein in midcalf and is shown here after one exercise movement. The opacified blood was seen to sweep down the varicose vein and enter the tibial deep veins. This is characteristic of the retrograde circuit in superficial vein incompetence.

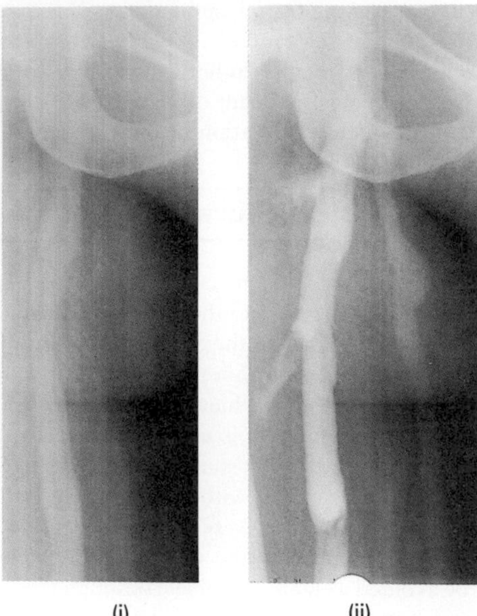

(i) (ii)

(b) (i) The deep veins have been opacified passively (80 ml of medium), with the patient standing still. The common femoral vein is weakly outlined. (ii) The patient is asked to make two exercise movements, rising on the toes and down again. The view shown here was taken immediately afterwards. Opacified blood has been pumped upwards and some has outlined an incompetent long saphenous vein as blood spills down it and to the deep veins of the leg made slack by the muscle contractions.

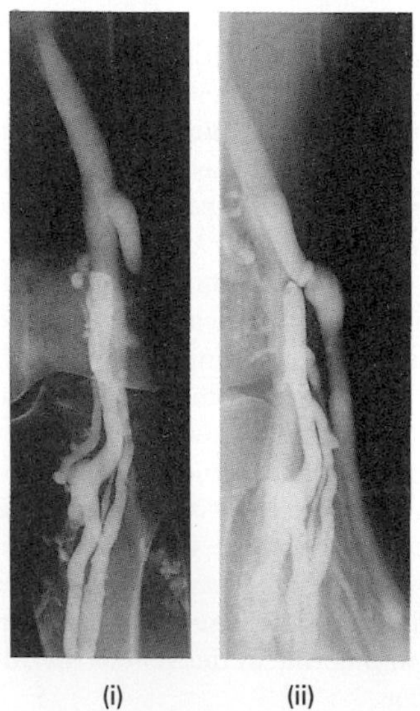

(i) (ii)

(c) Similar spillover and down an incompetent short saphenous vein. (i) Before exercise. (ii) After exercise.

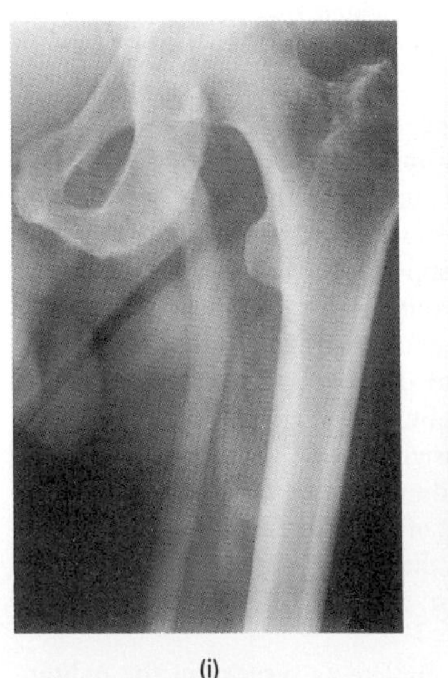

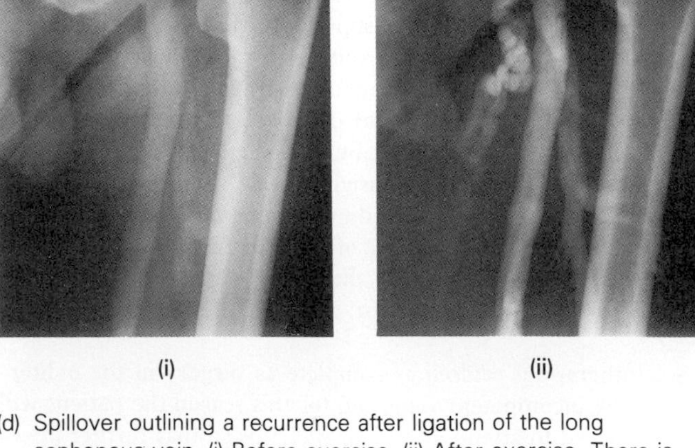

(i) (ii)

(d) Spillover outlining a recurrence after ligation of the long saphenous vein. (i) Before exercise. (ii) After exercise. There is increased density of medium in the femoral vein and a varicosed reconnection has been outlined by downflow to join an unstripped long saphenous vein.

Fig. 48 Functional phlebography (and see Fig 28). Patient in the near-vertical position.

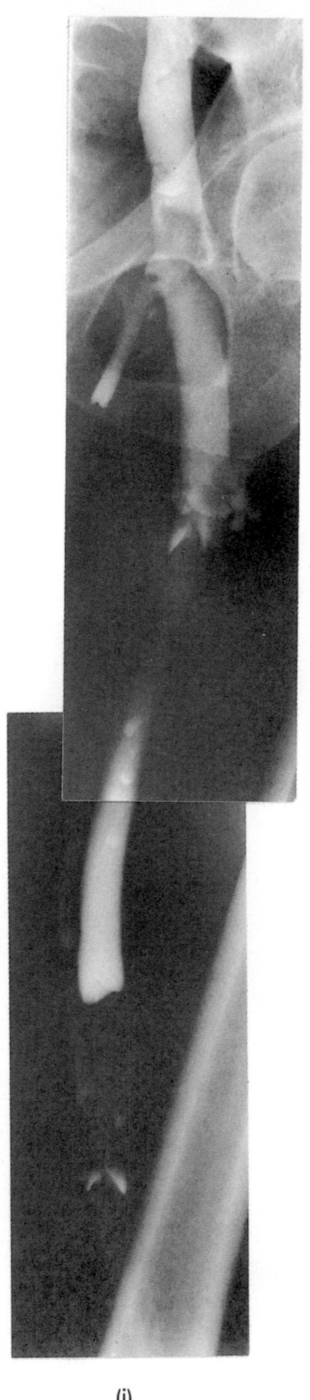

(i)

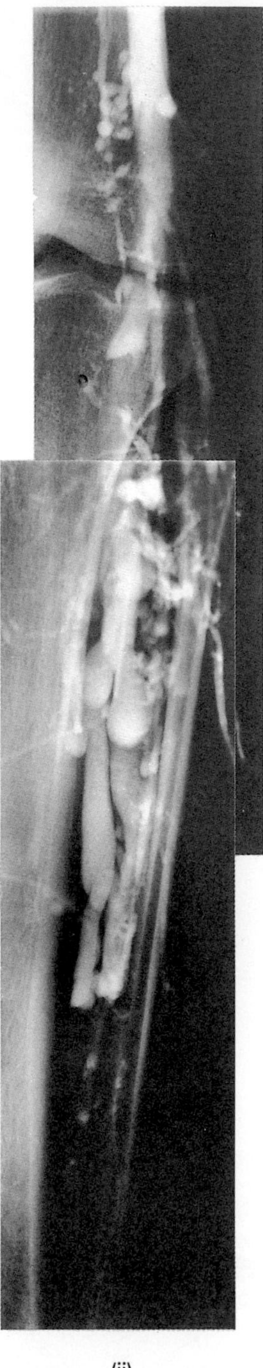

(ii)

(e) Assessment of valves in deep veins by the swill test. (i) Good valves shown in superficial femoral vein. A valve at the commencement of the profunda femoris is faintly shown and the upper long saphenous vein shows two competent valves. (ii) A series of valves displayed in the tibial veins.

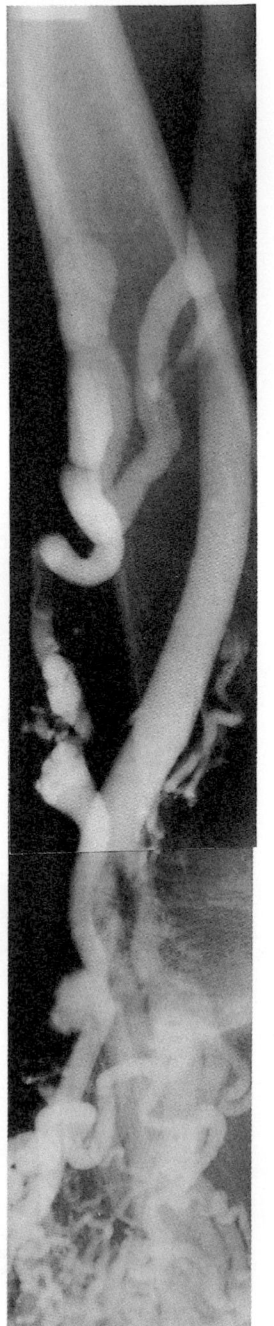

(f) Phlebogram displaying the short saphenous termination prior to surgery. This vein shows unexpected tortuosity and terminates at an unusually high level.

Treatment of varicose veins with venotensive changes and ulceration

When the characteristic skin changes of venous hypertension are evident and particularly when ulceration is present, care must be taken to be sure that the cause is simple incompetence in superficial veins and not a post-thrombotic deep vein impairment (Fig. 52). Surgery to the veins appropriate for the former may well be wholly inappropriate for the latter. Once unequivocal evidence has been obtained that the cause is superficial incompetence and the pathway of this has been accurately defined, treatment may be

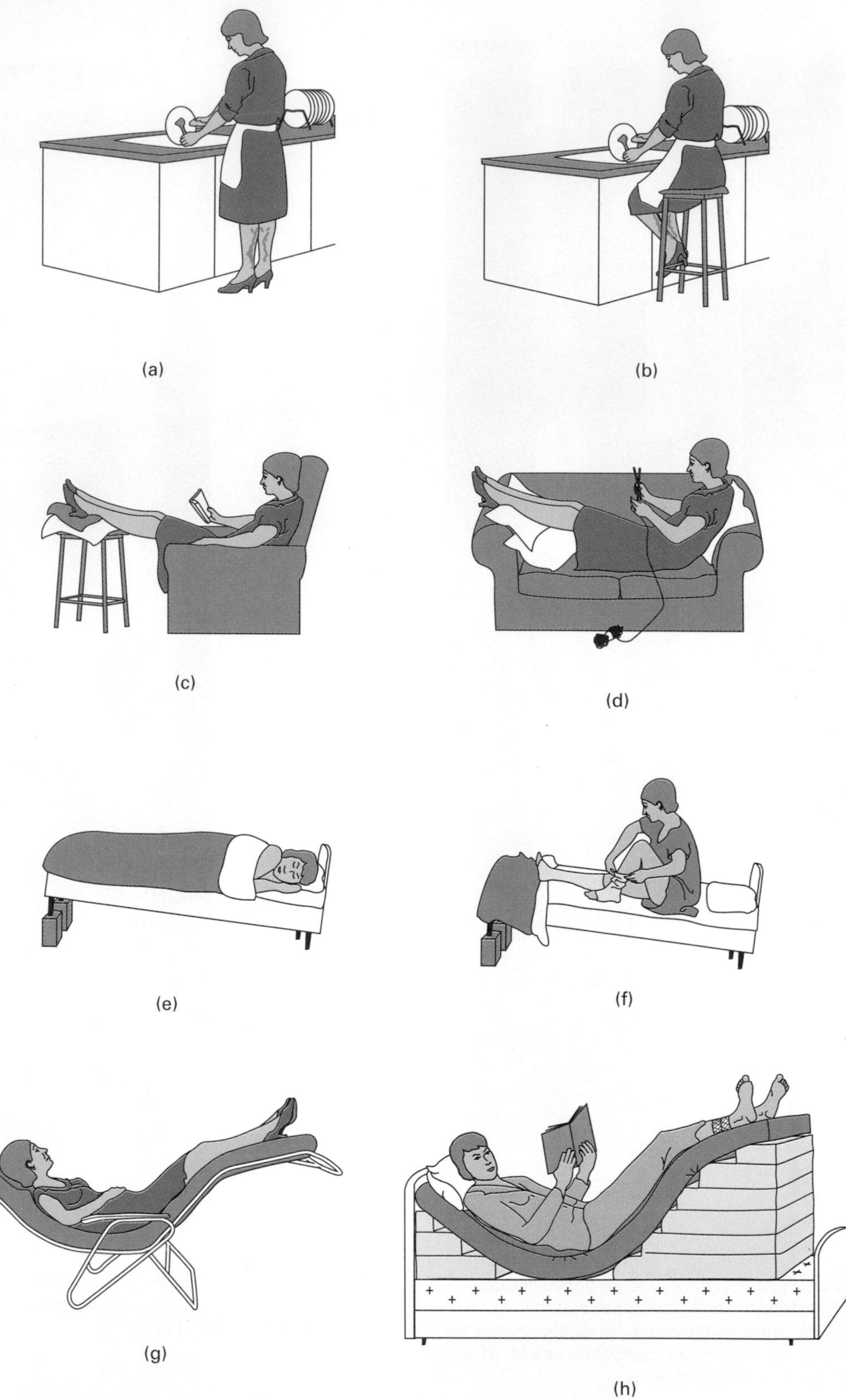

Fig. 49 Conservative management of venous disorders. General instructions for the patient, designed to minimize venous hypertension. (a) Avoid standing like this. (b) Sit whenever you can. (c) and (d) Make several opportunities during the day, and especially in the evening, to sit with legs raised high, above the level of your heart. (e) At night achievement of many hours of valuable elevation is possible by raising the foot of the bed. (f) Put on elastic stockings before getting up. (g) Investment in a specially designed chair may be better than improvisation, and will encourage maximal use. It should be remembered that every moment the legs are fully elevated they are improving, but when down, even with stockings, they are deteriorating, especially when standing still. The patient should be active, but take every opportunity to elevate, especially if ulceration threatens. (h) Sustained high elevation will be required for active venous ulceration. Blocks of 10 cm (4 inches) polyurethane foam can be used to form a shaped overlay on a bed. The limbs and feet should be moved frequently.

carried out as described above. The presence of venotensive changes indicates a severe state of incompetence probably best treated by surgery because the large incompetent veins likely to be present may soon reopen after sclerotherapy and more lasting benefit will be given by surgical removal of the source and pathway of incompetence, including the varicose veins themselves.

If the skin is unbroken, or even when a substantial 'clean' ulcer is present, there is no reason why surgery should not be performed without any preliminary treatment. However, if infection, such as cellulitis or an ulcer discharging pus, is present, then the patient should have a short period of treatment in hospital with the limb elevated and systemic antibiotics given. This is maintained until the ulcer enters a healing phase, that is, its base is covered with 'healthy' granulation tissue, pus is no longer being formed, pathogenic organisms such as *Staphylcoccus aureus* or *Streptococcus viridans* have been eliminated, and the skin edges slope smoothly to a thin, grey line of regenerating epithelium extending on to the granulation tissue. At this stage, now that the ulcer is 'clean', there is no need to delay surgery by waiting for the ulcer to heal completely; healing can continue concurrently with the patient's postoperative mobilization once the cause for venous hypertension has been removed. This policy would not be appropriate where superficial vein incompetence is accompanied by the more fundamental problem of primary valve deficiency (valveless syndrome—see below) because here the benefits to be expected of surgery may be so marginal that the ulcer could fail to heal without continued elevation.

Recurrent varicose veins

There is, undoubtedly, an appreciable recurrence rate for varicose veins and other expressions of superfical vein incompetence treated by sclerotherapy or surgery. The recurrences created by surgery can sometimes be more formidable than the original state. The causes of such failure in treatment may be summarized as follows.

Persistent varicose veins

Here it is soon apparent that the varicose veins have survived treatment. This may be due to one of the following factors.

Misdiagnosis of the original state where in fact the enlarged veins were, for example, not be due to simple varicose veins but deep vein impairment.

Incorrect identification of the source and pathway of incompetence.

Two separate sources feeding the same varicose veins were present originally and too limited a procedure has been carried out.

Removal of the pathway of incompetence and/or the varicosities has been inadequate and the remaining veins fill easily from a secondary source or by reflux through an enlarged perforating vein. This may respond to sclerotherapy or require a further operation to complete the first procedure.

True recurrence

The varicose veins at first disappear but then reappear in the same distribution within a year or two. The following reasons may account for this problem.

Inadequate removal of the source This will usually be due to failure to ligate a saphenous termination flush with the deep vein. The branches that survive re-establish the source. This is most likely to happen when the original main pathway of incompetence, usually a saphenous vein, has not been removed.

Failure to remove or obliterate the main pathway of incompetence It has already been pointed out that if a grossly incompetent saphenous vein is left intact it will act as a conduit directly communicating with the low pressure areas below the venous pumping mechanisms (the original key failure). During exercise, such as walking, the upper end of this large vein will then be at low pressure in close proximity to the relatively high deep vein pressure in the saphenous stump. This is a strong inducement for a vascular connection to be established from the high pressure vein to the low pressure vein. Two types of venous connecting network may be formed:

1. Anatomical reconnection, based on surviving side branches of a saphenous stump (Figs. 53(a) and see Fig. 53(d) (i)). This can be avoided by flush ligation with the deep vein and stripping the saphenous vein down to knee level.
2. Non-anatomical reconnection (re- or neovascularization). In recent years it has been repeatedly shown that, even when the saphenous vein has been ligated and divided above any branches, a plexus of small veins may form between the stump and an unstripped, incompetent saphenous vein (Fig. 53(b) and (c)). This process is not dependent on anatomical branches of the saphenous stump and can be avoided by removing the main pathway of incompetence, whether this is a saphenous vein or an enlarged branch, such as an anterolateral branch in the thigh. In the treatment of simple varicose veins it should be a fundamental principle that when the source of incompetence is surgically ligated the main pathway of incompetence should also be removed.

A latent second source has become active and surviving varicose veins have been taken over by this For example, if varicose veins are not removed at the time of long saphenous ligation and stripping, they form a ready-made, vacant pathway of incompetence which may be 'acquired' by a mildly incompetent short saphenous vein. This new source soon enlarges with the stimulus of unrestricted downflow (Fig. 53(d) (ii)). Alternatively, some other source, such as a midthigh perforator, may take over in similar fashion (Figs. 53(d) (iii) and see Fig. 41(b)). The possibility of a second source opening up in this fashion is considerably reduced if the varicose veins are effectively removed surgically or obliterated by sclerotherapy at the first procedure since otherwise they are a constant and visible invitation for an incompetent vein at higher level to send an ever increasing flow down to them. A second operation can give a good result provided that every effort is made to ensure accurate location of the source and, if there are any doubts, to confirm this by functional phlebography and varicography, or by ultrasonography.

A minority of recurrent varicose veins will arise in the states, described presently, of either primary valve deficiency or weak vein syndrome In the latter, varicose veins may proliferate within a few months after a good initial result. The surgeon should not conclude too quickly that treatment cannot succeed, perhaps condemning the patient to a lifetime of strong elastic stockings, but should assess the case in detail, including phlebography. This may show there is an opportunity for carefully planned surgery, based on accurate information, which can be very successful.

Fig. 50 Compression sclerotherapy; empty vein technique.

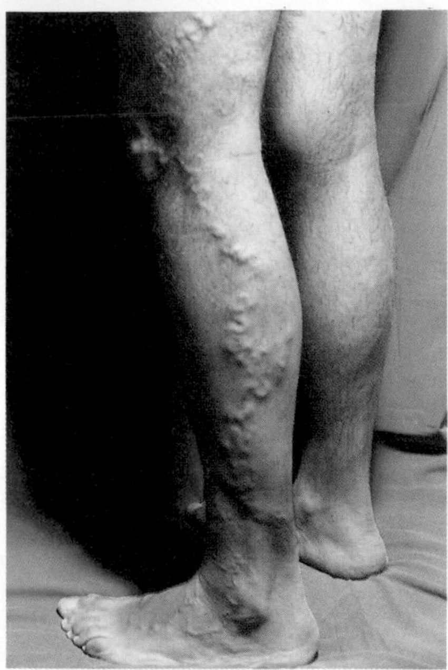

(a) Tortuous outlying varicose veins like this are ideal for compression sclerotherapy.

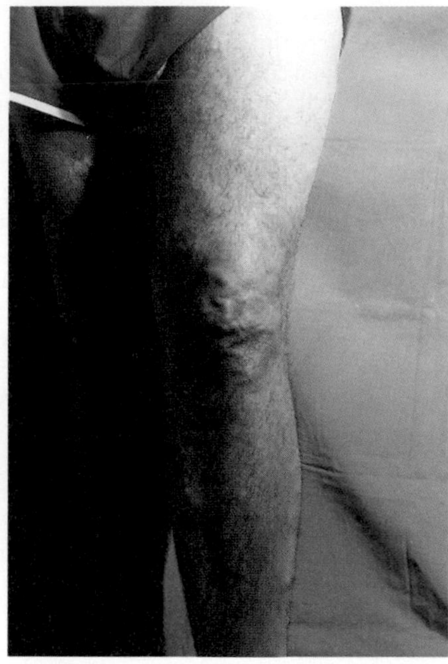

(b) All veins are identified and suitable sites for injection marked whilst the patient is standing.

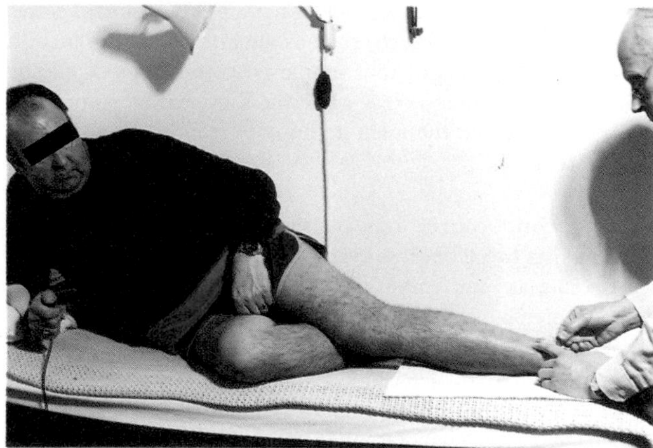

(c) Patient is repositioned on couch; sitting up helps to keep veins slightly distended.

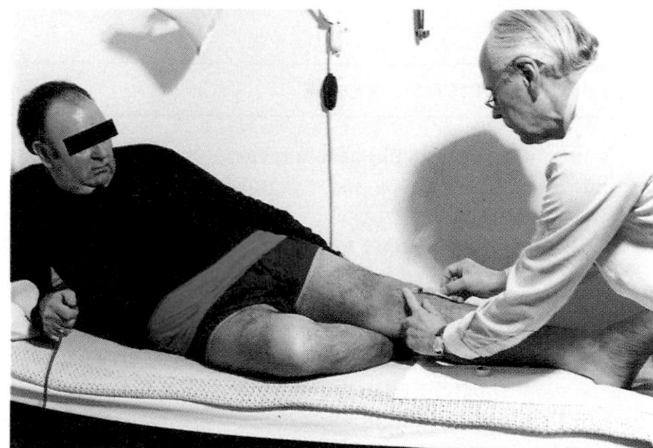

(d) Needle, with syringe containing 0.5 ml of sclerosant attached, is inserted into a selected vein.

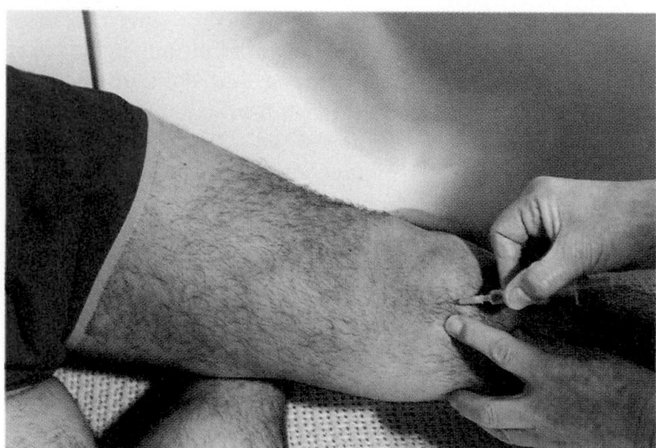

(e) Details of needle insertion. Skin is drawn down and needle inserted with lifting action of point to open vein lumen.

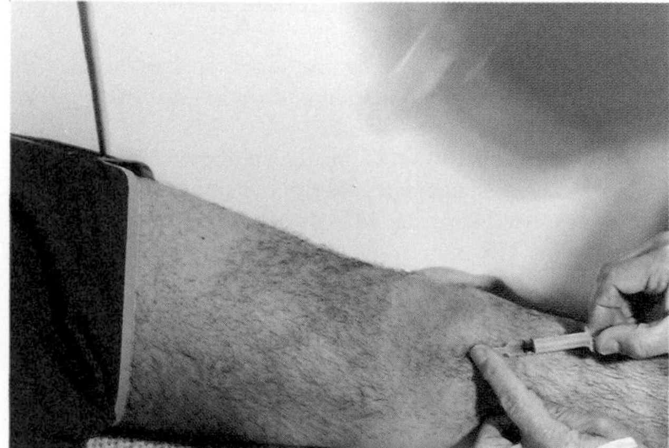

(f) Needle hub is steadied whilst slight suction withdraws a spot of blood to check correct entry into vein lumen. If there is any hint of arterial backflow reposition needle to vein nearby.

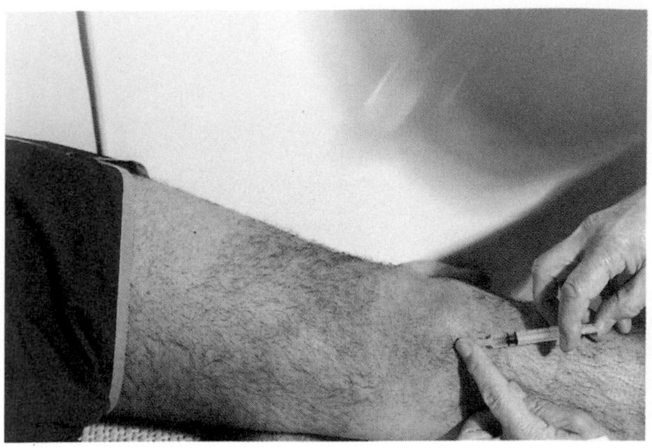

(g) Needle is cleared of blood by a small injection of sclerosant.

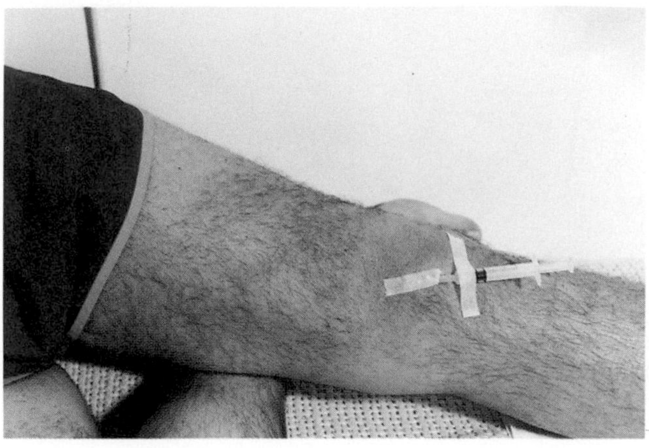

(h) Needle and syringe are taped to skin.

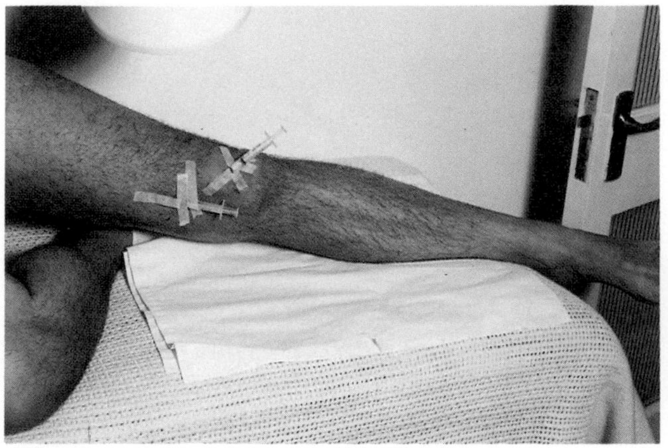

(i) This is repeated at selected sites.

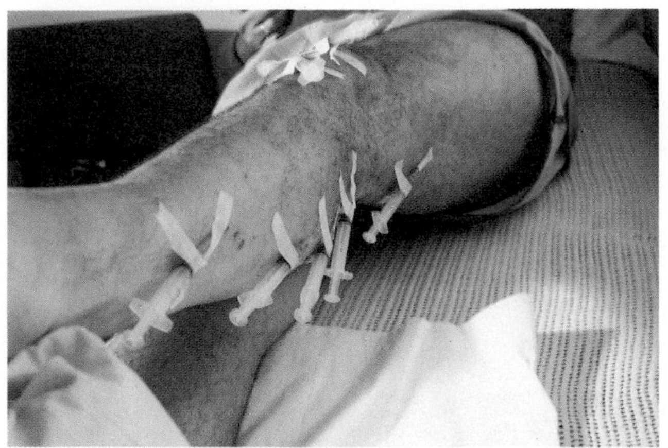

(j) Multiple syringes up the length of the varicose vein, all taped to skin; the foot is elevated to empty the veins.

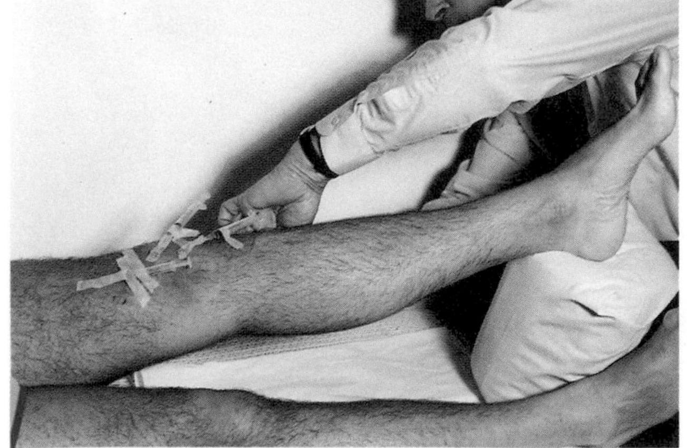

(k) Each syringe delivers chosen dose (0.5 ml or less, total dose in limb not exceeding 3 ml)

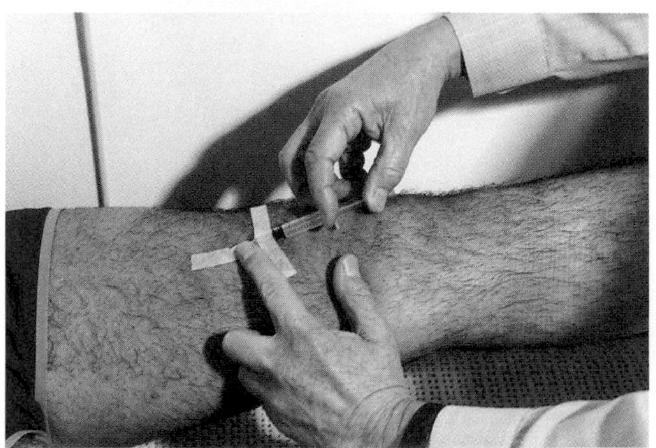

(l) Details of sclerosant delivery. Hub is steadied before plunger depressed.

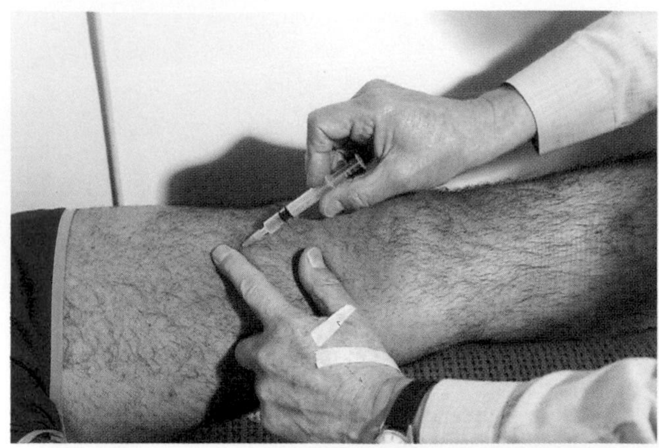

(m) Removing syringes. Tapes are removed and needle withdrawn with finger pressure over injection site.

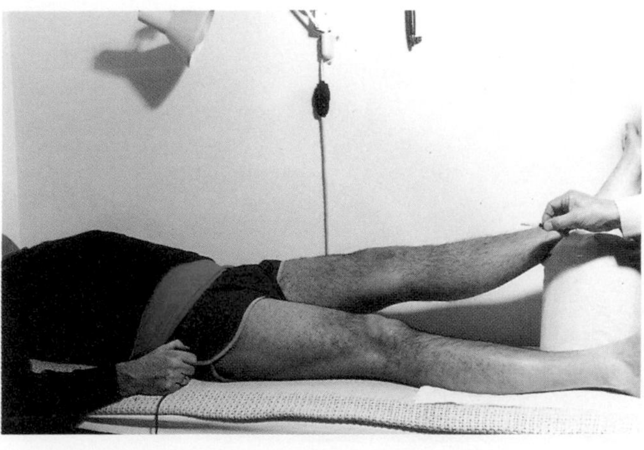

(n) All syringes removed. Limb remains in elevation.

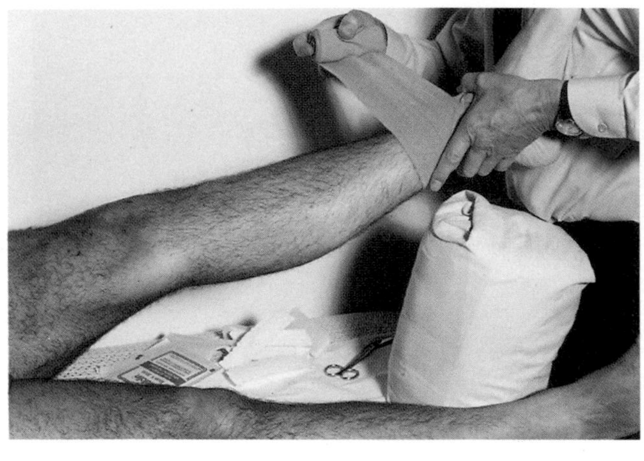

(o)

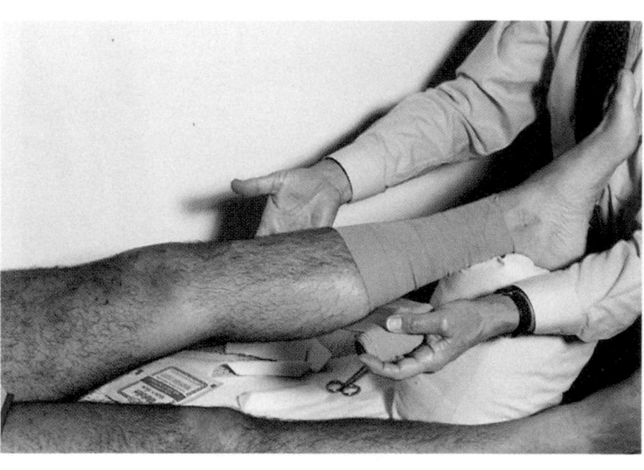

(p)

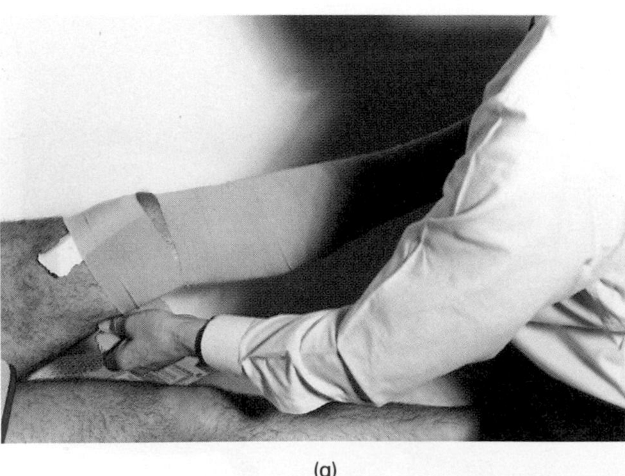

(q)

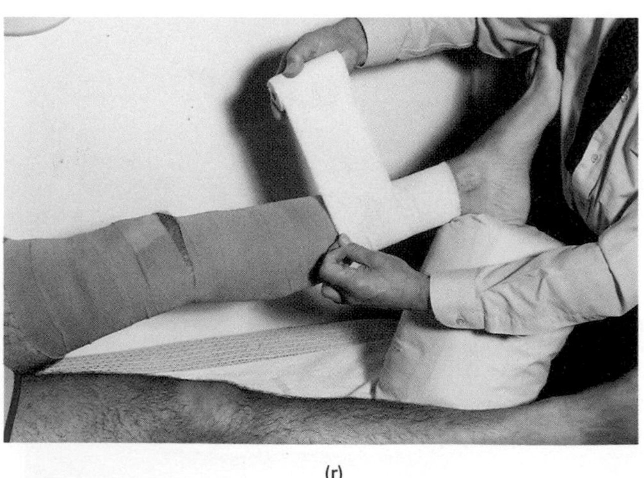

(r)

(o), (p), (q) Crepe bandage is applied over cotton pads at each injection site.

(r), (s), (t) The crepe bandage is now locked together by elastic adhesive bandage. A gap is left to permit knee flexion.

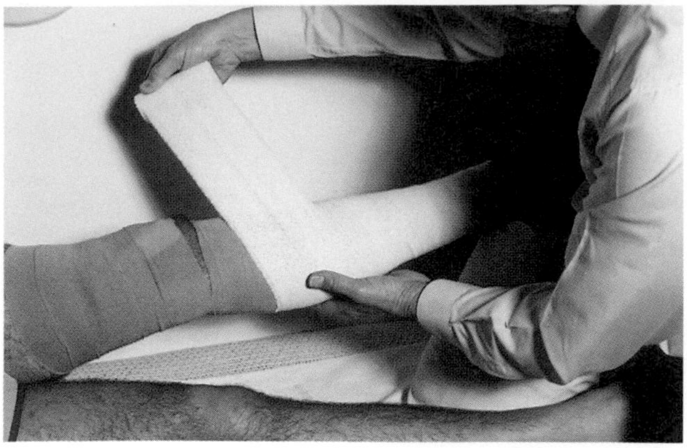

(s)

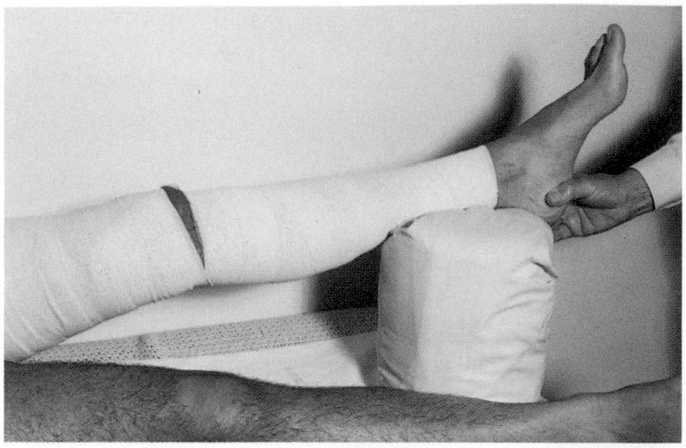

(t)

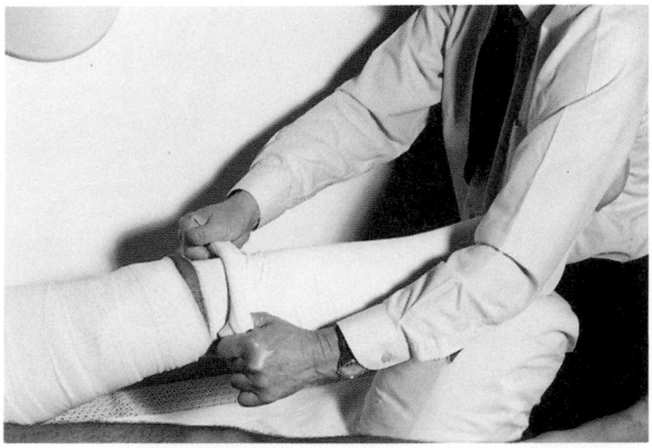

(u)

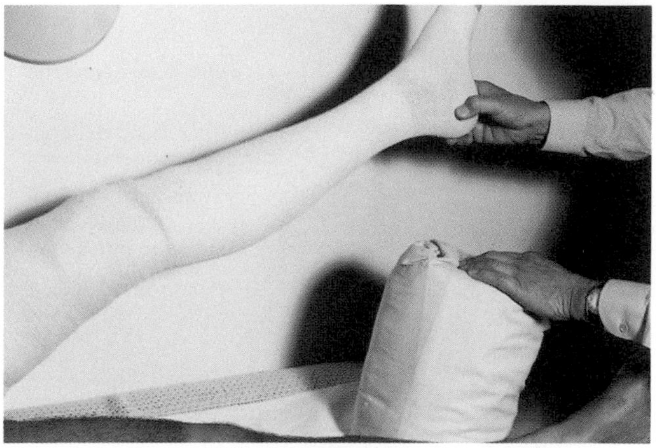

(v)

(u), (v) Final layer of elastic tubular bandage or elastic stocking is applied to ensure injected veins are kept as empty as possible. This remains in place for 3 weeks, followed by elastic support alone for 2 months.

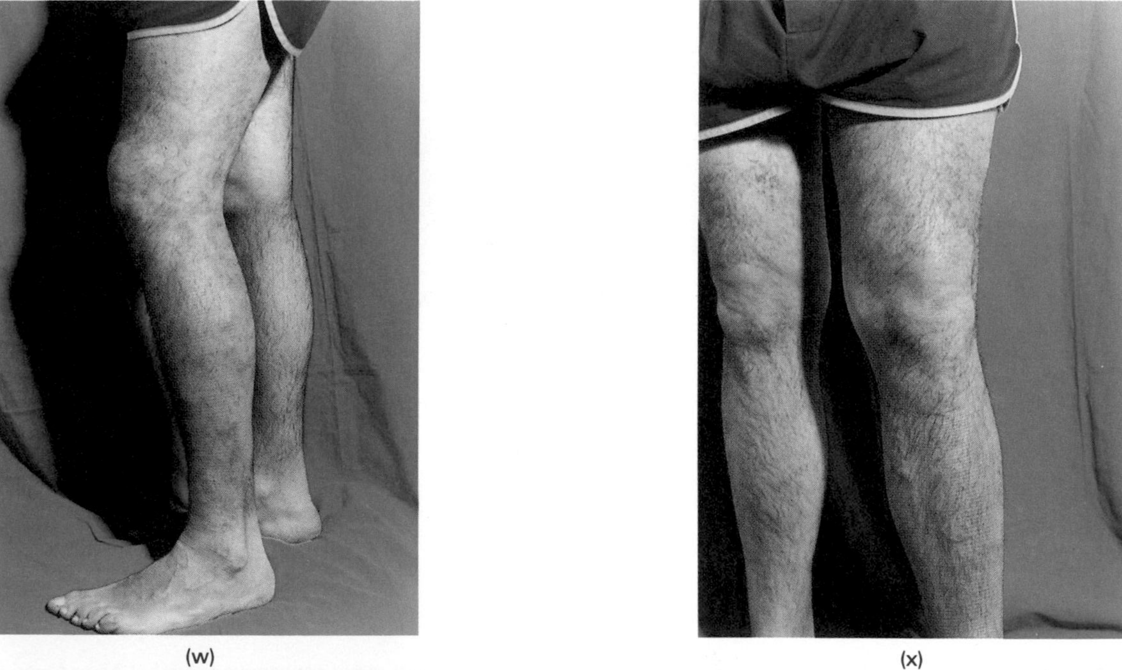

(w)

(x)

(w), (x) Result at 3 months. A slightly discoloured, firm cord has replaced the vein: this will slowly absorb over the next 6 to 9 months. This patient was seen 3 years later and the good result confirmed.

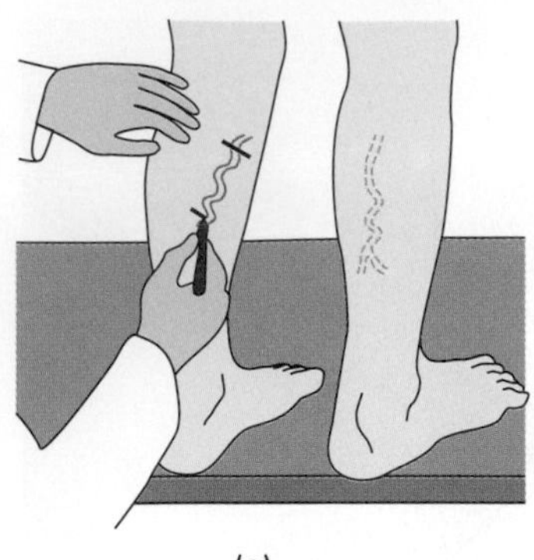

Fig. 51 Surgical technique in treatment of superficial vein incompetence.

(a) Planning the procedure before surgery. Preoperative 'marking out' of veins by an experienced person is essential to ensure easy identification of veins to be removed. There is no 'standard procedure'—the operation is planned individually for each patient.

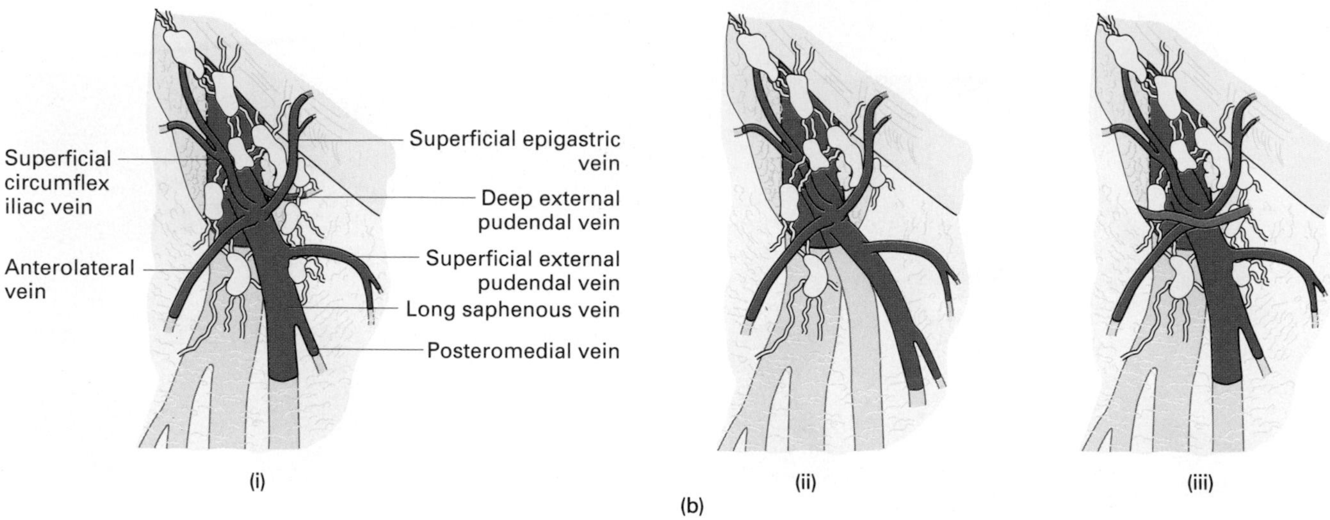

(b) Flush ligation of long saphenous termination. Some anatomical points. (i) A typical arrangement of saphenous termination and its branches. (ii) There are many variants. Shown here is a double long saphenous vein; either or both channels can be at fault. (iii) The superficial external pudendal artery may run over, shown here, or under the saphenous vein.

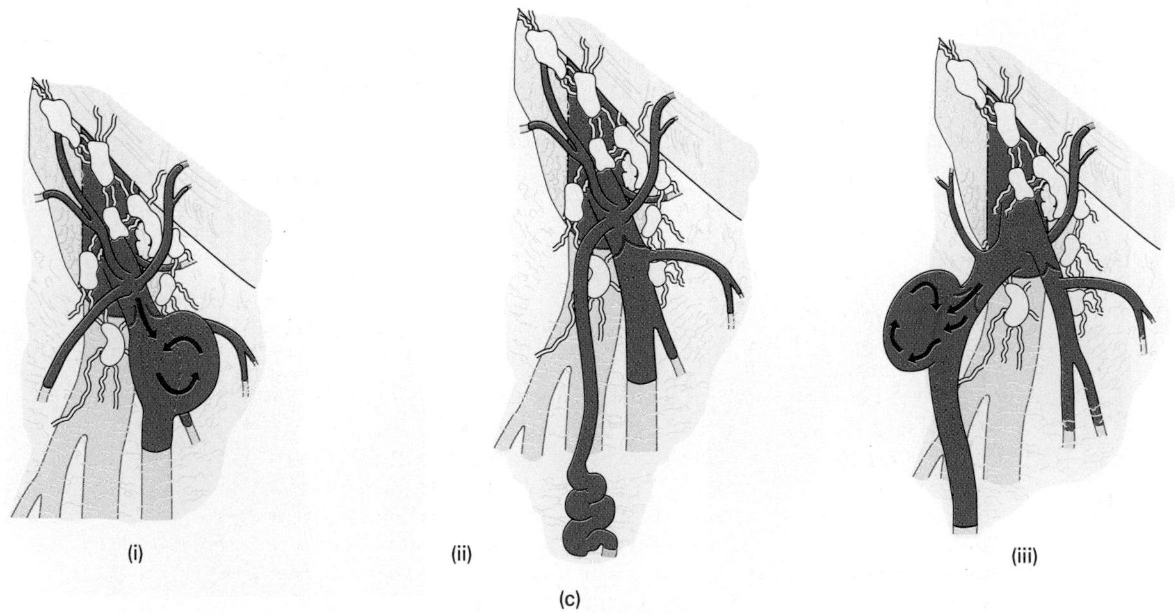

(c) Some features commonly present. (i) Saphena varix—a saccule below an incompetent upper saphenous valve but often found beneath any incompetent saphenous valve in the thigh. (ii) An anterolateral branch may be the main pathway of incompetence and downflow in it may bypass a competent upper long saphenous vein. (iii) Saccules are often present on an incompetent anterolateral branch.

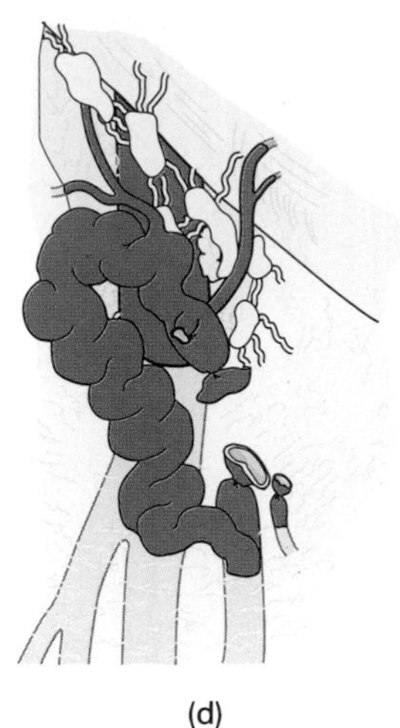

(d)

(d) 'Anatomical recurrence', caused by connection of surviving branches at saphenous termination with an unstripped saphenous vein.

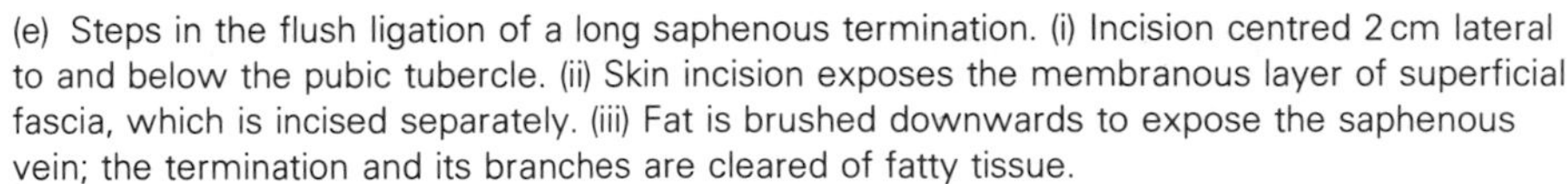

(e) Steps in the flush ligation of a long saphenous termination. (i) Incision centred 2 cm lateral to and below the pubic tubercle. (ii) Skin incision exposes the membranous layer of superficial fascia, which is incised separately. (iii) Fat is brushed downwards to expose the saphenous vein; the termination and its branches are cleared of fatty tissue.

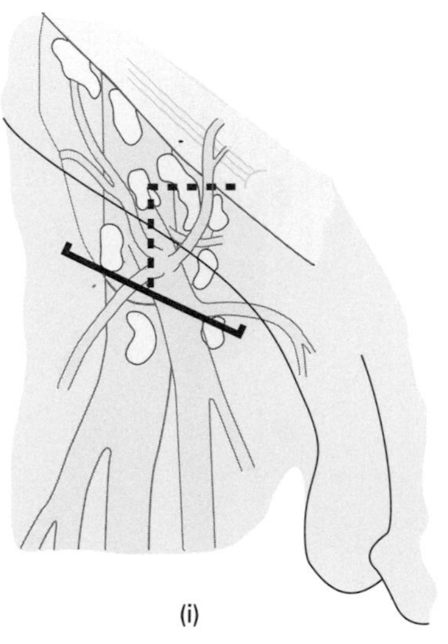

(i)

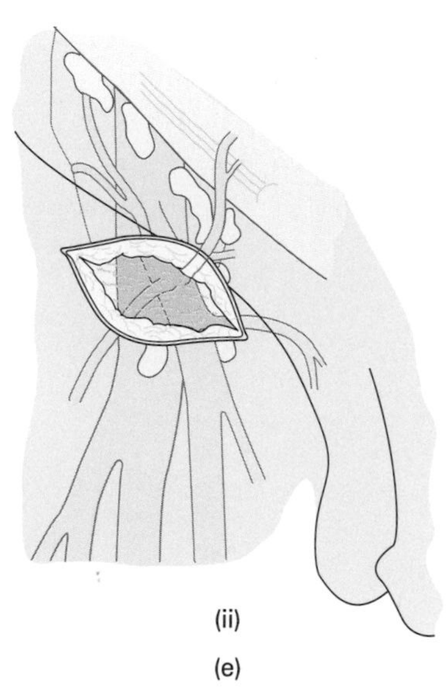

(ii)

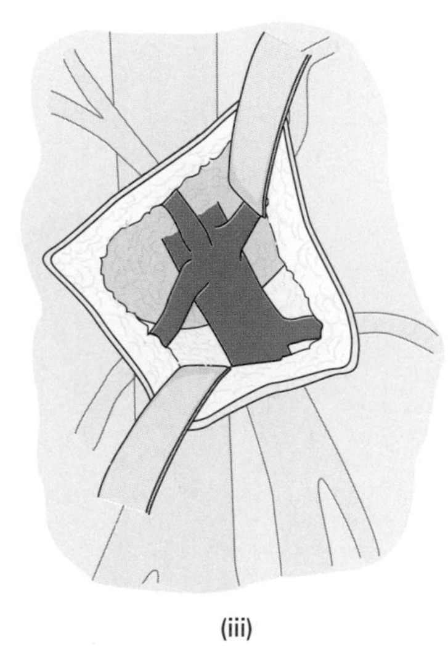

(iii)

(e)

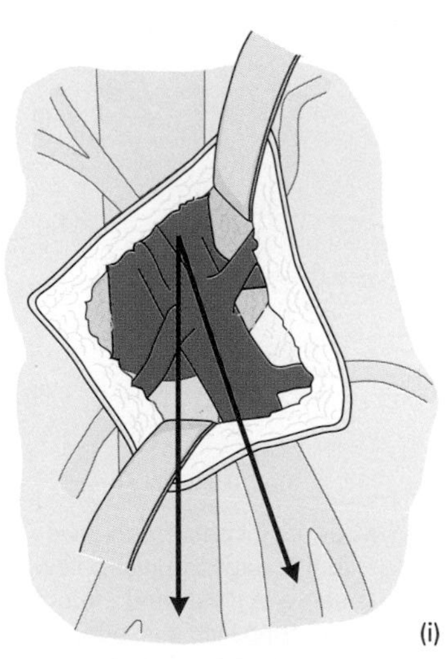

(i)

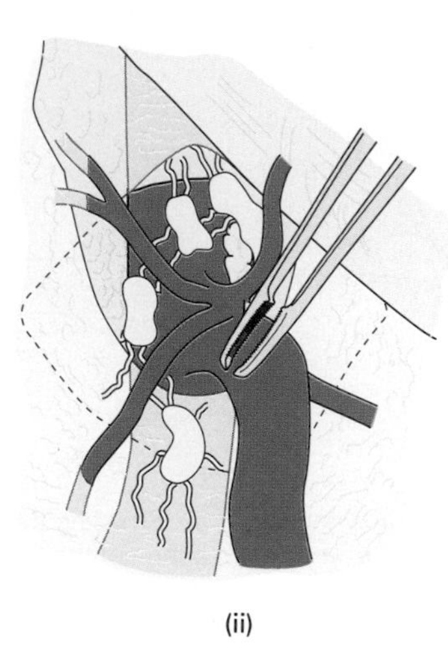

(ii)

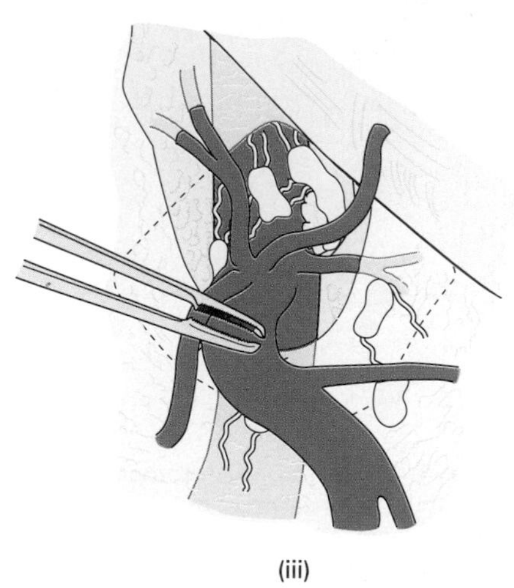

(iii)

(f)

(f) Checking correct identity of saphenous vein. (i) It is not axial to the limb but inclines to the medial aspect; several typical branches are always present at the true termination. (ii) and (iii) The junction with the common femoral vein must be seen beyond doubt from both medial and lateral aspects. (iv) Once certain of its correct identity, the saphenous vein is divided and drawn forward to facilitate division of its

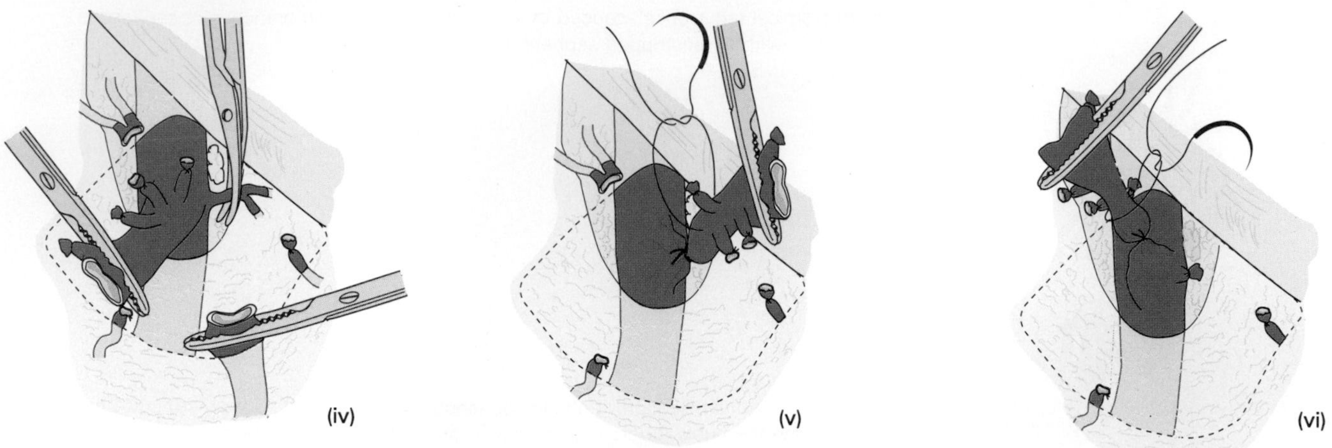

branches. (v), (vi), and (vii) When fully isolated, the saphenous stump is ligated flush with the common femoral vein and then again, more peripherally, with a transfixion stitch.

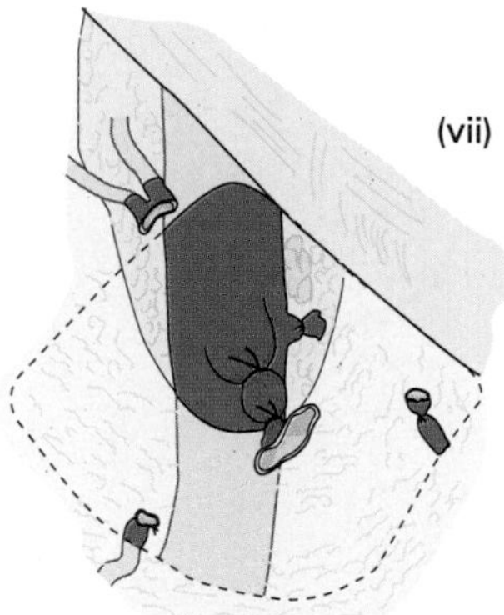

(vii)

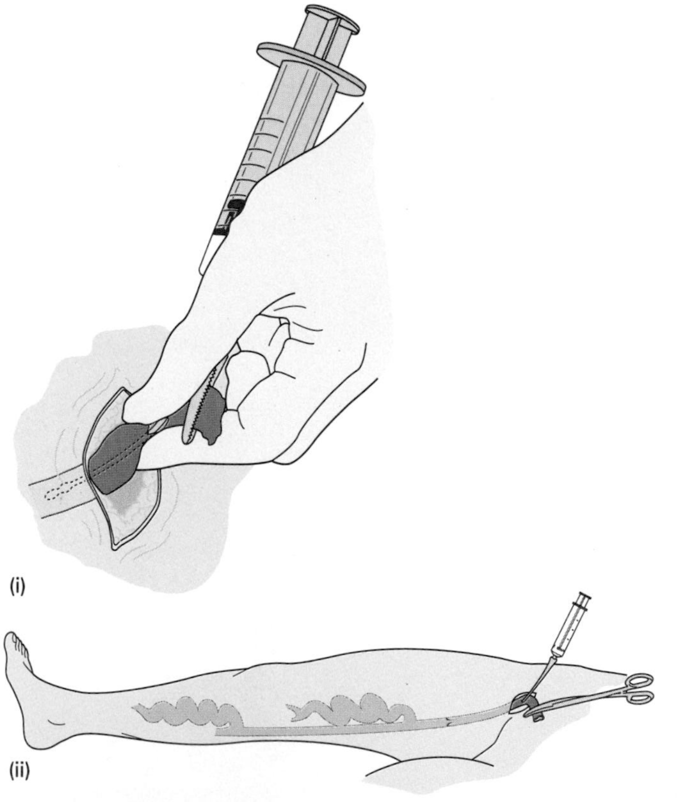

(i)

(ii)

(g)

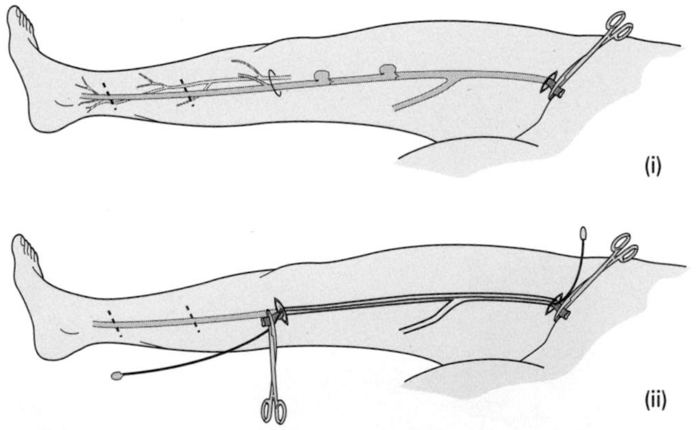

(i)

(ii)

(h)

(g) The syringe test for valve competence. (i) A cannula on a syringe filled with 20 ml of saline is introduced into the distal cut end of the saphenous vein. (ii) On emptying the syringe there should be no resistance and the varicose veins can be seen to bulge if the saphenous vein has no functioning valves. If there is resistance it is probable that this vein is not the pathway of incompetence which must be found elsewhere, for example, the anterolateral branch.

(h) Stripping the long saphenous vein when its incompetence has been confirmed. (i) The long saphenous vein is exposed just below the knee. The position of the saphenous nerve is illustrated; note its close proximity to the vein near ankle. (ii) A stripper is passed up to the groin. (iii) If there are special reasons, this may be done from the ankle but here the saphenous nerve is endangered by its proximity. Below the knee the posterior arch vein is often the main pathway of incompetence and the long saphenous vein is not at fault. (iv) The vein is double ligated around the stripper to prevent invagination of the stripper head. (v) The stripper emerging from the groin is now

(i) Clearing haematoma; postoperative support. (i) and (ii) At a late stage in the operation (to give time for haemostasis) haematoma in the track of the stripper is expelled by hand pressure and use of a sucker. (iii) A crepe bandage, or a light elastic stocking, up to midthigh, is sufficient support for the first 48 h; strong constrictive bandaging is most undesirable.

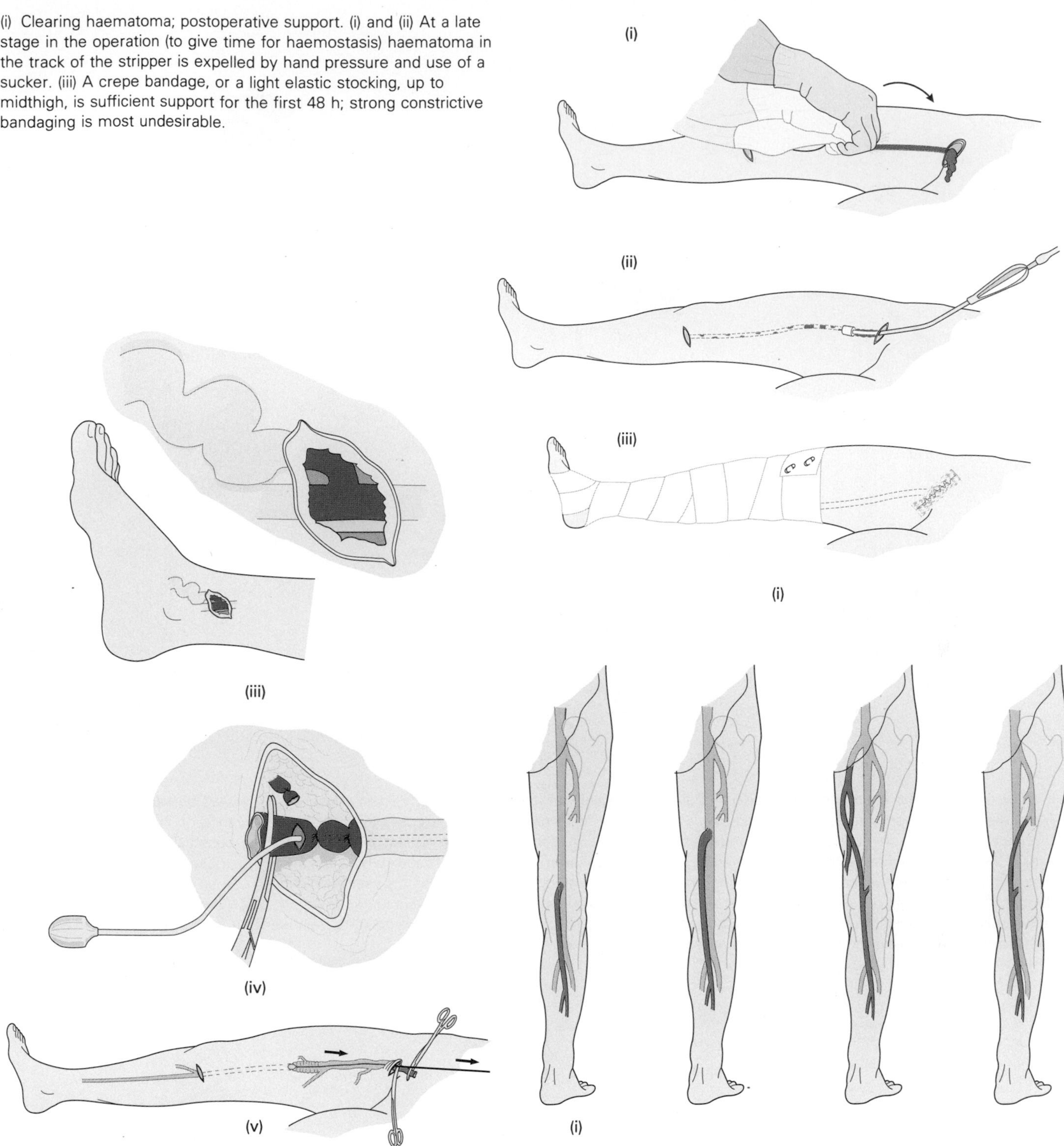

pulled upwards to strip the vein. A controlled, slow pull is best, with pauses when resistance and skin dimpling denote a branch is about to be pulled off; this gives time for these veins to contract before avulsion and minimizes bleeding from them. Note. Many surgeons prefer to pass the stripper downwards and strip in this direction. This is equally good but valve cusps may impede the stripper probe or it may enter side branches.

(j) Variations in termination of the short saphenous vein. Preoperative demonstration by phlebogram or ultrasonic imaging is strongly advised. (i) Usual level of saphenopopliteal junction. (ii) High level termination. (iii) Upward extension superficially to join the posteromedial branch of long saphenous vein. (iv) Upward extension deeply to profunda femoris.

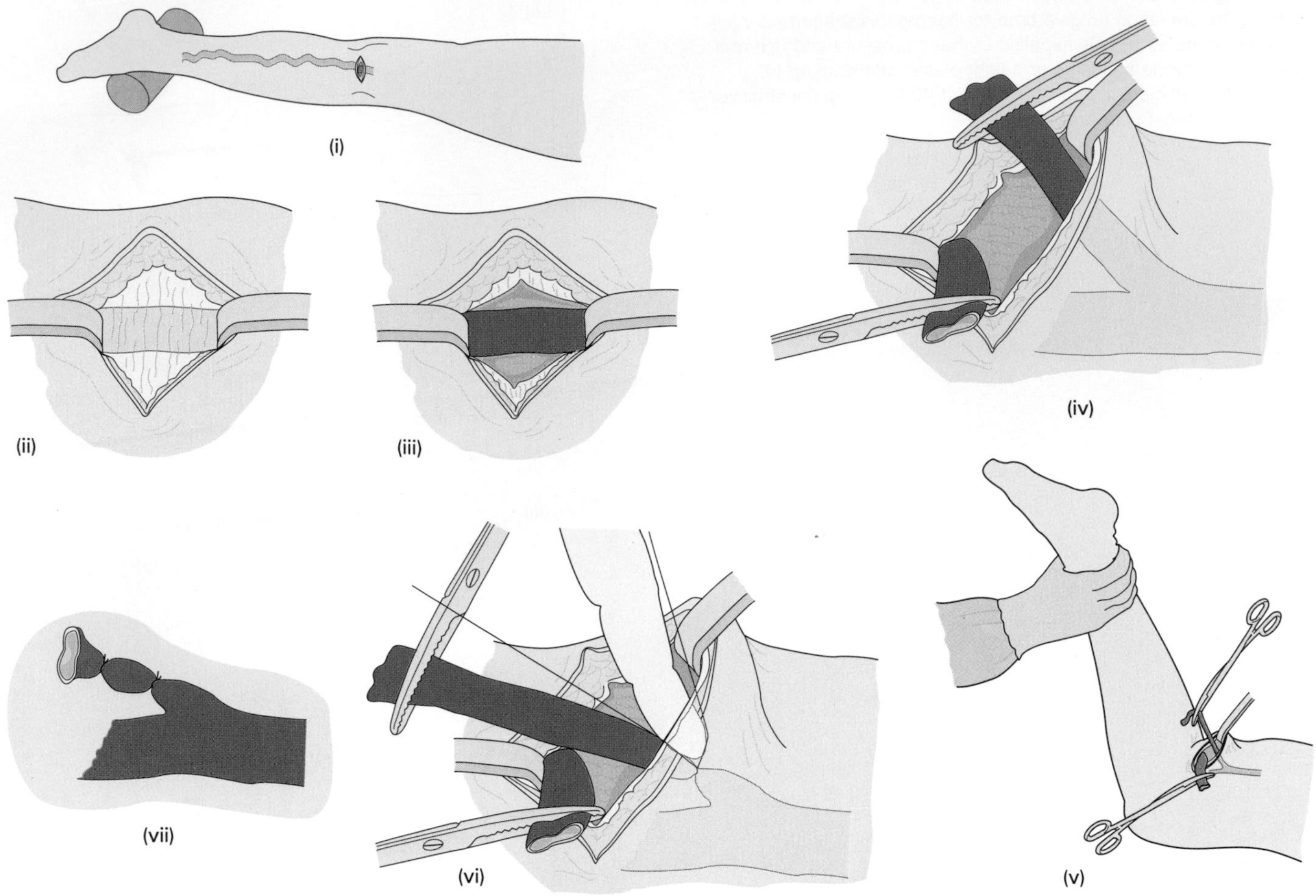

(k) High ligation of the short saphenous vein. (i) Patient is positioned face down, or nearly so, in a fashion that allows bending of knee. (ii) Transverse skin incision, at a level indicated by ultrasonic imaging or phlebography, exposes the deep fascia. (iii) Incision in the deep fascia. The short saphenous vein usually directly underlies it and is easily seen. Too deep a dissection may expose the popliteal vein and lead to a bad error if this is assumed to be the saphenous vein! If the popliteal artery can be felt immediately under the vein exposed then this is likely to be the popliteal vein—do not proceed! Passing the probe end of the stripper up the saphenous vein from midcalf can be a great help if identification is difficult, but is not infallible because it can occasionally enter the deep vein lower down. (iv)–(vii) When certain of identity, the saphenous vein is divided and followed upwards as far as possible to its junction with the popliteal vein where it is doubly ligated and the excess removed. Flexing the knee facilitates access.

(l)

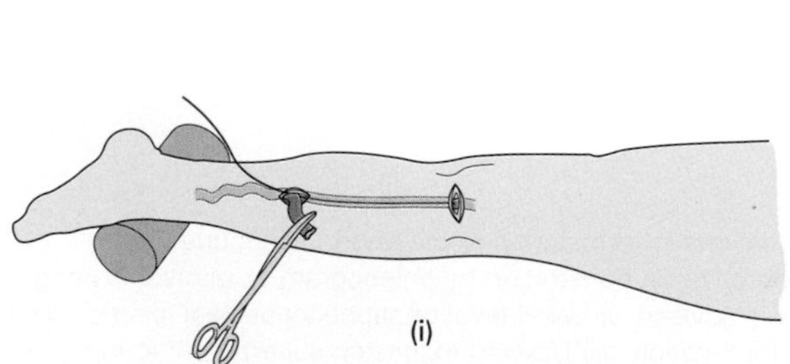

(l) Stripping the short saphenous vein. (i) A stripper is passed up from the point where the lowest varicosity takes off. (ii) Exposing the saphenous vein in the lower leg puts the sural nerve in danger as it is a sizeable structure applied closely to the vein. It must be identified and gently separated; the nerve has a distinctive vascular pattern on its surface.

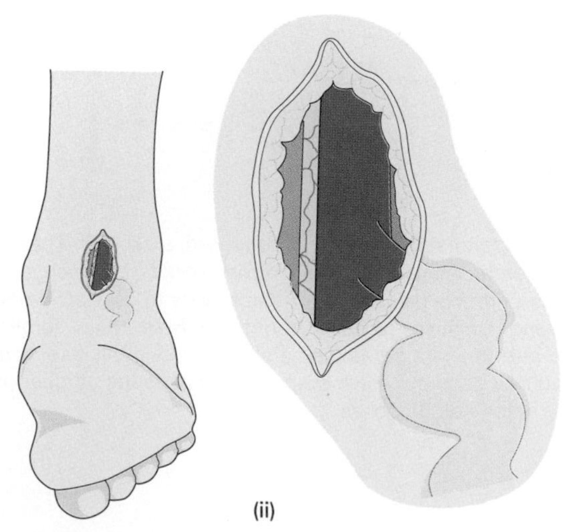

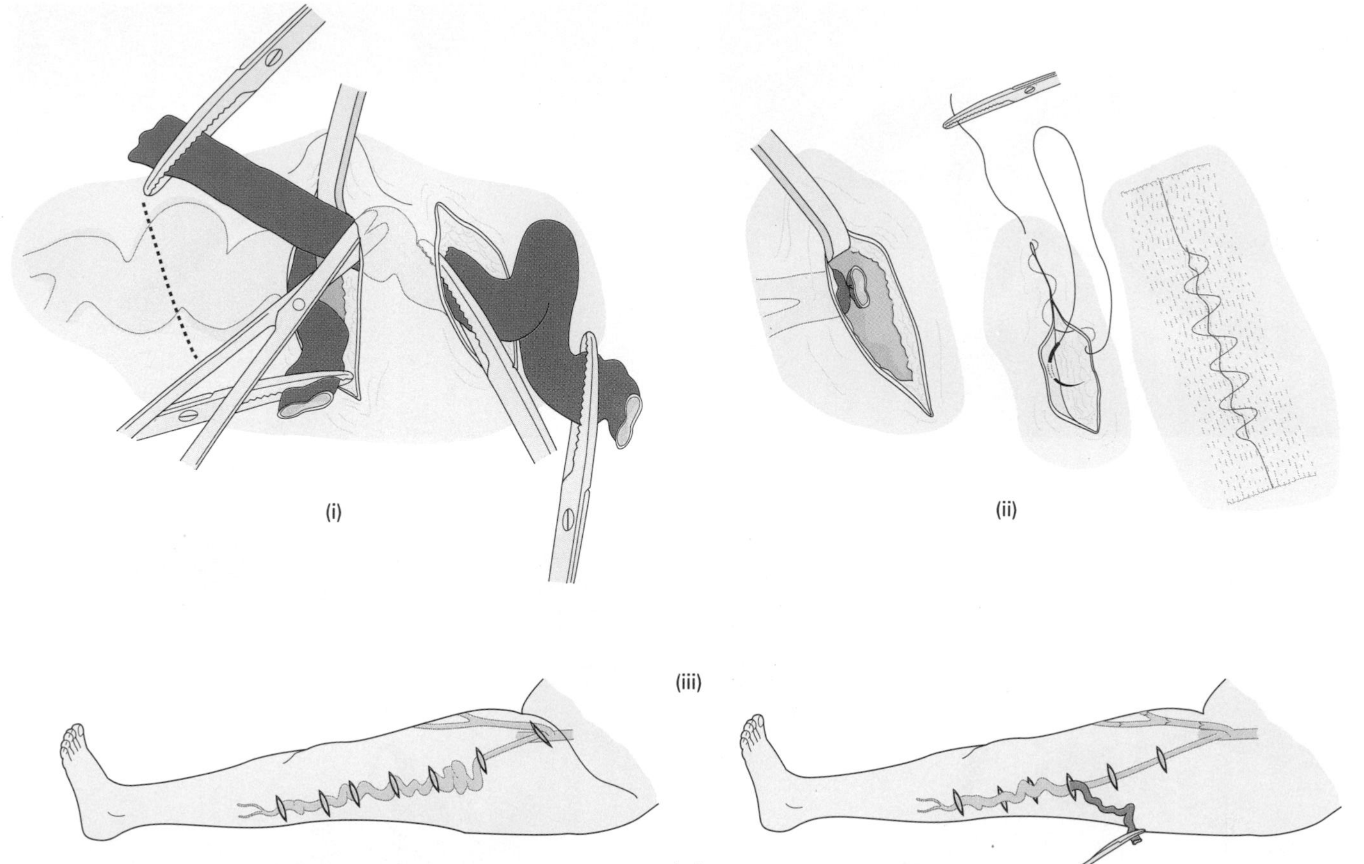

(i) (ii)

(iii)

(m)

(m) Removing outlying veins. (i) and (ii) Massive varicose veins can be removed by making small oblique incisions and tunnelling between them. Always use a subcuticular stitch for incisions. An unknotted monofilament, taped down with Micropore, withdrawn at 7 days, is ideal and avoids ugly cross-hatching of the scar. (iii) Less substantial veins can be removed by a series of small incisions tunnelling the vein out from one to the other, again closing with subcuticular stitch. Alternatively, most veins in this category are suitable for the stab-evulsion technique illustrated in Fig. 51(n).

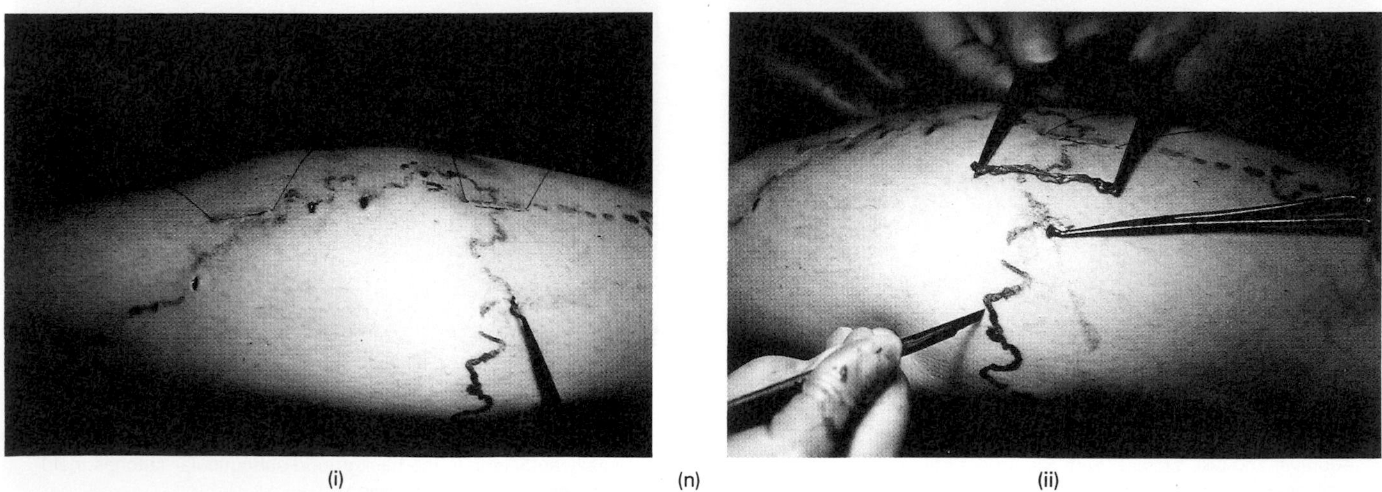

(i) (n) (ii)

(n) Photographs illustrating the stab incision and evulsion technique. In fact, the vein is coaxed and teased out rather than simply pulled upon, and the aim is to remove several centimetres from each stab incision. (i) The main incisions used for stripping a short saphenous vein have been closed with subcuticular stitches; several stab incisions already used can be seen. (ii) The portion of vein just removed from a stab incision is displayed. (iii) A further stab incision (about 2 mm across) is made. (iv) The underlying vein is picked up and teased out. (v) By pulling gently on the vein and pushing tissue away from its base with points of closed artery forceps, more and more of its length is freed. (vi) The

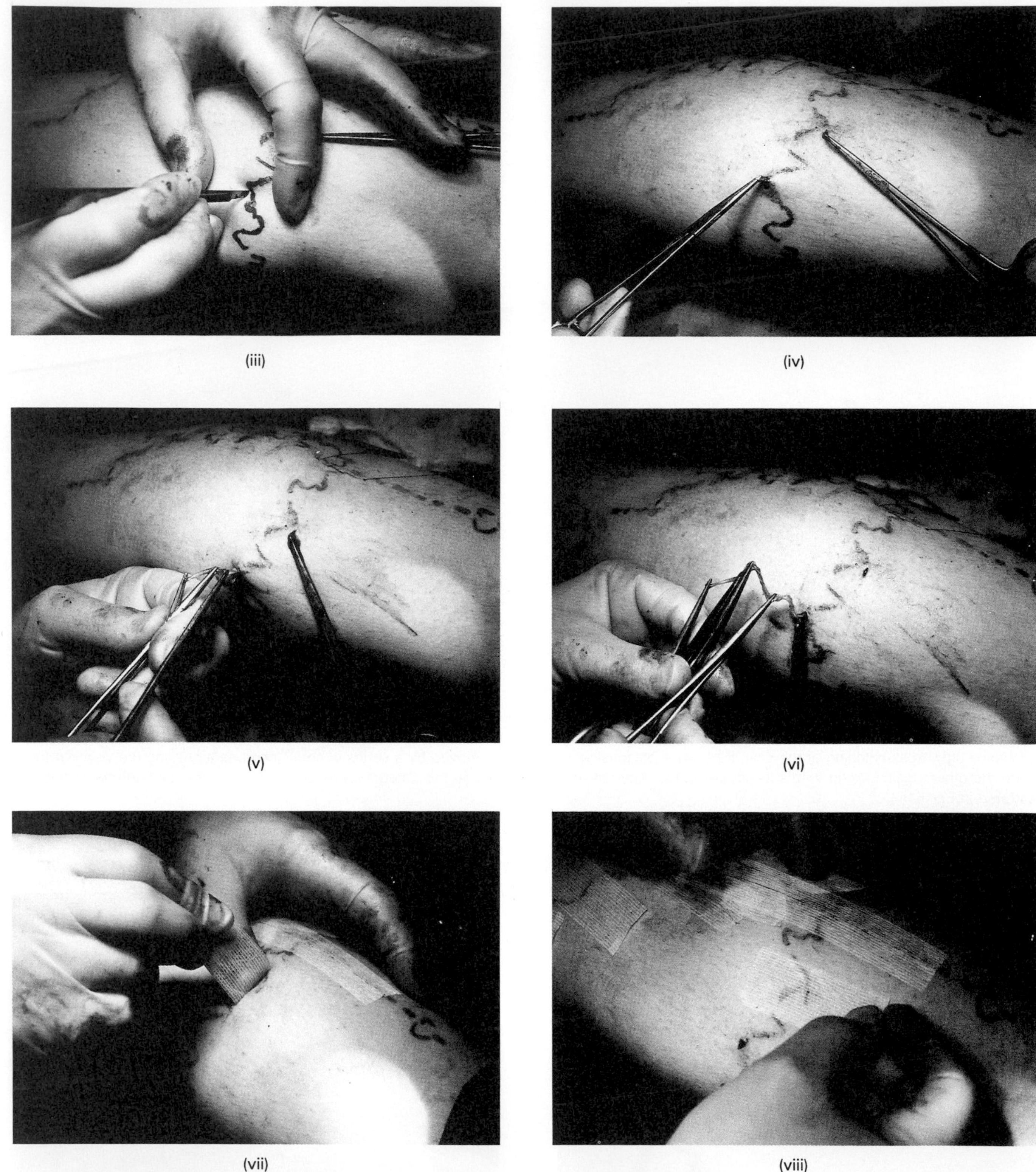

(iii) (iv) (v) (vi) (vii) (viii)

entire length, back to the previous stab incision, has been delivered and removed. This process can be repeated through further stabs as far as desired. (vii) and (viii) Closure with Micropore sterile tape, without any stitch, is usually sufficient. In the background subcuticular stitches, held in place only by adhesive strips (to allow expansion of tissues with oedema), can be seen at the main incisions.

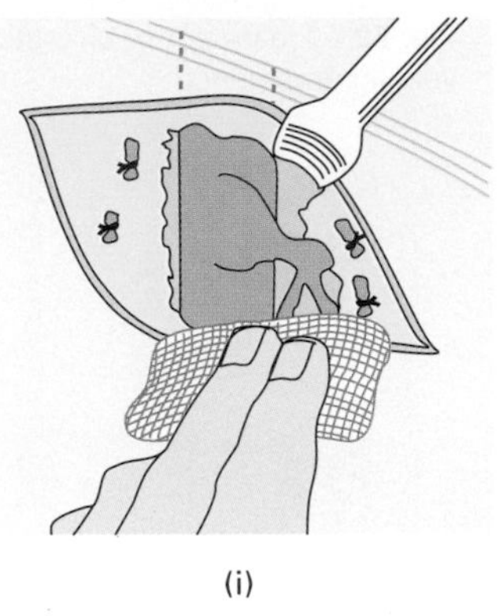

(i)

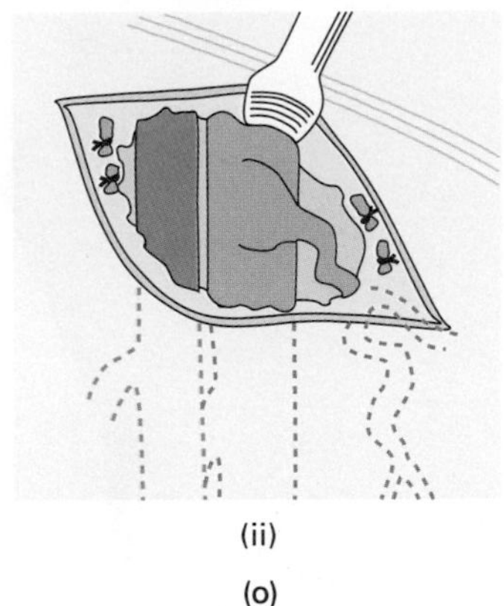

(ii)

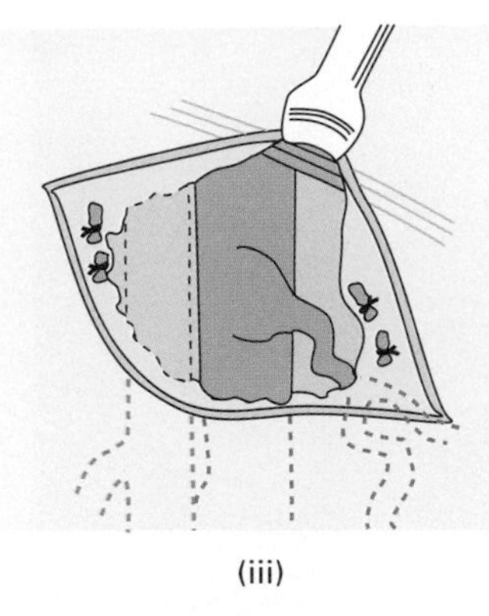

(iii)

(o)

(o) Recurrence from a long saphenous stump. Preliminary phlebography or ultrasonic imaging is essential. Scar tissue with varicose veins embedded in it can make operation difficult; lymphatics abound and damage to these may cause a lymph fistula. Use a transverse incision to skin but deepen this by a longitudinal incision to minimize injury to lymphatics. Three approaches are available. (i) Directly following local varicosities to the stump. These fragile veins amongst scar tissue break easily, but bleeding can be controlled by local pressure allowing progress elsewhere. It can prove difficult and the two approaches, given in (ii) and (iii), skirting the scar tissue may be preferable. (ii) The common femoral artery is exposed first and dissection is then moved medially to expose the neighbouring common femoral vein which is followed to the saphenous stump. (iii) The inguinal ligament is exposed first and then the common femoral vein, which is followed down to the stump.

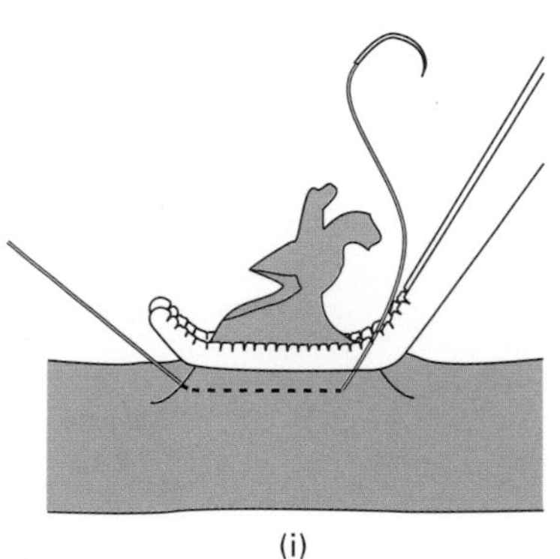

(i)

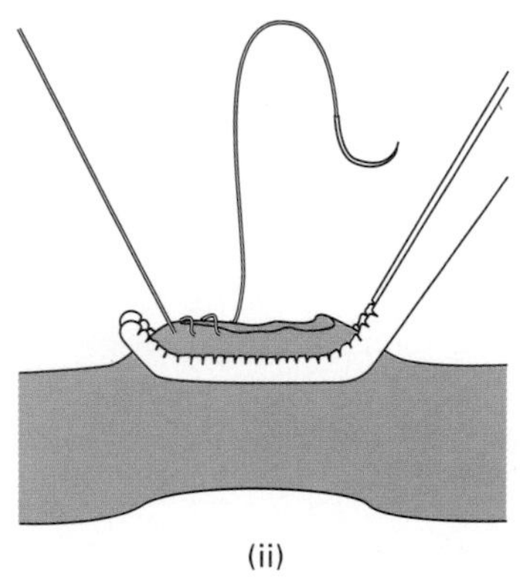

(ii)

(p) Removing the saphenous stump and repair of deep vein. (i) and (ii) Operation to remove a saphenous stump may involve repair of the deep vein. A suitable vascular clamp should be at hand and is invaluable if the need arises, as in the examples illustrated. Remember that using a sucker to clear a field of copious bleeding can soon exsanguinate the patient. Never continue using the sucker regardlessly—stop haemorrhage by finger pressure on a tight gauze pad and pause to think out another approach; one of those described above can allow the femoral vein to be exposed and a side clamp applied from a different direction.

Many varicose veins are labelled 'recurrent' when, in fact, they are due to a different set of veins, unrelated to the originals For example, several years after successful treatment of long saphenous varices a new set of varicose veins arising from the short saphenous vein may appear. This perhaps reflects widespread weakness in veins and valves, prone to incompetence and varicosis, but is not a contraindication to further treatment.

Hurried, inadequate treatment, insecurely based on an unproven source is a major factor in recurrent varicose veins. The source and pathway of incompetence must always be conclusively demonstrated by clinical tests and backed by Doppler flowmeter studies before surgery.

Compression sclerotherapy in the treatment of residual and recurrent veins after surgery

Residual varicose veins due to incomplete surgery or small veins that appear after an interval, are often best treated by compression sclerotherapy. There is a good prospect of response so that it is well worth a trial. This is no more than a completion of the original treatment, particularly when extensive varicosities have made complete elimination impractical at one operating session and survivors declare themselves later. Here, sclerotherapy is particularly valuable but in most cases adequate removal at surgery by multiple small incisions (Fig. 51(n)) makes this additional treatment unnecessary. Some surgeons, in order to reduce time on the operating table, have a deliberate policy of doing no more than 'high ligation and strip', leaving the varicose veins for treatment by sclerotherapy later; however, this is tedious for the patient and misses an ideal opportunity to complete treatment by a single procedure.

Treatment of major recurrences of varicose veins

Large recurrent varicose veins are often amongst the most difficult to treat. Previous surgery will have fragmented the anatomy of the superficial veins so that the new patterns are far less predictable. Some of the worst recurrences occur in the groin or behind the knee, over the site of saphenous ligation; there may be a history of several unsuccessful attempts to remove these but such attempts are always followed by early reappearance perhaps even larger and more uncomfortable than before. Such veins are unlikely to give more than a temporary response to sclerotherapy and surgery may be the only answer in spite of the previous failures. The problem is compounded by the fact that several sources of incompetence may be present and that the patient may suffer from a degree of weak

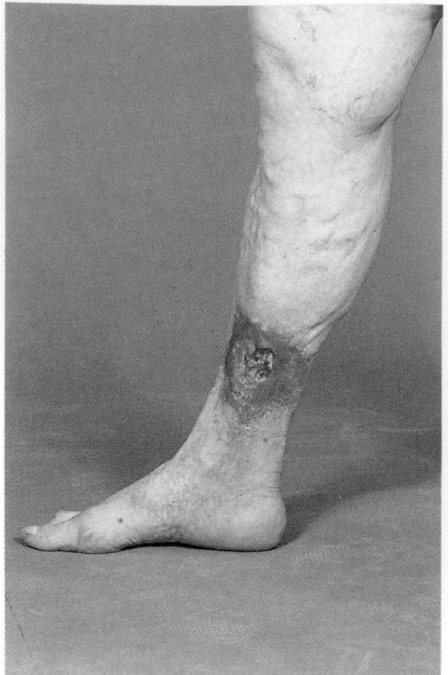

(a)

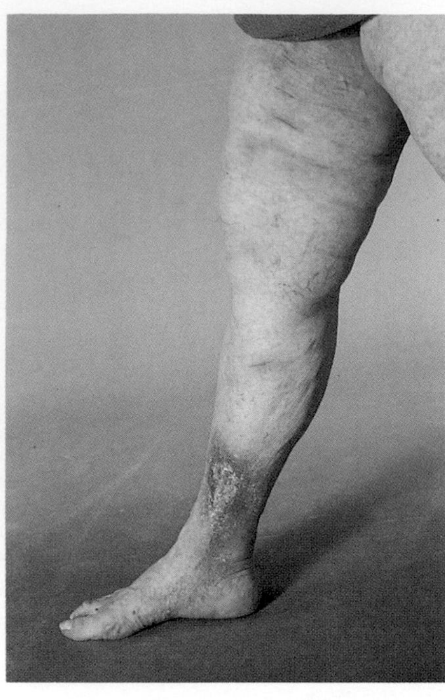

(b)

Fig. 52 Treatment of ulceration in superficial vein incompetence.

(a) This ulcer, in a middle-aged woman, was caused by massive incompetence in the long saphenous vein.
(b) The ulcer, now healed, 2 months after surgery with immediate postoperative mobilization. It remained well healed when seen a year later.

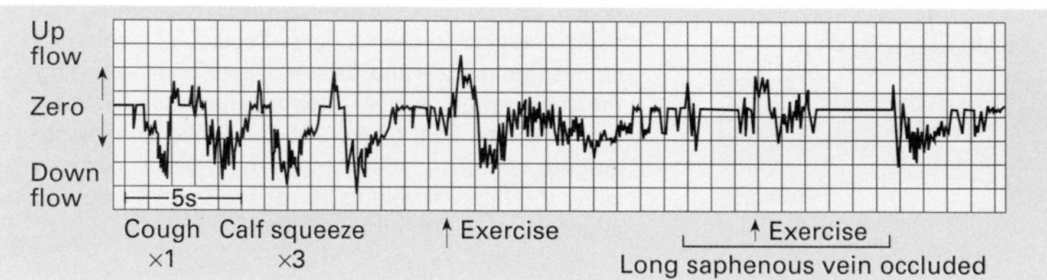

(c)

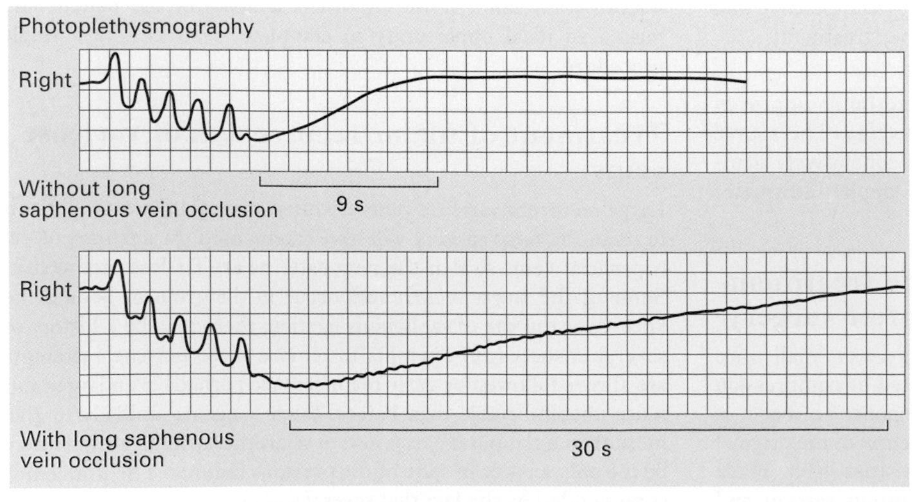

(d)

(c) and (d) Preoperative findings. All clinical tests strongly confirmed the diagnosis. Reproduced here, the Doppler flowmetry recordings showing downflow in the long saphenous vein after exercise, characteristic of simple incompetence; the photophlethysmograms showing refilling within 9 s, but restored to a normal 30 s when the long saphenous vein was temporarily occluded by fingertips.

vein syndrome. Nevertheless, with careful mapping out and study of flow patterns by Doppler flowmeter it is usually possible to understand the overall arrangement of the varicose veins, and the likely sources of flow down them from the deep veins. Guided by this information a combination of functional phlebography and varicography can give a good display of the key features, the sources, and pathways of incompetence upon which surgery can be based. No surgery should be considered without this detailed information and only a surgeon experienced in its interpretation and in carrying out such operations should embark on it; it is probable that exposure of the deep vein through dense scar tissue, traversed by large, fragile varicosities, will be needed in order to attain complete elimination of a leaking saphenous stump (Fig. 54) and this may involve repair to the deep vein (Figs. 51(d) and 51(p)). Any lesser effort is likely to bring yet another failure when in fact a most satisfying result may be attainable. An example of the complex patterns that may be encountered is given in Fig. 41(a). Such cases are not rare and require a special skill and perseverance. If weak vein syndrome is a factor, it may be wise to back up successful surgery with long-term use of elastic support up to the knee.

Having emphasized the difficulties of this aspect of venous surgery it must be stressed again that the best opportunity to carry out successful surgical treatment of varicose veins is at the first operation and the principles to be used in minimizing massive recurrence have been outlined in this section.

Complications of varicose veins

Two specific complications may arise in varicose veins as distinct from the changes caused by venous hypertension.

Haemorrhage

Varicose veins lying directly beneath the skin commonly become adherent to it and may so stretch it that it no longer provides adequate protective covering. Then, only the thinnest layer of skin and fragile, attenuated vein wall retain the blood, which shows inky blue through the membranous covering. This state is most likely to develop in varicose veins on the foot, ankle, and lower leg, particularly in elderly patients. The vein may burst with minor trauma or spontaneously when the patient is up and about. The ensuing haemorrhage can be copious but is easily stopped by finger pressure, or if the patient lies down with the foot elevated, and a firm pad and bandage applied. This can be an alarming experience for the patient and, although the aperture will be temporarily plugged with clot, it will soon bleed again (Fig. 55(a)). There is little natural tendency for it to heal because the underlying vein remains open and the unsupported, devitalized skin lacks the vascular base necessary for repair processes. Treatment must be completed by elimination of the affected varicosity and in an elderly person often this can be most simply achieved by compression sclerotherapy. However, the problem is usually more than a local one and whenever possible it is better to treat the accompanying superficial vein incompetence surgically and at the same time to excise the point of haemorrhage and its underlying varicose vein.

Veins liable to this complication can often be recognized and treated before haemorrhage occurs. Patients with such varicosities should be given clear instructions how to control haemorrhage if it should occur before treatment.

Phlebitis

Historical note

The term 'phlebitis' used to have a different and sinister significance before the introduction of asepsis towards the end of the 19th century. In the early part of that century surgeons thought of it as an inflammatory process in veins, with two types; one, fibrinous phlebitis, usually with a favourable outcome; the other, suppurative phlebitis, likely to prove fatal. The fibrinous variety corresponds to present day superficial or deep vein thrombosis, but it was not realized that in the deep vein it was far from benign and could cause death by pulmonary embolism until Virchow described this in the mid 19th century. Even so the dominant fear of the pre-Listerian surgeons was of suppurative phlebitis, which as we now know was a bacterial, infective state filling a vein with purulent clot liable to enter the bloodstream, causing pyaemia, with high fever, rigors, widespread abscesses and, inevitably, death. It was a well recognized complication to surgery of that time, especially when veins were ligated (with unsterile material in a septic operating field), trapping clot that had suppurated and could only escape by entering the circulation. For this reason surgery to varicose veins was greatly feared. However, when the bacterial cause was understood, and with the development of aseptic surgery, it ceased to be a serious problem. For a long time the purely thrombotic form, whether in superficial or deep veins, was assumed also to be bacterial. With the realization that this was not so the terms 'thrombophlebitis', 'phlebothrombosis', or, simply, 'vein thrombosis' were introduced to emphasize their essentially thrombotic nature and to distinguish them from the very different infective, suppurative type. It is important to realize that the latter is still a potential danger if ever the high standards of modern surgery should fail or when an uncontrolled infective cellulitis surrounding a vein creates a septic thrombosis within it. Fortunately, this is treatable with antibiotics and elimination of the source of infection, but surgery and medicine sometimes have to be practised in primitive conditions and the efficacy of modern methods should not allow past lessons to be forgotten. The old dragon of suppurative phlebitis has been subdued but not slain and its retreat to the shadows uncovered another formidable dragon, venous thrombosis, damaging and dangerous, with which we continue to grapple (see Section 8.2).

Superficial thrombophlebitis (phlebothrombosis)

Thrombosis in varicose veins is quite common and may be accepted as a complication without any very serious implications. However, when thrombosis occurs spontaneously in previously normal veins, it may well signify a serious background condition hitherto unsuspected. This includes malignancy (for example, in the pancreas or bronchus), leukaemia or polycythaemia, vascular disease (especially thromboangiitis obliterans), and disorders of blood clotting. Whether it appears as single episode or recurring episodes in different parts of the body (phlebitis migrans), it is a clear indication for full medical screening to identify the cause. Varicose veins in the lower limb, however, can be regarded as sufficient explanation for local thrombosis without necessarily searching further for an underlying cause.

Thrombosis within a varicose vein, or any superficial vein, is accompanied by a tender swelling, often red and slightly warm to the touch, and until quite recently this was commonly regarded as an inflammation of the vein caused by infection. As explained

Fig. 53 Recurrence at site of previous saphenous ligation.

(a) Anatomical recurrence; a renewed source from existing branches connecting with the original pathway of incompetence. (i) After long saphenous high ligation. A composite phlebogram showing a narrowed saphenofemoral junction with an otherwise intact but incompetent saphenous vein running down to the calf and filling varicosities (and gastrocnemius veins) there. A previous operation had removed only the superficial component of a double saphenous vein but had left the true termination narrowed but intact. (ii) and (iii) Clinical appearance and phlebogram of a recurrence after 'high' ligation of the short saphenous vein. A large varicosity arises from a surviving branch on the stump. This was confirmed at surgery which gave a good result.

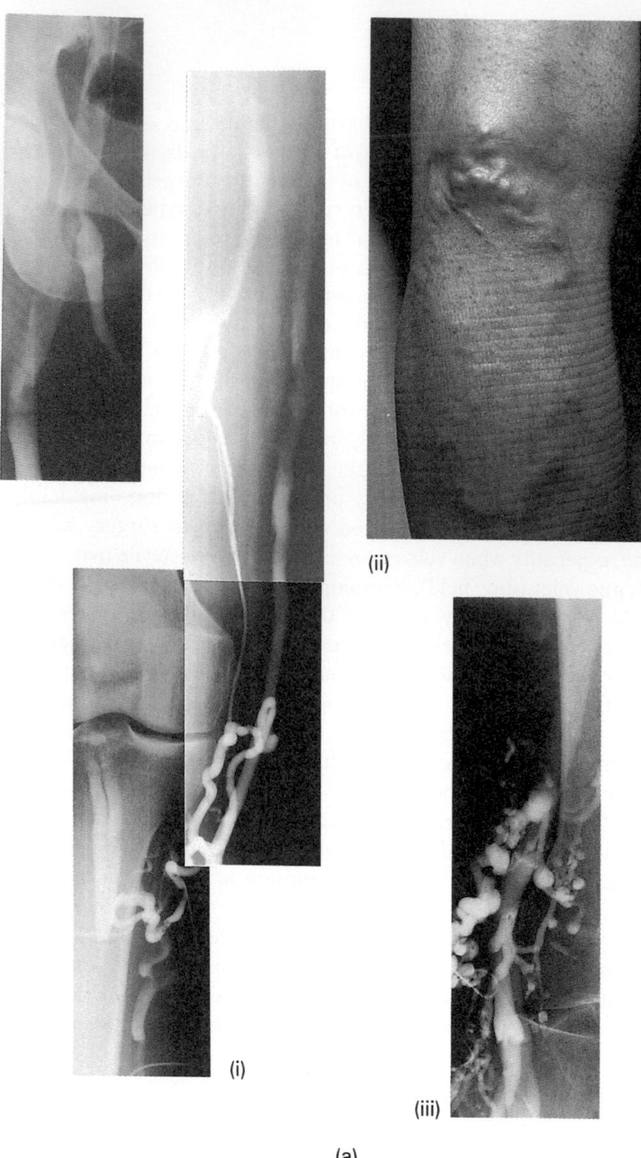

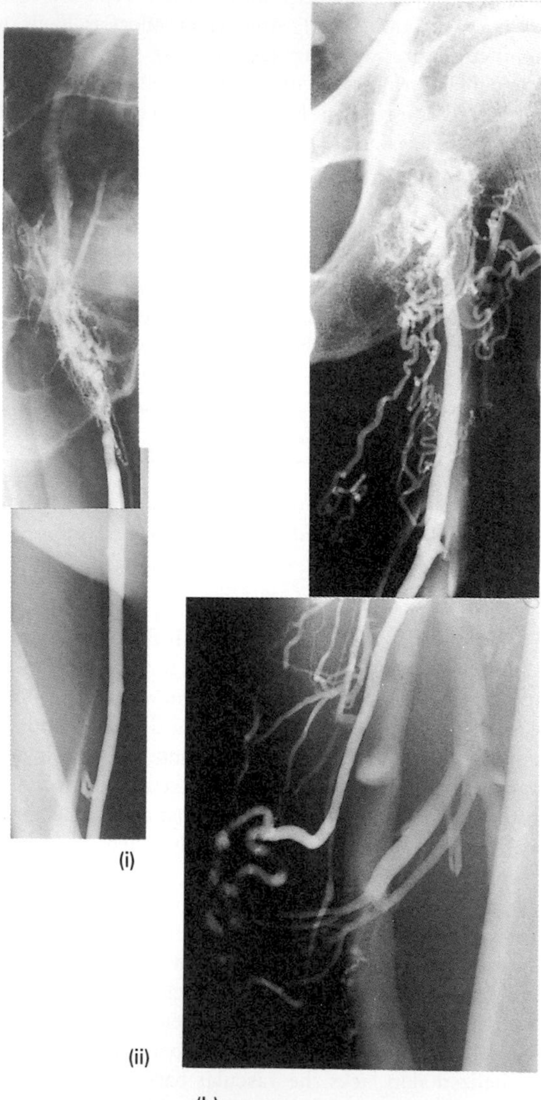

(b) Non-anatomical recurrence by revascularization of a long saphenous stump. Two examples are shown in different patients with reconnection between stump and an unstripped vein by a newly formed plexus of veins. (i) Connection with an unstripped incompetent long saphenous vein. (ii) Connection with a retained incompetent anterolateral branch.

(c)

(c) Non-anatomical revascularization at other sites of ligation. In this example, outflow has been re-established to the original pattern of varicose veins after ligation of a perforator in midthigh.

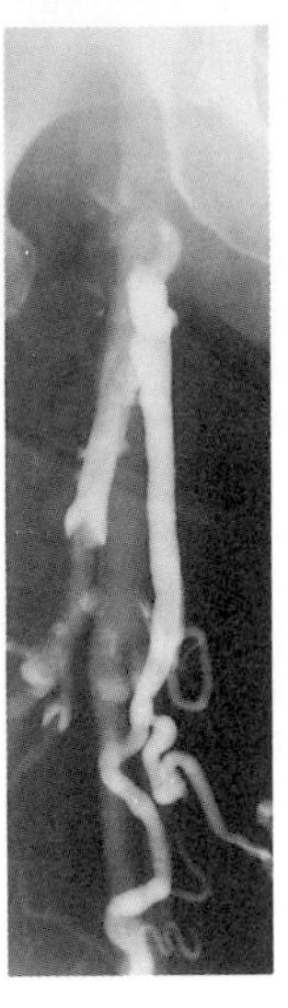

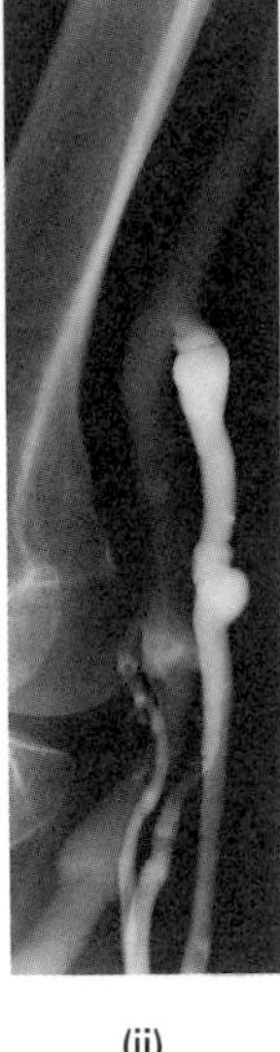

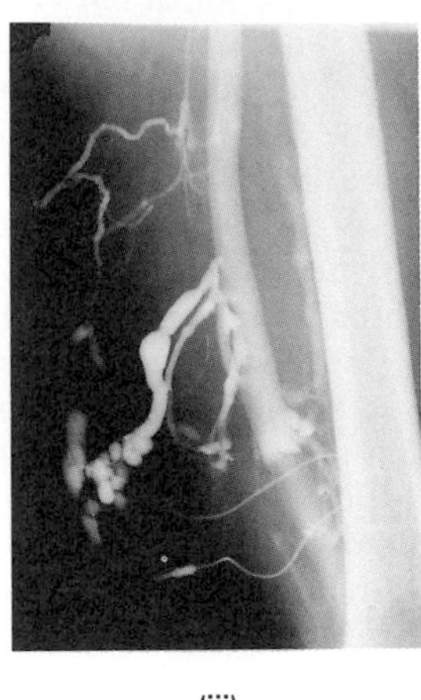

(i) (ii) (iii)

(d)

(d) Recurrence from a latent second source. Phlebograms after previous surgery to the long saphenous veins. (i) A small anatomical recurrence due to an incompetent anterolateral long saphenous branch is present. (ii) However, the major cause for renewed varicosities is from the short saphenous vein shown here. This became obvious only after the dominant long saphenous downflow had been reduced by previous operation. Surgery to both veins brought this elderly patient relief from long-standing discomfort. (iii) Phlebogram in another patient showing a typical midthigh perforator that has taken over remnants of the long saphenous system.

above, the old term of 'phlebitis' was retained until it was realized this was not so and that it must be distinguished from septic thrombosis in a vein secondary to a surrounding infection and which, by suppuration, is liable to cause a dangerous pyaemia. Now that it is recognized that the condition is a response to the thrombosis itself, the terms superficial thrombophlebitis or phlebothrombosis are used to denote this. Varicose veins are undoubtedly prone to thrombosis, partly because there are long periods of stasis in the unnaturally enlarged vein, for example when sitting, but also because production of fibrinolysin in the walls of a varicose vein is reduced. Even when quite a large thrombus has formed, blood continues to stream by it, continually depositing further thrombus so that the vein becomes progressively distended with clot. This does not, however, completely occlude the vein and studies by venography or by Doppler flowmeter show that, when the patient is upright and moving, blood continues to flow down the varicose vein, infiltrating its way round the clot and continually depositing further thrombus (Fig. 55(b)). The vein becomes painfully over-distended and shows an inflammatory reaction. This gives the key to treatment, which is to apply external compression to prevent blood from continuing to flow through the affected vein. The process may limit itself to a few centimetres of vein or may go on extending progressively to involve a considerable area, perhaps the entire calf, when it may be mistaken for a deep vein thrombosis. It may extend into the saphenous vein and along its full length, and in these circumstances, occasionally, may release a pulmonary embolus. Apart from this, it is seldom life-threatening although very troublesome to the patient.

Diagnosis

The tender red swelling on the leg, with an indurated cord of thrombosed vein is characteristic. The diagnosis can usually be safely made on clinical grounds alone but where deep vein thrombosis is seriously suspected, this should be checked by phlebography or ultrasonography rather than risk mistreating a life-threatening condition. Occasionally it is difficult to distinguish between superficial thrombosis in the long saphenous vein and a lymphangiitis but the latter condition will lack the firm cord of thrombosed vein and will be accompanied by high fever unlike the low pyrexia that may be present in superficial phlebitis.

Treatment

Traditional conservative treatment is by applying a firm compression bandage (as in sclerotherapy). An anti-inflammatory agent such as indomethacin may be used to relieve pain but antibiotics are not necessary. If the condition is unusually extensive it may be advisable to put the leg in high elevation (but check for ankle pulses beforehand), with the patient encouraged in active movements and maintained like this until the condition starts to recede; at this stage mobilization is commenced in a firm support bandage. In most circumstances anticoagulants need not be used but in extreme cases the condition will resolve more rapidly with a few days of heparin followed by oral anticoagulation for some weeks.

However, active intervention is often greatly to be preferred because it will bring immediate relief from pain and ensure a rapid recovery. If a substantial set of varicose veins are present and the circumstances allow it, the most effective course is to carry out the appropriate operation for this without delay and at the same time to excise the thrombophlebitic vein; this will be curative for the phlebitis and the varicose state that caused it. When this course is not possible, the simple procedure of evacuating the clot from the thrombosed vein is very effective and may be carried out under local anaesthesia by a single 2-mm skin incision into it. The clot is then extruded by firm finger pressure and a pad and bandage applied without skin suture. This gives complete relief and, provided firm compression is maintained for several weeks afterwards, will cure the phlebitis so that the overall problem of widespread varicose veins can be tackled at a more convenient time.

Thrombosis in deep veins is described separately in Section 8.2.

Syndromes of valve deficiency and weak vein walls

Valveless syndrome or primary valve deficiency

The majority of patients with incompetence in the superficial veins, described in the preceding section, fall into a clearly defined

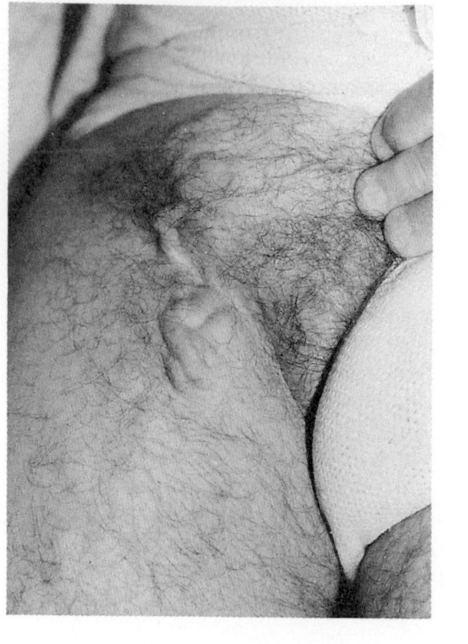

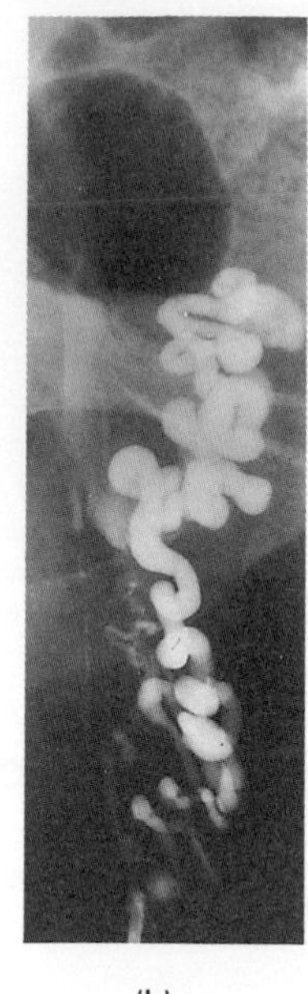

(a) (b)

Fig. 54 Repeated failure to eliminate a saphenous recurrence; the importance of preoperative assessment. (a) These varicose veins reappeared in the groin after three previous operations to remove them. Large varicose veins ran from here down the length of the limb and required a heavy full length elastic stocking to control them. (b) Phlebogram showing the origin from a shallow saphenous stump. Surgery exposing the common femoral vein allowed this to be closed off by direct suture of the deep vein (see Fig. 51(p)). The stump was negligible in size but gave considerable outflow through a venous plexus believed to be formed by revascularization. Surgery for this type of recurrence requires careful preparation including phlebography. This patient was seen 3 years later and there was no evidence of any further recurrence.

group that responds well to treatment. However, there is a group, about 8 per cent of venous disorders, in which a more widespread defect is present and treatment far less satisfactory. There is no sharp demarcation between the two groups but, rather, a spectrum of defect with, at one end, well defined superficial vein incompetence and, at the other end, a widespread deficiency of functioning valves in both superficial and deep veins. This deficiency of valves in the deep veins must not be confused with the post-thrombotic state described presently because the patients give no history suggesting previous deep vein thrombosis and, on phlebography, the deep veins are widely open without any evidence of post-thrombotic deformity or occlusion.

In the spectrum of valve deficiency, the 'well defined' states at one end have a normal complement of valves in superficial veins but these are incompetent; moving along the spectrum, valves in both superficial and deep veins become increasingly deficient in number. The absence of valves without any evidence of preceding thrombosis, suggests an inborn error in the development of valves. This is supported by the not uncommon finding of incompetent superficial veins in early teenage boys and girls, and the occurrence of valveless deep and superficial veins in well recognized states of congenital venous abnormality, such as Klippel-Trenaunay syndrome. Deficiency of valves in the deep veins leads to ineffective venous pumping so that venous hypertension easily develops, particularly if the superficial veins also have gross incompetence. Patients with well valved deep veins have a robust pumping mechanism which is not easily overwhelmed even by substantial superficial vein incompetence and this may explain why many patients have large varicose veins without any evidence of venous hypertension. By contrast, other patients with similar varicosities show obvious venotensive changes and ulceration, possibly because they lie halfway along the spectrum of change, with poorly valved deep veins and a relatively weak pumping mechanism, easily overwhelmed by superficial incompetence;

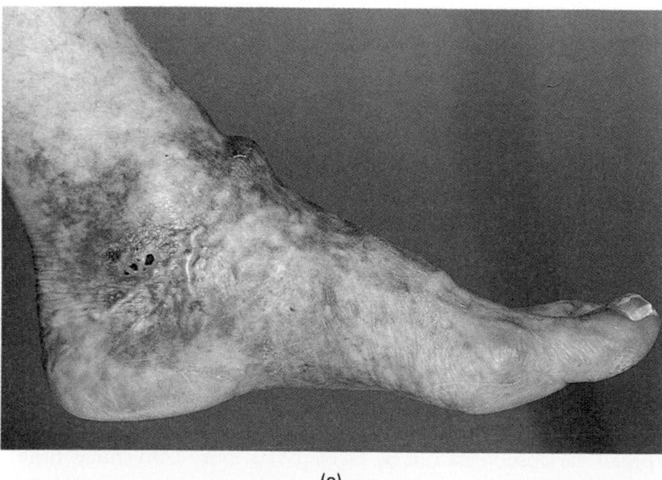

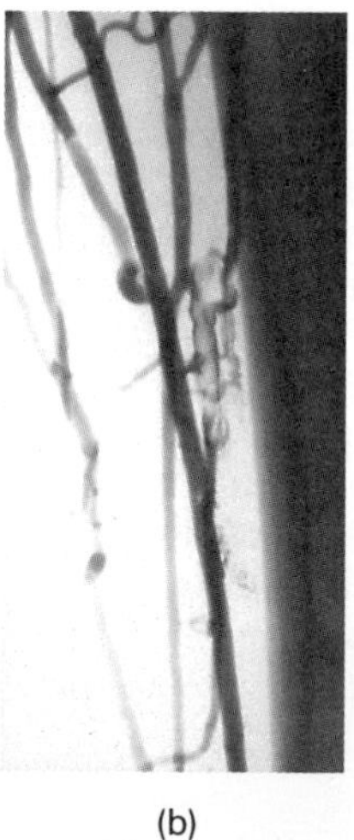

(a) (b)

Fig. 55 Complications of varicose veins. (a) Haemorrhage. Large varicose veins and venotensive pigmentation near the ankle, due to superficial incompetence in an elderly man. Just below the medial malleolus a scab can be seen marking the site of three episodes of severe haemorrhage; the veins nearby protrude through thin, fragile skin. Urgent treatment was necessary and sclerotherapy, advised because of the patient's infirmity, proved successful. (b) Thrombosis. Phlebogram of an area of superficial thrombophlebitis in a varicosity. Opaque medium can be seen streaming round the thrombus and Doppler flowmetry confirmed active downflow after exercise when standing. Use of a firm bandage to prevent such flow from causing a continuing build-up of thrombus is the basis of conservative treatment; this combined with expression of clot through a stab incision will bring immediate relief. Alternatively appropriate surgery to the incompetent superficial veins may be carried out with excision of the thrombosed vein.

surgery to the superficial veins can restore a precarious balance with healing of the ulcer, but requiring some care to keep it so. At the far end, the predominant failure is in the deep veins and causes a pump insufficiency too severe to be remedied by removing incompetent superficial veins. These patients suffer from intractable ulceration, not amenable to any form of surgery to the superficial veins (Fig. 56(a) (i)). For descriptive purposes this has been named here as the valveless syndrome but it is also known as primary valve deficiency and is, of course, one variety of chronic venous insufficiency. The main features of this state are summarized below.

There is no history of a previous deep vein thrombosis.

Gross saphenous incompetence is often present, or incompetence may come from multiple sources; obvious varicose veins are not necessarily present.

Selective Trendelenburg test does not control enlarged superficial veins because of the incompetence in deep veins.

Severe venotensive changes, often with ulceration, are present.

Doppler flowmetry to enlarged veins shows surge back and forth with little purposeful movement in either direction (Fig. 56(a) (ii)).

Photoplethysmography shows a short recovery time in keeping with an inadequate venous pump and incompetent valves; this is not improved by any manipulation of superficial veins.

Phlebography. The deep veins are widely open throughout with no evidence of previous deep vein thrombosis and few, if any, functioning valves can be demonstrated in them (Fig. 56(a) (iii)).

Ultrasonography. This will confirm substantial reflux and lack of valves in the deep veins.

Clinical presentation of these cases is very similar to post-thrombotic syndrome and the diagnosis is usually made from phlebography or ultrasonography.

Treatment

Provided that phlebography has shown the deep veins to be widely open but valveless, it is permissible to remove enlarged and valveless superficial veins. In borderline cases, this reduction in the load on the pumping mechanism may restore it to an adequate performance. In more severe examples it brings little or no benefit and treatment will have to rely upon the conservative measures of elevation whenever possible and the use of external support by elastic stockings.

Surgical restoration of valve function

As incompetence in deep veins is the main problem, it may be possible to improve this by one of the following methods:

Transposition of a deep vein into a neighbouring vein that is well valved, for example, implanting the upper end of a superficial femoral into the side of a valved profunda femoris vein nearby (Fig. 56(b)). This may be useful in congenital states of valve deficiency including Klippel-Trenaunay syndrome.

Transplantation of a suitable venous valve taken from elsewhere in the body and inserted as an autograft into an incompetent deep vein, for example, using a valve from the brachial vein, or a saphenous vein of the opposite side, to transplant into the upper popliteal vein (Taheri's operation) (Fig. 56(c)). Again, this may be of help in inborn states of valve deficiency.

Repair of prolapsing valve cusps by valvuloplasty (Kistner's operation). This procedure tightens up selected valve cusps when incompetence is caused by excessive length with one cusp prolapsing beneath the other (Fig. 56(d)). A small number of patients with severe venous insufficiency have this form of incompetence in the femoropopliteal deep veins and may be suitable for the procedure. The operation has yet to gain general acceptance although successful cases are reported.

Use of a tendon or silastic sling around the popliteal vein to act as a substitute external valve (Psathakis). This procedure has yet to be evaluated independently, and there is some indication that deep vein thrombosis and pulmonary embolism may be a problem.

Weak vein syndrome

This is a different state from that just described, although both may coexist. The patients often have a strong family history of varicose veins and develop unusually large, incompetent superficial veins leading down to equally large varicosities (Fig. 56(e)). With surgical treatment there is a strong tendency for further large, recurrent varicosities to appear within a year or two. Gross examples are seen following inadequate surgery, for instance, when the long saphenous vein has been ligated at too low a level or has not been stripped and the source of the recurrent varicosities is from surviving branches in a saphenous stump, perforators in the thigh, or interconnections between the saphenous systems. It is possible that extrinsic factors play a part; for example, some of the most severe cases are seen in people whose work involves prolonged standing and high consumption of alcohol, as in publicans and hoteliers. Clinical examination and phlebography gives a strong impression that the veins lack inherent strength and easily over-expand. This, indeed, may be the primary problem because weak vein walls will allow valve cusps to separate and become incompetent; deficiency of valves does not seem to be a cause because an adequate number may be present but grossly incompetent. Histological studies commonly find some degenerative changes in the vein walls of patients with varicose veins and in the state just described the primary defect may be an extreme form of this.

Diagnosis and treatment

If there has been no previous treatment all the usual features of simple incompetence will be found, including good control with a Trendelenburg test, although the veins are unusually large. This does not contraindicate surgery but is rather an encouragement for conscientious surgery; saphenous ligation must not leave any branches at the upper end, stripping of the long saphenous vein must be at least to upper calf, and all major varicosities must be removed.

If the patient presents with recurrent varicose veins, the massive size of these and their unusual pattern may be daunting. However, with careful mapping out and use of the Doppler flowmeter, the source and pathway of incompetence may be identified. Further surgery must be carefully planned and this will require detailed phlebography to guide the surgeon. A good long-term result may be obtained but in the very nature of the condition further recurrence is possible and, as a last resort, strong elastic stockings will be required to control the varicose veins as a long-term policy.

The two states just described, the valveless syndrome and the weak vein syndrome, are ill defined and ill understood. However, it would be unrealistic in describing the venous disorders to give the

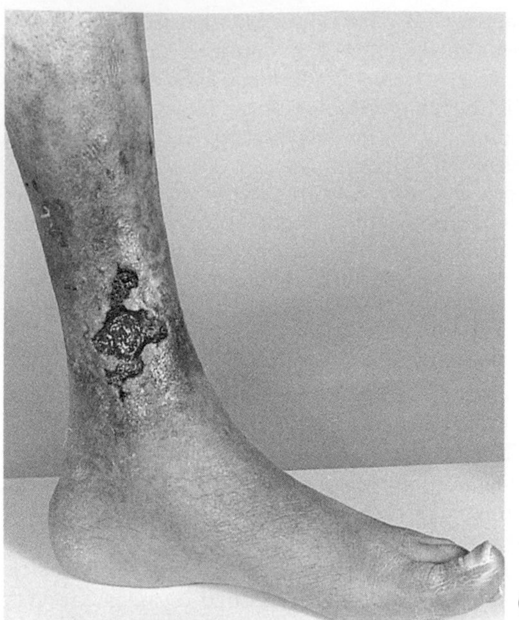

(i)

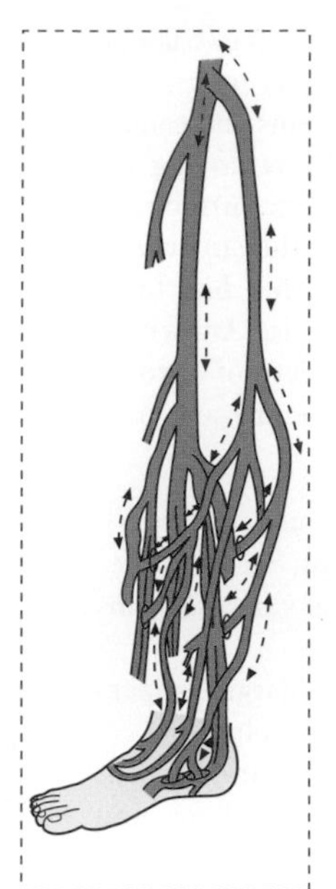

(ii)

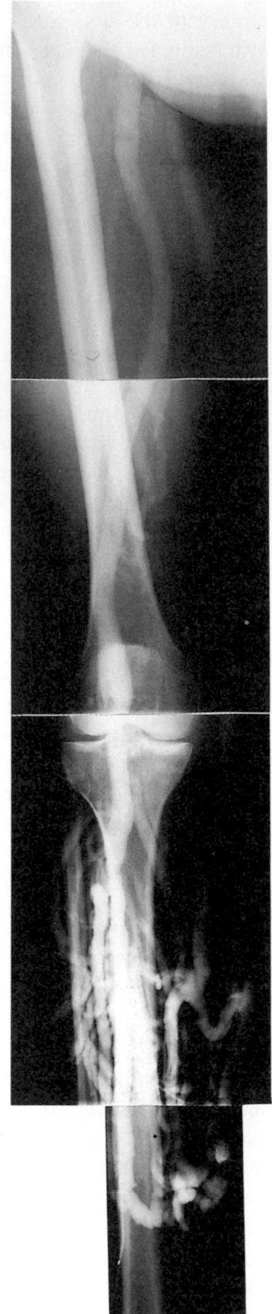

(iii)

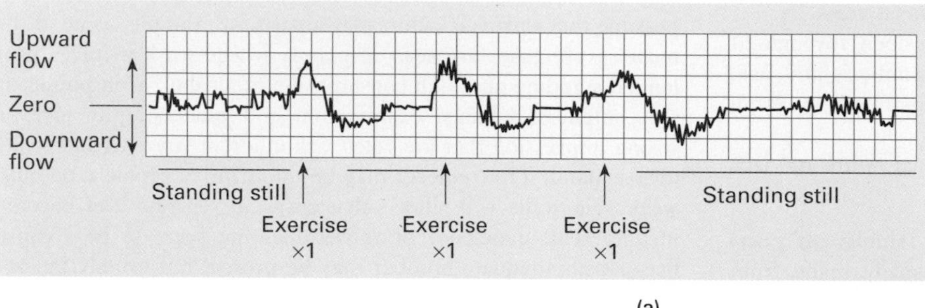

(a)

Fig. 56 Valve deficiency and weak vein states.

(a) Valveless syndrome. (i) Venous ulceration and surrounding venotensive pigmentation in an elderly patient with no history of a previous deep vein thrombosis. Superficial vein incompetence was not evident and a good arterial supply was present. This arises when there is a deficiency of functioning valves in the deep veins. (ii) In the valveless syndrome the musculovenous pump is ineffective and venous blood tends to surge back and forth with each muscular contraction. Doppler flowmetry may detect this; the phases of upflow and downflow with exercise are of equal duration and magnitude. (iii) Composite phlebogram in the valveless syndrome. Strong surge between tibial and superficial veins was evident on screening and, with a change of tilt from near-horizontal to near-vertical, opacified blood disappeared rapidly from higher levels as it shifted down valveless deep veins; no valves could be demonstrated.

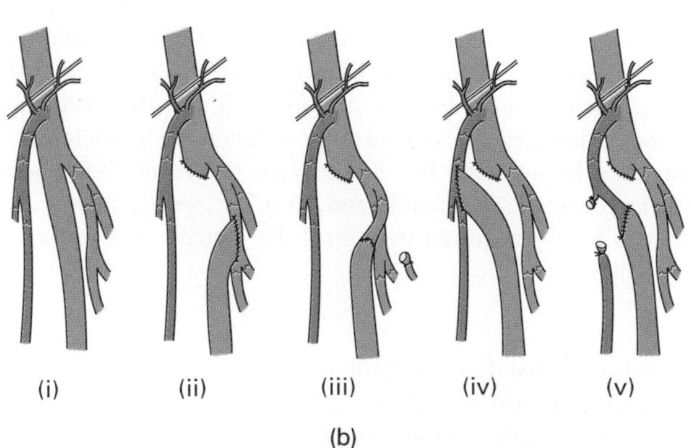

(b)

(b) Surgery for valve deficiency states. Transposition of a major vein to a well valved channel nearby. (i) A valveless femoropopliteal state but with good valves in the long saphenous or profunda femoris veins offers several opportunities for transposition. (ii) and (iii) End-to-side, or end-to-end, anastomosis with the profunda femoris vein or a tributary of it. (iv) and (v) End-to-side, or end-to-end, anastomosis with the long saphenous vein.

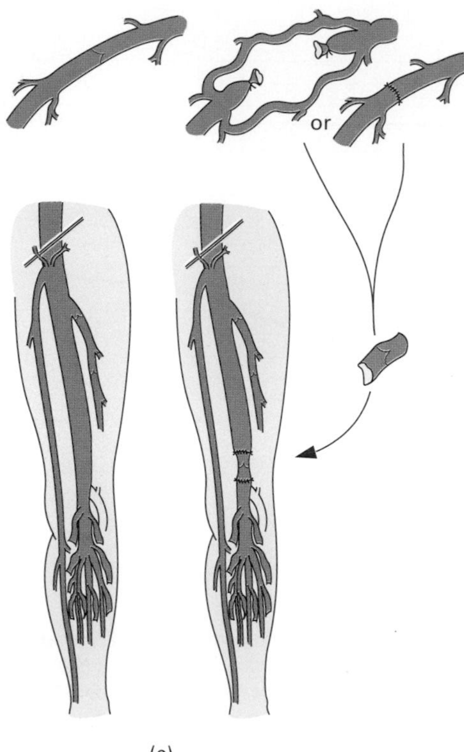

(c)

(c) Valve transplantation for femoropopliteal valve deficiency (Taheri). A good valve in the brachial vein is transplanted to the upper popliteal vein.

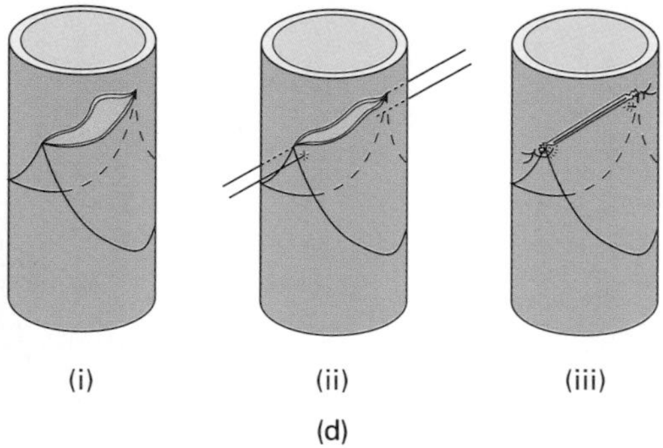

(i) (ii) (iii)

(d)

(d) Correction of prolapsing valve cusps (Kistner). The valve is exposed and the slack cusps tightened by appropriate stitches.

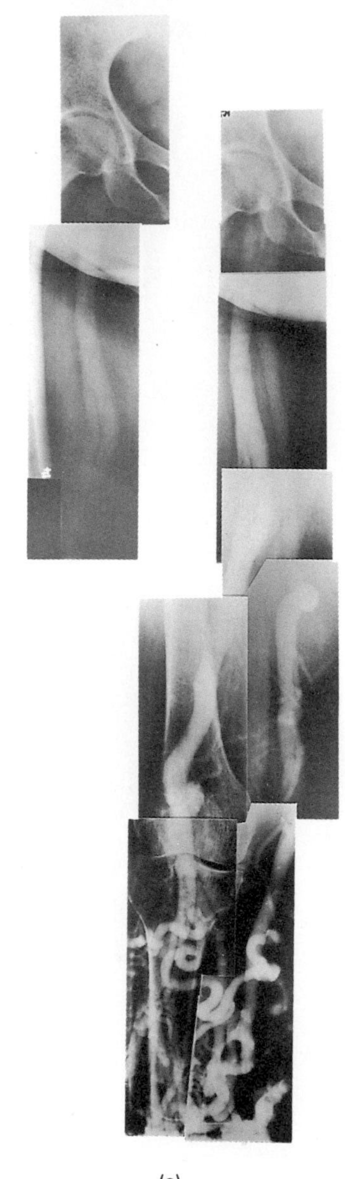

(e)

(e) Weak vein syndrome. Composite phlebogram in which superficial and deep veins show widespread weakening so that they have become massively enlarged, sacculated, or tortuous. This is accompanied by valve failure, caused by over-expansion of valve rings and separation of the cusps. Varicose veins in these patients are prone to massive recurrence after surgery.

impression that all categories are clear-cut and separate from each other. Certainly, most patients can be fitted into a well-defined category and rational treatment based upon this. In others, one of the ill-defined varieties just described may baffle the surgeon, or, it is possible for two separate categories of venous disorder both to be present in the same limb and give a very confusing picture. In these circumstances clinical expertise alone is not sufficient and the extra information provided by ultrasonic imaging and phlebography must be called upon to make sure that the best decision is made for the patient. Care must be taken to exclude the next category, the post-thrombotic syndrome.

Deep vein impairment. The post-thrombotic (post-phlebitic) syndrome

Thrombosis in the deep veins of the lower limbs is a common complication in serious illness, pregnancy, following surgical operations, and after severe injury, especially in fractures of lower limbs or pelvis. It may be localized to a small area or extend massively through both lower limbs; in its lesser forms it may pass almost unnoticed but in its major form causes severe illness and a threat to life through pulmonary embolism. In the affected limb(s)

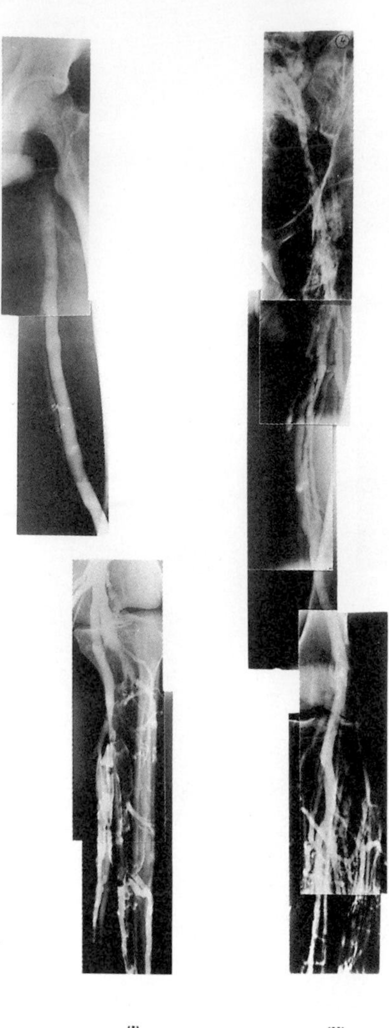

(i) (ii)

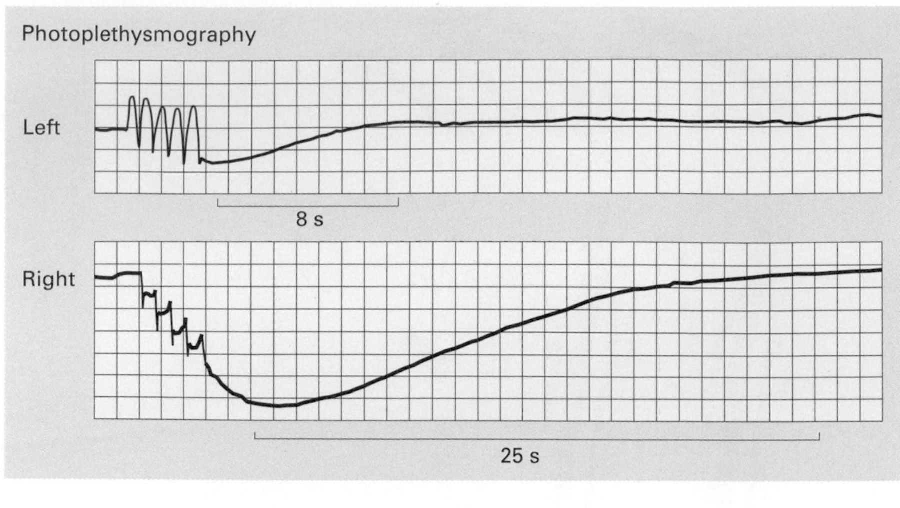

(iii)

(a)

Fig. 57 Post-thrombotic states.

(a) The consequences of deep vein thrombosis in a young man. (i) A phlebogram at time of left deep vein thrombosis. The tibial veins are filled with thrombus (tram-line sign), and the common femoral and iliac veins fail to fill. (ii) Three years later the patient has post-thrombotic syndrome with pigmentation, swelling, induration, and ulceration. Phlebograms show unsatisfactory tibial veins and extensive deformity in common femoral and external iliac veins. (iii) Photophlethysmography comparing the two sides. Left side (upper tracing) shows severely reduced refilling time at 8 s; unaffected right side is normal at 25 s.

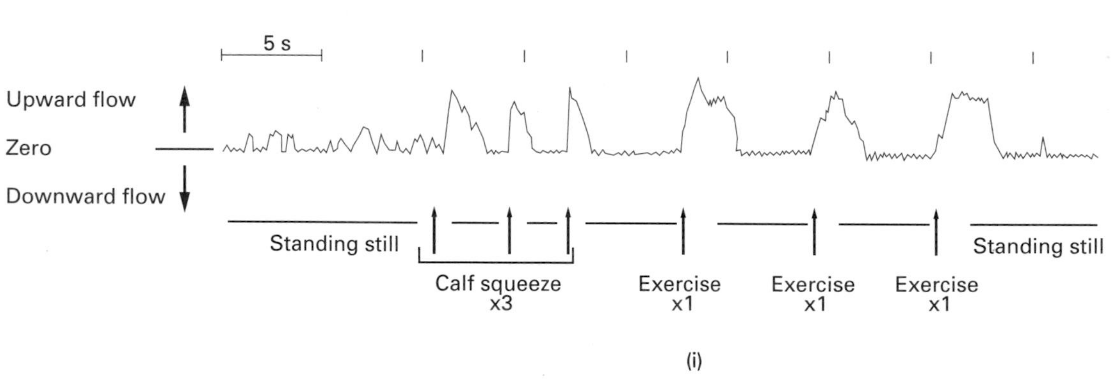

(i)

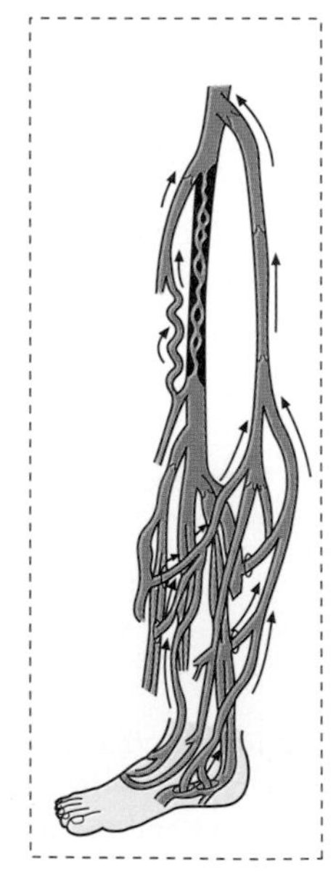

(b) Collateral flow in superficial veins compensating for deep vein obstruction. (i) A diagram of superficial veins taking the collateral flow past a deep vein obstruction. A Doppler flowmeter recording from the long saphenous vein of a patient with this condition shows upward flow, accentuated by exercise. (ii) Composite phlebogram in well-compensated post-thrombotic femoropopliteal obstruction, showing a short saphenous vein, and an upward extension of it, playing an important role in venous return. The long saphenous vein can be seen in the upper thigh also contributing to collateral return. This patient presented with slight swelling and prominent superficial veins some years after a fractured ankle and immobilization in plaster cast; conservative treatment was advised.

the severity of the resulting venous obstruction gradually subsides, partly due to absorption of thrombus and recanalization of the veins but also due to the progressive enlargement of collateral veins, both superficial and deep, providing an alternative pathway of venous return. However, neither of these changes reflects a return to true normality and venous flow in the limb is all too often permanently impaired with corresponding disability (Fig. 57(a)). The deep veins involved in this process will show the following changes in structure and function.

1. The vein may remain permanently obstructed, causing a persistently raised venous pressure beneath it and forcing other veins to act as collaterals (Fig. 57(b)).
2. The vein may recanalize but in this process it becomes severely deformed and the valves are rendered functionless. Not only does this channel offer resistance to venous return it lacks one of the essential characteristics of a vein, properly functioning valves (Fig. 57(c)). Thus, the ability to pump is lost and heavy reflux occurs down the vein. It cannot make any contribution to venous return against gravity and by reflux it will actively invalidate any return achieved by neighbouring veins.
3. Collateral vessels formed from vasa vasorum, lesser deep veins, perforators, and superficial veins will undergo great expansion with separation of the valve cusps so that the valves become disabled; eventually large channels without effective valves are formed which compensate for obstruction in the deep veins but are unable to prevent heavy reflux of blood down their length when the patient is standing (Fig. 57(d)). If only a small area is involved the effect may be insignificant but when major veins are extensively involved, venous return, which is adequate when the patient is horizontal, will suffer from the compounded difficulties of defective pumping units, resistance to venous outflow from exercising muscles, and heavy reflux in recanalized deep veins and collateral vessels when standing; this reflux rapidly reverses any benefit of venous return against gravity achieved by neighbouring undamaged parts of the venous system. The net result is a sustained high venous pressure in the limb, unrelieved by exercise, when the patient is up and about. This causes venous congestion and oedema, with the familiar changes of venous hypertension, pigmentation, induration of superficial tissues (dermatoliposclerosis), and, eventually, ulceration near the ankle. These long-term consequences of deep vein thrombosis are known as the post-thrombotic or postphlebitic syndrome and can give rise to severe disability in the limb. This is the commonest cause for chronic venous insufficiency but it is important to realize that similar venotensive changes can be caused by gross incompetence in the superficial veins, a state usually curable by surgery, in contrast with the post-thrombotic state which can be ameliorated but seldom cured (Fig. 57(e)).

There is great variation in the extent of changes such a limb will show and this will depend upon location, extent, and importance of the veins involved. Several patterns can be recognized but one or more of these may be present in the same limb (Fig. 57(f)).

1. Tibiopopliteal Here the deep veins below the knee are mainly affected. Small areas of thrombotic damage may give rise

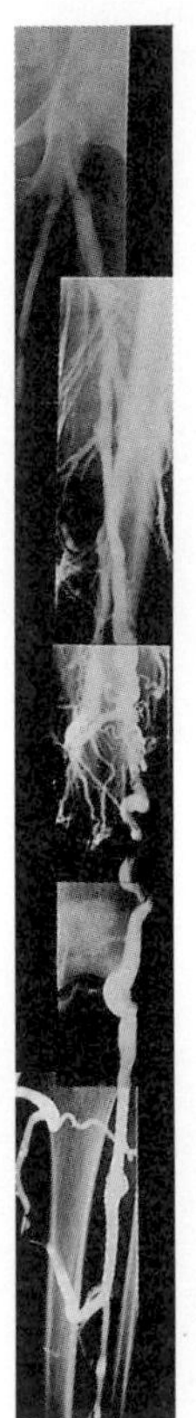

(ii)

(b)

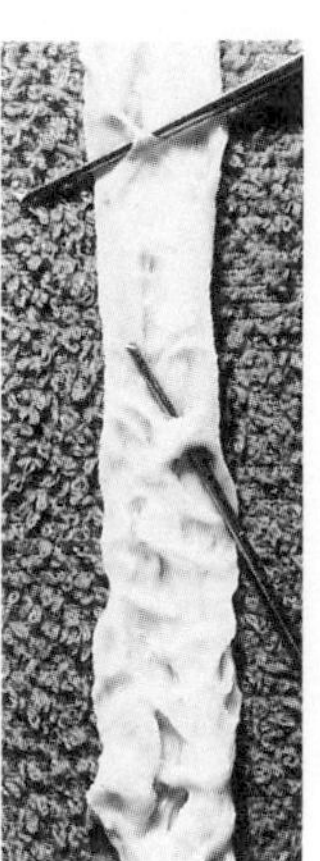

(c)

(c) Interior of a vein, recanalized after thrombosis. The lumen is irregular and deformed with synechiae stretching across it. A vein like this offers resistance to normal flow and lacks the valves essential to normal function.

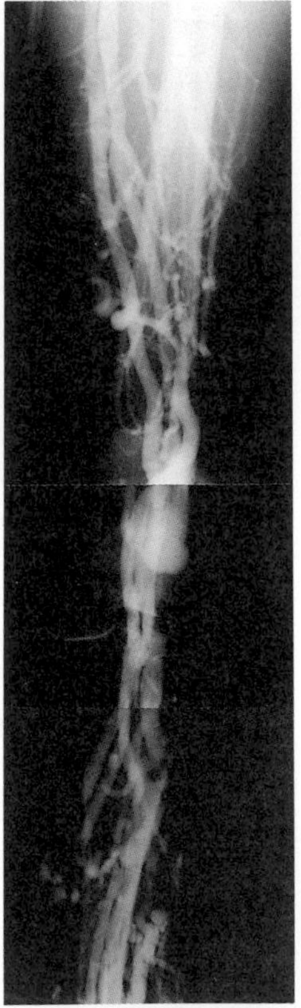

(d)

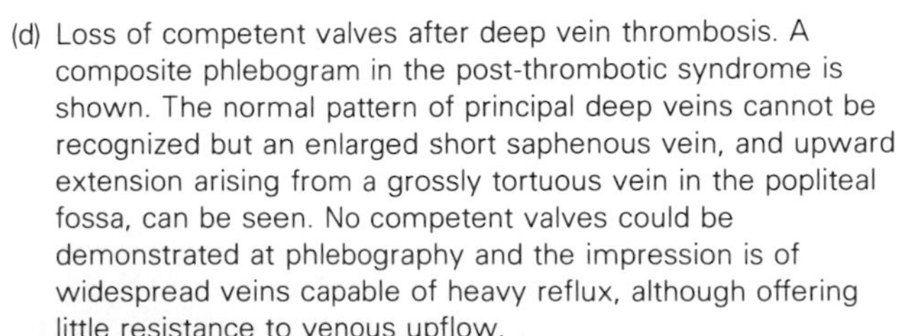

(d) Loss of competent valves after deep vein thrombosis. A composite phlebogram in the post-thrombotic syndrome is shown. The normal pattern of principal deep veins cannot be recognized but an enlarged short saphenous vein, and upward extension arising from a grossly tortuous vein in the popliteal fossa, can be seen. No competent valves could be demonstrated at phlebography and the impression is of widespread veins capable of heavy reflux, although offering little resistance to venous upflow.

to perforating veins forcibly ejecting blood outwards, but more diffuse patterns can disorganize the massive pumping mechanisms in the muscles below the knee sufficiently to create severe venous hypertension and all its complications (see Fig. 57(g)). The deep veins in this region are so numerous and complex that it is often difficult to define the defect precisely or to demonstrate it satisfactorily on phlebography or ultrasonography. Moreover, it may be difficult to say whether the state found is due to episodes of deep vein thrombosis, possibly multiple and silent, or whether there is a diffuse valveless state due to an inborn weakness or deficiency in the valves which has become progressively more severe as the years pass. As with all forms of deep vein impairment, the superficial and deep veins in the foot may respond to the excessive venous pressure by becoming greatly enlarged to form a venous pool in which blood is sequestered as the foot is raised from the ground but forcibly ejected upwards when it is put down again. This shift back and forth to the foot can only be an added burden to the already damaged pumping mechanism.

2. Femoropopliteal This is a common and more easily recognized form of post-thrombotic state (Fig. 57(b) (ii)). There is likely to be significant venous obstruction, with permanent swelling below the knee and all the undesirable effects of venous hypertension because the superficial veins, forced to act as collaterals, will ensure that venous hypertension is shared by the surface tissues. Added to this are all the undesirable effects of reflux in deep and collateral superficial veins.

3. Iliac The left common iliac vein is particularly vulnerable to thrombosis because it may be narrowed by the right common iliac artery passing over it. Thrombosis in this vein often fails to

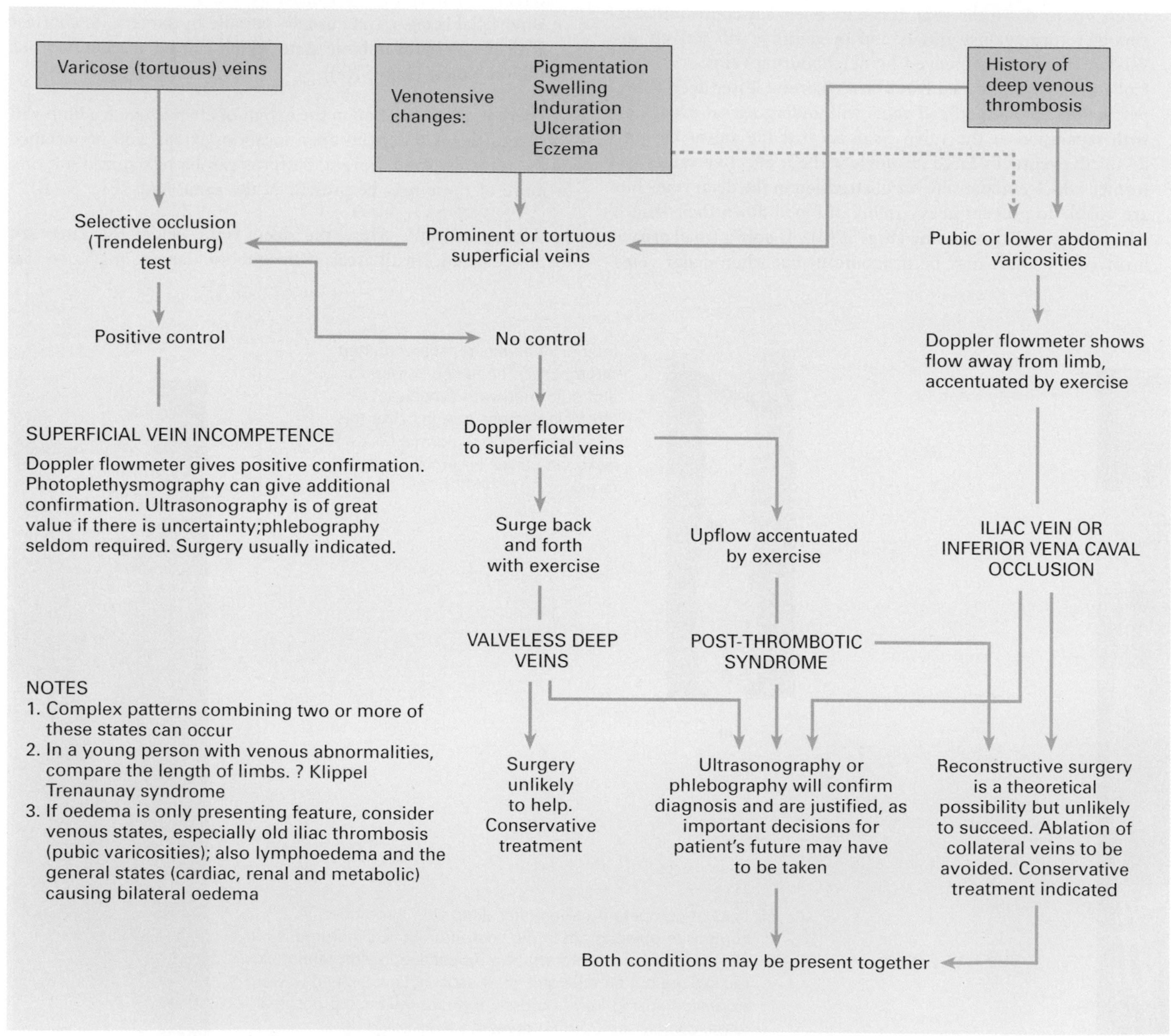

(e) Diagram of diagnostic pathways when venotensive changes are present. Treatment depends on the state causing venous hypertension and accurate diagnosis of this is essential. This requires more than clinical examination, and special investigation will be necessary.

(f) Patterns of post-thrombotic occlusion and some of the superficial veins used as collateral channels. In tibiopopliteal and femoropopliteal occlusion, long and short (and upward extension from it) saphenous veins and their branches are of paramount importance. In iliac vein occlusion, superficial veins (branches of external pudendal and superficial epigastric veins) cross the pubic region to the opposite side; many collateral deep veins within the pelvis will also be present. On phlebography demonstration of these veins, enlarged and tortuous, is important diagnostically.

(f)

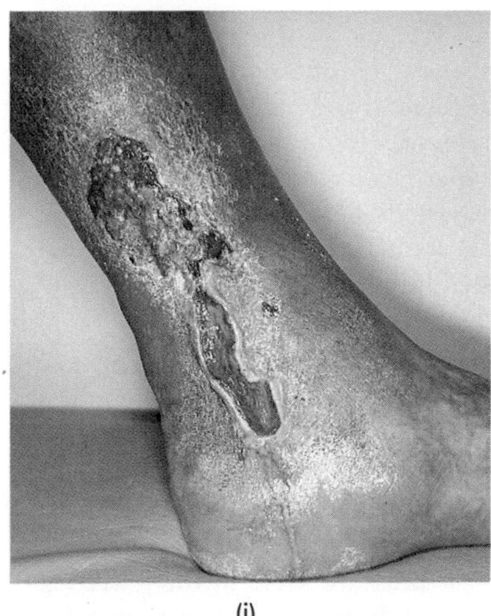

(i)

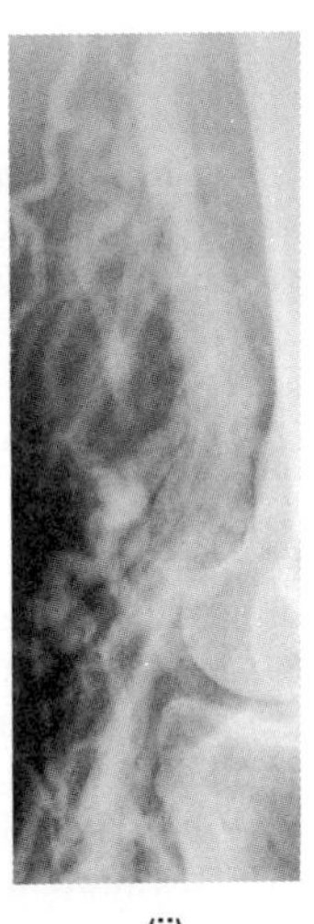

(ii)

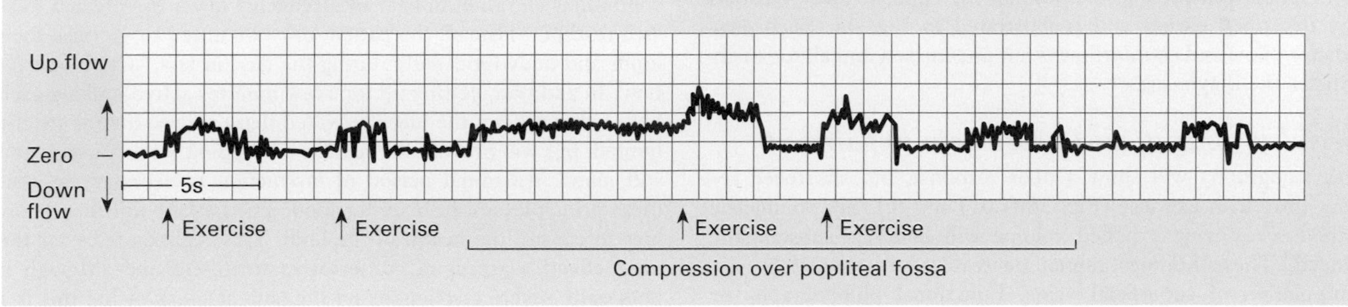

(iii)

(g) Chronic ulceration in severe post-thrombotic syndrome due to trauma, with occlusion of left popliteal vein. (i) Clinical appearance, showing the ulcer surrounded by typical, pigmented liposclerotic changes (see Fig. 63(c) for response to treatment). (ii) Phlebography was unable to demonstrate any filling in the popliteal vein but gastrocnemius veins and an unindentified tortuous vein substitute for it. (iii) Doppler flowmetry in the remnants of the left long saphenous vein. Exercise, or compression of the popliteal fossa (containing many collateral veins, shown on the phlebogram) accentuate upflow; there is no downflow. (iv) Photoplethysmography. On the left side, the response to exercise is poor and the refilling time is abnormally brief at 8 s; on the right side, the refilling time is normal at 20 s.

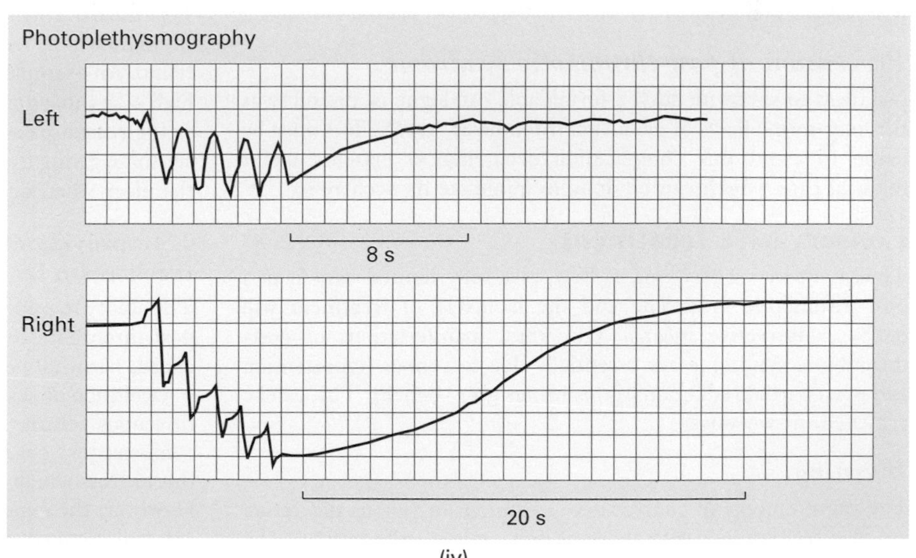

(iv)

(g)

recanalize so that the venous outlet to the limb remains permanently obstructed. If the limb below this is otherwise virtually undamaged, it may cause little more than slight swelling and the development of tortuous collateral veins crossing from the left to the right side of the pelvis, usually visible as varicosities in the pubic region (Fig. 58(a)–(h)). Beneath this it is possible for a typical long saphenous incompetence to develop, taking source from the pubic collateral veins, as described under the complex patterns referred to below. If this is not recognized, surgery to the saphenous system may damage important collateral veins in the groin.

4. Ileofemoral Iliac thrombosis is often accompanied by simultaneous thrombosis in the femoral and popliteal veins to give an ileofemoral post-thrombotic syndrome with a particularly severe pattern of venous hypertension combining the worst features of obstruction to the venous outlet, impaired pumping mechanism, and heavy reflux in recanalized deep veins and over-distended collateral veins (Fig. 58(d)–(h)).

Complex states

These can occur if the great pumping units in the muscles of the leg are substantially undamaged and able successfully to reduce venous pressure in the ankle and foot. In these circumstances it is possible to find the long saphenous vein acting as a collateral but giving off branches which set up a simple pattern of incompetence by allowing downflow to the low pressure areas in the lower leg and foot or, indeed, pubic collaterals may act as a source for incompetent downflow in the limb on the opposite side. This has been described earlier and is illustrated in Fig. 42. Such contradictory flow and counterflow is not uncommon and all too easily confuses the diagnosis.

Special investigations in deep vein impairment

Plethysmography will show a poor response and shortened refilling time with exercise (Fig. 58(f) (iv) and (g) (iii); volumetric methods measuring expelled volume will find this substantially reduced. These findings cannot be restored to normal by any manipulation of superficial veins. Functional phlebography or ultrasonography will confirm and define the state of the deep vein and valves. This is essential evidence before deciding that no cure is available, and only conservative management can be employed.

Prevention of post-thrombotic syndrome

Needless to say, with such a formidable catalogue of disability as the long-term effects of deep vein thrombosis, every effort must be made to avoid this complication occurring to patients under medical care. Much can be done to minimize its occurrence.

Conservative treatment

Treatment by surgery can, at best, give only limited benefit to a post-thrombotic syndrome and the mainstay of treatment will be by conservative means. The worst manifestations of post-thrombotic syndrome are essentially due to venous hypertension and even partial reduction of this brings great benefit. This can be achieved in two ways.

Warning

The requirements of conservative treatment in venous ulceration are in direct conflict with those of ischaemic manifestations. The treatment described below involves elevation or compression bandaging of the limb. In an ischaemic limb such treatment will severely aggravate its state and even cause its loss. Great care must be taken to ensure that such treatment is not carried out in these circumstances. If there is any doubt, the limb should not be raised above the horizontal and no form of compression bandage used until it has been proved that an adequate arterial supply is present.

1. Elevation of the limb above the horizontal

In this position venus return occurs by gravity without requiring any pumping mechanism. During elevation, with the feet above heart level, venous pressure in the extremity falls away and the higher the elevation the more complete this will be (Fig. 59(a)). Maintained in this position (Fig. 49(g),(h)) all the adverse changes will steadily recede. However, it is clearly not practical to keep a patient indefinitely immobilized in this fashion, so, as a compromise, there will be an initial period of continuous elevation in order to get the worst lesions, such as ulceration, healed. This is then followed by increasing mobility alternating with spells of elevation. Eventually the proportion of the day to be spent in elevation, necessary to keep the limb healthy, will be learnt and the patient will have to try to arrange his or her life within this limitation. Usually it is possible and this measure alone may be sufficient to maintain the limb in a reasonable state. If the patient becomes careless about spending sufficient time in elevation, deterioration of the limb soon gives a sharp reminder. Each patient will have to learn his or her own requirements in this respect. A programme of this sort, particularly during the time of continuous elevation, will bring the serious disadvantages of prolonged immobility, unless this is counteracted by a firm policy of exercise. The time of continuous elevation to heal an ulcer must never be referred to as 'bed rest' but, instead, the patient must be urged to exercise their limbs and body repeatedly during the day, in fact, 'activity elevation'. In addition, getting up for a few minutes active walking each hour will not harm the ulcer provided that exercise time is strictly limited, but will prevent the patient developing weak muscles and stiff joints. An initial period of instruction is necessary so that these principles are fully understood. The patient will then know how to control the health of the limb. This regimen is by far the most effective aspect of conservative treatment and although it puts quite severe restrictions on the patient's way of life this is a price most are prepared to pay to avoid the discomforts of uncontrolled venotensive changes. Clearly, in some patients the necessity to earn a living will prevent their following the programme they know to be necessary but even here ways of managing may be found. An example is that of a chef who worked every summer at a high salary in a top hotel, enduring steady deterioration in his limb as the season passed but then spent the winter in Mediterranean sunshine giving the limb proper care. He knew exactly how to heal the ulcer when opportunity allowed.

2. Improving efficiency of the damaged pumping mechanism by use of external support

The ability to pump blood upwards against gravity is impaired in a post-thrombotic limb by the following factors which may be influenced, harmfully or beneficially, by external compression.

Occlusion or severe deformity in major veins causes obstruction to venous return. Numerous lesser veins will dilate to provide a compensatory collateral mechanism but little can be done to assist this process which is a response to the venous changes in the limb. However, the superficial veins play a large part and any form of external compression, especially elastic compression, can impair this important mechanism. In superficial incompetence, firm compression of the superficial veins brings great benefit by pre-

Fig. 58 Post-thrombotic iliac vein occlusion.

(a) Iliac vein occlusion and superficial collateral veins. (i) Diagram of superficial veins likely to be involved. Many collateral veins also cross over deeply, within the pelvis. (ii) Doppler flow recording from a pubic varicosity in a patient with iliac occlusion. The predominant direction of flow is away from the occluded side and it is accentuated by exercise.

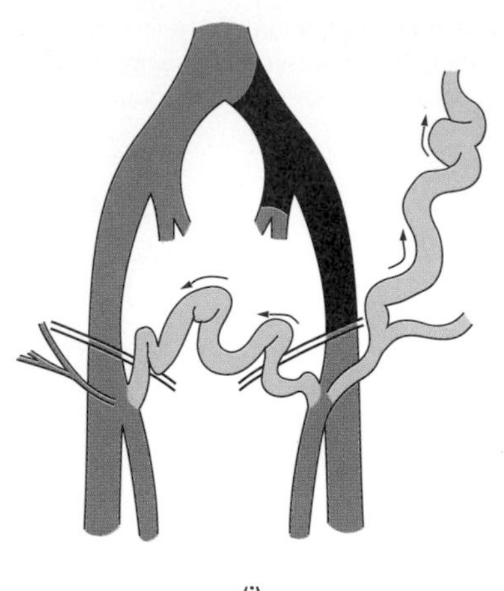

(i)

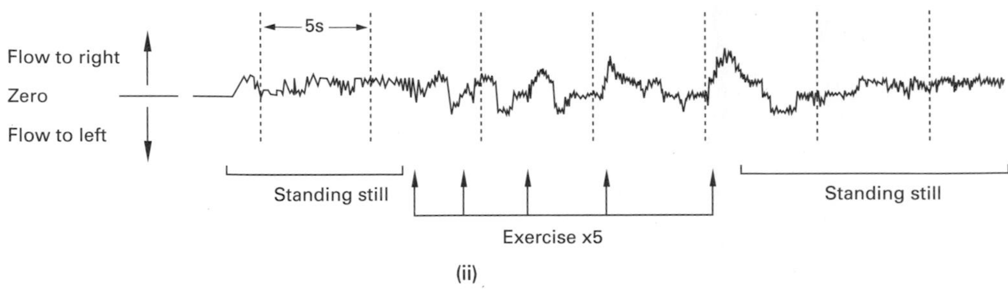

(ii)

(a)

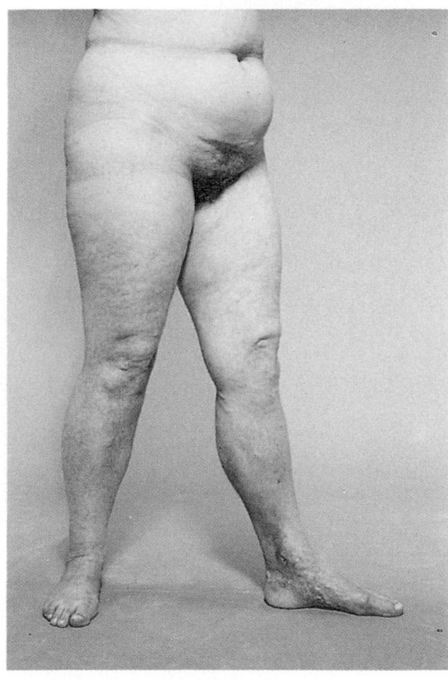

(b)

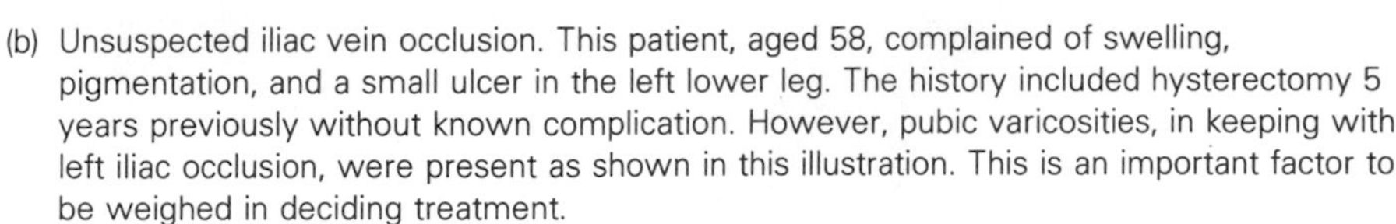

(b) Unsuspected iliac vein occlusion. This patient, aged 58, complained of swelling, pigmentation, and a small ulcer in the left lower leg. The history included hysterectomy 5 years previously without known complication. However, pubic varicosities, in keeping with left iliac occlusion, were present as shown in this illustration. This is an important factor to be weighed in deciding treatment.

(c) Minimal disturbance with isolated occlusion of the iliac vein. This patient noticed swelling of the left lower limb soon after the birth of twins 4 months previously and anticoagulant treatment had been maintained since then. Examination showed only 2 cm of swelling at calf level but no enlarged veins or obvious pubic varicosities. (i) Photoplethysmography showing a virtually normal refilling time. (ii) Phlebography showing occlusion of the left iliac vein with a large collateral vein running across the pelvis; the deep vein system below the inguinal ligament appears undamaged in keeping with the normal photoplethysmogram.

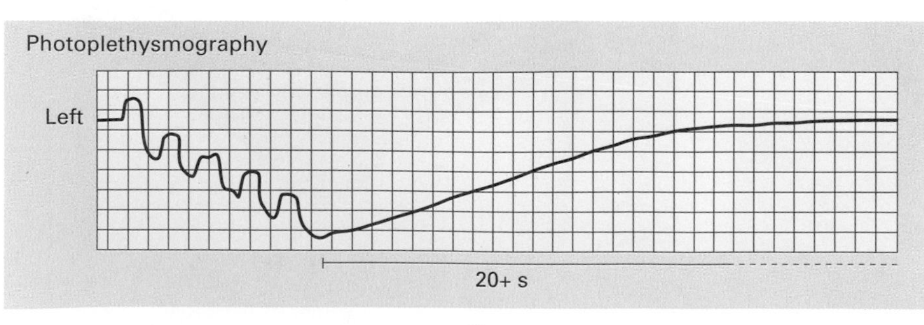

(i)

(c)

(ii)

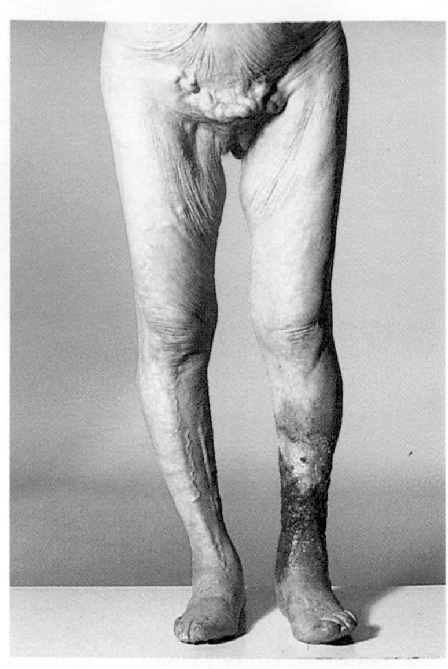

(d)

(d) The consequences of severe iliofemoral occlusion. In this elderly patient there is a huge chronic ulcer on the leg, with overall swelling of the limb. The massive pubic veins are clear evidence of iliac occlusion and part of a compensatory mechanism that should not be disturbed.

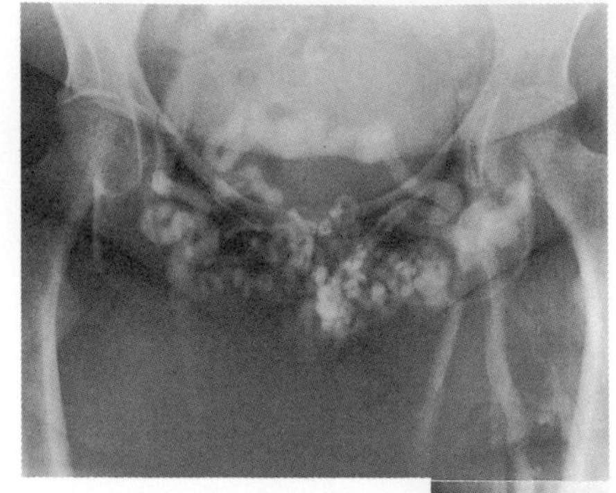

(e)

(e) Late consequences of iliofemoral thrombosis seen on phlebography. This patient gave a history of 'white leg' of pregnancy 30 years previously. The left iliac veins are occluded and extensive pubic varicosities can be seen compensating; the superficial femoral deep vein is occluded and venous return from below this occlusion is by the profunda femoris vein and the long saphenous vein. Apart from mild swelling this limb had given little trouble and her present complaint was of recurring phlebitis in varicose veins of the right limb due to long saphenous incompetence on that side arising from the pubic varicosities (see Fig. 42(b) (ii)).

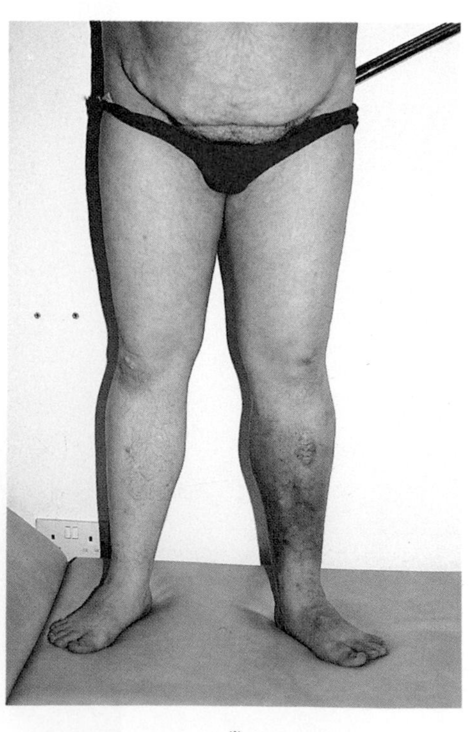

(i)

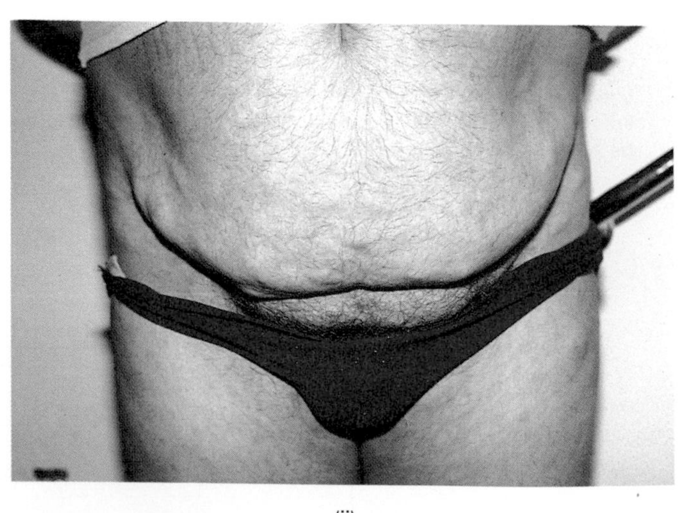

(ii)

(f)

venting heavy downflow in them but in post-thrombotic syndrome similar pressure in the upper calf or thigh can cause increased discomfort and deterioration in the limb by impeding collateral return. For this reason elastic support used in post-thrombotic syndrome must be carefully graduated to avoid compression where the main collaterals lie.

There is valvular incompetence because of widespread loss of effective valves, both in recanalized deep veins and in over-expanded lesser deep veins and superficial veins now acting as collaterals. No conservative measure can adequately restore valvular competence in these limbs. Any external compression designed to reduce reflux in these valveless veins may also impair their vital function of venous return and the advantages gained in controlling reflux will be lost by the disadvantages of restricting collateral return. Again, notice how this contrasts with superficial incompetence where elastic compression to the incompetent superficial veins brings no disadvantage because these veins are not acting as avenues of venous return. The elastic stocking so successful in superficial incompetence may be completely inappropriate to the post-thrombotic syndrome and this is a fundamental distinction between the two conditions.

Widespread over-expansion of the superficial and deep veins in the leg and foot is created by the sustained high venous pressure and, in effect, forms a large venous pool which constantly handicaps the venous pumping units that have survived undamaged. On muscle relaxation these healthy pumping chambers will be immediately flooded by blood from the unwanted venous pool and much of their effort is wasted on reducing a pool which has inexhaustible replenishment from above. In the case of the foot, when it is raised, blood which should be available to the pumping units cascades down to the underside at the very moment it should be entering the venous pumping chambers; on return of the foot to

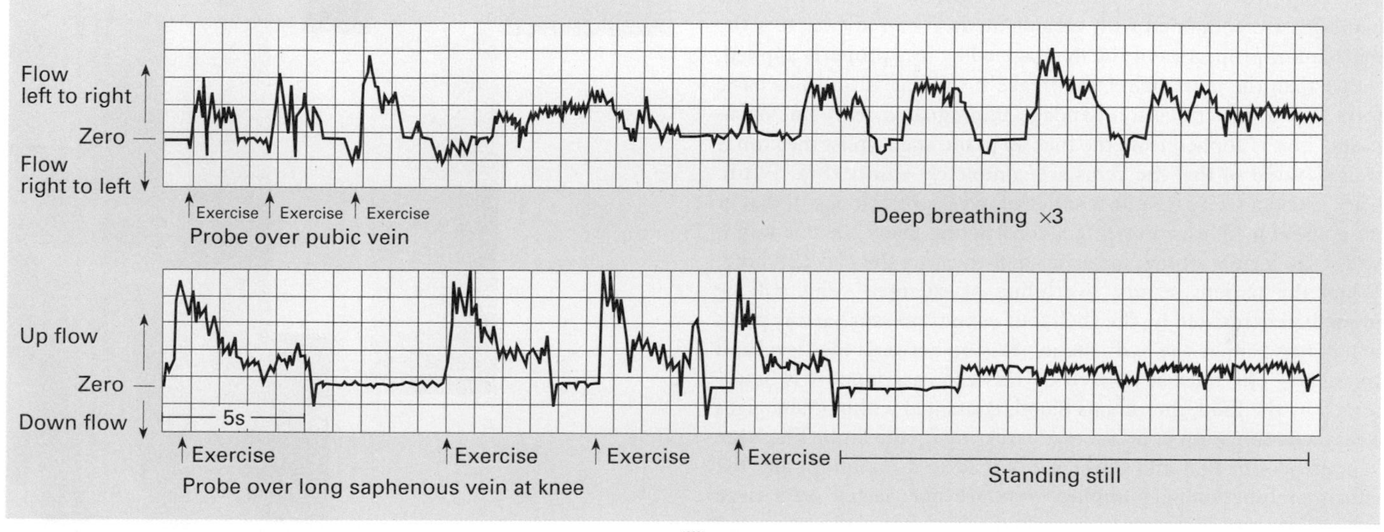

(iii)

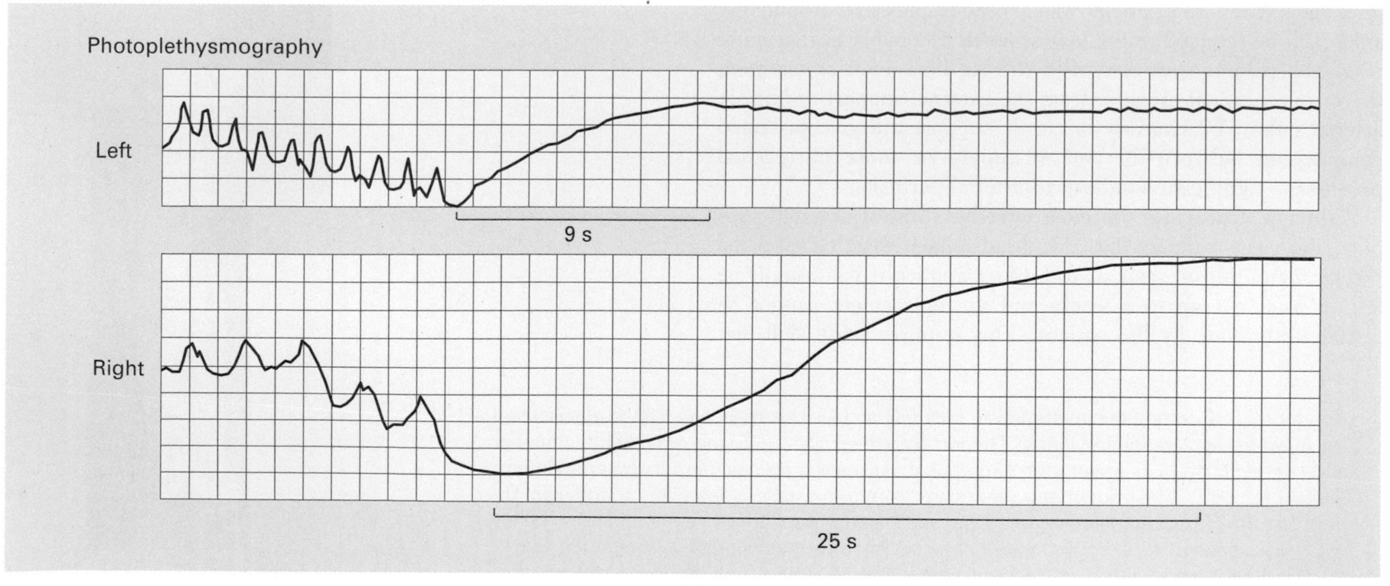

(iv)

(f)

the ground the blood is forced up again, giving a surge of high venous pressure in the lower leg. Reducing the venous pool by external support to the foot and lower leg, strong enough to resist the venous pressures, can take away this undesirable element and bring some relief to the overburdened pumping mechanism. Here external support can be of real benefit but if inexpertly applied can impede collateral return as explained above. It is quite wrong to think that crude compression is a virtue in the post-thrombotic limb—it must be used with discernment and then may bring benefit. There are two main forms of external support that can be used: inelastic containment and elastic compression by stocking or bandage.

Inelastic containment

This is the principle used in the paste bandage. This form of external support is often more successful than any other type in the ambulatory treatment and healing of a venous ulcer, and this is especially true in post-thrombotic syndrome. Although these bandages are combined with various medical ingredients, it is the mechanical properties of the bandage when it is properly applied, rather than the ingredients, that make it so successful. In its basic form it is a 7.5-cm cotton bandage impregnated with zinc oxide paste. This is applied from the toes up to the knee whilst the limb is well elevated so that the veins are completely empty (Fig. 59(b)). Care is taken to lay it on in a series of overlapping loops so that at no point is it tight or exerting a constricting effect. In this way it will set to form a strong, inelastic shell encasing the elevated limb. When the patient stands, overfilling of enlarged veins will be immediately resisted by the shell, but venous pressure at any point will not rise above the hydrostatic pressure between that level and the heart. The tension exerted by this external support is determined by the fluid, the venous blood, contained within it and gives a perfect graduation of pressure, decreasing up the limb. The large venous pool in foot and lower leg is held to a minimum and the efforts of functioning pumping units are not wasted on a large venous pool immediately replenished from above; the veins and capillary beds are prevented from excessive distension by the external support but at no point is the external pressure greater than that in the superficial veins so that collateral upflow will not be impeded. When the patient walks venous pressure around the ankle will be reduced to the lowest levels attainable in that limb; when the patient is at rest, with the leg horizontal or elevated, there is no residual pressure from the external support to impede arterial inflow. By contrast an elastic support will give sustained compression between 20 and 40 mmHg or more of residual pressure, a significant handicap to arterial perfusion.

Although it provides the most effective form of external support, the paste bandage has the disadvantage that it cannot be taken off and put on again at will. Once applied it will usually be left in place for up to 3 weeks and its replacement cannot be satisfactorily done by the patient. This requires some skill, not

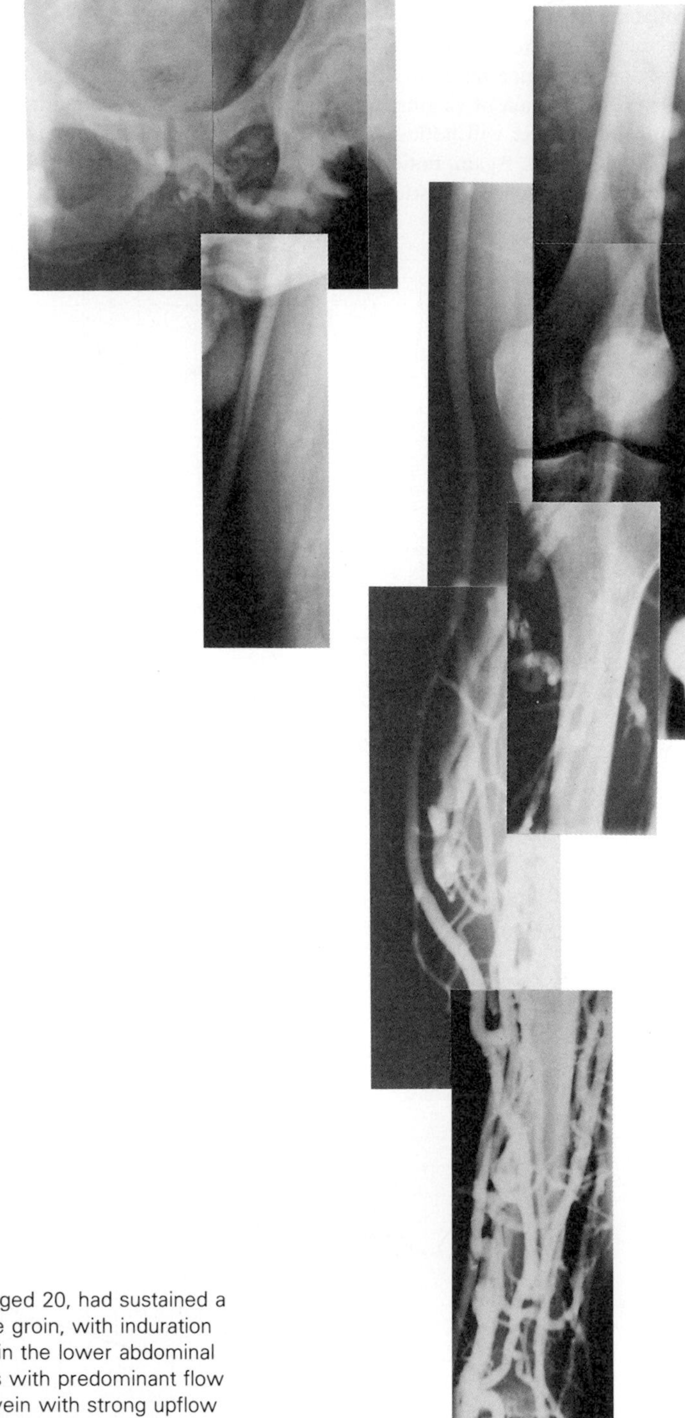

(v)

(f)

(f) Iliofemoral post-thrombotic state due to injury. (i) and (ii) This man, aged 20, had sustained a fractured pelvis 2 years previously. The left limb is swollen up to the groin, with induration and pigmentation in its lower part; large pubic varicosities are seen in the lower abdominal folds of fat. (iii) Doppler flowmetry recordings from pubic varicosities with predominant flow from left to right accentuated by exercise, and the long saphenous vein with strong upflow with peaks caused by exercise movements. (iv) Photoplethysmography. On the left side refilling time is only 9 s but on the right side is normal at 25 s. (v) Composite phlebogram showing the features of deformed and occluded deep vein at all levels, including the iliac veins; pubic and long saphenous veins, and an upward extension of the short saphenous vein form prominent collateral pathways of venous return.

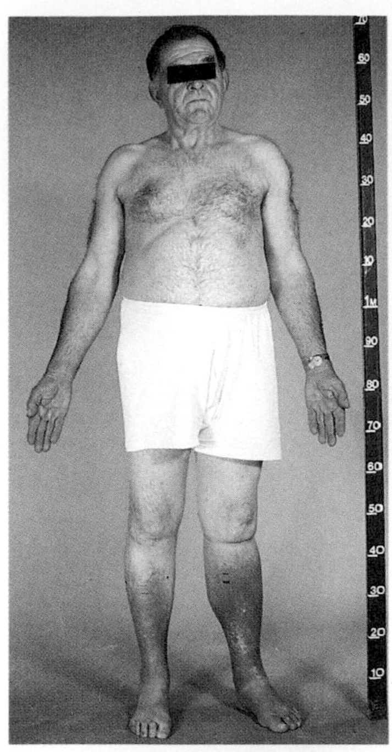

(i)

(g) Severe iliofemoral post-thrombotic syndrome after multiple fractures in road traffic accident. (i) The patient's left limb is swollen up to the groin and heavily pigmented below the knee. The right side is also pigmented but without obvious swelling. (ii) and (iii) Doppler flowmetry and photoplethysmography showing all the features of deep vein impairment on both sides. (iv) and (v) Phlebograms showing left iliac obstruction with collaterals crossing the pelvis and extensive failure in filling of deep veins of leg and thigh on both sides.

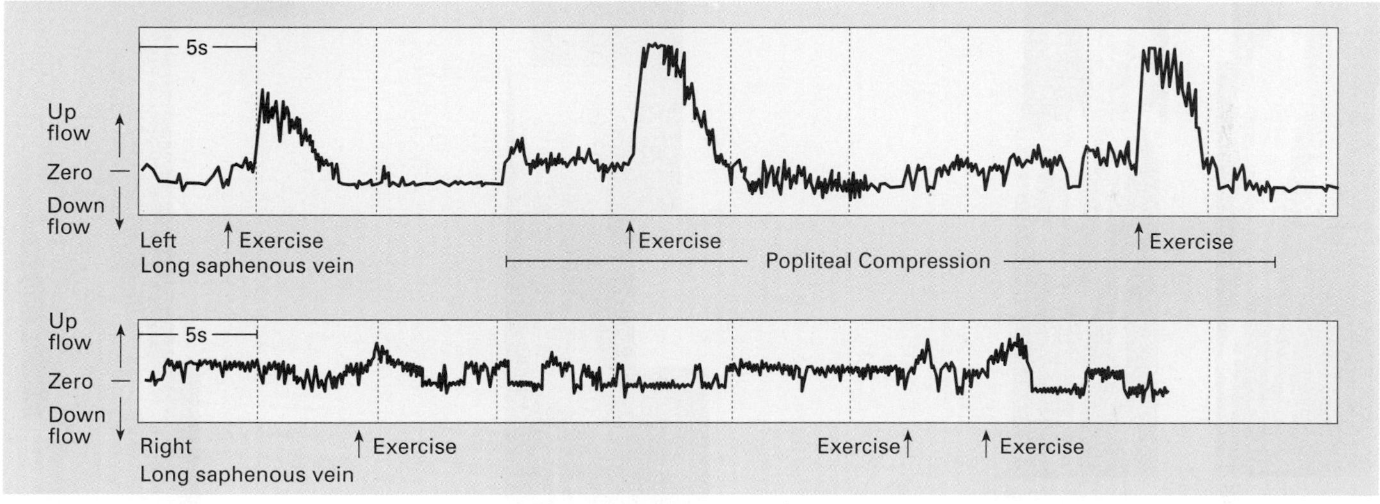

(ii)

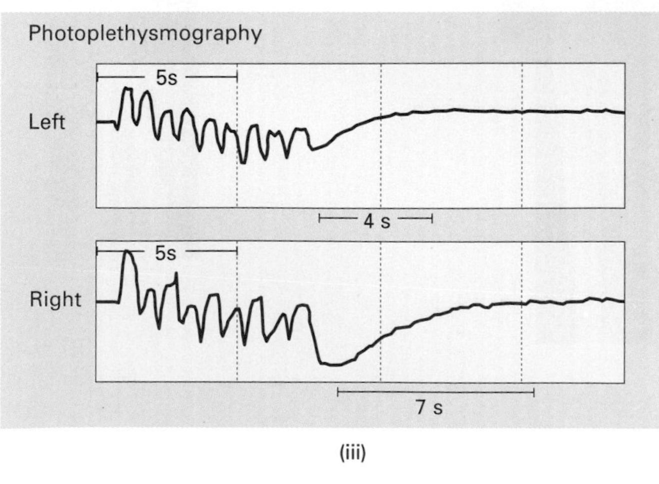

(iii)

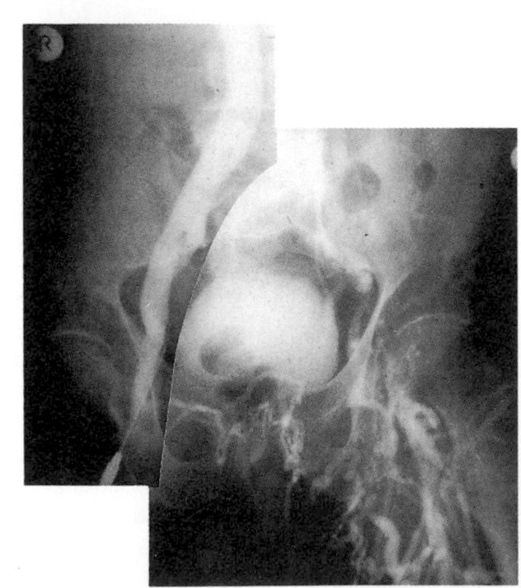

(iv)

(g)

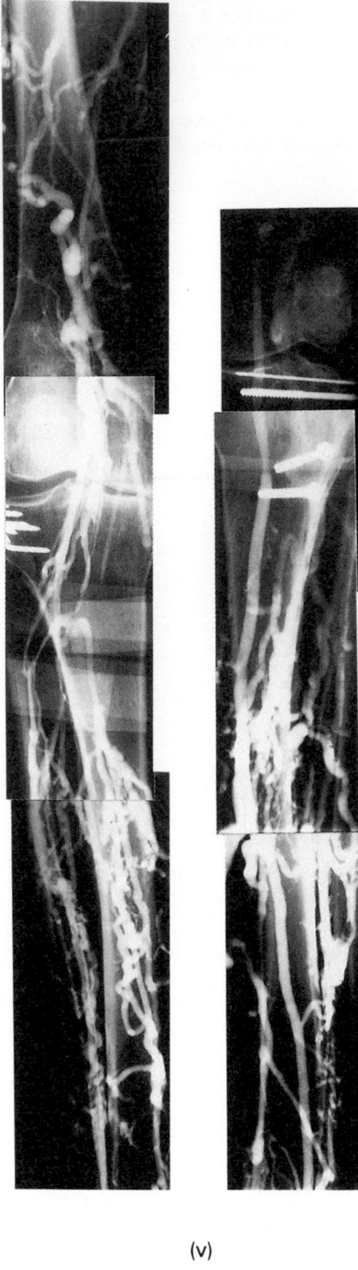

(v)

(g)

(h) Iliofemoral post-thrombotic syndrome is the most common cause for severe disability from chronic venous insufficiency. Two further examples are illustrated here by composite phlebograms. (i) This patient sustained deep vein thrombosis following fractured hip and prosthetic replacement. The long saphenous vein shows preferential collateral upflow and the deep veins are either severely deformed or fail to fill. (ii) This patient was known to have had a left deep vein thrombosis 3 years previously. Preferential collateral upflow is shown in the long saphenous vein which is interrupted in its upper part; a major role in venous return has been assumed by the short saphenous vein and an upward extension from it, winding round the posterior thigh to join remnants of the long saphenous vein. The iliac veins are occluded and pelvis collateral veins cross the pelvis.

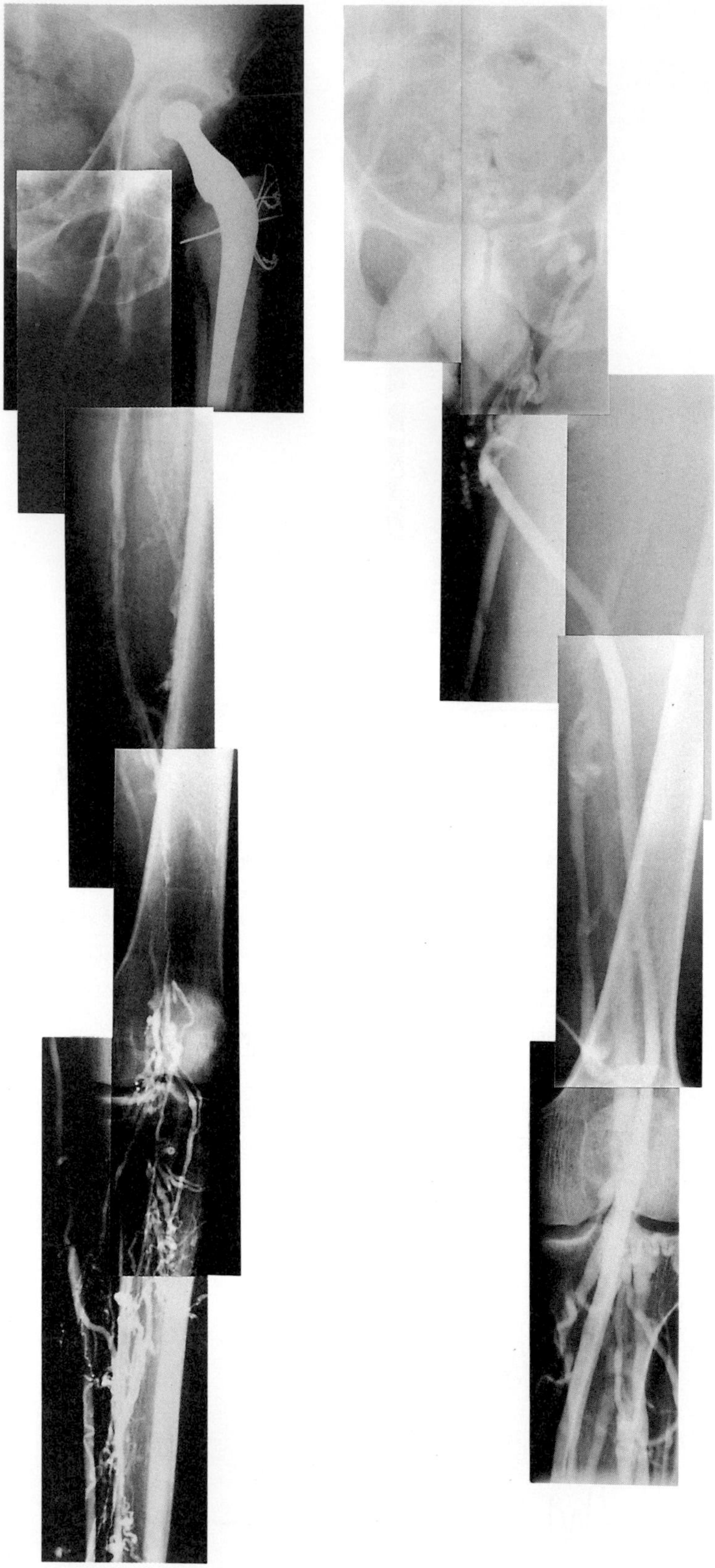

(i)

(ii)

(h)

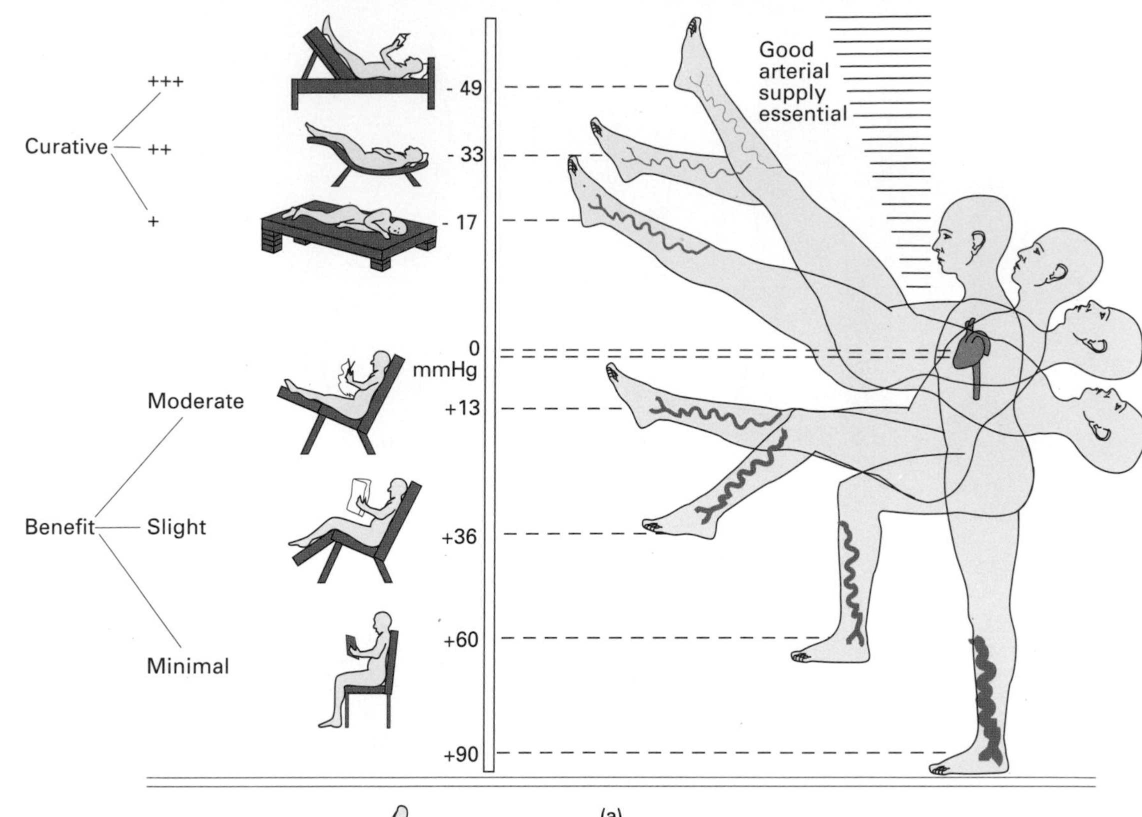

(a)

(i) (ii)

(iii) (iv)

(v) (vi)

(vii) (viii)

(ix) (x)

(b)

Fig. 59 Conservative management in post-thrombotic syndrome (chronic venous insufficiency).

(a) Elevation of the limbs is, by far, the most important measure. This is only truly effective when raised above the level of the heart because then there is no venous pressure in the extremity. This diagram shows various positions of elevation related to heart level and the resulting venous pressures in the lower leg. Elevation is only curative, for example in healing an ulcer, when it is well above heart level and maintained there for prolonged periods with minimal interruption. Lesser elevation brings some benefit and may be sufficient to protect a healed ulcer from recurrence. Always assess arterial supply before advising a policy of elevation.

(b) External support by bandage. In severe cases this may be necessary and a careful system of even application is essential, as illustrated here. This is best done with the limb horizontal or higher. The method shown is suitable for applying inelastic compression by paste bandage which is to remain in place for many days.

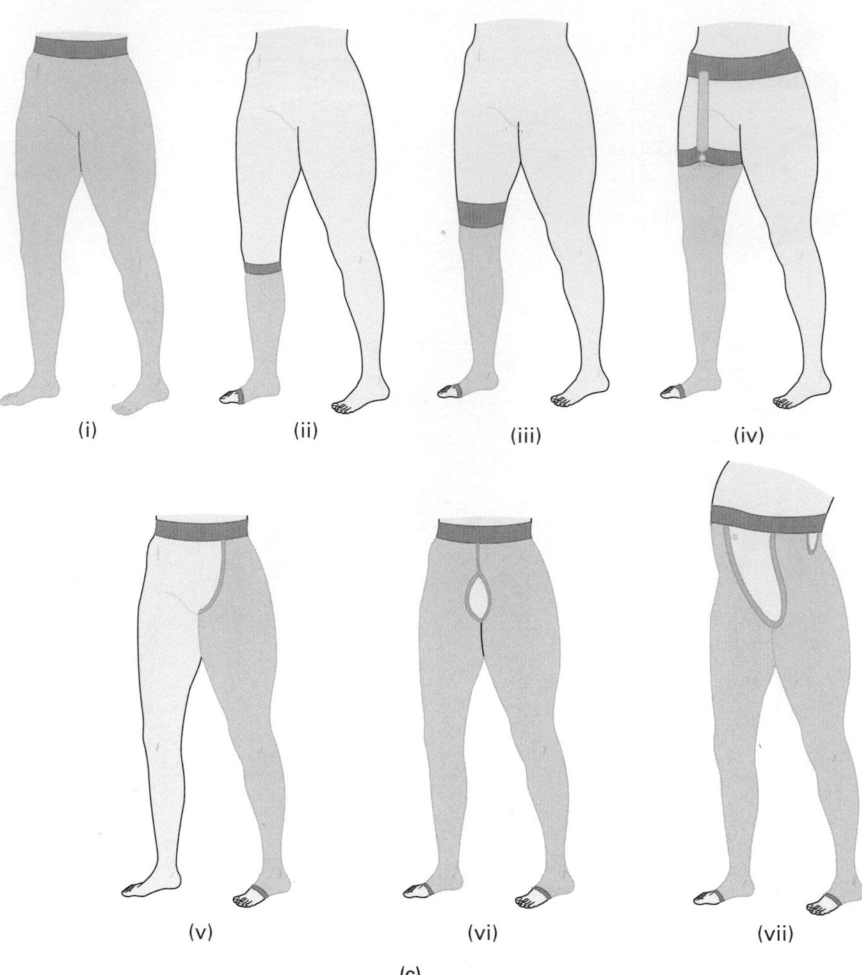

(c) Styles of elastic stocking commonly used. (i) Tights; widely used in lighter weights. (ii) Below knee; this requires a well rounded calf or use of one-way-stretch material to avoid riding down. (iii) Above knee (lower thigh); only suitable for a slim limb since otherwise it may not stay up. (iv) Thigh length (half or midthigh); requires suspenders. (v) Thigh length with waist attachment for support; used in special problems when extra strong support needed. (vi) Waist length for special bilateral problems requiring maximal support. (vii) Maternity stocking, as support tights or 'panty hose' stocking with adjustable top.

always easy for others in the family. For this reason it tends to be used only during the time necessary to heal an ulcer and has the great advantage that it allows this to occur while the patient is up and about. Once the ulcer has healed the external support can be changed to a more convenient elastic stocking, which may be sufficient to prevent recurrence.

Certain types of elastic stocking, skilfully fitted can come near to giving the same effect as a paste bandage. A strong one-way-stretch elastic stocking up to the knee, fitted accurately to give a snug fit but no compression when the limb is elevated, will immediately resist any expansion of the veins when the patient stands; this comes quite near to the principle of inelastic containment whilst having the advantage of being easily removable. Its elasticity is used to give accurate conformity with the limb and to allow it to be pulled on and off over the prominence of the heel, but, being one-way-stretch, it does not suffer from down-pull. Skilled fitting of this sort is not always available and the tendency is for the patient to be directed towards the convenience of easy fitting using a two-way-stretch stocking. Because of the need for the latter to grip the calf in order to resist down-pull, it is not suitable to provide inelastic containment. Strong elastic webbing bandage laid lightly around the elevated limb, without any compression, can also be used to give a form of inelastic containment, but this form of bandage is so often misused (see below) that it is best avoided unless the circumstances ensure proper use.

Elastic compression

A great variety of elastic stockings of various strengths are available. These may or may not envelop the toes, and extend from the foot up to the knee or to the thigh; depending on the strength required they may be fashioned as stockings or tights (Fig. 59(c)). The compression they give is graded so that light support gives 14–17 mmHg pressure (Class I in the United Kingdom), medium support gives 18–24 mmHg (Class II), and strong support gives 25–35 mmHg (Class III) compression at foot and ankle level. Above this level the stocking is so designed that the compression tapers off in parallel with the lessening venous pressure up the length of the limb when the patient is standing. In this way heavy compression in, say, the thigh, and constriction of venous outflow, is avoided. In most countries clear standards are laid down and in the United Kingdom the Drug Tariff of the National Health Service gives strict specifications for the various classes of graduated compression hosiery together with indications related to the severity of venous disorder and other conditions for which they are suitable. The manufacturers keep within these specifications and have succeeded in evolving knits that give compression with relatively little downwards pull but, nevertheless, the majority available are two-way stretch and will require support either by gripping the calf or, at higher levels, by suspender or as tights. In post-thrombotic syndrome the high venous pressures quickly generated when the patient is standing will require controlling with a relatively strong stocking giving 25- to 35-mmHg compression in foot and ankle. This has been found to be optimal but is really insufficient to resist full venous pressure; however, the stronger the stocking the higher the residual elastic compression when the limb is elevated and no longer needs compression. When a limb is raised above horizontal or when the patient is lying flat there is no significant venous pressure in the limb and any form of external support, inelastic or elastic, serves no useful purpose. An elastic support will, however, continue giving residual compression and this can be most undesirable by reducing arterial flow in the impoverished tissues near the ankle in post-thrombotic syndrome.

The importance of avoiding an elastic stocking which may impede collateral return through superficial veins has already been emphasized above. Many patients with post-thrombotic syndrome try various forms of elastic support but find they actually increase their discomforts and abandon their use. A stocking that brings comfort to the patient is likely to be beneficial but one causing discomfort may actually be doing harm. The patient must not be coerced into wearing stockings if the benefits are not apparent. With an active ulcer which is extremely tender and discharging purulent fluid, an elastic stocking is not in any way suitable; it will cause too much pain and within a short time will be saturated with exudate. An ulcer at this stage requires a spell of elevation to bring it to a healing phase, followed by ambulatory treatment in a paste bandage and, finally, healing maintained by a skilfully fitted elastic support. In the post-thrombotic limb it is often a matter of trial and error to see if the patient can be suited. In simple incompetence of the superficial veins (primary varicose veins) where all that is required is firm compression to stop the downflow in the incompetent veins, the fitting of elastic stockings is far less critical and often an ulcer will heal with their use. However, this is the very variety of venous disorder where surgery or sclerotherapy is highly successful and it should not be necessary to condemn these patients to the undoubted nuisance of permanent elastic support.

Conclusions

In post-thrombotic syndrome, a skilfully applied paste bandage is invaluable in healing a venous ulcer whilst the patient is ambulatory. An elastic stocking for the same purpose is less effective and often not tolerated by the patient. The principle of inelastic containment is far more desirable than elastic compression. However, external support of any sort is insufficient on its own and a policy of elevation whenever possible is essential.

Surgery to the veins in post-thrombotic syndrome

In this condition enlarged surface veins are usually acting as collaterals to underlying occluded deep veins. In these circumstances, not infrequently, a saphenous vein may have several competent valves along its length and is, therefore, a most valuable valved pathway of venous return that must be preserved. However, more often phlebography will have shown that it has no competent valves and it is tempting to consider its surgical removal in order to eliminate at least one cause for rapid build up of venous hypertension by reflux along its length. But this will also be destroying an important compensatory collateral mechanism and the disadvantages of this may outweigh the advantages of eliminating the component of incompetence. Moreover, Doppler flowmetry may show continuous upflow, accentuated by exercise, without reflux except briefly when the patient first stands. This implies that it is an important collateral which must not be removed without good evidence of alternative pathways of venous return. Phlebography may have supplied this, but useful confirmatory evidence may be obtained by phlethysmography during exercise with and without selective occlusion of the saphenous vein in question; occlusion may cause deterioration in the ability of the limb to reduce venous pressure by exercise and gives clear warning that the vein should not be removed. In true post-thrombotic syndrome there are few circumstances in which removal of the superficial veins will bring benefit. One such circumstance may be when there is an intractable ulcer directly overlying an enlarged perforator carrying collateral outflow, demonstrated by phlebography or ultrasonography. Elimination of this may redistribute collateral outflow and reduce the intensity of venous hypertension overlying the perforator and so enable the ulcer to heal. The use of phlethysmography with selective occlusion of the veins concerned, as just described, may support this procedure but without some such evidence it is not justifiable to remove enlarged superficial veins or perforators indiscriminately.

Surgical reconstruction of veins and valves

In post-thrombotic syndrome the real requirement is the replacement of occluded veins and valveless channels with good, well-valved veins. However, our ability in this respect is extremely limited but the following procedures may occasionally prove helpful.

1. Palma's operation

This is appropriate for the relief of oedema in post-thrombotic occlusion of an iliac vein, usually the left side, when the deep veins below the inguinal ligament are relatively undamaged. The long saphenous vein of the opposite limb is divided in the lower thigh and mobilized to swing it across to the affected side for anastomosis with common femoral or profunda femoris vein (Fig. 60(a) (i), (ii), and (iii)). If successful, this acts as an additional collateral vein providing a substantial venous outlet for the limb. Swelling may be considerably reduced but severe venotensive changes such as ulceration near the ankle are unlikely to be improved because these are the result of thrombotic damage at lower levels in the limb. A corresponding procedure using a PTFE vascular graft with external supporting rings, running extraperitoneally between the femoral vein on the affected side and the lower external iliac vein of the opposite side, and supported by a temporary arteriovenous fistula, has given a number of reported successes (Fig. 60(a) (iv)).

2. Popliteal to upper femoral vein bypassing (May-Husni operation)

This is designed to relieve the effects of deep vein obstruction in lower or midthigh. The long saphenous vein of the same limb is anastomosed to the lower popliteal or posterior tibial vein in order to provide a more effective outflow from the deep veins below the knee and taking it upwards to re-enter deep veins in the groin above the obstruction (Fig. 60(b)). This will be particularly effective if the saphenous vein is well valved and a number of successes have been reported. However, so often this vein is already acting as an effective collateral so that the rearrangement brings little improvement and, of course, it does not eliminate the heavy reflux in naturally occurring deep and superficial collateral veins throughout the limb which are so often grossly incompetent. This operation may be supported by a temporary arteriovenous fistula

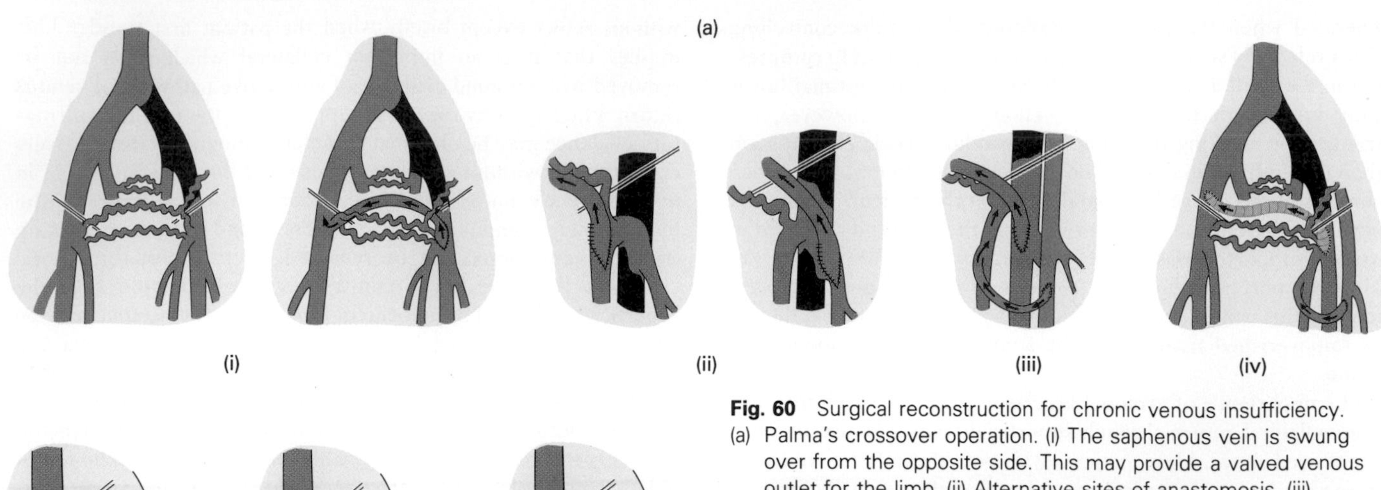

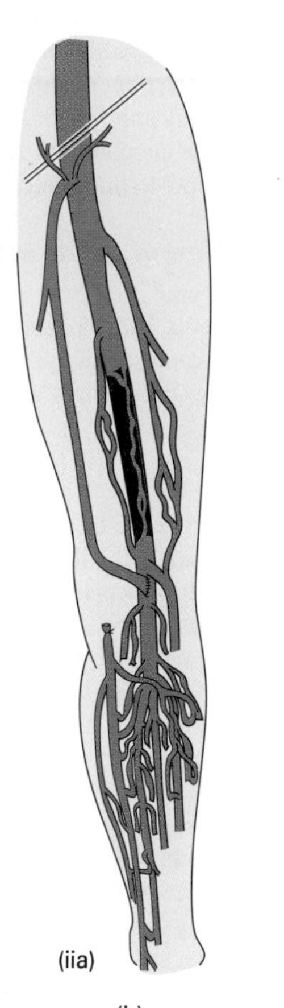

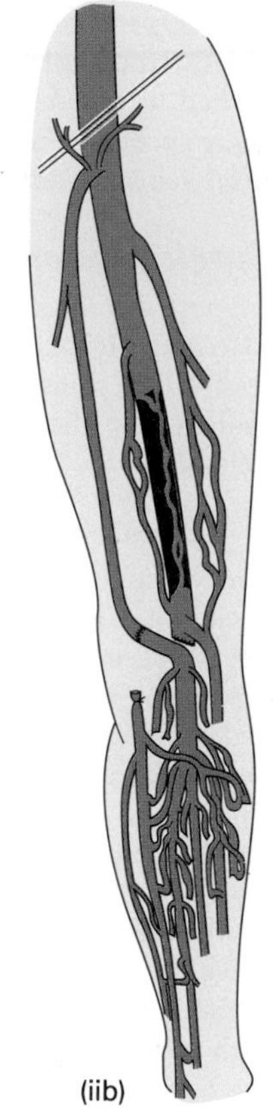

(i) (iia) (iib)

(b)

Fig. 60 Surgical reconstruction for chronic venous insufficiency.
(a) Palma's crossover operation. (i) The saphenous vein is swung over from the opposite side. This may provide a valved venous outlet for the limb. (ii) Alternative sites of anastomosis. (iii) Combined with a temporary arteriovenous shunt. (iv) Use of synthetic vascular graft (PTFE with supporting rings), combined with a temporary arteriovenous shunt. This conduit is not valved and its advantages can be offset by reflux.

(b) Popliteal to upper femoral bypassing procedure (May-Husni). (i) Preoperative state with femoropopliteal occlusion of deep veins. (ii) Long saphenous vein used as bypass from popliteal to common femoral vein: *a* by end-to-side anastomosis; *b* by end-to-end anastomosis. This procedure will give most benefit if the saphenous vein is well valved (often it is not) and if it is possible to eliminate reflux in other collateral channels.

to ensure the new venous channel is well distended with continuous flow and does not thrombose in the early postoperative healing period.

3. Restoration of valve function

If incompetence in a deep vein is the main problem, the following possibilities may be considered (previously illustrated in Fig. 56(b), (c), and (d)):

Transposition of a deep vein into a neighbouring vein that is well valved, for example, implanting the superficial femoral into a valved profunda femoris vein alongside, as described earlier. This is seldom applicable in post-thrombotic syndrome.

Transplantation of a suitable venous valve taken from elsewhere in the body. This is most unlikely to be appropriate in thickened, deformed post-thrombotic veins or in the multitude of collateral veins.

Repair of prolapsing valve cusps (Kistner's operation) is not in any way appropriate in post-thrombotic syndrome where the valve cusps are thickened, deformed, and adherent to neighbouring vein wall.

Various procedures with synthetic vein grafts, often supported by temporary arteriovenous fistulae, are under trial in the lower limb but these suffer from the serious defect that they are not valved (Fig. 60(a) (iv)). Attempts to evolve synthetic vein grafts for use in the lower limb are severely limited at present by inability to provide any satisfactory valve mechanism.

External valves. A sling may be used around a vein to act as a substitute valve. Psathakis has reported favourable results in over 200 patients using a tendon or silastic sling attached to flexor tendons of the knee and placed around the popliteal vein in patients with venotensive changes, including many with post-thrombotic syndrome, thought to be due to reflux in this vein. The theory is that when the flexor muscles contract whilst walking the sling tightens around the vein and prevents reflux in it. Its efficacy and the possible incidence of thromboembolism await independent evaluation.

Operations reconstructing the veins in post-thrombotic syndrome are very limited, with few suitable cases, and are best left to the experts specializing in this field.

Role of the perforator

The diagnosis of 'incompetent perforator' is frequently made but often incorrectly so. The following summary may help to put this into better perspective.

Inward flow to deep veins

Inward flow from the superficial to deep veins is normal but it is greatly enhanced in superficial vein incompetence as part of the retrograde circuit of gravitational downflow (see Fig. 30). This is an essential feature of the most common venous disorder, superficial vein incompetence, but the perforator is not at fault—it is performing its normal function in exaggerated fashion (see Fig. 61(a)). However, in many patients, there may also be a brief outward surge as the muscles contract or the foot is placed to the ground, alternating with the predominant downward and inward flow (Fig. 61(b)). This represents a degree of incompetence in one or more perforators, probably because they have been over-enlarged by heavy inflow from the varicose veins, but is not the primary fault. However, it can certainly be an aggravating factor if venotensive changes are present, and, after surgery to the varicose veins, may become the source of downflow to the foot. For these reasons an enlarged perforating vein showing surge is best eliminated at surgery when it is detected.

As a source of superficial incompetence and gravitational downflow

The upper termination of long and short saphenous vein (Figs. 48(b) and (c)), midthigh perforating veins (Figs. 53(d) (iii), and 61(c) (i)), and veins connecting between the pelvis and upper thigh (Fig. 39) are all examples of perforatoring veins which commonly become incompetent and act as the high level source for a pathway of simple incompetence. In similar fashion a perforator on the leg below the knee may act as a source of downflow to the foot (Fig. 61(c) (ii)). All the above are certainly 'incompetent perforators' and it is unfortunate that this term is also used to refer to heavy outward pumping through perforating veins below the knee and especially near the ankle.

Outward and upward pumping through low level perforators

Outward pumping may occur as part of a surge back and forth accompanying simple varicose veins as described above. Of far greater importance is its occurrence in the post-thrombotic syndrome as part of a collateral mechanism in venous return past occluded deep veins (Figs. 13, 57(b), and 61(d)). Here the perforator is playing a compensatory role and this must be recognized because it may be an important channel of venous return although inadvertently bringing high venous pressure to the vulnerable surface layers. There must not be an automatic response to remove an outward pumping perforator in the leg but instead the cause must be understood and its importance in collateral function assessed. Surgery removing this vein may sometimes be justifiable; for example, in post-thrombotic syndrome heavy collateral flow may be concentrated through one perforator and so increase local venous pressure that ulceration occurs over it. It is possible that removing this perforator will cause redistribution of collateral flow and dissipate the raised venous pressure over a wider area elsewhere in the leg. In this way the high venous pressure is no longer concentrated in one small area and the ulcer heals. The decision to do this rests on adequacy of alternative collateral pathways shown by radiography and the demonstration that recovery times at plethysmography are improved or, at least, not made worse by temporary occlusion of the perforator by finger pressure.

Incompetent gastrocnemius and soleal veins are perhaps the best examples of localized incompetent perforators capable of allowing passive reflux but on muscle contraction forcibly ejecting blood to the surface (Fig. 61(e)). This is being increasingly recognized and diagnosed by phlebography or ultrasonography. Suspicion of their presence is usually aroused by unusual discomfort, venotensive changes, and a pattern of radiating varicosities on the calf. Surgery ligating such veins in popliteal fossa, carefully selected by phlebography or ultrasonography, may prove very successful but does require experience.

Pseudoperforators

Certain arrangements of veins may be mistaken for direct leakage from the deep veins. In the midthigh, an upward extension of the short saphenous vein (Giacomini vein) may join the posteromedial branch of the long saphenous vein. In this way incompetence with its source in the short saphenous vein can give rise to long saphenous varicosities and may only be recognized when surgery ligating the long saphenous vein fails; even then it may be regarded as a midthigh perforator (Figs. 41(b) and 61(f)). In the upper calf a branch from an incompetent short saphenous vein may run across to the inner aspect and appear to be a true deep vein perforator (Fig. 61(g)). An incompetent long saphenous vein, or its posterior arcuate branch, may run down to the lower leg in concealed fashion and give off a large branch running to the surface near the ankle where it is interpreted as coming from a perforator.

CONGENITAL VENOUS DISORDERS

Venous anomalies in the lower limb

The venous system is subject to many minor aberrations such as duplicated deep veins, differing levels of short saphenous termination, or the presence of unusually large interconnecting branches between long and short saphenous systems in the thigh. All these variants originate in embryo during development of the venous system and, if the valves are inadequate, may account for unusual sources of incompetence but most are harmless and need not be detailed here. However, one particular abnormality deserves special mention. This is the persistence of the lateral vein of the lower limb to form a massive, valveless channel running superficially up the outer side of the leg and thigh, and terminating either in the profunda femoris or by running with the sciatic nerve into the pelvis to join the internal iliac vein (Figs. 62(a) and (b)).

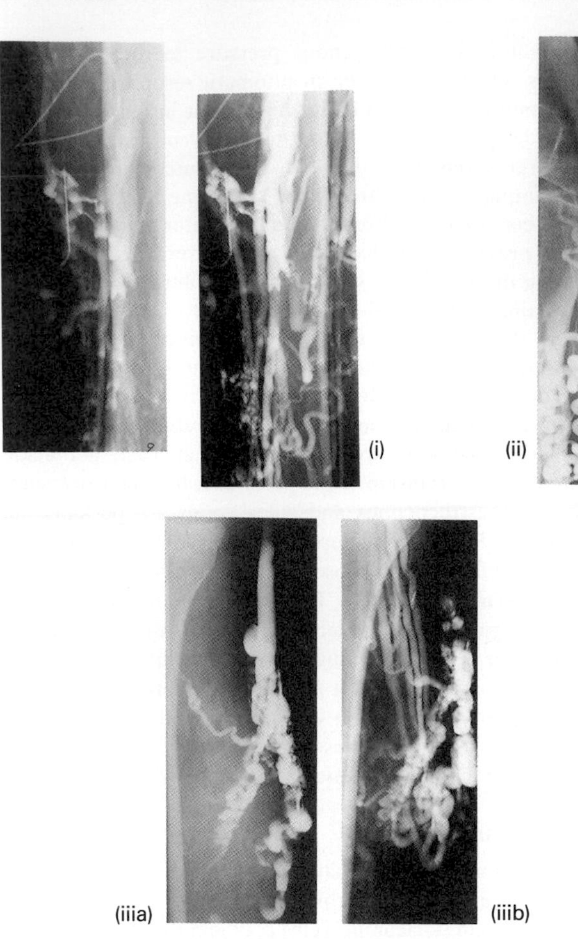

(a)

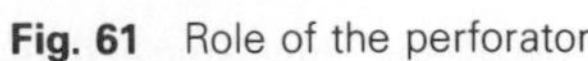

Fig. 61 Role of the perforator.

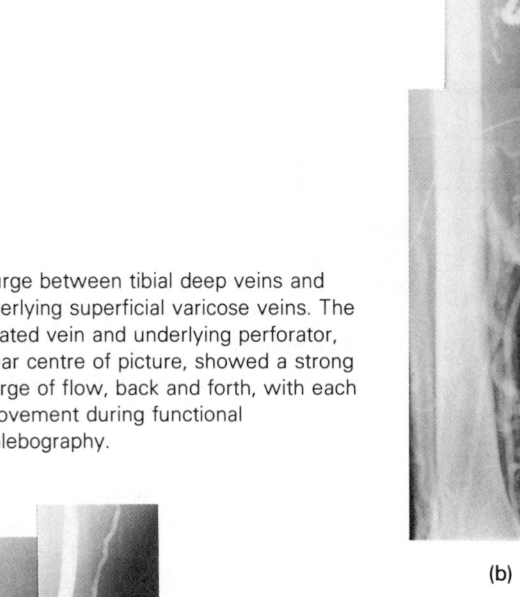

(b)

(b) Surge between tibial deep veins and overlying superficial varicose veins. The dilated vein and underlying perforator, near centre of picture, showed a strong surge of flow, back and forth, with each movement during functional phlebography.

(a) Inward flow. (i) Inward flow from superficial varicosities in lower leg filling deep veins progressively through a pair of perforating veins. (ii) Direct entry of flow from calf varicose veins into gastrocnemius venous sinuses. (iii) Flow from long saphenous varicosities into multiple gastrocnemius venous sinuses, *a* Before exercise, *b* After one exercise movement. As a single static picture, this can be misinterpreted as gastrocnemius vein incompetence but for full explanation of events in this illustration see Fig 61(c) (i).

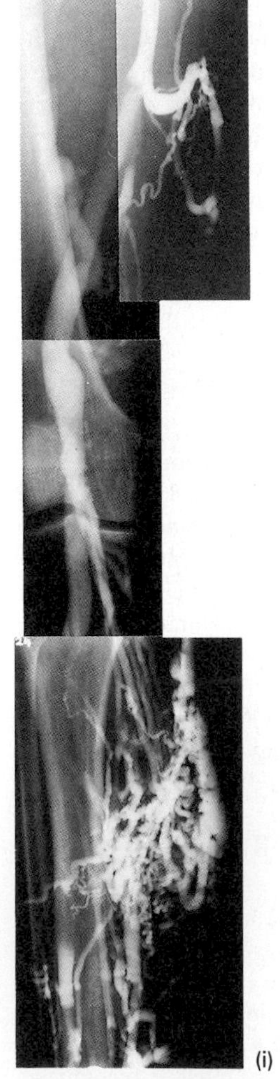

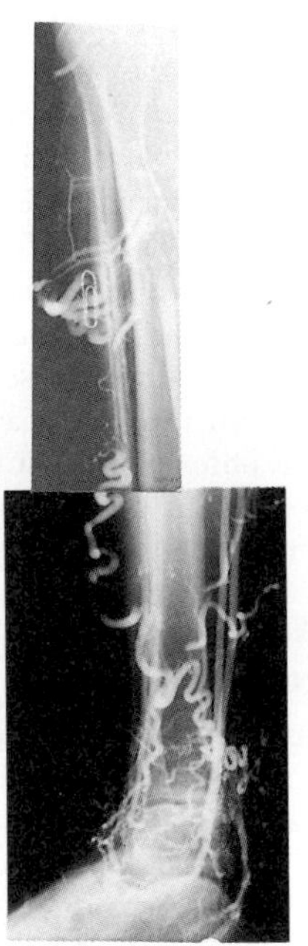

(c)

(c) Perforating vein outflow as a source of downflow in incompetent superficial veins. (i) Composite phlebogram of the veins partly shown in Fig. 61(a) (iii). The main origin of superficial downflow is from a midthigh perforator running to a portion of unstripped long saphenous vein in the thigh. (ii) Perforator outflow as a source of superficial incompetence may occur at any level from groin to lower leg. In this phlebogram, a pair of perforators are the source of outflow from anterior tibial veins to a varicose vein running down to the foot; a paperclip marks the point at which finger pressure controlled the vein.

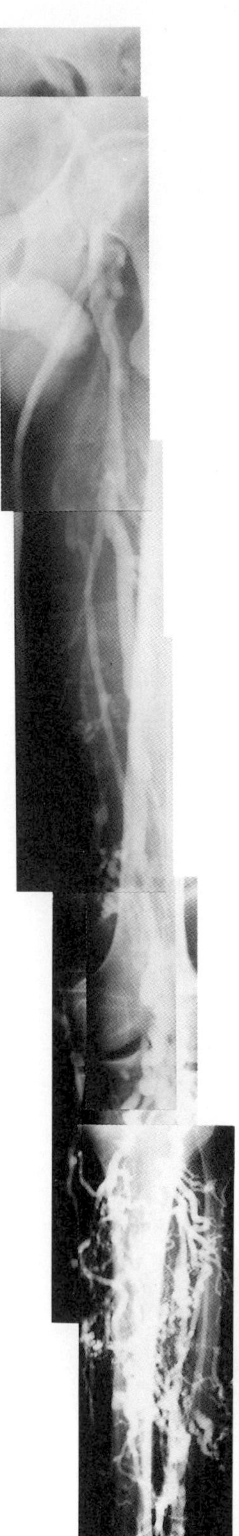

(d) Perforator outflow as part of a collateral mechanism. In this composite phlebogram, previous thrombosis has severely damaged the principal deep veins so that superficial veins are forced to act as collaterals up the length of the limb. The disorganized state of the leg veins is evident, with outflow from deep vein remnants at multiple points; this is well seen in the pair of dilated and tortuous perforating veins overlying the lower fibula.

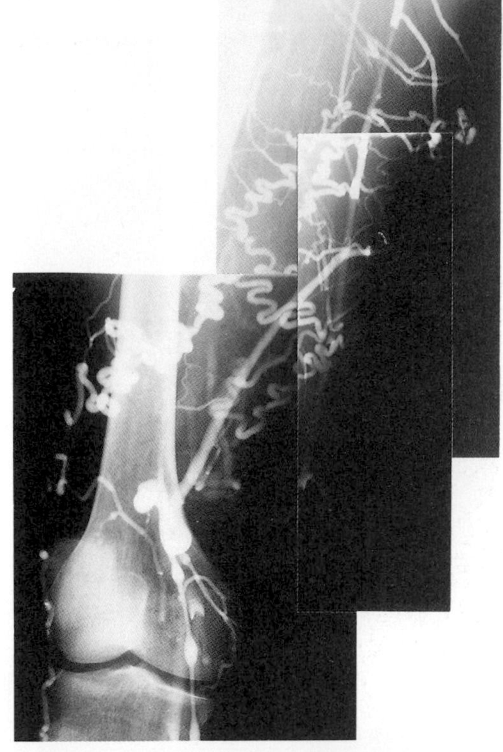

(f) Unexpected superficial interconnection mimicking a true perforator. In this composite phlebogram, a pseudoperforator, the source of incompetence in midthigh, is shown to arise from an upward extension of the short saphenous vein, running upwards posteriorly to join the long saphenous vein in midthigh. The commencement of this upward extension is dilated and tortuous but the short saphenous vein below this shows a series of effective valves.

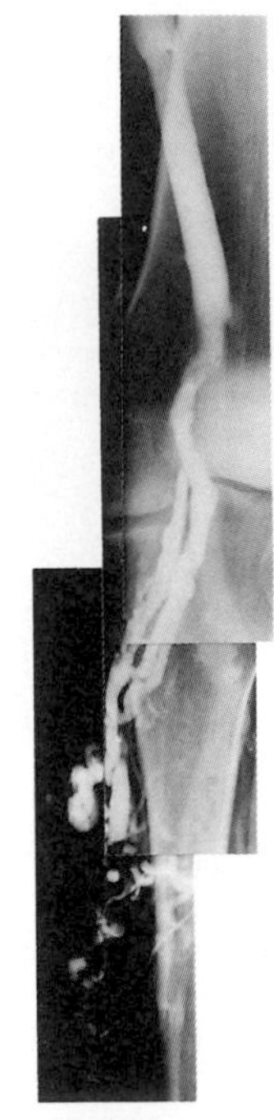

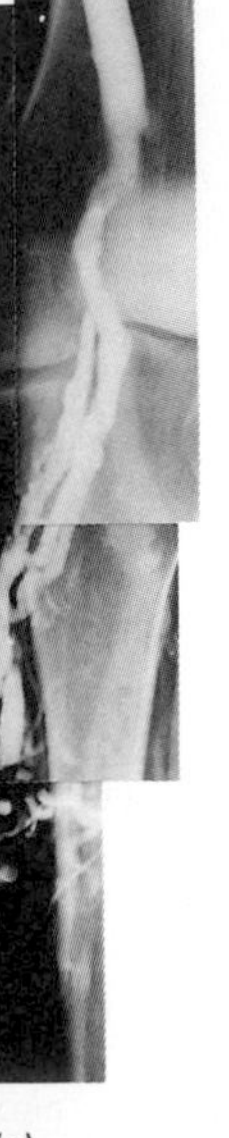

(e)

(e) Gastrocnemius vein incompetence and perforator outflow from a gastrocnemius venous sinus. This occurs as gravitational outflow when the muscle is relaxed or as forcible outward pumping on contraction. An example found at functional phlebography is shown here. Ultrasonographic colour imaging is probably the most effective way of demonstrating this.

(g) Interconnection in the upper calf between the two saphenous systems may be mistaken for a perforator. In the composite phlebogram shown here, a substantial, varicose branch of the short saphenous vein sends incompetent flow to remnants of the long saphenous system.

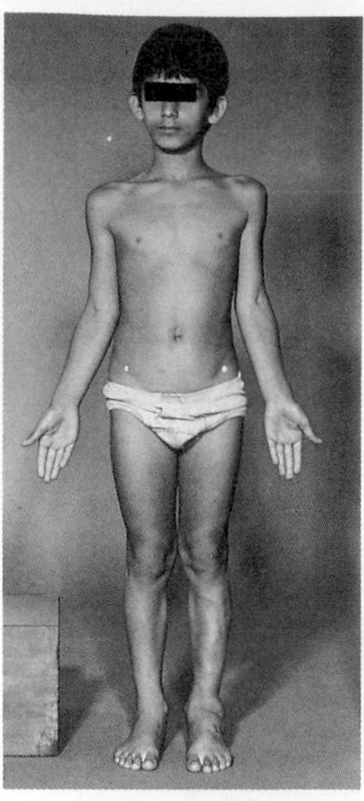

(i)

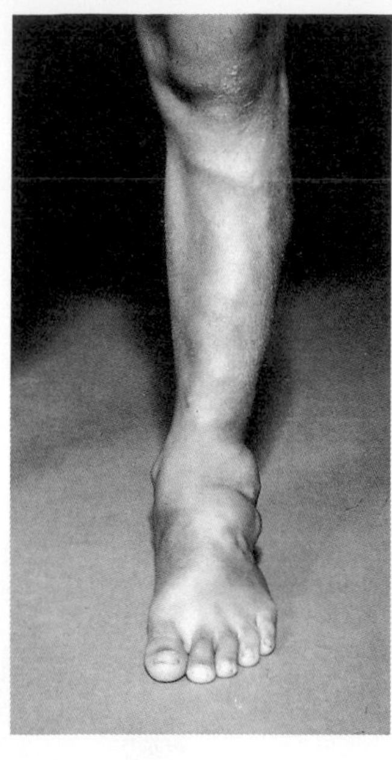

(ii)

(a)

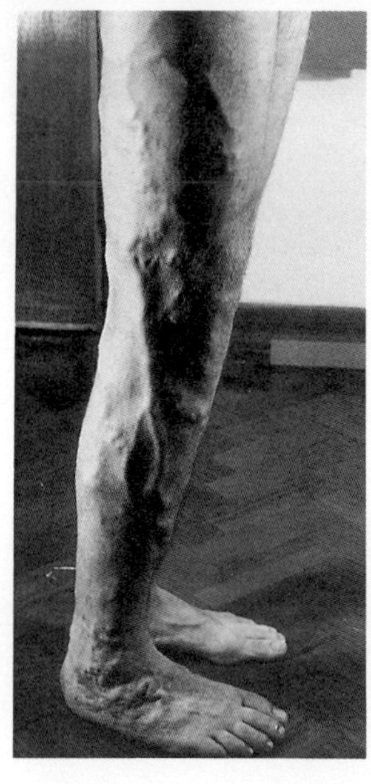

(i)

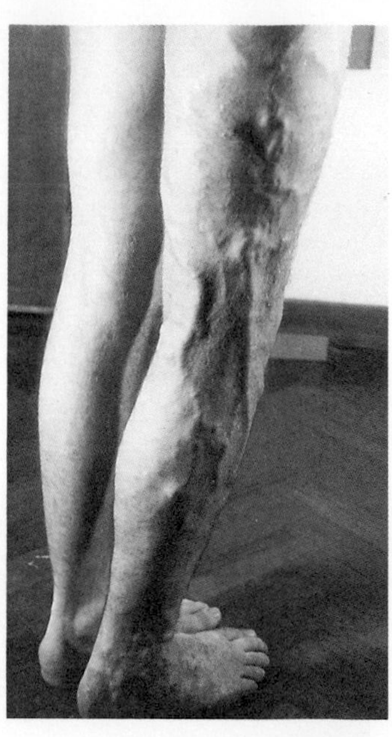

(ii)

(b)

(b) Persistence of the lateral vein of thigh in a young man with Klippel-Trenaunay syndrome. Two views of the right limb are shown with enlarged superficial veins (phlebectasia) running into a large persistent lateral vein. This terminated by joining the profunda femoris vein in the upper thigh and substituted in part for under-development of the deep veins. The right tibia showed 2 cm of lengthening compared with the normal left limb.

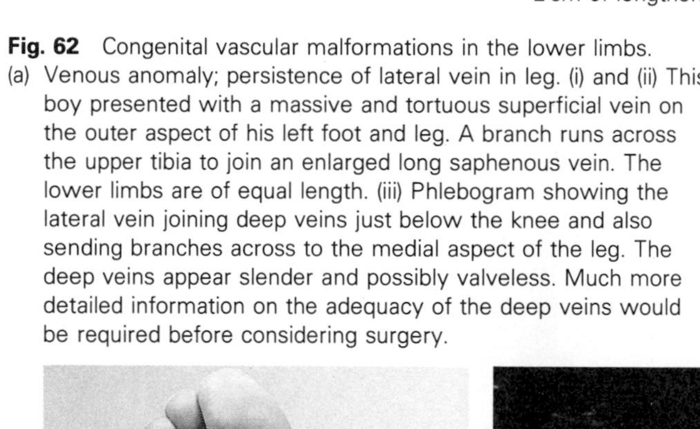

(iii)

Fig. 62 Congenital vascular malformations in the lower limbs.
(a) Venous anomaly; persistence of lateral vein in leg. (i) and (ii) This boy presented with a massive and tortuous superficial vein on the outer aspect of his left foot and leg. A branch runs across the upper tibia to join an enlarged long saphenous vein. The lower limbs are of equal length. (iii) Phlebogram showing the lateral vein joining deep veins just below the knee and also sending branches across to the medial aspect of the leg. The deep veins appear slender and possibly valveless. Much more detailed information on the adequacy of the deep veins would be required before considering surgery.

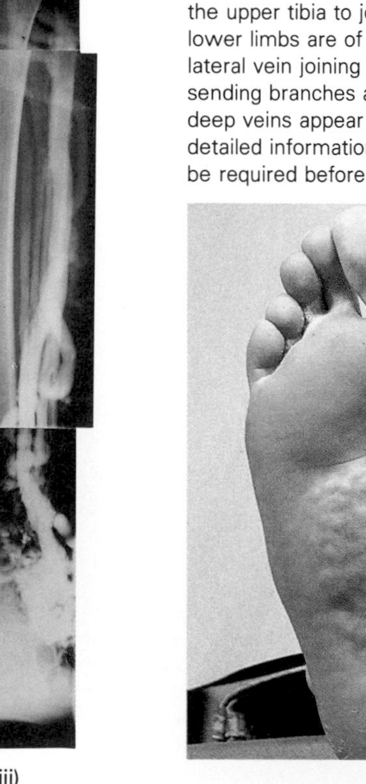

(i)

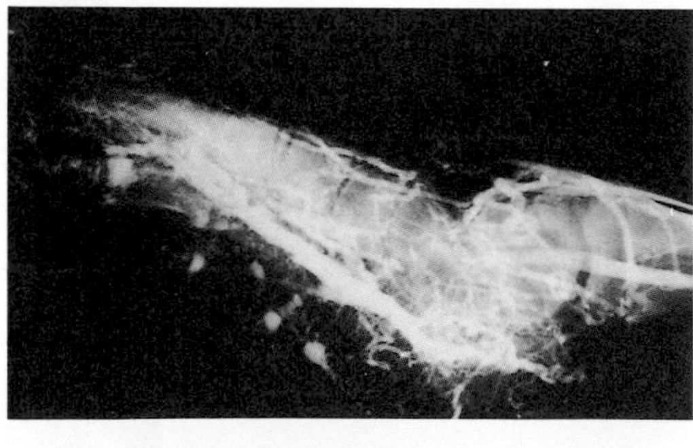

(ii)

(c)

(c) Localized cavernous angioma. (i) A large cavernous angioma causing discomfort under the foot of a young man. (ii) Angiogram in venous phase showing venous caverns in sole of foot and enlargement of plantar vein. It was possible to excise this angioma, and, although extensions through the plantar aponeurosis were not pursued, a good result was obtained.

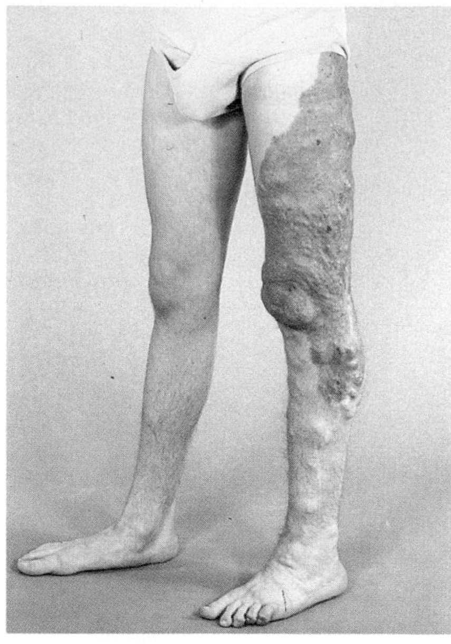

(d)

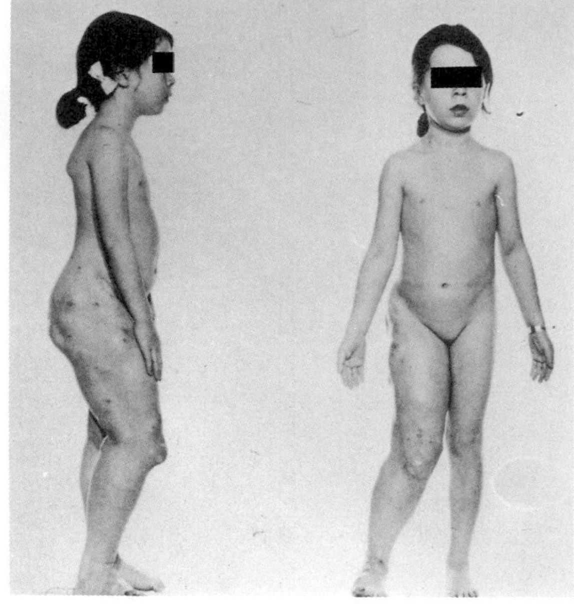

(e)

(d) Extensive venous angiomatosis (phlebangiomatosis and phlebectasia) without bone change. This 15-year-old boy had been followed over the previous 10 years. Massive superficial phlebangiomatosis involves the skin of upper calf, knee, and thigh; below this level extensive phlebectasia was present in the subcutaneous layers. Both limbs were of equal length; in the absence of any change in bone length this cannot be regarded as a full Klippel-Trenaunay syndrome. Various attempts at treatment by sclerotherapy and surgery met little success, largely limited by the vulnerability of the angiomatous skin which necrosed easily with any interference. The patient chose to avoid complex plastic surgery, prefering to wear strong elastic support to restrain excessive bulging of the abnormal vessels on standing. He was fully active in all sports including football.

(e) Klippel-Trenaunay syndrome in a child. Extensive phlebangiomatosis with considerable bone lengthening (hypertrophy) is shown and it is probable that the lymphatic system is also affected.

The importance of this is that there may be a concurrent failure in the development of the normal deep vein system so that the large, superficial channel forms the main venous return of the limb and inept surgery removing it may cause considerable embarrassment to venous return. Gross anatomical aberrations of superficial veins should always bring to mind the possibility of a corresponding failure in the deep veins which should be checked by phlebography before attempting any treatment.

Abnormal development of capillaries and veins

Localized vascular malformations

These take the form of angiomata of capillary or cavernous varieties. The former are made up of multiple enlarged capillaries and venules to give a dark red blemish (strawberry naevus), often present at birth and disappearing within a year or two. The

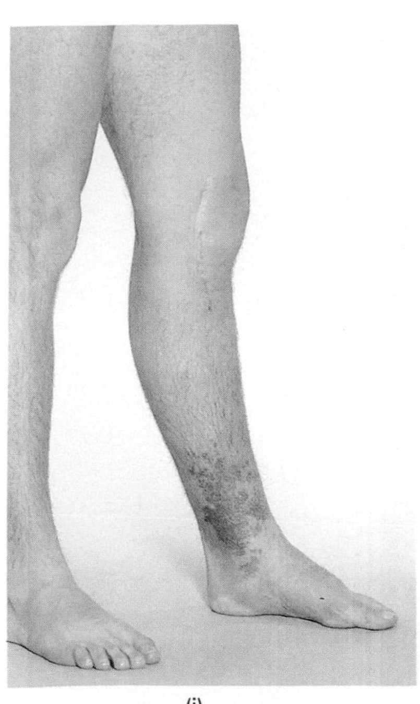

(i)

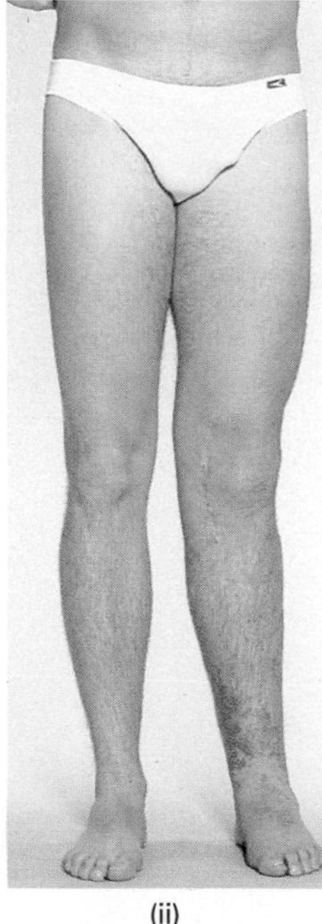

(ii)

(f)

(f) Klippel-Trenaunay syndrome in a young man. From childhood onwards the left limb had shown obvious enlargement in girth and, increasingly, in length. Epiphysiodesis had been carried out to control the overgrowth in length. The patient had played hockey at national level but in his early twenties developed discomfort and pigmentation in the lower leg, typical of venous insufficiency. Doppler flowmetry showed continuous upflow in superficial veins in keeping with deep vein deficiency (hypoplasia) and photoplethysmography indicated impairment of the venous pumping mechanism. Phlebography was not carried out as the patient was travelling from abroad, but his condition was explained to him, with advice on the general care of venous insufficiency and encouragement to keep active.

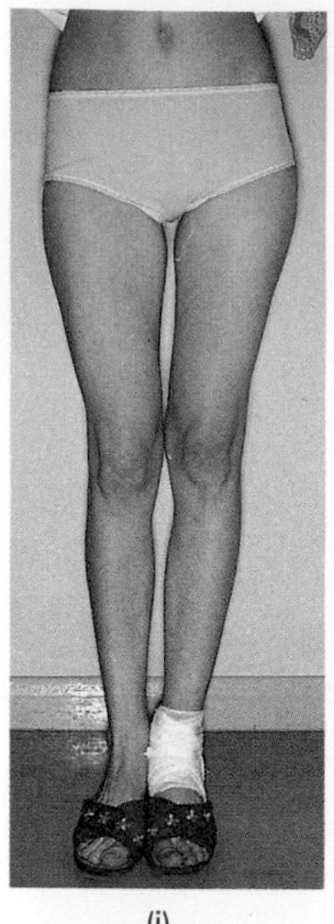

(i)

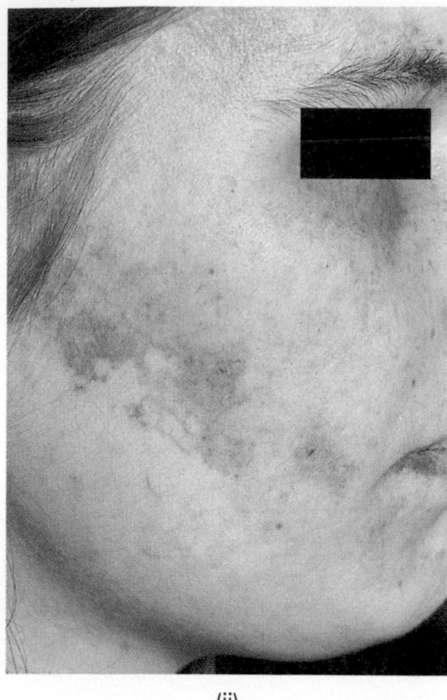

(ii)

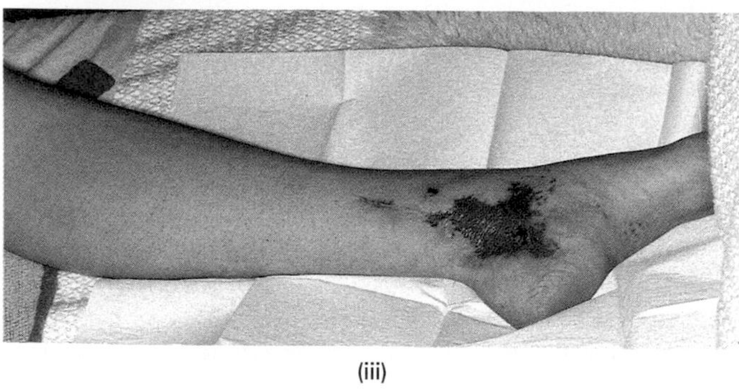

(iii)

(g)

(g) Klippel-Trenaunay syndrome in a young woman. This patient came for treatment of pigmentation and recurring ulceration at the left ankle, typical of venous hypertension. (i) The left limb was found to be 3 cm longer than the right. This photograph shows inequality in limb length, causing a tilted pelvis and different knee levels. (ii) Vascular markings were present elsewhere, here shown on the face. (iii) Venotensive pigmentation and healed ulceration seen at the left ankle. Phlebography showed extensive hypoplasia of deep veins, giving warning that interference with superficial veins could be harmful; conservative treatment succeeded in controlling the ulcer. There was no evidence of arteriovenous fistula.

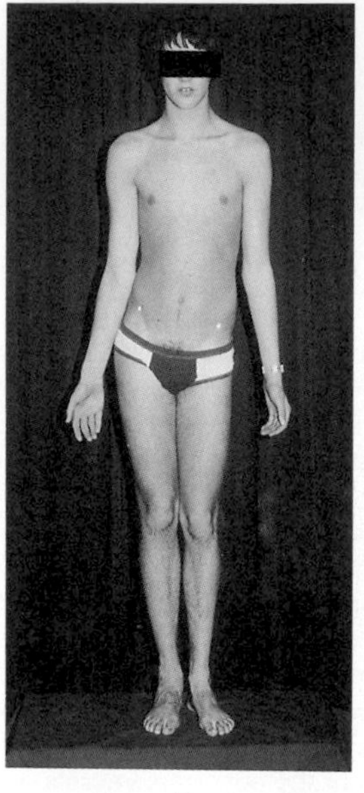

(i)

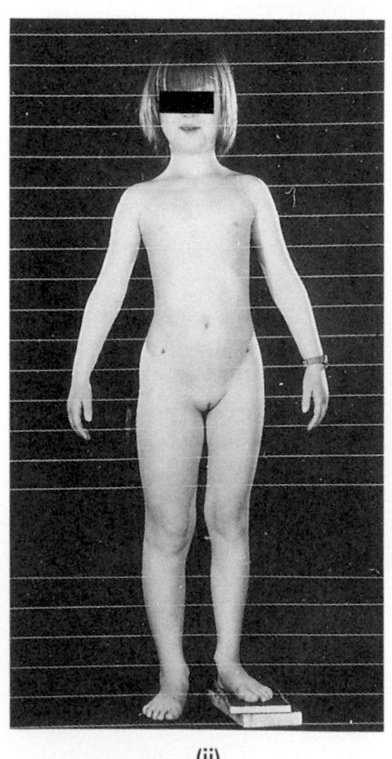

(ii)

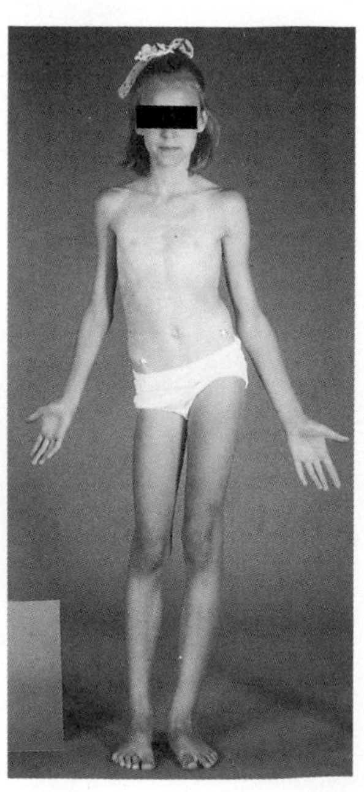

(iii)

(h)

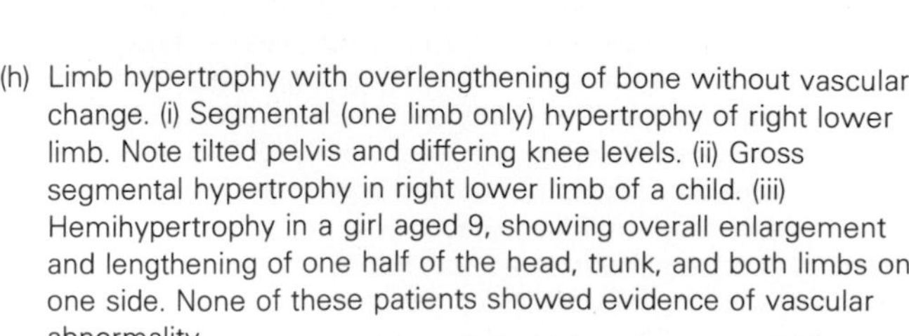

(h) Limb hypertrophy with overlengthening of bone without vascular change. (i) Segmental (one limb only) hypertrophy of right lower limb. Note tilted pelvis and differing knee levels. (ii) Gross segmental hypertrophy in right lower limb of a child. (iii) Hemihypertrophy in a girl aged 9, showing overall enlargement and lengthening of one half of the head, trunk, and both limbs on one side. None of these patients showed evidence of vascular abnormality.

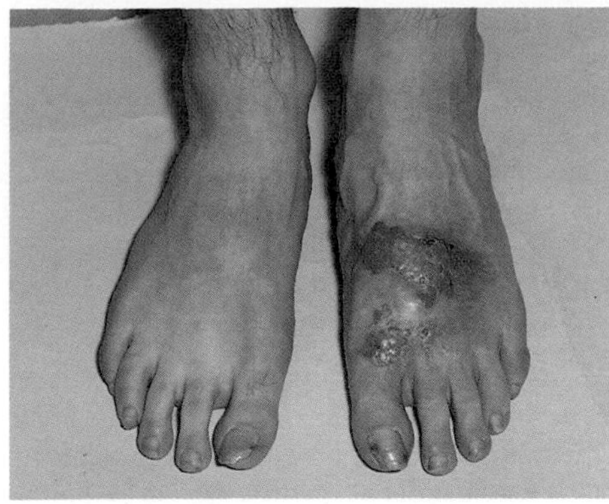

(i)

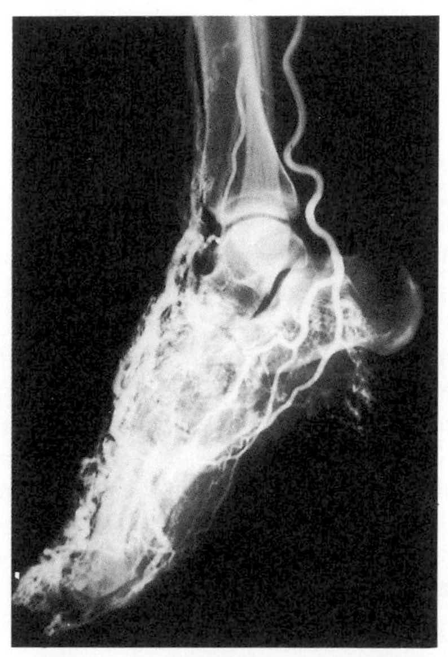

(ii)

(i) Localized congenital arteriovenous fistulae. (i) The foot of a boy aged 12 is shown. It is slightly enlarged and the veins are prominent; on the dorsum are areas of pigmentation and threatened ulceration, typical of venous hypertension. All the clinical features of multiple arteriovenous fistulae were present and angiography confirmed that these ramified through the foot so that local surgery was not feasible. A watchful policy, with strong external elastic support was advised; an amputation through normal tissue in the lower leg may become necessary eventually but only when circumstances make this essential. (ii) Arteriogram of a similar arteriovenous lesion in a young woman.

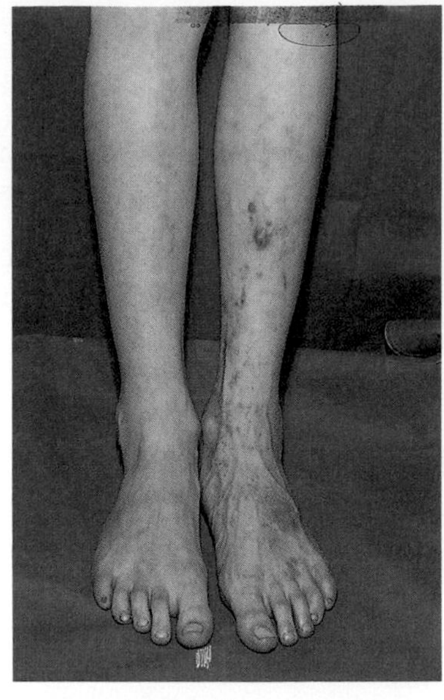

(i)

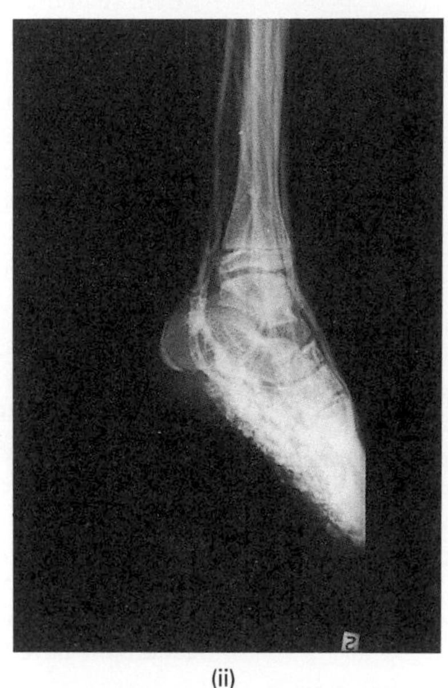

(ii)

(j) Multiple arteriovenous fistulae in foot and leg of a boy aged 9 (Parkes-Weber syndrome). (i) The features are essentially similar but more extensive to those in the preceding figure. The left tibia was 2 cm longer than the normal side, with a corresponding increase in the foot size. (ii) Arteriogram showing rapid perfusion into the vascular spongework of the foot and transit to the venous system.

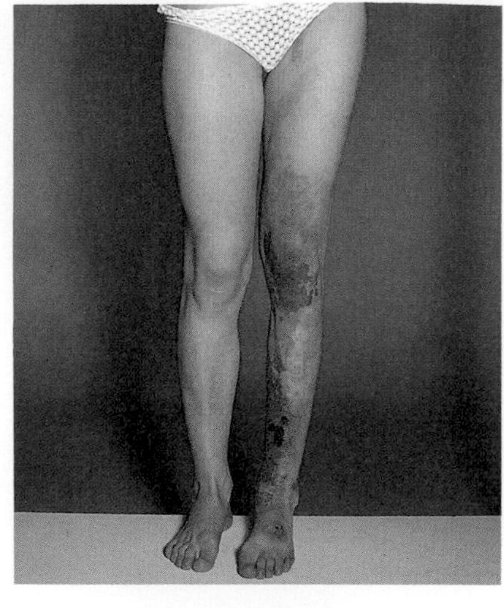

(i)

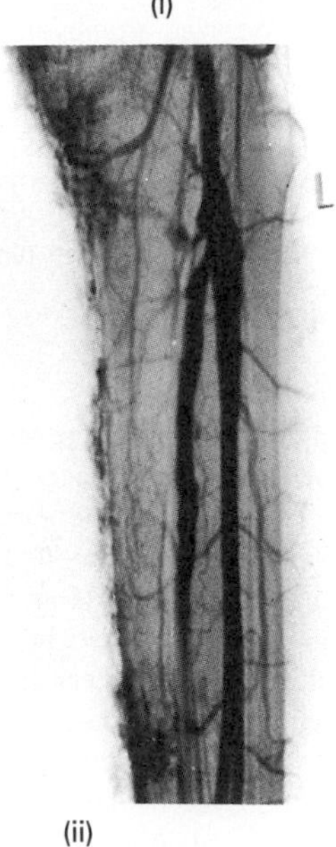

(ii)

(k) Multiple congenital arteriovenous fistulae involving an entire lower limb and neighbouring pelvis, in a young woman aged 18 (Parkes-Weber syndrome). (i) General view showing extensive pigmentation and ulceration from the knee downwards. Severe pelvic tilt due to 4 cm overlengthening of the limb is evident and the left knee is 2 cm higher than the right side because of tibial overgrowth. All the clinical features of diffuse arteriovenous fistulae were present, including cardiac hypertrophy and Branham's sign. (ii) Portion of arteriogram on this patient to show the distinctive spongework of multiple fistulae on the inner aspect of tibia. In the upper part, a large feeding artery can be seen running to an extensive area of fistulae. At a later stage, this artery was occluded by a Gianturco coil and this healed an overlying ulcer. This patient successfully went through two pregnancies without any apparent deterioration. For some years the ulceration has been controlled by strong elastic support and this conservative policy will be followed as long as possible.

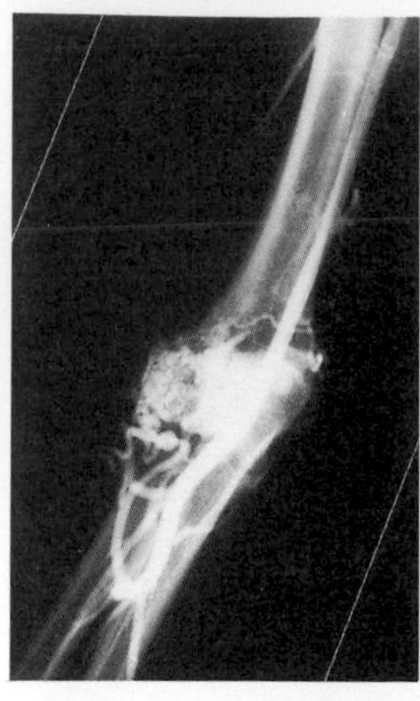

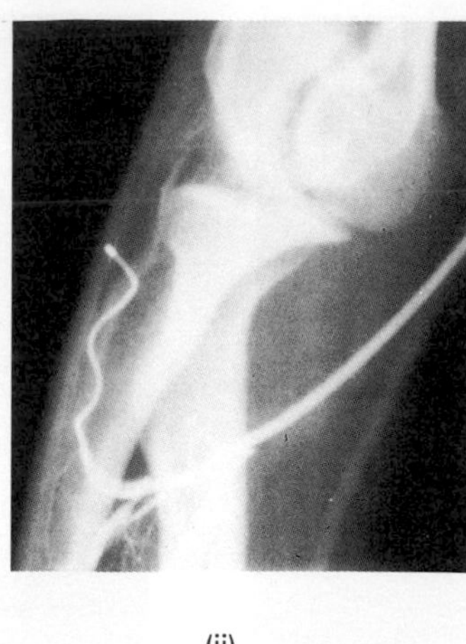

(i) (ii)

(l)

(l) Treatment of localized arteriovenous fistula by transluminal occlusion of its feeding artery. (i) Angiogram of fistula at the elbow of a young woman. The feeding artery to the fistulous area is clearly seen. (ii) Angiogram immediately after insertion of a Gianturco coil introduced by arterial catheter; all blood flow through the fistula has ceased. When reviewed a year later only a slight thickening was present with no evidence of persisting fistula.

cavernous angioma forms a protuberant swelling composed of large irregular blood-filled spaces. It usually proves persistent and may show apparent enlargement in childhood. Often it affects no more than skin and subcutaneous tissues but may extend deeply, lying in and amongst muscle (Fig. 62(c)). The boundaries of these lesions are not clearly defined but may be sufficiently limited to allow surgical removal. Surgery may require considerable skill as these angiomata cross anatomical boundaries and involve important structures which will require separating from the main mass by sharp dissection; the fringe of angioma that has to be left behind is usually unimportant. A small angioma may be treated by sclerotherapy or by laser.

Extensive venous angiomatosis

Cavernous angiomatosis may occur as a congenital defect extensively over a lower limb or elsewhere in the body (Fig. 62(d)). It is most obvious when the skin is involved, as a dark purple, irregular, compressible swelling but it often pervades the underlying layers extending into muscle and bone beneath. In the worst examples, this grossly abnormal venous state may be accompanied by severely defective deep veins which are either absent or lacking valves. A massive persistent lateral vein, referred to above, may be present. In such limbs venous return against gravity is likely to be severely defective and by the time adult life is reached venous hypertension causes a strong tendency to ulceration.

Klippel-Trenaunay syndrome

The extensive venous abnormality just described is often, but not always, accompanied by overgrowth in the bones to give increased length in the limb and this special variety is known as the Klippel-Trenaunay syndrome (Figs. 62(e), (f), and (g)). Because of the close association of severe venous malformation with overgrowth of the bones, any patient showing venous abnormality or angiomatosis should be examined for a change in the bone length. This change is usually made obvious by careful clinical examination comparing measurements between the bony points on the two limbs or simply by inspecting the patient in a standing position and looking for inequality in the levels of the corresponding bony prominences. Measurement by radiography is only necessary if study of progressive change over the years is required.

The significance of bony overgrowth in a limb (limb hypertrophy)

Over-lengthening of a limb may arise without any other abnormality and will then usually be seen in an orthopaedic clinic (Fig. 62(h)), but it is often found as a previously unnoticed accompaniment of gross vascular abnormality, as in Klippel-Trenaunay syndrome. Even if obvious vascular changes are not present the possibility of deep vein abnormality, perhaps with large, valveless channels causing venous hypertension and eventually ulceration in the limb must be borne in mind. The association with a large superficial lateral venous channel and defective or absent deep veins has already been mentioned above. Another cause for over-lengthening of bones is the presence of multiple arteriovenous fistulae (Parkes-Weber syndrome) but this condition should be regarded as separate from the venous states just described (see below). When bony overgrowth is found by a venous clinic it is important to place the young patient under orthopaedic care. Inequality in the length of the lower limbs with tilting of the pelvis should be compensated for by raising the shoe on the normal side since otherwise it may cause arthritis of the spine at an early age. Surgical correction of the bone length, either by epiphysiodesis whilst the bone is still growing or, better, by bone shortening as a young adult, may be necessary, if the vascular state allows this.

Relationship of congenital arteriovenous fistulae to Klippel-Trenaunay syndrome

It is well recognized that extensive congenital arteriovenous fistulae will cause overgrowth of bone in the vicinity. This leads to speculation that occult arteriovenous fistulae may account for bony overgrowth in Klippel-Trenaunay syndrome. This has not been demonstrated reliably and, although there are cases where both states undoubtedly coexist, the current view is that the two conditions have no direct relationship.

Congenital multiple arteriovenous fistulae in a limb (Parkes-Weber syndrome)

Congenital arteriovenous fistulae may be localized to, for example, part of the foot or leg (Fig. 62(i) and (j)), or multiple fistulae may extend over the whole limb and perhaps even the adjoining pelvis (Fig. 62(k)). There is a corresponding overgrowth of neighbouring bone, with enlargement of the bony structure of the foot if localized there, or, if the entire limb is involved, 5 cm or more increase in its length.

The communications between artery and vein are through sponge-like vascular formations, each supplied by a single large artery which breaks into multiple branches connecting with a leash of enlarged veins running from it. An obvious pulsatile swelling may be present with discoloration of the overlying skin and large veins radiating from it; with a stethoscope, a machinery pumping bruit can be heard extensively over the limb. Massive arteriovenous shunting may cause an increased pulse rate which drops back to normal when the main artery to the limb is temporarily occluded (Branham's sign). The constant struggle to maintain blood pressure and the premature return of a large volume of blood may cause considerable cardiac enlargement with eventual heart failure. Brown pigmentation and ulceration of the skin in the distal limb is often present, due to the sustained venous hypertension characteristic of this condition.

Diagnosis

The diagnosis is usually evident on clinical grounds and by finding that Doppler flowmetry shows strong pulsation within the superficial veins. Arteriography with serial pictures will confirm the diagnosis and often outline individual areas of fistulous communication and the arteries feeding them.

Treatment

Angiomata

Small lesions may be treated by laser therapy but others, if not too extensive, may be treated by sclerotherapy or by appropriate plastic surgery. It should be noted that the skin involved in angiomatous change may easily necrose if it is raised or undermined.

Klippel-Trenauney syndrome

Repeated sclerotherapy may bring considerable improvement in the cutaneous lesions. In some cases surgical excision and provision of skin coverage by a vascularized flap from the opposite limb may prove possible in order to give good skin coverage over, for example, the knee joint. However, the difficulties in doing this must not be under-rated; it is seldom possible to get beyond the angiomatosis and numerous vascular apertures may bleed copiously from the fringe that remains. Raising flaps of heavily involved skin may result in extensive necrosis and problems in skin coverage. Tissues involved in angiomatosis do not respond in a normal fashion if surgery is required and such problems are best left to surgeons with a special skill in this field.

If phlebography has shown that extensive valveless deep veins are present and causing venous ulceration, it is sometimes possible to reroute these veins by implanting them into a neighbouring major vein that is valved, for example, transposing a superficial femoral vein into a well-valved profunda femoris vein (Fig. 56(b)). Transplanting valves from brachial vein or the long saphenous vein of the opposite limb is a theoretical possibility but in practice is seldom a convincing form of treatment (Fig. 56(c)).

Conservative management

Usually a policy of conservative management will have to be followed. This will be by strong elastic support to compress the angiomatous lesions and to prevent progressive enlargement; special fitting of a full thigh length stocking with waist attachment may be required. In addition it is essential that a policy of elevation at every spare moment is followed in order to reduce venous hypertension and keep ulceration at bay.

Usually the limb is good in other respects and serves the patient well so that amputation must not be an option. With good conservative management a useful limb can be maintained indefinitely in a satisfactory state.

Congenital arteriovenous fistulae

Very localized lesions can be surgically excised after careful evaluation by arteriography. But even comparatively small lesions may be better treated by transluminal embolization described below. Amputation of a limb must not be resorted to except *in extremis*; it may not solve the problem which can continue in the stump.

Active treatment by transluminal occlusion

This requires expert planning and should be performed by an experienced vascular radiologist. A special indication for this is in cardiac failure when it is considered essential to reduce the arteriovenous shunting. The basis is occlusion of the feeding artery by transluminal introduction of an occlusive device, such as the Gianturco coil, under radiological control (Fig. 62(l)). This is far better than attempted surgical ligation. However, it is possible to cut off too much arterial supply and abruptly reduce arterial pressure below that of the abnormally high venous pressure so that capillary flow ceases, resulting in extensive ischaemic changes.

Conservative treatment

In most patients conservative treatment will be the mainstay of treatment. Very strong elastic containment and elevation of the limb at every spare moment will be essential. If ulceration or haemorrhage occur, inelastic containment, by paste bandage, maintained for many weeks, can be most valuable.

Many young patients reach adult life without mishap and continue successfully, even through pregnancy (Fig. 62(k)), using the methods outlined above. It is wrong to counsel anxious parents at an early age that the limb should be amputated either at that time or later, but rather to emphasize that every effort will be made to extend the useful state of the limb indefinitely.

ULCERS OF THE LEG

Chronic ulceration of the leg, often causing considerable disability, is a common problem with significant economic consequences for the individual and for society. In European countries nearly 90 per cent of these ulcers arise from one or other of the venous disorders described above but in the remainder there are many other causes; in these, treatment suitable for venous ulceration may be in direct conflict with that actually required and in the case of ischaemic ulceration may jeopardize the limb. Because of the prevalence of venous ulcer, it is all too easy to assume that this is the diagnosis and to give wholly inappropriate treatment. It is important to identify accurately the underlying cause in each case so that treatment may be correctly based on this. The diagnosis of 'leg ulcer' is totally inadequate and must always be qualified by a statement of the cause, backed by full evidence for this diagnosis. This requires an understanding of the range of leg ulcers that occur and the disease processes underlying them. The description that follows is appropriate for European countries but it must be remembered that the prevalence of leg ulcers has considerable variation geographically and within ethnic groups. Fortunately, venous ulceration has distinctive features that usually allow positive identification; the recognition and treatment of venous ulcers will be considered first.

Venous ulceration

For the reasons described earlier, venous disorders are liable, in varying degree, to develop venous hypertension. If this is sufficiently severe it causes excess capillary exudation and formation of a fibrin barrier around capillaries, with diminished nutritional exchange between capillary blood and the subcutaneous tissues and skin. An important phenomenon involved in this, recently recognized, is the deposition of leucocytes in capillaries affected by venous hypertension (white cell trapping). Endothelial cells, activated by hypoxia, cause leucocytes to become adherent and release injurious products which damage the endothelium with consequent migration of leucocytes into surrounding tissue to cause further harm there. It is as if the leucocytes with their defensive and scavenging properties, so valuable in an inflammatory reaction, are mistakenly attacking impaired capillary walls and neighbouring tissue. The destructive effect is enhanced by obstruction to capillary flow by the adherent layer of leucocytes and by thrombus resulting from activation of platelets. The precise sequence has yet to be established but 'leucocyte trapping' seems to play an essential part in the changes leading to venous ulceration. Oedema, induration, and fibrosis, accompanied by pigmentation of the skin develop progressively and, without treatment, culminate in tissue death and ulceration (Figs. 46(b), 47, 52, 56(a), and 63(a), (b), (c), (d)). The same characteristic changes also develop distal to arteriovenous fistula due to the common denominator in all these conditions, venous hypertension. A summary of the main features of typical venous ulcer is given below.

Position

The ulcer occurs where venous pressure is sustained at a high level and upon which unnaturally high peaks of pressure may be superimposed. Usually this is in the lower leg, occasionally on the upper aspect of the foot but never on its underside. Although the most common site is just above the medial malleolus it may occur almost anywhere on the leg according to the pattern of venous failure.

Age and distribution

No age of adult life is immune but the occurrence of venous ulcer increases with age probably due to progressive deterioration in the musculovenous pumping mechanisms with advancing years. Up to 1 per cent of the adult population may be affected by venous ulceration at some stage in their lives, with women affected slightly more frequently than men.

Manifestations

Ulceration is preceded by venotensive changes of local oedema, induration (liposclerosis), and brown pigmentation of the skin caused by extravasated haemosiderin. These changes are always found in the vicinity of a venous ulcer and if surrounding skin pigmentation is not present in a white skin the diagnosis is in doubt. However, haemosiderin is of a similar colour to the melanin in a black skin which may be increased locally around any long-standing skin lesion and, since the two pigments cannot be easily distinguished, increased pigmentation is not a reliable guide to venotension in black patients; moreover, melanin may be reduced in various circumstances, such as use of steroid cream, so that lack of surrounding pigmentation cannot be used to exclude a venous ulcer; nevertheless all the other evidence of venous insufficiency will be present and recognition of the cause should not be difficult.

Other forms of ulceration do not show these changes although they may be mimicked to some extent by a surrounding cellulitis. Fluid exudate is usual but, depending on prevailing bacteria and presence of necrotic tissue, may become purulent, possibly with an offensive odour. The ulcer causes variable discomfort and usually only harmless commensual organisms are found on bacterial culture; however, if it is infected by pathogens, such as *Staphylococcus aureus*, β-haemolytic streptococci, or anaerobic organisms, invasion of surrounding tissues may cause considerable pain. Pain is also characteristic of an ischaemic ulcer and the importance of distinguishing this from a venous ulcer is discussed below.

Diagnosis

Diagnosis is confirmed by the presence of substantial to severe accompanying venous disorder which is readily demonstrated by the usual clinical tests and by the special tests, including Doppler flowmetry, plethysmography, phlebography, or ultrasonography showing the characteristic abnormalities found in chronic venous insufficiency. Skin in the vicinity will show capillary stasis with laser Doppler rheography and a diminished oxygen tension.

Treatment

This will depend on the type of venous disorder causing ulceration. In superficial vein incompetence, surgery will have a major role by removing the pathway of incompetence but in most other cases conservative treatment by elevation and external support will have to be relied on, as discussed earlier. In the healing of a venous ulcer, counteracting venous hypertension is the most important measure and the most effective way of achieving this is elevation of the limb (Figs. 49(g)(h), 59(a) and 63(c)). Local applications to the ulcer itself are probably far less important. Strong antiseptics may actually be damaging and the ulcer is best cleansed by normal saline, and covered with an inert, non-adherent, moisture-preserving material such as a hydrocolloid gel. Steroid applications should be avoided since they may actually delay epithelialization and cause deterioration in the ulcer. Antibiotic preparations should not be used unless there is good reason, for fear of setting up a sensitization reaction in the surrounding skin which is particularly vulnerable to antibiotics (Fig. 63(e)) and to other materials commonly used in ointments and dressings. If pathogenic organisms have been demonstrated, any necrotic tissue should be excised, and an appropriate antibiotic given systemically for a few days. It must be emphasized that local treatment to the ulcer will not be effective unless venous hypertension is controlled by elevation for a good proportion of the day and all through the night. A sophisticated alternative to high elevation, particularly if oedema is troublesome, is the use of a pneumatic compression device acting sequentially upwards by multiple chambers enclosing the limb. These machines, often used in the control of lymphoedema, are widely marketed and can prove very successful in the healing and subsequent prevention of recurrence of ulceration in chronic venous insufficiency.

Most venous ulcers will heal with the regimen just outlined and often it may be combined with limited ambulation if external support with a paste bandage is used. If the ulcer is particularly large the process may be speeded up surgically by removing excess granulation tissue and applying some form of split skin graft. This should only be done when the ulcer has clearly reached a healing phase with sloping edges and a thin grey line of epithelial ingrowth. In cases where surgical control of venous hypertension is not possible, the ulcer will soon recur unless the patient has been instructed in an appropriate way of life which will include elevation of the limb whenever possible and the use of external support (Figs. 49 and 59(a), (b), and (c)). If a large ulcer proves intractable or it recurs repeatedly, a plastic procedure excising the ulcer and providing skin cover by a pedicle graft, or by a myocutaneous free graft vascularized by microvascular surgery, may give a fresh start

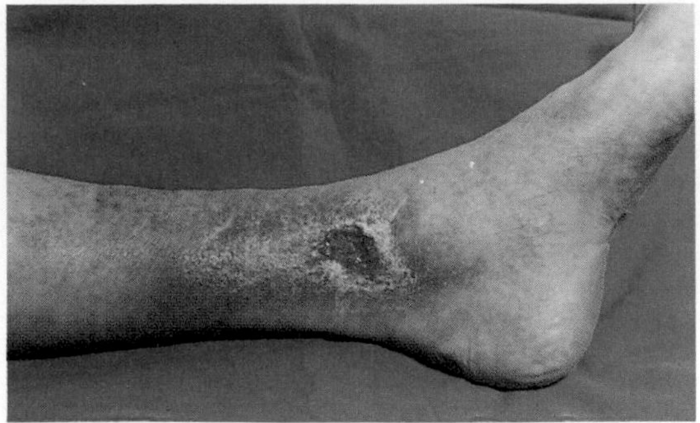

Fig. 63 Leg ulcers.
(a) Venous ulcer due to superficial vein incompetence. (i) Commencing venous ulceration. This patient had long neglected her varicose veins and ignored an increasing area of pigmented skin above the medial malleolus. She sought advice only when the shallow ulcer shown here had been present for several weeks. It soon healed with a programme of elevation and use of elastic support. She declined surgical treatment but had learnt how to prevent the ulcer from recurring.

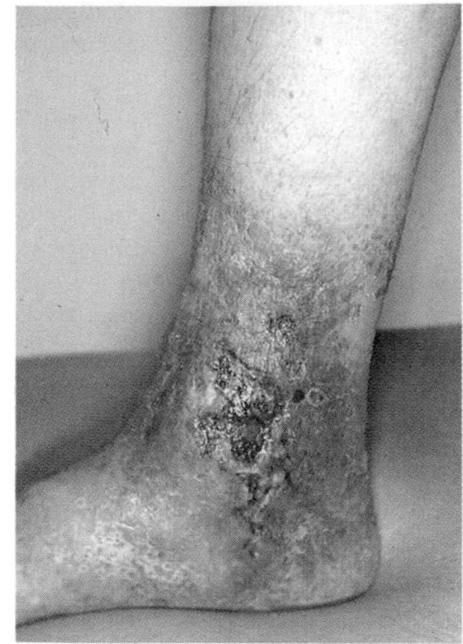

(b) Venous ulceration in valveless states. An ulcer in need of urgent treatment in an elderly patient. The extensive pigmentation and eczema shown here were due to a combination of superficial and deep vein insufficiency (valveless syndrome). The main ulcer is surrounded by satellite ulcers which will coalesce if treatment is not soon started. With a policy of elevation (arterial pulses were present) the ulcer healed. Stripping of the long saphenous vein was carried out subsequently to remove this factor and the patient urged to maintain a policy of elevation whenever possible and elastic support.

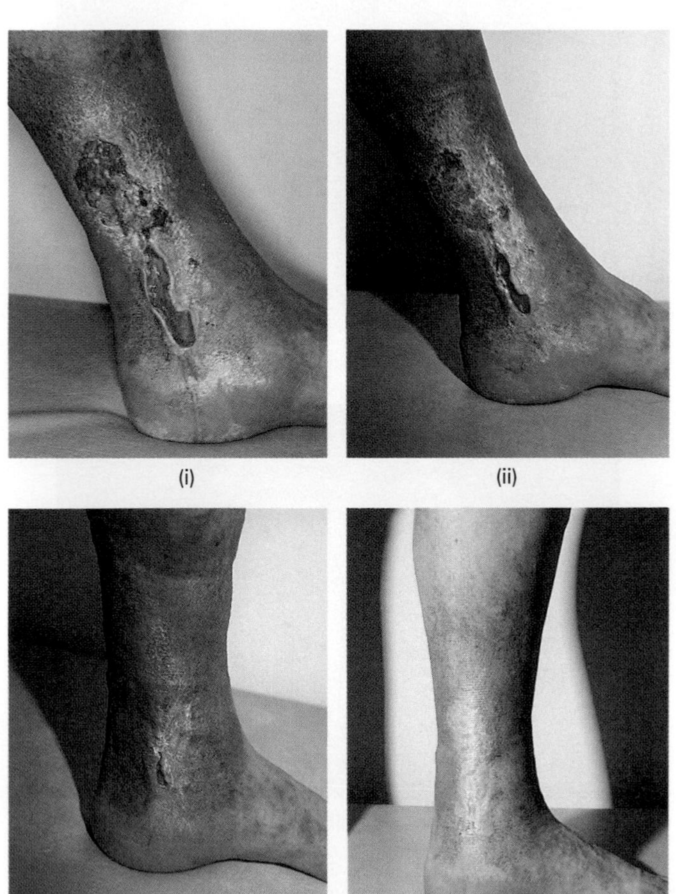

(i) (ii) (iii) (iv)

(c)

(c) Venous ulcer in severe post-thrombotic syndrome (and see Fig. 57(g)). This patient was unable to work because of a large, painful ulcer. The swelling, induration, and pigmentation surrounding the ulcer are typical of venous hypertension, in this case caused by incurable deep vein impairment so that only conservative treatment was feasible. Infection with *Staphylococcus aureus* was present and treated initially by systemic antibiotic. (i)–(iv) These pictures were taken over 4 months to show the gradual but impressive improvement in response to high elevation with active exercise, and eventual mobilization in inelastic (paste bandage) support; later, a knee-length one-way-stretch stocking was substituted. Prevention of recurrence in these circumstances can only succeed with sustained, conscientious effort by the patient; seen 2 years later, this patient was at work, with the limb in good condition.

but will require prolonged care to prevent eventual recurrence. In these circumstances it is imperative to make sure beforehand that ischaemia or malignancy is not the real cause for the ulcer's unsatisfactory response to treatment. The possible role of ligation of perforating veins is discussed earlier.

Others causes for leg ulcer

Ischaemic ulcer (arterial insufficiency)

This state is comparatively common and its management conflicts directly with that of venous ulcer so that distinguishing one from the other is of crucial importance. The ischaemia is usually due to atherosclerosis so that the older patient is most commonly affected but it can be encountered in young adults.

Main features

The ulcer is usually painful and situated on toes, foot, or leg; it is especially likely to occur over bony prominences, such as toe

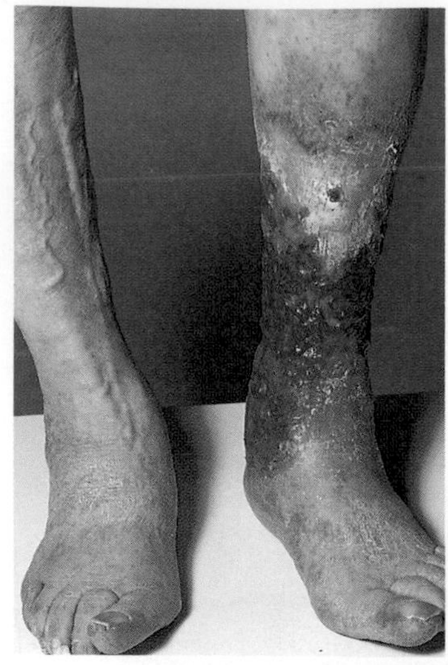

(d)

(d) Severe ulceration in iliofemoral post-thrombotic syndrome. This picture shows in more detail the ulcer illustrated in Fig. 58(d). Widespread atrophie blanche is present and indicates impoverished capillary beds. In an ulcer of this size severe anaemia may retard healing, and the possibility of malignant change must not be overlooked. The proliferative appearance suggests that ischaemia is unlikely to be a factor but this should be verified, and, as usual, metabolic factors such as diabetes must be excluded. Skin grafting with conservative treatment to counteract venous hypertension may heal the ulcer but, thereafter, constant vigilance will be needed to prevent recurrence.

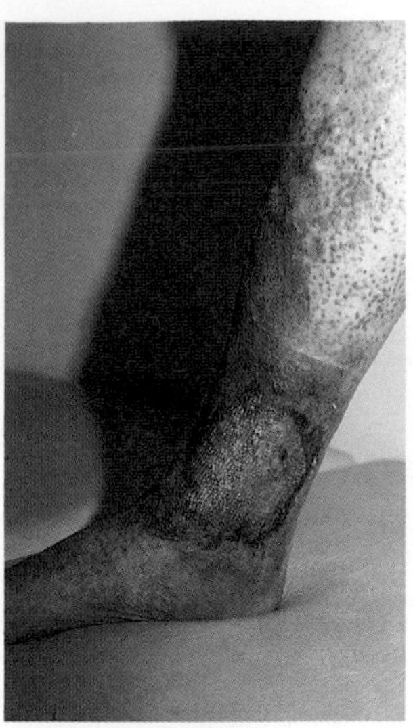

(e)

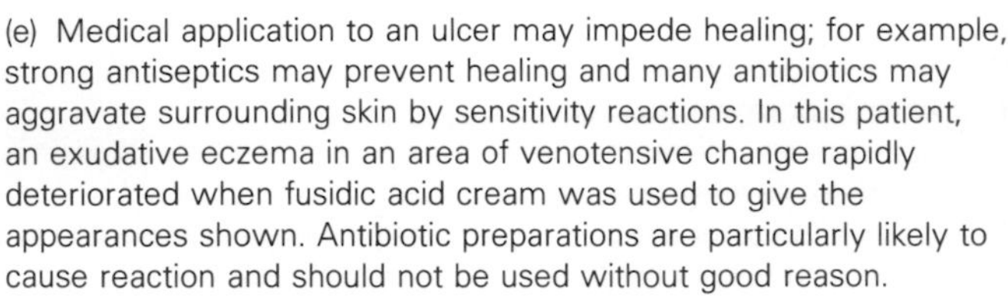

(e) Medical application to an ulcer may impede healing; for example, strong antiseptics may prevent healing and many antibiotics may aggravate surrounding skin by sensitivity reactions. In this patient, an exudative eczema in an area of venotensive change rapidly deteriorated when fusidic acid cream was used to give the appearances shown. Antibiotic preparations are particularly likely to cause reaction and should not be used without good reason.

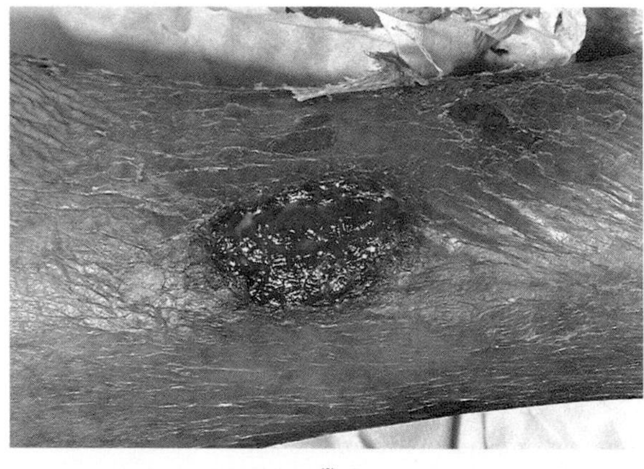

(i)

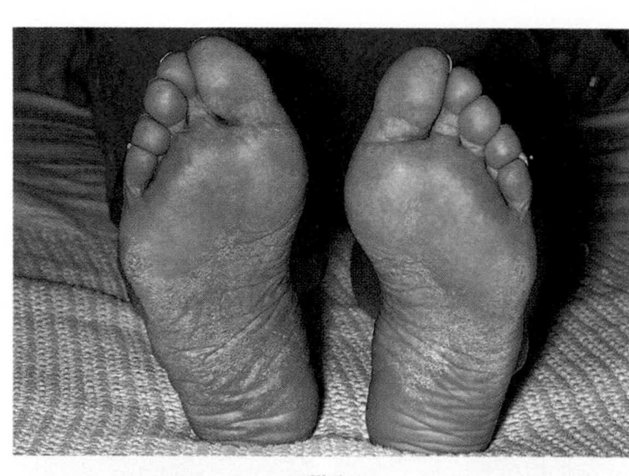

(iiia)

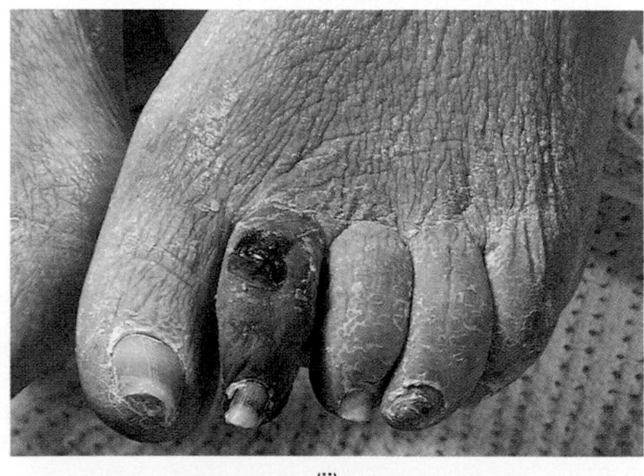

(ii)

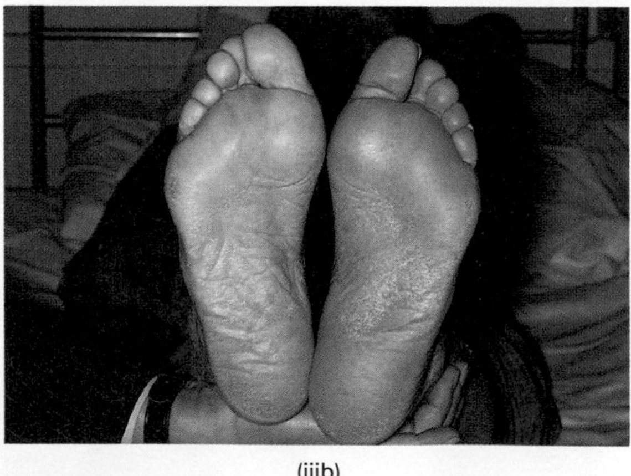

(iiib)

(f) Ischaemic ulceration. (i) An ischaemic ulcer is not surrounded by typical venotensive change and will be a dry ulcer with sparse granulation tissue. The illustration shows an ischaemic ulcer on the shin of an elderly person. (ii) Gangrene of toes is a common accompaniment of ischaemic ulceration. In this illustration, the wrinkled skin on the forefoot is due to recent subsidence of dependency oedema caused by the previous habit of hanging the leg out of bed to relieve rest pain. This is on the same limb as that illustrated in Fig. 63(f) (i). (iii) Critically ischaemic foot. *a* Colour is present in both feet when horizontal. *b* After 30 s of elevation the right forefoot and toes show obvious blanching because arterial perfusion pressure is insufficient to mount the gradient.

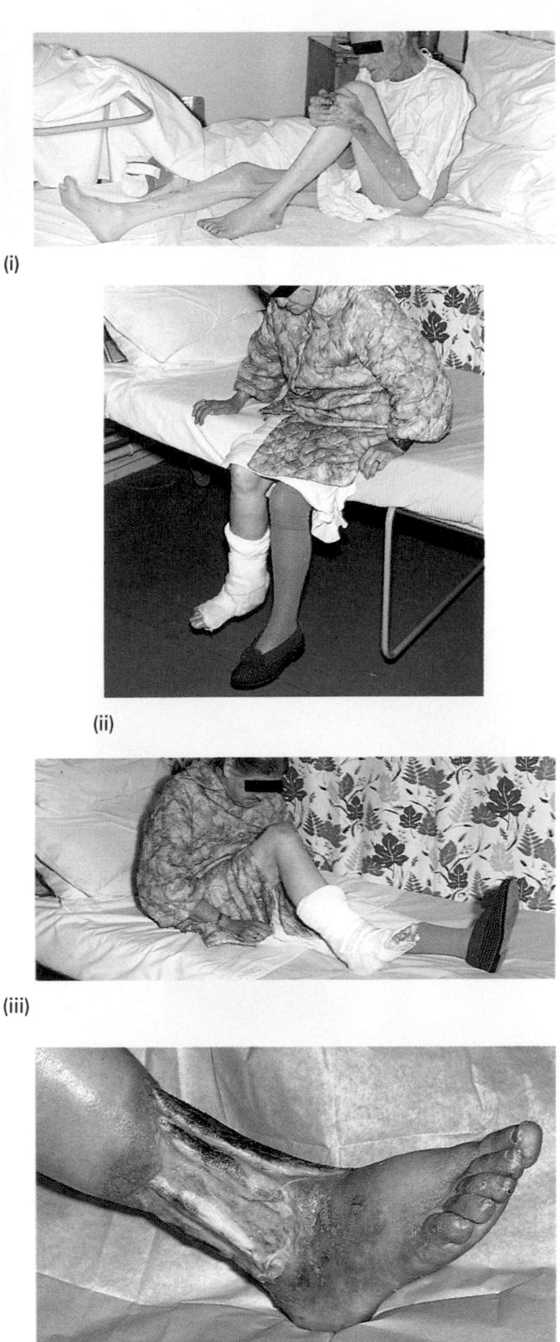

(i)

(ii)

(iii)

(iv)

(g)

(g) Characteristic postures of patients with ischaemic rest pain. (i) The typical 'knee-up' position of a patient with severe rest pain. This posture, or hanging the leg over the side of bed, brings a small measure of relief by using gravity to help arterial circulation at knee level down to the foot. (ii) and (iii) This elderly patient endured severe ischaemic rest pain for 3 months, sitting endlessly over the edge of the bed or in a 'knee-up' position. (iv) The massive ischaemic ulcer under the bandages of the last patient. Essentially, it is a dry ulcer, without granulation tissue or pus (there is not sufficient circulation to give inflammatory reaction) and with necrotic tendons exposed. A venous ulcer does not expose deeper tissues in this fashion. Amputation was necessary here, but arterial reconstruction to the left side succeeded in saving this limb when severe ischaemic rest pain developed a few months later.

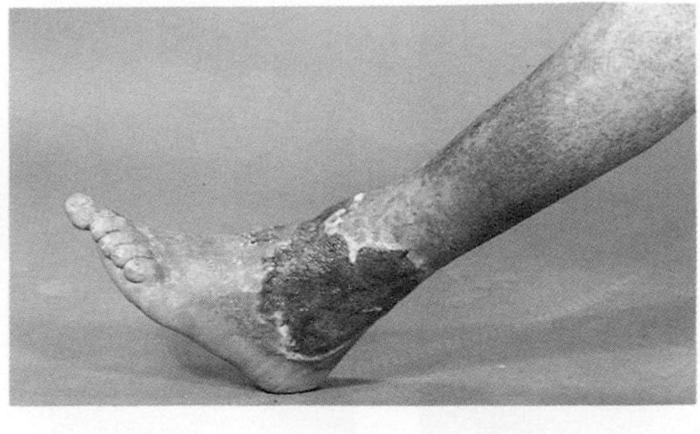

(h)

(h) Combination of chronic venous insufficiency and ischaemia. Illustrated here is massive ulceration in the left limb of a 65-year-old man. Originally, both lower limbs were similarly affected and it was found that gross long saphenous incompetence was present together with bilateral occlusion of the superficial femoral arteries. This gave opportunity to cure the venous incompetence by removing the long saphenous veins and using them as femoropopliteal grafts to restore arterial supply. One limb responded dramatically with healing of the ulcer; the other limb, shown in the illustration failed to do so and amputation was eventually resorted to, even though the arterial reconstruction remained open; it is possible that widespread occlusion of tibial and peroneal arteries caused this failure. Two years later the right limb remained in good condition with the patient actively using it.

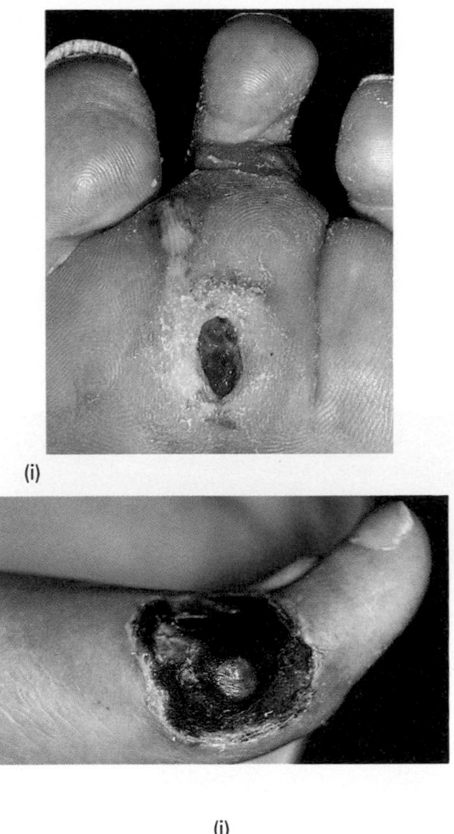

(i)

(ii)

(i)

(i) Diabetic ulcer and complications. (i) Typical neuropathic diabetic ulcers occur over bony prominences, as in this example over the head of the second metatarsal bone. Healing this ulcer might be possible but it would keep recurring unless the metatarsal head is removed. (ii) A similar ulcer over the head of the first metatarsal bone and opening into the joint. Stability was restored by removing the distal part of the first metatarsal and the great toe. Blood supply was ample to provide healing.

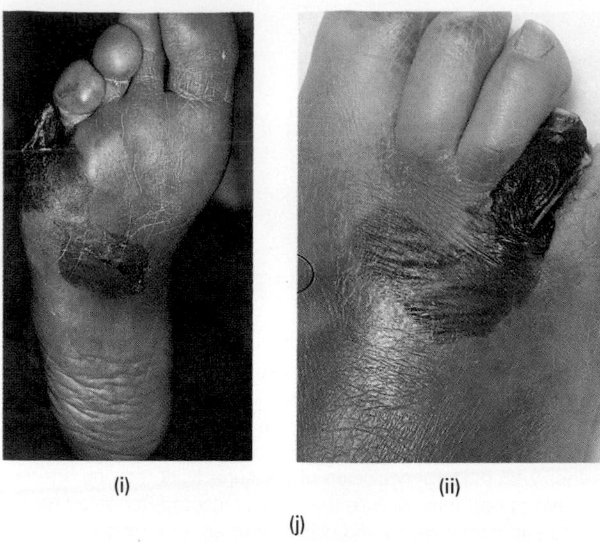

(i) (ii)

(j)

(j) Consequence of an open lesion in diabetic neuropathic foot; a painless, tunnelling gangrene likely to be ignored until it is too late to save the foot. (i) A lesion of the little toe has allowed infection to spread painlessly and insidiously into the deep compartments of the foot over the course of some weeks. The plantar tendons were found to be necrotic and surrounded by pus. In this patient there was inadequate healthy skin to permit a forefoot amputation. (ii) A similar lesion on the dorsum of the foot, again painless and very destructive in the deeper layers.

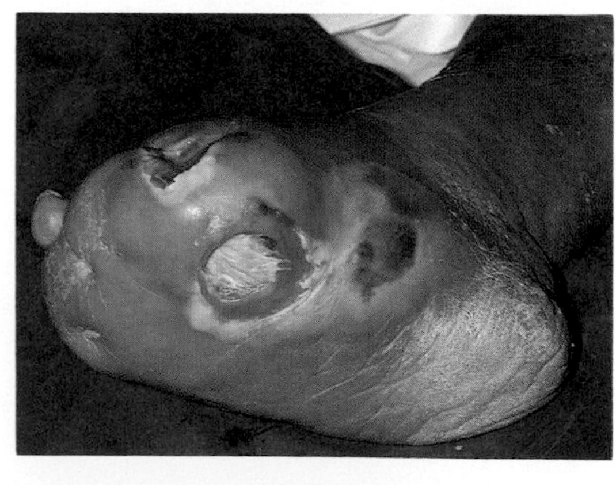

(k)

(k) The ultimate fate of a diabetic neuropathic foot. Over the course of many years the foot has been rescued from neuropathic ulcers by removing the heads of various metatarsal bones. In the illustration, further ulceration has occurred over the stumps of remaining metatarsals and has allowed infection to enter. This has tunnelled painlessly through the foot and into the lower leg, and was ignored by the patient as it spread slowly over the preceding weeks. The foot could not be saved but a below-knee amputation healed well.

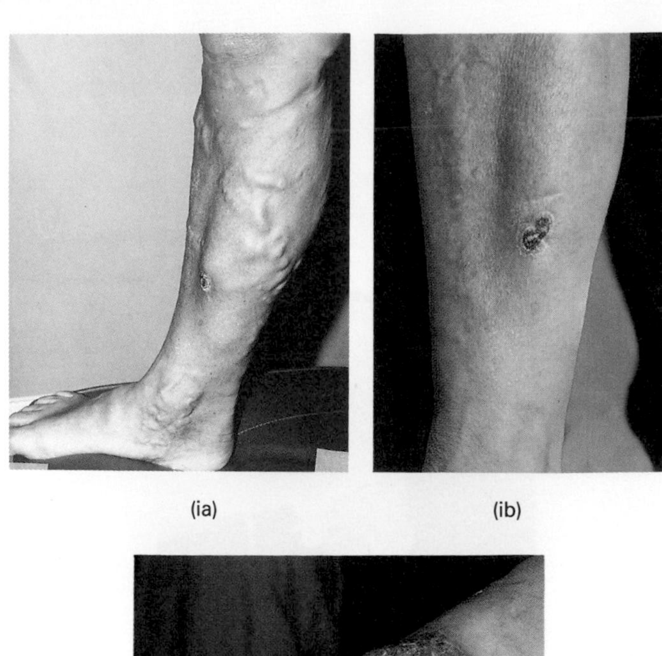

(ia) (ib)

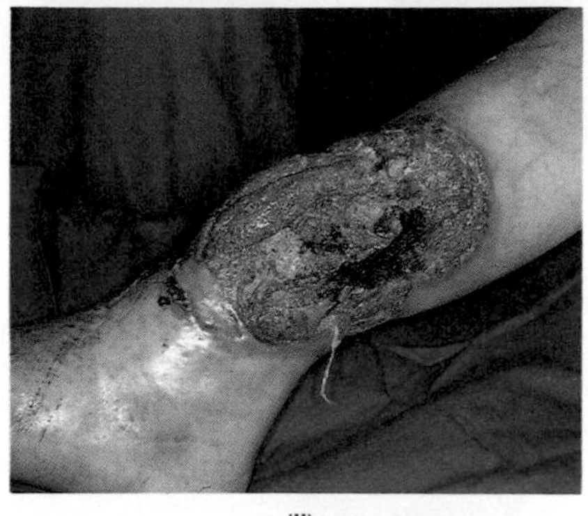

(ii)

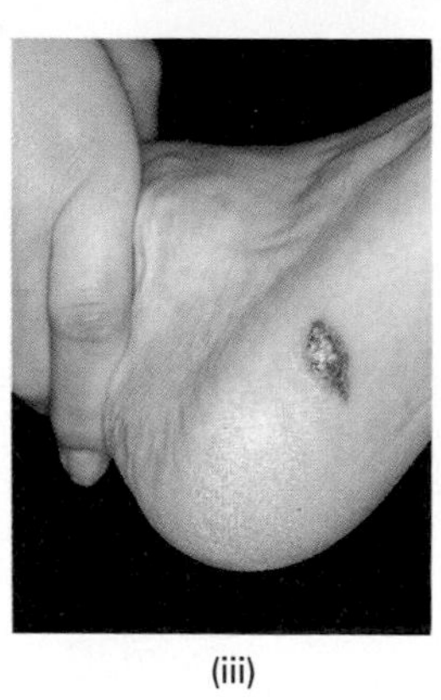

(iii)

(l)

(l) Malignant ulcers on leg and foot. (i) Basal cell carcinoma. *a* This small ulcer with surrounding pigmentation appeared over massive varicose veins due to long saphenous incompetence. There was some surrounding pigmentation and it was assumed to be venous. *b* Surgery to the veins gave a good result but the ulcer persisted, although pigmentation around it had gone. Its appearance 1 year later is shown and suggests a rodent ulcer. On excision, a basal cell carcinoma was confirmed. (ii) Squamous carcinoma; Marjolin's ulcer. In this patient, an ulcer had been present for many years, and was assumed to be venous. At the stage shown here, the first attendance at hospital, a massive, proliferative ulcer was present, involving underlying muscle and causing pathological fracture of the bone, and immediately recognizable as malignant. Biopsy confirmed a squamous carcinoma and amputation was the only feasible treatment. (iii) Malignant melanoma. The foot and toes are common sites for malignant melanoma and an example is shown here.

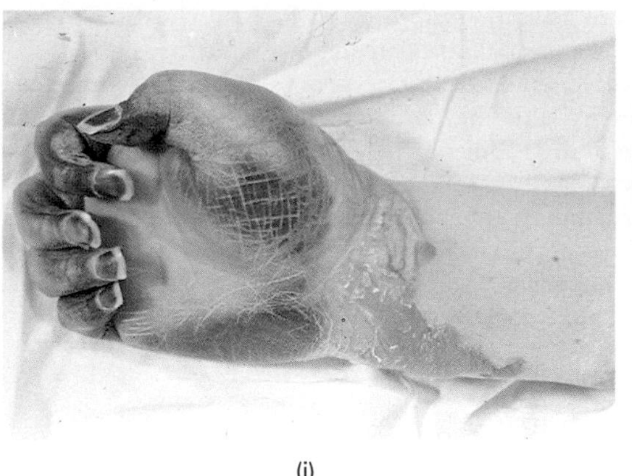

(i)

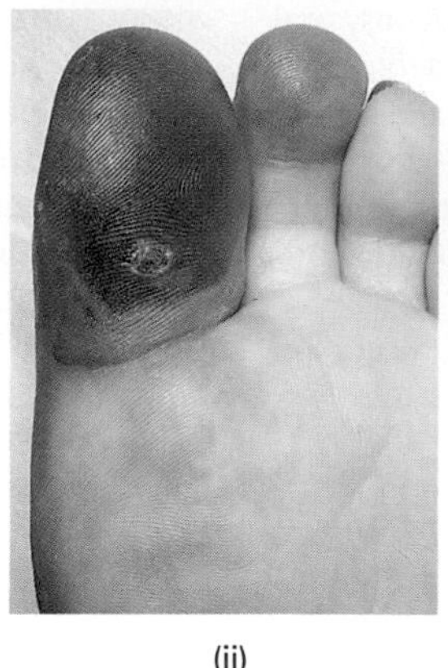

(ii)

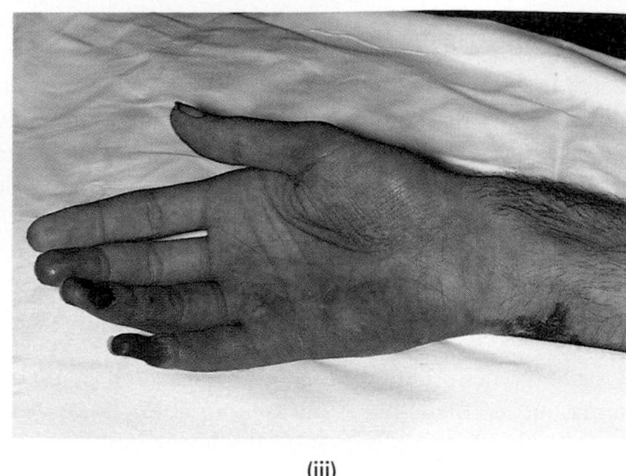

(iii)

(m)

(m) Lesions caused by intra-arterial injection. (i) Gangrene of a child's hand seen in the early days of intravenous barbiturate anaesthesia; in this case it was undoubtedly intra-arterial, a danger against which all anaesthetists take strict precautions. (ii) Gangrene of great toe following injection of a commonly used venous sclerosant (sodium tetradecyl sulphate) in the treatment of a plantar wart. The dosage was very small but sufficient to cause this damage by entering the artery supplying the wart. (iii) Ischaemic damage to tissues of wrist and hand, with gangrene in three fingers. This occurred in a drug addict and was caused by a misplaced self-injection of a barbiturate into the ulnar artery.

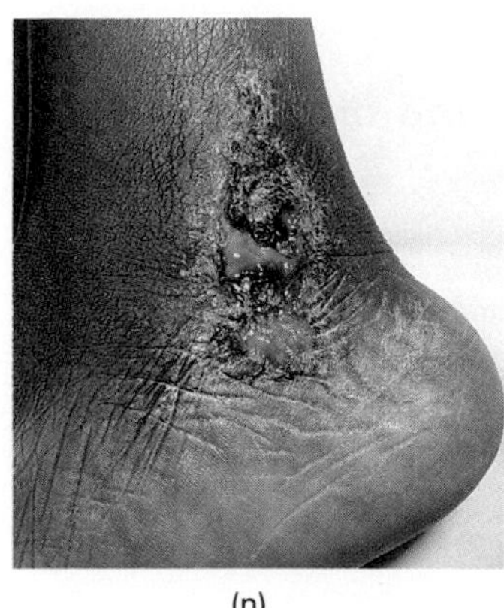

(n)

(n) Ulceration at the ankle in sickle-cell anaemia. Note the non-specific increase in melanin pigmentation around the ulcer which may be confused with the discoloration by haemosiderin around a venous ulcer. Other blood dyscrasias may cause ulceration, and severe anaemia from any cause will prevent healing.

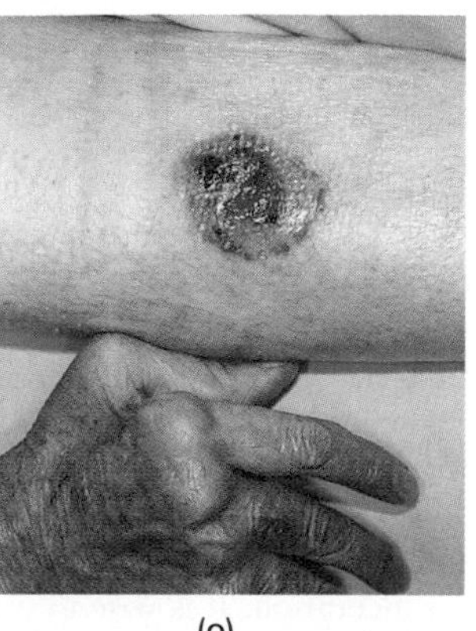

(o)

(o) Ulceration from vasculitis, seen here on the shin of a patient with rheumatoid arthritis.

joints, the malleoli, or the shin, where the impoverished skin is easily damaged by external pressure against the unyielding bone. The ulcer is 'dry', lacking exudate or pus because the circulation is insufficient to support inflammatory reaction (Figs. 63(f) and (g) (iii)). There will usually be a story of intermittent claudication, numbness of the toes and forefoot on walking, and a typical nocturnal ischaemic rest pain, relieved by sitting in knee-up position or hanging the foot out of bed (Fig. 63(g)), and made worse by elevation. The ankle pulses will be greatly reduced or missing and this is confirmed by Doppler flowmetry. Sensation may be reduced, and the toes and forefoot show pallor on elevation (Fig. 63(f) (iii)) with considerable delay in return of colour when the leg is placed horizontally again. Brown pigmentation of the surrounding skin, typical of venous ulceration, will not be present.

It is quite possible for venous ulceration to be accompanied by ischaemia, each condition aggravating the ill effects of the other (Fig. 63(h)). Treatment of ischaemic ulceration is considered elsewhere but it must be emphasized that elevation of an ischaemic limb can only reduce further its depleted arterial supply which has scarcely sufficient pressure to mount the gradient to the forefoot. To treat an ischaemic ulcer as a venous ulcer is a serious error. Pain in a leg ulcer, especially if it is made worse by elevation, should always suggest that ischaemia is present and the adequacy of arterial supply assessed. If there is any doubt the limb should not be raised above the horizontal.

Diabetic neuropathic ulceration

The most common cause for neuropathic ulceration is diabetes but other neurological conditions, including spina bifida, tabes dorsalis, syringomyelia, spinal cord or nerve injury, and even leprosy, should not be overlooked. The cause for ulceration here is loss of protective reflexes due to neuropathy. This leads to skin in the foot being given prolonged compression by body weight against bony prominences, such as the underside of a metatarsal head (Fig. 63(i)), the calcaneum, or the malleoli, without the patient being aware that damage is occurring. The arterial supply may be good and ischaemia is not usually a factor.

Diagnostic features

The ulcer is characteristically punched out and situated over a bony prominence. Evidence of the accompanying neuropathy may be provided by absent ankle jerks and diminished sensation in the toes and foot. In diabetes the diagnosis is easily confirmed by raised fasting levels of blood glucose.

These ulcers eventually allow entry of infection to surrounding tissues and set up a smouldering cellulitis that painlessly destroys the interior of the foot by necrosis of ligaments, tendons, and muscles (Figs. 63(j) and (k)). A diabetic ulcer is an unstable state which may eventually cause loss of a foot in this fashion and should not be allowed to continue unhealed. Healing is achieved by control of the diabetes and protection of the ulcer from external pressure, or by surgery to remove the underlying bony prominence, or, if need be, by forefoot amputation.

Diabetes may, of course, coexist with true venous ulceration and should always be excluded as a factor in leg ulcers.

Neoplastic ulcers

A primary neoplastic ulcer of the skin, such as malignant melanoma, or epithelioma is always possible. Basal cell carcinoma (rodent ulcer) is uncommon on the lower limb but the author has seen one case occurring in an area of venotensive change (Fig. 63(l) (i)). Malignant change in a long-standing venous ulcer is a well known possibility (Marjolin's ulcer) but even so there may be a long delay before this change is recognized (Fig. 63(l) (ii)). The foot and toes are a relatively common site for malignant melanoma which may ulcerate (Fig. 63(l) (iii)).

Tropical ulcers

Tropical ulcers, including cutaneous leishmaniasis and fungus infections, may be brought into temperate countries by travellers abroad.

Specific infection

Ulceration including tuberculosis and syphilis may be caused either as part of a systemic illness or as a localized infection. The possibility of lesions due to acquired immune deficiency syndrome (AIDS) should not be overlooked.

Blood dyscrasias

Any severe anaemia, sickle-cell anaemia, thalassaemia, hereditary spherocytosis, or leukaemia can provide obscure forms of chronic leg ulceration. It is wise to carry out routine blood examination at an early stage in the management of chronic leg ulcer.

Nutritional and metabolic disturbances

Vitamin and nutritional deficiencies, uraemia, and other metabolic disorders may cause or aggravate chronic ulceration.

Skin sensitivity or allergy

Skin sensitivity or allergy to materials at work, applied medicinally or for cosmetic reasons can either cause or aggravate ulceration. It is commonplace for leg ulcers to be exacerbated by inappropriate ointments, particularly antibiotics, cortisone, and antiseptics (Fig. 63(e)). A wide range of drugs taken internally may cause skin reactions and eventually ulceration but these lesions are likely to be widespread and not confined to a limb.

Trauma

Trauma as a single episode commonly sets off an ulcer in the presence of venous stasis, ischaemia, and in many of the generalized states referred to in this section. The skin of patients on corticosteroids becomes fragile and especially vulnerable to minor trauma.

Necrosis by injection of chemical, insect bite, or radiation

Misplaced injections during sclerotherapy may cause skin necrosis and prolonged ulceration. Many chemicals used medically or industrially can have the same effect. Particularly dangerous is inadvertent intra-arterial injection and many pharmaceuticals, including sclerosants and barbiturates, can cause extensive gangrene in the extremity; this may occur in medical procedures or by self-injection in drug addiction (Fig. 63(m)). High pressure injection of grease, used in servicing automobiles, can cause widespread destruction of subcutaneous tissue and skin. Insect bites may inject necrotoxins followed by unpleasant, prolonged ulceration. Insect bites may also implant parasitic or protozoal organisms which cause chronic lesions but these are uncommon in temperate climates.

Repeated trauma

Recurring trauma, either caused at work or self-inflicted in psychiatric disorders or malingering (dermatitis artefacta), can be an occasional cause for ulceration. Injury to the skin may occur from radiation or chemicals possibly without the patient realizing it.

Rheumatoid arthritis

Patients with rheumatoid arthritis may develop intractable ulceration on the legs or feet caused by vasculitis and this is sometimes mistaken for venous ulceration.

Systemic, autoimmune, and microvascular disease

Disorders such as systemic lupus erythematosus and polyarteritis can form lesions on the legs; these resemble the eczematous changes seen in venous disorder and eventually ulcerate.

The list of causes for leg ulceration given above is by no means complete but serves to illustrate the need to be constantly aware that one chronic leg ulcer in ten will not be venous in origin and will call for a special skill in diagnosis.

FURTHER READING

The following authoritative works give detailed accounts of the venous disorders and their treatment, together with comprehensive references to the most significant publications upon this subject.

Bergan JJ, Yao JST. *Surgery of the veins*. New York: Grune and Stratton, 1985.

Bergan JJ, Yao JST. *Venous disorders*. Philadelphia: W.B. Saunders, 1991.

Bradbury AW, Murie JA, Ruckley CV. Role of the leucocyte in the pathogenesis of vascular disease. *Br J Surg*, 1993; **80**: 1503–12.

Browse NL, Burnand KG, Lea Thomas M. *Diseases of the veins: Pathology, diagnosis and treatment*. London: Arnold, 1988.

Dodd H, Cockett FB. *The pathology and surgery of the veins of the lower limbs*. Edinburgh: Churchill Livingstone, 1976.

Gardner AMN, Fox RH. *The return of blood to the heart: venous pumps in health and disease*. London: John Libbey, 1989.

Lea Thomas M. *Phlebography of the lower limb*. Edinburgh: Churchill Livingstone, 1982.

May R. *Surgery of the veins and the pelvis*. Philadelphia: W.B. Saunders and Co. Stuttgart: Georg Thieme, 1979.

Negus D. *Leg ulcers*. Oxford: Butterworth-Heinemann Ltd, 1991.

Nicolaides A, Christopoulos D, Vasdekis S. Progress in the investigation of chronic venous insufficiency. *Ann Vasc Surg*, 1989; **3**: 278–92.

Nicolaides AN, Sumner DS. *Investigation of patients with deep vein thrombosis and chronic venous insufficiency*. London: Med-Orion Publishing Co, 1991.

Tibbs DJ. Varicose veins and related disorders. Oxford: Butterworth-Heinemann Ltd, 1992.

8.2 Deep vein thrombosis and pulmonary embolism

H. KIM LYERLY AND DAVID C. SABISTON

Deep venous thrombosis and pulmonary embolism are frequent causes of hospital admission, and an understanding of the complex mechanisms of thrombosis and thrombolysis is important in the prevention and management of patients with these disorders.

HISTORICAL ASPECTS

While pathologists had known for many years that thrombi at times formed in the peripheral veins, Virchow introduced the embolism concept as a result of his very cogent findings at autopsy. He observed that patients with pulmonary embolism often also had thrombi in the veins of the legs and pelvis. These thrombi were the same histological age as those found in the lungs. When thrombi were injected into the femoral veins of animals they ultimately lodged in the lungs. Virchow concluded that thrombi formed in the systemic veins and that thrombosis was caused primarily by three factors: reduced blood flow in the systemic veins, injury to the veins, and a state of hypercoagulability. These factors remain important in the pathogenesis of pulmonary embolism and are known collectively as Virchow's triad.

It is worth reviewing Virchow's original comments concerning the formation of thrombi in the peripheral veins. He stated quite succinctly:

'In the peripheral veins the danger proceeds chiefly from the small branches. By no means rarely do these become quite filled with masses of coagulum. As long, however, as the thrombus is confined to the branch itself, so long as the body is not exposed ... only the greater number of the thrombi in the small branches do not content themselves with advancing up to the level of the main trunk, but pretty constantly new masses of coagulum deposit themselves from the blood upon the end of the thrombus layer after layer; the thrombus is prolonged beyond the mouth of the branch into the trunk in the direction of the current of blood, shoots out in the form of à thick cylinder farther and farther, and becomes continually larger and larger. From a lumbar vein, for example, a plug may extend into the vena cava as thick as the last phalanx of the thumb. These are the thrombi that constitute the source of real danger; it is in them that ensues the crumbling away which leads to secondary occlusion in remote vessels.'

PATHOGENESIS OF THROMBOSIS AND THROMBOLYSIS

Thrombosis is usually initiated when alterations in the vascular endothelium cause platelets to adhere to subendothelial connective tissue. Collagen binds to platelet receptors to activate enzymes that catalyse the release of arachidonic acid. Cyclo-oxygenase converts arachidonic acid to thromboxane A_2 which increases phospholipase C activity and stimulates platelet activation and secretion. Cyclo-oxygenase is inhibited by aspirin and non-steroidal anti-inflammatory agents. Prostacyclin, in contrast to thromboxane A_2, is produced from arachidonic acid by endothelial cells and inhibits phospholipase C activity and platelet activation. Platelets release a variety of mediators after activation, including adenosine diphosphate which modifies the platelet surface, allowing fibrinogen to attach and link to adjacent platelets. Platelet-derived growth factor is also released, stimulating the growth and migration of fibroblasts and smooth muscle cells within the vessel wall.

The primary haemostatic plug is strengthened after several minutes by activation of the coagulation pathway which causes the production of thrombin and conversion of plasma fibrinogen to fibrin. The reactions require formation of a surface-bound complex and the activation of proteases by proteolysis: they are regulated by plasma and cellular cofactors and by calcium. For example, the local concentration of reactants is reduced by the flow of blood and increased by stasis. In addition, the absorption of coagulation factors to cellular surfaces and the presence of multiple inhibitors in plasma inhibit thrombosis.

Thrombolysis begins immediately after formation of the haemostatic plug. The principal physiological factor, tissue plasminogen activator, diffuses from endothelial cells to convert plasminogen absorbed to the thrombus into plasmin, which degrades the fibrin polymer. Plasmin can also degrade fibrinogen, but systemic fibrinolysis does not occur because tissue plasminogen activator activates plasminogen more effectively when it is absorbed to fibrin thrombi. Furthermore, excess plasmin is rapidly bound and neutralized by α_2-plasmin inhibitor, and endothelial cells also release an inhibitor of plasminogen activator.

A variety of factors may be responsible for the development of thrombosis in the absence of endothelial injury. Low blood flow increases local concentrations of coagulation reactants. This may result from venous varicosities, prolonged bed rest, or stasis during and after an operation or illness. Factors that diminish arterial blood flow include cardiac disease or shock. Congenital or acquired abnormalities in the fibrinolytic system and certain dysfibrinogenaemias also predispose to intravascular thrombosis. While the last two specific disorders are of extreme interest and help to elucidate the complex mechanisms of thrombosis formation, they are identified in only 10 per cent of patients with thrombosis.

Antithrombin forms complexes with all of the serine protease coagulation factors except factor VII. The anticoagulant effect of heparin is due to acceleration of the rate of formation of this complex. The most common antithrombin deficiency causes a mild defect in 1 of 2000 individuals. Patients with antithrombin deficiency can develop acute thrombosis or embolism which should be treated with intravenous heparin, since they usually have sufficient functional antithrombin to act as a heparin cofactor. Subsequent treatment with oral anticoagulants prevents recurrent thrombosis. Relatives of the patient should also be screened, and those found to have low antithrombin levels should receive proplylactic anticoagulation with heparin or plasma infusions prior to surgical procedures in order to raise the antithrombin III level and decrease the risk of thrombosis. Chronic oral anticoagulation is not recommended unless a clinical thrombotic episode occurs.

Protein C is converted to an active protease by thrombin after binding to thrombomodulin. Activated protein C inactivates plasma cofactors V and VIII and stimulates the release of tissue plasminogen activator from endothelial cells. The inhibitory function of protein C is enhanced by protein S. Patients with acute thrombosis and moderate protein C or S deficiency should receive heparin followed by oral anticoagulants, although treatment with warfarin may further reduce the concentration of both proteins C and S. Deficiency in proteins C or S may predispose to the rare but serious complication of warfarin-induced skin necrosis. Homozygosity for protein C deficiency is rare, but can be a cause of intravascular coagulation in the neonate. These patients may require periodic plasma infusions rather than oral anticoagulants to prevent recurrent intravascular coagulation and thrombosis. Defects in fibrinogen or plasminogen or decreased synthesis or release of tissue plasminogen activator have been described. Patients with these disorders, as well as those with abnormal plasminogen, have been successfully treated with heparin and oral anticoagulants.

In addition to the heritable disorders, many common conditions and illnesses are associated with an increased risk of thrombosis. Age is an important factor in the development of thrombosis, and pulmonary embolism primarily affects the middle-aged and elderly. Cardiac disorders, especially congestive heart failure, acute myocardial infarction, and atrial fibrillation, are particularly conducive to the development of pulmonary embolism. Metastatic malignancy, particularly carcinoma of the pancreas and prostate, is also associated with an increased incidence of pulmonary embolism. Patients undergoing major surgical procedures or suffering major trauma or burns also have an increased risk of venous thrombosis. Factors produced in damaged or ischaemic tissues or in patients with metastatic disease, together with venous stasis and endothelial injury, induce the formation of venous thrombi.

Pregnancy increases the risk of pulmonary embolism because pressure from the gravid uterus retards venous flow from the legs and pelvis. Postpartum infection may also predispose to septic thrombophlebitis and embolism, and oral contraceptives, which lower antithrombin III levels, are also associated with the occurrence of pulmonary embolism. Several haematological disorders which cause poorly defined abnormalities in circulating leucocytes and platelets predispose patients to venous thrombosis. Diseases which affect the endothelial cells, or the administration of drugs such as L-asparaginase, which inhibits production of multiple coagulation factors, may also predispose patients to thrombosis.

VENOUS THROMBOSIS

Haemostatic thrombi that form in veins when blood flow is reduced are richly endowed with fibrin and entrapped blood cells and contain relatively few platelets. These are often called red thrombi. The friable ends of these thrombi which form in leg veins often break off and cause emboli in the pulmonary circulation (Fig. 1). Thrombus formation is typically asymptomatic and the site does not usually become inflamed. Inflammation of a thrombus in a vein is called thrombophlebitis. The acute inflammatory response makes the developing thrombus firmly adherent to the intima of the vessel wall, making embolization uncommon.

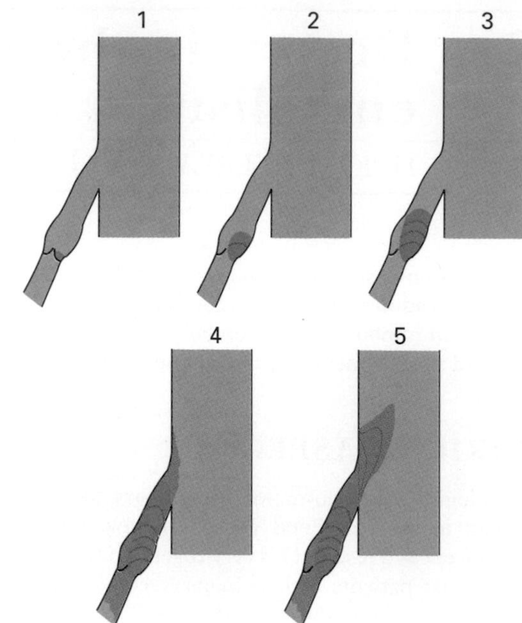

Fig. 1 Illustration showing propagation of deep thrombus arising in a valvular pocket with deposition of successive layers and ultimate extension of the non-adherent red thrombus into the lumen of a larger parent vein.

Venous thrombosis may involve the superficial or deep venous systems of the leg. When both systems are affected, thrombus formation usually begins in the deep veins and extends to the superficial system. Varicose veins are often associated with superficial thrombophlebitis of the lower extremities; other causes include occult malignant neoplasms, local trauma, and parenteral drug abuse. In a substantial number of patients the condition may be idiopathic.

The common clinical presentation of superficial thrombophlebitis is local pain, erythema, and induration, with tenderness of the thrombosed vein. When thrombophlebitis occurs below the knee, management consists of bed rest, leg elevation, and local application of heat to the affected veins. The disorder is usually self-limiting as obliteration of the affected part of the superficial venous system precludes subsequent attacks. The risk of thromboembolism is minimal and anticoagulation is not indicated. When thrombophlebitis extends above the knee, embolization may occur: such patients should be closely observed for cephalad progression of thrombus. Anticoagulation to prevent thromboembolism is indicated if the response to conservative management is poor.

Deep venous thrombosis is serious since the thrombus is much more likely to embolize to the lungs: when the thrombosis is proximal to the calf, there is a 50 per cent likelihood of pulmonary embolism, and up to 30 per cent of thrombi isolated to the calf veins embolize to the lungs. As many as 40 to 50 per cent of patients with deep venous thrombosis who develop pulmonary embolism have no symptoms of deep venous disease, causing a delay in the administration of appropriate prophylactic and therapeutic measures.

In patients who develop symptoms, mild oedema, superficial

venous dilatation, and pain in the calf are usually present. Palpation of the calf may disclose tenderness and occasionally a thrombosed vein can be felt at any site from the plantar aspect of the foot to the femoral triangle in the groin. A thrombosed vein is usually best identified by palpation in the popliteal space. Homans' sign (tenderness and tightness in the calf with hyperextension of the foot) provides further evidence of thrombosis, but it may be present with any type of calf muscle irritation and is not pathognomonic for thrombotic disease.

Most forms of deep venous thrombosis involve the popliteal vein and its tributaries, but occasionally the thrombosis extends proximally to the femoral or iliac veins. Swelling and pain in the distal thigh are more prominent if femoral vein thrombosis is present, but these signs may be absent. Phlegmasia caerulea dolens is the condition found when ileofemoral thrombosis is associated with massive swelling of the entire extremity to the inguinal ligament, severe pain, tenderness, and cyanosis. Ileofemoral arterial thrombosis with spasm is frequently present and is characterized by a pale cool extremity with diminished or absent pulses. Disease confined to the popliteal vein and its tributaries may be occult or confused with other conditions such as rupture of the gastrocnemius muscle or disorders involving the knee, particularly a ruptured Baker's cyst. It is therefore important to confirm objectively the presence of suspected deep venous thrombosis.

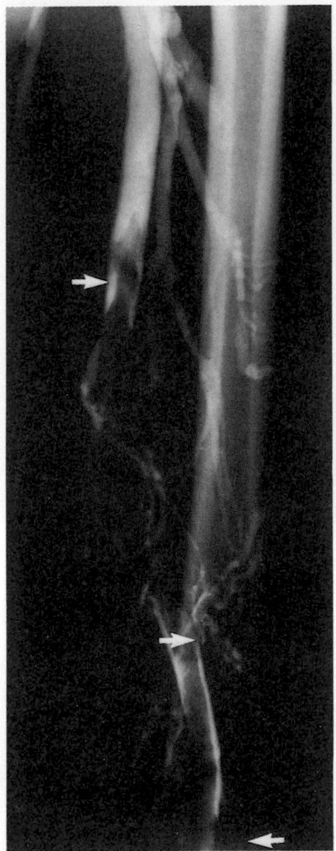
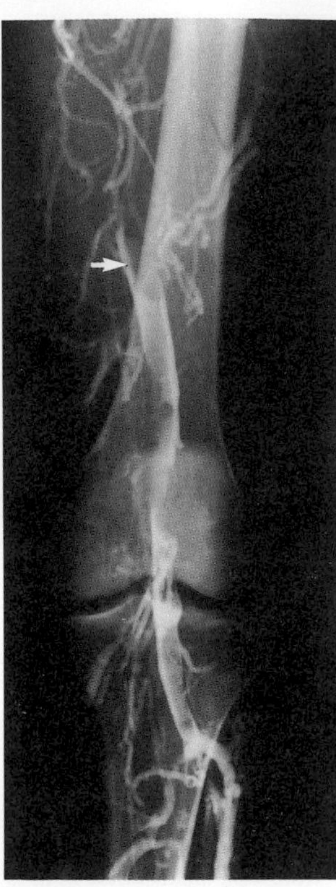

Fig. 2 Selected venograms showing 'intraluminal filling defects' which, in the vascular system, are diagnostic of acute thrombosis as outlined by radiographic contrast material (arrows). These are examples of extensive deep venous thrombosis involving the infrapopliteal veins of the calf, the popliteal vein, and the deep venous system of the thigh. The 'propagating tail' of the thrombus is identified in the mid-thigh.

Diagnostic tests

The most specific test for confirmation of the diagnosis of deep venous thrombosis is venography, in which contrast medium is injected into a vein on the dorsum of the foot to demonstrate the venous drainage through the popliteal, femoral, and iliac veins (Fig. 2). A normal result nearly always excludes the presence of venous thrombosis. However, venography may be complicated by venous thrombosis and extravasation of contrast media produces perivasculitis, cellulitis, and occasionally ulceration of the skin. Patients are, therefore, often initially screened with a non-invasive technique and undergo venography if the diagnosis remains in doubt. Venography using radioisotopes instead of contrast medium avoids complications, but although results with this technique are improving it is not in widespread use.

Real-time B-mode ultrasonic imaging combined with Doppler ultrasound (duplex scanning) is a practical, non-invasive method of assessment of blood flow in veins and valve cusp movement, and can differentiate between acute and chronic thrombosis. All of the major deep veins of the lower limb can be assessed; however, it cannot exclude the presence of thrombi in small veins and is less accurate in demonstrating thrombotic disease in the calf. With experience, it is both accurate and relatively inexpensive and can be used in patients requiring reassessment. Plethysmography is another non-invasive technique which is useful in the diagnosis of deep venous thrombosis. A calf plethysmograph measures volume changes and may detect the oedematous changes associated with thrombus formation. Like duplex scanning, plethysmography is helpful in demonstrating proximal thrombotic disease than that occurring in the calf.

Intravenous administration of radioactive fibrinogen is another sensitive non-invasive technique used to diagnose deep venous thrombosis. Following intravenous injection of [^{125}I]fibrinogen, the legs are scanned with a gamma-camera to detect the developing thrombus, which incorporates radioactive fibrinogen. This test is particularly accurate for detecting thrombosis in the calf, but high background radiation from the pelvic bones and urinary bladder means that it is not useful in assessing veins in the upper thigh. Any inflammatory condition also causes increased radioactivity, and results are not available for at least 12 h. Radioactive scanning of the lower extremities demonstrates deep venous thrombosis in as many as 54 per cent of patients following surgical treatment of a fractured hip, 50 per cent of patients following prostatectomy, and 28 per cent of general surgical patients over the age of 40. Scanning following injection of ^{111}I-labelled platelets may also be useful in the diagnosis of deep venous thrombosis.

Magnetic resonance imaging (MRI) is a reliable method of diagnosing venous thrombosis and can demonstrate thrombi in the pelvic veins (Fig. 3). MRI does not require the administration of intravenous contrast agents and can be used safely in patients with allergies to dye or with impaired renal function.

Treatment

Anticoagulation prevents the propagation of the original thrombus and the development of new thrombi while the existing thrombus is lysed by naturally occurring fibrinolysis. Intravenous heparin has rapid action and can be discontinued, or its effects reversed rapidly with protamine sulphate, to decrease the

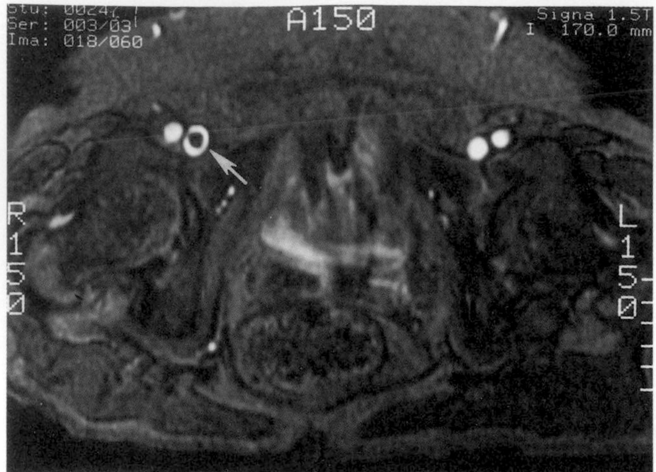

Fig. 3 Magnetic resonance image (33/13/60°) showing intraluminal thrombus (decreased signal) surrounded by flowing blood (high signal) in the right external iliac vein (arrow).

possibility of bleeding complications. Subcutaneous heparin is also effective.

Although anticoagulation is management of choice for most patients, fibrinolytics such as urokinase, streptokinase, and recombinant tissue plasminogen activator have been evaluated clinically. Fibrinolytics can completely lyse up to 70 per cent of existing thrombi, a feature that conventional anticoagulants lack. Among 108 patients with venographically verified deep venous thrombosis treated with streptokinase, total or partial thrombolysis was demonstrated angiographically in 60 (55.6 per cent). However, three died during treatment, all from pulmonary embolism, and six developed clinical signs suggestive of pulmonary embolism. Major bleeding was a complication in 16 patients (14.8 per cent), allergic reactions to streptokinase occurred in 23 patients, and one patient developed anaphylactic shock. Thus, although streptokinase was effective in the management of deep venous thrombosis, complications were significant and the routine use of fibrinolytic therapy has been prohibited by bleeding complications, especially in postoperative situations. In addition, lysis of thrombi more than 72 h old is reduced and fibrinolytics have no advantage over heparin in the prevention of recurrent venous thrombosis. Their role in managing deep venous thrombosis is therefore limited, although patients with extensive disease, such as in the iliofemoral system, may benefit from their use.

The surgical extraction of venous thrombi has been almost completely discontinued since the recurrence rate is high. Venous thrombectomy still has a role in the management of patients with extensive iliofemoral disease in which limb loss is imminent, such as in phlegmasia alba dolens.

Venous disorders of the upper extremities

With the increasing use of the intravenous route for infusion of fluid and pharmacological agents, the incidence of thrombophlebitis in the upper extremity has increased. Superficial thrombophlebitis is often associated with an indwelling venous catheter, and treatment is similar to that of superficial phlebitis in the lower extremity. If infection is suspected, the vein is aspirated with a large bore needle: if suppurative material is obtained the vein should be surgically excised. Antibiotics should be given, but anticoagulant therapy is usually not necessary since pulmonary embolism is an uncommon complication.

Thrombosis of the axillary and/or subclavian vein may occur when the upper extremity has been vigorously abducted at the shoulder, ceasing trauma to the vein. Venous obstruction may also occur when the vein is compressed between the clavicle and first rib, producing non-pitting oedema of the entire arm. Cyanotic mottling of the skin and distension of the superficial veins are also present. Axillary vein thrombosis may also be caused by congestive heart failure, indwelling venous catheters, external trauma, and neoplastic disease in the region of the axilla. The diagnosis is usually obvious after the history and physical examination and can be confirmed by venography. Treatment consists of arm rest in an elevated position and administration of anticoagulants. Venous thrombectomy may occasionally be performed, but rethrombosis is common. Subclavian vein occlusion may occur as an extension of axillary vein thrombosis or as a separate entity, and is commonly due to an indwelling venous catheter. Management is similar to that of axillary vein thrombosis. Recent series suggest that pulmonary embolism occurs in up to 12.4 per cent of patients with deep venous thrombosis of the upper extremity.

Occlusion of the superior vena cava may be caused by compression from a neoplasm or by lymphadenopathy. Trauma and/or infection from a central venous catheter may also cause thrombosis at this site. The superior vena caval syndrome includes cyanosis of the head and neck, with oedema of the upper chest and extremities and varying degrees of venous distension. Patients may complain of vertigo, headache, epistaxis, and occasionally fainting. Venography or MRI confirms and defines the level and extent of venous obstruction. Treatment includes anticoagulation and specific treatment of the underlying condition. Surgical excision of a neoplastic mass is occasionally indicated, and radiation therapy may be successful.

PULMONARY EMBOLISM

Pulmonary embolism is a common and sometimes fatal complication of deep venous thrombosis. Although it is recognized in the postoperative period, most patients develop pulmonary embolism secondary to non-surgical disorders, including congestive heart failure, cerebrovascular accidents, chronic pulmonary disease, systemic infections, carcinomatosis, and many chronic disorders.

Emboli that prove fatal are generally 1.5 cm or more in diameter and 50 cm or more in length, and are often fragmented (Fig. 4). The right pulmonary artery is more commonly affected than the left, and the lower lobes more often than the upper lobes. Emboli originate primarily in the systemic venous circulation—most arise in the iliac and femoral veins, but up to 20 per cent originate from other sources, including the inferior vena cava, the subclavian, axillary, and internal jugular veins, and occasionally the cavernous sinuses of the brain. Emboli due to neoplasms should also be considered in the differential diagnosis. Renal cell carcinoma metastasizes early in its clinical course, and direct extension to the renal vein and inferior vena cava may cause pulmonary embolism in 10 to 54 per cent of affected patients. Primary pulmonary neoplasms can also mimic pulmonary embolism. Cardiac tumours arising in the right atrium and right ventricle may be the site of extensive pulmonary emboli.

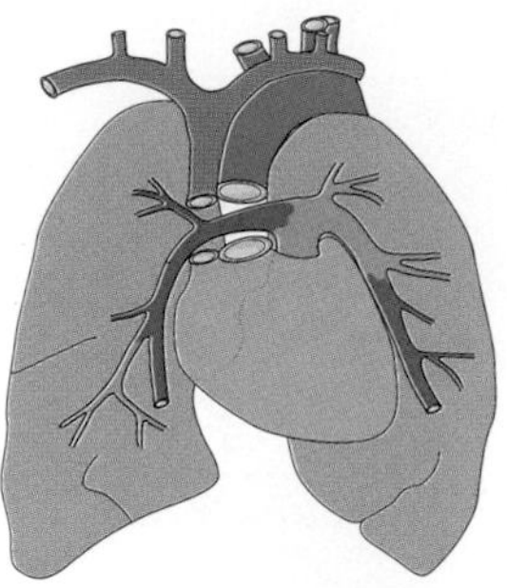

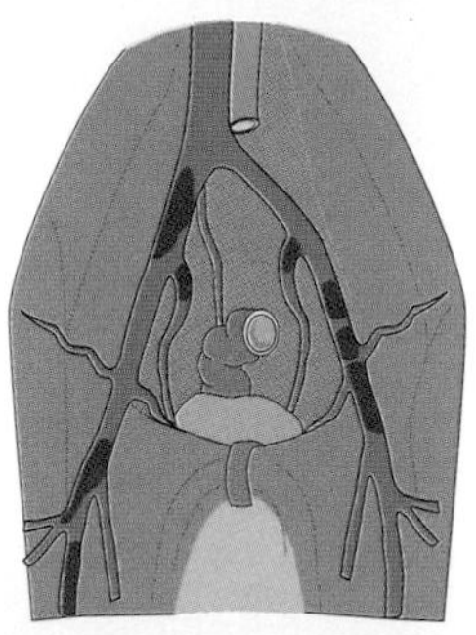

Fig. 4 Illustration of the findings in a patient with massive pulmonary embolism at the time of postmortem examination. Multiple thrombi are present in the iliofemoral system. The right pulmonary artery and its branches are totally occluded by emboli. The left lower lobar pulmonary artery is also occluded. Under these circumstances, the entire output of the right ventricle must pass through the left upper lobe, which greatly increases pulmonary resistance and right ventricular work. The sudden development of this degree of pulmonary arterial occlusion produces a clinical state of severe shock, since the left ventricle receives a much diminished amount of blood to supply the systemic arterial circulation. In otherwise normal patients, 50 per cent or more of the pulmonary arterial circulation must be occluded before serious cardiovascular manifestations are produced.

A primary feature of pulmonary blood flow is the low vascular resistance that enables flow in this bed to increase several-fold with minimal elevation of pulmonary arterial pressure. Physiological changes following pulmonary embolism are related to the size of the emboli and can be divided into those that produce microembolism (obstruction of terminal small arteries and arterioles) and those that produce macroembolism (occlusion of the large pulmonary vessels). Considerable reduction in the diameter of the main pulmonary artery and the primary branches (at least 50 per cent) is required to reduce pulmonary blood flow significantly or to produce pulmonary hypertension. Experimental thrombi of large diameter produced in the inferior vena cava and embolized to either the right or the left pulmonary artery 10 to 14 days after their formation produce minimal cardiovascular and respiratory responses. Occlusion of one pulmonary artery usually causes insignificant changes in the central venous pressure, right ventricular pressure, pulmonary arterial pressure, systemic arterial pressure, cardiac output, total oxygen consumption, and the electrocardiogram, despite occlusion of half of the pulmonary arterial circulation, provided the remaining lung is normal. If one lung is normal or nearly normal, removal of the opposite lung is relatively well tolerated: tidal volume and oxygen consumption at rest change only minimally. Similarly, ligation of one pulmonary artery or occlusion by an intraluminal balloon is accompanied by few cardiodynamic changes. During exercise similar occlusion causes an increase in pulmonary arterial pressure of only 12 to 50 per cent, while cardiac output may increase as much as three-fold. Such occlusion closely simulates the obstruction produced by large pulmonary emboli. It should be emphasized that these findings apply to healthy subjects: underlying cardiac or respiratory insufficiency alters this response appreciably. In patients with heart disease, exercise during unilateral occlusion of the right and left pulmonary artery by a balloon catheter produces a sharp elevation in pulmonary arterial pressure. Resection of less than one lung is followed by only minor changes in the pulmonary arterial pressure, whereas removal of a greater amount of pulmonary tissue is associated with elevated pulmonary arterial pressure.

Clearly, mechanical factors are the most important in determining the cardiodynamic effects of pulmonary embolism, but reflex effects may cause bronchoconstriction. Tachypnoea, pulmonary hypertension, and systemic hypotension have also been demonstrated following experimental embolization with small particles. This is probably not a common clinical problem, although it may occur after massive blood transfusion during which small emboli containing platelets, leucocytes, and fibrin may occlude the pulmonary microcirculation.

Clinical manifestations

A clinical diagnosis of pulmonary embolism may be difficult because of its similarity to a number of other cardiorespiratory disorders. Dyspnoea, chest pain, and haemoptysis are classic symptoms but are not sufficiently specific to establish a definite diagnosis. It should be emphasized that many patients have underlying cardiac disease, and dyspnoea and tachypnoea are the most frequent clinical findings. Accentuation of the pulmonary second sound is also common. Haemoptysis, pleural friction rub, gallop rhythm, hypotension, cyanosis, and chest splinting are present in no more than one-quarter of patients. Clinical evidence of venous thrombosis occurs in only one-third of patients. The signs and symptoms found in 1000 consecutive patients are shown in Table 1.

Table 1 Clinical manifestations in 1000 patients with pulmonary embolism

	Percentage
Symptoms	
Dyspnoea	77
Chest pain	63
Haemoptysis	26
Altered mental status	23
Dyspnoea, chest pain, haemoptysis	14
Signs	
Tachycardia	59
Recent fever	43
Rales	42
Tachypnoea	38
Leg oedema and tenderness	23
Elevated venous pressure	18
Shock	11
Accentuated P_2	11
Cyanosis	9
Pleural friction rub	8

Special examinations

In patients with acute pulmonary embolism and no other pulmonary disease, the plain chest radiograph is usually normal. Diminished pulmonary vascular marking at the site of embolism may be present (Westermark's sign). The ECG is not specific but significant changes can be confirmatory. No more than 10 to 20 per cent of patients subsequently proven to have pulmonary embolism show any alterations in the ECG, including disturbance of rhythm (atrial fibrillation, ectopic beats, heart block), enlargement of P waves, S-T segment depression, and T-wave inversion (particularly in leads III, AVF, V_1 and V_3), and of these, a smaller number show diagnostic abnormalities. The most common abnormality is S-T segment depression due to myocardial ischaemia, reduced cardiac output, and low systemic arterial pressures, as well as increased right ventricular pressure. Arterial blood gases are often normal, especially in young patients. Because clinical findings and routine examinations are non-specific, radioactive pulmonary scanning and pulmonary angiography are used to diagnose pulmonary embolism (Fig. 5). A schematic outline of the plan to be followed in establishing the diagnosis is shown in Fig. 6.

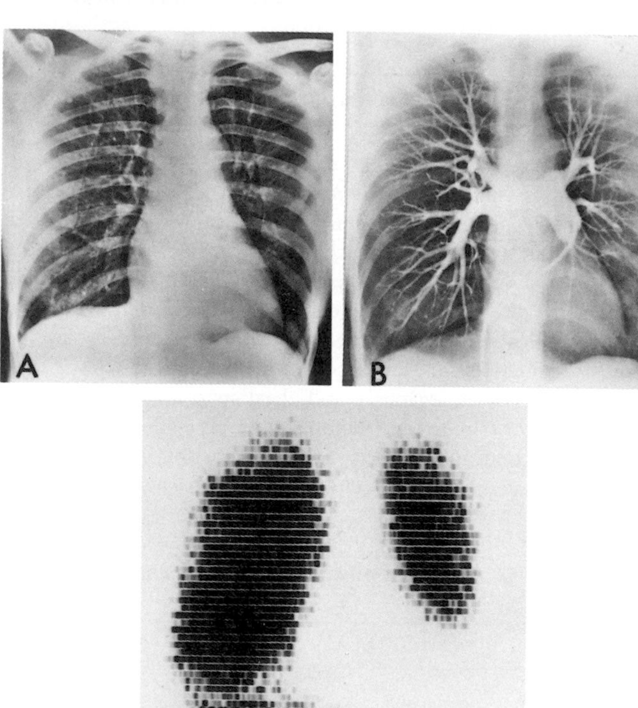

Fig. 5 Films from a patient with pulmonary embolism involving the left lower lobar pulmonary artery. (a) Slight diminution of the vascular markings to the left lower lobe is noted in comparison with those in the right lower lobe of the plain chest film (Westermark's sign). (b) Pulmonary arteriogram illustrating occlusion of the left lower lobe pulmonary artery. (c) Pulmonary scan showing absence of perfusion of the left lower lobe.

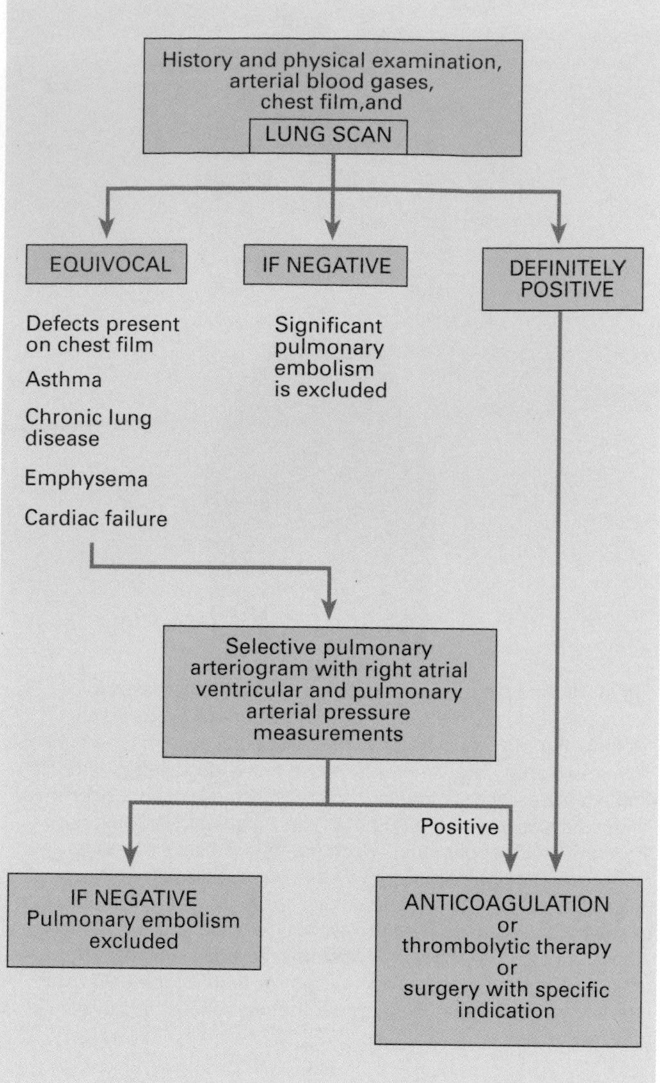

Fig. 6 A schematic outline of the plan to be followed in establishing the diagnosis of pulmonary embolism.

Radioactive pulmonary scanning

Radioisotope perfusion and ventilation pulmonary scans remain the most frequently employed technique in the diagnosis of pulmonary embolism. The method involves the detection of intravenously injected particles such as technetium–99m that become lodged in the pulmonary capillary bed.

The results of ventilation/perfusion scans are usually described in terms of the probability of embolism. High probability is indicated by segmental or greater perfusion defects with a normal ventilation scan (V/Q mismatch). Moderate probability is indicated by multiple subsegmental perfusion defects with a normal ventilation scan or segmental perfusion defects without a ventilation scan. Scans which are indeterminate show chronic obstructive pulmonary disease on the chest film or regions of perfusion scans, while subsegmental perfusion defects without a ventilation scan or matched perfusion and ventilation defects indicates a low probability of an embolism. High probability scans have a high positive predictive value for pulmonary embolism while low probability scans with low clinical suspicion are rarely associated with such emboli. Intermediate probability scans and low probability scans with high clinical suspicion are often associated with pulmonary embolism and indicate the need for arteriography to be performed.

Venograms or other non-invasive tests may be useful in establishing a definitive diagnosis of deep venous thrombosis, particularly in patients in whom the diagnosis is in doubt or when insertion of a vena caval umbrella is being considered.

The most definitive test for the diagnosis of pulmonary embolism is pulmonary arteriography. It is important that the appearance of the normal pulmonary angiogram is familiar in order that morphological and physiological changes can be appreciated. The arteries in the lower areas of the lung are normally larger because of a greater volume of pulmonary tissue. In most patients who survive the initial embolic episode the obstruction in the pulmonary arteries involves lobar or segmental branches. The defect should remain constant on several successive films in the series, and the flow may be sluggish, shown by a small pool of contrast medium that may persist in the artery above the obstruction after the venous phase of the angiogram. When pulmonary arteriography is performed later in the course of embolism, contrast medium may pass around the obstruction, causing delayed opacification of the artery distally. In some areas avascular segments resulting from unresolved thromboembolism may be seen. Oblique views of the pulmonary arteriogram should be obtained for maximal visualization and diagnostic accuracy. Pulmonary arteriography is safe when experienced radiologists use small diameter catheters and low osmolarity contrast agents.

MANAGEMENT

The importance of reaching an unequivocal diagnosis of pulmonary embolism before therapy is instituted warrants emphasis. The most reliable means of achieving absolute diagnosis are pulmonary scanning and arteriography. Because scanning is a simple, safe, and reliable technique, it is generally performed initially. If the pulmonary scan is to be used for definitive diagnosis, a concomitant plain chest film must show a normal pulmonary appearance in the area in which the scan demonstrates pulmonary arterial occlusion.

Prevention

Prophylaxis of deep venous thrombosis and pulmonary embolism is an important aspect of postoperative care. Nevertheless, no method or combination of methods completely prevents thromboembolism. Factors which reduce the risk include physical activity and elevation of the lower extremities for gravity drainage of venous return. Some consider compression of the legs by stockings or mechanical devices and prophylactic anticoagulation to be useful, but many disagree and these issues remain controversial. Early ambulation and resumption of physical activity after operation or bed rest for any reason has long been recommended.

Antiplatelet agents

Antiplatelet drugs play a role in the management of patients with thromboembolism. Non-steroidal anti-inflammatory drugs, including aspirin and dipyridamole, have also been shown to inhibit the platelet-release reaction secondary to ADP-induced platelet aggregation and adherence to collagen *in vitro*. Dipyridamole inhibits phosphodiesterase and raises intracellular cyclic AMP levels. The usual dose of 50 to 100 mg four times daily has no effect on platelet function, and it is usually administered in a combination with aspirin. Aspirin reduces the incidence of thrombosis from 20.4 per cent in controls to 12.5 per cent. In one study 1.2 g of aspirin daily was shown to be as effective as warfarin in preventing clinically diagnosed venous thrombosis and pulmonary embolism in a group of patients undergoing elective hip replacement. The incidence in the group receiving aspirin was 9 per cent, compared with 35 per cent in a previously studied control group. Studies of the overall effectiveness of antiplatelet drugs in the prevention of venous thrombosis and pulmonary embolism are continuing, because absolute certainty concerning their use has not yet been established. Dextran has also been used as an antiplatelet drug to prevent deep venous thrombosis.

Position and compression devices

Elevation of the legs with flexion of the knee as depicted in Fig. 7 causes a rapid runoff of the blood in the veins of the leg and thigh due to gravity. This is a simple, effective, and broadly applicable prophylactic measure. Pneumatic compression devices also decrease stasis and increase venous blood flow but are not widely used.

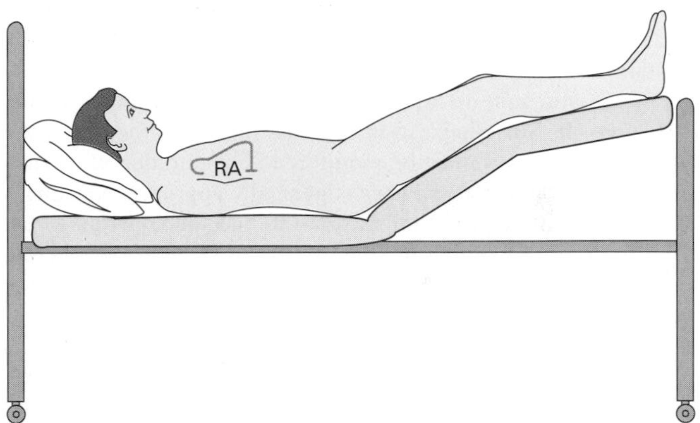

Fig. 7 Correct position for lower extremities in prophylaxis of pulmonary embolism. Note the additional break at the knee. It is important that the level of the veins in the lower extremities be above the mean level of the right atrium.

Prophylactic anticoagulation

While prophylactic anticoagulation may be beneficial, especially after trauma and in patients with orthopaedic disorders, the concept of low-dose heparin as a prophylactic measure remains controversial. The usual regimen is an initial dose of 5000 units subcutaneously, repeated every 8 to 12 h until the patient is fully ambulatory. Coagulation times are prolonged minimally, if at all, with a low risk of bleeding. The protection conferred, if any, may be due to the potentiation of a naturally occurring plasma inhibitor of activated factor X. A large number of trials with low-dose heparin given to surgical patients postoperatively have used ^{125}I-labelled fibrinogen scanning or venography, or both, for the demonstration of development of venous thrombosis. With some exceptions, these studies have generally indicated a decrease in the occurrence of deep venous thrombosis, compared with that in controls. The efficacy of low-dose heparin in the prevention of postoperative pulmonary embolism is less obvious. The most frequently quoted of these studies is a multicentre clinical trial involving more than 4000 patients. Another randomized study of a series of patients aged over 40 years undergoing intraperitoneal procedures under general anaesthesia lasting more than 30 min found that the incidence of calf vein thrombosis was reduced by low-dose heparin but that the incidence of proximal vein thrombosis and pulmonary emboli, which were detected by chest films, pulmonary function tests, and perfusion scanning, was not reduced.

Although low-dose heparin continues to be recommended by some to prevent thromboembolism, it is not frequently used. It appears to have limited value after prostatectomy, after myocardial infarction, and in major orthopaedic procedures, particularly repair of femoral fractures and reconstructive surgery of the hip and knee. Low-dose heparin prophylaxis is also inadequate for patients with an active thrombotic process. Finally, it may lead to heparin sensitivity and cause disseminated intravascular coagulation, a condition in which platelets aggregate into thrombi and which may result in gangrene of the extremities.

Anticoagulation therapy

Anticoagulation with heparin is the standard treatment for acute thrombosis and pulmonary embolism. Heparin is administered intravenously at an initial dose of 5000 to 10 000 units followed by constant infusion at a rate sufficient to raise the activated partial thromboplastin time to 1.5 to 2 times the control value, usually 1000 units/h. Since heparin is excreted mainly in the urine, the patient's renal status must be monitored. The duration of heparin therapy varies, but 5 to 10 days is generally appropriate as this is the time usually required for thrombi to become adherent to the venous wall. Oral coumarin therapy, begun several days before cessation of heparin therapy, allows adequate prolongation of the prothrombin time.

The major complication associated with heparin therapy is bleeding, especially from surgical sites and into the retroperitoneum. Aspirin therapy, poor platelet function, and intramuscular injections may contribute to the risk of significant bleeding. Although heparin anticoagulation can be rapidly reversed by the administration of protamine sulphate, this is not usually necessary as reduction or cessation of heparin often stops the bleeding. Delayed haemorrhage may occur in patients with recent prosthetic arterial grafts. Continuous lysis and resorption of old thrombus and its replacement with new thrombus occurs in suture lines until they are sealed by regeneration of new intima. Haemorrhage may occur up to 1 month after the placement of arterial grafts in patients maintained on heparin therapy. Contraindications to heparin therapy include internal bleeding, intracranial neoplasm, recent cranial surgery, trauma, or haemorrhagic stroke.

Thrombocytopenia occurs in about 10 per cent of heparin recipients: this may be severe, accompanied by intravascular platelet aggregation and arterial thrombosis. Recognition of this complication is critical since cessation of heparin can reverse this syndrome and may be life-saving. Commercial heparin preparations are heterogeneous and only about 20 per cent of the infused material has anticoagulant activity. Low molecular weight heparin fractions that retain anticoagulant activity are the treatment of choice in patients with heparin-dependent thrombocytopenia who require additional therapy. These fractions do not interact with platelets and may not cause thrombocytopenia. Administration of heparin for longer than 2 months is also associated with a risk of osteoporosis.

The coumarin anticoagulants (coumadin and warfarin), which prevent the reduction of vitamin K in the liver and induce a state analogous to vitamin K deficiency, are used to prevent the recurrence of venous thrombosis and pulmonary embolism. The average loading dose of coumadin is 15 to 30 mg on the first day and 10 to 20 mg on the second day. The maximal effect is usually reached in 36 to 48 h, and the average daily maintenance dose is usually between 5 and 10 mg (range 2–20 mg). Anticoagulation is easily achieved by administration of coumadin once daily, adjusting the dose until the desired prolongation of the prothrombin time is achieved.

The prothrombin time should be monitored regularly in patients receiving oral anticoagulants. Despite the most careful management, prothrombin time may fluctuate, and drugs that alter anticoagulant metabolism or degradation in the liver or which compete with albumin binding sites can increase or decrease their potency.

There is a direct relationship between the duration of anticoagulation and the risk of recurrent thrombosis. Although recommendations vary, most patients with a single uncomplicated thromboembolic event have maximal benefit after 3 to 6 months of anticoagulation. About 10 per cent of patients treated with an oral anticoagulant for 1 year have a serous complication requiring medical supervision and 0.5 to 1 per cent have a fatal haemorrhagic event, despite careful medical management. The anticoagulation effects of coumadin can be reversed by infusion of fresh frozen plasma or by the administration of vitamin K. In many patients reduction or omission of several doses improves haemostasis and stops haemorrhage. Despite the risk of bleeding, patients with prosthetic heart valves, severe mitral stenosis, cardiomyopathy, chronic congestive heart failure, recurrent or persistent atrial fibrillation, and an inherited prethrombotic disorder may require life-long anticoagulation.

Fibrinolytic therapy

Activators of the fibrinolytic system are frequently used to accelerate lysis of thrombi. These agents are either naturally occurring products or chemically modified derivatives, and they differ with respect to fibrin specificity and complications. Current indications for fibrinolytic therapy include patients with massive pulmonary embolism complicated by hypotension, severe hypoxaemia, and right heart strain or failure. In addition, fibrinolytic agents have been successfully administered to patients with extensive iliofemoral thrombophlebitis. While such therapy often resolves venous thrombi, there is no firm evidence that lytic therapy reduces the incidence of long-term complications. Fibrinolytic therapy may be of benefit in patients with thrombosis of the axillary vein, which does not respond well to conventional anticoagulation.

Two thrombolytic agents, streptokinase and urokinase, have been studied extensively. Both act by transforming plasminogen to plasmin but cannot discriminate between free and fibrin-bound plasminogen. Streptokinase is a soluble product of the metabolism of *Streptococcus pyogenes* (Lancefield Group A) which indirectly activates plasminogen. Patients who have suffered previous streptococcal infections may be allergic to streptokinase, clinically manifest as toxic reactions such as pyrexia, dyspnoea, tachycardia, and anaphylaxis. Urokinase is a product of renal epithelial and tubular cells which directly activates plasminogen. In a national co-operative study, urokinase combined with heparin therapy, compared with heparin alone, significantly accelerated the resolution of pulmonary thromboemboli at 24 h, as shown by pulmonary arteriograms, pulmonary scans, and right-sided heart pressure measurement. However, no significant differences in the recurrence rate of pulmonary embolism or in 2-week mortality were noted. Bleeding was a common complication, occurring in 45 per cent of patients receiving urokinase and heparin, compared with 27 per cent of those given heparin alone.

In a study of the long-term effects of thrombolytic treatment of acute and massive embolism, seven patients underwent pulmonary angiography with pressure measurements before and after intrapulmonary infusion of urokinase (average dose, 1724 units/kg.h) and heparin (average dose 17 units/kg.h). The treatment was monitored by daily measurements of pulmonary arterial pressure and was continued until normal pressure was achieved (an average of 6 days). Pulmonary angiograms showed massive obstruction before therapy, with improvement occurring within 6 days after treatment. The mean pulmonary arterial pressure declined from an average of 37 ± 9 to 13 mmHg after 6 days and to 15 ± 3 mmHg after 15 months. No recurrence of pulmonary embolism was observed. Mean pulmonary arterial pressure and total pulmonary resistance remained within normal limits in six of seven patients, at rest and during bicycle exercise in the supine position. All patients showed clinical signs of deep venous thrombosis early after treatment. Fifteen months later, four patients had normal deep veins, and three had phlebographic signs of old thrombosis. Normal pulmonary arteriograms were obtained in six of seven patients. The reserve capacity of the pulmonary vasculature assessed during heavy exercise was normal.

Streptokinase is usually given with a loading dose of 250 000: this may need to be repeated since patients may have antistreptococcal antibodies. Urokinase is given with a loading dose of 4400 units/kg body weight, administered over 10 to 30 min. A systemic lytic state develops with a decrease in fibrinogen levels, prolongation of the thrombin time, and prolongation of the euglobin lysis time. After the initial loading dose, 100 000 units of streptokinase or 4400 units of urokinase/kg body weight are administered hourly for 24 to 72 h. The lytic state is reversed by discontinuing the enzyme. Heparin therapy can be started after 6 h and is continued for 7 to 10 days. Fibrinolytic therapy should be initiated as soon as possible after the onset of thrombosis or embolism. The systemic fibrinolysis associated with the fibrinolytic agents may cause haemorrhage since essential haemostatic plugs are attached as well as pathological thrombi. Lytic therapy is therefore not recommended for patients with recent surgery or those with a history of a neurological lesion, gastrointestinal bleeding, or hypertension.

Recombinant tissue plasminogen activator is now available for general use. In one study, a group of patients with angiographically documented pulmonary embolism, all of whom had segmental or proximal pulmonary arterial obstruction within 5 days of the onset of symptoms or signs, were treated with 50 mg of recombinant tissue plasminogen activator every 2 h followed by an additional 40 mg every 4 h if required. Thirty-four of the 36 patients had angiographic evidence of thrombolysis by 6 h: clot lysis was slight in four, moderate in six, and marked in 24. Fibrinogen levels decreased by 30 per cent at 2 h and by 38 per cent at 6 h, with only two major complications. Infusion of recombinant tissue plasminogen activator via the artery does not offer significant benefit over administration by the intravenous route. Firm contraindications to the use of thrombolytic therapy include internal bleeding (recent or active), recent neurosurgery, insertion of an arterial prosthetic graft, cranial trauma, and a history of haemorrhagic cerebrovascular accident. Relative contraindications include a recent surgical procedure (within 7–10 days), cardiopulmonary resuscitation (within 7–10 days), or the presence of a coagulopathy.

Surgical management

While anticoagulant therapy of pulmonary embolism is usually successful, it may fail, and in this event the need for surgical management should be reviewed on an individual basis. Venous thrombectomy was previously recommended but is now rarely performed because of the high incidence of recurrent postoperative thrombosis. The presence of phlegmasia caerulea dolens with secondary arterial spasm is a rare indication for thrombectomy. Although thrombosis may recur in such patients, the venous lumen may remain patent for long enough to relieve the arterial spasm and prevent gangrene developing.

Although vena caval interruption was previously recommended for selected patients with pulmonary embolism, it is seldom performed today. A stainless steel umbrella designed by Greenfield and Michna can be inserted under local anaesthesia through the femoral or jugular vein. With this device a filter is fixed to the wall of the inferior vena cava by hooks (Fig. 8). Complications include distal migration to the bifurcation of the inferior vena cava, protrusion of the struts through the caval wall, formation of thrombus on the filter, misplacement of the device, retroperitoneal haemorrhage, perforation of the duodenum or ureter, and development of a thrombus proximal to the umbrella, producing emboli. The filter may also migrate into the iliac vein, renal vein, right atrium, right ventricle, or pulmonary artery, and such migration is occasionally fatal. The filter may also stimulate distal thrombosis in the vena cava and late occlusion may occur. Other filter types used are the Amplatz, Gunther, and birds nest.

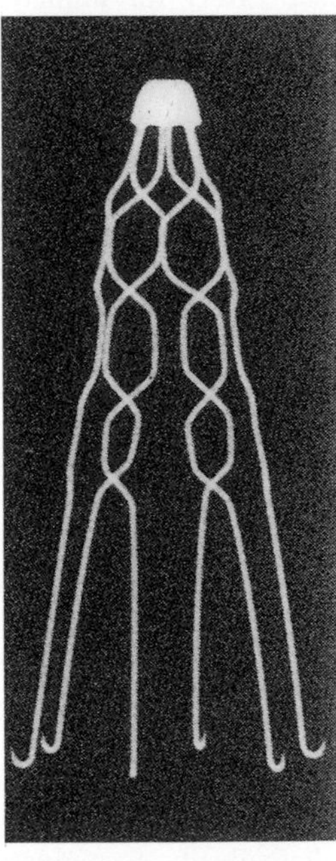

Fig. 8 Example of Kim-Ray Greenfield filter.

Pulmonary embolectomy

In 1908, Trendelenburg performed the first pulmonary embolectomy. He treated three patients with this procedure, the longest survival time being 36 h. In 1924, Kirschner performed the first successful pulmonary embolectomy associated with long-term survival. The first successful pulmonary embolectomy performed using extracorporeal circulation was reported in 1961: this is currently the preferred technique, since it permits continuous oxygenation of the body while the emboli are safely removed from the pulmonary arteries.

Persistent and refractory hypotension despite maximal resuscitation is the primary indication for pulmonary embolectomy, especially in a patient with massive embolism clearly documented by either a pulmonary scan or pulmonary arteriogram. Treatment includes systemic heparinization and the administration of vasopressors, inotropic agents, and endotracheal oxygen. The primary management should be by this approach, since many patients previously thought to require embolectomy respond favourably with intensive resuscitation. Usually, 1 or 2 h may be spent attempting to restore acceptable cardiopulmonary function, unless the clinical situation is desperate. An appropriate blood pressure should be maintained and embolectomy may be postponed, especially if renal and cerebral function is acceptable.

If pulmonary embolectomy is indicated, it is usually performed using cardiopulmonary bypass. A median sternotomy is made for exposure of the pulmonary artery. The main pulmonary artery is usually found to be free of emboli, although partial obstruction may be present. The emboli are removed from the right and left pulmonary arteries and from their major branches. Smaller emboli may be removed by passage of a Fogarty catheter and irrigation with saline. The pulmonary artery is closed and cardiopulmonary bypass is gradually discontinued, allowing the heart and lungs to resume normal function. An illustration of an embolectomy specimen and the patient's scan is shown in Fig. 9.

Patients with acute and severe cardiopulmonary collapse can be supported by partial cardiopulmonary bypass by a circuit from femoral vein to femoral artery for immediate resuscitation. If extracorporeal circulation is not available, a right or left thoracotomy with exposure of the most severely involved pulmonary artery can be performed, the side of predominant occlusion being determined by a scan or arteriogram. An anterior thoracotomy is appropriate for exposure of either the right or left pulmonary artery, which can be opened distally for removal of emboli while normal circulation to the opposite lung is maintained. A serious complication which may follow pulmonary embolectomy is massive endobronchial haemorrhage. Successful management involves endotracheal intubation for selective collapse of the lung and entrapment of the haemorrhage into the involved lung. Reperfusion pulmonary oedema may occur after pulmonary artery thromboendarterectomy, and prolonged mechanical ventilation is often required. The syndrome is a cause of postoperative hypoxaemia with local pulmonary infiltrate.

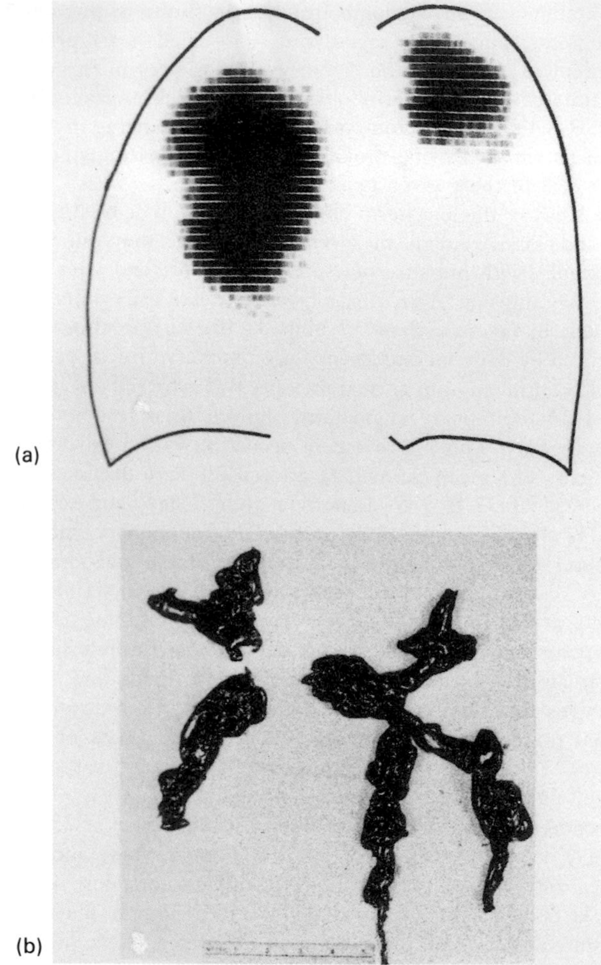

Fig. 9 Illustration from a patient with massive pulmonary embolism on the twelfth postoperative day following an orthopaedic operation and accompanied by intractable shock. (a) The pulmonary scan shows massive occlusion of the right lower and middle lobar pulmonary arteries as well as nearly all of the pulmonary arterial circulation of the left lung. (b) Emboli removed from both pulmonary arteries at the time of embolectomy.

Chronic pulmonary emboli

Most pulmonary emboli eventually resolve as a result of the action of the natural fibrinolytic systems. In a small number of patients, however, these emboli gradually accumulate in the pulmonary arterial system owing to inadequate fibrinolysis or recurrent episodes of embolism. Patients with chronic pulmonary emboli have a history of exertional dyspnoea progressing to severe respiratory insufficiency over several months or years. They may also complain of recurrent episodes of thrombophlebitis, haemoptysis due to the presence of large bronchial collaterals, and chest pain. Physical findings include signs of severe pulmonary hypertension, often combined with evidence of right ventricular failure; this may be manifested as a increased pulmonary second sound, a systolic murmur, hepatomegaly, and a S3 or S4 gallop. Medical management is usually unsatisfactory, and these patients have a poor prognosis.

Chest radiographs show a dilated pulmonary artery and oligaemic pulmonary fields in approximately half of these patients. Right ventricular enlargement is present in two-thirds and pleural effusion in approximately one-third of patients. Analysis of arterial blood gases in patients breathing room air reveals evidence of severe respiratory insufficiency, with hypoxaemia and arterial oxygen tension values of 55 to 60 mmHg and an arterial carbon dioxide tension ($P\text{aCO}_2$) of approximately 30 mmHg. The electrocardiogram is usually suggestive of chronic cor pulmonale, including right-axis deviation and right ventricular hypertrophy. Peripheral venography or MRI demonstrates venous thrombosis and indicates the source of the emboli.

Ventilation and perfusion radionuclide scans are consistent with the presence of pulmonary emboli, and perfusion defects correspond to oligaemic regions of the plain chest film and pulmonary arteriogram. Perfusion defects are usually noted bilaterally. Pulmonary arteriography allows documentation of emboli, determination of anatomical distribution of emboli, and recording of pulmonary artery pressure: the natural history is related to the magnitude of pulmonary arterial hypertension. If the mean pulmonary artery pressure is more than 30 mmHg, survival at 5 years is only 30 per cent, while only 10 per cent of those with mean pressure greater than 50 mmHg are alive at 5 years. Arteriography usually shows emboli in both lungs, with 55 to 75 per cent of the total pulmonary blood flow obstructed. Further preoperative studies include a thoracic aortogram with selective bronchial arteriography to demonstrate dilated and tortuous bronchial vessels. The bronchial circulation is often considerably dilated and communicates by collaterals with the distal pulmonary arteries.

Surgical management

Embolectomy may be performed on one or both pulmonary arteries. Either a right or left anterior thoracotomy can be undertaken when there is proximal occlusion of one vessel. Patients with bilateral pulmonary emboli, or with embolus of the main pulmonary artery, generally requires extracorporeal circulation during the procedure. These emboli are firmly attached to the artery wall and great care is required in the dissection. All distal emboli should be removed until there is adequate back-bleeding of bright red arterialized blood. Satisfactory distal back-bleeding can usually be predicted in advance from the information gained by selective injection of the bronchial arteries.

Postoperative complications include right ventricular failure in patients with long-standing cor pulmonale and pulmonary hypertension, haemorrhagic lung syndrome, which can be managed successfully by tracheal intubation with a dual lumen catheter and balloon occlusion of the affected lung, and phrenic nerve paresis, usually as a result of topical hypothermia. Psychiatric disturbances may also occur and are usually transient.

Embolectomy for chronic pulmonary embolism generally decrease pulmonary artery pressures and increases $P\text{aO}_2$ toward normal. In patients with proximal pulmonary arterial obstruction pulmonary embolectomy is likely to produce relief of respiratory insufficiency, a reduction in pulmonary hypertension, and an improvement of right-sided heart failure.

FURTHER READING

Bauer KA, Rosenberg RD. Congenital antithrombin III deficiency: insights into the pathogenesis of the hypercoagulable state and its management using markers of hemostatic system activation. *Am J Med* 1989; **87 (Suppl 3B)**: 39S–43S.

Bettman MA. Noninvasive and venographic diagnosis of deep vein thrombosis. *Cardiovasc Intervent Radiol* 1988; **11**: S15.

Broekmans AW, Vektkamp JJ, Bertina RM. Congenital protein C deficiency and venous thromboembolism: a study of three Dutch families. *N Engl J Med* 1983; **309**: 340.

Chitwood WR Jr, Lyerly HK, Sabiston DC Jr. Surgical management of chronic pulmonary embolism. *Ann Surg* 1985; **201**: 11.

Coon WW. Venous thromboembolism: prevalence, risk factors, and prevention. *Clin Chest Med* 1984; **5**: 391.

Ezekowitz MD, *et al.* Indium–111 platelet scintigraphy for the diagnosis of acute venous thrombosis. *Circulation* 1986; **73**: 668.

Hirsch J. Diagnosis of venous thrombosis and pulmonary embolism. *Am J Cardiol* 1990; 65: 45C.

Huisman MV, *et al.* Unexpected high prevalence of silent pulmonary embolism in patients with deep vein thrombosis. *Chest* 1989; **95**: 498.

Kelley MA, Carson JL, Palevsky HI, Schwartz JS. Diagnosing pulmonary embolism: new facts and strategies. *Ann Intern Med* 1991; **114**: 300.

Latham B, Kafoy EA, Barrett OJr, Gonzalez MF. Deficient tissue plasminogen activator release and normal tissue plasminogen activator inhibitor in a patient with recurrent deep vein thrombosis. *Am J Med* 1990; **88**: 199.

Loscalzo J, Braunwald E. Tissue plasminogen activator. *N Engl J Med* 1988; **319**: 925.

Makhoul RG, Greenberg CS, McCann RL. Heparin-associated thrombocytopenia and thrombosis: A serious clinical problem and potential solution. *J Vasc Surg* 1986; **5**: 522.

Maxwell RJ, Greenfield LJ. Effects of pulmonary embolism on survival of patients with Greenfield vena caval filters. *Surgery* 1987; **101**: 389.

Sabiston DC Jr, Wagner HN Jr. The diagnosis of pulmonary embolism by radioisotope scanning. *Ann Surg* 1964; **160**: 585.

Sabiston DC Jr, Wolfe WG. Experimental and clinical observations on the natural history of pulmonary embolism. *Ann Surg* 1968; **168**: 1.

Sandler DA, *et al.* Diagnosis of deep vein thrombosis: comparison of clinical evaluation, ultrasound, plethysmography, and venoscan with X-ray venogram. *Lancet* 1984; **ii**: 716.

Schafer AL. The hypercoagulable states. *Ann Intern Med* 1985; **102**: 814.

Thomas DP. Overview of venous thrombogenesis. *Sem Thromb Hemostasis* 1988; **14**: 1.

Virchow R. *Cellularpathologie in ihrer Begrudung auf physiologische und pathologishce Gewebelehre*. Berlin: A. Hirschwald, 1858.

White RH, McGahan JP, Daschbach MM, Harling RP. Diagnosis of deep-vein thrombosis using duplex ultrasound. *Ann Intern Med* 1989; **111**: 297.

Abnormalities of the lymphatic system

9

9 Abnormalities of the lymphatic system

KEVIN G. BURNAND

INTRODUCTION

The lymphatic system develops from four cystic spaces that appear on either side of the neck and in both groins. These large cisterns develop communications (lymphatic vessels or lymphangioles) which allow most of the lymph from the lower limbs and abdomen to be channelled through the cisterna chylae into the thoracic duct, which passes up on the left side of the bodies of the thoracic vertebrae before entering the internal jugular vein in the left hand side of the neck. A separate lymphatic trunk which drains lymph from the right upper limb and right side of the head and neck enters the right internal jugular vein. Lymph nodes develop as condensations along the course of these lymphatic pathways.

Abnormalities of development result in lymphatic aplasia, cystic hygroma, lymphatic and nodal hypo- and hyperplasia, and lymphangiomas.

FUNCTION

The lymphatic system has two main functions. The first is to remove macromolecules and excessive fluid from the interstitial space. Large molecules that escape into the tissue fluid have considerable difficulty in re-entering the vascular compartment. Proteins such as albumin, globulins, and fibrinogen that enter the interstitial fluid are usually returned to the plasma through the lymphatics. A number of coagulation factors and fibrinolytic activators also enter the lymph. Between 2 and 4 litres of interstitial fluid are returned to the vascular compartment each day by the lymphatics (Fig. 1).

The second major function of the lymphatics is to allow the circulation of lymphocytes from the lymph nodes into the bloodstream. Most exogenous antigens are presented to the central lymphoid system for the first time via the lymphatics. Recognition of antigens, with subsequent proliferation of specific clones of lymphocytes, takes place in the lymph nodes. Activated lymphocytes then pass into the circulation and thus to the other lymphatic tissues throughout the body.

PHYSIOLOGY

The interstitial space has a negative pressure and this, in combination with the hydrostatic pressures of the capillaries, encourages fluid to escape from the vascular compartment, overcoming the oncotic pressure of the plasma proteins which acts to suck fluid back into the circulation. The intraluminal pressure of the lymph system is similar to that of the interstitial fluid, and lymph capillaries must therefore actively absorb proteins through their pores. The mechanism by which this is achieved is unknown, but appears to require energy.

The lymphatic capillaries have large pores to allow large molecules to enter the lumen, and many valves that prevent the reflux of lymph and encourage its onward passage. Lymphatics have some circular smooth muscle in their wall and are capable of contraction. The combination of inherent contractility and valves ensure that lymph is propelled along the lymphatics and into the veins. Other factors that may influence lymphatic drainage include compression from surrounding arteries, and the negative pressure of the thoracic cavity sucking lymph upwards into the thorax from the abdomen.

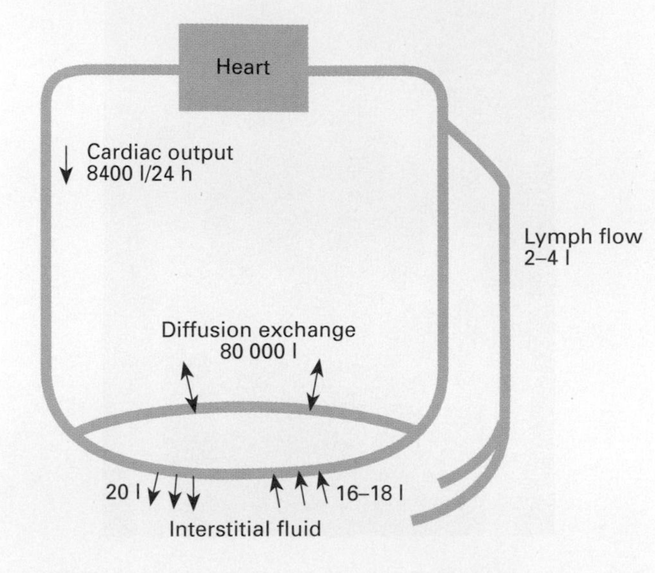

Fig. 1 The circulation passing through the interstitial fluid showing the contribution of the lymph circulation (2–4 l/day).

Content	Filtrate	Absorbate	Lymph
Fluid (l)	20	16–18	2–4
Protein (g)	80–200	0–5	75–195

LYMPHOEDEMA

This is defined as the excessive accumulation of interstitial fluid as a result of defective lymphatic drainage. The condition may be further subdivided into primary and secondary lymphoedema, secondary lymphoedema being the most common. Primary lymphoedema is three times more common in women than in men and has no known cause; secondary lymphoedema is the result of some recognized pathological process disrupting the lymphatic drainage.

Further subdivisions of primary lymphoedema have been made on the basis of the anatomical lymphatic abnormalities that are present. The lymphatic channels may be absent or severely hypoplastic (Fig. 2), being few in number and petering out more proximally. They may also be excessive in number (Fig. 3), though defective in function: such lymphatic hyperplasia is usually associated with excessive numbers of lymph nodes. The lymphatics may be dilated and ectatic (megalymphatics) (Fig. 4) and this abnormality is often associated with chylous ascites, chylothorax, and lymphatic reflux. Finally the lymphatics may be obstructed (Fig. 5); in primary lymphoedema this is often associated with fibrosis within the lymph nodes.

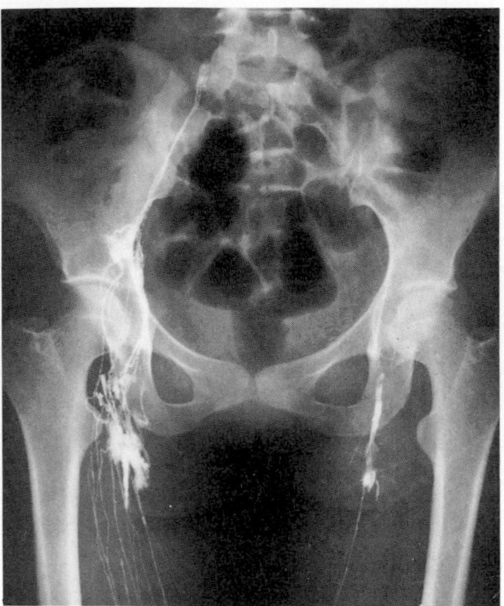

Fig. 2 A lymphangiogram showing severe hypoplasia of lymphatic channels in the left leg compared to normal numbers in the right leg. Proximal obstruction probably coexists in the nodes of the groin and left iliac region.

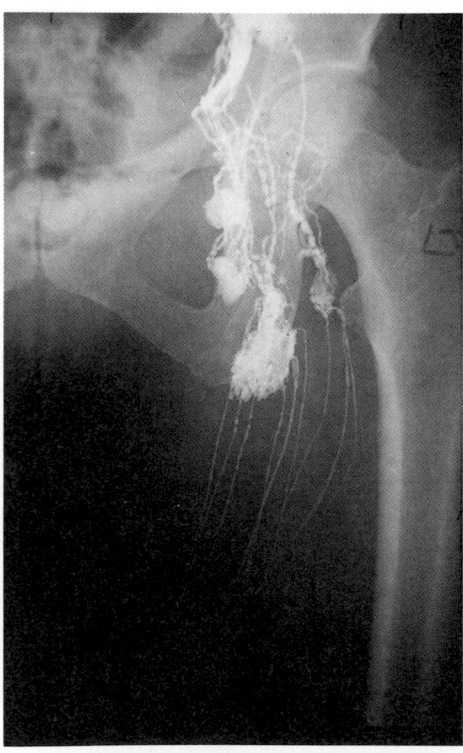

Fig. 3 A lymphangiogram demonstrating hyperplasia of the lymphatic channels with excessive numbers of lymphatics with enlarged lymph nodes in the groin.

Secondary lymphoedema

All patients presenting with lymphoedema must have a possible 'cause', excluded by careful examination and special tests where necessary.

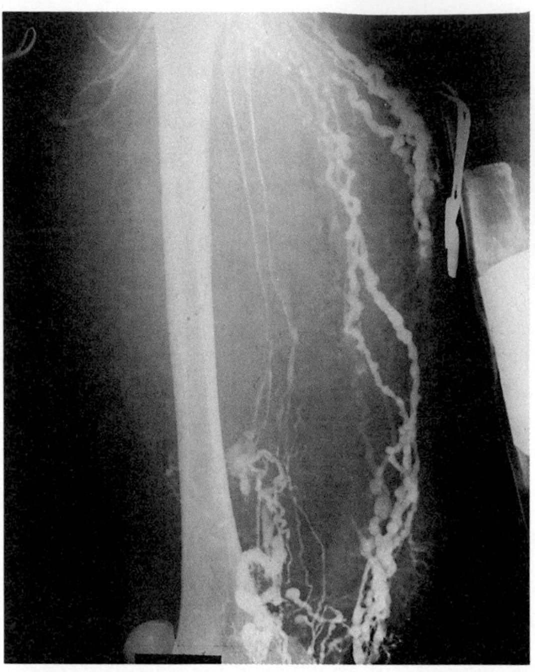

Fig. 4 Dilated ectatic lymphatics are present in the thigh without any competent valves.

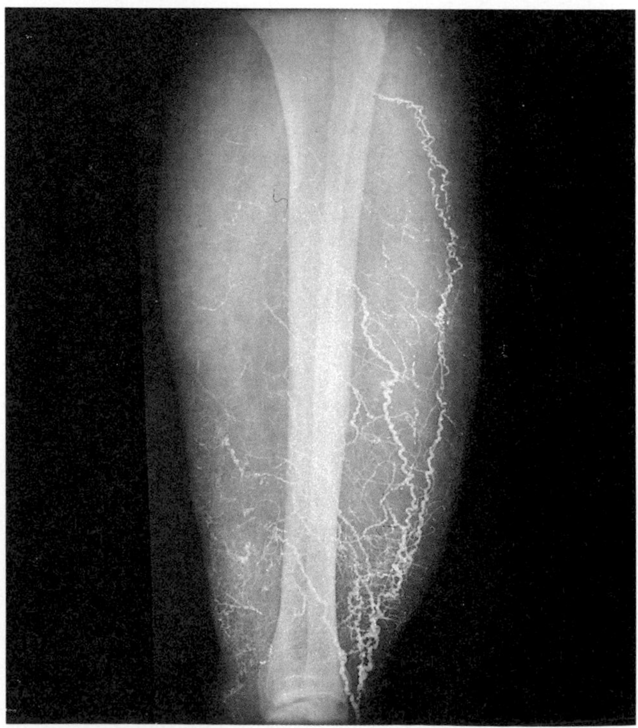

Fig. 5 Obstructed lymphatics in the calf with many extra lymphatics filling because of the proximal obstruction. The lymphatics are tortuous and fade out proximally.

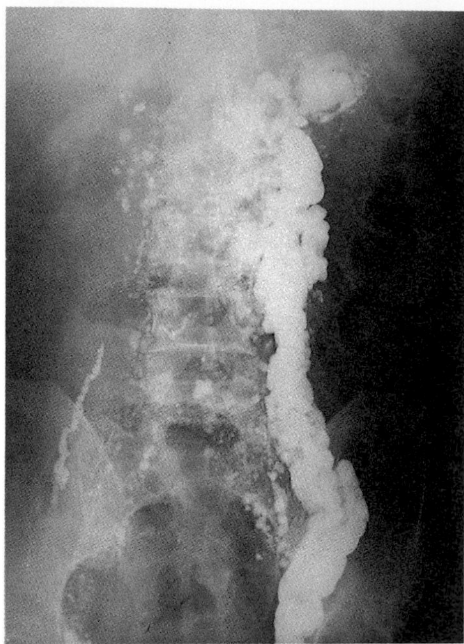

Fig. 6 A lymphangiogram showing massively dilated retroperitoneal lymphatic channels in a patient with filariasis.

Filariasis

This helminthic infection is a major global cause of lymphoedema. It is endemic in parts of Africa, especially the west coast, and is also common in India and parts of South America. The worm enters the lymphatics and lodges in the lymph nodes, where a severe fibrotic reaction causes obstruction to the lymphatic pathways, which are often grossly dilated (Fig. 6). This results in severe swelling of the limbs (usually the lower) called 'elephantiasis'.

The diagnosis is confirmed by finding microfilariae, which enter the blood in large numbers at night. To provide the maximum possibility of detecting filariae, a blood sample should be taken at midnight. A strongly positive complement fixation test suggests active or past filariasis.

Treatment with diethylcarbamazine destroys the filariae but does not reverse established lymphoedema; progression of the disease may, however, be slowed or prevented. Established lymphoedema is treated by the same methods as those used to treat primary lymphoedema.

Malignancy

Any malignant process that spreads to the lymph nodes can cause secondary lymphoedema, but this is more common after surgical resection or radiotherapy directed against nodal deposits of tumour. Hodgkin's disease and the non-Hodgkin's lymphomas can present with lymphoedema; this may also occur in patients with malignant melanomas and testicular seminomas (Fig. 7).

Surgical block dissection

This operation is invariably carried out to treat malignancies affecting lymph nodes, although in many cases it forms part of a staging or prophylactic procedure. The carcinomas commonly requiring block dissections are those of the breast and uterus. Malignant melanoma and testicular tumours are also often treated by block dissection or irradiation (Fig. 8a, b).

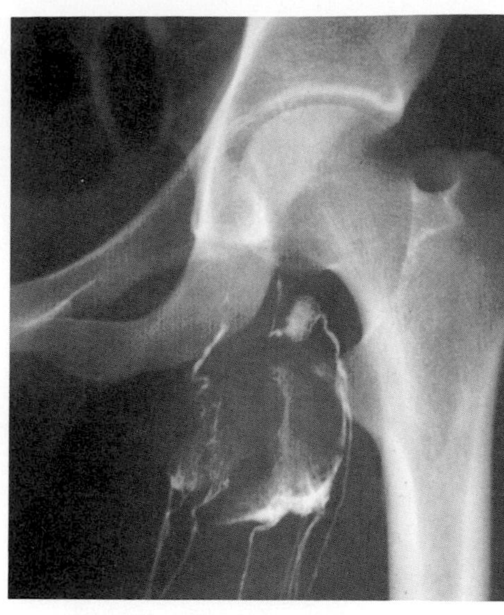

Fig. 7 A lymphangiogram showing massive nodal deposits in the inguinal nodes in a patient with secondary malignant melanoma.

Radiotherapy

Radiotherapy is a common cause of secondary lymphoedema of the upper limb in patients with breast carcinoma, especially when surgical block dissection has also been performed. Such combination therapy carries a higher risk of lymphoedema than either treatment in isolation. Radiotherapy results in nodal fibrosis, which can also cause obstruction of the lymphatic vessels. Recurrent tumour in an irradiated field may be responsible for lymphoedema developing some years after treatment of the primary disease.

Trauma

Severe trauma occasionally causes loss of tissue which includes lymph nodes or lymphatic channels. This is particularly seen after severe degloving injuries.

Chronic infection

Although tuberculosis has often been cited as a cause of lymphoedema, it is uncommon.

Chronic inflammation

At the St Thomas' lymphoedema clinic one or two patients are seen every year with severe rheumatoid disease (Fig. 9) or severe chronic eczema who develop mild lymphoedema. Chronic stimulation of the lymph nodes in these patients results in fibrosis and mild obstruction to the lymphatic drainage.

Acute infection

Severe cellulitis can occasionally damage the local subcutaneous lymphatics and cause mild lymphoedema. Patients suffering from subclinical primary lymphoedema may also develop a secondary cellulitis: the two presentations can be difficult to distinguish.

Self-induced

This quite common form of Munchausen's syndrome is produced by repeated tight application of a tourniquet. Total disuse of a limb can also cause swelling: this form of self-induced lymphoedema should be suspected if the limb cannot be moved passively

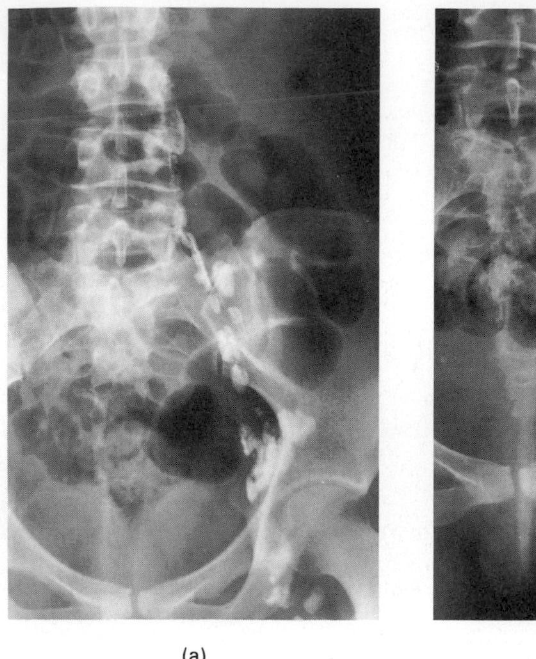

(a)

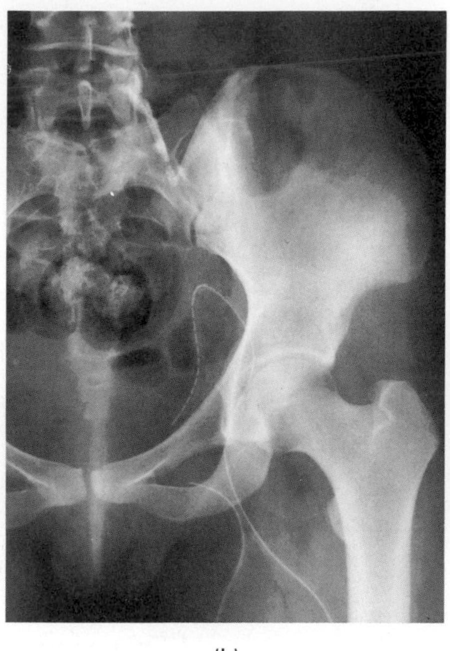

(b)

Fig. 8 (a) The lymphogram of a patient presenting with secondary deposits from a malignant melanoma within the iliac nodes. (b) The same patient after a lymphadenectomy showing that all the lymph nodes have been removed. A redivac drain is visible.

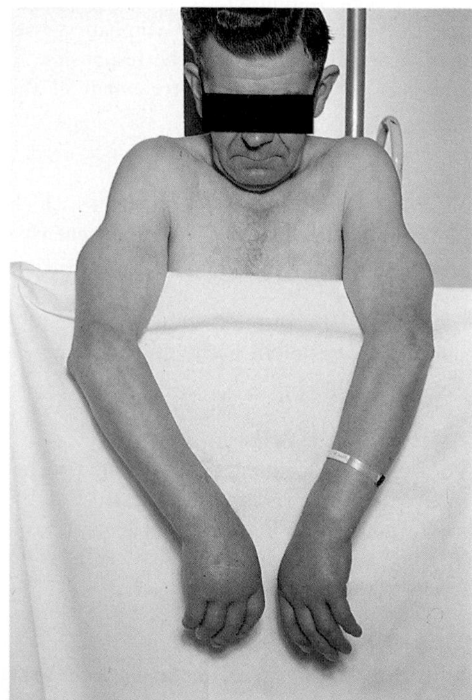

Fig. 9 A patient with lymphoedema of the upper limbs secondary to rheumatoid arthritis.

(Fig. 10). Lymphograms are usually normal or only mildly unusual. The cause should be suspected if there is a sharp cut-off to the lymphoedema and a rut due to application of the tourniquet. Patients should be told of the doctor's suspicions and referred for psychiatric advice.

Primary lymphoedema

Aetiology

Although by definition the cause of primary lymphoedema is obscure, some factors clearly influence its development. The small number of babies who have lymphoedematous limbs at birth usually have 'aplastic' and truly absent lymphatics. This condition

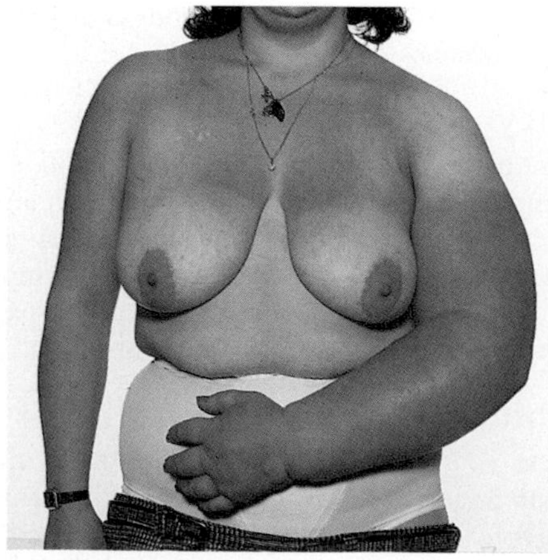

Fig. 10 A patient with 'self-induced' lymphoedema caused by disease of the arm. Notice the arm is held fixidly flexed at the elbow.

(Milroy's disease) has a clear genetic predisposition in some families. How, and why the lymphatic system is damaged or malformed, is not known, but other congenital abnormalities such as yellow nails, distercerciasis, and Pierre-Robin syndrome may coexist. Some degree of inheritance can be demonstrated in about one-third of all patients with primary lymphoedema. Congenital abnormality or absence of the lymphatics does not explain why lymphoedema develops relatively late in most patients, the most common age of onset being between 10 and 25 years of age.

It is possible that the constituents of the lymph draining through the lymphatics may damage the lymphangioles or lymph nodes. Lymph may contain large amounts of fibrinogen under certain circumstances, and this may coagulate and block the lymphatics; abnormal lymph may also cause nodal fibrosis which may lead to 'die-back', or disappearance of the lymphangioles. The primary disease may therefore be in the node, and this may cause the lymphatic hypoplasia. Anticoagulant therapy has been reported to produce improvement in patients with lymphoedema, lending some support to the concept that hypercoagulability of lymph may be harmful. Molecules as yet unrecognized within lymph may also be harmful to nodes and lymphatic vessels. None of these explanations accounts for the development of hyperplastic or dilated lymphatics.

Clinical features

Primary lymphoedema is much more common in the lower limbs than in the upper limbs: although this is partly explained by the influence of gravity, anatomical abnormalities are rarely present in the lymphatics of the upper limb.

The swelling may affect one or both lower limbs, the lower abdomen, the genital region, one or both upper limbs, and, rarely, the face or chest. In the lower limbs swelling usually develops around the ankle and on the dorsum of the foot, and spreads proximally (Fig. 11). In the majority of patients the oedema does not spread above the knee, but severe oedema of the whole limb including the buttock (Fig. 12) suggests a proximal nodal lymphatic occlusion. There are exceptions to this rule, however, and patients with proximal lymphatic occlusions may have no oedema of the ankle or foot. Because lymphatic oedema is chronic and has often been present for many years it stimulates a fibrotic reaction in the subcutaneous tissues, making them more resistant to deformation than is the case in acute oedema associated with cardiac failure or hypoproteinaemia. However, prolonged digital pressure will always produce a 'pit'. If such pitting cannot be demonstrated the diagnosis of lymphoedema must be questioned and another cause for the swelling should be sought.

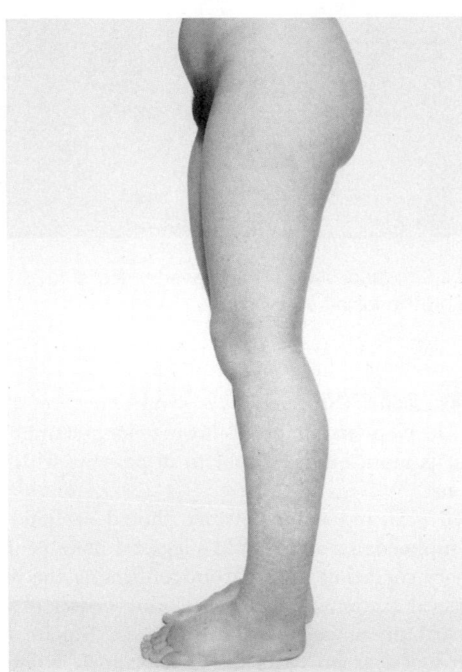

Fig. 11 Lymphoedema primarily affecting the dorsum of the foot.

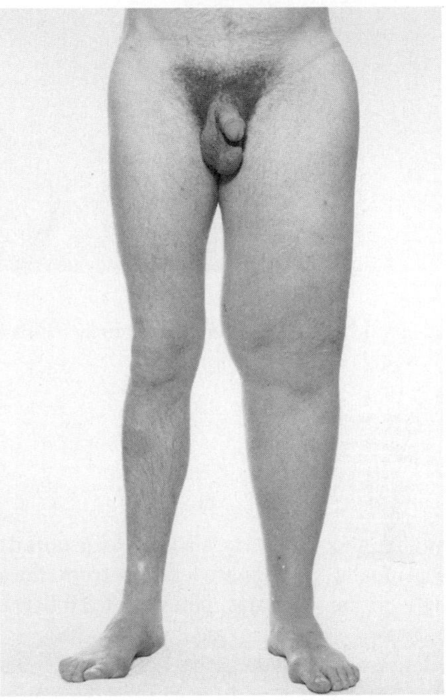

Fig. 12 Whole limb lymphoedema.

The onset of the swelling is usually insidious, and it may fluctuate. Even when lymphoedema becomes fixed all patients report that the swelling decreases during sleep and is maximal at the end of the day. Onset can occasionally be sudden, and progression rapid. This is often associated with cellulitis, which can be both a cause and a result of lymphoedema. Patients with sudden severe swelling usually have a proximal lymphatic occlusion and may have an underlying cause for the condition. Patients with malignant obstruction of both the veins and lymphatics often develop a severe brawny oedema of rapid onset that can cause intractable pain which may be very difficult to alleviate. Some patients develop marked cutaneous thickening which can progress to lymphatic warts (condylomata) and multiple coarse papillae. Other patients are troubled by repeated attacks of cellulitis. The infecting agent may enter through the hyperkeratotic skin or through cracks in the interdigital clefts which occur in athletes' foot.

Occasionally patients develop numerous vesicles in the skin which may leak clear lymph or, occasionally, chyle. These vesicles usually indicate that there are megalymphatics (Fig. 13) and lymphatic reflux. Vesicles usually arise over the upper thighs or on the

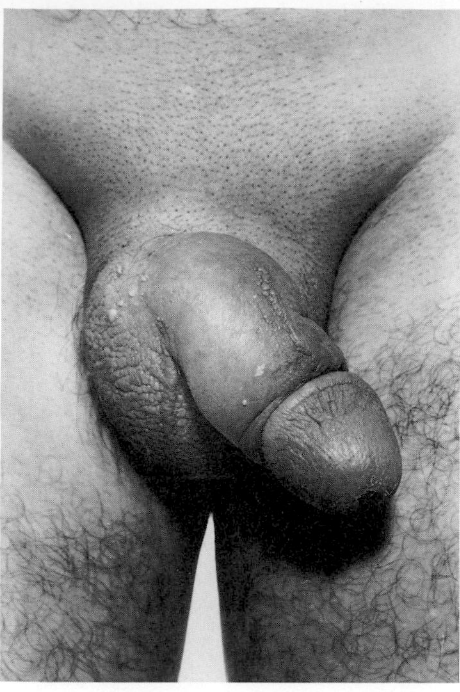

Fig. 13 Vesicles on the external genitalia usually indicative of megalymphatics and reflux.

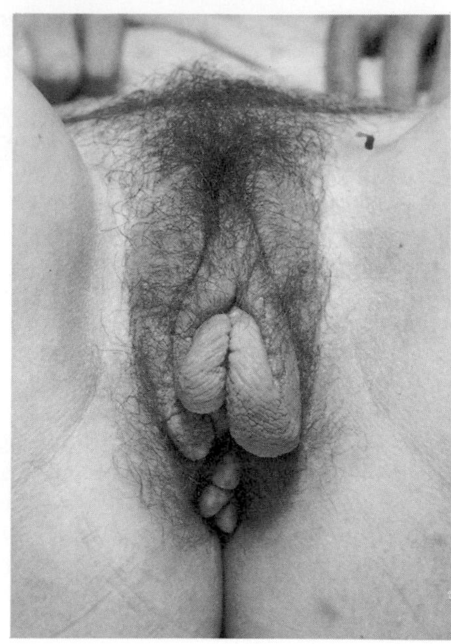

Fig. 14 Massive labial swelling due to lymphatic obstruction.

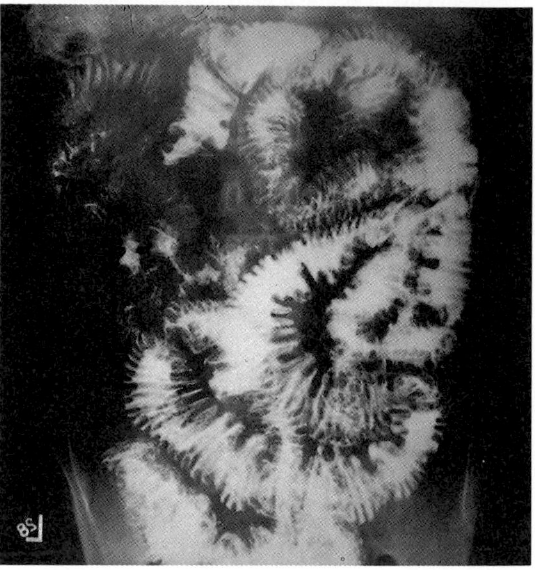

Fig. 15 A barium meal showing thickened mucosal folds in a patient with protein-losing enteropathy.

external genitalia, and they may also act as a portal of entry for bacteria. Occasionally the lymph leakage from these vesicles is severe enough to be a major source of embarrassment and irritation.

Severe oedema of the male genitals is both embarrassing and uncomfortable, interfering with work and sexual relationships. Penetration may be impossible and urination may be difficult when the penis is almost hidden inside a grossly swollen scrotum. Leaking vesicles and recurrent attacks of cellulitis often complicate the condition. Women with genital oedema usually have fewer problems but massive labial swelling can be uncomfortable and embarrassing (Fig. 14).

Lymph can leak into both the abdominal and pleural cavities, causing chylous ascites and pleural effusions. Patients present with abdominal distension, dyspnoea, or both. These problems are usually the result of leakage from refluxing megalymphatics; chyluria and chylous leakage from the vagina are rare complications. Protein-losing enteropathy can cause severe weight loss (Fig. 15) and chylous leakage from the serosal surface of the bowel may increase the ascites.

Lymphoedema may occasionally affect the upper limb, including the fingers (Fig. 16) and unilateral pectoral swelling can also occur. Oedema of the face usually presents as swelling of the eyelids, which are the most lax tissues in this region.

Patients with lymphoedema usually seek advice because they want to know the cause of the swelling, which causes major cosmetic embarrassment, even though it is often only of nuisance value. Severe swelling may make it impossible to buy shoes, and if the limb continues to swell its weight interferes with normal walking. Recurrent attacks of cellulitis may also be a major problem. Lymphangiosarcoma (Stuart Treves syndrome; Fig. 17) can infrequently develop in limbs following long-standing lymphoedema, but is more often a problem in patients with secondary lymphoedema.

A detailed past and family history should exclude secondary causes of lymphoedema and should suggest a possible inheritance of the primary condition. Apart from confirming the presence of pitting, physical examination excludes other causes of limb swelling and reveal any associated abnormalities. 'Square toes' often result when footwear prevents toe expansion. It is important to inspect the web spaces between the toes for athletes' foot, which is especially common in lymphoedematous limbs and is an important

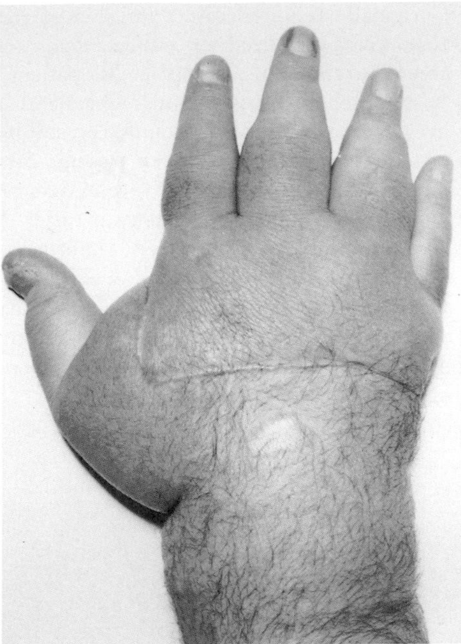

Fig. 16 Lymphoedema of the upper limb causing swelling of the fingers. Surgical reduction of the forearm has been performed. This lymphoedema was secondary to surgical removal of the axillary nodes and radiotherapy for a carcinoma of the breast.

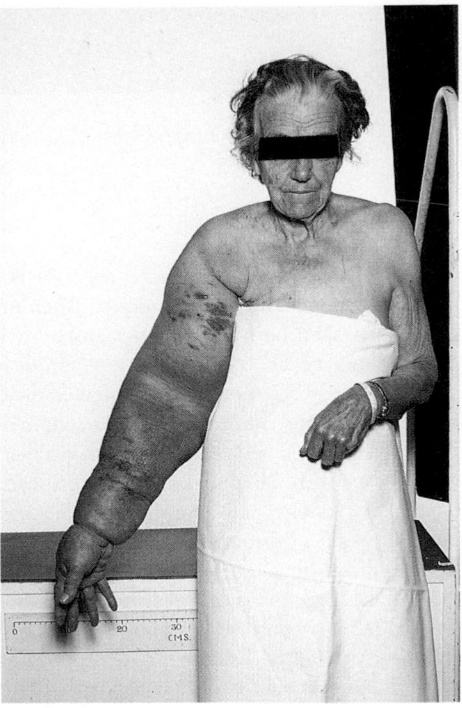

Fig. 17 A patient with chronic lymphoedema of the upper limb after mastectomy who developed lymphangiosarcoma in the affected limb—Stuart Treves syndrome.

portal of entry for bacteria that cause recurrent cellulitis. Yellow nail syndrome is occasionally associated with lymphoedema, as is distichiasis (two layers of eyelashes). Occasionally Pierre-Robin syndrome (micrognathia) and other skeletal abnormalities are present, and congenital cardiac anomalies are found also in patients with lymphatic hyperplasia.

The skin should be carefully examined for papillae and vesicles, and the limbs should be measured at fixed levels, above and below fixed bony points (Fig. 18), to allow both the natural history and the results of therapy to be evaluated. The length of the limbs should also be measured and the presence of any abnormal veins must be recorded. The abdomen and chest should be carefully examined for ascites or effusions. The groins and axillae should be palpated for pathologically enlarged lymph nodes. Rectal and vaginal examinations are indicated if a pelvic malignancy is suspected.

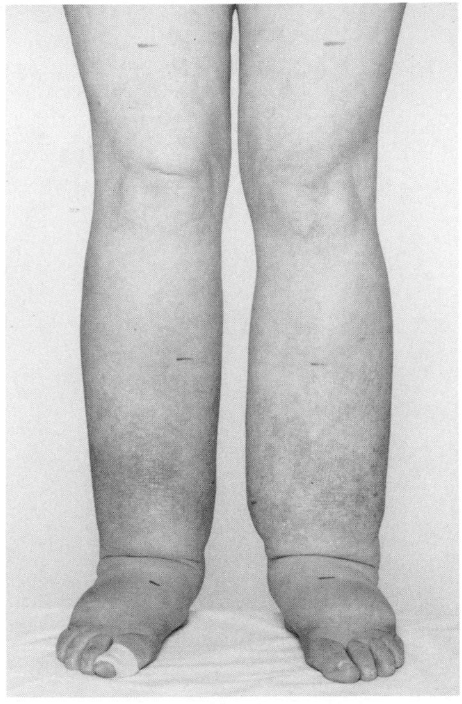

Fig. 18 Marks made at fixed levels on lymphoedematous limbs to allow measurements to be made of limb size for comparison in future years.

The physical examination should provide indications of whether the patient has primary or secondary lymphoedema, but unequivocal confirmation of the diagnosis is desirable. If the swelling is not the result of lymphoedema, other investigations are necessary.

Differential diagnosis

Venous oedema can sometimes be difficult to differentiate from lymphoedema, especially if it is caused by the iliac vein compression syndrome, when there is often little in the way of superficial venous engorgement. The presence of dilated collateral veins or varicose veins normally suggests venous oedema, as does a past history of deep vein thrombosis. Other causes of bilateral limb oedema include cardiac disease, nephrotic syndrome, hypoproteinaemia, fluid overload during intravenous therapy, and chronic liver disease. These disorders can be excluded by a careful physical examination and appropriate blood tests. Klippel Trenauney and Parks-Weber syndromes also cause limb enlargement: the former is occasionally associated with lymphoedema. True gigantism (Robertson's giant limb) also occurs, when all the tissues (muscles and bones) are hypertrophied. Abnormal fat deposition (lipoidosis or lipodystrophy) can be excluded by the fact that fat does not pit (Fig. 19). Periodic oedema experienced by women before menstruation is often difficult to separate from lymphoedema. Rapidly growing soft tissue sarcomata rarely cause diagnostic problems. Before making a diagnosis of one of these rare conditions, for which venography, CT scanning, and arteriography may be required, it is often simpler to exclude lymphoedema by isotope lymphography.

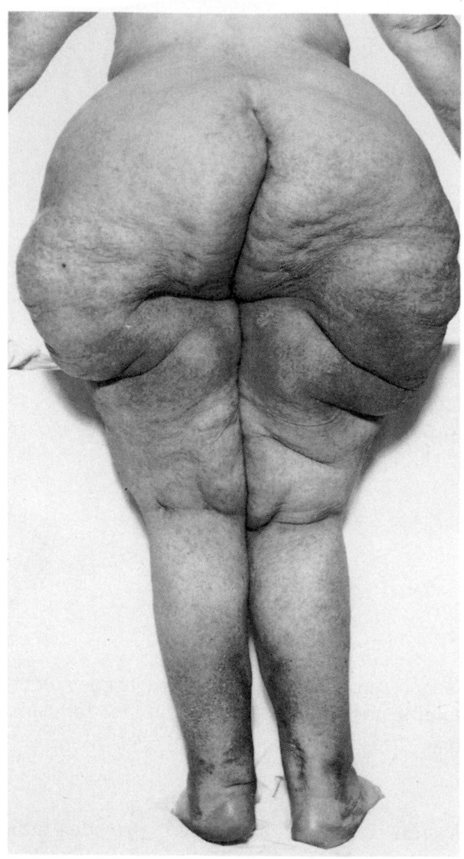

Fig. 19 A patient with massive fat deposition over the buttocks and thighs—lipodystrophy or lipoidosis.

Investigations

A full blood count, erythrocyte sedimentation rate, and chest radiographs are usually requested, but these investigations can be omitted. Measurement of serum protein, blood urea, creatinine, and electrolyte levels and liver function tests should be obtained in all patients.

Contrast lymphangiography

This is indicated to confirm the diagnosis and to determine, if possible, the type of lymphatic abnormality that is present. This investigation originally required direct infusion of contrast into lymphatics that were visualized by subcutaneous injection of patent blue green into the web spaces (Fig. 20): patients had to be admitted to hospital for the investigation, and general anaesthesia was usually necessary as few patients could keep still for the time required to obtain the radiographs. Such patients often require bed rest and leg elevation in hospital for several days to minimize foot oedema and make lymphatic cannulation easier. Lymphangiography does, however, provide precise information on the presence of hypoplasia, megalymphatics, and obstruction (including its site), and it still remains the 'gold standard' against which other techniques are judged. It is still essential before certain therapeutic options are considered, and is of some value in assessing prognosis.

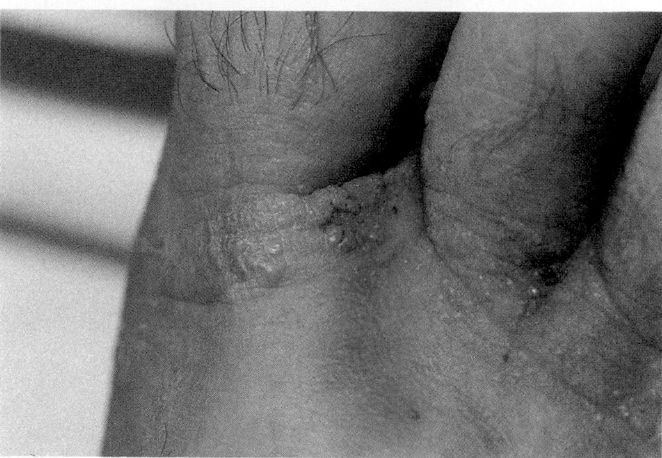

Fig. 20 Patent blue green injected into the web spaces to outline the lymphatics.

Isotope lymphography

Isotope lymphography has largely replaced contrast lymphangiography as the primary diagnostic technique. Rhenium sulphur colloid is specifically taken up by lymphatics and allows the presence of lymphoedema to be confirmed by a simple outpatient investigation. Normally, 0.3 per cent of the injected dose arrives in the groin within 30 min, and more than 0.6 per cent arrives within 1 h. In patients with venous oedema there is an excessive uptake, often above 3 per cent at 30 min, and this test can therefore distinguish between venous and lymphatic oedemas. Gamma-camera pictures provide information that the isotope is reaching the lymph node of the groin and delayed images may show a failure of progression, indicating proximal obstruction (Fig. 21). This should be confirmed by contrast lymphography, as should any equivocal findings. An attempt has been made to produce a special contrast media which was selectively taken up by the lymphatics from a subcutaneous injection. The prototype contrast material has not yet found its way into routine clinical practice.

Ultrasound imaging, CT scanning, and magnetic resonance scanning can all show enlarged lymph nodes, and guided biopsies of lymph nodes can be taken if malignancy is suspected. Needle or true-cut biopsies are probably safer as a preliminary procedure, since removal of large solitary fibrotic nodes may worsen pre-existing lymphoedema. A calcium chloride test may be helpful when protein-losing enteropathy is suspected.

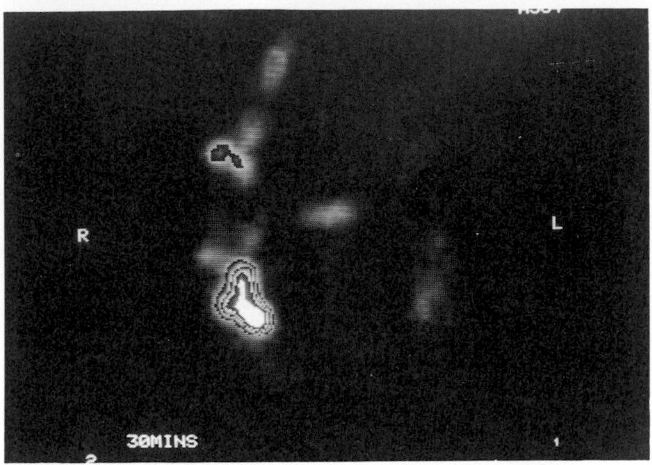

Fig. 21 A gamma-camera image of the groin and pelvis after injection of rhenium sulphur colloid showing uptake in the nodes of the right groin while activity is not reaching the nodes of the left groin.

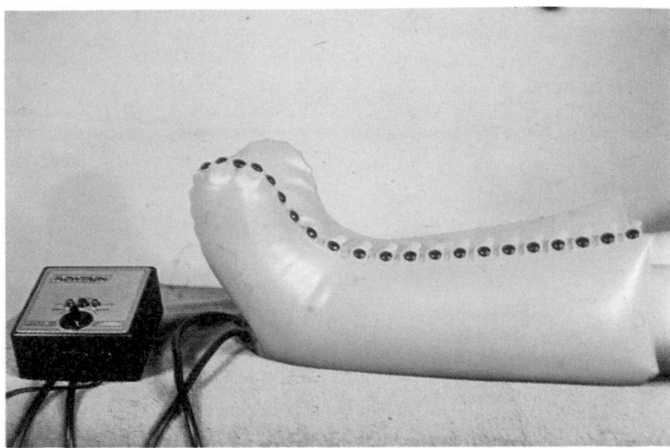

Fig. 22 Flowtron boots are a less expensive alternative to the lymphopress machine, which is very effective but costs approximately £1000.

Management

Many surgeons are content to diagnose mild lymphoedema from the history and physical findings without investigating the patient further. This clinical diagnosis can however be incorrect and isotope lymphography should be obtained if possible. This not only provides a firm diagnosis, but also allows an assessment to be made of prognosis and of possible problems that may be present in the contralateral limb. Young women with mild lymphoedema of gradual onset usually have distal lymphatic hypoplasia: there is prolongation of the time taken for the isotope to reach the groin nodes, but normal onward passage. This type of lymphoedema is often inherited (at least 30 per cent), and rarely becomes severe or extends above the knee. It is often bilateral but one limb may be affected several years before the other. Rarely, the upper limbs are also involved.

Physical methods

Patients with this condition rarely require surgery. They should be given advice on limb elevation, especially in the evenings and at night, and some patients benefit from regular massage or mechanical compression combined with wearing of graduated elastic compression stockings. Pneumatic massaging devices are obtainable, and sequential segmental machines such as the lymphopress (Fig. 22) are probably more effective than single chamber boots. These may be worn in the evenings or in bed at night, although they may interfere with sleep. Correctly graduated strong compression stockings (30–50 mmHg at the ankle, decreasing up the limb) only need to reach below knee level if the lymphoedema is distal in distribution. Elastic compression stockings do not cure lymphoedema, but they reduce fluid accumulation and often produce considerable symptomatic relief. They are poorly tolerated in warm climates and young women tend to be conscious of their appearance. Weight reduction is often beneficial and physical exercise is never harmful; concentrated compression therapy and massage may also reduce the size of lymphoedematous limbs.

Drug therapy

Diuretics are of little value in removing fluid from the whole body and may cause a number of problems when used unnecessarily for many years. Paroven (hydroxyrutosides) has some anecdotal support, as do the coumadins, but these compounds have not yet been tested in a well controlled clinical trial.

Antibiotics (flucloxacillin, amoxycillin, or one of the cephalosporins) should be prescribed for cellulitis and may be given in a low dose prophylactically if patients are troubled by repeated attacks. Athletes' foot must be eradicated by appropriate antifungal medication and creams. Careful attention to drying and powdering of the feet prevents infection and avoids an important portal of entry for virulent bacteria.

Surgery

Surgical reduction of severe whole limb lymphoedema that interferes with mobility or causes severe deformity (Fig. 23) is often appropriate. In a small proportion of patients preoperative contrast lymphangiography discloses a proximal lymphatic obstruction in the ileoinguinal region with normal distal limb lymphatics (Fig. 24). These patients (1–3 per cent of all those seen) can be expected to benefit from some form of lymphatic bypass operation.

Lymphatic bypass

A number of methods have been used to reunite obstructed lymphatics with the venous system. Many of these techniques, such as the skin bridge devised by Gillies and the omental pedicle, both of which were sutured to the obstructed lymph nodes in the groin, are only of historical interest. Direct anastomosis of lymph nodes to veins was originally performed by Niebulowitz, but fibrosis and low flow rates resulted in a high failure rate. Degni used a specially designed needle to insert lymphatics into the lumen of the vein, but the imprecise nature of this procedure has prevented its widespread acceptance. The advent of the operating microscope has made it possible to divide obstructed lymphatics and directly anastomose them into the side of the vein. However, the results have generally been disappointing. At least three of four lymphatics should be attached to the femoral vein in the groin in the hope that one or two anastomoses will remain patent.

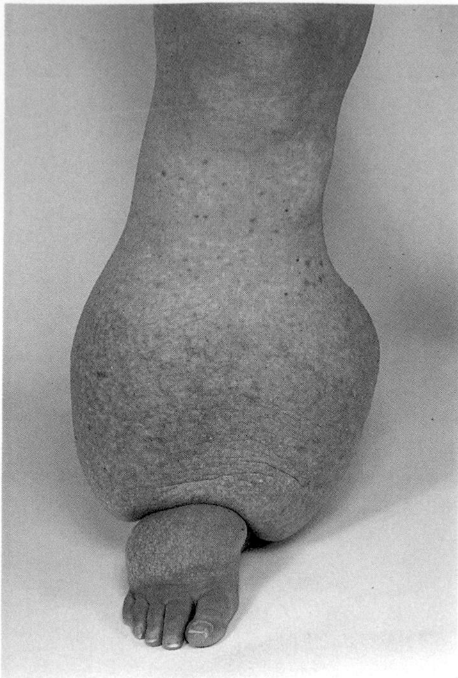

Fig. 23 This lymphoedematous limb is so large that it is interfering with mobility and should have its size reduced.

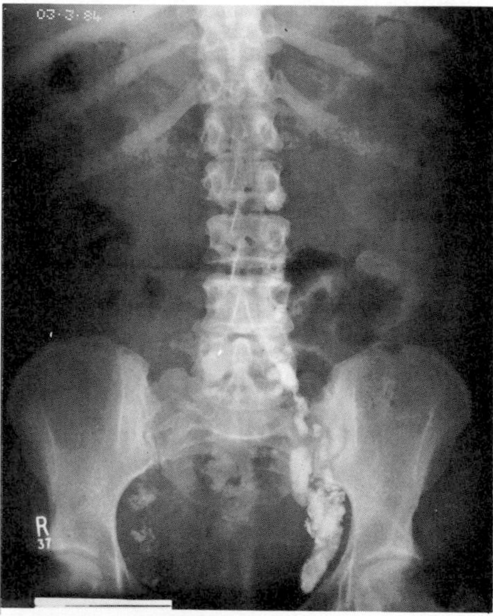

Fig. 24 A lymphogram showing lymphatic obstruction in the right inguinal region with contrast entering groin nodes but not passing up into the iliac chain although it does so on the left side.

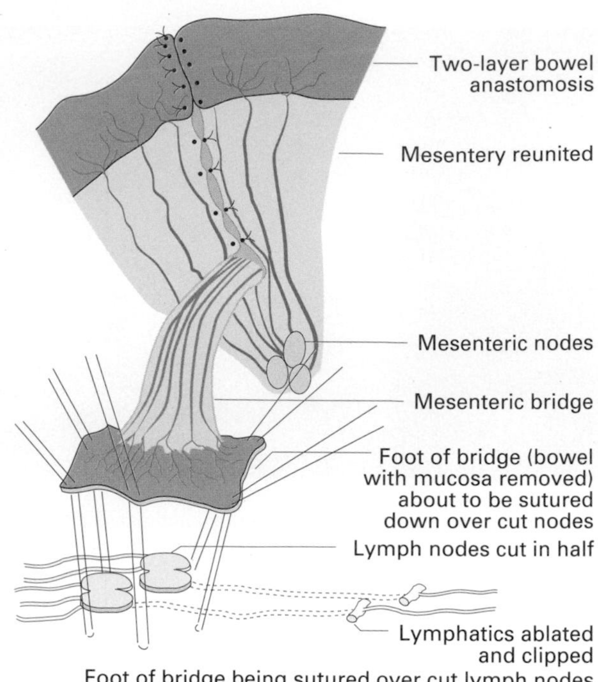

Fig. 25 A diagram to show the principles of the enteromesenteric bridge bypass operation. The pedicle of small bowel denuded of its mucosa is sutured over the bivalved lymph nodes below the level of obstruction.

Kinmonth and his associates developed the mesenteric bridge as an alternative to direct lymphovenous anastomosis. This operation uses the copious submucosal lymphatic plexus and the mesenteric lymphatics to drain the lymph from obstructed nodes in the ileoinguinal region. About 5 cm of the terminal ileum is resected on its mesenteric pedicle, as for an ileal conduit, taking great care to maintain the lymphatic drainage. The small bowel is reanastomosed behind the pedicle. The isolated segment is then opened along its antimesenteric border and the mucosa is stripped off the submucosa by a combination of sharp and blunt dissection after injection of a solution of adrenaline in saline (1:400 000). The isolated pedicle is then brought down to the first normal group of lymph nodes below the level of the obstruction, and sutured over them after they have been bivalved. Connections develop between the divided nodes and the submucosal plexus and lymph drains up the pedicle into the mesenteric lymph nodes, and eventually into the thoracic duct (Fig. 25).

This operation has been performed on over 40 patients at St Thomas' Hospital, London and has produced good results in more than half. Unfortunately there is no way of predicting those who will benefit from the procedure, although the careful selection of patients prevents inevitable failure. Young patients appear to fare better, and the distal limb lymphatics must still be functioning if a successful result is to be achieved. If limbs are too swollen resolution is poor, but swelling must be severe enough to justify major abdominal surgery. Perhaps for this reason surgery is appropriate for relatively few patients.

Reduction operations

Four types of excisional operation have been described to reduce the size of the limb. The Sistrunk operation involves excision of a large wedge or ellipse of skin and subcutaneous tissue which is then closed primarily. Homan elevated skin flaps from the subcutaneous fat, excising the underlying subcutaneous tissue before resuturing the skin flaps in place (Fig. 26). Thompson modified the Homan's operation by suturing one of the skin flaps to the deep fascia. Denudation of the superficial layers of the flap stops hair growth and prevents pilonidal sinus formation. The second flap is then sewn over the top of the denuded skin area (Fig. 27). This operation has largely been abandoned: it leaves unsightly scars, it is often

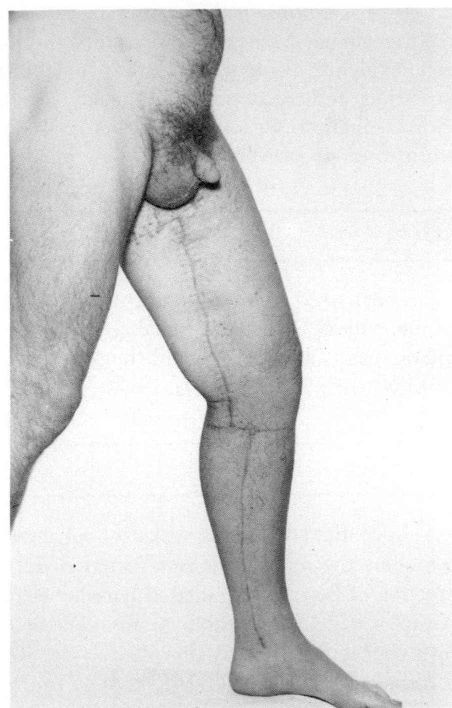

Fig. 26 A limb that has had a Homan's reduction of the lower leg and a Sistrunk excision of the thigh.

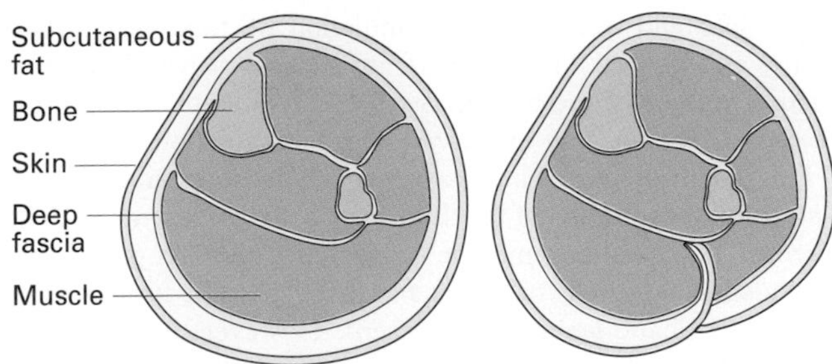

Fig. 27 The principle of the Thompson buried dermal flap operation—now largely obsolete.

complicated by pilonidal sinus formation, and the results appear to be no better than those of the simpler Homan's procedure.

Both Homan's and Thompson's operations can be complicated by skin flap necrosis and poor healing, particularly at the corners of the flaps. Great care needs to be taken to maintain the blood supply of the flaps, which must not be cut too thin. Flap reduction of the calf and foot is normally combined with a Sistrunk operation on the thigh if the whole limb is to be reduced in size (Fig. 26).

Charles invented an operation to remove the severely thickened skin in patients with filariasis. He excised all the diseased skin and the waterlogged subcutaneous tissue down to, and often including, the deep fascia from just above the ankle to just below the knee. The periosteum over the tibia was left intact and split skin grafts were then taken from normal donor skin (the opposite normal limb, or the abdomen, back, and buttocks) and used to cover the deep fascia or muscle. This operation produces the best reduction in limb size, but often at the expense of cosmesis. The ankle and knee area have to be carefully tailored to avoid a pantaloon effect (Fig. 28), and thigh reduction is also often necessary. Some patients have a poor acceptance of split skin grafts and require multiple operations to achieve complete healing. Other patients develop severe hyperkeratotic scars with warty excrescences, which produce severe deformity in the operated limb (Fig. 29). This can be treated by shaving off the warty nodules and thickened scars with a scalpel or skin graft knife; additional skin grafts are occasionally needed. However, final results are usually very satisfactory, especially in a grossly enlarged limb with very abnormal calf skin.

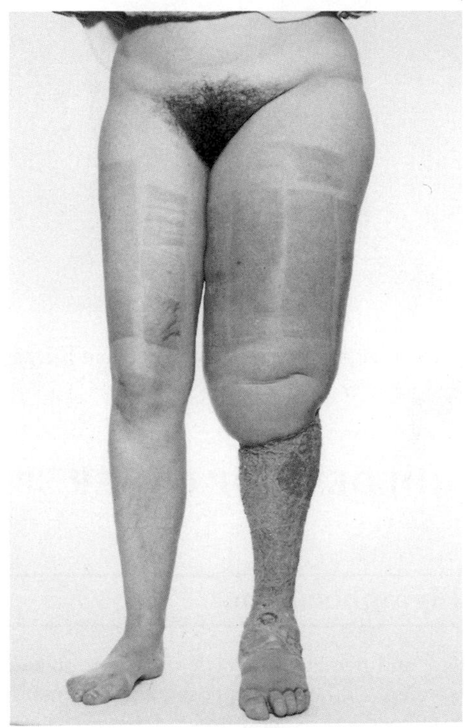

Fig. 28 A limb after a Charles reduction: the thigh has not been tapered enough, resulting in a pantaloon appearance.

Summary

The majority of patients can be managed conservatively. Few patients are suitable for bypass surgery: when surgery is indicatd an enteromesenteric bridge is probably the best form of bypass, having a spectacular effect in about half of the patients. Bypass surgery should be reserved for patients with gross limb swelling that interferes with limb function. Patients with really gross limb swelling and severe skin changes are best treated by a Charles reduction, combined with a local excision of enlarged thigh tissue. Homan's operation should be reserved for those with a moderate to severe degree of swelling. Patients with secondary lymphoedema caused by malignancy often have associated venous oedema. The results of reduction surgery under these circumstances are extremely poor.

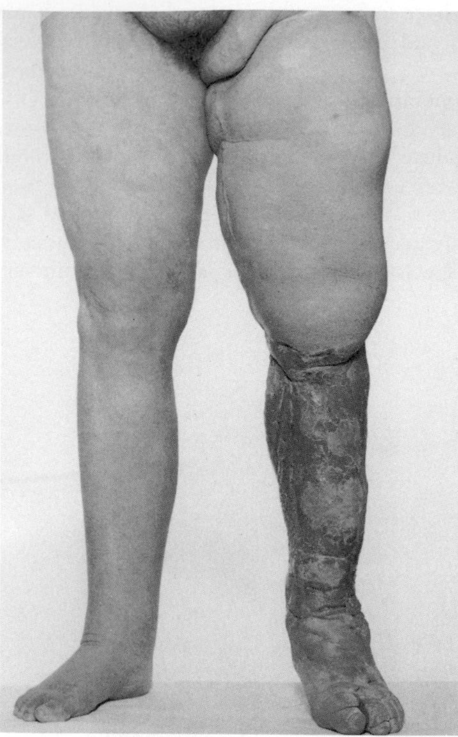

Fig. 29 A good Charles reduction, but the patient has developed eczema of the skin and hyperkeratotic scars.

LYMPHOEDEMA OF OTHER SPECIAL SITES

Genital lymphoedema

Minor scrotal and penile lymphoedema can be tolerated without specific treatment, although support garments may be helpful. Severe scrotal oedema is best treated by excisional reduction surgery in which a large central segment is excised from the scrotum, preserving the spermatic cords and testicles. The flaps are then primarily sutured using an absorbable material and the scrotum is drained. Mobilization of the testes with gentle abrasion of their surfaces may encourage adhesions to form, allowing lymph to drain via the testicular lymphatics, aiding the scrotal reduction.

The penis may be reduced by simple excisional procedures, combined with circumcision if necessary. Alternatively the skin and subcutaneous tissue can be stripped off the deep fascia and split skin grafts applied (a Charles operation of the penis). Both scrotal and penile reduction operations produce gratifying results for surgeon and patient.

Massive labial swelling can also be treated by excisional procedures.

Eyelids and upper limb

Eyelid swelling can be treated by lid reduction. Arm swelling can be treated by a Homan's type of limb reduction, which can be performed on both the inner and outer sides of the upper limb. Patients with postmastectomy oedema must be assessed carefully to ensure that the venous drainage is satisfactory and to be certain that there is no evidence of recurrent axillary nodal disease. Both venous obstruction and recurrent malginancy are contraindications to arm reduction. Postoperatively an elasticated sleeve should be worn to try to prevent recurrent swelling.

Liposuction

Liposuction has been used to remove subcutaneous fat in patients with mild lymphoedema. Anecdotal successes have been achieved but the cosmetic results are variable and the procedure should be used with caution.

Chylous reflux

Some patients have dilated (almost varicose) valveless megalymphatics which allow the reflux of lymph (often chyle) against the expected direction of flow. These dilated lymphatics often end in cutaneous vesicles which are visible in the skin or which may rupture into body cavities such as the pleura (see Section 35.9), peritoneum, kidney (see Section 41.16), bladder, uterus, and vagina. Rupture results in the accumulation of lymph or chyle in the relevant cavity (chylothorax, hydrothorax, chylous ascites, chyluria) and chylous discharge on to the skin surface or mucosa can also occur. Accumulation of chyle in the pleural and peritoneal cavities produces severe symptoms, and patients often become dyspnoeic and very distended. Patients with megalymphatics often also have a protein-losing enteropathy which can cause weight loss and exacerbate accumulation of fluid in the body cavities and tissues. This results from leakage of lymph from the mucosal surface of the bowel; associated lymphatic leakage from the serosal surface may exacerbate the accumulation of ascites.

The diagnosis of chylous ascites or chylothorax must first be confirmed by aspiration of the fluid, which is then tested for chylomicrons. The condition may be suspected if there is pre-existing lymphoedema of the extremities and it is especially likely if vesicles and lymphatic leakage are present. However, in quite a few patients the condition develops *de novo*. Chylothorax and chylous ascites must be distinguished from malignant ascites or a malignant effusion: cytological examination of the aspirate may help to exclude or confirm the presence of malignant cells. CT scan and ultrasound can demonstrate the presence of moderate or severe enlargement of the abdominal or mediastinal lymph nodes which suggests the possibility of a lymphoma or secondary malignant spread. Guided biopsy, laparoscopy, or laparotomy may be necessary to confirm these diagnoses. Contrast lymphography demonstrates lymphadenopathy, filling defects, or the presence of megalymphatics and is indicated if the diagnosis remains in doubt. Contrast lymphography may also demonstrate a lymphatic leak which can be surgically sealed.

Lymphoedema associated with megalymphatics rarely requires reduction surgery, but the complications of lymphatic vesicles, recurrent infections, lymphatic discharge on to the skin, chylous ascites, chyluria, and chylothorax often demand treatment. Leakage of chyle or lymph may be prevented by ligating or under-running the dilated lymphatic channels, but this carries the risk of lymphatic obstruction which will worsen the limb swelling. Despite this many patients benefit from ligation of dilated lymphatics, and sealing off of any obvious site of fistulation.

If a patient with chylous ascites or chylothorax has no obvious leak on the lymphangiogram, chromium chloride studies and a barium study of the small bowel may provide useful information before a laparotomy is performed. At laparotomy the posterior abdominal wall over the main lymphatic pathways must be carefully inspected for the presence of lymphatic leakage, and the whole of the intestine should be examined. If the surface of the small bowel is grossly abnormal and leaking lymph, the involved or most abnormal segment should be resected. If this simple approach fails, consideration must be given to shunting the ascites back into the venous system using a LeVeen or Denver shunt. Although these shunts often work well in patients with refractory ascites, chyle often blocks the plastic tubing, or the valve, and produces an early occlusion of the shunt. Many patients improve with simple avoidance of fat and prescription of medium chain triglycerides combined with diuretics.

Chylothorax may respond to aspiration but often recurs and is best prevented by some form of pleurodesis induced with talc, tetracycline, bleomycin, or pleural stripping. After these procedures some patients die from water- or lymph-logged lungs as the lymphatics draining the lung become obstructed when they are no longer able to empty into the pleural cavity. Nevertheless many patients with severe problems as the result of megalymphatics can be helped by some of the procedures outlined above. Cutaneous vesicles may be simply excised or touched with the diathermy or cautery, but they tend to recur. Recurrent infections should be treated by a prolonged course of broad-spectrum antibiotics.

Lymphangioma circumscriptum

These lesions are either considered as hamartomas or as localized abnormalities of the cutaneous lymphatic drainage. They present as a number of clear or slightly haemorrhagic cutaneous vesicles, often associated with subcutaneous thickening in the underlying fat (Fig. 30). Whimster thought that a lymphangioma circumscriptum was the result of defective lymphatic drainage from the subcutaneous tissue where a number of cisterns 'pump' lymph back into the overlying skin. These areas should be excised if they are unsightly or painful. They often occur on the trunk and it is important to excise a generous amount of subcutaneous tissue well beyond the ellipse of skin bearing the vesicles in order to remove the subcutaneous bladders described by Whimster. It is often quite difficult to excise all the skin lesions and they have a propensity to recur: excisional surgery is only required if they are symptomatic.

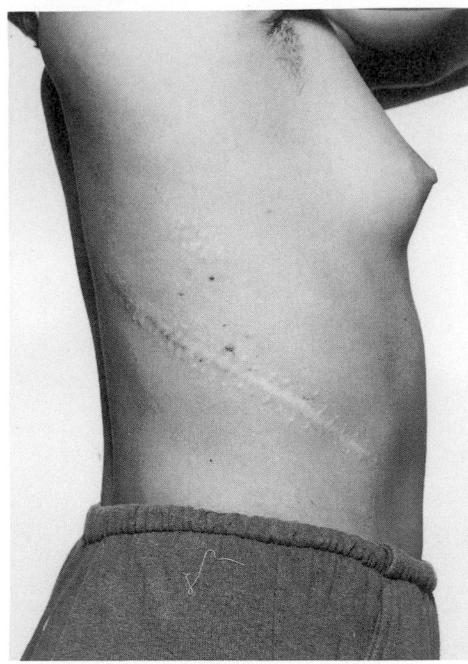

Fig. 30 A lymphangioma circumscriptum that has recurred after previous excision.

Cystic hygroma

In this developmental abnormality of the lymphatic system, lymphatic fluid collects in a cystic space which is often multilocular and situated in the base of the neck. Cystic hygroma commonly appears in childhood and presents as a soft, brilliantly translucent swelling in the base of the neck. Aspiration and injection of sclerosant may be attempted, but the swellings often recur and may require excision. Cystic hygromas must be dissected with great care as a number of important structures lie adjacent to them.

Mesenteric cysts

These localized lymphatic cysts within the mesentery appear as well-circumscribed mobile lumps within the abdomen. The diagnosis can be confirmed by ultrasound or CT scanning. They are treated by resection, often in association with the overlying area of small bowel. Although harmless, they may reach a considerable size if left untreated.

FURTHER READING

Browse NL, Stewart G. Lymphoedema: pathophysiology and classification. *J Cardiovasc Surg* 1985; **26**: 91–106.

Charles RH. *In a system of treatment*. Latham A, English TC, eds. London: Churchill, 1912; **3**: 516.

Degni M. New techniques of lymphatico-venous anastomosis for the treatment of lymphoedema. *J Cardiovasc Surg* 1978; **19**: 577–80.

Hawking F. *Diethylcarbamazine: a review of the literature with special reference to its pharmacology, toxity and use in the treatment of onchocerciasis and other filarial infections.* Geneva: WHO 1978; **78**: 142.

Kinmonth JB. Lymphangiography in man. *Clin Sci* 1952; **11**: 13–20.

Kinmonth JB. *The Lymphatics, Surgery, Lymphography and Diseases of the Chyle and Lymph Systems.* 2nd edn. London: Arnold, 1982.

Kinmonth JB, Patrick JH, Chilvers AS. Comments on operations for lower limb lymphoedema. *Lymphology* 1975; **8**: 56–61.

Nielubowicz J, Olsewski W. Surgical lympho-venous shunts. *Br J Surg* 1968; **55**: 440–2.

O'Brien BM. Micro lymphatico-venous surgery for obstructive lymphoedema. *Aust NZ J Surg* 1977; **47**: 284.

Sistrunk WE. Further experiences with the Kandolean operation of elephantiasis. *JAMA* 1918, **71**: 800.

Stewart G, Gaunt J, Croft DN, Browse NL. Dynamic and static lymphoscintography in the evaluation of chronic limb oedema. *Eur J Nucl Med* 1983; **8**: A40.

Thompson N. Surgical treatment of chronic lymphoedema of the arm and leg. *Br J Hosp Med* 1971; **1**: 395–408.

Thornton A, Pickering D. Abdominal lymphoscintography: an effective substitute for lymphography. *Br J Radiol* 1985; **58**: 603–10.

Wolfe JHN. The prognosis and possible cause of severe primary lymphoedema. *Ann R Coll Surg Engl* 1984; **66**: 251–7.

Zelikovski A, *et al.* Lympho-presse: a pneumatic device for the treatment of lymphoedema of the limbs. *Lymphology* 1980; **13**: 68–73.

Organ transplantation 10

10.1 Transplantation immunology and immunogenetics

HUGH AUCHINCLOSS AND PAUL S. RUSSELL

INTRODUCTION

Immunology and genetics have been among the most rapidly developing areas of science in the past few decades. It will be our purpose here to summarize basic information from these fields required for the work of the clinician who cares for recipients of transplanted organs. It is interesting to recall that the dawn of cellular immunology, as we now know it, and much of its early impetus to growth was generated by efforts to understand the behaviour of transplanted tissues.

The history of understanding of the fundamental processes of transplant rejection goes back further than is often appreciated. Much information, sometimes imperfectly interpreted, was gathered in the course of experiments in which samples of viable neoplastic tissue were transplanted to recipient animals which were immunogenetically different from those in which the tumours arose. This meant, as P. B. Medawar nicely put it, that investigators intending to 'study cancer by transplantation were actually studying transplantation with cancer'. Thus, the transplanted neoplastic cells were subject to rejection in all but highly compatible recipients.

Out of such experiments with transplanted tumours and increasingly with normal tissues, especially skin grafts, came fundamental information about the effect on transplant survival of the genetic relationship between donor and host, as well as a realization that the destructive process of rejection is indeed immunological in nature. Furthermore, a dawning of understanding regarding the immunological mechanisms that bring about rejection was emerging at just about the time of the first clinical trials of kidney transplantation in Boston and in Paris in the early 1950s. It was also known at this time that whole-body irradiation and treatment with certain chemical agents, especially cortisone derivatives, could significantly reduce the severity of the rejection response. In the prevailing atmosphere, attempts at organ transplants, making use of the safest possible surgical techniques were felt to be reasonable. Kidneys were attached, for example, to vessels in the groin and placed in subcutaneous pockets while urinary drainage to a leg bag was achieved by cutaneous ureterostomy. In some cases, partly as a direct kind of histocompatibility test, the new kidney was maintained in a sterile box and was attached to arm vessels by percutaneous conduits. The intent here was to determine the early outcome of an allogeneic transplant before placing the organ within the body of the recipient.

Initially, animal experiments established very clearly that prior exposure to nucleated cell injections or organized tissue transplants from a given donor would leave a recipient primed for a greatly accelerated reaction to later transplants from the same donor. This more vigorous reaction was accompanied by a much more rapid and intense invasion of migratory recipient cells into the grafted tissue. Observations such at this, coupled with the finding of Mitchison that the immunity induced by transplant rejection could be transferred to another recipient by transferring cells from lymph nodes draining the graft led to a generally held view that the immune response to transplanted tissues was mediated by activated recipient cells exerting their destructive effects directly upon the graft. However, evidence then began to accrue from a number of sources that humoral factors could, at least under some circumstances, have a dramatic and decisive impact on transplanted cells and tissues. One particularly striking observation was that certain kidney transplants were seen to be destroyed within minutes of receiving blood from their new hosts in a reaction called 'hyperacute' rejection. The character of the pathological changes seen in such transplants after their removal made it unlikely that the process could have been mediated by recipient cells and the emergence of techniques (originally following the important work of Peter Gorer) that could detect humoral antibodies directed toward cell surface antigens made it possible to show that hyperacute rejection was attributable to pre-existing humoral antibody directed to at least some of the antigens present in the transplant. This stimulated further exploration of the participation of humoral antibody in rejection reactions in animals, where such reactions had been extremely difficult to find by methods such as the passive transfer of serum to a new recipient from a previously immunized subject. It also suggested the advisability of testing the reactivity of a recipient's serum to donor cells in the presence of complement as a preliminary 'cross-match' test before a transplant is performed.

All these points have subsequently received much attention, and a great deal of refinement in our knowledge of how cellular and humoral immunity are generated has taken place. Discussion continues, as we will describe below, regarding the most appropriate tests for humoral antibody to donor cells, which will predict with certainty the destruction of a transplanted organ from the donor of those cells. Some uncertainty remains as to the types of donor cells that can be considered representative of a later organ transplant, and even, in the minds of some, whether the presence of cytotoxic antibody to donor T lymphocytes, for example, is regularly associated with harmful effects on certain organ transplants, especially livers and hearts.

Knowledge derived both from laboratory experiments and clinical observations continues to expand in this complex field. Differences of opinion, often leading to new advances, are bound to be present from time to time, but, as mentioned above, few would dispute the contention that the process of rejection, a direct manifestation of immunogenetic factors, is of central importance to the outcome of any living cell or tissue transplant. Accordingly, these processes are of great importance to surgeons and other clinicians who seek to help patients by the transplantation of living tissue and organs of any kind.

THE ANTIGENS THAT PROVOKE REJECTION

Activation of the immune system requires that receptors on B cells or T cells recognize foreign substances. Those structures having the right size and configuration to fit within these receptors are

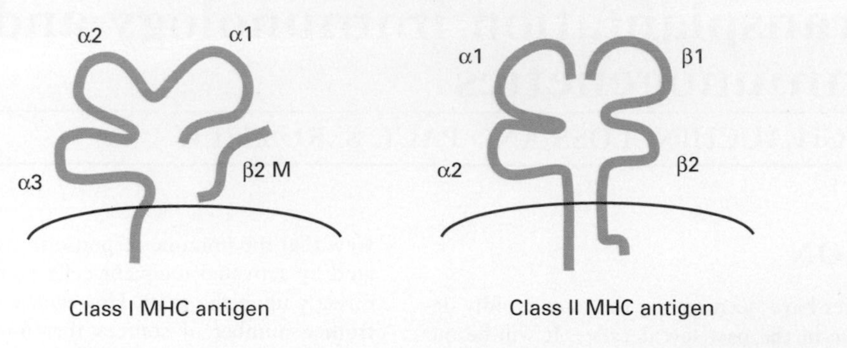

Fig. 1 Schematic diagram of MHC antigens, showing their domains.

called antigens. For the immune system as a whole, antigens may be soluble proteins or cell surface molecules, but only the cell surface antigens are capable of causing rejection of transplanted organs. Three types of surface antigens that are important in transplantation have been identified: (1) the major histocompatibility complex (MHC) antigens; (2) the minor histocompatibility antigens; and (3) the blood group antigens.

Major histocompatibility complex antigens

As their name implies, the major histocompatibility complex (MHC) antigens are the most important antigens causing graft rejection. Their presence was recognized from experiments using inbred strains of mice (see below) in which the products of one particular series of genes were found to be especially important in provoking graft rejection. The site within the genome which includes these genes is called the major histocompatibility complex. All species studied have been found to have MHC genes on a certain chromosome, and the antigens encoded within it have been well characterized in many of them.

Class I versus class II MHC antigens

Two types of MHC antigens have been identified and are now subdivided as class I and class II antigens. Over the years they have been given different names, as listed in Table 1. The class I MHC antigens are composed of two chains, one of which is very polymorphic (meaning that it varies from individual to individual) while the other, called β_2-microglobulin, is similar for all members of the species. The class II MHC antigens are composed of two polymorphic chains, called α and β. Class I antigens exist on almost all cells of the body, while class II antigens are less widely distributed, being expressed on macrophages, B cells, and other cells with 'antigen-presenting' function.

Table 1 Characteristics of human MHC antigens

Class I MHC antigens	Class II MHC antigens
Originally called SD antigens	Originally called LD or Ia antigens
Single polymorphic chain (associated with β_2-microglobulin)	Two polymorphic chains (the α chain is sometimes not polymorphic)
mol. wt. 45 000	mol. wt. 28 000 and 33 000
A, B, and C loci	DP, DQ, and DR loci
Expressed on almost all cells	Expressed on macrophages dendritic cells, B cells, and vascular endothelium

Structure

Despite the differences between the class I and class II MHC antigens, the two types of antigens probably have a similar tertiary configuration. In both cases, each chain has a short intracytoplasmic tail followed by a transmembrane portion with a relatively large extracellular portion which can be divided into regions called domains (Fig. 1). The β_2-microglobulin chain (molecular weight 12 000) is a constant chain with no polymorphism and is coded on a different chromosome to the MHC loci. It is necessary for the transport and expression of the class I MHC antigens on the cell surface.

Nomenclature and genetic organization

At least three different loci within the MHC of humans encode polymorphic class I antigens. Three other loci encode class II antigens. The expression of MHC antigens is codominant (the genes on both chromosomes of a pair are expressed) and therefore up to 12 different MHC antigens are expressed on the cell surface (six encoded on the chromosome inherited from the father and six on the chromosome from the mother).

In humans the three class I loci are designated A, B, and C and the three class II loci are called DP, DQ, and DR. These six loci are organized on chromosome 6 of humans such that the class I loci are together, as are the class II loci (Fig. 2).

Polymorphism and the MHC cleft

One of the cardinal features of the MHC antigens is that there is substantial variation in the fine structure of each antigen between individual members of the species. This occurs because there are many different alleles within each species that can encode the MHC antigen determined by any particular MHC locus. For example, there are at least 20 different MHC class I antigens that can be encoded within the A locus. This variation in the MHC antigens between individuals is called polymorphism.

Structurally, most of the variation between different MHC antigens occurs in the outer two domains of the molecule. Recent crystallographic data have revealed that these areas together form a 'cleft' in the exterior of the antigen and that this cleft on the different MHC antigens therefore has many slightly different configurations (Fig. 3).

HLA typing

The ability of the immune system to develop an antibody response against foreign MHC antigens has provided a tool with which the different antigens expressed by each individual can be characterized. The 20 or more class I antigens encoded in the A locus

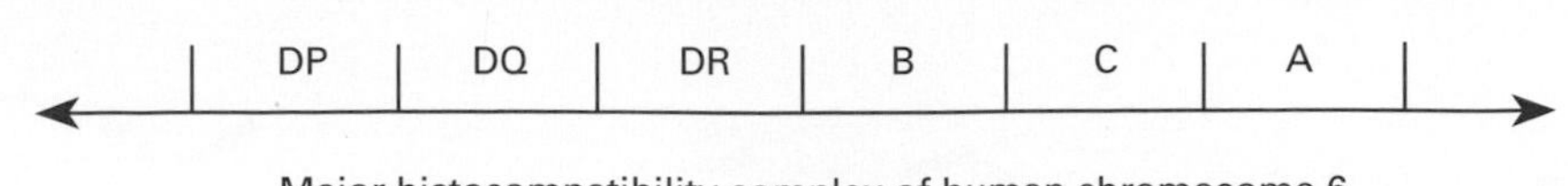

Fig. 2 Organization of the histocompatibility loci of the human MHC.

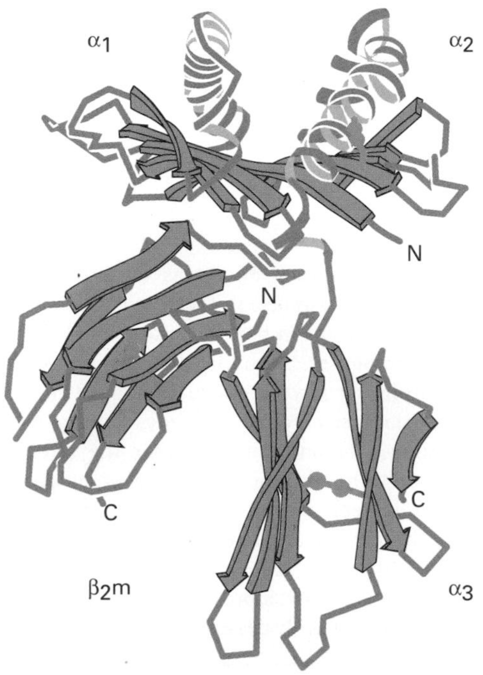

Fig. 3 Schematic representation of an MHC molecule.

have been given numbers such as A2, A3, etc. Similarly, numbers have been assigned to antigens of the other loci. In practice, the available reagents are not adequate to characterize all of the HLA antigens, and the current clinical practice is to define serologically only the HLA A, B, C, and DR antigens. Since there are two antigens (from two chromosomes) for each of the loci, one person's phenotype might be described as:

HLA-A2,3; B7,41; C1,4; DR1,4

The process of determining the HLA phenotype is called tissue typing. It is often confused with cross-matching, a procedure that tests not for compatibility but for the presence of pre-existing antibodies in a recipient, which can react with a donor's MHC antigens. The two techniques use similar methods but the implications of finding an HLA-matched kidney and one with a negative cross-match are completely different.

Inheritance of MHC antigens

In typical mendelian fashion, every person inherits one copy of the MHC from each parent. Each chromosome copy is called a haplotype. Unless the two parents express some of the same histocompatibility antigens, children will share half of their MHC antigens with each of their parents. This is called a one-haplotype match, and parents and children are often said to be 'haplo-identical'.

The sharing of MHC antigens between siblings is more variable. Since each parent has two MHC haplotypes and will pass on only one to each child, four possible combinations of haplotypes may be inherited. Thus, for a particular child the chance that another sibling will have inherited the same two MHC haplotypes is 1 in 4, in which case the siblings are genotypic 'HLA-identical'. The chance that the sibling will have inherited only one of the same MHC haplotypes is 2 in 4, in which case that sibling is 'haplo-identical'. The chance that another sibling will have inherited two different MHC haplotypes is 1 in 4, in which case that sibling is HLA mismatched. These odds are altered slightly by the possibility of genetic recombination occurring within the MHC (the incidence of which is 1 per cent), such that it is possible, for example, for a sibling to share 1½ MHC haplotypes (Fig. 4).

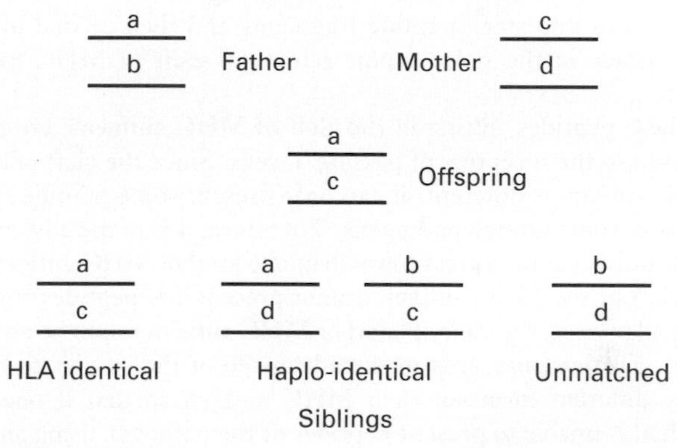

Fig. 4 Inheritance of MHC haplotypes. For a particular offspring seeking an organ transplant, 25 per cent of the siblings will be MHC identical, 50 per cent will be haplo-identical, and 25 per cent will be unmatched.

The function of MHC antigens

The presence of MHC antigens in every mammalian species and the strength of the immune response that they evoke suggests that they are important components of the immune system. However, despite their discovery in transplantation experiments and their importance in graft rejection, the MHC antigens probably do not exist in order to cause graft rejection since this would not offer survival benefit to the species. Despite this obvious point, it was not until the late 1970s that immunologists were able to assign a function to the MHC antigens beyond their role in transplantation.

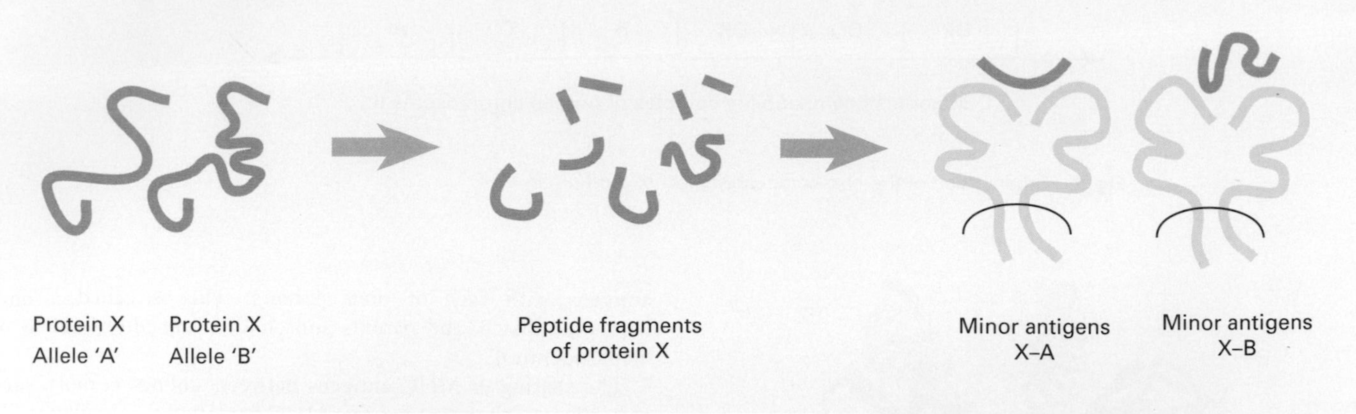

Fig. 5 Minor histocompatibility antigens are peptides of proteins with allelic variation presented in association with MHC molecules.

It is now believed that the MHC molecules serve as focusing elements which direct the cellular elements of the immune system to the site where they can do the most good. If one considers a viral pathogen, it would be inefficient to occupy an entire T cell in neutralizing one, or even several, tiny viral particles. This can be accomplished by the small, soluble, and abundant antibodies which are produced and secreted by B cells. The bulky machinery of T cells would be better used to eliminate the larger cells that have been damaged by viral infection or which have undergone neoplastic transformation.

The MHC antigens accomplish their purpose by acting as antigen-presenting structures. Invading pathogens are broken down within cells into small peptide fragments and then carried to the cell surface in the polymorphic structural cleft of MHC molecules.

These peptides, sitting in the cleft of MHC antigens, are then exposed to the receptors of passing T cells. Since the cleft of each MHC antigen is different, it can only present some peptide fragments of some foreign pathogens. Therefore, it is to the advantage of an individual to express more than one kind of MHC antigen. If the cleft of the MHC antigen cannot present any peptides from a particular virus, the cleft of another MHC antigen might be able to do so. Furthermore, it is to the advantage of the species to have many different forms of each MHC antigen so that if one individual is unable to present peptides of the pathogen using any of its MHC antigens, another individual expressing different MHC antigens might be able to do so. Thus the antigen-presenting function of MHC antigens explains the multiple loci within the complex and the polymorphism of the antigens encoded there.

While the MHC antigens serve to present the peptides of pathogens on the surface of infected cells, the goal of restricting T cells so that they recognize these peptides only in this setting requires an additional feature. This restriction is imposed on the immune system by selection during T-cell maturation only of cells with receptors that are triggered by peptide fragments presented in association with MHC antigens. Part of the T-cell receptor must recognize the peptide itself and part must recognize surrounding determinants formed by the MHC molecule. Because of this dual recognition by T-cell receptors, cell-mediated responses are said to require 'associative recognition'. The role that MHC antigens play in limiting the site of peptide recognition leads to their description as 'restriction elements'.

Although MHC antigens do not exist to prevent organ transplantation, nonetheless they do act as the stimulators and the targets of the immune response in organ rejection. These antigens are particularly important in part because they elicit both T- and B-cell immune responses. Secondly, because the MHC antigens are so polymorphic, it is very unusual to find two unrelated individuals whose antigens are not different. Thirdly, it is a peculiar feature of transplantation immunity that the strength of cell-mediated immunity to allogeneic (those from another individual) MHC antigens is very strong. For example, the precursor frequency of T cells that respond to a foreign MHC antigen is 100- to 1000-fold higher than the frequency of T cells that respond to the peptides of a pathogenic virus presented with an MHC molecule. This surprising finding is discussed further below.

Minor histocompatibility antigens

Minor histocompatibility antigens are simply defined as antigens that cause cell-mediated graft rejection but which are not major histocompatibility antigens. This definition by exclusion reflects the limited information available regarding the minor antigens, which are not, therefore, products of genes within the MHC. For many years they were pictured as similar in character but weaker in strength than the MHC molecules, but more recently this view has been replaced by a growing consensus that the minor antigens represent peptides of autologous proteins, which are presented on the surface of cells in association with major histocompatibility molecules. While such presentation of peptides probably occurs for many autologous proteins, minor histocompatibility antigens are formed when there is a genetically determined difference in a protein's structure between members of a species such that allelic variants among the peptide fragments can be presented in association with MHC antigens. As a hypothetical example, shown in Fig. 5, two different amino acid sequences for protein X (perhaps serum albumin) might exist such that a peptide of the protein from one individual, presented in association with an MHC molecule, will create a minor histocompatibility determinant which is foreign to the T cells of another individual.

The use of immunogenetics to estimate the number of minor antigens

The characterization of minor histocompatibility antigens described above suggests that there might be a large number of minor histocompatibility differences between any two members of

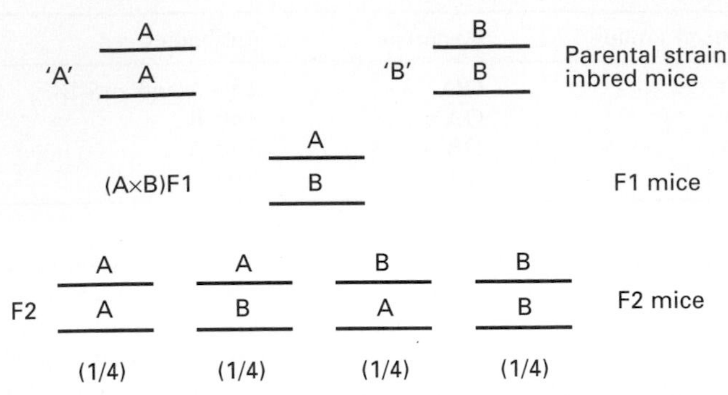

Fig. 6 Breeding inbred strains of mice to create F_2 generation.

a species. This does appear to be the case and this number has been estimated using inbred strains of mice and the principles of transplantation immunogenetics.

If one starts with two inbred mouse strains, 'A' and 'B', each homozygous throughout its genome, it is possible to generate F_1 offspring, called (A × B) F_1, by breeding A with B mice. All F_1 mice will be heterozygous for all polymorphic loci within their genomes. In addition, one can generate F_2 mice by breeding mice from the F_1 generation together. At any given locus, 25 per cent of F_2 mice will be 'AA', 50 per cent will be 'AB', and 25 per cent will be 'BB' (Fig. 6).

After breeding mice in the manner above, transplantation experiments can be performed between members of the generations. Such experiments have been carried out and the results summarized as the five 'laws of transplantation' (see Table 2). Although called 'laws', they were really experimental observations. They were described by Snell based on the work of C. C. Little and others at the Jackson Laboratory in Bar Harbor, Maine, United States.

Table 2 The five laws of transplantation

1. Grafts from strain A mice to strain A mice are accepted
2. Grafts from strain A mice to strain B mice are rejected
3. Grafts from A or B mice to F_1 offspring are accepted but grafts from F_1 mice to either parental strain are rejected
4. Grafts from F_2 mice to F_1 mice are accepted
5. Grafts from parental strain mice to F_2 mice are usually, *but not always*, rejected

C. C. Little recognized that these 'laws of transplantation' were the consequence of two fundamental principles:

(1) that graft rejection was determined by multiple histocompatibility loci with codominant expression of their products;

(2) that rejection would occur whenever the donor expressed products of histocompatibility loci which were not expressed by the recipient.

Little's insight identified the importance of histocompatibility loci in transplantation and initiated the experiments that identified what became known as the major histocompatibility complex of genes. He also recognized that the observation incorporated in the fifth 'law of transplantation' provided the means to determine the total number of histocompatibility loci.

To understand Little's reasoning, let us assume that there is only a single histocompatibility locus responsible for rejection, as shown in Fig. 6. Under these circumstances parental grafts from strain A to mice of the F_2 generation would be accepted by three-quarters of the offspring (those which were 'AA' or 'AB' at the important locus). If two histocompatibility loci were involved in graft rejection, then the probability of A strain graft acceptance by F_2 mice would be $(3/4) \times (3/4)$, or $(3/4)^2$. If the number of loci involved was larger still, then the probability (p) of graft acceptance would be:

$$p\ (\mathrm{P} \rightarrow \mathrm{F}_2) = (3/4)^n$$

where n is the number of histocompatibility loci. Since the fifth law of transplantation showed that P → F_2 grafts were usually rejected, Little concluded that n must be quite large. He also believed that it could be determined experimentally. In fact, the results of thousands of grafting experiments from parental to F_2 mice indicate that at least between 30 and 50 histocompatibility loci must exist. The major histocompatibility complex, encoding the MHC antigens discussed above, represents only one of these sites, and all the remaining loci encode minor histocompatibility antigens.

Associative recognition of minor histocompatibility antigens

One of the important ways in which minor transplantation antigens differ from major antigens is the requirement that T cells recognize minor antigens only when their peptides are presented in association with major histocompatibility molecules. Minor antigens are therefore similar to external pathogens, such as viruses, and the 'associative' recognition of minor antigens represents the normal process of T-cell recognition. In contrast, the direct recognition of allogeneic major histocompatibility antigens, without a requirement for antigen processing and presentation in association with other MHC molecules, represents an unusual T-cell response.

The peptides that form minor histocompatibility antigens can be expressed in association with either class I or class II MHC antigens. When in association with class II antigens, they generally activate a subpopulation of T cells that expresses a surface antigen called CD4. These T-cells function primarily to provide 'help' for other T cell responses. On the other hand, when presented in association with class I MHC antigens, they generally activate a subpopulation of T cells that expresses an antigen called CD8. These cells usually have cytotoxic function. Thus the response to minor histocompatibility antigens usually requires the function of both of the two major subpopulations of T cells. As will be discussed below, this requirement is in contrast to the response to major histocompatibility antigens.

The absence of an antibody response to minor antigens

Another important feature of minor histocompatibility antigens, in contrast to the MHC antigens, is that there is generally no detectable antibody response to these antigens. This feature, although surprising at first, when it was assumed that minor antigens were cell surface structures, similar to but weaker than MHC antigens, proved not to be so when it was recognized that the minor antigens probably do not exist independently on the cell surface in three-dimensional form but only as peptides presented with MHC molecules. Antibody responses to peptide fragments presented by MHC antigens have been generally difficult to detect. Without antibodies to the minor antigens, we lack one of the important tools to identify and characterize them.

Immunodominance in the response to minor antigens

Another feature of the response to minor histocompatibility antigens, called immunodominance (which is not the same as genetic dominance), is that in the face of multiple minor antigen disparities, the immune response may select only a few of these disparities as targets. Therefore, in some experimental cases where grafts differing by multiple minor antigens are exchanged, rejection of a second graft of a type expressing only one of the original minor antigens may not show evidence of sensitization to that antigen. An explanation for this phenomenon is that when multiple peptides are available for presentation by MHC molecules, some of them may associate preferentially with the available MHC antigens, excluding the other peptides. Thus the requirement for associative recognition of minor antigens is probably responsible for the phenomenon of immunodominance.

The H-Y minor antigen

One of many minor histocompatibility antigens has been studied extensively, namely the H-Y minor antigen, which can be detected by the rejection of skin grafts from male donors by female members of the same inbred strain of animal. As inbred females accept grafts from one another and inbred males accept grafts from females of the same strain, it appears that this graft rejection is due to expression of a minor antigen encoded on the Y chromosome. Some inbred strains of mice are capable of rejecting grafts exchanged between the sexes, while others are not. Therefore it is possible to investigate the requirements for a response to the H-Y histocompatibility antigen. Unfortunately this investigation has not provided simple answers. It appears that the ability to reject H-Y disparate grafts depends on multiple genes encoded both within the MHC and elsewhere.

The blood group antigens

The blood group antigens are carbohydrates and glycoproteins present on the surface of red blood cells and a few other cell types. They were identified and characterized because of their importance in blood transfusions, an early example of tissue transplantation.

Three major blood group antigens are commonly recognized, designated O, A, and B. In actual fact the situation is far more complicated than this simple designation implies, but for purposes of organ transplantation a simple picture is sufficient. In general, the different blood group antigens all arise from a single glycoprotein structure. The genes responsible for the several forms of this structure encode glycosylation enzymes which modify the core protein differently. Individuals of blood group O express the unmodified glycoprotein, those of blood group A express this glycoprotein with an additional external sugar, and those of blood group B express the core glycoprotein with a different additional external sugar. Individuals of blood group AB have the enzymes to add both additional sugar molecules. The inheritance of the major blood group antigens follows mendelian principles for a single locus with three allelic genes (O, A, B). The relationship between genotype and phenotype is shown in Table 3.

There is no T-cell mediated immune response to the blood group antigens, but there is an antibody response to these structures. The blood group antibodies are unusual in that they develop without prior exposure to foreign blood cells. Blood group antibodies are formed early in life, probably by exposure to cross-reactive determinants on common bacterial organisms. Since individuals do not form antibodies to structures that they express, individuals of blood group AB do not have antibodies to other blood group antigens while those of blood group O have both anti-A and anti-B antibodies. A and B individuals have antibodies to the antigen of each other.

Table 3 Blood group antigens

Blood group	Genotype	Antibodies
O	OO	Anti-A and anti-B
A	OA or AA	Anti-B
B	OB or BB	Anti-A
AB	AB	None

The issue of blood group antigens is complicated further by the existence of hundreds of other antigens on the surfaces of blood cells, which may prevent successful transfusion of blood. For transplantation of solid organs, however, only the ABO antigens need be considered since they are expressed on essentially all organs, especially on vascular endothelium. Therefore, as far as blood group antigens are concerned, O blood group organ donors are universal donors, AB donors can be used only for AB recipients, and A or B donors are suitable for recipients of their own blood group or AB individuals.

In the practice of organ transplantation three modifications of these general principles are noteworthy. First, not all organs are equally susceptible to antibody-mediated rejection by blood group antibodies, and transplantation of the bone marrow and liver in particular are sometimes performed across blood group barriers. Secondly, there are two subgroups of blood group A, called A_1 and A_2, and individuals of blood group O or B may not form antibodies which react with the A_2 determinant. Therefore it is sometimes possible to cross this blood group barrier in this special case (A_2 to O). Finally, removal of blood group antibodies from potential recipients by plasmapheresis before transplantation has occasionally allowed successful transplantation across blood group barriers. However, this approach is not widely applied, except for bone-marrow transplantation.

THE EXPRESSION OF TRANSPLANTATION ANTIGENS

Although essentially all cells of an individual share the same complement of genes, not all cells in the body express all of the transplantation antigens at all times. It is likely, therefore, that the factors affecting antigen expression will have an important effect on graft rejection. When considering these issues, 'constitutive' expression refers to the baseline level of antigen expression by a given cell type, while 'induced' expression refers to expression that occurs in response to various stimuli.

The tissue distribution of transplantation antigens

Class I MHC antigens are expressed constitutively on essentially every type of cell in the body. Only a few cell types, including spermatazoa and red cells, have unusually low expression of these antigens, which may be important in protecting them from immunological responses.

Class II MHC antigens are not constitutively expressed on all cells and are normally found on those types of cells that specialize in the uptake, processing, and presentation of soluble foreign antigens. These include B lymphocytes, macrophages, and dendritic cells (including Langerhans cells in the skin and Kupffer cells in the liver). Endothelial cells of vessels also express class II antigens, as do thymic epithelial cells; this is important for their role in positive and negative T-cell selection.

Because of the differences in tissue distribution, not all types of organs and tissues have equal expression of transplantation antigens and hence are not necessarily equal in their susceptibility to rejection. For example, experimental tail skin grafts from mice have fewer Langerhans cells than trunk skin grafts and therefore have fewer cells expressing class II antigens. This difference leads to significant differences in the strength of rejection for the two types of grafts. Clinically, it is not clear that sufficient differences exist between the commonly used organs in the destiny of cells expressing class II antigens to affect the outcome of organ transplantation, but it would not be surprising to find that such differences do exist, say between the heart and the liver.

The induction of transplantation antigen expression

The constitutive expression of class I antigens is sufficiently high that variations in the level of expression do not have an appreciable effect on the immune response to them. Variations in class II antigen expression, on the other hand, probably do have important consequences in transplantation immunology. Not only can the level of class II expression on antigen-presenting cells be increased, but in addition, cell types that do not normally express class II antigens can be induced to do so in response to several stimuli. γ-Interferon and interleukin-4 are especially important signals that include class II antigen expression.

In a normal immune response, the increased expression of class II antigens may amplify the immune response to antigens presented in association with class II molecules. In transplantation immunology, this effect has important implications regarding graft rejection. Since class II targets will only be expressed constitutively on certain cell types, many cells would avoid rejection aimed at these antigens unless induction occurs. Experimentally, class II induction can be prevented by antibodies against interferon and these antibodies can therefore be used to prolong graft survival in some cases of class II-only disparity. This experimental finding may explain the clinically recognized phenomenon that viral infections and other immune stimuli, such as vaccination, sometime induced rejection episodes. Perhaps the production of interferon or other lymphokines during infection induces the expression of class II antigens on the allograft, provoking previously dormant transplantation immunity.

The special role of antigen-presenting cells

The cell types that constitutively express class II antigens play a critical role in stimulating T cells. These cells are called antigen-presenting cells and they share the capacity to process foreign antigens, to present them in association with MHC antigens, and to secrete certain lymphokines which are required for T-cell activation. Thus it is more than just the expression of class II antigens that make these cells important.

The distribution of antigen-presenting cells in the body reflects the site where contact with foreign antigens will most likely occur or where immune responses can most powerfully be achieved. For example, the skin, intestinal tract, and lungs have large numbers of antigen-presenting cells and there are large numbers in liver, lymph nodes, and spleen. The function of the antigen-presenting cells in skin, where they are known as Langerhans cells, has been investigated in detail. Foreign antigens entering through the skin encounter abundant Langerhans cells at this site. These antigen-presenting cells, now known as 'veiled' cells because of their appearance, then carry the antigen from the skin to regional lymph nodes. At this site the antigen-presenting cells are known as 'interdigitating cells'. Inserted into lymph nodes, these antigen-presenting cells are in a good position to present peptides of the foreign antigens to the many recipient T cells that circulate through each lymph node. This process increases the likelihood that individual T cells will encounter each foreign antigen without requiring that every T cell circulate to the remote corners of the skin.

The consequences of this mechanism for antigen recognition and presentation for graft rejection are several. First, sensitization to allogeneic antigens may often occur not in the graft itself but rather in peripheral lymph nodes. This has been demonstrated experimentally using tissue grafts to vascularized sites that had been surgically deprived of lymphatic drainage. These grafts were not rejected. Secondly, the critical function of antigen-presenting cells suggests that without them graft rejection might not occur at all. Several experimental systems have shown this to be true, giving rise to the notion that rejection might be prevented by eliminating 'passenger leucocytes'. For example, under certain conditions tissue culture results in the selective loss of antigen-presenting cells from various endocrine tissues, including pancreatic islets, favouring the successful transplantation of these tissues without immunosuppression or with immunosuppression at reduced dosages. Unfortunately, the antigen-presenting cells of most organs include more than just leucocytes and it is difficult in clinical practice to eliminate all of the antigen-presenting cells from any organ.

Although prior removal of all antigen-presenting cells from donor organs is difficult to achieve, there is turnover of these cells in a donor organ after transplantation. Therefore, donor dendritic cells and macrophages are slowly replaced by cells arising from the recipient's bone marrow. In clinical transplantation, this exchange may contribute to a decline in the immunogenicity of a graft and of the frequency of rejection episodes over time.

MECHANISMS OF GRAFT REJECTION

So far this section has dealt primarily with the antigens that are the targets of the immune response. We will now consider features of the response itself. The presentation of this topic is confusing since there are two settings in which the mechanisms of graft rejection can be observed: the clinical and the experimental. While ideally the two sets of observations would be closely related by a clear understanding of the mechanisms involved, in fact that understanding is far from complete. Thus, not all features of graft rejection seen in one setting correlate clearly with observations in another.

Clinical patterns of rejection

Three main patterns of rejection are usually identified in clinical practice: (1) hyperacute rejection, (2) acute rejection, and (3) chronic rejection.

Hyperacute rejection

Hyperacute rejection is a form of rejection that occurs instantaneously after restoration of blood supply to the transplanted organ. Typically, the newly transplanted organ shows normal initial circulation followed by discoloration and then abrupt cessation of function as blood flow ceases throughout the organ. There is no known intervention that can do more than delay this process slightly.

In the mid-1960s investigators recognized that hyperacute rejection occurred when a recipient possessed antibodies in the serum before transplantation which were specific for donor antigens. With this information, it became possible to avoid hyperacute rejection by testing potential recipients for the existence of preformed antibodies, using a test called the cross-match, and thus to allow the selection of donors whose cells did not manifest any antigen against which the recipient had already formed antibodies.

As described above, preformed antibodies can arise from a number of causes. While blood group antibodies do not require prior exposure to blood cells of an incompatible donor, all other preformed antibodies to antigens of transplanted organs arise from prior exposure to foreign transplantation antigens. This can occur by blood transfusion, by pregnancy (which exposes the mother to the father's antigens expressed by the fetus), and by transplantation of organs. However, not every individual exposed to foreign antigens in these ways will necessarily form antibodies.

The correlation between the clinical pattern of hyperacute rejection and an immunological mechanism involving antibody-mediated rejection appears to be excellent. However, there is experimental evidence that an early rejection process resembling typical hyperacute rejection can occur in the absence of demonstrable antibody, presumably by cell-mediated mechanisms.

Acute rejection

Since hyperacute rejection can usually be avoided by use of the cross-match, the most commonly encountered clinical pattern of rejection is acute rejection. In this case, organs that have functioned well for a week or so then demonstrate diminished function over a period of several days. Biopsies at this time typically show a lymphocyte infiltrate. Without treatment, graft destruction will almost always occur but, unlike hyperacute rejection, acute rejection can often be treated and reversed by forms of immunosuppression that are effective against cellular immunity.

Variations in the histological picture of acute rejection can be detected. In some cases there is a dense eosinophilic infiltrate, which correlates with especially severe rejection. In other cases there is striking vascular destruction, leading to the description 'vascular rejection', often thought to imply that there is an antibody-mediated component to the rejection mechanism. However, the evidence for the association of specific histological findings with particular immunological mechanisms remains imperfect.

Acute rejection episodes tend to occur as discrete events, once or sometimes several times after transplantation. Most of these episodes take place during the first few months after operation, but episodes of sudden organ dysfunction which can be reversed by increased immunosuppression may occur months or even years after transplantation. Because of their sudden onset, rapid pace, and reversibility, these late episodes are also described as acute rejection episodes. They may be triggered by reduction or cessation of immunosuppression, but often have no clear aetiology.

Chronic rejection

Chronic rejection refers to a clinical picture of slow deterioration in organ function over months or years. The deterioration is difficult to control by standard immunosuppression. Pathological examination of organs suffering chronic rejection often reveals a relatively sparse lymphocyte infiltrate and may show a characteristic 'onion-skin' appearance with concentric cellular thickening and obstruction of flow in the small arteries of the graft, a finding that correlates well with the presence of antibodies in the recipient which are specific for donor antigens. These features suggest that chronic rejection may be caused by antibody-mediated mechanisms resulting from antibodies induced in the recipient after transplantation. It is unlikely, however, that all cases of chronic rejection are caused by humoral mechanisms alone.

Characterization of the clinical picture of graft rejection using the terms described above is extremely useful in the management of patients. Particular patterns respond to particular forms of treatment and the ability to judge the prognosis for survival of a transplanted organ is important in determining the vigour of the treatment effort. However, these characterizations can become misleading when they are used to imply a particular mechanism of rejection. This suggests a better understanding of the processes involved than actually exists and implies a scientific basis for the treatment employed, which has not yet been achieved.

Experimental studies of the mechanisms of graft rejection

Antibody-mediated rejection

Immediate rejection by preformed antibody

Numerous experiments demonstrate that antibodies can cause rejection which appears to be similar to the syndrome of hyperacute rejection recognized clinically. The antibodies must be present prior to the transplant and must be specific for antigens expressed on vascular endothelium. However, only certain vascularized organs are susceptible to immediate antibody-mediated rejection.

The pathophysiology of hyperacute rejection has been characterized in some detail. The initial step in the process involves binding of the preformed antibodies to the vascular endothelial cells of the new organ. This binding then initiates a series of interacting cascades. Complement fixation is involved, and activation of the classical complement system then activates the recipient endothelium, stimulates the clotting system, and triggers the kallikrein cascade. Within minutes there are substantial changes in the permeability and integrity of the endothelial lining, intense vascular constriction, and vascular thrombosis. These account for the clinical features and pathological findings of hyperacute rejection.

Some understanding of the mechanisms of hyperacute rejection has come from the many efforts to control it. Complement inhibitors, clotting inhibitors, and many other substances have been shown to delay the process. None of these interventions, however, is able to block the progression of hyperacute rejection in a clinically meaningful way. Once started, hyperacute rejection inevitably destroys the transplanted organ.

As a result of these findings, the principal effort in dealing with preformed antibody has been either to eliminate the preformed antibody prior to transplantation or to select donors or tissues which do not express the relevant target antigens. Elimination of preformed antibody by plasmapheresis or absorption, coupled with B-cell immunosuppression, has occasionally been successful in achieving successful transplantation across blood group barriers. In general, however, elimination of preformed antibody is an uncertain approach to transplantation when there is a positive cross-match. Some organs and tissues appear to resist rejection by antibody. Skin grafts do not suffer hyperacute rejection and can survive for long periods despite the presence of preformed antibody. The liver is quite resistant to antibody-mediated rejection, although liver transplants performed across a positive cross-match show inferior survival over the long term. Pancreatic islets, especially after periods of *in-vitro* culture, may also be resistant to antibody-mediated rejection.

Slow rejection caused by induced antibody

Even when antibodies specific for donor antigens are not present before a transplant, they may be induced by exposure to foreign antigens after the transplant has been performed. This antibody formation by B cells requires the help of T cells. The antibody tends to be specific for MHC antigens and to be IgG in class.

It is difficult to determine the role of induced antibody in causing rejection. This is partly because induced antibody is not formed unless T cells are present, making it hard to separate the contribution of direct cell-mediated graft destruction. In addition, there are examples where organs survive well despite the presence of measurable quantities of induced antibody. There are also some cases where antibodies specific for donor antigens actually seem to prevent rejection by T cells (a phenomenon called enhancement). Nonetheless, there is evidence that organ rejection can be caused by induced antibody responses. Clinically, we believe that there is a strong correlation between pathological recognition of an 'onion-skin' appearance of small donor arteries, the presence of induced antibody in the recipient, and slow, progressive graft destruction. Experimentally, there are examples of early xenograft destruction, occurring too late for hyperacute rejection, which take place despite high levels of T-cell immunosuppression and which correlate well with the appearance of induced antibody.

Cell-mediated graft rejection

In the absence of preformed antibody, the rejection of transplanted organs involves a cell-mediated mechanism that has three principal features. First, this rejection requires the function of T cells. This has been demonstrated by the indefinite survival of skin grafts on T-cell-deficient 'nude' mice. Secondly, the process shows immunological specificity and memory. This process has been demonstrated by showing that a second graft from the same donor is rejected more rapidly by a recipient than the first graft, while a second graft from an unrelated donor is not. Thirdly, the process is precisely targeted against the cells of the donor graft. This has been shown by skin graft experiments using 'tetraparental mice', formed by fusion of two embryos in the early stages of development. Mature tetraparental animals are composed of a mosaic of two different cell types interspersed throughout the body. For example, tetraparental mice originating from black and white parents show a speckled 'salt and pepper' coat colour. When skin from a mouse is transplanted to a recipient which is syngeneic with one parent but allogeneic to the other, only the allogeneic cells are rejected. The syngeneic cells survive the destruction of their allogeneic immediate neighbours.

Considerable effort has been devoted to determining the mechanisms by which T cells can cause graft destruction in a manner showing specificity, memory, and precise targeting. Several different experimental techniques have been used. First, there has been histological examination to determine the nature and distribution of T cells within a rejecting graft. Secondly, T cells within grafts have been removed and analysed for their type, function, and specificity. One way to achieve this has been to use 'sponge-matrix' allografts, which are inert sponges containing allogeneic target cells. These sponges can be removed from a recipient at any time after transplantation and the infiltrating cells squeezed out for analysis. Thirdly, T cells of different phenotypes have been transferred into T-cell-deficient animals to determine which types of cells are able to cause graft destruction. Fourthly, *in-vitro* assays of T-cell function, including proliferation interleukin-2 production, and cell-mediated cytotoxicity have been tested, seeking correlations between the development of these T-cell functions and the onset of graft destruction. All of these techniques for studying graft rejection have been refined by experiments using donors that differ from their recipients by only limited antigenic disparities and by using antibodies to T-cell antigens, such as the CD4 and CD8, which define subpopulations of the overall T-cell population.

Several conclusions have been generated from these studies. First, only a small portion of the T cells that invade an allograft are specific for the antigens of the donor. Secondly, only a small number of invading T cells are actually required for graft rejection. Thirdly, the T cells that invade a graft are generally of many types, with many functions, making it difficult to determine from this analysis the actual mechanism of graft rejection. Finally, there is an excellent correlation between the ability of the recipient to generate cytotoxic T cells *in vitro* against cells of a particular donor and the ability of that recipient to reject grafts from the same donor. These findings support the 'cytotoxicity hypothesis' that graft destruction is mainly caused by the development of cytotoxic T cells in a manner analogous to the *in-vitro* development of cell-mediated cytotoxicity.

The development of T-cell cytotoxicity

The development of T-cell cytotoxicity *in vitro* requires more than one T-cell function. According to the standard model (Fig. 7), the process begins with a random clustering of T cells around antigen-presenting cells based on the affinity of non-specific T-cell surface molecules for ligands present on these cells. One interaction is between a T-cell structure known as LFA-1 (for 'leucocyte function antigen') with a ligand called ICAM-1 (for 'intercellular adhesion molecule'). While this interaction promotes binding, it is not in itself sufficient to cause T-cell activation. Activation requires the specific binding of the T-cell receptor with determinants on the MHC antigens of the antigen-presenting cells. These determinants may be formed by the association of peptides derived from foreign proteins with self-MHC molecules or, in the case of graft rejection, by the presence of donor MHC antigens which are recognized directly.

In addition to requiring engagement of the T-cell receptor, T-cell activation is also augmented by other accessory molecules. Especially prominent are the interactions of the CD4 antigen, present on one group of T cells, with a determinant expressed on all class II MHC antigens, and those of the CD8 antigen, present on another group of T cells, with a determinant expressed on all

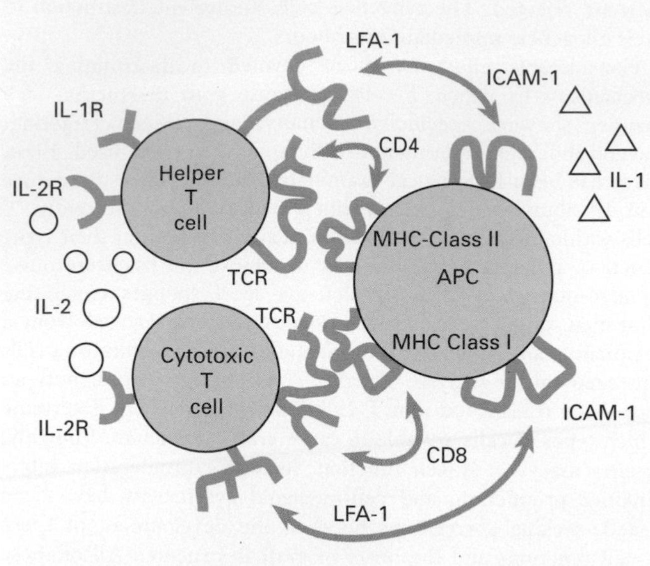

Fig. 7 Development of cytotoxic T cells. Multiple interactions between T cells and antigen-presenting cells and between helper and cytotoxic T cells are involved in the development of T-cell cytotoxicity. For abbreviations see text.

class I MHC antigens. These accessory molecules are responsible for the finding that $CD4^+$ T cells have specificity for class II MHC antigens, while $CD8^+$ T cells are specific for class I MHC antigens.

Finally, the standard model of T-cell activation also suggests that antigen-presenting cells secrete lymphokines, probably including interleukin-1 (IL-1), which bind to receptors on T cells to augment T-cell activation. One kind of T cell that is activated by these mechanisms is called a helper T cell. Once activated, helper cells begin to produce a lymphokine called interleukin-2 (IL-2), formerly described as T-cell growth factor, which contributes to the growth and maturation of activated cells. These activated T cells also express new receptors for IL-2, creating a positive feedback system which augments the helper response.

A second kind of T cell is a precursor of the cytotoxic T cell. It can also be activated by contact with antigen-presenting cells expressing foreign antigens. Proliferation and maturation of the cytotoxic T cell precursor into a functional cytotoxic T cell requires the IL-2 produced by helper cells. Once activated, these cytotoxic T cells can kill any cell expressing the same target antigens. Thus the development of T-cell cytotoxicity requires helper T-cell activity, precursors of cytotoxic cells, specific recognition of a foreign antigen, and the function of several non-specific cell surface molecules and soluble lymphokines.

The three cell cluster requirement for T-cell activation

The model of T-cell activation shown in Fig. 7 shows a helper T cell interacting with the same antigen-presenting cell as the precursor of the cytotoxic T cell. This 'three cell cluster' does appear to be an important requirement for T-cell activation *in vivo*. Apparently the IL-2 produced by a helper T cell can only provide help for cytotoxic T cells at a short distance. Thus lymphokines of this sort act like neurotransmitters rather than like hormones. *In vitro* the requirement for a three-cell interaction is not essential and excess IL-2 can be added to a culture, bypassing the requirement for the helper T cells in the generation of cytotoxic T cells.

Pathways of alloreactivity

The classic picture of T-cell activation usually shows the helper function being performed by $CD4^+$ T cells and the cytotoxic function being performed by $CD8^+$ T cells. This view has emerged because when both class I and class II antigenic disparities are present, $CD4^+$ T cells do tend to perform the helper function, while $CD8^+$ T cells tend to develop into cytotoxic T cells. Based on these findings, the designations '$CD4^+$' and 'helper' T cells are often used interchangeably as are '$CD8^+$' and 'cytotoxic' T cells. However, it is an important feature of alloreactivity that this association of phenotype and function is not absolute. $CD4^+$ T cells can show cytotoxic function and $CD8^+$ T cells can produce IL-2. Sometimes, these $CD8^+$ helper cells are also able to develop cytotoxic activity, leading to the designation 'helper-independent' cytotoxic T cells.

Because of this overlap of T-cell functions, careful analysis has been required to identify the multiple avenues by which alloreactive cytotoxicity can develop. Currently at least three pathways are recognized by which the necessary 'help' can be generated:

(1) $CD4^+$ T cells can recognize allogeneic class II MHC antigens directly;
(2) $CD4^+$ T cells can recognize peptides of alloantigens in association with self-MHC antigens;
(3) $CD8^+$ T cells can recognize allogeneic class I antigens directly.

In addition, three different populations of cytotoxic T cell precursors that can respond to alloantigens are now recognized:

(1) $CD8^+$ cytotoxic cells can recognize class I MHC antigens;
(2) $CD4^+$ cytotoxic cells can recognize class II antigens;
(3) $CD8^+$ cytotoxic cells, defying the association of phenotype with antigen specificity, can recognize and kill targets expressing a class II MHC antigenic disparity.

The pathways for generating 'help' and cytotoxic T cells are shown in Table 4. In most clinical transplant situations the number of antigenic disparities between recipient and donor is large enough that all of these potential pathways for the development of cytotoxicity are available.

Table 4 Pathways of alloreactivity

Source of help	Source of cytotoxic T cells
$CD4^+$ anti-allo. class II	$CD4^+$ anti-allo. class II
$CD4^+$anti-allo. class I presented by self-class II	$CD8^+$ anti-allo. class I
$CD8^+$ anti-allo. class I	$CD8^+$ anti-allo. class II

allo. = alloantigen

Other mechanisms of cellular graft rejection

Although there is strong experimental evidence that cytotoxic T cells represent an important mechanism of graft destruction, there are several experimental situations in which rejection correlates poorly with the development of cytotoxicity *in vivo*. First, the rejection of grafts expressing only minor histocompatibility antigen disparities has been reported to occur even when cytotoxic T cells specific for the donor have not been found in the recipient. Secondly, vigorous cell-mediated rejection of tissues transplanted between species is always seen, even though there is sometimes weak cell-mediated cytotoxicity measured *in vitro*. These exceptional cases raise the possibility that other mechanisms of rejection may be brought into play. Delayed-type hypersensitivity is a T-cell response that might be involved. In this case, lymphokines from T cells may activate macrophages to cause tissue destruction. Alternatively, the development of natural killer cells or lymphokine-activated killer cells might destroy foreign grafts. Both of these mechanisms would appear to lack the means to achieve the precise target specificity that is a feature of graft rejection, and thus their role in graft destruction remains uncertain.

Anti-T-cell immunosuppression

Since cell-mediated rejection is T-cell dependent, many forms of immunosuppression have been developed or selected because they interfere with T-cell function. For example, cyclosporin is a fungal product with a hydrophobic cyclic structure. It prevents the generation of interleukin-2 by T cells, blocking the generation of T-cell 'help'. OKT3 is a monoclonal antibody which is specific for the CD3 antigen, present on all T cells, and intimately associated with the T-cell receptor. This antigen is involved in the transduction of signals to the interior of a cell after engagement of the external receptor. Administration of OKT3 to patients eliminates all T cells from the circulation and then allows the return of T cells which lack the expression of the CD3 antigen. These cells are not functional without their signalling mechanism.

Because cyclosporin and OKT3 block a large portion of the T-cell response, their use leaves the recipient broadly immunosuppressed. Therefore efforts have been made to use antibodies specific for subpopulations of T cells or for other structures involved in the immune response. These include antibodies for CD4 or CD8 antigens, antibodies directed at the IL-2 receptor, and antibodies directed at the intercellular adhesion molecule on the antigen-presenting cell. Some of these will probably find a role in clinical practice, although that role has not yet been defined.

In addition to new monoclonal antibodies, new chemical immunosuppressive agents such as FK-506, 15-deoxyspergualin, and rapamycin are also being tested. Like cyclosporin, these are also non-specific reagents; however, their site of action may differ from that of cyclosporin.

Sensitized T cells in graft rejection

The scheme of T-cell activation leading to graft rejection described above starts with naive T cells that have never before encountered the donor antigens. While this process represents an important situation in graft rejection, it may not always reflect the situation in clinical transplantation. Just as B cells may have been activated before transplantation, so T cells may also have been sensitized by prior encounters with foreign MHC antigens. In addition, a majority of transplant recipients will experience an episode or more of graft rejection after their transplant, which will generate sensitized T cells. Thus the actual requirement in clinical transplantation may often involve the suppression of T-cell responses which have already been stimulated. The role of memory T cells, the factors that turn them from dormant to active cytotoxic T cells, and the difference between the requirements for immunosuppression before and after T-cell sensitization are all issues that require further study.

The strength of alloreactivity

The response of T cells to the alloantigens of donor grafts is expected since T cells would be expected to respond to any foreign antigen. What is not expected is that the allogeneic response should prove to be so powerful. The precursor frequency of T cells that respond to a single determinant of an allogeneic MHC antigen is in the range of 2 per 100 T cells. In contrast, the precursor frequency of T cells responding to determinants formed by a foreign virus or other extrinsic antigen presented in association with a self-MHC antigen is about 1 in 10 000. Thus, the allogeneic response is enormously powerful relative to the response to a pathogenic virus and, in fact, the allogeneic T-cell response is the most powerful immune response measured. Why should T-cell alloreactivity be so strong when the immune system presumably evolved to protect us from viruses and other pathogens and not to protect us from receiving kidney transplants from cadaveric donors? A clear answer to this question is not yet available. However, much has been learned recently about the selection of T cells to form the mature T-cell repertoire, removing some of the mystery of alloreactivity.

T-cell development depends on the presence of the thymus, hence the designation 'T' cell. In addition, T cells that can react with self-antigens are eliminated in the thymus prior to maturation. It is now also recognized that the thymus plays a critical role in positively selecting the T cells that are allowed to mature, by selecting those cells with high affinity for modified forms of self-MHC antigens in addition to removing the cells that can react with unmodified self-MHC antigens. This dual process is presumably useful because mature T cells will only encounter foreign antigens when peptides of those antigens are presented in association with self-MHC molecules. Therefore, the mature T-cell repertoire is chosen for its affinity for modified self-MHC antigens.

In addition to this understanding of the selection of the T-cell repertoire, it is now also recognized that allogeneic MHC antigens present determinants that look to T cells like modified self-MHC antigens. In immunology, this feature is referred to by the shorthand notation that

$$\text{Allo} = \text{Self} + \text{X}$$

where 'X' is the peptide of a foreign protein which is presented in association with a self-MHC antigen. Thus the mature T-cell repertoire, selected for the ability to recognize Self + X, also includes T cells capable of recognizing allogeneic MHC antigens directly.

The similarity of modified self-MHC antigens to alloantigens is sufficient to explain the ability of T cells to recognize allo-MHC antigens without a requirement that these antigens be processed and presented as peptides in association with self-MHC antigens. However, the selection process does not, in itself, explain why the alloreactive repertoire should be more powerful than that for modified self-MHC antigens. Why should the number of T cells reacting with a particular allogeneic determinant be so much larger than the number of T cells reacting with a particular Self + X determinant?

Several theories have been proposed to explain the strength of alloreactivity. First, the genes that encode T-cell receptors might be maintained especially because they encode specificity for MHC antigens. This germline encoding of MHC specificity would increase the efficiency of the T-cell selection process, since the thymus will only select those T cells that are able to recognize modified forms of self-MHC antigens. Those T cells without any affinity for an MHC antigen would always be wasted. According to this hypothesis, the high precursor frequency of alloreactive T cells occurs because the receptor genes actually encode an alloreactive repertoire. Some T-cell receptor genes have been identified which do show affinity for particular MHC antigens of their species, providing some support for this hypothesis.

A second theory to explain the strength of alloreactivity suggests that the high precursor frequency of alloreactive T cells does not result from more T cells recognizing allogeneic MHC determinants, but rather from the greater number of allo-determinants expressed on the surface of an allogeneic antigen-presenting cell. For example, an immune response to the measles virus requires that peptides of that virus be presented in association with self-MHC antigens on a self-antigen-presenting cell. But probably only a few of the MHC antigens on a given antigen-presenting cell are engaged in the process of presenting measles peptides, while the other MHC antigens are occupied with presenting other peptides of autologous proteins, forming determinants that do not stimulate autologous T cells. In contrast, every one of the allogeneic MHC antigens on an allogeneic antigen-presenting cell will be able to stimulate a T-cell response since these allo-MHC antigens can each be recognized directly. According to this hypothesis, the greater strength of alloreactivity is, in a sense, an artefact of our assay system: there are more of a particular allogeneic determinant on allogeneic antigen-presenting cells than of modified self-determinants on self-antigen-presenting cells. Therefore alloreactive T cells will be stimulated more easily than those that recognize modified self and their number will appear to be larger by precursor frequency analysis.

A third hypothesis is based on the notion that all MHC antigens are engaged in presenting peptides all of the time, but that most often these peptides are from autologous proteins, forming determinants that are considered self-determinants by T cells. For example, some MHC antigens may present peptides from serum albumin while others might present peptides from haemoglobin. According to this hypothesis, the MHC antigens of an allogeneic antigen-presenting cell also present these same peptides in association with the allogeneic MHC molecules. However, the association of an albumin peptide with an allo-MHC antigen or a haemoglobin peptide with that MHC antigen would not form a self-determinant. Therefore, a single allogeneic MHC antigen on an allogeneic antigen-presenting cell could present multiple new foreign determinants to responding T cells. Thus, a higher precursor frequency of alloreactive T cells would result from the large number of new determinants created out of a single MHC difference.

These hypotheses need not be mutually exclusive, and it is quite likely that each is correct to some degree. However, the relative role of these potential mechanisms, or of others, has not yet been determined. Nonetheless, the ability to generate such plausible explanations for the enormous strength of alloreactivity has removed some of the mystery from this phenomenon.

TOLERANCE

One of the cardinal features of the immune response is that it does not occur to self-antigens under ordinary conditions. This is called 'tolerance' and it is critical to an individual's survival. Tolerance is also a source of fascination to those interested in transplantation since its existence suggests that it ought to be possible to recapitulate nature, instructing the immune system to accept additional antigens (those of the donor graft) as 'self', thus avoiding the need for non-specific immunosuppression.

Immunologists have long assumed that tolerance is determined primarily in the thymus where T cells first develop. Recently, confirmation of the thymus's important role has been achieved by analysing the expression of T-cell receptors. First, there is now evidence that T-cell receptors are not expressed prior to the entry of precursor T cells into the thymus. Since tolerance requires specificity (and therefore the expression of the receptor), T cells cannot learn tolerance prior to arrival in the thymus. Secondly, analysis of receptor expression in the thymus has shown that T cells with specificity for self-MHC antigens do not mature in that organ. Thus there must be a mechanism in thymic T-cell maturation whereby cells reactive with self-MHC antigens are eliminated.

The thymus is able to prevent the maturation of T cells reactive with self-MHC antigens because that organ expresses all self-MHC antigens. On the other hand, many have wondered how tolerance to all self minor histocompatibility antigens can be achieved in the thymus when some of the peptides forming these antigens are probably expressed only in particular tissues. Thus it has been assumed that an extrathymic mechanism to achieve tolerance also exists. Recent experiments demonstrating such an extrathymic mechanism have made use of transgenic technology. Mice have been generated that express foreign MHC antigens, inserted into their genome along with tissue-specific promoter genes. Even when such mice do not express the foreign MHC antigen in the thymus, and do not delete the alloreactive population of T cells during T-cell maturation, they nonetheless fail to reject cells that do express the foreign MHC antigen. They also fail to generate a T-cell response *in vitro* to that alloantigen. Thus this alloreactive population of T cells has been inactivated by some peripheral mechanism after thymic maturation.

Another set of experiments has revealed that mature T cells can encounter foreign antigens in ways that trigger the cell, but which do not lead to immune activation. Helper T-cell clones stimulated by immobilized antigen, in the absence of the additional signals usually provided by antigen-presenting cells, can undergo transformation into blast cells and secrete some, but not all, of their lymphokines. Subsequent stimulation of these clones by normal antigen-presenting cells finds them inert to their stimulating signals. Thus it appears that incomplete stimulation of T cells can achieve their down-regulation under some circumstances.

Given the importance of self-tolerance to the survival of an animal, it is not surprising that the immune system should have more than one mechanism to avoid self-responses. In addition, most biological systems with activation responses have a regulatory system to prevent even appropriate responses from getting out of control. Thus efforts have been made to recreate nature's mechanisms. Two experimental techniques have been most successful in achieving this goal. First, in a notable series of experiments in the early 1950s, Billingham, Brent, and Medawar, consistent with the hypothesis advanced by Burnet, were able to show that foreign antigens, introduced sufficiently early in the maturation of an animal, are treated as self-antigens, allowing the induction of 'actively acquired immunological tolerance'. In mice the critical period extends for several days after birth, so that injection of allogeneic cells shortly postpartum induces 'neonatal' tolerance. Similar observations were made by the Czech biologist, Milan Hasek. Secondly, whole-body irradiation of adult rodents has been used to ablate the mature immune system, allowing reconstitution of the system by bone-marrow transplantation of cells expressing foreign antigens. This technique creates allogeneic bone-marrow chimeras, which are tolerant to both 'self' and to the foreign antigens. Although these two methods for achieving tolerance are useful experimentally, they require either too early or too drastic an intervention to be useful clinically.

Therefore, efforts to achieve tolerance in ways that might be clinically applicable have been undertaken.

Approaches to tolerance with clinical application

Transfusion

One approach aimed at specific downregulation of T-cell responses involves prior blood transfusion of allogeneic cells before organ transplantation. The use of this approach in clinical practice came about accidentally. Although some patients receiving blood transfusions before transplantation become sensitized to donor antigens, as might be expected, those recipients who had not become sensitized turned out to support subsequent graft survival better than expected. Experimental investigation suggests that this is partly due to a diminished T-cell response to the foreign antigens of the transplanted organ. The downregulation of T-cell responses as opposed to sensitization seems to depend on the intravenous route of antigen delivery and on the types of cells being transfused. Thus the finding of better graft survival after blood transfusion not only provided a clinical means of manipulating the immune system, but also stimulated investigation of means by which foreign antigens might be introduced in a non-stimulating way.

Depletion or inactivation of antigen-presenting cells

Part of the key to downregulating immune responses appears to be in avoiding the introduction of functional antigen-presenting cells. As discussed above, depletion of endocrine tissue antigen-presenting cells by tissue culture or by appropriate antibody treatment can achieve long-term graft survival. This technique may also achieve specific unresponsiveness to the antigens of the graft, such that subsequent grafts from the same donor, transplanted with the antigen-presenting cells still present, are not rejected. However, sufficiently strong stimulation of the immune system will often overcome this downregulation, causing rejection of the new and old grafts together. The survival of grafts depleted of antigen-presenting cells suggests again that antigens can be introduced into intact animals in a manner that downregulates rather than stimulates a T-cell response.

Clinically, depletion of antigen-presenting cells from donor organs has been difficult to accomplish. For example, it is not sufficient to remove only the leucocytes and lymph nodes from donor kidneys. Therefore, additional efforts have been made to inactivate donor antigen-presenting cells, rather than to remove them. One approach has been to use ultraviolet light to treat donor tissues. This has allowed successful tissue transplantation in some experimental situations where these cells are accessible to external illumination.

Clinical efforts toward chimerism

In addition to presenting antigens in a non-stimulating manner, efforts have also been made to achieve cellular chimerism, similar to that accomplished in bone-marrow chimeras, but using techniques that are less toxic than whole-body irradiation. Experimentally, lasting chimerism has been achieved by vigorous depletion of the mature immune system using several different monoclonal antibodies against T cells, low-dose irradiation of the recipient's bone marrow, and high-dose irradiation of the recipient's thymus. This is then followed by infusion of both donor and recipient bone marrow to reconstitute the immune system in the presence of foreign antigens. The technique has worked well in rodents and a few larger animals but has not yet been applied clinically. Some patients have been treated with antilymphocyte serum along with an infusion of donor bone marrow. However, lasting chimerism has not been achieved by this approach as yet.

The effort to achieve specific downregulation of T-cell responses and eventually of lasting tolerance represents a major area in which the immunological principles revealed by experimental methods and the achievement of their clinical application awaits completion. It seems that the tools are available to achieve specific immunosuppression and that appropriate modifications in techniques may well bring them to clinical practice. However, the potential for the introduction of such methods has been appreciated for several years. One reason for hesitating to embark on clinical trials of certain promising approaches, until they have been thoroughly explored in large animals trials, is the high level of success that is now being achieved with non-specific immunosuppressive agents. Nevertheless, the imperfections of our present approaches are clearly apparent and further progress is highly desirable.

PRACTICAL CORRELATES OF TRANSPLANTATION IMMUNOLOGY

This section has described some of the concepts in transplantation immunology, the science that underlies clinical organ transplantation. It is, of course, possible to perform clinical transplants quite successfully with little knowledge of these concepts. There are, however, some areas where a grasp of the relevant fundamentals of immunology can greatly facilitate one's understanding of clinical issues.

Antigen matching

One of the hotly debated questions in clinical transplantation is how important it is to achieve matching of transplantation antigens between donors and recipients. Although the question is controversial, the data related to this issue are reasonably well established. In the first place, organs and tissues can be exchanged between identical twins, who express identical transplantation antigens, without any rejection and without immunosuppression. Secondly, among living-related kidney donors, roughly 95 per cent of kidneys derived from HLA-identical siblings survive 1 year, compared to about 90 per cent of those from one-haplotype-matched family members. In comparison, about 85 per cent of kidneys from unrelated cadaveric donors survive for 1 year at the best institutions. Thirdly, the survival of kidneys from cadaveric donors varies according to the degree of MHC antigen matching. Studies comparing the outcome depending on the number of matched HLA antigens have suggested that there is some benefit from matching for DR antigens, but that the clearest benefit (in the range of 10 per cent improved 1-year graft survival) occurs only when there is matching for the products of the HLA-A, B, and DR loci (six antigens in all). This benefit probably increases somewhat as more time elapses following transplantation.

These data support the notion that antigen matching 'matters'. The controversy, however, arises between those who view the benefits of partial antigen matching as large, versus those who see them as relatively small in comparison to the disadvantages that occur when seeking better compatibility. Is it reasonable to subject living family members to surgery and the loss of a kidney to obtain better antigen matching? Is it better to gain a few percentage points in survival for a new patient whose name has recently been added to a long list of waiting recipients on the basis of a more favourable match, or to give that kidney to someone who has been waiting a year longer on dialysis? How much improvement in graft survival on the basis of compatibility will justify the cost of transporting kidneys over long distances and the negative effects of longer ischaemic times? These are difficult questions, which still lack precise answers and therefore generate substantial disagreement.

The cross-match

Antigen-matching is controversial and some are uncertain that any effort is necessary to achieve it. The cross-match, on the other hand, is a different issue entirely and is universally recognized to be important in kidney transplantation. A cross-match is performed by mixing serum from a prospective recipient with lymphocytes of a potential donor to determine whether the recipient has antibodies that are specific for the donor's antigens. If such antibodies are present, they bind to the donor's lymphocytes, causing lysis, when an exogenous source of serum complement, usually from rabbits, is added. A positive cross-match predicts with high accuracy that hyperacute rejection will occur if kidney transplantation is attempted between that donor and recipient, but there are exceptions in that not all antibodies in potential recipients are directed against HLA antigens. Not infrequently, autoantibodies are present as well as HLA antibodies and these may also be responsible for a positive cross-match, but in this instance the positive cross-match does not preclude transplantation.

Although simple in concept, there are practical difficulties with the cross-match which arise because the assay measures the presence of complement-fixing antibodies and not the initiation of hyperacute rejection. One problem is that not all antibodies fix complement equally well, but non-complement-fixing antibodies can cause hyperacute rejection. One approach to this problem is to amplify the assay by adding antibodies from another species that recognize and bind to the human antibodies of the recipient. If these recipient antibodies are bound to donor lymphocytes, the added antibodies will bind to them whether or not they are complement fixing, and these added antibodies, in turn, will fix complement to cause cell destruction. Another way to detect antibodies that do not fix complement is to use flow cytometry, which can detect antibody binding to cells even when they do not cause cell destruction. Both techniques increase the sensitivity of the cross-match assay, but both may be too sensitive, in some cases detecting antibodies that would not lead to hyperacute rejection. However, graft survival in highly sensitized recipients and retransplant patients are superior in those centres that use such sensitive procedures. Another problem with the cross-match is that the target cells (traditionally T lymphocytes from the donor) may not express all the target antigens of vascular endothelial cells that can elicit hyperacute rejection. Class II MHC antigens, in particular, are not usually expressed on human T cells, whereas antibodies against class II antigens can sometimes, but not always, cause hyperacute rejection. These antibodies can be detected using B lymphocytes as targets, a so-called 'B-cell cross-match'. However, not all patients with a positive B-cell cross-match suffer hyperacute rejection. Obviously it is difficult to know exactly how stringent to be in the interpretation of cross-match results, and different centres handle this problem differently.

Sensitization

Potential recipients of kidney transplants who do not have any antibodies in their sera that react with foreign lymphocytes are said to be 'unsensitized'. Those who have been exposed to foreign antigens may have antibodies against some or many different foreign antigens. These individuals are said to be 'sensitized'. The level of sensitization of prospective recipients is tested by reacting their sera separately with lymphocytes from many different individuals, who are selected because they express a broad range of the human HLA antigens. If the donor's serum causes lysis of 45 per cent of the panel of different target lymphocytes they are said to have a 45 per cent PRA (panel reactive antibody). Some prospective recipients have antibodies that kill lymphocytes from every individual in the panel. They are said to be 'highly sensitized' or '100 per cent sensitized'. Obviously, for high sensitized patients it is extremely difficult to find donor kidneys which will not generate a positive cross-match, although it is not really '100 per cent' impossible since a donor matched for all HLA antigens with the recipient should have a negative cross-match and, as mentioned above, some of these highly sensitized patients will have an autoantibody component.

The process of testing each individual against the panel is useful in predicting the difficulty of finding them a suitable kidney donor. It is also useful in identifying the specificity of the antibodies of the sensitized patient and therefore in determining which HLA antigens are most likely to generate a positive cross-match. This makes it possible to select kidneys that are most likely to be suitable for a highly sensitized recipient even before a cross-match, thereby increasing the efficiency of the screening and distribution process.

Many highly sensitized patients wait a long time for a negative cross-match, and some never receive transplants at all. As a result there has been great interest in the possibility of removing preformed antibodies from sensitized patients by plasmapheresis. Occasionally, successful transplants have been achieved in this manner, but the approach has generally been successful only in the case of ABO mismatched individuals. On the other hand, some highly sensitized patients show a gradual decline in both the percentage of 'panel reactivity' of their sera as well as the titre of antibody activity against individual cell samples from the panel, without any intervention. Some of these individuals have also developed antibodies against their own antibodies, which are referred to as anti-idiotypes. Why they develop in some but not other cases is not clear, but the possibility of using anti-idiotypes to remove the antibodies of highly sensitized patients remains intriguing.

Blood transfusions

Blood transfusions are one of the ways in which individuals may encounter foreign MHC antigens and thus become sensitized. Therefore it seemed reasonable in the early years of clinical transplantation to avoid transfusing prospective candidates for kidney transplantation whenever possible. Some patients were asked to struggle with very low haematocrits while waiting for an organ. Despite the sound rationale for this approach, data gathered during the mid 1970s indicated that patients who had received blood transfusions before transplantation and who were then given a cross-match-negative kidney transplant had better survival of their transplants than individuals who had never been transfused. Indeed, this issue was studied nearly 70 times between 1973 and 1984, almost always with the conclusion that blood transfusions were beneficial. Thus it became standard practice in many transplant centres to insist on a potential recipient receiving at least some blood transfusions prior to transplant, whether the potential recipient was anaemic or not.

Several explanations have been considered for the beneficial effect of blood transfusions. First, it is possible that viruses carried with blood transfusions cause chronic infections which are themselves immunosuppressive. Secondly, it may be that the introduction of multiple foreign MHC antigens before transplantation forces the eventual selection of a kidney donor that expresses the MHC antigens eliciting the weakest response from that particular recipient. This might occur because the antigens to which the recipient could react most strongly would have caused sensitization and therefore a subsequent positive cross-match when those antigens were expressed by a donor. In contrast, antigens to which the recipient was weakly reactive would not cause sensitization and hence would generate a subsequent negative cross-match. Thirdly, it is possible that the introduction of foreign MHC antigens intravenously may sometimes cause downregulation of the immune response to those antigens rather than stimulation, achieving a degree of specific tolerance. Each of these explanations is probably valid to some degree, but a great deal of scientific evidence suggests that downregulation by presentation of intravenous antigens is a factor in the better survival of transplants after transfusion. Although this finding encourages the hope of tolerance induction, it remains unclear exactly what mechanisms lead to downregulation in some cases and sensitization in others.

Although intentional transfusion of transplant candidates was the norm for many years, studies of the benefits derived from this approach, beginning in 1986, suggested that the advantage was becoming very small, and in some cases impossible to detect. This apparent change in an outcome that had been so repeatedly verified before was a startling event. The explanation for the shift probably lies in the improved results of transplantation for all recipients, whether transfused or not, derived from new immunosuppressive drugs and other technical advances. Thus, it was probably not that transfusions suddenly offered no benefit, but rather that the benefit was small compared to the strength of cyclosporin and OKT3 in preventing or reversing allograft rejection.

Even while the new data were being evaluated, a still more powerful influence caused a decline in the use of intentional blood transfusions before transplantation. The appearance of AIDS and the recognition that it could be transmitted by transfusion caused many patients to balk at transfusions offered in the absence of anaemia. Even when it became possible to assure patients that the risk of contracting AIDS was negligible, the new awareness by both patients and physicians of the risks of transfusion diminished enthusiasm for intentional transfusion. In recent years, the availability of recombinant erythropoietin for patients on dialysis has also decreased the need for blood transfusion to treat the anaemia associated with chronic renal failure. The number of patients coming to transplantation without ever receiving a blood transfusion has therefore increased during the past several years.

The shifting policies and standards regarding blood transfusions over the past 15 years is a fascinating story, revealing the way both scientific information and prevailing attitudes can alter clinical practice. The sequence reminds us that the most carefully considered rationale for our practices may not hold up with changing conditions and new insights. It is part of the special excitement of the field of transplantation that it is changing so rapidly, as both experimental and clinical studies provide new understanding.

FURTHER READING

Auchincloss H Jr, Sachs DH. Transplantation and graft injection. In: Paul WE, ed. *Fundamental Immunology*. New York: Raven Press, 1989: 889–922.

Barker CF, Billingham RE. The role of regional lymphatics in the skin homograft response. *Transplantation* 1967; **5**: 962.

Bevan MJ. High determinant density may explain the phenomenon of alloreactivity. *Immunol Today* 1984; **5**: 128–30.

Billingham RE, Brent L, Medawar PB. 'Actively acquired tolerance' of foreign cells. *Nature* 1953; **172**: 603.

Bjorkman PJ, Saper MA, Samraovi B, Bennett WS, Strominger JL, Wiley DC. Structure of the human class I histocompatibility antigen, HLA-A2. *Nature* 1987; **329**: 506–12.

Colvin RB. Immunopathology of renal allografts. In: Colvin RB, Bhan AK, McCluskey RT, eds. *Diagnostic Immunopathology*. New York: Raven Press, 1988: 151–97.

Cosimi AB, *et al.* Treatment of acute renal allograft rejection with OKT3 monoclonal antibody. *Transplantation* 1981; **32**: 535–9.

Doherty PC, Zinkernagel RM. H-2 compatibility is required for T-cell mediated lysis of target cells infected with lymphocytic choriomeningitis virus. *J Exp Med* 1975; **141**: 502.

Jeannet M, Pinn V, Flax M, Winn HJ, Russell PS. Humoral antibodies in renal allotransplantation in man. *N Engl J Med* 1970; **282**: 111–17.

Jenkins MK, Schwartz RH. Antigen presentation by chemically modified splenocytes induces antigen-specific T cell unresponsiveness *in vitro* and *in vivo*. *J Exp Med* 1987; **165**: 302.

Kahan BD. Cyclosporin. *N Engl J Med* 1989; **321**: 1725–38.

Lafferty K, Prowse S, Simeonovic C, Warren HS. Immunobioloby of tissue transplantation. A return to the passenger leucocyte concept. In: Paul WE, Fathman CG, Metzgar H, eds. *Annual Review of Immunology*. Palo Alto, California: Annual Reviews, Inc., 1983: 143–73.

Mason DW, Morris PJ. Effector mechanisms in allograft rejection. *Ann Rev Immunol* 1986; **4**: 119–45.

Merrill JP, Murray JE, Harrison JH, Guild WR. Successful homotransplantation of human kidney between identical twins. *JAMA* 1956; **160**: 277–82.

Mitchison NA, O'Malley C. Three-cell-type clusters of T cells with antigen-presenting cells best explain the epitope linkage and noncognate requirements of the *in vivo* cytolytic response. *Eur J Immunol* 1987; **17**: 1579–83.

Opelz G, Terasaki PI. Improvement of kidney-graft survival with increased numbers of blood transfusions. *N Engl J Med* 1978; **299**: 799.

Opelz G, Terasaki PI. International study of histocompatibility in renal transplantation. *Transplantation* 1982; **33**: 87.

Snell GD, Stimpfling JH. Genetics of tissue transplantation. In: Green E, ed. *Biology of the Laboratory Mouse*. 2nd edn. New York: McGraw-Hill, 1966: 457–91.

Williams GM, Hume D, Hudson R, Morris P, Kano K, Milgrom F. Hyperacute renal homograft rejection in man. *N Engl J Med* 1968; **279**: 611–18.

Winn HJ. Antibody-mediated rejection. In: Williams GM, Burdick JF, Solez K, eds. *Kidney Transplantation Rejection*. New York: Marcel Dekker, 1986: 17–28.

10.2 Organ procurement

FRANCIS L. DELMONICO

INTRODUCTION

The technical success of organ transplantation during the past decade has evolved in parallel with the surgical expertise which allows multiple organs to be obtained from a single cadaver donor. The procedure for multiple organ procurement has become widely adopted by transplant surgeons throughout the world, since this method was introduced by Starzl in 1983. Aside from the surgical advances however, the field of organ procurement has become the career interest of many medical personnel, who have functioned as co-ordinators of the organ donation process. This donation process now routinely entails a sequence of patient assessment and operative procedures, which includes determination of donor suitability, haemodynamic management prior to procurement, orchestration of operative events, and the preservation of the various organs.

THE SUITABLE CADAVER DONOR

Most organs for transplantation are procured from cadavers following the diagnosis of brain death. This diagnosis has facilitated the procurement of viable organs, free of the warm ischaemic injury seen when their removal follows the arrest of circulation. Nevertheless, the opportunity to salvage organs following cardiac asystole from otherwise suitable donors, remains inherently possible. Anaise has recently described an experimental procedure in dogs in which femoral vessel cannulation allows rapid exsanguination and installation of cold preservation fluid following cardiac arrest. Core visceral temperatures can be further decreased by continuous hypothermic perfusion of the abdominal cavity.

Following the cardiac death of many individuals, either in the emergency ward or on arrival at hospital, the Anaise method might allow sufficient *in-vivo* preservation, at least of the kidneys, to allow time for family permission to be obtained for organ removal. Thus far, this approach has received limited consideration because of the obvious public misunderstanding which might arise from its widespread implementation. However, these minimally invasive measures could be more comfortably initiated if individuals carried a donor card, indicating their prior consent to donation. They may also be applied in countries where consent for donation is presumed.

Clinical criteria of death

Although death may be defined in its simplest form as a permanent absence of brain function, this concept of death as it relates to brain activity is relatively new. Death was first characterized in terms of irreversible coma in 1968, following a report by an *ad hoc* committee of the Harvard Medical School, which was assembled to define brain death. Four essential criteria were necessary to establish coma as irreversible: unreceptivity and unresponsivity, no spontaneous movements or breathing, an absence of reflexes, and a flat electroencephalogram. These criteria have subsequently been modified to be less restrictive, but their accuracy has stood the test of extensive scrutiny. Prior to this report, death was only considered in terms of circulatory and respiratory function. With the development of sophisticated cardiorespiratory support systems, however, the notion of death based solely upon an absence of heartbeat became obsolete: arrest of heart activity could be considered a manifestation of death only by its terminal effect upon brain function. The routine resuscitation of patients following transient cardiac arrest forced a conceptual revision in the diagnosis of death.

Although Japan is a notable exception, the concept of brain death has become well accepted internationally during the past two decades. Homicide convictions have not been hampered by the brain death of a victim, and the medical progress report of brain death by Black greatly helped the medical profession to establish brain death as a diagnostic entity. Later, a commission of medical consultants to the President of the United States published guidelines for the determination of death, which acknowledged the concept of brain death and specified the criteria of brain death in terms of cerebral and brain-stem function. Many institutions subsequently adopted policies regarding brain death, with minor modifications appropriate for local medical practice, but incorporating the essential criteria of the presidential commission. For example, at the Massachusetts General Hospital, both clinical and laboratory criteria have been used to establish the essential elements of the diagnosis: cerebral unresponsiveness and brain-stem inactivity (Table 1). An apnoea test has become a standard method of confirming irreversible brain-stem damage, although the level of $P\text{CO}_2$ which must be attained may vary. However, absent brain-stem function is also recognized clinically when pupillary light, corneal, oculocephalic, and oropharyngeal reflexes are absent.

The absence of electrocerebral activity as revealed by an EEG can be supportive of the diagnosis of brain death; absence of cerebral blood flow as demonstrated by a radionuclide or angiographic procedure is an alternative. However neither of these investigations are required, as stressed by Pallis, provided a careful evaluation of brain-stem death has been performed (Table 2). In the United Kingdom the diagnosis of death is a diagnosis of brain-stem death.

A period of at least 24 h without neurological change is recommended before the diagnosis is made, especially for children less than 5 years of age. Screening for drugs which depress the central nervous system is also recommended. If the cause of coma is known with certainty and drug-related and metabolic causes have been excluded, a period of 6 h without clinical change is sufficient to allow a diagnosis of brain death in adults.

The use of barbiturates to reduce intracranial pressure and/or the seizure threshold, does not preclude the diagnosis of brain death, if the serum barbiturate level at the time of neurological examination is less than 1 mg per cent. The determination of brain blood flow may be useful in circumstances where barbiturate levels are higher.

The need to assess brain-stem activity for the diagnosis of brain death has precluded its application to anencephalic newborn infants, and to some irreversibly comatose individuals: these patient groups are both devoid of cerebral cortex activity, but show spontaneous breathing, which requires intact brain-stem function. An active debate has been waged as to whether brain-stem function

Table 1 Guidelines for determination of brain death (Massachusetts General Hospital): assessed upon: (a) the determination of a negative toxicological screen; (b) the presence of haemodynamic stability; (c) the absence of hypothermia

I. Clinical
- A. Cerebral unresponsiveness: no withdrawal to painful stimuli
  Spinal level movements do not preclude the diagnosis
- B. Brain-stem unresponsiveness:
  1. Apnoea test: the determination of severe medullary damage
     The patient should be removed from the respirator
     The arterial $P\text{CO}_2$ is brought to above 50 mmHg, and the pH to below 7.35
     Apnoea has been adequately demonstrated if no spontaneous respiration is observed
     During this test vital functions are supported by preoxygenation for 5 min with 100% O_2.
  2. Absence of other brain-stem functions:
     - (a) Pupils—at least 4 mm in diameter and unreactive to bright light. They should not be oval in shape since this demonstrates residual midbrain function
     - (b) Eye movements—there should be no spontaneous eye movement
       Oculovestibular testing with ice water irrigation of each ear separately should produce no eye movement
     - (c) Other—there should be no córneal external facial movement, or bulbar function such as gagging or coughing with tracheal stimulation

Spinal reflexes—the presence of deep tendon reflexes does not preclude brain death.

II. Laboratory testing
- A. Electroencephalogram: an EEG recording of at least 30 min duration should show no electrocerebral activity. Core body temperature should be above 90°F.
- B. Other ancillary testing: radionuclide or contrast angiographic demonstration of absent cerebral blood flow is a sufficient alternative to EEG

Table 2 Declaration of brain-stem death

1. Have the preconditions been met?
   Is the patient comatose and on a ventilator?
   Is there a positive diagnosis of structural brain damage?
   Have all possible attempts been made to remedy it?
2. Has proper attention been given to the necessary 'exclusions' (drug intoxication, primary hypothermia, major metabolic disturbances)?
3. The patient has been on the ventilator for several hours. Have each of two clinical examinations revealed;
   Absent brain-stem reflexes?
   Persistent apnoea (disconnection test)?
4. If so, the patient can be declared dead, even if the heart is still beating
5. Once the patient has been declared dead the respirator is ventilating a cadaver. It is no longer a 'life support system'
6. The patient is dead when the brain-stem is declared dead, not when the cadaver is disconnected from the respirator and the heart stops beating.
7. Neither EEG nor angiography are necessary for a diagnosis of brain-stem death

alone, irrespective of cerebral function, should imply the presence of 'life', and this has gained attention following the use of an encephalic donors of hearts and kidneys. At this time however, society has not accepted a diagnosis of death which disregards brain-stem function, that is a capacity to breath spontaneously, and the procurement of organs from anencephalics prior to death has not been sanctioned.

Age and medical restrictions

A detailed social and medical history should be taken from the donor's family by the organ procurement agency representative (either physician or co-ordinator) who obtains consent for donation. In addition to being aware of the donor history, procuring surgeons should perform an appropriate examination which might bear upon donor suitability. This includes looking for extremity lacerations which have become secondarily infected, or needle marks indicative of drug abuse, and a rectal examination in donors over 60 years of age.

The cause of brain death should be ascertained prior to its pronouncement and certainly prior to organ procurement. Irreversible brain injury is usually due to head trauma, subarachnoid or intracranial haemorrhage, brain hypoxia of known aetiology, drug overdose, or primary brain tumour (glioblastoma, astrocytoma, etc.). A history of any other malignancy should be ruled out; these include metastatic melanoma, choriocarcinoma, and renal cell carcinoma, which can cause spontaneous intracranial haemorrhage and may not be apparent as a cause of brain death. Primary malignancies such as lymphoma, renal cell carcinoma, choriocarcinoma have been transmitted unknowingly by liver and renal allografts resulting in the death of organ recipients.

All potential donors should be evaluated for the possibility of multiple organ donation. There are certain age restrictions which apply to the donation of individual organs (Table 3), although the persistent shortage of organ donors has led to these age limits being extended. Donor age has an impact upon successful transplantation, with recipients of organs from donors aged 16 to 65 years achieving the best clinical results. The use of kidneys from paediatric donors is controversial: children less than 3 years of age may not be suitable renal allograft donors unless *en bloc* paired kidneys are transplanted.

Table 3 Age restrictions to the multiple organ donor

Kidney	3–70 years
Liver	Newborn–65 years
Pancreas	Newborn–50 years
Heart	Newborn–40 years (male)
	Newborn–45 years (female)
Heart/lung	2–35 years
Lung	10–50 years

With no history of pre-existing organ disease.

Table 4 Laboratory testing

ABO blood type
Complete blood count (CBC)
Platelet count
Prothrombin time (PT)
Partial thromboplastin time (PTT)
Electrolytes (Na, K, Cl, CO_2)
Blood glucose
Blood urea nitrogen; creatinine (BUN, creat)
Bilirubin (total and direct)
Serum glutamic-oxaloacetic transaminase (SGOT)
Serum glutamic-pyruvic transaminase (SGPT)
Alkaline phosphatase
Amylase
Electrocardiogram
Echocardiogram
Creatinine phosphokinase-myocardial band (CPK-MB)
Chest radiograph
Bronchoscopic examination
Blood gases: Po_2, Pco_2, pH
VDRL or rapid plasma reagin test
Hepatitis B surface antigen
Serological testing for cytomegalovirus, hepatitis C virus, and HIV
Microbiology cultures: blood, sputum, drain effluents, and ureteral stump
Urine analysis

A past history of diabetes mellitus requiring treatment may not preclude organ donation; these patients should be evaluated on an individual basis and should not be excluded without consultation from local organ bank personnel (see Table 4). Similarly, a history of hypertension is no longer an absolute contraindication to donation, particularly of kidneys. If the hypertension is mild (diastolic pressure between 90 and 100 mmHg) and controlled with single agent therapy, a biopsy specimen during the period of renal preservation may be obtained and evaluated for the degree of intraparenchymal arteriosclerosis.

Potential donors with a history of autoimmune disorders must be carefully evaluated: the transmission of idiopathic thrombocytopenia purpura by liver transplantation has been reported. The 47-year-old recipient was subsequently cured by a second transplant.

Carbon monoxide poisoning from smoke inhalation can produce not only brain hypoxia but hypoxic myocardial damage that is not evident on echocardiography. Hearts obtained from victims of smoke inhalation have been observed to fail immediately following transplantation.

Infectious contraindications

Each potential donor must be assessed for carriage of infectious agents to prevent the transfer of micro-organisms to allograft recipients. Systemic infection transmitted by a cadaveric donor organ can result not only in a loss of the allograft, but also in death of the immunosuppressed recipient.

The history and physical examination of a potential cadaveric donor may reveal a systemic infection present prior to or associated with the patient's death: the latter may have been hospital acquired. The cause of death may promote an infectious complication: victims of drowning often eventually die of pneumonia, and burn victims may develop cutaneous sepsis.

Infections acquired prior to death

Viral infection

The presence of an active viral infection in the form of hepatitis, perineal herpes, encephalitis or meningitis, pneumonia, varicella zoster, or human immunodeficiency virus (HIV) infection, is an absolute contraindication to organ donation. A history of a specific viral infection does not preclude donation, however, but requires the exercise of clinical judgement, after a thorough gathering of historical information. Kidneys have been successfully transplanted from donors dying of Reye's syndrome, in which the influenza virus has been implicated. No adverse effects, in particular the development of Reye's syndrome, were evident in the allograft recipients.

A judicious approach is also applicable to potential donors with a history of hepatitis. Active viral hepatitis may be manifested by liver dysfunction at the time of donor death, and diagnosed either by the detection of hepatitis B antigenaemia, or serological reactivity to the hepatitis A or C viruses. The acquisition of the hepatitis B virus from renal allografts is well documented and patients positive for hepatitis B surface antigen should not donate their organs. However, a history of hepatitis B antigenaemia may not prohibit donation, if at the time of death the patient is hepatitis B antigen-negative and hepatitis B antibody-positive.

For many years, an unidentified viral pathogen (non-A, non-B hepatitis virus) had been implicated in the aetiology of hepatitis following transplantation, possibly transmitted from previously infected organ donors. Recently this elusive agent has been identified as hepatitis C virus. A flurry of clinical reports has documented the infectious potential of blood transfusions from hepatitis C antibody-positive donors. As a result, some blood banks have prohibited the transfusion of blood products from anti-HCV-positive donors. The question of transmission of hepatitis C virus to allograft recipients has also been raised, and organ procurement agencies have attempted to determine the prevalence of anti-HCV antibodies in their donor population. In a retrospective study of 716 consecutive donors to the New England Organ Bank between 1986 and 1990, 13 (1.8 per cent) of the donors tested were positive for antibodies to hepatitis C virus. Organs procured from these donors were transplanted into 29 recipients: hepatitis and/or liver failure was seen in 14 of the 29 (48 per cent) recipients (median onset 4.5 months after transplantation). Seroconversion for the virus occurred in four (29 per cent) of the 14 patients whose serum samples were available for testing before and after transplantation. All four patients developed liver disease. Thus, organ procurement agencies may restrict the acceptance of organs from donors positive for antibody to hepatitis C virus, unless the need of the recipient is so critical that transplantation is justified.

Since hepatitis A virus has not generally been considered a virulent pathogen for the allograft recipient, a donor history of hepatitis A virus infection has not been regarded as a contraindication to organ donation. A 3-month interval between active hepatitis A and death is accepted as sufficient to allow for organ donation, particularly if the serum titre of IgM antibodies to hepatitis A virus has returned to normal.

All potential organ donors should be assessed for HIV infection, as this virus can be readily transmitted by allografts. Screening for HIV by enzyme-linked immunoassay prior to organ donation is now routine; however, this assay for HIV antibodies may not detect recent onset HIV antigenaemia. Social circumstance must also be taken into account in the evaluation of potential cadaveric donors. A history of homosexuality or intravenous drug abuse may exclude a person from donation. Exclusion on the basis of social risk, may also be exercised for individuals who are homeless and alcoholic, prisoners, or immigrants from East Africa or Haiti, even if tests for hepatitis and HIV are negative.

Genital herpes virus infection at the time of death may raise a suspicion that the potential donor is a concomitant HIV carrier, even though the enzyme-linked immunosorbent assay does not reveal the presence of anti-HIV antibody. Aside from the implication of HIV infection, active herpes simplex may be transmitted through renal allografts to the immunocompromised recipient, and organ procurement from these individuals is best avoided.

Caution should also be exercised when potential donors have received multiple blood transfusions during resuscitation following trauma. HIV testing should be performed on a blood specimen obtained from the potential donor prior to the administration of transfusions since an infected individual may have a false-negative HIV test following repletion with multiple transfusions of blood.

Acute varicella zoster infection can be lethal in an immunosuppressed allograft recipient, and all potential allograft recipients should be screened for antibody to varicella-zoster virus prior to transplantation. Allograft recipients who are antibody negative are warned to avoid contact with individuals experiencing acute varicella, and individuals with primary or reactive varicella at the time of death should probably be excluded from donating organs.

Kidneys from donors shown to be serologically positive for cytomegalovirus may be the source of cytomegalovirus infection in allograft recipients, especially in seronegative recipients. Renal allografts may be preferentially disposed to transmission of this virus: a variety of cultured renal cell types will support growth of cytomegalovirus in culture, and donor-specific strains of the virus have been identified in renal allograft recipients by analysis of viral DNA. Cytomegalovirus has also been implicated in the rejection and atherosclerosis of cardiac allografts. Active cytomegalovirus infection, in the form of a pneumonia or hepatitis, therefore precludes organ donation. This type of cytomegalovirus infection may also raise the possibility of concomitant HIV infection, irrespective of the results of antibody testing.

Bacterial infection

Cystitis, as manifested by a positive culture of urine obtained through a Foley catheter, is not a contraindication to donation. If pyuria is observed, ureteral stump cultures may be obtained during the procurement procedure. While bladder contamination following Foley catheterization has not been associated with recipient infection following transplantation, a positive ureteral stump culture raises the possibility of active pyelonephritis, which is a contraindication to transplantation. Good surgical technique, with ligation of the distal ureters following ureteral transection, prevents potentially contaminated urine refluxing from the bladder into the open peritoneal cavity.

A history of pyelonephritis within 3 months of organ donation may increase the risk of transmission of bacteria to the recipient. Clinical judgement regarding the type of organism and verification of treatment should be exercised before recently infected kidneys are accepted for transplantation. *Pseudomonas aeruginosa* and *Staphylococcus aureus* have been reported to subsequently disrupt the vascular anastomosis of a renal allograft.

A history of chronic respiratory infection or acute pharyngitis does not exclude a patient from donating organs (with the exception of lung donation) unless a virulent organism such as *Staphylococcus aureus* is identified. If bacteraemia is not demonstrated by blood culture, donation may be considered to be safe.

Brain death due to mycotic aneurysm necessitates an evaluation of the cause: *Candida albicans* and *Staphylococcus aureus* are extremely dangerous to allograft recipients, and blood cultures from potential donors may be negative.

The death of a renal allograft recipient from disseminated tuberculosis transmitted through a cadaver kidney, obtained from a donor with unsuspected tuberculosis meningitis has been reported. The aetiology of the meningitis only became apparent several weeks after the donor's death, when mycobacteria grew in cultures of his cerebrospinal fluid. The donor's chest radiograph was normal. As well as documenting the transmission of tuberculosis via transplanted organs, this case underscores the danger of accepting organs from individuals with a diagnosis of meningitis of unknown aetiology.

A Venereal Disease Research Laboratory Test (VDRL) can detect non-specific antibodies directed against lipoidal antigens of *Treponema pallidum*. A VDRL or rapid plasma reagin test is routinely obtained on all individuals considered for organ and tissue donation. Although a positive test suggests exposure to *T. pallidum*, the lipoidal antigens used in the assay are found in a number of normal tissues, and a more specific test such as the fluorescent Treponema antibody absorption assay may be necessary to exclude a false-positive VDRL result. A positive reaction with the fluorescence assay is highly suggestive of infection.

Parasitic infection

Toxoplasma gondii is an indolent parasite, and infectivity of a potential donor may only become apparent after transplantation. Although toxoplasmosis may now be detected as an associated infection in patients with immunodeficiency syndromes such as AIDS, toxoplasmosis may be transferred from an unsuspected carrier who has died abruptly from trauma. In this latter circumstance detection of donor toxoplasmosis may only be accomplished retrospectively, following the detection of an elevated level of antibodies against Toxoplasma in stored donor blood. In general, retention of donor serum for such unforeseen developments may be prudent. Lethal toxoplasmosis has been transmitted to recipients of cardiac allografts from apparently healthy seropositive donors with unsuspected central nervous system disease. Thus, donor seropositivity to *Toxoplasma gondii*, identified in advance of transplantation, may be a contraindication to donation, especially for a seronegative recipient.

Fungal infection

Candida albicans frequently colonizes the vagina and perineum of patients who are maintained on broad spectrum antibiotics for a long period of time. Thereafter, the monilia may gain entrance to the bladder, through an indwelling Foley conduit. Wound infection and vascular disruption may follow transplantation of organs contaminated with Candida, especially to diabetic recipients. Fatal candidal mediastinitis has been reported in recipients of lungs from donors with a heavy growth of Candida in cultures from the trachea.

Histoplasma and Cryptococcus have been transmitted to renal allograft recipients by organs from donors who died of intracerebral pathology, without evidence of a pulmonary infection. These organisms are difficult to eradicate from the central nervous system unless a protracted course of antifungal therapy (amphotericin B) is administered. Even with careful documentation of proper therapy however, a history of fungal infection (also including cocciodiomycosis and blastomycosis) should exclude an individual from donation, despite the apparent absence of infection at the time of death.

Infections associated with terminal injury

Chest tubes are not a contraindication to organ donation unless culture of the pleural fluid is positive for an organism which poses a high risk to the recipient, such as *Pseudomonas aeruginosa* or *Staphylococcus aureus*.

Peritoneal drains contaminated with enteric bacteria may assume more significance, especially if they reflect current peritonitis due to injured or devitalized bowel. A retroperitoneal dissection of each kidney can be accomplished through separate flank incisions if necessary. This approach may also be used when gastrostomy tube leakage into the abdominal cavity is suspected in patients who have been nutritionally depleted and who display poor wound healing.

Although perforations of the bowel repaired within 1 week of brain death probably exclude a patient from consideration as a donor, prior repair of the intestine may not, provided that a Gram stain of peritoneal fluid reveals no organisms, blood cultures are negative, and appropriate antibiotic coverage has been administered during the interval.

Extremity fractures in a potential donor may pose a hazard for allograft recipients, if metal appliances have been placed to stabilize the fracture, and/or there is evidence of cellulitis adjacent to the cutaneous exit site of the appliance. Once again, antibiotics should have been administered for at least 48 h and blood cultures must be free of bacteria before organ procurement is undertaken.

Burn victims who sustain tracheobronchial injury from smoke inhalation are at risk of pneumonitis. Burn injuries also compromise the procurement procedure since incisions cannot be made through damaged skin. Nevertheless, if incisions can be fashioned through areas of skin which have not been burned, organs may be procured from burn victims within 48 h of injury. A longer interval between injury and death increases the risk of septic contamination of visceral organs, through either a compromised respiratory tract or through burned skin.

Infections acquired at the time of death

Cellulitis adjacent to antecubital or subclavian vein intravenous lines signal the possibility of line infestation, which can seed visceral organs with bacteria such as *Staphylococcus aureus*. Management prior to procurement surgery entails the removal of the intravenous line, administration of appropriate antibiotics for at least 24 h following line removal, and the determination of negative blood cultures.

Any untreated bacteraemia noted around the time of death creates a significant risk of bacterial transmission to allograft recipients. Organisms such as *Staphylococcus aureus* and *Pseudomonas aeruginosa* are especially virulent, and have been noted to disrupt anastomotic suture lines to the allograft. Systemic infection of the donor with these organisms (e.g. pneumonia) is generally a contraindication to donation.

Laboratory assessment

Traumatic injury to any visceral organ may initially be detected through laboratory testing of donor blood samples (Table 4). Unremitting functional impairment because of shock or trauma generally precludes procurement of the specifically injured organ.

Candidates for heart donation are usually free of cardiac murmurs and display a normal 12-lead ECG. Pathological Q waves suggestive of infarction are a contraindication to donation; other electrocardiographic abnormalities, such as ST segment changes, do not exclude donation. Echocardiography may be performed to assess myocardial function and potential valvular pathology in patients requiring pressor support, or in whom a murmur is audible. Mitral valve prolapse without mitral regurgitation is not uncommon and alone does not preclude heart procurement.

Candidates for lung or heart and lung donation should usually be free of a smoking history and have clear lung fields on chest radiographs. A Gram stain and culture of the tracheobronchial secretion should be performed. Blood gas assessment or respiratory function is determined by ventilating the donor with 100 per cent oxygen and no more than 5 cm of positive end-expiratory pressure: under these conditions, the arterial oxygen pressure of a blood sample should be greater than 300 mmHg.

Many transplant centres are willing to accept livers from donors whose liver function tests are not within normal range. A 2- or 3-s elevation in the prothrombin time, and/or mild elevations in transaminase levels are not necessarily a contraindication to procurement. A careful history and serological testing for hepatitis B surface antigen and antihepatitis C antibody are important elements in the decision.

Small liver lacerations may be observed at the time of organ procurement from victims of trauma with normal blood transaminase levels. A small laceration with no bleeding or bile leakage from the site may not represent a contraindication to liver transplantation.

Liver function is especially susceptible to hypoxia: haemodynamically unstable patients requiring pressor support, with marginal arterial oxygen pressure (<100 mmHg), may not be satisfactory candidates for liver donation, particularly if the oxygenation cannot be improved because of pulmonary oedema. Consequential impairment of liver function may be discerned by an increase of at least 5 s in the prothrombin time and a transaminase level that is twice normal.

A coagulopathy detected by thrombocytopenia, low fibrinogen level, and a marked elevation of the prothrombin and partial thromboplastin times, suggests a disseminated intravascular coagulopathy, which is known to be associated with head injury, but may also be the result of sepsis. Once again, clinical judgement must be exercised in determining any possible cause of sepsis, impairment of organ function, and the potential for transmission of bacterial organisms. A biopsy of the renal allograft prior to transplantation may be necessary to exclude the presence of microthrombi within the renal parenchyma. Pulmonary dysfunction is a frequent cause of irresolvable hypoxia in patients with disseminated intravascular coagulation because of the deposition of microthrombi in the lungs.

The standard determinations of serum creatinine, blood urea nitrogen, urinalysis, and urine output (>1 ml/kg.min) are used to assess satisfactory donor renal function. Creatinine levels above 2.0 mg per cent are not necessarily a contraindication to kidney donation if the cause of renal dysfunction is transient hypotension, and if the creatinine level falls with intravenous fluid repletion. Chronic renal insufficiency, as noted by a persistent creatinine level of greater than 2.0 mg per cent, combined with a urinalysis revealing proteinuria and/or sediment casts, contraindicate renal donation.

A history of diabetes mellitus precludes pancreas donation, but does not necessarily prohibit renal donation, especially if the serum creatinine level is less than 2.0 mg per cent. Mild elevations in serum amylase may not be a reflection of pancreatic injury or pancreatitis, since the enzyme may be derived from a salivary gland source following trauma. Neither mild hyperamylasaemia nor mild hyperglycaemia are contraindications to pancreas donation.

Lymph node procurement

Many organ procurement agencies have adopted a practice of extracting lymph nodes from the inguinal bed as soon as death has been declared and permission for organ donation has been granted. This practice has facilitated the identification of renal allograft recipients prior to kidney procurement, as accurate tissue typing from peripheral blood is usually difficult, and the subsequent preservation period of cold ischaemia.

A 6- to 8-cm incision is made below the inguinal ligament, along the course of the femoral vessels, using sterile technique. Three or four lymph nodes are more than sufficient for HLA typing, and these may be readily identified medial to the femoral vein.

Social considerations

In the same year in which the criteria were developed to determine brain death (1968), a Uniform Anatomical Gift Act (UAGA) was independently promulgated in the United States to facilitate the process of organ donation. The concept of the donor card was derived from the Uniform Anatomical Gift Act, as it permitted the decedent to certify an intent to donate, irrespective of the wishes of the surviving family. Nevertheless, a hierarchy of responsible family members was established for circumstances in which family approval would be requested. The order proceeded from spouse, to offspring, to parent, to sibling, and finally to guardian.

Unfortunately, few people have completed donor cards, even though renewal of a driver's licence affords a simple opportunity to do so. Moreover, the general policy of organ procurement agencies has been to obtain permission from the surviving family member, determined by the hierarchy noted above, even in instances where a donor card has been identified. Family wishes have prevailed despite properly indicated donor intent. It has also become a standard practice to obtain permission for organ procurement from the local medical examiner or coroner when potential donors have died from an unnatural cause. The medical examiner should be contacted in advance of organ procurement. The operative report may serve as evidence of the postmortem examination of the thoracic and abdominal cavities.

Measures such as the Uniform Anatomical Gift Act have not been successful in promoting a much needed voluntary organ donation. As a result, alternative approaches have been formulated to enhance the public awareness of the shortage of organs for transplantation. Legislation has been adopted, which makes a request for organ donation by hospital personnel mandatory in appropriate cases of brain death. However, this well-intentioned approach of 'required request' has not been successful in enlarging the donor pool in countries such as the United States, from the fixed rate of 16 donors/million population, to a rate estimated in some areas such as Austria to be as high as 38 to 50 donors/million population. This discouraging observation may mean that health care professionals have not accepted mandatory regulation and remain ambivalent about the concept of brain death and organ donation. The failure of 'required request' laws may also lead to the regulated process of consent being conducted by inconsistent and inexperienced personnel.

Presumed consent and financial incentives, although objectionable to many, remain options to boost the rate of organ donation in the future. Presumed consent for organ donation (organ removal takes place unless a surviving family member objects or the potential donor before death has objected) has been introduced in several European countries, resulting in an organ donation rate of approximately 25/million population.

MANAGEMENT OF THE CADAVER DONOR

Primary allograft function following transplantation is dependent upon careful maintenance of the donor after the declaration of brain death, the surgical technique of retrieval, and the duration and method of preservation.

Brain death elicits physiological responses which may lead to haemodynamic instability, including arrhythmias, a significant decrease in thyroid hormones (both T_3 and T_4), and a reduction in circulating adrenal cortical and insulin levels. Hypothermia is common, as central neurological control of body temperature is lost; the resulting shift from aerobic to anaerobic metabolism leads to acidosis, which may be exacerbated by the peripheral vasoconstriction arising from pressor support.

Hypotension may develop as a consequence of cardiac arrhythmia, brain-stem herniation, or hypovolaemia. Brain death may also induce diabetes insipidus and polyuria, which exacerbates hypotension through a reduced blood volume. Diabetes insipidus becomes apparent as the serum osmolality (>300 mosmol) increases. Hypovolaemia is also the expected result of resuscitative measures intended to minimize cerebral oedema, prior to the development of brain death.

The goals of donor management are the prevention of hypotension, hypothermia, and hypoxia. If not already instituted, central venous pressure and arterial lines should be placed, as well as a Foley catheter, to monitor blood pressure, blood volume repletion and hourly urine output.

Crystalloid replacement with Ringer's lactate solution should be given until a systolic blood pressure of at least 90 mmHg is achieved. Administration of synthetic arginine vasopressin (1–2 units/h) will reduce urine output, conserving intravascular water, and may also contribute to haemodynamic stability by an independent mechanism.

Following extensive research in brain dead experimental animals, Novitsky has proposed the routine administration of a hormonal cocktail consisting of triiodothyronine, insulin, and cortisol, to assure haemodynamic stability and minimize systemic acidosis, but this approach remains controversial.

The hypovolaemia associated with diabetes insipidus may be worsened by haemorrhage associated with traumatic injury: scalp lacerations are a frequent source of unsuspected blood loss. Blood transfusions may be necessary, particularly if the haematocrit has fallen to less than 25 per cent. Volume repletion should raise the central venous pressure, thereby optimizing intracardiac filling pressures and cardiac function. If these measures fail to restore a satisfactory blood pressure, dopamine may be given at an initial constant intravenous rate of 2 μg/kg.min. This may be increased to 10 μg/kg.min if necessary; more than this may reduce renal and mesenteric blood flow, as vasoconstrictive effects are predominant at higher doses.

Because of their vasoconstrictive properties, alternative pressors such as phenylephrine or levophed are not recommended. If a urine output of at least 1 ml/min is not achieved following volume and pressor resuscitation of the systolic blood pressure to greater than 100 mmHg, then mannitol (12.5–25 g) and/or frusemide (furosemide) (20–40 mg) may be given intravenously. Metabolic acidosis should be corrected by bicarbonate injection.

Monitoring of the donor following the determination of brain death, usually includes the sampling of blood and urine for bacterial culture, particularly in those who have been in hospital for longer than 48 h. The routine administration of broad spectrum antibiotics such as cephalosporin is advisable, even in the absence of bacteraemia.

OPERATIVE EVENTS

Following the transfer of the potential donor to the operating room, manually ventilated with 100 per cent oxygen, ventilator settings should be re-established to maintain the partial pressure of arterial oxygen at greater than 100 Torr. A warming blanket may be required to prevent the hypothermia (<32°C) associated with brain death, and its destabilizing effect upon cardiac function. The patient's arms should be maximally abducted, to permit a simultaneous dissection by thoracic and abdominal teams. Anaesthetic management of blood gases, central venous pressure, haematocrit, and urine output are essential for successful organ procurement. A haematocrit of less than 30 per cent should be restored by transfusion of warmed blood, especially if the patient is hypoxic or oedematous due to previously infused crystalloid solution. Bicarbonate administration may be necessary to correct metabolic acidosis.

A midline incision is made from the suprasternal notch to the pubis. As the sternum is split, bone wax is applied to minimize bleeding. If only intra-abdominal organs are being procured the sternal incision is omitted, and the midline incision is made from the xyphoid to the pubis. Some surgeons use a cruciate abdominal incision just above the umbilicus for extended exposure. Towel clips may be applied from the apex of each leaf of the abdominal incision, as it is folded to the opposing skin of the abdomen.

The organs of interest, whether thoracic or abdominal, must be inspected by the surgeon for unsuspected pathology or injury.

The thoracic teams generally begin the dissection by opening the pericardium and/or pleural cavities. The great vessels, including the vena cavae, the aortic arch, the innominate vessels, and the pulmonary artery are isolated. Both lungs may be mobilized and inspected by the division of the pulmonary ligaments.

The abdominal dissection may vary, depending upon the viscera to be procured. The liver is usually removed first, with the hepatic arterial circulation being established by dissection of the coeliac axis and superior mesenteric arteries. Replaced right or left hepatic arteries originating from the superior mesenteric or left gastric arteries must be preserved. When the donor is haemodynamically stable, the coeliac axis and superior mesenteric artery can be isolated to their branches. The portal vein is dissected and the inferior mesenteric vein may be cannulated to permit *in-situ* portal cooling, usually with Ringer's lactate solution. Alternatively, the splenic vein or superior mesenteric vein may be used for portal flushing if the pancreas is not required. The common bile duct is divided at the duodenal brim.

Pancreatic dissection may take place next. The spleen is dissected from its bed, and used as a handle to mobilize the tail and body of the pancreas. On the right side, a Kocher manoeuvre is used to dissect the C-portion of the duodenum and the head of the pancreas, again to the mesenteric vessels.

Each kidney and ureter is then mobilized by dissecting the poles beneath Gerota's fascia, the number and course of the left and right renal arteries being identified.

The donor is then anticoagulated systemically with 10 000 to 20 000 units of heparin, and the distal aorta above the iliac bifurcation is cannulated. Rarely, an iliac artery may provide a lower pole renal artery branch: this anatomical aberration must be carefully assessed before aortic cannulation, and if present the contralateral iliac artery can be cannulated for prograde aortic cooling. A cannula may also be placed into the inferior vena cava below the renal veins, to provide a controlled exit for visceral perfusate. Some surgeons prefer to transect the inferior vena cava and allow the perfusate to empty into the abdominal cavity.

In the thoracic cavity, cannulas are finally placed into the main pulmonary artery for cardiopulmonary-plegia and prostacyclin infusion, and into the proximal ascending aorta for cardioplegia. The superior and inferior vena cava are ligated and transected as the plegia solutions are given.

SEQUENCE OF EXCISION

Thoracic organs are excised first. Either cardiectomy is performed prior to lung removal (possibly as a double lung block); or the heart and lungs are removed *en bloc* and divided on a back table in the operating room. Alternatively the heart and lungs may be removed as a unit for transplantation to a single recipient. As the aortic arch is cross-clamped (usually with a staple device), perfusion of the intra-abdominal organs is begun through portal and aortic cannulas and this is continued during the thoracic excision.

Table 5 Sequence of procurement in multiple organ donation

Heart/lung or heart and lungs
Liver
Kidneys
Pancreas
Bones/tissues

The liver is the first intra-abdominal organ removed (Table 5). Although the simultaneous procurement of the liver and pancreas from a single cadaver donor was once considered to be technically impossible because of the same blood supply, it is now routinely accomplished. Transection of the portal vein, 2 cm cephalad to its bifurcation into the splenic and superior mesenteric veins, provides sufficient length of portal vein for transplantation with both the liver and pancreas. The arterial supply can be managed by providing a Carrel patch of aorta either to the coeliac axis of the liver, or to the coeliac axis and superior mesenteric artery of the pancreas. Usually however, the coeliac axis and aortic patch are retained with the liver, and the iliac bifurcation graft from the donor is anastomosed to the splenic and superior mesenteric arteries of the donor pancreas.

As the liver is removed, aortic perfusion of the kidneys and pancreas with preservation fluid is continued: approximately 2 litres of preservation fluid are usually given through the aortic cannula.

The method of whole organ pancreas transplantation which is most commonly employed uses a segment of duodenum to drain exocrine secretions into the bladder. Since the donor duodenum must be transected (usually with the staple device), the pancreas is removed following *en bloc* nephroureteroectomy, to avoid contamination of either kidney with enteric organisms. The pancreas preparation therefore consists of a segment of duodenum, the entire pancreas, and the attached spleen.

Finally, both kidneys are removed *en bloc* with a cylinder of aorta and inferior vena cava, and with attached ureters of at least 10 cm in length. Once removed the kidneys may be divided for separate packaging and cold storage preservation, or they may be placed separately (or *en bloc*) on to a pulsatile perfusion machine.

ORGAN PRESERVATION

The development of a consistently effective preservation fluid has dramatically changed the timing of renal, hepatic, and pancreatic transplant procedures. The preservation solution developed at the University of Wisconsin has extended the period of preservation to 48 h, permitting wider geographical sharing of renal allografts, which are allocated principally on the basis of HLA matching. The preservation time for liver and pancreas allografts has also been extended (Table 6).

Table 6 Preservation times

Organ	Hours
Heart	6
Lung	4
Liver	24
Pancreas	12
Kidney	60

The objective of organ preservation is to cool the core temperature of the organ parenchyma so that the demand for oxygen and the requirement for energy (in the form of ATP) can be markedly reduced. During this period of ischaemia, cellular integrity of the parenchyma is maintained. These goals can be achieved by flushing of the organs with one of several preservative solutions at a temperature of 47°C.

The constituents of the University of Wisconsin solution include hydroxyethyl starch and lactobionate which suppress cell swelling, glutathione and $MgSO_4$ to stabilize cell membranes during the cold ischaemic period, and allopurinol to scavenge oxygen free radicals associated with reperfusion injury, and to stimulate ATP synthesis after preservation.

The debate as to whether renal preservation is best achieved by pulsatile perfusion or cold storage has largely subsided. The simplicity of cold storage is a major cost-saving asset. In a randomized study conducted by the New England Organ Bank, renal allografts cold stored for less than 36 h functioned as well as the paired kidney preserved by pulsatile perfusion.

LIVING DONORS

Confronted with a persistently inadequate supply of organs from individuals who have died transplant clinicians have resorted to using living donors, not only for renal allografts but also for liver and pancreatic organs. Unrelated living donors of kidneys have been used when blood type compatibility and an emotional bond with the recipient exists. At one time, kidneys obtained from living related family members accounted for more than 30 per cent of renal transplants performed annually in the United States. The procurement of organs from living unrelated individuals in economically poor countries has been subject to unethical abuse. Nevertheless, living donation remains ethically accepted as a rewarding experience for the donor and a true benefit for the allograft recipient.

Improvements in immunosuppression and in the outcome of cadaver donor transplantation have reduced the proportion of organs obtained from living related donors in recent years. Between 1986 and 1990, 1753 (91.3 per cent) of the 1921 kidneys transplanted in Australia were from cadaver donors, 159 (8.3 per cent) were from living related donors, and 9 (0.5 per cent) were from living unrelated donors. In England, between 1989 and 1990, only 5.7 per cent of renal allografts were obtained from living donors. Thus, the number of living donors continues to fall far short of the demand of an increasing number of patients awaiting renal transplantation.

The operative risks of kidney donation during life are small; however, approximately 20 donors have died worldwide since the first successful living renal donation was performed in 1954.

Reports have appeared in the literature to suggest an increased incidence of hypertension in kidney donors many years after donation. However, although an increase in protein excretion and glomerular filtration has been noted immediately following removal of a kidney, renal function has remained well preserved, without evidence of long-term deterioration. In the past decade, complications have been observed in only five of more than 200 living donors at the Massachusetts General Hospital (two pulmonary emboli, one wound infection, one urinary tract infection, and one halothane hepatitis). All of these patients recovered without incident and there have been no deaths.

The success of organ transplantation is driving a continued research effort into the future use of xenografts. As immunosuppression improves, the possibility of successful xenografts will compel a social consideration of this approach. The persistent need for organs is unlikely to be resolved if only human donors are considered.

FURTHER READING

A Collaborative Study. An appraisal of the criteria of cerebral death. *JAMA*, 1977; **237**: 982–6.

Alexander JW, Vaughan WK. The use of 'marginal donors' for organ transplantation. *Transplantation*, 1991; **51**: 135–40.

Anaise D, *et al.* An approach to organ salvage from non-heartbeating cadaver donors under existing legal and ethical requirements for transplantation. *Transplantation*, 1990; **49**: 290–4.

Arras JD, Shinnar S. Anencephalic newborns as organ donors: a critique. *JAMA*, 1988; **259**: 2284–7.

Ascher NL, Bolman R, Sutherland DER. Multiple organ donation from a cadaver. In: Simmons RL, ed. *Manual of vascular access, organ donation and transplantation*. Berlin: Springer-Verlag, 1984: 105–43.

Bay WH, Hebert LA. The living donor in kidney transplantation. *Ann Intern Med*, 1987; **106**: 719–27.

Belzer FO, Glass NR, Sollinger HW, Hoffmann RM, Southard JH. A new perfusate for kidney preservation. *Transplantation*, 1982; **33**: 322–3.

Black P McL. Brain death (first of two parts). *N Engl J Med*, 1978; **299**: 338–44.

Black P McL. Brain death (second of two parts). *N Engl J Med*, 1978; **299**: 393–401.

Black P McL. Brain tumors (second of two parts). *New Engl J Med*, 1991; **324**: 1555–64.

Caplan AL. Ethical and policy issues in the procurement of cadaver organs for transplantation. *N Engl J Med*, 1984; **311**: 981–3.

Curran WJ, Hyg SM. The brain-death concept: judicial acceptance in Massachusetts. *N Engl J Med*, 1978; **298**: 1008–9.

Dakshinamurty KV, Date A, Jacob CK, Kirubakaran MG, Shastry JCM. Hepatitis in living-donor renal allograft recipients. *Transplantation*, 1988; **46**: 926–7.

Darby JM, Stein K, Grenvik A, Stuart S. Approach to management of the heartbeating 'brain dead' organ donor. *JAMA*, 1989; **261**: 2222–8.

Diethelm AG. Ethical decision in the history of organ transplantation. *Ann Surg*, 1990; **211**: 505–20.

Evans RW. Organ donation: facts and figures. *Dialysis Transplant*, 1990; **19**: 234–40.

Friedland GH, Klein RS. Transmission of the human immunodeficiency virus. *N Engl J Med*, 1987; **317**: 1125–34.

Goodman JL. Possible transmission of herpes simplex virus by organ transplantation. *Transplantation*, 1989; **47**: 609–13.

Gottesdiener KM. Transplanted infections: donor-to-host transmission with the allograft. *Ann Intern Med*, 1989; **110**: 1001–16.

Ho M, Suwansirikul S, Dowling JN, Youngblood LA, Armstrong JA. The transplanted kidney as a source of cytomegalovirus infection. *N Engl J Med*, 1975; **293**: 1109–12.

Iwai A, Sakano T, Uenishi M, Sugimoto H, Yoshioka T, Sugimoto T. Effects of vasopressin and catecholamines on the maintenance of circulatory stability of brain-dead patients. *Transplantation*, 1989; **48**: 613–17.

Kuo G, *et al.* An assay for circulating antibodies to a major etiologic virus of human non-A, non-B hepatitis. *Science*, 1989; **244**: 362–4.

Laquaglia MP, *et al.* Impact of hepatitis on renal transplantation. *Transplantation*, 1981; **32**: 504–7.

Levey AS, Hou S, Bush, Jr. HL. Kidney transplantation from unrelated living donors. *N Engl J Med*, 1986; **314**: 914–16.

Levin SD, Whyte RK. Brain death sans frontieres. *N Engl J Med*, 1988; **318**: 852.

Mani MK. Kidney transplantation from unrelated living donors. *N Engl J Med*, 1986; **315**: 714.

Marsh CL, Perkins JD, Sutherland DER, Corry RJ, Sterioff S. Combined hepatic and pancreaticoduodenal procurement for transplantation. *Surg Gynecol Obstet*, 1989; **168**: 254–8.

Medearis, Jr. DN, Holmes LB. On the use of anencephalic infants as organ donors. *N Engl J Med*, 1989; **321**: 391–3.

Merrill JP, Murray JE, Harrison JH, Guild WR. Successful homotransplantation of the human kidney between identical twins. *JAMA*, 1956; **160**: 277–82.

Novitzky D, Cooper DKC, Chaffin JS, Greer AE, DeBault LE, Zuhdi N. Improved cardiac allograft function following triiodothyronnine therapy to both donor and recipient. *Transplantation*, 1990; **49**: 311–6.

Olthoff KM, *et al.* Comparison of UW solution and Euro-collins solutions for cold preservation of human liver grafts. *Transplantation*, 1990; **49**: 284–90.

Pallis C. Brainstem death: the evolution of a concept. In: Morris PJ, ed. *Kidney Transplantation: Principles and Practice* 3rd edn. Philadelphia: W. B. Saunders, 1988; 123–50.

Pereira BJG, Milford EL, Kirkman RL, Levey AS. Transmission of hepatitis C virus by organ transplantation. *N Engl J Med*, 1991, **325**: 454–60.

Pirsch JD, *et al.* Living-unrelated renal transplantation: results in 40 patients. *Am J Kidney Dis*, 1988; **12**: 499–503.

Ploeg RJ. Kidney preservation with the UW and Euro-collins solutions. *Transplantation*, 1990; **49**: 281–4.

Prottas J. Shifting responsibilities in organ procurement: a plan for routine referral. *JAMA*, 1988; **260**: 832–3.

Rao KV, *et al.* Influence of cadaver donor age on posttransplant renal function and graft outcome. *Transplantation*, 1990; **49**: 91–4.

Ratner LE, Flye MW. Successful transplantation of cadaveric en-bloc paired pediatric kidneys into adult recipients. *Transplantation*, 1991; **51**: 273–5.

Report of the Ad Hoc Committee of the Harvard Medical School to examine the definition of brain death. A definition of irreversible coma. *JAMA*, 1968; **205**: 85–8.

Report of the Medical Consultants on the Diagnosis of Death to the President's Commission for the Study of Ethical Problems in Medicine and Biomendical and Behavioral Research. Guidelines for the determination of death. *JAMA*, 1981; **246**: 2184–6.

Ruder H, Schaefer F, Gretz, N, Mohring S, Scharer K. Donor kidneys of infants and very young children are acceptable for transplantation. *Lancet*, 1989; **ii**: 168.

Sadler AM, Sadler BL, Statson EB. 'The uniform anatomical gift act'. *JAMA*, 1968; **206**: 2501–6.

Shewmon DA, *et al.* The use of anencephalic infants as organ sources. *JAMA*, 1989; **261**: 1773–82.

Singer PA, *et al.* Ethics of liver transplantation with living donors. *N Engl J Med*, 1989; **321**: 620–2.

Southard JH, *et al.* Important components of the UW solution. *Transplantation*, 1990; **49**: 251–7.

Starzl TE, *et al.* A flexible procedure for multiple cadaveric organ procurement. *Surg Gynecol Obstet*, 1984; **158**: 223–30.

Stuart FP, Veith FJ, Cranford RE. Brain death laws and patterns of consent to remove organs for transplantation from cadavers in the United States and 28 other countries. *Transplantation*, 1981; **31**: 238–44.

Sutherland DER, Goetz FC, Najarian JS. Pancreas transplants from related donors. *Transplantation*, 1984; **38**: 625–33.

Task Force for the Determination of Brain Death in Children. Guidelines for the determination of brain death in children. *Ann Neurol*, 1987; **21**: 616–17.

Teperman L, *et al.* The successful use of older donors for liver transplantation. *JAMA*, 1989; **262**: 2837.

The Medical Task Force on Anencephaly. The infant with anencephaly. *N Engl J Med*, 1990; **322**: 669–74.

Truog RD, Fletcher JC. Anencephalic newborns—can organs be transplanted before brain death? *N Engl J Med*, 1989; **321**: 388–91.

Van Der Poel CL, *et al.* Infectivity of blood seropositive for hepatitis C antibodies. *Lancet*, 1990; **335**: 558.

10.3 Organ and tissue preservation

VERNON C. MARSHALL, PAULA JABLONSKI, DAVID SCOTT, AND BRIAN HOWDEN

OBJECTIVES OF PRESERVATION

Effective preservation is a requirement of techniques which involve transfer of viable organs and tissues. Graft damage must be minimized while the organ is still within the donor in preparation for graft procurement, during graft removal, during storage and transport of the graft, during the transplantation operation, and after reimplantation or revascularization. Some tissues, such as blood and skin, can be stored for several days or weeks. Vascularized autografts are usually reimplanted immediately, or within a few hours.

Allografts pose another problem. Not only must viability be maintained, but rejection of the grafts must be prevented by optimizing the match between donor and recipient tissue and by immunotherapy. These two objectives—preserving viability and preventing rejection—are closely linked. Optimal matching of antigens of graft and recipient requires a storage period of 24 h or more. Until recently storage for this length of time was only practicable for kidneys, but as prolonged storage becomes available for liver, pancreas, and heart, these grafts may also be allocated on the basis of improved tissue matching. Retrospective analysis has indicated that matching would improve the efficacy of cardiac transplants but this would require prolongation of the storage period beyond the current safe period of 6 h.

The process of clinical preservation usually begins with identification of the brain-dead, heart-beating cadaver donor. Effective preservation allows time for confirmatory tests of brain death, organization of operating teams for organ removal, typing and cross-matching of donor tissues against a pool of waiting recipients, excluding associated transplantable diseases such as infection or neoplasm in the donor, selecting and locating recipients and arranging their admission and preparation for surgery, arranging recipient operating teams, and time to transport organs over long distances, even between continents.

Good preservation also provides a window of diagnostic and therapeutic opportunity during the safe period of extracorporal storage. The time gained should be available for functional assessment of the graft to confirm its viability, and to predict early function after reimplantation. Good early function is obligatory in the case of heart and liver grafts. Immediate function of kidney and pancreas grafts, although not obligatory, is highly desirable and facilitates recipient management.

Effective immune manipulation of the recipient or of the graft itself during the period of storage is another (as yet largely unrealized) objective. Treatment of the stored organ to deplete it of antigen presenting cells, or other treatments to modify parenchymal and endothelial cell immunogenicity, could dramatically improve transplantation results.

HISTORICAL REVIEW

Attempts to preserve human tissues and organs from putrefaction and decay after death began in antiquity with the embalming and mummifying techniques which were developed to a fine art by the Egyptian dynasties.

In the 1930s the classical experiments of Carrel and Lindbergh (Fig. 1) applied perfusion techniques to preservation of organs for transplantation. They established ground rules for organ preservation by continuous *ex-vivo* perfusion—expert technology, perfect asepsis, and controlled biological conditions.

The Spanish Civil War marked the advent of blood banks and clinical application of tissue storage techniques. Cold storage was

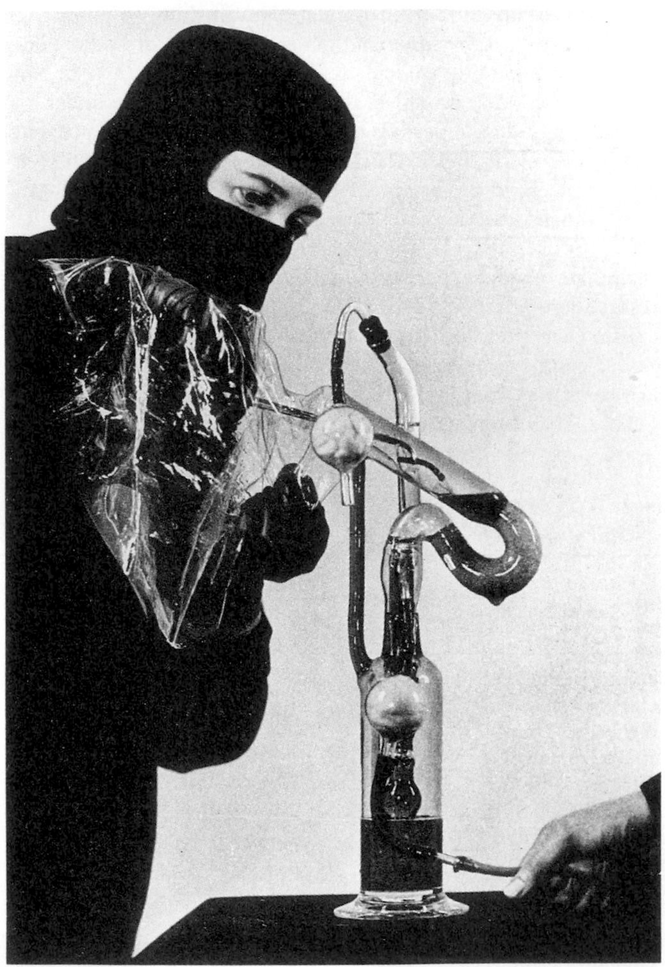

Fig. 1 Preservation apparatus of Carrel and Lindbergh.

used to diminish metabolic demand. Fortunately blood, the first widely preserved and transplanted biological substance, lent itself well to extended storage. Refrigerated storage was possible for 3 weeks.

The discovery of cryoprotectants by Polge and coworkers in 1949 ushered in a major extension of preservation times for a variety of simple cells and tissues. Blood cells and gametes (even embryos) could be stored after freezing. Weeks or months later, they could be thawed and successfully reimplanted as autografts or allografts. Such freezing was only successful for isolated cells or undifferentiated multicellular embryos: complex and heterogeneous organs were highly sensitive to freezing damage. The biophysical problems of freezing large organs were subsequently defined by Pegg and other workers. To date no consistent success has been obtained with the use of freezing to preserve organs such as kidneys, liver, or hearts. Concepts of frozen humans waiting revival at an appropriate future time on another planet or in an after-life remain in the realms of science fiction.

Hypothermic organ preservation, stopping short of freezing, has given more promising results for whole organs. Most early work centred on the kidney. Simple cooling and ice storage gave reliable protection for several hours only. In the 1960s Pegg and Calne showed that preservation could be improved by a cold intravascular flush. Initially the blood within the organ was replaced with fresh blood, plasma, or extracellular-like flushing solutions containing colloid. In 1969 Collins demonstrated the clear superiority of an 'intracellular' electrolyte flushing solution, high in potassium, magnesium, and phosphate, low in sodium and chloride, and without colloid. Kidney storage for 24 h became clinically practical, provided that the organ did not suffer too much damage due to periods of warm ischaemia prior to cooling. In the early 1970s Belzer *et al.* extended Carrel's work on recirculating machine perfusion. Machine storage extended the time during which kidneys could be reliably preserved from one day to 3 days. However, simple hypothermic storage (after flushing) and continuous machine perfusion gave equivalent results for 24-h preservation—particularly if warm ischaemia was avoided. It also became clear that flushing solutions did not need to mimic intracellular composition to be effective: other solutions, even simpler in composition, based on citrate and on sucrose were shown to be as effective as Collins' solution (Table 1). Clinical kidney preservation and transport could rely mainly on simple hypothermic storage after preliminary flushing with these solutions (Fig. 2); compact cold perfusion machines using modifications of plasma were also available for more extended storage times. Belzer *et al.* gave a further major stimulus to preservation research in 1987, demonstrating that a complex multicomponent solution (University of Wisconsin (UW) solution) gave significantly enhanced preservation of several organs (particularly pancreas and liver). With a new colloid—hydroxyethyl starch, the UW solution was suitable for both simple flushing and recirculatory machine perfusion. Current research in many centres is evaluating the efficacy of the numerous components of UW solution, and attempting to improve it further. Modifications of UW solution have been successful in extending the time of preservation of pancreas, liver, kidney, and heart.

Table 1 Organ preservation solutions (Collins', Citrate, phosphate buffered sucrose)

	EuroCollins	Isotonic citrate	Phosphate buffered sucrose
Sodium (mmol/l)	10	80	120
Potassium (mmol/l)	116	80	–
Magnesium (mmol/l)	–	40	–
Citrate (mmol/l)	–	55	–
Bicarbonate (mmol/l)	10	–	–
Chloride (mmol/l)	15	–	–
Phosphate (mmol/l)	58	–	60
Sulphate (mmol/l)	–	40	–
Glucose (mmol/l)	180	–	–
Sucrose (mmol/l)	–	–	140
Mannitol (mmol/l)	–	100	–
Osmolality (mmol/kg)	340	300	310
pH (at 0°C)	7.3	7.1	7.2

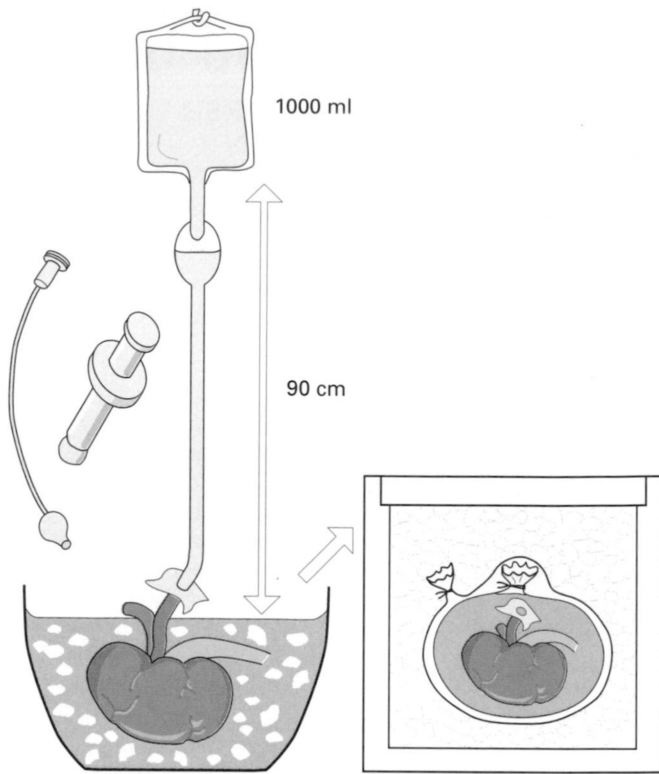

Fig. 2 Organ preservation by static ice storage after cold flushing.

THE PROBLEM: EFFECTS OF ISCHAEMIC HYPOXIA

Cells of normally functioning organs derive their energy from the oxidation of substrates obtained from the circulating blood (glucose, fatty acids, amino acids, or ketones); in the case of liver and muscle energy is obtained from breakdown of endogenous glycogen. Energy is stored within cells as phosphate bonds of adenosine triphosphate (ATP), creatine phosphate, and other nucleotides. Cellular composition is maintained in homeostasis by numerous enzymic reactions acting in concert under the directions of hormones or key compounds such as cyclic adenosine monophosphate.

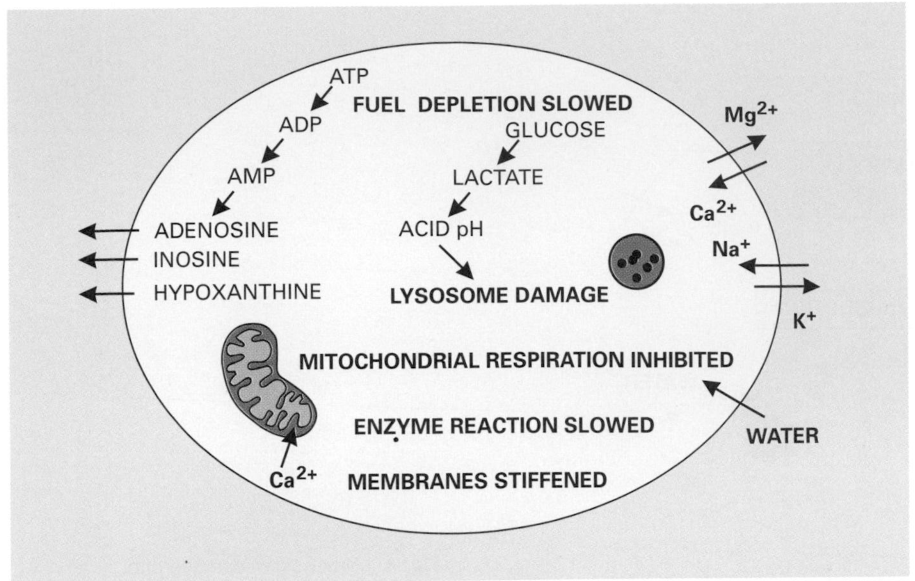

Fig. 3 Cellular effects of cold ischaemia.

Ischaemic damage

Ischaemia cuts off nutrients and oxygen supply to the organ. Continuing metabolic activity of the organ's parenchymal and other cells causes a cascade of events leading to irreversible cell damage and death. Metabolism becomes anaerobic; glycolysis causes depletion of high energy phosphate compounds. Degradation of ATP increases cellular levels of adenosine, inosine, and hypoxanthine. Depletion of the cell's energy stores inactivates Na^+-K^+-ATPase, the enzyme system controlling the sodium pump of the cell membrane. As fuel reserves disappear, sodium and chloride, freely permeable electrolytes which are normally actively excluded from the cell, diffuse into the cell down concentration gradients. As the osmotic force of non-permeable cellular proteins and anions is no longer balanced by the extrusion of sodium, water floods the increasingly swollen cell. Mitochondrial respiration is inhibited, and calcium enters the cytosol and mitochondria. Anaerobic metabolism temporarily uses glucose stores to generate ATP, but lactic acid is also produced, leading to progressive intracellular acidosis which activates lysosomal lytic enzymes leading to autolysis.

Most organs and cells can tolerate ischaemic hypoxia for 30 to 60 min without permanent damage. Parenchymal cells of most transplantable organs are generally similar in their tolerance to ischaemia. Rapidly metabolizing tissues are less tolerant: the heart is particularly vulnerable because it continues to beat until all energy reserves are depleted. Most organs are irreversibly damaged by 90 to 120 min of ischaemia at body temperatures. Vascular damage occurs along with the parenchymal effects: the cells of the vascular endothelial lining bear the brunt of this injury. These effects are slowed, but not reversed, by cooling (Fig.3).

Reperfusion damage (Fig. 4)

Reperfusion injury is an added hazard which contributes to irreversible damage. Accumulation of metabolic end products such as hypoxanthine, under anaerobic conditions, can set the stage for reperfusion injury. When blood flow is restored, oxygen influx leads to the formation of toxic compounds such as hydroxen peroxide, and superoxide and hydroxyl radicals. These active free radicals of oxygen produce further cellular, membrane, and microvascular injury. Under normal circumstances these harmful radicals are short lived, as they are rapidly cleared by endogenous scavenging mechanisms. Ischaemia depletes these endogenous mediators.

HYPOTHERMIC PRESERVATION: A PARTIAL SOLUTION

Static cold storage

Simple cooling markedly enhances ischaemic tolerance. All enzymic activity is temperature dependent—cooling diminishes metabolic activity, curtails oxygen demand, and slows degradation of energy stores. Hypothermia does not stop metabolism, but merely slows the metabolic clock and lessens the speed at which deterioration occurs. Cooling from 37°C (body temperature) to 0°C (storage temperature) extends the tolerance of most organs to ischaemia from between 1 and 2 h to about 12 h. Unfortunately cold does not slow all biological functions uniformly but causes discordance in a variety of metabolic processes which occur in concert at 37°C. Transmembrane passive diffusion of ions is not appreciably affected by hypothermia, while active transport mechanisms, such as those governed by Na^+, K^+-ATPase and Mg^{2+} Ca^{2+}-ATPase are inhibited below 10°C. Hypothermia alone cannot prevent cell swelling during storage (Fig. 3).

A major requirement for a cold flushing solution is therefore that it includes an impermeant to provide osmotic force to oppose cellular oedema (Fig. 5). Large anions such as lactobionate (molecular weight 358 Da), or non-electrolytes such as the saccharides raffinose (molecular weight 505 Da) or sucrose (molecular weight 342 Da), or chelates of citrate and magnesium (molecular weight approximately 1000 Da), can achieve this.

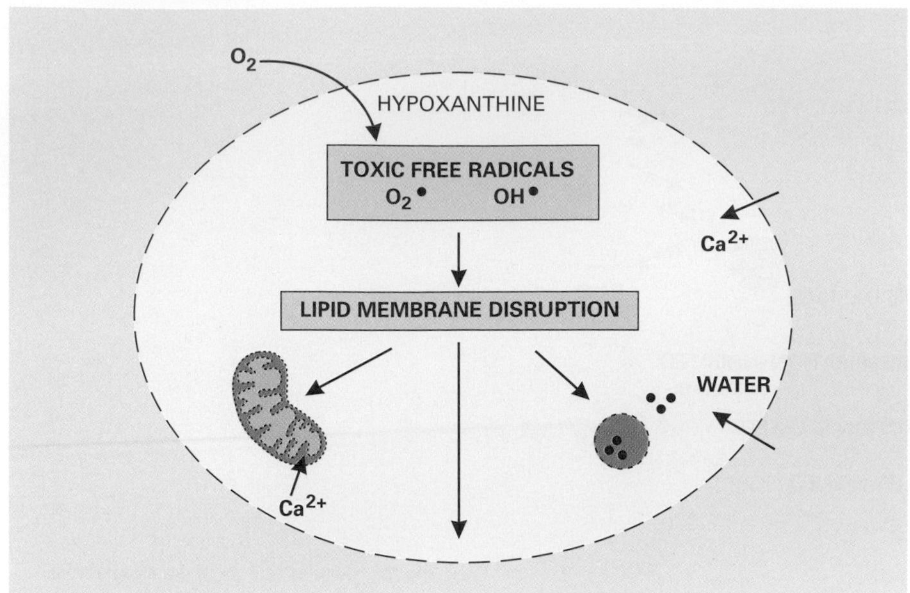

Fig. 4 Reperfusion damage after ischaemia.

Glucose (molecular weight 180 Da) can permeate the cell slowly and can stimulate an undesirable production of lactic acid and hydrogen ions by anaerobic glycolysis. Glucose in flushing solutions can be replaced by impermeant sucrose with benefit—especially for liver and pancreatic grafting, where cell membranes are even more permeable to glucose. An effective buffer (phosphate, citrate, or histidine) to counter intracellular acidosis is a second major requirement. The importance of these two mechanisms is indicated by the fact that a solution consisting solely of sucrose with an added phosphate buffer (PBS) is remarkably effective in kidney preservation—almost as effective as the very much more complex UW solution.

The electrolyte composition of flushing solutions can vary widely. The freely diffusible anion chloride is preferably replaced by an impermeant anion (lactobionate, gluconate, or chelated citrate). Flushing solutions often have high potassium (100–130 mmol/l) and low sodium (10–30 mmol/l) concentrations. Since the high potassium concentration is cardioplegic, these solutions cannot be used for early systemic intravenous use, and a systemic leak before the time of organ flushing and retrieval is highly dangerous. A high potassium concentration is also vasoconstrictive, slowing flushing rates and the rate of organ cooling. Solutions with the sodium/potassium ratio reversed (Na 130 mmol/l, K 10–30 mmol/l), have been shown to be virtually as effective, provided suitable impermeants and buffers are present in the solution, and chloride concentration is kept low.

Magnesium has proved to be a useful additive in many solutions since it forms chelates with lactobionate and citrate which cannot pass through membranes. By contrast, calcium levels are kept low, or even excluded since cell damage is associated with calcium

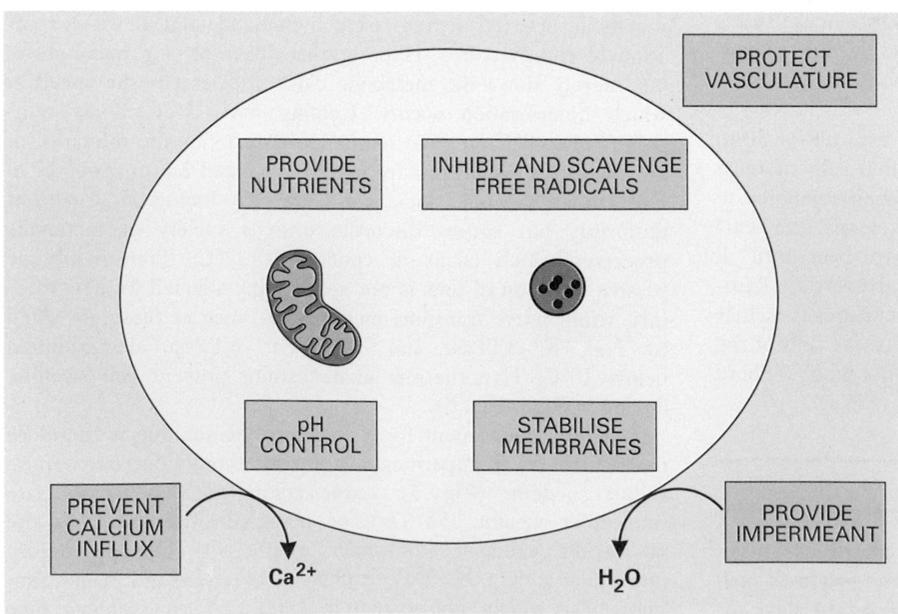

Fig. 5 Requirements of flushing solution for optimal organ preservation.

influx. Calcium (and magnesium) can precipitate in unstable solutions. Calcium is strongly chelated by lactobionate (and citrate), which may account partly for the usefulness of the latter substances in flushing solutions. This could be deleterious in heart preservation, contributing to harmful influx of calcium on reflow.

Preservation by simple hypothermic storage is limited by ultimate exhaustion of nutrients and accumulation of waste products. Preservation of kidneys can be extended to 3 days by simple storage using Collins, Citrate, PBS, and UW solutions. Preservation of liver and pancreas is more difficult, and was not consistently extended to 24 h until the advent of UW solution.

Table 2 UW preservation solutions

	UW solution	Modified UW solution (hydroxyethyl starch-free, Na/K reversed)
Lactobionate (mmol/l)	100	100
Raffinose (mmol/l)	30	60
Sodium (mmol/l)	30	125
Potassium (mmol/l)	125	30
Magnesium (mmol/l)	5	5
Chloride (mmol/l)	10	10
Phosphate (mmol/l)	25	25
Sulphate (mmol/l)	5	5
Adenosine (mmol/l)	5	5
Allopurinol (mmol/l)	1	1
Glutathione (mmol/l)	3	3
Insulin (units/l)	100	100
Dexamethasone (mg/l)	8	8
Hydroxyethyl starch (g/l)	50	–
Bactrim (ml/l)	0.5	0.5
Osmolality (mmol/kg)	320	320
pH (at 25°C)	7.4	7.4

University of Wisconsin (UW) Solution (Table 2)

The multiple factors influencing the effectiveness of preservation were analysed by Southard *et al.*, who produced a solution (UW) containing impermeants (raffinose, lactobionate), buffers (phosphate), free radical inhibitors and scavengers (glutathione, allopurinol), energy precursors (adenosine), vasoactive agents and hormones (steroids, insulin), and a colloid (hydroxyethyl starch). This complex solution was markedly more effective than other solutions (Collins', citrate, phosphate buffered sucrose) used for liver and pancreas preservation, and also for kidney and heart grafts. It was suitable both for cold-flush storage, and for continuous perfusion. Not all its components are equally important: hydroxyethyl starch can safely be omitted for cold flushing and simple hypothermic storage. High potassium levels are undesirable on several grounds, and reversing Na:K ratios does not significantly lower efficacy. Other additives, such as the buffer histidine, can improve preservation; the polysaccharide raffinose can be replaced by sucrose. Lactobionate is probably the most effective and most important component of UW solution. Gluconate (molecular weight 195 Da) appears slightly less effective as an alternative impermeant. Other adjuvants shown to be helpful include raffinose, glutathione, allopurinol, and adenosine. Steroids, insulin, and hydroxyethyl starch (HES) are of minor significance. Modified HES-free UW-derived solutions based on high concentrations of sodium lactobionate can give results similar or equal to the original UW solution.

Extension of experimental preservation by simple cold storage after flushing with modified UW solutions has been achieved for kidneys to 5 days, pancreas to 48 h, liver to 36 to 48 h, and for heart and lung towards 12 h. Recent clinical trials have confirmed the effectiveness of lactobionate-based UW solutions in preservation of kidney, liver, and pancreas; improved heart preservation for transplantation with UW flushing and storage has been demonstrated over standard cardioplegic solutions. Solutions with high concentrations of histidine, tryptophane, and α-ketoglutarate (Bretschneider-HTK) have also given improved organ preservation.

Other agents shown to be helpful additives to flushing solutions (and which hold promise for further extension of preservation times) include other energy sources and buffers, calcium channel blockers (verapamil, diltiazem, trifluoperazine), and stable prostacyclin analogues.

Continuous cold perfusion

Continuous cold perfusion by machine combines the benefits of hypothermia with continuous buffering, continuous washout of accumulating toxic metabolites, and continuous provision of oxygen and nutrients. Oxygen is more soluble at lower temperatures, and the reduced energy requirement of hypothermic organs can be provided by acellular perfusates. For all organs studied, viability has been maintained longest by continuous machine perfusion. A heat exchanger is needed to maintain temperature at 4 to 9°C, an atraumatic pump circulates the solution, and oxygenation is achieved either by simple surface diffusion or using a membrane oxygenator. An oxygen/carbon dioxide gas mixture, and an effective buffer are required to maintain a constant pH. A bubble trap and organ chamber complete the circuit (Fig. 6). Materials coming in contact with the fluid must be sterile, non-toxic plastics or metals. The perfusate must contain colloid to maintain intravascular volume and prevent development of an 'exploded' extracellular fluid space. Cryoprecipitated plasma or albumin was initially used, but albumin gradually leaks into the interstitium and leads to weight gain, so this has been replaced by other oncotic colloids (gelatin, dextrans, hydroxyethyl starch). Metabolic fuels improve long-term preservation—glucose has been the substrate most commonly used, while adenosine, other precursors, or ATP itself have been used as additional sources of energy. Organ reperfusion requires rapid renewal of membrane pump activity, and quick regeneration of cellular fuels. Addition of other substrates more specific to individual organs can also improve function after storage (arachidonic acid, essential amino acids, fatty acids). Fuel additives become increasingly important as preservation times are prolonged beyond 24 h.

Hypothermic cell swelling due to membrane pump inhibition still occurs with cold perfusion below 15°C unless chloride is replaced by impermeants.

Continuous perfusion becomes limited after about 5 days. By this stage considerable damage has usually occurred to the vulnerable vascular endothelium, leading to irreversible cellular damage on reperfusion. Research continues into ways of further prolonging safe preservation, and of protecting the microcirculation during perfusion.

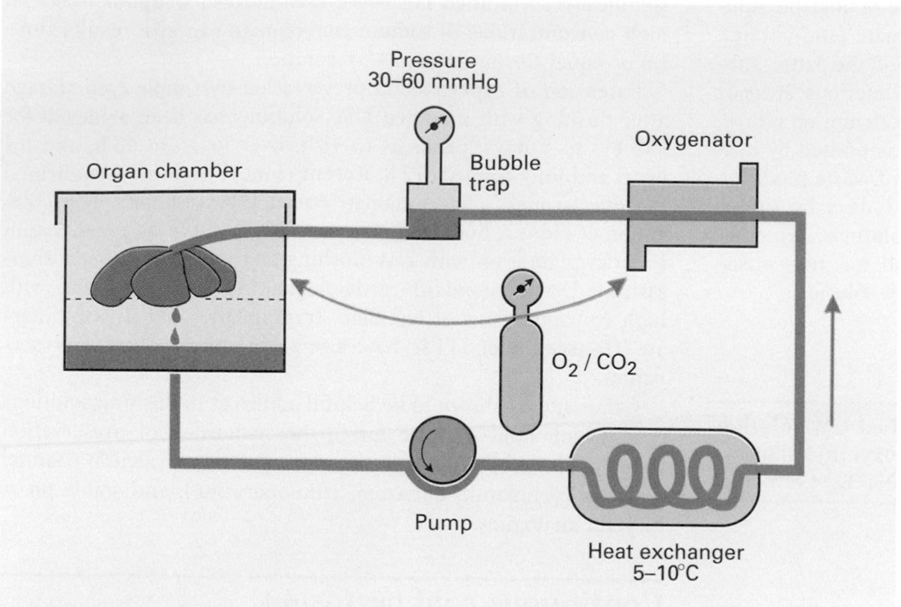

Fig. 6 Principles of continuous hypothermic machine perfusion.

Normothermic reperfusion

Organ perfusion at normal temperature can mimic normal function, but normothermic perfusion as a means of storage has not been possible for prolonged periods without seriously damaging the organ. Kootstra and his colleagues demonstrated that intermittent brief normothermic blood perfusion during cold storage improved preservation of both ice-stored and machine-perfused kidneys. The mechanisms of action are uncertain, but may relate to replenishing cellular energy stores and protecting the vasculature. The technique has not yet found clinical application.

Freezing and vitrification

Freezing is normally lethal to cells. Red cells, lymphocytes, spermatozoa, fertilized ova, embryos, and pancreatic islet cells can all be frozen and thawed satisfactorily in the presence of cryoprotectants. Simple tissues such as skin and cornea can also be preserved by freezing. Unfortunately freezing of organs, so attractive in concept in approaching true suspended animation and indefinite storage, has not proved feasible to date. The low surface area to volume ratio of organs compared to cells makes effective heat exchange a major problem. Cryoprotectants such as glycerol and dimethyl sulphoxide need to be present in high concentrations for adequate cryoprotection and this causes severe organ toxicity and vascular damage. Extracellular ice formation is innocuous when freezing cell suspensions, but can disrupt and severely damage the morphology of whole organs. The vascular system is especially vulnerable, and the attachment of vascular endothelial basement membrane is disrupted by freezing. Total vitrification of tissues is an alternative approach, but is also unsuccessful for whole organs. The tissue is first perfused with high concentrations of several cryoprotectants, so that on cooling neither intracellular nor extracellular freezing occurs. The solution vitrifies (i.e. solidifies into a glass state) at temperatures of approximately −120°C.

PHASES OF CLINICAL PRESERVATION

The donor

The function of the organ must be protected before and during procurement from the donor. Living donor grafts, such as kidney, are protected by maintaining blood and interstitial fluid volumes, by inducing a diuresis with mannitol during the operation, and by avoiding vascular trauma and vasospasm during mobilization and removal of the organ. Warm ischaemia is kept to a minimum.

Management of the brain-dead heart-beating organ donor follows similar protocols. Blood volume needs to be carefully maintained by transfusion and, when necessary, by central venous pressure monitoring. Diabetes insipidus is common in brain-dead patients; large volumes of fluid and careful monitoring are required. Over-transfusion and pulmonary oedema must be avoided in patients serving as heart and heart–lung donors. Renal support is given using dopamine (2–5 mg/kg.min). Systemic acidosis must be corrected. Mannitol 25 g, steroids 1 g, chlorpromazine 500 mg, and heparin 10 000 U are given just prior to *in-situ* aortic flush cooling. Nifedipine should be added if adrenaline or noradrenaline has been given to the donor. Expeditious and skilful organ removal from a well prepared, well hydrated cadaver donor with minimal warm ischaemia is the best guarantee of immediate organ function after grafting. The state of the organ prior to its removal in such instances becomes the best guide to subsequent early function.

Donors of multiple organs

In countries where kidney, heart, lung, liver, and pancreas transplantation is available up to 80 per cent of all cadaveric donors serve as donors of several organs. Criteria for the acceptance of donors for heart, lung, liver, and pancreas are more restricted than those for kidney transplantation. Transplanted hearts and livers

Table 3 Multiorgan donor: organ-specific criteria

	Kidney	Liver	Pancreas	Heart
Age limits (years)	<65	<45 (60)	<45	<45(60)
Exclusion	Pre-existing renal disease, diabetes	Pre-existing hepatobiliary disease, abdominal trauma, intoxication, cardiac arrest	Pre-existing diabetes, renal disease, hypertension, abdominal trauma, intoxication	Pre-existing heart disease, chest trauma, high dose inotropic drugs, cardiac arrest
Diagnostic tests	Serum creatinine, urinalysis, CMV status, HBsAg, HIV	ICU course <7 days, liver function tests normal, CMV status, HBsAg, HIV	ICU course <7 days, γ-glutamyl transferase normal, CMV status, HBsAG, HIV	ICU course <7 days, ECG, chest radiography, CMV status, HBsAg, HIV
Compatibility required for:				
Weight and size	No	Yes (possible to use cutdown liver)	No	Yes
ABO groups	Yes	Yes	Yes	Yes
HLA cross match	Yes	Only in sensitized patients	Only in sensitized patients	Only in sensitized patients

must function immediately to support life, whereas kidney recipients can be supported by dialysis while temporary tubular necrosis recovers. An example of criteria required for kidney, liver, pancreas, and heart grafts is set out in Table 3.

General criteria require a donor to be free from cancer (except for treated skin cancers and central nervous system malignancies). Systemic embolization of primary brain tumours can occur after ventriculoatrial shunting; such patients should not be used as donors. Donors should also be free from systemic sepsis which is particularly likely to occur in those given intensive care for more than 7 days, and negative for hepatitis B surface antigen (HBsAg), hepatitis C serology, and human immunodeficiency virus (HIV) antibodies. Any patient with a known or suspected history of homosexual activity or intravenous drug usage should be excluded—the patient may be in the latent period before HIV antibodies develop.

A full postmortem examination should be performed following cadaveric organ donation. Occasionally unsuspected disease in the donor such as tuberculosis indicates the need for a period of drug prophylaxis in the recipient. Occult cancers may also be identified.

Techniques of multiple organ retrieval are outlined elsewhere. The donor organs are skeletonized. All organs require induction of rapid hypothermia to restrict initial warm ischaemic damage. The heart is stopped by infusion of a cold cardioplegic solution and removed first; rapid cooling of other organs is initiated by *in-situ* cold flushing via the aorta and portal vein. Liver, pancreas, then kidneys, are removed in sequence during *in-situ* flushing. Once the organs have been cooled and removed, the dissection is completed in a bath of ice slush when the vascular pedicles of each organ are prepared for transplantation. Final washout with 1 to 2 l of the organ preserving solution (UW, Citrate, EuroCollins, PBS, HTK) is performed at this stage until the effluent is macroscopically clear and the organ uniformly pallid.

Non-heart-beating cadaver donors

Organ transplantation for end-stage disease is now well established worldwide in both developed and developing countries. Shortage of cadaver organs for transplantation remains a perennial problem, and is influenced by legal, ethical, cultural, and religious backgrounds of individual countries. The supply of organs from heart-beating brain-dead cadaver donors is inadequate to meet total demand. In developed countries the death rate from motor accidents has been lowered by public educational programmes, compulsory seat belt legislation, and other safety measures. Control of mortality from road crash epidemics has been an immensely impressive public health achievement; diminished numbers of brain-dead cadaver donors following road injury is an inevitable corollary.

Interest has thus rekindled in retrieval of organs from non-heart-beating cadavers. Organs from this source are unsuitable for liver, heart, or lung transplantation, but can be appropriate for kidney transplantation. Organ retrieval is facilitated by legislation governing early removal of organs after death, by public awareness of the problems, and by public support for organ transplantation. Kootstra and others in Europe and in the United States have shown that efficient organization in hospital emergency departments and in operating theatres can gain a significant number of adequately preserved kidneys from cadaver donors presenting with irreversible cardiac arrest. Special techniques include the insertion of aortic and caval balloon cannulae after groin cutdown, followed by rapid aortic delivery of large volumes of cold flushing solutions to provide *in-situ* cold perfusion of kidneys while preparations are being made for operative retrieval. Kidneys from these sources have provided very acceptable results; the frequency of delayed early function and of ultimately non-viable kidneys is higher than from heart-beating cadavers, but this additional source of cadaver organs has proved very valuable.

Extracorporeal storage

Simple cold storage

Most organs are subsequently immersed in cold preserving solution and stored at 0 to 4°C in a refrigerated container until reimplantation.

Kidneys are frequently transplanted within 24 h. This period can be extended safely for periods up to 36 to 48 h or longer, if such time is required to find and prepare an optimal recipient and to transport the refrigerated organ long distances. Liver and pancreas preservation with UW solution storage is effective for 12 to 24 h. Heart and heart–lung transplantation with current preservation solutions is restricted to a storage period of 5 to 6 h—increasing use of UW-derived solutions is likely to extend this time.

Perfusion storage

Organs are perfused continuously with a recirculating perfusate at 4 to 6°C. This technique is used less commonly now because of the increased effectiveness of preserving solutions for simple storage.

The recipient operation

While management of the donor is of great importance to subsequent graft function, factors operating in the recipient during operation and after reperfusion may be equally significant. Failure of blood flow to return uniformly to all portions of previously ischaemic tissues (no reflow phenomenon) is a recognized sequel of extended ischaemic damage to organs *in situ*, to autografts, and to allografts. This phenomenon has been described following ischaemia of kidney, heart, muscle, brain, and other tissues. In recent years much attention has therefore focused on potential damage suffered by the graft during the implantation operation, and in the early period after revascularization.

Delayed restoration of blood flow to the renal cortex after reperfusion can contribute significantly to delayed graft function. Reperfusion of the stored kidney, rather than marking the welcome end of its ischaemic insult, may exacerbate the effects of ischaemia and lead to further cellular damage and early acute tubular necrosis.

The severity of reperfusion injury is dependent on the events of retrieval and storage. Injury can follow prolonged warm ischaemia, or extended cold preservation by either static or perfusion storage. The pathophysiology relates to continuing effects or oligaemic (hypoxic) hypothermic events during organ retrieval and storage under the fresh stimulus of return of oxygenated blood flow (Fig. 4): pretreating the recipient, as well as the donor, can obviate some of these effects. Reperfusion injury can be exacerbated by gradual rewarming of the organ during reimplantation. Grafts should be kept cold with moistened cold packs during the recipient operation, and vascular anastomoses performed expeditiously. Addition of interposition arterial or venous jump grafts or other vascular repairs should be done as bench surgery on the preserved chilled organ. Technical failures of vascular anastomoses, requiring reclamping and revision, are potent contributors to reperfusion injury.

PRESERVATION OF INDIVIDUAL ORGANS AND TISSUES

Vascularized organs

Kidney

Simple hypothermic storage employs the following flush solutions: firstly, Collins' solution, with high concentrations of potassium, magnesium, phosphate, sulphate, and glucose. This extended preservation to 48 h, but precipitation of magnesium phosphate was a major problem. Subsequently, magnesium sulphate was omitted (EuroCollins solution) with no deleterious effect. Replacement of glucose by mannitol, sucrose, or raffinose improves function experimentally and in humans.

Citrate-based solutions, containing high concentrations of potassium, magnesium, citrate, sulphate, and mannitol were originally devised to overcome the limitations of Collins' solution. Both hypertonic and isotonic solutions are stable and provide successful clinical preservation for 48 h or more. High magnesium concentration is essential; magnesium citrate chelates provide the critical semipermeant component.

Recently, two other solutions have been shown to provide better renal preservation than the above which are nonetheless still widely used. These are phosphate buffered sucrose (PBS) and UW solution. The former is an isotonic solution containing only a phosphate buffer and sucrose, an impermeant solute. Clinically and experimentally this solution is highly effective. Preservation at 72 h was better with phosphate buffered sucrose than with Collins' or Citrate solutions.

UW solution was developed initially for pancreatic preservation. Subsequently, it was found to extend and improve preservation of the liver profoundly and became the preferred solution for multiorgan harvest, despite its higher cost. UW solution is highly effective in preserving dog kidneys for 72 h and rat kidneys for 48 h. Modifications of the solution, omitting the colloid (hydroxyethyl starch), are equally effective. High potassium concentration is not essential, and lactobionate can be replaced by gluconate. Clinically, a recent European Multicentre Trial indicated that kidneys preserved in UW solution produced a more rapid reduction of serum creatinine, higher creatinine clearance rate, and less dialysis when compared to EuroCollins (median preservation time 24 h, maximum 48 h). An additional advantage of use of UW solution was that sharing kidneys between centres to improve matching improved graft survival without any functional detriment for up to 48 h of storage. Other trials showed UW without HES to be equally beneficial.

Kidneys which have undergone more prolonged storage often exhibit poor early function for several days. Further extension of preservation requires additional resuscitative technology. Perfusion storage may resuscitate kidneys which have been subjected to adverse conditions before harvest or during storage. This could involve intermittent warm reperfusion with oxygen, nutrient amino acids, fatty acids, cofactors, and hormones. Normothermic reperfusion would be easier to apply clinically if a reliable synthetic perfusate could be developed.

Liver

Liver transplantation has been an established and effective treatment modality for end-stage liver disease since the early 1980s, but until recently livers were only able to be stored reliably for 12 h in Collins' or Citrate solutions. Preservation of the liver with EuroCollins or Citrate is less effective than preservation of the kidney for the hepatocyte is more permeable to glucose and mannitol, leading to reduced osmotic control and increased acidosis due to anaerobic glycolysis (EuroCollins). Pretreatment of the donor with chlorpromazine, or addition of chlorpromazine, diltiazem, or a stable prostacyclin analogue to the flush solution improves preservation.

A major advance in liver preservation occurred with introduction of UW solution. This solution provided effective preservation in the dog (48 h) and rat (30 h). Clinical preservation times have been safely extended to 24 h allowing procurement of liver grafts from distant cities, ample time for histopathological examination of the graft, more perfect recipient hepatectomy, and bench surgery of the graft to tailor adult grafts to fit one or more child recipients. The length of the preservation period within the range 4 to 24 h has not affected graft outcome in UW-preserved liver grafts. In contrast, the ischaemic period significantly affects EuroCollins livers preserved for this length of time.

Experimental studies have indicated that the essential ingredients of UW solution are the impermeant anion lactobionate, with additional osmolality provided by raffinose. Adenosine, allopurinol, and glutathione seem also beneficial. Omission of hydroxyethyl starch from UW solution is not detrimental to dog, rat, or human liver grafts. High potassium content has been shown to be unnecessary in 48-h preservation of the dog liver. Other buffers such as histidine can replace phosphate.

The hepatocyte is relatively insensitive to cold ischaemia; the primary damage is to the microvasculature and to the endothelial cells lining the sinusoid. Experimental studies indicate that although parenchymal cells remain viable during preservation for 48 h, a high proportion of endothelial cells are non-viable and this contributes to poor early function and mortality. UW solution helps to prevent cold-induced microcirculatory injury, but the mechanism of this protection is still speculative.

Prolonged preservation requires further refinement of solutions for static preservation, or development of perfusion preservation. Dog livers have been successfully stored for 72 h using continuous perfusion with modified UW solution: gluconate replaced lactobionate in this solution and calcium, adenine, glucose, and ribose were included.

Assessment of graft quality prior to implantation by measurement of ATP content, pH, energy charge, or morphology is not necessarily reliable; many of the detrimental changes occur after reperfusion. The volume and quality of bile flow, restoration of clotting, absence of lactate acidosis, blood amino acid clearance, and plasma concentration of bilirubin and aspartate aminotransferase can distinguish which grafts will recover.

During the recipient operation, it is advisable to replace the preservation fluid within the stored liver before releasing the suprahepatic caval clamp, by reflushing with balanced electrolyte solution, blood, or plasma, otherwise cardiac arrhythmias or arrest can occur due to the high concentrations of potassium, hydrogen ions, or pharmacological additives such as adenosine released into the circulation from the revascularized liver. Some centres use a warm rinse before release of the upper clamp; this avoids potential inhibition of cardiac activity from a large bolus of cold fluid.

Pancreas

Initial methods for pancreas preservation were based on those developed for kidney. The pancreas is more vulnerable to mechanical damage during retrieval, but is no more sensitive to either warm ischaemia or cold storage. The problems encountered in pancreatic grafting relate to its low circulatory flow rate and to vascular damage on storage and reperfusion. Thrombosis of vascular anastomses is more likely in organs subjected to poor preservation.

In early clinical studies, EuroCollins solution was successful, albeit for short periods of ischaemia: only about 10 per cent of grafts were preserved for longer than 12 h. Experimental preservation of the canine pancreas has been successful for 72 h (UW), and rat pancreas has been preserved for 48 h (UW, hydroxyethyl starch-free UW, and Citrate). Preservation times have been extended clinically using UW solution; this has markedly facilitated organization of transplant programmes. Clinically, graft survival has not been affected by extending preservation times to 24 h, although grafts stored for over 30 h show somewhat decreased graft survival. Retrospective analysis of transplant registry results showed that patients with better HLA-DR matching had significantly better graft survival. Prolonged effective preservation would allow allocation of grafts after matching.

Perfusion storage is inherently more difficult in the pancreas because of its low circulatory flow rate. Early studies using machinery designed for kidney perfusion were unsuccessful. Perfusion storage at low flow rates with UW-based solutions may in the future extend and improve pancreatic storage.

The interdependence of exocrine and endocrine cells has not been assessed. Ablation of the exocrine cells by polymer injection of the pancreatic duct does not appear to have any detrimental effect on 1-year graft survival, but long-term endocrine function may be compromised. Other transplant techniques involve reconstitution of pancreatic drainage via the intestine or the urinary bladder. Effective preservation of acinar cells helps minimize pancreatitis: elevated serum amylase is a common occurrence, and the level relates to preservation time. Acinar cell preservation provides a reliable and sensitive test of rejection. Monitoring of urinary amylase in bladder-drained pancreas transplants has become an accepted early indicator of rejection: falling urinary amylase indicates a need for more vigorous immunosuppression.

Heart

Heart preservation has employed simple static cold storage. As 85 per cent of the energy consumed by the heart fuels contraction of the myofibrils, cardioplegic arrest has been an essential feature of heart preservation. The development of heart transplantation from open heart surgery had a considerable influence on the strategies applied in heart preservation. Cardioplegic solutions developed for cardiac surgery provided safe preservation of myocardial function for only 5 to 6 h.

For transplantation, the heart is excised after induction of hypothermic cardioplegic arrest by *in-situ* flush with one of several standard cardioplegic solutions (Table 4). The graft is then stored cold in the flush-out solution or in EuroCollins solution. Sinus node dysfunction (usually transient) is common after transplantation and is related to the duration of ischaemia. Microvascular

Table 4 Cardioplegic solutions

	St Thomas's	Stanford	Wicomb
Sodium (mmol/l)	120	125	40
Potassium (mmol/l)	16	18	125
Magnesium (mmol/l)	16	–	5
Calcium (mmol/l)	1.2	–	–
Chloride (mmol/l)	160	98	–
Bicarbonate (mmol/l)	10	25	–
Phosphate (mmol/l)	–	–	25
Lactobionate (mmol/l)	–	–	100
Mannitol (mmol/l)	–	25	–
Glucose (mmol/l)	–	255	–
Raffinose (mmol/l)	–	–	30
Glutathione (mmol/l)	–	–	3
Procaine (mmol/l)	1	–	–
PEG 20M (g/l)	–	–	50
Osmolality (mmol/kg)	320	400	320
pH (0°C)	7.3	8.2	7.3

injury has been reported in the presence of well-preserved myocytes.

Flushing solutions commonly used for the preservation of other organs are also cardioplegic, but generally contain much higher concentrations of potassium (over 100 mmol/l instead of 20 to 30 mmol/l) and do not contain any calcium. Initial reluctance to apply such solutions to heart preservation stems from earlier studies indicating that potassium-induced contraction band necrosis occurred with potassium concentrations above 40 mmol/l, and that a 'calcium paradox' effect in cardiac preservation was important (cardiac muscle incubated in calcium-free medium undergoes severe irreversible damage when reperfused with calcium-containing medium due to a massive influx of calcium). Warm ischaemic damage enhances calcium influx. The occurrence of the calcium paradox during hypothermia is controversial; but removal of calcium from St Thomas's solution has been shown to be detrimental, and the calcium paradox phenomenon has been seen in experimental cardiopulmonary bypass.

Recently, modifications of UW solution have been used clinically in open heart surgery and for transplantation, and in experimental studies. The range of available experimental models include heterotopic transplants to the abdomen or neck in small animals, isolated perfused working heart models, metabolic tissue analysis and histology, nuclear magnetic resonance spectroscopy, and allograft function in larger animals. Specimens of human atrial myocardium can be obtained for study during open heart surgery. Successful orthotopic transplants have been reported after 12 h of preservation with UW solution in primates, and clinical trials with UW solution have given superior donor heart preservation over that obtained by Stanford and other solutions.

Maintenance of high energy phosphate levels (ATP and creatine phosphate) has been another goal, but no linear correlation exists between the concentration of adenine nucleotides in preserved heart and the functional outcome. When the level of these high energy compounds falls below a certain level no functional recovery occurs, but inadequate preservation may occur at normal levels. Addition of ATP or its precursors to preserving solutions can improve cardiac function, but this does not correlate with maintenance of tissue ATP levels and may have been due to the vasodilatory properties of the additives.

Generation of oxygen free radicals has been implicated in ischaemic heart disease and in reperfusion injury. Metabolic inhibitors and free radical scavengers have been used to pretreat the donor and as additions to the preserving solution. Improvements in left ventricular function, lipid peroxidation, and platelet aggregation have been demonstrated. Prostacyclins also dilate coronary vessels, inhibit platelet aggregation, and stabilize lysosomal membranes. A stable prostacyclin analogue added to the cardioplegic solution has been shown to improve ventricular function after clinical cardiac transplantation.

More prolonged myocardial preservation may depend on techniques. Perfusion at low flow rates with oxygenated perfusate improved preservation of rabbit hearts using a modified UW solution incorporating polyethylene glycol (PEG). A colloid is essential in such perfusates; PEG may prove a suitable alternative to hydroxyethyl starch.

Heart–lung

Simple cooling is sufficient for short-term preservation for heart–lung transplants. Lungs are flushed with cold EuroCollins solution via the pulmonary artery immediately after induction of cardioplegia. Flushing may be a source of injury and care must be taken to maintain pressure below that normally found in the pulmonary artery; lung distension is maintained by rhythmic ventilation at 50 to 70 per cent of normal inflation throughout the period of storage. Prostacyclin, superoxide dismutase, and catalase are beneficial when added to EuroCollins solution.

Clinically, treatment of the donor with prostaglandin E_1 followed by simple hypothermic flush with EuroCollins solution provides adequate 6-h preservation. In experimental heart–lung transplants in the dog, treatment of the recipient with superoxide dismutase also improved preservation. Use of a solution with lower potassium concentration may improve lung function: high potassium levels produce pulmonary vasospasm and may reduce the efficacy of the flush. Solutions containing colloid could be additionally beneficial in the lung.

Hypothermia and cardiopulmonary bypass with diluted blood is more complex, and has only been effective experimentally for 6 h. The addition of methylprednisolone, prostaglandin, and isoproterenol improved lung function.

Autoperfusion of heart–lung preparations at 30°C has afforded the longest lung preservation (12 h), but this procedure is cumbersome and limited in use. Adding metabolic substrates such as glucose or ribose enhances preservation, as does leucocyte depletion. Lung oedema, activation of complement, and subsequent pulmonary sequestration of leucocytes may play a role in lung dysfunction.

Lung

Transplantation of the lungs alone has met with increasing clinical success. Lung preservation using a EuroCollins flush is only successful for 5 to 6 h: after 12 h of storage pulmonary vascular resistance increases threefold and compliance is reduced; and after 24 h the lung is haemorrhagic and oedematous. Addition of methylprednisolone to the preserving solution and its administration to both the donor and recipient can allow storage to be extended to 12 h but not to 24 h.

The lung may require different preservation techniques from those used for other organs. Existing techniques have evolved primarily to maintain the viability of metabolically active cells (hepatocytes, myocytes, renal tubules). The maintenance of a well preserved microcirculation, essential for adequate lung function, may require a re-examination of available techniques. Blood perfusion at 25°C to 30°C with the addition of metabolites may afford optimum vascular preservation, without an irreversible energy deficit affecting parenchymal cells.

Small intestine

Clinical transplantation of the small intestine has not been widely applied, but several recipients of organ cluster grafts have survived for 12 months or more. The hazards of intestinal transplantation preclude it from being an alternative to home parenteral nutrition: the major problems are rejection and graft-versus-host disease.

Experimental preservation and transplantation of the small intestine was first attempted in the late 1950s. Storage for 24 h, after flushing both the vasculature and the lumen of the graft with EuroCollins' or histidine-based solutions, can maintain the physiological and pharmacological properties of the intestinal smooth muscle. Solutions containing dextrans have been equally effective. More prolonged preservation has not been successful. Treatment with free radical scavengers or allopurinol may improve preservation. The small intestine has the highest concentration of the enzyme xanthine oxidase: free radical damage has been implicated after warm ischaemic injury.

Composite tissues, limbs

Reconstructive surgery increasingly uses vascularized autografts of composite tissues (skin, subcutaneous fat, muscle, and bone) to fill large defects. Severed limbs and digits are often replaced as autografts. These complex operative procedures can take many hours. Storage of the grafts has predominantly relied upon simple cooling by refrigeration, and wrapping of the tissues in cold saline-soaked packs during implantation.

Supplementary vascular flushing has not been widely used for fear of damage to the small vessels requiring microvascular suture. Experimental studies have not indicated that flushing gives any significant improvement over simple hypothermic storage—which adequately covers the periods (usually less than 12 h) required in clinical practice. Tolerance of different tissues to ischaemia varies: muscle is more sensitive than skin and bone. Morphology and viability of skin, muscle, and bone can be preserved after several days of storage at 4°C using simple hypothermia in a moist environment. In whole-limb replacement, flushing with an organ preservation solution can aid cooling and potentially improve preservation. Before the circulation is restored to replanted limbs or other tissues of large bulk, any solution with high potassium levels should be flushed out with balanced electrolyte solution or plasma, otherwise fatal hyperkalaemic cardiac arrest can occur after release of clamps.

Tissue grafts

Cornea

Early in the 20th century it was realized that the cornea was not an inert transparent membrane, but a biologically active tissue needing careful handling if it was to survive the transplant operation. Pioneering efforts in the 1930s established the suitability of cadaver corneas for grafting and the feasibility of direct suturing of the graft to host tissues. The immunological privilege of the cornea was appreciated at an early stage. The cornea's function as a transparent reflecting and focusing complex requires the metabolic activity of a monolayer endothelium of mesodermally derived cells on the inner surface bathed by the aqueous humour.

For procurement from the cadaver donor, eyes are enucleated: this simple procedure can be done without elaborate preparation and need not be disfiguring. Originally corneas collected for transplantation were used immediately after the eye was removed, but storage in a moist environment at 4°C under sterile conditions allows penetrating (whole thickness) grafts to remain viable for up to 48 h after the death of the donor.

Intermediate storage times of up to 4 days can be achieved by the use of refrigerated tissue culture media. MK medium (developed by McCarey and Kaufman) containing dextran-40 and HEPES (*N*-2-hydroxyethylpiperazine-*N*-2-ethanesulphonic acid)-buffered tissue-culture fluid provides reliable preservation for 3 to 4 days. Storage in MK medium has achieved wide acceptance, but this still does not allow sufficient time for the ever more complex examinations required for the graft: examination of endothelial sheet integrity, disease screening (Creutzfeldt-Jakob syndrome, HIV antibodies, septicaemia), and tissue-typing, which may prove to be a valuable adjunct in corneal transplantation. Retrospective and prospective surveys have shown that results correlate with antigen matching. Further refinement of the tissue culture medium has resulted in the replacement of dextran-40 with chondroitin sulphate, which allows up to 14 days hypothermic preservation, with loss of only 3 per cent of the endothelial cells. Best preservation has been attained using 2.5 per cent chondroitin sulphate free of lower molecular weight moieties. Long-term storage can be achieved by cryopreservation of the isolated cornea. This technique was developed for prolonged eye banking, but has not gained universal acceptance.

Short-term hypothermic whole eye storage remains the most simple and convenient technique, particularly when there is no shortage of eyes, and in the United States this is still a common method of short-term banking of whole eyes. Tissue culture (MK) storage has gained acceptance by the majority of laboratories. A minority of departments use cryopreservation, and then only occasionally.

Pancreatic islets

Preservation and transplantation of pancreatic islet cells have been extensively studied experimentally. Intraportal transplantation of islet extracts is now achieving some clinical success. Cellular preparations, after collagenase digestion and purification, have been successfully preserved by tissue culture for 24 h at 37°C, by simple ice cooling for 24 h, or for more prolonged periods by freezing with addition of cryoprotectives.

Skin

Harvested split skin grafts used as autografts or allografts can be preserved for approximately 2 weeks by simple wrapping and rolling in packs moistened with saline or tissue culture fluid. These are then stored in the refrigerator at 4°C.

Xenografts of pig skin can be similarly prepared and have been widely used for temporary cover of denuded sites. More prolonged preservation can be provided by freezing, or by culturing epidermal cells which can subsequently be reimplanted as a monolayer.

Bone and cartilage

Autografts of fresh cancellous bone taken from iliac crest or other areas remain the most effective source of bone grafts, and provide viable osteoblasts and stimulate osteogenesis. Bone is a complex and active metabolic tissue, containing osteocytes bearing histocompatibility antigens nourished within a hydroxyapatite matrix. Stored allografts of bone can be cryopreserved for 12 months or more to provide a sterile source of bone matrix without viable cells. The biomechanical properties of bone do not seem affected by cryostorage, but preserved allografts are less active in stimulating osteogenesis than are fresh autografts.

Transplantation of large segments of cortical bone can provide a rigid bony matrix which is gradually replaced by creeping substitution of new bone. Transfer of viable cortical bone requires a vascularized graft which restores the bone's blood supply at its new site. Vascularized autografts of fibula and iliac crest can replace bony defects resulting from congenital anomalies, disease, or injury.

The metabolic needs of cartilage are chiefly met by diffusion of nutrients from synovial fluids; re-establishment of a blood supply is less critical than for bone. Chondrocytes also possess histocompatibility antigens and evoke an allograft rejection response. Intact cartilage survives better than isolated chondrocytes, showing the importance of the cartilage matrix. Experimentally, cartilage can be stored for 28 days in tissue culture medium at 4°C. The morphology of the cells and concentration of glycosaminoglycans and of collagen show no significant change, and the ability of cells to incorporate ^{35}S-sulphate into glycosaminoglycans does not diminish.

Cryopreservation at subzero temperatures with glycerol or dimethylsulphoxide produces a less favourable outcome, with loss of chondrocytes and conversion of hyaline cartilage to fibrocartilage. Isolated chondrocytes can be well preserved by freezing, suggesting poor penetration of cryopreservative.

Onlays or plugs of cadaveric articular cartilage fragments have been used as allografts in the management of degenerative arthritis. The methods remain experimental.

Bone marrow

Bone marrow transplantation is now the preferred treatment for aplastic anaemias and for many leukaemias. Marrow allografts usually require minimal preservation, other than that provided by simple hypothermia as for blood collection. Invariably, living donors have been used. Extension of bone marrow transplantation in the future using cadaver donors could involve cryoprotective techniques similar to those used for freezing of blood. There is also an increasing use of autologous marrow grafts in cancer, the patient's marrow being removed and preserved before intensive chemotherapy and/or irradiation is given. The preserved marrow is then returned to the patient.

Blood vessels

Autogenous veins are used to replace and bypass arteries in aortocoronary and peripheral vascular surgery. Occasionally autogenous arteries (such as the internal iliac) are used for short bypass procedures such as aortorenal grafts: in these situations the graft is a 'vital' one with the cellular tissues retaining their viability. The graft is usually prepared in heparinized saline at room temperature. Should the expected ischaemic period be longer than 1 h it is advisable to cool the vessel in iced saline. Blood vessels from cadaver donors are a very important source of extended arterial and venous conduits for renal, liver, and pancreatic allografts. These vessels are adequately preserved by simply hypothermic storage in standard flushing solutions. Vessels can be removed from cadaver donors, treated with glutaraldehyde, and stored indefinitely; they then become essentially collagenous tubes without apparent antigenic activity. This allografted non-living tissue does not cause a rejection reaction but will slowly degenerate, and a thrombosis or aneurysm can develop. It is an inferior option to the use of fresh autogenous vessels.

THE FUTURE

Preservation of organs and tissues for transplantation has entered a new and exciting phase with the development of multicomponent UW–lactobionate preserving solutions. The basic requirements of preservation remain rapid cooling aided by impermeants and buffers, but many other metabolic and pharmacological influences have been shown to enhance organ protection. Incorporation of such agents into preservation solutions, as well as their judicious use in preparation of the donor and in subsequent treatment of the recipient, has extended significantly preservation times of all organs and tissues. Although heart and heart–lung transplants still require rapid surgery with minimal storage times, prospects for extending safe preservation times for all vascularized organ grafts to 24 h or longer are now much closer. Research continues to look for more effective additives to preserving solutions, and to improve perfusion techniques, to extend safe preservation times even more. Preparation of the graft or cadaver donor by reduction of antigen presenting cells, as well as pregraft treatment of the recipient with selected monoclonal antibodies and other agents may also prepare the way for more successful transplantation. Advances in preservation will contribute significantly to such future developments.

FURTHER READING

Belzer FO, Southard JH. Principles of solid-organ preservation by cold storage. *Transplantation* 1988; **45**: 673–6.

Calne RY, *et al.* Renal preservation by ice-cooling: An experimental study relating to kidney transplantation from cadavers. *Br Med J* 1963; **2**: 651–5.

Carrel A, Lindbergh CA. *The Culture of Organs*. London: Hamish Hamilton Medical Books, 1938.

Collins GH, Bravo-Shugarman MB, Terasaki PI: Kidney preservation for transplantation: Initial perfusion and 30-hour ice storage. *Lancet* 1969; **2**: 1219–22.

Flye MW. *Principles of Organ Transplantation*. Philadelphia: WB Saunders, 1989.

Marshall VC, Jablonski P, Scott DF. Renal preservation. In Morris PJ, ed. *Kidney Transplantation. Principles and Practice*. 3rd edn., Philadelphia: WB Saunders Company, 1988: 151–82.

Polge C, Smith AU, Parkes AS. Revival of spermatozoa after vitrification and dehydration at low temperature. *Nature* 1949; **164**: 666.

Ross H, Marshall VC, Escott MO. 72-hour canine kidney preservation without continuous perfusion. *Transplantation* 1976; 21: 498–501.

Simmons RL, Finch ME, Ascher NL, Najarian JS, eds. *Manual of Vascular Access, Organ Donation, and Transplantation*. New York: Springer-Verlag 1984.

Todo S, Tsakis A, Starzl TE. Preservation of livers with UW or Euro-Collins solution. *Transplantation* 1988; **46**: 925–6.

Wahlberg JA, *et al.* 72-hour preservation of the canine pancreas. *Transplantation* 1987; **43**: 5–8.

10.4 Immunosuppression

PETER J. MORRIS

INTRODUCTION

The advances in organ transplantation, so evident in the other sections in this chapter, can be attributed to a great extent to the advances in immunosuppression over the last 40 years. In the 1950s total body irradiation was the only form of immunosuppression available and patients either died of marrow aplasia and overwhelming infection if given sufficient irradiation to prevent rejection of a renal transplant, or rejected the graft if given lower doses of irradiation. Nevertheless, some modest success was achieved in some patients at that time. The introduction of azathioprine in the early 1960s was a major advance in renal transplantation and was quickly applied in renal transplant units throughout the world. As graft survival could now be prolonged in many patients both in the medium and long term, there was a dramatic growth in the numbers of renal transplant units. Steroids were added to azathioprine firstly to treat rejection and then in combination with azathioprine to prevent rejection. Heterologous antilymphocyte globulin, usually made in horses at the time, was introduced to treat steroid resistant rejection in the 1970s, but basically the standard immunosuppressive therapy in all units was azathioprine and steroids for nearly 20 years until cyclosporin became generally available in the early 1980s.

Very quickly cyclosporin-based immunosuppressive protocols became standard therapy and remain so to this day. The introduction of cyclosporin led not only to a marked improvement in renal allograft survival (10–15 per cent), but also to a rapid improvement in liver and cardiac allograft survival. This led to a dramatic increase in the numbers of liver and cardiac transplants throughout the Western world.

During the next 10 years other immunosuppressive drugs will become available and some are already undergoing clinical trials, e.g. FK506 and RS61443. In addition the explosion in the production of monoclonal antibodies recognizing different cell surface markers on lymphocytes promises to add a new dimension to therapy with the hope of producing increased specificity of immunosuppression. Already OKT3, a pan-T-lymphocyte monoclonal antibody, is widely used to treat steroid resistant rejection and is also used as part of induction therapy in many centres. This agent is not a particularly specific antibody in that it recognizes all T cells but monoclonal antibodies against other lymphocyte targets should allow much greater specificity in immunosuppression to be achieved in clinical practice.

One of the major problems in clinical transplantation in the coming years will be the assessment of the large number of potentially valuable new therapies (both drugs and biological reagents) that will become available, remembering that the results of organ transplantation are now relatively good so that only large multicentre trials will be able to establish the true value or otherwise of new therapies. Furthermore, more sophisticated methods of analysis of outcome than mere graft survival will have to be developed.

DRUGS

Azathioprine

Azathioprine is a purine analogue, and is essentially an antiproliferative agent, inhibiting both DNA and RNA synthesis by preventing the synthesis of adenylic and guanylic acid from inosinic acid. For 20 years, in association with steroids, azathioprine provided the backbone of immunosuppressive therapy. In the cyclosporin era, azathioprine is still widely used in lower doses with cyclosporin on the assumption that it allows lower doses of cyclosporin to be used, hence decreasing the side-effects of both drugs. The major side-effect of azathioprine is leucopenia, and indeed regular white cell counts are the only method of monitoring the dosage. If used with steroids alone then the usual starting dose is 3.0 mg/kg daily reducing to maintenance levels of 2.0 mg/kg. However, when used as part of a cyclosporin-based protocol it tends to be used in doses of either 100 mg daily or 1.5 mg/kg daily.

Steroids

Prednisolone or prednisone are used routinely with azathioprine, and also in most cyclosporin-based protocols. Their mechanism of action in suppressing the alloreaction is unclear, but although immunosuppressive to some extent possibly their major action is an anti-inflammatory one. Certainly their concomitant use with azathioprine was essential to produce appropriate immunosuppression, but that is not clearly so in the cyclosporin era. When first introduced soon after azathioprine became available steroids were used in high doses and indeed most of the complications of transplantation in the 1960s and 1970s could be attributed to the use of high dose steroids, e.g. cushingoid changes, avascular necrosis of joints, peptic ulceration, infection, osteoporosis. The demonstration in controlled trials that low dose steroids were equally as effective in preventing rejection as high dose steroids quickly led to the general introduction of low dose steroid protocols, e.g. 20 mg daily during the first 2 to 3 months after transplantation reducing to maintenance levels of 10 mg daily, dramatically reduced the morbidity and mortality of renal transplantation.

High dose steroids are also used to treat rejection and a widely used protocol in this context is either 0.5 or 1.0 g of methylprednisolone given as an intravenous bolus daily for 3 days. This protocol successfully reverses the majority of acute rejection episodes of kidney, heart, and liver, and antilymphocytic globulin and/or OKT3 is reserved for steroid resistant infection.

Cyclosporin

Cyclosporin is a potent immunosuppressive agent, extracted from two strains of fungi imperfecti. It has a molecular weight of 1200 and comprises 11 amino acids (Fig. 1). Its major mechanism of

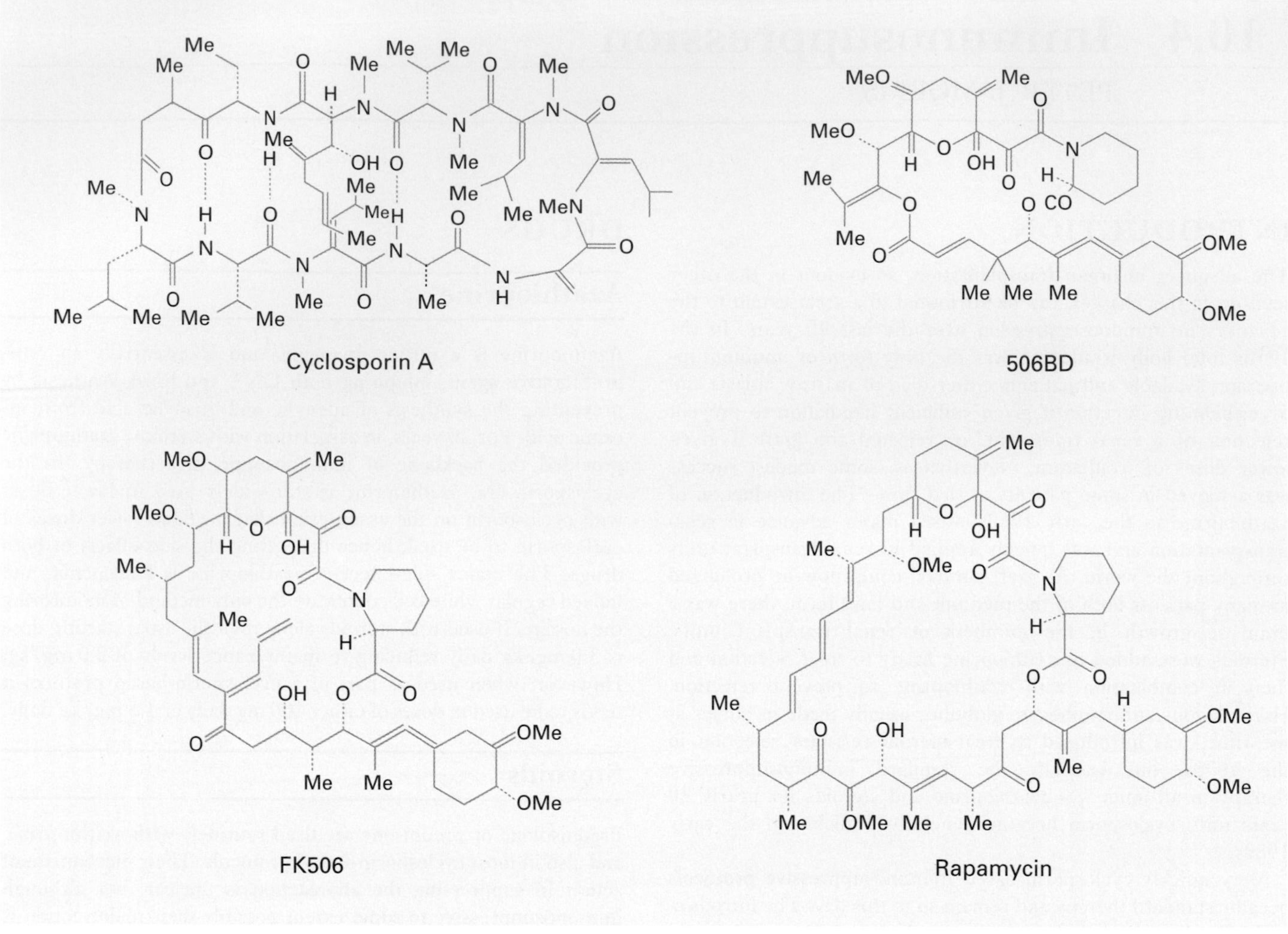

Cyclosporin A

506BD

FK506

Rapamycin

Fig. 1 The chemical structure of cyclosporin, FK506, rapamycin, and 506BD (an analogue of FK506).

action is to prevent the product of cytokines such as interleukin-2 (IL-2), which will be discussed in more detail later. When first introduced into clinical practice in renal transplantation and bone marrow transplantation it resulted in superior suppression of rejection and graft-versus-host disease respectively, which was reflected by better graft and patient survival. However side-effects soon became evident, the major ones being nephrotoxicity and hypertension (Table 1). Nephrotoxicity is a major problem of cyclosporin use in all forms of organ transplantation and bone marrow transplantation and although dose related to a great extent there is probably no effective dose of cyclosporin that is not nephrotoxic. The nephrotoxicity is due mainly to vasoconstriction of the afferent arterioles of the glomeruli, leading to a decrease in glomerular filtration rate, and these changes appear to be mediated by inhibition of vasodilator renal prostaglandin metabolites and increased production of thromboxane.

Because of the nephroxtoxicity and other dose related side-effects of the drug a number of cyclosporin-based protocols have evolved in an attempt to reduce the incidence of these side-effects (Table 2).

(i) Cyclosporin alone (monotherapy)

Although effective it is possible that higher doses of cyclosporin are required than if used with other agents.

Table 1 Side-effects of cyclosporin therapy

Renal	Nephrotoxicity; haemolytic-uraemic syndrome
Hepatic	Hepatotoxicity
Neoplastic	Lymphomas; fibroadenoma of breast; squamous cell carcinoma
Dermatological	Thickening; rashes, hypertrichosis
Gastrointestinal	Anorexia; nausea, failure to gain weight
Metabolic	Hyperkalaemia; hyperuricaemia; hypomagnesaemia; hyperglycaemia
Neurological	Tremor; convulsions; burning sensation in limbs; malaise; depression
Cardiovascular	Fluid retention; hypertension; hypercholesterolaemia; Raynaud's phenomenon; intravascular coagulation
Dental	Gingival hypertrophy
Haematological	Haemolytic anaemia

Table 2 Cyclosporin-based protocols

Cyclosporin ± steroids
Cyclosporin conversion to azathioprine after 3–12 months
Cyclosporin + azathioprine
Cyclosporin + azathioprine + steroids (triple therapy)
ATG/OKT3 + azathioprine + steroids → cyclosporin + azathioprine + steroids
ATG/OKT3 + cyclosporin + azathioprine + steroids

(ii) Cyclosporin and steroids

This is a commonly used protocol, but is not proven to be better than cyclosporin alone, although it has been suggested that the incidence of nephrotoxicity is lower when steroids are used.

(iii) Cyclosporin conversion therapy

Cyclosporin is used alone or with steroids and then at some given time after transplantation, e.g. 3, 6, or 12 months, cyclosporin is replaced with azathioprine and steroids preferably with some overlap. Undoubtedly renal function improves with conversion but the major drawback of these protocols is the risk of rejection occurring within the 1 or 2 months after conversion. Although these rejection episodes usually respond to steroid therapy, this type of protocol does require close supervision of patients after conversion. Nevertheless the financial aspects of this protocol as well as the improved renal function are attractive. Thus, this Oxford protocol, as it is often known, is widely used in developing countries.

(iv) Low dose cyclosporin, azathioprine, steroids (triple therapy)

This is a widely used therapy which produces very acceptable patient and graft survival (Fig. 2). It is not a more potent immunosuppressive protocol than other cyclosporin protocols, but it is relatively free of side-effects and easy to use. A typical protocol (as used in Oxford) would comprise cyclosporin 10 mg/kg.day reducing according to whole blood levels, azathioprine 100 mg/day, and prednisolone 20 mg/day reducing to a maintenance level of 10 mg/day, with the further aim of weaning patients off steroids altogether if renal function is stable at 1 year. Indeed our own experience of trials of steroid withdrawal in patients on triple therapy have shown benefits in levels of both hypertension and hypercholesterolaemia.

(v) Cyclosporin and azathioprine (double therapy)

This is not widely used and as the addition of steroids is required quite often in the early months it has no advantages over triple therapy.

(vi) Antithymocyte globulin (ATG) or OKT3, azathioprine, and steroids with introduction of cyclosporin as renal function is established (sequential therapy)

This type of protocol is widely used in North America in all forms of organ transplantation, but its use remains controversial both because improved graft survival has not been clearly established with the use of this type of protocol, and if subsequently steroid resistant rejection requires repeated treatment with either ATG or OKT3 then a substantial risk of developing a fatal acute lymphoproliferative disorder has been introduced. Nevertheless if there is no renal function after transplantation of a cadaveric kidney as a result of acute tubular necrosis, it is an attractive approach to the induction of immunosuppression, for there is reasonably good evidence that the use of cyclosporin in a patient with a non-functioning kidney delays the onset of function and also leads to long-term damage to the kidney.

(vii) ATG or OKT3, cyclosporin, azathioprine, and steroids (quadruple therapy)

This regimen is sometimes used in cardiac or liver transplantation. It probably represents an unnecessarily potent immunosuppressive protocol for most patients and is not recommended, except in the highly sensitized patient.

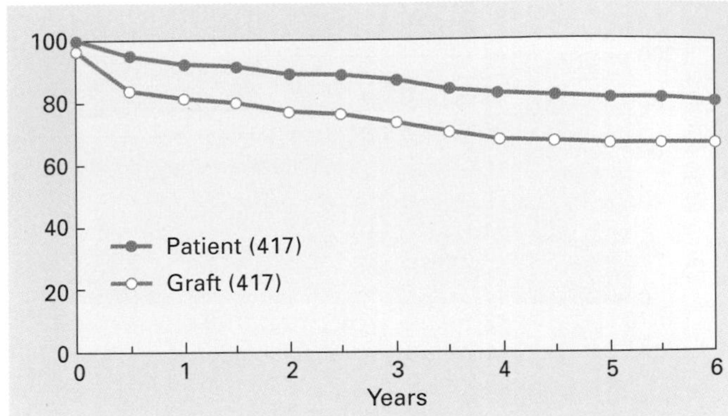

Fig. 2 Survival of patients and first cadaveric grafts treated with triple therapy (cyclosporin, azathioprine and steroids) in the Oxford Transplant Centre.

(viii) Monitoring of cyclosporin levels

A variety of techniques are commercially available but the most widely used techniques measure trough whole blood levels at either 11 or 24 h depending on whether the patient is taking cyclosporin twice daily or daily (there is no evidence that either dosing protocol is superior to the other). Trough levels are maintained at 200 to 400 μg/ml in the first 5 weeks and then at 100 to 200 μg/ml once stable graft function is established. Today most assays use monoclonal antibodies to cyclosporin A, the parent compound, which is essentially responsible for the immunosuppression and side-effects. High trough levels of cyclosporin are likely to be associated with toxicity and low levels with an increased incidence of rejection, but this is not inevitable and the trough levels must be used in association with other clinical, biochemical, and histological parameters.

FK506

Another potent immunosuppressive macrolide antibiotic, derived from *Streptomyces tsukubaensis*, FK506 has an entirely different structure to cyclosporin (Fig. 1) but its mechanism of action is similar in that it prevents the production of cytokines in response to antigen recognition (see later). On a weight for weight basis it is 10- to 100-fold more potent than cyclosporin. Its first clinical use in Pittsburgh was for the salvage of liver transplants undergoing rejection despite the use of high dose steroids and OKT3. In some 70 per cent of instances conversion from cyclosporin to FK506 resulted in improved liver function tests and survival of the liver allografts, an impressive debut. Its use as a primary agent with steroids has also been explored at Pittsburgh in liver, cardiac, and renal transplantation with excellent results in liver (Fig. 3) and cardiac transplantation. In contrast in a prospective controlled trial in renal transplantation, in which FK506 was compared with cyclosporin, no improvement in graft survival was observed and the same degree of nephrotoxicity was noted. Two large prospective controlled trials of FK506 in liver transplantation have been performed in North America and Europe and the results do show that FK506 is of value in liver transplantation. Thus, it would seem that this drug is going to represent a very useful addition to

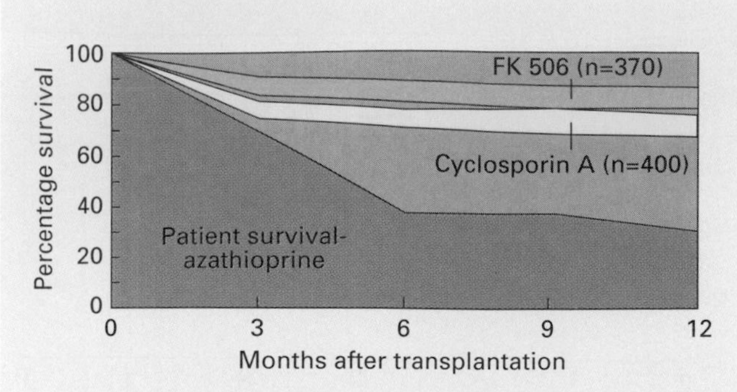

Fig. 3 Survival of patients and grafts after liver transplantation during the azathioprine era, and contrasting with patient and graft survival in Pittsburgh with cyclosporin or FK506.

our immunosuppressive armamentarium, especially in liver transplantation. In addition it has allowed a number of successful small bowel transplants in adults and children to be performed in Pittsburgh without a concomitant liver transplant, which does represent a significant advance in this area.

Rapamycin

Rapamycin is another macrolide antibiotic, with a very similar molecular structure to FK506 (Fig. 1), but in contrast an entirely different mechanism of action in that it inhibits the proliferation of the activated T cell. It is a potent immunosuppressive agent in experimental models but has not yet been used in clinical trials.

Mechanisms of action of cyclosporin, FK506, and rapamycin

There has been a marked increase in our knowledge of how these agents work, the implications of which are enormous in our understanding both of signal transduction after antigen recognition leading to T-cell activation and proliferation of the activated T cell. All three agents bind to a ubiquitous class of proteins within the cytoplasm known as immunophilins. Cyclosporin binds to cyclophilin while FK506 and rapamycin bind to a different immunophilin, FK binding protein (FKBP). These proteins are isomerases and it was first thought that the immunosuppressive action was due to inhibition of isomerase activity, but as it was realized that very small amounts of cyclosporin or FK506 were immunosuppressive although only binding to a portion of the total amount of isomerase available, other mechanisms were sought. Then another protein was found to be involved, namely calcinurin to which the complex of cyclosporin + cyclophilin and FK506 + FKBP bind, but not the complex rapamycin + FKBP; hence presumably the different effect of rapamycin. The drug–immunophilin complex and calcinurin inhibits the attachment of a protein, NFAT (nucleus factor in activated T cells), to the enhancer region upstream of the gene for IL-2, preventing its transcription and hence the production of IL-2 (Fig. 4). Just how this inhibition of NFAT occurs is not yet understood. It is not known what the complex of rapamycin + FKBP binds to but obviously as this binding prevents proliferation of the activated T cell, i.e. inhibiting the lymphokine-receptor signal, definition will further increase our knowledge of the response to alloantigens by T cells and allow the design of drugs with quite specific actions.

RS–61443

An ester of mycophenolic acid, this is an antiproliferative drug with a quite specific action in the purine pathway, namely the inhibition of the enzyme guanosine monophosphate. Thus it is relatively specific for lymphocytes. *In vitro* it has proved to be a powerful immunosuppressive agent especially when used together with cyclosporin; in addition it inhibits B-cell activity and hence antibody formation. Early experimental use and clinical trials suggest that this is a potent immunosuppressive agent. It is currently undergoing prospective randomized clinical trials in renal transplantation.

Cyclophosphamide

This antiproliferative agent is now seldom used but has been used as a replacement for azathioprine in the presence of hepatotoxicity considered to be due to this agent. It has also been used in India instead of azathioprine because it is cheaper, with success.

Mizoribine

Mizoribine, an imidazole nucleoside antibiotic which inhibits RNA and DNA synthesis via the purine biosynthesis pathway, has been used successfully instead of azathioprine in Japan for a number of years.

15-Deoxyspergualin

An antitumour antibiotic, it suppresses macrophage function and inhibits antibody production. It might have a place in sensitized patients but although used for a number of years, especially in Japan, no prospective clinical trials have been performed.

Brequinar sodium

This anticancer agent prevents all proliferation by inhibiting *de-novo* pyrimidine synthesis. In experimental models of transplantation it appears to be quite a powerful immunosuppressive agent, but as yet has not undergone clinical trials.

BIOLOGICAL AGENTS

Antilymphocyte or antithymocyte globulins

Heterologous antisera produced in another species, usually the horse or rabbit, have been used for many years primarily to treat steroid resistant rejection, but more commonly in recent years as inductive therapy to prevent rejection. In general the major action of antilymphocyte antisera is to reduce the T-lymphocyte count, but being heterologous antisera produced by immunization of

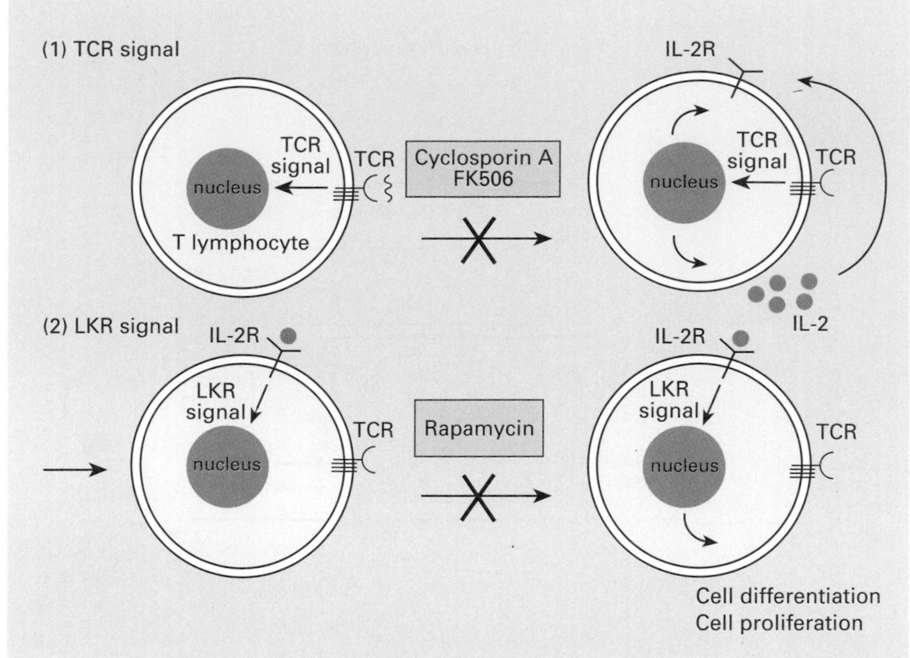

Fig. 4 Mechanism of action of cyclosporin, FK506, and rapamycin. Cyclosporin (CSA) and FK506 block the transduction of the signal from the T-cell receptor (TCR) after it has recognized antigen which leads to the production of lymphokines such as IL-2, while rapamycin blocks the lymphokine receptors signal, e.g. IL-2 + IL-2R which leads to cell proliferation.

horses or sheep with human splenocytes or thymocytes, they inevitably have some general antileucocyte action as well as some antiplatelet activity and may produce varying degrees of leucopenia or thrombocytopenia. However, a good biological agent, and several are available, will successfully reverse a steroid resistant rejection in 70 per cent of instances, with relatively few side-effects.

Monoclonal antibodies

Monoclonal antibodies are produced by immunizing either rats or mice with the particular antigen against which antibodies are required, e.g. T lymphocytes. Spleen cells from the rodent are then fused with a myeloma cell line to produce a hybridoma. The hybridomas are screened to find one producing the desired antibody, which can then be cloned, thus providing a source of only that highly specific antibody (Fig. 5).

Monoclonal antibodies can be produced against a variety of cell surface markers involved the cellular interactions of the immune response (Fig. 6) and hence allow the possibility of more specific approaches to immunosuppression. Unfortunately as the antibody is a rat or mouse immunoglobulin most patients develop anti-idiotypic or anti-isotypic antibodies against mouse globulin which makes them ineffective. However, genetic engineering has allowed chimaeric or humanized antibodies to be made, in which the antigen-binding part of the antibodies (variable part of Fab) is grafted on to the human constant parts of the heavy and light chains. Early experience suggests that immunization is much less likely in this situation.

OKT3

This represents a second generation of antithymocyte globulins, being a mouse monoclonal antibody directed against the CD3 molecule, which is intimately associated with the T-cell receptor, and hence it is a pan-T-cell antibody. It modulates the CD3 molecule with its T-cell receptor and is extremely effective in reversing a steroid resistant rejection in some 70 to 80 per cent of instances (but not necessarily more effective than a good antithymocyte globulin).

Two major disadvantages, one specific for OKT3 and the other of all monoclonal antibody therapies, are firstly the OKT3 syndrome, associated with the first one or two doses, and secondly the development of antibodies to either the idiotype or the isotype of the mouse globulin. The OKT3 syndrome is characterized by a high fever, dyspnoea, nausea, diarrhoea, and even anaphylactic shock, and is mediated in part by TNF. It can be diminished in intensity by prior administration of 1 g of methylprednisolone. Development of antibodies to OKT3 abrogates the effect of the antibody, and occurs in most patients, preventing its further use.

OKT3 is the only monoclonal antibody to be in widespread use but it is the forerunner of monoclonal antibody therapy in transplantation, where other antibodies are likely to be more specific in their actions.

Anti-CD4

Antibodies directed against the T-helper cell (CD4+) population, the pivotal cells in graft rejection, are potent in experimental models of transplantation where they may produce tolerance to an organ allograft. Clinical trials are in progress, but it will be surprising if such antibodies do not prove to have a role in transplantation.

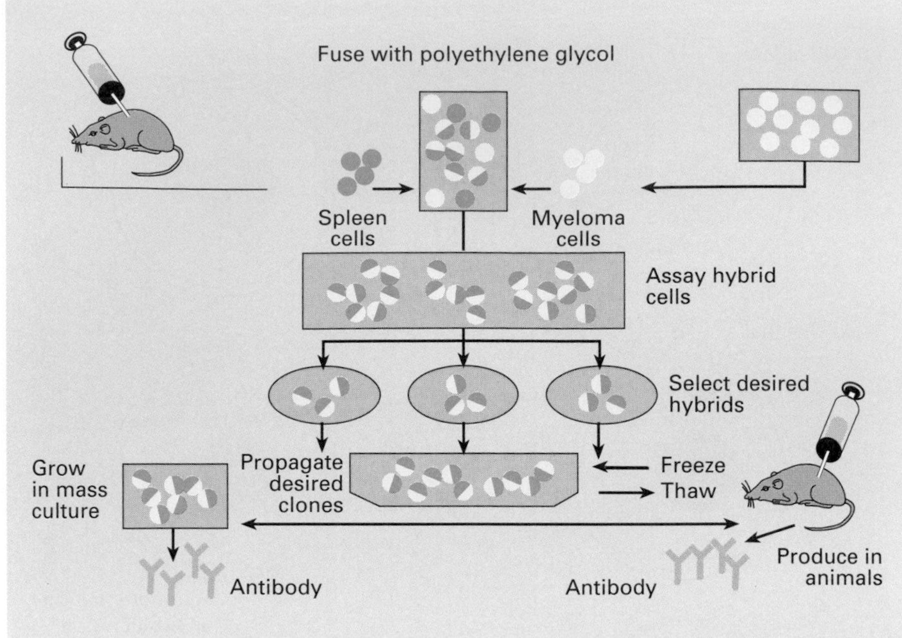

Fig. 5 A summary of the technology of monoclonal antibody production.

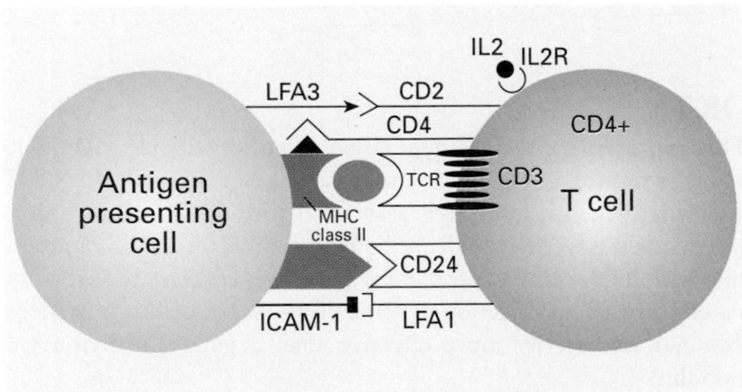

Fig. 6 Examples of the potential sites of action of monoclonal antibodies directed against targets on the cell surface of either the antigen presenting cell or the CD4 positive T-cell.

Anti-interleukin-2 receptor (IL-2R)

The IL-2R is expressed on activated T cells and antibodies against the appropriate epitope of the light chain of the IL-2R block the IL-2 driven proliferation of activated T cells. Such antibodies are extremely immunosuppressive in experimental rodent models, but clinical trials of anti-IL-2R antibodies used as prophylaxis during the first 10 days after transplantation have in general shown a very modest beneficial effect at best.

Anti-ICAM-1

One of a number of antibodies against adhesion molecules which are involved in the interaction between lymphocytes as well as between T-lymphocytes and endothelium, they have proved to be immunosuppressive in experimental models and are currently undergoing clinical trials in renal transplantation.

TOTAL LYMPHOID IRRADIATION

This is undoubtedly immunosuppressive in experimental models in the rodent and in primates where tolerance to organ allografts can be achieved. In clinical trials a course of total lymphoid irradiation before renal transplantation has proved to be effective in preventing rejection of renal allografts with the use of minimal immunosuppression after transplantation. Indeed there are several well documented cases of long-term survival in patients receiving no immunosuppressive drugs at all! However, the logistics of using total lymphoid irradiation (up to 21 daily treatments) before transplantation combined with dialysis and the advent of more potent immunosuppression with cyclosporin have led the centres pursuing this therapy to abandon it for the time being.

COMPLICATIONS OF IMMUNOSUPPRESSIVE THERAPY

Apart from the specific side-effects of the drugs or antibodies used in transplantation there are three major side-effects of immunosuppression. These are infection (especially viral infections), cancer, and cardiovascular disease. The increased incidence of cancer is particularly evident in those cancers with a putative viral aetiology—non-Hodgkin's lymphoma, squamous cell carcinoma of the skin, Kaposi's sarcoma, and cervical cancer in women—but all cancers show some increase in incidence. Aggressive atheromatous disease occurs in many transplant patients, and although associated with an increased incidence of hypertension and hyperlipidaemia, it may also be related to the long-term use of immunosuppressive drugs, a possible mechanism being unclear at this time.

FURTHER READING

Calne RY, *et al.* Cyclosporin A in patients receiving renal allografts from cadaver donors. *Lancet* 1978; **ii**: 1323–7.

Eugui EM, Almquist SJ, Muller CD, Allison AC. Lymphocyte-selective antiproliferative and immunosuppressive effects of mycophenolic acid *in vitro*: role of deoxyguanosine nucleotide depletion. *Scand J Immunol* 1991; **33**: 161–73.

Jones RM, Murie JA, Allen RD, Ting A, Morris PJ. Triple therapy in cadaver renal transplantation. *Br J Surg* 1988; **75**: 4–8.

Kahan B. Cyclosporin. *N Engl J Med* 1989; **321**: 1725–38.

Kohler H, Milstein C. Continuous culture of fused cells secreting antibody of predefined specificity. *Nature* 1975; **256**: 495–7.

Moller G, ed. Antibodies in disease therapy. *Immunol Rev* 1992; **129**: 5–201.

Morris PJ. Cyclosporin A. *Transplantation* 1981; **32**: 349–54.

Morris PJ. Low dose oral prednisolone in renal transplantation. *Lancet* 1982; **i**: 525–7.

Morris PJ. *Kidney Transplantation: Principles and Practice*, 3rd edn. Philadelphia: WB Saunders, 1988.

Morris PJ. Cyclosporin, FK506 and other drugs in organ transplantation. *Curr Opin Immunol* 1992; **3**: 748–51.

Morris PJ. *Kidney Transplantation: Principles and Practice*, 4th edn. Philadelphia: WB Saunders, 1994.

Morris RE. Rapamycins: antifungal, antitumor, antiproliferative and immunosuppressive macrolides. *Transplantation Rev* 1992; **6**: 39–87.

Ortho Multicenter Transplant Group. A randomized clinical trial of OKT3 monoclonal antibody for acute rejection of cadaveric renal transplants. *N Engl J Med* 1985; **313**: 337–42.

Salomon DR. Cyclosporin nephrotoxicity and long-term renal transplantation. *Transplantation Rev* 1992; **6**: 10–19.

Shapiro R, *et al.* Kidney transplantation under FK506 immunosuppression. *Transplant. Proc* 1991; **23**: 920–3.

Sollinger HW, Deierhoi MH, Belzer FO, Diethelm AG, Kaufmann ES. A phase I clinical trial and pilot rescue study. *Transplantation* 1992; **53**: 428–32.

Starzl TE, Todo S, Fung J, Demetris AJ, Venkataramman R, Jain A. FK506 for liver, kidney and pancreas transplantation. *Lancet* 1989; **ii**: 1000–4.

Thomson AW. FK506: profile of an important new immunosuppressant. *Transplantation Rev* 1990; **4**: 1–13.

Todo S, *et al.* Liver, kidney and thoracic organ transplantation under FK506. *Ann Surg* 1990; **212**: 295–305.

Waldmann H. Manipulation of T-cell responses with monoclonal antibodies. *Ann Rev Immunol* 1989; **7**: 407–44.

Winter G, Milstein C. Man-made antibodies. *Nature* 1991; **349**: 293–9.

White DJG, ed. *Cyclosporin A*. Amsterdam: Elsevier, 1982.

Wood KJ, Pearson TC, Darby C, Morris PJ. CD4: a potential target molecule for immunosuppressive therapy and tolerance induction. *Transplantation Rev* 1991; **5**: 150–64.

10.5 Kidney transplantation

PETER J. MORRIS

INTRODUCTION

Transplantation for the kidney has become the treatment of choice for end-stage renal failure in most age groups with perhaps the exception of the very young and the very old. That this has happened over the past 40 years represents one of the most significant developments in medicine in this century. Furthermore, advances in immunosuppression, histocompatibility, and organ preservation in the field of kidney transplantation have led to the successful transplantation of other organs, in particular the liver and heart.

The modern era of kidney transplantation began with the pioneer work of David Hume in Boston around 1950 with the transplantation of cadaver kidneys into non-immunosuppressed recipients. The kidneys were implanted in the thigh anastomosing the femoral vessels to the renal vessels with drainage of the ureter on to the skin. Some of these kidneys functioned for several weeks before being rejected. In 1954 Joseph Murray transplanted a kidney between identical twins where no immunosuppression was required, on this occasion placing the kidney retroperitoneally in the iliac fossa, essentially the technique as used today. This operation was a milestone in the field of transplantation as it confirmed that a successfully transplanted kidney in the absence of rejection was capable of essentially normal renal function.

Work continued in Boston, Paris, and the United Kingdom using total body irradiation of the recipient in an effort to prevent rejection of the transplanted kidney with some surprisingly good results in the short term, some kidneys functioning for several months. However, the discovery of the immunosuppressive properties of 6-mercaptopurine by Schwarz and Damashek in Boston in 1959 quickly led to the demonstration by Calne in England and Zukowski and Hume in Richmond, Virginia that this agent could prevent rejection of kidneys in dogs. Elion and Hitchings, who had produced 6-mercaptopurine at Burroughs Wellcome then developed azathioprine, of which 6-mercaptopurine is a metabolite. In further studies by Calne, working with Murray in Boston, azathioprine appeared to be perhaps less toxic than 6-mercaptopurine and very quickly was introduced as the standard immunosuppressive drug in clinical renal transplantation. Azathioprine, together with steroids, remained the conventional immunosuppressive therapy for 20 years until cyclosporin emerged on the clinical scene.

INDICATIONS FOR RENAL TRANSPLANTATION

Today it can be truly said that there are no absolute contraindications to renal transplantation, and all patients with end-stage renal failure are potential candidates for renal transplantation (Table 1). Of the metabolic disorders causing end-stage renal failure type I diabetes is by far the most common, ranging from 10 to 25 per cent of all patients coming to transplantation. Renal failure due to oxalosis has been considered an absolute contraindication to transplantation but recently successful transplantation has been reported in this condition by methods directed at prevention of the deposition of oxalate in the kidney by maintenance

Table 1 Indications for transplantation

Glomerulonephritis
1. Idiopathic and postinfectious crescentic
2. Membranous
3. Mesangiocapillary (type I)
4. Mesangiocapillary (type II) (dense deposit disease)
5. IgA nephropathy
6. Anti-GBM
7. Focal glomerulosclerosis
8. Henoch-Schönlein

Chronic pyelonephritis (reflux nephropathy)
Hereditary
1. Polycystic kidneys
2. Nephronophthisis (medullary cystic disease)
3. Nephritis (including Alport's syndrome)

Metabolic
1. Diabetes mellitus
2. Oxalosis
3. Cystinosis
4. Fabry's disease
5. Amyloid
6. Gout

Obstructive uropathy
Toxic
1. Analgesic nephropathy
2. Opiate abuse

Multisystem diseases
1. SLE
2. Vasculitis
3. Progressive systemic sclerosis

Haemolytic uraemic syndrome
Tumours
1. Wilms' tumour
2. Renal cell carcinoma
3. Incidental carcinoma
4. Myeloma

Congenital
1. Hypoplasia
2. Horseshoe kidney

Irreversible acute renal failure
1. Cortical necrosis
2. Acute tubular necrosis

Trauma

of a copious urine output and the administration of pyridoxine, phosphate, and magnesium solutions.

In addition the improved safety and decreased side-effects of modern immunosuppression allows the transplantation of young children and the elderly patient with very acceptable results at least in the short and medium term. In the case of infants born with renal failure due to congenital abnormalities of the urogenital tract, it is now considered preferable to maintain them on peritoneal dialysis until they are 2 or 3 years of age before giving them a renal transplant.

Recurrence of the original disease has not proved to be as big a problem as originally envisaged in the early years of renal transplantation. Although recurrence is relatively common in certain of the nephritides (e.g. mesangiocapillary–type II (dense deposit disease), IgA glomerulonephritis, and focal glomerulosclerosis), loss of the kidney due to the recurrence in these conditions is relatively uncommon (Table 2).

Table 2 Diseases with a high recurrence rate in renal allografts

	Approximate frequency of recurrence (%)
Primary kidney disease	
Focal segmental glomerulosclerosis	30
IgA nephropathy	50
Henoch-Schönlein purpura	80
Membranous nephropathy	10
Mesangiocapillary type I	25
Mesangiocapillary type II	95
Systemic disease with kidney involvement	
Haemolytic uraemic syndrome	50
Diabetes type I	100
Oxalosis	90
Amyloidosis	33

ORGAN DONATION

Living related donors

From the point of view of graft outcome living related transplantation still provides better long-term results than cadaver transplantation. In addition the ever-increasing shortage of cadaver donors means that living related transplantation remains an important option for the patient with end-stage renal failure. The selection of a donor from within a family is based firstly on the motivation of the potential donor(s) which should be truly altruistic without coercion from the patient or other members of the family, and secondly on the basis of blood group compatibility and the optimal HLA match in the presence of a negative crossmatch between recipient and donor (see later). The ideal combination is that between HLA identical siblings and next that between one HLA haplotype disparate siblings or parent to child (see Section 10.1). Having established that a family member is a suitable donor on the above psychological and immunological grounds, the donor must undergo an extensive medical evaluation, including a full investigation of renal function, and finally an angiogram to define the renal vasculature on each side.

The risks to the donor are not inconsiderable. There are first the risks associated with a major operation including a small risk of death, and second the long-term risk to a healthy donor of having one kidney. However, follow-up studies of donors for up to 20 years have revealed no excess risk of hypertension or renal failure over and above that of a normal age matched population.

Living unrelated donors

There is considerable controversy in this area and there is obviously opportunity for commercial exploitation, as seen in many developing countries. However, a case can be made for the use of living unrelated donors in exceptional circumstances where there is clearly a strong emotional relationship between donor and recipient, as for example between spouses. It should be remembered that in contrast to the family donor, the use of a living unrelated donor provides no greater chance of a successful outcome than the use of a cadaver donor, although there is some recent evidence suggesting that the outcome of living unrelated

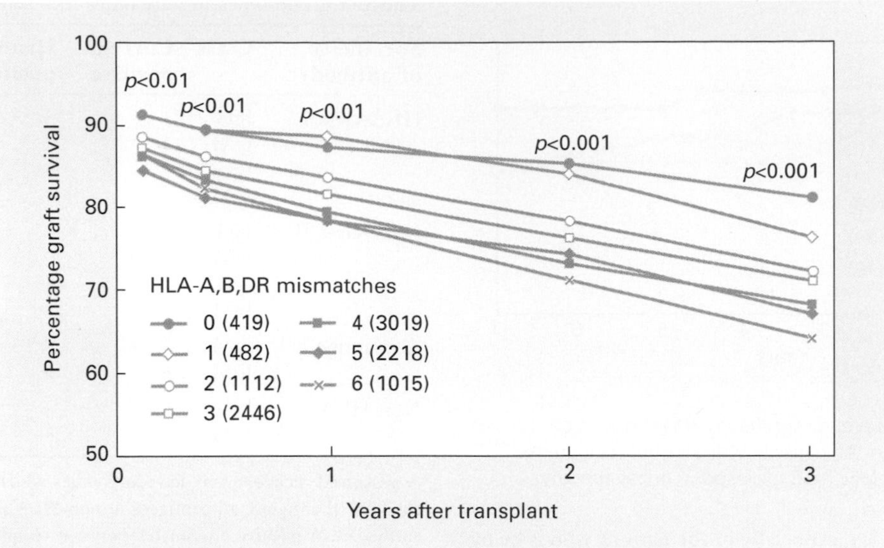

Fig. 1 First cadaver graft survival in white patients based on mismatches for HLA-A, B, and DR antigens.

transplantation is better than cadavar transplantation, and this is assumed to be due to the lack of any ischaemic damage to the kidney in the former.

Cadaver donor

Most kidney donors are cadaver donors in whom brain-stem death has been diagnosed while respiratory and cardiac function is being maintained on a ventilator. The usual cause of brain death is irreversible brain damage due to head injury or subarachnoid haemorrhage. It is important that renal function be normal and that urine output be maintained before and after the final diagnosis of brain death has been made. Most of the parameters of brain death reflect brain-stem death, for in the absence of brain-stem function respiratory and cardiac function cannot be maintained. The presence of widespread bacterial infection, cancer, or a positive test for hepatitis B, hepatitis C, or HIV would exclude a potential cadaver donor from further consideration. A history of hypertension or diabetes might be a relative contraindication to use of the kidneys but where doubt exists the kidneys can be removed and an immediate biopsy performed before a final decision is made. In general very young donors (less than 1 year) or very old donors (over the age of 70) are not considered suitable.

Removal of kidneys

In living-related kidneys the selected kidney (usually the left as it provides a longer renal vein) is removed either through a flank incision with the patient in the lateral position or transperitoneally through a midline abdominal incision.

Kidneys are removed from the cadaver donor *en bloc* following *in-situ* perfusion, with subsequent dissection and perfusion of the kidneys after removal. Today the removal of kidneys is usually part of a multiorgan retrieval procedure, and then the kidneys are the last organs to be removed.

ORGAN PRESERVATION

Although kidneys can be preserved by continuous perfusion with colloid solutions such as oxygenated human albumin for periods up to 72 h, machine preservation has been largely replaced by simple flushing of the kidney with one of a number of preservation solutions and storage in ice slush. This provides satisfactory preservation for up to 48 h, which is generally long enough for selection of the appropriate recipients on medical and matching grounds and transport of the kidneys within a national or even international network of organ exchange. The preservation solutions most widely used are Euro Collin's and hypertonic citrate, both solutions having in common a K^+ content similar to that within the cell. More recently the University of Wisconsin (UW) solution, the preservation fluid of choice in liver transplantation, has become more widely used in kidney transplantation as well. The important components of the UW solution are probably lactobionate and adenosine.

HLA MATCHING AND THE CROSSMATCH

Matching for HLA, the major histocompatibility complex (MHC) in man, presents major logistic problems in cadaver transplantation because of the genetic complexity of the HLA system. For this reason national or international organ exchange networks have developed, e.g. Eurotransplant, UK Transplant Support Service (UKTSS), and in the United States the United Organ Sharing scheme (UNOS), to try and ensure that as many recipients receive a beneficially matched kidney for the HLA-A, -B, and -DR antigens as possible. That this is worth trying to achieve is beyond question (Fig. 1), but even so many recipients with uncommon HLA phenotypes will be excluded on this basis from ever receiving a transplant. The approach to HLA matching can be simplified by matching just for HLA-DR which still provides an improved graft outcome not much less than that obtained by matching for the

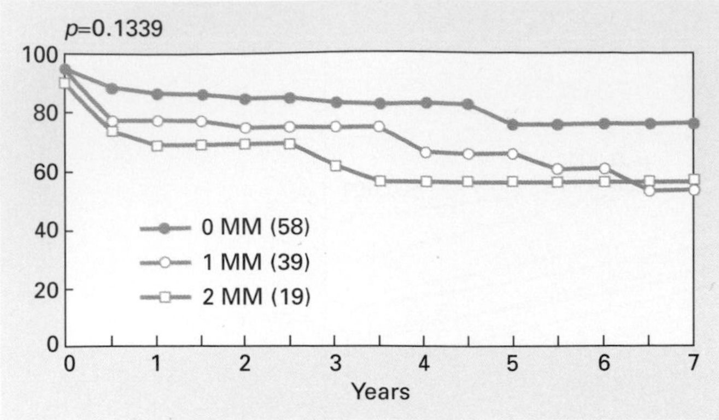

Fig. 2 Survival of 116 cadaveric regrafts in Oxford based on matching for HLA-DR alone. All patients were immunosuppressed with azathioprine, prednisolone, and cyclosporin (triple therapy).

whole of the MHC complex, especially in the patient who is being regrafted (Fig. 2). Nevertheless the benefits of matching in terms of graft outcome are modest in the case of a first graft, and for this reason failure to find an acceptable match for a recipient should not preclude that recipient from receiving a mismatched cadaver kidney with the more potent immunosuppression available today.

Perhaps the most important aspect of the matching procedure in cadaver transplantation is the crossmatch in which donor lymphocytes are added to serum from the recipient in the presence of rabbit serum as a source of complement. If the donor lymphocytes are lysed, this is known as a positive crossmatch. For many years, following the recognition of hyperacute rejection of a transplanted kidney in the presence of a positive crossmatch between donor and recipient, a positive crossmatch was considered to be an absolute contraindication to renal transplantation.

In more recent years the complexity of antibodies found in the sera of sensitized recipients has been recognized, and indeed not all antibodies are directed against HLA antigens. Thus an apparently sensitized recipient may have antibodies, e.g. autoantibodies which react with donor lymphocytes giving a positive crossmatch but which do not damage a subsequent kidney from that donor. As most patients who are sensitized by previous pregnancies, blood transfusions, or failed transplants have a mixture of antibodies including antibodies against HLA, it is important to define the class and specificity of these antibodies before transplantation as this helps in the interpretation of a positive crossmatch. Table 3 summarizes the types of antibodies in a sensitized recipient which may give rise to a positive crossmatch and whether a successful transplant is possible in the presence of that positive crossmatch.

Table 3 The types of antibodies in a sensitized recipient

Specificity of antibody	Class	Current positive	Historical positive	Transplant contraindicated
HLA-class I	IgG	+	+	Yes
	IgM	+	+	Yes
	IgG	−	+	Yes
	IgM	−	+	No
HLA-class II	IgG	+	+	Yes
	IgM	+	+	Yes
	IgG	−	+	?
	IgM	−	+	No
Autoantibody	IgM	+	+	No
	IgM	−	+	No
Non-HLA	IgG	+	+	No
	IgM	+	+	No

A sensitized recipient may have antibodies which are directed against HLA class I or II antigens, autoantigens or non-HLA antigen, or a mixture of these antibodies. A positive crossmatch between recipient serum and donor lymphocytes may be due to any of the above and may be obtained with serum taken at the time of transplantation (current positive) or at some earlier time, e.g. 6 months or a year before transplantation (historical positive). The specificity and class of antibody as well as the timing of the antibody appearance in relation to the transplant are important in determining whether a renal transplant is contraindicated in the presence of a positive crossmatch.

OPERATION

A renal transplant has been a very standard operation for many years now. The iliac vessels are exposed retroperitoneally through an oblique incision in one or other iliac fossa, the oblique muscles being divided in the line of the incision and the peritoneum reflected upwards and medially (Fig. 3). The renal vein is anastomosed end-to-side to the external iliac vein and the renal artery anastomosed either end-to-end to the divided internal iliac artery or, as is more usual with a cadaver kidney where the renal artery will have a cuff of aorta, end-to-side to the external iliac artery (Fig. 4).

The ureter is implanted in the bladder (ureteroneocystostomy) either through an anterior cystotomy with a submucosal tunnel to prevent reflux or as an extravesical procedure where the ureter is anastomosed to the mucosa of the dome of the bladder and then muscle is drawn over the ureter again with a view to preventing reflux. Whether the latter technique does prevent reflux is questionable. Another technique used successfully by some units (in particular at Massachusetts General Hospital) is to create a pyeloureterostomy in which the pelvis of the kidney is anastomosed to the recipient ureter.

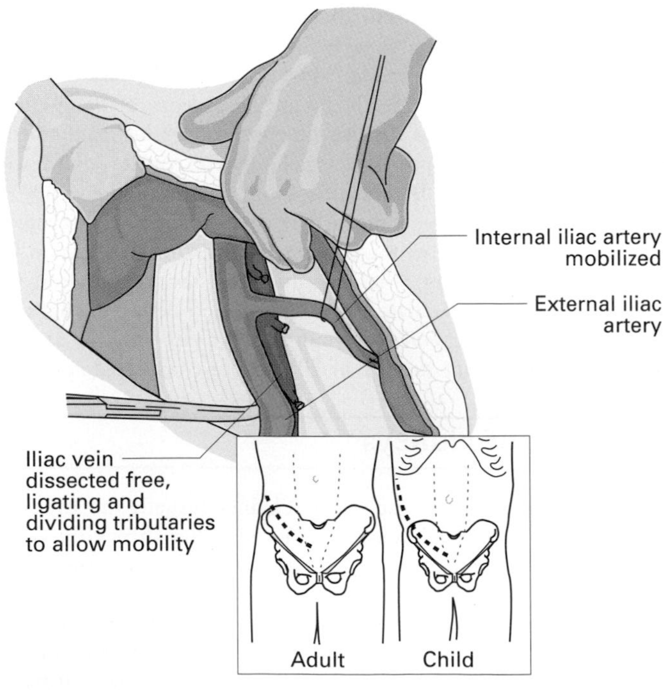

Fig. 3 Incisions for adult and child and the iliac arteries and vein exposed after reflection of the peritoneum upwards and medially.

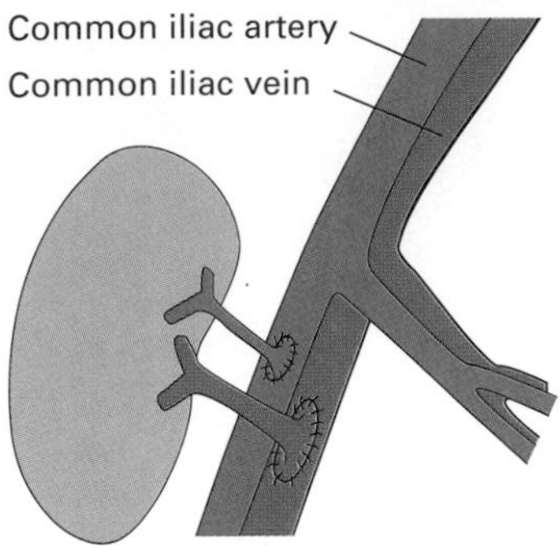

Fig. 4 The vascular anastomoses of a renal transplant showing an end-to-side anastomosis of the renal artery with a cuff of aorta to the external iliac artery and an end-to-side anastomosis of the renal vein to the external iliac vein.

Although not essential, usually a right kidney is implanted in the left iliac fossa and vice versa as this facilitates the vascular anastomoses. The wound is closed without drainage where possible, and an indwelling catheter left in the bladder for 1 to 5 days depending on the technique used.

POSTOPERATIVE COURSE

Immediate function

A kidney from a living related donor would always be expected to function immediately whereas only 60 to 80 per cent of cadaver kidneys will do so. Immediate function is usually associated with an osmotic diuresis and urine output over 24 h is anywhere from 5 to 25 l. This does require meticulous attention to fluid replacement and is made easier if there is a central venous pressure line in place over the first 48 h after surgery. After 48 to 72 h the kidney will begin to concentrate and the intravenous fluid replacement can be slowed and replaced by oral fluids.

Delayed or non-function of the transplanted kidney

In this situation which is usually due to acute tubular necrosis, other causes of delayed or non-function must be considered (Table 4). A renogram of the transplanted kidney will confirm the presence or absence of a blood supply. Ultrasound examination will demonstrate obstruction or a urine leak, while finally hyperacute rejection can be excluded by renal biopsy.

Table 4 Possible causes of delayed function or cessation of function in the first few days after renal transplantation

Acute tubular necrosis
Renal artery thrombosis
Renal vein thrombosis
Hyperacute rejection
Ureteric obstruction
Urine leak

Deterioration of function in a functioning graft

Where there is a functioning kidney with a falling or normal serum creatinine which then begins to rise, rejection is the most likely cause. This is confirmed by biopsy but an ultrasound examination will also exclude the presence of ureteric obstruction or leakage. If a renal vein or arterial thrombosis is suspected, both the ultrasound examination and a renogram will clarify the diagnosis.

Rejection

Four types of rejection may be seen after transplantation:

1. Hyperacute rejection

This is an immediate antibody mediated rejection occurring within the first 24 h of transplantation in the presence of a positive crossmatch due to HLA class I antibody or an ABO incompatible kidney. The classical hyperacute rejection (which is evident within 60 min of revascularization of the kidney) is not seen today, unless there has been an error in the interpretation of the crossmatch or rarely an incompatible ABO kidney is transplanted in error, but less florid examples are not uncommon and present as non-function of a kidney in a sensitized patient, more usually in a patient receiving a regraft.

2. Accelerated rejection

This is also rejection in a recipient specifically sensitized against the donor and is mediated by cells. It occurs between 2 and 4 days after transplantation, presenting with a deterioration of renal function often accompanied by a fever. A biopsy will show a florid cellular infiltration within the graft, often associated with arteriolar thrombosis and interstitial haemorrhage in severe cases.

3. Acute rejection

This is the outcome of the immune response to an allograft in a non-sensitized patient. Most commonly the first rejection episode will be apparent between 7 and 21 days after transplantation, but may present at any time after transplantation. Some 60 to 70 per cent of recipients of a cadaver allograft will have at least one acute rejection episode during the first 3 months after transplantation with current immunosuppressive protocols. In a classical example of an acute rejection episode the patient would present with a modest fever, the graft would be swollen and tender, and there would be a concomitant fall in urine output and a rise in serum creatinine. This picture is relatively uncommon today with current immunosuppression, where there may be a mild fever with minimal or no graft swelling and tenderness, the main feature being a deterioration in renal function as evidenced by a rise in serum creatinine. A biopsy will confirm the diagnosis. The differential diagnosis will be firstly cyclosporin nephrotoxicity and secondly ureteric obstruction. Blood levels of cyclosporin and an ultrasound respectively can be used to exclude these possibilities.

4. Chronic rejection

This is an insidious process represented by a steady deterioration in function at any time following the first few months of transplantation. A biopsy will confirm the diagnosis, but other diagnoses to be considered are ureteric obstruction, renal artery stenosis, and recurrence of the primary disease.

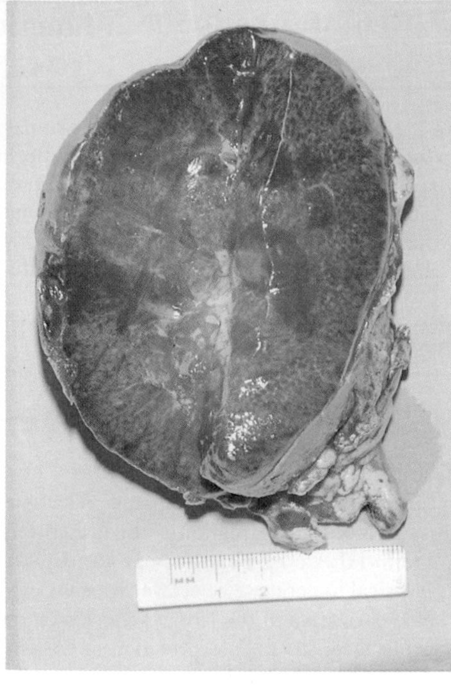

(a)

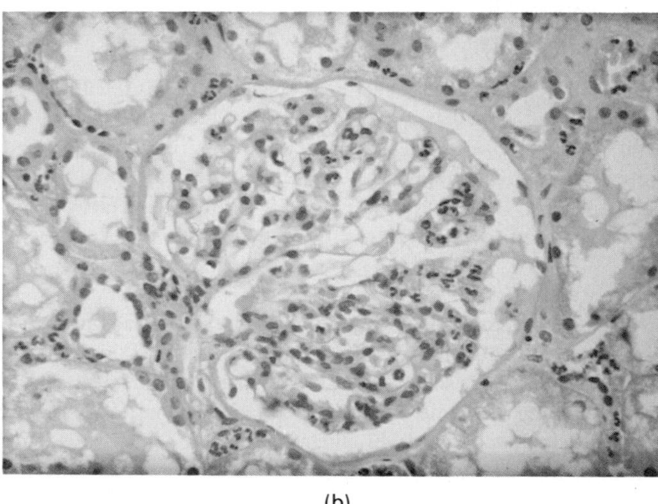

(b)

Fig. 5 (a) A hyperacutely rejected kidney on removal at 72+h. (b) A biopsy 20 min after revascularization showing an intense polymorphonuclear infiltrate within the kidney.

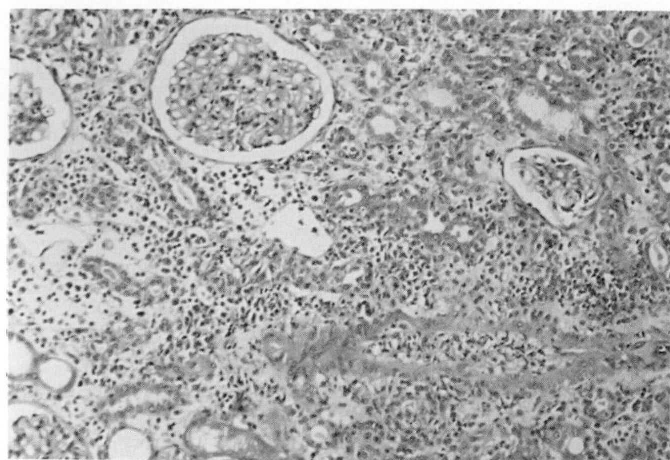

Fig. 6 Severe acute rejection with a dense mononuclear cellular infiltrate 10 days after transplantation.

Immunopathology of rejection

Hyperacute rejection

If a biopsy is taken from the kidney within 1 h of revascularization (i.e. before wound closure) this may reveal a marked infiltration of the kidney with polymorphonuclear leucocytes (Fig. 5). Subsequent biopsies at 24 h and later will reveal widespread glomerular capillary and arteriolar thrombosis with oedema, fibrinoid necrosis of arteriolar walls, and interstitial haemorrhage. Immunofluorescence will demonstrate deposition of IgM, IgG, and complement within the transplanted kidney.

Accelerated and acute rejection

The hallmark of these rejection reactions is the mononuclear cellular infiltrate, the density of which indicates the severity of the rejection, as does infiltration of the tubules themselves (Fig. 6). Associated with the cellular infiltrate are oedema and in severe cases interstitial haemorrhage and fibrinoid necrosis of arterioles. The cellular infiltrate contains approximately 65 per cent macrophages and 30 per cent T lymphocytes with CD8+ T lymphocytes being rather more prominent than CD4+ T lymphocytes. A small percentage of the infiltrate comprises natural killer (NK) cells and eosinophils. A smaller percentage of the T lymphocytes will exhibit activation antigens such as the IL-2 receptor. In addition there will be an induction of expression of MHC class II antigens on cells such as proximal tubular cells which do not express these antigens normally.

Chronic rejection

The major features of this chronic process are interstitial fibrosis within the parenchyma of the kidney and intimal hyperplasia of arteries within the parenchyma (Fig. 7).

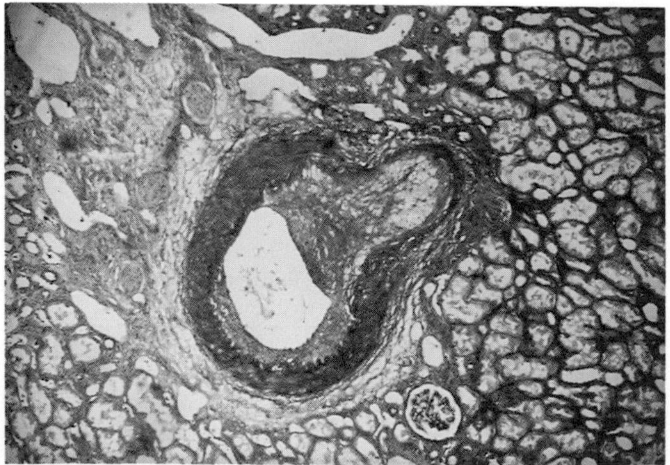

Fig. 7 Changes of chronic rejection in a medium-sized renal artery.

COMPLICATIONS OF RENAL TRANSPLANTATION

The complications of transplantation can be considered as technical or related to the immunosuppressive therapy itself, much of which is secondary to immunosuppression induced in the recipient.

Technical complications

Vascular complications

Renal artery thrombosis is very uncommon and usually presents within the first 2 weeks of transplantation as an abrupt cessation of renal function with no other clinical features. Renal vein thrombosis occurs much more commonly than hitherto, and may be related to the thrombogenic potential of cyclosporin. It usually occurs within the first few days of transplantation and is associated with an abrupt cessation of renal function associated with a painful, swollen, tender graft.

Renal artery stenosis may present at any time from several months to several years after transplantation, and although the stenosis may occur at the anastomosis it usually occurs just distal to the anastomosis. The patient presents with poorly controlled hypertension and deteriorating renal function (see later).

Urological complications

A urine leak, either from the bladder or the ureteric anastomosis occurs within the first 6 weeks of transplantation and is most commonly due to ischaemia of the lower end of the ureter due to a poorly removed kidney with skeletonization of the ureter or interruption of the ureteric blood supply within the hilum of the kidney. A bladder leak will heal with catheter drainage of the bladder, whereas ureteric necrosis is dealt with by excising the necrotic ureter and either reimplanting the ureter in the bladder over a ureteric stent or anastomosing the ureter to the patient's own ureter either end-to-side or end-to-end again over a stent.

Obstruction of the ureter presents at any time from weeks to years after transplantation and although the site of obstruction is usually in the lower one-third of the ureter, no doubt as a result of ischaemia, a significant number of pelviureteric obstructions are seen. Diagnosis is confirmed by ultrasound examination of the graft and an antegrade pyelogram. Immediate relief of the obstruction can be obtained by the insertion of a percutaneous ureteric stent or a percutaneous nephrostomy if this is not possible. Sometimes a stenosis can be dilated with a balloon, but otherwise corrective surgery is required, involving either reimplantation of the normal ureter if the stenosis is at the entry of the ureter into the bladder or a pelviureteric anastomosis using the patient's own ureter for a more proximal stenosis.

The incidence of urological complications after transplantation is now quite low in experienced units, being no higher than 5 per cent, which represents a marked improvement over that seen 15 to 20 years ago. This improvement is due to better techniques of kidney retrieval and implantation of the ureter, but in particular to the general use of low dose steroids after transplantation in more recent years.

Lymphocele

This is a collection of lymph around the graft, which arises from divided host lymphatics around the iliac vessels. This complication has also become relatively uncommon since it has been recognized that lymphatics must be ligated with silk rather than occluded with with diathermy. A lymphocele is retroperitoneal and as such produces symptoms from pressure on surrounding structures. Thus, it may present with deteriorating renal function due to pressure on the transplanted ureter, a swollen leg on the side of the graft due to pressure on the iliac vein, and tenesmus or strangulation due to pressure on the rectum and bladder respectively. The diagnosis is confirmed by ultrasound examination (Fig. 8). It is treated in the first instance by percutaneous drainage but if it recurs more than twice after percutaneous drainage it needs to be drained by fenestration into the peritoneal cavity. This can be done satisfactorily now by laparoscopic approach rather than an open operation.

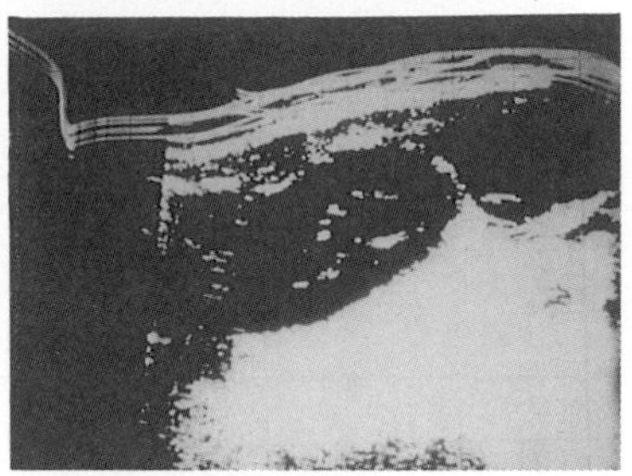

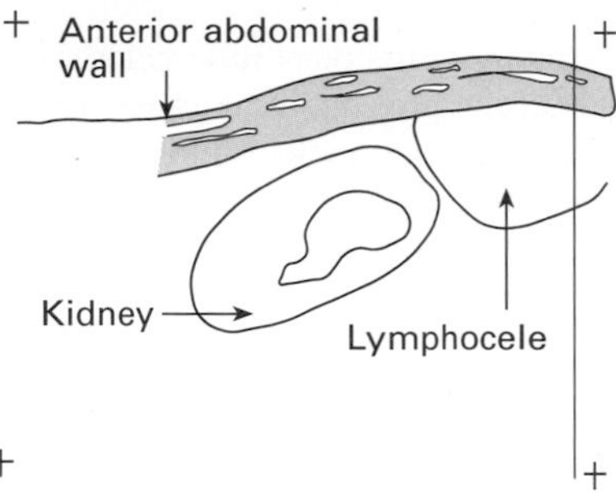

Fig. 8 A lymphocele adjacent to the renal transplant shown by ultrasound.

Immunological complications

Infection

Bacterial infections

Not only bacterial infections, but viral and protozoal infections may occur in transplant patients due in part or wholly to the immunosuppressive therapy given to prevent and treat rejection. The time at which an infection appears in relation to transplantation is important in arriving at a diagnosis, for viral (with the exception of herpes simplex) and protozoal infections are rare in the first month after transplantation. Pneumonia as a postoperative complication and urinary tract infections are common in the early weeks after transplantation. Asymptomatic urinary tract infections are relatively common due mainly to the indwelling catheter left in the bladder for several days after surgery. Wound infections are uncommon with an incidence of 1 to 2 per cent. A preventive antibiotic should be given with the induction of anaesthesia to cover contamination at the time of operation and in particular to cover the possibility of the transplanted kidney being

Table 5 Effect of donor CMV status on CMV infection in 306 renal allograft recipients at Oxford

	Recipient CMV seropositive		Recipient CMV seronegative	
	Donor CMV+	Donor CMV−	Donor CMV+	Donor CMV−
Group total	84	98	60	64
No. infected	52(62%)	52(53%)	38(63%)	0
	Reactivation or reinfection		Primary infection	

contaminated. An appropriate broad spectrum antibiotic is used, such as cefuroxime.

Of the mycobacterial infections tuberculosis is by far the most common and generally presents as a chest infection with fever, cough, and an infiltrate on radiography. However, tuberculosis may uncommonly present as an abscess or joint infection. Any patients who are from areas where tuberculosis is common, e.g. the Indian subcontinent, or who have a history of tuberculous infection in the past should receive prophylactic therapy for 1 year after transplantation (e.g. treatment with isoniazid).

Viral infections

The most common and potentially the most serious of the viral infections is cytomegalovirus (CMV) infection. This may be a primary infection in a CMV-seronegative recipient who receives a kidney from a seropositive donor or reactivation of the virus in a seropositive recipient. The likelihood of a CMV infection occurring is directly related to the potency of the immunosuppression used. The primary infection is more severe, but clinically in both instances the presenting feature will be a high fever (greater than 39°C) associated with a leucopenia. This high swinging fever may last 7 to 10 days and characteristically the patient feels unwell only during the time of the fever. Diagnosis of a primary infection is confirmed by seroconversion in a seronegative patient or a rise in titre in a seropositive patient, but this does not occur till several days after the onset of fever. More overt infection such as pneumonitis or hepatitis heralds a more serious problem and is potentially fatal in a primary CMV infection. For this reason it is desirable where possible to transplant a seronegative recipient with a seronegative kidney, for primary infection does not occur in this situation provided that the recipient only receives CMV seronegative blood if transfusion is required (Table 5). Vaccination of seronegative recipients before transplantation has been explored but the results of a large international multicentre trial are not yet available. Prophylactic administration of hyperimmune globulin has also been advocated but with little evidence to support its use in this way. Ganciclovir, an antiviral agent which has proved valuable in the treatment of an overt CMV infection, is now widely used prophylactically in patients at high risk of developing CMV infections, e.g. seronegative recipients given a seropositive kidney and then given ATG or OKT3 to prevent or treat rejection, where it is almost inevitable that a CMV infection will occur.

Herpes simplex infections around the mouth or less commonly the genitalia are frequent but resolve quickly with prompt treatment with systemic acyclovir. Acyclovir has been used prophylactically in patients with a history of herpes infections in the early weeks after transplantation when immunosuppression is at its highest level but is probably only justified in the case of a history of genital herpes.

Varicella zoster infections present rarely as chickenpox in recipients never previously exposed in which case the infection may be fulminating, but present commonly as shingles (Fig. 9). Acyclovir is the treatment of choice.

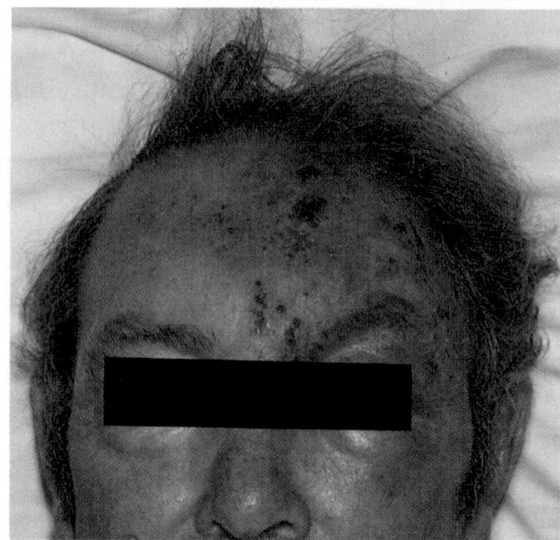

Fig. 9 Herpes zoster of the left side of the face in a man 2 years after renal transplantation.

Hepatitis B in the donor is a contraindication to transplantation, but it is not uncommon for recipients of a renal transplant to be hepatitis B positive. The outcome in those patients who are positive and immunosuppressed is uncertain in that liver failure may develop in some, but not all, patients after several years.

Hepatitis C, the cause of non-A, non-B hepatitis, in the donor is also a contraindication to transplantation, but is not uncommon amongst transplant recipients (approximately 5–10 per cent in some centres). It is unknown at this time whether this represents a longer-term risk of liver failure in the recipient when immunosuppressed following transplantation.

Protozoal infections

Pneumocystis carinii is the most important infection in this group and occurs at any time after the first month of transplantation, the patient usually presenting with a dry non-productive cough and a low grade fever. A chest radiograph may show patchy consolidation in one area of the lung at the early stages of the infection. A bronchoscopy and bronchial lavage should be carried out promptly if no alternative diagnosis is available, for cytological examination of the washings will inevitably confirm the diagnosis of pneumocystis. High dose septrin is the appropriate treatment. Pneumocystis is rare if prophylactic septrin (0.5 g/day) is used in the immunosuppressed patient and most units now use such a protocol at least for the first 6 months after transplantation.

Fungal infections

Candida infections of the mouth are not uncommon and prophylactic amphotericin lozenges are used during the first few months after transplantation. Aspergillosis is perhaps the most common of the other fungal infections, but is still relatively uncommon, and its common presentation is as a chest infection. Again the diagnosis is established by bronchoscopy and bronchial lavage.

Cancer

Although there is an increased incidence of most types of cancer in the immunosuppressed renal transplant recipient, this increased incidence is particularly dramatic in the case of tumours with a possible viral aetiology such as non-Hodgkin's lymphoma (100-fold increased incidence), squamous cell cancer of the skin (200-fold increased incidence), cervical cancer of the uterus (50-fold), and Kaposi's sarcoma (1000-fold). In countries with a high exposure to sunlight such as Australia some 50 per cent of patients will have developed at least one skin cancer within 10 years of transplantation, with a reversal of the normal basal cell to squamous cell cancer ratio of 2 : 1. Many of the squamous cell cancers are rapidly growing with an increased propensity to metastasize (Fig. 10). They also occur in unusual sites, e.g. perianal sites.

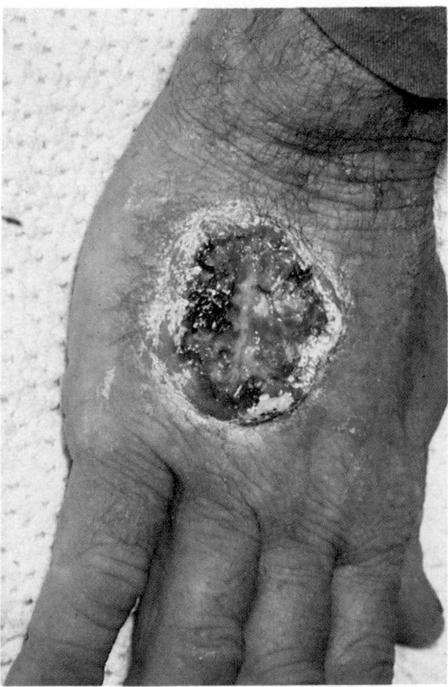

Fig. 10 A squamous cell carcinoma of the hand in a renal transplant patient. This lesion reached this size in 6 weeks.

The prevalence of lymphomas is greater with current immunosuppressive protocols, this undoubtedly being related to the potency of the immunosuppression. Two types of lymphoma are seen. The first is an acute lymphoproliferative disorder, usually occurring within the first year of transplantation, which may be associated with an increase in titre to Epstein-Barr virus (EBV). Its course tends to be rapidly fatal, but it may remit with reduction or cessation of immunosuppressive therapy together with a course of high dose acyclovir. Histologically that tumour is usually a polyclonal B-cell lymphoma. This acute lymphoproliferative disorder is more commonly seen in patients who have received ATG and/or OKT3 as part of their immunosuppressive protocol. The second type of lymphoma occurs at later times after transplantation and presents more typically with enlarged nodes. It may be a monoclonal B-cell lymphoma histologically and its response to conventional therapy is not dissimilar to that in a non-transplant recipient. Both types of lymphoma not uncommonly involve the base of the brain, which is an unusual site in lymphomas occurring in non-immunosuppressed patients.

Cardiovascular complications

As renal transplant recipients survive longer and become an increasingly more elderly population, ischaemic heart disease and cerebrovascular disease have become the major cause of death after transplantation. The major risk factors in the transplant population are hypertension and hyperlipidaemia. Hypertension requiring treatment after renal transplantation is common with current immunosuppressive protocols, and some 75 per cent of patients are on treatment at 1 year after transplantation. This incidence of hypertension has increased with the introduction of cyclosporin. Good control of hypertension is an essential part of the management of the transplant recipient, and often a combination of a diuretic, β-blocker, calcium channel inhibitor, and angiotensin converting enzyme (ACE) inhibitors is required to achieve control.

Poorly controlled hypertension, especially if associated with deteriorating renal function, should raise the question of a renal artery stenosis in the transplanted kidney (Fig. 11). An angiogram will be necessary to establish the presence of a renal artery stenosis, but even if present this does not mean that the stenosis is a functional one. The cautious introduction of an ACE inhibitor can be used as a diagnostic test in this situation for if renal function deteriorates and then returns to its previous level on cessation of the drug, this would strongly suggest that a radiological stenosis is a functional one. Renal vein renins from the transplanted kidneys and the host kidneys may be measured, but usually are not helpful.

Once the diagnosis of a functional renal artery stenosis is made then correction of the stenosis is indicated. In the first instance an

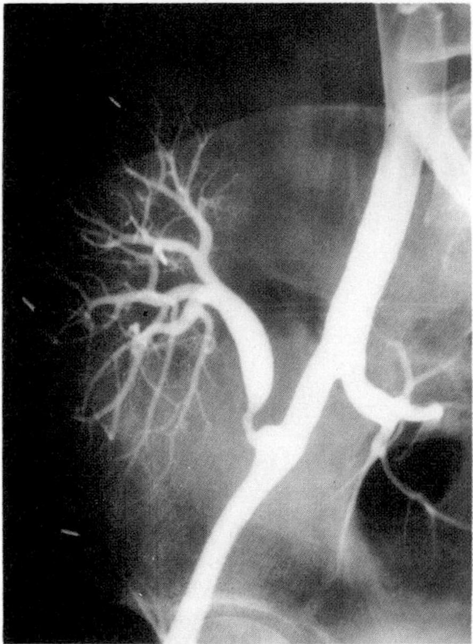

Fig. 11 A stenosis of the renal artery distal to an end-to-side anastomosis of the artery with a cuff of aorta to the external iliac artery.

attempt to dilate the stenosis by balloon angioplasty should be made. If this is unsuccessful then reconstructive surgery should follow, although the dissection of the renal vessels is usually difficult and requires considerable expertise in both vascular and transplantation surgery. Many types of reconstruction are possible but the most common are reimplantation of the renal artery distal to the stenosis into the iliac artery or insertion of a saphenous vein graft between the common iliac artery and the renal artery distal to the stenosis.

Ischaemic heart disease is common in the elderly and diabetic renal transplant population, but is managed in the same way as in the non-transplant patient. There is no contraindication to major cardiac surgery in these patients if this represents the most appropriate management.

A significant increase in cholesterol levels is seen in many patients after renal transplantation, the rise being essentially in the very low density lipoprotein fraction with a concomitant decrease in the level of high density lipoprotein, a major pattern of risk for ischaemic heart disease. The hypercholesterolaemia has been attributed to cyclosporin but may be more closely related to the use of steroids. In any case these patients should be treated energetically with a low cholesterol diet and where high levels of cholesterol remain then the introduction of cholesterol lowering agents is justified, although their place in this patient population is as yet unknown.

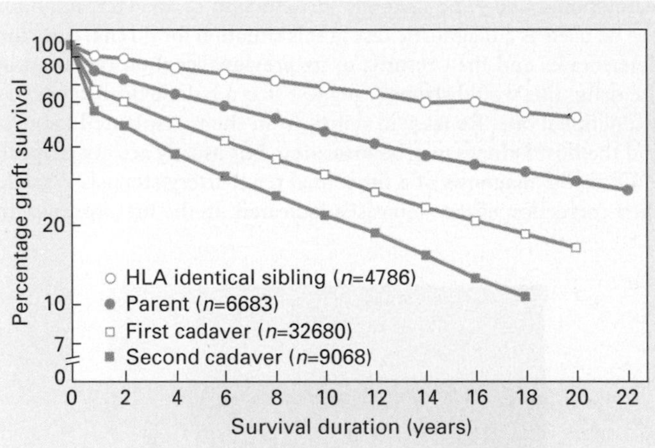

Fig. 12 Long-term graft survival of living related and cadaver transplants as recorded by the UCLA Registry.

RESULTS OF TRANSPLANTATION

Living related grafts

Apart from the rare instance in which transplantation between identical twins is possible, transplantation between HLA identical siblings provides not only the best short-term and long-term outcome graft survival (Fig. 12) but also as less immunosuppression is required there are fewer related problems. Living related donors and recipients sharing one HLA haplotype, i.e. parent to child or sibling transplant also have a better graft survival than cadaveric grafts. It now appears that living related and unrelated donors and recipients mismatched for both HLA haplotypes also have a better graft survival than cadaveric grafts, presumed due to the lack of ischaemic injury to the kidney in the living donor. Because of the better graft survival and also the shortage of cadaver kidneys, living related transplantation remains a justified procedure provided the donor has the appropriate motivation to be a donor without any financial or emotional coercion.

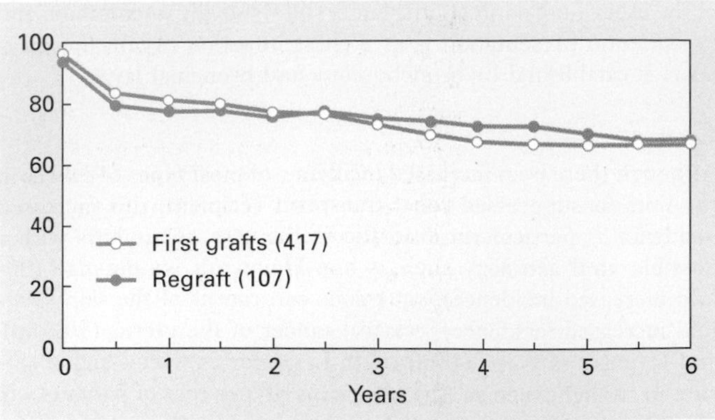

Fig. 13 The survival of cadaveric first grafts and regrafts in Oxford in patients immunosuppressed with triple therapy (azathioprine, prednisolone, and cyclosporin).

Cadaveric grafts

The bulk of renal transplants performed in the Western world are cadaveric (unlike in developing countries where the majority of transplants performed are still living related transplants). Graft survival has steadily improved over the last 20 years due to a variety of reasons so that around 80 to 85 per cent of grafts will be functioning at 1 year and around 65 per cent at 5 years (Fig. 13). Patient survival has not altered appreciably in recent years, being around 90 to 95 per cent at 1 year and 80 per cent at 5 years, and is unlikely to improve now that more elderly patients are being transplanted.

Factors influencing graft outcome

(1) Immunosuppression

Undoubtedly immunosuppression is the major factor in improving graft survival in recent years, with the introduction of cyclosporin resulting in a 10 to 15 per cent improvement in graft survival.

(ii) HLA matching

This has had a small but significant impact on cadaveric graft outcome (see earlier), while reliably predicting the outcome of living related transplantation.

(iii) Centre effect

The centre in which the transplant is performed remains a major determinant of graft outcome and still remains an unexplained phenomenon. It is not obviously associated with the experience of the unit, patient selection, or immunosuppressive protocols but no doubt reflects the influence of all of these and other unidentified factors.

(iv) Blood transfusions

That prior blood transfusions in the non-transfused recipient improved graft survival in the precyclosporin era is unquestioned, but today it is uncertain whether the transfusion effect exists or not, and many units are abandoning their deliberate transfusion policies in non-transfused recipients because of this and the small, but real, risk of transmitting HIV or non-A, non-B hepatitis (hepatitis C) by a blood transfusion.

(v) Age

The age of the recipient will influence graft outcome in that the elderly patient is more likely to have or to develop significant ischaemic heart disease and as a result the elderly recipient has a lower life expectancy than the younger recipient. However, the elderly recipient is less likely to lose a graft from irreversible rejection (Fig. 14). The age of the donor also has an impact on cadaveric graft survival in that kidneys from young (less than 10 years of age) or very old (over 65 years of age) donors show a poorer graft survival.

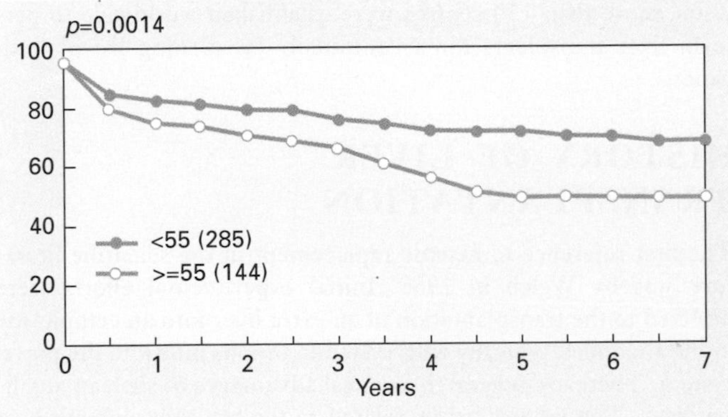

Fig. 14 Survival of first cadaveric grafts in Oxford in patients under or over the age of 55 at the time of transplantation. Graft survival is poorer in the older patient, but this is due primarily to a higher death rate with a functioning graft in the older recipient, mostly due to cardiovascular disease. All patients received triple therapy immunosuppression.

(vi) Race

The influence of the race of the donor or of the recipient remains uncertain. That a black patient in the United States has a poorer graft survival is undisputed, but distinguishing the possible genetic effect from the socioeconomic effect of a less privileged population has proved difficult. Nevertheless evidence has been provided that, after allowing for the socioeconomic influence, the black recipient does display a poorer graft survival than his white counterpart.

(vii) Non-compliance

Cessation of immunosuppressive drug therapy by the patient, either because of unacceptable side-effects or for financial reasons, is now one of the more common causes of graft failure.

(viii) Recurrence of the original disease

Although certain of the glomerulonephritides do recur (see earlier), loss of the graft as a result is relatively uncommon.

(ix) Other factors

Other factors such as the sex of the donor and recipient, blood group of donor and recipient, and parity of the recipient have little if any effect on graft outcome.

REHABILITATION

The patient with a successful transplant is in general restored to a normal existence with a quality of life as perceived by the patient being little different to that of the normal population. The majority of recipients of a successful graft will return to work, study, or managing the home within 6 months of transplantation.

Pregnancy after transplantation is possible whether the father or the mother is the transplant recipient. Although there is a higher level of spontaneous abortion in the transplant recipient, the incidence of developmental abnormalities in the live births that go to term, is not higher. Renal function may deteriorate during pregnancy where pre-eclampsia is more common, and rejection may occur after delivery. Provided that renal function is relatively normal there is no contraindication to pregnancy but careful monitoring of the fetus and renal function in the mother during and immediately after the pregnancy is essential.

FUTURE DEVELOPMENTS

As graft survival continues to improve with the introduction of more potent immunosuppression more attention will be paid to the side-effects of the immunosuppressive therapy and also to the prevention of cardiovascular disease. In addition, better and more specific immunosuppression may allow chronic rejection to be prevented, for this still remains a significant influence on long-term graft outcome.

FURTHER READING

Burdick JF, Racusen LC, Solez K, Williams GM. *Kidney Transplant Rejection: Diagnosis and Treatment*, 2nd edn. New York: Marcel Dekker, 1992.

Cicciarelli J, Cho Y. HLA matching: univariate and multivariate analysis of the UNOS Registry data. In: Terasaki PI, Cecka JM, eds. *Clinical Transplants 1991*. Los Angeles: UCLA Tissue Typing Laboratory, 1992; 325–33.

Hanto DW, Birkenbach M, Frizzern G, Gail-Poczalska KJ, Simmons RL, Schubach WH. Confirmation of the heterogeneity of post-transplant Epstein-Barr virus-associated B cell proliferations by immunoglobulin gene rearrangement analysis. *Transplantation* 1989; **47:** 458–64.

Mathew TH. Recurrent disease after renal transplantation. *Transplant Rev* 1991; **5:** 31–45.

Mickey R, Cho YW, Carnahan E. Long term graft survival. In: Terasaki PI, ed. *Clinical Transplants 1990*. Los Angeles: UCLA Tissue Typing Laboratory, 1991; 385–96.

Morris PJ, ed. *Kidney Transplantation: Principles and Practice*, 3rd edn. Philadelphia: WB Saunders, 1988.

Morris PJ. Immunological advances in clinical transplantation. *Transplant Proc* 1992; **24:** 2356–8.

Morris PJ, ed. *Kidney Transplantation: Principles and Practice*. 4th edn. Philadelphia: WB Saunders, 1993.

Murray JE. Human organ transplantation: background and consequences. *Science* 1992; **256:** 1411–16.

Penn I. Cancers following cyclosporin therapy. *Transplantation* 1987; **43:** 32–5.

10.6 Liver transplantation

A. BENEDICT COSIMI AND MICHAEL T. BAILIN

INTRODUCTION

The liver has a remarkable capacity to regenerate following even extensive necrosis. In some instances, however, progressive cirrhosis develops following injury induced by a variety of conditions, ranging from congenital biliary atresia to viral infections or alcohol abuse. In such patients, fatal complications of bleeding, infection, and progressive hepatic insufficiency can be reliably anticipated. Treatment with diet, various medications, immunosuppression, or even a few palliative operations is typically of short-term benefit at best. The only life-saving option for such patients, and also for some with acute fulminant hepatic failure, is replacement of the diseased liver with a healthy organ. Nevertheless, as recently as 1980, clinical liver transplantation still remained an investigational procedure which was being performed regularly in only two centres worldwide. Over the next 10 years, the practice of hepatology was completely transformed as hepatic replacement became accepted as not only a hypothetical possibility, but as the preferred therapeutic option that could be practically offered to a significant proportion of the thousands of patients who die annually from irreversible liver failure. As a result, decisions regarding the care of patients with liver disease should now be made with the perspective that future liver replacement may be required. Operative procedures in the portal area, such as portacaval shunts or complex biliary drainage manoeuvres, should generally be avoided since they greatly reduce the likelihood of a successful subsequent liver transplant. Similarly, holding the transplant in abeyance while awaiting the absolute terminal stages of hepatic failure significantly compromises the recipient's chances of survival and is no longer justified for suitable candidates with relentlessly progressive liver dysfunction.

This dramatic change in the recommended approach to the treatment of hepatic insufficiency is based upon the improvement in long-term survival and rehabilitation which has been achieved following transplantation. In marked contrast to the limited rehabilitation provided by other forms of intervention, over 80 per cent of the patients who survive transplantation return to full time employment, schooling, or homemaking. As described below, better definition of the most appropriate indications and timing for liver transplantation, improved methods of donor organ preservation, and refinements of surgical techniques and perioperative management, are among the factors which have contributed to the reduced morbidity and mortality. The availability of more selective, and therefore less toxic, immunosuppressive protocols, however, has been the most important development in the recent rapid growth of liver transplantation.

The almost simultaneous introduction into clinical trials of cyclosporin and monoclonal antibodies at the beginning of the last decade ushered in a new era of solid organ transplantation. Markedly improved results were immediately evident in patients following renal transplantation and even more dramatically, following liver transplantation where a doubling in 1-year survival was seen (Table 1). Stimulated by this encouraging change in clinical outcome, a Consensus Development Conference on Liver Transplantation was convened in the United States at the National Institutes of Health in 1983. Review of the results then being reported led the participants to conclude that liver transplantation was no longer an experimental procedure but a practical therapeutic approach. This determination encouraged a much wider application of the procedure, and over the next 8 years, more than 150 centres were established worldwide to perform liver transplants for a continually broadening list of indications.

Table 1 Recipient survival following liver transplantation

Era	Aetiology of liver failure	Proportion surviving	
		1 year (%)	5 years (%)
1963–1981	Benign	25–35	5–10
	Malignant	20–30	0–5
1982–1990	Benign	70–75	50–60
	Malignant	75–80	30–35
Candidates who fail to receive transplant		<10	

HISTORY OF LIVER TRANSPLANTATION

The first reference to hepatic replacement in the scientific literature was by Welch in 1955. Initial experimental efforts were directed to the transplantation of an extra liver into an ectopic site in the abdomen, typically with systemic venous inflow to the portal system. There are several theoretical advantages of such an auxiliary liver. The inherent risks related to the typically difficult host hepatectomy in the presence of severe portal hypertension and the instability that may develop during the anhepatic phase of the transplant procedure are avoided. In addition, any residual function of the retained native liver might provide a temporary supportive role during postoperative periods of compromised allograft function.

The early canine auxiliary allografts were rapidly rejected, making observations beyond a few days impossible. The more prolonged survival provided by the introduction of azathioprine immunosuppression revealed a rapid diminution of hepatic allograft mass beginning within 2 weeks after heterotopic implantation. The model thus led to the definition of the importance of hepatotrophic substances, including insulin, in the splanchnic venous blood. Techniques providing portal flow directly from the recipient's alimentary venous return into the transplanted liver proved essential for maintaining the long-term anatomical and functional integrity of the allograft. Perfection of these techniques led to the first clinical trial of auxiliary liver transplantation in November 1964. That attempt, and approximately 10 others over the next 4 years, all met with a fatal outcome, usually as a result of sepsis and hepatic failure. The first successful auxiliary liver transplant was performed in April 1969 at Memorial Hospital in New York. The procedure was performed in a 72-year-old patient with non-resectable cholangiocarcinoma. The allograft functioned normally for 9 months until the patient's death, secondary to infection in her own obstructed liver. The first heterotopic liver allograft to provide unquestionably prolonged survival was performed in 1972 by the same group for treatment of biliary atresia. That patient survived for more than 17 years. Nevertheless, overall clinical results following auxiliary liver transplantation have been poor: only two of 50 reported patients who had undergone the procedure by 1986 survived more than 1 year. Interest in the heterotopic procedure, however, has recently been renewed by reports of successful auxiliary partial liver transplantation in patients with complications of hepatic failure deemed to be so advanced that they were excluded from consideration for hepatectomy and orthotopic replacement.

The surgical techniques for orthotopic liver transplantation were first studied in canine experiments in 1956. Over the next 7 years, separate teams led by Moore, in Boston, and by Starzl, first at Chicago and then at Denver, independently identified the exacting technical requirements of the operation. Based upon these extensive studies, the first clinical attempt at liver replacement was undertaken at the University of Colorado in March 1963. Despite the experience of the surgical team, the procedure could not be completed due to massive haemorrhage. Over the next 4 years, isolated efforts to accomplish this formidable procedure at several institutions worldwide yielded no long-term successes. Hepatic failure leading to sepsis resulted from ischaemic damage and rejection in most of these recipients. It became clear that the successful clinical application of the technical skills already available would have to await the development of more effective immunosuppressive modalities. The addition of antilymphocyte serum to clinical protocols in 1966 helped to overcome this obstacle. With the use of triple-drug therapy including azathioprine, steroids, and antilymphocyte serum, improved results were first reported in renal allograft recipients. Soon afterwards the first human hepatic allograft recipient to achieve prolonged survival was given a new liver in Denver, in July 1967. This young patient, who underwent the procedure for treatment of an extensive hepatoma, lived with normal allograft function for more than a year before dying with recurrent cancer. Despite such occasional successes, however, frequent postoperative complications continued to plague the procedure and resulted in an early death rate of about 70 per cent. These results remained in stark contrast to the more satisfactory outcome which was being achieved following kidney transplantation. Most centres concluded that the technical complexity of the liver transplant operation would continue to limit its clinical relevance until more highly selective immunosuppressive agents, which would not render the host so vulnerable to infection, became available. Over the next 15 years, therefore, there was a virtual moratorium on the clinical application of liver transplantation except for continued efforts by the two teams in Colorado and Cambridge. As noted previously, more specific immunosuppresive agents, including cyclosporin and monoclonal antibodies, were eventually developed and after two decades of disappointments and tragic failures, these finally provided the effective immunosuppression that had been needed to demonstrate the clinical feasibility of hepatic replacement therapy. Further improvements in the management of rejection, such as the recent introduction of the experimental agent FK506, promise to continue to reduce the morbidity faced by liver allograft recipients and more widely extend the indications for the procedure.

Table 2 Indications for liver transplantation

I. Chronic advanced cirrhosis
  - A. Primarily parenchymal disease
    - (e.g.) Postnecrotic cirrhosis (viral, drug related)
      Alcoholic cirrhosis
      Cystic fibrosis
      Autoimmune liver disease
  - B. Primarily cholestatic disease
    - (e.g.) Biliary atresia
      Primary biliary cirrhosis
      Sclerosing cholangitis
      Cryptogenic cirrhosis
  - C. Primarily vascular disease
    - (e.g.) Budd–Chiari syndrome
      Veno-occlusive disease

II. Acute fulminant hepatic failure
  - A. Viral hepatitis
  - B. Drug-induced (e.g.) halothanes, sulphonamides
  - C. Metabolic liver disease (e.g. Wilson's disease, Reyes' syndrome)

III. Inborn errors of metabolism
  - (e.g.) Glycogen storage disease
    α_1-antitrypsin deficiency
    Wilson's disease

IV. Primary hepatic malignancies
  - A. Hepatoma ± cirrhosis
  - B. Cholangiocarcinoma
  - C. Unusual sarcomas arising within hepatic parenchyma

V. Retransplantation

INDICATIONS AND TIMING FOR LIVER TRANSPLANTATION

Since there is no effective alternative treatment available, liver transplantation should be considered for virtually any patient with advanced hepatic failure and a predicted survival of less than 1 year without hepatic replacement. Typical candidates can be divided into five broad groups, as outlined in Table 2. In infants and younger children, biliary atresia has been the most common indication. Initial management of these patients usually includes an attempted porticoenterostomy (Kasai procedure) during the neonatal period. Successful biliary diversion and stabilization can be accomplished in 50 to 75 per cent of these attempts, at least until some growth has occurred. This greatly increases the likelihood of a size-compatible liver donor becoming available. If the initial Kasai procedure fails, most centres now recommend immediate consideration for transplantation, since multiple attempts at revision of biliary drainage greatly compromise the likelihood of successful hepatectomy and liver treatment.

In later childhood, most candidates for transplantation have inborn errors of metabolism, postnecrotic cirrhosis, and hepatic neoplasms which are otherwise unresectable. In children with benign conditions, a fall-off from the established growth curve is often the major indication to proceed with transplantation. If permanent growth retardation is to be avoided, the optimal time for transplantation must often be at a much earlier stage in the evolution of deteriorating hepatic function than would be considered reasonable in adults.

In adults, the leading indication has been postnecrotic cirrhosis. Most of these patients have non-A, non-B viral hepatitis. Interestingly, there initially seemed to be little risk of significant disease recurrence following transplantation. With the recent development of a serological marker for hepatitis C, the clinical relevance of this disease in the allograft will be more accurately assessed. Patients who are chronically positive for hepatitis B surface antigen are highly likely to retain or redevelop their original serological markers of infection. Various perioperative manipulations, including treatment with immune globulin, interferon, or hepatitis B vaccine, have not clearly affected the incidence of recurrence. Some of these recipients have died with fulminant hepatitis in the allograft. However, the recurrent hepatitis B manifests with varying degrees of severity. Many patients enjoy prolonged symptom free-survival despite early post-transplant return of detectable serum levels of surface antigen. Thus, persistent pretransplant antigenaemia has not proved to be an absolute contraindication to transplantation. Potential candidates with hepatitis B virus e antigenaemia, which indicates a greater viral concentration, are at higher risk of developing clinically significant recurrence and are, therefore, more frequently excluded from consideration for transplantation. Hepatic replacement for other conditions leading to end-stage cirrhosis, including primary biliary or cryptogenic cirrhosis, sclerosing cholangitis, and autoimmune hepatitis, has been highly successful and is generally accepted as the appropriate therapeutic approach.

Despite the high prevalence of cirrhosis secondary to alcohol abuse, many of these patients are unsuitable for transplantation, both because they typically have multisystem disease, including severe cerebral atrophy, and because they are prone to precipitous clinical deterioration. In addition, non-compliance with essential medical therapy after surgery has been found to limit long-term success. As a result, application of hepatic transplantation for this indication has remained somewhat controversial. Nevertheless, the results of transplantation, combined with a multidisciplinary treatment programme for substance abuse in individuals with progressive liver dysfunction after discontinuing alcohol intake, are comparable to those for other accepted conditions. Thus, liver transplantation for selected patients with Laennec's cirrhosis is again being more widely evaluated.

The critical decision for all of these patients is the timing of the transplant. Until recently, the procedure was often considered so drastic that it was recommended only as a last resort when all other palliative measures had failed. Clearly, allowing these patients to deteriorate to the point of repeated gastrointestinal bleeding, malnutrition, sepsis, and coma, so compromises the chances of successful transplantation that it is no longer acceptable. The role of the hepatologist in choosing the optimum time for referral of the patient for transplantation is perhaps the most important determinant of survival following the procedure. Unfortunately, the natural history of these diseases proceeds at various rates in individual patients; the decision to proceed to transplantation cannot therefore be simply based on some predetermined clinical or biochemical profile. A combination of factors, including the nature and stage of the disease, the patient's age, quality of life, and history of any previous complications must all be considered. Appropriate candidates with primarily parenchymal conditions often present with hypoalbuminaemia, coagulopathy, variceal bleeding, or hepatic encephalopathy, while serum bilirubin levels are not markedly abnormal. Portacaval shunting should generally be avoided for management of variceal haemorrhage in potential transplant candidates from this group of patients. If bleeding cannot be controlled by conservative measures, including endoscopic sclerotherapy or bonding, it is reasonable to recommend splenorenal or mesocaval anastomosis for patients with Child's Class A cirrhosis. The long-term survival rate after portosystemic shunting in patients with more advanced cirrhosis is so inferior to that achieved by transplantation that appropriate candidates with class B or C cirrhosis should generally be considered for immediate liver replacement.

Severe hyperbilirubinaemia with intractable itching and the disabling complications of hepatic osteodystrophy may be the major indications for liver replacement for patients with cholestatic conditions. In contrast to the patients with primarily parenchymal disease, synthetic function is relatively preserved and there is often only limited evidence of portal hypertension when transplantation is, nevertheless, clearly appropriate.

Fulminant hepatic failure secondary to viral, toxin, or drug-induced sudden massive necrosis of a previously healthy liver represents a particularly difficult indication for transplantation. Although some of these patients recover, in those who progress to stage III–IV encephalopathy, a mortality rate of over 80 per cent can be anticipated. This unpredictable prognosis often leads to a delayed decision to proceed to transplantation. Hepatic replacement in these patients, in order to be successful, should be performed before stage IV coma and the sequelae of advanced cerebral oedema are established. Transplantation in patients at this point is associated with a mortality rate of greater than 50 per cent. Ominous earlier signs include persistent coagulopathy, hypoglycaemia, renal failure, rapid shrinkage of liver mass, and progressive encephalopathy despite maximal medical and nutritional support. At this stage, these patients should be referred for urgent liver replacement, hopefully before metabolic acidosis and sepsis develop. Transplantation prior to the development of these more grave signs could result in replacement of an occasional liver with reversible damage. Nevertheless, a survival rate of 60 to 75 per cent can now be achieved by transplantation, whereas at least 80 per cent of these patients will die with medical management alone.

A wide variety of liver-based congenital errors of metabolism can be successfully treated with liver replacement. Patients with an inborn metabolic defect such as haemophilia who require liver transplantation for other reasons (such as hepatitis), naturally, therefore, enjoy the additional benefit of complete correction of the underlying defect.

Primary malignancy of the liver involving both lobes or occurring in the presence of pre-existing cirrhosis which precludes even partial hepatic resection would appear to be an ideal indication for total hepatectomy and transplantation. Absence of the multisystem ravages of chronic liver failure and freedom from severe portal hypertension usually make these patients excellent surgical candidates. Although early survival following transplantation is good, cancer recurs within 1 year following liver replacement in over 50 per cent of the survivors. The results have been particularly discouraging in patients with cholangiocarcinoma in whom extrahepatic recurrences, typically as peritoneal or diaphragmatic implants or even intrahepatic metastases develop within months. The prognosis is more favourable following liver replacement for relatively small hepatomas presenting in a cirrhotic liver or for the slow growing fibrolamellar variant of hepatoma. Long-term disease-free survival has been observed in over 50 per cent of these recipients. Pretransplant assessment of patients with malignancy requires extensive diagnostic studies, often including exploratory laparotomy, in the effort to rule out occult metastatic disease. Clearly, however, more effective adjuvant therapy will have to be identified before liver replacement can be considered an appropriate approach, except for a few highly selected individuals, to hepatic cancer.

As the number of patients undergoing hepatic replacement has increased, the need for hepatic retransplantation has become more common. The reported frequency of retransplantation has varied between 5 per cent and 25 per cent among different centres. Overall survival rates following retransplantation are approximately 20 per cent lower than those following the primary procedure. Repeat liver transplantation is performed primarily in recipients whose initial graft is failing due to technical complications, primary non-function, or irreversible rejection. Retransplantation for uncontrolled acute rejection is uncommon: more typically, one observes relentlessly progressive chronic rejection which is manifested by worsening cholestasis and a histopathologic picture of 'vanishing bile ducts'. Retransplantation has generally been accepted as the only treatment available for these patients, although it has recently been suggested that the new immunosuppressive agent, FK506, may reverse these changes. Patients with primary graft non-function, secondary to unrecognized donor organ damage suffered during the agonal prerecovery period or to preservation injury, decompensate rapidly in the post-transplant period. As a result, they may be extremely unstable by the time a second donor is identified. The prognosis following retransplantation for this indication, therefore, is least favourable.

The selection from such a large patient population of the candidates most likely to benefit from liver transplantation relies primarily upon exclusion of coexisting conditions which have been found to increase the risks of early postoperative death unacceptably. Absolute contraindications (Table 3) include malignancy or uncontrolled infection outside the liver, secondary malignancies, life-limiting heart disease, or significant pulmonary disease. Currently active drug or alcohol addiction is also considered an absolute contraindication. As noted earlier, experience in patients with active addictions has emphasized that non-compliance with the post-transplant medical regimen almost inevitably leads to fatal complications.

Table 3 Contraindications to liver transplantation

I. Absolute
   - A. Uncontrolled infection outside the hepatobiliary system
   - B. Malignancy outside the hepatobiliary system
   - C. Secondary hepatic malignancy
   - D. Uncorrectable, life-limiting congenital anomalies
   - E. Active drug or alcohol abuse
   - F. Advanced cardiopulmonary disease

II. Relative
   - A. Age over 65
   - B. Portal vein thrombosis
   - C. Acute or chronic renal failure not associated with liver disease
   - D. Intrahepatic sepsis
   - E. Prior extensive hepatobiliary surgery
   - F. Hepatitis B surface antigen positive
   - G. HIV antibody positive

As surgeons have gained increasing experience with liver replacement, a number of factors which were previously felt to preclude successful transplantation have now been relegated to relative contraindications. These include, for example, age over 65 years (the oldest reported recipient of a liver was 76 years old at the time of transplantation), and portal vein thrombosis. Extensive clotting of the portal or even mesenteric veins, which previously made revascularization of the allograft impossible, can now be successfully managed through the use of vein grafts (see below). In patients with acute renal failure associated with hepatic decompensation (hepatorenal syndrome), renal function can be anticipated to improve rapidly following successful liver replacement. Patients with chronic renal dysfunction can be managed with simultaneous liver and kidney transplantation with only moderately increased risks.

DONOR SELECTION AND THE PROCUREMENT PROCEDURE

Donor selection

Most suitable kidney donors can also be liver donors. Ideally, one prefers a donor less than 65 years of age, though older donors have been used. There should be no previous history of alcoholism, neoplasia, except for brain tumours or skin cancer, or any current systemic viral or bacterial infection. The ABO blood group should be identical or compatible with the recipient. The chances of success with ABO incompatibility are, nevertheless, sufficient to occasionally justify the use of an incompatible liver in a critically ill individual who has no other available donor. Reasonable matching for body size between donor and recipient is essential in order to limit the technical difficulty of the reimplantation procedure. It is best to have a donor organ from a person whose weight is between 25 and 125 per cent of the recipient's: size constraints are particularly exacting for small individuals. Because of the rarity of potential donors in the paediatric population, one must often consider using older donors for transplantation into children. In some cases, the large size of the allograft has made successful reimplantation impossible. This obstacle is now being overcome by using adult livers, reduced in size to a single lobe or even segment (see below). Recently, this approach has been further extended to division of a single cadaver donor liver in such a way as to obtain two viable grafts for implantation into different recipients, or to procurement of a single lobe or segment from a living related donor for transplantation into a small child.

Histocompatibility testing currently plays little role in selecting recipients for liver transplantation. Typically, the urgency of the recipient operation precludes donor selection based upon tissue matching. Furthermore, retrospective analysis has not revealed a significant correlation between matching and results. Successful liver transplantation, in fact, has not infrequently been performed even in recipients with measurable serum levels of lymphocytotoxic antibodies reactive with donor histocompatibility antigens. Such a 'positive crossmatch' would be anticipated to result in hyperacute rejection of kidney allografts. This phenomenon has seldom been documented following liver transplantation, and only a modestly compromised long-term survival rate has been observed in hepatic recipients of such donor organs.

Allograft removal and preservation

The success of the multiple organ recovery involved during donor hepatectomy requires careful co-ordination among the teams to assure that there is no compromise in viability of any of the transplanted organs. In addition, it is critical to have anaesthesia sup-

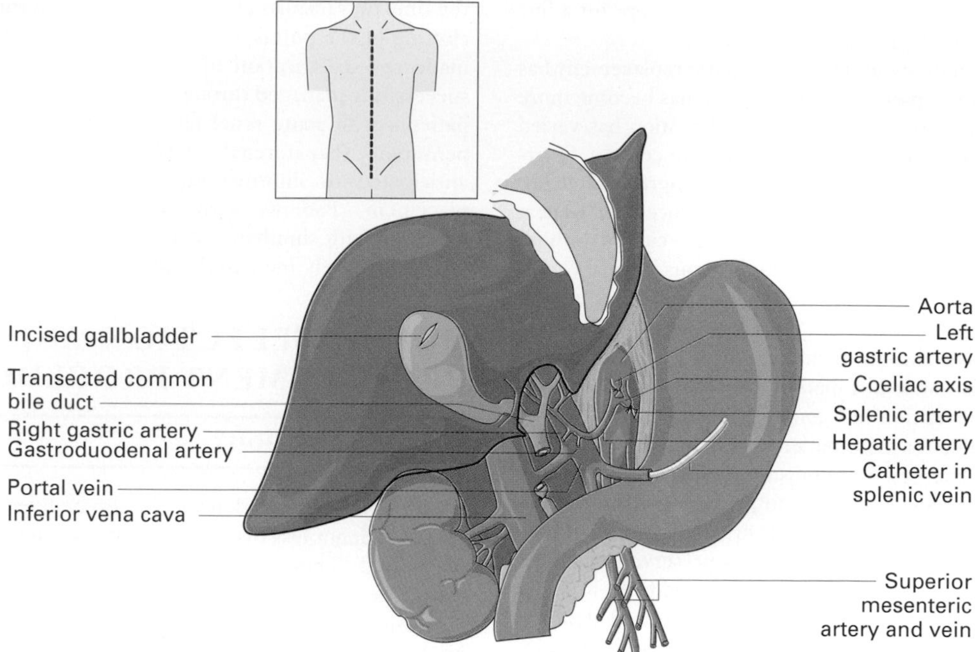

Fig. 1 Diagrammatic depiction of donor hepatectomy. (a) Exposure for multiple organ retrieval is through a long midline incision. (b) The portal area structures have been isolated and a perfusion catheter inserted into the portal vein via the transected splenic vein. For clarity the pancreas, which usually would be retracted inferiorly, has been omitted.

port to monitor and maintain cardiovascular integrity of the donor during the meticulous dissection, which may take 3 to 4 h.

Although the details will differ, depending upon the combination of organs to be removed, certain common principles prevail. These include wide exposure, dissection of each organ to its vascular connection while the heart is still beating, placement of cannulas for *in-situ* cooling, and removal of the organs while perfusion continues, usually in the order of heart and/or lungs, liver, kidneys, pancreas.

The organs are exposed through a midline incision extending from suprasternal notch to the pubis (Fig. 1(a)). Rapid inspection excludes unsuspected sepsis, neoplasia, or other significant pathology, and confirms the gross suitability of the organs to be procured. If the heart is to be used, it is usually mobilized as the first manoeuvre so that it can be quickly removed at any later stage should uncorrectable vascular instability occur during the dissection of other organs. The liver and often the pancreas are mobilized next. The coeliac axis is dissected to the aorta. If the pancreas is not to be used, the splenic and superior mesenteric arteries may be ligated and divided. The entire length of the coeliac axis, including a Carrel patch of donor aorta will be subsequently taken for anastomosis in the recipient. The common bile duct is transected and the gallbladder incised and flushed to prevent autolysis of the biliary epithelium. The portal vein is dissected to the confluence of the splenic and superior mesenteric veins where a cannula can be placed into the splenic vein for rapid portal perfusion (Fig. 1(b)). Skeletonization of the liver is completed by isolating the vena cava posteriorly, ligating and dividing the right adrenal vein, and freeing the suprahepatic vena cava.

If the pancreas is to be transplanted, the spleen is mobilized, the short gastric vessels are divided, and the spleen and pancreas retracted to the right. The body and tail of the pancreas are then carefully dissected free.

The kidneys and major abdominal vessels are next exposed by retracting the right colon and small bowel to the left. The kidneys are mobilized from the retroperitoneum, and the distal aorta and vena cava are completely freed. The donor is heparinized, after which a perfusion cannula is placed in the aorta and a venous drainage cannula into the vena cava.

Liver precooling, usually with 1 to 2 litres of crystalloid solution, is initially accomplished via the portal vein cannula. When the body core temperature falls to about 30°C, or earlier if haemodynamic instability occurs, the aorta is cross clamped at the diaphragm and *in-situ* aortic and portal vein flushing is begun using University of Wisconsin (UW) solution (Table 4). The cardioplegic infusion is next begun into the ascending aorta and cardiectomy is performed. The liver is removed next. Finally, the remaining mobilization of the kidneys is undertaken so that the entire block consisting of both kidneys, ureters, aorta, and inferior vena cava can be lifted out of the abdomen and placed in cooled perfusion solution. Segments of donor iliac artery and vein are also removed for possible use as vessel grafts during hepatic reimplantation. In donors from whom whole pancreaticoduodenal procurement is planned, we advise removing this organ block last in order to avoid possible contamination from the transected duodenum.

After completion of the donor hepatectomy, the allograft is further flushed through the portal vein and hepatic artery and then immersed in a sterile plastic bag containing UW preservation solution for storage on ice until transplantation. The anion, lactobionate, and the trisaccharide, raffinose, contained in this solution appear to be particularly effective impermeants for suppression of

Table 4 Composition of UW preservation solution

Constituent	Concentration	Function
K lactobionate	100 mmol	Impermeant
$NaKH_2PO_4$	25 mmol	Buffer
Adenosine	5 mmol	ATP stimulator
$MgSO_4$	5 mmol	Membrane stabilizer
Glutathione	3 mmol	Membrane stabilizer, antioxidant
Raffinose	30 mmol	Impermeant
Allopurinol	1 mmol	Radical scavenger
Insulin	100 U	Metabolic enhancer
Trimethoprim/ sulphamethoxazole	8 mg/40 mg	Antibacterial
Modified hydroxyethyl starch	50 g	Impermeant
Final concentration		
Na	30 mmol/l	
K	120 mmol/l	
pH	7.4	
Osmolarity	320–330 mmol/l	

hypothermia induced cellular swelling. The introduction of this preservation solution into clinical practice has extended the safe period of cold storage to as long as 24 h. This relatively prolonged preservation time increases the capability for more distant procurement and also relaxes the logistical constraints of the procedure. The recipient operation can now be scheduled on a semi-emergency basis, thus allowing more flexible use of operative rooms and personnel. Perhaps most importantly, the enhanced margin of safety has made possible the development of new techniques, such as reduced size liver transplantation, and has further minimized organ wastage by allowing donor hepatectomy to proceed even in circumstances where a recipient team is not immediately available.

THE RECIPIENT OPERATION

Anaesthetic considerations

One of the most important determinants of the perioperative mortality rate is the metabolic and resuscitative management by the anaesthesia team. The complexity of the procedure requires a number of extra access lines and pieces of equipment to provide adequate intraoperative monitoring and support. In addition to the usual anaesthesia machine, ventilator, and cardiac monitor with strip chart recorder, the operating room must usually have available a blood salvage device, separate pump systems for blood warming and rapid infusion, venovenous bypass, and a patient warming blanket, and often other special devices, such as the argon beam coagulator. Some attention, therefore, must be given to providing a reasonably compact and functional layout of the operative area. In adult recipients, access for infusion and monitoring is typically accomplished via a right radial arterial line, a large bore intravenous site in the right arm, and introducer catheters in each internal jugular vein, one for placement of the pulmonary artery catheter and one for connection to the rapid infusion pump. With this system, infusion rates as high as 2 l/min can be provided, if needed, during periods of rapid blood loss. Access sites in the legs are avoided since infusions would be unreliable during the period of vena cava occlusion. The left arm is avoided since the venovenous bypass return is usually via the left axillary vein. In small children, the use of pulmonary artery catheters is usually neither required nor practical. Adequate monitoring and infusion is provided by central venous pressure measurements and 14- or 18-gauge intravenous catheters.

Patients with hepatic failure are predisposed to developing hypoxia from atelectasis, due to ascites, and from intrapulmonary arteriovenous shunts. Thus, careful preoxygenation and rapid sequence induction anaesthesia are commonly used. An appropriately sized, low pressure cuff endotracheal tube is placed in anticipation of a possibly prolonged period of intubation. Adequate padding of the heels, sacrum, elbows, and head is provided to prevent pressure ulceration during the operation which not infrequently extends beyond 12 h. Hypothermia, resulting from the long duration of the procedure, extracorporeal blood circulation in the venovenous bypass, and the implantation of the iced allograft, must be anticipated. Measures to provide recipient rewarming are essential. These include warmed intravenous infusions, a heated ventilator circuit, a warming blanket on the operating table, and plastic drapes on the head and exposed extremities.

The selection of anaesthetic agents is governed by the high cardiac output, low peripheral vascular resistance state typically associated with end-stage liver disease. Isoflurane inhalational anaesthesia will reduce systemic resistance and may be used as tolerated. The preferred maintenance agent for haemodynamic stability is a narcotic anaesthetic employing fentanyl and/or morphine. Because some patients may not tolerate administration of routine anaesthesia, they are often given a benzodiazepine as well, to block memory. Lorazepam is frequently chosen, since this agent requires only glucuronidation for excretion.

Some of the intraoperative consequences of the transplant procedure are detailed in Table 5. The patients often develop metabolic acidosis, which should not be over-corrected with bicarbonate since they will also receive a large citrate load with administered blood products This will eventually be metabolized to bicarbonate and may lead to severe postoperative metabolic alkalosis. Although the determinants of need for packed red blood cells and fresh frozen plasma are independent, the patients typically require approximately equal volumes of each. Platelets are administered based upon pre- and intraoperative platelet counts and the number of blood volumes transfused.

Many of the occasionally catastrophic consequences of the

Table 5 Intraoperative consequences of orthotopic liver transplantation

1. Prolonged duration of surgery
   (Average 8 h; range 6–18 h)
2. Major blood loss
   (Average 15 units; range 1–10 blood volumes)
3. Unique problems during anhepatic phase
   (a) Lower body volume pooling
   (b) Coagulopathy
   (c) Hypocalcaemia, hypothermia, ? hypoglycaemia
   (d) Oliguria
4. Reperfusion problems
   (a) Hyperkalaemia, hypercarbia
   (b) Acidosis, hypoxaemia, hypothermia
5. Postperfusion events
   (a) Hypokalaemia
   (b) Coagulopathy

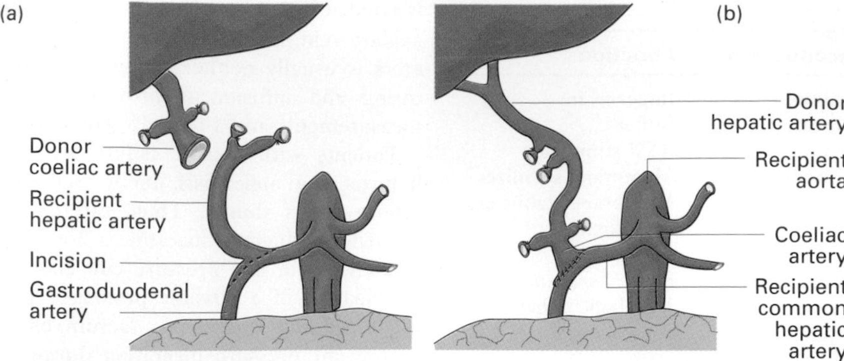

Fig. 2 Isolation of recipient coeliac axis for revascularization of liver allograft. (a) The recipient proper hepatic artery has been ligated distal to its bifurcation. (b) The subsequent arterial anastomosis is between donor coeliac axis (CA) or Carrel patch of donor aorta to the side of the recipient common hepatic artery at or proximal to the origin of the gastroduodenal artery.

anhepatic phase of the operation can be limited by use of venovenous bypass. Up to 40 to 50 per cent of the cardiac output can be returned to the heart from the lower body and viscera via the bypass. Continuous monitoring of central venous, pulmonary arterial, and systemic arterial pressures, and frequent determinations of cardiac output are required during this critical period. Hypotension may be caused by hypovolaemia, inadequate bypass return, air or thromboemboli from the pump, or myocardial depression secondary to hypothermia or to the hypocalcaemia resulting from citrate intoxication during the rapid transfusion of blood products. Although there is a theoretical possibility of hypoglycaemia developing during the anhepatic stage, typically the blood sugar remains normal to elevated, presumably from the anticoagulant in banked blood and from numerous glucose containing carrier infusions.

Another critical period occurs at the time of liver reperfusion. Despite prior flushing of the allograft, the sudden bolus of cold, hyperkalaemic, acidotic blood from the liver and lower body may cause severe pulmonary artery vasoconstriction with resultant hypotension. It is thus essential to stabilize the patient by correction of acid–base abnormalities and hypovolaemia. Administration of calcium chloride just prior to vena caval unclamping may be required to antagonize the imminent hyperkalaemia. As the allograft function improves later, following rewarming and arterial reconstruction, a major fall in serum potassium often occurs, as a result of both uptake into the revascularized hepatocytes and increased availability of ionized calcium as citrate metabolism begins in the liver. Potassium supplementation may be required. A significant bleeding diathesis may also develop at this stage, secondary to the accelerated fibrinolysis which appears in association with increased blood levels of fibrin degradation products. This consequence of hepatic ischaemia may lead to substantial blood loss. The importance of aggressive replacement of coagulation factors during the early reperfusion period, sometimes including antifibrinolytic agents, cannot be overemphasized.

Recipient hepatectomy

Removal of the diseased liver is a tedious process because of the coagulopathy inherent in patients with end-stage liver disease, the multiple venous collaterals and portal hypertension encountered, and the often dense adhesions from previous operations. Abdominal exploration in adults is carried out through bilateral subcostal incisions with a midline extension, usually including excision of the xiphoid. In children, this midline extension is seldom required. Meticulous haemostasis is obtained using a combination of electrocautery and suture ligation for essentially all dissection.

After entering the peritoneal cavity, the falciform and left triangular ligaments are divided, often requiring stepwise, silk ligatures for haemostasis. The gastrohepatic ligament (lesser omentum) is then exposed and similarly divided. If possible, the liver is left vascularized until the last stages, in order to retain as normal as possible levels of clotting factors and glucose control. In some patients with extensive bloody adhesions, it may be necessary to devascularize the liver earlier and then continue with the rest of the mobilization. The use of venovenous bypass at this point can help to stabilize the patients. Most teams, however, do not find the option of early bypass and rapid hepatectomy attractive.

The portal structures are generally isolated first. To maximize length for the subsequent biliary anastomosis, the recipient common bile duct is divided above the entrance of the cystic duct. If the patient has had a previous biliary enteric anastomosis, the anastomosis is taken down, protecting the portal area and the Roux loop which will be subsequently used for drainage of the donor liver. The proper hepatic artery is ligated and divided distal to the take-off of the gastroduodenal artery. The more proximal common hepatic artery is further exposed for subsequent anastomosis leaving the gastroduodenal artery intact (Fig. 2). Finally the portal vein is skeletonized, ligating and dividing tributaries including the coronary vein and any pancreatic veins which may be present. If the portal vein is found to be thrombosed, more proximal dissection beneath the pancreas to the area of confluence between the splenic and superior mesenteric veins will usually identify a suitable anastomotic site. Occasionally it is necessary to expose the superior mesenteric vein below the pancreas at the level of the middle colic vein to obtain a patent vessel with adequate flow for portal revascularization. In both of these instances, vessel grafts taken from the donor may be required to span the distance

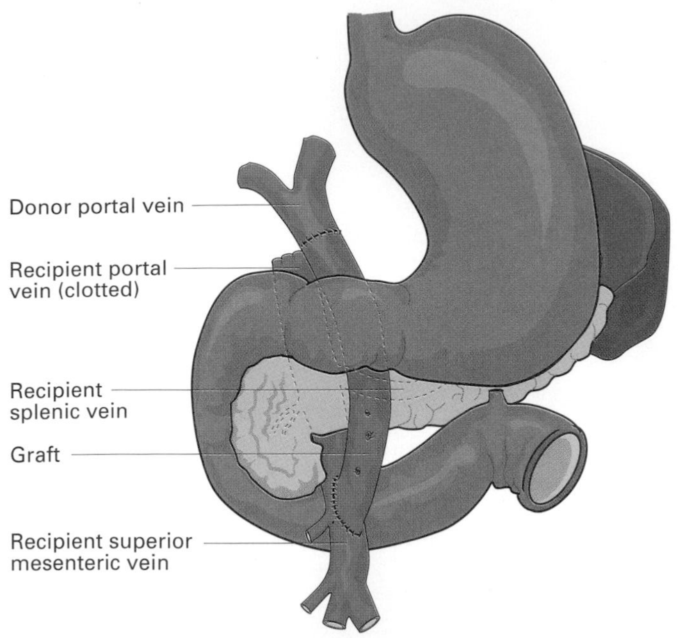

Fig. 3 Use of donor iliac vein to bypass thrombosed recipient portal vein. In patients with extensive thrombosis, the vein graft may have to be placed anterior to the pancreas to extend to a patent superior mesenteric vein. More commonly a suitable anastomotic site is found behind the pancreas at the confluence of the splenic and superior mesenteric veins.

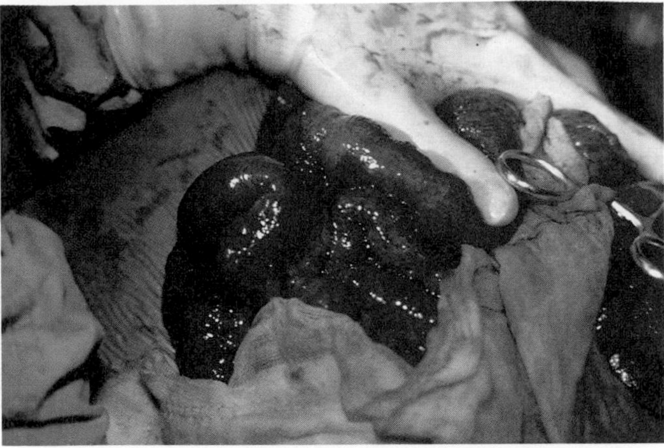

Fig. 4 Haemorrhage and oedema of bowel following portal vein occlusion without venovenous bypass. Although such severe splanchnic congestion is not inevitable, routine use of venovenous bypass during the anhepatic phase of the operation essentially eliminates this complication.

from the more proximal recipient vessel to the donor portal vein (Fig. 3).

Once the portal dissection has been completed, the infrahepatic vena cava is exposed. Because of extensive retroperitoneal collateral vessels, the tissues must often be divided between ligatures, as is practised in this dissection during portasystemic shunting. The inferior vena cava is carefully encircled at a level just above the right renal vein. The right adrenal vein is ligated and divided. The right lobe of the liver is elevated as the peritoneal and diaphragmatic attachments are coagulated or suture ligated. The bare area of the liver is separated from the diaphragm and any additional venous branches entering the vena cava from posteriorly are ligated and divided. Mobilization of a lengthy segment of suprahepatic vena cava is accomplished by encircling the cava close to its exit from the liver. By working at this level, the recipient phrenic veins are usually not encountered—being left attached to the cuff above the site where the vena cava will be divided. After this dissection, the mobilized liver is held in place only by its venous attachments.

Although venous bypass during the anhepatic phase of the procedure is not an absolutely essential component of the operation, severe splanchnic venous congestion can occur in its absence (Fig. 4), and many centres now use bypass for most adult recipients. Some of the potential benefits of venovenous bypass are summarized in Table 6. The haemodynamic stability provided by the high volume return of blood to the heart from otherwise obstructed venous beds allows revascularization of the donor liver in a less urgent fashion. A not insignificant advantage provided by such effective stabilization is the opportunity for training of inexperienced surgeons in this phase of the operation.

Heparin bonded catheters are inserted via a separate groin incision into the recipient's left femoral vein for decompression of the lower systemic venous bed. A second limb of the circuit is placed into the left axillary vein for blood return to the heart. An in-line centrifugal pump provides flow rates of 1 to 3 l/min (Fig. 5). Final resection of the recipient liver is then completed by clamping the portal vein and transecting it high in the hilum. Vascular clamps are placed on the infrahepatic and suprahepatic cavae. A long suprahepatic caval cuff is developed by incising the liver parenchyma and transecting the hepatic veins within the substance of the liver (Fig. 6). The infrahepatic cava is severed close to its junction with the caudate lobe. The liver is removed from the field and any major retroperitoneal bleeding sites are suture ligated. The third cannula of the venovenous bypass is then introduced into the lumen of the recipient portal vein to decompress the splanchnic venous system. This manoeuvre typically results in greatly diminished bleeding from the hepatectomy site. Final haemostasis can then be achieved by oversewing or cauterizing the exposed retroperitoneal tissues in the hepatic fossa (Fig. 7).

Orthotopic allograft revascularization

The suprahepatic vena caval cuff is tailored by opening the recipient hepatic veins into the caval lumen. Sutures are inserted at the corners of donor and recipient veins and the allograft is gently lowered towards the diaphragm. The posterior anastomosis is accomplished using everting mattress sutures placed from within

Table 6 Benefits of venovenous bypass

1. Improved haemodynamic stability
2. Preservation of renal function
3. Decreased blood loss
4. Decreased fluid requirements
5. Decreased risk of subsequent pulmonary congestion
6. Decreased gastrointestinal tract insult
7. Potential for earlier hepatic devascularization
8. Improved training opportunities

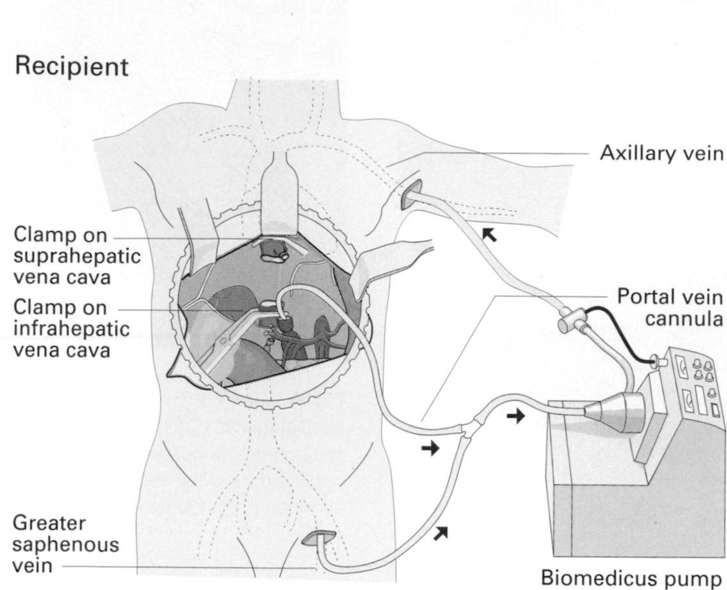

Fig. 5 Anhepatic stage of the transplant procedure with venovenous bypass. Lower body systemic venous blood and splanchnic blood are drained via the femoral and portal cannulae respectively. Blood is returned to the heart by the in-line centrifugal pump via the axillary vein cannula.

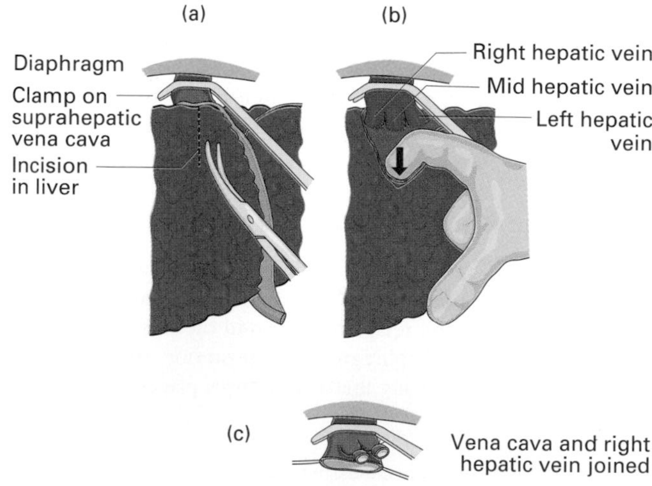

Fig. 6 Transection of recipient suprahepatic vena cava. A long cuff is developed by dividing the hepatic veins within the parenchyma of the liver. (a,b) The veins are then opened into the caval lumen to provide the anastomotic site (c).

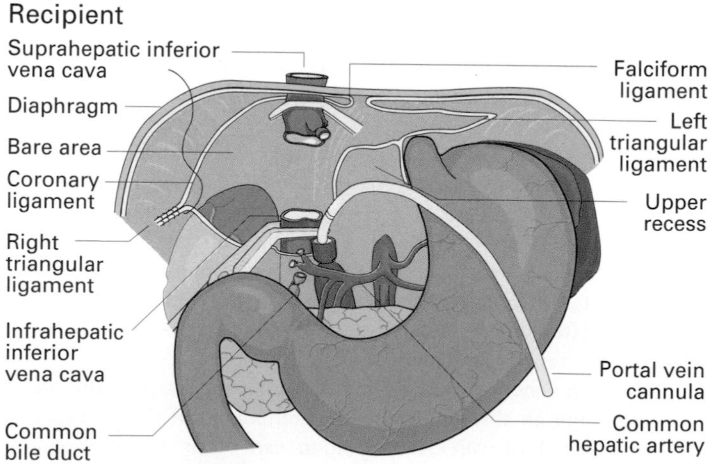

Fig. 7 Control of bleeding in retrohepatic tissues. The ligaments and retroperitoneal adhesions which had been divided to complete the recipient hepatectomy are fully exposed and can be oversewn or cauterized for complete haemostasis.

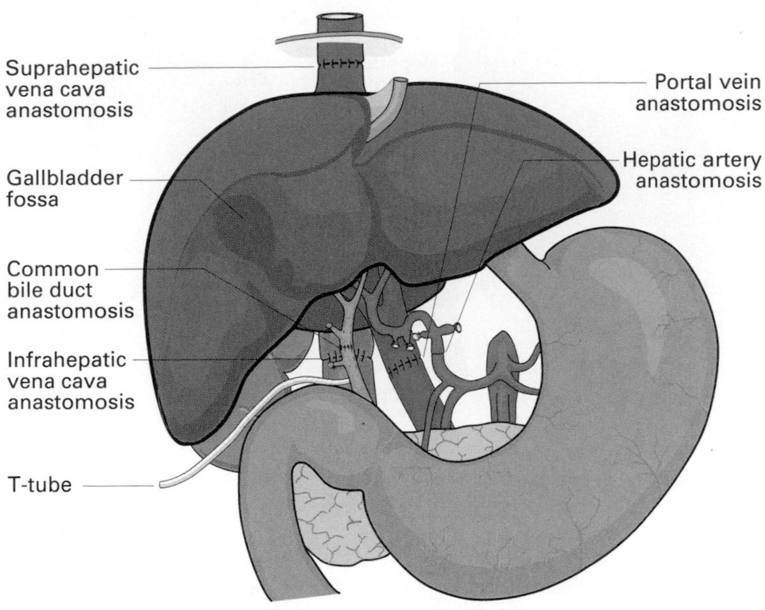

Fig. 8 Completion of the five anastomoses of orthotopic liver transplantation. The end-to-end suprahepatic vena cava, infrahepatic vena cava, and portal vein anastomoses are performed first to allow early reperfusion of the allograft. Arterial reconstruction may be to recipient proper hepatic artery as shown here or, more typically, to the common hepatic artery, as in Fig. 2. The biliary reconstruction is decompressed and stented with a T-tube.

the lumen. The anterior rim is completed in simple over and over fashion. The infrahepatic cava is reconstructed by usual end-to-end venous anastomotic techniques. Prior to completion of the anterior wall of this anastomosis, the allograft is flushed via the donor portal vein with cold Ringer's lactate solution. This important manoeuvre removes air and any remaining preservation fluid, which contains high concentrations of potassium and acidic radicals that have accumulated during the ischaemic interval, from the intrahepatic venous spaces.

Preparation for the portal vein anastomosis requires removal of the outflow limb of the bypass circuit from the recipient vessel. A running continuous suture approximates the ends of the widely spatulated donor and recipient portal veins. As noted earlier, this anastomosis may have to be placed at the confluence of recipient splenic and superior mesenteric veins or, in some instances, on to a vein graft. The suture for all of the venous anastomoses is tied leaving 1 cm or more of 'growth factor' between the knot and the vessell wall. This allows expansion of any purse-stringing effect and limits the likelihood of anastomotic stricture. At this point, most units favour release of the venous clamps to restore portal and vena caval flow through the liver. If the patient is stable, venovenous bypass is discontinued and the remaining catheters are removed to prevent intraluminal clotting.

The hepatic artery anastomosis is usually constructed by suturing the donor coeliac axis with attached aortic Carrell patch to the recipient hepatic artery at the level of the gastroduodenal take-off. Various arterial anomalies may require modifications in the method of reconstruction, even including insertion of donor iliac artery as a vascular graft to provide inflow directly from recipient infrarenal aorta.

Biliary reconstruction is begun after the donor gallbladder has been removed and adequate haemostasis of the operative area has been accomplished. End-to-end choledochocholedochostomy using interrupted absorbable sutures is performed in recipients whose native biliary tree is not diseased. The anastomosis is stented with an appropriately sized T-tube brought out through the recipient duct (Fig. 8).

Reconstruction is by choledochoenterostomy into a Roux-en-Y loop of jejunum for patients whose primary hepatic disease involved the biliary tree (such as biliary atresia, sclerosing cholangitis, cholangiocarcinoma). We favour stenting this anastomosis as well, using a small feeding tube brought out through the side of the Roux loop and the abdominal wall. This approach has the advantage of allowing postoperative radiographic studies of the anastomosis if any question of obstruction or leak develops.

Final haemostasis, placement of closed suction drains above and below the liver, and closure of the abdominal, axillary, and groin wounds, complete the operative procedure.

Partial or split liver transplantation

Because of the limited availability of suitably sized organ donors for the relatively large numbers of infants and small children with end-stage liver disease, a significant proportion of these candidates die before transplantation can be accomplished. This problem has been addressed by developing reduced size orthotopic liver transplantation. With this approach, livers from cadavers

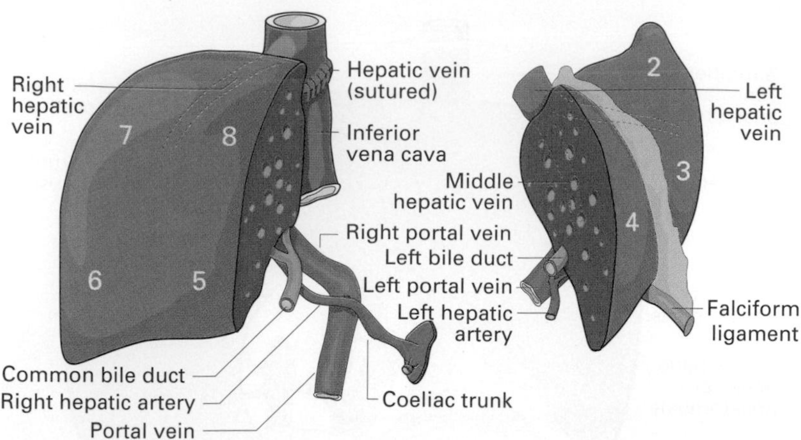

Fig. 9 Split liver preparation for transplantation into two recipients. The portal vein, coeliac trunk, common bile duct, and inferior vein cava remain attached to the right lobe. The left lobe will be revascularized and drained by lobar pedicles including the left portal vein, left hepatic artery, left bile duct, and middle and left left hepatic veins. Division of the allograft into true left and right lobes leaves the falciform and round ligaments (RL) attached to the left lobe. The numbers indicate hepatic segments.

weighing as much as 10 times that of the recipient can be successfully reduced in size and placed into paediatric recipients. Donor liver procurement is as described above. For partial liver transplantation, anatomic dissection of the graft is performed, *ex vivo*, to provide either a right or left lobe for reimplantation while discarding the resected portion. Growing experience with this technique has more recently progressed to partition of the vascular and biliary structures to obtain two viable grafts for use in two different recipients, the so-called split liver (Fig. 9). In patients receiving the right lobe graft, recipient hepatectomy and all vascular anastomoses are performed as described above. Biliary reconstruction is by choledochoenterostomy. Recipient hepatectomy in patients receiving the left lobe graft involves mobilization of the liver from the retroperitoneum as described but preservation of recipient inferior vena cava, suture closure of the right and accessory hepatic vein orifices, and use of the left hepatic vein for anastomosis to the graft. The short lengths of donor left portal vein and hepatic artery have generally necessitated the use of vessel grafts for revascularization in the recipient.

Auxiliary liver transplantation

Rarely, potential hepatic allograft recipients may be so unstable that they would be predicted not to be able to tolerate hepatectomy and orthotopic replacement. Transplantation of an auxiliary liver into a heterotopic position while leaving the diseased organ *in situ* could be a suitable alternative for such high-risk individuals. As noted above, long-term success following clinical attempts at heterotopic liver transplantation has been poor, primarily because of size constraints leading to technical complications and infection. Recent modification of the procedure, with reduction of the size of the graft by partial hepatectomy, may provide a satisfactory solution. For this approach, the donor liver is prepared *ex vivo* by removing the left lobe and reducing the vena cava to a short segment draining the right and middle hepatic veins. In the recipient, dissection is primarily limited to the portal area, as would be required for a portacaval shunt procedure. The infrarenal aorta is also freed over a length of 3 to 4 cm. The reduced size liver is oriented in the right subhepatic region with the donor vena cava overlying the recipient cava and the graft hilum facing the aorta (Fig. 10). Vascular anastomoses include donor vena cava to side of

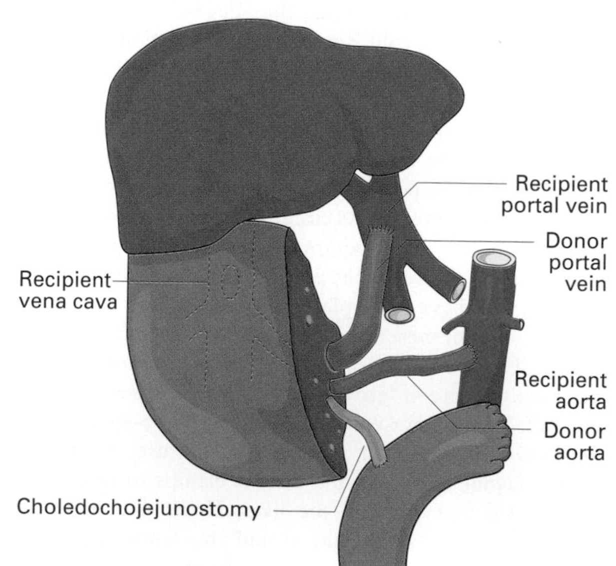

Fig. 10 Auxiliary partial liver transplantation. The donor right lobe is oriented in the subhepatic region with the hilum facing recipient aorta. Vascular anastomoses are: donor vena cava to side of recipient supra renal vena cava; donor portal vein to side of recipient portal vein; and Carrel patch of donor aorta to side of recipient aorta. Choledochojejunostomy using a Roux-en-Y loop provides biliary drainage.

recipient suprarenal vena cava; donor portal vein to side of recipient portal vein; and Carrel patch of donor aorta to side of recipient aorta. Biliary drainage is into a Roux-en-Y jejunal loop. Early experience with this approach appears promising but remains limited.

POST-TRANSPLANTATION MANAGEMENT, COMPLICATIONS

Non-immunological considerations

The early postoperative management of liver allograft recipients requires much more intensive monitoring and support than is required following kidney or pancreas transplantation. Because of their precarious pretransplant condition the prolonged operation and its attendant massive fluid shifts, and the coagulopathy and haemodynamic instability that can result if onset of normal allograft function is delayed, these recipients are initially cared for in a critical care unit. Satisfactory immediate postoperative cardiac output, maintenance of adequate renal function, and correction of abnormal clotting parameters may require aggressive blood and fresh frozen plasma replacement and support with vasoactive drug infusions. Other important aspects of the recipient's care can be considered as they relate to individual organ systems.

Hepatobiliary system

Satisfactory liver allograft function is manifested by the appearance of deeply pigmented bile in the drainage catheter and early restoration of clotting function. These recipients will typically have good renal function and will recover rapidly from anaesthesia so that successful extubation is possible within 12 to 48 h. If, however, there is minimal or watery depigmented biliary output ('white bile'), the early postoperative care will be more complicated. These recipients can be reliably predicted to require assisted ventilation, intensive infusion of fresh frozen plasma, and other complex resuscitative measures before adequate stabilization may be achieved. As noted above, retransplantation may be the only recourse for some patients with early graft dysfunction. Timely identification of those recipients with irreversible ischaemic injury is critical if retransplantation is to be successfully accomplished before fatal cerebral oedema develops. As in the pretransplant candidate with fulminant hepatic failure, uncorrectable coagulopathy (prothrombin time over 20 s), hypoglycaemia, acidosis, and new onset of renal failure are ominous. These findings, which usually prompt the urgent search for a second allograft, are typically encountered in less than 5 per cent of liver recipients, though this indication for retransplantation has been reported to be as high as 10 to 15 per cent by centres initially willing to accept more marginal donors.

Technical complications most commonly include intra-abdominal bleeding, vascular thrombosis, biliary duct problems, or infected fluid collections. The incidence of postoperative bleeding is directly related to the severity of intraoperative bleeding and the quality of immediate allograft function. Despite meticulous surgical technique and haemostasis in the operating room, diffuse capillary oozing may persist until hypothermia and inadequate plasma clotting factor levels have been corrected. If major blood loss persists despite reversal of the coagulopathy, emergency re-exploration is indicated to identify a probable surgically correctable cause. In patients whose early bleeding ceases, laparotomy is still often required, usually 36 to 48 h after the initial surgery, in order to evacuate perihepatic collections which may otherwise become secondarily infected.

Hepatic artery thrombosis, particularly in small children, should be suspected in all patients who have unexplained fever, a bile leak, or a positive blood culture for Gram-negative organisms. Doppler ultrasound or angiography will confirm the diagnosis. If the clinical presentation is one of fulminant liver failure, biliary leak, or relapsing bacteraemia, emergency retransplantation is the only viable therapy. The small proportion of patients who develop only mild liver dysfunction, without abscess formation, may be conservatively managed while arterial collaterals to the allograft develop.

The presenting symptoms of portal vein thrombosis are usually less devastating. Rarely, in the immediate postoperative period, this complication can produce severe biochemical abnormalities and even hepatic necrosis requiring retransplantation. More commonly, portal vein thrombosis is suggested by recurrent variceal bleeding, intractable ascites, or an unexplained elevation in prothrombin time. Successful management of this complication in patients without severe hepatic dysfunction is usually achieved by operative thrombectomy and correction of any technical abnormality encountered. In the late post-transplant period, a splenorenal shunt may be effective.

Bile duct problems, which historically accounted for the majority of postoperative complications, have greatly decreased in frequency since current reconstruction techniques became standardized. The routine use of a feeding or T-tube stent allows ready investigation of any suspected biliary tract complication. Anastomotic leak, usually manifested by appearance of bile in the abdominal drainage or an unexplained rise in serum bilirubin, occurs during the first several weeks after transplantation. Minimal, well drained leaks, not associated with hepatic artery thrombosis, will typically close spontaneously. More extensive bile collections require open drainage to create a controlled fistula or even resection and reanastomosis. Leaks secondary to arterial thrombosis are best managed by retransplantation. Biliary duct obstruction occurs more commonly in the later postoperative period, since the anastomoses are usually stented for several months following surgery. Short strictures can be dilated via endoscopic or percutaneous approaches. Surgical resection of the anastomosis and conversion to choledochojejunostomy may be required for more complex lesions. Earlier observations of diffuse obstruction by 'sludge' within the biliary tree are now seldom encountered. Control of this complication is presumably due to careful biliary flushing during the donor procedure and improved methods of reconstruction. An interesting and unusual cause of obstruction has been the development of a tension mucocele in a donor cystic duct remnant which shared a common wall with the bile duct, a phenomenon analogous to the 'Mirizzi' syndrome.

Postoperative hepatitis, usually caused by cytomegalovirus, can also cause graft dysfunction. Following serological or hepatic biopsy confirmation of the diagnosis, ganciclovir therapy is commonly instituted. Other viral infections, including recurrent hepatitis B or hepatitis C, for which interferon therapy may be indicated, can usually be histologically or serologically confirmed. Occasionally, differentiating these causes of allograft dysfunction from rejection may be difficult.

Pulmonary system

Aggressive efforts to prevent pulmonary complications are essential in all patients. Intensive chest physiotherapy, postural drainage, and endotracheal suctioning are routine. Flexible fibreoptic bronchoscopy may also be required to remove retained secretions causing segmental atelectasis. Right-sided pleural effusions are common in the early postoperative period and usually respond to diuretic therapy. Thoracentesis is rarely required to provide satisfactory lung re-expansion but should not be withheld when necessary, since even limited episodes of pulmonary dysfunction are poorly tolerated in these nutritionally depleted, debilitated, immunosuppressed patients. Attempted weaning from assisted ventilation is begun as soon as the recipient recovers from anaesthesia and demonstrates cough reflexes. If initial blood gases and mechanics are satisfactory, successful extubation can be accomplished usually within 12 to 48 h. Several unusual factors unique to liver allograft recipients may delay weaning. These include right diaphragmatic paralysis which may result from the intraoperative placement of the suprahepatic vascular clamp and the metabolic alkalosis which these patients often develop. Because the latter may contribute to compensatory hypoventilation, correction with potassium chloride, or rarely hydrochloric acid, may be necessary to allow successful early extubation.

Significant hypoxaemia resulting from development of intrapulmonary arteriovenous malformations in patients with chronic liver disease may persist into the early postoperative period. Although the prognosis for such patients is somewhat less favourable, such shunting, even advanced to the stage of digital clubbing, has been observed to reverse following successful liver transplantation.

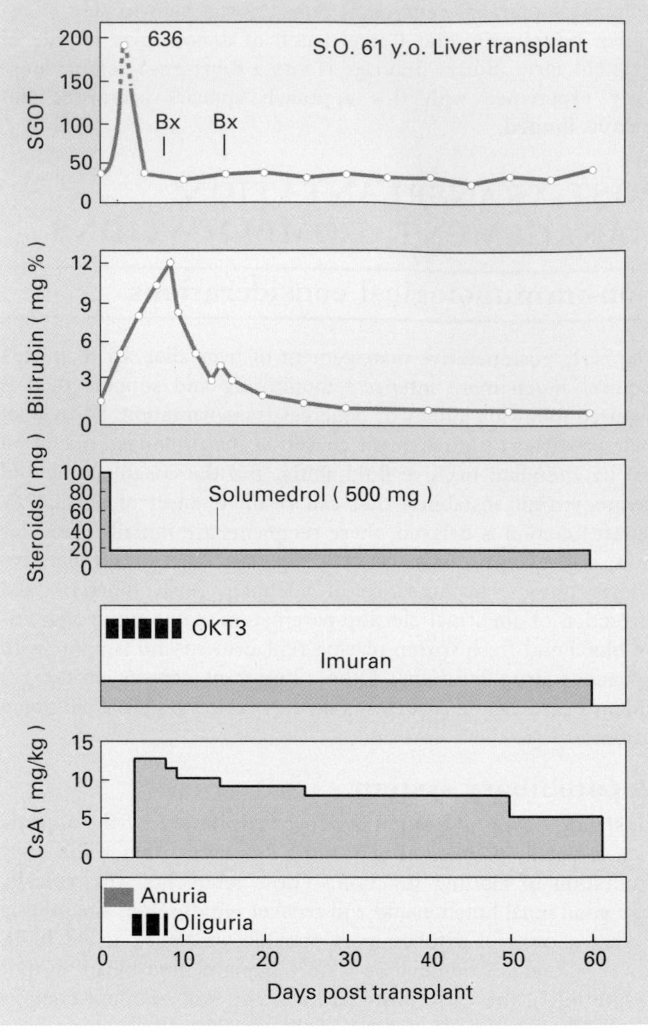

Fig. 11 Initial immunosuppressive management following liver transplantation in a 61-year-old patient. The patient developed anuric renal failure intraoperatively. Induction immunosuppression with OKT3 replaced intravenous cyclosporin during the immediate postoperative period. Oral cyclosporin administration was begun after renal function improved. Mild rejection (Biopsy (BX) proven) on day 18 was reversed with increased steroids.

Cardiovascular system

Initial haemodynamic stability is maintained by volume administration and the addition of inotropic, chronotropic, or vasoactive agents as guided by clinical findings and continuous invasive monitoring of usual cardiopulmonary variables. Not infrequently, significant hypertension develops in patients receiving intravenously administered cyclosporin. The increased risks of intracerebral haemorrhage and seizures require aggressive treatment of sustained hypertension. Nitroprusside is typically the agent of choice in the immediate postoperative period because of the rapid reversibility of its effect. Subsequent therapy may require a combination of diuretics, a vasodilator, such as hydralazine, and often a calcium-channel blocker, such as nifedipine, as well. Arrhythmias are unusual and are typically associated with hypoxaemia or severe electrolyte abnormalities.

Renal and metabolic systems

Acute renal failure may develop immediately postoperatively due to pre-existing renal insufficiency, intraoperative vena caval occlusion, extensive bleeding and hypotension, hepatic allograft dysfunction, and administration of nephrotoxic drugs, such as aminoglycoside antibiotics. All of these factors are exacerbated by the administration of cyclosporin, particularly via the parenteral route. Because survival is poor for patients who require dialysis, we attempt to limit the period of dysfunction by using induction immunosuppression with OKT3 rather than cyclosporin in recipients with persistent oliguria. As illustrated in Fig. 11, oral cyclosporin can be instituted after diuresis has resumed, and the biliary drainage tube has been clamped, parenteral administration of the drug being completely avoided. Extensive experience has established that in the presence of satisfactory hepatic allograft function, renal function regularly returns even in patients with pre-existing hepatorenal syndrome. Nevertheless, some patients with early acute tubular necrosis are left with persistently compromised renal function. Renal failure has gradually progressed, during chronic cyclosporin therapy, even to the need for renal transplantation in a few hepatic allograft recipients.

In addition to uraemia, other major metabolic derangements may require correction in the early postoperative period. These include hypothermia, hyperkalaemia, especially in the presence of poor hepatic and renal function, and hypocalcaemia and metabolic alkalosis resulting from citrate infusion.

Haematological system

Leucopenia and thrombocytopenia secondary to hypersplenism typically persist into the postoperative period. The leucopenia is usually of no clinical consequence; prolonged thrombocytopenia, however, may require platelet transfusions and limit the dosages of azathioprine that can be safely administered. The hypersplenism can be anticipated to resolve gradually over the first few weeks after successful liver transplantation. Haemolysis, at times requiring transfusion support, may occur 1 to 2 weeks postoperatively, most commonly in recipients of an ABO compatible, mismatched allograft. The haemolytic anaemia is the result of antirecipient isohaemagglutinins produced within the graft. Successful treatment has included transfusion, often using donor ABO group red blood cells, high dose steroids, and plasmapheresis during the typically transient period of haemolysis. Splenectomy has occasionally been required.

Another unusual haematological complication has been the development of aplastic anaemia in some patients who received a liver transplant for treatment of acute non-A, non-B viral hepatitis. The onset of aplastic anaemia has usually been within 1 to 6 months following transplantation and subsequent fatal infection is not infrequent. Some patients have had recovery of marrow function, either spontaneously or following antilymphocyte serum therapy, but the most effective therapeutic approach has not been defined.

Nutrition

Postoperative ileus usually resolves by the third or fourth day, after which progressive enteral alimentation is provided. In patients who remain obtunded, nasoenteric tube feedings are preferred to avoid the risks of aspiration. Some units routinely institute total parenteral nutrition in the immediate post-transplant period. Others, because of concerns over infection from the central line, reserve this approach for the few patients whose gastrointestinal tract cannot be used.

Neurological and psychiatric complications

Seizures and other neurological or psychiatric disorders, such as persistent obtundation, expressive aphasia, confusion, and transient psychoses, are common after liver transplantation. Some of the identified aetiological factors have included air embolism, cerebral oedema, intracranial bleeding, electrolyte disturbances, cyclosporin toxicity, and sleep deprivation. Air embolism has seldom been seen since the importance of flushing the liver prior to revascularization was recognized. Hypomagnesaemia and hypocholesterolaemia have been implicated as contributing factors in seizures associated with cyclosporin therapy and thus should be corrected when present. In patients with recurrent seizures, many centres prefer to replace cyclosporin with an antilymphocyte serum preparation until the patient stabilizes in the later postoperative period. Acute treatment for seizures is usually with diazepam or phenobarbital. Tegretol therapy is usually satisfactory for chronic prophylaxis. We try to avoid the repeated use of phenobarbitol or long-term dilantin administration because of the induction of cytochrome P-450 microsomal enzyme systems which rapidly decrease blood concentrations of immunosuppressive agents. An important aspect of these patients' care is the avoidance of excessively frequent monitoring of night-time vital signs and medication administration so the patient can have appropriate periods of sleep.

General surgical care

The perihepatic drains are removed, usually within 48 h following transplantation, except for the one at the portal area. This drain is left in place until cholangiography, 7 to 10 days postoperatively, confirms the integrity of the biliary anastomosis. The T-tube stent is usually tied off at this point and then left in place for 4 to 6 months. Earlier removal not infrequently leads to bile spillage and localized peritonitis due to the lack of a well-healed exit tract around the T-tube.

Immunosuppression and rejection

Conventional immunosuppressive regimens most commonly use a combination of cyclosporin, azathioprine, and steroids. Our protocol includes intravenous cyclosporin (4–5 mg/kg.day) started on the day of surgery with oral cyclosporin (10–12 mg/kg. day) being added as soon as it can be tolerated postoperatively. It is generally impossible to achieve therapeutic blood levels of the drug with oral therapy alone during the period of external biliary drainage. Methylprednisolone or prednisone is tapered by 40 mg decrements over 5 days from 200 mg/day to an initial maintenance level of 20 mg/day. Azathioprine is initiated at a loading dose of 5 mg/kg and then continued at 1 to 2 mg/kg. day. In patients with early renal dysfunction, we substitute OKT3 monoclonal antibody for cyclosporin during the period of oliguria (Fig. 11). More recently, some centres have replaced cyclosporin with the new macrolide antibiotic, FK506, with initial encouraging results.

Despite induction immunosuppression, 40 to 60 per cent of liver allograft recipients suffer one or more rejection episodes, usually beginning 5 to 14 days post-transplantation. Typical biochemical and clinical criteria suggesting rejection are listed in Table 7. Differentiating rejection from other disorders, such as allograft ischaemia, technical complications, or infection, can be difficult, and biopsy confirmation is frequently required. Histopathological changes of acute rejection include mononuclear cell infiltrates of portal tracts, subendothelial cells invading portal or central veins, cholestasis, bile duct damage, and variable hepatocellular necrosis. With more chronic rejection, manifested clinically by cholestatic jaundice, the hepatic artery intima is infiltrated by foamy macrophages which produce considerable narrowing of the vessel lumen. Interlobular bile ducts are often reduced in number and excess fibrosis appears in portal tracts. Unfortunately, many of the biopsy findings can also result from other conditions including cholangitis and viral hepatitis. Thus,

Table 7 Indicators of hepatic allograft rejection

Clinical
Fever
Right upper quadrant pain, back pain, anorexia, ascites,
Decreased bile output and bile pigment
Biochemical
Elevated serum bilirubin
Elevated transaminase
Elevated alkaline phosphatase
Elevated WBC
Cholangiogram
No leak
No obstruction
Doppler ultrasound
No collections
No ductal dilatation
Patent vessels
Biopsy
Portal inflammation
Hepatocellular necrosis
Endotheliitis

the ultimate diagnosis must take into consideration the entire constellation of clinical, biochemical, and histopathological findings lest overtreatment of multiple suspected rejection episodes exposes the patient to unacceptable risks of infection.

Rejection episodes are initially treated with increased steroid doses. If satisfactory reversal does not ensue, OKT3 monoclonal antibody or other antilymphocyte preparations are added to the regimen. FK506 may also prove to be effective in reversing rejection which has proved unresponsive to conventional therapy. As previously noted, retransplantation may be the only recourse for some patients with relentless chronic rejection.

The intensive immunosuppression required in these debilitated patients, who not infrequently also suffer technical complications, provides an ideal setting for invasive infection. The overall incidence of infection has been reported to range from 45 to 80 per cent, which greatly exceeds that observed in recipients of other solid organ allografts. These complications are the major source of morbidity and the most common cause of death in liver transplant recipients.

The major infections likely to be encountered are summarized in Table 8. Infections occurring in the early postoperative period may arise from agents transmitted with the allograft, pre-existing recipient conditions, or the typical bacterial complications of surgery. With currently employed donor screening for hepatitis B surface antigen and hepatitis C or HIV antibodies, transmission of these conditions has been essentially eliminated. More problematic are bacterial or Candida infections acquired during the preprocurement care of the donor. If terminal cultures become positive, intensive antimicrobial therapy is added to the routine perioperative antibiotic regimen. As noted above, patients with uncontrolled extrahepatic infection should be excluded from consideration for transplantation. In addition, some centres recommend selective bowel decontamination, particularly with respect to fungi, for potential liver recipients. Because of the uncertainty of the timing of the procedure, however, this approach is rarely practical, and post-transplant enteric administration of antifungal preparations is more commonly advised.

Table 8 Aetiology of common infections observed following liver transplantation

- I. Procedure related—usually bacterial
  - A. Transmission with the allograft
  - B. Technical complications (bleeding, vascular thrombosis, biliary problems)
  - C. Monitoring or infusion catheter contamination
  - D. Pulmonary complications (atelectasis, aspiration, pleural effusions)
  - E. Skin breakdown
- II. Hospital-related environmental hazards
  - A. *Aspergillus fumigatis*
  - B. Legionella
  - C. *Nocardia asteroides*
  - D. Bacterial colonization of nursing unit (Pseudomonas, Serratia, Staphylococcus)
- III. Community-related environmental hazards
  - A. Geographically limited (Histoplasmosis, Coccidioides, Blastomyces)
  - B. Ubiquitous saprophytes (Pneumocystis, Aspergillus, Cryptococcus, Nocardia)
  - C. Food, water contamination (*Listeria monocytogenes*, Salmonella)
- IV. Excessive immunosuppression or infection reactivation
  - A. Herpes group viruses
  - B. Hepatitis B, C
  - C. HIV
  - D. Influenza
  - E. *Mycobacterium tuberculosis*

Postoperative bacterial complications have most commonly been pneumonitis, abdominal or wound abscesses, or diffuse sepsis. The vast majority of these have been associated with technical complications, such as bleeding, arterial thrombosis, or biliary anastomotic problems. During the later (after 1 month) post-transplant period, viral and other opportunistic infections become more prevalent. Herpes group viruses are the most common: cytomegalovirus has been observed in 70 to 100 per cent of recipients, herpes simplex in approximately one-half, and herpes zoster in 5 per cent. Fortunately, the introduction of ganciclovir therapy has greatly reduced the morbidity and mortality due to these agents. Infection with the Epstein-Barr virus can produce conditions ranging from an infectious mononucleosis syndrome to a life-threatening lymphoproliferative disease similar to, or progressing to, B-cell lymphoma. This syndrome may regress if immunosuppressive dosages are decreased. Some groups recommend additional acyclovir therapy. As discussed above, reappearance of hepatitis B surface antigen is common in patients receiving liver transplants following hepatitis B. No effective therapy has been identified but the clinical course of the disease is not rapidly progressive in all patients. Interferon therapy appears to be effective in some patients who develop hepatitis C postoperatively.

Opportunistic infections are usually manifested as a primary infection of the lungs, most commonly due to Cryptococcus, Aspergillus, or Nocardia. During this later time period, pneumonitis caused by the protozoan *Pneumocystis carinii*, may also appear. Since these infections may progress rapidly or spread to other sites, aggressive efforts to identify the aetiologic agent and treat the infection are essential. These include examination of induced sputum, bronchoscopic brushings or biopsy, or even open lung biopsy, if necessary, to isolate the causative agent.

RESULTS AND REHABILITATION

As noted above, current overall success rates after liver transplantation in the current era are over 70 per cent at 1 year, with experienced centres reporting 5-year survival of approximately 60 per cent (Fig. 12). The expected long-term survival for these previously untreatable patients now exceeds that provided by modern care for many other commonly encountered conditions, including myocardial infarction and most solid tumours. Most deaths occur in the first 3 months after liver transplantation, early graft dysfunction or infection being the most common causes of failure

Table 9 Causes of death after liver transplantation

	Early (<3 months) (%)	Late (4–36 months) (%)
Infection	6	5
Hepatic failure	5	2
Technical complications	4	1
Rejection	2	3
Haemorrhage	2	–
Recurrent disease	1	3
Total	20	14

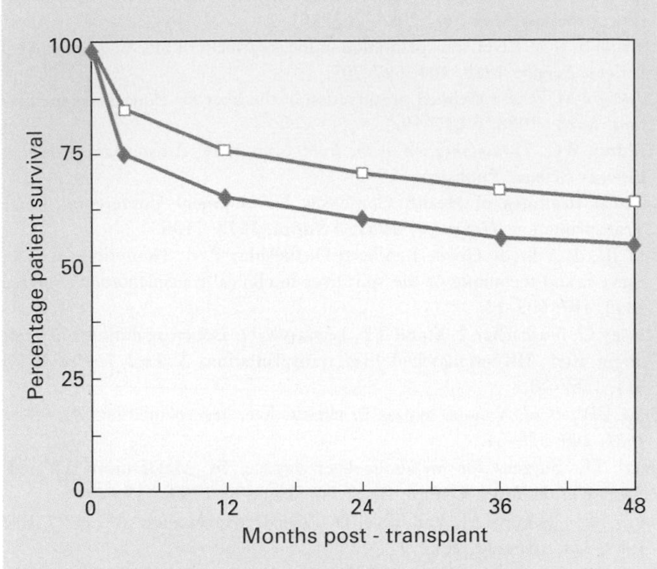

Fig. 12 Patient survival following orthotopic liver transplantation at Massachusetts General Hospital. Overall long-term survival since the programme's inception approximates 60 per cent. With increased experience and better definition of appropriate contraindications to transplantation the more recent survival rate continues to improve. □ 1986–90 (85 transplantations, 79 patients). ◆ 1983–90 (105 transplantations, 99 patients).

(Table 9). Rehabilitation in the majority of surviving patients is almost always excellent. In children, this includes a return of physical health and resumption of normal growth and development. In addition, emotional well being is restored so that these young recipients typically return almost immediately to their normally expected school level. Adult recipients are similarly able to return to a productive place in society: over 80 per cent resume their previous occupations or life-style and usually report that their performance is even more effective because of improved stamina and mental clarity.

Rehabilitation may be significantly delayed in some patients by the complications of osteoporosis which are commonly associated with chronic liver disease. Despite successful transplantation, the severe osteopenia which had developed preoperatively, consequent to altered vitamin D metabolism, may result in compression fractures, back pain, and prolonged disability. This condition generally stabilizes within 3 to 6 months following transplantation but again emphasizes the importance of the timely consideration of liver replacement before such secondary complications become too advanced.

Other limitations to complete rehabilitation include the side-effects of long-term immunosuppression, particularly nephrotoxicity and hypertension, development of recurrent or *de novo* malignancies, as may occur in all immunosuppressed patients, and chronic rejection, which may require retransplantation.

Because of the relatively recent development of liver transplantation, precise survival expectations beyond 5 years have not yet been established. Nevertheless, some of the earlier patients have now survived for over 20 years. Death in patients who survived at least 5 years after transplantation has occurred only rarely in such recipients. This suggests the prognosis for the 60 per cent of recipients currently expected to survive 5 years is indeed excellent.

CONCLUSIONS AND FUTURE OF LIVER TRANSPLANTATION

Liver transplantation has now come of age. The operation is technically difficult and many patients are in poor condition when they are referred for transplantation. Nevertheless, the procedure provides a chance for long-term survival and excellent rehabilitation for more than half of a group of patients whose lifespan would be measured in terms of months with any other therapy currently available. The identification of more selective and efficacious immunosuppression together with better means of preserving the donor allograft have been two of the most important factors that have made transplantation the preferred therapy for selected patients with end-stage cirrhosis or unresectable cancer limited to the liver.

Now that acceptable survival results have moved the procedure from the experimental arena to a truly therapeutic modality, other factors limiting its more widespread application must be addressed. The first of these is the question of cost effectiveness. The average cost of a liver transplant has been estimated to be between 100 000 and 200 000 US dollars. In fact, these costs probably do not greatly exceed those required to care otherwise for many chronically ill patients with advanced liver disease. These would include loss of income, costs of disability, medications, hospital admissions, palliative surgical procedures, and, predictably, terminal care. Nevertheless, new medical approaches such as organ transplantation, are constantly reviewed in terms of whether the funds being allocated, despite providing life-saving treatment, might not be more justifiably spent in other areas. In a dramatic example of the type of painful decision necessitated by limited resources, one United States state legislature recently voted to discontinue payment for all extrarenal transplantation. The not unexpected nationwide reaction to the death of a 7-year-old boy who was denied a bone marrow transplant subsequently led to review of the decision and the attempt to provide compromise solutions. Whether effective solutions can be identified remains unclear.

Interestingly, questions regarding cost effectiveness are generally being asked only of new medical therapies. In part, this is the fault of the medical community, which perhaps should be more active in identifying areas of established therapy that should be re-evaluated. It was rather incongruous, for example, to note that in the same journal issue in which the above state legislative decision was reviewed, a report appeared which indicated that the cost of treatment for moderate hypertension is estimated to be as high as 20 000 to 30 000 US dollars per year of life saved. While it is natural for new medical approaches to be the most likely targets for cost containment, scrutiny will probably soon extend to routinely accepted practices. As has been established in patients with end-stage renal failure, the new approach (transplantation) may be found to provide not only a better quality of life but also a more cost effective long-term treatment than the alternative (dialysis).

The second major issue limiting liver transplantation is the inadequate supply of donor organs. Currently, some patients die while waiting for a suitable organ, yet allografts are successfully transplanted from fewer than one-third of the estimated 12 000 to 18 000 people who die yearly in the United States in circumstances that could make organ donation feasible. Clearly, new approaches are needed to increase the number of organs available for transplantation and to improve upon the utilization of those organs procured.

The extent to which clinical liver transplantation will be applied, therefore, will be greatly influenced, at least in the short term, by economic and ethical issues. Ultimately, new approaches, including the use of non-human donor organs and more specific immunosuppressive regimens (for example, FK506 or more selective monoclonal antibodies), will undoubtedly make the procedure not only more available but also more effective and economically attractive.

FURTHER READING

Asher N, Stock PG, Bumgardner GL, Payne WD, Najarian JS. Infection and rejection of primary hepatic transplant in 93 consecutive patients treated with triple immunosuppressive therapy. *Surg Gynecol Obstet* 1988; **167**: 474–84.

Bismuth H, *et al.* Hepatic transplantation in Europe. *Lancet* 1987; **ii**: 674–6.

Brems JJ, Hiatt JR, Ramming KP, Quinones-Baldrich WJ, Busuttil RW. Fulminant hepatic failure: the role of liver transplantation as primary therapy. *Am J Surg* 1987; **154**: 137–41.

Broelsch CE, *et al.* Liver transplantation including the concept of reduced-size liver transplants in children. *Ann Surg* 1988; **208**: 410–20.

Calne RY. *Liver transplantation: the Cambridge/King's College Hospital experience.* 2nd edn. Orlando, Florida: Grune and Stratton, 1987.

Cosimi AB, Cho SI, Delmonico FL, Kaplan MM, Rohrer RJ, Jenkins RL. A randomized clinical trial comparing OKT3 and steroids for treatment of hepatic allograft rejection. *Transplantation* 1987; **43**: 91–5.

Cosimi AB, Jenkins RL, Rohrer RJ, Delmonico FL, Hoffman M, Monaco AP. Randomized clinical trial of prophylactic OKT3 monoclonal antibody in liver allograft recipients. *Arch Surg* 1990; **125**: 781–5.

Delmonico FL, *et al.* Procurement of a whole pancreas and liver from the same cadaveric donor. *Surgery* 1989; **105**: 718–23.

Evans RW. Cost-effectiveness analysis of transplantation. *Surg Clin North Am* 1986; **66**: 603–16.

Iwatsuki S, Gordon RD, Shaw BW, Starzl TE. Role of liver transplantation in cancer therapy. *Ann Surg* 1985; **202**: 401–7.

Iwatsuki S, *et al.* Liver transplantation in the treatment of bleeding esophageal varices. *Surgery* 1988; **104**: 697–705.

Kalayoghi M, *et al.* Extended preservation of the liver for clinical transplantation. *Lancet* 1988; **i**: 617–19.

Maddrey WC. *Transplantation of the liver.* New York, Amsterdam, London: Elsevier Science Publishers, 1988.

National Institutes of Health Consensus Development Conference. Liver Transplantation. *Hepatology* 1983; **4 Suppl**: 107S–110S.

Otte JB, de Ville de Goyet J, Alberti D, Balladur P, de Hemptinne B. The concept and technique of the split liver in clinical transplantation. *Surgery* 1990; **107**: 605–12.

Ramsey G, Nusbacher J, Starzl TE, Lindsay GD. Isohemagglutinins of graft origin after ABO-unmatched liver transplantation. *N Engl J Med* 1984; **311**: 1167–70.

Shaw BW, *et al.* Venous bypass in clinical liver transplantation. *Ann Surg* 1984; **200**: 524–34.

Starzl TE. Surgery for metabolic liver disease. In: McDermott WV, ed. *Surgery of the Liver.* Oxford: Blackwell Scientific, 1989: 127–36.

Starzl TE, Demetris AJ, Van Thiel D. Liver transplantation. *N Engl J Med* 1989; **321**: 1014–22, 1092–9.

Starzl TE, Iwatsuki S, Shaw BW, Gordon RD, Esquvel CO. Immunosuppression and other nonsurgical factors in the improved results of liver transplantation. *Semin Liver Dis* 1985; **5**: 334–43.

Starzl TE, *et al.* Evolution of liver transplantation. *Hepatology* 1982; **2**: 614–36.

Tarter RE, Erbs S, Biller PA, Switala JA, Van Thiel DH. The quality of life following liver transplantation. *Gastroenterol Clin North Am* 1988; **17**: 207–17.

Terpstra OT, Reuvers CB, Schalm SW. Auxiliary heterotopic liver transplantation. *Transplantation* 1988; **45**: 1003–7.

Tzakis A, Todo S, Steiber A, Starzl TE. Venous jump grafts for liver transplantation in patients with portal vein thrombosis. *Transplantation* 1989; **48**: 530.

Wall WJ. Liver transplantation: current concepts. *Can Med Assoc J* 1988; **139**: 21–8.

Williams JW, Peters TG, Vera SR, Britt LG, van Voorst SJ, Haggitt RC. Biopsy-directed immunosuppression following hepatic transplantation in man. *Transplantation* 1985; **391**: 589–96.

10.7 Heart and heart–lung transplantation

GEORGE V. LETSOU AND JOHN C. BALDWIN

HEART TRANSPLANTATION

History

Cardiac transplantation has become a useful treatment for a variety of patients with end-stage cardiac failure, offering such patients their only chance for dramatic improvement. The procedure has been used much more often in the past decade. More than 80 per cent of all heart transplants have been performed since 1984 and in 1990 more than 3000 were performed worldwide.

Pioneering work in cardiac transplantation was undertaken by Carrel and Guthrie in the early 1900s. In their heterotopic canine cardiac transplant model, a transplanted heart beat for approximately 2 h. The Soviet surgeon Demikhov, working in the 1950s, successfully performed 'heterotopic' canine cardiac transplants in which the donor heart was placed intrathoracically without removal of the native heart; he demonstrated the donor heart's ability to support the recipient by exclusion of the native heart from the circulation. Further advances followed the perfection of cardiopulmonary bypass techniques. The first successful long-term experimental 'orthotopic' cardiac transplants (in which the native heart is excised and replaced by the donor heart) were performed by Lower and Shumway in 1960; five of eight dogs survived for 6 to 21 days. They emphasized the need for excision of donor and recipient hearts at mid-atrial level, safe cardiopulmonary bypass, and topical hypothermia for cardiac preservation during excision and implantation. The first clinical cardiac transplant was performed in 1964 when Hardy and associates transplanted the heart of a chimpanzee into a human recipient, who lived for several hours. The first successful human to human orthotopic cardiac transplant was performed by Barnard in December, 1967 using techniques derived from laboratory work at Stanford University. The first cardiac transplant at Stanford was carried out 1 month later. Barnard's operation was sensational, widely publicized, and led to many other attempts. However, the results of many additional cardiac transplants performed in 1968 were dismal. Enthusiasm for the operation abated and in 1970 only 20 transplants were performed. Through persistent efforts in the 1970s, largely at Stanford University, improvements in recipient and donor selection, surgical technique, diagnosis of rejection, and postoperative care were achieved. A dramatic improvement in survival rates followed development of techniques for distant graft procurement in the mid-1970s and the introduction of the immunosuppressant cyclosporin in 1980. Presently, in excess of 3000 cardiac transplants are performed worldwide each year demonstrating the procedure's remarkable resurgence and success.

Current status and techniques

Recipient selection

Appropriate recipient selection is critical for optimal results. Recipients should have end-stage heart disease and a life expectancy of 6 to 12 months (i.e. New York Heart Association Class III or IV). All modes of conventional medical and surgical management should have been exhausted. Recipients are usually less than 60 years of age and without other irreversible systemic illness or organ dysfunction, not including prerenal azotaemia or passive hepatic congestion which are considered reversible. There should be no evidence of infection. All recipients should be emotionally stable, with a realistic attitude towards their illness, and must be able to comply with a rigid postoperative protocol requiring daily immunosuppressive medications for the remainder of their lives. These selection criteria were developed to identify the patient population most likely to survive and do well, given the limited supply of donor organs.

Relative contraindications include recent pulmonary infarction, insulin-dependent diabetes mellitus, and age 60 to 70. Recent pulmonary infarction is associated with an increased risk of haemorrhage during the systemic anticoagulation which is necessary for cardiopulmonary bypass. Insulin-dependent diabetes mellitus had been considered to increase morbidity, because an exacerbation of diabetes was expected with immunosuppressant steroids. However, recent reports indicate that cardiac transplantation can be successful in diabetics, although postoperative rejection episodes are more frequent. Although patients older than 60 have not traditionally been considered ideal recipients, cardiac transplantation is now being performed successfully in the 60- to 70-year-old age group.

Preoperative assessment of pulmonary vascular resistance is essential, since elevation increases perioperative mortality. The pulmonary vascular resistance is calculated during right heart catheterization (mean pulmonary artery pressure minus pulmonary capillary wedge pressure divided by the cardiac output in l/min) and should be less than 8 Wood units, as donor right ventricles are unable to function properly against higher pulmonary vascular resistance. During right heart catheterization, pulmonary vasodilators such as nitroprusside or prostaglandin E_1 may be administered in attempts to decrease the pulmonary vascular resistance. If resistance falls to less than 8 Wood units with such vasodilators, cardiac transplantation can be performed with acceptable mortality if similar vasodilators are administered in the postoperative period. Nevertheless, early and late mortality is increased; a 1 month mortality of 15 per cent and a 3 month mortality of approximately 50 per cent can be expected if baseline pulmonary vascular resistance is greater than 8 Wood units.

Idiopathic cardiomyopathy is currently the most common indication for cardiac transplantation and accounts for almost 50 per cent of the heart transplants performed yearly. Ischaemic coronary artery disease accounts for another 40 per cent of transplants. Less frequently, recipients suffer from valvular cardiac disease, congenital cardiac disease, or myocarditis. Approximately 3 per cent of transplants are repeat procedures performed for graft atherosclerosis. Much less common indications for cardiac transplantation include doxorubicin-induced cardiotoxicity, amyloidosis, Chagas' disease, cardiac tumours, and refractory arrhythmias.

Donor selection

Optimal results depend on proper donor selection. Appropriate donors are usually less than 45 years of age, have been certified brain dead by an appropriate physician under local laws, have not undergone prolonged cardiopulmonary resuscitation, and have normal electrocardiograms. Screening for communicable diseases such as HIV and hepatitis is performed routinely. No blood-borne infection should be present, although many donors have evidence of pulmonary bacterial colonization. If the status of the donor heart is questionable, further evaluation with central venous pressure monitoring, echocardiogram, or even coronary angiography may be necessary. If the potential donor suffered significant chest trauma, cardiac enzyme levels should be within normal limits.

Potential donors should not be less than 25 per cent of the recipient's weight. Relatively small donors are of greater concern when the pulmonary vascular resistance is elevated and larger donors should be sought since only more muscular hearts will be able to beat sufficiently strongly against the elevated resistance of the pulmonary bed. Care should also be taken when transplanting hearts from female donors into male recipients, as this has been associated with increased mortality.

Donors and recipients should be ABO blood group compatible. If a preoperative cyotoxic antibody screen using 50 to 100 random donor lymphocytes reveals more than 10 per cent to be cross-reactive, a preoperative lymphocyte cross-match is desirable. HLA matching is useful for research purposes. Retrospective analyses of grafts matched at the HLA-A and -B loci show slightly improved long-term survival and fewer infections, but no improvement in rejection rate, likelihood of death from rejection, or length of time to first episode of rejection. Donors and recipients matched for HLA-DR antigens have fewer episodes of rejection and also a slight increase in survival. However, these increases in survival are not sufficient to warrant preoperative HLA matching.

Operative technique

Donor and recipient operations have been largely standardized.

The donor operation is performed through a median sternotomy. If multiple organs are being procured, the chest portion of the operation is performed first or simultaneously with abdominal procedures. After the pericardium is opened, the heart is inspected for contusions or haematomas and is palpated to ensure absence of valvular or coronary artery abnormalities. Aorta, superior vena cava, and inferior vena cava are encircled and controlled. Once the abdominal viscera are dissected, preparations are made to remove all organs. The heart is removed first. Heparin is administered systemically and an ascending aortic cannula is placed for cardioplegia administration. The superior vena cava is ligated and divided. The inferior vena cava and left inferior pulmonary vein are incised, decompressing both ventricular chambers and preventing their distension. The heart is allowed to contract several times and empty completely. An aortic cross-clamp is then placed high on the ascending aorta, just proximal to the innominate artery, and cold crystalloid cardioplegia is infused via the ascending aortic cannula. Preservation is supplemented with topical cold saline. The heart is excised by dividing the aorta just proximal to the aortic cross-clamp; pulmonary veins and pulmonary arteries are divided at the pericardial reflection. The heart is packed in sterile saline at 4°C for transport. Other abdominal organs are subsequently harvested.

The recipient operation is also performed via median sternotomy. Aorta, superior vena cava, and inferior vena cava are encircled and controlled. After systemic heparinization, separate inferior and superior vena cavae cannulae are placed. The aorta is cannulated at the base of the innominate artery and cardiopulmonary bypass is initiated. Once the donor heart has arrived safely, systemic cooling to 26°C is initiated. An aortic cross-clamp and caval snares are applied. The native heart is excised at mid-atrial level. The aorta is divided just above the aortic annulus. The pulmonary artery is similarly divided at the supra-annular level and the native heart is removed. The donor heart is brought on to the operative field and is examined for a patent foramen ovale. The left atrium is opened with incisions connecting the pulmonary vein orifices. Aorta and pulmonary artery are separated. The heart is properly oriented and placed in the recipient's chest cavity. The left atrial anastomosis is performed first, with a running suture. Saline solution at 4°C is infused via an opening in the left atrial appendage and a similar solution is applied to the heart externally. The right atrial anastomosis is completed using running suture, and systemic rewarming is begun. The aortic anastomosis is completed and the cross-clamp is removed. The pulmonary artery anastomosis is completed with the heart beating. The pulmonary artery is decompressed and vented for at least 20 min prior to weaning the patient from cardiopulmonary bypass (allowing reperfusion of the new heart). Resuscitation with pressor support as necessary completes the procedure.

Immunosuppression

Many immunosuppressant regimens are currently in use, and most centres use at least three agents. Cyclosporin, a fungal metabolite, was introduced clinically in 1980 and is the mainstay of all regimens. Immediately before operation, 2 to 8 mg/kg are administered; a lower dose should be used in patients with renal insufficiency. The drug is continued indefinitely, maintaining a level of 200 to 300 ng/ml as measured by high pressure liquid chromatography. Nephrotoxicity is a common problem and renal function must be closely monitored.

Azathioprine has been used in all forms of transplantation as an antirejection treatment since the early 1960s. Currently, 2 to 5 mg/kg are given preoperatively, followed by a maintenance post-operative dose of 1 to 2 mg/kg.day. The white blood cell count must continuously be monitored: should this decrease or drop below 5000 cells/μl, the drug must be decreased in dosage or discontinued.

Corticosteroids are the third arm of most cardiac transplant immunosuppressive protocols. Many institutions give 500 mg of intravenous methylprednisolone on completion of the aortic anastomosis, and continue intravenous methylprednisolone for 24 h at a dose of 125 mg every 8 h. After 24 h, oral prednisone is started at a dose of 0.6 mg/kg.day and then tapered slowly over several weeks to a maintenance dose of 10 mg each day. Some institutions have successfully abandoned the use of steroids in maintenance immunosuppression, especially for children, because of their well known side-effects.

'Induction immunosuppression' with a fourth agent such as the monoclonal antibody OKT3 is gaining acceptance. Five milligrams of OKT3 are given each day during the initial 2 weeks following transplantation. Such four-drug regimens have decreased the frequency of rejection without increasing the likelihood of infection. No effect on overall survival has been documented.

Complications

In the first months following transplantation, rejection and infection are the most common complications: rejection accounts for 30 per cent of all deaths in cardiac transplant recipients and infections for 20 per cent. Seventy per cent of cardiac transplant recipients have an episode of rejection within the first 3 months after transplantation. After 1 year, the incidence of rejection decreases and less than 10 per cent of transplanted patients per year will have rejection episodes. The majority of rejection episodes respond to appropriate treatment. Approximately 50 per cent of recipients have an infection in the first year. The manifestations of severe systemic infection are often subtle, and monitoring for infection as well as for rejection is of paramount importance.

Rejection was difficult to diagnose in the early years, when a variety of criteria were used, including loss of QRS voltage, occurrence of supraventricular arrhythmias, and clinical signs of low cardiac output. The technique of endomyocardial biopsy revolutionized cardiac transplantation, allowing early treatment of rejection and improving survival. In the early postoperative period, endomyocardial biopsies are performed weekly. After 1 to 2 months, the frequency can be decreased. Usually, access to the right ventricular septal biopsy site is via the right internal jugular vein. Under fluoroscopic guidance, a biopsy forceps is manoeuvred to the septal region and at least four samples are obtained for pathological analysis. Right ventricular pressures and cardiac output are measured. Several scales have been developed for grading rejection: those most often used include the 'Texas system' and the 'Stanford system'. A new international grading system has recently been developed and is gaining acceptance (Table 1). The hallmark of rejection-requiring treatment is myocyte necrosis. An infiltrate of lymphocytes is indicative of lesser rejection; myocyte necrosis with extramyocardial haemorrhage is indicative of severe rejection and damage (Fig. 1).

If myocyte necrosis is detected, antirejection therapy should be begun immediately. Initial treatment at most centres is 1g of methylprednisolone intravenously for 3 days. Four days after

Table 1 A comparison of commonly used grading systems for rejection

Histologic findings	International grade	Stanford grade	Texas grade
No rejection	0	No rejection	0
Focal (perivascular or interstitial) infiltrate without necrosis	1A	Mild rejection	1
Diffuse but sparse infiltrate without necrosis	1B	Mild rejection	2 3
One focus only with aggressive infiltration and/or focal myocyte damage	2	Focal moderate	4 5
Multifocal aggressive infiltrates and/or myocate damage	3A	Low moderate	6 7
Diffuse inflammatory process with necrosis	3B	Borderline severe	8 9
Diffuse aggressive polymorphous infiltrate, ± oedema, ± haemorrhage, ± vasculitis, with necrosis	4	Severe acute	10

completion of this 'steroid pulse', endomyocardial biopsy is performed to assess treatment results. If significant rejection persists, monoclonal or polyclonal antibodies are administered. If rejection persists despite all treatments and progresses to haemodynamic instability, retransplantation should be considered. Since the introduction of cyclosporin, such refractory rejection has become uncommon.

Diagnosis of infection is difficult since immunosuppression obscures the usual manifestations, and findings are often subtle. Once infection is established, it can progress very rapidly and extremely aggressive, prompt treatment is necessary. An oral temperature over 100.5°F (38°C) must be considered presumptive evidence of infection despite the absence of clinical signs. Such a fever is an indication for thorough culturing, and aggressive evaluation.

Graft atherosclerosis is the most important late complication. It is felt to be a manifestation of chronic rejection based on immunological incompatibility, and manifests primarily as diffuse coronary artery narrowing. The distribution of coronary artery lesions is atypical in that most are distal lesions not amenable to treatment using conventional bypass or angioplasty techniques. Graft atherosclerosis is also atypical in that coronary artery lesions often develop extremely rapidly over several months. An association with cytomegalovirus infection has been documented, but antiviral treatment directed at this agent has not yet been shown to lessen the incidence of graft atherosclerosis. Retransplantation is the only therapeutic option.

Overall results

Cardiac transplantation is extremely effective for the treatment of end-stage cardiac failure. Survival rates in excess of 90 per cent at 1 year can be anticipated in younger patients with idiopathic or postpartum cardiomyopathies. An overall survival of 81 per cent at 1 year and 69 per cent at 5 years was documented by the registry of the International Society of Heart Transplantation in 1990 (see Fig. 2). Cardiac transplantation can no longer be considered experimental and should be offered to all patients who are appropriate candidates.

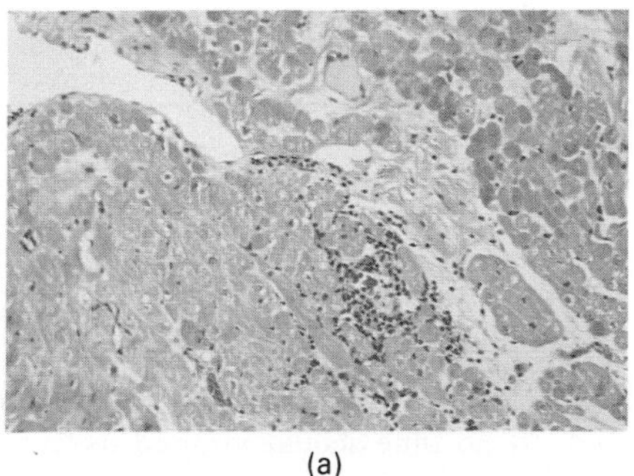

(a)

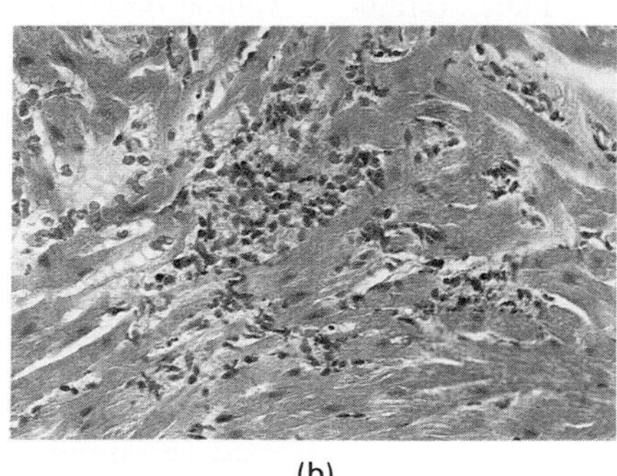

(b)

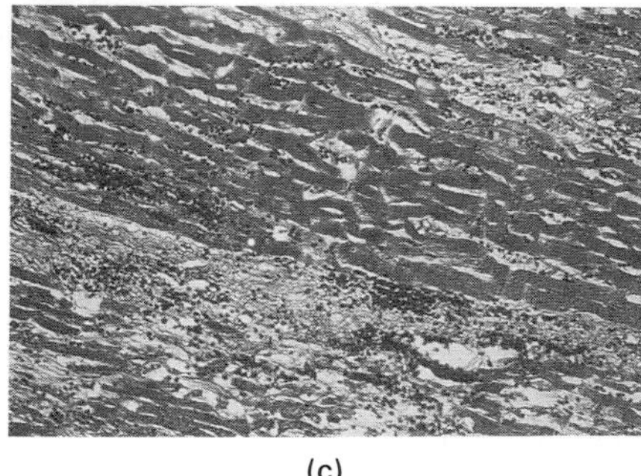

(c)

Fig. 1 Photomicrographs of endomyocardial biopsies. (a) Myocardial biopsy showing mild rejection. Note the perivascular infiltrates of lymphocytes. (b) Endomyocardial biopsy showing a moderate rejection with evidence of myocyte necrosis. Note the clusters of lymphocytes throughout the myocardial tissue with areas of myocyte destruction. (c) Endomyocardial biopsy specimen showing borderline severe rejection with a diffuse infiltrate of lymphocytes throughout the myocardium in one area in the upper left hand area of the total mycrograft showing diffuse and widespread myocyte destruction.

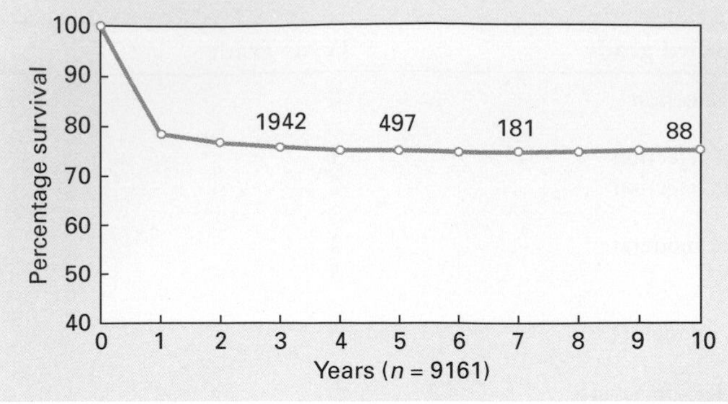

Fig. 2 Ten-year actuarial survival associated with orthotopic cardiac transplantation.

HEART–LUNG TRANSPLANTATION

History

The first attempts at cardiopulmonary transplantation date to the initial experiments of Carrel and Guthrie with cardiac transplantation. They performed heterotopic cardiopulmonary transplants in rats as early as 1905. Lower and Shumway performed canine cardiopulmonary transplants in conjunction with orthotopic cardiac transplants in the late 1950s and early 1960s. Canine cardiopulmonary transplants were complicated by the fact that dogs, unlike primates, require intact pulmonary innervation for normal respiratory function: subsequent experiments showed that primates could function normally with denervated lungs. The first human heart–lung transplant was performed in 1968 by Cooley in an infant who died after 14 h. With the development of successful cardiac transplantation at Stanford, further experimental work on cardiopulmonary transplantation as a means to circumvent the problem of elevated pulmonary vascular resistance resulted in the first successful clinical heart–lung transplantation programme in 1981. Since that time, cardiopulmonary transplantation has been initiated at many other centres. However, the donor pool for such transplants is small as both a normal heart and nearly perfect lungs are required. Thus, cardiopulmonary transplantation has not yet been as widely applied as cardiac transplantation.

CURRENT STATUS AND TECHNIQUES

Recipient selection

As in cardiac transplantation, appropriate recipient selection is critical. Recipients should be severely limited by their pulmonary and/or cardiac disease with a life expectancy of 6 to 12 months. All modes of conventional medical and surgical management should have been exhausted. However, transplantation of patients with end-stage disease requiring mechanical ventilation has rarely been successful. Generally, recipients should be less than 45 years of age and without other irreversible systemic illnesses or organ dysfunction, not including prerenal azotaemia or passive hepatic congestion which are considered reversible. Many potential recipients, especially those with cystic fibrosis, have evidence of pulmonary bacterial colonization, but there should be no active systemic infection. Mental stability is very important; all patients should be able to comply with a rigid postoperative immunosuppression protocol.

Previous full posterolateral thoracotomy is a contraindication to transplantation; this is associated with excessive bleeding after native heart–lung excision, which is difficult to control after implantation of the graft. More limited thoracotomies or previous open lung biopsy are relative contraindications. Recent pulmonary infarction is also associated with an increased risk of haemorrhage and is a relative contraindication. Insulin-dependent diabetes mellitus is a relative contraindication for the same reasons as in cardiac transplantation.

These criteria allow a substantial population to qualify for cardiopulmonary transplantation. As reported to the International Society for Heart Transplantation in 1991, 33 per cent of heart–lung recipients had primary pulmonary hypertension and Eisenmenger's syndrome accounted for 30 per cent (this includes many patients ineligible for orthotopic cardiac transplant due to combined end-stage left ventricular failure and elevated pulmonary vascular resistance). Cystic fibrosis accounted for 14 per cent of cardiopulmonary transplants and emphysema accounted for 7 per cent.

Donor selection

Criteria for the selection of appropriate donors are similar to those for cardiac transplantation, but, in addition, heart–lung transplant donors must have a Po_2 greater than 100 mmHg on 40 per cent inspired oxygen, normal lung compliance with a peak inspiratory pressure less than 30 to 35 mmHg, no major thoracic trauma, and a clear chest radiograph. Any history of smoking should be carefully evaluated. There should be no evidence of pulmonary bacterial colonization on sputum Gram stain or culture. A history of lung disease is unacceptable. These criteria are fairly strict due to problems inherent in pulmonary preservation and severely limit the donor pool. However, such criteria are essential if good clinical results are to be obtained.

Operative technique

Donor operation

Since pulmonary preservation is the limiting factor in cardiopulmonary transplantation, the donor operation assumes paramount importance. Throughout the donor procedure, the lungs must be carefully protected. At no time should inspired oxygen be greater than 40 per cent: if it is necessary to increase inspired oxygen above 40 per cent to maintain a Po_2 greater than 100 mmHg, consideration should be given to aborting the transplant. With the advent of multiorgan procurements, good communication between all procurement teams and the anaesthesiologist is essential. As little fluid as possible should be administered intravenously, as the lungs will not be able to clear fluid easily after transplantation. Heart–lung procurement is performed by median sternotomy. The pericardium is opened, the heart inspected and palpated, both anterior pleura incised, and the lungs inspected for contusion or haematoma. The aorta and both vena cavae are encircled and controlled. The main-stem trachea is controlled between the superior vena cava and the ascending aorta. After completion of the abdominal dissection, preparations are made to excise the heart–lung block. After systemic heparinization, a cannula for administration of cardioplegia is placed in the ascending aorta. A cannula is placed in the pulmonary artery for the administration of 'pulmoplegia' (modified Collins' solution with magnesium sulphate and dextrose added) after aortic occlusion. For 15 min prior to aortic occlusion, prostaglandin E_1 is administered intravenously in a slowly increasing dose from 20 ng/kg.min to 150 ng/kg.min. The superior vena cava is then ligated and divided. The inferior vena cava and left atrial appendage are incised, decompressing both ventricular chambers. The heart is allowed to contract several times and empty completely. The aorta is cross-clamped just below the innominate artery; cold crystalloid cardioplegia is infused through the ascending aortic root cannula and pulmoplegia is administered via the pulmonary artery cannula while gentle lung ventilation is continued, ensuring adequate pulmoplegia distribution. Preservation is supplemented with topical cold saline. The heart–lung block is excised beginning in the posterior mediastinum just anterior to the esophagus. The dissection is carried up the oesophagus from the diaphragm to the main-stem trachea. The aorta is divided just below the cross-clamp. The lungs are inflated to half their total volume and a stapling device placed across the main-stem trachea at least two cartilagenous rings above the carina. The heart–lung block is transported to the recipient at 4°C.

Recipient operation

A median sternotomy is used for the recipient operation. Safe removal of the native organs is technically challenging. Great care must be taken to protect phrenic, recurrent laryngeal, and vagus nerves. The aorta is cannulated at the base of the innominate artery; separate inferior and superior vena cavae cannulae are placed. After the donor organs have arrived safely, cardiopulmonary bypass is initiated. Atria are divided at the mid-atrial level, the aorta is divided at the supra-annular level, and the main pulmonary artery is divided. The native heart is removed. Pericardial pedicles preserving the phrenic nerves are created. A 3-cm cuff of pericardium is left anterior to the phrenic nerves, and the posterior incision for the phrenic pedicle is made just anterior to the pericardial reflection of the pulmonary veins. An incision is made in the remaining left atrium to separate the pulmonary veins from the posterior mediastinum. Care must be taken to avoid vagus nerve injury. After division of the left pulmonary ligament, bronchial collaterals to the native lung are divided and the bronchus is transected using a stapling device. The left lung is removed. The right lung is explanted in a similar fashion. At the procedure's conclusion, two pedicles containing the uninjured phrenic nerves remain.

The donor heart–lung block is then prepared for implantation. The tracheal staple line is excised and specimens of donor trachea are obtained for culture. A curvilinear incision is made in the right atrium, avoiding sinoatrial node injury. The recipient trachea is divided two or three rings above the carina in preparation for anastomosis to the donor, which is performed end-to-end using a running polypropylene suture. Right atrial and aortic anastomoses are performed sequentially with running suture, as in orthotopic cardiac transplantation. The new organs are reperfused for 20 to 30 min with the pulmonary artery decompressed and vented. Weaning from cardiopulmonary bypass is performed with resuscitation of the new heart and lungs, using pressors as necessary. Care must be taken to avoid administration of oxygen in excess of 40 per cent as the newly implanted lungs are exquisitely sensitive to oxygen. Early extubation is critical. Surgical interruption of pulmonary lymphatic drainage makes rigorous fluid restriction, early patient mobilization, and meticulous attention to respiratory care essential in the early postoperative period.

Immunosuppression

Immunosuppressant regimens are similar to those used in cardiac transplantation. However, following the initial dose of methylprednisolone steroids are administered for only 24 h. No further steroids are given for 3 weeks, while tracheal healing progresses. After 3 weeks, oral prednisone, 0.5 mg/kg.day, is begun and slowly tapered to 10 mg/day.

As in other solid organ transplants, cyclosporin is the mainstay of treatment. It is administered prior to operation in a dose of 2 to 8 mg/kg and then continued indefinitely in doses adequate to maintain a level of 200 to 300 ng/ml by high pressure liquid chromotography. Recipients must be monitored closely for nephrotoxicity.

Azathioprine is administered in a fashion similar to that in isolated cardiac transplantation. Some 2 to 5 mg/kg are given preoperatively; maintenance dosing at 1 to 2 mg/kg.day is instituted while the white blood cell count is monitored. During the initial postoperative period most centres administer another agent, such as rabbit antilymphocyte globulin, for additional protection in the period when steroids are not administered. Administration of OKT3 is not advocated because of its association with pulmonary oedema.

Complications

Technical complications are more common following cardiopulmonary transplantation than after cardiac transplantation. Operative mortality for heart–lung transplantation is still in excess of 10 per cent, as reported to the International Society for Heart Transplantation in 1991. Thirty per cent of deaths after cardiopulmonary transplantation can be attributed to technical causes, primarily bleeding and phrenic nerve injury. As experience increases, these complications are diminishing.

Rejection and infection are common, as in isolated cardiac transplantation. Twenty per cent of deaths are due to rejection and 30 per cent to infection.

Cardiac and pulmonary rejection may occur simultaneously or asynchronously. Cardiac rejection is less common than in patients undergoing isolated cardiac transplantation, although the reasons for this are unclear. Routine endomyocardial biopsy is, therefore, performed less frequently: usually, one or two endomyocardial biopsies are performed in the first month and subsequently only as clinically indicated. Cardiac rejection is graded using the previously described scales and is treated in the same fashion as isolated cardiac transplants. Pulmonary rejection is difficult to diagnose accurately. Although routine transbronchial endoscopic biopsies are performed at some centres, these have not yet demonstrated the same reliability as endomyocardial biopsies. Other techniques to detect rejection include broncheoalveolar lavage and radionuclide perfusion scanning, neither of which detects rejection reliably. The most reliable indicator of pulmonary rejection currently available is the appearance on chest radiograph, taken in conjunction with clinical suspicion of rejection and pulmonary function testing. If infiltrates develop that are not responsive to antibiotics or antiviral therapies, rejection must be considered and treated presumptively. Despite aggressive treatment of pulmonary rejection, bronchiolitis obliterans, a form of chronic rejection resulting in severely diminished lung function and a pattern of increased interstitial markings on chest radiograph, remains a formidable problem.

As in isolated cardiac transplantation, the diagnosis of infection is made with aggressive evaluation of any fever greater than 100.5°F (38°C) orally. Signs of infection are often subtle and appropriate treatment can only be instituted early if attempts at diagnosis are prompt and thorough.

Overall results

Combined heart–lung transplant is an effective treatment for primary pulmonary hypertension, Eisenmenger's syndrome, and cystic fibrosis. A survival rate in excess of 70 per cent can be expected at 1 year. Five-year survival data is not yet reliable, but is about 60 per cent.

FURTHER READING

Armstage JM, Hardesty RL, Griffith BP. Prostaglandin E_1: an effective treatment of right heart failure after orthotopic heart transplantation. *J Heart Transplant* 1987; **6**: 347–51.

Baldwin JC, *et al.* Distant graft procurement for combined heart and lung transplantation using pulmonary artery flush and simple topical hypothermia for graft preservation. *Ann Thoracic Surg* 1987; **43**: 670–3.

Barnard CN. The operation. A human cardiac transplant: an interim report of a successful operation performed at Groote-Schuur Hospital, Cape Town. *S Afr Med J* 1967; **41**: 1271–4.

Billingham ME. The postsurgical heart: the pathology of cardiac transplantation. *Am J Cardiovasc Pathol* 1988; **1**: 319–34.

Bristow MR, *et al.* OKT3 monoclonal antibody in heart transplantation. *Am J Kidney Dis* 1988; **11**: 135–40.

Burke CM, *et al.* Twenty-eight cases of human heart–lung transplantation. *Lancet* 1986; **i**: 517–19.

Frist WH, Oyer PE, Baldwin JC, Stinson EB, Shumway NE. HLA compatibility and cardiac transplant recipient survival. *Ann Thoracic Surg* 1987; **44**: 242–6.

Glanville AR, Imoto E, Baldwin JC, Billingham ME, Theodore J, Robin ED. The role of right ventricular endomyocardial biopsy in the long-term management of heart–lung transplant recipients. *J Heart Transpl* 1987; **6**: 357–61.

Grattan MT, Moreno-Cabral CE, Starnes VA, Oyer PE, Stinson EB, Shumway NE. Cytomegalovirus infection is associated with cardiac allograft rejection and atherosclerosis. *JAMA* 1989; **261**: 3561–6.

Higenbottam T, Stewart S, Penketh A, Wallwork J. Transbronchial lung biopsy for the diagnosis of rejection in heart–lung transplant patients. *Transplantation* 1988; **46**: 532–9.

Hunt SA, Schroeder JS. Managing patients after cardiac transplantation. *Hosp Practice* 1989; **24**: 83–100.

Kirklin JK, Naftel DC, Kirklin JW, Blackstone EH, White-Williams C, Bourge RC. Pulmonary vascular resistance and the risk of heart transplantation. *J Heart Transpl* 1988; **7**: 331–6.

Kreitt JM, Kaye MP. The Registry of the International Society for Heart and Lung Transplantation: eighth official report—1991. *J Heart Lung Transpl* 1991; **10**: 491–8.

Lower RR, Shumway NE. Studies on orthotopic transplantation of the canine heart. *Surg Forum* 1960; **11**: 18–29.

Pfeffer PF, Foerster A, Froysaker T, Simonsen S, Thorsby E. HLA-DR mismatch and histologically evaluated rejection episodes in cardiac transplants can be correlated. *Transplant Proc* 1988; **20**: 367–8.

Renlund DG, O'Connell JB, Gilbert EM, Watson FS, Bristow MR. Feasibility of discontinuation of corticosteroid maintenance therapy in heart transplantation. *J Heart Transpl* 1987; **6**: 71–8.

Rhenman MJ, Rhenman B, Icenogle T, Christensen R, Copeland J. Diabetes and heart transplantation. *J Heart Transpl* 1988; **7**: 356–458.

10.8.1 Experimental small bowel transplantation

ANDREW C. GORDON

INTRODUCTION

The era of experimental small bowel transplantation was heralded by the seminal paper of Dr Alexis Carrell, who in 1902 successfully transplanted segments of canine small bowel with vascular anastomoses to the great vessels of the neck. In 1959 Lillehei *et al.* successfully autografted autograft canine small bowel, using the mesenteric vessels to revascularize the bowel, whilst the first rodent model was described by Monchik and Russell in 1971.

The increasing technical success of renal transplantation in the late 1960s led to the establishment of several experimental small bowel transplantation programmes, but enthusiasm waned following the failure of all clinical attempts in humans. Interest was only reawakened by the improved immunosuppression offered by cyclosporin A in preventing rejection of renal allografts in the early 1980s, and there is now considerable activity in this field, with more clinical trials of small bowel transplantation being reported. At present the over-riding clinical problem is acute rejection of the graft, but many other potential problems are being addressed in the laboratory. These include:

1. Methods of reducing the incidence of rejection;
2. Early diagnosis and effective treatment of rejection episodes;
3. Graft-versus-host disease. Intestinal transplants contain more immunocompetent cells than any other solid organ graft, and if rejection can be prevented, graft-versus-host disease may become a problem;
4. Absorptive function of the graft. This depends on functional integrity of the gut wall, adequate venous and lymphatic drainage, and the establishment of effective peristalsis;
5. Techniques for optimal preservation of the graft;
6. The significance of the portosystemic shunt resulting from venous drainage directly into the systemic circulation;
7. The maintenance of the 'barrier' function of the gut mucosa against external pathogens following transplantation.

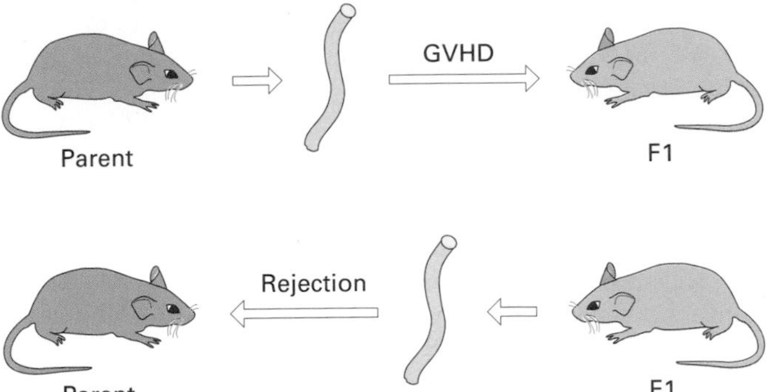

Fig. 1 Transplantation from parent to F1 hybrid results in graft-versus-host disease (GVHD) since host major histocompatibility antigens are recognized as foreign by the donor parental type lymphocytes transferred within the graft. Transplantation from F1 hybrid to parent results in rejection of the graft since major histocompatibility antigens displayed by the cells of the graft are recognized as foreign by recipient parental lymphocytes.

EXPERIMENTAL MODELS

Monchik and Russell used inbred rat strains and their F1 hybrid offspring (semiallogeneic combinations) to produce unopposed rejection or graft-versus-host disease (Fig.1). Recently there has been a tendency to study fully allogeneic models (in which both graft-versus-host disease and rejection may occur) as being more representative of the clinical situation. The use of mice has been limited to non-vascularized transplants of fetal tissue; pigs and dogs are used for studies in large animals. Fetal tissue can be transplanted as a non-vascularized graft, and is usually placed in the subcutaneous tissue of the back, from where it may subsequently be removed and anastomosed to the recipient's own gut. Although this allows the study of the immunological events following such a procedure, the relevance to clinical practice is limited.

Two basic experimental models of vascularized grafts are currently used: heterotopic, in which the ends of the graft are brought out to the skin of the anterior abdominal wall as a Thiry-Vella fistula, and orthotopic in which, after resection of most of the recipient's own gut, the proximal end of the graft is anastomosed to the recipient's duodenum and the distal end of the graft is anastomosed to the recipient's terminal ileum.

TECHNIQUES OF SMALL BOWEL TRANSPLANTATION

Part or all of the small intestine is removed, along with its vascular supply (portal vein and superior mesenteric artery with an aortic patch). The lumen is flushed to remove intestinal contents and the graft vasculature may be flushed with cooled saline. Using microvascular techniques, the donor aortic cuff is anastomosed to the recipient aorta. In the case of an orthotopic graft, venous drainage is established by anastomosis of the portal vein of the graft to that of the recipient. When the graft is placed heterotopically the venous drainage may either be into the recipient inferior vena cava or into the portal vein.

Portal venous drainage is favoured by some investigators: rat cardiac and renal allografts may show enhanced survival when venous drainage is directed into the portal circulation, and there is concern about the desirability of creating a portosystemic shunt in metabolically compromised patients. Whilst prolonged graft survival is documented in semiallogeneic rat models with portal venous drainage, this has not been observed in fully allogeneic combinations or in studies using larger animals. Present experimental evidence suggests that although metabolic disturbances can be detected if the venous drainage is into the systemic circulation, these may not be significant in clinical practice.

The recipient of an orthotopic graft depends on the transplanted gut for nutrition, making this model especially useful for nutritional and metabolic studies. The heterotopic model has the advantages that direct access to the graft lumen is possible via the stomata and that the nutritional state of the animal is independent of graft function. In the long term, however, the intestinal wall atrophies and the 'barrier' function of the mucosa is lost.

The technical failure rate of 10 to 30 per cent for small animal models is mostly due to vascular complications and intestinal anastomotic leaks. Despite the relative ease of creating vascular anastomoses in large animals, technical failure rates of 15 to 50 per cent are reported, to which intussusception and volvulus contribute significantly.

REJECTION

Histological examination of a rejecting graft at 6 to 7 days shows a diminution in the height of the villi and loss of villous epithelium. The brush border is lost and goblet cells are depleted. These changes are followed by widespread epithelial loss and infiltration of monocytes and macrophages into the lamina propria. Complete infiltration of the graft by inflammatory cells, with widespread destruction of the graft architecture, occurs by the ninth day. The nature of the infiltrating cells has been extensively studied using immunohistological techniques but the reported results are not particularly consistent.

There are several technical problems in the use of histology in both clinical and experimental practice. Firstly, a full thickness biopsy is essential if accurate assessment is to be made. Secondly, because of changes resulting from local trauma, biopsies from the stoma may not be representative of changes elsewhere. Thirdly, procurement of an adequate biopsy sample from the depths of the lumen of the graft may result in perforation and peritonitis. These problems have prompted the search for a simple, reliable, and rapid test to assess rejection. Although glucose, maltose, and xylose absorption are decreased during rejection, doubts have been expressed about the specificity of these observations and these changes are not seen until after the onset of histological evidence of rejection. The serum level of the mucosal enzyme *N*-acetyl hexosaminidase is increased during rejection, at the same time as or before the earliest detectable histological changes. This is a rapid biochemical assay which may prove to be useful in clinical practice. Intestinal absorption of low molecular weight polyethylene glycol (usually almost non-absorbable) can be assessed by measuring urinary levels. Increased levels are detected at the same time as or immediately before histological evidence of rejection becomes evident. The transmural potential difference across the graft wall is reduced during rejection. This decrease is apparent at the same time as the earliest histological changes. Monocyte procoagulant activity (a measure of the ability of peripheral blood monocytes to shorten the clotting time of human plasma) is enhanced during rejection and graft-versus-host disease, the effect just preceding histological changes. In rodents a simple and specific indicator of rejection which reliably precedes histological changes is the presence of an abdominal mass, caused by swelling of the graft and mesenteric lymph nodes.

LYMPHATIC AND NEURONAL RECONNECTION

A major concern (especially with regard to absorption of fat-soluble compounds such as cyclosporin A) is whether lymphatic drainage of intestinal allografts will be adequate. Studies in canine models have shown that lymphatic drainage commences at 2 weeks and is fully established by 4 weeks. In the rat drainage can be observed as early as 3 days after syngeneic transplantation, but full flow is not seen until 14 days. Drainage may be either by spontaneous lympholymphatic communication or development of lymphovenous anastomoses at the porta hepatis (as has been demonstrated in pigs).

It was shown in the 1960s that denervation of the canine intestine resulted in temporarily abnormal motility and gut function, whether the denervation resulted from autotransplantation or merely division of the splanchnic nerves. Myoelectrical activity returns on day 2 in unimmunosuppressed canine allografts and only ceases when the graft is destroyed by rejection. In immunosuppressed animals, however, electrical activity is maintained even in chronically rejected grafts. In canine allografts intraluminal pressure increases until day 6 or 7 and undergoes a marked reduction on day 8 post-transplantation, coinciding with the onset of overt rejection. In the rat, smooth muscle contractility and response to electrical stimulation and autonomic agonists is not impaired in syngeneic small bowel transplants. Since initiation and co-ordination of peristaltic activity takes place principally within the gut wall itself, it is likely that contractility and motility of small bowel transplants will be adequate (but not necessarily normal).

PREVENTION OF REJECTION

The effect of immunosuppressive regimens in the rat is very dependent on whether semi- or fully allogeneic strain combinations are used: it is much more difficult to obtain long-term survival in the latter. Prior to the introduction of cyclosporin A, conventional immunosuppression failed to prolong graft survival significantly in any model. Cyclosporin A monotherapy produces long-term survival, or at least marked prolongation of survival, in various semi-allogeneic and fully allogeneic rat models. The experience in large animal models has been less encouraging, with cyclosporin A significantly prolonging survival time, but producing few long-term dog or pig survivors. Whilst acute rejection is seen less often, chronic rejection is responsible for a considerable number of failures. The addition of other immunosuppressive agents such as azathioprine, antilymphocyte globulin, graft irradiation, portal drainage, and recipient splenectomy has not improved results significantly. The new macrolide immunosuppressive agent FK506 appears to be much more effective than cyclosporin A in preventing rejection of rat intestinal allografts, and its use in clinical small bowel transplantation in Pittsburgh appears encouraging.

Preoperative donor-specific transfusion in combination with cyclosporin treatment improves survival in some fully allogeneic rat combinations, but not in others. Treatment with monoclonal antibody directed against the interleukin–2 receptor prolonged survival in one semiallogeneic rat combination, an effect which was enhanced by concurrent administration of cyclosporin A.

GRAFT-VERSUS-HOST DISEASE

Graft-versus-host disease must be considered a potential problem in small bowel transplantation because of the vast numbers of immunocompetent cells transferred within the Peyer's patches and mesenteric lymph nodes of the graft. The disease may readily be seen in appropriate semiallogeneic rat models and also in certain fully allogeneic strain combinations. Graft-versus-host disease has been observed infrequently in dogs, and has never been reported in pigs. Graft-versus-host disease may be prevented either by reducing the lymphoid component of the graft or by the use of immunosuppressive agents, such as cyclosporin A or FK506. Three methods are available for reducing the amount of lymphoid tissue transplanted: surgical excision of the mesenteric lymph nodes (a relatively simple procedure in the rat); irradiation of the graft before implantation; or transplantation of only half of the donor small intestine.

GRAFT PRESERVATION

Although rat allografts may be stored safely for up to 24 h by a combination of intravascular and luminal flushing, canine experiments have suggested a maximum storage time of up to 12 h. Copious flushing of the graft lumen appears to be an essential part of any preservation protocol.

ABSORPTIVE AND BARRIER FUNCTION OF THE GRAFT

Present evidence suggests that, in the absence of rejection, absorption by the graft of all nutrients is adequate. Although subtle differences can be detected in water and electrolyte absorption by rat isografts and allografts, the animals remain healthy and gain weight normally. Similarly, in the absence of rejection the mucosal barrier is maintained.

Rejection (in which there is dramatic loss of the brush border and epithelial lining of the graft) results in marked reduction in absorptive function. The barrier function of the graft is severely compromised, allowing bacterial translocation into the host.

FURTHER READING

Carrel A. La technique operatoire des anastomoses vasculaire et la transplantation des visceres. *Lyon Med*, 1902; **98**: 859.

Lillehei RC, Goott B, Miller FA. The physiological response of the small bowel of the dog to ischemia including prolonged *in vitro* preservation of the bowel with successful replacement and survival. *Ann Surg*, 1959; **150**: 543–60.

Milland PR, Dennison A, Hughes DA, Collin J, Morris PJ. Morphology of intestinal allograft rejection and the inadequacy of mucosal biopsy in its recognition. *Br J Exp Pathol*, 1986; **67**: 687–98.

Monchik GJ, Russell PS. Transplantation of small bowel in the rat: technical and immunological considerations. *Surgery*, 1971; **70**: 693–702.

Schraut WH. Current status of small-bowel transplantation. *Gastroenterology*, 1988; **94**: 525–38.

10.8.2 Clinical small-bowel transplantation

A. BENEDICT COSIMI

INTRODUCTION

Recent improvements in total parenteral alimentation have significantly extended the survival for victims of short-bowel or severe malabsorption syndromes. Nevertheless, the long-term prognosis remains poor for patients whose residual bowel does not hypertrophy enough to allow at least partial enteral nutrition. Limiting factors for these individuals are recurrent infections that develop at venous access sites and the almost inevitable progressive liver dysfunction that results from prolonged high-calorie intravenous feeding. In such patients, the only viable alternative may be the attempted replacement of the diseased or absent bowel with a functioning allograft.

The number of patients who could benefit from bowel transplantation has been estimated to be approximately 1 or 2 per million of population per year. Suitable adult candidates are primarily patients who have survived massive bowel resection for treatment of benign conditions such as extensive Crohn's disease, vascular compromise, or trauma. Bowel transplantation has occasionally been recommended, as part of the multivisceral transplant used for reconstruction in patients whose extensive neoplasia was removed by 'upper abdominal exenteration'. In children, the short-gut syndrome typically results from conditions such as congenital neuromyopathy, extensive atresia, microvillus atrophy, or extensive resection following midgut volvulus or necrotizing enterocolitis.

Early attempts at clinical bowel transplantation using conventional immunosuppression with azathioprine, steroids, and antilymphocyte sera were extremely discouraging. Thus, by 1985, only seven such transplants had been reported. All recipients died, without adequate allograft function, within 3 months of the procedure. Unresolved obstacles, unique to bowel transplantation, were presented by the inescapable microbial colonization of the allograft, the immunological consequences of the large volume of immunocompetent donor lymphocytes necessarily transplanted into the recipient, an inadequate means of identifying rejection, and a high incidence of thrombotic complications. This bleak experience discouraged most transplant centres from pursuing additional clinical trials until further advances, including more effective and less toxic immunosuppressive agents, became available.

It was not until August of 1988 that the first successful clinical small-bowel transplant was performed in Kiel, Germany. The recipient had undergone total small-bowel resection for extensive mesenteric venous thrombosis. Ten weeks later, a 60-cm bowel segment was transplanted into the patient from an HLA-compatible sibling. Despite the excellent histocompatibility, multiple rejection episodes required aggressive immunosuppression with cyclosporin, steroids, and antithymocyte globulin. Life-threatening infectious complications, not unexpectedly, were encountered. Nevertheless, the recipient eventually became independent of parenteral nutrition and remains well over 4 years later.

In November 1988, successful transplantation of the liver and incontinuity small intestine was first accomplished in London, Ontario, Canada. The patient had suffered extensive bowel infarction secondary to a hypercoagulable state. The liver allograft corrected the coagulopathy and parenteral nutrition could be withdrawn from this patient 8 weeks after the transplant procedure.

These two cases established that small-bowel transplantation could provide a successful solution for the short-gut syndrome in patients with or without concomitant liver dysfunction. Nevertheless, the fact that a mere handful of successful cases has since been reported, from less than ten centres worldwide, emphasizes that this procedure is still not a realistic therapy, except for highly selected patients in whom all other treatment options have been exhausted.

DONOR MANAGEMENT AND ALLOGRAFT PREPARATION

As is true with kidney or pancreas transplantation, a suitable allograft for small-bowel replacement can be removed from a living donor but is more frequently obtained, in combination with other donor organs, from a cadaveric source. Specific considerations related to intestinal-tract procurement have been directed toward minimising microbial contamination from the bowel lumen and reducing the volume of lymphoid tissue retrieved with the allograft. Thus, provided there is time prior to organ retrieval, the donor is pretreated with a hyperosmolar cathartic in combination with non-absorbable antibiotics and antifungal agents. Based upon preclinical studies emphasizing that graft-versus-host disease (GVHD) can be induced by functional T cells in the intestinal transplant, donor lymphocyte depletion, using antilymphocyte globulin or the monoclonal antibody OKT3 prior to organ retrieval or irradiation of the excised allograft, have also been recommended. Interestingly, as discussed below, GVHD in human bowel transplant recipients has been encountered infrequently, making the necessity of these measures questionable.

The surgical technique of bowel allograft procurement depends upon the organs that are required. If the intestine is to be transplanted alone, a suitable segment is isolated, dividing the mesenteric vessels near their origin in cadaver donors, or more distally in a living donor. In the typical multiorgan procurement, the liver with the coeliac axis and proximal portal vein is separated from the intestine which remains in continuity with the distal portal vein and superior mesenteric artery (Fig. 1). For combined small bowel-liver transplantation, the donor jejunum, ileum, liver, and abdominal aorta containing the origins of the superior mesenteric and coeliac arteries are isolated. The liver and bowel, connected by the portal vein and aortic segment, are then perfused and removed, *en bloc*. The most complex procedure, in which a 'cluster' graft is required, involves *en-bloc* removal of the liver, pancreas, and variable amounts of duodenum and jejunum (Fig. 2).

Little information has been accumulated regarding the optimal method for preservation of human bowel allografts. Earlier studies suggested that continuous pulsatile perfusion might be required to maintain acceptable viability during *ex-vivo* storage periods of even 6 h. It is now clear, however, that adequate bowel preservation, at least for the short term, can be achieved by using an intracellular type of cold-storage fluid, such as Collin's or the University of Wisconsin solutions, which are employed for the other donor organs. Currently, successful bowel transplantation is accomplished after simple *in-situ* perfusion of the donor vessels followed, optionally, by *ex-vivo* flushing of the lumen of the excised bowel. Simple storage in the cold preservation fluid is effective for as long as 10 h. Whether more effective approaches can be devised to better maintain the integrity and, thereby, the early functional capacity of the allograft remains to be determined.

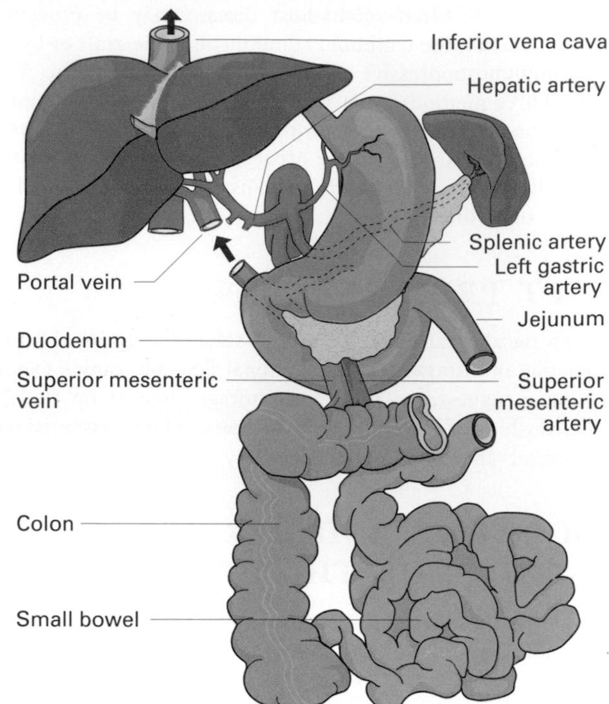

Fig. 1 Division of donor organs for separate liver and small intestine transplant procedures. The proximal portal vein is retained with the liver as is the hepatic artery in continuity with the coeliac axis. The distal portal vein arising from the confluence of the donor splenic vein and superior mesenteric vein are retained with the bowel graft. The superior mesenteric artery is usually taken with a cuff of donor aorta. The donor stomach, duodenum, pancreas, and colon will be resected from the small-bowel segment prior to transplantation.

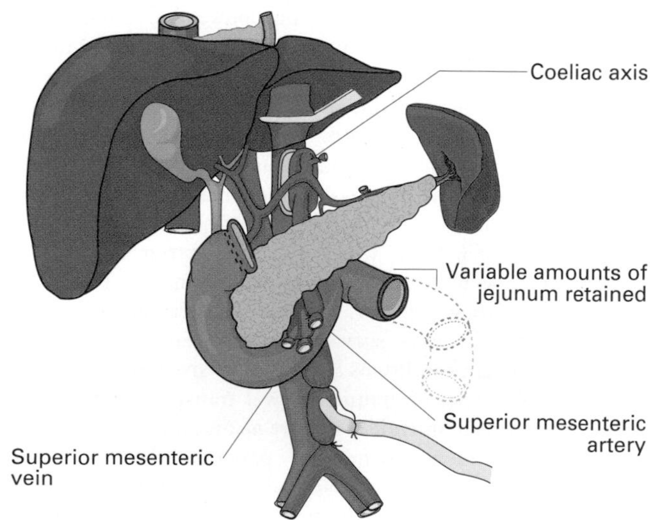

Fig. 2 'Cluster' tissue block procured to replace organs resected in upper abdominal exenteration procedure. The coeliac axis supplies duodenum and liver. The superior mesenteric artery and vein are shown ligated just below the pancreas in this specimen. These vessels would be retained with the bowel if the jejunum is transplanted into the recipient.

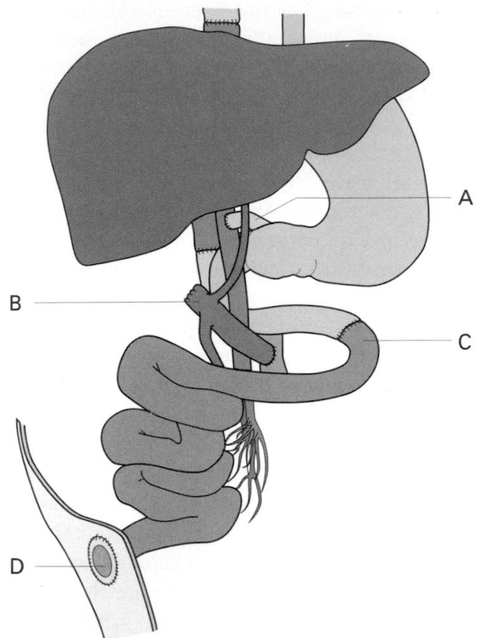

Fig. 3 Schematic diagram of combined liver–small bowel transplant (allograft tissues stippled). Donor supra- and infrahepatic venacavae have been anastomosed end-to-end with recipient. (A) End-to-side anastomosis of recipient and donor portal veins; (B) donor aortic conduit with coeliac axis to liver and SMA to bowel; (C) proximal jejunojejunostomy; (D) exteriorized donor distal jejunum. Not depicted is end-to-end anastomosis between donor and recipient common bile ducts.

RECIPIENT OPERATION

The technical aspects of bowel replantation alone are quite straightforward. Revascularization of the allograft is preferentially accomplished by anastomosing the donor portal or superior mesenteric vein to the recipient portal vein in the hepatic hilum or retropancreatic area. If it is not possible to construct a satisfactory portal–portal anastomosis, venous drainage can alternatively be provided into the recipient's systemic circulation. Arterialization is provided by anastomosis of the donor superior mesenteric artery to recipient aorta or iliac artery. For grafts that include the liver, which has been the more commonly performed procedure, revascularization is more complex (Fig. 3). The supra- and infrahepatic vena caval anastomoses are constructed end-to-end as for orthotopic liver transplantation. The transplant bowel portal venous drainage is through the non-transected donor portal vein; however, recipient portal venous drainage must also be provided. This may be accomplished by joining recipient and donor portal veins in end-to-side fashion, as depicted in Fig. 3, or by constructing a portacaval shunt between recipient vessels. Arterialization is provided by anastomosing the donor aortic conduit (Fig. 3) or a Carrel patch encompassing the origins of both the coeliac axis and superior mesenteric artery to the recipient infrarenal aorta. Complete restoration of continuity of the bowel is usually not undertaken at the primary transplant procedure. The distal end of the bowel is typically exteriorized to provide postoperative decompression and convenient access for the serial postoperative biopsies which are performed to evaluate the allograft status. Enteric anastomoses are subsequently performed when the allograft is known to be well vascularized and free of rejection.

POST-TRANSPLANT MANAGEMENT, COMPLICATIONS

Many of the technical problems that previously limited the success of bowel transplantation have been resolved with the use of current vascular techniques. Nevertheless, convalescence for these recipients is difficult, with recurrent rejection and septic episodes typically leading to protracted stays in hospital, even if no major surgical complications arise.

Unlike other organ transplants, the bowel allograft does not immediately regain normal function. Thus, total parenteral nutrition must be continued, sometimes for months postoperatively, when the attendant risks of catheter sepsis are even further increased because of the need for concomitant immunosuppression. Further complicating the post-transplant management is the erratic absorption, during periods of allograft dysfunction, of orally administered immunosuppressive agents.

At this stage of development of clinical bowel transplantation, the most efficacious postoperative immunosuppressive regimen remains undefined. Current reports indicate that substitution of the new macrolide immunosuppressant FK506 for conventional suppression provides a significantly improved outlook following intestinal transplantation. More than 30 patients treated with FK506 since 1990 have had successful bowel transplants.

In addition, there is no simple assay available for reliably detecting early bowel allograft rejection. Since rejection in experimental models is characterized by oedema, loss of villi, bleeding and ulceration of the mucosa, and submucosal mononuclear cell infiltrates, most centres have performed serial biopsies to monitor allograft status. However, histopathological examination of these partial-thickness biopsies does not always provide a reliable assessment of early rejection. Thus, immunohistochemical investigations, sequential measurement of intestinal permeability, and various measures of intestinal absorption are also being evaluated. A significant diagnostic advantage enjoyed by recipients of combined liver–small-bowel transplantation is the availability of better-defined functional and morphological criteria indicative of early rejection in the hepatic allograft. As a result, initiation of rejection treatment is typically undertaken on the basis of these criteria. This would also be expected to reverse any occult rejection that might be occurring simultaneously in the bowel. Acute rejection episodes following bowel transplantation are currently treated with high-dosage steroids and antilymphocyte preparations, such as ALG or OKT3, as in recipients of other organ allografts.

Although acute rejection episodes in human bowel allograft recipients have been encountered frequently, the incidence of graft-versus-host disease has been low. Only one documented transient episode of acute graft-versus-host disease has been reported. This resolved without any specific treatment and with no subsequent evidence of chronic graft-versus-host disease. Thus, the need for intensive lymphocytolytic treatment of the donor or the excised allograft is not clear.

Recipients of bowel allografts remain susceptible to the same infectious complications as other transplant recipients who are treated with comparable immunosuppressive regimens. Two specific problems have a particular impact on this group of patients. The first of these is bacteraemia and fungaemia due to translocation of these organisms from the bowel lumen as a result of an inadequate barrier function of the allograft mucosa. The primary microbial species responsible for these events are

Candida and the aerobic Gram-negative bacilli (Enterobacteriaceae and *Pseudomonas aeruginosa*) that normally populate the gut lumen. Of note, the anaerobic flora of the gut is rarely involved in such microbial translocation, and, indeed, provides some protection against superinfection—a phenomenon termed colonization resistance.

To counterbalance the inadequate barrier function of the bowel allograft, particularly in the first 6 months post-transplant, one of a variety of prophylactic regimens, which leaves the anaerobic flora intact, may be administered. Based upon experience in neutropenic cancer patients, either a fluoroquinolone (such as norfloxacin, ciprofloxacin, or ofloxacin), or a non-absorbable antibiotic combination (such as vancomycin, gentamicin, or polymyxin, plus fluconazole or amphotericin), is typically prescribed. Whatever the antimicrobial regimen chosen, the gut flora should be monitored, since any aerobic Gram-negative rods or yeast species colonizing the allograft will likely translocate to the bloodstream, necessitating revisions in the basic prophylactic regimen.

The second special infection-related problem in bowel transplant recipients is Epstein–Barr virus associated B-cell lymphoma, which occurs in over 10 per cent of long-term survivors of bowel allografts (as opposed to 1–5 per cent of other organ recipients). The pathogenesis of this process is complex and has to do with immunosuppression-induced Epstein–Barr virus reactivation (particularly by monoclonal or polyclonal antilymphocyte antibodies), secondary infection and immortalization of B cells, and failure of the normal surveillance mechanisms to eliminate these malignantly transformed cells. In addition, some investigators have suggested that the antilymphocyte regimens used to pretreat the donor in the effort to limit graft-versus-host disease might be causally related to the subsequent development of B-cell lymphomas in the recipient. The hope is that new protocols, including the addition of effective antiviral drugs to the immunosuppressive protocol, will create a therapeutic programme that is both safe and effective.

RESULTS AND FUTURE OF SMALL-BOWEL TRANSPLANTATION

There has been a resurgence of interest in transplantation of the small intestine since the first successful cases were reported in 1988. No official registry of bowel transplants has yet been established, making a complete summary of the experience in humans difficult. Communication with centres currently active in the field indicate that less than 100 of these procedures have been performed to date. Most of these have been undertaken since 1986.

The number of surviving bowel grafts which are sufficiently functional to allow withdrawal of all parenteral nutrition is small at this point, and the majority of these have been simultaneously transplanted with the liver. Whether this is because the intestine is less vigorously rejected when accompanied by the liver or simply because rejection is more easily diagnosed in liver allografts and therefore treated earlier, has not been established. Nevertheless, sporadic reports of chronically functioning isolated bowel allografts, including the world's first successful human transplant, are appearing. These successes indicate that, with further advances, it may soon be possible reliably to transplant the small intestine without the liver. Recently, at the University of Pittsburgh, an intensive clinical trial of bowel (with or without simultaneous liver) transplantation has been undertaken. The results, although preliminary, are encouraging.

In summary, small-intestinal transplantation represents a logical treatment for patients with short-gut syndrome whose survival is dependent upon total parenteral nutrition. Many unresolved obstacles, including inadequate immunosuppression, lack of a reliable means to maintain the allograft's functional barrier to infection, and the insensitivity of currently available diagnostic assays for rejection, have limited the applicability of the procedure. Nevertheless, the recent progress in this field will undoubtedly stimulate more widespread clinical trials in the near future. If bowel transplantation without simultaneous liver replacement can be performed with reliable success, it would be anticipated that this procedure will become the preferred treatment for most patients with short-gut syndrome. Successful small-bowel transplantation would obviate the considerable morbidity, mortality, and costs of total parenteral nutrition, and it would allow the patients to return to a relatively normal lifestyle. Moreover, unlike the situation with other organ transplants, the availability of suitable bowel allografts, from both living and cadaveric donors, should be more than sufficient to satisfy the need of all potential recipients who might benefit from small-intestine transplantation.

FURTHER READING

Deltz E, Schroeder P, Gebhardt H, *et al.* Successful clinical small bowel transplantation: report of a case. *Clin Transplantation* 1989; 3: 89–91.

Grant DR. Immunosuppression for small bowel transplantation. *Clin Transplantation* 1991; 5: 563–7.

Grant D, *et al.* Intestinal permeability and bacterial translocation following small bowel transplantation in the rat. *Transplantation* 1991; **52**: 221–4.

Grant D, *et al.* Successful small-bowel/liver transplantation. *Lancet* 1990; **335**: 181–4.

Hansmann ML, Hell K, Gundlach M, Deltz E, Schroeder P. Immunohistochemical investigation of biopsies in a successful small-bowel transplantation. *Transpl Proc* 1990; **22**: 2502–3.

Kirkman RL. Small bowel transplantation. *Transplantation* 1984; **37**: 429–33.

Revillon Y, Jan D, Goulet O, Ricour C. Small bowel transplantation in seven children: preservation technique. *Transpl Proc* 1991; **23**: 2350–1.

Schroeder P, Goulet O, Lear PA. Small-bowel transplantation: European experience. *Lancet* 1990; **336**: 108–111.

Starzl TE, *et al.* The many faces of multivisceral transplantation. *Surg Gynecol Obstet* 1991; **172**: 335–44.

Todo S, *et al.* Cadaveric small bowel and small bowel liver transplantation in humans. *Transplantation* 1992; **53**: 369–76.

Todo S, Tsakis A, Abu-Elmagd K, Reyes J, Starzl TE. Current state of intestinal transplantation. *Adv Surg*, 1994; **27**: 295–316.

10.9 Vascularized pancreatic transplantation

DAVID J. CONTI AND A. BENEDICT COSIMI

INTRODUCTION

At least 100 000 new cases of insulin-dependent (type I) diabetes mellitus appear worldwide each year. The discovery of insulin in 1921 provided the means to control the previously fatal complications of diabetic ketoacidosis. However this is only changed the natural history of the disease, since the extended survival which was suddenly provided by insulin treatment also allowed time for the degenerative secondary complications to develop.

Asymptomatic microangiopathic lesions develop in nearly all type I diabetics after 10 to 15 years of insulin-controlled hyperglycaemia. In nearly one-half of these patients, this progressive thickening of capillary basement membranes, together with accelerated atherosclerosis, results in clinically significant complications, typically first affecting the eyes, and then the peripheral nerves and vessels, the kidneys, and ultimately the heart and brain. Cardiovascular mortality in these patients is four times as great as that of the general population, cerebral vascular accidents are three times as frequent, and the prevalence of amputation is 20 times as high. Diabetes is the single most common cause of end-stage renal disease in the United States: approximately 30 per cent of patients who currently receive kidney transplants have diabetes. Despite successful renal transplantation, may of these recipients continue to suffer from the effects of other progressive complications of diabetes (Fig. 1). This dismal prognosis may not be inevitable, however, since experimental studies indicate that scrupulously tight control of glucose homeostasis may prevent or minimize the development of diabetic complications.

Currently, there are two possible approaches to achieving 'near-normoglycaemia': intensive regimens of exogenous insulin administration regulated by frequent glucose monitoring, and pancreas transplantation. The use of multiple daily insulin injections or insulin infusion pumps clearly maintains lower blood glucose levels than those which can be attained with standard insulin regimens. However, normoglycaemia is seldom achieved and a number of technical problems continue to limit the widespread application of these approaches. Obtaining frequent blood samples for monitoring of glucose by finger-pricks is a burden for many patients; subcutaneous abscesses may develop around the infusion devices; finally, not only does intermittent hyperglycaemia persist, but more importantly, there is a significant incidence of hypoglycaemic reactions, including occasional seizures and even sudden death. As a result, only the most motivated and compliant patients are able to follow these regimens. The attractiveness of pancreas transplantation arises form the expectation that a successful allograft will ensure complete euglycaemia, even without frequent blood glucose monitoring. The limitations are that, at least at present, this euglycaemia can be achieved only after a major surgical procedure, the life-long administration of immunosuppressive drugs, and reliance upon a limited supply of donor organs.

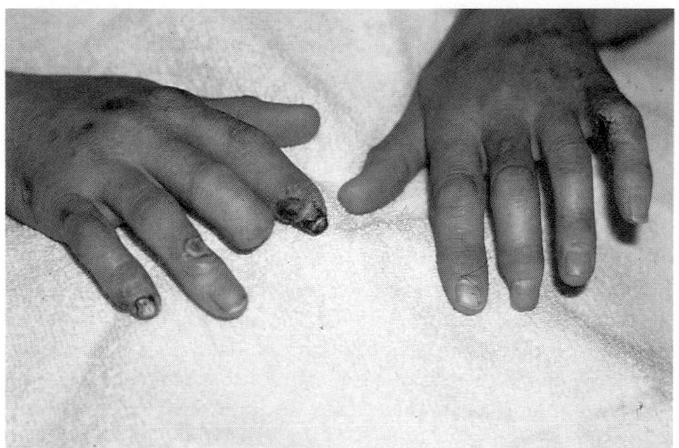

Fig. 1 Progressive peripheral vascular complications in a 29-year-old insulin-managed diabetic patient. End-stage renal disease had been treated by successful cadaver donor kidney transplantation 3 years earlier.

This work was supported in part from U.S.P.H.S. Grant HL-18646.

To avoid the surgical problems associated with the revascularization of the pancreas and the management of its exocrine secretions, transplantation of purified islet-cell preparations has been vigorously investigated. There is little doubt that, if islet-cell transplantation were to become a clinical reality, it would be the treatment of choice for insulin-dependent diabetes mellitus. The procedure itself would be minor, perhaps involving only a percutaneous intravenous injection, yet adequate islet-cell function would remove the need for exogenous insulin therapy. Recently, improved techniques for the isolation of islet cells, using continuous collagenase perfusion and more precisely defined density gradients for purification of the islet preparation have been developed. This has led to the first successful islet transplants with a handful of patients remaining normoglycaemic for over 6 months.

Until recently, trials using vascularized whole or segmental pancreas transplants were also largely unsuccessful (Table 1). However, refinements in the surgical procedure, together with advances in the immunosuppressive management of allograft recipients, now make it possible to achieve much more acceptable patient and allograft survival rates. In our experience, combined pancreatic and renal transplantation can now be accomplished with only a modest increase in risk over that associated with renal transplantation alone in diabetic recipients.

Table 1 Historical results reported worldwide following vascularized pancreas transplantation

Era	Reported no. of cases	Patient survival (1 year) (%)	Insulin independent (%)
1966–77	64	42	2
1978–82	201	72	21
1983–84	298	76	39
1985–86	438	83	44
1987–88	413	92	55

HISTORY

Pancreas transplantation was initially described in a large animal model in 1929. During the next four decades various investigators perfected the technical details of pancreaticoduodenal transplantation in dogs. This experimental background provided the setting for the first clinical pancreatic allograft performed by Kelly and Lillehei in December 1966, at the University of Minnesota. In that recipient, the pancreatic duct was managed by ligation. Over the next 7 years Lillehei and his associates performed another 13 pancreas allografts in diabetics, preserving exocrine function by anastomosing the donor ampulla of Vater or duodenal segment to a recipient jejunal Roux-en-Y loop. Only one of these pancreas allografts was still functional 1 year after surgery. Unacceptable mortality rates were encountered, predominantly because of septic complications. Since then, progress in pancreas transplantation has continued to lag well behind that of other solid organs, largely because of the unresolved technical difficulties related to management of the exocrine secretions. Of the 64 pancreaticoduodenal transplants performed between 1966 and 1977, only two grafts functioned for more than 1 year. Failures were the result of high infection rates, thrombosis, duodenal and/or pancreatic necrosis due to inadequate preservation, duodenal ulceration, and pancreatic or duodenal fistulae. As a consequence of these poor results, interest shifted from whole organ to segmental pancreas transplants, with multiple approaches to the management of the pancreatic duct, including ductal ligation, ductal obliteration by various polymers, free drainage of the exocrine secretions into the peritoneal cavity, or pancreatic duct-to-ureter anastomosis. None of these techniques proved completely satisfactory. Complications, including pancreatitis, pancreatic abscesses, fistulae, intractable pancreatic ascites, and diffuse pancreatic fibrosis, continued to limit their widespread application.

As a result, many groups, including our own, have refocused attention on whole organ transplantation (Fig. 2) using newer, more reliable approaches to exocrine drainage into the recipient's bladder. These whole organ techniques provide a number of advantages: a larger islet-cell mass is transplanted; the technical aspects of the vascular anastomoses are simplified as larger calibre vessels are used; venous drainage is enhanced, assuring greater blood flow through the allograft; and the use of a patch or short segment of donor duodenum for urinary exocrine drainage has proved to be relatively free of complications. The technique originally described suggested that urinary diversion of the pancreatic exocrine secretions could be best accomplished by using only a tiny patch of donor duodenum surrounding the ampulla of Vater. Because of the technical difficulty which may be encountered when dissecting the duodenum from the head of the pancreas, most groups have adopted the modification of retaining a 10- to 12-cm long segment of donor duodenum which can be anastomosed to the recipient bladder. These techniques allow free drainage of the pancreatic duct without the need for entering the recipient bowel, with the attendant potential for contamination. As described below, this approach also provides a means for serial monitoring of allograft exocrine function by simply measuring urinary pH and amylase concentrations.

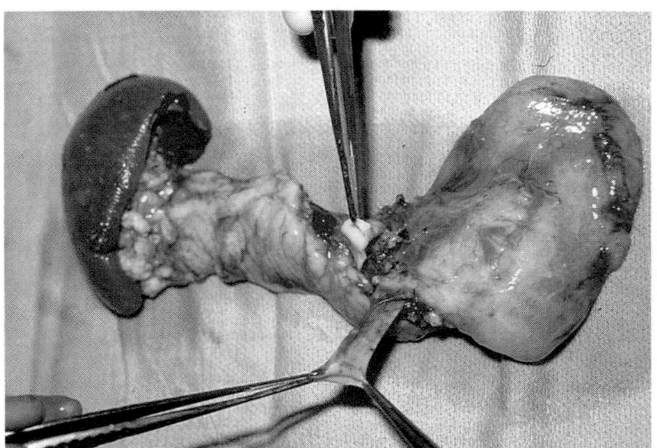

Fig. 2 Composite cadaver donor pancreaticoduodenal allograft prepared for transplantation. The single forceps grasps the donor aortic patch which encompasses the origin of the coeliac and superior mesenteric arteries. Two forceps demonstrate the donor portal vein segment.

DONOR AND PATIENT SELECTION

It is possible to remove the tail of the pancreas from a living donor and transplant it as a segmental graft. Because of the not insignificant risk to the donor, however, the great majority of pancreas grafts procured for transplantation have been from cadavers. As for any organ to be transplanted, active infection or malignancy in the donor, with the exception of non-disseminating intracerebral tumours, constitute generalized contraindications to pancreas procurement. In addition, since both hepatitis B and the acquired immune deficiency syndrome can be conveyed with the allograft, all donors must be shown to be hepatitis B surface antigen and HIV antibody-negative. Certain other conditions make the donor specifically unsuitable for pancreas donation. Diabetes (type I or II), a history of chronic pancreatitis, or traumatic pancreatic injury, are all contraindications to pancreatic retrieval. Suitable donors should be haemodynamically stable with adequate urine output, indicating sustained organ perfusion. Serum amylase, creatinine, and blood urea nitrogen levels should be near normal. A modest elevation in blood glucose does not necessarily preclude pancreatic donation: hyperglycaemia is not infrequently observed in cadaveric donors, and presumably results from the large volumes of intravenous solutions administered during resuscitative efforts and from the metabolic derangements induced by cerebral oedema and infarction. The administration of non-glucose containing intravenous solutions usually produces a normal blood sugar level over a period of 8 to 12 h. If adequate islet function is still in doubt, determination of glycosylated haemoglobin levels will confirm prior euglycaemia in the potential donor.

During the initial phases of pancreas transplantation, there was only one absolute requirement for histocompatibility, namely a negative T-cell crossmatch (absence of antibodies in recipient serum to donor HLA class I antigens). Retrospective analysis now suggests that graft survival rates may be improved if recipients are well matched with their donors at the HLA-DR loci. Worldwide results indicate a 71 per cent 1-year survival rate in recipients sharing two DR antigens, versus only 48 per cent allograft survival for those sharing one or no DR antigens with the donor. As new techniques for pancreas preservation are developed which allow sufficient time for more distant transport of the allograft, prospective matching of donor and recipient HLA-DR antigens will probably be more widely employed.

Table 2 Clinical status of 36 consecutive diabetic candidates for pancreas transplantation

Age	22–45 years
Diabetes duration	15–34 years
Daily insulin requirement	28–44 units
Glycosylated haemoglobin A levels	7.1–14.0%
Diabetic complications	
Nephropathy	100%
Retinopathy	75%
Enteric dysfunction	63%
Bladder dysfunction	55%
Peripheral vascular disease	50%

Currently, the typical candidate for pancreas transplantation has type I juvenile onset diabetes and significant renal dysfunction. The rationale for transplantation in such patients is that they are already candidates for renal transplantation and chronic immunosuppression. The additional surgical morbidity of the pancreas transplant only minimally increases the risks associated with renal transplantation. Contraindications include the presence of other advanced complications of diabetes, particularly coronary artery disease, blindness, or severe peripheral vascular disease. In our unit, we initially selected patients who were already dialysis dependent for simultaneous kidney and pancreas transplantation (Table 2). Although excellent survival can be achieved in this group of patients, the postoperative morbidity is greatly increased in those recipients with advanced diabetic complications prior to transplantation. In addition, there is little or no likelihood of reversal of these advanced complications despite persistent post-transplant euglycaemia. Currently, therefore, we favour combined kidney and pancreas transplantation for uraemic diabetic individuals who have not yet commenced dialysis. In some centres, the indication for pancreas transplantation has been extended even further to include patients with biopsy demonstrable diabetic nephropathy, but with good kidney function. Such patients would receive only a pancreas transplant. These patients should benefit most from a successful transplant, since their microangiopathic complications will be less advanced. However, because of the increased difficulties in diagnosing rejection in recipients of pancreas transplants alone (see below) and the lack of uraemia with its associated immunosuppression, current graft survival rates have proved less satisfactory than in kidney and pancreas graft recipients.

SURGICAL TECHNIQUES

Donor procedure

The composite pancreaticoduodenal allograft is isolated and perfused in the cadaver donor, nearly always in combination with kidney, liver, and heart procurement. The abdominal organs are initially exposed through a midline incision made from the suprasternal notch to the pubis (Fig. 3). Preparation of the pancreas allograft for removal is the most time consuming procedure, since extreme care must be takén to avoid operative trauma, which is probably the major factor leading to vasospasm and thrombosis of the pancreas after reimplantation. The spleen and tail of the pancreas are initially deflected medially by incising the peritoneum along the superior and inferior borders of the pancreas, to the level of the coeliac artery and superior meseneteric vessels, respectively. The inferior mesenteric vein can be cannulated for subsequent portal perfusion or ligated and divided along the inferior border of the pancreas. During this portion of the dissection excessive handling of the pancreas is avoided by using the spleen as a handle to manipulate the organ (Fig. 4). The arterial and portal vessels, shared by the liver and pancreas (Fig. 5) are divided at levels which will allow subsequent successful revascularization of

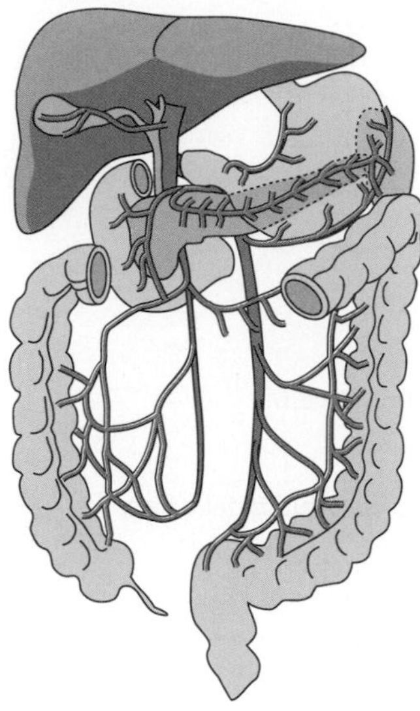

Fig. 3 Anatomy of upper abdominal organs and portal venous system to be isolated during multiple organ retrieval. For clarity, the omentum and transverse colon have been removed in this illustration though not in the actual surgical procedure.

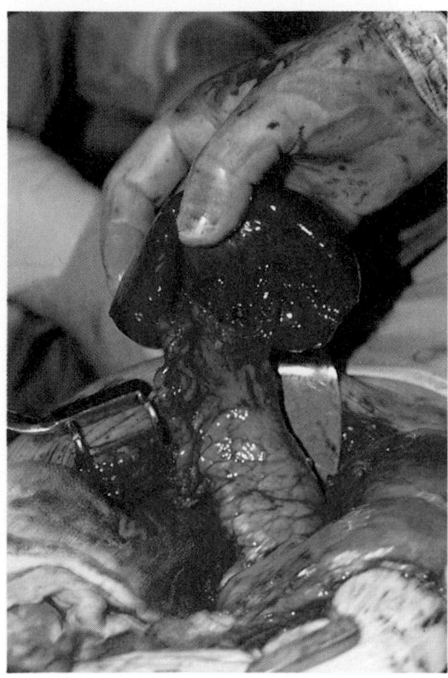

Fig. 4 Donor operation for removal of pancreaticoduodenal allograft. The tail and attached spleen have been reflected anteromedially using the spleen to manipulate the pancreas.

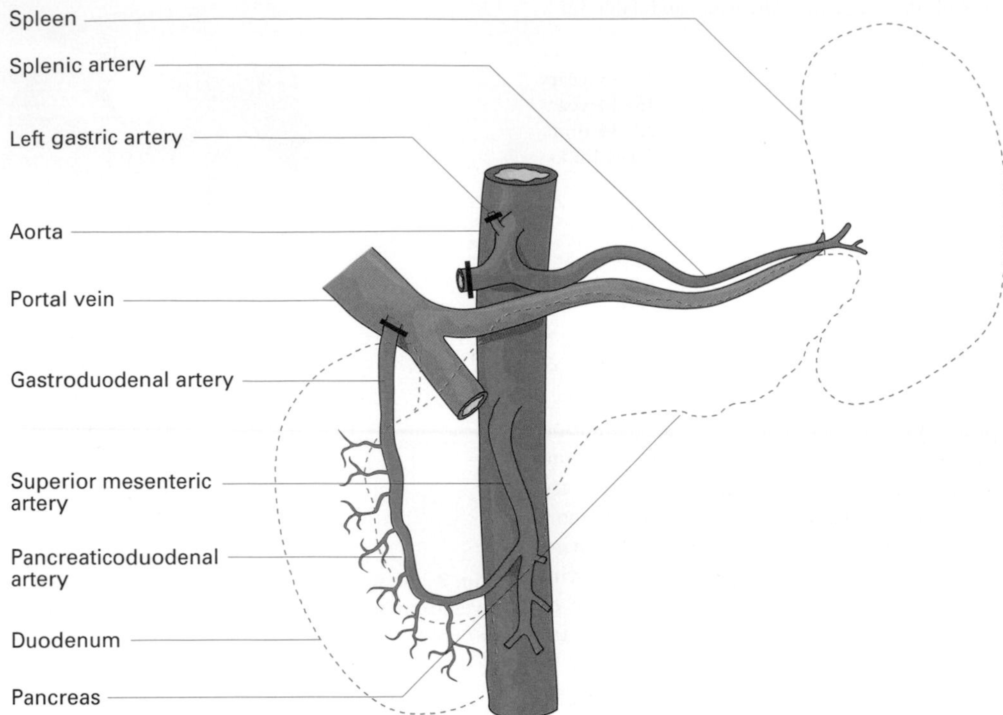

Fig. 5 Shared vascular anatomy of liver and pancreas donor organs. Sites for division of the vessels depend upon actual anatomic variations encountered at surgery. If the common hepatic artery and coeliac axis are taken with the liver, the splenic artery is usually reanastomosed end-to-side to the superior mesenteric artery prior to transplantation of the pancreaticoduodenal allograft.

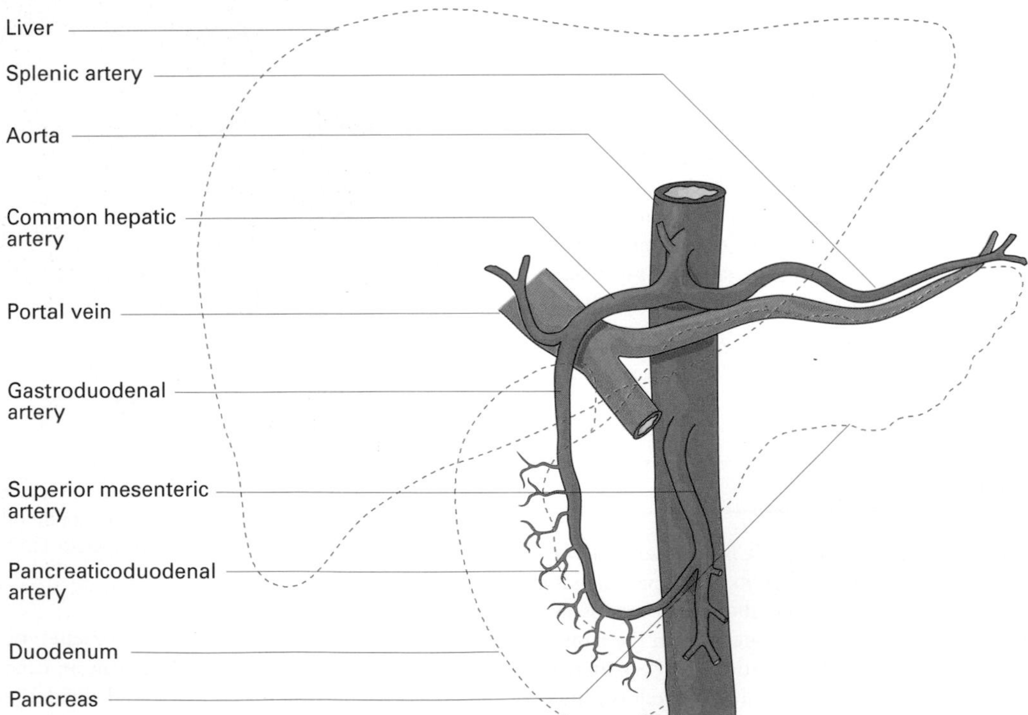

Fig. 6 Procurement of pancreaticoduodenal allograft with retained coeliac and superior mesenteric arteries. The common hepatic artery is transected at its origin from the coeliac axis for revascularization of the liver. The gastroduodenal and left gastric arteries are ligated and divided and the pancreaticoduodenal allograft is rearterialized using a cuff of donor aorta.

both allografts. The gastroduodenal artery is usually ligated and divided at its origin from the common hepatic artery. If the liver team is satisfied with the calibre of the common hepatic artery, it is divided at its origin from the coeliac axis (Fig. 6). If the hepatic artery is of inadequate size for hepatic revascularization, the splenic artery may be divided at its origin and the coeliac axis retained with the liver. The portal vein is typically divided at the level of the coronary vein. The superior mesenteric vein is divided as it crosses over the duodenum at the lower edge of the pancreas (Fig. 3). The distal superior mesenteric artery is also ligated at this level. Just prior to division of the vessels, the distal aorta is cannulated and the supracoeliac aorta is cross clamped as hypothermic perfusion via the aorta and portal vein is initiated. The liver and kidneys should be removed prior to division of the duodenum to avoid contamination by enteric flora. The duodenum is then divided with a stapling device just distal to the pylorus and approximately 5 cm distal to the ampullary region. The composite allograft is immediately placed into an iced solution (Fig. 2). The lateral wall of the duodenum is opened and the short duodenal segment irrigated with antibiotic and antifungal solutions. The arterial supply to the graft is further flushed with silica-gel filtered plasma or University of Wisconsin preservation solution and then the pancreas is placed in a sterile plastic bag for storage on ice until transplantation. This approach provides for a maximum safe ischaemic period of approximately 15 h.

For segmental pancreas transplantation, the tail and body of the pancreas are procured from a living, related donor by dividing the organ and the splenic vessels in a plane overlying the superior mesenteric vessels.

Recipient procedure

For simultaneous kidney and pancreas transplantation, the renal allograft is first placed usually into the left iliac fossa. Reconstruction of the urinary tract can be accomplished via a ureteropyelostomy or ureteroneocystostomy. The right iliac fossa is the preferred location for the composite pancreaticoduodenal allograft. If the donor coeliac axis was removed with the liver, the remaining splenic artery is usually anastomosed end-to-side to the superior mesenteric artery while the pancreatic allograft is still in the cold preservation solution. If the coeliac axis has been retained with the pancreas, the allograft is revascularized by anastomosing the donor portal vein and the aortic patch, which encompasses the origins of the coeliac and superior mesenteric arteries, to the recipient iliac vessels in an end-to-side fashion (Fig. 7). The vascular clamps are removed and perfusion is re-established with the donor spleen still attached. Currently, the preferred management of the exocrine secretions is by anastomosis of the donor duodenum to the dome of the recipient bladder. This is performed in a standard two-layer technique. Absorbable sutures are used for both layers of the bladder anastomosis to prevent subsequent stone formation on sutures which can erode into the bladder lumen. Exocrine secretions can alternatively be drained into a Roux-en-Y loop of recipient jejunum.

The spleen is removed after the duodenocystostomy has been completed and the vascular anastomoses have been inspected for patency and haemostasis. The rationale for temporarily leaving the spleen in place is that this provides the equivalent of a large arteriovenous shunt at the tail of the pancreas. This should encourage increased blood flow through the allograft during the early rewarming period, when the most intense vasospasm would be anticipated. Evidence supporting the validity of this hypothesis is provided by sequential measurements of arterial blood flow to the allograft, which reveal a 30 to 40 per cent decrease in flow after splenectomy is performed.

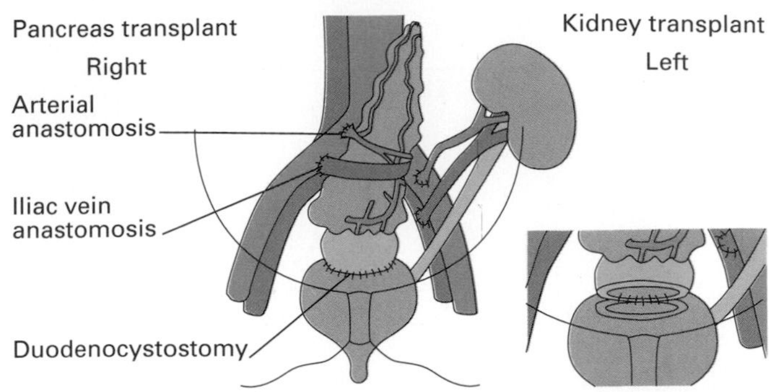

Fig. 7 Technique of simultaneous kidney and pancreas transplantation. The pancreas is usually placed into the right iliac fossa with vascularization to the recipient's iliac artery and vein. Exocrine secretion drainage is provided by duodenocystostomy performed with two layers of absorbable suture.

For segmental pancreas transplantation, revascularization is by simple end-to-side anastomosis of the donor splenic vessels to the recipient's iliac artery and vein. The pancreatic duct is managed either by occlusion with a synthetic polymer or by anastomosis of the duct into the bladder or a Roux-en-Y jejunal loop.

POST-TRANSPLANT MANAGEMENT

Although experimental studies of islet-cell transplantation suggest that endocrine pancreatic tissue is particularly immunogenic and so more likely to suffer rejection than other allografts, experience with vascularized segmental and whole pancreas transplantation do not confirm this concern, presumably because of the different nature of the grafts. Immunosuppression for pancreatic allograft recipients is, therefore, provided by protocols similar to those used in renal, hepatic, or cardiac transplantation. In our programme, initial immunosuppression includes a combination of cyclosporin administered orally (12 mg/kg.day, tapered to maintain plasma levels of 50–100 μg/l), prednisone (tapered over 5 days from 200 to 20 mg/day), and azathioprine (100 mg/day). Acute rejection episodes are initially treated with intravenous solumedrol. Patients whose rejection proves unresponsive to steroids are treated with OKT3 monoclonal antibody.

Because thrombotic complications historically accounted for up to 25 per cent of pancreatic allograft failures, many centres also recommend anticoagulation as part of the early postoperative regimen. We favour a protocol combining low molecular weight dextran (20 ml/h) and subcutaneous heparin (3000 U/8), beginning intraoperatively and continuing for 5 days postoperatively. Aspirin (325 mg/day) is initiated on day 1 and continued for 4 months unless haematuria necessitates earlier withdrawal. This approach, in conjunction with meticulous procurement techniques and temporary splenic retention following revascularization in the recipient, has resulted in only one instance of pancreatic vessel thrombosis in 36 consecutive recipients.

A cystogram is performed 5 to 7 days after transplantation to evaluate the duodenocystostomy. The Foley catheter is removed

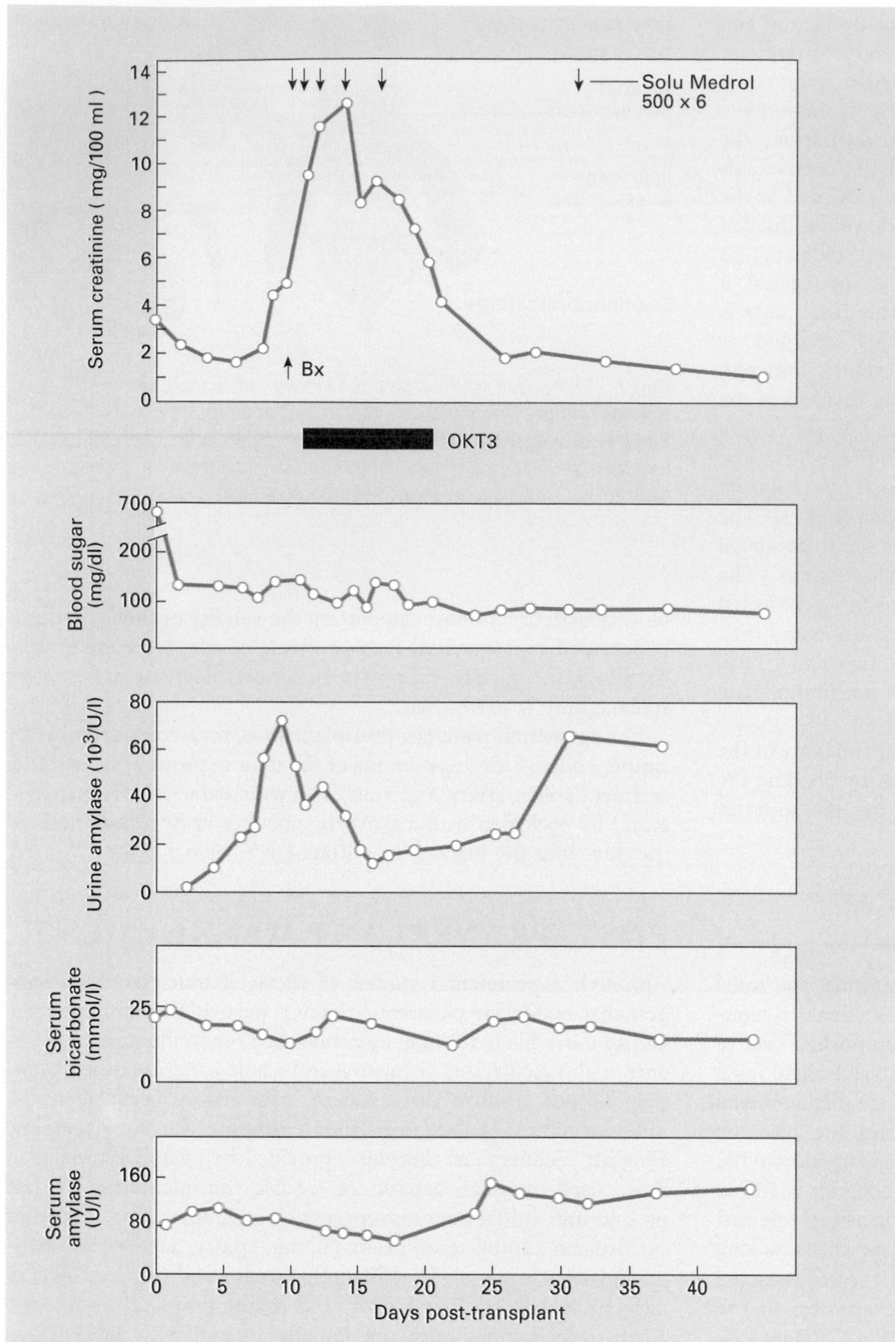

Fig. 8 Clinical course in a patient with renal allograft rejection beginning 10 days after simultaneous kidney and pancreas transplantation. Severe uraemia (serum creatinine >12 mg per cent) and depressed urine amylase levels were observed but significant hyperglycaemia did not occur even during high dosage steroid therapy. Following treatment with OKT3 monoclonal antibody, excellent function of both allografts returned and has persisted for over 3 years.

at this time, provided that the cystogram shows that the anastomosis is patent and without evidence of leakage. Renal and pancreatic function are serially monitored by serum creatinine and glucose levels. Unfortunately, the only completely valid clinical parameter indicative of pancreas rejection continues to be an elevation in the blood glucose level. Hyperglycaemia, however, is generally not manifested until rejection is well established, and at this late stage, the rejection process is often unresponsive to increased immunosuppressive therapy. This phenomenon results from the pathophysiology of pancreas destruction by rejection in which the early effector mechanisms primarily involve only the acinar tissue, with sparing of the islet-cells until quite extensive allograft damage has already occurred. Even at this late stage, hyperglycaemia is often not evident because of the large residual functional capacity of the islet cells: this clinical warning may not become evident until 80 to 90 per cent of the islet cell mass has been destroyed. Unfortunately, despite the much greater sensitivity of the acinar tissue to rejection, an elevated serum amylase level is also an unreliable diagnostic measure. Hyperamylasaemia in these patients may also result from perioperative trauma to the allograft, postoperative wound collections, and infection. Since rejection of renal allografts is usually detected at an early stage, serial monitoring of renal allograft function in recipients of kidney and pancreas transplants retrieved from the same donor, provides a reliable means of diagnosing rejection and initiates early treatment for a process presumably occurring simultaneously in both organs (Fig. 8). Furthermore, if the diagnosis is in doubt, percutaneous biopsies of the renal allograft can usually be obtained without difficulty. In our experience, renal allograft dysfunction secondary to rejection has always preceded any evidence of islet cell dysfunction.

One aspect of patient management unique to individuals who have received pancreatic allografts with urinary drainage of the exocrine secretions is that some indication of pancreatic allograft function can be obtained from measurements of urine pH (generally 7.5) and amylase levels (generally 30 000 units/24 h). A fall in urinary pH and amylase concentration often occurs during rejection crises (Fig. 8). However a disadvantage of urinary exocrine drainage is that these patients typically exhibit some degree of metabolic acidosis because of the bicarbonate loss. During periods of decreased renal function this can become severe and may require intensive oral or intravenous bicarbonate supplementation. Nevertheless, higher pancreas allograft survival rates are currently being observed in recipients of simultaneous kidney and pancreas transplants with bladder exocrine drainage than in recipients who receive a pancreas allograft after a previous kidney transplant, or in non-uraemic recipients of pancreas transplants alone (see below). This improvement in allograft survival is though to be due to the detection of rejection at an earlier, more treatable, stage.

RESULTS

As discussed above, early clinical results of vascularized pancreas transplantation were clearly unsatisfactory and the procedure properly remained experimental until the mid 1980s. Recent results, however, are more encouraging. Over 1200 pancreas transplants were reported worldwide between 1986 and 1989; 87 per cent of the recipients were alive at 1 year and 56 per cent of these patients were insulin independent. This improved success rate has been achieved even in recipients with advanced diabetic complications. Since the 1-year patient mortality rate following renal transplantation alone in this group of recipients is approximately 10 per cent, diabetic patients can now be honestly advised that the addition of pancreas transplantation does not significantly decrease their chances of survival. In some centres, the early survival rate for the pancreatic allograft itself is also approaching that for cadaver donor renal allografts, that is, approximately 80 per cent. Of our first 36 consecutive combined pancreas and kidney transplant recipients, 29 patients (80.6 per cent) remain independent of dialysis, 27 of whom (75 per cent) remain insulin free, at a mean follow-up of 28.4 months (Table 3).

Table 3 Post-transplant parameters in 36 consecutive kidney-pancreas allograft recipients

Observation period
Range: 1–50 months
Mean: 28.4 months
Insulin free: 27/36(75%)
Current fasting blood sugar: 68–150 mg %
Current glycosylated haemoglobin A: 4.0–6.7%
Dialysis free: 29/36 (80.6%)
Current serum creatinine 0.8–2.5 mg %
Aetiology of failures
Pancreas
Thrombosis: 1 day
Rejection: 2 weeks
Rejection/infection: 2 months
Death (infection): 4 months
Death (infection): 5 months
Death (ruptured bladder): 7 months
Death (hepatitis): 32 months
Death (cardiovascular): 36 months
Death (alcoholism): 41 months
Kidney
Functioning 23 months
Functioning 25 months
Rejection 2 months

METABOLIC EFFECTS

Factors that might delay a return to normal glucose metabolism during the immediate post-transplant period include: systemic rather than portal venous delivery of insulin from the allograft; denervation of the pancreas; intravenous infusions of large volumes of glucose-containing solutions during the perioperative period; immunosuppressive protocols using diabetogenic agents including steroids and cyclosporin; and ischaemic injury to the donor islet cell mass incurred either before death or during procurement and preservation. Despite these possibly adverse influences, the immediate clinical effects following successful pancreas transplantation are dramatic. Within the first 24 h, the allograft provides a self-regulating source of insulin: none of the recipients in our series required any intra- or postoperative exogenous insulin. Fasting blood glucose levels are typically mildly subnormal (60–90 ml/dl) because of the systemic venous drainage of the pancreas allograft. Interestingly, symptomatic hypoglycaemia has not been reported by these recipients. Glycosylated haemoglobin levels return to normal within 2 months after transplantation (Fig. 9), and the majority of recipients have normal responses to oral and intravenous glucose tolerance tests. Serum C-peptide and serum insulin levels are increased, both because of the systemic delivery of insulin and the decreased insulin sensitivity induced by steroid therapy.

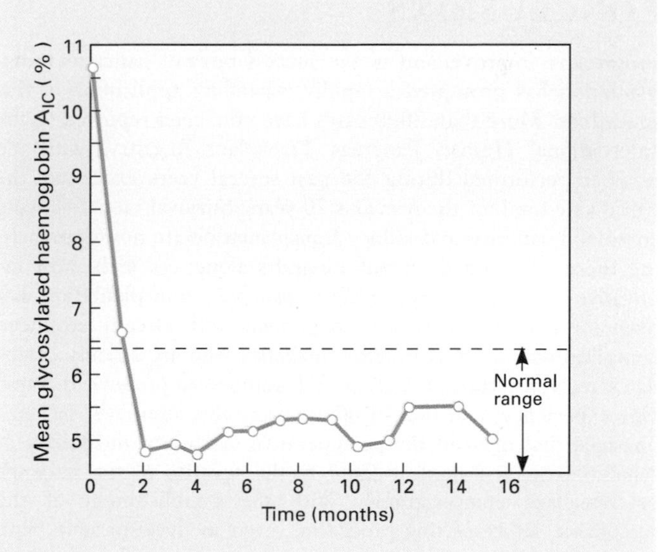

Fig. 9 Mean glycosylated haemoglobin A levels in diabetic recipients of simultaneous kidney and pancreas allografts. A dramatic fall to normal levels from regularly elevated pretransplant values was observed in all recipients within 2 months of pancreas transplantation.

Subjectively, the allograft recipients have been enthusiastic over their sense of well-being and freedom from years of insulin dependence and dietary restrictions. However, the precise impact of pancreas transplantation on the secondary complications of diabetes remains to be defined. While studies in laboratory animals have provided good evidence to suggest that pancreas transplantation can prevent and even reverse the early degenerative complications of diabetes, fewer data are available from humans. Most patients selected for pancreas transplantation to date have suffered from near end-stage diabetes, and advanced microangiopathic lesions are unlikely to regress substantially following correction of glucose metabolism. Nevertheless, some encouraging clinical evidence is beginning to accumulate, especially with regard to diabetic nephropathy. For example, pancreas transplantation prevents the simultaneously placed renal allograft from developing the histological lesions of diabetes which are typically seen after 1 to 3 years in diabetic patients receiving renal allografts only. Furthermore, in instances in which kidneys of a diabetic cadaveric donor have been transplanted into non-diabetic recipients, the microscopic lesions of mild nephropathy have been observed to reverse. Reversal of mild functional and morphological lesions in the kidneys of diabetic recipients without end-stage nephropathy has also been observed following pancreas transplantation. These observations indicate not only that diabetic glomerular lesions may be preventable, but also that early diabetic nephropathy may even be reversed if normal glucose homeostasis is provided. The progression of diabetic polyneuropathy has also been observed to cease once euglycaemia has been achieved by successful pancreas transplantation. Evaluation of this evidence is difficult, however, since correction of uraemia alone by a renal allograft often produces improvement in diabetic polyneuropathy. A number of investigators have reported stabilization or improvement in diabetic retinopathy in recipients of pancreas allografts, while others have failed to observe a consistently beneficial effect on established retinopathy.

CONCLUSIONS

Progressive improvement in the success rates of pancreas transplantation has prompted a rapidly expanding application of this procedure. More than 2000 cases have now been reported to the International Human Pancreas Transplant Registry, with the number performed during the past several years exceeding the worldwide total for the previous 20 years. Survival rates following combined pancreas and kidney transplantation are now approaching those achieved for renal allografts alone. As with most innovative therapeutic approaches, pancreas transplantation has been initially evaluated only in patients with already advanced complications, such as uraemic diabetics who are already candidates for renal transplantation and immunosuppressive therapy. Our experience, and that of others using this approach, has emphasized that most of the postoperative morbidity and failure of rehabilitation is directly related to the severity of the patient's pretransplant complications. With the establishment of the reasonable safety of this procedure, even in these patients with more severe disease, pancreas transplantation is now being offered to diabetics with less severe secondary complications.

Because only approximately half of the patient population with juvenile onset diabetes eventually develops clinically significant angiopathic complications, specific criteria are required to enable selection of appropriate candidates for pancreas transplantation. Unfortunately, it is impossible to identify at the time of onset of diabetes patients who will be most susceptible to the deleterious effects of deranged glucose metabolism. The most reliable early predictor of further complications continues to be renal dysfunction. Thus, we are currently recommending that combined kidney and pancreas transplantation be performed in patients with impaired renal function which has not progressed to dialysis dependence. We anticipate that the restoration of normal glucose metabolism at this earlier stage of the disease might be more effective in delaying or preventing the progression of microangiopathic complications. Obviously, if this expectation is realized and reliable means of diagnosing early rejection in the pancreas are developed, the logical approach would be to evaluate pancreas transplantation alone in patients with minimal albuminuria but normal renal function. In these patients, the expectation would be that euglycaemia might prevent the otherwise consistently predictable progressive renal failure and later need for kidney transplantation.

In summary, we and others have shown that vascularized pancreas transplantation can be preformed successfully, that such transplantation provides normal glucose metabolism, and that this can be accomplished with only a modest increase in risk over that of renal transplantation alone. In order to achieve the full therapeutic benefit of pancreas transplantation we still need to determine when in the course of the diabetic illness the procedure will be optimally effective in delaying or preventing secondary complications. Currently used procedures will almost surely become outmoded as islet transplantation is perfected or molecular approaches to regulation of insulin gene expression are defined. Meanwhile, it seems reasonable to continue exploration of the benefits of vascularized pancreatic transplantation in a gradually expanding population of insulin-dependent diabetics.

FURTHER READING

Abouna GM, Al-Adnani MS, Kremer GD, Kumar SA, Daddah SK, Kusma G. Reversal of diabetic nephropathy in human cadaveric kidneys after transplantation into non-diabetic recipients. *Lancet* 1983; **ii**: 1274–6.

Bilous RW, Mauer SM, Sutherland Der, Najarians JS, Goetz FC, Steffes MW. The effect of pancreas transplantation on the glomerular structure of renal allografts in patients with insulin-dependent diabetes. *N Engl J Med* 1989; **321**: 80–5.

Bohman SO, *et al.* Prevention of kidney graft diabetic nephropathy by pancreas transplantation in man. *Diabetes* 1985; **34**: 306–8.

Brooks J. Presidential address: Where are we with pancreas transplantation. *Surgery* 1989; **106**: 935–45.

Case Records of the Massachusetts General Hospital. Case 1–1988. *N Engl J Med* 1988; **318**: 31–40.

Corry R. Pancreatico-duodenal transplantation with urinary tract drainage. In: Groth CG, ed. *Pancreatic transplantation*. Philadelphia: WB Saunders, 1988; 147–53.

Corry RJ, Ngheim DD, Shulak JA, Beutel WD, Gonwa TA. Surgical treatment of diabetic nephropathy with simultaneous pancreatico-duodenal and renal transplantation. *Surg Gynecol Obstet*; 1986; **162**: 547–55.

Cosimi AB, *et al.* Combined kidney and pancreas transplantation in diabetics. *Arch Surg* 1988; **123**: 621–5.

Delmonico FL, Cosimi AB. Monclonal antibody treatment of human allograft recipients. *Surg Gynecol Obstet* 1988; **166**: 89–98.

Dubernard JM, Traeger J, Neyra P, Touraine JL, Tranchant D, Blanc-Brunat N. A new method of preparation of segmental pancreas grafts for transplantation. Trials in dogs and in man. *Surgery* 1978; **84**: 633–7.

Gliedman ML, *et al.* Clinical segmental pancreatic transplantation with ureter-pancreatic duct anastomosis for exocrine drainage. *Surgery* 1973; **74**: 171–80.

Goetz FC. Indications for pancreas transplantation. In: Toledo-Pereyra LH, ed. *Pancreas transplantation*. Boston: Kluwer Academic Publishers, 1988: 41–5.

Hanssen KF, Dahl-Jorgensen K, Lauritzen T, Feldt-Rasmussen B, Brinchmann-Hansen O, Deckert T. Diabetic control and microvascular complications: the near-normoglycemia experience. *Diabetologia* 1986; **29**: 677–734.

Kelly WD, Lillehei RC, Merkel FK, Idezuki Y, Goetz FC. Allotransplantation of the pancreas and duodenum along with the kidney in diabetic nephropathy. *Surgery* 1967; **61**: 827–37.

Kennedy WR, Navarro X, Goetz FC, Sutherland DER, Najarian JS. Effects of pancreatic transplantation on diabetic neuropathy. *N Engl J Med* 1990; **322**: 1031–7.

Landgraf R, *et al.* Fate of late complications in type I diabetic patients after successful pancreas-kidney transplantation. *Diabetes* 1989; **38**: 33–7.

Muhlhausser I. Near-normoglycemia and microvascular complications. *Diabetologia* 1987; **30**: 47–8.

Prieto M, Sutherland DER, Goetz FC, Rosenberg ME, Najarian JS. Pancreas transplant results according to the technique of duct management: bladder versus enteric drainage. *Surgery* 1987; **102**: 680–90.

Rabb HA, Niles JL, Cosimi AB, Tolkoff-Rubin NE. Severe hyponatremia associated with combined pancreatic and renal transplantation. *Transplantation* 1989; **48**: 157–9.

Ramsay R, *et al.* Progression of diabetic retinopathy after pancreas transplantation for insulin-dependent diabetes mellitus. *N Engl J Med* 1988; **318**: 208–13.

Sollinger HW, Pirsch JD, D'Alessandra AM, Kalayoglu M, Belzer FO. Advantages of bladder drainage in pancreas transplantation: a personal view. *Clin Transplantation* 1990; **4**: 32–6.

Sutherland DRR, Chow SY, Moudry-Munns KC. International Pancreas Transplant Registry Report. *Clin Transplantation* 1989; **3**: 129–49.

Sutherland DER, Goetz FC, Najarian JS. One hundred pancreas transplants at a single institution. *Ann Surg* 1984; **200**: 414–24.

Sutherland DER, *et al.* Pancreas transplantation in nonuremic, type I diabetic recipients. *Surgery* 1988; **104**: 453–64.

Tyden G, Brattstrom C, Haggmark A, Groth CG. Studies on the exocrine secretions of segmental pancreatic grafts in humans. *Surg Gynecol Obstet* 1987; **164**: 404–8.

The DCCT Research Group. Diabetes control and complications trial: results of feasibility study. *Diabetes Care* 1987; **10**: 1–19.

The Kroc Collaborative Study Group. Blood glucose control and the evolution of diabetic retinopathy and albuminuria. *N Eng J Med* 1984; **311**: 365–72.

van der Vliet JA, Navarro X, Kennedy WR, Goetz FC, Najarian JS, Sutherland DER. The effect of pancreas transplantation on diabetic polyneuropathy. *Transplantation* 1988; **45**: 368–70.

10.10 Pancreatic islet and fetal pancreas transplantation

DEREK W. R. GRAY

Although transplantation of isolated pancreatic islets in the insulin-dependent diabetic is not yet a routine clinical procedure, an extensive research literature exists and limited clinical trials are now in progress. Thus, this experimental area of transplantation needs to be considered in the context of vascularized pancreatic transplantation for type I diabetes.

RATIONALE

Transplantation of the vascularized pancreas has become increasingly respectable in terms of graft and patient survival, such that the results obtained now compare reasonably with those of other organ transplants. But the concept of transplanting an entire organ to cure a non-lethal condition when what is required is only a small fraction of the transplanted tissue would appear to be flawed. Although there is evidence that the complications of diabetes are caused by imperfect control of glucose metabolism and that improved glucose homeostasis would probably prevent their onset, there is also considerable evidence that transplantation of the endocrine pancreas at a late stage in the disease has relatively little effect on these complications. Therefore transplantation would have to be performed in the early years after presentation in order to influence the development of these microangiopathic complications of diabetes. Vascularized pancreatic transplantation with immunosuppression is never likely to be an acceptable therapy for the recently diagnosed young diabetic, but pancreatic islet transplantation could be, especially if this could be performed without the need for long-term immunosuppression, as might be possible (see below).

The idea of transplanting insulin-secreting tissue as a free graft for diabetes is older than the discovery of insulin, but little progress was made until relatively recently. In 1965 Moskalewski described the successful isolation of islets from the rodent pancreas using collagenase digestion, after which Lacy in 1967 perfected the isolation technique to produce sufficient islets for transplantation in rats. The enthusiasm raised by these early experimental results prompted several early attempts at human pancreatic islet allotransplantation and autotransplantation. Despite early claims to the contrary, it is now generally agreed that these early attempts failed, not least because the technique for islet isolation developed in the rat was not applicable to the human pancreas. These early clinical trials also emphasized the dangers of transplanting unpurified dispersed pancreatic tissue. Over the last 20 years techniques for isolation and transplantation of pancreatic islets have been developed in experimental animals. Significant technical advances in that period were the demonstration of successful transplantation of unpurified islet tissue in pancreatectomized dogs; the use of intraductal collagenase for islet isolation in the dog; and successful transplantation of purified islets in the dog. This work led to the successful development of techniques for islet isolation from the human pancreas. Further modifications continue to improve both the yield and purity of islets obtained from both human and other mammalian pancreases.

An alternative to the use of isolated adult islets is the transplantation of fetal pancreas, which arose out of observations by Coupland in 1960, namely that the endocrine tissue of the fetal pancreas is relatively well developed and survives transplantation while the exocrine tissue is poorly developed and undergoes atrophy after transplantation. However, it was the late Josiah Brown in 1974 who showed that transplantation of fetal pancreas would cure experimental diabetes in rodents.

ISOLATED PANCREATIC ISLET TRANSPLANTATION

Current techniques for pancreatic islet isolation

Although many techniques for islet isolation have been described in the past, varying from microdissection to dispersion with modified food blenders, almost all groups working with human pancreas, as well as the pancreas of other large mammalian species, now use a variant of intraductal collagenase digestion. The principle behind the technique is the delivery of the collagenase into an exocrine pancreatic duct, which allows selective digestion of the interacinar connective tissue (Figs. 1–3).

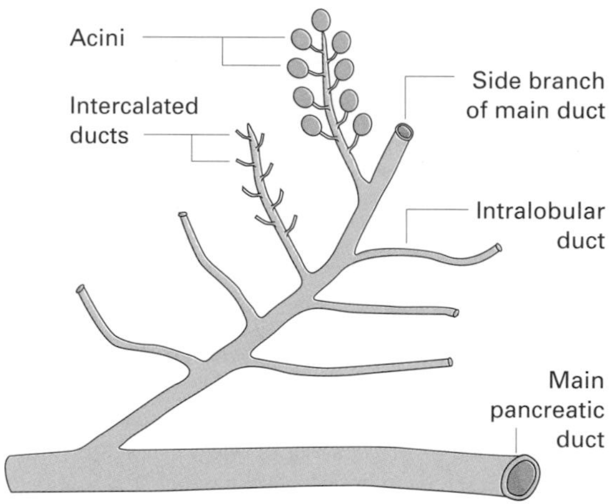

Fig. 1 The simple branch structure of the exocrine duct of the pancreas. Intralobular ducts arise from the length of the main duct and the acini are reached after two further divisions. This simple anatomical arrangement favours the dispersion of retrogradely injected fluids.

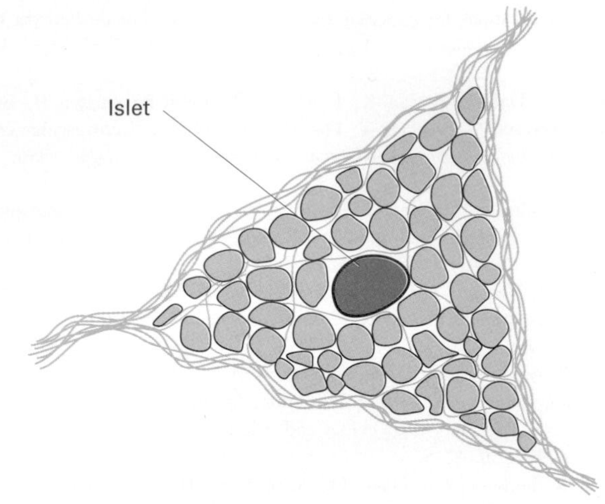

Fig. 2 The microscopic distribution of fibrous tissue (green) within the pancreas. A lobule with acini and a single islet (red) are shown. The fine interacinar islet collagen must be removed by the action of injected collagenase. The removal of the thicker interlobular and perivascular fibrous tissue would require longer digestion.

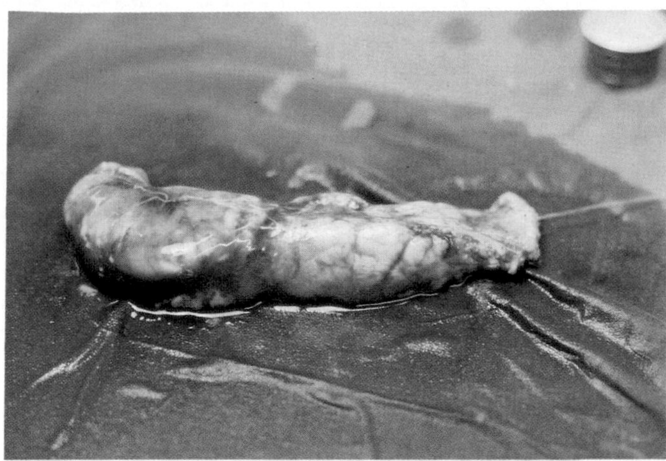

Fig. 3 Human pancreas distended by retrograde injection of collagenase into the pancreatic duct.

Under optimal conditions, for example, collagenase delivered at 39 °C, the interacinar fibrous tissue is removed within 10 to 30 mins. The digestion process can be stopped by cooling at this stage, but the thicker intralobular fibrous tissue remains largely undigested and to release the islets it is necessary to employ the gentlest possible mechanical dispersion. There are now a number of semiautomated machines that use the above principles to disperse human, porcine, and canine pancreas, liberating islets mixed with a large number of exocrine fragments. No entirely successful technique has been developed to separate the exocrine tissue from the islet tissue. The most successful technique relies on the differential density of islet and exocrine tissue, which allows separation of the tissues by centrifugation on a Ficoll or albumin density gradient (Figs. 4 and 5).

The prevention of rejection

Although some endocrine tissues are relatively non-immunogenic, there is no doubt that isolated pancreatic islets transplanted as a free graft are highly immunogenic. The mechanisms of rejection may be somewhat different to those of a vascularized organ allograft and more akin to those seen in skin allograft rejection. Although prolonged survival of islet allografts has been obtained with a number of immunosuppressive protocols in several animal models, permanent survival of grafts has been difficult to achieve, even in rodent models where tolerance to a vascularized graft has been produced. However, the introduction of cyclosporin, particularly using high-dose parenteral regimens, has resulted in the long-term survival of allografts in rat and dog models. Cyclosporin-based protocols, usually as part of a triple or

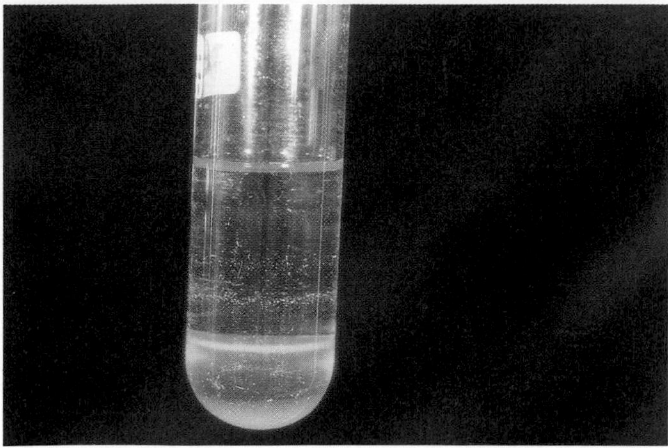

Fig. 4 Ficoll density gradient used to separate human islets from dispersed human pancreatic tissue. The dispersed pancreatic tissue is mixed with the densest layer, then progressively less dense layers of Ficoll are layered over this. After centrifugation the islets rise to a higher level than the bulk of the exocrine tissue.

quadruple therapy regimen, are currently being used for immunosuppression in clinical trials of isolated pancreatic islet transplantation.

One of the most exciting aspects of islet transplantation has been the possibility of abrogating the immune response to pancreatic islets by altering their immunogenicity before transplantation. This has been achieved experimentally by tissue culture for several days either in routine culture conditions or at room temperature, or by treatment with ultraviolet light, high oxygen tension, or antibodies specific for interstitial dendritic cells. Islet allografts treated in these ways have shown delayed or absent rejection in rodent and canine models. These studies have obvious clinical potential, allowing the treatment of diabetics by islet transplantation without the need for long-term immunosuppressive drug therapy. Another possible approach to the prevention of rejection is the microencapsulation of the islets in individual membranes that are impervious to larger molecules, for example antibiotics and lymphocytes, yet are permeable to nutrients and insulin secreted by the islets. Animal models suggest that this technique could allow transplantation without the need for immunosuppressive therapy, and might even allow the transplantation of islet xenografts from animals such as the pig.

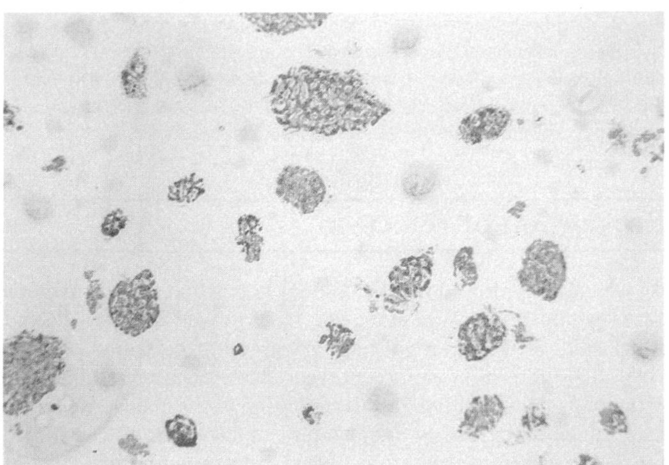

Fig. 5 Histological section of purified human islet tissue. Immunoperoxidase stain for insulin colours the islets brown. Several islets are seen to be intact yet completely separated from exocrine tissue. However, exocrine tissue is still present. Achieving full purification without an excessive loss of yield remains a problem.

Sites of implantation of pancreatic islets

Islets have been implanted in most possible sites in experimental rodent models with variable success, but studies in large animal models suggest that the most acceptable sites for clinical application are the liver (via the portal vein), the spleen (either via the splenic veins or by direct puncture), or beneath the kidney capsule (Fig. 6). At present the favoured site for clinical trials is the liver, using the portal vein. This appears to be safe, provided that the preparation is relatively free of exocrine contamination. However, impure preparations could cause portal hypertension with disseminated intravascular coagulation and should not be used in clinical trials.

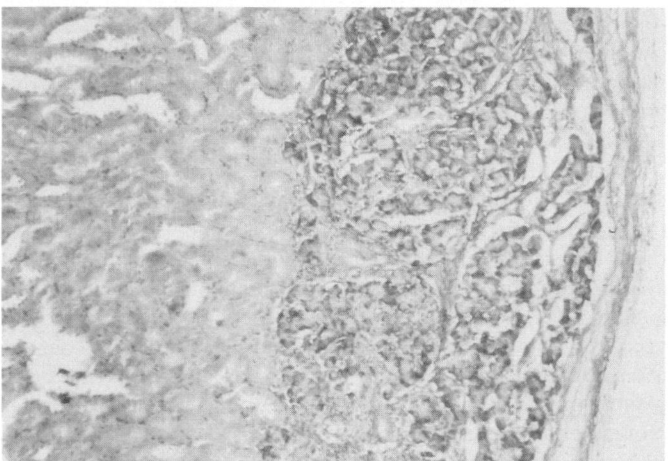

Fig. 6 Rat pancreatic islets transplanted beneath the kidney capsule (syngeneic transplant). The aldehyde-fuchsin stain for insulin is used to demonstrate insulin-containing β-cells, which stain dark mauve.

Prospects for long-term control of glucose metabolism

Transplantation of isolated pancreatic islets can produce virtually normal glucose metabolism in rodent models of experimental and autoimmune diabetes. But in larger animal models the blood sugar, although remaining within the normal range during normal nutrition, becomes abnormal in the presence of stress, probably due to a relatively reduced islet cell mass. Whether this abnormality would be important for prevention of the long-term complications of diabetes, which is the ultimate goal of islet transplantation, remains to be seen.

One disturbing feature of studies of autologous islet transplantation in the dog and monkey is that grafts have tended to fail after 1 to 3 years. This may be due to a process of exhaustion, related to a reduced islet cell mass and the site of implantation.

Recent reports in the dog model suggest that longer function is possible, but the definitive answer will probably only come from full clinical trials.

Clinical trials of isolated islet transplantation

As described above, the early trials of clinical islet transplantation were flawed by uncertainty about the viability and actual islet content of the tissue being transplanted. These experiments highlight a problem that has dogged islet transplantation research in general: how to express the actual quantity, the purity, the extent of exocrine contamination, and the viability of the isolated islet tissue in a standard format. Considerable progress has been made in producing more standardized methods of assessment that allow better comparisons between laboratories. Of particular importance has been the development of specific and rapid stains, such as dithizone, for the accurate identification of islet tissue. Over the past 5 years there have been further clinical trials from centres such as St Louis and Edmonton, where the mass of islet tissue, and the purity and viability of the tissue, have been better documented. Most transplants were performed in diabetic patients with renal failure who also underwent kidney transplantation at the same time, but more recent transplants have been performed in diabetic patients with stable long-term renal allografts. In current trials the intraportal route of implantation in the liver has been used, relying on cyclosporin-based immunosuppression with the addition of antithymocyte globulin to prevent rejection.

Some of the earlier transplants showed signs of function with elevated C peptide for a few weeks, but there was not sufficient function to allow the discontinuation of insulin. The islets used in these experiments were obtained from a single donor. More recently, several patients have had graft function sufficient to allow insulin to be discontinued for a period of several weeks to over 1 year, but islets from more than one donor were used in all but one of these cases. Thus this represents a major advance in islet transplantation but it is still far from becoming a routine therapy. Nevertheless, the situation could be compared to the earliest steps in kidney transplantation 40 years ago, when a few grafts functioned only for a few weeks or months after transplantation, but from which a successful method of treatment has grown.

FETAL PANCREAS TRANSPLANTATION

A major advantage of fetal pancreas transplantation over adult islet transplantation is that minimal processing of the islet tissue is required for transplantation. Although there is a potentially larger supply of human fetal pancreas than human adult pancreas (at least in those countries that permit abortion), several fetal pancreases are required in experimental models of diabetes to correct the diabetic state. Furthermore, the moral and ethical issues of using fetal tissue for transplantation are considerable. Another advantage of fetal pancreatic transplantation is the tremendous potential for growth of the fetal pancreas, unlike adult islets. However, immature fetal islet tissue does inhibit normal insulin secretion in response to glucose. For these reasons a long period of inadequate function is to be expected after transplantation of fetal pancreas into adult recipients, a prediction confirmed in rodent experiments.

Techniques of fetal pancreas transplantation

In comparison to adult islet transplantation, progress in fetal pancreas transplantation is less advanced. Functioning fetal pancreas transplants, both isografts and allografts, have been described and studied in detail in rodent models but, apart from successful fetal pancreatic transplantation in the pig, it has not been possible to repeat these findings in other large animal models. Some successful human cases have been reported from China, but none elsewhere. The fetal pancreas can be transplanted intact in the mouse, or in a few segments in the rat. The tissue is then small enough to survive as a free graft, the most successful site for implantation being under the kidney capsule (Fig. 7). In larger animals the fetal pancreas is too large to survive as a free graft and must be dispersed, either by sectioning the pancreas into small particles, or by digesting it with collagenase. The former provides less usable tissue, whereas it is possible to disperse the tissue fully using collagenase. After a period in tissue culture, which appears to favour islet tissue survival, the dispersed islet tissue forms 'pro-islets'. This process has proven particularly successful in the preparation of pig fetal tissue.

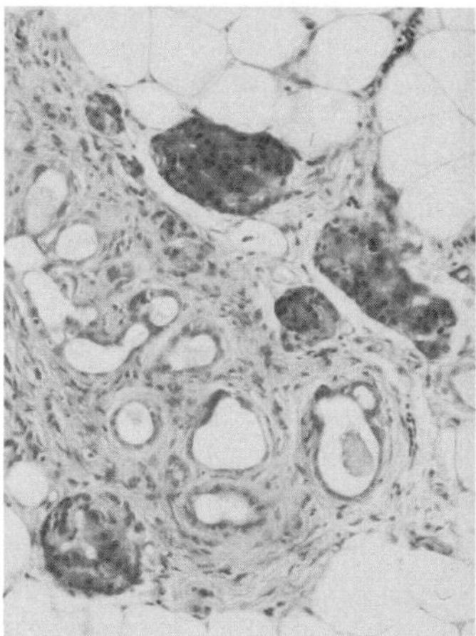

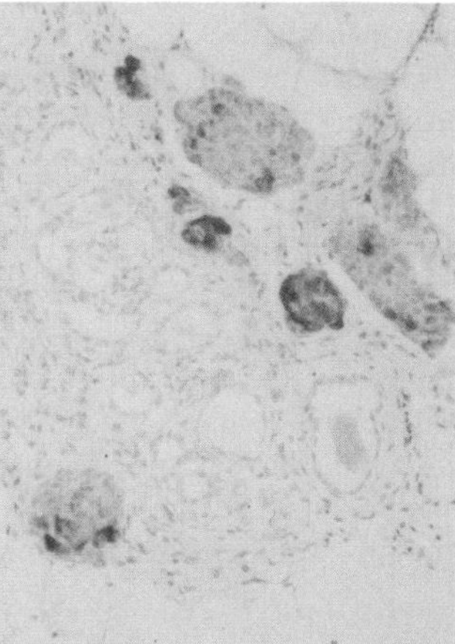

Fig. 7 Fetal rat pancreas transplanted beneath the renal capsule (syngeneic transplant). Adjacent sections are stained with haematoxylin/eosin and the immunoperoxidase stain for insulin. Note the well-preserved islets surrounded by fibrous tissue and ductal remnants. The acinar tissue has atrophied completely.

Prevention of rejection

As was the case for adult islets, initial hopes that fetal pancreatic tissue would be non-immunogenic have proved unfounded, and allografted or xenografted fetal pancreas is certainly rejected vigorously. Rejection can be prevented by various immunosuppressive protocols, although interpretation of these experiments is made difficult by the prolonged time it takes for the grafts to function after transplantation. Tissue culture in the presence of high oxygen tension has been used to reduce the immunogenicity of fetal pancreas grafts, as for adult islets. Long-term survival of allografted fetal pancreas grafts after culture has been described in mice, although this effect is markedly strain-dependent and has not been reproduced in the rat. Histological evidence that these culture techniques can prevent or delay rejection in large animals has also been presented, but there are no functioning models of fetal pancreas transplantation in large animals as a final confirmation.

Clinical trials of fetal pancreas transplantation

There have been a remarkable number of trials of fetal pancreas transplantation in man, stretching back some 15 years. Numerically the greatest number have been performed in China and the Eastern bloc countries, and despite claims of success in some patients, objective evidence of function has not been provided. Clinical trials have been undertaken in Sydney and Denver, as well as sporadic attempts elsewhere. The sites that have been used for transplantation include muscle pockets, the kidney capsule, and the intra-abdominal omentum. A combination of tissue culture prior to transplantation with a cyclosporin-based immunosuppressive protocol after transplantation has been used to try to prevent rejection. To date there has been no evidence of function either in terms of C peptide production or decreased requirements for insulin therapy.

FUTURE PROSPECTS FOR ISOLATED ISLET AND FETAL PANCREAS TRANSPLANTATION

That clinical development of isolated pancreatic islet transplantation to the point where definite, albeit short-term, function has been produced in a few patients is certainly an exciting advance. However, the function of these transplanted human islets has been less satisfactory than that obtained in animal models with an apparently equivalent transplanted mass. The reason for this difference needs elucidation, and, if the problem is solvable, this may result in functional one-to-one grafts. The problems of rejection, recurrence of disease (which has not been discussed here), and long-term function will then be the next hurdles to overcome before finally applying the technique to young diabetics.

Fetal pancreas transplantation needs development in a large animal model to answer some fundamental questions before application to the human is likely to succeed. There are moral and ethical issues involved that make general application of the technique seem unlikely at the present time.

FURTHER READING

Brown J, Molnar IG, Clark W, Mullen Y. Control of experimental diabetes mellitus in rats by transplantation of fetal pancreases. *Science* 1974; **184**: 1377–9.

Coupland RE. The survival and growth of pancreatic tissue in the anterior chamber of the eye of the albino rat. *J Endocrinol* 1960; **20**: 69–77.

Gray DWR, McShane P, Grant A, Morris PJ. A method for isolation of islets of Langerhans from the human pancreas. *Diabetes* 1984; **33**: 1055–61.

Gray DW, Morris PJ. Transplantation of isolated pancreatic islets. In: Groth CG, ed. *Pancreatic transplantation*. Philadelphia: W. B. Saunders, 1988: 363–90.

Horaguchi A, Merrell RC. Preparation of viable islet cells from dogs by a new method. *Diabetes* 1981; **30**: 455–8.

Lacy PE, Kostianovsky M. Method for the isolation of intact islets of Langerhans from the rat pancreas. *Diabetes* 1967; **16**: 35–9.

Mirkovitch V, Campiche M. Absence of diabetes in dogs after total pancreatectomy and intrasplenic autotransplantation of pancreatic tissue. *Transpl Proc* 1977; **9**: 321–3.

Morris PJ, Gray DWR, Sutton R. Pancreatic islet transplantation. *Br Med Bull* 1989; **45**: 224–41.

Moskalewski S. Isolation and culture of the islets of Langerhans of the guinea pig. *Gen Comp Endocrinol* 1965; **5**: 342–53.

Noel J, Rabinovitch A, Olson L, Kyriakides G, Miller J, Mintz DH. A method for large-scale high-yield isolation of canine pancreatic islets of Langerhans. *Metabolism* 1982; **31**: 184–7.

Sutherland DE. Pancreas and islet transplantation. I. Experimental studies. *Diabetologia* 1981; **20**: 161–85.

Sutherland DE. Pancreas and islet transplantation. II. Clinical trials. *Diabetologia* 1981; **20**: 435–50.

Warnock GL, Rajotte RV. Critical mass of purified islets that induce normoglycemia after implantation into dogs. *Diabetes* 1988; **37**: 467–70.

Warnock GL, *et al.* Continued function of pancreatic islets after transplantation in type I diabetes. *Lancet* 1989; **ii**: 570–2.

10.11 Xenogeneic transplantation

HUGH AUCHINCLOSS

INTRODUCTION

Xenogeneic transplantation is transplantation between members of different species. A discussion of xenogeneic transplantation, or 'xenografting', enters a textbook of surgery partly as history and partly as speculation, since clinical xenografting is not currently actually taking place. However, the notion that animals might donate organs to human beings has been a source of fascination since transplantation was conceived and the prospects for clinical xenografting being performed successfully in the future are good.

CLINICAL HISTORY

Xenogeneic transplantation has been attempted approximately 30 times in human beings. Although none of these transplants has survived for a full year, a kidney donated by a chimpanzee maintained good function for 9 months, until the patient died.

Reemtsma was the first to report a xenograft of a chimpanzee kidney to a human, in 1963; he went on to perform the procedure 12 times. Starzl reported a series of baboon kidney transplants to humans which started shortly afterward. Starzl also performed three chimpanzee to human liver transplants without success. A xenogeneic heart transplant was first reported in 1964 by Hardy. Several additional heart transplants were attempted including the case of 'Baby Fae' in 1985. All but one of these clinical efforts involved genetically closely-related primate donors and most were performed during the 1960s, when the immunosuppression available was less powerful than that used now.

ANTIBODY-MEDIATED REJECTION OF XENOGRAFTS

It was an historical accident that the first clinical attempts at xenogeneic transplantation were performed just as the phenomenon of hyperacute rejection was characterized. Hyperacute rejection is caused by pre-existing antibodies in a recipient's serum that are specific for donor antigens. Human beings may have antibodies specific for human blood group antigens; these antibodies can be induced by pregnancy, blood transfusion, or transplantation of other tissues. Human beings and other species also have 'natural' antibodies in their serum: these are specific for antigens of many other species and exist even without prior immunization. These natural antibodies may result in the hyperacute rejection of xenografts. Recognition of the importance of antibody-mediated rejection contributed to the decline in clinical xenografting, and the presence of natural antibodies is still the major obstacle to its widespread application.

Natural antibodies and their target antigens are not well characterized. Most of the antibodies are of the IgM subclass and probably react with endothelial glycoproteins. They may arise from cross-reactions with common environmental pathogens. In some respects natural antibodies are similar to the antibodies that react with ABO blood group antigens, although their target antigens are not the same. Very closely related species do not have natural antibodies reactive with each other: xenotransplantation between these so-called 'concordant' combinations is not followed by hyperacute rejection. The presence of natural antibodies causing hyperacute rejection defines 'discordant' combinations.

Although the existence of 'natural' antibodies hinders clinical xenografting, their presence makes xenotransplantation an excellent model to study the mechanisms and prevention of hyperacute rejection. Dozens of xenografting studies have been performed in which one or another substance has been used to delay rejection. These studies have provided information on the role of complement and vasoactive substances in hyperacute rejection, but their results have nonetheless been discouraging for clinical application. Whenever natural antibody has been present, hyperacute rejection has always occurred with only minimal delay after treatment. Even extensive absorption of antibody or its near-complete elimination by plasmapheresis, which have occasionally been successful in achieving allogeneic transplantation across blood group barriers, have not been successful in experimental xenotransplantation. The development of strategies to remove natural antibodies effectively is one of the major goals of research in xenografting.

While hyperacute rejection is a bigger factor in xenotransplantation than in allotransplantation it is still uncertain whether induced antibody responses to xenografts, which occur after transplantation, are also stronger than those induced by allografts. Some evidence suggests that they are. Since chronic graft rejection is thought to be frequently mediated by induced antibody, chronic rejection may prove an even greater problem for xenografts than for allografts, even if hyperacute rejection can be avoided by elimination of natural antibody. The induced antibody response to xenogeneic antigens probably does not reflect a secondary response of the natural antibodies, but rather a new response to xenogeneic antigens, including those of the major histocompatibility complex. Antibodies induced by concordant xenografting recognize the same determinants as those defined by allografting. Because of the likelihood that induced xenoantibody responses are stronger than those seen in allogenic combinations, strategies to achieve long-term clinical xenotransplantation will probably require forms of immunosuppression aimed at limiting this response.

CELLULAR IMMUNITY TO XENOGRAFTS

The special importance of antibody-mediated rejection in xenografting is in keeping with the simple notion that the more disparate a set of antigens is from those of the responding host the more powerful the immune response will be. When considering cell-mediated immune responses, however, the immunological discoveries of the past decade suggest that this simple dogma may not hold. The T-cell response to allogeneic MHC antigens is extraordinarily strong relative to the response to normal environmental pathogens. Late in the 1970s the basis of this strength was identified when immunologists realized that T cells recognize environmental pathogens as peptides of these antigens presented in association with 'self' antigens of the major histocompatibility complex and that developing T cells are selected for their ability to recognize such modified forms of self antigens. Allogeneic major histocompatibility complex antigens express determinants which are similar to those formed by the association of environmental pathogens and self antigens. The strength of the immune response to alloantigens therefore depends, in part, on their similarity to the responding host's own antigens. In the light of this concept, the possibility emerges that xenogeneic major histocompatibility complex antigens might be sufficiently dissimilar from those antigens of a responding species that they may not be well recognized by T cells. As a result, the cell-mediated response to xenografts may be weaker or of a different character compared with the response to allografts.

Three approaches have been used to test the strength of cell-mediated immunity to xenogeneic antigens in the absence of simultaneous humoral immunity. First, *in-vitro* assays of T-cell function, including mixed lymphocyte proliferation, interleukin-2 production, and cell-mediated cytotoxicity, have measured T-cell responses to xenogeneic stimulation. It is not certain, however, that these assays accurately reflect the processes of graft rejection. Secondly, *in-vivo* grafts exchanged between concordant species can test cellular immunity in the absence of preformed antibody, although not without induced antibody responses. Thirdly, certain kinds of *in-vivo* grafts may be resistant to antibody-mediated rejection, leaving them susceptible only to T-cell or other cell-mediated destruction. For example, skin grafts are very resistant to humoral attack, the liver is unusually resistant to antibody-mediated destruction, and cultured pancreatic islets may also be resistant to humoral immunity. Each of these approaches has been used to test the strength of cell-mediated responses to xenogeneic antigens.

In-vitro assays of T-cell responses to xenoantigens have provided mixed results. Some have suggested strong primary cellular responses to xenoantigens equivalent to those for allogeneic MHC antigens. In many cases, however, well-designed studies of T-cell immunity have shown substantially diminished responses to xenogeneic antigens compared with allodeterminants. For example, quantitative assays of cytotoxic T cells directed against xenoantigens have shown diminished precursor frequencies compared to those for alloantigens. In addition, assays of interleukin-2 production have shown absent or minimal responses to xenoantigens but strong responses to allodeterminants. The differences in these results may stem in part from the different species combinations and assay conditions used. Overall, however, evidence is emerging to support the notion that xenogeneic cellular immunity for some species combinations, as measured by *in-vitro* assays, is not as powerful as is that to allografts.

Additional analysis of the *in-vitro* cell-mediated response to xenoantigens has demonstrated that powerful secondary responses to xenoantigens can be generated after *in-vivo* priming, but that these secondary responses require the presence of antigen-presenting cells from the responding species. This result suggests that secondary recognition of xenoantigens involves recognition of peptides of these antigens presented in association with responder-type major histocompatibility antigens, on responder-type antigen-presenting cells, a mechanism similar to that used for recognition of environmental pathogens. These *in-vitro* studies, therefore, provide support for the notion that cell-mediated immunity directed against xenografts may not only be weaker, but also of different character to that directed against allografts.

Despite these *in-vitro* results, *in-vivo* experiments using concordant species to test the cell-mediated response to xenografts show that rejection is rapid. In addition, all standard forms of immunosuppression aimed at preventing cell-mediated rejection have been found to be less effective for xenografts than for allografts. Combinations of reagents have also been tested, in an attempt to produce optimal programmes for xenograft immunosuppression. Splenectomy, 15-deoxyspergualin, and other types of immunosuppression aimed at preventing B-cell responses, in addition to anti-T cell reagents, are often useful in achieving more prolonged xenograft survival. These results probably reflect a contribution of induced antibody in concordant xenograft rejection. It is difficult to tell whether *in-vivo* cellular immunity to xenoantigens is stronger or weaker than to alloantigens in these studies involving concordant species.

In-vivo studies of cell-mediated rejection of xenografts performed between discordant species have also been reported using skin grafts to avoid humoral rejection. Graft rejection without immunosuppression has again been rapid and poorly controlled by standard immunosuppression. However, antibody treatment of recipients to remove $CD4^+$ T cells has allowed prolonged survival of discordant xenogeneic skin and resulted in better survival of xenografts than of allografts placed on the same immunosuppressed recipients. These results demonstrate that *in-vivo* xenograft rejection is especially dependent on $CD4^+$ T cells and that the remaining cell-mediated response to xenografts is weaker than that to allografts, in the absence of $CD4^+$ cells.

The combined results of the *in-vitro* and *in-vivo* studies of cell-mediated xenograft rejection are difficult to interpret. On the one hand there appears to be a measurably weaker *in-vitro* T-cell response to xenoantigens in many cases and a particular requirement for $CD4^+$ T cells *in vivo*. On the other, cell-mediated xenograft rejection is rapid *in vivo* and is more difficult to control by standard immunosuppression than is allograft rejection. This apparent conflict may reflect imperfect measurement of T-cell mechanisms of xenograft rejection by *in-vitro* assays or the existence of other cellular processes of graft rejection which are dependent on $CD4^+$ T cell function, but otherwise independent of T cells. In either case, the results suggest that if B-cell responses to xenografts can be controlled or avoided, cell-mediated xenograft rejection may be prevented by more selective immunosuppression than is required for allografts.

TOLERANCE INDUCTION TO XENOGRAFTS

The ability to induce tolerance to xenoantigens has been studied by induction of neonatal tolerance and induction of tolerance in adult life by creation of bone marrow chimeras after whole body irradiation. The results of these studies have suggested that the ability to achieve tolerance to xenografts is similar to that for allografts in principle, but far more difficult to achieve in practice. This situation seems to result from the difficulty in achieving lasting survival of xenogeneic cells in the recipient even when the recipient is immunologically incompetent as judged by allogeneic cell survival. Perhaps the effector mechanisms of xenograft rejection arise earlier in development or are more resistant to whole body irradiation.

Both of these standard approaches to tolerance induction have practical limitations when considered for application to adult human patients. A modification of the technique for creating bone marrow chimeras has been developed in rodents to produce mixed chimeras, reconstituted (after whole body radiation) partially with syngeneic marrow cells and partially with donor (in this case xenogeneic) stem cells. In addition, the requirement for toxic whole-body irradiation has been avoided by using monoclonal antibodies, combined with more selective radiation, to prepare the recipient for marrow reconstitution. Further investigation of such practical strategies to achieve tolerance to xenoantigens may help make clinical xenografting possible.

NON-IMMUNOLOGICAL ISSUES IN XENOGRAFTING

Function in a xenogeneic environment

The difficulty in achieving long-term survival of xenogeneic cells in recipients of another species raises the possibility that there may be non-immunological incompatibilities which prevent some forms of xenografting. Animal organs may not function adequately in humans because of enzyme restrictions, receptor incompatibilities, differences in metabolic products, or for many other reasons. Little information is available regarding such possible incompatibilities. The kidneys of chimpanzees and baboons were capable of supporting human life for several months and pig livers were found to produce bile, to secrete porcine albumin, and perhaps to improve human neurological function when they were perfused with blood from patients with hepatic failure. Beyond these limited data, identification of the limits of xenograft survival and function will require control of immunological causes of graft failure. It is likely that such limitations do exist.

Sources of animal donors

Closely related to the question of xenograft function in a human host is the question of which species might prove the best donor for clinical xenogeneic transplantation. Presumably the more closely related species will show fewer incompatibilities of organ function. In addition, more closely related species are concordant to humans, thus avoiding the problem of natural antibodies. On the other hand, the subhuman primates, especially chimpanzees, are not available in large numbers, breed slowly in captivity, may have organs too small for human beings, and their use would present ethical problems today. Many investigators have therefore considered pigs as potential donors well suited for clinical xenotransplantation. These animals breed rapidly and are of appropriate size. However, man possesses natural antibody against pig antigens. Another consideration in selecting animal donors is whether endemic pathogens or non-pathogenic retroviruses of another species might prove dangerous to human beings.

Ethical issues

The idea of clinical xenotransplantation provokes much controversy regarding the ethical issues, as was demonstrated in the 'Baby Fae' case in 1985. The issues are of several kinds. From the point of view of the recipient, xenotransplantation would be entirely experimental and a successful outcome, as this chapter should indicate, cannot be confidently predicted. Thus appropriate informed consent for an uncertain undertaking would be necessary; obtaining informed consent would be particularly uncertain if the potential recipient were a child. With respect to the donor animals, ethical issues also arise. Some critics have objected especially to the use of subhuman primates because these animals have easily recognizable human characteristics. How can one know, however, where a line should be drawn that makes an animal too close for comfortable use by human beings. Others have objected to the breeding and use of any animals for the purpose of supporting human life by organ donation. In this case it is not clear how this would differ from the breeding of livestock for human food and clothing, an activity generally accepted by our society.

PROSPECTS FOR XENOGRAFTING

In many respects this chapter presents the uncertain prospects for clinical xenografting in the near future. Nonetheless, several approaches might result in successful xenogeneic transplantation being accomplished in this century. First, the many months of primate graft survival accomplished during the early 1960s makes it seem quite likely that some successful xenografts could be undertaken even today using closely related donors and modern techniques of immunosuppression. As still newer immunosuppressive agents become available, such as 15-deoxyspergualin and FK506, these prospects may become even better. Animal kidneys would probably not be used for humans as a first step, because dialysis can maintain most recipients satisfactorily until human organs become available. Patients with heart disease, however, might be saved in some circumstances by use of a primate donor, even if that were only a temporary bridge until allotransplantation could be performed. On the other hand, the limited number of animals available from concordant species will prevent widespread application of this approach, making it questionable whether it should be tried at all.

A second approach to xenotransplantation would be through achievement of better techniques to eliminate natural antibody and prevent humoral rejection, thereby allowing use of more disparate donors. Since successful allotransplantation across blood group barriers has been accomplished in a few cases, this approach may be feasible. Although plasmapheresis has never been sufficiently effective to achieve long-term xenotransplantation, the precise identification of the target antigens of natural antibody might allow more complete immunoabsorption. On the other hand, the effort to eliminate natural antibody has not been successful in over 20 years of work, making this approach to xenotransplantation very uncertain.

A third potential approach to achieve successful xenogeneic transplantation would be to achieve neonatal tolerance to xenogeneic antigens. For example, diagnosis of life-threatening cardiac birth defects *in utero* by ultrasound might provide the opportunity for prenatal introduction of xenogeneic cells, potentially rendering the newborn infant tolerant to antigens of this species. Sufficient experimental data to demonstrate the feasibility of this approach are not yet available.

A fourth potential approach would be to use xenogeneic tissues resistant to antibody-mediated attack. The liver might be one such organ, especially for children, who are at considerable risk of dying while awaiting a human donor. More likely, animal donors could provide pancreatic islets to treat diabetes mellitus: cultured pancreatic islets may be resistant to humoral rejection and they have the additional advantage of being depleted of antigen-presenting cells. There has been considerable difficulty in isolating large quantities of human islets, making the gap between the potential supply of human islets and the potential demand of thousands of diabetic patients very large. Since the cell-mediated response to discordant pancreatic islets may be more easily controlled than for allogeneic islets, this approach is promising.

While successful xenotransplantation has not yet been achieved, it is still not too early to imagine the use of xenogeneic tissues, not for their organ function, but rather as vectors to introduce the products of genes not normally carried by the animal donor. For example, techniques of molecular biology make it possible to imagine the creation of transgenic pigs expressing products of human genes which may be absent or defective in a human recipient. Transplantation of cells from these animals would avoid the malignant potential of long-term cultured human cell lines. It is also possible to imagine the selective breeding of herds of animal donors or the induction of genetic mutation so as to avoid expression of particular deleterious transplantation antigens. In these ways xenogeneic transplantation may be the key to a new era in the field of transplantation.

FURTHER READING

Auchincloss HJ. Xenogeneic transplantation. A review. *Transplantation* 1988; **46**: 1–20.

Auchincloss HJ. Xenografting: a review. *Transplant Rev* 1990; **4**: 1–7.

Calne RY. Observations on renal homotransplantation. *Br J Surg* 1961; **48**: 384.

Hardy MA. *Xenograft 25.* Netherlands: Elsevier Science Publishers BV (Biomedical Division) 1989.

Ildstad ST, Wren SM, Sharrow SO, Stephany D, Sachs DH. *In vivo* and *in vitro* characterization of specific hyporeactivity to skin xenografts in mixed xenogeneically reconstituted mice (B10 + F344 rat to B10). *J Exp Med* 1984; **160**: 1820.

Moses RD, Pierson RNI, Winn HJ, Auchincloss HJ. Xenogeneic proliferation and lymphokine production are dependent on CD4$^+$ helper T cells and self antigen-presenting cells in the mouse. *J Exp Med* 1990; **172**: 567–75.

Perper RJ, Najarian JS. Experimental renal heterotransplantation: I. In widely divergent species. *Transplantation* 1966; **4**: 377.

Pierson RN, Winn HJ, Russell PS, Auchincloss HJ. Xenogeneic skin graft rejection is especially dependent on CD4$^+$ T cells. *J Exp Med* 1989; **170**: 991–6.

Platt JL, Lindman BJ, Chen H, Spitalnik SL, Bach FH. Endothelial cell antigens recognized by xenoreactive human natural antibodies. *Transplantation* 1990; **50**: 817–22.

Reemtsma K. Renal heterotransplantation from nonhuman primates to man. *Ann NY Acad Sci* 1969: **162**: 412.

10.12 Neural tissue transplantation

RICHARD KERR

INTRODUCTION

The neuronal complement of cells within the central nervous system (CNS) is not capable of significant regeneration. For many neurological, especially neurodegenerative, disorders, effective therapy is either short acting or unavailable.

With the establishment in the mid-1980s of reliable methods of neural tissue transplantation came the rapid realization that this technique could be applied clinically. In a short period of time, many centres worldwide initiated programmes of neural tissue transplantation of either fetal tissue or autologous adrenal medulla into patients suffering from the neurodegenerative disorder, Parkinson's disease. Although these attempts have met with only limited success they have done much to stimulate research in the field of neural transplantation, a long neglected area of transplantation biology. This, together with our increasing knowledge of neurobiology will hopefully allow the full potential of this exciting area of transplantation to be established.

HISTORICAL BACKGROUND

The first published attempts at neural tissue transplantation date back to the late 19th century, but only following the work of the modern day pioneers, published in the early 1970s, has the field of neuronal transplantation progressed. Having defined the conditions required for graft survival and devised methods of graft identification, initially by histochemistry and more recently by immunohistochemistry, the stage was set for a rapid advance in the techniques of neural transplantation, and, to a lesser extent, in the understanding of the immune response to allogenic neural tissue. This was greatly assisted by the brain being considered a site of immunological privilege, a concept missing from a series of experiments using tumour grafts between animals of ill-defined genetic background. The survival of these grafts, together with the apparent lack of major histocompatibility complex antigen expression within the brain and the presence of the blood–brain barrier, meant that the question of rejection of allogenic tissue, one of the major stumbling blocks in all other fields of transplantation, did not have to be addressed, at least in theory.

A large variety of animal models, both functional and structural, have been devised to examine various aspects of neural tissue transplantation. The most widely used has been a movement disorder model of Parkinson's disease first described in 1973, induced by the injection of 6-hydroxydopamine into the substantia nigra of animals. This leads to a selective degeneration of the nigral projections to the striatum, similar to the changes seen in Parkinson's disease. The resultant neuronal degeneration causes a fall in the dopamine concentration in the striatum.

Administration of a dopamine agonist produces a characteristic movement disorder that is quantifiable. Insertion of fetal substantia nigra reduces this movement disorder, and considerable outgrowth of monoamine-containing neurones can be shown histochemically.

As an alternative, and by way of circumventing the putative ethical problems surrounding the use of fetal tissue, grafts of adrenal medulla (a source of dopamine) have also been used and appear to produce a similar improvement in the movement disorder.

Another, and perhaps widely under-used, functional model involves the selective reduction of the cholinergic input to the hippocampus by a lesion in the septohippocampal pathway. This induces a memory and behaviour abnormality that can be improved by the insertion of a septal graft rich in cholinergic neurones. Similar losses of specific populations of neuronal cells are seen in patients suffering from the neurodegenerative disorder, Alzheimer's disease.

Rather than inducing defects, congenital neuronal deficiency and the resultant deficit that this produces has provided a further way of examining the functional influence of a graft. One such model is the Brattleboro rat, which suffers from diabetes insipidus due to a deficiency of vasopressin-secreting neurones. Grafts of fetal anterior hypothalamus placed into the recipient third ventricle partially alleviate this deficiency.

Finally, a recently devised model utilizes the Purkinje cell degeneration mutant mouse, into which fetal cerebellar primordia are placed. The grafts appear to repopulate the deficient molecular layer of the cerebellum, synapses developing between the Purkinje cell-containing grafts and the host cell population.

In all these models, it is far from clear how the grafts exert their effect. Since there does appear to be synapse formation within the graft it is possible that a direct graft–host interaction is involved, but it may be that the grafts are merely acting as an exogenous source of the deficient neurotransmitter, or perhaps the source of a neurotrophic factor that is causing a degree of regeneration or repair of the host cells.

Whatever the exact mode of action, the reported success of grafts in these and many other studies, including autografts of adrenal medulla in a primate model, led to the clinical application of this technique to patients suffering from Parkinson's disease.

TECHNIQUES OF NEURAL TISSUE TRANSPLANTATION

Graft survival in any situation requires the implantation of viable tissue to an area of adequate blood supply with the minimum of trauma. For neural tissue transplantation, the use of young (fetal) tissue is essential. Fetal tissue appears to survive a short period of anoxia, while still retaining the capacity for continued growth and differentiation.

Neural tissue transplants may be of solid tissue or cell suspensions and can be placed directly into the host brain, into a preformed cavity or into the ventricle. The use of a cell suspension depends upon dissociation of the required area from the donor brain using trypsin, with subsequent stereotactic implantation into the host. Graft viability depends upon the origin of the tissue, the age, the mechanical trauma applied, and the use of trypsin. A graft containing viable cells is required to obtain good survival rates.

Similar parameters govern the implantation of solid tissue grafts, unless into a preformed cavity, where a delay in graft insertion may improve survival. The ventricular system offers a preformed cavity with a ready blood supply. However, this site only provides graft access to periventricular tissues and will not stop graft migration. Placement into the ventricle can be easily achieved stereotactically with minimal trauma.

CLINICAL APPLICATION OF NEURAL TISSUE TRANSPLANTS

In 1985, the results following the implantation of autografts of adrenal medulla in two patients suffering from Parkinson's disease were published. The initial symptomatic improvement noticed in these patients was very short lived, the grafts having been stereotactically placed into the head of the caudate nucleus. The publication of this work was met with initial scepticism, especially in view of the poor results. However, a subsequent report, published in 1987 from Mexico, described enormous success using adrenal medulla autografts in two young patients. This sparked off the clinical application of this technique in many centres worldwide.

Patients suffering from Parkinson's disease seemed the ideal starting place for studies on human neural tissue transplantation. Advantages include a specific neurochemical defect, together with the ability to use not only fetal cells, which show both good survival and extensive neurone outgrowth, but also autologous adrenal medulla as the graft material.

The preliminary rodent work utilizing these systems was applied directly to the human situation, and now in excess of 100 patients have received adrenal medulla to caudate autografts. Sporadic claims of success generated further interest. In general the results were disappointing, not only in terms of morbidity and mortality, but also due to a lack of symptomatic improvement. In 1988, questions were asked about the validity of the technique and a plea was made for extensive basic research before clinical trials proceeded any further. As an alternative to adrenal medulla, fetal tissue containing substantia nigra had also been used as a source of dopaminergic neurones. In the 1-methyl-4-phenyl-1,2,5,6-tetrahydropyridine-induced Parkinson's disease model in both rodents and primates, considerable success in amelioration of many motor deficits has been seen following such treatment. This naturally resulted in clinical trials using fetal mesencephalic tissue. Initial results, where such grafts have been placed into the putamen of the basal ganglia, rather than the caudate nucleus, appear encouraging.

The success of this work shows that human fetal dopaminergic-containing neurones can survive, grow, and continue to synthesize and store dopamine following allotransplantation into the putamen of immunosuppressed hosts. There are however, still many unanswered questions surrounding neural transplantation. Graft–host interaction is certainly not fully understood, although implied by the improvement of clinical signs. How long will the graft function, and if it fails, is this due to immune rejection or the underlying disease process? Is it that the graft is acting merely as a source of growth factor?

Future success and the ability to develop a robust system depends upon answers being established to these difficult questions.

FUTURE DIRECTIONS

Already, work is being directed towards the immune response to allogenic neural tissue. This is an area of major importance, for the criteria upon which the brain has for so long been considered a site of immunological privilege can no longer be substantiated. There are now several reports showing that neuroepithelium is capable of major histocompatibility complex antigen expression both *in vitro* and *in vivo*, and that neural tissue allografts are immunologically rejected. How this response is generated is uncertain, but it appears that it is only the glial population of cells that is capable of such antigen expression.

The question of how to overcome this response is therefore foremost. This may be achieved by the use of immunosuppressive drugs, but treatment with monoclonal antibodies directed against T-cell subsets involved in rejection also appears to enhance graft survival. The fact that the neuroepithelium can be dissociated into a single cell suspension and that alloreactivity appears to be related to only a small subpopulation of the cells may indicate that grafts devoid of those reactive cells will provide an alternative way to circumvent the rejection response. Initial studies using this technique suggest that allograft survival can be improved in this way.

The use of genetically engineered cells as a source of either growth factors or neurotransmitters offers a method of graft production that is not dependent upon tissue availability and would enable the development of grafts containing large populations of cells producing precisely what is required. Obviously, graft–host interaction would be limited, but this may be ideal in situations where only a source of growth factor or transmitter is required.

The biology of growth factors is expanding rapidly and the use of growth factors in the central nervous system has already been seen as a way of ameliorating many and varied neurodegenerative disorders. Neuronal cell degeneration appears to be arrested by direct injection of nerve growth factor. Cholinergic neurones, the cell type affected in patients suffering from Alzheimer's disease, appear to be especially sensitive to the effects of this factor. Careful optimism surrounds the future application of this finding and preliminary studies indicate that infusions of nerve growth factor actually reverse the atrophy of these neurones in the brains of aged rats.

Important structural studies, at both light and electron microscopic levels using more specific markers, continue in an attempt to detail the precise nature of the interaction between the graft and the host tissues.

CONCLUSION

That neural tissue can be successfully transplanted, and that the basic techniques are available has now been established. How to apply these techniques to best advantage, however, remains unclear. Future work must be directed towards more basic research, with judicious clinical application as a result of that research. In that way, the full potential therapeutic benefits may be realized and hopefully neural tissue transplantation will become widely available for the treatment of a variety of neurological disorders.

FURTHER READING

Borges LF. Historical development of neural transplantation. *Appl Neurophysiol* 1988; **51**: 265–77.

Fuchs HE, Bullard DE. Immunology of transplantation in the central nervous system. *Appl Neurophysiol* 1988; **51**: 278–96.

Backlund E-O, *et al.* Transplantation of adrenal medullary tissue to the striatum in Parkinsonism. *J Neurosurg* 1885; **62**: 169–73.

Sladek JR Jr, Shoulson I. Neural transplantation: a call for patience rather than patients. *Science* 1988; **240**: 1386–8.

Lindvall O, *et al.* Grafts of fetal dopamine neurons survive and improve motor function in Parkinson's disease. *Science* 1990; **247**: 574–7.

Bartlett PF, Rosenfeld J, Bailey KA, Cheesman H, Harvey AR, Kerr RSC. Allograft rejection overcome by immunoselection of neuronal precursor cells. *Prog Brain Res* 1990; **82**: 153–60.

Endocrine disease 11

11.1 The thyroid gland

NICHOLAS DUDLEY

SURGICAL ANATOMY

General orientations

The thyroid gland is situated in the anterior triangle of the neck, weighs approximately 20 g and consists of two lateral lobes (right and left), joined together by a midline isthmus. The small pyramidal lobe of Lalouette, of variable size, commonly joins the isthmus at its junction with the left lateral lobe by a fibrous band or strand of muscle fibres known as the levator glandulae thyroideae. The lobes measure approximately $5 \times 3 \times 1.5$ cm (slightly larger in women) and extend from the middle of the thyroid cartilage above to the sixth tracheal ring below. Each lobe fills the space between the trachea and oesophagus medially and the carotid sheath laterally. A strong condensation of vascular connective tissue, known as the suspensory ligament of Berry, binds the gland firmly to each side of the cricoid cartilage and it is this ligament, together with the pretracheal fascia which splits to invest the gland, which makes the thyroid move up and down on swallowing. The fascia (false or surgical capsule) sends fibrous septa into the gland substance, dividing it into numerous lobules. Each lobule consists of 30 to 40 follicles that contain colloid; these are the main secretory and storage elements.

Development of the thyroid

The thyroid gland develops from two distinct embryological structures: the primitive pharynx and the neural crest. A median pharyngeal downgrowth migrates between the first and the second arch components of the tongue and descends in a caudal direction along a line extending from the foramen caecum at the back of the tongue to the pyramidal lobe of the thyroid. In doing so, the track passes ventral to the hyoid bone and then loops behind it (Fig. 1). The track usually becomes obliterated but part occasionally persists, giving rise to a thyroglossal cyst or fistula. Rarely the thyroid bud fails to descend but develops *in situ* at the back of the tongue (lingual thyroid). Conversely, it may descend too far, causing a primary mediastinal or retrosternal goitre. Even less commonly the thyroid bud may fail to divide in two and appear as one lateral lobe, the left usually being absent. The parafollicular or C cells scattered between the cuboidal epithelial cells that line the thyroid follicles, are derived from the neural crest. They first migrate to the ultimobranchial bodies of the fourth and fifth branchial pouches and then to the thyroid (Fig. 2). These are the cells which in later life have the potential to undergo hyperplastic and malignant change, resulting in calcitonin-producing medullary carcinoma of the thyroid.

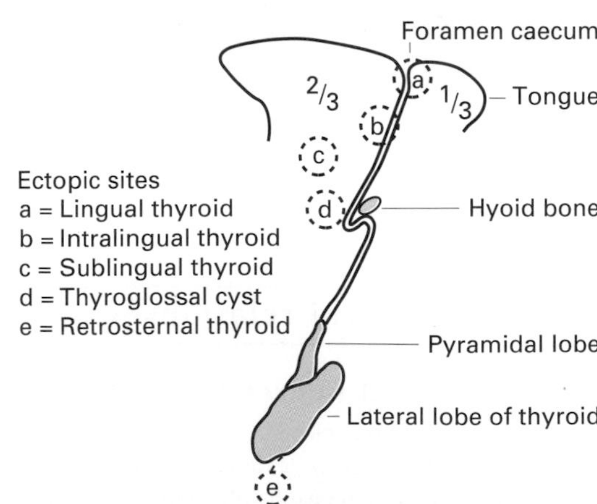

Fig. 1 Migration of the thyroid via the thyroglossal duct and possible ectopic sites of development and duct remnants.

Blood supply (Fig. 3)

The vascular supply of the gland is impressive and becomes more so in hyperactive thyroid states. The main supply is via two paired arteries; a third vessel occasionally supplies the lower pole of one

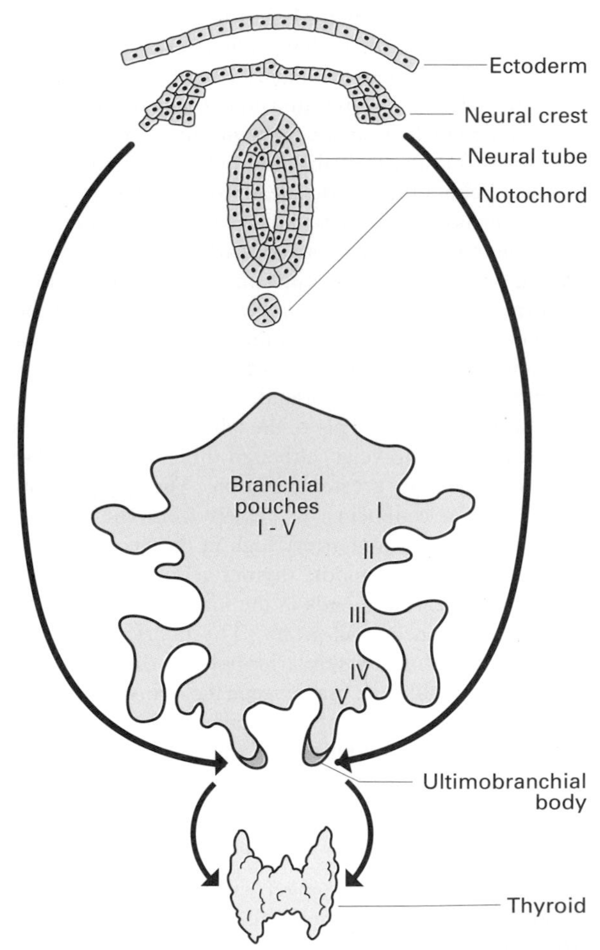

Fig. 2 Migration of the parafollicular C cells.

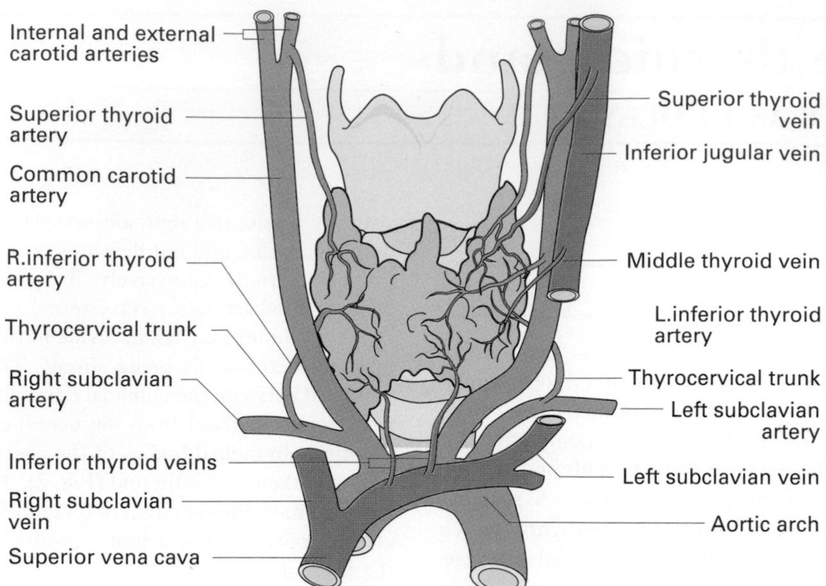

Fig. 3 Vascular supply to the thyroid.

or other lobe. The superior thyroid artery, the first branch of the external carotid, runs downward on the inferior constrictor to reach the apex of the lateral lobe, where it divides into a large anterior branch and a usually smaller, but important, posterior branch. Occasionally a tributary leaves high on the left to supply the pyramidal lobe near the midline. The inferior thyroid artery is generally much larger than the superior thyroid artery but is less constant, being absent or duplicated on one side or the other in 10 per cent of individuals. It arises from the thyrocervical trunk and passes upwards for a variable distance before looping down, running medially behind the carotid sheath to reach the posterolateral aspect of the gland at the junction of the middle and lower thirds. Numerous unnamed accessory arteries arise from the oesophagus and trachea, but the most frequently encountered is the thyroidea ima (Neubauer's artery), which courses up anteriorly on the trachea to reach the isthmus or one of the lower poles and originates from the aorta or brachiocephalic artery. In the absence of the inferior thyroid artery on one side, the thyroidea ima may be the principal source of blood supply to the lobe and therefore substantial. The named thyroid veins, although three in number like the arteries, are subject to greater variation. The superior thyroid vein, formed by a confluence of vessels from the upper pole, crosses the common carotid artery high in the neck to drain into the internal jugular. The middle thyroid vein, which overlies the inferior thyroid artery, also ends in the internal jugular vein after crossing the common carotid artery. The inferior thyroid veins descend from the isthmus and inferior poles of the lateral lobes to join the internal jugular or brachiocephalic veins in the anterior mediastinum and are intimately associated with the thyrothymic ligaments, which expand inferiorly as the lobes of the thymus.

Lymphatic drainage

The thyroid is generously supplied with lymphatics and a rich network ramifies throughout the gland. They drain primarily into mediastinal nodes inferiorly, tracheo-oesophageal nodes laterally, and the midline delphian nodes superiorly. Studies performed following injection of dye suggest that the majority of lymph from the thyroid returns to the thoracic duct without passing through the deep cervical lymph node chain or the nodes of the posterior triangle, although these pathways may open up secondarily (Fig. 4). This has implications for the assessment of patients with carcinoma of the thyroid, who may develop lymph node deposits outside the primary drainage areas, even on the contralateral side.

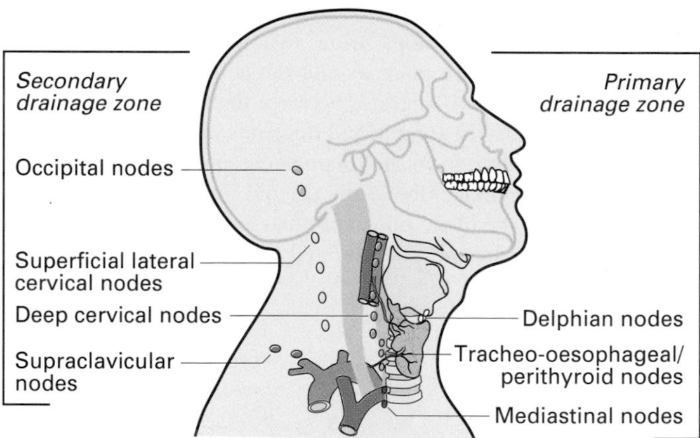

Fig. 4 Primary and secondary zones of lymphatic drainage of the thyroid.

Important anatomical relationships

Recurrent laryngeal nerves (Fig. 5)

There are several structures closely related to the gland with which a surgeon must be familiar. The most important of these is the recurrent laryngeal nerve on each side, which is a branch of the vagus. The latter, having entered the mediastinum, gives off the recurrent nerve, which returns to the neck having circled around

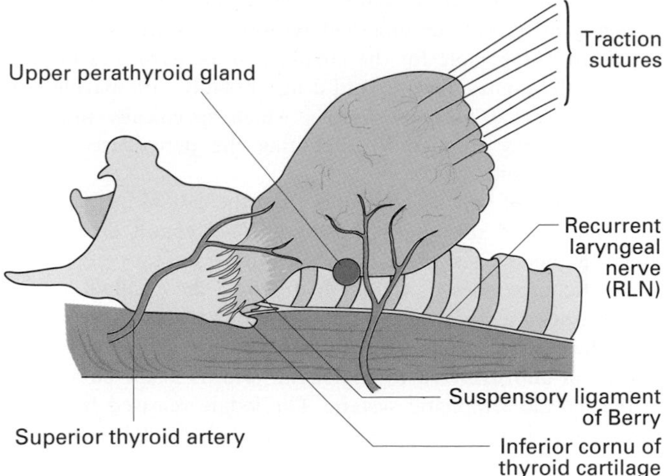

65% RLN passes medial to attachment of ligament of Berry
25% RLN passes through ligament of Berry
10% RLN passes through thyroid itself

Fig. 5 Course of the recurrent laryngeal nerve in the neck.

the arch of the aorta on the left and the right subclavian artery on the right. It ascends in the tracheo-oesophageal groove and has a variable relationship with the inferior thyroid artery on each side (Fig. 6). Occasionally the nerve itself divides early and branches around the artery (10 per cent of individuals). In approximately 0.25 per cent of individuals the recurrent laryngeal nerve on the right is non-recurrent but passes directly from the vagus to the cricothyroid muscles. As it takes the same course as the inferior thyroid artery, it is particularly vulnerable if its presence is unrecognized when this vessel is routinely ligated laterally.

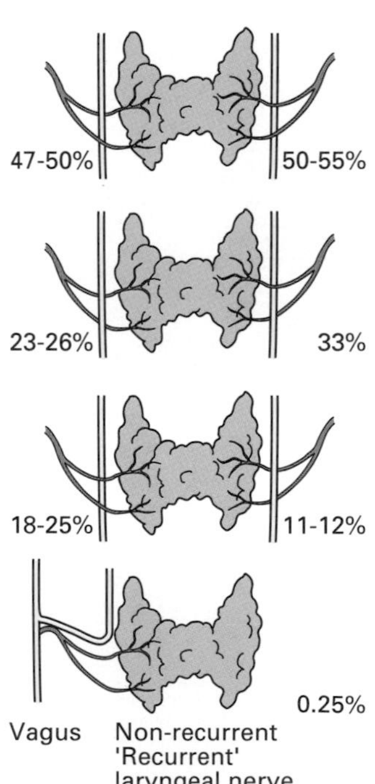

Fig. 6 Relationship of the recurrent laryngeal nerve to the inferior thyroid artery (right and left).

Whichever course the nerve takes, it ultimately enters the larynx posterior to the cricothyroid articulation passing under or through Berry's ligament. The nerve supplies all the intrinsic muscles of the larynx together with some sensory supply to the mucosa below the vocal cords. The principal effect of division of this nerve is paralysis of the vocal cord on that side.

The superior laryngeal nerve

This also arises from the vagus (inferior ganglion) and divides at the level of the hyoid bone into a large internal laryngeal nerve and a smaller external laryngeal nerve. The latter runs close to the superior thyroid artery but at a deeper plane, immediately above the superior pole of the thyroid. It terminates as the nerve supply to the cricothyroid muscle which acts as a tensor of the vocal cords on the same side.

The cervical sympathetic chain

This underlies the carotid sheath just medial to the vagus on the prevertebral fascia and is in close proximity to the inferior thyroid artery as it arches around medially.

Parathyroid glands

There are normally four parathyroid glands, the upper pair of which lie in close proximity to the dorsal aspect of the thyroid. They are usually found just above and medial to where the recurrent laryngeal nerve crosses the inferior thyroid artery, frequently tucked round behind its branches (Fig. 7). The lower parathyroid gland on each side is situated within a 2-cm radius of the lower pole of the thyroid typically on its surface anterolaterally and at a level below and medial to where the recurrent laryngeal nerve crosses the inferior thyroid artery (Fig. 8).

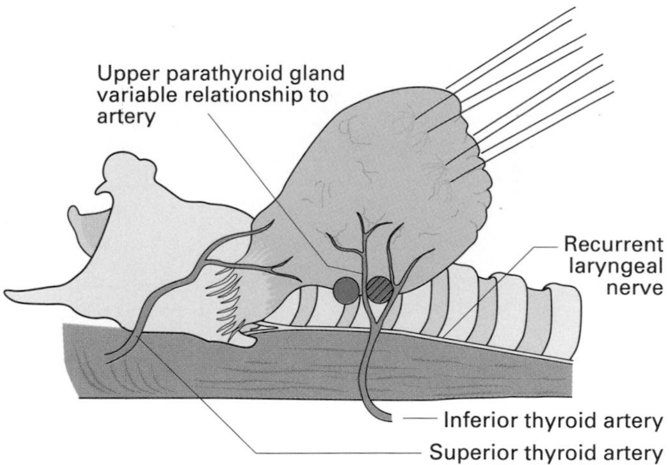

Fig. 7 Normal siting of the upper parathyroid gland.

PHYSIOLOGY

The thyroid, the largest endocrine gland in the body, produces three hormones, thyroxine (T_4), tri-iodothyronine (T_3) and calcitonin. T_4 and T_3 are both stored in the colloid, consisting primarily of thyroglobulin which is an iodinated glycoprotein. Thyroglobulin stores are dependent on adequate dietary iodine intake, which is essential for T_3 and T_4 synthesis. Iodine is derived mainly from milk and dairy products with a smaller proportion

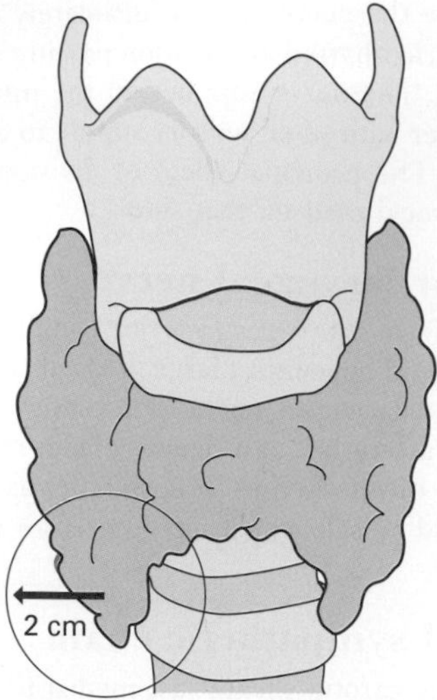

Fig. 8 Normal siting of the lower parathyroid gland.

from salt water fish and iodized salt. An average diet in the United Kingdom gives an intake of 100 to 150 μg of iodide daily—this is higher in North America, where iodine is added to a wider range of foodstuffs. Plasma levels therefore vary widely, depending on geographical locality. Iodides are absorbed in the stomach and upper gastrointestinal tract; approximately two-thirds is excreted via the kidneys, and one-third is trapped in the thyroid, where 95 per cent of the body stores of iodine are found. Hormone synthesis takes place only after the iodide has been oxidized to an active form by a peroxidase enzyme system, which is in turn generated by one of the cytochrome reductase systems. The activated iodine is bound covalently to tyrosine or monoiodotyrosine. The peroxidase system is also responsible for the coupling of iodotyrosines to produce iodothyronines. Antithyroid drugs, notably carbimazole, are rapidly converted to methimazole, which specifically prevents iodine becoming trapped by inhibiting the peroxidase system within the thyroid.

The release of thyroid hormones from the colloid begins when microvilli on the surface of the thyroid cell engulf droplets of colloid by pinocytosis; these then fuse with lysosomes containing proteolytic enzymes, which hydrolyse the colloid. The iodotyrosines are rapidly converted to iodide and thyroxine, which enters the blood stream via the thyroid capillaries (Fig. 9). A small quantity of unhydrolysed thyroglobulin returns to the circulation via the thyroid lymphatic system. The iodide released from the thyroid contributes to a much larger circulating iodide pool than the quite separate dietary iodide pool which delivers the element to the gland. Turnover is also slower.

Thyroid stimulating hormone (TSH) produced by the thyrotrophic cells of the anterior pituitary control the complex enzymatic reactions that trap iodine, convert it to T_3 and T_4 and release them into the circulation. When T_3 and T_4 levels rise above the normal range TSH production is shut down by a negative biofeedback loop (Fig. 10). Release of TSH is regulated by thyrotrophin releasing hormone (TRH), which is produced in the hypothalamus. TRH enters the capillary bed of the stalk median eminence passing via the portal veins and sinusoids to bathe the anterior pituitary cells. TSH biosynthesis shows a circadian rhythm, its secretion being maximal in the evening before the onset of sleep, remaining high overnight and falling to a low around midday. The pineal gland may be responsible for this rhythm.

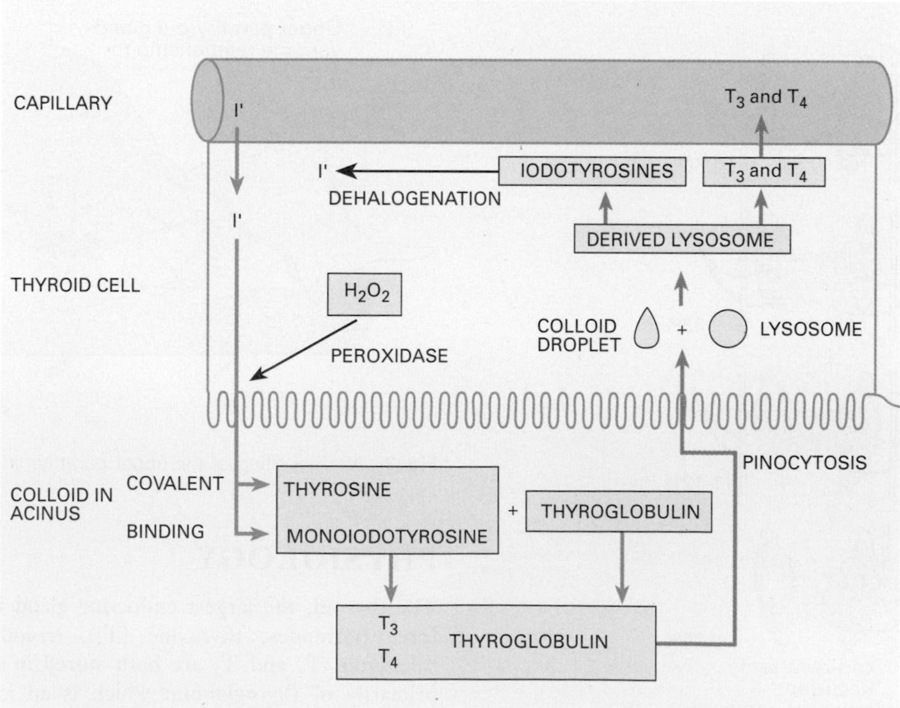

Fig. 9 Schematic representation of thyroid hormone synthesis and release into the bloodstream.

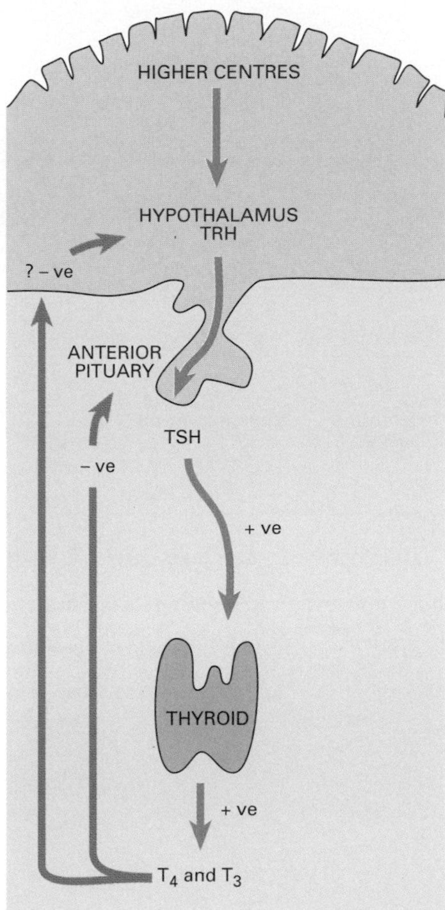

Fig. 10 Schematic representation of the hypothalamo-pituitary-thyroid axis.

The role of calcitonin in normal thyroid physiology has not been established in man, but it may be involved in the regulation of plasma calcium and phosphate concentration. However thyroidectomy which removes nearly all the parafollicular C cells causes no disturbance of calcium homeostasis. Medullary thyroid carcinoma, a tumour of the C cells which frequently results in gross hypercalcitoninaemia also rarely disturbs calcium levels in the plasma. The rise in plasma calcitonin which occurs during pregnancy and lactation appears to have no effect on the maternal skeleton, but calcium resorption may be prevented by a concommitant increase in the level of circulating cholecalciferol.

PATHOPHYSIOLOGY

Nearly all disorders of the thyroid result in some swelling of the gland itself and the non-specific term 'goitre' embraces them all. In clinical practice a working classification based on whether the gland is toxic or not and the nature of the enlargement is helpful. This enables a diagnosis to be made and appropriate action taken in the majority of patients (Fig. 11).

Non-toxic goitre

Diffuse/simple goitre

Physiological goitre

Enlargement of the thyroid is common during puberty and pregnancy, and at the menopause. This may be the result of increased physiological demand for thyroid hormone or as a response to growth hormone and variation in oestrogen levels. Increased levels of TSH are believed to be involved in the process but are not readily detectable in euthyroid patients.

Primary iodine deficiency/endemic goitre

The majority of 'endemic' goitres are due to low dietary intake of iodine (less than 100 μg a day). The worldwide geographical distribution of endemic goitre corresponds closely to alpine areas where glacial action has leached iodine from the soil and carried it away to the sea: endemic goitres are rarely seen in coastal areas. The response of high-risk populations to the addition of iodine to table salt or drinking water or to a depot injection of intramuscular lipiodol suggests that some patients with endemic goitres also have a metabolic defect in thyroxine synthesis which only declares itself when iodine is scarce.

Secondary iodine deficiency goitre

Dietary

Some endemic goitres are due to substances in the diet (goitrogens) which interfere with the trapping of iodine or the synthesis of thyroxine. These include the thioureas in uncooked vegetables of the brassica family—turnips, swedes, cabbages, Tasmanian weeds (used for cow feed), and soya beans. Excess dietary fluoride has been incriminated in the aetiology of goitre in the Punjab, while calcium excess has been implicated in Columbia, Cape Province, Burma, and Western China.

Drugs

The drugs most commonly responsible for thyroid enlargement of this type are the thioureas, especially when over-used in the treatment of thyrotoxicosis. Other drugs, including thiocyanates, iodine, *p*-aminosalicylic acid, resorcinol, lithium, and phenylbutazone, may all cause goitre if administered over a long period.

Genetic defects/dyshormonogenetic goitre

In a small proportion of patients the susceptibility to goitre formation is due to an autosomal non-sex-linked partially recessive gene defect. Five distinct biochemical defects resulting from the inheritance of a single gene abnormality have been described.

1. Inability to concentrate iodine in the gland;
2. Inability to bind iodine which if total results in congenital hypothyroidism. In some cases congenital deafness may be associated (Pendred's syndrome);
3. Inability to couple iodotyrosines to form iodothyronine (peroxidase and dehalogenase deficiency);
5. Inability to retain iodine in iodotyrosines due to the lack of the deiodinase enzyme. This results in loss of iodine in its organic form in the urine;
4. Abnormal protein binding of iodine in the plasma which is then unavailable to the normal process of hormone synthesis.

Although of academic interest it is not usually practical or helpful to investigate which of the above defects is responsible for a con-

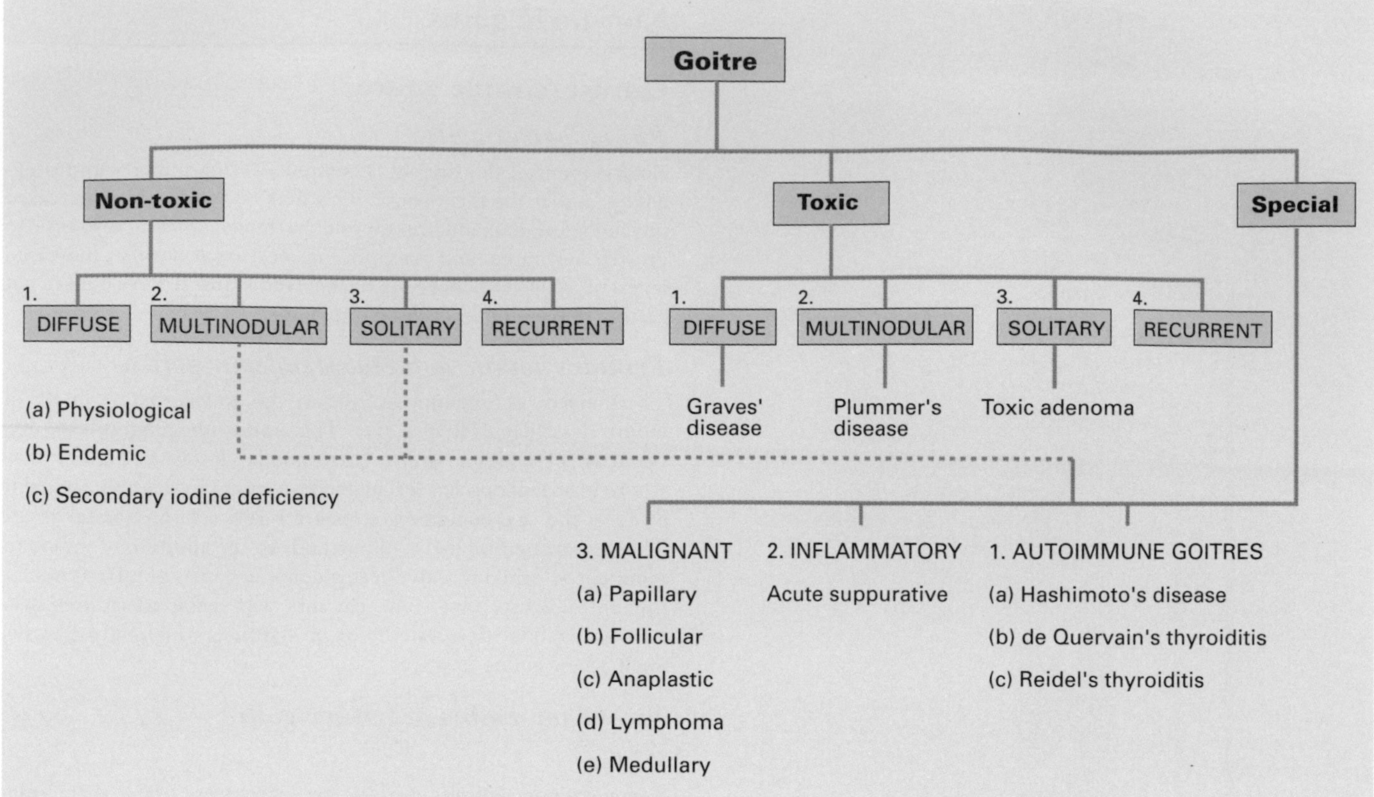

Fig. 11 Classification of goitres.

genital goitre. All of the above causes of dyshormonogenesis cause compensatory hypertrophy of the gland in an attempt to maintain physiologically appropriate serum levels of thyroid hormone. Under the influence of increased TSH stimulation the acini multiply in an even fashion throughout the gland, producing what is sometimes described as a parenchymatous goitre. When the process is controlled or the demand for thyroid hormone ceases colloid may collect in previously hyperplastic acini, resulting in a colloid goitre. This process is typically patchy, causing nodularity.

Multinodular non-toxic goitre

This type of thyroid enlargement most commonly affects middle-aged women and occurs sporadically: it may represent an acquired enzyme defect due to ageing. Many multinodular goitres develop from simple goitres, especially if iodine intake or availability is compromised. The initial diffuse hyperplastic process then becomes localized to one or several areas of disorganized thyroid metabolism in which the hyperplastic acini undergo colloid involution while others show haemorrhage, cystic degeneration, or necrosis. Fibrosis and calcification may supervene: a typical multinodular goitre shows all these macroscopic features.

Solitary nodular non-toxic goitre

Fifty per cent of goitres assessed clinically to be of this type are found to be multinodular on scanning or at surgery. Truly solitary nodules may be cystic or solid. The pathogenesis of solitary cysts is uncertain, but a minority are due to degeneration of a papillary carcinoma. A solitary solid nodule may be an adenoma, a degenerative nodule, a carcinoma, or may occasionally be secondary to thyroiditis. Four times as many females as males are affected, with a peak incidence in middle age. Ninety per cent of solitary nodules in this age group are benign, but at the extremes of life over 50 per cent are malignant.

Recurrent nodular goitre

This may occur after surgery for multinodular goitres or solitary nodules and usually represents progression of the original underlying process. It may be modified or prevented by administration of thyroxine to stop TSH release and suppress gland function.

Toxic goitre

Diffuse toxic goitre—Graves' disease/primary toxic goitre

The increase in size of the gland seen in patients with Graves' disease is typically due to epithelial proliferation, an increase in stromal vascularity, and lymphocytic infiltration. This may be due to a focal thyroiditis reflecting the production of autoantibodies. Occasionally this condition progresses with increasing fibrosis to become Hashimoto's disease. Graves' disease is not simply the result of the action of increased TSH levels secondary to a primary defect in the hypothalamus or pituitary, as was once thought. Genetic predisposition and psychological trauma have a role, and seasonality of the disease may result from variation in dietary intake of iodine. In populations with a high dietary iodine intake such as in the fish-eating Japanese, Grave's disease is more common. There is now general agreement that the hyperthyroidism and goitre of Graves' disease is caused by antibodies directed against the TSH receptor on the thyroid membrane:

these increase the action of TSH acting via the adenyl cyclase—cAMP system. This thyrotrophin receptor antibody was first isolated in 1956 from the serum of patients with Grave's disease as a substance which, on injection into guinea pigs pretreated with ^{131}I caused prolonged stimulation of radioiodine release. The nature of its action resulted in the name long-acting thyroid stimulator (LATS); this has subsequently been identified as a 7 S IgG molecule produced by lymphocytes. The presence of IgG, IgM, and IgE in the thyroid, the lymphocytic infiltration of the gland, the generalized lymphadenopathy frequently seen in Graves' disease and the IgG nature of the thyrotrophin receptor support its recognition as an autoimmune process. There is strong evidence of a genetic predisposition associated with the HLA-A1, B8, and DW3 antigens in Caucasians; Class II antigens of the D locus on chromosome 6 are believed to be associated with the gene coding for the abnormal immune response.

Toxic multinodular goitre/Plummer's disease/secondary thyrotoxicosis

Patients with long-standing nodular goitres often develop thyrotoxicosis. Excess thyroid hormones may be produced by the nodules themselves, by the paranodular tissue, or by a combination of both. Eye signs are usually slight and cardiac arrhythmias and cardiac failure more common than in Graves' disease; the reason for this is not known.

Solitary nodular toxic goitre/toxic adenoma/'hot' autonomous nodule

The distinction between multinodular and solitary nodular toxic goitres may be unnecessary but in approximately 5 per cent of thyrotoxic patients a single nodule consisting of hyperplastic epithelia and surrounded by acini in the resting phase is found. There is good correlation between the size of the nodule and the degree of hormone overproduction: overproduction of T_3 but not T_4 is common (T_3-toxicosis). Women are more likely than men to be affected with this type of goitre, and its maximum prevalence occurs between the ages of 40 and 60, although children may also be affected.

Recurrent nodular toxic goitre

Nodules associated with hormone overproduction may occur after thyroidectomy, suggesting that the causal factors are still prevailing.

Special goitres

Autoimmune thyroiditis

This term embraces a group of conditions that have in common the presence of circulating antithyroid antibodies; these may or may not have a causal relationship with the thyroiditis. Glandular enlargement due to lymphocytic infiltration is common.

Hashimoto's disease (lymphadenoid goitre)

This characteristically affects middle-aged women: the female to male ratio is approximately 15:1. Very high titres of thyroglobulin and antimicrosomal antibodies are common and the latter are usually associated with thyroid failure. The degree of lymphocytic infiltration of the thyroid correlates well with levels of these antibodies, especially in the fibrous variant, suggesting long-standing hyperimmunization. Microscopically the epithelial cells are enlarged and eosinophilic—these so-called Askenazy cells have been compared to hepatocytes. Lymphocytic infiltration of the stroma is intense, with the formation of lymphoid follicles. It seems probable that sensitization of these lymphocytes to thyroglobulin, mitochondria, and microsomes leads to the destructive fibrosis. A subacute variety of the condition causes transient pain and tenderness of the thyroid but in the majority of patients the thyroid enlargement changes over time from a rubbery consistency to stony hardness, associated with progressive hypothyroidism. The risk of lymphoma and primary thyroid neoplasia developing in a Hashimoto's gland is now considered to be low. Hashimoto's disease is not associated with antigen HLA-DR3 but is weakly associated with HLA-DR5; antithyrotrophin receptor antibodies are sometimes present and are likely to be responsible for the thyroid hyperplasia which is commonly seen. Some of these antibodies are biologically active, causing hormone overproduction.

de Quervain's thyroiditis/subacute thyroiditis

This condition is rare in Europe but is becoming more common in North America. The slightly tender thyroid enlargement is frequently preceded by an infection of the upper respiratory tract or by a viral illness such as mumps or coxsackie virus infection, suggesting an infective aetiology. Women in the 20- to 50-year age group are most commonly affected. Disruption of epithelial cells and extrusion of nuclei causes a pseudo-giant cell appearance. Inflammatory infiltration of the stroma by polymorphs, mononuclear cells, and lymphocytes can result in microabscesses and later fibrosis. Subsequent hypothyroidism is rare.

Reidel's thyroiditis/woody thyroid/ligneus thyroiditis

This is an extremely rare condition, and some even doubt its existence as a separate entity distinct from Hashimoto's and de Quervain's thyroiditis, both of which can produce a very hard and fibrotic gland. If the fibrosis is particularly dense and extends beyond the thyroid, tethering it to the trachea and strap muscles, the diagnosis of thyroid carcinoma must be considered. The cause is unknown but is probably one of a group of conditions, including fibrosing mediastinitis, retroperitoneal fibrosis, sclerosing cholangitis, and orbital pseudotumour, all of which are characterized by multifocal midline fibrosis.

Acute suppurative thyroiditis

This condition is now rarely seen due to the widespread use of antibiotics. The thyroid is usually infected by *Streptococcus pyogenes* or *Straphylococcus aureus*, originating from the bloodstream or from adjacent structures. The gland is enlarged, exquisitely tender, and there is surrounding induration. If not treated promptly with antibiotics the patient becomes acutely ill and an abscess will form. There is no disturbance of thyroid dysfunction, normal thyroxine and autoantibody levels being maintained.

Carcinoma of the thyroid

Malignancy of the thyroid is rare but the incidence appears to be rising: in the United Kingdom 25 cases occur per million of the population each year, with a death rate of six per million. Areas with a incidence of high endemic goitre (notably Columbia) also report a high prevalence of thyroid carcinoma, but there is no clear aetiological relationship. External radiotherapy administered to the head and neck in children (used in the past for the treatment of acne and tonsillitis) undoubtedly increases the risk of subsequent thyroid carcinoma (notably papillary) with an average latent interval of 10 years. Radioiodine therapy in children has also been associated with the subsequent development of low-grade malignant nodules. Papillary carcinoma is the most common malignancy in individuals exposed to modest radiation doses following atomic explosions. Familial thyroid carcinomas are rare. Intake of high levels of iodine predisposes to papillary carcinoma; and some races are more at risk. Follicular carcinoma, on the other hand is more common in areas where iodine intake is low; it appears to be TSH induced. The existence of an association between Hashimoto's thyroiditis and thyroid neoplasia is controversial; an important prospective study has not established a high incidence of the two conditions coexisting. Malignant thyroid tumours may be classified as primary and secondary, and their prevalence, major features, and prognosis are summarized in Table 1.

Papillary carcinoma

Papillary carcinomas account for 80 per cent of thyroid tumours in patients under the age of 40, reflecting its tendency to affect teenagers and young adults with a 2:1 female:male sex ratio.

In older patients this tumour may be associated with follicular lesions; in this case the papillary pattern of behaviour predominates, with a better prognosis. The typically unencapsulated pale homogeneous primary tumour (which commonly undergoes cystic degeneration) spreads via the lymphatics. If the whole of the gland is examined, micrometastases are present in 90 per cent of affected individuals. Multiple macroscopic deposits are found at operation in 20 per cent and spread to the regional lymph nodes occurs in 50 per cent of patients. Occasionally, the tumour within the thyroid is impalpable and less than 1.5 cm in diameter ('occult'). It may even be difficult to locate histologically. Whether or not a primary thyroid tumour is palpable the first evidence of a papillary lesion is frequently an enlarged deep cervical or posterior triangle lymph node, previously erroneously described as a lateral aberrant thyroid. Histologically, these tumours are characterized by papillary processes arranged like a Christmas tree, with variable colloid and follicular architecture. Laminated calcium-containing structures called psammoma bodies are often seen in well-differentiated papillary tumours.

Follicular carcinoma

This tumour affects three times as many women as men. It is associated with lack of iodine, and is therefore probably induced by TSH; this accounts for the fact that the tumour is more common in areas with a high incidence of endemic goitre. Macroscopically, the tumour is unifocal and encapsulated, with a pinkish cut surface which bulges. Capsular invasion is occasionally evident, and nodular components may develop to affect the whole lobe of the thyroid. Cystic degeneration is rare. The malignant potential of follicular carcinoma is dependent on the extent to which its capsule has been breached and the blood vessels invaded. This can only be assessed by examining the whole lobe with paraffin sections. Spread occurs via the bloodstream and the most common distant sites to be affected are the lung, bones, and brain. Lymph node involvement is unusual.

Anaplastic carcinoma

This tumour is noted for its speed of growth, local invasiveness, and early dissemination, but is fortunately rare. Its follicular cell origin is supported by the presence of small areas of differentiated thyroid carcinoma in a proportion of anaplastic carcinomas and probably accounts for its high prevalence in endemic goitrous areas. The histological appearance is varied, with spindle cell and giant cell patterns. If a patient diagnosed as having a anaplastic thyroid carcinoma survives for more than 1 year the histology should be reviewed: the diagnosis will invariably be revised to lymphoma.

Malignant lymphoma

This occurs mainly in elderly women and grows rapidly. Its association with long-standing Hashimoto's disease is now discounted. Histologically malignant lymphona may be confused with small round cell anaplastic carcinoma of the thyroid; this is resolved by monoclonal antibody studies.

Medullary thyroid carcinoma

This tumour has attracted considerable interest since it was first described in 1959, and now that clinical awareness has been aroused diagnosis is more frequent. It arises from the parafollicular C cells, which are distributed throughout the gland but are present in highest concentration in the upper poles, where most medullary thyroid carcinomas occur. If the tumour is solitary the disease is likely to be sporadic (80 per cent); if tumours are multiple the familial form is more likely (20 per cent). The latter shows a predominantly autosomal pattern of inheritance and men and women are equally affected; successive generations tend to develop tumours at a progressively earlier age. A chromosomal abnormality affecting chromosome 10 has been identified in individuals with the familial form of the disease and should prove helpful in identifying affected individuals in the future. Familial medullary thyroid carcinoma is also associated with tumours of the adrenal medulla (phaeochromocytoma) and with parathyroid

Table 1 Malignant thyroid tumours

	Type	Prevalence (%)	Average age at presentation	Spread	10-year survival (%)
Primary					
	Papillary	60	40	Via lymph nodes	80
	Follicular	25	50	Via bloodstream	60
	Anaplastic undifferentiated	10	60	Local and distant	0
	Malignant lymphoma	1	60	Local	?
	Medullary	5	50	Local	50
Secondary					
	Gastrointestinal } Breast	<1	60	–	0

hyperplasia—an endocrine triad categorized as multiple endocrine neoplasia Type IIA, or Sipple's syndrome. A distinct group of patients have a phenotypically different disease, characterized by medullary thyroid carcinoma and phaeochromocytoma but without parathyroid disease. This syndrome, called multiple endocrine neoplasia Type IIB, is also associated with characteristic facies, Marfanoid habitus, and submucosal neurofibromata of the tongue, eyelids, and lips (Fig. 12). This type is more aggressive in its behaviour than Type IIA and often rapidly fatal. The C cells of both sporadic and medullary carcinoma produce a near-specific tumour marker, calcitonin, which helps in its diagnosis and management.

Secondary thyroid carcinoma

Very rarely breast, renal, ovarian, and gastrointestinal cancers metastasize to the thyroid, where they present as a solitary nodule. It is surprising that metastases to the thyroid are not more common, considering the high percentage of the cardiac output relative to unit volume which circulates through the very vascular gland which must be considered a protected site.

INVESTIGATION FOR THYROID DISORDERS

There is no substitute for good history taking and careful clinical examination in the assessment of thyroid disorders. None of the available tests is infallible and misleading results may be obtained, especially if the patient is taking medication or has altered physiology, for example in pregnancy. Nevertheless major advances in the accurate measurement of hormones and antibodies either produced by or acting upon the thyroid have resulted in the development of an impressive array of tests to help confirm the clinical diagnosis and elucidate the more difficult diagnostic problems.

Tests of circulating thyroid hormone levels

Serum thyroxine (T_4) (normal range 55–150 nmol/l)

This measures the total protein-bound thyroxine and, provided that the patient is not on any drug or in a condition which might affect the serum levels of binding proteins, offers a good basic test for thyroid function, especially when myxoedema is suspected. Low levels are seen in patients with the nephrotic syndrome and falsely high levels occur in pregnancy and in those taking oral contraceptives. Some drugs, notably salicylates, phenytoin, and phenylbutazone, compete with T_4 for protein binding, resulting in falsely low levels.

Serum tri-iodothyronine (T_2) (normal range 1.2–3.1 nmol/l)

Serum levels of T_3, are also affected by changes in the thyroid binding proteins and are therefore subject to the same limits of interpretation. Serum T_3 falls more profoundly than T_4 in the elderly and in patients with non-thyroidal diseases. Enhanced secretion of T_3 is seen when the thyroid is deprived of iodine, making this assay unhelpful for the assessment of patients treated with drugs which block iodine uptake. The test is most useful in the confirmation of hyperthyroidism, especially when the clinical picture strongly supports a diagnosis of thyrotoxicosis but the levels of serum T_4 are normal.

Free thyroxine (normal range 8–26 pmol/l)

Since the introduction of a radioimmunoassay in kit form, it is now possible to measure the biologically active unbound circulating T_4 with precision and at relatively low cost. Drugs such as oral contraceptives or phenytoin have no effect on the results since protein

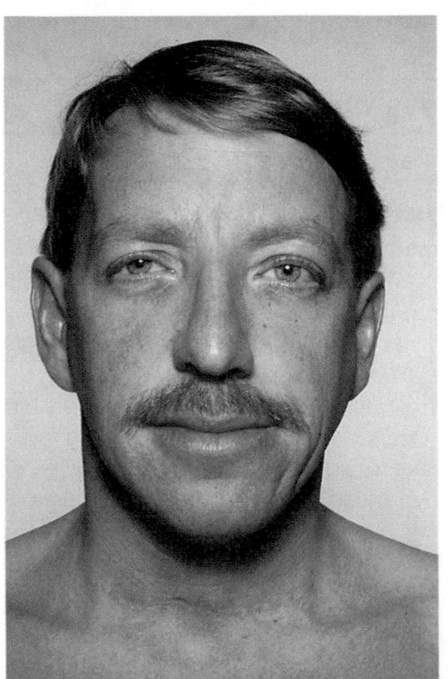

(a)

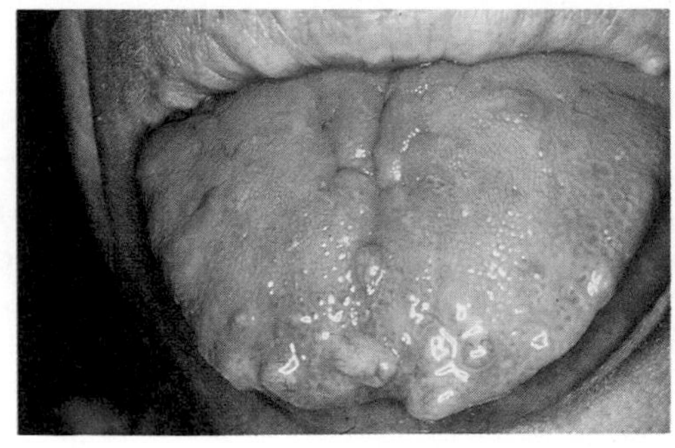

(b)

Fig. 12 Characteristic facies in multiple endocrine neoplasia Type IIb showing submucosal neurofibromata.

binding is not a factor. Levels of free T_4 do not appear to vary with age in healthy individuals.

Free tri-iodithyronine (normal range 3–9 pmol/l)

The free T_3 imino radioimmmunoassay has the same merit as the free T_4 assay, and is the best single test in the assessment of hyperthyroidism, providing the patient is not suffering from severe non-thyroidal illness. It is not helpful in the diagnosis of hypothyroidism.

Tests of hypothalamic–pituitary function

Thyroid stimulating hormone (normal range 0.5–5.0 mm/l)

Routine TSH assays lack sensitivity and cannot identify patients who may have subclinical hypothyroidism and might benefit from replacement therapy. New sensitive immunoradiometric assays (IRMA) probably represent the most helpful confirmatory test for both hypothyroidism when levels are high and hyperthyroidism when levels of TSH are undetectable. In severely ill patients or those in early pregnancy, however, falsely low TSH levels may be recorded, and hyperthyroidism can be missed.

Thyrotrophin releasing hormone test

Following the intravenous administration of 200 mg of thyrotrophin the patient's TSH levels are then measured in blood samples taken after 0, 20 and 60 min. An exaggerated response producing levels greater than 20 μU/l at 20 min is seen in patients with hypothyroidism. Little or no response ($<$ 1.8 mU/l) is seen in hyperthyroid patients. The test is being superseded by the immunoradiometric assay for TSH where this is available.

Dynamic tests of thyroid function

Radio-isotope uptake

Uptake measurements combined with thyroid scanning provide information about thyroid activity and also providing graphic information about the size and extent of the gland. This method is particularly helpful in showing the retrosternal extent of the gland (Fig. 13) and identifying which part of the gland is hyperactive (hot nodules) (Fig. 14). In North America, where radio-iodine therapy is more commonly employed for the treatment of thyrotoxicosis, a radio-isotope uptake study may identify clinically thyrotoxic patients with silent thyroiditis but low radio-iodine uptake. Ablative therapy should be avoided in such patients.

Tri-iodothyronine suppression test

T_3 administration normally suppresses pituitary TSH secretion and therefore reduces radio-iodine uptake in normal patients. Radio-iodine uptake is not so reduced in patients with Grave's disease, in whom the thyroid is being stimulated by antibodies rather than by TSH. The test is useful in distinguishing high radio-iodine uptake associated with iodine deficiency from that of hyperthyroidism, but can precipitate cardiac failure in the elderly. It has largely been superseded by the TRH test or immunoradiometric TSH assay.

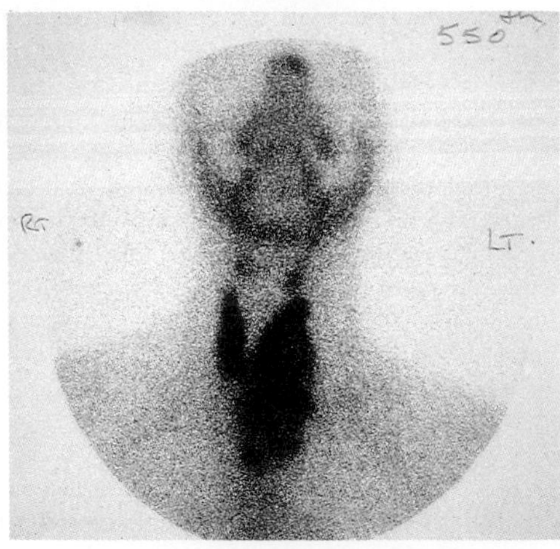

Fig. 13 ^{131}I scintiscan showing retrosternal extension of a goitre.

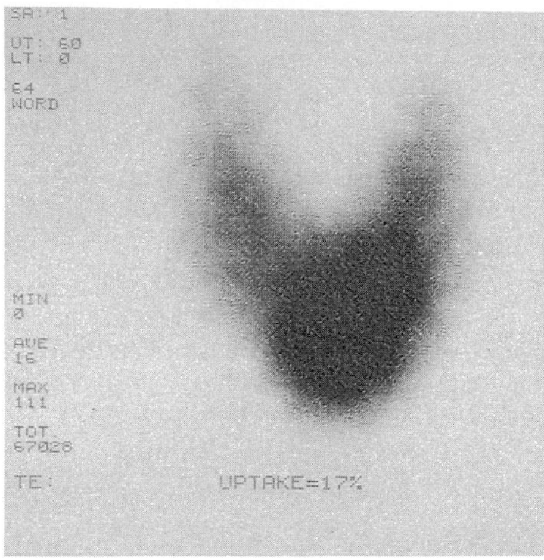

Fig. 14 ^{131}I scintiscan showing a solitary hyperactive 'hot' nodule.

Tests of thyroid dysfunction

Antithyroid antibodies (antithyroglobulin and antimicrosomal antibodies)

Very high titres of antithyroglobulin antibodies are seen in patients with Hashimoto's thyroiditis, especially in those with long-standing disease, when their presence strongly supports the diagnosis. Surgery should not usually be undertaken in patients with Hashimoto's thyrotoxicosis. The presence of antithyroglobulin antibodies in a hyperthyroid patient without eye signs suggests the diagnosis of Graves' disease. The presence of antimicrosomal antibodies indicates autoimmune thyroid disease of Hashimoto's type, and when found in patients who have already received thyroxine makes a presumptive initial diagnosis of thyroid failure more likely. This antibody is also seen in patients with thyroid malignancy.

Erythrocyte sedimentation rate (ESR)

The ESR is often modestly raised ($>$ 90 mm/h) in many patients with myxoedema and Hashimoto's thyroiditis, and is markedly elevated in de Quervain's thyroiditis.

Tests for suspected thyroid malignancy

Scintigraphy after radio-isotope administration

^{123}I has a half life of 13 h and is a gamma ray emitter; it gives a low radiation dose and is the isotope of choice. Areas of high uptake (hot nodules) are almost invariably benign. More than 50 per cent of nodules have low uptake rates, but only 10 per cent are subsequently shown to be malignant. The test discriminates poorly and is therefore hard to justify. The principal benefits of isotope scanning, other than those already mentioned, is to identify metastases or residual local disease after total thyroidectomy for follicular carcinoma (Fig. 15).

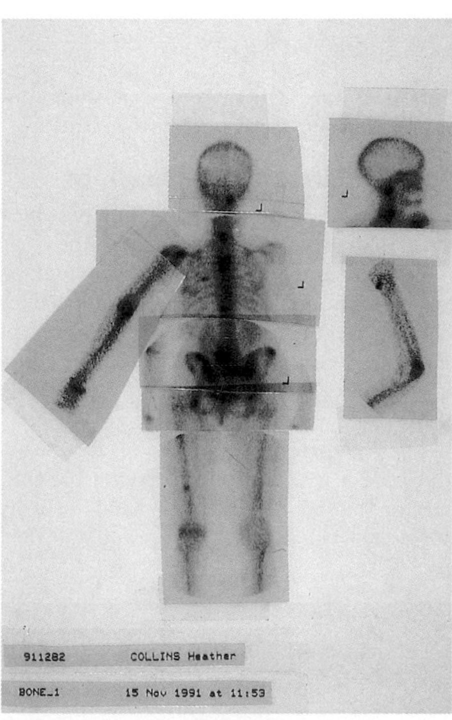

Fig. 15 Total body scintiscan showing metastases from follicular carcinoma.

Ultrasound scanning

This technique is helpful in identifying impalpable multiple nodules (multinodular goitre) which are much less likely to be malignant than is a solitary nodule. Justification for the use of this technique in the diagnosis of malignancy is, however, poor.

Fine needle aspiration or aspiration biopsy cytology

This technique promoted by the Karolinska Institute in Sweden for over 40 years, has only recently gained wider acceptance. A 25 gauge disposable needle on a 10-ml syringe enables cells to be aspirated from any suspicious area of the thyroid (Fig. 16). The procedure can be performed quickly and painlessly in the outpatient department without the need for local anaesthetic, providing a smeared specimen which is fixed and stained on a microscope slide. A high level of diagnostic accuracy can be achieved for the majority of thyroid conditions when the clinician and cytologist are experienced. The technique cannot distinguish benign from malignant follicular lesions since no information is available about capsular and vascular invasion; these lesions are best excised.

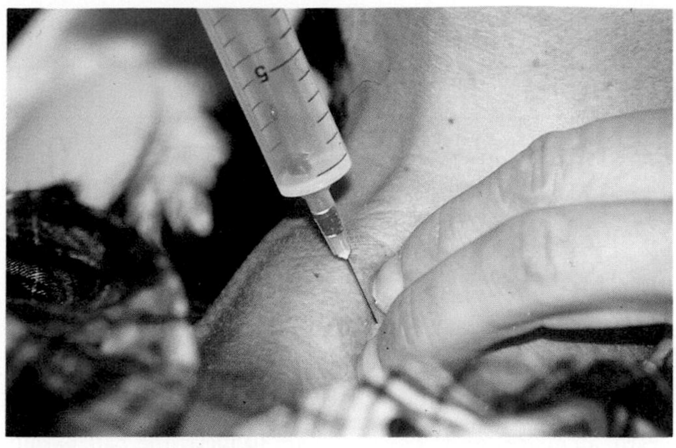

Fig. 16 Fine-needle aspiration from a thyroid nodule.

Serum calcitonin (normal range $<0.08\,\mu g/l$)

Elevated basal levels of this hormone produced by the parafollicular C cells are diagnostic of medullary thyroid carcinoma; serial measurements are also useful in predicting complete removal of the tumour or recurrence. Patients with Type II multiple endocrine neoplasia who have occult or premalignant medullary thyroid carcinoma (C cell hyperplasia) can be identified by a provocation test using a combination of pentagastrin (0.5 μg/kg body weight) and calcium gluconate (2.5 mg/kg body weight) infused IV over 30 s. Blood samples are drawn for calcitonin estimation prior to infusion and at 2, 5, 10, and 15 min post-infusion in a fasted subject. The test is safe and can be carried out in the outpatient department.

Serum thyroglobulin (normal range $<1\text{–}35\,\mu g/l$)

In patients who have undergone total thyroidectomy with or without radio-iodine therapy for differentiated thyroid carcinoma, levels of thyroglobulin above 50 μg/l indicate probable residual or recurrent tumour. Levels above 100 μg/l strongly suggest the presence of pulmonary or skeletal metastases.

Flow cytometry

Measuring the nuclear DNA content by flow cytometry offers the prospect of identifying diploid tumours, which have a good prognosis and aneuploid tumours, which have a poor prognosis . Data which have been accumulated from patients with papillary tumours correlate well with predicted outcome and should help decide the scale of surgical intervention.

SIGNS AND SYMPTOMS

Symptoms

There are two broad categories of symptoms related to thyroid disease: those occurring as a result of the enlargement of the gland itself and those related to its disordered endocrine activity. The history will establish whether one or both classes of symptoms are present, and examination then aims to elicit the relevant physical signs.

Neck symptoms

A lump in the neck

Nearly all goitres grow slowly and are painless; the patient only visits the clinician when the mass becomes a cosmetic problem. A rapid change in size of all or part of the thyroid may be caused by haemorrhage into a necrotic nodule, a fast growing carcinoma, or by one of the varieties of thyroiditis. When haemorrhage is the cause of a lump its appearance is invariably sudden (within 24 h) and it is usually painful. Malignant tumours only cause pain when local structures are involved. This occurs within weeks of development of an anaplastic carcinoma or within months or years for a papillary or follicular tumour.

Discomfort on swallowing

Thyroid swellings make swallowing uncomfortable but rarely obstruct the oesophagus, which easily moves out of the way or becomes stretched. Thyroiditis causes extreme pain on swallowing, radiating up into the jaw and ears. True dysphagia as a result of thyroid disease is a sinister symptom indicative of aggressive anaplastic carcinoma.

Dyspnoea

This most commonly arises as a result of deviation and compression of the trachea caused by asymmetrical thyroid enlargement. It may be accompanied by stridor when the patient has the head flexed forward or laterally to the side of the enlarged lobe.

Hoarseness of the voice

This symptom in association with a goitre is sinister and until proven otherwise should be considered secondary to a malignant process of the thyroid involving one of the recurrent laryngeal nerves. The hoarseness seen in hypothyroid patients derives more from mucus on the vocal cords than an inability to phonate.

Symptoms of hyperthyroidism and hypothyroidism

All bodily systems can be affected by altered thyroid activity. In hyperthyroidism increased metabolism is usually reflected in heat intolerance with a preference for cold weather coupled with increased sweating. The principal systemic symptoms of hyperthyroidism are shown in Table 2; hypothyroid symptoms are best summarized as the exact opposite.

Table 2 Symptoms of hyperthyroidism

Systems	Symptoms
Gastrointestinal system	Weight loss in spite of increased appetite, diarrhoea
Cardiovascular system	Palpitations and shortness of breath at rest or on minimal exertion, angina, and cardiac irregularity and failure in the elderly
Neuromuscular system	Undue fatigue and muscle weakness, tremor and shaking
Skeletal system	Increase in linear growth in children
Genitourinary system	Oligo- or amenorrhoea and occasional urinary frequency
Integument	Hair loss and pruritus
Psychiatric	Irritability, nervousness, and insomnia

Signs

Since examination traditionally follows functional enquiry the clinician will usually have a fairly strong impression of the patient's thyroid status and will know that attention needs to be directed primarily towards the thyroid itself. In those with thyroid dysfunction more specific signs need to be elicited.

Overall appearance of the patient

Euthyroid patients appear normal, apart from possible signs in the neck. Hyperthyroid patients are frequently noisy, agitated, and clearly nervous, but may be apathetic. Hypothyroid patients show little response to their environment, being subdued, slow in their movements, and frequently overweight. They typically have thickened and expressionless features and a 'peaches and cream' complexion (Fig. 17).

Examination of the hands

The hands provide a wealth of clues about a patient, and this is certainly true in thyroid disease. The hands of a hyperthyroid

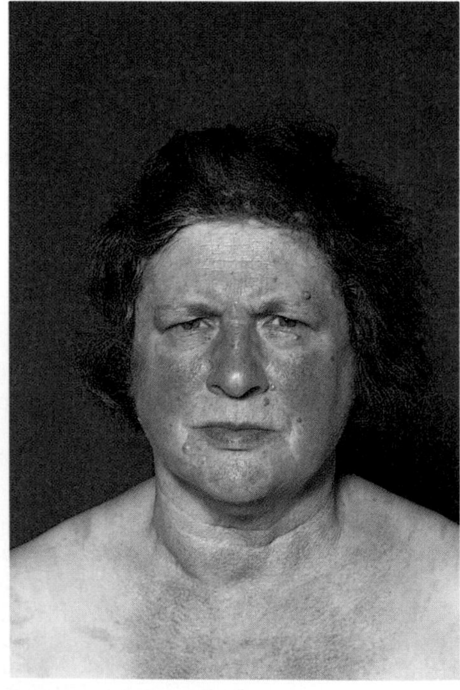

Fig. 17 Characteristic facies in myxoedema.

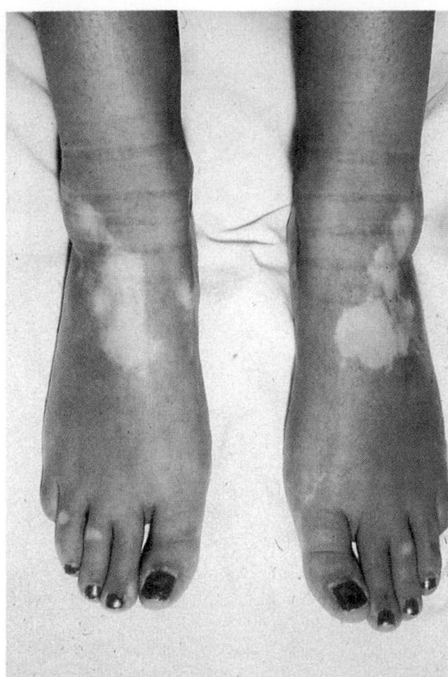

Fig. 18 Vitiligo in thyrotoxicosis.

patient usually show a fine tremor, which is accentuated by placing a sheet of paper on the back of the hand with the arms outstretched. Patchy depigmentation of the skin (vitiligo) surrounded by areas of increased pigmentation may be apparent (Fig. 18). Patchy subperiosteal deposition of new bone, simulating clubbing (thyroid acropathy) can occur. On shaking hands with the patient one is aware of increased temperature and sweating. Pulses at the wrist and at the bases of the fingers are easily felt due to increased systolic pressure; this is often accompanied by tachycardia greater than 80/min and irregularity.

The hypothyroid patient has cool, dry hands, and the palms are often pale yellow in colour. The increased bulk of the subcutaneous tissues cause the hands to look puffy and spadelike, and rings become tight. The nails are often fissured and cracked becoming separated from the nail bed (onycholysis or Plummer's nails). Bradycardia and a low volume pulse difficult to detect is characteristic of hypothyroidism.

Examination of the thyroid

Inspection

Confirmation that a swelling in the neck is arising from the thyroid is based on two observations—the site is anatomically correct and the swelling moves up and down on swallowing. Offering the patient a drink of water is helpful at this stage and subsequently aids more detailed examination by palpation. Much can be learned by simple inspection with the patient's neck properly exposed and with a good light source on one side. Prominent neck veins may indicate superior vena caval obstruction secondary to retrosternal extension of the goitre. Puckering of the skin, accentuated on swallowing, is seen with locally invasive thyroid cancer. Erythema of the skin is often present in patients with de Quervain's thyroiditis or suppurative thyroiditis. Deviation of the thyroid cartilage suggests asymmetrical enlargement of the thyroid.

Palpation

Palpation should be undertaken with the patient sitting comfortably in an upright chair with all clothes removed from around the neck. Standing behind with the thumbs placed on the patient's occiput to flex the head forward slightly, the clinician's hands encircle the neck and the right hand draws the sternomastoid muscle on the same side laterally whilst the fingertips of the other hand scan the surface of the underlying lobe (Fig. 19). The position of the hands is then reversed to evaluate the left lobe. The normal trachea should be in the midline of the suprasternal notch and not obscured by the thyroid isthmus. If there is any doubt about the relationship between anatomical features and any lump, or difficulty feeling below the lower pole of the lobe, the patient is asked to swallow. This will confirm whether the lump is part of the thyroid or whether retrosternal extension is likely to be present. If the head and neck becomes suffused (Fig. 20) with or without the onset of stridor, when the patient raises his arms above his head, retrosternal extension is present. In a patient with thyrotoxicosis careful palpation may detect a thrill. The overall neck circumference and precise measurements of any nodules should be recorded to provide a baseline if longer-term surveillance is indicated. The lymph nodes draining the thyroid should also be checked for any enlargement (see Fig. 4).

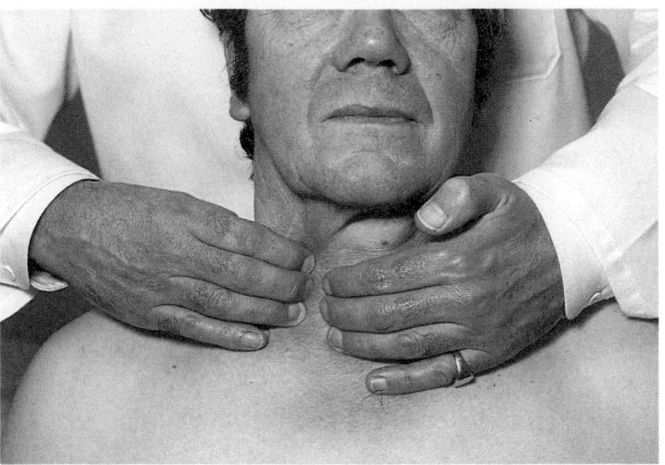

Fig. 19 Position of the hands for palpation of the thyroid—Lahey's grip.

Percussion

Testing for retrosternal extension of the thyroid by this method is considered to be of no value.

Ausculatation

A systolic bruit may be heard in Graves' disease and is an important sign of toxicity. It should not be confused with a transmitted systolic murmur secondary to aortic or pulmonary stenosis or from a venous hum that can be eliminated by pressure on the internal jugular vein at the level of the hyoid bone.

Special signs in hypothyroidism

The skin is characteristically dry and flaking with hyperkeratosis over the flexures. Coarsening of features and subcutaneous thickening, notably across the back of the neck and hands, are due

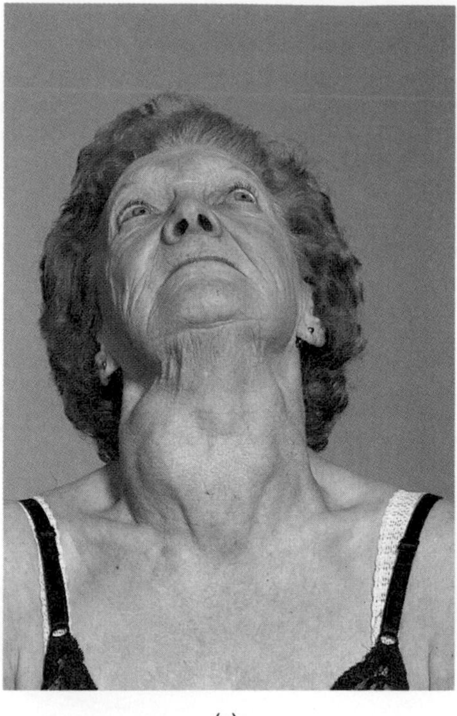

(a)

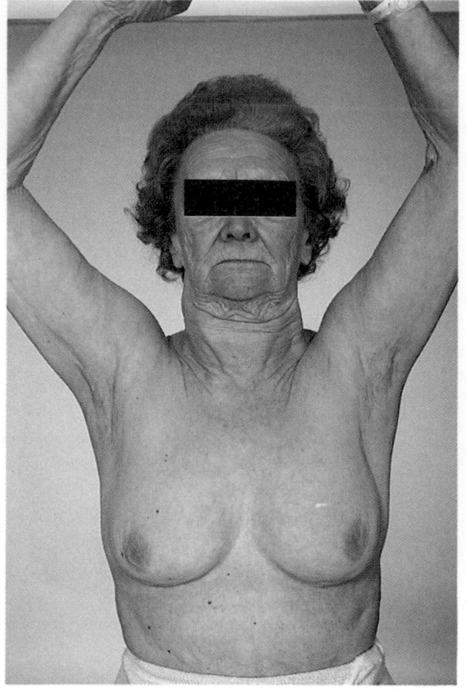

(b)

Fig. 20 Demonstration of superior caval obstruction due to retrosternal extension of a goitre accentuated by raising the arms.

to deposition of hygroscopic hyaluronic acid. This mimics oedema but does not pit on pressure. The hair is coarse, brittle, and falls out easily; loss of the outer one-third of the eyebrows is an unreliable sign of hypothyroidism, and is often seen in normal perimenopausal women. Macroglossia is often present and impairs speech. The reflexes are sluggish and their relaxation period is prolonged.

Special signs in hyperthyroidism

There are two main groups of physical signs, other than those affecting the thyroid: those confined to the eyes, and more general signs.

Eye signs

Swelling of the eyelids without exophthalmos is an indicator of dangerous congestive ophthalmopathy. Conjunctivitis and chemosis (Fig. 21) may be induced by a reduction in blinking rate and by an inability fully to close the eyelids whilst asleep. The conjunctivae are inflamed and prominent vessels are seen, especially at the lateral canthi. When oedema occurs (chemosis) the conjunctiva becomes thickened and wrinkled, and may actually prolapse between the lids. Excessive watering and photophobia occur.

Exophthalmos is caused by the eye ball being pushed forward by an increase in retro-orbital contents. In Graves' disease this is due to an increase in fat and bulkiness of the extrinsic muscles secondary to deposition of water and mucopolysaccharides combined with lymphocytic infiltration. The eyes may be affected asymmetrically. The single most crucial observation relates to the appearance of the white sclera below the inferior limbus of the cornea on forward gaze (Fig. 22). Accurate measurement of the degree of exophthalmos requires an exophthalmometer: an absolute reading of 18 mm or more or a difference of 2 mm between the eyes is considered significant. Looking down directly over the patient's forehead and observing the cornea in front of the supraorbital ridges is an easy bedside means of assessment but only reveals gross exophthalmos. The same applies when the patient can look upwards without wrinkling the forehead.

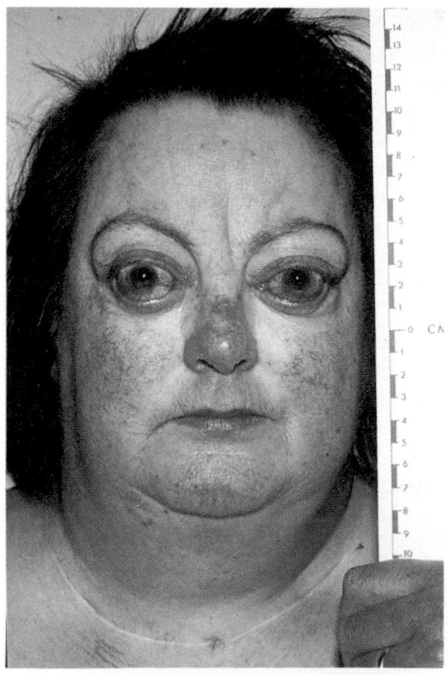

Fig. 21 Conjunctivitis and chemosis in hyperthyroidism.

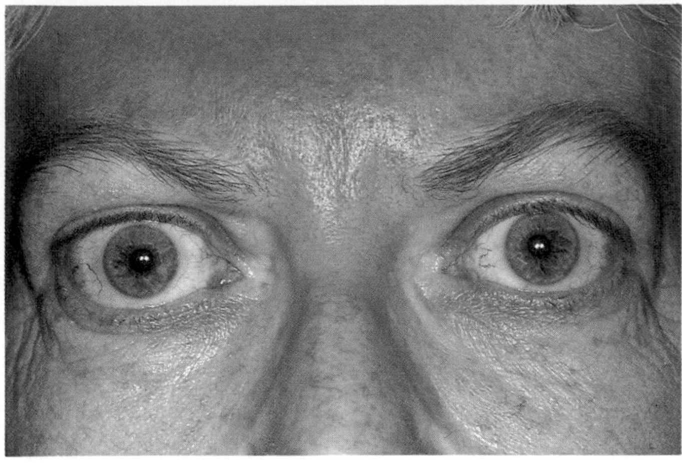

Fig. 22 Appearance of the eyes in a patient with exophthalmos, showing sclera visible beneath the iris.

Lid retraction is the result of spasm of the levator palpebrae superioris muscles, which causes the white sclera to appear between the upper lid and upper limbus of the cornea in all positions of gaze (Fig. 23). It prevents apposition of the eyelids during sleep and is a cause of conjunctival irritation and ulceration. This same spasm allows the sclera to become visible between the upper lid and cornea (lid lag) as a patient's eye follows the examiner's finger downwards (ideally an arm's length away from the patient's head). This test of lid lag is poorly reproducible and unreliable.

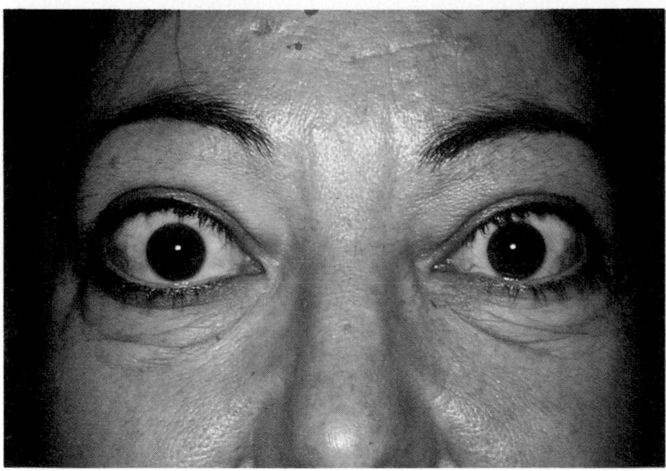

Fig. 23 Appearance of the eyes in a patient with lid retraction, showing sclera visible above the iris.

Disturbance of vision occurs as a result of oedema and lymphocytic infiltration affecting the extrinsic muscles of the eye, notably the superior rectus and inferior oblique. Diplopia commonly occurs on upward outward conjugate gaze, but upward inward gaze may also be affected. Both of these movements should be checked by asking the patient to follow the examiner's finger appropriately.

General signs

1. Proximal myopathy, producing wasting of the muscles of the shoulder girdle and pelvic girdle, may result in difficulty getting up from a chair or inability to carry a heavy shopping bag.
2. Hyper-reflexia.
3. Fine tremor of the tongue may also be present.
4. Pretibial myxoedema is seen in approximately 5 per cent of patients with Graves' disease, especially those with eye signs, and is due to deposition of mucopolysaccharides and hyaluronic acid. The skin is thickened, livid, with 'peau d'orange' appearance, typically extending over the front of the shins and occasionally over the dorsum of the feet (Fig. 24).
5. Splenomegaly is rare, but may be associated with generalized lymphadenopathy.

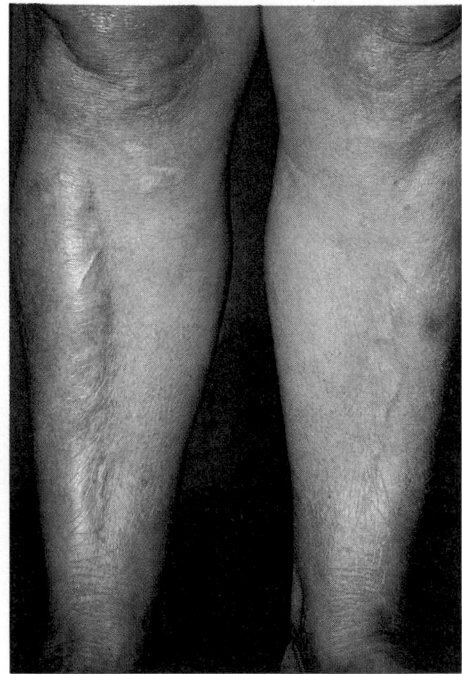

Fig. 24 Pretibial myxoedema seen in Graves' disease.

INDICATIONS FOR SURGERY

Non-toxic goitre

Diffuse non-toxic goitre

The incidental finding of a small soft goitre, especially if 'physiological' (see under pathophysiology), requires no treatment. Goitres occurring as a result of primary or secondary iodine deficiency rarely present until the condition is well established, but those detected at a small size may regress in response to iodine or eradication of the offending goitrogen in the diet. This process may be accelerated by giving thyroxine, which depresses the TSH drive to the gland. If there is no response partial thyroidectomy may be indicated on cosmetic grounds.

Multinodular non-toxic goitre

Large goitres of this type may well cause cosmetic disfigurement, pressure symptoms, and discomfort. All of these are good indications for surgery, the extent of which is dependent on the size and number of nodules present. Following surgery a small dose of thyroxine (0.1 mg daily) reduces the risk of recurrence.

Solitary nodular non-toxic goitre

Because of the high prevalence of solitary nodules (and even though over 50 per cent of those thought to be solitary are in fact part of a multinodular process) a policy of removing all of them surgically, although sound, is simply not practical. Fine-needle biopsy (aspiration biopsy cytology) has helped to reduce the incidence of surgical exploration of thyroid nodules by 25 per cent. It allows benign and malignant lesions to be identified with a high degree of specificity and sensitivity, and has the merit of being quick, painless, and easily performed as an outpatient procedure. All biopsy techniques are limited by the skill and ability of the operator to obtain a truly representative sample and by the experience and accuracy of the cytopathologist examining the specimen. The only serious limitation of this technique is failure to differentiate between a follicular adenoma and a follicular carcinoma: this can be done only by studying the overall histological pattern and, in particular, the presence or otherwise of capsular and vascular invasion. Unless the surgeon can depend on a cytology service which has a very low false-negative rate, total lobectomy (Fig. 25(a)) is advocated for all cases, especially in children and males under 40. Fine-needle biopsy quickly identifies a cystic nodule or simple cyst and, if less than 2 cm in diameter, drainage may be curative. Ideally the cyst wall should also be biopsied to ensure that a papillary carcinoma is not missed.

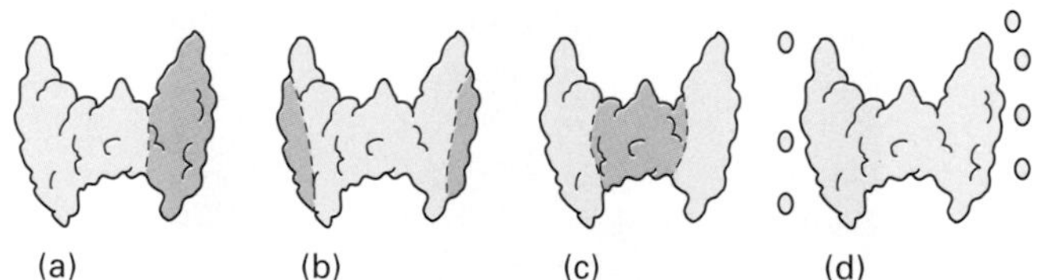

Fig. 25 Schematic representation of thyroid operative procedures. (a) Thyroid lobectomy. (b) Subtotal/near total thyroidectomy. (c) Isthmusectomy. (d) Total thyroidectomy and node clearance.

Thyrotoxicosis

There are three methods of treatment for this condition—antithyroid drugs, radio-iodine, and surgery. Over 50 years fashions have waxed and waned but a marked preference for radio-iodine persists in North America, while its use is more selective in the United Kingdom. The different treatments have their own advantages and disadvantages (Table 3). Ultimately it is for the patient to decide which treatment is most acceptable.

Surgery is most usually appropriate for the following conditions.

Large toxic multinodular goitre/Plummer's disease

The thyroid function of patients with large toxic multinodular goitre or classical Graves' disease is often very labile during treatment with antithyroid drugs, and relapse rates following withdrawal of medication are greater than 50 per cent. Unfortunately there is no reliable test to identify patients likely to relapse, although attempts to do so have been made on the basis of HLA status and levels of thyroid stimulating antibody. Radioactive iodine treatment is least suited for Plummer's disease as drug uptake is variable, there is minimal impact on the size of the gland, and response is slow. Surgery is best carried out sooner rather than later to avoid compromise of the airway and the cardiovascular system. The specific surgical procedure is a near total thyroidectomy, with the removal of at least 85 per cent of the gland (Fig. 25(b)), notably those parts shown to be 'active' on radio-iodine scanning.

Large diffuse toxic goitre (Graves' disease)

Patients affected with this condition are likely to have florid disease and cosmetic embarrassment. Prompt elective surgery should be performed after a course of treatment with antithyroid drugs and β-blockers. It is more debatable whether surgery should be undertaken when the gland is small, since the risks of hypothyroidism are greater than when a bulkier gland is the target.

Table 3 Disadvantages of antithyroid drugs, radioactive iodine, and surgery in the management of hyperthyroidism

Antithyroid drugs	Conservative ^{131}I	Surgery
Requires compliant and highly motivated patient to cope with variable drug regimen	Prospect of radiation therapy may be unacceptable to the patient	Prospect of neck surgery may be unacceptable to the patient
Needs close clinical and laboratory supervision over 18–24 months	Uncertainty about long-term carcinogenic effects of low radiation doses–known to be more oncogenic than high doses	Unsuited to patients of advanced age or poor medical status
Danger of over-treatment leading to hypothyroidism and thyroid enlargement	Uncertainty about teratogenic effects which restricts reproduction for (at least) 2 years after therapy	Scar inevitable with possibility of keloid formation
Risk of side-effects from drugs–rashes, nausea, and potentially dangerous marrow depression	Slow response to therapy (3–6 months) especially large multinodular goitres	Results are highly operator dependent
Poor response with large multinodular goitres	Not appropriate for cosmetically unacceptable toxic goitres	Small but definite risk of serious complications in skilled hands: recurrent laryngeal nerve damage $<1\%$; permanent hypoparathyroidism $<0.5\%$
Not appropriate for cosmetically unacceptable toxic goitres	Cumulative (high) hypothyroidism rate requiring long-term follow-up	Modest rate of hypothyroidism
High relapse rate		

However, in women, especially those in their reproductive years, who have relapsed after 12 to 18 months' treatment with antithyroid drugs, or in those in whom medication has proved impractical due to poor compliance or unacceptable side-effects, surgery is the first choice, providing it is acceptable to the patient and the necessary surgical skills are available. A sub-total thyroidectomy should be performed, which aims to leave one-eighth of the total mass (approximately 4 g) of thyroid tissue on each side.

Toxic solitary nodular goitre/toxic adenoma/autonomous 'hot nodule'

Surgical resection of the physiologically hyperactive part of a thyroid gland (demonstrable on radio-iodine uptake scan) is so straightforward that the other methods of treatment need not be seriously considered unless the overall medical state of the patient makes surgery inadvisable. Antithyroid drugs have the disadvantage of having to be taken for life, and radio-iodine therapy runs the risk of exposing surrounding normal tissue to irradiation. In addition, the nodule usually persists. The operative procedure indicated is subtotal lobectomy or isthmusectomy (Fig. 25(c)), depending on the location of the active nodule.

Childhood Graves' disease

Children with hyperthyroidism are prone to relapse after withdrawal of medical therapy and radio-iodine therapy is contraindicated due to the high incidence of benign and malignant nodules arising as a result of exposure to radiation. Unless medical therapy is effective quickly, surgery is the treatment of choice. Hypertrophy of thyroid remnants and recurrent thyrotoxicosis is common in children, and surgery therefore needs to be more radical. A surgeon experienced in operating on the thyroid gland in children can perform the operation avoiding high myxoedema rates and complications. Long-term follow-up is essential.

Thyrotoxicosis in pregnancy

This is rare, affecting 0.2 per cent of pregnancies, but can present a difficult management problem. Antithyroid drugs given to the mother cross the placental barrier and may cause hypothyroidism and goitre in the foetus (iatrogenic cretinism). Excretion of antithyroid drugs in the milk is at a level too low to cause comparable effects. Radio-iodine is never given in view of its possible teratogenic effects, especially in the first trimester or at the time when the fetal thyroid is trapping iodine. If maternal thyrotoxicosis is moderate or severe, and especially if cardiac symptoms herald possible cardiac failure late in pregnancy, elective subtotal thyroidectomy should be undertaken in the middle trimester, when it is safe and effective.

Special goitres

Hashimoto's disease/lymphadenoid goitre

A small goitre of this type in a euthyroid patient may require no treatment. As the goitre enlarges symptoms of pressure on the trachea and oesophagus are common; these may be relieved by exogenous thyroxine (0.1–0.2 mg/day) and prednisolone (20 mg/day). If there is still no response removal of the affected lobe or isthmus is indicated. Such goitres are relatively avascular and easily separable from the false capsule. Total lobectomy or total thyroidectomy is indicated in any patient with Hashimoto's disease in whom malignancy is suspected on clinical or cytological grounds.

De Quervain's thyroiditis

The acute pain associated with this condition can be alleviated by aspirin and a β-blocker. If this fails, 20 to 30 mg of prednisolone daily in divided doses for 1 month usually provides rapid relief. Thyroxine replacement may be required if hypothyroidism develops, but this is usually transient and treatment should be stopped after 6 months. Surgery is only required if the diagnosis is uncertain or equivocal on fine-needle biopsy.

Reidal's thyroiditis

Surgery is almost invariably required to exclude malignancy and to relieve the severe constriction of the airway. Relief can be obtained by dividing the thyroid isthmus, which is hard and brittle and can literally be snapped off the trachea with the fingers. Hypothyroidism frequently arises as the fibrosis progresses and needs to be treated indefinitely with thyroxine.

Thyroid cyst

Cysts less than 2 cm in diameter are treated by aspiration: the fluid should be examined cytologically, and the patient's condition monitored. Larger cysts are likely to recur and may well be cosmetically unacceptable. These carry a risk of sudden airways obstruction due to intracystic haemorrhage and are, therefore, best dealt with electively by thyroid lobectomy or isthmusectomy, according to site.

Carcinoma of the thyroid

The indications for and extent of surgery in carcinoma of the thyroid depend primarily on the histological type, but the age of onset and the mode of presentation will also influence management.

Papillary carcinoma

There is controversy about the extent of surgery required. The conservative approach to a solitary macroscopic tumour with no lymph node disease is a total lobectomy on the side of the tumour. The prognosis for the majority of patients is excellent if TSH is permanently suppressed by thyroxine (usually 0.1 mg/day). Total thyroidectomy is reserved for patients with macroscopic multifocal disease and/or demonstrable lymph node disease. Those who advocate a more aggressive strategy perform total or near-total thyroidectomy (Fig. 25(d)) for all cases, accepting the greater morbidity and higher incidence of hypoparathyroidism. The advantage of this approach is that multifocal tumour throughout the gland is always removed, the risk of anaplastic change in residual foci is excluded, and postoperative surveillance may be possible through serial thyroglobulin estimation. Deciding between the two strategies may be resolved by a scoring system devised to identify low- and high-risk patients based on four variables: age, grade, extent, and size (AGES); a higher score on each is associated with a poorer prognosis and the need for more radical surgery. DNA flow cytometry (possible on samples obtained at fine-needle aspiration) will also provide guidance on treatment, when the technique becomes more readily available. Surgery for papillary carcinoma should always include clearance of nodes in the primary lymphatic drainage zone. The thymus need not be disturbed unless obviously involved in the disease process, as ectopic parathyroids are frequently located in the thyrothymic ligament. Disease affecting lymph nodes in the secondary drainage areas may be suspected by their blue/black discoloration and often fleshy or cystic appearance. Clearance of all such nodes should be carried out by a modified neck dissection, only sacrificing the internal jugular vein and sternomastoid muscle if these are directly involved. The classical radical block dissection has been shown to confer no benefit in terms of reduced tumour recurrence rates or improved survival and leaves the patient disfigured and at risk of lymphoedema of the face. When disease recurs in lymph nodes, often years later (less than 10 per cent of cases treated by total lobectomy), the nodes are well encapsulated and can easily be excised 'berry-picking'. Even patients treated in this way for successive recurrences do not appear to have a compromised survival. When local invasion or distant spread not amenable to surgery occurs, radio-iodine may show uptake in approximately 20 per cent of papillary metastases and then the option of therapeutic radio-iodine can be considered.

Follicular carcinoma

This tumour typically presents as a non-toxic solitary nodule, and distant metastases rarely occur without a clinically impressive primary lesion. Most cases will be suspected on fine-needle biopsy and confirmed on examination of frozen sections after total lobectomy, as for papillary carcinoma. If there are unequivocal malignant features of capsular and vascular invasion, total thyroidectomy is the treatment of choice. Frequently, however, the pathological appearances are not clear-cut, and malignant features are easily missed because of sampling error, in which case it is best to wait until definitive paraffin sections are available. If these show minimal invasion suppression of TSH with thyroxine is all that is required. If, however, overt vascular or capsular invasion is seen, re-operation is strongly advised: total thyroidectomy should ideally be carried out within 7 to 10 days; beyond that time surgery becomes difficult due to new vessel growth and fibrosis. Although multifocal disease is not common, removal of the main 'iodine trap' enables distant metastases to be identified and ablated using radio-iodine. The usual routine is to withhold thyroxine after thyroidectomy until the patient becomes hypothyroid, usually within 3 to 6 weeks. The increased TSH drive then makes the secondaries avid for iodine and therefore more likely to be identified.

Anaplastic carcinoma

Surgery has little to offer for most patients, who are usually elderly, female, and infirm. The rare middle-aged patient may benefit from total thyroidectomy followed by external radiotherapy, although tumour cells may be implanted in the surgical incision. The surgeon's role is therefore mainly to establish the diagnosis beyond doubt. In view of the bulky nature of most anaplastic tumours a good representative sample can be obtained using a Trucut needle and local anaesthetic. Pressure on the trachea can sometimes be achieved by removal of the isthmus, but local radiotherapy often offers the only prospect of worthwhile palliation. The 12-month survival rate is zero and chemotherapy has so far failed to improve the dismal prognosis.

Malignant lymphoma

Some of these tumours, which mimic anaplastic carcinoma in their presentation and histology, arise in pre-existing Hashimoto's disease or as part of a generalized lymphomatous disease. Most are radiosensitive and regress following external beam radiotherapy; good 5-year survival figures have been reported. Chemotherapy is reserved for patients with disseminated disease. The role of surgery is therefore diagnostic and attempts to remove the lymphoma are rarely appropriate.

Medullary thyroid carcinoma

Total thyroidectomy is the procedure of choice in view of the high incidence of multicentric lesions in patients with both familial and sporadic disease. The upper poles and in particular the primary lymphatic drainage areas must be completely resected. The resection of lymph nodes in the central compartment should extend from the hyoid bone to the innominate vessels, since up to 75 per cent of them will be found to contain metastatic disease. Lymph nodes in the secondary drainage areas should be sampled and, if positive, removed in accordance with the modified dissection described for papillary carcinoma. When the diagnosis is suspected from the family history or confirmed by fine-needle biopsy a co-existing phaeochromocytoma or parathyroid tumour needs to be excluded: failure to attend to these endocrine tumours first may be catastrophic. A serial rise in serum calcitonin after thyroidectomy is a strong indicator of recurrent disease; this is detectable by pentavalent DMSA scanning. Metastases may be treated by surgery, radiotherapy, radio-iodine, or chemotherapy. Results are, however, often disappointing and calcitonin levels rarely return to normal.

Secondary thyroid carcinoma

Although rare, these most commonly arise from breast, kidney, ovary, or colon. Thyroidectomy may be indicated if the secondary deposits are confined to the thyroid and if the primary tumour is under control.

OPERATIVE SURGERY ON THE THYROID

Preoperative measures

Preparation is directed to ensure safe induction of anaesthesia and a trouble free intra- and postoperative course. Haemoglobin estimation, chest radiology, and an ECG are mandatory. Blood transfusion is rarely required: grouping and saving of serum is all that is required. If thyroid enlargement is massive or retrosternal, and if the patient shows clinical signs of respiratory embarrassment or superior vena caval obstruction, a CT scan of the neck and thoracic inlet (Fig. 26(a) and (b)) will indicate the possible need to enter the chest and potential problems which may be encountered on intubation. The vocal cords should always be examined by indirect laryngoscopy; this is especially important when the voice is compromised, malignancy is suspected, or when previous thyroid surgery has been undertaken. A small proportion of patients have unsuspected recurrent laryngeal nerve palsy; it is of clinical and medicolegal importance to both the patient and the surgeon to determine before surgery whether or not the vocal cords are moving normally. Thyrotoxic patients need to be rendered euthyroid or the peripheral effects of high circulating levels of thyroxine blocked. The majority of thyrotoxic patients referred for surgery have already received one or more courses of antithyroid drugs, but their condition remains unstable. Where residual toxicity is modest and surgery can be undertaken quickly it is standard practice in many centres to stop antithyroid drugs 10 days prior to operation and switch to oral propranolol in a dose of 30 to 120 mg every 6 to 8 h. The dose is adjusted to keep the patient's sleeping pulse at around 70 beats/min. Since the effective duration of action of propranolol is approximately 6 h it is important to administer medication right up to induction of anaesthesia

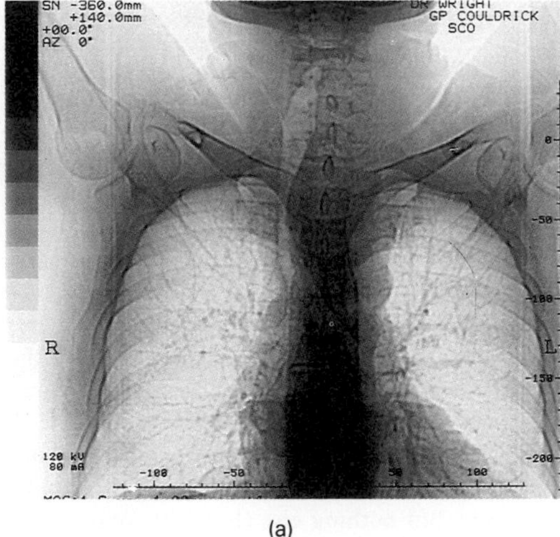

(a)

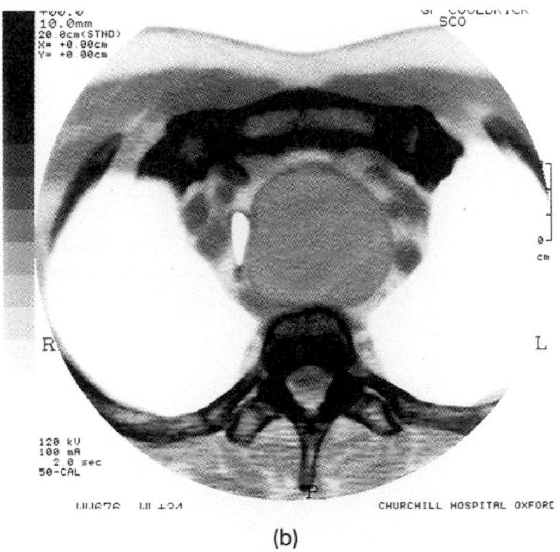

(b)

Fig. 26 Radiological assessment of a retrosternal goitre by (a) conventional chest radiograph and (b) CT scanning.

and to continue treatment thereafter, especially if the patient develops tachycardia. β-Blockers are contraindicated in patients with bronchial asthma, sinus bradycardia, or congestive heart failure. Patients with severe thyrotoxicosis who require relatively early surgery should receive a 6- to 8-week course of carbimazole (Neomercazole 10–15 mg 8-hourly). In the event of an adverse drug reaction propylthiouracil (100 mg three times daily) may be substituted for carbimazole. Extended use of thiourea drugs may cause prothrombin deficiency (hence the advisability of stopping the drug 10 days prior to surgery), leucopenia, or profound bone marrow depression. Full blood count and INR estimation should be checked if reduced resistance to infection or impaired haemostasis is suspected.

Standard surgical approach to the thyroid

The patient should be placed comfortably on the operating table and the surgical diathermy indifferent electrode securely attached to the thigh prior to placement of the surgical drapes. Good access to the anterior compartment of the neck is facilitated by placing a pillow under the shoulders to extend the cervical spine while supporting and stabilizing the head on a rubber ring or horseshoe. Failure to do so may result in severe postoperative pain and headache, especially in elderly patients with cervical spondylitis. In patients with a short stocky neck or a large goitre it is helpful to depress the shoulders by exerting gentle traction on the arms alongside the body and securing their position with foam wedges (Fig. 27). The table is then tilted 15° head-up to reduce engorgement of the neck veins. A flat board or magnetic pad

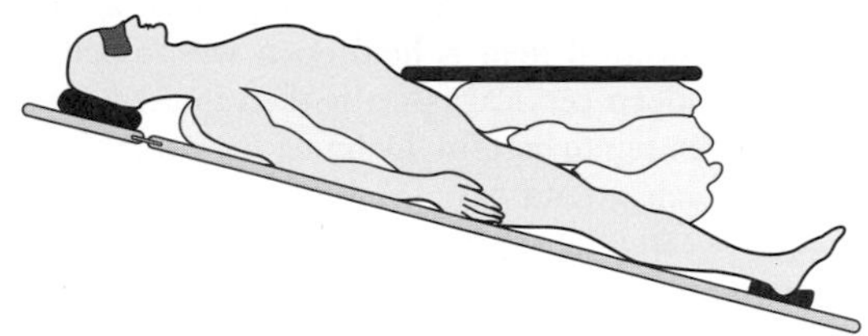

Fig. 27 Position of patient for operations on the thyroid gland.

supported by pillows placed on the lower chest and upper abdomen provides a convenient instrument tray. The skin is prepared with a suitable antibiotic solution and the operative field draped after gauze packs have been pushed well down into the recesses between the head support and the shoulder pillow on each side. These absorb blood loss at the lateral extent of the surgical excision and provide a good anchor for towel clips. The skin to be incised is now rarely infiltrated with 1 : 1000 adrenaline in saline solution, since much of the bleeding at the skin edge stops spontaneously. More persistent points of loss are best recognized and dealt with immediately, since extensive bruising and wound haematoma can develop after the vasoconstrictive effects of adrenaline have worn off.

The majority of thyroid procedures can be carried out through a Kocher collar incision which is placed in one of the natural skin creases (Langer's lines), approximately two finger breadths above the supraclavicular joint (Fig. 28). This may conveniently be marked before incision with a length of silk held taut against the skin around the convexity of the neck. The incision should be symmetrical: when the collagen in the scar matures it may contract unevenly if the stress lines are unequal, leading to a poor cosmetic result. Symmetry can be checked by the surgeon standing at the

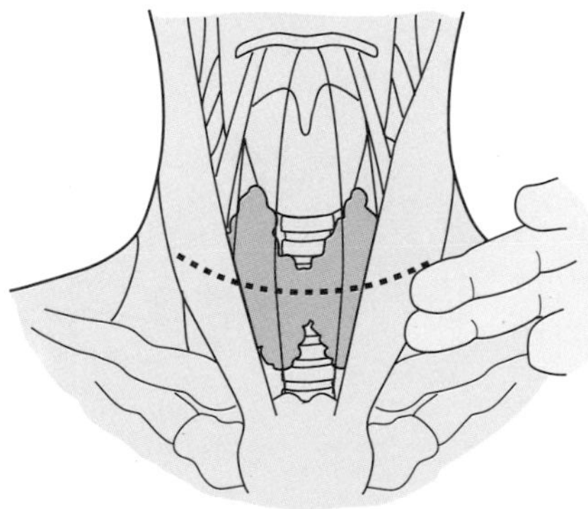

Fig. 28 Standard incision for operations on the thyroid gland.

head of the table and looking down on the proposed incision directly from above. Matching the skin flaps at the end of the operation is rarely a problem for an experienced surgeon, and the practice of cross-hatching the incision line with a needle, which carries the risk of provoking a keloid reaction, is undesirable. Deepening the incision through the subcutaneous fat and platysma muscle discloses the deep cervical fascia, investing the strap muscle centrally and the sternomastoid laterally. The anterior jugular veins course beneath the fascial layer on the anterior surface of the thyroid and, provided that the surgeon is careful and keeps to the plane between the platysma and fascia, blood loss is minimal. Mobilization is extended superiorly to the prominence of the thyroid cartilage and inferiorly to the suprasternal notch. The diamond-shaped surgical field is held open with a self-retaining retractor and the deep cervical fascia is then incised through the midline raphe from top to bottom. Defining the planes beneath the strap muscles which extend over the surface of the thyroid lobes laterally requires care: the sternothyroid muscle may be extremely thin due to compression by a greatly enlarged thyroid. Adherence of these layers is a feature of the inflammatory process seen in autoimmune thyroiditis and when thyroid malignancy extends outside the gland. Further exposure of the thyroid requires delivery of each lobe into the wound after division and ligation of the middle thyroid vein on each side. In most patients the strap muscles present no impediment to the forward dislocation of the lobes; if they do they should be divided since division or removal causes no detectable functional disability. In practice, a pair of long straight artery forceps inserted under the strap muscles at the junction of their upper one-third and lower two-thirds can define their lateral margin against the sternomastoid, allowing identification and preservation of the nerve of supply (the ansa hypoglossi) before the muscle is divided. Stay stitches to the upper and lower muscle flaps hitched over the joints of the self-retainer can act as a convenient retractor (Fig. 29).

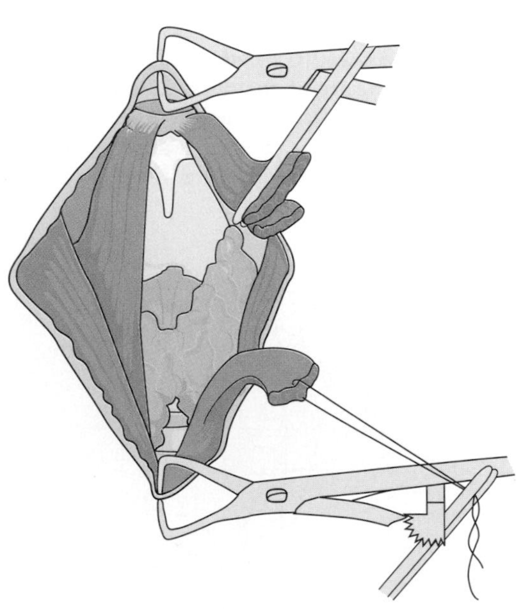

Fig. 29 Division and mobilization of strap muscles.

Specific thyroid surgical procedures

Subtotal thyroidectomy

The aim of this operation to remove sufficient thyroid tissue to cure hyperthyroidism yet preserve a posterior remnant of the gland on each side sufficient to maintain the patient in a euthyroid state. Most surgeons prefer to stand on the opposite side of the table to the lobe being delivered. Following mobilization of the lobe the upper pole vascular pedicle is identified below the adherent sternothyroid muscle. A thyroid director is then passed between the larynx and the thyroid pedicle just above the suspensory ligament. Damage to recurrent laryngeal nerve and the superior laryngeal nerve is avoided if the point of the director is aimed upwards and laterally; finger-tip pressure is sufficient to ensure that the point of the director is passing behind all of the upper lobe tissue, but nothing else (Fig. 30). With the director in

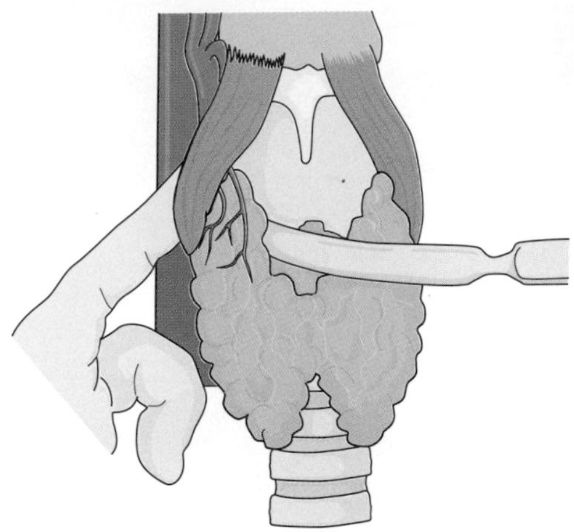

Fig. 30 Mobilization of superior pole of the thyroid gland.

place the pedicle is doubly ligated with a transfixion non-absorbable suture. The lobe is then grasped with a pair of tenaculum forceps and rotated medially. The inferior thyroid artery, identified by blunt dissection of the space between the trachea and common carotid artery, is under-run cleanly and precisely with a ligature mounted on an aneurysm needle. If this is placed laterally it is ready for tying in continuity avoiding involvement of the recurrent laryngeal nerve and parathyroids. Gentle traction on this ligature often throws the recurrent laryngeal nerve into prominence as it runs up at an acute angle from the mediastinum to reach the tracheo-oesphageal groove before assuming its intimate relationships with the branches of this artery. When the nerve is not evident an aberrant course should be suspected; this may be lateral or anterior to the trachea or even non-recurrent. The nerve can confidently be identified by its white colour, fine longitudinal surface vein, lack of pulsation, and lack of elasticity. Proceeding with the operation without having identified the nerve is hazardous. The thyroid lobe is freed inferiorly by isolating and dividing between ligatures the inferior thyroid veins, and the thyroidea ima artery where present. During this manoeuvre the recurrent laryngeal nerve should be kept in view and avoided at all times. The inferior parathyroid gland may be seen at this stage, especially if ectopic, lying in the thyrothymic ligament. This and its blood supply will be preserved if the veins are swept medially and secured close to the gland. In this form of thyroidectomy the parathyroids are not specifically identified; attempting to do so may jeopardize their blood supply. If a parathyroid gland seems to be inadvertently excised or devascularized it can be diced into 1 mm cubes and autotransplanted into the adjacent sternomastoid muscle. The surgeon then decides how much thyroid tissue to leave behind. The empirical formula of resecting seven-eighths and leaving one-eighth of the gland renders a large number of patients euthyroid. The merit of this approach is that it requires no modification for varying sizes of gland, but it has the disadvantage that it does not take into account the age of the patient (generally the younger the patient the more radical the resection needs to be) or the presence of antithyroid autoantibodies (which call for less radical excision). Attempts to standardized the size of the thyroid remnant to 3 to 4 g of tissue on each side, assessed by linear measurement or dental wax impressions, are not only highly inaccurate but meaningless. Having decided on the size of the thyroid remnant, small artery forceps are placed along the line of the incision on the posterolateral aspect of the surgical capsule of the gland. Placement above the level defined by the anterior surface of the trachea allows injury to the recurrent laryngeal nerve and parathyroids to be minimized. The gland is then incised with a scalpel blade directed obliquely down towards the trachea (Fig. 31). This procedure is then performed on the opposite side

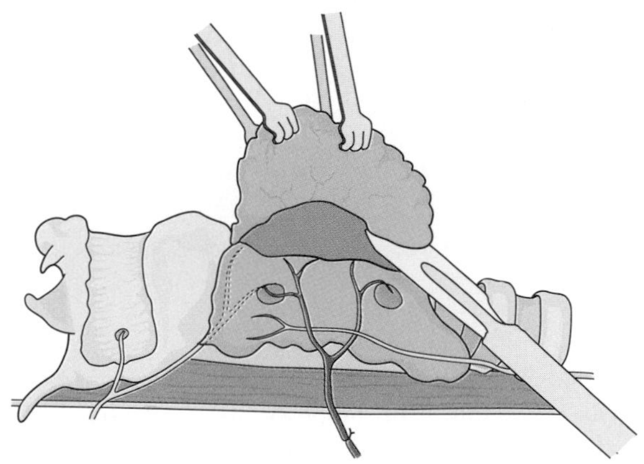

Fig. 31 Removal of thyroid lobe by sharp dissection, preserving parathyroid glands.

of the neck. Both lobes and isthmus having been freed the gland now remains attached only by the pyramidal lobe or fibrous remnant of the thyroglossal tract. This requires careful dissection upwards so that no additional thyroid tissue or blood supply is overlooked. The thyroid remnants are then sutured to the pretracheal fascia with a continuous absorbable suture in a herringbone fashion, picking up the surgical capsule and rolling the gland towards the midline and away from the recurrent laryngeal nerves (Fig. 32). As well as having an haemostatic effect, this ensures that the fibrotic reaction around the thyroid is well away from important structures, the neck requires further exploration at a later date. The thyroid bed should usually be drained on each side: where the dead space is modest a suction drain is ideal. After flexing the head the strap muscles, if divided, are rejoined by interrupted sutures and then approximated in the midline. Finally the platysma is closed and then the skin closed either with clips or a subcuticular suture.

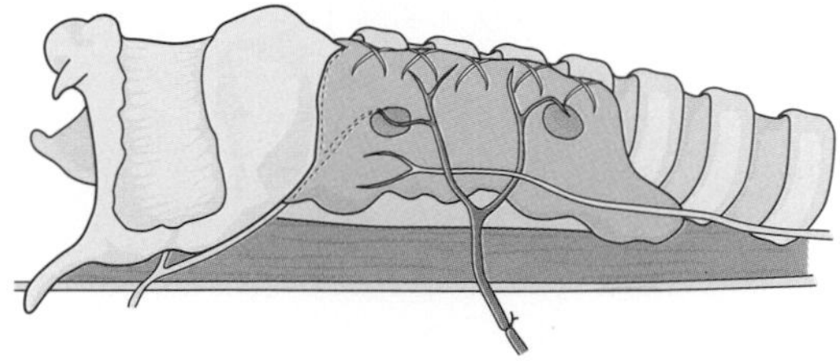

Fig. 32 Haemostatic suture of residual thyroid.

Partial thyroidectomy

This procedure is appropriate when a large multinodular goitre needs to be reduced in size. The standard exposure of the thyroid and subtotal excision is performed as described above. As much normal tissue as possible is left, consistent with a modest lateral remnant on each side which is not evident when the patient swallows. The isthmus or pyramidal lobe should be removed, even if apparently normal, since compensatory hypertrophy at that site is particularly unacceptable cosmetically.

Removal of a retrosternal goitre

Nearly all retrosternal goitres can be removed via a cervical incision, which should be placed lower than the conventional incision already described. However if preoperative symptoms and investigations indicate that the chest may need to be opened then the anterior chest wall is prepared and draped accordingly. In this instance the services of an experienced anaesthetist are imperative, especially if the airway is severely compromised. It is often safer to withhold sedative premedication and to rely on rapid intubation of the conscious patient, after spraying the vocal cords with local anaesthetic. Wholly or partially intrathoracic goitres derive their arterial supply from the superior and inferior arteries in the neck, and these should be secured in the usual way. Once the upper pole has been freed an attempt should be made to dissect the retrosternal portion of the lobe with the index finger, generally easing it upwards. Minimal force should be used to avoid damage to the recurrent laryngeal nerves, which cannot always be visualized. If this manoeuvre fails intracapsular enucleation of the retrosternal goitre may be appropriate; if retrosternal thyroid malignancy is suspected or if surgery is being performed for a recurrent goitre, formal splitting of the sternum is appropriate. An incision is made in the midline down to the periosteum, with cutting diathermy from the suprasternal notch to the xiphisternum (Fig. 33). The parietal pleura is freed in the midline and deviated laterally; the retrosternal goitre is then removed along routine lines and the chest closed by accurately reapproximating the sternum using wire sutures. A retrosternal drain is brought out superiorly and attached to an underwater seal to control any small pneumothorax which might be present.

Total thyroid lobectomy or total thyroidectomy

Thyroid lobectomy should always be for the treatment of a non-toxic solitary nodule which may prove to be malignant. If malignancy is confirmed on histological examination of frozen section total thyroidectomy may be appropriate, depending on cell type. The approach to the thyroid is standard but the subtotal excision technique described earlier differs in several important ways. At no stage is the gland grasped with tissue forceps for traction: this may rupture a malignant focus, with spillage of

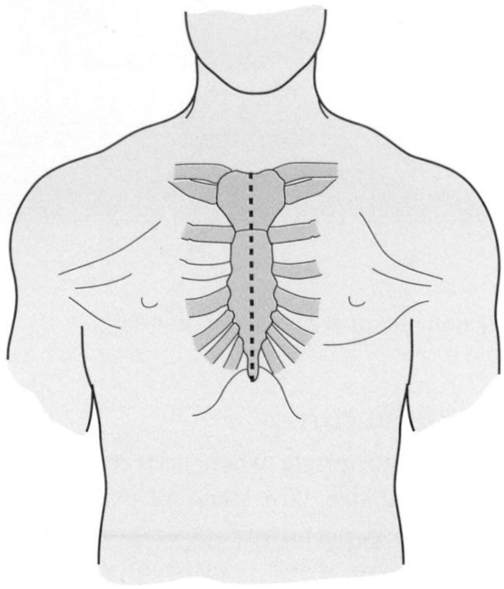

Fig. 33 Incision for partial or complete splitting of the sternum to gain access to a large retrosternal goitre.

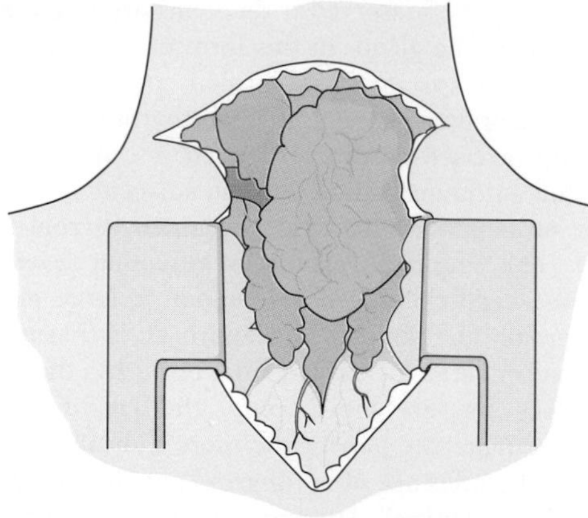

Fig. 34 Exposure of retrosternal goitre following splitting of the upper sternum.

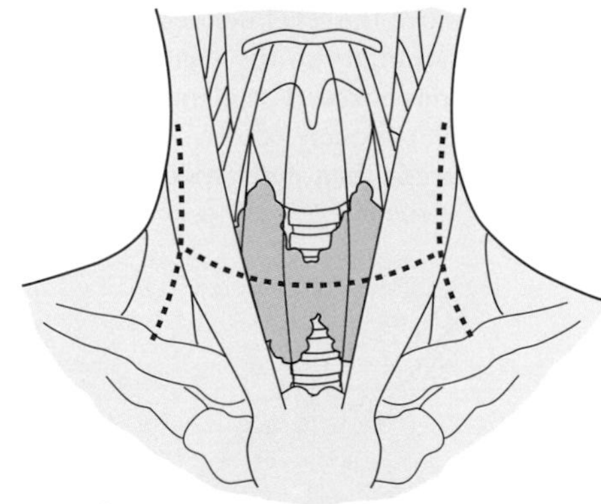

Fig. 35 Modification of thyroid incision to include bilateral lymph node dissection.

tumour cells. Multicentric tumour deposits or capsular invasion must be assumed to be present. The entire lobe, isthmus, and the midline portion of the contralateral lobe should therefore be removed, although if the recurrent laryngeal nerve or parathyroids may be compromised it is better to leave a small amount of thyroid tissue and ablate this later with radio-iodine. Blood is supplied to each parathyroid via an end artery arising from the inferior thyroid artery, but collaterals to this artery are probably picked up on the thyroid capsule from the oesophageal and tracheal vessels. It is better, therefore, not to ligate the inferior thyroid artery in continuity but to trace out each of its terminal branches and individually clip and divide these between mosquito forceps as they enter the false capsule. Concurrently, the recurrent laryngeal nerve is traced out along its course. As it traverses Berry's ligament to gain access to the larynx damage will be avoided by dissecting the nerve free under direct vision. Local invasion may prevent complete removal of thyroid malignancy, notably on the side of the larynx and oesophagus. In these circumstances the extent of the residual tumour should be marked with small clips to assist the radiotherapist in planning subsequent treatment fields.

Modified block dissection for thyroid carcinoma

The standard Kocher incision is extended on one or both sides (Figs. 34, 35) to allow routine exposure of the thyroid gland. If the malignancy involves the strap muscles or sternomastoid on one side these are resected *en bloc* with the thyroid, as described previously. The plane between the sternomastoid and strap muscles is opened up and the carotid sheath exposed. Involvement of lymph nodes of the internal jugular chain, extending to the posterior cervical and supraclavicular groups, can be detected if the sternal and clavicular heads of the sternomastoid are detached, and the muscle rotated upwards. This provides excellent exposure yet preserves the blood supply (occipital artery) and nerve supply (accessory). The muscle can be reattached on completion of the nodal dissection. Great care is needed when removing the upper and lower deep cervical nodes and their surrounding fat from the surface of the internal jugular vein. However, if the latter is heavily affected it too will require excision. The vagus and phrenic nerves are easily identified and preserved; however, the thoracic duct on the left and the main lymphatic duct on the right are easily damaged and if this occurs the affected duct should be tied off rather than repaired.

POSTOPERATIVE COMPLICATIONS

In competent hands thyroid surgery is associated with a low morbidity rate and no mortality. There are, however, local and specific complications which can severely compromise the outcome and be life threatening. The majority are avoidable with sound surgical technique and good preparation, particularly in thyrotoxic patients.

Haemorrhage

This is typically reactionary and is a potential problem in the first 24 h after surgery. Failure to secure the superior thyroid vessels efficiently, preferably with a transfixion suture, is associated with the risk of serious blood loss. Inadequate control of the inferior and middle thyroid vein may also have serious consequences. Major haemorrhage deep to the strap muscles must be recognized quickly: this may cause pressure on the airway within a confined space and rapid laryngeal and subglottic oedema. Medical and nursing staff need to be aware of the significance of pallor, respiratory difficulty, stridor, and swelling of the wound. The absence of blood loss from drains is not a reliable indicator of haemostasis since these can block easily. Any haematoma should be evacuated immediately, and intubation or tracheostomy may be necessary to avert a potentially life-threatening situation. Clip removers and a pair of artery forceps should be readily available at the bedside of all patients following thyroidectomy. These will allow the incision and the strap muscles to be opened. If stridor persists, skilled anaesthetic help is needed to perform intubation, which may be difficult in the presence of oedema. In the absence of such help a mini-tracheostomy or large medicut needle and cannula (No.12 blue) inserted percutaneously through the cricothyroid membrane or between the tracheal rings should stabilize the patient until haemorrhage can be arrested.

Recurrent laryngeal nerve damage

The incidence of permanent and transient damage to the nerve is low (less than 0.1 per cent and 2–4 per cent, respectively). It is largely avoidable if the surgeon routinely seeks to identify the nerve on each side during all operations on the gland. Loss of vocal power and huskiness is often evident for 2 or 3 days after surgery; this is most likely to be due to oedema and is relieved by local anaesthetic lozenges and/or humidified air. Persistence of symptoms may indicate neuropraxia, caused by stretching or crushing of the nerve; this is reversible and recovers over several weeks or months. Permanent damage will result if the nerve is divided or ligated and is more likely to occur when the anatomy is distorted, for example with recurrent or malignant goitres. Unilateral injury may be asymptomatic and will undetected due to compensatory hyperadduction of the unaffected cord unless routine postoperative laryngoscopy is performed. Symptomatic unilateral cord paralysis improves if the affected cord is stabilized in adduction by the submucous injection of Teflon under direct laryngoscopy. The effects of bilateral nerve injury are likely to be temporary but pose an immediate problem when the patient is extubated at the end of surgery since the unopposed adductor action of the cricothyroid muscles closes the glottis to such an extent that the least exertion results in airway obstruction. The patient must be promptly reintubated, paralysed, and ventilated whilst hydrocortisone is given 100 mg three times daily to combat the oedema and inflammatory response. The patient can usually be successfully extubated within 48 h; if this extubation fails tracheostomy is required. The permanent nature of laryngeal damage should not be accepted unless it lasts for more than 9 months. Exploration and resuture of the nerve, with grafting when necessary, is now feasible, as is the anastomosis of the hypoglossal and recurrent nerves.

Superior laryngeal nerve paresis

The true incidence of this injury is unknown due to the lack of any objective test of function until recently. A change in the voice, such as loss of pitch and inability to make explosive sounds, makes damage likely. Voice analysis using a Visipitch oscilloscope will help to confirm this damage, which may occur in up to 25 per cent of patients. The majority of patients will recover since the nerve has only been stretched. If no improvement is evident after 3 months, it is unlikely to occur. Bilateral damage results in a very flat, hoarse voice that tires easily.

Hypoparathyroidism

The serum calcium level should be monitored postoperatively since patients without overt hypoparathyroidism may develop vague lethargy and depression, insidious cataracts, mental deterioration, and psychosis. Hypocalcaemia due to parathyroid deficiency will usually be evident within 1 week of operation and should be suspected if the patient appears unduly agitated or depressed or hyperventilates. Circumoral tingling is generally the first and most sensitive indicator of a low serum calcium; paraesthesia in the fingers and toes preceding frank tetany is seen when hypocalcaemia is profound. Tapping over the facial nerve will cause contraction of the facial muscles (Chvostek–Weiss sign); however, this phenomenon may also be observed in 10 to 15 per cent of normal individuals. Carpopedal spasm, provoked by occlusion of the circulation to the arm (Trousseau's sign), indicates severe hypocalcaemia: intravenous infusion of 10 ml of 10 per cent calcium gluconate (given slowly to avoid cardiac arrest in systole) is required. This infusion may need to be repeated every 4 to 6 h. Oral effervescent calcium should also be administered 4 to 6 g daily, depending on response. If hypocalcaemia persists, vitamin D (calciferol 25 000–100 000 units) and 2 to 3 g oral calcium per day are given until a normocalcaemic state is achieved. Signs and symptoms of hypocalcaemia will recur in these patients at times of metabolic stress, such as pregnancy or the menopause.

Hypothyroidism and recurrent hyperthyroidism

The ability of the thyroid to produce sufficient thyroxine after thyroidectomy reflects not only the size of the remnant but also the pre-existing pathological processes within the gland. Hypothyroidism is inevitable after total thyroidectomy or malignancy, but is less predictable after, for example, a thyroid lobectomy to remove a benign solitary nodule. Avoiding hypothyroidism is one of the main challenges when operating for thyrotoxicosis. Factors affecting postoperative thyroid function include the severity of disease prior to surgery; the age of the patient; the presence of high levels of antithyroid autoantibodies before surgery; the size of the gland and evidence of lymphoid infiltration on histology; and how much of the gland is removed. An experienced surgeon can treat patients with resultant hypothyroidism rates of 10 to 15 per cent and persistent hyperthyroidism rates below 5 per cent. Hypothyroidism with rising TSH levels should be allowed to develop over 6 weeks after total thyroidectomy for malignancy (notably follicular lesions). A radio-iodine scan will then identify possible distant metastases, which can be ablated. Thereafter, T_3 (50–100 μg/day) is then administered in preference to T_4 by virtue of its shorter biological half-life (1 week), which enables repeat scans to be performed with minimal delay. Once isotope ablation of residual disease has been achieved conversion to T_4 is appropriate. The dose required shows great inter-individual variation, the majority only requiring 0.2 to 0.3 mg/day. Nearly all patients undergoing surgery for thyrotoxicosis become biochemically hypothyroid for 2 to 3 months after surgery; no correction is necessary as the majority will then stabilize in a euthyroid state. Clinical assessment should be maintained for at least 2 years, during which serum thyroxine and TSH levels should be monitored: a small percentage of patients will become clinically hypothyroid and require T_4 supplementation (0.1 to 0.2 mg daily). Routine administration of T_4 (0.1 mg daily) is recommended for all patients undergoing surgery for non-toxic, diffuse, or multinodular goitres since failure to suppress TSH drive can result in recurrent goitre, even if hypothyroidism is subclinical.

Tracheal collapse

Collapse of the trachea, the wall of which has become softened due to chondromalacia, occasionally occurs following removal of a long-standing goitre, especially if retrosternal. Such patients usually also suffer laryngeal oedema and reduced movement of the vocal cords, following difficult intubation and delivery of the lobes. Whenever the trachea is markedly soft and narrow, an elective tracheostomy should be performed.

Thyroid crisis

This is now very rare, with the improved methods of control of thyrotoxicosis, but when fully expressed, is characterized by high fever, tachycardia (atrial fibrillation), extreme restlessness, and delirium. High doses of antithyroid drugs (Neo Mercazole (carbimazole) 30 mg immediately and then 15 mg 8-hourly), plus 1 g of sodium iodide IV should be given promptly. Propranolol (2 mg) is slowly infused IV, with electrocardiographic control. Fluid replacement, ice pack cooling, and sedation may help to abort the crisis.

Cervical sympathetic damage

This rare complication results from deep, forceful retraction on the carotid sheath, producing Horner's syndrome. This is notable by the absence of the vascular dilatation component. The resulting myosis and ptosis are frequently permanent.

Wound complications

The deposition of excessive collagen in the scar to form a keloid is an unpredictable complication, but is said to be more prevalent in negroes, redheads, and in those undergoing surgery during pregnancy. Unless the scar can be excised and adapted to conform more readily to Langer's lines reoperation is unlikely to confer any improvement, but topical steroids and low dose irradiation may prevent recurrence. Infection is an uncommon complication and when it occurs a foreign body should be suspected; the most common offender is non-absorbable suture material. Rarely, sensitivity to the nickel clips used for skin closure results in blistering and breakdown.

FURTHER READING

Bäckdahl M, Wallin G, Aner G, Lundell G, Löwhagen T, Cranber PO. Cellular DNA content in thyroid tumours. A reliable factor for grading and prognosis. *Prog Surg*, 1988; **19**: 40–53.

Barnes HV, Gann DS. Choosing thyroidectomy in hyperthyroidism, *Surg Clin N Am*, 1974; **54**: 289.

Beahrs OH, Sakulsky SB. Surgical Thyroidectomy in the management of exophthalmic goitre. *Arch Surg*, 1968; **96**: 512–5.

Black EG, *et al.* Serum thyroglobulin in thyroid cancer. *Lancet*, 1981; **ii**: 443–5.

Crile G Jr. The fallacy of the conventional neck dissection for papillary carcinoma of the thyroid. *Ann Surg*, 1957; **145**: 317.

De Visschar M, ed. *The thyroid gland.* New York: Raven Press, 1980.

Duffy BJ Jr, Fitzgerald PJ. Cancer of the thyroid in children. *J Clin Endocrinol Metab*, 1950; **10**: 1296–1308.

Hall R, Besser M, eds. *Fundamentals of Clinical Endocrinology*. 4th edn. Edinburgh: Churchill Livingstone, 1989.

Hay ID, Grant CS, Taylor WF, McConahey WM. Ipsilateral lobectomy versus bilateral lobar resection in papillary carcinoma. A retrospective analysis of surgical outcome using a novel prognostic scoring system. *Surgery*, 1987; **102**: 1088–95.

Hedley AJ, *et al.* The effect of remnant size on the outcome of subtotal thyroidectomy for thyrotoxicosis. *Br J Surg*, 1972; **59**: 559–63.

Hollingshead WH. Anatomy of the endocrine glands. *Surg Clin N Am*, 1952; **32**: 1115–40.

Johnson IDA, Thompson NW, eds. *Endocrine Surgery*. London: Butterworth, 1983.

Kaplan EL, ed. Surgery of the thyroid and parathyroid glands. *Clinical Surgery International vol. 6*. Edinburgh: Churchill Livingstone, 1983.

Kark AE, *et al.* Voice changes after thyroidectomy: the role of the external laryngeal nerve. *Br Med J*, 1984; **289**: 1412–5.

Löwhagen T, Granberg PO, Lundell G, Skinnari P, Sunblad R, Willeum JS. Aspiration biopsy cytology (ABC) in nodules of the thyroid gland suspected of being malignant. *Surg Clin N Am*, 1979; **59**: 3–18.

McGregor AM, Rees-Smith B, Hall R, Petersen MM, Millar M, Dewer PJ. Prediction of relapse in hyperthyroid Graves' disease. *Lancet*, 1980; **i**: 1101.

Neil HB III, Townsend GL, Devine KD. Bilateral vocal cord paralysis of undetermined aetiology: clinical course and outcome. *Ann Otol Rhinol Laryngol*, 1972; **81**: 514–9.

Peden NR, Gunn A, Browning MCK. Nadolol and potassium iodine in combination in the surgical treatment of thyrotoxicosis. *Br J Surg*, 1982; **69**: 638–41.

Reeve TS, *et al.* Thyroid cancers of follicular cell origin. *Prog Surg*, 1988; **19**: 78–88.

Rose N. Investigation of post-thyroidectomy patients for hypoparathyroidism. *Lancet*, 1963; **i**: 124–7.

Russell CF, *et al.* The surgical management of medullary thyroid carcinoma. *Ann Surg*, 1983; **197**: 42–8.

Russell WO, *et al.* Thyroid carcinoma classification. Intraglandular dissection and clinicopathological study based upon whole organ section of 80 glands. *Cancer*, 1963; **16**: 1425–60.

Smith BR, Hall R. Thyroid stimulating immunoglobulins in Grave's Disease. *Lancet*, 1974; **ii**: 427–30.

Udelsman R, Dudley NE. Medullary carcinoma of the thyroid: management of persistent hypercalcitonaemia utilizing [^{99m}Tc] (v) dimercaptosuccinic acid scintography. *Br J Surg*, 1989; **76**: 1276–81.

Wade JSH. The management of malignant thyroid tumours. *Br J Surg*, 1983; **70**: 253–5.

Woolner LB, Beahrs OH, Black BM, McConahey WM, Keating FR. Classification and prognosis of thyroid carcinoma. *Am J Surg*, 1961; **102**: 354–87.

11.2.1 Hyperparathyroidism and the metabolic responses to parathyroidectomy

ALLAN R. BRASIER

INTRODUCTION

Primary hyperparathyroidism is a disorder of the parathyroid glands resulting in autonomous parathyroid hormone secretion and presents clinically as hypercalcaemia or the sequela of long-standing hypercalcaemia. Although the aetiology of this condition can be either sporadic or familial, surgical excision of the affected parathyroid glands represents the only curative treatment for primary hyperparathyroidism. In the appropriately selected patient, and in experienced surgical hands, cure rates of 90 to 95 per cent of patients for initial neck explorations can be expected. In these patients undergoing successful parathyroidectomy, abrupt changes in calcium balance can be expected. Because these patients may have impaired calcium homeostasis, special vigilance is warranted by the team responsible for the patient's care.

INCIDENCE AND AETIOLOGY

Primary hyperparathyroidism is an idiopathic disorder due to autonomous function of one or more affected parathyroid glands. Primary hyperparathyroidism is distinct from secondary hyperparathyroidism in that the latter condition represents excessive parathyroid hormone as a consequence of hypocalcaemic stimulus to the parathyroids. Tertiary hyperparathyroidism represents autonomous parathyroid function from long-standing secondary hyperparathyroidism and is usually seen in patients with end-stage renal disease.

The incidence of primary hyperparathyroidism peaks in the sixth decade of life in both men and women at 92 and 188 per 100 000 population, respectively. Data from North America, England, and Europe indicate that the prevalence of primary hyperparathyroidism is nearly 1:1000 with an age-adjusted incidence of 27.7 per 100 000 population. These data indicate that, as the population of developed countries continues to age, primary hyperparathyroidism will continue to be a common endocrinological problem.

Autonomous secretion of parathyroid hormone (PTH) can be the consequence of either idiopathic or genetic influences. The majority of cases of primary hyperparathyroidism (90 per cent) are sporadic cases (i.e., with no familial inheritance). Although a weak association has been made between a history of prior neck irradiation and subsequent development of primary hyperparathyroidism, the vast majority of patients will lack this history of exposure. In most series the female to male ratio is nearly 2:1. Molecular biological techniques have defined that in a given subset of patients, parathyroid adenomas are monoclonal in origin. Moreover, these parathyroid adenomas contain rearrangements of the PTH gene itself. Through unknown mechanisms, this clonal expansion of parathyroid tissue results in an alteration of the set-point between ionized extracellular fluid calcium and PTH release. Sporadic cases of hyperparathyroidism are usually the consequence of a single adenoma. These patients respond well to surgery.

Familial causes of primary hyperparathyroidism are seen in the multiple endocrine neoplasia (MEN) syndromes (types I and IIa), where hyperparathyroidism can be the presenting endocrinopathy. Familial parathyroid adenomas have also been described with other endocrinopathies, but this manifestation is extremely rare. Genetic rearrangements, including the q13 region of chromosome 11, have been described. The majority of cases of hyperparathyroidism in the MEN syndrome are associated with diffuse hyperplasia of all four parathyroid glands. Suspicion of a diagnosis of MEN syndrome is important not only for screening other family members, but also for determining the appropriate strategy for surgical exploration. Because all four parathyroid glands are likely to be hyperplastic, bilateral neck exploration is justified. Moreover, the expectations for postsurgical outcomes are different; parathyroidectomy can control hypercalcaemia in these patients, but rarely cures the condition.

PATHOPHYSIOLOGY OF PRIMARY HYPERPARATHYROIDISM

Maintenance of ionized calcium within the extracellular and intracellular fluids is critical to a variety of processes, including membrane polarization, neuromuscular activity, hormone release, and hormone action. In humans, calcium is found in three states in the extracellular fluid. Approximately 47 per cent of calcium is bound to circulating proteins. The major calcium binding protein is albumin, accounting for 70 per cent of protein-binding in serum, with 12 calcium binding sites per molecule. Ten per cent of extracellular calcium is found in complexes with bicarbonate and citrate. The remaining 43 per cent represents free ionized calcium which is the physiologically relevant form of calcium. Calcium in the serum is regulated within a narrow concentration range between 1.14 and 1.30 mmol/l. Because of the importance of albumin as a calcium binding protein, total calcium levels will vary as a function of albumin concentration. As an approximate rule, for every 1 g/dl drop in serum albumin, the total calcium concentration will drop 0.8 mg/dl, and the free ionized calcium will not be affected. This relationship is important in postoperative dilutional states where antidiuretic hormone (ADH) release and intravenous fluid administration can produce a significant dilutional hypoalbuminaemia that does not result in hypocalcaemic symptoms. In contrast, shifts between protein-bound and ionized calcium can be affected acutely by alterations in plasma pH. Under conditions of alkaline pH, a shift in the equilibrium between protein-bound and ionized calcium will occur, with more calcium being protein-bound and less available in the free fraction. In this manner, hyperventilation can cause hypocalcaemic symptoms, even in the presence of normal total serum calcium.

Parathyroid hormone (PTH) is the major extracellular calcium-regulating hormone in man. Parathyroid hormone is a classic pre-prohormone that is synthesized in the chief cell of the parathyroid gland. After the 21 amino acid amino terminal sequences (the pre-pro-sequences) are processed, parathyroid hormone is secreted as an intact 84 amino acid peptide. Intact PTH (1–84) is rapidly cleaved into N-terminal (1–33) and C-terminal (34–84) fragments that are biologically inactive. Intact PTH (1–84) has an estimated half-life of 5 min, whereas the biologically inactive metabolites are cleared much more slowly. These immunologically cross reacting fragments have hampered the development of precise radioimmunoassays for clinical use. PTH acts at three major target organs (kidney, bone, and intestine) directly and indirectly to regulate calcium balance. In the distal convoluted tubule of the kidney, PTH acts to stimulate calcium transport by increasing calcium resorption of the glomerular filtrate. In the proximal tubule, PTH increases the enzymatic activity of 1α-hydroxylase, an essential enzyme for the generation of the active metabolite of vitamin D, 1,25-$(OH)_2$-vitamin D. Independently, PTH produces phosphaturia and bicarbonaturia through a cyclic AMP-mediated mechanism, a process that accounts for the hypophosphataemia and metabolic acidosis clinically observed in patients with primary hyperparathyroidism. At the level of the bone, the second target organ for PTH effect, PTH mobilizes calcium from this reservoir through rapid effects on a calcium pool in equilibrium with the extracellular fluid and slower effects through induction of lysosomal enzymes in PTH-responsive osteoclasts. Almost paradoxically, PTH stimulates osteoblast activity and increases bone deposition as well, underscoring its important role as a regulator of bone remodelling. The third target organ, the intestine, is only indirectly affected by PTH. The action of PTH on the proximal tubule of the kidney results in elevated 1,25-$(OH)_2$-vitamin D production. This steroid hormone plays an important role in PTH action on bone, but also induces active calcium absorption in the small bowel. Under normal physiological situations, the three major target organs of PTH serve to normalize ionized calcium levels through increased kidney resorption, increased calcium mobilization from skeletal reserves, and increased dietary absorption in the gut.

Knowledge of the target organ effects of PTH applies to the pathological condition of primary hyperparathyroidism. In primary hyperparathyroidism affected parathyroid glands are functionally shifted in the calcium dose-response relationship of PTH release. These parathyroid glands have an altered 'set-point' and regulate ionized calcium concentrations at a level higher than desirable. Patients with primary hyperparathyroidism are hypercalcaemic due to PTH stimulus on the kidney to reabsorb calcium, on the bone to mobilize calcium, and from the gut to increase the fractional absorption of dietary calcium in spite of normal or even high total serum calcium levels. Although the direct effect of PTH on the kidney is to increase fractional reabsorption of calcium from the glomerular filtrate, the consequence of excess secretion of PTH is an elevated urinary calcium due to the high filtered load of calcium. Thus, the clinical consequences of long-standing autonomous parathyroid secretion are then predictable: renal disease due to nephrocalcinosis or nephrolithiasis, bone involvement (pain, pathological fractures, bone cysts) due to excessive bone resorption, and severe hypercalcaemia with neurological symptoms (anorexia, nausea/vomiting, and confusion).

Since the advent of simultaneous multianalyser (SMA) technology for routine analysis of serum calcium, the initial presentation of primary hyperparathyroidism has changed dramatically. Before 1960, the majority of patients presented with the classic clinical syndromes of bone disease (osteitis fibrosa cystica) or renal disease (nephrocalcinosis and/or nephrolithiasis). Now, the single largest category of patients are those diagnosed during the evaluation for asymptomatic (or minimally symptomatic) hypercalcaemia (50–80 per cent in most series).

DIAGNOSIS

The diagnosis of primary hyperparathyroidism is usually made during the evaluation for hypercalcaemia. Eighty per cent of patients are either asymptomatic or mildly symptomatic with non-specific constitutive symptoms such as fatigue, weakness, polydipsia, polyuria, arthralgia, and constipation. Although the majority of outpatients evaluated for hypercalcaemia (roughly 50 per cent) will be diagnosed as hyperparathyroid, other causes of hypercalcaemia must be considered. These include hypercalcaemia of malignancy (multiple myeloma, squamous cell carcinomas of head and neck), granulomatous disease (sarcoidosis), milk-alkali syndrome, endocrine disorders (thyrotoxicosis, adrenal insufficiency), vitamin D toxicity, drug use (thiazide diuretics, lithium), immobilization hypercalcaemia (particularly in patients with Paget's disease), and (benign) familial hypocalciuric hypercalcaemia. Hypercalcaemia on independent occasions in the setting of elevated levels of intact parathyroid hormone is diagnostic of primary hyperparathyroidism. However, this diagnosis must be made when thiazide diuretics or lithium-containing medications are withdrawn prior to evaluation, and when blood samples are taken with minimal venous occlusion to avoid artefactual hypercalcaemia due to haemoconcentration. The PTH assays available commercially are two-site immunoradiometric assays using one antiserum directed against the 1–34 amino acid portion of the PTH molecule and the second against the 39–84 amino acid sequence of the PTH molecule. Because this PTH immunoradiometric assay recognizes only intact PTH, cleavage fragments do not cross-react in the assay. Discrimination between hypercalcaemic patients with hypercalcaemia of malignancy and hyperparathyroidism is now quite good. Normal PTH values are reported between 10 and 65 pg/ml. Intact PTH values for patients with primary hyperparathyroidism will be in the high normal range or frankly elevated. In contrast, the majority of patients with hypercalcaemia of malignancy have suppressed PTH values (<1 pg/ml). Moreover, the advent of two-site assays for parathyroid hormone related peptide (PTHrp), the humoral agent implicated in humoral hypercalcaemia of malignancy, adds further discriminatory power to the work-up of the hypercalcemic patient.

In addition to calcium and PTH hormone assays, other evaluation of the patient with suspected primary hyperparathyroidism may be indicated. Albumin and ionized calcium concentrations help to determine the degree of ionized hypercalcaemia. Ionized calcium measurements are sometimes unreliable and generally only interpretable when specimen pH is concomitantly measured and is normal. Serum alkaline phosphatase may indicate underlying bone disease. Renal function assays, blood urea nitrogen, and creatinine may be useful to guide fluid and electrolyte therapy during the postoperative period, and may be helpful in predicting those patients prone to the development of postoperative hypocalcaemia and hypophosphataemia. Urinary calcium/creatinine ratios are sometimes helpful in differentiating primary hyperparathyroidism from patients with familial hypocalciuric hypercalcaemia.

INDICATIONS FOR PARATHYROIDECTOMY

Although the indications for surgical intervention in the truly asymptomatic patient are debated, parathyroidectomy represents the only curative modality available. Currently accepted indications for parathyroidectomy include patients with objective manifestations of primary hyperparathyroidism. Those include nephrolithiasis, reduced creatinine clearance, markedly elevated 24-h calcium excretion (250 mg/24 h), severe hypercalcaemia (greater than 12 mg/dl), recurrent pancreatitis, young patients (< 50 years of age), or patients in whom periodic assessment is not feasible. However, surgical intervention in the truly asymptomatic patient, in the absence of other considerations, is frequently justified on the basis of published series where 20 per cent of asymptomatic patients develop end-organ involvement within 5 years of the identification of hypercalcaemia, regardless of its severity.

PREOPERATIVE LOCALIZATION

Non-invasive preoperative localization has not had a significant impact on the 95 per cent success rate for initial neck exploration by the experienced parathyroid surgeon. Importantly, these anatomical studies are not used to make the diagnosis of primary hyperparathyroidism; they are used merely as a guide for the surgical exploration for patients in whom the diagnosis for primary hyperparathyroidism is established and in whom surgical intervention is contemplated. Localization techniques include the 10-MHz real-time ultrasonography with predictive accuracy of 75 to 80 per cent for enlarged parathyroid glands located in the neck. Ultrasound studies are not helpful for the localization of mediastinal parathyroid glands and do not discriminate parathyroid glands from hyperplastic lymph nodes well; however, they can be extremely useful for the evaluation of coexisting thyroid disease. Thallium-201 chloride–technetium–99m-pertechnetate scanning utilizes computer-aided subtraction to localize parathyroid glands with 75 per cent accuracy. This technique is particularly well suited for parathyroid adenomas located away from the thyroid gland. Magnetic resonance imaging (MRI) appears to be particularly helpful for mediastinal tumours and differentiating parathyroids from lymphatic or fatty tissue. CT scans require intravenous contrast and are prone to streaking artefacts in the supraclavicular region. Selective venous catheterization with PTH sampling is reserved for patients on whom reoperation is planned and in whom tumour localization is problematic. The selection of these localization techniques is due to the above considerations as well as the clinical picture, local radiological expertise, and, finally, preferences of the parathyroid surgeon. In general, however, the majority of these localization techniques are reserved for the uncured patient in whom repeat surgical exploration is planned.

FACTORS INFLUENCING SELECTION OF OPERATIVE TECHNIQUE

Experienced parathyroid surgeons appreciate the importance of understanding the embryology of the parathyroid gland as a determinant for successful parathyroid surgery. Because the parathyroid glands derive from the endodermal germ layers of the third and fourth branchial pouch and migrate caudally, the location of any individual gland can be highly variable. Nevertheless, the locations of the ectopic parathyroid gland follow the pathway of this caudal migration, and this knowledge facilitates the search for parathyroid glands (see Section 11.2.2).

The lower parathyroid glands originate from the third branchial pouch and migrate along with the thymus to assume a position at the lower poles of the thyroid gland. These lower glands can also be found associated with the thymus in the anterior mediastinum if the gland fails to disassociate from the thymus, or alternatively, can be localized cephalad to the upper pole of the thyroid sometimes still associated with thymic tissue. The upper parathyroid glands arise from the fourth branchial pouch. They remain almost stationary until they reach their final location at the upper pole of the thyroid. Consequently, these glands are the most predictable in their location; they receive their blood supply from the inferior thyroidal artery. With regard to the number of parathyroid glands, 87 per cent of patients have four, 6 per cent have fewer, and 6 per cent have five or more glands. Ninety per cent of glands are in the neck.

The majority of patients with primary hyperparathyroidism will manifest single parathyroid adenomas upon histological examination. Some 80 to 85 per cent of patients present with a single adenoma, usually chief cell histology, that varies in size between 100 mg and 40 g. Patients with large parathyroid adenomas represent a distinct abnormal entity. These patients have greater degrees of calcium elevation and are at greater risk for postoperative hypocalcaemia. Large excised glands also need to be carefully examined for the presence of mitotic figures and vascular or capsular invasion to exclude the possibility of parathyroid carcinoma (3 per cent of all cases). In 10 to 15 per cent of patients, depending on referral patterns, hyperparathyroidism is due to parathyroid hyperplasia. Microscopically, hyperplastic glands are also of the chief cell type. As a single gland, it cannot be distinguished from a parathyroid adenoma. The distinction between adenoma and hyperplasia is made upon the biopsy of an uninvolved gland. In the case of an adenoma, the uninvolved gland is histologically normal, with an increase in the fat content of both the chief and stromal cells. In the case of hyperplasia, an unsuspected gland may be smaller, but shows histological evidence of hypercellularity.

Controversy exists as to whether unilateral or bilateral neck explorations are indicated. Some argue that the findings of a unilateral adenoma and an atrophic gland on the ipsilateral side are sufficient evidence for the diagnosis of parathyroid adenoma. They cite an extremely low incidence of bilateral adenomas (< 1 per cent). Nevertheless, most experienced surgeons advocate selective bilateral neck exploration with identification of all four parathyroid glands and removal of only one adenoma and normal gland if only one abnormal gland is identified. Proponents of this approach cite a 10 per cent incidence of multiple adenomas or asymmetric hyperplasia. This approach is necessary for patients with suspected hyperplasia. In these patients, a subtotal resection of the smallest gland followed by removal of all remaining abnormal glands is recommended.

POSTOPERATIVE OUTCOME

As with many surgical procedures, the outcome and complications of parathyroidectomy vary with surgical expertise. In a review of primary hyperparathyroidism persistent hypercalcaemia was found in 6 per cent of cases in specialized centres compared with 15 per cent of cases in hospitals treating fewer than 10 cases per year. Likewise, the incidence of permanent hypoparathyroidism varied between 4 and 14 per cent. Additional complications include recurrent laryngeal nerve palsy (<0.1 per cent), mortality (<0.1 per cent), and exceedingly rare case reports of postoperative pancreatitis and obstructive ureteropathy. Captain Charles Martell, the first North American patient successfully surgically treated for hyperparathyroidism, died in 1932 of obstructive ureteropathy after surgery. Management of non-metabolic outcome to parathyroid surgery is discussed in Section 11.2.2.

METABOLIC RESPONSES TO PARATHYROIDECTOMY

Calcium homeostasis and PTH function after parathyroidectomy

In patients undergoing curative parathyroidectomy, an abrupt challenge to calcium homeostasis can be expected. Autonomously functioning hyperplastic or adenomatous parathyroid glands with an elevated calcium set-point suppress the normal parathyroid tissue by constant exposure to hypercalcaemia. This suppression is manifested by increases in fat content both of the chief cells and the stromal tissue of the normal, suppressed parathyroid glands. After the removal of the affected parathyroid glands, the normal glands must respond to the hypocalcaemic stimulus, and a lag phase is frequently seen for the recovery of the normal glands.

After successful parathyroidectomy, a rapid correction of most metabolic complications of primary hyperparathyroidism will be observed. The serum calcium begins to fall 4 to 12 h after surgery and its nadir is usually seen 48 to 72 h postoperatively. Immediately after parathyroidectomy, the urinary calcium level rises transiently until serum calcium falls; subsequently, urinary calcium becomes undetectable. Most patients report symptoms of hypocalcaemia 1 to 2 days before the nadir in serum calcium. These symptoms are usually circumoral or acral paraesthesiae. Total serum calcium falls 2 to 3 mg/dl within the first 24 to 48 h after successful surgery. This period is due to relative 'functional' hypoparathyroidism, and rarely lasts more than 2 to 3 weeks.

Numerous studies underscore the important relationship between excessive parathyroid gland biopsy and the incidence of transient hypocalcaemia. In one series, 37 per cent of patients with minimal biopsies became hypocalcaemic on postoperative days 2 to 3, whereas 62 per cent of patients with extensive biopsies of bilateral parathyroid glands became hypocalcaemic. This relationship is likely to be the consequence of injury or ischaemia to the remaining suppressed parathyroid glands, occurrences that delay their response to curative parathyroid surgery.

In addition to alterations in serum calcium, postoperative metabolic acidosis, declines in serum uric acid levels, and hypomagnesaemia have all been described during the immediate postoperative period. These changes are ascribed to either the lack of PTH hormone on the kidney, or the consequences of bone accretion (magnesium is deposited in the bone).

Since PTH acts via adenylate cyclase, detection of changes in nephrogenous cyclic AMP (NcAMP) have been used as indices for monitoring changes in PTH secretion after successful surgery for hyperparathyroidism. NcAMP falls to 50 per cent of preoperative values within 30 to 90 min after surgery, and is consistent with the estimated half-life of intact PTH in plasma. With the advent of the highly sensitive two-site PTH (1–84) immunoradiometric assays more detailed investigation of PTH dynamics in the postsurgical patient is now being undertaken. This assay can differentiate between normal and suppressed PTH values.

Evidence is accumulating that suppressed intact PTH (1–84) values during the early postoperative period are indicative of successful parathyroidectomy, and may be predictive of long-term cure in patients with intact parathyroid glands that remain after surgery. Some investigators have noted that extensive gland manipulation or biopsy can falsely elevate the intact PTH (1–84) values; caution should be used in interpreting detectable levels in the immediate postoperative period in those patients undergoing extensive neck explorations and gland biopsies.

How long the suppressed glands require to recover from long-term hypercalcaemic suppression has been addressed using the highly sensitive two-site PTH immunoradiometric assays. Functional hypoparathyroidism appears to be relatively brief, with demonstration of *de novo* PTH secretion by atrophic glands in more than 50 per cent of patients 20 h postoperatively, and 85 per cent of patients by 30 h postoperatively.

POSTOPERATIVE HYPOCALCAEMIA: PATHOPHYSIOLOGICAL MECHANISMS

We routinely measure total and ionized calcium, albumin, and magnesium daily or twice daily depending on the degree of suspicion for the development of hypocalcaemia. Severe postoperative hypocalcaemia, defined as hypocalcaemia on postoperative day 3 or later requiring supplemental calcium to prevent tetanic symptoms, occurs in 10 to 20 per cent of patients in reported series. The differential diagnosis is presented in Table 1, and includes functional hypoparathyroidism from suppressed or ischaemic parathyroid glands, hypomagnesaemia impairing PTH release, true hypoparathyroidism from surgical removal of all parathyroid tissue, or the 'hungry bones syndrome' due to remineralization of the skeleton.

Table 1 Differential diagnosis of hypocalcaemia after parathyroidectomy

1. Functional hypoparathyroidism
   (a) Suppressed parathyroid glands
   (b) Ischaemia/biopsy
   (c) Hypomagnesaemia
2. Permanent hypoparathyroidism (surgical)
3. 'Hungry bones' syndrome (skeletal remineralization)

Evaluation of the hypocalcaemic patient includes elicitation of physical signs as well as biochemical evaluation of serum. Classic physical signs of hypocalcaemia include the Chvostek's sign, the spasm of facial muscles innervated by the VIIth cranial nerve, produced by tapping the nerve as it exits the base of the skull. A Chvostek's sign can be non-specific, since 15 per cent of normal patients can have a positive test, so this sign is useful only if it was tested for and was not elicited preoperatively. Trousseau's sign is carpal spasm produced by elevating a blood pressure cuff above systolic blood pressure for 3 min. More serious forms of neuro-

Table 2 Laboratory values in differential diagnosis of hypocalcaemia†

	Ionized calcium	Phosphate	Magnesium	iPTH
Functional hypoparathyroidism	Low	Normal value, high	Normal, low[1]	Low[2], normal
Surgical hypoparathyroidism	Low	High	Normal value	Undetectable[3]
'Hungry bone' syndrome	Low	Low	Low	Low[4]

1. In patients with functional hypoparathyroidism due to hypomagnesaemia.
2. PTH hormone secretion is detectable within 20 h following unilateral adenomectomy, and seen in the majority of patients after 30 h.
3. Values of below 1 pg/l are consistently observed for patients with permanent hyperparathyroidism after postoperative day 3.
4. In the author's experience patients with 'hungry bone' syndrome have detectable levels of PTH (1–84); however, larger series are necessary before this criterion can be applied to patient care.

† Normal values: ionized calcium (1.14–1.30 mmol/l), inorganic phosphorus 2.6–4.5 mg/dl (0.84–1.45 mmol/l), magnesium 1.5–2.0 mEq/l (0.8–1.0 mmol/l), and intact PTH (1–84) 10–65 pg/ml.

muscular irritability include alterations in QT interval on electrocardiogram with ventricular irritability as well as seizures. These physical signs do not aid in the differential diagnosis of the different causes of hypocalcaemia, but do dictate the need and the urgency for therapeutic intervention.

Serum studies useful in the evaluation of the hypocalcaemic patient include total and ionized calcium, albumin (to assess the relative degree of protein binding), serum phosphate, magnesium, and when indicated PTH (1–84) by the two-site immunoradiometric assay. Anticipated laboratory values for the major causes of postoperative hypocalcaemia are tabulated in Table 2. Of the laboratory parameters, the most useful for separating functional from surgical hypoparathyroidism is the intact PTH immunoradiometric assay. By 3 days postoperatively all patients with functional hypoparathyroidism in our series had detectable PTH values. In contrast, patients with permanent surgical hypoparathyroidism had PTH values that were undetectable (<1 pg/ml). Serum phosphate measurements are the most reliable in distinguishing patients with hypoparathyroidism from those with ongoing remineralization of the skeleton ('hungry bones' syndrome). Because of the phosphaturic effect of PTH, patients with hypoparathyroidism tend to have normal–high serum phosphorus values. In the 'hungry bones' syndrome, however, extensive remineralization of the skeleton drives calcium, phosphate, and magnesium into healing bone, and patients become hypocalcaemic, hypophosphataemic, and hypomagnesaemic. In a recent retrospective study of unselected patients undergoing parathyroidectomy at a tertiary centre, patients manifesting hypocalcaemia and hypophosphataemia after curative parathyroid surgery constituted 12 per cent of the study population, indicating that although radiographically evident bone disease was not a prominent feature, the physiology of skeletal remineralization can still be seen. This is particularly evident after total parathyroidectomy, with or without implantation of part of a gland in the forearm, for secondary hypoparathyroidism in patients with chronic renal failure.

MANAGEMENT OF POSTOPERATIVE HYPOCALCAEMIA

The symptoms in most patients can be managed with institution of oral calcium carbonate 2 to 4 g/day (260 mg elemental calcium per 650 mg tablet) or a high calcium diet. A high calcium diet, also high in phosphate, is reserved for those patients with normal serum phosphate values. Functional postoperative hypoparathyroidism is transient, lasting from 3 days postoperatively to between 2 and 3 weeks postoperatively. The duration, in part, may depend on the extent of biopsy or manipulation of normal parathyroid glands. Patients undergoing bilateral neck exploration or reoperative procedures are at greater risk for permanent postoperative hyperparathyroidism, and these patients should be monitored accordingly. The incidence of permanent postoperative hypoparathyroidism varies from 0.3 to 14 per cent depending on the surgical expertise.

Severe hypocalcaemia, with symptoms or signs of tetany, needs to be more vigorously managed. Patients with severe hypocalcaemia (total calcium <6.5 mg/dl (<1.6 mmol/l)) demonstrating signs of neuromuscular or cardiac irritability (tetany) or those unable to take calcium by mouth may need to be treated with parenteral calcium. The goal of parenteral treatment of symptomatic hypocalcaemia is to provide 200 to 300 mg of elemental calcium acutely. The preferred treatment is two to three ampoules of 10 per cent calcium gluconate (93 mg elemental calcium/ampoule), while monitoring ECG and respiration, until tetany is controlled. Calcium gluconate is preferred to calcium chloride because of the lower incidence of thrombophlebitis with use of calcium gluconate. This can be followed by an infusion of 15 mg/kg elemental calcium over 4 to 6 h. Following acute parenteral therapy, oral therapy must be initiated (2–4 g/day elemental calcium). Vitamin D may also be necessary to increase oral absorption of calcium in patients with hypoparathyroidism or 'hungry bones' syndrome. In chronic renal failure patients, vitamin D therapy is standard practice and this should be continued after total parathyroidectomy.

In the presence of severe hypomagnesaemia and normal renal function, magnesium sulphate (1–2 g as 10 per cent solution) can be administered over a 6-min period. Because the normal magnesium concentration is necessary for normal PTH release, hypomagnesaemia should be considered and treated in the management of functional hypoparathyroidism. Moreover, because magnesium is deposited in the skeleton in the 'hungry bones' syndrome, magnesium replacement may also be necessary in this condition.

PREOPERATIVE RISK STRATIFICATION FOR COMPLICATIONS OF PARATHYROIDECTOMY

Several studies have implicated the extent of surgical biopsy as an important determinant of postoperative hypocalcaemia. Twice as many patients are likely to develop hypocalcaemia with bilateral neck exploration and multiple gland biopsy compared with matched controls undergoing unilateral neck exploration. Some 60 to 70 per cent of patients undergoing second operations because initial surgery failed are likely to develop permanent hypoparathyroidism. Importantly, the size of the parathyroid adenoma, as assessed by ultrasound volume or by the weight of excised parathyroid gland, is a strong indicator of greater degrees of preoperative hypercalcaemia and subsequent postoperative hypocalcaemia. In one study, this parameter was closely linked to postoperative hypocalcaemia and hypophosphataemia ('hungry bones' syndrome). Three additional preoperative variables of independent predictive value for the development of hungry bones syndrome identified by multivariate analysis were, in addition to the volume of adenoma (determined at surgery), the preoperative blood urea nitrogen, alkaline phosphatase, and patient's age. These patients had a significantly longer hospital stay than similarly treated counterparts. These data need to be verified on a prospective population, but raise the possibility that patients at risk for development of postoperative hypocalcaemia can be identified by routine preoperative screening. Identified patients could then be monitored more closely and treated more aggressively.

REVERSAL OF END-ORGAN COMPLICATIONS OF PRIMARY HYPERPARATHYROIDISM

Parathyroidectomy is expected to normalize serum calcium in uncomplicated patients undergoing initial neck exploration for parathyroid adenoma in 90 to 95 per cent of patients in active surgical centres. Patients with neuromuscular symptoms can be expected to improve after surgery. Evidence of type II muscle fibre atrophy was documented in a series of patients with proximal muscle weakness and primary hyperparathyroidism. After parathyroidectomy, their muscle strength improved. The incidence of recurrent nephrolithiasis is decreased, and some reports indicate an improvement in renal function in patients with declining glomerular filtration rate. The effect of parathyroidectomy on psychiatric symptoms of mental dullness and confusion is seen within days of surgery. However, anxiety, depression, and psychotic syndromes generally are not improved by surgical treatment.

Classic hyperparathyroid bone disease (osteitis fibrosa cystica) will heal rapidly and is one unambiguous indication for parathyroidectomy. Osteoporosis is used as a criteria for surgery; however, the response to surgery appears to be transient. Quantitative CT of vertebral density in one series demonstrated a non-sustained increase in bone density of 13 per cent after 4 months. In a separate study dual photon absorptiometry demonstrated a 10 per cent increase in vertebral or forearm bone density 3 months after successful surgery; there was no further increase in bone mass with time, however. Although more studies will be needed to clarify this issue, the effect of parathyroidectomy on the reversal of osteoporosis appears to be modest.

In summary, operative intervention in the patient with primary hyperparathyroidism can produce excellent results. With the appropriate preoperative evaluation to identify patients at risk for metabolic complications, and in experienced surgical hands, long-term cure rates of 95 per cent can be expected in patients whose hyperthyroidism is due to a parathyroid adenoma.

FURTHER READING

Abugassa S, Nordenstrom J, Eriksson S, Mollerstrom G, Alveryd A. Skeletal mineralization after surgery for primary and secondary hyperparathyroidism. *Surgery* 1990; **107**: 128–33.

Agus ZS, Wasserstein A, Goldfarb S. Disorders of calcium and magnesium homeostasis. *Am J Med* 1982; **72**: 473–85.

Anderberg BO, Gillquist J, Larsson L, Lundstrom B. Complications to subtotal parathyroidectomy. *Acta Chir Scand* 1981; **147**: 109–13.

Arnold A, Staunton CE, Kim HG, Gaz RD, Kronenberg HM. Monoclonality and abnormal parathyroid hormone genes in parathyroid adenomas. *N Engl J Med* 1988; **318**: 658–62.

Brasier AR, Nussbaum SR. Hungry bone syndrome: clinical and biochemical predictors of its occurrence after parathyroid surgery. *Am J Med* 1988; **84**: 654–60.

Brasier AR, Wang CA, Nussbaum SR. Recovery of parathyroid hormone secretion after parathyroid adenomectomy. *J Clin Endocrin Metab* 1988; **66**: 495–500.

Clark OH, Duh Q-Y. Primary hyperparathyroidism: a surgical perspective. *Endocrinol Metab Clin N Am* 1989; **18**: 701–14.

Heath DA. Primary hyperparathyroidism: clinical presentation and factors influencing clinical management. *Endocrinol Metab Clin N Am* 1989; **18**: 631–46.

Heath M III, Hodgsen SF, Kennedy MA. Primary hyperparathyroidism: incidence, morbidity and potential economic impact in a community. *N Engl J Med* 1980; **302**: 189–93.

Irvin SL 3rd, Dembrow VD, Prudhomme DL. Operative monitoring of parathyroid gland hyperfunction. *Am J Surg* 1991; **162**: 299–302.

Kanis JA. Disorders of calcium metabolism. In: Weatherall DJ, Ledingham JGG, Warrell DA, eds. *Oxford Textbook in Medicine*. Oxford: University Press, 1987: 10.51–10.69.

Kaplan EL., Bartlett S, Sugimoto J, Fredland A. Relation of postoperative hypocalcemia to operative techniques: deleterious effect of excessive use of parathyroid biopsy. *Surgery* 1982; **92**: 827–834.

Levin KE, Clark OH. Localization of parathyroid glands. *Ann Rev Med* 1988; **39**: 29–40.

Lloyd HM. Primary hyperparathyroidism: an analysis of the role of the parathyroid tumor. *Medicine* 1968; **47**: 53–71.

Netterville JL, Aly A, Ossoff RH. Evaluation and treatment of complications of thyroid and parathyroid surgery. *Otolaryngol Clin N Am* 1990; **23**: 529–52.

Nussbaum SR, Thompson AR, Hutcheson KA, Gaz RD, Wang CA. Intraoperative measurement of parathyroid hormone in the surgical management of hyperparathyroidism. *Surgery* 1988; **104**: 1121–7.

Nussbaum SR *et al.* Highly sensitive two-site immunoradiometric assay of parathyrin and its clinical utility in evaluating patients with hypercalcemia. *Clin Chem* 1987; **33**: 1364–7.

Scalzetti EM, Levinsohn EM, Numann P, Bassano DA. Vertebral mineralization after parathyroidectomy: measurement by quantitative CT. *Am J Roentgenol* 1988; **151**: 533–5.

Spiegel AM, *et al.* Intraoperative measurements of urinary cyclic AMP to guide surgery for primary hyperparathyroidism. *N Engl J Med* 1980; **303**: 1457–60.

Spiegel AM, *et al.* Urinary cAMP excretion during surgery: an index of successful parathyroidectomy in patients with primary hyperparathyroidism. *J Clin Endocrin Metab* 1978; **47**: 537–42.

Zamboni WA, Folse R. Adenoma weight: a predictor of transient hypocalcemia after parathyroidectomy. *Am J Surg* 1986; **152**: 611–15.

parenchymal cells and few lipocytes. Nodular hyperplasia is a feature strongly associated with the MEN syndrome.

Parathyroid carcinoma is the rarest cause of primary HPT (less than 3 per cent of cases) and its recognition depends more on the surgeon than on the pathologist since the diagnostic criteria are more clinical than histological. Typically a carcinoma is firm to hard, grey in colour, and adherent to adjacent tissues. The capsule of the gland eventually becomes invaded and metastases develop frequently in the local lymph nodes. Distant metastases in liver and bone are a late feature and indicate terminal disease.

(d) *Disturbance of physiology* This arises because of increases in both the circulating PTH and calcium. The production of PTH is said to have become 'autonomous' and fails to switch off as the plasma calcium rises. The hypercalcaemia causes the renal tubular absorption of calcium to be increased so that at any given filtered load more is lost in the urine and reflected in an increase in the 24-h urinary calcium. Bone turnover is also increased with reabsorption exceeding deposition, whilst more calcium is absorbed from the intestine because of stimulated calcitriol production in the kidneys.

Secondary hyperparathyroidism

(a) *Aetiology* This condition results from prolonged hypocalcaemia and is caused most frequently by chronic renal failure. Vitamin D deficiency and gluten-sensitive enteropathy are other provocative states.
(b) *Incidence* No precise figures are available but it is inevitable that patients with end-stage renal failure will develop secondary hyperparathyroidism unless prophylactic therapy with vitamin D analogues is given.
(c) *Pathology* Typically all four glands are enlarged and histologically they show the same features seen in hyperplasia due to primary HPT. The chief cells are the predominant cell type affected.
(d) *Disturbance of physiology* When the kidney starts to fail the reduction in glomerular filtration causes an increase in plasma phosphate. This in turn produces a reduction in the plasma ionized calcium to which the parathyroids respond by undergoing hyperplastic change.

Tertiary hyperparathyroidism

This condition identifies those patients with long-standing secondary HPT who develop the same sort of autonomous gland function described in primary HPT. The physiological sequelae are similar with hypercalcaemia coexisting with a raised PTH level. It is most frequently seen in patients on long-term dialysis for chronic renal failure and after renal transplantation. The glands are hyperplastic but may additionally produce adenomata, sometimes referred to as quarternary hyperparathyroidism.

Pseudohyperparathyroidism

This condition is mentioned because it gives rise to biochemical disturbances similar to those seen in primary HPT. Oat cell and squamous carcinoma of the lung, head, and neck, and carcinoma of the kidney and ovaries may all rarely produce parathyroid-like adenolate cyclase stimulating proteins. These interact with the PTH receptors and can mimic some of the effects of primary HPT.

CLINICAL FEATURES OF HYPERPARATHYROIDISM

The widespread use of multichannel autoanalysers for routine biochemistry screening has brought to light an increasing number of individuals with hypercalcaemia who on further investigation are shown to have HPT. Frequently the diagnosis is made so early that signs and symptoms have not had time to develop. Mildly symptomatic or asymptomatic patients identified in this way now account for more than 50 per cent of the total in most large series. In the 12 years prior to 1980, 54 per cent of the 200 patients coming to surgery in Oxford had originally presented with significant bone and renal disease. In the following decade a further 200 patients underwent surgery but the number of those with symptomatic bone and renal disease had fallen to 35 per cent. The time-honoured rhyme 'bones, stones, abdominal groans, and psychic moans' is still a useful prompt for the symptoms associated with HPT.

Bones

Disturbance of calcium metabolism causes vague bony aching and arthralgia especially in secondary HPT. It becomes acute and site specific if the weakened bone fractures. Very severe arthralgia is a feature of chondrocalcinosis (pseudogout) in which the surface of the articular cartilage becomes the site of metastatic calcification.

Stones

Long-standing severe hypercalcaemia may present with renal pain. The increased filtered load of calcium and the passage of alkaline urine leads to the formation of renal calculi. Less frequently nephrocalcinosis occurs with calcification of the renal parenchyma, i.e. outside the collecting system. The stones predispose to renal colic, urinary infection secondary to obstructive uropathy, and renal failure. Once established renal damage caused by HPT is irreversible and the stones tend to persist even after calcium homeostasis has been restored following successful surgery.

Abdominal groans

Mild abdominal pain is often due to large bowel colic related to the chronic constipation brought on by dehydration and hypercalcaemia. More severe epigastric pain arises in 5 to 10 per cent of patients with HPT due to peptic ulceration. This disorder may be causally related if the hypothesis is true that hypercalcaemia stimulates gastrin production and thereby increases basal gastric acid secretion. Certainly ulcer symptoms usually remit after successful parathyroid surgery and studies have shown that the gastric acid secretion returns to normal. There is a rare association in MEN type I patients with a Zollinger-Ellison type syndrome which probably represents an extreme gastrin response. Because surgical removal of the diseased parathyroid glands in such patients results in cure without the need for gastric surgery, the term pseudo Z-E syndrome has been proposed. The link between HPT and pancreatitis, both acute and chronic, is well described. It may be explained simply on the basis of metastatic calcification within the common bile duct causing acute pancreatitis (common channel theory) or throughout the pancreas in the chronic form. Alternatively it has been postulated that hypersecretion of glucagon by the α-cells of the inflamed pancreas causes hypoglycaemia which stimulates the parathyroids to become hyperplastic.

Psychic moans

Mental symptoms range from subtle mood change and behavioural disorder to marked organic psychosis and dementia. Loss of concentration, mild depression, and lassitude are frequent.

Hypercalcaemia *per se* induces anorexia, nausea, vomiting, and thirst, and is associated with polydipsia and polyuria. The most extreme form of hypercalcaemic syndrome is seen in acute hypercalcaemic crisis—a fulminating HPT state in which all the above symptoms are exaggerated. Unless this medical and surgical emergency is recognized and treated quickly the outcome can be fatal.

Physical signs

There are few signs associated with primary HPT but if the calcium is markedly elevated a parathyroid tumour in the neck may be palpable. Band keratopathy is occasionally visible on slit lamp examination of the cornea (Fig. 6). Proximal myopathy is a rare finding with related wasting and motor weakness. Diffuse osteitis fibrosa cystica first described by von Recklinghausen in 1891 with gross skeletal deformity, loss of height, etc., is unlikely ever to be seen again in developed countries due to earlier diagnosis. However focal swellings of bone, notably the lateral end of the clavicles due to the presence of 'brown tumours', are occasionally encountered (Fig. 7). In patients with secondary HPT soft tissue calcification especially in arteries, muscles, and subcutaneous tissues particularly around joints is common and scratch marks due to pruritus are frequent. The physical signs of tertiary HPT include all the foregoing, pruritus being even more severe with skin necrosis occasionally seen due to subcutaneous calcium deposition.

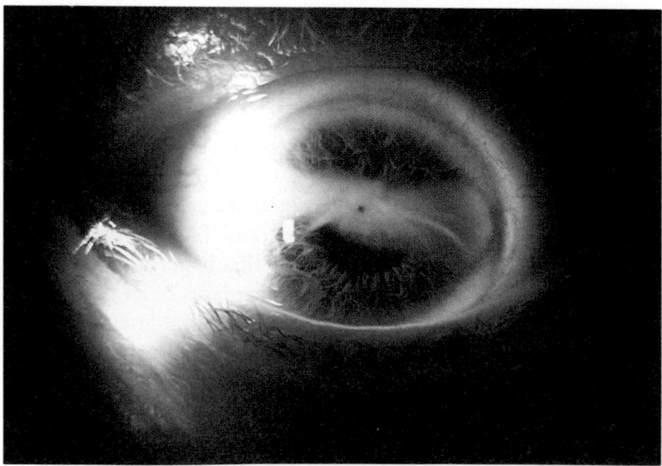

Fig. 6 Corneal calcification/band keratopathy in hyperparathyroidism.

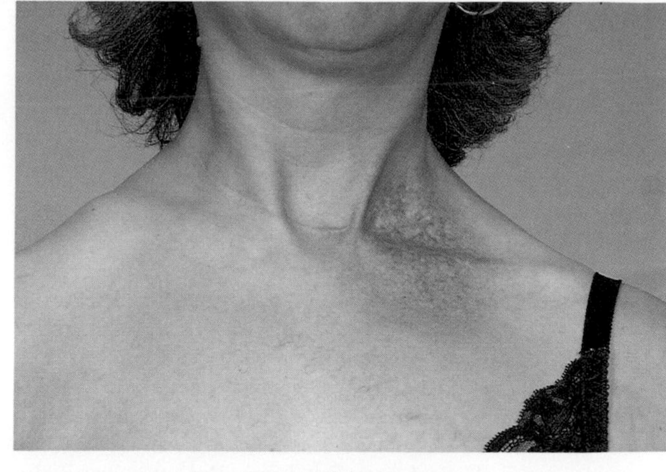

(a)

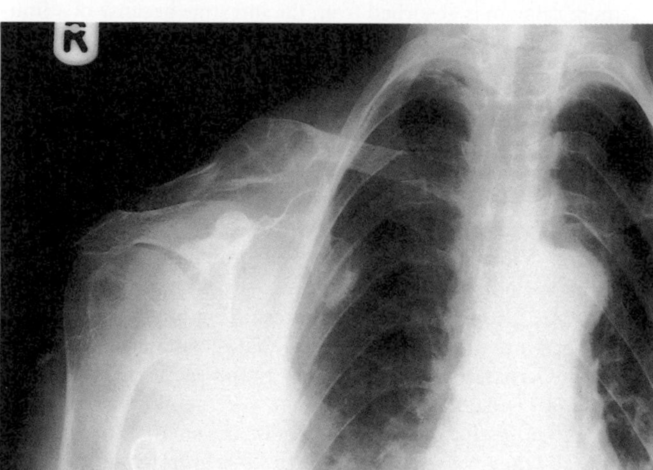

(b)

Fig. 7(a) and (b) Swelling of the clavicle due to a 'brown' tumour. Note previous radiotherapy to the neck which may have induced hyperparathyroidism.

INVESTIGATION OF HYPERPARATHYROIDISM

The single most important criterion for a diagnosis of primary HPT is a persistent and significant increase in the plasma calcium concentration. However primary HPT accounts for only approximately 20 per cent of all symptomatic patients with hypercalcaemia and a careful history and physical examination is necessary to exclude other causes, notably metastatic bone disease (primary breast, lung, etc.) and multiple myeloma. A more comprehensive list of causes of hypercalcaemia is summarized in Table 2. Distinguishing primary HPT from these other causes rests on three key biochemical tests.

1. *Plasma calcium (normal range 2.35–2.55 mmol/l)* A minimum of three estimations should be performed and where hypercalcaemia is modest it becomes more important to draw an uncuffed venous sample when the patient has been fasted. Normocalcaemic HPT is an accepted entity and tends to affect patients with recurrent renal stone formation. This small group

Table 2 Causes of hypercalcaemia (some conditions affect the plasma calcium by several mechanisms)

1. Raised PTH concentration in the peripheral circulation
   - Primary HPT—includes rare parathyroid carcinoma and MEN syndromes
   - Tertiary HPT
2. Production of PTH-like peptides
   - Renal cell carcinoma
   - Oat and squamous cell carcinoma of the lung
3. Excessive calcium absorption
   - Milk alkali syndrome
   - Hypervitaminosis D
   - Sarcoidosis (vitamin D hypersensitivity)—rarely in other granulomatous diseases, tuberculosis, and berylliosis
   - (Drugs)
4. Excessive bone resorption
   - Osteolytic metastases
     - Oat cell carcinoma of the lung
     - Carcinoma of the breast
   - Reticuloses
     - Malignant lymphoma
     - Multiple myelomatosis
   - Immobilization
     - Especially in growing children and those with Paget's disease
   - Thyrotoxicosis
5. Reduced urinary excretion of calcium
   - Benzothiazide drugs
   - Lithium
   - Familial hypocalciuric hypercalcaemia
6. Other rare causes—mechanism uncertain
   - Phaeochromocytoma
   - Vitamin A intoxication
   - Adrenal insufficiency

exhibits the rare biochemical profile of a calcium level usually towards the top of the normal range but with an inappropriately high PTH level.

2. *Plasma albumin (normal range 35–50 g/l)* This should be estimated at the same time and under the same circumstances as for plasma calcium. Albumin is the main calcium binding protein in the plasma so alternations in the albumin level have to be taken into account and the plasma calcium corrected appropriately. A simple and reliable method is addition of 0.02 mmol/l of calcium for every 1g/l of albumin below 40 and subtraction of 0.02 mmol/l for every 1 g/l above.
3. *Immunoradiometric intact PTH assay (IRMA) (normal range 0.9–5.4 pmol/l)* This should be estimated at the same time as the two foregoing tests. Two site IRMA assays measuring the level of the intact PTH molecule in the plasma have only recently become standardized and more readily available in kit form. In the past radioimmunoassays using antisera raised either against the mid, carboxy, or the *N*-terminal fragments of the PTH molecule could erroneously measure similar PTH polypeptides produced by some occult malignancies. Squamous and oat cell carcinoma of the lung and renal cell carcinoma as mentioned earlier are notable examples of tumours with this ability to elaborate PTH-like provoking hypercalcaemia in the absence of bony metastases.

Complementary tests that support the diagnosis and identify patients who have associated deleterious effects of HPT are as follows.

1. *Plasma phosphate (normal range 0.8–1.45 mol/l)* As the tubular reabsorption of calcium increases, that for phosphate decreases with more phosphate lost in the urine relative to calcium. The plasma level falls, notably in patients with advanced disease. Conversely, elevated plasma phosphate in the presence of hypercalcaemia and normal renal function suggest bony metastases or vitamin D intoxication.
2. *Plasma creatinine (normal range 70–150 mmol/l)* This is a useful indicator of renal function and if clearance falls significantly in a patient with HPT (> 30 per cent) in an otherwise asymptomatic patient, it signals renal damage and the need for surgical intervention.
3. *Alkaline phosphatase (normal range 80–250 i.u./l)* This is a useful indicator of bone disease; if in the normal range significant skeletal involvement is ruled out and there is no need for extensive radiological investigations of the skeleton.
4. *Plasma magnesium (normal range 0.75–1.05 mmol/l)* Hypomagnesaemia has been reported in up to 15 per cent of patients with primary HPT and may need to be corrected especially after the patient has been operated upon (see Section 11.2.1).
5. *Urinary calcium (normal range 2.5–7.5 mmol/l per 24 h)* An increase in the 24-h urinary calcium supports the diagnosis of HPT but a markedly elevated urinary calcium above 9 mmol/l characterizes non-PTH mediated hypercalcaemia. Perhaps the most important value of this test is to identify the rare patient with familial hypocalciuric hypercalcaemia. This condition frequently presents at a young age with symptoms of hypercalcaemia but the 24-h urinary calcium is less than 2.5 mmol/l and the patient has no parathyroid pathology. A relative who has undergone a failed neck exploration should alert one to the strong possibility of this condition.

The foregoing biochemical tests diagnose and quantify primary HPT in 95 per cent of suspected cases but the following tests are sometimes required to reinforce the diagnosis when the data are marginal or conflicting.

1. *Renal tubular absorption of phosphate (normal range 0.8—1.35)* This is a sophisticated method of identifying the effect of excessive PTH on the renal tubular absorption of phosphate. Simultaneous measurements of urinary phosphate, plasma phosphate, plasma creatinine, and urinary creatinine enable the relationship between filtered load and renal excretion of phosphate, i.e. phosphate clearance to be compared with creatinine clearance. It is expressed as a ratio, referring to a standard nomogram. In primary HPT the ratio is below 0.8.
2. *Urinary cyclical adenosine monophosphate (normal range < 2.5 nmol/100 ml of glomerular filtrate)* Raised levels have been claimed in nearly 90 per cent of patients with primary HPT in some series. False-positive and false-negative results reported by others limit the usefulness of the test.
3. *Hydrocortisone suppression/Dent test* This test has largely been rendered obsolete since the introduction of IRMA measurement of the intact PTH molecule. Administering high doses of hydrocortisone (40 mg three times a day for 10 days) does not usually lower the hypercalcaemia produced by primary HPT but if the corrected plasma calcium falls on day 4, 7, and 10 into the normal range or more than 0.25 mmol/l, the hypercalcaemia is likely to be due to causes other than primary HPT.

Radiological findings are rarely in themselves diagnostic of HPT and more usually complement the biochemical data. They may reinforce the need to offer surgery. The most frequent radiographic changes seen in both primary and secondary HPT are those affecting the skeleton.

1. *Bony radiographic changes* The overall picture is that of bone density loss (osteopenia) and subperiosteal reabsorption of bone. These are seen especially in the middle phalanges of the hand on the radial side together with loss of the terminal phalangeal tufts (Fig. 8). Subperiosteal absorption is seen in many other bones especially the lateral ends of clavicles, upper tibia, pubic symphysis, and sacroiliac joints. Localized areas of osteoclastic bone resorption with marrow fibrosis are seen in advanced bone disease. In the most severe form bone cysts and 'brown' tumours consisting of massive aggregations of osteoclasts (oestoclastoma) together make up osteitis fibrosa cystica (von Recklinghausen's disease) which as remarked earlier is now largely a medical curiosity. Generalized bone loss at a variety of sites has attracted some colourful descriptive nomenclature such as Rugger jersey spine (Fig. 9) and pepper-pot skull (Fig. 10), all of which aptly describe the osteoporosis and small osteolytic lesions. Absorption of the lamina dura around the teeth is reported but is an unconvincing radiological sign.

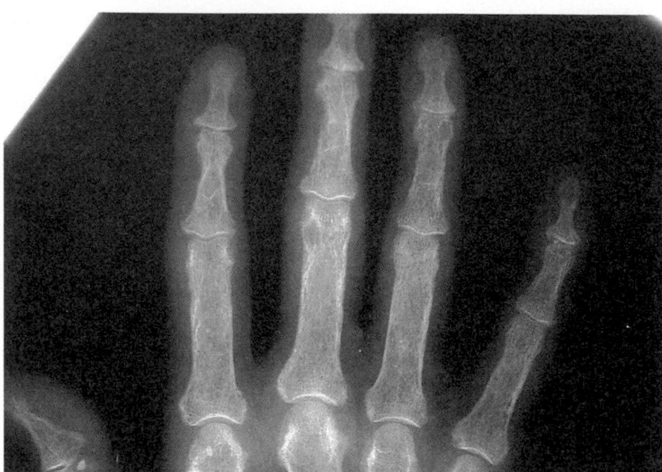

Fig. 8 Radiograph of the hand showing subperiosteal absorption of bone and loss of terminal phalangeal tufts.

2. *Renal radiographic changes* Discrete renal stones or diffuse calcification throughout the renal parenchyma (nephrocalcinosis) may be found and should be looked for on plain abdominal radiographs in patients with HPT even in the absence of symptoms. Sometimes the findings are unexpectedly dramatic (Fig. 11). An intravenous urogram may be indicated in the assessment of upper tract obstruction and overall renal function.
3. *Metastatic calcification* Mention has been made of the calcification which may be felt or seen radiologically in the skin and around blood vessels and joints. This phenomenon is readily confirmed on radiography of the relevant part.

LOCALIZATION OF PARATHYROID TUMOURS

Opinion is divided about the need to attempt localization of parathyroid tumours before the neck is explored surgically for the first time. In that situation an experienced surgeon can identify the

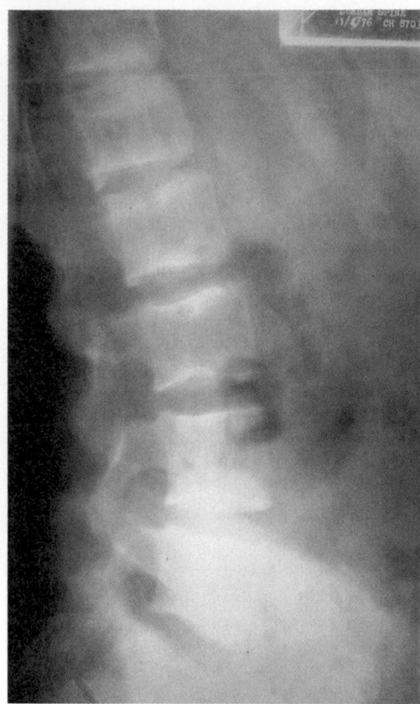

Fig. 9 Radiograph of 'rugger-jersey' spine.

pathology without any assistance in approximately 90 per cent of patients. None of the localization procedures to be described approach such a degree of accuracy and some are no better than 50 per cent accurate. Unfortunately localization techniques are least helpful when most needed, i.e. when the tumour is small (< 1 cm in diameter, < 100 mg in weight), ectopic (close to the heart and great vessels), or when the patient has a bulky neck due to obesity or coexistent thyroid enlargement. In view of the time and cost involved in such studies they are hard to justify except for patients who have had a previous unsuccessful neck exploration. The following localizing procedures are of proven value.

Selective venous sampling with PTH assay

This technique is the single most reliable method. It is based on the measurement of PTH concentration in samples obtained from

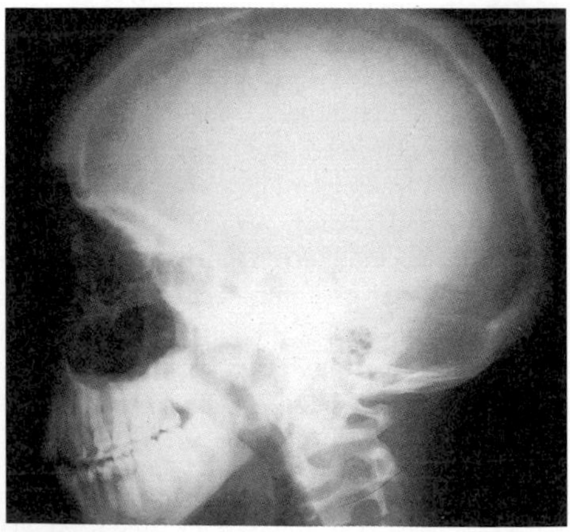

Fig. 10 Radiograph of 'pepper-pot' skull.

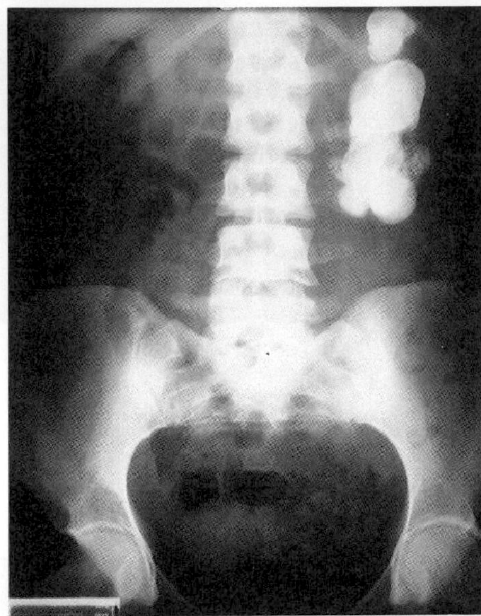

Fig. 11 Plain radiograph showing massive nephrolithiasis secondary to hyperparathyroidism.

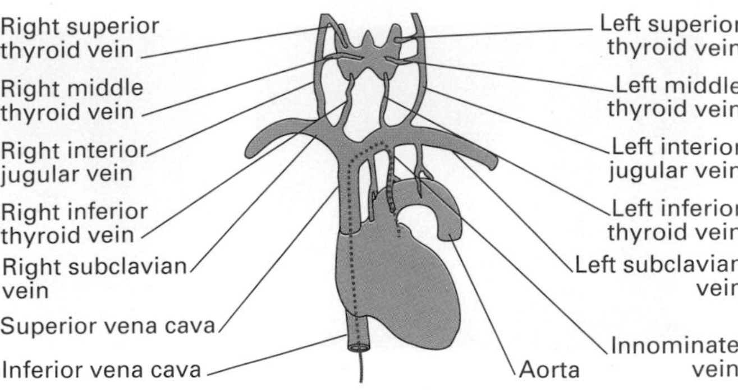

Sampling catheter threaded up via right femoral vein to anterior mediastinal vein just below aortic arch

Fig. 12 'Map' obtained by selective venography and hyperparathyroidism sampling showing site of adenoma under aortic arch.

PTH LEVEL INTACT ASSAY (pmol/l)

Sample no.	Level
1	17
2	400
3	18
4	20
5	20
6	21
7	16
8	1500
9	415
10	12
11	14
12	16
13	18
14	10

the superior vena cava, innominate vein, internal jugular, and the multiple small veins draining the thyroid and mediastinum. The sampling catheter is introduced via the femoral vein and each sample numbered with the site noted precisely. A map can then be constructed plotting the samples to look for the vein(s) draining the source of highest PTH concentration on radioimmuno assay (Fig. 12). Although good at lateralization in single gland disease (levels twice normal to that found in the background peripheral circulation being diagnostic) it cannot distinguish between an adenoma in the neck or one that has descended into the mediastinum leaving its venous drainage behind. Raised PTH concentration in all the thyroid veins suggest multigland hyperplasia. The drawback to this technique is that it is time consuming, expensive, and highly operator dependent.

Thallium/technetium subtraction scanning

A double tracer scintigram is performed using technetium–99m as sodium pertechnetate for imaging the thyroid and then thallium-201 (as thallous chloride) for imaging the thyroid and parathyroid glands simultaneously. A gamma-camera with on-line computer facilities substracts the pertechnetate image from the scatter corrected thallium image. Abnormal parathyroid tissue may then be demonstrated very convincingly (Fig. 13). However, the success rates reported from various centres have varied widely. False-positive results may be produced by thyroid adenomas and abnormal lymph nodes. False-negative results arise in cases of parathyroid hyperplasia and tumours close to the heart and great vessels which are lost in the normal high concentration of isotope in the central mediastinum.

Ultrasound

This technique has the merit of being quick and inexpensive but cannot scan behind the sternum and is confined to identification of parathyroids which may or may not be in the neck. It lacks the resolution to pick up small tumours (< 0.5 cm) but can raise suspicion with intrathyroidal tumours, those in the carotid sheath, and those between the trachea and oesophagus.

Computerized tomography (CT) and nuclear magnetic resonance imaging (MRI)

There is no consensus on which of these imaging techniques is best, but used in conjunction with selective venous sampling one or other may improve localization for the difficult reoperative case (Fig. 14).

INDICATIONS FOR SURGERY

Asymptomatic primary hyperparathyroidism

This is one of the controversial areas of HPT management and opinion is divided. Unfortunately only limited information is available about the natural history of primary HPT and although 20 per cent of asymptomatic patients in Purnell's series reported

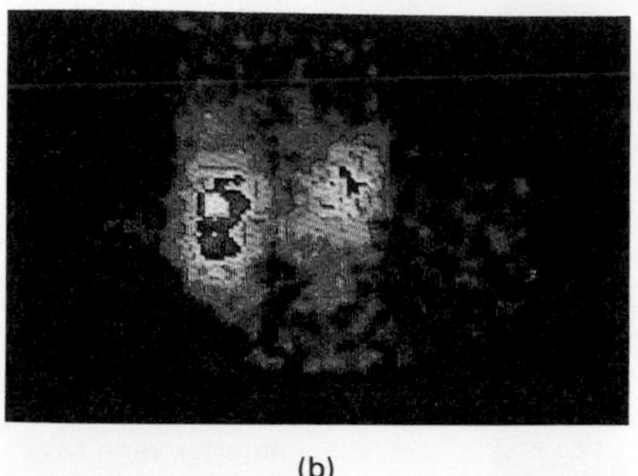
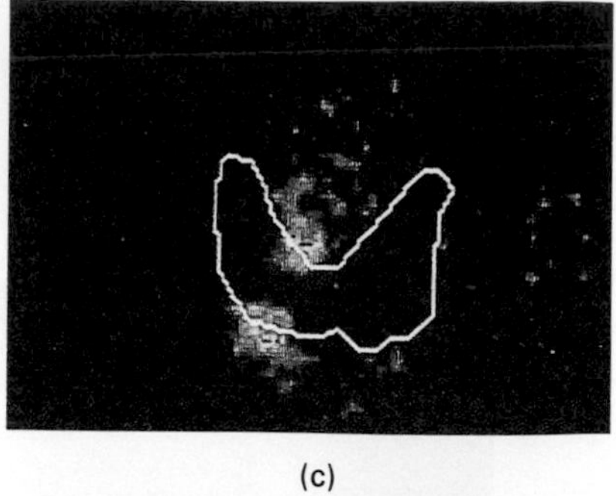

(a) (b) (c)

Fig. 13 (a) A technetium scan. (b) A thallium scan. (c) Subtracted image showing parathyroid adenoma.

from the Mayo Clinic came to surgery over a 10-year follow-up period, not all were operated upon because of the adverse effects of the disease. Over 50 per cent, indeed, showed no deterioration over 5 years. The longer-term effects on renal function, bone density, hypertension, and survival itself remain unclear. Meanwhile asymptomatic patients are being diagnosed with increasing frequency, as mentioned before, and in the absence of prospective trials randomizing patients to surgery or observation alone (attempted but failed in the United Kingdom) a policy has emerged in the United States and the United Kingdom that identifies those patients for whom surgery is most clearly indicated (Table 3).

Table 3 Indications for treatment in (mild) asymptomatic primary HPT

1. Persistent hypercalcaemia—corrected plasma calcium > 2.9 mmol/l
2. Osteopenia (bone densitometry) or alkaline phosphatase (bone origin) > 350 i.u./l
3. Renal calculi or nephrocalcinosis on abdominal radiograph
4. Renal impairment—creatinine clearance down 30 per cent
5. Patients under the age of 50 in whom long-term follow-up is impractical

Symptomatic primary hyperparathyroidism

There is good evidence that treatment is effective. The incidence of renal stones and infection decreases, osteitis fibrosa cysticica improves, subperiosteal resorption resolves, and patients with bone and joint pain are dramatically relieved. Where peptic ulceration is present it regresses and psychological disturbance may well resolve. Hypertension, which is found in 40 per cent of sufferers, is not in itself an indication for treatment and indeed deterioration after parathyroid surgery can occur. However, there should be no hesitation in advising surgery unless there are overwhelming medical contraindications. Alternative but less satisfactory options include embolization and CT or ultrasound guided laser or alcoholic destruction of an adenoma, if it can be confidently localized.

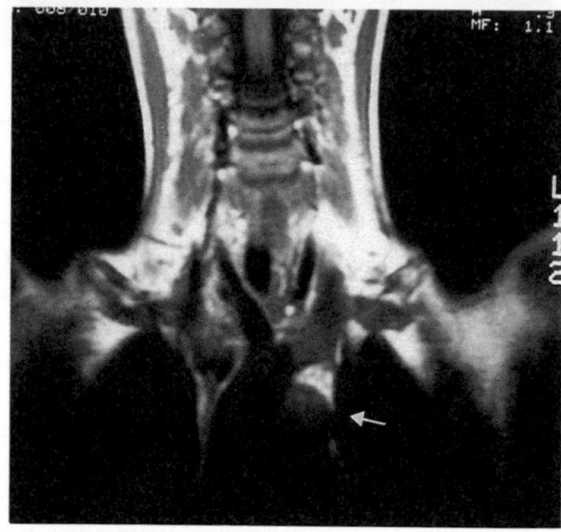

Fig. 14 MRI of the neck showing mediastinal adenoma.

Secondary and tertiary hyperparathyroidism

The majority of patients whose parathyroids undergo hyperplastic change in response to chronic renal failure, or rarely chronic intestinal malabsorption, can be controlled non-operatively. Correction of the hypocalcaemia with vitamin D which enhances calcium absorption from the gut, high calcium intake, restricted dietary phosphate, and the use of phosphate binding agents such as aluminium hydroxide are effective standard medical measures. Where the patient is undergoing dialysis secondary HPT can be controlled by increasing the level of calcium in the dialysate, having first lowered the serum phosphate to avoid ectopic calcification. Surgery is indicated when these measures fail and the patient has intractable bone pain, pruritus, or when soft tissue deposition has led to ischaemic skin necrosis and joint pain. Tertiary or autonomous HPT tends to be less responsive to the foregoing treatment and where the patient is not responding and is unlikely to receive a renal transplant, total parathyroidectomy is gaining momentum as the best treatment option. An alternative strategy is either to perform a subtotal parathyroidectomy and accept a high recurrence rate or to remove all the parathyroids in the neck and cryopreserve all but 60 mg of tissue which is then implanted into the forearm (see below for precise details of this technique). The hypercalcaemia seen following a successful renal transplant can usually be reversed by oral phosphate supplements and is slowly self-limiting.

OPERATIVE SURGERY ON THE PARATHYROIDS

Preoperative preparation

In general this is identical to the broad recommendations for thyroid patients (see Section 11.1) but the following special measures apply. Those with primary HPT and raised alkaline phosphatase and most renal bone disease sufferers (secondary) HPT should receive 2 to 4 μg per day of 1α-hydroxycholecalciferol 2 to 3 days prior to surgery. This practice helps to combat the profound hypocalcaemia and tetany that is unleashed when the parathyroid disease is removed and the 'hungry bones' then take up all available calcium. Grossly hypercalcaemic patients, some of whom may present in crisis with coma, delirium, anorexia, vomiting, and abdominal pain, pose a particularly difficult diagnostic challenge. Where rapid investigation excludes other possible causes of hypercalcaemia, fluid and electrolyte balance must be corrected as a matter of urgency. If large volumes of intravenous saline fail to reverse the dehydration oliguria and azotaemia provoked by the vomiting and polyuria, then a vigorous diuresis stimulated by frusemide or ethacrynic acid is appropriate. If renal function is severely compromised then peritoneal or haemodialysis may need to be considered.

Preoperative localization studies have already been discussed and are only advocated in those patients who have undergone a previous neck exploration. However, intraoperative localization is greatly assisted by giving the patient a vital dye, methylene blue, which selectively stains parathyroid tissue and makes recognition easier. It is given in a dose of 5 mg per kg body weight, diluted in 500 ml dextrose saline, infused over an hour prior to neck exposure. A larger dose up to 10 mg per kg body weight may be indicated in obese patients based on lean muscle mass but care is needed to avoid cardiotoxic effects. The intensity of staining is most impressive in four gland hyperplasia due to secondary HPT (Fig. 15) but many adenomas are equally recognizable appearing navy blue/purple depending on the degree of subcapsular haemorrhage (Fig. 16). Normal glands have a subtle pale greenish tinge.

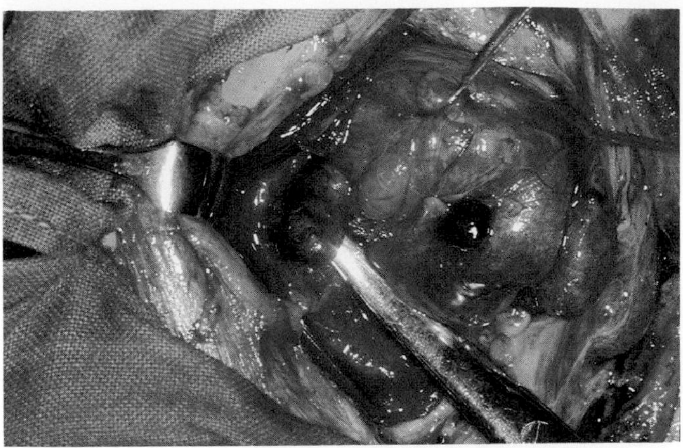

Fig. 15 Methylene blue staining of hyperplastic parathyroids.

Exposure and technique of exploration

This is identical to that described for the thyroid (Section 11.1) but is refined to meet the objective of identifying the four parathyroids and where they are all normal—a supernumerary abnormal gland. In meeting this objective there is no substitute for a patient systematic routine of neck exploration unconstrained by time. Meticulous haemostasis is crucial especially when the thyroid is freed from the strap muscles and the space is opened between the gland and carotid sheath. Where present the middle thyroid veins must be divided to allow full mobilization of the thyroid lobes forwards and medially. Finger retraction on a gauze swab is preferable to the use of grasping forceps which can traumatize the thyroid and lead to bleeding. If blood extravasates it stains the local tissues and makes identification of the parathyroids much more difficult. The inferior thyroid artery and recurrent laryngeal nerve are identified and gently retracted with linen or silastic vascular slings. These not only reduce the risk of damage to the nerve which may be adherent to the capsule of a parathyroid adenoma but also helps identification of the parathyroids which, as stated earlier, frequently derive their blood supply from one of the branches of this artery. Exposure of the superior parathyroid gland may require incision of the fascia binding the thyroid posteromedially to the trachea. If this is extended up to the level of the superior thyroid vessels the whole upper pole can be rolled forward. This manoeuvre also provides excellent access to ectopic superior parathyroid sites without the need to divide the superior thyroid pedicle. Some 90 to 95 per cent of upper parathyroids, however, are closely related to the inferior thyroid artery as it breaks up on the posterior surface of the gland,

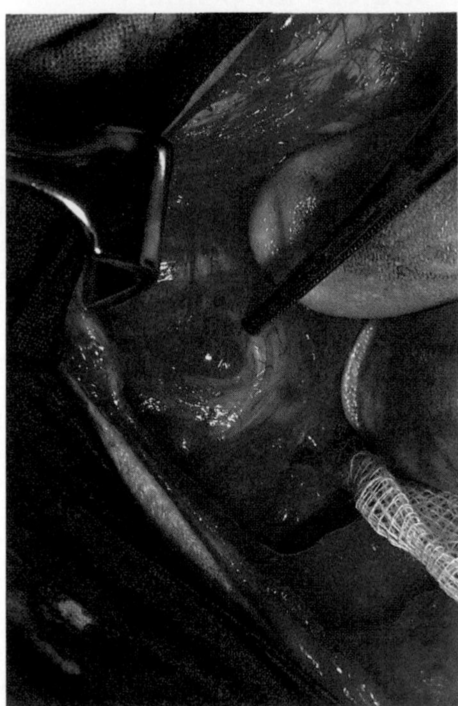

Fig. 16 Methylene blue staining of an adenoma.

i.e. within a 2-cm radius of this vessel. Not infrequently it is tucked round behind the upper branches (see Fig. 1). The inferior parathyroid glands are less constant in position but 80 per cent are still found within a 2-cm radius of the lower pole of the thyroid and many are quickly identified on the anterolateral aspect (see Fig. 3).

By this stage the experienced surgeon will usually have identified one or more normal parathyroids which narrows down the field of search for the missing pathological gland(s). Close inspection of the thyrothymic ligament which includes the inferior thyroid veins, lower polar fat, and the thymic horns as they extend into the anterior mediastinum will reveal the vast majority of these ectopic lower glands (20 per cent). If not, the next step is to search between the tracheo-oseophageal groove and behind the oesophagus. If a lower parathyroid is still elusive then it may lie within the thyroid (1–2 per cent of cases). Embryologically this is only possible if the parathyroid has become indented into a cleft in the thyroid so close inspection and palpation should detect a 'bulge' and opening up a cleft or incising the lower pole anterolaterally will display the missing gland without the need to do a blind thyroid lobectomy. Failing that, ectopic parathyroid may reside within the carotid sheath which should be opened right up to the carotid bifurcation near the angle of the jaw especially if a suspected abnormal upper parathyroid is still missing. A transcervical thymectomy is the last manoeuvre to be performed and may reveal the missing parathyroid when the thymus is sectioned. The entire routine described will have taken several hours but if unsuccessful (only 1—2 per cent of patients) a formal mediastinal exploration via a median sternotomy is not in the patient's best interest at this stage. When hypercalcaemia is severe it can always be moderated until urgent localization studies are performed. The basic requirement after sternotomy is to clear all remaining thymic and fatty tissue, notably around the innominate veins, great vessels, and within the aortopulmonary window.

Surgical strategy for primary hyperparathyroidism

In the majority of patients (80 per cent) a single adenoma is responsible for the condition and removing it will cure the patient. The tumour is removed with considerable care since there is a real danger of autotransplantation and recurrent disease if the capsule is ruptured and cells are split. When the pedicle can be located easily it is clipped between mosquito forceps and the gland then gently lifted up and dissected clear from the surrounding connective tissues with iris scissors. The pedicle is ligated with a non-degradable suture. Frozen section microscopy confirms the diagnosis. Two main strategies are then possible. (a) Identify the three other parathyroids which will involve exploration of the contralateral side and, relying on clinical judgement alone, conclude, if they look normal, that the patient has single gland disease and do nothing more. This strategy can be justified if the surgeon is experienced and acknowledges the fact that even if a macroscopically normal parathyroid appears hypercellular on biopsy this is of doubtful clinical importance. The majority of such patients are cured by removing the adenoma alone and more aggressive resection runs the risk of an increased incidence of hypoparathyroidism. If other macroscopically enlarged glands are found this raises the possibility of multigland disease and biopsy helps identify a second adenoma in 2 per cent of patients or genuine two to four gland hyperplasia in 10 to 15 per cent of patients with primary HPT. (b) Identify the other 'normal' gland on the ipsilateral side and submit it to frozen section. If normal the contralateral side of the neck is left undisturbed (Tibblin strategy). This strategy chooses to ignore the 1 per cent chance of another adenoma being present on the other side of the neck and neglects the chance to double check whether the patient might have multigland hyperplasia. For these reasons this strategy cannot be recommended.

When all four glands are enlarged due to hyperplasia, a subtotal (three and a half) parathyroidectomy is recommended. Initially the two largest glands are removed, and then one-half of each of the remaining glands is excised, ensuring that the half left behind has an intact blood supply. After a brief interval these two halves are inspected and the one which appears less viable is removed and the other is left *in situ* clearly marked with a titanium clip. If the patient becomes hypercalcaemic at a later date this facilitates recognition for further resection.

Surgical strategy for secondary and tertiary hyperparathyroidism

The challenge with these patients who require surgery is to identify all the hyperplastic glands (up to 6 per cent may have a supernumerary fifth gland), and excise sufficient parathyroid tissue to relieve the symptoms of renal osteodystrophy but leave an adequate amount to preserve normal parathyroid function. There is controversy about how this goal is best achieved. There are those who advocate subtotal parathyroidectomy and others who promote total parathyroidectomy. The disadvantage of subtotal parathyroidectomy, especially for patients with tertiary HPT whose calcium and PTH levels are both elevated, is the high recurrence rate. If renal transplantation is likely in due course, which would slowly correct the patient's hyperparathyroidism, then subtotal parathyroidectomy avoids the risk of unmasking vitamin D resistant osteomalacia which is sometimes encountered after total parathyroidectomy and is very difficult to treat. An alternative strategy that theoretically overcomes both these problems is to remove all the parathyroid tissue from the neck, implant 50 to 60 mg in the forearm, and to cryopreserve the rest. If the forearm transplant is too generous and hypercalcaemia persists or recurs then the surgeon has easy access to reduce the volume of transplanted tissue. If the patient becomes hypocalcaemic then the cryopreserved tissue is brought out of storage and some more is implanted. Whilst freshly transplanted parathyroid cells function well in over 90 per cent of patients, implanted cryopreserved tissue functions in no more than 70 per cent of patients. The precise technique is to remove all parathyroid tissue from the neck, confirm this histologically, and then dice one parathyroid on a flat surface into 1-mm cubes with a scalpel. Some 50 to 60 mg is transplanted into three or more separate muscle pockets in the brachioradialis muscle of the non-dominant forearm (Fig. 17). This is a delicate task requiring fine instruments to avoid crushing the fragments and haematoma which compromises the viability of the transplant. Each pocket is closed with a fine non-absorbable suture such as Prolene which prevents extrusion and is easily recognized if removal is required later. The rest of the parathyroid tissue from the other three or four glands is sectioned into 1 × 1 × 3 mm slices and placed in polypropylene vials containing tissue culture medium, antibiotics, dimethyl sulphoxide, and autologous serum. Freezing to −80°C is commenced quickly in a controlled manner after harvesting and the tissue is then stored in a liquid

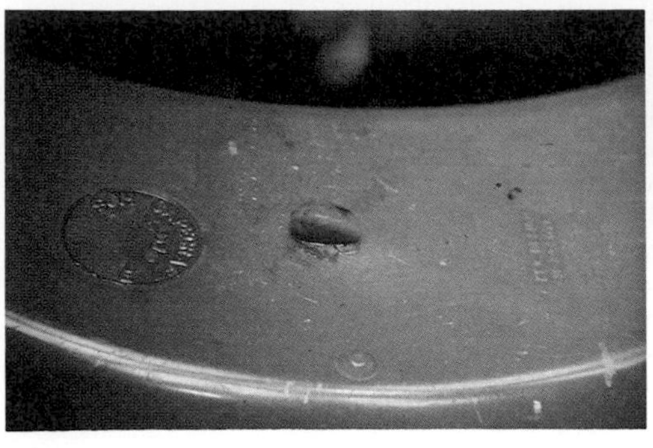

(a)

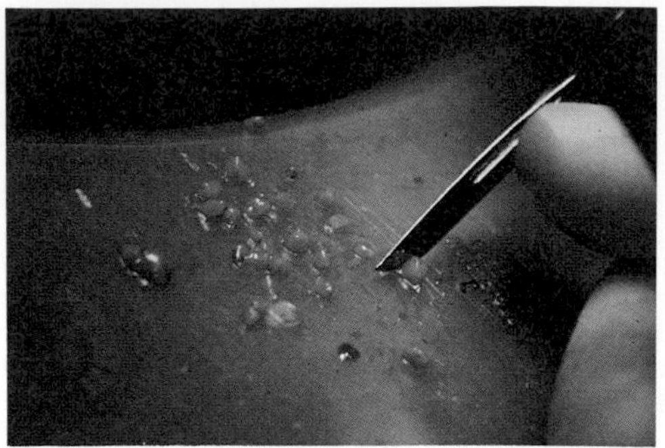

(b)

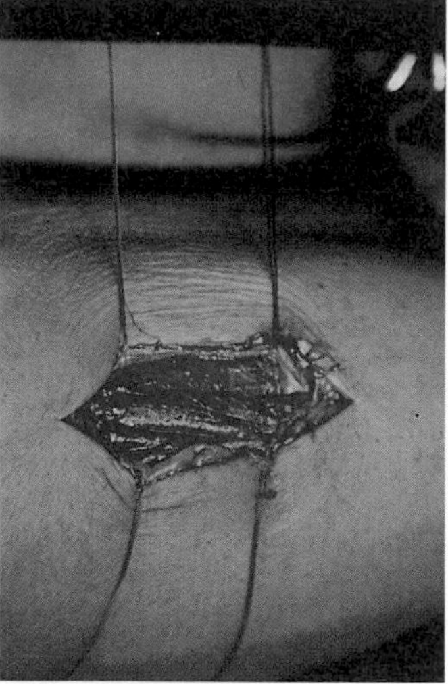

(c)

Fig. 17 (a),(b),(c) Preparation of parathyroid tissue for autotransplantation to non-dominant forearm.

nitrogen freezer. Reversing the process is done in a 37°C water bath and successful transplantation has been reported as long as 18 months after storage.

Surgery for parathyroid carcinoma

The surgeon should be alerted to the possibility of a parathyroid carcinoma if the plasma calcium is appreciably elevated above 3.5 mmol/l especially if recorded in the presence of a palpable neck mass. It is at operation, however, that suspicion should be raised if the affected parathyroid is firmer than normal, grey in colour, and adherent to the local tissues. Lymph node involvement is frequent. The surgical strategy is to perform an *en-bloc* resection of the tumour and surrounding soft tissue which usually implies an ipsilateral thyroid lobectomy and nodal dissection. Local recurrence may be eliminated by postoperative localized external beam radiotherapy.

Surgery for MEN syndromes

The MEN type I syndrome is characterized by asymmetrical hyperplasia of the parathyroids with a high percentage of supernumerary glands. Nearly all of these patients develop HPT eventually. Partial thyroidectomy and cervical thymectomy is therefore advocated to reduce the chance of recurrent hyperparathyroidism. The MEN type IIA syndrome, by comparison, only leads to hyperparathyroidism in approximately 30 per cent of sufferers and is due to adenomatous change in one or two glands. Removal of just one or two of these obviously enlarged glands is necessary to secure a normocalcaemic state.

POSTOPERATIVE RESULTS, COMPLICATIONS, AND MANAGEMENT

The care of a patient after exploration for HPT is identical to that described for a routine thyroidectomy in Section 11.1. The same potential complications can arise but the risk of haemorrhage and recurrent laryngeal nerve damage is much less. The metabolic responses to parathyroidectomy are discussed in detail in Section 11.2.1, but temporary hypocalcaemia is a frequent occurrence, especially in those patients with metabolic bone disease. As already described in the section on preoperative preparation, this can be treated expectantly with 1α-hydroxycholecalciferol which modifies the fall in the plasma calcium. Permanent hypoparathyroidism is a rare problem and affects 1 per cent of patients. In primary HPT an experienced surgeon will at the first operation successfully correct the hypercalcaemia in 95 per cent of patients with no recurrence over a 2-year period. Operative mortality approaches zero (0.2 per cent in the author's series). Eight per cent of patients undergoing subtotal parathyroidectomy for secondary and tertiary HPT, i.e. multigland involvement, have persistent or recurrent hyperparathyroidism. This figure rises to 30 per cent in those affected with the MEN I syndrome, who also suffer a greater risk of permanent hypoparathyroidism (4 per cent). Total parathyroidectomy with immediate autotransplantation of fresh parathyroid tissue achieves a functioning graft in over 90 per cent of patients. When the initial graft proves inadequate to maintain the level of plasma calcium, cryopreserved tissue can be successfully grafted after 18 months storage, but 35 per cent of these grafts fail.

Strategy after failed cervical exploration for hyperparathyroidism

Frequently patients in this category have had their primary surgery performed in a non-specialized unit. The validity of the diagnosis should be challenged with review of the original biochemical data. Whether there are discrepancies or not biochemical results will need to be rechecked. The possibility of familial hypocalciuric hypercalcaemia should be borne in mind as this syndrome has been implicated in 9 per cent of patients with failed neck exploration. The disease likewise should be reviewed in case multigland disease has been overlooked. Assuming the diagnosis is confirmed, the next crucial information to be checked is in the operation note. This should have recorded the precise location and appearance of all parathyroid tissue. When three normal glands have been found, the side of the missing fourth is established and the field of search narrowed. If four normal glands have been identified, the missing fifth is likely to be mediastinal. If there is incomplete documentation then a methodical re-exploration of the neck may be necessary unless localization studies have clearly shown the missing parathyroid(s) to be in the chest. The choice of localization study will depend on the local availability and expertise.

FURTHER READING

Bruining HA, *et al.* Results of operative treatment of 615 patients with primary hypoparathyroidism. *World J Surg*, 1981; 5: 85–9.

Clark OH, *et al.* Localization studies in patients with persistent or recurrent hyperparathyroidism. *Surgery*, 1985; **98**: 1083–94.

Dudley NE. Methylene blue for the rapid identification of the parathyroids. *Br Med J*, 1971; 3: 680.

Dunlop DAB, *et al.* Parathyroid venous sampling: anatomic considerations and results in 95 patients with primary hyperparathyroidism. *Br J Radiol*, 1980; **53**: 183.

Edis AJ, Beahrs OH, van Heerden JK, Akwari OE. 'Conservative' versus 'liberal' approach to parathyroid neck exploration. *Surgery* 1977; **82**: 466–73.

Gilmour JR. The gross anatomy of the parathyroid glands. *J Pathol Bacteriol*, 1938; **46**: 133–49.

Higgins RM, Richardson AJ, Retcliffe PJ, Woods CG, Oliver DD, Morris PJ. Total parathyroidectomy alone or with autograft for hyperparathyroidism *Q J Med*, 1991; **79**: 323–32.

Heath H III, Hodgson SF, Kennedy MA. Primary hyperparathyroidism. Incidence, morbidity and potential economic impact in a community. *N Engl J Med*, 1980; **302**: 189–93.

Kaplan RA, *et al.* Metabolic effects of parathyroidectomy in asymptomatic primary hyperparathyroidism. *J Clin Endocrinol Metab*, 1976; **42**: 415–26.

Lafferty FW, Hubay CA. Primary hyperparathyroidism: a review of the long term surgical and nonsurgical morbidities as a basis for a rational approach to treatment. *Arch Intern Med*, 1989; **149**: 789–96.

Law WM Jr, Heath H III. Familial benign hypercalcaemia (hypocalciuric hypercalcaemia): clinical and pathogenetic studies in 21 families. *Ann Intern Med*, 1985; **102**: 511–19.

Lilliemoe K, Dudley NE. Parathyroid carcinoma—pointers to successful management. *Ann R Coll Surg Engl*, 1985; **67**: 222–4.

McGeown MG. Effect of parathyroidectomy on the incidence of renal calculi. *Lancet*, 1961; i: 586–7.

Proye C. Exploration parathyroidienne pour hyperparathyroidie. *J Chir (Paris)*, 1978; **115**: 101.

Rothmund M. Wagner PK. Total parathyroidectomy and autotransplantation of parathyroid tissue for renal hyperparathyroidism. A one to six year follow-up. *Ann Surg*, 1983; **197**: 7–16.

Russel CF, Edis AJ. Surgical primary hyperparathyroidism. *Br J Surg*, 1982; **69**: 244.

Scholz DA, Purnell DC. Asymptomatic primary hyperparathyroidism: 10 year perspective study. *Mayo Clin Proc*, 1981; **56**: 473–8.

Shane E, Bilezikian JP. Parathyroid carcinoma: a review of 62 patients. *Endocrinol Rev*, 1982; **3**: 218–26.

Tibblin S, Boulesion AG, Ljungberg O. Unilateral parathyroidectomy due to a single adenoma. *Ann Surg*, 1982; **195**: 245–52.

van Heerden JA, *et al.* Primary hyperparathyroidism in patients with multiple endocrine neoplasia syndromes: surgical experience. *Arch Surg*, 1983; **118**: 533–5.

Wang CA. Surgical management of primary hyperparathyroidism. *Current Probl Surgery*, 1985; **22**: 1–50.

Wells SA, *et al.* Transplantation of the parathyroid glands in man. Clinical indications and results. *Surgery*, 1975; **78**: 33–44.

Wilder WT, Frame B, Haubrich WS. Peptic ulcer in primary hyperparathyroidism. An analysis of 52 cases. *Ann Intern Med*, 1961; **55**: 885–93.

Young AE, *et al.* Location of parathyroid adenomas by thallium-201 and technetium 99m subtraction scanning. *Br Med J*, 1983; **286**: 1384.

11.3 The adrenal gland

JUSTIN A. ROAKE

INTRODUCTION

One consequence of increasing subspecialization is that few surgeons now require a detailed knowledge of the disorders of the adrenal gland. Adrenal pathology is not only relatively uncommon but also tends to present with functional abnormalities due to excess or insufficient hormone secretion for which, most often, a physician will be consulted initially. Surgical involvement is usually limited to the management of conditions such as adrenocortical neoplasia or phaeochromocytomas at a stage when much of the diagnostic work-up has been completed. With this background in mind, this section has been written to provide core knowledge for the surgeon in training and a useful reference for the surgeon who may occasionally be called upon to manage the various disorders of the adrenals.

ADRENAL ANATOMY AND PHYSIOLOGY

The adrenal glands are paired structures located medial to the upper pole of each kidney. Normally each weighs between 4 and 5 g but after a prolonged illness they may increase substantially as a result of adrenocorticotrophic hormone (ACTH) stimulation. Rarely adrenal tissue may develop at an ectopic site which bears an embryological relationship to the urogenital ridge and its derivatives. Ectopic tissue has most frequently been documented in the testis or spermatic cord but it may be located anywhere in the retroperitoneum from the diaphragm to the pelvis; in most cases it consists almost entirely of cortex, but it can include medulla, especially when it is located in the region of the coeliac ganglion. The importance of ectopic adrenal tissue is that it may undergo hyperplasia in Cushing's disease or rarely it may undergo neoplastic change.

The adrenal cortex and medulla are anatomically and functionally discrete units. The steroid-secreting cortex originates from the mesoderm of the urogenital ridge and gains a distinctive yellow colour from its content of steroid precursors which include free and esterified cholesterol, triglycerides, and phospholipids. The catecholamine-secreting medulla on the other hand is derived from the neural crest and is thus closely related to the sympathetic nervous system and the extra-adrenal paraganglia. Primitive medullary cells develop along two lineages: the chromaffin cells which become phaeochromocytes and neuroblasts which mature into ganglion cells.

At birth the cortex consists predominantly of a wide fetal zone but after several months three clearly defined cortical zones can be identified. The subcapsular zona glomerulosa, which accounts for 10 to 15 per cent of the adult cortex, is the source of mineralocorticoids, the most important of which is aldosterone. The intermediate zona fasiculata which accounts for about 80 per cent of the adult cortex and the inner zona reticularis (5–10 per cent) produce glucocorticoids (predominantly from the zona fasiculata), the most active of which is cortisol, androgens (of which testosterone is the most significant), and small quantities of oestrogens. Cortisol and testosterone secretion is regulated by ACTH whereas aldosterone secretion by the zona glomerulosa is primarily regulated by the renin–angiotensin system and is largely independent of ACTH.

The adrenal medulla is extremely vascular and consists largely of a reticular network of catecholamine-secreting chromaffin cells with a closely related plexus of venous sinusoids intertwined amongst them that facilitates the release of catecholamines into the circulation. The gland has a rich nerve supply derived mainly from the coeliac and renal plexuses. The nerve endings terminate directly on the chromaffin cells which contain numerous electron-dense granules that have a role in the synthesis and storage of catecholamines. The predominant catecholamine produced and stored in the adrenal medulla is, as its name suggests, adrenaline but smaller quantities of noradrenaline are also produced.

DISORDERS OF THE ADRENAL CORTEX

Clinical disorders resulting from abnormal adrenocortical function can be considered to be of four types (Table 1). Hypofunction is most often a consequence of iatrogenic suppression or autoimmune destruction of the gland. Hyperfunction results from excessive production of adrenal hormones secondary to a functioning adrenal tumour or more commonly to overproduction of ACTH. Inborn errors of steroid synthesis may produce a mixed clinical picture of hyper- and hypofunction. Finally, non-functioning adrenal masses may present as an incidental finding or with symptoms unrelated to adrenal function.

In this section the various clinical syndromes associated with these disorders will be considered followed by an account of the diagnosis and management of adrenocortical tumours and the management of adrenal masses discovered incidentally during investigation of an unrelated condition.

Table 1 Disorders of the adrenal cortex and adrenal medulla

ADRENAL CORTEX
- Hypofunction
  - Congenital hypoplasia
  - Primary chronic adrenal insufficiency
  - Primary acute adrenal insufficiency
  - Secondary adrenal insufficiency
- Hyperfunction
  - Cushing's syndrome
    - Overproduction of ACTH
      - Pituitary micradenoma
      - Ectopic ACTH
    - Adrenal tumour
    - Hyperplasia
    - Iatrogenic
  - Conn's syndrome
    - Adrenal tumour
    - Hyperplasia
  - Virilization/feminization
    - Adrenal tumour
    - Inborn errors of metabolism
- Non-functioning adrenal masses
  - Cyst
  - Myelolipoma
  - Adrenocortical adenoma
  - Adrenocortical carcinoma
  - Metastasis

ADRENAL MEDULLA
- Medullary neoplasia
  - Neuroblastoma
  - Ganglioneuroma
  - Phaeochromocytoma
    - Benign
    - Malignant

Adrenocortical hypofunction

Congenital adrenal hypoplasia is a rare developmental anomaly which presents in the neonatal period. Two forms are recognized. The anencephalic type is associated with other serious congenital anomalies, usually including anencephaly, and these infants are usually stillborn or do not survive for more than a few days. The cytomegalic type may be genetically determined with a recessive pattern of inheritance and if recognized and treated appropriately with steroid replacement therapy long-term survival may result.

In later life adrenocortical hypofunction can be split into three categories: primary chronic adrenal insufficiency, primary acute adrenal insufficiency, and secondary adrenal insufficiency.

To the surgeon, secondary insufficiency is probably of greatest importance, or at least that most likely to be encountered. It is most frequently due to adrenal suppression resulting from chronic steroid therapy for a variety of conditions including autoimmune diseases or in the recipients of organ transplants. Alternatively it may be encountered following treatment of Cushing's syndrome by adrenalectomy or following removal of a functional adrenal adenoma. Secondary adrenal insufficiency may present with an 'adrenal crisis' especially during times of stress such as acute illness or following major surgery, unless adequate precautions are taken to prevent its occurrence (see below).

Primary chronic adrenal insufficiency (Addison's disease) is an uncommon condition which today is usually the result of autoimmune destruction of the adrenal cortex (previously tuberculosis was the most common cause). It is more common in women than men (M : F ratio approximately 3 : 1) and antiadrenocortical antibodies are demonstrable in the majority of cases, particularly in women. It may be associated with other autoimmune conditions and antibodies against the thyroid, parietal cells, or intrinsic factor are commonly found in these patients.

Primary acute hypoadrenalism may occur on a background of chronic adrenal insufficiency, for instance during 'adrenal crises' of addisonian patients or following too rapid withdrawal of steroids from patients with suppressed adrenals, or failure to increase replacement steroids in times of stress. More rarely it may be due to massive haemorrhagic adrenal infarction. In neonates, in whom the adrenal is relatively large, this may follow birth trauma and/or hypoxia. In adults, when it is known as Waterhouse–

Friederichsen syndrome, it is often related to acute bacteraemic infection, most commonly with the meningococcus, but it may also occur during pneumococcal, staphylococcal, or *Haemophilus influenzae* infections. It may also occur as a preterminal, agonal, event.

The symptoms and signs of primary and secondary adrenal insufficiency are similar except that primary chronic insufficiency may be associated with abnormal pigmentation, especially in the skin creases, scars, and inside the lips and cheeks. This is a consequence of chronic stimulation of the pituitary and overproduction of ACTH and β-melanocyte stimulating hormone which stimulate increased pigmentation.

Chronic cortisol deficiency commonly results in weight loss which is often associated with episodes of colicky non-specific abdominal pain, vomiting and diarrhoea, general malaise, and lack of energy and there may be marked postural hypotension. The features of 'adrenal crises' due to acute cortisol insufficiency include hypotension, shock, and hyponatraemia often associated with muscle cramps, myalgia, or unexplained fever.

The biochemical characteristics of hypoadrenalism are hyponatraemia, hyperkalaemia, and an elevated blood urea (8–15 mmol/l) all of which may occur in either primary adrenal insufficiency, in which both cortisol and aldosterone are deficient, or secondary insufficiency, where cortisol alone is deficient. These abnormalities tend to be most marked during acute adrenal crises. Proof of the diagnosis is not always easy since normal urinary cortisol excretion may be below the limits of detection and some urinary cortisol may be detected in hypoadrenalism. Likewise plasma cortisol levels in adrenal insufficiency are often in the low-normal range. A high plasma cortisol, however, especially during acute illness, effectively eliminates the diagnosis. Definitive proof of hypoadrenalism usually requires demonstration that the plasma ACTH is disproportionately high compared to plasma cortisol levels or that the adrenal fails to produce a normal secretory response following a challenge with exogenously administered ACTH.

The hypotensive patient with acute adrenal insufficiency requires immediate volume replacement with normal saline solution and steroid replacement, for example hydrocortisone 100 mg intramuscularly or intravenously, which should be administered prior to confirmation of the presumed diagnosis. Improvement should occur within 4 to 6 h if the diagnosis is correct. The patient should then receive regular steroid parenterally, for example hydrocortisone 100 mg intramuscularly or intravenously every 6 h for 2 or 3 days, and may subsequently require oral maintenance steroid replacement.

In primary chronic adrenal insufficiency both cortisol and aldosterone require replacement. This requires the equivalent of about 30 mg of cortisol per day (two-thirds administered in the morning and one-third in the evening) and the mineralocorticoid (for example fludrocortisone) dosage adjusted according to blood pressure and plasma renin. In secondary adrenal insufficiency only cortisol needs to be replaced. Patients should be advised to double the daily glucocorticoid dose during intercurrent illness, for example fever above 38°C, systemic infection, or trauma, and if vomiting occurs for more than 24 h parenteral replacement should be given. Prior to surgery patients should receive replacement therapy as for acute adrenal insufficiency, commencing 1 h before anaesthesia and converting to oral replacement therapy once reliable oral intake has been re-established.

Cushing's syndrome

Cushing's syndrome encompasses a group of disorders presenting with the symptoms and signs of exposure to excess glucocorticoids. Since the onset of symptom is usually insidious and the typical picture of the patient with all the features of the syndrome develops slowly, a relatively late clinical diagnosis is common.

Some features are more important than others diagnostically. These include skin atrophy producing skin which is palpably thin and the development of spontaneous purpura due to capillary fragility. Wasting affecting the proximal muscles, especially those of the pelvic girdle, and weakness which may be aggravated by hypokalaemia are also particularly characteristic. Osteoporosis, mainly affecting the axial skeleton and leading to spontaneous fractures of the ribs or vertebrae, and growth arrest in children are also important diagnostic clues. Other features of the syndrome which tend to be of less diagnostic value include central obesity, which predominantly affects the face ('facial mooning'), neck, and trunk and may contribute to the classical 'buffalo hump' appearance (Fig. 1), purple striae, poor wound healing and paper thin scars, facial hirsuitism, acne and plethora, oedema, moderate hypertension, glucose intolerance, amenorrhoea, and psychiatric manifestations such as depressive psychosis.

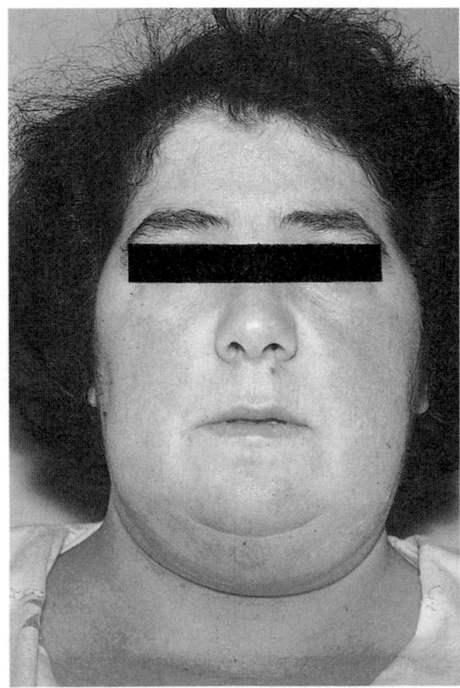

Fig. 1 The moon face of a patient with Cushing's syndrome.

Any of several underlying conditions of diverse aetiology may lead to Cushing's syndrome. Probably the most common cause today is iatrogenic Cushing's syndrome due to chronic administration of glucocorticoids to organ transplant recipients or patients with immune disorders. Cushing's syndrome due to primary adrenal disease or excessive exposure to ACTH is less common but collectively these conditions are of great importance because of the diagnostic challenge they pose and the potential for curative surgical intervention. Of these cases between 65 and 75

Table 2 Screening and diagnostic tests for Cushing's syndrome

Screening/diagnostic test	Cushing's disease	Ectopic ACTH	Adenoma (hyperplasia)	Carcinoma	Comments
24-h urinary free (unconjugated) cortisol	↑	↑ or ↑↑	↑	↑ or ↑↑	Screening test of choice. (May be ↑ with obesity, pregnancy, or oral contraceptive)
Plasma cortisol	↑	↑ or ↑↑	↑	↑ or ↑↑	Neither sensitive nor specific
Urinary 17-hydroxysteroid or 17-ketosteroid	↑	↑	↑	↑	Much overlap with normal subjects
Single-dose overnight dexamethasone suppression	No	No	No	No	Sensitive. Phenytoin or oestrogen may produce false-positive results
Low-dose dexamethasone suppression	No	No	No	No	Definitive diagnostic test
High-dose dexamethasone suppression	Yes	No	Most no (75% no)	No	Infrequently used today
Plasma ACTH	↑ or normal*	↑↑	Undetectable (↓ or normal)	Undetectable	Most useful test for determining the aetiology of Cushing's syndrome
Metyrapone 17-hydroxysteroid	↑ (Normal response)	↑ In 50%	↓ (↑ or ↓)	↓	
Metyrapone Plasma ACTH	↑	No response	No response	No response	
Steroid prodution >5000 nmol/day	Rare	Common	Rare	Common	

* Following bilateral adrenalectomy ACTH may be ↑↑.

per cent are attributable to an ACTH-secreting pituitary microadenoma which is often referred to as Cushing's disease as a tribute to Harvey Cushing who first described the condition in 1932. A further 10 to 15 per cent are due to ectopic sources of ACTH such as carcinoma of the lung (particularly small cell carcinoma), malignant pancreatic tumours, benign or malignant thymomas or (less commonly) carcinoids, phaeochromocytomas, medullary carcinoma of the thyroid, and rarely other primary carcinomas. Primary adrenal disease such as adenoma, adenocarcinoma, or micronodular adrenal hyperplasia account for the remaining 10 to 20 per cent.

Certain clinical features may give some indication as to the aetiology of Cushing's syndrome. Ectopic ACTH production by a rapidly growing malignant primary tends to produce very high levels of cortisol secretion with rapid development of a Cushing's syndrome in which features such as hypokalaemia and oedema predominate in addition to the clinical features of the primary disease. Cushing's syndrome resulting from ACTH secretion by benign tumours tends to have a more indolent course with gradual development of the clinical manifestations. Malignant tumours of the adrenal cortex may synthesize cortisol inefficiently and this may lead to excessive production of androgen precursors which in turn may produce hirsuitism and virilization, neither of which tends to be features of Cushing's syndrome induced by adrenal adenomas.

Investigation of patients suspected of having Cushing's syndrome is conducted in two phases: confirmatory screening or diagnostic tests followed by investigations to determine the underlying aetiology (Table 2). Probably the most useful screening test for hypercortisolism is the 24-h urinary free (unconjugated) cortisol excretion (the sensitivity and specificity of this investigation are approximately 95 per cent) but raised cortisol excretion may also be seen in obesity, during periods of stress, during pregnancy, or if oral contraceptives are being taken. The level of steroid overproduction may also give some guidance to the aetiology. Levels of more than 5000 nmol/day are commonly found in Cushing's syndrome due to ectopic ACTH or adrenal carcinoma but only rarely in other cases. Urinary 17-hydroxysteroid and 17-ketosteroid excretion reflects basal cortisol production but is less discriminating than free cortisol excretion and there is greater overlap with normal subjects. Plasma cortisol levels are more difficult to interpret because under normal circumstances there is great variability. However, loss of the normal diurnal variation with failure of the plasma cortisol level to fall at night is a useful and constant feature of Cushing's syndrome. Elevation of the midnight plasma cortisol is a sensitive test but it may also occur during pregnancy, stress, or in subjects taking oral contraceptives. A somewhat more definitive test for Cushing's syndrome depends upon the relative resistance to suppression by exogenous steroids. Dexamethasone is a potent steroid which normally suppresses pituitary derived ACTH and thus lowers plasma cortisol but in subjects with Cushing's syndrome suppression of cortisol secretion is resistant to low doses of dexamethasone and urinary excretion of 17-hydroxysteroids remains elevated. The single dose (overnight) dexamethasone suppression test, in which the morning plasma cortisol is measured after administration of 1 to 2 mg of dexamethasone at midnight, is associated with a low false-negative rate but a false-positive result may occur in the obese patient, in subjects taking oestrogens or phenytoin, or in the chronically ill. The so-called low-dose dexamethasone suppression test in which 24-h urinary 17-hydroxysteroids are measured during administration of 0.5 mg of dexamethasone 6-hourly may be more reliable.

The high-dose dexamethasone suppression test, in which 2 mg of dexamethasone is administered 6-hourly for 2 days and the 24 h urinary 17-hydroxysteroid excretion is measured during the second day, has been used to determine the underlying aetiology of Cushing's syndrome. In nearly all patients with Cushing's disease the 17-hydroxysteroid excretion is suppressed to less than 40 per cent of the baseline measurements but nearly all patients with adrenal tumours, most with adrenal hyperplasia and all with an ectopic ACTH source fail to show suppression. However, since suppressibility with dexamethasone is a matter of degree and subject to errors induced by natural biological variability, other, more reliable, diagnostic tests have tended to supersede the dexamethasone suppression tests. Determination of the plasma ACTH by radioimmunoassay of blood samples taken in the morning, when ACTH is usually detectable in normal subjects, is the most useful investigation for determining the cause of Cushing's syndrome. In primary adrenal disease the levels are undetectable (except occasionally in patients with micronodular adrenal hyperplasia in whom ACTH may be normal) whereas in Cushing's syndrome due to pituitary ACTH production the level is almost always elevated or normal. In cases of ectopic ACTH secretion plasma ACTH levels are always elevated and levels greater than 200 pg/l are virtually diagnostic. Note however that following adrenal ablation ACTH levels may be grossly elevated and this may be associated with Nelson's syndrome (see below).

Metyrapone is also useful in the determination of the aetiology of Cushing's syndrome. Metyrapone inhibits adrenal 11β-hydroxylation of 11-deoxycortisol to cortisol and thus leads to reduced cortisol secretion and a rise in ACTH and production and excretion of cortisol precursors. In cases due to primary adrenal adenoma, adrenal carcinoma, or ectopic ACTH production the pituitary is suppressed and no rise in ACTH or cortisol precursors occurs following administration of metyrapone but in 90 per cent of cases of Cushing's disease the pituitary does respond by increasing ACTH production.

Cushing's syndrome of non-adrenal origin

Diagnostic imaging and treatment of pituitary microadenomas is dealt with in detail elsewhere and will therefore be considered only briefly here. Untreated Cushing's disease commonly leads to death due to the complications of excessive exposure to cortisol including hypertension, stroke, and ischaemic heart disease. Although spontaneous remission has been documented this is an exception rather than the rule and therefore surgical treatment is generally recommended.

In the past permanent relief of hypercortisolism was achieved by total adrenalectomy but this was associated with a high operative morbidity and mortality, mainly as a consequence of chronic excessive exposure to steroids, and left the individual dependent upon life-long replacement therapy. Furthermore many patients developed very high ACTH levels, enlarged pituitary glands, and hyperpigmentation (Nelson's syndrome) often necessitating pituitary ablation. Today total adrenalectomy is reserved for the occasional patient in whom the pituitary lesion cannot be treated directly by surgical removal or irradiation.

In Cushing's syndrome secondary to ectopic ACTH secretion the ACTH secreting tumour should be sought and if possible removed. In the case of benign tumours, for example thymomas and some carcinoids, this may effect a surgical cure. When it is not possible to remove the source of the ACTH excessive cortisol secretion can usually be controlled with adrenolytic drugs such as metyrapone or aminoglutethimide which inhibits the conversion of cholesterol to Δ5-pregnenolone, thereby inhibiting production of cortisol, mineralocorticoids, and androgens. Occasionally surgical adrenalectomy may be considered if the ACTH source cannot be removed and the patient would otherwise have a good prognosis following relief of the hypercortisolism.

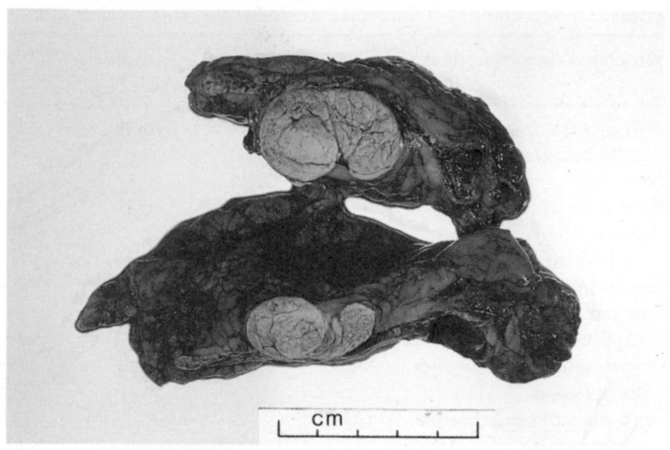

Fig. 2 A primary aldosterone secreting tumour (Conn's tumour) of the adrenal cortex.

Primary aldosteronism (Conn's syndrome)

Primary aldosteronism most commonly results from excessive and autonomous secretion of aldosterone by an adenoma of the adrenal cortex (Fig. 2) but less commonly may be due to bilateral micronodular hyperplasia involving the zona glomerulosa. Although the aetiology of the latter is unknown it has been suggested that it may represent tertiary aldosteronism, in which excessive renin secretion (subsequently suppressed) was the original stimulus, but this remains entirely hypothetical.

In 1955 Conn was the first to describe a patient with hypertension, neuromuscular symptoms, and renal potassium wastage which was associated with elevated aldosterone secretion and an adrenocortical adenoma. Excessive secretion of aldosterone produces hypertension, predominantly as a result of intravascular volume expansion secondary to aldosterone-induced salt and water retention, but as a primary cause of hypertension it is rare, and accounts for less than 0.5 per cent of cases. Primary aldosteronism is most commonly suspected when hypokalaemia is associated with alkalosis in the presence of hypertension but it must be distinguished from other (more common) causes of hypokalaemia associated with hypertension, particularly that induced by loop or thiazide diuretics, and by renin-induced secondary hyperaldosteronism. The latter is seen in hypertension due to renovascular disease and in severe essential hypertension. Primary aldosteronism without hypokalaemia is uncommon. Patients presenting with hypertension in whom studies to exclude Conn's syndrome should be undertaken include those with spontaneous hypokalaemia ($<$3.5 mmol/l), moderately severe hypokalaemia ($<$3.0 mmol/l) while taking diuretics or difficulty maintaining a normal potassium despite oral supplements or potassium sparing diuretics, and patients with hypertension refractory to treatment with no specific evidence of a secondary cause.

Confirmation of suspected primary aldosteronism can sometimes be difficult but most often the diagnosis is easily established by demonstrating elevated plasma aldosterone, or increased urinary excretion of aldosterone, despite adequate salt loading (confirmed by measurement of urinary sodium excretion) over several days. Hypokalaemia, inappropriate kaliuresis, and depressed plasma renin activity that fails to rise in response to salt and water depletion or the upright posture are supportive features but their absence does not exclude the diagnosis. In primary aldosteronism the plasma sodium is usually normal or elevated whereas, in contrast, hyponatraemia is often a feature of secondary aldosteronism. If the diagnostic tests are equivocal multiple measurements of aldosterone during salt loading may be needed.

It is important to distinguish between adrenal hyperplasia and an adenoma since the treatment of each condition differs. An adenoma is said to produce more pronounced biochemical abnormalities (higher aldosterone, and lower renin and potassium) than does hyperplasia but this is of little value in distinguishing the two and diagnostic imaging is required. Large adenomas (greater than 1 cm in diameter) may be detected reliably by computed tomography (CT) (Fig. 3) or magnetic resonance imaging (MRI) but since these investigations provide little or no information regarding the function of any abnormal tissue detected radionuclide imaging or selective venous sampling may be required to distinguish an adenoma from hyperplasia. Selective adrenal sampling for aldosterone and cortisol levels is an extremely valuable test in confirming the diagnosis and localizing a tumour. The cortisol levels allow the validity of the adrenal vein sampling to be established in comparison with peripheral samples (see adrenocortical tumours below).

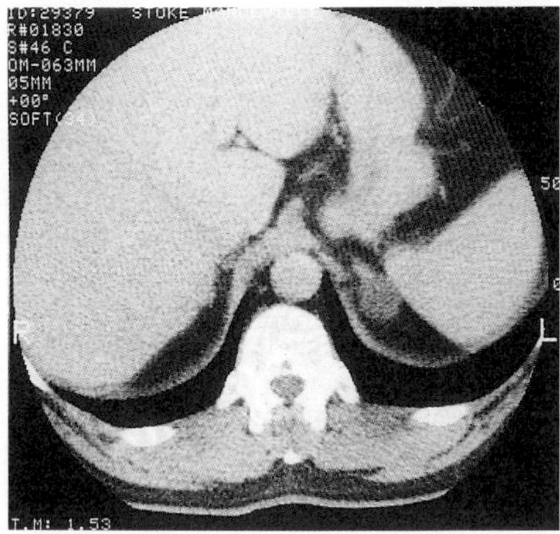

Fig. 3 A CT scan showing a Conn's tumour of the left adrenal gland.

Primary aldosteronism due to an adenoma is treated by surgical excision (adrenalectomy) once the hypertension and hypokalaemia have been corrected with spironolactone or amiloride. Surgical treatment of micronodular hyperplasia is much less satisfactory and the treatment of choice is long-term control with spironolactone or amiloride.

Virilization and virilizing or feminizing tumours

In children, virilizing tumours may present with precocious puberty, phallic enlargement, and development of secondary hair growth on the face, axillae, and pubes and the differential diagnosis includes congenital adrenal hyperplasia (see below), idiopathic hirsuitism, and other causes of precocious puberty. In the adult female, virilizing tumours present with deepening of the voice, hirsuitism, amenorrhoea, enlargement of the clitoris, increase in muscle bulk, and increased libido whereas, in the adult male, they may be relatively silent and may only be recognized as an incidental finding or, if malignant, by the development of metastases.

Virilizing adrenal tumours are most commonly diagnosed by finding an enlarged adrenal or adrenal mass on CT scan in association with appropriate biochemical abnormalities. Both adrenal and gonadal causes of virilization produce increased plasma androgens but elevated dehydroepiandrosterone (DHEA) which is secreted almost exclusively by the adrenal gland, suggests an adrenal cause for virilization. DHEA may also be elevated in some cases of idiopathic hirsuitism but this may be distinguished from an adrenal tumour biochemically by the dexamethasone suppression test: 17-ketosteroid secretion is not normally suppressed in cases due to adrenal tumours. In adrenocortical carcinoma producing virilization plasma DHEA and 17-ketosteroid levels tend to be very high.

Feminizing tumours are very rare and are almost always malignant. In men they may present with gynaecomastia and impotence before they have metastasized and curative resection may be possible but in women they tend to be advanced when first detected.

Congenital adrenal hyperplasia (androgenital syndrome)

This is a family of genetically controlled congenital disorders which have in common a complete or partial defect in the control of steroid biosynthesis producing elevated ACTH, excessive production of androgens and/or mineralocorticoids, and striking enlargement of the adrenals which reach 10 to 20 times their normal weight. Inheritance is by recessive genes with variable penetrance and the incidence is between 1 : 10 000 and 1 : 50 000 live births. Any one of several enzyme defects may be responsible but the most common is 21-hydroxylase deficiency in which cortisol and aldosterone production is defective and excessive secretion of pituitary ACTH results in high levels of adrenal androgen production that may produce virilization at birth or sexual precocity in males. Less commonly an 11β-hydroxylase deficit produces excess 11-deoxycortisol, a cortisol precursor with mineralocorticoid activity, which may produce hypertension in addition to increased androgen secretion. Other, less common, defects include 17-hydroxylase deficiency, 18-hydroxylase deficiency, and 3β-hydroxysteroid dehydrogenase deficiency.

There is a wide spectrum of clinical presentations but the diagnosis should be suspected in babies or children with abnormal genitalia (for example cryptorchidism, hypospadias, or ambiguous genitalia), clitoromegaly with or without pubic hair development in the female, or precocious puberty in the male or in children with hypertension. A family history of neonatal deaths, or siblings with hirsuitism or congenital adrenal hyperplasia helps to identify individuals with a relatively high risk.

The diagnosis is confirmed by laboratory investigations including 24-h urinary oxogenic- and oxosteroids and plasma cortisol (which maybe normal), ACTH, testosterone, and 17α-hydroxyprogesterone. Treatment is directed at correcting metabolic abnormalities (for example salt deficiency) followed by replacement of mineralocorticoid and cortisol, to suppress ACTH and reduce androgen overproduction. This should allow for emergence of normal gonadotriphic function at puberty and permit normal growth. Surgery for cryptorchidism or genital abnormalities may be required, often as staged procedures, and the perioperative period should be covered with increased steroid replacement as for adrenal insufficiency.

Adrenocortical tumours

Clinically detected adrenocortical neoplasms are roughly equally divided between benign and malignant. Most benign tumours secrete either glucocorticoids, mineralocorticoids, androgens, or oestrogens but, in contrast, carcinomas of the adrenal secrete large amounts of various biologically active and inactive steroids such that about half of them produce clinical features attributable to steroid secretion. Cushing's syndrome is the most common clinical presentation of adrenocortical tumours but they may also present with aldosteronism, virilization, or very rarely feminization. A mixed picture is characteristic of adrenocortical carcinoma and reflects the spectrum of steroids and biologically active steroid precursors produced by the tumour.

Diagnostic imaging and treatment of adrenocortical tumours

Following biochemical confirmation of a clinically suspected functional adrenal tumour localization and staging is required before planning surgical intervention. CT, the most commonly used imaging modality in the assessment of adrenal pathology, can identify almost all lesions greater than 1 cm in diameter and it has largely replaced investigations such as intravenous pyelography, retroperitoneal pneumography, nephrotomography, selective arteriography, or selective venography. Although CT is sensitive it is not specific and cannot, for instance, distinguish between adenoma, carcinoma, lymphoma, or haematoma. A CT scan may detect evidence of local invasion of the kidney or other adjacent structures and it may also demonstrate lymph node or liver metastases. Tumours more than 6 cm in diameter as assessed by CT should be suspected of malignancy and in these cases selective arteriography or venography may be useful to determine the degree to which local structures have been invaded, information which may be crucial in determining whether or not the tumour is operable. MRI is as sensitive as CT for detecting adrenal lesions but, in addition, it has been claimed that MRI may be capable of distinguishing an adrenal metastasis, carcinoma, or phaeochromocytoma from an adenoma, lipoma, or myelolipoma on the basis of tissue imaging characteristics but it remains unclear whether this claim can be substantiated. MRI does, however, demonstrate the relationship of adrenal pathology to adjacent vascular structures more clearly than CT and has therefore proved to be useful in the assessment of the local extent of suspected malignant tumours. CT and MRI should be treated as complementary investigations.

Isotope scans provide both anatomical and functional information and may be a useful adjunct to CT or MRI. In Cushing's syndrome the pattern of uptake of ^{131}I–6β-iodomethyl–19-norcholesterol (NP59) is dependent upon the underlying aetiology. Four distinct patterns are recognized. Lateralized increased uptake with non-visualization of the other side is virtually pathognomonic of an adrenocortical adenoma. However, there have been several reports of well differentiated cortisol secreting adrenocortical carcinomas which demonstrated intense uptake of NP59 and were initially thought to be benign on the basis of the NP59 scan. Adrenocortical carcinomas are usually unable to incorporate enough NP59 to be visualized by NP59 scintigraphy because of inefficient production of cortisol, and since pituitary ACTH is suppressed by the excessive cortisol production the contralateral gland is also suppressed, resulting in bilateral non-visualization. Thus, bilateral non-visualization in the presence of Cushing's syndrome is considered to be diagnostic of carcinoma. Androgen or oestrogen secreting tumours do not usually suppress ACTH and in these cases the pattern is one of bilateral uptake with marked asymmetry since the tumour itself is not visualized but the remainder of the ipsilateral gland and the entire contralateral gland are. In contrast, in Cushing's syndrome due to pituitary or ectopic ACTH the uptake is increased bilaterally and symmetrically. Micronodular hyperplasia of the adrenal may produce asymmetric bilateral increased uptake.

In primary aldosteronism radionuclide imaging, using radiolabelled cholesterol during dexamethasone suppression of cortisol secretion, can be used to detect functional tissue and may detect tumours as small as 5 mm in diameter. Selective adrenal vein catheterization and measurement of aldosterone on each side should reveal unilateral increased secretion with suppression of the other side if a functional adenoma is present but bilaterally increased secretion if aldosteronism is due to hyperplasia or is secondary to increased renin secretion. When radionuclide imaging is combined with selective adrenal vein catheterization a clear distinction between adenoma and hyperplasia should be achieved in most cases. Occasionally, however, a case for diagnostic surgical exploration can be made.

The preferred treatment for a functioning adrenocortical adenoma is surgical excision because the results of surgery are generally good and often produce a complete cure. Most adenomas coming to surgery are less than 4 cm in diameter and in selected cases it may be possible to preserve uninvolved adrenal tissue. Operations to resect adrenal adenomas causing Cushing's syndrome usually have excellent results but in the long term many patients remain obese and hypertensive. Surgical intervention in this group is, however, associated with a relatively high morbidity because of chronic exposure to excess glucocorticoids specifically resulting in poor wound healing, increased risk of infection, and a relatively high risk of pulmonary thromboembolism. Perioperative glucocorticoid supplementation is required because of chronic suppression of the contralateral gland and this must be continued, with graduated dosage reduction, for several months.

Following surgical removal of an aldosterone-producing adenoma the hypertension is cured in 70 to 80 per cent of cases and in the remainder surgery usually renders the hypertension more responsive to medical therapy. Several weeks before operation hypertension and metabolic abnormalities should be corrected medically. The hypertension is salt and water dependent and is best treated by sodium deprivation and potassium sparing diuretics. Postoperatively there may be a sodium diuresis and retention of potassium and close monitoring of plasma electrolytes is required in the first week. In some cases suppression of the contralateral gland results in postoperative aldosterone deficiency which may produce hyponatraemia with hyperkalaemia necessitating mineralocorticoid replacement until the remaining gland recovers.

Adrenocortical carcinoma

Carcinoma of the adrenal cortex is usually highly aggressive and has a poor prognosis. Fortunately it is a rare tumour with an incidence of about 1 per 1.5×10^6 population per year. It can occur in all age groups but most commonly presents in the fifth to seventh decades and it occurs roughly equally in both sexes.

The tumour may attain a very large size (>20 cm) and overall the median size at presentation is about 10 to 12 cm but relatively few (< 10 per cent) are less than 6 cm at presentation. Traditionally adrenocortical carcinomas are classified as functioning or non-functioning. Non-functioning tumours fail to produce clinical evidence of steroid synthesis but in most cases detailed studies indicate that these tumours do produce precursor steroids with little or no biological activity. The non-functioning tumours, which account for about 50 per cent of all carcinomas, often attain a very large size before detection and frequently present as an abdominal mass or with abdominal pain, weight loss, or fatigue. In some cases haemorrhagic necrosis of a large tumour may result in severe pain, fever, and even shock.

Functioning tumours may also be large at presentation because of inefficient steroid production by the malignant tissue and therefore relatively late development of endocrine manifestations. Commonly they present with symptoms and signs of cortisol, androgen, or oestrogen excess, often with a mixed picture, but clinical evidence of aldosterone excess is rarely a presenting feature and exclusive production of aldosterone by the tumour is very rare. Metastases to the local lymph nodes, liver, lungs, or less commonly bone are found in 70 to 75 per cent of patients at presentation and these may produce the initial manifestations of the disease.

Adrenocortical carcinomas usually appear lobulated and encapsulated and they frequently erode through their capsule and invade local structures such as the pancreas, kidney, and bowel. On cutting, areas of haemorrhagic necrosis are commonly found. Histologically it can be difficult to distinguish between a benign adenoma and a well differentiated carcinoma on the basis of cellular characteristics alone and it is often necessary to fall back upon the presence of local invasion and metastases as hallmarks of malignancy to make the diagnosis. The cellular DNA content may be useful diagnostically in that at least one study suggests that aneuploid tumours metastasize whereas euploid tumours do not. As CT-guided percutaneous fine-needle aspiration cytology is used more frequently in the assessment of adrenal masses, incorporating measurement of the DNA content may prove to be a powerful diagnostic approach.

Surgical eradication of the tumour offers the only chance of cure but even if complete resection is not possible because of invasion of vital structures, debulking of the tumour is important for palliation especially if the tumour is functional. In patients without demonstrable remote metastases a radical approach is generally advocated. Adrenocortical carcinomas are approached by a transabdominal or thoracoabdominal route and the tumour and adjacent involved organs are excised *en bloc*. In some cases even involvement of the inferior vena cava may not prevent complete resection provided the facilities for cardiopulmonary bypass are available. Lymph node metastases are excised with the tumour and liver metastases accessible for wedge resection should be removed. The operation must be covered with perioperative steroid replacement but in the case of non-functioning tumours this can be tapered relatively quickly over the first 1 to 2 weeks after the operation.

Chemotherapy may be used for inoperable or recurrent carcinomas or as an adjuvant to maintain remission following apparently complete excision. The agent with which there is the greatest accumulated experience in the treatment of these tumours is mitotane (*o,p'*-DDD), a derivative of DDT which produces selective necrosis of the zona fasiculata and zona reticularis. The effectiveness of mitotane is dependent upon the bulk of the tumour present and it is therefore important that surgical debulking is followed by early postoperative chemotherapy. Cortisol replacement therapy is invariably required and in some patients mineralocorticoid deficiency may also require treatment.

The clinical response to mitotane is rather variable and the side-effects (nausea, anorexia, neurotoxicity, ataxia, papilloedema, skin rashes, and cystitis) may lead to poor patient acceptance. However, the alternatives are limited as there is relatively little experience with other agents even though short-term responses to alkylating agents and doxorubicin have been reported. Treatments to reduce steroid production with aminoglutethimide or metyrapone may afford significant palliation but they do not produce tumour regression. Radiotherapy has not been systematically examined in the treatment of adrenocortical carcinoma but it has never been shown to be effective as a primary treatment or as an adjuvant for residual disease. However, it does appear to be effective for the relief of pain from bony metastases.

The prognosis correlates with the size of the tumour and the functional status, but overall the outlook is poor. Patients presenting with anaplastic tumours without laboratory evidence of steroid production have a median survival of about 6 months and the response to therapy is very poor. Differentiated carcinomas with hormone production are associated with a greater median survival (about 2 years) and in about 50 per cent there is objective evidence of a response to chemotherapy. Even in cases where surgical excision has been apparently curative long-term follow-up is required because late recurrence may occur.

'Incidentalomas' and non-functioning tumours

With wide application of sensitive non-invasive imaging of the abdomen the detection of an adrenal mass as an incidental finding during investigation for an unrelated condition has become an increasingly common clinical problem. For example, it has been estimated that approximately 1 per cent of upper abdominal CT scans performed for a variety of reasons will detect a clinically silent adrenal lesion. Although most solid lesions will be found to be non-functioning cortical adenomas they all require careful evaluation directed towards ruling out malignancy and detecting functional tumours which require excision. Other conditions such as myelolipoma may remain clinically silent, producing neither symptoms nor signs, but occasionally complications, such as bleeding into a cyst, may bring them to clinical attention.

The CT appearance may be diagnostic. Simple cysts, myelolipomas, and adrenal haematomas can usually be identified and managed appropriately on the basis of the CT image alone. Most cystic masses are benign endothelial-lined (lymphangiomatous or angiomatous) cysts or pseudocysts secondary to haemorrhage into a normal adrenal. Occasionally, however, cortical adenomas, adenocarcinomas, or phaeochromocytomas may undergo cystic degeneration. Following biochemical evaluation cystic masses should be aspirated, under ultrasonic or CT guidance, and the aspirate sent for cytological evaluation to confirm their benign nature. Suspicion of malignancy is an indication for operation. Adrenal haemorrhage may result from bleeding into an adrenal tumour and it should therefore be followed by a repeat CT scan.

Rarely the CT appearances will be diagnostic of primary adrenal carcinoma on the basis of size, lack of homogeneity, irregular borders, local infiltration, and evidence of metastases. Primary adrenal carcinomas are rarely found to be less than 6 cm in diameter and it has been estimated that in the absence of CT characteristics suggestive of malignancy fewer than 1 in 10 000 incidentally discovered lesions below 6 cm in diameter will be adrenocortical carcinomas. The likelihood that solid lesions 6 cm or more in diameter will be malignant is more difficult to estimate but it is probably in excess of 30 per cent. Metastatic carcinoma of the adrenal is also very uncommon but in the presence of a known primary malignancy elsewhere this becomes the most likely explanation for an incidentally detected solid adrenal lesion.

Careful clinical assessment is required to detect evidence of clinical or subclinical function but it is debated whether extensive biochemical evaluation is required in all cases. According to Ross and Aron, in the absence of certain clinical features of a functional tumour, biochemical exclusion of the diagnosis is unnecessary. For instance, virtually all patients with primary hyperaldosteronism have hypertension and in its absence biochemical exclusion is not required. Furthermore in hypertensive patients with an incidentally discovered adrenal mass the absence of spontaneous hypokalaemia has a 95 per cent negative predictive value for an aldosterone-producing adenoma and further biochemical exclusion is therefore not required. It is reasonable then to limit the initial studies directed towards the exclusion of function to plasma potassium, and 24-h urinary cortisol, catecholamine, and vanillylmandelic acid (VMA) excretion unless specific clinical evidence of function is present. In doubtful cases isotope scans such as NP59 and ^{131}I-MIBG* scans may also help to distinguish truly non-functional tumours from those with subclinical function. Evidence of hormone hypersecretion is an indication for operation.

The management of solid masses is controversial. It seems generally agreed that tumours 6 cm or more in diameter should be resected because they carry a high risk of malignancy and most surgeons would also agree that tumours less then 3 cm in diameter without biochemical evidence of function or any identifiable features of malignancy may be observed by CT. Evidence of growth should be an indication for operation but if they remain unchanged after repeated studies they are most likely to be benign, since carcinomas proliferate rapidly, and further studies are unnecessary. For tumours between 3 and 6 cm some surgeons advocate routine resection or selective resection based upon patient age (< 60 years for example) and operative risk but this policy involves high morbidity and expense with few patients benefiting from an earlier diagnosis of malignancy and it has not found general acceptance. Others routinely observe by repeated CT scans since the risk of malignancy is low and adenomas are not known to become malignant. MRI may help to distinguish adrenal metastases, phaeochromocytomas, and carcinomas from adrenal adenomas, lipomas, and cysts depending upon differences in signal intensities and may thus be helpful in determining whether operation should be advised. There is little evidence that MRI substantially improves diagnostic accuracy but it does increase the costs of investigation. One scheme for the management of 'incidentalomas' is presented in Fig. 4.

* *m*-Iodobenzylguanidine (MIBG) is an analogue of guanethidine that is structurally similar to noradrenaline and is taken up and concentrated in the adrenergic granules of the chromaffin cells in the adrenal medulla and sympathetic ganglia but it does not bind to postsynaptic receptors and therefore produces few pharmacological effects.

DISORDERS OF THE ADRENAL MEDULLA

The clinically important disorders of the adrenal medulla are tumours; the most important of these are neuroblastomas and phaeochromocytomas.

Neuroblastoma (see also Section 38.3.3)

Neuroblastomas occur almost exclusively in children and are the most common malignant tumours in neonates and infants less than 1 year old. The overall incidence is approximately 8 per million population per year with 50 per cent presenting within the first 2 years of life and about 75 per cent in the first 5 years. They arise from the neuroblasts of the adrenal medulla in roughly 50 per cent of cases or from the prevertebral or paravertebral ganglia from the neck to the pelvis.

The tumours have a variable appearance and may be irregular or nodular and range in size from 3 to 4 cm to massive retroperitoneal masses. They are very vascular, friable tumours and areas of haemorrhage, necrosis, and calcification are commonly found in larger examples. They tend to invade their capsule early and then infiltrate along tissue planes and perineural pathways. Frequently, however, the plane between an adrenal neuroblastoma and the kidney parenchyma remains intact and although structures such as the ureters, major vessels, and gut are often surrounded by tumour the lumen is rarely invaded. Neuroblastomas metastasize early to the prevertebral lymph nodes and by haematogenous spread to bone, bone marrow, and liver but pulmonary metastases are relatively rare. A peculiarity is that the bony orbit is frequently involved and this may produce proptosis and 'bruising' around the orbit.

A neuroblastoma may present with a wide range of symptoms and signs related to the varied sites of the primary and metastases. Abdominal pain may be a presenting symptom but it is often vague and difficult to assess in children. Sudden recognition of an abdominal mass, which is usually firm to hard, knobbly and irregular, and not particularly tender, is probably the most common mode of presentation. Some tumours produce biologically active peptides, for example VIP, which produce specific symptom clusters. The so called 'dumbbell' tumours may produce paralysis or other neurological signs in the lower limbs as a result of spinal cord compression or invasion. Metastases are present in over 50 per cent of cases at presentation and may produce symptoms including bone pain, or respiratory distress secondary to massive hepatomegaly.

Most tumours produce catecholamines and in 85 to 90 per cent of cases abnormal levels of urinary catecholamines or their metabolites may be detected. It should be noted however that benign ganglioneuromas can also raise the urinary catecholamine excretion. There are several serum tumour markers of neuroblastoma which may be particularly useful for monitoring disease activity. Neurone-specific enolase (NSE) is elevated in 95 per cent of cases with metastatic disease but only rarely so if the disease is localized, and high serum levels of the ganglioside Gd_2, which is expressed by virtually all neuroblastomas, are associated with active and advanced disease.

In investigation and staging of the tumour the minimum set of investigations should include liver and renal function tests, a chest radiograph and skeletal survey with orbital views, a bone scan, CT of the abdomen and pelvis, and a bone marrow aspirate. CT is

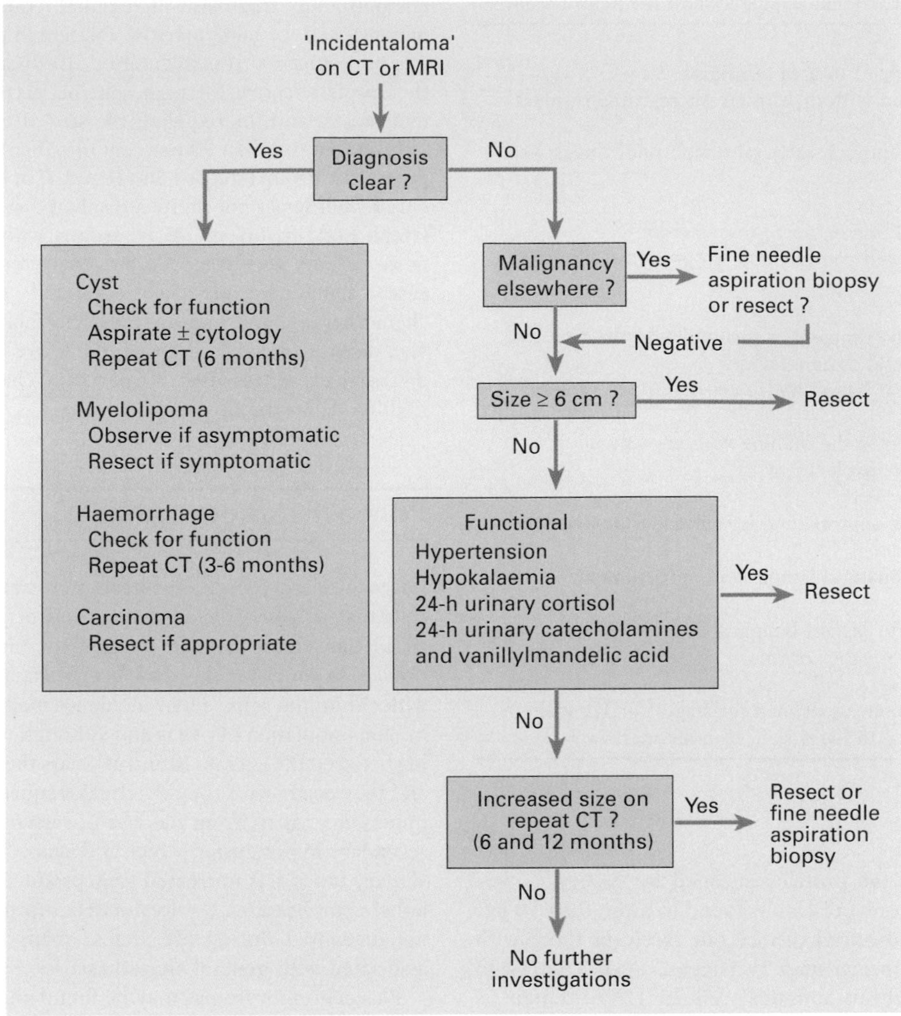

Fig. 4 A proposed management of adrenal 'incidentalomas'.

highly sensitive for abdominal masses and demonstration of lymph node involvement. MRI defines vessel encasement better than CT and provides superior imaging of the vertebral canal in the assessment of 'dumbbell' tumours. ^{131}I-MIBG scanning is also highly sensitive and is especially useful in the demonstration of metastases or recurrent tumour.

The prognosis in this condition is well known to be related to age and stage at presentation but other prognostic variables related to tumour biology have also been identified (Table 3). Tumours presenting in infancy have a relatively good prognosis even if they are relatively advanced and it is well documented that small tumours presenting during the first year of life have a fairly high incidence of spontaneous regression or maturation into a benign ganglioneuroma. Several staging systems have been used and that proposed by Evans in 1971 is perhaps the most widely used. However, this does not take into account the feasibility of surgical excision and more recently an international staging system for neuroblastoma (INSS) has been proposed which combines the Evans staging system and the results of surgical excision (Table 4). At all ages, stages I and II have a good prognosis and in infancy even stage III or IV disease is relatively favourable.

It is now recognized that up to 80 per cent of these tumours are associated with chromosomal abnormalities which have a bearing on the prognosis. Abnormalities of chromosome 1p are relatively common and associated with a relatively poor outcome. A single copy of the oncogene N-*myc* is normally present on the short arm of chromosome 2 but in many patients with a poor prognosis the N-*myc* gene appears to have been translocated to chromosome 1 and amplified resulting in the observed chromosome 1 abnormali-

Table 3 Prognostic factors in neuroblastoma

Factor	Good prognosis	Poor prognosis
Age	< 1 year	> 1 year
Stage	I and II all ages	III if > 1 year
	III and IVs if < 1 year	IV all ages
Chromosome 1p	Normal	Abnormal
N-*myc* oncogene	Single copy	Amplified
N-*myc* proteins	None detected	High levels
DNA content	Hyperploidy	Euploidy
Histology	Differentiated	Undifferentiated
		Stroma-poor
		Abnormal nuclear morphology
Urinary catecholamine metabolites	Low HVA:VMA	High HVA:VMA

Table 4 Proposed international staging system for neuroblastoma

Stage I
Localized tumour confined to area of origin
Complete gross excision with or without microscopic residual disease
Identifiable ipsilateral and contralateral lymph nodes negative microscopically
Stage IIa
Unilateral tumour with incomplete gross excision
Identifiable ipsilateral and contralateral lymph nodes negative microscopically
Stage IIb
Unilateral tumour with complete or incomplete gross excision with positive ipsilateral regional nodes
Identifiable contralateral lymph nodes negative microscopically
Stage III
Tumour infiltrating across the midline with or without regional lymph node involvement
or
Unilateral tumour with contralateral lymph node involvement
or
Midline tumour with bilateral lymph node involvement
Stage IV
Disseminated tumour to distant lymph nodes, bone, bone marrow, liver, and/or other organs
Stage IVs
Localized primary tumour as defined for stage I or IIa with dissemination limited to liver, skin, or bone marrow.

ties and high levels of the proteins encoded by N-*myc*. N-*myc* amplification and/or overexpression is found in more than 50 per cent of patients with advanced disease but rarely in those with stage I or II disease or special stage IV (stage IVs). In contrast to other tumours, in which an abnormal cellular DNA content is often associated with a poor outcome, in neuroblastomas hyperploidy is a favourable marker. Poorly differentiated tumours, especially those said to be stroma-poor and those with abnormal nuclear morphology, have a poor prognosis as do those with evidence of immature catecholamine synthesis as indicated by a high urinary homovanillic acid (HVA) to VMA ratio.

Treatment of a neuroblastoma usually requires a combined approach by surgeons and oncologists which is well planned and co-ordinated. Total surgical removal of localized disease is the most favourable outcome but when incomplete removal only is possible the tumour must be controlled with chemotherapy or radiotherapy. In disseminated disease surgery may initially be limited to establishing the diagnosis through biopsy of the primary and or metastases, although this may also be achieved by needle core biopsy. Delayed surgery may then be undertaken to assess the effectiveness of chemotherapy or radiotherapy and to excise residual tumour.

Chemotherapy seems to have made little impact upon advanced disease in older children even though cyclophosphamide, cisplatinum, doxorubicin, and tenopside have each been shown to produce complete or partial response rates of 35 to 45 per cent and some multidrug regimens have been curative in some patients with non-resectable localized disease. This is particularly disappointing given the dramatic results in the treatment of nephroblastoma and other tumours of childhood.

The use of radiotherapy has declined in recent times and currently it is used as primary therapy in combination with chemotherapy treatment of regional lymph nodes in infants or it may be used for bone marrow ablation in preparation for autologous bone marrow transplantation. In disseminated disease radiotherapy is effective for pain control, particularly that from bony metastases, and for reducing the size of troublesome metastases.

Overall more than 90 per cent of patients who fall into the good prognostic group (stages I and II and, if in infancy, stage III) can be cured whether or not there is residual disease following surgery or lymph node involvement. In groups with an intermediate prognosis (infants with stage IV, or older children with stage III disease) about 75 per cent respond to combined surgery, chemotherapy, and radiotherapy and more than 50 per cent survive disease free. Children over the age of 1 year with stage IV disease have a less than 20 per cent chance of survival despite multimodality therapy.

Phaeochromocytoma

Phaeochromocytomas are uncommon tumours of the chromaffin cells that secrete excessive quantities of catecholamines into the circulation. They are named from the Greek *phaeos* (dusky) and *chromos* (colour) for the dark brown staining of the tumour cells with chromium salts. Their incidence is approximately 1.5 to 2 per million population per year and although most commonly presenting between the ages of 20 and 50 years they may present at any age and they occur with roughly equal frequency in both sexes. Their importance, apart from the risk of malignancy, is that they cause secondary hypertension which if diagnosed early may be cured by surgery but if left untreated may produce serious and sometimes lethal complications. Unfortunately, up to one-third of cases are not diagnosed during life and in many of these cases death is associated with general anaesthesia for an unrelated procedure.

Phaeochromocytomas may be found anywhere from the neck to the pelvis, in the distribution of the neural crest-derived sympathetic/adrenal system. However, 80 to 90 per cent arise in the adrenal medulla and most extra-adrenal tumours (also known as paragangliomas) are intra-abdominal and arise in the region of the aortic bifurcation from the organ of Zuckerkandl. Overall only about 3 per cent of phaeochromocytomas are extra-abdominal and most of these are found in the paravertebral region in the chest but very rarely they may arise in the neck from the cervical ganglia.

The tumour may range in size from a few millimetres to a large cystic mass weighing approximately 3 kg but most tumours weigh less than 100 g, are between 3 and 5 cm in diameter, and are roughly spherical in shape. About 10 to 20 per cent are bilateral and this is more common in the familial varieties. Overall, 5 to 10 per cent are malignant and this is also more likely in familial phaeochromocytomas. In children phaeochromocytomas are less frequently malignant but a greater proportion are extra-adrenal, more are bilateral or multiple, and there is a greater chance of familial disease or an association with multiple endocrine neoplasia (MEN) syndromes.

Overall, between 10 and 20 per cent of phaeochromocytomas are familial and may be associated with some well known syndromes. These cases are more likely to present in childhood and are frequently (>50 per cent) multiple, or bilateral. In some, there is just a simple familial predisposition with an autosomal dominant pattern of inheritance without other associations. Others are associated with Sipple's syndrome also known as MEN type IIa (phaeochromocytoma, medullary carcinoma of the thyroid and C cell hyperplasia, and parathyroid hyperplasia or adenoma) or with MEN type IIb (phaeochromocytoma, medullary carcinoma of the thyroid and C cell hyperplasia, mucosal neuromata, and marfanoid features) both of which have an autosomal dominant pattern of inheritance. Approximately 5 per cent of patients with phaeochromocytoma have neurofibromatosis (von Recklinghausen's syndrome) that may be familial or sporadic but relatively few patients (approximately 1 per cent) with neurofibromatosis develop a phaeochromocytoma.

Phaeochromocytomas can present in many ways and this, combined with their relative rarity, explains why the diagnosis is often missed. Hypertension, which is commonly episodic, is the most consistent feature and is present in more than 90 per cent of cases. Two patterns are recognized: sustained hypertension with or without episodic rises which occurs in about 50 per cent of adults with phaeochromocytoma and paroxysmal attacks with normal blood pressure during the intervals. Most commonly both the systolic and diastolic pressures are elevated but if adrenaline is the major secretory product systolic hypertension and tachycardia may be associated with a normal or low diastolic pressure. A consistently normal blood pressure in the presence of a functioning tumour occurs in approximately 10 per cent of cases. It is not cost effective to screen all patients with hypertension since less than 1 per cent will have a phaeochromocytoma but hypertension in association with one or more of the other clinical features of phaeochromocytoma, or hypertension in children or young adults, should lead to appropriate screening tests.

The triad of headache, often sudden in onset and described as pounding, sweating, and tachycardia in a patient with hypertension is said to have high sensitivity and specificity (each in excess of 90 per cent) for phaeochromocytoma. Tremor, palpitations, and feelings of apprehension or anxiety are also common and the episodes may be associated with facial pallor or a mottled appearance to the skin. Attacks may occur several times per day or as infrequently as once a week. Most are short lived, lasting from 15 min to 1 h, and may be followed by feelings of exhaustion, weakness, and muscle aches. Various precipitating factors have been described which are often associated with a change in pressure on the tumour. In the case of abdominal phaeochromocytomas, straining at stool, lying in a particular position, bending over, or abdominal palpation have all been described as precipitating factors. Some drugs, for example metoclopramide, tricyclic antidepressants, or naloxone may precipitate dangerous hypertensive crises.

Other cardiovascular abnormalities are common and may be the first manifestation of a phaeochromocytoma. Patients may present with symptoms and signs of acute myocardial infarction, with myocarditis, with pulmonary oedema, or with arrhythmias that may be precipitated by anaesthesia, for unrelated surgery. Cardiovascular crises under anaesthesia especially, unexplained hypertension, tachycardia, oedema, or shock, should lead to performance of screening tests for phaeochromocytoma.

Neurological or psychiatric symptoms may also be presenting features as may strokes or seizures due to hypertension. Diabetes, due to the anti-insulin effect of catecholamines, and other endocrine abnormalities may occasionally dominate the clinical picture. Some phaeochromocytomas secrete parathyroid hormone, ACTH, or other biologically active peptides (for example VIP) each of which may produce an appropriate cluster of symptoms and signs. Some patients present with acute abdominal pain which is thought to be due to bowel ischaemia. Occasionally, however, abdominal pain may be due to haemorrhagic necrosis of the tumour which may precipitate marked hypertension followed by hypotension, shock, and even death as a consequence of sudden withdrawal of catecholamines resulting in arterial and venous dilatation in the presence of a shrunken intravascular volume.

Physical signs of phaeochromocytoma other than hypertension are relatively uncommon. In approximately 50 per cent of cases, hypertension is associated with postural hypotension that is probably a consequence of impaired orthostatic autonomic reflexes resulting from chronic overexposure to catecholamines. A large phaeochromocytoma may be palpable as an abdominal mass. Café-au-lait patches and neurofibromata may be associated with phaeochromocytoma and the thyroid should be examined for carcinoma.

Evaluation of suspected phaeochromocytoma

The most useful diagnostic tests for phaeochromocytoma are measurement of 24-h urinary excretion of noradrenaline, adrenaline, and their metabolites (normetadrenaline, metadrenaline and vanillylmandelic acid). Noradrenaline is generally the major secretory product but occasionally adrenaline, and rarely dopamine, may predominate. Although it has been suggested that adrenaline secretion may indicate an adrenal tumour it is clear that extra-adrenal phaeochromocytomas can also secrete adrenaline and thus the spectrum of catecholamine secretion is not a reliable guide to the site. In most cases excessive excretion of at least one catecholamine or metabolite will be detected but the pattern of abnormality is quite variable and assays of any one of them (for example vanillylmandelic acid) to the exclusion of the others may be misleading. In some cases repeated assays may be required to make the diagnosis especially when the symptoms are sporadic or if clinical suspicion is high in the presence of a negative or equivocal result. Ideally the urine collection should be begun immediately after an attack.

The place of assays for plasma catecholamines is disputed but there is evidence that small tumours may release predominantly unmetabolized catecholamines into the circulation and may be best diagnosed by direct measurement of circulating catecholamines. Overall, assays for plasma catecholamines, urinary metadrenaline and normetadrenaline, or urinary vanillylmandelic acid each have a very high positive predictive value but combinations of tests give the greatest diagnostic accuracy. False-positive results may occur in patients taking certain drugs (phenothiazines, methyldopa, or monoamine oxidase inhibitors, for example) or with excessive intakes of tea, coffee, or chocolate and rebound hypertension with high levels of circulating and urinary catecholamines may occur following withdrawal of clonidine.

Occasionally it may be necessary to distinguish between patients with a phaeochromocytoma and equivocally elevated plasma or urinary catecholamines and patients without a phaeochromocytoma who have excessive activity of the sympathetic nervous system. If clinical suspicion is high provocation or suppression tests may be performed but provocation tests must be undertaken with considerable caution because dangerous hypertensive crises may be precipitated. In the glucagon stimulation test, which is relatively free of adverse effects, a positive result is indicated by a clear increase in plasma catecholamines 1 to 3 min after administration of the drug. The clonidine suppression test relies upon the capacity of clonidine to inhibit neurogenically mediated catecholamine release. In patients with a phaeochromocytoma clonidine fails to suppress plasma catecholamine levels but the test should be administered with caution since clonidine suppression may result in hypotension and it should not be undertaken on patients with volume depletion or those already treated with β-blockers.

After the diagnosis has been established biochemically, localization of the tumour is important in order to confirm the diagnosis and to assist in the planning of the surgical approach. Modern non-invasive imaging can safely detect and localize virtually all tumours. CT of the abdomen and pelvis is the preferred modality since it will detect the majority of tumours. Whether it is positive or negative, however, a ^{131}I-MIBG scan provides useful additional anatomical and functional information and may locate occult second tumours or metastases to bone, liver, or lung. Preoperative CT and ^{131}I-MIBG together will locate more than 95 per cent of tumours. The place of MRI is less clear but it does have certain advantages over CT scan in relation to *in-vivo* tissue characterization. Phaeochromocytomas produce a high T_2-weighted signal intensity unlike other tumours in which the signal intensity is low and it may be possible to distinguish a phaeochromocytoma from other adrenal masses. Unfortunately malignant and benign phaeochromocytomas have the same MRI signal and cannot be distinguished. MRI can, however, distinguish tumour from surrounding vascular structures without the need for the administration of contrast and since there is no exposure to X-rays MRI is the investigation of choice in pregnancy. Older methods of localization, such as intravenous pyelography or venous catheterization and selective sampling at sites along the inferior and superior vena cavae, are rarely used today. Both are invasive and can provoke release of catecholamine and development of dangerous hypertensive crises. Occasionally venous sampling is used in subjects in whom clinical and biochemical tests strongly suggest phaeochromocytoma but radiological studies fail to identify the tumour. Several days before embarking upon this investigation adequate α- and β-adrenergic receptor blockade should be established.

Treatment

In most cases the appropriate treatment for phaeochromocytoma is surgery following medical therapy to prevent cardiovascular complications and reduce the risks of operative intervention. The medical preparation and anaesthesia is a critical aspect of surgery for phaeochromocytoma and is discussed in detail in Section 11.4.

The results of surgery are generally good with 75 to 90 per cent of patients cured of their hypertension and free of the risk of recurrent disease. However, the surgery is risky and close attention to management in the perioperative period is essential. In skilled centres the operative mortality is about 3 per cent. Several postoperative complications require special mention. Hypotension may result from marked arterial and venous dilatation following the sudden withdrawal of catecholamines and may be compounded by inadequate volume loading. The primary treatment here should be volume replacement rather than pressor agents. Hypoglycaemia may occur as a result of withdrawal of the anti-insulin effect of catecholamines and this may manifest as postoperative hypotension resistant to volume replacement and vasopressors. Finally if the arterial blood pressure does not return to normal within about 2 weeks of surgery evidence of residual phaeochromocytoma or metastases should be sought by checking urinary or plasma catecholamines. Persistent hypertension may be due to hypertensive vascular disease or coexistent essential hypertension and if the catecholamine levels remain elevated the clonidine suppression test should distinguish those cases in which the hypertension is under neurogenic control. Patients should generally be followed for life with annual blood pressure checks and catecholamine studies.

Malignant phaeochromocytoma

The diagnosis of malignancy depends upon clinical or macroscopic pathological evidence of local invasion or the presence of metastases (usually in the liver, lung, or bone) rather than on histological criteria. Histology may be misleading because the usual features of malignancy (nuclear pleiomorphism, giant cells, frequent mitotic figures, and capsular invasion) may all occur in tumours that subsequently follow a benign course. DNA ploidy, however, may prove to be a useful discriminatory test since it has been reported that benign phaeochromocytomas tend to have diploid DNA content whereas malignant tumours are hyperdiploid. High plasma or urinary dopamine levels are suggestive, but not diagnostic, of malignancy.

Malignant phaeochromocytomas tend to be slow growing tumours and evidence of recurrence, or of malignancy following excision of an apparently benign tumour, may occur many years after surgery. Following excision some patients survive for more than 20 years but the overall 5-year survival is about 45 per cent.

Whenever possible surgical excision or debulking of the tumour should be attempted. Some patients will be cured, and debulking facilitates the medical control of symptoms since the level of catecholamine secretion is proportional to the size of the tumour. If there is residual catecholamine secretion then medical therapy aims to control the effects of circulating catecholamines by α- and β-adrenergic receptor blockade, often supplemented with calcium channel blockade, and to inhibit the synthesis of catecholamines using α-methyltyrosine. This 'false' catecholamine precursor inhibits tyrosine hydroxylase which is the rate limiting enzyme for catecholamine synthesis.

Although malignant phaeochromocytomas respond poorly to chemotherapy or radiotherapy combination chemotherapy with cyclophosphamide, vincristine, and dacarbazine may produce temporary control in some patients and administration of ^{131}I-MIBG to ablate residual primary or secondary deposits has produced short-term remission or palliation in some cases but evidence of a significant long-lasting benefit is lacking.

SURGERY OF THE ADRENAL GLAND

The history of adrenal surgery begins in 1889 when Thornton resected a large adrenal tumour *en bloc* with the kidney in a young woman with hirsuitism. In 1914 Sargent performed the first planned operation to remove an adrenal tumour causing Cushing's syndrome and in 1926 César Roux in Lausanne and Charles Mayo in Rochester independently removed phaeochromocytomas. In the 1950s after the discovery of cortisone subtotal or total bilateral adrenalectomy was performed for adrenal hyperplasia and for pituitary dependent Cushing's syndrome. However, this procedure was associated with high surgical morbidity, 2 to 5 per cent operative mortality, and the need for life-long replacement therapy and has now been largely abandoned. Occasionally surgical ablation of the adrenals is still used in Cushing's disease or in the treatment of hormonally dependent tumours such as breast carcinoma.

Today the indications for adrenalectomy are largely restricted to resection of the various adrenal neoplasia. With modern imaging exploratory operations have become virtually obsolete and a carefully planned approach to adrenal surgery is almost always possible. There are several operative approaches to the adrenal glands and each has its own particular indications. The choice of approach depends upon the adrenal pathology and indications for operation, the size and shape of the patient, and the experience and familiarity of the surgeon with the various options.

The posterior extraperitoneal approach was first described over 50 years ago and is still used for selected patients. The original 'hockey stick' incision, however, is now rarely used and an oblique incision through the bed of the 11th or 12th rib is usually employed. The advantages of this approach are that it is direct, and relatively atraumatic, which minimizes postoperative pain, and both glands can be exposed simultaneously. The main disadvantage is that the operative field is relatively restricted which limits its usefulness to resection of small lesions such as adenomas less than 5 cm in diameter. It is not suitable for removal of large adrenal lesions (> 5 cm) or potentially malignant tumours. Retroperitoneal exposure of the adrenal through the flank is rarely indicated but it may be the preferred route in obese patients with Cushing's syndrome in whom only one gland needs to be explored.

The transabdominal approach, by an extended subcostal or bilateral subcostal incision, provides excellent exposure of both glands, if necessary, as well as the abdominal organs and the retroperitoneum. This approach is indicated for large lesions or potentially malignant tumours and it is mandatory for the resection of a phaeochromocytoma since it allows for early vascular control and for the possibility of bilateral, multiple, or extra-adrenal tumours. A midline approach may be used for extra-adrenal tumours in the organ of Zuckerkandl or the pelvis.

A thoracoabdominal approach provides outstanding exposure of the adrenal, but exposure of the contralateral gland is more difficult than by the anterior transabdominal route, and it is generally reserved for very large tumours that cannot be removed by the anterior approach.

FURTHER READING

Adrenal Surgery. *Urol Clin N Am* 1989; **16(3)**: 417–606.

Gajraj H, Young AE. Adrenal incidentaloma. *Br J Surg* 1993; **80**: 422–6.

Ross NS, Aron DC. Hormonal evaluation of the patient with an incidentally discovered adrenal mass. *N Engl J Med* 1990; **323**: 1401–5.

Smith EI, Castelbury RP. Neuroblastoma. *Curr Probl Surg* 1990; **XXVII(9)**: 573–620.

Thompson NW, Cheung PSY. Diagnosis and treatment of functioning and nonfunctioning adrenocortical neoplasms including incidentalomas. *Surg Clin N Am* 1987; **67(2)**: 423–6.

11.4 Preoperative preparation of patients with phaeochromocytoma

LEN E. S. CARRIE

There are two main dangers of operating on unprepared phaeochromocytomas.

1. Outpouring of catecholamines from the tumour due to preoperative anxiety, to anaesthesia or especially as a result of surgical handling of the tumour leading to severe hypertension or arrhythmias.
2. Profound hypotension as a result of sudden expansion of the vascular bed after clamping of the last venous drainage from the tumour.

Most phaeochromocytomas are predominantly noradrenaline secreting, but not only does the proportion of noradrenaline to adrenaline vary from case to case, but also the lability of the tumour, i.e. the readiness with which it secretes catecholamines. Because of this, some tumours appear docile even during handling at surgery, and case reports abound describing apparently successful regimens of preparation of the patient. However, phaeochromocytomas are unpredictable and it is better to use one basic, effective technique of preoperative preparation modified as appropriate to suit each case. This is best achieved by giving drugs which block the α- and β-adrenergic effects of catecholamines independently. The most useful long-acting α-blocking agent is phenoxybenzamine, which when given by mouth does not reach its peak effect for 12 to 24 h. Treatment with this drug should therefore be instituted at least 48 h before adding a β-blocking agent, as a surge of catecholamine output in the absence of β-adrenergic activity may result in a very high blood pressure due to lack of β-induced vasodilatation. There is a wider choice of β-blocking drugs, but one of the longer-acting, cardioselective agents such as atenolol or metoprolol may give smoother control. Labetalol, a mixed α- and β-blocking agent, can be used, but has the disadvantage of providing the α- and β-blockade in fixed proportions, with the latter predominating, the reverse of that required to treat the α-effects arising from the noradrenaline secreted by most tumours.

Some idea of the adequacy of α-blockade can be obtained by sequential haematocrit measurements, which fall as the blood volume expands. However, the most reliable method of assessing the adequacy of both α- and β-blockade is simply by charting the patient's pulse and blood pressure two-hourly (except during sleep) for several days. The blood pressure should be recorded both lying and standing, and use of different colours aids graphic representation. In addition, the pulse and blood pressure should be recorded if the patient has any symptomatic episode. The aim with effective treatment is a chart showing a steady pulse rate in the 60 to 70 beats/min range with no episodes of tachycardia and a blood pressure also devoid of surges, with a small postural drop. Because of the slow onset of adequate α-blockade and its associated increase in blood volume, at least a week is required for effective preoperative preparation. Changes in phenoxybenzamine should not be made more often than once daily. In a few cases, effective control of the blood pressure may be very resistant to adrenergic blocking drugs alone and other antihypertensive drugs, e.g. calcium channel blocking agents and ACE inhibitors may be added. α-Methyltyrosine, which inhibits tyrosine hydroxylase, the enzyme involved in the conversion of tyrosine to dopa—an essential step in the synthesis of both adrenaline and noradrenaline—may help stabilize blood pressure in difficult cases.

FURTHER READING

Brown MJ. Phaeochromocytoma. In: Weatherall DJ, Ledingham JGG, Warrell DA, eds. *Oxford Textbook of Medicine*. 3rd Edn. Oxford: University Press, 1994, in press.

Hull CJ. Phaeochromocytoma. Diagnosis, preoperative preparation and anaesthetic management. *Br J Anaesthesia*, 1986; **58**: 1453–68.

Sheps SS, Jiang N-S, Klee GG, Van Heerden JA. Recent developments in the diagnosis and treatment of pheochromocytoma. *Mayo Clin Proc*, 1990; **65**: 88–95.

The breast 12

12.1 Benign conditions of the breast

MICHAEL J. GREENALL

The demand for specialist treatment of patients with breast disease is increasing for several reasons. Firstly, the subject has become more complex, and an integrated approach involving not only surgeons but also radiologists, radiotherapists, pathologists, and medical oncologists is necessary. Secondly, the scope of the subject has increased dramatically. Not long ago the majority of surgeons who dealt with breast disease perceived their role as little more than differentiating benign conditions from malignancy and treating the latter. Patients now demand specific management of benign disorders which were previously ignored. Increased understanding of the relationship between benign and malignant disease has increased awareness of conditions previously dismissed as 'benign changes', mastitis or fibroadenosis. Finally, the development of new therapeutic and diagnostic methods such as screening, breast conservation, and adjuvant chemotherapy has increased the complexity of the management of breast cancer itself.

Many institutions have now developed specialized breast disease units, housing surgeons with a special interest and training.

ANATOMY AND PHYSIOLOGY OF THE BREAST

Development

The breasts are modified sweat glands in that they are embryologically derived from a downward growth of ectoderm into the underlying mesenchyme. The first stage of development occurs at 6 or 8 weeks of gestation, when two strips of thickened ectoderm, the mammary ridges, grow in a line extending from the embryonal axilla to the inguinal region. In many animals breasts develop along the whole length of this ridge, but in humans true breast tissue occurs only in the pectoral region.

Branching epithelial cords appear as 15 to 20 buds, which eventually become lactiferous ducts and associated alveoli. Each cord becomes surrounded by a connective tissue stroma of mesenchymally derived fat, connective tissue, and vascular tissue. These cords form the basis of the segmental pattern of the adult breast.

Towards the end of gestation the lactiferous ducts become canalized and open on to a pit in the epidermis. At the same time mesenchymal proliferation beneath the epidermis allows nipple development; failure to do so results in inversion.

Lobular development within the breast occurs particularly at puberty, with the ultimate development of 15 to 20 lobes, each of which drains into a single lactiferous duct; true secretory alveoli develop only during pregnancy and lactation.

Few changes occur in the early years of childhood. However, at the age of 10 there is growth of mammary tissue beneath the areola. This produces a characteristic protuberance on the chest wall called the breast bud or mound. True nipple development occurs at about the age of 12, followed 2 or 3 years later by further subareolar growth and formation of the bulk of the breast tissue. Finally, there is areolar recession, resulting in the classical shape of the adult breast. These changes at puberty are a result of the action of follicle stimulating hormone and luteinizing hormone, produced by hypothalmic stimulation of the pituitary gland on oestrogen production from the ovary.

THE ANATOMY OF THE ADULT BREAST

Gross anatomy

Although the adult breast varies greatly in size its base is fairly consistent anatomically, extending from the second to the sixth rib in the midclavicular line and overlying the pectoralis major, serratus anterior, and external oblique muscles. Medially, the breasts reach the sternal edge and laterally the mid-axillary line. The pyramidally shaped axillary tail extends into the axilla.

The fascial covering of the breast is of importance with respect to surgical technique. As it develops from the skin the breast is invested with superficial fascia which divides into two layers. The anterior layer provides a plane of dissection subcutaneously between the relatively small subcutaneous fat lobules and the larger lobules of mammary fat. The posterior layer of superficial fascia abuts against the deep fascia derived from the pectoralis major and serratus anterior, thus producing a potential space. This retromammary space is easily located surgically (Fig. 1).

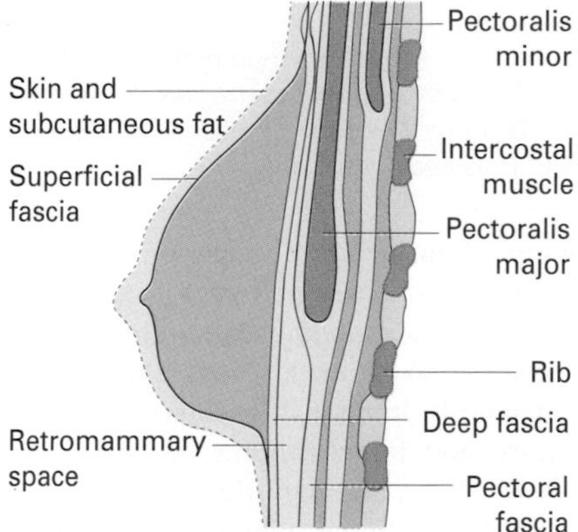

Fig. 1 The fascial coverings of the breast.

Between the two layers of superficial fascia there are condensations of fibrous tissue. These form the suspensory ligaments of Cooper which both divide the breast into lobes and act as a supportive framework.

Blood supply

The breast has a rich vascular supply from the internal mammary artery and from the thoracoacromial, subscapular, and lateral thoracic branches of the axillary artery. The main supply is via the second perforating branch of the internal mammary and lateral thoracic arteries; the former should be preserved during subcutaneous mastectomy.

The regional venous drainage forms a rich subareolar plexus which drains via the intercostal, internal mammary, and axillary veins.

Lymphatic drainage

The lymphatic drainage of the breast has obvious implications in the management of breast cancer and has been well documented in an elegant series of studies by Turner-Warwick.

Approximately 75 per cent of the lymphatic vessels drain to the 30 or so regional lymph nodes in front of and below the axillary vein. These nodes can conveniently be subdivided into three main groups according to their relationship with the pectoralis minor muscle; nodes at level 1 lie below the muscle, level 2 lymph glands lie behind it, and those of level 3 are in the apex of the axilla above the muscle. The majority of lymph drains from nodes at level 1 sequentially to those at levels 2 and 3; a small amount drains to the subscapular and interpectoral (Rotter's) groups of nodes. Extension of tumour to these latter nodes may imply retrograde spread and heavy involvement of axillary nodes by metastases (Fig. 2).

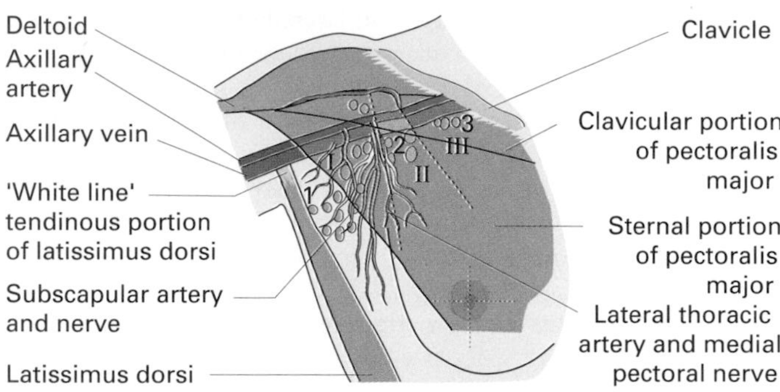

Fig. 2 The anatomy of the axilla showing lymph node groups, major vessels and nerves. (1) Most lateral border of level 1 at medial border of latissimus dorsi. (2) Central portion of level 2. (3) Most medial border of level 3 at Halstead's ligament.

A small amount of lymph drains from the superior aspect of the breast directly to the apical nodes. These pathways account in part for the well-documented, but relatively unusual, findings of nodal disease at level 3 but negative nodes in the lower axillary chain.

About 25 per cent of lymph drains to the internal mammary nodes in the second, third and fourth intercostal spaces. Such drainage is from the whole breast, although the majority of these pathways arise in its medial half. Some lymph drains to the opposite breast and down the rectus sheath. Drainage to the contralateral axilla and to intercostal nodes via the pectoral fascia is, however, minor. Similarly, there are few direct lymphatic communications between the breast and the lymph nodes above the axillary vein.

The distribution of major lymphatics accompanies the blood supply. The original description by Sappey in 1885 of a subareolar plexus which receives lymph centripetally and which then redirects it to the axilla has been discounted.

Innervation

The nervous supply to the breast is primarily by sensory and sympathetic nerves. Little parasympathetic innervation has been demonstrated. The nipple has a rich sensory supply whereas the majority of sympathetic innervation is to breast parenchyma.

Microscopic anatomy

The microscopic anatomy of the breast is a complex subject that has been the source of much controversy and confusion. Basically, there is a system of major ducts arranged in a segmental and radial pattern. These lead to the secretory component of the breast—the terminal ductal–lobular unit (TDLV). The breast is thus subdivided into lobes, although these are not precisely defined anatomically. The interlobar fascia (the most prominent of which are Cooper's ligaments) is dense and fibrous, whereas the periductal and intralobular connective tissue is much more loose and vascular. The connective tissue round the lobule is particularly loose, allowing expansion during pregnancy and lactation (Fig. 3).

The 'terminal ductule' of the terminal ductal-lobular unit has two components (Fig. 4). One lies outside the lobule and is known

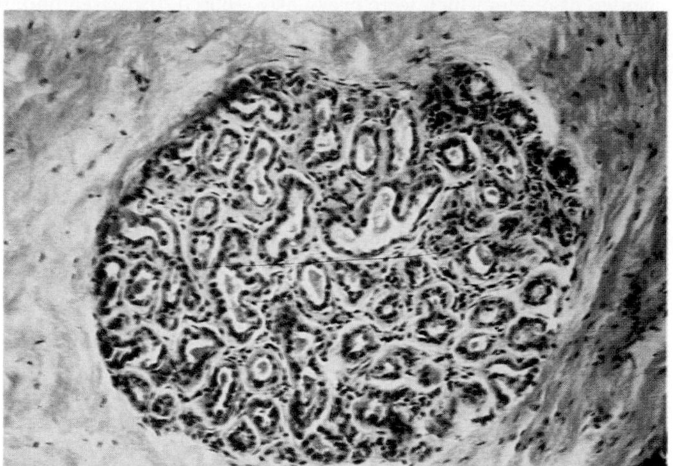

Fig. 3 A normal lobule composed of multiple acini with surrounding loose connective tissue. (By courtesy of Dr D. Tarin.)

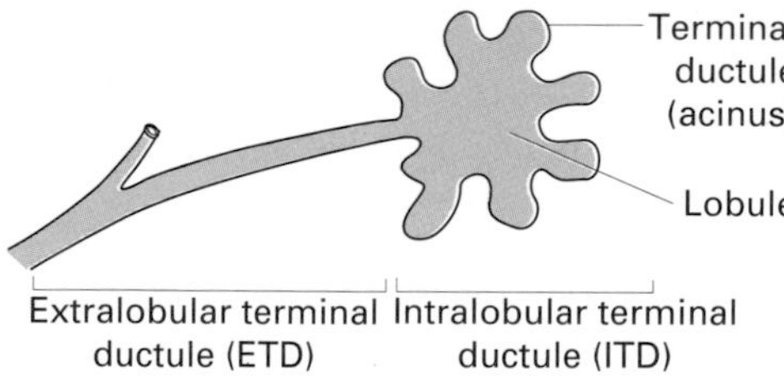

Fig. 4 The structure of the terminal ductal lobular unit (TDLU).

as the extralobular terminal ductule (ETD), whereas the other lies within the lobule (intralobular terminal ductule, ITD). The terminal ramifications of the latter form the secretory units of the breast (terminal ductules or acini), in a manner morphologically similar to the terminal units of respiratory alveoli in the lung.

The whole subject is complex because of difficulties with nomenclature. The term 'terminal duct' has been used for both the smallest epithelial unit in the lobule and the largest duct that opens on to the nipple surface. The same term has been used interchangeably with 'tertiary duct', 'ductule', and 'terminal ductule'. The problem is compounded by some authors wishing to retain the term 'acinous' only for those terminal units during breast feeding.

Histologically, that part of the duct system adjacent to the skin of the nipple is lined with stratified squamous epithelium. However, there is a sudden change to a double layer of columnar or cuboidal epithelium which characterizes the remainder of the duct system. The terminal ductules (acini) can undergo secretory changes and therefore have a role of both transport and secretion.

Between the epithelial cell layers and the basement membrane is a network of myoepithelial cells. These respond to oxytocin and are responsible for milk ejection during lactation.

PHYSIOLOGICAL CHANGES IN THE BREAST

Changes during the menstrual cycle

Despite widespread anecdotal belief to the contrary there is little evidence of substantial histological changes occurring in the breast throughout the different phases of the menstrual cycle. Retention of fluid may occur during the luteal phase, but this does not appear to be associated with morphological change.

Changes during pregnancy and lactation

The main histological change that occurs in the breast during pregnancy is lobular-alveolar growth and the development of new secretory units. This gives rise to the characteristic microscopic description of 'adenosis of pregnancy'. (Fig. 5). It is characterized

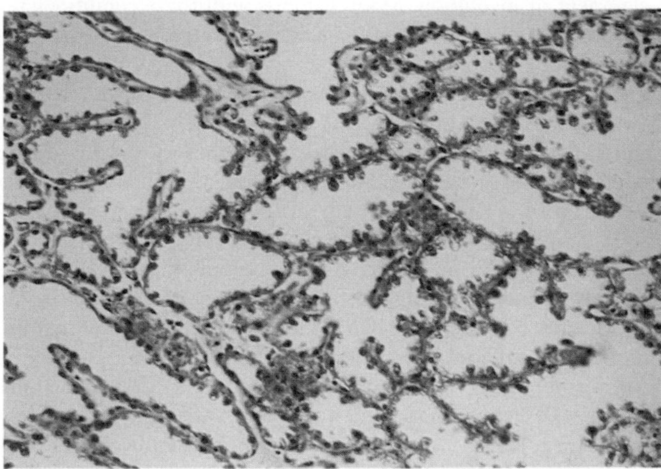

Fig. 5 Adenosis of pregnancy. There is alveolar dilation and additional secretory units (by courtesy of Dr D. Tarin).

histologically by alveolar dilatation and conversion of the resting two-layer epithelium to a monolayer, which demonstrates secretory changes within it. Colostrum formation, capillary growth, vascular engorgement, and myoepithelial cell hypertrophy are also apparent as pregnancy progresses. There is a doubling of breast weight from about 200 to 400 g, much of which is due to fluid retention. These changes occur under the influence of increased levels of luteal and placental sex hormones, placental lactogens, and chorionic gondotrophins.

Although some colostrum is formed within the breast during pregnancy true milk is not produced until about 2 days after parturition. This occurs due to the high postpartum levels of prolactin, which are maintained despite falling levels of other sex hormones which normally inhibit lactogenesis. During lactation the alveoli are distended with milk, the cells become cuboidal in shape and there is a resultant diminution of the intralobular space.

Following cessation of breast feeding there is gradual return to

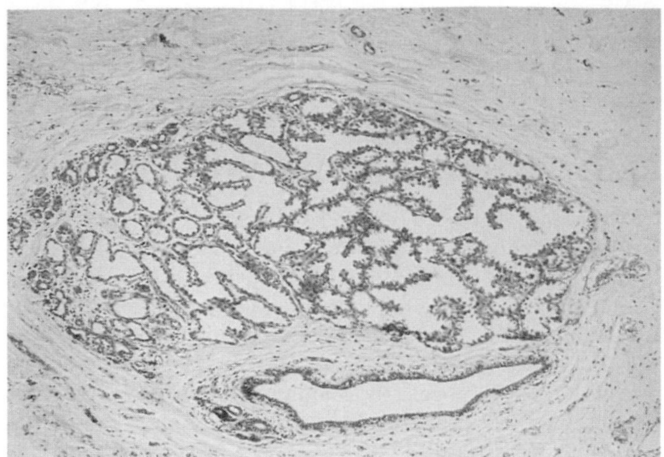

Fig. 6 Postlactational change. In one area of the lobule is adenosis of pregnancy. Elsewhere there is decrease in the number of acini, increased amount of fibrous tissue and lymphocytic infiltration (by courtesy of Dr D. Tarin).

the non-pregnant state. This process may take as little as 3 months, but in some individuals may take much longer. This process, known as post-lactational involution, is characterized histologically by lymphocytic infiltration and hyalinization of the lobules (Fig. 6). There is, however, little or no reduction in the number of ducts and lobules present.

Changes at the menopause

Involutional changes occur from about the age of 35, with regression of glandular tissue and its replacement by fat and fibrosis. Before the age of 50 this process is characterized by loss of some lobular tissue; in older women progression of this process results in the almost complete replacement of lobular tissue by collagen and fat. The end result is that although major duct systems are visible few lobules are seen. This is in contrast to post-lactational involution, which is characterized by minimal loss of lobular units.

Changes at the menopause have two important clinical implications. Firstly, fat infiltration of the breast produces the low density appearance of breast parenchyma seen on mammography, and thus makes this technique more successful in older woman. Secondly aberrations of this involutional change may explain some of the benign disorders that occur in this age group.

BREAST MILK

It is not the purpose of the present discussion to elaborate on the advantages and disadvantages of breast feeding. However, breast milk from a healthy mother allows normal development of an infant for 6 months or longer without need for any supplementation. In many underdeveloped countries breast feeding provides a major source of nutrition for the infant for up to 2 years. Breast feeding will continue despite a poor nutritional state of the mother.

Breast milk has a relatively low protein content; that which is present is in the form of casein and lactoglobulin. Carbohydrate is present as lactose, and fat as triglyceride. Human breast milk is rich in vitamins C and D and is a source of IgA. It is therefore important in helping provide an immune mechanism for the newborn.

A number of drugs are excluded in breast milk; this should always be taken into account when prescribing for breast feeding women. Of particular importance are alcohol, barbiturates, anticoagulants, tetracycline, and metronidazole.

BENIGN BREAST DISEASE

Until recently benign disorders of the breast were regarded as relatively unimportant: far more attention was focused on breast cancer. This has resulted in many patients with benign breast disease receiving rather scant attention from clinicians, and there has been relatively little academic investigation into this complex subject. Benign breast disease has also suffered from the major disadvantage of a hopelessly confusing terminology, inadequate classification, and poor correlation between clinical, radiological, and pathological features.

During the past decade there has been increasing interest in benign breast disease for a number of reasons. Firstly, patients demand investigation and treatment for symptoms of benign breast disease. This has, in turn, increased the number of women referred to specialist breast disease units; these have participated in scientific studies on the classification and treatment of their condition. Secondly there is the question of premalignant disorders and histological features which may imply an increased risk of breast cancer. Increasing understanding of these conditions may prove important in understanding the pathogenesis of breast cancer and in defining high risk groups in whom regular surveillance may be beneficial. Finally, the recently introduced breast screening programmes are likely to present pathologists and clinicians with as yet ill-defined histological entities which may be of importance in understanding the development of invasive cancer and its eventual treatment.

Classification of benign breast disease

There is no completely satisfactory classification of benign breast disease. Previous attempts have been based on a number of different factors such as clinical symptoms, patient age, histological features, or that part of the secretory system in which the abnormality has arisen. They all have inherent disadvantages. Firstly, there is poor correlation between clinical, pathological, and radiological features in any particular case. Secondly, benign breast disorders encompass a wide spectrum of clinicopathological features ranging from near normality to severe disease. Finally, the breast must be regarded as a physiologically dynamic structure in which cyclical variations are superimposed on changes of development and involution throughout the woman's life. These physiological changes may themselves be so extensive that they may fall outside what is regarded as the normal spectrum. The histological features of an individual abnormality must therefore be evaluated within the context of a wide range of normality.

It has therefore been suggested that the broad concept of benign breast disease should be reconsidered. Many so-called diseases of the breast might now be regarded more accurately as disorders that are based on aberrations of the processes of development, cyclical change and involution (ANDI). This does not mean that benign breast disease does not occur, but that the term should be reserved for disorders of such severity that they are frankly abnormal. This concept is, of course, rather ill-defined and will depend on interpretation and perception by both patient and clinician.

Aberrations of normal development and involution can account for many, if not all, benign breast disorders. A simplified system based on the various stages of physiological change (development, cyclical change, pregnancy, lactation, and involution) is shown in Table 1. It follows that most conditions listed under 'benign breast disorders' can be regarded as minor aberrations or normal development or involution. Many patients with these conditions require reassurance rather than specific treatment and explanation that they do not have a disease.

This approach is well demonstrated in patients with cyclical mastalgia and nodularity. The vast majority of premenopausal women experience a degree of breast discomfort and increasing nodularity prior to menstruation. For most, this amounts to little more than an inconvenience and is regarded as a normal physiological process. About 2 or 3 per cent of women are referred to a clinic with cyclical mastalgia, the symptoms of which are more severe, with distressing discomfort lasting a week or more. In the past all such patients, with either mild or severe symptoms, were described as suffering from 'fibrocystic disease' although there is little histological evidence of either fibrosis or cyst formation. Despite exhaustive investigation there is little evidence of any specific histological abnormality in women with cyclical breast pain, and if abnormal microscopic features are observed they correlate poorly with clinical features. Cyclical mastalgia and

Table 1 Classification of the pathogenesis of non-malignant breast disease based on the concept of aberration of normal development and involution

Physiological state of the breast	Normal	Benign disorder	Benign disease
Development	Duct development	Nipple inversion	Mammary fistula
	Lobular development	Fibroadenoma	Giant fibroadenoma
	Stomal development	Adolescent hypertrophy	
Cyclical change	Hormonal activity	Mastalgia and nodularity	
	Epithelial activity	Benign papilloma	
Pregnancy and lactation	Epithelial hyperplasia	Blood-stained discharge	
	Lactation	Galactocele	
Involution	Ductal involution	Duct ectasia, nipple retraction	Periductal mastitis with suppuration
	Lobular involution	Cysts, sclerosing adenosis	
	Involutional epithelial hyperplasia	Hyperplasia and micropapillomatosis	Lobular and ductal hyperplasia with atypia

Severe forms of the benign disorder may indicate a disease.

nodularity, like other benign breast conditions, must be regarded in their broadest terms.

Symptoms of benign breast disease

Despite the complexity of its classification there are relatively few presenting symptoms of benign breast disease. Symptoms fall into three main groups: breast pain, lumps, and disorders of the nipple and periareolar region. Infection of the breast causes further symptoms. As has been previously stated, attempts to correlate pathological and radiological findings with clinical features are a cause of much confusion and should be discouraged. A working clinical classification of benign breast disease is shown in Table 2, although it must be stressed that this does not imply whether the process is physiological or pathological, and in no way does it attempt to correlate symptoms with pathological features.

Table 2 Symptoms of benign breast disease

Breast pain (mastalgia)
- Cyclical
- Primary non-cyclical
  - Musculoskeletal
  - Sclerosing adenosis
  - Postoperative
  - Cervical root pain

Breast lumps
- Fibroadenoma
- Cyclical nodularity
- Cysts
- Galactocele
- Sclerosing adenosis
- Fat necrosis
- Lipoma
- Chronic abscess
- Normal structures (prominent rib, edge of previous breast biopsy, margin of breast tissue, etc.)

Disorders of the nipple and periareolar region
- Discharge
- Retraction
- Sepsis

Breast infection
- Lactational
- Non-lactational

Finally it must be remembered that the reason for many referrals is anxiety on the part of either the patient or her doctor. The accounts for the increasing number of patients seen with non-breast conditions, including skin rashes and chest wall pain. It is an important function of any breast clinic not only to treat symptoms but to allay the patient's fears of breast cancer.

Breast pain (mastalgia)

Pain is the most common reason for referral to a breast clinic and accounts for up to 50 per cent of patients seen. It is, however, the least understood of all breast symptoms, and the one whose management causes most controversy.

Literature on breast pain is often anecdotal, uncontrolled, and of poor quality. Nomenclature poses a major problem: a number of different terms such as mastitis, mastodynia, and mazoplasia, have been used to describe breast pain. Mastalgia has also been correlated with specific histological criteria, resulting in its description as 'fibrocystic disease', although this has lost favour for reasons described above.

It must be stressed that mastalgia is a symptom and does not imply any specific pathological process, any more than does pain in other sites of the body.

Classification of breast pain

Attempts to classify breast pain are surprisingly recent. There are two distinct group of patients with these symptoms (Table 2). One group of patients have symptoms which bear a definite relationship to the menstrual cycle (cyclical mastalgia); in the remainder there is no such correlation (non-cyclical mastalgia). Non-cyclical mastalgia has recently been reclassified to distinguish pain in the breast from that originating in surrounding tissues such as the chest wall.

Cyclical mastalgia

This is the most common type of breast pain, accounting for 40 per cent of all cases referred to a breast clinic. There is an important correlation with the menstrual cycle, with discomfort lasting for a varying period of time prior to menstruation. Because of this cyclical relationship to the menstrual cycle mastalgia is generally a condition of premenopausal women, who present at a median age of about 35 years. Characteristically, the features of cyclical mastalgia wax and wane. Episodes of discomfort may last for some months; there may then be years of freedom until symptoms begin again.

The pain of cyclical mastalgia is frequently, but not always, bilateral and is usually located in the upper outer quadrants. It is poorly localized and may radiate across the chest wall into the axillae or down the inside of the arm. The breasts are frequently described as being 'heavy' as if pregnant and many patients describe marked nodularity at the time of the discomfort.

There is a wide spectrum of symptoms in patients with cyclical mastalgia. The majority have only mild discomfort lasting 2 or 3 days prior to menstruation, and they are not unduly concerned by their symptoms. Such individuals are therefore best classified as having a breast 'disorder' (ANDI), rather than a disease. The small minority of women who have severe symptoms lasting throughout the cycle with relief only during menstruation are those to whom the term 'disease' may be applied.

There are no mammographic or pathological characteristics of cyclical mastalgia: indeed this lack of correlation between clinical, radiological and histological findings is one of the major characteristics of the condition. The mammograms shown in Fig. 7 are from patients with severe breast pain. In one there is almost complete replacement with fat, giving a translucent appearance, whereas the other is dense and nodular (Wolfe DY pattern).

Aetiology of cyclical mastalgia

The fact that symptoms of cyclical mastalgia correlate with the menstrual cycle implies a hormonal aetiology. Early investigations suggested that hormonal imbalance was the cause, the fundamental abnormality being relative hyperoestrogenism due to either increased oestrogen secretion or deficient progestogen production. However, the vast majority of studies have failed to demonstrate either abnormality in women with mastalgia.

More recently, abnormal prolactin secretion has been incriminated as an aetiological factor in cyclical mastalgia. Although

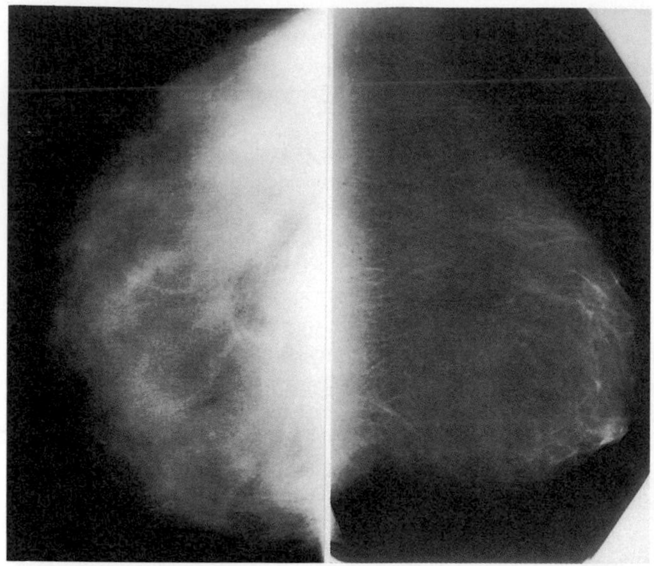

Fig. 7 Mammograms in patients with breast pain. In one the breast is radiologically translucent whereas the other is dense and nodular—Wolfe DY pattern (by courtesy of Dr B. Shepstone).

both random and basal levels of prolactin are normal in women with cyclical mastalgia, there is some evidence of impaired hypothalamic control of the release of this hormone in patients with severe symptoms. It should be appreciated, however, that the control of prolactin release is extremely complicated and that our current knowledge of its physiology is rather rudimentary.

The belief that cyclical mastalgia has a hormonal basis resulted in the suggestion that there would be an associated effect on fluid retention. However, despite a widespread belief that breast pain is due to water retention this has never been scientifically confirmed.

Other aetiological factors, including excessive caffeine ingestion or inadequate essential fatty acid intake, have been suggested. The latter is of particular interest as there is good evidence that essential fatty acid supplements can reduce the symptoms of cyclical mastalgia. The actual mechanism is unclear, but it may relate to a resulting deficit in prostaglandin E1 deficiency and a subsequent enhanced effect of prolactin on the breast.

Psychoneurosis has been widely incriminated as an important factor. However, there is no evidence of excessive anxiety, depression, or phobia in these patients when they are evaluated against appropriate control groups.

Treatment of cyclical mastalgia

More than 80 per cent of women attending a breast clinic with cyclical mastalgia require no treatment other than simple reassurance, particularly that such symptoms do not imply any form of neoplastic process. Fear of cancer drives many women to seek specific advice about breast pain, and the importance of such reassurance cannot be over-emphasized.

About 5 to 10 per cent of patients with cyclical mastalgia experience pain despite all reassurance. For those patients specific drug therapy may be considered. There is a sound theoretical basis for use of most agents which have been tried, apart from the fact that no constant physiological or pathological changes have been identified in this condition. Furthermore, no drug satisfies the criteria of being universally effective,free from side-effects, and freely available for use in patients suffering from benign breast disease. A large number of studies evaluating the efficacy of these drugs have been performed. However, because of the placebo effect of such treatment the results of many studies are inherently flawed, and reliance can only be placed on prospective, randomized, placebo controlled trials. A further problem of many studies is that they do not take into account the natural history of mastalgia. As a result a false impression of benefit may occur merely from natural remission, such as occurs in pregnancy or at the menopause.

Table 3 shows some of the agents widely used for the treatment of cyclical mastalgia, their possible modes of action, and common side-effects. Their overall efficacy is shown in Table 4.

Diuretics have been widely prescribed, although there is little rational basis for their use, and it is widely believed that much of their efficacy is due to a placebo effect. Similarly, there is no rationale for using antibiotics. The concept of relative hyperoestrogenism as a result of luteal deficiency has stimulated the evaluation of progestogens in cyclical mastalgia; the results have been generally disappointing in placebo controlled trials. Other widely adopted treatments of cyclical mastalgia are also of dubious value. Reduction in caffeine intake or administration of vitamins A or B_6 have failed to show any effect on cyclical mastalgia. Administration or oral contraceptives may reduce symptoms of cyclical breast pain, but total success can by no means be guaranteed.

Relative hyperoestrogenism can also be treated with the anti-oestrogen drug, tamoxifen. This was shown to be of benefit in a

Table 3 Drugs used for treatment of cyclical mastalgia

Class of agent	Mode of action	Drug and dosage side-effects	Incidence of side-effects (%)	More common side-effects
Diuretic	Reduction of body water	Diazide diuretic daily	Rare	Metabolic disorders, gout
Progestogen	Correction of luteal insufficiency	Medoxyprogesterone acetate 20 mg daily	20	Premenstrual symptoms, weight gain
Anti-oestrogen	Correction of hyperoestrogenism	Tamoxifen 10–20 mg daily	10	Hot flushes, weight gain, amenorrhoea, nausea, interference with anticoagulants
Dopamine agonist	Correction of hyperprolactinaemia	Bromocriptine 2.5 mg twice daily	20	Nausea, dizziness, headaches, postural hypotension
Antigonadotrophin	Suppression of FSH and LH	Danazol 200–400 mg daily	25	Weight gain, acne, amenorrhoea, hirsutism, voice change
Essential fatty acid (EFA)	Correction of EFA deficiency	Evening primrose oil 6 capsules daily	1	Nausea

Table 4 Efficacy of drugs used for cyclical mastalgia

	Response rate (%)
Tamoxifen*	90
Danazol	70
Bromocriptine	50
Evening primrose oil	45

* One study only.
Pyridoxine, diuretics and progestogens show no benefit compared to placebo.

single randomized trial, but as yet it only has a licence for use in malignant disease. Pain relief is provided by 10 mg tamoxifen daily; there seems little benefit in increasing the dose. Side-effects such as weight gain and hot flushes are troublesome and as it is contraindicated in pregnancy appropriate contraception is necessary.

Danazol probably acts as an antigonadotrophin by its action on the pituitary–ovarian axis. At a dose of 200 to 400 mg daily it depresses production of follicle stimulating hormone and luteinizing hormone and ovarian function. It significantly reduces breast pain, but is associated with side-effects in 20 per cent of patients. These include weight gain, acne, amenorrhoea, masculinization with hirsuitism, voice change, and reduction of breast size. Adequate non-hormonal contraception is necessary.

The suggestion of abnormal prolactin levels in patients with cyclical mastalgia, and the possibility that prolactin stimulates glandular breast tissue, led to hopes that the specific prolactin lowering agent, bromocriptine, would be useful in the treatment of cyclical mastalgia. This, a dopamine agonist, significantly reduced symptoms of cyclical mastalgia in benign breast disease. However, as is the case with danazol, its use has been curtailed by side-effects—such as nausea, postural hypotension, vomiting, and dizziness, which occur in up to 20 per cent of patients.

The suggestion that breast pain may be secondary to a deficit of essential fatty acids has led to its treatment with evening primrose oil, a mixture of linoleic and linolenic acids. Randomized studies have shown that it is effective and well tolerated in patients with cyclical breast pain. It is regarded as a natural homeopathic substance by many patients.

Patients with cyclical mastalgia should be treated initially with evening primrose oil, followed by danazol for patients refractory to treatment. Bromocriptine is a third choice, with activity similar to that of evening primrose oil but with a significant incidence of side-effects. The response rates tend to be lower for second and third lines of treatment. Tamoxifen has the drawback that it is not strictly registered for use in benign disease.

Responses to treatment are relatively short lived, usually of the order of 6 months. It is therefore our policy to treat for 3 months and then to see whether relapse occurs on cessation of therapy. Any relapse is an indication for restarting treatment, perhaps at a lower dose than originally used, or for a change in therapy if the initial response has been poor. Treatment is particularly difficult in young women, in whom mastalgia is often resistant to treatment, whose potential for breast pain may span several decades, and whose fertility must be considered. Bromocriptine and danazol are potentially teratogenic and require the use of a barrier form of contraception, as they interfere with oral contraceptives. Many younger women also dislike the amenorrhoea induced by tamoxifen and danazol.

Occasionally women with a long history of mastalgia unresponsive to all medical treatment demand consideration of mastectomy to release them from their discomfort. Although occasional patients may benefit from subcutaneous mastectomy, the general impression is that it should be avoided if at all possible.

Non-cyclical mastalgia

Non-cyclical mastalgia (Table 2) is even less well defined than its cyclical counterpart. It occurs in both pre- and post menopausal women, with a median age of presentation of 45. As well as having no close relationship to the menstrual cycle, non-cyclical mastalgia tends to be more chronic, unilateral, and located in the medial quadrants of the breast or the periareolar regions. It is not associated with lumpiness to the same degree as cyclical mastalgia and the pain is frequently described as burning or dragging rather than being a heavy feeling. The mastalgia is sometimes well localized; 'trigger spot zone' has been used in these individuals.

Attempts to classify non-cyclical mastalgia have been compromised by the dubious inclusion of other conditions that may cause breast pain. The best such example is that of 'duct ectasia/periductal/mastitis. The inclusion of this condition was based on the mammographic appearances of many patients with non-cyclical mastalgia, which showed widespread coarse calcification throughout the substance of the breast. This is also a feature of duct ectasia/periductal mastitis. However, the use of this term for patients with non-cyclical mastalgia has fallen into disfavour because of the principle of not mixing symptomatology with pathology, and because of the lack of evidence that pathological changes of duct ectasia correlate with breast pain.

Up to 50 per cent of patients with non-cyclical mastalgia have pain that arises not from the breast but from surrounding musculoskeletal structures (Table 2). A careful history and examination will identify such patients who, unlike those with true non-cyclical mastalgia, can be provided with relatively simple and effective therapy.

Aetiology of non-cyclical mastalgia

The aetiology of non-cyclical breast pain is unclear. However, some factors relating to cyclical mastalgia may also relate to non-cyclical breast pain.

Treatment

The management of true non-cyclical mastalgia is unsatisfactory. Many principles relating to the treatment of cyclical mastalgia may be applied to non-cyclical breast pain. However, overall response rates to various drug therapies are only about 50 per cent of those observed in patients receiving treatment for cyclical mastalgia. Both bromocriptine and evening primrose oil have shown particularly disappointing results. Response rates to the various drugs improve if patients with true non-cyclical mastalgia are differentiated from those with musculoskeletal pain.

Some success has been ascribed to surgical excision of 'trigger spot zones', but this approach has not been widely adopted.

Other causes of non-cyclical mastalgia

Musculoskeletal pain

This has previously been included as a cause of non-cyclical mastalgia, but has recently been demonstrated to be a separate entity. It is the most common cause of apparent pain in the breast originating from other sites. Musculoskeletal pain is often unilateral and localized along the lateral chest wall or the costochondral junction (Tietz's syndrome). Injection of local anaesthetic or steroids into the affected area produces good relief of symptoms.

Sclerosing adenosis

This may be found microscopically either as a single entity or in association with other abnormalities. It may be a minimal histological change or a macroscopically obvious entity. It is classified as an aberration of normal development and involution; microscopically it is characterized by proliferation of terminal duct lobules, myoepithelial cell proliferation, increased number of acini, and fibrous stromal change (Fig. 8). Multifocal and nodular types are described. Either may be painful and have been documented as a cause of mastalgia.

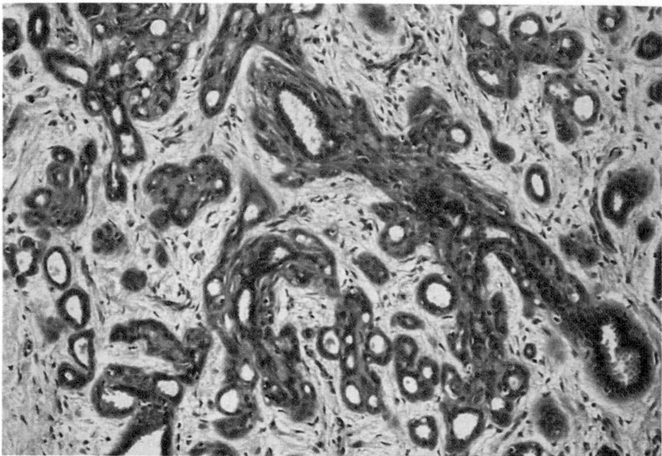

Fig. 8 Sclerosing adenosis. Note proliferation of duct lobules, increased number of acini and fibrosis (by courtesy of Dr D. Tarin).

The pain associated with sclerosing adenosis may be due to perineural invasion, and this may account for some patients with trigger spot zones. The main importance, however, is that macroscopically sclerosing adenosis may have a stellate appearance and may calcify—it may thus mimic carcinoma, both clinically and radiologically. The increased cellularity associated with sclerosing adenosis has been confused with carcinoma histologically, especially when examining frozen sections.

Previous surgery

A small number of patients continue to complain of pain after biopsy for benign breast disease. There is no clear reason for this phenomenon, although if the biopsy has previously been performed in an area subject to mastalgia it is likely that the original process will continue and be painful.

Cancer

Cancer is an uncommon cause of breast pain, although women do occasionally complain of discomfort, which may be more pronounced prior to menstruation, at the site of a tumour. The author has seen one young, intelligent woman complaining solely of breast pain, while failing to notice that the breast has been largely replaced by tumour.

Referred cervical root pain

This cause of pain in the breast should be considered in elderly patients in whom no other cause for mastalgia can be found.

Benign breast lumps

Approximately 40 per cent of all patients attending a breast clinic have a benign breast lump (Table 2). In the past there was a tendency to excise all lumps, and an excessive amount of unnecessary surgery was performed for benign disease. The main problem from the woman's point of view is fear that such a lump may be cancer. The clinician must therefore provide a high degree of diagnostic accuracy while at the same time ensuring that an excessive biopsy rate is prevented. It is now easier to exclude cancer with the development of diagnostic aids such as mammography, ultrasonography, and aspiration cytology.

The surgeon in the breast clinic has two important tasks when confronted with a patient with a breast lump. Firstly, he has to decide whether the lump is truly an abnormality or whether it can be regarded as being within the spectrum of normality. Secondary, if the lump is a true abnormality, he has to determine whether it is malignant.

The history is of particular importance. Enquiry should be made into the nature of the lump with respect to its duration, pain, change in size, and relationship to the menstrual cycle. The presence of menstrual irregularity and a previous history of similar problems should be sought. It is also important to enquire into the patient's risk factors for breast cancer, such as her age, number of children, age at first pregnancy, family history, and other potential predisposing factors such as hormone replacement therapy or oral contraceptive use.

Having established the risk or otherwise for breast cancer, the clinical impression must be confirmed by careful examination. Tethering of the skin, distortion of the breast, and nipple retraction are common features of malignancy, but they can also occur as a result of benign change. Mobility of the lump should be assessed: this is characteristic of a fibroadenoma and also quite obvious for cysts. Cancers tend to be more fixed, but are occasionally quite mobile.

Finally the surface of the lump should be assessed. Fibroadenomas have a lumpy, bosselated, surface whereas cysts are usually smooth and tense. Cancerous lumps are usually, but not always, hard. While a cancerous lump is likely to be hard, irregular, and fixed, it is not uncommon to see malignant tumours that are firm, quite regular, and which have a degree of mobility.

If there is any doubt a pathological diagnosis or biopsy is necessary; this should always be undertaken in any woman over the age of 25 with a solid discrete lump. In the majority of patients aspiration cytology is sufficient, but if this is in any way unsatisfactory or, if real doubt remains, then biopsy is mandatory. It is a brave clinician who does not remove a discrete breast lump from a 40-year-old nulliparous woman with a family history of breast cancer, even if fine-needle aspiration cytology is benign and mammography is reassuring.

Fibroadenomas and associated conditions

Fibroadenoma and related tumours are derived from the breast lobule and are characterized by both connective tissue and epithelial proliferation. They encompass a wide spectrum of conditions, ranging from the totally benign simple fibroadenoma to locally invasive and, rarely, frankly malignant tumours. There has been great confusion over their pathogenesis, particularly at the more malignant end of the spectrum. Such tumours are now

Table 5 Features of fibroadenoma and associated conditions

	Usual age at presentation (years)	Size	Characteristics of fibrous stomal element	Cellular atypia and pleomorphism
Benign simple fibroadenoma	16–40	<3 cm	Hypocellular	Absent
Giant fibroadenoma	15–18	>5 cm	Variable, some epithelial	Not prominent
(including juvenile fibroadenoma)	45–53		hyperplasia	
Phyllodes tumour	35–50	Variable	Hypercellular	Marked

commonly known as phyllodes tumours, but were previously described as cystosarcoma or phyllodes sarcoma. These descriptions are inappropriate because they imply a totally mesenchymal stromal origin whereas all of these tumours, whether benign, locally invasive, or malignant, also have an epithelial component. The major features of fibroadenomas and associated conditions are summarized in Table 5.

Benign simple fibroadenoma

Fibroadenomas are benign tumours showing evidence of both connective tissue and epithelial proliferation. They originate from the breast lobule and can be regarded as an aberration of normal lobular development rather than a true tumour. Their origin explains why fibroadenomas are common in young women at the time of lobular development, and why they are occasionally seen in combination with lobular carcinoma. The aetiology of a fibroadenoma is unknown; hypersensitivity to oestrogen within a lobule has been suggested.

The most important pathological aspect of a fibroadenoma is its connective tissue stroma. In the past great importance has been attached as to whether this stroma compresses adjacent ducts to form curved slit-like structures (intracanalicular pattern) or whether it simply surrounds a duct circumferentially (pericanalicular pattern). The fibrous stroma of such fibroadenomas has low cellularity and a regular cytology (Fig. 9). Occasionally there is histological evidence of fat, smooth muscle, squamous metaplasia, and infarction. The epithelial proliferation may be quite hyperplastic, but this is of no prognostic importance.

If the fibrous stroma shows a marked increase in both cellularity and atypia then the locally invasive and occasionally metastatic phyllodes tumour should be considered (see below). This entity can be regarded as the extreme end of the disease spectrum, simple fibroadenoma representing the other end.

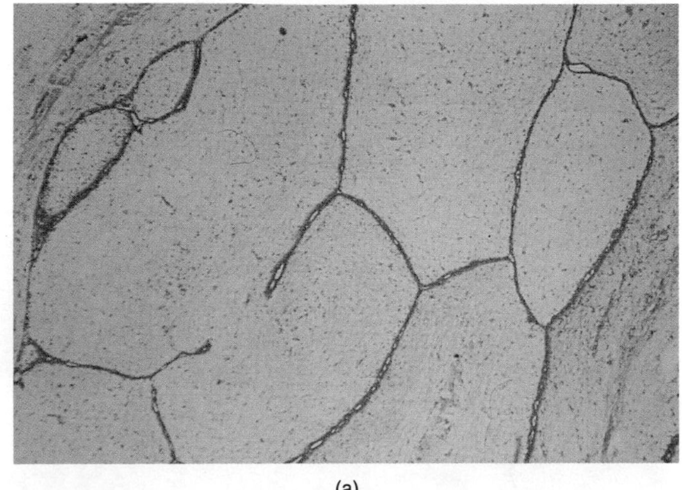

(a)

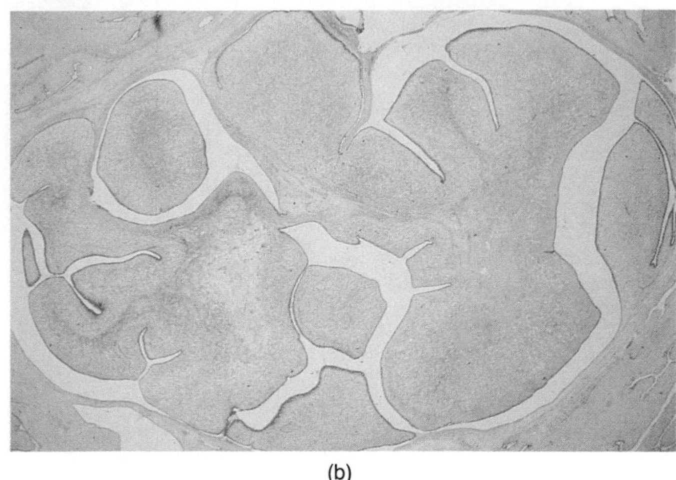

(b)

Fig. 9 Fibroadenoma and phyllodes tumour. Note the low cellularity and regular cytology of the benign fibroadenoma (a) but the hypercellularity, atypia, and abundant mitoses in the phyllodes tumour (b) (by courtesy of Dr D. Tarin).

Clinical features

Most fibroadenomas present in girls aged 16 to 24 years old. However, the use of pathological examination in the diagnosis of breast lumps in older women, the overall median age of presentation is nearer 30. They decrease in incidence after the menopause, when they undergo involution. During this time they may calcify and thus become apparent on mammography.

Fibroadenomas are smooth or slightly lobulated structures, usually measuring about 2 or 3 cm in diameter. With the exception of those adjacent to the nipple they are characteristically mobile. In young girls the term breast mouse is thus aptly applied. With increasing age the degree of mobility lessens because of the restraining effects of surrounding involuting fibrotic tissue. In the elderly they can still present as a small hardened mass which is still quite mobile.

About 10 per cent of all patients have multiple fibroadenomas on presentation,and occasionally one sees young women in whom the whole breast seems to be replaced by fibroadenotic tissue. Others present with multiple recurrent fibroadenomas. This occurs particularly among the black and oriental races.

Diagnosis

Up to the age of 25 a clinical diagnosis suffices. Thereafter pathological confirmation is required because of the need to exclude carcinoma. Fine-needle aspiration cytology provides an accurate method of diagnosis (Fig. 10) in older women, although hyperplastic epithelial cells can occasionally be mistaken for neoplasia. As fibroadenoma usually presents clinically in younger women, mammography has no place in its routine diagnosis. In older patients fibroadenomas appear as a solitary smooth lesion on radiography, with a density similar to or slightly greater than the surrounding tissue. With increasing age stippled calcification becomes apparent (Fig. 11).

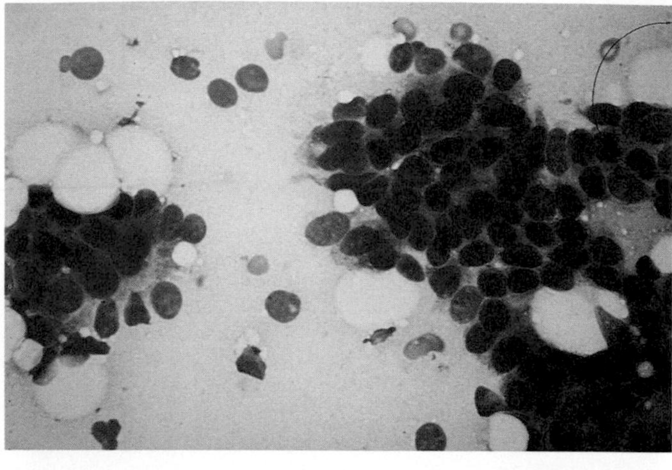

(a)

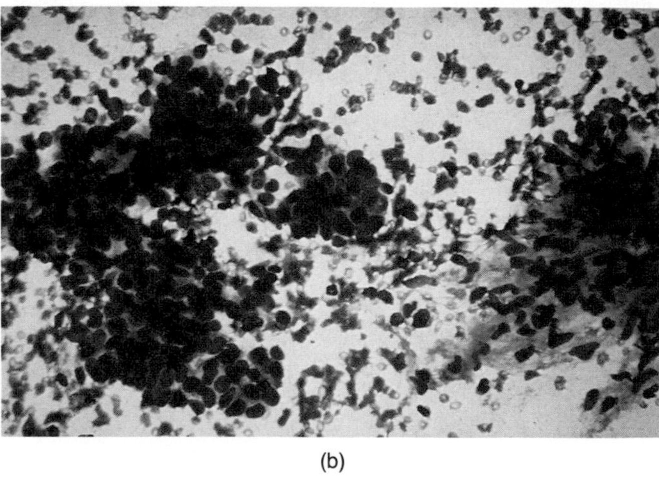

(b)

Fig. 10 Fine-needle aspiration cytology of fibroadenoma and phyllodes tumour. Note the regular groups of benign epithelial cells with associated bare nuclei in aspirate of fibroadenoma (a). The aspirate of the phyllodes tumour (b) shows gross cellularity, a hypercellular stroma and atypia (by courtesy of Dr I. Buley).

Management

The practice of surgically removing all fibroadenomas has now been condemned because of greater understanding of the natural history of this condition. If fibroadenomas are left untreated most will slowly increase in size from 1 to 3 cm in diameter over a period up to 5 years. The active growth phase is about 6 to 12 months, during which time there is a doubling of size. Thereafter they remain static or may (in up to one-third of cases) gradually become smaller.

In women under the age of 25 routine removal is unnecessary. This conservative approach may be recommended for woman under 35, provided that cytological examination rules out malignancy. This is, however, likely to result in a small number of cancers being missed, and removal of fibroadenomas is generally recommended after the age of 25. Such excision is best done under a general anaesthetic.

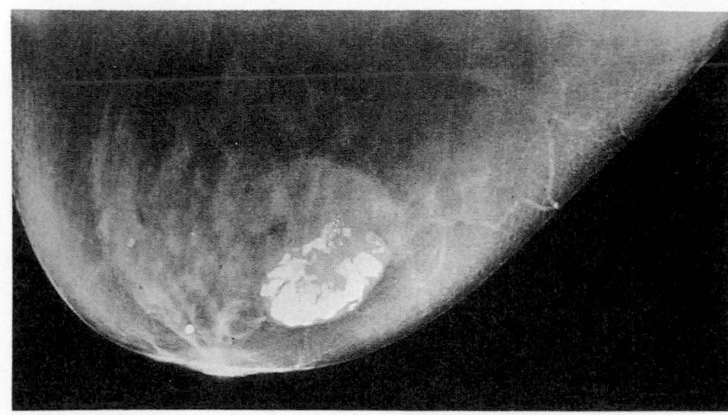

Fig. 11 Calcified fibroadenoma on mammography. Note the smooth opacity with coarse calcification within its structure (by courtesy of Dr B. Shepstone).

Recurrence of a fibroadenoma after removal is not uncommon. This may be due to a number of factors. Firstly, a truly metachronous fibroadenoma may develop. Secondly the original tumour may have been incompletely removed or missed at operation and, finally, it may be the mode of presentation of a previously undiagnosed phyllodes tumour.

Giant fibroadenoma

Giant fibroadenoma has a bimodal age of presentation at the extremes of reproductive life; those occurring in the younger age group have been described as juvenile fibroadenomas. They occur particularly in the 14 to 18 and the 45 to 50 age groups and are characterized by rapid growth to a large size. Giant fibroadenomas are, by definition, bigger than the common type of fibroadenomas, being at least 4 or 5 cm in diameter, and sometimes achieving a diameter size of 10 cm or more (Fig. 12).

Histologically, giant fibroadenomas contain the typical hypocellular stromal and epithelial components showing varying, though usually mild, degrees of hyperplasia and atypia; mitoses are uncommon. Such features are different from phyllodes

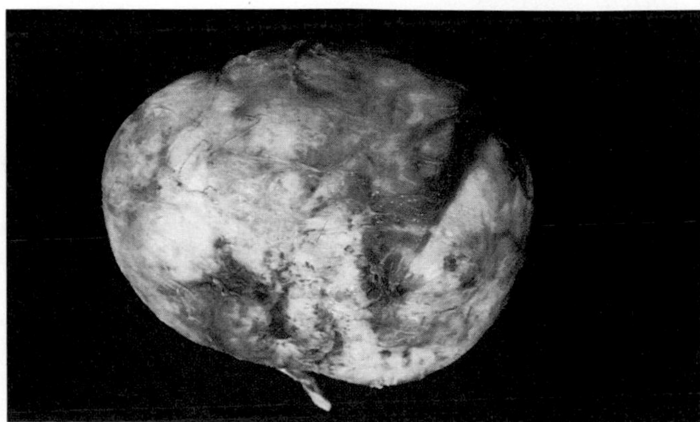

Fig. 12 A giant fibroadenoma 12 cm in size by (by courtesy of Dr D. Tarin).

tumours, which generally exhibit much more cellularity, pleomorphism, and mitotic activity. However there is some overlap of microscopic appearance between these two conditions (Table 5).

Clinical features

Giant fibroadenomas are more common in black and oriental races. Clinically patients present with pain in the breast associated with a rapid increase in size. On examination the breast is enlarged and the nipple may be displaced. The overlying skin frequently has a characteristic shiny appearance, and dilated veins may be apparent. In extensive, neglected cases skin necrosis can occur.

Occasionally girls may present with unilateral breast enlargement, and the fact that a mass is the cause is not appreciated. Giant fibroadenomas may be confused with virginal hypertrophy, although the latter is bilateral and not associated with cutaneous or venous changes.

Treatment

Management is by enucleation through an appropriately cosmetic incision. While this treatment initially results in some discrepancy in breast size the remaining breast tissue expands to virtual normality within a year or two. Wider excision or mastectomy is contraindicated.

Although some giant fibroadenomas can appear somewhat aggressive histologically and may even be confused with phyllodes tumour their clinical behaviour is completely benign. There is no evidence that they recur locally or metastasize.

Phyllodes tumour

Phyllodes tumours have been the cause of much misunderstanding and argument, partly related to their varied nomenclature. They have been described as phyllodes sarcoma, cystosarcoma, cystosarcoma phyllodes, and benign cystosarcoma. They have also been equated with giant fibroadenoma, but this is also misleading as it understates the malignant potential of the phyllodes tumour and implies similar histology. Conversely, terms such as cystosarcoma overstate the malignant potential and imply a false correlation with true mesodermally derived sarcomas. Phyllodes tumours show a wide spectrum of activity, varying from an almost benign condition to a locally aggressive, and sometimes metastatic tumour.

Phyllodes tumours appear well circumscribed but are characterized by irregular surface projections that may be cut during surgical excision, predisposing to recurrence. The cut surface is soft, brown in colour, and may exhibit cysts, necrosis, or haemorrhage. Histologically, both epithelial and fibrous stromal elements are present, with the stroma showing hypercellularity, much atypia and numerous mitoses (Fig. 9).

Clinical features

Phyllodes tumours occur in premenopausal women. They are usually seen in the 30 to 50 year age group, but are not uncommon in women aged about 20. They have the features of a common fibroadenoma but can grow rapidly to a large size and may involve much of the breast. The overlying skin may become reddened and, in advanced cases, can become frankly ulcerated. However, a degree of mobility is retained, even by large tumours. Axillary lymphadenopathy is uncommon; if it occurs it indicates an extremely aggressive form of the disease.

Despite the tendency to grow rapidly to a large size it is not uncommon for phyllodes tumours to present as a much smaller mass which is clinically indistinguishable from a simple fibroadenoma.

Treatment

Phyllodes tumours occurring in young women under the age of 20 are said to represent the benign end of the spectrum of this condition. As such, simple enucleation has been recommended, although the author prefers to excise the area more widely.

Older patients require wider excision with a 1 cm margin of normal breast tissue. Vary large tumours or those with aggressive histology may merit even wider excision, with quadrantectomy or even simple mastectomy and reconstruction for the largest tumours.

Even with an aggressive surgical policy of wide excision approximately 25 per cent of phyllodes tumours recur over a 10-year period. Such local recurrence should be widely excised. If recurrent tumours develop persistently mastectomy with reconstruction should be considered. A major worry with persistently recurrent phyllodes tumours is that they may metastasize, although this is a rare occurrence, being described in less than 5 per cent of patients.

Breast cysts

Breast cysts are among the more common reasons for referral to a breast clinic. They are frequently confused with more extensive cyclical nodularity. The description of cyclical nodularity as fibrocystic disease compounds the problem, and results in the false hope that many patients with cyclical nodularity can be treated by simple cyst aspiration.

True breast cysts are very common: up to 7 per cent of women develop a clinical cyst at some time during their lives. Postmortem studies show that a further 20 per cent of women have evidence of subclinical cysts in the breast, although many of these are only 2 or 3 mm in diameter.

As is the case with fibroadenomas, breast cysts can be regarded as an aberration of normal lobular physiology. The specific aetiology of this aberration is unknown, although there is some weak evidence that cyst formation may relate to hyperoestrogenism, such as may result from hormone replacement therapy. The pathogenesis of breast cysts is similarly unclear. Early workers suggested that they might simply be distended ducts or that they may result from cystic lobular involution. During this process lobules develop microcysts which eventually coalesce to become larger cysts; this process is potentiated by obstruction of lobular outflow and replacement of surrounding stroma by fibrous tissue.

More recent investigations have suggested that the aetiology of breast cysts is more complex than previously believed. There appear to be two distinct populations of macrocyst defined by their microscopic appearance, their biochemical profile, and clinical features (Table 6).

Aspirated fluid from simple uncomplicated cysts has a high $Na^+:K^+$ ratio (>3), similar to that found in plasma. The pH of

Table 6 Comparison of two types of breast cyst

	Simple	Apocrine
Lining epithelium	Simple cuboidal	Apocrine
Na^+/K^+ ratio	>3	<3
pH	<7.4	>7.4
Tendency to recurrence	Low	Moderate
Association with cancer	Not proven	Possible

this fluid is less than 7.4 and it is likely that the flat, rather featureless, epithelium of such cysts acts as a simple membrane through which interstitial fluid passively diffuses. These simple cysts tend to be single, not recurrent, and are unlikely to be associated with an increased risk of cancer.

The second type of cyst is lined by apocrine epithelium, characterized by large columnar cells resembling those found in apocrine sweat glands. The $Na^{+}:K^{+}$ ratio is less than 3, and similar to that of interstitial fluid. The pH of apocrine cysts is higher than that of simple cysts and their lining membrane secretes substances such as androgen conjugates. These observations suggest that apocrine epithelium actively secretes potassium into the cyst fluid. These cysts tend to recur as the balance between secretion of fluid and its reabsorption is in favour of reaccumulation. They may also be associated with an increased risk of breast cancer.

Other studies have shown that in the early stages of cyst development the microcysts are of the apocrine secretary type. It is only when macrocysts develop that differentiation into simple cysts occurs.

Clinical features

Cysts are classically seen in perimenopausal women between the ages of 45 and 52, although they frequently occur outside this age range, especially in individuals receiving hormone replacement therapy. They are usually single at presentation, but it is not uncommon to see multiple cysts in a breast. In the most extreme examples the whole breast seems to be composed of a number of cysts.

A characteristic of breast cysts is that they suddenly appear, even if they are quite large. The reason for this is that the cyst exists in a flaccid subclinical state prior to its presentation as a lump. The accumulation of a relatively small amount of fluid causes a disproportionate effect on intracystic pressure according to La Place's equation ($P = 2T/r$).

Cysts may be uncomfortable and are frequently frankly painful. There may be a vague relationship between discomfort and the menstrual cycle, with increasing pain prior to menstruation, although this is not a pronounced feature.

Cysts are frequently visible. However, their most characteristic feature is their smooth, tense nature on palpation. They have a degree of mobility but this is not as pronounced as that of fibroadenomas. The classic clinical appearances may be masked if the cyst is situated deep in the breast. Normal nodular breast tissue overlying the cyst may hide its classic smooth nature on palpation.

The diagnosis of a simple breast cyst is straightforward as cyst aspiration confirms the diagnosis. The amount of fluid aspirated is variable: it is usually about 6 or 8 ml, although occasionally cysts containing 60 or 80 ml of fluid are encountered. Cyst fluid varies in colour, ranging from pale yellow to almost black; sometimes the aspirate appears translucent whereas on other occasions it is thick and turgid.

Mammography and ultrasonography may aid diagnosis but these investigations are not essential, except as methods of screening these patients for cancer (Fig. 13). Little important information is gained from cytological examination of cyst fluid unless it is bloodstained.

Treatment

Breast cysts were previously treated by surgical excision. Such treatment is no longer recommended as simple aspiration will normally suffice. After aspiration the cyst remains as a lax impalpable structure which may still be seen on mammography. However, there must be no clinical evidence of a mass remaining after aspiration. If a mass does remain after aspiration, further investigation with fine-needle aspiration cytology or biopsy is indicated.

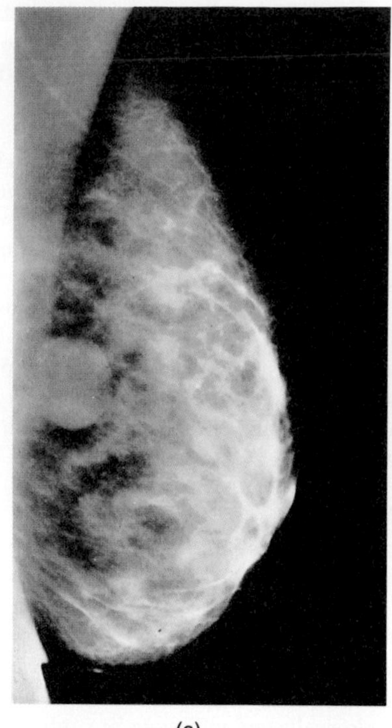

(a)

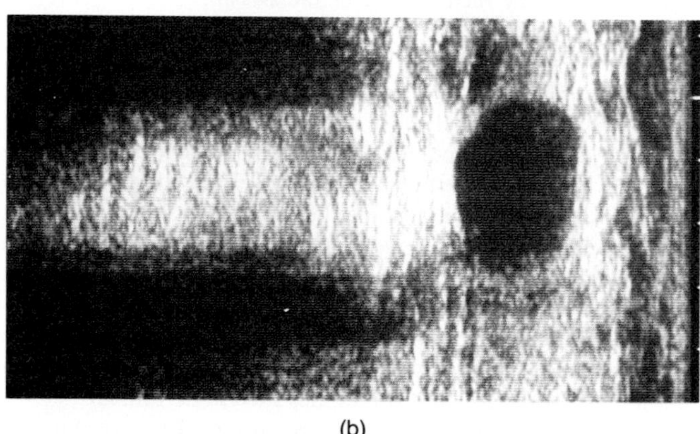

(b)

Fig. 13 Breast cyst on (a) mammography and (b) ultrasound. Note the well delineated homogenous opacity seen on both investigations (by courtesy of Dr B. Shepstone).

There are two main indications for surgical excision of the cyst. If the aspirate is blood-stained (as long as this is not due to direct trauma from the needle) an intracystic carcinoma may be present. The second indication, which is perhaps more contentious, is cyst recurrence. This may be simply due to inadequate aspiration and further such treatment may be attempted before excision. However, if the cyst recurs rapidly and more than once its excision is recommended.

Patients who develop persistently recurrent cysts throughout their breasts can present a difficult management problem. Recurrence is often at a different site from the presenting cyst. Up to 50 per cent of patients develop further cysts over 5 to 10 years, although the majority of individuals will only have one or two recurrences. However, a small number of women develop recurrences on a regular basis and may attend the breast clinic every 2 or 3 months for cysts to be drained. In the past some of these patients were treated by subcutaneous mastectomy. We now recommend danazol or tamoxifen treatment, although evidence in favour of this management is sparse and there are side-effects and limitations associated with the use of these drugs.

In theory, patients with breast cysts may be at an increased risk for breast cancer. Mammography should be performed on women presenting with cysts, although the yield of occult cancers is low. Patients with recurrent apocrine cysts may benefit from continued mammographic surveillance, although the evidence for their liability to breast cancer is conflicting. Patients with a solitary simple cyst do not require regular mammographic monitoring.

Cyclical nodularity

Many patients are referred to breast clinics with a lump that is really a manifestation of cyclical nodularity, but in a more localized and clinically discrete form. It is the mass, rather than the pain, which is the predominant feature. A careful history, however, will frequently reveal that the lump has been present for some time and that its size varies with the menstrual cycle. Many patients will also admit to discomfort or pain in the lump when it is most prominent.

A variation of this presentation is seen, particularly in teenagers and occasionally in older woman approaching the menopause. A large, diffuse, and frequently uncomfortable swelling develops suddenly, often, but not always, in the upper outer quadrant. Examination discloses a diffuse nodular swelling that may be somewhat tender. This changes usually resolves with the next menstrual cycle. If it persists, biopsy or aspiration cytology is indicated, together with mammography in older women.

As long as malignancy is excluded patients with cyclical nodularity presenting as a breast lump can simply be reassured.

Galactocele

Galactocele is well documented in older texts relating to breast disease, but they are perhaps less common than previously thought. Classically they present as a cyst in a woman who has recently stopped breast feeding, although they occasionally occur during lactation. Aspiration shows breast milk and is usually successful in resolving the problem.

The pathogenesis of galactocele is unclear; it may simply be a pre-existing simple cyst that fills with milk.

Sclerosing adenosis

Sclerosing adenosis is an uncommon cause of a breast lump. Clinically, it usually presents as a smooth, relatively mobile mass in the 30- to 50-year age group. It is frequently painful and can occasionally be a cause of mastalgia rather than of a mass.

Sclerosing adenosis can be regarded as an abnormality of normal development, characterized by lobular enlargement and distortion associated with fibrous stromal change.

Fat necrosis

Fat necrosis is another condition that has attracted more attention than it deserves, although it is a frequent cause of diagnostic difficulty in women with breast disease. This arises from delayed diagnosis of cancer in patients with a history of trauma, and the occasional mastectomy performed in patients with fat necrosis thought to be a tumour.

A history of trauma is easily provided by the patient. However, this is a trap for the unwary as many patients with cancer will try to attribute the lump to a previous injury.

By the time the patient presents at the clinic, any external evidence of injury has frequently disappeared. The lump can be small and hard and clinically may easily be confused with a carcinoma. Sometimes there is associated inflammation, tethering, and oedema.

Fine needle aspiration cytology is usually diagnostic (Fig. 14). Areas of fat necrosis are occasionally cystic, and aspiration can partially resolve the condition. However, in our unit we review patients diagnosed as having fat necrosis after 6 weeks, when the lump is excised if it has not disappeared. Mammography must be interpreted with care as fat necrosis can have radiological features similar to those of cancer (Fig. 15).

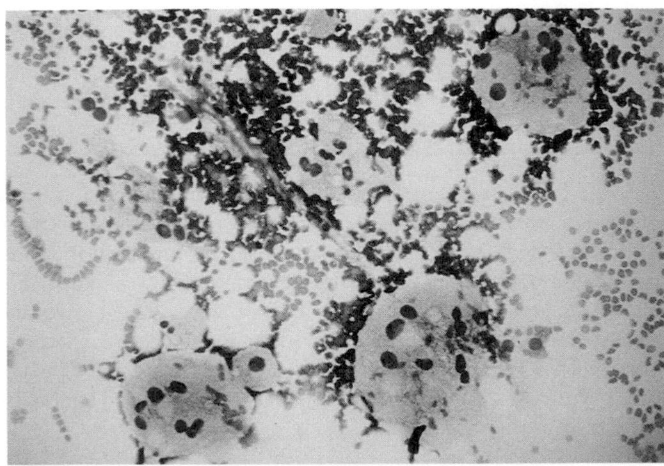

Fig. 14 Fat necrosis of the breast. Fine-needle aspiration showing characteristic foamy, fat-laden macrophages with few epithelial cells (by courtesy of Dr I. Buley).

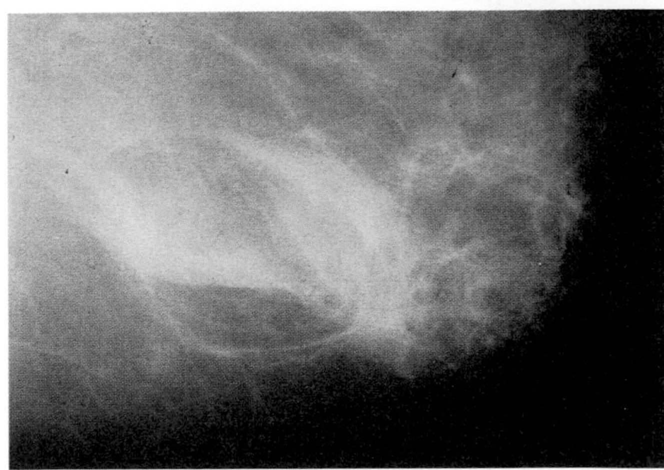

Fig. 15 Fat necrosis of the breast. Mammography showing a speculated opacity with calcification and features similar to a carcinoma (by courtesy of Dr B. Shepstone).

Lipoma, adenolipoma

Lipomas occur quite frequently in the breast, but not to the extent that might have been thought in view of the amount of fat that is present. They produce a soft mass which is best excised if there is any doubt as to its nature. The adenolipoma is a variation of lipoma. It sometimes has a marked fibrotic component and is best regarded as a hamartoma.

Chronic abscess

The increasing use of antibiotics as a treatment for inflammatory breast conditions occasionally results in a chronic sterile abscess. Treatment is by aspiration, or by open drainage with excision of the wall if recurrence develops.

Normal structures

Patients may present with the impression of a breast lump that may be due either to a normal structure, such as a rib, or a prominent area of breast tissue which may be made more obvious by the defect from a previous biopsy or from weight loss. Fatty replacement at the time of breast involution can also give the impression of a lump: at operation fibrotic fatty tissue is found.

Disorders of the nipple and periareolar tissue

Disorders of the nipple are no less controversial than other aspects of benign breast disease. There are the usual reasons for these difficulties, such as lack of consensus over terminology and poor correlation between clinical features, mammography, and pathological findings. The symptoms of disorders of the nipple and periareolar tissues are discharge, retraction, and the effects of periareolar sepsis (Table 7). There are multiple causes for each of these symptoms but one condition, duct ectasia/periductal mastitis, is of paramount importance.

Table 7 Disorders of the nipple and periareolar region

Nipple discharge
Physiological
Galactorrhoea
Duct ectasia
Papilloma and carcinoma
Cysts
Nipple inversion
Congenital
Nipple retraction
Duct ectasia
Cancer
Previous surgery

Duct ectasia/periductal mastitis

Duct ectasia and periductal mastitis has been described for more than a century but until recently it has been relatively ignored by both clinicians and pathologists. In the past it has been regarded as part of the spectrum of fibrocystic disease and because of its histological appearance it has been given a variety of names such as plasma cell mastitis, mastitis obliterans, and granulomatous mastitis. The clinical features of duct ectasia/periductal mastitis are extremely varied and, as histological or cytological confirmation is not always possible, diagnosis must sometimes be made on clinical grounds alone.

Pathogenesis

In 1951 Haagensen suggested that the primary change in patients with duct ectasia/periductal mastitis was simple dilatation of the larger periareolar ducts (duct ectasia, Fig. 16). It is unusual for all ducts to become dilated but such changes are frequently bilateral. The dilated ducts fill with a stagnant, thick green or creamy secretion (grumous). These stagnant secretions lead to loss of duct epithelial lining, and associated ulceration can cause further discharge, with bleeding from the nipple. There may also be a chronic inflammatory response (periductal mastitis) in the periareolar tissues because of leakage of the secretions through the damaged duct walls. Periductal mastitis may produce a painful mass or even a frank periareolar abscess; repeated inflammatory processes cause fibrosis and result in nipple retraction.

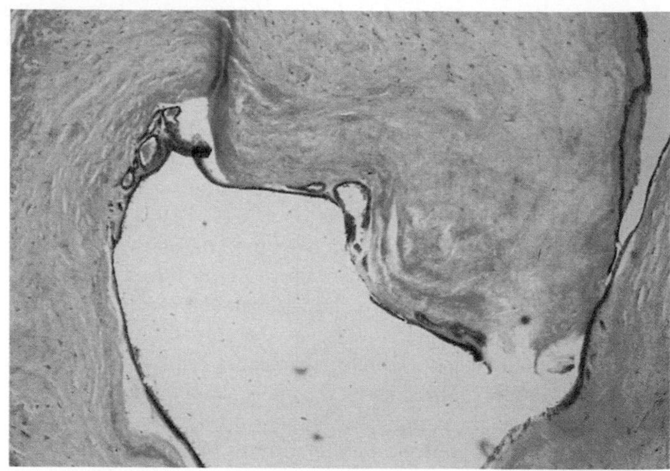

Fig. 16 Duct ectasia (by courtesy of Dr D. Tarin).

The various pathogenic processes of duct ectasia explain many of the symptoms associated with this condition. A difficult question to answer, however, is what causes the initial duct dilatation. Suggested possibilities include hormonally induced muscular relaxation of the duct wall, inadequate absorption of secretions, or obstruction of the system by squamous debris. Unfortunately, there is little scientific basis for these suggestions. An alternative theory is that the periareolar inflammation rather than the duct ectasia is the primary pathogenic process. Periareolar inflammation may result in secondary duct dilatation and the consequent discharge, fibrosis, and nipple retraction. This alternative theory explains why younger women tend to suffer the inflammatory complications of duct ectasia, whereas nipple inversion and discharge occur in older age groups.

Duct ectasia/periductal mastitis is, therefore, a complex disorder of uncertain aetiology. The wide variety of clinical symptoms associated with it can be best explained and understood by appreciating that there is more than one process in its pathogenesis.

The more severe symptoms of duct ectasia/periductal mastitis, such as abscess formation, can be regarded as a true benign breast disease. However, in all but its most severe form duct ectasia is best classified as a breast benign disorder originating from the normal process of duct involution with fibrosis.

Nipple discharge

Nipple discharge is a common symptom presenting to breast clinics (Table 7). The patient may fear cancer and the discharge may in itself be a cause of social embarrassment and annoyance. Treatment is therefore directed not only at diagnosing the cause of the discharge accurately but, if necessary, stopping the discharge itself.

Patients presenting with nipple discharge should be questioned as to whether it has been blood-stained, whether it is unilateral or bilateral, and whether it is associated with a lump. If a lump is present then diagnosis of the cause of the discharge becomes secondary to investigation of the lump.

Although inspection may reveal the source of discharge as one or more ducts, most patients have little visible abnormality. Excessive crusting may occasionally be seen on the nipple: this may simply be the dried products of secretion. Sometimes a skin disorder such as eczema may be found, the associated serous exudate producing the impression of nipple discharge.

Routine palpation of the breast must be followed by firm but gentle pressure around the areola. This will determine whether the discharge is unifocal or multifocal and whether it occurs in one or both breasts. It should also determine the nature of the discharge. Particular attention should be paid as to whether the discharge has the greyish shiny characteristic of human milk (galactorrhoea in the non-pregnant or non-lactating patient), whether it is watery, serous or, as is often the case, if it is of a thick opalescent nature which may vary in colour from cream to almost black. Of paramount importance, however, is whether the discharge contains blood. This may be bright red and fresh or much darker in colour due to the presence of degradation products.

Investigations

Our own experience in investigating nipple discharge radiologically and with cytology has been disappointing, although other authorities have reported success. Particular features of note on mammography are the intraductal microcalcifications of carcinoma *in situ* and dilated ducts associated with the secretory granules that indicate duct ectasia (Fig. 17). Ductography may demonstrate the presence of duct papillomas, but this investigation tends to be insensitive.

A number of centres recommend cytological examination of the discharge. This occasionally produces a positive finding although false negative results are common.

Causes of nipple discharge

There are a number of causes of nipple discharge (Table 7). Unfortunately it is difficult to correlate accurately the nature of the discharge with the cause, although certain features do act as a diagnostic guide. The presence of bright red blood in the discharge, a watery discharge, or drainage from a single duct are all factors that indicate a potentially serious cause and which require thorough investigation.

Physiological causes

Discharge of milk is a normal phenomenon during pregnancy and lactation. During pregnancy blood-staining is occasionally observed: this is of no significance and reassurance is all that is required. A milky nipple discharge may occur transiently in the neonate due to transplacental passage of luteal and placental hormones from the mother's circulation.

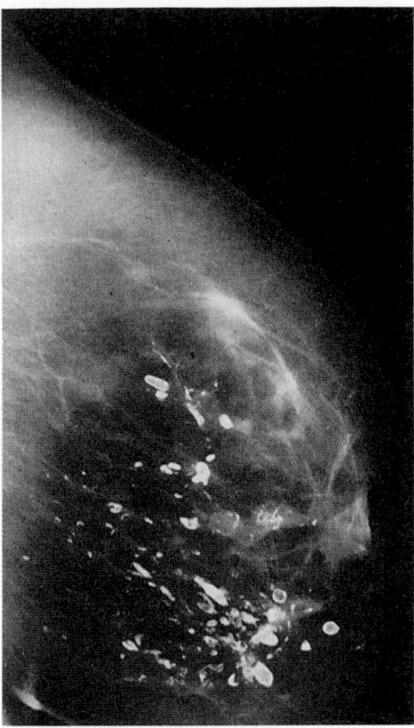

Fig. 17 Mammographic appearances of duct ectasia showing coarse calcifications of secretory granules in dilated ducts (by courtesy of Dr B. Shepstone).

Galactorrhoea

Galactorrhoea is secretion of milk not related to pregnancy or lactation, although in itself it can be a primary physiological process. Physiological causes include mechanical stimulation of the breast and stress. It may also occur for some years after cessation of breast feeding and may be seen as part of a normal physiological process at the menarche and menopause. Under these physiological circumstances simple reassurance is all that is required.

Galactorrhoea may also be a secondary phenomenon, occurring as a side-effect of drugs that enhance dopamine activity, such as chlorpromazine, haloperidol, metoclopromide, and methyldopa. Hyperprolactinaemia due to a primary prolactin-secreting tumour or from a secondary source, such as bronchogenic cancer, is an uncommon cause of galactorrhoea.

Duct ectasia

Duct ectasia is a common cause of nipple discharge. Characteristically it causes a multifocal, bilateral discharge which is thick and opalescent and of varying colours. However, the discharge of duct ectasia can be unifocal and frankly blood-stained, particularly in the perimenopausal and older age groups.

Duct papillomas

Papillomas are one of the more important causes of nipple discharge. The discharge is often from a single duct; it is frequently serous or serosanguinous and is frankly blood-stained in 50 per cent of cases. Papillomas also account for many of the relatively unusual cases of a watery discharge.

Most papillomas are solitary and are not considered to be premalignant. Occasionally two or three papillomas may be found in a single duct, and they are unlikely to have neoplastic potential (Fig. 18). Multiple papillomas, however, especially those

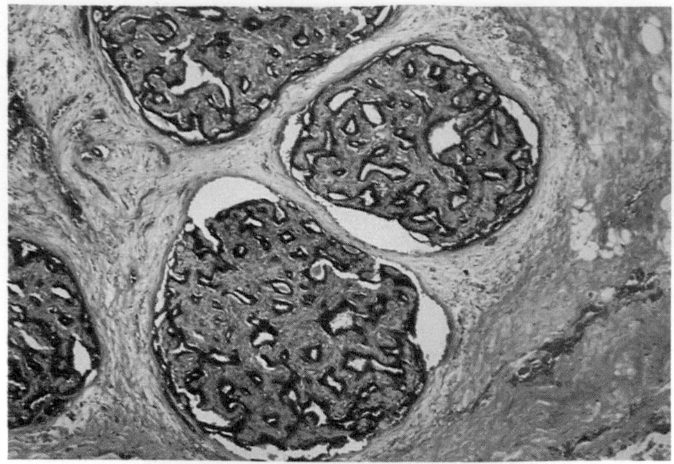

Fig. 18 Multiple intraduct papilloma (by courtesy of Dr D. Tarin).

occurring in the periphery of the breast and affecting more than one duct, carry an increased risk of malignant change. In one series, 15 or 39 such patients developed carcinoma. These peripheral lesions are more likely to cause a breast mass than a nipple discharge.

Carcinoma

As discussed below intraductal carcinoma, and even invasive cancer, can present as nipple discharge. This is usually from a single duct, is frequently watery or serous, and is generally frankly blood-stained.

Cysts

Cysts may be more common as a cause of nipple discharge than is generally appreciated. Some authorities regard cysts simply as dilated ducts and patients can occasionally produce a discharge simply by compressing an area of cystic change.

Idiopathic causes

Despite all attempts at establishing a diagnosis, even with biopsy, about 10 per cent of patients have no obvious pathological entity ascribed to the discharge. If the discharge has been blood-stained it must be considered that the cause has been missed. However, if the discharge was serous and non-blood-stained simple reassurance with careful follow-up will suffice.

Management of nipple discharge

If the nipple discharge is associated with a mass then treatment appropriate for the lump is constituted. If no mass is felt the management depends on the nature of the discharge.

1. Galactorrhoea causes such as mechanical stimulation and ingestion of drugs known to promote galactorrhoea should be excluded. If prolactin levels are normal simple reassurance is all that is required.
2. Discharge located to one duct but not blood-stained. Mammography should be performed in patients older than 35. All patients should undergo microdochetomy and in older women, who no longer wish to breast feed, a good case can be made for major duct excision.
3. Blood-stained discharge from a single duct. Treatment is the same as for a non-blood-stained discharge from a single duct. However, as a greater proportion of patients will have significant pathological findings exploration is even more essential. Bleeding often occurs only once or twice and there are no abnormal findings on firm palpation when the patient presents. Mammography should still be performed in patients over the age of 35, and all patients should be followed up for at least 6 months.
4. Multifocal and non-blood-stained discharge. Mammography should be performed in all women over the age of 35. If this is normal, simple reassurance is all that is necessary. If the discharge is excessive and causes social embarrassment major duct excision can be recommended. The usual cause of such discharge is duct ectasia. Operations for this condition have been associated with a high incidence of infection, and cephradine and metronidazole administration is recommended.
5. Multifocal and blood-stained discharge. Mammography with major duct excision is indicated, although many cases will be due to duct ectasia.

Surgery for nipple discharge remains somewhat controversial. The more conservative approach is microdectomy, which has the advantage that women should be able to breast feed after the operation. It is therefore probably the treatment of choice in younger individuals with a single duct discharge. However, as many patients with a single duct discharge will have a more widespread disorder, simple microdochetomy may be followed by recurrence of symptoms. A more appropriate operation for older women is major duct excision, which also allows easier nipple eversion if required.

Nipple inversion and retraction

The terms nipple inversion and retraction have been used interchangeably, and the distinction is somewhat arbitrary. Nipple inversion describes a congenital failure of eversion during development whereas retraction relates to a secondary process, usually due to duct ectasia or carcinoma.

Congenital nipple inversion

Congenital nipple inversion is a common problem occurring to a greater or lesser extent in up to 20 per cent of all women. Frank inversion causing difficulty with breast feeding is much less common: a degree of flattening of the nipple does not seem to interfere with the breast feeding process. This is hardly surprising because the nipple itself probably plays a relatively small part in anatomical aspect of suckling, since the infant creates a 'teat' from surrounding breast tissue as well as from the nipple itself.

Congenitally inverted nipples tend to be bilateral and patients can generally be reassured that there are few long-term sequelae from this condition. They should certainly be encouraged to breast feed. Women with congenitally inverted nipples have a higher incidence of duct ectasia/periductal mastitis.

Young women with congenitally inverted nipples often request surgical eversion. If possible this should be resisted, as the only satisfactory way of everting the nipple is to divide all the underlying ducts, which will prevent subsequent breast feeding. Furthermore, after such cosmetic surgery the nipples still have a rather flattened appearance rather than being protuberant.

Nipple retraction

The three main causes of nipple retraction are duct ectasia, carcinoma, and the effects of injudicious previous surgery.

Duct ectasia

Nipple retraction due to duct ectasia is characterized by bilateral changes and a characteristic linear transverse defect in its early stages. At this time it is possible to evert the nipple but as the process progresses digital eversion becomes more difficult. Other features of duct ectasia, such as a creamy multifocal discharge or stigmata of previous periareolar abscesses, are often present. An earlier belief that these changes often begin during pregnancy has not been confirmed.

Carcinoma

Retraction due to carcinoma is characterized by a shorter history and is unilateral. It is frequently associated with a mass. The effects of nipple retraction itself and any associated inflammation can make clinical assessment of the retroareolar area difficult. If there is any doubt, mammography and biopsy by major duct excision should be performed.

Postsurgical retraction

Injudicious surgery with inadequate care in reconstituting the breast can result in nipple inversion. This is often associated with an ugly periareolar defect and is difficult to rectify. It should be avoided by due attention to surgical technique.

Other disorders of the nipple and periareolar region

While discharge and retraction account for the majority of patients presenting with nipple disorders a number of other problems are occasionally encountered. Skin disorders, especially eczema, often affect the nipple and periareolar regions. Eczema must be differentiated from Paget's disease and is characterized by a long intermittent history, bilaterality, and its presence at other cutaneous sites. Features such as itching, serous discharge, and the nature of the periphery of the lesion are of little diagnostic significance. If there is any diagnostic doubt biopsy is required; a blind trial of topical steroids is to be condemned as Paget's disease can resolve temporarily in response to this treatment.

Fibroepithelial polyps present in adolescence and in young women. Excision, if required, can be performed under local anaesthetic. Chronic sebaceous cysts and retention cysts arising from Montgomery's tubercles are occasionally seen.

Nipple adenomas produce an uncomfortable mass beneath the nipple. They can cause ulceration and may be confused with Paget's disease. Simple excision will suffice; the condition is completely benign.

Pain and hypersensitivity in the nipples are difficult to explain. Sometimes this has a cyclical nature and enquiry will show a traumatic cause. Other patients describe hypersensitivity to cold, as in a Raynaud's type of phenomenon.

Infection of the breast

The majority of breast infections can be subdivided into those occurring during lactation and those which are a complication of duct ectasia/periductal mastitis. They have an entirely different aetiology, pathogenesis, and treatment, and may be considered completely separately.

Lactational breast abscess

Lactational breast abscesses occur during breast feeding, are generally somewhat peripherally situated, and are the result of infection by *Staphylococcus aureus*. Such abscesses tend to occur at the commencement of breast feeding when an inexperienced mother develops cracked nipples. They also occur at weaning when engorgement results from incomplete drainage of breast milk.

Cracked nipples resulting from the trauma of breast feeding are seen in the first week after delivery and again after about 6 months when the child's teeth first develop. There is acute pain in the nipple and examination reveals a linear fissure which may become secondarily infected.

Clinical features

The patient initially complains of discomfort in the breast, followed by painful swelling. The overlying skin may appear red and in extreme cases may undergo necrosis. Constitutional symptoms are common and by the time the patient presents she may have a high fever and be systemically unwell.

If ignored breast abscesses, like those elsewhere, will point and spontaneously discharge on to the skin surface.

Treatment

If lactational breast infection is seen prior to frank abscess formation, antibiotic treatment alone is often successful. Aspiration should be attempted to ensure that no pus is present. As many cases, especially those occurring in hospital, are due to penicillinase-producing staphylococci treatment must be with a penicillinase-resistant antibiotic such as a second-line penicillin or a cephalosporin. Such treatment will be successful in about 90 per cent of early cases.

If, on aspiration, pus is found or if other systemic features of an abscess are present drainage is necessary. However, some recent authorities have recommended repeated daily aspiration under antibiotic cover rather than formal surgical intervention. If formal drainage is performed, however, further antibiotic therapy is no longer required. The incision used to drain the abscess should limit any cosmetic deficit and allow drainage of pus under the influence of gravity. The majority of surgeons leave the wound open and pack it daily with antiseptic-soaked ribbon gauze, although primary closure under antibiotic cover has also been recommended.

An area of confusion is whether breast feeding should continue after treatment of a breast abscess. There is no place for suppression of lactation. The infant should be encouraged to feed from the contralateral breast while the affected side should be emptied either manually or with a breast pump. Cracked nipples should be washed gently and dried by dabbing rather than by rubbing. If there is evidence of nipple infection a nystatin-containing ointment should be applied topically.

Non-lactational breast abscesses

Non-lactational breast abscesses are entirely different from those occurring during breast feeding. They occur in the periareolar tissues, frequently recur, and the infecting organisms (if successfully cultured) are a mixture of bacteroides, anerobic streptococci and enterococci. Such non-lactational breast abscesses are a manifestation of duct ectasia/periductal mastitis and are usually seen in the 30- to 60-year age groups.

Clinical features

Patients with non-lactational breast abscesses often have a history of previous infective episodes in the periareolar region. Such abscesses often begin as a slightly tender periareolar mass. Spontaneous resolution is common but they often progress, with associated reddening of the overlying skin and increasing tenderness until the features of a frank abscess are present. Systemic upset is less pronounced than in patients with lactational abscesses. Scarring and distortion arising from treatment of similar such episodes may be present, and there may be other manifestations of duct ectasia/periductal mastitis, such as nipple retraction.

Treatment

If a non-lactational abscess is suspected the inflammatory mass should be aspirated and sent for both aerobic and anerobic culture. Initial treatment with metronidazole and flucloxacillin may be successful, although repeated aspiration may be required. Many patients will require drainage, although drainage should be avoided if possible. If drainage is necessary it should be performed through the smallest possible incision.

Definitive treatment requires duct excision and possible nipple eversion. This should be performed under appropriate antibiotic prophylaxis and only when the condition is quiescent. The majority of surgeons leave the wound open and leave it to heal secondarily although there is an increasing vogue for primary closure if local conditions are suitable.

Mammary fistula

Surgical or spontaneous discharge of an abscess from periductal mastitis may result in a mammary fistula with intermittent drainage of pus or serous fluid on to the areola. This may be superimposed on further episodes of periductal sepsis. Characteristically the breast demonstrates multiple incisions for drainage of previous abscesses, distortion, nipple retraction, and a fistula at the edge of the areola (Fig. 19). The basic cause is, again, duct ectasia/periductal mastitis.

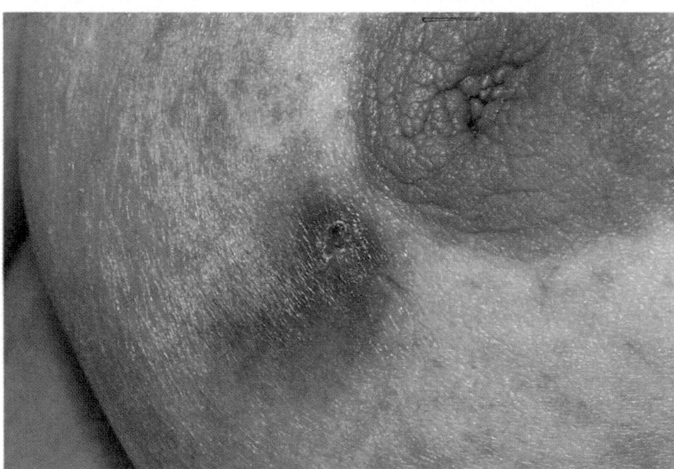

Fig. 19 Mammary fistula. Note the fistula opening on to the border of the areola.

Treatment is by fistulectomy, excision of the offending duct, and nipple eversion if required. If there is extensive periareolar disease or the nipple is grossly retracted a major duct excision should be performed. Most surgeons prefer to leave the wound open but again there is a growing trend for primary closure.

Fistula recurs in about 5 per cent of patients. The cause is variable, but includes continuation of duct ectasia/periductal mastitis in adjacent ducts and persistence of the proximal duct adjacent to the nipple because of an inadequate surgical technique.

Other causes of breast infection

Postoperative wound infections are relatively common after breast surgery, especially following surgical treatment of duct ectasia/periductal mastitis. Reasons for this include the relatively poor blood supply to fat, ischaemia resulting from deep sutures, and an accumulation of serum in the wound itself. Prophylactic antibiotics and drainage seem to have little impact in reducing the incidence of such problems; they are best minimized by meticulous technique.

The incidence of wound infection after surgery for duct ectasia/periductal mastitis has been so high in some centres that antibiotic prophylaxis with drugs such as combination metronidazole and flucloxacillin is now widely used.

Breast abscesses occasionally occur in neonates due to infection of milk induced by the transplacental passage of maternal hormones. If antibiotics do not help this condition great care must be taken during surgical drainage as damage to the breast disc at this age may lead to distortion in later life.

Tuberculosis, syphilis, hidradenitis, and pilonidal abscess have all been described as causing inflammation in the breast.

THE RELATIONSHIP OF BENIGN TO MALIGNANT DISEASE

General risk factors for breast cancer are discussed below. Preexisting benign breast disease is considered to be a risk factor, although the literature on the subject is conflicting. Studies have generally been based on selected populations who have had incomplete follow-up for an inadequate amount of time. A major problem has been lack of consensus between pathologists in ascribing individual terms to the various microscopic features and an obsession with the cancer risk associated with fibrocystic disease. The following terms require definition before further discussion.

Hyperplasia

This is cellular proliferation (Fig. 20). As far as the breast is concerned the normal ducts are lined by two layers of cells above the basement membrane. Hyperplasia is therefore defined as presence of three or more layers of cells, although individual cells may fill up or protrude into epithelial lined spaces. It is synonymous with the terms papillomatosis and epitheliosis.

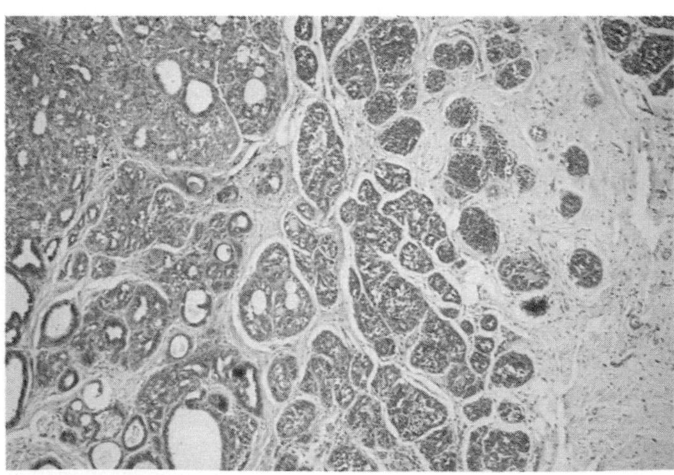

Fig. 20 Hyperplasia. Note the benign epithelial proliferation. Normal ducts are filled with hyperplastic cells (by courtesy of Dr D. Tarin).

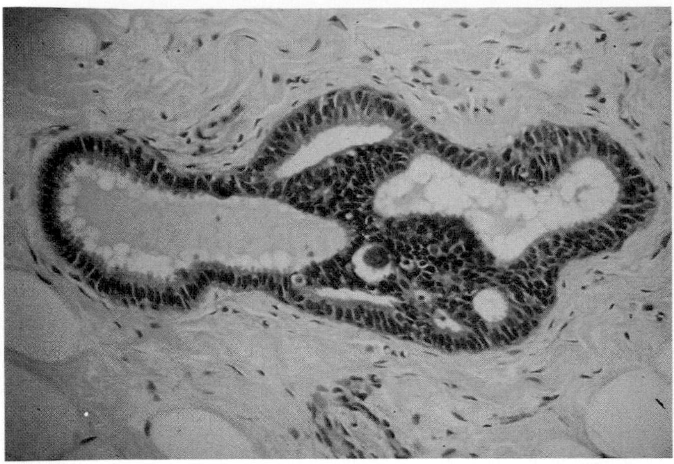

Fig. 21 Atypical ductal hyperplasia. Cells lining the duct show loss of polarity, nuclear pleomorphism, and atypia (by courtesy of Dr D. Tarin).

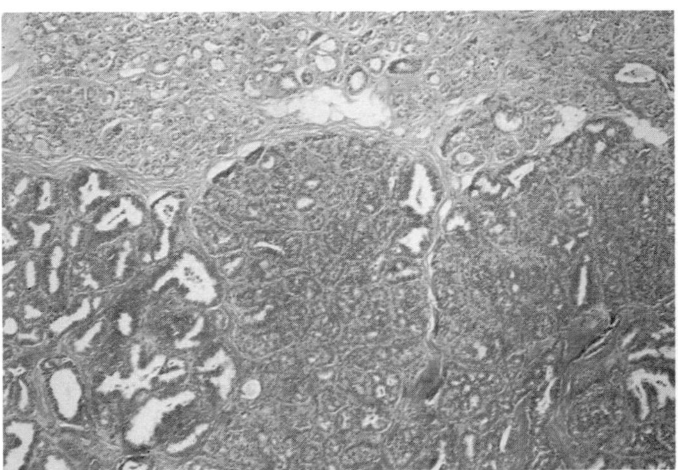

Fig. 22 Nodular adenosis (by courtesy of Dr D. Tarin).

Atypia

This occurs when hyperplastic cells exhibit bizarre or unusual features, either in the pattern of their cellular relationships or in the appearance of the nuclei (Fig. 21). The extent of atypia can be graded from 1 to 3, although this classification is empirical and subject to variation between pathologists.

Adenosis

This is an increase in the number of glandular elements. There is a normal relationship between cells and the basement membrane (Fig. 22).

Epitheliosis

This controversial term has found greater acceptance in the United Kingdom than in the United States. It has been used to describe the solid or semisolid benign epithelial proliferation which is found predominantly in the small ducts, ductules, and lobules. It has been implied that severe forms of epitheliosis amount to carcinoma *in situ*, although this point of view has been widely criticized. There has been a recent tendency to replace the term epitheliosis with hyperplasia.

Papillomatosis

This is also a controversial term which has found favour in North America. It has been criticized as it implies a derivation from the term papilloma, and the vast majority of examples bear no resemblance to a papillary pattern. Hyperplasia is being used instead of papillomatosis.

Studies of risk

The only study which has used accurate data to assess the risk of cancer in patients with benign breast disease is that of Page *et al.* The results of this study form the basis of an American Cancer Society consensus statement on the risk of breast cancer in patients with benign disease which was published in 1986 (Table 8). Cancer risk is defined as a liability to develop breast cancer in the ensuing 10 to 20 years, compared with development in age-matched women who have had no breast biopsy. It should be noted that these are not life-time risks.

Table 8 Relationship between benign and malignant breast disease

No increased risk
Sclerosing adenosis
Apocrine change
Duct ectasia
Mild hyperplasia
Fibroadenoma
Cysts
Apocrine metaplasia
Slight increased risk (1.5–2×)
Moderate or florid hyperplasia
Papilloma with fibrovascular core
Moderate increased risk (4–5×)
Atypical ductal hyperplasia
Atypical lobular hyperplasia
High risk (8–10×)
Ductal carcinoma *in situ*
Lobular carcinoma *in situ*

In their original study, Dupont and Page ascribed a slightly increased cancer risk to patients with sclerosing adenosis. However, other studies have not confirmed this finding and sclerosing adenosis is therefore currently considered as having no increased cancer risk.

The American consensus statement maintained that breast cysts were not associated with an increased cancer risk. Other studies have confirmed this opinion, but there is an increasing body of data suggesting that macroscopic cysts, especially those of the apocrine type, may be associated with an increased risk of breast cancer. Further work is required to clarify this question.

The inclusion of *in-situ* cancer may be criticized, as this diagnosis implies a neoplastic rather than a benign process. Conversely, multiple papillomatosis, not included in the above discussion, has been clearly demonstrated to be associated with an increased cancer risk.

The relative risk of developing invasive breast cancer following benign disease implies the existence of the classical pathway from normality to invasive cancer:

Normal → hyperplasia → atypia (grades 1–3) → carcinoma *in situ* → microinvasive cancer → clinically invasive cancer.

Care must be taken in interpreting this rather crude and perhaps naïve pathway. There is no evidence that the progression from normality to invasive cancer needs to pass through all the above stages. Furthermore once a certain point in the pathway has been reached there does not have to be further progression; in theory, regression may occur.

FURTHER READING

Dixon JM, Scott WN, Miller WR. Natural history of cystic disease: the importance of cyst type. *Br J Surg* 1985; **72**: 190–2.

Dupont WD, Page DL. Risk factors for breast cancer in women with proliferative breast disease. *N Engl J Med* 1985; **312**: 146–51.

Fentiman IS, Caleffi M, Hamed H, Chaudar MA. Dosage and duration of tamoxifen treatment for mastalgia: a controlled trial. *Br J Surg* 1988; **75**: 845–6.

Haagensen CD. Mammary duct ectasia—a disease the may simulate cancer. *Cancer* 1951; **4**: 749–61.

Hughes LE, Mansel RE, Webster DJT. Aberrations of normal development and involution (ANDI): a new perspective on pathogenesis and nomenclature of benign breast disorders. *Lancet* 1987; **ii**: 1316–9.

Hughes LE, Mansel RE, Webster DJT. *Benign Disorders and Diseases of the Breast: Concepts and Clinical Management*. London: Bailliere Tindall 1989.

Maddox PR, Harrison BJ, Mansel RE, Hughes LE. Non-cyclical mastalgia: an improved classification and treatment. *Br J Surg* 1989; **76**: 901–4.

Mansel RE, Dogliotti L. European multicentre trial of bromocriptine in cyclical mastalgia. *Lancet* 1990 **335**: 190–3.

Mansel RE, Wisbey JR, Hughes LE. Controlled trial of the antigonadotrophin danazol in painful nodular benign breast disease. *Lancet* 1982; **1**: 928–31.

Page DL, Anderson TJ. *Diagnostic Histopathology of the Breast*. Edinburgh: Churchill Livingstone 1987.

Thomas WG, Williamson RN, Davies JD, Webb AJ. The clinical syndrome of mammary duct ectasia. *Br J Surg* 1982; **69**: 423–5.

Turner-Warwick RT. The lymphatics of the breast. *Br J Surg* 1959; **46**: 574–82.

Winchester DP. American College of Pathologists Consensus Statement. The relationship of fibrocystic disease to breast cancer. *Am Coll Surg Bull* 1986; **71**: 29–31.

12.2 Cancer of the breast

MICHAEL J. GREENALL

Breast cancer is a major and important form of malignant disease in the Western World. In North America it was the most common malignancy among women, accounting for 27 per cent of all female cancers. Eighteen per cent of all cancer deaths are due to cancer of the breast, although since the mid-1980s the mortality from lung cancer has equalled and subsequently exceeded that of breast cancer as a cause of death in women. In the United States of America 130 000 new cases of breast cancer were diagnosed in 1987 and there were about 40 000 deaths from the disease. The equivalent figures from the United Kingdom are 30 000 and 15 000, respectively.

The risk of a woman developing breast cancer is a controversial subject and may be expressed in a variety of ways. In the Western world the cumulative risk (the proportion of a fixed group of women developing breast cancer over a set period of time) is about 7 per cent up to the age of 70. Thus, one in 14 women can expect to develop breast cancer.

DEMOGRAPHIC FEATURES

There is remarkable variation in the incidence of breast cancer between different countries. The rates in the United States and Canada are six times higher than those in Asia or black Africa. Rates nearly equal to those seen in North America occur in north European countries and in New Zealand. Intermediate rates occur in eastern and southern European countries, South America, and the Caribbean. Japan has a low incidence of breast cancer, although it is becoming more common.

The difference in breast cancer rates is not simply a function of genetic susceptibility. The incidence of breast cancer in black Americans parallels that of white Americans rather than that of black Africans, and the cancer incidence of offspring of migrants to the United States of America from Japan is similar to that of native Americans.

RISK FACTORS

The cause of breast cancer is unknown. However, epidemiological data indicate well-defined factors that indicate an increased liability to developing the disease. Such risk factors for breast cancer fall into three main groups: genetic, endocrine, and environmental; each may be of major, intermediate, or minor importance (Table 1). Many of the minor factors are the source of continued debate.

Major risk factors

Sex

Breast cancer is 100 times more common in women than in men. In strict epidemiological terms, therefore, female sex is a major risk factor for breast cancer, although it is often forgotten as such.

Age

As for other epithelial cancers the incidence of breast cancer increase with age. Breast carcinoma is only occasionally seen in the late teens but thereafter there is a rapid rise in age-specific rates. Up to the age of 40 the increase in age-specific cancer rate is very steep; the rate of increase then slows dramatically, although the overall breast cancer rate continues to rise until old age (Fig. 1). The cumulative risk of develop-

Table 1 Risk factors for breast cancer

Major factors
Female sex
Age
Previous breast cancer
Family history
Nulliparity
Benign breast disease (e.g. multiple papillomatosis)
Intermediate factors
Early menarche
Late menopause
Irradiation
Body weight
Benign breast disease (e.g. hyperplasia with severe atypia)
Minor or controversial faactors
Alcohol
Diet
Contraceptive pill and hormone replacement therapy
Benign breast disease (e.g. hyperplasia with moderate or mild atypia)

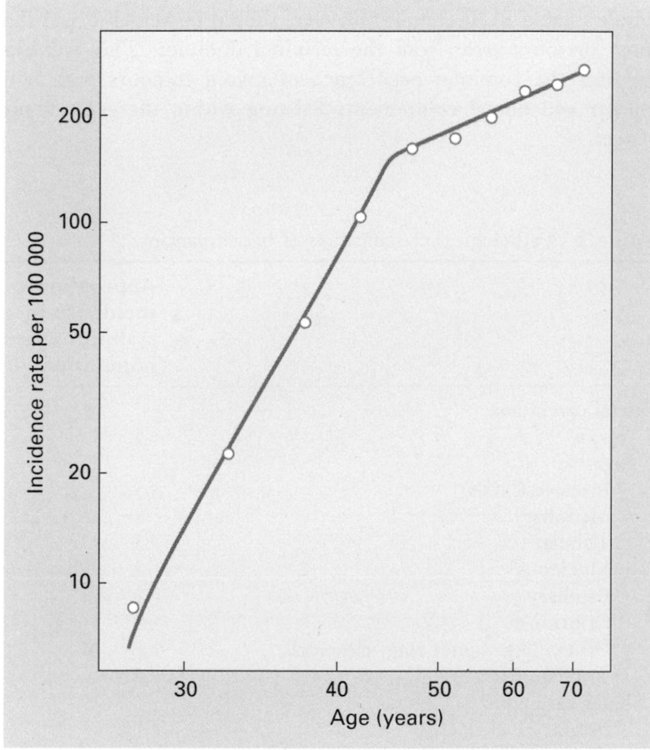

Fig. 1 Age specific breast cancer incidence. Note the rapid increase in age specific rate up to age 40.

ing breast cancer between the ages of 20 and 40 is 0.5 per cent whereas between 50 and 70 it is 5 per cent. This accounts for the fact that the majority of patients presenting with breast cancer are over the age of 50.

Previous breast cancer

The development of a second breast cancer may be a clinical manifestation of multifocal origin of the first cancer or may be an entirely new cancer. The risk of developing metachronous tumours has been addressed in a number of studies which have evaluated the development of cancer in the remaining breast after partial mastectomy. The incidence of such second cancers depends on whether or not synchronous bilateral cancers are included, but there appears to be an overall increased risk of 0.75 per cent to 1 per cent per year. Thus, the relative risk of developing a second non-synchronous primary 20 years after initial diagnosis of breast cancer is 1.2 to 1.5. This risk appears greatest in young women if their initial breast cancer is diagnosed before the age of 40.

Family history

A family history breast cancer is associated with an increased risk of the disease. The risk is greatest in patients with first-degree relatives (mother or sister) affected, especially if they were under the age of 50 when the disease developed. The relative risk of developing breast cancer is 1.7 to 2.5 in women with a history of breast cancer in a first-degree relative, and 1.5 among those with an affected second-degree relative. Whether the existence of multiple family members with breast cancer or the existence of bilateral disease in a relative indicates excessive risk is unclear, but such factors are likely to be of importance.

There is probably a direct genetic factor involved in the development of breast cancer in about 5 per cent of all patients.

Nulliparity

Nulliparity removes a protective effect against breast cancer. Single and nulliparous married women have a relative risk rate of 1.4 compared to parous women; however, this effect of parity is almost totally due to the protective influence of early age at first birth. Women who give birth to their first child before the age of 20 have a relative risk of 0.5 compared to nulliparous women; for those whose first birth occurred after the age of 30 there appeared to be virtually no protective effect, with a relative risk of 0.94. Some evidence suggests that women whose first birth is over the age of 35 may have an increased risk of breast cancer.

If the age at first birth is taken into account, subsequent pregnancies appear to have no influence on the risk of developing breast cancer. The protective effect occurs only if the pregnancy continues to full term.

Any protective effect of breast feeding is hard to assess as it is difficult to differentiate from the effects of pregnancy. However, recent data from one study indicated an independent protective effect of breast feeding, although other studies have failed to confirm this finding.

Benign breast disease

Benign disease is not usually recognized as a major risk factor, although multiple papillomatosis may be regarded as such.

Intermediate risk factors

Age of menarche and menopause

Women whose menarche occurs before the age of 12, have a relative risk of 2.30 compared to those starting menstruation after this age. This decreases as the age of onset of menstruation increases. The reduction in the age of the menarche over the past 100 years, especially in the Western world, probably results from improved nutrition and general health and may be important in the demographic variations in incidence of breast cancer.

The risk of developing breast cancer also relates to the age of the menopause. The relative risk of developing breast cancer is 0.5 per cent in those who cease to menstruate before the age of 45, compared to women who continue menstruating beyond age 55. Artificial menopause by oophorectomy or irradiation also reduces the risk of breast cancer.

Irradiation

An increased risk of breast cancer has been demonstrated in survivors of atomic explosions, women treated by radiation for postpartum mastitis, and patients receiving multiple chest radiographs during assessment of tuberculosis. This increased risk becomes apparent after a latent period of 10 to 15 years: the effect is most obvious in women exposed to irradiation when under the age of 35; there is little increased risk in women exposed after the age of 40.

Body weight

There is a strong relationship between body weight and breast cancer although this is critically dependent on age. In women under age 50 there is little correlation between risk of breast cancer and body weight. However, in the 60 to 69 age group an increase in weight from less than 60 to 70 kg or greater increases breast cancer risk to 1.8.

Benign breast disease

Severe atypia with hyperplasia is associated with a moderately increased risk of developing breast cancer.

Minor and controversial risk factors

Alcohol

Evidence for an association between consumption of alcohol and increased liability to breast cancer is becoming stronger, although the risk is small (1.5).

Diet

Although weight correlates with breast cancer risk the relationship between dietary factors such as fat or cholesterol intake have not been shown to be an important factor in the development of breast carcinoma.

Contraceptive pill

Some 15 case-controlled studies have evaluated the risk of breast cancer in women taking the contraceptive pill. The results are conflicting and if there is a risk it is small. Those most at risk are women taking oestrogen-based oral contraceptives early in life and taking them for at least 8 to 10 years.

Hormone replacement therapy

The data relating to cancer risk and hormone replacement therapy are conflicting. Small doses of exogenous oestrogen therapy for short periods of time in premenopausal women appear to be safe. However, when hormone replacements are taken for 8 years or longer there may be an increased risk of 1.5 to 2.0.

Benign breast disease

Some pathological entities, such as multiple papillomatosis and hyperplasia with gross atypia, are certainly associated with an increased risk of breast cancer (3.0). The risk is lower with lesser degrees of atypia. Patients with recurrent macroscopic apocrine cysts may also have a slightly increased risk of breast cancer.

The relationship between benign breast disease and risk of cancer is bedevilled by ascribing cancer risk to fibroadenoma and 'fibrocystic change'. There is no increased cancer risk for these two entities.

PATHOLOGICAL FEATURES OF BREAST CANCER

The histological assessment of breast cancer is of paramount importance in establishing the diagnosis of the tumour. It also helps determine the patient's prognosis and allows a greater understanding of the biology of the disease in any one particular case. Even relatively recently pathologists were satisfied in ascribing the term 'breast carcinoma' to all breast tumour specimens; the complexity of the subject is such that a more precise histological diagnosis is now required.

There are many methods of pathologically classifying breast cancer; most are based on whether the tumour is invasive or non-invasive and whether it is derived from the duct system or the lobule (Table 2). It should however, should be remembered that most tumours arise from the terminal ductules. This fact also explains the common occurrence of mixed tumours with both lobular and ductal components existing within the same breast cancer.

Table 2 Pathological classification of breast cancer

	Approximate incidence in symptomatic population
Ductal carcinoma	
In situ	5
Invasive	
Invasive (NOS)[a]	65
Medullary	5
Tubular	3
Mucinous	3
Papillary	3
Cribriform	3
Others (e.g. signet ring, clear cell, inflammatory)	3
Lobular carcinoma	
In situ	1
Invasive	10

[a] NOS, not otherwise specified.

Ductal carcinoma of the breast

This is the most common form of breast cancer accounting for 85 to 90 per cent of all cases. It can conveniently be subdivided into *in situ* and invasive types.

Ductal carcinoma in situ

Ductal carcinoma *in situ*, or intraductal carcinoma, is a preinvasive form of breast cancer. It is characterized by a proliferation of malignant breast epithelial cells, is confined to the duct system, and does not invade the basement membrane or surrounding tissues. In the unscreened population, ductal carcinoma *in situ* accounts for less than 5 per cent of all cases of breast cancer; in screening programmes the incidence increases to 15 to 20 per cent because it is associated with mammographically visible microcalcification. Postmortem studies show that the incidence of ductal carcinoma *in situ* is about 6 per cent in apparently normal breasts, but is as high as 40 per cent in mastectomy specimens associated with invasive cancer.

The most important aspect of ductal carcinoma is its malignant potential. The little that is known of the natural history of this entity comes from retrospective evidence of treating ductal carcinoma *in situ* by local excision alone. Such studies demonstrate a 30 to 50 per cent of ipsilateral invasive cancer, usually in the same quadrant, after an interval of some 10 to 15 years. The risk of developing invasive cancer depends on the extent of ductal carcinoma *in situ*.

There are five main histological types of intraductal carcinoma. The ducts, the terminal duct lobular units, and the lobules may be filled with malignant cells (solid type), the lesions may undergo central necrosis (comedo type), or they may have a sieve-like appearance (cribriform type). They may produce papillary projections (papillary or micropapillary types) or they may cling to the duct wall (clinging type). Comedo and papillary forms (Fig. 2) are the most common and are both associated with multicentric disease; comedo carcinoma is the most likely to become invasive and has the greatest expression of both DNA aneuploidy and of the C-*erb*2 oncogene.

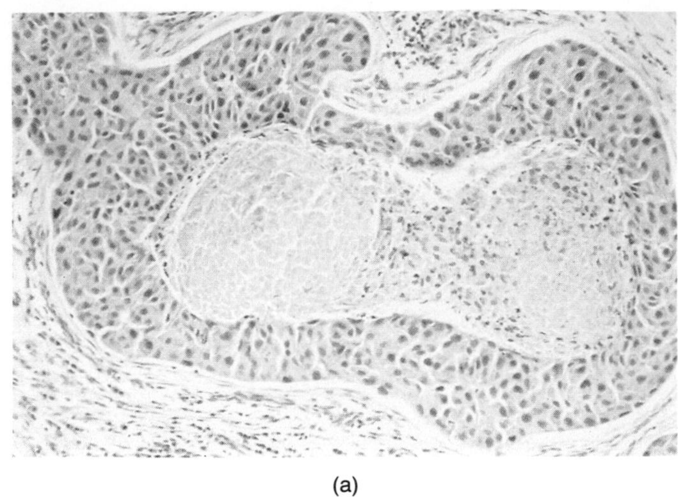

(a)

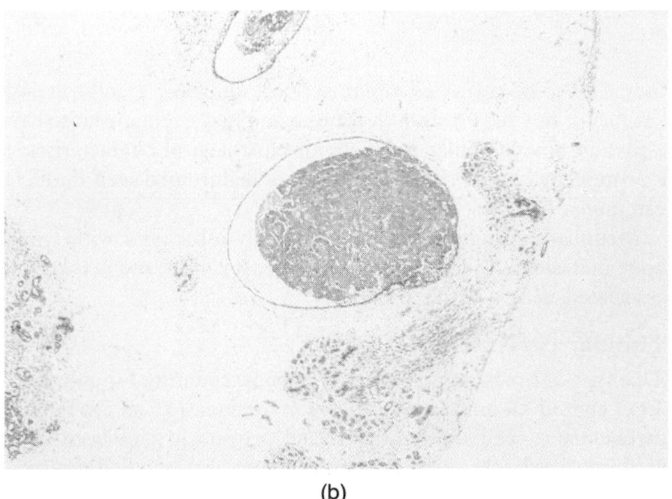

(b)

Fig. 2 Ductal carcinoma *in situ*. Duct distension with cancer cells and central necrosis (comedo type). (b) Papillary intraductal carcinoma distending the duct. In neither case is there evidence of invasion through the basement membrane. (By courtesy of Dr D. Tarin.)

Invasive ductal cancer

Once intraductal carcinoma has invaded the basement membrane of the duct it has demonstrated the most important prerequisite of all malignant tumours—the ability to infiltrate into surrounding tissue. The term 'invasive ductal cancer' therefore refers to the majority of tumours arising from the duct system. A large number of different morphological types of invasive duct cancer is apparent to the pathologist. Some have prognostic importance. However, they can be basically subdivided into those with specific histological features, and those in which there is no characteristic microscopic appearance. The majority of invasive ductal cancers fall into the latter group. These are described as infiltrating ductal carcinoma, not otherwise specified (NOS).

Infiltrating ductal carcinoma (NOS)

This is essentially a diagnosis for exclusion, but it accounts for about 65 per cent of all invasive mammary cancers. No specific gross or microscopic features allow recognition of this type of cancer: it is simply the lack of specific and consistent histological features that characterize lobular carcinoma and other special types of ductal cancer (Fig. 3). In a system of histological grading, infiltrating ductal carcinoma, not otherwise specified, would usually be classified as intermediate or high grade and, within the spectrum of invasive breast cancer, it has a relatively poor prognosis. However, other features such as tumour size and axillary nodal involvement are of more prognostic importance than histological features alone.

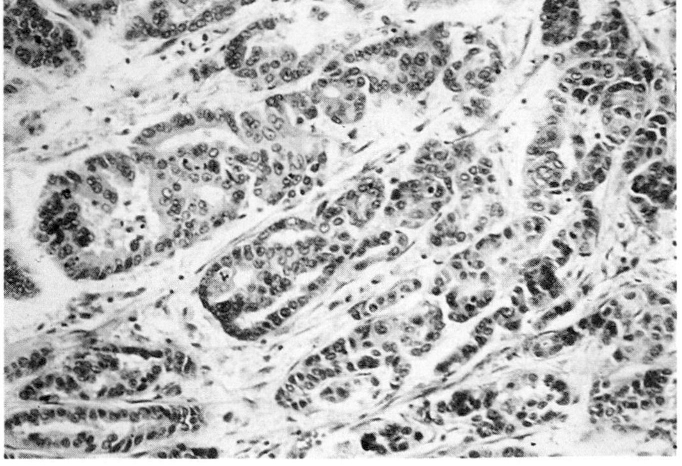

Fig. 3 Invasive ductal cancer (not otherwise specified). Malignant cells and poorly differentiated duct structures can be seen invading the surrounding stroma. (By courtesy of Dr. D. Tarin.)

Special types of infiltrating ductal carcinoma

Medullary carcinoma

Medullary carcinoma is a well recognized entity for about 6 per cent of all invasive mammary cancers (Fig. 4). Macroscopically

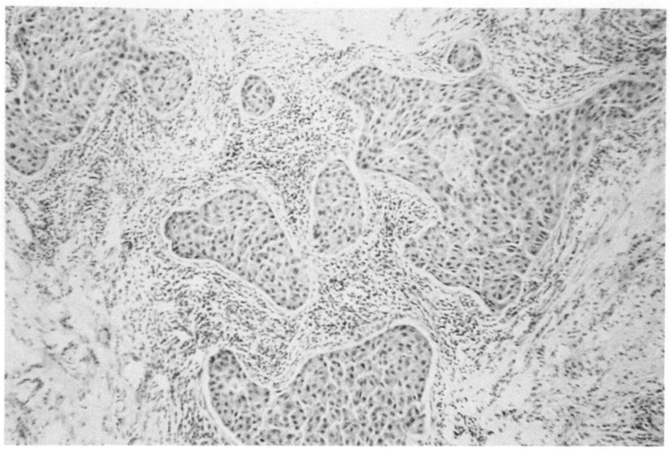

Fig. 4 Medullary carcinoma. Note associated lymphocytic infiltrate. (By courtesy of Dr D. Tarin.)

they tend to be soft, well circumscribed, and have a uniform consistency. They have a smooth contour and may even appear to have a pseudocapsule. Their most obvious histological characteristic is a prominent lymphocytic infiltration, a feature not seen in ductal carcinoma (NOS).

Medullary carcinoma is less frequently associated with lymph node metastases than other types of breast cancer and is therefore associated with a better prognosis.

Tubular carcinoma

This type of breast cancer is uncommon, accounting for only about 3 per cent of all infiltrating cancers of the breast (Fig. 5). Tubular carcinoma is well differentiated and previously had been often inappropriately classified in the not otherwise specified group.

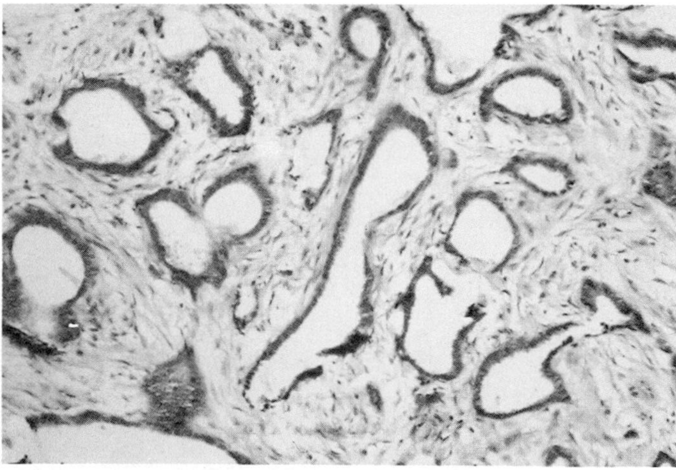

Fig. 5 Tubular carcinoma. Well differentiated tubular structures are apparent. (By courtesy of Dr D. Tarin.)

Most tubular cancers are small, being about 1 cm in diameter. They are hard and on section have a radial appearance. Histologically they form tubular structures with an open central space lined by a single layer of epithelium.

Recent interest in tubular carcinoma has been heightened by the impact of the breast screening programme. Not only is tubular carcinoma more frequently seen in screened individuals than in the symptomatic population but other abnormalities detected on mammography can cause diagnostic confusion. Of particular importance is the differential diagnosis between tubular cancer, sclerosing adenosis, and radial scar.

Patients with tubular carcinoma have a good prognosis and a 10-year survival rate in excess of 75 per cent. Nodal metastases, even when present, tend to be limited to one or two nodes only. It is uncommon for pure, well differentiated tubular carcinomas to metastasize to distant sites.

It is unclear whether special types of tumour such as tubular carcinoma dedifferentiate into more aggressive types of cancer as they progress (phenotypic drift). Such questions are of paramount importance when assessing the value of breast screening programmes.

Mucinous (mucoid) carcinoma

Mucinous carcinoma (Fig. 6) is characterized by a small rounded tumour which histologically demonstrates pools of mucous material in which are aggregates of cancer cells. This tumour accounts for about 2 or 3 per cent of all invasive cancer, but it has been associated with a survival rate which is appreciably better than that of ductal carcinoma (NOS). These tumours said to occur in older women and, like tubular carcinoma, rarely metastasize to lymph nodes.

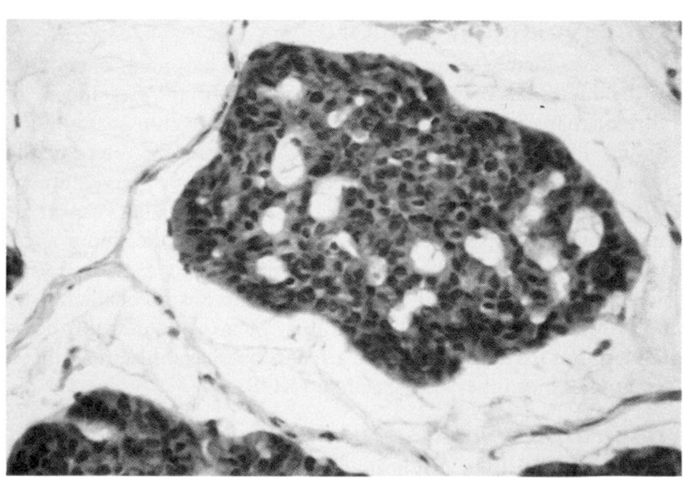

Fig. 6 Mucinous carcinoma. Tumour cells are lying in pools of mucinous material. (By courtesy of Dr D. Tarin.)

Papillary carcinoma

Unlike other subtypes of ductal carcinoma, papillary carcinoma can be easily subdivided into *in-situ* and invasive types. The non-invasive papillary carcinoma has the fronded structure of a papilloma. It is usually well delineated from surrounding breast tissue by a fibrous covering, hence the essentially inaccurate term of intracystic papillary carcinoma. As long as there is no extracapsular evidence of *in-situ* carcinoma simple excision of these 'intracystic papillary carcinomas' will suffice.

Invasive papillary carcinoma to account for only about 2 per cent of all breast cancers. Microscopically, they are usually well circumscribed and histologically demonstrate papillary formation. The prognosis is generally good.

Invasive cribriform carcinoma

This has only recently been recognized as a special type of invasive ductal carcinoma. It accounts for about 3 per cent of all breast cancers and may be more common in the screened population. It classically presents with a firm mass, but microscopy reveals characteristic stromal invasion with a cribriform pattern. They tend to be well differentiated and have a good prognosis.

Other types of invasive ductal carcinoma

The presence of signet ring cells in breast cancer is a rare but important phenomenon. Most of these tumours are diffuse and poorly defined. Histologically, for reasons which are unclear, they are often associated with lobular carcinoma and are characterized by signet ring cells with a peripherally placed nucleus and marked cytoplasmic vacuolization. Their prognosis is poor; they selectively metastasize to the peritoneal cavity and it becomes difficult to differentiate metastatic signet cell carcinoma from those originating in the gastrointestinal tract.

Clear cell tumours also have a poor prognosis. Their appearance is characteristic on haematoxylin and eosin staining; further selective stains demonstrate either a lipid-rich or glycogen-rich pattern.

Secretory carcinomas are rare. They are frequently small and are characterized by abundant intra-and extracellular areas of vacuolization. These tumours frequently occur in younger women and generally have a good prognosis; extremely rare breast cancers occurring in childhood are often of this type.

Inflammatory carcinoma has previously been ascribed to tumours occurring in pregnancy and lactation (mastitis carcinomatosis), although it is now apparent that it occurs in all age groups. The diagnosis of inflammatory cancer is dependent on the observation of tumour emboli in dermal lymphatics, giving rise to the red infiltrative appearance of this condition. It must be differentiated from peu d'orange which is simply due to lymphatic obstruction of the breast as a result of axillary nodal metastases from tumours of any type. Its prognosis is very poor.

Other rare types of infiltrating ductal carcinoma include those with carcinoid, adenocystic, and squamous features.

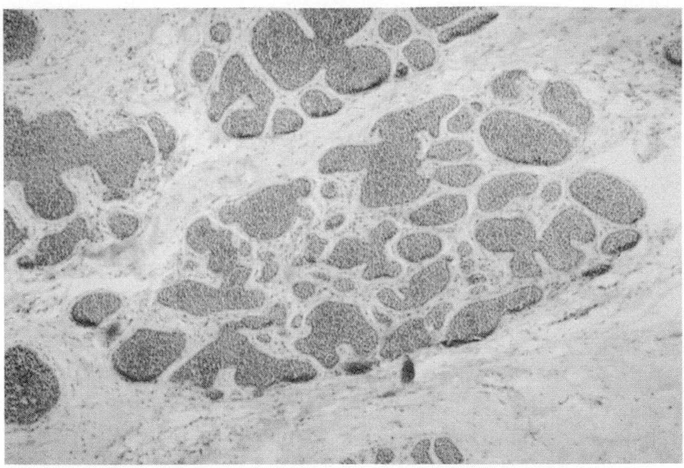

Fig. 7 Lobular carcinoma *in situ*. The acini are distended with a uniform population of malignant cells. There are no interstitial spaces. (By courtesy of Dr D. Tarin.)

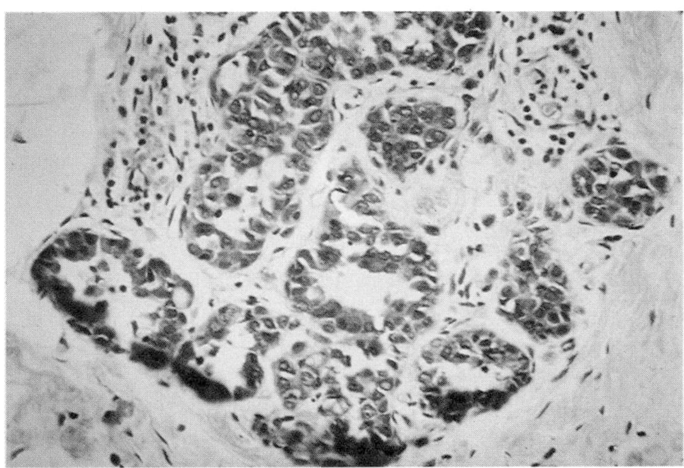

Fig. 8 Atypical lobular hyperplasia. The criteria for LCIS are not met. Only some acini are distended and interstitial spaces remain. (By courtesy of Dr D. Tarin.)

Lobular carcinoma of the breast

Lobular carcinoma can also be conveniently subdivided into *in-situ* and invasive forms, depending on whether the basement membrane of the lobule has been invaded by tumour.

Lobular carcinoma *in situ*

Lobular carcinoma *in situ*, like its intraductal counterpart, is also a preinvasive form of breast cancer. The term 'lobular carcinoma *in situ*' was used in its original description by Foote and Stewart in 1941; other terms, such as intra-acinous carcinoma and lobular neoplasia, have also been widely used.

The microscopic criteria for diagnosing lobular carcinoma *in situ* are well defined (Fig. 7). Within the lobule there must be a uniform proliferation of cells and, as a result, there should be no interstitial spaces and expansion of at least half of the acini in the lobular unit. If these criteria are not completely fulfilled then the term 'atypical lobular hyperplasia' is appropriate (Fig. 8). The term 'lobular neoplasia' was used by Haagensen to describe both atypical lobular hyperplasia and lobular carcinoma *in situ* although its use has been criticized as it implies that atypical lobular hyperplasia is a neoplastic process.

The most important aspect of lobular carcinoma *in situ* is its potential for becoming invasive. The risk of invasive lobular carcinoma developing following simple biopsy for lobular carcinoma *in situ* is only about 25 per cent over 20 years: this is a lower risk than that of ductal carcinoma *in situ*. Unlike ductal carcinoma *in situ*, lobular carcinoma *in situ* rarely expresses the C-*erb2* oncogene.

The biggest single study evaluating the malignant potential of lobular carcinoma *in situ* is that of Haagensen. As well as identifying the risk of frank malignant change, Haagensen made a number of important observations (Table 3). It is now generally agreed that as the risk of invasive cancer after diagnosis of lobular carcinoma *in situ* (relative risk, 10) relates equally to both breasts, it should be regarded as a risk factor for tumour development rather than a direct precursor. Atypical lobular hyperplasia carries a 4-fold increased risk for development of breast cancer.

Table 3 Features of lobular carcinoma *in situ*

Predominately premenopausal
Multifocal and bilateral
Does not metastasize
Is not palpable
Does predispose to invasive cancer
Invasive cancer develops in the contralateral breast in 50% of patients
The eventual cancers have a good prognosis

After Haagensen 1978.

In practice, lobular carcinoma *in situ* is usually discovered by chance. It has no mammographic features and is usually found on biopsy undertaken for other reasons.

Invasive lobular cancer

Invasive lobular cancer accounts for about 10 per cent of all cases of breast carcinoma, although its incidence varies quite widely. Up to 10 per cent of lobular cancers have a co-existing ductal component. Five main subtypes are described: classical, solid, alveolar, mixed, and pleomorphic. Their main pathological features are summarized in Table 4. The most common type, classical lobular carcinoma, is characterized by the 'Indian filing' of invading malignant cells, often in a 'targetoid' pattern (Fig. 9). The 'monotonous' features of individual cells along with lack of a specific histologic architecture results in difficulty in grading lobular carcinoma.

Table 4 Pathological features of invasive lobular cancer

Type	Pattern	Cell type
Classical	Indian filing, targetoid diffuse invasion	Small non-cohesive, regular, monotonous cell population
Solid	Sheet-like	
Alveolar	Globular aggregates	
Mixed	Mixture of above	
Pleomorphic	Diffuse infiltrate	Nuclear pleomorphism

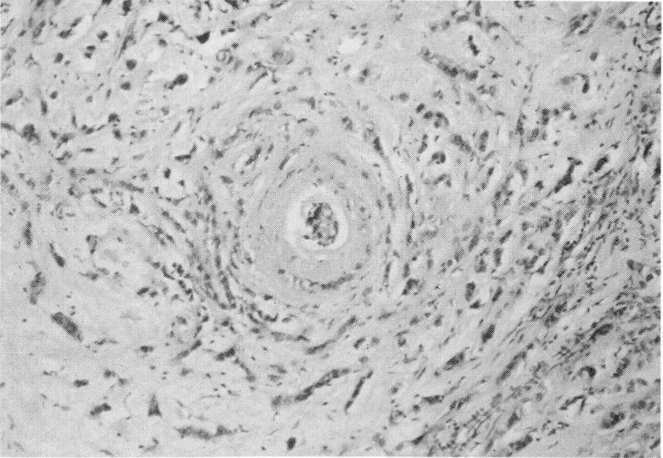

Fig. 9 Invasive lobular cancer. Indian filing of individual cells with a targetoid pattern is apparent. (By courtesy of Dr D. Tarin.)

Invasive lobular carcinoma is important with respect to its tendency to bilaterality and the fact that its clinical diagnosis may be difficult because of the diffuse infiltrative nature which frequently produces distortion of the breast rather than a lump. The prognosis of classic invasive lobular carcinoma is generally somewhat better than that of invasive ductal cancer. The other types of lobular carcinoma, especially its pleomorphic variant, have a worse prognosis than the classic form of this disease.

NATURAL HISTORY OF BREAST CANCER

The lay public, and indeed a number of medical practitioners, believe that transition from normality to breast cancer and thence to metastatic disease is a rapid process. The reverse is, in fact, the case. The natural history of breast cancer is normally characterized by long duration, but shows extreme heterogeneity between patients. Breast cancer is one of the more slowly growing tumours which therefore renders it suitable for screening programmes. The evolution of breast cancer, especially in its preclinical phases, can be measured in years or even decades, although there are exceptions to this rule in which the disease takes on a more aggressive form.

Our understanding of the preclinical phases of breast cancer is based on indirect observations of the morphological changes from normality to hyperplasia, atypia, carcinoma *in situ*, and finally to invasive cancer. It should be remembered, however, that this progression is by no means inevitable and, in theory, stages may be missed out. It is also possible that a given stage may be permanent or may even regress to a more normal state. Histological characteristics may be correlated with other biological factors, such as labelling index, doubling time, and growth fractions. Serial mammography has indirectly indicated that the doubling time for human breast cancer is usually of the order of 100 to 300 days, although exceptions to this are frequently seen. If it is also assumed that if a tumour of 1 cm size contains about 10^9 cells it would require about 30 doublings for a malignant cell to produce this volume. This does, of course, assume that there is no cell loss, that there is a linear growth rate, and that the tumour is initially derived from a single cell. Although these assumptions can be challenged, they do indicate that the preclinical phase of breast cancer would still be of the order of about 7 years and often much longer. Clinical observations of patients treated by biopsy alone for hyperplasia or atypia give some support for these figures.

The heterogeneity of breast cancer can also be appreciated from the percentage of cells that are undergoing cell division at any particular time (labelling index). Tumours with high labelling indices are associated with short doubling times and are therefore more aggressive. Overall, the median labelling index is about 3 per cent; the range extends from less than 1 per cent to approximately 40 per cent. High labelling indices are associated with poor prognostic factors such as premenopausal status and with a poor overall clinical outcome.

The natural history of clinically apparent breast cancer is also surprisingly slow. Historical observations on untreated breast cancer as recorded by the Middlesex Hospital, London, and the Connecticut Tumor Registry show an average survival of about 2.5 to 3 years without treatment. Such data can be criticized as they are historical and probably relate to a group of patients presenting with locally advanced rather than metastatic disease. They do, however, indicate the need for prolonged monitoring in patients with clinical breast cancer.

The spread of breast cancer

Once breast cancer is clinically apparent it will, by definition, tend to spread locally and to regional or distant sites. The extent and rate of spread varies greatly from one individual to another and is characteristic of the heterogeneity of the disease. Some tumours spread rapidly to regional nodes or distant sites while remaining small in the breast; others grow slowly to a large size without metastasizing. Clearly, those with the greatest metastatic potential have the worst prognosis.

Local spread within the breast

Within the breast there are three main mechanisms of spread. The most important mechanism is local spread by direct infiltration into the surrounding parenchyma. This occurs by the ramifying projections that give the characteristic macroscopic stellate appearance of breast cancer. If uncontrolled, direct infiltration of overlying skin or the underlying fascia occurs.

A second mode of local spread is by direct infiltration along ducts, although it is unclear whether this represents actual tumour growth or whether it reflects a field change of pre-existing *in-situ* disease. The presence of widespread *in-situ* cancer explains the phenomenon of multifocality in patients with breast cancer. Multifocality, or cancer within the same quadrant as the primary tumour, should be distinguished from multicentricity, which is defined as the presence of carcinoma outside the quadrant containing the primary tumour. In one study, 43 per cent of 246 patients with invasive breast cancer less than 4 cm in diameter demonstrated multifocality. In 43 per cent of these patients affected areas were more than 2 cm from the primary tumour; in 9 per cent additional foci of cancer were found more than 4 cm away. Such multifocal tumours are confined to the duct system in 66 per cent of patients, but the remainder demonstrate invasion into surrounding tissues. The incidence and extent of multifocality depends on the size of the primary tumour. These findings have obvious implications when treating breast cancer by conservative surgery.

Local lymphatic and vascular spread within the breast are also of prognostic importance. Of particular importance are those lymphatic pathways extending into the pectoral fascia and subareolar regions.

Regional spread of breast cancer

The regional spread of breast cancer is defined as that to the axillary, internal mammary, and supraclavicular nodes.

Axillary nodal spread

The axillary nodes represent the most important site of regional spread from breast cancer. Spread to axillary nodes is the most important prognostic indicator of breast cancer: approximately 45 per cent of all patients have nodal disease at presentation. The likelihood of axillary nodal spread is a function of the size of the breast primary, but even when correction is made for tumour size, disease in the axillary nodes remains the most important prognostic variable. For tumours less than 2 cm in diameter, the incidence of axillary nodal spread is less than 20 per cent. The incidence of axillary nodal disease is 35 per cent in those with tumours 2 to 5 cm in diameter, and 50 per cent of patients with tumours greater than 5 cm in size.

The clinical assessment of axillary nodes is notoriously unreliable. About 30 per cent of palpable and apparently diseased nodes are found to be histologically free of metastases; conversely, up to 30 per cent of apparently normal axillary nodes demonstrate histological evidence of metastatic disease.

The extent of nodal disease reported depends to a great extent on the pathological evaluation of the specimens. Not only is there a great variation from one centre to another in the surgical removal of nodes at axillary sampling or clearance, but there is also a marked difference between pathologists in retrieving and examining all the nodes provided in the surgical specimen. Techniques such as clearing the axillary fat with xylene to increase nodal yield and more thorough sectioning of the nodes themselves increase the positivity rate. However, few pathologists have adopted these methods.

The relationship between axillary nodal spread and prognosis depends on three factors: the number of nodes affected, the level of axillary nodal disease, and the extent of disease within the nodes themselves. Accurate appraisal of the nodes is therefore dependent on close liaison between the surgeon and pathologist with respect to orientation of the specimen at the time of axillary exploration.

Number of nodes involved

Survival rates based on the number of diseased lymph nodes show remarkable unity between studies. Results assessed by the American College of Surgeons have shown that the number of nodes affected by cancer provides valuable prognostic information. Documentation of nodal status as negative or positive for metastatic disease yields only qualitative data and fails to provide the prognostic information that can be obtained from full analysis of the number of nodes affected at axillary clearance. The number of negative nodes recovered on axillary clearance is of no prognostic importance, although some authorities claim that to ensure that the axilla is clear of metastases at least four, and possibly up to 10, negative nodes must be isolated. After 5 years women treated by mastectomy have an 82 per cent relative survival rate if no lymph nodes are involved and a 60 per cent survival rate if one or two lymph nodes are involved at the time of initial treatment. Women with five or six nodes affected have a 47 per cent survival rate; this is reduced to only 31 per cent if 11 or 12 nodes are involved. Women with more than 20 nodes involved have only an 8 per cent survival rate at 5 years.

Thus, according to studies made by the National Surgical Adjuvant Breast Project (NSABP), within the group of women with positive nodes, it is apparent that if one to three nodes are affected by the tumour the prognosis, while not good, can be relatively optimistic. However, women with four to 12 positive lymph nodes should be given a more guarded prognosis, and those with more than 13 axillary nodes affected have a decidedly poor outcome.

Level of disease

As previously described, the axillary nodes are conveniently divided into three groups depending on their relationship to the pectoralis minor muscle. Prognosis relates to the level of axillary node affected, although this is a less powerful factor than the total number of nodes affected by the tumour. Thus, Shottenfeld *et al.* showed that patients with disease in level I nodes had a 5-year survival rate of 65 per cent, those with disease at level II had a 5-year survival rate of 31 per cent, and no patients with disease affecting level III nodes survived for 5 years.

Patients with disease in level III nodes usually have a large number of affected lymph nodes. So-called skip metastases, in which metastatic deposits are found at levels II or III, but not at level I are found in only 2 per cent of patients. Thus, a dissection limited to level I alone is effective in determining the presence or absence of nodal disease but will tend to underestimate the degree of spread in many patients and will not provide accurate prognostic information.

The extent of disease in individual axillary nodes

The extent of disease within individual axillary nodes may also be of importance although, as is the case for level of involvement, there is a greater correlation with the number of nodes involved. Deposits less than 2 mm in size (micrometastases) can be detected only by histological methods. Such deposits usually occur in one node only; occasionally they are found in two, but their presence in a third is exceptional in the absence of macroscopic metastases. The prognostic significance of occult micrometastases is the subject of wide debate. They are probably far more common than is suggested by routine pathological examination of axillary nodes. The likelihood of detecting a micrometastasis during routine single section of an axillary node is about 6 per cent; this increases to 36 per cent if six equally spaced sections are taken through each lymph node.

The work involved in detecting micrometastases is extensive, and the question still remains as to their overall prognostic importance. It is likely that the presence of a single micrometastasis implies a slightly worse prognosis than for node negative disease, but improved survival compared to patients with a single pathologically obvious macrometastasis. This prognostic importance, however, is only applicable after at least 10 years; in practice the prognosis for patients with a single micrometastasis can be regarded as similar to those with node-negative disease.

In contradistinction to micrometastases, Haagensen and Stout down-staged their patients if nodal metastases were greater than 2.5 cm in diameter. Spread of metastatic disease outside the confines of the axillary nodes into surrounding fat is also a bad prognostic sign.

Internal mammary nodal spread

The internal mammary chain of lymph nodes lies at the anterior end of the intercostal spaces adjacent to the internal thoracic artery. Metastases in the internal mammary nodes are more commonly associated with medial or periareolar tumours and the overall incidence of such involvement is as high as 20 per cent. Disease affecting the internal mammary lymph nodes is rare in the absence of axillary nodal spread; only 8 per cent of patients have such disease if the axilla is clear.

Metastatic disease in the internal mammary nodes alone has the same prognostic implication as axillary nodal disease. However, if both the internal mammary and axillary nodes are affected the outlook is very poor, with a 25 per cent 10-year survival rate.

Because of the poor prognosis of patients with disease of the internal mammary nodes, various attempts at treatment have been adopted, including both surgical excision (in extended radical mastectomy) and radiation therapy. In some studies this aggressive approach has been associated with an improvement in survival in women with such metastatic disease. However, the routine excision of internal mammary nodes in all patients with breast cancer has not been associated with an overall improvement in survival.

It is unclear whether intramammary node disease, like supraclavicular node spread, should be regarded as regional or metastatic disease.

Supraclavicular nodes

Metastatic disease in the supraclavicular nodes implies extensive involvement of the internal mammary or axillary nodes. The frequent association with widespread metastatic disease means that supraclavicular nodal disease is associated with a poor prognosis.

Spread to distant sites

No site is immune to spread of the tumour, either at the time of presentation or later in the course of the disease. The most commonly affected sites are the bone, liver, and lung, but metastases to the brain, skin, and peritoneum are by no means uncommon.

Micrometastases in the bone marrow have been recognized for many years in patients with metastatic breast cancer. It is now becoming increasingly clear that such spread also occurs in up to one-third of patients with early, operable, breast cancer. The presence of micrometastases in bone marrow may correlate with other indicators of poor prognosis such as axillary lymph node metastases, tumour size, and oestrogen receptor status, but there is no clear evidence that they indicate a poor prognosis. In short, their relevance is unclear.

The clinical presentation of breast cancer

The majority of women presenting with breast cancer complain of a lump. Classically this is hard, painless, immobile, and demonstrates a degree of fixity to surrounding tissues, overlying skin, or the underlying pectoral muscle. The lump may be visible on inspection and may cause distortion of the breast on elevation of the arms or when tensing the pectoral muscles. Many tumours fail to demonstrate these classical characteristics, however. Not all breast cancers are hard: they are often described as being only firm. The degree of mobility can also vary: small tubular cancers can have a degree of mobility almost characteristic of a fibroadenoma. Finally, not all cancers are painless and occasionally patients describe the disconcerting symptoms of increased discomfort in the lump prior to menstruation. It is, therefore, advisable to undertake histological and cytological examination of any discrete lump in a woman over the age of 25. A diagnosis of a fibroadenoma or 'cystic change' without such confirmation is extremely dangerous.

Up to 15 per cent of women with breast cancer present with a more diffuse process within the breast, in which a lump is not necessarily the presenting feature. This is particularly common in younger patients with lobular carcinoma. The diffuse nature of the tumour produces distortion, puckering, and the eventual feeling of heaviness as the tumour extends through the breast. Later there may be nipple retraction and discomfort. A similar process occurs in patients who describe a thickening in the breast. Such symptoms can be difficult to differentiate clinically from those of benign breast disease.

Changes in the skin may be the sole presenting symptom; alternatively, they may be associated with other features of the cancer. Puckering may be pronounced and is often associated with the rather scirrhotic tumours of the elderly. However, this clinical sign is commonly observed in younger patients. Peu d'orange is a feature of advanced cancer. The cause of this characteristic clinical sign is oedema of the skin: this is not due to direct infiltration of the skin by tumour but represents lymphatic obstruction of the breast as a result of axillary metastasis. It must be differentiated from inflammatory breast cancer, in which cutaneous lymphatics contain tumour emboli. In advanced, untreated cases the skin may be broken, and tumour ulcerates through the skin, with associated haemorrhage and odour. Surrounding skin nodules are not uncommon in seriously neglected cases.

Presentation with changes at the nipple are not uncommon, but these primary tumours may be difficult to diagnose as they are often small and may be easily missed by mammography. Nipple distortion and inversion are not uncommon presenting features in patients with breast cancer. A unifocal or blood-stained nipple discharge is also indicative of malignant disease, often an intraductal carcinoma developing with the major duct system beneath the nipple. The discharge associated with intraductal cancer is characteristically watery and blood-stained, in contrast to the milk discharge of galactorrhoea and multifocal, tenacious, and coloured discharge of duct ectasia.

Paget's disease (Fig. 10) is usually a presenting feature of breast cancer in the elderly, although it is occasionally seen in other age groups. It usually represents an underlying intraductal carcinoma which may be quite extensive in the breast and which may also exhibit an invasive component. The origin of the characteristic, large, clear Paget cells remains an enigma. Whether they represent migration of tumour cells from the primary cancer or originate from the skin of the nipple itself remains unclear.

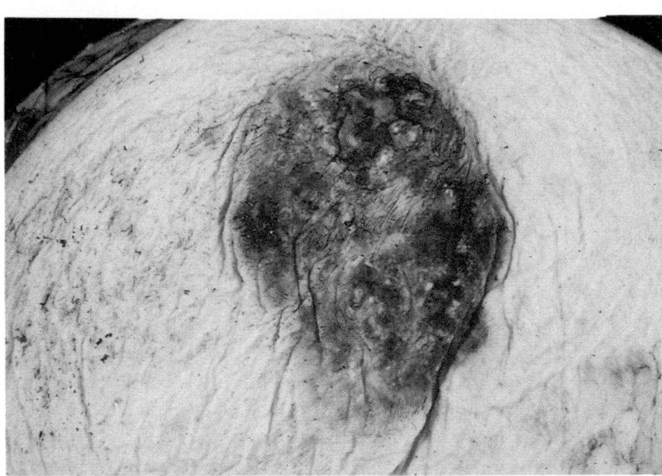

Fig. 10 Paget's disease of the nipple. The nipple is replaced by the classic exudative Paget's disease. (By courtesy of Dr D. Tarin.)

Finally, it should be remembered that breast cancer frequently presents with metastatic disease. This may be either to regional lymph nodes, such as those in the axilla or supraclavicular fossa, or to distant sites such as bone, lung, liver, or brain.

The diagnosis of breast cancer

There is no indication for a purely clinical diagnosis of breast cancer. The medicolegal consequences of an unnecessary mastectomy are such that there should be no doubt as to the diagnosis before embarking on definitive surgery.

Confirmatory diagnosis is by pathology and radiology, the former being by far the most important.

Pathological diagnosis

Fine needle aspiration cytology

This method has the advantages of being performed as an outpatient procedure and producing almost immediate results. The technique of aspiration is not difficult after an initial learning period, and it is relatively atraumatic. Its disadvantage is that it requires expert and specialized pathological interpretation. The false-negative rate is about 15 per cent, and false positive results occur in about 2 per cent of cases. False-negative results are due either to sampling errors as a result of missing the tumour at the time of aspiration or from failing to aspirate a particularly scirrhous acellular carcinoma. False-positives are uncommon but may be due to confusion with a hypercellular fibroadenoma or the effects of undisclosed hormone therapy, pregnancy, or lactation on normal breast tissue.

Aspiration cytology cannot differentiate *in-situ* or invasive cancer but can distinguish ductal from lobular carcinoma (Fig. 11).

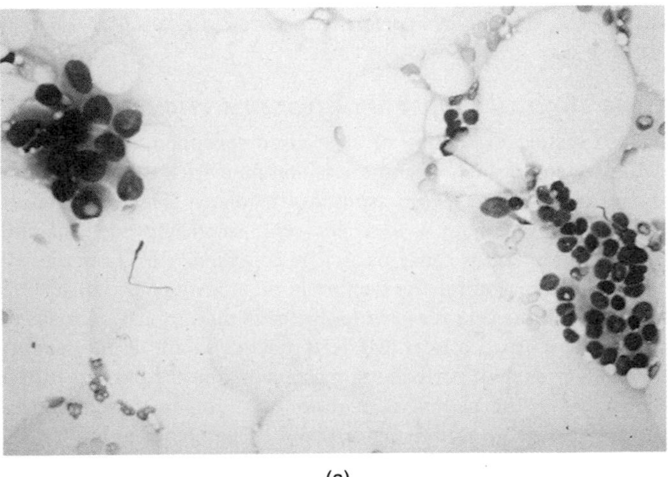

(a)

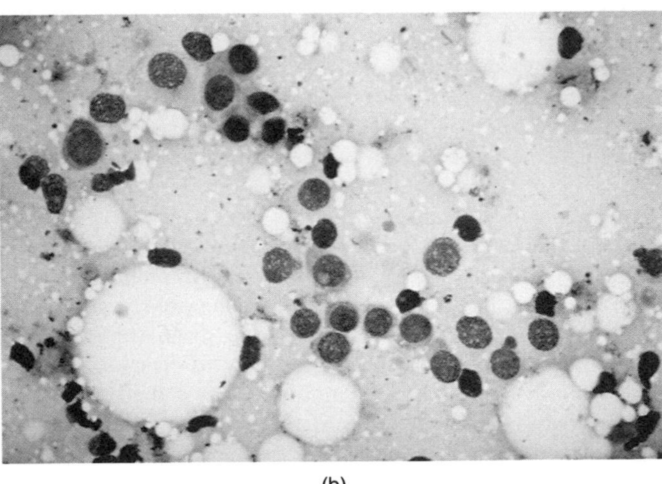

(b)

Fig. 11 Fine-needle aspiration cytology of breast cancer. Classic invasive ductal cancer; the cells are large, heterogeneous, and have irregular, dark-staining nuclei. A group of normal cells is also present. (b) The monotonous appearance of tumour cells typical of lobular carcinoma. (By courtesy of Dr I. Buley.)

Core biopsy

A variety of instruments can be used to provide a core of tissue in an outpatient procedure. This technique has to be performed under local anaesthetic, but it has the advantage that it produces a histological rather than a cytological specimen. The author has found the technique somewhat traumatic and liable to miss small scirrhotic tumours, although others have had great success with this method. As the core biopsy produces a histological rather than a cytological diagnosis, *in-situ* disease can be differentiated from invasive disease. Greater appraisal of the grade and type of tumour is also possible, although sampling errors are likely with such a small specimen.

Open surgical biopsy

Biopsy is required in patients who clinically are suspected to have a cancer yet in whom fine needle aspiration cytology or core biopsy fails to demonstrate malignant disease. It has the disadvantage of requiring hospital admission, although the majority of patients can be treated and discharged the same day. Its advantage is that it provides a definitive method of proving or excluding malignant disease. Open biopsy can occasionally be performed under local anaesthetic, but it is performed more easily under general anaesthesia.

Open surgical biopsy and frozen section

Frozen section evaluation of an excised specimen at the time of definitive surgery has become less common with the more widespread use of fine needle aspiration cytology. There is a false-positive rate of about 1 to 2 per cent: sclerosing adenosis and nipple adenoma can cause particular confusion with tumour.

A further reason for the decline in popularity of frozen section techniques is the very reasonable change in the surgical approach to women with breast cancer. Modern practice should avoid the outmoded approach of performing mastectomy on the basis of frozen section while the patient is anaesthetized and unable to discuss various treatment options determined by pathological findings.

Mammography

The last decade has witnessed a huge improvement in imaging methods for breast disease, and a high level of sensitivity and specificity is now available using modern mammographic techniques. The classic features of breast cancer on mammography are tissue asymmetry, mass effect, microcalcification, skin thickening, and nipple inversion (Fig. 12). One or more of these features may be present, the most reliable being a combination of mass effect with localized microcalcification.

Other methods of imaging such as ultrasonography, xerography, and thermography have also been successfully used in the diagnosis of breast cancer. However, for symptomatic masses which are amenable to fine needle aspiration cytology, good quality mammography alone should suffice as a diagnostic method.

Preoperative mammography is not only of diagnostic importance but also detects potential multicentricity and acts as a baseline for radiological evaluation of the breast in the years after initial diagnosis.

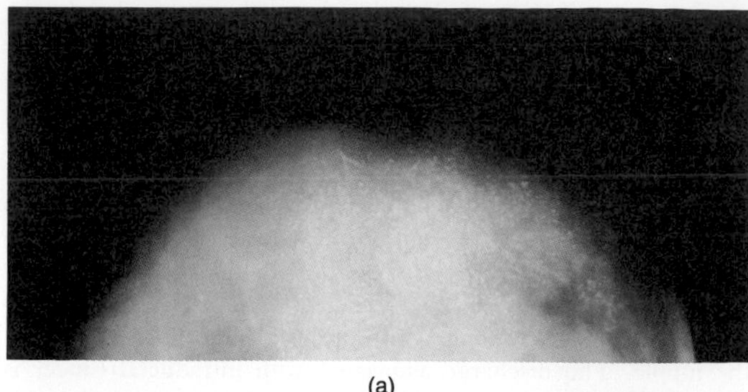

(a)

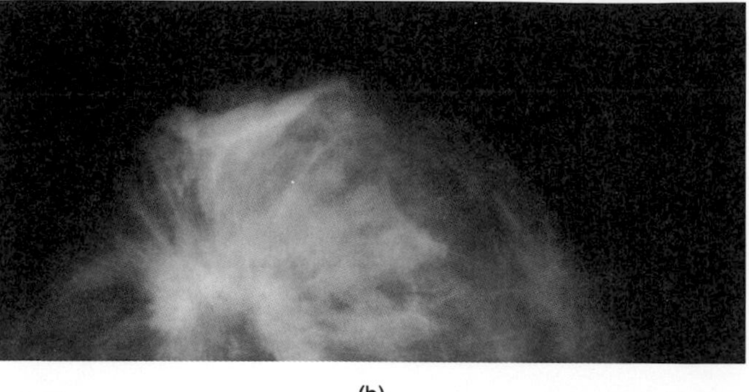

(b)

Fig. 12 Mammographic features of breast cancer. (a) Widespread microcalcification indicative of ductal carcinoma *in situ*. (b) A mass effect associated with distortion, skin thickening, and retraction. This is a classical feature of invasive ductal cancer. (By courtesy of Dr B. Shepstone.)

Evaluation of patients with breast cancer

Once the diagnosis of breast cancer has been made certain investigations are of value in subsequent management. All patients with breast cancer should undergo chest radiography and routine evaluation of haemoglobin, full blood count, electrolytes, and liver function tests. The value of other more sophisticated tests is open to doubt. There has been a vogue for performing bone, liver, and even brain scanning in all patients for the detection of asymptomatic metastases in patients who were felt to have early operable disease. In practice, however, there is a low incidence of true positive scans in 'operable' cancer. The positive yield for bone scanning, in patients with apparently localized disease is about 2 per cent, and approximately 50 per cent of these cases will be false-positives as a result of previous trauma or coexisting arthritis. There is an even lower positive yield with liver and brain scanning, some studies demonstrating a 100 per cent incidence of negative results following such investigations.

Although there is some disagreement over the usefulness of routine preoperative scanning, the overall incidence of positive results is low. However, patients with clinical stage III disease and those with symptoms suggestive of metastases should undergo further investigation. Brain scanning is of little value in patients with apparently operable breast cancer and the current recommendation is that if screening investigations are to be performed they should be limited to bone scintigraphy and ultrasonography of the liver.

Staging

Staging relates to the classification of breast cancer according to the anatomical extent of disease, each stage serving to aggregate cases having an approximately similar prognosis.

In essence, staging is somewhat simplistic as every variable in breast cancer is classified under a few simple categories. There is therefore loss of precision and wide variation within the stages. There is also the question of relating clinical to pathological staging. As discussed above there is a 30 per cent error rate in clinical evaluation of axillary nodes and the assessment of tumour size is similarly inaccurate. Pathological assessment of nodes and tumour size allows a greater accuracy of staging. However, since pathological staging can only be undertaken after surgical treatment it has obvious limitations in determining management.

Many staging systems have been proposed; none has been shown to be significantly better than others, although some have the advantage of simplicity. More commonly used systems are described below.

The Manchester system (1940)

Stage I. Tumour confined to breast. Any skin involvement covers an area less than the size of the tumour.

Stage II. Tumour confined to breast. Palpable, mobile axillary nodes.

Stage III. Tumour extends beyond the breast tissue because of skin fixation in an area greater than the size of the tumour or because of ulceration. Tumour fixity underlying fascia.

Stage IV. Fixed axillary nodes, supraclavicular nodal involvement, satellite nodules or distant metastases.

The TMN classification (UICC)

In 1954 the International Union against Cancer (Union Internationale Contre Cancere) attempted to classify breast cancer on a description based on the primary tumour (T), the regional lymph nodes (N), and distant metastases (M). This system has been modified on a number of occasions and has led to confusion and recent criticism. A simple modification is as follows:

T0—no evidence of primary tumour.
T1—tumour less than 2 cm in diameter.
T2—tumour 2 to 5 cm in diameter.
T3—tumour greater than 5 cm in diameter.
T4—tumour fixation to chest wall or skin

N0—axillary nodes not considered to contain tumour
N1—mobile involved axillary nodes
N2—fixed axillary nodes
N3—supraclavicular lymph node involvement or arm swelling.

M0—no distant metastases.
M1—distant metastases present.

The designation 'X' after T, N or M indicates inability to assess the clinical status of the tumour, nodes, or metastases. The correlation of the TNM System with stage is summarized in Fig. 13.

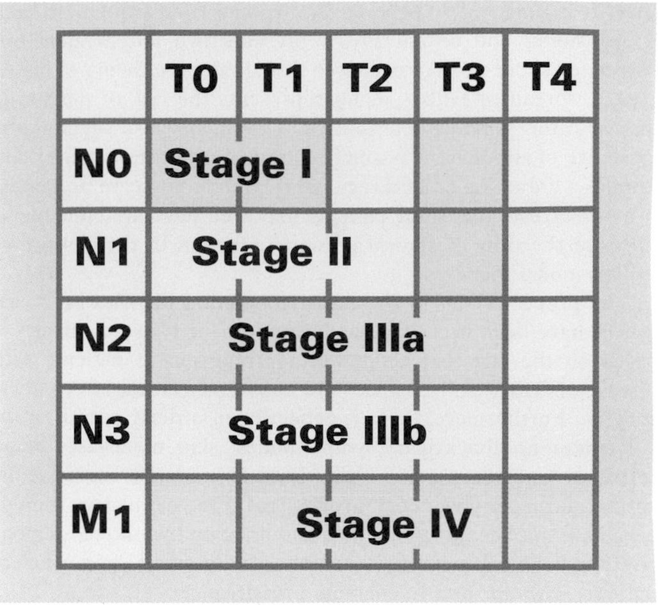

Fig. 13 A system of combining T, M, and N staging subsets with clinical stage.

The Columbia classification (Haagensen, Cooley, and Stout 1943, 1969)

Stage A—no skin oedema, ulceration, or fixation to chest wall, axillary nodes not clinically involved.

Stage B—clinically involved axillary nodes less than 2.5 cm in diameter and not fixed.

Stage C—grave signs of comparatively advanced carcinoma: oedema of skin, skin ulceration, fixation to chest wall, massive axillary involvement with nodes greater than 2.5 cm in diameter, and axillary fixation.

Stage D—advanced carcinoma including two or more signs in Stage E, satellite skin nodules, supraclavicular nodes, inflammatory cancer, arm oedema, or distant metastases.

Treatment of carcinoma of the breast

There has been a massive change in the treatment of breast cancer over the past 100 years. The past 20 years have witnessed fundamental changes in our approach, with decreasing reliance on radical surgical excision of the primary tumour and associated regional lymph nodes. This change of emphasis has resulted from a fundamental alteration in our philosophy of the spread of breast cancer, a greater appreciation of the systemic aspects of the disease, and increased realization that variations in local regional treatment are unlikely to alter prognosis.

Theories relating to the spread of breast cancer

Early concepts regarding the spread of breast cancer were proposed by Halsted. His opinion dictated the treatment of breast cancer for almost a century. He believed that breast cancer spread by direct permeation rather than embolization to the regional nodes. The nodes acted as a barrier to the further spread of cancer until they themselves were overladen with tumour, whereupon bloodborne metastases occurred. Such a concept of the spread of disease was the basis for performing *en-bloc* radical resection of the entire region in radical mastectomy and for the even more radical operations which followed that of Halsted.

A major flaw in Halsted's theory was, of course, that many deaths from metastatic disease occurred after radical surgery for small localized cancers. It thus became apparent that embolization, rather than permeation, of tumour cells is the predominant mode of simultaneous spread to both regional nodes and distant sites. It is now widely believed that spread from tumour to both lymph nodes and distant sites represents two independent but correlated processes. According to this alternative theory of breast cancer, spread to axillary nodes represents the risk of metastatic disease rather than its determinant. This theory also suggests the existence of an inherent systemic component to breast cancer and implies a limitation of local regional treatment alone on prognosis. It also suggests that some patients may well have systemic metastases at the time of clinical presentation even in the absence of axillary nodal metastasis.

The pros and cons of these two conflicting theories on breast cancer have been fiercely argued. Support for Halsted's theory is based on the fact that a significant proportion of patients with disease affecting axillary nodes are apparently cured after radical surgery. Furthermore, there is generally an orderly spread of involvement up the axillary lymph nodes, skip metastases being relatively uncommon, and there is little evidence for systemic spread accompanying nodal involvement. Free circulating tumour cells have not been demonstrated and imaging techniques demonstrate subclinical metastases in only a very small proportion of patients with apparently operable breast cancer.

The advocates of the alternative theory of breast cancer base their argument on both clinical and experimental evidence. There is no evidence to suggest that treatment of disease in axillary nodes is of any significance with respect to survival, although it does substantially improve the local control of tumour in that area. Further evidence for the alternative theory of breast cancer comes from experimental studies demonstrating failure of lymph nodes to filter tumour cells and from the existence of direct communications between afferent lymphatics and efferent veins around lymph nodes. Finally, studies of the natural history of breast cancer indicate that many tumours exist for several years before they become clinically apparent. Thus, there is ample opportunity for metastases to develop during this protracted period of occult growth. It has therefore been implied by some authorities that clinically apparent invasive breast cancer is never really curable.

The alternative theories of breast cancer are summarized in Table 5.

THE MANAGEMENT OF CANCER OF THE BREAST

The management of breast cancer requires a complex multidisciplinary approach involving surgeons, radiotherapists, medical oncologists, and pathologists, as well as other professionals such as counsellors and breast care nurses. For the sake of convenience the treatment of breast cancer will be discussed in three sections: the management of the breast itself, the axillary nodes, and potential micrometastases. However, it must be stressed that these three approaches have a final common aim—the successful treatment of patients with breast cancer. A properly co-ordinated approach by the various health professionals is required if optimal results are to be achieved.

Management of the breast

The importance of the management of the breast itself is to provide local tumour control and reduce any potential for metastasis to either local or distant sites. If this can be achieved using a surgical technique which allows conservation of the breast there is also the added bonus of improved cosmesis and, hopefully, a reduction in psychological trauma.

The traditional surgical treatment for breast cancer involved total removal of the breast. The various types of mastectomy describe those structures resected in association with the entire breast (Table 6). Up until the early 1970s breast cancer was treated by total mastectomy, in one or other of the forms described in Table 6. The most commonly performed operation was the Halsted radical mastectomy, although in Europe there had been a vogue for simple mastectomy with adjuvant radiotherapy since the early 1950s.

The second half of the 20th century witnessed increasing disillusionment with radical and mutilating forms of surgery for breast cancer. As a result the trend towards breast conservation has increased since the mid-1960s, although a number of centres had adopted this approach since before the Second World War. Again there are a number of different descriptions relating to breast conservation which has caused confusion. Tumourectomy, lumpectomy, tylectomy, segmental mastectomy, and quadrantectomy are all synonymous with a therapeutic procedure in which the primary tumour is removed and the breast is preserved. Unfortunately, these terms are not precisely defined, although they imply the removal of varying amounts of normal breast tissue in association with a primary tumour. The terms 'lumpectomy', 'tumourectomy', and 'tylectomy' imply removal of the tumour with a minimal or no margin of normal breast tissue around it. Segmental mastectomy implies excision of the tumour with a rim of associated normal breast tissue. However, this term is also

Table 5 Opposing theories of breast cancer

Halstedian	Alternative
1. Tumours spread in orderly manner based on mechanical considerations	1. There is no orderly pattern of tumour dissemination
2. Tumour cells traverse lymphatics to nodes by direct extension	2. Tumour cells traverse lymphatics by embolization
3. Positive lymph nodes indicate tumour spread and are the instigator of disease	3. Positive nodes indicate a tumour/host relationship which permits development of metastases rather than being their instigator
4. Regional nodes are barrier to passage of tumour cells	4. Regional lymph nodes are ineffective barriers to passage of tumour cells
5. The bloodstream is of little significance in tumour dissemination	5. The bloodstream is of considerable significance in tumour dissemination
6. The tumour is autonomous of the host	6. The host and tumour have a complex relationship
7. Operable breast cancer is a local–regional disease	7. Operable breast cancer is a systemic disease
8. The extent of surgical operation determines patient outcome	8. Variations in local–regional treatment do not substantially affect survival

Table 6 Anatomical structures removed in various types of mastectomy

	Structures removed												
	Skin	Most of gland	All of gland	Areola	Pectoralis minor muscle	Pectoralis major muscle	Some of low axillary nodes	Low axillary nodes (level 1)	Mid axillary nodes (level 11)	High axillary nodes (level 111)	Rotter's nodes (interpectoral)	Internal mammary nodes	Supraclavicular nodes	Mediastinal nodes
Subcutaneous		X												
Total (simple)	X		X	X										
Total with low node dissection (modified simple)	X		X	X				X						
Total with axillary dissection														
Modified radical (Auchincoloss)	X		X	X				X	X					
Modified radical (Scanlon)	X		X	X				X	X	X				
Modified radical (Patey)	X		X	X	X			X	X	X				
Radical mastectomy (Halsted)	X		X	X	X	X		X	X	X	X			
Extended radical (Urban)	X		X	X	X	X		X	X	X	X	X		
Extended radical (Dahl-Iversen)	X		X	X	X	X		X	X	X	X	X	X	
Super-radical (Wangensteen)	X		X	X	X	X		X	X	X	X	X	X	X

somewhat misleading as it implies that the breast is anatomically a segmental organ and that tumours occur in a localized segment. This is clearly not the case. The term 'quadrantectomy' denotes removal of a breast quadrant, and implies wider excision of normal breast tissue than segmental mastectomy. In practice, however, there is little distinction between these terms and although a number of authorities have recommended the adoption of a uniform nomenclature, none has found universal favour.

Once the questions regarding definition of terms and nomenclature have been addressed the simple, yet fundamentally important question which remains is whether breast conservation provides results as reliable in the treatment of breast cancer as total mastectomy. Furthermore, is there an additional benefit in terms of cosmetic and emotional adjustment? Finally, if breast conservation is justified, in which patients is this appropriate?

In terms of management of the breast the simplest approach would be to remove the tumour itself, preferably with a margin of normal tissue around it. In theory the more limited procedures of tumourectomy or lumpectomy are likely to be followed by a good cosmetic result but are more likely to be followed by local recurrence because of the likelihood of failure to excise the tumour completely. More extensive forms of conservative surgery such as quadrantectomy are more likely to provide good tumour control but are more liable to be followed by a less satisfactory cosmetic result because of the amount of breast tissue excised.

Studies evaluating simple excision of the tumour without adjuvant radiotherapy have produced somewhat disappointing results, with a local recurrence rate of approximately 30 per cent within 7 years. Local recurrence may result from positive margins of excision as a result of inadequate surgery or from development of further tumours either *de novo* or from pre-existing multifocal disease.

Failure of local excision alone to provide adequate tumour control in the breast led to the use of adjuvant radiotherapy to the remaining breast tissue. This combination of conservative surgery with adjuvant radiotherapy has now become a standard procedure for patients with breast cancer. A large number of studies have provided retrospective analysis of conservative treatment with surgery and irradiation for the treatment of this disease. The results have been generally encouraging with local recurrence rates of under 10 per cent, although in some centres 20 per cent of patients have developed locally recurrent disease after periods of 7 years of more.

Unfortunately, as the majority of studies relating to conservative surgery with adjuvant radiotherapy are retrospective, there are doubts about case selection. A more accurate appraisal can only be obtained from analysis of prospective randomized trials. There have been three major studies comparing conservative treatment with mastectomy which require more detailed discussion.

The Guy's Hospital studies

In the first study on breast conservation Atkins and his colleagues at Guy's Hospital, London, randomized patients over the age of 50 years with clinical stage I or II disease to either 'extended tylectomy' or classical radical mastectomy. Both operations were followed by axillary, supraclavicular, and internal mammary irradiation and the patients treated by tylectomy also underwent X-ray treatment to the residual breast tissue. Some patients received adjuvant thiotepa. Unfortunately, the dose of radiation used in this study was somewhat suboptimal.

After 10 years there was a significantly higher local recurrence rate in patients treated by breast conservation for both Stage I and II disease, although this had no impact on survival for patients with Stage I disease. Patients with Stage II disease treated by breast conservation had a worse prognosis.

A follow-up study from the same institution by Haywood and his colleagues randomized a further 258 clinical Stage I patients to the same regimens, but again with suboptimal radiation doses. On this occasion conservative treatment resulted not only in relatively poor local control but also decreased survival. Thus, the Guy's group provided inconsistent results following breast conservation, even in patients with Stage I disease.

The Milan study

A second important randomized study was that of Veronesi and his colleagues from Milan. Seven hundred and one women with tumours less than 2 cm in diameter and without palpable axillary nodes were randomized to either radical mastectomy or quadrantectomy, axillary dissection, and breast irradiation. Adjuvant chemotherapy was given to those patients with histologically proven lymph node metastases. Overall 13-year survival was 69 per cent and 71 per cent respectively, in the two groups. Local recurrence rates were similar in patients treated by radical mastectomy and in those treated by breast conservation.

The NSABP (protocol B–06) study

The third study evaluating breast conservation in the treatment of breast cancer was the protocol B–06 conducted by the National Surgical Adjuvant Breast and Bowel Project (NSABP). In this trial 1843 women were randomized to mastectomy or to segmental resection (lumpectomy), with or without radiation. All patients underwent axillary clearance, and those found to have positive nodes were given adjuvant chemotherapy. Patients found to have positive margins after breast conservation were converted to the mastectomy group—perhaps introducing some bias into the study.

After 8 years there was no significant difference in survival between patients treated with breast conservation and those with mastectomy. However, those patients treated by lumpectomy without radiation suffered a greater incidence of local recurrence in the ipsilateral breast.

Thus, two of these randomized studies clearly demonstrated that patients suitable for breast conservation have an equally good prognosis when treated by a conservative procedure with adjuvant radiotherapy rather than mastectomy. All the above studies may be also criticized in that case selection was still liable to exclude patients with more aggressive tumours, who may have not been selected for randomization. However, the other major criticism of these studies—that there has been inadequate follow-up—can now be answered, in that assessment for more than 8 years is now available.

Indications for breast conservation treatment

Patient choice is important. If a patient prefers to be treated by total mastectomy rather than breast conservation then, after appropriate counselling, her wishes should be adhered to. It is widely believed that women with breast cancer prefer to be treated by partial mastectomy. This is often, but not always, the case: many women who actually have the disease feel more secure after a total mastectomy, and other prefer to avoid irradiation treatment if at all possible. One recent study from the United Kingdom showed that 50 per cent of patients suffering from breast cancer actually prefer the concept of total mastectomy to breast conservation.

The other main indications for conservative therapy relate to tumour characteristics, the position of the cancer in the breast, and the nature of the breasts themselves. Tumour size is of paramount importance; most authorities recommend mastectomy if the tumour is more than 3 or 4 cm in diameter. The NSABP recommends partial mastectomy only if the tumour is less than 4 cm in diameter and when there is no fixation to the underlying muscle or overlying skin. Other surgeons pursue a more conservative approach and prefer to reserve breast conservation for tumours of less than 3 cm in diameter. Much will, of course, depend on the size of the breast. In small breasts a tumour 4 cm in diameter may require mastectomy, and conservation with good cosmetic results may only be a reality if the tumour is 2 cm or less in size. On the other hand breast conservation may be permitted for tumours greater than 4 cm in diameter if the breasts are large, although it must be remembered that heavy pendulous breasts may provide poor cosmetic results after conservation because of the oedema and fibrosis which may follow irradiation.

A further contraindication to breast conservation is multicentricity. Patients with a second tumour in the breast, whether it is clinically apparent or seen on mammography, should be considered for mastectomy if the tumours cannot be excised in continuity. Mammography is therefore an essential preoperative investigation to determine the presence of multicentric tumours.

Multifocality, as opposed to multicentricity, is present in up to 50 per cent of patients with breast cancer. Its extent depends on tumour size and it is this multifocality which may result in the unacceptable incidence of local recurrence if breast conservation is performed without adjuvant radiation therapy. It is yet to be determined whether adjuvant radiotherapy truly sterilizes multifocal disease or whether it simply delays recurrence to the very long term (10–20 years). Widespread multifocal disease certainly relates to local recurrence—its presence is a relative contraindication to breast conservation.

The question of multifocality is particularly important in patients with lobular carcinoma. It may be felt that this potentially multifocal and multicentric disease should be treated by mastectomy. However, as long as criteria relating to tumour size and type are adhered to there is no evidence that this particular type of tumour is any more likely to recur than is ductal carcinoma.

Centrally located tumours are a relative contraindication to breast conservation. Such tumours are often quite diffuse and they can be difficult to remove by segmental mastectomy. Furthermore, the end cosmetic result is often disappointing as many women perceive the nipple as being a fundamentally important part of the breast—both physiologically and psychologically. It is not uncommon for women to hold the view that if the nipple has to be removed then the treatment may as well be mastectomy. Despite this opinion many women are, in fact, pleased with the end cosmetic result, even though the nipple has to be removed in the treatment of a centrally located tumour. This is particularly true for those women with larger breasts, in whom a nipple reconstruction or prosthesis may be used.

Poor tumour differentiation is also a relative contraindication to breast conservation, although this is a somewhat empirical judgment in many cases. Moreover, an assessment of tumour grade is not possible until the cancer has actually been removed. Many poorly differentiated tumours are somewhat ill-defined and this specific clinical feature may be a further relative contraindication to breast conservation.

There have been doubts as to whether breast conservation is appropriate for patients with node-positive disease. As the presence of disease in axillary nodes indicates a higher risk of tumour dissemination there is, in fact, an argument in favour of breast conservation in these circumstances.

Despite the various contraindications to breast conservation this type of treatment has now become the management of choice for the majority of patients with breast cancer. However, there is still much variation from centre to centre, with some authorities recommending total mastectomy in up to 70 per cent of cases, whereas others recommend breast conservation for virtually all their patients.

Local recurrence after treatment of breast cancer

Local recurrence after either total mastectomy or breast conservation surgery is a major clinical problem. Locally recurrent disease must be distinguished from regional recurrence; the two are often confused. Local recurrence is that seen in the breast after conservative therapy or on the chest wall after mastectomy; regional recurrence denotes recurrent disease in regional lymph nodes. Local recurrence may be either localized or widespread. Both types, but particularly the latter, may be associated with widespread metastatic disease and it is therefore mandatory to stage all patients with either local or regional recurrence for distant metastases.

In general, the more radical the treatment the lower the incidence of local recurrence either on the chest wall after mastectomy or in the remaining breast tissue following breast conservation therapy. Thus, very minimal treatment such as lumpectomy alone is associated with a higher incidence of local recurrence than is partial mastectomy or quadrantectomy, particularly if associated with adjuvant irradiation. Similarly, there is a higher incidence of local recurrence after partial than total mastectomy. The lowest local recurrence rate (2 per cent for stage I disease) has been recorded after extended radical mastectomy.

The overall incidence of local recurrence after breast conservation with adjuvant radiotherapy is about 10 per cent, although some authorities have recorded figures in excess of 20 per cent in a period of 7 years or more. Local recurrence after total mastectomy has previously occurred in about 5 to 8 per cent of patients. However, in modern practice this incidence may be even greater because of selection of large, prognostically unfavourable tumours for this type of treatment.

Factors predisposing to local recurrence

Recurrent disease, either in the breast after partial mastectomy or on the chest wall after total mastectomy, is more common in patients with positive axillary nodes. It has therefore been suggested that as well as giving radiotherapy to all patients after partial mastectomy, the chest wall should be irradiated after total mastectomy if disease has spread to the nodes. Meta-analysis, however, has shown no improved survival in patients given adjuvant radiotherapy, although it reduces the local recurrence rate on the chest wall. Addition of radiotherapy to mastectomy may actually increase overall mortality because of an increased liability to myocardial infarction and lung cancer following irradiation.

Tumour size has also been shown in some studies to be associated with increased incidence of local recurrence after both total mastectomy and breast conservation. Some authorities therefore recommend adjuvant irradiation after both partial and total mastectomy if the primary tumour is large. Again, there is no evidence that this improves survival, although it reduces local recurrence.

Positive surgical margins following partial mastectomy would certainly be regarded as being an important risk factor for recurrence, although not all studies have confirmed this. Although positive surgical margins may relate to inadequate surgical technique they are also likely to occur in patients with extensive *in-situ* disease. It is therefore likely that widespread multifocality is an important factor predisposing to local recurrence.

Other factors such as high tumour grade, lymphatic or vascular invasion, and young age are also associated with recurrent disease.

Treatment of local recurrence after breast conservation

Local recurrence after breast conservation therapy can be treated by salvage mastectomy. Such treatment has been claimed to produce a 5-year survival rate of up to 50 per cent, and this may well be so for those patients with localized recurrence. Further breast conservation is sometimes feasible in these women. Unfortunately, however, up to 20 per cent of those who develop local recurrence in the residual breast tissue after breast conservation have advanced or unresectable disease. This is because local recurrence after breast conservation with adjuvant radiotherapy can occur as a 'field-change' throughout the irradiation field. Positive surgical margins may occur despite extensive surgical resection, musculocutaneous flaps, and skin grafts. Further local recurrence is not uncommon in these individuals, who face terminal illness with severe physical and psychological morbidity from uncontrolled and prolonged chest wall recurrence. Systemic treatment with tamoxifen or chemotherapy may alleviate symptoms but responses are often quite short-lived when recurrence is widespread.

Treatment of local recurrence after total mastectomy

Local recurrence after total mastectomy can present a difficult problem. Small focal areas of local recurrence can be surgically excised. If irradiation has not been previously used, X-ray therapy may prevent or delay further local recurrences. Similarly, adjuvant drug treatment with either chemotherapy or endocrine therapy may help reduce the risk of further recurrence.

Local recurrence after total mastectomy may present as a widespread area of recurrent disease. This is particularly difficult to treat. Surgical excision with associated transposed musculocutaneous flaps or skin grafting is often associated with positive margins, further local recurrence, and the rapid development of metastatic disease. Radiotherapy may be attempted if this has not already been used; chemotherapy or endocrine treatment may produce some regression of this somewhat remorseless process.

Reconstruction of the breast after total mastectomy

All women undergoing total mastectomy should be offered reconstruction, even if they have advanced disease. Although it was hoped that this would reduce the psychological sequelae of breast cancer this is not always so, although reconstruction can improve an otherwise miserable existence for some women. The increasing trend towards breast conservation should reduce the number of women requiring reconstruction after total mastectomy: if reconstruction is required after breast conservation therapy there must be doubts as to whether the original surgical operation was appropriate.

The two main questions relating to breast reconstruction are the timing and the technique. Breast reconstruction can be performed either at the time of initial surgery or delayed for, say, 1 to 2 years after diagnosis. The obvious advantage of immediate reconstruction is that women do not undergo a period of loss of the breast. Furthermore, only one surgical procedure is required. It must be remembered, however, that a reconstructed breast generally compares unfavourably with the original, and that immediate reconstruction can result in unfavourable comparison by the patient. It might also be argued that initial reconstruction, and its possible postoperative problems, should take second place to the actual treatment of the cancer. One of the author's personal fears is that if immediate reconstruction takes place and rapid local or distant recurrence occurs the patient may believe that surgical management of the cancer has taken second place to reconstruction. Finally, reconstruction may delay the early diagnosis of local recurrence, but data on this subject are lacking.

The advantage of delayed reconstruction is that the patient will compare, usually more favourably, the reconstruction with the mastectomy. Adjuvant therapy with chemotherapy or irradiation will have finished and the patient may be more psychologically attuned to her disease. Many women, however, defer or refuse delayed reconstruction on the basis that they and their partner have become quite used to the missing breast and that they have had enough medical treatment. This in part explains the author's experience that many younger women with children to look after tend to refuse reconstruction, whereas there is greater acceptance in women aged over 50.

Methods of reconstruction

There are numerous methods of reconstruction: no one method is perfect. Appropriate counselling is of particular importance before embarking on any reconstructive surgery. The patient should see photographs of both good and bad results to ensure a realistic approach. If possible she should talk to women who have previously undergone reconstruction. It is essential to stress the reconstruction will provide a 'mound' but that it will not feel or move like the original. Further counselling is required about nipple reconstruction, as this aspect is often forgotten.

The reader is advised to consult specialized plastic surgical texts on methods of reconstruction. However, for the sake of completeness some of the more widely used techniques are briefly discussed.

Reconstruction with subcutaneous or subpectoral implant

This is the easiest technique to perform, although skin necrosis and implant extrusion may occur, especially after irradiation and if a subcutaneous position is used. Most surgeons prefer to place the implant in a subpectoral position; the subcutaneous technique is mentioned only to be condemned as it frequently causes skin necrosis, extrusion, and a poor cosmetic result (Fig. 14).

When inserting the implant subpectorally care must be taken to ensure that the prosthesis is in an appropriate position. Since there is a tendency for such implants to migrate superiorly it is necessary to divide the tight fascial bands between the insertion of the pectoralis muscle and the rectus abdominus to allow appropriate positioning.

Two main cosmetic problems occur with this technique. The first is capsule formation, which is unsightly and also imparts a

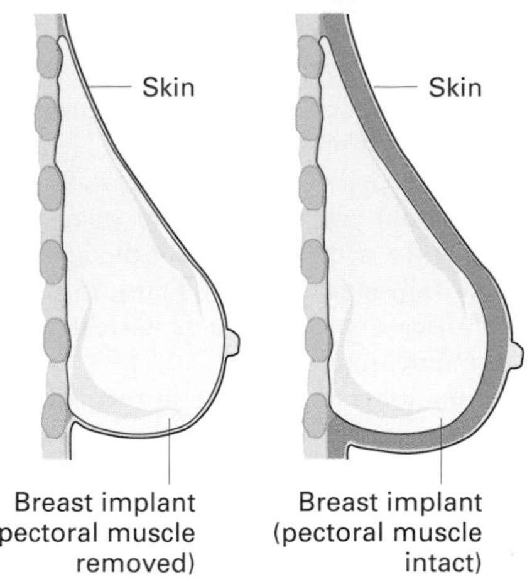

Fig. 14 Subcutaneous and subpectoral implants.

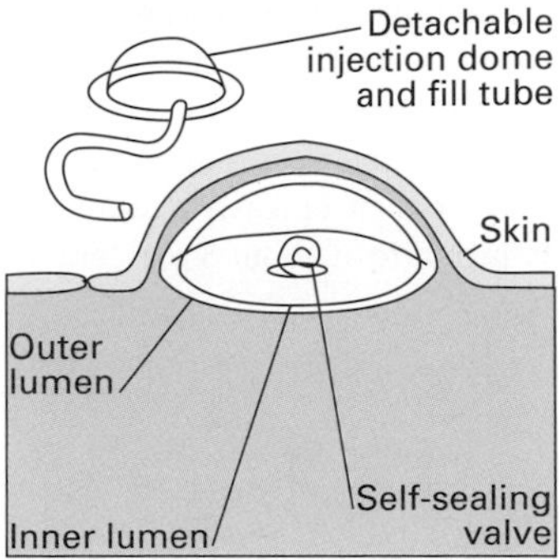

Fig. 15 The Becker combined expander/mammary prosthesis.

very hard texture to the breast. Capsule formation is less common if 'textured' implants are used. If excessive, the capsule can be surgically fractured or excised to improve appearance and to soften the reconstructed breast.

The second cosmetic problem with simple implants is lack of ptosis which occurs with the normal breast, especially with increasing age. The use of tissue expansion techniques can, to some extent, overcome this problem (see below), especially if performed in conjunction with one of the various plastic surgical procedures which enhance ptosis.

Most implants in current use are made of silicone gel. This material has the advantages that it is inert and has a relatively natural feel. Recent publicity regarding risk of cancer and autoimmune disease have been exaggerated. The alternative type of implant using saline gives a rather soft, striated and 'flabby' result. Furthermore leakage of saline can occur in the long term.

A major difficulty relating to this and other types of reconstruction is the fact that a nipple has to be recreated (see below). This problem can be avoided by performing a subcutaneous mastectomy, although many oncologists feel this is an inappropriate cancer operation because 2 to 10 per cent of the original breast tissue may be left behind following this technique.

Tissue expansion

Simple implants have limitations with respect to lack of natural ptosis and complications in irradiated skin. Both these problems can, to some extent, be overcome by gradual tissue expansion. Traditionally, this has been achieved by a tissue expander followed by insertion of a permanent prosthesis. The introduction of a combined tissue expander/permanent prosthesis has greatly simplified matters. The Becker expander/mammary prosthesis consists of an outer lumen filled with silicone gel and an inner chamber connected to a removable, self-sealing, side port (Fig. 15). This inner chamber is filled with saline and is gradually expanded to the desired volume over a number of weeks. The expansion eventually provided is substantially greater than the volume of the opposite breast. Once expansion is complete the saline chamber is aspirated to allow creation of a reconstructed breast of similar volume to that on the opposite side, while at the same time providing some ptosis. The self-sealing injection port can then be removed under local anaesthetic.

Pedicled and free myocutaneous flaps

The most commonly adopted technique has been the pedicled latissimus dorsi myocutaneous flap, because of its proximity, good blood supply, and ease of creation (Fig. 16). The bulk of muscle transposed, however, is often quite small and the technique frequently has to be combined with an implant. Some authorities report good results after immediate reconstruction with this technique, although it leaves a scar on the back and is often complicated by seroma formation.

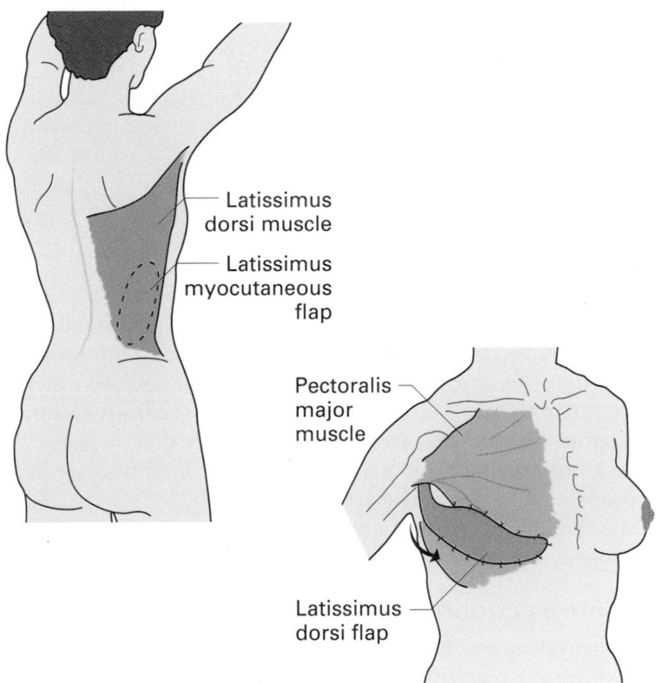

Fig. 16 The latissimus dorsi pedicled flap. The myocutaneous flap is swung on its axis anteriorly preserving its blood supply. The resulting flap can be sued to cover a defect after mastectomy for advanced disease or may be employed (in association with an implant) for reconstruction.

The most recent innovation has been the rectus abdominus myocutaneous flap. A longitudinal or transverse incision can be used. In the former a pedicle graft is swung on its axis to provide tissue bulk on the chest wall. Most authorities now prefer to use a transverse rectus abdominus flap in which a horizontal, elliptical, subumbilical incision is used for access (Fig. 17). Because of the rather precarious blood supply to this region many surgeons now recommend a free transverse rectus abdominus flap with microvascular anastomosis between epigastric and thoracodorsal vessels. There is a graft failure rate of about 8 per cent with this technique.

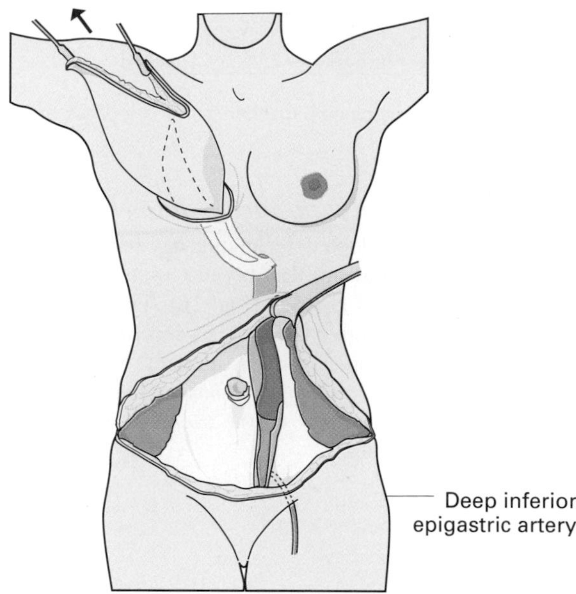

Fig. 17 The transverse rectus abdominus pedicled flap. The contralateral rectus muscle with associated skin is used to cover a defect on the chest wall. An alternative method adopts a free flap with microvascular anastomosis.

The cosmetic results of the free transverse rectus abdominus flap are such that they should be regarded as the 'gold standard' by which other methods of reconstruction are judged. Unfortunately, it is a time-consuming procedure and requires specific expertise with microvascular anastomosis. It is also relatively contraindicated in patients who are very obese or very thin, in those who have a pre-existing lower abdominal scar, in those who are heavy smokers, and in those who are above age 55.

All the above forms of reconstruction may require reduction mastopexy in the contralateral breast if equality is to be achieved.

Nipple reconstruction

For many women the nipple is the most important part of the breast, yet the majority of techniques described above fail to provide appropriate nipple reconstruction. Only subcutaneous mastectomy routinely preserves the nipple–areola complex; the disadvantages of this method are described above. Several methods of nipple reconstruction are available, using either any excessive skin on the reconstructed breast or a free graft from a distant site, such as the groin or thigh. An alternative approach is to use an adhesive prosthesis.

A difficulty with nipple reconstruction relates to pigmentation. If the reconstructed nipple is pale in comparison to that on the opposite side then simple tattooing may provide an appropriate effect.

Management of axillary nodes

The management of the axillary nodes is a controversial issue, and practice varies widely from centre to centre. However, the management of axillary nodes should provide certain well-defined end points. First it should act as a guide to staging and prognosis. Second, it dictates the need for adjuvant therapy with irradiation, chemotherapy or hormonal therapy. Third, it must provide good local control of disease in the axilla as untreatable axillary metastases can cause much morbidity.

Despite the importance of disease in the axillary nodes, however, there is no evidence that good therapeutic control of the axilla correlates with survival.

The major argument relating to management of axillary nodes concerns the extent of their surgical excision and the impact that this may have on staging, prognosis, and the subsequent control of axillary disease. The extent of surgical excision of the axillary contents can range from that of non-intervention to routine block clearance of all nodes in all patients. All approaches have their supporters and detractors.

The policy of non-intervention

Failure to assess axillary nodes has been rightly condemned. This approach has unfortunately been relatively common and has resulted in subsequent inability to prescribe rational local and systemic adjuvant therapy. Radiotherapy then has to be given blindly resulting in the needless irradiation of disease-free nodes. Similarly, it is impossible to provide a rational programme of systemic hormonal or chemotherapy if nodal status is not known.

Recently, however, there has been a resurgence of this rather negative approach to axillary nodes. This has resulted from appreciation that nodal control fails to correlate with prognosis and the wider use of adjuvant therapy. Supporters of non-intervention claim that if all patients receive systemic adjuvant therapy and careful monitoring, axillary nodal relapse can be treated as it occurs clinically. In fact, such axillary nodal relapse is relatively uncommon—a further point in favour of this approach. Whether this view will become more widespread is unclear.

The policy of axillary nodal sampling

Axillary nodal sampling, as opposed to full surgical clearance, has been widely practised in the United Kingdom although, like the policy of non-intervention, it has been criticized. A number of studies have failed to demonstrate adequate node retrieval using this technique, and staging is claimed not to be as accurate as with clearance. There are also doubts as to whether radiotherapy is as good as clearance in controlling axillary nodal disease.

A major problem relating to sampling is that it is poorly defined. There is no agreement as to the extent or boundaries of axillary surgery when sampling, although it is important to emphasize the necessity of removing enlarged or palpably hard nodes.

The supporters of axillary node sampling have answered all the above criticisms. Firstly, those studies which failed to demonstrate adequate nodal retrieval used inappropriate anatomic landmarks to define the axillary glands. Thus, the extent of dissection had been demarcated by landmarks such as the axillary tail of the breast or the intercostal–brachial nerve. When the axillary fat has been entered using appropriate anatomical dissection, sampling provides as good a qualitative assessment of the axilla as clearance. It must be admitted, however, that sampling fails to provide as much prognostic information in terms of a full nodal assessment, which may be performed after complete dissection of the nodes.

The supporters of sampling also claim that, if done properly, node-positive patients can be specifically targeted for adjuvant radiation therapy, whereas a full axillary dissection needlessly overtreats the 50 per cent of patients with negative nodes. The available data indicate that adjuvant radiotherapy provides as good overall control in the axilla as clearance. Such control does not, however, correlate with survival.

The whole question relating to sampling depends on how well it is done. When inappropriately performed it is rightly condemned. However, if done properly it provides qualitative data as good as those obtained from clearance, allows appropriate patients to be treated with radiotherapy, and provides a rational basis for systemic treatment. Such an opinion has been confirmed by Steele and his colleagues, who showed that surgical clearance provided no further qualitative data once adequate sampling had been performed.

The policy of axillary nodal clearance

Many of the criticisms relating to sampling are answered by axillary clearance. Block dissection of axillary nodes accurately stages the axilla, both qualitatively and quantitatively, and has the advantage that it provides a good mechanism for tumour control. The main criticism of clearance, however, is that the 50 per cent of patients with negative nodes do not require this treatment. There are also doubts as to the efficacy of clearance obtained with differing operative techniques. In some centres the pectoralis minor muscle is routinely removed or divided; in others it is merely retracted. This may explain the wide variation in nodal count between centres undertaking axillary clearance. The technical aspects of clearance may be compounded when it has to be performed through a separate axillary incision distant from the primary tumour site: in these circumstances access to the apex of the axilla may be limited.

Critics of clearance also suggest it may be followed by a higher incidence of arm lymphoedema than is sampling. However, as long as axillary clearance is not combined with radiotherapy there is little evidence that long-term morbidity after this more radical procedure is any worse than following sampling with adjuvant X-ray therapy.

Overall, there is little to choose between well-performed axillary sampling, with adjuvant radiotherapy treatment for patients with diseased nodes, and axillary clearance. Axillary clearance has the disadvantage that 50 per cent of patients undergo unnecessary dissection of their axilla, whereas radiotherapy is both time-consuming and expensive postoperatively. In the author's unit reliance is generally placed on axillary sampling followed with adjuvant radiotherapy for node-positive patients. However, if there is bulk nodal disease with metastases greater than 2 cm in diameter we prefer full surgical axillary clearance.

Treatment of potential micrometastases

Systemic metastatic disease in patients with breast cancer is a serious development, with a median survival after diagnosis of only about 14 months. Such metastases are particularly distressing when they occur in patients originally thought to have a relatively good prognosis by virtue of tumour size and negative axillary nodes. Earlier expectations of improved survival with either more radical surgery or adjuvant radiotherapy have not been realized. The systemic component of breast cancer, as described above, indicates that either the patient is cured by local treatment or that death occurs from metastatic disease at about the same time that she would have died without local intervention. This is because according to the non-Halstedian theory of breast cancer metastases are established prior to diagnosis and are outside the scope of even the most extensive local treatment.

The limitations of local treatment provided the initial rationale for the use of adjuvant systemic therapy at the time of, or following, initial surgical treatment of breast cancer. Such an approach was first adopted for breast cancer in 1948, when oophorectomy was suggested as an adjuvant treatment. Early studies produced conflicting results but indicated the need for a wider appraisal of the systemic approach which gradually developed over a 30-year period as more active chemotherapeutic and hormonal agents became available. As a result of numerous studies adjuvant systemic therapy is now regarded as an integral party of the primary treatment of breast cancer.

Adjuvant chemotherapy

The first large-scale studies evaluated single agent chemotherapy such as thiotepa, phenylalanine mustard, and cyclophosphamide. After a 12-year study Nissen-Meyer and his colleagues demonstrated a significant survival advantage in patients receiving a brief perioperative course of cyclophosphamide compared to untreated controls. Other experience with single agents was also encouraging, especially in patients with positive nodes, although there was some scepticism because of stratification within the trials and variations in treatment methods. Subsequent studies have evaluated a large number of chemotherapeutic regimens using a variety of agents and varying durations of treatment. A combination of cyclophosphamide, 5-fluorouracil, and methotrexate has been most widely used, because of its known activity in patients with overt metastatic disease and its relative ease of administration.

The initial study evaluating this combination therapy in breast cancer showed a 30 per cent reduction in mortality in patients receiving 12 cycles of treatment, but also showed that the effect was most clearly apparent in premenopausal women with 1 to 3 positive nodes. These results were regarded as a major advance in treatment of breast cancer, although other similar studies subsequently failed to confirm these findings. This discrepancy was compounded by occasional studies that even showed a worse prognosis in patients receiving adjuvant cyclosphosphamide, 5-fluorouracil, and methotrexate, although the majority of investigators demonstrated some benefit in selected groups of patients.

Because of the conflicting results obtained by various trials of adjuvant chemotherapy there was initially very little agreement as to the value of this form of treatment in patients with breast cancer. The matter was finally settled by adopting the statistical technique of meta-analysis of all randomized trials evaluating adjuvant chemotherapy for breast cancer. The results of this analysis were initially published in 1985 and 1988 but were subsequently updated in 1992 when 10-year monitoring was available.

More than 30 trials evaluating adjuvant polychemotherapy are now available for study, with a follow-up of up to 10 years. Meta-analysis has demonstrated a 25 per cent reduction in annual mortality in women aged under 50. This translates to an absolute reduction in 10-year mortality of about 10 per cent in node-positive patients, but only 4 per cent in those who are node-negative. Single agent chemotherapy does not have the same efficacy. The effect of chemotherapy in women under the age of 50 is almost completely manifest within 5 years of initial treatment, but continues for at least 10 years.

Combination polychemotherapy is also effective in women aged over 50, although not to the same degree as in younger patients. Meta-analysis demonstrates a 12 per cent reduction in annual mortality. The absolute survival difference is only 5 per cent for node-positive patients and even less for those who are node-negative.

As a result of the meta-analysis adjuvant polychemotherapy with cyclophosphamide, 5-fluorouracil, and methotrexate is now recommended for all node-positive women aged less than 50. A six-cycle course of treatment is now regarded as standard. Centres with a more aggressive treatment policy are also recommending this treatment for node-negative women aged less than 50, especially if there are other adverse factors such as large tumour size, poor differentiation, and oestrogen receptor-negative status. At the present time such chemotherapy has not been demonstrated to be associated with significant survival improvement. However, it is associated with prolonged time to initial relapse and it is argued that when monitoring has been continued for long enough a survival advantage will be truly demonstrated.

The 1992 overview analysis also demonstrated an adjuvant effect of cyclophosphamide, 5-fluorouracil, and methotrexate in node-positive women aged over 50. This effect was not apparent in the 1985 study and may relate to improved techniques now available for administering chemotherapy to older individuals. Some units are giving this combination chemotherapy to some node-positive patients over the age of 50, such as those who are oestrogen receptor-negative, as long as their overall performance status will allow this potentially toxic treatment.

A common side-effect of adjuvant chemotherapy in premenopausal patients is cessation of menses. Some authorities have therefore suggested that chemotherapy causes a pharmacological castration and ovarian ablation. Support for this concept is demonstrated in the most recent overview analysis of the positive effect of adjuvant oophorectomy in premenopausal women. However, even if the adjuvant effect of polychemotherapy is created by pharmacological ovarian ablation, this treatment also has an effect in node-positive postmenopausal patients. It is therefore likely that cylophosphamide, 5-fluorouracil, and methotrexate has a direct chemotherapeutic action in younger women as well as by potentially causing ovarian failure.

It is clear that adjuvant chemotherapy will be used more extensively in patients with breast cancer. Its use is likely to be extended to women less than 50 years old with node-negative disease. It is also likely to be used increasingly in patients over this age who have a poor prognosis and for whom adjuvant hormonal therapy may be inappropriate because of factors such as oestrogen receptor negativity.

Patients with a very poor prognosis, such as those with a large number of diseased nodes, may in future be considered for even more aggressive polychemotherapy such as provided by cyclophosphamide, Adriamycin, and 5-fluorouracil.

A further area of interest relates to 'neo-adjuvant' chemotherapy. Polychemotherapy prior to surgery may downstage the primary tumour and has a theoretical advantage of allowing early systemic treatment to potentially poor prognosis patients. However, it has yet to be determined whether this approach improves survival.

Adjuvant hormonal therapy

Hormonal manipulation is associated with almost as much controversy as adjuvant chemotherapy. However, its relative ease of administration and lesser toxicity has resulted in its more widespread application. Meta-analysis has now demonstrated very definite indications for its use.

Early studies evaluating hormonal manipulation adopted adjuvant oophorectomy in premenopausal women: these failed to show consistently any survival advantage. The introduction of tamoxifen produced an easily administered, relatively non-toxic form of oestrogen blockade, and this was, therefore, the natural agent to assess as an adjuvant treatment. Trials again produced conflicting results. Overview analysis, however, has subsequently demonstrated an overall reduction in annual odds of death of 17 per cent. The effect is greatest in patients age over 50 with positive nodes, in whom there is a 20 per cent reduction in annual mortality. This translates to an 8 per cent reduction in 10-year mortality. There is a small, yet still significant, effect in node-negative individuals. The effect of tamoxifen is less apparent in women aged under 50, whether node-negative or node-positive, with an overall delay in development of recurrence of 12 per cent. However, even in this group the results are described as 'non-significantly favourable'.

As is the case for adjuvant chemotherapy the effect of tamoxifen is found within the first 5 years but continues for at least 10 years after initial diagnosis. An important effect of adjuvant tamoxifen was the demonstration in the overview analysis that it reduces the risk of contralateral breast cancer by 39 per cent. This has obvious implications with respect to prophylaxis in high-risk groups of patients.

The role of adjuvant tamoxifen is now well established in women over the age of 50. The duration of treatment is, however, unclear: recommendations vary between 2 years, 5 years, and continued provision until relapse. Meta-analysis has demonstrated the best results for adjuvant tamoxifen when used for at least 2 years. Early fears relating to possible increased mortality from myocardial infarction and morbidity from osteoporosis have not been realized. It appears that, as far as cardiac and bony tissues are concerned, the oestrogenic effects of tamoxifen outweigh its anti-oestrogenic influence.

Despite meta-analysis the role of adjuvant tamoxifen remains a controversial issue. A number of authorities have expressed doubts as to its efficacy in oestrogen receptor-negative patients, although both overview analysis and some individual studies, contrary to expectations, have shown benefit in this particular subgroup. Similarly, some studies have shown a beneficial effect in women under the age of 50, although this has not been fully confirmed by overview analysis. Tamoxifen is not without side-effects, particularly in premenopausal patients, about 30 per cent of whom experience menopausal symptoms, nausea, weight gain, vaginal dryness, or discharge.

The most surprising finding of the 1992 overview analysis was a 24 per cent reduction in mortality in node-positive patients aged less than 50 following oophorectomy. The effect was as great as that of adjuvant chemotherapy and, as discussed above, gave credence to the concept that the cyclophosphamide, 5-fluorouracil, methotrexate regimen acts by providing a pharmacological oophorectomy. It is also likely that this drug treatment has inherent chemotherapeutic activity. It is as yet uncertain whether oophorectomy, rather than chemotherapy, should be used as an adjuvant in premenopausal breast cancer. It is also unclear whether oophorectomy, if used as an adjuvant treatment, should be performed surgically or whether reliance can be placed on either irradiation or administration of luteinizing hormone releasing hormone antagonists such as Zoladex to provide this effect. If performed surgically it is probable that oophorectomy could be performed using laparoscopic techniques.

Summary of current recommendations regarding adjuvant therapy in breast cancer

The following recommendations are based on the 1992 overview analysis. However, they are only guidelines and there will be variation in policy from centre to centre.

1. Six cycles of polychemotherapy with the cyclophosphamide, 5-fluorouracil, methotrexate regimen. All node-positive women aged less than 50. Possibly of value in node-negative women aged less than 50 and node positive patients over 50 if it can be tolerated in the latter group. This regimen in node-positive patients over age 50 is most likely to be of benefit if there are doubts as to the efficacy of adjuvant tamoxifen because of oestrogen receptor negativity etc.
2. A 2-year course of tamoxifen. All women over aged 50, particularly if node positive. The effect on women under 50 is small but probably valid especially if it is felt that adjuvant chemotherapy is not warranted.

Although there is a temptation to combine adjuvant chemotherapy with tamoxifen, there is no evidence that their effects are additive. Indeed, there is experimental evidence that tamoxifen inhibits the action of chemotherapy. Randomized trials are currently in progress evaluating combination chemotherapy with tamoxifen given either concurrently or sequentially.

SPECIAL PROBLEMS IN THE MANAGEMENT OF BREAST CANCER

Paget's disease of the nipple

The majority of patients with Paget's disease are elderly, although the author has seen one patient presenting with this condition in her twenties. The clinical presentation of Paget's disease with an itching, vesicular eruption involving the nipple is confirmed by biopsy and the subsequent demonstration of large cells with pale cytoplasm (Paget's cells) in the epidermis (Fig. 18). The origin and nature of Paget's cells are unknown, although they reflect an underlying ductal carcinoma. The ductal cancer may be either *in situ* or invasive and may or may not be associated with a mass. There is sometimes quite extensive disease within the breast.

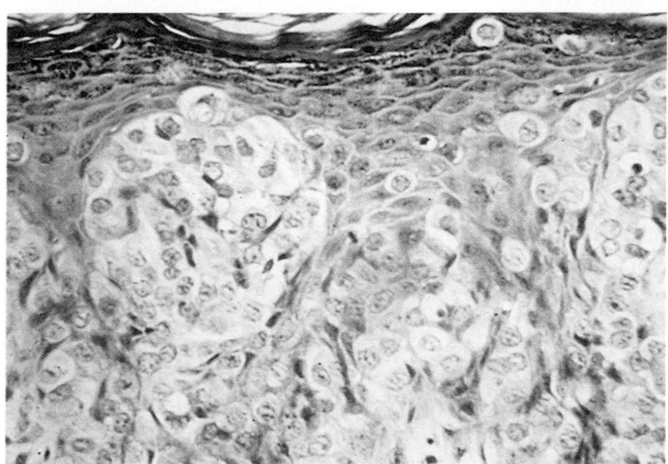

Fig. 18 Paget's cells. The large, clear Paget's cells are seen invading the epidermis. (By courtesy of Dr D. Tarin.)

The differential diagnosis is with eczema, which is usually bilateral and associated with disease elsewhere. Paget's disease of the nipple should also be distinguished from a frank tumour that is simply eroding the skin of the nipple and areola.

Paget's disease of the nipple has traditionally been treated by mastectomy with lower axillary clearance and is thought to have an excellent prognosis. If the cancer is of the *in-situ* type this is certainly true. Patients with more extensive disease associated with invasive cancer have a relatively worse prognosis.

Because so many patients with Paget's disease are elderly there has been a recent trend to treat this condition by wide local excision of the nipple and surrounding tissues. However, this may not be satisfactory treatment if positive margins result. Furthermore, excision of the nipple, especially in small breasts, may lead to a rather unusual cosmetic result. Treatment with tamoxifen or simple irradiation therapy alone has not been adequately evaluated.

Breast cancer in the elderly

Breast cancer is a common condition in very elderly women. Some, but not all, authorities claim that tumours in this age group are slowly growing, are associated with a high oestrogen receptor status, and have good prognosis. Treatment with the anti-oestrogen tamoxifen has therefore been advocated: randomized controlled trials have shown this to be as effective, in terms of survival, as surgery. Some authorities, however, have found an unacceptable incidence of local failure after this treatment and recommend mastectomy. Surgical excision is therefore still a good alternative and can be supplemented by adjuvant tamoxifen therapy.

The conservative approach using tamoxifen alone should be reserved for the very frail. It should also be remembered that not all elderly patients have good prognosis tumours. Presentation with axillary nodal involvement and the subsequent development of visceral metastases is common.

Breast cancer during pregnancy and lactation

Breast cancer during pregnancy and lactation is perhaps the subject *par excellence* in which opinion is based on anecdotal rather than proven scientific facts. It is fortunately rare, accounting for less than 1 per cent of all breast cancer cases. However, it is this rarity, along with difficulty in evaluating the pregnant or lactating breast, which makes diagnosis difficult and delayed treatment common.

The traditional view of breast cancer during pregnancy and lactation was that it was an inflammatory type of tumour with cutaneous erythema from intradermal lymphatic involvement (mastitis carcinomatosis). However, although inflammatory cancers do occur in pregnancy they are more common in other age groups. The majority of tumours seen in pregnant women are similar to those occurring in the non-pregnant state.

Those who believe breast cancer in pregnancy to be of an inflammatory type have also suggested that these tumours have a very bad prognosis. Anecdotal evidence implies that the prognosis is poor, although proper scientific appraisal of the available literature on the subject fails to confirm this belief totally.

Breast cancer occurring during pregnancy should be treated according to standard principles. Each case must be judged from its own merits regarding the indications or otherwise for breast conservation, adjuvant irradiation, and chemotherapy.

Previous recommendations regarding termination of pregnancy have been revised in the light of lack of evidence that it improves survival. However, as irradiation and adjuvant chemotherapy are contraindicated during pregnancy then a first trimester termination would be indicated for patients with locally advanced disease in whom these adjuvant treatments are necessary. The pregnancy can be continued, if the patient wishes, in those with apparently local diseases. The treatment of choice would be mastectomy and axillary clearance, as this would avoid need for adjuvant irradiation. If nodes were found to be positive then consideration would have to be given to termination of the pregnancy and provision of adjuvant chemotherapy.

If cancer is detected in the last trimester than surgical treatment can be provided using normal criteria. Adjuvant chemotherapy or irradiation can be delayed until after delivery.

For tumours occurring in the second trimester the choices of management are more difficult. A full discussion with the patient and partner is required and a treatment policy formulated which takes into account not only the state of the disease but also the patient's wish regarding the pregnancy.

Breast cancers occurring during lactation present special problems. Lactation should be suppressed with bromocriptine and treatment of the cancer based on standard principles.

One question asked by younger women previously treated for breast cancer is what the effect of a subsequent pregnancy may be on their well-being. Many authorities recommend that after the diagnosis of breast cancer pregnancy should be avoided for 2 and preferably 5 years. Such advice is again based on somewhat anecdotal evidence and is not widely supported in the literature. However, it is important to give honest advice to patients with a poor prognosis so that the consequences of an untimely pregnancy can be avoided.

Locally advanced cancer (Stage III)

Locally advanced tumours are defined as those more than 5 cm in diameter or those with fixed axillary nodes in which there is no evidence of distant metastases. The management of these cancers has been somewhat disappointing because of poor local tumour control and the high incidence of subsequent metastatic disease, resulting in an overall survival rate of 20 per cent or less.

The traditional treatment of locally advanced breast cancer, radical mastectomy, has produced disappointing results, with up to 40 per cent of patients developing local–regional recurrence within 2 years and low overall survival rates. As a result there has been enthusiasm for treatment with high-dose radiotherapy. Some studies, using doses in excess of 60 Gy, have obtained similar results to those achieved with mastectomy. Local recurrence rates could be reduced if the tumour was surgically debulked or if an even higher radiation dose was provided by an interstitial implant.

There is probably little to choose between mastectomy and primary irradiation in the management of locally advanced breast cancer. A combination of the two may produce improved local control, although this has yet to be demonstrated in prospective trials.

Recently there has been enthusiasm for adjuvant chemotherapy in patients with locally advanced tumours. Multiagent chemotherapy has been shown to improve disease-free survival in patients with locally advanced disease. A number of authorities now recommend neo-adjuvant chemotherapy to 'downstage' the tumour prior to treatment with surgery or irradiation. Not only does the main tumour shrink, but chemotherapy is delivered to potential micrometastases soon after diagnosis. However, no data are currently available which indicate whether this approach yields benefit in terms of either local control or overall survival.

Carcinoma *in situ*

Ductal carcinoma *in situ* (DCIS)

Ductal carcinoma *in situ* accounts for only about 5 per cent of all symptomatic breast cancers. It presents either with a mass or with nipple discharge, although it is occasionally a chance finding on biopsy for other reasons. In screening programmes, however, the incidence of ductal carcinoma *in situ* may be as high as 20 per cent and its relative importance has therefore increased over the last 5 years.

The natural history of ductal carcinoma *in situ* has been discussed. Most available data relate to symptomatic patients rather than those detected by screening, but it appears that the risk of developing invasive cancer in the former group is about 30 to 50 per cent over a 15-year period. The comedo variant of the tumour has a greater malignant potential than the cribriform, papillary, solid, and micropapillary types. Microinvasion is difficult to evaluate. Recent evidence suggests that this feature does not necessarily imply increased risk of frank malignant changes and may, in fact, be invariably present if searched for assiduously.

Further evidence relating to the malignant potential of ductal carcinoma *in situ* is available from studies which have found that this cancer occurs in the contralateral breast in up to 50 per cent of women previously treated for breast cancer. However, the risk of developing a frank invasive cancer is only about 20 per cent at 20 years after the diagnosis of the original primary tumour.

One unexplained feature of ductal carcinoma *in situ* is its high expression of the C-*erb2* oncogene. This is present in approximately 80 per cent of all such tumours, but in only 40 per cent of invasive tumours.

The treatment of ductal carcinoma *in situ* is controversial. When it is extensive in the breast, mastectomy is usually recommended. Such treatment provides local control and survival rates of almost 100 per cent. Treatment of smaller tumours, such as those detected by screening, is the subject of controversy. While some surgeons still prefer mastectomy, others recommend breast conservation and wide excision of the tumour. Adjuvant radiotherapy may reduce the risk of subsequent relapse; the same might also be true for adjuvant tamoxifen although there is no clear evidence to confirm this.

Despite the low incidence of axillary node disease in women with ductal carcinoma *in situ* it is always necessary to stage the axilla appropriately by limited dissection of its contents. A major drawback of performing local excision is the risk of inadequate resection and subsequent positive margins. Mammographic appearances do not provide a good guide to the extent of ductal carcinoma *in situ*: even a 2-cm margin of apparently normal breast tissue is associated with an unacceptable inadequate resection rate in screen-detected cancers. The supporters of local excision for ductal carcinoma *in situ* claim that even if margins of resection are positive for tumour a salvage mastectomy can be performed if relapse occurs. The flaw in this argument is that approximately 50 per cent of patients who develop relapse after wide excision will have invasive cancer. Although the impact of recurrence on survival is unknown, it is clearly a dubious principle to leave a patient with positive margins after local excision for ductal carcinoma *in situ*. Under these circumstances the author always recommends mastectomy with or without reconstruction.

Lobular carcinoma *in situ*

This has generated less interest than ductal carcinoma *in situ* in recent years because of the importance of the latter in screening programmes. Furthermore, its malignant potential is less than that of ductal carcinoma: only about 25 per cent of patients demonstrating invasion within 20 years of diagnosis. The risk of developing an invasive cancer is as great in the contralateral breast as in the side in which the original diagnosis was made. Lobular carcinoma *in situ* is now regarded, therefore, as a mark of cancer risk rather than a true premalignant tumour. It does not express the C-*erb*2 oncogene.

There are no clinical or radiological features of lobular carcinoma *in situ*, which is a chance histological finding following biopsy for some other condition. Recommendations for treatment vary from simple monitoring to mastectomy with contralateral mirror image biopsy because of its predisposition to bilaterality. The author suggests that wide excision should be performed. If the specimen obtained shows only a limited amount of fully excised tumour, routine observation is sufficient. If disease is extensive, and particularly if there are other risk factors for breast cancer, mastectomy with or without reconstruction must be considered. There is little merit in the contralateral biopsy.

Screen-detected cancer

Breast cancer is a common condition with a long natural history and there is evidence, perhaps controversial, that treatment at an earlier stage improves prognosis. In theory, therefore, breast cancer lends itself to earlier detection by mammography. The guidelines for successful screening have been laid down by the World Health Organization, and most of these criteria are fulfilled by breast screening programmes (Table 7).

Table 7 World Health Organization guidelines for screening

The condition must have a high prevalence
Its natural history must be known
It must have a well-defined early stage
There must be evidence that early treatment provides better results than treatment of later disease
There must be a suitable test
The test must be applicable
There must be facilities available for treatment of abnormality
The screening must do no psychogenic harm
It must be cost efficient

Unfortunately, there is no clear consensus as to the treatment of breast cancer, particularly for *in situ* subtypes of the disease. Mammography can be applied to populations of women, although it is technically sophisticated and may create anxiety. Whether breast cancer screening is truly cost beneficial in terms of overall health care has yet to be determined.

There are four main studies evaluating breast cancer screening: the Health Insurance Plan (HIP) study from New York, two studies from Sweden (the Two Counties and the Malmo studies), and one study from the United Kingdom. In addition there are case-control studies from Holland and Italy, and interim results from other centres such as those from Canada.

These studies provide conflicting results. The HIP study demonstrated a 30 per cent reduction in mortality in the screened group of patients although this was not detected until after 7 years. This study has been criticized in various ways, although it was a remarkable feat when it is considered that it was initiated in the early 1960s, when mammographic techniques were rudimentary. This may explain the small impact provided by mammography in detecting cancers in the screened group. Two hundred and ninety-nine cancers were detected in the study group; 167 of these were interval cancers in that they became clinically apparent between screening and 88 were clinically obvious at the time of screening. In only 44 patients was a mammographic abnormality found which was not clinically apparent.

The Two Counties Study from Sweden was based on randomization by geographic area and there are a number of statistical considerations which may be criticized. However, on balance, it is a large, well constructed study which provides good data in favour of screening.

The second Swedish study from Malmo failed to show a significant mortality difference between the screened and unscreened populations, although this was a relatively small trial and a true effect may have been missed. The United Kingdom study also failed to demonstrate a mortality difference between the screened and unscreened populations at initial observation times, although after 8 years a significant difference did become apparent.

Analysis of the above studies in conjunction with case-control studies and interim results from other trials indicates that screening may reduce the mortality of breast cancer by about 30 per cent. The effect is most obvious in women aged over 50. Few data support screening in women younger than 50, although a significant reduction in mortality did occur in this age group after prolonged observation in the HIP study.

National breast cancer screening programmes have now been initiated in a number of countries, particularly in northern Europe. The age range of women screened and the screening interval depends on the programme concerned. Generally, however, women between 45 and 65 are screened approximately every 2 years. In the United Kingdom, screening is undertaken over the age range 50 to 65, every 3 years. These criteria have been established to provide the maximum reduction in mortality for minimum cost. Initial screening is generally provided by a single oblique mammographic view; if an abnormality is found the patient is recalled for clinical examination and two-plane mammographic evaluation. Some programmes do not rely on clinical palpation as an initial mode of screening because of lack of evidence as to its efficacy.

Breast cancer screening has its critics. The reduction in mortality of 30 per cent translates to an improvement in survival of approximately 10 per cent. If these relative percentages are converted to absolute figures the number of patients in a given population whose lives may be extended by screening is small. Furthermore, the results of the studies on screening may have been influenced by bias. Lead-time bias is the time by which the diagnosis is advanced through screening: only the HIP study considered this factor. Lag-time bias is the tendency of screening programmes to detect tumours of low biological potential. Other biases, such as selection bias for inclusion in screening programmes and over-diagnosis bias (the diagnosis of an abnormality which might not otherwise have been diagnosed in the lifetime of the patient) should also be considered.

Critics of screening claim that its expense and relatively small effect on survival are not cost-effective. They claim that any improvement in survival may result from increased diagnosis of biologically favourable tumours such as ductal carcinoma *in situ* and those tumours of special type. In routine clinical practice ductal carcinoma *in situ* accounts for only 5 per cent of all cancers detected; in the screened population it accounts for about 20 per cent of all tumours diagnosed. Similar figures pertain to 'special' tumours with a good prognosis, such as tubular and medullary cancers. Whether these criticisms are justified cannot be addressed at the present time.

After the initial screen, in which 20 to 30 per cent of cancers can be clinically detected, screening is therefore particularly directed to the detection and treatment of small tumours with a favourable prognosis, and ductal carcinoma *in situ*. Lymph node metastases in this population should therefore be relatively uncommon: they occur in only about 15 per cent of patients as compared to 45 per cent in the unscreened population. However, as has been discussed above, there are doubts as to the ideal treatment of these screen detected cancers, especially ductal carcinoma *in situ*. Diffuse, extensive ductal carcinoma *in situ* is usually treated by mastectomy with or without reconstruction. Localised disease can be treated by wide excision; the role of adjuvant radiotherapy or tamoxifen after this treatment is, however, open to speculation and is currently the subject of a randomized trial in the United Kingdom. There are also doubts as to whether adjuvant radiotherapy is required following wide excision of small favourable tumours. This is also the subject of a randomized trial.

If breast cancer screening is to be successful it must be centrally controlled and funded, performed by specially trained personnel, and be associated with a quality assurance programme. Adequate public information is also of prime importance. If screening is performed in less than 70 per cent of the target population its impact is likely to be small. If performed properly with due attention to quality assurance, screening is likely to be of benefit to women in late middle-age.

FOLLOW-UP OF WOMEN WITH BREAST CANCER

The follow-up of women treated for breast cancer is generally somewhat haphazard with varying intervals of review, no protocol for investigation, and an arbitrary time of discharge—usually 5 years. This confusion is compounded by lack of evidence that prognosis is improved with an intensive, investigation—orientated, hospital observation compared to that of the primary care physician.

Breast cancer patients should receive emotional and psychological support as well as physical evaluation. The latter is directed towards the detection of local regional recurrence as well as distant metastases, although it should be appreciated that two-thirds of recurrences are symptomatic and noted by the patients between hospital visits.

The evaluation of local regional recurrence should include detection of new primary breast cancers. Mammography is therefore recommended every 1 to 2 years after initial diagnosis. Local recurrence in the breast or in regional lymph nodes can be treated or at least palliated with further surgery, irradiation, or chemotherapy.

Investigation for early, asymptomatic distant metastases is much less efficacious. Bony metastases are the most frequent type of relapse, and some authorities have recommended bone scintigraphy at yearly intervals, or less often. The yield of such investigations is low, the expense is considerable, and there is little evidence that detection and treatment of such asymptomatic recurrence improves the prognosis over that obtained when treatment delayed until the patient complains of symptoms. Furthermore, false-positive investigations provide a constant source of uncertainty. The argument for routine tests such as chest radiographs and liver scanning is even less convincing than that for bone scintigraphy.

In our own Unit we see patients at 3-monthly intervals for the first year. Stage I patients are then seen 6-monthly for a year and yearly thereafter. Stage II and III patients are seen 3-monthly for 2 years, 6-monthly for the third year, and then yearly. This is somewhat arbitrary. The time of discharge is also empirical, but for research purposes we monitor patients for 10 years, although the accumulation of large numbers of patients may well limit this ideal with the passage of time.

THE PROGNOSIS OF BREAST CANCER

The arbitrary description of the prognosis of breast cancer as a survival rate after an indeterminate amount of time is somewhat naïve. First, the natural history of breast cancer is uncertain and survival, even after the development of metastases, may be prolonged without treatment. Second, recurrence and subsequent death may occur as long as 25 years after the original diagnosis and, finally, if survival is prolonged death from other causes must be taken into account. Despite these limitations the analysis of survival demonstrates that about 80 per cent of patients with Stage I disease are alive after 5 years, whereas at 10 years this figure falls to 50 per cent. For Stage II disease survival rates are 50 per cent and 35 per cent, respectively. Overall survival, including those with Stage III and Stage IV disease at presentation, is likely to be less than 25 per cent after 10 years.

Critics of this method of survival analysis recommend an alternative method (Fig. 19). Curve A describes the survival characteristics in an age-matched population without breast cancer. Curve D is that of the population with breast cancer. Initially the mortality from breast cancer is excessive and curve D diverges from A. With the passage of time deaths from breast cancer become less common and the two curves become more parallel. True parallelism indicates that the risk of death in the population indicated by curve D is no greater than that of A and the group, as a whole, can be considered cured. Such analysis with long-term follow-up, however, shows an increased death rate from breast cancer even 30 years after initial diagnosis, although some of this long-term mortality is due to death from second breast cancers and the cardiopulmonary effects of irradiation.

Curve D describes the survival of two distinct groups. Patients in curve B have an intrinsically good prognosis. Curve C, however, represents the poor prognosis group. Unless their outlook can be improved it may be that the overall survival of symptomatic breast cancer patients will remain unaltered.

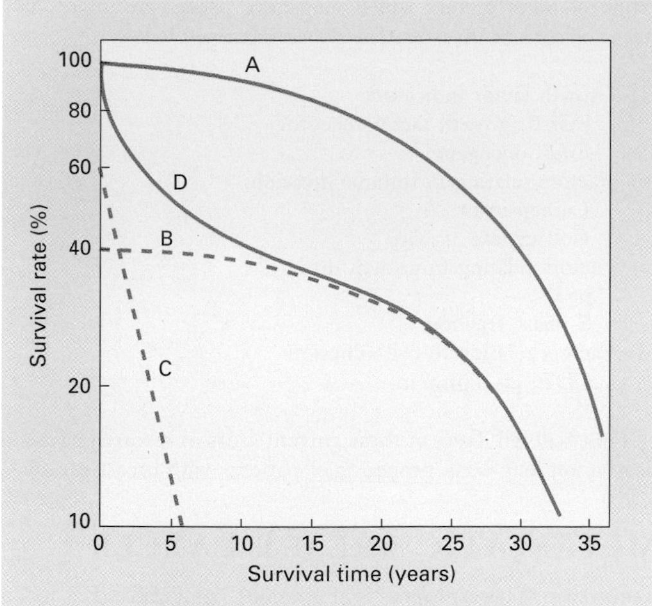

Fig. 19 Long-term survival in breast cancer (see text).

Prognostic factors in breast cancer

Prognostic factors have important implications for both the breast cancer patient and for her medical attendant. Not only do they act as a guide to overall prognosis, but they may also determine the need for adjuvant treatment. The latter is of current interest in that it may define a subgroup of patients with apparently favourable node-negative tumours who nonetheless have a poor prognosis and to whom adjuvant therapy may be specifically targeted.

The major arguments relating to prognostic factors are their inter-relationships and relative importance. The relative importance of clinical as opposed to pathological factors is also controversial: there is inherent inaccuracy in clinical assessment of features such as tumour size and axillary nodal involvement. Overall clinical stage is, therefore, only a relatively poor prognostic indicator, and is less important than specific pathological and certain biochemical parameters. Other clinical factors, such as patient age, menopausal status, obstetric history, and site of tumour in the breast have not been shown to be of much prognostic importance.

Prognostic factors can be determined by a multivariant analysis of the various clinical and pathological features of a group of patients with breast cancer. There is some discrepancy relating to the relative importance of prognostic features between studies although most show that axillary nodal disease, tumour size, and differentiation are the most important (Table 8).

The question of interdependence is difficult to address. An obvious example is tumour differentiation, which may be regarded purely as an expression of the inherent biology of the tumour. Thus a poorly differentiated tumour has unfavourable biological characteristics and is likely to be large at presentation, to be associated with axillary nodal involvement and negative receptor status, and to have a poor prognosis. On the other hand, many studies have shown that tumour differentiation is an independent prognostic variable in its own right and acts as a determinant independent of factors such as tumour size and nodal disease.

Table 8 Major prognostic determinants

1. Axillary nodal status
2. Tumour size
3. Histological grade
4. Hormone receptor status
5. Others (menopausal status, age, vascular invasion)

Lymph node metastases

Nearly all studies show that the presence of axillary lymph node metastases is the most important prognostic determinant. Prognosis is a function of the number of lymph node metastases, although other factors such as level of disease, extranodal spread, or size of tumour metastases may be of some minor significance. Thus, isolated tumour cells seen in axillary nodes using histochemical techniques represent the most minor degree of nodal involvement. The significance of these features is unclear. A single micrometastasis less than 2 mm in diameter is associated with an overall prognosis similar to that of node-negative disease. Disease affecting one node is also associated with a prognosis similar to that of node-negative disease, although after 10 to 12 years such spread may be associated with a worsening prognosis. Disease affecting up to three lymph nodes classifies the patient in a relatively favourable subgroup of stage II. Those with four to 12 nodes affected form an intermediate group; the prognosis is decidedly poor if more than 12 lymph nodes exhibit metastatic disease.

Tumour size

Tumour size is the second most important prognostic determinant. Although tumour size and lymph node metastasis are closely related they are also independent of each other in terms of prognosis. The influence of tumour size is most obvious when lymph nodes contain metastases and is probably of greatest importance in the first 5 years after the initial diagnosis.

Histological grade

The grading of invasive breast cancer has been regarded as notoriously difficult because of varying interpretation by pathologists. Some recent experience indicates that specialists in this field can, however, obtain a remarkable degree of agreement. Grade is classified as I, II, or III on the basis of tubule formation, nuclear pleomorphism, and mitotic rate. Mitotic rate is the most powerful factor.

About 20 per cent of cases are classified as well-differentiated (Grade I) although there is some variation between centres. Forty per cent of patients are classified as intermediate (Grade II), and the remainder demonstrate poor differentiation (Grade III). Investigations such as those of the Cancer Research Campaign and the Nottingham Tenovus Breast Cancer Study group clearly demonstrate a relationship between grade and prognosis, which is independent of other variables.

A difficult problem relating to histological grade is its correlation with the morphological type of the tumour, as there is a relationship between tumour type and prognosis. Special types of breast cancer such as pure tubular, mucinous, and invasive cribriform carcinoma have an excellent prognosis while infiltrating lobular and medullary carcinoma appear to have an intermediate prognosis between the first group and the common infiltrating ductal carcinoma of no special type. It could be argued that histological grading is appropriate only to invasive ductal cancer of no special type, but this would result in important prognostic information being unavailable for up to 25 per cent of patients.

The grading of classic lobular cancer is also difficult because of the nature of the tumour cells and lack of histological pattern in this particular type of cancer.

The importance of axillary nodal disease, tumour size, and differentiation has resulted in a number of successful attempts to define a 'prognostic index' using this information.

Hormonal receptor status

It has been known for many years that certain patients with breast cancer respond to endocrine therapy and have a more indolent form of the disease. Such endocrine sensitive tumours can be identified by measurement of oestrogen or progesterone receptors within the cancer itself. The oestrogen receptor is a cytosol protein that can be identified using a variety of methods. Previously, the most common method of detection involved the incubation of the supernatant fluid of a tissue homogenate with radiolabelled oestrogen. The unbound label is then removed by dextran-coated charcoal or sucrose density centrifugation and an assay performed. More recent methods use monoclonal antibodies against the receptor; such methods require smaller specimens although they are difficult to perform.

When cancer cells with intact and functional oestrogen receptors are exposed to oestrogen the latter is transported to the site of mRNA production in the nucleus. The result of this interaction includes the formation of additional oestrogen and progesterone receptors and other growth factors that help dictate cell characteristics.

The presence of oestrogen or progesterone receptors within the cell has been associated with an improved short-term prognosis in some, but not all, studies. Although they provide some prognostic information they are somewhat weak indicators of overall prognosis and not as important as tumour size, nodal status, or degree of differentiation.

Any improvement in prognosis of oestrogen receptor-positive tumours may be due to improved disease-free survival, improved survival after the first demonstration of metastases, or both. There is conflicting evidence as to whether oestrogen receptor status provides the differential information for premenopausal as opposed to postmenopausal women and for node-negative as opposed to node-positive disease.

The relative importance of oestrogen and progesterone receptors is difficult to assess. Some studies indicate that the presence of progesterone receptor is an inferior prognostic indicator compared to oestrogen receptor. On the other hand some authorities have demonstrated progesterone receptor to be as good a prognostic indicator as node status or tumour size. If oestrogen and progesterone receptors are both present the prognostic information is likely to be more powerful than if only one of these factors is present.

Other controversial factors

Other histological features such as vascular or lymphatic invasion in the breast, perineural invasion, tumour necrosis, or mucin production may be of prognostic importance although their clinical significance is open to doubt.

Current investigation of prognostic factors

The identification of high-risk patients and their potential for targeting this specific adjuvant therapy has resulted in the recognition of other factors which may have prognostic importance. Areas of current investigation are summarized below.

(a) Growth factor indicators:
- EGFR (growth factor receptor)
- *ErbB*$_2$ oncogene

(b) Factors relating to tumour invasion:
- Cathepsin D
- Collagenase activity

(c) Factors relating to growth rate:
- p53
- S-phase fraction

(d) Factors relating to cell adhesion:
- CD44 glycoprotein

Time will tell if any of these current areas of research have any bearing on long-term prognosis of patients with breast cancer.

METASTATIC BREAST CANCER

Recurrence of breast cancer is of ominous significance. It is incurable, with a median survival of about 15 months although there is a wide range lasting from only a few weeks to many years. The role of treatment in metastatic disease is two-fold: to alleviate symptoms and to prolong survival. Despite a plethora of new drugs and therapeutic options there is little evidence that overall survival has been improved once metastases have occurred, although the duration and quality of life in patients responding to therapy have improved.

The management of metastases demands a multimodality approach by surgeons, radiotherapists, and medical oncologists. The role of careful diagnostic radiology in assessing the extent of disease cannot be over-emphasized: appropriate counselling is particularly important, especially for mothers with young families, whose overall outlook must be frankly discussed.

Assessment of patients with metastatic disease

Once a patient has presented with recurrence it is necessary to determine the full extent of metastatic spread. This requires full and careful examination of the site of the original primary tumour and its regional lymph nodes. A full series of staging investigations, including chest radiography, abdominal ultrasound, and bone scintigraphy are also necessary to determine the presence of other sites of occult metastatic disease. Brain scanning is not recommended: the likelihood of this investigation detecting asymptomatic recurrence is small.

There is little evidence that tumour markers such as carcinoembryonic antigen have any significant role in assessment of metastatic breast cancer or the evaluation of response to treatment.

A full series of staging investigations helps to determine the appropriate therapy. It also allows a more accurate appraisal of response to treatment.

Prognostic indicators in metastatic disease

The most important prognostic indicator in metastatic disease is disease-free interval after diagnosis of the primary tumour. The median survival of women who relapse in a single site within 1 year

Table 9 Endocrine therapy in breast cancer

Mechanism of action	Drug	Dose	Side-effects
Anti-oestrogens	Tamoxifen	20 mg daily	Nausea, weight gain, hot flushes, vaginal bleeding, interference with anticoagulants, amenorrhoea
Progestogens	Megestrol acetate	160 mg daily	Weight gain, fluid retention
	Medoxyprogesterone	400 mg daily	Nausea, flushing, vaginal bleeding
Steroid hydroxylation inhibition	Aminoglutethimide	250 mg four times daily (with steroid)	Rash, dizziness, lethargy, cushingoid, addisonian states
LHRH agonists	Zoladex	3.6 mg subcutaneously monthly	Amenorrhoea, nausea, headache
Oestrogens	Diethylstilboestrol	15 mg daily	Vomiting, fluid retention, hypercalcaemia, thrombosis
Androgens	Fluoxymesterone	30 mg daily	Masculinization, nausea, weight gain

* Surgical therapy includes oophorectomy, adrenalectomy, and hypophysectomy. Problems include surgical complications and side-effects such as addisonian crises, diabetes instidus etc.
LHRH, luteinizing hormone releasing hormone.

of diagnosis is about 11 months; those who experience a disease-free interval of more than 5 years have a survival of up to 40 months.

The site of metastatic disease is also important: prognosis is more optimistic in patients with local regional or bony metastases than in those with recurrence in the liver or central nervous system. The number of metastatic sites is also a factor: survival of patients with three sites of metastases is only 50 per cent of those with one affected site.

Some prognostic information may be obtained from knowledge of oestrogen and progesterone receptor status, although this is not as important as the factors discussed above. However, such information may be important in determining treatment: patients positive for such receptors are more likely to respond to endocrine manipulation.

Treatment of metastases

The treatment of metastatic disease at individual sites is discussed below. However, as the majority of patients with metastases can be regarded as suffering from widespread systemic disease, the use of systemic therapy is nearly always appropriate. Breast cancer is relatively unusual in being responsive not only to radiotherapy and chemotherapy but also to various endocrine manipulations.

Endocrine therapy

The mechanism of response to endocrine therapy is unclear. The simplistic explanation is that breast cancer requires oestrogen for growth and that inhibition of this hormone's action will produce a response. This explanation, however, fails to explain why a given breast tumour can respond to both oestrogen withdrawal and addition. It also fails to explain how breast cancer may respond to other therapeutic manipulations involving progestogens, androgens, and corticosteroids, when there is little evidence that they are involved in tumour growth.

Despite the difficulties in understanding the mechanisms of endocrine therapy it appears that its effect is mediated by receptors, especially those for oestrogen. The overall response to endocrine therapy in breast cancer is about 30 per cent. However, it may reach 60 per cent in those positive for oestrogen receptors, or be as low as 10 per cent in those negative for such receptors. The higher the level of oestrogen receptors the greater the likelihood of response. If the level of progesterone receptors is also elevated the response rate is likely to be increased.

The choice of endocrine therapy

A wide range of endocrine therapies is available (Table 9). Some are pharmacological agents; others require surgical manipulation. The latter were frequently adopted up to the 1960s, but in the last 20 years oral agents have been used with increasing frequency. Apart from their ease of administration, pharmacological agents have a much broader application, as many of the surgical options were limited to premenopausal patients only.

In general there is little evidence that response rates to or survival benefit from one type of endocrine therapy are superior to those of any other, although androgens have fallen into disfavour because of their lower activity and side-effects. The choice of endocrine therapy is therefore based on ease of administration and freedom from side-effects. As a result the anti-oestrogen, tamoxifen, has become the treatment of choice for first-line endocrine therapy. Younger patients in particular, however, are prone to suffer hot flushes and weight gain with this treatment. Randomized trials have shown tamoxifen to be as effective as oophorectomy, aminoglutethimide, and progestogens.

Progestogens are as active as tamoxifen as a first-line agent. They are also a good second-line treatment after failure of response to tamoxifen in both premenopausal and postmenopausal patients. Side-effects, particularly weight gain, fluid retention, and nausea can be a problem.

Aminoglutethimide is as active as tamoxifen as a first-line treatment and, in some studies, has shown to be particularly effective against bone metastases. Dosage should be slowly increased but at the normal therapeutic dose (250 mg four times daily) supplemental hydrocortisone (30 mg daily) and even mineralocorticoid is required. Cushinoid and addisonian states can therefore accompany aminoglutethamide therapy. Other side-effects, such as rashes, nausea, and drowsiness somewhat limit its use, although it can be useful in premenopausal patients after failure of tamoxifen and progestogens.

Several authorities have recently described success with luteinizing hormone-releasing hormone agonists such as Zoladex. It is likely that this group of drugs will be used more often in premenopausal patients with metastatic breast cancer.

The success of the various oral agents has reduced enthusiasm for surgical endocrine therapy: adrenalectomy and hypophysectomy have almost disappeared from use. Some authorities still recommend oophorectomy with enthusiasm, and recent data relating to its potential role as an adjuvant in premenopausal Stage II disease suggests that its future may be assured. Whether oophorectomy will be replaced by the the newly introduced luteinizing hormone-releasing hormone agonists remains to be seen. The suggestion that a combination of endocrine therapies may improve survival has not been demonstrated in randomized studies, although higher response rates may be seen.

Tamoxifen is, therefore, the ideal first-line endocrine therapy, with an overall response rate of about 30 per cent (up to 60 per cent in those positive for oestrogen receptors). Failure to respond is an indication for abandoning endocrine therapy. Relapse following an initial response can be treated with a progesterone, although the response rate to such second-line treatment is only about half that seen with first-line therapy. Subsequent treatment failure may be treated by aminoglutethimide in premenopausal women and aminoglutethimide or oestrogen in postmenopausal patients, although response rates continue to diminish. Oestrogens must be used with care in patients with bone metastases because of the risk of hypercalcaemia. If oophorectomy has a role it is probably as a second-line treatment after a good response to tamoxifen in premenopausal patients. Androgens are now rarely used in patients with metastatic breast cancer.

A characteristic, but relatively unusual, feature of response to hormonal therapy is 'flare', the mechanism of which is unclear. It is characterized by an exacerbation of symptoms associated with erythema and swelling after the initiation of endocrine treatment. The symptoms resolve within 1 month.

Chemotherapy

About 60 per cent of patients with previously untreated metastatic breast cancer respond to appropriate chemotherapeutic protocols, although complete resolution of disease is seen in fewer than 20 per cent. The median duration of response is about 1 year, although this depends on the site of metastatic disease: better responses are seen in soft tissue and bone than in the liver or central nervous system. The time of response is also variable, depending on the site of disease. Cutaneous or lymphatic metastases may respond within 3 to 6 weeks; response may not be seen until after 4 or 5 months if metastases are in bone.

Chemosensitivity of breast cancer

Overall response rates to the more commonly used chemotherapeutic agents used in breast cancer are shown in Table 10. The most active agents are anthracyclines such as Adriamycin. In some, but not all, studies Adriamycin alone has produced a response rate approaching 60 per cent; in other investigations it has been shown to be as active as combination chemotherapy with cyclophosphamide, 5-fluorouracil, and methotrexate.

Table 10 Response rates to chemotherapeutic agents used for breast cancer

Adriamycin	45%
Cyclophosphamide	33%
Mitozantrone	33%
Methotrexate	25%
5-Fluorouracil	25%
L-Pam	20%
Vincristine	20%

Vincristine has been widely used in combination therapy for metastatic breast cancer but no advantage over regimens in which it is lacking has been demonstrated. Its advantage is that, unlike other commonly used agents, it is not myelosuppressive.

Mitomycin C demonstrates substantial activity against metastatic breast cancer and has even been shown to induce responses in tumours resistant to Adriamycin and cyclophosphamide. It is most commonly used in combination with methotrexate and mitozantrone (MMM) as a second-line treatment.

Combination chemotherapy has enhanced activity, albeit at the expense of a higher incidence of side-effects. The most commonly used regimen is the combination of cyclophosphamide, methotrexate, and 5-fluorouracil (CMF), which has an overall response rate of up to 60 per cent. The addition of vincristine and prednisone to this combination does not significantly enhance the response obtained. However, the substitution of methotrexate with Adriamycin (CAF) is associated with an increased response rate of prolonged duration, although with more side-effects.

Adriamycin, either alone or in combination with cyclophosphamide and 5-fluorouracil (AF), has been used mainly as a second-line treatment following failure of initial chemotherapy, or in the management of younger patients with a poor prognosis, such as those with liver metastases. Its toxicity precludes its use in older patients.

A more recently adopted combination is based on mitomycin C, methotrexate, and mitozantrone (MMM). This has potential value both as a primary management of metastatic breast cancer and a second-line treatment.

Combined chemoendocrine therapy

There has been a natural tendency to combine chemotherapy with endocrine treatment. Although response rates and duration of response may be enhanced the only overall benefit is small and as a result such combinations are not recommended. In theory at least the endocrine treatment may slow down the cell cycle, thus reducing the efficacy of the chemotherapy.

Management of metastatic disease at specific sites

Local regional recurrence

Recurrence in the remaining breast tissue after partial mastectomy or on the chest wall after total mastectomy has been discussed above. Local recurrence must be distinguished from regional recurrence: the latter relates to recurrent disease in the adjacent lymphatic field. Regional recurrence is always of clinical importance and implies a worsening of prognosis. However, it is particularly important if it occurs in a treated rather than an untreated field. The management of regional recurrence depends on the site of relapse. If it is in the internal mammary or supraclavicular areas radiation can be used, followed by endocrine or cytotoxic therapy as appropriate. Surgery has little part to play in the treatment of relapse at these sites.

Treatment of axillary relapse is by full surgical clearance, if this has not already been performed. Clearance of a previously irradiated axilla is likely to cause arm lymphoedema. Relapse occurring after clearance is treated by radiotherapy or systemic treatment.

Metastases in the gastrointestinal tract

The liver is a common site of metastatic spread of breast cancer. Such metastases are characteristically multiple and surgical resection has no role in their management. Resection is not even indicated in the unusual situation of a single hepatic metastasis. The prognosis of hepatic metastases is poor, and aggressive therapy is indicated. Hepatic metastases do not respond well to hormone therapy. In young patients with good performance status, combination chemotherapy, including Adriamycin, is appropriate as first-line therapy. Older patients may only be suitable for endocrine therapy, although this is not likely to be so efficacious.

Peritoneal metastases may cause acites or intestinal obstruction. Such metastatic spread is said to be particularly common in patients with lobular carcinoma. Systemic combination chemotherapy is required if it can be tolerated. Surgical intervention should be avoided if possible; it may be required to relieve obstruction, or for insertion of a peritoneal-systemic shunt if ascites becomes intractable.

Occasionally, isolated metastases are seen in the ovary or the adrenal gland. If the retroperitoneum is involved, however, it is usually a manifestation of widespread carcinomatosis including the peritoneal cavity. Renal failure due to obstructive uropathy is a common cause of death in these patients.

Pulmonary metastases

Metastatic disease to the lungs is often multiple and not amenable to surgical resection or radiotherapy. Systemic combination chemotherapy is indicated, although endocrine treatment is more appropriate for older poor-performance patients. Metastatic spread causing lymphangitis can cause distressing dyspnoea. The diagnosis can be difficult in its early stages because it produces few changes on chest radiographs. Combination chemotherapy should be instituted if possible, with the addition of steroids for symptomatic relief.

Widespread pleural metastases may cause an effusion; if recurrent and symptomatic they should be tapped. Pleurodesis is indicated if pleural effusions are persistent.

Bony metastases

Bony metastases are the most common form of secondary spread of breast cancer. These are usually at multiple sites, although it is not unusual for a solitary tumour metastasis to cause symptoms. Pain and pathological fracture are the most common forms of presentation.

A short course of radiotherapy will relieve the symptoms of bony metastases. Systemic therapy is indicated at the same time because of the high risk of developing recurrences at multiple sites, which may not be clinically or radiologically apparent. Endocrine therapy with tamoxifen is appropriate first-line treatment, especially in older patients; failure to respond is an indication for chemotherapy. Oestrogen therapy is contraindicated in patients with widespread bony metastases because of the risk of hypercalcaemia; conversely aminoglutethimide has been shown to be particularly active.

Pathological fractures require appropriate orthopaedic evaluation and surgical fixation where necessary. Widespread bony metastases, even if asymptomatic, may cause hypercalcaemia, with symptoms of fatigue, weakness, vomiting, and eventually coma with renal failure. Initial treatment involves rehydration with forced diuresis and administration of steroids to enhance calcium excretion in the urine. Resistant cases can be treated with either mithramycin or one of the diphosphonate drugs; both reduce serum calcium by inhibiting osteoclastic bone reabsorption.

Central nervous system metastases

Metastases may affect the brain itself, the cord, the meninges, or the epidural space, where they may cause cord compression. The symptoms resulting from such spread are therefore very varied, and central nervous system metastases must be considered in any patient with neurological signs or symptoms. Their treatment relies on radiation therapy. Surgery has a relatively small role, except for patients with cord compression: excision of brain metastases has no advantage over radiation therapy alone. Systemic therapy has not been widely used as most agents fail to cross the blood–brain barrier, although recent experience suggests that combination chemotherapy with steroids may have some activity in these patients.

Bone marrow metastases

The significance of occult bone marrow metastases is unclear. If symptomatic they are often associated with bony deposits. Treatment is complex because of potential leucopenia and thrombocytopenia resulting from both marrow replacement and the effects of chemotherapy. The choice of endocrine or chemotherapy is made on the basis of performance status, age, and ease of adminstration.

Ocular metastases

Acute presentation to the ophthalmologist with sudden painless blindness is not uncommon and may be due to a choroidal metastasis. Treatment is with local radiotherapy.

Other ocular symptoms may be produced as a result of metastatic disease to the bony orbit, the orbital contents, the optic nerve, or to the optic pathways within the brain itself.

Psychological sequelae following treatment of breast cancer

Women suffer psychiatric morbidity for at least 1 year after the diagnosis of breast cancer. Approximately 20 per cent of women demonstrate a significant departure from their normal mood 12 months after diagnosis compared with only 8 per cent of women who have undergone biopsy for benign disease.

The major symptoms relate to a combination of depression and anxiety, along with associated sleep disturbance, impaired concentration, fatigue, and various somatic symptoms such as headache and palpitations. About one in 10 of these patients have symptoms severe enough to warrant inpatient treatment.

Preoperative counselling and appropriate support in both the perioperative and postoperative periods is mandatory in the management of breast cancer. Specially trained health care professionals, including breast care nurses, social workers, and clinical psychologists should provide an integrated support network in conjunction with nursing and medical personnel. This is of particular importance if radiotherapy or chemotherapy are to be considered. The routine provision of such support results in improved quality of life; it may even favourably influence survival. Physiotherapy while in hospital reduces symptoms due to arm stiffness and may well speed rehabilitation. It is important to ensure that patients undergoing mastectomy without reconstruction are also introduced to surgical appliance specialists so that a prosthesis may be fitted while in hospital.

There is some controversy over the impact of a formal programme of psychological support in patients with breast cancer. Some controlled studies have failed to demonstrate a reduction in psychiatric morbidity following perioperative counselling. There is even some evidence that excessive counselling may lead to 'sensitization' of the patient and increased anxiety or depression, at least in the short term.

One area of particular interest relates to the psychological sequelae of mastectomy itself. It was hoped that partial mastectomy, with breast conservation, would reduce psychological morbidity. However, this does not appear to be the case: there is a similar incidence of psychological problems after both total and partial mastectomy. Fear of mastectomy is inextricably linked to that of the cancer itself, and variations in treatment have relatively little impact in reducing psychological morbidity. However, it must be remembered that mastectomy, as opposed to breast conservation, may devastate the lives of a substantial proportion of women.

PREVENTION OF BREAST CANCER

Breast cancer is nearly always a sporadic event; a true genetic factor is present in less than 10 per cent of cases. The majority of individuals with risk factors therefore do not develop breast cancer and the majority of patients with the disease are not at excessive risk. This makes prevention of breast cancer difficult.

Demographic studies show breast cancer to be particularly a disease of the Western world, and perhaps a result of the life-style adopted by those individuals in whom there is a high incidence. It is clearly difficult to change life-style factors such as age of having children, diet, and use of exogenous hormones, and attempts to reduce the incidence of breast cancer by influencing these factors may fail.

Two areas of prevention require special mention. It has been suggested that the low incidence of breast cancer in Japan may be secondary to the very low fat diet eaten in that country. In theory, reducting the amount of fat eaten by populations at risk may reduce the cancer incidence. However, it is very difficult for people of Western culture to reduce the amount of fat in their diet to that of endogenous Japanese.

Studies on adjuvant tamoxifen have shown a significant reduction in the incidence of contralateral breast cancer. Prophylactic chemosuppression with tamoxifen, especially for 'high-risk' patients, has therefore been suggested, and this is the subject of a number of trials currently in progress. An alternative method of reducing the incidence of breast cancer might be that of chemoprevention with agents such as the retinoids or selenium.

Occasionally very high-risk patients will ask their medical attendant for prophylactic mastectomy, with or without reconstruction, to avoid breast cancer. There is undoubtedly the occasional case where this is justified but if possible this rather aggressive approach should be avoided.

FURTHER READING

Atkins H, Hayward JL, Klugman DJ, Wayte AB. Treatment of early breast cancer: a report after ten years of a clinical trial. *Br Med J* 1972; **2**: 423–429.

Baum M. The curability of breast cancer. *Br Med J* 1976; **1**: 439–442.

Brinkley D, Haybittle JL. Long term survival of women with breast cancer. *Lancet* 1984; **1**: 1118.

Chu KC, Smart CR, Tarone RE. Analysis of breast cancer mortality and stage distribution by age for the Health Insurance Plan Clinical Trial. *J Natl Cancer Inst* 1988; **80**: 1125–1132.

Cuzick J, *et al.* Overview of randomised trials comparing radical mastectomy without radiotherapy against simple mastectomy with radiotherapy in breast cancer. *Cancer Treat Rep* 1987; **71**: 7–14.

Cuzick J, *et al.* Overview of randomised trials of post-operative adjuvant radiotherapy in breast cancer. *Cancer Treat Rep* 1987; **71**: 15–29.

Early Breast Cancer Trialists' Collaborative group. Effects of adjuvant tamoxifen and of cytotoxic therapy on mortality in early breast cancer. *N Engl J Med* 1988; **319**: 1681–1692.

Early Breast Cancer Trialists' Collaborative Group. Systemic treatment of early breast cancer by hormonal, cytotoxic, or immune therapy. *Lancet* 1992; **339**: 1–15.

Early Breast Cancer Trialists Collaborative Group. Systemic treatment of early breast cancer by hormonal, cytotoxic, or immune therapy. *Lancet* 1982; **33**: 71–85.

Fentiman I. Ductal carcinoma *in situ*. *Br Med J* 1992; **304**: 1261–1262.

Fentiman IS, Mansel RE. The axilla: a no-go zone. *Lancet* 1991; **337**: 221–223.

Fisher ER, *et al.* Pathologic findings from the NSABP (Protocol No.4). V. Significance of axillary nodal micro- and macrometastases. *Cancer* 1978; **42**: 2032–8.

Fisher ER, Sass R, Fisher B. Pathologic findings from the National Surgical Adjuvant Project for Breast Cancers (Protocol No.4). *Cancer* 1984; **53**: 712–23.

Fisher B, *et al.* Eight year results of a randomised clinical trial comparing total mastectomy and lumpectomy with or without irradiation in the treatment of breast cancer. *N Engl J Med* 1989; **320**: 822–828.

Haagensen CD, *et al.* Treatment of early mammary carcinoma: a co-operative international study. *Ann Surg* 1969; **170**: 875–78.

Haagensen CD, Lane N, Lattes R, Bodian C. Lobular neoplasia (so-called lobular carcinoma *in situ*) of the breast. *Cancer* 1978; **42**: 737–769.

Harris JR, Lippman ME, Veronesi U, Willett W. Medical Progress. Breast Cancer. *N Engl J Med* 1992; **327**: 319–327.

Hayward JL. The Guy's trial of treatments of early breast cancer. *World J Surg* 1977; **1**: 314–316.

Holland R, Veling SHJ, Mravunac M, Hendriks JHCL. Histologic multifocality of Tis, T1–2 breast carcinomas. *Cancer* 1985; **56**: 979–990.

McGuire WL. Adjuvant therapy of node negative breast cancer. DeVita VT. Breast cancer therapy: exercising all our options. *N Engl J Med* 1989; **320**: 525–529.

Page DL, Anderson TJ. *Diagnostic Histopathology of the Breast*. Edinburgh: Churchill Livingstone 1987.

Roberts MM, *et al.* Edinburgh trial of screening for breast cancer: mortality at seven years. *Lancet* 1990; **335**: 241–246.

Schnitt SJ, Silen W, Sadowsky NL, Connolly JL, Harris JR. Ductal carcinoma *in situ* (intraductal carcinoma) of the breast. *N Engl J Med* 1988; **318**: 898–903.

Shottenfeld D, *et al.* Ten year results of the treatment of primary operable breast carcinoma. *Cancer* 1976; **38**: 1001–1007.

Smith I. Adjuvant tamoxifen for early breast cancer. *Br J Cancer* 1988; **57**: 527–528.

Steele RJC, *et al.* The efficacy of lower axillary sampling in obtaining lymph node status in breast cancer; a controlled randomised trial. *Br J Surg* 1985; **72**: 368–369.

Tabar L, *et al.* Reduction in mortality from breast cancer after mass screening with mammography. *Lancet* 1985; **i**: 829–832.

Tabar L, Fagerberg G, Duffy S, Day N. The Swedish Two County Trial of mammographic screening for breast cancer: Recent results and calculation of benefit. *J Epidemiol Community Health* 1989; **43**: 107–14.

UK Trial of early detection of breast cancer group. First results on mortality reduction in the UK Trial of early detection of breast cancer. *Lancet* 1988; **ii**: 411–416.

Veronesi U, *et al.* Breast conservation is the treatment of choice in small breast cancer: long term results of a randomised trial. *Eur J Cancer* 1990; **26**: 668–670.

Wilson RE, Donegan WL, Mettlin C, Smart CR, Murphy GP. The 1982 National Survey of Carcinoma of the Breast in the United States by the American College of Surgeons. *Surg Gynecol Obstet* 1984; **159**: 309–318.

12.3 Needle localization and biopsy of non-palpable breast lesions

GLENN E. BEHRINGER AND DANIEL B. KOPANS

INTRODUCTION

Examination of the breast by mammography provides a sensitive method for early detection of non-palpable malignant tumours. Despite the fact that many breast cancers have been developing for some time before they can be detected by any method, earlier detection can improve the stage at which cancers are diagnosed and can reduce the absolute mortality from breast cancer by 30 to 40 per cent. The mammogram is the most important method of breast examination for detecting occult malignancy in asymptomatic women. Cancers detected by mammography alone are more likely to be at an earlier stage than those detected by physical examination or because of symptoms, with a correspondingly more favourable prognosis.

Mammography is unique in its ability to detect breast lesions that may represent cancers, but it is inaccurate in differentiating benign from malignant disease. Unfortunately, patterns of tumour growth and the breasts' response to them are frequently non-specific. Benign and malignant lesions may have similar morphology: characteristics such as smooth, well defined margins are statistically more common in benign lesions, but some cancers are sharply marginated. Even the classic lucent zone or 'halo sign' surrounding circumscribed masses does not guarantee a benign process. At the other end of the spectrum the spiculated architectural distortion of a radial scar, or area of fat necrosis is indistinguishable from the 'characteristic' morphological changes produced by breast cancer. Microcalcifications associated with cancer are frequently indistinguishable from those produced by benign processes.

Excision biopsy must therefore be carried out to establish a histological diagnosis on all suspicious non-palpable lesions demonstrated on screening mammography. Since 70 to 80 per cent of these anomalies will be benign upon biopsy examination radiologists must provide safe, accurate guidance for the surgeon to ensure that the lesion in question can be precisely excised with minimum cosmetic defect.

LOCALIZATION OF OCCULT LESIONS

Localization for biopsy examination cannot be successful unless the area in question can be demonstrated in three dimensions. Some lesions will be visible in one projection but not seen in a second. Most lesions are visible in the mediolateral view, but because of their proximity to the chest wall may require special rotated craniocaudal views to triangulate the lesion completely. If these manoeuvres fail, ultrasound examination or computer tomography (CT) can be used.

Since the majority of these lesions are benign, excision of a quadrant as a method of biopsy is contraindicated, not only because it is inaccurate, but because it also unnecessarily removes a large volume of tissue, leading to an unacceptable cosmetic result.

Skin markers are likewise not helpful unless the lesion is immediately beneath the skin.

The goal of accurate preoperative localization is the positioning of a needle within 5 mm of the lesion, if not directly through it. Many surgeons prefer that a guide be placed in an anteroposterior direction to facilitate surgery as this orientation parallels their operative approach. However, guides cannot be positioned from the front of the breast and directed back toward the chest wall under direct visualization, as mammograms can only be obtained orthogonal to this direction. There are many who appear to be quite skilled at this technique, although it generally requires repositioning of the guide to achieve 5 mm accuracy in placement. If an anteroposterior needle insertion is used it should be done with caution since needles introduced towards the chest wall can be inserted into the pectoralis muscles, or may pass into the pleural space, lung, or mediastinum. There have been instances of pneumothoraces caused by introducing needles in this direction and wires for localization placed in this fashion that were too short for the depth of the lesion have retracted into the breast when the patient sat up. A few wires have not only retracted completely into the breast, but when not retrieved were massaged by body motion into other anatomical areas.

Such complications are totally avoidable if placement of guidewires is carried out using paths of insertion parallel to the chest wall. The parallel approach is most accurate because the breast can be held firmly in the mammographic compression system during the procedure, with the lesion under direct visualization, allowing the exact relationship of the needle to the lesion to be determined.

Preoperative localization of cancers does not increase the risk of local recurrence when an approach parallel to the chest wall is used.

TECHNIQUE OF LOCALIZATION

Although the spot method, or injection of a vital dye in the vicinity of the lesion to stain the tissue has been successfully used to guide surgery, at the Massachusetts General Hospital a needle with a spring hook guidewire introduced parallel to the chest wall is used routinely. This configuration permits the hook to be completely contained in and pass through the needle lumen reforming to hook into the tissue when it is released from the needle tip. The introducing needle can thus be optimally positioned prior to engaging the hook. The guidewire can be afterloaded to anchor in the tissue. The guidewire also incorporates a thick segment just proximal to the hook. This area is positioned by the radiologist in proximity to the lesion so that the surgeon is alerted, during dissection of the wire, to the location of the suspicious area.

Most mammographic units have compression devices with openings that permit the breast to be held within the machine, while affording access to the volume of tissue into which the needle is to be placed. The procedure is begun by evaluating the location of the lesion on the screening mammograms. If the lesion is closest

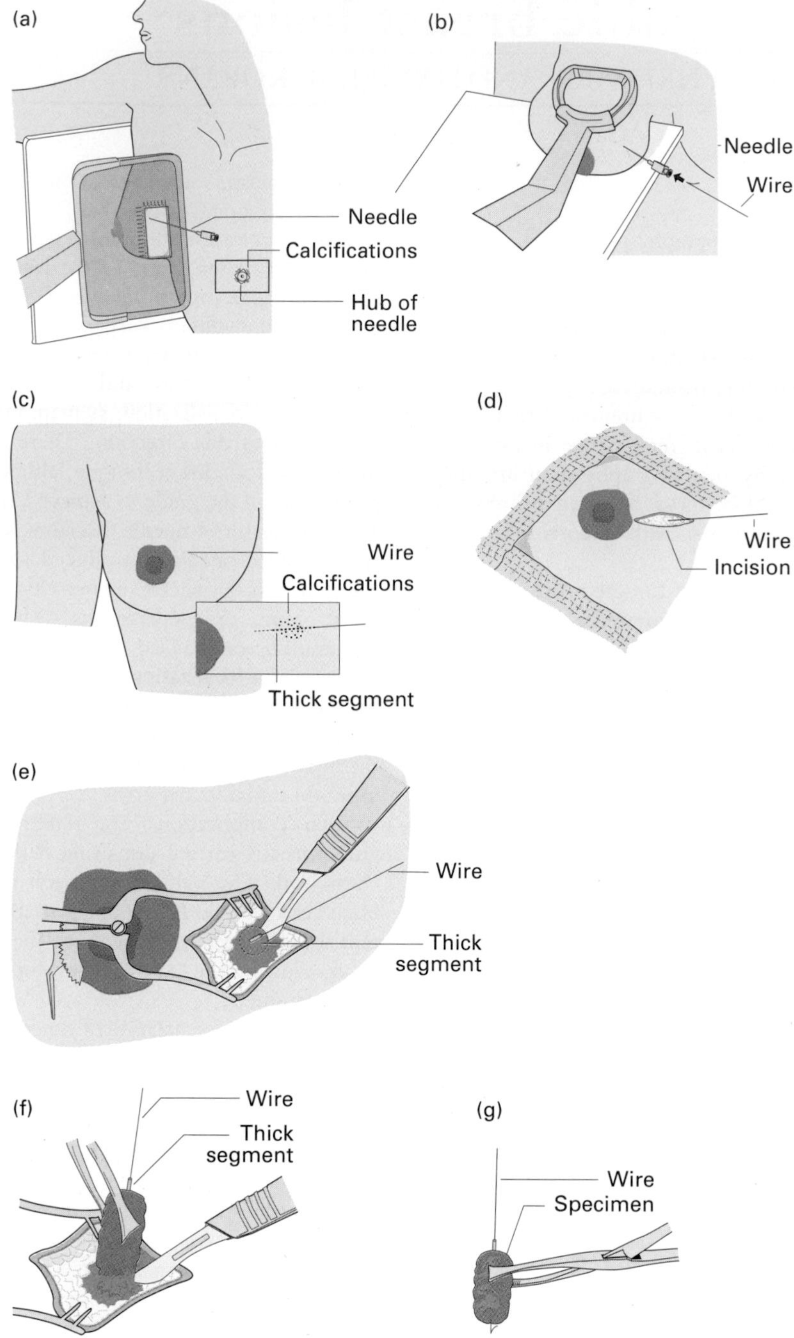

Fig. 1 (a) Localization of a medial lesion. The needle is inserted by mediolateral approach. (b) The guidewire is inserted after a confirmatory mammogram has been made. (c) The patient on arrival in the operating theatre. The guidewire protrudes from the breast. A mammogram shows good placement (inset portrays image of mammogram). (d) A linear incision is made along the course of the guidewire. (e) The incision to remove a core of tissue around the wire. (f) Traction is exerted on the specimen and it is amputated at its base. (g) A minimum volume specimen is obtained.

to the medial surface of the breast, initial needle positioning is accomplished by a mediolateral approach, inserting the needle from the medial skin surface. If the lesion is close to the lateral surface of the breast, a lateromedial approach is used. A lesion near the top of the breast is localized from the craniocaudal projection, while one at the bottom of the breast can be localized using a caudocranial projection.

Figure 1(a) demonstrates the localization of a lesion in the medial aspect of the right breast. The breast is compressed within the mammographic device so that a preliminary mammogram projects the lesion in the opening in the compression plate. Its co-ordinates are determined by marks around the plate opening.

A needle is introduced in the direction of the X-ray beam, passing through and beyond the suspicious lesion. Local anaesthesia is rarely required. If initial placement is suboptimal, it is possible to withdraw the needle partially, change the insertion angle, and reinsert without repuncturing the skin. A confirmatory mammogram is obtained through the compression plate. Ideally the hub of the needle should be superimposed on the shaft and on the lesion (Fig. 1(a) inset). The patient is then released from the machine with the needle in place, and the gantry is rotated 90° in preparation for depth determination. The fenestrated compression plate is replaced by a small spot compression device. The breast is recompressed, so that the X-ray beam will be perpendicular to the shaft of the needle, and another confirmatory film is made. If necessary, the needle position is adjusted so that the tip is positioned at the level where the hook will be placed. The hookwire is then inserted and the needle removed after a final radiograph showing the completed placement of the wire. Figure 1(b) shows the hookwire being inserted with the breast in craniocaudal position. The wire is then loosely taped to the skin with sterile tapes without traction. The patient leaves the mammography suite for the operating theatre.

NEEDLE-DIRECTED BIOPSY

Since only 15 to 29 per cent of lesions removed for biopsy examination on the basis of mammographic suspicion alone contain carcinoma, the goal of the surgeon is to obtain a specimen that will yield an unequivocal diagnosis with minimal risk to the patient in terms of complications and of cosmetic deformity. Accurate localization techniques, as described, permit the surgeon to remove a minimal volume core of tissue surrounding the wire guide that is adequate for diagnosis and does not create a breast deformity. The practice of performing a 'quadrantectomy' on all patients to obtain margins negative for cancer if the lesion is malignant is to be condemned since this procedure subjects the 80 per cent of patients with benign processes to the unnecessary removal of a large mass of tissue and to a resultant defect in the contour of the breast.

Figure 1(c) represents the patient upon arrival in the surgical suite. The guidewire protrudes from the skin of the breast and the confirmatory mammogram (inset) shows that the thick segment is centred in the lesion.

Local or general anaesthesia is used for the biopsy, which is performed as an outpatient procedure. After skin preparation and draping, a linear skin incision is made directly along the course of the guide (Fig. 1(d)). Dissection is carried down through the subcutaneous fat to the surface of the breast tissue. Meticulous haemostasis is maintained with the electrocoagulation unit.

Figure 1(e) shows the subcutaneous fat retracted and the thick segment of the wire just appearing at the surface of the breast tissue. The biopsy specimen is then obtained by plunging a No. 10 Bard Parker scalpel directly into the glandular tissue parallel to the guide wire, circumscribing the core of tissue to be removed.

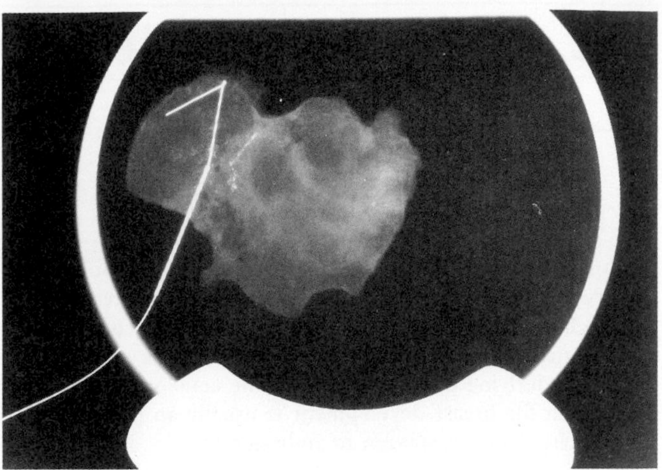

Fig. 2 Radiography confirms the lesion to be included in the specimen.

As shown in Fig. 1(f), after the first circular incision is made the core and wire are grasped with Allis' forceps and traction applied to the specimen so that it may be amputated at its base.

The specimen with contained wire (Fig. 1(g)) is placed in a plastic bag on ice (to preserve the level of oestrogen receptors) and is sent to the mammography department for radiological confirmation of the presence of the suspicious area. The specimen should be compressed in the radiographic device so that masses as well as calcifications can be seen. The specimen is then sent to the pathology department.

The diagnosis being confirmed (Fig. 2), haemostasis is completed. The biopsy site is closed with several interrupted absorbable sutures, and the skin is closed with a subcuticular suture of absorbable material.

FURTHER READING

Basset LW, Gold RH, Cove C. Mammographic spectrum of traumatic fat necrosis: the fallibility of 'pathognomonic' signs of carcinoma. *Am J Radiol* 1978; **130**: 119–22.

Brestal JB, Jones PA. Transgression of localizing wire into the pleural cavity prior to mammography. *Br J Radiol* 1981; **54**: 139–40.

Cohen MI, Matthies HJ, Mintyer RA, Keen ME, Murad T. Indurative mastopathies: a cause of false-positive mammograms. *Radiology* 1985; **155**: 69–71.

Collins VP, Loeffler RK, Tivey H. Observations on growth rates of human tumors. *Cancer* 1956; **9**: 988–1000.

Gallagher WJ, Cardenosa G, Rubens JR, McCarthy JA, Kopans DB. Minimal-volume excision of nonpalpable breast lesions. *Am J Radiol* 1989; **153**: 957–61.

Kopans DB, Meyer JE, Lindfors KK, Bucchianeri SS. Breast sonographgy to guide aspiration of cysts and preoperative localization of occult breast lesions. *Am J Radiol* 1984; **143**: 489–92.

Myer E, Kopans DB, Stomper PC, Lindfors KK. Occult breast abnormalities: percutaneous preoperative needle localization. *Radiology* 1984; **150**: 335–7.

Rosenberg AL, Schwartz GF, Feig SA, Patchefsky AS. Clinically occult breast lesions: localization and significance. *Radiology* 1987; **162**: 167–70.

Shapiro S, Venet W, Venet L, Roesser R. Ten to fourteen-year effect of screening on breast cancer mortality. *J Natl Cancer Inst* 1982; **69**: 349–55.

Swann CA, Kopans DB, Koerner FC, McCarthy KA, White G, Hall D. The halo sign and malignant breast lesions. *Am J Roentgenol* 1987; **149**: 1145–7.

Tabar L, Fayerberg CJG, Gad A, *et al.* Reduction in mortality from breast cancer after mass screening with mammography. *Lancet* 1985; **i**: 829–32.

12.4 Abnormalities of the male breast

LINDA J. HANDS

GYNAECOMASTIA

The male breast is normally vestigial but under certain hormonal and drug influences it may develop into a significant breast mound. Although gynaecomastia is a common condition, often with a physiological basis, it is important to consider the possible presence of underlying disease. Whatever the aetiology, the ultimate mechanism for breast development is usually an increase in the ratio of circulating oestrogen to androgen.

Clinical and histological appearance

A firm disc of breast tissue at least 2 cm in diameter underlies the nipple. Approximately 90 per cent cases are bilateral, although one side may be affected several months before the other.

Histological examination will show the early stages of duct development but if gynaecomastia persists for many months fibrous tissue replaces most of the breast tissue.

Physiological gynaecomastia

Physiological gynaecomastia occurs in the majority of men at some stage in their lives. Transient breast development appears in the neonate due to maternal oestrogens and returns in 40 to 70 per cent of boys at puberty. One-third of middle-aged men have some development of their breasts and the incidence gradually increases with age to about 60 per cent in the seventh decade.

The normal testis produces testosterone and small quantities of oestrogens. The adrenal gland also produces weak androgens, the bulk of which is removed by the liver. However excess adrenal androgens and some testosterone are aromatized to oestrogens in the peripheral tissues, particularly fat. At puberty a surge of gonadotrophins induces testicular activity. Oestrogen production reaches adult levels before that of testosterone thus increasing the oestrogen to androgen ratio, sometimes enough to stimulate breast development. This usually lasts a matter of months and in almost 75 per cent of cases it subsides within 2 years. Physiological gynaecomastia later in life is due to waning testicular function with a consequent increase in pituitary gonadotrophin, which favours relatively greater oestrogen production by the testis. At the same time, increased body fat leads to greater peripheral aromatization of androgens to oestrogens.

Pathological gynaecomastia

Drugs

This is the most common abnormal stimulant of breast development, especially in those over 50 years of age. Oestrogens, frequently given for prostatic carcinoma, often stimulate breast development (Fig. 1). It should be remembered that unprescribed oestrogens, especially those in industrial use, can be absorbed through the skin. Other drugs may have an oestrogen-like or anti-androgen effect but in many cases the mechanism behind drug associated gynaecomastia is unknown. Drugs used in the treatment of cardiac disease or hypertension are common causes: digitalis, spironolactone, calcium channel blockers, methyldopa, and captopril have all been associated with gynaecomastia. Also associated with breast development are cimetidine in high doses, the antifungal agent ketoconazole, tricyclic antidepressants, and even diazepam. Chemotherapy and radiotherapy, especially following orchidectomy for a testicular tumour, can also cause breast development, presumably because they suppress activity in the remaining testis. Abuse of drugs such as heroin and cannabis is known to cause gynaecomastia.

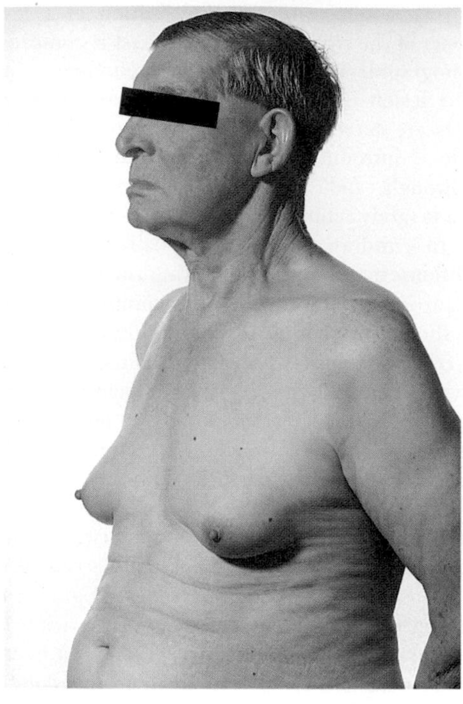

Fig. 1 Gynaecomastia due to oestrogen therapy for carcinoma of the prostate.

Tumours

Testicular tumours are an uncommon but important cause of gynaecomastia (Fig. 2). Ten per cent of malignant testicular tumours, usually teratomas, are associated with gynaecomastia; this is associated with a poorer prognosis. These tumours produce human chorionic gonadotrophin which stimulates testicular production of oestrogen and testosterone. Tumour tissue also converts androgens to oestrogens. Both these factors tend to increase the oestrogen: testosterone ratio. Occasionally a benign Leydig cell tumour of the testis causes gynaecomastia by producing excess oestrogen.

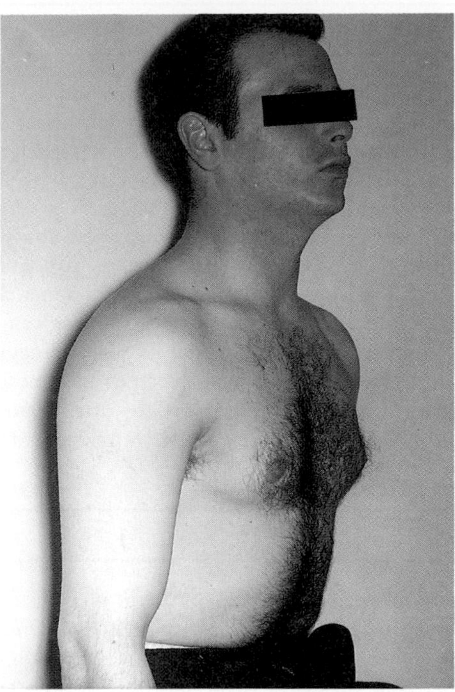

Fig. 2 Gynaecomastia due to a feminizing tumour of the testicle.

Even less commonly, other tumours, such as bronchial carcinoma and occasionally pancreatic and gastric neoplasms, produce human chorionic gonadotrophin and cause breast development. Adrenal tumours cause gynaecomastia by excessive production of androgens which are then converted to oestrogens. Liver tumours sometimes contain aromatases which increase the production of oestrogens from androgens and so lead to gynaecomastia.

Metabolic disease

Cirrhosis reduces the capacity of the liver to remove adrenal androgens from the circulation, leaving more available for peripheral aromatization to oestrogens, and this often results in gynaecomastia. Alcoholism causes gynaecomastia in the absence of cirrhosis by suppressing the pituitary testicular axis and therefore reducing testosterone production. Conversion of adrenal androgen to oestrogen becomes relatively more important in this situation. In renal failure and in starvation the pituitary adrenal axis is also suppressed and breast development occasionally occurs. However, it is a much more common symptom some months after starting dialysis or refeeding, probably because of resurgent testicular activity, similar to that occurring at puberty. Thyrotoxicosis is an important cause of gynaecomastia: it affects 30 per cent of hyperthyroid males, probably because of increased aromatase activity.

Hypogonadism

The failing testis is subjected to increased stimulation by pituitary gonadotrophins and responds by producing relatively more oestrogens, sometimes sufficient to cause breast development. Common causes of primary testicular impairment are ageing, maldescent of the testes, or damage from trauma or viral infection such as mumps. Chromosomal aberrations, particularly Klinefelter's syndrome, congenital enzyme deficiencies, and congenital anorchia are less common causes. Failure of the pituitary–testicular axis as a cause of hypogonadism and subsequent gynaecomastia has already been described.

Differential diagnosis

Carcinoma of the breast is considered later. Pseudogynaecomastia may occur, due to local fat deposition with no breast tissue development. The tissue lacks the firm, well-defined appearance of true gynaecomastia. It occurs in obese individuals and carries none of the implications of gynaecomastia.

Investigations

If growth indices are appropriate then pubertal gynaecomastia probably requires no further investigation. Approximately 50 per cent of the remaining patients with gynaecomastia will have a pathological or iatrogenic cause. A careful drug history is essential and evidence of liver and thyroid function should be sought on history and examination. The testes should be examined for atrophy or tumour and an ultrasound examination performed to exclude a small neoplasm, particularly in the patient under 40 years of age. A chest radiograph is also important. Thyroid and liver function tests, and measurement of serum human chorionic gonadotrophin, luteinizing hormone, oestrogen, and testosterone should be performed.

Treatment

Gynaecomastia itself requires no treatment unless it causes serious discomfort or embarrassment to the patient. The patient with physiological gynaecomastia often needs only reassurance. Any underlying pathology must obviously be treated and responsible drugs stopped if possible, but this does not guarantee resolution of breast development if it has been present for sometime.

In general, the results of hormone treatment are disappointing, although tamoxifen has been shown to help in some cases of pubertal and middle-aged breast development.,

Surgery is the mainstay of treatment. As a cosmetic operation it is important to leave the nipple/areola in the correct position, symmetrical with the other side, with minimal obvious scarring. Most patients have relatively modest breast development and a satisfactory subcutaneous mastectomy can be performed through an incision following the inferior margin of the areola. It is important to leave a smooth contour to the breast and avoid a central crater under the areola.

Occasionally breast development is so marked that excess skin has to be removed. Several techniques have been developed to do this while preserving the areola in position with an intact blood supply.

Liposuction can be a useful adjunct to leave an acceptable chest profile, but as it removes only fat and not breast tissue it cannot be the complete surgical answer in true gynaecomastia.

BREAST CARCINOMA

This is rare. About 1 per cent of all breast cancers occur in men, slightly more in the Middle East and Africa.

Presentation

Male breast cancer occurs most often in the seventh decade, slightly later than in women. Seventy-five per cent of patients present with a breast mass, the others with a bloodstained nipple discharge, nipple distortion, ulceration, or axillary lymphadenopathy. Despite the ease of examining the breast in a man in comparison to women, these tumours tend to present late, probably because of lack of concern regarding male breast symptoms. Inevitably most of these tumours arise beneath the areola, an unfavourable site for breast cancers. They are close to and often infiltrate both skin and muscle, and axillary spread is common by the time of presentation.

Histology

Most male breast cancers are ductal adenocarcinomas. Papillary tumours are uncommon, but occur more often than in women, hence the relative frequency of a nipple discharge at presentation. Over 80 per cent of these tumours are oestrogen receptor positive, a much higher percentage than in women, and this has implications for treatment. Beware the secondary deposit from tumour elsewhere, especially from prostate, which may be difficult to distinguish histologically.

Aetiology

There is strong evidence for a hormonal basis to the disease. Several studies, though not all, have shown significantly raised serum levels of oestrogens in men with breast carcinoma. There seems to be no increase in the incidence of breast tumours in men treated with oestrogens for carcinoma of the prostate, but the timing and duration of the hormone rise may be critical. Men who were much overweight in early adulthood have a greater chance of developing a breast tumour later in life, even if their weight subsequently falls. Obesity is linked to increased aromatase activity which increases the conversion of adrenal androgens to oestrogens. Male breast tumours are very common in patients with Klinefelter's syndrome, a condition in which there is impaired testicular function, and have also been described in association with long-standing hypopituitarism and hypogonadism, and with a history of orchitis. All these diseases would tend to increase the ratio of oestrogen: testosterone. Although similar influences have been described in the development of gynaecomastia there is no evidence that gynaecomastia itself leads to breast tumour.

A family history of male or female breast cancer is also important. Previous radiotherapy to the chest wall, certainly important in female breast tumours, has occasionally been associated with the development of male breast cancer.

Treatment

The proximity of the tumour to the chest wall and the frequency of axillary spread have led to a treatment by a radical or modified radical mastectomy in most centres. Simple mastectomy with postoperative radiotherapy has been advocated by some, but the local recurrence rate appears to be higher. Unfortunately the rarity of this tumour has precluded a prospective study comparing different treatments. Over 50 per cent of patients with disseminated disease respond to orchidectomy for a median period of nearly 2 years. On recurrence a further response can still be elicited by administration of tamoxifen or antiandrogens, such as cyproterone acetate: some centres elect to use these agents as first-line treatments in preference to orchidectomy. Many patients also respond to therapy with cytotoxic agents.

Prognosis

Overall about 50 per cent of patients die of their diseases in the 5 years following diagnosis. Stage for stage, the prognosis is probably similar to that in women: if no axillary nodes are involved then about 80 per cent survive 5 years, but only 30 to 40 per cent of those with axillary spread survive this long. Higher grade and larger tumours have a poorer outcome.

OTHER CONDITIONS OF THE MALE BREAST

Very rarely conditions relatively more common in the female breast such as fibroadenoma, fibrocystic disease, and phylloides tumour have been described in men.

FURTHER READING

Carlson HE. Gynecomastia. *N Engl J Med*, 1980; **303**: 795–9.

Erlichman C, Murphy KC, Elhakim T. Male breast cancer: a 13-year review of 89 patients. *J Clin Oncol*, 1984; **2**: 903–9.

Keddie N, Morris PJ. Male breast tumours. *Surg Gynecol Obstet*, 1967; **124**: 332–6.

Korenman SG. The endocrinology of the abnormal male breast. *Ann N Y Acad Sci*, 1986; **464**: 400–8.

Nuttall F. Gynecomastia as a physical finding in normal men. *J Clin Endocrinol Metab*, 1979; **48**: 338–40.

Nydick M, Bustos J, Dale JH, Rawson RW. Gynecomastia in adolescent boys. *JAMA*, 1961; **178**: 109–14.

Ribeiro G. Male breast carcinoma. *Br J Cancer*, 1985; **51**: 115–9.

Wilson JD, Aiman J, MacDonald PC. The pathogenesis of gynecomastia *Adv Intern Med*, 1980; **25**: 1–31.

Endoscopic surgery 13

13 Endoscopic surgery

JULIAN BRITTON AND HUGH BARR

INTRODUCTION

Surgeons have always wanted to look inside the human body but rigid and primitive instruments, poor illumination, and inadequate anaesthesia originally confined such procedures to the natural orifices. General anaesthesia and, at the end of the nineteenth century, the introduction of electric light and glass telescopes first made cystoscopy feasible and later bronchoscopy and laparoscopy. An angled telescope allowed the surgeon to see around a corner but the continuous curves of the bowel remained a barrier to further progress in gastrointestinal endoscopy until the development of flexible glass fibres. Gynaecologists were the first to appreciate the advantages of laparoscopy. Parallel developments in instrumentation and illumination soon meant that some therapeutic procedures could be performed although there were limitations because the operator was the only one who could see what he was doing and one of his hands was occupied holding the endoscope itself. Nevertheless laparoscopic sterilization and transurethral resection of the prostate have been standard operations for many years.

Minimally invasive or endoscopic surgery for a much wider range of operations has become possible as a result of the development of miniature television cameras which can be attached to any suitable telescope. The cameras are unobtrusive, light in weight, and provide a perfect and magnified colour image of the operative field on a television monitor. The surgeon has both hands free to manipulate instruments and any number of assistants can watch what is being done on separate monitors and operate as well. New instruments have been developed to overcome the limitations on access and movement within the body cavities and new ways of performing old and well established operations have also been devised. In that respect this chapter will be out of date by the time it is published but even so the basic principles of endoscopic surgery are already well established.

THE BASIC TECHNIQUE

Creating a space in which to work

Some endoscopic operations, such as those on the nasal sinuses, take place within a natural cavity so that no special methods are needed to obtain a space in which to work. But for operations within the chest or the abdomen it is first necessary to create a pneumothorax or a pneumoperitoneum. The most convenient way to introduce gas is to use the spring loaded Veress needle inserted through a small stab incision in the skin (Fig. 1). The needle has a sharp but flat bevelled point within which there is a blunt, hollow stylet through which gas flows from a distal side hole. As soon as the point of the needle penetrates the peritoneum or the pleura the stylet springs forward and pushes away the lung or the bowel thus lessening the risk of penetrating either structure.

The Veress needle can be introduced anywhere through the chest wall although the umbilicus is the most popular site in the abdomen. It is best to keep well away from any previous incisions as there are likely to be local adhesions. When creating a pneumoperitoneum it is wise, first, to be sure the bladder is empty and, after insertion, to test that the point of the needle is in the correct place. A hanging drop of saline in the hub of the Veress needle should fall easily into the peritoneum when the abdominal wall is lifted and once gas flow commences the intra-abdominal pressure should initially remain low whilst the gas flow rate should be high. Some surgeons prefer to introduce the first cannula under direct vision through a small skin incision and then to inflate the cavity. A gas-tight seal is obtained with a purse-string suture tied around the port. This is certainly a safe method if local adhesions are to be expected.

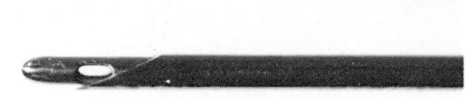

Fig. 1 The tip of a Veress needle to show the spring loaded blunt stylet with the side hole for carbon dioxide insufflation.

Carbon dioxide is the best gas to use; it is rapidly soluble should an embolism occur and it does not support combustion. The lung collapses spontaneously once gas is introduced into the pleural space and it is then only necessary to maintain a slight positive intrathoracic pressure. By contrast, maintenance of a pneumoperitoneum requires a constant intra-abdominal pressure of about 15 mmHg. Pressures in excess of this may lead to difficulties with ventilation whilst a fall in pressure will lead to a collapse of the pneumoperitoneum and the operative field will disappear from view. Modern high flow, electronically controlled, insufflators will maintain a preset intra-abdominal pressure and automatically correct minor leaks as well as the more substantial loss of gas that occurs every time an instrument is taken in or out of a port.

Artificial cavities can be created almost anywhere in the body by the forced insufflation of carbon dioxide into a natural tissue plane. The fibrous bands that cross these artificial spaces can be a nuisance and an alternative, in some circumstances, is to create the cavity by insufflating a balloon at an appropriate site within the tissues. The balloon is then removed but the cavity is maintained by the continued insufflation of carbon dioxide gas under pressure.

Obtaining a view of the operative field

The surgeon must be able to see what he is doing. Modern endoscopes are designed to carry light to illuminate the operative field and to pass the image back to the external television camera all within a single cylindrical metal tube (Fig. 2). The endoscope and the necessary instruments gain access to the operation site through cylindrical cannulae, or ports, placed through the body wall (Fig. 3). Where the cavity is only maintained by positive

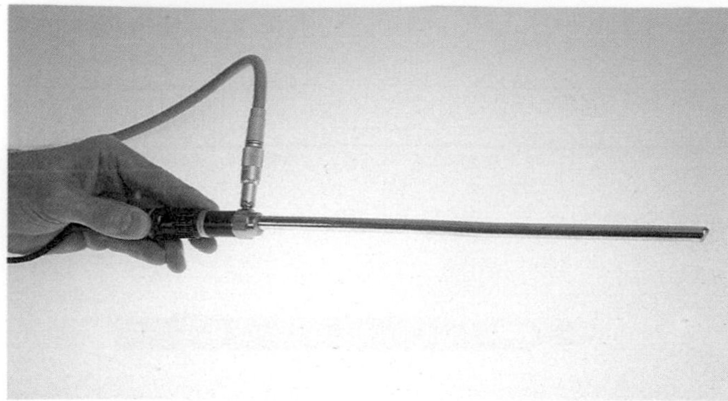

Fig. 2 An endoscope with video camera and light lead attached.

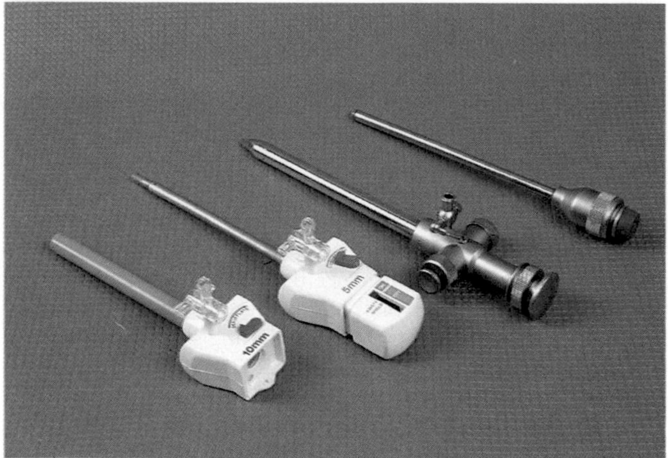

Fig. 3 A selection of endoscopic cannulae. From left to right: Disposable 11 mm and 5.5 mm ports and reusable 11 mm and 5.5 mm ports. The 11 mm reusable cannula has a trumpet valve whilst the other three cannulae have flap valves. Insufflation ports are provided on all except the 5.5 mm reusable cannula.

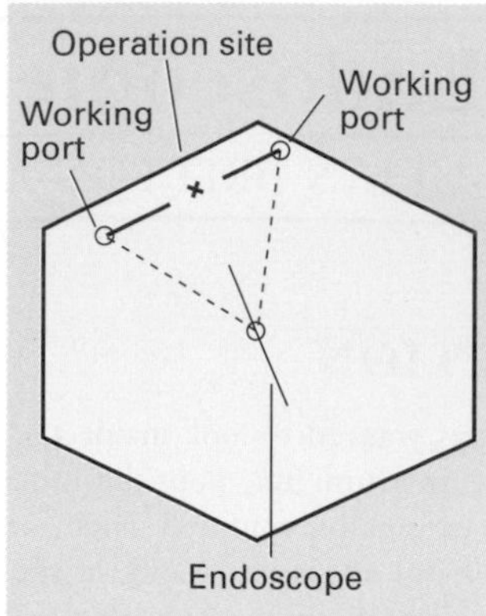

Fig. 4 Siting the ports. The endoscope is inserted at the umbilicus and the two working ports should be at the corners of an equilateral triangle. The operation site should lie midway between the two working ports.

pressure, as in the abdomen, these ports must be provided with valves to retain the gas within the cavity.

The telescope, the light source, and the television camera are essential for endoscopic surgery and are just as sophisticated as the operations for which they are used. Modern equipment is reliable and reusable but breakdowns do occur and will require expert repair so that spare equipment should be available in any large theatre suite. Most of the instruments are made either as reusable items that can be repeatedly sterilized or as single use disposable items. A few instruments, particularly those used to staple tissue together, are only available as disposable items. From the practical point of view either type of instrument is perfectly satisfactory and the choice is dictated purely by preference and cost.

Siting the ports

The proposed operation and the shape and size of the individual patient dictate the precise placement of the cannulae. The basic layout is two working ports and one port for the telescope. In general it is best if these three ports are placed at the apices of an equilateral triangle with the operative field midway along one side of the triangle (Fig. 4). Sometimes two sides have to be longer than the third but they should be equal and the endoscope should lie at the apex of the two long sides with the operative field midway along the short side. If this arrangement is followed then the tips of the working instruments will always lie at right angles across the field of view when they are being used. Additional ports, which are mostly used for retraction, should be placed outside the basic triangle.

The most common problem is for the operative field to lie further away from the endoscope than the midpoint between the two operating ports. If this happens the telescope and the instruments may touch each other which can make it impossible to work and to see what you are doing at the same time. Even if the endoscope and the instruments do not touch it may still be impossible to see the tips of the instruments as they are being used. This is inherently dangerous because the two-dimensional image makes the perception of depth very difficult. If scissors are being used it is a good rule that the manoeuvre should be abandoned unless the tips of the scissors can be clearly seen and it is absolutely certain that nothing unintended will be cut. An oblique viewing endoscope and instruments with curved blades can sometimes overcome both these difficulties.

Inserting the cannulae

Laparoscopic cannulae come in two standard sizes with an outside diameter of 5.5 mm and 11 mm (Fig. 3). They are designed to take 5 mm and 10 mm instruments respectively. Larger and smaller sizes are made for special purposes and reducing sleeves allow the use of small instruments through the larger ports. Most cannulae incorporate a gas-tight valve. Disposable cannulae and the smaller reusable ports use ball or flap valves whilst sliding trumpet valves are fitted to the larger reusable cannulae. Each cannula is fitted with a trocar which should have a sharp hollow-ground pyramidal point. When the trocar is rotated the sharp edges and the pyramidal shape of the point force the tissues apart and also cut some of the fibres so that less force is required to gain entry into a cavity.

To insert a cannula the whole assembly is held in the palm of the hand with the index finger lying along the shaft to prevent excessive penetration (Fig. 5). Each trocar and cannula is introduced through a small skin incision and then wound through the body wall with minimal pressure, thereby reducing the risk of a sudden

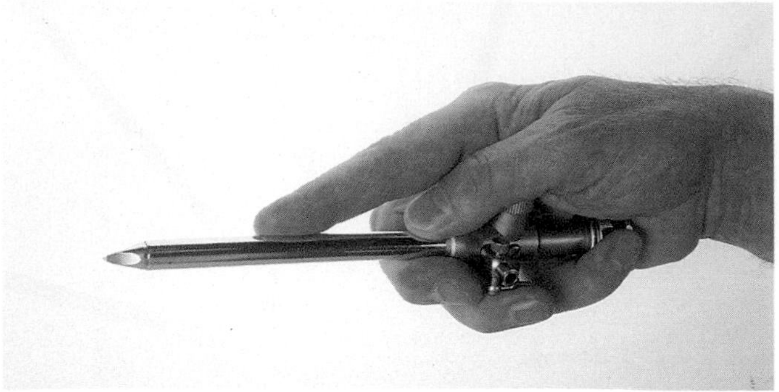

Fig. 5 How to hold the trocar and cannula. The index finger extended along the shaft of the cannula prevents excessive penetration.

uncontrolled entry into the cavity. Unless an open technique is used the first cannula is inserted blind and therefore carries the greatest risk of damage to underlying structures. Thereafter the entry of each subsequent cannula can be observed directly (Fig. 6) although it is still wise to angle the trocar away from any important structures.

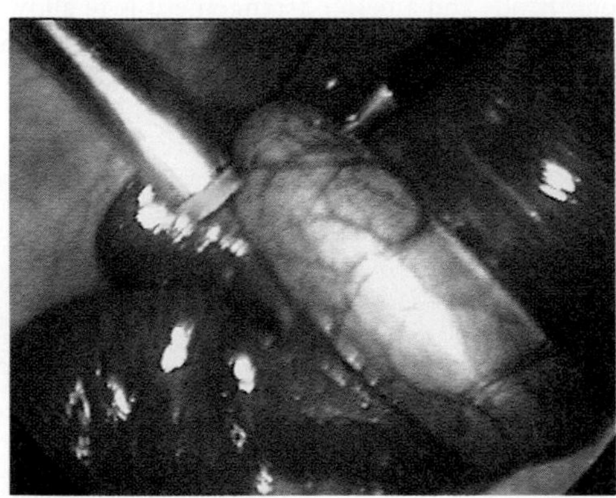

Fig. 6 A cannula within the peritoneal cavity. The gallbladder can be seen in the background.

Obtaining illumination

An external cold light source with an output of at least 250 W is essential for endoscopic surgery (Fig. 7). Light is conducted to the endoscope through a flexible fibreoptic cable and is automatically controlled by a feedback from the video camera so that more light is available as the field of view enlarges. Even so there are physical limits on the amount of light that can be delivered and losses should be reduced to a minimum. This means taking care not to break the glass fibres within the fibreoptic cable and removing blood, which absorbs light, from the operative field.

Acquiring an image

Endoscopes

The standard rigid endoscope is 10 mm in external diameter and contains the light cable and a glass rod-lens telescope (see Fig. 9). The illumination and the field of view, which is directly ahead

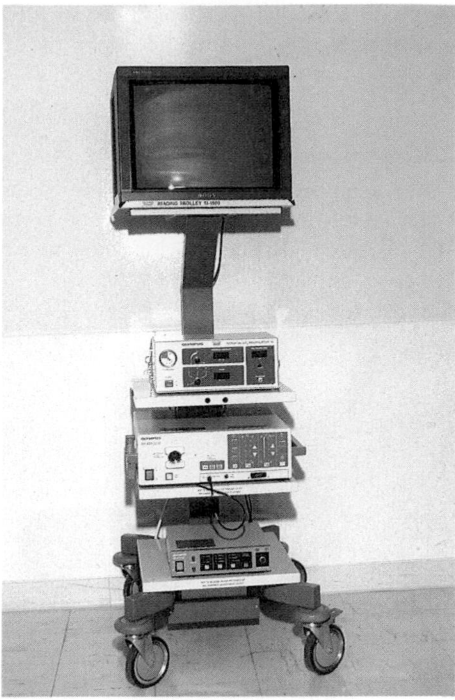

Fig. 7 A trolley for endoscopic surgery. From the top down: television monitor, electronic insufflator, light source, camera controller.

from the tip of the telescope (0° forward viewing), are exactly matched. A wide-angle lens at the tip of the telescope is the most useful for general purposes.

There are many variations in this basic design and forward-oblique viewing angles (30 and 45°) are certainly helpful in certain circumstances (Fig. 8). Endoscopes as fine as 0.7 mm in outside

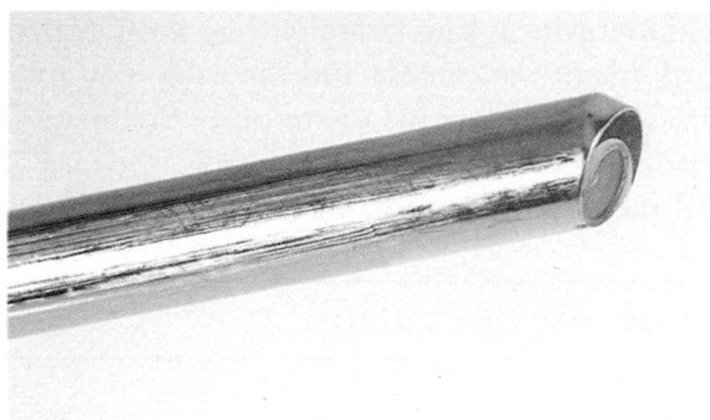

Fig. 8 This is a 30° 10 mm endoscope. The tip is angled and is clearly divided into two. The upper curved lens provides illumination and the lower circular lens carries the image.

diameter are available for intravascular work and for some operations the inclusion of an operating channel alongside the endoscope is an advantage. Endoscopes must be kept clean and undamaged. The camera and the endoscope should be carefully dried before they are put together to eliminate condensation and warming the endoscope and antifog solutions applied to the distal lens will reduce misting.

Endoscopes with a flexible end are already made and in the future the video camera may be placed at the tip of the larger instruments. Even stereoscopic endoscopes are under development.

The television camera

The colour television camera is externally mounted directly on to the end of the endoscope without the use of a beam splitter (Fig. 9). Any of the modern microchip cameras designed for endoscopic work are suitable although there are minor differences in colour reproduction and ease of use. All of them have a marker to indicate the orientation of the image and correct alignment of the camera and the endoscope is essential when a forward-oblique instrument is used. The cable from the camera leads back to a control box at the side of the operating table (Fig. 7). The electronic image is then fed to two or more monitors but it can also be recorded or transmitted over any distance, even to the other side of the world. Immersion in glutaraldehyde is the usual method of sterilization although the camera and the cable end must be protected from water. An alternative is to place the unsterile camera inside a sterile plastic sheath. This avoids the use of glutaraldehyde and the risk of water damaging the camera or its cable.

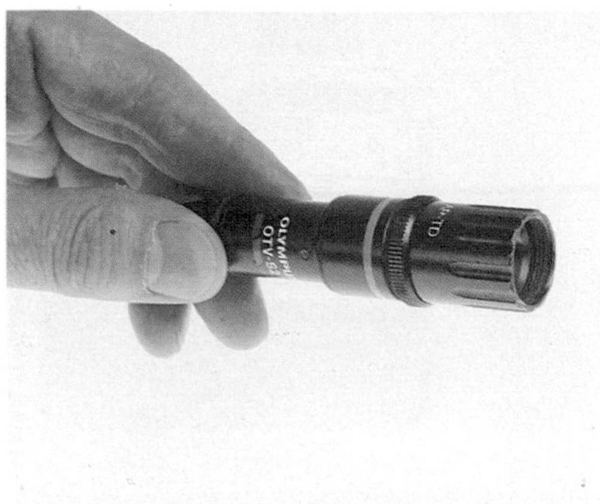

Fig. 9 A video camera which connects directly on to the end of the endoscope.

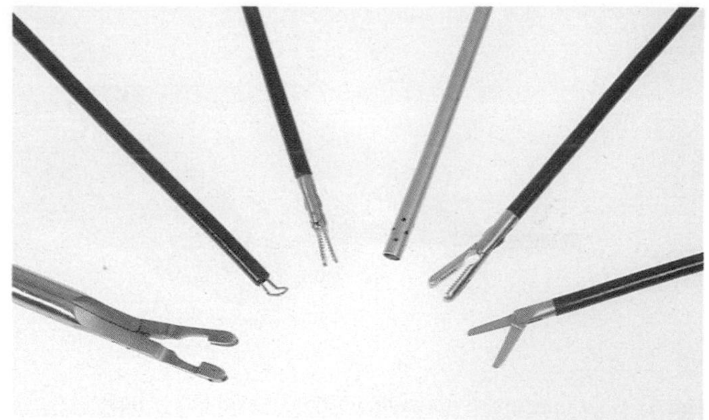

Fig. 10 A selection of endoscopic instruments. From the left: 10 mm polydioxanone clip applier, 5 mm insulated diathermy loop, 5 mm dissection forceps, 5 mm irrigator/sucker, 5 mm grasping forceps, 5 mm scissors.

Performing an operation

Instruments

The basic endoscopic instrument is either 5 mm or 10 mm in diameter and between 30 and 35 cm in length (Fig. 10). Shorter and thinner instruments are available for paediatric work and some stapling devices are 12 mm or more in diameter. Originally the working ends were simple adaptations of a conventional design which were attached by a long shaft to an ordinary handle but many of these instruments were not very easy to use in practice. A plethora of new instruments have now been developed specifically for endoscopic work although the demand for a long, narrow, and circular design does impose quite severe limitations on the engineer.

In an open operation there is complete freedom to move in any direction but an endoscopic instrument has only 3 degrees of movement. The shaft can move in or out (translation), the tip can rotate about the axis (axial rotation), or the whole instrument can rotate around the point of entry (relative rotation). These limitations and the fixed relationship of the working ends to the handle in most surgical instruments can impose impossible demands on the surgeons' hands and a better arrangement is to allow the shaft of the instrument to rotate on the handle (Fig. 11). There are also new designs of handle that can be used wherever they lie in the hand. Holding tissues in order to work on them is as essential in an endoscopic operation as it is in an open one but it can be difficult when the hinge of the forceps lies very close to the working end of the instrument. So far no entirely satisfactory design has been developed to overcome this problem but most of the available endoscopic graspers rely on refinements to the working surface of the blades usually by increasing the number or the size of the teeth in contact with the tissues. Conventional ratchets for securing an instrument to the tissues are almost impossible to release easily when they are positioned through an endoscopic cannula and screw threads on the handles (Fig. 12) or a trigger grip are better alternatives.

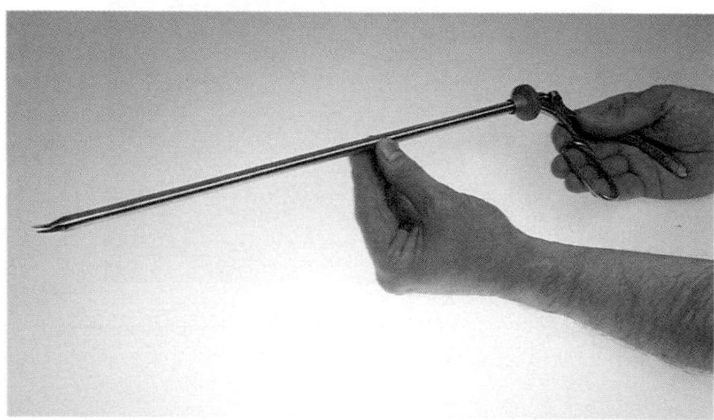

Fig. 11 This clip applier has a rotating shaft which makes manipulation much easier.

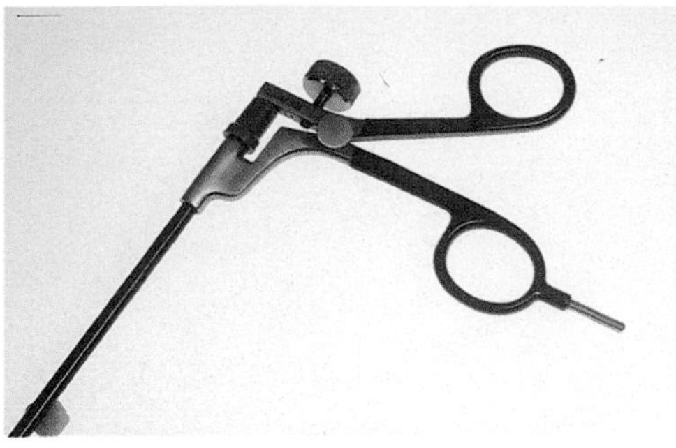

Fig. 12 A screw thread for holding the instrument closed is easier to use during laparoscopic surgery than a conventional ratchet.

The need to pass every instrument down a straight cannula imposes a limit on the curvature of the tips. This is a serious disadvantage when it is combined with the limitations on movement since it is commonly necessary to surround a structure before it is occluded and divided. It is true that the angle of approach can be infinitely varied if the curved tip can rotate on the shaft but it is still only possible to approach the structure from one general direction. A clever solution to this problem takes advantage of the memory that some metal alloys possess. The working end of the instrument is housed within a shaft of suitable diameter. When the end is pushed out of the housing the extension with the working end attached assumes a natural curve which makes dissection around a structure much easier. The end is then withdrawn into the housing before the instrument is removed.

In conventional surgery most instruments are designed for a single purpose and an efficient scrub nurse has always ensured that the surgeon has the instrument he needs immediately available. This is not so easy in endoscopic operations because every instrument has to be passed in and out of a cannula. This takes time and so there has been a move to devise instruments which do more than one thing. The most obvious adaptation has been the addition of diathermy to every suitable instrument so that both dissection and haemostasis can be accomplished without the need to change instruments (Fig. 13).

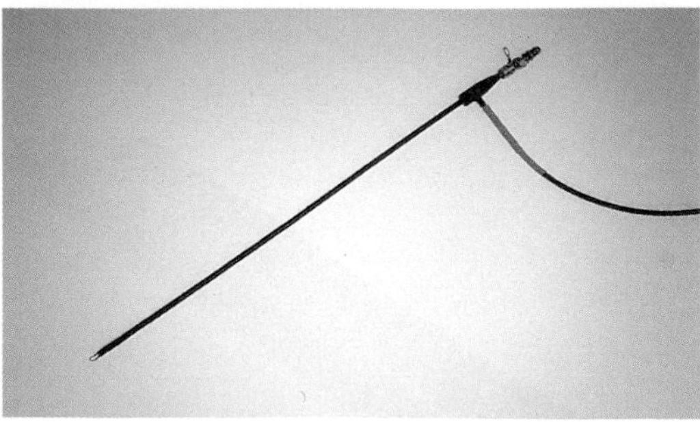

Fig. 13 An insulated wire loop dissector with diathermy attached.

Surgical technique

There are two fundamental parts to any surgical operation. Tissues and structures are first divided and are then joined back together again either in a different way or with part of the structure missing. In conventional surgery a scalpel and a pair of scissors are the basic tools for dissection and restoration is achieved with a needle and thread. Unfortunately neither the needle nor the knife adapt well to endoscopic work and alternative techniques have had to be developed.

Dissection

Dissection with a knife does not work in endoscopic surgery. Depth perception is difficult, the incisions always bleed and a sharp unprotected, and often invisible, blade could easily cause damage. Scissor dissection is not ideal either although it is sometimes essential. The tiny blades do not remain sharp for long particularly if they are also used for diathermy and the hinges become loose so that the tissues are not cut cleanly.

Gently tearing the tissues apart along the lines of least resistance either with a jet of water (aquadissection) or with a blunt instrument is useful. The dissection can be both accurate and precise because of the magnified image on the monitor even though the technique is not particularly attractive. Blunt instruments are safer when the tips cannot be seen and any small vessels can be occluded with diathermy as the dissection proceeds. Some oozing is inevitable and blood, which absorbs light, should be immediately sucked or washed away with warm saline solution. Even small amounts of blood can obscure the view during an endoscopic operation and so, whatever method of dissection is used, haemostasis is important.

Haemostasis

Coagulation

Coagulation of the tissues at the same time as they are divided is ideal and monopolar and bipolar diathermy, laser light, and ultrasound are all useful tools for dissection and adapt easily to the endoscopic environment. They minimize oozing and will stop haemorrhage from a visible vessel. When monopolar diathermy is used there should be a visible effect on the tissue the moment the current is passed (Fig. 14). If nothing happens there may be a short circuit and therefore the possibility of damage to another structure. The most common error is contact between the metal of an instrument and an uninsulated cannula outside the field of view. Lasers are also potentially dangerous if improperly used. The staff

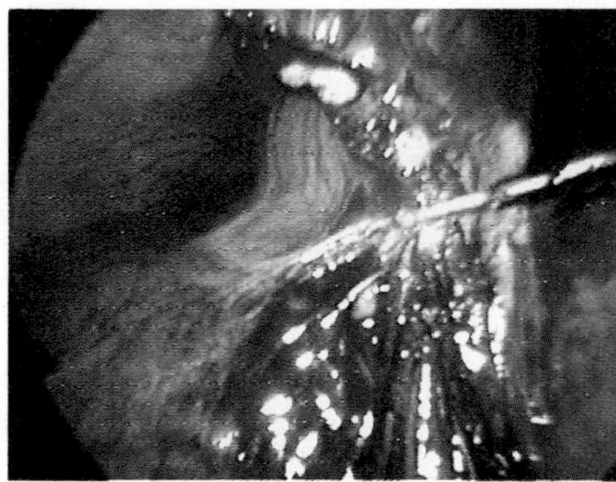

Fig. 14 A diathermy hook in use to dissect the gallbladder from the liver.

must wear eye protection and backstops may be needed on the instruments to ensure that structures beyond the intended target are not damaged by the beam.

Bipolar diathermy will occlude vessels the size of the appendicular artery but anything larger than this requires some form of mechanical closure. It is not practical to tie a conventional ligature through an endoscopic cannula but slip knots which can be placed around a structure and then pulled tight in a single movement are useful. The original Roeder knot (Fig. 15) was designed to be used with thick chromic catgut and there are modifications suitable for use with polyglactin and polydioxanone. All these knots are safe and reliable provided that they are properly constructed and correctly laid down. Every endoscopic surgeon should be able to tie them.

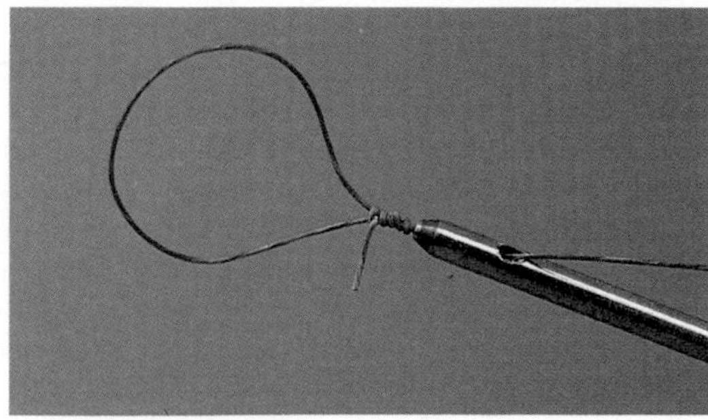

Fig. 15 A chromic catgut Roeder loop with a purpose designed ligature pusher for endoscopic ligation.

Clips

A more convenient method for occluding an artery or a duct is to apply a clip. Titanium metal clips are familiar and are available in multifire guns (Fig. 16) especially designed for endoscopic work. Polydioxanone clips (Fig. 17), which will eventually dissolve, have a locking mechanism which ensures that they are applied correctly. They can be difficult to close and have to be applied one at a time. Only one size of clip of either type is available at the present time.

Stapling

A vascular pedicle can be occluded and divided in one manoeuvre with a disposable stapler. The design is similar to the instruments used for intestinal anastomosis except that the staples are smaller and are placed closer together to ensure good haemostasis. Their use is limited by their cost.

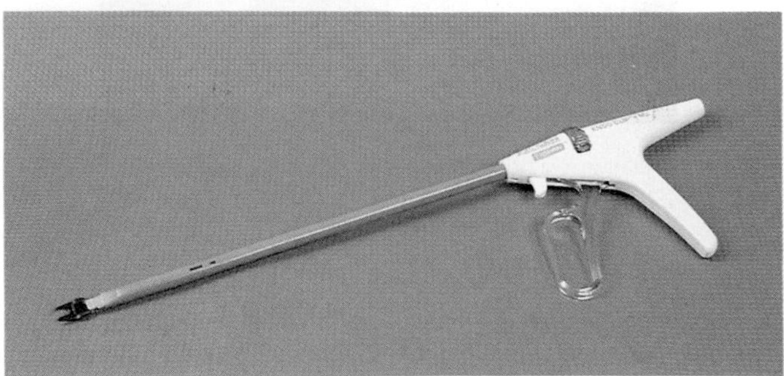

Fig. 16 A disposable multifire clip applier.

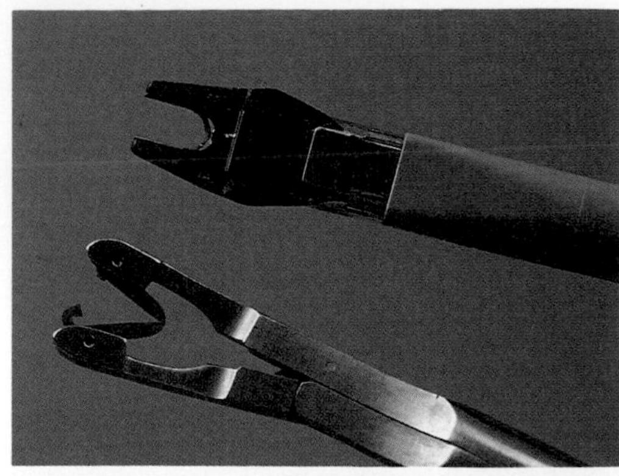

Fig. 17 Haemostatic clips. A polydioxanone clip is shown below the working end of the disposable multifire clip applier (Fig. 16) which places titanium metal clips. The polydioxanone clip has a locking mechanism and eventually dissolves but only one clip can be applied at a time.

Anastomosis

Endoscopic suturing requires time, constant practice, and considerable dexterity. Special ski needles are available (Fig. 18) and the knots can be tied externally and tightened with a pusher or internally with instruments. Quicker and easier but more expensive are the mechanical stapling devices that are becoming available (Fig. 19). Endoscopic adaptations of the larger stapling instruments which are in common use in conventional surgery are available although they are expensive. They will, in time, become the standard method for joining tissues together in an endoscopic operation.

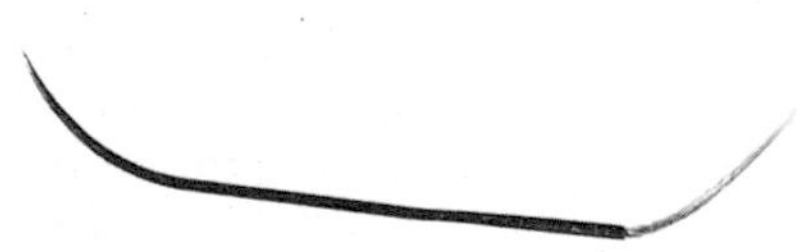

Fig. 18 A ski needle for endoscopic suturing. The shape is designed for ease of insertion through an endoscopic cannula whilst at the same time providing the advantages of a curved end for suturing.

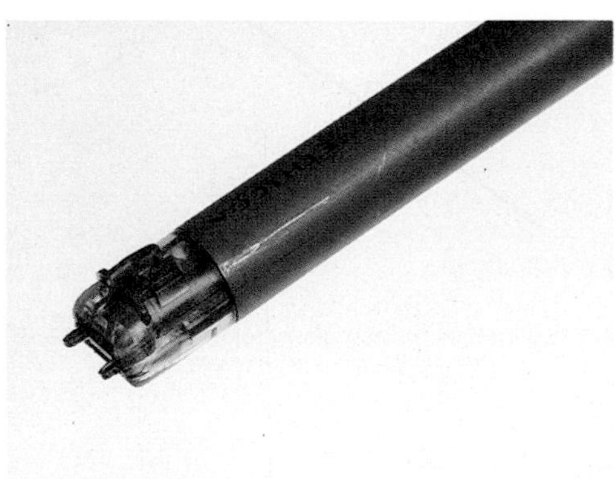

Fig. 19 A multifire endoscopic stapler. Single staples are inserted into the tissues with each squeeze of the trigger.

Removing the specimen

Most, but not all, endoscopic procedures require the removal of a specimen at the end of the operation. Small pieces of tissue can be easily removed through a large cannula. Larger specimens are more difficult. Some can be reduced in size by removing the contents and then the specimen either through a cannula or through the incision when the cannula is withdrawn. Large solid specimens are more difficult still. A few can be extracted through a natural orifice which is opened during the course of the operation but most must be reduced to smaller pieces and removed through one of the cannula sites. The specimen is placed inside a tough plastic bag introduced into the body cavity (Fig. 20). The bag is brought to the surface and the tissue is morcellated or liquefied with a special instrument within the bag inside the body. The pieces of tissue are removed or sucked away and the bag is then removed as well. The specimen is effectively destroyed so far as histological examination is concerned and suitable biopsies must be taken first.

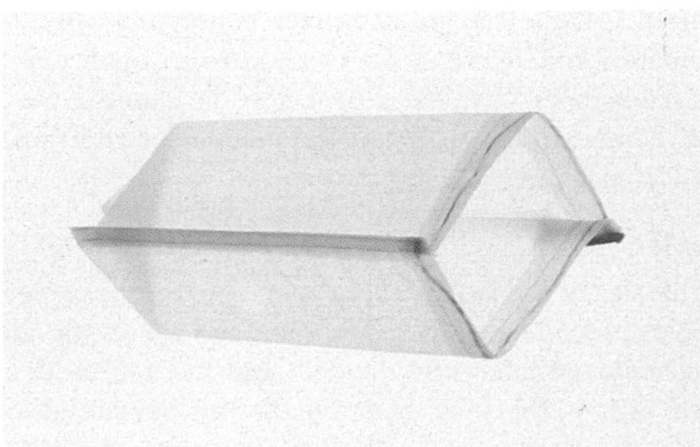

Fig. 20 A plastic bag designed for endoscopic use. The rolled up bag is inserted into the body cavity through a cannula. Tissue or stones are placed in the bag which is then extracted through one of the puncture sites.

Finally one of the cannula sites can be enlarged or a separate incision made specifically to remove the specimen. This obviously loses some of the advantages of the minimally invasive approach although the incisions are often smaller, more discreet, and less morbid than they would otherwise be.

Training the staff

Surgeons

Most surgeons are not familiar with endoscopic techniques but they can be used in every branch of surgery and in the future every surgeon will need endoscopic skills. Some initial training outside the operating theatre is useful for learning the basic manoeuvres that are needed. Flexible endoscopists are familiar with the two-dimensional image and the limitations of manipulation through an endoscope but everyone finds the reversed movement of endoscopic instruments as a result of the pivoting action of the body wall very strange to begin with.

Although more sophisticated training systems are now available, the most useful practice in our experience is to learn to peel a tangerine with scissors and forceps inside a box whilst watching the procedure on a television monitor (Fig. 21). This requires a team of two people, one to hold the camera and the other to operate on the fruit. It is easy to extend the idea to include learning to sew, tying a knot, or placing a clip. Once the basic technique is mastered it is then a question of assisting an experienced surgeon at a number of laparoscopic procedures and later starting to do parts of an endoscopic operation under supervision as with conventional surgical training. Every operation should be recorded for it is then easy to review and reconsider any difficulties that have been encountered.

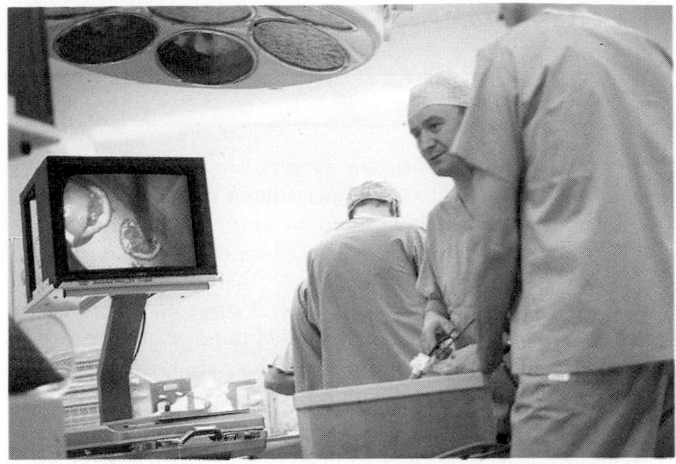

Fig. 21 Peeling a tangerine inside a training box. This teaches the necessary manual skills and is an essential preliminary before starting endoscopic surgery. It is easy to practise sewing and tying knots as well.

Anaesthetists

Anaesthesia for endoscopic surgery is little different to conventional anaesthesia for the same operation. Relaxation is needed for abdominal operations and the lung must be collapsed for procedures within the thorax. Excessive pressure within a body cavity will cause undesirable physiological effects but these are rare with the modern electronically controlled insufflators, although there is always the risk of a gas embolism. Some carbon dioxide will be absorbed during the course of a long operation but it is easily removed by increasing the ventilation rate. By its very nature there is less need for analgesia after an endoscopic procedure but it is worthwhile injecting bupivacaine around the small incision sites.

Theatre staff

Endoscopic procedures are popular with most theatre staff because everyone can easily see what is being done and there are obvious benefits for the patient. However, the scrub nurse can feel less involved than usual because there are fewer instruments to pass although the individual instruments often need particular attention. Hinge screws require regular tightening and the endoscope needs constant cleaning to ensure a clear image and there are many other similar little tasks so that an attentive and interested nurse will always make an operation run more smoothly.

Staff in the sterile supply department are involved too for the instruments are both delicate and hard to clean. They often contain fiddly little pieces which are essential for proper function but are easily lost when the instrument is taken apart. For example, trumpet valves must be oiled every time they are sterilized otherwise they will stick in use. Once again attention to detail can make all the difference in the operating theatre.

SPECIFIC OPERATIONS

Introduction

The development of endoscopic surgery can be compared in importance to the introduction of anaesthesia into surgical practice and the impact will be felt well into the next century. The enthusiasm for the endoscope now is in marked contrast to the rejection of the laparoscope in the past. It is true that gynaecologists have always used laparoscopy but few general surgeons embraced the technique, mostly because only a limited number of organs could be seen and not many abdominal operations are possible with one eye and one hand occupied with a laparoscope. It is the development of video equipment that has made the revolution possible.

It was also fortuitous and fortunate that the first operation to make endoscopic surgery a household word should have been cholecystectomy. The endoscopic operation is identical to an open procedure, it is not particularly difficult to do in most cases, and the benefits to the patient were, and still are, dramatic. There has been some evidence of overenthusiasm. A few obsolete operations have been resurrected because they are easy to do laparoscopically and a few serious complications have occurred but overall the advantages are obvious and patients themselves have been pressing to have an endoscopic operation where possible.

The intention in this section is to illustrate what is presently possible in detail for some operations and in outline for others. Many more endoscopic operations will have been described by the time this chapter is published and we shall leave the reader to discover more information either elsewhere in this book or in a specialist text.

The abdomen

The significant disadvantages of a major abdominal wound and the success of laparoscopic cholecystectomy has ensured the rapid development of endoscopic abdominal surgery. The retroperitoneal organs, with the exception of the kidney, are inaccessible at the moment and most of the operations, like cholecystectomy, are endoscopic adaptations of a conventional operation. A few procedures, for example hernia repair, explore new ideas and more of these can be expected.

Gastroenterology

Laparoscopic cholecystectomy

Laparoscopic cholecystectomy was first performed in 1987 by Phillipe Mouret in Lyons, France. The operation was immediately accepted by the surgical community and has been followed by a worldwide wave of enthusiasm for endoscopic surgery. The laparoscopic operation reduces the access required to an absolute minimum whilst at the same time achieving the same objective as a conventional open cholecystectomy.

Patient selection

Every patient who needs a cholecystectomy and is fit for a general anaesthetic should be suitable for the laparoscopic technique although pregnancy and portal hypertension might make the operation difficult. However, some of these patients will also have stones in the bile duct and, at the present time, laparoscopic exploration of the ducts is not widely available. It is important to identify these patients in advance and we select patients for preoperative endoscopic cholangiography on the basis of a history of jaundice, abnormal liver function tests, and dilatation of the bile ducts on ultrasound examination. Normal liver function tests virtually exclude the presence of ductal stones and only half the patients with an abnormal ultrasound will have an abnormal ERCP (endoscopic retrograde cholangiopancreatography). Any stones that are found on the preoperative cholangiogram can be removed, when appropriate, through an endoscopic sphincterotomy and the patient can then have a laparoscopic cholecystectomy at a later date. Preoperative intravenous cholangiography is preferred in some centres.

There are no absolute contraindications to a laparoscopic operation although the discovery of some unsuspected disease or problem during a preliminary laparoscopy may require a full laparotomy. Obesity is not a contraindication. The view of the operative field is just as good in a fat patient as it is in a thin one and the absence of an abdominal incision reduces the incidence of complications. Dense peritoneal adhesions, acute cholecystitis, severe chronic cholecystitis, and difficulty in identifying the anatomy in Calot's triangle can make continuing with a laparoscopic operation dangerous. Conversion to an open operation in these circumstances, which is necessary in about 5 per cent of patients, demonstrates good surgical judgement and must not be regarded as a failure.

Principles

The principles of the laparoscopic operation are the same as those in an open procedure. The cystic duct and the cystic artery are dissected out, occluded and divided, and the gallbladder is then dissected out of the liver bed. Diathermy haemostasis is used where necessary and the gallbladder is extracted from the abdomen through either the umbilical or the epigastric port.

In contrast to the open operation the common bile duct is not always seen and retrograde dissection is not really feasible because upward retraction of the fundus of the gallbladder is essential for exposure of Calot's triangle. Cholangiography can be done before the cystic duct is ligated and divided if necessary.

Operative technique

Preparation

General anaesthesia with full abdominal relaxation is essential and patients should receive the usual prophylaxis against wound infection and venous thrombosis. A urethral catheter is unnecessary provided that the patient empties his or her bladder before coming to the theatre and we only insert a nasogastric tube if the stomach is distended with gas. The patient lies flat on the operating table and the surgeon stands on the left side with the television monitors and the associated electronic equipment on either side at the head of the table (Fig. 22). Some surgeons prefer the patient in the Lloyd Davies position and stand between the legs to operate. The exposure of Calot's triangle is sometimes improved by elevating the head of the table and rotating the patient to the left.

Placing the cannulae

The Veress needle and the first 11 mm cannula are placed through the umbilicus (Fig. 23). We do not hesitate to adopt an open technique if there is any difficulty and we always do so if there is a paraumbilical hernia as this can be repaired at the end of the operation. The abdomen is inspected as soon as the forward viewing endoscope is inserted although only the gallbladder, the stomach, and the liver are well seen in most circumstances.

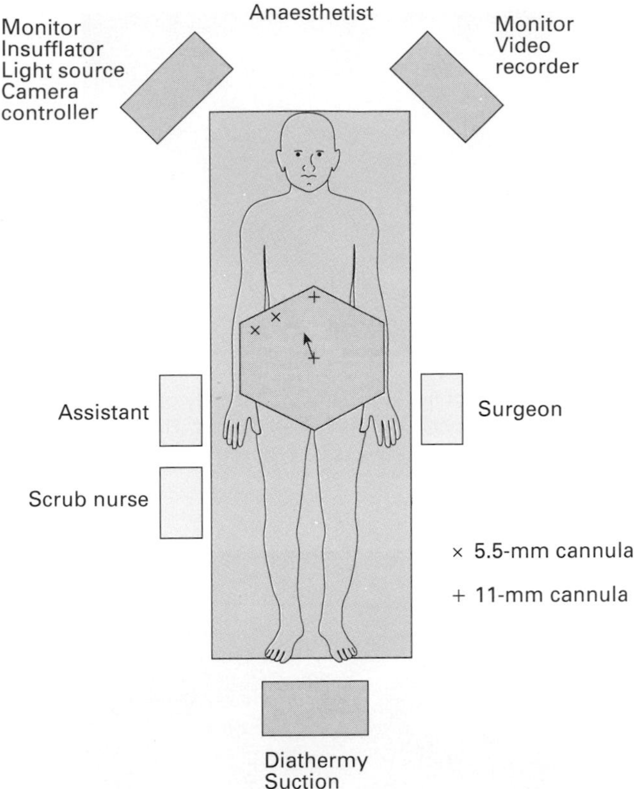

Fig. 22 The layout of the operating theatre during a laparoscopic cholecystectomy. The television monitors with the associated insufflator, light source, and camera controller are all located at the head of the operating table. The surgeon stands on the patient's left hand side and watches the monitor at the patient's right shoulder. The diathermy machine is most conveniently located at the patient's feet along with the sucker.

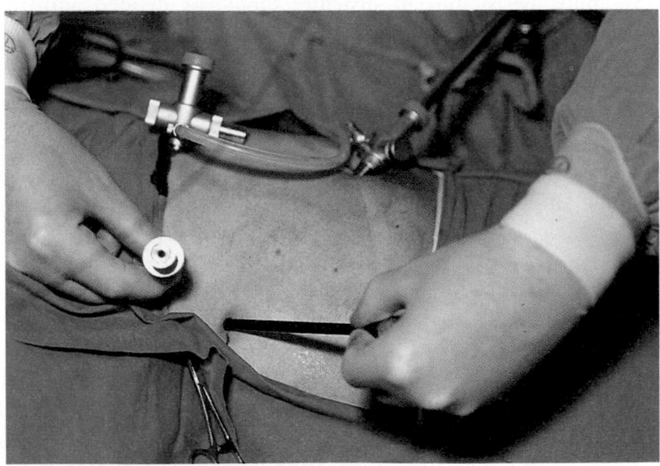

Fig. 23 Layout of the cannulae for a laparoscopic cholecystectomy. The picture is taken from the patient's right hand side with the head to the left. The endoscope is already inserted through the umbilicus and an 11 mm port is placed in the epigastrium and a 5.5 mm port under the costal margin. The surgeon is inserting the last 5.5 mm port laterally under the costal margin which will be used to elevate the fundus of the gallbladder. Gas insufflation is through the epigastric port.

Three further ports are needed and they should be placed under direct vision and after careful assessment of the anatomy of the individual patient. An 11 mm port is placed in the epigastrium and the tip should come through the right leaf of the falciform ligament. Two 5.5 mm ports are placed immediately below the right costal margin (Fig. 23). The medial one should complement the epigastric port and lie in the correct position in relation to the operative field whilst the lateral one is placed over the fundus of the gallbladder.

Occasionally in fat patients a fifth port to depress the duodenum and the colon is helpful and then a 5.5 mm cannula is inserted just to the left of the midline halfway between the umbilical and the epigastric ports. Cholangiography catheters and t-tube drains either come with their own special ports or are inserted through separate small incisions placed below the costal margin.

Dissecting Calot's triangle

A grasping forceps is placed through the right lateral port and is fixed to the fundus of the gallbladder. The gallbladder and the attached liver are then retracted upwards towards the patient's right shoulder. This opens up the subhepatic space (Fig. 24). Any adhesions to the gallbladder are divided and a second grasping forceps is attached to the neck of the gallbladder and pulled laterally to expose Calot's triangle.

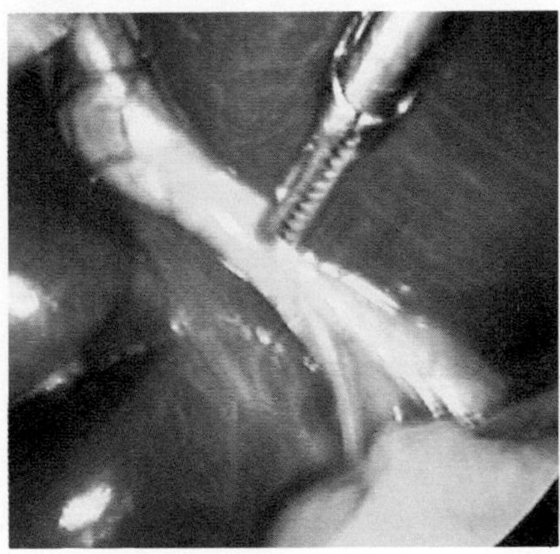

Fig. 24 Exposure of Calot's triangle. The fundus of the gallbladder is elevated and pushed up towards the patient's right shoulder. A grasping forceps is attached to the neck of the gallbladder and Calot's triangle is exposed. The bile duct, which cannot be seen, lies beneath the tissue in the bottom right corner of the picture.

Dissection through the epigastric port with the dolphin nosed forceps (Fig. 25) starts at the junction of the gallbladder with the cystic duct. The peritoneum, fat, and loose areolar tissue around the gallbladder is grasped and gently torn down towards the bile duct. This continues until the inferior aspect of the cystic duct is clearly seen. Any troublesome bleeding should be stopped at once with diathermy but care must be taken not to burn the bile duct. The superior aspect of the cystic duct is cleaned in the same way and eventually the duct is surrounded. Curved forceps can be useful for this (Fig. 26). The cystic duct is therefore clearly identified as a direct extension from the neck of the gallbladder and this is important because the junction of the cystic duct with the common bile duct is not always seen. Most of this dissection is done from the front but by varying the position and the placement

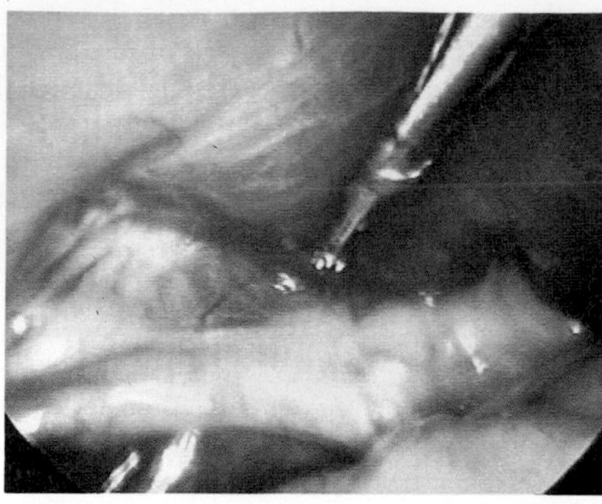

Fig. 25 Dissection of Calot's triangle. The dolphin nosed dissecting forceps are being used to strip the peritoneum and fat off the cystic duct and cystic artery.

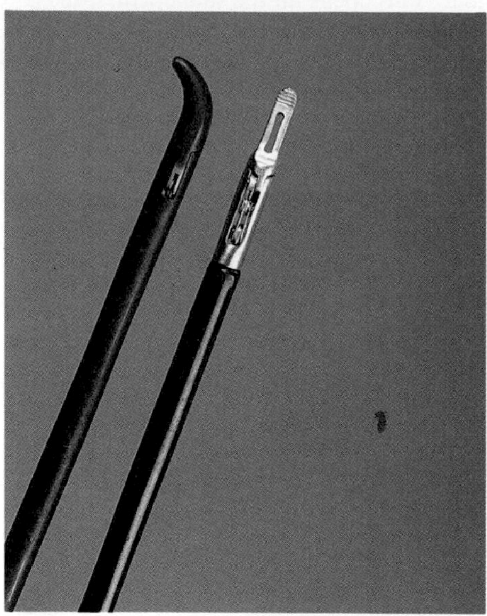

Fig. 26 A curved Petelin's dissector alongside the dolphin-nosed dissecting forceps. Note the grooves on the outside of the blades of the dolphin-nosed instrument which makes separation of the tissues easier.

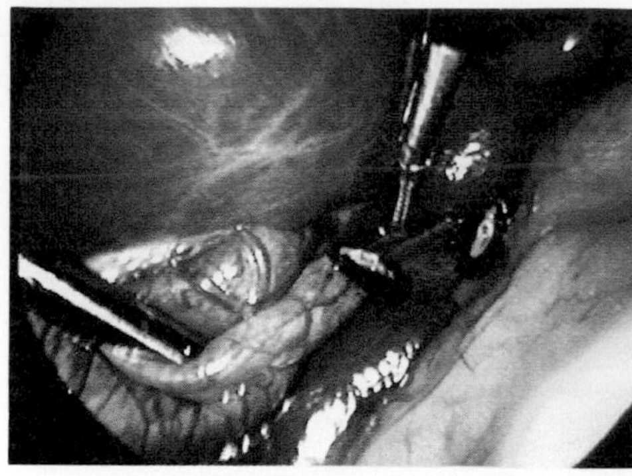

Fig. 27 Exposure of the cystic artery. The body of the gallbladder is on the left and the cystic duct has been divided. The cystic artery is clearly seen just in front of the dolphin-nosed dissecting forceps.

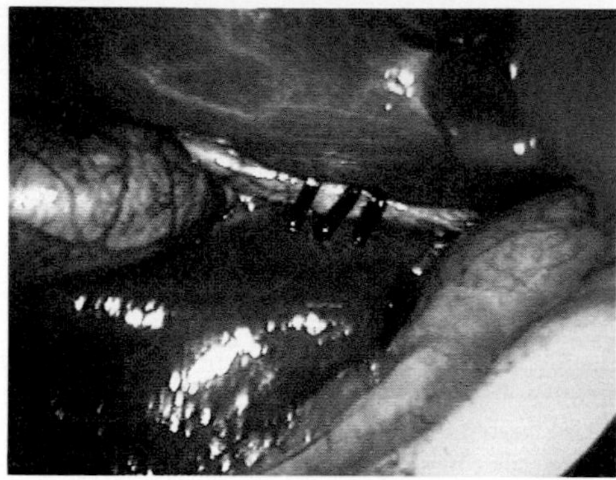

Fig. 28 Cystic duct clipped. The cystic duct will be divided with scissors and two polydioxanone clips will remain on the cystic duct stump.

of the forceps on the neck of the gallbladder it is often possible to expose the posterior aspect of Calot's triangle. The cystic artery is then exposed in the same way (Fig. 27). Both structures are clipped and divided (Fig. 28). Sometimes the cystic duct must be divided before the cystic artery can be safely dissected. Occasionally the cystic duct is too large to fit inside a clip. It must then be tied off with a Roeder knot.

The dissection is not always easy, particularly if there is a lot of fibrosis from chronic inflammation. The loss of tactile sensation is a disadvantage but there are some substitutes. Significant structures, such as an artery or a duct, contain elastic tissue and will twang if they are tweaked. Fibrous tissue has no such elasticity. As always it is important not to rush a difficult dissection because time often reveals the anatomy. Furthermore the variations in anatomy are no different from an open operation and the same rules therefore apply. No significant structure should be divided until the surgeon and his assistant are completely happy that they both understand the anatomy.

Peroperative cholangiography

The technique is identical to open cholangiography although it is rarely needed if a policy of preoperative cholangiography is adopted (Fig. 29). A cholangiogram will delineate the anatomy but if this is in doubt it is probably safer to convert to an open operation.

The cystic duct is occluded distally with a clip and a small proximal incision is made in the cystic duct with fine scissors. A catheter is guided into the duct and held there with a special instrument or a loosely applied titanium clip. Air bubbles must be excluded and the ports, which are radio-opaque, should be held out of the way while the radiographs are taken. We usually use a 1.3 mm umbilical catheter inserted through an intravenous cannula (size 14) although specially designed cholangiography catheters each with its own introducer are available.

Dissection and removal of the gallbladder

Once the cystic duct and the cystic artery are divided the free edge of the lesser omentum falls away. The midcostal grasper is repositioned just above the cystic duct clip and it is pulled upwards and away from the liver to expose the plane between the liver and the

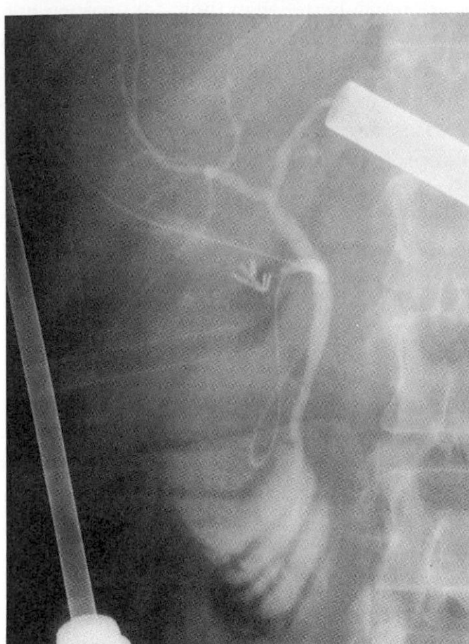

Fig. 29 A normal peroperative cholangiogram obtained during a laparoscopic cholecystectomy. The laparoscopic ports are not radio-opaque and must be held out of the way whilst the radiographs are taken.

gallbladder. The gallbladder is then dissected off the liver bed with scissors, diathermy, or a laser beam starting at the neck (Fig. 30). All the bleeding points on the liver bed are coagulated as dissection proceeds until the gallbladder is only just attached to the liver at the fundus. Any bile or blood that has accumulated is sucked away and, if necessary, a drain is placed in the gallbladder bed before this final strand is divided.

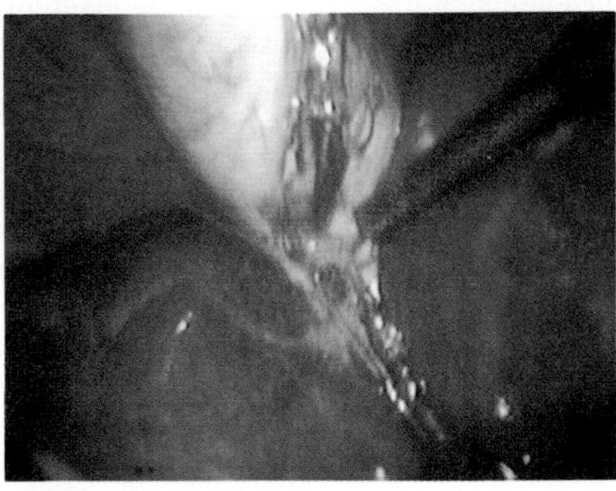

Fig. 30 Dissection of the gallbladder from the liver bed with a diathermy wire loop.

Dissection at the fundus is often difficult and simply requires patience and constant changes of position. If the gallbladder is perforated, and this is preferable to entering the liver itself, the bile and as many stones as possible should be removed. Nevertheless stones are often left behind in the peritoneal cavity where, somewhat surprisingly, they very rarely cause complications.

Once the gallbladder is free the cystic duct is drawn into one of the 11 mm ports and the port and the gallbladder are withdrawn together through the abdominal wall. Usually the fundus of the gallbladder and any contained stones remain within the abdomen and they must be manipulated through the wound. Crushing any large stones, sucking away the bile or extending the incision are sometimes necessary and all of these are easier to do if the gallbladder is inside a plastic bag.

A final inspection of the abdomen is appropriate before all the carbon dioxide gas is allowed to escape and the cannulae are removed. We only suture the abdominal wall if a wound has been enlarged and we prefer to close the skin with adhesive tape rather than with sutures.

Management of stones in the bile duct

The best management of bile duct stones in this new endoscopic era is not yet clear. We prefer to remove any stones from the bile duct at an ERCP procedure before embarking on a laparoscopic operation but this may not be appropriate and, sometimes, is impossible.

Large stones, which tend to occur in older patients with grossly dilated bile ducts, always cause difficulty at endoscopy but they are relatively easy to remove at a laparoscopic exploration of the bile ducts. In young patients it is best not to divide the ampullary sphincter and the duct must be explored surgically. The choice lies between a conventional open operation or one of the newer laparoscopic techniques.

Stones can be extracted from the bile duct through the cystic duct if it is first dilated with a suitable balloon. Instruments, including a narrow cholangioscope, can then be passed into the bile duct and the stones retrieved or broken up under direct vision. Stones in the hepatic ducts are difficult to find, particularly if the cystic duct enters the common duct low down behind the pancreas. A fine tube can be left in the cystic duct at the end to act as a drain and to permit later cholangiography. The precise place of this technique in endoscopic practice is not yet clear.

Direct endoscopic exploration of the bile duct is quite straightforward. A 30° forward oblique telescope gives the best view of the bile duct and a supraduodenal choledochotomy is easily made in the anterior surface of the duct with the diathermy hook and scissors. Stones can be washed out of the duct or removed with a balloon or a basket (Fig. 31). The ducts are then inspected with a choledochoscope and any remaining stones are removed. At the end a t-tube is sutured into the bile duct.

If stones are discovered in the bile ducts unexpectedly during the course of a laparoscopic cholecystectomy the surgeon is left in something of a dilemma. Small stones can probably be safely left to pass spontaneously. Larger stones need to be removed either immediately and surgically or at a later ERCP.

All three choices have disadvantages and deciding between them depends on the findings in the individual patient, the equipment available, and the skill and experience of the surgeon. If stones are left behind in the ducts it is probably wise to leave a drain down to the cystic duct stump in case it leaks. An ERCP should be done within a day or two of operation to remove any residual stones and as soon as retained stones are discovered.

Difficulties and complications

Inserting a cannula or the Veress needle can cause spectacular damage and invisible retroperitoneal aortic injury is one cause of an acute collapse during a laparoscopic operation. Such injuries are fortunately very rare.

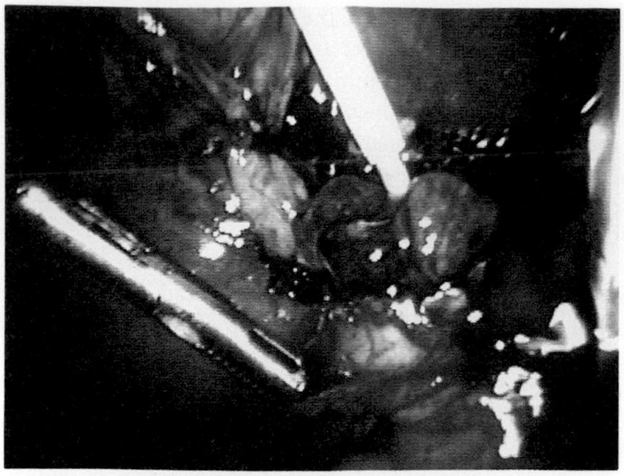

Fig. 31 Laparoscopic exploration of the common bile duct. Two large stones are being extracted from the bile duct with a balloon. A clip on the cystic duct can be seen at the top of the picture and the grasping forceps is holding the choledochotomy open.

Sudden severe haemorrhage is always a problem and it is best avoided in the first place. A torn cystic artery or a liver laceration are the common causes and haemorrhage from either can be difficult to stop. The usual general principles apply. Blood and clot are sucked or washed away and the best possible exposure is obtained whilst the surgeon applies local pressure to the bleeding area. The scrub nurse prepares the diathermy and a titanium clip applier and when everything is ready the pressure is removed and the bleeding point is identified and occluded. This is much more difficult to achieve with the limitations on movement in an endoscopic environment and there is sometimes no alternative to a laparotomy.

Every surgeon fears damaging a bile duct. In large published series the accident happens once in every 300 laparoscopic cholecystectomies. This is slightly more frequent than during an open operation and probably reflects the introduction of a new technique rather than a fundamental flaw in the operation. Great care should be taken to identify the anatomy correctly and to place any clips properly. It is very easy for a titanium clip to be placed so that the tips partially occlude the bile duct without the surgeon appreciating what has happened and any doubts about the anatomy should lead to an immediate laparotomy. The next most important aspect of a bile duct injury is that it should be recognized at the time. Late presentation of biliary damage is always associated with a poorer outcome. Exactly what is done depends upon the injury and when it is recognized but a laparotomy will usually be needed.

Reactionary haemorrhage is rare and generally requires a laparotomy although with increasing experience a repeat laparoscopy may be sufficient. Bile leaks from the cystic duct stump or the liver bed present with pain in the right upper quadrant, fever and a subhepatic collection on ultrasound. The bile is removed with a percutaneous drain and the leak is identified at an ERCP and is stopped by placing a stent in the bile duct. The drain remains until the drainage ceases and the stent is removed not less than 2 months later. Surprisingly a simple sphincterotomy will not allow the leak to close. A few patients present with a previously unidentified bile duct stone within a few months of their operation and the stone should be removed through an endoscopic sphincterotomy.

Benefits and results

The mortality rate following a laparoscopic cholecystectomy is about 0.1 per cent and the complication rate is about 4 per cent. Both figures are much better than those for an open operation and the cosmetic benefits of four small incisions are important to many patients. At the moment about 1 in every 20 patients needs a laparotomy although we can expect this figure to improve as experience increases. Patients must be warned about this beforehand and sign an appropriate consent form.

Most patients are mobile and can eat and drink later the same day. Some patients are troubled by nausea and vomiting but very few need opiate analgesia. Any drain can be removed after about 12 h and most patients can then go home. The majority are back at work within 2 weeks.

Laparoscopic appendicectomy

Laparoscopic appendicectomy combines the advantages of diagnosis and treatment in one procedure. The usual preoperative preparation is necessary and prophylactic antibiotics are given on induction of general anaesthesia. The patient must consent to an open operation should it be needed.

Placing the cannulae

The patient lies flat on the operating table and the bladder is emptied. After creating the pneumoperitoneum an 11 mm port and endoscope are placed through the umbilicus and the diagnosis is confirmed. Two further ports are needed on either side of the abdomen and should be placed in relation to the position of the appendix. An 11 mm port is placed in the right iliac fossa and a 5.5 mm port in the left iliac fossa.

Operative technique

Any local adhesions are gently divided and the tip of the appendix is grasped and drawn into the port in the right iliac fossa. The appendix mesentery is occluded with bipolar diathermy or a ligature around the appendicular artery and then divided. The base of the appendix is secured with a Roeder knot and then occluded beyond the ligature with bipolar diathermy. The appendix is divided across the burnt area and is removed through the right iliac fossa port. It is not necessary to bury the appendix stump. Free peritoneal fluid or pus can be sucked away and the peritoneal cavity washed although it is important not to flood infected fluid into the pelvis or the subphrenic spaces. It is easy to place a drain to the appendix stump if necessary and the pneumoperitoneum is then released and the ports removed.

Postoperative management

Most patients have less pain from the wounds than after a conventional appendicectomy but the recovery time is only slightly improved. Many patients are toxic from the infection and take time to recover whatever method is used to remove the appendix.

Complications

The only complication specific to the laparoscopic procedure is a low incidence of reactionary haemorrhage as a result of failure to occlude the appendicular artery properly. Septic complications occur just as with any other appendicectomy although wound infection is less serious.

Laparoscopic colectomy

Laparoscopic colonic resection is already possible for the techniques involved are no different to those used in a laparoscopic cholecystectomy or appendicectomy. However, tying and dividing the mesentery can be very tedious and the resection may not include all the important lymph nodes. It also takes a long time and considerable skill to construct a hand-sewn intraperitoneal anastomosis and although stapling guns can help they are presently too expensive for routine use. So a complete laparoscopic colonic resection is not really a practical option at the moment although this situation is unlikely to persist as new technological developments are introduced.

Nevertheless endoscopic techniques can be useful during colonic resection in certain patients. Division of the mesentery under laparoscopic vision is fairly straightforward (Fig. 32) and the segment of bowel can be delivered through a small discreetly placed incision, the resection and anastomosis being completed outside the abdominal cavity. The bowel is returned to the abdomen and any necessary drains are placed before all the ports are withdrawn and the incision closed. This approach minimizes the trauma to the patient and overcomes the problem of removing the specimen from the abdominal cavity.

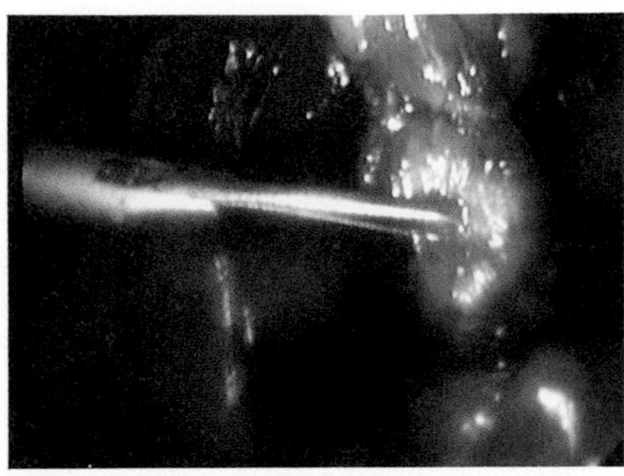

Fig. 32 Division of the ileocaecal artery following ligation with Roeder loop knots during a laparoscopically assisted right hemicolectomy.

Other gastrointestinal operations

Once the ideas and the concepts of an endoscopic operation are accepted it takes very little imagination to transfer almost every operation to an endoscopic procedure. Indeed most abdominal operations have already been done laparoscopically somewhere in the world.

Operations around the stomach, such as fundoplication and pyloromyotomy in neonates, are relatively easy to do although there is little demand for vagotomy. Small bowel resections are mostly required during emergency operations and although endoscopic techniques are described most surgeons will be naturally hesitant to embark on such procedures at the moment. The same remarks apply to splenectomy. Liver resections are clearly impractical at present but it is easy to deroof a liver cyst with a diathermy hook and bleeding from a liver biopsy site can often be controlled with a laparoscopic technique, thus avoiding a laparotomy. In both instances it is quite possible to suck away blood or other fluids lying in the peritoneal cavity.

Emergency laparoscopic surgery is still being developed. A perforated anterior duodenal ulcer is easy to close with an omental patch through the laparoscope as any surgeon who has done a laparoscopic cholecystectomy will appreciate. Laparoscopy for intestinal obstruction is difficult because of the distension but it is possible to decompress the bowel and then to divide an adhesive band. Some reports have also suggested that laparoscopy and laparoscopic surgical techniques are useful in patients with abdominal trauma.

Urology

Laparoscopic nephrectomy

This is the only laparoscopic procedure to remove a retroperitoneal organ although the kidney is approached across the peritoneum. The operation can take some time to do and at the moment it is probably best reserved for benign diseases of the kidney.

The patient is placed in the traditional lateral position and the endoscope is inserted at the lateral border of the rectus abdominis muscle level with the umbilicus. Three or four further ports are needed. The peritoneum on the lateral side of the colon is divided and the bowel falls away under gravity. The ureter is identified at the pelvic brim and traced up to the hilum of the kidney. The vascular pedicle is divided with a special stapling gun which inserts six rows of fine vascular staples and divides the tissues down the middle all in one action. The kidney is then freed from its surrounding attachments and removed from the abdomen within a laparoscopic organ bag.

Laparoscopic varicocelectomy

This is a straightforward day-case procedure that divides the testicular veins just above the internal inguinal ring. The endoscope is inserted through the umbilicus in the usual way and two 5.5 mm ports are required on either side of the umbilicus. The testicular vessels are easily seen through the peritoneum just inside the internal inguinal ring and it is a simple matter to divide the peritoneum with scissors, dissect out the testicular veins from the testicular artery, clip the veins, and excise a segment (Fig. 33). Even if the testicular artery is inadvertently included in a clip the testicle should still survive provided that the branches to the spermatic cord from the inferior epigastric artery are not damaged.

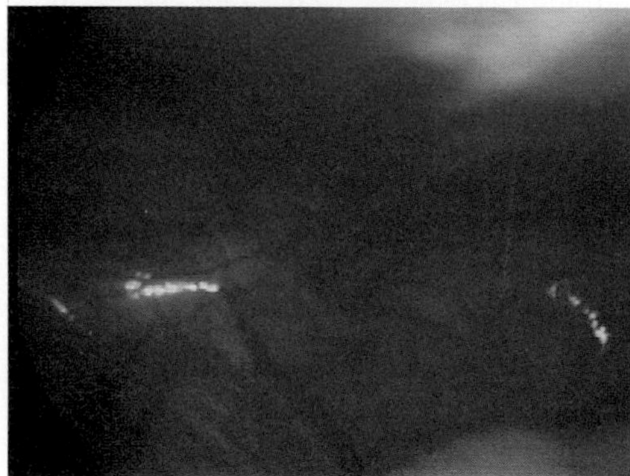

Fig. 33 Laparoscopic view of the left internal inguinal ring. The testicular vessels are visible beneath the peritoneum running inferiorly and to the left whilst the vas, which is white, runs medially over the iliac vessels down into the pelvis. It is a straightforward procedure to divide the peritoneum over the vessels, dissect out the testicular vein, clip both ends, and divide the vein to treat a varicocele.

Other urological operations

Peritoneal dialysis is widely used in the long-term treatment of chronic renal failure but the Silastic catheter is easily blocked by displacement of the tube out of the pelvis or with omentum wrapped around the side holes. It is easy to insufflate the abdomen through the catheter, remove any omentum adherent to the tubing, and to replace the coiled tip in the pelvis using the laparoscope and a suitable grabber passed though one 5.5 mm port. Transplanted kidneys are sometimes surrounded by collections of lymph (lymphocele) and if percutaneous drainage fails fenestration of the lymphocele into the peritoneal cavity is the best method of treatment. It is easy to cut a hole in the peritoneal wall of a lymphocele with a diathermy hook (Fig. 34). In both instances the benefit to the patient of avoiding a laparotomy is obvious.

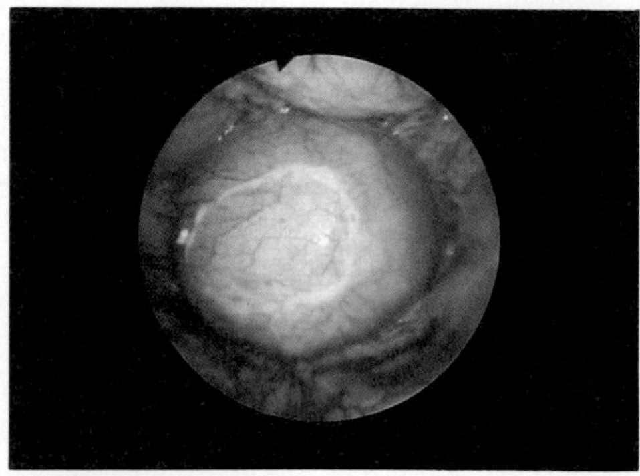

Fig. 34 Fenestration of a transplant lymphocele. The lymphocele can be clearly seen and a diathermy hook has marked out the circle of peritoneal wall which is to be removed.

Gynaecology

In some respects endoscopic surgery has not advanced so rapidly in gynaecology. This is partly because transcervical resection of the endometrium has reduced the need for hysterectomy but also because a laparoscopic hysterectomy, which is perfectly possible, is regarded by some gynaecologists as a rather more complicated version of a vaginal hysterectomy. Endoscopic operations on the fallopian tubes and the ovaries certainly have a place and are particularly valuable in preserving tubal function after the removal of an ectopic pregnancy for example. Laser ablation of endometriosis and the division of pelvic adhesions have been standard for many years and pelvic lymphadenectomy, which is a popular procedure in the United States, is an ideal operation for the endoscopist. For a detailed description of all these operations the reader is referred to a specialist text.

The abdominal wall

Laparoscopic inguinal hernia repair

Most inguinal hernias are repaired through a groin incision and approach the inguinal canal by division of the external oblique aponeurosis. The posterior or preperitoneal approach is also popular but it still involves an incision through the abdominal wall muscles. Either operation is decidedly uncomfortable and very few patients are back at work in less than a month. A nylon darn is the most popular method of repair but synthetic mesh is also used and seems to be particularly successful when it is placed in the preperitoneal plane. Laparoscopic hernia repair avoids the inguinal incision and combines the advantages of plastic mesh and the preperitoneal approach. As in paediatric surgery, where endoscopic hernia repair is not yet established, laparoscopy also identifies the patient with a hernia on the other side.

We describe below a transabdominal extraperitoneal mesh repair of an inguinal hernia which is one technique among many. We do not yet know which is the best, but it is certain that the operative anatomy is strange, the access is awkward, and the iliac vessels are alarmingly close to the operation site.

Principles

The basic objective of a laparoscopic inguinal hernia repair is to deal with the peritoneal sac and then to staple a sheet of plastic mesh over the muscular defect. A direct sac and a small indirect one can normally be easily pulled back into the abdominal cavity. A large indirect sac is best transected at the internal inguinal ring and the residual peritoneum left in the inguinal canal. The peritoneum must also be removed from a femoral hernia but it is then sufficient to plug the femoral canal with a roll of plastic mesh.

Operative technique

General anaesthesia with good relaxation of the abdominal wall is required and all our patients are given prophylactic antibiotics. The patient lies flat on the table although a little head-down tilt is sometimes helpful. A 10 mm endoscope is inserted through the umbilicus and the operation site inspected. Two further ports are needed, one on each side of the umbilicus at the lateral edge of the rectus abdominis. A large 12 mm port to take the stapler is placed on the side of the hernia and a 5.5 mm port on the other side (Fig. 35).

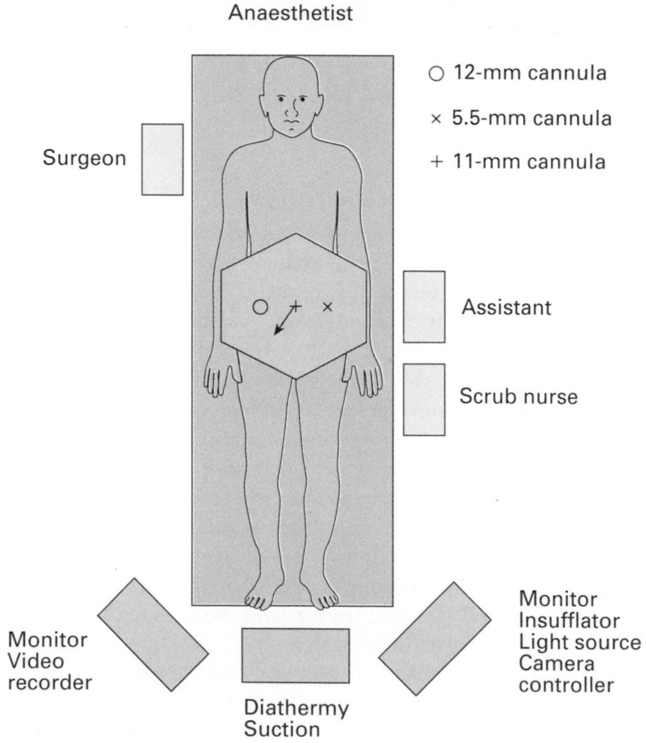

Anaesthetist
○ 12-mm cannula
× 5.5-mm cannula
+ 11-mm cannula
Surgeon
Assistant
Scrub nurse
Monitor
Video
recorder
Diathermy
Suction
Monitor
Insufflator
Light source
Camera
controller

Fig. 35 The layout of the operating theatre for a laparoscopic hernia repair on the right side. All the equipment stands at the foot of the table and the surgeon operates from the side of the hernia. The 10 mm endoscope is inserted through the umbilicus as usual. A 12 mm cannula to accommodate the angled stapling gun (see Fig. 37) is inserted at the lateral border of the rectus sheath level with the umbilicus on the side of the hernia and a 5.5 mm cannula is placed in a corresponding position on the other side.

An indirect hernia is very different in appearance from a direct one. The direct sac is a wide necked defect straight through the anterior abdominal wall flanked on the lateral side by the inferior epigastric vessels and medially by the umbilical ligament. An indirect hernia clearly runs obliquely through the abdominal wall muscles and the end of the sac cannot usually be seen. The testicular vessels are visible in the inferolateral corner of the sac at the internal inguinal ring whilst the vas appears as a white cord slipping out of the inferomedial corner and running down over the iliac vessels into the pelvis (Fig. 36).

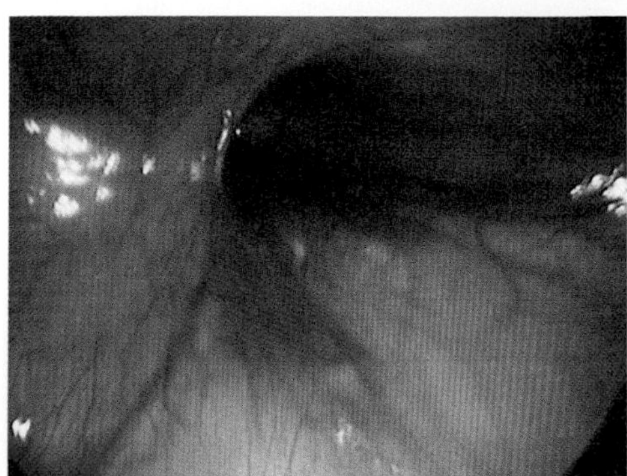

Fig. 36 Laparoscopic view of the internal inguinal ring in a patient with an indirect inguinal hernia on the right hand side. The testicular vessels are clearly seen through the peritoneum running into the inguinal canal. The vas emerges from the inferior and medial portion of the hernia sac and runs over the iliac vessels down into the pelvis.

The operation starts well lateral and superior to the hernia sac by dividing the peritoneum. The peritoneal incision continues horizontally across the top of the internal ring and up to, and sometimes into, the umbilical ligament. The peritoneum is then dissected downwards and is thus pulled out of the hernia although sometimes the sac is best circumcised at its neck.

The testicular vessels and the vas are often rather adherent and the dissection can be somewhat difficult at this stage. The abdominal wall muscles and the inferior epigastric vessels should then be cleaned of any fatty tissue.

At this point the anatomy of the whole area should be apparent. Medially the pubic tubercle should be palpable with Cooper's ligament running away posteriorly and laterally. Anteriorly and laterally the posterior aspect of the conjoint tendon should be visible spreading behind the inferior epigastric vessels. The inguinal ligament is rarely identified. A 10 cm by 5 cm sheet of Prolene mesh is rolled up and passed into the peritoneal cavity through the 12 mm port. It is unravelled, manipulated to cover the margins of the hernia defect, and stapled in place. Medially the inferior margin of the mesh can be stapled to Cooper's ligament but laterally great care must be taken not to damage the testicular vessels, the vas, and the femoral nerve. An angled stapling gun helps to place the staples correctly (Fig. 37).

Finally the original peritoneal layer is lifted back up over the mesh and stapled back to the peritoneum on the anterior abdominal wall. Deflating the abdomen can make this easier. The ports are then removed and the muscles at the site of the 12 mm port are sutured if necessary.

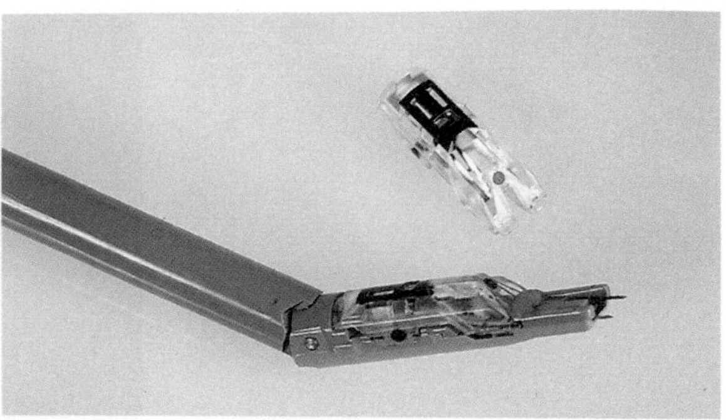

Fig. 37 A multifire angled stapling gun for use in laparoscopic hernia repair with a spare cartridge of staples.

Postoperative management

Most patients are up and about later the same day and many of them can go home. There is no reason to restrict their activity in any way as the repair does not depend on muscles healing together and although most patients experience some discomfort in the groin they do not need much analgesia. Most patients are back at work within 2 weeks.

Complications

One alarming development is gross gaseous distension of the scrotum at the end of the operation. Fortunately the carbon dioxide is rapidly absorbed with no serious consequences. An inguinal haematoma is a nuisance and damage to the femoral nerve is a cause of persistent pain in the wound. Infection around the mesh is rare. So far as recurrence is concerned this type of laparoscopic operation appears to have recurrence rates very comparable to the open operation, but only time will tell if the conjecture is true.

The chest

Transthoracic cervical sympathectomy

All the conventional open approaches to the cervical sympathetic trunk are unsatisfactory, either because of poor access and inadequate exposure, or the proximity of important structures. In contrast, the endoscopic operation is easy and safe and the surgeon has an excellent view of the sympathetic trunk. The procedure itself is simple, elegant, and quick.

A pneumothorax with carbon dioxide is created with the patient fully anaesthetized and lying flat on the operating table with the arms abducted to 60°. A 5 mm endoscope is introduced into the chest in the fourth intercostal space at the anterior axillary line and the cervical sympathetic trunk is immediately visible under the parietal pleura on the necks of the 2nd, 3rd, 4th, and 5th ribs (Fig. 38). The stellate ganglion is sometimes seen superiorly. Through a separate port in the fifth intercostal space it is a simple matter to divide the sympathetic trunk just below the stellate ganglion and either to excise a segment or obliterate the chain with diathermy over the second, third, and fourth ribs. A special port with a channel for the endoscope and one for the instruments is available and means that the operation can be done with only one puncture. Both sides can be done at the same time and most patients can go home the next day.

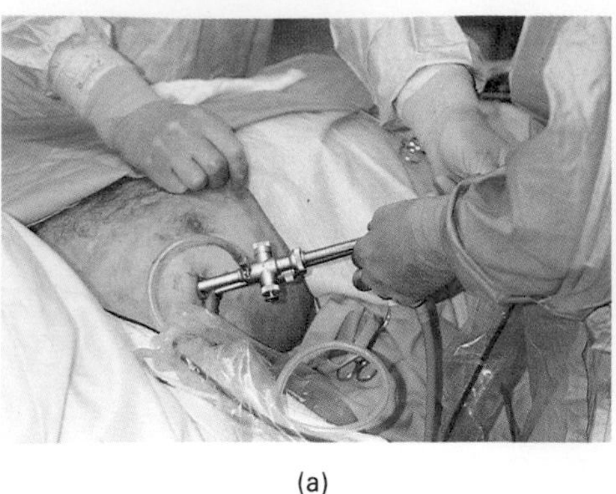

(a)

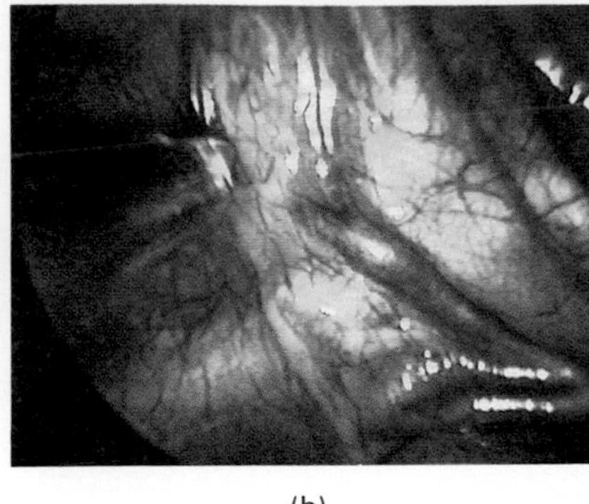

(b)

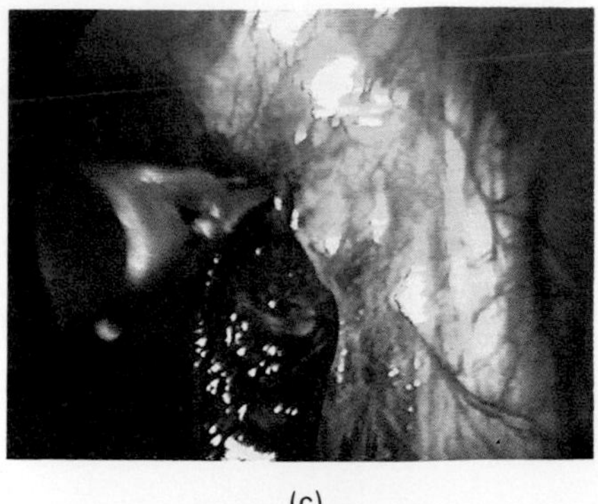

(c)

Fig. 38 (a) Position of trochars for a right thoracoscopic sympathectomy (patient's head is to left side). (b) Thoracoscopic view of sympathetic chain overlying necks of second and third ribs. The metal probe points to the sympathetic chain as it crosses the superior intercostal vein. The apex of the lung is visible in the lower part of the field. (c) The sympathetic chain has been divided on the neck of the second rib after opening the pleura. The upper end of the chain is being held up by grasping forceps.

Other thoracoscopic operations

Any technique that avoids a painful thoracotomy is to be welcomed and the new stapling instruments make any form of endoscopic pulmonary resection relatively easy although the specimen has to be removed within an organ bag.

Mediastinal operations and oesophageal resections are also feasible. There are two approaches to oesophageal resection. In one technique the abdominal and cervical dissections take place through conventional incisions but the thoracic oesophagus is mobilized endoscopically across either pleural cavity. The oesophagus and stomach are pulled up into the cervical incision, the tumour resected, and then continuity is restored.

An alternative approach is to mobilize the oesophagus within the mediastinum by dissection under endoscopic vision using a specially designed instrument which is inserted through a cervical incision and slowly advanced down the mediastinum alongside the oesophagus. The stomach is mobilized laparoscopically and, once again, everything is drawn up into the neck where the resection and the anastomosis are performed.

CONCLUSION

Endoscopic techniques are already widely used in other surgical specialties that we have not discussed. Arthroscopy has revolutionized operations on the knee in orthopaedics, for example, and nasal operations are much more accurate when viewed through an endoscope. Every branch of surgery will be influenced in due course and even now fine endoscopes are being made that can be inserted through a tiny burr hole into the subarachnoid space to examine the surface of the brain. It will not be long before neurosurgical operations are possible without the need for a craniotomy.

New operations and new ways of performing old operations are being developed with astonishing speed and endoscopic surgery is still in its infancy. Many future developments will depend on advances in technology but they will also depend on surgical skill. It is also of critical importance that proper evaluation of these developments takes place continually, not only in assessing the quality of the results of endoscopic surgery, but also the cost effectiveness of these procedures.

FURTHER READING

Alain JL, Grousseau D, Terrier G. Extramucosal pyloromyotomy by laparoscopy. *J Pediatr Surg* 1991; **26**: 1191–2.

Barkun JS, *et al.* Randomised controlled trial of laparoscopic versus mini cholecystectomy. *Lancet* 1992; **340**: 1116–9.

Byrne J, Walsh TN, Hederman WP. Endoscopic transthoracic electrocautery of the sympathetic chain for palmar and axillary hyperhidrosis. *Br J Surg* 1990; **77**: 1046–9.

Coptcoat MJ, Wickham JEA. Laparoscopy in urology. *Min Invas Ther* 1992; **1**: 337–42.

Cuschieri A, Berci G. *Laparoscopic biliary surgery*. Oxford: Blackwell Scientific Publications, 1990

Cuschieri A, *et al.* The European experience with laparoscopic cholecystectomy. *Am J Surg* 1991; **161**: 385–7.

Cuschieri A, Buess G, Perissat J, eds. *Operative manual of endoscopic surgery*. Berlin: Springer-Verlag, 1992.

Dandy DJ. The present state of arthroscopy. *Min Invas Ther* 1991; **1**: 51–6.

Gotz F, Pier, A, Bacher C. Modified laparoscopic appendectomy in surgery. A report on 388 operations. *Surg Endosc* 1990; **4**: 6–9.

Holohan TV. Laparoscopic cholecystectomy. *Lancet* 1991; **338**: 801–3.

Hunter JG. Laparoscopic transcystic common bile duct exploration. *Am J Surg* 1992; **163**: 53–8.

Larson GM, *et al.* Multipractice analysis of laparoscopic cholecystectomy in 1983 patients. *Am J Surg* 1992; **163**: 221–6.

Loh A, Taylor RS. Laparoscopic appendicectomy. *Br J Surg* 1992; **79**: 289–90.

Macintyre IMC. Laparoscopic herniorrhaphy. *Br J Surg* 1992; **79**: 1123–4.

Martin IG, *et al.* Laparoscopic cholecystectomy as a routine procedure for gallstones: results of an 'all-comers' policy. *Br J Surg* 1992; **79**: 807–10.

Masters A, Rennie JA. Endoscopic transthoracic sympathectomy for upper limb hyperhidrosis. *Min Invas Ther* 1992; **1**: 325–8.

Miller SS. Laparoscopic operations in paediatric surgery. *Br J Surg* 1992; **79**: 986–7.

Myers WC, *et al.* A prospective analysis of 1518 laparoscopic cholecystectomies. *N Engl J Med* 1991; **324**: 1073–8.

Paterson-Brown S. Emergency laparoscopic surgery. *Br J Surg* 1993; **80**: 279–83.

Sackier J, Berci G, Phillips E, Carroll B, Shapiro S, Paz-Partlow M. The role of cholangiography in laparoscopic cholecystectomy. *Arch Surg* 1991; **126**: 1021–6.

Sutton C. Operative laparoscopy. *Br J Hosp Med* 1993; **49**: 312–27.

Wilson RG, Macintyre IMC, Nixon SJ, Saunders JH, Varma JS, King PM. Laparoscopic cholecystectomy as a safe and effective treatment for severe acute cholecystitis. *Br Med J* 1992; **305**: 394–6.

The oesophagus 14

14.1 Dysphagia

J. SHAPIRO

PHYSIOLOGY

For purposes of study, the swallow has been divided into three phases: oral, pharyngeal, and oesophageal.

Oral phase

Prior to the onset of the oral phase, the major portion of a food bolus is formed into a cohesive mass and is held between the anterior tongue and the hard palate. The soft palate is pulled anteriorly and rests against the back of the tongue, which is slightly elevated, closing the oral cavity. The oral phase begins when the tongue moves the bolus posteriorly and ends when the bolus passes the anterior tonsillar pillars. During this phase, the tongue elevates in an anterior to posterior direction. An anterior labial seal and a lateral buccal seal keep the bolus in proper position (Table 1).

Table 1 Oral phase

Begins:	tongue moves bolus posterior
Ends:	bolus passes anterior pillars
Time:	<1 s
Components:	tongue elevates anterior to posterior
	tongue forms central groove
	labial seal anterior
	buccal seal lateral
Control:	peripheral nervous system, voluntary

Pharyngeal phase

The pharyngeal phase begins when the food bolus passes the anterior tonsillar pillars and ends when the bolus passes through the upper oesophageal sphincter into the oesophagus. During this phase the palate elevates and retracts, closing the nasopharynx. The laryngeal valves close and the suprahyoid muscles elevate the larynx under the base of the tongue. The bolus is propelled through the pharynx by the backward motion of the base of tongue and contraction of the pharyngeal constrictor muscles. When the upper oesophageal sphincter opens it creates a negative pressure in the hypopharynx, facilitating passage of the bolus into the oesophagus. During the pharyngeal phase respiration is inhibited. The exact trigger for initiation of this phase of the swallow is unknown; it may be related to the position of the base of the tongue (Table 2).

Oesophageal phase

The oesophageal phase begins when the bolus enters the oesophagus and ends when it passes through the lower oesophageal sphincter into the stomach. A sequential peristaltic wave in the oesophagus propels the bolus. The lower oesophageal sphincter relaxes as the bolus passes into the stomach (Table 3).

Table 2 Pharyngeal phase

Begins:	bolus passes anterior pillars
Ends:	bolus passes through upper oesophageal sphincter into oesophagus
Time:	<1 s
Components:	velum elevates and retracts—nasal passage closed
	bolus propelled through pharynx
	larynx closes and elevates
	respiration inhibited
	upper oesophageal sphincter relaxes
Control:	peripheral nervous system involuntary

Table 3 Oesophageal phase

Begins:	bolus enters oesophagus
Ends:	bolus passes through lower oesophageal sphincter into stomach
Time:	8–20 s
Components:	sequential peristaltic wave propels bolus
	relaxation of lower oesophageal sphincter
Control:	autonomic nervous system involuntary

The upper oesophageal sphincter is a zone of high pressure between the pharynx and the oesophagus that prevents air from entering the oesophagus and helps prevent oesophageal contents from refluxing into the pharynx. The muscles which form the upper oesophageal sphincter are the cricopharyngeus and either the lower fibres of the inferior pharyngeal constrictor or the upper fibres of the cervical oesophagus.

At rest the sphincter is closed, and closure is maintained by both tonic contraction of the intrinsic sphincter muscle and passive elastic forces. Inhibition of the intrinsic musculature contraction of the sphincter and contraction of the suprahyoid muscles creates anterosuperior displacement of the cricoid cartilage, thereby opening the sphincter (Fig. 1).

PATHOPHYSIOLOGY

Dysphagia, or difficulty in swallowing, is a common complaint. For purposes of discussion, abnormalities in swallowing can be divided into dysfunction in each of the separate phases. In reality, these phases are so inter-related that the abnormalities are often in more than one phase.

Oral phase dysfunction

In some patients the tongue holds the bolus too far forward on the palate, resulting in anterior leakage. Weakness of the labial or cheek muscles leads to malpositioning of the bolus either out of the oral cavity or into the lateral sulci. Any decreased sensation in the oral cavity makes it much more difficult to manipulate the bolus

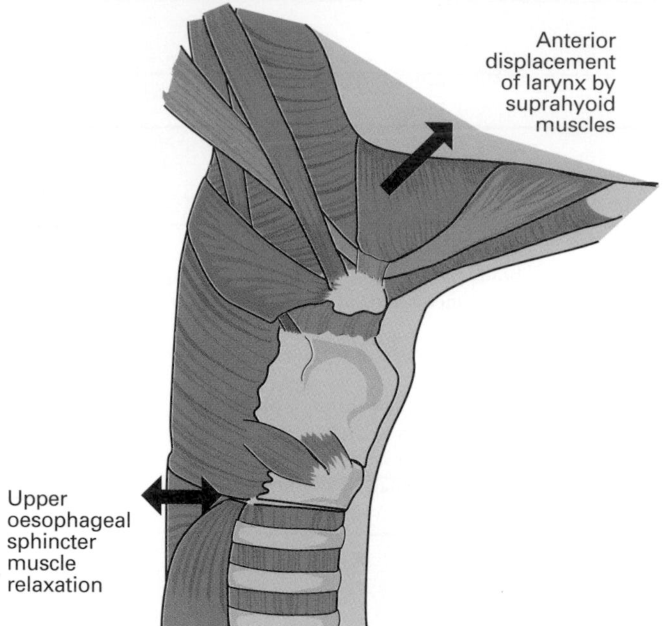

Fig. 1 Opening of the upper oesophageal sphincter requires relaxation of the upper oesophageal muscles and anterior displacement of the larynx by contraction of the suprahyoid muscles.

into proper position. Tongue dysfunction may be due to either tethering of the tongue or decreased tongue movement. Many patients have a inco-ordination of the normal anterior to posterior tongue motion. This inco-ordination can be a devastating problem because it leads to difficulty in initiating the pharyngeal phase of the swallow.

Pharyngeal phase dysfunction

In the pharyngeal phase, limitation in palatal motion leads to nasal regurgitation of the bolus. A frequent abnormality is decreased propulsion of the bolus by the pharynx. This response may be secondary to poor function of the tongue, decreased pharyngeal constrictor muscle activity, or dysfunction in opening of the upper oesophageal sphincter. Decreased laryngeal elevation may compromise the opening of the upper oesophageal sphincter or may result in poor laryngeal protection due to reduced epiglottic deflection or because the larynx is not positioned properly under the base of the tongue. Failure of the vocal cords to close during the swallow will also leave the larynx unprotected. Many patients have a delay in the onset of the pharyngeal phase of the swallow.

Aspiration

Aspiration is a symptom of dysphagia; it can result from dysfunction in either the oral or pharyngeal phases. Aspiration itself is divided into three components: that occurring before, during, or after the swallow. Aspiration before the swallow is caused by presentation of the bolus to the pharynx before the larynx has closed and elevated, probably because of either poor oral control, causing spillover of the bolus into the pharynx or delay in the onset of the pharyngeal phase of the swallow. Aspiration during a swallow occurs because of abnormalities in the pharyngeal phase such as poor laryngeal elevation or closure, or both. Aspiration after a swallow results from inability of the pharynx to clear the bolus during the pharyngeal phase. This leaves residue in the pharyngeal recesses that is subject to spillover into the pharynx at a time when the larynx is unprotected.

Factors contributing to dysphagia

Insertion of a tracheotomy tube exacerbates dysphagia by limiting laryngeal elevation and decreasing normal vocal fold reflexes. Hyposalivation makes it difficult to initiate a swallow. Radiation therapy often causes hyposalvation and may also lead to tissue oedema and fibrosis, affecting both the oral and pharyngeal phases of the swallow. The effect of medications on swallowing function is not well known, but drug therapy may play an important role in dysphagia.

HISTORY

A precise history is essential when evaluating a patient with dysphagia. The distinction between dysphagia and odynophagia must be made: odynophagia is pain on swallowing, and is often associated with either neoplasia or infection. The presence of referred pain, such as otalgia, may be caused by a hyopharyngeal lesion.

When a patient complains of dysphagia, specific symptoms must be known and the consistencies of food or liquid which exacerbate the symptom must be defined. Patients may describe a bolus as being 'stuck' or 'caught'. The location of this sensation and the kind of manoeuvre used by the patient to dislodge the bolus are all helpful points. Regurgitation of the bolus is common in patients with a major oesophageal obstruction.

Aspiration in a patient with normal laryngotracheal sensation causes coughing; the timing of this cough can help to indicate the timing of the aspiration. For example, patients with Zenker's diverticulum often aspirate anywhere from several minutes to some hours after the meal, when the contents of the filled diverticulum spill over into the unprotected pharynx. Nasal regurgitation and voice change may indicate problems with palatal and vocal cord function, respectively. Change in diet and weight loss can reflect the degree of severity of the swallowing abnormalities.

Because dysphagia is often associated with other systemic disorders, a thorough clinical history must be obtained. Neurological abnormalities such as change in mental status, dysarthria, and diplopia are all potentially relevant. Gastrointestinal symptoms might include dyspepsia or acid regurgitation. Rheumatological manifestations include diffuse muscle weakness or skin disorders. Psychosocial factors that may have either precipitated or exacerbated the dysphagia should be investigated.

PHYSICAL EXAMINATION

Physical examination should include the muscles of facial expression, tongue mobility and strength, and palatal elevation and sensation. The correlation between the gag reflex and dysphagia is not known and may not be clinically important. A full examination of the nasopharynx, hypopharynx, and larynx is important to determine whether there are any structural or neurological lesions.

VIDEOFLUOROSCOPY

Videofluoroscopy is a radiological technique used for evaluating dysphagia. The patient is seated in an upright position and given small quantities of barium in liquid, paste, and solid forms. A camera is focused on the oral and pharyngeal regions throughout the swallow, recording the images on videotape. If a swallowing abnormality is seen, various manoeuvres, such as change in bolus texture, head position, and breathing, are used to attempt to correct the abnormality.

The specific events evaluated during fluoroscopic examination include oral transit time, pharyngeal transit time, the presence and degree of residue in the pharyngeal recesses, the extent of laryngeal elevation, the presence and timing of aspiration, degree of upper oesophageal sphincter relaxation, the effect of various bolus textures and position on the swallow, and the integrity of cervical oesophageal peristalsis.

Swallowing videofluoroscopy is indicated for almost all symptomatic dysphagia patients who are able to co-operate to some degree. The small quantities of barium used carry minimal risks, even for a patient with gross aspiration. There have been no reported complications from this test. The test is also particularly helpful in any patient in whom aspiration is suspected, whether or not the patient is subjectively aware of the problem. Videofluoroscopy does not accurately demonstrate structural abnormalities, and subtle oesophageal abnormalities may be missed.

BARIUM SWALLOW

The barium swallow is a cineradiographic study of the oesophagus. Following administration of a large quantity of liquid barium to the supine patient, the fluoroscopy camera follows the bolus from the upper oesophageal sphincter to the lower oesophageal sphincter. Suspected reflux can be accentuated by procedures such as the Valsalva manoeuvre.

A barium swallow should be performed in any patient with odynophagia. If the laryngoscopic examination is normal, the barium study reveals the source of the odynophagia. If the laryngoscopy reveals any infection, such as candidiasis, or a tumour, the extent of oesophageal disease needs to be assessed. Any patient with dysphagia for solid foods should also undergo a barium swallow since a structural lesion may not be visualized on videofluoroscopy. A standard barium swallow is often used as one method for detecting gastro-oesophageal reflux. Patients whose symptoms localize to the lower neck or sternum are likely to have oesophageal disease and they should also undergo a barium swallow. Any unexplained dysphagia in a patient in whom a swallowing videofluoroscopy is normal should be further studied with a standard barium swallow.

ENDOSCOPY

Endoscopic examination performed under anaesthesia might include direct laryngoscopy, nasopharyngoscopy, oropharyngoscopy, oesophagoscopy, and bronchoscopy. In patients with head and neck cancer it is important to delineate the exact site of the lesion and also to rule out any other synchronous primary lesions. Flexible fibreoptic oesophageal endoscopy is indicated for patients with suspected oesophageal disease. Endoscopy may be combined with a dilatation in patients with a known stricture.

OTHER TECHNIQUES

Techniques such as scintigraphy, sonography, and electromyography are being developed and refined so that they may have more applicability in the clinical sphere.

DISORDERS ASSOCIATED WITH DYSPHAGIA

Many disorders can cause dysphagia (Table 4). Neurological deficits may be associated with cerebral vascular accidents, head trauma or cranial nerve neuropathies and often result in gross swallowing inco-ordination. Muscular disorders such as polymyositis can affect the laryngopharyngeal musculature, resulting in severely reduced ability to propel a bolus. Oculopharyngeal muscular dystrophy is a rare genetic disorder which affects people of French Canadian descent. The two symptoms, bilateral ptosis and dysphagia, usually present after age 50. There is progressively poor bolus propulsion and aspiration.

Table 4 Disorders associated with dysphagia

Neurological:	CVA, trauma, Parkinson's disease, amyotrophic lateral sclerosis (ALS), myasthenia gravis, multiple sclerosis (MS), cerebral palsy, Huntington's chorea
Muscular:	oculopharyngeal muscular dystrophy, connective tissue disease
Co-ordination:	cricopharyngeal achalasia, Zenker's diverticulum
Structural:	neoplasia, strictures, webs, rings, laryngopharyngeal or oral resections

Zenker's diverticulum is an outpouching of the pharynx, usually between the upper border of the cricopharyngeus muscle and the lower border of the inferior constrictor muscle (Fig. 2). Dysfunc-

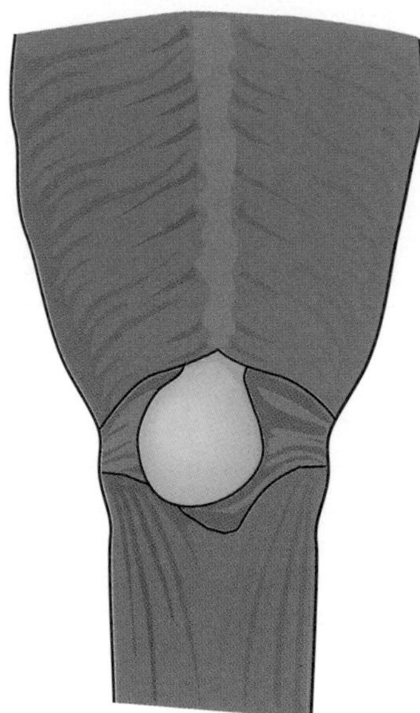

Fig. 2 Zenker's diverticulum. Most common location is between the upper border of the cricopharyngeus and the lower border of the inferior constrictor.

creased relaxation, may contribute to its aetiology. In this condition, the food bolus collects in the diverticulum, and spills over into the unprotected larynx, causing aspiration. Cricopharyngeal achalasia is a rare entity defined as isolated incomplete relaxation of the cricopharyngeus muscle without disfunction of the other pharyngeal constrictor muscles (Fig. 3). Structural lesions, such as oesophageal webs, rings, or strictures, often cause solid food dysphagia.

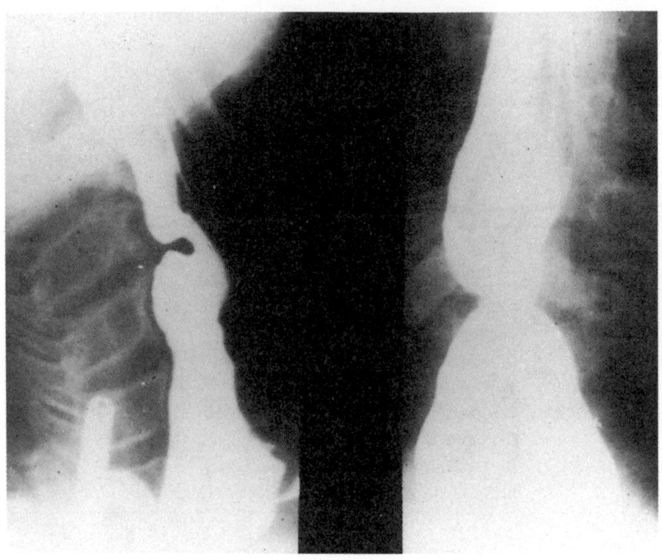

Fig. 3 Prominence of the cricopharyngeal muscle seen on anterior–posterior and lateral views of barium swallow.

Treatment

Dysphagia is sometimes relieved by treating the underlying disorder with specific drugs. For example, Parkinson's disease may respond to Sinemet and polymyositis may respond to oral steroids. Oesophageal lesions such as strictures or webs are treated by dilatation.

The indications for upper oesophageal sphincterotomy (often called a cricopharyngeal myotomy) are unclear. Isolated cricopharyngeal achalasia and oculopharyngeal muscular dystrophy respond well to a sphincterotomy; for achalasia occurring in conjunction with diffuse pharyngeal dysfunction, however, the benefit of a myotomy is questionable. Of the several surgical approaches to Zenker's diverticulum, the most frequently performed is diverticulectomy through a left lateral cervical incision. A myotomy should always be performed concurrently or the diverticulum is likely to öccur.

Patients with disorders that do not respond to medication or surgery may benefit by 'swallowing therapy'. After the swallowing abnormalities are identified on videofluoroscopy various manoeuvres are tried to see which facilitates the most nearly normal swallow; for example, patients with a supraglottic laryngectomy, who often aspirate postoperatively, must be taught a 'supraglottic swallow', which involves flexing the neck, holding the breath on inspiration, swallowing, coughing, and then exhaling.

If none of the above treatment options results in the ability to swallow without aspiration and to maintain nutritional status, the patient requires a non-oral feeding route, such as a gastrostomy tube or a jejunostomy tube.

FURTHER READING

Logman J. *Evaluation and treatment of swallowing disorders*. San Diego: College-Hill Press, Inc., 1983.

McConnel FMS. Analysis of pressure generation and bolus transit during pharyngeal swallowing. *Laryngoscope*, 1988; **98**: 71–8.

Shapiro J, Goyal R. Disorders of the upper esophageal sphincter. In: Fried MP, ed. *The larynx*. Boston: Little Brown and Co., 1988: 293–317.

Sokol EM, Heitman P, Wolfe BS. Simultaneous cineradiographic and manometric study of the pharynx, hypopharynx and cervical esophagus. *Gastroenterology*, 1966; **51**: 960–74.

14.2 Perforation, Boerhaave's syndrome, and Mallory-Weiss syndrome

LUC A. MICHEL AND JEAN-MARIE COLLARD

INTRODUCTION

Oesophageal perforation can be caused by external trauma or any instrument, device, or foreign body reaching the hypopharynx.

Laceration and rupture of the lower oesophagus or the gastro-oesophageal junction are also associated with forceful or prolonged emesis. Since the original description of Boerhaave, the term 'spontaneous' rupture of the oesophagus has been used almost routinely in the literature to include all perforations involving the entire thickness of the oesophageal wall and associated with emesis. Mallory and Weiss described another syndrome of acute postemetic lacerations of the gastric cardia as a source of major haemorrhage following an alcoholic debauch. The decision for surgical or non-surgical management of oesophageal perforation from any aetiology remains difficult.

AETIOLOGY AND PATHOPHYSIOLOGY OF OESOPHAGEAL PERFORATION

Iatrogenic perforation

Because perforations occur during oesophagoscopy, gastroscopy, and oesophageal dilatation, frequent contemporary use of upper gastrointestinal fibreoptic endoscopy has increased the actual number of perforations. The most common area of perforation from an endoscopic examination is the region of the crico-pharyngeus muscle. The perforation rate of 0.11 per cent in a 1988 survey of 35 412 endoscopic examinations is unchanged by comparison with the 0.13 per cent rate reported in a 1974 survey of 211 410 endoscopic examinations.

Dilatation of the oesophagus carries a risk of perforation because it is usually performed for relief of stricture resulting from reflux oesophagitis, postoperative stenosis, or achalasia. Even bouginage under endoscopic control gives a false sense of security, as perforation can occur without the operator's knowledge when the bougie is pushed ahead of the endoscope. Early dilatation after a caustic burn may also predispose to perforation because it is performed through friable tissues.

Forceful hydrostatic or pneumatic dilatation for achalasia carries a 4 per cent incidence of oesophageal perforation with mediastinal sepsis versus only a 1 per cent incidence after oesophagomyotomy. Dilatation with semiflexible bougies (Eder–Puestow or Savary type bougies), which have a hollow centre and can be threaded on to an endoscopically inserted guide wire, or with mercury filled bougies is even less dangerous (<0.5 per cent) and does not have to be performed under fluoroscopy. To obtain an upper gastrointestinal series before endoscopy or dilatation is, however, a wise step if the patient has an history of dysphagia, regurgitation, reflux oesophagitis, or previous oesophageal surgery.

Celestin plastic tubes passed transorally through an unresectable carcinoma of the oesophagus as a palliative procedure have also been incriminated in iatrogenic perforation. Sengstaken–Blakemore tubes and Linton tubes for tamponade of oesophageal varices can cause oesophageal disruption when they are kept inflated too long or when an agitated patient extracts them while they are still inflated. Oesophageal perforation occurs also after sclerotherapy (either by puncture of needle or necrosis from sclerosant) for variceal haemorrhage, and endoscopic laser therapy of advanced oesophageal carcinomas.

Traumatic endotracheal intubation usually perforates the oesophagus just below the cricopharyngeus muscle, generally in the dorsal midline at an area of weakness where the mucosa is supported only by fascia (Lannier's triangle). Para-oesophageal operations such as hiatal hernia repair, vagotomy, and radical pneumonectomy are also responsible for oesophageal perforation. Simple monitoring devices such as the oesophageal stethoscope or the oesophageal obturator airway included in some cardio-pulmonary resuscitation kits have caused oesophageal perforation.

Boerhaave's syndrome

Patients with postemetic spontaneous perforations of the oesophagus are properly classified as examples of Boerhaave's syndrome. The adjective 'spontaneous' does not imply the absence of predisposing factors or of underlying oesophageal disease; rather this term means perforation not resulting from iatrogenic trauma, foreign body, or direct external trauma. Spontaneous rupture of the oesophagus and acute postemetic lacerations of the gastric cardia (Mallory–Weiss syndrome) are probably related, since vomiting causes both syndromes. The precise physical and clinical conditions that are prerequisites for rupture or laceration are often unknown, however. Perhaps the lack of muscularis mucosa in the wall of the lower oesophagus may be one anatomical explanation.

Oesophageal perforation caused by foreign bodies

Jackson and Jackson reported the classic account of 2733 foreign bodies lodged in the oesophagus; of these 526 were bones and 535 coins. The frequency of bones is not surprising as they can be present in food. In adults, the wearing of artificial dentures may inhibit feeling an object before swallowing and can be the indirect cause of swallowing or inhaling a foreign body. Pieces of artificial denture may also be swallowed. Endoscopic removal of the foreign body should be performed under general anaesthesia, especially in the paediatric age group. Severe perforations can be caused by attempted removal of foreign bodies, either by a poorly trained endoscopist or by one who tries to push the foreign body ahead of the endoscope into the stomach too vigorously. Whenever possible, a duplicate of the foreign body should be obtained in order to select accurately the proper endoscope and forceps to use. The duplicate can also afford an opportunity to study possible presentations of the object in the oesophageal lumen. Considering the elasticity of a normal oesophagus, the surgeon faced with impaction of a smooth foreign body should suspect a pre-existing oesophageal stricture.

External trauma

Because of the protected location of the oesophagus, penetrating injuries are rare and are generally associated with injuries to other surrounding structures. In a 1979 review of 125 consecutive penetrating wounds of the chest (54 per cent stab wounds and 46 per cent gunshot wounds) oesophageal perforation was disclosed at early thoracotomy in only three cases. Reference to earlier series shows that penetrating wounds of the thoracic oesophagus carry a mortality of 47 to 57 per cent compared with 11 to 17 per cent for cervical oesophageal wounds.

DIAGNOSIS OF OESOPHAGEAL PERFORATION

Although 7 per cent of patients may be asymptomatic, oesophageal perforation usually causes severe thoracic pain, followed by fever, dysphagia, mediastinal and subcutaneous emphysema, and ultimately dyspnoea and systemic sepsis. Shock and empyema are more frequent after perforation of the thoracic oesophagus than after perforation of the cervical oesophagus. The presence of one or several of these symptoms or signs after clinical events such as oesophagogastric endoscopy, instrumentation, or insertion of tubes should lead to early diagnosis of oesophageal perforation (or at least to early suspicion of such a diagnosis).

As a rule, preoperative confirmatory evidence of oesophageal perforation should be obtained by chest radiography and a Gastrografin (meglucamine ditrizoate) swallow study, followed eventually by barium study if the Gastrografin swallow is negative. Computed tomographic scan of the mediastinum after contrast swallow is sometimes useful to visualize a tiny oesophageal perforation that has been missed by conventional radiographic study. A radiograph of the cervical spine is helpful in some patients suspected of having perforation of the cervical oesophagus. Air is often evident in the prevertebral tissue planes. A widened retropharyngeal space seen on a lateral cervical radiography (Fig. 1) or a computed tomographic scan (Fig. 2) due to an abcess, gives a definitive answer. The disappearance of normal cervical spinal lordosis and appreciable anterior displacement of the oesophagus and the upper airways are other useful diagnostic elements.

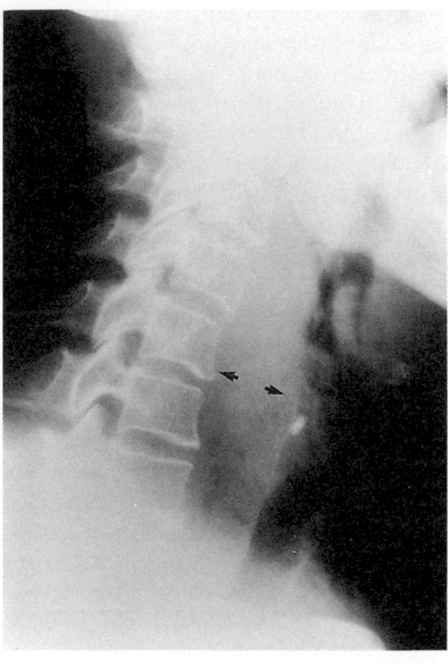

Fig. 1 Lateral radiograph of the neck showing a widened retropharyngeal space (black arrows).

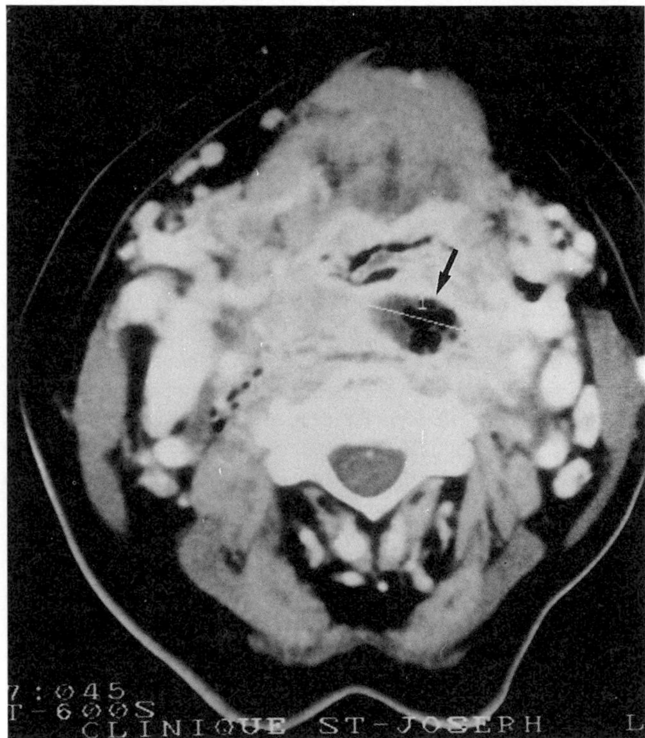

Fig. 2 Computed tomographic scan of the neck region showing a retropharyngeal abscess (black arrow) related to instrumental perforation of the cervical oesophagus.

To localize a radio-opaque foreign body, radiographs of the neck (anteroposterior and lateral views) should be made in hyperextension, since the normal position of the clavicular shadow hides the oesophageal inlet. Hyperextension of the neck raises the larynx and the oesophageal inlet, making them visible in the lateral projection. If the suspected object is not radio-opaque (the pull-tab of a drinks can is a frequent example in children), a contrast examination with thin barium solution is also indicated.

Widening of the superior mediastinum, cervical subcutaneous emphysema in a patient with a neck wound, and increased distance between the trachea and the vertebrae (prevertebral shadow) are the main radiographic signs of traumatic cervical oesophageal perforation. Widening of the entire mediastinum, mediastinal emphysema, and hydropneumothorax are the most common findings in thoracic oesophageal perforation (either iatrogenic or spontaneous). All patients who are seen with haematemesis or bloody drainage from the nasogastric tube following trauma to the chest should be studied promptly with Gastrografin oesophagography to ascertain the presence of perforation. All cervical wounds penetrating the platysma muscle should be explored to rule out oesophageal injury or injury to other cervical structures.

TREATMENT OF OESOPHAGEAL PERFORATION

Five modes of treatment are proposed: non-operative conservative treatment, drainage alone, suture repair of the perforation (supported or not by local tissue flap), early oesophagectomy, and oesophageal exclusion.

Conservative treatment

The non-operative approach can be attempted early after instrumental perforation occurring in a hospital environment with a patient in fasting conditions who has minimal systemic symptoms and no evidence of clinical sepsis. Such a conservative treatment includes massive antibiotic therapy (against aerobic and anaerobic bacteria), intravenous hydration, withdrawal of all oral intake, and eventually nasogastric drainage and total parenteral nutrition. However, in the early stage after an instrumental perforation of the cervical or thoracic oesophagus it is impossible to determine whether a tiny transmural perforation will lead to massive pleural contamination with subsequent shock and adult respiratory distress syndrome (or will remain contained within the mediastinum).

Operative treatment

Absolute indications for emergency operation are the presence of hydropneumothorax, pneumoperitoneum, empyema, systemic sepsis, shock, and adult respiratory distress syndrome. The surgical option (drainage alone, suture repair, oesophagectomy, oesophageal exclusion) depends on the site of injury (cervical, thoracic, or abdominal).

Cervical perforation

Suture and drainage by placement of Penrose or Jackson–Pratt drains are performed through an incision anterior to the sternocleidomastoid muscle.

Thoracic perforation

Simple pleural drainage or drainage through a paravertebral rib resection is sometimes indicated for the poorest surgical risks (elderly patients with several complicating factors, physical status corresponding to classes 4 and 5 in the classification of the American Society of Anesthesiologists). The mortality rate after simple drainage is 50 per cent; even in these difficult situations, we recommend early thoracotomy and closure of the perforation. However, releakage following suture repair continues to be the principal cause of postoperative morbidity and mortality. The degree of inflammatory change in the muscular wall of the oesophagus is such that layered closure may be impossible or technically unsatisfactory, especially when the diagnosis has been delayed. For this reason, the suture should be supported with a local tissue flap, including pericardium, diaphragm, intercostal muscles, and gastric wall (Fig. 3).

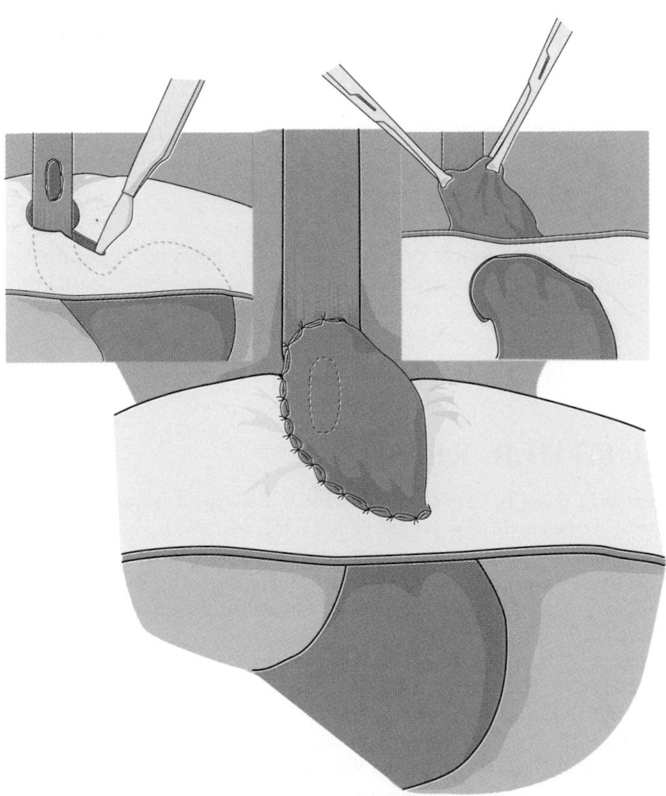

Fig. 3 Closure of oesophageal perforation supported with a local tissue flap made of stomach wall. The gastric fundus is applied over the perforation and sutured to the oesophagus wall.

Another simple way of dealing with the problem of delayed recognition of oesophageal perforation consists of flapping or wrapping a pedicled pleural flap (Fig. 4) on or around the oesophagus, suturing it firmly over the area of leakage and around its margin. This procedure has the virtue of permitting closure of the perforation and complete cleansing of the pleural space, with decortication of exudate from the lung surface and avoidance of a second operation. Drainage gastrostomy and sometimes feeding jejunostomy are performed concurrently.

Early oesophagectomy followed by re-establishment of gastrointestinal continuity by a left colon bypass or oesophagogastrostomy is indicated in the presence of obstructing lesions of the thoracic oesophagus (such as cancer, caustic burn with stricture, severe stricture related to hiatal hernia with reflux). In these situations, it is better to resect both the perforation and the original lesions, rather than to rely on repair and drainage alone. Oesophagectomy should be performed within a few hours after perforation: greater delay, and the presence of local and systemic infection, requires the resection to be made in badly contaminated tissues with potential risks to the anastomosis.

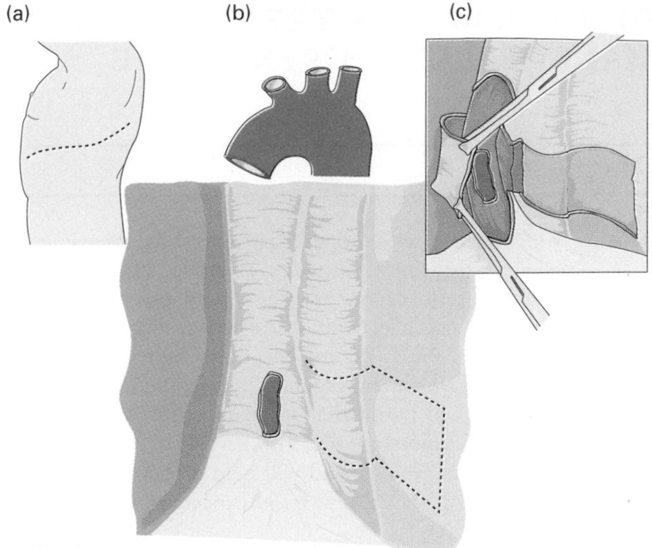

Fig. 4 Diagram of the pleural flap technique following late diagnosis of thoracic oesophagus perforation. Exposure through bed of left seventh rib. Pedicled pleural flap wrapped around the oesophagus and sutured over the area of perforation.

Exclusion–diversion of the oesophagus, when the diagnosis has been delayed or the primary treatment has failed, is the only way to control persistent mediastinal and pleural infection. The principle underlying exclusion–diversion has long been applied to the treatment of fistulae of other portions of the intestinal tract. For perforation of the thoracic oesophagus, the technique consists of suturing the oesophageal perforation, instituting mediastinal and pleural drainage, and placing an umbilical tape or a large ligature around the oesophagus above the cardia and deep to the vagus nerves. Temporary oesophageal exclusion using the stapling technique has also been described; a cartridge of the TA 55 stapler is applied to the oesophageal wall just above the cardia. Repermeation of the oesophagus can occur within 30 days following stapling.

Diversion of the upper oesophagus is then accomplished by cervical oesophagostomy. A gastrostomy is performed for feeding. At a time of election after healing of the perforation, a thoracotomy is performed and the oesophageal ligature above the cardia is removed. The cervical oesophagostomy is also closed.

Abdominal perforation

Perforation of the abdominal portion of the oesophagus generally occurs after vagotomy or hiatal hernia repair, and can be treated by primary suture repair and drainage of the upper abdomen. The suture of the perforation can be supported with a local tissue flap made of stomach wall (Fig. 3) as recommended for thoracic perforation.

DIAGNOSIS AND TREATMENT OF MALLORY–WEISS SYNDROME

Diagnosis

Patients who present with upper gastrointestinal bleeding and have a recent history of vomiting or retching, especially when associated with recent alcohol intake, should be endoscopically examined for presence of lacerations of the gastric cardia or the gastro-oesophageal junction, which are indicative of the Mallory–Weiss syndrome. Emergency endoscopic examination is mandatory in order to locate the site of bleeding accurately and assess its severity. Endoscopy will also reveal other synchronous upper gastrointestinal lesions, and will help direct the surgeon to the responsible lesion should a surgical procedure be required to control the haemorrhage.

Treatment

Bleeding from Mallory–Weiss lacerations is controllable by non-operative therapy in the majority of these patients. Resuscitative measures that should be carried out before and during the emergency endoscopic procedures include immediate assessment of the clinical and haemodynamic status, maintenance of intravascular volume, and gavage with ice water using a No. 36 F Ewald[R] tube. In many instances, bleeding from Mallory–Weiss lacerations is so minor that gavage with ice water controls the bleeding.

Balloon tamponade for the treatment of Mallory–Weiss syndrome is contraindicated, since the inflated balloon may cause tears in a gastric hiatal hernia, which is commonly found in patients with Mallory–Weiss Syndrome.

Ten units of vasopressin diluted in 10 ml of saline solution injected intravenously over a 10-min period will induce vasoconstriction if no coronary artery disease is evident. The vasopressin injection can be repeated at intervals of 1 to 2 h, or (preferably) a constant intravenous infusion of 0.3 to 0.4 units per minute can be started. However haemodynamic function and urine output must be monitored carefully, since tachyphylaxis and an antidiuretic effect can develop.

Indications for the surgical treatment of Mallory–Weiss syndrome are decreasing, and no definite study has demonstrated the value of one surgical procedure over another. The surgical technique generally used to control massive bleeding from a Mallory–Weiss laceration that remains refractory to all conservative measures is oversewing the lacerations with a running suture of 2–0 catgut through an anterior gastrotomy (Fig. 5). The best exposure is obtained through gastrostomy made in the middle one-third of the stomach and by using a large Deaver retractor while pulling upward on the nasogastric tube. This allows the cardia to be brought into view and exposes the folds at the oesophagogastric junction.

For lacerations that extend higher into the lower oesophagus, left thoracotomy may be necessary to expose the bleeding tears by opening the oesophagus. If unremitting haemorrhage from associated gastritis complicates the situation, truncal vagotomy should be coupled with a generous gastrectomy.

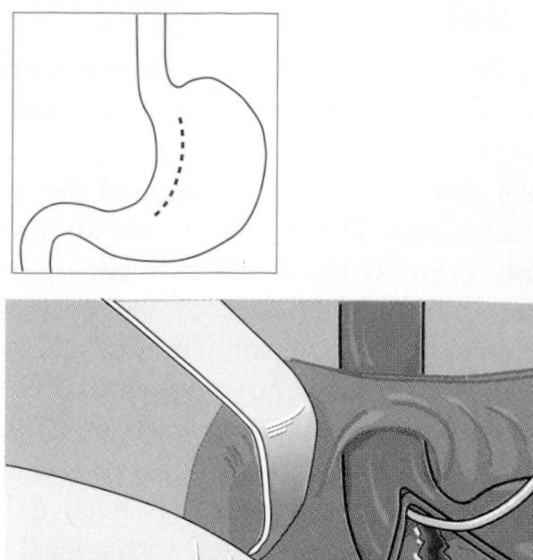

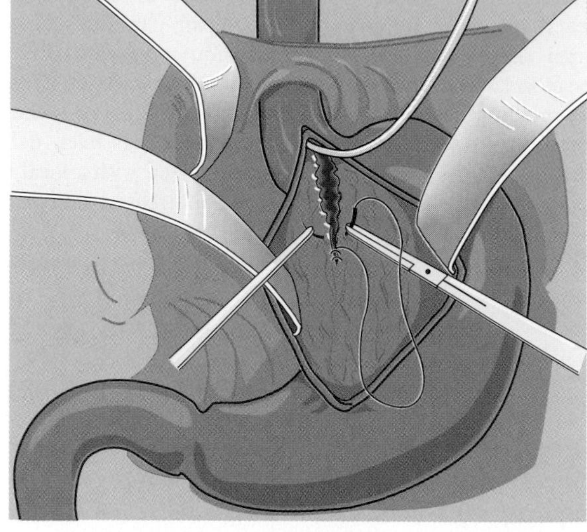

Fig. 5 Surgical treatment of Mallory–Weiss syndrome. Exposure obtained through a wide gastrostomy made in the middle one-third of the stomach. Deaver retractors used to visualize the lesions while the nasogastric tube unfolds the oesophagogastric junction.

FURTHER READING

Ancona E, Gayet B. Esophageal perforations. Etiology, diagnosis, localization and symptoms. In: Siewert JR, Hölsher AH, eds. *Diseases of the esophagus. Pathophysiology, diagnosis, conservative and surgical treatment*. Berlin: Springer Verlag, 1988: 1327–30.

Baue AE. Bleeding from lacerations of the cardia: the Mallory–Weiss syndrome. *JAMA* 1963; **184**: 325–8.

Caamano A, Dumon JF, Meric B, Noirclerc MJ. Foreign bodies in the esophagus. In: Jamieson GG, ed. *Surgery of the esophagus*. New York: Churchill Livingstone, 1988: 383–6.

Cameron JL, *et al*. Selective nonoperative management of contained intrathoracic esophageal disruptions. *Ann Thoracic Surg* 1979; **27**: 404–8.

Conn HO. Hazards attending the use of esophageal tamponade. *N Engl J Med* 1958; **259**: 701–7.

Gouge TH, Depan HJ, Spencer FC. Experience with Grillo pleural wrap procedure in 18 patients with perforation of the thoracic esophagus. *Ann Surg* 1989; **209**: 612–17.

Grillo HC, Wilkins EW, Michel LA, Malt RA. Esophageal perforation. The syndrome and its management. In: De Meester TR, Skinner DB, eds. *Esophageal disorders. Pathophysiology and Therapy*. New York: Raven Press 1985: 493–9.

Hankins, JR, *et al*. Palliation of esophageal carcinoma with intraluminal tubes: experience with 30 patients. *Ann Thoracic Surg* 1979; **28**: 224–9.

Hendren WH, Henderson BM. Immediate esophagectomy for instrumental perforation of the thoracic esophagus. *Ann Surg* 1968; **168**: 906–1003.

Herman B, Reiter JJ, Manegold BC, Barth H, Schoorn HD. Endoscopic perforation of the esophagus. Treatment and results. In: Siewert JR, Hölsher AH, eds. *Diseases of the esophagus. Pathophysiology, diagnosis, conservative and surgical treatment*. Berlin: Springer Verlag, 1988: 1340–1.

Jara FM. Diaphragmatic pedicle flap for treatment of Boerhaave's syndrome. *J Thoracic Cardiovasc Surg* 1979; **78**: 931–3.

Johnson J, Schwegman CW, MacVaugh H. Early esophagogastrostomy in the treatment of iatrogenic perforation of the distal esophagus. *J Thoracic Cardiovasc Surg* 1968; **55**: 24–9.

Kassels SJ, Robinson WA, O'Bara KJ. Esophageal perforation associated with the esophageal obturator airway. *Crit Care Med* 1980; 8: 386–7.

Kuwano H, Matsumata T, Adachi E, Ohno S, Matsuda H, Mori M, Sugimachi K. Lack of muscularis mucosa and the occurrence of Boerhaave's syndrome. *Am J Surg* 1988; **158**: 419–22.

Loop F, Groves LK. Esophageal perforations (collective review). *Ann Thoracic Surg* 1970; **10**: 571–87.

Michel LA, Grillo HC, Malt RA. Operative and nonoperative management of esophageal perforations. *Ann Surg* 1981; **194**: 57–63.

Michel LA, Serrano A, Malt RA. Mallory–Weiss Syndrome. Evolution of diagnostic and therapeutic patterns over two decades. *Ann Surg* 1980; **192**: 716–21.

Okike N, *et al.* Esophagomyotomy versus forceful dilation for achalasia of the esophagus: results in 899 patients. *Ann Thoracic Surg* 1979; **28**: 119–23.

Oparah SS, Mandal AK. Operative management of penetrating wound of the chest in civilian practice: review of indications in 125 consecutive patients. *J Thoracic Cardiovasc Surg* 1979; **77**: 162–8.

Silvis SE, Nebel O, Rogers G, *el al.* Endoscopic complications: results of the 1974 American Society for Gastrointestinal Endoscopy survey. *JAMA* 1976; **235**: 928–30.

Skinner DB, Belsey RH. Surgical management of esophageal reflux and hiatus hernia: long-term results with 1030 patients. *J Thoracic Cardiovasc Surg* 1967; **53**: 33–9.

Soderlund C, Wiechel KL. Oesophageal perforation after sclerotherapy for variceal haemorrhage. *Acta Chir Scand* 1983; **149**: 491–5.

Thal AP, Hatafuka T. Improved operation for esophageal rupture. *JAMA* 1964; **188**: 826–8.

Urschel HC, *et al.* Improved management of esophageal perforation: exclusion and diversion in continuity. *Ann Surg* 1974; **179**: 587–91.

Wirthlin LS, Malt RA. Accidents of vagotomy. *Surg Gynecol Obstet* 1972; 135: 913–16.

Wirthlin LS, VanUrk H, Malt RB, Malt RA. Predictors of surgical mortality in patients with cirrhosis and nonvariceal gastroduodenal bleeding. *Surg Gynecol Obstet* 1974; **139**: 65–8.

14.3.1 Reflux disease and hiatal hernias

MICHAEL G. W. KETTLEWELL

Disorders of the oesophageal hiatus cause considerable morbidity ranging from that of an intermittent nuisance to serious disabling disease. Diagnosis is often difficult and treatment mostly medical. Surgical treatment must be judicious and carefully selected to be effective.

ANATOMY

The oesophagus is a muscular tube connecting the pharynx and the stomach and traversing the posterior mediastinum. The lining is normally squamous epithelium which is surrounded first by circular and then longitudinal smooth muscle. The whole lies in the loose connective tissue of the posterior mediastinum. The vagal plexus is closely attached to the oesophagus and coalesces on the distal third to form the anterior and posterior vagal trunks. The distal 4 to 6 cm of the oesophagus passes into the abdominal cavity through the crura of the left diaphragm just anterior to the aorta and posterior to the left lobe of the liver. Connective tissue to the right becomes the lesser omentum while that to the left forms the gastrophrenic ligament. The blood supply to the oesophagus in the neck is from the thyroid vessels while in the thorax the arterial supply is both directly from the aorta and from the bronchial arteries. Venous drainage is to the azygos system. The left gastric vessels supply the distal oesophagus. Lymphatic drainage is to peri-oesophageal nodes and thence to the thoracic duct which lies between the oesophagus and the vertebra column.

The nerve supply is autonomic via the vagus and the thoracic sympathetic chain. There are, therefore, cholinergic, adrenergic, and also nitrergic nerves, the last being crucial in relaxation of the distal oesophagus.

FUNCTIONAL PHYSIOLOGY

A bolus of food or fluid is propelled from the pharynx into the oesophagus. The larynx is raised, the epiglottis tilted posteriorly, and the cords are closed to prevent food entering the trachea. The superior oesophageal sphincter at the level of the cricoid cartilage relaxes to receive the bolus which is carried down the oesophagus by a peristaltic wave preceded by a wave of relaxation. Relaxation is mediated through nitrergic nerves while peristalsis is cholinergic (see also Section 14.1).

The pressure within the thoracic oesophagus is negative with respect to the abdomen and reduces still further with each breath, yet food generally stays within the stomach once there. This is a function of the distal oesophageal high pressure zone. Manometric studies show a pressure inversion point between the abdomen and the thorax at the crura. The distal 3 cm of oesophagus have an even higher luminal pressure suggesting a functional sphincter even though there is no obvious anatomic structure. It is this high pressure zone in achalasia which is at a particularly high pressure and cannot relax because of loss of nitrergic nerves, possibly as the result of previous Herpes zoster infection. The functional integrity of the high pressure zone is important for continence between the stomach and the oesophagus. Continence is probably also enhanced by the obliquity of the cardia and its position distal to the apex of the gastric fundus creating a type of flutter valve. The fundus, when full and distended, also exerts some pressure upon the abdominal oesophagus. The diaphragmatic crura appear to play no part in gastro-oesophageal continence at rest but are important at moments of sudden rises in intra-abdominal pressure, for example during coughing and straining, when contraction of the diaphragm pinches the oesophagus tightly shut.

Absolute continence of the cardia would be disastrous since it is necessary to vomit and release gas from time to time. Selective incontinence is achieved by contracting the longitudinal muscle to shorten the oesophagus and open the angle at the cardia. Gas is then released by relaxation of the high pressure zone while vomiting is accompanied by vigorous reverse gastric peristalsis against a closed pylorus.

A number of substances affect the high pressure zone either enhancing the pressure or inducing relaxation (Table 1). Some may be important in normal physiological function or the pathophysiology of reflux disease, although some of the effects may be pharmacological.

Table 1 Factors affecting the high pressure zone

Increase pressure	Decrease pressure
Gastrin, pentagastrin	Anticholinergic drugs
Acetylcholine	Somatostatin
Histamine	Nicotine
Alkali	Acid
	Cholecystokinin

PATHOPHYSIOLOGY OF REFLUX

The most important disease state is caused by disorders of the oesophageal hiatus that produce pathological reflux of gastric contents into the distal oesophagus. Some reflux must be considered normal and therefore pathological reflux is defined as more reflux than the 95 per cent confidence limits for the normal population. Translated into numerical terms; reflux is pathological if the distal oesophageal lumen is at a pH below 4 for more than 4 per cent of a day or there are more than 10 reflux episodes per 24 h (see also Section 14.6). An acid reflux episode is defined as a drop in luminal pH below pH 4. The much rarer alkaline reflux of duodenal contents raises the pH above 7.5. Physiological reflux is rapidly cleared from the oesophagus back into the stomach by successive peristaltic waves until the pH is restored to 7. Prolonged exposure of the oesophagus to acid may be caused not only by frequent episodes of reflux but also by large volume reflux and defective oesophageal clearance, or a combination of all three.

Anatomic changes at the oesophageal hiatus such as a sliding hiatus hernia or resection of the distal oesophagus make incompetence of the continence mechanism more likely (Fig. 1). Obesity is a frequent concomitant of sliding hiatus hernias and may be aetiological by inducing a chronic rise in intra-abdominal pressure displacing the stomach in a cephalad direction into the thorax. Age is also important for reflux is commoner at either extremes of age. The gastro-oesophageal mechanism is not fully mature in infancy and becomes incompetent again in senescence. Furthermore, oesophageal peristalsis, and therefore clearance, is less efficient. In old age these defects are commonly accompanied by a hiatus hernia making pathological reflux even more likely. A hiatus hernia *per se* does not always induce reflux. Gastric emptying may also be slower than normal and therefore contribute to reflux.

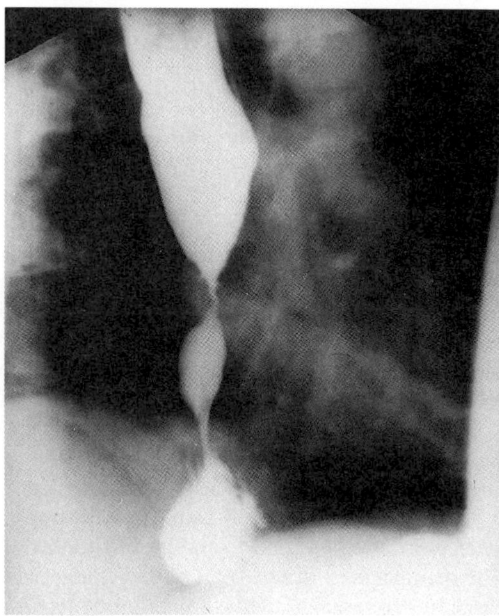

Fig. 1 Barium meal demonstrating a sliding hiatus hernia.

Reflux is both painful and damaging to the oesophagus. Gastric contents are corrosive and 'burn' the oesophageal squamous epithelium. Gastric and duodenal juices together are more destructive than either alone indicating that the damage is not purely pH dependent. The refluxate causes inflammation and loss of the squamous epithelium which, in severe cases, may produce deep chronic ulceration and/or peptic strictures. In some patients the oesophageal squamous epithelium is replaced by columnar metaplasia, the so-called Barrett's oesophagus, which has either gastric or intestinal characteristics. The oesophagitis is graded macroscopically from normal (grade 0) to grade 4 which is severe confluent oesophagitis with ulceration, stricture formation, or columnar metaplasia (Table 2). There is surprisingly poor correlation between the severity of inflammation and the symptoms although the severity of the oesophagitis is a combination of the corrosive content of the refluxate and the length of time of the exposure. Grade 4 oesophagitis therefore represents the most severe reflux, although it is not clear why some patients produce strictures and others a columnar-lined Barrett's oesophagus. The latter may represent a local change in epithelial cell differentiation induced by reflux but whether this is an idiosyncratic response, or one to a particular pattern of reflux, is not clear. Barrett's oesophagitis tends to occur in younger patients with severe daytime reflux while strictures usually form silently in elderly patients who tend to have nocturnal reflux and diminished oesophageal clearing. Such patients present with dysphagia and seldom complain of reflux or heartburn.

Table 2 Grading oesophagitis

Grade 0	Normal
Grade 1	Minimal oesophagitis
Grade 2	Streaky oesophagitis
Grade 3	Confluent oesophagitis
Grade 4	Ulceration
	Stricture
	Barrett's oesophagitis

An important complication of Barrett's oesophagitis is the propensity for developing adenocarcinoma within the columnar epithelium. The risk is about 1 per 100 patient years but the risk is greater in those patients with intestinal metaplasia. It is, therefore, sometimes suggested that the risk is sufficiently great to warrant endoscopic surveillance annually but the cost for each life saved is high.

Symptom complex

Retrosternal burning pain (heartburn) is the most common symptom of reflux. Mild symptoms are frequent, and almost normal, after meals, particularly if people stoop a lot soon after a heavy meal. Symptoms may however be severe, persistent, and unrelated to posture and may also be accompanied by acid brash (an acid taste in the mouth). Nocturnal reflux may be sufficiently painful to wake a patient from sleep and occasionally food may be regurgitated into the mouth. Such patients often complain of a foul taste in the mouth on waking. Nocturnal reflux may present in the elderly as recurrent respiratory tract infections as a result of frequent aspiration, and in rare cases reflux may be responsible for attacks of asthma in younger patients. Whether the asthma is caused by inhalation of acid gastric juice or is a reflex bronchospasm induced by acid in the distal oesophagus is uncertain. Odynophagia (painful swallowing) may also be a manifestation of oesophagitis and occasionally reflux may cause diffuse oesophageal spasm which produces severe crushing chest pain mimicking angina or a myocardial infarct.

Peptic strictures usually present in older patients with gradually progressive dysphagia, first for solids then liquids, but with surprisingly little weight loss and often no heartburn. In contrast, patients with carcinoma of the oesophagus usually present with rapidly progressive dysphagia and marked weight loss despite the brevity of the history.

Diagnosis (see also Section 14.6)

The history is the most important indication for the diagnosis which is confirmed by endoscopy (Table 3). This demonstrates the oesophagitis or the columnar transformation of the distal oesophageal mucosa (Figs. 2 and 3). A sliding hiatus hernia is often visible with the squamocolumnar junction of the oesophagus and the stomach at a variable distance above the crura of the diaphragm. When oesophagitis is absent but the history is strongly suggestive of reflux, 24-h oesophageal pH measurement may demonstrate pathological reflux and a temporal correlation between reflux episodes and the symptoms (Fig. 4). If the symptoms are atypical then an acid infusion test (Bernstein test) may help correlate the retrosternal pain with acid in the oesophagus. The test is positive when the patient consistently complains of pain when 0.1M hydrochloric acid is infused into the oesophagus and the pain reliably goes when the infusate is changed to saline.

Table 3 Diagnostic methods

First line	Second line
History	24-h pH recording
Endoscopy	Barium meal
	Acid infusion test
	Manometry
	Cineradiography
	Electrocardiogram

Rarely oesophageal manometry is helpful in the diagnosis of diffuse oesophageal spasm, produced by acid reflux, as a cause of non-cardiac chest pain and in the presence of a normal electrocardiogram and exercise test.

Barium contrast studies may demonstrate a hiatus hernia but are little value in the diagnosis of reflux. A barium swallow is, however, an important, non-invasive first investigation of dysphagia for three reasons: (a) to diagnose a pharyngeal pouch which

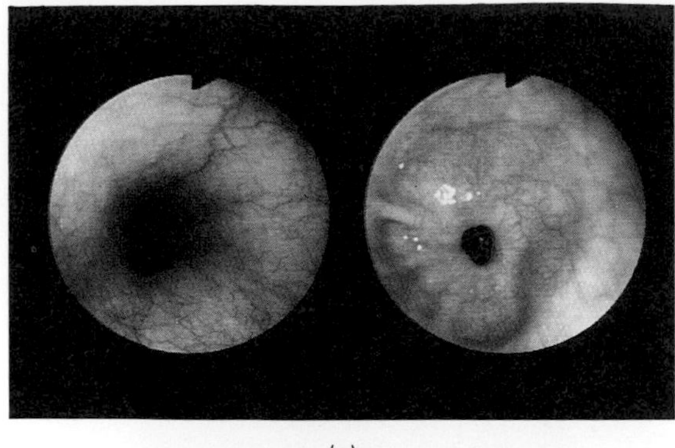

(a)

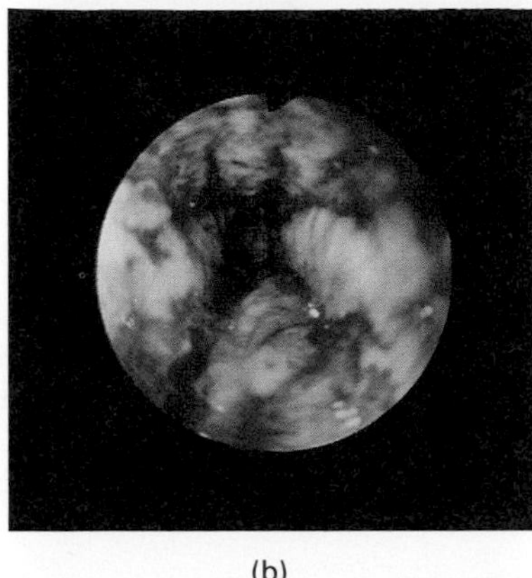

(b)

Fig. 2 (a) and (b) Endoscopic appearances of oesphagitis gráde 3.

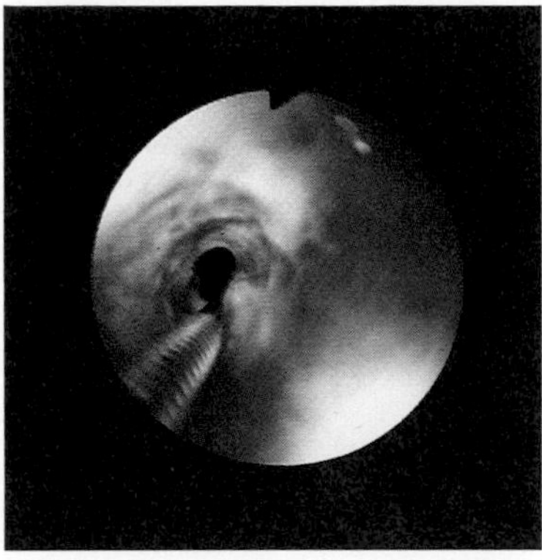

Fig. 3 Endoscopic appearances of a peptic oesophageal stricture.

is a hazard for the endoscopist; (b) to give an anatomical reference point should surgery be necessary; and (c) so that endoscopy can be arranged for a suitable occasion when dilatation or laser therapy is available. Cineradiography is, however, valuable in the diagnosis of dysphagia caused by neurological or pharyngeal muscular disorders, some of which may be secondary to pathological reflux.

Treatment

Initial management of reflux calls for the adaption of a number of important general corrective measures such as weight reduction;

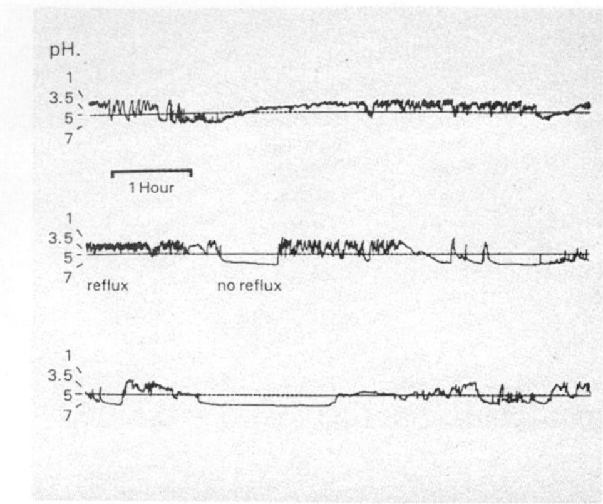

Fig. 4 An example of intra-oesophageal pH recording showing reflux episodes coinciding with symptoms of heartburn.

avoiding heavy meals just before retiring to bed or doing heavy work; stopping smoking; avoiding anticholinergic drugs and excess alcohol, and taking antacid alginates for relief of symptoms. Antacid alginates are better at providing relief than antacids alone because the alginate lines the oesophageal epithelium and provides added protection from contact with acid. These measures alone are sufficient for most patients with mild symptoms and an important adjunct for all patients with pathological reflux (Table 4).

Table 4 Treatment options

General
Weight reduction
Stop smoking
Dietary changes
Sleep propped up
Avoid stooping
Medical
Antacid alginates
H_2antagonist
Proton pump inhibitor
Prokinetic drugs
Surgical
Fundoplication
Antrectomy and Roux-en-Y

More severe symptoms and oesophagitis require more specific therapy such as acid suppression, initially with H_2 antagonists or if that is insufficient then a proton pump inhibitor, such as omeprazole or lansoprazole, which provides more complete acid suppression. Symptomatic volume reflux may persist even after adequate acid suppression and may require regular medication with a prokinetic drug such as metoclopramide, domperidone, or cisapride to enhance gastric emptying and oesophageal clearing.

Surgery is reserved for the few patients who remain severely symptomatic with proven reflux resistant to medical therapy or younger patients who require continuous long-term specific medication to control symptoms. For the latter patients there is some unease about prescribing drugs for a lifetime.

The essence of surgical management is to increase distal oesophageal pressure and prevent excess reflux while allowing physiological reflux. The majority of operations are performed through the abdomen and are based on the fundal wrap originally described by Nissen (Fig. 5). This operation is usually performed through a supraumbilical midline incision but laparoscopic techniques are now being developed and applied successfully. The oesophagus is mobilized from the hiatus and the stomach reduced into the abdomen if there is a hiatus hernia and the oesophagus is sufficiently long. The hiatus is narrowed by suturing the crura together to restore a normal anatomic size. The greater curve of the stomach is then mobilized by dividing the short gastric vessels and the fundus wrapped around the distal oesophagus. The stomach is sutured to itself around the oesophagus with about four stitches above the hepatic branches of the vagus nerve. The wrap is loosely fashioned over a 48 FG oesophageal bougie passed down the

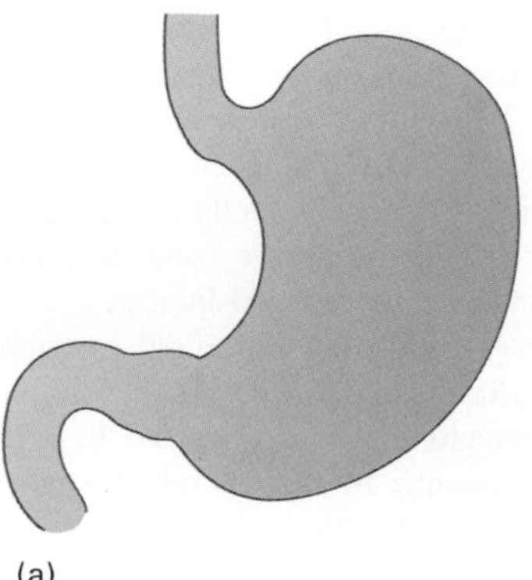

(a)

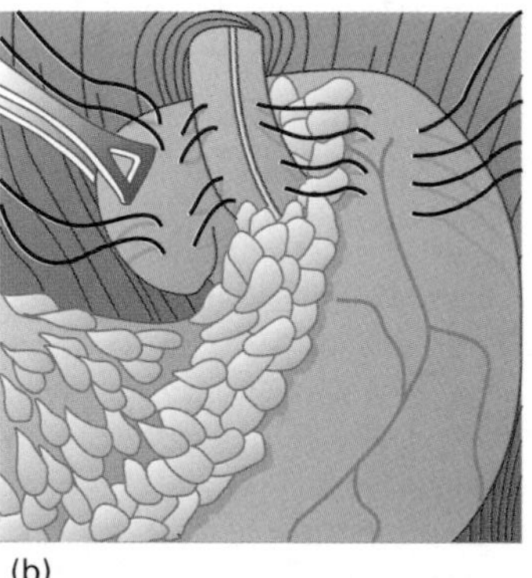

(b)

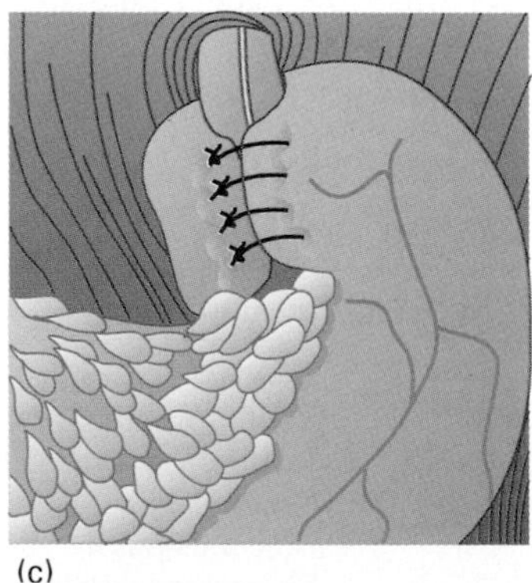

(c)

Fig. 5 Technical details of Nissen's fundoplication.

oesophagus and is only 2 cm long. Too tight a wrap produces marked and lasting dysphagia and too long a wrap induces gastric bloat by making the gastro-oesophageal junction too competent, so preventing belching or vomiting.

The Nissen fundoplication is a 360° fundal wrap. Numerous modifications have been expounded by surgeons, mainly varying the amount of wrap to as little as 180° around the distal oesophagus. In general the efficacy in preventing reflux increases with the circumference of the wrap as do the risks of gas bloat and dysphagia. If the oesophagus is substantially shortened a transthoracic approach is appropriate and either a Nissen fundoplication is fashioned within the chest or a Belsey operation performed (Fig. 6). Belsey's procedure invaginates the oesophagus into the fundus of the stomach, like an old-fashioned inkwell, and includes the diaphragm. In effect this operation produces a 270° wrap which is effective but is associated with the greater trauma of a thoracic incision.

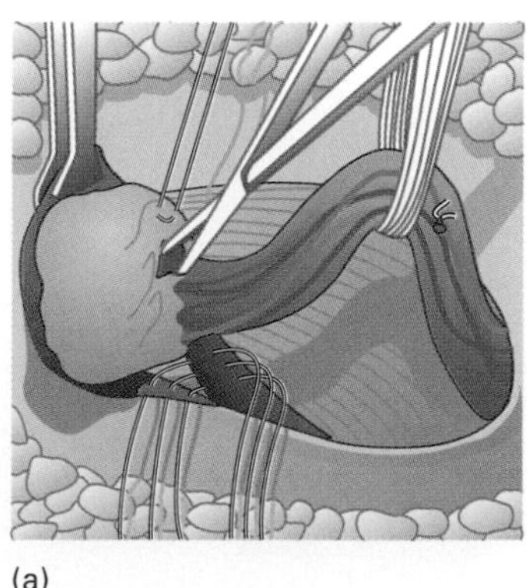

(a)

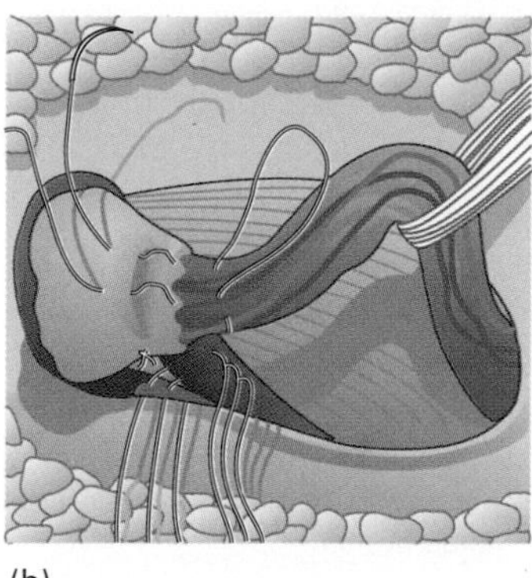

(b)

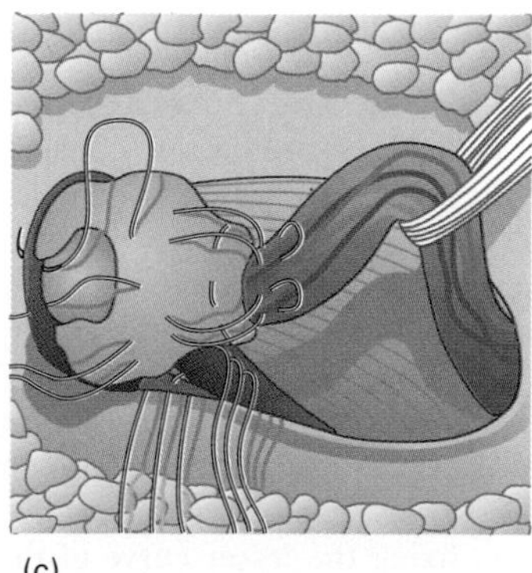

(c)

Fig. 6 Technical details of Belsey Mark 4 hiatus hernia repair.

A simple and novel operation to increase lower oesophageal pressure was devised by Angelchik in the United States. A silicone ring prosthesis, somewhat like a small doughnut, is tied around the abdominal oesophagus. The operation is quick easy and readily repeatable and although it is as effective in restoring the high pressure zone and controlling reflux as a well performed fundoplication, the greater long-term morbidity from migration of the prosthesis is unacceptable.

STRICTURES (see also Section 14.3.2)

The great majority of patients with peptic oesophageal strictures can be managed successfully by endoscopic dilatation under sedation followed by continuous treatment with a proton pump inhibitor. It appears that omeprazole therapy will reduce the need for and frequency of redilatation which is required, on average, every 15 to 18 months with simple antacid or H_2 antagonist therapy. Between one-third and one-half of the patients with strictures need only one dilatation but a small number, who have transmural fibrosis, restricture rapidly and require frequent dilatation or need to self dilate regularly using a mercury weighted bougie. Men with strictures respond significantly less well than women and relapse quicker and more frequently.

Some younger or fitter patients should have antireflux surgery after dilatation to prevent relapse or the need for continuous medical therapy. Rarely the strictures are so fibrotic and unyielding, and restenosis so rapid, that resection of the stricture is necessary.

'Bile' diversion by antrectomy and Roux-en-Y has been shown to be useful in some patients with intractable reflux and is advisable after resection of a stricture because a vagotomy is performed of necessity. Vagotomy produces gastric outlet obstruction which in turn needs gastric drainage, but a pyloroplasty would potentiate 'bile' reflux and therefore the Roux-en-Y is the best drainage procedure (Fig. 7). It is important to make the duodenojejunal anastomosis at least 45 cm distal to the gastrojejunostomy, or bile will reflux into the stomach and thence into the oesophagus.

PARA-OESOPHAGEAL HIATUS HERNIAS

Para-oesophageal or rolling hiatus hernias are less common than the sliding variety but are potentially more serious. The anatomic difference from the sliding hernias is that the distal oesophagus and cardia remain in their normal intra-abdominal position while the fundus and body of the stomach roll through the widened hiatus to lie in the posterior mediastinum, beside the oesophagus. In extreme cases the entire stomach and pylorus may lie within the chest (Fig. 8). The condition is fairly common in the old and very elderly and is often totally asymptomatic. Occasionally there is a combination of a rolling hernia with a sliding hernia.

Three serious problems may occur as a consequence of the stomach rotating into the chest.

1. Patients may suffer intermittent respiratory and cardiac embarrassment, particularly postprandially, because of pressure from a distended intrathoracic stomach.
2. Patients may get acute gastric dilatation or gastric volvulus and become acutely and seriously ill.

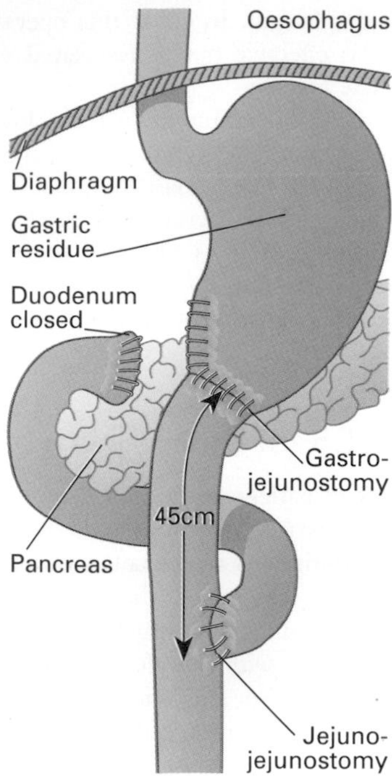

Fig. 7 Antrectomy with Roux-en-Y bile diversion.

3. Gastric ulceration is relatively common in rolling hernias and the ulcer may penetrate mediastinal structures such as the aorta or pericardium.

While most para-oesophageal hernias are usually asymptomatic and are diagnosed from chest radiographs taken for other reasons, some patients present with intermittent epigastric or chest pain, particularly after meals, accompanied by quite marked shortness of breath. Sometimes intermittent dysphagia or vomiting are the presenting symptoms. Sudden severe upper abdominal and chest pain with cyanosis and progressive cardiovascular collapse herald gastric volvulus or acute gastric dilatation. Because of the rotation and angulation of the stomach in these cases, vomiting is usually impossible and the stomach becomes progressively distended and ischaemic. The stomach may perforate as a consequence of the ischaemia but death may supervene earlier unless the patient is resuscitated rapidly and the stomach decompressed by passing a nasogastric tube or endoscope. Urgent surgical correction is also essential.

Rarely a patient may present with dyspepsia, or the complication of haematemesis and melaena, because of a gastric ulcer. If the ulcer erodes the aorta or left atrium the haemorrhage is catastrophic and rapidly fatal.

Diagnosis is usually by a plain anteroposterior chest radiograph which shows a large gastric bubble and fluid level behind the heart. Barium contrast studies may occasionally provide useful additional information (Fig. 9). Endoscopy is difficult because the stomach is full and rotated, and it is often impossible to get out of the stomach and into the duodenum. The endoscopic diagnosis is, therefore, usually gastric outflow obstruction rather than intrathoracic gastric volvulus because the endoscopist is seldom aware that everything is in the thorax. The endoscopist must also be careful to decompress the stomach at the end of the procedure lest the gas distension precipitates an acute gastric dilatation. Computed tomography is also diagnostic but has no advantages over a chest radiograph or a barium meal.

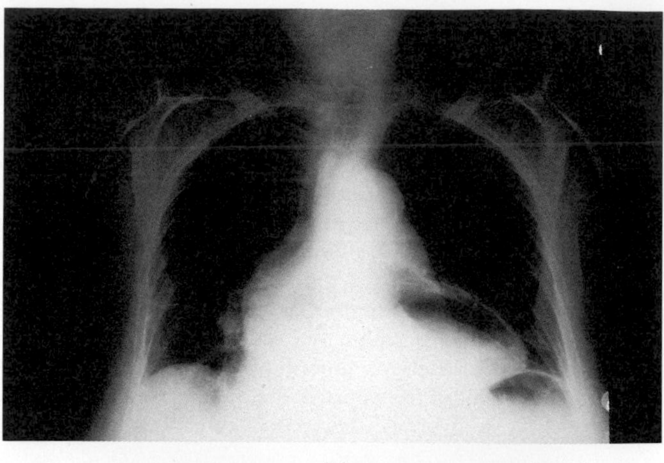

(a)

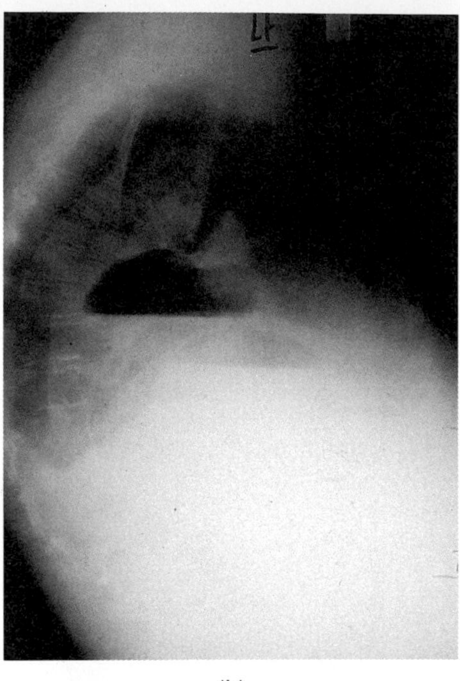

(b)

Fig. 8 (a) and (b) Chest radiographs demonstrating a large para-oesophageal hiatus hernia.

Treatment

Medical treatment is of no value. Surgical correction is necessary if the patient is disabled by symptoms or is acutely ill. Rapid fluid replacement, gastric decompression, oxygen therapy, and intravenous antibiotics are important preoperative measures for the acutely ill patient with gastric volvulus.

An elective operation in an old patient is usually best performed through an upper midline abdominal incision. The stomach can usually be reduced easily through the hiatus into the abdomen. The hernial sac is excised and the crura approximated, with non-absorbable sutures, to close the hiatus around the oesophagus. An anterior gastropexy, fixing the lesser curve of the stomach to the anterior abdominal wall with three or four sutures, prevents any possible recurrence. A posterior stapled gastroenterostomy pro-

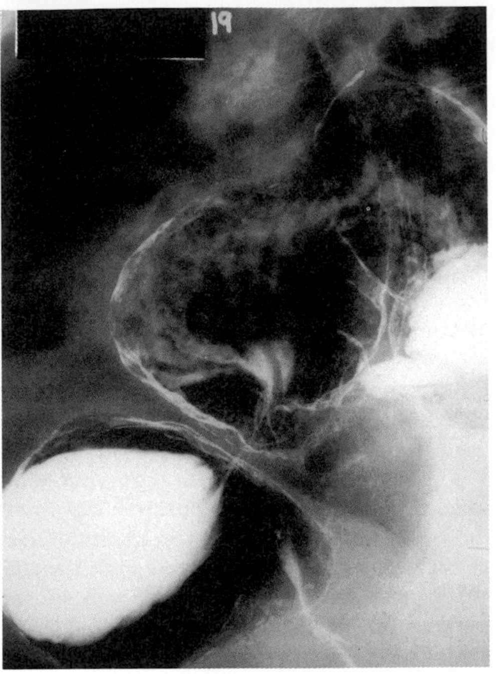

Fig. 9 Barium meal of a large para-oesophageal hernia.

vides alternative or additional fixation for the stomach and ensures adequate gastric drainage. A gastroenterostomy alone, which can be performed quickly and easily through a very small incision, may be quite sufficient for some frail patients.

It is dangerous to attempt to deliver the stomach from the thorax through an abdominal incision in acute cases or those with a penetrating peptic ulcer because of the risk of gastric rupture. For these cases a left thoracotomy through the 7th or 8th rib is the best approach and provides good access to decompress and mobilize the stomach. Peptic ulcers may be excised or a partial gastrectomy performed. The hiatus is then repaired after excising the hernial sac and returning the stomach into the abdomen. This operation is however much more traumatic for elderly or frail patients and carries a greater risk of complications.

FURTHER READING

Progress Symposium—gastro-esophageal reflux disease: surgical viewpoint. *World J Surg*, 1992; **16**: 287–363.

Dehn TCB. Surgery for uncomplicated gastrooesophageal reflux. *Gut*, 1992; **33**: 293–4.

DeMeester TR. Prolonged esophageal pH monitoring. In Read NW, ed. *Clinical Applications of Gastrointestinal Mortality*. London: Wrighton Biomedical Publishing, 1989.

Stoker DL, Williams JG. Alkaline reflux oesophagitis. *Gut*, 1991; **32**: 1090–2.

Ireland AC, Holloway RH, Toouli J, Dent J. Mechanisms underlying the antireflux action of fundoplication. *Gut*, 1993; **34**: 303–8.

14.3.2 Benign oesophageal strictures

BRYAN F. MEYERS AND JOHN C. WAIN

INTRODUCTION

Stricture is commonly the result of acute oesophagitis followed by chronic transmural oesophagitis and subsequent fibrosis. Reflux of gastric juices is responsible for 90 per cent of benign strictures of the oesophagus. Less frequent causes include infection, trauma, and congenital malformations (Table 1).

Table 1 Aetiology of benign oesophageal strictures

Gastro-oesophageal reflux
Postoperative (anastomotic)
Corrosive ingestion
Nasogastric tube trauma
Pill impactions
Moniliasis
Radiation therapy
Viral infections
Congenital
Miscellaneous

Painless dysphagia is the typical presenting symptom of oesophageal strictures. Diagnostic dilemmas are frequent because of the similarity in the signs, symptoms, and radiological findings for benign and malignant oesophageal disease. Once a benign stricture is diagnosed, treatment selection must be made from an array of medical and surgical therapies. With most reports identifying the mean age of a stricture patient as 75 years, appropriate treatment must weigh the benign nature of the disease against the symptomatic impairment, general health, and estimated longevity of the patient.

REFLUX STRICTURES

Reflux or peptic strictures are a complication of severe gastro-oesophageal reflux disease (Fig. 1). Three factors influence the severity of this process: a mechanically defective lower oesophageal sphincter, inefficient oesophageal clearance of refluxed acid, and abnormal gastric emptying resulting in an excess of acid available for reflux. Reflux strictures occur just above the squamocolumnar junction, the anatomical location of which varies depending on the presence or absence of Barrett's epithelium. Strictures may arise in 35 per cent of patients with Barrett's epithelium (Allison-Johnstone stricture) or may result from nighttime pooling of gastric acid below the cricopharyngeus muscle (cricopharyngeal web).

Peptic stricture does not occur in all cases of gastro-oesophageal reflux disease. Strictures arise in 10 per cent of adults treated for reflux symptoms and 12 per cent of paediatric patients having antireflux surgery. When stricture occurs during medical treatment of gastro-oesophageal reflux disease, it signifies failure

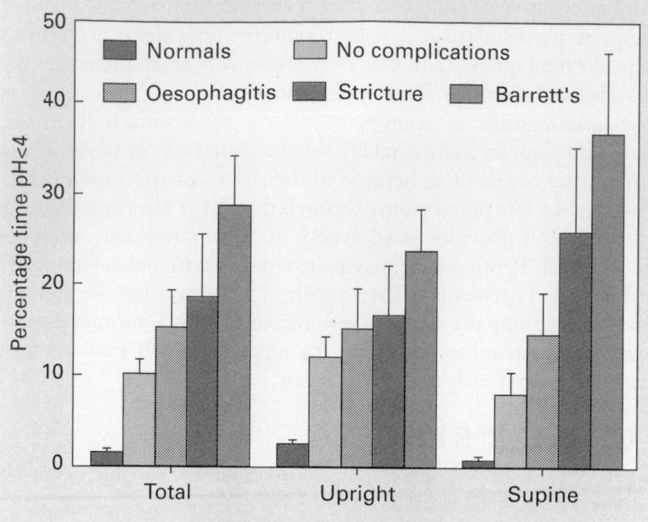

Fig. 1 Acid exposure in the distal oesophagus expressed as a percentage of total time and time in the upright and supine position in which pH was less than 4. Worsened reflux in stricture patients is consistent with the thesis that stricture occurs in an aggressive form of gastro-oesophageal reflux.

of conservative therapy. Symptoms of gastro-oesophageal reflux disease typically precede symptoms of stricture by months to years. The spontaneous resolution of previously severe reflux symptoms may signify the development of a stricture. However, 50 per cent of patients with reflux strictures may present themselves with only dysphagia and no prior history of reflux. In a small fraction of cases, adults enter urgently with an acute food bolus impaction.

The Schatzki–Inglefinger ring is a sharply defined fibrous narrowing of the distal oesophagus at the squamocolumnar junction, forming the proximal edge of a sliding hiatal hernia. The ring consists only of mucosa and submucosa and is well treated with bougie dilatation. Surgery is warranted only if intractable reflux becomes evident after dilatation.

Scleroderma may cause a particularly difficult reflux stricture. The fibrous replacement of oesophageal smooth muscle in scleroderma results both in inefficient oesophageal peristalsis and a decreased resting pressure of the lower oesophageal sphincter. Fewer than 50 per cent of patients with scleroderma-related strictures obtain relief when treated conservatively. Frequently, early resection and intestinal interposition are required.

NON-REFLUX STRICTURES

Infectious causes

Infections are rare causes of oesophageal stricture, but may be increasing because of the prevalence of immunosuppressed patients with the AIDS virus. *Candida albicans* is the most frequent pathogen, accounting for nearly half the cases. Also cited are infections with Herpes simplex virus (HSV) and cytomegalovirus (CMV), mucormycosis, histoplasmosis, and tuberculosis.

Initial treatment is directed at the underlying pathogen. Intravenous fluconazole and amphotericin have been recommended for severe candidal infections. Intravenous gancyclovir is advised for HSV or CMV infections. Additional treatment such as bougie dilatation should be delayed to allow resolution of the underlying infection. Dilatation may be unnecessary when acute inflammatory oedema mimics a stricture. Furthermore, the acute nature of these infections makes dilatation more dangerous. The oesophagus lacks the chronic thickening of peptic strictures and is more apt to rupture during dilatation. Exceptions to this rule are the strictures caused by mucormycosis, histoplasmosis, and tuberculosis. These strictures are less likely to respond to antimicrobial drugs or dilation and may require resectional therapy.

Trauma

Localized injury to the oesophagus can cause transmural inflammation, which results in stricture. Caustic burns from ingested alkali or acids are the most frequent examples of this class of stricture. Other causes include prolonged nasogastric intubation, radiation therapy, or pill impaction. Pill injuries are rare in patients with an otherwise normal oesophagus. The finding of such an injury should prompt a search for an underlying cause such as a neoplasm or a motility disorder. Old age and sustained release pills are additional risk factors for pill induced stricture. Potassium chloride and quinidine are the most common agents. Aspirin, ascorbic acid, phenytoin, and tetracycline have also been cited as causes.

An increasingly frequent problem is post-sclerotherapy stricture, reported in 4 to 50 per cent of patients who have received sclerotherapy for oesophageal varices. Studies reveal no evidence of gastro-oesophageal reflux disease in these cases. Fibrosis caused by the sclerosant is the most likely aetiology.

Congenital

Congenital causes for oesophageal stenosis such as oesophageal atresia and tracheo-oesophageal fistulae are most frequently identified in neonates and infants. Both of these developmental foregut abnormalities may result in late oesophageal stricture despite initial surgical correction. Tension at the repair site, subclinical anastomotic leaks, acid reflux, and abnormal distal oesophageal motility all predispose for perianastomotic stricture. A related problem is residual tracheobronchial remnants within the oesophagus after correction of congenital tracheo-oesophageal fistula. Surgical intervention is rarely required for anastomotic stricture but may be necessary for tracheobronchial remnants.

Oesophageal webs (thin fibrous membranes in the mid or upper oesophagus) are covered by normal squamous epithelium on both sides and are successfully treated with bougienage.

Miscellaneous causes

Rare systemic illnesses have been reported to cause oesophageal stricture including pemphigus, Stevens–Johnson syndrome, toxic epidermonecrolysis, Behçet's syndrome, chronic granulomatous disease of childhood, Crohn's disease, Plummer Vinson syndrome, and epidermolysis bullosa dystrophica recessive. Treatment consists of therapy of the underlying disease and gradual dilation. Resection with oesophageal replacement is required in rare cases in which the strictures do not respond to conservative therapy.

DIAGNOSTIC TESTS (see also Section 14.6)

The goals of diagnostic testing are to exclude malignancy, to assess the severity and aetiology of the stricture, and to search for associated underlying conditions. One of the first steps to evaluate the patient with dysphagia is to obtain a barium swallow. Barium oesophagography is a simple, inexpensive examination which can assess the diameter and length of the stenosis as well as provide clues to other causes of dysphagia. A hiatal hernia with free reflux to the level of a short distal oesophageal stricture suggests a diagnosis of peptic stricture. Strictures longer than 20 mm, 'apple core' lesions, upper or mid-oesophageal location, and the absence of reflux all raise the suspicion of neoplasm rather than stricture. In either case, the barium swallow serves as a guide to the subsequent endoscopic examination.

Endoscopic biopsy and cytological brushings are essential to exclude malignancy in the early assessment of oesophageal stricture. Endoscopy allows a careful assessment of the length and location of the stricture relative to the squamocolumnar junction, the gastro-oesophageal junction, and the diaphragmatic hiatus. Biopsy and brushings should be taken of the stenosis, and any oesophageal mucosa of abnormal appearance. Initial dilation of the stricture is generally performed at the time of endoscopy.

Pressure manometry is an important step in the evaluation of patients with stricture. Manometry can assess the status of the lower oesophageal sphincter and oesophageal motility. A low or normal lower oesophageal sphincter pressure is typical of gastro-oesophageal reflux disease. Manometry can also facilitate selection of operative therapy. Some authors rely on manometric indications (e.g. mean lower oesophageal sphincter pressure less than 6 mmHg, intra-abdominal length of the lower oesophageal sphincter less than 1 cm, and total length less than 2 cm) to select patients for surgery (Fig. 2). When poor distal motility is noted, a partial fundoplication (i.e. Belsey wrap) would be advised to avoid postoperative dysphagia. This is in contrast to the recommended use of a total fundoplication (i.e. a Nissen wrap) when motility is normal.

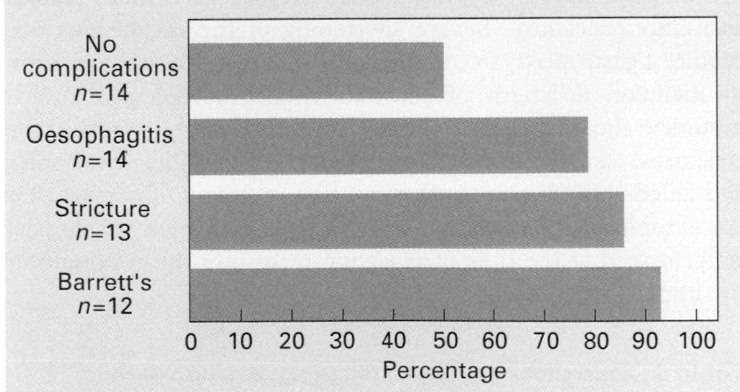

Fig. 2 Prevalence of a mechanically defective lower oesophageal sphincter, defined as a pressure of 6 mmHg or less, abdominal length shorter than 1 cm, overall length shorter than 2 cm, or any combination of these, in patients with progressive severity of oesophageal injury.

Oesophageal pH studies, typically 24-h continuous lower oesophageal pH monitoring, have high sensitivity and specificity for diagnosing gastro-oesophageal reflux disease as a cause of oesophageal stricture. It is important that such studies be performed after adequate dilatation of the stricture and temporary discontinuation of H_2-blocking medications.

CONSERVATIVE THERAPY

After a diagnosis of benign oesophageal stricture is made, most patients respond to a course of conservative therapy consisting of intensive medical treatment with concurrent dilation of the stricture.

Standard medical therapy for reflux stricture includes simple measures such as elevation of the head of bed, avoiding eating before bedtime, and the use of antacids. Histamine receptor antagonists (H_2-blockers) such as cimetidine, ranitidine, famotidine, and nizatidine are the mainstays of medical therapy. A 6-week course of H_2-blockers at standard dosages allows healing of oesophagitis and erosions in 50 to 75 per cent of patients. However, maintenance treatment with H_2-blockers has not been shown to prevent recurrence of oesophagitis.

Omeprazole is a potent sodium-potassium ATPase inhibitor that decreases acid production in the stomach. It is very effective against gastro-oesophageal reflux disease, with 75 to 95 per cent healing of oesophagitis at a daily dosing of 20 to 40 mg. Maintenance therapy, however, shows relapse rates of 11 to 26 per cent.

Metoclopramide, domperidone, and cisapride increase the lower oesophageal sphincter pressure and improve gastric emptying, correcting two factors responsible for gastro-oesophageal reflux disease. These agents may be used with H_2-receptor blockers or omeprazole for maximal medical therapy.

Intralesional steroid (triamcinolone acetate) has been used endoscopically to avoid resection of caustic and anastomotic strictures that have failed to improve with other medical therapy. However, controlled trials will be necessary to prove the safety and efficacy of this method.

DILATION THERAPY

Dilation plays an important role in stricture management. The primary therapeutic goal of dilation is to break up the fibrous stricture and improve dysphagia and alimentation. Dilatation is frequently required to allow endoscopic inspection and biopsy, manometry, and pH monitoring for diagnosis. When a stricture is non-dilatable, treatment requires stricture resection and oesophageal reconstruction.

Although clinical improvement in some patients may last months or years, objective results of dilation are transient, with manometric improvement lasting less than 12 weeks. Increases in lumen size after dilation are smaller than the subjective improvement in swallowing would suggest, a finding explained by the fact that forceful dilation disrupts the stricture but creates localized muscular spasm.

Many dilators are used for treating benign oesophageal strictures. Axial dilators, or bougies, forcefully break the fibrous stricture as they are passed from proximal to distal. Balloon dilators, on the other hand, are positioned through the stricture prior to inflation and exert a radial force (Fig. 3). No trials have shown a significant difference in the dilating capabilities of axial bougies and radial balloon dilators. Disposable balloon dilators are more expensive than reusable alternatives.

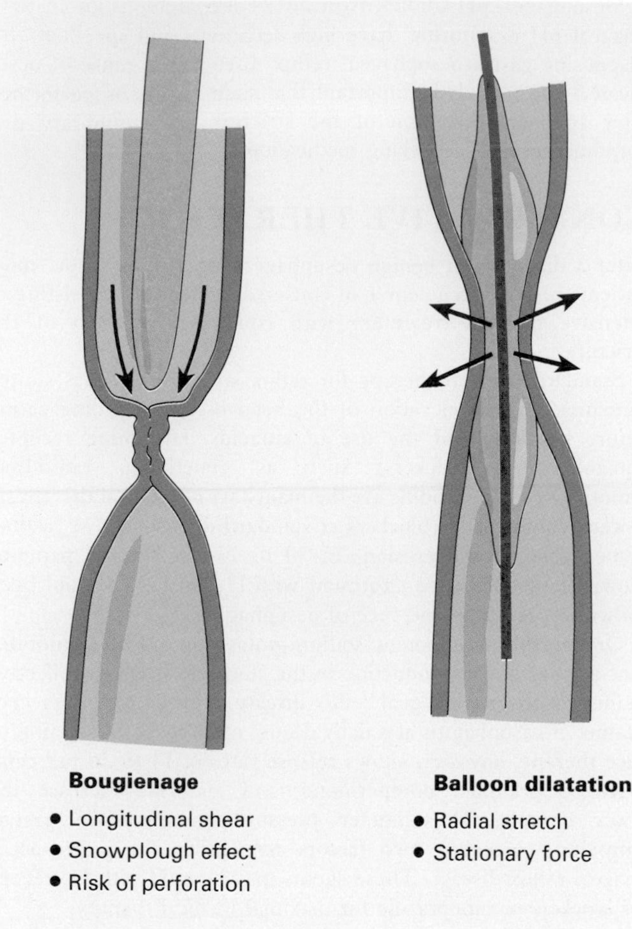

Fig. 3 Schematic representation of the different dilating forces generated by bougienage technique versus balloon dilation. Despite theoretical differences, no studies have definitively shown either method to be safer or more effective.

Maloney and Hurst dilators are mercury-filled rubber bougies that are easy, economical, and safe to use. The bougies are passed manually, with topical anaesthesia, but without fluoroscopic control; they are safe enough for selected patients to use them independently at home. Eder–Puestow dilators consist of a flexible guidewire which is passed through the stricture and over which a series of metal olives are passed. The Savary–Gilliard dilator resembles the Eder–Puestow bougie in that it consists of a spring-tipped guidewire over which tapered plastic bougies (6–17 mm diameter) are passed. Trials have described more effective and longer-lasting results when Eder–Puestow style dilators are compared with rubber bougies. Less frequently used axial dilators include the Tucker string-guided dilator which requires a gastrostomy, and Hegar dilators which may be used at laparotomy.

Balloon dilations are performed by positioning the proximal aspect of the balloon at the proximal limit of the stricture. The balloon is inflated to 35–60 mmHg and the inflation is held for 1 min. The use of balloon dilators may be better in selected short strictures. Examples include the Rigiflex TTS system, the Gruentzig balloon, and the Browne–McHardy pneumatic dilator.

RESULTS OF CONSERVATIVE THERAPY

The results of conservative treatment combining medications and dilation have been reported by numerous investigators. Overall, conservative therapy results in relief of dysphagia, satisfactory alimentation, and an infrequent need for maintenance dilations in 60 to 75 per cent of patients. In one large series, 46 per cent needed one dilation, while 75 per cent needed three or less to achieve long-term relief from dysphagia. Perforations occur in 1 per cent of procedures and in 3 per cent of patients over a prolonged course of dilations.

Patients receiving conservative therapy include a selected population of patients who would fare poorly with surgery because of their age or underlying conditions. Selecting non-surgical therapy means accepting the attendant risks of repeated dilations for an indefinite time. There is controversy regarding the appropriateness of prolonged conservative therapy, particularly for patients with Barrett's epithelium.

SURGICAL THERAPY

Surgical therapy for benign oesophageal strictures is reserved for the patient who fails to improve with conservative management or who suffers complications from dilations. Table 2 lists the indications for referring a patient with stricture to surgery. The choice of operation is best made with consideration of the ability to dilate the stricture preoperatively as well as knowledge of the propulsive force of the oesophagus and the degree of anatomical shortening that has occurred.

Table 2 Indications for surgery of benign stricture of the oesophagus

Non-dilatable strictures
Excessively frequent dilations (more than 1 per month)
Complications of dilations
Persistent reflux leading to recurrence
Physician preference

Commonly performed operations are listed in Table 3. In a patient with a dilatable stricture and minimal shortening of the oesophagus, a satisfactory result may be obtained by performing preoperative and intraoperative dilations together with a standard antireflux procedure. Severe shortening of the oesophagus may require a gastroplasty in conjunction with the antireflux procedure to maintain a length of intra-abdominal oesophagus and to minimize the chance of a slipped antireflux wrap. Non-dilatable strictures, severe primary oesophageal dysmotility syndromes, and failed antireflux procedures require resection of part or all of the oesophagus. Reconstruction with jejunum, colon, or stomach is performed at the time of resection to restore the continuity of the upper gastrointestinal tract.

Table 3 Operations performed for peptic stricture of the oesophagus

Dilation and antireflux procedure (Nissen, Belsey, Hill)
Collis gastroplasty and fundoplication (Belsey, Nissen)
Resection and interposition (jejunum or colon)
Resection and gastric pull-up

Non-resectional surgery

The first level of surgical intervention is dilation in conjunction with a standard antireflux procedure such as a Nissen, Belsey, or Hill repair. With some variations depending on the type of operation being performed, the gastro-oesophageal junction is placed intra-abdominally and may be wrapped with gastric fundus. (Figs. 4, 5, 6) These operations create good or excellent results in 70 to 85 per cent of patients with less morbidity and mortality than is seen with resection. Dilation and an antireflux procedure should be reserved for patients with abnormal 24-h oesophageal pH

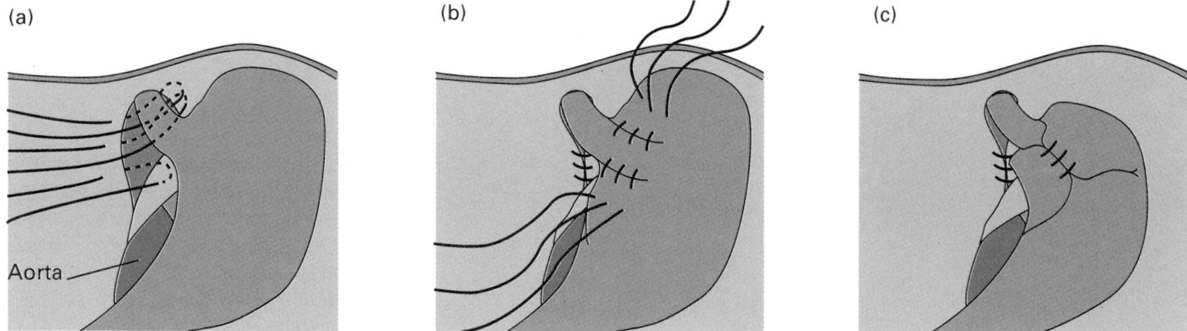

Fig. 4 The technique for performance of a Nissen fundoplication. The suture line is 2 to 3 cm in length. (a) The oesophagus and fundus have been mobilized and sutures placed in the oesophageal hiatus. (b) The hiatus is closed. The fundus has been rotated behind the oesophagus and the fundoplication sutures placed. (c) The completed fundoplication.

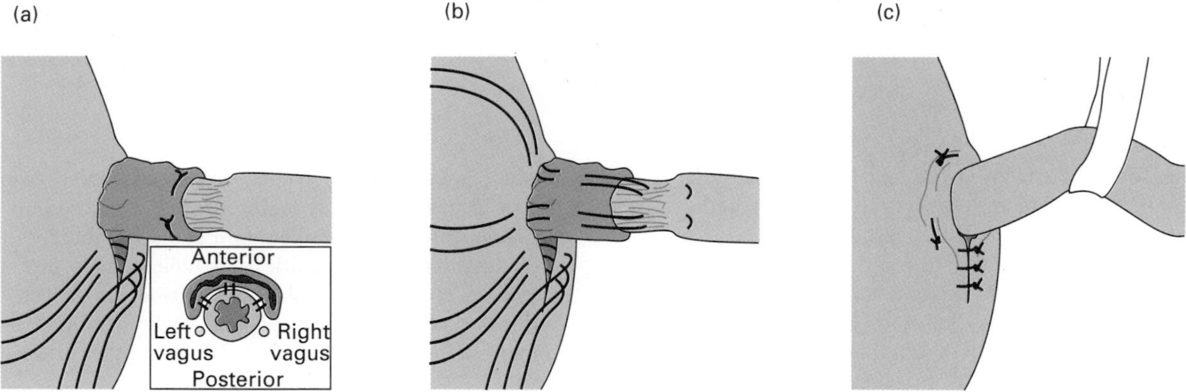

Fig. 5 The technique for performance of a Belsey fundoplication. (a) Through a left thoracotomy, sutures are placed in the hiatus and the first row of the fundoplication is complete. The inset shows the 240° wrap which is created. (b) The second row of sutures. (c) The final appearance.

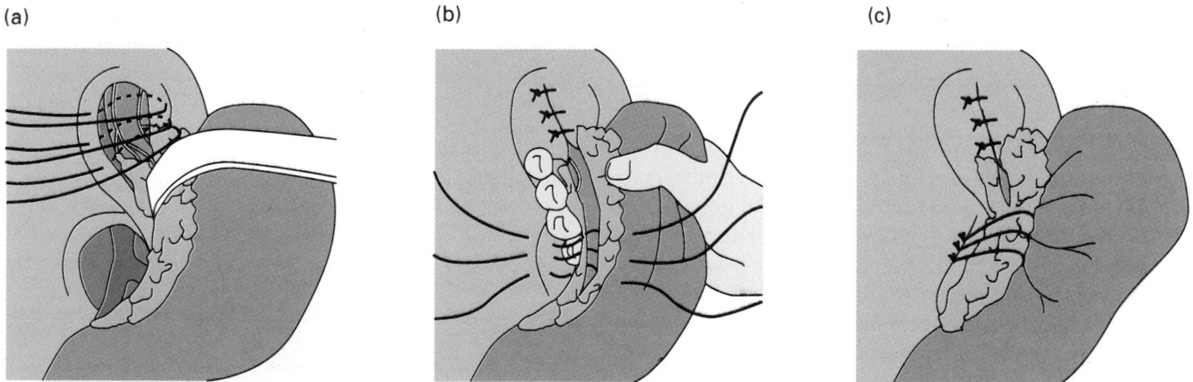

Fig. 6 The technique for performance of a Hill gastropexy. The distal oesophagus is imbricated within the lesser gastric curve. The cardia is anchored to the median arcuate ligament. (a) The cardia has been dissected and sutures placed for closure of the hiatus. (b) The sutures from the median arcuate ligament to the phrenoesophageal bundles are demonstrated. (c) The completed repair.

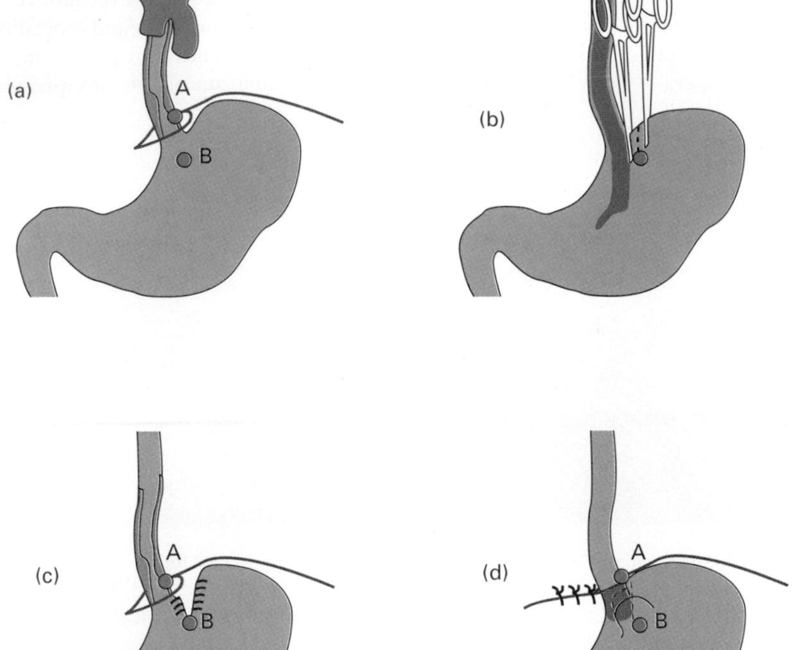

Fig. 7 The technique for performance of a Collis-Belsey gastroplasty. The oesophagus is mobilized from its mediastinal bed between the hiatus and aortic arch. Acquired oesophageal shortening precludes adequate reduction of the oesophagogastric junction (point *A*) below the diaphragm. After gastroplasty, point *B* is treated as the new oesophagogastric junction. (a)–(d) Diagram to illustrate a Belsey hiatus hernia repair. Some 3 to 5 cm of distal oesophagus is secured in the abdomen below the diaphragm. (b) Diagram illustrating gastroplasty combined with a Belsey hernia repair. (c), (d) The additional length of 'false oesophagus', created from the lesser curve of the stomach, acts as the lower oesophageal segment which is replaced in the abdomen below the diaphragm.

monitoring, diminished lower oesophageal sphincter tone on manometry, proven relief of dysphagia after dilation, and evidence of adequate peristalsis in the distal oesophagus.

For patients with a reflux stricture and a shortened oesophagus, gastroplasty combined with dilation and fundoplication is indicated. The so-called Collis–Belsey or Collis–Nissen operations consist of a Collis gastroplasty to lengthen the shortened oesophagus and a partial or complete antireflux wrap of the neo-oesophagus with gastric fundus (Fig. 7). One study described 93 per cent of patients experiencing good long-term results. In patients with motility disorders, the results are less dramatic, with only 54 per cent experiencing good results. A Nissen 360° wrap has also been used in conjunction with gastroplasty, but may be complicated by recurrent dysphagia if distal oesophageal motility is suboptimal.

Resectional surgery

There are instances in which oesophageal resection and reconstruction for benign stricture is advisable despite the greater risk attendant with this procedure. Patients who have undergone one or more previous antireflux operations, patients with severe reflux stricture and a primary dysmotility syndrome, and patients with non-dilatable strictures are candidates for resection.

Resection of the strictured oesophagus allows several alternatives for reconstruction: jejunal interpostion, colon interposition, or gastric pull-up. If resection can be limited to a short distal segment, jejunal interpostion grafting can provide a safe and effective conduit. Jejunal grafts are based on more reliable blood supply than are colonic grafts, especially in the elderly. Furthermore, jejunal grafting avoids the necessity for vagotomy and gastric drainage which is required when a gastric pull-up is used for reconstruction. When jejunum is not suitable for oesophageal reconstruction, isoperistaltic left colon may be successfully employed in the same fashion. The stomach remains a suitable substitute for resected oesophagus, but reflux and postvagotomy complications make it less desirable than other alternatives.

FURTHER READING

Hands LJ, Papavramidis S, Bishop H, Dennison AR, McIntyre RL, Kettlewell MGW. The natural history of peptic oesophageal strictures treated by dilatation and antireflux therapy alone. *Ann R Coll Surg* 1989; **71:** 306–10.

Little AG, Naunheim KS, Ferguson MK, Skinner DB. Surgical management of esophageal strictures. *Ann Thoracic Surg* 1988; **45:** 144–7.

McCord GS, Clouse RE. Pill-induced esophageal strictures: clinical features and risk factors for development. *Am J Med* 1990; **88:** 512–18.

Mansour KA, Malone CE. Surgery for scleroderma of the esophagus: a 12-year experience. *Ann Thoracic Surg* 1988; **46: 513–14.**

Mercer CD, Hill LD. Surgical management of peptic esophageal stricture: twenty-year experience. *J Thoracic Cardiovasc Surg* 1986; **91:** 371–8.

Parente F, *et al.* Opportunistic infections of the esophagus not responding to oral systemic antifungals in patients with AIDS: their frequency and treatment. *Am J Gastroenterol* 1991; **86(12):** 1729–34.

Patterson DJ, *et al.* Natural history of benign esophageal stricture treated by dilatation. *Gastroenterology* 1983; **85:** 346–50.

Pearson FG, Cooper JD, Patterson GA, Ramirez J, Todd TR. Gastroplasty and fundoplication for complex reflux problems: long-term results. *Ann Surg* 1987; **206(4):** 473–81.

Penagini R, Al Dabbagh M, Misiewicz JJ, Evans PF, Trotman IF. Effect of dilatation of peptic esophageal strictures on gastroesophageal reflux, dysphagia, and stricture diameter. *Dig Dis Sci* 1988; **33(4):** 389–92.

Schatzki R, Gary JE. Dysphagia due to a diaphragm-like localized narrowing in the lower esophagus ('lower esophageal ring'). *Am J Roentgenol* 1953; **70(6)**: 911–22.

Shemesh E, Czerniak A. Comparison between Savary-Gilliard and balloon dilatation of benign esophageal strictures. *World J Surg* 1990; **14**: 518–22.

Siewert JR, guest editor. Gastro-esophageal reflux disease: surgical point of view. *World J Surg* 1992; **16**: 288–363.

Stirling MC, Orringer MB. The combined Collis–Nissen Operation for esophageal reflux strictures. *Ann Thoracic Surg* 1988; **45**: 148–57.

Waring JP, Talbert GA, Austin J, Sanowski RA. Gastroesophageal reflux and sclerotherapy strictures. *Am Surgeon* 1990; **56(11)**: 662–4.

Zaninotto G, DeMeester TR, Bremner CG, Smyrk TC, Cheng SC. Esophageal function in patients with reflux induced strictures and its relevance to surgical treatment. *Ann Thoracic Surg* 1989; **47**: 362–70.

14.4.1 Oesophageal diverticula

HENNING A. GAISSERT AND JOHN C. WAIN

INTRODUCTION

Diverticula are acquired, focal pouches of oesophageal wall consisting of mucosa and variably attenuated muscular coat. They may occur anywhere in the oesophagus between the pharyngo-oesophageal junction and the lower oesophageal sphincter. Adults are usually affected, the incidence increasing with age.

Two different types of diverticula are recognized on the basis of their pathogenesis. Pulsion diverticula form as localized herniations due to increased luminal pressure in patients with motility disorders or chronic oesophageal obstruction, and provide an 'escape route' for pressure and swallowed food. Traction diverticula develop at the level of tracheobronchial lymph nodes as a result of granulomatous inflammation with secondary involvement of the adjacent oesophagus and subsequent contracture of scar tissue. Diverticula occur predominantly in three anatomical locations. Zenker's or pharyngo-oesophageal diverticulum is a pulsion defect of the posterior mucosa between the inferior pharyngeal constrictor muscle and the cricopharyngeal sphincter due to simultaneous inco-ordinate contraction. Mid-oesophageal lesions are typically traction diverticula and lie close to subcarinal, paratracheal, or hilar lymph nodes. Epiphrenic diverticula are found in the lower oesophagus above the diaphragm, and are also of the pulsion type. The upper thoracic oesophagus is rarely affected by diverticula. Pulsion defects are more likely to interfere with oesophageal function and produce symptoms. As a result, symptoms occur regularly in Zenker's diverticula, often in epiphrenic diverticula, and rarely in traction diverticula.

PHARYNGO-OESOPHAGEAL DIVERTICULA

Some 70 to 80 per cent of all oesophageal diverticula requiring surgical therapy are Zenker's diverticula. The principal physiological defect leading to formation of a pharyngo-oesophageal diverticulum is a loss of co-ordination during the second stage of swallowing. The oblique course of the inferior pharyngeal constrictor muscle and the horizontal direction of the cricopharyngeal sphincter create an unsupported triangular region devoid of muscle in the posterior wall (Fig. 1). Normally, the cricopharyngeal sphincter relaxes during contraction of the pharyngeal constrictors, allowing propulsion of food. In patients with Zenker's diverticulum the sphincter is closed during the pharyngeal contraction. Although not every swallow may demonstrate this discoordinate pattern, its cumulative effects expose the muscle-free area to high pressures, eventually leading to the formation of a pouch. It is unclear whether this disorder arises from a primary or secondary dysfunction of the cricopharyngeal sphincter. Gastro-oesophageal reflux, although suspected to cause reflex contraction of this muscle, is not associated with increased cricopharyngeal pressures.

Symptoms occur early in the course of pouch formation and are progressive. Patients complain of dysphagia and gurgling noises during swallowing. As food is retained in the pouch, fetor oris and spontaneous regurgitation of its undigested contents develop. Respiratory complications are frequent, including aspiration, asthma, pneumonia, and, occasionally, lung abscess. Pressure of the pouch on the recurrent laryngeal nerve may cause hoarseness. As the pouch increases in size, a soft mass may be palpated in the neck. Neglect of symptoms may result in weight loss, cachexia, and respiratory compromise. Perforation is rare and usually due to iatrogenic injury. One-third of patients have associated oesophageal functional disorders, such as hiatal hernia, diverticula elsewhere in the oesophagus, achalasia, or diffuse spasm. Nevertheless, radiographic contrast studies (Fig. 2) are usually sufficient to arrive at the diagnosis and to delineate the rest of the oesophagus: motility studies are generally not required. Oesophagoscopy is indicated when there is complete obstruction or if malignancy is suspected, since cancers occasionally occur in the pouch.

Zenker's diverticulum requires treatment regardless of diverticulum size. Symptoms do not improve with other forms of therapy, and the hazards of regurgitation and aspiration increase with pouch enlargement. Myotomy and diverticulectomy are the two elements of successful surgical therapy. If the pouch is small, cricopharyngeal myotomy alone relieves symptoms. The cricopharyngeal muscle is divided vertically in the posterior midline, dissecting the mucosa over half the circumference to prevent recurrent obstruction. If the pouch is well developed, diverticulectomy is performed during the same operation to remove the cause of regurgitation (Fig. 3). Care must be exercised to avoid over-excision of oesophageal mucosa and creation of a defect too large to close without tension or stenosis. Some surgeons prefer diverticulopexy with fixation to the prevertebral fascia to obliterate the lumen of the sac.

Myotomy and diverticulectomy produce excellent results. In a follow-up study from the Mayo Clinic, over 90 per cent of patients were asymptomatic. Operative mortality was 1.2 per cent and complications, including recurrent laryngeal nerve palsy, usually of transient nature, and oesophagocutaneous fistula arising from

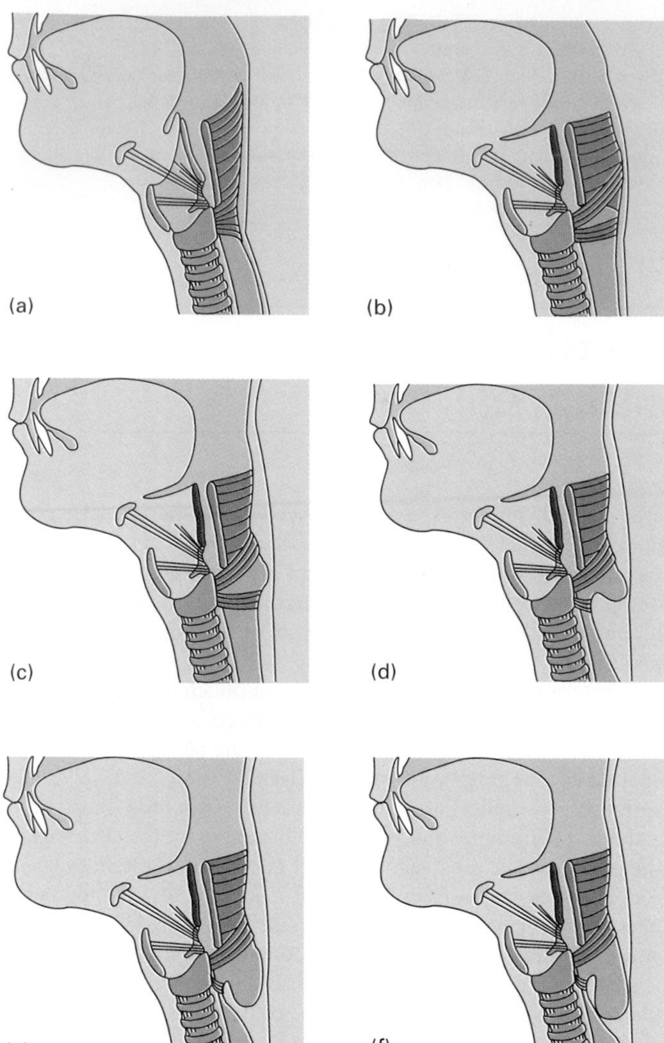

Fig. 1 Development of a pharyngo-oesophageal diverticulum. (a) and (b) Normal movements of larynx and pharynx during swallowing. (c) to (f) Formation of a pouch. (a) Respiration with descended larynx and relaxation of its sphincters. The cricopharyngeal sphincter closes the oesophagus with forward displacement of the posterior pharyngeal wall. The pharyngeal constrictors are relaxed. (b) During deglutition, the larynx is pulled upward and forward to the hyoid. The pharyngeal constrictors begin a peristaltic wave, and opening of the cricopharyngeus allows food to pass into the oesophagus. (c) Failure of the cricopharyngeus to relax appropriately delays passage of the food bolus. (d) A small pouch is formed in the bare area and is passively enlarged by food. (e) Further enlargement of the pouch separates the oesophagus from the prevertebral fascia and aligns pharynx and diverticulum in a vertical axis, while the oesophageal opening is moved to an oblique position. (f) Pressure on the oesophagus by the large pouch causes further obstruction.

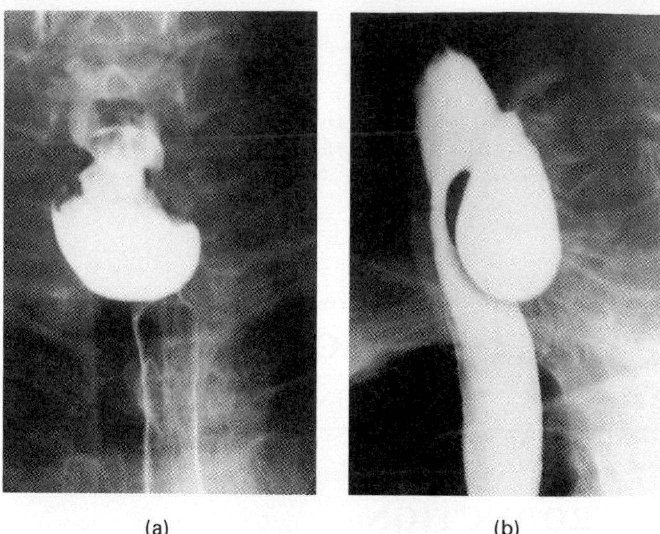

Fig. 2 Barium swallow in a patient with Zenker's diverticulum. Sagittal (a) and lateral (b) view of a large pharyngo-oesophageal pouch.

the suture line, which closed spontaneously with adequate drainage, affected 4.9 per cent of patients.

EPIPHRENIC DIVERTICULA

This entity is relatively uncommon, representing 10 to 20 per cent of all oesophageal diverticula. The male to female ratio is 2 : 1. Epiphrenic diverticula occur usually in the lower oesophagus within 10 cm of the diaphragm and project as solitary lesions into the right chest; left-sided or multiple lesions may be encountered. The resulting pouch is from 2 to over 10 cm in diameter and often has a narrow neck. Most epiphrenic diverticula are associated with functional motor disturbances, and some cause organic obstruction. Symptoms due to the diverticulum, however, develop in fewer than half of all patients. Patients present with dysphagia, regurgitation, and epigastric or chest pain. Occasionally, examination is prompted by aspiration with choking or coughing. Because these complaints are frequently associated with other benign oesophageal disorders, symptomatic patients should undergo complete evaluation including barium swallow (Fig. 4), motility studies, and endoscopy.

Appropriate therapy in patients with symptoms consists of surgical resection of the diverticulum and alleviation of underlying motor or organic disorders (Figs. 5 and 6). Access to the oesophagus is provided by posterolateral thoracotomy, usually on the left. The diverticulum is exposed and resected, closing the defect in the oesophagus. Distal obstruction should be excluded preoperatively, because it jeopardizes the closure of the oesophagus and may result in recurrence of the diverticulum. In most cases, an oesophageal myotomy extending from the site of the diverticulum distally to the lower oesophageal sphincter is required. If motility studies demonstrated motor dysfunction due to diffuse spasm, a long myotomy extending from the lower oesophageal sphincter to the aortic arch is performed. Any associated hiatal hernia is repaired, albeit cautiously because of the risk of recurrent obstruction. The individualized operative approach to each of these conditions emphasizes the need for a thorough preoperative understanding of the pathophysiology based on motility and other functional studies. Postoperatively, the oesophagus remains decompressed with a nasogastric tube until a Gastrografin study after 1 week has confirmed the absence of a leak.

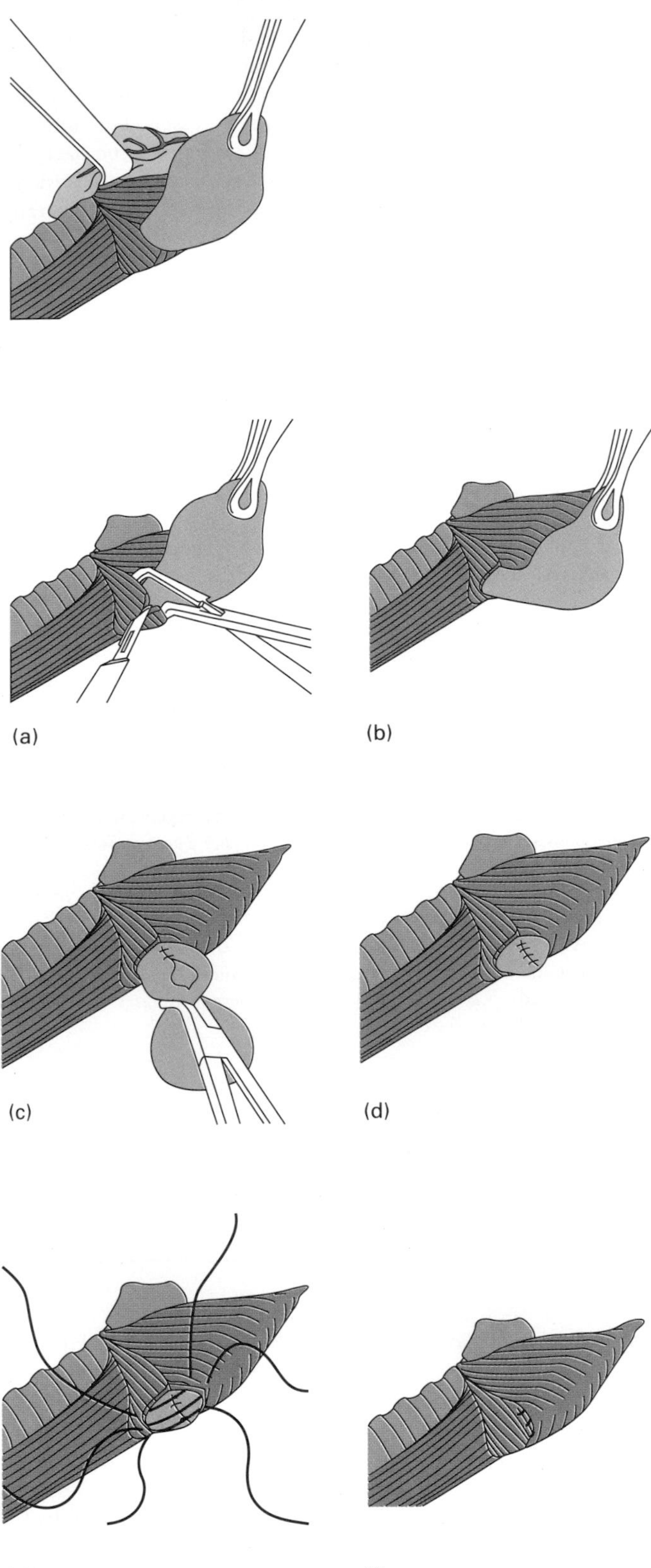

Fig. 3 Technique of cricopharyngeal myotomy and diverticulectomy. The oesophagus is exposed through an incision anterior to the sternocleidomastoid muscle. (a) and (b) The myotomy is performed in the posterior midline. (c) and (d) The diverticulum is clamped and excised, closing the oesophagus transversely with inverted, interrupted sutures. (e) and (f) The oesophageal closure is protected with transverse closure of the muscularis. If the sac is small and only a myotomy is performed, the muscle layer is left open.

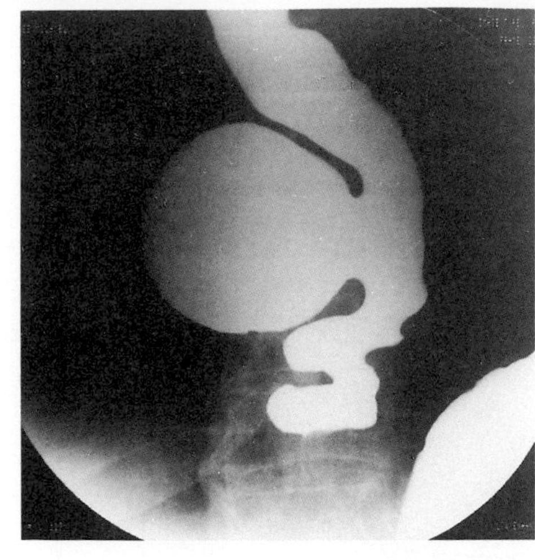

Fig. 4 Barium swallow in a patient with an epiphrenic diverticulum.

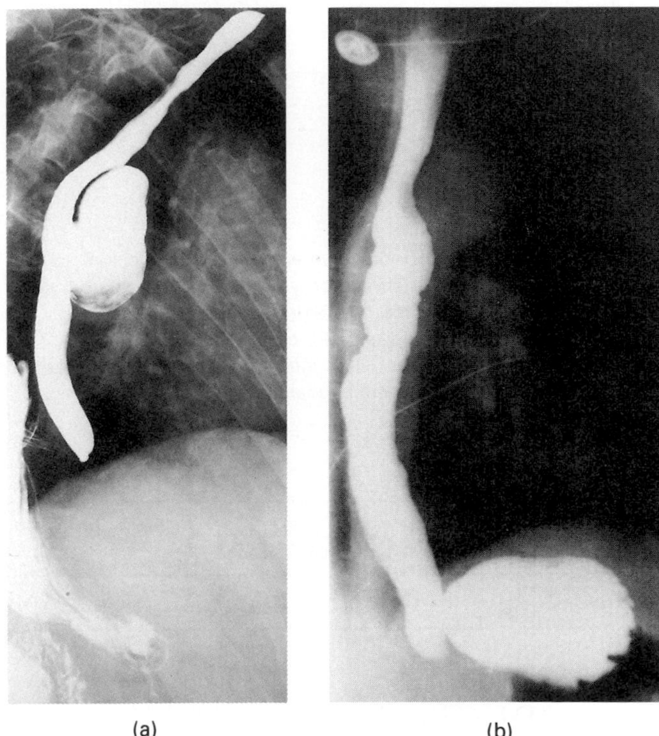

Fig. 5 Mid-oesophageal pulsion diverticulum. (a) Preoperative view. (b) Postoperative view after excision of diverticulum and distal oesophageal myotomy.

TRACTION DIVERTICULA

These diverticula occur as a result of granulomatous necrosis of tracheobronchial lymph nodes due to tuberculosis or histoplasmosis. The oesophagus is involved because of its proximity to the inflammation. Fixation of a transmural segment of oesophageal wall, followed by cicatricial contraction of the involved nodes and peristaltic extension of the surrounding oesophagus results in the formation of a true diverticulum. The sac is typically located on the left side, has a broad neck, and points upward. For this reason,

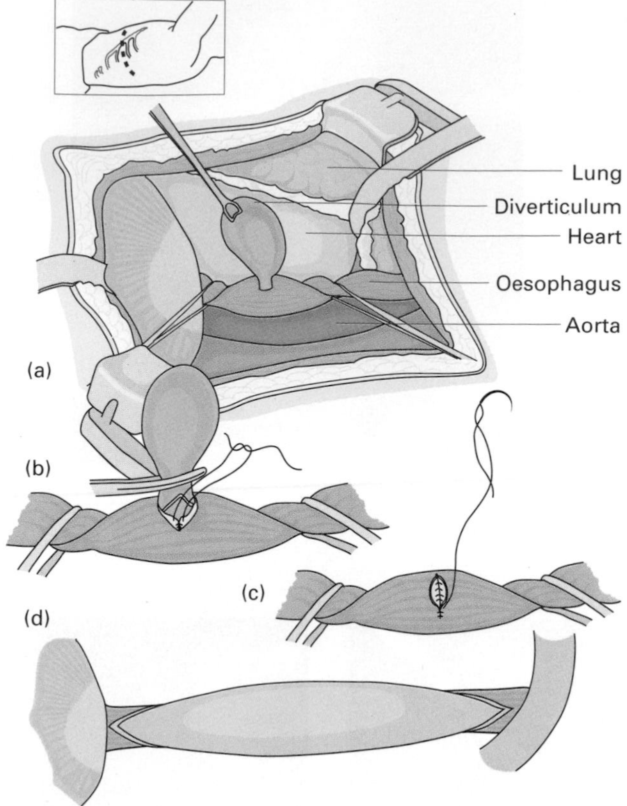

Fig. 6 Technique for excision of an epiphrenic diverticulum. (a) Surgical approach via left thoracotomy. The oesophagus is turned around its axis to expose the right-sided diverticulum. (b) The diverticulum is clamped and excised, closing the mucosa with inverted, interrupted sutures. (c) Closure of the muscularis. (d) Long myotomy opposite to the oesophageal closure.

it is rarely filled with food particles and rarely causes symptoms. Fistulization to the airway and haemorrhage are rare complications. Bleeding into the oesophagus originates most often from erosion of small bronchial or oesophageal vessels, but communication with the superior vena cava and exsanguination have been reported. Symptomatic patients should undergo local excision of the diverticulum with closure of the oesophagus and separation from the tracheobronchial tree with a vascularized tissue flap of intercostal muscle or pericardial fat.

FURTHER READING

Allen TH, Clagett OT. Changing concepts in the surgical treatment of pulsion diverticula of the lower esophagus. *J Thoracic Cardiovasc Surg*, 1965; **50**: 455–62.

Cheitlin MD, Kamin EJ, Wilkes DJ. Midesophageal diverticulum. Report of a case with fistulous connection with the superior vena cava. *Arch Intern Med*, 1961; **107**: 252–9.

Debas HT, Payne WS, Cameron AJ, Carlson HC. Physiopathology of lower esophageal diverticulum and its implications for treatment. *Surg Gynecol Obstet*, 1980; **151**: 593–600.

Ellis FH, Schlegel JF, Lynch VP, Payne WS. Cricopharyngeal myotomy for pharyngo-esopphageal diverticulum. *Ann Surg*, 1969; **170**: 340–9.

Habein HC, Kirklin JW, Clagett OT, Moersch HJ. Surgical treatment of lower esophageal pulsion diverticula. *Arch Surg*, 1956; **72**: 1018–24.

Habein HC, Moersch HJ, Kirklin JW. Diverticula of the lower part of the oesophagus. A clinical study of one hundred forty-nine nonsurgical cases. *Arch Intern Med*, 1956; **97**: 768–77.

Huang BS, Payne WS, Cameron AJ. Surgical management for recurrent pharyngoesophageal (Zenker's) diverticulum. *Ann Thoracic Surg*, 1984; **37**: 189–91.

Negus VE. Pharyngeal diverticula. Observations on their evolution and treatment. *Br J Surg*, 1950; **38**: 129–46.

Payne WS, Pairolero PC, Trasatek VF. Cervical and thoracic esophageal diverticulum. In: Grillo HC, Austen WG, Wilkins EW, Mathisen DJ, Vlahakes GJ, eds. *Current Therapy in Cardiothoracic Surgery*. Philadelphia: Dekker, 1989: 243–5.

14.4.2 Achalasia

HENNING A. GAISSERT AND JOHN C. WAIN

INTRODUCTION

Achalasia is a motility disorder of the oesophagus characterized by failure of the lower oesophageal sphincter to relax in response to swallowing and absence of peristalsis in the oesophageal body. The disease is most often progressive, leading to gradual dilatation of the oesophagus above the sphincter. Patients typically present with dysphagia, regurgitation, and substernal chest pain. Surgical or pneumatic disruption of the lower oesophageal sphincter relieves the obstruction and effectively restores swallowing.

The earliest available description of the disease and a successful treatment was provided in 1674 by Thomas Willis who treated a man with perpetual vomiting. Willis fashioned a sponged-tipped rod made of whale bone that the patient used to force open his cardia after meals for the following 15 years. Russell first reported treatment of the constricted sphincter by inflation of a silk-covered rubber balloon in 1887. Von Mikulicz introduced the term cardiospasm in 1904 and described dilatation of the gastro-oesophageal junction through a gastrostomy. In 1913 Heller performed surgical division of the muscular narrowing by means of two myotomies on the anterior and posterior surface of the lower oesophagus, through an abdominal incision. Plummer developed a successful method of forcefully dilating the sphincter with hydrostatic pressure using a rubber bag passed over a thread; he reported his personal experience with 301 cases in 1921. Modifications of the procedures introduced by Heller and Plummer are the mainstay of effective therapy today.

EPIDEMIOLOGY

The incidence rate of radiologically confirmed cases of achalasia in population studies from Great Britain and the United States averages between 0.4 and 0.6 cases/10^5 population/year, although peak rates as high as 2 cases/10^5 have been observed. The disease is known in most races and on all continents. In Europe and the United States, men and women are affected in equal proportions, although some series show a slight male predominance. Most patients present between the third and fifth decade of life, and less than 5 per cent of patients have the infantile type of disease. In South America, particularly in Brazil, mega-oesophagus is most frequently a manifestation of Chagas' disease, caused by *Trypanosoma cruzi* infection. Chagas' disease resembles achalasia because of the diffuse ganglion cell involvement and similar abnormalities of oesophageal motility. Patients with Chagas' disease, however, develop disease of multiple organs, including cardiomyopathy, megacolon, and megaureter. It can be diagnosed by specific serological tests.

PATHOGENESIS

The primary abnormality causing chronic constriction of the lower oesophageal sphincter and loss of peristalsis remains unknown. Potential aetiologies are a primary disease of the oesophageal wall, a disorder affecting the peripheral or central autonomic motor neurones, and autoimmune or inflammatory disease. Various experimental procedures, including selective ischaemic or toxic injury to the oesophagus and bilateral cervical vagotomy, result in conditions similar, but not identical, to achalasia.

The earliest documented histological finding in achalasia is degeneration of ganglion cells in the myenteric plexus of Auerbach. A reduction in number or absence of ganglion cells, predominantly in the oesophageal body but also in the distal narrowed oesophageal segment is noted. These changes are generally more pronounced in advanced disease. Recent studies have found a selective impairment of postganglionic inhibitory neurones in the circular layer of the lower oesophageal sphincter. As a result, cholinergic agonists produce an accentuated tightening and the lower oesophageal sphincter relaxant cholecystokinin produces a paradoxical contraction of the sphincter. Neural damage occurs at two further levels. Abnormalities similar to Wallerian degeneration occur in both myelinated and non-myelinated fibres of the vagus nerve. Nerve cells in the dorsal motor nucleus of the vagus nerve in the brain-stem are diminished in number or absent.

Ultrastructural studies of oesophageal muscle fail to demonstrate a specific injury in achalasia. In advanced disease, gross observation of the oesophagus demonstrates a 1.5 to 4.5 cm distal narrowing with normal wall thickness. The wall of the oesophageal body is thickened due to an increase of the circular muscle layer. The lumen is enlarged, elongated, and tortuous. Diverticula or pseudodiverticula of the mid-oesophagus occur occasionally. The mucosa demonstrates typical lesions of chronic stasis, including oesophagitis and ulcerations.

EVALUATION

A gradual onset of symptoms over months to years is characteristic of achalasia. Over 90 per cent of all patients have symptoms for longer than 1 year, and half are symptomatic for more than 3 years. Some may have symptoms for several decades. In addition to obstruction of swallowing, patients complain of regurgitation or vomiting of undigested food. Ellis and Olsen described how a typical patient copes with his eating problem.

> He shuns company while eating and is unwilling to dine in public. He learns quickly which foods will pass most easily and hence often avoids cold foods or solids such as meats or apples. He knows that he must not eat before retiring for fear of regurgitation, choking, and coughing. Some patients with advanced achalasia develop techniques for forcing food through the cardia. Merely drinking large quantities of water will sometimes overcome the resistance at the cardia [. . .]. Others learn to execute a "Valsalva maneuver", [. . .] thus increasing intrathoracic pressure until the lower sphincter gives way. In the process the patient usually stands in a crouched position, often holding on to a mantelpiece or stair rail.

Weight loss is present in 60 per cent of patients. Substernal chest or epigastric pain occurs in one-third of all patients. Nocturnal regurgitation may lead to aspiration, and pneumonia is present in 10 per cent of patients. In infants respiratory problems may be the first symptom to prompt evaluation and diagnosis.

Typical findings on plain chest radiograph include widening of the mediastinum and a posterior mediastinal air-fluid level. Chronic aspiration may cause abnormalities of the lung fields. Barium swallow demonstrates the characteristic dilatation of the oesophagus with a narrowing at the gastro-oesophageal junction (bird's beak deformity) in over 85 per cent of patients (Fig. 1). The size of the oesophageal body on contrast studies provides an approximation of disease severity: a diameter of less than 4 cm is termed mild disease, 4 to 6 cm moderate, and greater than 6 cm severe ('mega-oesophagus'). Further indicators of disease severity are the amount of retained food and degree of peristalsis observed on fluoroscopy.

Oesophageal manometry confirms the clinical diagnosis and reliably separates patients with similar symptoms due to other motility disorders, such as diffuse oesophageal spasm (Fig. 2). Four criteria are characteristic of achalasia: elevated lower oesophageal sphincter pressure, incomplete or absent relaxation of the lower oesophageal sphincter, absence of peristalsis in the oesophageal body, and elevated intra-oesophageal pressure. Absence of co-ordinated peristalsis is required for diagnosis, but weak simultaneous contractions are often observed early in the course of the disease. A subgroup of patients have 'vigorous achalasis', a hyperdynamic disco-ordinate motility pattern with simultaneous, high amplitude contractions of the oesophageal body. The latter condition may be accompanied by epiphrenic diverticula.

Complete endoscopic examination of oesophagus and stomach should be part of the initial evaluation, to detect disease complications, such as ulceration, and to rule out carcinoma. The oesophagus is often patulous and contains food particles and secretions. The mucosa exposed to these contents is frequently inflamed. The lower sphincter is closed, but provides little or no resistance to the endoscope which is easily advanced into the stomach.

DIFFERENTIAL DIAGNOSIS

Two conditions mimic the radiological and manometric features of achalasia. Chagas' disease occurs uncommonly outside South America and generally also affects other organs. Pseudoachalasia is the rare presentation of a carcinoma at the gastro-oesophageal junction with gradually worsening dysphagia, narrowing at the lower sphincter, and manometric findings characteristic of achalasia. Patients typically have symptoms for less than 1 year, and weight loss predominates. Inhalation of amyl nitrate leads to sphincter relaxation in achalasia, but not in pseudoachalasia. The diagnosis of pseudoachalasia is made by endoscopic examination and biopsy, but findings are subtle and require a high index of suspicion and often, serial examination.

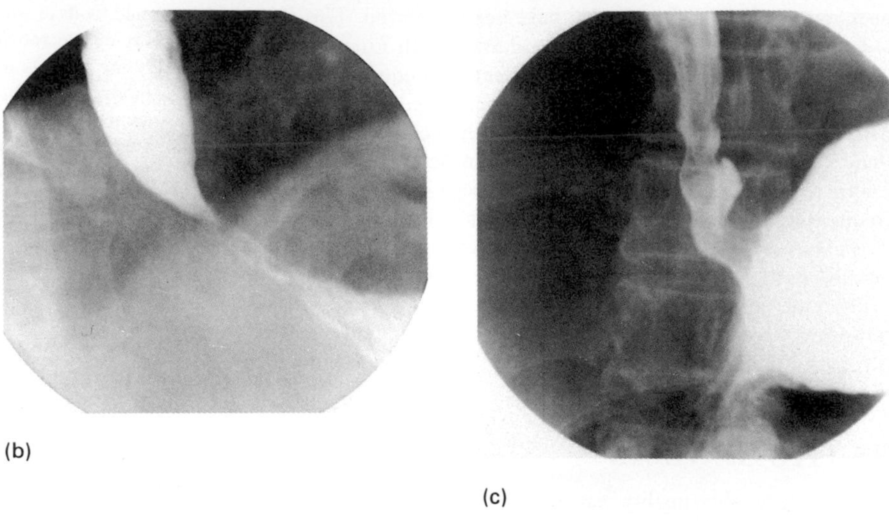

(a)

(b)

(c)

Fig. 1 Barium swallow in a patient with achalasia. (a) Retained food, moderate oesophageal dilatation, and bird's beak deformity of distal oesophagus. (b) The gastro-oesophageal junction before oesophagomyotomy. (c) Same region after oesophagomyotomy.

Diffuse oesophageal spasm may present with symptoms similar to those of early achalasia. Indignation of this condition are diffuse narrowing or segmental contractions of the oesophagus on radiological examination and motility studies demonstrating relaxation of the lower oesophageal sphincter in diffuse spasm. A peptic stricture that occurs as a complication of scleroderma may imitate achalasia on contrast studies, but concomitant systemic manifestations usually indicate the diagnosis.

TREATMENT

Successful therapy consists of judicious weakening of the lower oesophageal sphincter by forceful dilatation or oesophagomyotomy to allow gravity drainage of food while avoiding chronic gastro-oesophageal reflux. Therapy does not restore the normal anatomy of the sphincter or co-ordinated peristalsis of the oesophageal body. Sphincteric disruption, however, relieves dysphagia and regurgitation in most patients. Therapy with calcium channel blockers and nitrates decreases lower oesophageal sphincter pressure transiently. Although patients with mild and moderate symptoms of achalasia experience improvement of swallowing, these drugs do not produce lasting relief and no information on disease progression during treatment is available. Drug therapy should therefore be used for extended periods only in patients unable to undergo standard treatment.

Pneumatic dilatation

Forceful dilatation is accomplished with an expandable balloon made of silk-covered rubber or polyurethane, inflated with water or air, and advanced either over thread, an olive-tipped bougie, or under radiographic control. Pneumatic dilatation using a polyurethane balloon and fluoroscopy is the currently preferred method. The dilator is typically placed through the narrowed segment and the balloon is rapidly inflated for a period ranging from seconds to a few minutes. If the result is unsatisfactory repeated attempts or a larger balloon is required. The patient can leave the hospital on the same day or after overnight observation. If the first treatment produces no improvement, another dilatation may be considered after 3 months.

Approximately 70 per cent of patients improve after the procedure. Advantages of dilatation are the avoidance of general anaesthesia and the painful incision. Treatment cost are lower. Further dilatations are required in approximately 16 per cent of patients and a myotomy in 8 per cent. Disadvantages include a high incidence of gastro-oesophageal reflux disease (20 per cent of patients) and a 1 to 10 per cent risk of oesophageal perforation. Appropriate treatment of acute perforation consists of thoracotomy and primary repair of the oesophagus.

Oesophagomyotomy

In principle, this is derived from the duplicate Heller myotomy by the abdominal approach. However, many modifications of oesophagomyotomy for achalasia have evolved with the aim of reducing the postoperative complications of reflux and recurrent obstruction.

Thoracic or abdominal access

When operating through the abdomen, division of the phreno-oesophageal ligament is required to expose the lower oesophagus. The added effects of a weakened sphincter and a dissected hiatus are followed by high incidence of reflux, making a routine fundoplication necessary. Thoracotomy offers direct access to the lower sphincter without obligatory injury to the diaphragmatic attachments and risk of reflux (Fig. 3). In the future, laparoscopic or thoracoscopic approaches may reduce perioperative discomfort and hasten recovery, but effectiveness and safety of these procedures await confirmation.

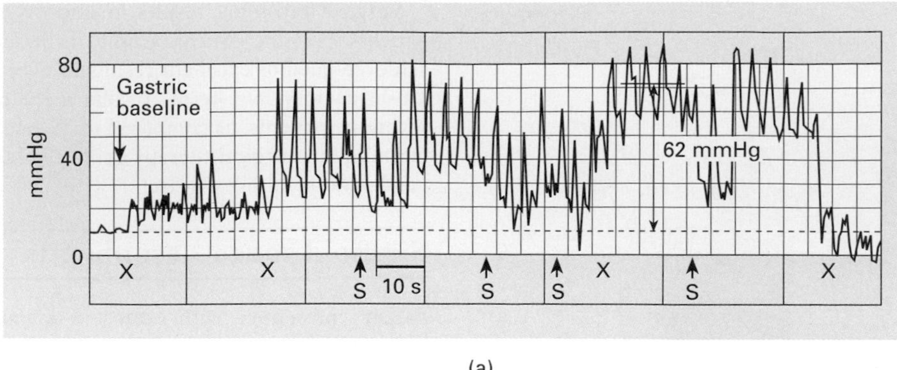

(a)

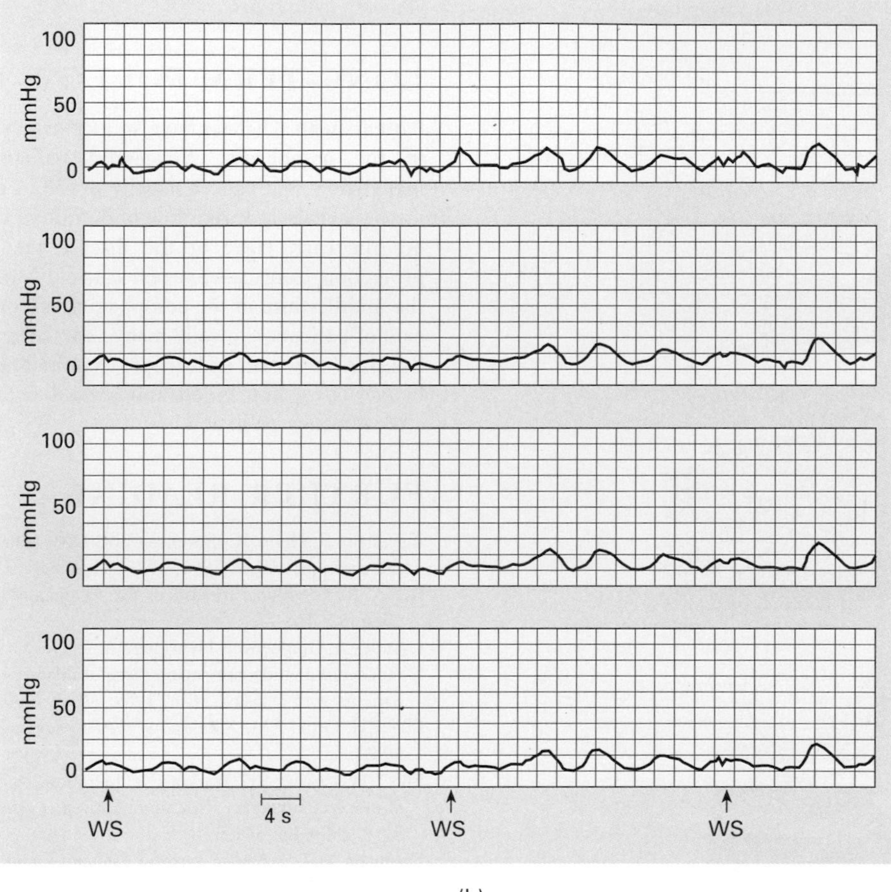

(b)

Fig. 2 Oesophageal motility tracing of a patient with achalasia. (a) The catheter is moved through the maximum high pressure zone. The lower oesophageal sphincter is hypertensive with incomplete relaxation during swallowing. x, catheter moved up 0.5 cm. S, swallow. (b) The oesophageal body demonstrates total absence of peristalsis. Contractions are simultaneous, of low amplitude, and resemble respiratory artifact. WS, wet swallow.

The extent of myotomy

The longitudinal incision into the muscle must divide all circular fibres on the lower oesophagus and reach proximally to all dilated oesophagus. Any remaining constriction will lead to persistent dysphagia. However, extending the incision too far on to the gastric wall results in free reflux. The myotomy should therefore continue for less than 1 cm on to the stomach, where the presence of transverse cardiac veins is first noted. Exact execution of this step is probably the most critical determinant of postoperative results.

Addition of antireflux procedure

While those who perform only myotomy restrict a fundoplication to specific indications, i.e. the presence of a hernia, others consider it routine. They argue that a widely dissected hiatus provides improved exposure and believe that the incidence of postoperative

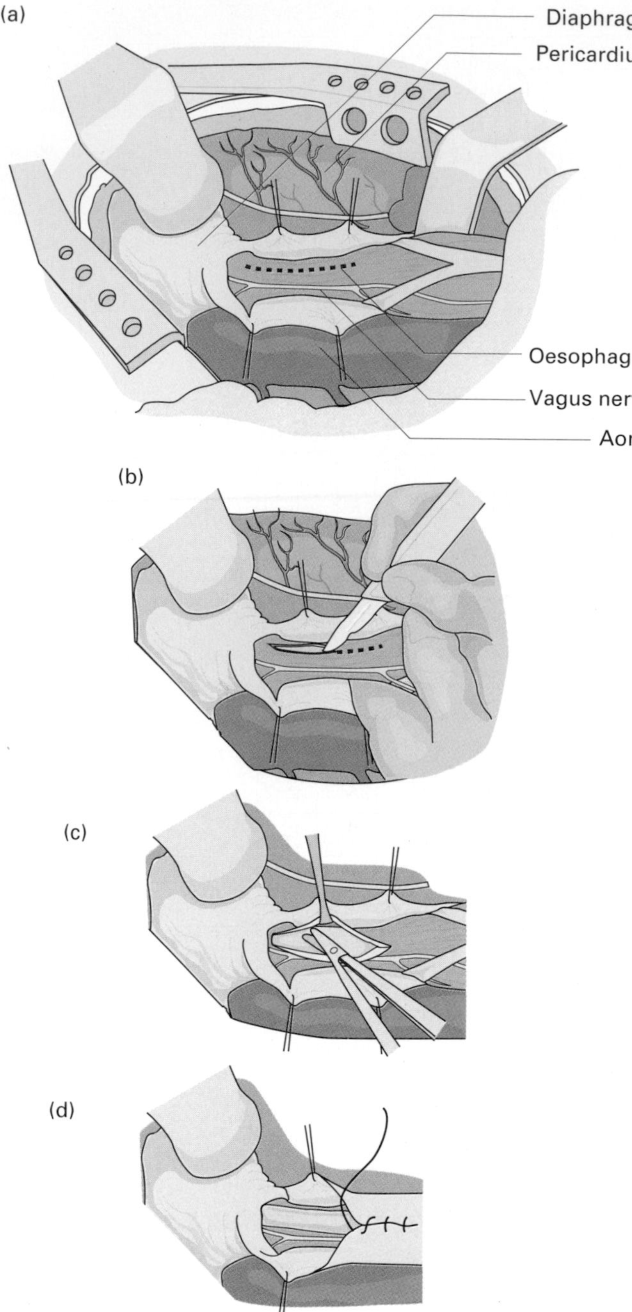

Fig. 3 Oesophagomyotomy via left thoracotomy. (a) Operative exposure. Dotted line indicates extent of myotomy. (b) Incision of the muscularis. (c) Separation of mucosa and muscularis over half the oesophageal circumference. (d) Suture narrowing of the hiatus in the presence of a hernia.

reflux is reduced. However, the rate of failure after fundoplication is 10 to 15 per cent, which equals the overall incidence of postoperative reflux after myotomy and raises doubt regarding the benefit of adding this procedure in all patients. If reconstruction of the hiatus is required, the lack of oesophageal peristalsis often results in recurrent obstructive symptoms which require oesophageal dilatation and long-term observation. Total fundoplication is therefore avoided, and 'loose' Belsey and 'floppy' or incomplete Nissen repairs are preferred.

Surgical myotomy results in improvement in 90 per cent of patients. In the Mayo Clinic experience, simple myotomy achieved good or excellent results in over 90 per cent of patients. Unsatisfactory long-term, results were noted in 6 per cent of myotomy patients, as compared to 19 per cent after forceful dilatation. Thus surgical therapy produces better results with risk of postoperative reflux disease.

Sigmoid mega-oesophagus

Patients presenting with extensive dilatation of the oesophageal body or unrelenting post-treatment reflux may respond poorly to conventional therapy. Replacement of the oesophagus with stomach or intestinal interposition should be considered to alleviate symptoms.

LONG-TERM FOLLOW-UP

Patients with achalasia have an increased risk of dying from cancer of the oesophagus. Successful palliation does not prevent malignancy, but cancer usually develops in patients who had advanced achalasia at the time of definitive therapy. Treatment during the early stage of the disease may thus afford a relative protection from oesophageal cancer. Most frequently located in the middle-third of the oesophagus, tumours develop in 5 to 8 per cent of patients, typically many years after diagnosis or treatment. Routine long-term endoscopic examination with brush cytology or biopsy is recommended and should continue indefinitely, even after effective palliation.

FURTHER READING

Aggestrup S, Holm JC, Sorensen HR. Does achalasia predispose to cancer of the esphagus? *Chest*, 1992; **102**: 1013–16.

Belsey R. Functional disease of the esophagus. *J Thoracic Cardiovasc Surg*, 1966; **52**: 164–88.

Csendes A, Braghetto I, Henriquez A, Cortes C. Late results of a prospective randomised study comparing forceful dilatation and oesophagomyotomy in patients with achalasia. *Gut*, 1989; **30**: 299–304.

Ellis FH, Olsen AM. *Achalasia of the Esophagus*. Philadelphia: WB. Saunders, 1969.

Ellis FH, Crozier RE, Watkins E. Operation for esophageal achalasia. Results of esophagomyotomy without an antireflux operation. *J Thoracic Cardiovasc Surg*, 1984; **88**: 344–51.

Ferguson MK. Achalasia: current evaluation and therapy. *Ann Thoracic Surg*, 1991; **52**: 336–42.

Ferguson TB, Burford TH. An evaluation of the modified Heller operation in the treatment of achalasia of the esophagus. *Ann Surg*, 1960; **152**: 1–9.

Kahrilas PJ, Kishk SM, Helm JF, Dodds WJ, Harig JM, Hogan WJ. Comparison of pseudoachalasia and achalasia. *Am J Med*, 1987; **82**: 439–46.

Little AG, Soriano A, Ferguson MK, Winans CS, Skinner DB. Surgical treatment of achalasia: results esophagomyotomy and Belsey repair. *Ann Thoracic Surg*, 1988; **45**: 489–94.

Okike N, Payne WS, Neufeld DM, Bernatz PE, Pairolero PC, Sanderson DR. Esophagomyotomy versus forceful dilation for achalasia of the esophagus: results in 899 patients. *Ann Thoracic Surg*, 1979; **28**: 119–25.

Shimi S, Nathanson LK, Cuschieri A. Laparoscopic cardiomyotomy for achalasia. *J R Coll Surg Edin*, 1991; **36**: 152–4.

Skinner DB. Myotomy and achalasia. *Ann Thoracic Surg*, 1984; **37**: 183–4.

Slater G, Sicular AA. Esophageal perforations after forceful dilatation in achalasia. *Ann Surg*, 1982; **195**: 186–8.

Topart P, Deschamps C, Taillefer R, Duranceau A. Long-term effect of total fundoplication on the myotomized esophagus. *Ann Thoracic Surg*, 1992; **54**: 1046–52.

14.5 Benign and malignant tumours

CAMERON WRIGHT, HENNING A. GAISSERT, FRANCESCO PUMA, AND DOUGLAS MATHISEN

INTRODUCTION

Oesophageal cancer is an uncommon and often lethal malignancy. Unfortunately, symptoms rarely occur until late in the clinical course. The goal of surgical treatment remains relief of dysphagia and cure. Combined modality treatment represents a new approach to oesophageal cancer and may·offer improvements in survival of selected patients.

EPIDEMIOLOGY

There is considerable variation throughout the world in the incidence of squamous cell carcinoma of the oesophagus. The incidence ranges from 5 per 1000000 in the United States to 100 per 100000 in Linxian, China (Table 1). There is also a marked difference in death rates within each country. The peak age of occurrence is between the ages of 50 and 70 years with a median age of death of 66 in the United States. In Western nations, oesophageal cancer is much more common in men than in women (about fivefold). Oesophageal cancer is more common (threefold) in black than in white subjects in the United States. In 1980 squamous cell carcinoma represented 90 per cent of oesophageal cancers and adenocarcinomas only 10 per cent. Recent reports indicate an increase in incidence of adenocarcinoma. In some reports, adenocarcinoma has accounted for more than half of all cancers of the oesophagus. Many of the adenocarcinomas have occurred in Barrett's mucosa, largely in caucasian males.

Table 1 Oesophageal cancer incidence among males around the world

Geographic area	Incidence rate per 100000
Linxian China; Caspian region of Iran	100+
Transkei, South Africa; parts of Kazakhstan; Rhodesia; Brittany, France	50–99
Parts of South Africa; Shanghai	20–49
Hong Kong; Singapore (Chinese); most areas of China; Miyagi, Japan; India; Caribbean Islands; Brazil; France; United States (blacks)	10–19
Most areas of Japan; United Kingdom; New Zealand; Southern Europe	5–9
Canada; United States (whites); Australia; Israel; Western Africa; Scandinavia; Central and Eastern Europe	0–5

RISK FACTORS

Alcohol

Many epidemiological studies confirm that heavy alcohol users have an increased risk of oesophageal cancer and that the risk is substantial in very heavy drinkers. When combined with cigarette smoking, the risk is even greater.

Tobacco use

Studies confirm that smoking leads to an increased risk of oesophageal cancer also in a dose dependent fashion. Moderate smokers have a fivefold increase in risk. This is true for cigar and pipe smoking as well as for cigarette smoking.

Nutritional deficiency

The geographical variability of oesophageal cancer strongly correlates with areas that have poor nutritional status. Nutritional factors beyond malnutrition that have been implicated include soil deficiencies in zinc, molybdenum, magnesium, and iron. The clearest relationship exists with molybdenum deficiency in the soil, which leads to accumulation of nitrates and nitrites in plants in turn leading to nitrosamines, a known oesophageal carcinogen. Plummer–Vincent (Patterson–Kelly) syndrome is associated with carcinoma of the upper third of the oesophagus and is associated not only with iron deficiency anaemia, but also vitamin B deficiencies. Coeliac disease (non-tropical sprue) is associated with an increased risk of oesophageal cancer perhaps due to the malabsorption syndrome that leads to multiple nutritional deficiencies.

Chronic oesophageal irritation

Oesophageal disorders associated with an increased incidence of carcinoma include chronic lye strictures, achalasia, and perhaps oesophageal diverticuli. Long-term use of spicy and hot drinks may also predispose to chronic irritation and are implicated in the pathogenesis of oesophageal carcinoma. Tylosis is a rare autosomal dominant disease associated with an increased risk of carcinoma of the oesophagus.

PATHOLOGY

Until recent years, the majority of oesophageal cancers were squamous in histology. For purposes of classification, the oesophagus may be divided into three anatomic areas: the upper, middle, and lower third. The upper third (cervical oesophagus) extends from the cricopharyngeal sphincter to the thoracic inlet, the middle third from the thoracic inlet to 10 cm above the gastro-oesophageal junction and the lower third from 10 cm above the gastro-oesophageal junction to the cardia of the stomach. About 15 per cent of squamous cell cancers occur in the upper one-third, 50 per cent in the middle third, and 35 per cent in the lower third.

Three gross patterns of growth are commonly seen. The ulcerating type has a well-defined ulcer with raised irregular edges. The fungating type has a large intraluminal growth component with an irregular surface. The infiltrating type has extensive intramural growth, often circumferential, with minimal ulceration. There is often a significant submucosal extension of tumour far from the visible edge of mucosal tumour (longitudinal spread), more so in a cephalad fashion than a caudad one. In one study, cancer was present 6 cm cephalad from the primary tumour in 22 per cent of patients and 9 cm from it in 11 per cent of patients. The caudad growth was rarely more than 5 cm distal. These data underlie the importance of wide resection of the oesophagus and frozen section analysis of resection margins to ensure complete removal of the tumour.

Transmural tumour penetration (vertical growth) is present in the majority of cases that come to surgery. Lack of a serosal covering of the oesophagus may explain the early invasion of mediastinal structures. Mediastinal structures commonly invaded include the trachea and left main bronchus, aorta, pericardium, and pleura. A malignant airway–oesophageal fistula occurs more commonly than an aorto-oesophageal fistula.

Lymph node metastases are common and correlate with the depth invasion of the tumour. For lesions limited to the submucosa (T1) there is only a 14 per cent incidence of positive nodes. (For discussion of staging, see below.) The incidence of nodal metastases rises from 30 per cent for lesions limited to the muscularis propria (T2), 50 per cent for lesions up to the adventitia (T3) and 75 per cent when the tumour invades the peri-oesophageal tissues (T4). Lymph node metastases may be found at a distant site from the primary tumour because of the extensive longitudinal spread of tumour via the submucosal lymphatic vessels. The lymphatic drainage of the oesophagus is primarily longitudinal rather than segmental, further complicating the surgical treatment of oesophageal cancer. Akiyama has convincingly demonstrated that lymph nodes are often positive at the opposite end of the oesophagus from the carcinoma regardless of whether the cancer is in the upper or lower oesophagus (Table 2). Visceral metastases involving the lung, liver, bone, kidneys, pleura, and brain are common at death.

BIOLOGY

The natural history of oesophageal cancer may be inferred on the basis of extensive mass screening studies done in China on high-risk populations. Screening was performed primarily by abrasive cytology utilizing a swallowed balloon that is inflated and pulled back through the oesophagus thus collecting a representative sample of epithelial cells. Dysplastic cells are almost always found in association with cases of early carcinoma. Furthermore, dysplasia can progress to carcinoma although not invariably so. In one study of over 1500 patients followed for up to 12 years, 15 per cent developed carcinoma if severe dysplasia was present. Only 1 per cent developed oesophageal cancer with mild dysplasia and no carcinomas were found in the control group with normal cytologies. In a separate study of 14 000 subjects, the average age of those with severe dysplasia was 52, whereas those with carcinoma was 57, suggesting a 5-year lag time in developing carcinoma once severe dysplasia develops. Not all patients with dysplasia will develop carcinoma; in one study 45 per cent of mildly dysplastic and 40 per cent of severely dysplastic cells returned to normal over several years. In patients with early cytologically diagnosed carcinoma who refused treatment and were followed, about one-half remained asymptomatic in the early stage of the disease for a mean period of 75 months. The other one-half developed symptomatic late carcinoma an average of 55 months after diagnosis. Thus, the development of symptomatic carcinoma takes many years and allows for ample time for early diagnosis. Surgical treatment of early, cytologically diagnosed, asymptomatic cancers in China provides a greater than 90 per cent survival at 5 years, emphasizing the importance of early diagnosis.

Once overt symptoms occur, the average survival without treatment is 9 months. The most common cause of death is bronchopneumonia. Patients usually procrastinate in reporting their symptoms, leading to a further delay in diagnosis of often 3 to 4 months. Metastases to lymph nodes and visceral organs as well as mediastinal invasion have often already occurred precluding the

Table 2 Location of positive lymph nodes according to position of tumour

	Location of tumour		
Group of lymph nodes	Upper oesophagus	Middle oesophagus	Lower oesophagus
Thoracic			
Superior mediastinal	29	11	10
Middle mediastinal	27	21	14
Lower mediastinal	29	18	27
Abdominal			
Superior gastric	32	33	62
Coeliac axis nodes	0	4	21
Common hepatic artery lymph nodes	0	2	10
Splenic artery lymph nodes	0	6	15

Percentage of positive lymph nodes.

chance for a surgical cure. Mass screening programmes in areas of low incidence are not cost effective.

STAGING

The current TMN staging system was developed by the American Joint Committee on Cancer (AJCC) in conjunction with the International Union Against Cancer (UICC) (Table 3). The primary determinants of survival in surgically treatable oesophageal cancer are the depth of invasion and the presence of lymph node metastases. This staging system incorporates these two critical variables. Survival is stage dependent. Stage I cancer is rare in the Western world. Although postsurgical staging can be accurately performed, presurgical staging is still suboptimal because computed tomographic scanning does not reliably determine the depth of invasion by tumour or the status of the regional nodes. Endoscopic ultrasound may play an important role in the future in this regard.

Table 3 Staging of oesophageal carcinoma

T Primary Tumour			
TX	Primary tumour cannot be assessed		
TO	No tumour		
Tis	Carcinoma-*in–situ*		
T1	Tumour invades the lamina propria or submucosa		
T2	Tumour invades the muscularis propria		
T3	Tumour invades the perioesophageal tissue		
T4	Tumour invades adjacent structures		
N Regional lymph nodes			
NX	Regional nodes cannot be assessed		
NO	No regional lymph node metastasis		
N1	Regional lymph node metastasis		
M Distant metastases			
MX	Distant metastasis cannot be assessed		
MO	No distant metastasis		
MI	Distant metastasis		
Staging groups			
Stage 0	Tis	NO	MO
Stage 1	T1	NO	MO
Stage IIA	T2	NO	MO
	T3	NO	MO
Stage IIB	T1	N1	MO
	T2	N1	MO
Stage III	T3	N1	MO
	T4	Any N	MO
Stage IV	Any T	Any N	M1

SYMPTOMS

Dysphagia, first to solids then liquids, is the most common presenting symptom. This is a late symptom and usually indicates that two-thirds of the circumference is involved. Patients often adjust their diet to soft solids and flush their foods through with liquids to accommodate their dysphagia. Weight loss is common and at times disproportionate to the duration of dysphagia. Odynophagia or painful swallowing is often seen. Steady deep chest pain often indicates mediastinal invasion.

Cough or hoarseness is common in upper oesophageal tumours as a result of a direct invasion of the airway or the recurrent laryngeal nerve. Aspiration pneumonia may be present either as a result of overflow obstruction or due to a malignant oesophageal–airway fistula. Patients with a fistula usually have severe paroxysms of coughing immediately after swallowing liquids.

SIGNS

Physical examination is usually unrewarding. Cervical adenopathy is rarely palpable. Evidence of weight loss is usually apparent.

LABORATORY DATA

Laboratory data are rarely helpful in making the diagnosis, although they may be of some benefit in staging (i.e. elevated alkaline phosphatase for bone or liver metastases). Laboratory data also help in assessing the risk of oesophagectomy (i.e. renal and hepatic function). Pulmonary function testing and arterial blood gas measurement are helpful to quantify the extent of chronic obstructive pulmonary disease. Patients with underlying coronary artery disease should have an echocardiogram to assess left ventricular function and a stress test to assess the extent of ischaemic myocardium.

RADIOLOGY

Chest radiographs

Chest radiographs are usually unremarkable. Possible abnormalities include an oesophageal air–fluid level, infiltrates suggesting aspiration, pleural effusion suggesting pleural dissemination, mediastinal widening (due to the tumour or lymphadenopathy), and pulmonary nodules suggesting lung metastases.

Barium oesophagram

The barium swallow is the mainstay of radiological diagnosis (Fig. 1). Abnormality of the oesophageal axis (angulation of a long axis of the oesophagus) strongly suggests mediastinal invasion and thus helps predict unresectability.

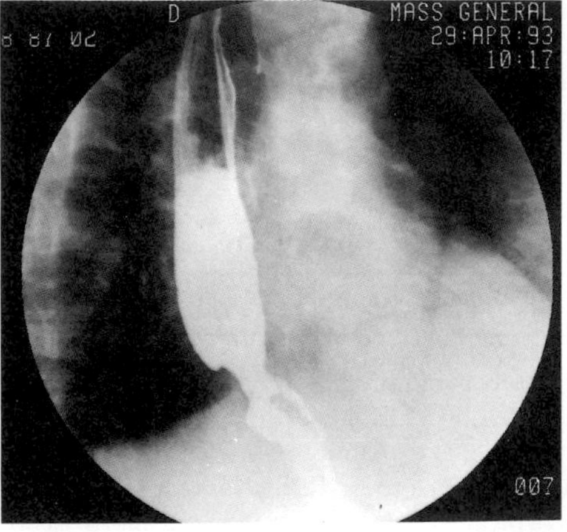

Fig. 1 Barium swallow demonstrates the typical annular defect of the lower oesophagus in a patient with an adenocarcinoma of the oesophagus.

Computed tomography of the chest and abdomen

Computed tomography (CT) displays the oesophageal wall and mediastinal structures clearly and in addition, allows evaluation of the common relevant metastatic sites (liver, lymph nodes, adrenal glands, lungs, and kidneys) (Fig. 2). All patients should undergo CT evaluation, but CT does not accurately predict invasion. Gross distortion of a mediastinal structure indicates invasion; the presence of a fat plane between the tumour and the structure predicts the absence of invasion. Evaluation of tumours at the gastro-oesophageal junction is very difficult although it is improved by distension and contrast opacification of the stomach. Evaluation of lymph nodes is suboptimal; enlargement does not always predict metastases and most excised positive lymph nodes are of normal size.

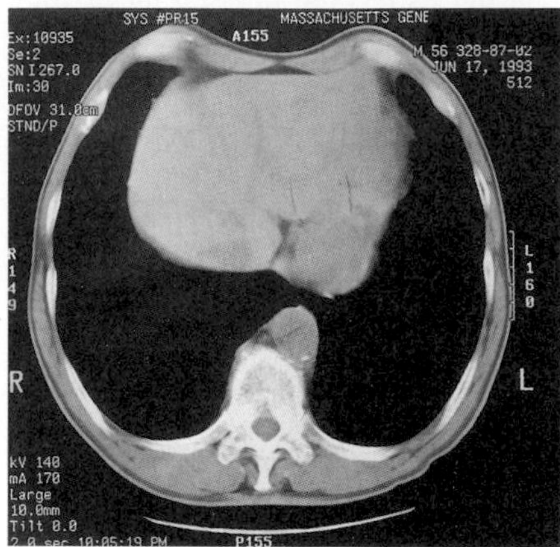

Fig. 2 Computerized axial tomogram demonstrates large retrocardiac mass in a patient with an adenocarcinoma of the distal oesophagus.

Radionucleotide scans

Bone scans are performed for clinical suspicion of bone metastases based on either a history of bone pain or an elevated alkaline phosphatase. Liver scans are inferior to CT in determining the presence of liver metastases.

ENDOSCOPY

Oesophagoscopy

Oesophagoscopy is required in the assessment of all patients with dysphagia and allows histological (or cytological) confirmation of suspected carcinoma. It is important to measure the length of the lesion and the distance from the incisors for staging and treatment planning. Typical tumours are friable and bleed easily. Multiple biopsies from suspicious areas should be performed. The ability to make a histological diagnosis is increased by taking multiple biopsies. Brush cytology is often very helpful. About 10 per cent of biopsies are non-diagnostic and repeat oesophagoscopy and biopsy is required. The stomach, pylorus, and duodenum should also be examined to assess any additional pathology and to evaluate the stomach for use as an oesophageal substitute.

Bronchoscopy

Bronchoscopic examination of the airway is necessary in all upper and middle third carcinomas. Transmural spread of tumour can be confirmed by visual inspection and biopsy. Bulging of the airway indicates abutment, but does not usually signal direct invasion of the airway.

Laparoscopy

Laparoscopy can allow reliable assessment and biopsy of the superficial aspect of the liver, perigastric lymph nodes, and the peritoneum, if indicated by previous staging examinations.

Thoracoscopy

Thoracoscopy can be used to confirm invasion into local structures or to sample lymph nodes for staging. The role of video-assisted thoracoscopy for oesophagectomy needs to be defined.

Endoscopic ultrasound

Endoscopic ultrasound improves the ability to determine wall penetration and abnormal lymph nodes. Thus endoscopic ultrasound may improve preoperative staging. Five distinct wall layers can be identified that correspond to the mucosa, lamina propria, muscularis mucosa, muscularis propria, and adventitia. Carcinoma appears as an irregular hypoechoic mass (Fig. 3).

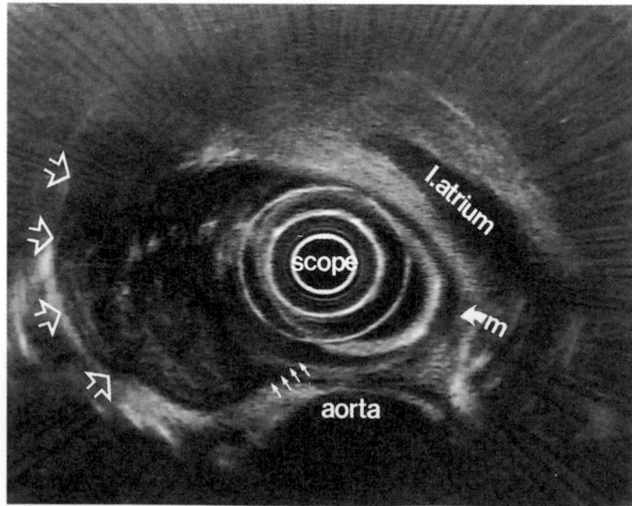

Fig. 3 Endoscopic ultrasound image of an oesophageal mass in the mid-esophagus. Note the adjacent structures in the mediastinum, aorta, and the left atrium. The wall structure of the oesophagus is also evident; the thickest hypoechoic layer is the muscularis propria (m). The tumour has extended beyond the muscularis layer (see small arrows) and into the mediastinum (large arrows).

Depth of penetration of the wall can be accurately assessed. Regional lymph nodes can be identified and metastases predicted on the basis of size and appearance. The use of endoscopic ultrasound is limited to those neoplasms that allow passage of the probe. However, the presence of a tight malignant stricture is an excellent (90 per cent) predictor of a stage III tumour. Its exact role in the management of oesophageal cancer is uncertain. Its greatest use may be in improved staging for patients undergoing preoperative adjuvant therapy.

TREATMENT OPTIONS FOR CARCINOMA OF THE OESOPHAGUS

The goal of treatment in carcinoma of the oesophagus is twofold: palliation of dysphagia and cure of the cancer. The standard of therapy is oesophageal resection. Resection quickly restores swallowing ability to normal and palliates dysphagia. As a single therapy, surgery offers the greatest chance for cure. Cure rates vary from institution to institution. A cumulative review of all published reports in English for surgical resection of squamous cell carcinoma of the oesophagus by Muller demonstrates the magnitude of the problem and summarizes the experience with 76 900 patients. Only 56 per cent of patients have resectable disease at first presentation. Resection was associated with an operative mortality of 13 per cent. Survival was 27 per cent at 1 year, 12 per cent at 2 years, and only 10 per cent at 5 years. Recent reports from selected institutions have shown a decrease in operative mortality and increase in 5-year survival. Many centres have reported mortality rates under 5 per cent and 5-year survivals around 20 per cent with surgery alone for squamous cell carcinoma of the oesophagus.

Oesophageal resection

There are many surgical approaches available for oesophageal resection. The main determinants of the operation chosen are the surgeon's preference and level of the tumour. The three most common approaches currently in use are the Sweet left thoracoabdominal approach, the Lewis laparotomy and right thoracotomy approach, and the Grey–Turner transhiatal oesophagectomy as popularized by Orringer. Excellent clinical results have been obtained for each technique in centres experienced in their use. There is little difference in morbidity or mortality between any of these approaches. Other techniques include the radical *en-bloc* oesophagectomy, an exclusive left thoracic approach (the stomach mobilization is done through a diaphragmatic incision), and the right thoracoabdominal approach.

The Sweet approach

The Sweet left thoracoabdominal approach is best employed for gastro-oesophageal junction carcinomas or low oesophageal carcinomas. Tumours 35 cm or more from the incisors are ideally suited to this approach. A double lumen endotracheal tube is used to block and deflate the left lung, enhancing exposure. The patient is placed in the right lateral decubitus position. An oblique left upper quadrant laparotomy is performed to explore the gastro-oesophageal junction area and the liver. If there is no contraindication to resection, a thoracoabdominal incision through the sixth or seventh interspace is performed. The diaphragm is incised circumferentially to avoid injury to the phrenic nerve branches. The stomach is mobilized on the right gastric and gastroepiploic arteries. The omentum is divided, preserving the right gastroepiploic artery. The left gastric artery is double ligated. The gastrohepatic omentum is divided with care taken to identify accessory arteries to the left lobe of liver. The hiatus is dissected. A pyloromyotomy or pyloroplasty is then done according to the surgeon's preference. The oesophagus is then dissected in *en-bloc* fashion from the pericardium to aorta. The level of anastomosis should be at least 5 cm above gross tumour to ensure adequate margins. If a higher level of intrathoracic anastomosis is desired, dissection can be easily performed below the arch of the aorta and then above it, allowing a supra-aortic anastomosis to be made lateral to the aortic arch. If exposure is limited, a second interspace thoracotomy can be made usually through the fourth interspace, allowing better access for anastomosis. The main advantage of this approach is the excellent exposure of the gastro-oesophageal junction and the ease of mobilizing the stomach, especially in obese patients. It offers the best exposure for the most complete abdominal lymphadenectomy. The limiting factor to this exposure is the position of the heart and aortic arch while doing the anastomosis. This can be partially overcome by choosing a second higher interspace as discussed. The largest negative factor about this approach is the fact that the aortic arch is in the way of the surgeon, thus limiting access to the total thoracic oesophagus and encouraging an anastomosis below the aortic arch.

Lewis approach

The Lewis right thoracotomy and laparotomy approach is best for mid- or lower-third lesions. An upper midline laparotomy is performed and the upper abdomen explored. If there are not contraindications to resection, the stomach is mobilized as previously described. It is important to enlarge the hiatus to prevent compression of the stomach when it is brought into the chest. As much of the lower oesophagus is mobilized as can be accomplished from the abdomen since this can be difficult through a high right thoracotomy. A table mounted type of retractor facilitates the dissection of the hiatus and lower oesophagus. The patient is then positioned for a right thoracotomy. The right lung is collapsed and the azygos vein ligated and divided. There is excellent exposure to the entire thoracic oesophagus which is dissected from pericardium to vertebral body. Care should be taken to ligate tissues in between the aorta and oesophagus to avoid injury to the thoracic duct. The stomach is then elevated up into the chest and a high intrathoracic anastomosis is made at the apex of the right chest. Care should be taken to avoid pulling too much of the stomach into the chest. If pulled too tightly a relative obstruction can be created at the hiatus. Excessive stomach will tend to fall into the costophrenic sulcus and impair emptying. The advantage to this approach is excellent exposure of the thoracic oesophagus and ease of anastomosis. It is easy to obtain a wide margin on the tumour because of the excellent exposure of the superior aspect of the oesophagus. The main difficulty encountered with the Lewis approach is lack of exposure of the gastro-oesophageal junction and hiatus especially in obese patients.

Transhiatal oesophagectomy

Transhiatal oesophagectomy is best used to remove upper-third or lower-third neoplasms. It is relatively difficult to remove stage III midoesophageal tumours with this approach. The operation is done in a supine position with a single lumen endotracheal tube. A laparotomy is performed first and the abdomen is explored. The stomach is prepared as an oesophageal substitute. It is helpful to open the hiatus anteriorly as described by Pinotti. This facilitates exposure of the distal oesophagus almost to the level of the carina. Vessels can be ligated under direct vision. The side of left neck is opened and the oesophagus exposed; care is taken to avoid retractor injury to the recurrent laryngeal nerve in the tracheo-oesophageal groove. The upper third of the oesophagus can be dissected under direct vision. If a transmural tumour is present in this area and if additional exposure is required, a partial upper sternal split can be performed as first described by Scannell. The sternal split facilitates exposure in this area. The area around the carina is often difficult to expose and usually has to be done in a 'blind' fashion. The oesophagus is removed and the stomach is brought up through the posterior mediastinal oesophageal bed and a cervical anastomosis performed.

Perceived advantages to transhiatai oesophagectomy are the avoidance of a thoracotomy and a cervical anastomosis. Anastomotic leaks occur more commonly in the cervical area, but can be easily drained and are rarely associated with the devastating complications of thoracic leaks. Although avoidance of a thoracotomy allows greater tolerance of the procedure as compared with transthoracic techniques, any advantages are difficult to prove. The major drawbacks are the limited *en-bloc* resection, the 'blind' area around the carina, and the possibility for an increased incidence of injury to nearby structures (thoracic duct, azygous vein, trachea, and recurrent laryngeal nerves). No randomized studies have been done comparing transhiatal with transthoracic oesophagectomy. Non-randomized studies have failed to demonstrate less morbidity, mortality, or hospital stay with the transhiatal technique (Table 4).

Fate of the pylorus

Most surgeons favour a drainage procedure with oesophagectomy. A small number of controlled trials have been performed comparing the results of no pyloric drainage procedure versus using a drainage procedure. No clear advantage has been shown. The incidence of gastric outlet obstruction with no drainage has been under 10 per cent, and the need for reoperation has been under 2 per cent. Dumping is a recognized side-effect of a drainage procedure and is one reason that some surgeons prefer not to perform one. If postoperative gastric outlet obstruction fails to respond to conservative measures, reoperation can be difficult. This is the primary reason that surgeons prefer to perform a pyloromyotomy or pyloroplasty.

Anastomotic technique

In 1942, Churchill and Sweet described a triple-layer technique of oesophagastrostomy and conventional *en-bloc* resection of the cancer and adjacent lymph nodes. Five years later, Richard Sweet published his initial experience with surgical management of carcinoma of the oesophagus in 141 patients. Operating in an era without sophisticated postoperative monitoring devices, mechanical ventilation, or broad-spectrum antibiotics, his results were remarkable: an operative mortality of 15 per cent, anastomotic leaks in 1.4 per cent of patients, and overall 5-year survival of 11 per cent. This served as a standard for many years. Much of the success is directly attributed to the reliability of the anastomosis and remarkably low anastomotic leak rates. Sweet emphasized the details of technique and warned against factors predisposing to anastomotic leak. The lack of an oesophageal serosal layer and the segmental blood supply of the oesophagus make oesophageal anastomosis more demanding than other intestinal anastomoses. Atraumatic handling of the tissues, preservation of the blood supply of both the oesophagus and stomach, avoidance of the use of crushing clamps, lack of tension on the anastomosis, use of fine interrupted sutures, cutting with a knife or other sharp instrument, and tying sutures gently but firmly to avoid cutting tissues are all important details in the performance of an anastomosis. Few modifications have been made from the technique Churchill and Sweet proposed 45 years ago. Preservation of the blood supply is crucial when mobilizing the stomach and oesophagus. The blood supply of the stomach will be from the right gastric and right gastroepiploic arteries. The oesophagus should not be mobilized beyond a few centimetres above the proposed level of the anastomosis to avoid interference with the segmental blood supply. A circle approximately 2 cm in diameter is scored on a portion of the serosa of the stomach (Fig. 4). The circular defect in the stomach should be 2 cm away from the stapled edge of the stomach to avoid compromise of the blood supply. Individual vessels are identified and ligated with fine silk sutures. This minimizes bleeding while the anastomosis is performed and allows for precise placement of sutures.

Interrupted horizontal mattress sutures of fine suture material (we use 4–0 silk) are used to construct the back row of the anastomosis. Corner stitches are placed first, and the remaining sutures are evenly spaced between them. The sutures on the stomach involve the seromuscular layers and those on the oesophagus, the longitudinal and circular muscle layers. The oesophageal sutures should be deep enough to include both the longitudinal and

Table 4 Comparison of transhiatal (THE) and transthoracic (TTE) oesophagectomy

Author, year	Operative mortality (%)		Respiratory complication (%)	Anastomotic leaks (%)
Shahian, 1986	THE (30)	13.3	21.4	15.4
	TTE (65)	6.2	16.9	1.8
Hankins, 1989	THE (26)		8.0	54
	TTE (52)	6.0	38	5.9
Streitz, 1991	THE (17)		5.9	
	TTE (43)	2.3		2.3
Daniel, 1992	THE (77)		8.0	
	TTE (24)	8.0		4

Number of patients in parentheses.

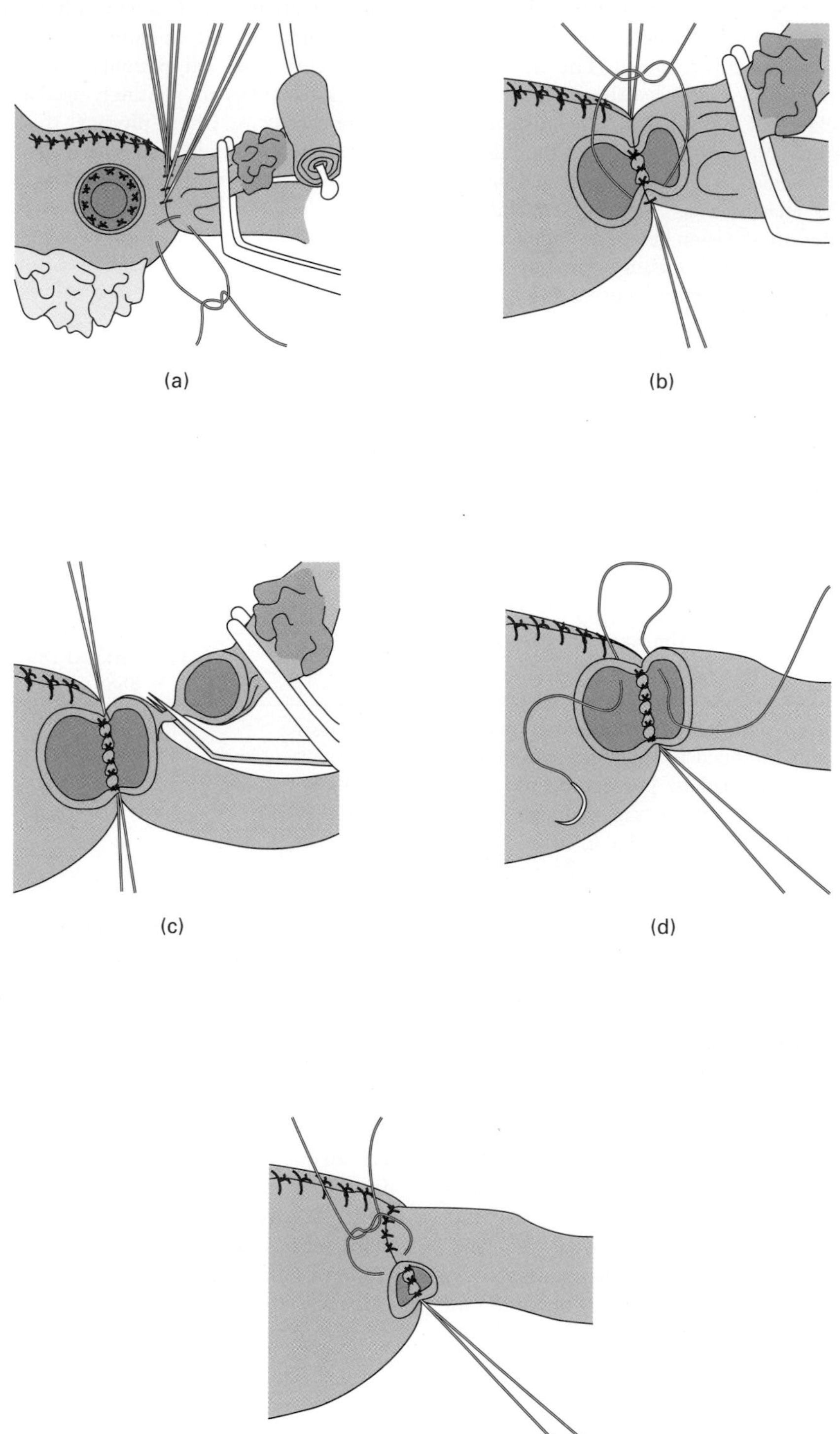

Fig. 4 Surgical technique. (a) The serosa of the stomach has been scored, and the vessels have been ligated. The back row of the sutures has been completed. (b) The button of stomach has been removed and the anterior wall of oesophagus, opened. (c) The back row of the inner layer is completed, and the oesophagus is transected. (d) The remainder of the inner layer is completed. A Connell stitch is used for closure of the final opening. A nasogastric tube is advanced across the anastomosis under direct vision before the inner layer is completed. (e) The outer layer is nearly finished.

circular muscles of the oesophagus. The sutures should not be tied too tight, to avoid necrosis or cutting through the muscle.

The oesophagus is opened sharply from one corner stitch to the other. The circular button of stomach is removed. The inner layer is completed with simple sutures including just the mucosa of the oesophagus and the full thickness of the stomach. The knots are on the inside, thereby allowing inversion or turning-in of the mucosa of both the oesophagus and stomach. This is accomplished for the entire circumference of the anastomosis. A nasogastric tube is passed into the stomach under direct vision before a single Connell stitch is placed for closure of the final opening. Healing of the inverted mucosa is an important feature in preventing leakage, and the location of the knots on the luminal side minimizes foreign body reaction within the actual tissues of the anastomosis. The outer row is completed using horizontal mattress sutures as described for the back row of the outer layer.

The omentum mobilized with the stomach is placed over the anastomosis anteriorly to provide an additional layer of coverage. The posterior part of the anastomosis lies between the oesophagus and the more proximal stomach. A few sutures are placed between the stomach and the mediastinal pleura to avoid tension on the anastomosis when the patient is upright, particularly if the stomach is full.

Viability of tissues on each edge of the anastomosis is best maintained if trauma is avoided. The edges are never crushed with clamps and, indeed, are handled with forceps as little as is possible. Once the first stitch is placed and tied, traction on it permits placement of the next without the need for grasping the mucosa with instruments. The sutures are tied by positioning the index finger cephalad to the anastomosis, lifting the stomach to the oesophagus, and avoiding pulling down on the fixed and more fragile oesophagus. Delicacy in suturing is especially important for the outer layer of the anastomosis because the oesophagus lacks a peritoneal surface.

A nasogastric tube passed through the anastomosis for a short time avoids distraction at the suture line by a distended stomach. Gentle, periodic irrigation of the tube ensures its patency. Temporary gastric decompression more than compensates for any potentially deleterious effect of an intraluminal foreign body lying against the suture line for a short period.

We have published our experiences with this technique on a consecutive series of 104 patients. There were three postoperative deaths (2.9 per cent). Two deaths were attributable to pneumonia and respiratory failure (patients aged 59 and 73 years). Both patients smoked at least one pack of cigarettes per day preoperatively. The third death was also due to pneumonia and respiratory failure. This 76-year-old patient had an emergency operation for massive gastrointestinal bleeding. Dilatation was necessary in five patients for anastomotic stricture 3 to 6 weeks postoperatively. One dilatation-to-three dilations were required for successful resolution of dysphagia. Delayed anastomotic stricture was not apparent in this group of patients. All patients had postoperative barium swallows. There were no anastomotic leaks, even of localized type. These results have been reported by others using a similar two-layer technique.

POSTOPERATIVE MANAGEMENT

Patients are usually returned to the intensive care unit intubated and are electively ventilated overnight and extubated the following morning. Use of thoracic epidural anaesthesia with a combination of narcotic and local anaesthetic is routinely used and greatly ameliorates postoperative pain. Pulmonary artery catheters are not routinely used unless clinically indicated. Fluid status is carefully monitored and an indwelling bladder catheter is employed for several days. All patients receive perioperative antibiotics. Nasogastric tubes are routinely used and are removed when bowel function returns. Chest physical therapy and nebulized aerosols are routinely administered to improve pulmonary toilet. Jejunostomy tubes are placed in high-risk patients or those who are nutritionally depleted. Enteral feeding is begun usually on the second or third postoperative day. A Gastrografin swallow is obtained to check the anastomosis when bowel function returns. An oral diet is then begun and advanced to a soft solid diet.

Morbidity and mortality

Pulmonary complications are the most common postoperative complication encountered regardless of the approach used (Table 5).

Table 5 Pulmonary complications after oesophagectomy

	Transhiatal (%) (n = 8886)	**Transthoracic (%)** (n = 2436)
Atelectasis	21	26
Pneumonia	27	13
Respiratory insufficiency	23	10

The most feared complication following oesophagectomy is anastomotic leak. Leak rates as high as 10 to 15 per cent are commonly reported. Many series, however, do report leak rates under 5 per cent. These are usually associated with a two-layer anastomosis. Cervical anastomotic leaks usually present themselves with fever and a painful, swollen neck incision. The neck incision should be reopened and adequate drainage established. Healing will usually occur with provision of drainage, antibiotics, and adequate nutrition. A stricture may develop, requiring several dilatations to restore normal swallowing. Cervical anastomotic leaks are rarely fatal. Intrathoracic anastomotic leaks are much more serious. Mortality rates of 50 per cent or higher are still reported following free intrathoracic leaks. They demand prompt aggressive treatment. If the leak occurs in the first few days following operation, re-exploration is necessary to exclude the possibility of gastric necrosis. If that is found, the stomach should be debrided, closed, and returned to the abdomen. A cervical oesophagostomy should be performed and wide mediastinal and pleural drainage should be carried out. Reconstruction of the gastrointestinal tract can be done at a later date. Leaks detected after 1 week are best treated by immediate dependent drainage. Drainage should be converted to open drainage with a rib resection at an appropriate time. The critical issue is to establish adequate drainage of all infected material immediately after the diagnosis is made. Failure to achieve adequate drainage may lead to erosion of the airway or mediastinum. Small asymptomatic contained leaks can be seen as well. If they are indeed contained, treatment antibiotics, withholding of oral intake, and adequate nutrition eventually lead to healing. At least 1 week should pass before the patient is restudied. Anastomotic leaks remain the source of greatest morbidity and mortality. They require great judgement and immediate action to avoid a fatal outcome. These facts underscore the need for meticulous attention to detail in performing the oesophagogastric anastomosis.

Survival following oesophagectomy

At the Massachusetts General Hospital in the era prior to multimodality treatment of oesophageal carcinoma, survival following resection in all patients was as follows: 2 years, 31 per cent, 3 years 24 per cent, and 5 years 21 per cent. In a large series of Japanese patients who were grouped according to stage, 5-year survivals were as follows: stage I 60 per cent, stage II 30 per cent, stage III 20 per cent, and stage IV 5 per cent. There is no proof that there is any difference between radical *en-bloc* oesophagectomy, transthoracic oesophagectomy, or transhiatal oesophagectomy even though they obviously involve removal of different amounts of oesophagus and surrounding tissues as well as different degrees of lymphadenectomy (Table 6).

RADIATION THERAPY

Radiation therapy remains as one of the possible primary treatment modalities for squamous cell carcinoma of the oesophagus. Numerous large studies have been published facilitating comparison of results with surgical treatment. Unfortunately, 5-year survival statistics in many large series in which patients are treated with a curative intent with high dose radiation therapy show a survival of only 5 to 10 per cent at 5 years. The best results with primary radiation therapy obtained are in cervical carcinomas. Local control and survival are greatest in those patients with early stage I or stage II lesions and are poorest with advanced lesions. Radiation therapy usually does not control the local disease. There is an approximate 70 per cent failure rate after radical radiotherapy at the local site. The majority (75 per cent) of the local failures occur in the first year, thus prohibiting effective palliation for the majority of the patients. However, temporary palliation can be achieved with lower doses of radiation therapy which can be of help in patients who are not expected to live long.

Adjuvant radiotherapy

Hancock has recently reviewed the results of preoperative radiation therapy in over 1000 patients. Unfortunately, the average 5-year survival was only 6 per cent overall, which is not a significantly different rate from results of either surgical treatment or radiation therapy alone. In a highly selected group of patients who completed both radical radiotherapy and resection, the 5-year survival rate was approximately 14 per cent, not significantly different from historical surgical 5-year survival rates. Additionally, some groups have reported worse results with preoperative radiation therapy, primarily because of the toxicity associated with radical radiotherapy, leading to greater postoperative complication rates. There have been three well conducted prospective trials involving preoperative radiation therapy (Table 7). In no trial was a significant difference noted in median survival or in 5-year survival compared with surgical treatment alone. Preoperative treatment with radiation therapy is not recommended. One well designed randomized trial was reported of postoperative radiation therapy following oesophagectomy and again no significant difference was noted in long-term survival. Routine use of postoperative radiation therapy is therefore not recommended.

ADJUVANT CHEMOTHERAPY

Adjuvant preoperative chemotherapy has been reported, the majority of reports being pilot studies using cisplatin-based regimens. Partial and complete response rates up to 66 per cent have been reported. Other agents used included 5-fluorouracil, etoposide, bleomycin, and vincristine. Responders note a significant improvement in their dysphagia. Treatment toxicity in most series has been mild. Complete clinical response is usually associated with residual microscopic evidence of tumour, underlining the need for oesophagectomy. Complete clinical response has been associated with improved long-term survival in most series. The current programme at the Massachusetts General Hospital for squamous cell carcinoma of the oesophagus involves two cycles of preoperative cisplatin and 5-fluorouracil followed by resection and selective postoperative radiation or chemotherapy. A complete response has occurred in 37 per cent, a partial response in 40 per cent, and no response in 23 per cent. Operative mortality was 4 per cent. Seven per cent of the patients had no tumour in the resected specimen. Postoperative treatment included radiation therapy in 27 per cent, chemotherapy in 31 per cent, both therapies in 16 per cent, and no therapy in 27 per cent. Actuarial 5-year survival for the entire group of patients is 41 per cent. Complete responders had a 5-year survival of 68 per cent whereas partial and no responders had a 5-year survival of 20 per cent. A group of 27 patients followed for a minimum of 5 years now has an absolute 5-year survival of 42 per cent. A national trial is under way to randomize prospectively patients in an attempt to verify this observation.

Preoperative chemotherapy and radiation therapy

Steiger from Wayne State University reported the first combined modality series. Their treatment programme included 3000 cGy

Table 6 Survival following oesophagectomy

Technique	Author	Year	Number	Three-year survival (%)
Historical	Sweet	1952	284	22
Transthoracic	Katlic	1982	142	24
Transhiatal	Orringer	1986	147	23
Radical (*en bloc*)	Skinner	1986	80	24

Table 7 Results of preoperative radiation therapy

Author, year	*n*	Dose (Gy)	Resected %	5-year survival (%)
Launois, 1981	67	40	70	10
	67	0	50	11
Gignoux, 1987	102	33	73	11
	106	0	81	10
Wang, 1989	104	40	93	35
	102	0	85	30

n = number of patients.

of radiation in combination with chemotherapy (one-half of the patients received 5-fluorouracil and mitomycin-C and one-half received cisplatin and 5-fluorouracil). Their treatment programme had a significant treatment mortality rate, which approached 30 per cent. No evidence of tumour was found in 31 per cent of patients. Those patients having a complete response appeared to have prolonged survival. Others have reported similar results.

ADENOCARCINOMA OF THE OESOPHAGUS

Adenocarcinoma of the oesophagus is reported with increasing frequency from many institutions in the United States. Many authors now report more adenocarcinomas than squamous cell carcinomas in surgical series. A recent epidemiological study by Blot in the United States has shown that incidence rates between 1976 and 1987 were fairly stable for squamous cell carcinoma, but increased more than 100 per cent for adenocarcinoma among men. From 1984 to 1987, adenocarcinomas accounted for 34 per cent of all oesophageal cancers among white men. The corresponding percentages for black men, white women, and black women were 3, 12, and 1 per cent respectively. The rate of increase during the 1970s and 1980s surpassed that of any other cancer. The much higher rates among white compared with black subjects suggest that cigarette smoking and alcohol intake, risk factors that are more commonly present in black subjects, are not major risk factors as they are for squamous cell carcinoma of the oesophagus.

Most of the adenocarcinomas are in association with a columnar-lined oesophagus (Barrett's oesophagus). Other possible sites of origin include the superficial mucosal glands which occur in either end of the oesophagus, the deep submucosal glands which are distributed throughout the oesophagus, and areas of ectopic gastric mucosa. Barrett's oesophagus is thought to be an acquired condition due to severe gastro-oesophageal reflux. The development of adenocarcinoma arising in the columnar-lined mucosa was first described in 1952 and the tendency for this columnar-lined epithelium to develop adenocarcinoma was first reported by Naef in 1975. Barrett's mucosa is found in about 10 per cent of all patients who undergo endoscopic examination for symptoms of gastro-oesophageal reflux. Barrett's mucosa can become dysplastic and when high grade dysplasia develops there is a substantial risk for developing adenocarcinoma. Estimates of risk of malignant change in patients with simple Barrett's oesophagus are about one case per 300 patient years from the time of diagnosis. Compared to a matched population, the risk of developing adenocarcinoma in a patient with Barrett's mucosa is approximately 40 times higher.

Barrett's oesophagus with dysplasia

Dysplasia is present in the majority of patients who undergo resection for Barrett's adenocarcinoma, lending support to the hypothesis suggesting that dysplasia leads to high-grade dysplasia and hence to invasive carcinoma. Dysplasia is graded using criteria established by the inflammatory bowel disease–dysplasia morphology study group. Low-grade dysplasia consists of mildly dysplastic nuclei confined to the lower half of the epithelium. High-grade dysplasia consists of either severe nuclear dysplasia or dysplastic nuclei extending through the entire thickness of the epithelium. High-grade dysplasia is synonymous with carcinoma-*in-situ*.

Patients with Barrett's oesophagus should undergo surveillance endoscopy approximately every year to screen for the development of dysplasia or carcinoma. Four-quadrant biopsies should be taken every 1 to 2 cm until normal squamous epithelium is reached. Special attention should be paid to subtle alterations in the appearance of the epithelium, as these areas are more likely to show advanced disease. If low-grade dysplasia is diagnosed, surveillance should be increased to every 3 to 6 months and intensive medical therapy instituted. Dysplasia has regressed with medical therapy in the majority of patients so treated. However, carcinoma has developed during intensive medical therapy for low-grade dysplasia. There is no proof that an antireflux operation can prevent adenocarcinoma from developing.

Once high-grade dysplasia develops, oesophagectomy should be performed. Approximately one-half of patients have invasive carcinoma in the resected specimen (Table 8). The majority of patients so treated are either stage 0 or I. The 5-year survival approaches 100 per cent in stage 0 patients.

Table 8 Oesophagectomy for high-grade dysplasia in Barrett's oesophagus

Author	Year	No. of patients	Adenocarcinoma (%)
Altorki	1991	9	45
Pera	1992	19	50

Barrett's adenocarcinoma

Eighty per cent of the neoplasms are in the lower third and 20 per cent are in the middle third of the oesophagus. Patients who present themselves with dysphagia have neoplasms that are usually transmural with regional lymph node metastases. There is extensive submucosal spread of the tumour similar to squamous cell carcinoma. Resection remains the best therapeutic option. The entire extent of Barrett's mucosa should be removed at the time of oesophagectomy as second adenocarcinomas occur in residual Barrett's mucosa. The 5-year survival rate with oesophagectomy approaches 10 per cent. Survival rates approach 90 per cent among those who have early cancer limited to the mucosa recognized by surveillance endoscopy.

PALLIATION OF DYSPHAGIA

Dysphagia is the primary clinical symptom of patients with oesophageal carcinoma that requires palliation. Although palliative resection is recommended by many, it is associated with higher postoperative morbidity and mortality compared with those patients who undergo 'curative' oesophagectomies. Oesophageal bypass is considered by some surgeons to provide appreciable palliation of dysphagia in those for whom resection is not possible. Morbidity rates of 50 per cent and mortality rates of 25 to 30 per cent are commonly reported. Median survival following palliative bypass is usually less than 6 months. Most surgeons have abandoned this approach. Use of the Nd-YAG laser may relieve dysphagia, but several treatment sessions are usually necessary to restore an adequate lumen. Repeat treatment sessions are not usually necessary as patients usually die before the tumour regrows. There is a low incidence of perforation with this approach and the ability to swallow is usually quickly restored.

There has been a renewed interest in oesophageal bypass tubes. The older rigid tubes, usually inserted by open techniques, were associated with high mortality rates and frequent complications. The newer silastic tubes are inserted by dilating the oesophagus and pushing the tube in place. The incidence of complications, perforation, and high mortality rates have been low in most series. The distal end is ideally situated above the gastro-oesophageal junction to avoid reflux. These prostheses allow swallowing of liquids and some soft solids. This approach allows quick restitution of swallowing and satisfactory palliation. Average median survival is 3 to 6 months following tube insertion.

UNUSUAL OESOPHAGEAL NEOPLASMS

Small cell carcinoma

About 150 cases of oesophageal small cell carcinoma have been reported with striking morphological and biological features similar to small cell carcinoma of the lung. These tumours contain cells with characteristic cytoplasmic granules (neurosecretory type) which are argyrophilic. Because both the lung and oesophagus are derived from the embryological foregut, argyrophilic neurosecretory cells can be expected in the oesophagus. These cells have indeed been found in small cell carcinoma of the oesophagus. Their clinical course is remarkably similar to that of small cell carcinoma of the lung. The tumours are typically fungating and polypoid with surface ulcerations and are commonly found in the middle and lower third. Widespread metastases are common. Multimodality therapy with chemotherapy and radiation is the treatment of choice with little role for surgery. There are a few long-term survivors.

Melanoma

Melanoblasts have been reported in the oesophageal mucosa and are typically scattered throughout the oesophagus. Oesophageal melanosis is a benign condition seen in approximately 5 per cent of people with apparently normal oesophaguses, but is associated with malignant melanoma of the oesophagus in approximately one-third of all reported cases. Melanoma of the oesophagus is a rare tumour and fewer than 150 cases have been reported. The average age is about 60 and males predominate. Melanomas typically are polypoid and often can grow large. The tumour may be black, brown, or grey; most melanomas are ulcerated. Patients present themselves with dysphagia and when first seen appear to have localized resectable disease. Regional lymph node metastases are quite common. Surgical resection is the treatment of choice although long-term survival is rare. Chemotherapy and radiation therapy have not proved effective.

Leiomyosarcoma

Leiomyosarcoma is the most common sarcomatous tumour of the oesophagus. Males predominate and the typical age at presentation is 60. Most present themselves in the middle or lower thirds of the oesophagus and have a characteristic pedunculated appearance on radiological examination. The tumour often achieves a large size before obstructive symptoms occur. Myosarcomas are typically well localized and resectable and in general do not invade adjacent mediastinal structures until later in their course. Surgical resection is the treatment of choice and has produced long-term survivors. Although radiation therapy may provide palliation, surgery appears to offer superior cure rates.

BENIGN TUMOURS OF THE OESOPHAGUS

Leiomyoma

Autopsy studies confirm that these are extremely rare tumours. Reports have ranged from 1/1000 postmortem examinations to 2/36000 postmortem examinations. Leiomyomas occurring in the oesophagus represent about 10 per cent of all gastrointestinal leiomyomas. Leiomyomas rarely occur in the cervical region, but are equally distributed between the middle and lower third levels. Less than 5 per cent of the leiomyomas are multiple. Leiomyomas are usually found in men (ratio of 2:1). There is a wide age distribution between 20 and 70 years. The tumours are usually intramural and well circumscribed. Unusual configurations of leiomyomas with a horseshoe pattern are not uncommon. Leiomyomas rarely undergo malignant transformation. The growth rate of these tumours appears quite slow as the duration of reported symptoms often can be quite long. Dysphagia and odynophagia are the most common presenting symptoms. They are frequently found as incidental findings during assessment for other gastrointestinal complaints. Barium oesophogram typically shows a smooth semilunar defect with sharp borders and an intact mucosa. Horseshoe type leiomyomas characteristically produce obstruction. Oesophagoscopy should be performed, but typically only a bulging mass is seen. The overlying mucosa is usually intact, and should not be biopsied. All symptomatic leiomyomas should be removed. Small asymptomatic tumours should be left in place. For mid-third lesions, a right thoracotomy is chosen whereas lower third lesions are best approached through a left thoracotomy. The tumour can be enucleated from the oesophageal wall. Care must be taken to avoid entering the oesophageal mucosa. The incision in the oesophageal musculature is closed with interrupted sutures.

Benign polyp

Benign polyps of the oesophagus are rare, but are notable for their sometimes dramatic presentation with regurgitation of the polyp into the mouth which can produce airway obstruction. The polyps are usually solitary and are frequently quite long and cylindrical in shape. Because of constant peristaltic action, elongation frequently occurs which then can permit regurgitation into the mouth. Marked dilatation of the oesophagus can occur because of gradual enlargement of the polypoid mass. Polyps are typically composed of vascular fibroblastic connective tissue, covered by normal mucosa. Dysphagia is the predominant symptom, but occasionally the patient will relate a history of intermittent regurgitation of a mass into the mouth. The barium oesophagogram is often diagnostic, showing a long intraluminal filling defect with a rounded lower border. Oesophagoscopy confirms results of barium studies. These lesions usually occur in older men and usually arise from the cervical oesophagus. Treatment is always surgical, both to relieve symptoms and to rule out malignancy. Occasionally small polyps have a base that can be readily seen and the stalk can be endoscopically divided and the base cauterized. Larger polyps require oesophagotomy on the side opposite to the tumour. This can be done through a cervical approach for high lesions or upper sternotomy or lateral thoracotomy for lower lesions. The oesophagus is closed in layers.

FURTHER READING

Aikiyama H, *et al.* Principles of surgical treatment for carcinoma of the esophagus. Analysis of lymph node involvement. *Ann Surg*, 1981; **194**: 438–46.

Blot WJ, *et al.* Rising incidence of adenocarcinoma of the esophagus and gastric cardia. *JAMA*, 1991; **265**: 1287–9.

Burt M, *et al.* Malignant esophogorespiratory fistula: management options and survival. *Ann Thoracic Surg*, 1991; **52**: 1222–9.

Cusumano A, *et al.* Push-through intubation: effective palliation in 409 patients with cancer of the esophagus. *Ann Thoracic Surg*. 1992; **53**: 1006–9.

Daniel TM, *et al.* Transhiatal esophagectomy: a safe alternative for selected patients. *Ann Thoracic Surg*. 1992; **54**: 686–90.

Delarue NC, Wilkins E Wassel, Wong J, eds. *International trends in general thoracic surgery*, Vol. 4. *Esophageal cancer*. St. Louis: C. V. Mosby CO, 1988.

Earlom R, Cunha-Melo JR. Oesophageal squamous cell carcinoma. II. A critical review of radiotherapy. *Br J Surg*, 1980; **67**: 457–61.

Earlom R, Cunha-Melo JR. Oesophageal squamous cell carcinoma. I. A critical review of surgery. *Br J Surg*, 1980; **67**: 381–90.

Gignoux M, *et al.* The value of pre-operative radiotherapy in esophageal cancer: results of a study of the EORTC. *World J Surg*, 1987; **11**: 426–32.

Hancock SL, Glatstain E. Radiation therapy of esophageal cancer. *Semin Oncol*, 1984; **11**: 144–58.

Hankins JR, *et al.* Carcinoma of the esophagus. A comparison of the results of transhiatal versus transthoracic resection. *Ann Thoracic Surg*, 1989; **47**: 700–5.

Hilgenberg AD, *et al.* Pre-operative chemotherapy, surgical resection, and selective post-operative radiation therapy for squamous cell carcinoma of the esophagus. *Ann Thoracic Surg*, 1988; **45**: 357–63.

Launois B, *et al.* Pre-operative radiotherapy for carcinoma of the esophagus. *Surg Gynecol Obstet*, 1981; **153**: 690–2.

Lewis I. The surgical treatment of carcinoma of the oesophagus. *Br J Surg*, 1946; **34**: 18–31.

Mathisen DJ. *Seminars in Thoracic and Cardiovascular Surgery—Esophagus*. 1992; **4**.

Mathisen DJ, *et al.* Transthoracic esophagectomy: a safe approach to carcinoma of the esophagus. *Ann Thoracic Surg*, 1988; **45**: 137–43.

Moon BC, Woolfson IK, Mercer CD. Neodymium: yttrium–aluminum–garnet laser vaporization for palliation of obstructing esophageal carcinoma. *J Thoracic Cardiovasc Surg*, 1989; **98**: 11–15.

Muller JM, *et al.* Surgical therapy of oesophageal carcinoma. *Br J Surg*, 1990; **77**: 845–57.

Pera M, *et al.* Barett;s esophagus with high-grade dysplasia: an indication for esophagectomy? *Ann Thoracic Surg*, 1992; **54**: 199–204.

Rice TW, *et al.* Esophageal carcinoma: esophageal ultrasound assessment of pre-operative chemotherapy. *Ann Thoracic Surg*, 1992; **53**: 972–7.

Roth, JA, Ruckdeschel JC, Weisenburger TH, eds. *Thoracic oncology*. Philadelphia: W. B. Saunders, 1989.

Shahian DM, *et al.* Transthoracic versus extrathoracic esophagectomy: mortality, morbidity and long term survival. *Ann Thoracic Surg*, 1986; **41**: 237–46.

Skinner DB. *En bloc* resection for neoplasms of the esophagus and cardia. *J Thoracic Cardiovasc Surg*, 1983; **85**: 59–71.

Streitz JM Jr, *et al.* Adenocarcinoma in Barrett's esophagus: clinicopathologic study of 65 cases. *Ann Surg*, 1991; **213**: 122–5.

Streitz JM, Williamson WA, Ellis FH. Current concepts concerning the nature and treatment of Barrett's esophagus and its complications. *Ann Thoracic Surg*, 1992; **54**: 586–91.

Steiger Z, *et al.* Eradication and palliation of squamous cell carcinoma of the esophagus with chemotherapy, radiotherapy and surgical therapy. *J Thoracic Cardivasc Surg*, 1981; **82**: 713–19.

Sweet RH. Surgical management of carcinoma of the midthoracic esophagus. *N Engl J Med*, 1945; **233**: 1–7.

Turner GG. Excision of thoracic oesophagus for carcinoma, with construction of extra-thoracic gullet. *Lancet*, 1933; **ii**: 1315–16.

14.6 Surgical oesophageal disease: diagnostic considerations

CHERYL J. BUNKER

Diagnostic testing of the oesophagus is indicated in three settings: (1) initial evaluation of a symptomatic patient; (2) in the preoperative patient to ensure successful surgery; and (3) in the postoperative patient with new or residual symptoms following surgery.

GASTRO-OESOPHAGEAL REFLUX

Initial diagnosis

Diagnostically, the 24-h pH probe is considered to be the gold standard for documenting gastro-oesophageal reflux. A small-calibre catheter is passed through a nostril into the oesophagus, and is taped in place so that the distal tip of the probe is 5 cm above the upper margin of the lower oesophageal sphincter. The probe is attached to a recording box, which documents the oesophageal pH, confirming the number of episodes of acid reflux and the length of time needed to clear acid from the oesophagus with each reflux episode. The catheter remains in place for 24 h, while the patient is eating, sleeping, and performing his or her usual daily activities. During this time, the patient keeps a diary to correlate symptoms, meals, and sleep with the record of acid reflux generated by the pH probe. Established criteria are used to ascertain whether or not truly pathological reflux is present. Alternative or complementary studies are available, but none, other than the 24-h pH probe, provides an actual recording of reflux episodes in the 'real life' setting.

When use of a pH probe is not feasible, an oesophageal scintigraphy study offers a reasonable alternative. Scintigraphy entails ingesting an isotope-labelled liquid meal; radioactive counts are recorded over the oesophagus and stomach. A shortcoming of this method, however, is that it evaluates the patient over a very limited period in an artificial setting. Patients who primarily have reflux postprandially or nocturnally may, therefore, have a false-negative scintigraphic scan. From the patient's perspective, scintigraphy has the advantage of not needing to swallow a catheter. Often patients who will not tolerate a catheter are receptive to drinking the radioactively labelled liquid.

The traditional barium upper gastrointestinal series serves two purposes in gastro-oesophageal reflux. First, it can document the presence of reflux, and second, it can identify complications of reflux such as strictures, oesophagitis, oesophageal ulcers, or tumours (Table 1). The limitation is the short length of time over which the patient is evaluated. To help compensate provocative manoeuvres may be attempted to elicit gastro-oesophageal reflux. Manual pressure over the stomach, increasing intra-abdominal pressure by straight-leg raising, or altering the patient's position from supine to prone (or prone to supine) all increase the likelihood of detecting reflux on a barium series. Unfortunately, neither the sensitivity nor the specificity can approach that of the 24-h pH probe in detecting reflux.

Upper gastrointestinal endoscopy does not provide a means of quantitating reflux directly, but does permit an assessment of mucosal injury that can result from reflux (Table 2). Biopsies demonstrating basal cell hyperplasia or an excessive number of eosinophils strongly imply pathological gastro-oesophageal reflux.

Table 1 Diagnostic studies in gastro-oesophageal reflux

To confirm the diagnosis
24-h pH probe
Oesophageal scintigraphy
Barium upper gastrointestinal series
Bernstein acid perfusion test
To identify complications
Barium upper gastrointestinal series
Upper gastrointestinal endoscopy
To identify contributing factors
Oesophageal motility study (manometry)

Table 2 Signs of gastro-oesophageal reflux on upper gastrointestinal endoscopy

On gross inspection
Oesophagitis
Oesophageal ulceration
Appearance of Barrett's mucosa
On microscopic examination
Basal cell hyperplasia
Increased number of eosinophils
Barrett's mucosa

Finally, there is the Bernstein acid perfusion test designed to determine whether a patient's symptoms result from exposing the oesophagus to acid. The Bernstein test entails infusing normal saline as a baseline, followed by 0.1 M hydrochloric acid into the mid or distal oesophagus in a single-blinded fashion such that the patient does not know he or she is receiving the acid. The acid is dripped in until the patient begins to experience heartburn or chest pain, or until 30 min have passed. Saline is then reinfused, to document resolution of symptoms, and for a few minutes as a 'control' before acid is reinfused as a second challenge. A test is considered positive if symptoms are elicited on two separate acid infusions. Although, this study does not document gastro-oesophageal reflux, it provides presumptive evidence that acid exposure of the oesophageal mucosa leads to the patient's symptoms.

Preoperative evaluation

Preoperatively, confirming the diagnostic suspicion of gastro-oesophageal reflux with a laboratory test such as a 24-h pH probe is valuable in reassuring both patient and surgeon that an antireflux procedure will indeed bring relief of symptoms. Additional studies to rule out confounding diagnoses, such as gastritis or cholelithiasis, may be warranted if the symptoms or diagnostic studies are equivocal.

Determining whether or not complications of refractory gastro-oesophageal reflux have occurred is a prudent preoperative measure, as such a finding might influence the surgical procedure selected. The evaluation should include an upper endoscopy with biopsies of the distal oesophagus to eliminate the possibility of Barrett's oesophagus with dysplasia. A barium swallow or an upper gastrointestinal endoscopy will also identify patients with reflux-induced strictures. A tight stricture or severe dysplasia in the setting of Barrett's oesophagus might indicate the need for resecting the involved segment of oesophagus, and thus, would alter the surgical plan.

Verifying normal peristalsis in the oesophageal body preoperatively is vital, as antireflux surgery essentially creates a barrier to the passage of material through the gastro-oesophageal junction. Inadequate strength of contractions or poorly co-ordinated contractions in the oesophageal body preoperatively, can leave the patient with dysphagia postoperatively. Advance knowledge of such a motility disorder might alter the decision to proceed with surgery. A barium swallow provides a gross estimate of oesophageal peristalsis. An oesophageal motility study, however, is a much more precise evaluation of peristalsis, and should be obtained preoperatively if possible.

An oesophageal motility study takes approximately 20 min and involves inserting a slender nasogastric catheter through which precise measurements are made. Two types of catheters are available: solid state, or water-perfused. Currently, manometry provides the most accurate measurements of the strength of contractions as well as the timing and co-ordination of peristaltic waves down the oesophagus. Specific criteria have been set in terms of the amplitudes, durations, and timing of contractions in the body of the oesophagus, as well as normal ranges for the resting tone, percentage relaxation, and timing of relaxation of the upper and lower oesophageal sphincters. These measurements are used to define the various oesophageal motility disorders. A preoperative motility study is also useful in determining the exact location of the lower oesophageal sphincter.

Postoperative considerations

Patients who have undergone an antireflux procedure may present themselves with three primary categories of postoperative problems that relate to oesophageal function: (1) continuation of the original reflux symptoms, (2) the new onset of dysphagia, or (3) the inability to belch. In patients who have symptoms of continued reflux postoperatively, studies should be initiated to determine whether or not the surgery has truly failed. A barium swallow, specifically to document passage of both barium liquid and tablets through the oesophagus, is essential. If this is not revealing, a 24-h pH probe, as was suggested for before surgery, should be obtained. If significant reflux is present, another operation may be indicated.

Persistent dysphagia following antireflux surgery generally indicates either inadequate peristalsis in the body of the oesophagus, or too tight a wrap at the base of the oesophagus. A barium swallow is the best initial study, using barium in both liquid and tablet form to assess bolus progression through the oesophagus. An oesophageal motility study provides the most precise measurements of oesophageal peristalsis, as well as the resting tone and function of the distal oesophagus in the region of the surgical wrap. If peristalsis is inadequate or if the wrap is too tight, dilatation of the distal oesophagus (or in certain cases, a second operation) may be required.

The inability to belch after antireflux surgery (the 'gas-bloat syndrome') suggests that the distal oesophagus may have been wrapped too tightly. As with dysphagia in the postoperative setting, a barium swallow and possibly oesophageal manometry are indicated.

ACHALASIA

Initial diagnosis

Nearly 100 per cent of patients with achalasia present with dysphagia. The evaluation of oesophageal dysphagia generally begins with a traditional barium swallow to differentiate motility disorders such as achalasia from anatomical disorders such as strictures or webs. The classic radiological findings in achalasia include a dilated oesophageal body with the absence of peristaltic contractions, and a tapering of the distal oesophagus known as a 'bird's beak' which represents the tightly contracted lower oesophageal sphincter. Retained food often is present in the oesophagus due to delayed oesophageal clearance (Fig. 1). Achalasia can

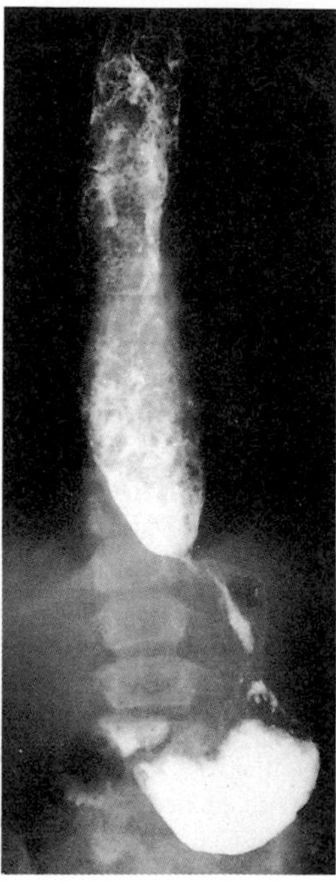

Fig. 1 Typical features of achalasia on barium oesophagram.

also be staged according to the findings on a barium oesophagram. In Stage 1 disease the oesophageal body has a maximal diameter of less than 4 cm. In Stage 2 disease the maximal diameter is 4 to 6 cm; in Stage 3 disease, the diameter is greater than 6 cm. In the more advanced cases, the oesophageal body may progress into a sigmoid configuration. The proximal oesophagus generally appears normal, as it is comprised of striated muscle, and, therefore, is not affected by the disease process.

Ideally, oesophageal manometry to confirm achalasia is carried out. Although there are variants, the classic manometric findings in achalasia are low amplitude, non-peristaltic contractions in the oesophageal body, with an elevated resting tone of the lower oesophageal sphincter. Typically, the lower oesophageal sphincter also does not relax appropriately in response to swallows.

Preoperative evaluation

When achalasia is suggested on a barium oesophagram, upper endoscopy is indicated. Typically, a dilated oesophagus, often filled with debris, is found on endoscopy. Retroflexion in the stomach to view the gastro-oesophageal junction is essential to eliminate the possibility of a gastric tumour in the cardia. The high-pressure lower oesophageal sphincter of achalasia does not obstruct the passage of an endoscope into the stomach. Difficulty passing an endoscope into the stomach may signify a more serious problem, such as a tumour in the gastric cardia. Finding a neoplasm would clearly alter the therapeutic approach.

Postoperative considerations

Following surgery for achalasia, nearly 20 per cent of patients experience gastro-oesophageal reflux. Diagnostic testing is generally not necessary, but would include a barium swallow or 24-h pH probe to document the reflux if there were any question about the aetiology of the patient's symptoms. An upper gastrointestinal endoscopy may be warranted in certain individuals to assess the presence or extent of reflux-induced oesophagitis.

FURTHER READING

Bernstein LM, Baker LA. A clinical test for oesophagitis. *Gastroenterology*, 1958; **34**: 760–81.

Fisher RS, Malmud LS, Roberts GS, Lobis IF. Gastroesophageal (GE) scintiscanning to detect and quantitate GE reflux. *Gastroenterology*, 1976; **70**: 301–8.

Henderson RD. Achalasia of the oesophagus. In: *Esophageal manometry in clinical investigation*. New York: Praeger 1983: 140–63.

Ismail-Beigi F, Horton PF, Pope CE. Histological consequences of gastroesophageal reflux in man. *Gastroenterology*, 1970; **58**: 163–74.

Johnson LF, DeMeester TR. Twenty-four-hour pH monitoring of the distal esophagus. *Am J Gastroenterol*, 1974; **62**: 325–32.

Katzka DA. Barrett's esophagus: detection and management. *Gastroenterol Clin N Am*, 1989; **18**: 339–57.

Ogorek CP, Fisher RS. Detection and treatment of gastroesophageal reflux disease. *Gastroenterol Clin N Am*, 1989; **18(2)**: 293–313.

Reynolds JC, Parkman HP. Achalasia. *Gastroenterol Clin N Am*, 1989; **18**: 223–55.

The stomach and duodenum 15

15.1 Peptic ulcer—stomach and duodenum

JOHN P. WELCH AND CLAUDE E. WELCH

INTRODUCTION

About 10 per cent of the population in the United States and Great Britain suffer from gastric or duodenal ulcers at some time. Most of these ulcers are not serious or chronic and those that do not heal spontaneously respond to medical therapy. Hospital admission and surgery are required by only a small proportion of people with these diseases. For example, in the Massachusetts General Hospital there were about 500 admissions per year for gastric or duodenal ulcer in 1973; a decade later there were only 300 per year. About 25 per cent of patients admitted with these ulcers now undergo surgical procedures.

Statistics concerning the frequency of the diseases must be regarded with some scepticism. Barium contrast studies cannot identify the many small superficial ulcers that come and go within a space of a few days. Endoscopy now discloses many of these ulcers; however, it may also produce false-negative results if the stomach and duodenum are distorted by a previous surgical procedure or by hypertrophic gastric mucosa. The true incidence of ulcer disease is, therefore, higher than is shown in most statistics.

Although the term peptic ulcer is frequently applied to all of these lesions, it is really a misnomer. Duodenal and stomal ulcers are due primarily to gastric acid. Gastric ulcers have several causes; they may either be benign or malignant and must be regarded with suspicion. There are also other less common lesions, such as stress ulcers, Cushing's ulcer, Curling's ulcer, and ulcers due to hypergastrinaemia that must be considered. At present about 60 per cent of the operations or diagnoses made on surgical wards for ulcer disease are due to duodenal ulcer, 35 per cent to gastric ulcers, and 5 per cent to less common causes.

Recent investigations have led to the conclusion that *Helicobacter pylori* is the cause of the majority of cases of duodenal and gastric ulcer. In a study by Hentschel *et al.*, eradication of this infection has led to freedom from symptoms and apparent cure in 84 per cent of cases of duodenal ulcer. Therapy has included combinations of antibiotics (amoxicillin and metronidazole) and ranitidine for 6 weeks. Graham has used other antibiotics; he concludes that the major causes of peptic ulcer at the present time are *H. pylori* infection, excessive use of non-steroidal anti-inflammatory drugs, and hypersecretory states.

HISTORICAL NOTES

The earliest operations involving extirpation of the stomach were performed for cancer. Although the French surgeon Jules Péan performed a pylorectomy for cancer in 1879, the patient died 5 days later. Rydigier, the great Polish surgeon, had a similar unsuccessful case. Billroth was the first surgeon to report survival of a patient following excision of the distal portion of the stomach in 1881; he anastomosed the stomach to the duodenum, thereby establishing what has been known ever since as the Billroth I procedure. The patient lived for 4 months before dying from disseminated cancer. In 1885 his assistant, Wölfler, operating on a patient with gastric cancer, performed a preliminary gastrojejunostomy and, at a second stage, removed the distal stomach and closed the duodenal stump; thereafter this operation was known as the Billroth II. The first gastrojejunostomy for an obstructing cancer was performed in 1891 by Wölfler.

In the last two decades of the nineteenth century duodenal ulcers were rare, although benign gastric ulcers were recognized with increasing frequency. Rydigier, in 1881, performed a gastric resection for a benign gastric ulcer, and the patient survived. He received wide criticism; the editor who published the paper (entitled *The first gastric resection for gastric ulcer*) added the comment 'And hopefully the last' to the article.

The first operation for duodenal ulcer—a gastrojejunostomy—according to Herrington, was performed by Codivilla in 1893. This quickly became the procedure of choice for both duodenal and gastric ulcers. Twenty years later, extensive gastrectomies, fostered by von Haberer and by Finsterer began to displace pylorectomies, which were the earlier operations of choice. Angry controversies developed between proponents of gastroenterostomy and those supporting gastric resection. It was not until the 1930s that it was recognized that a large number of gastrojejunal ulcers appeared after gastrojejunostomy; thereafter gastric resection, as popularized by Finsterer, was finally accepted. Nevertheless, occasional gastrojejunostomies were performed in major clinics in the United States for benign ulcers even as late as 1945.

The heyday for gastric resection in the United States lasted until 1943. At that time Dragstedt and Owens reintroduced bilateral truncal vagotomy for the treatment of duodenal ulcers. This operation had been used before. Brodie, from London, had studied it experimentally in 1814; Latarjet had combined it with a conservative gastric resection in 1922; Schiassi had combined vagotomy with drainage in 1925. However, Dragstedt had undertaken many important laboratory experiments that showed the potential of vagotomy had great potential. His recommendation, made in a two-page report, was based upon only two patients who had been followed for 2 months after operation. Nevertheless, his experiments were so convincing that the course of gastric surgery was immediately and completely changed.

Bilateral truncal vagotomy, performed either through the abdomen or the chest, was soon found to be unsatisfactory: the stomach often failed to empty, and early recurrences occurred in one-third of the patients. Hence, an accompanying drainage procedure either by pyloroplasty or gastrojejunostomy (Dragstedt's operation) became the favourite procedure for duodenal ulcer.

Dissatisfied with the results of radical resections of the stomach for duodenal ulcer, and the obvious successes of vagotomy, two separate groups of surgeons almost simultaneously proposed the operation that combined a partial resection of the stomach with truncal vagotomy. The first of these operations was carried out by Smithwick and Farmer in Boston in October 1946; they called the operation 'hemigastrectomy and vagotomy'. In January 1947, Edwards and Herrington, in Nashville, unaware of Smithwick's operation, performed the same procedure. They called it 'conservative gastrectomy' or 'antrectomy and vagotomy'. Both groups found a spectacular reduction in acid production because of the elimination of antral gastrin and of parietal cell stimulation. This method essentially eliminated the major problem that followed many previous operations—recurrent ulcer.

Thereafter, attention was diverted from recurrence and was focused on other side-effects of operations for duodenal ulcer disease; as a result proximal gastric vagotomy was developed. Clinical use of this procedure was begun in 1965. Because there have been variations in the technique of this operation the method is discussed in detail below.

Arguments for and against various operations will be discussed below. Suffice it to say here that surgeons are not unanimous in their selection of the best operation for duodenal ulcer. Meanwhile, gastric ulcers continue to be treated with satisfaction by some type of gastric resection, often combined with truncal vagotomy.

DEMOGRAPHY

Gastric and duodenal ulcers are common throughout the world, although supporting evidence from many countries is unreliable. The incidence and severity of peptic ulcer is decreasing in the Western world; the number of deaths from this cause have declined steadily in the past 60 years in the United States. The number of deaths due to ulcers of the stomach and duodenum has decreased from 6.0 per 100 000 population in 1930 to 5.5 in 1950, 3.7 in 1972 (this period was still before widespread use of H_2-receptor antagonists) and to 2.7 in 1986.

A complete survey of all hospitals in Sweden showed that in 1950 there were 64 elective admissions for ulcer operations per 100 000 hospital admissions, compared with 11 in 1986. The number of operations decreased from 9.4 per 100 000 admissions in 1956 to 6.6 in 1986. Gustavsson *et al.* observed that the dramatic decrease in peptic ulcer surgery started long before the advent of fibreoptic endoscopy, H_2-receptor antagonists, and highly selective (proximal gastric) vagotomy. They also concluded that the falling incidence of perforation indicates that the ulcer prevalence (or severity) has diminished.

Taylor, commenting on the changing picture of peptic ulcer disease in Great Britain up to 1989, stated that in the 10 years since H_2-receptor antagonists have become available no reduction occurred in the number of deaths due to this disease in England and Wales. Instead, deaths have now shifted to older age groups: 95 per cent of the deaths occur in patients over 55 years of age.

Our studies of ulcer disease from 1974 to 1985 show a sharp decline in elective operations for duodenal ulcer to approximately 10 per year. The number of cases as well as the death rate in those patients operated on for acute massive haemorrhage and acute perforation have remained nearly constant during the entire period.

In summary, operations for peptic ulcer now are chiefly undertaken for massive haemorrhage and acute perforation. Because poor-risk elderly patients are frequently the victims of these catastrophes, the hospital mortality is increased in contrast to the overall reduction in mortality of peptic ulcer in the United States.

PATHOPHYSIOLOGY OF GASTRIC AND DUODENAL ULCER

Ulcers of the stomach and duodenum are caused chiefly by the effects of hydrochloric acid, produced by the parietal cells of the stomach, and by lack of protection of the mucosa against this acid. Acid production is by far the most important factor as far as duodenal ulcer is concerned, but cannot be the only factor, since the severity of duodenal ulcers and their responses to therapy do not vary directly with the amount of gastric acid secreted.

Additional factors are important in the production of gastric ulcers. Gastric contents can be retained for a much longer period than duodenal contents and are not neutralized as rapidly as by duodenal chyme. The mucous membrane of the stomach must normally be protected continuously from the damaging effect of the hydrochloric acid which it secretes. This protective layer consists of an adherent layer of mucus which is separated from the gastric mucosa by a bicarbonate layer that normally neutralizes any hydrochloric acid diffusing back through the mucous layer. The mucous layer also protects the gastric mucosa against other noxious agents such as bile, alcohol, and aspirin and other irritating drugs.

Secretion of acid by the parietal cells of the stomach is influenced by several mechanisms. Stimulation by the vagus nerves accounts for about 50 per cent of acid secretion. Gastrin that is secreted by the antral mucosa causes 40 to 45 per cent of the secretion and the remaining 5 to 10 per cent is due to gastrin that comes from the intestinal tract from various APUD cells.

Production of gastric mucus should presumably vary according to the blood supply of the organ (Fig. 1). Experimental studies have shown that prostaglandins increase the mucosal blood supply and increase the bicarbonate level and thickness of the mucous layer; they may, therefore, play an important role in the protection of the gastric mucosa.

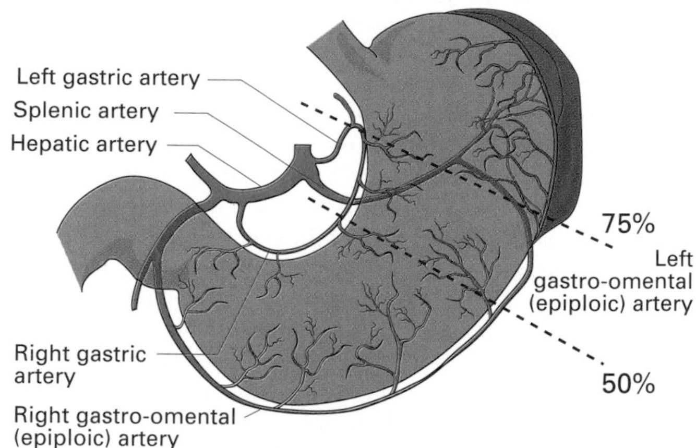

Fig. 1 Blood supply of the stomach. The stomach is supplied by the left and right gastric, the right and left gastroepiploic arteries and the vasa brevia which arise from the splenic artery. The most important of these arteries is the left gastric since most major gastric bleeding arises from this vessel. The main artery supplying the duodenum is the gastroduodenal which arises from the hepatic and anastomoses freely by means of its two terminal branches—the superior pancreaticoduodenal and the right gastroepiploic arteries.

The stomach contains several types of glands. Mucus-secreting glands are located throughout the stomach; gastrin-producing cells occur in the antrum and in an area that often runs along the lesser curvature up nearly to the oesophagus. Chief cells, located mainly in the upper half of the stomach, secrete pepsin. Parietal cells secrete hydrochloric acid and also are located almost entirely in the fundus.

The stomach is supplied by both sympathetic and parasympathetic nerves. Although the function of the sympathetic nerves is not of great importance to surgeons, during the 1940s it was noted that patients with ulcers who underwent bilateral lumbodorsal sympathectomies for essential hypertension lost their ulcer pain immediately after the operation.

The parasympathetic supply comes from the vagus. Section of both vagus trunks at the oesophagogastric level not only reduces a major stimulus to the secretory activity of the parietal cells but also produces major changes in the motility of the stomach. The secretion of gastrin by antral cells may also be diminished.

The cause of a partial return of acid secretion after bilateral truncal vagotomy remains a mystery. True regeneration of the nerves has never been demonstrated in the stomach, although Nyhus did describe 'budding' of minor branches. Parasympathetic fibres probably run together with the sympathetic nerves along other major arteries such as the right gastroepiploic artery or the splenic artery and they may become more active after vagotomy.

Causes of gastric ulcers vary in importance depending upon the location of these ulcers. In 1965 Johnson observed the different behaviour of ulcers in different portions of the stomach and classified them into three groups. In patients with type 1 ulcers, located in the body of the stomach, gastric acid secretion as determined by secretory tests is low. Here inadequate mucosal protection and back-diffusion of hydrochloric acid through the protective bicarbonate and mucous layer into the gastric mucosa seem to be involved in the disease. Silen suggested it is in this location that alternating waves of gastric acid from above and refluxing alkaline secretions from the duodenum destroy the protective layer of mucus.

Johnson's type 2 gastric ulcers (those combined with a present or past duodenal ulcer) and type 3 (those in the prepyloric area) behave more like duodenal ulcers; here the effects of acid production appear to be more important.

Ulcers that develop after the formation of anastomoses of the stomach with the intestine, or ulcers which recur after various operations for duodenal or gastric ulcers are due to persistent secretion of hydrochloric acid.

Extragastric lesions can lead to increased levels of serum gastrin and consequent acid production, followed by ulceration in the stomach, duodenum, or intestine. The prime example is the gastrinoma—the usual cause of the Zollinger–Ellison syndrome.

DIAGNOSIS

The diagnosis of a gastric or duodenal ulcer is made from protean symptoms and signs. If the ulcer is acute and uncomplicated, epigastric pain occurs typically about 3 a.m. and an hour or more after meals. Pain is located in the mid-epigastrium to the right of the midline with duodenal ulcers, and in the midline or slightly to the left of the midline with gastric ulcers. The pain is relieved by food or antacids. Slight nausea or epigastric fullness is common. Vomiting is uncommon unless pyloric obstruction supervenes.

Physical examination is negative except for slight tenderness, usually sharply localized to the area in which the pain is felt. Confirmatory evidence is obtained by endoscopy and, particularly in the case of a gastric ulcer, by biopsy examination. A gastric ulcer should be considered to be malignant unless scrupulous biopsy examination of a large specimen indicates otherwise and unless the ulcer heals on medical therapy. In more chronic cases, barium contrast studies are also helpful. The stool should be examined for occult blood; blood counts should be made to rule out anaemia.

Any complication of ulcer disease raises the question of surgical therapy. Some severe complications occur without previous symptoms, but others may be treated medically, at least for a certain time. Close co-operation between physicians and surgeons is necessary in the care of such cases. These complications, all of which may lead to operative procedures, are acute perforation, bleeding (either massive, repetitive, or occult), pyloric obstruction, intractability, and fistula formation.

Acute perforation is accompanied by the abrupt onset of severe epigastric pain and shock, with hypotension and sweating. There is often a brief period in which the patient feels somewhat better, but the pain recurs with greater intensity. An abdominal radiograph taken 6 h after perforation with the patient upright shows gas beneath the diaphragm in 60 per cent of the patients. In questionable cases, Gastrografin can be injected through a nasogastric tube to determine whether or not there is a perforation. Determining whether or not the patient had previous ulcer symptoms is important: the choice of operation may depend upon this single factor.

Acute massive haemorrhage is defined clinically by the requirement of five units of whole blood to restore normal vital signs and blood counts. The patient vomits blood and exhibits signs of shock. In the great majority of cases there is a history of intake of some drug such as aspirin that irritates the gastric mucosa.

Occult bleeding, characterized by tarry stools or merely by positive guaiac stools, may occur in patients with duodenal ulcers. Diagnosis is obtained most readily by endoscopy.

Obstruction is diagnosed by repeated vomiting, hyponatraemia, and hypochloraemia. If there is accompanying ulcer pain, the obstruction is probably due to oedema about an active ulcer; if there is no accompanying pain, it is probably a result of fibrosis and scar. On examination a greatly distended stomach is palpable. Peristaltic waves can be observed in thin patients, running from left to right. Diagnosis is made by the insertion of a nasogastric tube and confirmed later by barium studies and endoscopy to exclude or confirm the presence of an obstructing tumour.

Intractability refers to chronic ulcers that have not responded to treatment with various medications. Many patients have symptoms that suggest ulcers, but no objective evidence of abnormalities on endoscopy or barium studies. Vigilance is essential before an operation is undertaken since patients in whom objective evidence of ulcer disease is minimal and in whom no relief is obtained on standard medications are apt to do poorly after an operation.

The differential diagnoses in these patients include a variety of possibilities, ranging from functional abnormalities to hiatus hernia with reflux oesophagitis, gallstones, pancreatitis, and coronary disease.

MAJOR TYPES OF PEPTIC ULCER

The three major types of peptic ulcers—gastric, duodenal, and stomal (anastomotic)—have certain distinguishing characteristics in addition to those noted above.

Gastric ulcer (Fig. 2)

Gastric ulcers occur most commonly in elderly women, with the highest incidence between 55 and 60 years of age; duodenal ulcers, in contrast, are more common in men at a younger age.

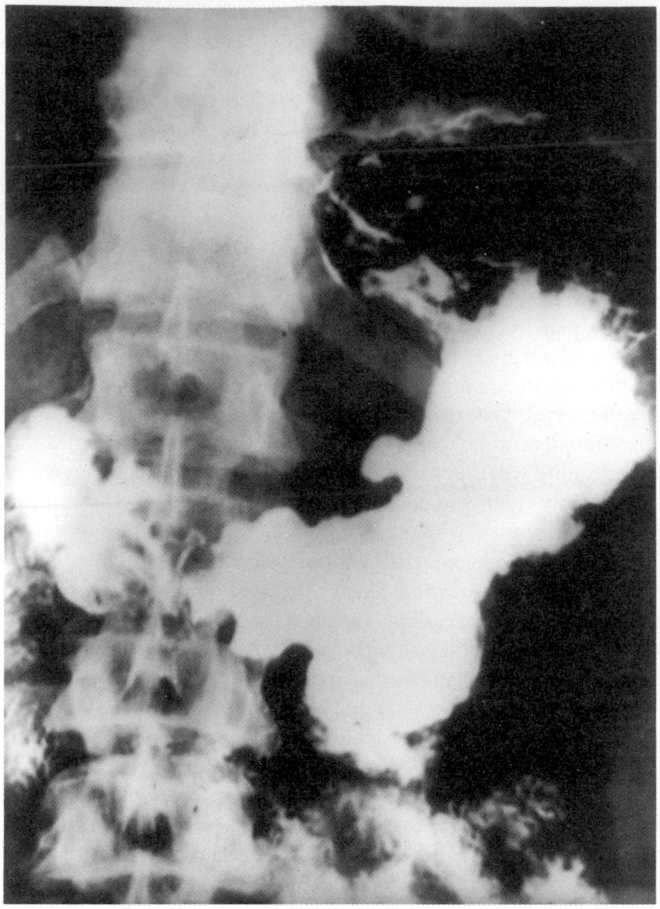

Fig. 2 Gastric ulcer (Type 1, Johnson). The ulcer is located on the lesser curvature at the annulus.

If preoperative acid studies are undertaken in patients with type 1 ulcers, gastric pH levels approach those indicative of achlorhydria and are distinctly higher than those with types II or III or with duodenal ulcers.

A benign ulcer must be distinguished from an ulcerating cancer. The location of an ulcer in the stomach is not helpful, although ulcerating lesions on the greater curvature are rare and appear to be as likely to be due to cancer as to benign disease. Both advanced age and comparative hypochlorhydria are also characteristic of gastric cancer. A good clinical rule is to suspect that every gastric ulcer is malignant initially. Diagnosis cannot be considered adequate until the results of endoscopy and biopsy are known. Even if these studies suggest the lesion is benign, failure of the ulcer to heal or its recurrence must be regarded as danger signs and an indication for operation.

The symptoms of a gastric ulcer are similar to those of a duodenal ulcer except that in gastric ulcer the epigastric pain tends to be slightly more to the left. Bleeding occurs more commonly and perforation less frequently than is the case with duodenal ulcers: most perforations occurring in what appears to be the immediate prepyloric area are actually duodenal ulcers. Massive haemorrhage from a gastric ulcer is more likely to be fatal than that from a duodenal ulcer.

An unusual complication of a perforation occurs when ulcers on the greater curvature penetrate into the colon, producing a gastrocolic fistula. The usual causes of such fistulae are cancers of the colon or stomach penetrating into the neighbouring viscus. Surgical intervention is necessary.

Duodenal ulcer

Duodenal ulcers characteristically occur in young men aged 20 to 50 years, but they may appear at any age. They are usually initially diagnosed clinically by pain in the epigastrium just to the right of the midline. The pain varies in nature and in intensity; it often is described as 'burning' and is most likely to occur at night and several hours after eating. The pain is reduced rapidly by intake of food or antacids. Less common symptoms include heartburn from oesophageal reflux, and nausea and vomiting.

Duodenal ulcers are usually located in the first portion of the duodenum, known as the bulb. Although benign ulcers are found lower in the duodenum, cancer must be suspected if ulcerating lesions are found in this unusual location.

The diagnosis of a duodenal ulcer with only minimal symptoms is made on the basis of the typical pain and response to food or drugs that reduce acid secretion or protect the mucosa. In such cases neither endoscopy nor barium contrast radiographs are necessary. Diagnosis in more severe cases is preferably made by endoscopy; repeated endoscopies to monitor healing are not indicated unless the patient responds poorly. Barium contrast studies are helpful, particularly if an operation is contemplated, because the extent of the duodenal deformity can be delineated.

Perforations of the duodenum are usually due to anterior ulcers. Chronic perforations are rare; they usually arise from the posterior wall and are contained by the head of the pancreas. Occasionally, fistulae to other organs, such as the biliary tree or colon, occur.

Stomal (anastomotic) ulcer

Stomal ulcers have many characteristics that distinguish them from gastric and duodenal ulcers, and provide difficult diagnostic and technical problems for surgeons. They develop following gastric resection or other procedures, such as gastroenterostomy, that involve the anastomosis of the stomach to some other portion of the gastrointestinal tract. In such cases an ulcer develops near the stoma; it is almost invariably in the efferent limb of the intestine, not in the stomach.

These ulcers are due to the effects of gastric acid on the susceptible intestinal mucosa. There appears to be a direct relationship between vulnerability to acid and distance of the intestine from the pylorus. For example, technical errors have at times led to gastroileal or gastrocolic anastomoses: they are much more likely to be followed by stomal ulcers than are gastroduodenal or gastrojejunal stomas.

Stomal ulcers are nearly always associated with high levels of acid secretion and hence occur after operations for duodenal ulcer, or for type 2 or 3 gastric ulcers. If the previous operation was apparently adequate to reduce acid, the possibility of hypergastrinaemia resulting from the retained antrum syndrome or from a gastrinoma should be considered: serum gastrin levels should be measured. Rarely, such ulcers may be confused with cancer arising in the gastric mucosa near an anastomotic line.

Diagnosis may be difficult. Endoscopy is essential, but may fail to disclose an ulcer after a gastrojejunostomy if the ulcer is remote from the stoma. Barium studies are helpful if the ulcer is in the duodenum, but not after Billroth II resections. If bleeding is a symptom, selective angiography can often confirm the diagnosis.

The symptoms of such ulcers include pain, haemorrhage, and perforation. Pain is usually similar to that associated with the previous ulcer, but occurs more to the left in the epigastrium if the complication follows gastroenterostomy. Medical therapy, similar to that for duodenal ulcer, has been used frequently for this symptom. Although some observers have reported favourable results, most cases recur when therapy is stopped. The indications for surgical therapy are therefore broader than for other types of ulcer disease, and include the presence of a stomal ulcer as well as all of the other standard indications for ulcer surgery.

A serious complication of a stomal ulcer that develops after a Billroth II gastrectomy or a gastrojejunostomy is a gastrojejunocolic fistula. Patients may have relatively little pain, but have sudden uncontrollable diarrhoea. The faeces contains undigested food and vomiting of faeces may occur, with a persistent foul smell on the breath. Loss of weight and malnutrition occur unless prompt surgical relief is provided. A barium enema or upper gastrointestinal series will confirm the diagnosis.

The operation that is required includes resection of the stomach, intestine, and colon involved in the fistula. Antibiotic preparation, both orally (neomycin and erythromycin base) and parenterally (metronidazole and ampicillin, for example, or cefotetan and gentamicin) is necessary, and the colon must be cleansed by administration of laxatives or a polyethylene-glycol based cathartic. After an adequate gastric resection and vagotomy, the continuity of the jejunum is restored, and a new gastrojejunostomy is made. If the patient is in generally good medical condition, continuity of the colon is also restored, but if the patient is badly malnourished both ends of the resected colon can be brought out at colostomies, continuity being restored at a later date.

The operative procedure for a stomal ulcer depends upon the original operation for ulcer disease. If the previous procedure was a gastroenterostomy alone, gastric resection and bilateral vagotomy are necessary in addition to reconstruction of jejunal continuity. If a gastric resection and vagotomy had been performed previously, the duodenal stump must be exposed to ensure that the entire antrum was removed, and any residual intact vagal fibres or trunks must be identified and divided. If the previous resection and vagotomy was apparently adequate, a higher gastric resection is required.

Because the operative field in the abdomen is often obscured by numerous adhesions, a secondary vagotomy may be very difficult or dangerous. A transthoracic vagotomy is advisable in these circumstances.

MEDICAL THERAPY OF GASTRIC AND DUODENAL ULCER

The medical therapy is similar for both gastric and duodenal ulcer and includes the use of specific medications and elimination of known gastric irritants. Attempts to relieve social problems that include irregular habits of eating, working, and sleeping are also made.

Gastric irritants include tobacco, alcohol, caffeine, aspirin, ibuprofen, indomethacin, and salicylates, as well as many other non-steroidal anti-inflammatory drugs. Although the exact mechanism by which cigarette smoking is related to ulcer disease is not known, experience has shown that smoking leads to the development and prevents healing of ulcers. Alcohol is a severe irritant that promotes the formation of ulcers. Patients who have portal hypertension and are believed to be bleeding from oesophageal varices actually often have ulcers of the stomach or duodenum. Aspirin is also a direct irritant: its effect on platelet adhesiveness means that it not only causes ulcers, but leads to bleeding from them. Ibuprofen and the numerous proprietary drugs in which it is present are also irritants. Orange juice is irritating because it contains citric acid.

For many years diet was considered to be closely related to ulcer disease. Elaborate concoctions, relying chiefly on milk and cream, were considered to be essential in acute stages of the disease. These specific diets are not essential: regular food, taken at regular intervals, is best. Because food tends to reduce the action of acid on the mucosa, small, frequent meals are desirable in acute episodes. A drink of milk or a flavoured milk drink and a few crackers are valuable as a snack prior to bedtime and for rapid control of pain that appears in the middle of the night, despite the secretogenic stimulus of milk on gastric acid secretions.

Specific medications to control ulcers include antacids, H_2-receptor antagonists, mucosal coating agents, omeprazole, and prostaglandins. Pharmacies offer a host of antacid preparations. They contain such compounds as sodium bicarbonate, magnesium carbonate, and aluminium hydroxide. The calcium content of some of these agents potentiates acid secretion, however. In 1973 compounds available as over-the-counter preparations were graded for safety and efficiency by a panel set up by the Food and Drug Administration (FDA): Mylanta II was the most effective.

The most common prescription drugs are the H_2-receptor antagonists, particularly cimetidine (300 mg four times daily) and ranitidine (150 mg twice daily), although several others are being developed.

The most effective mucosal coating agent is sucralfate (1 g four times daily). Omeprazole acts upon the intracellular proton pump and can eliminate gastric acid production altogether.

Among their numerous other properties, prostaglandins increase the blood supply to the gastric mucosa and decrease the damaging effects of non-steroidal anti-inflammatory drugs. The only prostaglandin approved to date by the FDA is misoprostol.

Controlled studies in which various drugs were tested and compared with placebos indicated that antacids, H_2-receptor antagonists, sucralfate, and omeprazole were equally effective in so far as relief for pain was concerned. Using pain control and endoscopy as elements for comparison, about 80 per cent of ulcers healed within 1 month, although healing time was longer with gastric ulcers and in aged patients. The recurrence rate within 6 months was high. A gastric ulcer that either fails to show definite evidence of healing within 1 month or that recurs after therapy has ceased should always be regarded with suspicion, even if biopsy specimens show no sign of cancer. These ulcers should be considered for surgical removal.

SURGICAL THERAPY OF PEPTIC ULCER DISEASE

Up to 1970 surgical therapy was chiefly undertaken in patients with painful gastric or duodenal ulcers who failed to respond to medical measures. These so-called 'intractable' cases are now rare, not only because better therapeutic drugs have been found, but because ulcers are less virulent than they were in the past.

Major attention must now be paid to patients who present as emergencies, with either acute massive bleeding or acute perforations. Both of these catastrophes demand surgical salvage; medical therapy is not an option.

Recommended operations for gastric, duodenal, and stomal ulcers (Table 1)

Gastric ulcer

The essential features of an elective operation for gastric ulcer are: (1) preliminary endoscopy and biopsy of the lesion; (2) partial gastrectomy that includes the entire antrum and the ulcer; (3) the addition of bilateral truncal vagotomy except for type 1 ulcers; (4) for juxtaoesophageal ulcers, intragastric biopsy of the lesion, followed by antrectomy and Billroth II anastomosis, leaving the ulcer *in situ* (Madlener procedure). For ulcers complicated by massive haemorrhage or perforation a distal gastrectomy that includes the ulcer is preferred.

Table 1 Preferred operations

	First choice	Second choice
Duodenal ulcer		
Perforation	VA, B I or II	Plication
Massive haemorrhage	VA, ligation	VP, ligation
Obstruction	VA, B I or II	GR, B I or II
Intractability	VA, B I or II	PGV
Gastric ulcer		
Perforation	VA, B I	GR
Massive haemorrhage	VA, B I	GR
Obstruction	VA, B I	GR
Elective		
Type 1	GR, B I	VA, BI
Types 2, 3	VA, B I	VA, B II

B I = gastric resection, gastroduodenostomy.
B II = gastric resection, gastrojejunostomy.
GR = two-thirds gastric resection, no vagotomy.
PGV = proximal gastric vagotomy.
VA = truncal vagotomy, antrectomy.
VP = truncal vagotomy, pyloroplasty.
(These are rough guides. B I is preferred to B II if the duodenum is not badly deformed. See text for further details.)

Duodenal ulcer

In elective operations performed for intractable pain, antrectomy and bilateral vagotomy is preferred; proximal gastric vagotomy or pyloroplasty and bilateral truncal vagotomy are acceptable, according to criteria specified below. Selection of operations for patients with a massive haemorrhage or acute perforation are discussed below.

Stomal ulcer

Serum gastrin levels should be measured to ascertain the presence of a gastrinoma. If the previous operation was a gastroenterostomy or pyloroplasty, a Billroth II resection and bilateral truncal vagotomy are performed. If the previous operation was a Billroth II gastrectomy, a bilateral truncal vagotomy or higher gastric resection plus vagotomy is recommended.

Indications and preparation for operation

The major indications for surgical treatment of peptic ulcer include acute perforation, acute massive haemorrhage, gastric outlet obstruction, and intractability. Less common indications include repeated episodes of minor bleeding and fistula formation (gastrocolic, duodenocolic, or from the duodenum into any portion of the biliary tree). Intractability in the case of a gastric ulcer means delayed healing or recurrence after healing, even in the absence of pain: such apparently benign ulcers can actually be malignant.

Preparations for operation may need to be limited to 'essentials' in patients who present as emergencies with acute perforation or massive haemorrhage. Nasogastric decompression prior to induction of anaesthesia, intravenous or intramuscular administration of antibiotics, establishment of intravenous lines for administration of electrolytes, and a supply of compatible blood are essential.

In patients likely to require surgery, but in whom there is no emergency, time may be taken for necessary diagnostic measures. Suction on an inlying nasogastric tube is necessary if there is any evidence of obstruction. Thorough medical evaluation, including haematological studies, may indicate the need for preoperative transfusions.

In the remainder of this section each of the indications for surgery is discussed in detail.

Acute perforation

Perforated duodenal ulcers

The diagnosis of an acute perforation of a duodenal ulcer is suggested by the sudden onset of severe epigastric pain followed by a variable degree of shock and often slight vomiting. In the untreated patient, the condition tends to improve after a few hours, to be followed shortly thereafter by increasing prostration, pain spreading throughout the abdomen, and cardiovascular collapse. Physical examination typically reveals a board-like abdomen, with tenderness most marked in the mid- or right epigastrium. Peristalsis is absent. The temperature in the first few hours after perforation is normal.

Six hours after onset of symptoms an abdominal radiograph taken in the sitting position shows free air beneath the diaphragm in about 60 per cent of cases (Fig. 3). If the diagnosis is in doubt, Gastrografin injected through an inlying nasogastric tube will show evidence of extravasation through the perforation.

The differential diagnosis includes acute cholecystitis, acute pancreatitis, strangulating intestinal obstruction, acute appendicitis, perforation of some other portion of the intestinal tract, and mesenteric thrombosis. A past history of ulcer disease is predictive, since the chances that the present episode is due to a perforated ulcer are greatly increased in such patients.

Occasionally, a perforated ulcer seals spontaneously and the patient will continue to improve. However, these 'formes frustes' are rare, and delay before an operation, other than to institute nasogastric suction, antibiotics, and intravenous administration of fluids and electrolytes, is dangerous.

Exploratory laparotomy is often necessary to confirm the diagnosis. The size of the perforation may vary greatly, from a diameter of only 2 to 3 mm to a hole 2 to 5 cm across.

When the abdomen is opened, the perforation may have sealed spontaneously, covered in most cases by adjacent omentum. Such

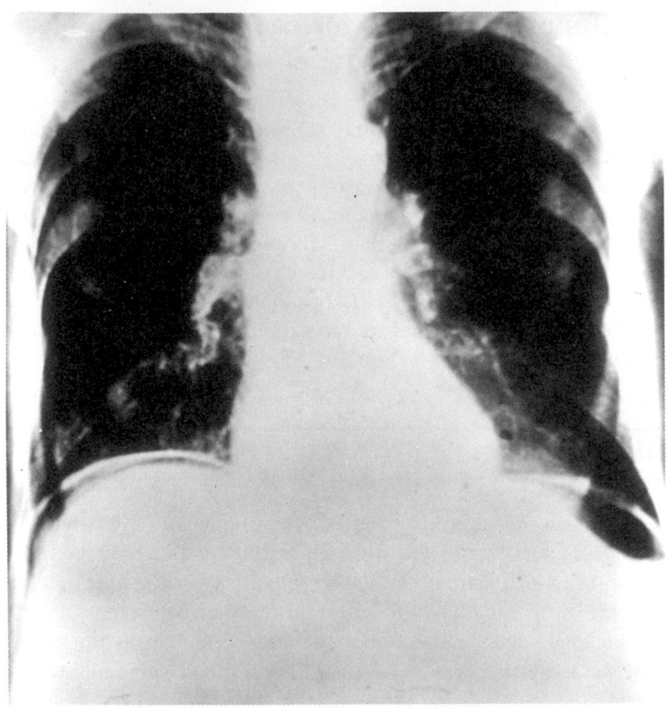

Fig. 3 Subphrenic gas secondary to perforation of a duodenal ulcer. Note gas located beneath both diaphragms. The film is taken with the patient erect.

a finding has led some surgeons to advocate the non-operative treatment of what is believed to be an acutely perforated ulcer, such treatment consisting of nasogastric suction, antibiotics, and intravenous fluids and electrolytes. The diagnosis of an abdominal catastrophe may be missed and this approach must be abandoned if the patient's condition appears to be deteriorating. This injunction means that such patients must be watched carefully and that operation may be necessary at an unfortunate hour.

Although this method of therapy may produce satisfactory results in young, vigorous patients, older persons often have other serious diseases such as mesenteric thrombosis; they cannot withstand the effects of peritonitis, and spontaneous sealing of the perforation does not occur as often as in younger patients. The main indications for such treatment include patients with recent coronary occlusion or those in whom the diagnosis has been delayed and in whom the ulcer has apparently sealed spontaneously.

At the time of operation for an acutely perforated duodenal ulcer the surgeon must choose between a simple closure of the perforation or a definitive procedure designed to prevent future recurrences of ulcer disease. Simple closure may be effected with a few interrupted sutures, an omental or round ligament patch, or by suture closure reinforced with omentum. Care must be taken to avoid obstructing the duodenum with the sutures.

In certain instances a more radical operation is necessary. Such cases include a giant perforation that cannot be closed by suture, a large posterior ulcer, a perforated ulcer on the anterior wall, or perforation accompanied by profuse bleeding. As was noted above, the most important indication for a definitive operation is a history of a previous ulcer.

Definitive operations can be carried out successfully at the time of the great majority of operations for perforation. Appropriate procedures include gastric resection (with or without truncal vagotomy), pyloroplasty and bilateral truncal vagotomy, and proximal gastric vagotomy. Opinions vary concerning the choice of these procedures. Our preference has been for bilateral truncal vagotomy and antrectomy, although some surgeons opt for proximal gastric vagotomy.

Unless operating conditions are optimal, the surgeon must choose a simple closure of a perforation as a life-saving method; if necessary a definitive procedure can be performed later. Follow-up studies after simple plication show that nearly one-third of all patients remain free of symptoms, and about half of those with recurrent symptoms requires a definitive operation for ulcer disease later. In the last Massachusetts General Hospital series of 107 patients, 21 per cent received a definitive operation within 5 years after simple plication.

Perforated gastric ulcers

The great majority of perforated gastric ulcers are located in the immediate prepyloric area. They behave in the same way as perforated duodenal ulcers, and the same considerations are applicable. However, perforations of ulcers elsewhere in the stomach introduce the possibility of malignancy, and immediate definitive resections of the stomach are recommended. If the patient's condition is poor, and only a simple closure is contemplated, biopsy specimens should be taken of the margins of the ulcer.

Acute massive haemorrhage

A patient who has required 5 units of blood during a single hospital admission by definition has a massive haemorrhage. When a patient enters with serious upper gastrointestinal bleeding, the source can usually be determined with reasonable certainty on clinical grounds. Nearly two-thirds of all cases of severe upper gastrointestinal haemorrhage are due to ulcers of the stomach or duodenum. A past history of ulcer disease, a recent history of ingestion of gastric irritants such as aspirin or ibuprofen, sudden profuse vomiting of blood, and later haematochezia are typical. The other major causes of massive upper gastrointestinal bleeding—portal hypertension and oesophageal varices—can usually be eliminated by history and physical examination, but the frequency of concomitant ulcer disease makes other early diagnostic procedures essential. At times, a bleeding duodenal ulcer is manifested merely by tarry stools.

Early upper gastrointestinal endoscopy is the most valuable diagnostic study. However, profuse bleeding may make it useless, since such patients must be taken directly to the operating room. If an Ewald tube is passed into the stomach and irrigation with saline solution is continued until the bleeding slows to a trickle, the time is ripe for endoscopy, and the source can usually be determined.

Selective angiography can be helpful but is not always available. On the other hand injection of 99 m-technetium-labelled erythrocytes is not useful because of the heavy background radiation in the upper abdomen. Although barium contrast studies often show the ulcer, they should not be used before angiography because residual barium might prevent further imaging studies.

The diagnosis of the source of bleeding must often be made by laparotomy. An adequate incision and careful observation of the abdominal contents should indicate the probable site of bleeding. A wide gastrotomy incision that extends across the pylorus, if necessary, gives the best exposure to help find the source.

Therapeutic measures for acute massive bleeding include injection of vasopressin into a peripheral vein, irrigation of the stomach for removal of blood clots, continued nasogastric suction, elimination of oral intake, and intravenous replacement of blood, fluid, and electrolytes. Until an operation is performed or the patient recovers, a careful chart of the vital signs and repeated assays of the haematocrit are essential.

Massive bleeding is not well tolerated in patients over 60 years of age: under that age, mortality is not increased by delay and attempts to control the bleeding by endoscopic techniques such as electrocoagulation or laser.

Older patients respond much better to early operation. As shown in a controlled series by Morris *et al.*, delay of definitive treatment by over 48 h increases the mortality rate in patients 60 years of age or over from 2 per cent to 15 per cent. Such delay did not increase mortality in younger patients, however.

Early operation is indicated in patients bleeding from the gastroduodenal artery or a gastric ulcer. Angiographic embolization of the gastroduodenal or the left gastric arteries may be effective, but there are dangers involved. A foreign body may slip from the gastroduodenal into the hepatic artery and lead to hepatic necrosis; one in the left gastric artery may lead to necrosis of the upper portion of the stomach.

Operations for massively bleeding duodenal ulcers

The site of bleeding must be determined. If the source is the gastroduodenal artery, it must be ligated as the first step. This procedure involves suture of the artery, either above the duodenum as it emerges from the hepatic artery or within the duodenal lumen, suture of the caudal portion of the artery within the duodenum or of the two major branches—the superior pancreatoduodenal and the right gastroepiploic—and of the transverse pancreatic artery. Heavy, non-absorbable sutures are used.

In other instances the duodenum may be boggy and bleeding from multiple areas; in such instances it may be impossible to identify single vessels to ligate.

As soon as bleeding has been controlled, a definitive operation can be carried out. We believe that hemigastrectomy and truncal vagotomy followed by a Billroth II anastomosis is best; others prefer the simpler pyloroplasty and truncal vagotomy. A major determinant in the selection is the experience of the surgeon. Gastric resection is more difficult, but gives slightly better control of bleeding because it removes areas of gastritis and duodenitis that are potential sources of postoperative bleeding.

Operations for bleeding gastric ulcers

Gastric resection is preferred for bleeding gastric ulcers. A truncal vagotomy should be added if the ulcer is in the prepyloric area or if the patient has a history of a duodenal ulcer. Either a Billroth I or II anastomosis can be made.

In some patients who are very poor operative risks, a local excision of the ulcer may be performed. However, the chances of recurrence within a year approach nearly 50 per cent.

The most difficult stomach ulcer to treat is one located in the proximal portion. In older patients who are poor risks, a distal resection, ligation of the left gastric artery, and intragastric plication of the ulcer is recommended.

Some surgeons have approved simple plication for all bleeding gastric ulcers. We have had no experience with this method. The only patient treated in this way in the Massachusetts General Hospital in the last decade required a second operation within 24 h for recurrent bleeding; he did well after a gastric resection.

Results of operations for massive bleeding from gastric and duodenal ulcer

The reported results of such operations vary greatly. In the Massachusetts General Hospital the mortality in the last study was 22 per cent; many of these patients had bled after other serious operations such as coronary artery bypass. Other groups have reported mortality rates as low as 10 per cent. It is impossible to compare surgical results with other methods of therapy; endoscopy is rarely attempted in such cases and arteriography is used infrequently. Furthermore, patients in whom other methods of therapy have failed are relegated to surgeons in the hope that they can solve the problem.

Obstruction

Gastric outlet obstruction is one of the important indications for surgery for an ulcer of the stomach or duodenum. Such complications must be regarded with care, because gastric cancer may be present, but is difficult to diagnose in these circumstances.

Duodenal ulcers cause obstruction for two reasons: in young patients acute ulcers are associated with much surrounding inflammation and oedema; in the elderly fibrosis develops about an old ulcer. Differentiation between the two modes of obstruction usually can be made by observation during several days of nasogastric suction, intravenous administration of H_2-receptor antagonists, and intravenous alimentation. Oedema usually subsides within a few days, while fibrotic obstruction continues to produce large quantities of gastric aspirate.

In either case the prognosis is poor without operation. However, obstruction due to oedema that subsides rapidly can be treated conservatively for a few weeks, at which time the operation will be much easier and safer.

The operation chosen depends on the condition of the patient. Gastric resection combined with vagotomy is our preference in young patients, although vagotomy and gastroenterostomy may be performed if inflammation about the pylorus is severe. Proximal gastric vagotomy is contraindicated.

Older patients in poor condition who are considered to have fibrotic obstruction and burned-out ulcers, can be treated if necessary by gastroenterostomy under local anaesthesia. A gastric resection will generally be tolerated, but the addition of a vagotomy may lead to a prolonged period of gastric atony, and should be avoided.

Obstructing gastric ulcers should be treated by gastric resection combined with truncal vagotomy.

Intractability

Intractability implies that a patient with an ulcer has been treated with the best available medical therapy but is still symptomatic. Such ulcers are usually duodenal or prepyloric. It is important that a gastrinoma is ruled out by appropriate tests. The patient should undergo endoscopy while symptoms are most severe; if an ulcer is present, and further medical therapy only leads to temporary relief, a standard ulcer operation should be performed.

There are many patients who complain of ulcer-like symptoms, but in whom no objective evidence of an ulcer can be found: other causes of epigastric distress should be investigated. These patients should be examined carefully by endoscopy and by barium contrast radiography before an operation is undertaken. To do otherwise may mean that the operative findings will be unimpressive and that the patient will complain of the same symptoms postoperatively.

In these patients full medical therapy is recommended before embarking on any possibly curative operation. Under these circumstances the least that can be done is the best. A proximal gastric vagotomy will be the least likely to subject the patient to new, more serious postoperative symptoms, provided that the procedure is uncomplicated.

Few operations are performed for intractability. In the Massachusetts General Hospital about 10 operations for persistent or recurrent gastric ulcer and 10 for recurrent or persistent duodenal ulcer are performed per year. The number is likely to be considerably higher in countries where continued medical therapy is impossible and where operations are performed for less strict criteria.

Minor haemorrhages

Repetitive minor haemorrhage is another indication for operation. The source of such bleeding is more likely to be ulcer disease associated with gastritis or duodenitis; major vessels, such as the left gastric or gastroduodenal are not involved. The symptoms usually consist of repeated episodes of tarry stools, which may not be associated with pain.

Other sites of occult bleeding may need to be investigated, and endoscopy during a bleeding episode is essential to confirm the diagnosis. Otherwise, this difficult diagnostic problem may require such measures as preoperative arteriography and intra-operative endoscopy.

When the symptoms are not controlled by medical measures, operation is necessary. Gastric resection with bilateral truncal vagotomy is preferred; the antrum should be completely excised. Careful examination of the entire gastrointestinal tract at the time of operation is essential.

Fistulae secondary to ulcer disease

Gastric ulcers can perforate into the transverse colon, producing a gastrocolic fistula, the symptoms of which include vomiting of faeces and severe diarrhoea. Exactly the same type of fistula and symptoms can occur if the underlying disease is either gastric or colonic cancer. The diagnosis of a fistula may be made by barium contrast radiographs or endoscopy. However, endoscopic observation and biopsy to rule out cancer are indicated. If the lesion is benign, gastric and colonic resections are necessary; malignancy of either the stomach or colon requires more extensive resection.

Duodenal ulcers may penetrate into the common bile duct or the ascending or transverse colon; involvement of any other organ is rare. Although the general principles of therapy are the same as for gastric ulcers, choledochoduodenal fistulae furnish special problems. This problem may arise either from a duodenal ulcer in the second portion of the duodenum or from primary disease of the biliary tree. If biliary tract disease can be ruled out and the dissection promises to be dangerous, a low ulcer can be treated by a Billroth II resection; the duodenal stump can be closed cephalad to the fistula, leaving it in place. A vagotomy is added.

Operations for peptic ulcer disease

Antrectomy (hemigastrectomy) and bilateral vagotomy

This operation is the favourite procedure employed by many surgeons for the treatment of both duodenal and gastric ulcers because of its superiority in elimination of gastric acid, a low recurrence rate, and the absence of most of the troublesome sequelae of more radical gastrectomies.

Indications for operation

The indications for the use of this operation include any of the complications of duodenal ulcer, and gastric ulcer located in the pylorus or prepyloric area, or gastric ulcer combined with duodenal ulcer. It also can be used for all other peptic ulcers of the stomach.

This is an operation of considerable complexity and severity. It carries a higher risk of postoperative complications than pyloroplasty and vagotomy, proximal gastric vagotomy, or gastric resection alone. Even skilled surgeons may have to adopt different procedures in very ill or aged persons.

Operative procedure

The operation is a combination of bilateral truncal vagotomy and distal gastrectomy. The procedure is completed by either a Billroth I gastroduodenostomy (Fig. 4) or a Billroth II gastroenterostomy (Fig. 5). Antrectomy and hemigastrectomy are considered to be synonymous for practical purposes.

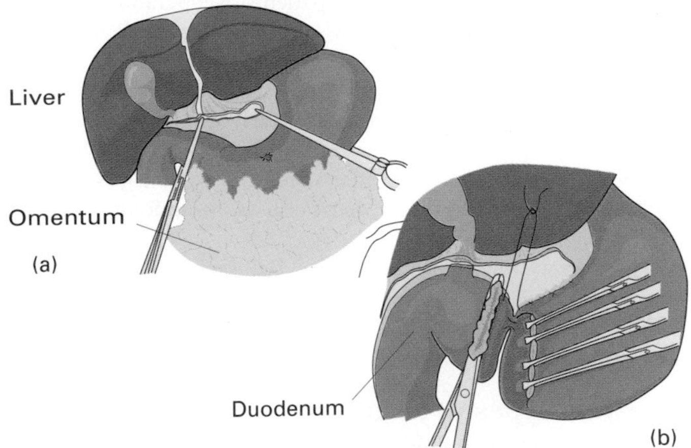

Fig. 4 Hemigastrectomy and gastroduodenostomy (Billroth I resection). Distal gastric resection (antrectomy or hemigastrectomy) is followed by an end-to-end gastroduodenostomy. This operation is satisfactory for type 1 gastric ulcers, but must be accompanied by bilateral truncal vagotomy when used for duodenal ulcers, gastric ulcers that are prepyloric, gastric ulcers associated with duodenal ulcers, and pyloric ulcers.

Results of operation

The outstanding feature of this operation is that the incidence of recurrent ulceration is less than 1 per cent after 5 years in all large series. Furthermore, long-term data are now available, and indicate no increase in the rate of recurrence.

In the last Massachusetts General Hospital study, the operative mortality in elective cases was 0.5 per cent; this increased when

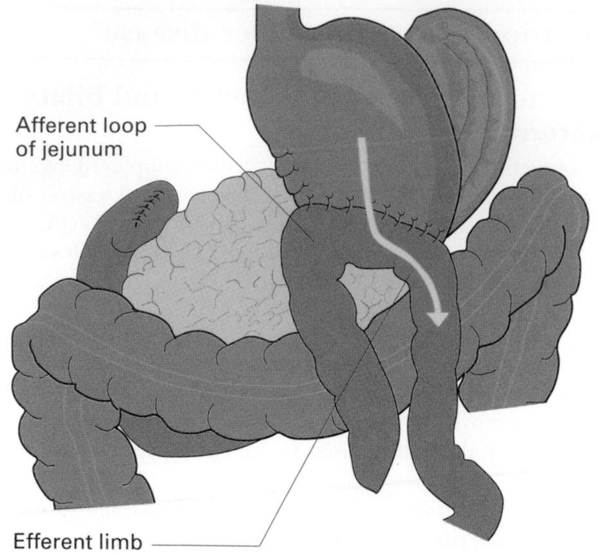

Fig. 5 Hemigastrectomy and gastrojejunostomy (Billroth II resection). This procedure must be accompanied by a bilateral truncal vagotomy. If a vagotomy is not performed, a more extensive (75 per cent) gastric resection is necessary.

the indications for operation were acute massive haemorrhage or acute perforation. Morbidity from early complications led to reoperation in 8 per cent of cases; reoperations for recurrent ulcer were necessary in 0.3 per cent of patients. Reoperations for other reasons (chiefly alkaline gastritis or motility problems) were necessary at a late period in 5 per cent of patients.

Smithwick found in his early studies that reduction in fasting and stimulated acid secretion was nearly complete, that long-range dumping symptoms occurred in about 5 per cent but were disabling in only 1 per cent, that significant weight loss occurred in 3 per cent, and persistent diarrhoea was troublesome in 3 per cent.

Herrington reported that in his last series of 341 patients treated between 1975 and 1984 65 per cent obtained an excellent result, 20 per cent a good result, 12 per cent a fair result, and 3 per cent a poor result.

Various types of vagotomy

Three types of vagotomy require consideration. Bilateral truncal vagotomy denervates the entire stomach and the gastrointestinal tract to the midcolon (Fig. 6). When combined with other operations it is extremely effective in reducing the number of recurrent ulcers. However it does carry some deleterious side-effects, reducing the ability of the stomach to empty and being followed by other late motility disturbances, occasional vagus diarrhoea, and reflux alkaline gastritis.

Selective vagotomy denervates the entire stomach but leaves nerves to the gallbladder, pylorus, and bowel intact. From a practical point of view this operation is more difficult and time-consuming than truncal vagotomy, appears to have nearly equivalent results, and has attracted few supporters.

Proximal gastric vagotomy, the most recently developed type of vagotomy, has received enormous support and is the only type of vagotomy that can be used without pyloroplasty, gastroenterostomy, or antrectomy.

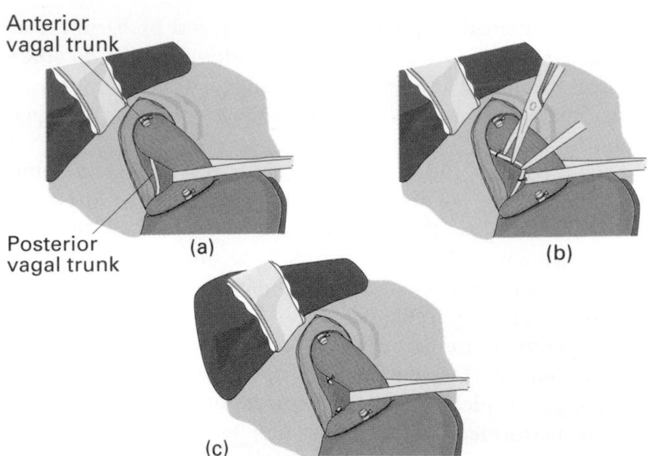

Fig. 6 Truncal vagotomy. The oesophagus is exposed at the hiatus by retracting the left lobe of the liver. (a) The anterior nerve has been divided. (b) The posterior nerve is divided and a 2- to 3-cm section is removed for biopsy. (c) A search is made for any residual fibres.

Historical notes

This surgical procedure, which many observers today believe is the best available operation for duodenal ulcer, was developed relatively recently. Conceived in America, first tried in Germany in combination with procedures designed to reduce spasm of the pyloric muscle, and used shortly afterward without any interference with the pylorus simultaneously in Denmark and England, it has a peculiarly international flavour. For this reason, the operation first had several different names, and differences in technique led to acrimonious exchanges between various pioneers.

The world was looking for a superior operation for duodenal ulcer when, in 1957, Griffiths and Harken in Seattle, performed the original laboratory investigations in dogs that proved the feasibility of the operation. Truncal vagotomy alone at that time was known to lead to gastric paresis, with severe gastric retention and accentuation of the gastrin factor, actually leading to an increase in the activity of a duodenal ulcer unless an emptying procedure—either pyloroplasty or gastroenterostomy—was added. The new operation, which allowed the retention of motor function in the antrum and a functioning pylorus, appeared to be the answer.

When Holle, in Munich, first described the procedure in 1965, he was concerned that the antrum would not empty properly, and performed additional procedures, such as section of the pyloric muscle. Such additions were viewed with alarm by Amdrup and Jensen in Copenhagen and Johnston in Leeds; their publications in 1970 included descriptions of the operation as it is now performed. They believed that Holle's additions were actually types of pyloroplasty, and that the known evils of pyloroplasty of dumping and bile reflux would be repeated. However, it should be recognized that pyloric obstruction is now considered as a contraindication for proximal gastric vagotomy. The term proximal gastric vagotomy now is used in preference to its synonyms—highly selective vagotomy, superselective vagotomy, selective proximal vagotomy, or parietal cell vagotomy.

Indications for proximal gastric vagotomy

Proximal gastric vagotomy has been used for the treatment of uncomplicated duodenal ulcers, in combination with closure of an acute perforation, or in combination with ligation of the gastroduodenal artery for massive haemorrhage. We propose a limited role for the procedure: namely, a procedure to be undertaken in thin, poorly nourished patients who require surgery because of pain unresponsive to medical therapy. It is contraindicated for duodenal ulcers causing obstruction, for pyloric ulcers, and for gastric ulcers. Although nearly all surgeons agree it is contraindicated for any gastric ulcer, Jordan has combined proximal gastric vagotomy with ulcer excision in selected patients.

Description of the operation

The operation comprises division of the branches of the anterior and posterior vagus nerves to the stomach, identified from the lower 7 cm of the oesophagus down to the 'crow's foot'—the vagal branches in the distal 8 cm of the stomach (Fig. 7). The operation is meticulous and time-consuming.

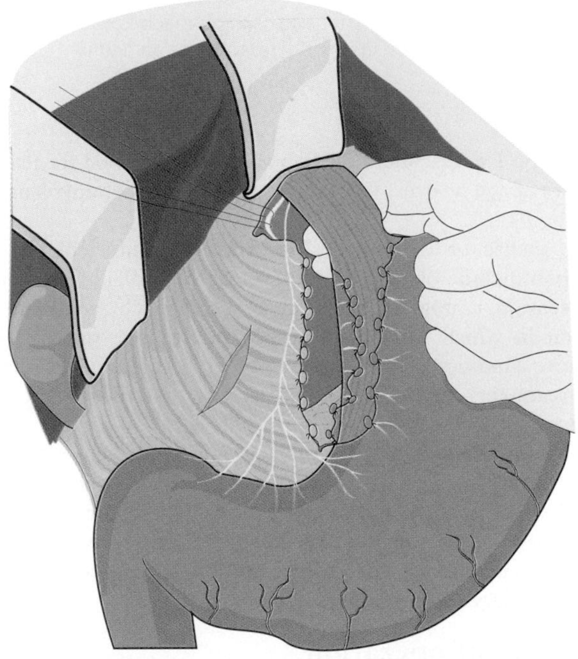

Fig. 7 Proximal gastric vagotomy. The branches of both anterior and posterior vagus nerves running from the main trunks to the lower 7 cm of oesophagus and the upper stomach down to 8 cm above the pylorus have been divided. The main trunks are left intact.

Because of the high rate of recurrent ulceration, many modifications of the procedure have been suggested. Operative proof of section of the nerves has been demonstrated by stimulation of the denervated lower oesophagus or by intragastric measurements of pH. Dissection of the vagal trunks from the lower 7 cm of oesophagus is necessary to eliminate the 'criminal nerve of Grassi'; otherwise, appreciable vagal innervation would remain. The nerves running along the right gastroepiploic vessels are also divided by some surgeons, but this has met with little favour. Taylor prefers a posterior truncal vagotomy and an extramucosal division of the branches of the anterior vagus down as low as the crow's foot by means of a long incision through the serosa and mucosa of the anterior stomach wall near the lesser curvature.

Results

The results of this operation have been studied extensively in the laboratory and in clinical practice. One of the most careful and complete investigations was carried out by a collaborative group in Switzerland, France, and Germany under the direction of Allgöwer and Muller. Five years after the original operation, complete investigations were carried out and these were repeated at the end of 10 years. There was an 85 per cent follow-up after 5 years, and three-quarters of the patients also underwent endoscopy. One of their most important findings was a high incidence of asymptomatic ulcers on endoscopy, although the significance of this finding is not clear.

From their observations as well as those of others the following conclusions seem justified. Firstly, the operative mortality is extremely low (<0.5 per cent), and postoperative complications are rare. The development of gastric ulcers can be prevented by careful closure of the peritoneum over the area from which vagal branches have been removed. Secondly, when proximal gastric vagotomy is performed for the indications listed above, the recurrence rate at the end of 5 years is about 10 per cent, although the recurrence rate continues to rise thereafter and, according to Jensen in Copenhagen, is 39 per cent at the end of 15 years.

In 1942 Visick established criteria for judging postoperative results that, after minor modifications, have been widely accepted. They are: Visick I, totally asymptomatic; Visick II, minor symptoms, not interfering with daily activities; Visick III, periods of inability to perform daily tasks, or continuous symptoms interfering with life; Visick IV, totally incapacitated, or secondary operation required for relief of symptoms. Results reported by some surgeons indicate that 5 years after proximal gastric vagotomy 95 per cent of patients are rated Visick I or Visick II. Other observers are not so optimistic: 90 per cent is a more common figure.

Preoperative studies of gastric secretion are of little or no value, except to exclude patients with Zollinger–Ellison syndrome. Postoperatively, basal acid reduction is reduced by about 60 per cent, and secretion due to pentagastrin stimulation by about 50 per cent. Postoperatively, weight loss is uncommon, and weight gain often occurs, blood studies are normal, with no evidence of anaemia, serum calcium levels remain normal, and dumping syndrome, diarrhoea, and bile gastritis are rare. Recurrences are usually associated with only minor symptoms, and most of them can be treated medically. An operation is necessary in about 3 per cent of cases, and antrectomy is safe and has excellent results. In the Basle series, there was a clinical recurrence rate of about 5 per cent symptomatic, asymptomatic recurrences in a total of 14.9 per cent, and later gastric resection in 2 per cent of all patients.

The continued presence of gastric acid prevents colonization of the stomach with Gram-negative bacilli and may be a deterrent to later development of cancer of the stomach.

Pyloroplasty and truncal vagotomy

Pyloroplasty and vagotomy is the simplest surgical treatment for duodenal ulcer and in selected instances it can be used in the treatment of bleeding, obstruction, perforation, and intractability. It also allows a stomach that failed to empty after bilateral vagotomy of any type to drain more effectively. The operation carries low morbidity and mortality rates.

With so many recommendations, it is no wonder that pyloroplasty-vagotomy was the favourite procedure for duodenal ulcer for many years after Dragstedt's popularization of vagotomy. However, as is usual with most operations for peptic ulcer, late complications have reduced its popularity.

The operation usually consists of a Heineke–Mikulicz procedure (Fig. 8). A longitudinal incision is made across the distal stomach and the proximal duodenum and closed transversely, so that the action of the pyloric valve is obliterated. In other cases, when the proximal duodenum is badly deformed by scar, a Finney procedure (essentially a side-to-side gastroduodenostomy) or a Jaboulay procedure (gastric resection plus side-to-side gastroduodenostomy) is used.

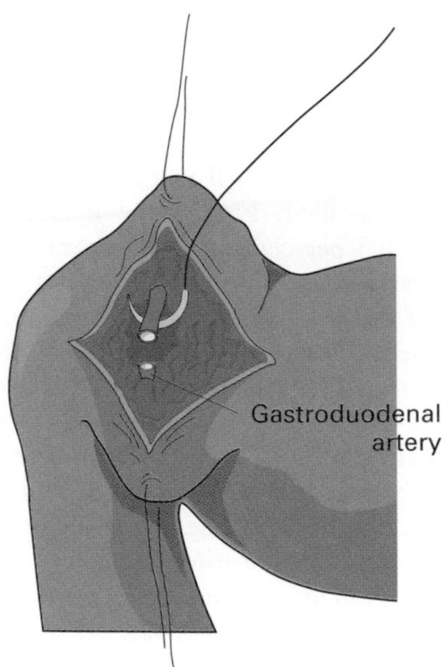

Fig. 8 Pyloroplasty, vagotomy, and ligation of gastroduodenal artery for massive bleeding. A Heineke-Mikulicz pyloroplasty is done by making a 5-cm horizontal incision that crosses the pylorus. After ligation of the bleeding artery with stout non-absorbable sutures, the pyloroplasty is completed by closing the incision in a vertical fashion with two layers of sutures. Bilateral truncal vagotomy is performed.

Some surgeons report a recurrence rate of 5 per cent. Others found it to be much higher. Herrington's figure was 18 per cent, and the average is about 10 per cent. If reoperation is necessary, the dissection is difficult because of the proximity of the pancreas and the common bile duct. The great majority of surgeons find it unsatisfactory for the treatment of gastric ulcer. The absence of a pylorus leads to a high incidence of alkaline gastritis; this is increased if a simultaneous cholecystectomy is done. Dumping syndrome and diarrhoea are common sequelae. The popularity of this operation has waned, and it has been succeeded by proximal gastric vagotomy or by vagotomy and antrectomy.

Partial gastrectomy without vagotomy

The usual procedure involves resection of the distal two-thirds of the stomach followed by either a Billroth I or a Billroth II anastomosis (Fig. 9). In our opinion the operation is neater and more accurate when sutures are inserted by hand, although stapling instruments can be used.

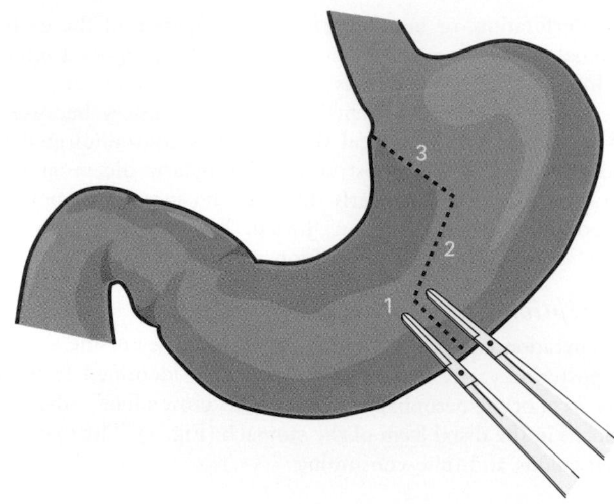

Fig. 9 Operation for high gastric ulcer. Whenever possible a high gastric ulcer should be excised together with a distal gastrectomy. If a vagotomy appears to be dangerous because of inflammation, a two-thirds gastrectomy is performed. The stomach is divided sequentially as shown by the numbers, to leave an adquate reservoir.

For type 1 gastric ulcer this is a standard operation for patients 70 years of age or over. In younger patients a vagotomy is usually added.

For gastric or duodenal ulcer, relative indications for this operation include obesity, an abnormally high diaphragm, portal hypertension, emergency operations for massive bleeding, or perforation in which a definitive procedure is wise but in which operative conditions are less than optimal. It is also performed for the treatment of long-standing pyloric obstruction in aged patients.

The main disadvantages of this operation include a recurrence rate of at least 2 to 3 per cent of cases, and a weight loss that averages 4 kg in men and 6 kg in women. The recurrence rate is lower than that of any of the standard operations other than vagotomy-antrectomy. Late complications such as motility problems secondary to vagotomy are also avoided.

Selection of operation

Surgeons vary in their preference of an elective operation for duodenal ulcer. There is an indication for each of the four operations described above: our preference is usually vagotomy-antrectomy.

There are definite contraindications to proximal gastric vagotomy, as noted above, while contraindications to vagotomy-antrectomy are rare, except that the surgeon should avoid resective procedures, when possible, in thin, malnourished patients, and in those in whom subjective symptoms appear to be out of proportion to objective findings. Women also do less well than do men, particularly in so far as weight loss is concerned.

When a patient apparently has a long life ahead, or one that might take him to countries where drug therapy is not available in case of recurrent symptoms, vagotomy-antrectomy is more likely to fill his needs (Fig. 10). Neurotic patients who magnify symptoms do better with proximal gastric vagotomy.

Patients must be informed of the side-effects of both operations and the high incidence of recurrent ulcer after proximal gastric vagotomy compared with vagotomy-antrectomy.

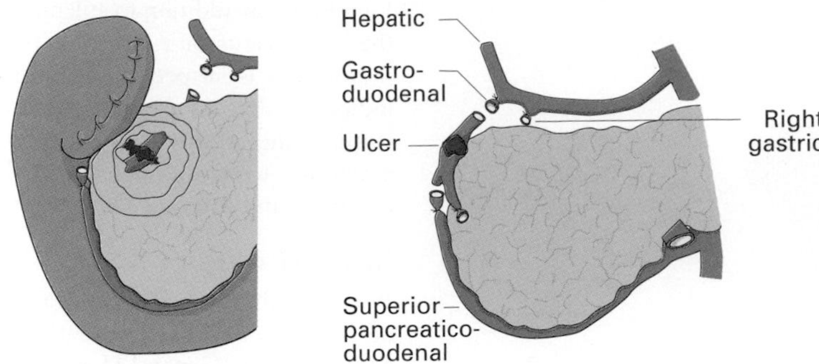

Fig. 10 Gastrectomy and gastroenterostomy with ligation of gastroduodenal artery for massive bleeding. Control of the bleeding gastroduodenal artery is secured by proximal and distal ligation. The duodenal stump is closed leaving the open bed of the ulcer on the pancreas. Hemigastrectomy (antrectomy), gastroenterostomy (preferably antecolic), and bilateral truncal vagotomy complete the operation.

POSTOPERATIVE COMPLICATIONS

Postoperative complications may be divided into two major groups—early and late. Early complications follow within a month after the date of initial surgery. Late sequelae occur after that time.

Early postoperative complications

In addition to relatively uncommon problems involving the cardiovascular, pulmonary, hepatic, or renal systems, there are certain complications referable to specific operative procedures on the stomach or duodenum. They include postoperative haemorrhage, suture line leakage, damage to adjacent tissues or organs, and stomal delay.

Postoperative haemorrhage

If there are signs of postoperative bleeding such as falling blood pressure, rising pulse rate and fall in haematocrit soon after operation the surgeon must consider several possibilities. If there is no blood in the aspirate from a nasogastric tube, extragastric bleeding is likely. Splenic rupture or damage to the vessels in the hilum are the most likely causes, particularly following a vagotomy.

If there is blood in the nasogastric aspirate, other causes must be considered. The initial bleeding site may not have been identified or adequately controlled by the first operation. If the initial site has been treated satisfactorily, bleeding from another area in the mucosa is not uncommon in the presence of extensive gastritis. The bleeding may have originated from a suture line. Bleeding from the site of insertion of a gastrostomy tube is not infrequent.

Bleeding usually occurs within the first few hours or the first day after the original operation. Whether or not a second laparotomy must be carried out depends upon the patient's response to conservative measures, including continued nasogastric tube irrigation and aspiration, and intravenous replacement of fluids, electrolytes, and blood. Severe or continued bleeding is an indication for re-exploration. Following a gastrectomy, the stomach is opened, previous suture lines are inspected, and the gastric remnant is examined for other bleeding sites. If a source is not discovered in the stomach, the duodenum is explored.

If all findings, including oesophageal and distal duodenal endoscopy are negative, and the patient has been vomiting blood, haemorrhage probably arose from the stomach. Tiny gastric ulcers or cirsoid aneurysms are the most likely causes, and a generous subtotal gastrectomy (75 per cent) is indicated. This is one of the few cases in which a so-called 'blind gastrectomy' has to be performed in the hope that the bleeding lesion will be excised to save the patient's life.

Suture line leakage

By far the most common problem is duodenal stump leakage following a Billroth II gastrectomy. This catastrophe occurs in 1 per cent of such operations; unless a remedial operation is undertaken immediately, the mortality rate rises to nearly 50 per cent.

Leakage can be avoided or minimized by several methods. If a gastrectomy is planned, but the inflammation about the duodenum appears particularly severe, the surgeon should consider performing a vagotomy and gastroenterostomy. A controlled duodenal fistula can be made at the time of the original operation by catheter duodenostomy (Fig. 11). Alternatively, a drain may be placed near the duodenal stump; if a leak occurs it will probably track into the site of the drain.

Drainage from an incompletely sutured duodenal stump or rupture of the suture line may occur at any time after the operation but is rare after 7 days. Rupture is diagnosed by the sudden onset of severe pain and tenderness in the right upper quadrant. If a drain is already in place, spontaneous drainage of duodenal contents may occur. If no drain has been inserted at the time of operation, the treatment of such a leak is immediate operation and the insertion of drains near the duodenal stump. Attempts to identify the site of drainage in the stump may lead to further damage. A catheter can occasionally be placed in the stump itself.

A leak from a gastroduodenostomy or a gastrojejunostomy is suggested by unusually severe postoperative local pain and tenderness. If it is detected at an early stage, the opening can be repaired and the suture line can be bolstered with omentum; at a later stage, a fistula is almost certain to develop. Fistulae with only a small output may heal spontaneously if nasogastric suction and hyperalimentation are used. Other fistulae will require surgical repair.

Damage to adjacent tissues or organs

Gastric resections for duodenal ulcer may be followed by pancreatitis if the pancreas has been damaged. Fortunately, pancreatitis is usually mild and subsides after conservative treatment. Vagotomy

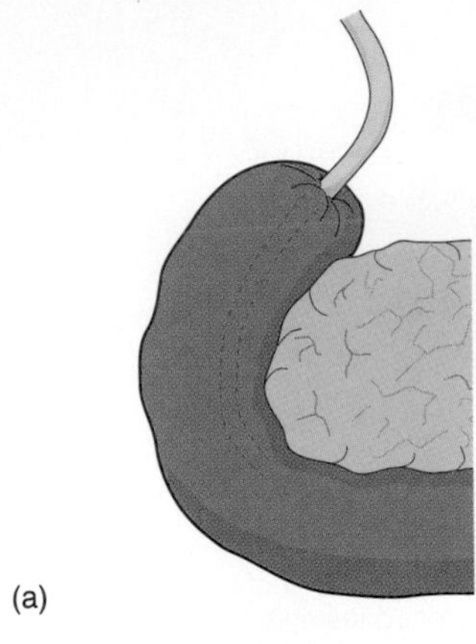

(a)

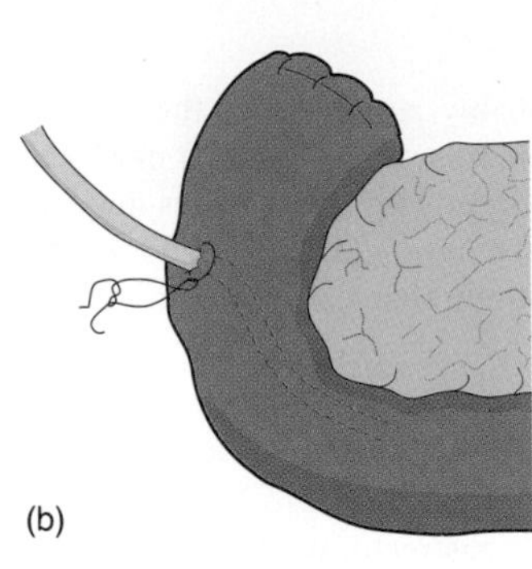

(b)

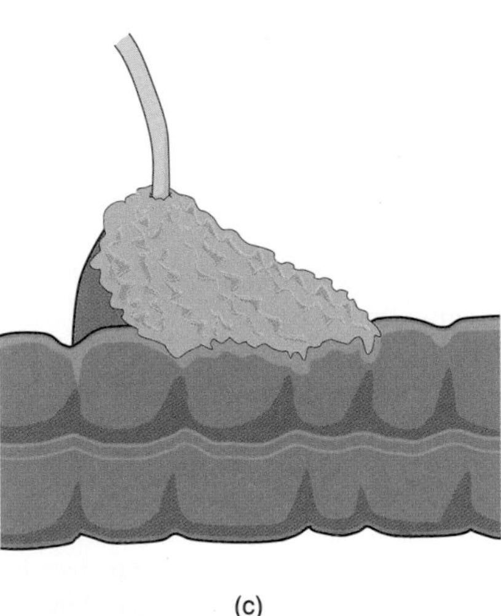

(c)

Fig. 11 Catheter duodenostomy. When a Billroth II resection is contemplated, and the duodenal stump is likely to be difficult, as much normal duodenum as possible should be left *in situ*. Dissection along the head of the pancreas should be minimal. If there is massive haemorrhage from the gastroduodenal artery, haemostasis is secured. A 16-gauge French whistle-tip catheter is inserted into the duodenum and sutured firmly in place. The catheter must irrigate freely and must be water-tight. End duodenostomy ((a) and (c)) is necessary for very difficult duodenums, and lateral duodenostomy (b) for duodenums in which closure is possible, but less than completely satisfactory.

Vagotomy, in addition to splenic injury, may lead to perforation of the oesophagus or rupture of the diaphragm. If an oesophageal perforation is suspected, an immediate drink of Gastrografin is indicated. An oesophageal perforation requires closure by overlapping the gastric fundus or by suturing a pleural flap or omentum over the defect. Wide drainage of the left upper quadrant and often of the left pleural cavity is essential.

Stomal delay

If a gastroduodenostomy or gastrojejunostomy is not functioning normally 10 days after operation, the patient has stomal delay. A Massachusetts General Hospital study showed this to occur after gastric resection in 4.7 per cent of patients; the addition of truncal vagotomy increased the incidence to 8.6 per cent. Function is likely to be regained slowly in elderly patients who received preoperative treatment with cimetidine, who have had a long period of obstruction, or who have had a vagotomy combined with a procedure on the stomach. A low serum potassium or albumin level can lead to malfunction. Starch peritonitis has also been implicated; fat necrosis in a large omentum, and mechanical obstruction from adhesions just distal to a gastrojejunostomy are other causes.

Endoscopy should be performed to ascertain that the anastomosis is patent; some authors have reported that gentle passage of the scope into and down the efferent loop produces immediate improvement (Fig. 12). The patient is usually treated with central alimentation and careful observation; medications such as bethanecol (Urecholine) or metoclopramide tend not to be helpful. Reoperation is recommended if there is no improvement in 2 weeks.

Acceptable mortality rates are 0.5 per cent for elective proximal gastric vagotomy and 1 per cent for gastric resections.

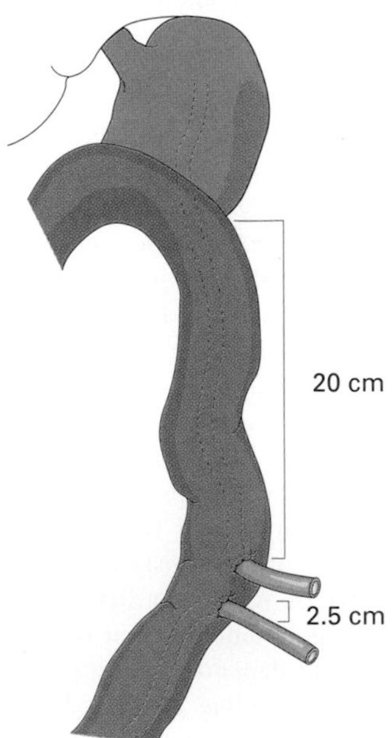

Fig. 12 Double jejunostomy. This procedure, popularized by Allen and Donaldson, essentially prevents problems with stomal obstruction following gastric resection and gastrojejunostomy. A 16-gauge French soft catheter is inserted through the jejunum in a retrograde fashion into the stomach; this is a gastrostomy tube. A second catheter is passed distally and can be used if necessary for alimentation.

Late sequelae

The late sequelae of operations for duodenal and gastric ulcer vary, depending upon the substance of the original procedure. The majority follow some type of gastrectomy; others are due to vagotomy or to loss of the pyloric sphincter. They can be roughly classified into three groups—those chiefly of historical significance, those that occur today but are rare, and those that occur today in 5 per cent or more of patients or are of current interest.

Sequelae of historical interest that are unusual today

These include the afferent loop syndrome, a mechanical problem that arises when a long jejunal afferent loop is used for a Billroth II resection or as a result of an inadequate anastomotic opening. Typical symptoms are sudden attacks of severe vomiting of bile, unmixed with food in acute cases. Persistent dilatation of the afferent loop leads to retention of duodenal contents, secondary proliferation of bacteria, and symptoms, such as anaemia and malnutrition, suggestive of a blind loop syndrome. Surgical conversion to a Billroth I anastomosis is curative.

Sequelae due to technical errors, such as gastroileostomy rather than gastrojejunostomy, are also of historical interest. They result in severe diarrhoea and late defects in absorption of food, including vitamins. A beri-beri syndrome has been reported. The error is most likely to occur when there is non-rotation of the small intestine and there is no ligament of Treitz.

Microcytic anaemia was common when the duodenum was bypassed and the oral intake of iron was poor. Macrocytic anaemia can follow high subtotal resections; it is universal after total gastrectomy because the loss of intrinsic factor prevents the absorption of vitamin B_{12}. Regular injections of cyanocobalamin (vitamin B_{12}) are necessary for the remainder of the patient's life.

Absorption of fats, proteins, and/or carbohydrates decreases directly with an increase in the amount of stomach resected. Iron absorption can be diminished following construction of Billroth II anastomoses since the duodenum is a major site of iron absorption. Calcium can be lost due to persistent diarrhoea, with consequent osteoporosis. An increased incidence of certain diseases such as tuberculosis has been reported after extensive gastrectomy in poorly nourished patients.

For the interested reader a detailed discussion of these problems was made in 1963 by Stammers and Williams. Their careful studies served to reduce the standard amount of stomach that was resected for ulcer disease.

Sequelae that occur today but are rare

These include technical errors: an unusually small gastroduodenostomy can result in symptoms of partial obstruction with epigastric fullness, heartburn, and episodes of vomiting; conversion of a Billroth I to a Billroth II anastomosis relieves symptoms. An inadequate gastrojejunostomy also requires a secondary operation.

Vagal diarrhoea is a complication in which the aetiology is not clear, but severe, almost uncontrollable explosive diarrhoea occurs after about 1 per cent of bilateral truncal vagotomies. Other causes of diarrhoea, such as colonization of the stomach with Gram-negative bacilli or giardiasis, must be excluded. Herrington and Sawyers have successfully employed a reversed loop of the jejunum for the treatment of a few such patients.

A patient with dental plates and a Billroth II anastomosis may unknowingly swallow a large amount of undigestible material such as orange pulp, and develop intestinal obstruction from a bezoar. After truncal vagotomy, endoscopy may disclose undigested masses of vegetable material in the stomach; most are of no significance.

Small gastric reservoirs can lead to malnutrition. Such operations are now rarely performed for ulcer disease, except when total gastrectomy is necessary for hypergastrinaemia, when they are usually tolerated well. In some instances Scott has proved the value of a gastric pouch fashioned with two to three loops of jejunum: this can improve the ability of a patient to eat larger meals.

Important sequelae

Some sequelae occur today in 5 per cent of patients or are of current interest. These are of variable significance and range from potentially serious, such as a persistent or recurrent ulcer (Table 2), to those in which symptoms appear to be functional with no accompanying pathological change. Precise definition of some of these syndromes is difficult and the relative emphasis placed upon them by different observers differs. We prefer to emphasize persistent or recurrent ulceration because of its potential for future serious problems and because it can be confirmed by objective rather than by subjective evidence.

Table 2 Recurrence rate of ulcer disease after various operations

Operation	Author	Rate (%)	Date
Duodenal ulcer			
Gastroenterostomy	(Average, estimated)	25	1932
Subtotal gastrectomy	Visick	5	1948
Subtotal gastrectomy	Stammers, Williams	2.5	1963
Subtotal gastrectomy	Welch, Rodkey	8	1963
Billroth I	Wallensten	12	1957
Billroth II	Wallensten	4	1957
Billroth I, vagotomy	Paul Jordan	1	1985
Billroth II, vagotomy	Smithwick	<1	1970
Billroth II, vagotomy	Herrington	0.6	1973
Roux-en-Y, vagotomy	(Estimated)	1	1989
Pyloroplasty, vagotomy	Mayo Clinic	12	1980
Pyloroplasty, vagotomy	Herrington	18	1976
Drainage, vagotomy*	McGregor, McVay	3	1978
	Woodward	6	1986
Proximal gastric vagotomy	Hoffmann	39	1989
	Jordan (Paul)	8	1985
	Sawyers, Herrington	10	1985
	Goligher (proved)	4.3	1978
	Goligher (possible)	15	1978
	Muller (clinical)	6	1985
	Muller (total)*†	14	1985
Gastric ulcer			
Gastric resection	Paul Jordan (Type 1)	2.8	1986
Billroth I, vagotomy	George Jordan	1	1986
PGV (Pyloric)	Muller (clinical)	9	1985
	Muller (total)†	15	1985
(Prepyloric)	Muller (clinical)	16	1985
	Muller (total)†	29	1985
(Prepyloric)	Clark	35	1977

* Vagotomy and pyloroplasty in 65 per cent; vagotomy and gastroenterostomy in 28 per cent.

† Includes all ulcers proved by endoscopy.

Postoperative symptoms (mild or moderate)

Careful questioning of patients who have undergone gastric surgery uncovers a large number of symptoms, many of which can also be elicited from individuals who have never had an operation. The incidence and significance of dyspeptic symptoms, such as postprandial fullness, weight loss, loss of appetite, and nausea, that are secondary to the operative procedure is, therefore, hard to assess.

Satisfaction after an operation for duodenal ulcer is usually about 90 per cent, regardless of the procedure performed. Many patients do, however, have minor symptoms that put them into Visick grade II. Müller found that 64 per cent of patients were grade I (asymptomatic) following proximal gastric vagotomy, while 28 per cent were grade II (minor symptoms). Hoffman found that 15 per cent of patients were Visick class II, regardless of the type of vagotomy used.

The percentage of patients in Visick class II appears to be nearly the same after vagotomy-antrectomy as after proximal gastric vagotomy, truncal vagotomy-pyloroplasty, and selective vagotomy with pyloroplasty. It is only in the proportion of more unfavourable results (Visick III or IV) that there is a variation between the results of different procedures.

Recurrent ulcer

For many years postoperative recurrent ulcers have been regarded as the cardinal sign of an unsuccessful operation. Some doubt has been cast upon this conclusion by the fact that many recurrences following proximal gastric vagotomy can be treated successfully with H_2-receptor antagonists. Such treatment may, however, not be readily available in developing countries, where the first operative procedure needs to be curative.

Absolute figures concerning recurrences after the same type of operation often show wide variations, and these depend upon factors that are impossible to analyse. Some of these variations are shown in Table 2. However, certain generalizations are warranted.

The recurrence rate after gastric resections for type 1 gastric ulcer, even without vagotomy, is negligible; other late sequelae are also minimal. Pyloric ulcers, prepyloric ulcers, and gastric ulcers associated with duodenal ulcers do not respond well to proximal gastric vagotomy; they should be treated by antrectomy plus bilateral truncal vagotomy.

The recurrence rate after gastric resection and bilateral truncal vagotomy is 1 per cent or less after 5 years and does not appear to increase later. The highest rate of recurrence is after proximal gastric vagotomy, and this appears to rise with time.

Billroth I and II gastric resections have a similar rate of recurrence if a bilateral truncal vagotomy is added; without a vagotomy, the recurrence rate after a Billroth II is lower.

Endoscopic examination 5 years after proximal gastric vagotomy shows that active ulcers are present in approximately twice as many individuals as those who have symptoms. The fate of these silent ulcers is not known.

Recurrent ulcers after proximal gastric vagotomy can be successfully treated by a gastric resection.

Dumping syndrome

This syndrome consists of a combination of one or more of the following: fall in blood pressure, sweating, pallor, abdominal distension, cramps, diarrhoea, weakness, and a desire to lie down. Early dumping occurs within 15 to 30 min after eating; late dumping occurs about 2 h after eating.

Early dumping occurs in some persons who have not had an operation. However it is accentuated by any mechanism that destroys the action of the pyloric valve, so that gastric contents are discharged rapidly into the duodenum or jejunum. Liquids with a high osmolality, such as a chocolate milk shake, are most likely to initiate symptoms. It is most common after gastric resections and least common after proximal gastric vagotomy. It occurs in about 25 per cent of patients who have had a gastric operation other than proximal gastric vagotomy in the early weeks after operation and tends to disappear with time.

Preoperative administration of a hypertonic glucose solution may identify those who are likely to suffer from postoperative dumping. The mechanism is believed to be the rapid fluid and electrolyte shift into the intestinal lumen in response to this challenge. Increased activity of hormone secreting cells in the intestine also may be a factor.

Medical therapy of the syndrome consists of solid rather than liquid meals, small but repeated servings, and a low intake of carbohydrates and of dairy products. Additional aids, such as separate intake of solids and liquids, and avoidance of very warm or very cold liquids, can help. After a patient finds that certain foods are tolerated well, others may be added one at a time.

Surgical treatment has generally been unsatisfactory. The operation most likely to succeed consists of an interposition of a retroperistaltic 10-cm loop of jejunum between the distal end of the stomach and the duodenum; a vagotomy must be added if one has not already been performed.

Because dumping symptoms tend to disappear after months or even several years, a conservative attitude is warranted in the treatment of these patients.

Late dumping occurs 2 to 3 h after eating, and affects only 2 per cent of patients. The symptoms are also related to carbohydrate ingestion; 2 h after eating the hyperglycaemia induces an oversupply of insulin which then leads to a reactive hypoglycaemia attended by symptoms of prostration and sweating. Moderation of carbohydrate intake usually controls the symptoms.

Alkaline gastritis

The causes and classification of postgastrectomy symptoms are severe enough to interfere with an individual's lifestyle and are extremely difficult to analyse. Nowhere is the problem more difficult than with alkaline gastritis.

This syndrome arises because of regurgitation of bile and duodenal contents back into the stomach. The existence of such a syndrome is proven by the fact that diversion of bile relieves the symptoms, yet no individual symptoms or objective findings serve to distinguish the syndrome prior to operation. Epigastric distress, particularly after eating, nausea, and occasional vomiting and/or diarrhoea are common but totally non-specific. What appears to be obvious gastritis to the endoscopist is often normal according to the pathologist.

In an attempt to find some preoperative test that would help to make the diagnosis, Warshaw injected various solutions into the stomach through a nasogastric tube. Patients with the syndrome developed pain after injection of a strong alkali solution, but not after saline or acid infusion. Such patients appeared to have better results from a reparative operation than others who had a negative test.

The syndrome is most common after a Billroth II gastrectomy, but is nearly as common after a Billroth I or pyloroplasty. It occurs rarely after a proximal gastric vagotomy. Since the symptoms often tend to diminish with the passage of time, a conservative approach is indicated.

To detour upper intestinal contents from the stomach, a Roux-en-Y anastomosis is made (Fig. 13). The jejunum must be divided and the proximal end anastomosed to the descending jejunum 45 cm below the stomach. Although this procedure received great enthusiasm when it was first introduced, a satisfactory result is found in less than two-thirds of patients treated in this way. Some of those with unsatisfactory results prove to have motility problems that may be helped with a higher or even a total gastric resection. However, a large proportion of the unsatisfactory results occur in patients with multiple psychiatric complaints. In some of these the original operation appears to have been performed after inadequate evaluation.

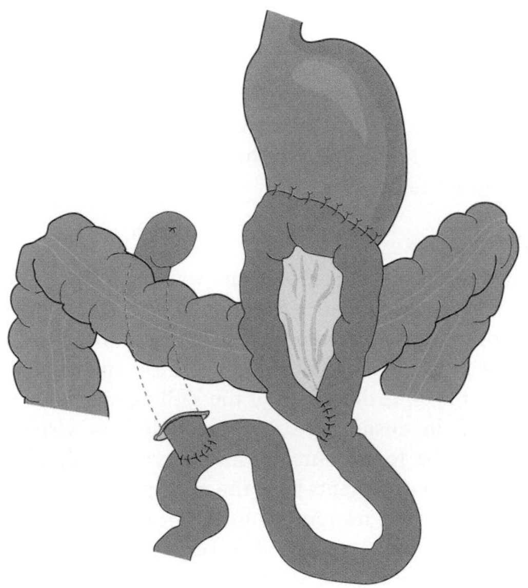

Fig. 13 Tanner operation no. 19 (modification of Roux-en-Y anastomosis). This procedure was performed for alkaline gastritis following truncal vagotomy, hemigastrectomy and Billroth II anastomosis. The afferent limb of the gastrojejunostomy is divided; the upper segment of the jejunum is anastomosed to the descending limb of the jejunum a short distance below the gastrojejunostomy. The open end of the proximal jejunum is then anastomosed end-to-side to the jejunum 40 to 50 cm below the gastrojejunostomy.

Motility problems

Disturbances of the normal motility of the stomach and/or duodenum can lead to unduly rapid emptying or to paresis. Rapid emptying, known as dumping, is considered above. Slow emptying of the stomach can lead to stomal delay, obstructive vomiting, the formation of gastric bezoars, poor nutrition, and loss of appetite and weight.

Primary motility problems involving the stomach are rare, but they often appear after surgery, particularly when a vagotomy has been performed. In patients who have not undergone any operative procedure, diseases such as diabetes, scleroderma, amyloid disease, central nervous system abnormalities, and Chagas' disease must be considered. In this section disturbances secondary to operations for gastric or duodenal ulcer will be described.

Motility of the stomach is activated by the vagus nerve. Little peristalsis is demonstrable on radiographic studies of the fundus, even in normal persons. One or more pacemakers near the lower portion of the fundus initiate impulses which lead to antral peristalsis and emptying of the stomach. Because the pacemakers are activated by the vagus nerves, vagotomy without pyloroplasty or gastroenterostomy often causes emptying of the stomach to become unco-ordinated and weak, and marked gastric dilatation can occur.

When food reaches the duodenum another pacemaker in the proximal portion institutes peristaltic waves that progress smoothly down through the duodenum and the jejunum. Interruption as, for example, by a Roux-en-Y loop of jejunum, creates an additional factor that leads to poor gastric emptying. If any of the necessary anastomoses are technically inadequate, a mechanical factor contributes to the problem.

The diagnosis of inadequate emptying of the stomach can be made at an early stage by barium studies. Radionuclides may be mixed with food and the amount and rate of emptying quantitated.

Treatment includes small meals at regular intervals. Urecholine (bethanechol) is occasionally effective. We have not found metoclopramide particularly valuable, but have had no experience with domperidone. Erythromycin has proved valuable in treatment of diabetic gastroparesis and could be helpful in some cases.

Surgical therapy is required only rarely. Vogel has advised the use of a higher subtotal gastrectomy with a Roux-en-Y anastomosis. We have had one patient in whom a total gastrectomy provided a spectacular cure after repeated high resections and anastomoses had failed.

Cancer of the stomach after gastric operations

Several operations on the stomach lead to reflux of intestinal contents into the stomach or the stomach remnant. 'Intestinalization' of the mucosa of the stomach (a change from the histologic picture of gastric mucosa to that of intestinal mucosa) follows in many instances and is believed to be a precursor to the development of cancer.

Cancer of the gastric stump (colloquially called 'stump cancer') has been studied extensively. Although there is an increased risk of developing gastric cancer in patients who have had a gastrectomy, compared with the risk of the normal population, this increase is not great and, in view of the rarity of gastric cancer in the United States today, presents no important threat. Stump cancer does not appear for at least 10 years after a gastrectomy, and the appearance of most cases is even more delayed. Stump cancer is not frequent enough to warrant routine endoscopies.

OTHER TYPES OF ULCER DISEASE

Several distinct types of ulcers can be identified in the group of lesions called stress ulcers.

Cushing's ulcer

These lesions were described originally by Harvey Cushing in 1932. They consist of deep, frequently perforated ulcers that arise in the oesophagus, stomach, or duodenum. They occur most typically after neurosurgical illnesses.

Curling's ulcer

These are typical duodenal ulcers which essentially occur in burned patients. When they were first described (1842) duodenal ulcers were uncommon. Whether they represented previous ulcers activated after the burn, or whether they are associated with true stress ulcers is not clear.

Ulcers due to gastric irritants

Aspirin is a prime example of an irritant. In addition to its effect on platelet adherence, it directly irritates the gastric mucosa and leads to superficial ulcerations. Ibuprofen and alcohol provoke similar local injuries. Accidental or suicidal ingestion of acids or alkalines can lead to rapid mass destruction and perforation of the oesophagus and/or stomach. Alkalis exert their effect mainly on the oesophagus and acids mainly on the body of the stomach.

Ulcers due to steroid therapy

Whether or not steroids lead to ulceration of the stomach is controversial. However, there appears to be a clear association between such therapy and perforations of the colon.

Stress ulcers

True stress ulcers are superficial lesions that appear after burns, sepsis, severe trauma, protracted hypotension, or serious operations. They may involve only the mucosa (and are often therefore called mucosal erosions), or they may penetrate into the submucosa. Perforation is rare; massive bleeding is the usual complication. Stress ulcers are always found in the fundus, but many also occur throughout the stomach and proximal duodenum.

Prevention of these ulcers is important: bleeding carries a high mortality rate. Treatment includes prevention of gastric distension (usually by nasogastric intubation and suction), respiratory care, and the administration of either antacids, H_2-receptor antagonists, or mucosal protectants. Controlled studies suggest that antacids are the most effective treatment, but intravenous cimetidine is easier to use and is more economical of nurses' time. Another factor that still needs investigation is whether attempts to make the stomach achlorhydric and hence, poorly resistant to growth of bacteria, can lead to colonization of the normally sterile stomach with enteric organisms. If so, aspiration of gastric contents could lead to devastating pneumonitis.

Diagnosis of stress ulcers can be made by endoscopy. The endoscope can also be used to treat bleeding ulcerations, by electrocoagulation which is safer than the laser beam.

Selective arteriography shows extreme dilatation of arterioles particularly in the fundus of the stomach. However, embolization or even selective perfusion with vasopressin is dangerous because of the possibility of necrosis of the gastric wall.

Surgical therapy of these ulcers has been quite unsatisfactory for several reasons, not least of which is the fact that the patients are already very ill. A high subtotal gastrectomy and vagotomy is usually preferred, but even this may be followed by bleeding from the gastric remnant. The alternative, total gastrectomy, is an operation of considerable magnitude but must be chosen if the condition cannot be controlled by less radical measures.

Gastric ulcers secondary to malignancy

Fifty years ago ulcerating cancers of the stomach frequently were confused with benign ulcers. Today endoscopic examinations and biopsies have augmented barium contrast studies of the stomach, and the incidence of cancer of the stomach has declined spectacularly in frequency in the United States as well as in western Europe. This problem of diagnosis now arises only rarely. Nevertheless, endoscopists have been known to miss a lesion in the gastric fundus or may fail to obtain a satisfactory biopsy.

Complete healing of an ulcerating cancer occurs rarely, if ever. There is no evidence that a benign gastric ulcer can degenerate into cancer. Therefore, it is necessary to be certain that a gastric ulcer that appears to be benign actually heals. Furthermore, if a gastric ulcer recurs after therapy the possibility of underlying malignancy is increased.

Malignant lymphomas of the stomach are prone to develop superficial ulcers; however some may be deep and may perforate. Because these ulcers may respond to the medical therapy for a benign ulcer, unless biopsy specimens are taken, the diagnosis may be missed. Barium studies may show a thick-walled stomach with hypertrophic mucosal folds. A CT scan may demonstrate enlarged lymph nodes in the area of the coeliac axis. The preferred treatment is gastric resection followed by radiation and/or chemotherapy.

Hypergastrinaemia

The definition of hypergastrinaemia rests on laboratory studies which show an elevated serum gastrin level. Gastrinomas and the retained antrum syndrome are the only common causes that are surgically important.

Gastrinomas

The first description of such lesions was made by Zollinger and Ellison in 1955, who reported patients with the combination of severe peptic ulcers, often located in unusual locations, excessive amounts of gastric secretion of high acidity, and non-β-cell pancreatic tumours. The definition of the Zollinger–Ellison syndrome was modified in ensuing years to include less virulent ulcers. Tumours may be found outside the pancreas or duodenum, and about 25 per cent of patients have the multiple endocrine neoplasia type I syndrome and no tumour in the peripancreatic area.

Clinical symptoms typical of severe peptic ulcer disease—epigastric pain, weight loss, and vomiting—occur in 90 per cent of patients; severe diarrhoea occurs in one-third. The symptoms may progress slowly or very rapidly. The most important laboratory finding is an elevated serum gastrin level: the upper normal limit is 150 pg/ml, but patients with the Zollinger–Ellison syndrome may have levels over 350 pg/ml at some time of the day. Additional diagnostic evidence is provided by determination of the basal acid output of the stomach, which is not normally over 4 mEq/h for women and 6 mEq/h for men. Although the normal maximal acid output after stimulation by Histalog (a histamine analogue) is 30 mEq/h for women and 40 mEq/h for men, a level of over 15 mEq/h raises the suspicion of a gastrinoma. The diagnosis is confirmed if the injection of intravenous secretin elevates serum gastrin to at least 200 pg/ml. According to Townsend and Thompson, various other causes of hypergastrinaemia, including G-cell hyperplasia, retained antrum, pyloric obstruction, pernicious anaemia, and duodenal ulcers, do not cause this rise after injection of secretin. Gastrin levels may also be elevated after treatment with H_2-receptor antagonists and omeprazole.

Since over 60 per cent of peripancreatic gastrinomas are malignant, and the major symptoms arise from the severe ulcer disease, the treatment of gastrinomas for many years consisted of total gastrectomy. However, excision of some gastrinomas may result in permanently normal gastrin levels, and cure of the patient without any procedure on the stomach. The tumour may be located preoperatively by CT scanning, ultrasound, selective angiography, and selective venous sampling. These measures generally fail to identify small tumours, such as the micropolypoid gastrinomas, only 1 to 8 mm in diameter, which are found in the duodenum.

Symptoms associated with excessive acid secretion have been controlled by the administration of H_2-receptor antagonists or omeprazole; such medical therapy has to continue throughout the life of the patient. At the present time, the pendulum has swung back to surgical therapy since a gastrinoma may be discovered and the patients may be cured by its excision.

If the tumour cannot be found or if liver metastases are present, some type of surgery must be undertaken on the stomach; these procedures have ranged from proximal gastric vagotomy to total gastrectomy. Total gastrectomy is the procedure that is most likely to succeed: postoperatively, patients often gain weight. Townsend and Thompson are strong advocates of total gastrectomy for all of these patients; there were no operative deaths in their series. Even in the presence of metastatic disease, progression of the tumour may be retarded by chemotherapy consisting of 5-fluorouracil and streptozotocin; somatostatin analogues are also effective.

Retained antrum syndrome

An easy solution to the problems of the difficult duodenum encountered in Billroth II resections has eluded many surgeons. As explained previously, our preference is to make a catheter duodenostomy.

In 1895, von Eiselsberg suggested that the treatment of inoperable cancer should involve exclusion and closure of the antrum, which is left *in situ*. This relatively simple exclusion procedure was later applied by some surgeons to the treatment of peptic ulcer; unfortunately antral exclusion was followed by a high incidence of gastrojejunal ulcers. In a personal series treated by Allen in the late 1930s, seven out of eight patients with duodenal or prepyloric ulcers developed anastomotic ulcers within a year.

The same problem proved to be a serious argument against the two-stage gastrectomy of McKittrick. Such patients underwent Billroth II resections with antral exclusion at the first stage, and excision of the antrum at the second. If the second operation was not performed within 6 weeks, nearly all of these patients developed a gastrojejunal ulcer.

Dragstedt proved that the antrum, when it was in an alkaline rather than an acid medium, produced unusually large amounts of gastrin. If a vagotomy had not been performed, stimulation of the parietal cells resulted in excess acid production and a new ulcer.

Even the addition of bilateral truncal vagotomy to the two-stage operation, as carried out by Waddell and Bartlett, proved to be dangerous. Other complications such as intussusception of the antrum followed and the operation was discarded.

The conclusion is clear: a retained antrum is ulcerogenic, and whenever a patient who has undergone a previous gastric resection for ulcer disease is operated on for a recurrent ulcer, the surgeon must look carefully and must excise any antral tissue that remains proximal to the duodenum.

Other causes of hypergastrinaemia

In addition to gastrinomas and the retained antrum syndrome there are many other unusual causes of hypergastrinaemia. G-cell hyperplasia is characterized by increased production of gastrin by the antral mucosa because of an increase in number of gastrin-producing cells. To establish the diagnosis, other unusual causes of hypergastrinaemia, such as pernicious anaemia, achlorhydria, atrophic gastritis, renal failure, and treatment with H_2-receptor antagonists must be eliminated; the reasons for the hypergastrinaemia seen in these conditions is not clear.

FURTHER READING

Donahue PE, Bombeck CT, Condon RE, Nyhus LM. Proximal gastric vagotomy versus selective vagotomy with antrectomy: results of a prospective, randomized clinical trial after four to twelve years. *Surgery*, 1984; **96**: 515–91.

Edwards LW, Herrington JL Jr. Vagotomy and gastroenterostomy—vagotomy and conservative gastrectomy. *Ann Surg*, 1953; **137**: 873–83.

Emås S, Fernstrom M. Prospective, randomized trial of selective vagotomy with pyloroplasty and selective proximal vagotomy with and without pyloroplasty in the treatment of duodenal, pyloric and prepyloric ulcers. *Am J Surg*, 1985; **149**: 236–43.

Farmer DA, Howe CW, Porell WJ, Smithwick RH. The effect of various surgical procedures upon the acidity of the gastric contents of ulcer patients. *Ann Surg*, 1951; **134**: 319–31.

Fischer AB. Twenty-five years after Billroth II gastrectomy for duodenal ulcer. *World J Surg*, 1984; **8**: 293–302.

Goligher JC. A technique for highly selective (parietal cell or proximal gastric) vagotomy for duodenal ulcer. *Br J Surg*, 1974; **61**: 337–45.

Goligher JC, Hill GL, Kenny TE, Nutter E. Several standard elective operations for duodenal ulcer. Ten to 16 year clinical results. *Br J Surg*, 1978; **65**: 145–51.

Graham DY. Treatment of peptic ulcers caused by *Helicobacter pylori*. *N Engl J Med* 1993; **328**: 349–50.

Hentschel E, *et al.* Effect of ranitidine and amoxicillin on the eradication of *Helicobacter pylori* and the recurrence of duodenal ulcer. *N Engl J Med*, 1993; **328**: 308–12.

Herrington JL Jr. Historical aspects of gastrointestinal surgery. In Scott HW Jr, Sawyers JL, eds. *Surgery of the stomach, duodenum and small intestine*. London: Blackwell, 1987: 3–24.

Hoffmann J, Jensen H-E, Christiansen J, Olesen A, Loud FB, Heauch O. Prospective controlled vagotomy trial for duodenal ulcer; results after 11–15 years. *Ann Surg*, 1989; **209**: 40–5.

Johnson HD. Gastric ulcer. *Ann Surg*, 1965; **162**: 996–1004.

Jordan PH Jr. Duodenal ulcers and their surgical treatment: where did they come from? *Am J Surg*, 1985; **149**: 2–14.

Muller C, Martinoli S. *Die proximal-selektive vagotomie*. Berlin: Springer-Verlag, 1985.

Nyhus LM, Wastell C. *Surgery of the stomach and duodenum*. 4th edn. Boston: Little Brown and Co., 1986.

Scott HW Jr, Sawyers JL. *Surgery of the stomach, duodenum, and small intestine*. London: Blackwell, 1987.

Stammers FAR, Williams JA. *Partial gastrectomy*. London: Butterworths, 1963.

Tanner NC. The surgical treatment of peptic ulcer. *Br J Surg*, 1964; **51**: 5–23.

Taylor T. Lesser curve superficial seromyotomy—an operation for chronic duodenal ulcer. *Br J Surg*, 1979; **66**: 733–7.

Townsend CM Jr, Thompson JC. Up-to-date treatment of the patient with hypergastrinemia. *Adv Surg*, 1987; **20**: 155–81.

Visick AH. A study of the failures after gastrectomy. *Ann R Coll Surg Engl*, 1948; **3**: 288–94.

Welch CE. *Surgery of the Stomach and Duodenum*. 5th edn. Chicago: Yearbook Publishers, 1973.

Welch CE. Gastric Resection for duodenal ulcer. In Scott HW Jr, Sawyers JL. *Surgery of the Stomach, Duodenum, and Small Intestine*. Ch. 35. London: Blackwell Scientific Publications, 1987: 681–95.

Welch CE, Rodkey GV, Gryska PR. A thousand operations for ulcer disease. *Ann Surg*, 1986; **204**: 454–67.

15.2 Non-operative management of perforated peptic ulcer

ARTHUR K. C. LI AND S. C. SYDNEY CHUNG

Immediate operative repair is the most widely practised therapy for duodenal perforations and would seem to be the only conceivable course to recommend for most patients. However, most surgeons have encountered patients who refuse operations for their perforated ulcers and still recover. At operation the perforation has sometimes already been sealed off by omentum or adjacent organs and has to be reopened before it can be repaired. Indeed, the fact that non-operative treatment for perforated peptic ulcers may be successful has been recognized since 1870. In 1964 Herman Taylor reported the conservative treatment of 256 patients with perforations: only 21 patients required surgery and the overall mortality rate was 11 per cent. Seely and Campbell reported seven deaths in 139 patients treated conservatively, a mortality rate of 5 per cent. These results are better than those of surgical repair at the time and are comparable to most present day series. A more recent series from Dublin confirmed that conservative treatment can have acceptable results. The only randomized controlled comparison between non-operative treatment and surgery was performed in Hong Kong. This study indicated that an initial period of expectant treatment does not increase the mortality or morbidity in patients with perforated ulcers. More than 70 per cent of patients in the expectant treatment group recovered without an operation.

Non-operative management should only be employed if an experienced surgeon interested in this form of treatment is willing to personally supervise the patient's progress. Once the diagnosis of a perforated ulcer is made a nasogastric tube should be inserted as early as possible to empty the stomach and to reduce the leakage of gastrointestinal contents. The success of conservative treatment of perforated ulcer depends on keeping the stomach empty by nasogastric suction. Leakage from the perforation is kept to a minimum so that the omentum and surrounding organs have a chance to seal the perforation. Much attention to detail on the part of the medical and nursing staff is necessary to ensure that the tube is properly positioned in the stomach and that the stomach is properly emptied. Intravenous fluid is administered at a rate depending upon the degree of dehydration to maintain a urine output of at least 30 ml/h. In elderly patients and those in shock, central venous pressure measurements allow a more accurate assessment of fluid replacement. Broad spectrum antibiotics are also administered. The patient is carefully monitored and should be examined at least 12-hourly by the surgeon who made the initial assessment. Improvement is indicated by decrease in the pulse rate, temperature, and abdominal tenderness and by an improvement in the general well being of the patient. The surgeon must be prepared to abandon conservative management and to undertake operative intervention without delay if the patient fails to improve. The majority, however, will dramatically improve within 12 to 24 h. Oral fluids may be started when all signs of peritonitis disappear and intestinal activity returns. Normal diet is resumed within a few days. The patient should be treated with H_2-receptor blocking drugs. Upper gastrointestinal endoscopy is performed 6 weeks later: evidence of healed duodenal ulceration will be seen in the great majority of patients. A decision is then made, depending on the individual circumstances, to stop medical treatment or to continue long-term maintenance H_2 blockade.

An upper gastrointestinal series using water-soluble contrast material is a useful adjunct for the definitive diagnosis and treatment of these patients. The demonstration of an ulcer crater without leakage in a patient with a typical history and peritonitis is reassuring and provides circumstantial evidence that the cause of peritonitis is indeed a perforated ulcer. It also suggests that spontaneous sealing has probably occurred. Contrast meals fail to detect persistent leakage in about 10 per cent of patients. One should rely on the overall clinical picture rather than the result of the contrast meal. Free leakage of contrast into the peritoneal cavity indicates that the crisis is not yet over and a high degree of vigilance needs to be maintained. Leakage shown on the contrast meal by itself do not mandate immediate surgery. In our experience perforations seal without operation in about 60 per cent of patients in whom leakage is detected on the contrast meal.

The importance of close supervision by an experienced surgeon cannot be overemphasized. The definitive diagnosis of patients with peritonitis can be difficult; some patients may have conditions such as colonic perforation, for which early operation is essential. Six to 12 h after the onset of peritonitis, the patient enters the so-called 'stage of delusion', which may deceive the unwary. The patient feels subjectively better, the acute pain eases, and the board-like rigidity of the abdomen disappears. In such cases there may be continued leakage. Unless an experienced surgeon is prepared to examine and supervise these patients on admission and at short intervals thereafter, it is likely that any deterioration in the patient's condition will be detected too late to be reversed. In fact, an expectant policy is much more demanding on the surgeon's time, skill, and judgement than is an immediate operation. To undertake such treatment without the close involvement of a skilled surgeon committed to conservative treatment would be foolhardy.

It was hoped that conservative treatment may improve the outlook for frail elderly patients who may be too ill to withstand general anaesthesia. Unfortunately this is not so: perforations are less likely to seal spontaneously in elderly patients. The greater omentum is atrophic in the elderly and is presumably less effective in sealing perforations. In addition, the elderly patient withstands continued intra-abdominal sepsis poorly. Early laparotomy after adequate resuscitation offers the best chance of recovery in these high risk patients.

In patients with perforated peptic ulcers, an initial period of non-operative treatment with careful observation may be safely allowed except in the elderly. The use of such an observation period can obviate the need for emergency surgery in more than 70 per cent of patients. Definitive ulcer surgery may then be reserved for patients who have frequent relapses of ulcer disease and other complications while receiving H_2-receptor blocker treatment.

FURTHER READING

Crofts TJ, Park KGM, Steele RJC, Chung SCS, Li AKC. A randomized trial of nonoperative treatment for perforated peptic ulcer. *N Engl J Med* 1989; **320**: 970–3.

Keane TE, Dillon B, Afdhal NH, McCormack CJ. Conservative management of perforated duodenal ulcer. *Br J Surg* 1988; **75**: 583–4.

Redwood TH. Two cases of perforation of the stomach; one recovery. *Lancet* 1870; i: 647.

Seely SF, Campbell D. Nonoperative treatment of perforated peptic ulcer: a further report. *Surg Gynecol Obstet* 1956; **102**: 435–6.

Taylor H. Aspiration treatment of perforated ulcer. *Lancet* 1951; i: 7–12.

15.3 Carcinoma of the stomach

HUGH BARR AND MICHAEL J. GREENALL

The ancient Egyptian papyrus Ebers describes a patient with dysphagia in whom the stomach had the appearance of a shrivelled fetal face. This may well represent the first description by Egyptian physicians of a gastric carcinoma, a disease that is now a major health care and surgical problem.

INCIDENCE AND EPIDEMIOLOGY

As is the case with many neoplasms there is a widespread variation in the incidence of gastric carcinoma around the world. Gastric cancer occurs in almost epidemic proportions in Japan with an incidence 70 per 100 000 males and a cumulative risk of developing the disease by the age of 75 of 11 per cent. It is said to be the 'national disease', accounting for nearly 52 per cent of deaths from malignancy in men and 38 per cent in women in 1960. Other countries with a high incidence of the disease (over 30 per 100 000 males) include Chile, Costa Rica, Hungary, Poland, Portugal, Iceland, Rumania, Indonesia, and Italy. There is a particularly low incidence in some central African countries (Uganda).

Marked regional variations have been reported. In Columbia, an incidence of 50 per 1 000 000 males occurs in the inland city of Cali, compared with 12 per 100 000 males on the coast at Cartagena. The rural population in Poland is at greater risk than the urban population, in contrast to the situation in other cancers.

In the United States and the United Kingdom the overall incidence has fallen over the last 50 years. In the United States the age adjusted mortality (per 100 000) for men fell from 28 in 1935 to 9.7 in 1967 and to 8.2 in 1986. This decline has occurred in all racial groups and in both sexes, and reflects the change in incidence and not earlier diagnosis, better treatment, or changes in definition. Although a falling incidence has been noted in most countries, there has been no decline in Poland or amongst Japanese men. There has been an increase in the number of deaths reported in both men and women in Portugal.

Carcinoma of the stomach is closely correlated with age, occurring predominantly between the fifth and seventh decade and in people in the lower socioeconomic groups (social class III and IV). In countries with a high incidence of disease the peak incidence tends to occur at an earlier age than is seen in low-risk areas. It is universally more common in men than women. In the United Kingdom the male : female ratio is 1 : 1 for young adults, rising to 2 : 1 in the sixth decade. Variations in geographical incidence are not incompatible with environmental factors playing an important role: first-generation migrants sustain the risk rate of their country of origin, but the mortality rate in subsequent generations of Polish and Japanese immigrants to the United Stares falls to an intermediate level.

SITE OF GASTRIC CARCINOMA

As well as a fall in the incidence of gastric carcinoma in the United States and United Kingdom there has been an impression that the tumour is moving proximally, with a rising incidence of adenocarcinoma of the cardia. In one series from the United Kingdom the number of carcinomas reported in the upper third of the stomach rose from 17 per cent (1951–55) to 39 per cent (1981–85). This was accompanied by a reduction in tumours of the middle third (31 per cent to 19 per cent) and lower third of the stomach (51 per cent to 47 per cent). Similarly in Japan, the proportion of proximally located cancer has increased from 10 per cent to 40 per cent of diagnosed tumours. However, antral and prepyloric tumours remain the most common, followed by those in the body and fundus. There is some evidence that tumours in the fundus are more aggressive, with a greater tendency to submucosal invasion regardless of the histological type. The gross morphological difference in the fundus that may explain this is the thinner muscularis mucosa and the presence of tightly packed glands that might block lateral growth. In addition signet ring carcinoma is more common in the fundus. Proximally placed tumours generally have a worse prognosis than those placed distally. This phenomenon may be a result of the features described above or because they tend to be at a more advanced stage at presentation.

AETIOLOGICAL FACTORS

Genetic

There is clear evidence of familial clustering of carcinoma of the stomach, the most famous being that of the Bonapartes. Napoleon, his father, his grandfather, brother, and three sisters died of gastric carcinoma. However, only 4 per cent of patients have a family history of the disease, and there is slightly greater correlation between identical rather than fraternal twins.

Aird, in 1953, described an association between blood group A and gastric carcinoma: the relative risk over patients with blood group O is 1.2 times. This difference has been related to the nature of mucopolysaccharide secretion in the stomachs of group A patients, and greater susceptibility to ingested carcinogens. The cancer that develops is of the diffuse type (Lauren classification), there being no increased incidence of the intestinal type.

Environmental and dietary

Although genetic factors may be important, environmental and dietary agents are of far greater importance. Various foodstuffs have been implicated in the aetiology of the disease, predominantly low quality diets poor in milk, animal protein, and vitamins but rich in starch. Heavily salted pickles favoured in Japan (tsukemono) have been implicated, as have the smoked fish and meats eaten in Iceland and Scandinavia: these smoked meats contain polycyclic hydrocarbons (such as benzopyrene) which are probable carcinogens. The decline in the incidence of the tumour in the United States has been attributed to the widespread use of refrigeration with a decline in food preservation by smoking or salting.

Much interest has been devoted to the role of nitrosamines, which have been shown to be carcinogenic to the gastric mucosa in experimental situations. It is suggested that ingested nitrates and nitrites present in some high protein diets, as food preservatives, or in water and soil may be converted to nitrosamines (*N*-nitroso compounds) by the action of gastrointestinal bacteria. The presence of atrophic gastritis and associated achlorhydric stomach may predispose to the production of these *N*-nitroso carcinogens. High gastric pH encourages bacterial overgrowth in the stomach; these organisms are able to reduce dietary nitrates and convert the nitrites to carcinogenic nitrosamines in the presence of dietary protein. This sequence may only be one factor and defects in the mucosal barrier associated with diseased mucosa in patients with atrophic gastritis is likely to facilitate carcinogen penetration.

Other ingested agents implicated are neat spirits favoured by some Scandinavian countries, Japanese saki, and contaminated whisky. Cigarette smoking and elevated levels of zinc and lead in drinking water have been implicated, as has talc and asbestos in the atmosphere. Groups of workers which have been shown to be at high risk include metal industry workers, painters, printers, fishermen, and ceramic and clay workers.

Premalignant conditions

This group of conditions includes those that, if untreated, become malignant, as well as disorders of the stomach that may predispose to gastric cancer. In particular patients with hypogammaglogulinaemia (50-fold excess) and pernicious anaemia (three-fold excess) are at high risk.

Chronic atrophic gastritis and intestinal metaplasia

Patients with hypogammaglobulinaemia and pernicious anaemia have chronic atrophic gastritis and the incidence of gastric cancer is said to be higher in patients with this condition. Certainly achlorhydria results from the chronic atrophic gastritis and 75 per cent of patients with gastric carcinoma are achlorhydric. Strickland has divided chronic atrophic gastritis into two subgroups: type A, which is associated with pernicious anaemia, predominantly affects the fundus and body and is autoimmune in origin, while type B gastritis affects the antrum and is related to environmental factors. This type is also found in the stomach some years after gastrectomy for benign peptic ulcer disease and may be regarded as a failure of the gastric mucosa to respond to repeated injury. Both types predispose to cancer.

Intestinal metaplasia of the gastric mucosa is commonly found in association with gastric cancers, and epidemiological studies have confirmed that populations with a high incidence of carcinoma of the stomach also have a high incidence of intestinal metaplasia. However, mucosal atrophy and intestinal metaplasia are common phenomena, their incidence increasing with increasing age, and they are particularly common in elderly populations. Some suggest that the intestinal type of gastric cancer results from gastric mucosa that has undergone a sequence of mutations and defined histopathological changes that may start in the first decade of life. The first lesion is atrophic gastritis followed by progressive intestinalization of the mucosa to intestinal metaplasia, then dysplasia and finally carcinoma. The finding of some of these precursor conditions alone cannot at present be regarded as definitely premalignant unless dysplastic mucosa is found.

Recently, gastric cancer has been associated with *Helicobacter pylori* infection. This organism is associated with antral inflammation and gastritis. It is proposed that infection and inflammation may result in the production of an epidermal growth factor which may have an oncogenic action on gastric mucosa.

Benign gastric ulcers

The relationship between benign gastric ulcer and gastric cancer is controversial. There is debate over whether benign chronic gastric ulcers have malignant potential; the suggestion is that the regenerating mucosa around an ulcer is prone to become malignant. The issue is further clouded since some ulcerating gastric cancers can mimic benign gastric ulcers closely, sometimes healing in response to medical treatment. Approximately 4 to 10 per cent of all gastric cancers behave in this way, and 70 per cent of early gastric cancers may heal as part of the 'lifecycle of the malignant ulcer'. Improvements in endoscopy with biopsy have improved detection of both benign and malignant disease, and it appears that the development of cancer in the edge of a benign gastric ulcer is rare. There is no clear description of a proven benign ulcer turning malignant. The stable incidence of gastric ulcer with a decline in the incidence of gastric carcinoma supports the view that gastric ulcer is not a premalignant condition. Similarly the location of benign and malignant disease is different, with most benign gastric ulcers (50–70 per cent) occurring on the lesser curve. It is now accepted that the most important question on finding a gastric ulcer is to decide whether it is benign or malignant from the outset.

Gastric polyps

Gastric polyps are found in 0.5 per cent of individuals undergoing autopsy. Most (65–90 per cent) are hyperplastic polyps that are regenerative, non-neoplastic lesions and usually smaller than 2 cm. Only two patients have been reported in whom a carcinoma was found in association with a hyperplastic polyp. There is no strong relationship with gastric carcinoma and these polyps should not be regarded as premalignant.

In contrast adenomatous polyps are truly premalignant. They are often larger (80 per cent greater than 2 cm) and are tubulovillous or villous on microscopic examination. The frequency of malignant change increases with increasing size. In a large series, 38 per cent of patients with gastric adenomatous polyps had gastric carcinoma. Similarly 34 per cent of post-gastrectomy specimens removed for gastric cancer contain adenomatous polyps, and severe dysplasia with carcinoma *in situ* has been found in over 20 per cent of removed polyps.

Previous gastric surgery

As early as 1922 Balfour reported a gastric cancer occurring in the residual stomach after surgery for benign peptic ulcer disease. The term 'stump cancer' was soon used since carcinoma seemed to occur more frequently after Billroth I and II gastrectomy than after vagotomy with pyloroplasty or gastroenterostomy. A large postmortem study demonstrated that gastric cancer was less frequent in patients who had undergone gastric surgery 15 years prior to death, but six times greater in those who had surgery 25 years earlier. In a historical prospective cohort study in Denmark from 1955 to 1982, the risk of gastric cancer immediately, and for 15 years after, peptic ulcer surgery was less than expected. This was attributed to patients having less gastric mucosa exposed to carcinogen following gastrectomy. However, the risk of cancer was 2.1 times greater than the general population 25 years after surgery. The greatest risk (3.2 times) was in male patients who had had a Billroth II gastrectomy. Patients who had simple suture of a perforated ulcer had no increased risk, indicating that peptic ulcer disease was not a risk factor. The pathogenesis of gastric stump cancer has been shown experimentally to be related to operations that promote duodenogastric bile reflux, achlorhydria, and atrophic gastritis. Overall, the risk of developing gastric cancer following gastrectomy has been reported as between 3 and 10 per cent. The decline in surgery for peptic ulcer disease means that there is every prospect that in 20 or 30 years stump cancer may become a rare phenomenon.

Ménétrier's disease and hyperplastic gastropathy

Gastric carcinoma has been described as a complication of Ménétrier's disease, but the magnitude of risk is unknown. In Ménétrier's disease, there is giant hyperplasia of the gastric mucosal folds and the condition can be difficult to distinguish from gastric polyposis or lymphoma (see Section 15.6). The mucosal abnormality associated with Ménétrier's disease results in hyperplasia of mucus glands, whereas the parietal cell mass falls. Thus gastric secretion is rich in protein and mucus but is often hypochlorhydric. Hypersecretory conditions, including Zollinger–Ellison syndrome, may be associated with hyperplastic rugal folds and excessive acid secretion without increased risk of gastric cancer.

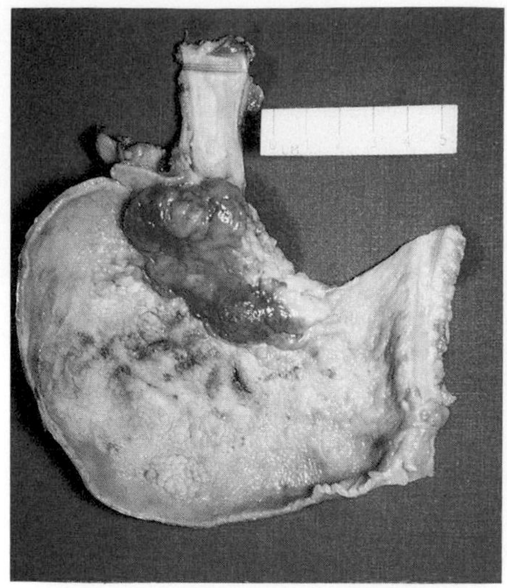

Fig. 1 Polypoid carcinoma of the gastric cardia causing oesophageal obstruction.

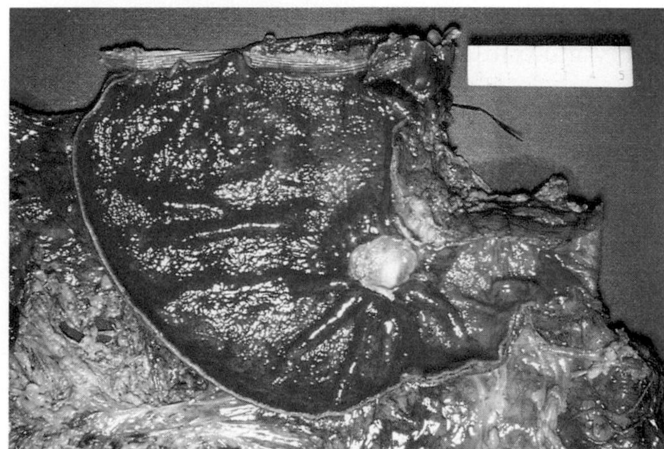

Fig. 2 Ulcerating cancer of the gastric antrum.

PATHOLOGY

Macroscopic appearance

Advanced gastric ulcer

Marked variations in the gross appearance of operative and excised specimens have been described in the Western literature and by the Japanese, using the endoscopic descriptions of predominantly early gastric cancers. Approximately 10 per cent of these tumours are polypoid fungating tumours, with a nodular polypoid surface with superficial ulceration (Fig. 1). This group of cancers has a relatively good prognosis after aggressive surgical management, many being well-differentiated adenocarcinomas. Ulcerating or penetrating cancers, which occur in more than 50 per cent of patients (Fig. 2), are sessile and may have the appearance of a benign gastric ulcer. Superficial spreading carcinoma is more unusual (6 per cent of tumours). This tumour is diffusely infiltrative over a wide area, although it is predominantly confined to the mucosa and submucosa; 50 per cent have metastasized to the perigastric lymph nodes at the time of presentation and operation. A further subgroup of diffusely infiltrative cancer is the linitis plastica (leather bottle) carcinoma (Fig. 3), which is characterized by extensive infiltration of the submucosa and muscular layers with a marked fibroblastic/desmoplastic reaction around columns of malignant cells. Endoscopic recognition of this neoplasm may be difficult and superficial biopsy of mucosa alone may prove negative. Extension into the oesophagus and mesentery may occur and advanced tumours may involve the entire stomach. Superficial erosions are common but deep ulceration is unusual. Although spread of gastric cancer beyond the pyloric ring is generally considered to be rare, up to 25 per cent of diffusely infiltrative tumours may involve the first part of the duodenum. This tumour carries a particularly poor prognosis.

The morphology of advanced gastric cancer can be divided into three strict morphovolumetric types. The ratio of the amount of muscle invasion to mucosa affected defines a funnel type (mucosal involvement greater than muscle: ratio less than 0.75), column type (equal involvement: ratio 0.75 to 1.25), and the mountain type (muscle greater than mucosal involvement: ratio over 1.25).

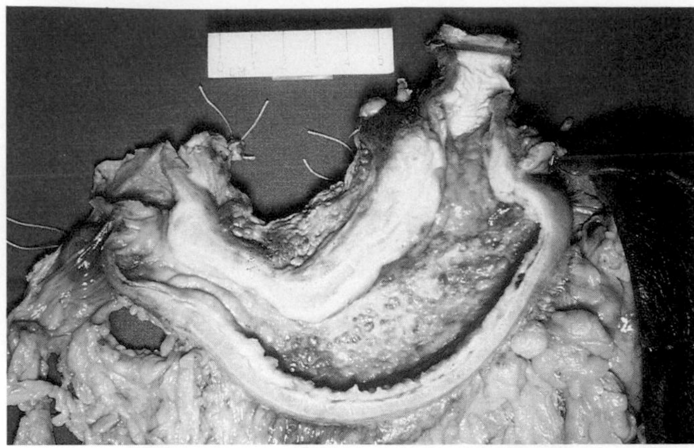

Fig. 3 Linitis plastica of the stomach.

The metastatic characteristics of these tumours are variable: the funnel type carry the best prognosis, with 62 per cent lymph node involvement, followed by the column type (80 per cent lymph node metastasis), and finally the mountain type (lymph node metastasis in 85 per cent).

Early gastric cancer

The great interest in the detection of early cancer by endoscopy has produced a separate classification based on endoscopic appearance. The term early gastric cancer is used to describe tumours confined to the gastric mucosa and submucosa, irrespective of nodal status: there is a close correlation between the depth of invasion at microscopic examination and postoperative survival. Early carcinoma of the stomach is divided into three main groups, type I—protruding, type II—superficial, and type III—excavated (Fig. 4). Type II is divided into three subgroups, elevated (a), flat (b), and depressed (c). There is undoubted overlap between the protruded (I) and superficial elevated (IIa) types, and also between excavated (III) and superficial depressed types (IIc). As well as these basic types there are three combined types which exhibit features of two different types, type I and IIa (III), type IIa and IIc, and type IIc and III.

The precise classification of early gastric cancer by the Japanese and the use of vigorous investigation has increased its detection rate from 5 to 40 per cent of all gastric cancers over the past 20 years. In the West early gastric cancer accounts for 9 per cent of all cancers detected and 19 per cent of resected tumours; the rate of detection does not appear to be increasing. Comparison of the clinical, morphological, and histological features of early gastric cancer reveals remarkable similarity in the disease between Japan and the United Kingdom.

There are few data on the natural history of early gastric cancer, since it is usually actively treated. One study has shown that 50 per cent of cases progress to advanced cancer within 3 years from the time of endoscopic diagnosis, and almost all patients develop advanced disease within 5 years. Recently, the definition of early gastric cancer has been challenged, since the 5-year survival is 99 per cent if there are no lymph node metastases, but falls to 73 per cent if lymph nodes are involved.

Multiple synchronous gastric cancer

Multiple synchronous gastric cancer was described by Moertel, who defined strict criteria for diagnosis. Each lesion must be

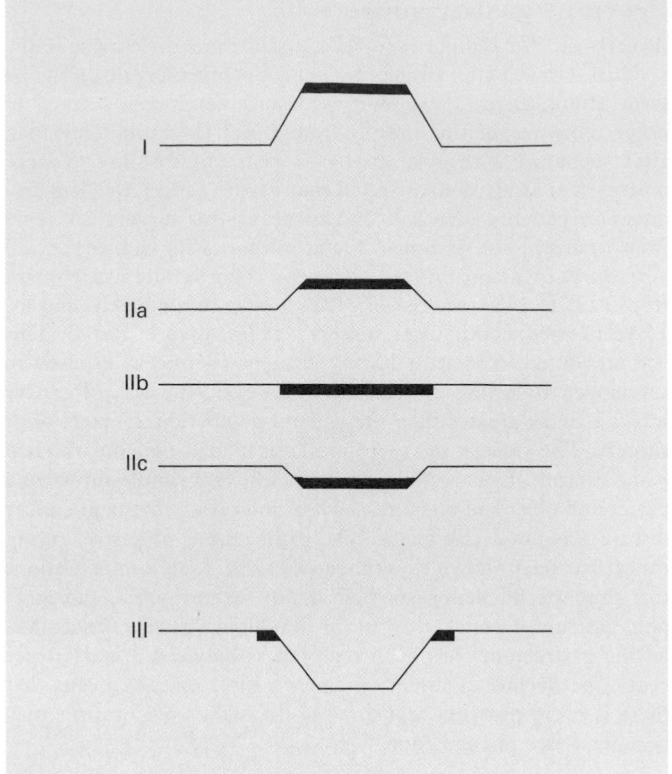

Fig. 4 Schematic diagram of the Japanese classification of early gastric cancer.

proved histopathologically to be malignant, all lesions must be separated by normal gastric wall, and the possibility that the lesions represent a local extension or metastasis must be ruled out beyond reasonable doubt. It is sometimes difficult to verify this last criterion, and attention is paid to the extent of venous and lymphatic invasion surrounding each tumour. If there is extensive invasion a diagnosis of multiple gastric cancer is inappropriate. The incidence was originally thought to be 2 per cent of all gastric cancers, but with advances in diagnostic techniques it appears to be between 6 and 9 per cent.

Microscopic appearance

The great majority of gastric cancers are adenocarcinoma; other tumours are rare. Classification is difficult, primarily because different histological features may coexist in one tumour mass. The WHO classification based on morphology divides gastric cancer into five types: adenocarcinoma, adenosquamous carcinoma, squamous cell carcinoma, undifferentiated carcinoma, and unclassified carcinoma. The adenocarcinomas are divided into four patterns; papillary, tubular, mucinous, and signet ring, which may be divided by degrees of differentiation. In tumours presenting a mixed picture with varying degrees of differentiation in the same tumour, classification is based on the predominant type.

A simpler classification by Lauren recognized an intestinal type similar to colon adenocarcinoma and a diffuse type that did not form glands. The intestinal type is defined by the cellular architecture, and the diffuse by its pattern of growth: polypoid and superficial spreading carcinomas are of the intestinal type, whereas linitus plastica is diffuse. Ulcerative tumours fall into either group. The intestinal type carries the more favourable prognosis and is more common in areas with a high incidence of the disease. In general, intestinal cancer is said to arise within intestinalized mucosa and the diffuse tumour is thought to originate from normal epithelium without evidence of a preceding lesion. Synchronous cancers are more commonly of the intestinal type of tumour. Some carcinomas fall into a mixed or unclassified category.

A similar classification for advanced carcinoma invading beyond the muscularis propria was proposed by Ming in 1977. Cancers were divided into an expanding type that produces nodules that compress adjacent tissue (similar to Lauren's intestinal type), and the infiltrative type that does not form masses (Lauren's diffuse type). The best concordance for tumour classification by different pathologists examining the same specimens is with Lauren's classification and this is the most widely used.

Considerable interest surrounds the prognostic significance of histological evidence of host defence against the tumour. Infiltration of the tumour by macrophages, polymorph leucocytes, lymphocytes, and plasma cells is a favourable sign, as is evidence of a host response in draining lymph nodes, characterized by sinus histiocytosis and follicular hyperplasia.

The microscopic appearance of early gastric cancer is strongly correlated with the macroscopic appearance (Lauren classification). Type I and IIa are of the intestinal type whereas type IIc and III are all diffuse type: this is not surprising since intestinal type carcinomas have an expansile growth pattern leading to polypoid growth. The prognosis of early gastric cancer is predominantly related to the depth of invasion and this greatly over-rides any histological classification.

One of the characteristics of gastric cancer is the tendency of the tumour to spread intramurally via lymphatic channels. Thus the surgical resection margins must be at some distance from the palpable edge of the tumour. The extent of intramural spread is related to the depth of invasion of the tumour. Lateral extension of tumour confined to the muscularis propria lateral does not extend beyond 3 cm, but significant numbers of tumours penetrating this layer show intramural spread beyond this distance, although never beyond 6 cm.

Patterns of spread and metastasis

In Western series between 40 and 60 per cent of patients have obviously incurable and often disseminated disease at presentation. In Japan the number who can be offered curative resection with excision of all macroscopic tumour is much higher at 75 to 80 per cent. The poorly differentiated mucinous and signet ring tumours are more invasive, although in series from the United Kingdom most tumours are large and advanced at presentation and have spread, and the degree of differentiation is of little relevance. In Japan up to 40 per cent of patients have early gastric cancer with tumours confined to the mucosa and submucosa: those with poorly differentiated carcinomas are more subject to metastasis and have decreased survival.

Penetration of the gastric serosa

The depth of invasion of the cancer through the gastric wall has a marked effect on the prognosis. If the muscularis propria and then the serosa are breached the prognosis following treatment becomes considerably worse. Lymph node metastasis occurs in 18 per cent of patients in whom the serosa is not penetrated and over 50 per cent survive for 5 years following resection. If the serosa is penetrated 80 per cent of patients have lymph node metastases, with a correspondingly poorer prognosis. Once the serosa of the stomach has been breached the tumour is likely to spread by transcoelomic implantation of shed cells. If the area of serosa involved is less than 10 cm^2, free viable intraperitoneal malignant cells can be found in 22 per cent of patients, compared with 72 per cent if the area is greater than 20 cm^2. Implantation of these cells characteristically occurs in the ovary, producing Krukenberg tumours (bilateral ovarian tumours from a signet ring carcinoma), or in the pelvis to produce a shelf which is palpable on rectal examination (Blummer's shelf). It must be emphasized that penetration of the gastric serosa is the most important prognostic indicator.

Gastric tumours may spread by direct extension and invasion of adjacent structures including liver, pancreas, and spleen. In postmortem studies from the United States the peritoneum, mesentery, and omentum are invaded in over 40 per cent of patients.

Lymphatic drainage and lymph node involvement

The involvement of lymph nodes and the pattern of spread is particularly important for gastric cancers. In Western series some form of lymph node involvement is present in 70 per cent of patients undergoing resection of gastric tumours. Even in Japanese series, mucosal cancer is associated with a 3 per cent incidence of lymph node involvement; this rises to 15 per cent if the submucosa is involved. The anatomical classification of lymph nodes varies in the West and Japan, and confuses the interpretation of the results of surgery. In the Western literature four zones of lymph drainage corresponding to the blood supply are identified. Zone 1 is located in the gastrocolic omentum along the right gastroepiploic vessels, draining the pyloric portion of the greater curve and draining to the pylorus and then to coeliac and aortic nodes. Zone 2 is in the gastrocolic and gastrosplenic omentum around the left gastroepiploic vessels draining from the upper half of the greater curve. From here drainage is to the pancreaticosplenic lymph nodes and to the aortic nodes. Zone 3 has efferent channels from the proximal two-thirds of the stomach and the upper lesser curve and surrounds the left gastric artery. Some lymph from this area drains into perioesophageal lymph nodes. The distal portion of the lesser curve and pylorus drains to Zone 4, situated above the pylorus and going to the hepatic artery and para-aortic lymph nodes. However, according to Western data, the lymphatic drainage of the stomach is unpredictable and radical resection must include lymph nodes from all zones.

The Japanese have adjusted and stratified the classification of lymph drainage (Fig. 5). Group I (N1) are perigastric lymph nodes, group II (N2) nodes along and at the roots of the major vessels, group III (N3) are lymph node at the root of the superior mesenteric artery, in the hepaticoduodenal ligament, and behind the pancreas. Group IV (N4) are distant lymph nodes. It is clear that this definition may not be adequate for planning surgical resection along strict oncological principles, since a perigastric node (N1) at the antrum is a distant node (N4) if the cancer is in the cardia. Thus the lymph nodes can be given station numbers (Table 1 and Fig. 5) and the node status and surgical excision planned according to the node station in relation to the site of the primary tumour (Table 2). The Japanese have found that there is an orderly spread to regional lymph nodes which is clearly related

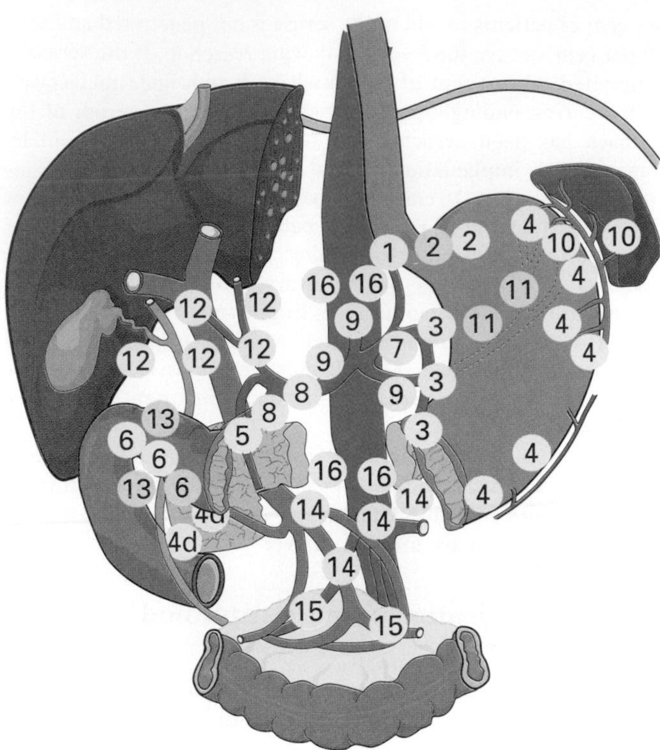

Fig. 5 Lymph node stations defined by the Japanese Research Society for gastric cancer.

Table 1 Numbering of the gastric and upper abdominal node stations (see also Fig. 5)

Station number	Anatomical location
1, 2	Adjacent to the cardia (perigastric)
3, 4	Adjacent to lesser and greater curve
5	Suprapyloric (right gastric artery)
6	Infrapyloric
7	Left gastric artery
8	Common hepatic artery
9	Coeliac artery
10	Hilium of the spleen
11	Splenic artery
12	Hepaticoduodenal ligament
13	Behind pancreatic head
14	At the root of the mesentery (superior mesenteric artery)
15	Middle colic artery
16	Para-aortic

to the position of the tumour. These data have not been confirmed in Western studies. The difference may, in part, relate to the difference between advanced gastric cancer in the West and the greater incidence of potentially curable patients identified in Japan. However, skip lesions to distant lymph nodes do undoubtedly occasionally occur; N2 nodes are involved without N1 (perigastric) nodal involvement in 11 per cent of patients.

Carcinoma at the cardia presents a distinct problem, for it may involve lymph nodes in the mediastinum. In a review of over 400 patients neoplastic involvement of paracardial nodes occurred in 48 per cent and para-oesophageal nodes were affected in 37 per cent of patients.

Table 2 Node stations related to location of the tumour to define nodal status and extent of nodal dissection

	Location of gastric cancer			
Node station	Antral/body	Body	Cardia	Total stomach
1	N2	N1	N1	N1
2	N3	N2	N1	N1
3,4	N1	N1	N1	N1
5,6	N1	N1	N2	N1
7–9	N2	N2	N2	N2
10,11	N3	N2	N2	N2
12–14	N3	N3	N3	N3
15,16	N4	N4	N4	N4

In general, any involvement of the lymph nodes is a poor prognostic indicator, as is the number of nodes involved, invasion of four or more lymph nodes being unfavourable compared with fewer being involved. This statement implies that an adequate lymphadenectomy has been performed to sample these nodes. The number of lymph nodes to be found at each station is very variable. If stations 1 to 11 are removed (R2 gastrectomy) an average of 27 nodes should be removed. If stations 1 to 16 are cleared (R3 gastrectomy) the mean number rises to 43.

Distant metastasis

The most common sites for distant metastatic spread are the liver (49 per cent), lung (33 per cent), ovary (14 per cent), bones (11 per cent), and cervical and supraclavicular (Virchow) nodes (8 per cent). Patients with distant metastases have a poor prognosis: 95 per cent of patients with liver involvement will die within 1 year, irrespective of the primary cancer.

Staging for gastric carcinoma

As with all neoplasms a uniform staging system is required to allow the results of treatment to be compared. The TNM system of staging can be applied to gastric cancer and is summarized in Table 3. Another widely used staging system based on the results following excision and pathological examination is somewhat simpler (Table 4). For cancers that are locally resectable the most important prognostic sign that can be assessed at laparotomy is penetration of the wall of the stomach by the carcinoma.

CLINICAL PRESENTATION

The symptoms of gastric carcinoma are often vague, non-specific, and attributed to non-specific dietary indiscretion or indigestion. By the time the diagnosis is made, the tumour is often incurable or non-resectable. This was elegantly illustrated by Theodor Storm's (1888) poem 'Beginn des Endes' describing his death from gastric carcinoma. ''Tis a prick, 'tis scarce a pain ... indeed 'tis naught; ... it is too late'. Unfortunately 100 years later this experience is still common. Definite symptoms do not usually occur until the tumour is large enough to obstruct the lumen or cause disordered gastric function by invading a large segment of the wall, or until it bleeds. Over 70 per cent of patients have had some symptoms for greater than 6 months prior to seeking advice, the most common of

Table 3 Summary of TNM system for the staging of gastric carcinoma

T stage	Tumour status in relation to penetration of gastric wall
T1	Confined to mucosa
T2	Involving all layers to serosa
T3	Penetrating serosa, with or without direct invasion of adjacent tissues and organs
T4	Diffuse infiltration of gastric wall
TX	Degree of involvement unknown
N stage	**Lymph mode involvement**
N0	No lymph nodes involved
N1	Perigastric nodes adjacent to tumour involved
N2	Metastasis to nodes on both curvatures or regional areas
NX	Lymph nodal status unknown
M stage	**Distant involvement**
M0	No metastasis
M1	Distant metastasis, distant lymph node involvement beyond regional lymph nodes

Table 4 Staging system for gastric cancer

Stage	Definition
1a	Tumour confined to gastric mucosa only (T1, N0, M0)
1b	Tumour extending to but not through the serosa (T2, N0, M0)
1c	Tumour extending through the serosa with or without local invasion (T3, N0, M0)
II	Diffuse involvement of gastric wall (T4, N0, M0), or any involvement of gastric wall in association with tumour deposits in the perigrastric lymph nodes (T1–T4, N1, M0)
III	Any degree of gastric wall with involvement of perigastric lymph nodes distant from the tumour or on both gastric curvatures (T1–T4, N2, M0)
IV	Distant metastasis

which are vague indigestion or upper abdominal/epigastric pain, followed by weight loss, nausea and vomiting, haematemesis and malaena, profound anorexia, early satiety, and flatulence. The pain may mimic angina pectoris, or may exhibit periodicity and be relieved by food, mimicking benign gastric disease. Interestingly true postprandial pain is relatively unusual in patients with gastric carcinoma. If the tumour is at the cardia, over 60 per cent of patients will present with dysphagia, indicating a greater than 80 per cent obstruction of the oesophageal/gastric cardia lumen. Weight loss may be quite insidious and although most patients have lost significant amounts few complain of this directly.

Early gastric cancer presents with symptoms similar to those of dyspepsia. Purely mucosal gastric cancers are symptomatic in 50 per cent of patients, and early endoscopy is advised for patients over the age of 40 years with persistent dyspeptic symptoms. If these patients have dysplastic changes then regular endoscopy is necessary. Some recommend resection for severe dysplastic changes in young, otherwise healthy, patients. The duration of symptoms prior to surgery in those with early gastric cancer ranges from 3 to 72 months; surprisingly, this is little different from those who present with advanced cancers. There are generally few physical signs in patients with early gastric cancer, although epigastric tenderness is present in 10 per cent, the remainder having a normal physical examination. It is not possible to be highly specific about important symptoms and no symptom correlates with extent of disease. The presence of an epigastric mass is a poor prognostic sign, but is not in itself an indication of inoperable disease.

Approximately 10 per cent of patients in Western series present with palpable cervical lymph nodes, ascites, jaundice, a palpable abdominal, or a pelvic mass. Sister Joseph's nodule, named after a nurse at the Mayo Clinic who discovered the phenomenon, a visible and palpable secondary deposit at the umbilicus due to spread along the lymphatics around the falciform ligament, is not an uncommon presentation of advanced disease. In patients presenting with this sign, the primary tumour is most commonly in the ovary, followed by the stomach and colon. It is a poor prognostic sign and the mean survival of patients in whom the primary lesion is gastric is only 3.5 months. Troisier's sign, an enlarged lymph node in the left supraclavicular fossa (Virchow node), indicates lymphatic spread via the thoracic duct. Armand Trousseau (1801–1867), a Paris physician, first suspected he had a gastric cancer when he developed superficial thrombophlebitis on the legs (Trousseau's sign), but Trousseau's sign is also associated with pancreatic cancer.

INVESTIGATION

Laboratory

Routine biochemical and haematological tests may disclose anaemia which is common in these patients. This is usually of an iron deficiency type, being microcytic and hypochromic reflecting blood loss and is not only a feature of advanced disease, since 20 per cent of patients with early gastric cancer will be anaemic. Testing of the stools for occult blood may well be positive. Approximately two-thirds of patients with gastric cancer have achlorhydria but this is of little diagnostic relevance. The level of carcinoembryonic antigen in the serum is elevated in 30 per cent of patients with advanced tumours but fails to detect early disease. Similarly oncofetal antigen is elevated in some benign inflammatory gastric disorders as well as in malignancy.

Radiography

The mainstay of diagnosis for many years was barium contrast studies of the upper gastrointestinal tract. In Japan the double contrast air/barium study has been perfected and used for mass population screening. Air and barium are introduced together to coat the mucosa with a thin layer of barium and enhance mucosal detail. The technique can be further refined by using high density barium, carbon dioxide, simethicone for gas dispersion, and glucagon to induce gastroparesis. In Western countries endoscopy is more sensitive than radiography, but some Japanese studies using modern photographic techniques have found the diagnostic accuracy of these methods to be similar. Computerized tomography, ultrasonography, and magnetic resonance are most helpful in the diagnosis of metastatic disease. These methods identify enlarged lymph nodes and tumour deposits but do not differentiate tumour from benign change. In early gastric cancer, metastases are usually confined to the perigastric lymph nodes, which are difficult to detect. Attempts to improve the accuracy of preoperative lymph node involvement include localization with monoclonal targeted isotopes, endoscopic lymphography, endoluminal ultrasound, and dynamic CT.

Endoscopic ultrasonography discloses perigastric lymph nodes greater than 3 mm in diameter in 70 per cent of patients. If the examination is preceded by the oral administration of an oil-in-water emulsion uninvolved nodes can be identified by echo enhancement at their margin, whilst metastatic nodes show no enhancement. The sensitivity of this test in Japanese hands reaches 92 per cent with a specificity of 100 per cent for nodes greater than 3 mm. Endoscopic lymphography following submucosal injection of contrast can identify metastatic filling defects in involved lymph nodes. Dynamic CT has only slightly improved the diagnostic accuracy of conventional CT and some lymph nodes regions cannot be clearly seen.

Endoscopy and biopsy

The development of fibreoptic, flexible forward viewing endoscopes with a controllable tip has been a major advance, allowing direct visualization of the stomach and accurate biopsy of any lesion which is identified. Endoscopy is observer dependent and visual endoscopic interpretation, even in experienced hands, is often incorrect in deciding on the nature of a lesion in over 10 per cent of cases. If up to 10 biopsies are taken from each lesion the diagnostic accuracy reaches 100 per cent. The accuracy of biopsy is now clearly been shown to be related to the number of biopsies taken. The working recommendation is that four to six biopsies should be taken from each lesion, and from the inner border of the edge of any ulcer.

Improvements in endoscopic techniques include dye-spraying, fluorescence endoscopy, magnified endoscopy, electronic endoscopy, and endoscopic ultrasonography. This last technique can differentiate early gastric cancer from advanced tumours in 80 per cent of patients, but has so far failed to allow preoperative differentiation of mucosal from submucosal cancer because of the problems of fibrosis in the muscular propria and submucosa that may surround ulcerated early gastric cancers.

Cytology

Cytological study of gastric aspirate for exfoliated malignant cells has been reported for patients with advanced disease, but has a variable accuracy of between 40 and 90 per cent. The cytological specimen may be collected by gastric washing, washing with addition of a mucolytic agent, and the passage of a balloon. Cytological analysis of brushings of suspicious lesions collected directly has an accuracy of 81 per cent; combination with biopsy improves the accuracy to 91 per cent. The principal limitation of both cytology and biopsy is failure to obtain an adequate sample. Interpretation problems may be posed by atypical cells associated with regeneration around an ulcer. Immunocytochemical stains such as fetal sulphaglycoprotein may be useful for cytological preparations.

Laparoscopy and laparotomy

Laparoscopy may be valuable as an initial operative assessment to exclude extensive disease, since hepatic, peritoneal, ovarian, or extensive local disease may be assessed. Laparotomy is necessary in all patients with local disease. The presence of extensive nodal disease excludes patients from curative surgery. Some advocate biopsy and frozen section of a lymph node from the infracoeliac periaortic region prior to commencing radical resection. In Japan, peritoneal washings are taken at initial laparotomy for cytological examination, and lymph node sampling with frozen section is performed prior to deciding whether a curative resection is feasible. Locally invasive disease may be excised curatively only if it is minimal.

POPULATION SCREENING

Government-subsidized mass screening has been introduced in Japan, using predominantly radiological methods, with photofluorographic radiology performed at designated centres or by mobile units. Approximately 5 million people are screened every year. After 25 years of screening, the rate of gastric cancer had decreased from causing over 50 per cent of all deaths from malignant disease in men to 33 per cent. Similarly, deaths in women have been reduced from 38 per cent to 28 per cent. The incidence/detection of early gastric cancer has risen from under 2 per cent in 1945 to 63 per cent in some centres. The overall 5-year survival from gastric cancer has risen to over 50 per cent. There are clear shortcomings in using survival rate in evaluating the effectiveness of screening. In particular there is concern at the definition of early gastric cancer and its distinction from dysplasia, or 'worrying mucosal appearance'. Also most studies report 5-year survival and there may well be a lead time bias. Recently, a detailed follow-up has demonstrated that two-thirds of patients with cancer detected by screening in Osaka were cured of their disease 15 years after resection.

Screening of asymptomatic patients is not considered feasible except in Japan, where 25 per cent of gastric cancers are identified by screening programmes. Despite the wider use of the flexible endoscope in the West, the detection of early stage I cancers has not increased. Screening of some high-risk groups is feasible: certain centres have introduced programmes to allow early endoscopy of dyspeptic patients over the age of 40 years, and serial endoscopy until healing of all patients with gastric ulcer. Patients with atrophic gastritis, dysplasia, or adenomatous polyps are offered endoscopy on an annual basis. Among 2659 patients examined in this scheme, 57 cancers have been identified, 20 per cent of which were early gastric cancers, but only 60 per cent of these were suitable for attempted curative surgery.

The excellent results of surgery obtained in Japan have fuelled debate as to whether the disease there is different from that in the West. In all countries Stage I disease is associated with a relatively good prognosis. Yet the overall 5-year survival in Europe, for this stage of disease, was reported as 70 per cent compared with 98 per cent in Japan (Table 5), suggesting differences in biological

Table 5 Comparison of the 1-, 2-, and 5-year survival (per cent) in patients treated in the United Kingdom and Japan with a 'curative' resection for stage I, II, and III

Stage	United Kingdom Year			Japan Year		
	1	2	5	1	2	5
I	86	82	72	95	93	84
II	72	55	32	90	85	65
III	52	26	10	80	60	35
IV	10	5	1	20	15	5

behaviour of the tumour. A detailed review of tumour classification has clarified this issue. The British Society of Gastroenterology reviewed the histology of 319 patients from 41 hospitals with histopathological findings of dysplasia and early gastric cancer. Although there was good agreement between pathologists on the difference between dysplasia and cancer, over one-third of patients thought to have early gastric cancer were found to have more advanced disease on reassessment. The true 5-year survival rate of the group redefined as having early gastric cancers was 90 per cent, compared with 75 per cent of the group initially defined as early gastric cancer. Thus European survival rates for the disease approach those in the East if strict Japanese criteria are used. Unfortunately, the issue cannot yet be regarded as completely resolved. In Japan there is a higher incidence of better prognosis tumours and some tumours do behave differently in the East and West; however, when direct comparisons are made between like tumours the results appear similar.

TREATMENT AND RESULTS

Historical considerations

Historical references to what appears to be gastric carcinoma can be found in the writings of Hippocrates, Galen, and Avicenna. However, it was not until the nineteenth century that Jean Cruveilhier attempted to distinguish between benign and malignant gastric lesions, and gastric cancer was initially referred to as 'la maladie de Cruveilhier' by French physicians. A treatise in 1839 by Bayle clearly described the detailed pathology of gastric cancer and suggested treatments. Resection was attempted by Jules Péan (France) in 1879 and 1 year later by L. Rydygier (Poland). Reconstruction was undertaken using catgut to form a gastroduodenostomy. Both operations were unsuccessful, the patients dying shortly after the procedure as a result of peritonitis from gastric leakage. It appears that an inadequate number of sutures were used. It has been reported that a French surgeon in Arras attempted gastric resection 1 year prior to Péan but details are not available. Theodor Billroth (1829–1894) believed that a safe technique could be developed for the excision of gastric cancer and dispatched Carl Gussenbauer and Alexander Winwater to the postmortem room and the laboratory to investigate the possibility. They found after examining the records of the Vienna Pathological Institute that over 40 per cent of pyloric tumours were amenable to surgical resection and did not appear to be associated with distant metastases. They developed the procedure of the Billroth I gastrectomy in the dog: two of seven dogs treated survived for a prolonged period and two others died of anastomotic dehisence.

Billroth's first gastrectomy for gastric cancer was performed on Frau Therese Heller in 1881, under chloroform anaesthesia, using antiseptic precautions. The gastroduodenal anastomosis was performed with carbolized silk sutures. Unfortunately, a few hazelnut sized mesenteric lymph nodes were found and histological examination confirmed tumour involvement. The patient survived for 4 months, and died of recurrent disease.

Immediately after the initial success of the Billroth I operation, Wölfler (Billroth's assistant) was instructed by his superior to devise a palliative operation to relieve gastric outlet obstruction for unresectable tumours. Thus the technique of bypass gastroenterostomy was devised in 1881, and used clinically later that year. In January 1885, Billroth performed a resection of the distal stomach, closing the transected duodenum and stomach and restoring continuity by a gastroenterostomy to the posterior wall of the stomach. The patient survived for 18 months and the Billroth II operation was born (Fig. 6).

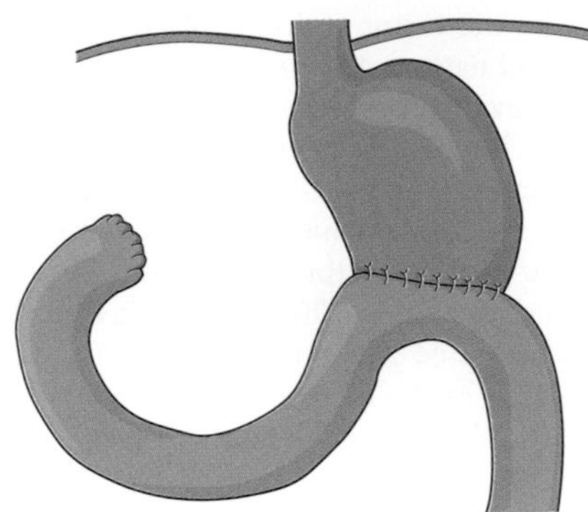

Fig. 6 The reconstruction of a Billroth II or polya operation after resection of an antral carcinoma of the stomach.

By 1890, 41 resections for gastric cancer had been performed at the Billroth clinic with a successful outcome in 19; by 1894 the overall mortality was reported as 55 per cent. These results prompted Welch in 1885 to write that no instances of prolonged recovery or cure followed operation for gastric cancer despite the 'great sensation' produced by Billroth's operative achievements. Extended surgery was explored as a means of improving survival: Carl Schlatter (1897) performed total gastrectomy with end-to-side oesophagojejunal anastomosis. Brigham (1898) also excised the entire stomach in a patient who survived for 18 years and died of other causes. The fact that this patient survived longer than 3 years prior to the identification of gastric intrinsic factor (in 1929 by W.B. Castle) and when vitamin B_{12} supplements were not available may indicate that the gastrectomy was not total.

Billroth's initial gastroduodenal anastomosis with partial closure of the gastric lesser curve was soon found to be associated with leaks at the junction of the lesser curve and the duodenal anastomosis. This area was called the 'jammer ecke' (crying corner) and a further inverting triangular suture was subsequently inserted in this area. It is appropriate to acknowledge the work of the Budapest surgeon Eugen Polya (1876–1944), which was first recognized by William Mayo. He devised the retrocolic anastomosis of the entire width of the gastric segment to the jejunum after gastrectomy (Fig. 6).

There are now many distinguished names associated with various forms of gastrectomy. There was an extended period of debate in the 1940s as to whether the jejunal anastomosis should be isoperistaltic, retroperistaltic, antecolic, retrocolic, with a long or short afferent loop, to the entire gastric stoma, or whether a valve was necessary. Various modifications allowed the attachment of an eponym to each modification of gastrectomy, often with a strongly held anecdotal belief of its superior merits. At present most surgeons favour partial closure of the gastric stoma as described by Hofmeister, with an antecolic anastomosis for reconstruction and a short afferent loop after a cancer resection. The precise form of reconstruction is of little relevance.

The oncological approach: factors affecting prognosis

Since Billroth's first resection, gastrectomy has been the mainstay of therapy. However, the optimal surgical management is still a subject of intense debate. The controversy lies between the predominantly Western belief that the pathological stage of disease is the crucial prognostic factor and the widespread Eastern opinion that the extent and nature of the resection, combined with adjuvant therapy, are major factors in improving the results. Predetermined factors such as location of the tumour and the extent of nodal and, in particular, serosal involvement undoubtedly affect survival, but the manner in which the resection is performed can have a significant impact on the prognosis. Thus one view must not be exclusive of the other. The importance of early detection is now universally accepted and in the absence of distant metastasis, aggressive resection of the carcinoma is justified.

Poor prognostic factors in relation to the presentation of the tumour are serosal invasion, presence of lymph node metastasis, presence of free carcinoma cells in the peritoneum, Lauren's classification (intestinal better than diffuse), cardial tumour, histological invasion of lymph vessels, tumour stage, tumour depth and size, and the patient's age. The poor prognostic variables that relate to surgery are positive resection margins, inadequate lymphadenectomy, and the need for an associated splenectomy. The most important single prognostic factor is serosal invasion. It is now clearly demonstrated that the number of lymph nodes affected or the extent of resection does not affect the prognosis if the serosa is involved.

The basic oncological approach for resection of mucosal cancers is wide excision of the primary tumour with *en-bloc* removal of the lymphatic drainage and network of lymph nodes. This approach has undergone re-evaluation for some tumours, with lesser resection in combination with other means of treatment providing a more conservative and equally effective option. At present our understanding of the biological behaviour of gastric carcinoma, in particular with regard to the very limited effectiveness of radiotherapy and chemotherapy, means that radical excisional surgery probably offers the best chance of cure.

Radical and attempted curative surgery

The problems of definition of radical excision in treatment of gastric cancer confuse the interpretation of the results of surgery. The main areas that must be addressed are the extent of gastric resection, and the extent of lymph node resection.

Extent of gastric resection

Adequate gastrectomy implies surgical margins in the stomach free of tumour. Gastrectomy may therefore be partial or subtotal if the tumour is distal or total if it is more proximal. Adequate resection margins in the stomach are defined as an 8- to 10-cm proximal and distal clearance in the unstretched stomach. Failure to resect the stomach widely with microscopic clear margins is highly detrimental to survival. If the resection margin is not confirmed to be free of microscopic diseasee, the prognosis of a Stage II tumour falls to that of a Stage IV tumour. The specific operation for a gastric carcinoma depends somewhat on its site. There is a widespread belief that subtotal gastrectomy is associated with poor local control. However, total gastrectomy appears to have no advantage over adequate gastrectomy for local tumours. A prospective controlled study comparing total and subtotal gastrectomy (with the same node dissection) for carcinoma of the gastric antrum demonstrated no survival difference between the two groups. At Memorial Sloan-Kettering Cancer Center total gastrectomy was found to be detrimental to survival, not because of the extent of resection, but predominantly because splenectomy was associated with this operation. It is recommended that an exclusive policy of elective total gastrectomy when the tumour can be widely resected by a subtotal gastrectomy is incorrect. For patients with synchronous multiple gastric cancers, logic suggests that a total gastrectomy is essential. Paradoxically the survival after total gastrectomy does not exceed that after partial gastrectomy, and it has been suggested that small synchronous lesions may regress after resection of the main tumour, although there is no evidence for this. In general, multiple cancers should be treated by total gastrectomy where possible.

Lesions in the body and fundus of the stomach present different problems. Total gastrectomy is often advocated in patients with such lesions because the small amount of stomach that remains after more conservative surgery has little reservoir capacity. Both total and proximal gastric resection require the creation of an oesophagoenteric anastomosis and the operative mortality is 5 per cent. Theoretically, total gastrectomy carries a lower risk of recurrence or a second gastric cancer in long-term survivors. Total gastrectomy with a Roux-en-Y reconstruction is also superior to proximal gastrectomy since these patients are less subject to alkaline reflux. These tumours are often far advanced at presentation because they reach considerable size before producing symptoms. They have a less favourable prognosis than tumours in the antrum.

The preferred method of reconstruction after total gastrectomy is as a Roux-en-Y with a 60-cm Roux to prevent bile reflux. The creation of a pouch to act as a reservoir to prevent early satiety has been advocated. The Hunt-Lawrence pouch (Fig. 7) is created

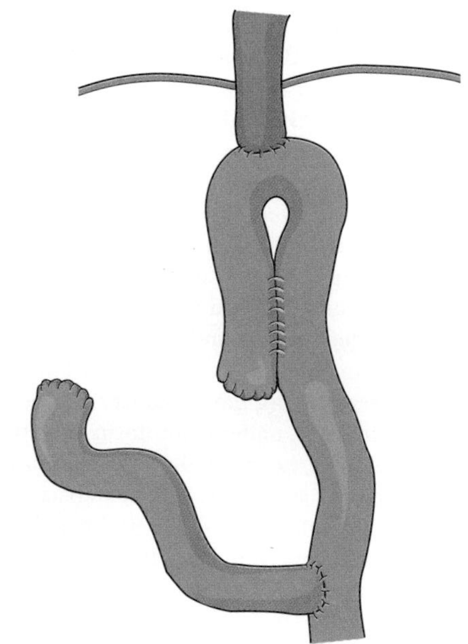

Fig. 7 Following total gastrectomy a Hunt-Lawrence pouch is created from a long Roux loop with an enteroenteric anastomosis at 80 cm.

from a long Roux loop with an enteroenteric anastomosis at 80 cm. It is simply folded on itself and a 10-cm side-to-side anastomosis created below the oesophageal anastomosis. A partial gastrectomy is best reconstructed as an antecolic polya type of gastrectomy (Fig. 6).

Gastric cancer at the cardia represents a special management problem. At presentation only 10 per cent of patients have disease restricted to the stomach, and only 2 per cent are early cancers. The tumour may infiltrate the lower oesophagus, and a 10-cm oesophageal clearance is advised to be certain of clear resection margins. Thus surgery involves principles of gastric as well as oesophageal surgery, and in certain respects it should be regarded as a separate entity.

Extent of lymphadenectomy

The benefit of lymphadenectomy in the treatment of gastric cancer has been emphasized by the Japanese. This concept is not new in oncology. Wide lymphadenectomy encompassing one or more echelons of uninvolved lymph nodes improves survival in the small number of patients with limited nodal involvement seen in Western series. The Japanese Research Society for gastric cancer defines a curative resection as one in which patients without peritoneal, serosal, or hepatic involvement have a gastric resection with a lymph node dissection one level beyond that of pathological lymph node involvement.

The Japanese classification of the type of gastrectomy corresponds to how radical the operation is in terms of removing the groups of lymph nodes, according to the Japanese classification (N0–N4). R0 gastrectomy does not remove any lymph node group, R1 gastrectomy removes those nodes in group I (N1), which are predominantly perigastric lymph nodes, but leaves a large portion of the greater omentum. No formal lymphadenectomy is performed during this resection. A hybrid form of this resection, a traditional radical gastrectomy including omentectomy and partial lymphadenectomy is predominantly performed in the West. The Japanese results suggest that in most circumstances the radical R2 gastrectomy gives the best chance of prolonged survival, and this operation is predominantly performed in that country.

R2 gastrectomy carries the same criteria for adequate gastric removal but includes lymphadenectomy to remove Group II (N2) nodes *en bloc* with stomach. The precise tissues removed depends on the site of the cancer. In general the entire greater omentum is removed, with the superior leaf of the transverse mesocolon, pancreatic capsule, and lesser omentum. Lymph node dissection starts by removing the nodes along the gastroduodenal artery to its origin at the hepatic and is continued laterally to the porta hepatitis along the common hepatic artery. The nodes are cleared medially along the common hepatic artery to the coeliac axis which is cleared and continued along the splenic artery to the hilum of the spleen. Clearance in this area is facilitated by mobilization of the distal pancreas. R3 gastrectomy attempts to remove nodes in Group III (N3) and involves pancreatic and splenic resection. The overall Japanese results demonstrate a corrected 5-year survival following R0, R1, R2, and R3 resections of 26 per cent, 42 per cent, 50 per cent, and 40 per cent. Thus the Japanese have adopted R2 gastrectomy as the usual form of treatment for operable early gastric and advanced gastric cancer. The justification for the use of this radical operation in early tumours is the finding that N1 lymph nodes are involved in 1 to 5 per cent of mucosal and 11 to 19 per cent of submucosal cancers. The rates of metastasis in N2 lymph nodes is 0 to 2 per cent for mucosal and 2 to 9 per cent for submucosal cancers. Metastasis to Group N3 and N4 nodes is unusual. A selective policy could be adopted if the depth of the primary could be accurately assessed preoperatively. Indeed there is no difference in survival after R1 and R2 gastrectomy for mucosal cancer without lymph node metastasis, but a significant survival advantage in patients undergoing R2 resection if lymph nodes are involved. R2 and R3 gastrectomy are performed remarkably safely by Japanese surgeons, with an operative mortality of 1 to 3 per cent.

Resistance to, and failure to adopt the R2 gastrectomy in the West, has occurred because a clear advantage over the traditional Western radical resection has not been demonstrated, predominantly because of varying experience. In the West, the R2 operation is associated with a longer duration of surgery, greater blood loss, longer postoperative hospital stay, and greater morbidity. The Japanese surgeons have demonstrated no difference between postoperative mortality and the level of nodes dissected.

Lesions at the gastric cardia tend to metastasize to all the regional lymph nodes and extended total gastrectomy (R3) is required to encompass all the lymph nodes, in addition to mediastinal dissection. This carcinoma has such a dismal prognosis that almost any surgical procedure is palliative and often a more simple proximal gastric resection is most appropriate.

The treatment of stump cancer should follow the same principles for radical excision. The pattern of lymph node spread is different. The previous resection has often left lymph channels along the left gastric vessels, and lymph drainage from the greater curve and into the jejunal mesentery are more important. Radical excision usually implies total gastrectomy and excision to the origin of the jejunal artery supplying the gastroenterostomy.

The mortality and morbidity of the operation is related to the nature of resection, with distal partial gastrectomy being safest, followed by subtotal gastrectomy, and then total gastrectomy. Factors that are significantly related to postoperative complications, apart from operative procedure, are age, sex, and splenectomy. Men and patients of more advanced age are more prone to complications, as are those who have a splenectomy. In general the mortality of surgical resection of gastric cancer in Western countries is falling, from less than 10 per cent in the 1970s to 2 per cent in the 1990s, and is approaching the results that are obtained in Japan.

The results of surgery are summarized in Table 5, which compares series from Japan and the United Kingdom. Overall the survival results are substantially better in Japan than in the United Kingdom.

Palliative surgery

In the West very few patients present with early gastric cancer; in one large series only 90 of 13 000 patients with gastric cancer fulfilled the criteria. Approximately 55 per cent of patients with gastric cancer are suitable for laparotomy, with curative resection in only 21 per cent. The remainder will have no procedure (15 per cent), palliative resection (10 per cent), or bypass (9 per cent). Unfortunately, laparotomy and palliative surgery carry a significant mortality (10–30 per cent) and morbidity, and before embarking on palliative excision it is important to define the goals of this form of surgery. Symptoms due to obstruction, such as dysphagia, vomiting, and obstructive pain may be relieved by

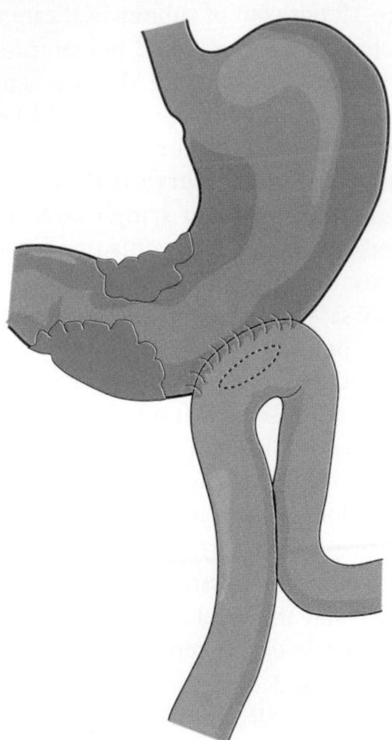

Fig. 8 Palliative gastroenterostomy to bypass an obstructing distal carcinoma of the gastric antrum.

surgical resection or bypass (Fig. 8). Bleeding can be relieved by resection. If at laparotomy curative resection is impossible, the alternatives are a palliative resection, a bypass, or no procedure. The consensus is that palliative non-radical resection may provide the best chance of relief of symptoms, and some patients (6 per cent) show prolonged survival after this procedure. Palliative bypass procedures do not increase survival times and are only necessary if there is obstruction. The benefit on the quality of life is highly questionable, and the mean survival for patients is 5 months. There are various methods of non-operative palliation, including laser therapy and intubation for dysphagia, and interstitial laser therapy for bleeding gastric cancers.

The role of radiotherapy

Local and regional recurrence occurs in 80 per cent of patients with distant metastases, and at death 16 to 22 per cent have locally recurrent disease only. 'Second look' laparotomy in asymptomatic patients without evidence of distant metastasis reveals local recurrence in 69 per cent. These findings have been used to suggest a role for adjuvant radiotherapy. Gastric adenocarcinoma has generally been regarded as radioresistant and, although it is less sensitive than squamous cell carcinoma, useful response and tumour shrinkage has been achieved in patients given palliative radiotherapy for malignant dysphagia. The major limitation to radiotherapy has been the problem of achieving a dose that will spare adjacent normal tissue, including the liver and the small intestine. Intraoperative radiotherapy may overcome some of these problems. In some Japanese centres, after attempted curative resection, intraoperative radiotherapy is administered to the coeliac axis and the tumour bed. There is some evidence to suggest that patients with stage III and IV disease undergoing this therapy have a prolonged survival compared with historical controls. Radiotherapy delivered postoperatively to patients following palliative and curative resection seems to have little influence on survival.

The benefits of radiotherapy are best if bulk disease is controlled by other means. Unfortunately, patients with gastric cancer may have large and unresectable tumours at presentation. It has been suggested that preoperative radiotherapy may be used to shrink the tumour and allow subsequent resection. Unfortunately accurate radiotherapy planning is difficult preoperatively, and there is little evidence that preoperative radiotherapy is beneficial.

The role of chemotherapy

Systemic

The rationale for the use of adjuvant chemotherapy in gastric cancer is clear, since surgery is only potentially curative, and 70 per cent of patients with cancer confined to the gastric wall on pathological examination will die of the disease. Although the disease is apparently localized it has, therefore, in fact extended beyond surgical resection or is already disseminated and systemic therapy is required for any attempt to eradicate the disease. Gastrointestinal cancers are generally unresponsive to chemotherapy, but gastric cancers appear to be more sensitive than most and in particular respond better than colorectal cancer. Despite evidence to suggest that combined chemotherapy is better, most studies have been performed with single agents. Mitomycin C, doxorubicin, 5-fluorouracil, and the nitrosoureas will produce tumour shrinkage in up to 30 per cent of patients with advanced disease. The combination of 5-fluorouracil, doxorubicin, and mitomycin C at present represents the most effective regimen for advanced gastric cancer, with 40 per cent of patients showing a partial response, although only 5 per cent will have a complete response. The translation of a response in advanced cancer into an effective adjuvant regimen in less advanced disease has proved difficult. Again there is differing experience between Western series and the positive Japanese studies. In the extensive European and American trials, no survival benefit has been demonstrated with combinations of fluorouracil, mitomycin, and methyl CCNU, and with 5-fluorouracil, doxorubicin, and mitomycin C administered after potentially curative surgery. The Japanese have demonstrated some survival advantage in patients treated with mitomycin C, alone or in combination, when given intraoperatively or in the very early postoperative period. The trials have been criticized because the survival benefit has been demonstrated by the retrospective formation of subgroups. Overall there is no convincing evidence that cytotoxic chemotherapy is of use after resection for gastric cancer. General application of adjuvant chemotherapy cannot be recommended. The role of preoperative (neoadjuvant) chemotherapy has to be established, but may increase the resectability rate. The combination of postoperative chemotherapy with radiotherapy has also failed to improve survival in this disease.

Regional

Since malignant cells are shed into the peritoneum by the tumour, various local methods have been developed to eradicate localized intraperitoneal disease. Local instillation of cytotoxics, or hyperthermic peritoneal perfusion with cytotoxic agents initially appeared effective but no survival benefit was demonstrated in a randomized clinical trial. Palliation of advanced tumours with endoscopic regression and some long-term survival can be achieved by local arterial infusion of cytotoxics, but this remains inappropriate for most patients.

FURTHER READING

Abe S, Shiraishi M, Nagaoka S, Yoshimura H, Dhar DK, Nakamura T. Serosal invasion as the single prognostic indicator in stage IIA (T3N1M0) gastric cancer. *Surgery* 1991; **109**: 582–8.

Adam YG, Efron G. Trends and controversies in the management of carcinoma of the stomach. *Surg Gynecol Obstet* 1990; **169**: 371–85.

Alcobendas F, Milla A, Estape J, Curto J, Pera C. Mitomycin C as an adjuvant in resected gastric cancer. *Ann Surg* 1983; **198**: 13–17.

Allum H, Powell J, McConkey C, Fielding WL. Gastric cancer: a 25 year review. *Br J Surg* 1989; **76**: 535–40.

Boku T, *et al.* Prognostic significance of serosal invasion and free intraperitoneal cancer cells in gastric cancer. *Br J Surg* 1990; **77**: 436–9.

Craanen ME, Dekker W, Ferwerda J, Blok P, Tytgat NJ. Early gastric cancer: a clinicopathologic study. *J Clin Gastroenterol* 1991; **13**: 274–83.

De Dombal FT, *et al.* The British Society of Gastroenterology early gastric cancer/dysplasia survey: an interim report. *Gut* 1990; **31**: 115–20.

Dent DM, Madden MV, Price SK. Randomized comparison of R1 and R2 gastrectomy for gastric carcinoma. *Br J Surg* 1988; **75**: 110–12.

Fielding JWL. Gastric cancer: different diseases. *Br J Surg* 1989; **76**: 1227.

Hioki K, Nakane Y, Yamamoto M. Surgical strategy for early gastric cancer. *Br J Surg* 1990; **77**: 1330–4.

Husemann B. Cardia carcinoma considered as a distinct clinical entity. *Br J Surg* 1989; **76**: 136–9.

Kampschoer GHM, Nakajima T, van de Velde CJH. Changing patterns in gastric cancer. *Br J Surg* 1989; **76**: 914–16.

Lauren P. The two main types of gastric carcinoma: diffuse and so-called intestinal-type carcinoma. *Acta Pathol Microbiol Scand* 1965; **64**: 31–49.

Lawrence M, Shiu MH. Early gastric cancer: twenty-eight year experience. *Ann Surg* 1991; **213**: 327–34.

Maruyama K, Gunven P, Okabayashi K, Sasako M, Kinoshita T. Lymph node metastases of gastric cancer. General pattern in 1931 patients. *Ann Surg* 1959; **210**: 596–602.

Mitsudomi I, Wantanabe A, Matsusaka T, Fujinaga Y, Fuchigami T, Iwashita A. A clinicopathological study of synchronous multiple gastric cancer. *Br J Surg* 1989; **76**: 237–40.

Oota K, Sobin LH. *Histological typing of gastric and oesophageal tumors.* International Histological Classification of Tumors. 18. Geneva: WHO, 1977.

Paterson IM, Easton DF, Corbishley CM, Gazet J-C. Changing distribution of adenocarcinoma of the stomach. *Br J Surg* 1987; **74**: 481–2.

Schlag P. Adjuvant chemotherapy in gastric cancer. *World J Surg* 1987; **11**: 473–7.

Shiu MH, *et al.* Influence of the extent of resection on survival after curative treatment of gastric carcinoma. *Arch Surg* 1987; **122**: 1347–51.

Toftgaard C. Gastric cancer after peptic ulcer surgery. A historic prospective cohort investigation. *Ann Surg* 1989; **210**: 159–64.

Yasuna O, Hayashi S. Factors influencing the postoperative course of 113 patients with early gastric cancer. *Jpn J Clin Oncol* 1986; **16**: 325–34.

15.4 Duodenal diverticula and duodenal tumours

WOLFRAM TRUDO KNOEFEL AND DAVID W. RATTNER

DUODENAL DIVERTICULA

Introduction

Duodenal diverticula are found in up to 25 per cent of patients, but rarely cause symptoms. When complications occur, early diagnosis is essential if treatment is to be successful. Duodenal diverticula can be classified into the common extraluminal type and the rare intraluminal type, according to their pathogenesis and clinical presentation.

Extraluminal duodenal diverticula

The first well documented report of a duodenal diverticulum was made by Morgagni in 1762. Although only 100 cases were reported during the next 150 years the introduction of radiological evaluation of the gastrointestinal tract led to duodenal diverticula becoming recognized as a common anatomical abnormality. Earlier this century many patients underwent diverticulectomy for uncertain indications with ambiguous results. Diverticula cause symptoms in only a minority of patients, but their presence should not be ignored in the differential diagnosis of acute abdominal events.

Aetiology

The aetiology of primary duodenal diverticula is unknown. They are in fact pseudodiverticula (because they are not composed of all layers of the bowel wall) and resemble 'pulsion' type diverticula seen in other parts of the gastrointestinal tract. These diverticula tend to occur adjacent to the papilla of Vater, perhaps because of a local weakness in the duodenal wall. Embryologically diverticula could result from a *locus minoris resistentiae* in the musculature, as this is the site of budding and fusion of the pancreatic anlagen in the duodenal fenestrum.

Secondary diverticula are true diverticula, consisting of all layers of the bowel wall. They are caused by adhesions or extraluminal scarring often related to peptic ulcer disease, and are consequently most common in the first part of the duodenum. They account for less than one-fifth of all extraluminal diverticula and do not cause symptoms.

Anatomy

Most duodenal diverticula are solitary and occur in the second portion of the duodenum. The major papilla is usually located close to the rim of the diverticulum; in rare instances, it may lie deep within the diverticulum. Occasionally, diverticula are found around the minor papilla of Santorini. About 10 per cent of diverticula occur in the third or fourth portion of the duodenum. Juxtapapillary duodenal diverticula are more likely to cause symptoms than do diverticula in other parts of the duodenum.

Epidemiology

Although extraluminal duodenal diverticula are rare in young patients, their frequency increases with age. There is no sex predilection. At autopsy, primary extraluminal duodenal diverticula occur in up to 22 per cent of individuals, depending on the technique employed and the mean age of the autopsy subjects. The frequency of diverticula in radiologic series is between 0.16 per cent and 5.76 per cent while endoscopic studies show an incidence as high as 23 per cent. Endoscopic and radiological examinations are performed only in patients with symptoms attributed to the upper gastrointestinal tract, and therefore do not necessarily represent the general population. The assumption is that extraluminal duodenal diverticula are rare in those under the age of 30, but may be present in up to 20 per cent of the general population with increasing age.

Clinical presentation

Ninety per cent of duodenal diverticula are asymptomatic and are detected incidentally during radiological or endoscopic investigation of the upper gastrointestinal tract for an unrelated disease. In 10 per cent of patients, duodenal diverticula are responsible for symptoms; symptomatic diverticula are more common in the elderly. Distension of the diverticulum may cause pain and nausea. Because the symptoms are non-specific they are often attributed to cholelithiasis or gastritis. Some patients may have undergone cholecystectomy and dietary trials without relief. Only after elimination of all other more common causes of upper abdominal pain and nausea are the patient's symptoms attributed to the duodenal diverticulum.

Although complications of duodenal diverticula are rare, they can be devastating. (Table 1). The most common complication is diverticulitis with perforation. Extraluminal diverticula may infarct and rupture if a gallstone or an enterolith obstructs the orifice into the duodenum. Foreign bodies such as fish bones are also prone to perforate the attenuated diverticular wall. However, whether perforation actually results from occlusion of the orifice by an enterolith or from stasis due to the lack of a muscular wall remains unclear. Retroperitoneal abscess and fistula are the most common sequelae of perforation (Fig. 1). Rarely, perforation may lead to a duodenocolic fistula with diarrhoea as the main symptom.

Table 1 Complications of duodenal diverticula

Inflammation
Diverticulitis and peridiverticulitis
Perforation
Abscess formation
Fistula formation
Obstruction
Common bile duct
Pancreatic duct
Duodenum
Haemorrhage
Recurrent cholangitis
Pancreatitis

Because diverticula are located in the retroperitoneum, the development of symptoms is insidious, and diagnosis is often delayed. Abdominal or back pain and fever are the most common presenting symptoms. Because of the delay in diagnosis of diverticular perforation, mortality rates can be as high as 50 per cent. Even intraoperatively, the diagnosis may be obscure unless the duodenum is fully mobilized and the retroperitoneum is explored. Intraoperative findings such as bile staining of tissues, retroperitoneal emphysema, and oedema suggest a perforated extraluminal duodenal diverticulum.

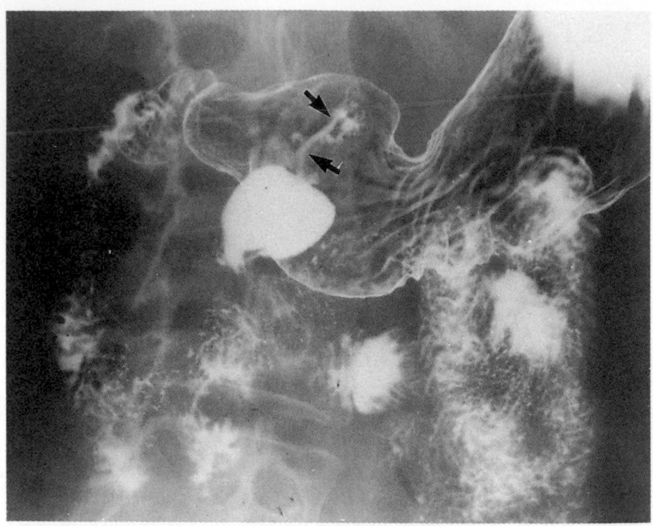

Fig. 1 Perforated extraluminal duodenal diverticulum of the fourth portion of the duodenum with retroperitoneal fistula (arrows).

The relationship between cholelithiasis, choledocholithiasis and juxtapapillary diverticula is well established. Duodenal diverticula predispose patients to gallstone formation. Even after cholecystectomy, choledocholithiasis is more common in patients with diverticula than in the general population. Juxtapapillary diverticula may compress the distal common bile duct and cause dysfunction or incompetence of the choledocho-duodenal sphincter. Bile cultures from patients with diverticula demonstrate a 70 to 80 per cent incidence of bacterial colonization. Intestinal bacteria are able to split conjugated bilirubin into unconjugated bilirubin and glucuronic acid by the action of the hydrolytic enzyme β-glucuronidase. Unconjugated bilirubin then combines with calcium in the bile to precipitate and form calculi. Since pigment gallstones are the most common stones in patients with diverticula, a causal relationship is assumed.

Juxtapapillary diverticula are also associated with an increased incidence of pancreatitis. While many of these patients have gallstones, pancreatitis may occur in the absence of biliary lithiasis: this may be due to reflux of duodenal contents through the incompetent ampullary sphincter or even compression of the distal pancreatic duct by the diverticulum.

Haemorrhage occurs if the diverticular wall is ulcerated due to diverticulitis. Bleeding is rarely massive, but patients may present with haematemesis, melaena, and anaemia. Because the bleeding site is within the diverticulum, diagnosis may be difficult. Diverticulectomy is generally required to obtain hemostasis.

Diagnosis

Most asymptomatic duodenal diverticula are diagnosed by duodenoscopy; however, upper gastrointestinal series is the diagnostic tool of choice if perforation or a fistulization of a duodenal diverticulum is suspected. Computer assisted tomography may also be helpful in detecting perforation of a duodenal diverticulum. Haemorrhage is best localized by duodenoscopy. Extraluminal diverticula often extend into the pancreas and therefore may be overlooked at autopsy and during surgery.

Treatment

An uncomplicated duodenal diverticulum does not warrant surgical intervention. In patients with symptoms due to distension of diverticula, relief may be obtained if the patient assumes a position which allows dependent drainage of the diverticulum. The position can be determined by fluoroscopy. Acute obstruction of a diverticulum, which may be the cause of acute pancreatitis or biliary stasis, can be relieved by endoscopic clearance of the diverticulum. If acute obstruction recurs, diverticulectomy should be considered. Some authors have recommended cholecystectomy for silent gallstones in patients with duodenal diverticula to prevent later biliary complications, but there is no firm evidence that this prescription is beneficial for patients who otherwise would not require surgery.

One per cent of patients with diverticula require surgical treatment of a complication. To expose the diverticulum, a Kocher manoeuvre should be performed, as most diverticula are juxtapapillary. Those in the third part of the duodenum, proximal to the superior mesenteric vessels, may be visualized by a wide Kocher manoeuvre and mobilization of the hepatic flexure of the colon. The duodenum distal to the superior mesenteric vessels may be exposed by opening the ligament of Treitz at the base of the mesocolon. The simplest surgical treatment is invagination of the diverticulum into the duodenum without opening the duodenum. This is possible only in small, non-inflamed diverticula. Simple resection of the diverticulum is warranted in almost all cases in which the anatomy permits control of the biliary and pancreatic duct. A transduodenal or combined extraduodenal and transduodenal approach my be necessary to achieve this goal. If a large residual defect remains after resection it should be closed perpendicular to the long axis of the bowel. Primary closure can usually be performed, because the neck of the diverticulum and the duodenal wall are separate from the acute inflammatory process. Resection, however, may be difficult in cases where the diverticulum is buried in the head of the pancreas or the papilla lies deep within the diverticulum. Therefore, in cases in which a direct approach to the diverticulum seems too hazardous, division of the duodenum 2 cm distal to the pylorus with drainage by a Roux-en-Y duodenojejunostomy may be performed. Another method of bypassing a diverticulum is 'diverticulization' of the duodenum (antrectomy, vagotomy, choledochostomy, and Billroth II anastomosis). Choledochoduodenostomy or choledochojejunostomy alone do not relieve problems arising from the pancreatic duct and are therefore rarely indicated.

Postoperative deaths and complications are primarily caused by advanced spread of retroperitoneal infection and duodenal fistulae. The only way to prevent extensive spread of retroperitoneal infection is early diagnosis and adequate drainage. Less frequent postoperative complications such as pancreatitis and haemorrhage result from over-aggressive attempts to dissect the diverticulum from the pancreas. A transduodenal approach without the necessity for dissection of the pancreas or Roux-en-Y duodenojejunostomy is often the safest approach.

Intraluminal duodenal diverticula

Intraluminal duodenal diverticulum is a rare entity, less than 100 cases being reported in the world's literature. In contrast to extraluminal duodenal diverticula, however, most patients become symptomatic. There is a high incidence of coexisting congenital gastrointestinal and extraintestinal anomalities.

Aetiology and anatomy

In the fifth week after conception proliferation of the duodenal epithelium nearly obliterates the lumen of the second to fourth portions of the duodenum. Early in the sixth week vacuoles start to coalesce and form two channels, and by the eighth week both channels are normally consolidated. Intrinsic duodenal obstruction can develop when the duodenum is incompletely recanalized. Duodenal atresia, stenosis, obstructing mucosal diaphragm, or duodenal duplication may develop.

Intraluminal duodenal diverticula arise either from an incomplete duodenal duplication or from a duodenal diaphragm. Incomplete recanalization of one of the two channels may result in a communicating incomplete duplication of the duodenum that ends blindly and is attached to only a small part of the duodenal wall. A duodenal diaphragm may be transformed into a pulsion intraluminal diverticulum with circumferential attachment by the continuous force of the intestinal stream.

Most intraluminal diverticula originate in the second part of the duodenum. As the diverticulum is not innervated it cannot generate peristaltic waves, nor can it cause pain *per se*. The diverticulum is lined on both sides by epithelium and also contains fibrous tissue with a few smooth muscle cells of the muscularis mucosae. It is poorly vascularized and therefore prone to necrosis if the pressure inside the diverticulum increases. The diverticulum may then slough with no residual defect.

Clinical presentation

Intraluminal diverticula cause symptoms of partial intestinal obstruction. Unlike duodenal stenosis due to a duodenal diaphragm or to duodenal duplication, which cause symptoms early in life, symptoms occur mainly between the third and fifth decade of life, when the diverticular sac has enlarged sufficiently to obstruct the duodenum. Asymptomatic periods occur when the duodenum is empty and the diverticulum collapses. Postprandial epigastric pain and fullness, vomiting, gastrointestinal bleeding, and weight loss are common. Epigastric tenderness may be present and pancreatitis occurs in 10 to 20 per cent of cases. Rarely, intussusception may occur.

Diagnosis

Diagnosis is established either by radiological or endoscopic means. Duodenoscopy is superior to radiological examination in localizing the papilla of Vater and determining the important relationship between the diverticulum and ampulla. The typical radiological appearance is that of a barium coated pouch within the duodenum (Fig. 2). If the sac is not filled with barium (in cases where the opening is very small) it may appear as a pedunculated polyp and the diagnosis may be hard to establish even endoscopically. The exact location has to be determined before surgery since there are no visible changes on the serosal surface of the duodenum and the diverticulum tends to collapse after duodenotomy making palpation quite difficult.

Treatment

All intraluminal diverticula require treatment unless the patient is too frail to undergo even endoscopic therapy. Without removal of the diverticulum recurrence of symptoms is certain. Curative treatment consists of removal of the diverticulum by laparotomy and duodenotomy or by endoscopy. Care must be taken to avoid injury to the papilla, which is usually located in the immediate vicinity of the diverticulum. If the diverticulum is not circum-

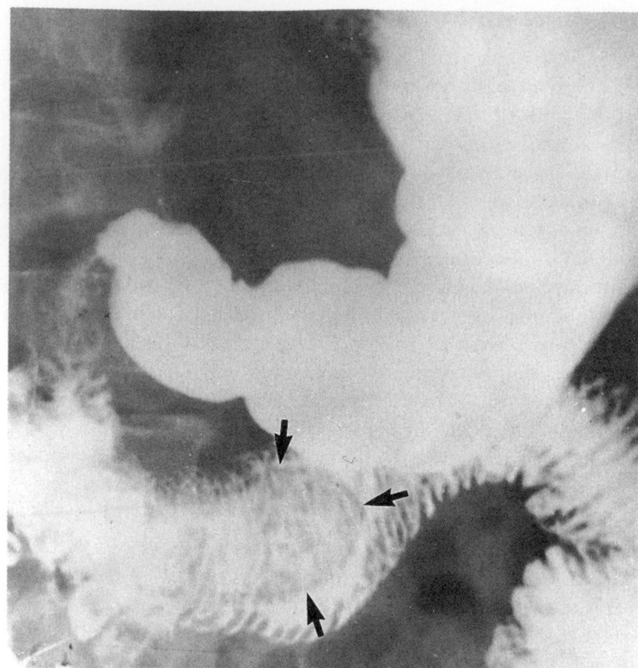

Fig. 2 Intraluminal duodenal diverticulum. The barium coated pouch extends from the second to fourth portion of the duodenum (arrows). (By courtesy of Joseph T. Ferrucci Jr., M.D.)

ferentially attached, it can be resected endoscopically with an electrocautery snare. If the diverticulum is attached circumferentially, it can be inverted with the endoscope and then partially resected to create an opening in the blind end measuring at least 1 cm in diameter. When the papilla, common bile duct, or pancreatic duct cannot be clearly identified and intubated for an endoscopic procedure, duodenotomy should be performed. If at the time of duodenotomy the papilla cannot be identified, choledochotomy and placement of a bile duct probe to localize the papilla should be performed prior to resection of the diverticulum. The blind end of the diverticulum has to be identified before resection to rule out complete duplication of the duodenal lumen. Less than 10 bypass operations such as gastrojejunostomy or duodenojejunostomy have been reported to treat intraluminal duodenal diverticula. None of these operations diverted the intestinal stream successfully because diverticulization of the duodenum was not performed and the diverticulum filled again slowly after the operation, leading to recurrence of symptoms.

Duodenal duplication

Incomplete recanalization of the duodenum may result in complete duodenal duplication without connection to the duodenum. Most patients become symptomatic within the first decade of life presenting with nausea and vomiting as signs of partial duodenal obstruction. The radiographic appearance is that of an ovoid, smooth, non-pedunculated filling defect on the medial wall of the duodenum. When the duplication of the duodenum is complete, the common bile duct and pancreatic duct are often involved in the common wall, making complete excision impossible. Treatment in this instance is by generous fenestration of the dividing wall, avoiding the common bile pancreatic duct.

DUODENAL TUMOURS

General considerations

Primary tumours of the duodenum are uncommon. Their peak incidence is between the sixth and eight decade of life, and symptomatic benign and malignant duodenal tumours occur with equal frequency and a near equal sex distribution. The aetiology of duodenal tumours is unknown. The low incidence of these tumours in comparison with adenocarcinoma of the colon and stomach has lead to speculation about the existence of protective factors, such as secretory immunoglobulins, small intestinal hydroxylases that could inactivate potential carcinogens, alkalinity in the duodenum that could prevent formation of potential carcinogens, rapid transit of liquid bowel contents, and lack of bacteria.

Symptoms are related to the tumour location and result from either obstruction of the ampulla, partial duodenal obstruction, or from bleeding caused by the tumour. Nausea and vomiting, pain, jaundice, anaemia, pancreatitis, haematemesis, melaena, palpable mass, duodenal obstruction, weight loss, intussusception, and acute bacterial cholangitis may all occur. Neuroendocrine tumours present with symptoms due to the effects of hormone production.

The diagnosis is often made on upper gastrointestinal series and is confirmed by endoscopy. These two tests provide complementary information: the former defines the precise location and extent of the tumour and detects lesions in the third and fourth portion of the duodenum that are not routinely detected endoscopically. Endoscopy affords the opportunity to delineate the relationship of the tumour to the ampulla and also permits biopsy to be undertaken for tissue diagnosis. Although CT scanning may detect the presence of nodal or liver metastases, it seldom alters management.

Annular pancreas, a relatively common congenital abnormality may be confused with annular carcinoma. It is differentiated by its endoscopic appearance, which shows intact duodenal mucosa, and by computed tomography.

Benign duodenal tumours

Adenomas

Adenomas are the most common benign tumours in the duodenum and present either as adenomatous polyps, Brunner's gland adenomas, or villous adenomas. The last have a high rate of malignant transformation and are therefore discussed under malignant tumours.

Adenomatous polyps

Adenomatous polyps are sessile, nodular, or pedunculated. Although most are asymptomatic, periampullary lesions may cause intermittent jaundice or pancreatitis. Anaemia may also occur secondary to chronic blood loss.

Duodenal adenomatous polyps are common in familial polyposis coli, Peutz–Jegher's syndrome, and Gardner's syndrome, when they may undergo transformation into villous adenomas and adenocarcinomas. However, prophylactic pancreaticoduodenectomy is not recommended. Instead these patients should undergo periodic upper gastrointestinal endoscopies with numerous biopsies and endoscopic removal of suspicious polyps (large lesions, ulcerated or bleeding lesions, lesions with white or firm areas, and lesions found to have tubulovillous components). If an invasive carcinoma is detected radical resection is indicated.

Patients who present with a limited number of adenomatous polyps should undergo endoscopic resection if this is technically feasible. If a suspicious lesion cannot be removed endoscopically, duodenotomy and complete excision is required. If a solitary adenoma is histologically proven to be benign, no further treatment or particular follow-up is necessary. Periodic endoscopy is recommended in patients with multiple polyps.

Brunner's gland adenomas

Brunner's gland adenomas may present as pedunculated polyps, circumscribed nodular hyperplasia, or diffuse nodular hyperplasia. They differ neither in location nor in histology from normal Brunner's glands and produce alkaline mucus. The malignant potential of Brunner's gland adenomas is extremely low. Most patients remain asymptomatic; symptoms which may occur include epigastric pain, bleeding, and obstruction of the duodenum. Endoscopic or local open resection are curative. After surgery patients should receive a treatment with H_2-receptor antagonists if a substantial amount of Brunner's glands have been removed.

Lipomas

Lipomas are smooth submucosal masses with a characteristic yellow appearance on endoscopy. Most remain fairly small, but some may become pedunculated, obstruct the duodenum and cause pain. Intussusception may occur in younger patients. Mucosal erosion may cause bleeding. Enucleation or local excision is sufficient treatment for symptomatic lesions.

Other benign tumours

Haemangiomas and lymphangiomas are well circumscribed submucosal masses, composed of blood vessels or lymphatic vessels, respectively. Bleeding from haemangiomas may be massive enough to require emergency laparotomy. Both tumours tend to be multifocal. Neurofibromas and schwannomas are poorly circumscribed lesions with wavy, fibrillary elements and are identical to those seen elsewhere in neurofibromatosis. However, duodenal involvement is uncommon in von Recklinghausen's disease and less than 20 per cent of neurofibromas are associated with this syndrome. Bleeding is the most common presenting symptom. Symptomatic lesions should be excised. Leiomyomas are discussed together with leiomyosarcomas because they are not easily differentiated from their malignant counterparts.

Malignant duodenal tumours

In contrast to other gastrointestinal malignancies,up to 25 per cent of duodenal malignant tumours are associated synchronously or metachronously with other primary malignancies. These are most often other adenocarcinomas of the intestinal tract, but breast and prostatic adenocarcinoma, bladder carcinoma, and lymphomas have also been associated with adenocarcinoma of the duodenum. Common aetiological factors may be responsible and since the duodenum is a rare site of tumours it has been postulated that there is an underlying defect in immune surveillance which allows malignant tumours to develop in other locations as well. Close monitoring of all patients with duodenal tumours is therefore warranted (Table 2).

Table 2 Prognosis of malignant duodenal tumours

Tumour	5-year survival (%)
Adenocarcinoma	20–40
Villous adenoma	90–100
Neuroendocrine tumours	50–75
Lymphoma	40
Leiomyosarcoma	40–50

Adenocarcinoma

Primary adenocarcinomas of the duodenum are rare, accounting for less than 0.5 per cent of all carcinomas of the gastrointestinal tract. However, the duodenum is the most common site of carcinoma in the small bowel, accounting for 50 per cent of all cases. Virtually all carcinomas of the duodenum are mucin-producing adenocarcinomas originating from glandular epithelium. Macroscopically their appearance ranges from ulcerating and infiltrating to polypoid. Adenocarcinomas most frequently occur in the periampullary region, and approximately 20 per cent of duodenal adenocarcinomas arise in villous adenomas. Rarely, adenocarcinomas are found in a duodenal diverticulum or in patients with non-tropical sprue.

Clinical symptoms of adenocarcinoma of the duodenum depend on the location of the tumour. Fifty per cent of patients present with jaundice and up to 75 per cent of patients have occult blood in their stool. Other common symptoms are frank gastrointestinal haemorrhage and anaemia, abdominal pain, nausea and vomiting, weight loss, pancreatitis, duodenal obstruction, and acute bacterial cholangitis. Although most patients will present with at least one of these symptoms, they are all non-specific and non-diagnostic.

Duodenoscopy is the most sensitive diagnostic procedure because it detects small lesions that may not be visualized by upper gastrointestinal series (Fig. 3) or hypotonic duodenography. If the diagnosis is established endoscopically, however, an upper gastrointestinal series should be performed to search for synchronous jejunal and ileal lesions. It is of utmost importance that the entire duodenum be visualized as the distal duodenum is more often affected than the first portion of the duodenum. One should not be lulled into a false sense of security if endoscopic biopsies fail to reveal carcinoma in a suspicious lesion: the entire lesion should be removed for definitive evaluation. Computed tomography allows assessment of extraluminal spread, involvement of lymph nodes and distant metastasis. Carcinoembryogenic antigen levels tend to be slightly elevated before surgery and should decline after surgery, but they are an unreliable marker for both initial diagnosis and subsequent studies.

The treatment of choice in patients with adenocarcinoma of the duodenum is pancreaticoduodenectomy. Only small tumours in the fourth portion of the duodenum should be treated with distal duodenectomy and duodenojejunostomy. In these cases it may be advisable to place the duodenojejunostomy to the right of the superior mesenteric vessels to avoid placing the anastomosis in the tumour bed. Small tumours of the proximal duodenum in poor risk patients can be resected by extended antrectomy with Billroth II reconstruction. Extreme care should be taken to avoid injuring the accessory pancreatic duct and the common bile duct in these patients.

Both staging and grading have prognostic value. Patients with carcinoma *in situ* have a near 100 per cent 5-year survival provided

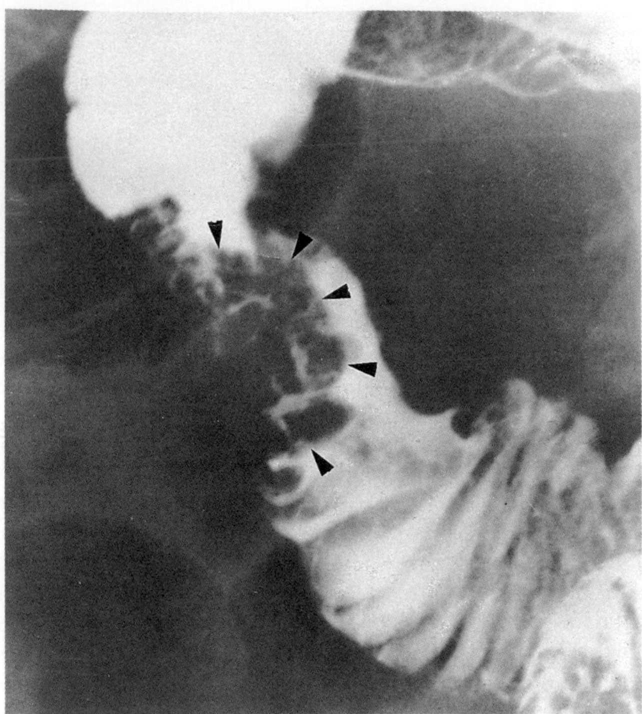

Fig. 3 Polypoid adenocarcinoma of the second portion of the duodenum stenosing the duodenal lumen. (By courtesy of Joseph T. Ferrucci Jr., M.D.)

that the tumour is completely resected. Few lesions are diagnosed at this early stage, but 30 per cent of lesions are discovered before lymph node involvement occurs. Curative resection in these patients carries a 50 to 70 per cent chance of 5-year survival. In patients with resectable lymph node involvement, however, the 5-year survival is only 20 per cent. Up to half of all patients with adenocarcinoma of the duodenum have unresectable lesions, and only occasionally survive for more than 1 year. Patients with well differentiated Grade I or II carcinomas have a 5-year survival greater than 50 per cent. In contrast Grade III lesions carry a 20 per cent 5-year survival and no patient with Grade IV lesions has yet been reported to survive 5 years. When palliative procedures are necessary, biliary obstruction can be relieved with endoprostheses or surgical bypass. Gastrojejunostomy is generally required to relieve duodenal obstruction. Rarely a palliative resection can be completed to treat ongoing haemorrhage. Adjuvant therapy for adenocarcinoma of the duodenum has been of little value. Chemotherapy has shown no significant effect and the side-effects of radiation to the duodenum outweigh its benefits.

Villous adenoma

Some 40 to 50 per cent of villous adenomas of the duodenum harbour adenocarcinoma. In contrast to villous adenomas of the colon, size is not related to their malignant potential (Fig. 4). Villous adenomas may be discovered incidentally on endoscopy or may cause biliary obstruction, bleeding, or duodenal obstruction. The majority of tumours are located around the papilla of Vater and therefore present with symptoms earlier than other duodenal tumours. Although duodenoscopy yields excellent results in visualizing the lesion, up to 50 per cent of carcinomas in villous adenomas are missed by endoscopic biopsy. To obtain a definite diagnosis the entire tumour has to be examined histologically after complete removal. The presence of obstructive jaundice implies malignancy in virtually all cases.

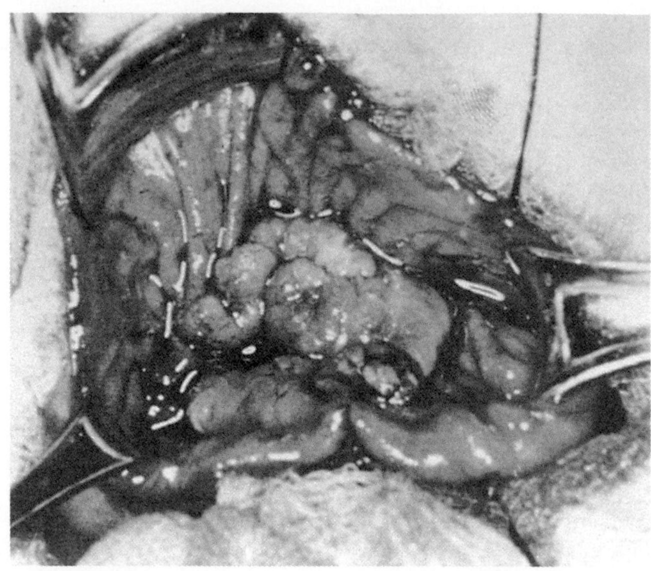

Fig. 4 Villous adenoma of the ampulla, seen through the opened duodenum.

In the few cases with a tumour which is small and pedunculated, endoscopic resection is possible. In all other cases duodenotomy is required. Benign villous adenomas can be locally excised (Fig. 5). For lesions histologically proven to be benign and carcinoma *in situ* removed endoscopically with free margins, close follow-up with frequent duodenoscopy is adequate treatment. Local recurrence occurs in 20 to 50 per cent of patients, making close surveil-

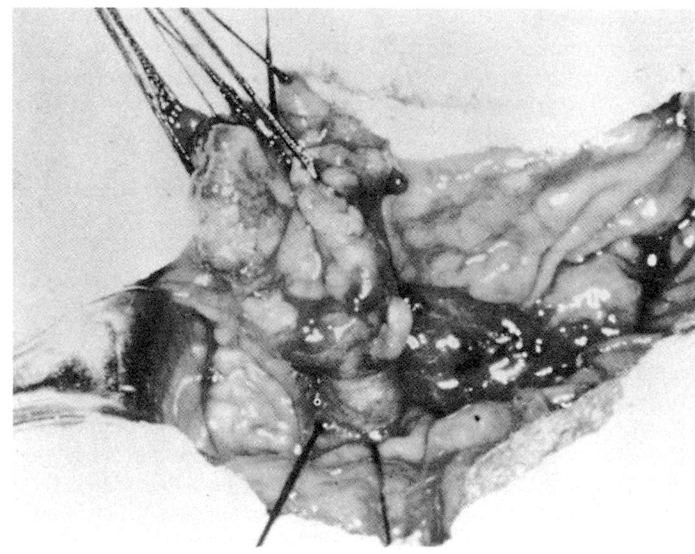

Fig. 5 Submucosal excision of a benign villous adenoma.

lance mandatory. In centres with experience in performing pancreaticoduodenectomies, where the operative mortality is less than 5 per cent, pancreaticoduodenectomy is preferred to local excision. Since one cannot be certain when invasive adenocarcinoma is present, pancreaticoduodenectomy is the treatment of choice.

Carcinoid

Carcinoid tumours are the second most common malignant lesion in the duodenum after adenocarcinomas. They often occur in conjunction with multiple endocrine neoplasia types 1 and 2, von Recklinghausen's neurofibromatosis, and phaeochromocytoma. They may present as adenocarcinoid tumours with glandular and neuroendocrine differentiation. Most tumours measure less than 1 cm in diameter; tumours larger than 1.5 cm are generally malignant and over 90 per cent have metastasized at the time of diagnosis. Few patients ever become symptomatic with carcinoid syndrome from these tumours, and carcinoids are often incidental findings at duodenoscopy or autopsy. However, there is some controversy as to the definition of a carcinoid in the duodenum. For this Section we have considered only serotonin-containing tumours.

Surgical resection is the only therapy for duodenal carcinoid. Local excision is sufficient for benign tumours less than 1.5 cm in diameter; for larger or invasive tumours the rules for resection of adenocarcinoma apply. Trials with radiotherapy and chemotherapy have been disappointing. The prognosis is better than for patients with adenocarcinomas, with overall 5-year survival rates 50 to 75 per cent.

Leiomyoma and leiomyosarcoma

Leiomyomas of the duodenum are the most frequent non-epithelial benign tumours, accounting for about 20 per cent of all benign duodenal tumours. Leiomyomas and leiomyosarcomas occur in all portions of the duodenum. They are well circumscribed, intramural tumours with whorls of smooth muscle closely resembling normal muscularis but usually lacking a true connective tissue capsule. The malignant counterpart, leiomyosarcoma, is not easily distinguished by gross appearance. If the tumour is found to invade adjacent structures or if metastases are found, the malignant nature of the tumour is clear. If the lesion is isolated, only histological evaluation can establish the nature of the tumour. The presence of more than one mitosis per high power field establishes the diagnosis of malignancy.

When symptoms occur, bleeding is the most common complaint. Sarcomas tend to be hypervascular tumours, and haemorrhage, which can occur from central necrosis of the tumour as well as from erosion of the mucosa, may be massive. Large lesions may cause partial duodenal obstruction. Endoscopically, the tumours appear as a smooth, submucosal mass over which the mucosal folds are stretched and effaced. Benign lesions in the distal duodenum can be treated by segmental duodenal resection; if, however, the lesion is close to the papilla, enucleation with preservation or reimplantation of the ampulla is required. If there is any doubt as to the malignancy of the lesion pancreaticoduodenectomy is recommended. Leiomyosarcomas undergo haematogenous spread to the liver and lungs. In selected cases, distant metastases are not a contraindication to surgery as some low grade leiomyosarcomas grow slowly and many patients seem to benefit from aggressive resection of metastatic disease. The role of adjuvant radiotherapy and chemotherapy is under investigation. Generally, sarcomas are much more radiosensitive than adenocarcinomas. Palliative combination chemotherapy with doxorubicin, cyclophosphamide, vincristine, and imidazole carboxamide has yielded response rates over 65 per cent. The long-term prognosis for leiomyosarcomas is intermediate between adenocarcinoma and carcinoid, with 50 per cent of patients surviving 5 years.

Lymphoma

Although primary lymphoma of the duodenum is rare, the duodenum may be involved in systemic lymphoma. Only 5 per cent of all lymphomas are primary intestinal lymphoma and less than 10 per cent of these are located in the duodenum. The only way to establish the diagnosis of primary lymphoma is to exclude the presence of the disease in other organs. Most duodenal lymphomas are non-Hodgkin's lymphomas of B-cell origin. Only a few reports exist of Hodgkin's lymphomas or T-cell lymphomas. Involvement of the mesentery and the draining lymph nodes is common.

Lymphomas are difficult to distinguish from carcinoma preoperatively, though they tend to be larger than carcinomas. Often endoscopic biopsies are non-diagnostic as lymphomas arise in the submucosa. In advanced disease (Fig. 6), however, perforation and multiple lesions are more common in lymphomas than in adenocarcinomas of the small bowel.

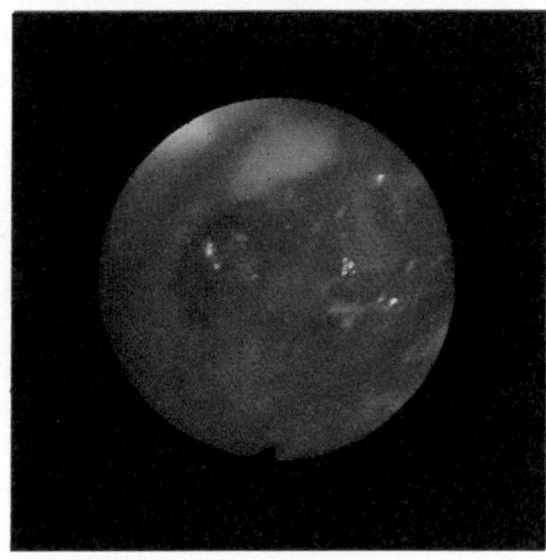

Fig. 6 Advanced B-cell lymphoma with multiple erosions. (By courtesy of Stefan A. Müller-Lissner, M.D.)

Lymphomas cause symptoms similar to those of duodenal and pancreatic carcinomas, and their appearance on computed tomography may be confused with pancreatic cancer. Primary lymphoma of the duodenum can be cured by complete resection in only 40 per cent of patients. The role of adjuvant radiotherapy and chemotherapy has not yet been firmly established, but for the more common jejunal and ileal lymphomas a benefit has been shown. In patients who survive 5 years, recurrence is extremely rare and prognosis is excellent. In patients with unresectable lymphoma, radiotherapy and chemotherapy are the primary therapeutic modalities, surgery being used only to treat complications.

FURTHER READING

Chappuis CW, Divincenti FC, Cohn IJr. Villous tumors of the duodenum. *Ann Surg* 1989; **209**: 593–599.

Donald JW. Major complications of small bowel diverticula. *Ann Surg* 1979; **190**: 183–188, 1979.

Heilbrun N, Boyden EA. Intraluminal duodenal diverticula. *Radiology* 1964; **82**: 887–894.

Hiraoka T, Nakamura M, Ohno K, Imagawa M, Ishida M. Endoscopic excision of intraluminal duodenal diverticulum. *Dig Dis Sci* 1985; **30**: 274–281.

Joesting DR, Beart RW, vanHeerden JA, Weiland LH. Improving survival in adenocarcinoma of the duodenum. *Ann J Surg* 1981; **141**: 228–231.

Komoroswki RA, Cohen EB. Villous tumors of the duodenum: a clinicopathological study. *Cancer* 1981; **47**: 1377–1386.

Løtveit T, Skar V, Osnes M. Juxtapapillary duodenal diverticula. *Endoscopy* 1988; **20**: 175–178.

Pinotti HW, Tacla M, Pontes JF, Betarello A. Surgical procedures upon juxta-ampullar duodenal diverticula. *Surg Gynecol Obstet* 1972; **135**: 11–16.

Ryan DP, Schapiro RH, Warshaw AL. Villous tumors of the duodenum. *Ann Surg* 1986; **203**: 301–306.

Spigelman AD, Williams CB, Talbot IC, Domizio P, Phillips RKS. Upper gastrointestinal cancer in patients with familial adenomatous polyposis. *Lancet* 1989; i: 783–785.

Williamson RCN, Welch CE, Malt RA. Adenocarcinoma and lymphoma of the small intestine. Distribution and etiologic associations. *Ann Surg* 1983; **197**: 172–178.

Wilson JM, Melvin DB, Gray G, Thorbjarnarson B. Benign small bowel tumor. *Ann Surg* 1975; **18**: 247–250.

15.5 Gastritis

THOROLF SUNDT III

Gastritis may be an acute or chronic condition. The acute form may be precipitated by the ingestion of chemicals such as salicylates, non-steroidal anti-inflammatory agents, acid, and alkali. Other possible causes include thermal injury, ionizing radiation, uraemia, generalized stress, and shock following infection by Gram-negative bacteria. Damage to the gastric mucosal barrier results in acute inflammation, with oedema and polymorphonuclear infiltration of the mucosa, submucosa, and lamina propria. In severe cases this process can lead to ischaemia, followed by sloughing of necrotic mucosa and by erosive gastritis or frank ulcer formation. For the most part, acute gastritis is self-limiting and is amenable to medical therapy alone; operative intervention is required in only a small percentage of cases. Appropriate surgical treatment of the complications of acute gastritis may involve simple oversewing of ulcerations, vagotomy and pyloroplasty, or even total gastric resection, as dictated by the nature of the specific case.

The common forms of chronic gastritis—chronic superficial gastritis, atrophic gastritis, and gastric atrophy—exist as a spectrum of disease with respect to both mucosal inflammation and glandular atrophy. The inflammatory infiltrate typically seen in chronic gastritis is composed predominantly of lymphocytes and plasma cells, and may be limited to the mucosa or extend into the muscularis. The degree of glandular cell atrophy is not related to the intensity of the infiltrate in a simple fashion, little inflammation typically being seen in patients with complete gastric atrophy. Chronic superficial gastritis is characterized by limitation of the inflammatory infiltrate to the foveolar region of gastric mucosa without appreciable glandular atrophy. In chronic atrophic gastritis a variable degree of parietal loss of chief cells is seen. In true gastric atrophy glandular elements are entirely lost, although mucus-secreting cells are retained in the gastric pits. The gross pathological and endoscopic appearance of atrophic gastritis is that of a friable, grey mucosa with reduced or absent folds. Chronic superficial gastritis may be difficult to recognize grossly, endoscopic biopsy being required for diagnosis.

Functional alterations associated with atrophic gastritis include reduction in both basal acid output and maximal acid response, which may exceed that predicted on the basis of the degree of glandular cell loss observed histologically. Decreased secretion of pepsinogen and intrinsic factor are also observed. Because most of these abnormalities are asymptomatic, chronic gastritis is often diagnosed as an incidental finding during evaluation of an acute episode. Frank pernicious anaemia occurs only with the development of autoantibodies to intrinsic factor, as well as to parietal cell components. Only a fraction of patients producing such antibodies suffer inadequate cobalamin absorption, however, and functional assessment is required to establish the diagnosis.

Two forms of chronic atrophic gastritis have been defined on serological, morphological, and functional grounds. Type A is characterized by the presence of antibody to parietal cells. Mucosal abnormalities typically affect the corpus of the stomach diffusely, resulting in severe impairment of acid secretion. The antrum is spared and gastrin secretion is frequently elevated. It is this form that may progress to pernicious anaemia. Parietal cell antibody is not detectable in patients with type B gastritis. Patchy mucosal changes of the corpus with only moderate secretory impairment and extensive antral involvement are characteristic; serum gastrin levels are often low. This is the more common form and has been referred to as antral gastritis.

The pathogenesis of chronic gastritis remains unclear. Ageing is a factor; the condition appears to be quite common among the elderly, which is associated with Hashimoto's thyroiditis, hyperthyroidism, hypothyroidism, insulin-dependent diabetes mellitus, hypoparathyroidism, and addisonian hypoadrenalism. An increased incidence of pernicious anaemia among first-degree relatives of those with the condition further suggests that autoimmune response genes may be involved. The development of type B gastritis may be related to repeated episodes of acute gastritis or to chronic irritation due to duodenal reflux. Infection with the spiral Gram-negative bacterium *Helicobacter pylori* has been associated with gastric and duodenal ulcer, dyspepsia, and gastritis of the antral form. There is mounting evidence that *H. pylori* infection the cause, not the consequence, of chronic gastritis. Chronic superficial gastritis resulted after an investigator intentionally ingested the organism, and improvement in symptoms has been observed following treatment for such infection. Unfortunately, effective antimicrobial therapy is hindered by the acid environment of the stomach. It is likely that antral gastritis. shares aetiological factors with gastric ulcer. Alternatively it may be a precursor lesion: such ulcers are often associated with type B gastritis.

The sequelae of chronic gastritis include haemorrhage and carcinoma, and both are apparently more common in patients with type B gastritis than in those with type A disease. The incidence of both approaches 10 per cent, but the true risk of carcinoma in patients with atrophic gastritis is difficult to estimate, as rates of gastric cancer vary greatly between populations, and the prevalence of chronic gastritis is uncertain. Since atrophic gastritis is common, routine surveillance endoscopy is not generally recommended for patients with chronic gastritis among populations in which the incidence of gastric malignancy is low.

Metaplasia is often seen in atrophic gastritis and may be intestinal or pseudopyloric in type, the latter being more commonly associated with antral gastritis. Although metaplasia is not necessarily premalignant, atrophic gastritis with intestinal metaplasia is often found in patients with adenocarcinoma. Experimental models of gastric carcinoma in rats using *N*-methyl-*N'*-nitro-*N*-nitrosoguanidine demonstrate both cancer and intestinal metaplasia, suggesting an association with similar causative factors, if not progression from one to the other.

Multiple carcinoids and endocrine cell micronests can occur in the fundal mucosa of patients with Type A atrophic gastritis. This phenomenon may be related to the trophic action of gastrin, which is present in high levels in patients with this form of atrophic gastritis. Because such tumours can metastasize, excision is recommended for isolated carcinoid tumours. Multifocal disease requires either total gastrectomy or careful endoscopic surveillance.

There may be an increased risk of carcinoma following gastric resection. Experimentally, an increased risk of malignancy has been demonstrated, possibly resulting from the development of atrophic gastritis and intestinal metaplasia secondary to chronic bile reflux. There is increased cell turnover and development of carcinoma following a gastrectomy and Polya reconstruction (which is associated with bile reflux) in experimental animals fed *N*-methyl-*N'*-nitro-*N*-nitrosoguanidine.

In a recent comparison of patients who underwent Billroth I, Billroth II, or Roux-en-Y reconstructions following gastric resection, atrophic gastritis and intestinal metaplasia seemed more common following the Billroth operations. Metaplasia was generally moderate, and no evidence of carcinoma occurred in this series. Because patients were usually symptomatic following Roux-en-Y reconstructions, however, there was no clear mandate against the Billroth operation.

The less common forms of chronic gastritis include chronic cystic gastritis, in which flattened epithelial cells line dilated gastric glands deep in the lamina propria. Granulomatous gastritis related to tuberculous infection, sarcoid, or Crohn's disease is characterized by antral and duodenal involvement with mucosal inflammation and ulceration that may lead to gastric outlet obstruction. Eosinophilic gastritis is a rare condition in which eosinophils infiltrate the distal stomach and the proximal small bowel to a variable extent, resulting in enlargement of antral folds and simulating the giant hypertrophic gastritis characteristic of Ménétrier's disease. Although this condition may lead to obstruction, it is generally amenable to medical therapy alone.

FURTHER READING

Graham DY, Klein PD. *Campylobacter pyloridis* gastritis: the past, the present, and speculations about the future. *Am J Gastroenterol*, 1987; **82**: 283–6.

Houghton PWJ, Mortensen NJMcL, Williamson RCN. Effect of duodenogastric reflux on gastric mucosal proliferation after gastric surgery. *Br J Surg*, 1987: **74**: 288–91.

Ihmäki T, Saukkonen M, Siurala M. Long-term observations of subjects with normal mucosa and superficial gastritis: results of 23–27 years' follow-up examination. *Scand J Gastroenterol*, 1978; **13**: 771–5.

Itsuno M, *et al.* Multiple carcinoids and endocrine cell micronests in Type A gastritis: their morphology, histogenesis, and natural history. *Cancer*, 1989; **63**: 881–90.

Ovsaka JT, Ekfors TO, Luukkonen PE, Lempinen MJ. Histologic changes in the gastric stump mucosa and late clinical results after Billroth I< Billroth II and Roux-en-Y operations for peptic ulcer disease. *Ann Chir Gynaecol*, 1988; **77**: 1–5.

Strickland RG, MacKay IR. A reappraisal for the nature and significance of chronic atrophic gastritis. *Am J Dig Dis*, 1973; **18**: 426–40.

15.6 Ménétrier's disease

THOROLF SUNDT III

The condition which is called hypertrophic gastropathy, hypertrophic gastritis, or hyperplastic gastropathy, is uncommon and is characterized by massive enlargement of rugal folds in the body and fundus of the stomach (Fig. 1). It is most widely known by its eponymic title, Ménétrier's disease. Ménétrier (1859–1935) did not define a syndrome; rather he reported in 1888 the postmortem observations of two patients showing extraordinary gastric pathology in association with gastric cancer. The stomachs of both patients were filled with tenacious mucus and demonstrated similar microscopic pathology. One patient had ascites and peripheral oedema; the other had recently suffered a major cerebral infarction. Although Ménétrier acknowledged that others had observed patients exhibiting such giant enlargement of gastric folds before him, his name has been linked with this condition.

DIAGNOSTIC CRITERIA

Although conceptions of the disorder differ widely in detail, there is agreement that the finding of enlarged gastric rugae in the body and fundus, largely sparing the antrum, and exclusive of those of granulomatous or neoplastic origin, is central to the diagnosis of Ménétrier's disease. Radiological criteria reflecting this gross pathology are similarly broadly accepted. Microscopically, the foveolar compartment is typically expanded with elongated and branched gastric pits, often with focal cystic dilatation. The deep compartment may be hyperplastic, normal, or atrophic, with cystic dilation of gastric glands. Ming has attempted to define three microscopic patterns of hypertrophic gastropathy: mucous cell predominant, glandular cell predominant, and a mixed mucous–

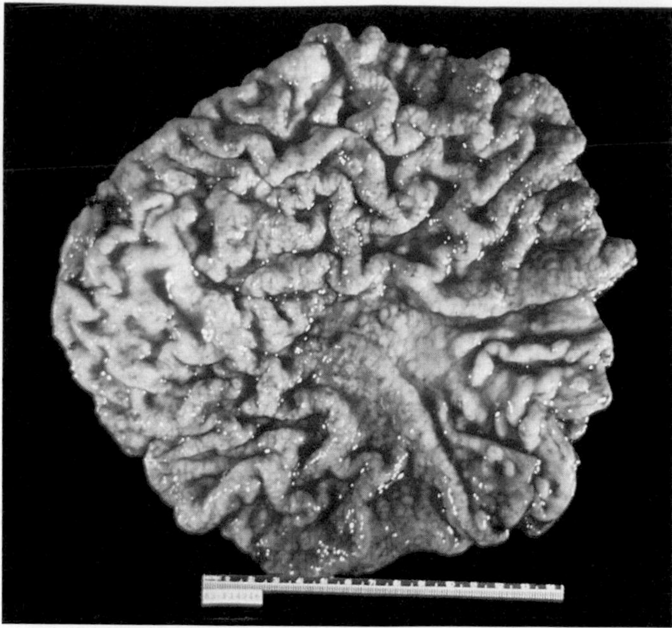

Fig. 1 Massive enlargement of rugal folds in the body and fundus of the stomach in Ménétrier's disease.

glandular type. Some authors have suggested that only the mucous cell type should be considered representative of Ménétrier's disease, but Ming made no such claim; in fact he suggested that the patient reported by Ménétrier probably had the mixed cell type hyperplasia.

In the middle of this century several studies identified hypoproteinaemia and hypochlorhydria as frequently associated findings in patients exhibiting pathological findings similar to those reported by Ménétrier. Since then, some authors have applied one or both of these as diagnostic criteria, but this policy is far from universal.

Attempts to subdivide hypertrophic gastropathies on the basis of such criteria have resulted in a plethora of descriptive labels, but have been largely unsuccessful in clarifying the disorder because of overlap among groups of patients. There is poor correlation between acid secretion and serum protein levels. Furthermore, there is an imperfect relationship between these parameters and the mucosal histology as defined by Ming's criteria. Additional confusion stems from inconsistencies in evaluation of cases of suspected Ménétrier's disease, making it difficult to be certain that all are in fact *bona fide*. In a recent review of 125 cases diagnosed as Ménétrier's disease over a 26-year period, sufficient data to merit an unequivocal diagnosis were available for only six patients.

This quagmire is best avoided by focusing on the hallmarks of each case. As each of the diagnostic features appears to lie along a spectrum which may vary not only between patients, but possibly over time within the same individual, we have suggested the rubric *trivalent gastropathy*, emphasizing the importance of defining these parameters in each instance and without arbitrarily implying relationships among these aspects. In all cases of suspected Ménétrier's disease measurement of serum albumin and gastrin levels (to rule out the Zollinger-Ellison syndrome, which can also produce gastric mucosal hypertrophy), gastric acid secretion studies, and a full-thickness gastric biopsy are mandatory.

TREATMENT

Therapy is directed to relieving pain (present in over 80 per cent of cases) blood loss (34 per cent), and symptoms of hypoproteinaemia (40 per cent). Anticholinergic therapy may diminish acid secretion and possibly tighten gastric cell junctions, reducing protein losses via this route. H_2-receptor blockers may have similar effects. These are only temporary measures, however, and do not address the risk of gastric carcinoma. Furthermore, it is unclear whether they have any effect on the hypercoagulable state often associated with Ménétrier's syndrome.

Surgical resection offers a definitive solution. Distal subtotal gastrectomy with a Billroth I or Billroth II reconstruction is to be discouraged, as it would entail anastomosis of abnormal stomach to normal intestine with the attendant risks of anastomotic leakage and obstruction. Vagotomy and pyloroplasty avoids such an anastomosis and offers a reduction in acid output, but fails to address the risk of neoplasia. Total gastrectomy is the best therapeutic solution to Ménétrier's disease and is generally well tolerated. Employing only normal tissues in the reconstruction, all abnormalities are corrected, and the risk of gastric neoplasia is removed.

The risk of gastric cancer in the setting of Ménétrier's disease is difficult to quantify. Retrospective analyses have found neoplasia in 10 to 15 per cent of reported cases; prospective studies are difficult, given the rarity of the condition. The increased cell proliferation essential for carcinogenesis in most epithelial systems might be expected to create a fertile field for the development of carcinoma in hyperplastic gastric mucosa. In two of the six cases we have recently reported, gastric carcinoma developed years after the initial diagnosis of Ménétrier's disease and, in another, the full spectrum of preneoplastic to malignant epithelial changes was seen. The safety of medical management with routine endoscopy is uncertain, because the sensitivity of such surveillance with random biopsy in the setting of such a diffusely abnormal organ is unknown. The association of adenocarcinoma with Ménétrier's disease appears real and makes the argument for total gastrectomy stronger.

FURTHER READING

Sundt TM III, Compton CC, Malt RA. Ménétrier's disease: a trivalent gastropathy. *Ann Surg* 1988; **208**: 694–701.

15.7 Gastric volvulus and acute gastric dilatation

HUGH BARR

GASTRIC VOLVULUS

Introduction

Gastric volvulus is an abnormal rotation of the whole or part of the stomach. The terminology does not distinguish between 'torsion', which is simple rotation, and true volvulus, which implies luminal obstruction. Little attention is paid to the difference, although volvulus is more dangerous because of the risk of necrosis and perforation. Berti first described the condition in 1866: he reported the postmortem findings in a 60-year-old female of 'an entire mass of organs making two complete horizontal turns, the oesophagus and the duodenum were interlaced'. Subsequently Berg described the successful operative treatment of gastric volvulus in two patients in 1895 and 1896. The detailed review and observations in 1930 by Buchanan clarified the anatomical variants associated with this rare condition, and aetiological factors were clearly addressed by Tanner (1968).

Anatomy and aetiology

The stomach is maintained in its normal position by four ligaments. The lesser curve and liver are joined by the gastrohepatic ligament, the greater curve is attached to the spleen and transverse colon by the gastrosplenic and gastrocolic ligaments, and the cardia is held fixed by the phrenicoesophageal ligament. Some form of ligament abnormality (extreme laxity, absence, or disruption) is essential to allow rotation; the direction of rotation is determined by which ligaments are lax and which points remain relatively fixed. The condition can be broadly classified into two groups.

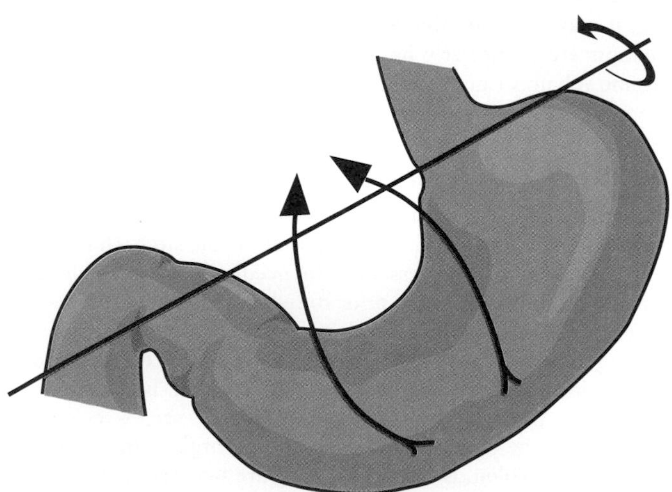

Fig. 1 Organoaxial volvulus with axis of rotation.

Organoaxial volvulus (Fig. 1)

The pylorus and oesophagogastric junction remain relatively fixed and rotation occurs around a line between these two. There are two subgroups of this condition. In the first (posterior organoaxial) the stomach rotates through 180° left to right, such that the anterior surface is facing backward. The posterior surface presents under the abdominal wall and is covered by the mesocolon when, as is usual, the transverse colon has participated in the rotation. In some patients the colon remains in an inferior position due to extreme laxity or rupture of the gastrocolic ligament. Thus two further subgroups of posterior organoaxial volvulus can be defined, dependent on the position of the stomach in relation to the colon, the infracolic and the supracolic. The spleen and pancreas may also be displaced with the stomach.

The second, and rarer type is anterior organoaxial volvulus. The greater curve passes backwards and presents in the lesser sac, resulting in the anteriorly facing posterior gastric wall being covered by the gastrohepatic ligament. Rotation cannot usually proceed beyond 180°. This type of volvulus is often partial. In a number of patients the cardia remains in place while only the antral portion of the stomach rotates. This abnormality may be seen in association with an hourglass stomach in which a large antral pouch has formed, which is able to pivot on its margins.

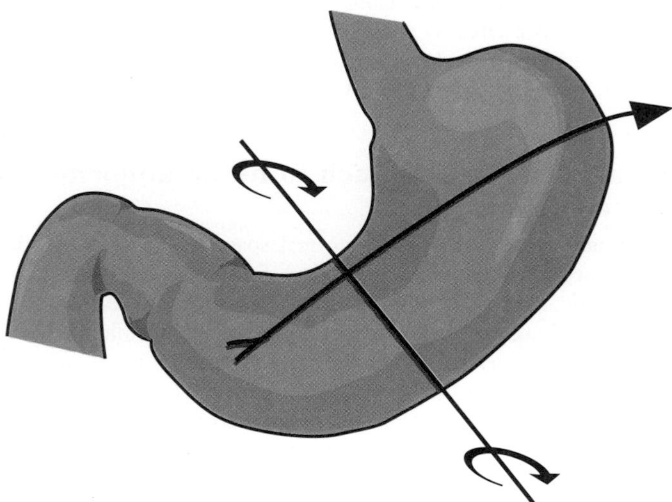

Fig. 2 Mesenteroaxial volvulus with axis of rotation.

Mesenteroaxial volvulus (Fig. 2)

Rotation from right to left around a vertical line at right angles to the axis of rotation of organoaxial volvulus. The cardia remains in position and a mobile pylorus rotates anteriorly or posteriorly until it is in juxtaposition with the cardia. The anterior wall is sharply kinked and folded on itself, while the posterior wall is covered by a lax gastrocolic ligament. The right half of the transverse colon is carried up in front of the volvulus towards the splenic flexure. The remainder of the abdominal organs remain undisplaced.

Organoaxial volvulus is most common in adults, accounting for 50 per cent of reported cases. Mesenteroaxial volvulus accounts for 29 per cent, and a combination is reported in 2 per cent. The remainder have not been classified. In infants and children, however, mesenteroaxial volvulus accounts for 53 per cent of reported cases, with organoaxial volvulus in 35 per cent and a combination in 5 per cent.

Predisposing factors

Although ligamentous laxity must be present there are a number of conditions that are associated with the development of volvulus. These can be divided into three groups.

1. Abnormalities of the stomach
2. Abnormalities of the surrounding viscera
3. Rotation of the stomach to fill an abnormal space

Abnormalities of the stomach

These include conditions that produce acute or chronic distension. Pyloric stenosis and duodenal obstruction result in elongation of the ligaments and gastric ptosis. A heavy bolus lying in the lower part of the greater curve may act as a lower fixed point around which mesenteroaxial rotation can occur. In infants, absence or attenuation of ligaments may be a result of failure of fusion of fetal visceral mesenteries, and the presence of congenital bands may predispose to volvulus.

Abnormalities of the surrounding viscera

Splenomegaly, producing elongation of the gastrosplenic ligament, has been cited as an aetiological factor. Other conditions that are associated include volvulus of the transverse colon and midgut, and dislocation and hypoplasia of the left lobe of the liver.

Rotation of the stomach to fill an abnormal space

The stomach may enter an abnormal space in association with a para-oesophageal hernia, in other forms of hiatus or diaphragmatic hernia, or with congenital or acquired eventration of the diaphragm. Approximately 65 per cent of children with gastric volvulus have an associated eventration or hernia of the left hemidiaphragm. In a study of infants younger than 12 months, 81 per cent had one of these anomalies. In adults the most common association is an organoaxial volvulus in a large paraoesophageal hernia: in one series, 15 per cent of 138 surgically treated para-oesophageal hernias contained an intrathoracic gastric volvulus.

Diagnosis

The clinical presentation of gastric volvulus is entirely dependent on whether it is acute with complete obstruction and/or strangulation, or chronic and associated with partial obstruction and no ischaemia. An acute event may occur in a stomach that has had a chronic volvulus.

Acute volvulus

A diagnostic triad of vomiting followed by non-productive retching, localized epigastric pain, and failure to pass a nasogastric tube are symptoms which indicate obstruction of the gastro-oesophageal junction. True vomiting is unlikely to occur: instead frothy white material and saliva is regurgitated. In the initial phase there is likely to be few abdominal physical signs, although gastric distension may occur and signs of peritonitis and perforation follow strangulation.

The classic triad is often difficult to interpret in infants, since pain and retching are non-specific, and the failure to pass a nasogastric tube may be difficult to interpret. In older patients the condition can be difficult to distinguish from myocardial ischaemia: an electrocardiogram is often helpful. The plain radiograph appearance is often dramatic in both adults and children, with a hugely dilated stomach and a double fluid level on the erect film. In patients with eventration or diaphragmatic hernias the inverted stomach may be seen in the chest. Contrast studies are often unhelpful, since retching renders the study dangerous and will only demonstrate obstruction with no contrast entering the stomach.

Chronic volvulus

Chronic or recurrent volvulus presents a clinical picture that may be mistaken for gallbladder disease, gastritis, or peptic ulceration. Pain is often mild and episodic, although bouts of upper abdominal colic and vomiting can occur. Dysphagia may be present if the oesophagogastric junction is distorted, and eructation of swallowed air can be difficult. After meals gastric peristalsis may be noisy and cause embarrassment, a situation that is relieved by lying down. There are no characteristic physical signs. In contrast to acute volvulus radiographs using contrast media may demonstrate the abnormality.

Treatment

Acute volvulus requires immediate preoperative resuscitation followed by urgent laparotomy. The stomach must be derotated, gangrenous areas resected, and the stomach fixed with repair of any associated defects. Although passage of a nasogastric tube will deflate the stomach and occasionally produce spontaneous reduction, it may perforate the oesophagus or stomach, and persistent attempts are particularly hazardous in infants. The treatment of chronic volvulus can proceed more slowly, with careful preoperative evaluation and assessment of the risks of surgery.

Decompression and derotation

An upper midline incision provides adequate access in adults; a transverse incision is required in children. If the stomach is massively distended decompression with needle, trochar, or gastrotomy aspiration is necessary prior to reduction. If a gastronomy is performed it should be closed immediately, since the gastric opening may migrate to an inaccessible position on reduction. Careful inspection of the stomach for areas of ischaemia, including the posterior wall through the lesser sac, is essential. Resection of the stomach and surrounding organs, in particular the transverse colon, is required if they are non-viable. Once the stomach is reduced the remainder of the procedure aims to prevent a recurrence.

Fixation and prevention of recurrence

Conditions predisposing to volvulus should be dealt with directly, and this may be all that is required. In patients without a predisposing cause or where the causative defect does not lend itself to surgical correction, or when this is inappropriate in an ill frail patient, some form of gastropexy should be performed. The simplest involves the formation of a gastrotomy: this technique is particularly suitable in children, tethering the stomach to the anterior abdominal wall. However, recurrence is common following simple fixation. It must be remembered that most infants have a diaphragmatic defect that requires correction. Gastroenterostomy and partial gastrectomy should be restricted to patients with peptic ulcer disease, who require definitive surgery for this. Tanner recommended gastropexy with colonic displacement in patients with eventration of the left diaphragm. The colon is detached from the stomach and placed under the left hemidiaphragm to fill the space; the lesser curve of the stomach is then sutured to the edge of the liver and falciform ligament. This form of gastropexy carries the lowest recurrence rate. An operation devised by Opolzer, comprising a side-to-side fundus to antral gastrogastrostomy is not to be recommended, since it allows the volvulus to remain and oesophageal and pyloric obstruction can still occur. Following surgery, prolonged gastric stasis may occur and a gastrostomy is useful to maintain decompression.

ACUTE GASTRIC DILATATION

In modern surgical practice this is a rare disorder, but it can produce profound circulatory disturbance and death. It is akin to paralytic ileus and the same factors are often the cause. Acute gastric dilatation may occur following gastric or abdominal surgery, trauma, retroperitoneal haematoma, hypoxia, or electrolyte disturbance. It appears to be slightly more common in women and children, and may be seen in sedated patients receiving oxygen via nasal catheters.

Presentation

The clinical presentation is sufficiently distinct to allow differentiation from paralytic ileus. The patient develops tachycardia, and may become shocked; hiccups are common and may be followed by belching, and enormous and effortless vomiting. The vomitus has a characteristic appearance that was described by Hamilton Bailey as the colour of 'storm water of a peat laden stream'. There may be upper abdominal distension. The condition can be suspected clinically and the distended stomach can often be outlined by percussion. The diagnosis is confirmed by the passage of a nasogastric tube and the aspiration of copious volumes of fluid. A plain abdominal or chest radiograph will demonstrate a hugely distended stomach. The condition can be fatal since vomitus may be aspirated and the hypovolaemia from fluid loss is considerable.

Treatment

The stomach is decompressed by nasogastric suction and the fluid and electrolyte loss replaced intravenously. An underlying cause should be sought and corrected if present, but this is generally not the case, and following decompression for several days spontaneous recovery of gastric function occurs.

FURTHER READING

Buchanan J. Volvulus of the stomach. *Br J Surg*, 1930; **18**: 99–108.

Cole BC, Dickinson SJ. Acute volvulus of the stomach in infants and children. *Surgery*, 1971; **70**: 707–15.

Haas O, Rat P, Christophe M, Friedman S, Favre JP. Surgical results of intrathoracic gastric volvulus complicating hiatal hernia. *Br J Surg*, 1990; **77**: 1379–81.

Tanner NC. Chronic and recurrent volvulus of the stomach. *Am J Surg*, 1968; **115**: 505–15.

Wastell C, Ellis H. Volvulus of the stomach: a review with a report of 8 cases. *Br J Surg*, 1971; **58**: 557–62.

15.8 Foreign bodies and bezoars

MICHAEL N. MARGOLIES

FOREIGN BODIES

Ingested foreign bodies occur most often in children under the age of 3 years, in patients with psychiatric disorders, in patients who use excess alcohol and drugs, among convicts, and in denture wearers. More than 99 per cent of ingested foreign bodies are asymptomatic: the principal risk associated with foreign body ingestion in children is oesophageal impaction and injury. More than 95 per cent of objects that reach the stomach pass through the gastrointestinal tract without ill effect, and guilt and anxiety of the parents often require more attention than does the child who has swallowed an object. The role of the surgeon is to identify the occasional patient in whom surgical treatment is needed. The history may or may not be reliable, depending upon parental observation of objects held by the infant. The majority of potentially harmful objects are radio-opaque. Radiographs should encompass the entire gastrointestinal tract from pharynx to anus. Non-radio-opaque objects may be further localized using contrast studies. Endoscopy is useful to differentiate intragastric objects from neoplasms.

Foreign bodies in asymptomatic patients for the most part should be allowed to progress through the gastrointestinal tract spontaneously, monitored by serial radiographs. Foreign bodies are frequently missed on stool examinations, which are not usually sufficiently assiduous. Unless a particular object has a known capacity for causing mischief, or outpatient observation is not reliable, children need not be kept in hospital.

The indications for operative removal of gastric foreign bodies include: signs of obstruction, perforation, or bleeding; accumulation of multiple foreign bodies in the stomach; certain large or long sharp objects; objects known to result in toxicity; failure of the foreign body to leave the stomach, and impaction.

Gastric outlet obstruction due to a foreign body is not encountered as frequently as is small bowel obstruction. Haemorrhage may occur following local mucosal ulceration at the site of impaction. Ulceration secondary to prolonged foreign body retention usually heals once the foreign body is removed. Perforation of the stomach and duodenum often presents as a fistula into adjacent organs, including the liver in the case of gastric perforations and the right kidney or inferior vena cava in the case of sharp objects in the adjacent duodenum. Late perforations complicating toothpick, chicken, or fishbone ingestion are insidious and associated with much morbidity; they are rarely identified preoperatively.

Smooth objects are innocuous in the stomach, and considerable patience should be exercised to permit their passage. Even remarkably large objects such as scissors or tableware can pass through the gastrointestinal tract in the adult. Gastric retention of foreign bodies may be related to pre-existing pyloric stenosis. If after 4 weeks the object remains, or if the object is larger than the duodenal loop, or long and sharp, removal using fibreoptic endoscopy is indicated. A variety of grasping forceps and snares have been devised for removal. For ferrous metal objects successful removal using a magnet attached to a nasogastric tube is useful in paediatric patients, and anaesthesia is not required. Endoscopic removal carries the risk of oesophageal damage or impaction upon withdrawal; endoscopic devices should be equipped with a protective sheath drawn over the object at the time of withdrawal. One might argue that if a foreign body can be safely extracted by endoscopy it can usually be left to pass naturally.

Objects likely to cause perforation or impaction include those that are long, sharp, and pointed, such as open safety pins or hair grips in children under 2 years, toothpicks, needles, and toothbrushes, as well as objects with a configuration likely to prevent passage thorugh the pylorus or through the second portion of the duodenum. Of all gastrointestinal tract perforations due to foreign body one-quarter to one-half occur in the stomach or duodenum. Alkaline disc batteries are innocuous unless there is radiographic evidence of disruption of the battery case, which may result in leakage and caustic damage to the stomach wall. In the case of narcotic packet ingestion for purposes of smuggling, endoscopic removal is contraindicated as intragastric breakage of the package may prove fatal (Fig. 1).

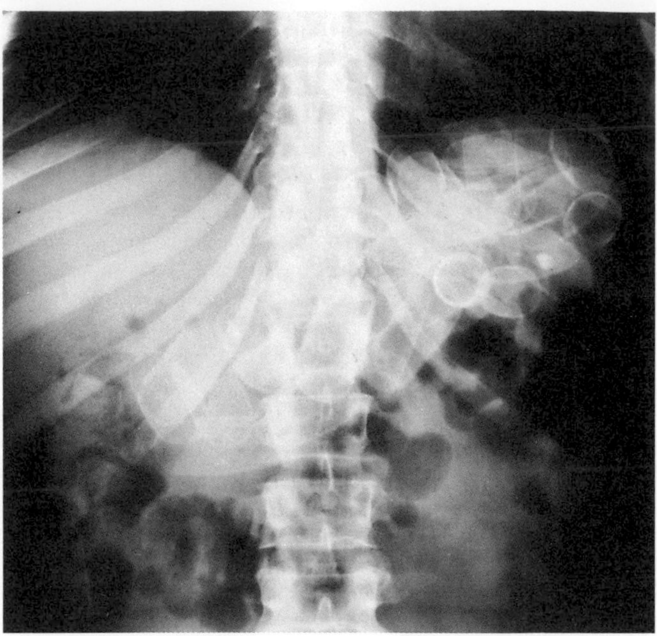

Fig. 1 Abdominal radiograph of a 35-year-old male who swallowed multiple heroin packets.

If endoscopic removal fails or there is evidence of obstruction, perforation, or bleeding, surgical gastrotomy should be performed. It is important to obtain an immediate preoperative film to be sure that the object has not migrated. Removal of non-impacted duodenal foreign bodies may be simplified by manually replacing the object into the stomach; otherwise duodenotomy is necessary. If multiple foreign objects are present the small bowel should always be examined.

BEZOARS

Bezoars are concretions of ingested material, originally described in animals. They are of considerable historical and now clinical interest. Bezoar is a transliteration of the Arabic *badzehr* or the Turkish *panzehr*, meaning antidote. The oriental bezoar is found in the stomach and intestine of the bezoar goat *Capra aegagyrus* or that of the gazelle, *Antelope dorcas*. Bezoar stones were prized until the eighteenth century as cures for a variety of diseases—a large bezoar stone set in gold was included in the inventory of the crown jewels at the time of the ascension of James I to the English throne in 1662.

The classification of bezoar into four types is somewhat arbitrary in that the term is usually reserved for concretions of ingested food or chemicals; high fibre food boluses are close relatives.

Trichobezoars consist of a mass of ingested hair combined with other fibres, and usually occur in young women (90 per cent), including some with psychiatric difficulties. The hair forms a black cast of the stomach with a glistening mucoid appearance and a foul odour (Fig. 2).

The most common type of phytobezoar, concretions of botanic origin, occur following the ingestion of persimmons (*Diospyros virginiana*). In the south-eastern United States this bezoar occurs typically in hunters who eat this fruit when unripe. Related

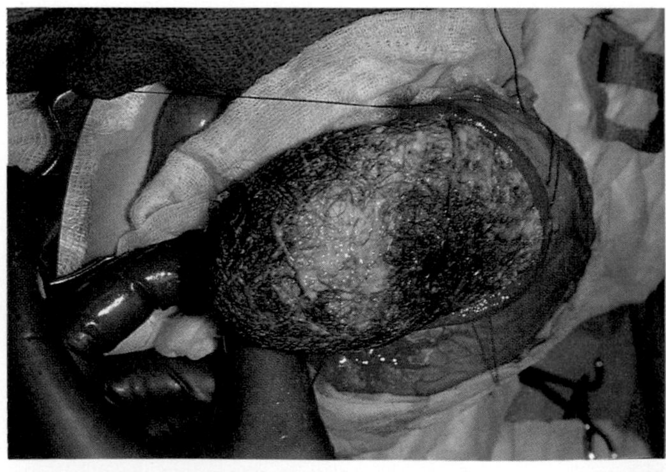

Fig. 2 Gastric trichobezoar at gastrotomy in a young girl.

members of the same genus are found in Israel, Japan, Korea, India, and Zimbabwe. Unripe persimmons contain large amounts of a soluble phlobatannin which coagulates in the stomach to form a tenacious glue that entraps fibres. This type of bezoar is also known as a '*diospyrobezoar*'. A second common type of phytobezoar follows ingestion of citrus fruits, although an immense variety of other vegetable matter has also been implicated. Incompletely chewed citrus segments are hygroscopic and expand in the small bowel, sometimes causing obstruction. Trichophytobezoar is a combination of the two forms mentioned above.

Bezoars may also be formed by concretions of medications or chemicals. The shellac bezoar occurs in furniture workers who imbibe an alcoholic solution of shellac; the shellac precipitates in the stomach, particularly when this cocktail is followed by water. The relative incidence of neonatal lactobezoar and antacid bezoar has increased, the former being associated with prematurity, and the latter with intensive antacid therapy in high-risk hospital inpatients, particularly those in renal failure.

Factors predisposing to bezoar formation include both diet and pre-existing gastroduodenal pathology. In addition to the binge eating of persimmons or citrus fruits, monotonous high fibre diets during famine or following periods of religious fast or at harvest time in the tropics may produce bezoars. During the past several decades the most common form of bezoars in developed countries has been found in patients who have undergone gastric surgery. These phytobezoars, 90 per cent of which are composed of citrus fruits, occur several months to many years after any surgical procedure with the potential for altering gastric emptying. They occur in 5 to 14 per cent of postgastrectomy patients. Postgastrectomy bezoars occur in patients with poor dentition, high fibre intake, reduced gastric acid production and gastric stasis with or without partial gastric outlet obstruction. An increased incidence of bezoar may also occur in patients with diabetic gastroparesis or other neurological conditions affecting the stomach, such as autonomic neuropathy and myotonic dystrophy.

Gastric bezoars may be asymptomatic and found only incidentally. When symptoms occur they are due to the size of the bezoar and its complications—most commonly obstruction, and less often bleeding or perforation. Large masses may cause a sensation of epigastric fullness and early satiety. Nausea, vomiting, and abdominal pain are common due to the size of the mass or obstruction, or associated ulceration. Gastric outlet obstruction is uncommon in phytobezoar but can certainly cause partial outlet obstruction after gastrectomy. However, small bowel obstruction due to migration or fragmentation of a gastric bezoar is common. Obstruction may follow attempts at endoscopic fragmentation. Intestinal obstruction due to bezoar is seen in patients with an intact gastrointestinal tract, as well as in those who have undergone gastric surgery.

Patients with a large trichobezoar may suffer weight loss, anaemia, gastrointestinal bleeding, and obstructive symptoms. Trichobezoars may extend from the stomach into and through the entire small intestine, the so-called 'Rapunzel syndrome'. A history of trichophagia may be elicited. The physical findings include palpable epigastric mass, alopecia, and halitosis. 'Daughter' trichobezoars may result in intestinal obstruction. Gastric ulceration with haemorrhage or frank perforation due to trichobezoar carries significant mortality.

Bezoars may be visible on plain films as mottled densities in the left upper quadrant. Phytobezoars are frequently missed (75 per cent) during contrast studies: they appear as a mobile foreign body of varying size that may become infiltrated with barium. Trichobezoars form a cast of the stomach outlined with barium. Small bowel bezoar is occasionally seen directly on plain films, but more commonly the findings are those of small bowel obstruction; the bezoar may be identified on antegrade contrast studies of the small bowel.

The principal differential diagnosis of gastrobezoar is neoplasm, particularly when the bezoar is fixed in position. Endoscopy can serve to differentiate the two; bezoars are often discovered incidentally at endoscopy performed during evaluation of symptoms following gastrectomy. Endoscopy should be undertaken in all cases of suspected bezoar to detect associated abnormalities, as gastroduodenal ulceration is present in 10 to 40 per cent of patients.

Uncomplicated gastric phytobezoar can usually be managed without operation. Digestion of the bezoar using repeated doses of oral cellulase has greater reported success rates (>83 per cent) than the use of the proteolytic enzyme papain or the mucolytic agent acetylcysteine. Gastric emptying may be promoted by the use of metoclopramide. Occasionally simple gastric lavage is sufficient. If these measures are unsuccessful, bezoars may be fragmented and removed endoscopically using biopsy forceps or stone baskets, or disrupted using streams of water. Ulcerations at the site of an impacted bezoar usually heal following removal of the foreign body, although bezoars can occur in patients with preexisting ulceration at the gastric outlet. Surgical gastrotomy is reserved for patients with large phytobezoars or those that are symptomatic. In contrast, trichobezoar should always be managed surgically (Fig. 2), as conservative measures and endoscopy are of no avail; untreated trichobezoar carries a significant morbidity and mortality. Prophylactic antibiotics should be given; trichobezoars are typically putrefied.

Small bowel bezoars are treated surgically if obstruction supervenes. At laparotomy, attempts should be made to advance the bezoar into the colon manually. If these efforts are unsuccessful, enterotomy and extraction are necessary. One must guard against the not infrequent occurrence (4 to 17 per cent) of multiple bezoars by examining the stomach and the entire small bowel at laparotomy. Preoperative endoscopy is of value in cases of small bowel obstruction due to bezoar in order to identify unsuspected gastric or duodenal bezoar and extract or fragment these if possible, as they may be readily missed upon attempted palpation at laparotomy when there has been previous gastric surgery.

After successful bezoar removal, attention must be directed towards prevention of recurrence. Intake of high fibre foods, especially citrus fruits, should be avoided and adequate dentition assured. Chronic prophylactic oral enzyme therapy and the use of metoclopramide may reduce the incidence of recurrence. Tachyphylaxis to metoclopramide is rapid, however. The paradox of the bezoar is that while they were treasured in antiquity, much effort now is spent in ridding ourselves of them.

FURTHER READING

Buchholz R, Haisen AS. Phytobezoars following gastric surgery for duodenual ulcer. *Surg Clin N Am* 1972; **52**: 341.

Carp L. Foreign bodies in the intestine. *Ann Surg* 1927; **85**: 575.

DeBakey M, Ochsner A. Bezoars and concretions. A comprehensive review of the literature with an analysis of 303 collected cases and a presentation of 8 additional cases. *Surgery* 1938; **4**: 934–63, 1939; **5**: 132–60.

Diettrich NA, Gau, FC. Postgastrectomy phytobezoars—endoscopic diagnosis and treatment. *Arch Surg* 1985; **120**: 432–5.

Goldstein SS, Lewis JH, Rothstein R. Intestinal obstruction due to bezoars. *Am J Gastroenterol* 1984; **79**: 311–18.

Groff DB. Foreign bodies and bezoars. In: Welch KJ, Randolph JG, Ravitch MM, O'Neill JA, Rowe MI, eds. *Pediatric Surgery*. vol 2, 4th edn. Chicago; Year Book Medical Publishers, 1986; pp 907–11.

Hashmonai M, Kaufman T, Schramek A. Silent perforations of the stomach and duodenum by needles. *Arch Surg* 1978; **113**: 1406–9.

Henderson FF, Gaston EA. Ingested foreign body in the gastrointestinal tract. *Arch Surg* 1938; **36**: 66–95.

Hines JR, Guerkink RE, Gordon RT, Weinermann P. Phytobezoar: a recurring abdominal problem. *Am J Surg* 1977; **133**: 672–74.

James AH, Allen-Mersh TG. Recognition and management of patients who repeatedly swallow foreign bodies. *J R Soc Med* 1982; **75**: 107–10.

Joseph AE, Crampton AR, Agha FP, Tsang T-K. Impacted foreign bodies in the duodenum. *Am J Gastroenterol* 1987; **82**: 1074–7.

Kaplan O, Klausner JM, Leluck S, Skornick Y, Hammar B, Rozin R. Persimmon bezoars as a cause of intestinal obstruction: pitfalls in their surgical management. *Br J Surg* 1985; **72**: 242–3.

Kirk AD, Bowers BA, Moylan JA, Meyers WC. Toothbrush swallowing. *Arch Surg* 1988; **123**: 382–4.

Krausz MM, Moriel EZ, Ayalon A, Pode D, Durst AL. Surgical aspects of gastrointestinal persimmon phytobezoar treatment. *Am J Surg* 1986; **152**: 526–30.

Macmanus JE. Perforations of the intestine by ingested foreign bodies. Report of two cases and review of the literature. *Am J Surg* 1941; **52**: 393–402.

Margolies MN, Galdabini J. Abdominal pain relieved by vomiting in a 55-year-old woman with peptic ulcer disease. Case records of the Massachusetts General Hospital, Clinico-Pathologic Conferences. *N Engl J Med* 1978; **298**: 1301–7.

Miller SF. Foreign body ingestions. *J Am Fam Phys* 1975; **11**: 123.

Moriel EZ, Ayalon A, Eid A, Rachmilewitz D, Krausz MN, Durst AL. An unusually high incidence of gastrointestinal obstruction by persimmon bezoars in Israeli patients after ulcer surgery. *Gastroenterology* 1983; **84**: 752–5.

Pellerin D, Fortier-Beaulieu W, Guegen J. The fate of swallowed foreign bodies. Experience of 1250 instances of subdiaphragmatic foreign bodies in children. *Prog Pediatr Radiol* 1969; **2**: 286–302.

Rider JA, *et al.* Gastric bezoars: treatment and prevention. *Am J Gastroenterol* 1984; **79**: 357–9.

Roesch W, Koch H, Fruehmorgen P, Classen M. Operative endoscopy of the upper gastrointestinal tract. *Gastrointest Endosc* 1974; **20**: 108–9.

Schwartz GF, Polsky HS. Ingested foreign bodies of the gastrointestinal tract. *Am Surg* 1976; **42**: 236–8.

Schwartz JT, Graham DY. Toothpick perforation of the intestines. *Ann Surg* 1977; **185**: 64–6.

Spitz L. Management of ingested foreign bodies in childhood. *Br Med J* 1971; **4**: 469–72.

Suita S, Ohgami H, Nagasaki A, Yakabe S. Management of pediatric patients who have swallowed foreign objects. *Am Surg* 1989; **55**: 585–90.

Webb WA, Jones, McD. Foreign bodies of the upper gastrointestinal tract: current management. *South Med J* 1984; **77**: 1083–6.

Winkler, WP, Saleh J. Metoclopramide in the treatment of gastric bezoars. *Am J Gastroenterol* 1983; **78**: 403–5.

Zarling EJ, Thompson LE. Nonpersimmon gastric phytobezoar. A benign recurrent condition. *Arch Intern Med* 1984; **144**: 959–61.

The small intestine 16

16.1 Small bowel obstruction

LESLIE W. OTTINGER

GENERAL CONSIDERATIONS

Presentation

Whatever its site and cause, small bowel obstruction leads to rapid accumulation of fluid and gas in the lumen proximal to the site of obstruction. This event is the result both of swallowed air and of intestinal fluid excretion. Peristalsis causes distension in the distal obstructed segment first, with gradual proximal accumulation of air and intestinal fluid. With so-called high obstruction, in areas such as the proximal jejunum, vomiting may supervene early, relieving the distension. When obstruction is distal, vomiting may not occur until late in the course of the disease.

In typical cases of acute obstruction there is initial active peristaltic activity proximal to the site. Most patients complain of crampy pain. Within a few hours this activity declines, and oedema and increasing distension mark the end of peristaltic activity; there may be no cramps or only occasional cramps. Persistent, steady pain usually indicates ischaemia or perforation. A change in the characteristics of small bowel contents is also characteristic of the later stages of obstruction. Bacterial overgrowth and stagnation make the fluid feculent, with an increase in opacity and a foul odour. Appearance of fluid of this type in the vomitus or from a nasogastric tube confirms the diagnosis of obstruction.

Obtaining a detailed history and performing a thorough examination will provide a diagnosis of underlying cause in more than three-quarters of cases. It is especially important to identify abdominal wall hernias, which frequently strangulate when surgery is delayed.

Laboratory tests are of little value beyond helping to rule out other causes of abdominal pain. The exception to this rule is the plain radiograph of the abdomen, which is especially helpful in confirming the clinical impression of obstruction, and can also, when interpreted by an experienced clinician, add additional useful information as to completeness, site, and aetiology of obstruction. Upright films may show air in the biliary or portal system and beneath the diaphragm; these are important observations with respect to timing of surgery.

Aetiology

A list of the causes of intestinal obstruction is long, even if those normally only encountered during infancy and childhood are excluded. (Table 1). In geographic areas where life expectancy is long and surgical care readily available, at least half of the cases are the result of adhesions, usually postoperative. Hernias, whether of the abdominal wall or internal organs, are the second leading cause. Other important general causes are primary and metastatic tumours, local inflammatory processes such as appendicitis or diverticulitis of the colon, and various strictures, such as those seen in Crohn's disease. The causes and their relative incidence vary widely with geographic region.

Table 1 Usual causes of small bowel obstruction

Adhesions	Obturation-strictures
Postsurgical	Ischaemic
Inflammatory	Radiation
Radiation	Inflammatory
Meckel's diverticulum	Gallstone-bezoar
Hernias	Intussusception
Abdominal wall	Benign neoplasm
Internal	Meckel's diverticulum
Neoplasms	Volvulus
Primary	Superior mesenteric artery syndrome
Benign	
Malignant	
Metastatic	

The mechanism of the obstruction is more important than the specific aetiology, since this factor bears on the likelihood of bowel compromise. There are four general mechanisms: most dangerous are, first, volvulus with torsion and, second, incarceration in a confined space. Although volvulus can be the result of a failure of fixation of all or the distal part of the small bowel it is more commonly the result of twisting around a fixed point, as from an adhesion or tumour nodule. This event can rapidly lead to vascular compromise and infarction.

Incarceration in a fixed space is usually due to an abdominal wall hernia. Intra-abdominal defects and traps, congenital or acquired, are also sites of potential incarceration. Once entrapped, impaired venous return and torsion may rapidly lead to infarction of the segment.

Obturation of a segment of bowel, usually narrowed by a pathological process such as fibrosis or tumour growth, is the third mechanism. Such obstruction may be intermittent because of the repeated gradual passage of a bolus of intestinal contents through the stricture. A large bezoar or gallstone may obstruct a normal segment of bowel, usually the distal ileum, by this mechanism. Vascular compromise is unlikely in obturation obstruction.

The last mechanism is intussusception. In adults, it is almost always due to an intramural or mucosal lesion. It does not usually lead to ischaemia and infarction.

Non-operative measures

As a rule, mechanical small bowel obstruction is an urgent indication for surgical intervention. This practice reflects the risks of strangulation and perforation, the fact that persistence of obstruction will eventually require an operation in many cases, and the likelihood of recurrence even with spontaneous resolution.

Preoperative assessment of fluid status with rapid replacement of deficits is important. A patient whose obstruction has been identified many hours from its onset, when there has been vomiting or sequestration of large amounts of fluid in the lumen, intestinal wall and peritoneal cavity, may require administration of several litres of fluid. In these cases, restoration of an adequate urine output serves as a useful general index of adequate replacement. In older patients, especially those with a history of cardiac disease, central venous or pulmonary artery pressure monitoring may be needed. Concurrent, sometimes exacerbated, medical problems such as diabetes mellitus and cardiac impairment must be considered and managed separately.

Nasogastric suction relieves distension from air swallowing and reduces fluid passage into the small bowel; it should be instituted early in management. The use of long intestinal tubes has less justification. They do not pass readily, do not empty the stomach, and delay more definitive management. Generally, they have no useful role in the management of acute obstruction. Although exceptions may be cited, an efficiently functioning nasogastric tube is clearly preferable in most cases.

Surgical intervention

Though sometimes easy, operative intervention may be complex. The procedure requires the management of the segment of intestine at the site of obstruction, the distended proximal bowel and the underlying cause of obstruction.

If the patient has had a previous surgical incision which, with enlargement, will afford a portal for complete abdominal exploration, it should be used. This approach allows repair of all associated hernias and easy access to the most frequent site of obstruction by adhesions, which is the incision itself. It is usually wise to enter the abdomen through an extension into normal tissues to avoid injury to adherent loops.

In patients with late obstruction and in the elderly, the distended segments should be handled with care as they may easily be torn. The object is to find the junction of dilated and collapsed bowel. Though it may be preferable to follow collapsed loops proximally, this is not usually possible.

Decompression of dilated loops may be desirable to facilitate an anastomosis or closure of the abdominal wound. Closed methods of accomplishing this goal include the milking of contents back into the stomach with aspiration through a nasogastric tube. This method is usually possible without excessive trauma to the bowel only in young children. Alternatively, a long tube may be advanced from the stomach by digital manipulation into the distended loops. Finally, a sump suction device may be passed directly into the distended loops through an enterotomy controlled with a 'purse string' suture. Even with careful attention to prevention of local soilage, direct aspiration of enteric contents is associated with an increase in postoperative wound sepsis. Unless clearly needed, the best policy often is to omit decompression altogether.

When indicated, a simple resection of small bowel and direct anastomosis, even when the proximal bowel is distended, is safe enough. Sometimes, as with carcinomatosis or extensive pelvic adhesions, a side-to-side bypass is the better choice. Parenteral administration of antibiotics, begun preoperatively, decreases the incidence of septic complications when resection or bypass is performed.

The determination of the viability of a segment of intestine is a common problem. Generally, the opinion of an experienced surgeon after 10 to 20 min of observation suffices. To prevent early perforation or late strictures, a resection is the best choice when doubt exists. Although fluorescein injections with illumination of the surface with a Wood's lamp and detection of surface flow by Doppler devices provide scientific approaches to the diagnosis, they are neither necessary nor commonly available at the moment they are needed.

When obstruction is due to adhesions the question of whether all or only the offending adhesions should be released is unresolved. Generally, adhesions can be expected to recur when there has been any trauma to serosal surfaces. Thus, as a rule it is probably wise to divide only those adhesions involving the bowel at the site of obstruction and those that prevent restoration of the proximal and distal segments to their normal place of residence in the abdominal cavity.

Reduction of abdominal wall hernias before operation is desirable when easily accomplished. An exception is a hernia in the inguinal or femoral area; prompt operation is required. The surgeon may prefer to be able to examine the incarcerated segment of bowel through the herniorrhaphy incision before it is dropped back in. Another exception is the presence of local signs of inflammation that may indicate strangulation or perforation.

Prevention

Any laparotomy should be performed with operative measures that minimize adhesion formation, decreasing the incidence of small bowel obstruction. All reasonable steps to minimize serosal trauma should be utilized, including gentle handling and packing of intestine and avoiding the unnecessary introduction of foreign material into the peritoneal cavity. Sutures and ties involving the serosa cause small areas of tissue ischaemia and necrosis which can cause adhesions. Serosal defects should not be repaired if the underlying muscularis and submucosa are intact.

The second preventive measure, of course, is the repair of abdominal wall hernias. Any inguinal hernia that is symptomatic or is the site of occasional temporary bowel incarceration should be repaired, as should all incisional hernias.

COMPLEX PROBLEMS

Postoperative obstruction

Mechanical small bowel obstruction can complicate the postoperative course after any operative entry into the peritoneal cavity. The diagnosis is obscured by ileus and the symptoms and signs that are a usual accompaniments of a laparotomy incision.

Normally, paralysis of peristaltic function resolves within 72 h after a laparotomy involving handling of the intestine. There is then an absence of distension, and the patient reports a return of appetite along with expulsion of flatus and faeces. In cases of obstruction, normal peristaltic function may never return, or may do so only to be interrupted by an episode of obstruction. The superimposition of the signs and symptoms of obstruction on those of convalescence after laparotomy makes the diagnosis elusive.

Most cases are the result of adhesions and involve the ileum. Although the extent of adherence of peritoneal surfaces to each other is variable, the time course usually is not. By 72 h after laparotomy, extensive soft adhesions will have formed. These seem most extensive at about 10 days to 2 weeks, by which time they become dense and vascular. A gradual process of resolution then occurs; this may go on for many years, accounting for appearance of obstruction at remote times. This process of adhesion formation in some cases is abnormally vigorous and may then reflect peritoneal reaction to foreign material introduced during the operation. Sterile peritonitis can be an important contributor

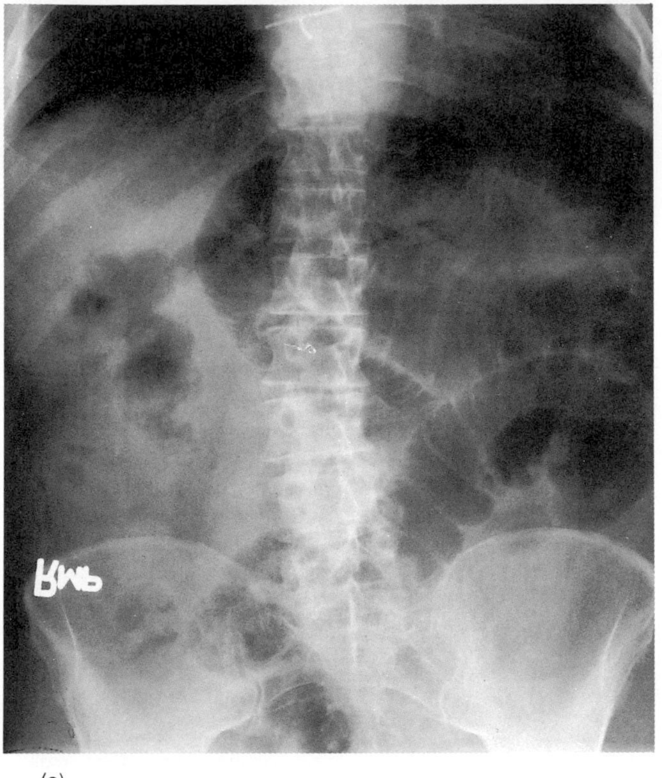

(a)

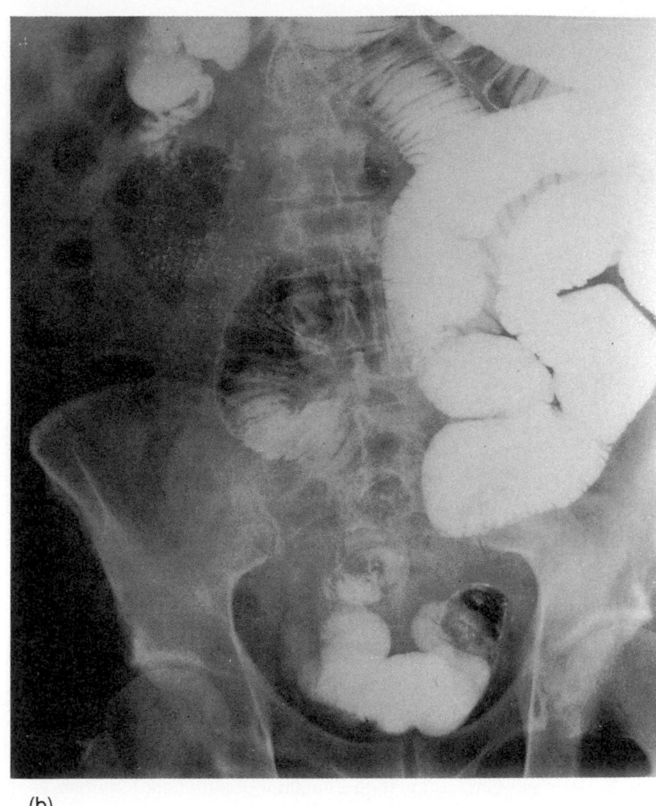

(b)

Fig. 1 (a) Plain film suggesting intestinal obstruction. Sixty-two-year old male 14 days following a pelvic exenteration. (b) Oral barium study showing complete obstruction in the pelvis 16 h after administration.

to a course of delayed resumption of intestinal function without actual mechanical obstruction. Obstruction by adhesions in the early period is usually the result of kinking and tensions on adherent loops of intestine rather than of obturation. The presence of a stoma or intestinal tube may contribute to these mechanical problems by offering a fixed cicatricial point. Other causes of obstruction include internal hernias and peritoneal defects after partial dehiscence of the deep layer of a wound or the peritoneal floor. An abscess involving adjacent segments of intestine can cause obstruction or can lead to localized ileus.

The clinical problem is to distinguish between cases of mechanical obstruction and those that reflect ileus prolonged by a sterile peritonitis or other factors, such as chronic narcotic use. Fortunately, except when there is a peritoneal defect, strangulation of an obstruction is rare in a postoperative patient. Careful repeated observation of the patient is paramount. Radiography offers the next best help: plain films show gas throughout the small and large bowel in most cases of ileus. In difficult cases, the use of barium will sometimes provide important information (Figs. 1, 2).

Careful replacement of fluid and electrolytes is needed, and nutritional support may facilitate overall recovery. It is generally believed that nasogastric decompression is essential and that decompression through a long tube may be helpful; passage of such tubes is most likely to succeed in those patients with mechanical obstruction. The usefulness of long tubes in the overall management of patients is estimated to be high by some surgeons, but many do not find them useful.

The timing of surgical intervention is difficult. Although it is important to relieve mechanical obstruction promptly, operations on patients with profound ileus and in those with extensive non-obstructing adhesions are fruitless and delay recovery. No simple rule can be offered. Generally, complete obstruction, evidence of sepsis, and an unacceptably prolonged course dictate an exploratory operation. An unacceptably long course is the least useful indication.

Recurrent obstruction

The risk of strangulation and the likelihood of early recurrence usually dictate prompt operation at the first episode of obstruction. An operation for obstruction due to adhesions carries a higher likelihood of recurrence than a laparotomy for other indications. This is of the order of 20 per cent. When obstruction recurs, the possibility of a cause other than adhesions is lower, and there is perhaps more justification for a non-operative management, in the form of decompression with a nasogastric tube and careful parenteral replacement of lost fluids and electrolytes.

During any period of observation, there will be continued concern about the possibility of bowel compromise. The nature of pain is the best indicator of this complication. Plain and contrast studies are helpful in ruling out complete obstruction, which also serves as an indication for surgical relief. If the obstruction resolves, there is generally no reason for a laparotomy in the patient with recurrent obstruction due to adhesions.

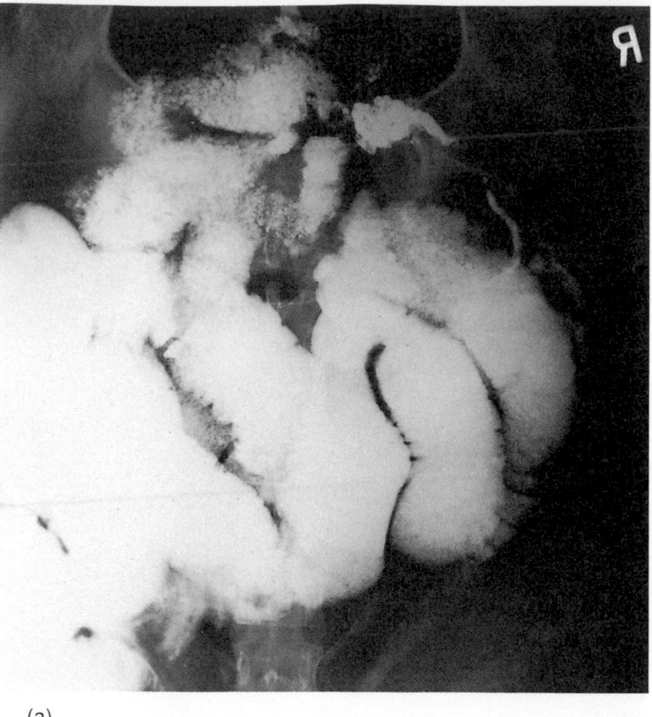

(a)

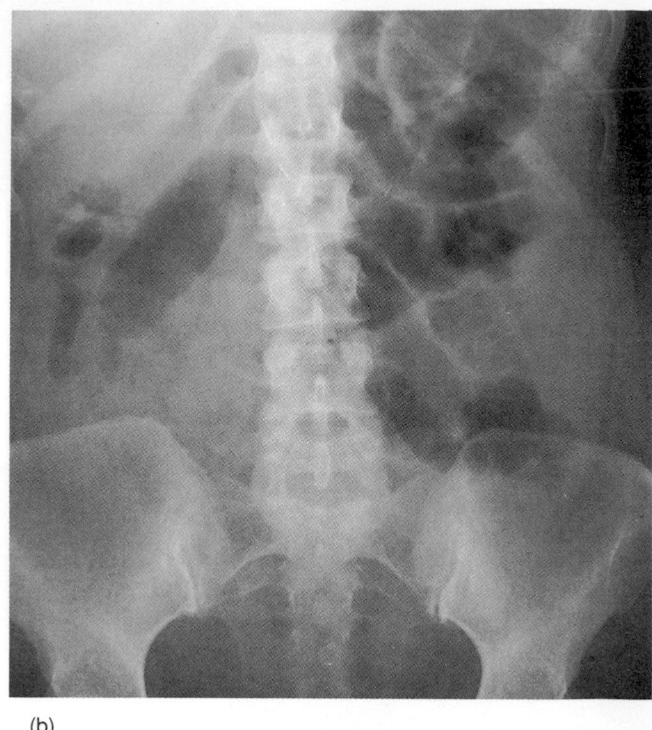

(b)

Fig. 2 (a) Plain film, suggesting intestinal obstruction. Fifty-one-year old female 17 days following a hysterectomy, salpingoophorectomy and omentectomy. (b) Oral barium showing progression of barium into the colon 12 h after administration. No operation was required.

There is no good way to prevent the recurrence of adhesions. Some authorities have suggested that plication of the wall or mesentery of the small bowel to form a ladderlike configuration may be helpful: there is no good evidence for the efficacy of these measures, and few surgeons use them. An in-lying long enteric tube may also produce a configuration of loops less prone to obstruction from adhesions. Such tubes should be left in place for at least 2 weeks, but their efficacy has not been clearly established.

Radiation enteritis

Injuries to the small intestine may follow radiation to any part of the abdominal cavity: many result from therapy for pelvic tumours. Although these injuries may lead to perforation with abscess formation of fistulae, the most common complication is intestinal obstruction.

During the actual course of radiation treatment, damage to the mucosa may lead to ulceration and oedema. Delayed damage to small blood vessels causes more serious complications such as progressive arteritis and eventual thrombosis. Infarction and perforation may ensue, but the more frequent result is the induction of dense adhesions containing collateral vessels, and the occurrence of fibrous strictures. Serosal surfaces of injured intestinal segments acquire a characteristic thickened, scarred, hypervascular appearance.

The cause of acute complete obstruction can only be established at the time of operation. Segments of intestine with a grossly abnormal appearance may not heal; when used for anastomosis, there is a high incidence of failure. A segment with a nearly normal appearance and satisfactory bleeding on transection can be used confidently. Microscopic examination adds little to the surgeon's impression in selecting bowel for anastomosis. Resection is the preferred management. If dissection of radiation-damaged loops of bowel out of the pelvis offers an unacceptable risk, a bypass may be selected. It is better to transect the bowel above the obstruction for an end-to-side anastomosis than to perform a side-to-side bypass in continuity.

A trial of non-surgical management is reasonable when a prior history or contrast study has established the diagnosis of radiation enteritis and obstruction is not complete. Some episodes due to obturation or oedema will resolve and may not recur. Parenteral nutrition may aid the process of resolution.

Metastatic malignant tumours

Peritoneal seeding sometimes leads to multiple narrowed segments and consequent obturation obstruction; this may occur in the absence of other terminal manifestations of the tumour. Strangulation is rare, since the loops are relatively fixed. Retroperitoneal or mesenteric deposits may contribute to the impaired motility.

Patients tend to have intermittent episodes of obturation obstruction. A minimal residue diet may reduce symptoms and acute obstruction usually clears on nasogastric suction. In patients with a relatively good prognosis, there may be a role for surgical intervention for bypass or even resection of obstructed sites. Careful evaluation with contrast studies allows selection of the smallest feasible procedure, to be performed through a limited field. Wide exploration of the abdomen is likely to be both unnecessary and counterproductive.

Superior mesenteric artery syndrome

Obstruction of the distal duodenum due to its compression between the artery and posterior structures, either the aorta or vertebral bodies, has been termed the superior mesenteric artery syndrome. Findings on plain film and contrast studies are dilatation of the stomach and duodenum with a termination by obstruction with a linear configuration at the level of the artery.

The syndrome may follow weight loss, immobilization in bed, and various operative procedures, but it also may occur spontaneously. It is seldom seen in obese patients. There appears to be a component of impaired motility in some patients and abnormalities of fixation of the ligament of Treitz have also been cited. The onset is often insidious with the gradual appearance of nausea and vomiting.

Though conservative measures should first be tried, the majority of patients eventually require surgical relief. Simple gastrojejunostomy does not relieve symptoms. Various measures can be used to adjust the position and fixation of the duodenum and proximal jejunum. Duodenojejunostomy performed through the mesocolon in a side-to-side fashion is most likely to succeed. The jejunum just beyond the ligament of Treitz should been employed in the anastomosis.

FURTHER READING

Baker JW. Stitchless plication for recurring obstruction of the small bowel. *Am J Surg* 1968; **116**: 316–24.

Bizer LS, Liebling RW, Delany HM, Gliedman ML. Small bowel obstruction: the role of nonoperative treatment in simple intestinal obstruction and predictive criteria for strangulation obstruction. *Surgery* 1981; **89**: 407–13.

Bulkley GB, Zuidema GD, Hamilton SR, O'Mara CS, Klacsmann PG, Horn SD. Intraoperative determination of small intestine viability following ischemic injury: a prospective controlled trail of two adjuvant methods (Doppler and fluorescein) compared with standard clinical judgment. *Ann Surg* 1981; **193**: 628–37.

Hines JR, Gore RM, Ballantyne GH. Superior mesenteric artery syndrome. Diagnostic criteria and therapeutic approaches. *Am J Surg* 1984; **148**: 630–2.

Lee CS, Mangla JC. Superior mesenteric artery compression syndrome. *Am J Gastroenterol* 1978; **70**: 141–50.

McCarthy JD. Further experience with the Childs–Phillips plication operation. *Am J Surg*. 1975; **130**: 15–19.

Noble TB Jr. Plication of small intestine as prophylaxis against adhesions. *Am J Surg* 1937; **37**: 41–4.

Schofield PF, Holden D, Carr ND. Bowel disease after radiotherapy. *J R Soc Med* 1983; **76**: 463–6.

Smith DH, DeCosse JJ. Radiation damage to the small intestine. *World J Surg* 1986; **10**: 189–4.

Wolfson PJ, Bauer JJ, Gelernt IM, Kreel I, Aufses AH Jr. Use of the long tube in the management of patients with small intestinal obstruction due to adhesions. *Arch Surg* 1985; **120**: 1001–6.

16.2.1 Crohn's disease of the small intestine

D. P. JEWELL

Strictures of the small intestine, not obviously due to tuberculosis, have been recognized since at least the sixteenth century. In the late nineteenth century, amongst the case histories of patients with supposed ulcerative colitis, there are those who also had gross ileal involvement. In 1913 Dalziel recognized that ileal inflammation could occur as a disease entity. He described the macroscopic appearances at surgery and the histological features of a chronic granulomatous inflammation predominant in the submucosa, which he distinguished from tuberculosis. However, little attention was given to this description until Crohn, Ginsberg, and Oppenheimer published their classical description of 'regional ileitis' in 1932. Later, in the 1930s, it became apparent that the disease often affected the right colon in continuity with terminal ileal disease, but primary disease of the colon was not accepted until the description of Lockhart-Mummery and Morson in 1960.

The presence of disease in the colon made the term regional ileitis or terminal ileitis inappropriate. Subsequently, regional enteritis or granulomatous enteritis has been used, but the eponymous term 'Crohn's disease' is preferable, since it does not imply an anatomical site nor the presence of granulomata.

DEFINITION

Crohn's disease may affect any part of the alimentary canal from mouth to anus, although ileal, ileocolonic, or colonic involvement are the most common patterns. The disease is characteristically discontinuous, or in other words, the disease may affect a number of segments with relatively normal intestinal mucosa in between. The inflammation is often transmural but is predominantly submucosal and is associated with a chronic inflammatory infiltrate, fissures, ulcers, and fibrosis, which may lead to stricturing. Granulomata, with giant cell formation, are the hallmark of the disease but are not always present.

EPIDEMIOLOGY

Crohn's disease has a worldwide distribution, although there is considerable variation in its actual incidence. In northern Europe and the United States of America, the annual incidence is about 3 to 5 per 100 000 of the population, with a prevalence of about 40 to 60 per 100 000. In Japan the disease appears to be about 10 times less common, and it is rarer in developing countries. However, diagnostic difficulties are considerable in those parts of the world where intestinal tuberculosis is still common.

The incidence of the disease in Britain, Scandinavia, and Israel increased during the 1950s and 1960s (Table 1), but it may now have reached a plateau. The incidence of the disease may be increasing in children. Ethnic differences also influence the incidence, with particularly high incidence rates in Ashkenazi Jews and a low incidence in Americans of African descent. Some series show a slight female preponderance, but this is not marked. The peak age of onset is in young adults (20–40 years of age), but the disease may present at virtually any age.

The pattern of the disease appears to be similar wherever it occurs in the world, although extraintestinal manifestations are

Table 1 Incidence rates (per 100 000 population) of Crohn's disease

Country	Time period	Incidence
USA		
Baltimore	1960–63	1.2
	1977–79	3.1
Olmsted County	1965–75	13.5
	1978–82	3.9
UK		
Aberdeen	1955–57	1.2
	1961–63	2.8
	1967–69	4.5
	1973–75	2.6
Scandinavia		
Stockholm	1955–59	1.5
	1965–69	3.6
	1970–74	4.5
	1975–79	4.1
Copenhagen County	1961–69	1.3
	1970–78	2.7
Israel	1971–75	0.5
	1976–80	1.8

probably more common in Caucasians. Ileal disease is particularly interesting in Japan, since it is often associated with very extensive longitudinal ulcers. These can be seen in Western patients but they are rare.

GENETICS

The familial incidence of Crohn's disease varies widely between series, but is probably 10 to 15 per cent. First-degree relatives are mainly affected and may have Crohn's disease or ulcerative colitis. Nevertheless, it has not been possible to describe the inheritance in classical mendelian terms. There is 20 to 30 per cent discordance in monozygotic twins. It is exceptionally rare for both husband and wife to be affected. No clear association with any of the HLA antigens has been found, although in Japan there is a weak association with HLA-DR2.

AETIOLOGY

The presence of granulomata suggested a mycobacterial aetiology to the clinicians of the 1930s, but no evidence for such an organism could be found.

However, in 1984 isolates of *Mycobacterium paratuberculosis* from Crohn's tissue were reported and the isolated organisms induced intestinal inflammation when given, by mouth, to newborn goats. Since then, several more isolates have been made in different countries and using DNA probes, most of these have been shown to be identical with *M. paratuberculosis*. Nevertheless, the significance of these isolates remains very doubtful, since less than 10 per cent of tissues cultured have proved positive. Secondly, the clinical response of Crohn's disease to antimycobacterial therapy has not been overwhelmingly successful and, in controlled trials, no effect has been seen. At the present time, several groups are attempting to identify *M. paratuberculosis* DNA in tissues, using the polymerase chain reaction to amplify the DNA. Despite the extreme sensitivity of this technique, findings have been essentially negative.

Many other infectious agents have been implicated (viruses, cell-wall-deficient pseudomonads) but no convincing evidence for them has accumulated. However, several lines of evidence suggest that luminal factors may be important. Active disease often responds to the use of elemental diets, which appear to be as effective as corticosteroids. Colonic disease, resistant to medical treatment, frequently subsides following defunctioning of the colon by means of a split ileostomy. Challenging the defunctioned colon with ileostomy effluent will trigger an inflammatory response, although this is not seen if an ultrafiltrate of the effluent is used. Thus, luminal bacteria may have some influence on the course of the disease, although the effects of elemental diets and defunctioning may equally well implicate a biochemical or metabolic alteration in the luminal environment.

Many studies have now shown that patients with Crohn's disease are more likely to be smokers, and this is in sharp contrast with ulcerative colitis, which is found more often in non-smokers. Thus smoking confers a relative risk of 3 to 4 for Crohn's disease. The reasons for this are completely obscure. Smoking is known to affect the synthesis of colonic mucus and mucosal blood flow. It also effects arachidonic acid metabolism and some immunological effector mechanisms. However, whether any of these mechanisms can explain the opposite associations between smoking and ulcerative colitis or Crohn's disease remains speculative.

There may be an increased incidence of Crohn's disease in young women receiving oral contraceptives. However, the association, if it exists, is weak and largely disappears when the data are adjusted for smoking habits and social class.

PATHOGENESIS

There is considerable evidence to suggest that immunological mechanisms play a role in the pathogenesis of mucosal inflammation. Thus, intestinal macrophages and T cells are activated within the inflamed intestine and release a wide variety of cytokines as well as inflammatory mediators. These soluble mediators have profound local and systemic effects, which include altering epithelial cell permeability and ion flux, initiating fibrosis by activating fibroblasts, damaging endothelium resulting in local ischaemia, and stimulating an acute-phase response (Table 2).

Table 2 Pathogenesis of Crohn's disease—the potential role of soluble mediators released during immune activation

1. Fever, weight loss, hypoalbuminaemia acute phase response	IL-1, IL-6, TNF
2. Increased epithelial permeability (contributing to diarrhoea)	λIFN, C', LTB4, PAF, $O^{\cdot-}$
3. Endothelial damage (ischaemia)	IL-1, TNF, IL-2, LTB4, PAF, $O^{\cdot-}$
4. Increased collagen synthesis (fibrosis)	IL-1, IL-6, TNF, TGFβ1
5. Increased epithelial cell proliferation (causing decreased villous height)	TGF-α

IL, interleukin; TNF, tumour necrosis factor; TGF, transforming growth factor; γIFN, γ-interferon; LTB4, leukotriene B4; PAF, platelet activating factor; $O^{\cdot-}$, reactive oxygen metabolites; C', activated complement.

The more difficult question is whether Crohn's disease represents a specific immunological disturbance. For example, does the chronic inflammatory nature of the disease reflect an abnormality in the regulation of the mucosal immune response? So far, evidence to support such a hypothesis is lacking. Assays for T-cell suppressor or helper function, whether using peripheral blood or mucosal lymphocyte populations, have produced variable results. However, recent data suggest that patients with Crohn's disease, in common with patients with ulcerative colitis, may have an impaired ability to induce suppressor cells to specific antigens. This inability is present in patients whose disease is in remission and on no therapy, suggesting that there may, indeed, be an underlying problem in immunoregulation.

Deficient immunoregulation would allow an immune response in the intestinal mucosa to proceed unchecked and might explain why these patients exhibit humoral and cellular immune responses to a wide variety of luminal and epithelial antigens. A particularly interesting finding is that, although patients with active ulcerative colitis or Crohn's disease may show a rise in total serum IgG concentration, the patients with Crohn's disease show a predominant rise in the IgG2 subclass whereas those with ulcerative colitis have a predominant increase in IgG1. This difference could indicate that different antigens are involved in each disease, since protein antigens are associated with an IgG1 response whereas carbohydrate or bacterial antigens stimulate an IgG2 response. Equally, it could represent a genetic difference between the two diseases.

PATHOLOGY

Crohn's disease affects the small intestine in at least 70 per cent of all patients with the disease. Of these, about half have ileal involvement alone and the rest will have associated colonic disease—usually affecting the right colon. However, 30 per cent of patients with ileal disease alone will show a proctitis on sigmoidoscopy.

Macroscopically, the affected segment of small intestine is thickened due to oedema and fibrosis, which can be severe enough to cause a stricture. The mucosa is inflamed and may have a 'cobblestone' appearance, due to a combination of submucosal oedema and fissuring ulcers (Fig. 1). In mild disease, small aphthoid ulcers may be visible on the mucosa. In more severe disease, these ulcers become larger and coalesce. Ulceration is often serpiginous, especially on the mesenteric border. On the serosal surface, Crohn's disease may have a fairly characteristic appearance, with creeping fat and marked vascularity.

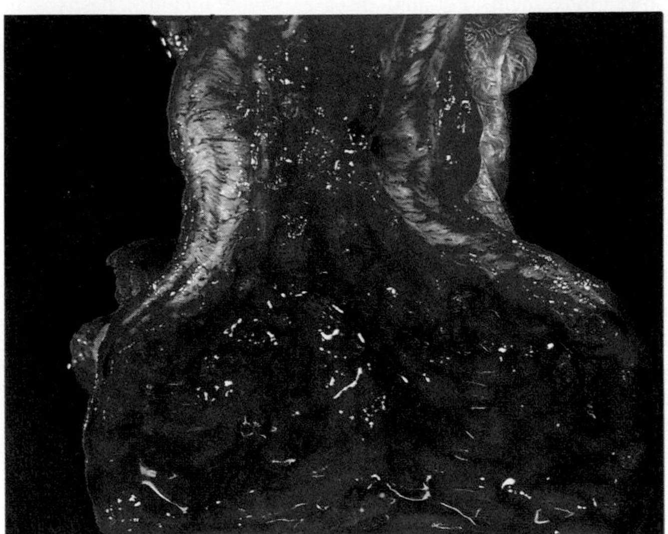

Fig. 1 Macroscopic appearances of ileal Crohn's disease, showing thickening of the wall and extensive ulceration.

The predominant histological feature is a chronic inflammatory infiltrate of lymphocytes and plasma cells in the lamina propria and submucosa (Fig. 2). There is usually shortening of villous height with increased crypt depth, and there may be evidence of 'pyloric metaplasia'.

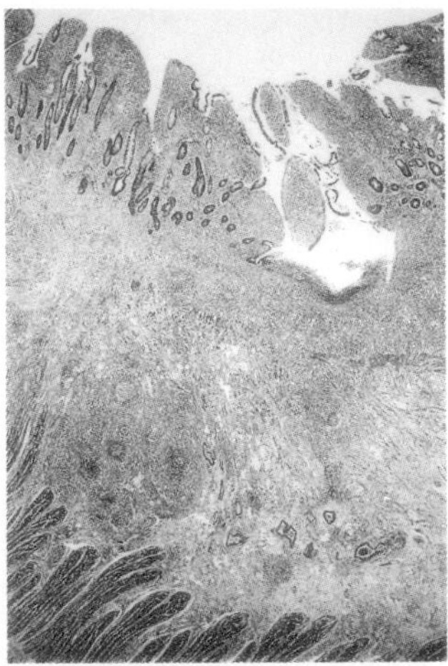

Fig. 2 Low-power views of ileal Crohn's disease, showing expansion and inflammation of the submucosa and a fissure ulcer in the mucosa.

This last finding has been investigated recently and represents a novel lineage of cells budding from the adjacent crypts. This appears to be part of a normal mucosal repair mechanism and may develop under the influence of epidermal growth factor.

When the Crohn's disease is active there is also an increase in neutrophils and eosinophils, and there is usually ulceration of the surface epithelium. One characteristic feature is the fissure ulcer, which often penetrates deep into the mucosa (Fig. 3). These

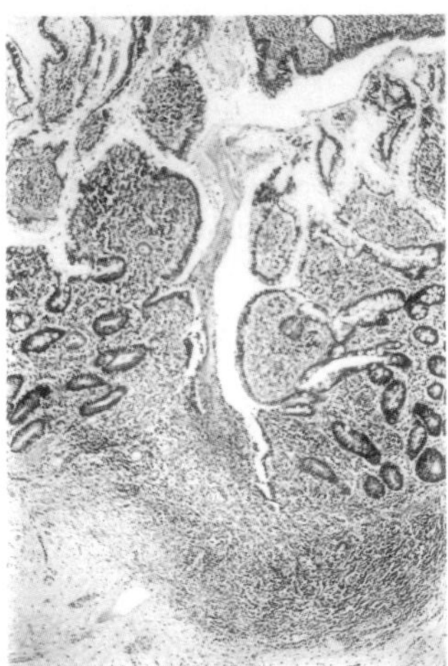

Fig. 3 High-power view of a fissure ulcer overlying a lymphoid aggregate.

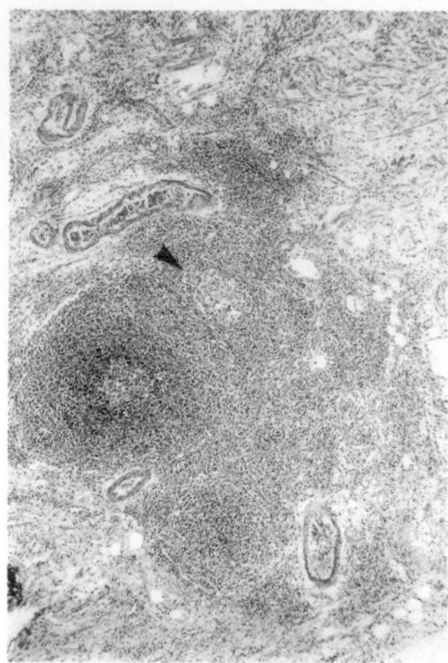

Fig. 4 A granuloma containing a multinucleated giant cell in the submucosa of the ileum.

fissures are lined by macrophages and lymphocytes and may be associated with granulomata and multinucleated giant cells (Fig. 4). Fibrosis is another prominent feature, especially in the submucosa. The inflammation of Crohn's disease is often transmural and therefore it is common to see chronic inflammatory changes with granuloma formation on the serosal surface.

Lymphoid follicles are prominent and there may be small, localized areas of ulceration in the overlying epithelium. It has been postulated that these lesions represent the earlier lesion of Crohn's disease, but this remains a speculative, though attractive, hypothesis.

Granulomata occur with variable frequency, partly depending on the number of sections examined and the time spent searching for them. However, they are probably present in no more than 65 per cent of patients with ileal disease, and some series quote only 30 per cent. Certainly there appear to be fewer granulomata in ileal disease than in colonic Crohn's disease, the frequency increasing as the disease becomes more distal. Granulomata are often associated with blood vessels or lymphatics, and some recent experiments, using operative specimens injected with intra-arterial resins, have shown that the granulomata are actually within the walls of arterioles. Although the presence of granulomata has been claimed to indicate a good prognosis, subsequent studies have not confirmed this.

Neuronal hypertrophy is another histological feature that is frequently present. Nerve endings, in particular, become prominent and stain strongly for vasoactive intestinal polypeptide, but whether this is specific for Crohn's disease, or whether it is merely associated with the neural hypertrophy known to occur proximal to obstructive lesions, is not known.

CLINICAL FEATURES

Symptoms

The most common symptoms of small intestinal Crohn's disease are diarrhoea (90 per cent), abdominal pain (55 per cent), anorexia, nausea, and weight loss (22 per cent). Malaise, lassitude, and the symptoms of anaemia are frequently present.

The diarrhoea usually consists of the passage of frequent loose or watery stools. Nocturnal diarrhoea may occur. Frank blood in the stool is not usually seen, although small amounts of blood may be passed in patients with an accompanying proctitis. A few patients may have a steatorrhoea but the passage of pale, bulky stools which are difficult to flush away is uncommon.

The pain may either be a dull ache, often located to the right iliac fossa, or a periumbilical colicky pain. Both types of pain can radiate into the back.

Some patients present with general symptoms of vague ill health, with few, if any, abdominal symptoms; this usually leads to a considerable delay in diagnosis and is seen particularly in children, in whom failure to thrive or growth failure are common presentations.

The symptoms of small intestinal Crohn's disease may be caused by active inflammation, intestinal obstruction, or both. Patients with previous ileal resections may have a watery diarrhoea due to malabsorption of bile salts, or their symptoms of anaemia may be due to vitamin B_{12} deficiency. Partial obstruction from stricturing disease may cause bacterial overgrowth, which may cause steatorrhoea, bloating, excess wind, weight loss, and a general malaise.

Thus, the symptomatology of Crohn's disease is complex, and an awareness of the differing causes of symptoms is important in making an accurate clinical assessment.

Physical signs

Many patients look well, are well nourished, and have few abnormal physical signs. However, evidence of weight loss, anaemia, and signs of iron deficiency and clubbing of the nails are common. Peripheral oedema may occur if hypoalbuminaemia is present. In very sick patients, there is often marked cachexia, proximal myopathy (from hypokalaemia or vitamin D deficiency), easy bruising, and pigmentation.

Abdominal examination may be normal, but right iliac fossa tenderness is common. Thickened loops of ileum or a frank abdominal mass may be palpable. Visible peristalsis usually denotes obstruction but, in cachectic patients, may just be normal small-bowel movement. Perianal disease, which includes fleshy skin tags, fissures, or fistulae, can occur in up to 14 per cent of patients with ileal disease. Rectal examination may demonstrate tender pelvic loops of inflamed intestine.

Acute presentation

Although the majority of patients complain of symptoms which have been present for weeks or months, a few (less than 10 per cent) present with a more acute history. This often consists of right iliac fossa pain, fever, and malaise over a few days. These patients are frequently diagnosed as having acute appendicitis, and the true diagnosis is only revealed at operation. Nevertheless, a careful history often reveals more long-standing symptoms, and investigation often shows a mild anaemia or a lowish albumin. Thus, however classical the clinical picture for acute appendicitis appears to be, a full history, together with documentation that signs of chronic disease are absent, documentation of a normal anus, and a normal haemoglobin, should be essential before proceeding to appendicectomy.

Diagnosis

The diagnosis of small intestinal Crohn's disease is made by barium contrast radiology. When available, the technique of enteroclysis (small-bowel enema) should be used, as this allows much better definition of the mucosal pattern than a conventional barium meal and follow through. Thus, scattered aphthoid ulcers are much more likely to be seen on a small-bowel enema, and it also allows a much better assessment of strictures. More advanced disease will be associated with the appearance of fissure ulcers, mucosal oedema, and narrowing of the intestinal lumen (Figs 5, 6). Fistulae to other loops of bowel or to other organs may be visualized (Figs 7, 8).

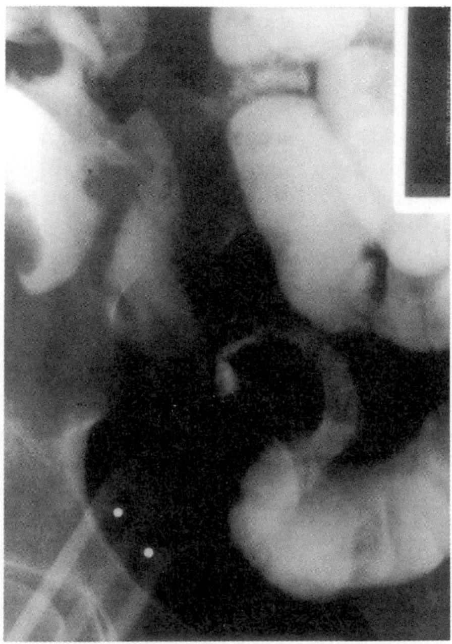

Fig. 5 Small-bowel enema, showing Crohn's disease of the terminal ileum. The ileum is thickened, strictured, and shows mucosal oedema. There is proximal dilatation, indicating obstruction.

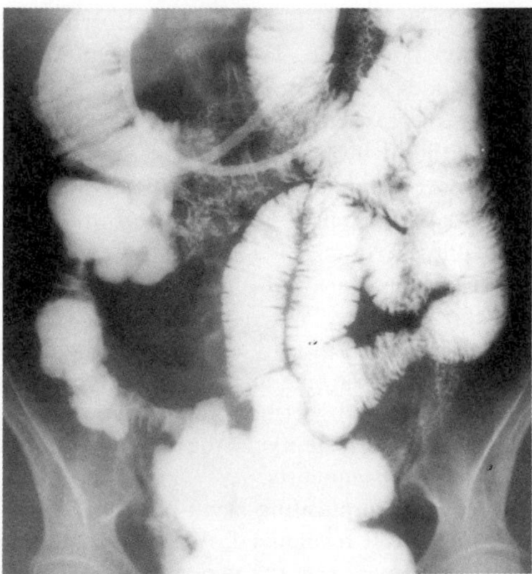

Fig. 6 Ileal Crohn's disease, shown by a small-bowel enema, illustrating fissure ulcers and characteristic asymmetry.

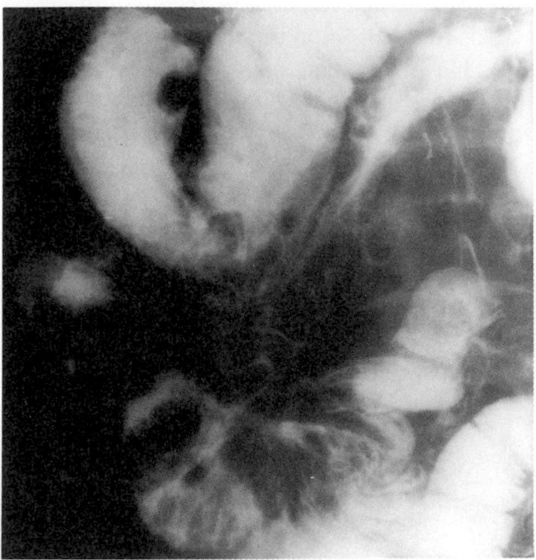

Fig. 7 Severe ileal Crohn's disease with multiple fistulae into neighbouring loops.

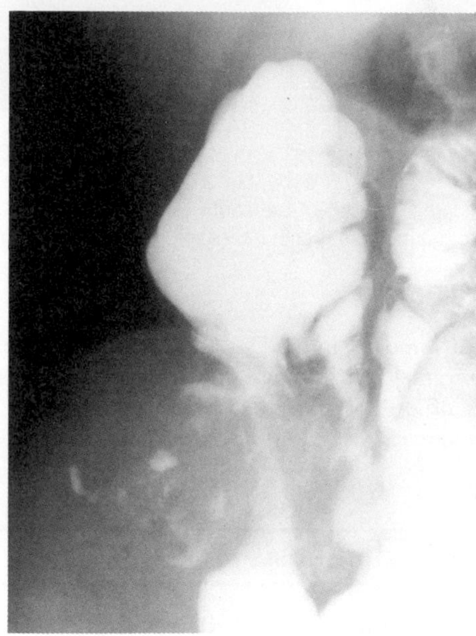

Fig. 8 Crohn's disease of the terminal ileum, associated with a large abscess resulting from fistula formation and perforation.

When a small-bowel enema confirms Crohn's disease, a full examination of the colon should always be made. It is usually sufficient to perform a sigmoidoscopy with rectal biopsy and a double-contrast barium enema. Nevertheless, the barium study will miss scattered aphthoid lesions in the colon and so, for a full assessment, colonoscopy should be performed. The importance of taking biopsy specimens cannot be overemphasized since focal inflammation and even granulomata can be seen histologically in 25 to 30 per cent of patients in whom the macroscopic appearance of the mucosa is normal. Colonoscopy may also allow terminal ileal biopsy specimens to be obtained, which can be helpful in cases where the radiological appearances are suggestive but not diagnostic.

White-cell scans (using indium- or technetium-labelled granulocytes) may also be helpful in determining the extent of the disease (Fig. 9). However, their major use is in assessing patients where symptoms are more severe than would be expected from the barium radiological appearances and in excluding local perforation with abscess formation.

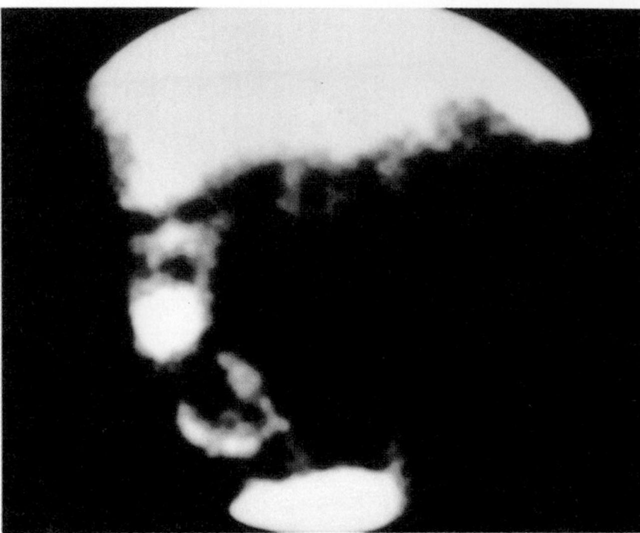

Fig. 9 ^{99}Tc-labelled white-cell scan in a patient with ileal Crohn's disease. The liver is seen clearly, but, in addition, the white cells have accumulated in loops of the ileum and the ascending and transverse colon, indicating active disease in these segments.

Computed tomography (CT) scans, especially following contrast medium, may demonstrate thickening of the intestinal wall, but they are of low specificity. CT scans and magnetic resonance imaging can be very useful in the assessment of fistulae or pelvic abscesses.

Differential diagnosis

As already mentioned, an acute ileitis frequently mimics an acute appendicitis. Nevertheless, only a small proportion of patients with an acute ileitis have Crohn's disease, on the grounds that only about 10 per cent will have recurrent disease on prolonged follow-up. The remainder are assumed to have an infective cause, and *Yersinia enterocolitica* or *Y. pseudotuberculosis* account for a few. These organisms can be isolated from stool cultures, but a rise in serum antibody titre is the most reliable method of making the diagnosis.

For more chronic disease, the differential diagnosis includes lymphoma, Behçet's disease, tuberculosis, actinomycosis, and tumours (adenocarcinoma, carcinoid). A small-intestinal lymphoma may be difficult to distinguish from Crohn's disease, except following laparotomy. The presence of focal colonic disease at colonoscopy, and the appearances on an abdominal CT scan, may be helpful. Behçet's disease of the small intestine is primarily a vasculitic process and virtually always occurs when there is evidence of disease elsewhere (for example, ocular or genital ulceration, deep vein thrombosis, neurological involvement). Ileal perforation is not uncommon in Behçet's disease but is very rare in Crohn's disease of the small intestine. Radiation enteritis may also mimic Crohn's disease, but a history and radiological appearances make the diagnosis clear.

The most difficult differential diagnosis is intestinal tuberculosis when Crohn's disease is suspected in patients at high risk from tuberculosis (for example, Asian patients). Stool culture and serum antibody titres are unhelpful. Radiologically, tuberculosis often affects a very short segment of the ileum and is not usually associated with cobblestoning or asymmetry, which are so characteristic of Crohn's disease. Skip lesions are uncommon in tuberculosis. Colonoscopy with multiple biopsies may be helpful, as caseating granulomata containing acid-fast organisms can be found in a few patients. Finally, laparoscopy may show serosal or peritoneal tubercules.

Obviously, active tuberculosis elsewhere (such as lungs and kidney) makes the diagnosis of the intestinal disease, and hence the management, straightforward.

Complications

Perforation, acute dilatation, and massive haemorrhage may all occur in small-intestinal Crohn's disease but they are rare, being much less common than in Crohn's disease of the colon. Obstruction due to fibrous strictures is the most common local complication and the strictures may be multiple. Fistulae to neighbouring loops of small or large bowel or to other organs such as the bladder or vagina occur in 10 to 17 per cent of patients.

Gallstones are more frequently found in patients with ileal Crohn's disease, particularly if an ileal segment has been excised, than in a healthy population. The mechanism is the interruption of the enterohepatic circulation of the bile salts, with eventual depletion of bile salts.

Renal stones are also more commonly present in patients with Crohn's disease. They are usually oxalate stones, secondary to hyperoxaluria. This occurs when there is steatorrhoea since the fat binds intraluminal calcium. Thus the normal precipitation of calcium oxalate does not occur, leaving free oxalate to be absorbed from the colon and excreted through the kidneys. Another renal complication is the involvement of the right ureter in the inflammatory process occurring in the terminal ileum and caecum. This may give rise to a recurrent pyelonephritis or, more commonly, a right hydronephrosis.

Amyloidosis is a rare but well-recognized complication of long-standing Crohn's disease. When it occurs, it is often present throughout the intestinal mucosa and may also affect the kidney, leading to nephrotic syndrome and renal failure. If renal amyloid occurs, it is important to get the Crohn's disease into remission (that usually means resection) as the amyloid has been documented to regress subsequently.

Adenocarcinoma complicating small-intestinal Crohn's disease is very rare but is well recognized. A review of the 58 reported cases up to 1982 showed that the majority occurred in the ileum; 18 occurred in a bypassed loop. Most patients died within a year of diagnosis, presumably indicating the difficulty of making the diagnosis in a patient who already has Crohn's disease and abnormal radiological appearances of the small intestine.

Extraintestinal manifestations

Small-intestinal Crohn's disease, in contrast to colonic disease, is rarely associated with erythema nodosum, uveitis, or an acute arthropathy, which occur in no more than 1 per cent of patients with ileal disease. If these extraintestinal manifestations represent deposition of immune complexes, and the evidence for this is only suggestive, then it is possible that the greater antigenic load within the colonic lumen may explain their association with colonic disease. These manifestations occur when the intestinal disease is active.

Pyoderma gangrenosum may also complicate active Crohn's disease but, again, it is very rare when there is no colonic involvement.

Sacroiliitis occurs radiologically in 10 to 12 per cent of patients, although only a small proportion will complain of low back pain. Unless the patient has the HLA-B27 haplotype, sacroiliitis does not develop into a full-blown ankylosing spondylitis. This last condition occurs in about 1 per cent of patients with Crohn's disease who, almost exclusively, have the HLA-B27 haplotype. It is more commonly seen in patients with colonic involvement than in those with only ileal disease. Ankylosing spondylitis may present long before intestinal disease is suspected and is characterized by progressive stiffness of the back, leading ultimately to a rigid spine. The natural history of the back condition is independent of the Crohn's disease and, therefore, the presence of disabling back symptoms is not an indication for extensive surgical resection of the Crohn's disease.

Fatty liver may occur in any patient who is severely ill from Crohn's disease and is reversible once remission is achieved. During these severe attacks there may be transient rises in serum concentrations of transaminases or alkaline phosphatase, but they have no clinical significance.

Isolated granulomata may occur within the liver. Primary sclerosing cholangitis seems to be much less common in Crohn's disease than in ulcerative colitis, and is usually diagnosed on the basis of a persistently raised serum alkaline phosphatase. Liver biopsy may reveal the classical periductular fibrosis with chronic portal inflammation, but the appearances range from a chronic active hepatitis picture with portal inflammation and piecemeal necrosis, to gross fibrosis with obliteration of the bile ducts. The definitive diagnostic test is endoscopic retrograde cholangiopancreatography (ERCP), which will show the distribution of the disease—intrahepatic, extrahepatic, or a combination. Occasionally, there is a predominant stricture in the extrahepatic bile duct which can be worth dilating or stenting if the patient has an obstructive jaundice. Cholangiocarcinoma, a well-recognized complication of sclerosing cholangitis in patients with ulcerative colitis, is very rare in Crohn's disease and very few properly documented cases have been described. Whether this relates just to the low incidence of sclerosing cholangitis in Crohn's disease or whether other mechanisms are operating is unclear.

Assessment of disease activity

Since patients with Crohn's disease may have symptoms relating to active inflammation, bacterial overgrowth, obstruction, or as a result of previous surgery, assessment of the activity of the disease is difficult and a clinical assessment by itself can be misleading. Laboratory data frequently help and should include the haemoglobin, platelet count, albumin, and erythrocyte sedimentation rate (ESR). When available, serum concentrations of the acute-phase proteins, C-reactive protein and orosomucoid are particularly good indicators of active inflammation.

A large number of activity indices have been devised in order to standardize activity assessment. The Crohn's Disease Activity Index is the most widely used, as well as the Harvey–Bradshaw simplification of the Crohn's Disease Activity Index. However, the calculation of activity indices is subject to wide variation and their use is mainly for clinical trials rather than in routine clinical practice.

Labelled white-cell scans are often useful in patients when there is still doubt about whether symptoms are primarily inflammatory or obstructive. The distinction is obviously important for management decisions.

MEDICAL MANAGEMENT

Since Crohn's disease cannot be cured, the role of the clinician is to control the inflammation, to correct nutritional deficiencies, and to ameliorate symptoms. These aims will frequently involve surgery and, indeed, 70 to 75 per cent of patients will require at least one operation during their lifetime. Thus, management of these patients requires close co-operation between physicians and surgeons. In general, medical treatment should be dictated by symptoms. Large doses of corticosteroids or immunosuppression are not indicated in asymptomatic patients who have active disease shown only by laboratory data.

Nutrition and diet

Patients with severe disease are often malnourished and will require both nutritional replacement and support during the acute illness. Nutritional support may be parenteral or enteral, the latter being administered through a fine-bore nasogastric tube.

Parenteral nutrition by itself has no primary effect on the disease process, but several trials have now shown that elemental diets are as effective as corticosteroids in obtaining remission. However, the unpalatability of elemental diets makes for poor patient compliance and there is some evidence that relapses occur more quickly after dietary therapy than following corticosteroids. In the long term, patients should be advised to eat a normal well-balanced diet, avoiding only those foods which they know upset them.

A few patients with extensive small-bowel disease may have hypolactasia and will benefit from a lactose-free diet. The use of elimination diets is still unproven. However, a low-residue diet is advisable for patients with stricturing disease.

For most patients who have intermittent relapses of distal ileal disease, vitamin supplements are unnecessary, provided a serum vitamin B_{12} concentration is measured regularly (an annual measurement should be sufficient unless the value is progressively falling). However, patients with more extensive disease may benefit from folic acid, iron, B vitamins, and calcium. Magnesium and zinc deficiencies may also occur, and serum concentrations should be measured in patients with extensive disease that is chronically active. Oral iron is frequently poorly tolerated by these patients, and a total dose of iron given by slow intravenous infusion is often indicated. There is a potential danger of anaphylaxis but this occurs very rarely. Nevertheless, it is a wise precaution to have adrenaline and hydrocortisone readily available and the patient closely monitored while the infusion is in progress.

Treatment of mild to moderate disease

Patients with mild symptoms and with only minor changes in their inflammatory markers (such as platelet count, C-reactive protein, ESR) can be treated initially with sulphasalazine (1 g twice a day) or mesalazine for 4 to 6 weeks. These drugs have been shown to be effective in clinical trials, especially for colonic disease. Metronidazole (400 mg three times a day) may also be beneficial for mild disease. Alternatively, patients can be given oral prednisolone (20 mg daily) for 4 to 6 weeks.

For more active disease, or when initial treatment with sulphasalazine or mesalazine has not controlled symptoms, larger doses of prednisolone should be used. This usually implies starting with an oral dose of 40 to 60 mg daily, tapering to 20 mg over a period of 2 to 3 weeks. Patients are then treated for a further 4 weeks before the prednisolone is tailed off completely. If the disease is going to respond to cortocosteroids, that is usually complete by 6 weeks of therapy. In formal clinical trials, there has been no advantage in combining corticosteroid therapy with sulphasalazine.

Treatment of severe disease

Severe Crohn's disease is defined as a patient with symptoms of active disease (diarrhoea, abdominal pain, anorexia, weight loss) who has evidence of systemic disturbance (tachycardia, fever, anaemia). An abdominal mass may be present. These patients are best admitted to hospital, and they respond well to intravenous corticosteroids (for example, hydrocortisone, 100 mg every 6 h; or prednisolone, 20 mg every 8 h), intravenous fluids, and electrolyte and blood replacement. Intravenous metronidazole (500 mg every 8 h) is also often given, although there is no firm evidence to support its use. The majority of patients settle rapidly on this regimen and can be started on a light diet after a few days.

For patients with severe ileal disease complicated by stricturing or fistulae, intravenous corticosteroids and metronidazole should be given initially to allow much of the inflammation to settle before proceeding to surgery.

Parenteral nutrition, while not indicated for all patients requiring intravenous corticosteroid therapy, should be considered for each patient, especially if complications such as fistulae are present and if surgery seems a likely outcome.

Chronic active disease

Some patients go into a satisfactory remission and become symptomatic when their prednisolone dosage falls below 15 or 10 mg daily. Yet other patients rapidly relapse once prednisolone is withdrawn completely. These patients can be considered to have chronic active disease and it is this group that may benefit from immunosuppressive therapy.

In Europe, azathioprine (2 mg/kg) is usually used, but in the United States of America 6-mercaptopurine is more commonly used (azathioprine is metabolized to 6-mercaptopurine in the liver). Some patients respond well to these drugs and it is then possible to withdraw the corticosteroids. The exact mode of action of these drugs is not known but their beneficial effect, if it occurs, is seen over a period of several weeks. If a patient responds well, the problem then is to know how long to continue treatment. There are no data on this point but most clinicians would treat for 1 to 2 years before stopping the immunosuppressives.

Side-effects are fairly uncommon, with nausea and diarrhoea being the most frequent. However, regular blood counts (every 1–2 months) should be done, as marrow suppression occasionally occurs. Minor elevations of transaminase and an acute pancreatitis are other potential adverse reactions.

Recently, cyclosporin A has been used for chronic active disease at a dose of 5 mg/kg. Its role in therapy is still being evaluated in clinical trials. It is not recommended for general use at the present time since adverse reactions, in particular nephrotoxicity, are common. Methotrexate is also being evaluated but, so far, experience is limited to anecdotal reports only.

Symptomatic treatment

Diarrhoea in patients with Crohn's disease is best treated by treating the cause (active disease, bacterial overgrowth, etc). Patients with a bile salt-induced diarrhoea following ileal resection may benefit from cholestyramine but this must be used sparingly if more than 100 cm of terminal ileum has been resected as it will exacerbate fat excretion. However, a few patients will continue to complain of diarrhoea when all treatable causes have been identified and corrected. Antidiarrhoeal drugs (loperamide, codeine phosphate, diphenoxylate hydrochloride) may then have a role.

Maintenance of remission

In contrast to ulcerative colitis, there is very little evidence that sulphasalazine is useful in maintaining remission, although a recent multicentre trial from Canada provides some support for the effectiveness of mesalazine. Several trials have tested the hypothesis that sulphasalazine or mesalazine might reduce the relapse rate following surgical resection. However, the results have been variable, with only some trials showing benefit. Therefore, until unequivocal evidence emerges for or against maintenance therapy with 5-aminosalicylic acid drugs, the decision whether to use such treatment remains an individual one. Certainly, there is no general case to the made for maintenance therapy with corticosteroids, although in the American National Cooperative Study, patients who went into remission on prednisolone appeared to stay in remission more frequently if low-dose corticosteroids were continued, compared to those who receive placebo maintenance therapy.

Dietary studies have shown that the subsequent course of the disease is not influenced by the amount of dietary fibre or sugar consumed.

PROGNOSIS

Crohn's disease is a disease of high morbidity and low mortality. Nevertheless, despite recurrent relapses or, indeed, surgical operations, the majority of patients lead full and active lives if there has been good nutritional support, regular follow-up, and judicious use of medical and surgical treatment.

Following ileal resection, at least 45 per cent of patients will have a recurrence within 5 to 10 years, which tends to be less than the recurrence rate following ileocolonic resection. Of those that do relapse, approximately half will require further surgery. However, the risk of requiring further resections is probably not increased by previous resections, although this point is debated.

Recently, endoscopic examination of the 'neoterminal ileum' has shown recurrent inflammation in 65 to 80 per cent of patients during the 6 months following ileocolonic resection. Endoscopic appearances range from diffuse inflammation to aphthoid ulceration to confluent ulceration. However, it is not yet entirely clear whether the severity of these endoscopic recurrences predicts the subsequent clinical course.

Survival curves drawn by actuarial methods have shown that mortality tends to increase with the length of history. For the first 15 years of the disease, mortality is no different from a matched control population, but then tends to increase above that expected.

CROHN'S DISEASE IN PREGNANCY

Female patients with Crohn's disease are as fertile, in general, as a control population. However, patients should avoid conceiving when the disease is active as there tends to be a high incidence of miscarriage. Apart from this, pregnancy seems to have little effect on the Crohn's disease and therefore patients should not be discouraged from having children if they wish. Should a relapse occur during pregnancy, it should be treated as vigorously as if the patient was not pregnant. Corticosteroids and sulphasalazine should be used as indicated, and should in no way be withheld. Patients conceiving while on treatment should be reassured that the developing fetus is not at risk, and the drugs should only be withdrawn as dictated by the activity of the disease. Some patients conceive while on azathioprine. Once again, there is no hard evidence that this will harm the fetus, although it is probably wise to stop the drug. However, if the Crohn's disease has been difficult to control and has only recently gone into remission with the introduction of azathioprine, the drug should be continued. A recent audit on the outcome of pregnancies in women with Crohn's disease who were receiving azathioprine has not shown an increased incidence of congenital abnormalities.

CROHN'S DISEASE IN CHILDREN

The disease can occur rarely within the first few months of life, but the frequency then increases after the age of 2 years. Epidemiological studies in the United Kingdom suggest that the incidence of Crohn's disease in children is increasing at a time when it has levelled out, or even fallen, in the adult population. The anatomical distribution of the disease is similar to that seen in adults. Symptomatically, the presentation may also be similar to that in adults, but some children will present with growth failure as the only manifestation. There is frequently a considerable delay in diagnosis, either because of the absence of gastrointestinal symptoms or because the children are labelled as having 'toddler's diarrhoea', 'growing pains', milk allergy, or even a functional syndrome. Once the diagnosis is suspected, it should be confirmed with full gastrointestinal assessment as described for adults.

Treatment should follow the same guidelines as those outlined for adults, with appropriate modification in the dosage of the drugs. Nutritional support is perhaps even more important than in adults, and a dietitian should document the child's dietary intake at regular intervals. Growth charts should be in the hospital notes, and recordings of height and weight should be made at each visit. Dietary supplements may be necessary to maintain an intake of at least 2000 kcal with 15 g nitrogen daily.

FURTHER READING

Allan RN, Keighley MRB, Alexander-Williams, J, Hawkins C, eds. *Inflammatory bowel diseases.* 2nd edn. Edinburgh: Churchill Livingstone, 1990.

Alstead EM, Ritchie, JK, Lennard-Jones JE, Farthing MJG, Clark ML. Safety of azathioprine in pregnancy in inflammatory bowel disease. *Gastroenterology* 1990; **99**: 443–6.

Jewell DP, ed. Pathogenesis of inflammatory bowel disease. *Eur J Gastroenterol Hepatol* 1990; **2**: 235–65.

Kirsner JB, Shorter RG, eds. *Inflammatory bowel disease.* 3rd edn. Philadelphia: Lea and Febiger, 1988.

Lowes JR, Jewell DP. The immunology of inflammatory bowel disease. *Springer Semin Immunopath* 1990; **12**: 251–68.

16.2.2 Surgery for Crohn's disease of the small intestine

NEIL MORTENSEN

INTRODUCTION

Opinion on the nature of surgery for small bowel Crohn's disease has varied since the earliest operations described by Crohn and colleagues. At first wide resection was the treatment of choice, but high relapse rates led to a period when bypass procedures were popular. In due course these patients appeared to have a high incidence of septic and fistula complications from their bypassed segments and there was a return to radical surgery once more. Since Crohn's disease is a diffuse intestinal problem, and the majority of patients undergo surgery at some time during the course of their disease, there has been a move towards minimal or conservative surgery. The rate of recurrence increases with the length of follow-up, and there is a group of patients who require repeated resections at increasingly frequent intervals. It is this group who are at greatest risk of developing a surgically induced short-bowel syndrome and malnutrition. Recurrence of Crohn's disease is independent of the presence of microscopic disease at the resection margins and, as yet, there is no successful adjuvant medical therapy to decrease the incidence of recurrence following surgery.

Strictly speaking, there is no such thing as a surgical recurrence of Crohn's disease, but rather a recrudescence of a previously quiescent focus of Crohn's disease at a different site.

THE AIMS OF SURGERY

Since Crohn's disease cannot be cured by wide surgical excision, surgical management is reserved for the complications of Crohn's disease. The main indications are to:

(1) remove or relieve an area of stenosis causing persistent or recurrent obstructive symptoms;
(2) treat enterocutaneous or enterovesical fistulae;
(3) drain an intra-abdominal abscess—this role is now being achieved increasingly by percutaneous radiological techniques;
(4) control acute or chronic blood loss, though this is rare;
(5) treat free perforation, but this is exceedingly uncommon.

Since the risk of recrudescence of Crohn's disease is sufficient to require the treatment of approximately 6 per cent of cases a year, many patients will need a number of operations during a lifetime. It is important when operating to deal only with the specific complication which has been the indication for the procedure, and bowel should not be removed just because it is affected by Crohn's disease. Surgery should be as conservative as possible, but stenosed bowel, even in a defunctioned segment, should not be left untreated. The greatest care must be taken with surgical technique, ensuring well-vascularized, tension-free anastomoses and the avoidance of inadvertent damage to adjacent loops of the bowel.

CROHN'S DISEASE AT SPECIFIC SITES IN THE SMALL INTESTINE

Gastroduodenal

Gastroduodenal disease is rare and almost always occurs in association with disease elsewhere. It can cause bleeding or stenosis, and disease in the duodenum most frequently produces clinical symptoms (Fig. 1). At endoscopy it can be difficult to distinguish between peptic ulcer and Crohn's disease. Peptic ulcers almost always respond to H_2-receptor antagonists, whereas Crohn's disease does not.

Resection of the duodenum is not feasible and therefore this is the one area of the small bowel in which bypass is the preferred treatment. At one time gastrojejunostomy was thought to be the treatment of choice. However, in some patients who have already had extensive small-bowel resection, gastric hypersecretion may result, and it has been customary to add a vagotomy to reduce the high risk of stomal ulceration. This vagotomy may, in turn, compound the patient's problem with diarrhoea.

A selective vagotomy has the theoretical advantage that diarrhoea is less likely to occur. With the advent of H_2-receptor antagonists and omeprazole it is possible to control gastric secretion in Crohn's disease patients. Where possible, a strictureplasty should be carried out on pyloric or duodenal disease to save the patient the complications of a gastroenterostomy. There

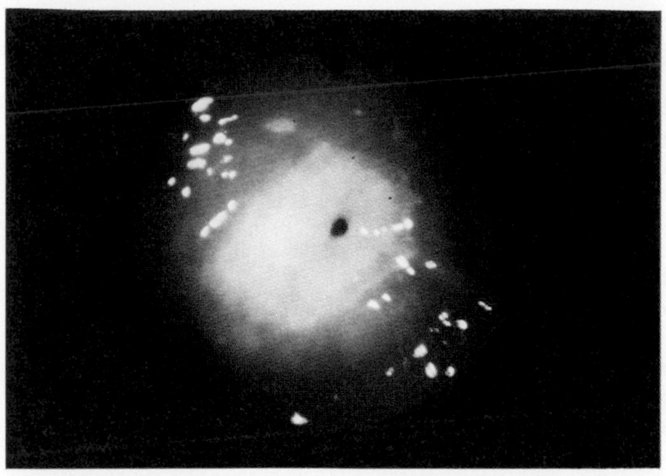

Fig. 1 Endoscopic appearance of Crohn's disease at the pylorus. There is pinpoint gastric outlet with surrounding ulceration.

are preliminary reports of the use of balloon dilatation for duodenal stenosis caused by Crohn's disease, but it is too early to judge its success.

Jejunum and ileum

The most commonly affected site is the terminal ileum. However, there may be multiple foci throughout the small bowel (Fig. 2) and here it is often difficult to tell exactly which lesion is responsible for the patient's symptoms. The most common indication for surgery in Crohn's disease of the small bowel is recurrent intestinal colic, provoked by solid food. Presentation is often insidious or subacute and may or may not be associated with diarrhoea. Weight loss is a major symptom. The patient may be anorexic, or be literally frightened to eat for fear of pain.

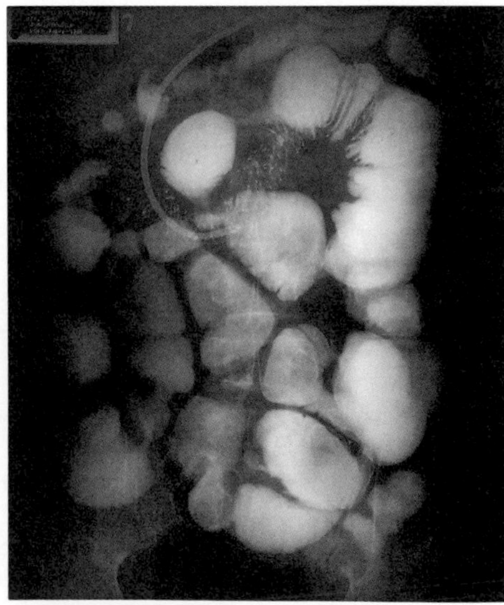

Fig. 2 Small bowel enema demonstrating multiple strictures and dilated areas in diffuse small bowel Crohn's disease.

SURGERY

General principles

It is wise to give the patient full bowel preparation just in case there is any colon involvement. Routine antiembolus measures are taken, including stockings and low-dose subcutaneous heparin. Since there is good evidence that patients with Crohn's disease have organisms in lymphatics and lymph nodes outside the bowel wall, antibiotic prophylaxis with a cephalosporin and metronidazole is given for between 2 and 5 days. In this situation the antibiotics are probably being used for established infection rather than to prevent inoculation of a clean abdominal operation site. We usually give intravenous steroid cover (hydrocortisone 100 mg thrice daily) for the operation, introducing oral steroids when the patient is taking fluids by mouth. This is reduced to a dose of 10 mg, on which the patient is maintained until review. Although many surgeons would operate on a patient flat on the operating table, ileosigmoid or ileorectal fistulae in Crohn's disease are common and, in complicated cases, access to the rectum may be necessary. Therefore I usually operate on patients in the modified lithotomy Trendelenburg position used for colorectal surgery. A full laparotomy is carried out, carefully examining the whole length of the intestine for external macroscopic features of Crohn's disease.

Ileocolic disease

This is best treated with a conservative ileocaecal resection to include a short margin of macroscopically normal gut on each side of the resection specimen (Fig. 3). In patients with severe disease, however, the presence of minor macroscopic evidence of Crohn's disease at the anastomotic site is not important and the emphasis should be on preserving gut length. There has been some controversy over the use of various suture materials and the precise type of anastomosis used, and their possible effect on disease recrudescence. There is no definite evidence of an effect of either of these; I usually carry out a straight end-to-end ileocolic anastomosis, using absorbable suture material (3-0 Vicryl). It is helpful to mark the site of the anastomosis with metal clips so that future radiological investigations can localize new disease.

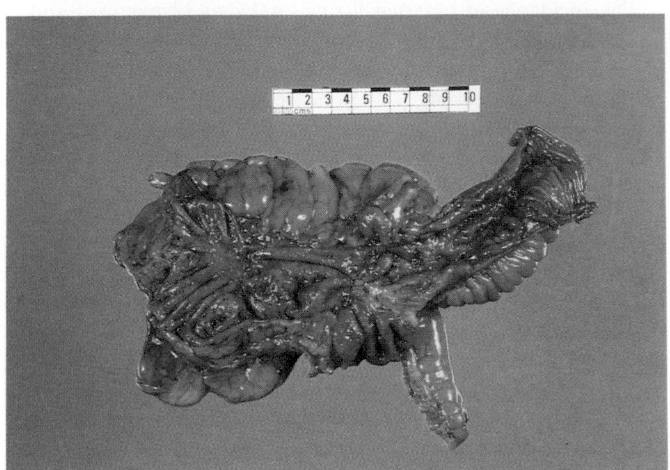

Fig. 3 Resection specimen of ileocolic Crohn's disease.

Results of surgery for ileocolic disease

Actuarial methods are now widely used for the effective comparison of results of treatment between various centres because they correct for the varying lengths of follow-up between individual patients.

The cumulative operation rate for patients with distal ileal disease at 5 years from the time of diagnosis is 80 per cent. Cumulative reoperation rate after the first resection for distal ileal Crohn's disease at 5 years after the first operation is 25 per cent and at 10 years this rises to 35 per cent. If an ileocolic anastomosis is inspected carefully by colonoscopy, aphthous ulceration can be seen on the ileal side of the anastomosis as early as 6 months after surgery. There is no evidence that age at the time of initial diagnosis has any effect on recurrence rate.

Although recurrent disease is therefore very common, surgical treatment of distal ileal disease rapidly restores the patient with chronic persistent symptoms to good health. On average, patients have an operation once every 10 years, so they could expect to have 3 or 4 operations over a lifetime.

Multisite small intestinal disease

Lee pioneered the concept of treating Crohn's disease strictures by strictureplasty. He operated on patients with intestinal obstruction and malnutrition in whom excisional surgery was thought to be contraindicated because of diffuse small bowel involvement or a short-gut syndrome resulting from previous excisions. Lee proposed the concept of minimal surgery to overcome sites of obstruction. In some places this would be a mini-resection, and in others strictureplasty. In a subsequent report of 10 years' experience of strictureplasty for obstructive Crohn's disease, including the first patients operated on by Lee in Oxford, 24 patients had 86 strictureplasties at 30 separate operations. There were no deaths, fistulae, or wound infections related to the operation site and patients made positive weight gains in the postoperative period.

Ten further operations for obstructive symptoms were carried out in four patients 18 months after their previous strictureplasties. All but one of the previous strictureplasties in the additional operations were found to be widely patent and not the cause of the recurrent obstruction. Alexander Williams carried out 198 strictureplasties in 64 patients. In addition to using the technique in short stenoses, he has used a Finney pyloroplasty-like method for stenotic areas of more than 10 cm in length. Major complications developed in five patients who developed enterocutaneous fistulae, a clinical leak rate of 2.5 per cent. At 6 months 80 per cent had an excellent symptomatic response, being free of pain with improvement in general well-being.

Another study looked at the site-specific recurrence rate in 41 patients treated by strictureplasty, and reported that no recurrence occurred in those patients. A control group continued to be treated by small-bowel resection and there was no difference between the two groups. There is no evidence as yet that disease remaining at the strictureplasty site precipitates early recrudescence.

Operative technique

In multifocal disease it is essential to identify every stricture. Even though a stricture may not look very narrow from the outward appearance, this can be misleading (Fig. 4). I usually choose the middle stricture and open it on the antimesenteric border, along

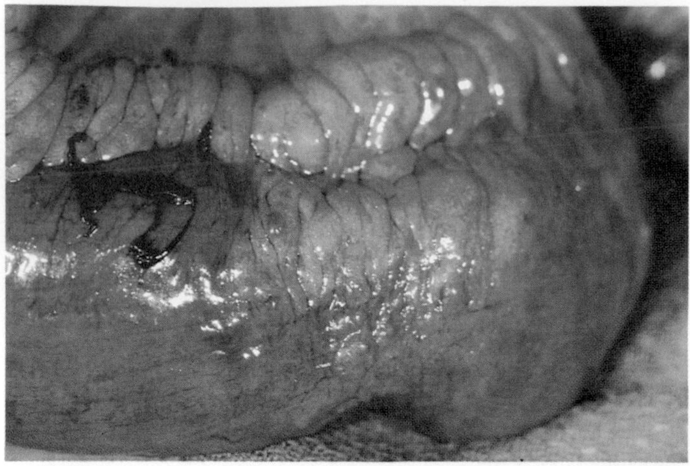

Fig. 4 A typical short segment of ileal Crohn's disease. Note the narrowing and fat wrapping. The external appearance of a stricture like this can be misleading with much more luminal narrowing than expected.

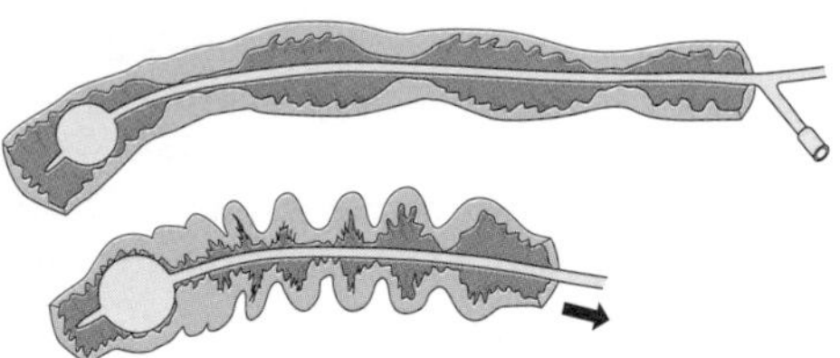

Fig. 5 Balloon catheter characterization of small bowel Crohn's disease strictures.

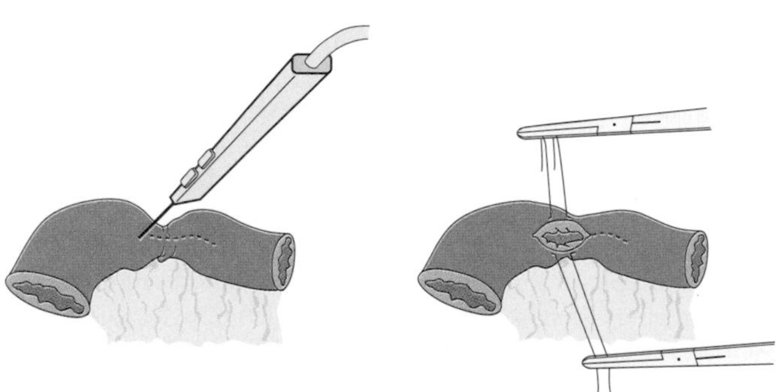

Fig. 6 Strictureplasty—a longtitudinal incision is made between stay strictures with diathermy.

the long axis of the small intestine. A 20 French gauge Foley balloon catheter is inflated with saline to give balloon diameters of 15, 20 and 25 mm (Fig. 5). The intestine is then characterized from the duodenojejunal flexure to the caecum by passing the catheter along the gut lumen and then inflating the balloon, allowing it to impact at each stricture site as it is slowly withdrawn. This ensures that no strictures are undetected and prevents the dangerous scenario of obstruction downstream from a suture line. The diameter is recorded and its position marked with a suture. A stenosis of less than 20 mm diameter is usually treated by strictureplasty. The stricture site is held in stay sutures and a longitudinal incision made by diathermy (Fig. 6). The bowel is opened out, and, if the appearance is suspicious, a biopsy should be taken to exclude the possibility of cancerous change, although we do not do this routinely. The stricture site is then closed transversely in the manner of a Heinecke-Mickulicz pyloroplasty (Fig. 7), although some slightly longer strictures have been anastomosed in the manner of Finney. We use a continuous absorbable suture in a single layer. In our experience the median length of the strictureplasty has been 3 cm. Simultaneous intestinal resections have been undertaken for longer sections of disease, but we make these mini-resections as far as possible. Multiple strictureplasties can be carried out at any one sitting and the strictureplasty sites are usually marked with metal clips for future reference. A stapling technique has been described using a GIA stapler, but the resulting anastomosis looks more like a side-to-side than a strictureplasty.

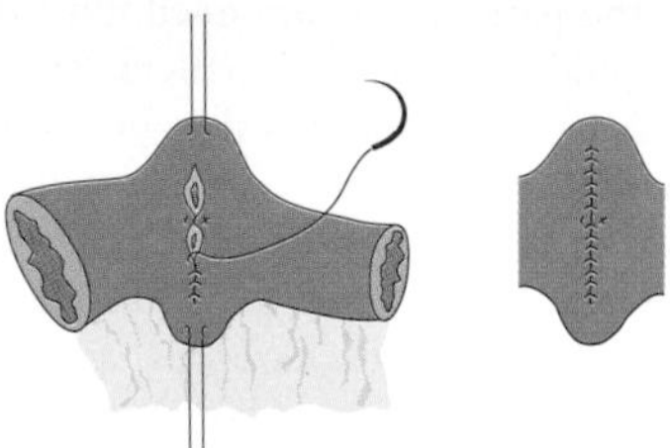

Fig. 7 Strictureplasty—the structure site is sutured transversely.

What happens at the strictureplasty site?

There is some evidence that disease may heal, or at least not progress. Removing the obstructive element, even though the original triggering factors are likely to be present, may modify the progression of the disease. Once obstruction has occurred, a chain of events is precipitated resulting in mucosal leakiness, transmural fissuring, and, eventually, abscess and fistula formation.

FISTULA AND ABSCESS

Small-bowel Crohn's disease can be complicated by enteroenteric, enterovesical, or enterocutaneous fistulae. It is important to emphasize that postoperative fistulae may be due to an anastomotic breakdown, and not associated with any residual or recurrent active Crohn's disease.

The incidence of external fistulae is 17 to 22 per cent and of internal fistulae, 9 to 25 per cent. Preoperative abscess as a complication of Crohn's disease occurs in some 10 per cent of patients and, following resection, postoperative abscess is found in 14 per cent, of which a third occur in patients with a preoperative abscess. The organisms involved are usually enteric, including *Escherichia coli*, *Bacteroides fragilis*, and enterococci. Wound infection and intra-abdominal abscesses are common problems in patients with Crohn's disease.

These abscesses may be primary or secondary. They probably occur at the site of a transmural fissure and may be the first stage in the development of a fistula as the abscess tracks to another loop of gut or the abdominal wall. The common sites for an abscess are the pelvis, abdominal wall, and psoas sheath, or around the segment of affected bowel. Abscesses penetrating posteriorly into the psoas produce symptoms of fever, weight loss, and a flexion deformity of the hip. They can point at the groin or buttock (Fig. 8). Drainage of the abscesses invariably results in a fistula. Secondary abscesses

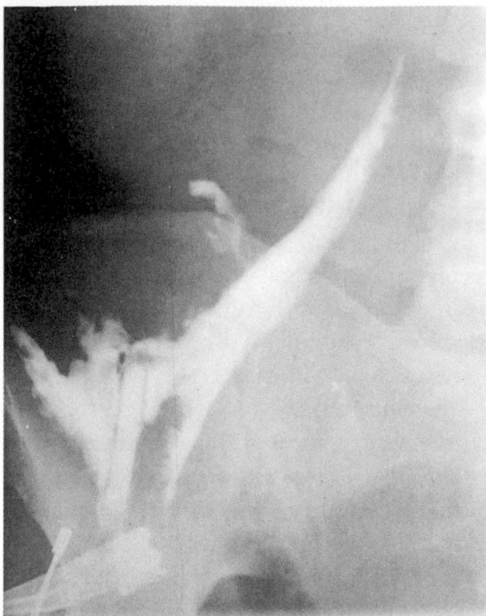

Fig. 8 Sinogram through a sinus in the right inguinal region showing a psoas abscess secondary to ileocaecal Crohn's disease.

are more common and follow surgical procedures, often in malnourished septic patients. They may also occur slowly and present many months later.

Most external fistulae pass through the site of a previous surgical incision, and a spontaneous fistula through the abdominal wall is rare.

Appendicectomy and fistula

An external fistula following appendicectomy usually arises from a segment of ileum actively involved with Crohn's disease rather than the appendix stump. If Crohn's disease is found at a laparotomy for presumed 'appendicitis' the appendix should be removed. This will ensure that future attacks of pain can be managed without confusion. Where there is extensive caecal involvement, an ileocaecal resection is preferred.

Free perforation

This is surprisingly rare from small-bowel Crohn's disease. Sudden onset of pain in a patient with an exacerbation of Crohn's disease treated with steroids should be regarded as a possible perforation until proven otherwise.

Fistula and abscess: investigation

Fistula and abscess go hand in hand, and fistula cannot be treated successfully without the elimination of any concurrent abscess.

History and examination

Fever, weight loss, diarrhoea, and abdominal pain are the usual symptoms of an internal fistula, although some enterenteric fistulas can be entirely asymptomatic. A discharge sinus is the hallmark of an external fistula, although only about 50 per cent may discharge faeces, the rest producing gas or pus (Fig. 9). There may be a mass or area of tenderness to suggest an abscess.

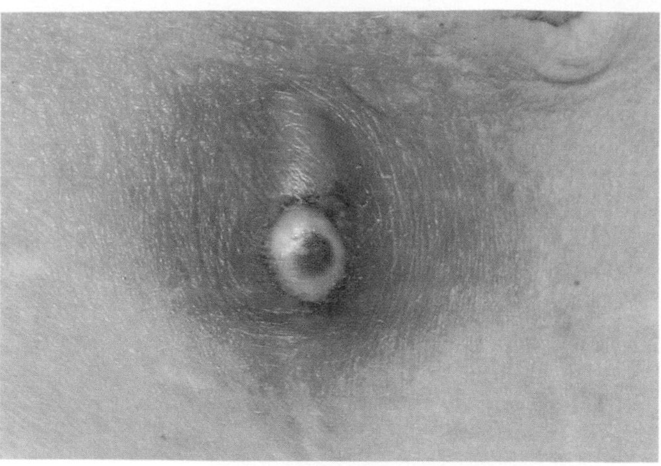

Fig. 9 An enterocutaneous fistula complicating Crohn's disease pointing through an old laparotomy scar.

Investigations

Nutritional and biochemical assessment should include haemoglobin, serum albumin, body weight, lymphocyte count, and liver function tests. Barium contrast studies, especially a small-bowel enema, are best for demonstrating areas of small-bowel disease, a fistula, and even an abscess (Fig. 10). Fistulography provides important information about the complexity of a track. Ultrasound and computerized tomography (CT) scans are the best methods for demonstrating an abscess, and CT-guided percutaneous drainage of abscesses is becoming increasingly successful (Fig. 11). Endoscopy will help to define the extent of mucosal disease and the presence and nature of a stricture, but rarely identifies a tiny fistula track, for example at an ileocolic anastomosis.

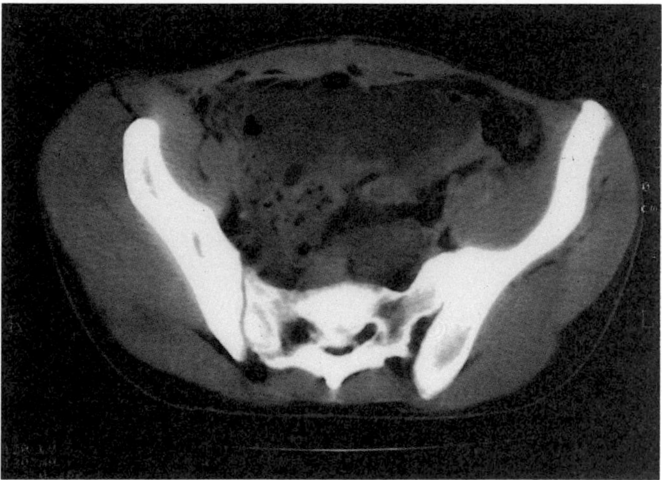

Fig. 10 A small bowel enema showing ileal loops separated by a mass—an abscess.

Treatment of abscesses and fistulae

Many internal fistulae are asymptomatic and often a chance finding at laparotomy. Any area of active small-bowel Crohn's

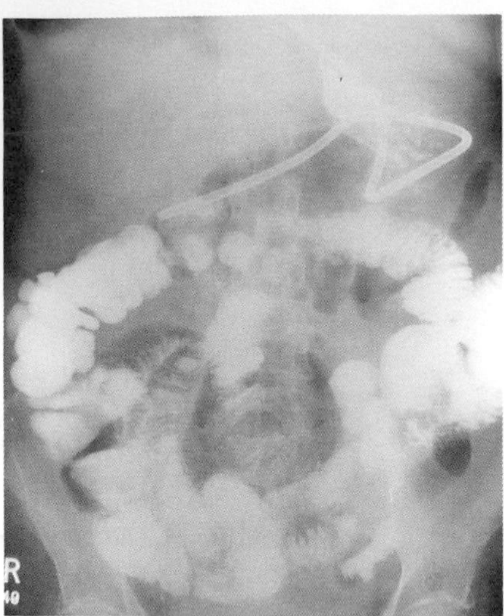

Fig. 11 CT demonstrating an intra-abdominal abscess.

disease adherent to an adjacent organ should be regarded as a fistula until proven otherwise. Disease is usually on the small-bowel side of an enterocolic fistula. This can be pinched off and the hole in the colon closed. Formal resection is seldom necessary. Enterocutaneous fistulae usually arise at an anastomosis or in a segment of non-involved bowel damaged at surgery. The management of these can be very challenging and requires a team approach. Within the first 24 hours, fluid and electrolyte problems must be corrected and the skin protected with stomadhesive and a wound-management appliance. Intravenous nutrition should next be established through a dedicated central venous line. If there is an abscess it must be drained, preferably by a percutaneous technique. Broad-spectrum antibiotics are given for a defined period and are not a substitute for adequate drainage. Then the fistula anatomy can be defined. It is reasonable to try a period of conservative management, and some 60 to 70 per cent of postanastomotic fistulae will heal spontaneously.

Spontaneous enterocutaneous fistulae rarely heal. Although medical trials with azathioprine, 6-mercaptopurine, and cyclosporin have been reported, surgical exploration and resection of the fistula with anastomosis is usually necessary.

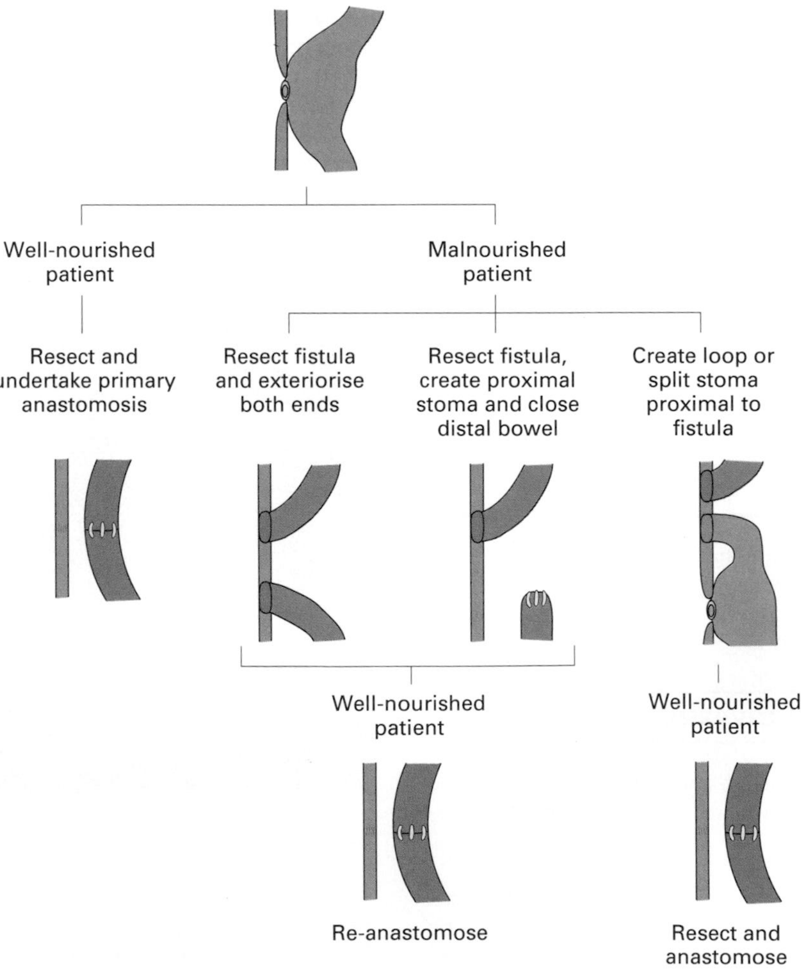

Fig. 12 Diagram showing the strategy for managing an enterocutaneous fistula complicating Crohn's disease.

Surgical closure

Operative treatment can be successful in experienced hands, provided there is not extensive sepsis or profound hypoalbuminaemia, and distal obstruction must be carefully excluded. If the patient is grossly hypoalbuminaemic or septic, the procedure of choice is resection and exteriorization of both bowel ends or, less optimally, a proximal bypass leaving the disease and fistula in place. When the patient is well and the sepsis drained, a second procedure to restore continuity is permissible. It may be necessary to wait for many weeks until a patient is fit enough for a further operation. Where the patient is well, resection and primary anastomosis are indicated (Fig. 12).

Abscess

An abscess pointing at the skin surface should be drained but is usually followed by a fistula. The introduction of ultrasound and CT have not only improved diagnosis and localization of abscesses, but percutaneous drainage techniques have largely replaced open laparotomy with all its hazards in a sick patient. The drainage of an intra-abdominal abscess is an absolute priority and undrained sepsis can be lethal. Antibiotics should be given in short effective courses, taking into account bacteriological reports on any swabs taken from an abscess.

Enterovesical fistula

Repeated urinary tract infections, turbid urine, and pneumaturia suggest an enterovesical fistula. This is not an absolute indication for surgery but they seldom heal and eventually come to surgery.

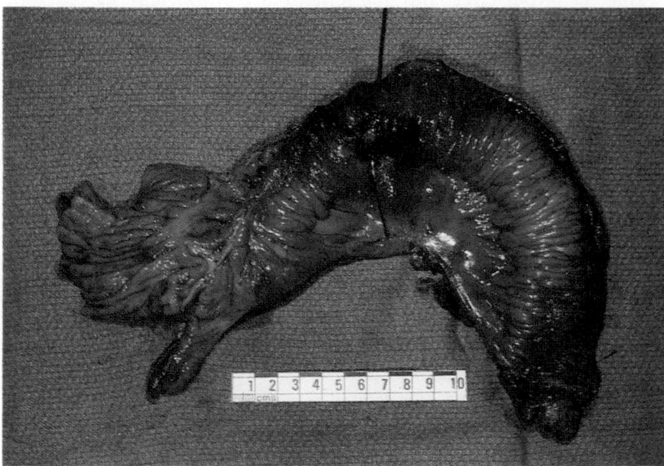

Fig. 13 Ileocolic resection specimen from a patient with an enterovesical fistula. The probe indicates the site of the fistula which has been 'pinched off' the bladder.

The small bowel can usually be 'pinched' off the bladder and resected (Figs. 13, 14). The bladder itself only requires curettage and careful closure. A catheter is left in the bladder for at least a week.

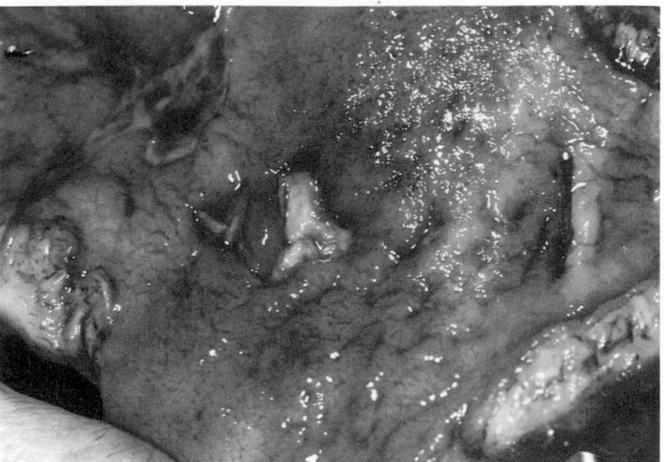

Fig. 14 Mucosal surface of the same specimen showing the discrete ulceration characteristic of Crohn's disease. The large ulcer in the middle was the internal opening of the enterovesical fistula.

FURTHER READING

Alexander Williams J, Irving M. *Intestinal fistulas.* Bristol: Wright, 1982.

Alexander Williams J. The technique of intestinal strictureplasty. *Int J Colorect Dis* 1986; **1**: 54–7.

Allan RN, Keighley MRB, Alexander Williams J, Hawkins C., eds. *Inflammatory bowel diseases.* 2nd edn. Edinburgh: Churchill Livingstone, 1990.

Coutsoftides T, Fazio VW. Small intestine cutaneous fistulas. *Surg Gynecol Obstet* 1979; **149**: 333–6.

Dehn TCB, Kettlewell MGW, Mortensen NJMcC, Lee ECG, Jewell DP. Ten-years experience of strictureplasty for obstructive Crohns disease. *Br J Surg* 1989; **75**: 339–41.

Fazio W, Galandiuk S. Strictureplasty in diffuse Crohns jejun ileitis. *Dis Colon Rect* 1985; **28**: 512–18.

Greenstein AJ, *et al.* Perforating and non perforating indications for repeated operations in Crohn's disease. *Gut* 1988; **29**: 588–92.

Keighley MRB, Eastwood D, Ambrose NS, Allan RN, Burdon DW. Incidence and microbiology of abdominal and pelvic abscess in Crohn's disease. *Gastroenterology* 1982; **83**: 1271–5.

Lee ECG, Papionnu N. Minimal Surgery for chronic obstruction in patients with extensive or universal Crohn's disease. *Ann R Coll Surg Eng* 1982; **64**: 229–33.

Sayfan J, Wilson DAL, Allan A, Andrews H, Alexander Williams J. Recurrence after strictureplasty or resection for Crohn's disease. *Br J Surg* 1989; **76**: 335–8.

Williams JG, Wong WD, Rothenberger DA, Goldberg SM. Recurrence of Crohn's disease after resection. *Br J Surg* 1991; **78**: 10–19.

16.3 Small bowel fistulae

LESLIE W. OTTINGER

A fistula is an abnormal communication between a hollow viscus and some other organ or structure, including the skin. To be classified as such, it is understood that the communication remains open for long enough to present a clinical problem. Some fistulas are complex, with multiple tracts and associated abscess cavities. Others are simple and heal spontaneously. The subject of this chapter is fistulae originating in the duodenum, jejunum, or ileum.

CLASSIFICATION

There are several ways to classify fistulae and these are useful in selecting measures for management and for comparison of therapeutic approaches. The first is descriptive, and includes the sites of origin and termination: examples are jejunocutaneous or ileovesical fistulas. A second classification is internal versus external; internal fistulae include ileocolic or ileoileo fistulae; external fistulae include duodenocutaneous or ileovaginal. Thirdly, external fistulae can be classified by output. A useful practical separation is into low output fistulae that produce less than 200 ml of discharge per day and high output fistulae that discharge more than that amount. Finally, it is helpful to classify fistulae into those originating from normal intestine and those associated with an abnormality such as Crohn's disease or radiation enteritis.

CAUSES

Almost all external fistulae develop as an early complication following surgical procedures. A few of these are the result of technical errors in bowel anastomoses or repair; more frequently, they result from sepsis in the region of a suture line. In either case, they present as an abscess draining through the recent incision followed by the establishment of a fistula. A few external fistulae occur at the site of an old surgical incision, and are associated with a foreign body, usually mesh used in the repair of a fascial defect, recurrence of inflammatory bowel disease, or a tumour. Rarely, external fistulae are spontaneous and occur at the site of drainage of an abscess originating from a bowel perforation. These can be caused by a tumour or inflammatory bowel disease.

Internal fistulae differ in that they seldom follow a surgical procedure, but are usually the result of a local perforation of diseased bowel. An abscess forms that affects an adjacent structure. In most cases this is a loop of small intestine or colon but it can be part of the urinary tract or even the biliary system.

PRINCIPLES OF MANAGEMENT

Spontaneous rapid closure of fistulae is seen regularly on removal of a draining or feeding tube from the duodenum or jejunum. This rapid healing can be expected when the fistula originates from normal intestine, is made up of a narrow cicatricial tract, and is not associated with active sepsis. There must also be a satisfactory capability for normal healing, which implies an adequate nutritional status.

The factors contributing to failure of spontaneous closure are largely implied in the foregoing paragraph. They include origin of the fistula in abnormal intestine, such as a segment involved by Crohn's disease, radiation enteritis, or a tumour. Other intrinsic factors preventing spontaneous healing are an extensive defect in the intestine, such as dehiscence of a suture line or the presence of distal obstruction.

The absence of a narrow cicatricial tract is frequently the result of local sepsis. Thus, the internal intestinal opening empties into a cavity or cavities which then drains through the abdominal wall. The presence of a foreign body may prevent the local control of sepsis and the formation of such a tract. Finally, the junction of mucosa of the intestine with that of another loop of intestine or the skin can prevent healing. This is an especially important factor in internal fistulae.

In patients severely depleted by an underlying illness or chronic fluid and electrolyte losses, healing also may be impaired. In the chronically ill patient, a loss of 15 per cent of body weight and a low serum albumin furnish useful clues to the specific need for extra nutritional support.

Measures to decrease fistula output not only simplify management, but also allow more rapid closure and simplify the management of skin inflammation and erosion.

The basic steps in the management of fistulae are outlined in Table 1. Experience and judgement are important in reaching decisions about the need and timing of surgical intervention. The goal is to achieve permanent closure of the fistula in the shortest time and with the lowest possible risk to the patient. Individual management based on sound principles is the key.

Table 1 Steps in the management of intestinal fistulae

1. Replenish blood volume and electrolytes
2. Initiate measures for local skin care
3. Perform studies to demonstrate site of origin and aetiology
4. Initiate measures to decrease volume output (if high)
5. Evaluate need for and initiate nutritional support
6. Control local sepsis
7. Decide on need and timing for surgical intervention

General measures

Some patients with fistulae present with serious acute problems that include fluid and electrolyte depletion and uncontrolled sepsis. Aggressive management to correct these decreases the chance of secondary complications such as renal failure and metastatic sepsis. The measures to be employed do not need further discussion here.

Prevention of skin breakdown is much easier than its management: sump catheters may be required for the management of a large wound. Later a collecting bag should be used as a means for protecting the skin and quantitating output. The assistance of an enterostomal therapist or nurse skilled in the various possible approaches to this is ideal, but devoted nursing care is the major element in success.

Once these two steps have been accomplished, studies should be undertaken to determine the site of origin of the fistula, the condition of the intestine at that point, and whether there is an associated abscess cavity. Generally, a fistulogram, using a water soluble radio-opaque medium, is a good first choice, perhaps combined with an ultrasound study or CT scan. If there is no cavity, barium studies can then be used to gain further detail and to opacify the intestine at and below the fistula. Orally administered barium will usually give the most information, including information about the size of the leak, the absence of distal obstruction and the presence of a tumour, or extent of inflammatory changes in the intestine itself.

Steps to decrease fistula output may simplify management and increase the rate of spontaneous closure. The initial measure is the placement of a nasogastric tube or if long-term use may be indicated, a gastrostomy tube. Sometimes this can be placed at the time of another operative procedure. The nasogastric tube is, however, a cause of discomfort, and it can increase the tendency toward aspiration and pulmonary sepsis in older and debilitated patients and may also induce an oesophageal stricture. Pharmacological means of decreasing output include the administration of H_2 blockers without antacids and somatostatin analogues.

The status of the patient or anticipation of a long period of starvation may indicate a need for nutritional support. Central parenteral hyperalimentation will allow the intestinal tract to be placed completely at rest. This has special benefits in the patient with Crohn's disease, in whom regression of the extent and severity of the disease is commonly observed. A few fistulae in such patients may actually heal simplifying later surgical intervention.

A second approach uses elemental diets. These can be completely absorbed and require no digestion. They are poorly tolerated orally because they are so unpalatable but can be instilled through a small nasogastric feeding tube, a gastrostomy tube or a jejunal feeding tube. Continuous rather than bolus infusion is better tolerated. They are most useful in patients with a very distal fistula or in those who have a feeding tube in place distal to a proximal fistula.

Finally, especially with a low output fistula, oral feedings are sometimes well tolerated. The output of the fistula should be monitored. If it is not much increased by eating, this can provide the least expensive and safest form of nutritional support.

Early surgical intervention usually involves only measures to gain better control of the fistula and increase the likelihood of spontaneous closure. In addition to the placement of draining and feeding enterostomy tubes, this includes steps to promote the formation of a single narrow drainage tract. Abscess cavities must be unroofed or drained and placing a catheter adjacent to or even in a fistula opening may be useful. Simple closure of the fistula opening with sutures at this stage is, however, almost certain to fail.

The definitive treatment of fistulae that do not close spontaneously is surgical resection. Most external fistulae associated with Crohn's disease require such treatment. In almost all cases a segment of intestine is removed with anastomosis, the sutured bowel being placed in an area not affected by inflammation or other abnormality. A bypass may be all that can be accomplished. Duodenal fistulae are an exception: segmental resection is seldom feasible, and the surgical measure most likely to succeed is Roux-en-Y limb anastomosed over the fistula, converting it to a permanent internal fistula (Fig. 1). If direct closure seems possible, the suture line should be protected by bringing up a loop of intact small intestine as a 'serosal patch'. This condition meets the need of providing a normal local environment for healing.

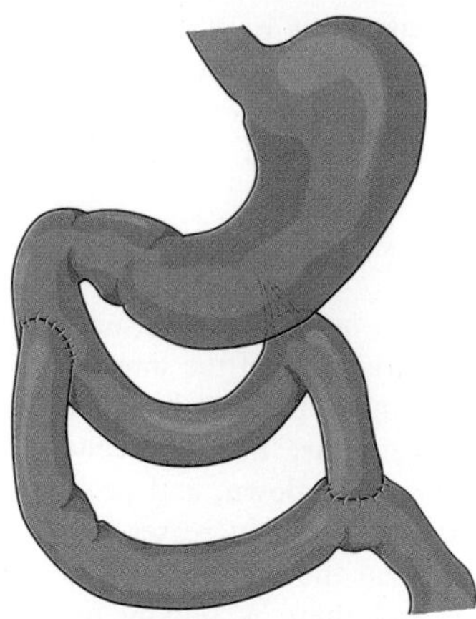

Fig. 1 Use of a jejunal limb to convert a duodenocutaneous fistula to an internal fistula.

Timing of surgical intervention requires judgement and experience. Factors that enter into the decision are size and location of the fistula, condition of the patient, nature and extent of intestinal abnormality, presence of obstruction, fistula output, and likelihood of eventual spontaneous healing. The surgeon must also consider the likelihood of accomplishing a satisfactory operation. The acute obliterative peritonitis that follows complicated operations is likely to be an important factor in reoperation between 10 days and 6 weeks after the original operation. The tendency at the present time is to delay too long rather than operate too soon. Medical management has largely eliminated the necessity for urgent resection of fistulae but can also contribute unnecessarily to the period of disability and expense by lengthening the stay in hospital.

LOW OUTPUT FISTULAE

These fistulae drain small amounts of fluid, arbitrarily up to 200 ml/day. The drainage often has the appearance of mucous or infected material that does not suggest an intestinal origin. Acute low output postsurgical fistulae are the result of trivial injuries to the intestine, as in closing the abdominal wall or a small leak from an intact bowel anastomosis or repair, and almost always heal spontaneously. Obtaining adequate local drainage and a short period of parenteral fluid support facilitates closure.

Persistence of a low output fistula usually indicates the presence of a foreign body, typically heavy sutures or mesh, or an intrinsic abnormality of the intestine at the site of origin. The use of fine absorbable suture material can prevent some of these fistulae. Synthetic mesh that comes in contact with a segment of intestine eventually causes perforation, an abscess, and, typically, a low output chronic fistula. Sometimes only part of the mesh need be removed to secure healing: removal of all of the mesh creates the difficult additional problem of dealing with the resulting fascial defect at the time of operation.

The lack of urgency in the setting of a low output fistula allows complete evaluation of the intestine proximal and distal to the site of origin. The management of Crohn's disease, other inflammatory conditions, radiation enteritis, and tumours is usually not specifically altered by the presence of the fistula. Other factors dictate the timing and nature of surgical intervention.

HIGH OUTPUT FISTULAE

The presence of a high output fistula usually indicates either the diversion of a substantial part of the intestinal contents or a very proximal origin, and many patients have partial or complete obstruction or extensive suture line dehiscence. The likelihood of sepsis, extensive skin breakdown, and problems related to fluid loss and nutritional depletion increases with output. Successful management centres on the methodical application of measures already described, and there is seldom need for urgent direct surgical intervention. Some high output fistulae heal spontaneously, but many will be best managed by an elective resection under optimal conditions. The principles important to successful surgery have already been listed. The fact that local closure with limited exposure seldom succeeds is worth emphasis: the operation should be broad enough in scope to achieve an optimal repair. It is often better to enter the abdomen through a new incision and to begin by exposing the uninvolved loops of intestine. Patience and skill in dissection are needed. Any intestinal suture line must be placed in contact with normal serosal surfaces: leaving it in an area of chronic inflammation invites formation of a new fistula. Wide exposure will facilitate accomplishment of this objective and permits management of multiple fistulae or residual pockets of infection. Drains should be avoided unless considered absolutely necessary. Consideration should be given to the placement of draining gastrostomy and feeding jejunostomy tubes in complicated cases.

INTERNAL FISTULAE

Internal fistulae are almost always the result of chronic inflammation of the intestine. Perforation and abscess formation leads to communication with an adjacent loop of bowel or viscus. A few fistulae follow trauma or surgical misadventures.

Ileoileal and ileocolonic fistulae are relatively harmless and often asymptomatic—obstruction or sepsis rather than the fistula itself are the usual reasons for resection. Fistulae to the bladder or, rarely, to other parts of the urinary system, lead to recurrent bouts of urinary sepsis; for this reason they usually require resection. Duodenocholedochal fistulae, a rare complication of duodenal ulcer disease, are often asymptomatic, but may lead to episodes of biliary sepsis.

The first principle in management is to resect the segment of diseased bowel that gave origin to the fistula. Unless the intestine or viscus at the other end of the fistula is intrinsically diseased, a resection is not necessary. When the duodenum is the site, as in an ileoduodenal fistula from Crohn's disease, the closure should be buttressed with a loop of normal intestine. Simple closure is sufficient for fistulae to the vagina, uterus, or urinary bladder.

FURTHER READING

Aguirre A, Fischer JE, Welch CE. The role of surgery and hyperalimentation in therapy of gastrointestinal-cutaneous fistulae. *Ann Surg* 1974; **180**; 393–401.

Bury KD, Stephens RV, Randall HT. Use of a chemically defined, liquid, elemental diet for nutritional management of fistulas of the alimentary tract. *Am J Surg* 1971; **121**; 174–83.

Coutsoftides T, Fazio VW. Small intestine cutaneous fistulas. *Surg Gynecol Obstet* 1979; **149**; 333–6.

Edmunds LH, Williams GM, Welch CE. External fistulas arising from the gastro-intestinal tract. *Ann Surg* 1960; **152**; 445–71.

Greenstein AJ. The surgery of Crohn's disease. *Surg Clin N Am* 1987; **67**; 573–96.

Halasz NA. Changing patterns in the management of small bowel fistulas. *Am J Surg* 1978; **136**; 61–5.

Hill GL, Bourchier RG, Witney GB. Surgical and metabolic management of patients with external fistulas of the small intestine associated with Crohn's disease. *World J Surg* 1988; **12**; 191–7.

Nubioloa-Colonge Badia JM, Sancho J, Gil MJ, Segura M., Sitges-Serra A. Blind evaluation of the effect of octreotide (SMS 201–995), a somatostatin analogue, on small bowel fistula output. *Lancet* 1987; **ii**; 672–4.

Pettit SH, Irving MH. The operative management of fistulous Crohn's disease. *Surg Gynecol Obstet* 1988; **167**; 223–8.

Soeters PB, Ebeid AM, Fischer JE. Review of 404 patients with gastrointestinal fistulas. Impact of parenteral nutrition. *Ann Surg* 1979; **190**; 189–202.

16.4 Diverticular disease of the small bowel

MICHAEL N. MARGOLIES

MECKEL'S DIVERTICULUM

Meckel's diverticulum is a congenital diverticulum arising from failure of embryonic obliteration of the omphalomesenteric (vitelline) duct connecting the fetal gut to the yolk sac, that normally occurs during the fifth to seventh week of gestation. In contrast to other small-bowel diverticula, Meckel's diverticulum contains all intestinal layers and is antimesenteric. It is the most common congenital anomaly of the small intestine, found in 0.5 to 3.0 per cent of the population at postmortem examination. It is most often found within 1 metre of the ileocaecal valve and rarely up to 180 cm from the valve; the length of the diverticulum is usually less than 12 cm but can vary from 0.5 to 56 cm.

Meckel's diverticulum has a blood supply independent of that of the contiguous ileum, distinguishing it from ileal duplication; in addition, ileal duplication usually arises from the mesenteric border. The embryonic blood supply of the vitelline duct is by paired vitelline arteries, of which the right forms the superior mesenteric artery, while the left artery involutes. The blood supply to the diverticulum is derived from a remnant of one of these arteries. A mesodiverticular band may connect the diverticulum to the ileal mesentery; the contained vessel is often obliterated.

Associated anomalies

Simple Meckel's diverticulum represents the most common end-result among a set of omphalomesenteric duct anomalies, in which the entire duct is obliterated and is absorbed, with the exception of several centimetres attached to the small intestine (Fig. 1). Other associated abnormalities of duct obliteration include the following:

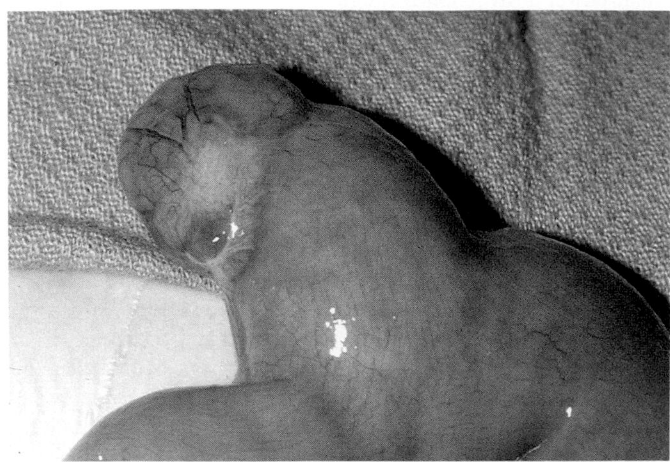

Fig. 1 Meckel's diverticulum in an 11-year-old male with rectal bleeding. Note the pale area near the top, signifying underlying heterotopic tissue.

(1) the entire vitelline duct persists, resulting in a fistula between the ileum and the umbilicus;

(2) the distal end of the duct persists as a sinus opening at the umbilicus or as an umbilical polyp;

(3) the duct lumen is obliterated but not absorbed, forming a fibrous band attached to the umbilicus, to other viscera, or with a free end;

(4) a segment of the duct remains patent, forming a cyst or 'enterocystoma' along its course;

(5) the mesodiverticular band described above;

(6) heterotopic tissue, usually consisting of gastric epithelium, is found in 30 to 50 per cent of cases, but may include pancreatic (5 per cent), colonic, jejunal, or duodenal elements;

(7) the diverticulum may be buried in an intramesenteric position or have a separate mesentery.

Radiological diagnosis

Meckel's diverticulum can be identified preoperatively by radionuclide scanning, barium contrast studies, arteriography, and occasionally by computerized tomographic scanning, with varying degrees of success. The pertechnetate anion ($^{99}Tc^{m}$) is selectively taken up and is secreted by gastric mucosal parietal cells in their normal and aberrant locations, as well as by thyroid and salivary glands and the choroid plexus. Thus, the demonstration of Meckel's diverticulum by abdominal scanning (Fig. 2) as an extragastric localized area of uptake, which increases temporally in parallel with gastric mucosal uptake, depends on the presence of ectopic gastric mucosa. Scanning is most successful in cases of bleeding due to associated peptic ulceration in children. In the most experienced centres, the sensitivity of detection is 85 per cent and specificity is 95 per cent. However, $^{99}Tc^{m}$ scanning may be less accurate than generally believed, particularly in adults, where the sensitivity is lower. A negative scan at any age does not exclude the diagnosis. Moreover, false-positive scans occur, ascribed to such unrelated conditions as small-bowel tumours, small-bowel obstruction, hydronephrosis, enteric duplication, and arteriovenous malformations.

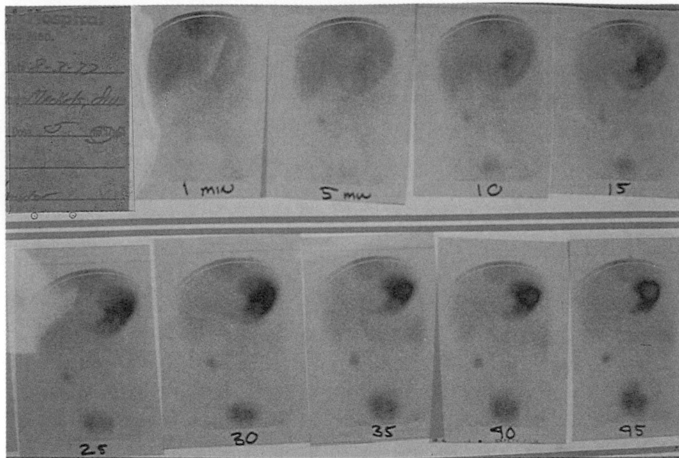

Fig. 2 Serial $^{99}Tc^{m}$ scans in an 11-year-old male with rectal bleeding. Note that the isotope uptake at a site in the right side of the abdomen corresponding to a Meckel's diverticulum increases simultaneously with gastric uptake. The large round area of uptake at the bottom represents the urinary bladder.

The diagnosis of Meckel's diverticulum is occasionally suggested on plain abdominal films on the basis of an enterolith or radio-opaque foreign body in the right lower quadrant or a persistent right lower quadrant or subumbilical gas collection. On antegrade small-bowel barium studies, the diverticulum is sometimes directly visualized, or suspected by virtue of the mass effect on the adjacent ileum or frank obstruction. Because the diverticulum may only fill transiently, careful fluoroscopy is necessary. The diagnostic yield is increased by use of a small-bowel enema or enteroclysis, in which contrast is given following nasoduodenal or nasojejunal intubation. Barium enema examination may identify ileocolic or even ileo-ileal intussusception as the basis for obstruction. During episodes of major gastrointestinal bleeding due to Meckel's diverticulum, barium studies should not be done. Occasionally, extravasation of contrast dye is seen on mesenteric arteriography in actively bleeding patients, but the diagnostic yield is low.

Clinical syndromes due to Meckel's diverticulum

The manifestations of Meckel's diverticulum are protean. The pathological complications of the diverticulum are related directly to the particular pattern of accompanying vitelline duct abnormalities. Thus they can mimic many intra-abdominal conditions. Meckel's diverticulum should be considered as a possible cause of any intra-abdominal disease in which the diagnosis is not evident.

The complications of Meckel's diverticulum include bleeding, obstruction, diverticulitis, enterolith, and tumours, in addition to associated anomalies. The diagnosis is seldom made preoperatively (less than 4 per cent of cases), except in cases of lower gastrointestinal bleeding in the paediatric population. The pain or tenderness from inflammatory or obstructive complications of the diverticulum do not necessarily occur in the right lower quadrant, but may be located in other abdominal quadrants or vary in location due to small-bowel motility and the position of the diverticulum relative to the ileocaecal valve. Sixty per cent of Meckel's diverticula become symptomatic before the age of 10 years. The pattern of complications is also age-related, with bleeding most common in children (75 per cent of complications before 10 years of age) and rare after age 30. Small-bowel obstruction may occur at any age, but in children intussusception of the diverticulum is a more likely cause of obstruction. In children, obstruction and bleeding account for approximately equal proportions (30 to 35 per cent) of symptomatic cases. Diverticulitis accounts for 20 per cent of cases, with a peak incidence in older children. Persistent umbilical fistula is seen in neonates. Neoplasms and the hernia of Littré occur in older adults. The incidence of complications of the diverticulum is also related to gender. Although the anomaly is found equally among males and females, complications are observed 2 to 3 times more frequently in males.

Peptic ulceration and haemorrhage

Meckel's diverticulum is the most frequent cause of painless, major, lower gastrointestinal bleeding in a previously healthy infant. One-half of cases occur before 2 years of age. More than 95 per cent of bleeding Meckel's diverticula contain ectopic gastric mucosa, causing mucosal ulceration either in the diverticulum near the heterotopia or in the adjacent ileal mucosa. Bleeding may be intermittent or continuous, appearing as melaena or exsanguinating bleeding with frank blood and clots. The bleeding has sometimes been described as 'brick red'. The bleeding is occasionally associated with pain, presumably due to the peptic ulceration. Spontaneous cessation of bleeding usually occurs. There may be chronic bleeding of lesser magnitude. The differential diagnosis includes juvenile polyps, arteriovenous malformation, intestinal haemangiomas, and blood dyscrasias. Diagnostic manoeuvres include haematological examination, sigmoidoscopy, and, when appropriate, contrast radiological studies, which are useful only to exclude other sources of bleeding. The sodium $^{99}Tc^{m}$ pertechnetate scan, if positive, is usually diagnostic (Fig. 2).

Treatment choices include surgical resection of the diverticulum or of the involved small bowel. Care must be taken not to miss a diverticulum adherent to the ileum. If diverticulectomy is elected, attention should be directed to removing any peptic ulcer in the adjacent ileum. At present the complication rates from small-bowel resection and diverticulectomy with closure are likely to be similar; in earlier reports diverticulectomy was assumed to be safer.

The diagnosis of peptic ulceration of Meckel's diverticulum in the absence of bleeding ('dyspepsia Meckelii') is uncommon. There may be episodes of abdominal pain in the right lower quadrant or in the region of the umbilicus with a temporal pattern similar to gastroduodenal peptic disease, but not directly relieved by alkali. Pain may be relieved by food intake in a delayed fashion.

Obstruction

The precise preoperative diagnosis of small-bowel obstruction due to Meckel's diverticulum is seldom made in the absence of a characteristic antecedent history of episodes of intermittent obstruction manifested by abdominal pain and vomiting and of peptic symptoms occurring in the absence of demonstrable upper gastrointestinal ulceration. Meckel's diverticulum may cause small-bowel obstruction through several different mechanisms:

1. Two per cent of cases of intussusception are due to Meckel's diverticulum. Intussusception occurs more frequently in children with heterotopic tissue acting as the leading point. The intussuscepting mass may also be due to diverticulitis or contained enterolith. Symptoms include abdominal pain, vomiting, and abdominal tenderness. In addition, rectal bleeding may occur and an abdominal mass may be appreciated. Obstruction may be intermittent, suggesting a reduction of the intussusception. In adults with intussusception due to the diverticulum, neoplasm in the diverticulum is a more likely cause; symptoms may be chronic and recurrent.
2. A persistent, obliterated vitelline duct attached to the umbilicus may serve as a fixed point for volvulus, or cause entrapment as an internal hernia.
3. The diverticulum may be attached by a band to another viscus, resulting in an internal hernia or serving as a fulcrum for volvulus.
4. Similarly, obstruction may occur due to herniation of the small bowel beneath a mesodiverticular band or volvulus.
5. The mesodiverticular band can cause obstruction by direct ileal compression.
6. Adhesive obstruction may arise secondary to prior inflammation of the diverticulum.
7. A diverticulum which becomes enlarged due to diverticulitis, or by obstruction of the mouth of the diverticulum, may cause obstruction by compression of the adjacent ileum.
8. The diverticulum may become inverted into the ileal lumen, causing an obturating obstruction.
9. The inguinal or femoral hernia described by Littré, mainly in the elderly, contains a strangulated diverticulum. Up to one-quarter of cases occur in umbilical hernias.
10. Rarely, an axial volvulus of the diverticulum occurs, resulting in infarction.
11. In one case of a very long diverticulum, obstruction was due to the formation of a true knot involving another viscus.
12. Obstruction may occur in neonates due to extrusion or prolapse of the ileum through the umbilicus via the patent vitelline duct.

Surgical treatment of obstruction found to be due to Meckel's diverticulum includes division of offending bands if present, and small-bowel resection or simple diverticulectomy, as well as resection of non-viable segments that may occur in volvulus or intussusception.

Diverticulitis

Acute diverticulitis may result from peptic ulceration associated with gastric heterotopia, contained enteroliths or foreign body, or obstruction or narrowing of the mouth of the diverticulum. The symptoms of abdominal pain, fever, and vomiting with signs of abdominal tenderness, sometimes in the right lower quadrant, are usually indistinguishable from the presentation seen in acute appendicitis. Abdominal tenderness may be located elsewhere than in the right lower quadrant. Meckel's diverticulitis is potentially more serious than appendicitis, because the process is not contained as often. Perforation and generalized peritonitis may ensue. When the inflammatory process involves an adjacent viscus, a fistula may form. Surgical resection and administration of antibiotics are dictated by the same considerations that apply to appendicitis.

Enteroliths and foreign bodies

Enteroliths are rare complications, forming in narrow-necked diverticula where there is stasis (see Section 16.10). True foreign bodies may lodge in the diverticulum. Both enteroliths and foreign bodies may be associated with diverticulitis, may result in bowel obstruction, or can cause haemorrhage from local pressure necrosis. Plain abdominal films that show calculi as well as small-bowel obstruction may cause diagnostic confusion with gallstone ileus.

Neoplasms

Approximately 1 per cent of Meckel's diverticula developed neoplasms, which occur more often in men. These account for 1 per cent of the complications of Meckel's diverticulum and may be benign or malignant. In contrast to the small intestine *per se*, where adenocarcinoma is the most common histological type, carcinoid (34 per cent) and leiomyosarcoma (18–44 per cent) are most commonly identified in Meckel's diverticulum, while 12 to 20 per cent of tumours are adenocarcinomas. Among benign tumours, leiomyoma is the most frequent. Although the majority of carcinoids are incidental findings, 20 per cent are associated with metastases. Neoplasms of Meckel's diverticulum become apparent when they produce obstruction, sometimes as the leading point for intussusception, or when they cause haemorrhage (sometimes occult) or inflammation.

Management of the incidental Meckel's diverticulum

Whether or not to remove a Meckel's diverticulum when it is found incidentally at laparotomy is a source of controversy. Early series of cases, based on autopsy or pathological materials or on retrospective clinical studies that were often anecdotal, resulted in the conclusion that up to 34 per cent of patients with a diverticulum would suffer a complication. Surgery for complications of Meckel's diverticulum appeared to result in a higher incidence of mortality and morbidity than did incidental resection when an uncomplicated Meckel's was found at laparotomy, particularly in the elderly. Opinions regarding incidental diverticulectomy are based on:

(1) knowledge of the incidence of the anomaly in the population;
(2) the likelihood in that population of complications that may be related to age and gender or to the anomalous anatomic findings at laparotomy;
(3) The morbidity and mortality attributed to resection of a non-diseased diverticulum versus that for a complicated Meckel's diverticulum.

Whether the incidence in a population is 1 per cent or 2 per cent, and whether the complication rate is assumed to be 5 per cent or 10 per cent, would result in opposing recommendations.

A substantially larger percentage of Meckel's diverticula remain innocuous. From a study of a large population, Soltero and Bill concluded that at birth there is a 4.2 per cent risk of complications from Meckel's diverticulum over the lifetime of a patient, and that such risk was age-related, falling to 1 per cent at age 50 and to near zero in the elderly. Furthermore, the current mortality of surgery for complicated Meckel's diverticula is lower than in the past. On the other hand, the mortality for excision of incidental Meckel's diverticulum in youth is virtually nil, while the morbidity associated with small-bowel resection or enterotomy remains.

Nonetheless, certain guidelines may be offered. The most important factor is the age of the patient. The majority of surgeons would remove an incidental Meckel's diverticulum in children under 2 years of age, but most would not interfere with this lesion in patients over 30 to 40 years of age in the absence of complicating pathology. Relative indications for resection include diverticula in men and the nature of the pathological process that prompted the laparotomy, such as the presence or absence of appendicitis or peritonitis. Thus, in children or youths undergoing elective surgery, removal of an incidental Meckel's diverticulum is reasonable. Since ectopic tissue is found in 40 to 50 per cent or more of patients with complications of Meckel's diverticulum (compared with 6–10 per cent of patients with bland diverticula), the presence of palpable heterotopia may be an indication for resection. However, up to one-half of heterotopia may not be appreciated on palpation, although the larger ones usually are. There is insufficient evidence to argue that diverticula with a narrow orifice should be removed. Longer diverticula may be more likely to cause difficulties. Findings at surgery indicating prior diverticulitis, including scarring or adhesions, would dictate excision. The presence of a band to the umbilicus or other viscus would require, as a minimum, division of the band at any age.

ACQUIRED DIVERTICULA OF THE SMALL BOWEL

In contrast to Meckel's diverticulum, small-bowel diverticula, like colonic diverticula, are acquired; they occur along the mesenteric border and usually lack muscular layers. The reported incidence of small-bowel diverticulosis varies between 0.2 and 4.6 per cent in autopsy series, no doubt dependent on the age of the population under study and the degree of enthusiasm of the prosector for their detection, using bowel insufflation. The mean age for detection is in the seventh decade. The diverticula may be single, but are usually multiple, and are confined to the jejunum in 80 to 90 per cent of cases, the remainder being in both jejunum and ileum or confined only to the ileum (Fig. 3). Jejunal diverticulosis is associated (in 33–75 per cent of cases) with diverticula elsewhere in the gastrointestinal tract, particularly in the colon.

Small-bowel diverticulosis has been associated with disorders of intestinal motility in which there is 'intestinal pseudo-obstruction' due to myopathy or neuroenteric disorders; these pulsion diverticula, due to increased intraluminal pressure acting at weak points in the lumen, are proposed to represent the end-stage of a chronic intestinal motility disorder. At surgery the jejunal musculature may be thickened, with relative dilatation of the proximal bowel.

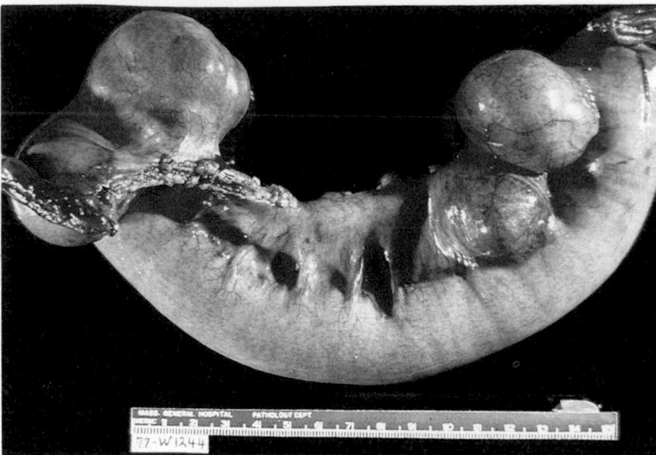

Fig. 3 Operative specimen of a segment of jejunum inflated to show three large diverticula which were the source of gastrointestinal bleeding in a 53-year-old man. This patient had melaena, requiring 13 units of blood, with negative preoperative endoscopic and angiographic examinations

Diagnosis

Because of an ageing population, the diagnoses of small-bowel diverticulosis and its complications are being made more frequently. Vague epigastric or periumbilical pain, bloating, and early satiety have been ascribed to small-bowel diverticulosis. However, these symptoms allow a specific diagnosis only by exclusion. The triad of anaemia, epigastric distress, and air–fluid levels on plain abdominal films may be a clue to the diagnosis. Small-bowel diverticulosis is most often discovered as a result of more dramatic complications. Except in the case of malabsorption, the cause is not often identified preoperatively.

Jejunal diverticula may be detected by barium studies of the small bowel, particularly on delayed films. Jejunal dyskinesia can be seen during fluoroscopy, where barium is not propelled normally, but moves in and out of the diverticula, associated with partial obstruction. The diagnostic yield is enhanced by small-bowel enteroclysis, in which the duodenum/jejunum is intubated and the bowel is insufflated and examined by the radiologist during compression.

Complications of small-bowel diverticulosis and their treatment

Pathological consequences of small-bowel diverticulosis include diverticulitis, haemorrhage, obstruction, and malabsorption. The formation of enteroliths, fistulae to surrounding organs, asymptomatic pneumoperitoneum, and malignant tumours are less common complications.

Diverticulitis

The pathogenesis of small-bowel diverticulitis parallels that of colonic diverticulitis. The common presenting complaints are pain, nausea, vomiting, signs of sepsis, and abdominal tenderness. Occasionally a mass is palpable. The diagnosis is rarely made preoperatively, as the process may be localized in virtually any abdominal quadrant. Perforation may occur into the mesentery, can be walled off by adjacent organs, or may result in free perforation with generalized peritonitis. Older anecdotal reports of high mortality rates for perforated diverticulitis treated by surgical resection are no longer valid.

Obstruction

In addition to the 'pseudo-obstruction', or motility disorder, associated with small-bowel diverticulosis, frank mechanical obstruction may occur from diverticulitis, adhesions associated with the inflammatory process, enteroliths arising in a diverticulum, and volvulus about surrounding adhesions. Relief of the obstruction should include resection of the segment involved with diverticulitis. Enteroliths, usually composed of choleic acid, form in diverticula where there is stasis, and may lead to obstruction due to local diverticulitis or to obturation in more distal small bowel. Enterotomy to remove enteroliths is sufficient treatment, although resection of diverticula, if localized, may be advocated. When jejunal diverticulosis is found incidentally at laparotomy, resection should be carried out if there are signs of pseudo-obstruction of the involved segment (thickened bowel wall and proximal dilatation).

Haemorrhage

Haemorrhage from jejunal diverticulosis presents as massive rectal bleeding in more than two-thirds of instances, occasionally accompanied by haematemesis; bleeding is often recurrent. Initial endoscopy serves to exclude other sources. Arteriography is the procedure of choice thereafter for localization of the bleeding site, although sometimes the tagged red blood cell scan is useful. When preoperative localization of the bleeding site fails and laparotomy is still required, cross-clamping of the bowel above and below the bleeding site may be useful to define the segment which fills with blood, thus dictating resection. When bleeding cannot be localized in this way and the patient, usually elderly, has concurrent colonic diverticulosis, thought preoperatively to be a likely source, both colon resection and resection of the small-bowel segment involved with diverticulosis should be done.

Malabsorption

Small-bowel diverticulosis is one possible cause of the 'blind loop' or 'stagnant bowel syndrome', in which there is stasis of intestinal contents, resulting in bacterial overgrowth. The metabolic consequences of bacterial overgrowth include megaloblastic anaemia, due to bacterial uptake of vitamin B_{12}, and to steatorrhoea, due to decreased bile salts as a result of bacterial hydrolysis of conjugated bile salts, with impaired micelle formation. In addition, there may be diarrhoea, weight loss, neuropathy, hypoproteinaemia, and mild abdominal pain associated with jejunal dyskinesia. In addition to laboratory evidence for malabsorption, stasis is also indicated by the presence of colonic bacteria in duodenal aspirates and by radiological detection of the diverticula. Initial treatment includes vitamin B_{12} parenteral supplementation and broad-spectrum antibiotics. Twenty-five per cent of patients do not respond to this treatment, and in these cases resection of the segment containing the diverticula is required. Because diverticula are usually in the jejunum, extended resections are relatively well tolerated.

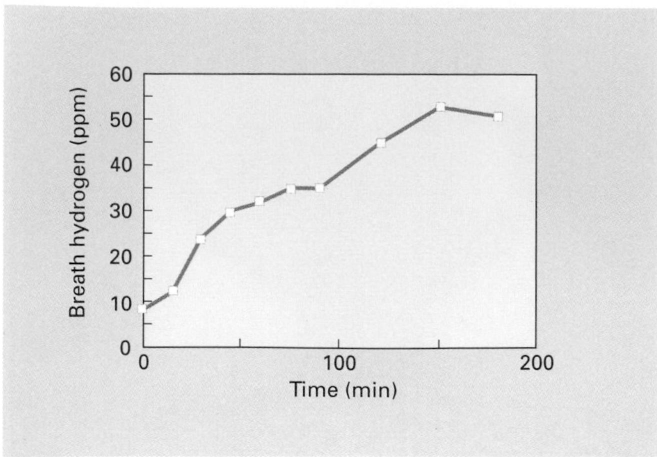

Fig. 4 The results of a lactulose breath test in a patient with jejunal diverticulosis. There is an early rise in breath hydrogen (expressed as parts per million) beginning at 10 min. The colonic peak occurs at 150 min.

aspirate is required to diagnose the free α-chains characteristic of α-chain disease.

CAUSES OF MALABSORPTION

There are numerous causes of malabsorption and it is convenient to divide them into those involving a failure of intraluminal digestion and those where there is a failure of mucosal absorption. Table 2 lists some of the major causes.

Failure of intraluminal digestion

Cholestasis

This may be due to intrahepatic or extrahepatic causes: the former include primary biliary sclerosis, alcohol, drugs or viral hepatitis, the latter benign or malignant biliary strictures, ampullary or pancreatic tumours, and bile-duct stones. Chronic pancreatitis may also result in obstruction of the lower end of the common bile duct, giving rise to a typical 'rat-tail' stricture which can be seen at endoscopic retrograde cholangiopancreatography (ERCP). Primary sclerosing cholangitis can involve both intrahepatic and extrahepatic ducts. Whatever the cause of cholestasis, malabsorption is caused by bile salt insufficiency, and patients therefore develop steatorrhoea and the accompanying malabsorption of the fat soluble vitamins (A, D, K).

Table 2 Causes of malabsorption

Failure of intraluminal digestion
Cholestasis
Pancreatic insufficiency
Poor mixing
Bacterial overgrowth
Drugs
Failure of mucosal absorption
Coeliac disease
Tropical sprue
Whipple's disease
Hypogammaglobulinaemia
Lymphoma, α-chain disease
Infections
Radiation damage
Mesenteric ischaemia
Enzyme deficiencies
Crohn's disease
Short bowel syndrome

Pancreatic insufficiency

This is usually caused by chronic pancreatitis or by proximal obstruction to the pancreatic duct by tumour, and results in steatorrhoea and malabsorption of the fat soluble vitamins. The secretory capacity of the pancreas has to be reduced to less than 10 per cent of normal before malabsorption develops.

Poor mixing

Inadequate mixing of food with bile and pancreatic secretions may occur after a Polya gastrectomy, gastroenterostomy, or a Roux-en-Y procedure. This may give rise to a degree of maldigestion but, if frank malabsorption occurs, other factors such as bacterial overgrowth may also be involved.

Bacterial overgrowth

The mechanisms involved in fat malabsorption caused by bacterial overgrowth are discussed above. Bacteria may also compete with the host for vitamin B_{12}, resulting in the development of a megaloblastic anaemia. The proximal small intestinal flora is usually less than 10^4 organisms/ml: bacterial counts greater than this constitute bacterial overgrowth. This is found in many small bowel diseases, including Crohn's disease, jejunal diverticulosis, strictures, autonomic neuropathies, or other causes of pseudo-obstruction. Bacterial overgrowth will also complicate a 'blind-loop' such as the afferent limb of a Polya gastrectomy or an end-to-side anastomosis (Fig. 5), or internal enteric fistulae (especially gastrocolic or ileocolic). Recently, it has been recognized that elderly patients may develop bacterial overgrowth and malabsorption in the absence of any demonstrable anatomical abnormality. In some patients with bacterial overgrowth (for example, those with jejunal diverticulosis) the small bowel mucosa may show some loss of villous height and a chronic inflammatory infiltrate, but this is never as severe as the mucosal changes seen in coeliac disease.

Jejunal diverticulosis (Fig. 6) occurs in the elderly and is usually asymptomatic unless bacterial overgrowth is sufficient to cause steatorrhoea. When this occurs antibiotics should be given, as for any cause of bacterial overgrowth. Metronidazole is the drug of choice, but since many of these patients will require repeated courses, which may induce resistant organisms, doxycycline and neomycin can be used in rotation with metronidazole. The complications of jejunal diverticulosis, in addition to malabsorption, are a silent perforation (which needs no specific treatment) and volvulus (which requires resection). Only very rarely does an acute diverticulitis develop; this should, in the first instance, be treated with intravenous fluids and antibiotics.

Autonomic neuropathy of the intestine is usually seen in association with diabetes mellitus but other causes include vincristine, spinal cord injury, Shy–Drager syndrome, amyloidosis, and systemic sclerosis. Other signs of autonomic neuropathy, such as postural hypotension and a fixed R-R interval on a Valsalva manoeuvre, are nearly always present. Apart from controlling

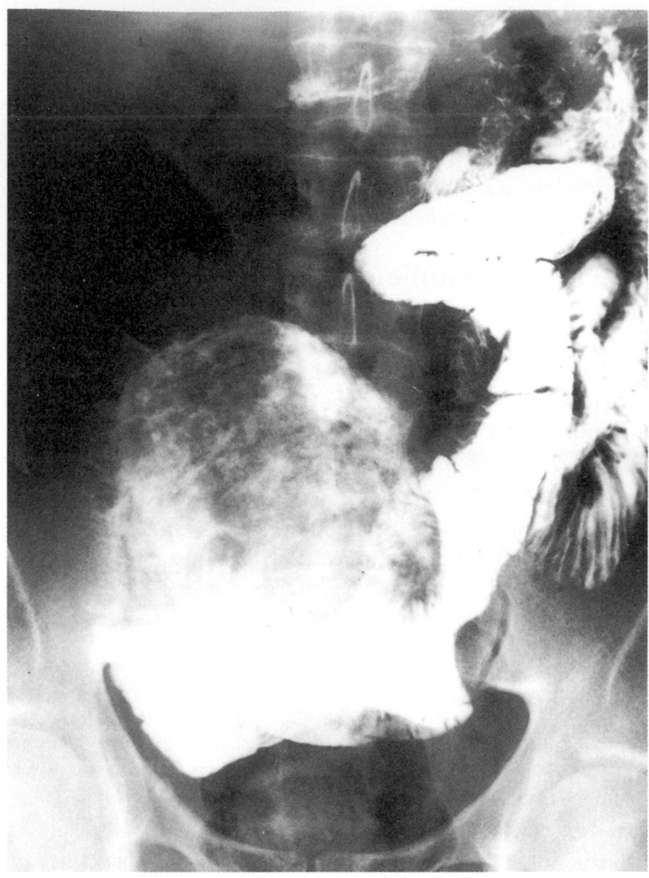

Fig. 5 A large blind loop as a result of an end-to-side anastomosis in the small intestine (by courtesy of Dr D. J. Nolan).

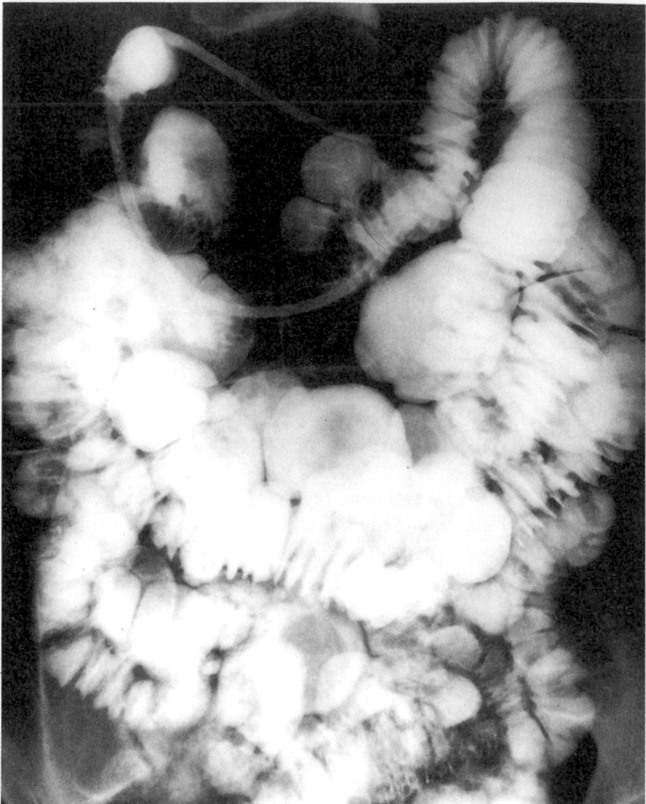

Fig. 6 Small bowel enema demonstrating jejunal diverticulosis (by courtesy of Dr D. J. Nolan).

bacterial overgrowth, management consists of symptomatic control of diarrhoea and nutritional support.

Drugs

The drug in common usage which may rarely cause malabsorption is neomycin, which appears to cause steatorrhoea by precipitating bile salts. Cholestyramine can also increase fat excretion by binding bile salts.

Failure of mucosal absorption

Coeliac disease

Coeliac disease predominantly affects children and young adults, although it may occur at any age. The incidence varies considerably, being present in about 1 in 5000 to 7000 of the population in the West but being exceptionally rare in other parts of the world. This distribution may be explained by the very close association of coeliac disease with HLA antigens. Approximately 95 per cent of patients with coeliac disease are HLA-DQ2 and over 80 per cent have the haplotype B8, DR3, DQ2. Thus, the aetiology of coeliac disease represents an interplay between genetic factors and the ingestion of gluten. Nevertheless, the fact that there is 30 per cent discordance amongst monozygotic twins suggests that other factors are important in initiating the disease. Recently, there has been considerable interest in the role of adenovirus 12 as an initiating factor because there is sequence homology between an epitope in an 'early protein' (E1b) of the virus and a surface epitope of a gliadin fraction (gliadin is prepared from gluten by alcohol extraction). Coeliac patients show cellular immune responses to both viral and gliadin epitopes and the gliadin epitope has been shown to be toxic in *in-vivo* challenge studies. Hence, it is possible that exposure to this virus in a person with the genetic susceptibility to develop coeliac disease may break oral tolerance to gluten and allow a harmful mucosal immunological reaction to occur.

Although patients with coeliac disease may still present with the classical clinical picture of weight loss, anorexia, steatorrhoea, and the signs of nutritional deficiency, the majority of patients are now diagnosed at a much earlier stage: unexplained iron deficiency anaemia or the symptoms of an irritable bowel syndrome are the most frequent presenting features. Any patient who presents with a variable bowel habit, abdominal pain, distension, and wind, who has lost weight or who also complains of aphthous ulcers of the mouth should undergo a small intestinal biopsy. This will show severe villous atrophy with crypt hyperplasia in affected individuals. Treatment consists of a gluten-free diet. Patients should be instructed by dietitians and, ideally, should also become members of a national coeliac society, which continually provides their members with information on the gluten status of new food products and disseminates knowledge about the disease. A repeat biopsy should be obtained after 3 to 4 months of dietary treatment to check that the mucosa has returned towards normal. The strict definition of coeliac disease requires a gluten challenge with repeat biopsy, but this is usually reserved for patients in whom the diagnosis may be in doubt. Patients will need to be on a gluten-free diet for life and should adhere to it strictly. A visit to a specialized clinic is recommended at least once a year.

Adherence to a strict diet not only achieves maximal histological remission, but may avoid the long-term complications of coeliac disease, namely an ulcerating jejunoileitis or a mucosal T-cell lymphoma. Carcinomas of the gastrointestinal tract, especially the oesophagus, are also associated with coeliac disease but whether strict dietary control influences the incidence of carcinoma is less clear.

Patients who have clear evidence of nutritional deficiencies (e.g. iron, folate, vitamins K or D) will need replacement therapy initially, but once the jejunal mucosa returns to near normal there should be no need for long-term supplements. If the coeliac disease is severe, affecting a substantial part of the small intestine (indicated by a marked steatorrhoea) patients may also benefit from lactose withdrawal until the brush border of the enterocytes have recovered on the gluten-free diet.

Some patients (<10 per cent) who appear to have coeliac disease do not show histological recovery on gluten withdrawal even after many months. The usual reason is lack of dietary compliance. However, if this has been excluded, other conditions should be considered. These include collagenous sprue (the biopsy shows >12 μm subepithelial collagen band and, usually, hypoplastic crypts), lymphoma, hypogammaglobulinaemia, amyloidosis, tropical sprue, chronic ischaemia, or Whipple's disease. Other conditions such as Crohn's disease, tuberculosis, systemic sclerosis, and radiation enteritis may also be associated with a flat mucosal biopsy but there is usually obvious evidence of these diseases on barium radiology.

Hypogammaglobulinaemia

IgA deficiency is the most common immunodeficiency disorder, and may be symptomless or associated with recurrent upper respiratory tract infections, sinusitis and skin sepsis. It also affects about 10 per cent of patients with coeliac disease.

Common variable hypogammaglobulinaemia, in which there is a variable depression of serum IgA, G, and M, is also associated with a flat small intestinal mucosa which does not usually respond to gluten withdrawal. Many of these patients develop giardiasis or cryptosporidiosis, and bacterial overgrowth is common. Treatment involves eradication of infection and patients may benefit from a lactose-free diet.

AIDS is associated with a lack of mucosal $CD4^+$ cells in parallel with the fall in circulating $CD4^+$ lymphocytes. Hence, degrees of mucosal abnormalities are common in these patients and opportunistic infections may contribute to the mucosal damage and subsequent malabsorption.

Lymphoma

Intestinal lymphomas are of three main types.

1. The so-called Western lymphoma is usually a focal tumour (Fig. 7). It is a B-cell lymphoma, mainly centrocytic or centroblastic in type.
2. A diffuse lymphoma (Mediterranean type). This usually causes 'α-chain' disease, in which the abnormal clone of B cells gives rise to plasma cells which synthesize and release free α chains of IgA without the accompanying light chain. The disease causes profound malabsorption. Diagnosis is made by a small intestinal biopsy and by the demonstration of free α chains in serum, saliva, jejunal aspirate, or urine.
3. T-cell lymphoma may also complicate coeliac disease.

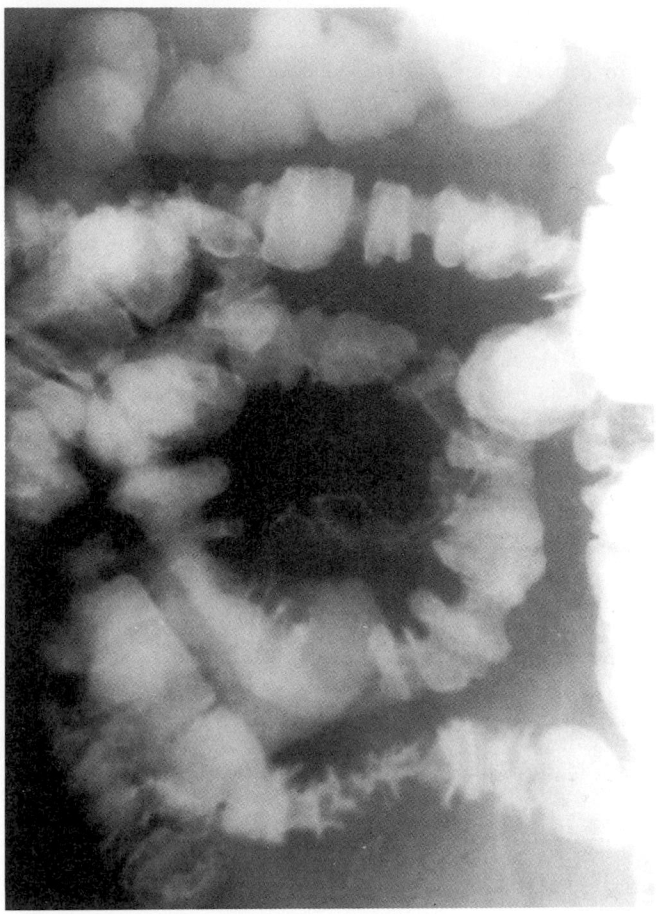

Fig. 7 Lymphoma of the ileum as seen on a small bowel enema (by courtesy of Dr D. J. Nolan).

SHORT BOWEL SYNDROME

This usually results from massive surgical resection following mesenteric infarction or from repeated resections for Crohn's disease. Malabsorption occurs because there is loss of absorptive surface. However, there may be bacterial overgrowth or there may be a degree of mucosal abnormality leading to hypolactasia.

Management involves correction of bacterial overgrowth, a lactose-free diet (if necessary, and diet may need to be low in disaccharides generally if there is severe brush border damage), and full dietary supplements, together with intramuscular administration of vitamin B_{12} (250 μg every 3 months). Some patients will require home parenteral nutrition to maintain body weight and an adequate intake of minerals and vitamins.

MANAGEMENT OF MALABSORPTION

The primary management is to treat the cause of the malabsorption: pancreatic enzymes must be given for pancreatic insufficiency, a gluten-free diet for coeliac disease, antibiotics for bacterial overgrowth. In these instances, there is usually no need for long-term nutritional supplements provided the malabsorption is corrected adequately. However, in the acute stage replacement with vitamins, iron, calcium, magnesium, and zinc may be necessary.

For patients in whom the cause of malabsorption cannot be corrected, management may require oral supplements of B vitamins, iron and folate. All patients with ileal resections are at risk from vitamin B_{12} deficiency and may need supplementation—250 μg vitamin B_{12} given intramuscularly every 3 months is sufficient. Patients with continuing steatorrhoea, including those with prolonged cholestasis, extensive mucosal atrophy of the small bowel, and those with a short bowel syndrome, will suffer from malabsorption of vitamins A, D, and K. Monthly intramuscular injections of these fat soluble vitamins may be needed (e.g. vitamin A 10 000 U, vitamin D 100 000 U, vitamin K 10 mg). Dietary management will include a low fat diet, for those with prolonged steatorrhoea, and supplements of carbohydrate and protein. However, if there is extensive villous atrophy these supplements will need to be in the form of glucose and tri- or dipeptides which can be absorbed directly without requiring enzymatic digestion. Medium chain triglyceride should also be given as a way of providing fat in a steadily absorbable form.

FURTHER READING

Bouchier IAD, Allan RV, Hodgson HJF, Keighley MRB. The small intestine. In *Textbook of Gastroenterology*. London: Bailliere Tindall, 1984; Ch. 8: 339–640.

Romano TJ, Dobbins JW. Evaluation of the patient with suspected malabsorption. *Gastroenterol Clin N Am* 1989; **18**: 467–83.

Teh LB, *et al.* Assessment of fat malabsorption. *J Clin Pathol* 1983; **36**: 1362–6.

16.6 Short bowel syndrome

JACK COLLIN

I have finally kum to the koncluzion that a good reliable sett of bowels is wurth more tu a man than enny quantity ov brains.

Josh Billings, 1818–85

DEFINITION

The short bowel syndrome is characterized by:

1. Inadequate length of intestine
2. Diarrhoea
3. Steatorrhoea
4. Weight loss
5. Nutritional deficiency
6. Rapid intestinal transit
7. Hypergastrinaemia.

The syndrome can result from congenital deficiency of the intestine or may follow surgical resection for infarction or otherwise incurable disease (Table 1). The majority of cases occur at the extremes of life: the most common cause in neonates is necrotizing enterocolitis, and in the elderly, mesenteric vascular occlusion.

Table 1 Causes of short bowel syndrome

Neonates and infants
Necrotizing enterocolitis
Congenital anomalies
Volvulus neonatorum
Intestinal aplasia
Aganglionosis
Meconium ileus
Intussusception
Neoplasia
Adults
Mesenteric vascular occlusion
Arterial thrombosis or embolism
Venous thrombosis
Dissecting aortic aneurysm
Trauma
Intestinal strangulation
Inflammatory bowel disease
Intestinal neoplasia
Radiation enteritis
Tuberculosis

HOW MUCH INTESTINE?

The mean length of the adult small intestine in life has been estimated at 450 cm but it is 200 cm longer when measured at autopsy. Precise measurement is impossible because of constant variations in tone and contractility, which can be modified by drugs and by stretching, particularly along the antemesenteric border. Repeated measurements at laparotomy on the same patient invariably produce a different answer each time, so any claim to precision is entirely illusory. This fundamental problem has led to various opinions about both the length of intestine that can be resected without producing any detectable effects on intestinal absorption and the minimum length required to support life. Such claims are intrinsically pointless: much depends on the actual segments of bowel resected, the presence of an intact ileocaecal valve, and the colon and also on the normality or otherwise of the remaining intestine. As a general rule 50 per cent of the small intestine can be resected without causing severe or persistent malabsorption. As more intestine is removed the effects of malabsorption become progressively more severe, and lifelong dependence on medical support is inevitable for any patient with less than 100 cm of small intestine.

MASSIVE INTESTINAL RESECTION

Resection is the only lifesaving option for patients with intestinal infarction, but intestine of doubtful viability can be conserved initially, a final decision being made at a planned laparotomy 24 h later. If more than half the small intestine is being resected such a 'second look' policy can save valuable inches of intestine and make a great difference to the long-term well-being of the patient. When the gut is diseased, but viable, the indications for intestinal resection are often relative: when the disease process is so extensive that less than 200 cm of intestine remain unaffected abnormal but functionally useful intestine can be conserved. In patients with Crohn's disease the recognition that limited resections and strictureplasties through diseased small intestine can be accomplished with uncomplicated healing has saved a number of patients from massive gut resection in the last 5 years. The more widespread use of such techniques would undoubtedly be beneficial, since prevention of the short bowel syndrome is preferable to its treatment.

The operative mortality for massive intestinal resection is high, particularly in the very young and old. Mortality is partly a consequence of the seriousness of the underlying pathology; acute mesenteric vascular occlusion still carries an overall mortality rate of more than 90 per cent. Intestinal resection is technically simple and many lives can be saved by adequate perioperative resuscitation and postoperative intensive monitoring and care. An understanding of the functional disturbances to be expected will allow appropriate corrective therapy to be instituted.

Physiological consequences of massive intestinal resection

The pathophysiological changes that occur after massive resection of the small intestine can conveniently be considered in the three clinical phases which are commonly described: the acute, adaptive and chronic phases. Although this scheme is helpful in understanding the problems encountered in this complex disorder the phases are by no means distinct or exclusive and have many features in common.

Acute phase

This phase begins as soon as the postoperative ileus has recovered and lasts for about 4 weeks. Its characteristic feature is profuse watery diarrhoea with the passage of 5 to 10 litres of fluid daily per rectum or through the stoma. Severe fluid and electrolyte depletion is liable to occur and unless the loss is replaced as it takes place, a life-threatening situation can rapidly develop. These problems, which basically arise as a consequence of acute loss of much of the intestinal surface area and rapid intestinal transit, are particularly severe if the ileocaecal valve has been removed or if there has been associated colonic resection, since most normal fluid and electrolyte absorption occurs in the colon. The problem is compounded by gastric hypersecretion secondary to the hypergastrinaemia which commonly occurs. A large volume of acidic fluid is presented for intestinal absorption and delayed gastric emptying may result in vomiting or nasogastric aspiration of large volumes of fluid, causing further fluid and electrolyte depletion. Acute peptic ulceration (stress ulcer) is liable to develop and routine prophylaxis with H_2- receptor antagonists and antacids is a sensible precaution.

In the early part of this phase the patient will also experience the catabolism which always occurs as part of the normal metabolic response to severe trauma. Fluid losses gradually diminish and, provided there has been adequate replacement of water and electrolytes, together with maintenance of calorie and nitrogen balance by parenteral nutrition, the patient will survive to enter the adaptive phase.

Adaptive phase

Intestinal adaptation to massive gut resection is a complex process which can take up to 2 years. The process is more effective in the ileum after proximal resection but occurs to a lesser extent in jejunum after distal intestinal resection. The changes affect the whole of the remaining bowel but are most marked in the small intestinal mucosa. Teleologically the process can be regarded as an attempt to increase total mucosal surface area and thereby increase intestine absorption. There is an increase in the circumference of the intestine, but only minimal increase in length. Villous height and crypt depth also increase due to epithelial hyperplasia, producing an increased number of absorptive cells, although the number of crypts and cells per unit area is unchanged. There is an increase in total mucosal cell turnover with an increased rate of migration of epithelial cells from crypt bases to the tips of the villi, but the life of an individual cell appears to remain the same. These changes are more marked in the ileum than in the jejunum, possibly because in the intact bowel the jejunum is already adapted for maximal absorption, whereas the ileum provides a reserve capacity to be called upon in the event of incomplete absorption of nutrients from the jejunum.

The terminal ileum serves a special role in the absorption of bile salts and vitamin B_{12}: this function is unique and is irreplaceable if the terminal ileum has been resected. Reduced bile salt reabsorption interrupts the enterohepatic circulation and causes a reduction in the bile salt pool. Gastric hypersecretion may reduce the pH of jejunal contents, allowing bile salt precipitation and inactivating pancreatic lipase. Pancreatic fibrosis can also arise as a consequence of massive intestinal resection, and all of these factors combine to cause steatorrhoea and reduced absorption of fat soluble vitamins.

Intestinal adaptation requires the presence of food in the intestinal lumen; together with bile and pancreatic secretions this appears to exert a trophic effect on intestinal mucosa. Humoral factors also play an essential part, along with gastrin and enteroglucagon, although the exact role of these and other hormones is unknown. Heterotopic autotransplants of intestinal mucosa in animals subjected to massive intestinal resection show hypertrophy, as does intestinal mucosa in parabiotic animals. Serum from animals with the short bowel syndrome also exerts a stimulatory effect on mucosal cells in tissue culture.

Chronic phase

This lifelong phase begins when all of the adaptive changes which can occur have taken place. It is an intrinsically unstable state which is easily disturbed by relatively minor gastrointestinal upsets or intercurrent illness. Acute disturbances in the form of diarrhoea and fluid and electrolyte depletion may still occur, with intravenous fluid replacement being required even by patients who are usually able to survive on enteral nutrition alone. The characteristic problems of this phase are the long-term maintenance of a sufficient intake of calories and nitrogen and the prevention and correction of deficiencies of minerals, essential amino acids, fatty acids, vitamins, and trace elements which are liable to develop. The recognition of these deficiencies has become easier as experience with increasing numbers of patients surviving to this stage has built up.

The objective of management is to maximize the degree to which enteral nutrition contributes to the patient's total intake. Some individuals are able to maintain their health with an oral diet alone, others require frequent or intermittent supplementation by parenteral infusions. The most severely disabled will require total long-term parenteral nutrition: in these patients the preservation of venous access sites and prevention of cannula sepsis is a major priority.

A number of interesting specific problems are liable to develop in the chronic phase. Gallstones may form as chronic bile salt depletion results in the secretion of lithogenic bile and the precipitation of cholesterol in the gallbladder. There is also an increased incidence of urinary calculi, particularly oxalate stones. Oxalates in the diet are normally precipitated by calcium, but in patients with the short bowel syndrome calcium coprecipitates with unabsorbed fatty acids, leaving oxalate to be absorbed. This problem can be overcome by restriction of dietary oxalate intake and the administration of additional calcium supplements.

CURRENT TREATMENT OF THE SHORT BOWEL SYNDROME

Enteral and parenteral nutrition

These form the mainstay of treatments in this condition and are dealt with in detail in Section 000.

Drug therapy

Drugs have a limited role, apart from certain specific indications. H_2-receptor antagonists may be required to control acid secretion in patients in whom persistent hypergastrinaemia is a problem. Their availability has largely removed the need for vagotomy, which is fortunate since in some patients the associated gastric drainage operation exacerbated diarrhoea by producing an incontinent stomach.

Antidiarrhoeal agents, particularly those which exert their effects by reducing gut motility, are frequently prescribed but any benefit produced is likely to be marginal, except in patients who have retained a useful length of colon.

Antibiotics may be required to treat gut or catheter sepsis but can have a deleterious effect on intestinal absorption by producing changes in the intestinal bacterial flora. They should be used with caution.

Surgical treatment

Many surgical procedures have been designed to treat the short bowel syndrome; most are experimental although several have been used in patients. The large number of operations described bears tribute to surgical ingenuity, although several procedures border on the fanciful. Attempts to slow intestinal transit and increase the duration of contact between gut contents and the absorptive mucosa have included interposing segments of stomach, small intestine, and colon, either isoperistaltic or reversed; construction of intestinal valves, baffles, or strictures; recirculating intestinal loops of various designs; attempts to provide a framework for the growth of intestinal neomucosa, and the use of retrograde electrical pacing of the intestinal myoelectrical activity.

Three surgical procedures may have some role to play in the practical clinical management of patients with the short bowel syndrome.

Reversed intestinal segment

The optimum length of small intestine to reverse is around 10 cm: longer lengths increase the likelihood of development of intestinal obstruction. The effect of reversal has been assumed to be due to a delay in transit, with increased time available for absorption of nutrients from intestine proximal to the reversed segment. There may also be some increase in absorption from the reversed segment itself since retrograde perfusion of intestine has been shown to increase intestinal absorption. The usefulness of this operation will remain limited by technical difficulties and the reluctance to sacrifice even a small segment of intestine in patients who have so little.

Intestinal lengthening (the Bianchi operation)

This ingenious operation relies on the fact that the final distribution of blood supply from the mesenteric arcade is arranged so that each side of the intestine is independently vascularized. It is possible to separate the leaves of the mesentery, with its contained vessels, and divide the intestine longitudinally; anastomosis of the two tubes end to end doubles the length of intestine, while halving its circumference (Fig. 1). Increase in intestinal absorption is predicted from the known fact that intestinal adaptation results in intestinal dilatation but little increase in length. This operation has been used to improve intestinal function in a number of infants.

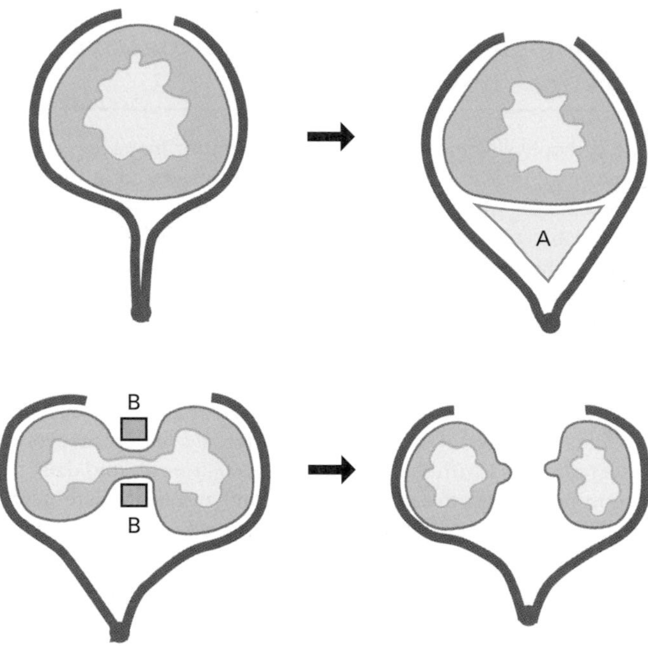

Fig. 1 The Bianchi operation. A, plane of cleavage of mesentery; B, jaws of stapling device.

Intestinal allotransplantation

Experimental intestinal allotransplantation has been investigated for more than 30 years, but the results of clinical application have, until recently, been disappointing. This treatment, which is discussed in detail elsewhere, holds out the best hope for the future of finally achieving a cure for patients with the short bowel syndrome (see Section 10.8.2).

FURTHER READING

Mitchell A, Watkins RM, Collin J. Surgical treatment of the short bowel syndrome. *Br J Surg* 1984; **71**: 329–33.

Williamson RCN. Intestinal adaptation. *N Engl J Med* **298**: 1393–1402; 1444–50.

16.7 Radiation enteritis

CHRISTOPHER G. WILLETT

INTRODUCTION

With the increased application and efficacy of radiation therapy in the management of patients with gastrointestinal, genitourinary, and retroperitoneal malignancies, normal tissue response to this treatment is important. Intestinal tolerance is a major factor limiting radiation treatment of tumours of the abdomen and pelvis. Small and large bowel complications (both acute and long-term) are closely related to radiation therapy techniques. Acute complications are correlated with volume of bowel irradiated and fraction size, while long-term complications are related not only to the volume of bowel treated and fraction size but also to total dose of radiation administered. Table 1 summarizes the incidence of long-term severe small bowel complications stratified to the parameters of total dose, fraction size, and volume and design of the radiation fields from a number of different series. As the data show, severe small bowel complications occur with high frequency in patients treated with large fields and high doses of radiation. Limiting small bowel irradiation to 45 to 50.4 Gy in 1.8 Gy fractions and large bowel irradiation to 55 to 60 Gy in 1.8 Gy fractions, with the use of carefully designed fields and technique, should limit complications to less than 5 per cent of patients. Other reported predisposing factors to long-term radiation injury include obesity, diabetes mellitus, hypertension, pelvic inflammatory disease, prior abdominal or pelvic surgery, and the use of concurrent chemotherapy during radiation therapy. Acute and long-term complications occur with distinct clinical courses and pathological manifestations.

ACUTE COMPLICATIONS

Gastrointestinal symptoms are common during the course of radiation treatment to the pelvis and/or abdomen. Large bowel symptoms consist of an acute proctocolitis with diarrhoea and tenesmus. Sigmoidoscopy during treatment frequently shows an inflamed, oedematous, and friable mucosa. Acute small bowel reactions may result in nausea, abdominal cramps, and watery diarrhoea, primarily due to the depletion of actively dividing cells in what is otherwise a stable cell renewal system. In the small bowel, loss of the mucosal cells results in malabsorption of various substances including fat, carbohydrate, protein, and bile salts. In the large bowel, failure of fluid adsorption results in watery diarrhoea.

Although occasionally severe, these symptoms are usually self limited and managed by the use of antispasmodic and anticholinergic medications. Some patients with symptoms refractory to these drugs may respond to a bile sequestrating agents (such as cholestyramine), although such reports are anecdotal. In a double blind placebo controlled trial, buffered acetysalicylate was effective in improving gastrointestinal symptoms in patients who had undergone curative radiotherapy for malignant gynaecological disease. The prevalence and severity of radiation induced diarrhoea may also be reduced by using an elemental diet or total parenteral nutrition during therapy.

LONG-TERM COMPLICATIONS

Long term complications include obstruction, perforation, bleeding, malabsorption, and fistulae. The latent period between completion of radiation therapy and the subsequent development of these complications is usually 6 to 24 months but chronic radiation enteritis can occur many years after the original treatment. Colicky abdominal pain is the most common symptom, and generally precedes bloody diarrhoea, tenesmus, steatorrhoea, and weight loss. Less commonly, patients present with an acute obstruction or perforation of the small or large bowel.

Table 1 The incidence of long-term severe small bowel complications

Study	Total dose/fraction size	Technique	Severe small bowel complications
Roswell Park: cervix cancer/ paraortic nodes	60 Gy/2 Gy/7–8 weeks (split course)	AP/PA: Para-aortics (to T12) Pelvis	6/21(29%)
M. D. Anderson: cervix cancer/ paraortic nodes	55 Gy/1.7 Gy/6–7 weeks	AP/PA Extended field to L4 or T12 Pelvis	18/120(15%)
M. D. Anderson: Postoperative/ adenocarcinoma of rectum	40–50 Gy/1.8 Gy/5 weeks	AP/PA Pelvis (below L5)	10/89(11%)
Massachusetts General Hospital: Postoperative/ adenocarcinoma of rectum	45–55 Gy/1.8 Gy/5–6 weeks	4 fields: PA/AP and laterals Pelvis	4/97 (4%)

Pathological study of bowel affected by chronic radiation enteritis demonstrates obliterative endarteritis of the small vessels in the intestinal wall, submucosal fibrosis, and lymphatic dilatation. Perhaps the injury sustained by endothelial and connective tissue in the intestinal wall leads to progressive ischaemia of the intestinal wall. Ischaemia then leads to mucosal ulceration, necrosis of the intestinal wall with subsequent bleeding, perforation, stricture, and fistula formation, alone or in combination.

Radiation enteritis can also be progressive: in a series of 51 patients reported by Galland, only 24 patients remained symptom free after the first manifestation and treatment, whereas 20 patients developed second, third, or more gastrointestinal problems. Bleeding appeared to be a less ominous presentation: no new complications followed a bleeding episode, while 33 per cent of those with stricture and 89 per cent of those with perforation or fistula later manifested new lesions.

The medical and surgical treatment of chronic radiation enteritis is complex and requires individual management. Isolated damage to the rectum or rectosigmoid junction can often be managed with a low residue diet and steroid suppositories, but damage to the large intestine is frequently associated with significant injuries to the distal part of the small intestine. In the management of lesions of the small intestine, antispasmodics, anticholinergics, broad spectrum antibiotics, cholestyramine, and salicylazosulphapyridine have been used but responses to these agents have been anecdotal and based on a small number of patients. The use of a low fat diet, a low residue diet, or a gluten and lactose free diet with low fat as well as elemental diets have all been reported to be useful in selected patients with chronic radiation enteritis. A randomized study comparing total parenteral nutrition, with or without methylprednisone, with enteral nutrition for patients with severe chronic small bowel radiation enteritis found the former to be beneficial, with improvement in nutritional, radiological, and clinical parameters. The efficacy of total parenteral nutrition administration appeared to be enhanced by use of methylprednisone.

Before definitive surgical treatment is embarked upon, the status of the original malignancy and the extent of radiation damage should be assessed. Sepsis, malnutrition, and biochemical abnormalities should be corrected. Although wide resection and primary anastomosis may be appropriate for patients with single, discrete areas of radiation induced pathology manifested as obstruction, perforation, or bleeding, the majority of patients have more generalized radiation damage. Those who present with radiation induced perforation of the small bowel should be treated as emergencies, with avoidance of primary anastomosis. Exteriorization of the involved segments may be the optimal procedure in this situation, even though a further operation will be necessary to reconstitute the alimentary tract. An enteric fistula can sometimes be managed conservatively but such management is rarely successful. Gastrointestinal bypass without extensive resection of the involved bowel has less mortality and a higher success rate.

SUMMARY

Abdominal and pelvic radiotherapy is increasingly used in the curative treatment of many abdominal and pelvic malignancies. Bowel tolerance is a major limitation to this treatment. Long-term complications occur less frequently than acute complications but are substantially more serious. Efforts must be made to minimize long-term bowel complications: these include the use of modern radiation treatment planning and techniques. Surgical measures to exclude the small bowel from the radiation field—absorbable mesh, ectopic implant, cystopexy, and omental flap—have shown encouraging results in reducing the amount of small bowel in the radiation field and thus reducing the incidence of small bowel injury.

FURTHER READING

Galland RB, Spencer J. Natural history and surgical management of radiation enteritis. *Br J Surg* 1987; **74**: 742–7.

Gunderson LL, Martenson JA. Gastrointestinal tract radiation tolerance. *Frontiers Radiat Ther Oncol* 1989; **23**: 277–98.

Gunderson LL, Russell AH, Llewellyn HJ, Doppke KP, Tepper JE. Treatment planning for colorectal cancer: radiation and surgical techniques and value of small-bowel films. *Int J Radiat Oncol Biol Phys* 1985; **11**: 1379–93.

Hoskins RB, *et al.* Adjuvant postoperative radiotherapy in carcinoma of the rectum and rectosigmoid. *Cancer* 1985; **55**: 61–71.

Kinsella TJ, Bloomer WD. Tolerance of the intestine to radiation therapy. *Surg Gynecol Obstet* 1980; **151**: 273–84.

Loiudice TA, Lang JA. Treatment of radiation enteritis. *J Gastroenterol* 1983; **78**: 481–7.

Mennie AT, *et al.* Treatment of radiation-induced gastrointestinal distress with acetylsalicylate. *Lancet* 1975; 942–3.

Minsky BD, Cohen AM. Minimizing the toxicity of pelvic radiation therapy in rectal cancer. *Oncology* 1988; **2**: 21–5.

Piver MS, Barlow JJ. High dose irradiation to biopsy confirmed aortic node metastases from carcinoma of the uterine cervix. *Cancer* 1977; **39**: 1243–6.

Sher ME, Bauer J. Radiation-induced enteropathy. *Gastroenterology* 1990; **85**: 121–8.

Smith DH, DeCosse JJ. Radiation damage to the small intestine. *World J Surg* 1986; **10**: 189–94.

Taylor Whartor J, Facog WJ III, Facog TGD, Facog FNR, Fletcher GH. Preirradiation cellotomy and extended field irradiation for invasive carcinoma of the cervix. *Obstet Gynecol* 1976; **49**: 333–8.

Vigliotti A, Richard TA, Romsdahl MM, Withers HR, Oswald MJ. Postoperative adjuvant radiotherapy for adenocarcinoma of the rectum and rectosigmoid. *Int J Radiat Oncol Biol Phys* 1986; **13**: 999–1006.

Yeoh EK, Horowitz M. Radiation enteritis. *Surg Gynecol Obstet* 1987; **165**: 373–9.

16.8 Hamartomas and benign neoplasms of the small bowel

JOHN G. N. STUDLEY AND ROBIN N. WILLIAMSON

The small bowel, which comprises the duodenum, jejunum, and ileum, represents approximately 75 per cent of the length of the gastrointestinal tract. The duodenum is about 25 cm long, the jejunum 200 cm, and the ileum 300 cm. This varies widely, and the length of the normal adult small bowel ranges from 300 cm to 850 cm. Since the small bowel provides 80 to 90 per cent of the surface area of the gastrointestinal tract, it might be expected to harbour most of the neoplasms. In fact, more lesions occur in the oesophagus, stomach, colon, and rectum, although the disparity is less for benign tumours than for malignant tumours. Hamartomas are randomly scattered through the gut.

To set the incidence of tumours in perspective, only 1.5 to 6 per cent of all gastrointestinal tumours arise in the small intestine and 20 to 25 per cent of these are found in the short duodenal segment. The population incidence of benign tumours is approximately 0.1 to 0.8 per cent.

Several hypotheses have been advanced to explain the relative scarcity of small bowel neoplasia, including the fluid nature of the contents and their rapid transit, decreasing exposure to ingested carcinogens; a low concentration of bacteria and alkaline pH, which might reduce the endogenous formation of carcinogens; detoxification of carcinogens by enzymes such as benzopyrene hydroxylase which are present in the mucosa; and the presence of protective immune factors, notably IgA, which is secreted especially in the ileum.

PRESENTATION

At least half of all benign enteric lesions are asymptomatic and are found incidentally at laparotomy or autopsy. Innocent lesions may also be observed during investigation of the gastrointestinal tract. Symptoms caused by the remainder vary from non-specific complaints, such as nausea, dyspepsia, discomfort in the epigastrium or right upper quadrant, fatigue, bloating, and weight loss, to haemorrhage or obstruction.

Obstruction is the presenting feature in 40 to 70 per cent of cases. Although often partial and recurrent, it can be sudden and complete. Intussusception is a frequent type of obstruction, with the tumour acting as the apex of the intussusceptum. In other instances obstruction may be due to a mass effect of the lesion or to volvulus. Rarely, stenosis of the bowel occurs, due to the local effects of vasoactive peptides secreted by a carcinoid tumour.

Haemorrhage, which is the presenting feature in 20 to 50 per cent of cases, is frequently occult and causes anaemia, but major bleeding can lead to both haematemesis and melaena. More than 90 per cent of gastrointestinal haemorrhagic events stem from the oesophagus, stomach, proximal duodenum, and colorectum. It is important to consider small bowel lesions once these more accessible sources have been excluded. Occasionally mucocutaneous pigmentation (in Peutz–Jeghers syndrome), café-au-lait spots (neurofibromatosis) or telangiectasia (Osler–Rendu–Weber syndrome) will alert the clinician to the presence of small bowel lesions.

Periampullary lesions can cause jaundice or pancreatitis, or a large tumour may be palpable. Serosal lesions may perforate, bleed, or fistulate, and gastrinoma presents with intractable ulceration.

INVESTIGATION

Duodenal lesions are more amenable to accurate diagnosis than are jejunoileal lesions. Upper gastrointestinal endoscopy is the mainstay for detecting lesions in the first and second parts of the duodenum, and has the added advantage of allowing biopsies to be taken. Among contrast studies hypotonic duodenography is preferable to simple barium meals for detecting small lesions.

The jejunum and the ileum are the least accessible parts of the gut to evaluate without recourse to laparotomy. Radiographic options are a barium meal and follow-through examination, or an intubated small bowel meal (small bowel enema), which gives superior pictures; contrast is instilled rapidly through a transpyloric tube. The terminal ileum can frequently be seen on a barium enema and is visible in 20 to 30 per cent of colonoscopies. Many vascular lesions lie within the wall of the small bowel and will escape detection unless superior mesenteric angiography is performed.

In patients with active haemorrhage isotope scanning should also be considered, using Tc-99m-labelled sulphur colloid or Tc-99m-labelled red blood cells. Such techniques allow bleeding rates as low as 0.1 ml/min to be detected, while 0.5 to 1 ml/min is usually necessary to enable a lesion to be localized angiographically. A careful search should be made on the arteriogram for the vitelline artery of a Meckel's diverticulum and for the early filling vein of an angiodysplasia. Laparotomy is an important investigation in small bowel disease and should not be overly delayed. Most actively bleeding lesions are readily seen or felt. In obscure cases, cross-clamping the bowel at various levels may localize the source. Lastly, operative enteroscopy can be undertaken by passing a colonoscope either by mouth or through a small enterostomy or, in a retrograde direction, from a caecostomy. Transillumination of the bowel wall from within may be more productive than endoscopic inspection of the mucosa (Fig. 1).

Small bowel endoscopy (enteroscopy) in the conscious patient has recently been described. A 5-mm diameter endoscope is introduced into the gastrointestinal tract transnasally and passes down the small intestine, with the help of peristalsis. In one study the endoscope reached the distal ileum or colon in 36 of 60 patients examined in this way. Average intubation time was 6 h, and a possible site of bleeding was identified in 20 patients.

Another technique currently undergoing assessment is percutaneous endoscopy. Access is achieved through the abdominal wall into the stomach or caecum, using the same technique as that for endoscopic insertion of feeding gastrostomies. Examination of the bowel can be achieved by introducing an endoscope through the created fistula. Further evaluation is needed.

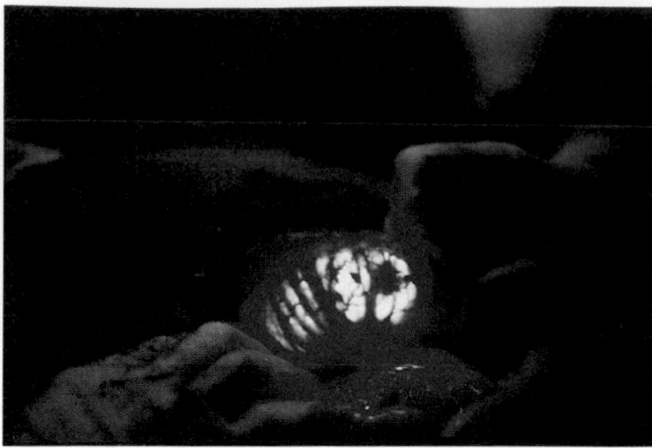

Fig. 1 On-table enteroscopy. Transillumination of the small-bowel wall shows a small angiodysplastic focus that had been causing intermittent haemorrhage.

Ultrasound, computerized tomography (CT), and magnetic resonance imaging have all been used in assessing small bowel lesions: at present CT is the most productive, especially for lesions in the duodenum. Lipomas can be differentiated from other tissues throughout the gastrointestinal tract when CT is combined with intraluminal contrast; this information may prevent unnecessary laparotomy. The efficacy of ultrasound is limited by the presence of bowel gas, while the accuracy of magnetic resonance imaging is reduced by poor resolution due to respiratory movements and peristalsis.

HISTOPATHOLOGY

The intestinal wall is composed of mucosa, submucosa, muscularis and serosa; the autonomic nerve supply is found chiefly in the submucosal and muscular layers. The proximal duodenum is distinguished by the presence of Brunner's glands while the ileum has a relative abundance of lymphoid follicles. The mucosa contains villi and crypts. Villi are lined by columnar cells, which are absorptive in nature, and mucus-secreting goblet cells. Each villus has a central stroma containing blood and lymphatic vessels. Crypts are lined by undifferentiated cells, which develop as they grow on to the villus, by enteroendocrine cells, which secrete a variety of biologically active peptides, and by occasional Paneth cells.

Classification of small bowel tumours is not straightforward. The distinction between hamartomas and true neoplasms is often unclear, and the malignant nature of some lesions is controversial. For our purposes, lesions will be discussed under three main headings: benign neoplasms, intermediate neoplasms, and hamartomatous lesions (Table 1). Frankly malignant tumours are discussed elsewhere. Intermediate neoplasms are lesions that have a definite malignant potential but can be difficult to classify histopathologically. The clearest example is an endocrine tumour (jejunoileal carcinoid or duodenal gastrinoma). Villous adenoma and smooth muscle tumours may also be difficult to classify as clearly benign or malignant, but are considered to be 'benign' in this classification. For completeness, heterotopic tissues and duplications within the small bowel will be briefly considered (Table 1).

Table 1 Non-malignant tumours of the small intestine

1. Benign neoplasms
   - Epithelial
     - Tubular adenoma
     - Villous adenoma*
     - Polyposis syndromes (adenoma)
     - Brunner's gland adenoma
   - Stromal
     - Adipose tissue
       - Lipoma
     - Connective tissue
       - Smooth muscle tumours*
       - Neurogenic tumours
       - Fibroma
     - Endothelium
       - Vascular tumours
       - Lymphatic tumours
2. Intermediate neoplasms* (endocrine tumours)
3. Hamartomatous lesions
   - Peutz-Jeghers syndrome
   - Other polyposis syndromes (hamartoma)
4. Heterotopic tissue
   - Localized
   - Disseminated
5. Duplications

* Villous adenoma and leiomyoma have a strong malignant potential and could also be regarded as intermediate neoplasms.

BENIGN NEOPLASMS

The low prevalence of these lesions has already been stressed. Among benign tumours, leiomyomas, lipomas, adenomas, and haemangiomas are relatively common, while others are rare.

Epithelial

Tubular adenomas

These lesions are generally polypoid, whereas most villous (papillary) adenomas are sessile. Tubular adenomas are relatively common in the duodenum and much less so in the distal small bowel. They are usually single but may be multiple. The symptoms that they cause include abdominal pain and varying degrees of obstruction or haemorrhage, depending on the position and size of the polyp. A lesion near the major pancreatic papilla may cause obstructive jaundice.

There are numerous reports of malignant change occurring in these neoplasms, a situation that is thought to reflect the adenoma–carcinoma sequence in the colon. The incidence of malignant change increases with the size, site, and number of lesions as well as with histological type. In one series the mean diameter of benign polyps was 2.65 cm, compared with 3.7 cm for those containing both benign and malignant elements. The average diameter of jejunal carcinomas was 4.3 cm and of ileal carcinomas 4.7 cm. Malignant change is more likely to occur in periampullary lesions than elsewhere in the duodenum or jejunoileum. Villous adenomas are more likely to undergo malignant change than are tubular adenomas, and multicentricity increases this risk.

Adenomas should be removed, in view of their premalignant potential. Histological examination of the whole specimen will then allow an accurate assessment of actual or potential

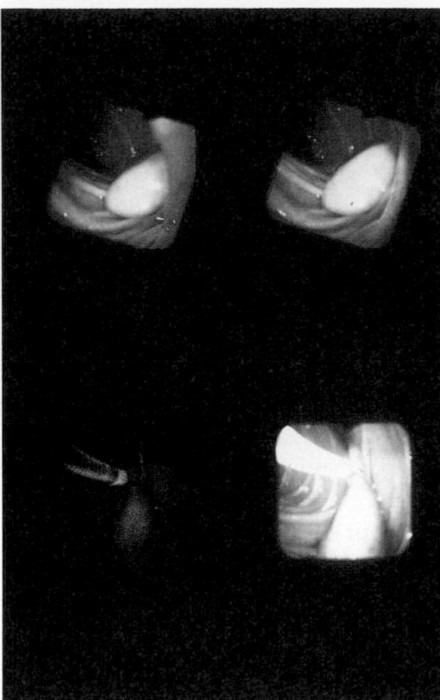

Fig. 2 Endoscopic snaring of a tubular adenoma in the duodenum (by courtesy of Mr J. Spencer).

malignancy. The best treatment for jejunal and ileal polyps is unclear: some clinicians believe that local enterotomy with excision of the lesion is adequate, but others favour segmental resection. Duodenal polyps less than 2 cm in diameter may be removed endoscopically in one piece (Fig. 2). Formal laparotomy and duodenotomy are required for adequate excision of larger lesions. The adenomas of familial polyposis are considered below.

Villous adenomas

Although these interesting lesions are rare, they have been identified in the duodenum with increasing frequency during recent years. The distinction between tubular and villous adenomas is not always clear cut: some adenomas have both tubular and villous elements ('tubulovillous adenoma'), as occurs in the large bowel. The mean age at presentation of a villous adenoma is 60 years, and there is no sex preponderance. Common symptoms include obstructive jaundice, obstruction, and occult bleeding. Most lesions arise within the second part of the duodenum, and the mean diameter is approximately 4 cm.

The crucial feature of these tumours is their strong propensity for malignant change, which mimics their behaviour in the colon and rectum (Fig. 3). Carcinoma has been reported in 35 to 63 per cent of lesions, and size is a poor predictor of malignant transformation. Tumours in the proximal duodenum can be identified by endoscopy, but hypotonic duodenography or other contrast studies are usually necessary to demonstrate distal lesions.

Proper management of these tumours requires accurate detection and assessment of any malignant change; unfortunately, this is often not possible before excision. Distant metastases obviously indicate malignancy, but endoscopic biopsy can give false negative results in 25 to 56 per cent of patients with localized lesions, probably because of the large size of the lesion and hence the sampling error. Computerized tomography may indicate invasion into surrounding tissues. In many instances, however, definitive diagnosis can only be obtained after removal of the whole lesion and histological examination.

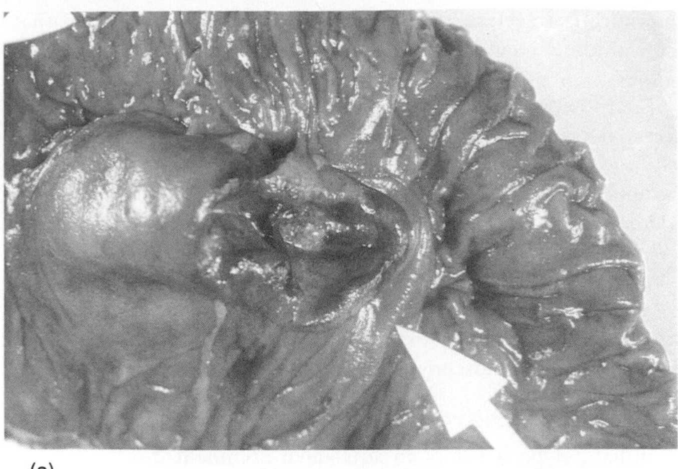

(a)

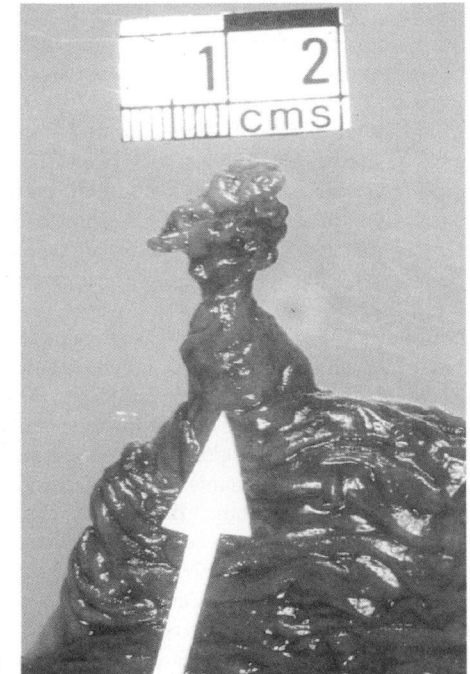

(b)

Fig. 3 Villous adenoma and carcinoma of the duodenum. (a) Ulcerating adenocarcinoma of the duodenum (arrowed) arising at the papilla in a 34-year-old man who presented with obstructive jaundice. (b) Origin of the carcinoma from a villous adenoma is strongly suggested by the fact that a concomitant (benign) villous adenoma was found in the third part of the duodenum in the resection specimen.

At laparotomy, distant metastases must be excluded, and the duodenum should then be assessed; if there is obvious infiltration or induration a diagnosis of malignancy is likely. Frozen section biopsy at this stage may indicate malignant change, in which case radical resection should be entertained in the form of a pancreatoduodenectomy. If the diagnosis is still unclear a duodenotomy can be performed and submucous resection undertaken. If the lesion lies close to the ampulla, local excision of the ampulla with reimplantation of the ducts or sphincteroplasty has been described. If peroperative (or subsequent) histological analysis demonstrates malignant change, a more extensive resection can be considered. There is a local recurrence rate of 28 per cent after submucous resection; as a consequence it has been argued that radical resection of all villous tumours should be undertaken in fit subjects.

Snare endoscopic removal can be undertaken in patients unfit for major surgery. However, this technically difficult procedure often leads to piecemeal resection and incomplete retrieval of the tumour. Endoscopic laser ablation has also been used successfully. Damage to the ampulla from either of these therapies can be avoided with an endoscopic stent. Lesions distal to the ampulla can be removed by segmental resection of bowel.

The follow-up of these patients should be determined by the final histology and the extent of resection. For locally excised lesions regular endoscopy is mandatory.

Polyposis syndromes (adenoma)

Familial polyposis coli is an autosomal dominant disease characterized by the presence of multiple adenomatous polyps in the colon and rectum. Patients with Gardner's syndrome have additional extracolonic manifestations; these are currently considered to be different expressions of the same disease due to variable penetration of the abnormal genes.

It is now clear that polyposis coli is not confined to the colon: in the last 20 years gastroduodenal polyps have been described, and the term familial adenomatous polyposis is often preferred. Most gastric polyps are hyperplastic and will not be considered further, except to state that we have recently encountered one patient with this condition who developed metachronous carcinomas of the stomach and duodenum.

Adenomatous polyps have been reported in the duodenum of 24 to 93 per cent of patients with familial adenomatous polyposis. These lesions, which are usually multiple and occur mainly in the second part of the duodenum, share the affinity of sporadic solitary adenomas for the periampullary region. The consensus of opinion is that these polyps are premalignant: there have been many reports of periampullary carcinoma developing. Indeed, this malignancy is the most common extracolonic carcinoma in familial adenomatous polyposis, occurring in 2 to 12 per cent of patients. In those with abdominal colectomy it may actually be more common than carcinoma of the rectum.

The natural history of these polyps is unclear. A recent report indicated no progression of duodenal lesions in 14 of 17 patients over an average observation period of 7.1 years. It is interesting that in one further patient a 1.7-cm polyp in the duodenal cap was overlooked and 22 months later a carcinoma was present.

All patients with familial adenomatous polyposis require upper gastrointestinal endoscopy at some stage. Hypotonic duodenography and an intubated small bowel meal may be needed for further delineation of duodenal or jejunoileal disease. Biopsy specimens should be taken from the periampullary region to detect microscopic lesions in 'normal' mucosa. Tumours less than 0.5 cm in diameter may either be observed or destroyed endoscopically, but larger lesions should be removed. Regular surveillance is indicated.

Jejunoileal polyps have also been reported. Although there are few data regarding their natural history, the risk of carcinoma appears low. Excision must still be considered, especially when the chance of malignant change is increased, as it is in the tubulovillous or villous types of adenoma.

Brunner's gland adenoma

These rare lesions are confined to the duodenum and three forms have been described: polypoid and isolated or diffuse nodular hyperplasia. Adenomas usually arise proximal to the papilla and are less than 1 cm in diameter (although there is one report of a lesion 12 cm in diameter). Many small lesions will be asymptomatic, but larger ones can present with non-specific upper abdominal gastrointestinal symptoms, occult or major haemorrhage, or obstruction. There is one report of duodenal malignancy originating from Brunner's glands. Treatment is removal, either by endoscopy (for small lesions) or surgery (for larger lesions). Concomitant microcarcinoids were recently reported in one resection specimen.

Circumscribed nodular hyperplasia is characterized by sessile projections in the duodenal cap, whilst in the diffuse form the lesions are found throughout the duodenum. Although the underlying reasons are unclear, the incidence seems to be higher in patients with chronic renal failure. Presentation is often incidental, as the condition is usually asymptomatic; vague discomfort, haemorrhage, or obstruction can occur. Diagnosis requires endoscopy or a barium meal, which demonstrates a cobblestone mucosal appearance. Provided a confident diagnosis can be made, no treatment is usually necessary.

Stromal

Adipose tissue—lipoma

These lesions become apparent in the sixth and seventh decade and are usually pedunculated, intraluminal lesions, although some are submucosal. They vary from 0.5 to 8 cm in diameter. Some reports indicate that lipomas are more common in the ileum than in the duodenum or jejunum.

Most lipomas are small and asymptomatic, but once they exceed 4 cm in diameter symptoms such as intussusception or (rarely) bleeding from surface ulceration can develop. Even lipomas less than 1 cm in diameter can cause serious haemorrhage.

Lipomas almost certainly have no malignant potential, although a solitary case of liposarcoma of the ileum has been described. Symptomatic lesions should be removed either endoscopically or surgically, and there is also a case for removing asymptomatic duodenal lipomas because of their potential for causing obstruction, obstructive jaundice, and haemorrhage.

Connective tissue

Smooth muscle tumours

Leiomyomas are common small bowel neoplasms which usually present in the fifth or sixth decade and probably have an equal sex distribution. Macroscopically they appear either as extraluminal, intramural, dumb-bell lesions or as intraluminal lesions; most are extraluminal (Fig. 4). They occur throughout the small bowel, but predominantly in the jejunum and ileum.

Intraluminal lesions usually present with haemorrhage secondary to mucosal ulceration (Fig. 5), but obstruction can arise from intussusception or due to a mass effect. Extraluminal lesions can become enormous and undergo central necrosis with a risk of haemorrhage; these tumours may be palpable. Unusual presentations include volvulus, perforation, and fistula formation.

Leiomyomas are vascular and may be demonstrated by angiography. Extramural lesions can also be detected by CT scan, whereas intraluminal forms are more likely to be visible on contrast studies, when they appear as lesions with a central crater. Leiomyomas have a definite malignant potential, and histological distinction between benign and malignant forms can be difficult:

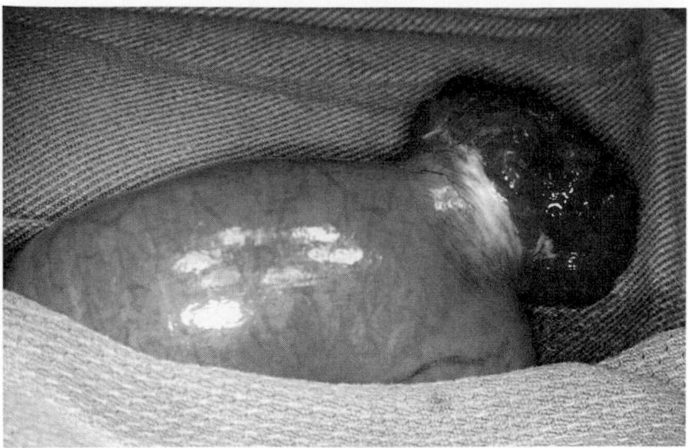

Fig. 4 Large extraluminal leiomyoma of the jejunum.

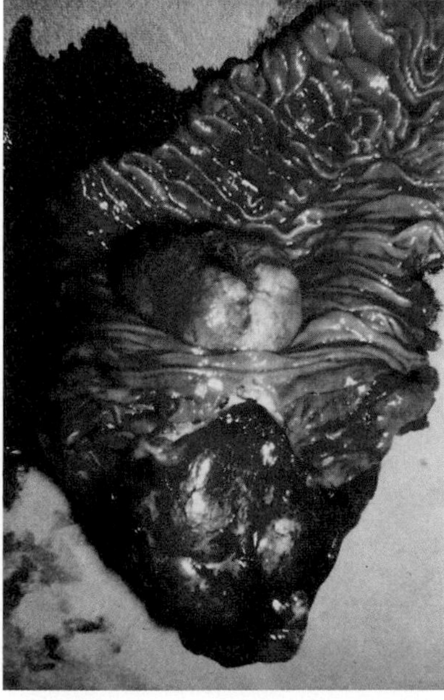

Fig. 5 Leiomyoma of the small bowel with ulceration causing haemorrhage (by courtesy of Mr J. Spencer).

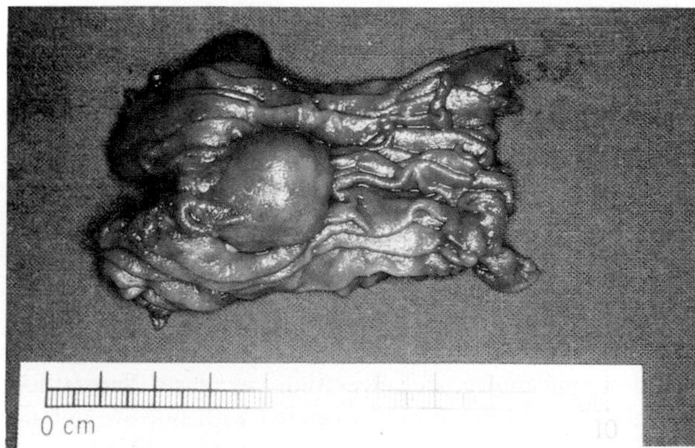

Fig. 6 Intraluminal leiomyoma of the small bowel treated by local excision (mucosal aspect).

although the frequency of mitoses can be a distinguishing feature it is not pathognomonic. For this reason, leiomyomas should be resected with a clear margin of tissue (Fig. 6).

Neurogenic tumours

Neurofibromas, schwannomas, gangliocytic paragangliomas, paragangliomas, and ganglioneuromas are included in this category. All are derived from nervous tissue, either the nerve sheath, paraganglia, or ganglia.

Neurofibromas are the most common subtype. Most of them are not associated with other diseases, but 11 to 25 per cent of patients with von Recklinghausen's disease develop lesions in the gastrointestinal tract. Isolated neurofibromas tend to occur in the ileum, whereas in neurofibromatosis the jejunum and stomach are preferentially involved, followed by the ileum and duodenum. Lesions are usually subserosal, but they can be intramural or intraluminal. Ulceration leading to bleeding is the usual presentation, but bowel obstruction can occur. Schwannomas may present in a similar manner. Some 15 to 20 per cent of neurofibromas are reported to be malignant, and treatment is by excision of the affected bowel.

Gangliocytic paragangliomas are rare. Lesions are polypoid, appearing predominantly in the second part of the duodenum but sometimes in the distal duodenum or jejunum (Fig. 7). In a review of 39 cases the mean age of presentation was 52 years; symptoms included haemorrhage (62 per cent) and abdominal pain (21 per cent), but a few tumours were asymptomatic (13 per cent). Paragangliomas and ganglioneuromas are rare.

Fibroma

These rare lesions develop within the wall of the small bowel and are usually asymptomatic, although they may present with intussusception and obstruction. The histological diagnosis can be confused with inflammatory lesions or with smooth muscle tumours or neurogenic tumours.

Endothelium

Vascular tumours

Three forms are recognized: capillary haemangiomas, cavernous haemangiomas, and multiple telangiectasia. Simple capillary lesions can be single or multiple (Fig. 8), while cavernous haemangiomas are usually single. Most appear as a polypoid mass (Fig. 9), but a diffuse infiltrating form has also been described. Symptoms include haemorrhage or, more rarely, obstruction. In patients with multiple telangiectasia numerous lesions 1 to 5 mm in diameter are evident in the bowel: a hereditary form of this condition is Osler–Weber–Rendu disease. Occasionally these lesions are part of a generalized haemangiomatosis. Malignant change is extremely rare in haemangiomas, and it is important not to confuse multiple lesions with metastases.

Investigation includes radiological contrast studies, which may demonstrate either polypoid or stenosing lesions. Selective mesenteric angiography can identify abnormalities, but the technique is more likely to be productive when bleeding is active. If operation is required, transillumination of the bowel may demonstrate small lesions, but the technique can be difficult when there is blood in the lumen. Intraoperative endoscopy may also be helpful. Symptomatic neoplasms should be treated by simple excision. If multiple abnormalities are present, only bowel associated with the lesion should be excised so as to conserve intestine.

There are also vascular abnormalities of the small bowel which, although not true neoplasms, should be considered in the differential diagnosis of gastrointestinal bleeding. Differences of

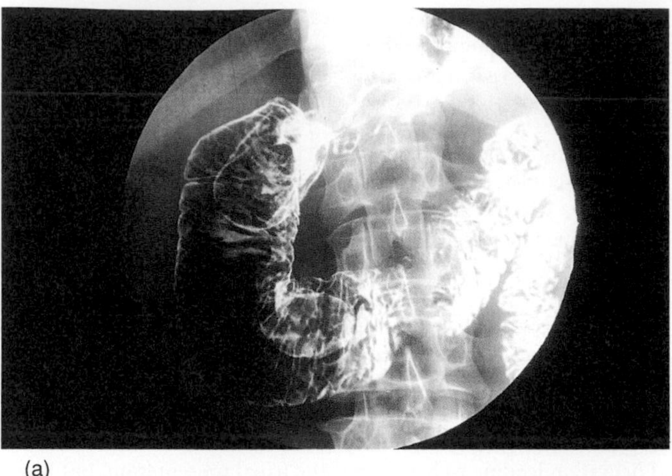
(a)

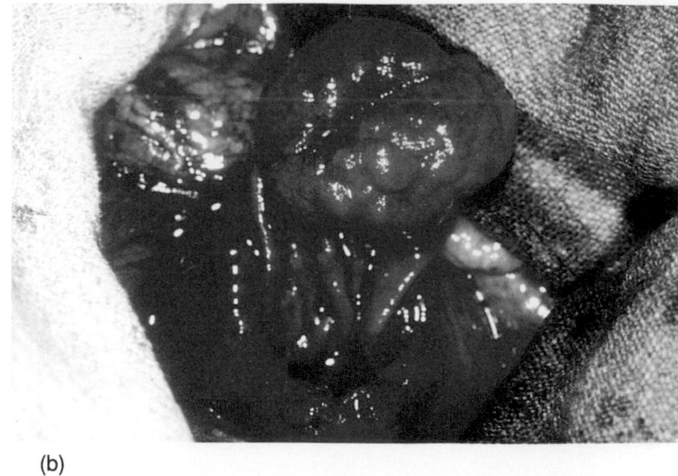
(b)

Fig. 7 Duodenal paraganglioma. (a) Barium meal examination undertaken for mild dyspepsia in a man of 64 years shows a tumour in the third part of the duodenum. (b) At operation a circumscribed lesion was found at this site and locally excised.

opinion exist regarding their nomenclature: arteriovenous malformation, angiodysplasia, vascular malformation, and ectasia have all been used to describe these vascular abnormalities. Intestinal lesions have been classified into three groups: Group 1 comprises solitary lesions in the right colon, usually occurring in patients over 55; Group 2 contains lesions in the small bowel in younger patients, thought to be congenital; and Group 3 comprises patients in whom multifocal lesions exist, as in hereditary haemorrhagic telangiectasia. An alternative classification includes congenital arteriovenous malformations, which can present at any age, or idiopathic angiodysplasia, which is acquired in later years.

Although the overall prevalence of these lesions is low, they are a common cause of obscure gastrointestinal bleeding. They arise within the submucosa, and erosion through the mucosa is required to produce detectable haemorrhage. They occur predominantly in the right colon, but can also be found in the jejunum and ileum, stomach, and duodenum in decreasing frequency.

The preoperative investigation of choice is selective mesenteric angiography, which may even demonstrate lesions that are not bleeding at the time. Radiological features include localized vascular tufts and opacification of early draining veins. In patients with active bleeding, an indication of the part of the bowel that is responsible can be obtained by isotope scanning with labelled red blood cells. Identification of these lesions at laparotomy may require endoscopy or peroperative radiographic localization.

A resection specimen of bowel thought to include the lesion may not contain any histological abnormality. If at all possible localization should be attempted by injecting the specimen with a barium gelatin mixture or latex material.

Lymphatic tumours

These occasional lesions include lymphangiomas, lymphatic cysts, and lymphangiectasia. Lymphangiomas are composed of multiple lymphatic channels and appear as smooth round lesions protruding into the lumen of the bowel. Lymphatic cysts can be recognized as small yellow nodules on the mucosal or serosal surface (Fig. 10). Both lymphangiomas and lymphatic cysts are benign and rarely cause symptoms. Treatment is by simple excision.

Primary lymphangiectasia is probably a congenital disease in which the lymph vessels of the bowel are abnormally dilated. Patients present with hypoproteinaemia and protein-losing enteropathy, and a low serum albumin. Secondary lymphangiectasia is thought to be an acquired form of the condition and is associated with diseases such as lymphoma, carcinoma, and sarcoidosis.

INTERMEDIATE NEOPLASMS (endocrine tumours)

Knowledge of these lesions is developing at a rapid pace and a full discussion of endocrine tumours is beyond the scope of this text: relevant features only have been summarized.

Carcinoid tumours develop from neural crest cell lines and are included in the APUDoma group of lesions (APUD = amine precursor uptake and decarboxylation). In the bowel they may be classified in accordance with their derivation from the foregut (including the duodenum), midgut (including the jejunoileum), and hindgut. The foregut and midgut lesions can be identified microscopically by staining with ammoniacal silver nitrate (argentaffin). Midgut carcinoids are argentaffin positive: high levels of 5-hydroxytryptamine (serotonin) are secreted. By contrast, foregut carcinoids are argentaffin negative and secrete low levels of serotonin. These lesions may also secrete a variety of peptides including gastrin, somatostatin, and glucagon.

The appendix is the most common site of carcinoid tumour, followed by the ileum, jejunum, rectum, and duodenum. Most ileal lesions are found distally, while the more unusual duodenal carcinoids are concentrated proximally in the first and second part of the duodenum. Rare associations between duodenal carcinoid tumours (often somatostatinomas) and neurofibromatosis, alone or in combination with phaeochromocytoma, have been reported. Twenty to 30 per cent of carcinoids are multicentric.

Lesions typically appear as submucosal nodules which grow slowly towards either the mucosa or the serosa; they may become polypoid in appearance, and ulceration can occur. Serosal lesions in the jejunum and ileum are associated with fibrosis and subsequent stenosis, owing to local vasoconstrictor peptides secreted by the tumour (Fig. 11). This phenomenon may cause obstruction.

Clinical presentation is usually during the fifth decade and both

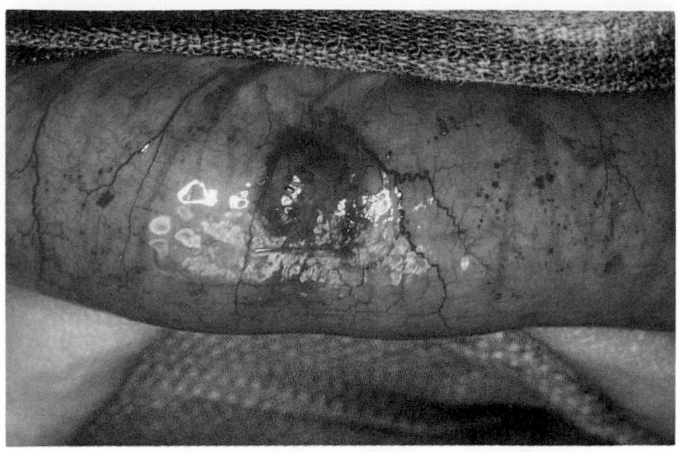

(a)

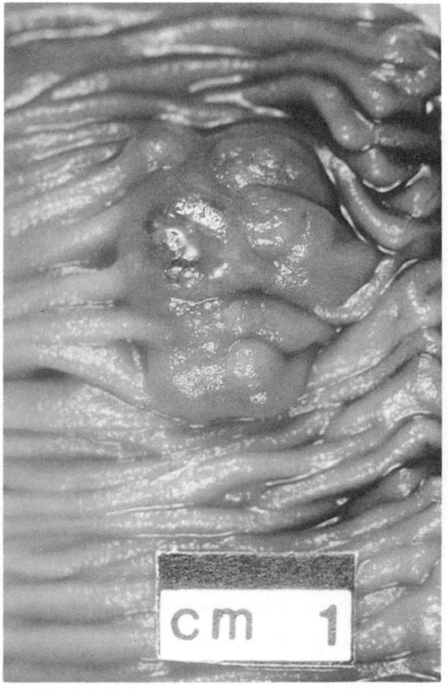

(b)

Fig. 8 Capillary haemangioma of the small bowel in a woman of 62 years who had persistent anaemia from occult gastrointestinal haemangioma. (a) Serosal aspect of tumour. (b) Mucosal aspect showing ulceration over the lesion.

sexes are affected equally. Some 70 to 80 per cent of jejunal and ileal tumours are asymptomatic, and symptoms that do occur are often non-specific. However, episodes of obstruction can result from intussusception or kinking of the bowel due to local fibrosis, and bleeding is a rare presenting feature.

Carcinoid syndrome is not a feature of local, non-metastasizing lesions in the gastrointestinal tract, since 5-hydroxytryptamine is metabolized in the liver. The syndrome may be evident if carcinoids drain directly into the systemic circulation, for example if the primary lesions are in the bronchus or ovary, or if liver metastases are present.

Eighty per cent of duodenal lesions cause symptoms due to ulceration, obstruction, and jaundice; their presence may also be heralded by the effects of vasoactive secretions, including gastrin, somatostatin, and glucagon.

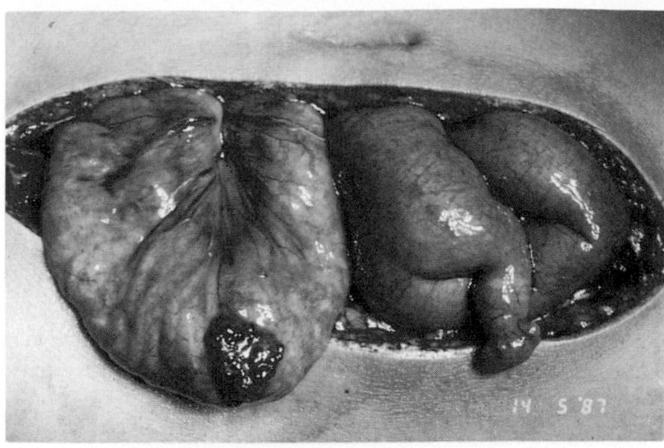

Fig. 9 Cavernous haemangioma of the small bowel. Note coincident Meckel's diverticulum (by courtesy of Mr J. Spencer).

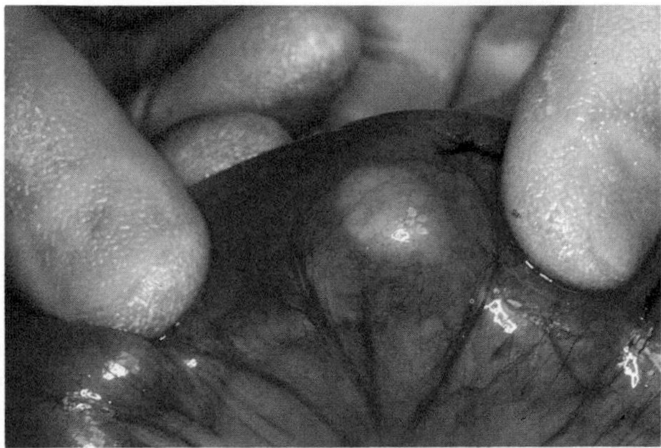

Fig. 10 Lymphatic cyst of mid small bowel: incidental finding at operation.

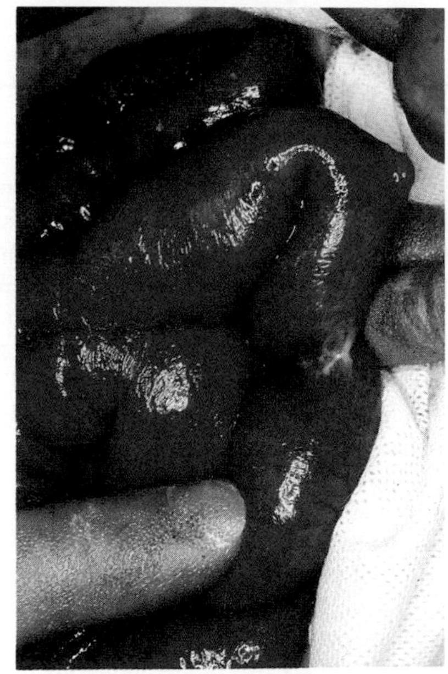

Fig. 11 Ileal carcinoid tumour causing luminal stenosis. Multiple carcinoids were found with nodal metastases, and side-to-side bypass of the small bowel has been performed (by courtesy of Mr J. Spencer).

Some authorities believe that carcinoid tumours are benign with a malignant potential, while others consider that they are all malignant. Once the primary tumour exceeds 2 cm in diameter, there is an 80 to 90 per cent chance of metastases developing; thus size is the dominant factor determining malignant change.

Although wide excision is preferable for carcinoids in view of the malignant potential, treatment depends on the site of the lesion. A full laparotomy is always necessary to exclude the presence of multicentric lesions. Lesions in the jejunum and ileum can be managed by wide local excision, including the draining mesenteric lymph nodes. Treatment of terminal ileal tumours may require a right hemicolectomy. An intense vasospastic reaction can be provoked by handling larger carcinoids during surgery. Small duodenal neoplasms may be dealt with by local excision, but pancreatoduodenectomy is indicated for large tumours. Small duodenal lesions have been treated conservatively in patients with a high operative risk.

Duodenal gastrinomas are present in 13 to 38 per cent of patients in whom the tumour is located. These tumours may be small (2 mm diameter) and only detectable by duodenotomy and eversion of the mucosa to allow adequate visualization and palpation. Forty to 60 per cent are not associated with lymph node metastases and consequently have a good prognosis.

HAMARTOMATOUS LESIONS

A hamartoma is best defined as 'an excessive focal overgrowth of mature normal cells and tissues in an organ composed of identical cellular elements'. As previously indicated, histopathologists disagree over the classification of many enteric lesions. Among those already discussed in the preceding sections, Brunner's gland adenoma, neurofibroma, gangliocytic paraganglioma, haemangioma, and lymphangioma have all been described as hamartomas. Several lesions are generally accepted as hamartomas and these will now be described.

Peutz–Jeghers syndrome

This is the most common syndrome affecting the small intestine and is inherited in an autosomal dominant fashion. Multiple polyps, either pedunculated or sessile, can occur throughout the intestinal tract, but the small bowel is mainly affected: usually the jejunum, but sometimes the ileum or duodenum. Polyps are usually 0.5 to 1 cm in diameter but may be larger. Groups of polyps can appear in different areas sequentially. The disease is associated with mucocutaneous pigmentation, notably on the face, lips, buccal mucosa, palms, and soles.

Most patients present within the first three decades of life. The two main features are obstruction and haemorrhage: recurrent episodes of colic are commonly due to intussusception, and haemorrhage can lead to anaemia. Malignancy may occur in 2 to 3 per cent of patients and is most common in the duodenum. In the colon malignant change may be due wholly, or in part, to carcinoma developing in coexistent adenomatous polyps, but this has not been reported in the small bowel.

Treatment should generally be conservative. If surgery is required for complications, local resection is sensible as repeated procedures may be needed in the future.

Other polyposis syndromes (hamartoma)

These are rare conditions. Juvenile polyposis syndromes have been reported to affect both the small and the large bowel. Malignant change has not been reported in juvenile polyps of the small bowel in these conditions.

The Cronkhite–Canada syndrome is characterized by polyposis throughout the gastrointestinal tract, causing diarrhoea and steatorrhoea. Associated ectodermal changes include alopecia, nail dystrophy, and skin hyperpigmentation.

HETEROTOPIC TISSUE

Tissue identified in a site at which it is not usually present is referred to as heterotopic. In the small bowel this abnormality may be either localized or disseminated.

Localized

Gastric mucosa can appear in the duodenum or in developmental abnormalities of the small bowel, such as Meckel's diverticulum or duplications. Gastric heterotopia in the duodenum seems to be of little clinical significance: it is detected endoscopically only if the lesion appears as a polyp (which can occasionally cause symptoms) or a prominent fold, but both these are rare. Gastric (oxyntic) mucosa in a Meckel's diverticulum may be associated with a peptic ulcer which can bleed or perforate. Treatment is by Meckelian diverticulectomy. Since technetium is taken up by oxyntic mucosa, scintigraphy may localize the source of haemorrhage.

Heterotopic pancreatic tissue can occur in the duodenum and upper jejunum or in a Meckel's diverticulum (Fig. 12). The appearances are usually of a nodule within the submucosa or muscularis, although polypoid forms have been reported. Most of these ectopic masses are asymptomatic. Small lesions at the ampulla can cause biliary obstruction, mimicking periampullary cancer, and large lesions can produce obstruction or haemorrhage from mucosal ulceration. Symptomatic lesions should be locally removed, as should incidental lesions discovered at laparotomy if the surgeon is in diagnostic doubt. Combinations of heterotopic tissues are rare, but gastric mucosa and pancreatic tissue have been observed both in the duodenum as a submucosal mass and in Meckel's diverticulum.

Disseminated

Endometriosis can affect the small bowel, albeit rarely. In a review of over 7000 cases, only 12 per cent involved the gastrointestinal tract, of which 72 per cent affected the sigmoid colon and rectum; small bowel was affected in only 7 per cent. In the small bowel the ileum is most often affected.

Diagnosis is difficult. It may be suggested by symptoms indicating varying degrees of obstruction, including nausea, vomiting, colic, and diarrhoea, which are more prominent on a cyclical basis, in line with menstruation. It must be remembered however that patients with endometriosis may develop obstructive symptoms due to adhesions secondary to the disease itself. Most cases of small bowel endometriosis will be diagnosed at laparoscopy or laparotomy as an incidental finding, rather than as a cause of small bowel symptoms.

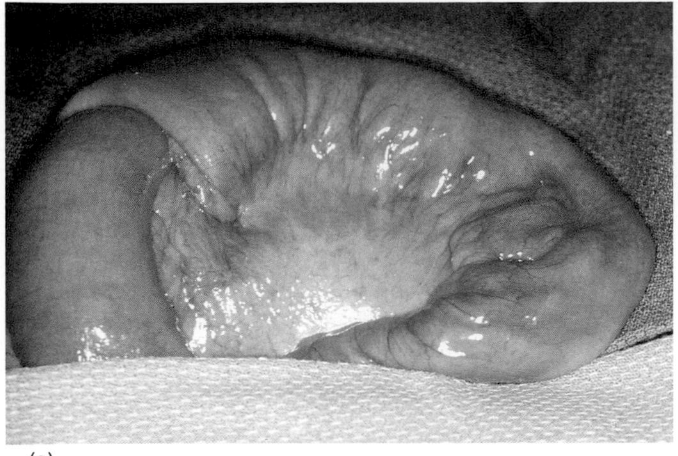

(a)

(b)

Fig. 12 Invaginated Meckel's diverticulum containing heterotopic pancreatic tissue. Barium enema had shown a filling defect in the terminal ileum of a 47-year-old man with a short history of diarrhoea. (a) At laparotomy an intussuscepting tumour of the ileum was found. (b) An ulcerated nodule of ectopic pancreas at the tip of an invaginated Meckel's diverticulum formed the apex of the intussusception.

If symptomatic, the affected segment of bowel should be resected. If asymptomatic lesions are present and malignancy can be excluded, current developments in the management of the endometriosis, including endocrine therapy or laser ablation, may preclude the necessity for bowel resection.

DUPLICATIONS

Half of these rare intestinal lesions affect the jejunum or ileum. They appear within the mesentery of the bowel in two main forms: cystic with no communication with the lumen of the bowel, or tubular, connected with the bowel lumen either proximally or distally. The lumen of the duplication is lined with intestinal epithelium plus part or all of the normal muscle components. Gastric heterotopia occurs in 15 to 36 per cent of cases.

Up to 85 per cent of patients present in infancy (before 2 years), but symptoms can occur in later years. The presentation is usually with an abdominal mass or obstruction, and rarely by ulceration of heterotopic gastric mucosa or adjacent small bowel mucosa, causing bleeding or perforation.

Treatment is by excision of the affected segment of bowel. The lesion cannot usually be removed from adjacent bowel, owing to the common blood supply. If the duplication is extensive, surgical options include opening both ends of the lesion into the bowel, coring out mucosa through multiple incisions or attempts at local removal, which may be facilitated in the rare event of a separate mesentery.

FURTHER READING

Ashley SW, Wells SA, Jr. Tumors of the small intestine. *Semin Oncol* 1988; **15**: 116–28.

Chappuis CW, Divincenti FC, Cohn I Jr. Villous tumors of the duodenum. *Ann Surg* 1989; **209**: 593–9.

Dial P, Cohn I Jr. Tumors of the jejunum and ileum. In: Scott HW Jr, Sawyers JL, eds. *Surgery of the stomach, duodenum and small intestine*. Boston: Blackwell Scientific Publications, 1987: 937–51.

Feldman JM. Carcinoid tumors and syndrome. *Semin Oncol* 1987; **14**: 237–46.

Frimberger E, Hagenmuller F, Classen M. Endostomy: a new approach to small-bowel endoscopy. *Endoscopy* 1989; **21**: 86–8.

Herbsman H, *et al.* Tumors of the small intestine. *Curr Probl Surg* 1980; **17**: 127–82.

Kaplan EL, *et al.* Gastrinomas: a 42-year experience. *World J Surg*1990; **14**: 365–76.

Lewis BS, Waye JD. Chronic gastrointestinal bleeding of obscure origin: role of small bowel enteroscopy. *Gastroenterology* 1988; **94**: 1117–20.

Monk JE, Smith BA, O'Leary JP. Arteriovenous malformations of the small intestine. *South Med J* 1989; **82**: 18–22.

Morson BC, Dawson IMP, Day DW, Jass JR, Price AB, Williams GT. Benign epithelial tumours and polyps. In L Morson BC, Dawson IMP, eds., *Morson and Dawson's gastrointestinal pathology*. 3rd edn. Oxford: Blackwell Scientific Publications 1990: 351–9.

Morson BC, Dawson IMP, Day DW, Jass JR, Price AB, Williams GT. Malignant epithelial tumours. In: Morson BC, Dawson IMP, eds. *Morson and Dawson's gastrointestinal pathology*. 3rd edn. Oxford: Blackwell Scientific Publications 1990: 360–71.

Morson BC, Dawson IMP, Day DW, Jass JR, Price AB, Williams GT. Non-epithelial tumours. In: Morson BC, Dawson IMP, eds. *Morson and Dawson's gastrointestinal pathology*. 3rd edn. Oxford: Blackwell Scientific Publications, 1990: 372–87.

Perey BJ. Neoplasms of the duodenum. In: Scott HW, Jr., Sawyers JL, eds. *Surgery of the stomach, duodenum and small intestine*. Boston: Blackwell Scientific Publications, 1987: 571–84.

Perzin KH, Bridge MF. Adenomas of the small intestine: a clinicopathologic review of 51 cases and a study of their relationship to carcinoma. *Cancer* 1981; **48**: 799–819.

Sarre RG, Frost AG, Jagelman DG, Petras RE, Sivak MV, McGannon E. Gastric and duodenal polyps in familial adenomatous polyposis: a prospective study of the nature and prevalence of upper gastrointestinal polyps. *Gut* 1987; **28**: 306–14.

Stahl C, Grimes E. M. Endometriosis of the small bowel. Case reports and review of the literature. *Obstet Gynecol Surv* 1987; **42**: 131–5.

Wander JV, Das Gupta TK, Neurofibromatosis. *Curr Probl Surg* 1977; **14**: 1–81.

16.9 Nutrition for small bowel disorders

ADRIAN SAVAGE

Disorders of the small bowel are the most common indication for parenteral nutritional support. Among a series of patients requiring total parenteral nutrition (TPN) at the Massachusetts General Hospital in the period 1 November 1988 to 1 November 1989, prolonged postoperative ileus or intestinal obstruction, sometimes associated with intra-abdominal sepsis or anastomotic leakage, formed the single largest group of patients requiring TPN (Table 1). Enterocutaneous fistula was a relatively uncommon indication for TPN. Other conditions of the small bowel necessitating TPN were mesenteric infarction, massive small bowel resection, malabsorption syndromes, and inflammatory bowel disease.

NUTRITIONAL ASSESSMENT

Four questions need to be addressed when assessing a patient for nutritional support. First, the degree of malnutrition must be estimated: the more malnourished the patient, the more urgent nutritional support becomes. Second, the prognosis or outcome of the disease must be assessed. The need for nutritional support is greater if the underlying condition is unlikely to resolve quickly. Third, an assessment of the patient's calorie, protein, and fluid and electrolyte requirements is a prerequisite to appropriate nutritional support. Finally, the route of administration of nutritional support must be assessed. Parenteral nutrition should only be administered if nutrition cannot safely be administered by the gastrointestinal tract.

Malnutrition may pre-exist in patients presenting for surgery, and the higher risks associated with surgery in such patients are well known. These may not be preventable by preoperative TPN. Alternatively, malnutrition may develop insidiously because of delay in the institution of oral feeding after surgery. The development of malnutrition under these circumstances may be difficult to recognize.

Many methods for documenting nutritional depletion have been described. The simplest is based on the change in usual body weight and the serum albumin estimation. Patients who have lost more than 10 per cent of their usual body weight as a result of illness in less than 2 months may be considered malnourished. A loss of 25 per cent or more of the usual body weight indicates severe malnutrition. The serum albumin estimation below 35 g/l indicates malnutrition if there is no protein losing enteropathy and no nephrotic syndrome. Anthropometric measurements such as arm muscle circumference and triceps skinfold, estimation of the serum transferrin, and skin tests of delayed hypersensitivity have limited application in routine clinical assessment of nutritional status.

Patients undergoing major abdominal surgery suffer few ill effects from a 3- to 5-day period of starvation while awaiting resolution of the paralytic ileus. In such patients, the risks of administering parenteral nutritional support are greater than the benefits. However, in the small minority of patients who develop postoperative complications which prevent the restitution of oral intake, parenteral nutritional support should be considered after 7 days, and even earlier if sepsis develops.

ASSESSMENT OF CALORIE REQUIREMENTS

The administration of insufficient calories to meet the needs of the patient will fail to reverse catabolism and the main goals of nutritional support, wound healing, maintenance of skin integrity, and the prevention of loss of lean body mass will not be achieved. Overfeeding may also be hazardous. The over-administration of protein may precipitate the requirement for dialysis in patients with borderline renal failure. Hyperglycaemia resulting from infusion may be difficult to control with insulin. Overfeeding increases CO_2 production and may make it difficult to wean patients from ventilatory support. Hyperalimentation is associated with fatty change of the liver. Finally, patients on long-term TPN may become obese if overfed.

The Harris–Benedict equations (Table 2) are one of the earliest methods for determining the calorie requirements at rest. These formulae take into account the height, weight, age, and sex of the

Table 1 Indications for TPN at the Massachusetts General Hospital from November 1988 to November 1989.

Gastrointestinal indications		Other indications	
Postoperative ileus	110	Aspiration pneumonia	12
Intestinal obstruction	47	Burns	21
Intraperitoneal sepsis	28	Major trauma	29
Enterocutaneous fistula	18	Liver failure	13
Mesenteric infarction	17	Multisystem organ failure	83
Small bowel resection	15	Chylothorax	1
Inflammatory bowel disease	17		
Pancreatitis	94		
Postoperative cholecystitis	10		
Malabsorption	3		
Oesophagitis	10		
Gastrointestinal bleeding	33		
Total	402		156

Table 2 The Harris–Benedict equation for basal energy expenditure (BEE)

Men	(BEE) = 66 + (13.7 × W) + (5 × H) − (6.8 × A)
Women	(BEE) = 655 + (9.6 × W) + (1.8 × H) − (4.7 × A)

W = weight in kg, H = height in cm, A = age in years.

patient. Tall heavy young men require almost three times as many calories as small elderly thin women. The basal energy expenditure that this equation calculates must then be multiplied by a stress factor (Table 3). For patients who are severely catabolic due to burns or septicaemia, this stress factor is 2. This method of assessing calorie requirements has been compared to the results of indirect calorimetry and found to be on the generous side.

Table 3 Factor by which the basal energy expenditure is multiplied for varying disease states

1.2	Mild starvation Postoperative
1.5	Peritonitis Long bone fracture
1.7	Severe infection Multiple trauma Multiorgan failure 30% burn
2.0	50% + burn

Having assessed the patient's energy needs, an attempt at estimating the protein requirement should also be made. Patients who are severely catabolic will require up to 2.5 g of protein/kg body weight/day while a patient who is well will only require 1 g protein/kg.day. Patients in renal failure in whom it is hoped to avoid the requirement for dialysis, should have their protein restricted to 40g/day, mainly in the form of essential amino acids. Patients with liver failure may respond to over-administration of protein with a rise in the serum urea and a worsening of hepatic encephalopathy.

The protein component of TPN is administered in the form of amino acid solutions. There is little to choose between the different types of amino acid solutions for patients with disorders of the small bowel except that glutamine, as yet not routinely available, may be an important substrate for maintenance of the gastrointestinal mucosa. In enteral feeds, the source of nitrogen in polymeric diets is whole protein derived from caseinates, soy isolate, and egg white. Predigested or elemental enteral diets are also available, in which the protein is provided as free amino acids or oligopeptides. Elemental diets are expensive and relatively unpalatable and should be reserved for patients who are not able to digest and absorb polymeric diets.

The remaining calorie requirement may be made up by the administration of a combination of dextrose solutions and fat emulsions. Up to 60 per cent of total calorie intake, but not more than 2 g/kg body weight, may be made up of intralipid. Since fat has a respiratory quotient of 0.7, compared with 1.0 for carbohydrates, the use of intralipid as a main source of calories in ventilator dependent patients will result in production of less CO_2 than is the case if the calories are made up predominantly with dextrose, and this may aid weaning from the ventilator. For other patients, 500 ml of 10 per cent intralipid twice a week will meet the requirements for essential fatty acids, and the remaining calories may be made up with dextrose. In enteral feeds, fat is derived commonly from corn or soybean oil and carbohydrates from hydrolysed corn starch. The majority of enteral diets are lactose free; some patients develop transient lactose intolerance postoperatively.

The average patient requires between 2 and 3 litres of free water a day with between 90 and 150 mmol/l sodium, and between 60 and 100 mmol/l potassium. For a patient maintained on TPN, a 2000-kcal, 80-g protein diet is made up of a 4 per cent amino acid and 25 per cent dextrose solution, administered via an intravenous catheter placed in a central vein. Losses from the gastrointestinal tract, for example from a high output fistula or nasogastric aspiration, must be replaced by increasing the free water and electrolyte composition of the TPN solution as appropriate. The majority of enteral diets are made up to 1 kcal/ml, a 2000-kcal diet being provided in a volume of 2 litres.

Most TPN regimens include sufficient vitamins to meet the patient's daily requirements, but these will not make up a deficit in the vitamin depleted patient. While it is possible to measure the levels of most vitamins, it is often easier to treat empirically any suspected deficiencies.

ROUTE OF ADMINISTRATION

Parenteral administration is more expensive, prone to a greater complication rate and may be less effective at reversing nutritional loss than enteral nutrition. Parenteral nutrition also results in atrophy of gastrointestinal mucosa, while enteral nutrition reduces bacterial translocation and maintains mucosal integrity. There is, therefore, every reason to administer nutrition enterally rather than parenterally, if at all feasible.

POSTOPERATIVE ILEUS

Ileus following abdominal surgery affects the stomach and colon rather than the small bowel, whose motility and function is often normal in the immediate postoperative period. Nutrients can be administered into the jejunum in the immediate postoperative period, but this is associated with a high incidence of nausea, bloating, vomiting, abdominal pain, and diarrhoea. There is also a risk of aspiration of enteral feed if vomiting occurs, especially in drowsy patients. Carefully selected patients with prolonged ileus, for example, following pylorus-preserving pancreatoduodenectomy, may be successfully nourished by jejunostomy feeding. Enteral nutrition is contraindicated in patients with mechanical intestinal obstruction, intra-abdominal sepsis, and anastomotic leakage. In practical terms, any patient whose postoperative ileus has not resolved within 7 days after surgery should be considered for TPN. The development of intra-abdominal sepsis, anastomotic leakage or Gram-negative septicaemia results in severe catabolism and rapid loss of lean body mass. In such patients, TPN should be given early.

ENTEROCUTANEOUS FISTULAE

Enterocutaneous fistulae develop as a result of Crohn's disease, radiation enteritis, or following surgery, and may develop more commonly in malnourished patients than in those with a normal nutritional status. Intestinal enterocutaneous fistulae may be divided into two types; high output fistulae, which produce more than 500 ml/day, and low output fistulae. High output fistulae usually arise from the small bowel while low output fistulae commonly communicate with the colon, and both types may be associated with intra-abdominal abscess. Enterocutaneous fistulae will close provided that there is no distal obstruction to the gastrointestinal tract, that intra-abdominal sepsis is adequately drained, and that the nutritional status of the patient is good.

Nutritional problems are common in patients with enterocutaneous fistulae. In the early stages, fluid and electrolyte balance is often unstable and care must be taken to replace electrolytes, including magnesium. Continuing intra-abdominal sepsis may result in a requirement for more calories than expected. Later, specific deficiencies, especially in calcium, the fat-soluble vitamins A, D, E, and K, and vitamin B_{12} may occur, and supplementation in addition to the vitamin preparation routinely added to TPN may be required. Once sepsis has resolved, selected patients may be managed by enteral feeding. Patients with low output fistulae may be managed on low residue enteral feeds. For patients with high output fistulae, enteral feeding may be possible if access to the distal gastrointestinal tract is available.

INFLAMMATORY BOWEL DISEASE

Patients with inflammatory bowel disease are often malnourished. This is manifested by loss of weight, hypoalbuminaemia, and growth retardation in children. In addition, patients with inflammatory bowel disease may be malnourished as a result of the complications of surgery, including enterocutaneous fistulae and short bowel syndrome. Remission of disease has been reported with bowel rest and total parenteral nutrition, but oral nutritional supplementation may be equally effective. Enteral nutritional supplementation with elemental diets such as Vivonex or Vital HN are useful if the small bowel is extensively affected by Crohn's disease. TPN should probably be reserved for patients with intra-abdominal sepsis, fistulae, or short bowel syndrome.

Specific nutritional deficiencies occur in patients with inflammatory bowel disease. The predilection of Crohn's disease for the terminal ileum may cause vitamin B_{12} depletion. Fat malabsorption related to both Crohn's disease and a lack of bile acids in the enterohepatic circulation may lead to deficiency in the fat-soluble vitamins A, D, E, and K. Folate deficiency may occur in association with the administration of sulphasalazine.

SHORT BOWEL SYNDROME

Resection of more than 50 per cent of the small bowel, as a result of mesenteric infarction or multiple resections for Crohn's disease, may result in an inability to maintain nutritional status, although some patients with as little as 25 per cent of the small bowel remaining may eventually adapt to enteral nutrition. Much depends on whether the colon is in continuity with the residual small bowel. Terminal ileal resection has a greater effect on the nutritional status since the jejunum is not able to adapt to absorb bile salts and vitamin B_{12}, while the ileum will adapt to absorb nutrients after jejunal resection. The nutritional deficit which results from massive small bowel resection is compounded by fluid and electrolyte loss. This may be exacerbated by diarrhoea, secondary loss of bile salts, and fatty acids into the colon.

TPN should be administered while the transition to oral fluids and nutrients is made gradually: adaptation of the residual bowel may continue for up to 2 years, and oral intake should be instituted slowly. Some patients require life-long TPN supplementation. Fluid and electrolyte depletion secondary to diarrhoea or high ileostomy output may be helped by glucose–electrolyte replacement solutions or by adding salt to the diet. Many patients are able to tolerate a normal diet but many require enteral supplementation since more calories are needed to compensate for malabsorption. The standard polymeric diets are often more useful than elemental diets, whose high osmolarity may exacerbate intestinal fluid loss. Special attention must be paid to replacement of calcium and vitamin D, the fat-soluble vitamins A, E, and K whose absorption may be impaired along with dietary fats, and vitamin B_{12}, whose specific absorption mechanism may have resected.

MONITORING

The progress of patients on TPN must be monitored according to clinical indications. Daily estimation of fluid balance, weight, and plasma electrolytes and glucose are essential in the early stages of instituting nutritional support. Weekly estimation of calcium, liver function, albumin level, the haematological profile, and trace element level are also important. A decline in weight, the development of muscle wasting, the failure of wounds to heal, or the development of pressure sores should indicate that nutritional support needs to be reviewed.

FURTHER READING

Alexander JW, Nutrition and translocation. *J Parenteral Enteral Nutr* 1990; **14 (suppl)**: 170–4S.

Benedict FG. *Lectures on Nutrition*. Philadelphia: W B Saunders & Co, 1925: 31–54.

Daly JM, Bonau R, Stofberg P, Bloch A, Jeevanandam M, Morse M. Immediate postoperative jejunostomy feeding: clinical and metabolic results in a prospective trial. *Am J Surg* 1987; **153**: 198–204.

Detsky AS, Baker JP, O'Rourke K, Goel V. Perioperative parenteral nutrition: a meta-analysis. *Ann Intern Med* 1987; **107**: 195–203.

Greenberg GR, Fleming CR, Jeejeebhoy KN, Rosenberg IH, Sales D, Tremaine WJ. Controlled trial of bowel rest and nutritional support in the management of Crohn's disease. *Gut* 1988; **29**: 1309–15.

Harris JA, Benedict FG. *A Biometric Study of Basal Metabolism in Men*. Publication No. 279. Washington DC: Carnegie Institute of Washington, 1919.

Jeejeebhoy KN. *Energy metabolism in the critically ill*. London: John Libbey & Co Ltd; 1985: 93–101.

Mann S, Westenskow DR, Houtchens BA. Measured and predicted caloric expenditure in the acutely ill. *Crit Care Med* 1985; **13**: 173–7.

Matuchansky C. Parenteral nutrition in inflammatory bowel disease. *Gut* 1986; **27**: 81–4.

Michel L, Serrano A, Malt RA. Nutritional support of hospitalized patients. *N Engl J Med* 1981; **304**: 1147–52.

Rombeau JL, Rolandelli RH. Enteral and parenteral nutrition in patients with enteric fistulas and short bowel syndrome. *Surg Clin N Am* 1987; **67**: 551–71.

Souba WW, Herskowitz K, Salloum RM, Chen MK, Austgen TR. Gut glutamine metabolism. *J Parenteral Enteral Nutr* 1990; **14** (suppl). 45–50S.

Studley HO. Percentage of weight loss; a basic indicator of surgical risk in patients with chronic peptic ulcer. *JAMA* 1973; **106**: 458–60.

Veterans Affairs total parenteral nutrition cooperative study group. Perioperative total parenteral nutrition in surgical patients. *N Engl J Med* 1991; **325**: 525–32.

Wells C, Tinckler L, Rawlinson K, Jones H, Saunders J. Postoperative gastrointestinal motility. *Lancet* 1964; **i**: 4–10.

16.10 Foreign bodies

MICHAEL N. MARGOLIES

The variety of intestinal 'foreign bodies' is enormous and is limited only by the imagination and appetites of patients. Although ingestion of foreign bodies is common, the symptoms from ingestion are not: the diagnosis is only made by history, if available, or following the appearance of a complication. The definition of foreign body is problematic, as certain 'foreign bodies' such as a food bolus, or phytobezoar would be considered food, whereas other 'foreign bodies' such as enteroliths and gallstones originate within the digestive system of the host (Table 1). However, all these are included as foreign bodies by virtue of the complications that may arise from their presence in the gut lumen.

Table 1 Foreign bodies of the small intestine

1. True foreign bodies: metal, wood, plastic, etc.
2. Narcotic packets
3. Bezoars
4. Food bolus
5. Enteroliths and gallstones
6. Concretions
7. Intestinal parasites

The complications of small intestinal foreign bodies requiring surgical treatment include obstruction, perforation, and bleeding. In the absence of a history of unusual ingestion or of the finding of a radio-opaque foreign body, the specific cause is rarely identified preoperatively. The clinical presentation and the indications for surgery in patients with complications of foreign body ingestion are indistinguishable from other causes of obstruction, perforation, and bleeding.

Only 1 to 2 per cent of all cases of acute small bowel obstruction are due to obturation by a foreign body. The site of obstruction is most commonly in areas of narrowing: the distal ileum, the ileocaecal valve, or sites of preexisting inflammatory disease with stricture, neoplasm, or diverticula. Choices of operative treatment include manual displacement of the intraluminal object, if safe, into the colon, removal via enterotomy, or resection if the object is imbedded or has caused transmural necrosis. Perforation due to presence of a foreign body may result in diffuse peritonitis, but more commonly it presents itself as contained sepsis with a localized abscess or as fistulization into an adjacent viscus or parenchymatous organ. Treatment includes, in addition to antibacterial agents, removal of the foreign body, closure of the enterotomy or resection as dictated by the local findings, and drainage of abscess if it is present. Bleeding from a small bowel foreign body arising through mucosal pressure necrosis and ulceration is infrequent.

The management of patients with an ingested foreign body in the absence of the above complications is dictated by the nature of the foreign body. Once objects have left the stomach more than 95 per cent of them proceed through the small intestine and colon unimpeded and without untoward effects. The population of patients suffering foreign body ingestion includes children, those with psychiatric disorders, alcoholics, prisoners, and denture wearers who have diminished palatal sensation. A relative, although controversial indication for surgery, is failure to pass a foreign body as evidenced by lack of progress on serial radiographs. In children, the average time for passage of an object through the small intestine is 5 days. If their parents are reliable, children can be managed as outpatients to await passage confirmed by observation of stools or occasional radiographs.

Certain categories of foreign objects have special features that may dictate surgical removal.

TRUE FOREIGN BODIES

Repeated and multiple ingestion of metallic objects

Certain patients with severe psychiatric disorders or incarcerated felons repeatedly ingest an astonishing variety of objects, including pins, eating utensils, bedsprings, razor blades, bolts, and scissors. Evidence of self mutilation and drug use is common. Once these objects reach the small bowel they are likely (>90 per cent) to further traverse the gastrointestinal tract safely. Perforation or obstruction occurs in only 0.5 per cent of instances. Inasmuch as these patients have a remarkable propensity for eating their environment, as manifested in particular by ingesting parts of hospital beds, if surgery becomes indicated, radiographs should be obtained immediately prior to exploration.

Miniature battery ingestion in children

Although alkaline disc batteries can potentially leak their caustic contents in the stomach, other types of batteries (mercury, lithium, silver) are innocuous; the risk of mercury poisoning is low. Once such smooth round batteries reach the small intestine virtually all will pass.

Other objects

In contrast to metallic foreign bodies, pointed wooden objects such as splinters or toothpicks, and fish or chicken bones are more hazardous owing to their length and sharp ends, which make them more likely to perforate the bowel wall. Up to one-third of such objects which reach the small bowel may cause perforation. These patients most often present with an acute abdomen, radiographs and history being unrevealing. Perforation usually results in intra-abdominal abscess or fistula: this may occur at any site in the bowel wall but in particular in the ileocaecal region, including Meckel's diverticulum, where the differential diagnosis includes more common inflammatory lesions. Toothpick perforations are particularly prone to produce fistulae with late septic complications.

NARCOTIC PACKET INGESTION

A popular method of narcotic smuggling involves the placement of drugs, commonly cocaine or heroin, in latex packages or condoms into body cavities or by swallowing, their retention being favoured by the use of constipating agents. In addition to the risk of obstruction (6 per cent), acute narcotic toxicity and death has occurred. The fatal oral dose of cocaine is 1 to 3 g; a single packet of cocaine contains 3 to 12 g, and carriers ingest many packets. The likelihood of ruptured packets and resultant mortality has decreased, however, as smugglers have grown more sophisticated, and immediate surgery is no longer mandatory. Mild cathartics may be used and patients may be discharged when proved free of packets by radiological and serial stool examinations. Older types of packets (containing loose cocaine covered by two to four layers of condoms or latex) are more prone to rupture. If this type of packaging can be identified by history or by recovery of packets from the rectum or stool, or if toxicity is present, surgical removal is indicated. Packets are frequently visible on plain films.

BEZOARS

Small intestinal obstruction due to bezoar is a common form of obturating obstruction, usually occurring as a late sequela of gastric surgery. Bezoars consisting of concretions of vegetable fibres (phytobezoar) reach the small bowel either directly through the pylorus or through a gastroenterostomy, or after fragmentation consequent upon attempted gastroscopic removal. Caution must be exercised at laparotomy not to overlook other bezoar fragments in addition to the one provoking the obstruction. Small bowel bezoars may also originate in duodenal or jejunal diverticula, as well as in Meckel's diverticulum. Trichobezoar may involve the small bowel by extension for a considerable distance distal to a large gastric hairball.

FOOD BOLUS OBSTRUCTION

Although not true foreign bodies, large boluses of certain foods may cause small intestinal obturating obstruction. These include masses of citrus fruit fibres, desiccated fruits, any high fibre food such as coarse bread at times of famine or following religious fasts, turtle eggs, and grasshoppers. Food bolus obstruction in non-temperate zones can often be managed without laparotomy, as the obstruction is usually partial. Additional factors that predispose to food bolus obstruction include prior gastric surgery and inadequate dentition. In cases of obstruction by food bolus or bezoar, postoperative education of patients to avoid binge eating, modification of fibre intake, and fitting of dentures may be useful in preventing recurrence. The operative management of obstruction by food bolus or by bezoar is similar, with attempts to squeeze the mass or fragment into the colon. When firmly impacted, an enterotomy may be needed.

GALLSTONES AND ENTEROLITHS

Enteroliths or intestinal calculi are presumed to form *de novo* in the bowel lumen. They consist of calcium or magnesium salts or, contain cholesterol and bile acids. They were, in earlier reports, considered to be common 'foreign bodies'. Their appearance is, however, rare, and a specific diagnosis preoperatively is rarer still. They may form in the stagnant milieu of duodenal or jejunal diverticula, in blind loops, and in areas of Crohn's disease or tuberculosis.

CONCRETIONS OF MEDICATIONS OR CHEMICALS

Small bowel obstruction may result from medications, including antacids and boluses of hydrophilic colloid laxatives, which absorb water and swell into a gelatinous mass. Antacid obstruction is seen particularly in patients undergoing haemodialysis. Concretions in the small bowel can also occur in those with more bizarre forms of ingestion, such as drinking alcoholic solutions of shellac, and cement powder used for producing mortar or concrete.

INTESTINAL PARASITES

Infestation by the round worm *Ascaris lumbricoides* accounts for 10 to 15 per cent of cases of intestinal obstruction in endemic tropical areas in Africa and Asia. Following appendicitis, ascariasis is the second most common cause of acute abdomen in children in those area. Massive ascariasis can cause low grade intestinal obstruction, which can often be managed conservatively with fluids, gastric drainage, and repeated doses of antihelmintics. However, acute complete obstruction may occur, sometimes following the use of a vermifuge. The dead or dying worms impacted in the terminal ileum and right colon are capable of causing tissue necrosis and perforation. In addition to the presenting symptoms of small bowel obstruction the masses of worms may be palpable or visible on plain films. Worms may be present in the vomitus or stool. Although intestinal obstruction may be due to obturation, volvulus, or intussusception, irritative intestinal spasm due to the worms may contribute. At surgery, if the obstructing bolus of worms cannot be advanced distally, resection may be necessary, particularly if local gangrene, volvulus, or intussusception has occurred.

FURTHER READING

Ashby BS, Hunter-Craig ID. Foreign-body perforations of the gut. *Br J Surg* 1967; **54**: 382–4.

Brown WM, Pearson PF, Smerdon GR, Burkitt R. Ingested foreign bodies in childhood. *Br Med J* 1971; **4**: 620–1.

Caruana DS, Weinbach B, Goerg D, Gardner LB. Cocaine-packet ingestion. *Ann Intern Med* 1984; **100**: 73–4.

Case records of the Massachusetts General Hospital. Case 12–1966. *N Engl J Med* 1966; **274**: 570–5.

David TJ, Ferguson AP. Management of children who have swallowed button batteries. *Arch Dis Child* 1986; **61**: 321–2.

Devanesan J, Pisani A, Sharma P, Kazarian KK, Mersheimer WL. Metallic foreign bodies in the stomach. *Arch Surg* 1977; **112**: 664–5.

Freed TA, Sweet, LS, Gauder PJ. Case reports: balloon obturation bowel obstruction: a hazard of drug smuggling. *A J R* 1976; **127**: 1033–4.

Hacker JF, III, Cattau EL, Jr. Management of gastrointestinal foreign bodies. *Am Fam Phys* 1986; **34**: 101–8.

James AH, Allen-Mersh TG. Recognition and management of patients who repeatedly swallow foreign bodes. *J R Soc Med* 1982; **75**: 107–10.

Lancashire MJ R, Legg PK, Lowe M, Davidson SW, Ellis BW. Surgical aspects of international drug smuggling. *Br Med J* 1988; **296**: 1035–7.

Louw JF. Abdominal complications of *Ascaris lumbricoides* infestation in children. *Br J Surg* 1966; **53**: 510–21.

Miller SF. Foreign body ingestions. *Am Fam Phys* 1975; **11**: 123–6.

Schwartz JT, Graham DY. Toothpick perforation of the intestines. *Ann Surg* 1977; **185**: 64–6.

Spitz L. Management of ingested foreign bodies in children. *Br Med J* 1971; **4**: 469–72.

Ward-McQuaid N. Intestinal obstruction due to food. *Br Med J* 1950; **1**: 1106–9.

16.11 Pneumatosis cystoides intestinalis

ANDREW MITCHELL

Pneumatosis cystoides intestinalis is an uncommon condition characterized by the presence of submucosal and/or subserosal gas-filled cysts in the intestinal wall. These cysts, which may reach several centimetres in diameter, contain largely nitrogen or hydrogen and occur in the small bowel more commonly than in the colon and rectum.

Pneumatosis cystoides intestinalis was first reported as a post-mortem observation by Du Vernoi in the eighteenth century. The condition is commonly asymptomatic and discovered incidentally at laparotomy or on radiological investigation of an unrelated symptom, but it can also produce abdominal pain, subacute intestinal obstruction, intussusception, or rectal bleeding. Its aetiology remains obscure. Favoured theories include the intramural penetration of gas-producing organisms, excessive intraluminal fermentation, and the forcing of gas under high pressure into the bowel wall, either from the lungs via the mediastinum and mesentery in patients with pulmonary disease, or from the intestinal lumen after surgery or biopsy has left a mucosal breach. Each of these theories is supported by clinical and experimental observations. The condition is well recognized in pigs and some other animals.

Pneumatosis cystoides intestinalis is most common in men between the ages of 30 and 50 years, and has an association with peptic ulceration and pyloric stenosis, intestinal bypass surgery for morbid obesity, and chronic lung disease. A plain abdominal radiograph may show a linear arrangement of gas collections, or pneumoperitoneum, without clinical signs of peritonitis. Contrast studies distinguish this condition from polyposis by demonstrating radiolucent defects in the bowel wall which extend outside the column of barium (Fig. 1).

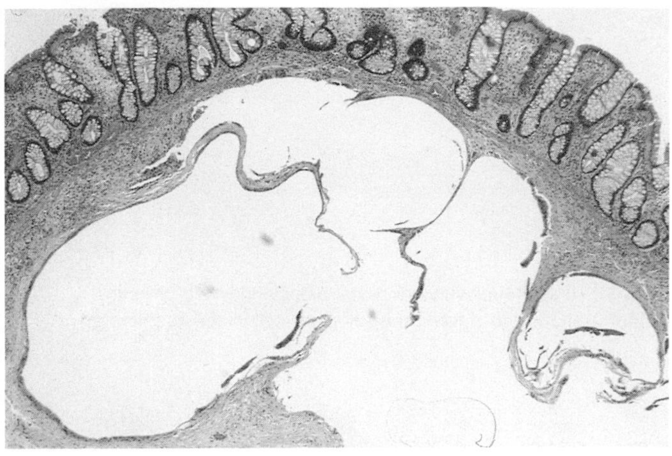

Fig. 2 Rectal biopsy showing normal mucosa with multiple cysts in the submucosa.

Accurate diagnosis prevents unnecessary surgery. The occasional familial occurrence of the condition increases the risk of confusion with familial polyposis coli and, therefore, of inappropriate colectomy. Biopsy should be performed, when the cyst will sometimes rupture with a hissing sound. Histology is diagnostic (Figs. 2 and 3).

No treatment is necessary for the 85 per cent of patients who are asymptomatic. Oxygen therapy has been used successfully for symptomatic patients and is thought to work by inducing the

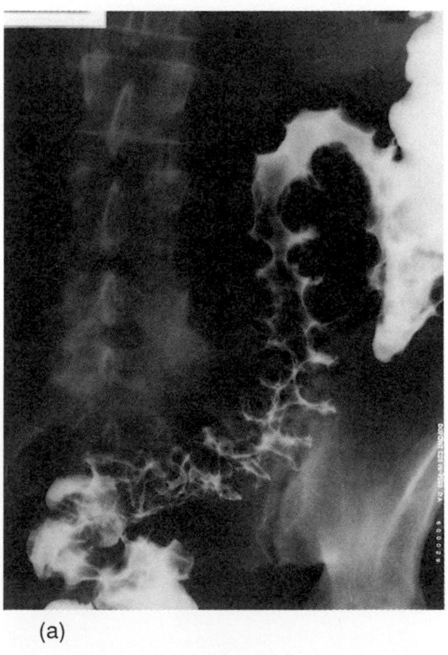

(a)

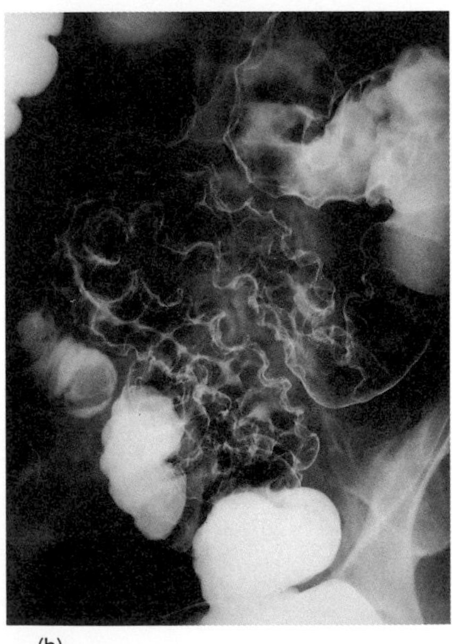

(b)

Fig. 1 (a and b) Barium enema appearances of pneumatosis coli.

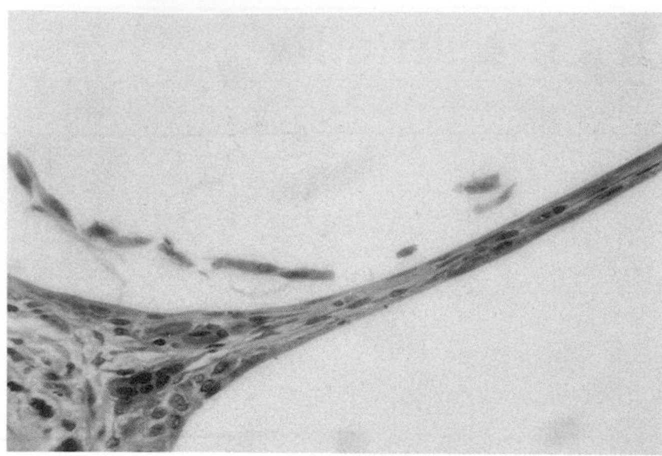

Fig. 3 High-power view of rectal biopsy showing chronic inflammation with a foreign body giant cell in the cyst lining.

exchange of inert gases from the cysts for oxygen, which is later absorbed. Good results have been reported after inhalation of 70 per cent oxygen, achieving a Po_2 of 250 mmHg for 5 days and after hyperbaric oxygen therapy at 2.5 atmospheres (252.5 kPa) for 150 min on each of 3 successive days. Dietary treatment has been successful in selected patients.

Intestinal resection should be reserved for patients with complications or severe refractory symptoms. The results of surgery in these cases are good.

FURTHER READING

Case WG, Hall R.Surgical treatment of pneumatosis coli. *Ann R Coll Surg Engl* 1985; **67**: 368–9.

Elberg JJ. Oxygen therapy for pneumatosis coli. *Acta Chir Scand* 1985; **151**: 399–400.

Galandiuk S, Fazio VW. Pneumatosis cystoides intestinalis. A review of the literature. *Dis Colon Rect* 1986; **29**: 358–63.

Spigelman AD, Williams CB, Ansell JK, Rutter KRP, Phillips RKS. Pneumatosis coli: a source of diagnostic confusion. *Br J Surg* 1990; **7**: 155.

van der Linden W, Marsell R. Pneumatosis cystoides coli associated with high H_2 excretion: treatment with an elemental diet. *Scand J Gastroenterol* 1979; **14**: 173–4.

Surgery for obesity 17

17 Surgery for obesity

RONALD A. MALT AND JOHN G. KRAL

Fat stores increase when energy intake exceeds energy utilization; they decrease when utilization exceeds intake. Although that is invariant physics, the reasons why some people form more fat cells or more efficiently fill their fat stores is more obscure. Irrespective of why a variation in fat storage occurs, excess storage is a disease with high comorbidity and wide prevalence in the industrialized world.

GENETICS

Seventy per cent of obesity may be hereditary. The genetic contribution to obesity is great enough to enable infants who burn energy sources efficiently at 3 weeks of age to be discriminated from those who do not and who will be overweight at 3 months of age. In a study of adopted Danish children the major correlate of body weight was the weight of biological parents. In Swedish children familial obesity and the degree of overweight in puberty were the best predictors of adult overweight and excess mortality. Southwestern American Indians (the Pimas) are genetically predisposed to converting ingested calories to fat and to have a genetic inability to generate heat after a meal or during exercise. Studies of twins and families in Canada have conclusively demonstrated that the capacity for thermogenesis is inherited.

DIET

Although a fat person seeking to lose weight is always fighting his genes, he is not unable to reduce his weight. Historically, the masses of people were thin: European peasants and artisans of the 18th century lived on the edge of starvation, eating bread and grains as their chief foods. Surprisingly few English and Scots ate cheese, milk, and eggs, even when these were available. In the 18th century, the average consumption of meat was about 240 g per year, chiefly on feast days, a notable exception in the 16th century being a cannibalistic family of Scottish brigands who subsisted on travellers to the point of hanging their flesh to cure.

Obesity in times past must have been more often a consequence of Falstaffian indulgence in alcohol than of overeating. Shakespeare recognized that the grave did 'gape thrice wider', for Falstaff 'than for ordinary men': an increased mortality rate for the grossly obese could naturally explain the leanness of the masses. Social stigmatization and ostracism, then as now, probably contributed to underestimation of the prevalence of obesity.

BODY IMAGE

When food became more easily available, Victorian *embonpoint* was the reaction. Curves were desired; angles were anathema. Today the main reason why 'overweight' people want to lose weight is to conform to the angular fashion of the time. Although women are more concerned with that goal than men, for both sexes appearance is a more important stimulus for regulating body weight than is the potentiation of cancer, cardiovascular disease, non-insulin dependent diabetes, renal disease, disorders of respiration and sleep, pseudotumor cerebri, joint disease, masking of intra-abdominal disease, and interference with the activities of daily living caused by obesity (Fig. 1). Indeed, 'life changes'—meaning stressful events initiating the search for a new start—often precipitate searching for a surgical treatment for obesity.

SOCIAL STIGMATA

Obesity inflicts handicaps other than disease and appearance. Obese men in Denmark have lower social standing, and, hence, lower income, than men of normal weight. As a determining variable, obesity is independent of parental social class, intelligence, and education: only 30 per cent of obese Danish men reach the social class of a semiskilled labourer or lorry driver, compared with 51 per cent of normal-weight controls. Several reasons for this situation have been proposed: a negative attitude of normal weight people toward the obese, of personal conflicts in the normal-weight people who would be fat in the absence of coercion to be thin, and the public's stereotype that fat people have lost control of themselves. Negative attitudes toward obesity, documented as early as kindergarten, continue into adult life.

IDEAL WEIGHT

Life insurance statistics unequivocally demonstrate increased mortality in those who are overweight as well as in those who are

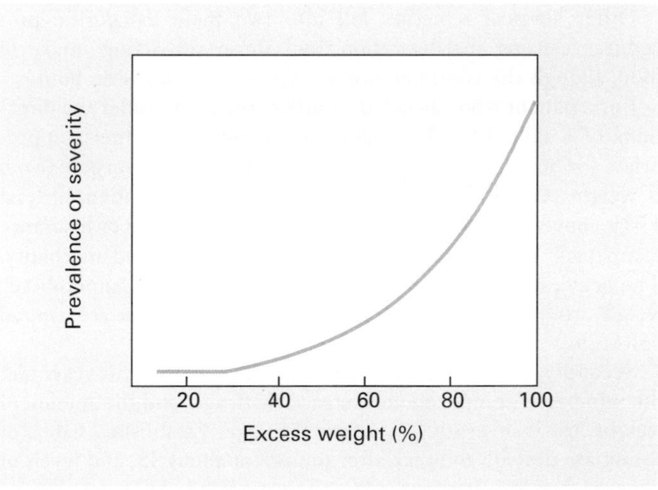

Fig. 1 Prevalence of morbidity and mortality and severity of disease increase exponentially as weight exceeds the desirable or 'ideal' level. At 60 per cent there is a threshold beyond which sudden death, diabetes, hypoventilation, heart failure, thromboembolism, and hypertension increase precipitously.

underweight. The criticism that such studies are flawed by being limited to people who can afford insurance has been amply met by large national population studies in Norway, the United Kingdom, and the United States. Obesity is an independent risk factor for cardiovascular disease, diabetes, respiratory insufficiency, some forms of cancer, stroke, and sudden death. The risks of comorbidity increase exponentially with increasing weight in all groups studied: young men aged 23 to 34 years who were twice or more ideal weight had a 12-fold increased incidence of death in a Veterans' Administration study in Los Angeles.

Data emerging during recent years demonstrate that the distribution of fat is of greater importance than is the magnitude of obesity. People whose deposits of fat are in the trunk or abdomen (android obesity) have greater morbidity and mortality rates than those with a more typically female distribution on the hips and buttocks. In fact, the distribution of adipose tissue, which is hereditary, is a determinant of dietary thermogenesis and resting energy requirements. Sex steroids and hepatic metabolism are strongly implicated in the morbidity associated with abdominal distribution of fat.

SURGERY

People become so desperate to look as they wish they did—or as others think they should—that they will resort to operations to lose weight or to lose specific areas of fat. This point is reached after lesser remedies have been exhausted, including, sometimes, supervised diets of 400 to 600 calories daily for many months in a hospital losing weight, only to regain and overshoot their former weight in a short period of time.

The logical surgical extension of the semistarvation approach is to keep the fat person's jaws closed with interdental wires to prevent eating. This method generally works, but only so long as the wires remain in place. Once the wires are removed, the rate of recidivism is over 90 per cent, as it is in every other form of self-controlled dietary programme or after use of intragastric balloons. As well as the potential problems of dental damage there is also non-compliance despite mandibular wiring: consumption of high calorie liquids is not impeded by dental fixation alone.

Other surgical remedies fall into two main categories: procedures causing malabsorption, and those restricting intake of food, though the common gastric bypass procedures do both.

For a patient who has failed all other treatment under the directions of a skilled family practitioner or internist, criteria appropriate for being accepted into a program of bariatric surgery (*baros* = weight [Greek]) are, firstly, morbid obesity—a patient at least 45 kg above the weight for height specified by charts of insurance companies, or the presence of severe obesity-related morbidity. The heaviest patients seeking surgical treatment, the 'superobese', weigh around 200 to 300 kg; typical mean weights are around 130 kg in women.

Secondly, patients should preferably be less than 50 years old: the number of complications increases with age, and the amount of weight lost is inversely proportional to age. Established habits of eating are difficult to break after the age of about 35, and levels of physical activity decrease. On the other hand, lack of sufficient maturity and understanding usually excludes patients in or below the early twenties.

Thirdly a normal psychological balance, and ability to cooperate and understand the importance of follow-up care is also important. Psychiatric consultation should be obtained when there is doubt. A history of psychiatric hospitalization, remarkably, is a predictor of medical complications of the surgery. Alcoholism is a contraindication. Fourthly, the patient must have a commitment to adhere to regular follow-up visits to his physician and surgeon, ideally for his lifetime. A surgical setting in which patients are part of a long-term investigative programme and in which surgeons perform at least two such operations a month is the ideal, as is a hospital with the multidisciplinary resources to manage the perioperative and postoperative needs of the morbidly obese.

Operative procedures

Operations that cause malabsorption or speed the passage of food, or both, are intestinal bypass and, to a certain extent, gastric bypass. Operations limiting the amount of solid food that can be ingested or passed through the upper intestinal tract are the various methods of stapling the stomach and of restricting the size of the gastric orifice through which food must pass before it can reach the small intestine. Gastric bypass does both.

However well these operations are performed, failures are inevitable. The walls of the stomach are smooth muscle; hence they expand with time; compensatory hypertrophy and hyperplasia of the intestine increase absorptive capacity technical failures of staple lines and stomal reinforcement occur and, probably most important, (mal)adaptive eating behaviour by the patient defeats the purpose of the operation. There is, therefore, less correlation between weight loss and the size of stomas and pouches than there might be if only laws of physics prevailed.

Obese patients are at increased risk of perioperative complications such as wound infections, herniae, pneumonia, and thromboembolism. Development of techniques for preventing these complications have appreciably reduced these risks in centres specializing in this type of surgery (Table 1), and these techniques are applicable to any operation on obese patients.

Table 1 Perioperative management of obese patients

A. Preoperative measures
   1. Stop smoking (for at least 6 weeks)
   2. Stop oral contraceptives (1 month) minimizing risk of pulmonary embolism
   3. Reduce sugars in diet
   4. Physical therapy, incentive spirometer
   5. Antibacterial showers
   6. Prophylactic antibiotics routinely—(e.g. 1–2 g cefazolin)

B. Intraoperative measures
   1. Antibiotics, paper drapes, irrigation
   2. Antithrombotic measures: heparin, stockings, intermittent compression, haemodilution
   3. Pulmonary precautions—reverse Trendelenburg position, empty the stomach, anaesthetist provides intermittent hyperinflation ('sigh'), immediate extubation
   4. Surgical technique—exposure (retractor system), avoid subcutaneous sutures

C. Postoperative procedures
   1. Early ambulation (within 4 h)
   2. Nasal oxygen
   3. Surveillance—central venous pressure to facilitate and assess fluid administration, blood gases, glucose monitoring to treat frequent hyperglycaemia
   4. Semirecumbent position

The processes listed above have variable effects, and similar patients given apparently identical operations can have disparate results. Long-term assessments can be difficult because patients tend to move away and to take up new lives, whether fat or not. Thus, for intelligent assessment and application of bariatric surgery, most of it should be done by surgeons committed to well-controlled trials of all the variables.

Types of bariatric operations

Small bowel resection

The original bariatric operations were inspired by observations of weight loss in patients with extensive resections for vascular compromise, inflammatory bowel disease, or cancer. Unwillingness to perform irreversible procedures for obesity led to abandonment and development of a host of bypass operations. The severe debility and hepatic dysfunction following jejunocolostomy, for example, quickly made this procedure obsolete.

Jejunoileal bypass (Fig. 2)

A short-bowel syndrome can be created by joining the end of about 35 cm of proximal jejunum either to the side of the distal ileum about 10 cm proximal to the ileocolic junction or to the end of the transected ileum, attaching the blind stump of bypassed intestine to the colon. Despite this prescription and adoption of other formulae of length and mode of bypass, none gives consistent results. Although almost every patient loses appreciable weight, and about 15 per cent reach ideal weight, the complications of hepatic dysfunction (presumably from nutritional cirrhosis, portal bacteraemia, or both); hypokalaemia, hypocalcaemia, and hypomagnesaemia; renal lithiasis from fat malabsorption, oxaluria, and dehydration; cholelithiasis; a peculiar form of enteroarthritis; pneumatosis intestinalis; and prevalent diarrhoea are considered to be too high a price to pay, though patients uniformly are more satisfied than physicians. Weight loss following these operations is probably most dependent upon aversive conditioning with concomitant decreased food intake—every episode of gorging being followed by diarrhoea, cramping, and flatulence.

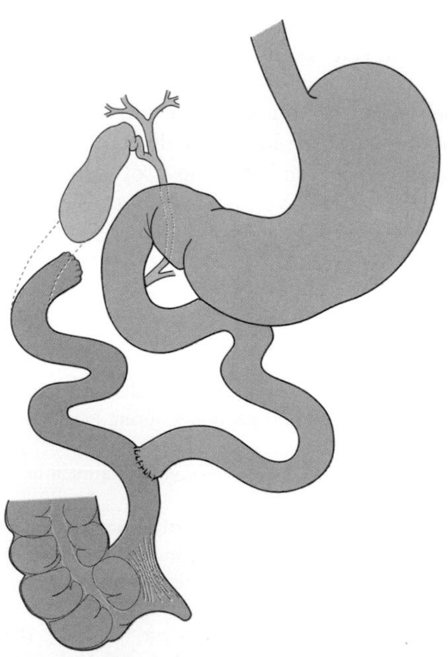

Fig. 2 End-side jejunoileostomy, attaching 35 cm of proximal jejunum to the terminal ileum, 10 cm before the ileocaecal valve.

With knowledge of management and prevention of complications and technical improvements, there is possibly still a minor role for jejunoileal bypass in selected patients: for example, a 300-kg patient who ideally requires a bariatric operation on the stomach might be brought to a more manageable weight for gastric surgery by preliminary jejunoileal bypass.

Biliopancreatic bypass (Fig. 3)

These operations have not been widely accepted. They aim at producing malabsorption by diverting the flow of bile or pancreatic juice, or both to a more distal site.

As originally developed, this operation consisted of resection of at least two-thirds of the stomach, emptying being provided by Roux-en-Y gastroileostomy. This short circuit bypasses half of the small intestine, which is drained into the distal ileum 50 cm before the ileocaecal valve. It is aimed at producing maldigestion and malabsorption; indeed, it predisposes to frank protein–calorie malnutrition unless it is meticulously managed. The biliopancreatic bypass has been modified by excluding most of the stomach without resecting it, as in gastric bypass (below). Biliopancreatic bypass procedures must be reserved for very highly selected patients in research centres.

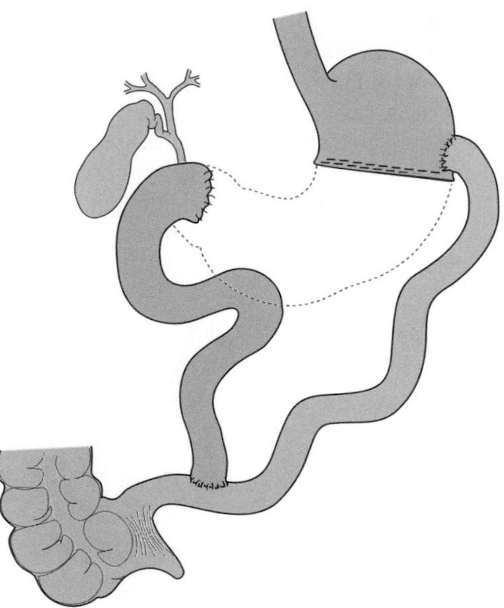

Fig. 3 Roux-en-Y gastric bypass with a 20-ml proximal stapled pouch drained via a 40-cm minimum efferent jejunal limb. In biliopancreatic diversion the limb is longer than 200 cm, as is the afferent limb which is attached 50 cm before the ileocaecal valve.

Gastric bypass (Fig. 3)

Using an upper midline incision, a small gastric pouch is created by firing a surgical stapling apparatus across the stomach, immediately below the oesophagogastric junction. The gastric pouch is drained by a Roux-en-Y gastrojejunostomy.

A large self-retaining retractor system fixed to the operating table provides exposure. A surgical stapler puts four parallel rows of staples across in a single firing of the device. Because there has to be a means of egress of food and secretions from the stomach, a Roux-en-Y limb of jejunum is joined to the pouch. Deficiencies of iron, calcium, thiamine, vitamin B_{12}, and of folic acid must be prevented after gastric bypass. Marginal (stomal) ulcers are rare complications.

Vertical banded gastroplasty (Fig. 4)

This operation aims to create both a small gastric pouch and an outlet that does not dilate. These goals are accomplished by placing four rows of staples parallel to the lesser curvature of the stomach, creating a gastric tube with a capacity of 15 ml or less. A 32 F Ewald orogastric tube passed by the anaesthetist serves as a template for creating the pouch. Banding of the outlet is done by stitching a 15-mm wide strip of polypropylene or nylon mesh to itself through a hole stapled through both stomach walls using an entero-entero-anastomotic type stapler (EEA®) with a diameter of 25 or 28 mm. In the latest modification of the vertical banded gastroplasty, the length of the strip is 4.75 cm. A 4.5-cm circumference adds complications, but does not produce superior weight loss.

The Silastic® ring vertical gastroplasty is an improvement over the vertical banded gastroplasty. It avoids the creation of a stapled hole through the stomach, which has occasionally been the site of fatal postoperative leaks. A nylon suture passed through a silicone tube is stitched through both walls of the stomach adjacent to the lowest portion of the vertical staple line. Because of the risk of erosion of the foreign material in the band or ring into the stomach, we band the outlet with strips of linea alba fascia harvested before entering the peritoneal cavity.

Staple-line disruption, the other technical complication of the procedure, has been vastly diminished since the introduction of broad, four-row staplers. The most serious complications are perforations of the oesophagus and stomach, either from lacerations during freeing of the oesophagogastric junction or from perforations or leaks caused by the stapling. Mortality rates are generally below 1 per cent in centres specializing in this type of surgery.

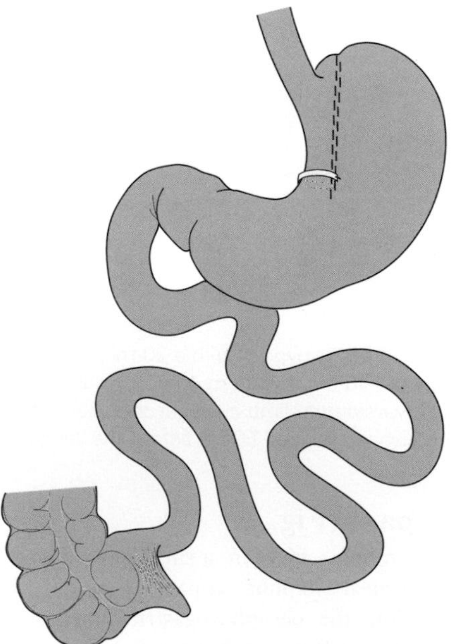

Fig. 4 Vertical gastroplasty with a 45–50 mm external band to limit the internal diameter of the egress from the 20-ml pouch to 9–12 mm.

Failure of weight loss after gastric surgery for obesity is troubling. Patients who eat sweets habitually lose less weight after gastroplasty than after gastric bypass (55 per cent versus 70 per cent of excess weight). Presumably the aversive conditioning from the dumping syndrome after gastric bypass helps reduce intake of calorically dense sweet liquids. Comparisons between purely gastric restrictive operations and gastric bypass have consistently revealed greater weight loss with gastric bypass. The bypass operations take longer, entail more perioperative complications, and cause more long-term deficiencies. Reoperations for failure of weight loss after gastric restriction are hazardous. The 40 to 50 per cent of gastroplasty patients who fail to lose weight over the long term and who require reoperation should have an operation with a component of malabsorption, such as gastric bypass or even an intestinal bypass.

Ancillary procedures

The gallbladder is often removed during any bariatric operation because of the risk of developing cholecystitis or forming stones during weight loss. Treatment with ursodeoxycholic acid can prevent gallstones from forming during weight loss. The gastric restrictive procedures in themselves, as well as the weight loss they achieve, are effective against gastro-oesophageal reflux disease in hiatus hernia. Some surgeons remove a fibroid uterus, or one that is otherwise abnormal or perform tubal ligation, or do both, at the time of bariatric surgery. Patients with a large panniculus adiposus ('apron') can benefit from lipectomy and abdominoplasty at the time of their bariatric procedure. Many patients require reduction of redundant skin and adipose tissue after weight loss.

Results of antiobesity surgery

The goal of bariatric surgery, to reduce weight, is fulfilled at least temporarily in the majority of patients. Around 30 per cent of preoperative body weight is lost during the first 1 to 2 years after most types of procedures. Long-term maintenance, however, is elusive, as many patients disappear from follow-up examination.

From a medical standpoint, however, the surgery is a resounding success. Not only is it vastly superior to diet, exercise, drugs, hypnosis, behaviour modification, or any non-operative treatment, but it dramatically improves diabetes, hypertension, respiratory insufficiency, and the host of comorbid conditions associated with obesity. Well-controlled studies are needed to determine the effects on longevity. Patients attest to the fact that quality of life is better.

FURTHER READING

Broomfield PH, *et al.* Effects of ursodeoxycholic acid and aspirin on the formation of lithogenic bile and gallstones during loss of weight. *N Engl J Med* 1989; **319**: 1567–78.

Carey LC, Martin EW, Mojzisik C. The surgical treatment of morbid obesity. *Curr Probl Surg* 1984; 78

Eckhout GV, Willbanks OL, Moore JT. Vertical-ring gastroplasty for morbid obesity. Five year experience with 1463 patients. *Am J Surg* 1986; **152**: 713.

Hall JC, *et al.* Gastric surgery for morbid obesity. *Ann Surg* 1990; **211**: 419–27.

Harrison GG. Height-weight tables. *Ann Intern Med* 1985; **103**: 989–94.

Hirsch J, Leibel RL. New light on obesity. *N Engl J Med* 1988; **318**: 509–10.

Ismail T, Kirby RM, Crowson MC, Baddeley RM. Vertical silastic ring gastroplasty: a 6-year experience. *Br J Surg* 1990; **77**: 80–2.

Knapp VJ. Major dietary changes in nineteenth-century Europe. *Persp Biol Med* 1988; **31**: 188–93.

Kral JG. Morbid obesity and related health risks. *Ann Intern Med* 1985; **103**: 1043–7.

Kral JG. Surgical treatment of obesity. *Med Clin N Am* 1989; **73**: 251–64.

MacLean LD, Rhode BM, Forse RA. Late results of vertical banded gastroplasty for morbid and superobesity. *Surgery* 1990; **107**: 20–7.

Mason EE. Morbid obesity: Use of vertical banded gastroplasty. *Surg Clin N Am* 1987; **67**: 521–37.

Mossberg H-O. 40-year follow-up of overweight children. *Lancet* 1989; **ii**: 491–493.

Naslund I. The size of the gastric outlet and the outcome of surgery for obesity. *Acta Chir Scand* 1986; **152**: 205–10.

Pasulka PS, *et al.* The risks of surgery in obese patients. *Ann Intern Med* 1986; **104**: 540.

Roberts SB, Savage J, Coward WA, Chew B, Lucas A. Energy expenditure and intake in infants born to lean and overweight mothers. *N Engl J Med* 1988; **318**: 461–6.

Sonne-Holm S, Sørensen TIA. Prospective attainment of social class of severely obese subjects in relation to parental social class, intelligence, and education. *Br Med J* 1986; **292**: 586–9.

Stricker EM, Verbalis JG. Control of appetite and satiety: insights from biological and behavioral studies. *Nutr Rev* 1990; **48**: 49–56.

Stunkard AJ, *et al.* An adoption study of human obesity. *N Engl J Med* 1986; **314**: 193–8.

Sugerman HJ, *et al.* Weight loss with vertical banded gastroplasty and Roux-Y gastric bypass for morbid obesity with selective versus random assignment. *Am J Surg* 1989; **157**: 93–102.

Vasudeva R, Holt S, Taylor TV. Obesity: medical and surgical management. *Curr Opin Gastroenterol* 1989; **5**: 865–9.

Weststrate JA, *et al.* Resting energy expenditure in women: Impact of obesity and body-fat distribution. *Metabolism* 1990; **39**: 11–17.

Colon and rectum 18

18.1 Diverticular disease: diverticulitis, bleeding, and fistula

GRANT V. RODKEY

DEFINITION

Diverticula of the intestinal tract are pockets or protrusions deriving from the lumen and extending through the wall of the gut. Diverticula that are enclosed by all layers of the bowel (serosa, muscle, and mucosa) are called 'true'; those that lack muscle as a component of the sac are termed 'false'. True diverticula are usually congenital, while false diverticula are acquired and usually secondary to pulsion forces within the gut. Diverticula may arise in both the small and large bowel, but this discussion will be limited to colonic diverticula.

Diverticula of the colon are generally multiple and, in the absence of inflammation, are collectively described as 'diverticulosis'. In the presence of inflammation, the condition is termed 'diverticulitis'. While this distinction is clear when the colon is examined surgically or histologically, symptoms of colonic dysfunction due to diverticulosis sometimes mimic those of diverticulitis. Thus, clinical distinction between the two conditions is often blurred. The term 'diverticular disease of the colon' may be applied to all stages of the disease from diverticulosis and its complications.

HISTORY

Diverticular disease of the colon has been recognized relatively recently and understanding of its manifestations has been dependent upon the twentieth century development of diagnostic radiology. Cruveilhier in 1849 described the gross anatomical findings in colonic diverticulosis, as did Habershon in 1857. Ball discussed the gross pathology of intermittent inflammation of diverticula and ascribed two cases of sigmoidovesical fistula to this cause. Graser identified oedema, fibrosis, thickening of the bowel wall and narrowing of the bowel lumen associated with inflamed diverticula that he called 'peridiverticulitis'. Beer analysed 15 cases of diverticulitis and described associated stenosis of the sigmoid, free perforation with peritonitis, localized peritonitis with abscess formation, and sigmoidovesical fistulae. Mayo and associates reported a series of five patients who underwent resection of the colon for complications of diverticulitis; they recommended that the inflamed bowel should be resected before complications occur. They established external drainage for abscesses, constructed 'artificial anus' (colostomy) for obstruction and defined the terms 'diverticulitis' and 'peridiverticulitis'.

In 1910 Keith contributed the important observation that the primary change in diverticular disease appears to be thickening and foreshortening of the muscular layers of the gut. Contrast meals or enemas were used for radiographic demonstration of colonic diverticula by Abbe, deQuervain, Case, and Spriggs and Marxer. Case and deQuervain independently used the term 'diverticulosis' to denote diverticula without evidence of inflammation. Smithwick introduced modern concepts of surgical treatment of diverticular disease.

PATHOPHYSIOLOGY

The pathophysiology of diverticular disease is complex, involving abnormalities of anatomy and neuromuscular function, physical principles of pressure relationships within cylinders and spheres, the virulence of mixed bacterial flora of the colon, and inflammatory processes within the peritoneal cavity and in the retroperitoneal space.

Colonic muscular changes in diverticular disease first noted by Keith were further studied by Celio, Edwards, Morson, and Hughes. Thickening and foreshortening of the taeniae occur, as well as foreshortening and clustering of the circular muscle fibres with relatively weak areas in the intertineal regions and between fascicles or bands of circular fibres. Diverticula tend to extrude through these weak areas, and as Noer pointed out, these may be intimately associated with mesenteric vessels perforating through to the submucosal layers of the bowel and with the epiploic appendages.

The nature of the colonic muscular changes in diverticular disease is poorly defined. One suggested explanation has been that the bowel muscle develops work hypertrophy secondary to abnormal neuromuscular irritability. The sigmoid is the narrowest portion of the colon and functions as a partial sphincter. Its motor activity is increased by a variety of stimuli including emotional and psychological tensions, ingestion of food, cholinergic drugs, morphine, and the absence of mechanical distension. Its muscular contraction is inhibited by anticholinergic drugs and by mechanical distension. Physiological studies by Painter and his associates and by Arfwidsson and Koch have demonstrated increased irritability of the sigmoid in patients with diverticular disease, compared to normal controls. This same pattern of increased motor activity was observed by Lumsden and associates in patients with the irritable colon syndrome (Fig. 1).

As the most irritable and narrowest segment of the colon, the sigmoid develops the highest intraluminal pressure per unit of muscular wall tension (Laplace's Law). Painter and Truelove have shown that patients with diverticular disease develop sigmoid globular segmentation and intraluminal pressures of 90 mmHg in response to emotional stress and also in response to the injection of morphine. These observed patterns of increased motor activity and intraluminal pressure in the sigmoid correlate well with the observed distribution of diverticula, which usually occur first in the sigmoid and propagate proximally over a period of years. Diverticulosis of the colon is accompanied by disease in the sigmoid in approximately 95 per cent of patients.

Histological and histochemical studies of the intrinsic nerves and muscle layers of the bowel in diverticular disease have not confirmed abnormal neural architecture, muscle hyperplasia, or muscle hypertrophy. Light and electron microscopy show normal muscle cells in colonic diverticular disease, neither hypertrophy nor hyperplasia being detected. These studies identified an increase in elastin content in the taeniae coli to more than 200 per cent of the level seen in normal controls. The elastin content in

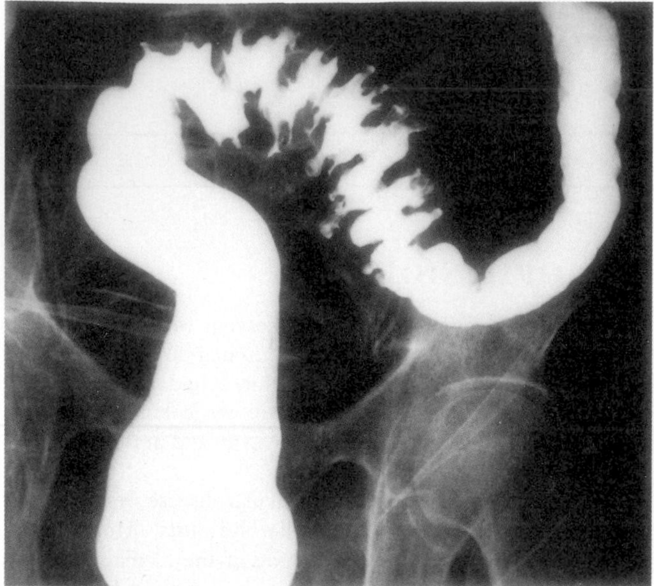

Fig. 1 Barium enema showing diverticulosis localized to the sigmoid.

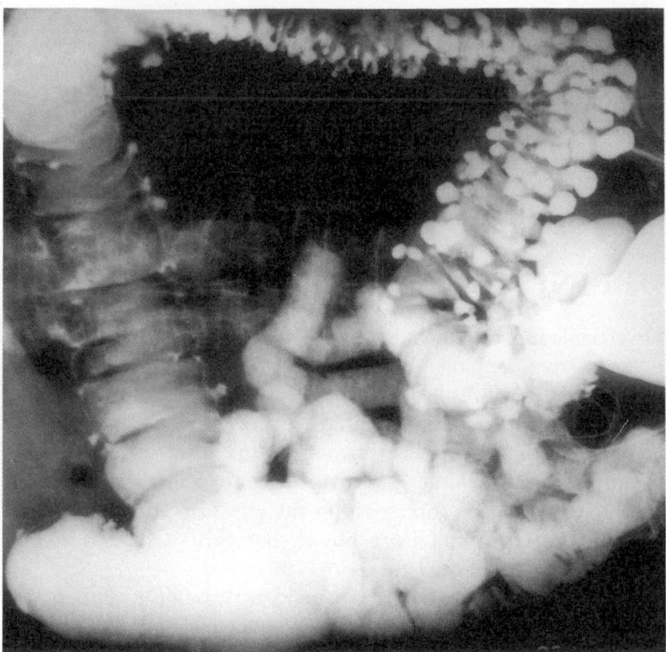

Fig. 2 Diffuse diverticulosis of the colon.

circular muscle was not appreciably different in diseased and normal bowel. It has been suggested that this elastosis is the basis for the foreshortening of the taeniae observed in diverticular disease.

Stimulated by the observation that some patients with diverticular disease have diffuse colonic disease with relatively less muscular abnormality in the sigmoid, Ryan has suggested that there may be a variant form of diverticular disease related to a diffuse connective tissue disorder distinct from the muscular abnormality of the sigmoid. There has been no histological confirmation of this theory, but the clinical pattern described requires further study (Fig. 2).

The physical principles of pressure–tension relationships within the tubular colon or its globular segments also play an important role in the development and progression of diverticular disease. Laplace defined these relationships as follows:

$$T = PR \text{ (or } P = T/R\text{)}$$

where T is tension in the gut wall, P is intraluminal pressure, and R is radius of the cylinder or sphere.

Thus in the sigmoid, where the lumen of the gut is small, muscular tension generates maximum pressures within the lumen of the bowel. These high pressures promote the extrusion of diverticula through weak areas in the gut wall: points of blood vessel penetration and the intermuscular spaces between circular smooth muscle fasicles in the inter-tineal intervals. Diets low in fibre do not distend the sigmoid and appear to promote these changes. Life-long low-residue diets in rats and rabbits produce diverticulosis of the colon, and broad-based population studies also seem to indicate a protective effect of high fibre diets on diverticular disease in man. Dietary factors may therefore play a significant role in the development and progression of diverticular disease of the colon.

The mixed and virulent bacterial flora of the colon may include *E. coli*, Pseudomonas, Serratia, Enterobacter, Citrobacter, Bacteroides, Enterococci, and Clostridia, most of which are facultative or obligate anaerobes. Depending upon the degree of extraluminal spread of these bacteria there may be localized inflammation with tissue necrosis, general peritonitis, or septicaemia with septic shock.

The propensity to develop diverticular disease is also partly inherited. Some families have a particularly high incidence of diverticula. Identical twins have been observed to develop diverticula at an early age and patients with multiple endocrine neoplasia syndrome type II B are prone to colonic diverticulitis. Oriental populations are more prone to right colonic diverticular disease, and diverticular disease of the colon occurs three times as frequently in Sweden as in neighbouring South Finland. The incidence of diverticular disease among young people (under age 40) may also be an expression of genetic predisposition to the condition.

INCIDENCE

The true incidence of colon diverticular disease is unknown and varies in different countries, depending upon factors such as genetic predisposition, diet, and age of the population. Among Western countries diverticular disease is uncommon before the age of 40; about 5 per cent of the population are estimated to have the disease by age 50 and approximately 70 per cent by age 85. Among those developing the disease before the age of 50 males predominate while above this age the majority of patients are female. However, there is a statistical bias since more females than males survive into the later decades of life.

In one large series, 94.6 per cent of cases of colonic diverticular disease were located in the sigmoid, while the descending colon was affected in 0.7 per cent; transverse colon, 1.0 per cent; ascending colon, 2.2 per cent; and caecum 1.5 per cent. In the same series, the age-specific incidence was 1.2 per cent in the third decade, 4.5 per cent in the fourth decade, 10.6 per cent in the fifth, 21.1 per cent in the sixth, 29.4 per cent in the seventh, 25.3 per cent in the eighth, 7.4 per cent in the ninth, 0.4 per cent in the tenth and 0.1 per cent in the eleventh decade of life among 688 cases requiring surgical treatment.

The apparently lower incidence of colonic diverticular disease in countries where high fibre diets are customary has already been mentioned. Among Oriental populations colonic diverticular disease is predominantly right-sided and the absolute frequency is lower than among western populations. However, among Orientals living in western countries the pattern of diverticular disease seems to shift more toward left-sided predominance.

CLINICAL FEATURES

The clinical manifestations of diverticular disease cover a broad spectrum. Many patients remain asymptomatic for long periods. The most frequent early symptoms are those of functional colonic disturbance—distension, cramps, diarrhoea or constipation, and local pain in the left lower abdomen. Concomitant bacterial inflammation (diverticulitis) may be associated with increased pain, left lower abdominal tenderness, palpable mass, fever, dysuria, urinary frequency and, occasionally, pneumaturia. General peritonitis and septicaemia signify more serious infection or perforation of a diverticulum. Rarely, the disease may present as septicaemia with pylephlebitis and gas in the portal venous system, or as a retroperitoneal infection dissecting upward to present as pneumomediastinum. More commonly, retroperitoneal infection tracks into the scrotum on either side, into the abdominal wall, the perineum, or into the left upper thigh. Attachment of small bowel loops to the inflammatory process in the colon may result in small bowel obstruction or development of a fistula into the small bowel. In females, diverticulitis may be associated with creation of fistulae into the fallopian tubes, uterus, or vagina, as well as into the urinary bladder (Figs. 3, 4).

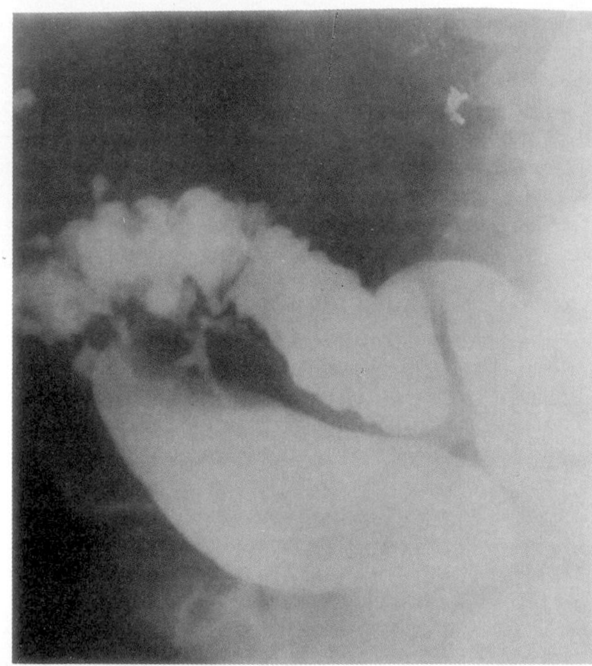

Fig. 4 Barium enema with diverticulitis of sigmoid and fistula into barium-filled urinary bladder, lateral view of pelvis.

Diverticular disease presenting as massive rectal haemorrhage is usually seen in patients who have diffuse diverticular disease throughout the colon (Figs. 5, 6). Rarely, diverticular disease may present with acute colon obstruction or with a tender, palpable mass due to a giant diverticulum of the sigmoid.

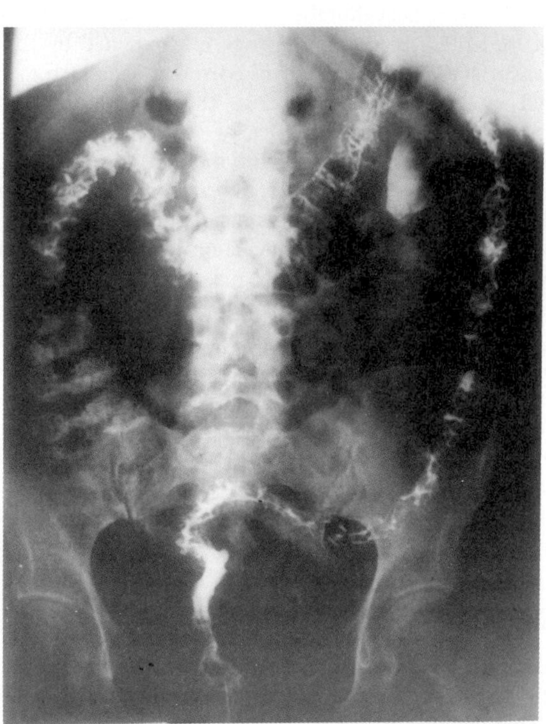

Fig. 3 Barium enema showing perforated diverticulitis of descending colon with retroperitoneal abscess.

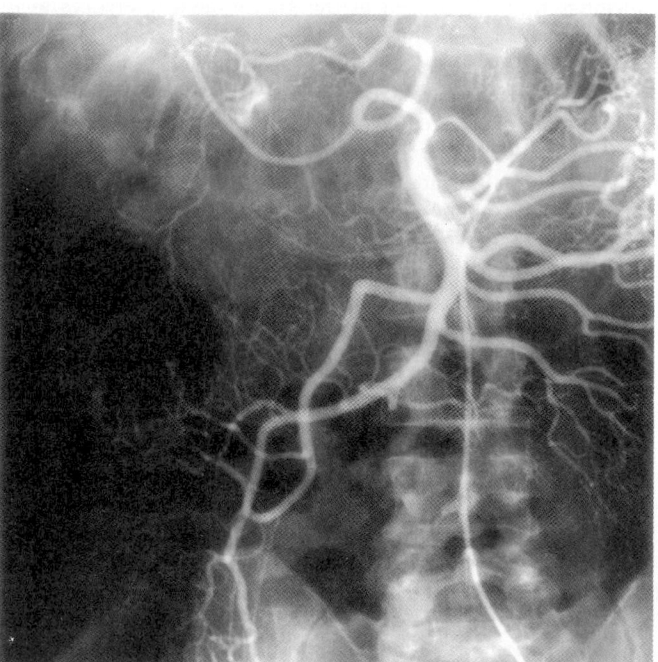

Fig. 5 Superior mesenteric angiogram showing extravasation of contrast medium into a diverticulum of right transverse colon.

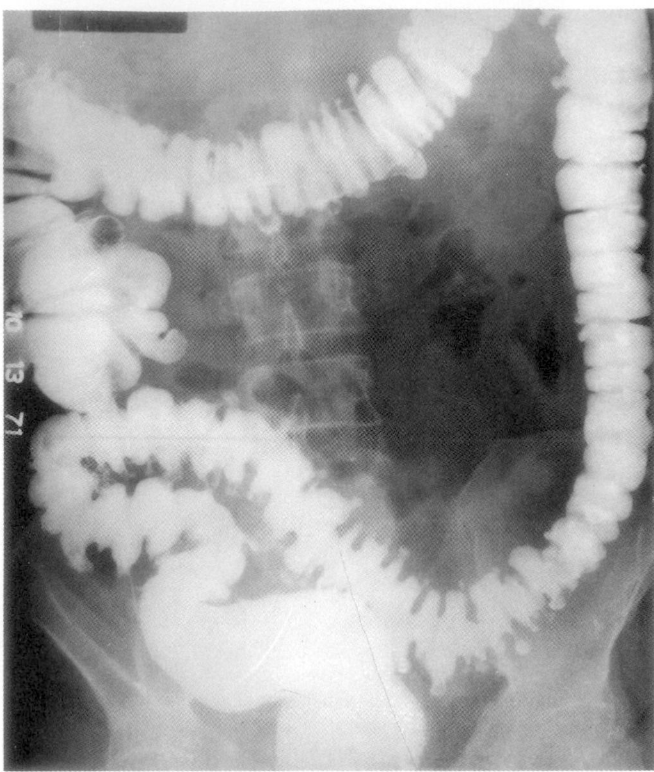

Fig. 6 Same patient as in Fig. 5, barium enema showing diffuse colonic diverticulosis.

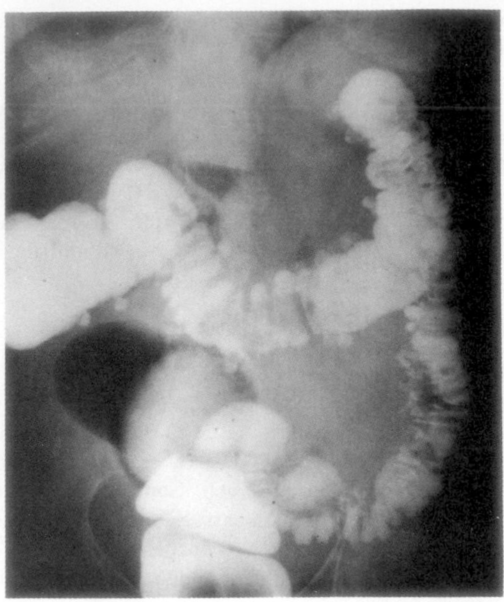

Fig. 7 Barium enema showing a giant diverticulum projecting upward and to the right from the sigmoid colon.

DIVERTICULOSIS AND DIVERTICULITIS

Diverticulosis is the presence of non-inflamed diverticula, or outpouchings from the lumen of the gut through interstices in its muscular wall, which consist of mucosa, attenuated submucosa, sparse muscular fibres, and serosal covering. Initially, these diverticula are microscopic in size but continued rhythmic peaks of intraluminal pressure due to peristaltic contractions cause them to enlarge slowly, until they become globular nodules projecting from the external surface of the bowel. These globules are usually not larger than about 1 cm in diameter, but they may become larger. Diverticula of 3 cm or more in size are called 'giant diverticula'; these gas-filled protuberances have been recorded with a diameter of 35 cm (Fig. 7). The globular diverticula communicate with the bowel lumen by a very narrow neck, through which gas usually can pass freely; a valve-like mechanism may contribute to the formation of giant diverticula. Diverticula frequently fill with faecal material extruded from the lumen that may then become inspissated and firm. This process usually begins in the sigmoid and spreads proximally over the course of several years.

Infection and inflammation of individual diverticula is called 'diverticulitis'. The incidence of such inflammation among patients with diverticulosis has been estimated at 15 to 25 per cent, but is not accurately known.

Factors that initiate diverticulitis are speculative. Pressure necrosis or erosion from inspissated faeces in the diverticulum has been implicated as a causative mechanism. Transmitted pressure from peristaltic contraction may cause ballooning of the diverticulum and subsequent microscopic or macroscopic rupture. Inflammation generally occurs first at the apex of the diverticulum, which is the area of poorest circulatory perfusion and is often (or perhaps always) associated with micro- or macroperforation. Gross perforation results in immediate general faecal contamination of the peritoneum. More frequently, the perforation is contained by tissues in the wall of the colon or its mesentery or is buttressed by inflammatory adhesions to the abdominal or pelvic wall or adjacent viscera; a localized abscess then forms. This may rupture back into the lumen of the colon, track along the wall or mesentery of the bowel, may be contained by the pelvic visceral surfaces or adherent small bowel loops, attach to the abdominal wall, or may dissect into the retroperitoneal tissues (Fig. 3). The abscess may resolve by local healing, persist as a localized collection, rupture free into the peritoneal cavity, or may dissect through tissue planes to drain externally by fistulization to bowel, genitourinary tract, abdominal wall, or perineum.

The mixed bacterial flora of the colon causes severe inflammation with extensive tissue necrosis and very dense scar formation on healing. Repeated bouts of localized diverticulitis may thus result in ligneous inflammatory swelling and scarring of the sigmoid and its mesentery with foreshortening and partial chronic obstruction of the bowel diminishing the efficiency of its peristaltic activity. In addition, shortening of the muscular wall of the sigmoid throws the mucosa into ridges of redundant folds that further inhibit effective stool transit. The symptomatic manifestations of diverticulitis are diverse and complex and, on clinical grounds, not always distinguishable from those of diverticulosis.

COMPLICATIONS

The complications of diverticular disease include sepsis, fistula (usually as a result of healed sepsis), bleeding, obstruction, and intractable painful disturbance of bowel function.

Septic complications of diverticular disease include localized inflammation within the bowel wall or mesentery, localized pelvic abscess, perforation with diffuse bacterial and/or feculent peritonitis, adherence to adjacent visceral or peritoneal surfaces, septicaemia, and septic shock. Sepsis is the indication for surgery in approximately 35 per cent of patients requiring operative treatment of colonic diverticular disease.

Fistulae form as the result of spontaneous drainage of an abscess into an adjacent viscus or to the external surface of the body. A channel communicating with the lumen of the bowel is thus created. Because of inflammation and continuing faecal contamination, fistulae rarely heal spontaneously; about 5 per cent of all operations required for diverticular disease involve treatment of fistulae.

Bleeding is intermittent and slight in approximately 10 per cent of patients with diverticular disease: this must be distinguished from bleeding caused by adenocarcinoma of the colon. Acute, massive haemorrhage from diverticular disease is of greater significance: this is not due to diverticulitis, and generally occurs in individuals with diffuse diverticulosis affecting the colon. Erosion of a small blood vessel by inspissated faeces in the diverticulum has been suggested as a cause for massive haemorrhage. An alternative mechanism may be traction and tearing of the relatively inelastic vessels when the diverticulum stretches during peristaltic contraction. Massive bleeding is the indication for surgery in approximately 10 per cent of patients requiring operative treatment of diverticular disease.

Colon obstruction secondary to diverticular disease may be partial and chronic or complete and acute. The acute presentation may be accompanied by concurrent small bowel obstruction, and should always be suspected. Operations for obstruction are somewhat less frequent than those required for massive bleeding, about 9 per cent of cases.

Patients with intractable disturbance of bowel function (distension, cramps, diarrhoea, or constipation) and persistent pain may require surgical treatment even in the absence of the more defined complications listed above. These patients require careful clinical evaluation and judgment, and comprise about 25 per cent of those undergoing surgery for diverticular disease.

ASSOCIATED PATHOLOGY AND MORBIDITY

Diverticular disease occurs predominantly in elderly patients who have associated diseases that complicate diagnosis and influence treatment. Adenocarcinoma and polyps of the colon may coexist with diverticular disease, although a causal relationship is not recognized. Chronic ulcerative colitis or regional enterocolitis (Crohn's disease) may also occasionally affect patients with colonic diverticular disease.

Ischaemic colitis due to segmental arterial inflow restriction leading to mucosal necrosis without infarction of the muscular layers may cause pain, diarrhoea, and rectal bleeding. These changes may be confused with or may coexist with diverticular disease. Angiodysplasia, abnormal arteriovenous shunts in the colonic submucosa, especially in the right colon, may cause massive haemorrhage that must be differentiated from haemorrhage due to diverticulosis. Many patients who have colonic angiodysplasia also have diverticulosis.

Many medical diseases of the elderly weaken the immune response, predisposing patients with diverticulitis to its septic complications. These conditions include obesity, diabetes, chronic corticosteroid therapy, chronic alcoholism, asplenism, radiation therapy, cancer chemotherapy, prosthetic implants, post-transplantation immunosuppression, and AIDS. These conditions make prompt, accurate diagnosis and effective treatment of diverticular disease even more critical.

DIAGNOSIS

The symptoms of colon diverticular disease are diverse, and depend upon the stage of the disease. Diverticulosis may cause abdominal distension, cramps, constipation, diarrhoea, lower abdominal pain, and, rarely, massive rectal bleeding. Diverticulitis may present any or all of the above symptoms with the exception of massive rectal bleeding. Abdominal pain may be increased and fever, nausea, vomiting, dysuria, urinary frequency, pneumaturia, and external faecal fistulae may be noted. Patients with complications of diverticulitis may have chills, high fever, generalized abdominal pain, and septic shock. Symptoms may be suppressed in patients receiving chronic steroid therapy, causing significant delay in diagnosis.

Physical signs of colon diverticular disease vary according to the stage. Abdominal distension, tenderness, a palpable and tender lower abdominal mass, and normal peristaltic sounds are often observed. Fever may or may not be present. Patients with diffuse peritonitis may have diffuse abdominal tenderness, spasm, and rebound tenderness, and they are usually febrile. Rectal examination may reveal high rectal tenderness or a mass; it may also be normal.

Diagnosis may be aided by faecal occult blood test, urinalysis, leucocyte count, haematocrit, and liver function tests. If all of these tests yield normal results, however, the diagnosis of colon diverticular disease is not excluded. Patients with right-sided colon diverticulitis may have symptoms, signs, and laboratory findings indistinguishable from those of acute appendicitis.

Endoscopy has limited value in the diagnosis of acute diverticulitis, although rigid sigmoidoscopy may identify tenderness and fixation at the rectosigmoid junction. Colonoscopy is useful in identifying associated colitis, polyps, or adenocarcinoma, but spasm of the sigmoid may limit the effectiveness of the examination. Patients suffering from massive haemorrhage are not suitable candidates for colonoscopic study.

Radiographic examination is the main diagnostic technique in colonic diverticular disease. In patients with chronic or subacute symptoms, a barium enema examination may confirm the presence of diverticula, provide evidence for or against the diagnosis of diverticulitis, and help to exclude the presence of adenocarcinoma or other associated disease of the bowel. If partial obstruction of the colon is found diverticular disease may usually be distinguished from adenocarcinoma by the greater length of affected tissue, intact mucosa, muscular spasm, taper rather than blunt ends to the narrowed segment, and the presence of diverticula in the former. Diagnosis may be confirmed by colonoscopic examination.

Suspected acute diverticulitis or its complications should be investigated initially with plain and upright abdominal films and chest radiographs. Colon and/or small bowel distension may indicate obstruction. Free gas in the peritoneal cavity, retroperitoneal tissues, bladder, or portal venous system is a sign of acute diverticulitis with perforation and is a clear indication for early surgical intervention. Plain films frequently yield no diagnostic clues, and performance of a barium enema carries the risk of perforation of an inflamed diverticulum or barium contamination of the peritoneal cavity if a perforation is present. Computed tomography of the abdomen following oral administration of contrast medium (Gastrografin 10 ml in 300 ml water hourly for 3 or 4 h prior to examination) has therefore become the most reliable examination for diagnosing diverticulitis of the colon. Diagnostic findings include visualization of diverticula, thickening of the bowel wall, thickening or 'stranding' fibrosis in the mesentery, thickening of adjacent viscera (bowel, bladder), and extraluminal mass, sinus tract, or abscess with fluid and/or gas (Figs. 8–12).

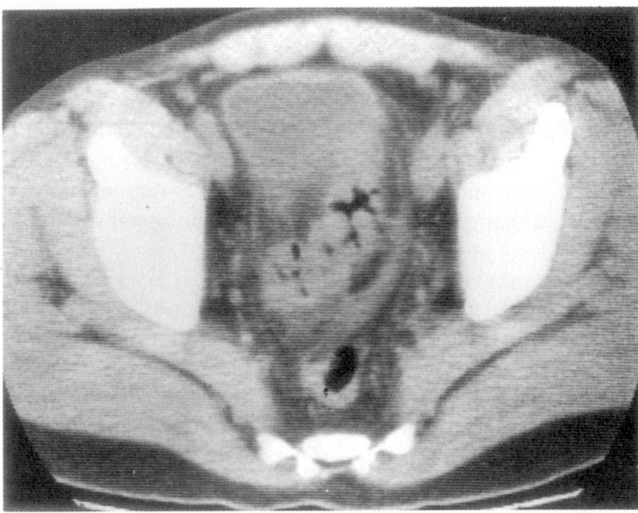

Fig. 8 Pelvic CT scan showing sigmoid diverticula, thickening of the bowel and mesentery, small amount of pelvic fluid and increased density in pelvic fat—all consistent with acute diverticulitis without abscess.

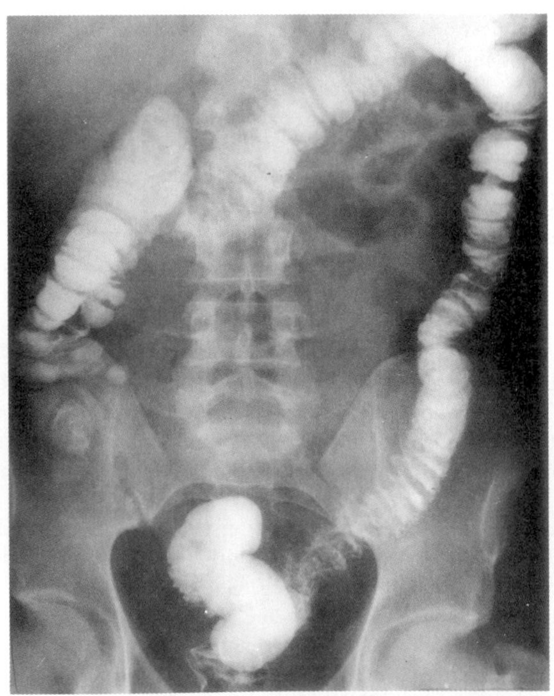

Fig. 9 Same patient as in Fig. 8, barium enema showing only early muscular changes of diverticular disease.

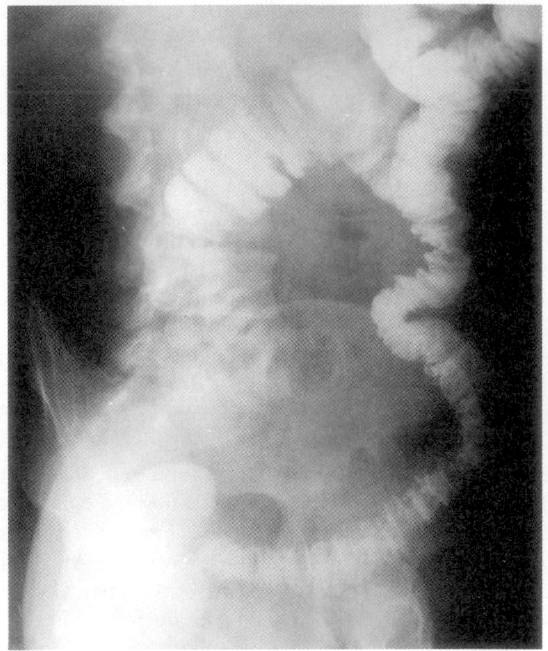

Fig. 10 Same patient as in Fig. 8, lateral view of pelvis.

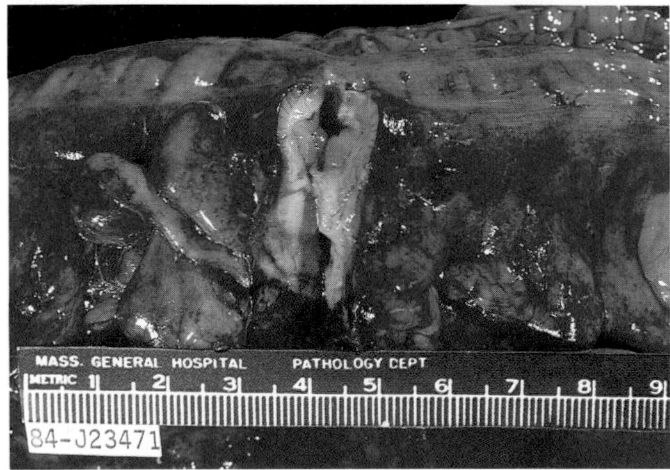

Fig. 11 Same patient as in Fig. 8, resected specimen showing acute diverticulitis with perforation and localized peritonitis.

Radiographic studies are important in locating the site of massive haemorrhage from the colon. Selective catheterization of superior and inferior mesenteric arteries and intra-arterial administration of contrast may disclose the site of haemorrhage, and whether this is due to diverticulosis, angiodysplasia, or other causes. Fully one-half of these bleeding points are located proximal to the splenic flexure. Intra-arterial infusion of vasopressin (0.2 U/min) will control 50 per cent of such haemorrhages and permits elective study and treatment. If haemorrhage is not controlled by vasopressin, the site of the bleeding may be identified prior to emergency resection of the appropriate bowel loop.

If fistulization to the genitourinary tract is suspected, diagnostic studies should include urine culture, intravenous pyelography, and cystoscopy.

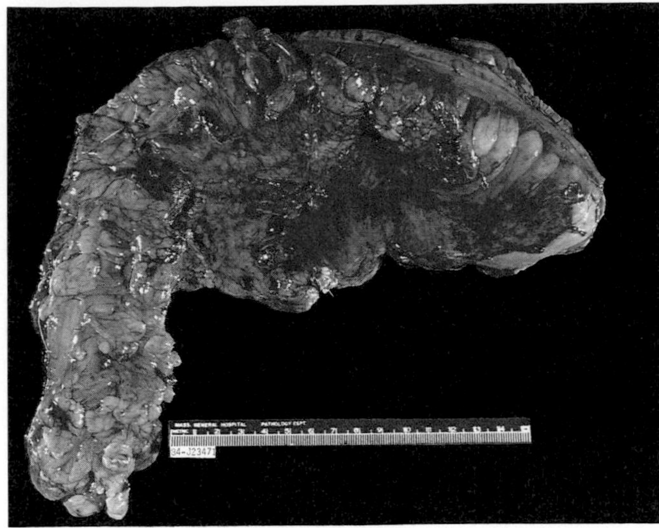

Fig. 12 Same specimen as in Fig. 11, incised to show site of perforation. Note thickening and fibrosis of pericolonic fat.

MANAGEMENT OF UNCOMPLICATED COLON DIVERTICULAR DISEASE

Uncomplicated diverticular disease can be managed by dietary manipulation, including provision of supplementary dietary fibre, stool softeners, and anticholinergic drugs to inhibit peristaltic cramps. High fibre intake results in a larger, softer stool which distends the colon and undergoes more rapid transit through the gut. The extra force is optimally provided by a diet rich in fruit, vegetables, and whole grain cereals, with generous water intake. Supplementary bulk may be supplied with 10 to 20 g of wheat bran daily. Softening and moisturization of the stool may be aided by ingestion of powdered psyllium seed husks (5–10 g daily). Drugs that may inhibit peristalsis (such as propantheline bromide 7.5–15 mg thrice daily) may give symptomatic relief. Morphine causes increased intracolonic pressure and should be avoided: if narcotic medication is required, meperidine hydrochloride (50–75 mg) may be used.

TREATMENT OF COMPLICATIONS OF COLON DIVERTICULAR DISEASE

The pathophysiology, symptoms, complications, and methods of diagnosis of diverticulitis and its sequelae have been discussed in preceding sections and diverticulitis itself will be regarded here as a complication of diverticular disease. The accurate diagnosis of complications such as sepsis (including fistula as a late manifestation), bleeding, obstruction, and intractable pain with functional bowel disturbance is essential to enable effective treatment. Many methods of treatment, both surgical and non-surgical, have been used in the past and have been found to be inadequate or have been replaced by more effective procedures. In this section emphasis will be given to treatments that are currently considered safest and most effective.

Septic complications

Patients with acute diverticulitis should be treated by restriction of oral intake and by intravenous administration of fluids and antibiotics with a broad spectrum of activity against enteric pathogens. A regimen including cefotetan, 1.0 g every 12 h and metronidazole, 250 mg every 6 h intravenously is appropriate; other combinations of appropriate antibiotics may be equally effective. Many patients treated in this manner will improve rapidly, with resolution of the signs of local inflammation and ileus within a few days. When the gut function is restored (as marked by passage of flatus or stool) it is safe to resume oral feeding and, usually, to switch to oral administration of metronidazole (250 mg every 6 h). Following resolution of the local inflammation, a barium enema examination should be performed to assess the disease more accurately. The patient should be placed on a high fibre diet. Such treatment is sufficient in approximately 65 per cent of patients admitted to hospital for acute diverticulitis; the remainder will require some kind of surgical intervention.

Patients who remain febrile and tender and exhibit evidence of systemic illness after 12 to 24 h of treatment as outlined above should be re-examined: fever, leucocytosis and abdominal or rectal tenderness or mass are highly suggestive of a pericolic or pelvic abscess. Ultrasonography or repeat CT scan are useful for confirmation (Fig. 13) but on clinical grounds, such a patient is a candidate for surgical exploration.

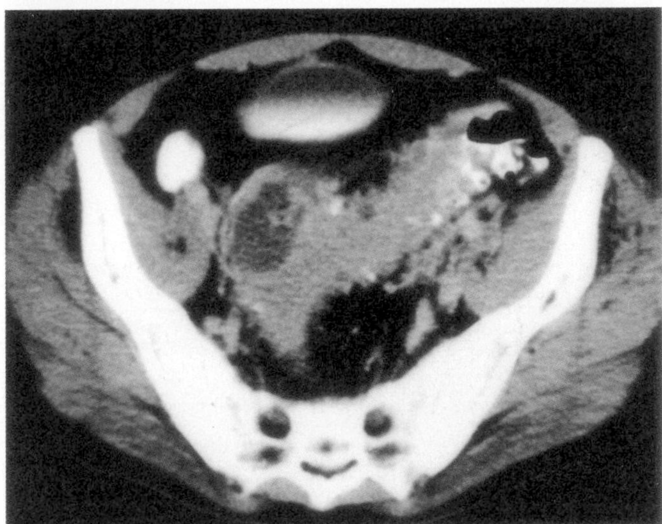

Fig. 13 CT scan showing sigmoid diverticulitis with pelvic abscess.

If the abscess is wholly contained within the bowel wall and mesentery and can be extirpated with a segmental resection, and if the (unprepared) bowel is relatively empty and free of inflammation, a one-stage resection and end-to-end anastomosis may be considered. Such patients are uncommon, and a safer course is to resect the inflamed segment of bowel, close the distal resected end (usually rectum), and pull the proximal resected end through the abdominal wall as a colostomy. Drains may or may not be left in the pelvis, depending on the clinical indications. Patients who are treated in this way are candidates for anastomosis after they have made a complete recovery—generally in 3 months.

An alternative treatment that may be considered when the facilities are available is initial CT-guided percutaneous drainage of the abscess, continued antibiotic treatment, and resection of the involved segment with primary end-to-end anastomosis 7 to 10 days later (Figs. 14, 15). If severe inflammation or residual abscess is found at this time the anastomosis should be abandoned in favour of resection, rectal turn-in, and colostomy. About 40 per cent of patients who require operations for diverticular disease have localized or pelvic abscesses. The expected mortality rate among such patients is approximately 2.5 per cent.

The most serious septic complication of diverticular disease is free perforation of the colon with bacterial or faecal peritonitis. The majority of patients presenting with this clinical picture have coexisting severe illnesses, and many are immunosuppressed. In addition to cefotetan and metronidazole these patients should receive an aminoglycoside such as gentamicin, 1 to 1.5 mg/kg intravenously every 8 h, and serum levels (peak 8–12 µg/ml, trough < 2 µg/ml) should be monitored daily until they are stable. Patients with general peritonitis must be closely monitored for respiratory, renal, and liver failure, septic shock, and for coagulopathy. Patients receiving chronic steroid therapy should be given increased supplementary doses (hydrocortisone, 300 mg/day) and intravenous fluids should be administered to assure adequate urine output (approximately 50 ml/h). As soon as the patient is haemodynamically stable resection of the perforated bowel segment, rectal turn-in and end-colostomy of the descending colon should be performed. All pus and debris should be irrigated from the peritoneal cavity. If there is gross contamination, delayed primary closure of skin and subcutaneous fascia decreases the risk of wound sepsis.

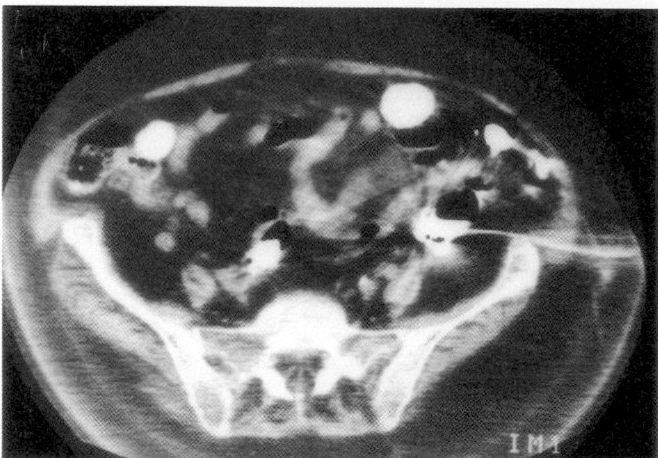

Fig. 14 CT scan showing drainage of pelvic abscess via percutaneous catheter.

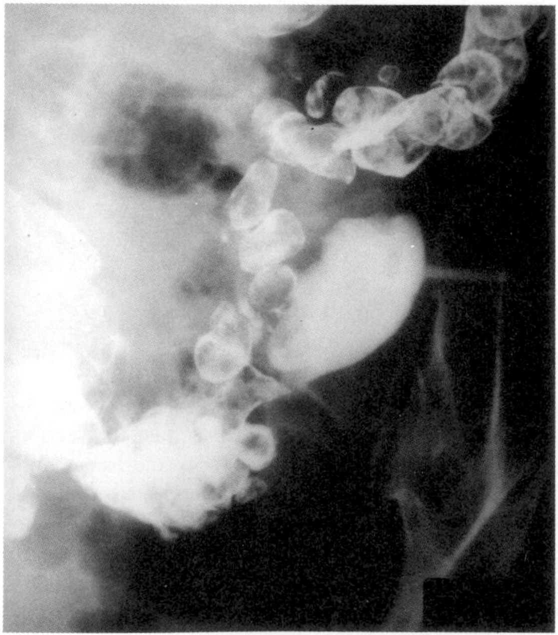

Fig. 15 Same case as in Fig. 14 with injected contrast medium filling the abscess cavity and entering the sigmoid lumen.

Postoperatively, these patients require intensive monitoring and support of all vital systems. However, removal of the septic focus usually results in prompt improvement as long as this has been treated soon after perforation. Delay is associated with increased morbidity and mortality. Patients with general peritonitis comprise about 10 per cent of those requiring operation for diverticular disease; their expected mortality is approximately 45 per cent.

Fistulae are late manifestations of septic complications of diverticular disease and represent the end-stage of spontaneous drainage of an abscess into adjacent viscera or to the skin surface. In descending order of frequency, fistulae may be colovesical, coloenteric, colovaginal, colocutaneous (abdominal wall), colouterine, colosalpingeal, colocolonic, coloureteral, or colocutaneous (perineum or thigh). Operations for fistula are elective and permit preliminary mechanical and antibiotic preparation of the colon. An effective regimen is the administration of 240 ml of magnesium citrate by mouth 2 days prior to and on the day before operation. On the day preceding surgery erythromycin base 1.0 g and neomycin 1.0 g are given by mouth at 12 noon, 1.00 p.m. and 9.00 p.m. An enema is given on the night before surgery.

Intravenous cefotetan and metronidazole are administered just prior to surgery, and these may be continued for 24 h or more postoperatively, depending upon the surgical findings. During the operation the degree of inflammation and scarring in the sigmoid and at the site of the fistula is assessed. A one-stage resection of the sigmoid colon, including the fistula and a segment of the fistulized organ (bladder, small bowel, etc.), with primary anastomosis of the colon and suture of the fistulized viscus, can be performed in about 25 per cent of patients. In the remainder, it will be safer to perform a loop colostomy in the right transverse colon, close the incision, and allow 3 months for the pelvic inflammation to subside. A second stage operation is then required to resect the sigmoid colon and the fistula and to create an anastomosis between the descending colon and the rectum. After another month a barium enema should be performed to assure the integrity of the anastomosis. Thereafter, the colostomy may be closed. Operations for fistula account for about 9 per cent of operations required for diverticular disease. The expected mortality rate in this group of patients is less than 1 per cent.

Massive colonic bleeding

Massive bleeding is the indication for approximately 9 per cent of operations for colon diverticular disease. Patients with this presentation often have diffuse diverticulosis and usually do not have associated diverticulitis with pain and tenderness as localizing markers. Confounding conditions such as angiodysplasia and ischaemic colitis may also obscure the diagnosis. Endoscopy is not generally helpful in such cases and it is better to proceed promptly with selective angiography of the superior and inferior mesenteric arteries. If bleeding continues at a rate of 0.5 ml/min the locus of bleeding can frequently be identified. With the arterial catheter in the feeding artery, infusion of vasopressin (0.2 U/min for 24–48 h) may control the haemorrhage. If the patient recovers and only diverticular disease is present, appropriate treatment is a high fibre diet, as for chronic diverticular disease; if bleeding is not controlled or recurs, surgical intervention is required.

When the bleeding site is identified, a segmental resection with end-to-end anastomosis is the operation of choice. If the site cannot be located, subtotal colectomy with ileorectal anastomosis should be performed as an emergency procedure. Since there is no time for preoperative preparation of the bowel, these patients should receive broad-spectrum antibiotics intravenously pre- and postoperatively, as well as appropriate blood replacement. The expected mortality rate in this group of patients is approximately 10 per cent.

Obstruction

Obstruction in colonic diverticular disease may be chronic, due to postinfection scarring as well as to muscular narrowing of the sigmoid. Acute obstruction is usually associated with active diverticulitis or associated abscess and may be accompanied by obstruction of adherent small bowel loops.

Patient with chronic obstruction generally tolerate preoperative mechanical and antibiotic preparation of the bowel and may undergo semi-elective surgery. One-stage resection and anastomosis under intravenous perioperative antibiotic cover may be performed in most of these patients.

Acute colonic obstruction is usually superimposed on acute diverticulitis and, as described, is frequently associated with abscess or small bowel adhesions. These seriously ill patients require nasogastric suction, broad-spectrum triple antibiotics, intravenous fluids, and prompt surgical intervention. The optimum operative procedure in these patients is lysis of the small bowel adhesions, drainage of abscesses, resection of the inflamed strictured segment, rectal turn-in, and end-descending colostomy. Bowel continuity should be restored at a second procedure after an interval of 3 months.

Colon obstruction is the indication for about 8 per cent of operations for diverticular disease, and the mortality rate is about 2 per cent. Acute obstruction occurs in one in eight of such patients.

Intractable colon dysfunction and pain

Many patients with colon diverticular disease have chronic lower abdominal pain, distension, cramps, and diarrhoea, or constipation, with the last two sometimes alternating. Barium enema will confirm the presence of diverticulosis and may show marked irregular deformity of the sigmoid and descending colon due to muscular thickening and shortening. Although there is no organic stricture, symptoms may suggest partial functional obstruction. Colonoscopy may help to exclude other causes of symptoms such as inflammatory bowel disease or adenocarcinoma, but spasm and narrowing of the sigmoid often make the procedure difficult and of limited value.

Dietary management, anticholinergic medication, and stool conditioners may fail to provide relief, and some patients will require surgical resection of the affected bowel. Since the operation in these cases is semi-elective, preoperative mechanical and antibiotic preparation of the bowel can be undertaken. Perioperative intravenous antibiotics should be administered. Primary resection and anastomosis should be performed in nearly all of these patients. However, if unexpected inflammation or scarring make the dissection dangerous the bowel should be divided, with the proximal end converted to a colostomy and the distal end turned in. Re-resection and anastomosis should be planned after an interval of 3 months.

Resection for intractable dysfunction and pain accounts for about 25 per cent of patients undergoing surgery for diverticular disease. The expected mortality rate for these patients is less than 1 per cent.

Diverticulitis in proximal colon segments

Although 95 per cent of operations for diverticular disease are performed in the sigmoid and descending colon, in 1 per cent of cases the transverse colon is affected and in 2 per cent each the ascending colon and the caecum is affected. The same principles of bowel preparation and antibiotic usage that have been discussed previously also apply in these instances. When operation is required local excision of the inflamed diverticulum may occasionally be feasible, but in most instances segmental resection and primary anastomosis preferable. Diverticulitis of the caecum may mimic acute appendicitis except that the clinical course may be less fulminant and nausea less common. If a caecal inflammatory mass is encountered ileocaecal resection to remove the mass *en bloc* with primary reanastomosis of the bowel is the preferred treatment.

ELECTIVE COLON RESECTION FOR DIVERTICULAR DISEASE

Complications for diverticular disease and their associated mortality rates are so severe that attempts have been made to define groups of patients who should benefit from elective colon resection to pre-empt these complications. These include patients with

(1) recurrent attacks of local inflammation (two or more);
(2) persistent tender abdominal mass;
(3) narrowing or marked deformity of the sigmoid on radiographic examination;
(4) dysuria associated with diverticulosis;
(5) rapid progression of symptoms from time of onset;
(6) clinical or radiographic signs that do not definitely exclude carcinoma;
(7) relative young age.

The age of the patient is particularly important in considering elective operation. All patients less than 50 years of age may be expected to suffer from repeated attacks of diverticulitis and progressive complications. These patients should therefore be encouraged to undergo resection of the affected segment as an elective procedure under the safest possible conditions.

The few patients who present with giant diverticula should also be treated by elective colon resection. Candidates for organ transplantation who have diverticular disease should be considered for elective colon resection prior to the transplantation procedure. Overall mortality rates for emergency operations for diverticular disease exceed those for elective operations by more than 5 to 1.

TECHNICAL CONSIDERATIONS

Operative treatment of colon diverticular disease is technically demanding and should be undertaken only by experienced surgeons. Sepsis, scarring, foreshortening, thickening and narrowing of the bowel, associated abscesses, obstruction, and fistulae present challenges that require both technical expertise and mature judgement. In addition, decisions have to be made regarding avoidance of injury to adjacent structures, the length of bowel to be resected, primary anastomosis or diversion of the faecal stream, the security of bowel anastomosis, the advisability of colostomy proximal to an anastomosis, and the appropriateness and placement of drains.

The spleen and the left ureter are particularly at risk of damage during operations for diverticular disease. Accidental splenic injury and subsequent splenectomy create a risk of venous thromboembolic complications and may permanently impair immunity. The left ureter may be adherent to the sigmoid mesentery or bound in dense scar in the region of the pelvic brim, sometimes with partial ureteral obstruction. Preoperative placement of a left ureteral catheter as a stent may help to identify the ureter in an area of inflammation or dense scar. Ureteral injury can be avoided by dissecting the mesentery of the descending colon from Gerota's fascia, identifying the ureter near the renal pelvis, then dissecting downward through the difficult area, keeping the ureter in a posterior position and always in view.

The choice of abdominal incision is important for a safe and convenient resection of the left colon. Although a midline or a left paramedian incision is the more conventional approach, an oblique curved incision that begins at the lateral border of the right rectus muscle 4 cm above the symphysis pubis crosses both rectus muscles and curves upward to the costal margin in the left flank gives ideal exposure of both the spleen and the depths of the pelvis. The use of the Trendelenberg position and tilting of the table to the right permit the small bowel to be packed into the right upper abdomen, leaving the field clearly exposed from the splenic flexure to the cul-de-sac. Closure of the wound in layers and reapproximation of the rectus muscles by figure-of-eight synthetic absorbable sutures gives reliable and comfortable healing and essentially removes the risk of incisional herniation. If a sigmoid or descending colostomy is required the bowel may be brought through a separate incision above and medial to the incision to create a stoma at the level of the umbilicus. Transverse colostomy may be accomplished easily by lifting the abdominal wall with the left hand within the abdomen and making a transverse right upper quadrant incision through which a loop of right transverse colon may be drawn (Figs. 16–19).

The length of colon to be resected depends upon the extent of muscular abnormalities in the gut wall as well as the extent of the inflammatory changes. The distal resection margin should be at the level of the intraperitoneal rectum, which is usually the distal extent of diverticular disease. The rectum may be effectively brought upward by blunt retroperitoneal dissection from the hollow of the sacrum, making division and anastomosis technically easier. The resected specimen should include all the narrowed and inflamed segment, as well as the area of muscular thickening and foreshortening: in most instances this will require resection of a length of at least 25 cm. The splenic flexure should be freed and

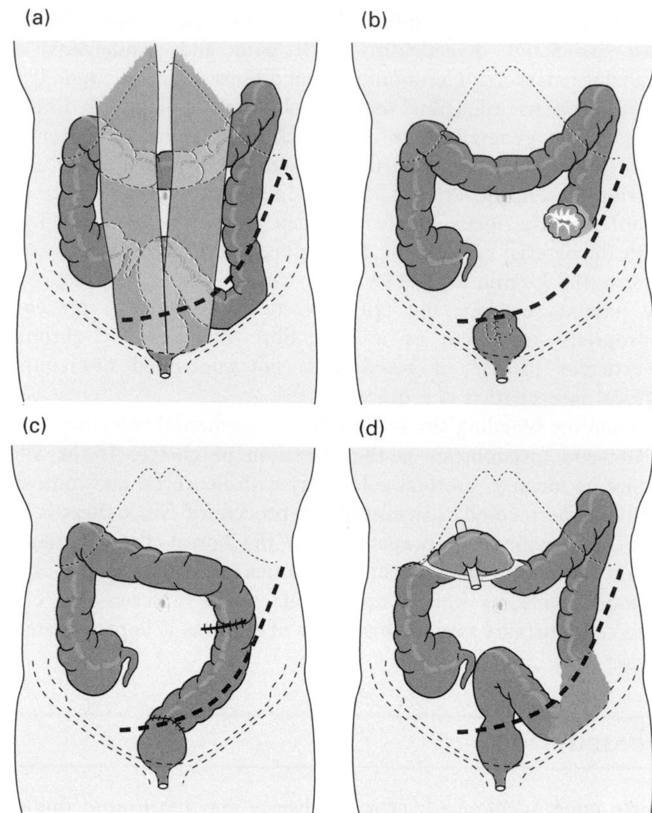

Fig. 16 (a) Preferred incision for left colectomy involves transverse division of rectus muscles two fingerbreadths above symphysis pubis, oblique extension from left rectus border to costal margin in the line of fibres of the external oblique muscle. (b) Resection of inflamed sigmoid with rectal turn-in and proximal end colostomy (Hartmann procedure). (c) Delayed repair after Hartmann procedure with excision of colostomy and additional colon affected by diverticulosis, end-to-end colorectal anastomosis. (d) Diverticulitis with severe local inflammation and fibrosis making primary resection of the disease hazardous, managed by right transverse colostomy delayed left colon resection.

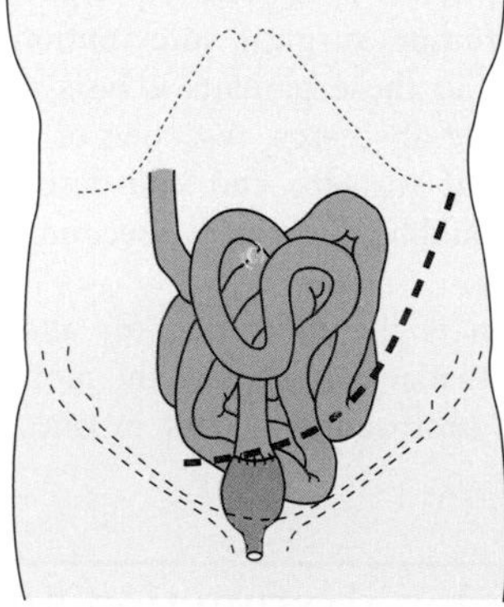

Fig. 17 Subtotal colectomy with ileorectal anastomosis for massive haemorrhage in diffuse diverticulosis, site of bleeding not identified.

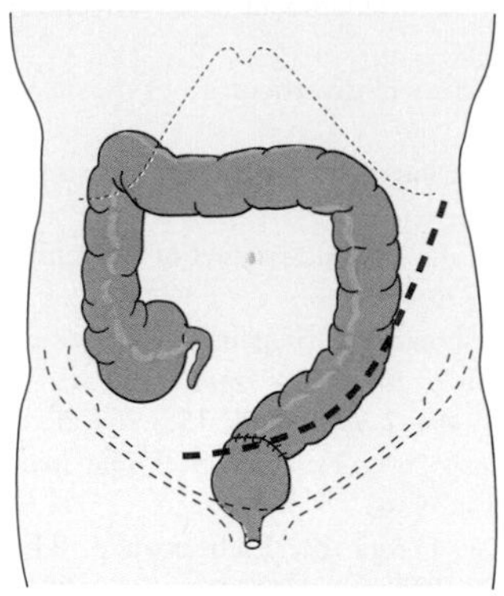

Fig. 18 One-stage resection and primary anastomosis for sigmoid diverticular disease.

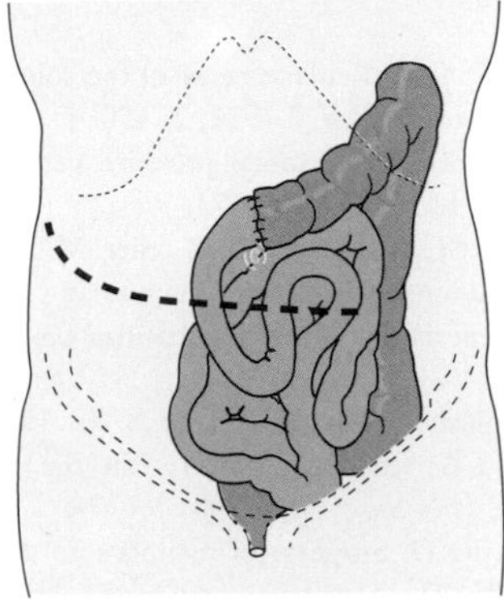

Fig. 19 Right colectomy with ileotransverse colostomy for caecal diverticulitis. Note transverse incision which is ideal for this procedure.

the left colic artery and vein divided and ligated near their origins to permit the splenic flexure or left transverse colon to be brought to the rectum without tension. The anastomosis may be stapled or hand-sewn but must be accurate, without tension and in well perfused bowel. If the anastomosis is not technically perfect, a right transverse colostomy should be added and, in selected cases, pelvic drainage will be required.

COMPLICATIONS FOLLOWING TREATMENT

Operative complications of treatment of colonic diverticular disease include splenic injuries (2 per cent), intraoperative haemorrhage (2 per cent), colonoscopic perforation (1 per cent), and ureteral injury (0.6 per cent).

Postoperative complications include respiratory failure (6 per cent), wound abscess (4 per cent), anastomotic leak (2.5 per cent), renal failure (2 per cent), peritonitis (2 per cent), incisional hernia (2 per cent), haemorrhagic shock (2 per cent), ileus (2 per cent), thrombocytopenia (2 per cent), small bowel obstruction (1.5 per cent), and sigmoidocutaneous fistula (1 per cent). Many other conditions occur with a frequency of less than 1 per cent.

Anastomotic leak is a serious postoperative complication which needs to be identified promptly and is treated by abdominal re-exploration, transverse colostomy, and external drainage of the contaminated area. All such patients are gravely ill and require triple antibiotic coverage (metronidazole, ampicillin, and gentamicin) with careful metabolic monitoring and support. There is a 10 per cent mortality rate associated with this complication. All patients who recover have long, complex, and costly illnesses necessitating multiple additional operative procedures. Re-resection of the area of failed anastomosis is mandatory and effective healing should be demonstrated by barium enema prior to attempted closure of the transverse colostomy.

Postoperative abscesses may be subphrenic, pelvic, or intermesenteric. These abscesses can often be treated by percutaneous catheter drainage; if treatment is not successful, open drainage is required.

Intestinal obstruction should be treated by nasogastric decompression and intravenous administration of fluids, including intravenous hyperalimentation. This will permit resolution of the obstruction without re-exploration in most instances. If pain, distension, and leucocytosis do not resolve quickly, surgical re-exploration of the abdomen should be carried out.

Intravenous hyperalimentation by means of a central line is an important adjunct to treatment of postoperative complications in patients in whom oral feedings must be restricted for more than 5 to 7 days. Nutrition, effective antibiotic therapy, fluid intake to maintain renal function, defunctioning of the bowel, and adequate drainage of sepsis are critical to the recovery of such patients.

RESULTS OF TREATMENT

Overall mortality rates for patients requiring operation for colon diverticular disease are in the range of 5 per cent. Mortality among patients requiring emergency surgery for complications of the disease is more than five times greater than among those undergoing elective procedures. Patients need an average of 1.5 operations for successful treatment, but those with severe complications often require several staged procedures before recovery.

Complications of operations are frequent (approximately 30 per cent overall), often serious, and usually related to sepsis. Multiple organ failure may follow septic shock, which occurs either as a manifestation of the primary disease or as a postoperative complication. Morbidity among patients with postoperative complications tends to be prolonged, often lasting for several months.

The high mortality and morbidity rates among patients treated for complications of diverticular disease support the recommendation that those who are at high risk of developing complications should undergo elective colon resection. Unfortunately, 50 per cent of those who require emergency operations for complications of diverticular disease have had symptoms for less than 30 days at the time of the presenting illness.

Long-term results of colon resection for diverticular disease are excellent. Most patients are relieved of their chronic bowel complaints and all the septic sequelae of the disease, although they tend to have slightly more frequent stools (2–3 per day) as compared to their preoperative status. Patients who require ileorectal anastomosis for massive haemorrhage may have troublesome diarrhoea that generally responds to medical management. Recurrent diverticulitis is rare following adequate resection of the diseased bowel segment, and affects less than 5 per cent of patients overall. However, among patients who have had incompleted staged operative treatment and who may be left with a colostomy and defunctioned sigmoid or rectum, the disease and its complications may continue in the defunctioned segment.

SUMMARY

Diverticular disease of the colon is a disease increasing in frequency as the average age of Western populations increases. While its causes are multifactorial, at least one prophylactic measure appears to be the provision of a diet high in fibre, causing a relatively short transit time of stool in the gut.

The complications of diverticular disease are severe and are associated with significant morbidity and mortality. Surgical resection of affected colon segments is effective treatment but is hazardous if sepsis is present.

Improved results of treatment depend upon skilled judgment, technical expertise, and effective antibiotic and metabolic management. Elective operation should be considered for patients with repeated attacks of diverticulitis, those under the age of 50, and for patients with diverticular disease who have reduced immunological competence or who may be candidates for organ transplantation.

FURTHER READING

Abbe R. A case of sigmoid diverticulitis simulating malignancy. *Weekly J Med Surg Rep* 1914; **86**: 190–1.

Arfwidsson S, Kock NG. Intraluminal pressure in the sigmoid colon of normal subjects and patients with diverticular disease of the colon. *Acta Chir Scand* 1964 (Suppl); **342**: 47–55.

Athanasoulis CA, *et al.* Mesenteric artery infusion of vasopressin for haemorrhage from colonic diverticulosis. *Am J Surg* 1975; **129**: 212–16.

Beer E. Some pathological and clinical aspects of acquired (false) diverticula of the intestine. *Am J Med Sci* 1904; **128**: 135–45.

Carlson AJ, Hoelzel F. Relation of diet to diverticulosis of the colon in rats. *Gastroenterology* 1949; **12**: 108–15.

Celio A. Zur Pathologie der chronischen Stenosierenden. Diverticulitis coli-Sog. diverticulitis tumor. *Helv Chir Acta* 1952; **19**: 93–118.

deQuervain F. Zur diagnose der erworbenen dickdarmdivertikel und der sigmoiditis diverticularis. *Deutsche Z Chir* 1914; **128**: 67–85.

Edwards HC. *Diverticula and Diverticulitis of the Intestine.* Baltimore: Williams & Wilkins, 1939: 335.

Fleischner FG, Ming S, Henken EM. Revised concepts on diverticular disease of the colon. *Radiology* 1964; **83**: 859–72, and 1965; **84**: 599–609.

Graser E. Uber multiple falsche Darmdivertikel in der flexura Sigmoidea. *Munch Med Wochenschr* 1899; **46**: 721–3.

Havia T, Manner R. The irritable colon syndrome: a follow-up study with special reference to the development of diverticula. *Acta Chir Scand* 1971; **137**: 569–72.

Horner JL. Natural history of diverticulosis of the colon. *Am J Dig Dis* 1958; **3**: 343–50.

Hughes LE. Postmortem survey of diverticular disease of the colon. *Gut* 1969; **10**: 336–51.

Keith A. Diverticula of the alimentary tract of congenital or of obscure origin. *Br J Med* 1910; **1**: 376–80.

Labs JD, Sarr MG, Fishman EK, Siegelman SS, Cameron JL. Complications of acute diverticulitis of the colon: improved early diagnosis with computerized tomography. *Am J Surg* 1988; **155**: 331–6.

Lumsden K, Chaudhary NA, Truelove SC. The irritable colon syndrome. *Clin Radiol* 1963; **14**: 54–63.

Morris J, Stellato TA, Haaga JR, Lieberman J. The utility of computed tomography in colonic diverticulosis. *Ann Surg* 1986; **204**: 128–32.

Morson BC. The muscle abnormality in diverticular disease of the sigmoid colon. *Proc Roy Soc Med* 1963; **56**: 798–800.

Mueller PR, *et al.* Sigmoid diverticular abscesses: percutaneous drainage as an adjunct to surgical resection in 24 cases. *Radiology* 1987; **164**: 321–5.

Noer RJ. Haemorrhage as a complication of diverticulitis. *Ann Surg* 1955; **141**: 674–83.

Painter NS, Burkitt DP. Diverticular disease of the colon: a deficiency disease of Western civilization. *Br Med J* 1971; **2**: 450–4.

Painter NS, Truelove SC. Intraluminal pressure pattern in diverticulitis of the colon. *Gut* 1964; **5**: 201–13, 365–73.

Painter NS, Truelove SC, Adrian GM, Tucher M. Segmentation and the localization of intraluminal pressures in the human colon with special reference to the pathogenesis of colonic diverticula. *Gastroenterology* 1965; **49**: 169–77.

Pohlman T. Diverticulosis. *Gastroenterol Clin N Am* 1988; **17**: 357–85.

Rodkey GV, Welch CE. Changing patterns in the surgical treatment of diverticular disease. *Ann Surg* 1984; **200**: 466–78.

Rothenberger DA, Wiltz O. Surgery for complicated diverticulitis. *Surg Clin N Am* 1993; **73**: 975–92.

Ryan P. Changing concepts in diverticular disease. *Dis Colon Rect* 1983; **26**: 12–18.

Schoetz DJ. Uncomplicated diverticulitis: indications for surgery and surgical management. *Surg Clin N Am* 1993; **73**: 965–74.

Smith TR, Cho KC, Morehouse HT, Kratka PS. Comparison of computed tomography and contrast enema evaluation of diverticulitis. *Dis Colon Rect* 1990; **33**: 1–6.

Smithwick RH. Experiences with the surgical management of diverticulitis of the sigmoid. *Ann Surg* 1942; **115**: 969–83.

Whiteway J, Morson BC. Elastosis in diverticular disease of the sigmoid colon. *Gut* 1985; **26**: 258–66.

Wolf AV. Demonstration concerning pressure-tension relations in various organs. *Science* 1952; **115**: 243–44.

18.2.1 Inflammatory disorders

NEIL MORTENSEN

When a patient presents with diarrhoea, two broad groups of diseases must be considered—specific and non-specific inflammatory bowel disease (Table 1). Although it is not the purpose of this section to describe specific infectious diseases in detail, it is important to bear them in mind when considering the management of patients with severe diarrhoea so that inappropriate surgery can be avoided. Conversely, although altered bowel function with blood in the stool in an African, Asian, or Arab patient undergoing investigations in the West is more likely to be due to bacillary or amoebic dysentery or schistosomiasis, other problems such as ulcerative colitis must be considered. With the increase in travel to tropical countries by Western patients, infectious diseases must always be ruled out first.

AMOEBIC DYSENTERY (see also Section 41.1)

This disease is caused by the protozoan *Entamoeba histolytica* which, when ingested as a cyst, invades the large intestine, pro-

Table 1 Inflammatory bowel disease of the colon

Specific inflammatory bowel disease	Non-specific inflammatory bowel disease
Infective	
Amoebic dysentery	Ulcerative colitis
Bacillary dysentery	Indeterminate colitis
Schistosomiasis	Crohn's disease
Tuberculosis	
Campylobacter enterocolitis	
Yersinia enterocolitis	
Enterobius vermicularis	
Non-infective	
Radiation enterocolitis	
Ischaemic colitis	
Eosinophilic gastroenteritis	

ducing colonies in the colonic wall and ulceration, which may occasionally bleed briskly. Intestinal amoebiasis usually presents as a fluctuating bleeding diarrhoea, amoebic appendicitis, or an amoeboma. Rectal amoebic ulceration can mimic a carcinoma (Figs. 1, 2). Barium enema may show deformity of the caecum at the site of an amoeboma (Fig. 3).

Fresh stool specimens must be examined quickly for protozoa. Treatment with metronidazole has a rapid effect, and surgery is rarely necessary.

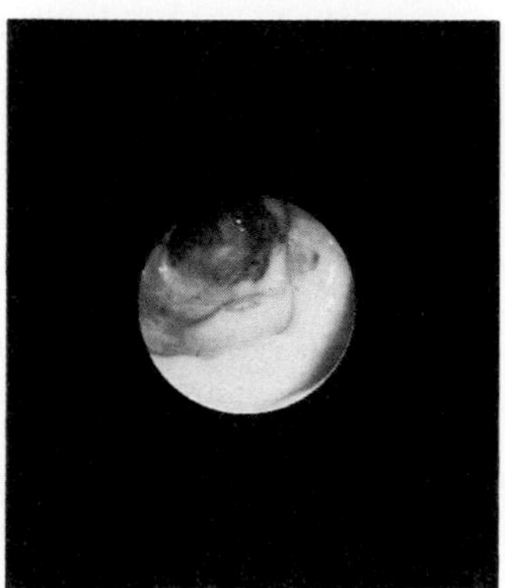

Fig. 1 Sigmoidoscopic view in amoebic colitis showing mucosal ulceration.

BACILLARY DYSENTERY (SHIGELLOSIS)

This is often an epidemic disease and a contact history can usually be obtained. Shigella multiplies rapidly in the colon, producing endotoxins which can cause a coagulopathy or haemolytic anaemia when infection is severe. Inflammation of the colon leads to necrosis of epithelium and desquamation, with formation of a membrane and discrete ulcers. Diagnosis is usually made by stool culture. Most cases will settle with conservative and supportive measures, but antibiotics are usually required for infection with *Shigella shiga*.

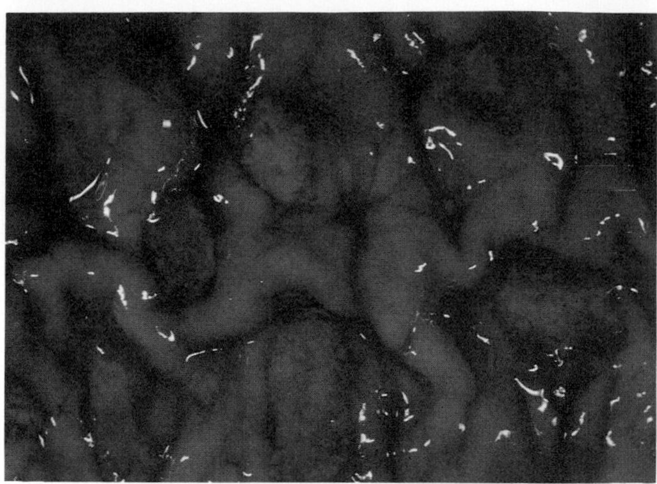

Fig. 2 Macroscopic appearance of colonic surface showing amoebic ulcers.

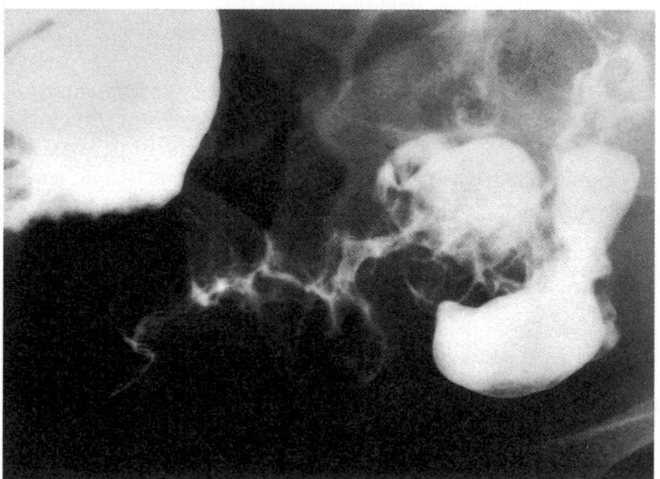

Fig. 3 Barium enema showing an amoeboma in the ascending colon.

SCHISTOSOMIASIS (see also Section 41.9)

This infection is acquired when contaminated fresh water containing the cercariae of *Schistosoma mansoni*, *S. intercalatum*, or *S. japonicum* come into contact with skin. Once inside the human bloodstream the adult worms pass through the liver and portal system and lodge in the wall of the large intestine. Granulomatous reactions to the parasite result in ulceration, bleeding polyps, and fibrosis. Intestinal symptoms are a late occurrence, with exacerbations of colitis occurring intermittently. Hepatic infestation and portal hypertension may also cause intestinal bleeding. Repeated stool specimens have to be examined for parasites; sigmoidoscopy may show ulceration and a rectal biopsy is helpful. Barium enema shows an immobile, irregular colon. Serological tests are valuable around 4 weeks after infection. Treatment is most commonly with niridazole.

TUBERCULOSIS (see also Section 41.3)

In tropical counties, ileocaecal tuberculosis is an important and often underdiagnosed cause of intestinal disease. Colonic or anal tuberculosis alone is very rare.

OTHER SPECIFIC COLONIC INFECTIONS

Campylobacter enterocolitis and *Yersinia enterocolitica* may infect the small intestine, but usually cause a colitis with a characteristic infective clinical picture. Campylobacter and salmonellae are the most common cause of bloody diarrhoea. In immunocompromised patients, cytomegalovirus, herpes simplex virus, and *Mycobacterium avium intestinale* can all cause colitis.

Oxyuriasis caused by the threadworm or pinworm is a common infection in children and may affect whole families. Ova are ingested in contaminated food or drink or from hands contaminated with faeces. Female larvae migrate to the caecum or colon, and as their ova are shed they pass through the anus on to the perianal skin. These cause intense pruritus ani, resulting in scratching and reinfection. There may be an eosinophilia. The worms can be seen on sigmoidoscopy in the anal canal, and the ova identified in scrapings from perianal skin. Treatment, usually for the whole family, is with piperazine or mebendazole.

Rarely, *Enterobius vermicularis* can cause appendicitis or a perianal abscess.

SPECIFIC NON-INFECTIVE CONDITIONS

Radiation enterocolitis

Gastrointestinal symptoms develop in 10 per cent of patients receiving 50 Gy or more for abdominal or pelvic disease. Either the small bowel or large bowel can be damaged.

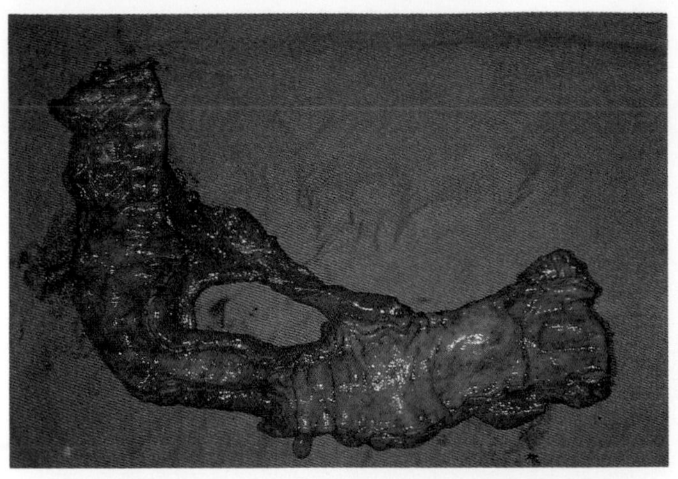

Fig. 4 Stricture in the sigmoid colon due to irradiation.

Acute proctitis

After 1 to 2 weeks, a diarrhoeal illness with bleeding and tenesmus results from damage to rapidly dividing cells. At this stage there may only be a mild inflammation of rectal mucosa. Delayed symptoms some weeks later result from ischaemia caused by obliteration of submucosal small vessels, and there may be ulceration or necrosis.

Late symptoms

Six months or many years after the original radiotherapy continuing ischaemia may occur due to small vessel changes with secondary fibrosis. Ulceration, abscesses, fistulae, or strictures can occur and the mucosa looks pale with telangiectasia (Fig. 4). There is no specific treatment, but a course of local or systemic steroids may be worthwhile. Surgery is avoided if possible because of the poor healing and high incidence of complication.

OTHER SPECIFIC CONDITIONS

A number of other conditions can mimic inflammatory bowel disease, including irritable bowel syndrome, diverticular disease, and ischaemic disorders. Eosinophilic gastroenteritis is a rare condition of unknown aetiology which may affect any part of the gastrointestinal tract, and which presents with diarrhoea, abdominal pain, and bleeding. An eosinophilia is present in biopsies and peripheral blood. Corticosteroid treatment is often effective.

18.2.2 Pathology of non-specific inflammatory bowel disease

NEIL J. MORTENSEN

The only two absolute distinguishing pathological features between Crohn's disease and ulcerative colitis are the presence of significant small bowel disease and the finding of giant cell granulomata in the former.

ULCERATIVE COLITIS

Ulcerative colitis is a mucosal disease that almost invariably involves the rectum and spreads proximally. The extent of the disease may increase and, rarely, decrease again, giving recognizable periods of activity and remission. Inflammation is limited to the mucosa, except in acute and severe colitis. There may be little visible from the serosal aspect of the bowel on gross inspection. The mucosa is usually congested and friable, with a velvety texture; there may be varying degrees of ulceration. The left side of the colon is usually affected and improvement following steroid enemas can produce an artificial sparing of the rectum or sigmoid. True sigmoid sparing or right-sided disease is rare.

Microscopy shows a diffuse infiltration of acute and chronic inflammatory cells limited to the mucosa (Fig. 1). The glandular pattern is distorted with goblet cell depletion, and crypt abscesses are numerous. In inactive disease, glands may be shortened and atrophic. Long-standing disease may be associated with dysplasia of the epithelium, which can be graded as mild, moderate, or severe. Severe dysplasia (precancer) is frequently associated with cancer elsewhere in the colon and when detected in rectal or colonoscopic biopsies, proctocolectomy must be considered. It is now also accepted that Crohn's disease is associated with an increased risk of cancer even in bypassed small intestine.

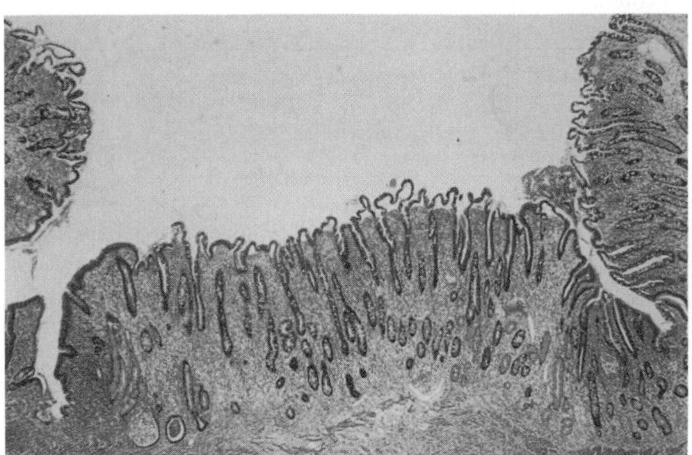

Fig. 1 Photomicrograph showing typical appearance of ulcerative colitis, with flattened mucosa, ulceration, and glandular depletion.

CROHN'S DISEASE

Crohn's disease of the large intestine has been recognized as a separate entity since the definitive description of Lockhart Mummary and Morson. Since then, many cases previously labelled as ulcerative colitis have been reclassified as Crohn's disease of the large intestine. Crohn's disease is restricted to the colon in some 20 per cent of patients; another 60 per cent have ileocolonic involvement. It is usually a right-sided disease but limited left-sided disease can occur, especially associated with anal disease in the elderly.

In the colon, Crohn's disease is characteristically a granulomatous condition with transmural aggregates of inflammatory cells and penetrating fissuring ulceration (Fig. 2). The bowel wall is thickened and the serosa opaque. Strictures and fistulae occur between bowel segments and there are large fleshy lymph nodes in the mesentery or pericolic fat. The mucosa is oedematous and characteristically traversed by linear ulcers, giving a cobblestone appearance to the surface. Areas of non-involved bowel separate

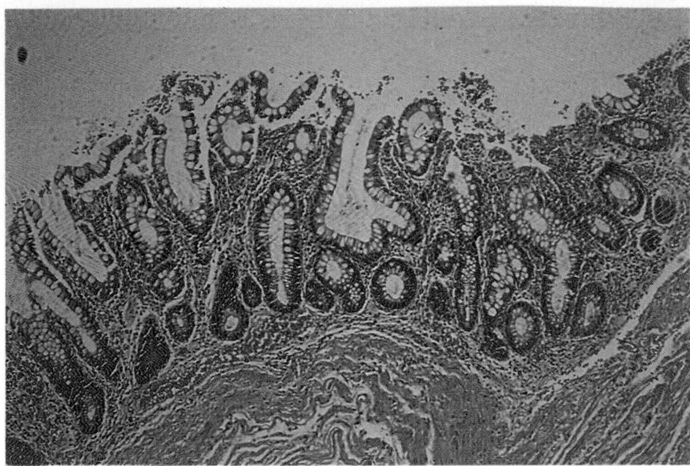

Fig. 2 Photomicrograph showing typical appearance of Crohn's colitis, with deep fissures, focal inflammation, and a granuloma in the submucosa.

the disease segments (skip lesions), although there may be cases with diffuse disease. Careful inspection of normal looking mucosa may reveal tiny aphthoid ulcers, which start as ulcerating lymphoid follicles; these may be the initial lesion in the disease. Rectal sparing and anal disease are common features. The key distinguishing feature on microscopy is the granulomata which are scattered throughout the bowel wall, together with fissuring, ulceration, and a regular glandular pattern with a normal goblet cell population. Granulomata are only found in 60 per cent of patients, however, and fissures are seen in only 30 per cent. Fibrosis in the submucosa is common; there may be neural proliferation, pyloric gland metaplasia, and a vasculitis.

BIOPSY AND NON-SPECIFIC INFLAMMATORY BOWEL DISEASE

Rectal biopsy is often more helpful in establishing a diagnosis in ulcerative colitis than in Crohn's disease, because of the problems of sampling error. A normal rectal biopsy is strong evidence against the diagnosis of ulcerative colitis, but it must be stressed that normal appearances on sigmoidoscopy do not imply normal histology. In Crohn's disease the chance of obtaining an abnormal specimen on biopsy increases as the diseased segment becomes closer to the anal canal, but even when disease is restricted to the ileum, abnormal rectal biopsies can be found in up to 12 per cent of patients. Multiple colonscopic biopsies make it possible to document precisely the extent and distribution of colonic disease, particularly in those with mild ulcerative colitis and Crohn's disease. Because of the small size of the colonic biopsies granulomata are detected less frequently than in rectal biopsies.

Histopathology in severe colitis

Distinction between Crohn's disease and ulcerative colitis is most difficult when the disease is severe. Ulcerative colitis can become transmural, with deep ulceration and fissures. The irregularity in goblet cell depletion is then less obvious and the histopathology can be confusingly similar to that of Crohn's disease. Occasionally this distinction is not made, even after study of the operative

Table 1 Clinical differences between Crohn's disease and ulcerative colitis

	Crohn's disease	Ulcerative colitis
Symptoms		
Bleeding	Sometimes	Very common
Abdominal pain	Common	Sometimes
Urgent defecation	Sometimes	Very common
Abdomen		
Abdominal mass	Sometimes	Rare
Spontaneous fistulae	Sometimes	Never
Anal region		
Ulceration	Common	Rare
Infection	Common and complicated	Occurs
Lesions preceding bowel symptoms	Sometimes	Never
Endoscopy		
Rectal involvement	50%	95%
Appearance	Oedema, ulcers, normal patches	Uniform continuous granular friable
Prognosis		
Medicine	Inadequate in 80%	80% successful cure
Surgery	Liable to recur	Cure possible
Cancer	Slight	Definite

specimen, and the diagnosis can only be finally resolved when the rectum is removed or when disease appears in the small intestine. In some cases the features overlap so much that the disease has to be labelled 'indeterminate colitis'.

CLINICAL DIFFERENTIATION BETWEEN ULCERATIVE COLITIS AND CROHN'S DISEASE

The differences in distribution and histological appearances of the two diseases make it convenient to recognize ulcerative colitis and Crohn's disease as separate entities. The main clinical differences are shown in Table 1. Differences are seen in anatomical distribution, in the type of ulceration, and the continuity or discontinuity of the disease. Fibrosis is not a feature of ulcerative colitis and fibrous strictures rarely occur (Table 2).

In Crohn's disease, fibrosis can cause fibrotic strictures with obstructive symptoms. Since ulcerative colitis causes a severe diarrhoea, there may be secondary or thrombosis of haemorrhoids. Crohn's disease tends to affect adjacent structures with fistulation into the bladder, fallopian tube, ureter, or other intra-abdominal structures. A chronic retroperitoneal abscess can spread to the psoas sheath, and the characteristic anorectal lesions of Crohn's disease can spread to the external genitalia or give rise to a rectovaginal fistula. All types of non-specific inflammatory bowel disease can give rise to extraintestinal manifestations, usually associated with an exacerbation of inflammation in the gut.

Table 2 Extraintestinal manifestations of ulcerative colitis and Crohn's disease of the colon

Those occurring transiently during disease activity	
Skin	Erythema nodosum, pyoderma gangrenosum
Mucous membranes	Aphthous ulcers of mouth and vagina
Eyes	Iritis
Joints	Flitting arthritis of large joints
Persistent irrespective of disease activity	
Joints	Sacroileitis, ankylosing spondylitis
Liver	Chronic active hepatitis, cirrhosis
Biliary system	Sclerosing cholangitis, bile duct carcinoma
Renal	Amyloidosis in Crohn's disease

FURTHER READING

Lockhart Mummery HE, Morson BC. Crohn's disease (regional enteritis) of the large intestine and its distinction from ulcerative colitis. *Gut* 1960; 1: 87–105.

Morson BC, Dawson IMP. *Gastrointestinal Pathology*. 2nd edn. Oxford: Blackwell 1979.

Price AB. Overlap in the spectrum of non-specific inflammatory bowel disease—colitis indeterminate. *J Clin Pathol* 1978; 3: 567–77.

18.2.3 Ulcerative colitis

NEIL MORTENSEN

EPIDEMIOLOGY AND INCIDENCE

The highest incidence of ulcerative colitis occurs in temperate climates and in Caucasians, the populations of Europe, Australasia and North America being the most commonly affected. Annual incidence rates combined with the number of new cases diagnosed per 100 000 population per year vary between 3.3 and 6.5. Ulcerative colitis is about two to three times more common than Crohn's disease, and there is little evidence to suggest that its incidence is increasing, although most studies show an increasing incidence of Crohn's disease. Improved awareness of Crohn's disease and its distinction from ulcerative colitis are not sufficient to account for this increase.

Age distribution

Both ulcerative colitis and Crohn's disease are usually diagnosed in patients between 15 and 40 years of age. The actual age of peak incidence varies between series and there is a second peak in later years.

Sex

Ulcerative colitis is more common in men, whereas Crohn's disease is more common in women. Both diseases have a higher incidence among Jewish people.

Prevalence

The number of patients with the disease per 10^5 population at risk varies between 37.4 and 79.9 for ulcerative colitis.

AETIOLOGY OF ULCERATIVE COLITIS

Genetic factors

There is an increased incidence of ulcerative colitis in the close relatives of patients with the disease. Ankylosing spondylitis can occur in the same families, with or without inflammatory bowel disease. The histocompatibility antigen HLA B27 is found in most patients with colitis and ankylosing spondylitis, but no histocompatibility antigen is clearly associated with inflammatory bowel disease alone. The familial tendency of the disease has been interpreted as being due to similar childhood environment or inherited factors, but the rarity of ulcerative colitis in spouses and its recurrence in different generations in widely separated branches of the family make this less likely.

Immune mechanisms

Circulating humoral antibodies to an antigen present in colonic epithelial cells and to certain bacteria can be demonstrated in the peripheral blood of some patients with ulcerative colitis. Antibody-dependent cytotoxicity against colonic epithelial cells can also be demonstrated in tissue culture. Normal lymphocytes become cytotoxic after incubation with a serum of a patient with colitis. Immune complexes can be demonstrated both in the circulation and within the mucosa. Immune complexes in the lamina propria may cause activation of the complement pathway, with attraction of leucocytes and local tissue damage. Local sensitivity to one or more food antigens has been suggested as a factor. The presence of antibodies to milk protein does not correlate with the duration or severity of disease. However, normal permeability of the intestinal wall to these antigens may be increased when the mucosa is inflamed and the presence of circulating antibodies to food or bacterial antigens may be a secondary effect.

Microbiology

There are no striking differences between normal stool and the faeces of patients with ulcerative colitis. It is possible that normal bacterial flora may play a role in the aetiology of the disease, although no specific antigen has been identified. Cross-reactivity between a bacterial antigen and a mucopolysaccharide present in colonic epithelial cells may precipitate a self-perpetuating autoimmune reaction resulting from a sensitivity to the bacterial antigen. Local mucosal antibodies to anaerobic organisms can also be demonstrated. A first attack of ulcerative colitis can follow a bowel infection, supporting the idea that contact with bacterial antigens due to damage of normal mucosal defences can play a role in the development of the condition.

Environmental factors

The rarity of ulcerative colitis in Africa and the Far East and its relative prevalence in the Western world suggests that environmental factors may be important, but no specific dietary components have been implicated.

CLINICAL FEATURES

Bloody diarrhoea in an otherwise fit patient is the most common presenting symptom. Patients with a limited proctitis may complain of either tenesmus or constipation. Severe disease may cause most constant diarrhoea with cramping abdominal pain, urgency, and episodes of incontinence. The well recognized extraintestinal manifestations of ulcerative colitis are listed in Table 2 in Section 18.2.2.

Examination of the patient may reveal nothing of note in the abdomen or, occasionally, some tenderness in the left iliac fossa and signs of anaemia. Rectal examination reveals blood and mucus on the glove, and the mucosa may feel velvety. Sigmoidoscopy shows a confluent proctitis with contact bleeding, ulceration, and granularity (Fig. 1). It is important to assess the upper limit of disease. Rectal biopsies should be taken from the posterior wall of the rectum below the peritoneal reflection to avoid iatrogenic perforation.

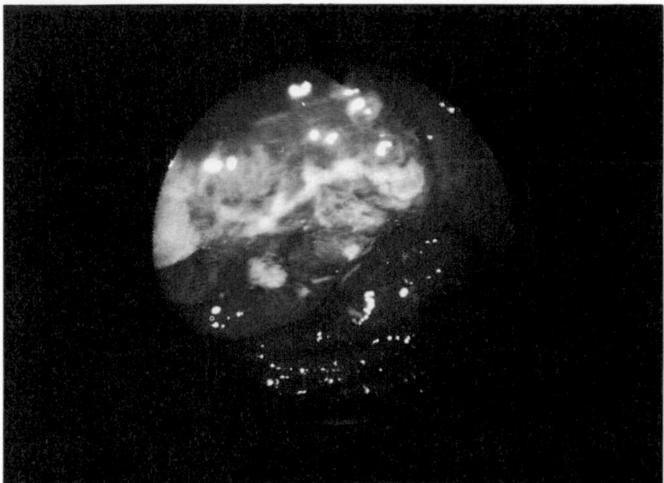

Fig. 1 Typical appearance of a mild to moderately severe proctitis.

Investigation

Although a double-contrast barium enema will demonstrate the full extent of macroscopic disease (Fig. 2), colonoscopy is the most useful investigation. The characteristic appearance on colonoscopy is of an erythematous mucosa, with or without ulceration which may bleed on contact (Fig. 3). A normal vascular pattern is lost and there may be blood and pus in the lumen. Even when the mucosa appears normal, biopsy specimens should be taken to define the exact limit of disease. Ulcerative colitis is worse in the rectum and extends more proximally, but treatment with local steroids may give an appearance of relative rectal sparing. Great care should be taken in conducting either a barium enema or colonoscopy in patients with severe colitis to avoid perforation. Blood samples should be taken to allow the presence of anaemia and signs of systemic inflammation to be assessed. Other tests should include measurement of ESR or viscosity, C-reactive protein albumin, and to assess nutritional status.

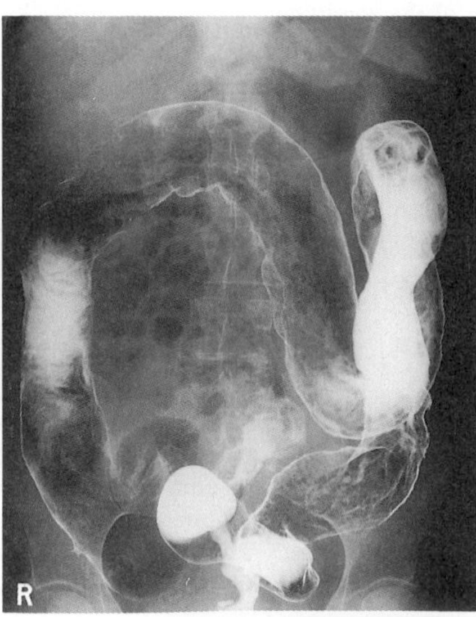

Fig. 2 Double contrast barium enema demonstrating a tubular left colon and ulceration in a total colitis.

MEDICAL MANAGEMENT

Good medical management is vital to prevent progression of disease and severe relapses. It is aimed at reducing inflammation, pain, and diarrhoea. A combination of aggressive medical treatment and conservative surgery ensures the best joint management of patients with severe disease.

Corticosteroids

Controlled trials have shown that corticosteroids have a therapeutic effect in ulcerative colitis. Severely ill patients can be given intravenous prednisolone, while in those with less severe disease oral prednisolone is effective, usually starting with a dose of 40 to 60 mg. Topical preparations in the form of foam or retention enemata, can be used when the inflammation is limited to the distal colon and rectum.

Sulphasalazine

Sulphasalazine is a combination of sulphapyridine and 5-aminosalicylic acid. It is poorly absorbed in the small intestine and is split in the colon by a bacterial action to liberate the active 5-aminosalicylic acid. This reduces inflammation and is used to prevent relapse. Sulphapyridine is, however, responsible for side-effects such as dyspepsia, skin rashes, and azoospermia. Intolerant patients can be given an enteric-coated preparation or one of the more recently developed 5-aminosalicylate preparations, such as mesalazine or olsalazine.

Azathioprine

Azathioprine either in combination with steroids or alone can be used to reduce steroid doses needed for maintenance and prolongation of remission. Side-effects include bone marrow depression, skin rash, and febrile reactions. Azathioprine is usually reserved for the patients with the most resistant chronic disease.

Antibacterial agents

There is no evidence that antibacterial agents have any effect in ulcerative colitis, but intravenous antibiotics may be administered to some patients with severe ulcerative colitis prior to surgery.

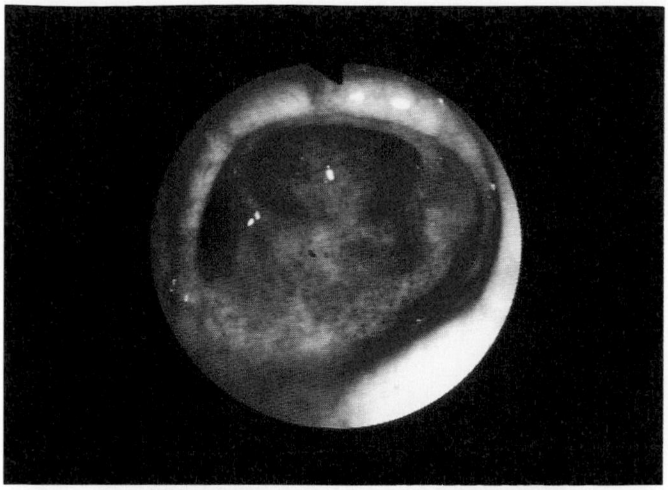

(a)

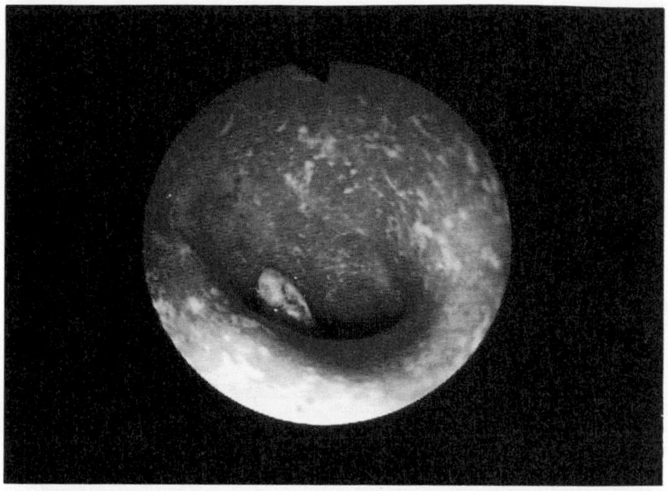

(b)

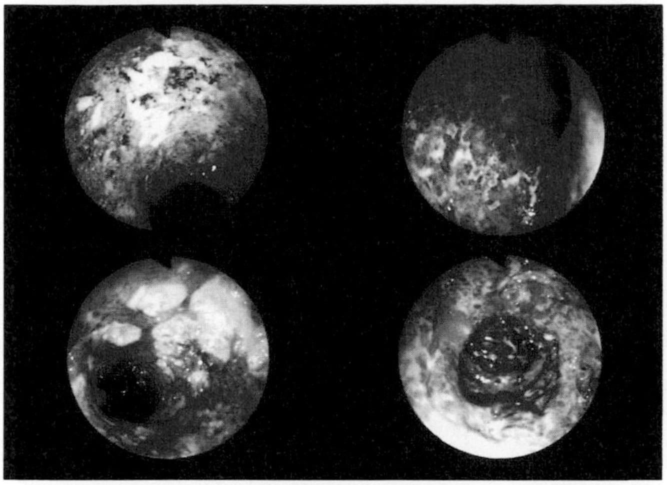

(c)

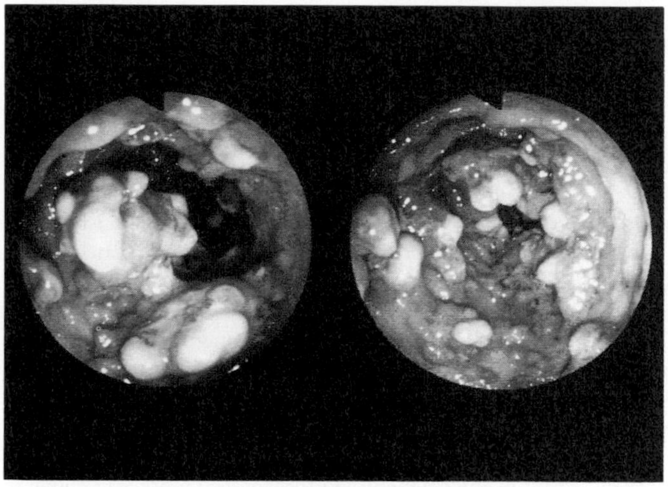

(d)

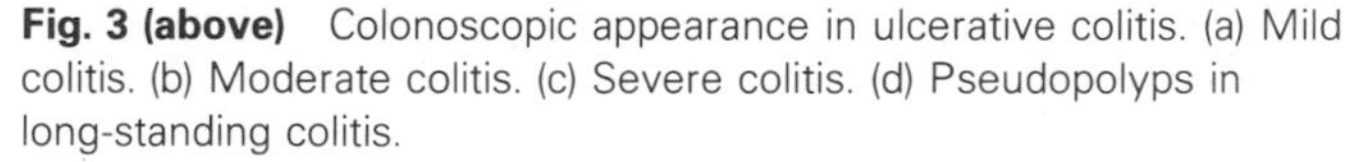

Fig. 3 (above) Colonoscopic appearance in ulcerative colitis. (a) Mild colitis. (b) Moderate colitis. (c) Severe colitis. (d) Pseudopolyps in long-standing colitis.

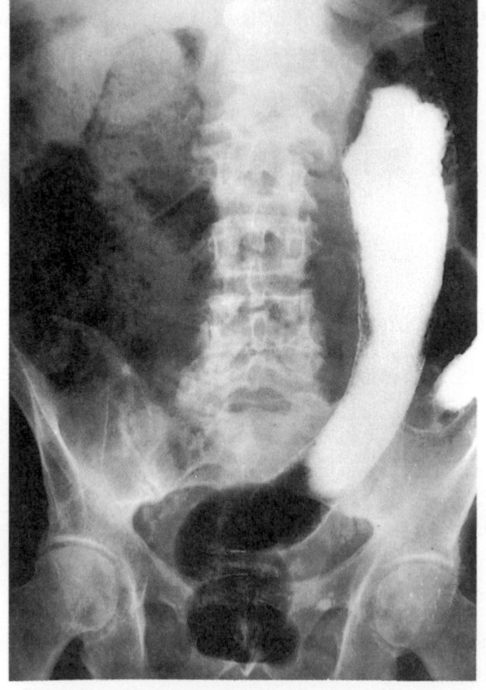

Fig. 4 (left) Plain abdominal film. Paradoxical right-sided constipation in a patient with left-sided ulcerative colitis.

Symptomatic treatment

Treatment with loperamide, codeine phosphate, or diphenoxylate decreases stool frequency and water and electrolyte losses, but it is not recommended. It may mask signs of severe disease and may precipitate a toxic dilatation. If the proximal colon is normal, hard constipated stool may accumulate proximal to the diseased left colon and treatment with a stool softening or bulking agent may be necessary (Fig. 4).

18.2.4 Surgical management of ulcerative colitis

NEIL MORTENSEN AND TERENCE O'KELLY

INDICATIONS FOR OPERATION

Although most patients with ulcerative colitis escape surgery, 2 per cent of those with distal colitis and up to 33 per cent of those with extensive disease will require an operation.

Acute illness

Severe acute colitis is characterized by the passage of more than six loose, bloody motions per day, together with systemic signs, including tachycardia, fever, and hypoalbuminaemia. The crucial points in management are early recognition, aggressive medical therapy, and regular review by a joint medical and surgical team. Stool is cultured to rule out a specific bacterial cause or the rare case of amoebic colitis. Corticosteroids are administered intravenously (400 mg hydrocortisone or 64 mg methylprednisolone daily) and rectally (100 mg hydrocortisone in 100 ml normal saline, infused into the rectum over 15–20 min). The patient is allowed only sips by mouth; fluids are given intravenously.

This treatment is successful in 75 per cent of patients, whose illness resolves within 5 to 7 days. They will feel well, passing two to three semiformed, bloodless motions each day. The remaining 25 per cent either deteriorate despite treatment or fail to recover completely; they may suffer a relapse when a normal diet is resumed. In both of these instances urgent surgery is indicated, since these patients will all require surgery in the subsequent few weeks and there seems little point in delay. A surgical procedure that does not result in a permanent ileostomy is also more acceptable to anxious and ill patients. The administration of antibiotics or steroids at a higher dosage has no therapeutic advantage and is not recommended. Early studies suggested a possible use for cyclosporin in the treatment of acute colitis, but the results of controlled trials are awaited.

If within the first 24 h of admission the patient has a pulse rate greater than 100 beats/min, a temperature over 38°C, or passes more than nine stools per day, or if mucosal islands are visible on a plain abdominal radiograph (Fig. 1), surgery will probably be required. Perforation and colonic dilatation (the upper normal limit of colon diameter is 5 cm) that fails to resolve rapidly when medical treatment is started or that develops during treatment is an indication for emergency surgery. Massive colorectal bleeding may also require emergency surgical intervention. Intraoperative colonic lavage and colonoscopy can help locate the source of bleeding and may obviate the need for proctocolectomy.

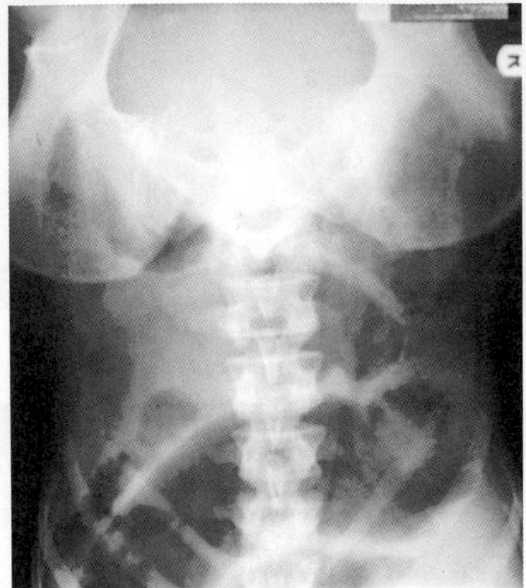

Fig. 1 Plain abdominal radiograph in a patient with severe ulcerative colitis showing dilatation of the transverse colon and mucosal islands.

Chronic illness

The main indication for elective surgery is chronic illness that responds poorly to medical treatment or that is punctuated by frequent episodes of severe acute colitis. The threshold for referral by physicians and the degree of debility which many patients are prepared to tolerate has been reduced with the advent of restorative proctocolectomy. Physical, social, and employment factors should all be considered in the evaluation of a patient, as these can be affected by symptoms of the colitis or by the medication used in its treatment. The patient's age and the duration of illness are also important considerations when deciding on the appropriateness of surgical intervention.

Benign colorectal strictures produced by ulcerative colitis, and some extraintestinal manifestations such as extensive pyoderma gangrenosum (Fig. 2) and iritis (but not sclerosing cholangitis or ankylosing sponylitis), are rare indications for surgery.

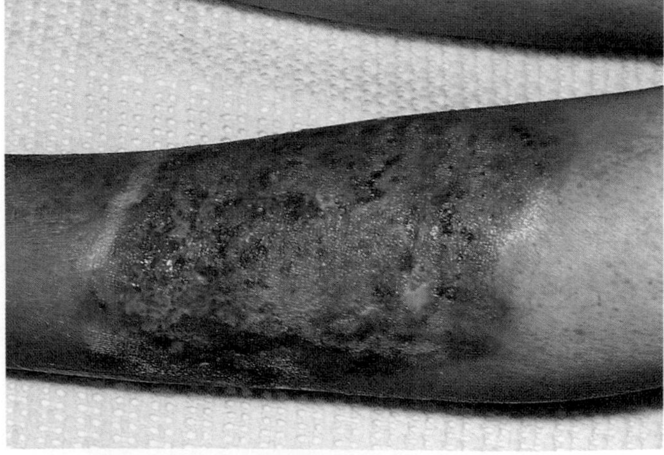

Fig. 2 Pyoderma gangrenosum on the lower leg of a patient with ulcerative colitis. This healed after proctocolectomy.

The risk of carcinoma

Patients with ulcerative colitis have an increased risk of developing colorectal carcinoma (Fig. 3). This situation is particularly true for those who have chronic total colitis which started as a severe first attack in childhood. A precancerous stage is indicated by the finding of dysplasia in colorectal biopsy specimens. Surveillance programmes have been established to examine the large bowel at colonoscopy every 2 years when the disease has been present for 10 years. Biopsy specimens are taken either of specific lesions or from random sites of the mucosal field, as dysplasia in one area can indicate the presence of an unsuspected malignancy elsewhere.

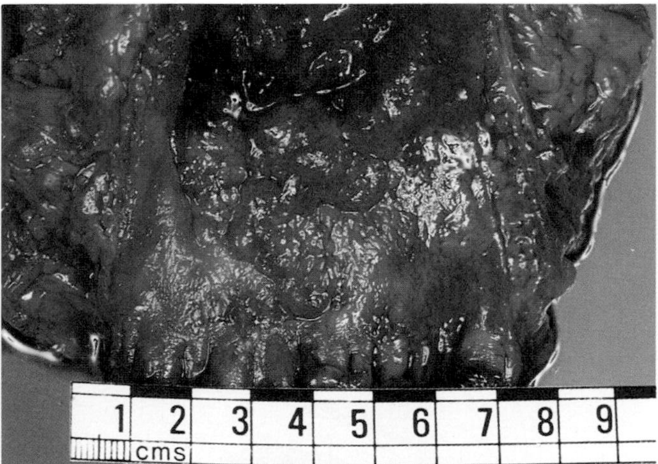

Fig. 3 Colectomy specimen from a patient with a carcinoma in the rectum complicating ulcerative colitis.

Results from these programmes suggest that the probability of developing a carcinoma is 3 per cent at 17 years, 5 to 7 per cent at 20 years and 9 to 1 per cent at 25 years. Very few, if any, cancers develop before a 10-year-history of colitis.

Unfortunately, dysplasia is not an ideal marker of malignancy. Its detection is subject to observer variation, and cancer can develop in the absence of changes at a distant site. Identifying dysplastic changes, however, is the only currently available method for detection of a precancerous state, and is most reliable when severe or high-grade changes are found in a biopsy from a villous or polypoidal lesion (Fig. 4). A similar degree of dysplasia from an area of flat mucosa is less likely to be associated with synchronous carcinoma. The finding should be verified by a second, independent, pathologist and colectomy should be advised only if dysplastic change is present at two sites in the colon. Surgery is also recommended when low-grade dysplasia is found in a raised lesion; its presence in flat mucosa is an indication for increased vigilance only.

Until a more sensitive and specific marker of premalignancy is found, the true value of screening for colorectal cancer in ulcerative colitis remains uncertain.

SURGICAL OPTIONS

Until quite recently, complete proctocolectomy (or panproctocolectomy) was the best operation for patients with ulcerative colitis who required surgery. This position has, however, been challenged by the advent of restorative proctocolectomy which, with few exceptions, is now considered the first-choice elective surgical treatment for this condition. Restorative proctocolectomy has also forced a re-evaluation of the recommended management for those undergoing urgent or emergency operations. The various options available and their indications are shown in Table 1.

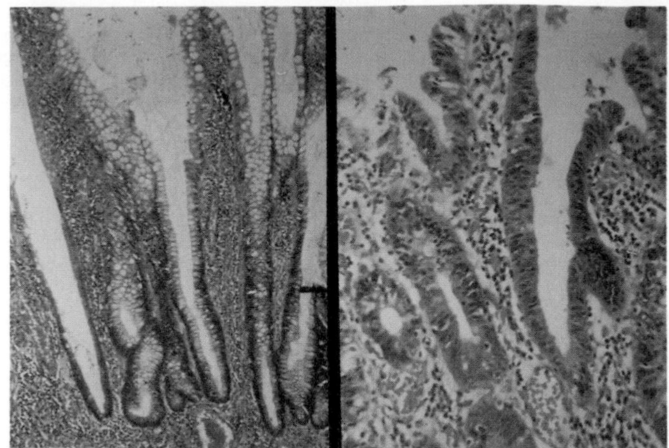

Fig. 4 Photomicrograph of a section from a colonic biopsy showing severe dysplasia complicating ulcerative colitis.

Complete proctocolectomy

Until the development of the Brooke ileostomy and advanced materials for stoma appliances, surgery was a last resort. In the 1950s, however, proctocolectomy became the established procedure.

This operation has several advantages: all diseased tissue is excised at one operation, it removes the risk of cancer, it is a well tried and usually uncomplicated procedure, and the patient can return to normal activities expeditiously. Unfortunately, the patient is left with a permanent ileostomy, which may have serious social and psychological consequences. In the long-term the ileostomy may require revision and small bowel obstruction may develop due to adhesions. Chronic perineal sinus occurs in 5 to 10 per cent of cases and delayed healing of the perineal wound is not uncommon. Sexual dysfunction arising from damage to pelvic autonomic nerves occurs in 0.5 to 1 per cent of male patients. Dyspareunia may be a result of adhesions in female patients.

With the advent of restorative surgery, this procedure is currently indicated only in elderly patients, particularly those with weak anal sphincters, and in those unwilling to subject themselves to a more complicated operation with the possibility of additional morbidity and a longer hospital stay. In Oxford, one-quarter of our patients elect to have a complete proctocolectomy; the majority choose the restorative procedure.

Procedure

With the patient in the modified lithotomy Trendelenburg position, the abdomen and perineum are prepared. The rectum is

Table 1 Comparison of the three operations most commonly used in the treatment of ulcerative colitis

	Proctocolectomy and Brooke ileostomy	Colectomy with ileorectal anastomosis	Total proctocolectomy with ileal pouch–anal anastomosis
Advantages	Curative, one operation	Sphincter unchanged; evacuation 2–4 times day; no stoma; no bladder or sexual dysfunction	Curative; continent
Disadvantages	Incontinence, external ileostomy appliances; need to empty 4–8 times per day	Not curative; cancer risk persists; proctectomy for cancer or disease in 5–50%	Failure 10%; need to evacuate 4–8 times per day
Complications	Stoma revision 10–25% Perineal wound 10–25% Small bowel obstruction 10–20% Bladder dysfunction minimal Sexual dysfunction minimal	Small bowel obstruction in 10–20%; potential anastomotic leak with disease	Pouch fistulas; sepsis; stenosis small bowel obstruction in 10–20%; pouchitis; bladder dysfunction minimal; sexual dysfunction minimal; anal excoriation
Contraindications	None	Sphincter incontinence; severe rectal disease; rectal dysplasia; rectal cancer	Crohn's disease; rectal cancer in distal half

washed out with an antiseptic and a close perianal purse string is placed. The previously marked ileostomy site is trephined. The abdomen is opened through a long mid-line incision, the colon mobilized and the vessels divided comfortably near the bowel, from the caecum to sigmoid. The pelvic dissection can be carried out in the close rectal or mesorectal plane (Fig. 5). The perineal operator meanwhile makes a close perianal incision and develops the intersphincteric plane. Infiltration with dilute adrenaline may aid this dissection. The specimen is removed through the perineal wound. The perineum is closed in layers with absorbable sutures. Suction drains are placed from above.

The terminal ileum is delivered through the stoma trephine and everted to make a 2- to 3-cm spouted (Brooke) ileostomy. The lateral space is closed to prevent small bowel herniation.

Complications include pelvic bleeding and intra-abdominal sepsis. Small bowl adhesion obstruction occasionally requires laparotomy. Stoma protraction or retraction requiring revisional surgery occurs in 5 to 10 per cent of patients.

Stomatherapy

Specialist nurse support in stomatherapy is essential. The stomatherapist will mark the appropriate stoma site, and provide information, counselling and postoperative care in stoma management.

Colectomy with the formation of a Kock continent ileostomy

This procedure retains the advantages of a complete proctocolectomy and replaces the spouted Brooke ileostomy with a flush, continent stoma and an intra-abdominal reservoir constructed of ileum (Fig. 6). Early technical problems, particularly with the nipple valve, have been resolved, but the advent of restorative proctocolectomy has virtually abolished the indications for this procedure. It could be considered in a patient who has already had a complete proctocolectomy and who expresses a strong wish to be rid of the ileostomy.

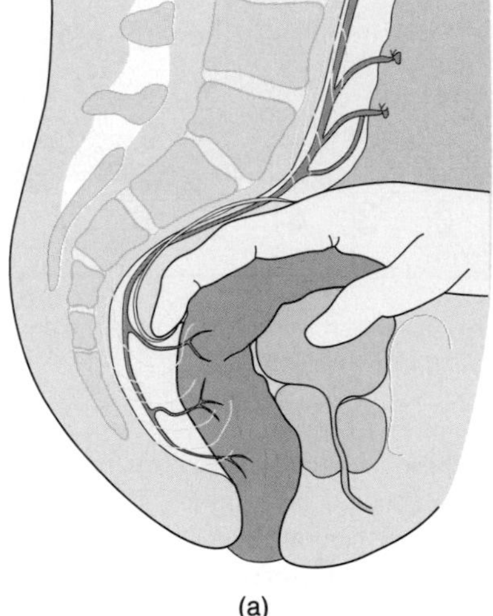

(a)

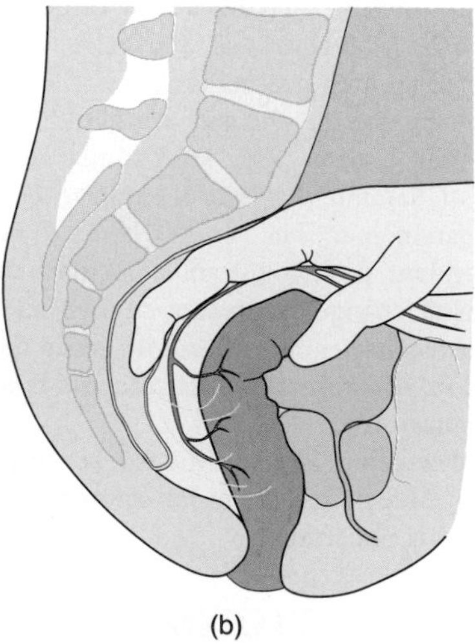

(b)

Fig. 5 Diagram to show the difference between the close rectal (a) and the mesorectal (b) plane used in pelvic dissection.

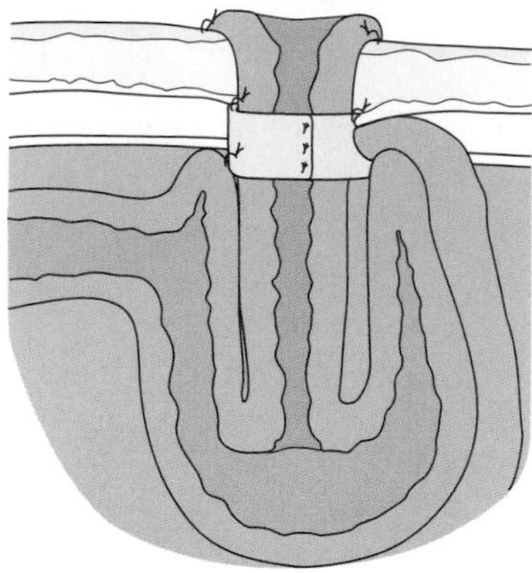

Fig. 6 Kock pouch continent ileostomy showing a Marlex mesh collar reinforcing the nipple valve.

Colectomy with ileorectal anastomosis

This procedure is attractive because it is relatively quick and straightforward, and it can be associated with a good functional outcome. However, its use remains controversial because, by leaving behind the rectum it is associated with a continuing risk of carcinoma. It might be considered in a patient with a compliant rectum which is relatively spared from disease. The presence of a functioning sphincter is essential, and the patient must be reliable as life-long monitoring is required. Coexisting sclerosing cholangitis or portal hypertension, which would make rectal dissection hazardous, are also indications for this operation. It is also an option, in children, allowing them to pass through adolescence without a stoma or until a pouch is indicated.

Restorative proctocolectomy

This is the procedure of choice for the elective treatment of ulcerative colitis. It is not indicated in the presence of Crohn's disease, a lower-third rectal cancer (a high early cancer does not exclude restorative proctocolectomy if local tumour clearance can be achieved without sphincter excision), or poor anal sphincter function. Current operations involve the creation of an ileal reservoir of various designs, followed by an anastomosis to the anal canal.

Emergency surgery for severe acute colitis

Both complete proctocolectomy and subtotal colectomy, with formation of an ileostomy and mucous fistula, have been used in the treatment of acute colitis. However, with the possibility of later restorative surgery, subtotal colectomy has become the procedure of choice. Timing of surgery is obviously critical, and with careful management the 'late case' should be avoidable. Turnbull introduced the principle of 'blow hole' colostomy, in which the thin friable perforating colon was managed by multiple ostomies to the abdominal wall. This avoided the hazardous resection of a difficult colon, but it is rarely required nowadays. The splenic fixture is usually the most dangerous area in an emergency colectomy, and this part of the procedure must be undertaken with great care, packing off the area in case of an inadvertent perforation. If omentum is adherent to the colon it should be left in place and should not be preserved.

The best way to manage the mucous fistula remains undecided. It can be sewn to the skin at the lower end of the laparotomy wound should the rectum break down or, less conventionally, closed and placed subcutaneously. This will avoid creation of a second stoma but allow for discharge of blood and pus through the wound should the rectum break down. In either case, subsequent identification of the rectum is straightforward. Closure of the rectum at the peritoneal reflection (as in Hartmann's procedure) carries the risk of possible perforation of the inflamed stump and abscess formation. Conservative proctocolectomy which includes removal of the rectum to the level of the pelvic floor is not advised. Proctocolectomy is associated with a high degree of morbidity and may make any subsequent pelvic dissection technically difficult. It is only indicated in the rare patient with colitis and rectal bleeding. The various options for managing the rectum after subtotal colectomy are shown in Fig. 7.

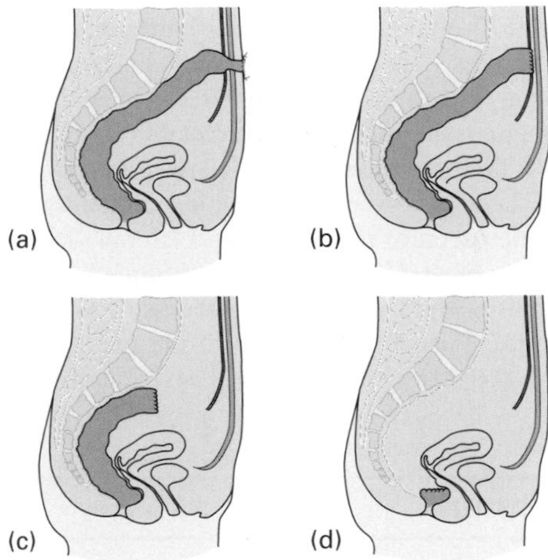

Fig. 7 Options for the management of the retained rectum after subtotal colectomy for ulcerative colitis. (a) Conventional mucous fistula. (b) Subcutaneous closure. (c) Hartmann's. (d) Conservative proctocolectomy.

RESTORATIVE PROCTOCOLECTOMY

Historical background

In 1947, Ravitch and Sabiston demonstrated that in both animals and humans it was possible to remove the rectal mucosa and leave denuded but functional rectal muscle. This mucosal proctectomy could be followed by creation of an ileoanal anastomosis, pulling the ileum through the rectal muscle cuff and sewing it to the modified skin of the anal canal. Ravitch performed this operation in two young adults with ulcerative colitis, who were subsequently continent. Although the technique was tried by a number of other surgeons over the following decade, the procedure never gained widespread acceptance because of operative complications, incontinence, intolerable frequency, and perianal dermatitis. However, the considerable success of mucosal proctectomy and pull-through procedures for children with Hirschsprung's disease tempted some paediatric surgeons to try a similar approach in young patients suffering from ulcerative colitis, with encouraging results.

A better understanding of the mechanisms of normal continence and defecation, together with the introduction of the Kock pouch, were the stimuli for the development of the pelvic ileal reservoir. The use of a single narrow tube of ileum as a replacement for rectum resulted in very poor reservoir function. Parks and colleagues introduced a pelvic triple-loop ileal reservoir, which was sewn to the anus after mucosal proctectomy. Utsunomiya in Japan and Fonkalsrud in the United States developed similar procedures shortly afterwards.

Parks' original operation has undergone considerable modifications since it was first described. Several of these, together with other important issues surrounding restorative proctocolectomy, are discussed below.

The plane of rectal dissection

Many patients suffering from ulcerative colitis are young and sexually active. Preservation of the pelvic nerves, and in particular the nervi erigentes, is of great importance. Early proctocolectomy was associated with a 10 per cent incidence of impotence, but adoption of a perimuscular plane for rectal dissection reduced the incidence of this complication to below 0.5 per cent. Similar results have been achieved by dissection in the avascular plane around the mesorectum posteriorly and laterally but close to the bowel wall anteriorly (Fig. 5). This technique is reported to be quicker and associated with less blood loss; it is widely used in North America. Formal comparison of the two methods and information on the relative incidences of sexual dysfunction are not available.

Pouch design

The pouch originally described by Parks and Nicholls was a triple-loop S pouch with a long efferent limb which emptied poorly and frequently required intubation to effect complete evacuation. This problem has been overcome by shortening the length of the efferent segment. A two-loop J pouch, four-loop W pouch, and lateral isoperistaltic or H pouch have also been described. These pouches can be hand-sewn or stapled and use approximately 40 to 50 cm of terminal ileum. The various designs are illustrated in Fig. 8; their function is compared below. Figure 9 shows a triplicated S pouch *in situ* in the pelvis.

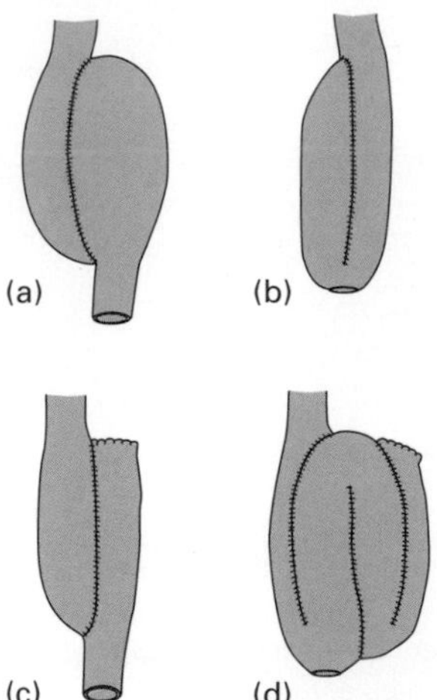

Fig. 8 The four pouch designs. The J and W pouches are most often used now. (a) Triplicated or S. (b) Duplicated or J. (c) Lateral or isoperistaltic. (d) Four-loop or W.

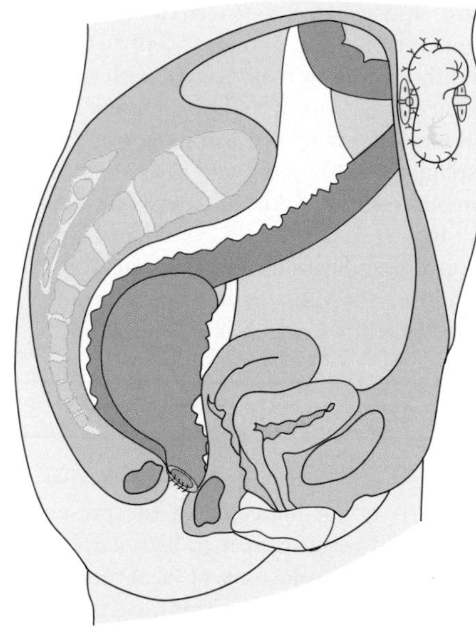

Fig. 9 Triplicated S pouch in the pelvis with a covering loop ileostomy. Care has to be taken not to make the efferent limb too long in this design.

The ileal pouch–anal anastomosis

Is mucosectomy necessary?

When restorative proctocolectomy was first introduced, the rectum was transected 10 cm above the pelvic floor and the mucosa striped off the underlying muscle by a tedious endoanal dissection up from the dentate line. This achieved the aim of excising all potentially diseased mucosa, but also removed the anal transitional zone, an area of cuboidal rather than columnar mucosa which extends for approximately 1.5 cm above the dentate line and has a rich sensory nerve supply.

The rectal muscle cuff has not been shown to be essential for the appreciation of pouch fullness; indeed it may increase the incidence of pelvic sepsis if left in place. On the other hand, the anal transitional zone is thought to play an important role in sensory discrimination as well as incontinence. The postoperative functional results of restorative proctocolectomy are better if this mucosa is preserved. However, there is a long-term risk from leaving behind potentially diseased mucosa and retention of the anal transition zone is not universally accepted. Pathological changes suggestive of ulcerative colitis have been found in anal canal mucosa from patients undergoing proctocolectomy. Even more worrying are reports of dysplasia and adenocarcinoma in this zone. In Oxford, no dysplasia has been found in a review of over 50 consecutive specimens, and clinical carcinoma arising in this area in patients with long-standing ulcerative colitis is virtually unheard of.

Based on the current balance of information, O'Connell and Williams advise against mucosectomy in the absence of rectal mucosal dysplasia. However, mucosectomy should be carried out if rectal dysplasia is diagnosed preoperatively or is found on subsequent histological examination of the surgical specimen which must, for this reason, be meticulous. Figure 10 illustrates the possible levels of ileoanal anastomosis.

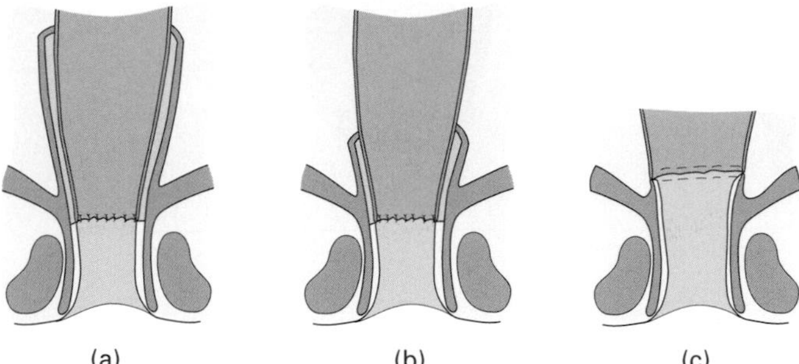

Fig. 10 The evolution of the ileoanal anastomosis from a long muscle cuff and mucosectomy (a), short muscle cuff and mucosectomy (b), and flush transection at the pelvic floor without mucosectomy and preserving the anal transitional zone (ATZ) (c).

A sutured or stapled anastomosis?

The question of whether the ileoanal anastomosis should be hand-sutured or stapled is less controversial. Minor defects in continence are not uncommon after manual endoanal anastomosis. Such deficiencies may be caused by retraction and dilatation injury to the anal sphincters at the time of operation. Certainly, impaired internal sphincter function has been noted. It was hoped that circular stapling devices would improve continence, as they produce minimal mechanical sphincter damage. However, objective evidence suggests that a significant fall in internal anal sphincter activity still occurs after stapled anastomosis, although the cause of this problem remains obscure. The only demonstrable improvement in pouch–anal function after stapling the anastomosis is a reduction in nocturnal evacuation. However, stapling devices do have the advantage of speed and can produce a great saving in time if used throughout the operation (Fig. 11). Four-loop W reservoirs cannot be constructed easily with staplers.

Is a temporary ileostomy always needed?

Until quite recently, all authors agreed that the reservoir and ileoanal anastomosis should be temporarily defunctioned with a loop ileostomy. This accepted practice has now been challenged. If the surgeon is familiar with the technique of pouch surgery, the operation is technically straightforward, and if the patient was not maintained on high-dose steroids preoperatively, the ileostomy can be omitted as, based on present evidence, this does not seem to be associated with additional morbidity. This avoids a subsequent surgical procedure which has its own attendant complications and which requires hospital admission.

Postoperative management and course

If a defunctioning ileostomy is formed, a period of 6 to 8 weeks is allowed to elapse before closure. If an ileostomy is omitted, the pouch is intubated with a wide-bore balloon catheter for at least 7 days to divert the faecal stream. The perianal region should be protected by barrier cream and a careful record must be kept of fluid balance. Patients can be allowed home 10 to 14 days postoperatively if they are well and confident. Early review is sensible in order to monitor and advise on pouch function. Constipating medication will reduce stool frequency in the first few months.

Very few deaths have been reported after restorative proctocolectomy, no doubt as a result of careful patient selection. However, there is appreciable morbidity which declines as the surgeon becomes increasingly familiar with the techniques involved. Pelvic sepsis, with or without anastomotic breakdown, develops in 8 to 25 per cent of cases and can be difficult to manage as it cannot drain freely. Healing by fibrosis can impair the eventual functional result. Adhesion obstruction also occurs frequently and further laparotomy is needed in up to 15 per cent of patients. Strictures are seen in 10 per cent of patients, but usually respond to simple dilatation. Fluid and electrolyte loss from the defunctioning ileostomy can produce a dehydration syndrome which may be exacerbated by steroid withdrawal.

Overall, 75 per cent of patients recover uneventfully and 25 per cent experience serious morbidity.

Functional results

Following restorative proctocolectomy, most patients defecate spontaneously about five to seven times every 24 h, and will be able to defer defecation without urgency. Few patients suffer frank incontinence, but minor imperfections such as spotting or soiling occur in up to 33 per cent during the day and 56 per cent at night. Some 20 per cent of patients use codeine phosphate or loperamide hydrochloride.

The determinants of ileoanal pouch function have recently been reviewed. The best clinical results are associated with a large capacity, compliant pouch which empties completely and which sits above normally active anal sphincters. Total daily stool volume, postoperative pelvic sepsis, and pouchitis are also important. Some evidence suggests that three and four-loop pouches produce the lowest stool frequency because they are more capacious than those formed from two loops of ileum. However, this is disputed. It is recognized that the pouch functions in part by modifying terminal ileum motility, but the relationship between this, capacity, and compliance remains unexplained.

Outright failure which requires pouch excision occurs in only 5 per cent of patients and is caused by persistent pelvic sepsis, undiagnosed Crohn's disease, or unacceptable stool frequency.

Long-term mucosal changes

The long-term health of the pouch mucosa is of more concern and has recently been the subject of extensive review. Early studies on Kock pouches showed chronic inflammation as well as villous atrophy, and similar changes are seen in most pelvic reservoirs. Colonic metaplasia has been noted on histological examination and is supported by studies using histochemical and immunological markers. The cause of these changes is not known, but probably involves bacteriological and immunological factors. The risk of future dysplasia and even frank malignancy cannot be ignored but, to date, no such occurrence has been reported in either a pelvic or a Kock pouch.

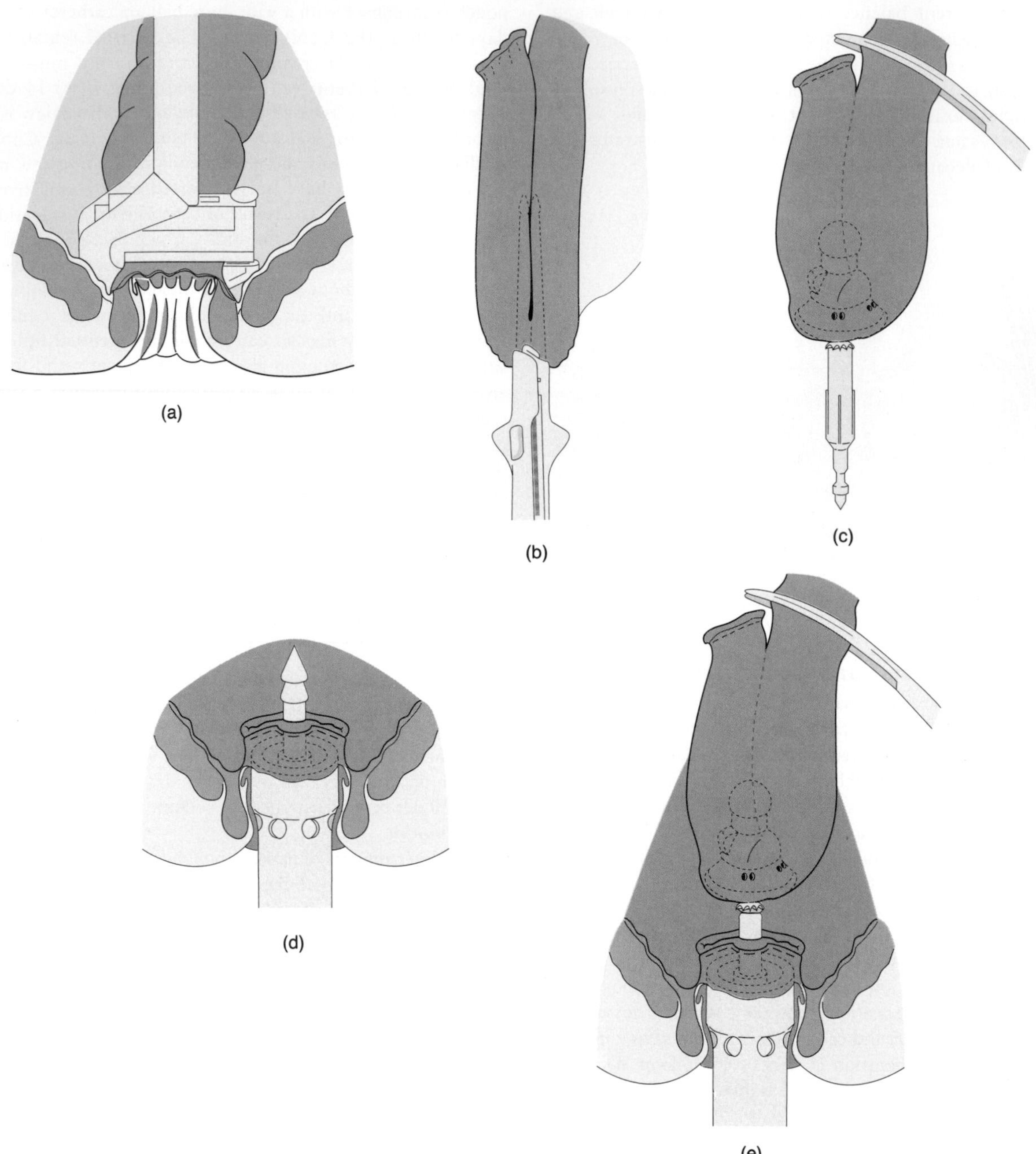

Fig. 11 Steps in the stapled construction of an ileoanal reservoir. (a) The rectum is transected at the top of the anal canal. (b) The two-loop reservoir is constructed. (c) An opening is made at the most dependent point in the pouch and the anvil shaft complex placed inside with a purse string. (d) The anastomosing gun is placed in the anal remnant and the trocar advanced. (e) The two parts of the anastomosing gun are docked and the stapled anastomosis completed.

More acute inflammatory changes also occur and can produce pouchitis—a condition which is characterized by diarrhoea in the presence of endoscopic and histological features of acute inflammation (Fig. 12). It has only been diagnosed unequivocally in patients who had ulcerative colitis, affecting between 10 and 20 per cent of those undergoing restorative proctocolectomy. Pouchitis is more common in patients who had extensive disease than in those whose colitis was left-sided or distal. The pathogenesis of pouchitis is not known and is almost certainly multifactorial. Contact between the pouch mucosa and ileal contents with stasis and bacterial overgrowth are essential features. The importance of genetic predisposition, the presence of specific bacterial strains, epithelial defects, and immunological abnormalities is uncertain, but these have all been implicated as causative agents. Outlet obstruction, pouch ischaemia, and Crohn's disease are important differential diagnoses which should be excluded.

In the absence of a controlled therapeutic trial, the treatment of pouchitis is empirical. Metronidazole is probably the most commonly used agent and may function as an immunosuppressive agent as well as an antibiotic. Enemas containing steroid or 5-

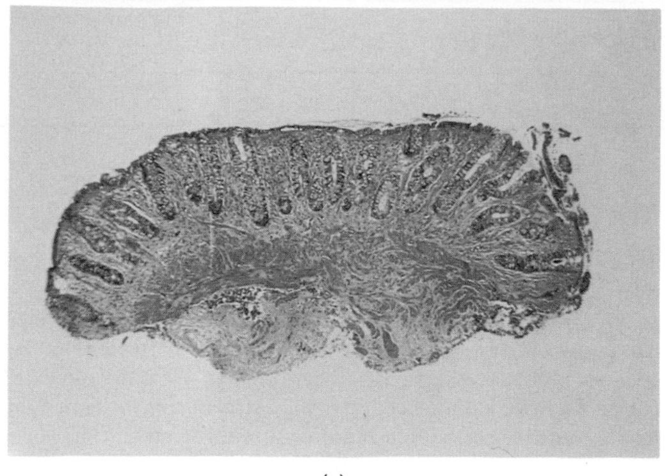

(a)

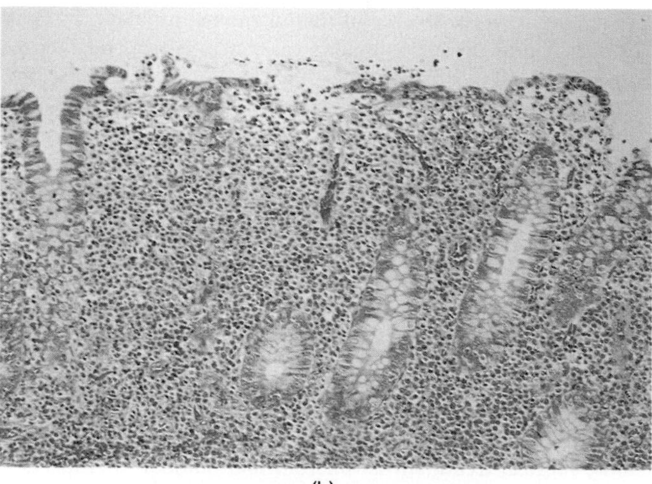

(b)

Fig. 12 (a) and (b) Photomicrograph showing the typical change which occurs in the pouch mucosa.

aminosalicylic acid derivatives, oral sulphasalazine, and short courses of oral steroids can also be used. Most episodes of pouchitis will resolve when treated with one or a combination of these agents. Very rarely, pouchitis is unresponsive and must be treated by the formation of a defunctioning ileostomy or even pouch excision.

Other long-term considerations

Almost all patients undergoing restorative proctocolectomy are satisfied with the outcome of their operation and over 90 per cent prefer the pouch to a permanent ileostomy because of increased self-confidence, cleanliness, sexual self-image, lack of interference with social and sports activities, and ease at work. Impaired sexual function is related to the proctocolectomy rather than the pouch.

No serious long-term nutritional sequelae have emerged after restorative proctocolectomy, but a mild microcytic anaemia associated with a low serum iron concentration is seen in up to 30 per cent of patients. Serum vitamin B_{12} levels may be marginally lowered but serum folate concentration is normal, and there is no abnormality of fat and fat-soluble vitamin absorption or of liver function.

FURTHER READING

Berry AR, De Campos R, Lee ECG. Perineal and pelvic morbidity following perimuscular excision of the rectum for inflammatory bowel disease. *Br J Surg* 1986; **73**: 675–7.

de Silva HJ, Kettlewell M, Mortensen NJ, Jewell DP. Acute inflammation in ileal pouches (pouchitis). *Eur J Gastroenterol Hepatol* 1991; **3**: 343–9.

Everett WG, Pollard SG. Restorative proctocolectomy without temporary ileostomy. *Br J Surg* 1990; **77**: 621–2.

Fazio V. W. The role of anastomosis for ulcerative colitis. In: Allan RN, *et al.* eds. *Inflammatory Bowel Disease*. Edinburgh: Churchill Livingstone, 1990; 433.

Fonkalsrud EW. Endorectal ileoanal anastomosis with isoperistaltic ileal reservoir after colectomy and mucosal proctectomy. *Ann Surg* 1984; **199**: 151–7.

Hulten L, Svaninger G. Facts about the continent iloesotomy. *Dis Colon Rect* 1984; **27**: 553–7.

Jewell DP. Medical management of severe ulcerative colitis. *Int J Colorectal Dis* 1988; **3**:186–9.

King DW, Lubowski DZ, Cook TA. Anal canal mucosa in restorative proctocolectomy for ulcerative colitis. *Br J Surg* 1989; **76**: 970–2.

Lennard-Jones JE, Ritchie JK, Hilder W, Spicer CC. Assessment of severity of colitis: a preliminary study. *Gut* 1975; **16**: 579–84.

Lennard-Jones JE, *et al.* Precancer and cancer in extensive ulcerative colitis: findings among 401 patients over 22 years. *Gut* 1990; **31**: 800–6.

Nicholls RJ, Lubowski DZ. Restorative proctocolectomy: the four loop (W) reservoir. *Br J Surg* 1987; **74**: 564–6.

O'Connell PR, Williams NS. Mucosectomy in restorative proctocolectomy. *Br J Surg* 1991; **78**: 129–30.

Parks AG, Nicholls RJ. Proctocolectomy without ileostomy for ulcerative colitis. *Br Med J* 1978; **ii**: 85–8.

Shepherd NA. The pelvic ileal reservoir: apocalypse later? *Br Med J* 1990; **ii**: 886–7.

Utsonomiya T, *et al.* Total colectomy, mucosal proctocolectomy and ileo anal anastomosis. *Dis Colon Rect* 1980; **23**: 459–66.

Watts JMcK, de Dombal FT, Goligher JC. Longterm complications and prognosis following major surgery for ulcerative colitis. *Br J Surg* 1966; **53**: 1014–23.

Williams NS. Restorative proctocolectomy is the first choice elective surgical treatment for ulcerative colitis. *Br J Surg* 1989; **76**: 1109–10.

18.2.5 Crohn's disease of the colon

NEIL MORTENSEN

CLINICAL FEATURES

These depend upon the site affected. There are three typical patterns. Small bowel disease usually affects the ileocaecal segment. The patient presents with colicky abdominal pain, diarrhoea, and weight loss (see Section 18.2.4). Colonic disease may present as colitis with bloody diarrhoea, urgency, and frequency, similar to that of ulcerative colitis. Discontinuous disease with fibrosis and stenosis may, however, cause diarrhoea without bleeding or colonic obstructive symptoms. Fistulation to adjacent organs may give rise to the distinct clinical feature of a colovesical or rectovaginal fistula. Ileocolic fistula between the ileum and the sigmoid colon is usually due to ileal disease. Colonic disease is secondary and may cause an increase in diarrhoea or no symptoms at all. Perianal disease is a particular feature of Crohn's disease: a chronic anal fissure may be the first presenting symptom.

INVESTIGATION

Barium enema may show areas of discontinuous disease. In patients with stricture (Fig. 1), in whom the diagnosis may be in doubt, a colonoscopy will show mucosal changes, and information from multiple biopsies will allow the exact distribution of disease to be documented (Fig. 2). Colonic stricture should be carefully investigated since it may indicate occult malignancy. Blood tests, including measurement of ESR or viscosity and C-reactive protein levels will give an indication of disease activity. Serum albumin levels indicate nutritional status.

MEDICAL MANAGEMENT

There are two clinical pictures which must be distinguished in the management of colonic Crohn's disease. Administration of steroids, and occasionally azathioprine, is appropriate treatment for disease flares, which give rise to mucosal ulceration and oedema. This treatment is similar to that used for ulcerative colitis. Fibrosis and thickening, with obstruction or formation of a fistula and an abscess often requires surgical treatment, however. Before surgery is undertaken nutritional status must be assessed. Patients with extensive gut disease or sepsis may be severely nutritionally depleted: serum albumin level and weight loss history are a rough guide to the degree of the nutritional problem. Intravenous nutrition or, in some suitable cases, nasoenteric feeding may be necessary.

INDICATIONS FOR SURGERY

As with small intestinal disease, the management of Crohn's disease of the colon is medical unless a specific complication is present (Table 1).

Specific surgical treatment for colonic disease

Although Crohn's disease of the colon may behave like ulcerative colitis, surgical treatment is different in a number of respects.

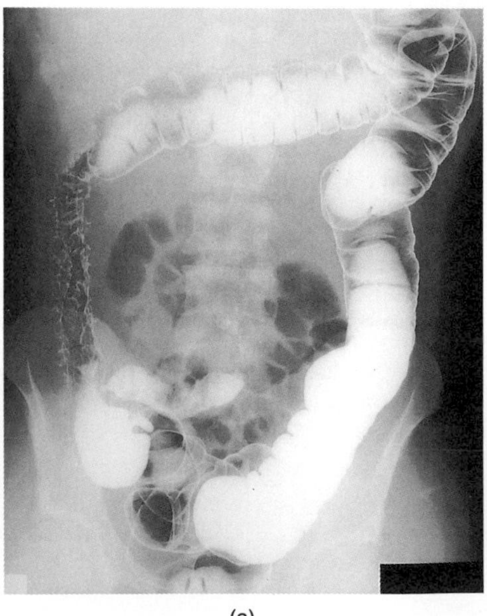

(a)

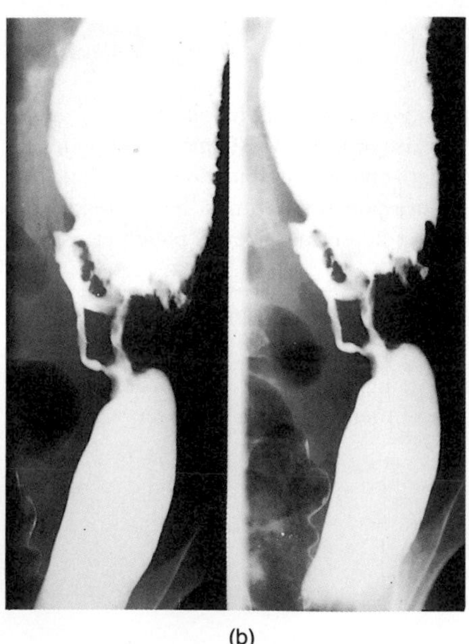

(b)

Fig. 1 Barium enema showing (a) a segment of Crohn's disease in the right colon with normal mucosa elsewhere. (b) Views of the left colon in a patient with colonic Crohn's disease. There is a stricture with fistulation.

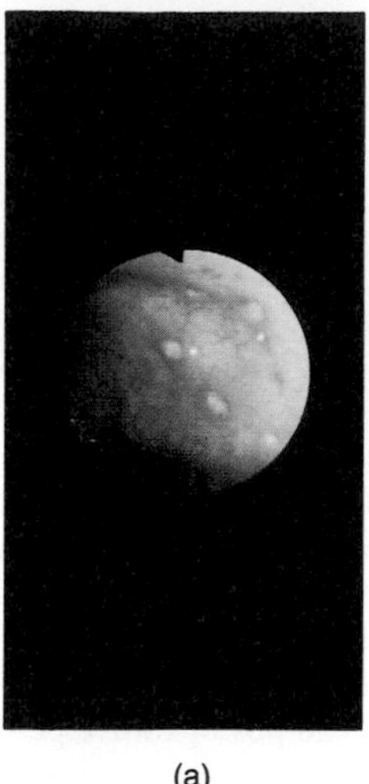

(a)

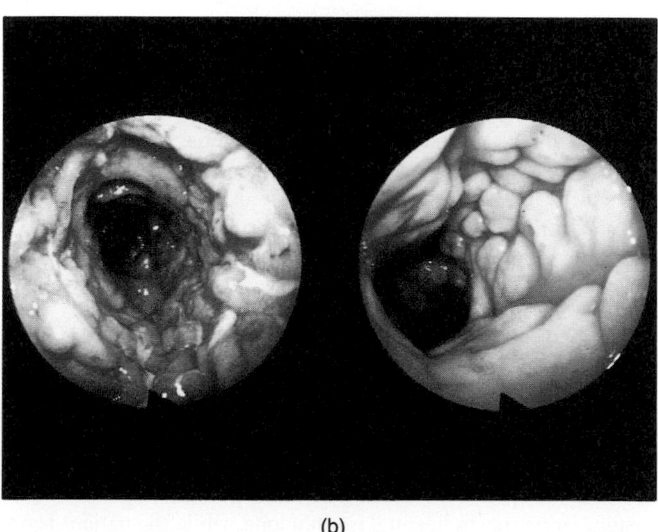

(b)

Fig. 2 (a) Colonoscopic appearance of early Crohn's disease with aphthous ulceration. (b) Colonoscopic appearance of severe Crohn's colitis.

Table 1 Complications of Crohn's disease

Dangerous acute complications
Perforation, dilatation
Severe haemorrhage
Chronic subacute complications
Abscess
Fistula
Obstruction
The failure of a severe acute attack of Crohn's colitis to respond to drug therapy
Chronic disability or ill health
Risk of developing carcinoma, though this is less common than in ulcerative colitis

Emergency surgery

The usual indication is acute fulminating Crohn's colitis with bleeding, toxic dilatation, or perforation. It is important to note that the perforation can occur without toxic dilatation. The procedure of choice is usually a subtotal colectomy with formation of an end ileostomy. A mucous fistula may be constructed initially if there is relative rectal sparing. Oversewing of the rectal stump at the level of the peritoneal reflection is advised only if the rectum is normal, since in the presence of active Crohn's disease there is the risk of breakdown and intra-abdominal sepsis. The formation of a mucus fistula also has the advantage of allowing topical steroid irrigation of the defunctioned distal rectum.

There is a limited place for primary resection and ileorectal anastomosis as an emergency procedure, for example in patients who are fit, in whom there is no pre-existing sepsis, and when the rectum is spared. If the operative field is contaminated, the risk of dehiscence, leakage, or fistula formation is high and it would be wise to employ a proximal loop ileostomy in these cases. The indications for a primary proctocolectomy in emergency situations are also limited. If there is severe bleeding from the rectum there may be no choice, but secondary rectal excision is best performed at a later date, when the patient's general condition has improved.

Use of an emergency defunctioning loop or split ileostomy should be considered. Defunctioning of diffuse or multiple site colonic disease may allow it to resolve, and in about one-third of patients gut continuity can be restored without resection. A loop ileostomy has the advantage that closure does not require a laparotomy, but the disadvantage that, unless constructed properly, overspill occurs and defunction of the distal bowel is not complete.

Following an emergency operation for Crohn's colitis the patient is usually left with a mucus fistula or oversewn rectal stump. Patients in whom restoration of intestinal continuity may be possible have to be carefully selected. An ileorectal anastomosis is only advised where there is rectal sparing, minimal small bowel disease, and quiescent anal disease. They must therefore be carefully investigated by a rectal examination, proctoscopy, and anal manometry. Continuing inflammation in the rectal stump can be due to defunction colitis as well as Crohn's disease, and this should be borne in mind when interpreting rectal biopsies.

Elective surgery

Segmental colectomy

In some patients with colonic Crohn's disease a single localized segment is affected, causing either a stricture, fistula, or abscess. It is reasonable to perform a limited resection with an immediate colocolonic anastomosis in these patients. This preserves macroscopically normal colonic tissue and may have a functional advantage in preserving colonic water handling. Allan *et al.* have reported their experience in 36 patients treated by segmental colectomy. The 10-year reoperative rate for recurrent disease was 66 per cent, compared with 53 per cent among patients undergoing subtotal colectomy and ileorectal anastomosis. There was no clinical evidence of an anastomotic leak in 29 patients, suggesting that the procedure can be safe.

Subtotal colectomy and ileorectal anastomosis

This is indicated in patients with severe diffuse colonic disease and rectal sparing. It is particularly indicated in younger patients, since it allows them to complete their education, start a career, and begin a family without the risk of sexual dysfunction or the disability associated with a stoma and perianal wound. This operation is contraindicated if the anal sphincter has been damaged as a result of previous perianal surgery or severe perianal disease, or if the patient has extensive rectal disease. In the presence of extensive small bowel disease, recurrence rates after ileorectal anastomosis may be high.

The majority of patients have a good functional result with an ileorectal anastomosis, provided that the reservoir function of the rectum can be maximized by anastomosis at the rectosigmoid junction. The majority of patients will have less than six bowel actions a day and troublesome diarrhoea is unusual. The worst functional outcome is seen in patients who have obvious macroscopic disease of the rectum.

The major early complication is anastomotic dehiscence, which occurs in between 5 and 30 per cent of patients. A covering loop ileostomy may reduce the incidence of this complication, although if this is thought necessary it may not be wise to perform the ileorectal anastomosis at all. The operative mortality ranges from 0 to 5 per cent. Recurrence rates are shown in Table 2: these seem to be higher than those in similar patients undergoing proctocolectomy and ileostomy.

Recurrence of disease does not always mean that a proctocolectomy and ileostomy is inevitable. Recurrence at the ileorectal anastomosis can be dealt with medically or by a further resection and ileorectal anastomosis.

Total colectomy with formation of an end ileostomy and mucous fistula

Total colectomy with formation of an end ileostomy and a mucous fistula or oversewing of the rectal stump has the advantage of safety and reduces the risk of recurrence proximal to an anastomosis. The recurrence rates in the ileum and ileostomy are similar to those seen after a proctocolectomy. The main indication is as an emergency procedure for severe colitis, but subsequent restoration of continuity is often not possible. This operation can also be used for the treatment of severe proctitis or severe perianal disease in patients likely to suffer delayed perianal wound healing or persistent perineal sinus. Continuing sepsis in the perineum, however, often means that the rectal stump has to be removed later. Operative mortality is of the order of 8 per cent and recurrence proximal to the stoma in the ileum is 13 per cent over 10 years.

Total proctocolectomy

This is indicated for extensive colonic disease involving the rectum, with or without perianal disease. It is also indicated in patients with severe anorectal disease, even in the presence of an apparently normal upstream colon. Recurrence rates in the proximal colon and the problem of a liquid flush end colostomy are considerable. A permanent end ileostomy is therefore preferable.

The incidence of stomal dysfunction is high. Complications associated with the stoma include retraction, prolapse, fistula formation, and obstruction. Most of these can be managed by local revision, but in the presence of recurrent Crohn's disease, laparotomy and resection is often necessary.

There is a high incidence of delayed perianal wound healing with resulting long-term morbidity and a persistent perianal sinus. Healing rates are slower if the wound is left open than is the case in patients treated with suture and suction drainage. Healing rates range from 63 per cent by 12 weeks to 33 per cent by 6 months. If there is faecal contamination and the risk of sepsis is high, the perineal wound should be left open. Perianal wounds which show delayed or non-healing are associated with high fistula in ano, faecal contamination, and postoperative perineal wound infection.

Management of the unhealed perineal wound

Management should be conservative initially, but if after a few months the perineal wound is recurrently discharging or has exuberant granulation tissue around the sinus it should be explored. Primary causes of long-term failure to heal include a foreign body such as a stitch, a pilonidal sinus, hydradenitis, an enteroperineal fistula, retained rectal mucosa, and malignancy. A large number of procedures have been suggested, such as currettage, suture and excision, muscle grafting, and skin grafting; all are associated with a variable success rate.

Other problems

A significant number of patients develop urinary and sexual dysfunction as a result of nerve injury and perineal fibrosis. The incidence can be reduced by a perimuscular excision of the rectum and an intersphincteric excision of the anus.

Proctocolectomy is associated with the lowest recurrence rate but it has an operative mortality of between 3 and 9 per cent. The postoperative stay in hospital is often long, while the patient learns to care for their stoma, and also due to delayed perineal wound healing. Recurrence rates following proctocolectomy are about half of those seen after restorative surgery (see Table 2). Recurrent disease is usually located in the distal ileum.

Proctectomy

In a small proportion of patients with Crohn's disease only the rectum is involved, often associated with severe perianal disease. If the disease cannot be controlled medically a permanent end colostomy may be suitable for selected patients. Particular indi-

Table 2 Recurrence rates after resection of colonic Crohn's disease

Study	Length of follow-up (years)		Recurrence rate after proctocolectomy (%)			Recurrence rate after colectomy and ileorectal anastomosis (%)			Recurrence rate after segmental colectomy (%)		
	Range	Mean	*n*	5 years	10 years	*n*	5 years	10 years	*n*	5 years	10 years
New Haven	–	8.5	34	27	40	–	–	–	–	–	–
Cleveland	–	11.5	127	13	28	–	–	–	–	–	–
St Mark's	1–28	9.5	107	5	10	40	38	56	–	–	–
Leeds	7–25	15	162	10	15	45	52	60	–	–	–
Birmingham	–	–	74	19	24	63	28	43	–	–	–
Birmingham	0–37	15–5	–	–	–	63	33	53	36	48	65

cations for this procedure include a high fistula or rectovaginal fistula, together with narrow anorectal strictures. Problems of perineal wound healing should be borne in mind, together with the difficulty in managing a liquid colostomy experienced by some patients.

External faecal diversion

Faecal diversion (loop ileostomy) has been advocated by the Oxford group as an alternative to conventional surgical management in the following circumstances.

1. To achieve colonic healing and allow intestinal continuity to be restored without resection where the disease is diffuse but not severe enough to warrant a proctocolectomy.
2. To facilitate major resection in those with poor health.
3. To limit resection in patients with diffuse disease.
4. To avoid growth retardation in children with diffuse colitis requiring colectomy.
5. To protect or avoid a primary anastomosis, and after small bowel resection in patients with persistent colonic disease.
6. In the management of refractory perianal disease as a means of delaying or even preventing proctocolectomy.

It is associated with a high incidence of early disease remission.

A limited number of patients are suitable for this form of management. The percentage of patients in whom intestinal continuity can be restored varies from over 60 per cent to less than 30 per cent, and relapse after restoration of continuity ranges from 28 to 60 per cent. Nevertheless, a proximal loop ileostomy is a relatively minor procedure and in the debilitated patient may buy time before definitive surgery is contemplated.

PERIANAL DISEASE

Over 50 per cent of patients with Crohn's disease have anal lesions; these are most common in those with rectal disease. Fissure in ano is the most common lesion and may be asymptomatic. Such a fissure can heal with medical management or may become chronic and the site of subsequent fistula formation, probably by distorting anal glands. These fissures are often painless, but if there is an associated submucosal or intersphincteric abscess pain is so severe that proximal defunction is necessary (Fig. 3a). Anal surgery for fissure should be avoided as far as possible. A fistula in ano may develop either directly as a result of Crohn's disease or

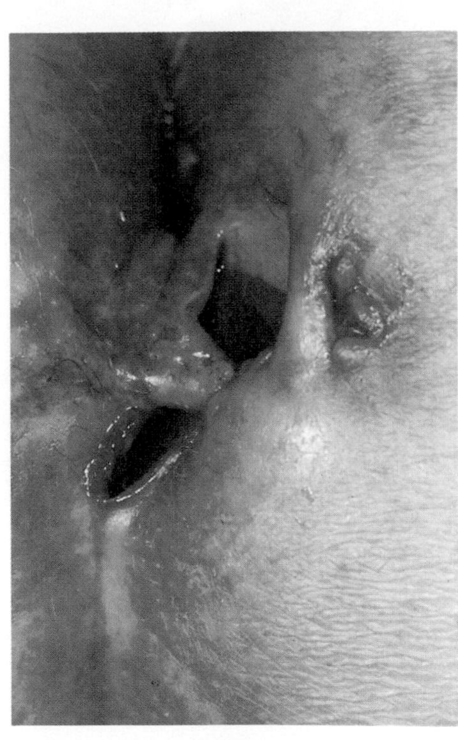

(a)

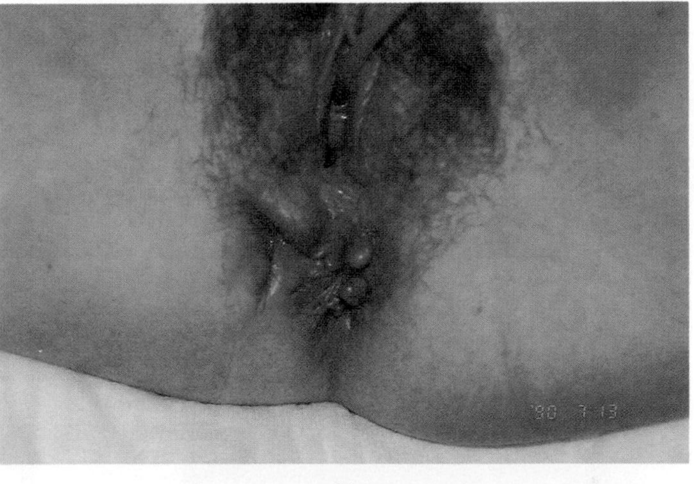

(b)

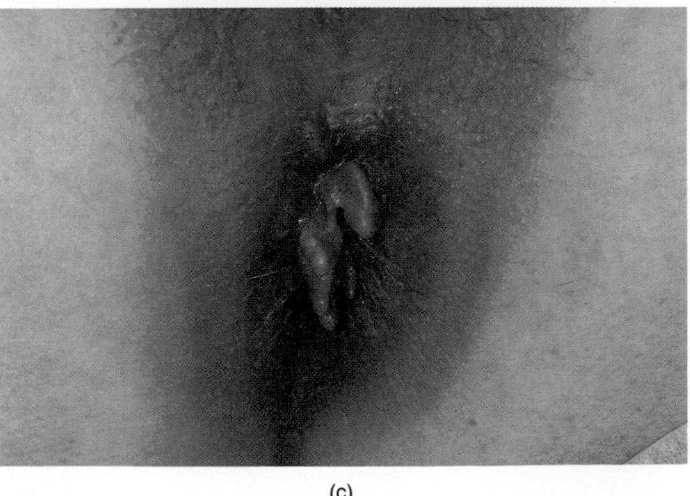

(c)

Fig. 3 Typical appearances of perianal Crohn's disease. (a) Deep perianal ulceration; (b) perineal fistulae; (c) large oedematous skin tags.

Table 3 Perianal lesions in patients with Crohn's disease

Perianal lesions	Secondary lesions	Incidental lesions
Anal fissure	Skin tags	Piles
Ulcerated oedematous pile	Anal/rectal stricture	Perianal abscess/fistula
Cavitating ulcer	Anovaginal/rectovaginal fistula	Cryptitis
	Carcinoma	

secondary to its effect upon the anal gland anatomy; fistulae are sometimes multiple and complex (Fig. 3(b)). Associated abscesses have to be drained but every attempt should be made to conserve any sphincter muscle. The key note to management is to be conservative.

Medical management

Since many of these fistulae are asymptomatic or only intermittently symptomatic, treatment with metronidazole, steroids, and occasionally azathioprine can have dramatic effects on control of progress of disease, provided that no undrained pus is present.

Surgical management

Proper assessment is difficult in the clinic and symptomatic patients should undergo an examination under anaesthesia. Fistula tracts are carefully probed and curretted; if associated abscesses cannot be drained without division of muscle a seton can be left in place, often for many weeks or months, to control symptoms. A long-term indwelling seton functioning as a drain can often prevent or delay the need for proctectomy. I usually use a 2-mm diameter coloured plastic vessel loop tied loosely rather than tightly (Fig. 4). If the disease is progressive or fails to respond to conservative management despite repeated examinations under anaesthesia it is worth considering a proximal diversion (see above). Proctectomy is necessary for the treatment of severe disease unresponsive to conservative therapy. Bear in mind that longstanding fistula in ano may undergo malignant change in patients with Crohn's disease.

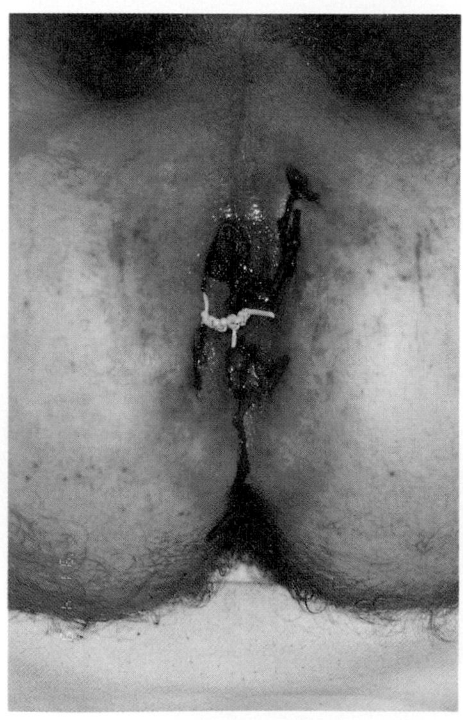

Fig. 4 Perianal disease managed with a seton.

RECTOVAGINAL FISTULA

These may be quiescent, but can be very troublesome (Fig. 5). Asymptomatic patients need no treatment, and low fistulae can be laid open. A chronic indwelling seton can be used for drainage, as for perianal fistula, and where there is no severe rectal disease or proximal disease, repair of a fistula by a vaginal flap can be successful. Patients with intractable disease and those developing incontinence require a proctectomy.

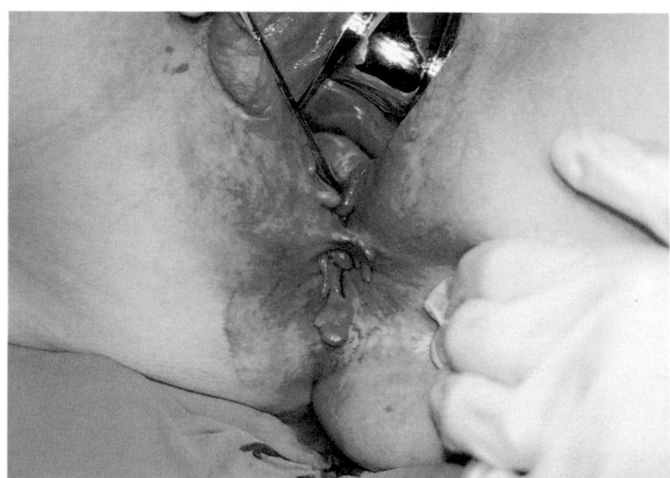

Fig. 5 Rectovaginal fistula complicating perianal Crohn's disease.

HAEMORRHOIDS

Great care must be taken in treating haemorrhoids in patients with Crohn's disease. A haemorrhoidectomy should be avoided as far as possible; symptoms will generally settle spontaneously or following local steroid applications (Table 2).

FURTHER READING

Allan A, Andrews H, Hilton CJ, Keighley MRB, Allan RN, Alexander Williams J. Segmental colonic resection is an appropriate operation for short skip lesions due to Crohn's disease in the colon. *World J Surg* 1989; **13**: 611–16.

Lee ECG. Surgery for Crohn's disease. *Gut* 1984; **25**: 217.

Williams JG, Wong WD, Rothenberger DA, Goldberg SM. Recurrence of Crohn's disease after resection. *Br J Surg* 1991; **78**: 10–19.

18.2.6 Pseudomembranous colitis

NEIL MORTENSEN AND TERENCE O'KELLY

This diarrhoeal illness, of variable severity, is caused by *Clostridium difficile*. The condition derives its name from yellowish-white plaques which are found throughout the colon and rectum in its severe form.

AETIOLOGY

Pseudomembranous colitis is caused by a cytotoxin produced by *C. difficile*, a Gram-positive, anaerobic, spore-forming bacillus. The bacterium is not normally present in the colon and infection only occurs in individuals with diminished resistance to colonization. Although pseudomembranous colitis has been reported in patients with chronic obstruction and in association with cancer chemotherapy, it most commonly occurs as a complication of antibiotic treatment, especially in patients with diminished host resistance. All antibiotics in common medical use have been reported to precipitate pseudomembranous colitis; the link is strongest with lincomycin, clindamycin, ampicillin, amoxycillin, and cephalosporins.

HISTOPATHOLOGY

This is an acute, exudative, inflammatory process. If present, plaques are multiple but not confluent, 2 to 5 mm in diameter, and they adhere to the underlying mucosa. Microscopically, they consist of fibrin, mucous, polymorphs, and epithelial debris (Fig. 1).

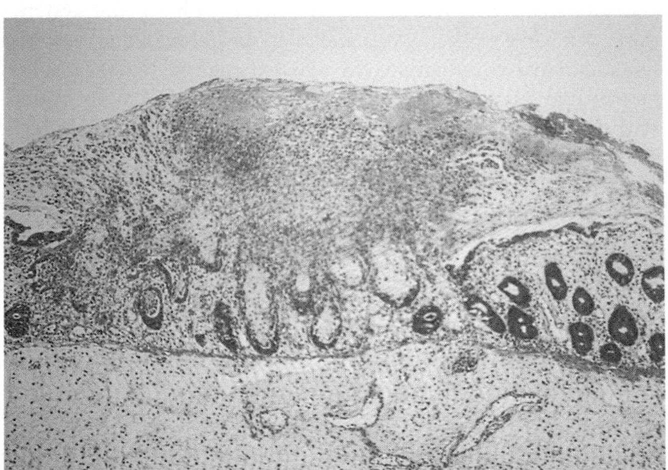

Fig. 1 Rectal biopsy showing a 'pseudomembrane' consisting of fibrin, mucous, polymorphs, and epithelial debris (×40).

CLINICAL FEATURES

The most common presenting features are watery diarrhoea of variable severity and a low grade fever. These can occur from 2 days to 3 weeks after antibiotic treatment, including antibiotic chemoprophylaxis before surgical procedures. Colicky abdominal pain, bloody diarrhoea, and toxic megacolon are recognized but infrequent complications. Sigmoidoscopy usually discloses rectal plaques in severely affected patients. The mucosa between plaques appears normal.

Diagnosis is established by demonstrating the presence of *C. difficile* toxin in the stools of symptomatic individuals. The organism can be cultured and its presence may be demonstrated in the absence of measurable toxin production. Under these circumstances, alternative diagnoses should be considered and these are outlined in Table 1.

Table 1 The differential diagnoses which should be considered in cases of suspected pseudomembranous colitis

Non-specific inflamatory bowel disease
Ulcerative colitis
Crohn's disease
Specific inflammatory bowel disease
Infections
Salmonella
Shigella
Campylobacter
Entamoeba histolytica
Ischaemia

TREATMENT

Fluid and electrolyte resuscitation should be instituted if necessary, and urgent surgical opinion sought in patients with toxic megacolon in whom perforation is imminent or has actually occurred. Otherwise, pseudomembranous colitis is managed conservatively. Symptomatic patients whose stools contain *C. difficile* toxin, should be treated with oral metronidazole 250 mg or vancomycin 125 mg every 6 h. If possible, other antibiotics should be withdrawn. In addition, barrier nursing is required to prevent spread of the organism to other patients, as it is highly contagious. Clinical improvement should be noted within 48 h, but relapse may occur, due to either reinfection or the failure of initial treatment to eradicate the bacteria completely.

Treatment is not recommended if toxin production cannot be demonstrated, despite positive *C. difficile* cultures. Antibiotic therapy may be instituted in spite of this if a patient is symptomatic and other causes of diarrhoea have been excluded.

FURTHER READING

Burdon DW. Bacterial infections: Clostridia and gastrointestinal disease. *Curr Opin Gastroenterol* 1987; 3: 127–9.

Keighley MRB, Burdon DW. Pseudomembranous colitis. In: Marston A, ed. *Vascular Disease of the Gut*. London: Edward Arnold, 1986; 86–102.

18.2.7 Ischaemic colitis

TERENCE O'KELLY AND NEIL MORTENSEN

Ischaemic colitis is an inflammatory condition produced by interruption of the blood supply to the colon insufficient to cause full thickness tissue death. It most commonly affects those in the sixth to the eighth decades of life and is thus being seen with increasing frequency in our progressively elderly population.

AETIOLOGY

Ischaemic colitis may be caused by occlusion of a major artery, small vessel disease, venous obstruction, 'low flow' states, or intestinal obstruction (Fig. 1). In each case, the mucosa and submucosa are predominantly affected, the extent of injury being determined by the severity and longevity of the insult. Ischaemia reduces the integrity of the mucosa and allows invasion by pathogenic organisms such as clostridia, which are normal constituents of colonic flora. These processes produce inflammation and mucosal ulceration which may resolve completely. Alternatively the insult can result in permanent injury with healing by fibrosis and subsequent stricture formation. Rarely, necrotizing colitis develops, which can spread to affect areas of the colon which are not ischaemic.

Although any part of the colon can be affected, the splenic flexure is particularly susceptible to ischaemic injury because it is the site of the watershed between the superior mesenteric artery, supplying the transverse colon, and the inferior mesenteric artery which supplies the descending colon. These vessels are linked by a marginal artery, but this is frequently absent or poorly developed at the splenic flexure. Occlusion of either major artery or their feeding branches (middle colic artery from the superior mesenteric artery and left colic artery from the inferior mesenteric artery) can therefore result in ischaemia. This point is of particular relevance during aortic and colorectal surgery if the inferior mesenteric artery is ligated. During aortic surgery it is important to confirm pulsatile flow in the superior mesenteric and marginal arteries prior to ligating a patent inferior mesenteric artery. If this is absent or if doubt exists then the inferior mesenteric artery should be reimplanted into the graft.

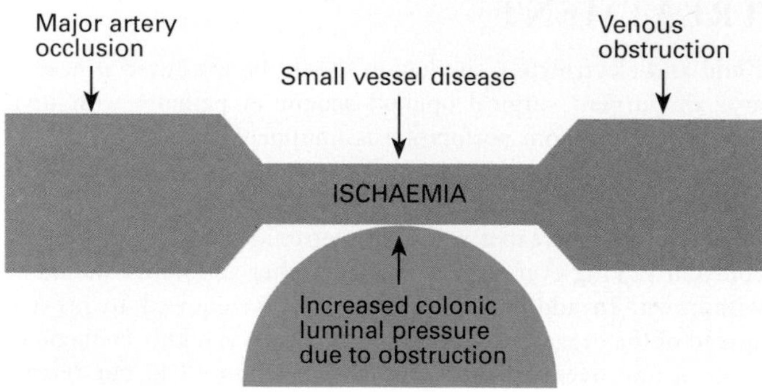

Major artery occlusion
- Thrombosis
- Embolism
- Trauma
- Iatrogenic

Small vessel disease
- Polyarteritis nodosum
- Systemic lupus erythemotosus
- Buerger's disease
- Rheumatoid arthritis
- Diabetes mellitus
- Radiation

Low flow
- Cardiogenic
- Hypovolaemic
- Iatrogenic

Venous obstruction
- Widespread thrombosis
- Oral contraceptive pill

Fig. 1 Aetiological factors responsible for ischaemic colitis.

CLINICAL FEATURES

History

A typical patient is 50 years of age or more and complains of left-sided abdominal pain which is acute in onset and started in the left iliac fossa. Loose stools, which characteristically contain dark blood as well as clots, may be passed. There may be a history of previous similar episodes, or of peripheral or cardiovascular disease, or collagen vascular disease, especially if the symptoms are atypical.

Examination

As ischaemic colitis is predominantly a disorder of colonic mucosa and submucosa it is not usually associated with a major systemic upset, but a low grade pyrexia and tachycardia should be expected. On abdominal examination, the affected colon is tender and may be palpable. Dark blood will be present *per rectum*. Signs of peripheral vascular disease or other associated conditions should be sought.

INVESTIGATION

It is important to first establish the diagnosis and then determine the presence of any treatable aetiological factors.

Radiological investigations

A plain abdominal radiograph and a contrast enema are the most useful investigations in the initial stages of this disorder. 'Thumbprinting' is diagnostic and is most often seen at the splenic flexure (Fig. 2). It is present at an early stage (from 3 days) and is the result of submucosal oedema and haemorrhage which produce swellings that project into the bowel lumen. These are clearly seen in contrast studies.

Later, mucosal ulceration and irregularity may develop and these can resemble the appearances of ulcerative colitis or Crohn's disease. However, ulcerative colitis invariably affects the rectum and there is loss of the normal colonic haustral pattern while in Crohn's disease deep ulcers resemble 'rose thorns' and areas of

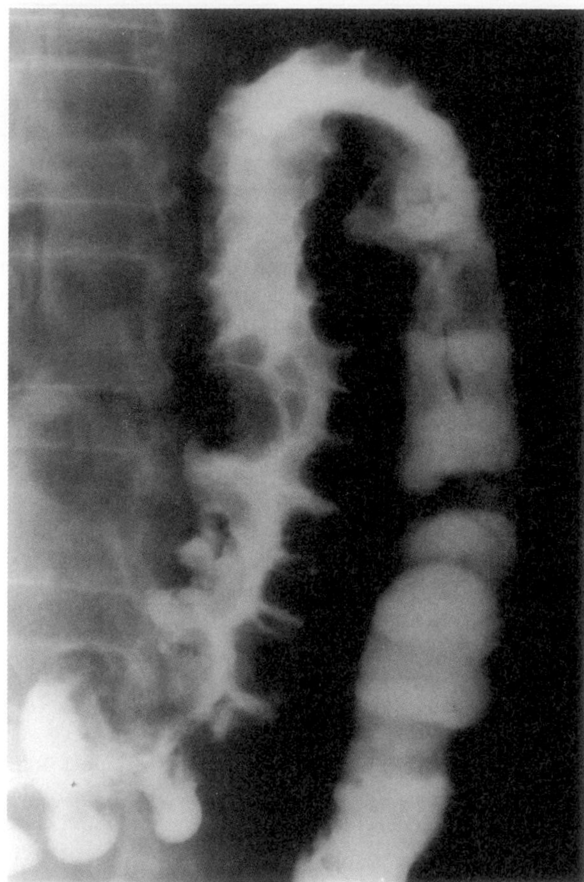

Fig. 2 A barium enema showing the typical 'thumb printing' sign of ischaemic colitis. Note that this is most marked at the splenic flexure. The appearances are the result of oedematous mucosal folds caused by ischaemia.

affected colon are separated by normal bowel. These features are not seen in ischaemic colitis.

Although many of the features of ischaemic colitis are reversible, stricture formation, if it occurs, is not and causes further diagnostic problems. Ischaemic strictures are often long, uniform and have smooth, gradual beginnings and ends, an appearance called 'funnelling'. However, these findings do not exclude carcinoma; this diagnosis should be considered, particularly if only a short segment of colon is affected. The role of angiography is not established. Although it can be valuable in isolated cases where significant, symptomatic occlusive lesions are revealed, there is generally no correlation between the appearance of vessels at angiography and the integrity of the colonic blood supply.

Endoscopy

Ischaemic lesions are usually beyond the reach of the rigid sigmoidoscope, but colonoscopy can be used to visualize and biopsy affected colon. In the early stages of ischaemia, the mucosa will be heaped up, oedematous, and bluish purple (the 'thumbprints' seen radiologically). It will bleed on contact with the endoscope or other instruments. Later, ulceration as well as strictures may be seen.

DIFFERENTIAL DIAGNOSIS

The differential diagnosis is outlined in Table 1. It should be noted that some of these diagnoses, for example carcinoma, are also possible aetiological factors for ischaemic colitis.

TREATMENT

This will be determined by the mode of presentation, which in turn reflects the underlying stage of the ischaemic process. Conservative management is the mainstay of treatment for those seen with acute symptoms. The patient is rested in bed and given intravenous fluids. Broad-spectrum antibiotics are often administered, although there is no conclusive evidence to suggest that they influence outcome. There is no place for anticoagulation or steroid administration unless this is indicated by an underlying disorder such as vasculitis.

It is very rare for ischaemic colitis to progress to frank colonic gangrene, but all patients should be monitored frequently to assess progress. If the injury is transient then resolution occurs after a few days to a week. More severe insults lead to stricture formation. These require investigation and treatment if they produce symptoms or if there is diagnostic doubt. Excision followed by end-to-end anastomosis is safe, although it is essential to ensure the viability and vascularity of the resection margins. If malignancy is excluded, then the resection can be limited to the affected segment but a more radical excision should be performed if there is continuing diagnostic uncertainty.

Table 1 Ischaemic colitis: differential diagnosis

Disorders of the gastrointestinal tract	
Inflammatory bowel disease	
Non-specific	Ulcerative colitis
	Crohn's colitis
Specific	Pseudomembranous colitis
	Amoebic dysentery
	Bacillary dysentery
	Others, e.g. Campylobacter infection
Carcinoma	
Diverticular disease	
Pancreatitis	
Disorders outside the gastrointestinal tract	
e.g. Urinary calculus	
Urinary sepsis	
Gynaecological sepsis	
Abdominal aortic or iliac artery aneurysm	

FURTHER READING

Marston A. Vascular disease of the colon. In: Marston A, ed. *Vascular Disease of the Gut*. London: Edward Arnold, 1986: 158–70.

18.3 Colorectal cancer and benign tumours of the colon

M. G. W. KETTLEWELL

Cancer of the colon and rectum is the second most common cancer after lung cancer in the Western world, though it is less common than gastric cancer worldwide. It therefore contributes considerably to morbidity and mortality in Western societies. Until the last decade treatment had been limited to excisional surgery; the generally poor outcome showed little sign of improving.

New information from epidemiological studies, molecular biology, and imaging, together with surgical innovations and trials of adjuvant therapy offer possibilities for preventing some cancers, diagnosing others earlier, and improving both quality and duration of survival for the majority of patients while avoiding unnecessary mutilation for those with no prospect of cure. A thorough understanding of the disease and the options for management are therefore more necessary than ever.

EPIDEMIOLOGY

The incidence of large bowel cancer varies between and within countries, which strongly suggests an environmental cause. The incidence is almost equal between the sexes, with some differences in risk ratio for cancers of different parts of the large bowel. Rectal cancers are twice as common among men but for the rest of the large bowel the male : female ratio is about 0.8 : 1 with right-sided cancers even more common in women.

The incidence of bowel cancer is high in the urban 'western' world but is rare in Asia, Africa, and parts of South America (Table 1). There are also apparent geographical differences in incidence within countries. For example the incidence is higher in Scotland than in England, and higher in northern Italy and the northern United States than in the southern parts of the same countries. This mirrors changes in incidence of coronary heart disease. This north/south divide is not a fundamental association with latitude: the incidence of bowel cancer among the Finns and the Eskimos is low, suggesting the differences are more likely to be due to differences in social and dietary behaviour, perhaps induced by climatic changes. The incidence is also different among different cultural groups within countries, for example, 18/100 000 white South Africans have colonic cancer while the incidence amongst their black compatriots is about 6/100 000. The proportions in New Zealand whites and Maoris are similarly 3 : 1, though the incidence is about twice that of South Africa.

Table 1 Approximate incidence per 100 000 people

Africa	2
Asia	15
South America	15
West Europe	40
USA	35

These differences in incidence among racial groups and within different areas of countries suggest that genetic or cultural factors are dominant in the genesis of the tumours. However, several studies of different religious and cultural groups who live in the same place but who have different lifestyles, have shown that environmental and cultural differences are mainly responsible for the variable incidence of large bowel cancer. Furthermore, migrants, such as the Japanese moving to the United States via Hawaii, show the cancer incidence of their adopted country within a generation. Colon cancer is also more common in urban areas, for example in Hong Kong, Singapore, and urban Brazil. Lifestyle therefore appears a more important factor in causing colon cancer for whole populations than geography or genetic make-up. However, individuals or families may also have a strong genetic predisposition to develop colon cancer.

The peak incidence for the disease is in the seventh decade, some 5 years later than the corresponding peak for colonic adenomatous polyps, which suggests that prolonged exposure to weak environmental carcinogens is necessary to induce tumours and that most, possibly all, pass through the benign phase before turning malignant. The epidemiology of proximal and distal or rectal cancer is not the same worldwide. The ratio of rectal to colonic cancer varies from 1 : 3 in white South African males to 1 : 1 in Finns and Maoris. There is also some evidence that right-sided cancers are becoming more common in the United Kingdom and the United States of America which suggests that there are qualitative differences in the aetiology of cancers at each end of the colon.

AETIOLOGY AND PATHOGENESIS

Genetic factors

The epidemiological evidence so far suggests that environmental factors predominate in the genesis of large bowel cancer within populations, but it would be surprising if inherited genetic factors did not play a numerically small yet important role in the formation of some colon cancers (see also Section 42.1).

Colonic cancers, in common with all other tumours, show qualitative and often quantitative changes in the chromosomes when compared to normal cells. Many colon cancer cell lines show chromosome distortion, with trisomy of some or many chromosomes, sometimes to the point of aneuploidy. There is evidence to suggest that tumours with a poor prognosis have a more bizarre chromosomal configuration with a greater proportion of aneuploid cells.

Many cancers also express oncogenes of various types, in particular the *ras* and *myc* classes. Oncogenes were first identified in RNA viruses capable of inducing cancers, but it is likely that these 'viral oncogenes' found in colon cancers are an expression of part of the normal cellular genetic material responsible for growth and not a new viral infection. Growth genes are counterbalanced by genes responsible for restricting growth and perhaps inducing differentiation. These apparently viral genomes were probably incorporated into the genomes of animals very early in evolution, in much the same way that symbiotic intracellular organisms became mitochondria. It is self-evident that very local environmental changes in the embryo induce expression or inhibition of the growth and regulator genes to produce the entire organism. Carcinogens may similarly enhance the 'oncogene' expression or inhibit the regulators when inducing carcinomas or their adenoma precursors.

Some genes or gene deletions may also provide some protection against the development of cancer, in much the same way that possession of the recessive sickle-cell or thalassaemia genes protect against malaria to some extent. It seems that the cystic fibrosis gene deletion, Delta F 508 codon, which is carried by about 1 in 27 people, may protect against colon cancer and some other tumours.

A small number of colonic cancers have a definite inherited genetic cause. These take the form of familial adenomatous polyposis syndromes and the familial cancer syndromes (or hereditary non-polyposis colonic cancer). Familial adenomatous polyposis syndromes account for as little as 0.5 per cent of all colonic cancers but they are important as a biological model for other cancers and as a model for constructing algorithms of therapeutic management based on sound biological principles (Table 2).

Table 2 Polyposis syndromes

Colonic manifestations	Extracolonic lesions
Familial adenomatous polyposis syndromes	
Familial adenomatous polyposis	Retinal pigmentation
Gardner's	Osteomas, desmoids, other gastrointestinal cancers
Oldfield's	Sebaceous cysts
Turcot's	Intracranial tumours
Hamartomas	
Peutz Jegher's	Perioral freckles
Juvenile polyps	

Familial adenomatous polyposis is an inherited propensity to develop numerous adenomas throughout the colon, some of which become malignant in time. The condition is inherited as an autosomal dominant with high penetrance but variable expression, and approximately half the children of the index case inherit the condition. The polyps appear at around puberty, and nearly all patients manifest polyps by their early 30s. There are a few reports of patients presenting later, but the chance of being affected if a sigmoidoscopy is normal are 1 per cent or less after the age of 35 years.

Recent work has shown that the genetic abnormality in familial adenomatous polyposis is a deletion of genetic material on the long arm of chromosome 5. The absence of this gene or cluster of genes seems responsible not only for the colonic polyps but also neoplasms in other parts of the gastrointestinal tract, the mesenchyme, and occasionally the brain. There appears to be a general derangement of cell protein formation common to many tissues. Gardner's syndrome with osteomas, desmoids, gastric hamartomas, and a propensity for gastric, pancreatic, and small bowel tumours, is the most severe form of the syndrome. Patients with the more common familial adenomatous polyposis seldom have clinically obvious extraintestinal manifestations. The least severe manifestation, Turcot's syndrome, is characterized by fewer colonic polyps, but affected patients also have intracranial tumours, which are more lethal. While it is likely that Turcot's cases are part of the familial adenomatous polyposis spectrum and therefore exhibit the same DNA abnormality, it has yet to be proved.

Peutz-Jegher syndrome and juvenile polyposis are not strictly part of the familial adenomatous polyposis syndromes, but for convenience they may be considered alongside. These conditions are rarer and the polyps fewer in number, but the trait is inherited in a dominant fashion. The polyps are hamartomas, which often have adenomatous changes around them. This adenomatous change predisposes to malignant transformation and increases the risk of colon cancer. It is likely that the genetic abnormality of these two conditions is quite different from that of familial adenomatous polyposis.

Hereditary non-polyposis colonic cancer is more common but less obvious than familial adenomatous polyposis. The inheritance is again autosomal dominant, but the appearance of the cancer is clinically similar to sporadic cases of colorectal cancer, although it occurs at a younger age. In these cases, which account for some 5 per cent of all colorectal cancers, the genetic abnormality is usually on chromosome 17 or 18. Two subtypes of the syndrome have been recognized: site-specific colonic cancer, where individuals of a family are susceptible to colonic cancer but not cancers of other organs (Lynch type 1), and cancer family syndromes where female members of the family are prone to breast and uterine cancers as well as colonic tumours (Lynch type 2). The tumours may all develop in the same individual but, more commonly, the three types of cancer appear in different members of the family. Occasionally tumours of other organs are found (the Muir-Torre syndrome).

It is interesting that the cancers in patients with Lynch type 1 and 2 syndromes develop in early middle life rather than in the seventh and eighth decades, as do sporadic cases. The cancers occur predominately on the right side of the colon and are of low malignancy, again in contrast to the sporadic cases. While the two Lynch syndromes appear different there may be but a single genetic abnormality exhibiting pleiotropy.

Environmental factors

The most important environmental factors in the aetiology of colon cancer are likely to exert their influence within the lumen of the colon. The strongest evidence is for a role of diet in the induction and growth of tumours. The significant association between diet and the prevalence of colonic cancer and heart disease suggests that a diet rich in fat and meat is a common factor in both diseases (see also Section 42.2).

Fat, cholesterol, and bile acids

Epidemiological studies, case–control studies, cohort studies, and animal experiments provide strong evidence that a diet rich in fat, and particularly in animal fat, is associated with a high incidence of colon tumours and, in animals, with the promotion of malignancy. While fat is the major environmental factor so far identified, fat itself is not a carcinogen. Animal experiments suggest that all fats are mutagenic in very high concentrations, but unsaturated fats are more likely to induce progression from adenomas to cancer. Luminal fat, and in particular its oxidation products, promote colonic epithelial cell proliferation and an increase in crypt cell production rate, yet ketone bodies are also an important source of nutrition for the mucosa. Diets high in animal fats are rich in cholesterol, which is a major substrate for bacterial degradation, and there is a correlation between the incidence of colon cancer and the amount of cholesterol in the faeces. It is unlikely that cholesterol *per se* is a carcinogen, but its metabolites probably are. Some metabolites may also have an endocrine action which is an aetiological factor for some colonic cancers. For example: some HNPCC cases are associated with oestrogen dependent breast and uterine tumours: familial adenomatous polyposis patients develop their adenomas at or after puberty when sex hormone levels are high.

Probably the most important action of dietary fat is to stimulate choleresis, thereby increasing the levels of faecal bile acids which are, in turn, metabolized by bacteria to the secondary bile acids lithocholic and deoxycholic acid, which are powerful tumour promotors. Other situations which increase faecal bile acid concentrations, such as cholecystectomy, gastric surgery, and terminal ileal resection, are also associated with an increased risk of colon cancer.

Calories and protein

Colon cancer is more common in human populations with a high total calorie intake or a high protein intake, though the two are usually associated. There appears to be a general promoting effect of calories in carcinogenesis but it is difficult, in man, to separate the effect of calories from that of fat and the lack of fibre or resistant starch. Some protein breakdown products and amino acids enter the colon to be degraded by bacteria into compounds such as the *N*-nitrosamines, which are powerful carcinogens. The relative load of protein products entering the colon is, however, small compared with that of cholesterol. Nevertheless it is increased in patients with intestinal hurry and may contribute to the carcinogenic effects of cholecystectomy, gastric surgery, and ileal resection.

Fibre

Western food is notoriously low in dietary fibre and resistant starch, with a consequent increase in intestinal transit time. Epidemiological studies show a negative correlation between the amount of fibre in the diet and the prevalence of colonic and rectal cancer which, though it may be an epiphenomenon, suggests a causal relationship.

Dietary fibre consists of many different substances with different properties, from soluble compounds such as pectins and hemicellulose, to insoluble celluloses and lignins. Resistant starches may also be considered part of dietary fibre because they are indigestible. Indigestible fibre increases the bulk of stool, principally by retaining water, and decreases the colonic transit time in most people (but increases it in patients with colonic irritability and pathologically rapid transit). Fibre alters the colonic bacterial flora both qualitatively and quantitatively, and is partially degraded by these bacteria to produce numerous luminal products, such as flatus. Fibre also dilutes and absorbs luminal toxins. The combination of these factors may have conflicting effects upon the colonic epithelium, but the net result is to reduce the carcinogenic capacity of the luminal contents. Animal experiments provide conflicting data: some components of dietary fibre promote colonic carcinogenesis while others are protective. The combined effects of dietary fibre deficiency on the stool content, consistency, and transit may account for the well-known association of colonic carcinoma with diverticular disease, constipation, and haemorrhoids.

Minor dietary constituents

A number of dietary constituents have been found to inhibit carcinogenesis, including selenium, vitamins C and E, retinoids, β-carotene, and plant sterols. Diets low in vitamin C and β-carotene also tend to be low in dietary fibre. Selenium is an essential trace element which, experimentally, has been shown to inhibit carcinogenesis in rats. Endemic selenium deficiency is rare but does occur in New Zealand, which might account for the particularly high incidence of colonic and rectal cancer among those of European stock and the relatively high incidence among Maoris compared to other natives of the Pacific basin.

Bacteria

Bacteria are a major constituent of stool and are important contributors to the colonic luminal environment. The two bacterial enzymes so far shown to be important are β-dehydroxylase, which breaks down harmless primary bile acids into the mutagenic secondary bile acids lithocholic acid and chenodeoxycholic acid, and 4,5-nuclear dehydrogenase, which desaturates bile acids to produce substances that are both tumour initiators and growth promoters.

The close correlation between the incidence of colonic carcinoma and faecal secondary bile acid concentration is a clear indication of the importance of bacterial activity upon the colonic epithelial environment. Furthermore there is a correlation between the carriage of nuclear dehydrogenase-producing Clostridia in the colon and the incidence of colonic cancer. These bacteria also require a neutral pH and hydrogen acceptors for optimal activity and high-risk populations have been shown to have higher pH and hydrogen acceptor levels than controls. It is likely that further studies will yield more important information in the search for luminal carcinogens, growth promotors and growth inhibitors.

Irradiation

X-rays are important mutagens. It is therefore hardly surprising that intracavity irradiation in the treatment of carcinoma of the cervix uteri is associated with a small increased incidence of rectal cancer within the field of irradiation. The cancers appear some 5 to 15 years later. There is, however, no known increased risk of colonic cancer in people living in areas with higher background levels of radiation, nor after abdominal radiation for conditions such as testicular tumours or Hodgkin's disease.

Inflammatory bowel disease

Ulcerative colitis has, for a long time, been known to increase the risk of colonic cancer. The risk increases almost exponentially with time some 10 years after the onset of the disease, particularly in patients who have total colitis, those with a severe first attack, those who develop the disease in childhood, and those patients whose disease follows a relapsing course. Patients with mild distal colitis have no greater risk of developing rectal cancer than the normal population, while patients with severe long-standing disease have a 1 in 2 chance of developing colonic cancer after 30 years. Colonic epithelial dysplasia seems to be the precursor lesion, though progression of a particular area of dysplasia is not inevitable. Areas of dysplasia may be scattered throughout the colon, which explains the greater likelihood of multiple cancers among those with colitis. The tumours are seldom polypoid or exophitic but usually flat and infiltrating, which makes diagnosis more difficult. The prognosis of these colitic cancers was originally thought to be particularly poor but more recent data suggests that stage for stage there is no difference in prognosis compared to sporadic cancers.

Crohn's colitis is also associated with an increased risk of cancer in the diseased segment as well as in other areas of the digestive tract. The risk is, however, less than that associated with severe ulcerative colitis. It is uncertain whether the chronic inflammation is the main predisposing factor for carcinogenesis in these two conditions or whether genetic make-up or bile acids and their metabolites are more important.

Surgical procedures

Surgical injury in the form of an anastomosis increases the risk of a cancer developing at the site of injury both in experimental models and as a site of implantation in man after resection of a colonic cancer. There has been some debate about the effect of different suture materials upon the risk of implantation but the data are conflicting and the evidence inconclusive.

Cholecystectomy is also associated with an increased risk of colonic cancer, in particular right-sided lesions among women. The risk is similar after gastric surgery in man but not in experimental animals. Both operations may exert their effect by increasing the delivery of bile acids to the colon, thereby increasing the concentration of secondary bile acids within the colon.

Ureterosigmoidostomy, performed for urinary diversion, is particularly associated with the development of colonic cancer at, or near, the ureterocolic anastomosis. Why this should be so is not certain but it may be caused by the effect of phenols, cresols, and other compounds from cigarette smoke, excreted in the urine, upon the colonic epithelium (Table 3).

Table 3 Cancer promoters and inhibiters

Promoters	
Genetic	Familial adenomatous polyposis
	Hereditary non-polyposis colonic cancer
	Peutz-Jegher's
	Juvenile polyposis
Diet	Fat
	Bile acids
Bacteria	Nuclear dehydrogenase-producing Clostridia
Operations	Cholecystectomy
	Gastric surgery
	Ureterosigmoidostomy
Irradiation	
Diseases	Ulcerative colitis
	Crohn's disease
Inhibitors	Fibre
	Selenium
	Vitamins C and E
	-Carotene

Colonic polyps

The association between colonic polyps and colonic cancer has been known for a long time. The incidence of malignant change increases with both the size of the polyps and the degree of dysplasia. Tubular adenomas are less prone to malignancy than are villous adenomas, which may also be very large. It is now believed that most, if not all, colonic cancers originate within an adenoma, and while most polyps do not become malignant it is clear that a polyp which has been growing for some years to achieve considerable size is more likely to do so. Equally clearly some pass through the adenoma phase quickly, underlying the dual process of tumourigenesis and malignant transformation.

The prevalence of adenomas and the prevalence of colonic cancer run in parallel in epidemiological studies. Polyps are also frequently found in close proximity to cancers. The distribution of adenomas around the colon is the same as that of colonic cancers and some adenomas snared endoscopically disclose microscopic foci of cancer. The transformation of a benign adenoma into a cancer is thought to take, on average, about 5 years; the mean age of patients at diagnosis with polyps is 5 years less than that of patients presenting with a colonic cancer.

Immunosuppression

Long-term immunosuppression, either for the prevention of transplant rejection or as a consequence of HIV infection, predisposes to cancer. Lymphomas, which may affect the colon as well as the small bowel, are the most common abdominal neoplasm in immunosuppressed transplant patients. Squamous cell carcinoma of the anus is not uncommon among transplant patients and is usually associated with human papillomavirus infection. Small cell carcinomas of the colon, which are rare in the otherwise healthy population, have been reported in AIDS patients. However, there appears to be no association between adenocarcinomas of the colon and immunosuppression.

Neoplasms themselves induce some degree of immune suppression, either directly through products of the malignant cells or indirectly through malnutrition and cachexia. Some, but not all, colon cancers induce a vigorous local immune response with an intense cellular infiltrate within the tumour, or a histiocytic reaction in the draining lymph nodes. Suppression of this immune response is probably mediated by secretion of soluble suppressor factors such as the retroviral protein p15E, which is also responsible for the immunosuppression induced by retroviruses and is present in a number of tumours including colon cancer.

PATHOLOGY, STAGING, AND PROGNOSIS

Colonic cancers, in common with most epithelial tumours, are polyclonal with clones of cells exhibiting differing degrees of 'malignancy'. The more undifferentiated or more 'malignant' clones are more likely to spread and metastasize. A tumour's biological behaviour is the main determinant of the tumour's propensity to spread locally and to metastasize and, therefore, indicates the ultimate prognosis. This in turn is reflected to some extent by the histopathological features of a cancer. There is little doubt that, in the near future, other phenotypic characteristics, identified by molecular biological methods, will provide even more accurate prognostic information. For example, tumour cells that stimulate angiogenesis or have fewer surface adhesion molecules are more likely to metastasize and therefore to have a worse prognosis. Tumour secondaries, which are often derived from selected clones of a polyclonal primary, are unlikely to behave in the same way as the primary tumour and will generally be more malignant.

Tumour biology is very much reflected by the stage of the

disease, and therefore the amount of spread, at presentation. It is no surprise that there is a significant inverse relation between the length of history and the stage of the disease at diagnosis. Quicker growing tumours usually present with a short history and are advanced at the time of treatment. Although the clinical and pathological stage is a 'snapshot' in the life of a tumour, it provides the most accurate prognostic index; this may be refined further by the histopathological features. Several staging methods are in use throughout the world, and each has strengths and weaknesses. The most commonly used are the Dukes' classification and derivations of it, or the Union Internationale Contre Cancer (UICC) TNM classification. The former has the advantage of great simplicity but considerable disadvantages from lack of precision: it does not reflect accurately the depth of tumour penetration, the extent of spread outside the bowel, the number of lymph nodes affected by tumour, or the presence or absence of metastasis, all of which have an important bearing upon prognosis. Derivations such as the Astler-Coller and Australian classifications refine the Dukes' staging but do not provide the flexibility of the TNM method which enables useful division into subsets without being unduly complex. It is therefore most appropriate that surgeons adopt the UICC TNM classification as a suitable international standard (Table 4 and Fig. 1).

Table 4 Cancer staging—Dukes' classification

A	Tumour confined to bowel wall
B	Tumour involving or through serosa
C	Lymph nodes involved
	C1 Apical node clear
	C2 Apical node involved

The anatomical site of the cancer has an influence on the stage of the disease and an independent effect upon prognosis. Right-sided colonic cancers tend to be at a more advanced pathological stage at the time of presentation, but the prognosis is generally no worse than is that of left-sided tumours. Stage for stage, right-sided lesions have a better prognosis; this may reflect subtle differences in aetiology. Rectal tumours have a generally better prognosis, because of earlier presentation and easier accessibility.

Staging gives information about prognosis in general, but particularly indicates the probability of occult hepatic metastasis, which is the major factor affecting survival. Patients with Dukes' C tumours are more likely to have occult hepatic metastases than those with Dukes' B tumours, while patients with Dukes' A lesions are most unlikely to have hepatic metastases. Occult hepatic metastases account for the majority of deaths from colonic cancer: while only about 20 per cent of patients die from local spread of the disease, which is also reflected in the clinical stage.

Age generally has little effect on the behaviour or prognosis of colonic tumours, except for patients under the age of 40 years, who appear to have a particularly poor prognosis.

HISTOPATHOLOGICAL GRADING AND TYPING

Grading depends upon subjective interpretation of the degree of tumour differentiation at histological examination. Various grading systems have been proposed, but grading into two broad groups, low or average grade tumours which are well to moderately differentiated and high grade or undifferentiated, reduces the variation between observers while at the same time providing useful prognostic information. Patients with high grade

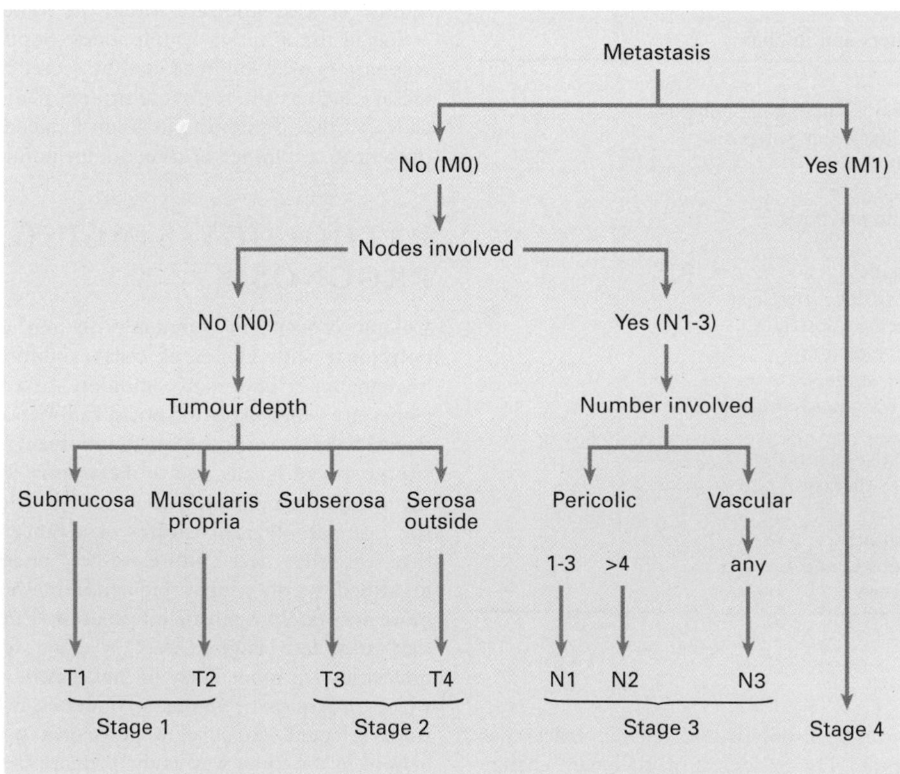

Fig. 1 UICC TNM classification (after Hermanek 1989).

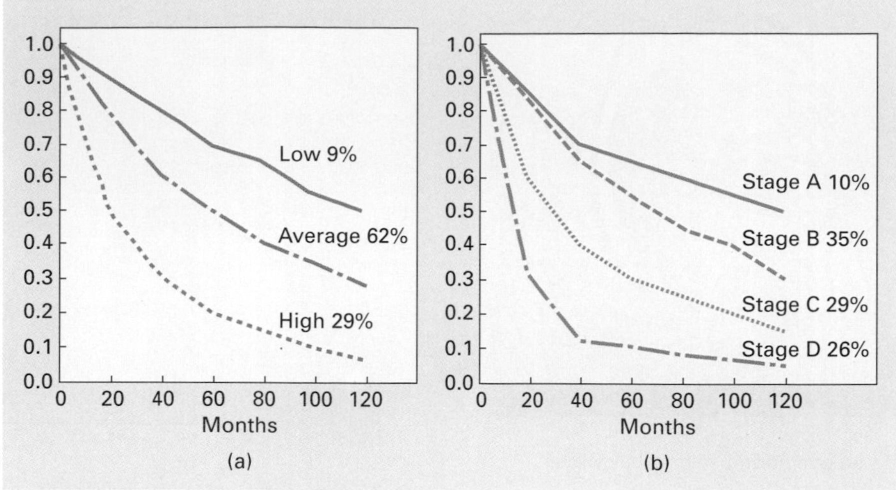

Fig. 2 Survival by (a) histological grade. Very few tumours are truly low grade. The main distinction is between average and high grade. (b) Dukes' stage and survival. A few patients with advanced disease have a long survival. (After Chapuis *et al. Br J Surg* 1985; 72:698–702.)

cancers fare worse than do those with well differentiated lesions after taking account of the tumour stage (Table 4 and Fig. 2).

Typing, on the other hand, reflects the cellular characteristics. Mucinous, signet cell, and small cell tumours are variants of the more common adenocarcinoma and the frankly undifferentiated cancers. Again typing may give some useful additional prognostic information. Signet cell and small cell tumours have a worse prognosis than adenocarcinoma, while mucinous lesions tend to recur locally. Occasionally rectal cancers turn out to be squamous cell types which are more responsive to chemotherapy and irradiation. Melanomas, which have a particularly poor prognosis, are found rarely in the rectum. Both of these tumours are, however, more common at the anus.

Histological features such as vascular, lymphatic, or perineural invasion are prognostically unfavourable. By contrast, lymphocytic infiltration of the tumour and a histiocytic reaction in the regional lymph nodes are minor favourable prognostic features.

Identification of surface tumour antigens, such as carcinoembryonic antigen, oncogene expression and DNA ploidy, add potential refinement, but these are not yet in routine use. Full characterization of the molecular biological features of cancer cells will in the future probably provide more important prognostic and therapeutic information than histological typing and grading. It may appear academic at present to stage patients and their tumours, but it will become clinically important as the place of adjuvant chemotherapy and irradiation becomes clearer, particularly when chemotherapy improves. In the mean time it is important to collect pathological data accurately to allow clinical studies and the audit of surgical performance. The latter cannot be judged in the absence of good histopathological information.

Figures 3 to 12 show the pathological features described above.

PROGNOSIS

Stage remains the most important indicator of prognosis (Table 5). The prognosis of patients with adequately treated Stage 1 cancers is little different from that of an otherwise healthy

Table 5 Prognosis

TNM stage			Percentage 5-year survival	
			Rectal cancer	Colon cancer
T1	N0	M0	100	100
T2	N0	M0	80	100
T3	N0	M0	65	90
T4	N0	M0	50	70
anyT	N1	M0	55	65
	N2	M0	35	50
	N3	M0	30	35
	any N	M1	10	10

After Hermanek 1989.

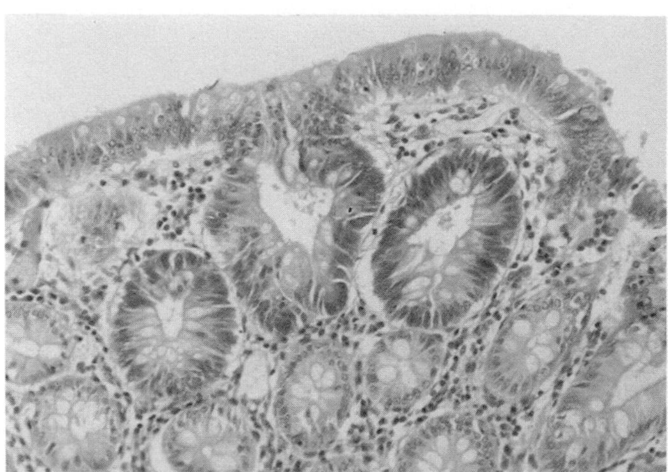

Fig. 3 Microadenomatous change in three crypts in a case of familial adenomatous polyposis.

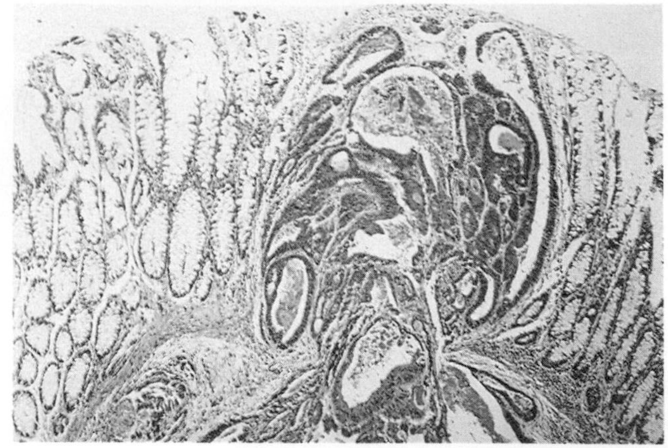

Fig. 4 A focus of cancer in an otherwise benign tubulovillous adenoma.

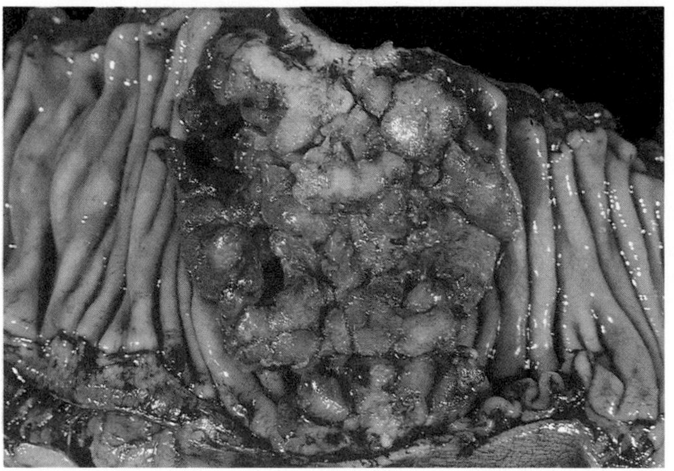

Fig. 5 Cancer of the rectum in a fresh resection specimen.

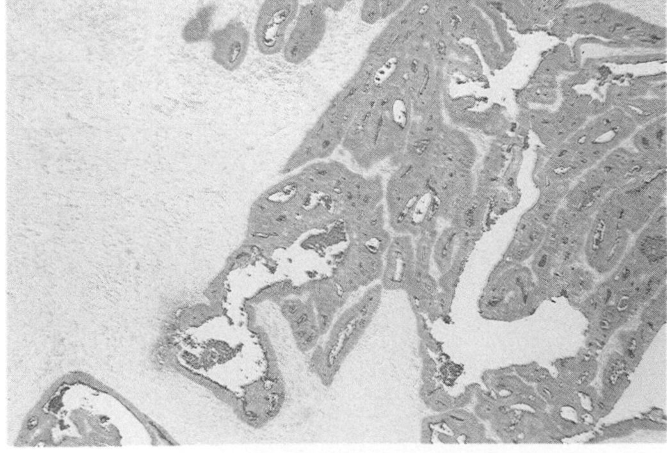

Fig. 6 A well differentiated adenocarcinoma invading the muscle coat and showing a brown carcinoembryonic antigen positive immunoperoxidase stain.

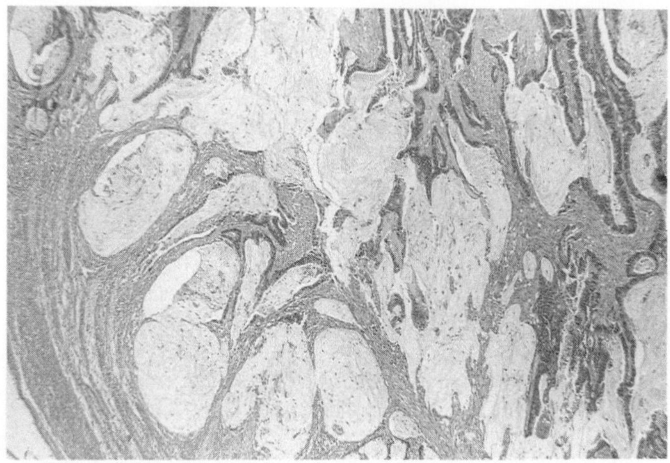

Fig. 7 A mucinous adenocarcinoma of the colon.

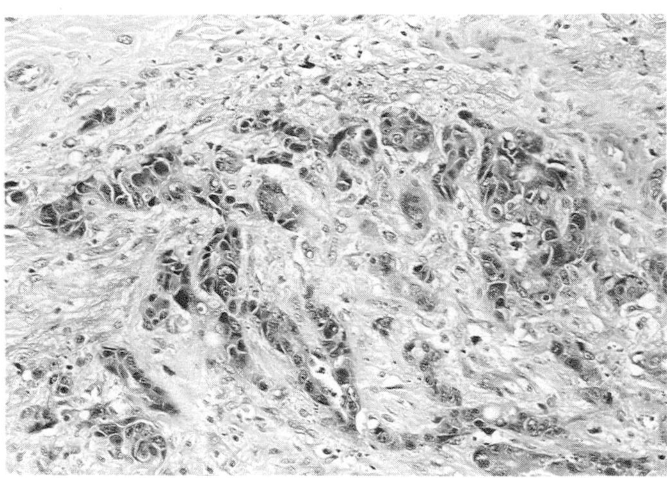

Fig. 8 A poorly differentiated carcinoma with little tubular formation and marked cytological dysplasia. There is no inflammatory response.

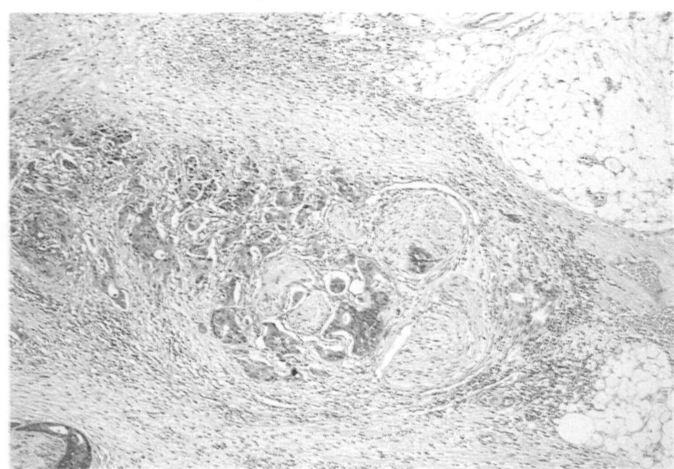

Fig. 9 Perineural invasion by colon cancer.

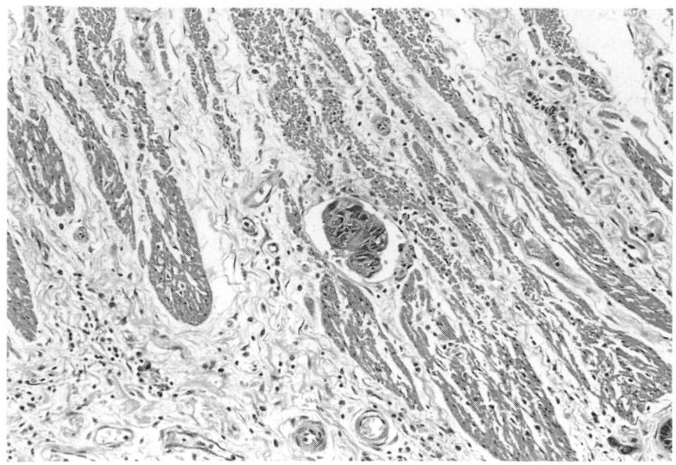

Fig. 10 Lymphatic invasion by colonic cancer.

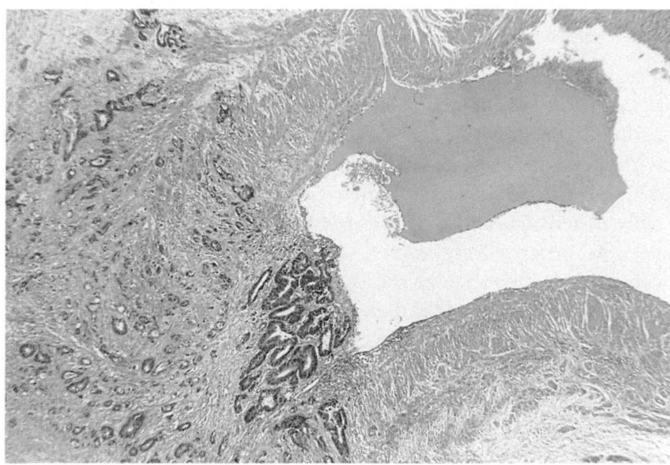

Fig. 11 Venous invasion by colon cancer.

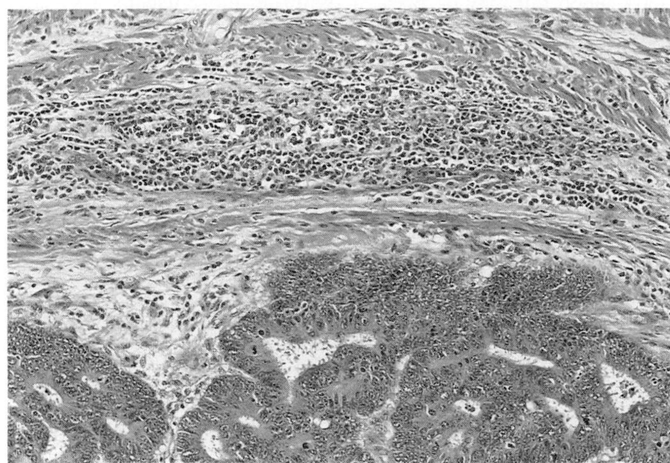

Fig. 12 A marked inflammatory infiltrate around a moderately differentiated colon cancer.

population of the same age; 95 to 100 per cent live 5 years or more after resection. Patients with cancer spread through the serosa only have a 40 to 60 per cent chance of living 5 years, although the prognosis is more favourable if the tumour is only just through the serosa and is correspondingly worse if adjacent structures are invaded. Lymph node metastasis further adversely affects prognosis, with only about 30 per cent of patients surviving 5 years. Subclassification is useful: 60 per cent of N1 patients may live 5 years while less than 30 per cent of N3 patients will survive. A few patients, some 5 to 10 per cent, live 5 years even with hepatic metastases, although 85 per cent of such patients die within 1 year of diagnosis.

The survival curve of patients with colonic and rectal cancer treated by resection is curvilinear, reaching a nearly flat plateau. Few patients develop metastatic disease 5 to 10 years after surgical treatment of the primary lesion. Many patients are therefore cured of their cancer. This suggests that large bowel cancer is somewhat unusual, because metastasis occurs relatively late in the lifespan of the tumour; many other cancers, such as cancer of the breast, lung, or melanoma, metastasize early. Natural survival with metastases then depends very much on the symbiotic relationship between the tumour and host.

CLINICAL PRESENTATION (Table 6)

Patients with colonic and rectal cancer have a broad range of clinical presentation which can be subclassified according to the anatomical site of the primary. Distribution of cancers and adenomas is uneven around the colon. Caecal and right-sided tumours account for about 20 per cent of large bowel cancers, while 70 per cent occur distal to the splenic flexure and about 45 per cent are at or below the rectosigmoid junction (Fig. 13).

Table 6 Presenting symptoms

Right colon	Anaemia Right iliac fossa pain Central abdominal colic Diarrhoea Pyrexia of unknown origin Weight loss Appendicitis
Left colon	Left iliac fossa pain Lower abdominal colic Constipation/diarrhoea Blood ± mucus Obstruction Peritonitis Weight loss
Rectal cancer	Blood and mucus per rectum Diarrhoea Tenesmus Incomplete evacuation Sacral/perineal pain

Caecal and right-sided carcinoma

Right-sided tumours are often remarkably silent and many patients present with only the symptoms and signs of iron deficiency anaemia from protracted occult blood loss, a fact which is

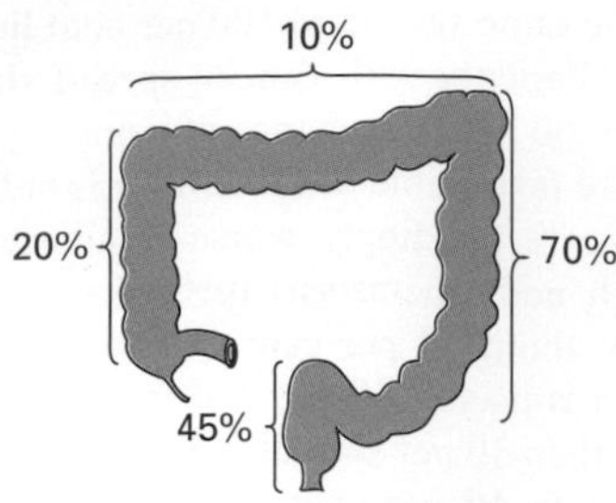

Fig. 13 Distribution of colonic adenomas and cancers around the colon.

all too often forgotten or ignored. Rarely the blood loss is copious, particularly in patients who are receiving anticoagulants.

The faeces entering the caecum are liquid, and obstruction is a relatively late presentation. As the lumen becomes narrowed the patient complains of intermittent central or right iliac fossa colic, which is often postprandial, stimulated by the gastrocolic reflex. The pain is often followed by the onset of intermittent diarrhoea, possibly the consequence of faecal fermentation and the accumulation of bacterial toxins within the bowel lumen. Typical distal ileal obstruction occurs if the tumour obstructs the ileocaecal valve, or if the ileocaecal valve becomes incompetent in the face of complete caecal obstruction. Waves of central abdominal colic occur with progressive central abdominal distension and borborygmi. Visible peristalsis, faeculent vomit, and dehydration are late manifestations. Not infrequently a palpable mass is the presenting symptom, though more commonly the mass is felt during clinical examination.

Elderly patients occasionally present with acute appendicitis when the carcinoma occludes the appendicular orifice. It is therefore always wise to consider the diagnosis of caecal carcinoma in any older person who presents with acute appendicitis. The diagnosis may not be obvious at the time the appendix is removed and must be sought subsequently by barium enema examination. Quite commonly the tumour penetrates the bowel wall posteriorly, producing a sealed perforation and an abscess in the psoas muscle. Such patients present with the symptoms and signs of infection accompanied by a painful mass in the right iliac fossa. The pain may radiate down into the leg or hip, particularly if the femoral nerve is involved in the abscess, or if the abscess tracks down below the inguinal ligament to appear in the femoral triangle. Similarly the pain may radiate posteriorly if the abscess erodes the lumbar muscles to point in the loin. Occasionally an anterior tumour may produce a free perforation of the caecum or right colon to produce peritonitis with severe generalized abdominal pain, a silent abdomen, and percussion rebound tenderness.

Occasionally, right-sided colon cancers present with general symptoms of malaise and lack of well being, sometimes with a pyrexia of unknown origin. These symptoms are either the result of a small occult abscess or are due to tumour burden, usually from metastases. The symptoms and signs of metastases are legion, but are usually accompanied by pain and tenderness over the liver, which is the most common site of metastasis. These symptoms are usually produced by rapid growth of the secondaries distending the liver capsule. Metastases tend to grow much more rapidly than the primary because they are 'aggressive' selected clones from a polyclonal tumour. The metastases may also outgrow their blood supply, partially infarct and undergo necrosis. Haemorrhage into the necrotic metastasis may then occur as a secondary event. Either situation will produce pain, malaise, and perhaps a pyrexia which will resolve spontaneously. Many patients with hepatic metastases are quite asymptomatic in the early stages, when hepatomegaly may be the only physical sign.

Caecal tumours may spread locally and transperitoneally before causing bowel symptoms. As the tumour burden increases, cytokines released from leucocytes may cause the loss of well being, anorexia, and weight loss: these are common features of carcinomatosis. Cytokine release is thought to be the mediator that alters the patient's metabolism and ultimately causes cachexia. Local spread of tumour throughout the peritoneum and into the omentum may produce a protein-rich ascites. Infiltration of the small bowel mesentery sometimes produces pseudo-obstruction, or chylous ascites by obstruction of lacteals. Occasionally distension due to ascites is the presenting feature.

Rarely, patients present with signs or symptoms of widespread tumour dissemination such as leucoerythroblastic anaemia from marrow infiltration, a persistent cough from pulmonary secondaries, generalized lymphadenopathy or a hard tumour nodule at the umbilicus, the so-called Sister Marie Joseph sign.

Left-sided and sigmoid lesions

The stool dehydrates and becomes harder as it reaches and passes through the left colon to be stored in the sigmoid before defaecation. Patients with a left-sided colonic cancer commonly present with a change in bowel habit, often constipation alternating with diarrhoea, usually accompanied by lower abdominal colic, possibly distension, and a desire to defecate. The symptoms tend to become progressively severe, and this may serve to distinguish cancer from diverticular disease or colonic irritability. The irritable colon syndrome is usually seen in younger adults; if a middle-aged or older patient presents with a change in bowel habit the symptoms should be assumed to be caused by a colon cancer until proved otherwise. Progressive constipation or diarrhoea are less common changes of bowel habit, either of which may end in complete large bowel obstruction.

Change in bowel function is often accompanied by the passage of altered blood, and sometimes mucus, in the stool or on its surface, particularly in the case of distal sigmoid lesions. Occasionally patients present with colonic bleeding as an isolated symptom. The loss is usually intermittent, with small amounts of dark blood but may be brisk, a symptom more usually associated with diverticular disease. Brisk bleeding from a colonic cancer is more likely to occur in a patient treated with anticoagulants.

A few patients present with a pain or mass in the left iliac fossa, but a mass is often palpable in the abdomen on physical examination. A palpable carcinoma of the splenic flexure must be distinguished from an enlarged spleen or kidney.

Some patients, surprisingly, have remarkably few symptoms until they present with massive abdominal distension due to complete large bowel obstruction. In these circumstances the caecum becomes very distended. Unless distension is recognized and treated rapidly, or unless the ileocaecal valve becomes incompetent, caecal perforation leads to faecal peritonitis. If the ileocaecal valve is incompetent, the obstructed large bowel decompresses into the ileum to produce a mixed clinical picture of large and small bowel obstruction. Occasionally the tumour itself will perforate, causing sudden acute abdominal pain and peritonitis. More commonly the tumour becomes attached to adjacent organs and may invade them. A sigmoid cancer may invade the lateral abdominal wall and form an abscess, or invade a loop of small bowel and either produce an ileocolic fistula with severe diarrhoea or small bowel obstruction. Neoplasms of the splenic flexure or descending colon invading the jejunum sometimes present with severe intestinal haemorrhage. Sigmoid cancers commonly invade either the uterus, ovaries, or the bladder. Colonic cancer is the second most common cause of colovesical fistulae after diverticular disease, and patients usually present with haematuria and recurrent urinary tract infections initially, and later with pneumaturia or faecaluria. Similarly a sigmoid cancer fixed in the pelvis may fistulate into the vagina to produce an offensive irritating discharge that changes to frank faecal incontinence *per vaginam*.

Left-sided lesions may sometimes present from the start with anaemia or the symptoms and signs of dissemination but this event is less common than with right-sided lesions.

Rectal cancer

Rectal cancers are a particular subset of left-sided lesions, important for two reasons. Firstly, the accessibility of the lesions should enable the diagnosis to be made at an early and favourable stage, and secondly the diagnosis is often needlessly delayed while the symptoms are attributed to haemorrhoids or an anal fissure.

Most patients with rectal cancer present with bleeding. While the blood is often dark and mixed with the stool or coating the surface, it may be bright and quite separate from the faeces. For this reason the symptoms are often attributed to haemorrhoids. Minor changes in bowel habit, such as increased frequency of defaecation, mucus with the stool, or mucus diarrhoea are also quite common. Mucus diarrhoea is particularly associated with large villous adenomas which have often become malignant. The mucus is rich in potassium and may be sufficiently profuse to produce dehydration and coma. Tenesmus, the continuous urge to defecate, is a grave symptom produced by an advanced rectal tumour inducing a permanent sense of fullness. Tenesmus may give way to continual sacral pain, sometimes radiating down the inner thighs, as the tumour invades the sacrum and the sacral plexus of nerves. Anal pain, initially on defecation and later continuous, may occur as a low rectal cancer invades the anal canal. Incontinence supervenes when the anal sphincters are destroyed. Proctalgia fugax (fleeting perineal pain) is a rare presenting symptom and therefore when it occurs *de novo* in later life, rectal cancer must be considered as a possible diagnosis.

Few patients present with disseminated disease though this may occur in younger people with rapidly progressive tumours or in those whose rectal symptoms are ignored for a long time. Similarly large bowel obstruction is a rare and late mode of presentation of rectal cancer.

Rectal cancers generally cause symptoms early in their course. The tumours are accessible and this translates into a better prognosis than that seen with cancers of the rest of the colon. Biological features may also contribute to the better prognosis but these have yet to be identified convincingly.

INVESTIGATION

The importance of a good history and a careful physical examination cannot be overstressed. The completion of the physical examination should always be a digital rectal examination to feel for a mass, assess the mobility and position of the mass, and to feel for enlarged extra rectal lymph nodes. The examination is completed by an immediate study of the stool for occult blood using the Hemoccult® test or something similar. A proctosigmoidoscopic examination of the rectum and anus should follow.

Tests for occult blood in the faeces are still being improved, but in general the greater the specificity of the test the less its sensitivity. The most widely used test at present is the Hemoccult®, a guaiac test which depends on the peroxidase-like reaction of haematin, a degradation product of haemoglobin, to produce a blue colour on the test paper. The test is not particularly sensitive and so avoids detecting blood shed from the mouth or upper gastrointestinal tract, but it is quite specific for left-sided cancers. The overall accuracy is about 60 per cent in the presence of a colon cancer. Laboratory guaiac tests are usually more sensitive but less specific with more false-positive, but less false-negative results. Antibody tests for human haemoglobin in the stool are being developed but have yet to replace the simple and robust Haemoccult test as the most useful out-patient investigation.

There is a debate whether the proctosigmoidoscopic examination should be performed with a rigid or flexible fibreoptic instrument, in prepared or unprepared bowel, in the left lateral or prone jack-knife position. While it is largely a matter of tradition and individual preference, it is also to some extent governed by the information sought. A flexible sigmoidoscope can reach much higher up the colon, in comfort, than the rigid 30 cm instrument, but the examination requires a phosphate enema preparation. The diagnostic yield is also much better, mainly because more bowel is examined. The rigid instrument is nevertheless useful for inspecting the unprepared rectum. The mucosa, faeces, blood, and mucus can be examined in their natural state quickly and easily with the patient in the left lateral position. It is particularly useful to see whether blood is mixed with faeces and also if it is coming down from the sigmoid colon. An enema may wash away much of the 'evidence', and also makes the mucosa hyperaemic, stimulating it to secrete mucus as though inflamed.

Both the rigid and flexible instruments can be used easily in the left lateral position, most popular in Great Britain, or the prone jack-knife position using a special tilting table, which is the custom in the United States. Rigid sigmoidoscopy requires some care to avoid rectal perforation, but needs less experience than the fibreoptic method to obtain useful diagnostic information. Both instruments must only be advanced when the lumen is seen clearly. The investigation should be painless or at worst produce only mild discomfort. Blind intubation is a recipe for disaster ranging from pain to perforation.

It is possible to employ either method of sigmoidoscopy selectively to use the patient's and clinician's time most efficiently. When a patient presents with symptoms and signs of rectal pathology an unprepared rigid proctosigmoidoscopy is preferable. If, however, the history suggests that the problem lies more proximally, flexible sigmoidoscopy is more practical.

Barium enema and colonoscopy (see also Section 6.4)

There is much futile debate about the relative merits of barium enema and colonoscopy as the better method of investigating the colon, for each investigation provides different but complementary information. The barium enema gives good anatomical and topographic information which not only may be quite sufficient to diagnose a polyp or carcinoma but demonstrates the site and configuration of the lesion. The anatomical position of a

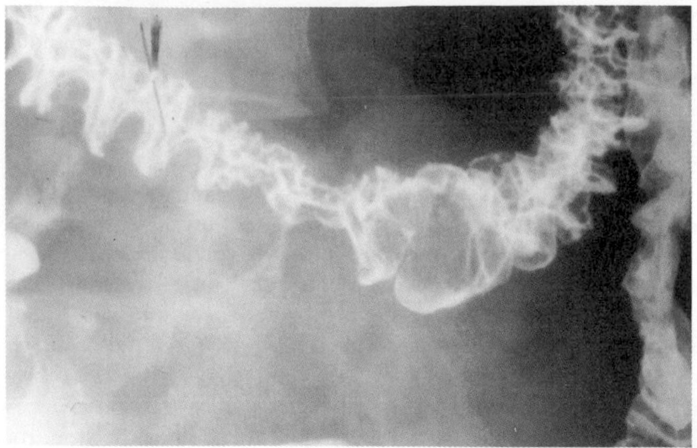

Fig. 14 Barium enema showing a large tubular adenoma of the transverse colon.

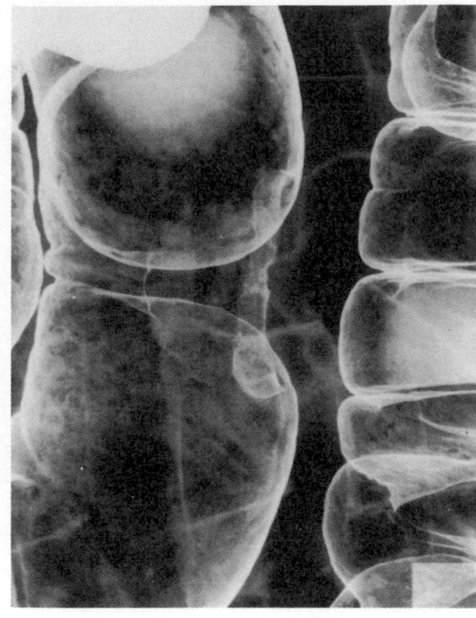

Fig. 16 Double contrast barium enema with a small ulcerative colonic cancer.

cancer is clearly of great importance to a surgeon planning an operation. The discrimination for small lesions and mucosal abnormality is considerably enhanced by the double contrast technique compared to the single contrast enema. The air insufflated after the barium shows clearly the mucosal destruction from an ulcerated carcinoma or the mucosal coating of both adenomatous polyps and polypoid carcinomas (Figs. 14–17).

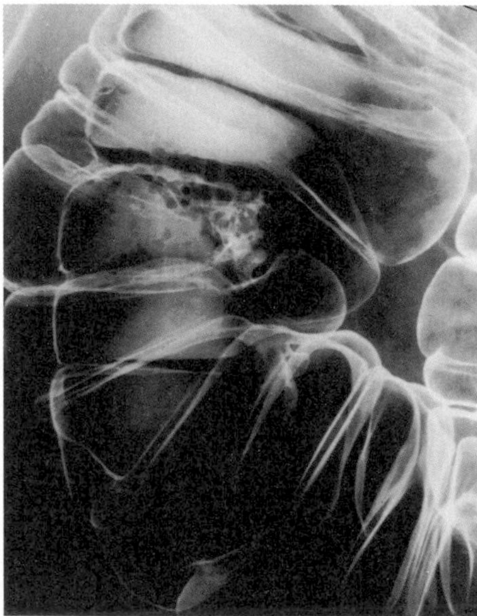

Fig. 15 Double contrast barium enema showing a caecal villous adenoma.

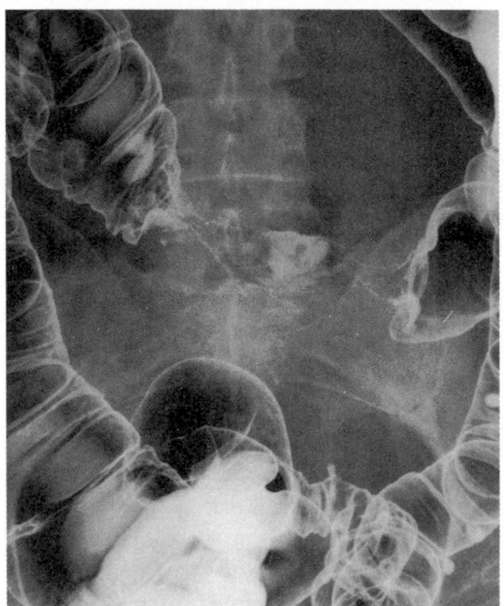

Fig. 17 Double contrast barium enema of a long applecore malignant stricture of the transverse colon.

Colonoscopy requires the same meticulous bowel preparation as a double contrast barium enema, but the patients also need some sedation. Colonoscopy is therefore more invasive, and the patients need both time to recover and somebody to take them home. There is also a small risk, about 1 : 1500, of colonic perforation during endoscopy. Nevertheless colonoscopy enables a more detailed study of the mucosa, visualizing lesions of less than 0.5 cm. The principal advantage over radiology is that lesions can be biopsied, or removed by snare cautery if they prove to be adenomatous polyps or a small polypoid carcinoma (Fig. 18). The main dis-

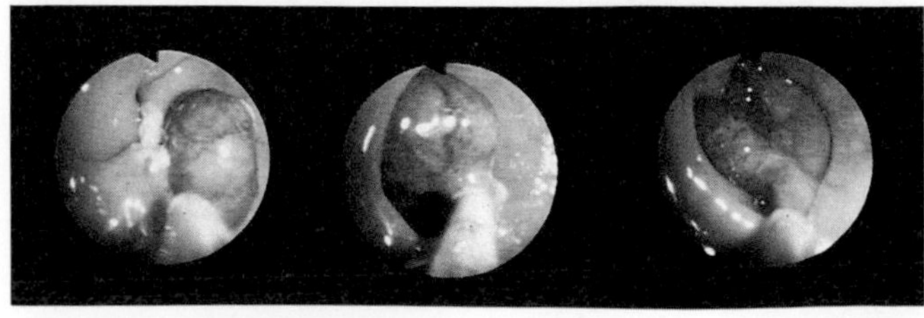

Fig. 18 Colonoscopic pictures of an adenoma being snared.

advantages are that anatomical localization is too poor to plan an operation as to where a skin crease incision may be used; there is seldom a complete permanent record of the investigation to refer to, and it is quite possible to miss lesions behind haustra.

Both investigations may be necessary to reach a diagnosis and plan therapy, but it is reasonable to start with a barium enema when patients present with a change in bowel habit and abdominal pain, with or without abdominal distension. If the main symptom is bleeding or anaemia, then colonoscopy is the investigation of choice because it enables identification of other bleeding lesions such as angiodysplasia, which are impossible to identify radiologically. Treatment such as polypectomy and laser therapy is also possible. Biopsy specimens of a cancer or inflammatory bowel disease provides confirmation of the diagnosis and enables confident planning of treatment.

Intrarectal ultrasound

Small endoluminal ultrasound instruments have recently added refinement to the diagnosis and preoperative staging of tumours, particularly of the rectum. Ultrasound probes mounted on a colonoscope are expensive and seldom used, but rigid rectal ultrasonography is now an established means of assessing the depth of penetration of the bowel wall by the tumour (Fig. 19). Enlarged lymph nodes can also be identified, but confirmation of node metastasis is less reliable (Fig. 20). This improved diagnostic information is essential when considering local treatment for a rectal cancer, and sometimes when choosing between an abdominoperineal excision of the rectum or a low anterior resection.

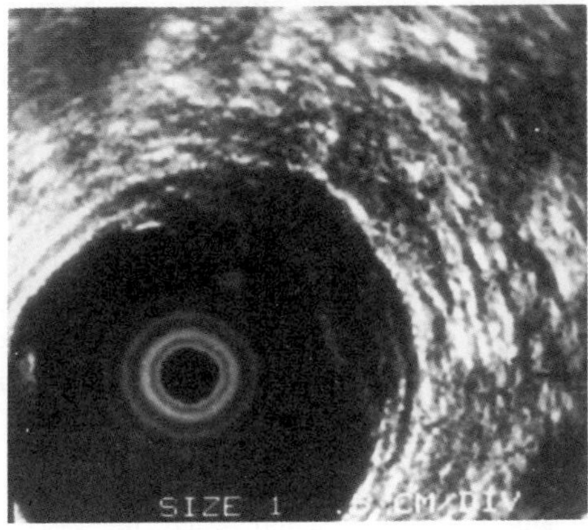

Fig. 19 Intrarectal ultrasound of a T2 tumour. The dark outer rectal muscle wall is intact.

Ultrasound and CT

Once the diagnosis of carcinoma of the colon or rectum is made secondary investigations are necessary to plan and organize treatment. Preoperative detection of metastasis is clearly crucial to allow treatment to be modified. It is quite possible to perform a whole battery of investigations which is both a burden for the patient and unnecessarily expensive. Tests should be efficient and yield maximal information at minimal cost. The liver is the most common site for metastasis followed by lung, retroperitoneum,

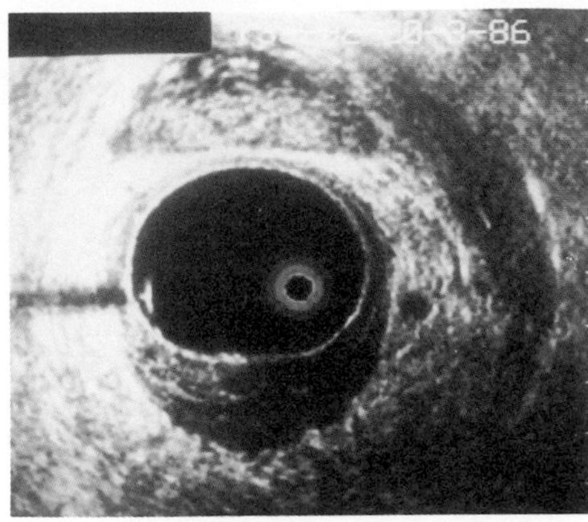

Fig. 20 Intrarectal ultrasound. T3 tumour posteriorly obliterating the dark rectal muscle band. An enlarged lymph node is also visible (T3, N1). The prostate is seen anteriorly.

ovary, peritoneal cavity, and, rarely, adrenal glands; abdominal ultrasonography and a plain chest radiograph are both useful and economic. However ultrasonography is very operator dependent and the investigation tends to vary in quality. The hard copy of the study is not so helpful as the real-time examination, and so review is not particularly useful. Transabdominal ultrasound can seldom detect metastases less than 1 cm in diameter. Abdominal computed tomography (CT) provides better discrimination for smaller hepatic lesions and can distinguish angiomata from metastases as small as 0.5 cm diameter, after contrast enhancement. CT also provides more information about lymphadenopathy and invasion of surrounding structures but at greater cost (Fig. 21).

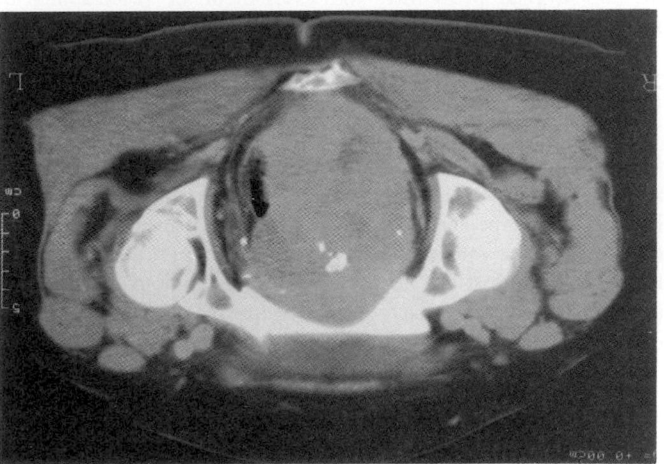

Fig. 21 CT of a rectal leiomyosarcoma filling the pelvis, arising from the rectal muscle and compressing the lumen (left).

Either investigation is excellent for detecting small volumes of ascites, ovarian enlargement, and hydronephrosis from retroperitoneal spread to the ureters. CT or ultrasound-guided biopsy or fine-needle aspiration cytology may be particularly useful in confirming or excluding the presence of metastasis. Abdominal ultrasound is the investigation of first choice to screen for metastases and CT is then reserved for cases where more information is

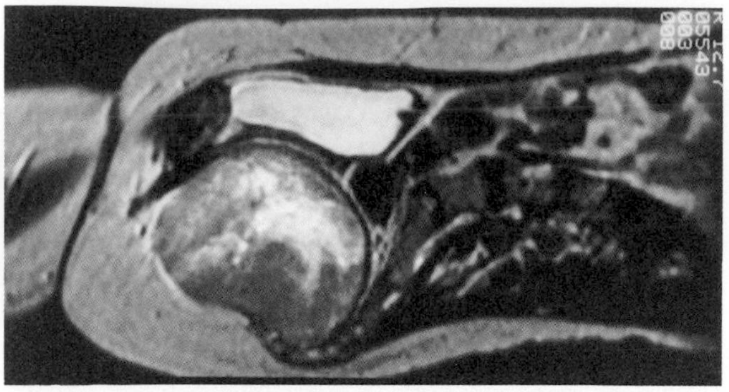

Fig. 22 MRI of a different rectal leiomyosarcoma behind the rectum which is pushed forward, compressing the bladder. The rectal muscle merges with the tumour.

required, so justifying the additional costs. Magnetic resonance imaging (MRI) can also identify tumours and metastases but adds little to the investigation of most cases of colonic cancer. However it may provide useful additional information in patients with large sarcomas of the colon or rectum (Fig. 22).

Intraoperative hepatic ultrasound is a recent and particularly useful method of detecting hepatic secondary deposits, locating their anatomical site in the segments of the liver, and determining the number of metastases. Histological confirmation of metastasis can then be made by direct needle biopsy and frozen section histology. The investigation is easily performed using a flat ultrasound probe in the palm of the hand and systematically moving it over the liver surface. The anatomical detail of the liver is excellent, the discrimination is much better than transabdominal ultrasonography and probably better than CT, and allows sensible modification of the surgical procedure and assessment of resectability of hepatic secondaries.

Blood tumour markers

Measurement of circulating antigens released by the tumour, such as carcinoembryonic antigen or, less commonly, α-fetoprotein have frequently been advocated but they have proved to be of little diagnostic value and have not passed into general use. They are, however, of limited use in studies of tumour biology and in prospective studies, particularly of follow-up practice, and in the use of second look laparotomy to treat occult tumour recurrence.

General investigations

Any patient being considered for an operation requires some preoperative investigations to confirm fitness for the procedure and to pre-empt postoperative problems. These investigations should include an electrocardiogram, simple lung function studies, particularly in people with a history of pulmonary problems, and a haemoglobin estimation. Renal function and state of hydration is satisfactorily monitored by estimation of blood urea, creatinine, and electrolyte concentrations. If an ultrasound examination suggests ureteric obstruction an excretion urogram should be performed to demonstrate its site. It is also most important to make a formal estimation of the nutritional state preoperatively, for postoperative morbidity is greatly increased in malnourished patients. The best estimation of nutritional state is by history of diet intake and weight loss, and physical examination, looking for the features of malnutrition. The level of serum albumin is the best single blood marker of malnutrition despite the many other causes of hypoalbuminaemia.

TREATMENT

Treatment has two objectives: firstly to treat the patient's symptoms without causing more problems than the cancer, and secondly to cure the patient of his cancer without putting the patient at undue risk. These two aspects of therapy are not necessarily the same and may, in fact, be in conflict. The patient's best interests will be served by his wishes and expectations, the demands of therapy and the presence or absence of serious comorbidity. For example a frail, elderly, infirm patient with rectal cancer causing few symptoms, but who has severe cardiac disease, may require little or no treatment for the rectal lesion when otherwise major resectional surgery with or without adjuvant therapy would be appropriate for a younger, fitter patient.

Surgical cure of colonic cancer requires excision of all the cancer. The principle that the tumour should be excised with an adequate margin of surrounding tissue, and as much of the vascular supply as is practical to ensure generous clearance of the local and regional lymph nodes, has stood the test of time and is agreed upon by all surgeons. There is, however, a considerable debate about what constitutes adequate margins and sufficient lymph node clearance. It is rare for a tumour to spread up or down the bowel as much as 2 cm from the primary unless it is undifferentiated or a signet cell tumour. Little bowel therefore needs to be removed on either side of the cancer to provide an adequate clearance. For rectal tumours, a 5 cm margin of clearance is satisfactory, though this may be reduced safely to as little as 2 cm for small, well differentiated lesions. Usually more colon is resected but this is determined by the vascular and lymphatic anatomy. Spread is likely to be more extensive into contiguous tissues such as the mesorectum, the lateral rectal ligaments, the bladder, the abdominal wall, the omentum, or the small bowel. Lateral margins therefore need to be generous to obtain adequate clearance. Where a tumour is invading adjacent structures and is resectable, all involved structures should be resected *en bloc* to avoid tumour dissemination. The prognosis for patients where the tumour has been resected piecemeal is significantly poorer.

A no-touch technique was advocated by Turnbull of the Cleveland Clinic Foundation, Ohio, where the vascular pedicle was ligated and divided before the tumour was handled or mobilized on the theoretical assumption that mobilization would shed malignant cells into the portal vein and increase metastasis formation. Although the technique was widely adopted, only one objective study has lent any support to the practice and it is indeed surprising how few systemic metastases occur, even when malignant cells are infused directly into the circulation through peritoneovenous shunts used to treat malignant ascites.

It is customary to remove the entire mesentery, ligating the vessels supplying the involved colon at their origin in order to achieve a radical removal of the draining and potentially diseased lymph nodes. Lymph node metastases occur along the pericolic arcade as well as down the main vascular pedicle. Ligation of the vascular supply and the need to remove the territory of bowel supplied by those vessels principally determines the amount of colon removed on either side of the cancer. While the prognosis is appreciably worse if the apical lymph node is involved by the cancer this does not necessarily imply that removal of all the draining lymph nodes will improve the prognosis for any or all patients. Traditional oncological surgical thinking was essentially anatomical, namely that tumours spread sequentially down an anatomical pathway and therefore it was necessary to remove the pathway to ensure cure. In an anterior resection for a mid-rectal cancer, for example, it was considered essential to ligate the inferior mesenteric artery at its origin from the aorta and also remove the ascending left colic artery. Resection in turn necessitated removal of the left colon because the marginal arcade around the splenic flexure is frequently incomplete. It seems irrational, from a biological standpoint, to think that ligation of the inferior mesenteric artery 2 cm more distal, so sparing the ascending left colic artery, would make any difference to the prognosis, and there is now evidence to show that high ligation provides no significant survival advantage. The nodal involvement indicates the malignant potential of the tumour and hence the probability of occult distant metastases and has no real bearing on the surgery, which should be directed to controlling the local and regional disease. High ligation should be reserved for those cases where the proximal nodes are clinically involved with tumour. Accurate lymph node staging may become as important as it is for breast cancer when adjuvant chemotherapy becomes more effective.

Another important general principle is that the ends of colon to be anastomosed after resection should have a good blood supply and be seen to bleed arterial blood, for ischaemia is the main cause of anastomotic failure and subsequent leakage. Tension on the anastomosis and overtight sutures are other important avoidable technical errors which may lead to failure of the anastomosis.

The material with which the anastomosis is made does not seem to be of critical importance. Colocolic anastomoses were, until fairly recently, fashioned in two layers, an outer seromuscular layer with a non-absorbable suture such as linen or silk and an inner absorbable, all coats, layer of 'catgut'. The outer layer was usually interrupted, while the inner layer was often a continuous suture. Randomized studies have demonstrated that a single layer interrupted, all coats, anastomosis performs better than the two-layer technique and most surgeons now use a single layer of slowly absorbable suture material, such as polyglactin or polyglycolic acid, when performing a hand-sewn anastomosis. Interrupted sutures are probably safer than a continuous suture in the left colon where the stool is solid, because they cause less stenosis before the sutures have disintegrated. If the mucosa is everted the anastomosis is more likely to leak and it is therefore important to ensure that the mucosa is inverted by the sutures. While it is quite easy to do this with an all layers interrupted suture Matheson has introduced the serosa/submucosal modification which avoids the mucosa, inverts satisfactorily, and has been shown to have a very low leakage rate (Fig. 23).

Stapling instruments, first developed in Russia, are now widely used to perform anastomoses. Construction of a side-to-side anastomosis using linear stapling devices is suitable if the bowel can be delivered on to the abdominal wall. End-to-end anastomosis using a circular stapler is most useful for low pelvic anastomoses. The instruments certainly shorten operating time, particularly when performing a low anterior resection of the rectum, but they are much more expensive than sutures. Controlled studies do not show any convincing differences in leakage rates between hand-sutured anastomoses and stapled anastomoses, provided the surgeon is equally competent with either technique. Selection of method is one of surgeon preference and economics. Concern has been expressed about steel staples potentiating anastomotic recurrence of the cancer, for which there is some experimental support. However, controlled clinical comparisons show that stapled anastomoses are significantly less likely to develop tumour recurrence.

BOWEL PREPARATION

Bowel preparation is generally accepted to be necessary before performing an anastomosis, though this surgical dogma was questioned in a recent prospective series of colon resections. However there is convincing evidence that reducing the faecal load, and with it the colonic bacterial load, reduces both wound and anastomotic problems. Mechanical preparation is the most important means of producing a 'socially clean colon'. Earlier studies also suggested that further reduction in bacterial flora with preoperative oral non-absorbable antibiotics such as sulphonamides, neomycin, and erythromycin base, conferred additional reductions in septic complications. However, the therapeutic effect appears to have been systemic from small amounts of antibiotic absorbed, and greater efficacy is achieved by using therapeutic doses of systemic antibiotics. Luminal antibiotics offer no additional advantage to mechanical bowel preparation provided systemic antibiotic prophylaxis is used.

Numerous methods of preparation have been proposed, tried, and used with little evidence of superiority, as measured by anastomotic or wound problems. Saline or osmotic purges such as Picolax® or Golytely® are currently the most widely used, give an acceptably clean colon in most patients, and are reasonably tolerated by most patients. Picolax preparation involves taking two sachets of non-absorbable sodium and magnesium salts dissolved in water and 2 l or more of clear fluid through the day on the day before operation. Golytely produces purgation with polyethylene glycol in about 4 l of fluid. The large volume of fluid required to produce a good preparation nauseates some patients.

Preoperative preparation is impossible in some patients with obstruction or perforation; in these circumstances a clean colon can be produced by intraoperative antegrade lavage of the colon after resection of the cancer. A small Foley catheter is introduced through the appendix stump or into the distal ileum, which is occluded proximally with a soft intestinal clamp. Warmed saline is then irrigated through the colon until it is perfectly clean. The effluent is collected by tying a large bore plastic tube, such as anaesthetic gas scavenging tubing, into the cut end of the bowel and placing the distal end in a suitably large bucket. The proximal end of the colon is then freshened before creation of the anastomosis. Closed collecting systems have been devised which are more aesthetic to use but are neither necessary nor economic. There are clear clinical and economic advantages if a primary resection and anastomosis can be performed safely in the acute situation, rather than a preliminary stoma or a resection and stoma with subsequent re-anastomosis.

ANTIBIOTIC PROPHYLAXIS

Sepsis bedevilled colonic surgery for many decades and was the cause of much morbidity and occasional mortality. Systemic

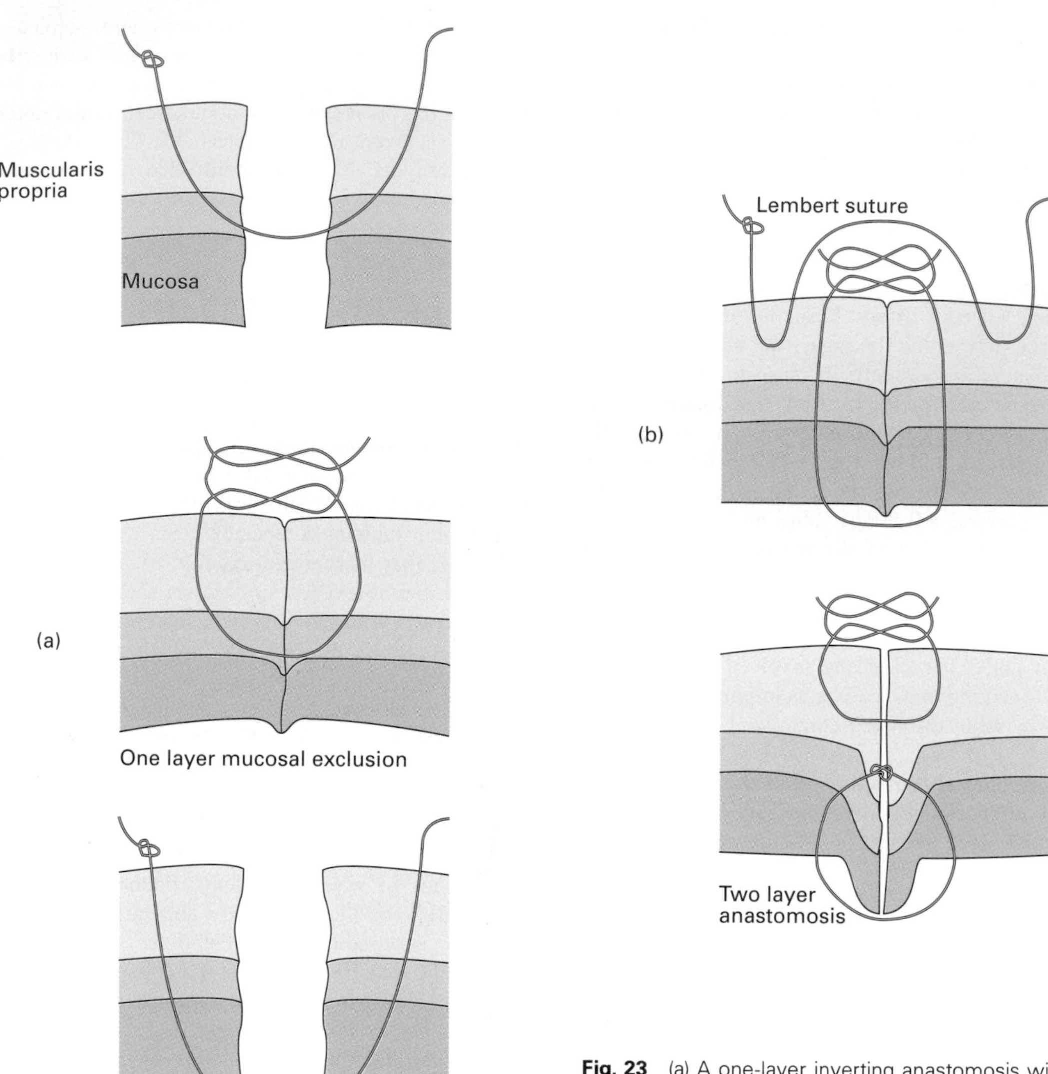

Fig. 23 (a) A one-layer inverting anastomosis with mucosal exclusion. (b) A two-layer inverting anastomosis. The inner layer traverses all coats while the outer layer is a seromuscular suture.

broad-spectrum antibiotic prophylaxis aimed against aerobic and anaerobic bowel pathogens has revolutionized colorectal surgical practice. Wound infection rates have been reduced from as high as 70 per cent to less than 10 per cent, while serious intra-abdominal sepsis has been reduced from as much as 20 per cent to less than 5 per cent.

Second-generation cephalosporin drugs active against Gram-negative organisms, in combination with metronidazole or tinidazole, active against anaerobic bacteria, are effective and widely used. Different drugs used singly and in combination for prophylaxis, provide numerous study data but little therapeutic advantage. The essential for effective prophylaxis is a high tissue level of antibiotic at the time of operation and, therefore, of potential tissue contamination. The antibiotics should be administered intravenously at the induction of anaesthesia; if the operation lasts longer than 3 or 4 h a repeat dose should be given to maintain therapeutic tissue levels. A delay of four or more hours after operation before giving the antibiotic provides no prophylaxis against infective complications and is as good as no prophylaxis at all. Good tissue levels of metronidazole can be achieved from intrarectal metronidazole suppositories; this is acceptable for proximal colonic resections but not for rectal resections.

There is some debate over the number of doses of antibiotic required to provide effective prophylaxis, but there is definitely no advantage in giving more than three doses of most antibiotic regimens, while one good dose may well be as effective and more economical. The loading dose required may be higher than that used to treat an established infection. For example, cefuroxime 1.5 g and metronidazole 1 g is a very common regimen for prophylaxis. If the patient has an abscess or infection at the time of resection it is clearly prudent to treat the infection with a full course of antibiotic therapy. Unnecessary continuation of treatment or the use of inappropriate antibiotics, such as clindamycin, predisposes to *Clostridium difficile* infection and pseudomembranous colitis, a severe and sometimes fatal complication when not recognized early. Severe persistent postoperative diarrhoea is the commonest symptom and the diagnosis is confirmed by identifying the organism or toxin in the stool. Treatment with vancomycin is usually effective.

THROMBOEMBOLISM PROPHYLAXIS

Elderly patients with malignancy are particularly liable to venous thrombosis and pulmonary embolism, a sometimes fatal and often preventable complication of surgery. Additional risk factors are obesity, varicose veins, and a previous history of thrombosis or embolism. It is therefore necessary to consider perioperative prophylaxis for patients undergoing resection for colonic cancer. Subcutaneous heparin, 5000 i.u. three times daily until the patient is fully mobile, is the most common method of prophylaxis and the one for which there is most supporting data. Blood loss may be greater than usual if the thrombin time is increased. Perioperative Dextran 70 infusion is an alternative method, but allergic reactions to the Dextran occasionally occur. Compression stockings and active calf exercises are also commonly used while the patient is bedbound, but evidence for their efficacy is scant. Intraoperative calf muscle stimulation is claimed to provide effective prophylaxis, but again the evidence is unconvincing.

RESECTIONS

Carcinoma, caecum, and right colon

Right hemicolectomy is the standard operation for cancers of the caecum and ascending colon, removing as little of the terminal ileum and as much of the ileocolic artery as is possible while still maintaining the blood supply to the terminal ileum. More terminal ileum may need to be removed for tumours near the ileocaecal valve, but vitamin B_{12} deficiency and bile salt diarrhoea are common complications if more than 50 cm is resected. The ascending right colic artery is also ligated at its origin from the ileocolic artery. The distal extent of colon removed depends upon the site of the tumour. The resection may need to extend to the mid-transverse colon for cancers near the hepatic flexure. The terminal ileum is then anastomosed to the proximal transverse colon in one or two layers (Fig. 24). On the other hand the caecum may be preserved when resecting tumours at the hepatic flexure and a colocolic anastomosis fashioned, thus preserving the reabsorptive capacity of the caecum and reducing the risk of postoperative diarrhoea (Fig. 25).

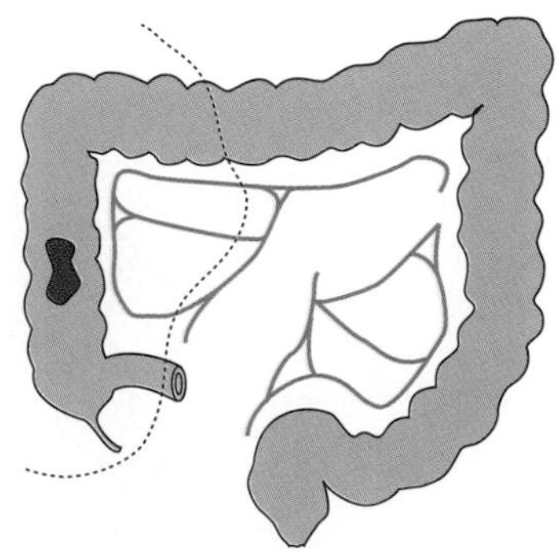

Fig. 24 Right hemicolectomy.

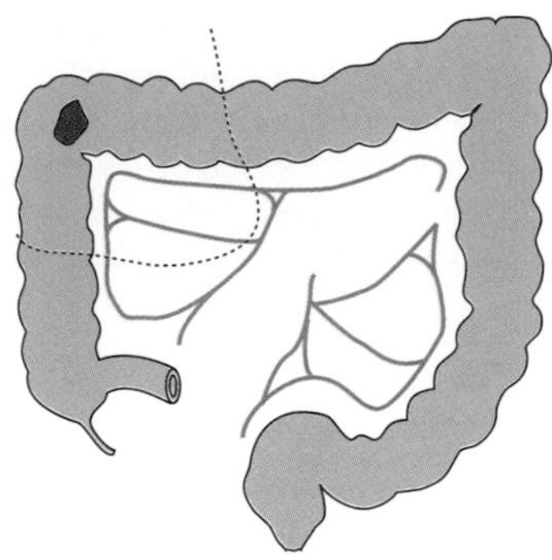

Fig. 25 Hepatic flexure resection.

A midline incision is the most common approach, but small cancers are readily resected through horizontal or oblique (Rutherford-Morison) muscle cutting incisions. The latter approaches cause less pain because tension on the wound is less and the nerve supply to the wound is easily blocked with bupivicaine to provide immediate postoperative analgesia. Furthermore the wound heals with less spread or keloid scarring and is therefore more cosmetically acceptable. A midline incision is, however, easier to extend should more resection be necessary. Endoscopic techniques for colonic resection are already being developed in order to minimize the trauma and pain of the abdominal wall incision. The entire operation, including the anastomosis, can be performed endoscopically. Alternatively the colon can be mobilized endoscopically before delivering the bowel and tumour through a small abdominal incision where the resection and anastomosis are completed by hand. These new techniques look promising and may reduce hospital stay but are more time consuming and have still to be refined and tested rigorously against conventional operations.

Transverse colectomy

The most usual approach is through an upper midline incision that may extend a little below the umbilicus, though a transverse muscle cutting incision provides excellent exposure for the transverse colon. The lymphatic drainage for cancers of the transverse colon is along the middle colic vessels to the root of the superior mesenteric artery. Resection therefore removes most of the colon supplied by the middle colic artery and in particular the splenic flexure where the pericolic vascular arcade is often incomplete (Fig. 26). If lymph nodes along the ascending right colic artery are

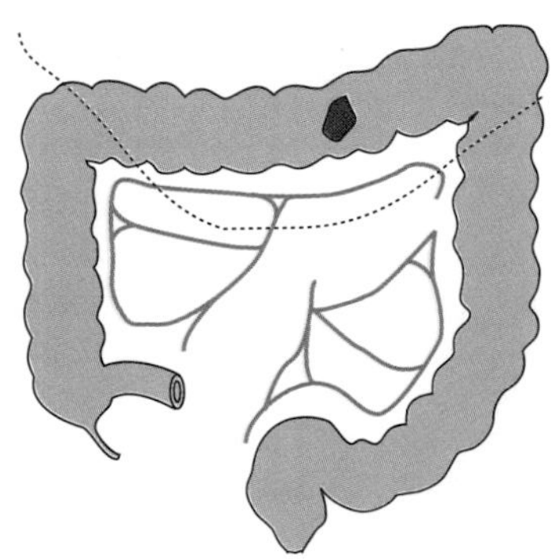

Fig. 26 Transverse colectomy.

enlarged and potentially cancerous, the resection may need to be extended to include part of the ascending colon. The omentum is removed *en bloc* with the tumour leaving the gastroepiploic vessels. Resection of part of the stomach or jejunum may be required if the colonic tumour is invading either organ. The resection is completed by an end-to-end colocolic anastomosis.

Left hemicolectomy

Generous exposure is necessary to provide good access to the splenic flexure, which is often high and attached to the spleen, and so again a midline incision, extending above and below the umbilicus, is most often used, though some surgeons prefer an oblique Rutherford-Morison incision. Careless traction on the colon while mobilizing the splenic flexure may tear the spleen and produce haemorrhage sufficient to require splenectomy which increases the risk of thromboembolism in the immediate postoperative period and the risk of overwhelming infection in the future, a complication therefore to be avoided. The proximal resection should include the splenic flexure because the ascending left colic artery is ligated at its origin and the pericolic anastomosis is often inadequate to ensure a good blood supply to the anastomosis. The transverse colon is mobilized sufficiently to perform a tension free anastomosis. The distal resection extends into the sigmoid colon preserving one of the distal sigmoid arteries and the pericolic vascular arcade. The inferior mesenteric artery is seldom ligated at its origin but should it be necessary to take this vessel because of node metastases, the distal resection should be extended to the proximal rectum which is adequately supplied from the middle rectal artery (Fig. 27).

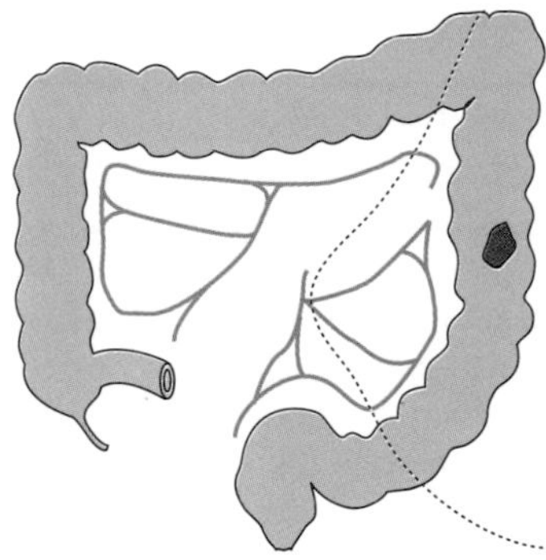

Fig. 27 Left hemicolectomy.

Sigmoid colectomy

Three-quarters of all large bowel cancers lie distal to the splenic flexure and most are found in the sigmoid colon. This is readily approached through either a lower midline incision or a Rutherford-Morison incision. The sigmoid colon has the advantage of usually being mobile and on a generous mesentery and therefore the dissection seldom needs to be extensive. If the sigmoid colon is also affected by diverticular disease, mobilization needs to be more extensive to provide a tension-free anastomosis, particularly when there is inflammation and fibrosis. The sigmoid vessels are ligated as they arise form the inferior mesenteric (Fig. 28), preserving the ascending left colic and superior rectal vessels. If the proximal mesenteric nodes are involved then the inferior mesenteric artery may need to be taken at its origin and an extended left hemicolectomy performed to provide sufficient tumour clearance for adequate local clearance and control.

Sigmoid cancers often invade surrounding structures such as the abdominal wall, ovary, uterus, bladder, or small bowel. In such cases *en bloc* removal of the invaded organs is necessary. If the tumour is stuck to the abdominal wall, the peritoneum and muscle are excised, preferably using diathermy. Care must be taken to identify and preserve the ureter; preservation may be difficult, particularly when there is considerable pericolic inflammation. If the ureter is invaded then the involved segment may be removed and the ureter re-anastomosed obliquely with fine catgut or polyglactin, thereby reducing the risk of ureteric stricture. If too much ureter has been removed to restore continuity the proximal ureter may be joined end-to-side to the contralateral ureter producing a crossed ureteroureterostomy. Left oophorectomy or hysterectomy may also be required to give sufficient clearance for local control of the cancer. The bladder is more commonly invaded in males, and partial cystectomy may be necessary. The bladder is then closed in one or two layers of absorbable sutures and drained with a catheter for about 10 days to ensure adequate healing.

Rectal cancer

Rectal cancer presents a challenge for the surgeon both technically and in clinical judgement. About 25 per cent of large bowel cancers develop in the rectum; since the prognosis is generally more favourable than that for more proximal tumours, cure should more often be the rule. Some 30 years ago nearly all patients with rectal cancer were treated by excision of the rectum and anus and left with a permanent left iliac fossa end colostomy, because it was considered both dangerous and therapeutically inadequate to remove less and to attempt a restorative anastomosis. Improvements in operative technique and careful clinical studies have shown both premises to be incorrect, at least for most lesions of the midrectum and all in the proximal rectum. The skill and judgement comes in selecting patients for restorative resection, local excision, abdominoperineal excision or, sometimes, non-operative methods when palliation is the sole objective.

The distance of the tumour from the anal canal is central in deciding upon an anterior resection of the rectum with anastomosis, because sufficient clear margin is required beyond the cancer to minimize the chance of local recurrence, while satisfac-

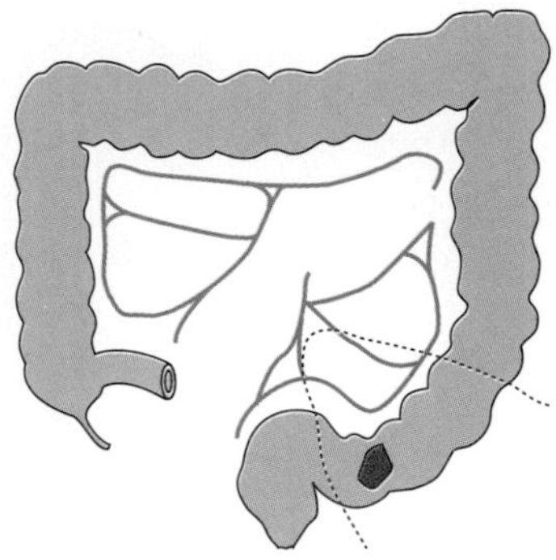

Fig. 28 Sigmoid colectomy.

tory long-term function is better with a greater residual rectal reservoir. Radical resection close to the anus not only reduces the rectal reservoir but also impairs internal sphincter tone, thereby reducing anal control and continence. It used to be said that a clear margin of at least 5 cm distal to the tumour was essential to prevent anastomotic or local recurrence; more recent data suggest that cancers seldom infiltrate the bowel wall as much as 1 cm beyond the macroscopic margin, and a 2-cm margin is therefore both ample and safe, provided that the cancers are well or moderately well differentiated. Poorly differentiated or undifferentiated tumours may spread further along the bowel wall and a margin of at least 5 cm is advisable. What appears more important is that tumours that have extended through the bowel wall may spread more extensively within the mesorectum or laterally around the middle rectal vessels. All the mesorectum should therefore be removed, and the lateral clearance should be at least as far as the sacral parasympathetic nerves to prevent local recurrence. The obvious extension of this concept is that a complete pelvic node dissection, similar to that of a Wertheim's hysterectomy would improve survival, but it is disappointing that *en bloc* internal iliac lymph node removal adds nothing but morbidity and confers no survival advantage.

Tumour stage remains, at present, the most important factor in deciding upon the surgical approach for the patient; tumour differentiation is a useful subsidiary factor. For example a T3, N1 undifferentiated tumour is biologically less favourable, requiring greater margins of clearance to prevent local recurrence, than a T1, N0 well differentiated lesion. The latter may be quite suitable for local excision if the tumour is small enough.

Anterior resection

Anterior resection is now the standard radical operation for cancers of the upper and mid-rectum and for the more favourable tumours of the distal rectum when a 2-cm margin of clearance is possible while still leaving the anal transition zone intact.

The usual approach is through a lower midline incision, which may extend above the umbilicus if the splenic flexure requires mobilization. A few surgeons advocate a subumbilical horizontal muscle cutting incision as an alternative. Early ligation of the vascular pedicle before the tumour is handled or dissected, originally advocated by Turnbull, may reduce the incidence of hepatic metastases, though the evidence is not yet conclusive. Flush ligation of the inferior mesenteric artery at its origin from the aorta is still practised by many surgeons for cancer clearance, although it is not based on a proper perspective of tumour biology and there are no satisfactory data to support the manoeuvre. Ligation just distal to the origin of the ascending left colic artery, which is my own preference, does not compromise survival and ensures a good blood supply to the left colon which may be lost by a flush ligation of the inferior mesenteric artery (Fig. 29). If the apical node is involved a flush ligation is necessary to control the local disease although the overall prognosis is poor.

Pelvic dissection requires accuracy firstly to avoid cutting too close to the tumour and secondly to spare the autonomic nerves to the bladder and penis. Posteriorly, the dissection is carried caudad behind the mesorectum but anterior to the sympathetic *nervi erigentes*. Laterally, the middle rectal vessels are secured on the side wall of the pelvis but medial to the parasympathetic plexus supplying the bladder. As the rectum and tumour are mobilized out of the pelvis, the surgeon must avoid dissecting too close to the

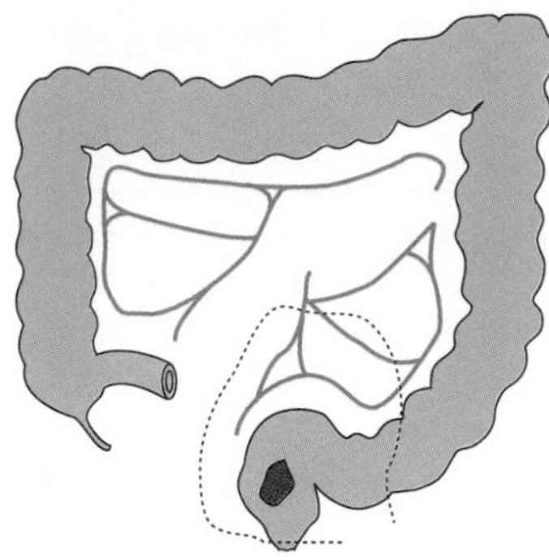

Fig. 29 Anterior resection of the rectum.

cancer, thereby compromising the prospect of cure. Cutting close to the tumour is a common mistake particularly when traction is applied to the rectum and the surgeon is inexperienced. When the rectum is fully mobilized the mesorectum is cleaned from the bowel wall and a cross-clamp is applied just proximal to the proposed site of the anastomosis and the rectum is irrigated with 1 per cent chlorhexidine solution, povidone iodine solution, or perchlorate of mercury, to kill any viable tumour cells that have been shed into the bowel lumen and which could implant into the anastomosis. Shed neoplastic cells are a potential cause of local recurrence of cancer, particularly at the suture line, though most local pelvic recurrences arise from residual tumour in the mesorectum, in the lateral ligaments, or on the side wall of the pelvis. These recurrences may then invade the anastomosis to appear at the suture line.

The anastomosis is either fashioned manually with sutures or mechanically with stapling instruments. Each method is equally effective, provided the surgeon is adept at either technique although there is some evidence to suggest that tumour recurrence may be less in patients with staples. There are numerous minor technical modifications to suit individual surgical idiosyncrasies but the essentials common to all are a good blood supply to the cut ends of the bowel and an anastomosis free from tension. Poor blood supply and tension at the suture line are likely to cause anastomotic leakage, sepsis, and sometimes peritonitis. For this reason many surgeons insist that the splenic flexure should be mobilized fully, but there are no objective data to support this practice in all cases. Repeated taeniamyotomy proximal to the anastomosis, originally used to treat diverticular disease, will also increase the length of the colon, and reduce tension on the anastomosis and colonic contraction. However, the incidence of anastomotic leakage and local tumour recurrence after anterior resection has been shown to depend upon the surgeon's skills almost as much as the tumour biology and to vary four-fold from the best to the worst results. Each surgeon must audit his performance to ensure that his technique is unimpeachable.

The functional results of anterior resection are usually good, sometimes moderate, but occasionally poor in terms of stool frequency, urgency, and continence, particularly when the colon is anastomosed to the upper anal canal. Internal anal sphincter function is often impaired by the necessary cancer clearance, probably due to damage to the nerve supply. External anal sphincter function usually remains normal but is insufficient to maintain complete continence, particularly when the stool is loose and the proximal colon is not compliant. Bowel function continues to improve spontaneously for 12 to 18 months, but early functional results can be improved by fashioning a small colonic pouch to increase colonic compliance and then anastomosing the pouch to the anus.

Abdominoperineal excision of the rectum

This operation is now largely reserved for larger T2–3, N 0–3 tumours of the distal rectum and those which are poorly differentiated, when a safe anastomosis is not practicable. The original operation described by Miles is for surgeons operating single-handed. The rectum is mobilized down to the pelvic floor through a subumbilical midline incision. The bowel is divided and the distal sigmoid brought out as a left iliac fossa colostomy. The distal colon is oversewn and is folded down into the pelvis before closing the pelvic peritoneum over the rectum. The abdominal wound is then closed and the colostomy is matured using catgut or polyglactin sutures. A marginally better mucocutaneous junction is produced if the sutures are placed at a subcuticular location rather than through the skin, in the manner described by Turnbull. The patient is then turned on to the left lateral side for the perineal dissection. A perianal elliptical incision is made to mobilize and deliver the anus and distal rectum. The most common error in the perineal dissection is to dissect too close to the rectum, and therefore to the tumour, defeating the prime objective of controlling the local disease. To avoid this mistake the initial dissection is carried well into the ischiorectal fossa, dividing the pudendal vessels supplying the anus before dividing the levator ani muscles laterally. The tip of the coccyx may also have to be removed to give adequate clearance of posterior cancers. Anteriorly, the dissection in males is constrained by the urethra, prostate, and seminal vesicles, though the last can be removed if necessary. A Cluttons sound or urethral catheter provides a useful landmark to prevent damage to the urethral bulb. Mobilization is much easier in females, for the back wall of the vagina can be removed with the rectum, providing a particularly useful manoeuvre for clearing anterior tumours. The perineal tissues are then closed loosely over a drain. There is much discussion in the medical literature on the merits of different methods and types of drain with no clear consensus, which leaves surgeons to exercise their preferences: mine is to use an 8-mm tube drain through the perineal wound.

Abdominoperineal resection is now more commonly performed with the patient in the modified lithotomy Trendelenberg position and two surgeons operating simultaneously. The perineal part of the operation is often, wrongly, delegated to the less experienced operator, which may account for the unacceptably high rates of local recurrence in some series. It is my contention that the perineal operator should be the more experienced, or if a trainee is operating then it must be with direct supervision to avoid the mistake of cutting close to the tumour or damaging the urethra. The principles of the operation are otherwise similar to those of the Miles procedure.

Hartmann's operation

Hartmann's operation is, in essence, an anterior resection of the rectum without an anastomosis. The proximal bowel end is brought out as a left iliac fossa colostomy and the rectal stump is oversewn deep in the pelvis. The operation is seldom performed electively or for cure and is usually reserved for palliation, or sometimes as a preliminary procedure for acute cases. The surgeon preparing to perform an anterior resection may be faced with a much more advanced tumour with pelvic peritoneal tumour seedlings and perhaps extension to the side wall of the pelvis or even more widespread metastases. Good palliation may be provided by removing the primary cancer to relieve intolerable bowel symptoms, but the certainty of early local recurrence and failure to palliate precludes creation of an anastomosis. Patients presenting with acute malignant colonic obstruction or peritonitis from perforation of a rectal cancer may also be unsuitable candidates for resection and primary anastomosis. Perforation of a cancer implies incurability because of pelvic seeding with malignant cells. Pelvic sepsis increases the chance of anastomotic breakdown and leakage, and may also encourage local recurrence. Safer palliation is therefore achieved by resection without anastomosis. However, for acute colonic obstruction the colon can be prepared satisfactorily by intraoperative antegrade colonic lavage to produce a clean bowel which may be anastomosed safely as an alternative to Hartmann's operation, provided the disparity between the ends to be joined is not large. A temporary defunctioning proximal stoma may give additional safety.

Local excision

Some small early well differentiated rectal cancers (T1–2, N0) may be managed by local treatment with the expectation of cure. However, less than 10 per cent of patients are likely to be suitable for such treatment, although the precise proportion of patients with such lesions is unknown. Numerous techniques have been advocated: their proponents claim success but there are no satisfactory comparative studies to support such claims. Local recurrence of the cancer because of inadequate clearance or tumour implantation is the principal problem which may jeopardize alternative methods of treatment. *Per anum* disc excision of the rectal tumour, with a margin of more than 0.5 cm and suture of the defect in the rectum, is the technique most commonly used and one that provides an excellent specimen for histological assessment. This method, however, requires wide dilatation of the anus with the risk of subsequent faecal incontinence from damage to the anal sphincters, and is inadequate for lesions higher in the rectum because of inaccessibility. The method has been refined and the operating range extended by Buess using a specially modified operating proctoscope with binocular magnified vision and endoscopic instruments inserted through side ports in the proctoscope. The operating field is maintained by continuous CO_2 insufflation, magnification provides accuracy, and the anus is not forcibly dilated, but the technical skills require practice. Nevertheless the method looks promising, especially for small cancers and villous adenomas.

Alternatively lesions can be electrocoagulated, using conventional surgical diathermy apparatus, the charred tissue being curetted until soft healthy tissue is reached. Good results have been reported but again the anus requires forceful dilatation and no specimen is provided for histological examination. Endoscopic resection, using a modified urological instrument, glycine irrigation, and the same techniques used to resect bladder tumours or the prostate, overcomes these problems but the resected specimen is less easy to stage than a disc excision because of fragmentation. The results of endoscopic resection appear comparable to those of major resection for similar biologically favourable tumours. Both these local methods are simple and can be repeated whenever necessary. Larger cancers in frail elderly patients, unsuitable for major surgery, can be treated by endoscopic resection with the objective of symptom and tumour control rather than cure

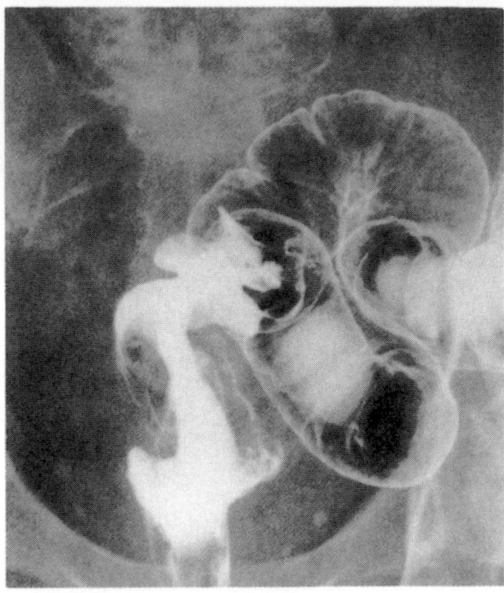

Fig. 30 A large rectal cancer controlled by endoscopic transanal resection in a frail elderly man. Minimal residual disease and no symptoms 2 years after initial treatment.

(Fig. 30). A few tumours regress and disappear with repeated resection while a similar proportion, particularly undifferentiated lesions, continue to grow and metastasize. The majority are contained.

Irradiation and, in particular, high-dose interstitial irradiation has also been claimed to give good results although there is an increased risk of carcinogenesis in the long term.

Laser therapy may also have a place in the treatment of smaller rectal and colonic tumours. The laser light is delivered through a colonoscope or flexible sigmoidoscope which allows treatment to be given to an outpatient under intravenous sedation. The most widely used laser is the neodymium YAG laser which vaporizes and coagulates the tissue to a depth of 5 mm. Small cancers can be destroyed but larger lesions are difficult to treat satisfactorily even with energies as high as 40 kJ. Photodynamic therapy also looks promising, but again for small lesions. This method requires pre-treatment with a light-sensitive haematoporphyrin derivative which is selectively retained in tumours. Laser light, of the correct wavelength to be absorbed by the haematoporphyrin derivative, is delivered by a copper or gold vapour laser. The absorbed energy induces release of oxygen free radicals, which in turn produce local tissue damage and destruction within the tumour. The main complication of the treatment is a skin rash induced by exposure to sunlight. Patients therefore need to remain indoors and keep the skin covered for a few days after taking the haematoporphyrin derivative.

Transrectal ultrasonography appears an important method for selecting patients and tumours for local therapy and also for monitoring progress. Ultrasound provides good images of the rectal wall and therefore the depth of tumour invasion (Figs. 19, 20). It is also able to image enlarged lymph nodes.

ACUTE PRESENTATIONS

Nearly one-fifth of patients with colon cancer still present acutely with either obstruction or perforation and have a worse prognosis, stage for stage, than those presenting electively.

Colonic obstruction

Approximately 15 per cent of patients in large unselected series present with acute large bowel obstruction. About half are left-sided cancers which suggests that proportionately more right-sided cancers present with obstruction since 75 per cent of colon cancers occur distal to the splenic flexure. This is not surprising because the stool is liquid in the caecum, which accounts for the later presentations with anaemia or obstruction; any stenosis in the left colon is likely to produce a change in bowel habit which prompts presentation to the doctor. In general, obstructing cancers are more advanced than those presenting electively which accounts for some, but not all, of the poorer prognosis.

The history of patients presenting with acute colonic obstruction is often surprisingly short, with rapidly progressive constipation, abdominal distension, abdominal pain, and the inability to pass flatus. Vomiting is a common consequence of the abdominal pain, but faeculent vomiting is a late symptom and only occurs when the ileocaecal valve is incompetent.

The physical signs depend on the site of the obstruction. Right-sided lesions usually present with what appears to be distal small bowel obstruction; patients suffer central abdominal colic, distension, borborygmi and later, faeculent vomit. Tenderness is not a common feature unless the obstruction is prolonged, but dehydration, hypotension, and tachycardia occur early because large volumes of fluid and electrolytes are sequestered in the ileum and are lost as vomit. A plain abdominal radiograph confirms the diagnosis of distal small bowel obstruction with gross gaseous distension of the small bowel and little or no gas in the colon. A contrast study of the colon is seldom required before surgical treatment.

Left colonic obstruction more commonly presents with gross distension limited to the colon: the ileocaecal valve remains competent in about 60 per cent of patients. Very high intraluminal pressures are generated, reducing circulation to the colon and, in particular to the thin-walled caecum, which is in danger of ischaemic rupture. Clinically, the distension is more in the flanks. Tenderness over the caecum is an early sign and signifies impending rupture, faecal peritonitis, and endotoxaemia, which often progresses to multiorgan failure and death. Obstructed bowel sounds are not a dominant feature: a secondary ileus with scant tinkling sounds is more usual. The plain abdominal radiograph shows gross colonic distension and there is often a sharp cut-off at the point of obstruction, with an airless distal colon. A contrast study of the colon is, however, essential to confirm the diagnosis, identify the site of obstruction, and exclude conditions such as pseudo-obstruction, acute myxoedematous colonic obstruction, and ischaemic colitis.

Acute colonic obstruction requires urgent surgical relief, but before going to the operating theatre the patient needs rehydration and re-expansion of the circulatory volume. If there are signs of peritonitis, antibiotics should also be given parenterally.

Obstructing right and transverse colon cancers are relatively easily treated by an immediate right hemicolectomy or extended right hemicolectomy, respectively, and an end-to-end ileocolic anastomosis which rids the patient of the primary and treats the obstruction at one operation. Left colonic and rectal obstruction, however, presents more of a problem and surgical strategies are still evolving. It used to be considered that emergency left colonic resection in obstructed, unprepared bowel carried too high a mortality rate and that the obstruction was best relieved by a caecostomy or transverse loop colostomy. The patient was then restored to better health, the bowel prepared by washouts, and the left colon resected and anastomosed at an elective procedure 2 or 3 weeks later. The colostomy was sometimes closed at the same time as the resection but more usually later when the patient had recovered fully from the resection, so completing a three-stage operation. The cumulative mortality and morbidity of the three stages is high, particularly in elderly patients. The length of hospital stay is also long, which substantially increases the costs of treatment. Such multistaged resections are now seldom performed in modern hospitals, but an emergency colostomy still has a place if the patient is far from good medical help.

Over the last 20 years evidence has accumulated which supports definitive single-stage treatment for the obstructed left colon. The present choice is between an extended or subtotal colectomy and ileosigmoid or ileorectal anastomosis, removing all the obstructed colon, and a more limited colonic resection, with on-table colonic lavage to decompress and clean the obstructed colon, and a colocolic, or colorectal anastomosis. There are no convincing comparative data to decide the issue. Early evidence suggested that limited colonic resection and anastomosis was liable to leak because the bowel was unprepared, there was great disparity between the ends to be joined, and the vascular supply to the obstructed colon was suspect; therefore resection of all the obstructed colon became fashionable. Mortality and morbidity was certainly lower but at the expense of poorer long-term, bowel function. With on-table colonic lavage, systemic antibiotics, and better suture material, anastomotic techniques, and postoperative support, the pendulum has swung back to more conservative resections with satisfactory results. The obstructed colon is more readily mobilized if it is first decompressed by inserting a 19 gauge needle into the lumen and attaching it to suction. The anastomosis may be protected by a caecostomy or loop ileostomy for added safety.

Rarely a Hartmann's operation is performed for an obstructing left colon cancer with the intention of subsequent re-anastomosis. The operation is usually reserved for palliation when pelvic peritoneal metastases would make an anastomosis hazardous or risk recurrent obstruction.

Perforation

Perforation is less common than is obstruction, occurring in about 5 per cent of patients. The site of perforation is usually within the tumour and is not associated with obstruction but is the consequence of tumour necrosis. The patient presents with severe, often sudden, abdominal pain and signs of peritonitis. Rapid cardiovascular collapse and endotoxaemic shock usually signify a major leak and faecal peritonitis, rather than a small perforation with purulent peritonitis, but may also follow delay in diagnosis. Because the perforation occurs through the tumour, malignant cells are disseminated throughout the peritoneum, making cure unlikely. Good palliation is therefore the paramount aim and long-term survival is an unanticipated bonus.

The patient requires pain relief, rapid fluid and colloid resuscitation, and systemic antibiotic therapy before moving to the operating theatre. Delay in diagnosis and definitive treatment greatly increases the risk of subsequent multiorgan failure and death. The surgical judgements are similar to those required for obstruction, with the caveat that as few tissue planes as possible should be opened in order to reduce the risk of abscess formation. Resections should be conservative rather than radical, and the ends of the bowel should either be brought out as a stoma and mucous fistula, or, if a primary anastomosis is fashioned, a loop ileostomy should be made because an anastomosis is more likely to leak in the presence of severe sepsis. In addition the peritoneal cavity should be lavaged well with saline alone or containing antibiotics effective against enteric organisms. Tube drains should be inserted into the pelvis and subphrenic spaces. Systemic antibiotic therapy should be continued for at least 5 days. Occasionally it is wise to leave the abdominal wound completely open as a laparostomy to allow peritoneal exudates to drain freely and to enable easy, and if necessary repeated, access to spaces where pus may collect. Many patients will require inotropic support, visceral vasodilator drugs, and careful surveillance of cardiovascular function, and will therefore need to be in an intensive therapy unit postoperatively.

ADJUVANT THERAPY

Evidence from treating other types of cancer suggests that adjuvant therapy should be successful, and is most likely to be effective against minimal disease and micrometastases. Such treatments should, in theory, be used postoperatively and in patients at greatest risk of having residual but microscopic disease (T3 and N2 lesions). Chemotherapy, immunotherapy, and irradiation have all been tried as adjuvant treatments before and, more often, after surgery without unequivocal success. Meta-analysis of many randomized trials of both irradiation and chemotherapy suggest some small survival advantage in some groups of patients for each method of treatment. Such evidence has been the stimulus for a large multicentre study in the United Kingdom (AXIS) to try to establish the roles of chemotherapy and irradiation. Very large numbers of patients are required to provide convincing proof because of the many clinical and pathological variables that affect outcome and must be accommodated.

Radiotherapy may be administered either before or after removal of the primary tumour with different aims in view. Patients with large T3 or T4 rectal cancers fixed to the pelvis on clinical and CT examination and therefore not usefully removable may have their tumours 'downstaged' sufficiently to convert an irremoveable lesion into one that is resectable some 6 weeks after a radiation dose of 50 to 60 cGy. Such pelvic irradiation slightly but significantly reduces the risk of local recurrence after resection, but this is not yet translated into a corresponding survival advantage. Postoperative irradiation of the tumour bed of less advanced resectable T3–4 cancers, particularly of the rectum and caecum, may also reduce the risks of local recurrence, which in turn could produce a 5 to 10 per cent improvement in 5-year survival rates. Lack of convincing evidence in favour of radiotherapy will, for the present, encourage surgeons to be selective and to restrict adjuvant irradiation to such patients judged clinically to be at particular risk of local recurrence where there may be a small but useful clinical yield.

Similarly, postoperative adjuvant chemotherapy, principally with 5-fluorouracil as a single agent, may provide a small survival advantage in selected patients, such as those with N2 tumours, who are at particular risk of occult hepatic metastases. The most promising results are from infusion of 5-fluorouracil into the portal vein to provide a high therapeutic dose directly to the micrometastases. Experimental and clinical studies suggest that the incidence of hepatic metastases is slightly less after portal vein infusion, but the differences are not yet sufficiently large or certain to warrant widespread use. Other agents such as Adriamycin, mitomycin C, doxorubicin, and cisplatin have been tried but are toxic and have, at present, no useful role as adjuvant chemotherapeutic drugs for colorectal cancer. Irradiation has been tried in combination with 5-fluorouracil and semustine as adjuvant therapy in patients with rectal cancer with apparent improvement in survival but at the cost of increased toxicity. The addition of folinic acid however improves the efficacy of 5-fluorouracil while reducing the toxicity. There is, however, little doubt that chemotherapy and irradiation, perhaps in conjunction with biological modulators such as interferons or cytokines, will in the future, play an increasingly important role in the treatment of patients with Dukes' B and C lesions.

Adjuvant immunotherapy with agents such as BCG and *Corynebacterium parvum* have been tried in patients with more advanced colon cancers with the objective of stimulating the immune system non-specifically, but sufficiently to produce a lethal effect on micrometastases. The theory is that immune surveillance can affect tumour survival and, indeed, those cancers with a marked lymphocytic and macrophage infiltration, and a histiocytic response in the adjacent lymph nodes have a better prognosis. Unfortunately the results of clinical trials have been disappointing. Levamisole, a non-specific immune stimulant, has also been tried both alone and in combination with 5-fluorouracil with mixed results. One study of 5-fluorouracil and levamisole appeared sufficiently encouraging for the combination to be widely used for adjuvant therapy in the United States although the control comparison was questionable.

PALLIATION

Many patients present with incurable colonic cancer, or suffer a recurrence after surgery. This situation makes management difficult, for the burden of treatment must be weighed carefully against the potential gain, not only in length of life but, more importantly, in the relief of symptoms and the quality of the time remaining. The prospect of cure to some extent justifies radical therapy but the aims of palliation must be different and therefore the measures modified to achieve those aims. The options open to the surgeon are surgery, irradiation, chemotherapy, and drug management of symptoms.

Surgery

Surgery may be directed to the primary lesion or to the secondaries, for example in the liver or small bowel (Table 7).

Table 7 Surgical options for palliation

Surgery to primary	Surgery to metastases
Resection ± stoma	Hepatic resection
Bypass Ileocolic Colocolic	Hepatic artery Embolization Cannulation Ligation
ETAR	Interstitial laser therapy
Laser therapy	Small bowel Resection Bypass
Cryotherapy	Ureteric stenting

Patients often present with symptoms from the primary colonic cancer and totally asymptomatic metastases. In these circumstances it is obvious that the patient is, in general, best served by removing the primary, provided that the burden for the patient is not too great compared to the expected survival. Reducing the tumour load appears to provide better palliation than leaving it *in situ*. If, for example, a patient has a readily removable caecal cancer causing obstruction and has hepatic metastases, the best procedure is to perform a right hemicolectomy. However, if the caecal cancer is invading the abdominal wall and there are also widespread peritoneal metastases then the obstruction is best relieved by performing an ileotransverse anastomosis. Resection is usually an easier choice for most colonic cancers, but palliative removal of rectal, and in particular low rectal cancers, poses problems: the risks of purely palliative surgery are greater and the functional results worse in the short term. In these cases alternatives to resection may be more appropriate and careful clinical judgement becomes crucial. Occasionally a palliative abdominoperineal resection or a low anterior resection with a coloanal anastomosis is justified provided that the primary is readily removable. If the tumour has infiltrated the pelvis widely, local recurrence is almost inevitable and after an abdominoperineal excision of the rectum may fungate through the perineal wound, or vagina, making the patient's position worse rather than better. Therefore a palliative endoscopic transanal resection (ETAR) or laser therapy is often more appropriate. Endoscopic resection debulks the tumour and provides good relief of symptoms such as diarrhoea, bleeding, urgency, incontinence, and tenesmus, but provides less relief of the pain produced by the tumour infiltrating the pelvic nerves. Similar results can be obtained with a neodymium YAG laser using 30 to 40 kJ of energy at each session. The main difference between endoscopic transanal resection and laser therapy is that laser treatment requires more frequent repetition at about 6-week intervals while the latter only needs repeating every 3 to 4 months. Occasionally, endoscopic transanal resection or laser therapy may be combined with an end left iliac fossa colostomy, when the cancer has invaded the anal sphincter or fistulated into the vagina producing faecal incontinence. The colon can easily be approached and divided through the small incision made for the stoma.

Cryotherapy using liquid nitrogen probes can produce tumour destruction but it appears slower and less effective than laser therapy. Photodynamic treatment using copper or gold vapour lasers with systemic haematoporphyrin derivative to concentrate the laser energy in the tumour, may destroy small anastomotic recurrences of cancer or cutaneous metastases. The laser is expensive and the haematoporphyrin derivative produces quite marked light sensitivity, so that treatment must be matched to the patients symptoms.

A very few patients present with an isolated secondary in one or other lobe of the liver which is suitable for removal either by excision of a hepatic segment or a hepatic lobectomy. Hepatic metastases draw most of their blood supply from the hepatic artery, in contrast to normal hepatocytes which receive 80 per cent from the portal vein. This physiological fact enables a selective attack to be made on the metastases by obliterating the arterial supply to the secondaries or delivering cytotoxic agents via the hepatic artery. Arterial blood flow can be stopped effectively by arterial embolization with fibrin clot or gelfoam. Alternatively the hepatic artery may be ligated at operation, although this is a much more invasive procedure and is therefore usually combined with resection of the primary. Symptomatic metastases can also be successfully treated with interstitial laser therapy. Several laser fibres are inserted into the metastases with ultrasound guidance under local anaesthesia and some sedation. Low energy Nd YAG laser light is then passed into the tumour for 2 to 3 min to produce gentle heat coagulation of tissue for a radius of 1 to 2 cm around the fibre tip.

Irradiation

Gastrointestinal tumours are generally considered to be radioresistant, but the symptoms produced by an unresectable rectal cancer can often be relieved by external beam irradiation. Useful palliation may be obtained at the relatively low dose of 35 cGy, but increasing the dose to 55 cGy improves the response without greatly increasing the morbidity, although some radiation cystitis may occur. Pain in particular, is better relieved than by either endoscopic transanal resection or laser therapy. Resection and radiation can be used in combination to produce rapid relief of symptoms but an indolent ulcer may follow endoscopic transanal resection performed some months after higher dose irradiation. Irradiation is seldom used for intra-abdominal colon cancer primaries or metastases and is ineffective for hepatic metastases.

Chemotherapy

Colonic cancers are relatively resistent to current chemotherapeutic agents, both singly and in combination. Nevertheless useful subjective and objective responses can be obtained even though the therapeutic margin is small. 5-Fluorouracil is the most widely used agent, either alone or in combination, and provides an objective response rate of about 15 per cent for metastatic disease when infused intravenously at a dose of 20 mg/kg day over 5 to 7 days, repeated every 4 to 6 weeks providing there is continued evidence of a reasonable clinical response. The response to 5-fluorouracil is enhanced by the addition of high dose folinic acid: partial response rates as high as 45 per cent have been claimed with no increase in toxicity. Semustine may also improve the response to 5-fluorourcil though at the expense of increased morbidity. The principal adverse reactions are nausea and bone marrow suppression, producing leucopenia and thrombocytopenia. However, these complications are time- and dose-dependent, and can be reduced easily by adjusting the delivery schedule. When palliation is the objective it would seem reasonable to withhold treatment until metastases cause symptoms, but there is evidence that treatment at the time of diagnosis, before symptoms appear, improves both survival and palliation.

Many other chemotherapeutic agents, such as the platinum compounds mitomycin C, and doxorubicin, have been used and useful responses claimed but usually at the cost of more adverse reactions and no convincing evidence of improved therapeutic efficacy.

Immunotherapy has a long but rather disappointing history in the treatment of advanced cancers, particularly with agents such as *Corynebacterium parvum* or BCG, but recent advances in molecular biology, recombinant technology, and immunology promise exciting therapeutic possibilities. For example, lymphokine-activated killer lymphocytes are to some extent tumouricidal in a non-specific manner, while specifically activated tumour infiltrating lymphocytes are many times more active against malignant cells. The cytokine interleukin-2, which activates lymphocytes, has been infused alone and in combination with other growth regulators such as the interferons or chemotherapeutic drugs in the treatment of cancers. Encouraging results have been obtained in some tumours, including colonic cancers, but with unpleasant side-effects. These cytokines, with the macrophage product tumour necrosis factor, are also responsible for many of the paraneoplastic phenomena such as anorexia, malaise, and cachexia, which are the main side-effects of treatment. Cytokines may also promote tumour angiogenesis, metastasis formation, and hypercalcaemia, so that therapeutic potential is mixed.

There is, however, little doubt that a therapeutic revolution which will substantially improve the outlook for patients with colorectal cancer and affect the way in which such patients are managed lies just round the corner.

LIVER RESECTION

The diagnosis of hepatic metastases usually signifies incurability but occasionally a metastasis is isolated and situated within the liver at a site suitable for resection with some expectation of prolonged survival and possibly cure. The results of liver resection are good where the metastasis is solitary, but poor when multiple, even when the metastases are confined to one lobe of the liver.

There is, at present, no convincing evidence that resection improves survival, even in the few patients with a single metastasis, for there are no controlled trials of hepatic resection. A possible explanation, if a little cynical, is that solitary slow growing metastases merely represent favourable biology with a naturally long survival while multiple metastases indicate the opposite. Hepatic resection is technically feasible with a low risk of morbidity and mortality in experienced units, providing the remaining liver has a good vascular supply and venous drainage as well as normal bile ducts. Ideally, the metastasis should be peripheral and confined to one hepatic segment, making segmental resection practical. Hepatic lobectomy may be necessary for large or multiple metastases affecting one lobe of the liver. Intraoperative ultrasonography is an essential prerequisite for resection to exclude metastases and to establish the hepatic anatomy. However, resection should probably be limited to patients with isolated secondaries until better systemic therapy becomes available, when surgical debulking of tumour may become a more worthwhile proposition.

Patients who have what appears to be a single small metastasis should be monitored carefully with CT or ultrasound examinations at approximately 3- or 4-monthly intervals to assess the growth rate of the metastasis and the development of other metastases. Most often patients who, at first, appear to have a solitary secondary tumour rapidly develop radiologically obvious multiple metastases and are therefore not suitable for hepatic resection. It is clearly important to allow time for occult metastases to become overt and so avoid subjecting patients to unnecessary operations. Fortunately there is no convincing evidence that hepatic metastases will generate further metastases within the liver, or elsewhere, which makes a reasonable delay both safe and practical.

FOLLOW-UP

It is a hallowed tradition in many units to review patients in the outpatient clinic at regular, if infrequent, intervals after colonic cancer resection. While these visits may provide a pastoral service to patients and an educational experience for the surgeon there is little evidence that they are therapeutically useful if the review is

Table 8 Follow-up

Strategy (a)	Strategy (b)		
	Tumour T1,2	Tumour T3,4;N1+	Tumour M1
Colon clear at postoperative clinic visit ↓ Colonoscopy at 5-year intervals and review if symptomatic Treat recurrence	↓ Colonoscopy 5 yearly and review if sympotomatic	↓ Review 3-monthly CEA, ultrasound Treat if positive ↓ Review response Repeat CEA and ultrasound ↓ Repeat cycle	Treat ↓ Review ↓ Repeat cycle?

confined to a clinical examination and a proctosigmoidoscopy. The theoretical rationale for such clinical review, that recurrence or metastases will be detected early and that the results of subsequent treatment will be better, has not been borne out because most patients who develop recurrence present with symptoms in the intervals between clinic visits and the results of treatment have in the past not produced any survival advantage. The main reason for the lack of yield from routine clinical review is that the sensitivity for detecting small potentially treatable disease is too low. However, some recent studies that suggest improved survival and better palliation from treating patients with cancer recurrence before they become symptomatic give some hope that review may be useful if it is more directed.

Clinical review should be directed to detecting minimal disease recurrence in those patients at greatest risk of developing metastases (T3,4 N1–3; Dukes' B and C), and to diagnosing metachronous colonic polyps and cancers, which occur in about 10 per cent of patients (more if the first cancer develops at a young age). The latter is quite simply achieved by colonoscopy at 5-yearly intervals, up to the age of 75 years, once the colon has been shown to be clear of polyps or cancers. The detection of minimal disease requires more than clinical examination. Serum carcinoembryonic antigen is a sensitive indicator of recurrence or residual cancer in many, but not all patients. A postoperative rise in serum carcinoembryonic antigen has been used as a reason for a 'second look' laparotomy with the hope of removing small recurrences, but unfortunately with disappointing results. Hepatic ultrasound and CT scanning will also detect small metastases, particularly in the liver, while rectal endosonography will diagnose local extrarectal recurrence after anterior resection. Large controlled studies are, however, required to overcome the problems of lead time bias and length bias and to prove that the additional costs of such routine investigations can be reliably translated into useful benefit for patients. It is therefore reasonable to suggest that such detailed and structured review is confined to centres undertaking studies of treating minimal recurrent disease while others may reasonably restrict review to patients who become symptomatic (Table 8).

Colonoscopy should be performed within a year of operation if the colon has not been visualized clearly preoperatively. If polyps are identified and removed, colonoscopy is repeated annually until the colon is clear of adenomas, before extending to 5-yearly. The improbability of developing a further colon cancer after the age of 75 years in a colon free of adenomas makes this a useful age to discontinue colonoscopy.

SCREENING

Screening has been introduced enthusiastically throughout the developed world for breast and cervical cancer in women, using mammography for the former and cervical cytology for the latter. By contrast routine chest radiographs have long since been abandoned as a means of screening for lung cancer which highlights the central issues for screening programmes.

For screening to be useful the disease must be fairly common, detectable fairly easily and economically by simple means, early treatment must carry a significant survival advantage, and the cost of each life saved must be a reasonable burden on the community.

A priori, colorectal cancer would appear to be an ideal disease for which to screen. It is the second most common cancer in the Western world; treatment is relatively straightforward and cheap in its early stages, and survival after treatment of early disease is excellent. Furthermore the colonic mucosa is accessible throughout its length both to inspection and sampling. Colonoscopy is clearly the best method of diagnosing and even treating the cancer precursors, adenomas, and small early cancers, but it is too invasive and expensive to be an acceptable means of screening the whole population at risk. Colonoscopy may reasonably be reserved to screen those people with a particularly high risk of developing colonic cancer (Table 9) when the expense and unpleasantness become worthwhile.

Table 9 Colonoscopy screening for high risk groups

Familial adenomatous polyposis syndromes
Juvenile polyposis
Peutz-Jegher's symdrome
Familial cancer syndromes Lynch type 1 and 2
Ulcerative colitis (>10 years; total colitis; severe first attack)
Crohn's colitis?
Ureterosigmoidostomy
Previous colonic cancer
Previous colonic adenomas

Screening colonoscopy should be repeated every 4 to 5 years provided the patient remains free of adenomas or, in the case of colitis, dysplasia, when endoscopy should be repeated at least annually. Patients with colitis and colonic dysplasia are at such a high risk of developing invasive cancer or of having an occult cancer elsewhere in the colon that some clinicians advocate repeat colonoscopy at 6-month intervals, while others advise colectomy.

Populations with a lower risk of developing cancer require a simple, non-invasive, cheap and acceptable method of screening. Over the age of 50 years the incidence of colon cancer begins to rise quite sharply. Fortunately most polyps and early cancers shed blood into the lumen, which allows the blood itself, or degradation products such as haematin, to be detected in the stool. Testing the stool therefore provides a theoretically ideal means of screening for colonic cancers and polyps. However healthy individuals shed about 1 ml of blood into the gastrointestinal tract daily; patients with colon cancer may shed from 1 to 75 ml per day, and there are also numerous other sources of pathological bleeding into the gut.

Tests that are very sensitive lose specificity because they detect blood shed normally into the gut and blood ingested with food. By contrast, less sensitive tests may be highly specific but miss too many lesions to be useful for screening. The ideal test, which has yet to be produced, must be a compromise between sensitivity and specificity to be the highest predictor. The most widely used test at present which fulfils these criteria, Hemoccult®, detects haematin and may therefore miss very low lesions because insufficient blood has been degraded, or caecal cancers because the blood has been completely degraded beyond haematin. The sensitivity and positive predictive value of the test is increased if stools are sampled on three separate occasions. While Hemoccult® provides the best positive predictor currently available, other chemical and immunological tests are being developed which may supersede Hemoccult® in the near future. People who are positive for faecal occult blood are then selected for further investigation by flexible sigmoidoscopy or colonoscopy.

Screening not only presents profound logistical problems but also statistical problems in proving the efficacy of early treatment because of potential bias. Patients whose stools test positive may be from a biologically distinct population with an inherently favourable prognosis while people who refuse screening may bear unfavourable tumours. Interval cancers, which present and are diagnosed between screening, appear to be more aggressive and rapidly growing with a poorer prognosis. Selection bias is therefore important. Screening occurs at intervals and is therefore more likely to detect slower growing tumours producing a length bias on the outcome of screening. If early treatment does not cure the disease or affect the ultimate outcome—something that appears unlikely for colorectal cancer—then detection earlier in the natural lifespan will only give an apparent increase in survival time, producing the so-called lead time bias. Death occurs at the same time: it is merely the time of diagnosis which has moved. The expectation and hope is that time to death also moves significantly but this has yet to be proved for screen-detected colorectal cancer.

The Nottingham screening project is the largest and most comprehensive study of its kind addressing these difficult issues in relation to colonic and rectal cancer. The early results indicate that more and earlier cancers are being detected in the screened population. Allowing for non-responders and the interval cancers, cautious anticipation suggests that a useful survival advantage will be provided at an acceptable cost.

MISCELLANEOUS MALIGNANT COLONIC TUMOURS

Sarcomas and lymphomas of the colon are rare in comparison to adenocarcinomas. Leiomyosarcomas are, however, more common in the colon than the small bowel, while the reverse is true for lymphomas, presumably because of the greater concentration of lymphoid tissue in the small intestine. Sarcomas usually present with a mass, which increases in size slowly if the lesion is low grade but quite rapidly if it is high grade. Surgical removal may be challenging and local recurrence is common (Figs. 21, 22). The prognosis of high-grade tumours is particularly poor and not materially improved by adjuvant treatment.

BENIGN TUMOURS OF THE COLON

Benign tumours can arise from each component of the colon but, with the exception of mucosal adenomas, they are rare. Adenomas share the same uneven distribution as cancers around the colon. Not only are they common, they are also important because of their association with, and their propensity to become, colon cancers. The aetiology and epidemiology of adenomas and their relationship to cancers has already been described.

Adenomas

Adenomas are usually polypoid and vary considerably in size, shape, and histological differentiation. All adenomas start life as a neoplastic change in a single crypt (microadenomas) which gradually increases in size. Well-differentiated tubular adenomas are the most common and are more often pedunculated, particularly when larger. The stalk may be 3 or 4 cm long and the shape of the polyp may sometimes be quite bizarre (Fig. 31). By contrast, the less differentiated villous adenomas are less common and invariably sessile, often extending as a carpet over many centimetres of colon. Tubulovillous adenomas lie between the two both in frequency and morphology. They are usually polypoid but sessile, with a fairly broad base or a short stalk. Why the different types of

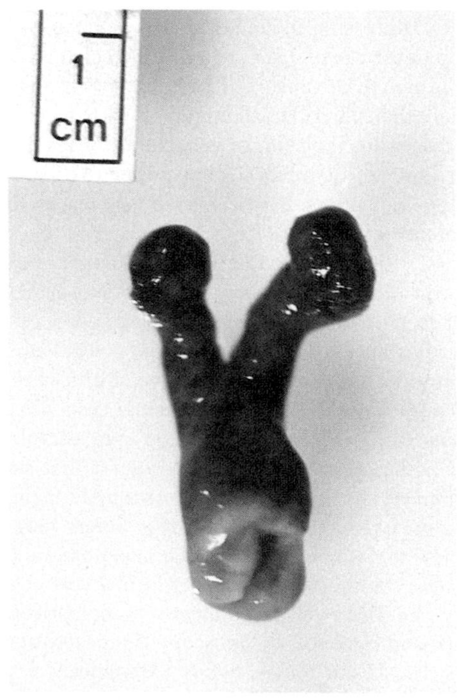

Fig. 31 A double-headed pedunculated tubular adenoma removed colonoscopically.

adenoma have such different morphology is not clear but it is possible that the tubular adenomas are sufficiently slow growing for the peristaltic action of the colon, pulling the polyp down the lumen, gradually to produce a mucosal stalk by traction, whereas the faster growing villous adenoma expands laterally faster than a stalk can develop and produces less luminal mass to induce intussusception. The incidence of malignant change in an adenoma increases with the size of the tumour and the histological dysplasia, such that foci of cancer are common in large villous adenomas (Table 10).

Most adenomas are silent and are diagnosed during the investigation of other bowel symptoms. They may be detected by faecal occult blood screening, but when larger the blood in the stool may be clinically obvious. Bleeding is often episodic, small in volume, dark, and mixed in the faeces. However bleeding can occasionally be brisk, bright, and copious, particularly when a large polyp partially sloughs from its pedicle. Villous adenomas may also present with intermittent bleeding, but more often presents with the passage of mucous, which may be of sufficient volume to produce mucous diarrhoea. Large rectal lesions, replacing as much as 20 cm of mucosa, can cause enough mucus diarrhoea, rich in potassium, to induce dehydration, collapse, and hypokalaemic confusion. Urgency and urge incontinence are also common symptoms of these large villous adenomas.

There is much useless debate about the best method of diagnosing polyps. A good double contrast barium enema can reliably detect polyps 0.5 cm or more in diameter. Colonoscopy can detect smaller lesions and has the added advantage of allowing simultaneous treatment, but it is also only about 95 per cent accurate. Use of the two investigations together increases the overall accuracy to nearly 100 per cent. From an economic point of view however, colonoscopy is the method of first choice if a polyp is suspected. Treatment for very small adenomas is biopsy cautery. Bigger polyps are snared and those larger than 5 cm are snared piecemeal, using electrocautery to coagulate and destroy the base. Complications of colonoscopic polypectomy are uncommon with proper care, but the most serious are perforation and haemorrhage. The frequency of perforation in skilled hands is about 1 per 1000 polypectomies and the respective incidence of bleeding sufficient to require transfusion is about 1 per 300. Vapourization using a Nd-YAG laser has been used to destroy adenomas, but this method carries a greater risk of perforation and does not produce a specimen for histological examination. Photodynamic therapy has also been used effectively for small adenomas but has little apparent advantage over the simpler and less expensive snare polypectomy.

Patients require endoscopic monitoring after polypectomy, and most authorities advise repeat colonoscopy at annual intervals until the colon is clear of polyps, when the interval may be increased to 4 or 5 years. Faecal occult blood screening may be advised for the intervening years. The incidence of polyps at subsequent endoscopy is 25 per cent when one polyp was found initially and 50 per cent when two or more polyps were snared.

Large sessile rectal villous adenomas are not suitable for colonoscopic removal and sometimes present the surgeon with a formidable challenge particularly in the very elderly patients most likely to have such a tumour. The choice of procedures is listed in Table 11.

Table 11 Methods of removing rectal villous adenomas

1. Peranal disc excision
2. Trans-sacral excision (Kraske; York Mason)
3. Peranal submucous dissection (Parks)
4. Electrocoagulation (Madden)
5. Nd-YAG laser vaporization
6. Peranal endoscopic excision (Buess)
7. Endoscopic transanal resection
8. Anterior resection of rectum

Small low lesions may be readily removed through the dilated anus by excision of a disc of rectal wall, or resection of mucosa alone if one can be sure there is no malignant change. The dissection of the mucosa is made much easier by infiltrating 1 in 200 000 noradrenaline solution into the submucosa. Small mucosal defects do not require closure and rapidly re-epithelialize, but defects resulting from a full thickness excision need to be sutured. The main advantage of this technique is that a good specimen is provided for easy histological examination. The Buess endoscopic technique of operating through a large proctoscope with the rectum insufflated with CO_2 is an extension of this method which provides better access to the proximal rectum but requires the skills of stereotactic operating. The instrumentation is expensive and the skills are not yet widely available. Both anterior resection

Table 10 Association between adenomas and malignancy
(a) Histology and malignancy

	Percentage of total	Percentage carcinoma *insitu*	Percentage invasive carcinoma
Tubular	64	12	3
Tubulovillous	27	11	8
Villous	9	14	9

(b) Size and malignancy

Size (cm)	Total (%)	Tubular (%)	Tubulovillous (%)	Villous (%)	Carcinoma *in situ* (%)	Invasive carcinoma (%)
<0.9	29	40	9	8	5	0.5
1–1.9	47	46	50	48	13	5
2–2.9	17	12	31	19	18	10
>3.0	7	2	10	25	27	13

Adapted from Shinya and Wolff 1979.

and trans-sacral resection are major operations with major risks of morbidity, which may be justified for younger patients with large adenomas but not for the frail and debilitated. Parks devised the method of removing large villous adenomas *per anum* by infiltrating the submucosa with noradrenaline solution and excising a tube of rectal mucosa. The resulting large defect was then closed by plicating the rectum like a concertina. The technique is not easy and needs considerable dilatation of the anus, which is best avoided in elderly patients with already weakened sphincters. Deep electrocoagulation effectively destroys adenomas but produces no specimen and also requires considerable anal dilatation. Laser therapy avoids anal dilatation but again provides no specimen; however it is most useful for treating more proximal lesions, such as caecal villous adenomas, in patients unfit for resection. Endoscopic transanal resection, with continuous glycine irrigation, is in many ways ideally suited for the removal of small and large villous adenomas. The anus is not dilated, operation is quick with a low morbidity, can be repeated, and provides a reasonable, if fragmented, specimen for examination. However the operation does require the skills and experience of urological endoscopic surgery.

Patients with familial adenomatous polyposis syndrome require total colectomy and ileorectal anastomosis or a restorative proctocolectomy at some time in the later teens or early twenties because of the inevitable development of invasive cancer in one or more of the adenomatous polyps with the passage of time. The timing of surgery may reasonably be fitted around important social and educational events provided the colon is kept under annual endoscopic surveillance. The functional results of colectomy and ileorectal anastomosis are better than those of restorative proctocolectomy but the distal rectum of patients so treated must be inspected regularly to ensure that the residual polyps do not grow and become malignant. For reasons that are not clear the rectal polyps usually regress in size and number after colectomy and ileorectal anastomosis.

Hamartomas

Two types of hamartoma are found in the colon: juvenile polyps (Fig. 32) and Peutz-Jegher's polyps which may be single or multiple (Fig. 33). There is a strong family history, particularly in patients with multiple hamartomas. Presentation is similar to that of adenomas but, like the familial polyposis coli syndromes, at a younger age than sporadic adenomas. The importance lies in the observation that the hamartomas are frequently associated with adenomatous change and, therefore, a risk of malignant transformation. Treatment is usually by colonoscopic polypectomy, unless the polyps are very numerous when colectomy and ileorectal or pouch-anal anastomosis is preferable.

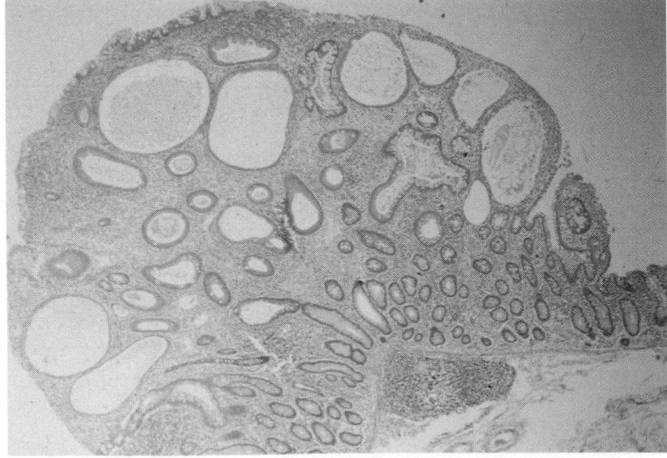

Fig. 32 Histological appearances of juvenile hamartomatous polyp.

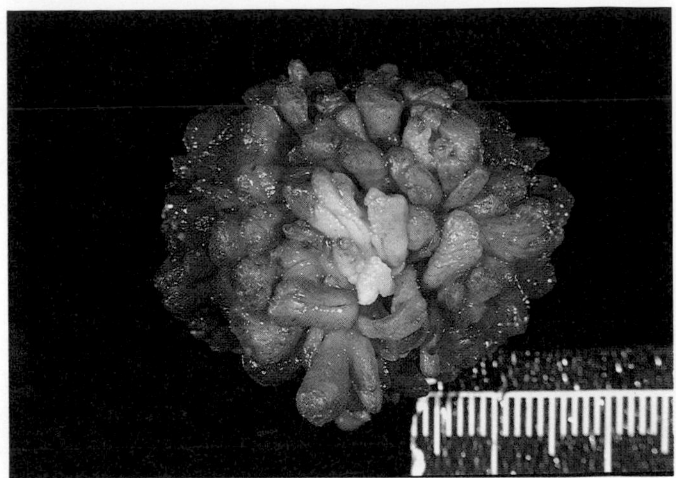

Fig. 33 A Peutz-Jegher's polyp snared endoscopically.

Mesenchymal tumours

Lipomas are not uncommon and are usually a chance finding at colonoscopy, although some may acquire a stalk and intussuscept, causing obstruction and pain. The appearances are obviously different from an adenoma. The polyp is smooth, usually dome shaped, and covered with normal looking mucosa. When large and intussuscepting the leading point may infarct (Fig. 34). Most lipomas need no treatment, but when large they are best removed. Colonoscopic snare removal is often possible but there is a real risk of perforation if the base is broad. Removal may be incomplete if the polyp extends into the colonic wall. In these cases the snare cuts slowly because of the insulating properties of fat.

Leiomyomas of the colon are uncommon and are usually asymptomatic chance findings. Recognition is, however, important. Like lipomas the polyp is dome-shaped and covered by normal mucosa. Unlike gastric leiomyomas there is little risk of haemorrhage. Haemangiomas also occur in the colon and present with intermittent and sometimes severe colonic haemorrhage. They are benign and are readily treated by segmental resection after diagnosis by colonoscopy or angiography.

Carcinoid (neurendocrine) tumours

Gut endocrine tumours occur in the colon but, though uncommon, are often multiple. Many are benign but larger lesions are usually malignant and present and metastasize in much the same way as an adenocarcinoma. The rectum is the more common site for malignant 'carcinoids'. Treatment is similar to that of rectal cancer, although more bowel should be removed to encompass the multifocal nature of the disease. Colonic 'carcinoids' do not secrete 5-hydroxytryptamine and therefore do not produce the

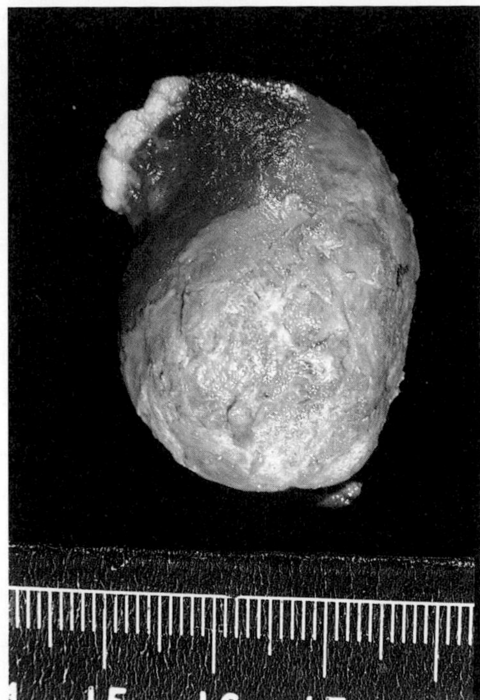

Fig. 34 A pedunculated colonic lipoma which was causing an intussuception and was removed colonoscopically.

syndrome associated with ileal carcinoids. Immunological staining identifies the microscopic tumours and shows that colonic 'carcinoids' contain a wide variety of neuroendocrine substances rather than a single gut hormone. The prognosis for malignant carcinoids' is poor; less than 30 per cent of patients survive for more than 5 years.

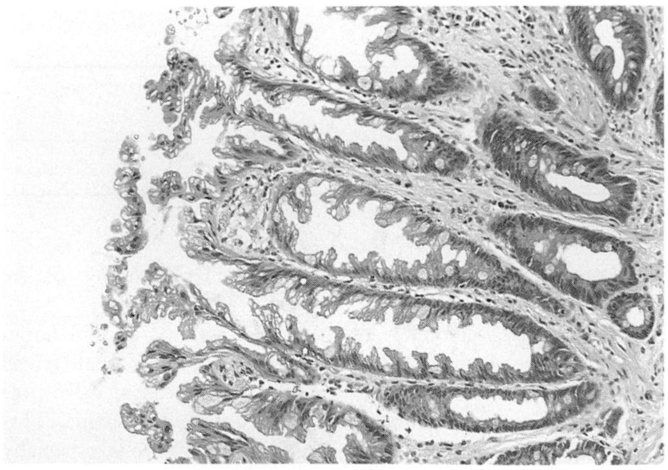

Fig. 35 Histology of a metaplastic polyp. Note the sawtooth appearances.

Metaplastic/hyperplastic polyps

Metaplastic polyps, which are synonymous with hyperplastic polyps, are the most common small polyps seen in the rectum and distal sigmoid colon. They are often multiple, usually about 5 mm or less in diameter, and are slightly raised above the surrounding normal mucosa. They are pale and uniform, which readily identifies them macroscopically from adenomas. The histological appearances are also distinctive (Fig. 35). Their importance lies in distinguishing them from adenomas for the former are quite innocent, with no malignant potential, and cause no symptoms. While their aetiology is unknown there is a statistical association between metaplastic polyps and adenomas, probably because both are more common in older patients. Some clinicians therefore suggest that all patients with metaplastic polyps should at least undergo a flexible sigmoidoscopy to exclude adenomas. If no adenomas are found then the patient needs no further endoscopic surveillance.

FURTHER READING

General reading

Deans GT, Parks TG, Rowlands BJ, Spence RAJ. Prognostic factors in colorectal cancer. *Br J Surg* 1992; **79**: 608–13.

Goligher JC. *Surgery of the Colon, Rectum and Anus.* 5th Edn. London: Balliere Tindall, 1983.

Mortensen N, ed. *Colorectal Cancer.* Clinical Gastroenterology vol 3. No 3. Balliere Tindall, London, 1989.

Progress Symposium. Carcinoma of the large bowel. *World J Surg* 1991; **15**: 561–622.

World Progress in Surgery—Management of Adenocarcinoma of the Low Rectum. *World J Surg* 1992; **16**: 428–515.

Aetiology and epidemiology

Clarke PJ, Dehn TCB, Kettlewell MGW. Changing patterns of colorectal cancer in a regional teaching hospital. *Ann R Coll Surg Eng* 1992; **74**: 291–3.

Kingsnorth AN, Lumsden AB, Wallace HM. *Br J Surg* 1984; **71**: 791–4.

Stephenson BM, Finan PJ, Gascoyne J, Garbett F, Murday VA, Bishop DT. Frequency of familial colorectal cancer. *Br J Surg* 1991; **78**: 1162–6.

Biology and pathology

Appleton GVN, Davies PW, Williamson RCN. Effect of defunction on cytokinetics and cancer at colonic suture lines. *Br J Surg* 1990; **77**: 768–71.

Clausen MR, Bonnen H, Mortensen PB. Colonic fermentation of dietary fibre to short chain fatty acids in patients with adenomatous polyps and colonic cancer. *Gut* 1991; **32**: 923–8.

Hermanek, P. Colorectal carcinoma: histopathological diagnosis and staging. In: Mortensen N, ed. *Clinical Gastroenterology* Vol. 3, No 3. Balliere Tindall, London. 1989.

Lofberg R, Brostrom O, Karlen P, Ost A, Tribukair B. Carcinoma and DNA aneuploidy in Crohn's colitis—a histological and flow cytometric study. *Gut* 1991; **32**: 900–4.

Rew DA, Wilson GD, Taylor I, Weaver PC. Proliferation characteristics of human colorectal carcinomas measured *in vivo*. *Br J Surg* 1991; **78**: 60–6.

Screening

Dunlop MG. Screening for large bowel neoplasms in individuals with a family history of colorectal cancer. *Br J Surg* 1992; **79**: 488–94.

Hardcastle JD, Armitage NC, Chamberlain J, Amar SS, James PD, Balfour TW. Fecal occult blood screening for colorectal cancer in the general population. *Cancer* 1986; **58**: 183–4.

Ultrasound

Charnley RM, Morris DL, Dennison AR, Amar SR, Hardcastle JD. Detection of colorectal liver metastases using intraoperative ultrasound. *Br J Surg* 1991; **78:** 45–8.

Roubien LD, *et al.* Endoscopic ultrasonography in staging rectal cancer. *Am J Gastroenterol* 1990; **85:** 1391–4.

Surgery and survival

Chapuis PH, Dent OF, Fisher R, *et al.* A multivariate analysis of clinical and pathological variaties on prognosis after resection of large bowel cancer. *Br J Surg* 1985; **72:** 698–702.

Phillips RKS, Hittinger R, Blesovsky L, Fry JS, Fielding LP. Large bowel cancer: surgical pathology and its relationship to survival. *Br J Surg* 1984; **71:** 604–10.

Surtees P, Richie JK, Phillips RKS. High versus low ligation of the inferior mesenteric artery in rectal cancer. *Br J Surg* 1990; **77:** 618–21.

Liver resection

Doci R, Gennari L, Bignami P, Montalto F, Morabito A, Bozzetti F. One hundred patients with hepatic metastases from colorectal cancer treated by resection: analysis of prognostic determinants. *Br J Surg* 1991; **78:** 797–801.

Scheele J, Stangl R, Altendorf-Hofmann A. Hepatic metastases from colorectal carcinoma: impact of surgical resection on the natural history. *Br J Surg* 1990; **77:** 1241–6.

Chemotherapy

Goldberg JA, Kerr DJ, Wilmott N, McKillop JH, McArdle CS. Regional chemotherapy for colorectal liver metastases: a phase 2 evaluation of targeted hepatic arterial 5-fluorouracil for colorectal liver metastases. *Br J Surg* 1990; **77:** 1238–40.

Hunt TM, Flowerdew ADS, Birch SJ, Williams JD, Mullee MA, Taylor I. Prospective randomized controlled trial of hepatic arterial embolization or infusion chemotherapy with 5-fluorouracil and degradable starch microspheres for colorectal liver metastases. *Br J Surg* 1990; **77:** 774–82.

Scheithauer W, Rosen H, Kornek G-V, Sebasta C, Depisch D. Randomised comparison of combination chemotherapy plus supportive care with supportive care alone in patients with metastatic colorectal cancer. *Br Med J* 1993; **306:** 752–5.

Obstruction and perforation

Runkel NS, Schlag P, Schwarz V, Herfarth C. Outcome after emergency surgery for cancer of the large intestine. *Br J Surg* 1991; **78:** 183–8.

Stomas

Karanjia ND, Corder AP, Holdsworth PJ, Heald RJ. Risk of peritonitis and fatal septicaemia and need to defunction low anastomosis. *Br J Surg* 1991; **78:** 196–8.

Polyps

Madden MV, *et al.* Comparison of morbidity and function after colectomy with ileorectal anastomosis or restorative proctocolectomy for familial adenomatous polyposis. *Br J Surg* 1991; **78:** *789–92.*

Minopoulos GJ, McIntyre RLE, Lee ECG, Kettlewell MGW. Colonoscopic polypectomy in a regional teaching hospital. *Br J Surg* 1983; **70:** 51–3.

Shinya H, Wolff WI. Morphology, anatomic distribution and cancer potential of colonic polyps. *Ann Surg* 1979; **190:** 679–83.

Palliation

Berry AR, Souter RG, Campbell WB, Mortensen NJMcC, Kettlewell MGW. Endoscopic transanal resection of rectal tumours—a preliminary report of its use. *Br J Surg* 1990; **77:** 134–7.

18.4 Obstruction of the colon

LESLIE W. OTTINGER

Obstruction of the colon as a separate clinical entity is singled out for discussion for two reasons. Firstly, it brings its own serious complications (the most dramatic being perforation), which are not directly related to the underlying cause. Secondly, it introduces special elements that influence the timing and limit the selection of procedures in managing the actual cause of obstruction.

GENERAL CONSIDERATIONS

Obstruction of the intestine at any level leads to progressive distension of the proximal bowel with fluid and gas. In the small intestine, distension may result in early vomiting if the site is proximal or in the sequestration of large amounts of fluid if it is more distal. Neither distension nor sequestration is an important elements in the presentation and course of obstruction of the colon.

The obstructed colon has less peristaltic activity, and dilatation tends to cause fewer and less severe cramps than small bowel obstruction. In the majority of patients the ileocaecal valve prevents decompression of the colon into the small intestine. This situation results in closed loop obstruction, which is especially hazardous because it can result in massive dilatation of a segment of the colon without the signs and symptoms usually associated with intestinal obstruction. Secondary dilatation of the small intestine with its consequences may follow, but it is slow to develop and is usually unimportant.

Colon obstruction presents as an emergency, especially because of the associated complication of perforation. Even when intraluminal pressure is constant, the tension on a segment of colon wall increases with an increase in diameter; the relatively larger diameter and thinner wall of the caecum and ascending colon make these the most frequent sites of perforation. In the final stages before perforation there is an embarrassment of circulation, which can also contribute to rupture of the wall. The site of perforation may be in a more distal segment of the colon, usually just proximal to an obstructing lesion such as a carcinoma.

During barium studies under the fluoroscope the normal ascending colon dilates readily up to only about 9 cm in diameter. In chronic obstruction, much larger degrees of distension may nevertheless be quite harmless. Still, when plain radiographs show distension of the ascending colon beyond 10 cm, the possibility of rupture must be considered as imminent. If the capacity of the right colon is exceeded, the serosa between the taeniae splits, perforations, usually punctuate, appear in the mucosa, and patches of haemorrhage and even infarction are also commonly observed. Perforations of this type initially lead to progressive contamination of the peritoneal cavity, but may not actually decompress the obstructed colon.

The clinical course of colon obstruction is often quite insidious. Up to 80 per cent of cases are caused by a carcinoma. Many of these patients will have experienced prior episodes of partial obstruction and may not be aware that complete obstruction has developed until 2 or 3 days have passed. Although lower abdominal cramps are usually reported, these may be mild. Cessation of the passage of stool or gas is the most frequent complaint, and an observant patient will also report abdominal distension. Physical examination shows a quiet abdomen with obvious tympany and distension, sometimes most pronounced over the ascending colon. There may be tenderness over compromised bowel, the caecum or the area proximal to a tumour. Rectal examination may disclose a low rectal tumour as the cause of obstruction. More commonly, the rectum feels capacious and empty. In the presence of a tumour or compromised bowel, there may be traces of blood. The physical examination should include a careful search for abdominal wall hernias, especially in any old surgical incisions.

Plain radiographs of the abdomen are usually helpful in colon obstruction. They may confirm or support the diagnosis and point to the site and aetiology; they can also suggest the presence of perforation by showing free air and can demonstrate a dangerously distended right colon. If an expeditious barium study is obtained, it will help identify the actual site and nature of obstruction (Fig. 1). The barium enema examination should be done without preparation and care must be taken not to push barium above the obstruction.

In practice, it is difficult to assess the likelihood of colon perforation. When obstruction is partial, sequential evaluation of symptoms and the presence and degree of tenderness over the right colon can suggest impending perforation. If obstruction is complete, and especially if decompression into the small intestine is absent, urgent surgical exploration with decompression is the first consideration.

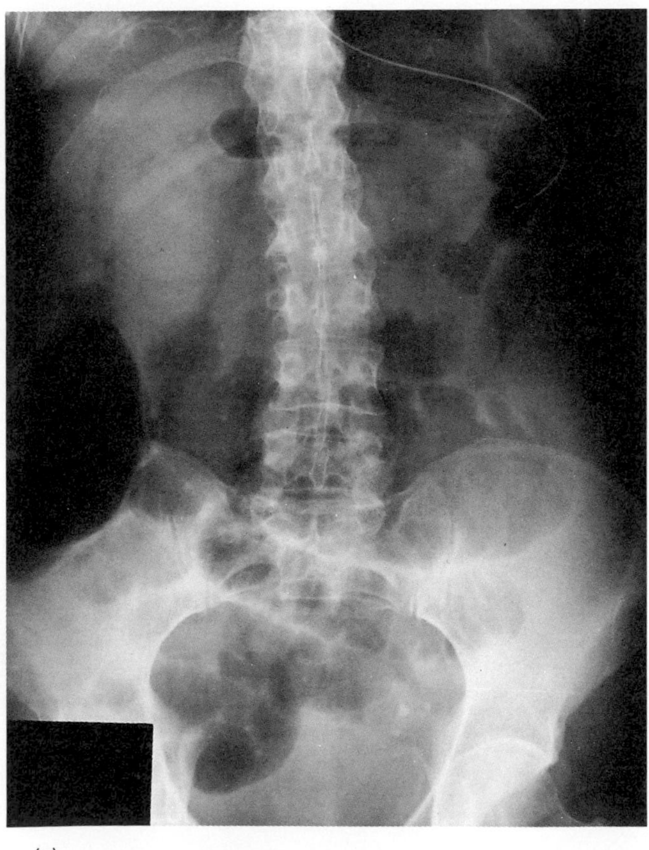

(a)

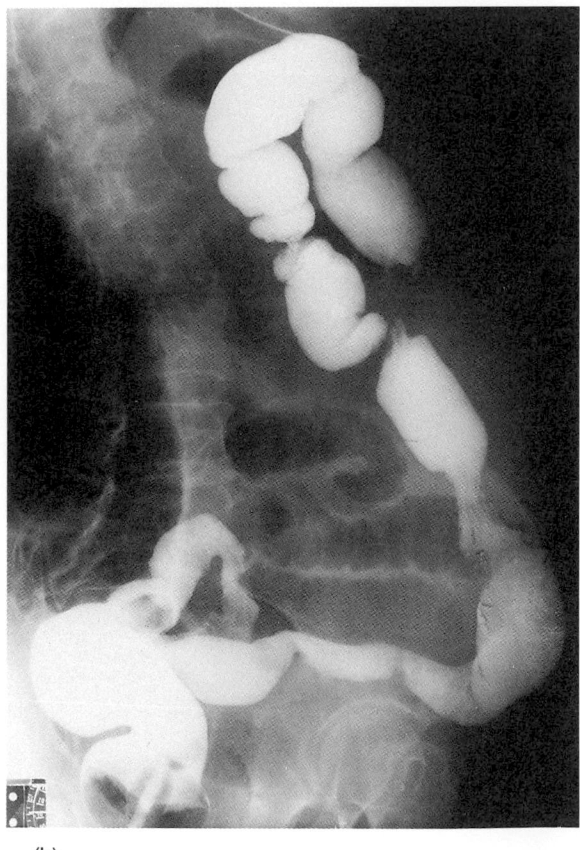

(b)

Fig. 1 (a) Plain radiograph in a patient with a 3-day history of obstipation showing distension of both small and large bowel. (b) Barium enema in the same patient (oblique view). There is complete obstruction by a carcinoma just proximal to the splenic flexure.

CAUSES OF COLON OBSTRUCTION

Carcinoma

In the more economically developed areas of the world, carcinoma is by far the most frequent cause of colon obstruction. Carcinomas of the left colon are the most likely to lead to obstruction, although those in other areas also cause obstruction, the least frequent being those of the rectum. Most patients in whom the obstruction involves the distal colon have a presentation that includes an initial period of symptoms of partial obstruction. Final obstruction reflects obturation of the narrow residual channel by faecal material. Obstruction in the right or transverse colon is more likely to occur without preceding symptoms, perhaps because of the liquid nature of the stool.

The prognosis of treated obstructing carcinomas is not very different from that of non-obstructing lesions of similar location and extent. Prognosis may be estimated by use of the Dukes' or other classification. The early operative risk is much higher in these patients especially with respect to perforation.

Diverticulitis

Complete acute colon obstruction is rarely caused by diverticular disease, although it sometimes occurs due to obturation of a strictured oedematous segment. Incomplete obstruction is more usual, and there may be associated partial or complete obstruction of an adherent loop of small intestine.

Differentiation between a carcinoma and diverticular disease of the sigmoid may be very difficult and can lead to an incomplete or delayed resection in a patient incorrectly diagnosed as having diverticulitis.

Volvulus

Volvulus of either the ileum, caecum and right colon or of the sigmoid colon almost always leads to acute obstruction. The twist of 180° or more around the mesenteric axis imparts a similar twist in the longitudinal axis; this is the immediate cause of obstruction. Because vascular compromise may result, there is a danger of perforation in neglected cases. Expert interpretation of the plain radiograph will usually establish the diagnosis. Contrast enemas may be needed when there is considerable dilatation of the proximal colon or small intestine (Fig. 2). Volvulus of the right colon generally reflects a failure of fixation of the colon. Sigmoid volvulus is probably an acquired abnormality but is usually observed in patients with an elongated colon. Spontaneous reduction of all forms of volvulus will often occur, relieving obstruction; recurrence is the rule.

Other causes

Only a few cases of colon obstruction are due to causes other than cancer diverticulitis, and volvulus. The uncommon causes include

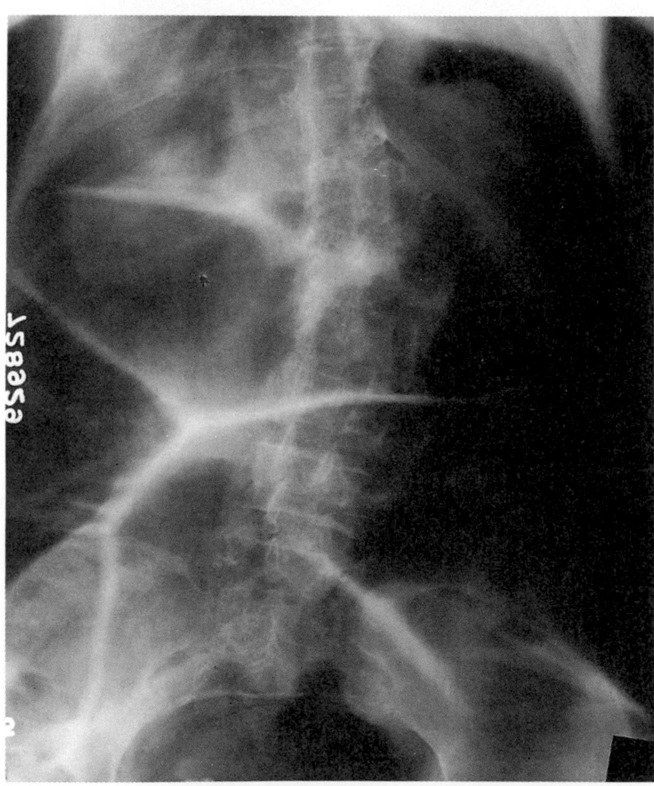

(a)

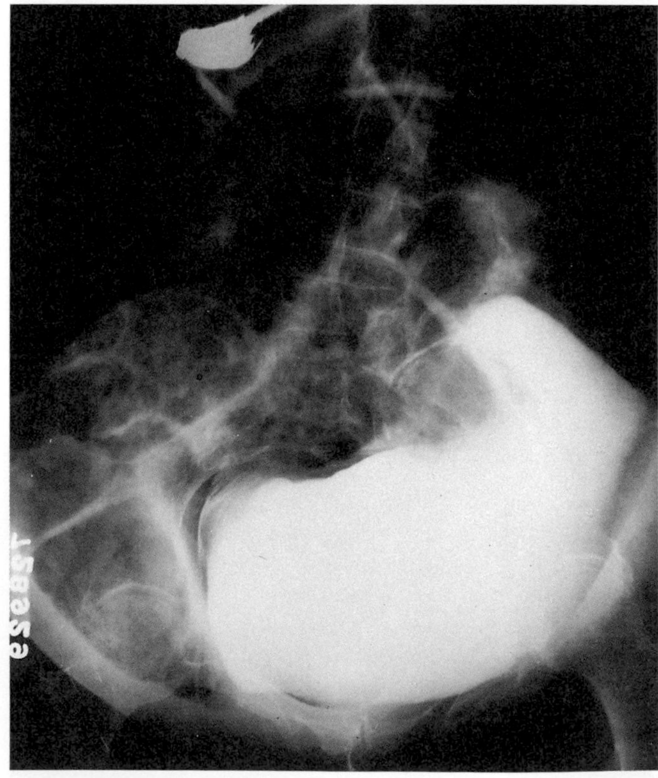

(b)

Fig. 2 (a) Plain radiograph of a patient with abdominal distension, tympany, and obstipation but otherwise without symptoms. (b) Barium enema in the same patient, demonstrating volvulus of the sigmoid colon.

incarceration in hernias, strictures such as those that follow vascular compromise, metastatic malignant tumours, especially those of pelvic origin, radiation strictures, and various inflammatory conditions. Adhesions, although a common cause of small bowel obstruction, are a rare cause of colon obstruction.

MANAGEMENT

General principles

Management should be directed at relief of obstruction before perforation occurs. Secondary objectives include treatment of the underlying cause and restoration of the continuity of the colon with the smallest number of operations in the shortest time feasible. Choices between the various surgical alternatives reflect the urgency of the situation, the condition of the patient, the state of the bowel to be used for anastomosis, and the potential for cure of a malignancy. Impending or actual rupture of the right colon is another major modifying factor. As with anastomosis in elective resections, tension, impaired circulation, and local contamination may all dictate a staged procedure. An anastomosis between distended ileum and normal colon is usually safe: one between distended and normal colon much less so.

Carcinoma of the colon

In the treatment of obstructing tumours in the caecum, ascending or right transverse colon, a right colectomy extended across to the transverse colon as needed is the usual procedure. Even if the colon is distended, an adequate dissection for cure is feasible, and an anastomosis of the ileum to normal and usually empty collapsed distal colon is safe. If the caecum is perforated or when other factors make the risk exceptionally high, a resection with ileostomy carries less immediate risk, although a second stage is required for reanastomosis.

If the obstructing lesion is in the region of the splenic flexure and down to the mid-sigmoid colon, a right colectomy with extension to include the lesion (a subtotal colectomy) with ileocolonic anastomosis may still be selected. In the young and healthy patient seen by an experienced surgeon subtotal colectomy is an acceptably low risk and troublesome diarrhoea afterward is the exception. A segmental resection with direct anastomosis using distended and unprepped proximal bowel carries a high risk. The safe procedure is to perform a resection with an end colostomy and with reanastomosis as a second stage. A proximal transverse colostomy or a caecectomy and ileostomy for caecal perforation with staged later section may be dictated by the general or local operating conditions. Recent reports suggest that antegrade intraoperative irrigation may be used in selected cases to establish safe conditions for a direct anastomosis.

When a tumour is present in the distal sigmoid colon or upper rectum, a single stage operation is seldom feasible. If a satisfactory dissection can be carried out under the operating conditions, a resection with an end proximal colostomy should be done. Otherwise, a proximal defunctioning colostomy alone is done. If the defunctioning colostomy can be carried out in the sigmoid colon rather than in the transverse colon, a single subsequent operation may be possible: many surgeons consider it unsafe to have two separate colon suture lines because of an increased risk of postoperative leakage. A prior colostomy remote from the operative anastomoses makes a third stage necessary.

When the obstructing tumour is at or below the peritoneal reflection, fortunately an unusual site for obstruction, a two- or three-stage operation is generally the best choice because a satisfactory dissection for the resection of a malignant tumour is often neither feasible nor safe under these conditions. If hepatic or other unresectable metastases are present, however, a Hartmann procedure (resection of the tumour with closure of the rectum and an end sigmoid colostomy) is a good single stage choice. Alternatively, a proximal transverse colostomy must be performed as a first stage, with resection of the tumour deferred until proper conditions can be secured.

In the presence of colonic obstruction there is always a risk when the caecum is not directly examined: severe damage to the wall caused by distension can result in perforation occurring even after distal decompression. Most operations should therefore include visualization of the caecum. Some minor transmural injuries can be managed by imbrication or by the placement of a caecostomy tube. Right colectomy is necessary with more advanced injuries or perforation. The site of colon obstruction and its management and the general condition of the patient determine whether an ileostomy or an ileocolonic anastomosis is indicated.

Diverticulitis

Complete obstruction from diverticulitis is, in fact, rare. In most cases, obstruction is incomplete, and an element of inflammation and oedema will respond to antibiotics and to 'putting the colon at rest'. When non-surgical treatments fail, a primary resection can almost always be performed safely. An extensive dissection of mesenteric nodes is not necessary.

Conditions for a primary unprotected colonic or colorectal anastomosis often cannot be met. A safe colon anastomosis is one that can be left in a clean, normal field: there must be no gross faecal contamination, nor any exudate and purulent material from an abscess. Most cases of obstructive diverticulitis are best managed by primary resection and end colostomy. Continuity is restored at a second operation several weeks later. When there is a large abscess or the local inflammatory reaction precludes a safe dissection, a defunctioning transverse colostomy with drainage of the abscess as a first stage may be the only safe alternative. Another alternative in selected patients is percutaneous drainage of the abscess, with later resection if obstruction resolves.

Volvulus

Obstruction due to volvulus of the ileocaecal area requires prompt diagnosis and management in order to avoid the otherwise common complication of perforation. The diagnosis can be made on plain radiograph, but a contrast study is usually obtained. Once the diagnosis is established, an urgent laparotomy is needed. Although colonoscopic decompression or reduction by a column of barium may be feasible, the possibility of mural compromise and the likelihood of recurrence make resection with primary anastomosis the favoured management in almost all cases. In the presence of perforation with extensive peritoneal contamination or when other factors dictate a more expeditious procedure, resection with ileostomy and later reanastomosis may be the best choice.

When the caecum is intact and undamaged, caecopexy offers an alternative to resection. A long segment of the ascending colon should be secured to the left abdominal wall by raising a peritoneal flap and forming a retroperitoneal track for the colon, fixing the cut edge of the peritoneum to the anterior aspect of the colon with multiple sutures.

The management of sigmoid volvulus is in some ways quite different from that of a caecal volvulus. Perforation is rare and decompression through a rigid sigmoidoscope, perhaps by inserting a well lubricated tube through the lumen, is easily accomplished in most patients. The tube can be left in place. In chronically debilitated patients, simple decompression by this technique, when needed, may be the best choice.

If decompression is successful and definitive treatment is selected, the procedure would be an elective sigmoid resection after routine bowel preparation. An unprotected primary resection and anastomosis can usually be undertaken safely. Fixation of the sigmoid colon without resection is usually not successful because of marked redundancy and the adjacent location of the colon segments in the proximal and distal ends of the volvulus.

When decompression fails or when there is evidence of infarction or perforation, management is difficult. Reduction of the loop at operation can result in perforation and massive faecal contamination of the peritoneal cavity. If a tube is placed in the rectum before surgery, it can sometimes be manipulated into the loop by the surgeon for decompression. Primary anastomosis is seldom feasible after emergency resection. Most surgeons perform an end sigmoid colostomy with staged restoration of colon continuity. An alternative in the absence of perforation or of bowel infarction would be intraoperative decompression with the rectal tube, followed by an elective resection after proper preparation of the colon and patient.

Volvulus of the transverse colon is rare, and principles of management are the same as for caecal volvulus.

Miscellaneous causes

Numerous other anatomical and pathological causes of acute colon obstruction are encountered (Table 1). Although certain principles for their management can be re-emphasized, the surgeon is left to analyse and resolve each as an individual problem. Whatever the primary site of obstruction, the possibility of caecal perforation should be considered; failure to visualize the caecum always carry a risk. Healing of any anastomosis is uncertain when it cannot be placed in a normal, uncontaminated area of the peritoneal cavity. Even a diverting proximal colostomy will not ensure healing of a questionable anastomosis. The additive risks of staged operations favour a one-stage procedure, but only under near optimal conditions of anastomosis. Finally, bypassing an obstructed segment of colon does not always preclude the risk of subsequent perforation, especially when an ileocolonic bypass is used.

Table 1 Unusual causes of colon obstruction

Strictures
Radiation
Ischaemic
Infections
Schistosomiasis
Lymphogranuloma
Actinomycosis
Tuberculosis
Amoebiasis
Obturation
Gallstone
Bezoar
Extrinsic
Pancreatitis
Endometriosis
Metastatic carcinoma
Inflammatory adhesions

FURTHER READING

Albers JH, Smith LL, Carter R. Perforation of the cecum. *Ann Surg* 1956; **143**: 251–5.

Ballantyne GH, Brandner MD, Beart RW Jr, Ilstrup DM. Volvulus of the colon. Incidence and mortality. *Ann Surg* 1985; **202**: 83–92.

Howard RS, Catto J. Cecal volvulus. A case for nonresectional therapy. *Arch Surg* 1980; **115**: 273–7.

Koruth NM, Krukowski ZH, Younger GG, Hendry WS, Logir JR, Jones PF. Intra-operative colonic irrigation in the management of left-sided large bowel emergencies. *Br J Surg* 1985; **72**: 708–11.

Morgan JP, Jenkins N, Lewis P, Aubrey D. Management of obstructing carcinoma of the left colon by extended right hemicolectomy. *Am J Surg* 1985; **149**: 327–9.

Saini S, Mueller PR, Wittenberg J, Butch RS, Rodkey GV, Welch CE. Percutaneous drainage of diverticular abscess. An adjunct to surgical therapy. *Arch Surg* 1986; **121**: 475–8.

Savage PT. Immediate resection with an end-to-end anastomosis for carcinoma of the large bowel presenting with acute obstruction. *Proc R Soc Med* 1967; **60**: 207.

Wolmark N, Wieand HS, Rockette HE, Fisher B, Glass A, Lawrence W. The prognostic significance of tumor location and bowel obstruction in Dukes B and C colorectal cancer. Findings from the NSABP clinical trials. *Ann Surg* 1983; **198**: 743–52.

Wright HK. The functional consequences of colectomy. *Am J Surg* 1975; **130**: 532–4.

18.5 Volvulus of the colon

ALAN R. BERRY

INTRODUCTION

Acute volvulus of the colon is a surgical emergency and although accounting for not more than 5 per cent of all cases of large bowel obstruction in the Western world (Fig. 1), it is a much more common cause of large bowel obstruction in other parts of the world. The incidence of the various types of colonic volvulus is shown in Fig. 2: sigmoid volvulus is by far the most common, accounting for about two-thirds of all cases. Caecal volvulus accounts for most of the remaining cases, while volvulus of the tranverse colon and splenic flexure are very rare indeed. A simultaneous volvulus of the sigmoid and right colon has been reported. Together sigmoid and caecal volvulus represent over 90 per cent of cases of colonic volvulus.

The presence of an elongated mesentery about which the bowel can rotate is fundamental to the pathogenesis of colonic volvulus. Although a mesentery is a normal feature of the sigmoid colon, a caecal volvulus can only occur if the usual fixation of the caecum in the right iliac fossa has not occurred during development. Although many of the features of the different kinds of colonic volvulus are similar, important differences exist and so they are best considered separately.

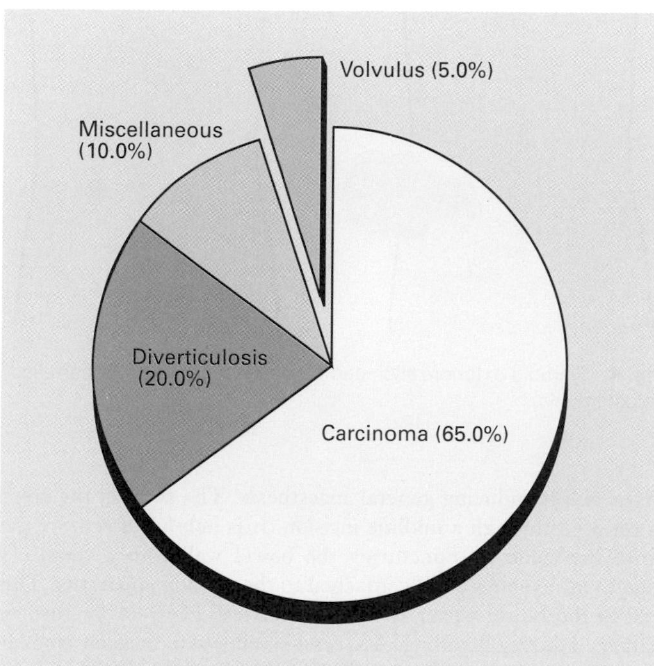

Fig. 1 The causes of colonic obstruction.

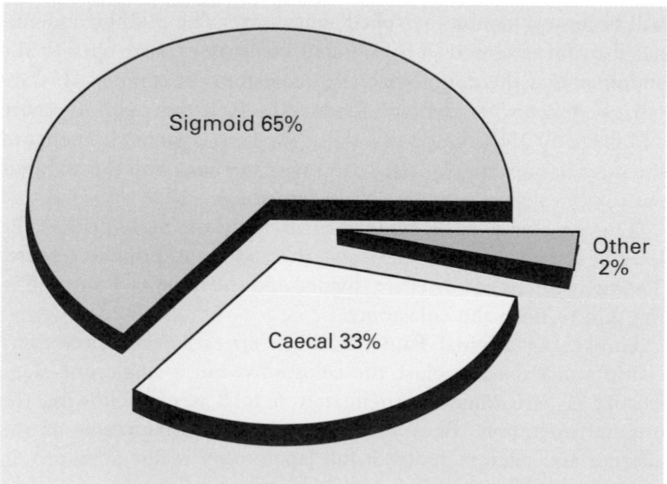

Fig. 2 The types of colonic volvulus.

VOLVULUS OF THE SIGMOID COLON

Incidence and pathogenesis

Sigmoid volvulus is common in the continents of India, Africa, parts of South America, and in Eastern Europe, where it has been shown to be responsible for up to 50 per cent of all cases of intestinal obstruction. In Western Europe and North America, however, it is uncommon, accounting for about 5 per cent of all cases of large bowel obstruction. The incidence in one large reported series in New York was 1.3 per 10 000 hospital admissions.

It is thought that the major contributing factor in those parts of the world where there is a high incidence is the high dietary fibre content. Other factors which are recognized to be important are a long redundant colon, an acquired megacolon, chronic constipation, and a narrowly based mesentery.

The peak age incidence of sigmoid volvulus is in the eighth decade, with 70 per cent of patients presenting after 70 years of age and up to 40 per cent of patients being over 80 years old. A high proportion of patients presenting with acute sigmoid volvulus (up to 60 per cent) are institutionalized. The condition is particularly common in elderly patients suffering from psychiatric and chronic neurological diseases such as stroke or multiple sclerosis. Other conditions with which it tends to be associated include cardiovascular disease and diabetes.

Presentation and clinical features

The condition usually presents with acute colicky abdominal pain, almost invariably associated with distension and, in one-half of all patients, with constipation. These features in an elderly person with a chronic psychiatric or neurological complaint should immediately raise the possibility of sigmoid volvulus. On examination, the most striking finding is of a tensely distended, tympanitic, 'drum-like' abdomen. The rectum is empty of stool. Bowel sounds are often increased but signs of peritoneal inflammation such as rebound tenderness or guarding are unusual. When these signs are present they suggest that colonic infarction or gangrene has occurred. Signs of dehydration may be apparent if presentation has been delayed and these should always be sought.

Radiology

The most useful investigation of patients suspected of having a sigmoid volvulus is a plain supine abdominal radiograph. This alone may be diagnostic in 70 to 80 per cent of patients. The typical appearance is that of a single grossly distended loop of colon arising out the pelvis and extending towards the diaphragm. Haustral markings are usually lost (Fig. 3).

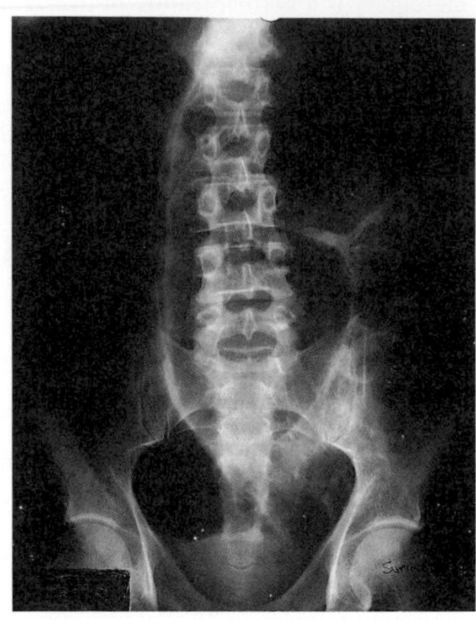

Fig. 3 Plain supine radiograph showing sigmoid volvulus.

Investigation by a contrast enema such as dilute barium or a water-soluble contrast medium will increase the diagnostic yield of radiology to over 90 per cent of patients. If gangrenous bowel or perforation is suspected a water-soluble contrast must be used rather than barium, as the latter will produce a severe peritonitis. The pathognomonic sign on a contrast enema is described as a 'birds beak' or 'ace of spades' appearance, produced as the upper end of the barium column tapers into the spirally twisted distal sigmoid colon.

Treatment

Most patients can be treated initially by non-operative means. Careful rigid sigmoidoscopy and the passage of a flatus tube via the sigmoidoscope is successful in up to 90 per cent of cases, and is well worth trying in the first instance. Protective clothing is recommended as the results of a successful decompression are usually explosive. A mortality of between 1 and 4 per cent is reported for the treatment and great care is essential if colonic perforation is to be avoided. Following a successful deflation, the flatus tube should be left in place for at least 48 h, and some would recommend as long as 5 days. Unless this is done the likelihood of an early recurrence is very high (50–90 per cent).

The alternative to endoscopic deflation is emergency surgery, but this is associated with a mortality of up to 40 per cent. Mortality is higher for sigmoid resection (52 per cent in one reported study by Welch and Anderson in 1987) than for operations aimed at fixing the mobile colon (colopexy) which had a 2.8 per cent mortality. However, the 28 per cent incidence of recurrence reported to follow sigmoid colopexy mitigates against it as an approach. In the minority of patients who have signs of infarction and peritonitis, emergency surgery should not be delayed, but in most cases early treatment should be non-surgical, surgery being reserved for those in whom this fails.

The emergency operation of choice is sigmoid exteriorization and resection, using a modification of the Paul–Mickulicz technique (Fig. 4). After resuscitation with intravenous fluids, antibiotic prophylaxis (such as a cephalosporin and metronidazole) is given before inducing general anaesthesia. The twist in the colon is reduced through a midline incision. It is helpful to remove gas from the colon by puncturing the bowel wall with a small (19 gauge) intravenous needle attached to the suction apparatus. This makes the bowel easier to handle and less likely to be torn or damaged during handling. A second smaller skin incision is made in the left iliac fossa through which the collapsed, freely mobile, sigmoid colon can easily be exteriorized. At this stage the future afferent and efferent loops of colon should be opposed and sutured together close to the abdominal wall, preparing the bowel for what will become a 'double-barrelled' colostomy. The midline abdominal incision is closed. The sigmoid colon is excised outside the abdomen and the double-barrelled colostomy is completed. Care must be taken when dividing the mesentery at this point to secure and ligate all of the blood vessels, as the large sigmoid branches of the inferior mesenteric artery can easily slip back into the abdominal cavity causing troublesome haemorrhage.

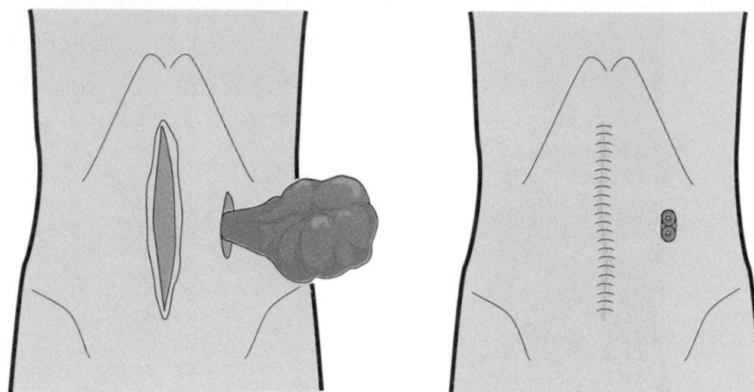

Fig. 4 Sigmoid exteriorization and resection with a double-barrelled colostomy.

This problem can be avoided by dividing the mesentery at the level of the abdominal wall, inside the abdomen, prior to closure. The two lumens of bowel are divided and the mucosa is sutured to the skin to form the colostomy.

Unlike the original Paul–Mickulicz operation an enterotomy clamp is not used to close the colostomy, but a single one-stage closure is performed approximately 6 to 8 weeks following the original operation. Because of the close approximation of the afferent and efferent limbs, a full laparotomy is not necessary in order to do this.

An alternative operation in the emergency situation is the

Hartmann procedure, in which the distal bowel end is closed within the pelvis following sigmoid colectomy. This operation has no advantages in the management of sigmoid volvulus when the distal and proximal ends of bowel can be easily approximated. It has the disadvantage that the second operation to reanastamose the bowel is very difficult. Sigmoid colectomy and primary anastomosis is not usually recommended in the emergency situation, but may be an alternative for an experienced colonic surgeon using 'on-table' antegrade colonic irrigation via caecal intubation to clean the bowel of faeces before anastomosis. Patients who develop recurrent volvulus after non-operative, or rarely after emergency operative treatment should be offered elective surgery, as there is a reported mortality of over 20 per cent for patients who continue to be managed conservatively. The operation of choice is sigmoid colectomy and primary anastomosis after a suitable preoperative bowel preparation. This can be achieved by giving patients clear fluids only by mouth for 48 h before surgery and two doses of sodium picosulphate on the day before operation.

An algorithm for the management of patients with sigmoid volvulus is shown in Fig. 5.

VOLVULUS OF THE CAECUM

Caecal volvulus is much less common than volvulus of the sigmoid colon, accounting for less than 1 per cent of all cases of intestinal obstruction and up to 40 per cent of all cases of colonic volvulus. In a reported series from Scandinavia the incidence was 3 to 6 per million per year. It carries a mortality of 20 per cent. In this condition the caecum remains mobile and shares a common mesentery with the ileum. It is therefore free to rotate, usually clockwise, out of the right iliac fossa to the mid- or left side of the upper abdomen (Fig. 6), producing a closed loop obstruction of the ascending colon and distal ileum.

Presentation and clinical features

Caecal volvulus may present as a fulminant condition with intestinal strangulation secondary to mesenteric torsion or, less dramatically, with features of intestinal obstruction. Rarely it is a chronic intermittent condition. The peak age of presentation is 30 to 40 years of age—much younger than that for sigmoid volvulus, and it is more common in females. There often appear to have been a triggering event, such as a recent laparotomy and it is well recognized following gynaecological procedures. Occasionally it can occur secondary to an obstructing colonic carcinoma and, like sigmoid volvulus, it may be related to a high fibre intake. The presenting symptoms are usually non-specific. Abdominal pain is almost invariably present and nausea, vomiting, constipation, and distension will occur in about one-third of patients. In thin

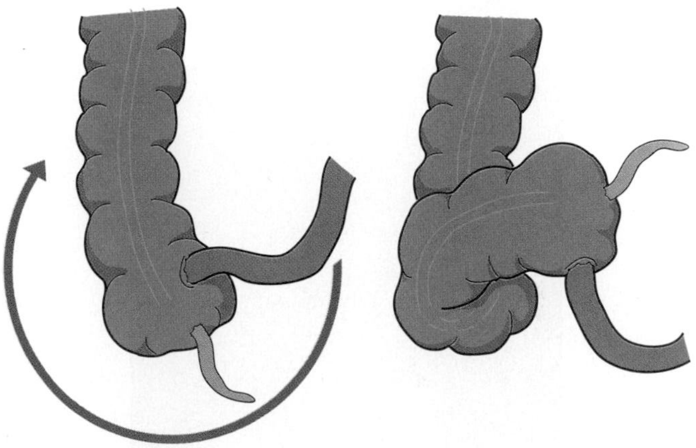

Fig. 6 The mechanism of caecal volvulus.

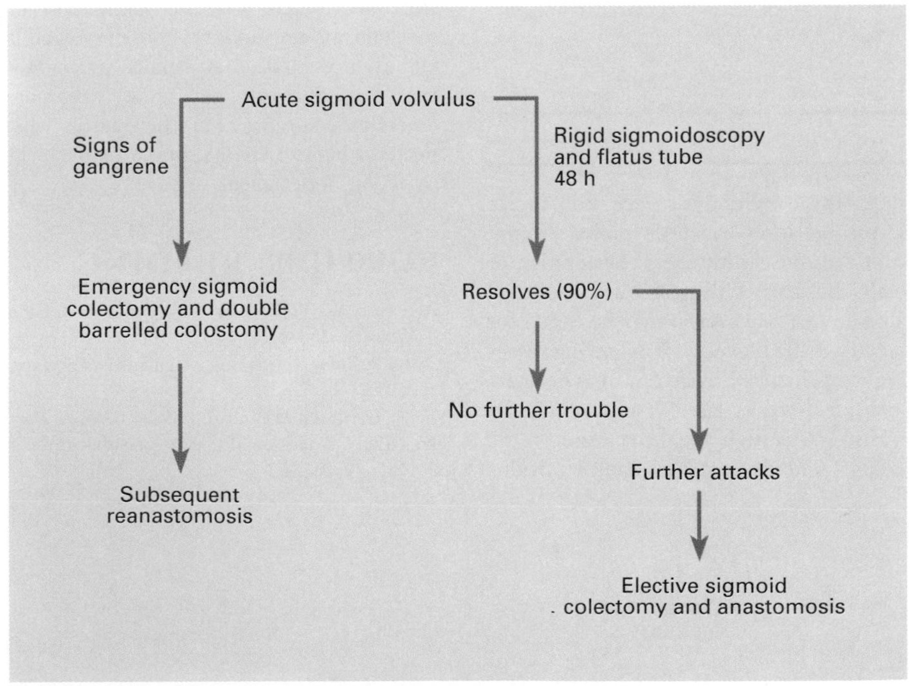

Fig. 5 Algorithm for the management of sigmoid volvulus.

patients it may be possible to palpate the resonant distended caecum in the central or upper abdomen while the right iliac fossa is empty.

Radiology

The key to the diagnosis of caecal volvulus, as with sigmoid volvulus, is the plain abdominal radiograph. The caecum typically assumes a gas-filled 'comma shape' facing inferiorly and to the right (Fig. 7). In a retrospective analysis Anderson and Mills (1984) found that the diagnosis was evident on the plain abdominal radiograph in 40 out of 45 patients with caecal volvulus. The diagnosis is usually made in around 50 per cent of patients however. Other radiological appearances are of non-specific colonic obstruction or of small bowel obstruction. A barium enema may be useful to exclude any other predisposing colonic lesion and on occasions it has been effective in reducing the volvulus.

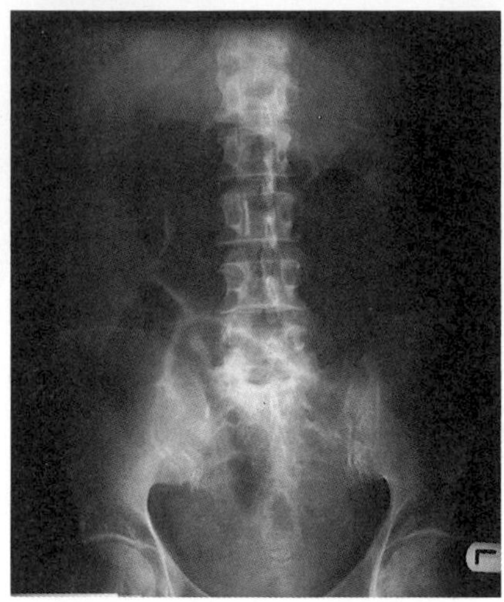

Fig. 7 Plain supine radiograph showing caecal volvulus.

Treatment

The mainstay of treatment for this condition is surgery and, unlike sigmoid volvulus, endoscopic deflation has little place. Prompt caecal resection is mandatory in those with caecal perforation or infarction and this is usually possible with a primary ileocaecal anastomosis. In severely ill patients, however, it may be expedient to exteriorize the proximal and distal bowel ends following resection, as an ileostomy and mucous fistula. These can then be anastomosed at a second operation 6 weeks later. The mortality in patients with gangrenous bowel is as high as 40 per cent.

The management of patients who present with caecal volvulus without evidence of strangulation is less clearly defined. Fixation of the caecum (caecopexy) to prevent recurrent torsion has its advocates. This is best achieved by combining suture fixation to the lateral abdominal wall with stripping of the parietal and visceral peritoneum to create raw surfaces that will stick firmly and permanently together. Unfortunately the technique has a recurrence rate of up to 20 per cent. The addition of a tube caecostomy has been advocated in addition to caecopexy and this has been shown to reduce the recurrence rate. However this addition is associated with an increase in surgical morbidity, mainly from septic problems from leakage, such as cellulitis, wound infection, and occasionally necrosis of the abdominal wall. The caecostomy tube can be removed after 1 week and the tract will normally close spontaneously within a few days. Occasionally, however, discharge of ileal contents persists, requiring further surgery formally to close the hole or resect the caecum.

The definitive treatment of caecal volvulus, even when the bowel is viable, is caecal resection and primary ileocolic anastomosis. If the surgeon has sufficient experience this is the preferred management. Whichever method is chosen, and the differing opinions would suggest that there is little between the options, prompt treatment is essential to prevent bowel strangulation.

OTHER TYPES OF COLONIC VOLVULUS

Volvulus of the splenic flexure is extremely rare, accounting for less than 1 per cent of colonic volvuli, and it results from a congenital absence of one or more of the ligaments which normally fix that part of the bowel. The patients present with acute intestinal obstruction usually with a preceding history of chronic constipation. The diagnosis is made by diagnostic enema. Endoscopic deflation is often possible, but the patient should undergo definitive bowel resection to prevent recurrence.

Transverse colon volvulus is also very rare. It occurs when a degree of malrotation exists and can also result from chronic constipation, which leads to elongation of the mesentery. The mechanisms are similar to those involved in sigmoid volvulus. The clinical presentation is usually subacute or chronic but patients can present with an acute fulminant condition requiring emergency surgery. For this reason when the diagnosis is suspected a barium enema should be performed and prompt elective resection undertaken.

FURTHER READING

Anderson JR, Welch GW. Acute volvulus of the right colon. *World J Surg* 1986; **10**: 336–42.

Bak MP, Boley SJ. Sigmoid volvulus in elderly patients. *Am J Surg* 1986; **151**: 71–5.

Tejler G, Jiborn H. Volvulus of the caecum. *Dis Colon Rect* 1981; **31**: 445–9.

Welch GH, Anderson JR. Acute volvulus of the sigmoid colon. *World J Surg* 1987; **11**: 258–62.

18.6 Chronic constipation in adults

NEIL MORTENSEN

INTRODUCTION

An increasing number of adult patients with severe constipation who have not responded to the usual dietary measures and laxatives are being seen in surgical practice. This is not a trivial symptom and the patient's life both at home and at work is often severely restricted by abdominal pain, distension, a poor sense of well-being, and decreased bowel frequency. The symptom of constipation cannot be precisely defined. Patients have a problem with defecation and may be worried by infrequent and/or hard stools which are difficult to pass. Different types of severe constipation have a different cause and require a different therapeutic approach.

ASSESSMENT

Patients with minor, easily treated symptoms do not require sophisticated investigation. A careful history of the exact nature of the constipation, together with any history of sexual or psychiatric problems, is essential. Abdominal examination will reveal the presence of a palpable faecal mass. Weakness of the pelvic floor is indicated by extreme descent of the perineum on straining. Laxity of the anal sphincter and perianal soiling is usually associated with gross faecal impaction in the rectum.

Patients can generally be divided into those with a colon of normal width and those with an abnormally wide or capacious rectum and/or colon: a barium enema defines into which of these two groups the patient falls. In those patients with rectal impaction, an unprepared radiograph using a water-soluble contrast material will illustrate the rectum and the distal colon with the impacted stools still in place. The rate of transit of contents through the colon can be estimated by a single abdominal radiograph taken 5 days after the patient has swallowed 20 radio-opaque markers. In specialist units, information about evacuation disorders can be obtained by recording the appearance of the rectal and anal canal on video tape or fast film sequences as the patient expels a barium gel or paste. Simple manometric studies can be used to test rectal sensation and the rectoanal inhibitory reflex by distending a balloon in the rectal ampulla.

ADULT HIRSCHPRUNG'S DISEASE

A small proportion of patients with Hirschprung's disease do not present until adolescence or young adult life. Elliot and Todd reported 39 such patients treated at St Mark's Hospital, London, between 1965 and 1984. There were 26 males and 13 females with a mean age of 23 years. The Duhamel operation produced good results, with complete continence, and daily evacuation, in 36 patients; the remaining three patients had poorer results, with occasional incontinence. Investigation of this disorder should include a barium enema which will reveal the characteristic junction between the dilated proximal colon and the aganglionic segment (Fig. 1). Anorectal physiology studies will show an absent rectosphincteric reflex, and full thickness rectal biopsy will demonstrate the absence of ganglion cells in the myenteric plexus. A frozen section biopsy of the normal colon during the operation will ensure that normally innervated bowel is brought down behind the aganglionic rectum.

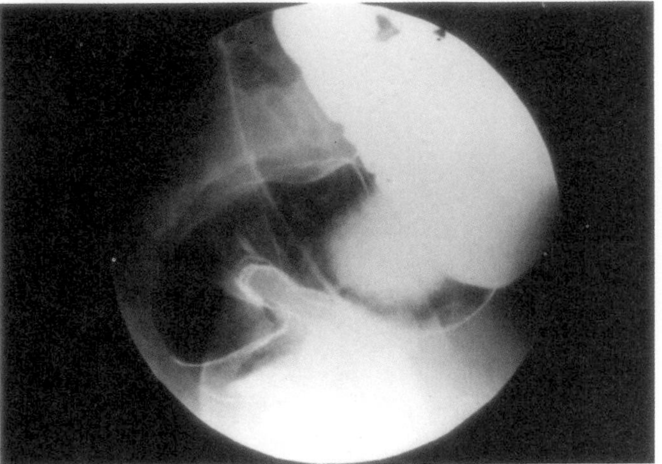

Fig. 1 Lateral radiograph of the pelvis. Barium enema demonstrating the narrowed area in Hirschprung's disease at the junction with the aganglionic segment.

IDIOPATHIC MEGARECTUM AND MEGACOLON

Once Hirschprung's disease and metabolic and other secondary causes of a dilated colon have been excluded there remains a group of patients with a dilated large bowel of unknown cause. This condition affects males and females equally and it may commence in childhood or adult life. Recurrent faecal impaction is the usual presentation, though in childhood it may present with soiling. The nerve plexuses and muscle coats appear grossly normal on histological assessment and the aetiology of this condition remains unknown. The rectal diameter is usually greater than 6.5 cm. In two-thirds of cases the rectum alone is affected, but in one-third of cases the dilation extends into the sigmoid colon (Fig. 2).

It is worth trying medical treatment initially, prescribing a combination of enemas, suppositories, and osmotic laxatives which will keep the rectum empty. If laxatives are poorly tolerated or are ineffective and it seems unlikely that the grossly dilated bowel will recover, surgery is indicated. It is not clear which is the best procedure to offer these patients. The alternatives include a preliminary loop ileostomy followed by either a Duhamel procedure or a resection and coloanal anastomosis. In those with a moderately dilated colon a colectomy with ileorectal anastomosis may offer a reasonable compromise. In a recent series of 40 patients undergoing a colectomy for this condition 80 per cent achieved normal bowel frequency and most were relieved of the need for laxatives. A third of the patients, however, continued to experience some abdominal pain. Ileorectal anastomosis produced

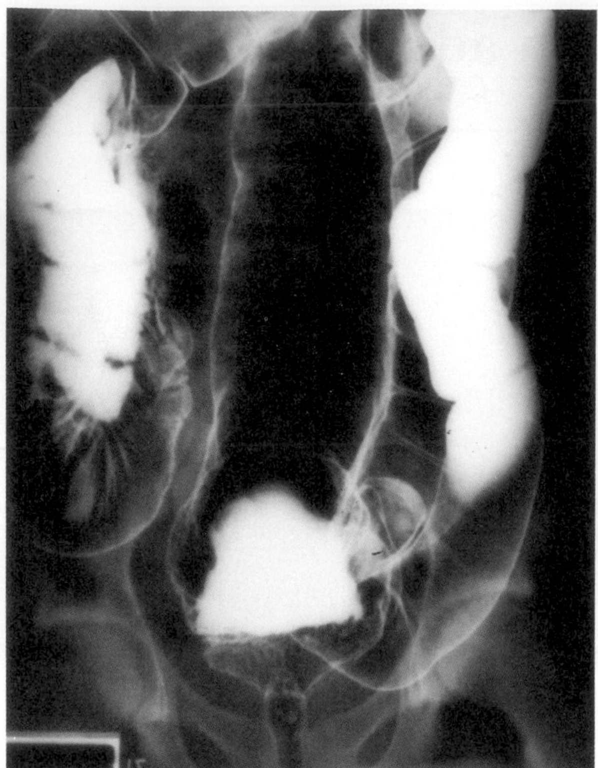

Fig. 2 Barium enema. Megarectum and megasigmoid.

results superior to those of a caecorectal anastomosis or a sigmoid resection: these last operations had a higher incidence of persistent constipation. In patients with a grossly dilated rectum the most commonly performed procedure was the Duhamel operation. It seems however that results in this situation are less satisfactory than those obtained in patients with Hirschprung's disease. In a series of 20 patients reported by Stabile only half achieved a normal bowel frequency. Seven patients remained constipated and of these five required further surgery. The other alternative is a resection of the grossly dilated rectum and a coloanal anastomosis. This usually has to be performed using a hand suturing technique because of the thickness of the rectal stump. There are no reliable data on the outcome of this procedure.

The patient who remains constipated despite colectomy may be treated by creation of a stoma, bringing out proximal bowel of normal diameter. If there is progressive dilatation of the proximal colon an ileostomy may be necessary and, in very selected cases, a restorative proctocolectomy would be an alternative approach.

Severe idiopathic slow transit constipation

Preston and Leonard Jones (1986) reported a series of 64 women complaining of severe constipation. The patients passed about one stool weekly with the aid of laxatives and were greatly troubled by abdominal pain, bloating, malaise, and nausea to the extent that their symptoms were an increasing social disability. A decrease in bowel frequency and other symptoms were often noticed around the age of puberty and slowly became worse until they were at their most severe by the third decade. In a few patients the symptoms appeared suddenly after an abdominal operation or an accident.

A barium enema in these patients shows a normal rectal and colonic diameter; on large bowel transit studies, less than 80 per cent of the 20 shapes or radio-opaque markers ingested on the first day have been passed on the fifth day (Fig. 3). The recto-sphincteric reflex is normal, and a full thickness rectal biopsy is not normally required, though in doubtful cases it is sensible to exclude Hirschprung's disease.

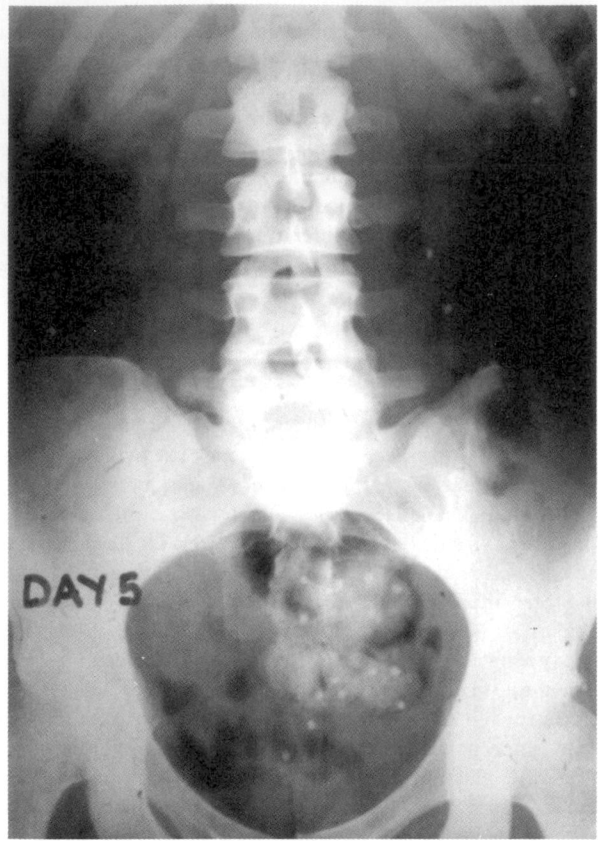

Fig. 3 Plain radiograph 5 days after the ingestion of 20 radio-opaque markers. More than 80 per cent are still present, indicating slow transit.

As is the case in patients with megarectum, it is as well to institute medical therapy for as long as possible, aimed at emptying the rectum with osmotic laxatives, suppositories, or enemas. These patients have usually tried the whole range of laxatives and many of them become increasingly constipated despite quite high doses of concurrent laxative medication. Interestingly, high fibre diets often make their symptoms worse.

The surgical options include a segmental colectomy, a colectomy and caecorectal anastomosis, colectomy and ileorectal anastomosis, a proctocolectomy and ileoanal reservoir, or an ileostomy. It is now generally believed that segmental colectomies have nothing to offer: patients tend to become progressively constipated within a year or so of this operation. The most widely used operation is colectomy and ileorectal anastomosis. In a series reported by Kamm *et al.* (1988) of 44 patients, all female with a median evacuation frequency of once every 4 weeks, 22 patients were reported to be normal, 17 had diarrhoea, and 5 had recurrent constipation after this procedure. A worrying feature was the fact that 71 per cent of the patients had continuing abdominal pain. In the series reported by Roe *et al.* (1988) 22 patients underwent colectomy and ileorectal anastomosis. There were four failures, two with pain and bloating, one with continuing constipation, and one patient had recurrent adhesions. In the study by Kamm *et al.* (1988) 10 patients needed psychiatric treatment for severe psychological disorders. While many of these patients are completely normal there is a small subgroup with severe and often occult psychological problems who need to be very carefully investigated and managed prior to surgery. If a colectomy and ileorectal anastomosis fails there is the possibility of creating a stoma. Van der Syp *et al.* (1990) reported 37 such patients; those who improved most following creation of a stoma were those with idiopathic constipation who had not undergone previous surgery. Of the 10 patients who had had a failed ileorectal anastomosis only 50 per cent were improved by a colostomy. A number of these patients continued to have pain and bloating and a continued use of laxatives. There is the possibility, however, in the colostomy group of colostomy irrigation, and even a colostomy plug.

Chronic idiopathic intestinal pseudo-obstruction

This is a rare group of patients who have severe constipation and a dilated colon, but also dilatation of the upper intestine. In one-third of patients the disorder shows Mendelian inheritance. Histological studies have demonstrated abnormalities of nerve plexuses and smooth muscle in most patients. Treatment is usually with prokinetic agents to increase intestinal motility. A number of patients also require nutritional support.

Evacuatory disorders

Some patients will give a clear history of an evacuatory disorder. Despite what seems to be a normal propulsive effort by the colon with stool in the rectum, the patient is unable to expel it. Evacuatory disorders have been given a number of names including outlet obstruction, anismus, pelvic floor spasm, the solitary ulcer syndrome, rectal intussusception, and the descending perineum syndrome.

The patient gives a characteristic history of evacuatory difficulty. This may involve long periods of time sitting straining at stool, manipulation of the anal margin, pressure on the perineal body, and, in female patients, pressure on the posterior wall of the vagina. In some patients the distress becomes so extreme that the anal canal is digitated and the faecal material manually removed.

The cause of this condition is not known: there may be a number of underlying problems ranging from an inappropriate contraction of the pelvic floor to an occult rectal intussusception. Physiological studies usually show a normal anal sphincter and rectum but the key investigation is the evacuation proctogram. A mixture of some form of starch and barium or a dilute barium paste is inserted into the rectum and the patient is then asked to strain as at stool. The time taken to expel the simulated stool is noted and any abnormalities in the architecture of the rectal wall recorded (Fig. 4).

The surgical options include rectal prolapse repair, anorectal myectomy, lateral division of the puborectalis, repair of a rectocele, and colostomy. The demonstration of spasm of the pelvic floor led Kamm *et al.* (1988) to use lateral division of the puborectalis muscle for the treatment of 15 patients with this condition: four of them improved while three had mild incontinence. The operation has now largely been abandoned. Pinho *et al.* (1989) used a variation of a procedure advocated for patients with Hirschprung's disease. A long myectomy of the internal anal sphincter and the rectal smooth muscle wall was made in the midline, posteriorly. There is, however, no evidence that these patients have an abnormality of the smooth muscle of either the anal sphincter or the rectum. In 63 patients with a 30-month follow-up there was no functional improvement in 70 per cent and 10 per cent of the patients developed mild incontinence. When an occult rectal intussusception is found on evacuation proctogram it is tempting to think that a rectopexy rather as for a rectal prolapse procedure would solve the problem. However, in a group of 17 patients reported by Roe *et al.* (1986), only four treated by rectopexy required no further treatment, five went on to require a subtotal colectomy, two had an ileostomy, and one a sphincterotomy. Only two patients had a successful result. This is an extremely difficult group of patients to manage satisfactorily. Often a careful explanation of the problem and reassurance that digitation for example does not do any harm will suffice. When it is impossible to distinguish between slow transit constipation and an evacuation disorder a loop ileostomy will allow time for further evaluation. If it is quite clear that there is an evacuatory disorder it is worth creating a colostomy and using colostomy irrigation as a semipermanent solution.

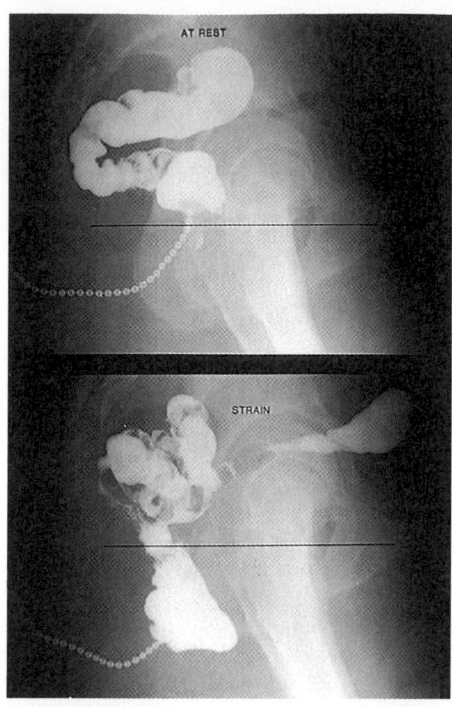

Fig. 4 Evacuation proctogram. The patient is straining and unable to pass any barium paste from the rectum.

FURTHER READING

Bartolo DCC, Roe AM, Virjee J, Mortensen NJMcC. Evacuation proctography in obstructed defaecation and rectal intussusception. *Br J Surg* 1985; 72 (suppl): 111–6.

Elliot MS, Todd IP. Adult Hirschprung's disease: results of the Duhamel procedure. *Br J Surg* 1985; **72**: 884–5.
Hinton JM, Lennard Jones JE, Young AC. A new method for studying gut transit times using radio opaque markers. *Gut* 1969; **10**: 842–7.
Hosie KB, Kmiot WA, Keighley MRB. Constipation: another indication for restorative proctocolectomy. *Br J Surg* 1990; **77**: 801–2.
Kamm MA, Hawley PR, Lennard Jones JE. Outcome of colectomy for severe idiopathic constipation. *Gut* 1988; **29**: 969–75.
Pinho M, Yoshioka K, Keighley MRB. Longterm results of anorectal myectomy for chronic constipation. *Br J Surg* 1989; **76**: 1163–4.
Preston DM, Lennard Jones JE. Severe chronic constipation of young women: 'idiopathic slow transit constipation'. *Gut* 1986; **27**: 41–8.
Roe AM, Bartolo DCC, Mortensen NJMcC. Diagnosis and surgical management of intractable constipation. *Br J Surg* 1986; **73**: 854–61.
Stabile G, Kamm MA, Hawley PR, Lennard Jones JE. Results of the Duhamel operation in the treatment of idiopathic megarectum and megacolon. *Br J Surg* 1991; (b) **78**: 661–3.
Stabile G, Kamm MA, Hawley PR, Lennard Jones JE. Colectomy for idiopathic megarectum and megacolon. *Gut* 1991: **32**: 1538–40.

18.7 Angiodysplasia

PAUL C. SHELLITO

INTRODUCTION

Angiodysplasia is an acquired submucosal arteriovenous malformation which may cause lower gastrointestinal bleeding in elderly patients. It is often difficult to diagnose, and many aspects of the disease are unclear; reported statistics about incidence and results of treatment therefore differ widely. Angiodysplasia has been reported to account for between 2 and 60 per cent of adult patients with lower gastrointestinal bleeding; it probably causes the majority of incidents of massive lower gastrointestinal bleeding in older patients, with diverticulosis accounting for most of the remainder. There is also little agreement about the prevalence of angiodysplasia in adults; estimates range from 1 to 30 per cent, but the true figure is probably 1 to 5 per cent.

Typical angiodysplastic lesions are 0.5 to 1.0 cm in diameter, bright red, flat or slightly raised, and covered by very thin epithelium (Fig. 1). Between 70 and 90 per cent of the lesions appear in the right colon, although they may also be found in the distal colon, and can also occur, less often, anywhere else in the gastrointestinal tract. Most patients have two or three lesions. Angiodysplasia probably accounted for many episodes of what were in the past thought to be diverticular bleeds. Thus, there is only partial truth to the maxim that diverticulitis is predominantly a left-sided disease, and bleeding diverticulosis a right-sided disease.

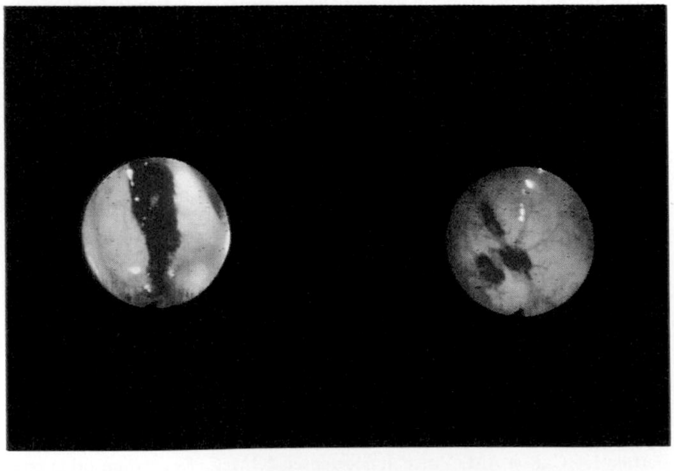

Fig. 1 Typical angiodysplasia lesions in the caecum. At right, prompt bleeding after slight surface trauma is seen.

AETIOLOGY

Theories of aetiology abound, but it is probably an acquired degenerative lesion resulting from chronic, intermittent, partial low grade obstruction to submucosal venous outflow within the muscular bowel wall, due to contraction and distension of the colon. This in turn causes dilatation first of submucosal veins, and then capillaries and precapillary sphincters, leading to a small arteriovenous malformation. Since the right colon has the widest diameter in the large bowel, the law of LaPlace predicts that wall tension is greatest there. Thus, the intramural venous obstruction would also be maximal in that location, which could account for the right-sided predilection of angiodysplasia. Alternatively, but less convincingly, the lesions might appear because of low mucosal blood flow leading to chronic submucosal shunting. The relatively low mucosal perfusion could be accounted for by high right colon wall tension with or without chronic constipation, as well as by cardiac valvular disease. The least likely explanation is that it may simply arise because the thin wall of the right colon provides minimal support for the microscopic vasculature, leading to foci of dilatation which degenerate into arteriovenous malformations. It has been suggested that an abnormal pulse wave pattern in the ileocaecal artery due to cardiac valve disease contributes to this degeneration. Numerous accounts have documented an association with 'cardiovascular disease' (50–100 per cent), and especially aortic valve disease (20–30 per cent). Not all studies have revealed a correlation with valve lesions, however, and assertions of cause and effect are conjectural. There are major methodological deficiencies in all reports of correlation between angiodysplasia and heart valve disease.

Inherited gastrointestinal arteriovenous malformations such as hereditary haemorrhagic telangiectasia or Osler–Weber–Rendu syndrome are similar but unrelated. Unlike angiodysplasia, hereditary haemorrhagic telangiectasia is familial, tends to affect younger patients, and produces many more lesions which are much more widely dispersed throughout the gastrointestinal tract as well as in the skin and mucous membranes. Unlike haemangiomas, angiodysplasia is not neoplastic.

CLINICAL PRESENTATION AND COURSE

Gastrointestinal bleeding is the only clinical manifestation of angiodysplasia, and patients are usually over 60 years old. The most common result of bleeding lesions is gross haemochezia or maroon stools, and sometimes melaena, although some reports claim that 30 to 50 per cent of patients show only anaemia and guaiac-positive faeces. Less than 10 per cent is a more likely proportion. The natural history of angiodysplasia is uncertain. Because the bleeding occurs from tiny capillaries and venules covered by very thin epithelium, episodes tend to be self limiting, but chronic and recurrent. Massive haemorrhage with hypotension is unusual. In contrast, diverticular bleeding, which comes from one or two larger eroded arterioles, is more likely to be acute and massive. After clot has formed around the responsible diverticular vessel, recurrent bleeding is less likely than with angiodysplasia. Patients with angiodysplasia may have a long history of recurrent idiopathic gastrointestinal bleeding, with multiple unrevealing prior investigations, possibly including laparotomy. The arteriovenous malformations are too small to cause haemodynamic changes (in the absence of bleeding), pain, or perforation.

DIAGNOSIS AND PATHOLOGY

Angiodysplasia has largely been recognized and characterized only since the advent of colonoscopy and mesenteric angiography. Because the lesions are small, flat, and not transmural, they are overlooked by barium enema radiography or inspection of the serosal surface at laparotomy. Even pathological examination will usually miss angiodysplasia unless special injection techniques are used. The mesenteric vessels of the specimen may be injected with barium followed by radiography, or the vessels may be perfused with silicone rubber followed by tissue clearing with methyl salicylate (Fig. 2), so that only the vascular network remains opaque. Specialized pathological examinations reveal tortuous, enlarged, thin walled submucosal veins communicating with clusters of dilated mucosal capillaries (Fig. 3). Endoscopic biopsies are rarely helpful, however, because the mucosal lesion is variable,

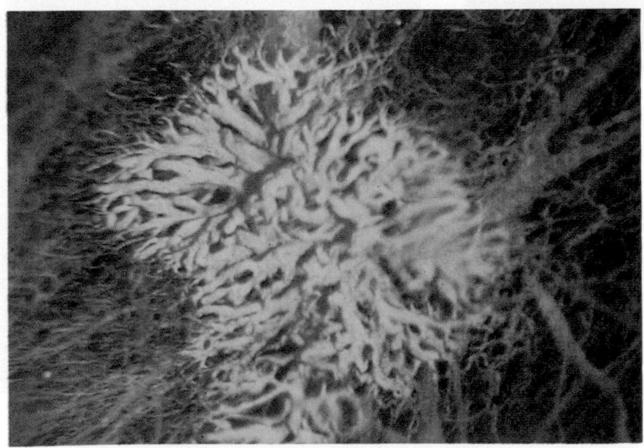

Fig. 2 Angiodysplasia after silicone injection and tissue clearing. A dense collection of abnormal submucosal vessels is demonstrated.

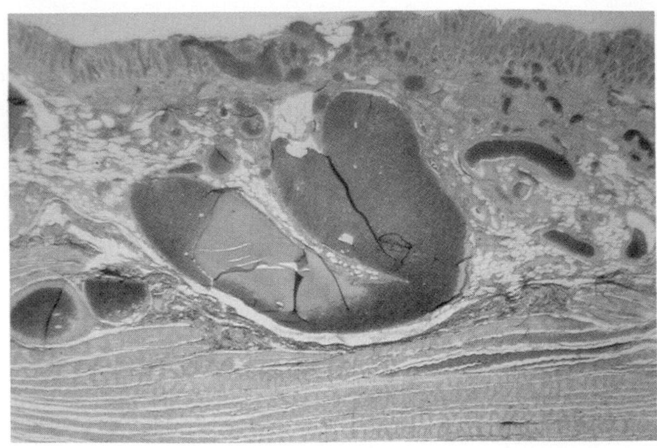

Fig. 3 Histopathology of angiodysplasia. Barium has been injected intravascularly, which stains dark brown in this slide. Submucosal veins are seen, as well as an overlying smaller plexus of mucosal vessels.

and the biopsy forceps do not usually reach as deep as the abnormal submucosal veins.

The appearances at angiography reflect the theory of pathogenesis. In 90 per cent of cases a large, tortuous, slowly draining submucosal vein is found; a mucosal vascular tuft is seen in 70 per cent; 60 per cent of cases show an early draining dilated vein, which correlates with the final stage of formation of the arteriovenous malformation. Small angiodysplasias can be quite inconspicuous on angiography, unless active haemorrhage is taking place and extravasation of contrast is demonstrated. Unfortunately, because bleeding from angiodysplasia is typically episodic, extravasation is not often demonstrable at angiography.

The colonoscopic appearance is pathognomonic (Fig. 1). The lesions are flat or slightly raised, bright red, and 0.5 to 1.0 cm in diameter. Because of the magnification afforded by the colonoscope, the tiny dilated mucosal vessels in and around the lesion can frequently be seen on close inspection, although these small malformations can be overlooked on endoscopy unless the colonic mucosa is quite clean. Polyethylene glycol gut lavage solutions clean out the colon more effectively than older laxative and enema preparations, and make discovery of angiodysplasia more likely. Care must be taken not to confuse angiodysplasia with traumatic ecchymoses (which are seen on withdrawal but not insertion of the colonoscope), and prominent veins (which are bluish, not bright red). Angioplastic lesions may be almost hidden behind a mucosal fold in the right colon, or just proximal to the ileocaecal valve. The diagnosis can be made 80 to 90 per cent of the time using either colonoscopy or angiography. Endoscopy is probably the more sensitive and specific technique, but opinions differ, depending upon local expertise, and upon which method is accepted as the standard by which to judge the other. Both angiography and colonoscopy may produce false positive results. Colonoscopy is less invasive than angiography, and also has the advantage of providing biopsies if desired. Furthermore, the entire colon and sometimes the terminal ileum can be meticulously assessed to exclude other diseases or detect synchronous angiodysplasia. A growing array of endoscopic therapeutic manoeuvres are also possible, including fulguration and polypectomy.

MANAGEMENT

Treatment is indicated for an angiodysplasia that has bled, because of its tendency to cause chronic recurrent haemorrhage. The choice is between surgical resection and endoscopic coagulation. Both treatments are fairly uncomplicated; the most difficult challenge is to make an accurate diagnosis, using the methods discussed above, in order to direct therapy appropriately. Other possible sources of bleeding must be ruled out, and care must be taken not to overlook synchronous angiodysplasia spots. Since angiodysplasia is usually found in the right colon, right hemicolectomy is often curative (or removal of whatever bowel segment is responsible). Rebleeding occurs in 15 to 25 per cent of surgically treated patients, usually because of overlooked arteriovenous malformations in other areas of the bowel, or an error in diagnosis. If preoperative evaluation has reasonably convincingly demonstrated right-sided angiodysplasia, and left-sided diverticulosis is found at laparotomy, it is still acceptable to limit the resection to the right colon. If no specific treatment is undertaken at least half of the patients with angiodysplasia will rebleed.

Despite satisfactory results with surgery, the modern treatment of angiodysplasia is endoscopic coagulation, unless the lesions are large or quite numerous. Either laser photocoagulation (Fig. 4) or electrocoagulation may be used. Photocoagulation is preferable: the use of 'hot biopsy' forceps allows the target to be grasped, the mucosa drawn up off the underlying bowel wall, coagulating current applied, and the lesion released (Fig. 5). The technique minimizes the risk of perforation, which is an important consideration in the thin walled caecum (in contrast to coagulation of bleeding ulcers in a duodenum or stomach thickened by chronic inflammation). No actual biopsy of the arteriovenous malformation is required, since the diagnosis may be made by inspection alone. If a laser is to be used, argon is preferable to neodymium-yttrium aluminium garnet (Nd:YAG). The light wavelength from an argon unit is preferentially absorbed by red pigment and also penetrates more superficially than does light from a Nd:YAG machine. Both characteristics are nicely suited to treatment of superficial blood vessel malformations. Whether using laser photocoagulation or hot biopsy electrocoagulation, it is best to start at the periphery of the lesion and progress toward the centre.

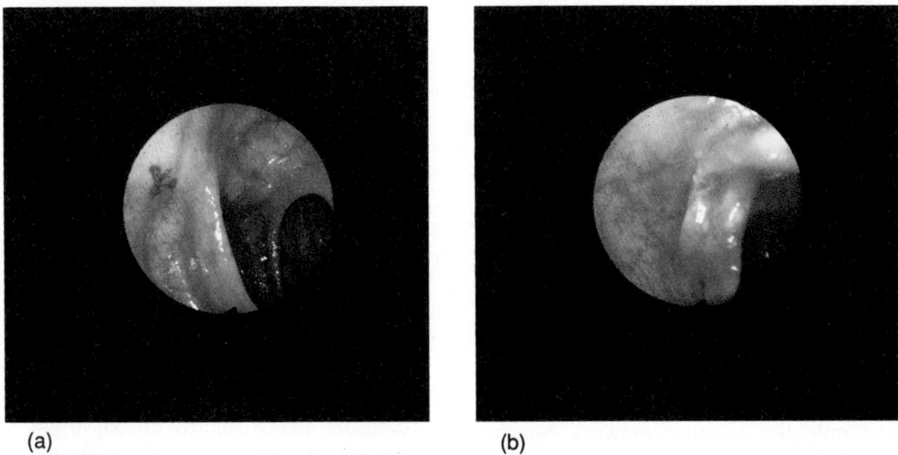

(a) (b)

Fig. 4 Nd:YAG laser photocoagulation of angiodysplasia. (a) Right colon angiodysplasia. (b) After cauterization.

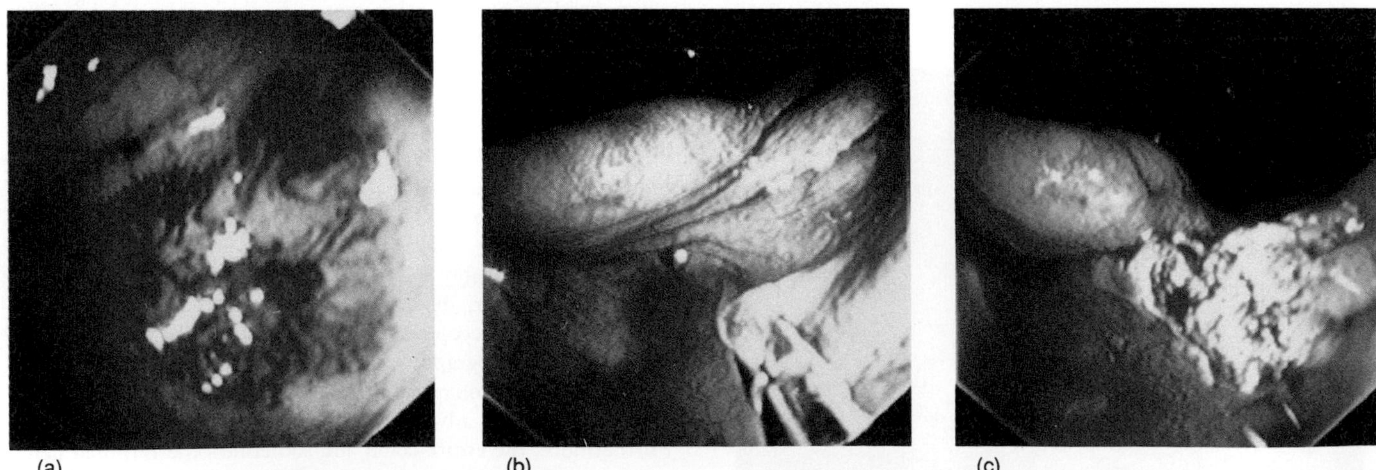

(a) (b) (c)

Fig. 5 Hot biopsy coagulation of angiodysplasia. (a) Close up view of the lesion. (b) The angiodysplasia has been grasped and pulled up by the biopsy forceps, while electrocoagulation is carried out. (c) The mucosa has been released (without biopsy), leaving white coagulated mucosa visible. The ileocoecal valve is just above and to the left of the coagulated area.

The mucosa should be cauterized until it is white, not black. Coagulation of large angiodysplasias should be carried out in stages, several weeks apart, to minimize the risk of perforation. The colon and terminal ileum should be searched carefully for synchronous lesions. Rebleeding occurs in only 10 to 30 per cent of patients, and this is usually from lesions overlooked or incompletely coagulated, making early follow-up colonoscopy is prudent. Nevertheless, even in patients who rebleed after endoscopic treatment of arteriovenous malformation of the gastrointestinal tract the frequency of haemorrhage episodes and number of transfusions declines. Perforation follows in up to 7 per cent of treatments, usually when a Nd:YAG laser is used. The best treatment for an asymptomatic angiodysplasia lesion that has been found incidentally during colonoscopy is unclear. The risk of later haemorrhage is unknown but is probably low; it is therefore reasonable to leave quiescent lesions alone. Experienced endoscopists, however, may justifiably prefer to eliminate the uncertainty.

FURTHER READING

Baum S, *et al.* Angiodysplasia of the right colon: a cause of gastrointestinal bleeding. *Am J Roentgenol* 1977; **129**: 789–94.

Boley SJ, *et al.* On the nature and etiology of vascular ectasias of the colon. *Gastroenterology* 1977; **72**: 650–60.

Boley SJ, *et al.* Vascular ectasias of the colon. *Surg Gynecol Obstet* 1979; **149**: 353–9.

Danesh BJZ, *et al.* Angiodysplasia, an uncommon cause of colonic bleeding. *Int J Colorect Dis* 1987; **2**: 218–22.

Emanuel RB, *et al.* Arteriovenous malformations as a cause of gastrointestinal bleeding. *J Clin Gastroenterol* 1985; **7**: 237–46.

Gostout CJ, *et al.* Mucosal vascular malformations of the gastrointestinal tract: clinical observations and results of endoscopic Nd-YAG laser therapy. *Mayo Clin Proc* 1988; **63**: 993–1003.

Greenstein RJ, *et al.* Colonic vascular ectasias and aortic stenosis: coincidence or casual relationship? *Am J Surg* 1986; **151**: 347–51.

Imperiale TF, Ransohoff DF. Aortic stenosis, idiopathic gastrointestinal bleeding and angiodysplasia: is there an association? *Gastroenterology* 1988; **95**: 1670–6.

Price AB. Angiodysplasia of the colon (review). *Int J Colorect Dis* 1986; **1**: 121–8.

Richter JM, *et al.* Angiodysplasia: natural history and efficacy of therapeutic interventions. *Dig Dis Sci* 1989; **34**: 1542–6.

Richter JM, *et al.* Angiodysplasia: clinical presentation and colonoscopic diagnosis. *Dig Dis Sci* 1984; **29**: 481–5.

Talman EA, Dixon DS, Gutierrez FE. Role of arteriography in rectal hemorrhage due to arteriovenous malformations and diverticulosis. *Ann Surg* 1979; **190**: 203–13.

Tedesco FJ, Griffin JW, Khan AQ. Vascular ectasia of the colon: clinical, colonoscopic, and radiographic features. *J Clin Gastroenterol* 1980; **2**: 233–8.

Trudel JL, Fazio VW, Sivak MR. Colonoscopic diagnosis and treatment of arteriovenous malformations in chronic liver gastrointestinal bleeding. *Dis Colon Rect* 1988; **31**: 107–10.

18.8 Prolapse of the rectum

PAUL C. SHELLITO AND NEIL MORTENSEN

The term 'rectal prolapse' implies a full thickness circumferential descent of the rectum through the anus. A prolapse of only the rectal mucosa is called incomplete or mucosal prolapse. A variant of complete rectal prolapse has been described in which the upper rectum prolapses into the middle or lower rectum without actually reaching the anal canal. This is called an internal prolapse, or intussusception of the rectum.

INCIDENCE

Rectal prolapse occurs at the extremes of life. Complete rectal prolapse is found chiefly in elderly female patients: 85 per cent of adults with full thickness rectal prolapse are women and the incidence is maximal in the fifth decade and upwards. Many patients are of very advanced age, being in their eighties or nineties. In men, though the incidence is much lower, rectal prolapse presents throughout the age range or may be more common in the second and third decades of life. Mucosal prolapse is most common in young children.

The increased incidence in female patients might imply an effect of childbirth on the pelvic floor, but in many series half of the patients are childless. Furthermore, uterine and rectal prolapse only rarely occur together.

AETIOLOGY

Partial prolapse

In children there is usually some promoting factor such as diarrhoea, constipation, or bad defecatory habits. A chronic cough or severe coughing attacks can cause a rectal prolapse. In adults prolapsed mucosa is associated with third-degree haemorrhoids, and in older patients it may occur as a result of a weak anal sphincter. Parks *et al.* described the descending perineum syndrome in which the anterior wall of the rectum causes an evacuatory disorder.

Complete prolapse

Anatomical findings

Complete rectal prolapse is associated with a collection of distinct anatomical changes (Table 1). The most striking of these is the abnormally deep rectovaginal, or in males rectovesical, pouch. This gave rise to the earliest theory of the cause of rectal prolapse, namely that it was a form of sliding hernia, the pouch of Douglas being the hernial sac pressing the anterior rectal wall into the rectal lumen.

Table 1 Anatomical findings in complete rectal prolapse

Diastasis of the levators
Deep pouch of Douglas
Redundant rectosigmoid
Lax lateral and posterior attachments
Loss of horizontal lie
Elongated mesorectum

Broden and Snellman described the radiographic changes seen when an intussusception was the lead point of a rectal prolapse found at 6 to 8 cm from the anal verge. In 60 per cent of patients this was anterior, in 32 per cent annular, and in 8 per cent posterior. An enterocele developed late, if at all (Fig. 1).

Most patients with complete prolapse have a weak atonic anal sphincter, and many also have a weak pelvic floor. It is not clear whether this is a cause or an effect of the prolapse: some patients have a large prolapse, but a normal anal sphincter once the prolapse has been reduced, while others with prolonged marked changes in the pelvic floor may have had a rectal prolapse for only weeks or months.

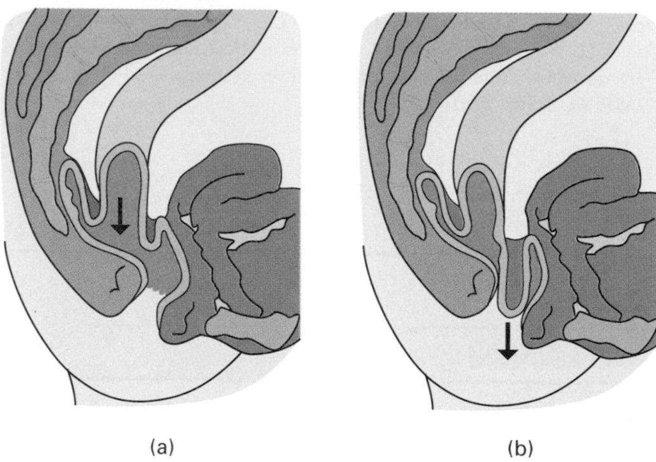

Fig. 1 Diagram showing a rectal intussusception (a) passing into the anal canal (arrow) to become a full thickness rectal prolapse (b) arrow.

Although rectal prolapse may occur in patients with cauda equina lesions, most patients with rectal prolapse have no obvious neurological abnormality. Studies of anorectal physiology show a reduction of resting anal pressure and maximum voluntary contraction pressure, impaired rectal sensation, absence or abnormalities of the rectosphincteric reflex, an increase in pudendal nerve latency, and histological evidence of muscle denervation in the external anal sphincter. These changes are most apparent in those patients who have a combination of prolapse and incontinence. Denervation of the voluntary sphincter muscles may be due to stretching of the pudendal nerves during descent of the rectum in the course of prolapse.

Since the intussusception described by Broden and Snellman starts well above the pelvic floor, these changes are probably a result of the rectal prolapse rather than the cause of it. Of 250 patients with anterior mucosal prolapse 20 per cent developed a full thickness rectal prolapse within 10 years.

The aetiology of rectal prolapse is still not clear. Known initiating factors include diarrhoea, constipation, and disorders of the pelvic floor which, acting together with predisposing factors such as a deep pouch of Douglas, a redundant sigmoid colon, and a weak pelvic floor, together bring about intussusception as the first stage in the genesis of a rectal prolapse.

CLINICAL FEATURES

Prolapse in children

Rectal prolapse in a child usually becomes apparent during defecation. It may reduce itself spontaneously sometimes, while at other times it may need to be replaced digitally. There is sometimes discomfort and a slight discharge of mucus or blood, but the child is usually perfectly well and normally continent.

On examination the prolapse consists of a ring of mucosa projecting 2 to 4 cm beyond the perianal verge. Gentle palpation between finger and thumb usually reveals that the prolapse consists of only two layers of mucosa. Very little pressure is required to reduce the prolapse and the anal sphincter appears normal. If there is only a history of prolapse, it is important for the surgeon to see the prolapse occurring in the clinic. Rarely the prolapse may be a complete rectal prolapse. Differential diagnosis includes a prolapsed rectal polyp or the apex of an intussusception. In the latter case it is possible to pass the tip of an examining finger along the slit between the intussuscepted bowel and the wall of the anal canal.

Prolapse in adults

Symptoms include those due to the prolapse itself and those due to the weakness of the anal sphincter. The prolapse first becomes apparent during evacuation or during episodes of raised intra-abdominal pressure. When the bowel wall is prolapsed mucus and blood may soil underclothes. There is also a degree of incontinence of faeces and flatus, giving rise to urgency and soiling episodes. Patients often have coincident constipation which aggravates the prolapsed condition.

The anus is usually patulous and there is a degree of mucosal prolapse evident at the anal orifice. Distraction on the anal margin causes the anus to open widely and the patient will often be able to push down a prolapse if it is not immediately apparent (Fig. 2). On

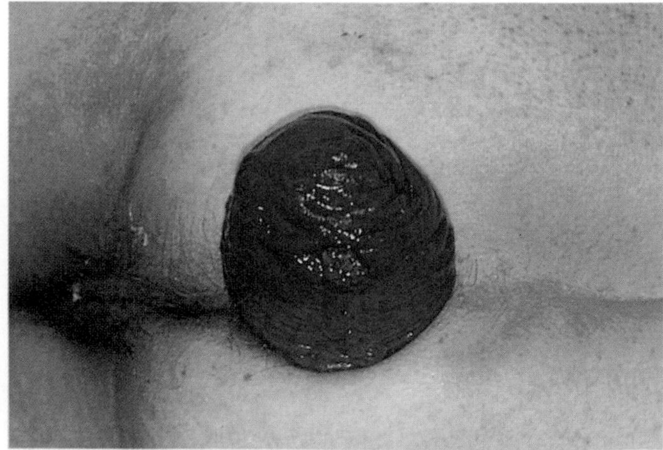

Fig. 2 A full thickness rectal prolapse.

palpation the anal sphincter is usually very weak. Voluntary contraction is usually poor and there is blunting of anal and rectal sensation. The mucosa on the apex of the prolapse may show some granularity or even superficial ulceration from repeated trauma caused by contact with underclothing.

When the prolapse is produced with the patient straining, palpation between finger and thumb reveals the double thickness of tissue; this is especially evident anteriorly where the deep pouch of Douglas and any possible contained loops of small intestine may add to the bulk of the prolapsing rectum. Most prolapses over 5 cm in length are complete but it can sometimes be difficult to tell whether a shorter prolapse is simply mucosa or a complete procidentia. If the patient is unable to produce a prolapse on the examination couch the diagnosis can be made on allowing the patient to adopt the usual squatting position secluded in a toilet. Some patients may find it easier to produce the prolapse in these circumstances than in the clinic.

On reducing the prolapse it is important to carry out a sigmoidoscopic examination to exclude any other abnormality within reach of the instrument.

Differential diagnosis

Large third-degree haemorrhoids, a large polypoid tumour of the rectum, sigmoid colon prolapsing and emerging at the anus, or a purely mucosal prolapse must all be differentiated from a complete procidentia.

Complications

Most patients can reduce the prolapse readily, although urgent admission may be required if the bowel becomes oedematous and cannot be reduced. It may be possible to reduce such a prolapse manually in the clinic with the patient lightly sedated. In the rare situation of a gangrenous rectal prolapse an emergency perineal rectosigmoidectomy may be necessary. Proctitis, ulceration, and rarely severe haemorrhage can occur but these are not usually clinically important.

TREATMENT

Prolapse in children

Rectal prolapse in children is a self-limiting disease and usually responds to conservative measures. Correction of bowel habit and small doses of laxatives may be all that is necessary. Occasionally a submucosal injection of phenol or alcohol may be required to secure fixation of the prolapse.

Rectal prolapse in adults

Partial prolapse

Minor mucosal prolapse can be treated in the same way as third-degree haemorrhoids, either by conservative measures or surgical excision. In older patients, in whom a partial prolapse complicates a weak anal sphincter a postanal repair operation may be necessary.

Complete prolapse

Innumerable methods for fixing a rectal prolapse have been described in the surgical literature, and they can be divided into perineal, sacral, and abdominal procedures. A procedure should be chosen with consideration for the age and fitness of the patient. There is perhaps no single ideal operation, and the art of prolapse management is to match the procedure to the patient.

Perineal procedures—partial excision of the rectum through the anus

Delorme's operation

This operation is becoming increasingly popular. With the bowel fully prolapsed a circular incision is made through the mucosa of the prolapse 1 cm from the dentate line (Fig. 3). Infiltration with dilute adrenaline solution helps indicate the submucosal plane.

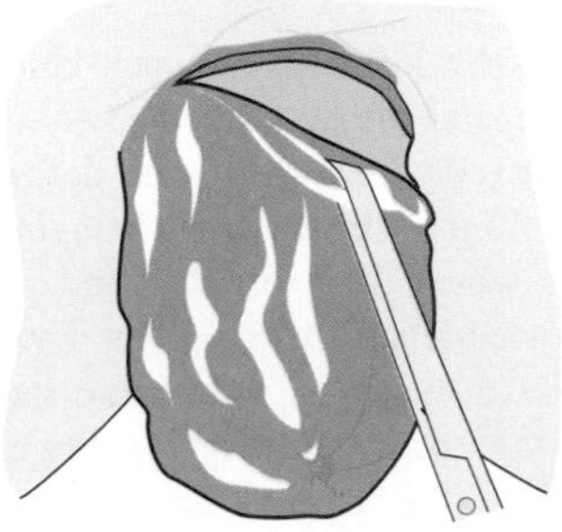

Fig. 3 Delorme's operation. An incision is made in the mucosa 1 cm above the dentate line with the rectum fully prolapsed.

The mucosa is then dissected from the underlying muscle coat as a sleeve until the apex of the prolapse is reached, and the dissection is carried on down into the prolapse as far as possible (Fig. 4). This leaves the outer aspect of the prolapse without any mucosal covering. The underlying muscle coat is imbricated with a series of longitudinal sutures to bunch up or reef it and bring the edges of the mucosa together (Fig. 5). The mucosa is then sutured with absorbable sutures and the prolapse gently reduced. Christiansen and Kirkegaard have advocated this operation for elderly frail patients. It has a particular place in this group and the procedure can also be used in patients with rectal prolapse complicating chronic ambulatory peritoneal dialysis.

Where there is coincident anal sphincter weakness it is possible to carry out a postanal repair at the same time. Only a small series

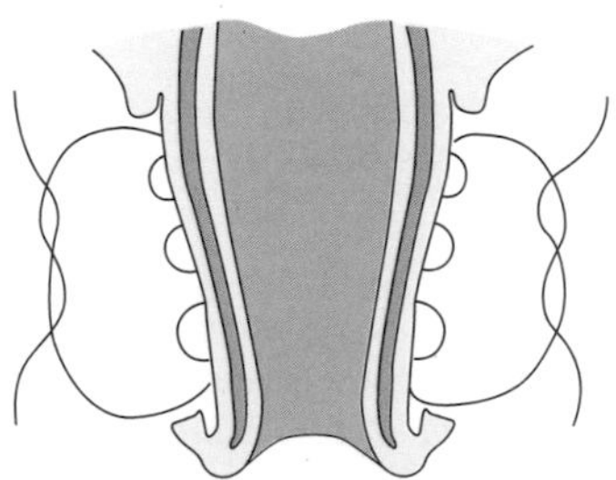

Fig. 4 Delorme's operation. The mucosa is stripped off the underlying muscle as far up as possible.

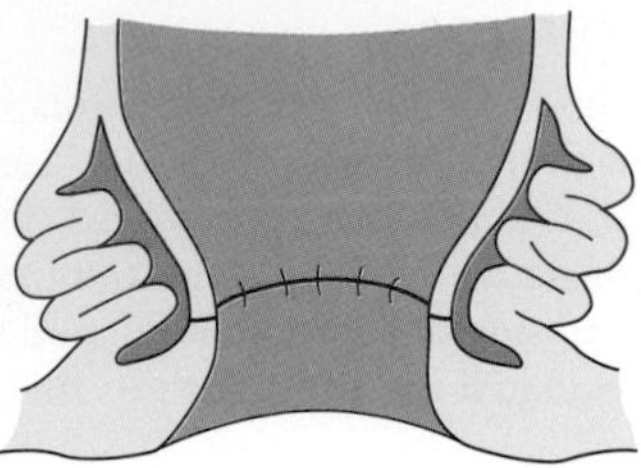

Fig. 5 Delorme's operation. The muscle coat is imbricated with a series of longitudinal sutures.

of cases have been reported. Delorme's procedure is a compromise operation and if recurrence does occur then the procedure can simply be repeated. It may also have a further advantage in that it does not cause constipation or an evacuation disorder, and there is no danger of pelvic nerve damage.

Rectosigmoidectomy

With the patient in the lithotomy or jack-knife position the prolapse is pulled down, and the outer of the two tubes of rectal wall is divided circumferentially just above the dentate line. The inner tube of rectum can then be drawn down bringing the distal sigmoid to the anal canal, where it is divided and sutured to the anal remnant with absorbable sutures (Fig. 6). The specimen resected should be 15 to 20 cm in length, leaving no slack rectum or distal colon to allow further prolapse (Fig. 7). Popularity for this procedure has waned in the United Kingdom, but it is still very popular in the United States.

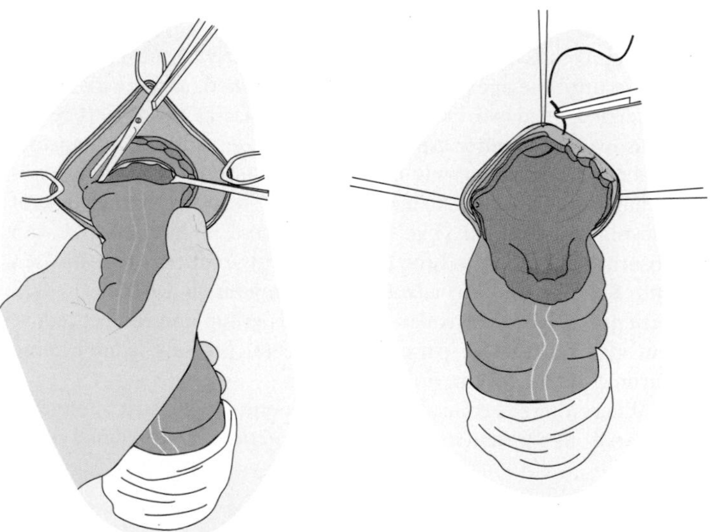

Fig. 6 Perineal rectosigmoidectomy. The inner tube of rectum can be brought down bringing the distal sigmoid to the pelvic floor.

Experience in the United Kingdom in the 1960s was disappointing with a high recurrence rate. Altermeier has modified the procedure to include suturing of the levator muscles anterior to the rectum. This is a plication of the puborectalis sling which attempts to improve sphincter function postoperatively and to reduce the incidence of recurrence. Long-term recurrence rates are not

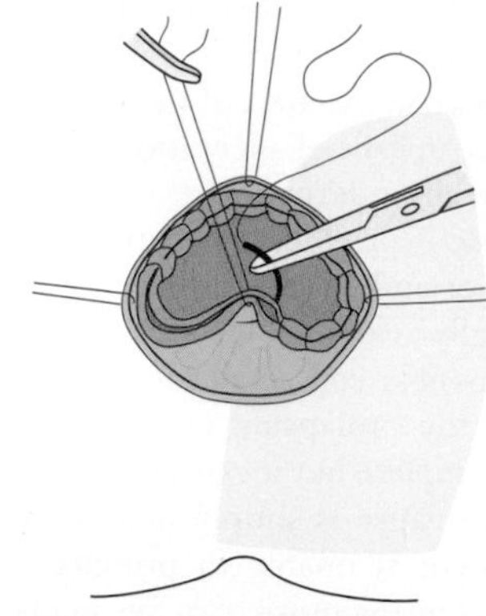

Fig. 7 Perineal rectosigmoidectomy. The rectosigmoid is divided and sutured to the anal remnant leaving no slack for further prolapse.

known, and removal of the reservoir function of the rectum must have considerable physiological effects.

Encircling the anal orifice with foreign material

Variations of this procedure have been popular because of their simplicity.

The Thiersh operation

Incisions are made in front of and behind the anal margin to allow the passage of wire, stout nylon, or even silastic around the anal sphincter. It is usually overlapped and sewn together anteriorly to provide the right amount of tension (Fig. 8). The procedure can be carried out under regional or local anaesthesia in elderly frail patients. In principle, the technique works by supporting the reduced prolapse and causing a local reaction which induces fibrosis and stenosis of the anal canal.

In our experience this procedure can work quite well for small prolapses, but if the prolapse is large the wire or nylon tends to

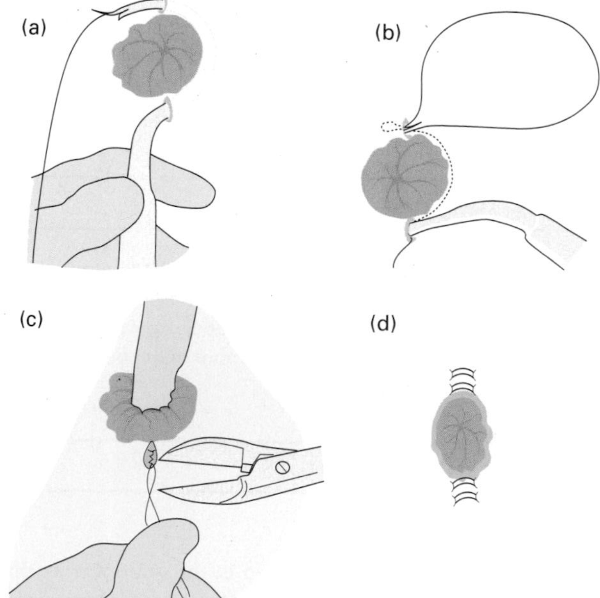

Fig. 8 The Thiersch operation. Incisions are made in front of and behind the anus and an encircling suture placed under correct tension.

migrate and cut through the skin. Recurrences are common and the Thiersh operation cannot be regarded as anything more than a temporary solution.

Variations on the technique have been described, including placing a silastic band around the top of the external sphincter below the levator muscles, but there is no evidence that this produces better results.

Postanal repair and perineorrophy

In patients with a weak anal sphincter and marked symptoms of incontinence it is tempting to use a sphincter plication procedure to hold in the prolapse. Unfortunately this is rarely successful for long and the technique can only be used for small prolapses.

Sacral procedures

A number of operations have been described which exploit the Kraske approach alongside the coccyx and behind the sacrum. With the patient in the jack-knife position an incision is made over the coccyx and parasacral area, giving access to the presacral and postrectal space. The rectum is mobilized, shortened by imbricating sutures, and foreign material is placed in the presacral space. None of these procedures has stood the test of time and become particularly popular.

Abdominal procedures

The general principle of these operations is to repair the prolapse by mobilizing the rectum and fixing it to the sacrum. Repair of the pelvic floor is sometimes performed simultaneously.

Ripstein's operation

The mobilized rectum is fixed to the sacral hollow by means of a sling of Teflon mesh 5 cm wide. This is passed around the rectum and the ends are sutured behind it to the fascia on the front of the sacrum, just below the promontory. In addition, a few sutures are passed between the edges of the Teflon and the anterior and lateral rectal walls. Jurgeleit *et al.* reported 55 patients treated in this way at the Lahey clinic. There were no operative deaths, and there was a 7.5 per cent recurrence rate. In a postal survey of members of the American Society of Colon and Rectal Surgeons the recurrence rate was 2.3 per cent and significant problems with constipation and faecal impaction occurred in 6.7 per cent of patients. Stricturing at the site of the sling occurred in 2 per cent of patients. A modification of this operation, placing the mesh behind the rectum, has been reported by Keighley *et al.*

Ivalon rectopexy

Following early experience with the use of polyvinyl alcohol sponge in the repair of herniae, Wells used a 3-mm thick sheet of Ivalon measuring 10 × 15 cm. After a full mobilization of the rectum the Ivalon is placed behind it, partially wrapping the full circumference of the rectum, and resutured, fixing it and the sponge to the sacral hollow. In 101 cases reported by Penfold and Hawley from St Mark's Hospital there were no operative deaths but four patients developed postoperative sepsis and the Ivalon had to be removed in one of these: sepsis in the implanted foreign body is a recognized hazard of this procedure. After 2 to 10 years, three patients had developed a recurrence and 31 suffered mucosal prolapse. Continence was improved in about 30 per cent of the patients postoperatively. Reasonable results have also been reported in a group of young patients with rectal prolapse treated by the same operation.

Presacral rectopexy and simple suture

An alternative to the use of an implant of either Teflon or Ivalon is simply to mobilize the rectum and fix it to the sacral promontory. No major series has been reported, but six recurrences were noted in 79 patients treated in this way.

The Pemberton–Stalker operation

In this procedure the mobilized rectum is lifted out of the pelvis and the sigmoid colon is then fixed in an elevated position to the peritoneum of the anterior abdominal wall or the pelvic bone, and in female patients to the uterus. The procedure was popularized at the Mayo Clinic in the 1940s and gave a recurrence rate of 35 per cent.

The Frykman Goldberg procedure

Here the rectum is fully mobilized preserving the lateral ligaments which are pulled up and made taught. These tight bands are then sutured to the presacral fascia to keep the bowel up out of the pelvis. After mobilizing the descending colon the sigmoid loop is resected. Watts *et al.* reported 138 patients treated in this way, with a recurrence rate of 1.9 per cent.

Anterior resection

Some surgeons favour a straight anterior resection. When the anal sphincter is very weak an abdominoperineal excision would be justified.

The Roscoe–Graham procedure

Variations on this procedure have been described by a number of surgeons. The rectum is fully mobilized but in addition the pelvic floor is plicated either in front of or behind the rectum. The aim of this part of the procedure is to maintain the rectum in an elevated position and to improve postoperative continence. Goligher felt that it provided no more than a temporary buttress which after several months could no longer be palpated.

Technique

There are a number of abdominal rectopexy techniques, but this is perhaps the most widely used.

Patients should undergo a full bowel preparation in case the rectum is damaged during mobilization. Prophylactic intravenous antibiotics should be given. The patient is placed in Lloyd-Davis stirrups, a urinary catheter is passed and a lower abdominal incision is made. A head down tilt makes access to the pelvis easier. The small bowel is packed off, and the uterus is hitched up with stay sutures. Peritoneal cuts are then made to mobilize the rectum, starting on the right side of the base of the mesosigmoid but a little way up the mesentery so that the peritoneum can be preserved and closed over the repair. The incision is carried down to the bottom of the often deep pouch of Douglas, crossing anteriorly and joining a similar cut on the left side. The presacral space is opened, identifying and preserving the presacral nerves posterolaterally and the left ureter. The posterior dissection can now be carried right down to the pelvic floor (Fig. 9). Anteriorly, the plane between the posterior vaginal wall and the rectum is opened and dissected with a combination of blunt and sharp dissection. There is debate over whether the lateral ligaments should be divided: some evidence suggests that bilateral division results in abnormal rectal function.

A 15 × 10 cm sheet of implantable material (Ivalon sponge, Marlex, Mersiline, or Teflon) is fixed to the presacral fascia, care being taken not to puncture middle sacral vessels or pelvic veins (Fig. 10). The use of several sutures increases the risk of damage

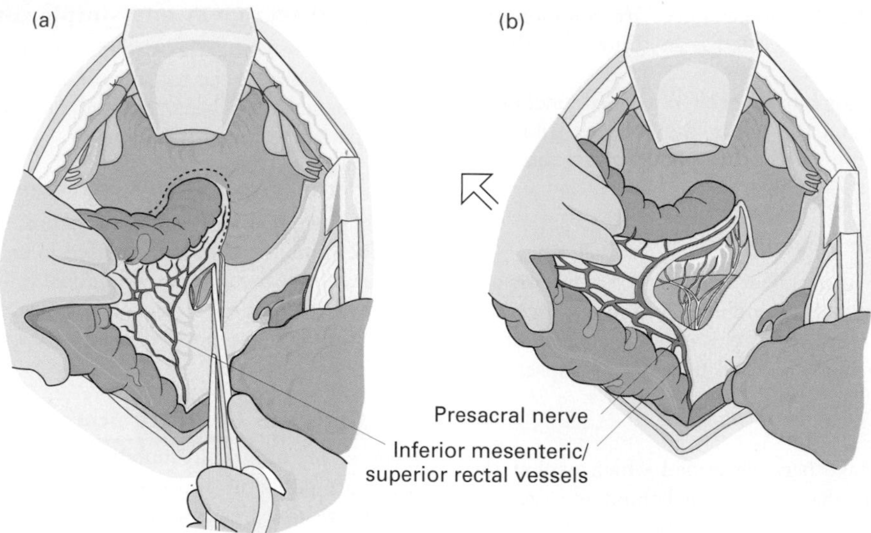

Fig. 9 (a and b) Abdominal rectopexy. Mobilization of the rectum in the mesorectal plane down to the pelvic floor. The lateral ligaments have not been divided.

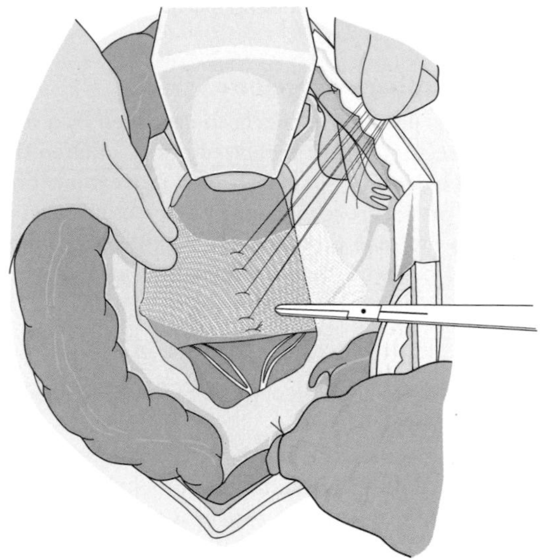

Fig. 10 Abdominal rectopexy. The mobilized rectum is drawn up and a sheet of implantable material is sutured to the sacral promontory.

to sacral veins: two or three probably suffice. Once the implanted material has been attached to the sacral promontory and presacral fascia either the same sutures or a new set of sutures can be used to attach this in turn to the fully mobilized and stretched up mesorectum, taking in a section of the serosa of the rectal wall at the same time. The implant is then partially wrapped around the lateral sides of the mobilized rectum (Fig. 11), leaving one-third of the anterior circumference of the rectal wall uncovered to minimize the risk of stenosis or functional constipation. Sutures are then placed to fix this in position. The pelvic peritoneum can then be covered over all of this, leaving two suction drains in the cavity to prevent a haematoma.

Variations on this procedure include the use of a transverse abdominal incision and limited peritoneal incisions gaining access to the presacral space and the mesorectal plane.

The procedure is usually well tolerated, even by elderly patients. Intravenous fluids should be given for 48 h since some patients suffer marked postoperative paralytic ileus. A mild laxative is prescribed from the second or third postoperative day to prevent constipation and straining at stool. There is often an irregularity of bowel habit and continence in the immediate 2 or 3 weeks postoperatively.

DESCENDING PERINEUM SYNDROME

During straining the anal canal should not descend more than 2 cm below a line joining the ischial tuberosities. In patients with

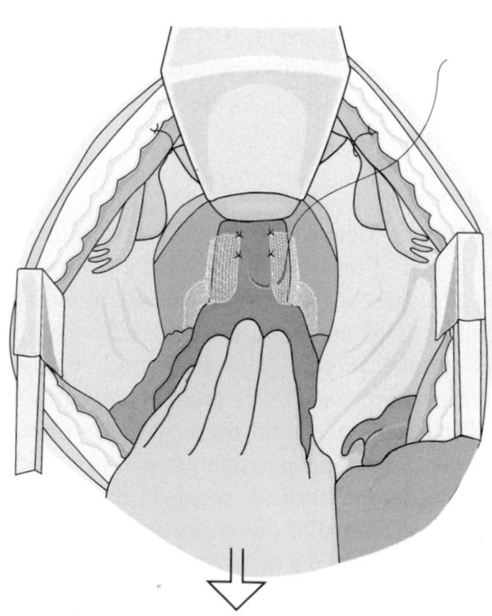

Fig. 11 Abdominal rectopexy. A partial wrap around half the posterior circumference of the rectum fixes it to the sacrum.

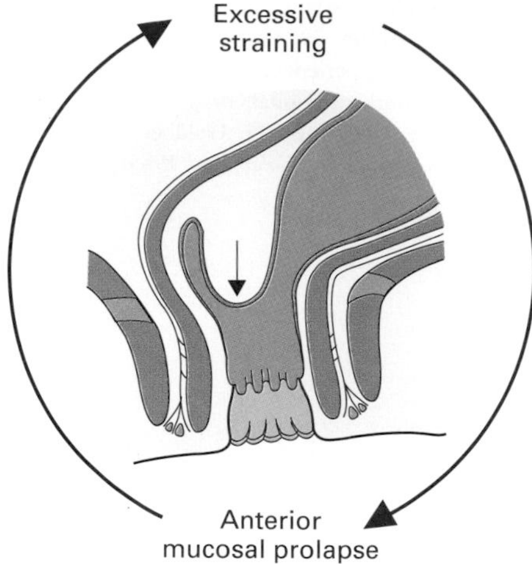

Fig. 12 The vicious circle causing anterior mucosal prolapse and solitary rectal ulcer.

descending perineum syndrome the anal canal at rest lies at a lower level; straining causes the perineum itself to balloon well below the lower margin of the bony pelvis. It is more common in women and may occur at any age, although it is rare before the third decade.

Aetiology

It is probable that excessive straining weakens the pelvic floor muscles and stretches the pudendal nerves supplying the pelvic floor, which then bulges and allows the anterior wall of the rectum to prolapse into the upper anal canal (Fig. 12). This anterior mucosal prolapse results in a feeling of incomplete evacuation, to which the patient will respond by further straining efforts.

Gross perineal descent on its own does not always cause symptoms and some patients remain continent.

Clinical features

The patient's main symptoms are of intractable tenesmus but there may also be the passage of mucus and blood. There is often a past history of haemorrhoidectomy, inappropriately performed for what was thought to be haemorrhoidal symptoms. There may be anorectal incontinence, and others have a dragging perineal pain. Physical examination usually reveals reduced resting anal tone and descent of the perineum at rest and on straining. Proctoscopy may reveal an anterior rectal mucosal prolapse, and in intractable cases a solitary ulcer of the rectum may develop (see below).

Management

Treatment consists of avoiding further straining by alterations in diet and the administration of bulking agents, suppositories, and enemata.

Anterior mucosal prolapse or prolapsing haemorrhoids can be treated by injection therapy or band ligation. Great care must be taken with surgical excision, since the haemorrhoidal tissue may be an important component of the patient's remaining continence.

SOLITARY ULCER SYNDROME

The solitary ulcer syndrome is often, but not always, associated with the descending perineum syndrome. It rarely takes the form of a single large depressed ulcer, and is more commonly an area of mucosal change on the anterior wall of the lower rectum. This may be ulcerated in places, but the mucosa is oedematous, heaped up, and bleeds easily on contact. Sometimes these appearances can extend around the whole rectal circumference. Histologically, there is replacement of the lamina propria by fibroblasts and smooth muscle cells, typically arranged at right angles to the muscularis mucosa.

Clinical features

It is now thought that these changes are the result of mucosal trauma. The lower, anterior ulcers are usually associated with the mucosal prolapse, while higher ulcers are associated with intussusception of the rectum. The mucosal changes probably result from a straining effort in the presence of a contracting sphincter muscle which then pinches and damages the prolapsing mucosa. This gives rise to the common symptoms of the passage of mucus and blood, and the thick, ridged, oedematous mucosa gives a sense of anal obstruction and pain, resulting in prolonged and excessive straining. There may be multiple fruitless attempts at defecation.

These symptoms and the appearance of a rectal ulcer can be easily mistaken for a carcinoma and it is important to obtain a biopsy sample.

Treatment

This is usually conservative. Straining efforts are discouraged. If symptoms become intractable they may be improved by an abdominal rectopexy, fixing both the anterior and posterior walls of the rectum.

FURTHER READING

Allen Mersh TG, Henry MM, Nicholls RJ. Natural history of anterior mucosal prolapse. *Br J Surg* 1987; **74**: 679–82.

Altemeier WA, Schowengerdt C, Hunt T. Nineteen years' experience with the one stage perineal repair of rectal prolapse. *Ann Surg* 1971; **173**: 993–1006.

Boulos PB, Stryker SJ, Nicholls RJ. The longterm results of polyvinyl alcohol (Ivalon) sponge for rectal prolapse in young patients. *Br J Surg* 1984; **71**: 213–14.

Broden B, Snellman B. Procidentia of the rectum studied with cineradiography: a contribution to the discussion of causative mechanism. *Dis Colon Rect* 1968; **11**: 330–47.

Christiansen J, Kirkegaard P. Delorme's operation for complete rectal prolapse. *Br J Surg* 1981, **68**: 537–8.

Goligher JC. *Diseases of the Colon, Rectum and Anus*. London: Balliere Tindall, 1984.

Henry MM, Swash M. *Coloproctology and the Pelvic Floor*. London: Butterworth, 1989.

Ihire T, Seligson U. Intussusception of the rectum internal procidentia. *Dis Colon Rect* 1975; **18**: 391–6.

Keighley MRB, Fielding JWL, Alexander Williams J. Results of Marlex mesh abdominal rectopexy for rectal prolapse in 100 consecutive patients. *Br J Surg* 1983; **70**: 229–32.

Neill ME, Parks AG, Swash M. Physiological studies of the anal sphincter musculature in faecal incontinence and rectal prolapse. *Br J Surg* 1981; **68**: 531–6.

Parks AF, Porter NH, Hardcastle J. The syndrome of the descending perineum. *Proc R Soc Med* 1966; **59**: 477–82.

Penfold JCB, Hawley PR. Experiences of Ivalon-sponge implant for complete rectal prolapse at St Mark's Hospital. *Br J Surg* 1972; **59**: 846–8.

Watts JD, Rotherburger DA, Buls JG, Goldberg SM, Nivatvongs S. The management of procidentia. *Dis Colon Rect* 1985; **28**: 96–102.

The appendix 19

19.1 Acute appendicitis

CHARLES M. FERGUSON

INTRODUCTION

The diagnosis of appendicitis can be difficult, occasionally taxing the diagnostic skills of even the most experienced surgeon. Likewise, the judgemental decisions in the management of patients with appendiceal inflammation or abscess can be difficult. The patient with appendicitis must first recognize that he has an episode of pain that is unique, and then present to a physician who recognizes the condition. Delays in diagnosis arise from errors on the part of either patient or physician, and all delays complicate the illness.

HISTORY

Patients with appendicitis generally present with a typical pattern of distress. The most common initial symptom is pain, typically diffuse, epigastric, or periumbilical in distribution and gnawing in character. Some patients have no pain, but feel unwell, with a severe upset stomach. Shortly after the initial pain, anorexia, nausea, and occasionally, vomiting develop. Anorexia is the most constant symptom of appendicitis. If it is absent, the diagnosis should be questioned. Vomiting, if present, occurs early in the attack, usually several hours after the initial pain. Vomiting occurring before the onset of pain, makes a diagnosis of appendicitis questionable, and a viral illness more likely.

The initial pain is due to the early obstruction, dilation, and infection of the appendix. As this visceral pain is mediated through visceral pain fibres, it is poorly localized. When the infection in the appendix becomes established and transmural, the serosa of the appendix and parietal peritoneum are involved, causing a localized pain from somatic pain fibres in the abdominal wall at the area of the appendix. Because the appendix is generally located one-third of the way from the anterior, superior iliac spine to the umbilicus (McBurney's point), the area of greatest pain is generally in the right lower quadrant.

Patients may present with localized pain in the right upper quadrant from a long appendix, in the left lower quadrant if malrotation is present, and in the anterior wall of the rectum if the appendix is located in the pelvis. The most common location of 'atypical' somatic pain is the right flank in patients with a retrocaecal appendix. Somatic pain reflects the location of the appendix; if the development of symptoms and signs suggest appendicitis, an atypical location of maximal pain does not rule out the diagnosis.

Many patients with appendicitis have pain on motion and pain present during the trip to hospital may abate when motion ceases. These events do not mean that their illness is resolving: pain on motion is caused by motion of the inflamed appendix against the peritoneum. The patient presenting after perforation of the appendix complains of generalized pain. The history is usually a sequence of generalized pain that became localized to the right lower quadrant and later became generalized.

Less common symptoms include diarrhoea, which may occur early or late in the course of appendicitis. Early in the course of appendicitis patients may have one or two loose bowel movements, or they may have an episode of massive evacuation of normal stool. This sequence represents a response to visceral pain and is usually limited to one or two episodes, rather than the persistent diarrhoea caused by viral or bacterial infection. Later in the course of appendicitis, diarrhoea may return because of irritation of the rectum by an inflamed pelvic appendix. This diarrhoea is mucoid and persistent; it is accompanied by tenesmus and can easily be mistaken for gastroenteritis if proper attention is not paid to the history. Testicular pain or retraction of the testes may occur at any time in the course of appendicitis, the appendix and testicle both being innervated by the tenth thoracic spinal segment.

The concept of recurrent appendicitis is gradually being accepted in the United States, and patients often describe previous episodes of pain that were the same as the present in all aspects except severity. Surveys suggest that this sequence occurs in about 25 per cent of patients.

PHYSICAL FINDINGS

Tenderness over the site of the appendix is the *sine qua non* of appendicitis. However, tenderness may be absent early in the course of the illness or unelicitable in obese individuals. Tenderness over the appendix is due to inflammation of the serosa of the appendix and the overlying parietal peritoneum; so early in appendicitis there may not be enough inflammation to cause this diagnostic finding, although it is unusual for patients to present this early in the course of their illness. More commonly, difficulty in eliciting tenderness over the appendix arises from its retrocaecal location. Patients with a retrocaecal appendix may experience some mild right-sided or right flank tenderness. In extremely obese people, localizing tenderness is difficult, simply because palpation of the abdomen is cushioned by subcutaneous fat. In addition, the entire panniculus of the abdomen may be caudal to the peritoneal cavity. When the abdomen is palpated in such a patient, the normal topographic anatomical landmarks must be ignored.

While much has been made of tenderness at McBurney's point, this is not as reliable as the presence of tenderness at some point in a patient with a suggestive history. Classically, the area of maximal tenderness will be one-third of the way from the anterior superior iliac spine to the umbilicus, but in fact it will be wherever the appendix is in the individual patient.

Many surgeons rely on the demonstration of local muscular rigidity to make a diagnosis of appendicitis. This muscular rigidity is produced by inflammation of the parietal peritoneum overlying the appendix, and thus takes longer to develop than local tenderness. Many patients with early appendicitis demonstrate little or no rigidity of the abdominal wall. Subtle rigidity can be demonstrated by palpation of the left lower quadrant while talking with the patient. The palpating hand is slowly moved toward the right lower quadrant (or area of maximal pain), which is gently palpated. This sequence helps to differentiate true rigidity from the voluntary spasm that occurs from nervousness. Similarly, Rovsing's sign, or pain in the right lower quadrant upon palpation of the left lower quadrant, is a sign of local peritonitis. Severe, well-established rigidity of the abdominal wall is a sign of well-established local peritonitis and of impending (or previous) perforation.

Another useful sign to establish the presence of local peritonitis is the shake test. Most surgeons perform this by grasping the iliac wings and shaking the pelvis from side to side. The patient complains of pain at the site of the appendix if local peritonitis is present. It is more helpful to kick or push the stretcher gently while watching the patient's face: a grimace is a sure sign of local peritonitis.

The elicitation of signs of local peritonitis may be difficult in patients with a retrocaecal or pelvic appendix. The psoas sign, pain caused by extending the thigh to stretch the psoas muscle, is generally positive in patients with a retrocaecal appendix and local peritonitis. If the appendix is adjacent to the obturator internus muscle, stretching of this muscle by external rotation of the hip elicits severe pain and spasm. With a true, inflamed pelvic appendix, the only signs of local peritonitis may be found on rectal examination in men or vaginal examination in women. It is often impossible to differentiate pelvic appendicitis from pelvic inflammatory disease by physical examination alone, but accurate history will generally solve the dilemma.

Patients who present late with appendicitis may have only generalized tenderness and rigidity. This is a sure sign of perforation, but without an accurate history, the diagnosis remains obscure.

Hyperaesthesia or dysaesthesia may occur in patients with non-perforated appendicitis. Although these are inconstant findings, when present they occur on the right side of the abdomen, in the distribution of the tenth, eleventh, and twelfth thoracic nerves. Paraesthesiae are best elicited by light scratching with a sharp sterile needle.

Fever is a late physical finding in appendicitis. Before perforation, body temperature is usually no more than 39 to 39.5°C, but with perforation may rise to 40 to 41°C. If fever has been present since the onset of the illness, consider other causes.

LABORATORY EXAMINATIONS

Laboratory examinations are rarely helpful in the diagnosis of appendicitis. Leucocytosis is common, usually in the range of 11 000 to 17 000 mm^3. However, this occurs once appendicitis is well established, and the illness should generally be diagnosed before it develops. A leucocytosis over 20 000 mm^3 suggests perforation of the appendix or another diagnosis. Urinalysis is unhelpful in the diagnosis or exclusion of appendicitis. Mild pyuria may occur due to irritation of the bladder by a pelvic appendix or irritation of the ureter by a retrocaecal appendix. Thus, in patients with symptoms suggestive of either appendicitis or urinary tract infection, urinalysis is not diagnostic of either condition.

Radiographic techniques have been recommended in the evaluation of patients with possible appendicitis. Plain abdominal films demonstrate a faecalith in the area of the appendix in 10 per cent of patients with appendicitis. This finding is highly suggestive of appendicitis in a patient with a compatible history and physical examination. Plain abdominal films may reveal other abnormalities, such as localized ileus in the right lower quadrant, soft tissue density in the right lower quadrant, or free intraperitoneal air. These are so non-specific as to be of no value in the diagnosis of appendicitis.

Barium enema has long been recommended for the evaluation of possible appendicitis. Findings suggestive of appendicitis include spasm of the terminal ileum or caecum, external compression of the caecum, and non-filling or partial filling of the appendix. While several series suggest diagnostic accuracy rates of 90 per cent, review of these studies discloses that about one-quarter of patients with an abnormal barium enema have a normal appendix at the time of exploration. Probably the best case that can be made for barium enema is that if the entire appendix is filled, appendicitis is virtually ruled out.

Ultrasound and computed tomography (CT) have recently been used in the evaluation of patients with suspected appendicitis. Ultrasound is performed with high resolution linear array transducers and gentle but thorough compression of the abdomen, with the goal of eliminating any gas-filled bowel between the transducer and the appendix. Ultrasound criteria for the diagnosis of appendicitis are a non-compressible appendix, surrounded by a hypoechoic thickened wall more than 2 mm in diameter. In addition, the maximal diameter of the visualized appendix should exceed 6 mm. Using these criteria, sensitivity rates of 75 per cent and specificity rates of 100 per cent have been reported. The sensitivity is usually considerably lower in patients with perforated appendicitis, as the rigidity of the abdominal wall prevents its adequate compression. Realistically, a sensitivity of only 75 per cent is too low to be acceptable in a diagnostic test. Ultrasound has not, therefore, become widely used in the diagnosis of appendicitis, although a totally normal appendix visualized by ultrasound makes appendicitis unlikely. CT has been touted by radiologists but has not been widely accepted by surgeons for the diagnosis of appendicitis. CT findings suggestive of appendicitis include pericaecal increased density of pericolic fat, appendicoliths, a thickened appendix, and a periappendiceal abscess. Oral contrast media are necessary to enable adequate evaluation of the gastrointestinal tract. Reported sensitivity and specificity are approximately 80 per cent, making the test of limited value in establishing a diagnosis. Its real value is in the evaluation of patients with atypical pain that is not particularly suggestive of appendicitis, and in the evaluation of possible appendiceal abscess.

DIFFERENTIAL DIAGNOSIS OF APPENDICITIS

In evaluating a patient with abdominal pain suggestive of appendicitis, other possible causes of abdominal pain must be considered. From a management viewpoint, the various diagnoses can be divided into those that require surgery and those that do not. The former include perforated carcinoma of the right colon, perforated right colonic diverticulitis, perforated ulcer (with tracking of visceral contents along the right gutter to the right lower quadrant), sigmoid diverticulitis (especially with a mobile sigmoid colon), Meckel's diverticulitis, ectopic pregnancy, and ovarian torsion. Any of these disorders may be indistinguishable from appendicitis at presentation, but as each usually requires surgery for resolution, their differentiation from appendicitis is not crucial.

Surgery has limited value in the management of many other disorders which are almost indistinguishable from appendicitis. These include pelvic inflammatory disease, Mittleschmerz pain (from ruptured ovarian follicular cyst), 'mesenteric adenitis', viral gastroenteritis, bacterial gastroenteritis, acute Crohn's ileitis, and typhoid. Pelvic inflammatory disease is more likely than appendicitis to occur during the proliferative phase of the menstrual cycle. It has a longer duration of symptoms, higher fever, greater leucocytosis, and less well localized pain, with more pelvic pain and cervical motion tenderness than appendicitis. Mittleschmerz pain can usually be diagnosed by its occurrence at ovulation and by the fact that most patients have experienced painful ovulation before. Although fever is uncommon, tenderness and leucocytosis may occur. The diagnosis is usually made by exclusion—the patient is observed and the pain resolves. 'Mesenteric adenitis' is also a diagnosis of exclusion; the patient has all the typical features of appendicitis, but at exploration is found to have a normal appendix and some enlarged lymph nodes in the mesentery of the distal ileum. The cause of the illness is obscure. Viral and bacterial gastroenteritis are indistinguishable clinically, and the diagnosis of bacterial gastroenteritis is made only when the results of stool cultures become available (usually after the patient has been treated or the illness has resolved spontaneously). Viral and bacterial gastroenteritis may usually be differentiated from appendicitis by the massive diarrhoea present in typical gastroenteritis. Diarrhoea associated with appendicitis is rarely massive or prolonged. Most patients with gastroenteritis present with diffuse abdominal pain that rarely becomes well localized; if any tenderness develops, it is usually mild and generalized. It is most unusual to find a patient with true right lower quadrant tenderness due to gastroenteritis.

DIAGNOSIS IN DIFFICULT CIRCUMSTANCES

Retrocaecal appendicitis

The symptoms and signs of appendicitis are altered when the appendix is retrocaecal. Pain is generally not as severe as that in patients with an abdominal or pelvic appendix, and pain rarely becomes well localized to the right lower quadrant. Many patients with a retrocaecal appendicitis have a history of generalized abdominal pain, fairly constant for several days, never localizing, and never really interfering with normal activities. Occasionally, the pain becomes localized to the right flank or to the right upper abdomen. Patients with retrocaecal appendicitis have tenderness in the area of the appendix, provided that the area can be palpated. In true retrocecal appendicitis, the area of tenderness is in the flank or costovertebral angle, simulating pyelonephritis. Occasionally the tenderness is subcostal, because the tip of the appendix is located at or near the hepatic flexure. In an obese patient tenderness can often not be elicited since the retrocaecal appendix is so well encased in retroperitoneal fat that it cannot be felt.

The combination of abdominal pain, more or less localized to the right side of the abdomen, with some aspect of nausea or anorexia, and no other suggestive diagnosis should raise the suspicion of retrocaecal appendicitis. The presence of fever or leucocytosis makes the diagnosis of retrocaecal appendicitis even more likely. Unfortunately, most such patients are dismissed by physicians as having gastroenteritis, a most unusual occurrence in the absence of significant diarrhoea. Eventually, such patients present with a retrocaecal abscess due to perforation of the appendix (Fig. 1).

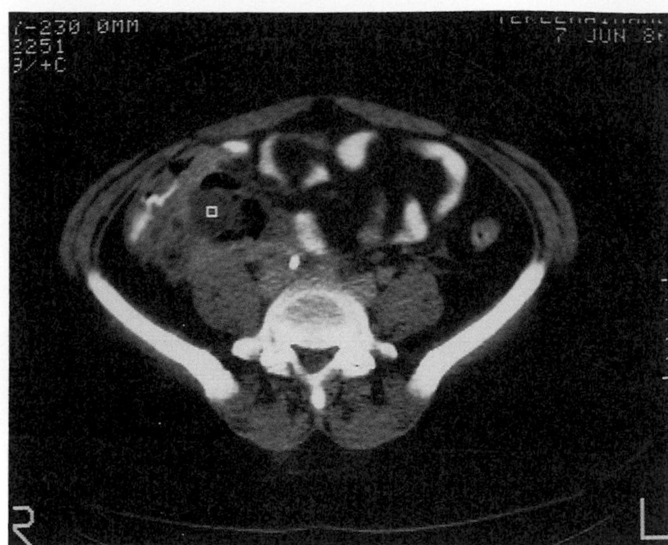

Fig. 1 CT scan demonstrating retrocaecal appendiceal abscess (marker).

Appendicitis in the elderly

Elderly patients tend to present late in the course of appendicitis and with less well-defined symptoms; the incidence of perforation is therefore higher. Most elderly patients with appendicitis have a history of several days of poorly defined abdominal pain, anorexia, and fever. Rarely is the pain well localized to McBurney's point; rather, it is generally described as being in the right side of the abdomen. Most old patients have fever and abdominal tenderness at the time of presentation with appendicitis. Tenderness is either in the right lower quadrant, the right flank, or is diffuse from the effects of free perforation. The psoas sign and obturator sign are unhelpful in old patients because almost every manoeuvre is equally uncomfortable.

Appendicitis in pregnancy

The diagnosis of appendicitis in pregnancy is difficult because the appendix is displaced by the gravid uterus. Early in the course of pregnancy the appendix remains in its normal position, and diagnosis is routine. By the middle of the second trimester of pregnancy, however, the appendix becomes displaced superiorly, attaining a position in the right upper flank or epigastrium. Appendicitis may be easily mistaken for pyelonephritis or cholecystitis.

The abdominal wall is lifted from the appendix by the gravid uterus, and muscular laxity occurs: the abdominal findings associated with peritoneal irritation by the inflamed appendix may therefore be fewer than one might expect in the non-pregnant individual. Leucocytosis is a normal physiological response of pregnancy (up to 12 500 leucocytes/mm^3) and cannot be relied upon to help confirm the diagnosis of appendicitis. White blood cell counts as high as 25 000 leucocytes/mm^3 are not unusual in pregnant women with appendicitis.

MANAGEMENT OF APPENDICITIS

The management of non-perforated appendicitis is surgical removal. If the diagnosis is clear, an incision should be made over the point of maximal tenderness, generally at McBurney's point. Many surgeons favour a true McBurney's incision, with an oblique skin incision at McBurney's point and splitting of the external and internal oblique muscles in the line of their fibres; others prefer a transverse skin incision with muscle splitting. The skin incision need be only 3 to 6 cm long (depending on the patient's build), and can be easily extended by cutting the rectus fascia and retracting the rectus muscle medially. The taenia of the colon are followed to the base of the appendix, and blunt dissection is used to free the appendix from its surrounding inflammatory tissue. The mesoappendix is divided between clamps and ligated with an absorbable suture. The base of the appendix is divided and is also ligated with absorbable suture material. The base of the appendix may be inverted using either a purse-string suture or a 'Z-stitch' (Fig. 2),

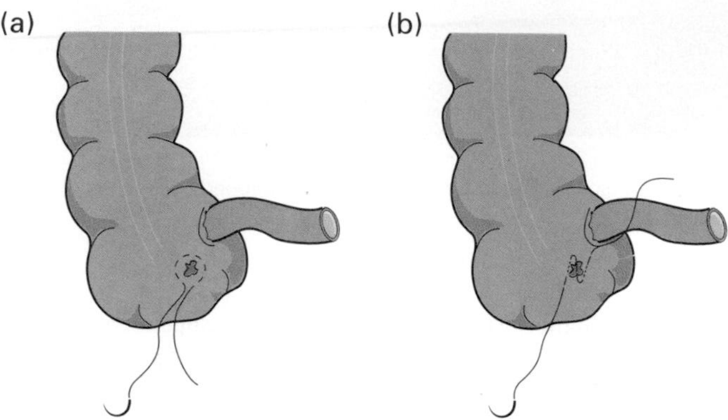

Fig. 2 (a) Purse string stitch at base of appendix. (b) 'Z-stitch' used for closing base of appendix.

although there are no firm data to suggest that inversion of the stump produces better healing than simple ligation. The muscle layers of the abdominal wall are closed with absorbable suture; the skin is closed with a monofilament suture that should be placed deep enough to eliminate dead space in the subcutaneous tissue (Fig. 3).

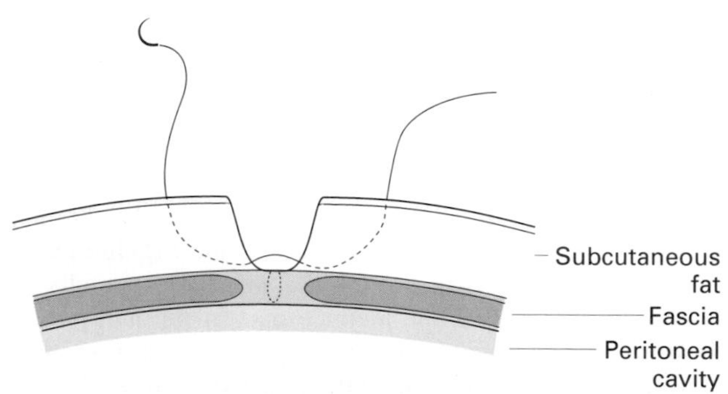

Fig. 3 Placement of cutaneous stitch to eliminate dead space.

For patients in whom the diagnosis of appendicitis is suspected, but not definite, several options are available. The most attractive of these is simply to admit the patient to the hospital for further observation. Over the course of 12 to 24 h one should be able to characterize the course of the illness well enough to determine whether an exploration for possible appendicitis, further tests (for example, computerized tomography), or discharge is in order. Although there is some risk of perforation of the appendix during this period of observation, if the patient is re-examined frequently, one should be able to avoid this complication. The risk of perforation is low in the first 24 h of symptomatic appendicitis; it is therefore safe to observe patients early in the course of their illness, when physical findings may not be well developed.

Another option is laparoscopy. This examination is commonly used in patients with symptoms and signs suggestive of both appendicitis and pelvic inflammatory disease. To exclude the diagnosis of appendicitis by laparoscopy, the entire appendix must be seen and must be normal. If the appendix is retrocaecal, mobilization of the right colon and retraction of the appendix will be necessary. In a patient with an unclear diagnosis, laparoscopy may be performed as both a diagnostic and a therapeutic manoeuvre. The technique for laparoscopic appendectomy is straight forward. A high flow rate laparoscopic insufflator, video camera and monitor, and adequate assistance are required. The abdomen is filled with carbon dioxide, a large trocar (10, 11, or 12 mm) is placed infra-umbilically and the laparoscope with camera is placed through it. A large trocar is placed through the left rectus sheath, avoiding the inferior epigastric vessels, halfway between the pubis and the umbilicus. An additional (5 mm) trocar is placed suprapubically. Through these trocars, the appendix is freed from surrounding tissues. Once free, it is usually helpful to place an additional small trocar in the right upper quadrant to hold the appendix up toward the abdominal wall. The mesoappendix is dissected and bleeding is controlled with clips or suture. The base of the appendix may be controlled with pretied suture loops, sutures, or endoscopic staples. The laparoscope is moved to the left-sided large trocar, and the appendix is removed through the umbilical trocar by widening the fascial opening in the abdominal wall.

MANAGEMENT OF THE APPENDICEAL MASS

Patients seen late in the course of appendicitis often have a palpable mass in the right lower quadrant. These account for about 3 per cent of patients, and traditionally they have been managed with antibiotics and bed rest, reserving surgery for those who do not respond to such conservative therapy. Non-operative therapy is successful in 80 to 90 per cent of patients; causes of failure include sepsis, unresolved abscess, and small bowel obstruction from adhesions to the inflammatory mass. The rate of failure of non-operative therapy is higher in patients with a well defined abscess at presentation than in those with diffuse inflammation, and abscess can be reliably diagnosed using CT. If an abscess is found, operative drainage or CT-directed drainage is indicated. Percutaneous, radiologically guided drainage is successful in 85 per cent of patients and avoids the need for operative intervention in patients with active sepsis. Most patients treated in this way can be discharged from the hospital in 7 to 10 days.

Traditionally, all patients with an appendiceal mass underwent appendectomy 6 to 8 weeks following their acute illness. However only 20 per cent of patients develop another episode of appendicitis following treatment of an appendiceal abscess or diffuse inflammation, prompting some surgeons to abandon interval appendectomy. The morbidity associated with interval appendectomy is so low, however, that there is a case for it being performed in patients for whom surgery does not pose a risk because of coexistent medical illnesses. If an interval appendectomy is not performed, patients beyond young adulthood should undergo a barium enema examination or colonoscopy to exclude the possibility of a locally perforated right colon carcinoma.

ANTIBIOTICS IN APPENDICITIS

All patients with suspected appendicitis should receive broad-spectrum antibiotics preoperatively. The duration of antibiotic therapy is the subject of some controversy, but it should be governed by the severity of the appendicitis. In the patient with early, acute appendicitis, without purulence or gangrenous changes, 24 to 48 h of antibiotic therapy should suffice. In those with perforated appendicitis, appendiceal abscess, or gangrene of the appendix, 7 to 10 days of antibiotic therapy seems prudent. The choice of antibiotics seems to be less important in the prevention of wound infection than the timing of their administration. Effective regimens include cefoxitin alone, ampicillin-sulbactam, ampicillin-clavulanic acid, cefotetan, cefoperazone, an aminoglycoside with metronidazole, aminoglycoside and clindamycin, and imipenem.

FURTHER READING

Balthazar EJ, Megibow AJ, Hulnick D. CT of appendicitis. *Am J Roentgenol* 1989; **153**: 687–91.

Bauer T, Vennits B, Holm B. Antibiotic prophylxasis in acute nonperforated appendicitis. *Ann Surg* 1989; **144**: 338–40.

Berry J, Malt RA. Appendicitis near its centenary. *Ann Surg* 1984; **200**: 567–75.

Burns RP, Russell WL. Appendicitis in mature patients. *Ann Surg* 1985; **201**: 695–704.

Crabbe MM, Norwood SH, Robertson HD. Recurrent and chronic appendicitis. *Surg Gynecol Obstet* 1986; **163**: 11–13.

Ferzli GE, Ozuner G, Davidson PG. Barium enema in the diagnosis of acute appendicitis. *Surg Gynecol Obstet* 1990; **171**: 40–2.

Fisher KS, Ross DS. Guidelines for therapeutic decisions in incidental appendectomy. *Surg Gynecol Obstet* 1990; **171**: 95–8.

Gotz F, Pier A, Bacher C. Modified laparoscopic appendectomy in surgery. *Surg Endosc* 1990; **4**: 6–9.

Horowitz MD, Gomez GA, Santiesteban R. Acute appendicitis during pregnancy. *Arch Surg* 1985; **120**: 1362–7.

Puylaert JBCM, Rutgers PH, Lalisang RI. A prospective study of ultrasonography in the diagnosis of appendicitis. *N Engl J Med* 1987; **317**: 666–9.

Silen W. *Cope's Early Diagnosis of the Acute Abdomen*. New York: Oxford University Press, 1991.

19.2 Primary appendiceal malignancies

ROBB H. RUTLEDGE

INTRODUCTION

Although primary appendiceal malignancies make up only about 0.5 per cent of all intestinal tumours, they are important because they are rarely diagnosed preoperatively or intraoperatively.

The four main types of appendiceal neoplasms are carcinoid, mucinous cystadenocarcinoma, colonic adenocarcinoma, and adenocarcinoid tumours (Table 1). They have different clinical presentation and prognosis and require different therapy, but are alike in that they all carry a 15 to 20 per cent chance of a second malignancy developing, concurrently or subsequently, usually in the gastrointestinal tract.

Table 1 Primary appendiceal malignancies

Type of tumour	Frequency (%)
Carcinoid	85
Mucinous cystadenocarcinoma	8
Colonic adenocarcinoma	4
Adenocarcinoid	2
Others	1
Lymphosarcoma, paraganglioma, and granular cell tumours	

CARCINOID TUMOURS

Although the vast majority of appendiceal carcinoids behave in a benign fashion, they are considered malignant because they all have the potential for invasion, metastasis, and production of physiologically active substances.

Carcinoids occur in about 0.5 per cent of appendectomy specimens and account for about 85 per cent of appendiceal malignancies. At least 50 per cent of all carcinoid tumours originate in the appendix. They are most common in young adult women, probably because they are discovered accidentally among the large number of incidental appendectomies performed in association with hysterectomies and cholecystectomies.

At least 80 per cent of carcinoid tumours are incidental findings discovered during surgery for other indications. Sometimes they are found as coexisting disease in patients with acute appendicitis, and occasionally they are actually the cause of the acute appendicitis. Rarely do they present as metastatic disease or the malignant carcinoid syndrome.

Pathology

Carcinoids are small, yellow-white firm, well circumscribed, but unencapsulated tumours. Most are spheroidal or elliptical; some diffusely involve the appendiceal wall. Many carcinoids are unrecognized grossly being seen only on microscopic section. About 70 per cent are located in the tip of the appendix, 22 per cent in the body of the appendix, and 8 per cent in the base of the appendix.

Seventy per cent of carcinoids are less than 1.0 cm in diameter, and only about 15 per cent are larger than 2.0 cm in diameter before fixation: larger tumours tend to occur in younger patients. Since size is the most important factor in determining treatment, measurements should be recorded *in vivo*, because after fixation shrinkage of 35 per cent can occur.

Carcinoids are composed of nests of small, uniform, argyrophilic cells with occasional acinar formation. The different microscopic patterns are of little practical importance because there is little correlation between the microscopic appearance and the biological malignancy of the tumour. Debate exists as to whether the cells arise in the base of the crypts of Lieberkuhn or from neuroendocrine cells in the lamina propria beneath. Although mitoses are infrequent, the muscularis and subserosal lymphatics are often invaded. The mesoappendix is frequently involved, but spread to regional lymph nodes and distant sites is rare. Spread to the liver may be associated with the carcinoid syndrome.

Treatment

Size is the most important guide in considering the malignant potential of appendiceal carcinoids. Distant metastases and death occur only in patients with tumours larger than 2.0 cm in diameter (1.5 cm in a fixed specimen). Treatment for good risk patients is outlined in Table 2. Carcinoids in the base of the appendix should have enough caecum removed to leave margins free of neoplastic disease but a right hemicolectomy is not required merely because of the location of the tumour.

Table 2 Carcinoid tumours

Size*	Percentage of patients	Treatment
⩽1 cm	70	Appendectomy
1.0–2.0 cm	15	
Mesoappendix and lymphatic −		Appendectomy
Mesoappendix and lymphatic +		Right hemicolectomy
⩾2 cm	15	Right hemicolectomy

*2.0 cm fresh = 1.5 cm fixed.

Controversy exists with regard to proper treatment for patients with carcinoids between 1.0 and 2.0 cm in diameter. Moertel feels that an appendectomy with removal of the mesoappendix is adequate for nearly all patients in this group. Others are more aggressive and advise a right hemicolectomy if lymphatic permeation and mesoappendiceal invasion are present since regional lymph node involvement is more likely. Sufficient data to enable this question to be settled are not available.

Prognosis

The 5-year survival for patients with appendiceal carcinoids is 99 per cent. Recurrences are found only in those patients with large tumours or in those who had intra-abdominal spread at the original surgery. All intra-abdominal disease should be resected if possible, primarily or at a later operation if there is a recurrence. In patients in whom all recurrent disease can be resected the 5-year survival rate is about 75 per cent.

Metastatic disease in the liver is rare with appendiceal carcinoid tumours, but when present in association with the carcinoid syndrome medical treatment with 5-hydroxytryptamine (serotonin) antagonists or debulking of the tumour mass, either at laparotomy or by hepatic arterial embolization, is indicated.

MUCINOUS CYSTADENOCARCINOMA

Although mucinous cystadenocarcinoma is included with colonic adenocarcinoma as adenocarcinoma, it is considered separately here because of its different behaviour. Cystadenocarcinoma is both the second most common appendiceal malignancy and one of the few that can be diagnosed preoperatively, allowing elective preoperative preparation.

There is no sexual predilection; patients are usually younger than the typical adenocarcinoma patient. Cystadenocarcinoma is nearly always symptomatic, causing a variant of acute appendicitis and a palpable right lower quadrant mass. A barium enema may show a non-filling appendix with a globular mass; computed tomography shows a mass of near water density with calcium in its wall. About 50 per cent of patients have intra-abdominal metastases, with concomitant ascites, intestinal obstruction, and pseudomyxoma peritonei.

Pathology

Mucocele is a term used to describe an appendix with a diffuse globular swelling, a dilated lumen with large amounts of mucus, and occasional mucinous intraperitoneal collections. A mucocele can be caused by obstruction of the appendiceal lumen, by mucosal hyperplasia, by mucinous cystadenomas, and by mucinous cystadenocarcinomas. Because the term has no aetiologic or prognostic significance, it is gradually being discarded from current classifications.

Mucinous cystadenomas and cystadenocarcinomas may be indistinguishable grossly, and resemble each other microscopically. Both neoplasms contain mucus-secreting epithelial mucosal cells with varying degrees of atypia, mitoses, and papillary configuration. As the intraluminal mucus secretion continues, the wall becomes thin, ulcerated, and calcified. The mucin eventually penetrates the wall and appears in the periappendiceal and retroperitoneal areas.

The distinction between malignant mucinous cystadenocarcinoma and its benign counterpart is based on two histological features: the first is the invasion of the appendiceal wall by atypical glands; the second is the identification of epithelial cells in any intraperitoneal mucinous collection.

Rupture of appendiceal mucinous cystadenomas and cystadenocarcinomas accounts for about 33 per cent of pseudomyxoma peritonei cases. Although gelatinous ascites *per se* is innocuous, the implanted mucin-producing malignant cells cause peritoneal irritation, recurrent ascites, and intestinal obstruction.

Treatment

The distinction between mucinous cystadenomas and mucinous cystadenocarcinomas is important. Cystadenoma is cured by simple appendectomy, even in the presence of periappendiceal fluid collections, while a right hemicolectomy is the best treatment for a malignant mucinous cystadenocarcinoma in a good risk patient.

Since many cystadenocarcinomas are associated with intra-abdominal metastases, aggressive debulking, omentectomy, drainage of mucin collections, and oophorectomy are often needed. Multiple surgical procedures are more beneficial for recurrences than are chemotherapy and irradiation.

Prognosis

Because mucinous cystadenocarcinomas are slowly progressive, patients have a better prognosis than do those with an adenocarcinoma. Both appendectomy and right hemicolectomy are used for curative therapy: 5-year survival rates are about 70 per cent with both methods. When 10-year survival is considered however right hemicolectomy proves itself clearly superior, yielding a 65 per cent survival rate compared to 37 per cent after appendectomy. Even patients with metastases and pseudomyxoma peritonei have 50 per cent 5-year and 20 per cent 10-year survival rates.

COLONIC ADENOCARCINOMA

Colonic adenocarcinomas are much less common than carcinoids, occur in older patients, and are nearly always symptomatic. Most patients present with acute appendicitis, frequently with a periappendiceal abscess. The correct diagnosis is almost never made preoperatively, only occasionally intraoperatively, but commonly after the microscopic examination is complete. Further operative therapy must then be considered.

Pathology

There are no distinctive gross features of this type of carcinoma. Most are near the base of the appendix and appear as a firm nodularity or diffuse swelling that quickly occludes the appendiceal lumen. A few have been reported in a previously invaginated appendiceal stump. Microscopically the picture is a typical colonic adenocarcinoma. Since the appendiceal muscle walls are thin, any malignancy that involves the submucosa is essentially subserosal. Mesenteric and lymphatic involvement is common, most tumours being Dukes' B and C stages.

Therapy

Since the lymphatic drainage of the appendix is identical to that of the caecum, only a right hemicolectomy can accomplish a wide removal of the tumour with an adequate dissection of the regional lymph nodes. Although a rare Dukes' A tumour may be cured by an appendectomy, a right hemicolectomy is preferred for all good risk patients with localized disease, even if the appendix has perforated. If the correct diagnosis is known intraoperatively, a right colectomy is performed primarily. If not, a secondary right hemicolectomy must be undertaken within several weeks. An accompanying oophorectomy may be added in postmenopausal women.

Prognosis

The outlook is less favourable for patients with the colonic type of adenocarcinoma than for those with mucinous cystadenocarcinoma and similar to the prognosis of other colonic carcinomas, stage for stage. Survivors are few if regional lymph nodes contain cancer. Adjunctive therapy with 5-fluorouracil and levamisole will improve the prospects.

ADENOCARCINOID TUMOURS

This recently described tumour is a rare appendiceal malignancy that has both carcinoid and adenocarcinoma features. It is also called goblet cell carcinoid, mucinous carcinoid, and crypt cell carcinoma. Because it is more aggressive than the typical carcinoid but less so than an adenocarcinoma, the term adenocarcinoid seems to describe it best. Adenocarcinoids are mixtures of tubuloglandular structures and goblet cells that arise from the base of the glands and spare the luminal mucosa. They stain positively for acid mucin and argyrophilic granules and commonly invade perineural and lymphatic structures.

Adenocarcinoids are nearly always symptomatic, show no sexual preference, and usually present as acute appendicitis. Since this tumour has an unusual propensity to spread to the ovaries, the patient may present with ovarian masses (Krükenberg tumour).

Pathology

Adenocarcinoid tumours are inconspicuous and do not have a characteristic gross appearance. They are usually less than 2.0 cm in diameter involve all parts of the appendix equally, and are diffusely infiltrative. Unlike the situation with ordinary carcinoids, size is not a reliable guide to their clinical behaviour.

Debate exists about the histogenesis of adenocarcinoid tumours. Adenocarcinomas derive from primordial endodermal elements, while carcinoids develop from neural crest cells. There might be a simultaneous malignant transformation of the two stem cell types. Alternatively crypt base stem cells may be the origin, since they have the potential to differentiate into either cell type.

Metastatic disease may or may not be of the same type as the primary tumour. Frequently, the ovarian metastases will be pure signet ring carcinoma.

Treatment

A right hemicolectomy is the best treatment for nearly all patients with localized disease. Because the diagnosis is nearly always made postoperatively, right hemicolectomy is performed as a secondary procedure, along with an oophorectomy in most cases. If the patient has intra-abdominal metastases, aggressive resection is usually helpful.

Some patients with a Krükenberg tumour (usually bilateral) will have no obvious gastrointestinal source. A concomitant appendectomy should be undertaken to avoid overlooking a small primary appendiceal adenocarcinoid.

Prognosis

Adenocarcinoids lie between ordinary carcinoids and adenocarcinoma in malignant potential. Adenocarcinoids with a primarily tubular pattern fare better than those with a goblet cell pattern. The overall 5-year survival is about 80 per cent. Nearly all survivors are those with the tumour localized to the appendix. Patients with intra-abdominal spread and ovarian metastases have a poor prognosis.

SUMMARY AND RECOMMENDATIONS

1. A frozen section examination should be performed whenever the appendiceal findings are atypical. A diagnosis of an appendiceal malignancy can then be made intraoperatively, allowing appropriate surgery to be performed primarily.
2. All patients with an appendiceal malignancy should be followed, since 15 to 20 per cent of them develop a second malignancy.
3. Although surgery has been the main treatment for appendiceal malignancies, chemotherapy and radiation therapy should be helpful in the future.
4. Appendectomy is recommended for patients whose appendiceal carcinoids are 1.0 cm in diameter, before fixation and for many whose tumours are between 1.0 and 2.0 cm in diameter. Right hemicolectomy is recommended in good risk patients whose tumours are 2.0 cm or more in diameter, or between 1.0 and 2.0 cm if there is evidence of lymphatic permeation and mesenteric invasion.
5. Benign mucinous appendiceal tumours are treated by appendectomy while a right hemicolectomy is best for mucinous cystadenocarcinoma. Aggressive surgical treatment for intra-abdominal metastases and pseudomyxoma peritonei can allow long survival.
6. Most of the colonic forms of appendiceal adenocarcinomas are Dukes' C stage, require a right hemicolectomy, and have the same prognosis as do other colon adenocarcinomas.
7. Adenocarcinoids are a rare appendiceal malignancy of dual cell origin that have a predilection for producing ovarian metastases and have a malignant potential between that of carcinoids and adenocarcinomas. A right hemicolectomy, with concomitant oophorectomy in postmenopausal women, is the recommended therapy.

FURTHER READING

Anderson A, Bergdahl L, Boquist L. Primary carcinoma of the appendix. *Ann Surg* 1976; **183**: 53–7.

Aranha GV, Reyes CV. Primary epithelial tumors of the appendix and a reappraisal of the appendiceal mucocele. *Dis Colon Rect* 1979; **22**: 472–6.

Berardi RS, Lee SS, Chen HP. Goblet cell carcinoids of the appendix. *Surg Gynecol Obstet* 1988; **167**: 81–6.

Bowman GA, Rosenthal D. Carcinoid tumors of the appendix. *Am J Surg* 1983; **146**: 700–3.

Conte CC, Petrelli NJ, Steele J, Herrera L, Mittelman A. Adenocarcinoma of the appendix. *Surg Gynecol Obstet* 1988; **166**: 451–3.

Edmonds P, Merino MJ, Li Volsi VA, Duroy PH. Adenocarcinoid (mucinous carcinoid) of the appendix. *Gastroenterology* 1984; **86**: 302–9.

Gilhome RW, Johnston DH, Clark J, Kyle J. Primary adenocarcinoma of the vermiform appendix: report of a series of ten cases and review of the literature. *Br J Surg* 1984; **71**: 553–5.

Higa E, Rosai J, Pizzimbono CA, Wise L. Mucosal hyperplasia, mucinous cystadenoma, and mucinous cystadenocarcinoma of the appendix. *Cancer* 1973; **32**: 1525–41.

Lundquist M, Wilander E. A study of the histopathogenesis of carcinoid tumors of the small intestine and appendix. *Cancer* 1987; **60**: 201–6.

Lyss AP. Appendiceal malignancies. *Semin Oncol* 1988; **15**: 129–37.

Moertel CG, Weiland LH, Nagorney DM, Dockerty MB. Carcinoid tumors of the appendix: treatment and prognosis. *N Engl J Med* 1987; **317**: 1699–701.

Rosai J. *Ackerman's surgical pathology*. 7th edn. St Louis: CV Mosby Co, 1989; 563–71.

Stephenson JB, Brief DK. Mucinous appendiceal tumors: a clinical review. *J Med Soc NJ* 1985; **82**: 381–4.

Syracuse DC, Perzin KH, Price JB, Wiedel PD, Mesa-Tejada R. Carcinoid tumors of the appendix. *Ann Surg* 1979; **190**: 58–63.

Warkel RL, Cooper PH, Helwig EB. Adenocarcinoid, a mucin-producing carcinoid tumor of the appendix. *Cancer* 1978; **42**: 2781–93.

19.3 Pseudomyxoma peritonei

HUGH BARR

Pseudomyxoma peritonei is a clinical condition in which a large quantity of mucinous fluid or more gelatinous material accumulates in the peritoneal cavity. The term was first used by Werth in 1884 to describe a specific pathological entity that followed the rupture of a pseudomucinous cyst of the ovary, with subsequent implantation of the cyst contents on to the peritoneal surface followed by massive production of gelatinous material. Subsequently, Frankel in 1901 reported pseudomyxoma peritonei found at autopsy, presumed to have occurred following the rupture of a mucocele of the appendix. The term is now more generally used to describe the clinical condition, but it is not a single pathological entity with a uniform prognosis.

The mucinous material is an acid mucopolysaccharide (pseudomucin) that may be relatively cell free or may contain benign or frankly malignant appearing cells. It is generally thought that the pseudomucin is produced following implantation of cells from a primary tumour or organ. However, it is suggested that metaplasia of the peritoneal cells stimulated by the mucinous fluid may produce local spread and further production.

At present, the condition should always be regarded as potentially malignant, although identification of frankly malignant disease may be difficult and take several years. The myxomatous process is usually confined to the peritoneum with no lymphatic, parenchymal, hepatic, or extraperitoneal spread. Tumours of the ovary, in particular cystadenocarcinomas (16 per cent of which will produce pseudomyxoma peritonei) or less commonly cystadenomas, and appendiceal adenocarcinomas are the usual cause. Other sites of origin have been reported, including carcinomas of the uterus, colon, common bile duct, pancreas, and duplication cysts, and carcinoma of urachal cysts. Pseudomyxoma peritonei following rupture of an appendiceal mucocele is usually associated with an obstructing appendiceal adenocarcinoma. Benign mucoceles produced by experimental ligation of the appendix stump do not produce the condition following their perforation. This has led some to conclude that the obstruction has to be produced by a mucin-producing adenocarcinoma, and reports of the condition occurring after rupture of a benign mucocele may be incorrect.

The presentation is dependent on the underlying cause. The relatively benign behaviour of the tumour responsible often produces a prolonged clinical course: the patient presents with increasing abdominal distension and there is a marked disparity between the physical signs and the general well-being of the patient. Pain due to distension may occur but weight loss is unusual, and in most patients there is little impairment of their usual activities. Anaemia, elevation of the erythrocyte sedimentation rate, and hypoglycaemia have been reported. Pseudomyxoma is occasionally only identified at operation. Diagnosis may be suggested prior to laparotomy by a plain abdominal radiograph showing masses with annular areas of calcification. Ultrasound scanning shows multiple echogenic areas similar to multiseptate ascites but the bowel does not float in fluid. CT reveals dense homogeneous material with the intestines displaced to the side, unlike the situation in ascites.

A wide variety of possible treatments has been advocated, and the role of surgery is still contentious: randomized trials of comparative therapy are not available since the condition is very unusual. In some patients the disease runs a very benign course and aggressive therapy is inappropriate. However, there is evidence that surgical removal of the pseudomucin and underlying tumour, if necessary by repeated laparotomy, improves the prognosis. In particular, if the disease is localized, radical excision with peritoneal toilet offers the best prospect of cure. The use of 5 per cent dextrose solution during operation as a mucolytic agent may prevent recurrence. If surgery is incomplete, the prospect of a response to chemotherapy is improved if radical cytoreductive surgery has been performed. Intraperitoneal and systemic chemotherapy with a variety of agents including thiotepa, melphalan, cisplatin, 5-fluorouracil, mitomycin C, and chlorambucil, is well tolerated and is worthwhile. Although responsive to radiotherapy, the complications of total abdominal radiotherapy and the difficulties of surgery in these circumstances means that radiotherapy should be deferred until the response to chemotherapy has been assessed. However, radiotherapy should not be withheld if patients fail to respond to other treatment.

The prognosis of this condition is very variable, partially associated with the histological type of the underlying tumour but more so with the degree of dissemination of the myxomatous process. There is a very good outlook for prolonged symptom-free survival in patients with this condition, generally associated with radical surgery followed by adjuvant chemotherapy and radiotherapy.

FURTHER READING

Little JM, Halliday JP, Glenn DC. Pseudomyxoma peritonei. *Lancet* 1968; ii; 659–63.

Fernandez RN, Daly JM. Pseudomyxoma peritonei. *Arch Surg* 1980; **115**:-409–14.

Anus 20

20.1 Haemorrhoids

W. HAMISH THOMSON

INTRODUCTION

Haemorrhoids have been diagnosed and treated since the dawn of civilization and yet both their cause and nature, and even their symptomatology, remain hotly debated. The student's path to understanding is further hindered by a confusing terminology, a legacy of folklore, and, most tellingly, anatomical accounts which at best simply ignore pivotal morphological features, and at worst occasionally perpetuate unfounded, though persuasive, myths. Here is a journey to embark upon with both faulty and inadequate maps, and a set of muddling signposts.

The author's task therefore is to guide the reader, for the road is there all right; all that is needed is clearer cartography. He will hope to show that haemorrhoids are not some sort of variocosity, that there is no reason why they should by themselves be particularly itchy or painful, and that the various manifestations of their 'attacks' are logically attributable to basic pathological processes; finally he hopes to clarify what exactly the various labels 'internal', 'external', 'thrombosed', 'strangulated', and 'sentinel', mean.

Piles being a morbid change from the normal, the normal must first be mastered. The anatomy is therefore the key and must be studied in some detail.

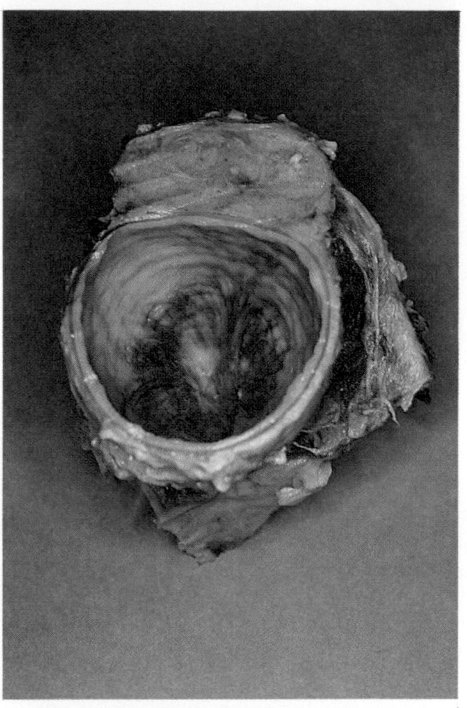

Fig. 1 The view from above: on looking down into the rectal ampulla and beyond the (closed) anal canal the horizontal folds of rectal mucosa can be seen to give way to the vertically disposed 'columns of Morgagni' lining the upper anal canal. The transected prostate, staining light blue, is seen adjoining the rectum anteriorily.

ANATOMY OF THE ANAL LINING

The anal canal's interior is usually described as a sphincteric tube, 4 to 5 cm in diameter, lined in its upper two-thirds by mucosa thrown into vertical folds and in the lower one-third by the appendageless squamous epithelium of the sensitive anodermal cuff, the two meeting at the dentate line. This view arises from the routine method of preparing the specimen for dissection. It provides no clue, however, to those intricacies of its infrastructure which explain the almost inevitable, and inherently diverse, vagaries of its average existence.

An anorectum removed from a fresh cadaver and fixed by distension with formalin appears much as described above (Fig. 1). However, if a specimen is prepared in exactly the same way, but after the veins have been filled (retrogradely through the superior rectal vein), the appearance is quite different (Fig. 2). The anal lining now bulges as three main pads, more or less subdivided by vertical folds, or 'columns' of Morgagni. These are the anal cushions. It is their existence and their curious and unique structure which provide the key to the understanding of piles.

The anal cushions

Contemporary anatomical accounts of the anal lining may be inadequate, but many of its special features were noticed more than a century ago. The anal submucosa was likened to cavernous tissue because of its thickness and rich vascularity. Only in recent years, however, was its discontinuous grouping into three main masses observed. These pads, extending above and below the dentate line, are the anal cushions. Morgagni's folds more or less subdivide their mucosal part. Slitting open a specimen prepared as in Fig. 2 shows them *en face* (Fig. 3), so belying the traditional anodyne description. At microscopic level these anal cushions exhibit some intriguing features.

Blood supply

The cushions receive a very rich intercommunicating supply from the superior, middle, and inferior rectal (synonymously called haemorrhoidal) arteries. Between five and eight branches of the superior rectal artery pass from the mesorectum through the rectal ampullary wall to descend into the anal submucosa, where they anastomose with the other branches emerging through the muscle wall. Local mucosal excisional procedures inevitably encounter substantial branches from any or all three sources. The profuse arterial supply communicates with the venous system not only through capillaries but also by direct arteriovenous shunts. These provide for a mechanical function (see later) which probably explains the richness of supply.

The veins of the anal lining are distinguished by discrete dilations along their course, particularly below the dentate line in the subanodermal tissues (Fig. 4 (a, b)). These were once thought to result from disease but are in fact normal, being found in all adults and at birth (Fig. 5). The veins drain mainly into the superior

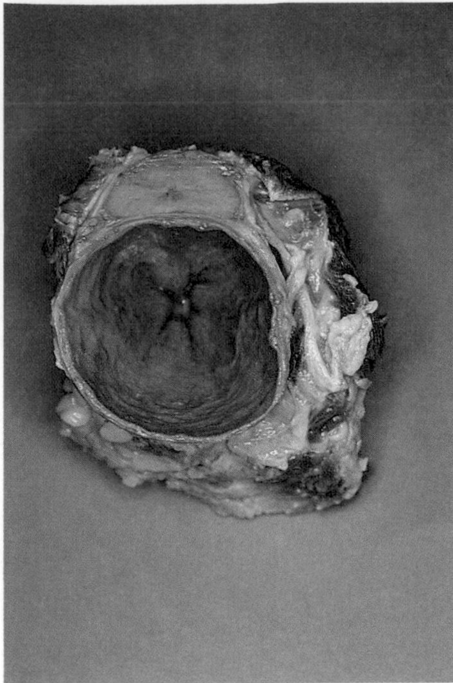

Fig. 2 The same view as Fig. 1, now with the veins filled with a coloured suspension of barium sulphate demonstrating the shape, position and existence of the anal cushions conferring a stellate cross section to the anal lumen. The finer folds of Morgagni have been more or less erased, and subdivide the anal cushions. Again the prostate is seen anteriorly.

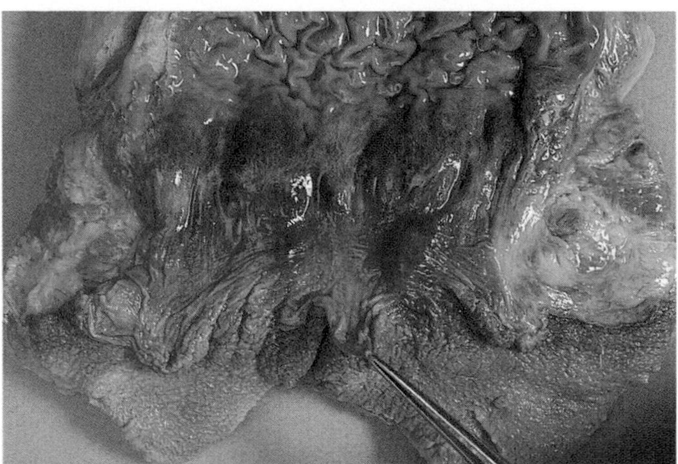

Fig. 3 An anal canal, prepared to demonstrate the anal cushions as in Fig. 2, slit open to show the interior. The anal cushions can be seen dark in their mucosal part with blood pushed down ahead of the barium sulphate suspension injected into the superior rectal vein.

rectal vein but also through and below the sphincter into the systemic circulation. Dissection preparations suggest that their infrasphincteric communications become increasingly tenuous in adult life (Fig. 4(a)). If so postdefecatory anal verge engorgement, a problem in some patients, and the oedema and discomfort of some prolapsed piles, may be explained.

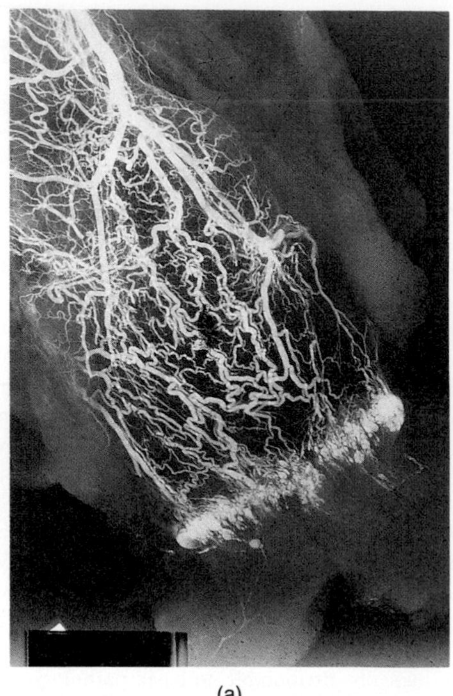

(a)

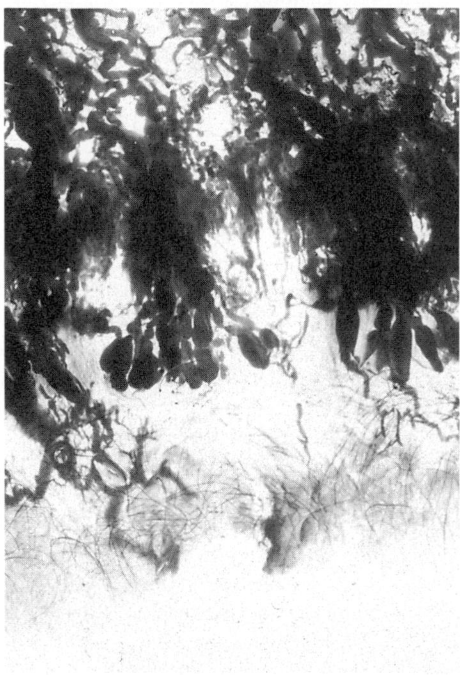

(b)

Fig. 4 (a) Radiograph of an anorectal specimen prepared by filling the superior rectal vein with a warm barium/gelatin mixture which on cooling sets in the veins. The specimen has been slit open. The venous saccules are easily filled from above but drain poorly inferiorly into the subcutaneous perianal tributaries of the inferior rectal vein, a feature often noted in adult specimens. (b) Close-up of the slit open anal canal from an adolescent, viewed with transmitted light. The veins have been filled with latex and the tissues rendered translucent. Drainage into the inferior rectal tributaries is freer than in later life.

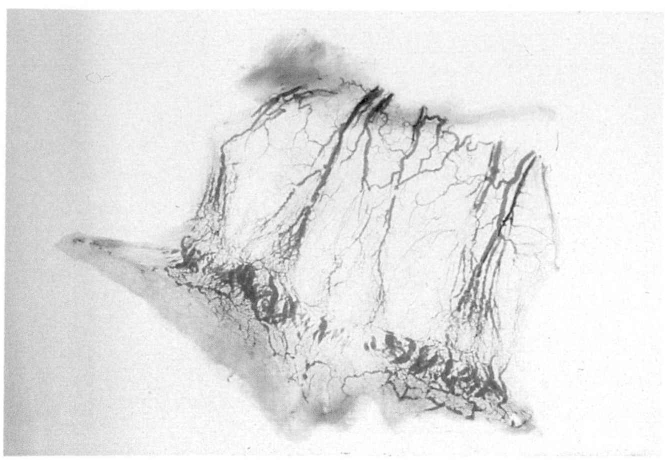

Fig. 5 Venous saccules in an infant anorectum demonstrated by (blue) latex injection and a tissue clearing technique. In babies drainage into the perianal veins below the anal sphincter is more readily demonstrable than in adult specimens.

Support

The cushions are supported against the shearing, extruding forces of defecation by smooth muscle—the musculus submucosae ani—and by elastic tissue. Discovered by Treitz (1853) and variously described and labelled since, this has for some reason sunk, like the venous saccules, into contemporary oblivion. The musculus submucosae ani descends from the internal sphincter in separate bundles (Fig. 6(a)) which coalesce beyond the dentate line under the anoderm, to form a dense stroma around the venous saccules there (Fig. 6(b)). A longitudinal section (Fig. 7) shows its full extent and demonstrates how the looser submucosal part of the cushions is supported by the tougher more strongly secured anodermal component, and how the muscle's contraction during defecation both flattens the cushions and holds them up against the internal sphincter.

Function

Being composed of a sacculated venous plexus with a rich arterial network the anal cushions provide a spongy variable volume 'washer' on which the sphincter can contract, thereby assisting its closure. Their looser textured nature above, supported by the tougher subanodermal part below, is designed to help provide a watertight seal.

THE NATURE OF PILES

The anal cushions can be seen viewed from above in a specimen (Fig. 2), from below with a proctoscope (Fig. 8), by transverse histological section (Figs. 9(a, b)), or by holding the anal lining up to the light (Fig. 10). The one constant feature is their regular arrangement in the left lateral (3 o'clock), right posterior (7 o'clock), and right anterior (11 o'clock) sectors of the anal circumference: this is, of course, where piles occur. It is logical to conclude therefore that piles are the clinical expression of their internal disruption and downward displacement. It is certainly what they resemble (Fig. 11(a)), while anal varices, a rare finding, look to be what they are (Fig. 11(b)).

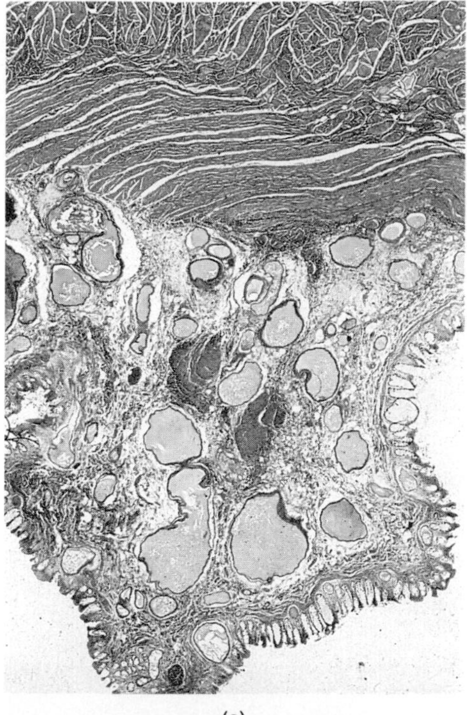

(a)

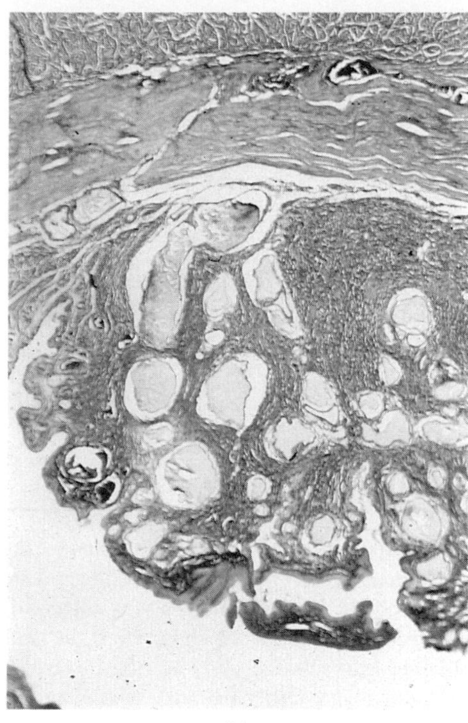

(b)

Fig. 6 (a) Transverse section of anal cushion above the dentate line, stained with haematoxylin and eosin. The venous saccules are distended with faintly pink staining barium sulphate suspension. Two separate bundles of deep pink staining smooth muscle of the musculus submucosae ani are seen amongst the venous saccules in the submucosa. (b) Transverse section of an anal cushion below the dentate line where the vein saccules are now surrounded by dense deep pink staining smooth muscle. There is also abundant elastic tissue and collagen, not demonstrated by this stain, all providing much firmer support for the subanodermal part of the anal cushions.

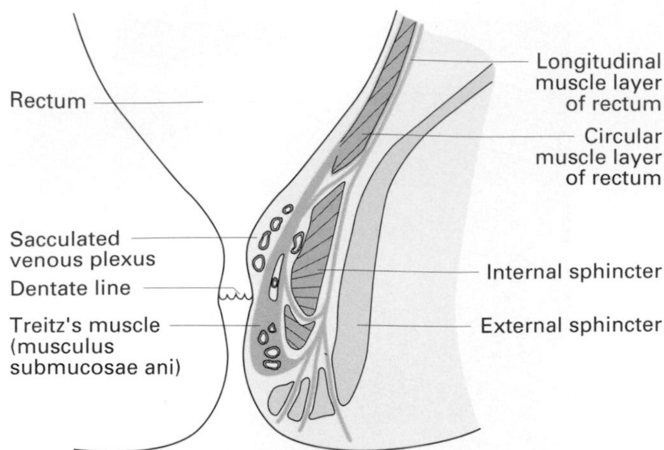

Fig. 7 Diagrammatic longitudinal section of anal canal illustrating the derivation and distribution of Trietz's muscle (muscularis submucosae ani).

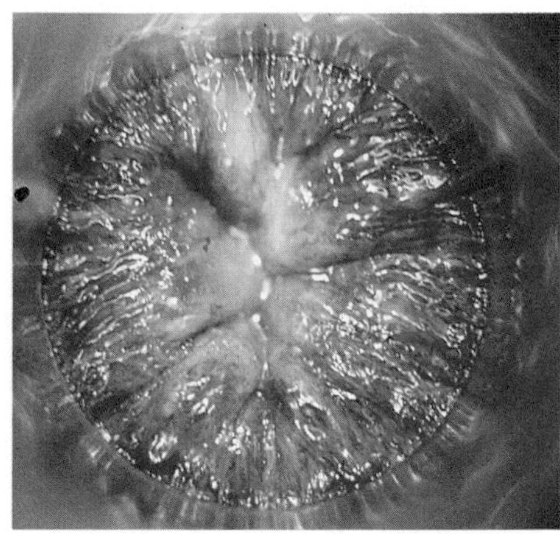

Fig. 8 The proctoscopic appearance of normal anal cushions.

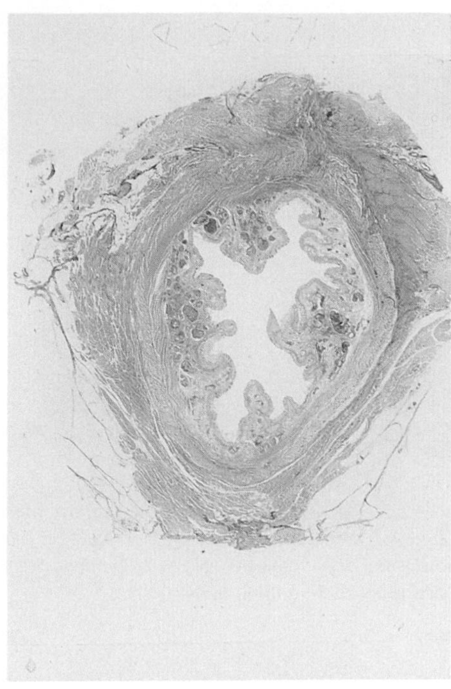

(a)

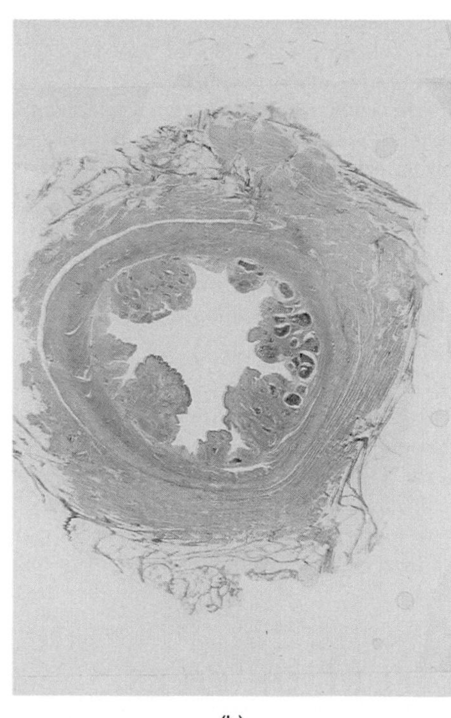

(b)

Fig. 9 Transverse sections of the anal canal prepared to demonstrate the cushions, above (a) and below (b) the dentate line.

Pathology

The anal cushions are disrupted to produce piles by the forces of defecation. For many sufferers defecatory habits and stool consistency are probably to blame. The Valsava effect of excessive straining engorges the cushions, which have lost the support of the external sphincter as it relaxes. The shearing force of hard stools will increase the damage. Other patients, who claim a lifetime of regular easy bowel actions, may have a congenital deficiency in the supporting tissues of the anal cushions. Weakness arising from the influence of progesterone on smooth muscle and elastic tissue probably explains the predisposition to haemorrhoids in pregnancy, although a general increase in pelvic vascularity also contributes. Many women date their haemorrhoids not to actual pregnancy, but to parturition, when the supporting tissues of the anal cushions may be stretched and torn.

Histological examination often shows larger vascular spaces than normal and more prominent connective tissues but no changes not accounted for by the effects of disruption.

Classification

The terms ‘internal’, ‘external’ and ‘intero-external’ are often used but serve no great purpose and are confusing, meaning different things to different people. It is better to stick to the basic premise

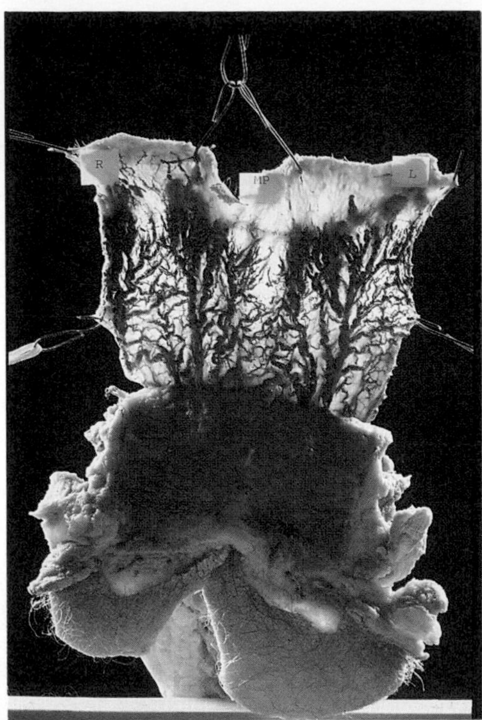

Fig. 10 The anal lining dissected from the internal sphincter and held up to the light.

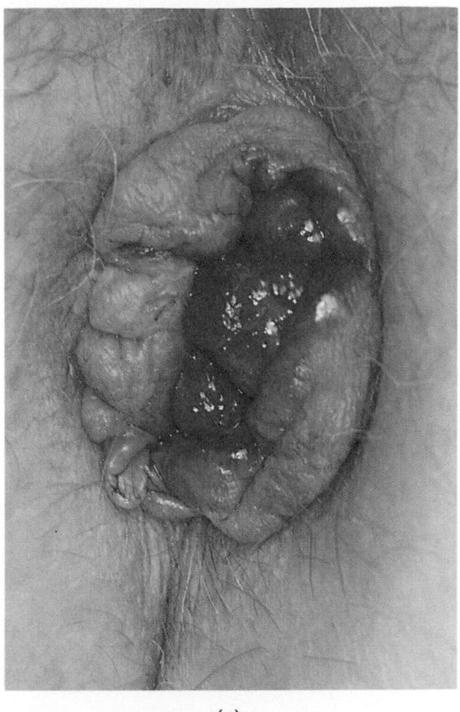

(a)

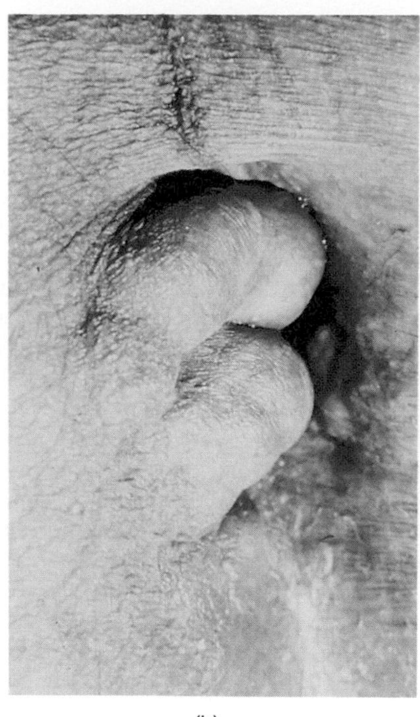

(b)

Fig. 11 (a) Prolapsed piles. (b) Anal varices in portal hypertension.

that piles are disrupted cushions and then observe whether the firmly tethered anodermal part is also involved, or whether, as commonly occurs, there is a superimposed skin tag instead.

It is customary to classify haemorrhoids by degree: first degree, only bleeding announces their presence; second degree, spontaneously reducing prolapse at defecation; third degree, prolapse requiring manual replacement; fourth degree, permanent prolapse. However, while a classification is required for the purpose of comparing different treatment techniques scientifically, the degree of any particular patient's piles may vary with time and may be misleadingly represented: indeed one may find gross pile protusion in patients quite unaware of prolapse.

SYMPTOMS

Although the underlying lesion in piles—disruption of the supporting and anchoring tissues of the cushions—means that prolapse is inherent in their nature, patients, are often either unaware of it or unconcerned. Bleeding is much more worrying and is the usual reason for seeing a doctor. Prolapse is, however, the other unequivocal symptom. Pain, itching, and anal dysfunctional effects are less reliable diagnostic criteria.

Bleeding

The capillaries of the lamina propria are only protected by a single layer of epithelial cells, and little trauma is required to breach them. Since it is the more lax-textured, upper part of the anal cushion which mainly prolapses, dragging the mucosa to the outside, trauma due to wiping or contact with clothes often occurs. Repeated trauma produces a chronic inflammatory response, making the damaged mucosa a brighter red and granular (Fig. 12), and so more friable and likely to bleed.

A great deal of unnecessary investigation, which is costly, inconvenient, uncomfortable, and occasionally even hazardous for the patient, can be avoided by time spent unravelling exactly what is meant by bleeding per rectum. Patient and courteous attention to detail in taking a history is always amply repaid, but never more

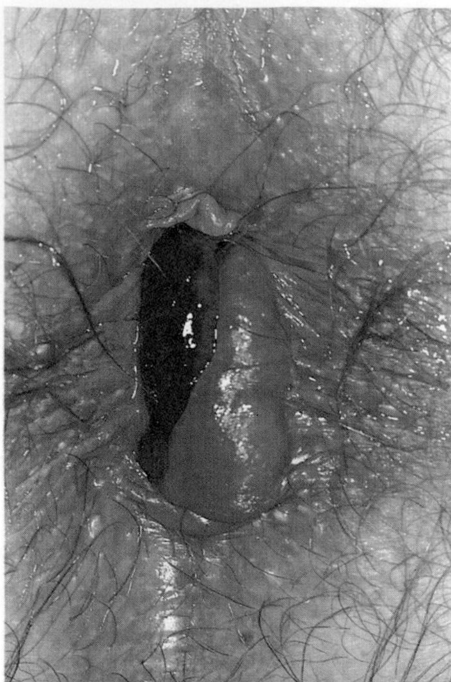

Fig. 12 Inflamed permanently prolapsed pile.

so than in anal bleeding: haemorrhoids are very common, and yet bleeding may also be indicative of a more serious condition. First and second degree piles, which remain intra-anal except at defecation, bleed with the bowel movement. Being capillary blood it is bright red. If enquiry reveals that it occasionally drips, an anal origin is certain, because the anus remains closed by tonic contraction of the sphincter except at the moment of defecation. Blood that drips into the pan, after passage of the stool, must originate from extruded anal mucosa, or from a fissure in the anoderm. The only other, and extremely uncommon, possibility is a rectal polyp on a long enough stalk. Blood smeared on the stool in the pan is ominous and unlikely to be coming from piles, since freshly shed blood ought to disperse straight away into the water. The fact that it remains on the stool suggests either that it has congealed there, or is mixed with mucus, indicating a higher lesion.

Passage of clotted blood also demands exculpation of a colorectal source, and a careful history may provide a useful clue. Piles may still be the explanation if questioning reveals that the clots were only seen on the paper and looked fresh; such clotting can have occurred in freshly shed blood lying at the anal verge. It is very rare for a large pile to bleed back into the rectum and proclaim itself by passage of older clots at stool. Third and fourth degree piles may bleed into clothing, sometimes dramatically. Occasionally a patient's claim to passing dark blood is found to derive from seeing it on clothing after it has dried and deepened in colour.

Prolapse

Patients may be quite unaware of protruding anal cushions, even when they are fourth degree, and surprisingly few report for treatment for this symptom alone. Descriptions of a fleshy lump or prolapse usually have to be elicited by questioning. For some, however, life is plagued by a pile which prolapses on exertion, making them uncomfortable, exuding mucus, and generally restricting their work or leisure. Others have to lie down after defecation to reduce the protusion.

Pain

Pain is a contentious issue in pile symptomatology. Although claimed to be a prominent and attributable problem, there seems to be no good reason why a disrupted anal cushion should actually be painful. When trapped outside the closed anus, distortion combined with oedema and congestion from lymphatic and venous impairment may well cause discomfort. In many causes pain on defecation is due to an easily overlooked fissure. Some patients nevertheless do experience relief from pain after simple treatment of their undoubted piles.

Episodes of painful irreducible swelling which last a week or so can be most unpleasant. Often given the inaccurate epithet 'strangulated' piles, they are usually due to greater or lesser degrees of infarction resulting from obstruction of venous drainage by thrombosis and consecutive clotting in the sacculated venous plexus. 'Infarction' is used here in its proper sense, denoting an intravascular and interstitial 'stuffing with blood', and not in its common contemporary misusage implying necrosis. Although necrosis would supervene if circulatory impairment by venous blockage were sufficient, the usual outcome is spontaneous resolution as the clot shrinks and lyses and venous circulation is restored. This condition is discussed more fully below.

Itching

When the patient's main concern is itching, piles are seldom, if ever, to blame: a local skin condition is usually responsible. Although treatment of coexisting piles may help relieve itching it is unwise to encourage a patient greatly bothered by pruritus to believe that relief will be produced from curing piles.

Rectal dysfunction

Defecatory derangement can result from excitement of a disrupted anal cushion, causing a sensation of incomplete evacuation, particularly when the cushion is engorged by fruitless straining, which further congests the cushions and worsens the problem. Unsatisfied defecation is also a feature of other anorectal conditions, including rectal tumour.

Soiling

Blood and serum from the exposed inflamed mucosal part of a pile dries dark on underclothing and may be thought faecal. Only very rarely, however, do third and fourth degree haemorrhoids allow minor conduction of rectal contents to the surface. Mucus may also exude from the exteriorized mucosa of piles and can be the presenting symptom.

EXAMINATION

When a meticulous history suggests piles and the findings agree examination can be confined to the anorectum. The only equipment required is proctoscope, sigmoidoscope, light source, and biopsy forceps.

SIGNS

There are several dynamic influences on a pile's presentation—the vigorous arterial supply, the presence and possibly changing diameter of the arteriovenous shunts, the variability of cushion bulk due to capacity of the venous saccules, and the effects of cushion displacement and anal sphincter contraction on venous and lymphatic drainage. As a result, not only does the appearance change from time to time in the same patient, but the same symptom may have different causes in different patients. For instance, whereas most patients complaining of prolapse have a simple displaced pile (Figs. 11(a), 12) a 'lump' felt by others may be due to engorgement of the subanodermal veins due to impairment of drainage (Fig. 13) or transient post-defecatory anodermal oedema (Fig. 14).

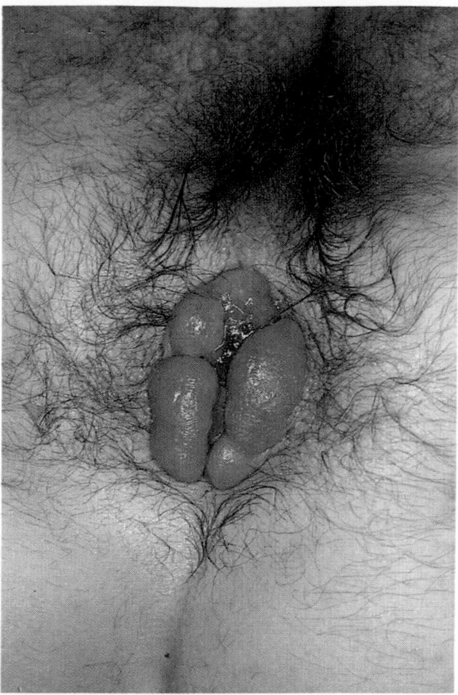

Fig. 14 Postdefecation oedema also occasionally contributes greatly to the bulk of 'prolapse', and must result in some way from impairment of either venous or lymphatic drainage.

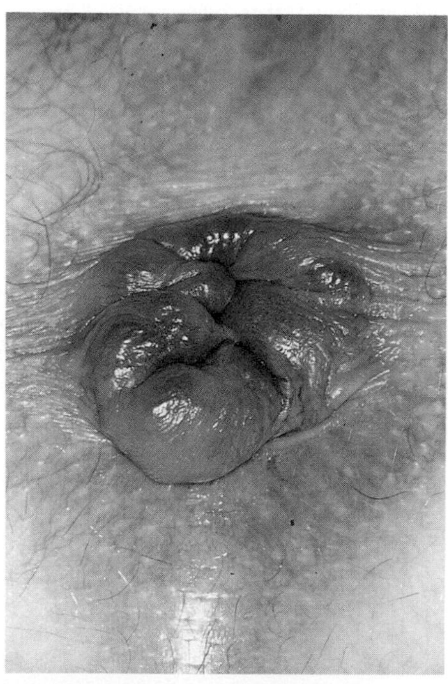

Fig. 13 Engorgement of the subanodermal veins masquerades as prolapse in some patients. Paucity of drainage of the venous saccules trapped outside by sphincteric closure (Fig. 4(a)) may explain this phenomenon.

Piles that are transiently displaced suffer little trauma, but when the mucosal part is frequently exposed it becomes inflamed (Fig. 12). Thrombosis and clotting in the vein sacs (when blood flow may be turbulent) also influence the appearance of the pile, but as an indication there will be associated discomfort or, depending on the extent of clotting and consequent infarction, frank pain. Solidification of a small part of the venous plexus causes an uncomfortable attack of swelling of the pile, with oedema but little infarction. Greater degrees of obliteration of venous drainage embarrass the circulation accordingly (Fig. 15). The fully infarcted pile (Fig. 16), despite its appearance, usually settles uneventfully. Many patients who seek medical attention because

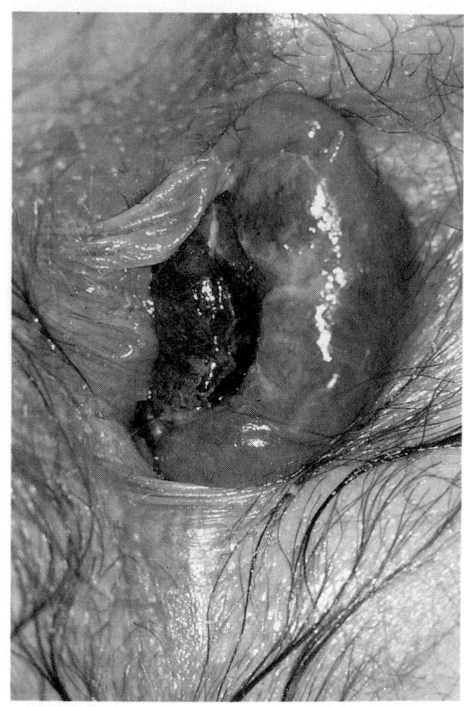

Fig. 15 Early venous clotting in an anal cushion. Individually clotted saccules can be seen through the subanodermal oedema.

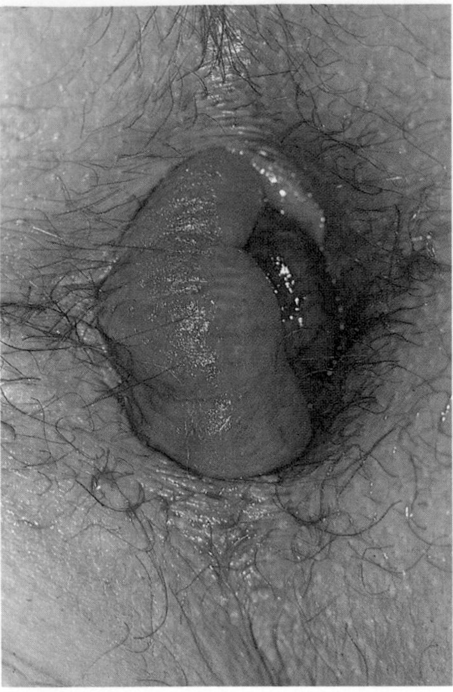

Fig. 16 Later effects of clotting of the sacculated venous plexus with infarction of the pile.

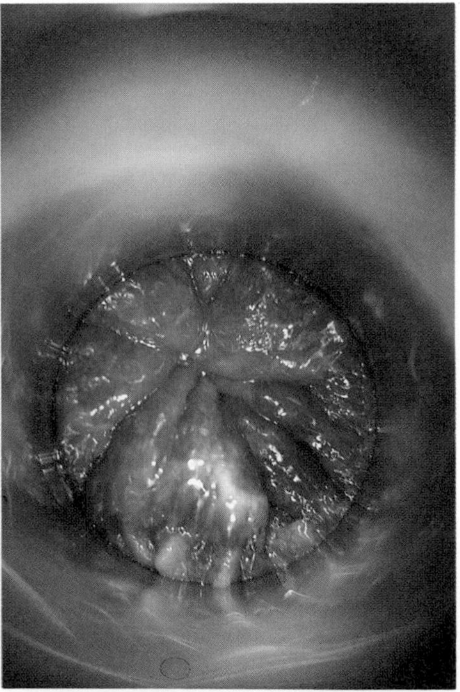

Fig. 17 Proctoscopic appearance of a disrupted anal cushion.

of such an attack of saccular clotting, and who graphically describe the severity of the condition, have recovered by the time of specialist consultation. The term 'strangulated piles' may be misapplied to this condition, causing inappropriate and inevitably unsuccessful efforts at supposedly therapeutic replacement.

A disordered cushion may, therefore present in one of several ways as a lump at the anal verge. In most cases, however, external inspection provides no clue to their presence, and nothing abnormal is found on anal digitation, since uncomplicated piles are impalpable. A nodular induration is felt if clotting has occurred and this may occasionally become firm due to fibrosis. In most patients, the diagnosis is suggested by the history and confirmed by proctoscopy. Interpretation of the proctoscopic appearance is not straightforward. Since anal cushions are normal structures (Fig. 8), their distinction from piles (Fig. 17) is only one of degree. Bright red granularity of the mucosal part of a cushion is certain evidence of its disruption, and the extent to which the cushions bulge into the instrument's end on straining and follow it out on withdrawal, provide a valuable guide.

Sigmoidoscopic exclusion of rectal disease is an essential part of the establishment of the diagnosis. Because piles are common finding them does not rule out another condition higher in the rectum causing the symptoms. There is, however, no evidence for the claim still occasionally made that haemorrhoids can result from rectal carcinoma or pelvic masses (an erroneous idea originating from the belief that piles resulted from venous obstruction).

DIFFERENTIAL DIAGNOSIS

Anal tags

Many patients mistake anal tags for piles, and indeed the disrupted anodermal part of a cushion may have a similar appearance. Anal tags are cutaneous protruberances at the junction of the anoderm and perianal skin. They are of uncertain origin, but possibly result

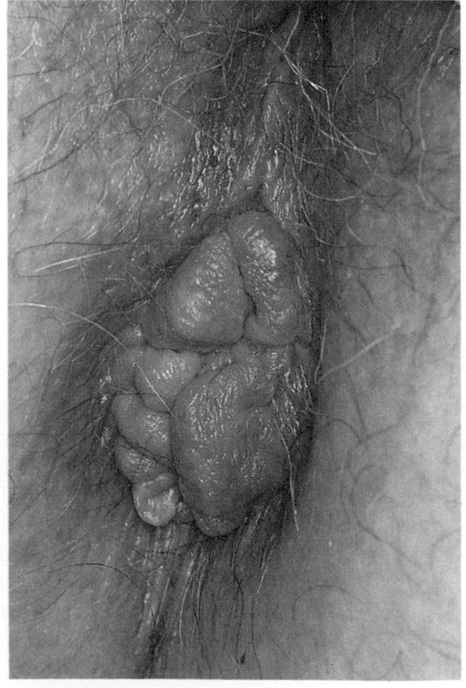

Fig. 18 Skin tags.

from local derangement of lymphatic drainage, as their occasional disarming partial reformation soon after excision suggests. They can be solitary and discrete, or form a circumferential irregular fringe (Fig. 18).

Fibrous anal polyp

These are club-like protruberances from the dentate line and seem to be hypertrophied anal papillae, again possibly due to lymphatic obstruction (Fig. 19).

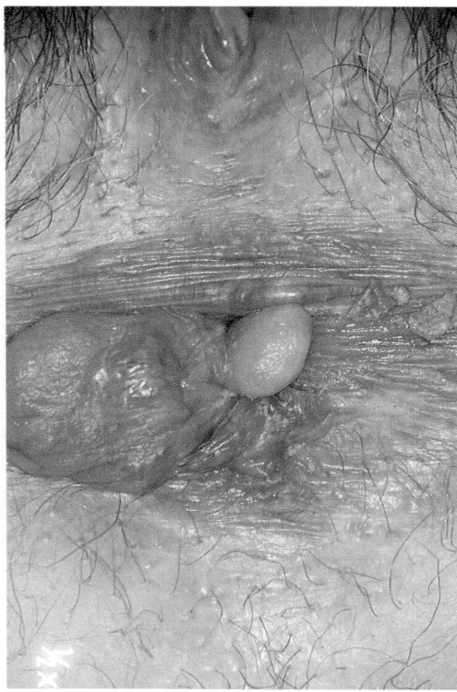

Fig. 19 A fibrous anal polyp, in this case surmounting a pile which consists, unusually, entirely of the disrupted anodermal component of the cushion.

Sentinel pile

This misnomer is given to a skin tag marking the distal end of an anal fissure, found usually in the posterior midline (Fig. 20).

Fissure

A patient described as having 'painful itchy piles' may well be suffering from an anal fissure, particularly if this is associated with a sentinel tag masquerading as a pile. The deep burning pain of a fissure on and after defecation and the associated itching are quite unlike the discomfort which might accompany a pile.

Dermatitis

Eczematous, psoriatic, and fungal dermatitis causes anal discomfort which often promotes referral as a case of haemorrhoids.

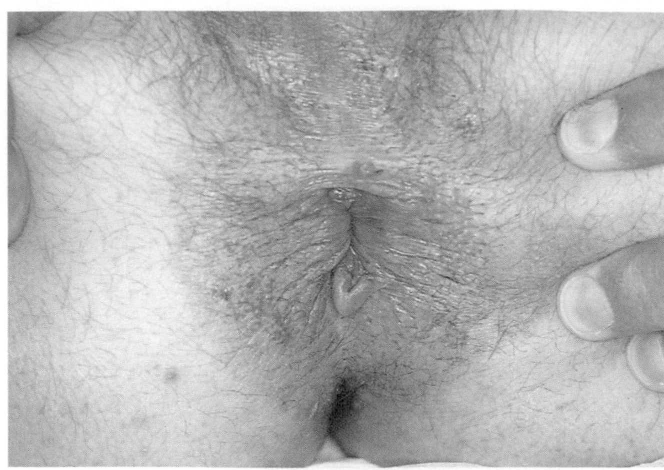

Fig. 20 A midline oedematous tag, or 'sentinel pile', at the lower end of a posterior fissure. Note also the perianal dermatitis with punctate excoriations, perhaps in this case iatrogenously arising from a reaction to locally applied anaesthetic cream.

Hyperkeratosis (seen as pale slightly soggy or glazed skin), punctate excoriations, and hairline radiating skin cracks will suggest the correct diagnosis.

'Perianal haematoma'

Perianal haematoma is one of the many local misnomers applied to anal disorders. It appears as a dark, tender, berry-like lump at the anal verge which is in fact a clotted subanodermal venous saccule (Fig. 21). Its other name, also inaccurate, is 'thrombosed external pile', a term which, to add to the confusion, is also applied to infarcted piles.

Rectal prolapse

Early rectal prolapse may be confused with piles. If the patient is inhibited from straining sufficiently to produce the lesion, the prolapse may look like an anterior pile. Full prolapse, however, has an unmistakable appearance. It is rare in men.

Rectal tumour

Rectal tumours can easily be missed by insufficient attention to the history and a careless digital examination, for it is not so much the length of the finger which matters, as the amount of thought behind it. Because of the rectum's curvature even upper-third tumours may be palpable. Even when nothing is felt or seen, if the patient's symptoms do not accord with the findings, further investigation is required. Ominous symptoms are old blood, particularly if slimy or clotted, unsatisfied defecation, deep discomfort, and 'wet' flatus.

Proctalgia fugax, proctitis, descending perineal syndrome, fistula, and warts

All of these may masquerade as 'piles'.

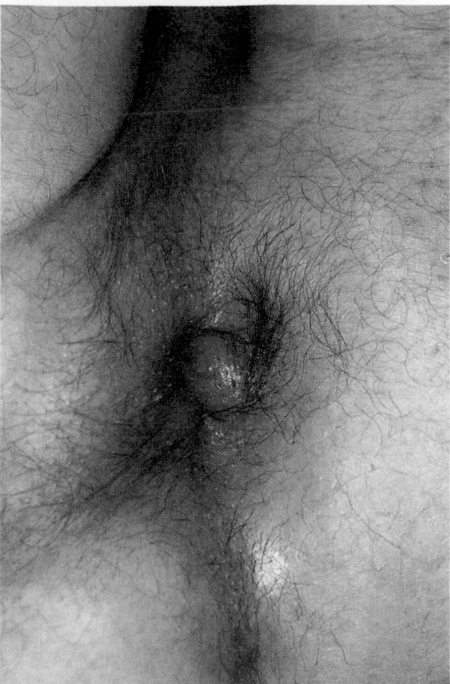

Fig. 21 So called 'perianal haematoma'; in fact a single venous saccule greatly distended with clot.

TREATMENT

Piles should be treated on their merits, tailoring the procedure to the patient's predicament and complaint. Only rarely are piles a threat to health in causing anaemia, so treatment should be suggested, not urged, and directed by symptoms rather than the attendant's obsession with neatness. Surgery is the replacement of one lesion by another; the aim is to ensure that the second is preferable to the first.

Management is either conservative or interventional, the latter being divided into those techniques aimed at reducing tissue volume and promoting adhesion of the remainder, and those claiming to work by other means.

Only by returning to the principle that piles are disrupted anal cushions can the beginner make any sense of the bewildering array of treatments available. At the dawn of this era of diversity, the *Lancet* aptly mocked the dilemma produced by the advent of yet another proclaimed method by heading the editorial: 'To tie, to stab, to stretch; perchance to freeze'.

Conservative treatment

As the fluctuating severity and intermittent nature of symptoms suggest, piles in their early stages are not an all-or-nothing complaint. For many patients advice to increase dietary fibre to bulk and soften stools, removal of literature from the lavatory, avoidance of excessive straining, and prompt manual replacement, may be sufficient to prevent marginally disrupted cushions from being much of a nuisance. Bulk laxatives may be helpful, as may simple suppositories, which certainly lubricate the adjacent surfaces so that the piles replace more readily and may in addition have some unknown emollient effect on the piles themselves, as their protagonists believe.

Interventional treatment

Outpatient procedures

Rubber band ligation

This works by strangling a 'polyp' of the insensitive mucosal part of a pile with a small elastic O-ring. It is mounted on a ligating device and snapped on to the pile through an anoscope by a releasing trigger, the grasped tissue having been first pulled into place. The strangled tissue withers and falls away in a few days, leaving a small ulcer which usually heals within a month. No anaesthesia is required.

Infrared photocoagulation and bipolar diathermy

Both of these cause tissue destruction by heat. The instruments are applied through an anoscope to coagulate a predictable volume of adjoining tissue. The mucosal part is treated; no anaesthesia is required.

Sclerotherapy

An irritant chemical solution, usually 3 ml of 5 per cent phenol in arachis oil, is injected into the submucosa at the base of each pile. When the varicose vein theory of piles prevailed it was thought to act by inducing fibrosis to constrict the superior rectal venous drainage, so, it was thought, deterring transmission of the supposed high pressures from the portal system. In fact it probably causes some shrinkage of tissue by necrosis, and adhesion as a result of the ensuing inflammatory reaction.

Cryotherapy

A liquid nitrogen probe is placed against the pile for 3 min, and causes cold necrosis. Local anaesthesia at least is said to be needed.

Inpatient procedures

Haemorrhoidectomy

Here, the offending bulk is excised. 'Open' and 'closed' methods are used. The ligation/excision technique of Milligan and Morgan, which is safe and well tried, leaves an open wound at the site of the pile, the ligated pedicle of which, containing branches of the superior rectal artery, lies alongside. When the pedicle has separated the wound heals by secondary intention.

Primarily closed wounds however can be safely achieved both by the submucosal dissection haemorrhoidectomy, whereby excess tissue is excised from under raised mucosal and anodermal flaps which are then stitched back, or simply by diathermy excision of the pile within a longitudinally disposed ellipse, achieving haemostasis by diathermy coagulation and then wound closure with absorbable stitches.

Forcible anal dilation

This was widely practised as a treatment for piles in the last century. The nineteenth century French surgeon, Verneuil, again reconciling its effect with the varicose vein theory, thought it improved venous drainage by stretching the rectal muscular button holes which convey the anal tributaries of the superior rectal vein. When reintroduced some years ago, it transiently displaced the surgical standby of the time, haemorrhoidectomy, but was later shown to have limited application. It probably helps patients who have discomfort and difficulty in defecation by easing the effort of evacuation, so reducing the congestion of the cushions from excessive straining.

Pile stitching

This has been advocated. Absorbable sutures are placed above the dentate line to attach the cushion back to the internal sphincter. Obliteration of its blood supply also reduces bulk.

COMPLICATIONS

Vasovagal reaction

Some patients faint after banding and occasionally after injections.

Pain

Pain is inevitable after haemorrhoidectomy, whatever the technique. Band ligation also causes pain, but this is unpredictable and many patients suffer little discomfort. Clotting in the adjacent sacculated venous plexus is occasionally precipitated by banding, causing severe, prolonged pain. Combining banding with an anal stretch seems to increase this risk and is not recommended. Because of pain and the possibility of fainting it is sensible to warn the patient in advance against driving home unaccompanied after such outpatient procedures.

Haemorrhage

All methods except injection, stretching and perhaps haemorrhoidectomy by primary closure techniques leave a moist open wound to heal by secondary intention and thereby carry the irreducible risk of secondary haemorrhage. Although rare it is most worrying for the patient. Anxiety is reduced by explaining the possibility beforehand and the methods by which it can readily be managed—traction on a balloon catheter inflated in the rectum, say, or suturing the bleeding point. As a wise precaution, procedures carrying a risk of secondary haemorrhage should not be undertaken within 3 weeks of a trip abroad or to remote parts.

Infection

Sepsis seldom complicates either haemorrhoidectomy or ambulatory procedures. When it occurs it is managed with antibiotics and drainage where appropriate. Haemorrhoidectomy, even by banding, can be followed by infection in the immunocompromised patient.

Impairment of continence

Over-vigorous stretching, particularly in the elderly, can have this disastrous consequence. The procedure should always be performed in a controlled way using the finger tips, gauging the force used to the strength of contracture of the tissues, rather than according to an arbitrary numerical formula. The stretch should be distributed equally around the circumference by changing direction.

Given the anal cushion's function, removal of excess tissue during haemorrhoidectomy can be expected to impair continence, particularly since most of the tissue excised is anodermal. When the procedure is necessary, therefore, the amount of tissue excised should be kept to the minimum compatible with relief of symptoms.

Urinary symptoms

Haemorrhoidectomy is notorious for causing transient difficulty in voiding in men. Banding may also induce curious bladder symptoms.

COMPARISONS OF TREATMENT

A generation ago the choice was simple: piles classed as first or second degree were injected, and third and fourth degree cases underwent haemorrhoidectomy. Little was done properly to test the efficacy of either. With the introduction of ambulatory tissue-reducing techniques and the advent of the now ubiquitous clinical trial, the scene has entirely changed. Haemorrhoids make an excellent subject for trials. The supply is inexhaustible and the effects of treatment can be assessed both subjectively and objectively. There are also many different treatments to evaluate.

Conservative treatment has been compared with band ligation; bulk purgatives or high fibre diet with sclerotherapy, stretching, sphincterotomy, band ligation, and freezing. Banding has also been compared with sclerotherapy, haemorrhoidectomy, stretching, and infrared photocoagulation. Photocoagulation has been compared with bipolar diathermy, and one type of haemorrhoidectomy has been judged against another. Excellent and praiseworthy though such trials are they suggest a 'rivalry', when in fact no one treatment is best for all patients. Their greater merit is in showing prospectively and with careful control and monitoring, that benefit can be derived from each measure, so allowing us an informed choice of the possible treatments.

Haemorrhoidectomy still has a place when gross disruption of the sensitive anodermal part of the cushion is the main problem. A trial has shown that simple ligation/excision is in fact no more painful than submucosal dissection. When the shape and size of the pile is appropriate, closed methods of haemorrhoidectomy have much to recommend them. The obvious drawback of haemorrhoidectomy is its requirement for admission, anaesthesia, and a longer recovery time. Cryodestruction is a messy, prolonged, and anatomically less accurate way of achieving the same end as haemorrhoidectomy. Infrared coagulation has the same beneficial effect as banding. Since it causes less pain and requires fewer days off work, it has greater patient acceptability. Band ligation, however, achieves its objective in significantly fewer treatment sessions and the instrument is both a great deal cheaper and more robust. The discomfort of banding can be rendered more tolerable, particularly in the light of more immediate benefit, if the patient is adequately warned beforehand and provided with analgesic tablets, and something to keep the motions soft. Forcible anal dilation may have a limited adjunctive place in the treatment of piles but would no longer be advanced as an alternative management. Sclerotherapy can be effective, but the improvement is not so reliably maintained as with other methods. Its undoubted advantage is cost and convenience.

Management of infarcted ('strangulated') piles

Although some clinicians advocate emergency anal stretching and others haemorrhoidectomy, in the author's experience the majority of cases settle spontaneously. Previous symptoms improve, presumably due to fibrosis. Management therefore is simply bed rest as required, stool softeners, and analgesia. Local anaesthetic preparations have variable effects but may be helpful. Surgery in areas of such compromised tissue may be unwise and excessive, and recovery is no quicker. In the rare event of infarction progressing to necrosis, however, and in the occasional patient suffering severe and prolonged pain, debridement haemorrhoidectomy (cutting away the dead tissue) speeds recovery and certainly relieves the pain dramatically.

CONCLUSION

Once one understands the detailed anatomy of haemorrhoids and their pathological possibilities, their management is straightforward, and the treatment effective, acceptable, and reasonably trouble free. The important part is diagnosis. The patient's preconception that piles are responsible for their symptoms must not cloud the clinician's mind. Uppermost must be the question whether reducing the bulk of the anal cushions and mooring them more firmly will logically address the presenting problem. If not, then in a 19th century surgeon's words, 'in such cases prudence equally forbids the rash interposition of unavailing art, and the useless indulgence of delusive hope'.

FURTHER READING

Ambrose NS, Hares MM, Alexander-Williams J, Keighley MRB. Prospective randomised comparison of photocoagulation and rubber band ligation in treatment of haemorrhoids. *Br Med J* 1983; 286: 1389–91.

Dehn TCB, Kettlewell MGW. Haemorrhoids and defaecatory habits. *Lancet* 1989; i: 54–5.

Dennison AR, Whiston RJ, Rooney S, Morris DL. The management of haemorrhoids. *Am J Gastroenterol* 1989; **84**: 475–81.

Dennison, A, Whiston RJ, Rooney S, Chadderton RD, Wherry DC, Morris DL. A randomised comparison of infrared coagulation with bipolar diathermy for the outpatient treatment of haemorrhoids. *Dis Colon Rect* 1990; **33**: 32–4.

Editorial. To tie, to stab, to stretch, perchance to freeze. *Lancet* 1975; **ii**: 645.

Gibbons CP, Trowbridge EA, Bannister JJ, Read NW. Role of anal cushions in maintaining continence. *Lancet* 1986; **i**: 886–8.

Greca F, Hares MM, Nevah E, Williams JA, Keighley MRB. Randomised trial to compare rubber band ligation with phenol injections for treatment of haemorrhoids. *Br J Surg* 1981; **68**: 250–2.

Haas PA, Fox TA, Haas GP. The pathogenesis of haemorrhoids. *Dis Colon Rect* 1984; **27**: 442–50.

Hosking SW, Smart HL, Johnson AG, Triger DR. Anorectal varices, haemorrhoids, and portal hypertension. *Lancet* 1989; **i**: 349–52.

Jensen SL, Harling H, Arseth-Hansen P, Tange G. The natural history of symptomatic haemorrhoids. *Int J Colorect Dis* 1989; **4**: 41–4.

Marshman D, Huber PJ, Timmerman W, Simonton CT, Odom FC, Kaplan ER. Haemorrhoid ligation. *Dis Colon Rect* 1989; **32**: 369–71.

Murie JA, Mackenzie I, Sim AJW. Comparison of rubber band ligation and haemorrhoidectomy for second and third degree haemorrhoids. *Br J Surg* 1980; **67**: 786–8.

Murie JA, Sim AJW, Mackenzie I. The importance of pain, pruritus and soiling as symptoms of haemorrhoids and their response to rubber band ligation. *Br J Surg* 1981; **68**: 247–9.

Roe AM, Bartolo DCC, Locke Edmunds J, Mortensen NJ McC. Submucosal versus ligation excision haemorrhoidectomy. *Br J Surg* 1987; **74**: 948–51.

Templeton JL, Spence RA, Kennedy TL, Parks TG, Mackenzie G, Hanna WA. Comparison of infrared coagulation and rubber band ligation for first and second degree haemorrhoids: a randomised prospective clinical trial. *Br Med J* 1983; **286**: 1387–9.

Thomson WHF. The nature of haemorrhoids. *Br J Surg* 1975; **62**: 542–52.

Thomson WHF. Non-surgical treatment of haemorrhoids. *Br J Hosp Med* 1980; **24**: 298–301.

Thomson WHF. The one-man bander: a new instrument for elastic ligation of piles. *Lancet* 1980; **ii**: 1006–7.

Thomson WHF. The real nature of 'perianal haematoma'. *Lancet* 1982; **ii**: 467–68.

Senapiti A. A randomised controlled trial of injection sclerotherapy with bulk laxatives. *Int J Colorect Dis* 1988; **2**: 124–6.

20.2 Pruritus ani

CHRISTOPHER G. MARKS

Pruritus is defined as itching of the skin, especially without visible eruption (*The Oxford English Dictionary*). When this is confined to the perianal area it is known as pruritus ani. Individuals vary in their capacity to feel itching; some hardly notice an extensive dermatitis while others suffer greatly from an eruption that does not usually cause itching. Within a single individual the threshold of itching also varies with the state of concentration, tiredness, or boredom.

AETIOLOGY

Generalized medical diseases

Generalized itching is a common complaint. In the initial investigation, parasitic diseases such as scabies and infestation with body lice must be excluded. A number of organic diseases, including

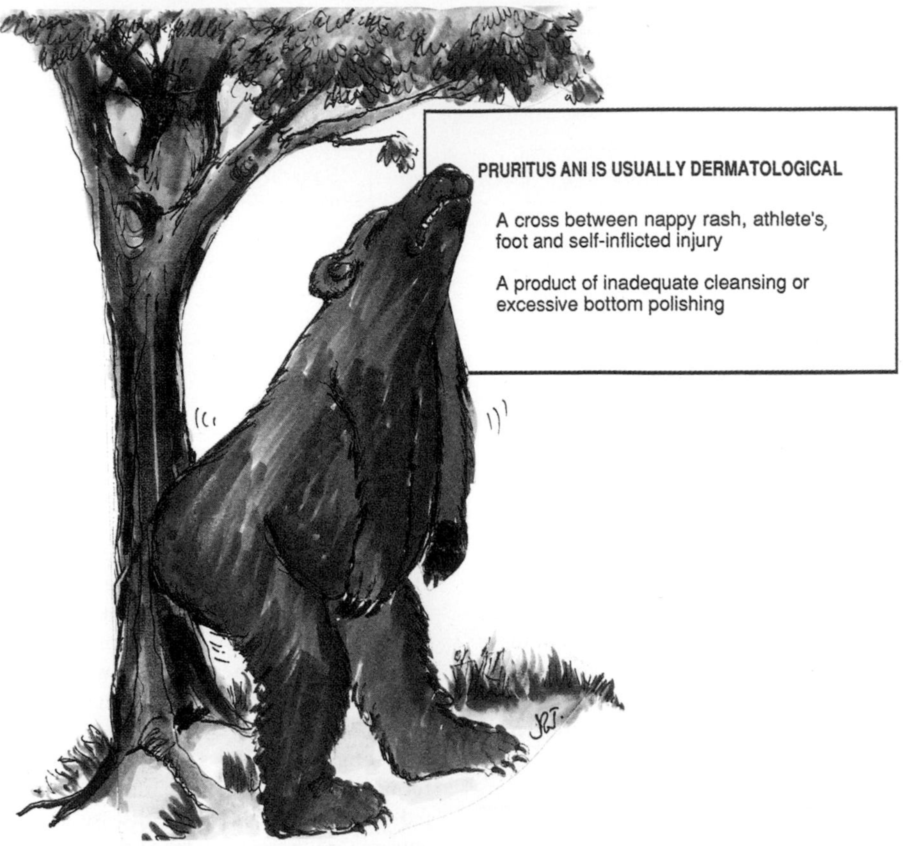
PRURITUS ANI IS USUALLY DERMATOLOGICAL
A cross between nappy rash, athlete's foot and self-inflicted injury
A product of inadequate cleansing or excessive bottom polishing

Fig. 1 Pruritus ani.

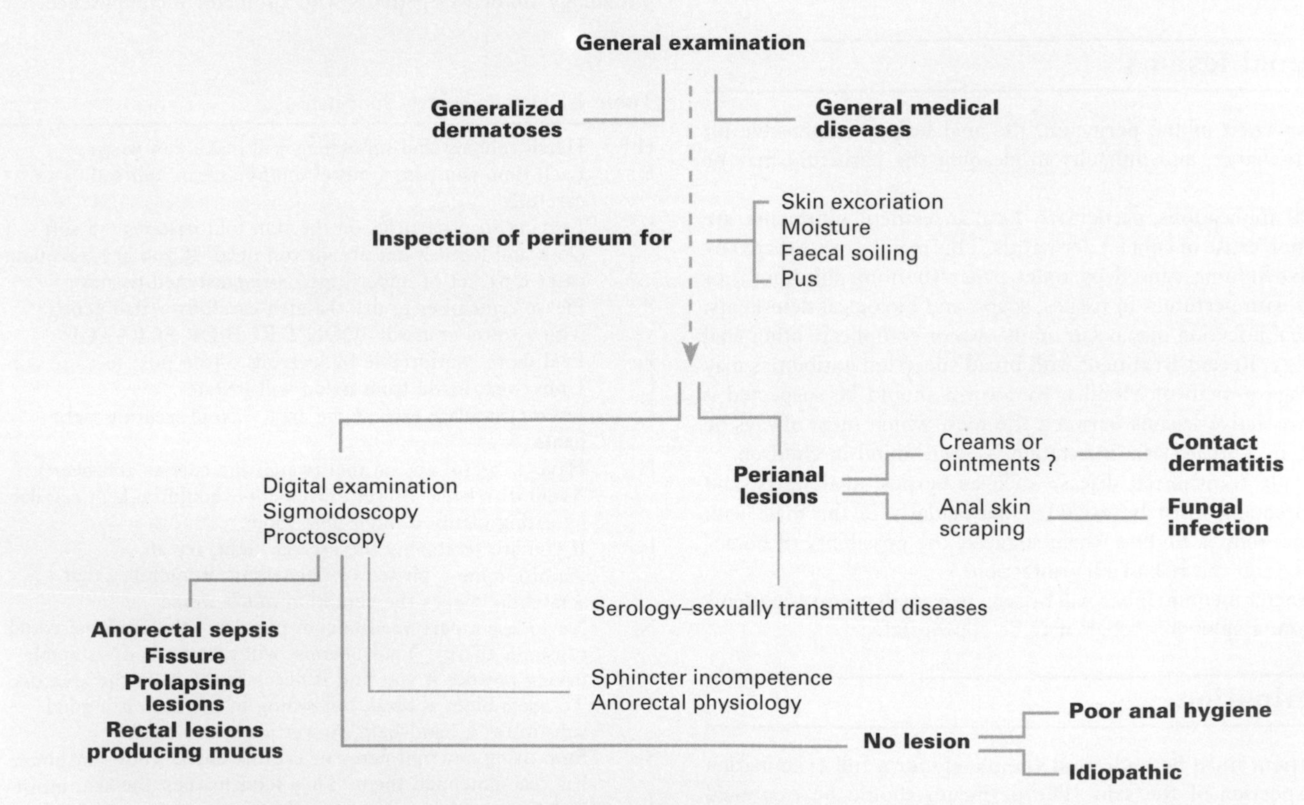

Fig. 2 Diagnosis of pruritus ani.

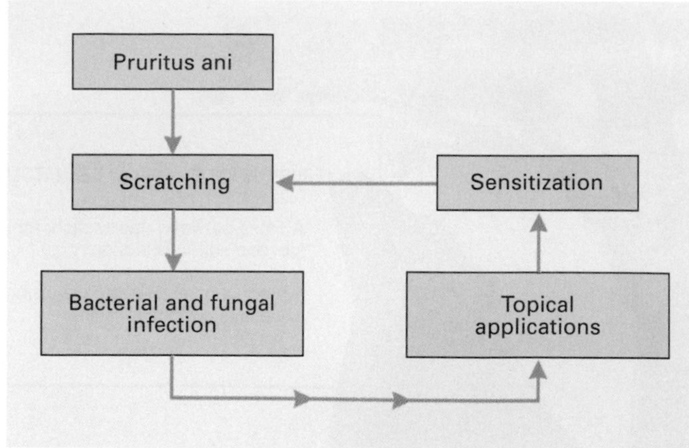

Fig. 3 The vicious circle.

anaemia, uraemia, diabetes, liver disease, and reticuloses, may present with itching. Normal results of biochemical examination of urine and serum and full blood counts will exclude most of these conditions. In the absence of organic disease or local skin disorders a diagnosis of psychogenic irritation may be made. The most common site for intractable localized itching is the anogenital region.

General dermatoses

Eczema, psoriasis, lichen planus, seborrhoeic intertrigo, and allergic eruptions are encountered most frequently in patients with pruritus ani.

Perianal lesions

On inspection of the perineum, the anal lesions responsible for pain, discharge, and difficulty in cleaning the perineum may be seen.

Local applications, particularly local anaesthetic ointments, are a common cause of contact dermatitis. This may be exacerbated by excessive trauma caused by toilet paper (bottom polishing!), or contact with perfumes in tissues, soaps, and biological detergents.

Fungal infection may occur on its own or complicate other anal pathology. Recent treatment with broad spectrum antibiotics may encourage growth of Monilia. Ringworm should be suspected if there are active lesions between the toes, which must always be inspected. Threadworm infestation is often found in children.

Sexually transmitted disease such as herpes, anal warts, and HIV infection, must be excluded, particularly in the male with poor anal tone, a finding which suggests the possibility of homosexuality and the risk of HIV infection.

Sphincter incompetence will be seen in a small group of patients for whom a sphincter repair may be appropriate.

Examination

The patient must be undressed completely for a full examination and inspection of the skin. The perineum should be examined carefully for moisture and soiling, skin maceration and excoriation, a skin eruption, perianal lesions, and prolapse. Separation of the buttocks will demonstrate the presence of a gaping anus due to poor anal tone, and digital examination will confirm this. Digital examination together with sigmoidoscopy and proctoscopy will also identify sphincter incompetence, fistulae, haemorrhoids, and rectal lesions.

If fungal infection is suspected, skin scrapings should be taken for microbiological examination. Serological tests must be requested if sexually transmitted disease is suspected. Microscopy and culture are necessary to exclude specific infections by agents responsible for diarrhoea. Worm infestation can be diagnosed by the presence of ova on microscopic examination of a swab from the perianal skin. Rectal lesions should be biopsied and anorectal physiology studied in patients with sphincter incompetence.

Table 1 How to control your itch

H	Harsh rubbing and scratching will make you worse
E	Each time you pass a bowel motion, clean yourself carefully
L	Leaving soap particles on the skin fold irritates – a soft cloth and tepid water are all you need. If you are travelling carry a packet of unperfumed, premoistened tissues
P	Please remember to dry the area carefully – dab gently with a towel or tissue. DON'T RUB OR SCRATCH
F	Feel more comfortable by wearing cotton next to your skin
U	Underwear made from nylon will irritate
L	Let air circulate around the area – avoid wearing tight pants
H	Have a careful eye on diet (watch the curries and beer!) Avoid diarrhoea. Bowel movements should be kept regular by eating plenty of high fibre food
I	If you are scratching the area at night, try an antihistamine – piriton or phenergan. Remember that scratching makes the condition much worse
N	Never use a perfumed talcum powder – the perfume could cause an allergy. Your chemist will recommend a suitable drying powder if you find it necessary to keep the area dry
T	To use a bidet is ideal, but sitting in the bath is a good substitute. A hand-held shower jet is also useful
S	Stop using any ointments or creams unless your consultant has recommended them. They tend to keep the skin moist and soggy and can cause an allergy

TREATMENT

In severe pruritus a vicious circle becomes established whereby the pruritus causes scratching which leads to secondary bacterial or fungal infections, which are treated by a multitude of topical applications, often containing local anaesthetic, which in turn produces more sensitization and more scratching, making the pruritus ani worse.

The first step is to control infection and then to stop all topical applications. A cream containing low-dose hydrocortisone (1 per cent) combined with an antifungal agent (miconazole nitrate 2 per cent) should be applied to the perianal area. If severe inflammation and infection are present, a stronger steroid is used, for example a cream containing triamcinolone acetonide 0.1 per cent, gramicidin 0.025 per cent, neomycin 0.25 per cent, and nystatin 100 000 units/g. These creams should be used for approximately 2 weeks, and sparingly thereafter. In the long term a patient with very dry skin may be helped by moisturizing cream or lotion (Johnson's Baby Lotion® for example); conversely, a powder will dry excessively moist skin.

Despite the topical application of medications, itch at night may continue to be a major problem. An antihistamine (promethazine hydrochloride 10–25 mg) will control this, although it may cause drowsiness. Anal lesions which require surgery should be excised after the pruritus has improved. Using this approach the majority of patients with pruritus will be cured, although most understand that a lasting cure requires a great deal of effort on their own behalf. At the end of the first consultation, the patient should be given general advice on anal hygiene, which is reinforced by a leaflet giving a list of 'do's and don't's. This leaflet is a good way of ending the consultation and providing the obsessional patient with a well defined strategy.

20.3 Fissure-in-ano

THOMAS C.B. DEHN

Fissure-in-ano is a common disorder, characterized by exquisite pain (proctalgia) during and following defecation. It results from a longitudinal tear in the squamous epithelium of the anal canal, frequently precipitated by the passage of a constipated stool, although, in a small proportion of patients, it may follow an episode of diarrhoea. The disorder is more common in males and has a peak incidence in the second decade in females and the third decade in males, although it may also occur in infancy and in old age. In 75 to 94 per cent of cases the fissure is situated at the posterior anal margin: anterior fissures are more commonly encountered in women and may follow parturition or gynaecological procedures. Fissure may coexist with haemorrhoids (Fig. 1).

PATHOPHYSIOLOGY

Acute anal fissures are superficial and are not normally associated with skin tag formation. Chronic anal fissure is associated with the development of both anal tags and polyps as a result of inflammatory oedema. Chronic subepithelial infection at the fissure results in fibrosis and, in rare instances, anal stenosis. The torn edges of the anal epithelium become undermined and the ulcer deepens, exposing fibres of the internal sphincter muscle. A vicious cycle ensues (Fig. 2) in which subepithelial inflammation causes spasm of the internal sphincter, inhibiting free drainage of the infected fissure and permitting continued inflammation, resulting in a small, chronic, inadequately drained abscess. The reflex relaxation of the internal sphincter that normally follows defecation is lost in patients with anal fissure; instead contraction of the internal sphincter occurs.

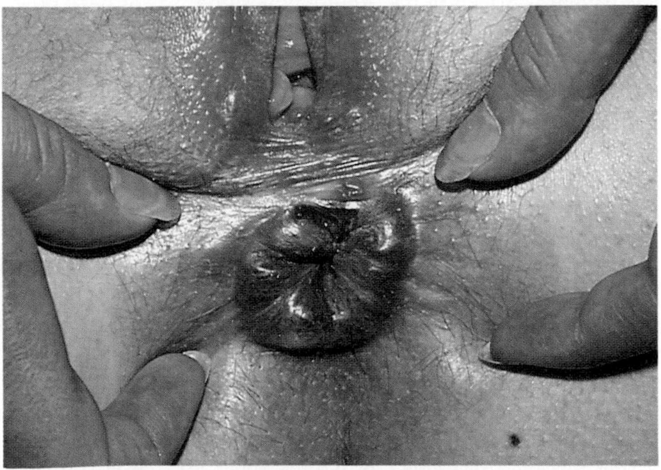

Fig. 1 Anterior anal fissure in a female patient with coexisting haemorrhoids.

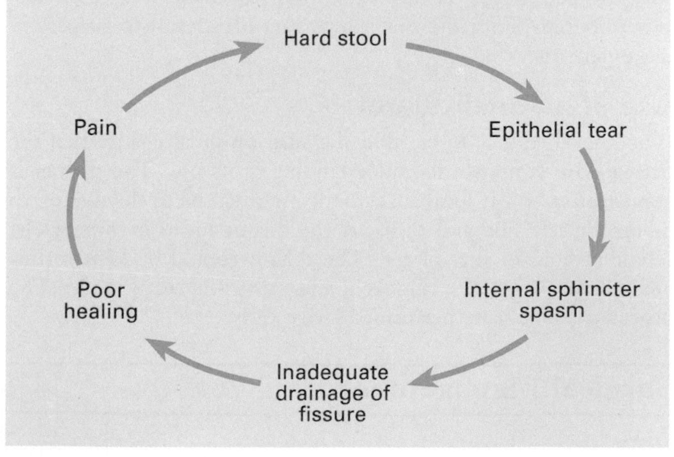

Fig. 2 Diagram illustrating cycle of development of anal fissure.

SYMPTOMS

Pain during and shortly after defecation occurs in 73 to 100 per cent of patients; bright rectal bleeding is seen in between 75 and 100 per cent of cases and mucous anal discharge and pruritus ani are also common. The clinical history of chronic anal fissure is typically cyclical; periods of acute pain are followed by temporary healing, only to be succeeded by further acute pain.

DIAGNOSIS

The patient should be examined in the left lateral position. Visual examination may disclose a posterior oedematous tag and, on parting the buttocks, an associated fissure may be seen. Discomfort may be severe enough to prevent a digital rectal examination being performed. At some stage in the patient's treatment sigmoidoscopy should be undertaken, under anaesthesia if necessary, to exclude specific causes of fissure, including inflammatory bowel disease (especially Crohn's disease), anal syphilis, anal herpes, anal carcinoma, lymphoma, anoreceptive intercourse (with or without HIV infection), and, in children, sexual abuse.

MANAGEMENT

The principle of management is to break the vicious cycle, thus allowing the fissure to heal by reducing internal anal sphincter spasm.

Conservative management

Acute fissures may heal following alteration of stool consistency. Warm sitz baths and dietary bran produce better symptomatic relief than either hydrocortisone cream or lignocaine gel applied locally in patients suffering from a first attack of posterior anal fissure. Continued consumption of unprocessed bran (15 g/day) may also reduce the recurrence rate. Healing rates of 80 per cent have been reported following 3 weeks' treatment with Proctosedyl ointment (cinchocaine anaesthetic 0.5 per cent and hydrocortisone 0.5 per cent).

The need for regular use of an anal dilator and local anaesthetic gel is debatable. Although this regimen has produced healing rates of 54 per cent, other studies were unable to demonstrate any improvement in the healing of anal fissures when a dilator was used in addition to locally applied lignocaine gel. The presence of anal tags and polyps has been cited as contraindication to conservative therapy since there is a high rate of referral to surgery in these patients.

Use of an anal dilator

If an anal dilator is to be used the surgeon must ensure that the patient can demonstrate understanding of its use. The patient is instructed to smear local anaesthetic ointment on to the dilator, to lie on the left side and to insert the dilator up to its hilt, whilst retaining hold of the dilator. The dilator should be kept in this position for 30 to 60 s, removed, and washed in soapy water. The procedure should be performed twice daily.

Surgical management

Surgical management aims to reduce internal sphincter spasm either by maximal anal dilatation or by internal sphincterotomy.

Maximal anal dilatation

This procedure was first suggested by Recamier in 1838, but became popular following its use by Lord in 1968. It may be performed under local or general anaesthesia. Maximal anal dilatation produces immediate relief from proctalgia in between 75 and 95 per cent of patients, but the recurrence rate is around 10 per cent. Early postoperative complications include bleeding and prolapsing haemorrhoids, and there may be a temporary impairment of control of flatus and faecal soiling.

Internal sphincterotomy

This operation was first described by Eisenhammer, who divided the sphincter in the posterior position. The recurrence rate following posterior sphincterotomy and fissurectomy is equal to that following lateral sphincterotomy, but the time taken for the wound to heal is double that of lateral sphincterotomy and there is also a greater incidence of postoperative faecal soiling, which is reported to occur in around 25 per cent of patients following posterior sphincterotomy.

Lateral sphincterotomy

Parkes described open lateral sphincterotomy in 1967. Postoperative pain and incontinence are less common following this procedure than after posterior sphincterotomy. The procedure was modified by Notaras in 1969, who described the technique of lateral subcutaneous sphincterotomy: this produces immediate relief of proctalgia in 90 to 100 per cent of patients, healing of the fissure within 2 to 4 weeks in 80 to 98 per cent, and fissure recurs in less than 5 per cent. The operation may be performed under local or general anaesthesia, but better results are obtained when general anaesthesia is used.

Lateral subcutaneous sphincterotomy causes temporary impairment of control of flatus in no more than 10 per cent of patients, while faecal soiling occurs in less than 7 per cent. Three randomized prospective studies comparing anal dilatation and lateral subcutaneous sphincterotomy have demonstrated markedly superior results following the surgical procedure.

Operative technique—lateral subcutaneous sphincterotomy

No special preoperative preparation is required and surgery may be undertaken as a day-case procedure under general anaesthesia. The patient is placed in the lithotomy position; 15° of head down tilt is advantageous and the perianal area is shaved. Digital and sigmoidoscopic examination is undertaken if it has not previously been performed.

A lubricated anal retractor (of the Eisenhammer or Park's variety) is inserted into the anal canal and the blades positioned to allow exposure of the anal canal in the lateral (3 or 9 o'clock) position. The groove between the internal and external sphincter muscles can readily be palpated when the retractor is opened (Fig. 3). If desired, 5 to 10 ml of 1 per cent xylocaine and adrenaline (1/200000) solution may be infiltrated into the intersphincteric and submucous spaces (Fig. 4). Using a size 15 scalpel blade a 0.5 to 1 cm radial incision is made in the lateral position over the internal sphincter, exposing the distal edges of the internal and external sphincter muscles (Fig. 5). Holding the medial end of the incised epithelium with forceps, the blades of the dissecting forceps (McIndoe's or Lahey type) are passed into the submucosal space and the handles parted to open up the space. The blades of the scissors are then reinserted into the space

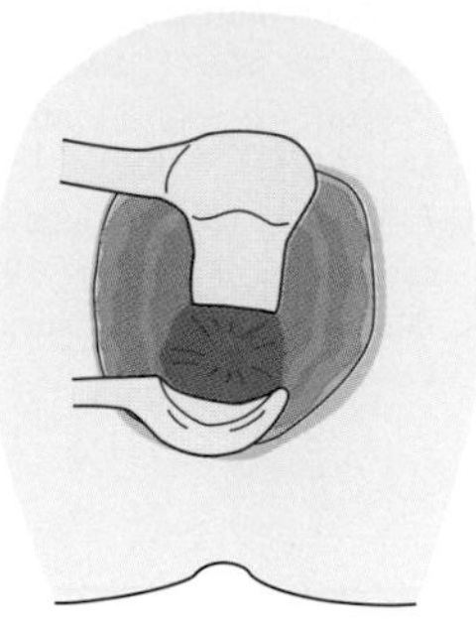

Fig. 3 Line drawing illustrating anal retractor in place and the groove palpable between internal and external anal sphincters.

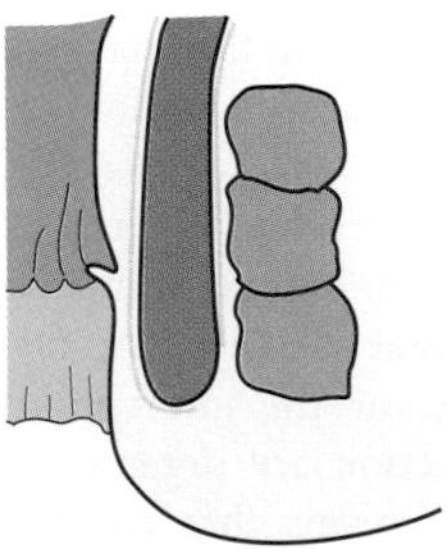

Fig. 4 Cross-section of anal canal illustrating anal sphincter, intersphincteric, and submucous spaces.

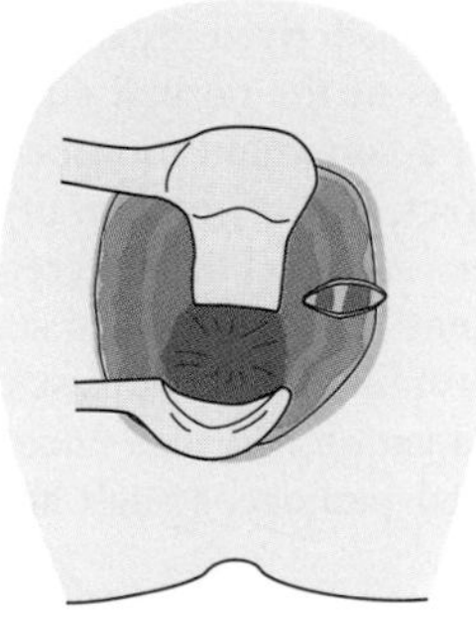

Fig. 5 Line drawing illustrating radial incision exposing internal and external sphincters.

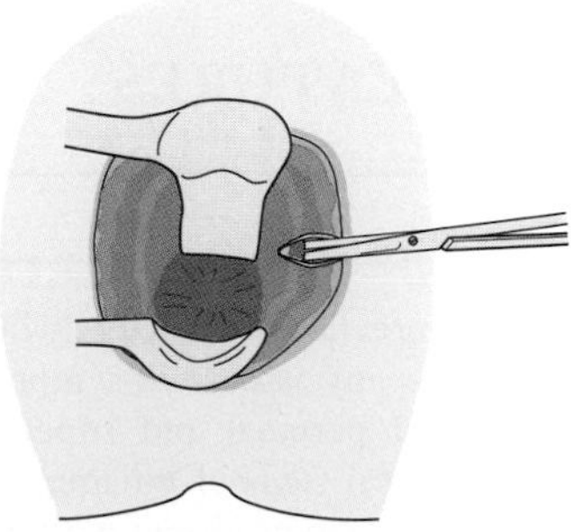

Fig. 6 Line drawing illustrating scissor method of opening submucosal and intersphincteric plane.

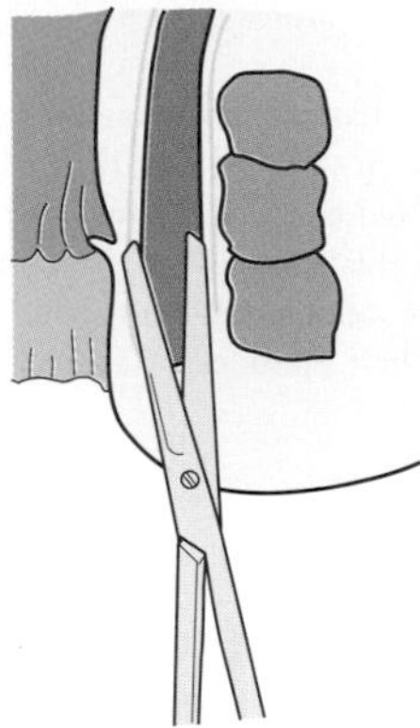

Fig. 7 Cross-section of anal canal illustrating proximal limit of division of internal sphincter muscle.

between the internal and external sphincter muscles and the handles parted to open up this plane (Fig. 6). The scissors are then withdrawn and introduced with the blades parted, one to lie in the intersphincteric space, the other to lie in the submucous space. The index finger of the left hand of the operator is inserted into the anal canal, the finger tip being placed at the level of the dentate line, and the scissor handles closed to divide the internal sphincter muscle from this point distally (Fig. 7). Associated tags and polyps can be excised. A dry gauze dressing is placed over the wound. Stool softeners and bulking agents should be administered from 48 h preoperatively and during the postoperative period and mild oral analgesia may be necessary for 24 to 48 h postoperatively, when slight perianal bruising may be observed.

Treatment in special situations

Children

Acute fissure-in-ano in children usually responds to treatment with stool softeners (lactulose), bulking agents, and locally applied anaesthetic ointment. In rare instances, gentle anal dilatation with Hegar's dilators or lateral sphincterotomy may be required. It is important to remember that painful diarrhoea in children may be the presenting symptom of anal fissure, since proctalgia may result in faecal retention and spurious diarrhoea.

Crohn's disease

Fissure-in-ano may account for 26 per cent of new referrals for patients with Crohn's disease. Medical treatment of the disease usually results in healing of the fissure, as does surgical excision of intestinal Crohn's disease. Extreme caution is advised when undertaking local anal surgery: examination under anaesthesia and drainage of local sepsis may be all that is necessary to relieve symptoms. Sphincterotomy is extremely hazardous since this may be followed by widespread pelvic sepsis and fistula formation.

FURTHER READING

Bennett RC, Goligher JC. Results of internal sphincterotomy for anal fissure. *Br Med J* 1962; **ii**: 1500–3.

Gough M, Lewis A. The conservative treatment of fissure-in-ano. *Br J Surg* 1983; **70**: 175–6.

Hawley PR. The treatment of chronic fissure-in-ano, a trial of methods. *Br J Surg* 1969; **56**: 915–8.

Hoffman DC, Goligher JC. Lateral subcutaneous internal sphincterotomy in treatment of anal fissure. *Br Med* J 1970; **iii**: 673–5.

Jensen SL, Lund F, Nielsen OV, Tange G. Lateral subcutaneous sphincterotomy vs anal dilatation in the treatment of fissure-in-ano in outpatients: a prospective randomized study. *Br Med J* 1984; **289**: 528–30.

Jensen SL. Treatment of first episodes of acute anal fissure: a prospective randomised study of lignocaine ointment versus hydrocortisone ointment or warm sitz baths plus bran. *Br Med J* 1986; **292**: 1167–9.

Lock MR, Thomson JPS. Fissure-in-ano: the initial management and prognosis. *Br J Surg* 1977; **64**: 355–8.

McDonald P, Driscoll AM, Nicholls RJ. The anal dilator in the conservative management of acute anal fissures. *Br J Surg* 1987; **70**: 25–6.

Sweeney JL, Ritchie JK, Nicholls RJ. Anal fissure in Crohn's disease. *Br J Surg* 1988; **75**: 56–7.

20.4 Anorectal abscess

TERENCE O'KELLY AND NEIL MORTENSEN

A clear understanding of anorectal anatomy and pathology are essential for the successful management of this common surgical problem.

ANATOMY

The anal canal and rectum are surrounded by a number of potential tissue spaces, and anorectal abscesses are classified according to which of these they occupy (Fig. 1). Perianal and ischiorectal abscesses are encountered most frequently, representing 80 per cent of cases. Intermuscular and perirectal abscesses are much less common. It should be remembered that sepsis can spread with time and more than one space can therefore be affected simultaneously.

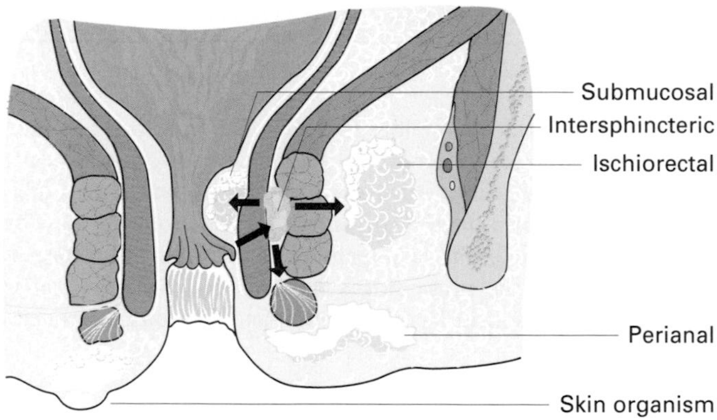

Fig. 1 The anatomy and classificiation of anorectal abscess.

AETIOLOGY

In about 20 per cent of patients with anorectal abscess there is a clear predisposing cause, such as inflammatory bowel disease (especially Crohn's disease), anorectal cancer, anal fissure, complicated haemorrhoids, or local trauma. Perirectal abscesses, lying between the levator ani and the pelvic peritoneum, can occur secondary to infection of another pelvic structure such as a fallopian tube or the prostate. In the majority of cases, however, no obvious cause can be demonstrated, and sepsis arising in an anal gland is frequently, but not invariably the culprit. There are 6 to 10 such glands distributed around the anal canal which drain into the base of the anal crypts. Glands commonly ramify into the internal anal sphincter and can extend as far as the intersphincteric plane. Perianal infection may develop when a gland fails to drain adequately. If this results in abscess formation, then the communication with the anal canal often leads to involvement of either the internal anal sphincter or the intersphincteric plane (or both). Other sources of infection are organisms that invade from the perianal skin, and organisms that enter from a distant site by haematogenous spread. The former is the more common of these.

BACTERIOLOGY

Culture of pus from an anorectal abscess generally discloses one of two populations of pathogens whose presence correlates with the underlying aetiology: skin-derived organisms such as *Staphylococcus aureus* and members of the normal gut flora. The former are rarely associated with a communication between the abscess and the gastrointestinal tract, whilst isolation of the latter makes such a communication very likely. This difference has an important bearing on management: it is essential to send a specimen of pus for microbiological examination in all cases of anorectal abscess. Microbiological investigation may also uncover infection with less commonly encountered pathogens such as *Mycobacterium tuberculosis* or Actinomyces.

AGE AND SEX

Anorectal abscesses affect both sexes but are 2 to 3 times more common in men than women. Abscesses can occur at any age, but are most common in the fourth to the sixth decades of life.

CLINICAL FEATURES

History

The position of an anorectal abscess largely determines its mode of presentation as well as any associated symptoms. Pain is a prominent initial feature of perianal and superficial ischiorectal abscesses, followed by local signs of inflammation. Such symptoms are less evident or may even be absent with deep infections, which tend to develop insidiously with pyrexia and systemic upset. This can lead to diagnostic confusion.

In all cases, it is important to establish whether there is a history of previous episodes of anorectal sepsis and how these were treated. The possibility of a predisposing cause should be explored.

Examination

Superficial lesions produce obvious signs of acute inflammation. In the case of a perianal abscess, there is a localized, fluctuant, red, hot, and tender swelling close to the anus. Such signs are more diffuse in patients with ischiorectal sepsis, where fluctuance is a late finding. Other features that might be noted are skin necrosis, if there is gross swelling, and crepitus if a gas-forming organism is present.

Deeper infections produce less obvious abnormalities, and these are only apparent on digital rectal examination. The diagnostic clue in such instances is the presence of a tender mass or an area of induration. Fluctuance may be detected. It is important to ascertain the position of such lesions with respect to the gut tube and the pelvic floor as this can have an important bearing on subsequent management.

INVESTIGATION

In most instances, diagnosis is established from the history and examination. Where doubt remains, endoluminal ultrasound (anal and rectal) as well as computerized axial tomography (CAT) may be helpful. Examination under anaesthesia as a primary diagnostic procedure may be required.

If the clinical findings suggest a predisposing condition, it should be investigated on its own merits. Locally invasive procedures such as sigmoidoscopy should be performed under general anaesthetic to prevent undue discomfort to the patient.

TREATMENT

Relief of symptoms and prevention of further tissue damage

This is achieved by incision and drainage after the patient has been examined under an appropriate anaesthetic. The site of drainage will generally be dictated by the clinical findings, but should be placed over the most dependent part of the abscess, as close to the anal canal as possible. Linear incisions are recommended as these cause minimum tissue damage. The abscess cavity should be examined for possible extensions and all loculi must be broken down. The cavity should be curetted and necrotic tissue excised. Additional treatment with antibiotics is not usually required.

Investigation of an underlying cause

It is clearly important to establish whether there is a communication between the abscess and the gastrointestinal tract. A specimen of pus should be sent for microbiological examination and the anal canal and abscess cavity should be examined for the presence of a fistula. Gentle pressure on the abscess may cause release of pus into the anal canal, demonstrating the site of an internal opening. If a fistula (see Section 20.5) is thought to exist, its path can be explored with a Lockhart–Mummery probe, and it can either be laid open, if it is very low, or it can be marked with a seton for subsequent definitive treatment. If a fistula cannot be demonstrated then no further immediate measures are required.

Action in cases where a fistula is not found at the first operation

Further intervention is not indicated if the pus specimen contains skin flora only. However, additional measures are recommended if gut-derived organisms are cultured, since the possibility of an underlying fistula remains. Ideally, the patient should be reviewed under anaesthetic 7 to 10 days after the initial procedure. This should be a sufficient delay to allow inflammation to subside and so increase the chance of demonstrating any fistula that may be present. A detailed account of fistula management is given in Section 20.5.

Treatment protocols for anorectal abscesses include simple drainage only and drainage followed by primary closure combined with systemic antibiotic therapy. Such measures can be effective but they reduce the chance of demonstrating an underlying communication with the gut and thus increase the possibility of future anorectal sepsis.

FURTHER READING

Goligher J. Anorectal abscess. In: Goligher J, ed. *Surgery of the Anus, Rectum and Colon*. London: Bailliere Tindall, 1984: 167–177

Grace RH, Harper IA, Thompson RG. Anorectal sepsis: microbiology in relation to fistula-in-ano. *Br J Surg* 1982; **69**: 401–3.

Grace RH. The management of acute anorectal sepsis. *Ann R Coll Surg* 1990; 72: 160–2.

20.5 Fistula-in-ano

NEIL MORTENSEN

A fistula-in-ano is an abnormal communication between the anal canal or rectum and the perianal skin. This simple definition is complicated, however, by the fact that there may be no internal opening, there may be no external opening, and the track itself may be very complex. The most common cause of fistula in ano is anal gland sepsis (Fig. 1(a and b)). A resulting perianal abscess may drain through the perianal skin and heal spontaneously or may persist as a fistula-in-ano. A small number of such fistulae-in-ano are caused by trauma, anal surgical injury or, in the case of extrasphincteric fistula, diverticular disease or foreign body

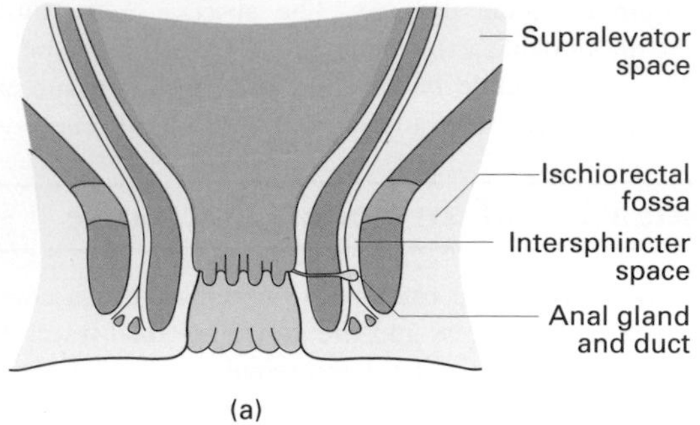

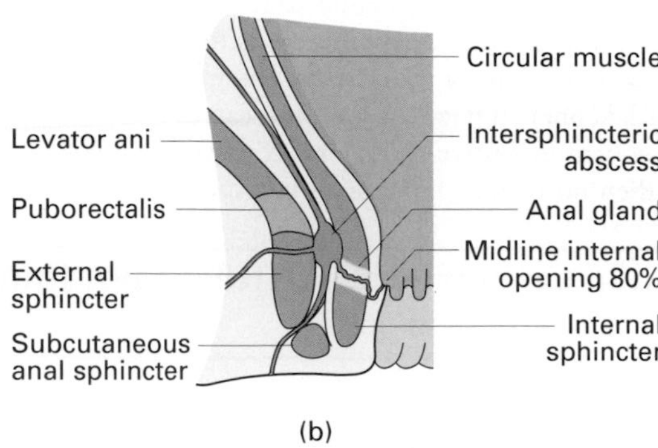

Fig. 1 (a) Anatomy of the anal canal showing an anal gland in the intersphincteric space, with the glandular duct opening in the anal canal at the dentate line. (b) Coronal section of anal canal, showing the relationship between the anal gland, an intersphincteric abscess and the possible paths fistula tracks can take within the sphincter complex.

perforation of the rectosigmoid. In addition, diseases such as ulcerative colitis, Crohn's disease, tuberculosis and, occasionally, anal canal carcinoma may cause an irregularity or distortion of the opening of the anal glands, predisposing to a fistula with ensuing cryptoglandular infection. Rarely the threadworm *Enterobius vermicularis* may cause anal gland infection and fistula formation.

CLASSIFICATION

The most widely used classification is that of Parks *et al.* (1976); that of Eisenhammer (1978) is very similar. These classifications emphasize the relationship between the fistula and the external sphincter muscle. The frequencies of the various types of fistula are shown in Table 1.

Table 1 Classification of 769 fistulae (Marks and Ritchie 1977)

Superficial	16.4%
Intersphincteric	55.9%
Trans-sphincteric	21.3%
Suprasphincteric	3.4%
Extrasphincteric	3.0%

PRINCIPLES OF MANAGEMENT

The management in fistula in ano aims to eradicate the sepsis in the anal gland whilst preserving the maximum amount of anal function (Table 2).

Table 2 Management of anal fistula

Definition of anatomy
Surgical drainage of abscess and tracks
Eradication of anal gland origin
Preservation of sphincter function
Postoperative care of the wound

Table 3 Anal fistula: methods of assessment

Palpation for induration
Examination under anaesthesia
Palpation
Probes
Lockhart–Mummery
Lacrimal
Injection
Methylene blue
H_2O_2
Lay open/currettage–granulation tissue
Imaging techniques
Fistulography
Anal ultrasonography
CT
MRI

Assessment

The first step in successful management is careful assessment (Table 3). Inspection of the perianal area may or may not reveal an obvious perianal sinus representing the external opening of a fistula (Fig. 2). On palpation there is the important sign of induration, not only in the skin around the external opening, but also along the course of the fistula track. Any degree of sepsis in the intersphincteric plane will cause considerable thickening in that region. Induration at the junction between the pelvic floor and the upper anal canal, so called 'supralevator induration', is an important physical sign of uncontrolled sepsis spreading up to the supralevator space from the intersphincteric plane. Goodsall's law may be helpful, indicating the most likely position for the internal opening (Fig. 3). It is worth remembering that the abscess in the intersphincteric plane can extend in a horseshoe around the circumference of the anal canal. The anal canal and rectum should be carefully examined by rectoscopy and proctoscopy to exclude any other local lesion. Occasionally an internal opening, sometimes disclosed by a small bead of pus will be seen, but this is unusual.

Examination under anaesthesia

Palpation should be repeated under anaesthesia and the extent of the tracks defined using probes designed by Lockhart Mummery:

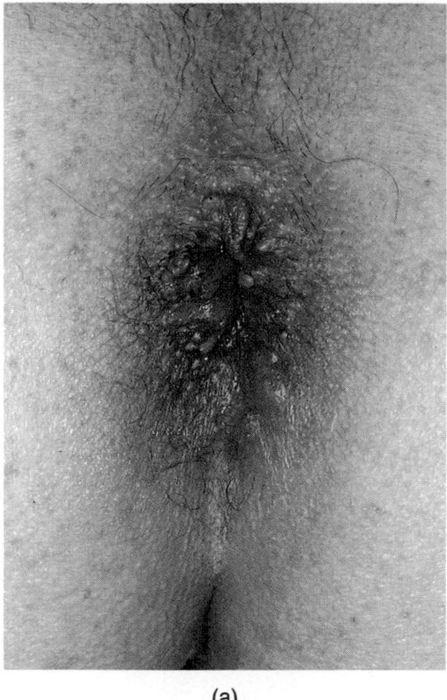
(a)

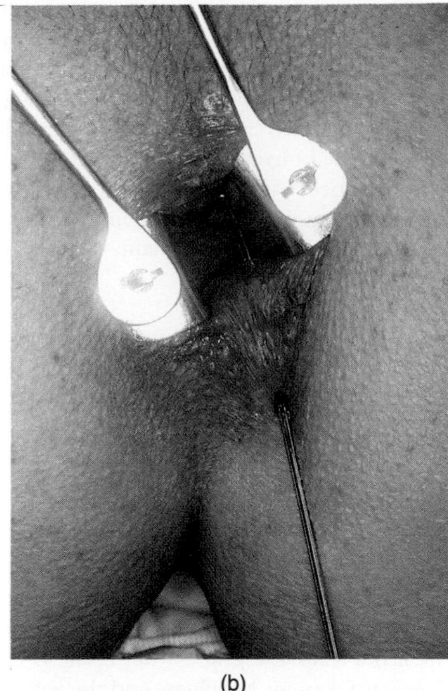
(b)

Fig. 2 (a) Typical appearance of the external opening in a fistula in ano. (b) Probe passed through fistula.

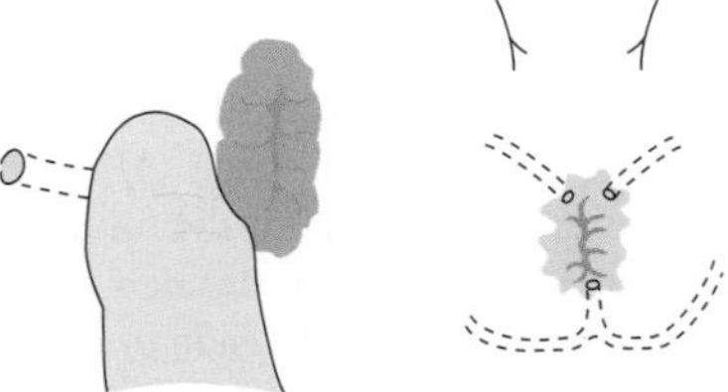

Fig. 3 Goodsall's law. Anterior to a line bisecting the perianum transversely fistula tracks pass radially directly into the anal canal. Posterior to the line fistulae pass backwards tending to enter the anal canal in the midline posteriorly.

lacrymal probes are too soft (Fig. 4). A probe should be passed through the external opening whilst 'feeling' with the examining index finger in the anal canal (Fig. 5). Injection of methylene blue has the disadvantage that staining of tissues may make appreciation of the true extent of the tracks more difficult. Injection of hydrogen peroxide into the external opening of the fistula will not stain tissues, but the appearance of bubbles in the anal canal with an anal retractor in place will confirm a fistula and define the position of the internal opening. If probing does not reveal the extent of the track the superficial part of the fistula should be laid open, looking for the characteristic granulation tissue of the lining of the track. The opened track is probed again, and if necessary the incision is extended until the anatomy of the fistula is clear.

Imaging techniques

A number of imaging techniques have been introduced but these are still being developed and are no substitute for careful palpation. Fistulography may be helpful in the investigation of the rare

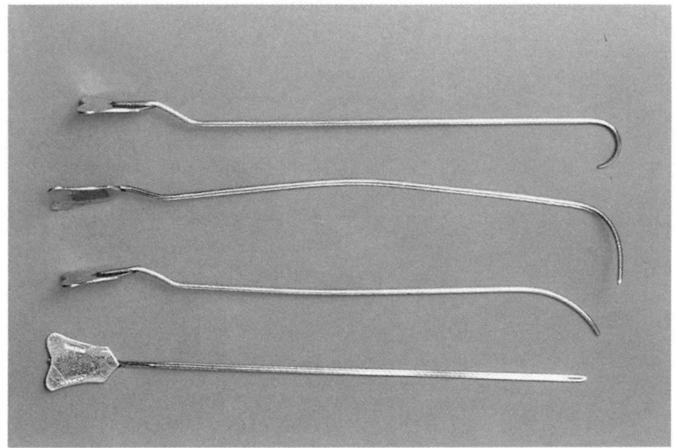

Fig. 4 Lockhart-Mummery fistula probes. The varying angulation of the fistula tip gives a choice of probes for difficult parts of the track and for different types of fistula. The 'umbrella' probe is particularly useful for identifying an internal opening.

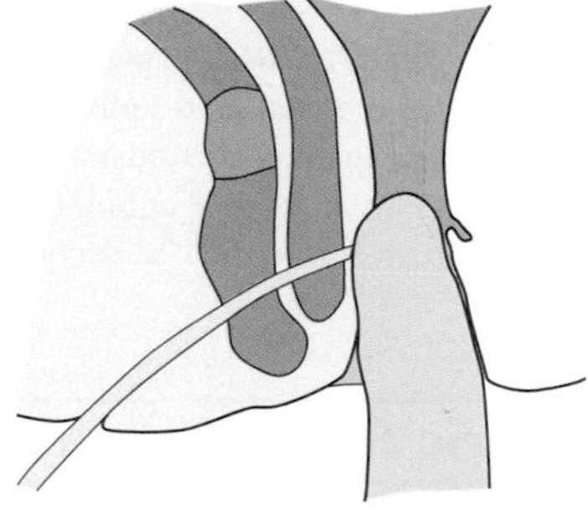

Fig. 5 Probe in the fistula track, examining finger in the anal canal. 'Feeling' for the fistula track internal opening.

extrasphincteric fistula, but is rarely necessary in simpler fistulae. CT and magnetic resonance imaging scanning have both been used in the assessment of fistula-in-ano but without any convincing evidence of improvement in management. Anal ultrasonography is not yet widely available, but can demonstrate secondary tracks and abscesses, and the use of hydrogen peroxide to show up bubbles in the fistula track which have a characteristic echo-rich appearance may improve its accuracy. Breaches in the internal sphincter and changes in the intersphincteric plane can be seen.

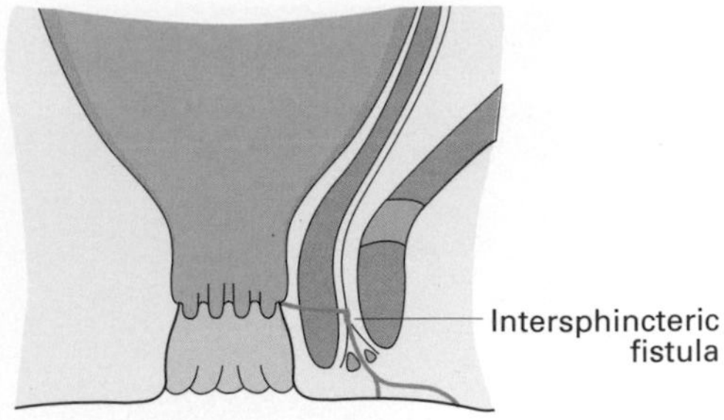

Fig. 7 Intersphincteric fistula.

TREATMENT OF FISTULA-IN-ANO

Superficial fistula-in-ano

A superficial fistula is treated simply by laying it open (Fig. 6): at the most this may involve dividing the distal internal anal sphincter. Care is needed in the midline posteriorly, where the guttering caused by this partial sphincterotomy can sometimes cause problems with incomplete closure of the anal canal and soiling. Having laid open the track the granulation tissue is carefully curetted out, a biopsy is taken for histology, and the wound is cleaned and dressed with a superficial dressing rather than by tight packing. Postoperative care is just as important as the operation: the patient should take daily baths and the anal wound should be reviewed soon after the procedure.

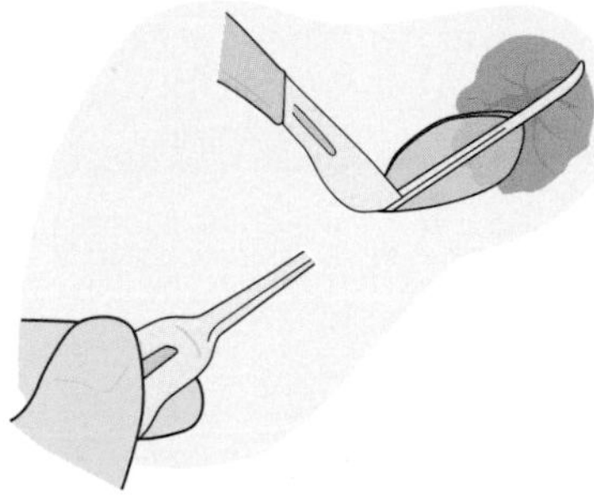

Fig. 6 The simple lay open operation over a fistula probe for superficial fistula-in-ano.

Intersphincteric fistula-in-ano

The standard treatment (Fig. 7) is to lay open the intersphincteric track by dividing the distal internal anal sphincter, curetting out the anal gland and then draining any secondary tracks. Again, care must be taken in dividing the internal sphincter in the midline posteriorly to avoid guttering and subsequent continence problems.

Trans-sphincteric fistula-in-ano

Similar principles apply in the management of trans-sphincteric fistula (Fig. 8). The intersphincteric abscess should be drained, together with any secondary tracks. Occasionally a secondary track passes upwards to the top of the ischiorectal fossa or through the pelvic floor to the supralevator space. A primary track below the anal valves should be drained by dividing the external anal sphincter; if above the anal valves it is drained using a seton. Great care must be taken in the judicious division of muscle. In the study by Marks and Ritchie (1977) 164 of 796 fistulae in ano were trans-sphincteric; 7 per cent of these had tracks below the anal valves, and in 14 per cent the primary track was at or above the level of the anal valves.

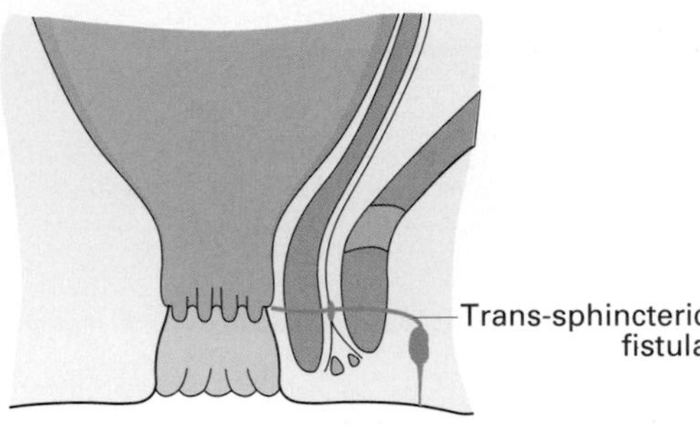

Fig. 8 Trans-sphincteric fistula. An abscess can present either in the intersphincteric plane or the space outside the external sphincter.

Suprasphincteric fistula-in-ano

These are fortunately rare. The track passes straight upwards in the intersphincteric space, over the puborectalis muscle and down through the ischiorectal fossa to the skin. There may be an associated horseshoe abscess in the supralevator space (Fig. 9).

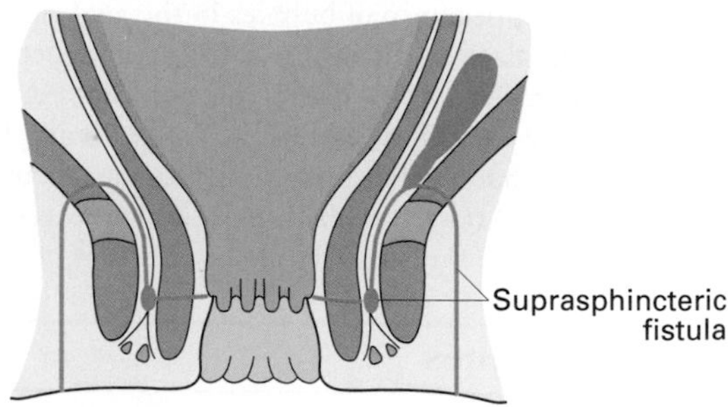

Fig. 9 Suprasphincteric fistula. The track encompasses all the muscles of continence. Note the supralevator space abscess that may be present.

Division of the track would result in certain incontinence. The intersphincteric space is drained and the anal gland curretted out. A seton is then passed around the external anal sphincter. Healing may take many months.

The place of a seton in management

Linen, silk and nylon thread have been used as a seton but a brightly coloured soft plastic vessel loop is easy to identify and comfortable for the patient to sit upon. There is some debate over the method of action of a seton: some clinicians feel that it works as a slow elastic ligature and therefore must be tightened periodically. A second school feel that the seton acts by ensuring chronic drainage of the fistula track (Fig. 10). In a series reported by Thomson and Ross (1989) the sphincter was preserved in 44 per cent of patients after a prolonged period of seton drainage. The seton could then be removed and the fistula healed. In the other 56 per cent, the external sphincter was divided after prolonged seton drainage allowing subsequent healing. A seton certainly allows time for any sepsis and induration to settle before a decision about further treatment is made. As a general principle it is important to leave the seton in place for many months and to be prepared to perform repeated examinations of the area under anaesthesia when the anatomy of the fistula is not clear. Some have suggested that the use of a seton in the management of less complex fistulae may avoid any muscle division at all, but recurrence rates after this approach have not been reported.

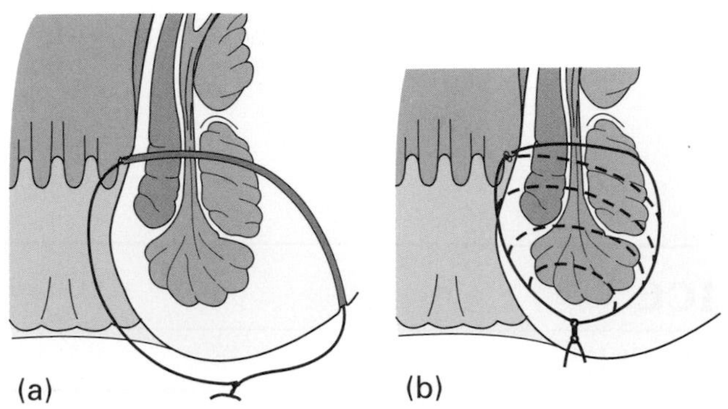

Fig. 10 Mechanism of action of a seton. (a) Chronic drainage. (b) Slow elastic ligature.

Flap techniques

There are two further alternative approaches to the trans-sphincteric or suprasphincteric fistula that allow for optimum preservation of sphincter muscle. Aguilar *et al.* (1985) have described a technique which preserves the internal sphincter by using an endoanal flap advanced over the internal opening (Fig. 11). The intersphincteric abscess is, of course, drained and the external part of the track in the perianal area is cleaned out. Wedell *et al.* (1987) used a flap including muscle while Mann and Clifton (1985) have described a procedure in which the external sphincter is divided and the fistula rerouted inside it. The external sphincter is immediately repaired to allow for complete excision of the fistula without the undivided support of any sphincter muscle (Fig. 12).

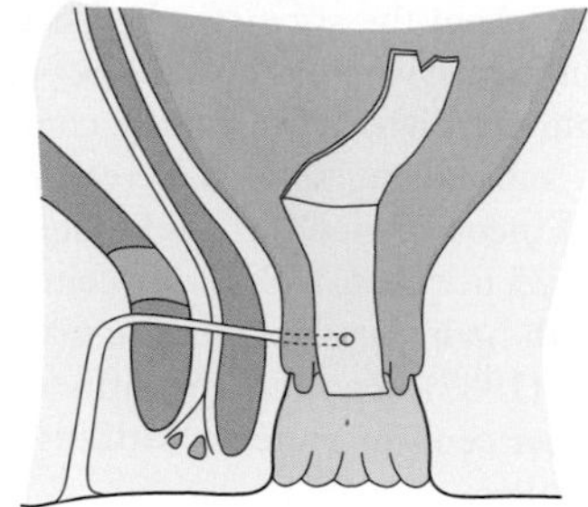

Fig. 11 Flap advancement technique for trans-sphincteric fistula. The external fistula component has been excised and curretted. The external anal sphincter has been closed. A flap has been raised to be sutured over the defect.

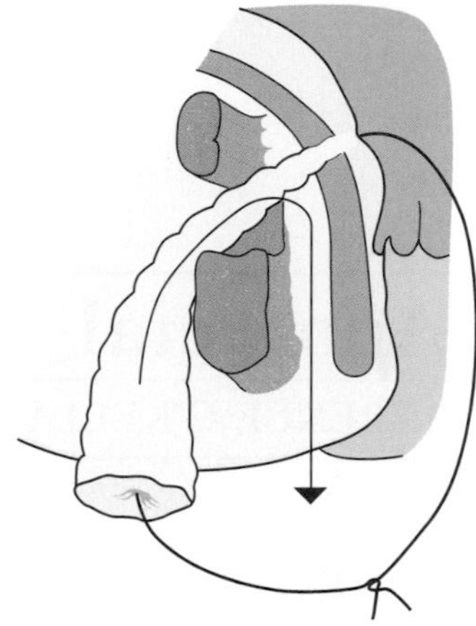

Fig. 12 Rerouting technique. The cored out trans-sphincteric track is displaced inside the external anal sphincter which is repaired primarily. The fistula can then be excised in the intersphincteric plane or transposed submucosally to allow immediate repair of the internal anal sphincter.

Patients treated by these procedures have not been followed for long periods, but there is an increasing trend towards maximum preservation of sphincter muscle in fistula surgery.

Colostomy

A defunctioning colostomy is not necessary in the management of most fistula patients but they should undergo meticulous bowel preparation and systemic antibiotics. Where uncontrolled sepsis complicates a trans-sphincteric or suprasphincteric fistula, a colostomy may be indicated.

Anal continence

The two crucial outcomes of fistula surgery are anal sphincter function and recurrence of the fistula. In a study by Belliveau, *et al.* (1983) anal canal pressures in a group of patients in whom the external sphincter had been divided were compared with a group in whom the external sphincter had been preserved and with a control group. The resting anal canal and voluntary contraction pressures were significantly diminished after external sphincter division. Of those in whom the sphincter had been preserved, 83 per cent had full continence whereas only 32 per cent of those who had undergone sphincter division were fully continent, and some of these needed a subsequent sphincter repair. In a study by Girona *et al.* (1987) incontinence for solids, liquids, and gas was seen in 4.3 per cent, 25 per cent, and 21 per cent respectively, of a group of patients with high trans-sphincteric fistulae 3 years after treatment. Parnaud (1987) reported incontinence rates varying between 16 and 26 per cent for patients with intersphincteric and trans-sphincteric fistulae.

Fortunately these difficult trans- and suprasphincteric fistulae are seen in a minority of patients, but expert surgical management is required in order to avoid recurrence and postoperative incontinence.

FURTHER READING

Aguilar PS, Plasencia G, Hardy TG, Hartmann RF, Stewart WRC. Mucosal advancement in the treatment of anal fistula. *Dis Colon Rect* 1985; **28**: 496–8.

Belliveau P, Thomson JPS, Parks AG. Fistula in ano. A manometric study. *Dis Colon Rect* 1983; **26**: 152–4.

Eisenhammer S. The final evaluation and classification of the surgical treatment of the primary anorectal cryptoglandular intermuscular (intersphincteric) fistulous abscess and fistula. *Dis Colon Rect* 1978; **21**: 237–54.

Girona J. Symposium. Fistula in ano. *Int J Colorect Dis* 1987; **2**: 51–71.

Mann CV, Clifton MA. Re-routing of the track for the treatment of high anal and anorectal fistulae. *Br J Surg* 1985; **72**: 134–7.

Marks CG, Ritchie JK. Anal fistulae at St Mark's Hospital. *Br J Surg* 1977; **64**: 84–91.

Parks AG, Gordon PH, Hardcastle JD. A classification of fistula in ano. *Br J Surg* 1976; **63**: 1–12.

Parnaud E. Symposium: Fistula in ano. *Int J Colorect Dis* 1987; **2**: 51–71.

Thomson JPS, Ross AH McL. Can the external anal sphincter be preserved in the treatment of trans-sphincteric fistula in ano? *Int J Colorect Dis* 1989; **4**: 247–50.

Wedell J, Meier ZN, Eissen P, Banzhaf F, Kleine L. Sliding flap advancement for the treatment of high level fistulae. *Br J Surg* 1987; **74**: 390–1.

20.6 Anorectal incontinence

TERENCE O'KELLY AND NEIL MORTENSEN

INTRODUCTION

Anorectal incontinence is a relatively common and profoundly disabling complaint, which can be defined as the inability to delay discharge from the anal canal until a suitable moment arises. In the community, the prevalence of anorectal incontinence increases with age such that 1.1 per cent of men and 1.3 per cent of women over 65 years of age are affected. Some groups, notably long-stay geriatric and psychogeriatric patients, are more commonly affected, with up to 60 per cent suffering leaks of faeces each day.

THE MAINTENANCE OF NORMAL ANORECTAL CONTINENCE

This is achieved by the interplay of functional sphincters, anorectal sensitivity, rectal compliance, and stool composition. Of these, the smooth muscle internal anal and striated muscle external anal sphincters are of prime importance. Both are tonically active at rest but the internal anal sphincter is responsible for 80 per cent of tone in this state. The internal sphincter relaxes in response to rectal distension (the rectosphincteric reflex) and its importance in normal and disordered continence is being increasingly recognized.

The external sphincter encircles the internal anal sphincter and is innervated by the pudendal nerve (sacral roots S3 and S4). Its activity is recruited when continence is threatened, either by raised intra-abdominal pressure (coughing or straining) or when the internal sphincter relaxes and defecation is not planned. Superiorly, the external and sphincter blends with puborectalis. The forward pull of this, the most medial part of the levator ani, produces angulation at the anorectal junction and luminal occlusion. The puborectalis therefore functions as a sphincter, enhancing continence to solids. It does not, however, act as a 'flap valve' as was previously thought.

The anal canal has a rich sensory innervation that is able to discriminate between gas, liquids, and solids. Sensory nerve endings may be brought into contact with the contents of the rectum in a process called anorectal sampling. Sampling occurs subconsciously several times each minute and is facilitated by internal sphincter relaxation which abolishes the pressure gradient between the rectum and upper anal canal (Fig. 1). Mechanoreceptors that lie in the muscles of the pelvic floor and side walls subserve the sensation of rectal fullness.

Even if the motor and sensory components of the anal canal function normally, continence can still be threatened by the arrival of copious amounts of fluid stool, especially if rectal compliance is diminished, as it is in patients with inflammatory bowel disease or following irradiation.

THE CAUSES OF ANORECTAL INCONTINENCE

Anorectal incontinence can occur when any facet of the normal continence mechanism is defective. The causes of such abnormalities are outlined in Table 1, and some are discussed below.

Faecal impaction

This common cause of incontinence should always be considered in the elderly and patients in institutions. Those affected show diminished anorectal sensation combined with a failure of the

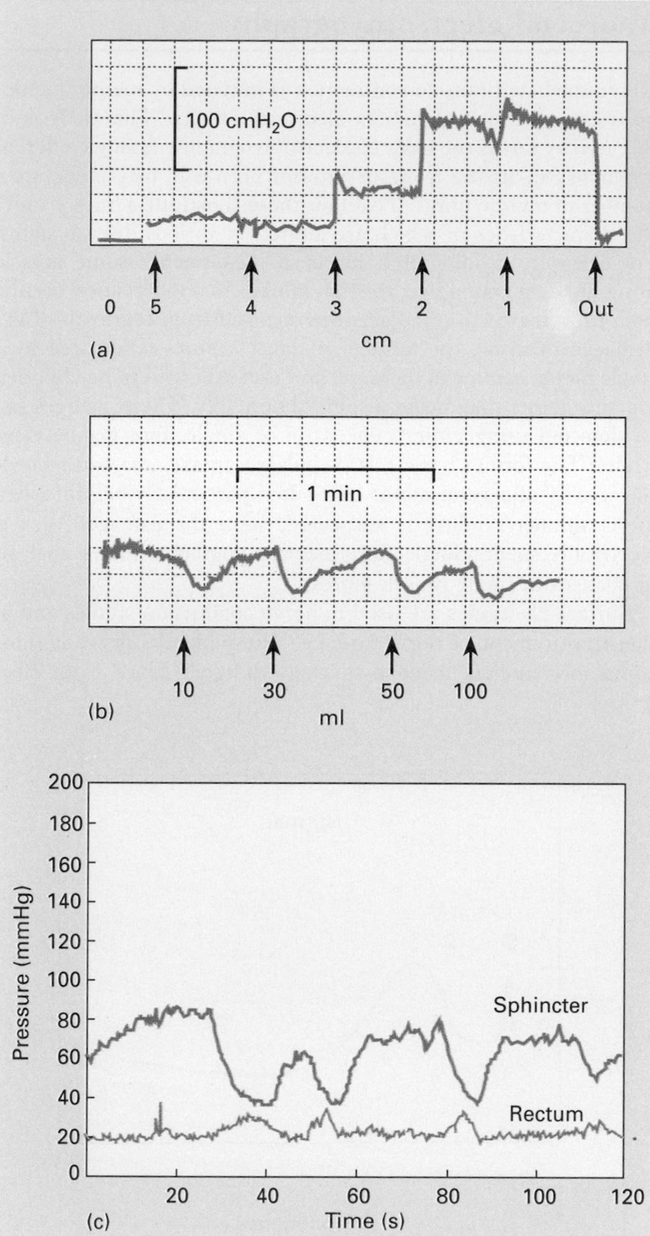

Fig. 1 Anorectal manometry recordings in the resting state showing (a) the anal canal pressure profile on withdrawal of a balloon tipped catheter from the rectum, (b) relaxation of the internal anal sphincter as the rectum is progressively distended by an air filled balloon (the rectosphincteric reflex), and (c) episodic relaxations of the internal and sphincter which equalize rectal and anal canal pressures and facilitate anorectal sampling.

external sphincter to respond to internal sphincter relaxations. In addition, the internal sphincter relaxes at lower levels of rectal distension when compared with normal age-related individuals.

Direct sphincter injury

The sphincters may be divided erroneously at the time of anorectal surgery or may be damaged by accidental injuries. Direct sphincter injury also occurs during childbirth, making this a significant and potentially preventable cause of incontinence. Patients who sustain anal sphincter injuries during childbirth should be offered elective caesarian section in subsequent pregnancies to prevent further damage.

Table 1 The causes of anorectal incontinence.

Incontinence with normal sphincters
Severe diarrhoea
Inflammatory bowel disease
Faecal impaction
Fistula
Dementia or mental retardation
Incontinence with abnormal sphincters
Direct sphincter injury
Surgical
Trauma
Obstetric
Sphincter neuropathy
Upper motor neurone lesions
Cerebral-tumour, stroke, trauma
Spinal-demyelination, tumours
Lower motor neurone lesions
Idiopathic
Cauda equina lesions
Pelvic tumours
Demyelination
Diabetes
Congenital abnormalities
Rectal prolapse
Anorectal carcinoma

Idiopathic anorectal incontinence

This is the most common cause of primary anorectal incontinence seen in adult surgical practice, and it particularly affects middle-aged women. Histological and electrophysiological examination of the striated muscle components of the continence mechanism indicate the presence of a denervation/reinnervation injury which is probably caused by stretching of the pudendal and pelvic nerves. Such stretch injuries may occur first during childbirth and are then compounded by subsequent, chronic straining at stool. As well as striated muscle weakness, affected patients may have diminished anal sensation, abnormal anorectal sampling and weakness of the internal anal sphincter.

CLINICAL FEATURES

History

All patients attending coloproctology or gastroenterology clinics should be asked directly about anorectal incontinence as this may be a hidden symptom. Many patients complain of diarrhoea when they in fact have urgency and incontinence. The character and frequency of the leakage should be determined and careful attention paid to defecatory, previous medical, and obstetric histories. Neurological symptoms must be documented.

Examination

It is important to perform a complete examination since incontinence can be a manifestation of disease outside the anorectum.

Particular attention should be paid to the abdomen and the innervation of the perineum and lower limbs. Inspection of the perineum, anus, and rectum should be performed with the patient in the left lateral position at rest and while performing the Valsalva manoeuvre. The presence of soiling, scarring, the external opening of a fistula, a patulous anus, perineal descent, and prolapse should be noted. The integrity of perineal innervation should be determined by testing pin-prick sensation and the anocutaneous reflex. Digital anorectal examination allows qualitative assessment of the resting anal pressure as well the changes which occur on voluntary contraction and coughing. Indeed, digital examination performed by an experienced physician may be as good as formal anal manometry in assessing anal sphincter function. The presence of impacted faeces, other masses, and tenderness should be noted. All patients should undergo proctoscopy and sigmoidoscopy to exclude neoplasia, inflammatory bowel disease, fistulae, fissures, mucosal prolapse, and haemorrhoids.

INVESTIGATIONS

A thorough clinical assessment will usually disclose reveal a diagnosis without recourse to specialist investigations. These may, however, be required and are outlined here.

Anorectal manometry

Measurement of anal canal pressures allows assessment of the function of both sphincters. A variety of pressure measuring devices which use perfused, balloon-tipped (air- or water-filled) or microtransducer-tipped catheters is now available. These are inserted into the rectum and then gradually withdrawn. Once the high-pressure zone of the sphincters is reached, the distance from the anal verge is noted and the pressure recorded at 1-cm intervals (stations) as the catheter is removed. The pressure produced by the internal sphincter (maximum resting pressure) and the resting sphincter length can thus be measured (Fig. 1). The procedure is then repeated with the patient attempting to close the anal canal as tightly as possible so that a measure of external sphincter performance is derived (maximum voluntary contraction pressure).

The integrity of the rectosphincteric reflex can be assessed by measuring anal pressures during incremental inflation of a rectal balloon (Fig. 1). Inflation of a balloon in the rectum allows measurement of rectal sensation (recording when distension is first perceived as well as the maximum tolerated volume) and rectal compliance. These features can also be assessed by the saline continence test in which up to 1500 ml of warmed saline is infused into the rectum while anal and rectal pressures are recorded. The volume at which leakage occurs provides another measure of external sphincter function.

Anorectal sensation

Sensation within the anal canal is routinely quantified by measuring anal mucosa electrosensitivity. A constant current of increasing strength is applied between two platinum electrodes mounted on a catheter placed within the anal canal, and the level (mA) at which it is first perceived (a tingling or pulsing sensation) is recorded for the upper, middle, and lower zones of the canal. Sensation is reduced in some patients with anorectal incontinence.

Anorectal electromyography

Nerve-mediated muscle contraction is initiated by membrane depolarization, which generates electrical activity. The analysis of this activity forms the basis of electromyography. A single efferent motor nerve, arising from an anterior horn cell, may innervate a number of muscle fibres. Together these constitute a 'motor unit', the characteristics of which are altered in various disease states. For example, in idiopathic anorectal incontinence some muscle fibres are denervated by a traction injury. As reinnervation occurs, both from ingrowth of adjacent nerves and from regrowth of the damaged neurone, the number of muscle fibres innervated by a single motor nerve will increase, and they will tend to be clumped together rather than being dispersed normally. These changes can be detected using either concentric or single fibre needle electrodes. The former has a relatively large uptake area and records the activity of several motor units. It is particularly helpful when direct sphincter injury is suspected, since the damaged area is electrically silent. Single fibre electromyography allows analysis of changes in single muscle fibres.

Surface electrodes are used in nerve conduction studies and in the measurement of nerve latency. The pudendal nerve is most commonly studied, using a specially designed glove, with elec-

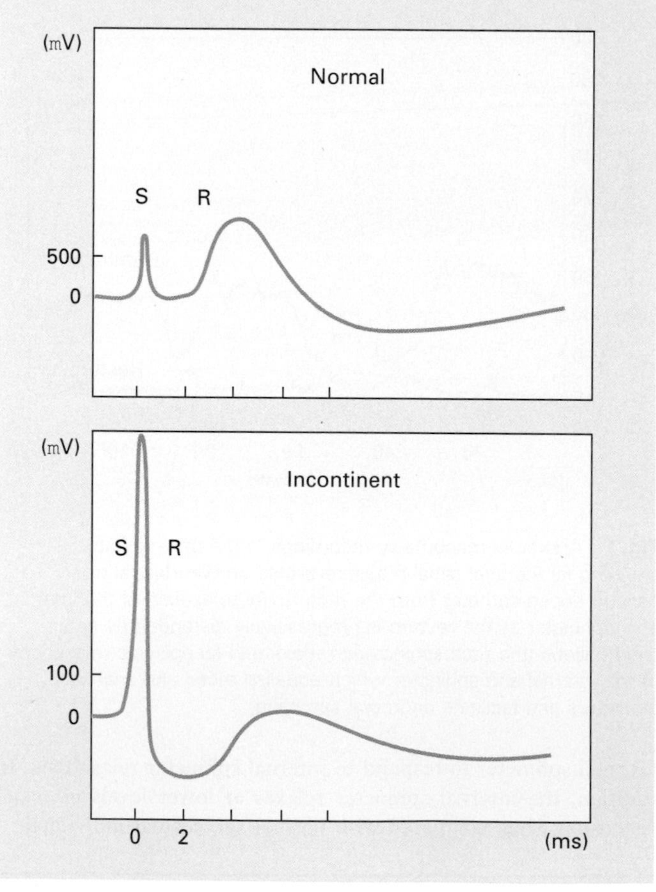

Fig. 2 A comparison of electromyographic recordings from the external anal sphincter in a normal subject and a patient suffering from idiopathic anorectal incontinence after pudendal nerve stimulation (S). In the incontinent patient, nerve conduction is slower and the resulting signal (R) is of diminished amplitude, indicating that there is damage to the nerve.

trodes attached to the tip of the finger. These stimulate the pudendal nerve at the ischial spine and additional electrodes positioned more proximally on the finger detect the resulting contraction of the external sphincter. The speed with which the nerve conducts impulses can thus be measured: this is slowed in idiopathic anorectal incontinence (Fig. 2). Similar studies, using transcutaneous nerve stimulation, can be performed to assess the integrity of the cauda equina.

Anorectal radiology

In most patients with anorectal incontinence it is wise to assess the entire large bowel to ensure that there is no proximal contributory lesion such as an unsuspected carcinoma. A colorectal survey can be achieved either by barium enema or by colonoscopy; it can be difficult to achieve adequate bowel preparation since incontinent patients have difficulty retaining preparatory enemas. The anorectum can also be assessed at proctography, by endoluminal ultrasound and by magnetic resonance imaging (MRI).

Anal ultrasonography yields high resolution images of both sphincters. Defects in the external sphincter caused by direct sphincter injury correspond with areas of electrical silence on electromyography. Damage to the internal sphincter can also be assessed.

Magnetic resonance imaging has several advantages. It does not rely on ionizing radiation, it allows images to be generated in multiple planes, and it provides good soft tissue characterization. MRI is of great value in assessing patients with congenital anorectal anomalies, either when they first present or later when they suffer from poor anal function and when further surgery is contemplated.

Are anorectal investigations useful?

Investigations are useful when they aid diagnosis, direct management, or if they can predict the outcome of a particular treatment. To a large extent anorectal investigations are useful because they aid diagnosis and objectively measure abnormalities but, as yet, they do not have a more extended role in management. Although they have been used to assess the effects of treatment in clinical research, they do not generally predict outcome in individual patients. Electromyography and MRI are, however, useful in the management of congenital anorectal anomalies, while anal endosonography and concentric needle electromyography is of use in the diagnosis of sphincter tears. Nerve conduction studies are useful if they define a treatable cauda equina lesions such as a disc prolapse.

TREATMENT

Conservative measures

Conservative treatment should be tried in all patients, except when the clinical features and results of investigations suggest an

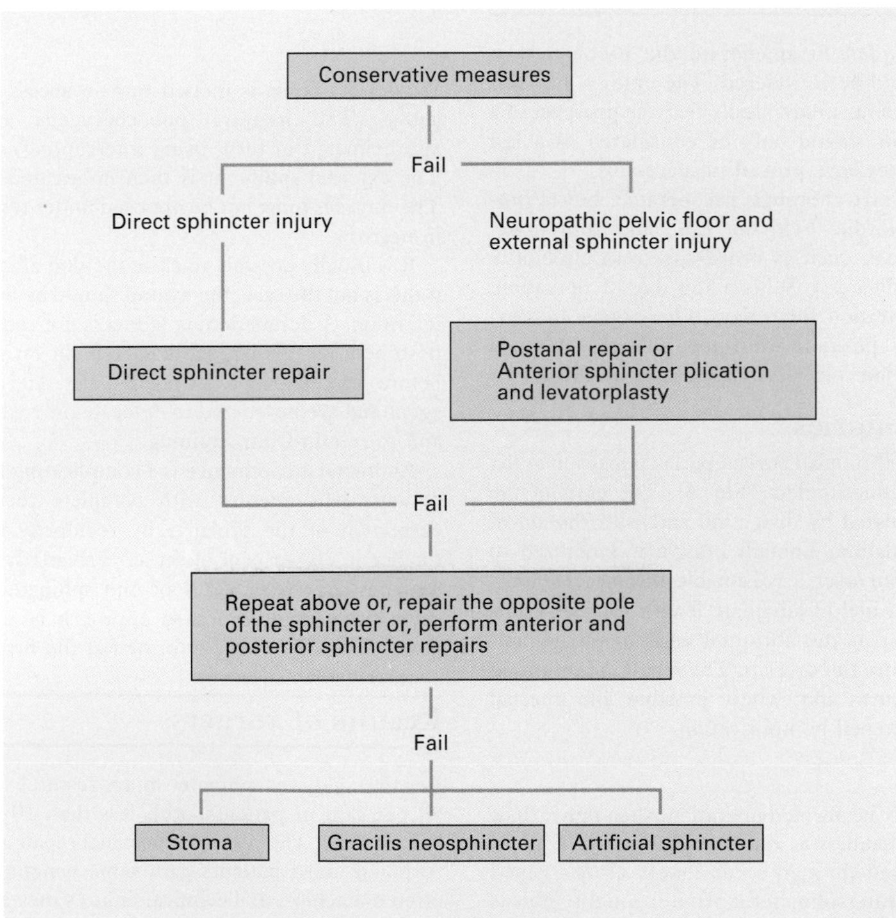

Fig. 3 Surgical management of anorectal incontinence.

underlying pathology such as inflammatory bowel disease, carcinoma or prolapse when appropriate treatment is required. Counselling of patients should aim at production of a solid stool once each day. Codeine phosphate or loperamide may be helpful and a low fibre diet is recommended. Such measures will be most beneficial in patients with mild symptoms. If their problem is transient or intermittent, or if they are satisfied with conservative treatment, nothing further need be done. A successful outcome can be expected in up to 40 per cent of patients treated by diet and drugs alone.

Other non-operative therapies include pelvic floor physiotherapy, biofeedback conditioning, and electrical stimulation. Promising early results have recently been reported in patients given repeated stimulation of the pudendoanal reflex arc, and biofeedback conditioning has been used successfully in some centres. These techniques are, however, time-consuming and have not yet proven to be of long-term benefit. In addition to these, we are currently investigating the use of an anal plug which is made of specially coated synthetic sponge. Plugs are inserted into the anal canal like a conventional suppository and expand once inside. Initial trials have shown that a 'tulip' shaped plug is tolerated best and is, on average, retained for 11 to 12 h. They are comfortable, easy to insert and remove, and only 20 per cent of plugs allow leakage whilst in use. Once available, it is hoped that plugs will be used alone or as an adjuvant to other measures.

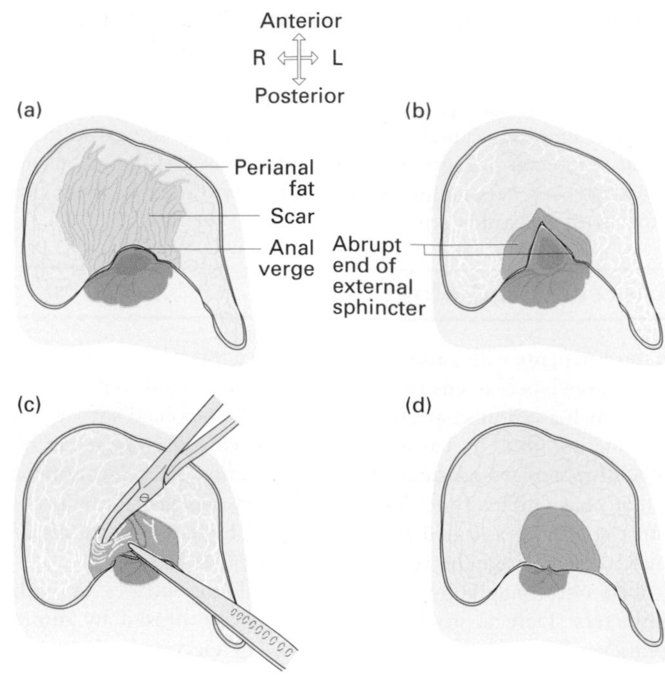

Fig. 4 Repair of direct sphincter injuries. (a) The scar is explored through a curved perianal incision. (b) The scar is excised leaving the abrupted ends of the external sphincter. (c) The ends of the external sphincter are mobilized. (d) The mobilized sphincter is overlapped and secured in place, so reconstructing the muscle ring.

Principles of surgery in anorectal incontinence

If conservative measures fail to ameliorate the problem then surgical intervention should be considered. The options available are outlined in Fig. 3. Patients undoubtedly fear the prospect of a permanent stoma and this should only be considered as a last resort when other measures have proved unsuccessful.

All patients should receive thorough preoperative bowel preparation with Picolax (Nordic, Feltham, UK) and appropriate antibiotic chemoprophylaxis, such as broad-spectrum antibiotics administered intravenously every 8 h on the day of operation, followed by oral administration for 6 days. Operations are performed in the lithotomy position, with the buttocks strapped apart. Adrenaline can be injected locally to reduce bleeding.

Direct sphincter injuries

These should be explored through a curved perianal incision in the area of the previously defined defect (Fig. 4). The ends of the external sphincter are isolated by dissection and with the aid of peroperative nerve stimulation. Enough muscle is mobilized to allow an overlapping repair over a reasonable distance cranially (3–4 cm) so that an anal canal of adequate length can be reconstructed. The fibrous scar at the abrupted ends of the injured muscle can be used to secure the overlap. The repair is performed using non-absorbable sutures and, where possible, the internal anal sphincter is also tightened by imbrication.

Postanal repair

This is the most commonly performed operation when pelvic floor and external sphincter weakness is due to neuropathy (Fig. 5). The sphincters are exposed through a curvilinear or 'V'-shaped postanal incision and the intersphincteric plane is sought. This is the bloodless anatomical key to the operation which, when entered and followed superiorly, leads up to the pelvic floor, where Waldeyer's fascia is incised to gain access to the presacral space above. The levators—pubococcygeus and puborectalis—are approximated in turn, using interrupted non-absorbable sutures. The external sphincter is then imbricated with a similar suture. The muscles must not be opposed under tension as this may result in necrosis.

It is usually possible to close the skin after both procedures but, if this is not the case, the wound should be left to heal by secondary intention. A defunctioning stoma is not required routinely. In the postoperative period, patients remain on fluids only for 2 days before commencing a low residue diet. All receive a stool softening agent and are instructed to defecate only when they have the urge and to refrain from straining.

Anorectal incontinence is a complicating factor in 75 per cent of patients who present with complete rectal prolapse. Surgical correction of the prolapse by rectopexy fails to relieve incontinence in 30 per cent of these, particularly when there is marked weakness of the pelvic floor and sphincteric striated muscle. In such instances a combined approach is advised, rectopexy and postanal repair being performed at the first operation.

Results of surgery

Repair of a direct sphincter injury restores full continence in 78 to 90 per cent of patients, with less than 10 per cent achieving no benefit at all. The results of postanal repair are outlined in Table 2. Although most patients gain some benefit, perfect continence is often not achieved. Technical failures may arise in the presence of concomitant proximal disease such as the irritable bowel syndrome or due to continuing neuropathy. It was formerly thought

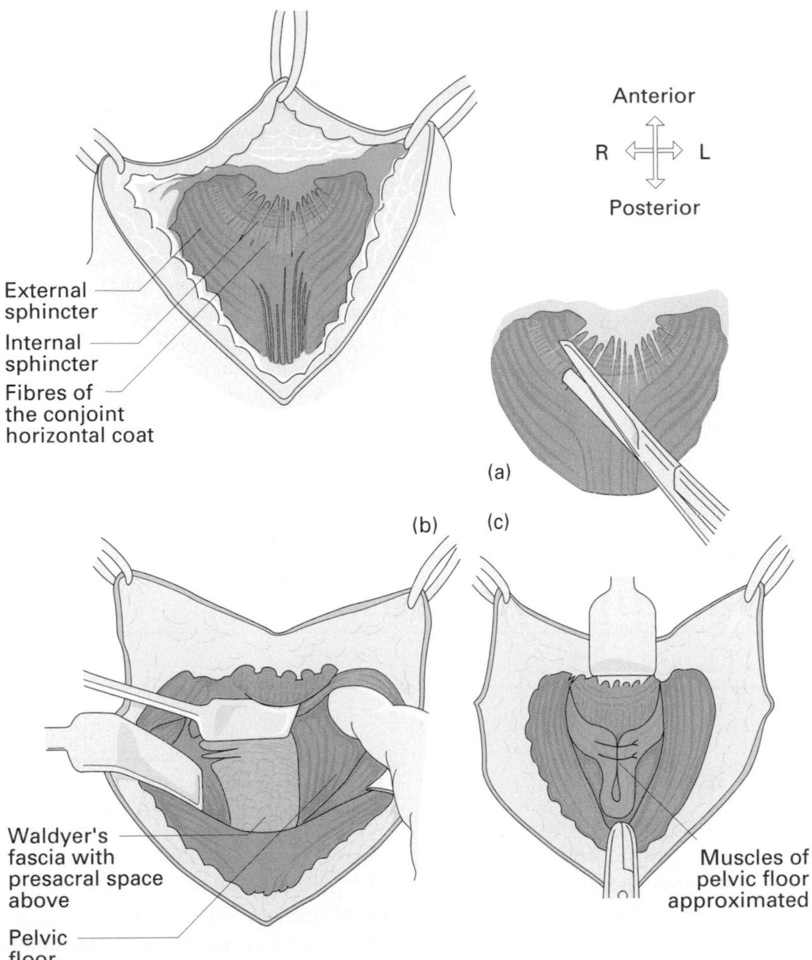

Fig. 5 Postanal repair. (a) The sphincters are exposed through a curvilinear or 'V' shaped postanal incision and the intersphincteric plane sought. The fibres of the conjoint longitudinal coat may be seen. The plane is relatively bloodless and is developed cranially to the pelvic floor. (b) At the pelvic floor, Waldeyer's fascia is incised to gain access to the presacral space above. (c) The muscles of the pelvic floor are approximated in turn (without tension) using non-absorbable sutures.

Table 2 The outcome of postanal repair for anorectal incontinence.

	Fully continent	Improved but not fully continent	Not improved
Keighley and Fielding 1983 (n=39)	27 (69%)	6 (15%)	6 (15%)
Browning and Parks 1983 (n=42)	8 (19%)	26 (62%)	8 (19%)
Womack *et al.* 1988 (n=16)	6 (37%)	8 (50%)	2 (12.5)
Miller, *et al.* 1988 (n=17)	10 (59%)	4 (23%)	3 (18%)
Scott *et al.* 1990 (n=62)	28 (45%)	23 (37%)	11 (18%)

that the success of postanal repair is determined by restoration of anorectal angulation; however, it has now been shown that success is related to increasing sphincter pressures and enhancing anal canal sensation. Similar results are achieved with anterior sphincter plication and levatorplasty.

Patients who fail to benefit from these procedures are difficult to manage. A repair can be repeated or, if there has already been a posterior repair, an anterior repair can be performed. Anterior and posterior repairs can be undertaken simultaneously in patients with very weak sphincters. These procedures can be technically difficult and may again be unsuccessful. Alternative approaches which have been suggested, include the construction of a neosphincter by transposition of the gracilis muscle and the implantation of an artificial sphincter based on a device used in urinary incontinence. Gracilis transposition has been combined with prolonged neurostimulation, with the effect of converting it from a fast twitch to a slow twitch muscle. Problems arising from muscle necrosis and electrode instability seem to have been overcome. These techniques are still in their developmental phases, but hold promise for the future.

FURTHER READING

Bartolo DCC, *et al.* Flap valve theory of anorectal continence. *Br J Surg* 1986; 73: 1012–4.

Browning GGP, Motson RW. Results of Parks operation for faecal incontinence after anal sphincter injury. *Br Med J* 1983; **286**: 1873–5.

Browning GGP, Parks AG. Postanal repair for neurogenic faecal incontinence: correlation of clinical result and anal canal pressures. *Br J Surg* 1983; **70**: 101–4.

Henry MM, Swash M, eds. *Coloproctology and the Pelvic Floor*. London: Butterworths, 1985.

Keighley MRB, Fielding JWL. Management of faecal incontinence and results of surgical treatment. *Br J Surg* 1983; **70**: 463–8.

Lubowski DZ, Swash M, Henry MM. Neural mechanisms in disorders of defaecation. Clin Gastroenterol 1988; **2**: 201–23.

Miller R, *et al.* Ano-rectal sampling: a comparison of normal and incontinent patients. *Br J Surg* 1988; **75**: 45–7.

Miller R, *et al.* Prospective study of conservative and operative treatment for faecal incontinence. *Br J Surg* 1988; **75**: 101–5.

Read NW, Abouzekry L. Why do patients with faecal impaction have faecal incontinence? *Gut* 1986; **27**: 283–7

Roe AM, Bartolo DCC, Mortensen NJMcC. A new method for assessment of anal sensation in various anorectal disorders. *Br J Surg* 1986; **73**: 310–2.

Scott ADN, Henry MM, Phillips RKS. Clinical assessment and anorectal manometry before postanal repair: failure to predict outcome. *Br J Surg* 1990; **77**: 629–30.

Speakman CTM, Kamm MA. The internal anal sphincter—new insights into faecal incontinence. *Gut* 1991; **32**: 345–6.

Williams NS, *et al.* Construction of a neoanal sphincter by transposition of gracilis muscle and prolonged neuromuscular stimulation for the treatment of faecal incontinence. *Ann R Coll Surg Engl* 1990; **72**: 108–13.

Womack NR, Morrison JFB, Williams NS. Prospective study of the effects of postanal repair in neurogenic faecal incontinence. *Br J Surg* 1988; **75**: 48–52.

20.7 Perianal pilonidal disease

R. G. SOUTER

PILONIDAL SINUS (Fig. 1)

Pilonidal disease affects young adults after puberty and is unusual after the age of 40. The condition is painful and unpleasant, typically affecting overweight patients in their second and third decades, who are dark haired and often have poor personal hygiene. Treatment is sought either because of pain, persistent offensive discharge, or the development of major secondary infection, such as a pilonidal abscess.

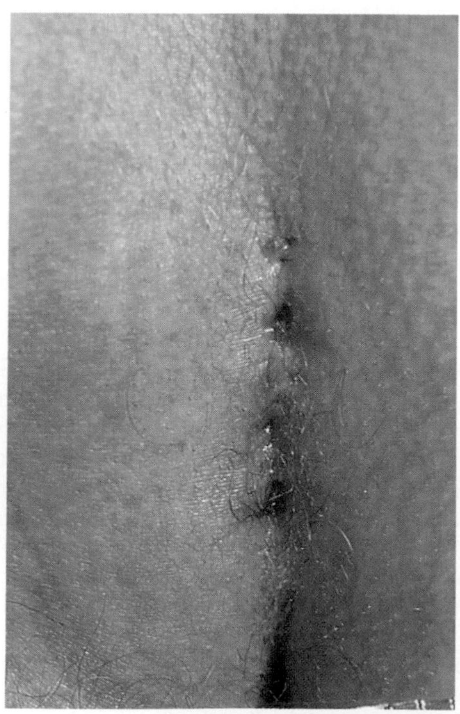

Fig. 1 Pilonidal sinus.

Incidence

Sacrococcygeal pilonidal disease was found in 365 of 31 497 men (1.1 per cent) and in 24 of 21 367 women (0.11 per cent) in a survey of Minnesota college students. A higher proportion of females attend for treatment giving a treatment ratio of four males to every female. The condition is more common in Caucasians than in Asians or Africans.

Aetiology and pathology

Pilonidal sinus is an acquired disease due to obstruction of hair follicles in the natal cleft, often associated with ingrowth of hair. Subcutaneous hair acts as a foreign body, initiating a reaction which is often complicated by varying degrees of infection. Ingrowth is enhanced by the rolling or sucking action of the obese buttock, or by prolonged sitting and vibration, as illustrated by the epidemic of pilonidal disease seen in American military personnel during the Second World War (jeep drivers' disease).

The sinus is pit lined with epithelium and sometimes containing hair. It is centrally placed and 4 to 8 cm cephalad to the anus. When the pilosebaceous follicle has been obstructed a cavity lined with granulation tissue forms, with the subsequent development of secondary tracks; these may rupture lateral to the midline creating secondary openings. These tracks may become complex, and as the diseases progress treatment becomes increasingly difficult.

Treatment

The ideal treatment leads to rapid recovery with a short hospital stay, a low possibility of recurrence, and minimal pain. Infection is the main cause of treatment failure.

Simple pilonidal sinus

This can be defined as a central sinus, with a small cavity and minimal secondary tracks where the openings are not far from the midline.

The sinus, associated granulation tissue, and secondary tracks should be excised. Whether the patient is prone with the buttocks strapped apart, or in the left lateral position, is a matter of preference. It is advisable to administer a preoperative bolus of a broad spectrum antibiotic, active against aerobic and anaerobic bacteria: cefuroxime 1.5 g IV and metronidazole 1 g IV would be appropriate for most patients. Having excised the area and secured haemostasis, the wound is closed with three or four deeply placed mattress sutures of 1 nylon, which are introduced about 1 cm away from the skin edges, and pass right through the fat to the level of the sacral fascia. More superficially placed sutures of 2/0 or 3/0 nylon can be added to 'tidy up' the wound and to ensure that the skin edges are accurately approximated.

Tension sutures and pressure dressings cause wound ischaemia and hinder healing, and are not indicated. If there is concern that the excised area will ooze, causing an accumulation of blood and serum beneath the skin flaps which could prejudice healing, a fine bore suction drain should be inserted. This is removed when drainage is minimal, usually by the second or third postoperative day. The superficial 'fine' sutures are removed after 1 week and the deeper sutures after 10 days. If the wound becomes obviously infected during this period, the sutures are removed early, and the opened wound packed with antiseptic impregnated gauze.

Traditional treatment involved excision of the affected area and daily packing of the open wound. Time to healing averaged over 40 days, with considerable patient discomfort and prolonged nursing time. Primary closure in selected cases gives healing in over 90 per cent of patients in 2 weeks. In those patients in whom the wound has to be reopened, time to healing is not likely to be in excess of those treated traditionally with excision and an open wound. Covering the operation with prophylactic antibiotics, or even a full course of seven days treatment may improve the results, but this is not proven.

Complex pilonidal sinus

Lord's procedure offers the prospect of treating complex sinus tracks on an outpatient basis. Treatment involves excision of the follicle opening and the passage of small brushes down the tracks on a weekly basis, removes granulations and encourages free drainage, permitting healing to take place. Other treatments have included the injection of phenol solution into the tracks to stimulate fibrosis. In expert hands this treatment produces healing in an average of 42 days, but it has never been popular. This may be because of the need for regular outpatient visits and the careful supervision required.

Radical excision of the area is not indicated: this takes months to heal and is very painful. The long-term recurrence rate is disappointingly high.

Complex tracks can be laid open and packed individually. Alternatively a skin flap can be used to cover the defect, keeping the scar from the midline and creating a flattened natal cleft. The greatest experience of this is provided by the 'advancing' flap operation proposed by Karydakis. This operation gave primary healing and long-term cure in the vast majority of a very large series of Greek army personnel treated for pilonidal sinus. Whether this would be reproduced by others is questionable. More complex flap operations have been described, but there is no evidence to suggest that these give better results.

Preventing further ingrowth of hair whilst the wound remains immature is important, and the patient is advised to keep the area scrupulously clean and free of hair by the use of depilating agents or by shaving.

Pilonidal abscess

Drainage of the abscess under general anaesthetic rapidly relieves pain. All infected granulation tissue and tracks should be excised at the same time and the wound packed with antiseptic impregnated ribbon gauze. The pack is changed daily until healing is complete. The aim is the creation of a saucer shaped wound, which should heal from its base without the development of epithelial bridges to prevent proper packing. Most patients will be allowed home on the third postoperative day, with further supervision of packing on an outpatient basis. Healing can be achieved in about 60 per cent of patients treated in this way in 10 weeks. The remainder will either take much longer to be cured or will be left with a pilonidal sinus; 40 to 60 per cent of these will need further treatment.

Primary closure after drainage of the abscess and local installation of antibiotic gel has given excellent results in some hands, and over 80 per cent of wounds so treated have been reported to undergo primary healing with an extremely low rate of recurrence. However there is no convincing evidence that this is the correct method of treatment.

FURTHER READING

Allen-Marsh TG. Pilonidal sinus: finding the right track for treatment. *Br J Surg* 1990; **77**: 123–32.

Bascom J. Pilonidal disease: long term results of follicle removal. *Dis Colon* Rect 1983; **26**: 800–7.

Buire LA. Jeep disease. *South Med J* 1944; **37**: 103–9

Courtney SP, Merlin MJ. The use of fusidic acid gel in pilonidal abscess treatment: cure, recurrence and failure rates. *Ann R Coll Surg Eng* 1986; **68**: 170–1

Dwight RW, Maloy JK. Pilonidal sinus—experience with 449 cases. *N Engl J Med* 1953; **249**: 926–30.

Karydakis GE. New approach to the problem of pilonidal sinus. *Lancet* 1973; **ii**: 1414–14.

Lord PH. Anorectal problems: etiology of pilonidal sinus. *Dis Colon Rect* 1975; **18**: 661–4.

Maurice BA, Greenwood RK. A conservative treatment of pilonidal sinus. *Br J Surg* 1974; **51**: 510–2.

20.8 Cancer of the anus

MICHAEL J. GREENALL

INTRODUCTION

The most common type of cancer arising in the anus is squamous or epidermoid carcinoma (Table 1). This is, however, a rare tumour, and is 20 to 30 times less common than colorectal cancer. Of the other tumours that occasionally arise in the anus, only malignant melanoma is seen with any frequency; this is eight times less common than epidermoid carcinoma. Other tumours are so rare that there is only anecdotal experience of their treatment.

Table 1 Anal cancer

1. Epidermoid anal cancer
   (a) At the anal margin
   (b) In the anal canal
2. Melanoma
3. Adenocarcinoma. Either arising *de novo* from anal glands or fistula or from downward spread of rectal adenocarcinoma
4. Basal cell carcinoma
5. Bowen's disease
6. Paget's disease

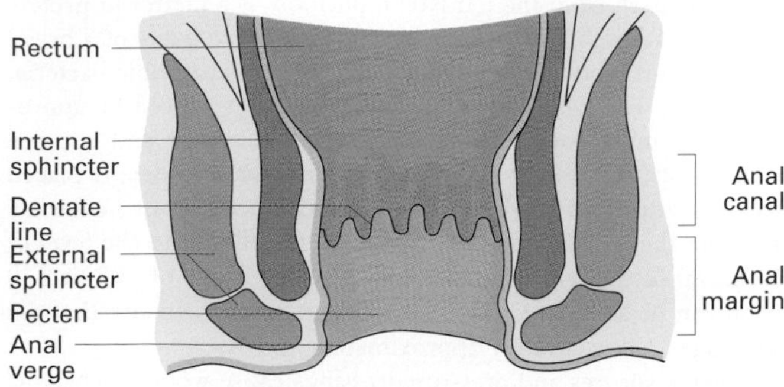

Fig. 1 The anatomy of the anal canal and anal margin.

EPIDERMOID CANCER OF THE ANUS

Anal epidermoid cancer is sensitive to both chemotherapy and irradiation. This has led to reappraisal of the surgical treatment for this condition, with a trend away from abdominoperineal resection to a much more conservative surgical approach that allows preservation of the anal sphincter mechanism.

Much of the early information on anal cancer was derived from small, retrospective studies that used a variety of pathological terms and staging systems. Other studies combined their results with other types of anal cancer such as melanoma, adenocarcinoma, etc. Data were therefore conflicting. In addition, there has never been any agreement as to the anatomical boundaries which distinguish the anal canal from its margin; epidermoid cancers arising at these two sites have, therefore, not been accurately differentiated. As epidermoid cancer arising in the canal differs fundamentally in its clinical presentation, pathological features, treatment, and prognosis from that at the margin, distinction between the two conditions is mandatory.

Anatomic considerations

Anatomists regard the anal canal as that part of the alimentary tract distal to the rectal ampulla. However, this definition does not correlate with the clinical and pathological characteristics of anal cancer in that region. Although there is general agreement that the proximal end of the anal canal correlates with the anorectal ring, its distal limit is more poorly defined; both the dentate (pectinate) line and the anal verge have been used (Fig. 1). Similarly, there is no clear definition of the lateral border of the anal margin, although one authority has recommended that it lies within a 5-cm radius of the verge itself.

The definition of the distal limit of the anal canal as the dentate line or the anal verge is of paramount importance since the anatomical boundary used to differentiate between the anal canal and its margin determines the relative incidence of tumours at these two sites. When the anal verge is used as the boundary, less than 15 per cent of cancers are ascribed to the margin, whereas those authorities using the more proximal dentate line claim that 30 per cent of tumours occur at this site.

The dentate line itself is a cause of confusion. It corresponds to the site of the anal valves and represents the junction of the post-allantoic gut with the proctodeum. It is described as the 'anal transitional zone' because of its transitional cell appearance with characteristics of both the cuboidal rectal mucosa above and the modified squamous epithelium of the pecten below. The transitional zone does not, however, correspond to the macroscopic limits of the dentate line. Transitional epithelium, with islands of squamous cells within it, extends up to 2 cm above the line, explaining how tumours of this epithelial type occur in the more proximal anal canal.

Pathology

Epidermoid carcinoma of the margin accounts for only about 15 to 30 per cent of all squamous anal cancers. Eighty-five per cent are well differentiated and produce keratin. Basaloid features are rare and presumably result from the development of an invasive squamous component within a pre-existing basal cell carcinoma.

Epidermoid cancers of the canal are usually more poorly differentiated, and only about 30 per cent produce keratin. Basaloid (cloacogenic or transitional) features, found in about 40 per cent of tumours, imply derivation from the anal transitional zone. When basaloid features are present there is usually a squamous component as well: classification as squamous or basaloid is based on the predominant cell type, although this is somewhat academic and subject to differences in interpretation.

Clinical features

The most common presenting features of anal cancer are pain, bleeding, change in bowel habit, and pruritus ani. Less common presentations include inguinal lymphadenopathy from secondary spread to that site, and as an unexpected histological finding in a haemorrhoidectomy specimen.

About 60 per cent of patients with epidermoid anal cancer at the anal margin have associated perianal conditions, including condylomata, chronic fistula, leucoplakia, or the effects of previous irradiation. Such features are found in less than 10 per cent of patients with tumours arising in the anal canal.

An area of particular interest lies in the relationship of anal cancer to sexually transmitted disease. Earlier studies suggested an association with lymphogranuloma venereum and syphilis, although this was not subsequently confirmed. However, more recent epidemiological data have provided evidence in support of the hypothesis that a sexually transmitted agent is involved in the pathogenesis of anal squamous cancer, especially in the homosexual population. Human papilloma virus type 16 DNA has been detected in more than 50 per cent of patients with anal cancer, indicating that this may be the transmissible agent involved.

Diagnosis

Epidermoid anal cancer is diagnosed on the basis of examination of biopsy specimens. The differential diagnosis includes conditions such as rectal adenocarcinoma, Bowen's disease, Paget's disease, condyloma acuminata, leucoplakia, Crohn's disease, and certain intrinsic skin disorders such as lichen sclerosus et atrophicus. At the time of diagnosis it is necessary to determine accurately the stage of the disease. Difficulties encountered in staging on a clinical basis have been overcome by the increasing use of local ultrasound to assess muscle invasion. Computerized tomography or MRI imaging may also help determine the presence of local invasion or metastatic disease.

Treatment

Epidermoid cancer of the anal margin

Local excision is sufficient treatment in the majority of patients with epidermoid cancer of the anal margin, giving a 5-year survival rate in excess of 80 per cent, although large tumours may require skin grafting. The prognosis may be determined by the depth of invasion.

Abdominoperineal resection has not been widely adopted for patients with tumours at the anal margin. When it has been used it has been usually reserved for deeper infiltrative tumours or for patients with persistent recurrence; the survival rate of about 50 per cent is therefore somewhat less than that obtained after simple local excision. A potential advantage of abdominoperineal resection is that inferior mesenteric nodal metastases will be resected, although such spread is rare in cancers arising at the margin.

There are few data on primary irradiation or combined chemotherapy and irradiation of epidermoid cancer of the anal margin. Although responses have been observed there seems little need for this approach as simple local excision will suffice in the vast majority of patients.

If recurrence occurs after local excision of anal margin cancer, further simple excision may be attempted. If this is not possible, radiotherapy, using either external beam irradiation or an implant, may be considered. Occasional patients require abdominoperineal resection although good local tumour control may be difficult to achieve if there is persistent recurrence.

The good survival following local excision of epidermoid cancer of the anal margin results from the relatively benign characteristics of the tumour. These relatively well differentiated, keratinizing squamous tumours therefore behave rather like other primary skin cancers arising elsewhere on the body.

Epidermoid cancer of the anal canal

Epidermoid cancer of the anal canal has a worse prognosis and requires more complex treatment than its relatively benign counterpart at the margin.

A wide variety of treatments have been adopted for patients with tumours in the anal canal, ranging from local excision to preoperative neoadjuvant chemotherapy and radiotherapy followed by abdominoperineal resection. It is its potential for chemo- and radiosensitivity that has caused much interest in the past few years.

Local excision

Simple local excision alone is only rarely applicable to patients with epidermoid cancer of the anal canal. When performed the prognosis has been relatively good, with a 5-year survival of up to 65 per cent: this presumably reflects the early stage of disease for which the operation was performed. It is probably only suitable for those superficially invasive tumours that are less than 2 cm in diameter, and is not generally recommended.

Abdominoperineal resection

Abdominoperineal resection has been the standard treatment for epidermoid cancer of the anal canal, with a 5-year survival rate of 50 per cent. A wide perineal phase of the operation is recommended; if inguinal lymph nodes are involved, inguinal lymphadenectomy is required as a secondary procedure. Survival depends on tumour size, histological grade, depth of invasion, and overall staging. Earlier suggestions that predominantly basaloid tumours have a better prognosis than the more usual squamous type have not been substantiated.

Primary radiotherapy

Primary irradiation has been used in the treatment of epidermoid anal cancer for over 50 years. In the past the various radiotherapeutic techniques were inadequate and produced disappointing results in terms of both tumour control and local morbidity. However, more modern megavoltage X-ray therapy has produced encouraging results, with 5-year survival rates in excess of 50 per cent, and with the added advantage of allowing anal sphincter preservation. Interstitial techniques have also been used with success in some centres.

Primary irradiation therapy may sometimes be associated with severe local morbidity and patients may require a colostomy because of anal necrosis or stenosis.

Neoadjuvant chemoirradiation

The original, somewhat empirical, observation by Nigro and his colleagues in 1974 of the effects of preoperative treatment of epidermoid anal cancer with combination chemotherapy and irradiation attracted much attention. Their use of 5-fluorouracil and mitomycin C was somewhat arbitrary, although both had demonstrated cytotoxic activity against a wide range of gastrointestinal tumours and also exhibited properties of radiosensitization.

The chemoirradiation regimen now currently used varies between institutions. Most give mitomycin C on day 1 of the treatment followed by infusion of 5-fluorouracil over a 5- to 7-day period. Irradiation starts either concurrently with chemotherapy or 3 days after the mitomycin C has been given. The average radiation dose is about 30 to 50 Gy, given over 3 to 7 weeks, a lower dose than is usually recommended for patients treated by radiation alone. These regimes are associated with side-effects such as radiation-induced proctitis and dermatitis, leucopenia, thrombocytopenia, stomatitis, and diarrhoea.

In most centres patients are re-examined about 4 to 6 weeks after completion of radiotherapy: About 70 per cent will show a complete response to their treatment and in only 10 per cent is there no effect. Those patients who fail to respond require abdominoperineal resection. The major question is whether after a complete response simple excision of residual scar tissue will suffice, or whether these patients should be treated by abdominoperineal resection. Current data provide no real answer, but do indicate that neoadjuvant chemoirradiation may reduce the need for abdominoperineal resection. Whether it improves survival is less clear. These questions are currently being addressed by randomized controlled studies.

MALIGNANT MELANOMA

Malignant melanoma of the anus is rare and has a poor prognosis. Whereas one can usually expect a 50 to 70 per cent 5-year survival for cutaneous melanoma occurring elsewhere in the body the average 5-year cure rate reported in the literature for malignant melanoma in the anal region is only 6 per cent.

Malignant melanoma of the anal region usually presents with bleeding or a mass. It often appears as a slightly pigmented lesion, although amelanotic melanoma is recognized at this site. Unfortunately, many patients have disease affecting the inguinal lymph nodes at the time of presentation.

Because of its rarity, virulence, and poor prognosis the treatment of this tumour has varied from simple local excision to radical abdominoperineal resection with bilateral prophylactic groin dissection. Adjuvant chemotherapy and radiation treatment seem to provide little benefit.

The majority of long-term survivors have been treated by abdominoperineal resection. There seems to be little benefit of prophylactic inguinal node dissection, although staging by nodal biopsy at the time of abdominoperineal resection may be clinically useful.

ADENOCARCINOMA OF THE ANUS

Adenocarcinoma of the anal canal may result from downgrowth of a primary rectal tumour or from carcinoma developing *de novo* in an anal gland or fistula. Such tumours are rare, the prognosis is poor, and treatment is by abdominoperineal resection.

BASAL CELL CARCINOMA

Basal cell carcinoma is another rare anal condition. Experience is anecdotal but full thickness local excision appears to assure a cure.

BOWEN'S DISEASE

Bowen's disease is an intraepithelial *in-situ* squamous cancer of the skin and is seen more commonly on the trunk, hands, and face than in perianal and genital areas. It is associated with synchronous and metachronous cancers at other sites.

Clinically, it appears as a slowly growing, minimally elevated, erythematous plaque-like lesion. The histological picture is that of an *in-situ* squamous cancer; above an intact basement membrane the cells demonstrate loss of polarity, acanthosis, and an inflammatory infiltrate. The characteristic Bowenoid cells have large hyperchromatic nuclei, with vacuoles providing a haloed effect.

The treatment of Bowen's disease is wide local excision, with skin grafting if necessary: special attention must be paid to the margin of excision. Long-term follow-up is necessary because of the possibility of recurrent disease in an area predisposed to the development of this condition.

PAGET'S DISEASE

Extramammary Paget's disease is an extremely rare intraepithelial neoplasm. Unlike its counterpart in the breast it is not always associated with frank underlying malignancy. The clinical appearance of Paget's disease is that of a pale grey, crusting, scaly lesion. The diagnosis is confirmed by demonstrating the characteristic Paget cells with their large pale cytoplasm that stains positively with aldehyde-fuscin. Any associated invasive cancer arises from a skin appendage such as a sweat gland rather than from rectal mucosa.

If no frank cancer is present then simple excision is suitable treatment for Paget's disease. Negative margins of resection must be obtained or recurrence is likely. If there is underlying malignancy then a deeper, wider excision is needed, but the outlook is generally poor.

FURTHER READING

Fenger C. The anal transitional zone. Location and extent. *Acta Pathol Microbiol Immunol Scand* (A) 1979; **87**: 379–86.

Greenall MJ, Quan SHQ, DeCosse JJ. Epidermoid cancer of the anus. *Br J Surg* 1985; **Suppl**. S97 – S103.

Greenall MJ, Quan SHQ, Stearns MW, Urmacher C, DeCosse JJ. Epidermoid cancer of the anal margin: pathologic features, treatment and clinical results. *Am J Surg* 1985; **149**: 95–101.

Nigro ND, Vaitkevicius VK, Considine B. Combined therapy for cancer of the anal canal: a preliminary report. *Dis Colon Rect* 1974; **17**: 354–56.

Palmer JG, *et al.* Anal cancer and human papillomavirus. *Dis Colon Rect* 1989; **32**: 1016–22.

Peritoneum and intraperitoneal abscesses 21

21.1 The peritoneum and peritonitis

D. L. McWHINNIE

THE PERITONEAL CAVITY

The peritoneal cavity is lined by the peritoneal membrane that consists of a single layer of mesothelial cells supported by loose connective tissue. The membrane comprises two components in continuity: the visceral peritoneum covers the abdominal organs and the parietal peritoneum lines the abdominal wall (Fig. 1). The cavity is thus a closed sac except for the fimbriated ends of the fallopian tubes. The mesothelial cells secrete serous fluid which provides a lubricant to allow gliding movements of the viscera. In the normal healthy adult the peritoneal cavity contains about 100 ml of serous fluid, secreted from a total peritoneal surface area of approximately 2 m^2. This large surface area of thin semipermeable peritoneal membrane can be utilized for peritoneal dialysis.

(a)

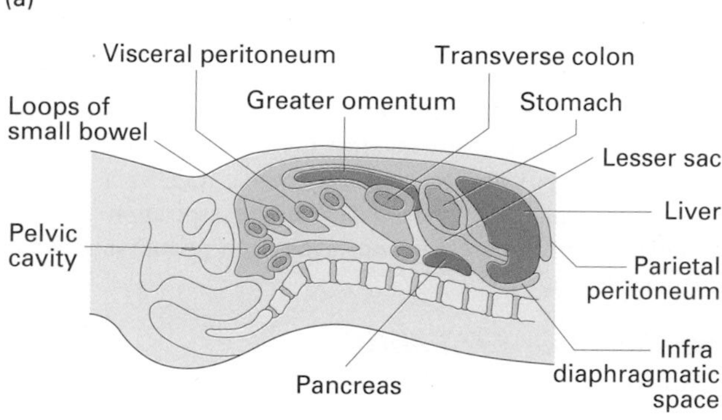

(b)

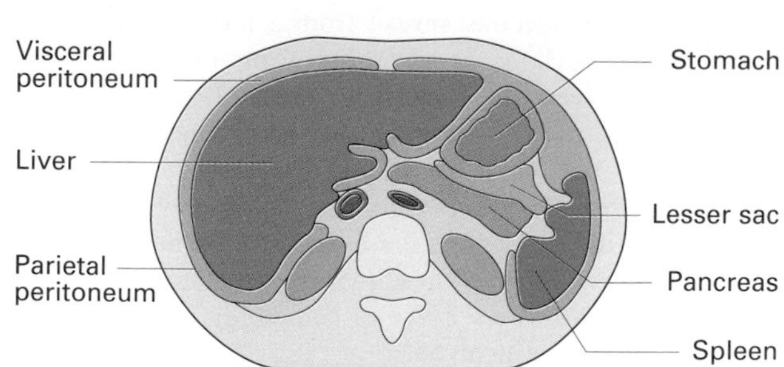

Fig. 1 Peritoneal cavity. (a) Coronal section; (b) transverse section showing the dependency of pelvic cavity and infradiaphragmatic space in the recumbent patient. The visceral and parietal peritoneum are shown lining the abdominal organs and abdominal wall.

The technique of peritoneal dialysis has been used in the treatment of renal failure since the late 1940s but was of limited intermittent application until the development of the implanted Tenckhoff silicon rubber catheter in 1968 (see Section 7.16). This allowed peritoneal dialysis to be performed continuously and safely for longer periods commonly of several years' duration. Dialysis fluid is stored in sterile PVC bags and during an 'exchange' the bag is connected to the Tenckhoff catheter by PVC tubing. The dialysate is encouraged to enter the abdominal cavity by gravity, through elevation of the bag. Between three and five exchanges of 1 to 2 litres of peritoneal dialysate are performed daily. Clearance of particular electrolytes is achieved by reducing their concentration in the dialysate. Fluid balance is monitored by the measurement of daily weights and measured by altering the proportion of 'hypertonic' (3.8 per cent glucose solution) and 'isotonic' (2.36 per cent glucose solution) exchanges. While the dialysis fluid is in the peritoneal cavity, the uraemic toxins diffuse from the blood supply of the mesentery and peritoneum. At the end of each dialysis cycle the dialysate is drained by gravity and returned to the bag. This simple technique of continuous ambulatory peritoneal dialysis (CAPD) has been adopted in many dialysis centres as initial therapy for renal failure in diabetics, in young patients with the prospects of any early transplant, and in those patients with poor vascular access.

The pattern of innervation of the visceral and parietal peritoneum determines the pattern of abdominal pain that occurs when the peritoneum is inflamed. As the visceral peritoneum receives only afferent innervation from the autonomic nervous system, stimuli from the visceral peritoneum are localized only to the foregut, midgut, or hindgut in the midline. The visceral nerves do not mediate pain or temperature but respond to distension, traction, or pressure. In contrast, the parietal peritoneum is innervated by both somatic and visceral afferent fibres which allows the accurate localization of pain when the parietal peritoneum is inflamed.

The anatomy of the abdominal cavity determines the pattern of fluid movement within the abdomen. Functionally, four compartments exist within the peritoneal cavity: the pelvis, the right and left paracolic gutters, and the infradiaphragmatic space (Fig. 1). As the paracolic gutters slope into the infradiaphragmatic space superiorly and over the pelvic brim inferiorly, fluid in the recumbent patient collects under the diaphragm and in the pelvis, the common sites for abscess formation (see Section 21.2).

PERITONITIS

Localized or generalized peritonitis

Peritonitis is defined as inflammation of the peritoneal cavity, where the peritoneal fluid increases in volume with the passage of a transudate rich in leucocyte polymorphs and fibrin. Initially, peritoneal inflammation is often localized and the affected area contained by a wrapping of greater omentum, adjacent bowel, and fibrinous adhesions. If the inflammatory focus is part of an ongoing process, or if host defences are lowered, localized peritonitis may progress to life-threatening generalized peritonitis. There is massive exudation of inflammatory fluid into the peritoneal cavity causing hypovolaemia, often compounded by toxaemia from absorbed products and septicaemia if infection is present. Diffuse peritoneal irritation causes peristaltic paralysis with the cessation of bowel motility.

Signs and symptoms

The clinical features of peritonitis are dependent on both the aetiology and the progression of the inflammation. The early manifestations of peritonitis following disease of an abdominal viscus are characterized by the primary disease process itself and a detailed discussion can be found in the appropriate chapter. An overview of the signs and symptoms of the acute abdomen are detailed in Chapter 28. In summary, the signs and symptoms of peritonitis secondary to a diseased abdominal viscus are as follows: initial inflammation of the visceral peritoneum overlying the damaged organ results in poorly localized abdominal pain, through stimulation of the visceral autonomic nerves. Irritation of the nearby parietal peritoneum results in localization of the pain. Associated symptoms include malaise, nausea and vomiting, and an associated low-grade fever. The four cardinal signs of peritonitis, consisting of tenderness, guarding, rigidity, and rebound tenderness may also be elicited. When the peritonitis is generalized the patient is clearly unwell, with marked fever and dehydration and absent bowel sounds. Pain is diffuse throughout the abdomen and is exacerbated by even the slightest movement. Shoulder-tip pain is diagnostic of diaphragmatic inflammation.

Acute peritonitis

Acute peritonitis may be classified as (a) primary (spontaneous), where an infection has arisen *de novo* within the peritoneum or (b) secondary where the inflammatory process involving the peritoneum is the result of an identifiable primary process (Table 1).

Table 1 Aetiology of peritonitis

Acute peritonitis
(a) Primary (spontaneous)
(b) Secondary
Acute suppurative
Granulomatous
Chemical (aseptic)
Interventional
Traumatic
Drug-induced
Chronic (sclerosing) peritonitis
Infectious
Drug-induced
Chemical
Foreign-body
Carcinomatosis

Primary (spontaneous) peritonitis

Idiopathic peritonitis is uncommon, constituting about 1 per cent of all cases of peritonitis and occurs when no obvious source for the peritoneal infection can be demonstrated. It was classically described in young girls where the port of entry was presumed to be through the fallopian tube or via haematogenous spread. Formerly, pneumococci were implicated but in recent years haemolytic streptococci, *Escherichia coli*, and *Klebsiella* spp. are now more frequently cultured.

Other causes of spontaneous peritonitis are associated with patients suffering intercurrent disease. Pneumococcal infection is well recognized in the postsplenectomy child and in those who have nephrotic syndrome. Adults with cirrhosis are prone to a wide variety of spontaneous bacterial infections because of the proteinaceous nature of the ascitic fluid which provides an excellent culture medium for blood-borne bacteria to proliferate. Successful treatment of primary peritonitis, without resorting to laparotomy is rare. Only when peritoneal tap and culture of peritoneal fluid reveals a non-enteric organism can conservative antibiotic therapy be instituted with caution.

Secondary peritonitis

Acute suppurative peritonitis

This is the most common form of peritonitis encountered by the surgeon and results from the perforation of a viscus (e.g. appendix, peptic ulcer, colonic diverticulum, or gallbladder), ischaemia of an intra-abdominal organ (e.g. strangulated hernia, volvulus, mesenteric artery occlusion), or extension of an existing infection of an abdominal organ (e.g. appendix abscess, liver abscess, pyosalpinx). Surgical intervention is the treatment of choice and in most cases is mandatory, being aimed at the primary disease process. Supportive therapy before laparotomy includes opiate analgesia, antibiotic therapy (against both aerobes and anaerobes), correction of hypovolaemia and electrolyte imbalance by intravenous fluid replacement, and nasogastric aspiration to reduce abdominal distension and prevent aspiration pneumonia through inhalation of vomit.

Granulomatous peritonitis

The presence of chronic granulomata within the abdominal cavity in association with peritonitis is the result of infection, most commonly with tuberculosis but occasionally with fungi such as *Candida albicans*. Tuberculous peritonitis is usually associated with a tuberculous focus within the abdomen (e.g. intestine, mesenteric lymph node, fallopian tubes) but occasionally can develop by haematogenous spread from a focus outside the abdominal cavity, such as in the lung. The causative agent is *Mycobacterium tuberculosis*, nowadays usually of the human rather than the bovine strain, following widespread pasteurization of milk. Although the incidence of the disease is low in Western countries, occurring in the chronically ill or malnourished patient, the disease is still prevalent in the Indian subcontinent and in the Far East. Immigrants from these locations remain susceptible to the condition. Females are twice as commonly affected as males but all age groups are involved.

Pathologically, tuberculous peritonitis may present with ascites or with intra-abdominal adhesions but there is often considerable overlap between the two forms of the disease. Clinical presentation is insidious with vague generalized abdominal pain, low-grade fever, anorexia, and weight loss. The ascitic patient may also present with gross abdominal distension while those with intra-abdominal adhesions may present with pain and distension or bowel obstruction. Preoperative diagnosis is uncommon. Tuberculous ascites is difficult to differentiate from other forms of ascites. The leucocyte count may demonstrate a lymphocytosis and lymphocytes also predominate in the ascitic fluid. Centrifugation and direct microscopy of the ascitic fluid rarely demonstrate the tubercle bacillus. Culture of ascitic fluid is positive for tuberculosis in less than one-half of all cases. At laparotomy, the entire peritoneal cavity is usually studded with tuberculous nodules and the initial differential diagnoses include carcinomatosis, starch peritonitis, and widespread fat necrosis. In the patient who presents with subacute or acute bowel obstruction, widespread fibrinous adhesions with matting of intestines and omentum predominate. Here the differential diagnoses includes other forms of sclerosing peritonitis (see under Chronic Peritonitis). Confirmation of tuberculous peritonitis is made by histopathology and treatment consists of combination chemotherapy (rifampicin, isoniazid, and ethambutol) for up to 12 months.

Chemical (aseptic) peritonitis

Aseptic peritonitis refers to the peritoneal inflammation from substances other than bacteria but bacterial contamination and overgrowth soon follow. A perforated peptic ulcer provides the most severe and common form of chemical peritonitis with gastric juice and bile contaminating the peritoneal cavity. Biliary peritonitis alone may follow gangrene and perforation of the gallbladder, or, after cholecystectomy, may be the result of unrecognized division of an accessory hepatic duct, an insecure ligature on the cystic duct remnant or displacement of a T-tube following exploration of the common bile duct. Blood in the peritoneum is also a cause of peritoneal irritation after slow bleeding (e.g. a ruptured graafian follicle or following splenic injury) rather than from a catastrophic haemorrhagic event such as a ruptured aneurysm where the primary pathology itself overshadows the peritoneal irritation. Meconium and urine may also precipitate chemical peritonitis.

Interventional peritonitis

Endoscopy of the gastrointestinal tract may precipitate acute peritonitis through colonoscopic perforation of a diverticulum or inadvertent perforation of the oesophagogastric junction during oesophageal dilatation. Similarly, the urinary bladder may be perforated during diagnostic or therapeutic cystoscopy leading to a urinary leak within the abdomen. The recent expansion of interventional radiological procedures has precipitated a multitude of assaults on the abdominal cavity, such as CT guided biopsy and drainage of abscesses, mesenteric angiography and therapeutic embolization, and percutaneous transhepatic cholangiography and stenting, all providing further potential for peritonitis.

Peritonitis may follow abdominal surgery where bowel and gastric contents, blood, and urine escape into the abdominal cavity following anastomotic dehiscence. In patients with renal failure treated by continuous ambulatory peritoneal dialysis, a permanent indwelling catheter in the abdominal cavity provides a portal of entry for exogenous bacteria despite the use of stringent aseptic techniques during dialysis exchanges (see Chapter 8).

Traumatic peritonitis

Abdominal trauma may produce acute peritonitis in several ways. Penetrating wounds of the abdomen without visceral injury may provide a route for exogenous bacterial contamination. Penetration of a visceral organ may precipitate the spillage of visceral contents into the peritoneal cavity. Severe blunt trauma may disrupt intra-abdominal organs directly or indirectly through disruption of their vascular supply.

Drug-induced peritonitis

Warfarin anticoagulation can cause peritoneal irritation and peritonitis through leakage from a spontaneous retroperitoneal haematoma. The symptoms of acute peritonitis have also been described during treatment with the antituberculous agent, isoniazid.

Chronic (sclerosing) peritonitis

Chronic or sclerosing peritonitis is the end result of a heterogenous group of conditions (Table 1). Classically, sclerosing peritonitis is characterized by dense adhesions, especially between loops of small bowel, and in the most extreme cases the entire small bowel and even the large intestine and liver is cocooned in a dense adhesive membrane of fibrous tissue (Fig. 2). The classical description of sclerosing peritonitis relates to the β-adrenoceptor blocker practolol. This drug was first introduced in 1970 but the first reports of thickening of serosal membranes appeared 4 years later and the drug was withdrawn from general use in 1976. During this 6-year period, approximately 200 patients worldwide were diagnosed as having sclerosing peritonitis. Patients presented with subacute small bowel obstruction or acute-on-chronic small bowel obstruction. Treatment consisted of surgical stripping of the cocoon of fibrous tissue from the underlying intestine and was a long and tedious procedure. Intra-abdominal fistula formation and death was not uncommon. In the early 1980s sclerosing peritonitis made a reappearance in patients undergoing continuous ambulatory peritoneal dialysis. Patients presented with impaired ultrafiltration capacity due to the deposition of the fibrous membrane on the peritoneum, and the clinical features of bowel obstruction, either acute or chronic. Epidemiological studies demonstrated that the sclerosis was due to the chlorhexidine and alcohol solution used to sterilize the connectors of the CAPD catheters at the time of peritoneal dialysis 'exchanges'. Approximately 1 ml of antiseptic solution was able to enter the peritoneal cavity at the time of each exchange causing irritation to the peritoneal membrane. Other mechanisms which may precipitate

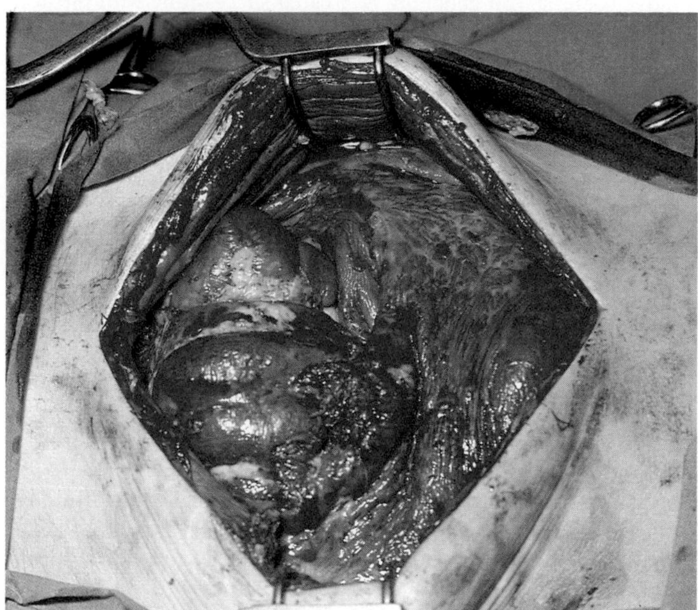

Fig. 2 Sclerosing peritonitis following CAPD. The small bowel, large bowel, and liver are cocooned in a fibrous membrane. (By courtesy of Dr B. Junor.)

sclerosing peritonitis in CAPD patients include the presence of acetate in the dialysate and recurrent CAPD peritonitis with fibrin deposition over the peritoneal membrane.

Foreign-body granulomatous peritonitis was not uncommon in patients who had undergone laparotomy, in the days before the introduction of 'talc-free' surgical gloves. The main component of surgical talc is starch and starch peritonitis was first described in 1956 and is due to starch sensitivity. Some 2 to 6 weeks after an initial laparotomy from which the patient usually makes an uneventful recovery, the patient would represent with either ascites or signs and symptoms of bowel obstruction. At laparotomy, multiple nodules are seen over the parietal and visceral peritoneum, mimicking malignant deposits with dense adhesions between loops of bowel. Treatment consists of lysis of adhesions and the diagnosis is confirmed by histology where birefringent granules are observed. Administration of steroids is ineffective in preventing intestinal adhesions.

Other forms of chronic peritonitis which may form dense adhesions include the adhesive form of tuberculous peritonitis (see under acute peritonitis) and carcinomatosis.

FURTHER READING

Brown P, Baddeley H, Read AE, Davies JD, McGarry J. Sclerosing peritonitis, an unusual reaction to a β-adrenergic-blocking drug. *Lancet*, 1974; ii: 1477–81.

Ellis H. The hazards of surgical glove dusting powders. *Surg Gynecol Obstet*, 1990; 171: 521–7.

Kittur DS, Korpe SW, Raytch RE, Smith GW. Surgical aspects of sclerosing encapsulating peritonitis. *Arch Surg*, 1990; **125**: 1626–8.

Maddaus MA, Ahrenholz D, Simmons RL. The biology of peritonitis and implications for treatment. *Surg Clin N Am*, 1988; **68**: 431–43.

Saklayen MG. CAPD peritonitis. Incidence, pathogens, diagnosis and management. *Med Clin N Am*, 1990; **74**: 997–1010.

Willcox CM, Dismukes WE. Spontaneous bacterial peritonitis. A review of pathogenesis, diagnosis and treatment. *Medicine (Baltimore)* 1987; **66**: 447–56.

21.2 Intra-abdominal abscesses

MARK S. PASTERNACK AND MORTON N. SWARTZ

PATHOGENESIS OF INTRA-ABDOMINAL ABSCESSES

Generalized bacterial peritonitis and focal intra-abdominal abscesses are extremes in the spectrum of intra-abdominal infection. Primary bacterial peritonitis (not secondary to a perforated viscus), particularly when due to a single species of aerobic or facultative bacteria, can generally be treated successfully with medical therapy alone. In contrast, the intra-abdominal abscesses require drainage in addition to antibiotic therapy.

Investigations in rodent models of intra-abdominal infection have identified polymicrobial infection, specifically with a mixture of aerobic and anaerobic bacteria, and foreign matter as key requisites for the development of intra-abdominal abscesses. When Enterobacteriaceae such as *E. coli* are the sole pathogens, the acute mortality rate due to bacteraemia is high, but survivors do not develop late intra-abdominal abscesses. Surprisingly, intra-abdominal infection with the anaerobic Gram-negative *Bacteroides fragilis* does not lead to early death or subsequent abscess development. However, an infection with the combination of these pathogens is remarkably effective in generating abscesses in surviving animals, even when antibiotic therapy effective against *E. coli* is administered acutely, preventing early deaths from bacteraemia. The presence of foreign matter facilitates the development of progressive infection. These requisites are readily met in clinical practice, where a perforated viscus is the most common risk factor for the development of intra-abdominal abscess, where polymicrobial infection is the rule, and when luminal contents or devitalized tissue provide a suitable nidus for infection.

The acute inflammatory response is ineffective in overcoming such mixed infections, and may even promote the development of abscesses. The presence of bacteria within the normally sterile peritoneal cavity leads to an influx of acute inflammatory cells and the ingress of plasma across the inflamed vascular bed. Omentum and fibrinous adhesions localize the site of infection, producing a phlegmon, but the hypoxic environment characteristic of such mixed infections facilitates the growth of anaerobes, and impairs the bactericidal activity of granulocytes. The degradation of cellular and bacterial debris by granulocytic hydrolases creates a hypertonic fluid that expands in response to osmotic forces, and the abscess cavity enlarges. This process can continue until a lethal complication such as bacteraemia, or erosion of a viscus or blood vessel develops, or until the host succumbs to the debilitating chronic inflammatory process.

ANATOMICAL CONSIDERATIONS

Intra-abdominal abscesses tend to develop in one or more discrete locations. The subphrenic spaces (in relation to both the right and left hemidiaphragms), subhepatic space (particularly the posterior aspect of the subhepatic space), the parocolic gutters located posterolaterally in the concavities between the spine and the lateral abdominal wall, and the pelvic peritoneum are the most commonly encountered sites of abscess formation. In addition to pooling in these dependent spaces, the respiratory movement of the diaphragms produces negative intra-abdominal forces that draw fluid to the subphrenic spaces. Abscesses in the lesser sac generally develop as a consequence of severe pancreatitis or perforated gastric or duodenal ulcers, or as complications of gallbladder or gastric surgery. Localized abscesses may develop in relation to a gangrenous viscus, resulting in periappendiceal, subhepatic, pericholecystic, or interloop abscesses, localized by the gut mesentery and adjacent loops of bowel.

MICROBIAL AETIOLOGY

The microbial flora of the digestive tract shift from small numbers of aerobic streptococci (including enterococci) and facultative Gram-negative bacilli in the stomach, duodenum, and jejunum to larger numbers of these species together with a great excess of anaerobic Gram-negative bacilli (particularly *Bacteroides* spp.) and anaerobic Gram-positive flora (streptococci and clostridia) in the distal ileum and colon. Intra-abdominal abscesses usually contain multiple pathogens, and almost always a mixture of aerobic and anaerobic organisms. The yield obtained from abscess cultures depends on the prior or concurrent administration of antibiotics, the care with which cultures are transported in a truly anaerobic environment (preferably a capped syringe of abscess contents, cultured promptly), and the diligence with which cultures are processed both aerobically and anaerobically.

Occasionally, yeasts such as *Candida* species may be recovered from abscess fluid. Patients who develop intra-abdominal abscesses after prolonged hospital admission or prior antibiotic therapy may be colonized by a variety of nosocomial pathogens. Abscesses that follow penetrating trauma may also include skin flora such as staphylococci, or non-fermenting Gram-negative bacilli such as *Pseudomonas* species acquired from the environment.

UNDERLYING CAUSES

Perforation of a viscus (complicating peptic ulcer disease, appendicitis, diverticulitis, cholecystitis, Crohn's disease, adenocarcinoma of the colon); progressive ischaemia and infarction of the gallbladder, pancreas, or intestine, including typhlitis in the setting of profound neutropenia; penetrating injuries to the abdominal viscera; or leakage of intestinal contents during abdominal surgery are the usual antecedent events which lead to the development of intra-abdominal abscesses. Although abscesses may localize in close relation to the site of initial peritoneal contamination, the anatomical considerations described above regularly lead to the development of subphrenic or pelvic abscesses distant from the primary lesion.

CLINICAL FEATURES

An abscess is readily suspected in a patient with a predisposing primary intra-abdominal disease or whose postoperative course is complicated by abdominal pain, focal tenderness, progressive fever, leucocytosis, and intermittent polymicrobial bacteraemia. However, many of these classic features may be absent, and patients with an intra-abdominal abscess may present with persistent ileus, abdominal distension, mild liver function abnormalities, an unexplained and persistent pleural effusion, or an entirely non-localizing debilitating illness with or without fever. Pelvic abscesses may be associated with urinary frequency, diarrhoea, or tenesmus. Fever, malaise, and associated symptoms may emerge only after the completion of antibiotic therapy for a postoperative pneumonia or superficial wound infection. Occasionally, symptoms may develop indolently months after an initial presentation, and the relationship between the current illness and prior abdominal surgery may be overlooked. Rarely, the symptoms may suggest a primarily intrathoracic process (empyema, purulent pericarditis, or pneumonia) as a result of extension of a subphrenic abscess through the diaphragm. A pneumonia-like presentation may result from slow spread through the diaphragm with necessitation directly into a bronchus rather than the more frequent extension into the pleural space.

DIAGNOSIS

Abnormal haematological parameters accompanying progressive inflammation such as leucocytosis, anaemia, and thrombocytosis are frequently present, but debilitated and elderly patients often fail to mount a reactive leucocytosis. Polymicrobial bacteraemia strongly implicates the presence of an intra-abdominal abscess. In many patients receiving antibiotic therapy, only a single species may be recovered on blood culture, but other foci of infections (urinary tract, intravascular catheter, pneumonia) should also be considered.

Modern cross-sectional imaging techniques have greatly facilitated the diagnosis of intra-abdominal abscesses, and have revolutionized their therapy (Fig. 1): simply considering the possibility of such a complication and initiating the appropriate imaging studies become crucial factors in confirming the diagnosis. Conventional abdominal plain films may indicate the presence of an abscess by demonstrating abnormal (extraluminal) collections of gas, air–fluid levels, or mottled material. More subtle findings may include pleural effusion, elevation of the diaphragm, or mass effect displacing the stomach or other viscera. The use of iodinated soluble oral contrast agents with CT scanning provides information on displacement or obstruction of viscera by an inflammatory mass or abscess, and has largely supplanted barium contrast studies in such evaluations.

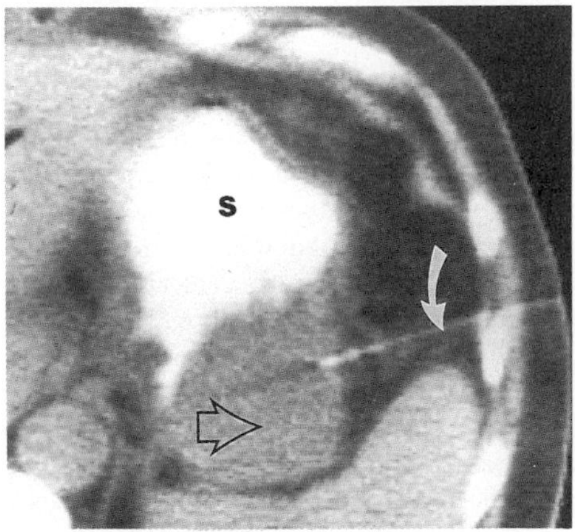

Fig. 1 Lesser sac abscess following partial gastrectomy visualized by abdominal CT scanning. The homogeneously appearing abscess (hollow arrow) is posterior to the contrast-filled stomach remnant (S) and anterior to the spleen. This collection could not be distinguished from haematoma except by percutaneous aspiration. The position of the percutaneous drainage catheter (curved arrow) is easily confirmed in this CT image. (By courtesy of Peter Mueller, MD.)

Ultrasound and CT scanning provide independent approaches for the detection of intra-abdominal abscesses. Both show established abscesses to have an ellipsoid shape and to displace adjacent viscera, and some have a discernible abscess wall or rind. Volumetric estimates can be extrapolated directly from the images. The sequence of imaging studies depends largely on an individual institution's resources and experience. Ultrasound instruments are mobile and may be transported to the bedside of a critically ill patient, allowing rapid imaging without X-irradiation. The quality of such studies is somewhat dependent on the skill of the operator, the sensitivity of the instrument used, and the interpretation skills of the consulting radiologist. The most important limitations, however, are the need for a sonolucent 'window' to image the region of interest, and the interference created by overlying bowel gas, dressings, and drains. Pelvic, subphrenic, and relatively superficial intra-abdominal collections abutting the abdominal wall are readily visualized by ultrasound. The ultrasound appearance of intra-abdominal abscesses varies from homogeneous hypoechoic fluid to more complex echogenic collections. A visualized collection may be sterile (bile, haematoma) or infected, and aspiration is usually required to document the presence of an abscess.

CT scanning requires transport of the patient to the scanner, and is routinely performed after the administration of both oral and intravenous contrast material; this limits its utility in patients with profound ileus or renal insufficiency. Serial images are obtained from the level of the diaphragm to the pelvis; these images are particularly helpful in identifying an occult abscess, and in excluding multiple abscesses. In addition to identifying a low-attenuation extraluminal mass, CT scans can document inflammatory oedema in the adjoining fat (obliteration of fat planes) and hyperaemia in the abscess capsule (enhancement). CT imaging is particularly well-suited for investigation of small or deep intra-abdominal collections.

Ultrasound and CT imaging techniques have limited the role of radionuclide scanning in the diagnosis of intra-abdominal abscesses. Gallium-67 citrate is administered intravenously, and binds to lactoferrin released by leucocytes at sites of inflammation. Indium-111 oxine is used to label the patient's granulocytes *ex vivo*, which are then re-infused intravenously. Although each method is effective at identifying intra-abdominal abscesses, the images provide insufficient resolution to guide needle drainage. Gallium-67 scanning is limited by its excretion by the colon, delaying scanning for 1 to 3 days before the background level is satisfactory to image intra-abdominal collections. It also lacks specificity, since Gallium-67 is concentrated by neoplasms and sterile inflammatory processes. Indium-111 labelling of granulocytes is laborious, the labelling and scanning process requires 6 to 12 h, and leucocyte uptake may also lack specificity. False-positive findings suggesting an abdominal abscess can result from a pulmonary infection from which indium-111-labelled leucocytes have been coughed up in sputum, swallowed, passed through the gastrointestinal tract and pooled temporarily in the caecal area. The use of such techniques is now largely limited to patients in whom intra-abdominal abscesses are strongly suspected but whose ultrasound or CT images fail to provide adequate diagnostic information.

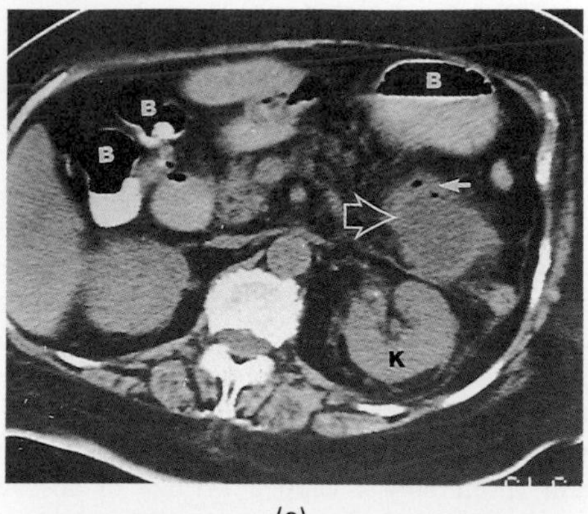

(a)

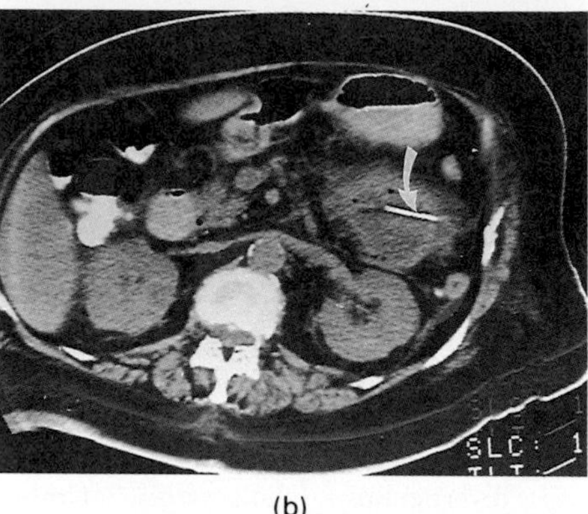

(b)

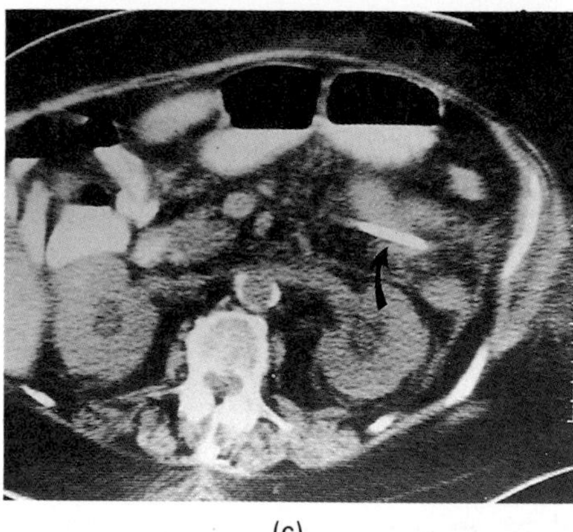
(c)

Fig. 2 Use of CT scanning to identify and drain an intra-abdominal abscess. (a) An abscess (hollow arrow) containing fluid and air (small solid arrow) is present anterior to the left kidney (K). Several loops of contrast-filled bowel are visible (B). (b) The position of the percutaneous drainage catheter (curved arrow) within the abscess cavity is confirmed. (c) Scan performed prior to catheter removal demonstrates resolution of the abscess. (By courtesy of Peter Mueller, MD.)

THERAPY

Once an intra-abdominal abscess has been defined radiologically, a drainage procedure is necessary. Over the past decade percutaneous catheter drainage procedures based on cross-sectional imaging techniques have become increasingly important. Ultrasound or CT study localizes the collection and defines safe access for catheter placement, avoiding adjoining viscera and blood vessels, and facilitating dependent drainage (Fig. 2). An initial diagnostic needle aspiration is frequently performed to document access to the suspected abscess, to provide fluid for Gram stain and culture, and to facilitate placement of a larger bore drainage catheter. The highest rates of successful catheter drainage have been associated with single, unilocular abscesses. Multiple or complex abscesses, such as those which are poorly defined, multilocular, or septated containing necrotic material, or associated with a visceral fistula, have lower cure rates (about 50 per cent) when managed by catheter drainage alone. Initial percutaneous drainage often offers important benefits to the critically ill patient, even when the abscess is complex. Such manoeuvres may control sepsis, improve haemodynamics, and stabilize the patient prior to definitive surgical treatment. Initial catheter drainage may also drain peridiverticular or other local abscesses sufficiently to make single-stage resection and internal anastomosis possible, rather than traditional multiple-stage procedures.

After placement of a suitable percutaneous catheter and gentle aspiration of abscess contents, repeat imaging should be performed to confirm catheter position and to estimate the size of the residual cavity. Subsequent cessation of drainage may be due to effective obliteration of the cavity, or occlusion or dislodgement of the catheter. Catheters may be gently irrigated with 5 ml of sterile saline; if this procedure is unsuccessful in re-establishing drainage, catheters may be manipulated or replaced during repeat imaging. The duration of drainage is usually 1 to 2 weeks, and is accompanied by resolution of fever, signs of toxicity, and leucocytosis. Persistent drainage usually reflects the presence of an enteric fistula—this can be documented by sinography under fluoroscopic control.

Surgical exploration is largely restricted to patients who have failed to improve despite percutaneous drainage, or in whom collections are not amenable to catheter drainage. Ideally, direct surgical drainage should be performed via an extraperitoneal approach, to limit the risk of further contamination of the peritoneal cavity. After thorough debridement and irrigation of the abscess, multiple soft drains should be placed, facilitating dependent drainage. In some instances transabdominal exploration is necessary. When pancreatic abscesses or large collections develop in association with extensive necrotizing pancreatitis, particularly involving the lesser sac, surgical exploration is inevitable, and in some centres surgical drainage is undertaken directly. Interloop abscesses are also difficult to drain percutaneously and may be multiple; they generally require transabdominal drainage. Pelvic abscesses are often palpable as tender bulging masses impinging on the vagina or rectum. Drainage is achieved transvaginally or transrectally, with incision, digital exploration, and thorough irrigation.

Antibiotic therapy plays an adjunctive role in the management of abscesses, but medical treatment alone never represents definitive therapy. Since abscess fluid generally contains a mixture of aerobic or facultative organisms as well as anaerobes, initial empirical therapy must be effective against a broad range of pathogens. Simple and effective therapy against all of the recovered pathogens is sometimes problematic, and with adequate abscess drainage it is not usually necessary to treat every organism with maximally potent antibiotics. Fortunately, currently available antibiotics offer several options for empiric therapy.

Clindamycin and gentamicin have become a 'gold standard' of empirical therapy for intra-abdominal infections. However, the combination of ampicillin, gentamicin, and metronidazole is a more cost-effective regimen that provides therapy against enterococci as well as Gram-negative bacilli and anaerobes. In selected circumstances, such as in critically ill patients with bacteraemia due to ampicillin-resistant Gram-negative bacilli, or in neutropenic patients, a variety of newer β-lactam agents (piperacillin; second generation cephalosporins such as cefotetan or cefoxitin; third-generation agents such as cefotaxime, ceftriaxone, or ceftazidime; or imipenem) or agents combined with β-lactamase inhibitors (ampicillin-sulbactam or ticarcillin–clavulanic acid) may be used in place of ampicillin. When one of these agents provides adequate activity against anaerobic bacteria, metronidazole or clindamycin may be omitted. Careful monitoring of blood levels of gentamicin is important to minimize the risk of nephrotoxicity. When *Candida* species appear to play an important aetiological role, based on its presence in abundance on Gram stain, subsequent candidaemia, and the patient's immune status, therapy with amphotericin B is indicated, although its use may be supplanted in selected patients by the less toxic antifungal agent fluconazole.

Special considerations in the management of subphrenic abscesses

The importance of intra-abdominal catastrophes such as suppurative appendicitis and perforation of the stomach and duodenum requiring emergency laparotomy as antecedent causes for the development of subphrenic abscesses has waned; prior surgical procedures, particularly of the biliary tract, stomach, and colon are now the most frequent causes of subphrenic abscess. The growing frequency of left subphrenic abscesses, as high as 40 per cent in some series, has reflected this change in aetiology. The falciform ligament divides the left and right subphrenic spaces and limits the frequency of bilateral subphrenic abscesses. However, multiple synchronous intra-abdominal abscesses including subphrenic collections are rather common, and failure to identify and drain these additional abscesses is frequently responsible for adverse outcomes. The coexistence of infected and non-infected loculated collections adds to the complexity of this situation. Occasionally, right subphrenic abscesses develop in relation to a hepatic visceral abscess, particularly amoebic abscess. Since amoebic disease is cosmopolitan and ubiquitous, this diagnosis should always be considered in acutely ill individuals with parenchymal hepatic abscesses and subphrenic collections.

The deep location of these infections leads to a paucity of localizing signs and symptoms beyond the systemic findings discussed above. Ultrasound readily displays the diaphragm and is particularly valuable in distinguishing between pleural effusions and subphrenic collections. CT scanning is helpful in defining the precise localization of a subphrenic abscess and identifying the presence of additional intra-abdominal collections. Traditional open drainage of subphrenic abscesses through the bed of the twelfth rib used extraperitoneal and extrapleural approaches whenever possible, to minimize the risk of spreading infection within the abdomen and certainly within the pleural space: complicating empyemas were often fatal. Percutaneous catheter drainage is effective in draining most subphrenic abscesses, and a transperitoneal approach is most commonly used, reducing the risk of pneumothorax associated with transthoracic approaches. The risks associated with open transabdominal drainage of such abscesses have fallen greatly, and this approach allows synchronous collections to be treated at the same time. The management of individual patients depends on the antecedent causes of abscess formation, the precise anatomical location of the abscess, the availability of skilled interventional radiologists, and the presence of additional lesions.

Special considerations in the management of pelvic abscesses

Women can also develop abscesses following infection of the pelvic viscera as part of the spectrum of pelvic inflammatory disease.

Neisseria gonorrhoeae and *C. trachomatis* are the primary pathogens responsible for salpingitis in sexually active women. These organisms are frequently recovered by endocervical culture or rapid diagnostic methods, but progression to tubo-ovarian abscess is often accompanied by polymicrobial infection with aerobic and anaerobic bacteria. Intrauterine contraceptive devices and altered local resistance factors accompanying menses are considered to be risk factors for the development of salpingitis. The spectrum of clinical presentation can be broad, but tubo-ovarian abscesses should be considered in patients with persistent fever and pelvic pain and tenderness despite appropriate initial intensive parenteral antibiotic therapy, such as cefoxitin and doxycycline (Fig. 3). Pelvic ultrasound is valuable in corroborating the clinical diagnosis, and distinguishing frank abscess from phlegmon; laparoscopy can be performed if there is diagnostic uncertainty. Surgical drainage (usually via colpotomy) is indicated in patients who fail to respond to initial medical therapy. In patients with a ruptured tubo-ovarian abscess, laparotomy with unilateral salpingo-oophorectomy is required. In some centres, percutaneous catheter drainage is attempted prior to surgical exploration.

In addition to polymicrobial tubo-ovarian abscesses, intrauterine devices have also been associated with pelvic actinomycosis. This indolent process often produces few clinical manifestations until a pelvic mass is appreciated. The extensive inflammatory mass is usually associated with tubo-ovarian abscess formation and surrounding woody induration, and can produce ureteral and/or bowel obstruction. There is obliteration of normal tissue planes, and the lesion may be mistaken for widespread malignancy. Initial resection is not feasible, and patients require prolonged parenteral therapy (6–12 weeks of penicillin) prior to definitive resection.

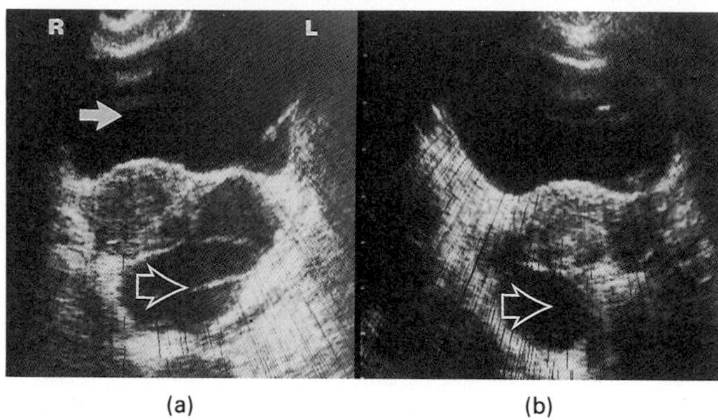

(a) (b)

Fig. 3 (a), (b) Two transverse ultrasound views of a multiloculated tubo-ovarian abscess (hollow arrows). Septations within the abscess are best seen in (a). The filled bladder appears as a large echo-free space (solid arrow). (By courtesy of Peter Mueller, MD.)

FURTHER READING

Altemeier WA, Culbertson WR, Fullen WD, Shook CD. Intra-abdominal abscesses. *Am J Surg*, 1973; **125**: 70–9.

Boyd DP. The subphrenic spaces and the emperor's new robes. *N Engl J Med*, 1966; **275**: 911–7.

Centers for Disease Control. Pelvic inflammatory disease: guidelines for prevention and management. *MMWR* 1991; **40**: 1–25.

Clark RA, Towbin R. Abscess drainage with CT and ultrasound guidance. *Radiol Clin N Am*, 1983; **21**: 445–59.

Halasz NA. Subphrenic abscess: myths and facts. *JAMA*, 1970; **214**: 724–6.

Mueller PR, Simeone JF. Intra-abdominal abscesses: diagnosis by sonography and computed tomography. *Radiol Clin N Am*, 1983; **21**: 425–43.

Mueller PR, *et al.* Percutaneous drainage of subphrenic abscess: a review of 62 patients. *Am J Roentgenol*, 1986; **147**: 1237–40.

Mueller PR, vanSonnenberg E. Interventional radiology in the chest and abdomen. *N Engl J Med*, 1990; **322**: 1364–74.

Ochsner A, Graves AM. Subphrenic abscess: an analysis of 3,372 collected and personal cases. *Ann Surg*, 1933; **98**: 961–90.

Onderdonk AB, Bartlett JG, Louie T, Sullivan-Seigler N, Gorbach SL. Microbial synergy in experimental intra-abdominal abscess. *Infect Immun*, 1976; **13**: 22–6.

Papanicolaou N, *et al.* Abscess-fistula association: radiologic recognition and percutaneous management. *Am J Roentgenol*, 1984; **143**: 811–5.

Rotstein OD, Pruett TL, Simmons RL. Mechanisms of microbial synergy in polymicrobial surgical infections. *Rev Infect Dis*, 1985; **7**: 151–70.

Sanders RC. The changing epidemiology of subphrenic abscess and its clinical and radiological consequences. *Br J Surg*, 1970; **57**: 449–55.

vanSonnenberg E, *et al.* Temporizing effect of percutaneous drainage of complicated abscesses in critically ill patients. *Am J Roentgenol*, 1984; **142**: 821–6.

Wang SMS, Wilson SE. Subphrenic abscess: the new epidemiology. *Arch Surg*, 1977; **112**: 934–6.

The liver 22

22.1 Surgical anatomy of the liver and biliary tree

ADRIAN SAVAGE

SURGICAL ANATOMY OF THE LIVER

The external appearance of the liver shows its division into two lobes by the umbilical fissure and falciform ligament. Further subdivisions are made on other superficial features. The quadrate lobe is a subdivision of the right lobe and lies to the left of the gallbladder fossa and to the right of the umbilical fissure. The transverse hilar fissure forms the posterior boundary of the quadrate lobe and divides it from the caudate lobe posteriorly (Fig. 1). These features and names are of historical interest only.

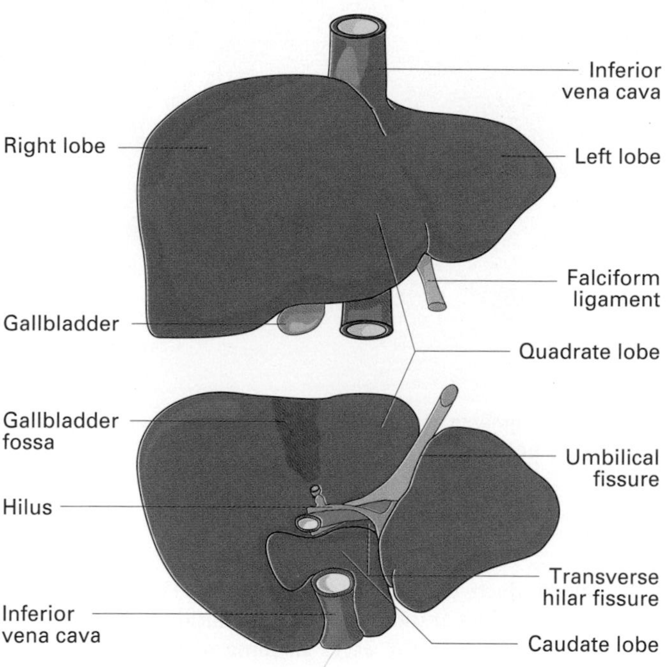

Fig. 1 Divisions of the liver by its external features.

The internal architecture of the liver bears only a superficial relationship to its external appearance. Cast studies of the biliary tree and portal venous radicles show that the liver is divided into right and left halves, according to the territories of drainage of the right and left hepatic ducts and areas of supply of the right and left branches of the portal vein and hepatic artery. This principal division is called Cantlie's line, after its first description in 1898, but it is not readily visible on external examination. It runs from the medial edge of the gallbladder fossa to the inferior vena cava posteriorly. The nomenclature of hepatic anatomy has become confused by the use of the term 'lobe' which has been applied to both the division of the liver by its external features and the territories of drainage of the right and left hepatic ducts.

Glisson's capsule, a peritoneal and fibrous covering, invests the liver. The reflections of the capsule on to the right hemidiaphragm form the coronary ligament and right triangular ligament, and the reflection from the left liver on to the left hemidiaphram forms the left triangular ligament. Glisson's capsule is also reflected over the falciform ligament. The structures at the hilum of the liver are invested in dense fibrous tissue continuous with Glisson's capsule; here this covering is known as the hilar plate. The hilar plate is continuous with the peritoneal layers investing the common hepatic and common bile duct, cystic duct, and gallbladder.

The liver is supplied by blood, 80 per cent of which comes from the portal venous system and 20 per cent of which is delivered by the hepatic artery. Venous drainage is by three large short hepatic veins that pass posteriorly to the inferior vena cava, which is close to the posterior surface of the liver. Drainage of bile occurs from the left and right hepatic ducts to the common hepatic and bile duct and then to the second part of the duodenum.

The portal vein is formed by the confluence of the superior mesenteric vein and the splenic vein in front of the inferior vena cava and behind the neck of the pancreas. The portal vein runs behind the pancreas to the free border of the lesser omentum where it traverses the hilum of the liver in the hepatoduodenal ligament behind the common bile duct and to the right of the hepatic artery. At the hilum of the liver, the portal vein divides into left and right branches. The vein with its accompanying branches of the biliary tree and hepatic artery, are invested in a fibrous sheath continuous with the hilar plate.

The common hepatic artery usually arises from the coeliac axis and travels across the posterior abdominal wall to lie just above the pylorus. Here it gives off the gastroduodenal artery before continuing as the hepatic artery proper which then runs in the gastroduodenal ligament medial to the common bile duct and anterior to the portal vein to the hilum of the liver. The hepatic artery divides into the left and right hepatic artery well below the hilum of the liver. Sixteen per cent of individuals have an aberrant right hepatic artery, which arises from the superior mesenteric artery and runs in the groove to the right of the portal vein and common bile duct. Less commonly, the arterial supply to the left half of the liver comes from the left gastric artery.

The venous radicles in the liver give rise to three hepatic veins: the right, middle, and left hepatic veins which are short and large. The middle hepatic vein usually joins the left hepatic vein before entering the inferior vena cava. In addition, a number of unnamed short veins enter the inferior vena cava directly. These arise in the caudate lobe which, because of is embryological development from the dorsal mesogastrium, could be expected to have a different venous drainage.

SEGMENTATION OF THE LIVER

The three hepatic veins divide the liver into four sectors, each of which is further subdivided into two segments. The whole liver is therefore divisible into eight segments: four are in the right half, and three in the left half (Fig. 2). The remaining segment is the caudate lobe, which should be considered separately because of its different embryology, variable blood supply, and venous drainage. Two differing descriptions are in common use regarding segmentation of the liver; that of Couinaud and that of Goldsmith and Woodburne. These differ mainly in nomenclature, and the description of Couinaud will be used here.

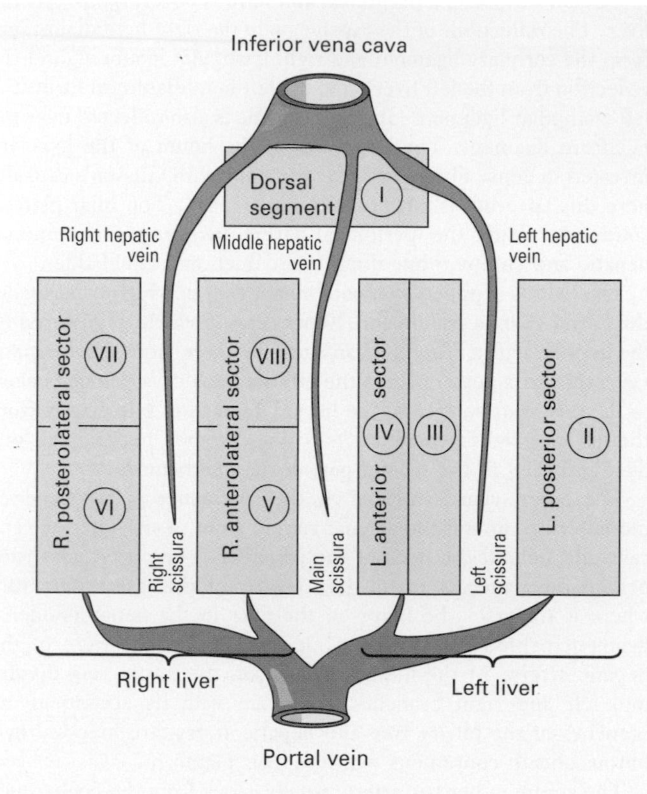

Fig. 2 Schematic representation of the segmentation of the liver.

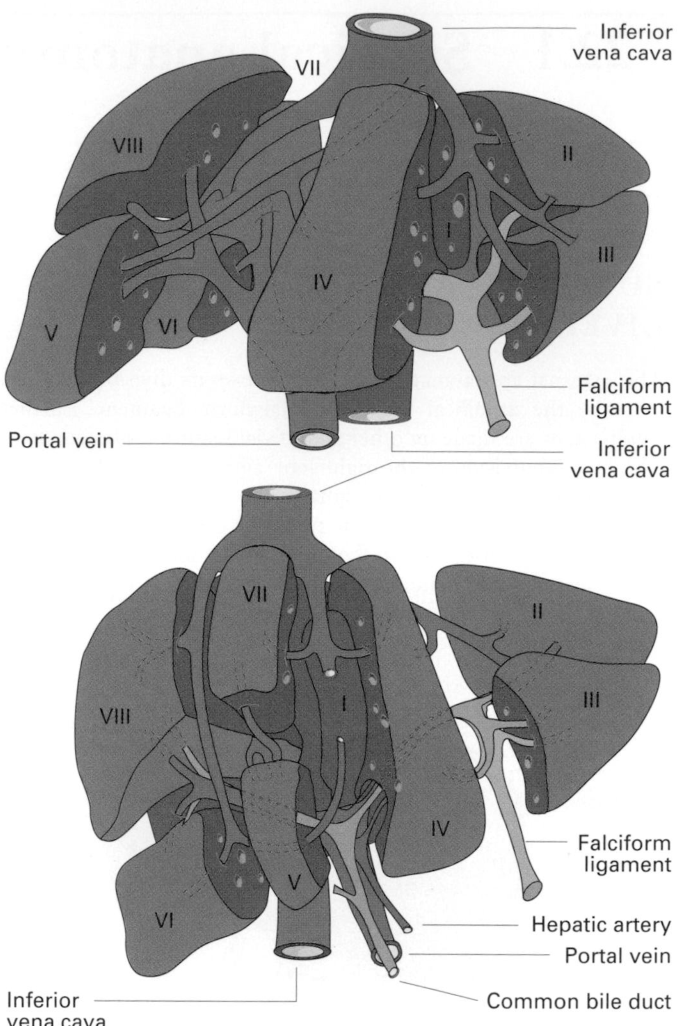

Fig. 3 The segments of the liver showing the segmental biliary tree and venous drainage.

The segments are numbered anticlockwise I to VIII starting with the caudate lobe (Fig. 3). Each segment is supplied by a named portal venous radicle and is drained by a segmental bile duct, forming the smallest anatomical unit of hepatic resection. Removal of segments II to IV is described as 'left hepatectomy' and removal of segments V to VIII, 'right hepatectomy'. Removal of segment IV (the quadrate lobe) in addition to right hepatectomy is described as extended right hepatectomy. The use of this nomenclature avoides the confusion inherent in the use of the terms 'hepatic lobectomy' and 'trisegmentectomy'.

THE INTRAHEPATIC BILE DUCTS

The interlobular bile canaliculi join to form segmental bile ducts that eventually drain into the right or left hepatic ducts. On the right, ducts from segments VI and VII join to form the right posterior sectoral duct which runs horizontally across the gall-bladder fossa, where it is surgically accessible after localization by needle puncture or intraoperative ultrasound. The right anterior sectoral duct runs more vertically and is formed by the confluence of the ducts from segments V and VIII.

Segmental ducts from segments II, III, and IV merge to form the left hepatic duct at the base of the umbilical fissure. Although there are variations in the exact anatomy of this confluence of segmental bile ducts, these are of little clinical relevance. The duct from segment III is surgically accessible by dissection in the groove to the left of the umbilical ligament, where it lies anterior to its accompanying branch of the portal vein and hepatic artery. The left hepatic duct runs from the base of the umbilical fissure to the hilum in the transverse hilar fissure, invested by the fibrous tissue of the hilar plate with the left portal vein lying posterior and the left hepatic artery lying inferior. The left duct is surgically accessible by division of the peritoneal fold under the quadrate lobe (segment IV), a procedure known as lowering the hilar plate.

At the hilum of the liver, the right and left hepatic ducts join to form the confluence of the bile ducts. Anatomical variations of both the intrahepatic and extrahepatic biliary tree are so common that a 'normal', pattern is seen in less than 60 per cent of individuals (Fig. 4). In 57 per cent, the right anterior and posterior sectoral ducts join to form a right hepatic duct, whereas in the remainder, the right anterior and posterior sectoral ducts join the confluence individually, or join one or other of the right sectoral ducts. The fact that the right posterior sectoral duct may join either the common hepatic duct or the cystic duct in 6 per cent of individuals is surgically important, since this may alter the approach for cholecystectomy.

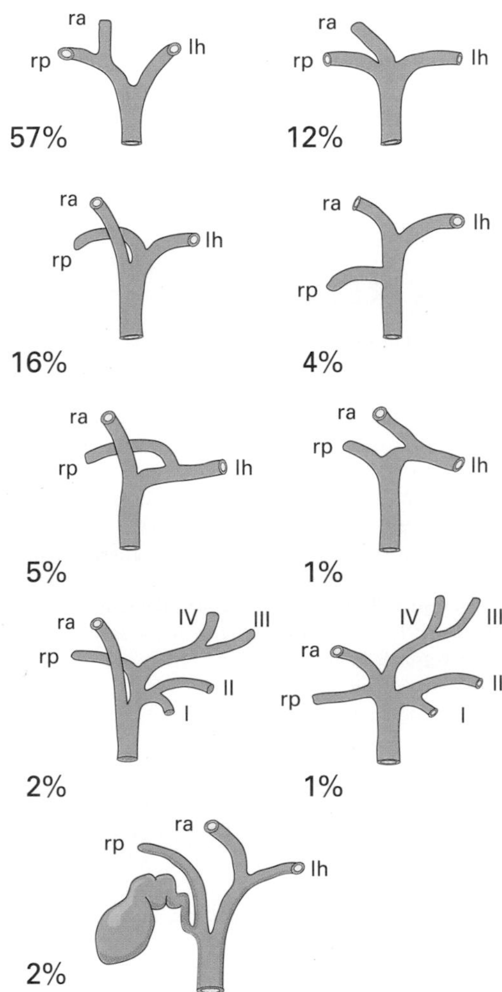

Fig. 4 Anomalies of the confluence of the bile ducts. ra = right anterior sectoral duct, rp = right posterior sectoral duct, lh = left hepatic duct and roman numerals refer to hepatic segments.

THE GALLBLADDER

The gallbladder lies in a fossa on the lower surface of the liver. Four parts of the gallbladder are described: the fundus, the body, the infundibulum, and the neck. In addition, a Hartmann's pouch often develops as a pathological feature in the neck and infundibulum of the gallbladder in the presence of gallstones. Various congenital abnormalities have been described, including double, bilobed, and intrahepatic gallbladder, and congenital absence. The occasional presence of a long mesentery is of significance since it may allow torsion. The gallbladder drains by the cystic duct to the junction of the common hepatic duct and common bile duct. The mucosa of the cystic duct forms crescentic folds known as the spiral valve of Heister which tend to block the passage of a gallstone and of some cannulas used for operative cholangiography.

CALOT'S TRIANGLE

Calot's triangle is formed by the common hepatic duct to the left and the cystic duct below. Although the original description of this area gave the cystic artery as the superior border, the inferior surface of the liver is now accepted as this border. The cystic artery usually arises from the right hepatic artery behind the common hepatic duct and runs behind the right hepatic duct and through Calot's triangle to the gallbladder. In 20 per cent of individuals the cystic artery arises from a right hepatic artery that runs anterior to the common hepatic duct, and the right hepatic artery forms a loop or 'caterpillar hump' with the cystic artery originating from the apex in 7 per cent of individuals. In the latter case, the right hepatic artery may be mistaken for the cystic artery during cholecystectomy. In 10 per cent of individuals the cystic artery arises proximally from the right hepatic artery and runs anterior to the common hepatic duct, while the right hepatic artery runs posterior to this duct.

Two other major anomalies may be encountered during the course of dissection in Calot's triangle for cholecystectomy. An aberrant right hepatic artery from the superior mesenteric artery occurs in 16 per cent of individuals, running in the groove between the common hepatic duct and the portal vein. It can be seen in the medial border of Calot's triangle in 90 per cent of such patients. The right posterior or anterior sectoral ducts may also run through Calot's triangle and may be mistaken for the cystic duct.

THE BILE DUCTS

From the confluence of the bile ducts, the common hepatic duct runs for some 2.5 to 3.5 cm down to its confluence with the cystic duct, resulting in the formation of the common bile duct. This junction is variable: the cystic duct opens directly into the confluence of the bile ducts in 2 per cent of individuals, and extends down behind the duodenum before joining the common hepatic duct in another 15 to 20 per cent (Fig. 5).

The common hepatic and bile ducts are supplied by arteries that originate from the right hepatic, gastroduodenal, and retroduodenal arteries. The major arteries supplying the bile duct run axially at three o'clock and nine o'clock. Other small arteries run axially in the mesentery around the bile duct and form a plexus over the bile duct. It is not established whether injury to the blood supply will result in a postoperative bile duct stricture. However, it is reasonable to assume that extensive dissection around the bile duct will impair the vascular supply of the bile duct.

The common bile duct passes behind the first part of the duodenum. It may be exposed by division of the peritoneal fold over the superior aspect of the first part of the duodenum and by drawing the duodenum downwards. It then runs either in a groove in the back of the head of the pancreas or in the loose areolar tissue behind the head of the pancreas. Here it may be exposed by Kocher's manoeuvre, that is, division of the peritoneum lateral to the

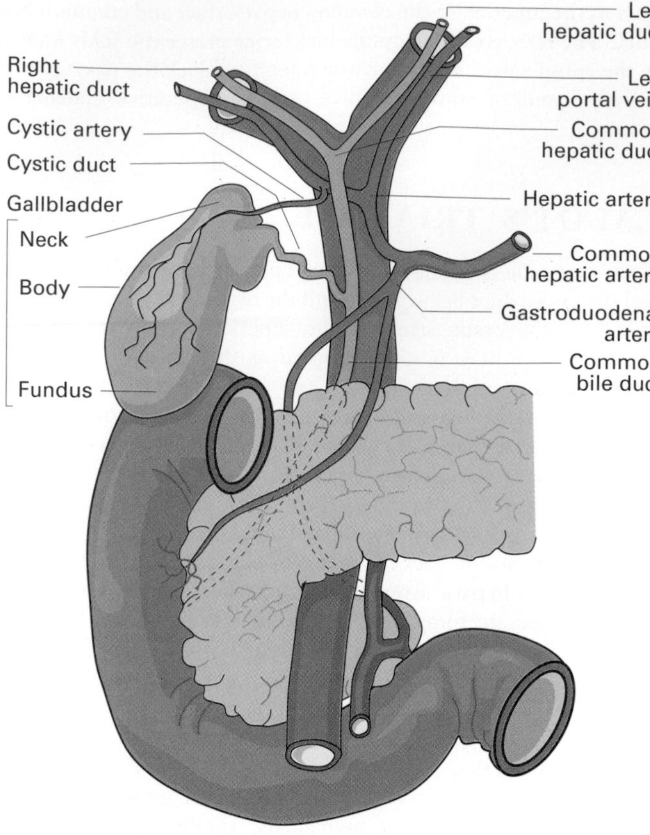

Fig. 5 The relations of the extrahepatic biliary tree.

duodenum and reflection of the duodenum and head of the pancreas medially. It curves to the right to enter the medial duodenal wall about 2 cm below the duodenal cap, where it is joined by the main pancreatic duct of Wirsung to form the sphincter of Oddi, which discharges into the duodenum through the ampulla of Vater.

Some 2 cm of the terminal portion of the common bile duct lies within the wall of the duodenum where it is surrounded by the smooth muscle fibres of the sphincter of Oddi. The pancreatic duct may be closely applied to the common bile duct at this point and may similarly be invested in smooth muscle of the sphincter of Oddi. The exact anatomy of the terminal common bile duct and pancreatic duct follows one of three patterns. They may unite outside the wall of the duodenum and traverse the duodenal wall to the papilla as a common channel. They may join within the duodenal wall and have a short common terminal channel. Separate orifices have been described.

FURTHER READING

Bismuth H. Surgical anatomy and anatomical surgery of the liver. *World J Surg* 1982; **6**: 3–9

Couinaud C. Lobes et segments hépatiques. Notes sur l'architecture anatomique et chirurgicale du foie. *Presse Med*, 1954; **62**: 709–12.

Couinaud C. *Le Foie: Etudes Anatomiques et Chirurgicales*. Paris: Masson 1957: 9–12

Goldsmith NA and Woodburne RT. The surgical anatomy pertaining to liver resection. *Surg Gynecol Obstet* 1957; **195**: 310–18.

Northover JMA, Terblanche J. A new look at the arterial supply of the bile duct in man and its surgical implications. *Br J Surg* 1979; **66**: 379–84.

Smadja C, Blumgart LH. The biliary tract and the anatomy of biliary exposure. In Blumgart LH, ed. *Surgery of the liver and biliary tract*. Edinburgh: Churchill Livingstone 1988; **1**: 11–22.

22.2 Hepatic trauma: principles of management

RONALD A. MALT

The liver is effectively an intrathoracic organ (Fig. 1). It is protected from external forces, except for those severe enough to break ribs or to split the diaphragm (Fig. 2). Twenty-five per cent of blunt injuries and 5 per cent of penetrating injuries are fatal. If kinetic forces have rent the liver nonetheless, other organs are likely to have been be injured, and a Budd-Chiari syndrome may result from herniation of the liver through the diaphragm.

Recognize potentially lethal injuries in remote organs

Little's cartoon (Fig. 3) shows that in 120 cases of liver injury the brain was injured 15 times (10 fatally), the spleen 21 times (6 fatally), and bones 45 times (14 fatally). It is important to deal immediately with remote injuries that have the potential to become lethal, even if at the moment they don't seem dangerous. Otherwise they'll be forgotten.

Gain exposure by a midline xiphoid-to-pubis incision

Only wide exposure permits examination and treatment of the liver and of other organs, such as the right colon and the pancreas. Elevate the patient's left arm on an 'ether screen' or other atraumatic means of support to facilitate exposure when a sternotomy or a thoracoabdominal incision is demanded (Fig. 4). Figure 5 illustrates an abdomen that was explored for bleeding through a low-transverse incision without avail. When that incision was converted to a proper incision (the vertical component) the haemorrhage was stopped easily. Lyse the coronary and the triangular ligaments to mobilize the liver in all directions for inspection and repair (Fig. 6).

Control or observe low-pressure bleeding

Although until recently all liver injuries were handled as if they were incipient catastrophes, CT scans show that in many of these

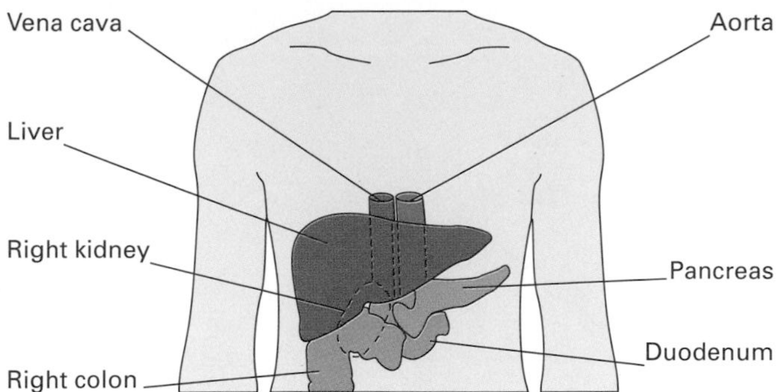

Fig. 1 Relation of liver to adjacent organs.

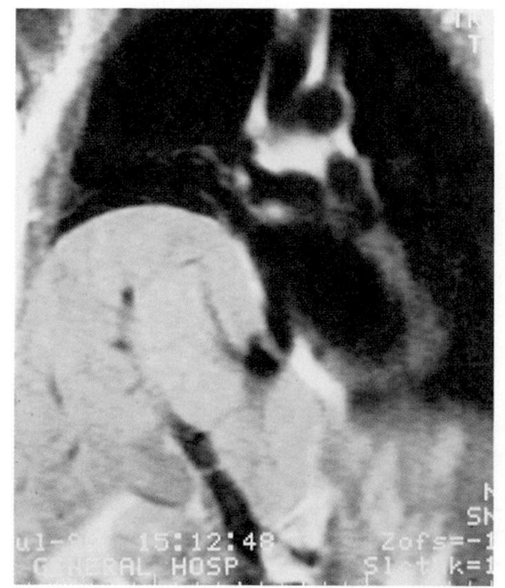

Fig. 2 Herniation and entrapment of liver through ruptured right hemidiaphragm.

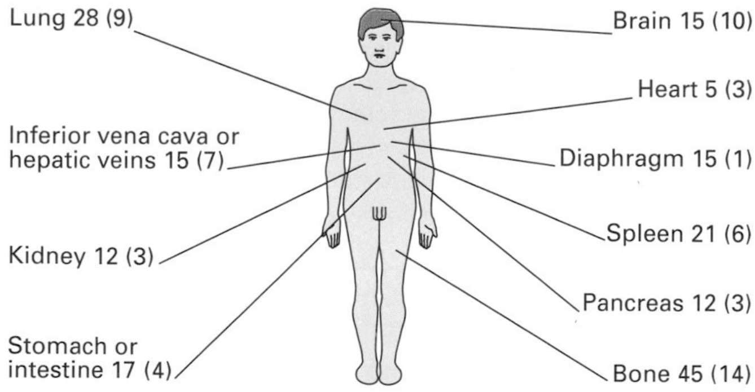

Fig. 3 Injuries to remote organs and incidence of death (number in parentheses).

injuries blood loss is less than 500 ml; for these stable and relatively minor injuries observation alone is satisfactory. Indeed, 60 per cent of blunt injury and 90 per cent of penetrating injury can be managed conservatively provided that CT examination ascertains that the hepatic flexure of the colon and the right kidney are not damaged. To the contrary, unstable patients do not benefit from

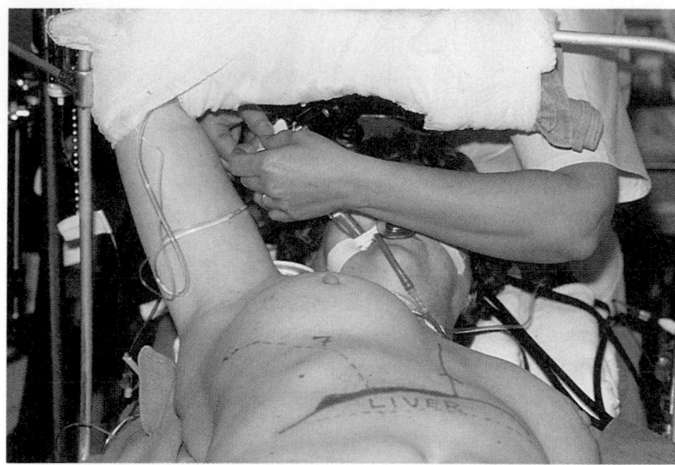

Fig. 4 Facilitating trans-sternal or thoracoabdominal access to the liver.

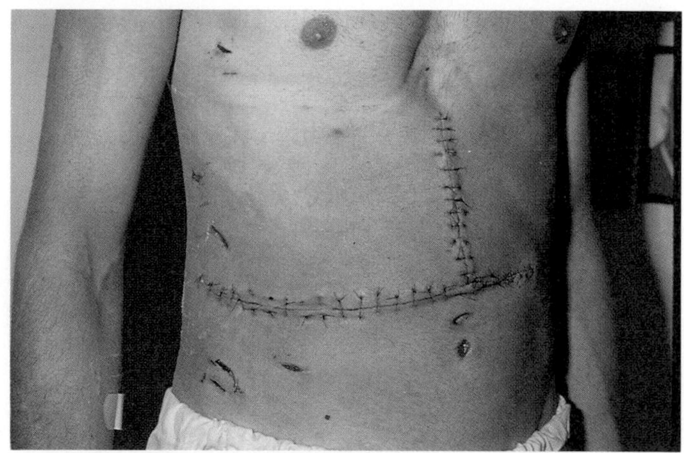

Fig. 5 Urgent exposure gained through a previously made transverse supraumbilical incision was inadequate for proper exposure, but a midline incision permitted rapid control of an arterial injury. Multiple stab wounds are visible.

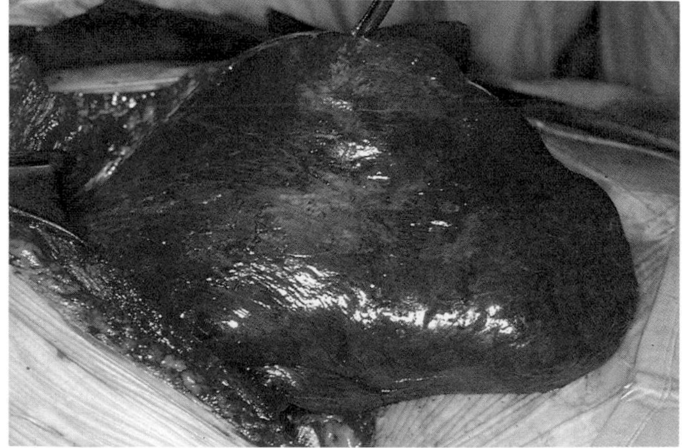

Fig. 6 Although one can infrequently raise the liver to the abdominal wall for emergent optimal exposure, it is sometimes possible.

the use of CT scans because the interval from arrival in the emergency department to the time of surgery is too long for safety. Unstable patients need an urgent laparotomy.

One must be aggressive if the patient deteriorates or if the magnitude of bleeding increases. Control intravascular losses by infusing volume-expanding solutions and blood products through a 14-G needle in a major vein of each upper extremity or through a subclavian vein cannula. Do not use lower extremity veins for this purpose because the inferior vena cava might have to be cross clamped, blocking blood flow cephalad. Although one might imagine that controlling haemorrhage in a fragmented liver would be a formidable task, even if the liver is semipulped manual pressure to the liver against the diaphragm generally stops haemorrhage because bleeding is usually from hepatic veins, and their pressure is low. Two dozen Mikulicz pads for tamponade are a further aid, however.

Maintain core temperature and prevent heat loss

Although one cannot pump heat into a patient, who normally generates the heat of a 60-W light bulb, he or she can be kept from losing heat by having the room temperature above 26°C from the start. If this temperature, or a higher one, can be maintained, and if the patient's skull is covered with an internally reflecting aluminium cap, the core temperature will probably stay within a physiological range, allowing normal enzymic processes to work, particularly those associated with coagulation of blood. The Bair Hugger®, recently introduced, facilitates thermoregulation in patients at risk of hypothermia because it permits a controlled flow of warm air to stream over body surfaces enveloped in plastic manifolds and designed specifically for warming truncal and axial organs.

Remember occult vena caval bleeding

When bleeding persists and its site of origin is undiscoverable, think first of a tear in the inferior vena cava, especially if blood drips from the diaphragm or emerges from behind the liver and is present in the lesser sac. Use a disposable 18-F Frazier aspirator to clear the field of blood. It is without price in every operation associated with the likelihood of major blood loss.

In principle, try to get the liver on to the abdominal wall, just as in mobilizing a spleen for splenectomy. When a rent in the vena cava or in a proximate vein declares itself, apply local pressure until instruments and help arrive. The most important instruments are Judd–Allis vascular forceps (clamps). Apply five or more Judd–Allis clamps to the lips of the rent to set the stage for undersewing them or using them to approximate the posterior vein wall through an open anterior wall.

Atriocaval shunts

The need to insert an atriocaval shunt is rare (Fig. 7). Occasions for its insertion are so infrequent that few surgeons have an opportunity to use it regularly. In our hospital a single insertion was successful in the 1960s; no further use of it has been recognized or undertaken. Even in Houston, Texas, only 31 patients were treated with an atriocaval shunt over a period of nearly 10 years. At San Francisco General Hospital, where the shunt was devised, shunts were inserted in only 27 patients over a span of about 20 years. Survival of 12 patients gave a mortality rate of 55 per cent.

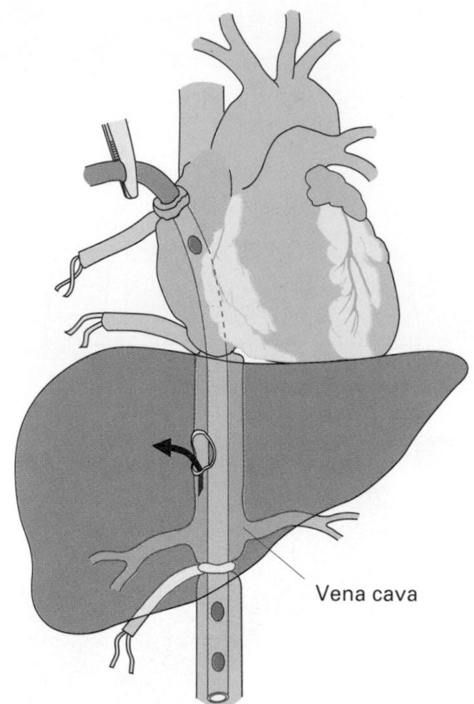

Fig. 7 Schema of Shrock–Blaisdell shunt.

Air embolism kills surreptitiously

A decrease in end tidal $P\text{CO}_2$ is the most specific sign of air embolism, except for a windmill murmur in the heart. Depending upon the patient's size, his position on the operating table, and the degree of cardiovascular compensation, an air embolism of 20 ml, or less, can kill. Although the commonly invoked remedy is to turn the patient left side down to permit air to rise into the right heart, this action is seldom a specific because air is certainly already in the cardiac ventricles. Having a defibrillator at ready is more important, because attempts at removal of air from the right heart by aspiration through a jugular or subclavian central line are less successful than might be anticipated and because air often enters the cannula during fruitless efforts at removing intra-atrial froth.

Prevent haemodilution

This is the great dichotomy between surgeons and anaesthesiologists. The surgeon would like the blood to clot on demand. The anaesthesiologist is imbued with the need to deliver a plethora of lactated Ringer's solution to support physiological processes. An initial appropriate compromise is for the anaesthesiologist to administer not more than 2 litres of Ringer's solution unless massive volume replacement has to be undertaken with only Ringer's solution at hand. Otherwise, the formula should be to transfuse both 10 units of platelets and 5 units of packed cells for every 5 units of blood given after the first five. Once haemodilution has occurred there is no use trying to correct the situation at the operating table. Pack the abdomen and restore homeostasis in an intensive care unit.

Facilitate haemostasis

Although Pringle's manoeuvre (compression of the hepatic vascular triad) is sometimes touted as a sovereign remedy for bleeding of all sorts in hepatic trauma, even Pringle's attempts to make compression work were virtually unavailing, and matters are often little better today. Notwithstanding, compress the liver against the diaphragm as described above and use Pringle's manoeuvre for the fastest and the most effective ways of dealing with fragmented liver and torrential bleeding from an unknown source. The problem is that accessory and replaced right and left hepatic arteries are common; the ability to compress aberrant blood vessels outside of the portal triad is a matter of luck. Occlusion of the infradiaphragmatic vena cava is sometimes helpful, but impeded venous return to the heart is often more than the patient can stand. Although a normal liver can withstand an hour of arterial ischaemia during an elective resection to remove a neoplasm, the tolerance of a burst and bleeding liver is far less.

Given that major tears of the parahepatic vena cava and of the right hepatic vein are usually fatal, devote attention to local haemostasis in the parts of the liver under your control: namely, the shattered hepatic parenchyma and the major and minor intrahepatic veins liable to bleed or to suck air, or both. Drain the liver bed with suction catheters above and below. Although drainage is sometimes frowned upon by the experts, experts won't be reading this chapter.

Place bolsters of Teflon felt approximately 4 cm long and 1 cm wide over and under regions of hepatic bleeding. Coapt the Teflon felt with no. 1 chromic catgut insofar as is possible, avoiding nearby structures in the portal triad (Fig. 8). Felt does not extrude, even in the presence of sepsis. If a ragged surface of liver presents itself, try converting it to a fishmouth contour to make closure easier, with or without Teflon bolsters.

When minor, persistent bleeding thwarts efforts to clear the field of blood, spray the sites with thrombin solution; then place a Hemopad® of crystalline collagen on the raw surface, followed by a rubber dam of appropriate size. When the dam is eventually removed, the thrombin and collagen layer remain. Although thrombin glue may work the same way, it is not approved for use in America because of the risk of hepatitis C contamination.

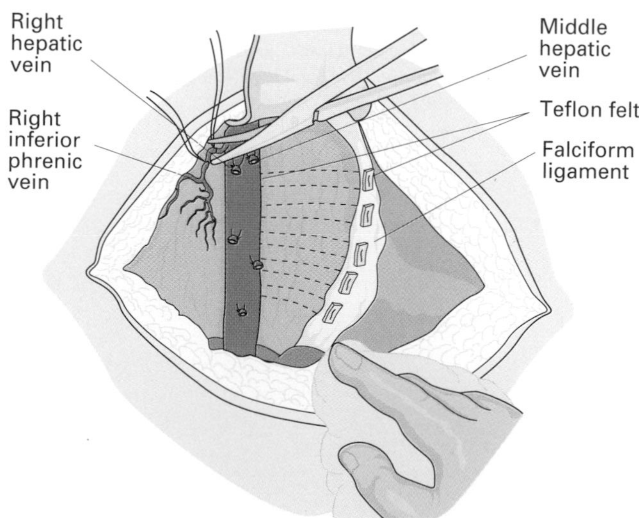

Fig. 8 Cinching bolsters of Teflon felt to achieve haemostasis.

Types of injury

Deal with the five common types of injury as follows.

Subcapsular haematomas If they do not expand or burst, let them heal themselves as the blood and plasma are absorbed.

Stab wounds not bleeding when they are examined in the operating room require only observation initially. Do not drain them or stir them up.

Partial major amputations Do not try to mate them to their former locations. Because it contains growth factors that probably facilitate haemostasis and healing, pack omentum into major crevices in the liver and tie it in place with non-strangulating heavy chromic catgut.

The burst liver Try to preserve an artery to any segment or segments provided that the portal vein blow flow is normal and that collateral blood vessels are intact. Otherwise pack the liver with gauze pads beneath, above, and around itself. Wrapping and compressing the liver with polyglactin mesh is a potential solution, but not one commonly applied. Arteriography after homeostasis is gained is a reasonable option in some instances to identify post-traumatic false hepatic artery aneurysms (Fig. 9).

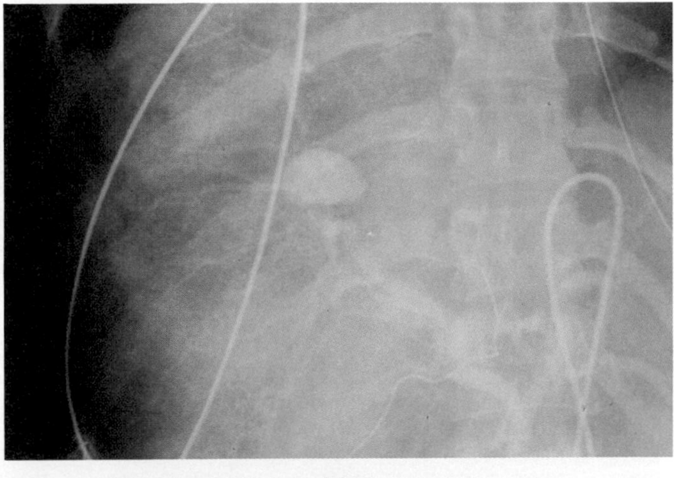

(a)

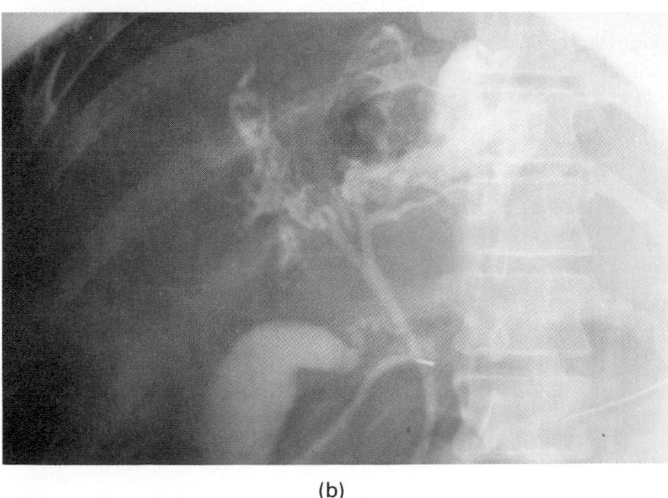

(b)

Fig. 9 (a) Ruptured false aneurysm of liver secondary to a shotgun wound. (b) Haemobilia. Radiographic contrast substance mixed with blood, filling the biliary system.

Deal with false aneurysms in the radiology suite, not in the operating room. (Figure 10 shows the result of haemobilia, made clear after an injection of radiographic contrast medium, i.e., blood filling the biliary system.)

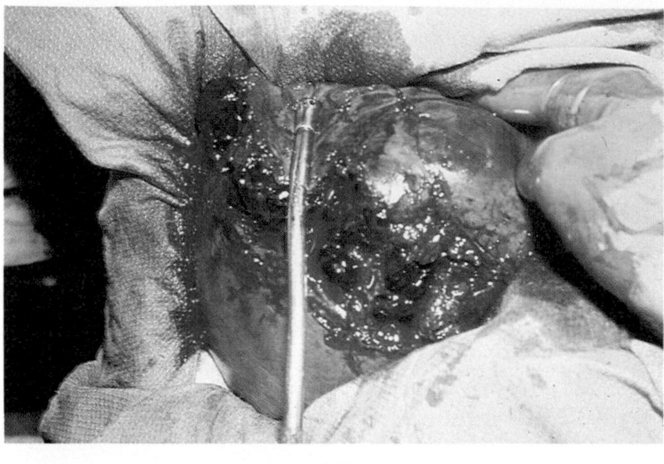

(a)

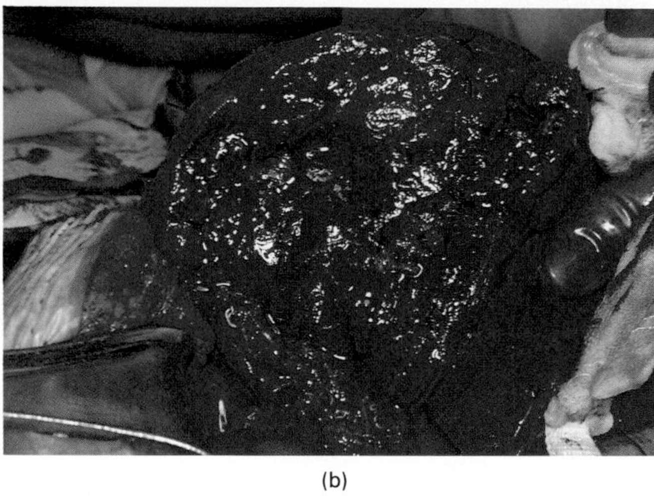

(b)

Fig. 10 (a) Shattered liver capsule stitched futilely with chromic catgut. Haematoma was allowed to remain. The only action needed for completion was to cut through Glisson's capsule posteriorly. (b) A clean, dry surface at the conclusion of the operation.

Therapeutic embolization with thrombin and Gianturco–Wallace coils may be appropriate. If injury demands occlusion of a major branch of the portal vein, use Doppler duplex ultrasonography to be certain that the portal vein, carrying 80 per cent of oxygen to the liver, is patent and functional.

Practically, the vena cava is part of the liver, even if it is not anatomically recognized as being so. Thus, the final aspect of recognizing and treating hepatic trauma is again to be alert to associated vena caval injury.

Remember that gauze packing of an injured liver is a practically foolproof way even for surgeons of little experience in hepatic trauma to deal with a potentially lethal situation. Ignore the smell of *Pseudomonas* and *Proteus* species. They seldom require specific treatment. When packs are removed after 12 or 24 h, following restoration of homeostasis, if the surgeon does not consider his experience adequate to deal with a complex problem, the patient can generally be transported to another hospital easily and with no hazard.

In extremis, consider the possibility of liver transplantation.

FURTHER READING

Burch JM, Feliciano DV, Mattox KL. The atriocaval shunt. Facts and fiction. *Ann Surg*, 1988; **207**: 555–68.

Ciresi KF, Lim RC Jr. Hepatic vein and retrohepatic vena caval injury. *World J Surg*, 1990; **14**: 472–7.

Dobson DE, *et al.* 1-Butyryl-glycerol: a novel angiogenesis factor secreted by differentiating adipocytes. *Cell*, 1990; **61**: 223–30.

Feliciano DV. Surgery for liver trauma. *Surg Clin N Am*, 1989; **69**: 273–84.

Hollands MJ, Little JM. Non-operative management of blunt liver injuries. *Br J Surg*, 1991; **78**: 968–72.

Hollands MJ, Little JM. The role of hepatic resection in the management of blunt liver trauma. *World J Surg*, 1990; **14**: 478–82.

John TG, *et al.* Liver trauma: a 10-year experience. *Br J Surg*, 1992; **79**: 1352–6.

Krige JEF, Bornman PC, Terblanche J. Therapeutic perihepatic packing in complex liver trauma. *Br J Surg*, 1992; **79**: 43–6.

Pachter HL, *et al.* Significant trends in the treatment of hepatic trauma. Experience with 411 injuries. *Ann Surg*, 1992; **215**: 492–502.

Reed RL, *et al.* Continuing evolution in the approach to severe liver trauma. *Ann Surg*, 1992; **216**: 524–38.

Schweizer W, *et al.* Management of traumatic liver injuries. *Br J Surg*, 1993; **80**: 86–8.

Sharp KW, Locicero RJ. Abdominal packing for surgically uncontrollable haemorrhage. *Ann Surg*, 1992; **215**: 467–75.

Sheldon GF, Rutledge R. Hepatic trauma. *Adv Surg*, 1989; **22**: 179–94.

Stevens SL, Maull KI, Enderson BL. Total hepatic mesh wrap for hemostasis. *Surg Gynecol Obstet*, 1992; **175**: 181–2.

22.3 Abscesses—pyogenic and amoebic

PATRICIA L. HIBBERD AND ROBERT H. RUBIN

PYOGENIC ABSCESSES

Epidemiology

The incidence of pyogenic liver abscess in developed countries has not changed appreciably over the past 50 years, being estimated at 8 to 16 cases/100 000 admissions, with a prevalence at autopsy of 0.3 to 1.5 per cent. A slight male predominance of cases has remained during this period, and no ethnic group appears to be at increased risk (Table 1).

Table 1 Liver abscesses—epidemiology

	Pyogenic abscesses	Amoebic abscesses
Incidence/100 000 hospital admissions (1980s)		
USA	10	2
India	30	90
Change in incidence, 1900s versus 1980s	None	Increase
Age	43–60	28–48
Sex ratio (male:female)	1.4:1	Up to 19:1
Risk factors	Biliary tract disease	Immigrants from Mexico
	Malignancy	Travellers from endemic regions
	Diabetes mellitus	Homosexual males
	Cirrhosis	Residents of Indian reservations
	Immunosuppressed patients	Institutionalized patients

What has changed over this time are the age of the patients and the underlying cause of the liver infection. Fifty years ago, the majority of patients were under the age of 40 and appendicitis was the leading cause of the disease; today the average age is between 43 and 60, with an increasing proportion of cases over age 60. This change corresponds to the finding that appendicitis has been replaced by biliary tract disease as the most common underlying aetiology. The increasing age of patients has been associated with an increased incidence of malignancy in patients with liver abscesses. In younger patients with liver abscess related to biliary tract disease the underlying process is usually benign, such as biliary tract calculi; in the elderly, malignancies invading or compressing the biliary tract are common.

Aetiology and pathogenesis

Pyogenic liver abscesses may be divided into two general categories, based upon the size and distribution of the focal sites of inflammation, the acuity of clinical presentation, and the nature of the therapy that is required. Macroscopic abscesses are usually restricted to one lobe of the liver, are frequently single or confluent, present subacutely with symptoms of several days to weeks' duration, and require some form of primary drainage. Microscopic abscesses are multiple, widely distributed throughout the hepatic parenchyma, usually manifest themselves acutely over a few days, and require primarily medical therapy, with any surgery that is carried out being aimed at the underlying process, rather than the hepatic parenchymal inflammation.

Focal infection within the liver can be divided into six general categories, based upon the pathogenetic route by which infecting organisms were introduced into the liver (Table 2).

Table 2. Aetiology of pyogenic liver abscesses

Biliary tract disease
Portal vein pylephlebitis
Hepatic arterial infection, secondary to bacteraemia
Post-traumatic, from blunt or penetrating injuries
Direct extension from a contiguous source of infection
Miscellaneous (including cryptogenic)

Biliary tract disease

Hepatic abscess may arise due to cholangitis whenever bile flow is obstructed. In general, total obstruction is associated with elevated pressure within the biliary tree, an acute septic course, and miliary microabscesses throughout the hepatic parenchyma—a process that has been termed 'acute suppurative cholangitis'. Infection associated with less complete obstruction is associated with normal biliary tract pressure, a subacute course, and macroscopic abscesses.

Portal vein pylephlebitis

Liver abscess may arise because of suppurative thrombophlebitis in the portal venous system that is secondary to such intra-abdominal inflammatory processes as appendicitis (the classical cause), diverticulitis, infected haemorrhoids, or any other cause of intra-abdominal or pelvic infection that impacts upon the portal venous system. A clinical curiosity which remains unexplained is that although portal vein bacteraemia is common in patients with inflammatory bowel disease, hepatic abscess is uncommon.

Hepatic arterial infection

Two subcategories of liver abscess should be considered. Systemic bacteraemias may occasionally seed the liver, resulting in either macroscopic abscesses (usually in the setting of some form of antimicrobial therapy that permits the individual to survive, although not to be cured of the systemic process) or, more commonly, miliary microabscesses. Typically, such infections occur in children with such underlying conditions as chronic granulomatous disease, leukaemia, or other disturbances of granulocyte number or function, and are caused by such organisms as *Staphylococcus aureus*. In other patients the primary process affecting the hepatic artery is thrombosis, with hepatic injury then becoming superinfected with micro-organisms of local or systemic origin. With the increasing prevalence of liver transplantation, particularly in young children in whom the hepatic arterial anastomosis is especially vulnerable, this entity is becoming more common.

Post-traumatic

Both penetrating and non penetrating trauma to the liver can result in liver abscess formation. The common denominator is hepatic necrosis, intrahepatic haemorrhage, and intraparenchymal bile extravasation. Such areas of devitalized tissue commonly become infected, even if they are initially sterile, resulting in macroscopic abscesses. Prevention of this form of hepatic abscess is dependent upon an aggressive surgical approach to devitalized hepatic tissue, wide excision of such necrotic tissue being essential.

Direct extension of infection

Contiguous sites of infection involving the gallbladder, subphrenic space, or pleural space and disease processes in which gastric or intestinal perforation occur directly into the liver can result in macroscopic hepatic abscesses. Malignancy is often present in patients with bowel perforation.

Miscellaneous causes

The aetiology of the liver abscess remains obscure in about 5 per cent of patients, even after extensive evaluation. Presumably, a minor injury to the liver renders such individuals susceptible to seeding by a transient bacteraemia. Other unusual causes of liver disease, such as cysts, intrahepatic malignancy, amoebic abscesses, and hydatid disease, may become secondarily infected, resulting in a pyogenic liver abscess. The common denominator, as in the post-traumatic cases, is the microbial seeding of a *locus minoris resistentiae* within the liver.

Bacteriology

The majority of the organisms that invade the liver to cause hepatic abscesses are derived from the gastrointestinal tract: gastrointestinal flora account for more than 75 per cent of these abscesses (Table 3). Polymicrobial infection occurs in 22 to 64 per cent of cases, usually involving both aerobic and anaerobic flora of gastrointestinal origin. *Escherichia coli* is the most common aerobic organism isolated from liver abscesses, being demonstrated in specimens from 35 to 45 per cent of patients, with *Klebsiella pneumoniae* being the second most frequent isolate in this category. Other aerobic Gram-negative bacteria, including *Proteus* spp., *Enterobacter cloacae*, *Citrobacter* spp., *Pseudomonas aeruginosa*, *Morganella morganii*, *Serratia marsecens*, and *Acinetobacter* and *Eikenella* spp. may also be isolated, usually in association with other gut flora. Those are particularly common in patients with biliary tract disease.

Anaerobic and microaerophilic organisms, either alone or in conjunction with aerobic organisms, are isolated from up to 60 per cent of pyogenic liver abscesses. *Bacteroides fragilis* (particularly spp. *fragilis*) is the most common anaerobe isolated, but such others as other *Bacteroides* spp., *Fusobacterium* spp., anaerobic streptococci, *Clostridium* spp., and *Actinomyces* spp. may be found on occasion. An important group of organisms are the microaerophilic streptococci, particularly *Streptococcus milleri*. If appropriate microbiological techniques are employed (especially the provision of an environment enriched with CO_2 microaerophilic streptococci may be found to be the most common causes of pyogenic liver abscess. *S. milleri* is especially virulent and likely to cause suppuration of the liver and other organs.

Other Gram-positive organisms account for less than 25 per cent of isolates. *Staphylococcus aureus* and group A streptococci occur most commonly after trauma and in children with the previously delineated granulocyte disorders. Seeding of the liver in these individuals usually is secondary to a systemic bacteraemia.

Focal candida infection of the liver and/or spleen has been reported in an increasing number and variety of patients, most notably in those undergoing chemotherapy for leukaemia or liver transplantation. In the leukaemic patient in particular a subacute–chronic entity that has been termed hepatosplenic candidiasis has been defined. This is characterized by persistent fevers and macroscopic abscesses due to *Candida* spp., most notably *C. albicans* and *C. tropicalis*. This process is usually initiated when the patient is neutropenic due to chemotherapy, presumably due to the entrance of the yeast into the portal vein through mucosal ulcerations induced by the chemotherapy. The abscesses and the clinical symptoms persist, however, even after haematological remission has been achieved.

Table 3 Bacteriology of pyogenic liver abscesses

	Percentage of all cultures
Single organism	22–64
Enteric Gram-negative bacteria	
Escherichia coli	35–45
Klebsiella pneumoniae	8–27
Others	8–40
Anaerobic bacteria	
Bacteroides fragilis	Up to 60
Others	2–36
Gram-positive bacteria	
Staphylococcus aureus	Up to 25
Streptococcus pyogenes group A	2–3

Clinical presentation

Patients with microscopic liver abscesses usually have an acutely septic clinical presentation, with fever, rigors, and, not uncommonly, hypotension, as well as right upper quadrant discomfort that can be quite severe. Other manifestations depend upon the underlying condition producing the microabscesses: rapidly progressing jaundice in the presence of biliary tract disease, congestive heart failure if the systemic sepsis is associated with endocarditis.

In contrast, the clinical presentation of macroscopic liver abscesses is more subacute, developing over several days to weeks, with fever, night sweats, anorexia, weight loss, and malaise far more common than rigors and hypotension. Fever is present in 90 per cent of these patients, nausea, vomiting, and abdominal pain occur in 50 to 75 per cent, and symptoms such as pleurisy, diarrhoea, dyspnoea, and cough are seen in 5 to 25 per cent of patients.

Other than fever, abdominal tenderness, usually localized to the right upper quadrant, is the most common physical finding, being demonstrable in 50 to 75 per cent of affected individuals. Hepatomegaly is demonstrable in approximately 50 per cent of patients with macroscopic liver abscesses. Jaundice is uncommon, unless biliary obstruction is present.

Almost all patients with pyogenic hepatic abscesses have abnormal haematological and liver function tests. Leucocytosis, usually of a moderate extent, is noted in 70 to 80 per cent, an elevated ESR in at least 90 per cent, and anaemia in 50 to 65 per cent of patients with liver abscess. The most characteristic liver function test abnormality observed in patients with hepatic abscess is an elevated alkaline phosphate level, which is observed in more than 75 per cent of these individuals. An elevated serum bilirubin level is seen in 40 per cent of patients, with elevated transaminases being found in approximately 30 per cent. Other abnormalities that are not uncommon include a prolonged prothrombin time and a raised serum vitamin B_{12} level. Laboratory abnormalities associated with a poor prognosis include an elevated bilirubin and a serum albumin level of 2 g/dl.

Positive blood cultures are obtained in approximately 50 per cent of all patients. Although up to 65 per cent of abscesses are polymicrobial when aspirated pus is cultured from the liver, it is unusual to retrieve more than one organism from the blood cultures.

Chest radiographs are abnormal in about 50 per cent of patients, usually because the inflammatory process within the liver impinges on the diaphragm, producing a variety of 'sympathetic' responses. These include a right pleural effusion, right lower lobe atelectasis and pneumonitis, and elevation of the right hemidiaphragm. Occasionally, if a gas-forming organism is present in the abscess, air–fluid levels are discernible on chest or abdominal radiographs. Rarely, a liver abscess presents by discharging itself into the chest, with both clinical symptoms (cough, haemoptysis, dyspnoea) and chest radiographic appearances which reflect this.

Diagnostic evaluation

Clinical suspicion of a liver abscess (either pyogenic or amoebic) is aroused when a patient has fever, right upper quadrant abdominal pain and tenderness, and abnormal liver function tests (Fig. 1). The differential diagnosis includes acute cholecystitis, cholangitis, subphrenic or subhepatic abscess, malignancy, and hepatitis.

Ultrasonography is the initial procedure of choice to assess a suspected liver abscess because it is non-invasive, 80 to 90 per cent accurate, and capable of delineating liver lesions as small as 2 cm in diameter. Ultrasound is more useful than computed tomography (CT) for distinguishing solid masses from cystic lesions. However, ultrasonography may miss lesions in the dome of the right liver lobe or multiple microscopic abscesses. Fatty infiltration can produce an echogenic liver, making detection of small abscesses difficult. Although some features of amoebic abscesses differ on ultrasound from those of pyogenic origin, the differences are not sufficient to permit a specific diagnosis.

Abdominal CT can detect intrahepatic collections as small as 0.5 cm in diameter and can be particularly useful in identifying multiple small abscesses or abscesses located near the hemidiaphragm. The diagnostic accuracy of CT is 90 to 95 per cent. Another advantage of CT is that it may identify other abdominal pathology responsible for the pyogenic liver abscess.

Although radionuclide scans of the liver have a sensitivity comparable to that of ultrasonography in detecting liver abscesses, nuclide scans have largely been replaced by ultrasonography and by CT, at least in part, because either sonography or CT allows the clinician to proceed directly to percutaneous aspiration for either diagnosis or therapy. Any material obtained by aspiration should be examined microscopically after Gram staining, cultured aerobically and anaerobically, and, if there is any suspicion clinically or epidemiologically, submitted for examination for *Entamoeba histolytica* trophozoites. Fungal and mycobacterial cultures should also be carried out, particularly in immunosuppressed patients.

Treatment

The traditional approach to the therapy of pyogenic liver abscesses has been open surgical drainage of the abscess, correction, whenever possible, of the underlying pathology that led to the abscess, and a 4- to 6-week course of parenteral antibiotics (Fig. 2). Such antibiotics have usually included a β-lactam, an aminoglycoside, and either metronidazole or clindamycin (aimed at the anaerobic organisms), but treatment could be modified on the basis of microbiological results. Over the past decade, the majority of patients with macroscopic pyogenic abscesses have been managed with antibiotics and percutaneous drainage, thus avoiding more surgery in typically debilitated patients.

Percutaneous drainage is carried out under CT or ultrasound guidance, with the insertion of a pigtail catheter using the Seldinger technique. Samples are then withdrawn for microbiological examination, the abscess cavity is gently irrigated with saline, and the catheter is left in place to provide continuing drainage. More than one catheter may need to be placed to provide complete drainage. Such percutaneous aspiration and drainage does not correct the problem in 10 to 30 per cent of patients, and open drainage is then necessary. Failure to achieve drainage may be due to poor catheter placement, to the presence of a multiloculated abscess, to excessive viscosity of the abscess contents causing plugging of the drainage catheters, to thick abscess walls that do not collapse with drainage, and to inadequate anatomical localization of the abscess. Follow-up ultrasonography or CT scanning is necessary to ensure complete resolution of the process.

Percutaneous drainage is less likely to be of value when there are multiple abscesses, a known intra-abdominal source of infection that requires surgical correction, and abscess of unknown cause, ascites, or when the abscess requires a transpleural drainage route.

Patients with biliary tract disease, diverticulitis, and appendicitis as the source for their liver abscesses are better treated with open surgical drainage, than by percutaneous drainage. Guidelines other than those mentioned to recommend percutaneous or an open surgical approach to these patients are still being formulated.

Mortality rates of patients with macroscopic liver abscesses reported in the 1960s and early 1970s were 65 to 79 per cent. Recent studies have noted a marked improvement, with mortality rates being as low as 11 per cent. Such improvement is due to the widespread availability of ultrasonography and CT scanning and hence earlier diagnosis, and the utility of the percutaneous approach to drainage, especially in debilitated patients, who tolerate conventional surgery poorly. The major determinants of mortality are the nature of the underlying process causing the abscess, the anatomy of the intrahepatic infection, and the presence or absence of such comorbidity factors as cancer, diabetes, heart disease, and renal failure.

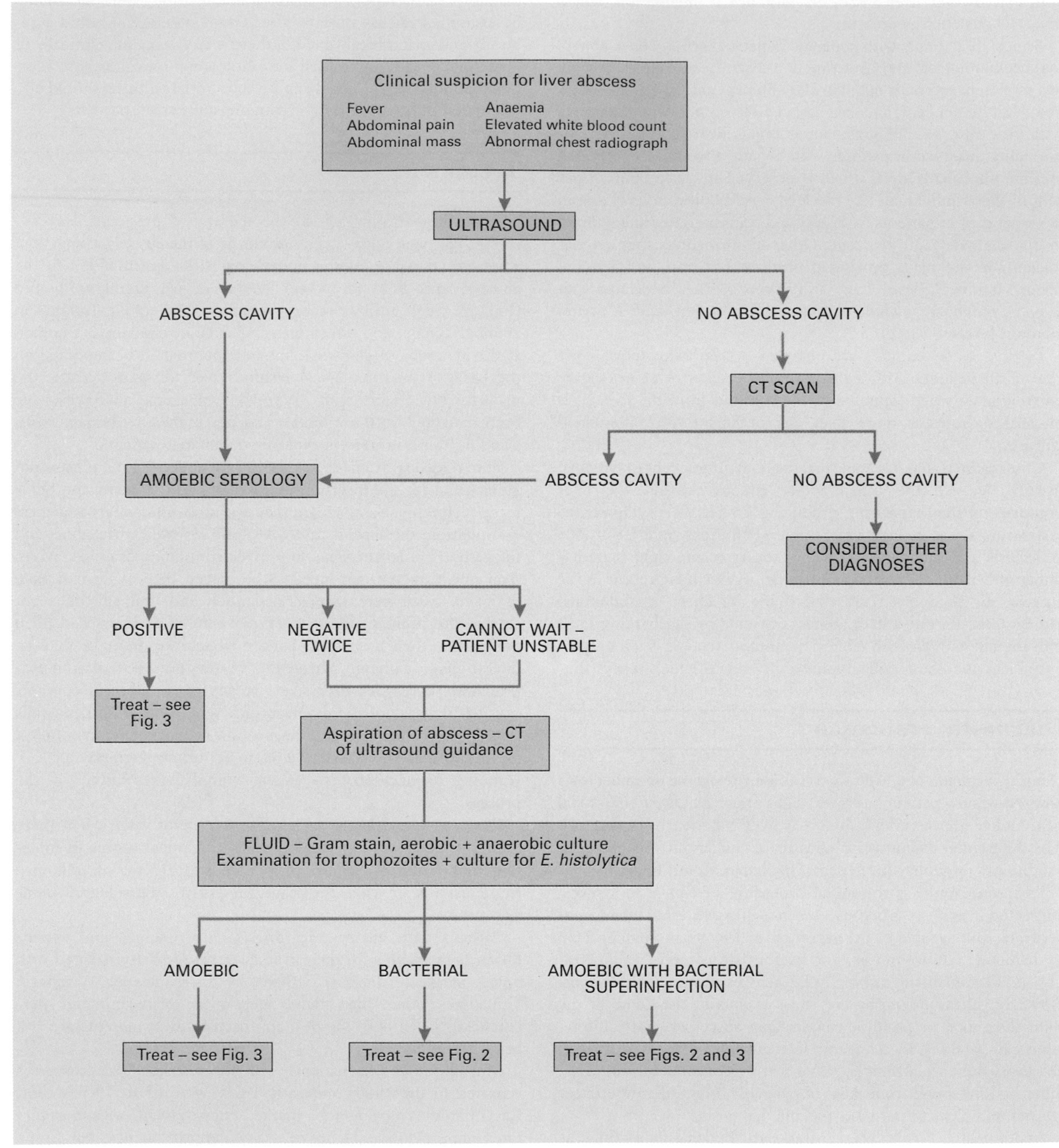

Fig. 1 Diagnostic scheme for suspected liver abscess.

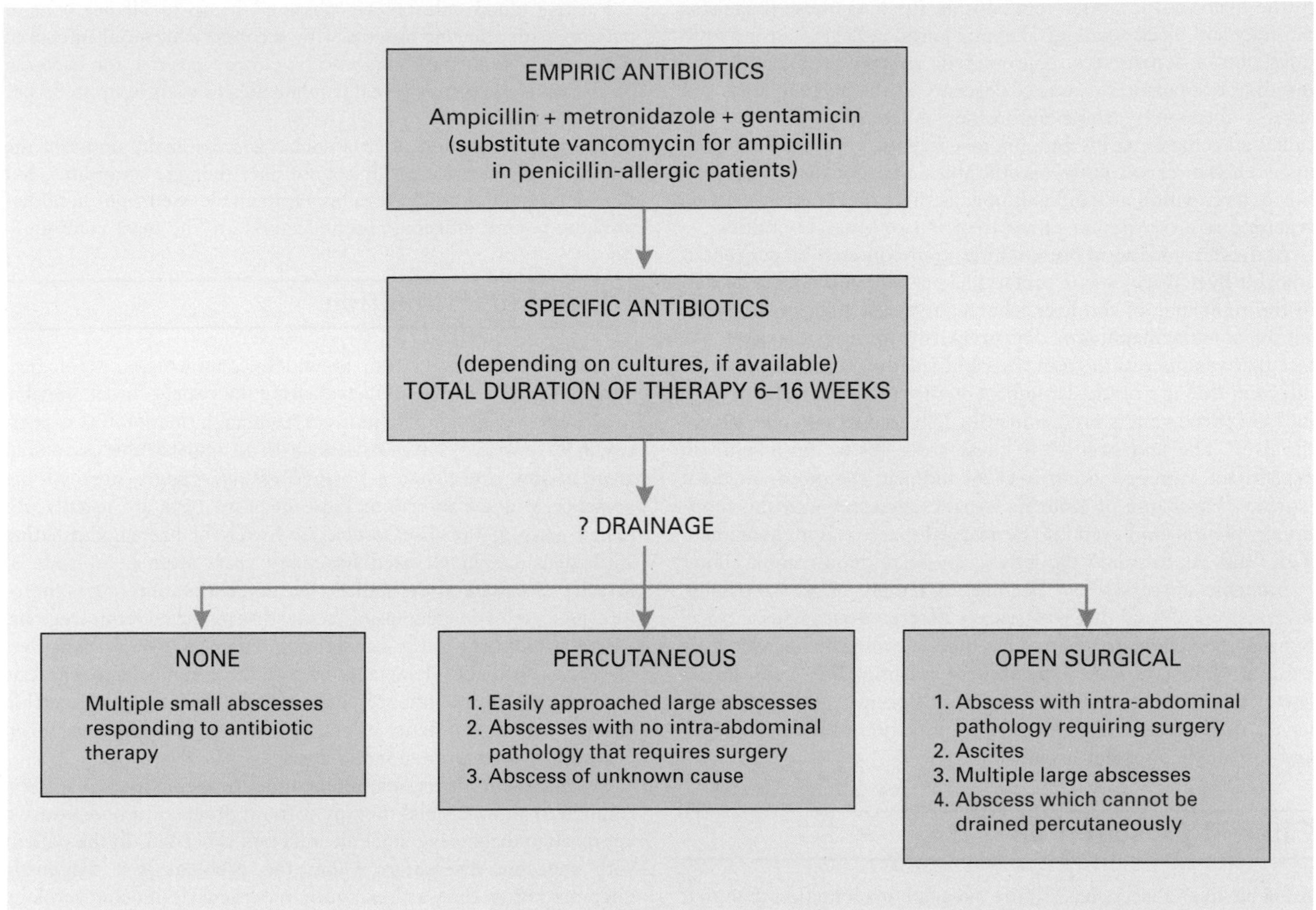

Fig. 2 Treatment of pyogenic liver abscesses.

AMOEBIC ABSCESSES

Epidemiology

Entamoeba histolytica infection affects an estimated 10 per cent of the world's population, with the great majority of such infections occurring in people living in sub-Saharan Africa, the Indian subcontinent, Asia, and parts of Central and South America. In these endemic areas approximately 50 per cent of the population is infected, with 90 per cent or more being asymptomatic cyst passers. In more developed countries, amoebic infection occurs predominantly in immigrants or travellers returning from endemic areas, in sexually active male homosexuals, in residents of Indian reservations, and in people institutionalized for mental or emotional disability. The common denominator in these last groups is an increased opportunity for person-to-person spread via the faecal–oral route.

Amoebic liver abscess occurs in less than 10 per cent of individuals infected with this organism. Whereas amoebic infection of the liver is far less common than is pyogenic infection in the United States, in areas of the world such as India, amoebic abscesses are 3 to 5 times as frequent as pyogenic liver abscesses. The average age of patients with amoebic liver abscess is between 28 and 48 years, which is significantly younger than patients with pyogenic infection (Table 1). Although infection rates are similar in men and women, there is a striking male predominance (up to 20:1) in patients who develop hepatic abscesses from amoebiasis. Particularly severe invasive disease occurs in patients with compromised cellular immunity, in young infants, in the malnourished, in pregnant women, and in patients receiving corticosteroids.

Aetiology and pathogenesis

Amoebiasis is initiated by the ingestion of *E. histolytica* cysts. Once these cysts reach the small intestine, motile trophozoites are released and migrate to the colon, where they proliferate along with the resident bacterial flora. In most cases the organism becomes a commensal. There is some evidence that virulence of different strains can be correlated with a particular isoenzyme pattern of key enzymes which can be isolated from the trophozoites. Other important determinants of invasiveness probably include the inherent virulence of the organism, diet, the constituents of the bacterial flora of the gut, and both humoral and cell-mediated host resistance.

Once intestinal infection is established, amoebae may be carried to the liver via the portal vein. Within the liver these organisms multiply and block small intrahepatic portal radicals, causing focal infarction of hepatocytes. A proteolytic enzyme produced by the invading trophozoites causes coalescence of the invaded areas and abscess formation. Some authorities differentiate between so-called amoebic hepatitis and amoebic hepatic abscess, depending upon whether or not a macroscopic abscess has formed. We regard this differentiation as a difficult one, as this process might best be regarded as a continuum rather than as two separate entities.

At the time of clinical presentation, approximately 80 per cent of amoebic liver abscesses are solitary; 83 per cent of them are located in the right lobe of the liver, characteristically high in the dome subjacent to the diaphragm. The propensity for this site reflects the fact that venous return from the right side of the colon (amoebic infection having a particular impact on the caecum and right colon) into the portal vein is predominantly delivered to the right lobe of the liver. The juxtaposition of these abscesses to the diaphragm explain the common occurrence of thoracic symptoms in these patients. Discharge of amoebic hepatic abscesses into the subphrenic, pleural, and even into pericardial spaces is not uncommon, with frank rupture into the lung as an uncommon complication.

Amoebic abscesses can become extremely large, containing several litres of fluid that is classically described as 'anchovy sauce' but may be yellow or green. This fluid is primarily necrotic liver tissue and blood, with a paucity of inflammatory cells unless bacterial superinfection has occurred. Because bile appears to have a deleterious effect on amoebae, infection of the gallbladder and bile ducts does not occur.

Clinical presentation

Amoebic liver abscess has a more subacute presentation than that of pyogenic liver abscess. Symptoms typically evolve over a few weeks to months (as opposed to several days to weeks for a pyogenic process) before medical attention is sought. Initial symptoms are non-specific: fever, anorexia, night sweats, malaise, anorexia, nausea and vomiting, and weight loss. As the disease becomes established, right upper quadrant abdominal pain becomes a dominating symptom in at least two-thirds of these patients. Approximately 25 per cent of patients exhibit thoracic symptoms, such as pleurisy, non-productive cough, right shoulder pain, and/or hiccups as an important part of the symptom complex. Characteristically, simultaneous intestinal complaints such as dysentery or diarrhoea are not present. Uncommonly, patients may have a more acute presentation, suggesting an acute abdominal surgical emergency.

The patients typically appear chronically ill, with fever, abdominal tenderness, and hepatomegaly. Chest findings (râles, decreased breath sounds, dullness to percussion, impaired diaphragmatic movement) are observed in 50 per cent of patients. Jaundice is rare (less than 15 per cent of individuals).

Anaemia and an elevated erythrocyte sedimentation rate are present in at least 80 per cent of patients, as well as a moderate leucocytosis in 60 to 75 per cent. More extreme white blood cell responses suggest the presence of bacterial superinfection. Eosinophilia is not observed in patients with amoebic liver abscesses; if present, another explanation should be sought. Normal liver function tests do not exclude the diagnosis of an amoebic abscess, although slight to moderate elevations of the alkaline phosphatase, reduction in the serum albumin, and minimal changes in transaminase values are generally observed.

Positive blood cultures are obtained in up to 20 per cent of patients with amoebic abscess with secondary bacterial infection. Aspirated abscess fluid may also be culture positive for bacteria. Stool examination may reveal trophozoites or cysts in up to 25 per cent of patients.

The typical location of an amoebic abscess in the dome of the right lobe of the liver produces not only thoracic symptoms, but also abnormalities on chest radiograph: an elevated right hemidiaphragm, pleural effusion, and atelectasis are the most common.

Diagnostic evaluation

In areas of the world free of endemic amoebiasis, serological testing is extremely useful in evaluating the patient for an amoebic liver abscess (Fig. 1). The indirect haemagglutination test is positive in 90 to 95 per cent of patients with an amoebic abscess, and in areas of low prevalence a positive result strongly suggests the presence of acute infection. False-negative tests are usually obtained early in the disease course. Levels of haemagglutinating antibodies remain elevated for many years after an episode of invasive disease, and the indirect haemagglutination test is therefore less useful in diagnosing acute disease in endemic regions, where 50 per cent of the general population may be seropositive. Levels of antibodies detectable by counterimmunoelectrophoresis and indirect immunofluorescence usually become undetectable within 6 months of acute infection; they may be more useful in evaluating patients in endemic areas.

Since amoebic abscesses, unlike most pyogenic liver abscesses, respond to antimicrobial therapy without drainage, a non-invasive approach to diagnosing amoebic infection is needed. In the patient with subacute disease in whom the problem is a diagnostic dilemma rather than a therapeutic emergency, amoebic serology should be performed and a therapeutic trial is initiated if the patient has an appropriate epidemiological history. If the patient is unstable, if there is reason to suspect a pyogenic component to the illness on the basis of clinical or epidemiologic findings, if the amoebic serology is negative, or if the patient has failed to respond clinically to several days of antiamoebic therapy, a percutaneous needle aspiration should be performed.

Treatment

Most amoebic abscesses are cured with a regimen of metronidazole 750 mg orally or intravenously three times per day, for 10 days, followed by treatment with an agent that is effective in eradicating the cysts which may persist in the intestine after treatment with metronidazole (Fig. 3). Agents effective in the treatment of such luminal disease include iodoquinol 650 mg orally three times per day for 20 days, diloxanide furoate 500 mg orally three times per day for 10 days, or paramomycin 25 to 30 mg/kg.day orally in three divided doses for 7 days.

Most patients show a prompt therapeutic response to metronidazole, with defervescence and decreased abdominal pain within 3 or 4 days. This response is useful for differentiating amoebic and pyogenic abscesses in situations where serological testing is unavailable or uninterpretable. Fewer than 10 per cent of patients with amoebic liver abscess fail to respond to metronidazole therapy. Treatment in the non-responders is with dihydroemetine (1–1.5 mg/kg.day, maximum dose 90 mg/day intramuscularly for 5 days) plus chloroquine phosphate (600 mg base/day for 2

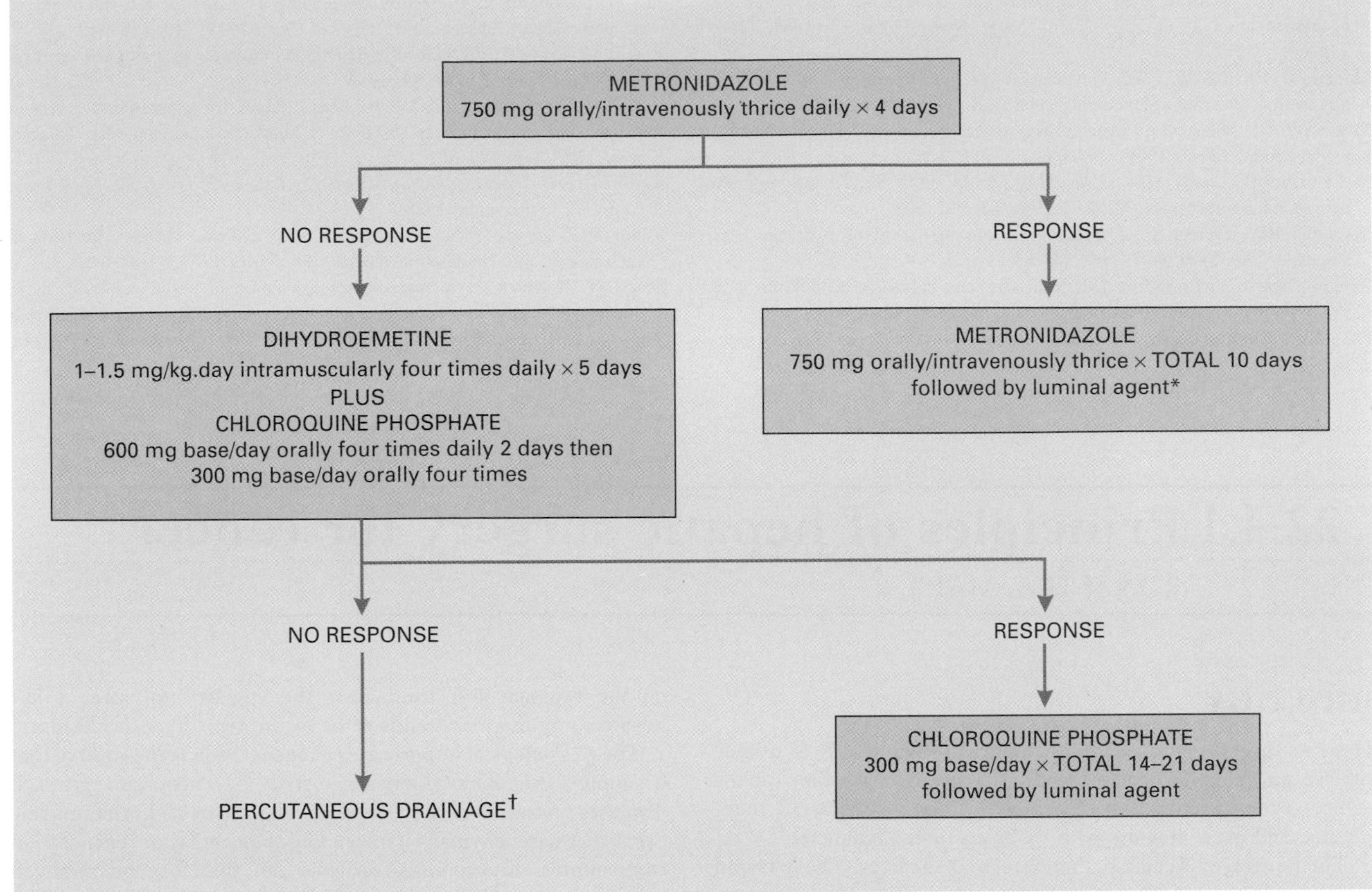

Fig. 3 Treatment of amoebic liver abscesses. *Luminal agents include: iodoquinol 650 mg orally thrice daily × 20 days; diloxanide furoate 500 mg orally thrice daily × 10 days; paramomycin 25–30 mg/kg.day orally in three divided doses × 7 days. †Other indications for percutaneous drainage are abscess in the left lobe of liver and a possible large abscess. Indications for open surgical drainage are perforation to peritoneum, possible bacterial superinfection, and if the diagnosis is uncertain and percutaneous drainage is impossible.

days, followed by 300 mg of chloroquine base orally daily for 2–3 weeks). This regimen should be followed by treatment with an agent active against luminal disease.

Considerable controversy surrounds the role of percutaneous drainage in the management of amoebic liver abscesses. Proposed indications for such drainage include liver abscesses in the left lobe of the liver, because of the risk of rupture into the pericardial sac, drainage of large abscesses to facilitate more rapid healing with chemotherapy, and lack of response to metronidazole therapy. However, because of the risk of introducing bacteria during catheter drainage, we reserve a drainage procedure for patients in whom the differentiation between pyogenic and amoebic infection is unclear, for acutely ill patients, for patients who have failed to respond to therapy, and for patients whose infection has spread into adjoining structures.

Treatment of an amoebic hepatic abscess is usually successful, mortality being associated only with delayed diagnosis or complications such as bacterial superinfection, or rupture into adjoining structures.

FURTHER READING

Ahmed L, Rooby AE, Kassem MI, Salama ZA, Strickland GT. Ultrasonography in the diagnosis and management of 52 patients with amebic liver abscess in Cairo. *Rev Infect Dis* 1990; **12**: 330–7.

Barnes PF, DeCock KM, Reynolds TN, Ralls PW. A Comparison of amebic and pyogenic abscess of the liver. *Medicine*, 1987; **66**: 473–83.

Bertel CK, van Heerden JA, Sheedy PF II. Treatment of pyogenic hepatic abscesses (surgical vs. percutaneous drainage). *Arch Surg* 1986; **121**: 554–8.

Bowers ED, Robison DJ, Doberneck RC. Pyogenic liver abscess. *World J Surg* 1990; **14**: 128–32.

Cohen JL, Martin FM, Rossi RL, Schoetz DJ. Liver abscess. (The need for complete gastrointestinal evaluation). *Arch Surg* 1989; **124**: 561–4.

Conter RL, Pitt HA, Tompkins RK, Longmire WP Jr. Differentiation of pyogenic from amebic hepatic abscesses. *Surg Gynecol Obstet* 1986; **162**: 114–20.

DeCock KM, Reynolds TB. Amebic and pyogenic liver abscess. In: Schiff L, Schiff ER, eds. *Diseases of the liver*. 6th edn. Philadelphia: JB Lippincott Company, 1987: 1235–53.

Farges O, Leese T, Bismuth H. Pyogenic liver abscess: an improvement in prognosis. *Br J Surg* 1988; **75**: 862–5.

Greenstein AJ, Barth J, Dicker A, Bottone EJ, Aufses AH Jr. Amebic liver abscess: a study of 11 cases compared with a series of 38 patients with pyogenic liver abscess. *Am J Gastroenterol* 1985; **80**: 472–8.

Gyorffy EJ, Frey CF, Silva Jr. J, McGahan J. Pyogenic liver abscess (diagnostic and therapeutic strategies). *Ann Surg* 1987; **206**: 699–705.

Holdstock G, Balasegaram M, Millward-Sadler GH, Wright R. The Liver in infection. In: Wright R, Millward Sadler GH, Alberti KEM, Karran S, eds. *Liver and biliary disease*. 2nd edn. London: Baillière Tindall WB Saunders Company, 1985: 1077–119.

Johnson RD, *et al*. Percutaneous drainage of pyogenic liver abscesses. *Am J Roentgenol* 1985; **144**: 463–7.

Klatchko BA, Schwartz SI. Diagnostic and therapeutic approaches to pyogenic abscess of the liver. *Surg Gynecol Obstet* 1989; **168**: 332–6.

Maharaj B, Bhoora IG, Patel A, Maharajh J. Ultrasonography and scintigraphy in liver disease in developing countries. *Lancet* 1989; **ii**: 853–6.

McCorkell SJ, Niles NL. Pyogenic liver abscesses: another look at medical management. *Lancet* 1985; i: 803–6.

McDonald MI, Corey GR, Gallis HA, Durack DT. Single and multiple pyogenic liver abscesses. *Medicine* 1984; **63**: 291–302.

Miedema BW, Dineen P. The diagnosis and treatment of pyogenic liver abscesses. *Ann Surg* 1984; **200**: 328–35.

Pineiro-Carrero VM, Andres JM. Morbidity and mortality in children with pyogenic liver abscess. *Am J Dis Child* 1989; **143**: 1424–7.

Pitt, HA: Liver abscess. In Shackelford RT, Zuidema GD, eds. *Surgery of the alimentary tract*. Vol 4. Philadelphia: WB Saunders Co, 1983: 465–97.

Pitt HA, Zuidema GD. Factors influencing mortality in the treatment of pyogenic hepatic abscess. *Surg Gynecol Obstet* 1975; **140**: 228–34.

Prasad M, Arora A. Problem of pyogenic liver abscess in a tropical country. *Am J Gastroenterol* 1989; **84**: 1466.

Ralls PW, Barnes PF, Radin DR, Colletti P, Halls J. Sonographic features of amebic and pyogenic liver abscesses: a blinded comparison. *Am J Roentgenol* 1987; **149**: 499–501.

Ravdin JL, ed. *Amebiasis: human infection by Entamoeba histolytica*. New York: Churchill Livingstone, 1988.

Rubin RH, Swartz MN, Malt R. Hepatic abscess: changes in clinical, bacteriologic and therapeutic aspects. *Am J Med* 1974; **57**: 601–10.

Singh JP, Kashyap A. A comparative evaluation of percutaneous catheter drainage for resistant amebic liver abscesses. *Am J Surg* 1989; **158**: 58–62.

Thompson JE, Forlenza S, Verma R. Amebic liver abscess: a therapeutic approach. *Rev Infect Dis* 1985; **7**: 171–9.

22.4.1 Principles of hepatic surgery for cancer

RONALD A. MALT

BIOLOGY

Hepatic surgery is based on anatomical principles. It is usually precise and can be nearly bloodless. Cure or palliation can be achieved for patients with unicentric primary or metastatic neoplasms, and even in some with multicentric malignancies.

The lungs are resectable, therefore, so is the liver. The liver and lungs are plethoric: afferent and efferent blood vessels intertwine. Each organ drains into a carina. In the lung the carina is at the bifurcation of the trachea. In the liver it is at the confluence of the bile ducts. During surgery certain conduits must be controlled in each of the organs. In the lungs these are the bronchii; in the liver, the bile ducts.

When haemostasis is perfect and cut bile ducts are closed or are drained into the small bowel, there is scarcely a limit to the extent of hepatic surgery, provided only that enough parenchyma is left to synthesize clotting factors, to detoxify, to conjugate metabolic products, and to perform the other functions of the liver.

REGENERATION

While the lung, after resection, lies almost passive in the chest, cytologically speaking, the liver contains a population of long-lived normal cells that can be recruited to undergo mitosis when lost parenchyma must be replaced. Although the replacement of parenchymal mass is commonly termed regeneration, it is not. Regeneration means regrowth of an organ. This is seen in the ability of a newt to produce a new limb from the scar of an amputation stump, or in the annual sprouting of a stag's antlers. Hepatic regeneration is less complex, being characterized only by compensatory hypertrophy and hyperplasia of existing cells, which are mysteriously signalled to begin growth and are equally mysteriously stopped when the demand for new cells is met. Transforming growth factor-β_1, a polypeptide, may be one mediator of these events. Hepatic growth factors also participate.

The anatomical importance of 'regeneration' is that new parenchyma grows only in the mass of existing parenchyma. After a right hepatectomy the patient's regenerative mass is centred on the remnant left liver, near the epigastrium; after a left hepatectomy the mass tends to be in the right hypochondrium.

The physiological importance of regeneration is the reserve that it supplies after a neoplasm is resected. As a neoplasm grows, it displaces normal liver tissue: it does not destroy it. In the unlikely event that parenchyma is damaged by the neoplasm, regeneration compensates. Enormous neoplasms can therefore be removed from the liver with little compromise of parenchymal mass. The same mass that was sustaining life before surgery is the parenchymal mass available for homeostasis afterwards.

The usual surgical mythology that Prometheus ('forethought') was chained to a rock for stealing fire from the gods is too simplistic. In actuality, Prometheus, son of the Titans Iapetus and Clymene, made man from clay, and stole fire from heaven (or from the forge of Hephaesteus) as revenge for Zeus's having deprived man of fire. Furthermore, when animal sacrifices were made, Prometheus tricked Zeus and other gods into choosing tough meat, while men got the better parts.

To punish Prometheus, Zeus had him chained to a rock in the Caucasus mountains, exposed to a vulture (or eagle), who feasted on Prometheus' liver by day, the liver regrowing nightly. (Perhaps this was the phase of his life in which Prometheus invented numbers.) Torture continued until Hercules freed Prometheus, or, in another version, until Prometheus revealed the secret of Thetis.

Prometheus knew that Thetis would have a son more powerful than his father, Zeus. Although Zeus loved Thetis, he knew also that he would be in danger from one of his sons, but not which one. Prometheus knew the secret, but he would not reveal it until he was freed, nor would he accept Pandora as a bride. Thetis was then married to Peleus, a mortal, so that her son would not be immortal. The son was Achilles.

The liver injured by trauma is less able to defend itself: the signal for the initiation of regeneration comes too late. Despite the belief that 90 per cent of the liver can be lost with impunity, the patient usually dies, from a combination of blood loss and coagulopathy. A patient who survives massive loss of parenchyma following resection of neoplasia is likely to experience chronic fatigue, since regeneration is finite.

ANATOMY AND NOMENCLATURE

The structural analogy between the lung and the liver proposed above is not just a pedogogic device, but practical knowledge: it ultimately determines both how to divide and resect the liver and how to identify functional units exactly.

A plane erected between the medial aspect of the gallbladder bed and the axis of the inferior vena cava splits the liver into two unequal parts.

Just as the right and left bronchi split at a carina to provide the architecture for moving air in and out of the right and left lungs, the liver may be divided bloodlessly, or nearly so, along the plane from the gallbladder bed to the vena cava, historically called Cantlie's line. Bile drains into the right and left hepatic ducts from the respective halves of the liver at a carina: namely, the confluence of the bile ducts. The right and left lungs are matched by the right and left liver. Just as a right or a left pneumonectomy is possible, so is a right or left hepatectomy. There are no true lobes in the liver. Thus, there can be no lobectomies, only hepatectomies and segmentectomies.

The liver is comprised of eight segments, each of which has both dedicated arteries and branches of the portal vein that nourish them and specific hepatic veins that drain them into the three major hepatic veins: right, middle, and left. (see Section 22.1) The nutrient sources of a segment are so invariable that during a hepatectomy a confident surgeon, in principle, does not need to ligate the bile duct, the portal vein branch, and the hepatic artery branch separately. Because the vessels are all within a single peritoneal investment (the Walaesian sheath), a single ligature around the contents of the sheath could be satisfactory. The small portion of liver lying on the intrahepatic portion of the inferior vena cava and draining direct to the vena cava is imprecisely, but probably irrevocably, called the caudate lobe (segment I). The imprecise term 'trisegmentectomy' recently introduced into surgical cant should be expunged.

ELECTIVE RESECTIONS

Imaging studies

With the exception of hepatic neoplasms such as carcinoid or glucagonoma that may secrete an unmistakable hormone, spot diagnoses of specific neoplasms are difficult; they were practically impossible before the advent of sensitive and specific means of imaging. Of all the methods of diagnostic imaging the most useful and economic is a CT scan enhanced by intravenous injection of a contrast medium.

The magnetic resonance image is an excellent adjunct, because the T_2-weighted image uniquely displays haemangiomas and other tissues high in water content. MR is also the most sensitive way to detect metastatic disease in the liver.

Arteriography shows the arteries and delineates vascularized neoplasms. The experienced hepatic surgeon needs only to feel the arteries at the operating table to learn almost everything he needs to know about their distribution.

Exception to this argument is taken by some who support the need to identify and to treat in some special manner a replaced right hepatic artery or other arterial anomalies. These concerns usually are of little moment: a replaced right hepatic artery supplies the right liver and the gallbladder. Since these are highly likely to be the targets of surgery the replaced artery will have to be divided. Even if a replaced right hepatic artery were to be cut by accident, necrosis of the liver rarely develops, as long as portal vein dynamics are normal. The main advantages of arteriography are in disclosing vascular hepatic metastases, which are poorly detected by other means, and in illuminating the anatomy of neoplasms involving the inferior vena cava, the right renal vein, the extrahepatic portions of the hepatic veins, or the portal vein.

Intraoperative ultrasonography to identify hepatic metastases is rarely better than the experienced surgeon's hand. The principal exception concerns detection of hepatic cell carcinomas less than 4 cm in diameter, which are elusive without sonographic localization. Less importantly, sonography defines the route of intrahepatic veins and permits balloon occlusion and removal of a segment containing a small cancer in a cirrhotic liver.

Nuclear scans

Because hepatoadenomas are true neoplasms, they are supposed to lack Kupffer cells. In principle, they should not take up $^{99}Tc^{m}$ sulphur-colloid. Focal nodular hyperplasia, not being a neoplasm, should be able to take up the colloid. Unfortunately, the specificity with which a differential diagnosis can be made is poor.

BIOPSY EXAMINATION

Knowledge of the histopathology of a neoplasm before surgery is only helpful when a neoplasm is suspected to be so disseminated that excisional surgery is useless, or when the liver is likely to be so diseased that the possibility of recovery is remote. Otherwise, focal hepatic neoplasms are routinely removed with a rim of normal liver tissue 1 or 2 cm thick, irrespective of the cell type.

Biopsy specimens are likely to be interpreted erroneously because of sampling error. If that were not the case, and if the possibility of encouraging peritoneal implantation of neoplastic cells or of precipitating haemorrhage from a haemangioma or from a vascular carcinoma could be dismissed, biopsy examination might theoretically be helpful in determining whether a tumour-like growth such as focal nodular hyperplasia or benign neoplasms such as hepatic cell adenoma could be spared. Imaging studies are generally safer and are specific enough for most purposes.

OPERATIVE EXPOSURE

A right thoracoabdominal incision leaves nothing to chance, but causes unnecessary morbidity. Aside from the discomfort of a transected ensiform cartilage, closure of the diaphragm must be perfect to avoid bilothorax. A retrospective study of hepatic resections over a 27-year interval (1962–1988) indicated that a fall in the use of a thoracic incision from 57 per cent to 19 per cent was associated with a fall in the mortality rate from 19 per cent to 9.7 per cent; improved standards of care were obviously responsible for some of this decline. Resections of paracaval or of retrocaval neoplasms are practically the only indication for the thoracoabdominal approach. An abdominal approach is usually both adequate and feasible. Any requirement for more room, if the patient is short or fat, or both, or where the neoplasm is paracaval, is easily met by a modest median sternotomy. The patient's arm is suspended over his right chest wall to provide unlimited exposure. Nonetheless, an extensile abdominal exposure is required to take advantage of the elevated rib cage provided by a retractor fixed to the operating table. Much better mechanical advantage in elevating the thorax is provided by the bariatric surgery crossbar of a retractor such as the Omni-Tract^{R} than by that of simple, fixed retractors pulling in the plane of the abdominal wall. When a bilateral subcostal incision is used in conjunction with a 'wishbone' Omni-Tract retractor^{R}, exposure is not only less good, but closing the incision is more difficult because one of the elements to be sewn is cut muscle that is fixed to an unyielding rib cage. Moreover, a subcostal incision often heals with the contracting, caudad portion of the incision heaped above the level of the cephalad skin. At least four intercostal nerves on each side are also cut. The extensile exposure cuts only the intercostal nerves on one side, and the vertical line of the incision facilitates the use of both manual and mechanical retractors.

HEPATIC NEOPLASMS

About half of a Finnish adult male population examined in forensic autopsies had benign liver neoplasms or tumour-like nodules, such as cholangioadenomas, focal nodular hyperplasia, and haemangiomas. The sizes of these neoplasms ranged from those that were only a few millimetres in diameter to those over 2 cm in diameter. There is no reason to suppose that other populations are different. Presumably, these tumours account for the unexpected lumps sometimes felt by meticulous surgeons who examine the liver routinely during a laparotomy for another reason. Such lumps should be ignored, unless an experienced surgeon regards one or more of them as being exophytic or umbilicated, and consequential.

Types of neoplasms

Cholangioadenomas

Cholangioadenomas, also called bile-duct rests or hamartomas, are so common as to be ignored, even in postmortem examinations.

Haemangiomas

Although cavernous haemangiomas are frequent, they are rarely important. Those less than 8 cm in diameter seldom need treatment, except when an ill-advised biopsy provokes haemorrhage. Even then they generally bleed less than expected. Intervention is required only when the haemangioma (usually diagnosed best by MR imaging) causes symptoms of a mass lesion, displacing or irritating other organs, or if it ruptures. Leaks and ruptures are uncommon, however: fewer than 50 cases of ruptured haemangioma seem to have been recorded. All those that rupture are over 8 cm in diameter (about 270 cm^{3}); a few smaller ones have leaked. Why one haemangioma 8 cm in diameter should leak, while another five times larger remains intact is a mystery. Perhaps the amount, the distribution, and the strength and compliance of the connective tissue are important considerations.

The common haemangioma is resectable along non-anatomical lines by any method favoured by the surgeon. Most, including giant haemangiomas, can and should be enucleated rather than resected, unless only a bridge of intact hepatic parenchyma has to be divided. There is no cause for concern if the resection margin of an enucleated or resected haemangioma contains evidence of haemangiomatous tissue, since they do not recur, except for rare instances in which concurrent oestrogen therapy potentiates growth.

Hepatic adenoma

These used to be regarded as a nosological curiosity. The initial paper showing that rupture of hepatic adenomas into the peritoneal cavity might be caused by the use of oral contraceptives was rejected, as being improbable.

Contemporary publicity has now alerted physicians and patients to the role of oral contraceptives in fostering the development of adenomas, although both pristine liver cell adenomas and the ruptured variety are infrequent. It is not yet determined whether hepatic adenomas progress to carcinomas. Although the risk is small, some adenomas, without doubt, undergo carcinomatous transformation.

Two-thirds of the liver parenchyma is right liver: most neoplasms, including adenomas (or colorectal metastases for that matter) are, therefore, located in the right liver. No one can predict which adenomas will rupture, nor why. When adenomas in the right liver burst, they are often deep-seated neoplasms, and an immediate hepatectomy, with its attendant risks, is sometimes required.

From a clinical viewpoint, any source of steroidal stimulation should be withdrawn from a hormone-treated man or woman thought to have a hepatic adenoma. If the neoplastic mass regresses by 50 per cent over the next 3 months, no treatment is likely to be needed. Adenomas that do not regress upon stopping hormonal therapy should be removed. Because of the possibility of carcinomatous transformation, albeit small, imaging studies at 3-month intervals for a total of 1 year should probably be pursued to assess the possibility of malignant growth.

Focal nodular hyperplasia

This is a 'condition', not a disease or a neoplasm. It is probably a fibrogenic response to idiopathic ingrowth of blood vessels. If, because of its central scar and characteristic spherical or oblate shape the inferential diagnosis of a space-occupying mass is focal nodular hyperplasia, there is no indication for its removal, in the absence of symptoms. Concentration of $^{99}Tc^{m}$-labelled sulphur colloid in the tumour may help, or at least guide, diagnosis, but specificity is low: liver cell adenomas, formerly thought to be unable to concentrate the colloid, often do so.

Cystadenoma

Like focal nodular hyperplasia, cystadenoma is a tumour-like condition, not a neoplasm. Cystadenoma probably represents growth of a bud of bile-duct primordium. Fewer than 75 cystadenomas have been reported, the majority in women: they are four times more common in women than in men. Although hepatic cystadenomas produce all the discomfort and other effects of an intrahepatic mass, they do not cause jaundice unless they happen to compress a major bile duct. If symptoms persist, hepatic cystadenomas must be removed both for cure and to avoid confusion with the rare hepatic cystadenocarcinomas. Cystadenomas can usually be enucleated.

Hepatocellular carcinoma

Hepatocellular carcinoma is by far the most common and important visceral neoplasm in the world, but it could be virtually eliminated by wide-scale inoculation against hepatitis B virus, provided that the level of protection afforded by the vaccine were high. The efficacy of the vaccine decreases in those over age 50 years, and people in third-world countries do not avail themselves of the vaccine, irrespective of their age. In transgenic mice injected with hepatitis B virus, intracellular progression of liver tissue from inflammation to carcinoma is unmistakable. Alcohol, aflatoxin, and male sex are other putative carcinogens or cocarcinogens.

Because multicentric hepatic cell carcinoma on a substrate of a liver ravaged by alcoholic cirrhosis is common in the Western world, resection is usually impractical, except for those who harbour encapsulated, unicentric cancers. Even though the best 5-year survival rate after resection is only about 35 per cent, aggressive surgical removal of a limited hepatic cell carcinoma is worthwhile, because there is otherwise no effective adjunctive therapy, although arteriographic chemotherapeutic embolization of the neoplasm may be beneficial.

The fibrolamellar variant hepatocellular carcinoma should also be treated surgically. This tumour is encapsulated and occurs mostly in women (but sometimes also in steroid-treated men); it can usually be resected, with a survival rate as high as 40 per cent after 4 years.

Minimal hepatocellular carcinomas (those <4 cm in maximal diameter) are rare in the United States, but common in the 'hepatic cancer belt' of Africa and Asia and in France also, as a result of historical referral patterns. In the 'cancer belt', screening programmes identify these neoplasms as a matter of routine: first, by assaying for abnormally high levels of α-fetoprotein in the blood and, second, if those are high, by ultrasonographic scans of the liver.

Even in patients with considerable cirrhosis, hepatitis, and hepatic dysfunction, minimal cancers can be removed by a bloodless resection of the neoplasm with a few millimetres of apparently normal parenchyma as described above. Asanguineous conditions are met either by occlusion of portal blood flow from the hepatic segment harbouring the neoplasm or by total occlusion of blood flow to the liver.

Because hepatocellular carcinomas invade the bile ducts and the hepatic and portal veins, deposits of cancer in the bile ducts may produce obstructive jaundice. Neoplasm in the hepatic and portal veins may cause portal hypertension and Budd-Chiari syndrome, manifested by bleeding oesophageal varices.

Cystadenocarcinoma

This is a rare, idiopathic, and limited cancer which is sometimes curable by resection. By analogy with hepatic cystadenomas, cystadenocarcinomas are thought to originate from bile duct primordia.

Cholangiocarcinoma

Cholangiocarcinomas probably originate from cells in the lining of bile ducts; the entity of biliary papillomatosis may represent one of its stages. Cholangiocarcinomas mimic some of the behaviour of hepatocellular carcinomas in that they may coexist in a parenchymal (or 'peripheral') phase and a 'central' phase, invading bile ducts widely and producing symptoms of bile duct obstruction as the chief manifestation of disease.

Bile ducts can sometimes be freed of cancer, and regions of the biliary system not amenable to 'thrombectomy' of the neoplasm can be resected, yielding palliation of symptoms for several years. Parenchymal multicentricity is normally inexorable; however, one of our patients is alive 4 years after resection of all the hepatic segments except segments I, II, and part of segment V, combined with thrombectomy of the ducts from segments V and VI, which were drained into a Roux-en-Y loop.

Sarcoma

Angiosarcomas are interesting because they are rare and incurable, but mainly because their aetiology is usually specific and obvious. They usually arise following injection of Thorotrast decades ago (a radioactive imaging substance that emits thorium daughters), following arsenic exposure of agricultural workers, especially in the vineyards of the Moselle Valley, following testosterone in boys with Fanconi's syndrome, and after exposure to vinyl chloride (the monomer of many plastics). Sarcomas otherwise are rare.

Although angiosarcoma is incurable, leimyosarcomas and embryonal rhabdomyocarcomas may be curable by excision and adjuvant chemotherapy. Because some fibrosarcomas and leiomyosarcomas secrete an insulin-like growth factor, they initially manifest themselves by causing hypoglycaemia.

Metastases (see Section 22.4.2 for full discussion)

Countless metastases lodge in the liver: few grow, and only the minority are worth removing. Nevertheless, huge, indolent metastases from exotic sources, such as mesonephric duct carcinoma, are sometimes resectable with the expectation of cure or of long-term palliation.

Colorectal primary cancers contribute the greatest number of resectable metastases to the liver; these are often indolent. Metastases originating in the right colon tend to be myriad and biologically aggressive; those from the descending colon and rectum are more likely to be solitary, or at least enumerable. An estimate has been made that only seven of 1750 patients with untreated hepatic metastases from the colon and rectum have ever survived 5 years.

By removing metastases the hypothesis is that the patient will be shifted from membership of a group about to die into a group that has a 25 to 35 per cent 5-year survival rate. However, no one is certain of the natural history of untreated colorectal metastases. Some remain static for years, having a growth period of 2 to 3 years before they become obvious.

Resection of four or fewer metastases is appropriate, including any satellites clustered around the central neoplasm. Resection of more than four metastases is generally futile, because with that degree of metastatic spread, both deposits in the liver and occult lymphatic and vascular metastases are often widespread.

The hope that removal of an enormous mass of metastatic colorectal cancer by a major hepatectomy will relieve pain and discomfort is often unrealized.

FURTHER READING

Chisari FV, *et al.* Molecular pathogenesis of hepatocellular carcinoma in hepatitis B virus transgenic mice. *Cell*, 1989; **59:** 1145–56.

Franco D. Malignancy of the liver. *Curr Opin Gastroenterol*, 1990; **6:** 447–53.

Franco D, *et al.* Resection of hepatocellular carcinomas: results in 72 European patients with cirrhosis. *Gastroenterology*, 1990; **98:** 733–8.

Ishak KG, Malt RA. Sarcomas of the liver and spleen. In: Raaf JH, ed. *Management of Soft Tissue Sarcomas*. Chicago: Year Book Medical Publishers 1992: 165–80.

Karhunen PJ. Benign hepatic tumours and tumour-like conditions in men. *J Clin Pathol*, 1986; **39:** 183–8.

Savage AP, Malt RA. Elective and emergency hepatic resection: determinants of operative mortality and morbidity. *Ann Surg*, 1991; **214:** 689–95.

Stocker JT, Ishak KG. Focal nodular hyperplasia of the liver: a study of 21 pediatric cases. *Cancer*, 1981; **48:** 336–45.

Takayama T, *et al.* Malignant transformation of adenomatous hyperplasia to hepatocellular carcinoma. *Lancet*, 1990; **ii:** 1150–3.

Wanless IR, Mawdsley C, Adams R. On the pathogenesis of focal nodular hyperplasia of the liver. *Hepatology*, 1985; **5:** 1194–200.

22.4.2 Metastatic carcinoma of the liver

ADRIAN SAVAGE

Metastatic carcinoma of the liver is far more common than primary malignant hepatic tumours. Until 1980, the treatment of metastatic carcinoma of the liver was largely expectant. The last 12 years have, however, seen a dramatic change in the management of this disease. Patients who have developed liver metastases are now assessed with a view to resection or chemotherapy. In addition, patients who have undergone curative resection for colorectal cancer and who are at risk of developing metastatic liver cancer are now routinely screened by sonography and serial estimation of carcinoembryonic antigen to detect hepatic metastases before they have developed beyond curative hepatic resection.

Because of the portal venous circulation, blood-borne metastases from gastrointestinal carcinomas usually appear first in the liver; spread of other carcinomas, such as those originating from breast and lung to the liver is usually indicative of widespread disseminated disease. Hepatic metastases from colorectal cancer are common, sometimes solitary, and slow to progress; they may occur without evidence of dissemination elsewhere. For this reason, patients with metastases from colorectal cancer form a special group. This is also true of patients with metastases from carcinoid or neuroendocrine tumours of the gastrointestinal tract and pancreas, in whom disabling symptoms attributable to the secretion of peptides and other vasoactive substances may occur. In patients with the carcinoid syndrome, hepatic resection to relieve symptoms may be indicated, while chemotherapy and embolization may are often effective in the treatment of the Zollinger–Ellison and VIPoma syndromes.

THE NATURAL HISTORY OF HEPATIC METASTASES

Although patients with unresectable hepatic metastases occasionally survive for more than 5 years, the median survival is under 6 months. Much depends upon the site and nature of the primary tumour and the extent of disease at the time of presentation.

Site

Metastases from cancer of the colon and rectum are slower to develop than metastases from carcinomas elsewhere. The median survival of patients with hepatic metastases from colorectal cancer is 177 days compared with 75 days for patients with metastases from carcinoma of the stomach and 54 days for patients with metastases from carcinoma of the pancreas. The survival of patients with hepatic metastases from carcinoid tumours and other tumours of neuroendocrine differentiation may be very prolonged.

Extent of metastatic disease of the liver

As would be expected, the greater the proportion of the liver affected by metastases the shorter the survival of the patient. The extent to which the liver is affected by metastatic disease can be assessed by ultrasound or CT imaging, or by palpation at laparotomy. In either case, it is important to assess the approximate proportion of the liver that is replaced by metastases and whether the distribution of the metastases is such that curative resection may be contemplated. Three groups are described, according to the percentage of liver tissue replaced by metastases: less than 25 per cent replacement, 25 to 75 per cent replacement, and greater than 75 per cent replacement of the liver parenchyma. For patients with liver metastases at the time of resection of a colorectal cancer, the mean survival is 3.4 months for those with greater than 75 per cent hepatic replacement compared with 6.2 months for patients with less than 25 per cent hepatic replacement. Similarly, patients with widespread metastases have a mean survival of 3.1 months, compared with 10.6 months for patients with multiple but potentially resectable metastases and 16.7 months for those with solitary metastases.

Histology

The grade of the tumour also has a bearing on the prognosis. The mean survival of patients with metastases from colorectal cancer that are well or moderately differentiated on histological examination is 13 months, compared with 7 months for patients with poorly differentiated tumours. The histological grade of hepatic metastases, determined by Broder's classification confirms a mean survival of 11 months for grades 1 and 2 compared with 7.6 months for grade 3 and 5.5 months for grade 4.

CLINICAL FEATURES

Hepatic metastases may be an incidental finding during the preoperative assessment or at laparotomy in a patient with a carcinoma. The presence of hepatic metastases is a contraindication to surgical resection of gastric, pancreatic, or oesophageal carcinoma. The presence of hepatic metastases increases the morbidity and mortality of surgical resection for colorectal cancer. The operative mortality rate may be as high as 22.7 per cent for patients undergoing resection of a carcinoma of the colon or rectum in the presence of liver metastases compared with 4.6 per cent for those without liver metastases.

Some patients may develop symptoms and signs attributable to the liver metastases. Acute abdominal pain from necrosis of or haemorrhage into a hepatic metastases may be confused with acute cholecystitis, right ureteric colic, or appendicitis. Hepatic metastases may also present with a mass, fever malaise, jaundice, and pruritus.

The presence of hepatomegaly, ascites, and peritoneal spread adversely affects the prognosis of hepatic metastases. The survival of patients with hepatomegaly is 7.7 months, compared with 14.3 months if the liver is not palpable. Ascites, if present, is associated with a survival of 3.8 months compared with 13 months if absent. Of the biochemical estimations, the serum alkaline phosphatase is the most important with regard to prognosis. The survival of patients with colorectal cancer liver metastases is 2.8 months if the alkaline phosphatase level is elevated compared with 6.2 months if normal.

Hepatic metastases detected as a result of routine screening after apparently curative resection of a colorectal cancer are associated with a better prognosis, first because the early detection of hepatic metastases gives the best chance of surgical resection and the only hope of cure and second, because the earlier the metastases are detected, the longer the patient will survive with his metastases. The best method of screening is as yet undetermined. Examination of the liver by ultrasound at yearly intervals is currently the favoured method. However, it is interesting to note that the majority of patients undergoing hepatic resection for metastases from colorectal cancer are detected on investigation of an elevated carcinoembryonic antigen level, and very few from isotope or sonographic imaging.

TREATMENT OF METASTASES FROM COLORECTAL CANCER

Resection

The majority of patients with hepatic metastases present with disease that has spread beyond surgical resection: only about 5 per cent of patients with hepatic metastases from colorectal cancer are suitable for surgical resection. The survival of patients undergoing resection of hepatic metastases is 25 per cent at 5 years, and 1 to 2 per cent of patients with colorectal cancer could therefore be cured by resection of their hepatic metastases. As 24 000 patients a year are registered with a diagnosis of colorectal cancer in England and Wales, approximately 1200 patients may benefit from resection of hepatic metastases and 300 patients a year could be expected to be cured.

Resection, or some other new modality, such as alcohol ablation, are the only hopes of cure. Hepatic resection for metastases is, however, associated with an operative mortality of 5 per cent and serious morbidity of up to 30 per cent. While the postoperative stay may be as short as 13 days, it may be several months before the patient regains his preoperative strength and vigour. Before considering hepatic resection, the potential benefits must be weighed against the risks. The patient must be in good general health and fit enough to withstand major abdominal surgery. Advanced age in its own right is not a major contraindication to hepatic resection for colorectal cancer metastases, although few such resections have been performed in patients over the age of 80. Local recurrence and metastases other than those in a resectable portion of the liver are also a contraindication to hepatic resection. Several studies have analysed subgroups of patients undergoing hepatic resection for colorectal metastases in order to identify factors which may indicate a better prognosis.

Features relating to the primary colorectal carcinoma have proved disappointing in determining the prognosis after resection of hepatic metastases. Hepatic metastases from Duke's A colorectal carcinomas are very rare. Opinion is divided as to whether patients with liver metastases from Dukes' C colorectal carcinomas fare worse than those with metastases from Dukes' B carcinomas (Table 1).

The histological grade of the primary tumour or its metastases would be expected to have a bearing on the prognosis. The mean survival after resection of metastases from poorly differentiated tumours is 7.1 months compared with 17.9 months for moderately or well-differentiated tumours. In another series, none of nine patients with poorly differentiated tumours undergoing resection of hepatic metastases survived to 3 years while the 5-year survival of 77 patients with well or moderately differentiated tumours was 20 per cent. However, as few patients with poorly differentiated tumours undergo resection of hepatic metastases, statistical significance is difficult to demonstrate. The primary site, whether colon or rectum, the age and gender of the patient, and the preoperative carcinoembryonic antigen level do not have any significant effect on prognosis following resection of hepatic metastases. Patients with symptomatic hepatic metastases fare worse than patients whose disease is asymptomatic. However, as patients who have developed symptoms from their metastases may be presumed to have more advanced disease, the better survival of asymptomatic patients may be attributable to a lead time bias.

The success of resection of metastases from colorectal cancer depends on the technical ability to resect with a wide margin the portion of the liver containing the disease. Most reports show trends towards a better prognosis in patients with solitary metastases compared with those with multiple metastases, or less than four metastases compared with more than four. Similarly, survival is marginally better in patients with metastases less than 5 cm in diameter. However, failure to resect all the metastatic cancer, direct involvement of adjacent structures by the hepatic metastases, or involvement of the portal triad lymph nodes is associated with a significantly worse prognosis. Similarly, the 5-year survival of patients whose hepatic resection margin is less than 5 mm is 9 per cent, compared with 23 per cent for patients with a greater resection margin.

Following resection of hepatic metastases, approximately one-third of patients develop recurrence in the liver alone. Such patients should be reassessed with a view to a second resection; several successful repeat hepatic resections have been performed.

Table 1. Survival after resection of hepatic metastases from colorectal carcinoma

Study	Dukes' 'B'	Dukes' 'C'	*p* value
Butler *et al.* 1986	55% 5-year	10% 5-year	$p < 0.001$
Registry of Hepatic Metastases 1988	47% 5-year	23% 5-year	$p < 0.001$
Hughes *et al.* 1989	35% 5-year	28% 5-year	?
Morrow *et al.* 1982	36% 5-year	25% 5-year	?
Gennari *et al.* 1986	No significant difference		NS
August 1985	No significant difference		NS
Logan *et al.* 1982	26.3 months	28.2 months	NS
Coburn 1987	29% 5-year	26% 5-year	NS
Savage and Malt 1992	22% 5-year	16% 5-year	NS

Resection of metastases from sites other than the colorectum

Resection of metastases from carcinoma of the lung, stomach, or pancreas carries a poor prognosis and is not justified. Resection of metastases from carcinoma of the breast may be justified if the patient is symptomatic and if hormonal therapy or chemotherapy fails to control symptoms; long-term survival has been reported. Patients with metastases from carcinoid tumours and other neuro-endocrine tumours may benefit greatly from palliative resection to alleviate symptoms due to the secretion of vasoactive substances and peptides. Such metastases may have a well-defined plane around them which allows the metastasis to be enucleated. Although such resection is palliative, the survival may be measured in years and the relief of symptoms dramatic.

Chemotherapy

Despite two decades of intense clinical investigation, colorectal cancer metastatic to the liver remains highly resistant to systemic chemotherapy. Only the fluoropyrimidines (5-fluorouracil (5-FU) and flurodeoxyuridine) have shown a consistent therapeutic activity, and numerous studies have not demonstrated any other agent to be superior to these drugs. A large number of trials have evaluated the efficacy of combination chemotherapy but often promising initial results have not been reproduced. A report of 10 different chemotherapeutic treatments in 848 patients with colorectal cancer showed that none was superior to 5-FU. Systemic 5-FU induces an objective response in 15 to 20 per cent of treated patients, without prolonging life. A similar response rate of 23 per cent for hepatic metastases has been observed.

There is substantial evidence, mainly for tumour cell cultures studies, to suggest that antitumour agents have a steep dose–response relationship. Hepatic artery or portal venous cannulation and regional chemotherapy will result in higher regional concentrations of chemotherapeutic agents in the liver. Thus, hepatic artery or portal venous infusion of 5-FU may be indicated in patients with unresectable liver metastases in whom there is no evidence of local recurrence or dissemination elsewhere. Although the metastases in the liver are thought to originate from dissemination via the portal venous circulation, once developed, they derive their chief blood supply from branches of the hepatic artery. One prospective randomized trial has reported a response rate of 34 per cent following hepatic artery infusion of 5-FU compared with 23 per cent following intravenous administration of 5-FU. However, no effect on survival has yet been demonstrated.

In distinction to the treatment of patients with metastases from colorectal cancer, chemotherapy may have an important role in their prevention. A trial, of postoperative portal venous perfusion of 1 g of 5-FU compared with no adjuvant treatment in 257 patients suggests that untreated patients are at twice the risk of dying than treated patients. The results of a multicentre trial of adjuvant perioperative 5-FU are awaited.

Embolization

Liver metastases can be treated by embolization of their blood supply. A cannula is introduced into the femoral artery and advanced until the coeliac axis has been cannulated. An angiogram is then performed and the vessels supplying the metastases identified. If possible, these vessels are then superselectively cannulated. Absolute alcohol, gelfoam, or steel coils may be introduced to occlude the blood supply.

Embolization is most effective for patients with hepatic metastases from neuroendocrine tumours since it reduces the symptoms attributable to the secretion of vasoactive substances. Embolization via the hepatic artery has not been shown to improve survival of patients with metastases from carcinoma of the colorectum and other gastrointestinal malignancy.

Apart from occasional complications of arterial puncture, haematoma formation, arterial dissection, and thrombosis, embolization of a hepatic metastasis may result in pain, fever, and leucocytosis. This post-embolization syndrome affects up to 50 per cent of patients undergoing this procedure and may last for a week. Septicaemia or hepatic abscess may develop in up to 10 per cent of patients.

Radiotherapy

The efficacy of radiotherapy in the treatment of metastases in the liver is limited by the radiosensitivity of normal hepatocytes and the relative insensitivity of metastatic carcinomas. The maximum dose which can be administered before inducing radiation hepatitis is 35 Gy; this dose is too low for curative irradiation of metastatic carcinomas. Radiotherapy is occasionally useful in the palliation of severe pain from hepatic metastases but does not prolong survival.

Interruption of blood supply

Because hepatic metastases derive their blood supply mainly from the hepatic artery, simple ligation of the hepatic artery or full arterial devascularization of the arterial supply to the liver has been attempted in the treatment of patients with liver metastases. Metastases that are highly vascular, such as carcinoid tumours, may show a better response. A transient decrease in tumour size without improved survival has been reported following hepatic artery ligation and devascularization. The rapid re-establishment of arterial flow through collateral supply limits the efficacy of this technique.

FURTHER READING

Adson MA, van Heerden JA. Major hepatic resections for metastatic colorectal cancer. *Ann Surg* 1980;**191**:576–83.

August DA, Sugarbaker PH, Ottow RT, Gianola FJ, Schneider PD. Hepatic resection of colorectal metastases. *Ann Surg* 1985;**201**:210–218.

Bengtsson G, Carlsson G, Hafström L, Jönsson P-E. Natural history of patients with untreated liver metastases from colorectal cancer. *Am J Surg* 1981;**141**:586–589.

Bradpiece HA, Benjamin IS, Halevy A, Blumgart LH. Major hepatic resection for colorectal liver metastases. *Br J Surg* 1987;**74**:324–326.

Butler J, Attiyeh FF, Daly JM. Hepatic resection for metastases of the colon and rectum. *Surg Gynecol Obstet* 1986;**162**:109–113.

Cobourn CS, Makowka L, Langer B, Taylor BR, Falk RE. Examination of patient selection and outcome for hepatic resection for metastatic disease. *Surg Gynecol Obstet* 1987;**165**:239–246.

Ekberg H, *et al.* Determinants of survival in liver resection for colorectal secondaries. *Br J Surg* 1986;**73**:727–731.

Finan PJ, Marshall RJ, Cooper EH, Giles GR. Factors affecting survival in patients presenting with synchronous hepatic metastases from colorectal cancer: a clinical and computer analysis. *Br J Surg* 1985;**72**:373–377.

Fortner JG, Silva JS, Golbey RB, Cox EB, Maclean BJ. Multivariate analysis of a personal series of 247 consecutive patients with liver metastases from colorectal cancer: 1. Treatment by hepatic resection. *Ann Surg* 1984;**199**:-306–316.

Foster JH. Survival after liver resection for secondary tumors. *Am J Surg* 1978;**135**:389–394.

Gennari L, Doci R, Bozzetti F, Bignami P. Surgical treatment of hepatic metastases from colorectal cancer *Ann Surg* 1986;**203**:49–54.

Grage TB, *et al.* Results of a prospective randomized study of hepatic artery infusion with 5-fluorouracil versus intravenous 5-fluorouracil in patients with metastases from colorectal cancer: a Central Oncology Group Study. *Surgery* 1979;**86**:550–555.

Holm A, Bradley E, Aldrete JS. Hepatic resection of metastasis from colorectal carcinoma: morbidity, mortality and pattern of recurrence. *Ann Surg* 1989;**209**:428–434.

Hughes K, Scheele J, Sugarbaker PH. Surgery for colorectal cancer metastatic to the liver. *Surg Clin N Am* 1989;**69**:339–359.

Iwatsuki S, Starzl TE. Personal experience with 411 hepatic resesctions. *Ann Surg* 1988;**208**:421–434.

Jaffe BM, Donegan WL, Watson F, Spratt JS Jr. Factors influencing survival in patients with untreated hepatic metastases. *Surg Gynecol Obstet* 1968;**127**:1–11.

Lavin P, *et al.* Survival and response to chemotherapy for advanced colorectal adenocarcinoma. *Cancer* 1980;**46**:1536–1543.

Logan S, Meier SJ, Ramming KP, Morton DL, Longmire WP Jr. Hepatic resection of metastatic colorectal carcinoma. *Arch Surg* 1982;**117**:25–28.

Morrow CE, Grage TB, Sutherland DER, Najarian JS. Hepatic ressection for secondary neoplasms. *Surgery* 1982;**92**:610–614.

Pestana C, Reitmeier RJ, Moertel CG, Judd ES, Dockerty MB. The natural history of carcinoma of the colon and rectum. *Am J Surg* 1964;**108**:826–829.

Pittam MR, Thornton H, Ellis H. Survival after extended resection for locally advanced carcinomas of the colon and rectum. *Ann R Coll Surg Engl* 1984;**66**:81–84.

Registry of Hepatic Metastases. Resection of the liver for colorectal carcinoma metastases: a multi-institutional study of indications for resection. *Surgery* 1988;**103**:278–288.

Savage AP, Malt RA. Elective and emergency hepatic resection: determinants of operative mortality and morbididity. *Ann Surg* 1991;**214**:689–695.

Savage AP, Malt RA. Survival after hepatic resection for malignant tumours. *Br J Surg* 1992;**79**:1095–1101.

Segall HN. An experimental anatomical investigation of the blood and bile channels of the liver. *Surg Gynecol Obstet* 1923;**37**:152–178.

Taylor I. Colorectal liver metastases—to treat or not to treat. *Br J Surg* 1985;**72**:511–516.

Taylor I, Machin D, Mullee M. A randomized controlled trial of adjuvant portal vein cytotoxic perfusion in colorectal cancer. *Br J Surg* 1985;**72**:359–363.

Wood CB, Gillis CR, Blumgart LH. A retrospective study of the natural history of patients with liver metastases from colorectal cancer. *Clin Oncol* 1976;**2**:285–288.

22.5 Asian perspective on hepatocellular carcinoma (HCC)

NAOFUMI NAGASUE

Hepatocellular carcinoma (HCC) is common in Oriental countries. It is one of the most malignant tumours, and carries a poor prognosis without treatment because of a high incidence of associated liver cirrhosis and its propensity to invade the portal or hepatic veins and to spread rapidly to the entire liver. Most of hepatocellular carcinomas in the East develop on a substate of underlying cirrhosis caused by hepatitis virus.

Although the resectability of the tumour is low because of this high incidence of associated cirrhosis and late diagnosis, the routine use of serum α-fetoprotein estimation and ultrasonography in patients with chronic liver disease has increased the rate with which tumours smaller than 5 cm in diameter are detected. Most physicians recommend monthly estimation of serum α-fetoprotein and an imaging study every 3 months for patients with chronic liver disease.

DIAGNOSIS

A sharp, steady rise in serum α-fetoprotein is highly diagnostic for hepatocellular carcinoma. However, it is noteworthy that serum α-fetoprotein is normal in 43 per cent of patients with tumours smaller than 3 cm in diameter. Ultrasonography is extremely useful to cover the weakness of α-fetoprotein measurements. Small hepatocellular carcinomas are usually hypoechoic, but may be hyperechoic if the tumour contains fat. The weak point of this method is that lesions in the right hepatic dome are often missed because of its blind angle. Another problem is that the ultrasonographic probes currently available can rarely detect lesions smaller than 1 cm in diameter.

Angiography is more sensitive for the detection of minute hepatocellular carcinomas, as they are usually hypervascular even if they are tiny. However, tumours in segments II and III (Couinaud classification) can occasionally be missed even by superselective arteriography. Computed tomography (CT) without contrast media is not so effective in detecting small tumours developing in cirrhotic livers, although enhanced CT has a higher detection rate. Magnetic resonance imaging of the liver is accurate only when the tumour is more than 2 cm in diameter, when the detection rate is 97.5 per cent compared to 33.3 per cent for tumours less than 2 cm in diameter.

The most important approach for the early detection of minute hepatocellular carcinomas is to combine two or three of the methods described above.

Differential diagnosis

Recent advances in diagnostic methods have increased the chances of detecting asymptomatic tumours of the liver. However, qualitative differentiation of space-occupying lesions is not necessarily easy, particularly when the lesions are small. One of the lesions which needs to be differentiated from hepatocellular carcinoma is adenomatous hyperplastic nodule in the cirrhotic liver. This occasionally contains tiny nodules of hepatocellular carcinomas within it, or both conditions may develop synchronously or metachronously in the same cirrhotic liver. Although this lesion is usually discovered by ultrasonography its sonographic features are similar to those of hepatocellular carcinoma. CT is usually negative but may show the presence of a low-density lesion if fatty change is prominent; angiography is usually negative. Another lesion to be differentiated from hepatocellular carcinoma is haemangioma. Small haemangiomas are hyperechoic on ultrasonography and may or may not be depicted by angiography. Ultrasound- or CT-guided needle biopsy is necessary to obtain a definitive diagnosis.

TREATMENT

Early detection of small hepatocellular carcinomas makes resection possible, even in the presence of liver cirrhosis, because such small tumours can be removed by a minor hepatic resection. In a series of 22 cirrhotic patients with hepatocellular carcinoma smaller than 3 cm in diameter, the 3-year survival rate was only 12.8 per cent without anticancer treatment. Higher survival rates are obtainable by partial wedge or segmental resection.

Limited resection of the cirrhotic liver with minute hepatocellular carcinomas can be safely undertaken using intraoperative ultrasonography: this will reveal the many small tumours embedded in the liver parenchyma which are both invisible and impalpable during surgery.

Resection of the cirrhotic liver is technically demanding because portal hypertension and coagulation disorders are usually present to some degree in those with liver cirrhosis. The Pringle manoeuvre (compression of the portal triad), with or without temporary occlusion of the hepatic vein trunk, is useful to prevent severe haemorrhage and to reduce postoperative morbidity and mortality. The operative mortality rate is usually below 5 per cent after limited resection of the cirrhotic liver. The long-term survival rate is 30 to 50 per cent.

It is not known whether liver transplantation produces a better result than conventional resection in the treatment of hepatocellular carcinoma in the Orient. However, the results from Cambridge, Hanover, and Pittsburgh indicate a possibility that many patients benefit more from liver transplantation than hepatic resection because preclinical small tumours with advanced cirrhosis seem to represent a more favourable indication for transplantation.

FURTHER READING

Arakawa M, Kage M, Sugihara S, Nakashima T, Suenaga M, Okuda K. Emergence of malignant lesions within an adenomatous hyperplastic nodule in a cirrhotic liver: observations in five cases. *Gastroenterology* 1986; **91**: 198–208.

Chang Y-C, Nagasue N, Kimura N, Ota N, Yukaya H. Ultrasonographic features of hepatocellular pseudotumour in the cirrhotic liver. *Clin Radiol* 1988; **39**: 635–8.

Ebara M, *et al.* Diagnosis of small hepatocellular carcinoma: Correlation of MR imaging and tumour histologic studies. *Radiology* 1986; **159**: 371–7.

Ebara M, *et al.* Natural history of minute hepatocellular carcinoma smaller than three centimetres complicating cirrhosis: a study in 22 patients. *Gastroenterology* 1986; **90**: 289–98.

Kanematsu T, Takenaka K, Matsumata T, Furuta T, Sugimachi K, Inokuchi K. Limited hepatic resection effective for selected cirrhotic patients with primary liver cancer. *Ann Surg* 1984; **199**: 51–6.

Kobayashi K, *et al.* Screening methods for early detection of hepatocellular carcinoma. *Hepatology* 1985: **5**: 1100–5.

Kubo Y, Okuda K, Musha H, Nakashima T. Detection of hepatocellular carcinoma during a clinical follow-up of chronic liver disease: observation sin 31 patients. *Gastroenterology* 1978; **74**: 578–82.

Kudo M, *et al.* Small hepatocellular carcinomas in chronic liver disease: detection with SPECT. *Radiology* 1986; **159**: 697–703.

Lee C-S, *et al.* Surgical treatment of 109 patients with symptomatic and asymptomatic hepatocellular carcinoma. *Surgery* 1986; **99**: 481–90.

Liau Y-F, *et al.* Early detection of hepatocellular carcinoma in patients with chronic type B hepatitis: a prospective study. *Gastroenterology* 1986; **90**: 263–7.

Nagasue N, Yukaya H, Hamada T, Hirsoe S, Kanashima R, Inokuchi K. The natural history of hepatocellular carcinoma: a study of 100 untreated cases. *Cancer* 1984; **54**: 461–5.

Nagasue N, Yukaya H, Ogawa Y, Akamizu H, Kimura N, Takahashi M. Diagnosis and treatment of minute hepatocellular carcinoma in the cirrhotic liver: report of 21 cases. *Chir Epatobil* 1984; **3**: 11–20.

Nagasue N, Yukaya H, Suehiro S, Ogawa Y. Tolerance of the cirrhotic liver to normothermic ischemia: a clinical study of 15 patients. *Am J Surg* 1984; **147**: 772–5.

Nagasue N, Yukaya H, Ogawa Y, Hirose S, Okita M. Segmental and subsegmental resections of the cirrhotic liver under hepatic inflow and outflow occlusion. *Br J Surg* 1985; **72**: 565–8.

Nagasue N, *et al.* Appraisal of hepatic resection in the treatment of minute hepatocellular carcinoma associated with liver cirrhosis. *Br J Surg* 1987; **74**: 836–8.

Nagasue N, Yukaya H, Chang Y-C, Kimura N, Ota N, Nakamura T. Hepatocellular pseudotumour (regenerating nodule) in the cirrhotic liver mimicking hepatocellular carcinoma. *Br J Surg* 1988; **75**: 1124–8.

Nagasue N, *et al.* Intraoperative ultrasonography in resection of small hepatocellular carcinoma associated with cirrhosis. *Am J Surg* 1989; **158**: 40–2.

Okuda K, *et al.* Natural history of hepatocellular carcinoma and prognosis in relation to treatment: study of 850 patients. *Cancer* 1985; **56**: 918–28.

Sheu J-C, *et al.* Early detection of hepatocellular carcinoma by real-time ultrasonography: A prospective study. *Cancer* 1985; **56**: 660–6.

Sheu J-C, Lee C-S, Sung-J-L, Chen D-S, Yang P-M, Lin T-Y. Intraoperative hepatic ultrasonography: an indispensable procedure in resection of small hepatocellular carcinomas. *Surgery* 1985; **97**: 97–103.

Sumida M, Ohto M, Ebara M, Kimura K, Okuda K, Hirooka N. Accuracy of angiography in the diagnosis of small hepatocellular carcinoma. *Am J Roentgenol* 1986; **147**: 531–6.

Takashima T, Matsui O, Suzuki M, Ida M. Diagnosis and screening of small hepatocellular carcinomas: comparison of radionuclide imaging, ultrasound, computed tomography, hepatic angiography, and α_1-fetoprotein assay. *Radiology* 1982; **145**: 635–8.

Takayasu K, *et al.* Angiography of small hepatocellular carcinomas: analysis of 105 resected tumours. *Am J Roentgenol* 1986; **147**: 525–9.

Tan Z-Y, *et al.* Surgery of small hepatocellular carcinoma: analysis of 144 cases. *Cancer* 1989; **64**: 536–41.

Terada T, Kadoya M, Nakanuma Y, Matsui O. Iron-accumulating adenomatous hyperplastic nodule with malignant foci in the cirrhotic liver: histopathologic, quantitative, and magnetic resonance imaging *in vitro* studies. *Cancer* 1990; **65**: 1994–2000.

22.6 The Budd-Chiari syndrome

TIMOTHY C. WANG AND JULES L. DIENSTAG

DEFINITION

The Budd–Chiari syndrome is a loose term used to designate disorders characterized by hepatic venous outflow obstruction. The pathological features of hepatic vein thrombosis were first described by Budd in 1845. In 1899, Chiari reported the clinical syndrome of hepatomegaly, ascites, and abdominal pain, and coined the eponym Budd–Chiari syndrome. The clinical features and treatment of the disorder depend on the site of obstruction. Hepatic venous outflow obstruction can result from thrombotic or non-thrombotic occlusion of the major hepatic veins or the inferior vena cava. Occlusion at either site interrupts the blood flow from the liver, leading to a marked elevation of sinusoidal pressure, intense congestion of the liver, and destruction of hepatic parenchyma.

CLINICAL PRESENTATION

Although the Budd–Chiari syndrome is rare in the United States, it is common in Northern India, South Africa, and the Orient. The syndrome can occur at any age, but generally presents in the third or fourth decade of life and is slightly more common in women. Budd–Chiari syndrome can present either as an acute, rapidly evolving illness, or as a disorder that progresses slowly and insidiously over a period of months to years. The majority of patients have rapidly developing liver disease, with signs and symptoms of less that 3 months' duration: the classic triad is the sudden appearance of ascites, hepatomegaly, and abdominal pain. Other common symptoms such as nausea, anorexia, vomiting, and diarrhoea are fairly non-specific. Clinical jaundice is rare, and splenomegaly is found in fewer than one-third of patients. Rarely, patients may present with fulminant hepatic failure and shock. In patients with long-standing Budd–Chiari syndrome, portal hypertension develops, and patients may present with progressive ascites and wasting, bleeding oesophageal varices, hepatic encephalopathy, and hepatorenal syndrome.

PATHOGENESIS

The Budd-Chiari syndrome most often occurs as a result of an underlying illness known to be associated with thrombotic complications, although there may be no apparent predisposing factor in up to one-third of cases (Table 1). In large compilations of patients from the United States, the most common predisposing conditions are myeloproliferative disorders, polycythaemia rubra vera, and paroxysmal nocturnal haemoglobinuria. Polycythaemia rubra vera is the single most common cause of the Budd–Chiari syndrome in the United States. Many patients at initial presentation of the condition have a normal haemoglobin and haematocrit but a markedly elevated red cell mass. Studies have suggested that patients with paroxysmal nocturnal haemoglobinuria may have a progressive disease, with early thrombosis of only small hepatic veins and minimal or no symptoms, followed later by complete occlusion of large hepatic veins and a life-threatening course.

Table 1 Causative factors in Budd–Chiari syndrome

Idiopathic
Membraneous webs
Haematological disorders
Polycythaemia rubra vera
Paroxysmal nocturnal haemoglobinuria
Myeloproliferative disorders
Tumours
Hepatocellular carcinoma
Adrenal carcinoma
Renal cell carcinoma
Hypercoagulable syndromes
Antithrombin III deficiency
Protein C deficiency
Lupus anticoagulant
Oral contraceptives
Pregnancy and postpartum state
Infections
Amoebic abscess
Echinococcus infection
Aspergillosis
Syphilis
Trauma
Connective tissue disorders
Miscellaneous

Modified from Maddrey WC, *Semin Liver Dis* 1987; 7: 32–8.

Other myeloproliferative disorders such as essential thrombocythaemia, agnogenic myeloid metaplasia, and chronic myelogenous leukaemia have also been reported in association with the Budd–Chiari syndrome.

A number of tumours in and around the liver, particularly hepatocellular, adrenal, and renal carcinomas, but also Wilms' tumour, leiomyosarcoma of the inferior vena cava, right atrial myxoma, and carcinoma of the lung, pancreas, and stomach, may cause the Budd–Chiari syndrome either by direct invasion of the inferior vena cava or by increasing the tendency toward thrombosis.

Budd–Chiari syndrome may develop during pregnancy or in the postpartum state, within a few weeks or months after delivery. Many cases occur in women taking oral contraception. Although a definite causative link has not been shown, a multicentre case-control study has suggested that the relative risk of hepatic vein thrombosis among recent users of oral contraceptives compared with that of non-users was 2.37 ($p < 0.02$), a risk similar to that of stroke, myocardial infarction, or venous thromboembolism.

A number of infectious processes may be associated with the Budd–Chiari syndrome, the most common being amoebic abscesses, aspergillosis, hydatid cyst, and syphilis. Trauma, most commonly blunt abdominal trauma, is also a common cause of Budd–Chiari syndrome. Hypercoagulable states that have been reported in patients with Budd–Chiari syndrome include antithrombin III deficiency, protein C deficiency, and the presence of lupus anticoagulant (antiphospholipid antibody). Most of the connective tissue disorders, including systemic lupus erythematosus, mixed connective tissue disorder, and scleroderma have been reported as possible causes. Rare causes of the Budd–Chiari syndrome include Behçet's syndrome, ulcerative colitis, α_1-antitrypsin deficiency, sarcoidosis, and idiopathic hypereosinophilic syndrome.

In the Orient, the Middle East, and South Africa, a membranous web or a long segmental obstruction of the inferior vena cava is the most common cause of the Budd–Chiari syndrome. The origin and pathogenesis of these webs remains controversial. Hirooka and Kimura conducted a detailed study of 205 patients with Budd–Chiari syndrome reported in the Japanese literature, and found that a membranous web accounted for 73 (35 per cent) of cases. They classified the membranes into seven types, based on embryological studies, concluding that the webs resulted from a developmental anomaly or congenital malformation. In 1986, however, a patient had a mural thrombus that evolved over 2 years into a membranous web, suggesting that membranous webs can be a sequel of thrombosis. Although membranous webs have been considered rare in the United States, a series of 35 patients with Budd–Chiari syndrome, out of whom 8 patients (23 per cent) had idiopathic membranous obstruction of the inferior vena cava was reported from Los Angeles; most of these were immigrants from the Far East.

The cause of the Budd–Chiari syndrome is unknown in approximately 30 per cent of cases. However, a latent myeloproliferative disorder, despite the absence of peripheral blood changes, may be demonstrated in a majority of these patients by the spontaneous formation of erythroid colonies in the absence of erythropoietin.

DIFFERENTIAL DIAGNOSIS

Many disorders can be mistaken for the Budd-Chiari syndrome and should be considered in the differential diagnosis. Liver disorders with features similar to the Budd–Chiari syndrome include alcoholic hepatitis, viral hepatitis, cirrhosis, and hepatic malignancy. Disorders outside the liver that resemble the Budd–Chiari syndrome include constrictive pericarditis, tricuspid insufficiency, right atrial myxoma, and right-sided heart failure. All of these conditions, however, rarely present a diagnostic problem. Hepatic veno-occlusive disorder, on the other hand, mimics the Budd–Chiari syndrome and may be part of the same disease spectrum. Veno-occlusive disorder is characterized by non-thrombotic obstruction at the level of the sublobular and terminal branches of the hepatic veins in the liver. Although initially described as a complication of poisoning with pyrrolizidine alkaloids present in Jamaican bush teas, the disease is now seen as a complication of high dose chemotherapy and radiation therapy in patients receiving bone marrow transplantation.

The diagnosis is established by demonstrating radiographically the patency of the major hepatic veins and inferior vena cava, and/or by liver biopsy.

DIAGNOSIS

Budd–Chiari syndrome is generally difficult to diagnose on the basis of clinical criteria alone, and routine laboratory testing is not particularly helpful. The aminotransferases are usually only slightly elevated and are of little diagnostic value. These enzymes may reach concentrations greater than 1000 IU in acute, severe Budd–Chiari syndrome or when hepatic vein thrombosis occurs in association with thrombosis of the portal vein. Serum alkaline phosphatase activity is usually elevated by a factor of 1.5 to 2; the serum bilirubin level is usually less than 5 mg/dl. The characteristics of the ascites fluid are highly variable: ascites fluid protein usually ranges from 1.5 to 3.0 g/dl, although exudative ascites with a protein concentration of greater than 3.0 g/dl is not uncommon.

Because the physical findings and routine liver chemistry tests are non-specific in suspected Budd–Chiari syndrome, imaging studies play an important role in the diagnostic evaluation. Hepatic scintigraphy has been used extensively in the past; some patients show decreased uptake in the left and right lobes, with retained uptake in the caudate lobe, resulting in the so-called 'central hot spot.' More often, however, hepatic scintiscanning shows a diffuse, inhomogeneous pattern of tracer uptake, and other imaging modalities, such as ultrasonography, computed tomography, and magnetic resonance imaging, are therefore used. All three of these techniques can reveal non-specific abnormalities such as hepatomegaly, ascites, inhomogeneity of the liver parenchyma, as well as the more specific findings of absence of hepatic veins and 'common-shaped collaterals.' Magnetic resonance imaging has certain advantages in evaluating the hepatic vasculature because of its depiction of blood vessels as regions of absent signal, the 'flow-void phenomenon', but the technique is expensive and not widely available. Compared with other modalities, real-time Doppler duplex ultrasound has the advantage of low cost and easy availability and at present is probably the screening test of choice. In addition to showing thrombosis or occlusion of the major hepatic veins or inferior vena cava, Doppler ultrasound can often demonstrate the actual level of obstruction. Moreover, recent studies suggest that colour-flow Doppler ultrasound is superior to duplex imaging and can give a real-time overview of all vascular structures within the liver. Both colour-flow Doppler ultrasound and magnetic resonance imaging (MRI) are useful in evaluating shunt patency in patients with the Budd–Chiari syndrome who have undergone portasystemic shunting; both compare favourably with venography. In the future, colour-flow Doppler imaging may become the initial screening technique in patients with a suspected diagnosis of Budd–Chiari syndrome.

For most patients, venography and liver biopsy remain the standards for diagnosis. Inferior vena cavography, performed by introducing a catheter into the femoral vein, can demonstrate the site of obstruction as well as provide access for pressure measurements. The venogram can show occlusion or marked narrowing of the major hepatic veins; characteristically, there is difficulty in catheterizing the hepatic veins in patients with Budd–Chiari syndrome, but the catheter can often be advanced a short distance, and injection of dye in the wedged position may reveal a spider web pattern of intrahepatic collaterals. The inferior vena cava may be shown to be patent, or occluded by tumour, thrombus or web, or compressed and narrowed by an enlarged caudate lobe. Pressure measurements should be taken in the right atrium and the inferior vena cava to determine whether a pressure gradient is present across the diaphragm. Portal venography, from superior mesenteric arteriography with examination of the venous phase, should also be performed if portal vein thrombosis is suspected. Concomitant portal vein thrombosis occurs in up to 20 per cent of patients with hepatic vein thrombosis.

The diagnosis of Budd–Chiari syndrome is supported by a percutaneous needle biopsy of the liver. The classic pathological findings include sinusoidal dilation and centrilobular congestion, followed later in the disease course by centrilobular necrosis, cell dropout and atrophy, scant inflammation, and extravasation of red blood cells into the space of Disse. Eventually, in patients with long-standing Budd–Chiari syndrome, fibrosis of a 'nutmeg' liver develops. Blind percutaneous liver biopsy is often difficult or dangerous because of the presence of ascites or coagulopathy; however, ultrasound or CT directed biopsy can be performed with relative safety in most patients.

The suspicion of the Budd–Chiari syndrome demands rapid and aggressive diagnosis. Patients should undergo urgent evaluation, with non-invasive imaging followed by venography. Some authorities urge prompt liver biopsy examination in patients with suspected Budd–Chiari syndrome in order to assess the degree of hepatic injury and to identify patients with Rappaport Zone III necrosis who may require immediate surgery. However, the diagnosis can be established with venography alone in most patients.

NATURAL HISTORY

The natural history of the Budd–Chiari syndrome is variable, depending on the rapidity and extent of the hepatic venous outflow occlusion. For the majority of patients who do not undergo surgical or angiographic intervention, however, the prognosis is poor; relentless deterioration and death ensue. Although spontaneous resolution is described, these cases are rare and unlikely to occur except in the very early stages of the disease. On the other hand, some patients with mild disease may be clinically stable for years. These patients often respond to diuretics for a while, especially if an underlying hypercoagulable state (e.g. myeloproliferative disorder) can be treated as well. A small proportion of patients with very early hepatic vein thrombosis respond to transluminal angioplasty or thrombolytic therapy. The majority of patients, however, if treated non-operatively die within months of the onset of symptoms. Survivors of the acute phase almost invariably develop cirrhosis of the liver and die within a few years from hepatic failure, bleeding oesophageal varices, or other complications of chronic liver disease. The overall mortality rate exceeds 50 per cent at 2 years.

TREATMENT

The therapeutic approach to patients with the Budd–Chiari syndrome depends on the severity, duration, and cause of the obstruction. Patients with suspected Budd–Chiari syndrome should undergo an urgent evaluation, and those with severe, acute disease or a liver biopsy that shows severe Zone III necrosis or fibrosis should immediately be considered for surgical intervention. Medical therapy is useless in patients with severe disease and in those in whom hepatic vein thrombosis is fully established. However, patients with mild, non-acute Budd–Chiari syndrome, and those in whom a liver biopsy shows no necrosis or fibrosis, can be considered for a trial of medical therapy and close observation.

Medical therapy

Diuretic therapy is sometimes useful in relieving the intense ascites (Table 2). Although anticoagulant therapy is probably not effective in promoting clot resolution, it may be useful in preventing further clot formation. The underlying disorder should be treated: for example, patients with a chronic myeloproliferative disorder can be treated with hydroxyurea or α-interferon. Women taking oral contraceptives in whom the Budd–Chiari syndrome develops often do well with simple discontinuation of their medication.

Table 2 Treatment of the Budd–Chiari syndrome

Medical
Treatment of underlying disorder
Chemotherapy (hydroxyurea)
Discontinuation of oral contraceptives
Diuretics
Anticoagulants
Thrombolytic agents
Streptokinase
Urokinase
Percutaneous transluminal angioplasty
Surgical
Portacaval shunts
Side-to-side portacaval shunt
Mesocaval shunt
Mesocaval H graft
Portoatrial shunts
Mesoatrial shunt
Portoatrial shunt
Cavosplenoatrial shunt
Transcardiac membranotomy
Inferior vena cava reconstruction
Transposition of spleen into pleural cavity
Peritoneovenous shunt
Hepatic transplantation

Modified from Maddrey WC, *Semin Liver Dis* 1987; 7: 32–8.

In patients with a possible reversible component to their thrombosis, a trial of a thrombolytic agent is worthwhile. Many patients with acute hepatic vein or inferior vena cava thrombosis are treatable with streptokinase or urokinase. Thrombolytic therapy, however, is probably effective only if given within 72 h of clot formation; it is not useful in patients with established obstruction. Furthermore, thrombolytic therapy carries a risk of severe haemorrhagic complications.

Another medical alternative is the use of percutaneous transluminal angioplasty. Initially, Fogarty balloon catheters were employed in this technique, which involves pulling the inflated balloon through the web. The Gruentzig catheter is now the device of choice. Balloon angioplasty is especially useful for relieving membranous obstruction of the inferior vena cava or hepatic veins and is probably the treatment of choice in this setting. Transluminal angioplasty has also been used to treat hepatic vein thrombosis, although there may be a high rate of reocclusion.

Surgical therapy

Surgery plays an important role in the treatment of the Budd–Chiari syndrome. Most uncontrolled studies suggest that surgically treated patients do better than those treated medically. The liver damage in Budd–Chiari syndrome results from pressure necrosis secondary to a marked elevation in sinusoidal pressure. Most surgical approaches to reverse the blood flow in the portal vein, transforming the portal vein into an outflow tract for the congested liver. Portal decompression reduces sinusoidal pressure, prevents further injury to the hepatocyte, and allows liver regeneration. Serial liver biopsies following portasystemic shunts show complete or nearly complete return to normal liver architecture and histology; however, the reversibility of the hepatic damage is related directly to the extent and duration of hepatic venous outflow obstruction. Therefore, early surgical decompression would be expected to result in more successful reversal of parenchymal abnormalities.

If the patient has severe, acute Budd–Chiari syndrome and/or the liver biopsy reveals significant centrilobular necrosis, but not severe fibrosis, the patient is a good candidate for an immediate portasystemic shunt. The exact approach depends on the results of angiography and the status of the inferior vena cava. Pressure measurements should be made in the right atrium and the suprahepatic and infrahepatic inferior vena cava. In the absence of caval obstruction, the traditional surgical approach has been a side-to-side portacaval shunt or one of its variants, such as a mesocaval shunt or mesocaval H graft (Table 2). These shunt operations are very effective and carry a low operative mortality. Side-to-side portacaval shunt for hepatic vein thrombosis effectively lowers portal pressure, relieves ascites, returns liver chemistry to normal, relieves hepatosplenomegaly, improves liver architecture, and improves long-term survival. Portasystemic encephalopathy is rarely a complication. The mesocaval shunt and the mesocaval H graft are haemodynamically equivalent but may be associated with a higher incidence of thrombosis or occlusion.

Patients with the Budd–Chiari syndrome may suffer obstruction of the inferior vena cava by thrombosis, tumour or web, or compression by an enlarged caudate lobe. Portal decompression in these patients must be performed by means other than the standard portacaval shunt. As discussed earlier, patients with isolated membranous obstruction of the inferior vena cava can be treated with percutaneous transluminal angioplasty or, failing that, can undergo a surgical transcardiac membranotomy. For those with hepatic vein thrombosis and infrahepatic occlusion of the inferior vena cava, a mesoatrial shunt is the therapy of choice. This technique, first described by Cameron and Maddrey in 1978, involves anastomosis of a long Dacron or Gore-Tex graft to the superior mesenteric vein, which is tunnel led anterior to the liver and into the chest (bypassing the obstructed inferior vena cava, and its anastomosed to the right atrium. Results with the mesoatrial shunt have been encouraging but, over the long term, a 25 to 30 per cent occlusion rate occurs. Warren and others have suggested a two-stage approach for obstruction of the inferior vena cava resulting from compression by a hypertrophied caudate lobe. Patients first undergo a mesoatrial shunt for hepatic and caval decompression; several months later, the patients undergo a second operation, in which the mesoatrial shunt is taken down and a definitive side-to-side portacaval shunt is performed.

Another alternative is the retrohepatic inferior vena cavoplasty or reconstruction and side-to-side portocaval shunt; this is also useful in the setting of recurrent thrombosis of a mesoatrial shunt. A portoatrial shunt is another alternative to the mesoatrial shunt and is useful in patients with Budd–Chiari syndrome with an obstructed inferior vena cava and superior mesenteric vein. Other reported variations on the standard shunt operation include the cavosplenoatrial shunt, and transposition of the spleen into the pleural cavity (to create a portapulmonary shunt). Efficacy of the splenopleural shunt is sporadic.

The peritoneoatrial (LeVeen) shunt does little to alter the underlying pathophysiology of the ascitic syndrome. Its use is limited to patients who are not candidates for either a portasystemic shunt or hepatic transplantation.

For patients with the Budd–Chiari syndrome and hepatic decompensation, liver transplantation is the treatment of choice. A number of patients with advanced hepatic failure resulting from the Budd–Chiari syndrome have undergone transplantation. Early results with orthotopic transplantation of the liver indicated 1- and 3-year survival rates of 71 per cent and 54 per cent respectively; however, five patients have had recurrence of thrombosis in the hepatic veins or the portal vein of the hepatic graft. More recent attempts at hepatic transplantation for treatment of the Budd–Chiari syndrome have included early anticoagulant therapy by using low-dose heparin, followed by coumadin. A 3-year survival of 88 per cent has been observed. The presence of a chronic myeloproliferative disorder is not believed to be a contraindication to liver transplantation, as long as there is adequate therapy for the underlying condition (e.g. hydroxyurea).

A major area of controversy is the question of shunt surgery in patients with Budd–Chiari syndrome who may need a liver transplant later. For patients who have end-stage liver failure orthotopic liver transplantation is clearly required. For patients who have less severe fibrosis and liver damage, the decision is less clear, because liver transplantation is technically difficult and the operative mortality is higher after a portacaval shunt. Practically, however, most patients with early Budd–Chiari syndrome respond well to a portasystemic shunt, and this is therefore the surgical treatment of choice. Patients treated with surgical decompression and those treated non-operatively should be followed closely with serial biochemical studies and non-invasive vascular imaging. Patients who have undergone portasystemic shunting and who have progressive disease should be considered for transplantation (Table 3). Likewise, patients who have been followed closely on medical therapy who show signs of progressive hepatic vein occlusion or centrilobular necrosis should undergo portasystemic shunting.

Table 3 Approach to the Budd–Chiari syndrome

Diagnosis
Clinical suspicion
  Abdominal pain
  Hepatomegaly
  Ascites
Diagnostic evaluation
  Non-invasive imaging (ultrasound, CT, MRI)
  Venography
  Liver biopsy

Therapy
Non-acute Budd–Chiari syndrome
1. Diuretics
  ↓ if unsuccessful
2. Portasystemic shunt
  ↓ if liver failure present
3. Transplantation

Acute Budd–Chiari syndrome
1. Percutaneous transluminal angioplasty vs. thrombolysis
  ↓ if unsuccessful
2. Portasystemic shunt vs. transplantation

FURTHER READING

Campbell DA, *et al.* Hepatic transplantation with perioperative and long-term anticoagulation as treatment for Budd–Chiari syndrome. *Surg Obstet Gynecol* 1988; **166**:511–17.

Grant EG, Perella, R, Tessler FN, Lois J, Busuttil R, Budd–Chiari syndrome: the results of duplex and color doppler imaging. *Am J Roentgenol* 1989; **152**: 377–81.

Henderson JM, *et al.* Surgical options, hematologic evaluation, and pathologic changes in Budd–Chiari syndrome. *Am J Surg* 1990; **159**: 41–50.

Hirooka M, Kimura C. Membranous obstruction of the hepatic portion of the inferior vena cava. *Arch Surg* 1970; **100**: 656–63.

Maddrey WC. Hepatic vein thrombosis (Budd–Chiari syndrome): possible association with the use of oral contraceptives. *Semin Liver Dis* 1987; **7**: 32–8.

Millikan WJ, *et al.* Approach to the spectrum of Budd–Chiari syndrome: which patients require portal decompression? *Am J Surg* 1985; **149**: 167–76.

Mitchell MC, Boitnott JK, Kaufman S, Cameron JL, Maddrey WC. Budd–Chiari syndrome: etiology, diagnosis, and management. *Medicine* 1982; **61**: 199–218.

Murphy FB, Steinberg HV, Shires, GT, Martin LG, Bernardino ME. The Budd–Chiari syndrome: a review. *Am J. Roentgenol* 1986; **147**: 9–15.

Orloff MJ, Girard B. Long term results of treatment of Budd–Chiari syndrome by side to side portacaval shunt. *Surg Obstet Gynecol* 1989; **168**: 33–41.

Sparano J, Chang, J, Trasi S, Bonanno C. Treatment of the Budd–Chiari syndrome with percutaneous transluminal angioplasty. Case report and review of the literature. *Am J Med* 1987; **82**: 821–8.

Terabayashi H, Okuda K, Nomura F, Ohnishi K, Wong P. Transformation of the inferior vena cava thrombosis to membranous obstruction in a patient with the lupus anticoagulant. *Gastroenterology* 1986; **91**: 219–24.

Valla D, *et al.* Primary myeloproliferative disorder and hepatic vein thrombosis. A prospective study or erythroid colony formation *in vitro* in 20 patients with Budd–Chiari syndrome. *Ann Intern Med* 1985; **103**: 329–34.

Valla D, Le MG, Poynard T, Zucman N, Rueff B, Benhamou JP. Risk of hepatic vein thrombosis in relation to recent oral contraceptives: a case-control study. *Gastroenterology* 1986; **90**: 807–11.

Warren WD, Potts JR, Fulenwider JT, Millikan WJ, Henderson JM. Two stage surgical management of the Budd–Chiari syndrome associated with obstruction of the inferior vena cava. *Surg Obstet Gynecol* 1984; **159**: 101–7.

22.7 Surgery for Budd–Chiari syndrome

RONALD A. MALT

Glisson's capsule is to the liver what the tunica albuginea is to the testis and the dura mater is to the brain: an enveloping, tough, collagenous sac that maintains the form of the organ, and perhaps some elements of function, but which strangulates its contents if they expand.

Litres of hepatic artery and portal vein blood normally flood the hepatic sinusoids and fill the hepatic veins on their way out of the liver to the inferior vena cava just below the diaphragm. In the Budd–Chiari syndrome (Fig. 1), when the normal outflow pathways are lost (Figs 2, 3), hepatic compliance decreases. So does the flow of blood, frequently leading to self-perpetuating ischaemia of hepatic tissue and to cell death. In severe cases the entire centrilobular architecture of the portal unit collapses, causing what is called zone III necrosis.

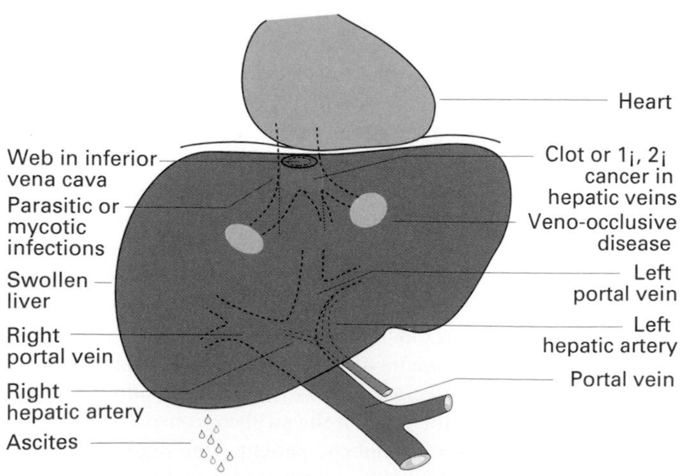

Fig. 1 Causes and consequences of the Budd-Chiari syndrome and sites of occlusion.

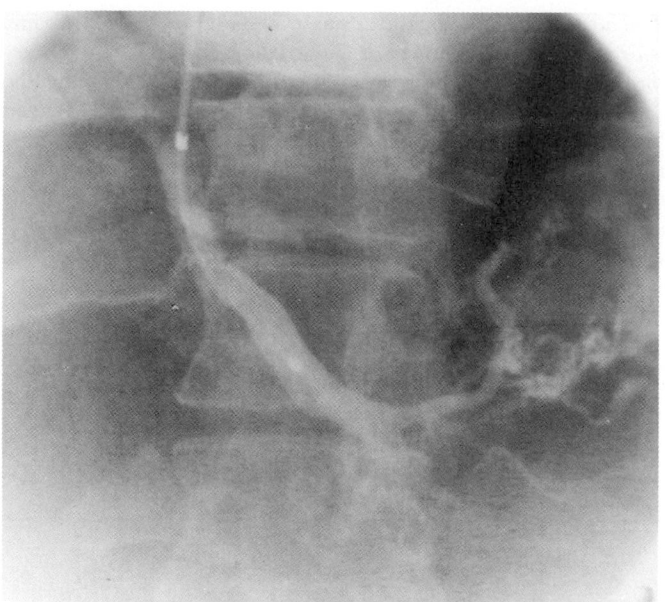

Fig. 2 Angiographically injected delineation of a partially occluded hepatic vein.

Dogs, raccoons, and seals normally have smooth muscle around the exits of their hepatic veins. Minor degrees of hypoxia and other deviations from homeostasis cause these veins to be throttled by the smooth-muscle 'valves', which stop the egress of blood and

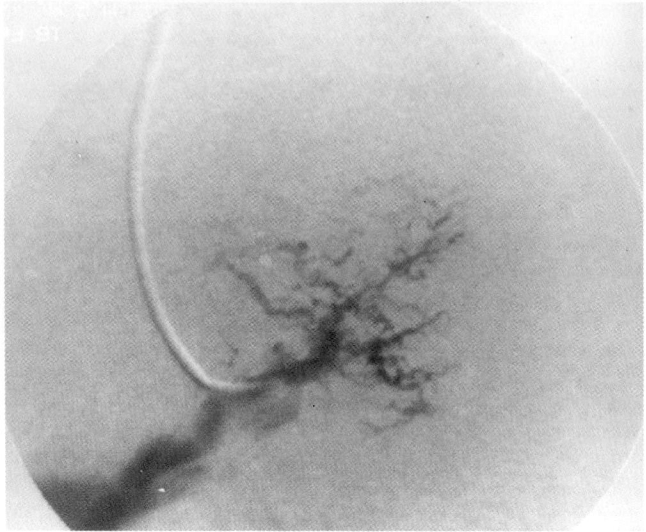

Fig. 3 Almost total distal occlusion of a hepatic vein.

Table 2 Liver in normal haemostasis

Synthetic
Prothrombin complex (II–VII–IX–X)
Fibrinogen (factor I)
Labile factor (factor V)
Surface factors (factors XI + XII)
Inhibitors of activators of plasminogen
Factor VIII (25–50%)
Proteins C and S
Antithrombin III
Degradative
Removes fibrin degradation products from circulation
Removes fibrin monomers from circulation
Removes activated factors VII_a–IX_a–X_a

From Tullis JL: Hematologic problems of liver disease: coagulopathies and hypersplenism. In: McDermott WV Jr, ed. *Surgery of the Liver*. Cambridge: Blackwell Scientific Publications, 1989: 390. Reprinted by permission of Blackwell Scientific Publications.

Table 3 Abnormalities of haemostasis in liver disease

Portal congestion
Venous distension (varices and haemorrhoids)
Hypersplenism with thrombocytopenia
Peripheral congestion
Vena cava constriction (hepatomegaly and ascites)
Reduced arterial Po_2 with endothelial anoxia
Hypoalbuminaemia and oedema
Toxic
'Hyperbilirubinaemia with decreased platelet function
Elevated bile salts with increased thrombin action on plasminogen
Decreased reticuloendothelial function
Delayed clearance of monomers
Delayed clearance of fibrin degradation products
Decreased hepatocyte function
Diminished synthesis of factors I, II, V, VII, IX, X, II, XIII
Diminished synthesis of inhibitors of activators of plasminogen
Diminished synthesis of antithrombin III

often provoke a fracture of the liver. These peculiarities of the species explain why so little written about the canine liver in shock has any relevance to the human situation.

AETIOLOGY

The most frequent idiopathic cause of the Budd–Chiari syndrome is clotting within the lumen of the hepatic veins (Table 1). Therefore speculation is rife that loss of natural anticoagulants might be causal. In fact, three natural anticoagulants are present in human liver: antithrombin III, protein C, and protein S. Antithrombin III is so potent that 1 ml is enough to antagonize all the thrombin in the circulating blood (Tables 2, 3). Cigarette smoking and the use of oestrogens, which are known aetiological agents of the Budd–Chiari syndrome, antagonize antithrombin III rapidly.

Table 1 Major causes of the Budd–Chiari syndrome

Thrombosis of hepatic veins
Vena cava neoplasm or clot
Chemical veno-occlusive disease (chemotherapy)
Embolic veno-occlusive disease (bone-marrow transplantation)
Membranous occlusion of vena cava

SYMPTOMS AND SIGNS

In its most virulent form, the victim of acute Budd–Chiari syndrome, usually a woman, is seized with abdominal pain, followed by abdominal swelling with bloody ascites. Hepatomegaly is detectable if the abdomen is lax. Figure 1 and Table 1 describe the causes of the syndrome.

DIAGNOSIS

As soon as the diagnosis is suspected, and provided that renal function is good enough to sustain the injection of angiographic contrast media, angiographic studies of the major veins at risk must be done to delineate the anatomy of the disease and to estimate whether blood clots are present and whether or not they might be extractable or dissolvable (Figs 2, 3). A liver biopsy specimen must be secured as the major indicator of the state of parenchymal integrity. In the assessment of blood flow, Doppler duplex ultrasound scanning and magnetic resonance data may eventually be as accurate as angiographic examinations, but without their attendant risks.

Pressure measurements within the veins are interesting, but are not essential, except to determine whether or not the pressure in the inferior vena cava is too high to prevent its use for decompression. Actually, measurements of portal venous and hepatic venous pressures tend to be specious because of artefacts induced by the volume of ascites and the mass of the swollen liver pressing on the inferior vena cava in a recumbent patient. One might have suspected that the narrowed inferior vena cava in Fig. 4 would be associated with a high intraluminal pressure; in fact, the pressure was low.

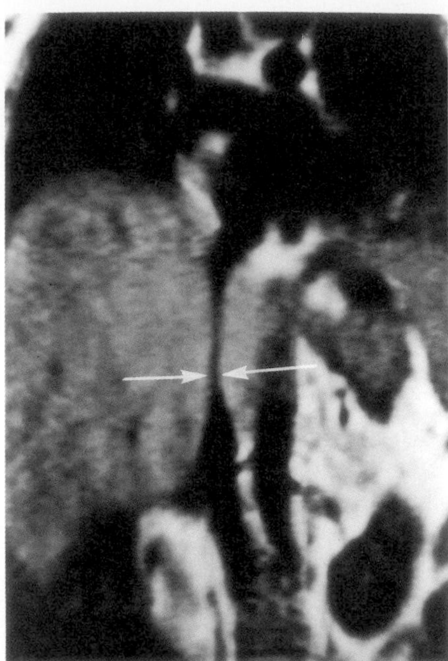

Fig. 4 Magnetic resonance image of the inferior vena cava (coronal view; arrows) showing ostensible, severe compression of the inferior vena cava, but a normal or low pressure within it, as assessed at the operating table.

TREATMENT

Although the best time to see and treat a patient with Budd–Chiari syndrome is as soon as the diagnosis is entertained, a number of medical specialists generally consider the patient before a surgeon is called. The first judgement to be made is whether the disease is in an early stage, and, if so, whether it is likely to respond to thrombolytic therapy or to physical extraction of the clots (if that is the cause of the problem) by surgical or radiological means.

By the time the surgeon operates, the task is unenviable. For fear of immunological disaster, haematologists sometimes forbid the use of fresh frozen plasma, even if it is the only means of remedying intraoperative hypocoagulability, and massive doses of methylprednisolone are often given to counteract the immunological ravages of thrombogenic diseases (such as paroxysmal nocturnal haemoglobinaemia), making normal tissue fragile and diaphanous. On the other hand, high-protein ascites within the peritoneal cavity may be transformed into a thick peel adherent to the intestines and enveloping them in a shell of fibrous tissue called a small-bowel cocoon. Small-bowel obstruction is to be expected, and enteric leaks during surgery are common because of the inability to distinguish enveloping adhesions from the normal small-bowel wall.

Although a peritoneal–atrial prosthetic shunt of plastic tubing from the peritoneal cavity to the superior vena cava (LeVeen or Denver shunt) (Fig. 5) may relieve the massive ascites accompanying the Budd–Chiari syndrome, the proteinaceous fluid within the tubing has a natural propensity to clot, making long-term patency of the shunt problematic.

On occasion, surgical thrombectomy is successful. Lysis of clots with streptokinase or urokinase, by either systemic administration or direct instillation into the affected veins, may be successful but is unpredictable. Radiologically guided dilatation of the stenosed hepatic veins is sometimes worthwhile. There is no body of experience to gauge the comparative worth of lysis and radiological dilatation against that of the surgeon.

If these 'lesser' techniques are inappropriate or fail to relieve intravenous obstruction, three other approaches are possible:

1. Converting the portal vein or another splanchnic vein into an outflow tract for the liver;
2. Fracturing a membrane in the inferior vena cava, if one exists;
3. Transplanting a new liver.

Obstructive membranes in the inferior vena cava above the orifices of the hepatic veins are a genetic or acquired disease of Oriental populations; once a membrane is recognized, it is easily broken with a finger or a dilator inserted into the inferior vena cava (Fig. 6). An expandable metal stent inserted into the vena cava under radiological guidance might help to assure patency of the fractured membrane.

But for the shortage of donor livers and the prudent caution exercised because of the problems that could face a transplant recipient, hepatic transplantation would be the best remedy for all cases of the Budd–Chiari syndrome, except those caused by membranous obstruction of the vena cava or those in which extraction of clot or neoplasm from around the orifices of the hepatic veins is feasible.

Portacaval shunt

If the hepatic veins alone are occluded, but the portal vein and the inferior vena cava are patent, the simplest way of using the portal vein as an outflow tract is to make it one limb of a side-to-side portacaval shunt (Fig. 7). These circumstances, unhappily, are rare. In the Budd–Chiari syndrome the difficulty with any procedure requiring mobilization of the portal vein is that the nearby caudate 'lobe' is turgid; it encroaches on the operative site. Furthermore, in every instance the inferior vena cava and the portal vein have to be mobilized so that they can be joined on an obliquity (somewhat like a side-to-side choledochoduodenostomy).

For the inferior vena cava to reach the portal vein, it may be necessary to cut both the several lumbar veins behind the vena cava and those in the region of the right renal vein and cephalad to it, allowing one to free the inferior vena cava liberally. For the portal vein to reach the vena cava, mobilization from the bifurcation of the vein just before entry into the liver to a variable caudad distance behind the convexity of the pancreas is required. A good result can be expected from a side-to-side shunt in these conditions if the surgery goes well. Unfortunately, the presence of a portacaval shunt increases the difficulty of connecting blood vessels in a subsequent liver transplantation.

H-grafts

To avoid problems of mobilization, H-grafts are sometimes used. The advantage of an H-graft is that the portal vein and the inferior vena cava remain *in situ*, being connected with a segment of Dacron or Teflon vascular prosthesis, reinforced externally with plastic rings to keep it from collapsing (Fig. 8). Occasionally a segment of autogenous vein is used, but the result is unpredictable. The problem is that the bulk of the liver is often so great that even if the shunt looks perfect, shifting anatomy produces a kink.

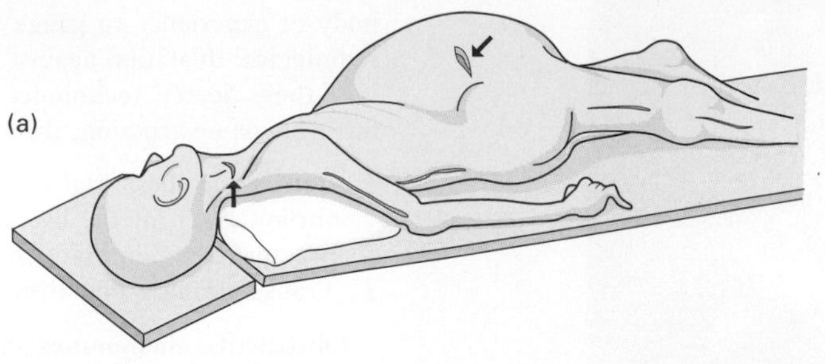

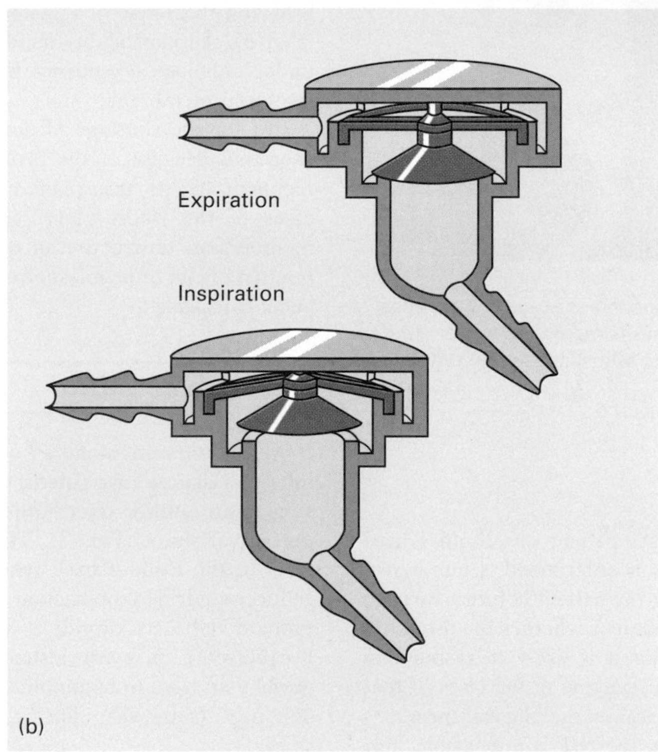

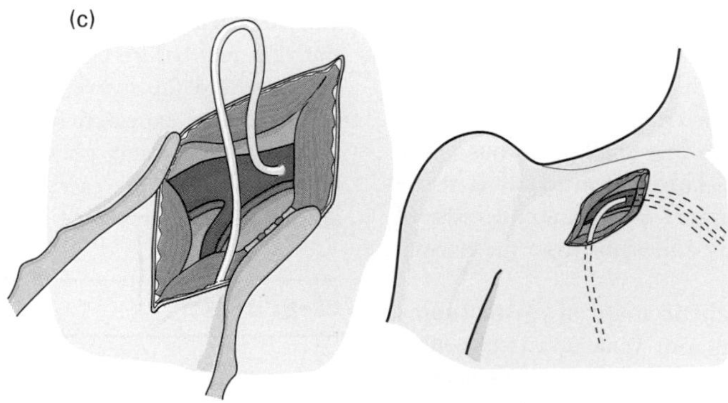

Fig. 5 Peritoneal-atrial prosthetic shunt. (a) Position of patient; arrows indicate sites for insertion of abdominal and cervical cannulas. (b) LeVeen peritoneal–atrial shunt. The valve must have low resistance and must open when 3–5 cm of water pressure is applied to it. It must then seal rapidly and perfectly. If it does not, blood from the superior vena cava will flow retrograde into the abdomen. The Denver shunt (not shown) is more streamlined; its mechanism involves basically a pair of sensitive flutter valves within a plastic capsule. (c) Infraclavicular insertion of the cannula into the subclavian vein, avoiding the formation of kinks over clavicle.

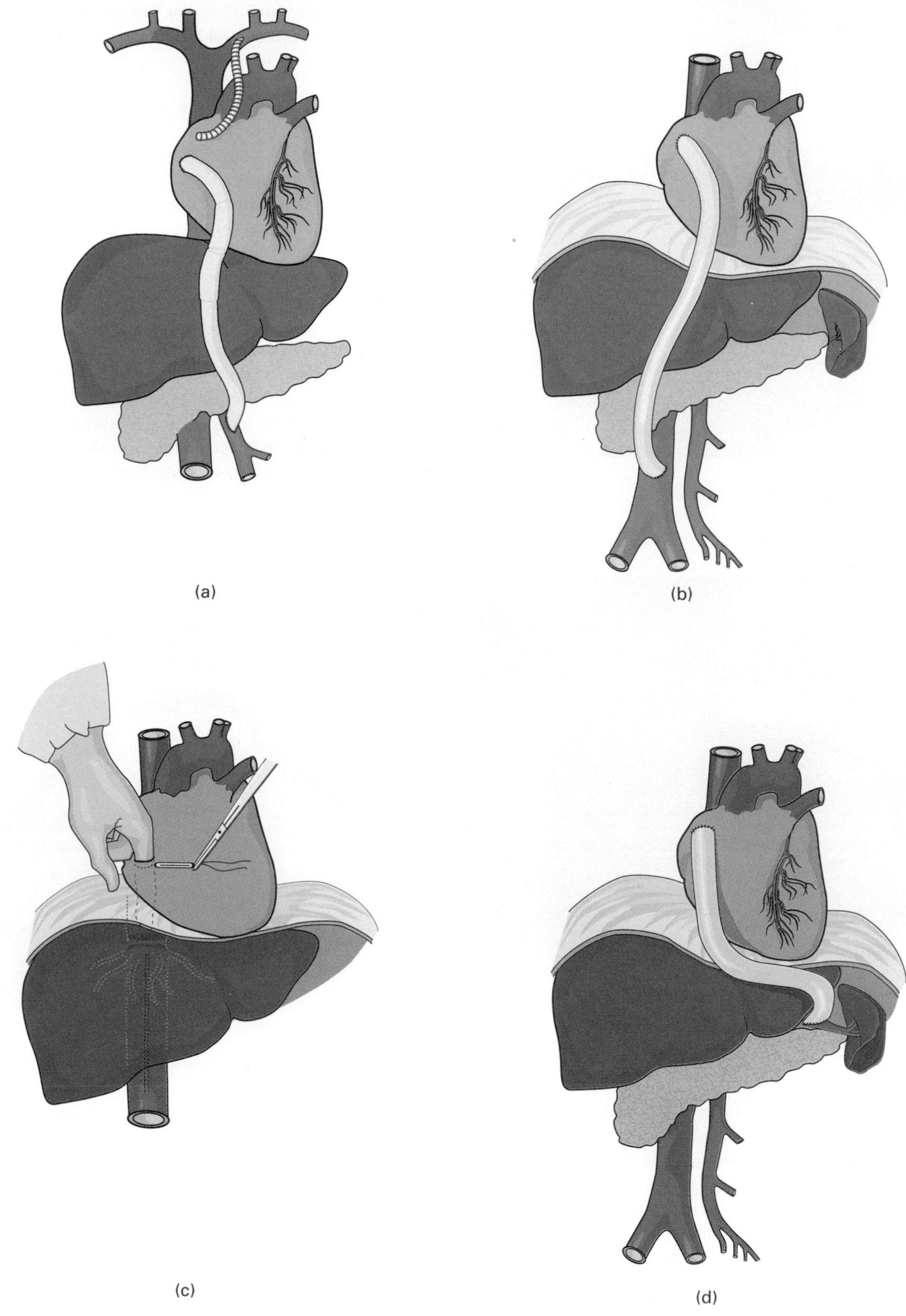

Fig. 6 Varieties of transdiaphragmatic shunts designed to bypass the blocked hepatic veins and to restore hepatic venous outflow. (a) A mesoatrial shunt and innominate–atrial shunt. Note use of double layer of graft in middle portion to increase stiffness. (b) An inferior vena cava–atrial shunt. (c) Transcardiac membranotomy with finger fracture technique (d) A splenic–atrial shunt.

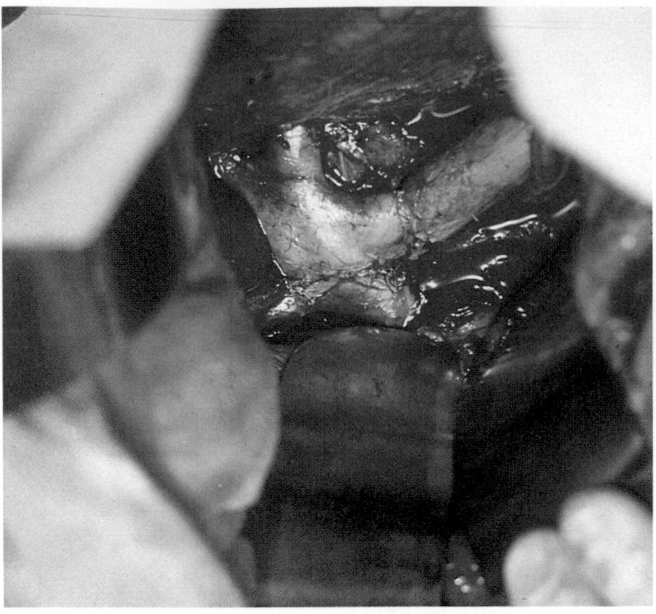

Fig. 7 Side-to-side portacaval shunt; native veins.

These are the best answers to a difficult dilemma, excepting only hepatic transplantation. Originally, Fonkalsrud used a Dacron prosthesis as a bypass from the splenic vein to the inferior pulmonary vein. Cameron and others have extended the prosthesis to the right atrium (Fig. 6), and have developed a number of practical variations.

The first was a mesocaval C-shunt, using the superior mesenteric vein as the outflow tract and a clot-free retroduodenal inferior vena cava as the decompression conduit, provided that a pressure gradient of more than 20 mmHg was not present between the right atrium and the inferior vena cava. Recently, Cameron's mesoatrial shunt (Fig. 6) has proved more practical, provided the prosthesis is made of externally supported Gore-Tex and a more unyielding cylinder of Silastic or a sleeve of Dacron prosthesis is passed over the portion of the conduit at risk of compression in its substernal route to the heart.

If radiological incursions continue to be successful, the need for surgical splanchnic venous shunts will be reduced. A flexible, expandable, tube made of fine wire Wallstent® can sometimes be passed under radiological guidance through the superior vena cava, through the liver, and then into the portal vein, effectively creating a portasystemic venous shunt (Fig. 9).

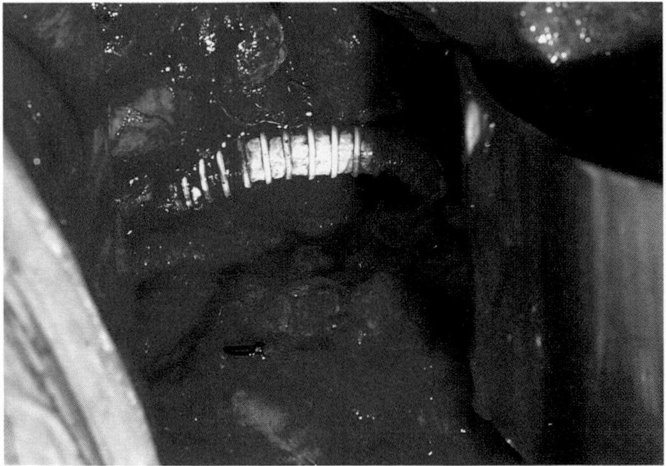

Fig. 8 Prosthetic portacaval H-graft of externally supported (ringed) expanded polytetrafluoroethylene (PTFE). Massive hepatic turgidity disappeared in a few days.

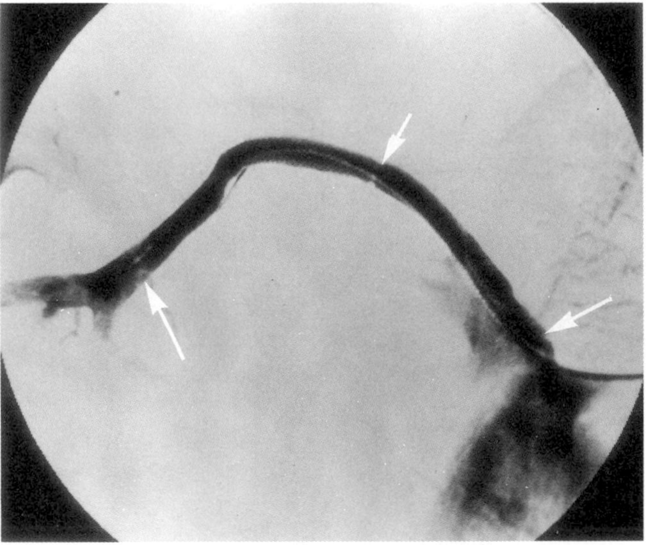

Fig. 9 Transjugular portal venogram. Two expandable mesh metal stents (Wallstent®) were placed end to end to conduct hepatic venous blood to the inferior vena cava over a distance of 68 mm from the portal vein, effecting a portacaval shunt. Arrows indicate the location of the stents and the site of their abutting. The portal vein pressure was 68 mmHg before the stents were placed, but only 19 mmHg afterwards. Patency for over 6 months has been documented. The patient takes coumadin.

Buckling of the prosthesis is sometimes a problem even when an externally supported (ringed) prosthesis is used, because the rings that one counts upon to support the otherwise floppy conduit can also serve as fulcrums, over which the fabric bends. Keeping the prosthesis short (perhaps only 3.5 cm long) and cutting the hoods of the prosthetic graft to ensure that they correspond perfectly to recipient orifices in the portal vein and in the inferior vena cava 90° away from each other are the keys to success.

Abdominothoracic shunts

In these operations, too, decompression of the liver is gained by allowing native structures to remain in place, but making them serve as an outflow conduit to the inferior vena cava or to the heart.

FURTHER READING

Ahn SS, Yellin A, Sheng FC, Colonna JO, Goldstein LI, Busuttil RW. Selective surgical therapy of the Budd–Chiari syndrome provides superior survivor rates than conservative medical management. *J Vasc Surg* 1987; **5**: 28–37.

Bismuth E, Hadengue A, Hammel P, Benhamou J–P. Hepatic vein thrombosis in Beçhet's disease. *Hepatology* 1990; **11**: 969–74.

Cambria RP, Shamberger RC. Small bowel obstruction caused by the abdominal cocoon syndrome: possible association with the LeVeen shunt. *Surgery* 1984; **95**: 501–3.

Cameron JL, *et al.* The Budd-Chiari syndrome: Treatment by mesenteric–systemic venous shunts. *Ann Surg* 1983; **198**: 335–46.

Halff G, Todo S, Tzakis AG, Gordon RD, Starzl TE. Liver transplantation for the Budd–Chiari syndrome. *Ann Surg* 1990; **211**; 43–9.

Hay JM, *et al.* Syndrome de Budd–Chiari avec thrombose de la veine cave inférieure: traitement par une derivation mesenterico-innominé. *Gastroenterol Clin Biol* 1988; **12**: 755–8.

Henderson JM, *et al.* Surgical options, hematologic evaluation, and pathologic changes in Budd–Chiari syndrome. *Am J Surg* 1990; **159**: 41–8.

Klein AS, Cameron JL. Diagnosis and management of the Budd–Chiari syndrome. *Am J Surg* 1990; **160**: 128–33.

Louis JJ, *et al.* Budd-Chiari syndrome: treatment with percutaneous transhepatic recanalization and dilation. *Radiology* 1989; **170**: 791–3.

Ludwig J, Hashimoto E, McGill DB, van Heerden JA. Classification of hepatic venous outflow obstruction: ambiguous terminology of the Budd–Chiari syndrome. *Mayo Clin Proc* 1990; **65**: 51–5.

Malt RA, Dalton JC, Johnson RE, Gurewich V. Side-to-side portacaval shunt versus nonsurgical treatment of Budd-Chiari syndrome. *Am J Surg* 1978; **136**: 387–9.

Martin LG, Henderson JM, Millikan WJ Jr, Casarella WJ, Kaufman SL. Angioplasty for long-term treatment of patients with Budd-Chiari syndrome. *Am J Roentgenol* 1990; **514**: 1007–10.

Nakao K, Adachi S, Kawashima Y, Okamoto E, Manabe H. A radical operation for the Budd–Chiari syndrome associated with obstruction of the inferior vena cava: A report of six patients. *J Cardiovasc Surg* 1984; **25**: 216–21.

Oldhafer KJ, Ringe B, Wittekind C, Pichlmayr R. Budd–Chiari syndrome: Portacaval shunt and subsequent liver transplantation. *Surgery* 1990; **107**: 471–4.

Orloff MJ, Girard B. Long term results of treatment of Budd–Chiari syndrome by side to side portacaval shunt. *Surg Gynecol Obstet* 1989; **168**: 33–41.

Rollins BJ. Hepatic veno-occlusive disease. *Am J Med* 1986; **81**: 297–306.

Tullis JL. Hematologic problems of liver disease: coagulopathies and hyperspplenism. In: McDermott WV Jr, ed. *Surgery of the liver*. Boston: Blackwell Scientific, 1989: 389–95.

Wang Z, *et al.* Recognition and management of Budd–Chiari syndrome: report of 100 cases. *J Vasc Surg* 1989; **10**: 149–56.

The biliary tract 23

23.1 Benign diseases of the biliary tract

JULIAN BRITTON, KENNETH I. BICKERSTAFF, AND ADRIAN SAVAGE

INTRODUCTION

Benign diseases of the biliary tract are one of the most common surgical problems in the world. Gallstones affect millions of people in the West, while oriental cholangitis is common in the East. Surgery plays an important part in treatment: over half a million cholecystectomies are performed each year in the United States of America. New percutaneous techniques avoid the need for a conventional abdominal incision; they are playing an increasing role in treatment but a thorough understanding of the basic anatomy, physiology, and pathology of the biliary tract is required.

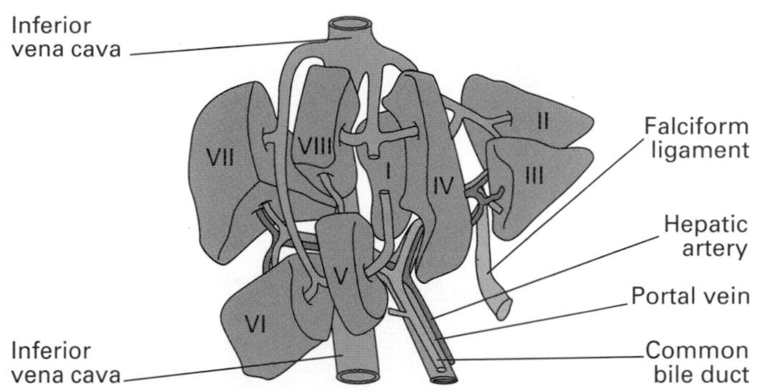

Fig. 1 Segmental biliary and hepatic anatomy.

ANATOMY

Development

The liver and the biliary tract are derived from the foregut. The liver first appears in the 3-week embryo as a hollow endodermal bud from the distal foregut. This bud, the hepatic diverticulum, consists of rapidly proliferating cells that penetrate into the ventral mesogastrium. These cells eventually develop into the liver; the connection between the hepatic diverticulum and the foregut is preserved to form the bile duct. A ventral outgrowth of the bile duct gives rise to the gallbladder and the cystic duct. As the intestine rotates the entrance from the bile duct into the duodenum moves to a posterior position and the common bile duct comes to lie behind the duodenum and pancreas.

Within the developing liver the bile ducts are distributed in a segmental fashion. Bile is secreted by the liver cells into bile canaliculi. The canaliculi drain into ductules and on into larger segmental bile ducts which are tributaries of either the left or the right hepatic ducts. The left hepatic duct drains segments II, III, and IV; segments V, VI, VII, and VIII drain into the right hepatic duct. The caudate lobe (segment I) lies astride the inferior vena cava posteriorly and drains into both the right and the left hepatic ducts. This segmental anatomy of the liver and its ducts is important in liver and biliary tract surgery (Fig. 1) and is discussed in more detail in Section 22.1.

Extrahepatic bile ducts

The right and left hepatic ducts join to form the common hepatic duct at the hilum of the liver. The confluence usually lies outside the liver itself and in front of the right portal vein. The left hepatic duct has a relatively long extrahepatic course on the posterior aspect of the quadrate lobe (segment IV) where it is accessible to the surgeon, whereas the right hepatic duct enters liver tissue almost immediately. In fact this normal arrangement only occurs in 60 per cent of individuals. There are a large number of anatomical variants. The most common (20 per cent) is for one of the main tributaries of the right duct, usually the right anterior duct, to enter the common hepatic duct directly (Fig. 2). In 12 per cent of individuals there is a triple confluence formed by the right posterior, right anterior, and left hepatic ducts. One important variation is the presence of an anomalous subvesical duct, the duct of Luschka, which runs in the gallbladder fossa. It is found in 12 to 50 per cent of individuals, drains a variable portion of the right liver and is potentially vulnerable during a cholecystectomy.

The main bile duct runs from the confluence of the hepatic ducts to the papilla of Vater (Fig. 3). It is normally 10 to 12 cm in length and about 6 mm in diameter in anatomical specimens. In life, the upper limit of normal diameter on ultrasound is 7 mm. On direct cholangiography, when the duct is deliberately distended, it is up to 12 mm. The entrance of the cystic duct divides the bile duct into the common hepatic duct above the entrance and the common bile duct below. The supraduodenal portion of the bile duct lies in the free edge of the lesser omentum, anterior to the portal vein and to the right of the hepatic artery. The right hepatic artery normally crosses the common hepatic duct posteriorly, but occasionally it lies in front of the duct. Inferiorly the bile duct curves laterally away from the portal vein and passes behind the first part of the duodenum. It then runs across the posterior part of the head of the pancreas, either in a groove or in a tunnel within the gland. As the bile duct traverses obliquely through the wall of the duodenum it is joined by the main pancreatic duct of Wirsung. The exact arrangement of this junction is variable. Normally both ducts unite to form a common channel of variable length and enter the bowel through the papilla of Vater on the posteromedial wall of the second part of the duodenum. In about 10 per cent of individuals there is no common channel and each duct enters separately. There are very few muscle fibres in the wall of the bile duct, but the proximal bile and pancreatic ducts and the common channel are surrounded by circular and longitudinal smooth muscle. This muscle complex is known as the sphincter of Oddi and the muscle fibres are structurally, embryologically, and functionally distinct from the musculature of the duodenum (Fig. 4).

The authors are grateful to Dr Roger Chapman for his help with the section on primary sclerosing cholangitis.

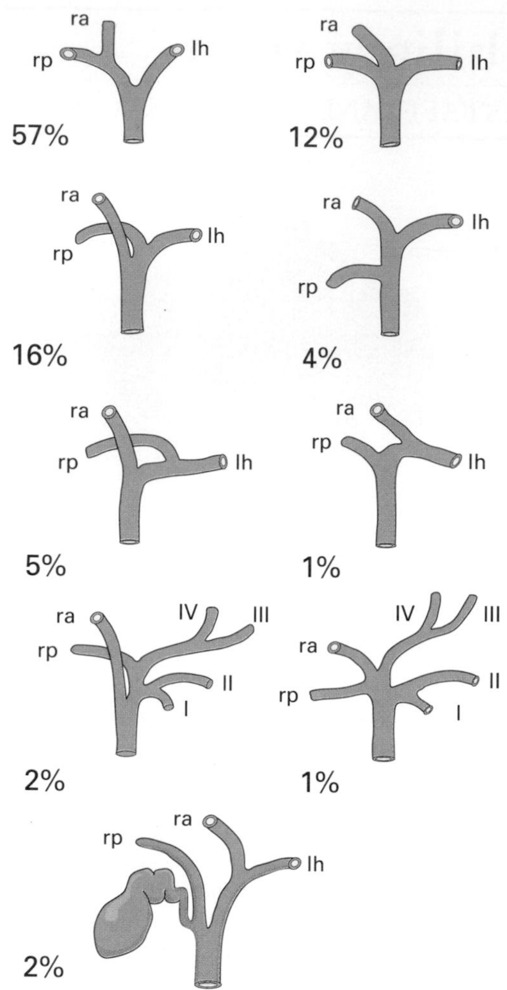

Fig. 2 Variations in the confluence of the bile ducts at the porta hepatis. The bottom illustration shows the rare but important anomaly when the cystic duct joins the right posterior hepatic duct. ra, right anterior hepatic duct; rp, right posterior hepatic duct; la, left hepatic duct. I, II, III, IV—bile ducts from liver segments I, II, III, IV.

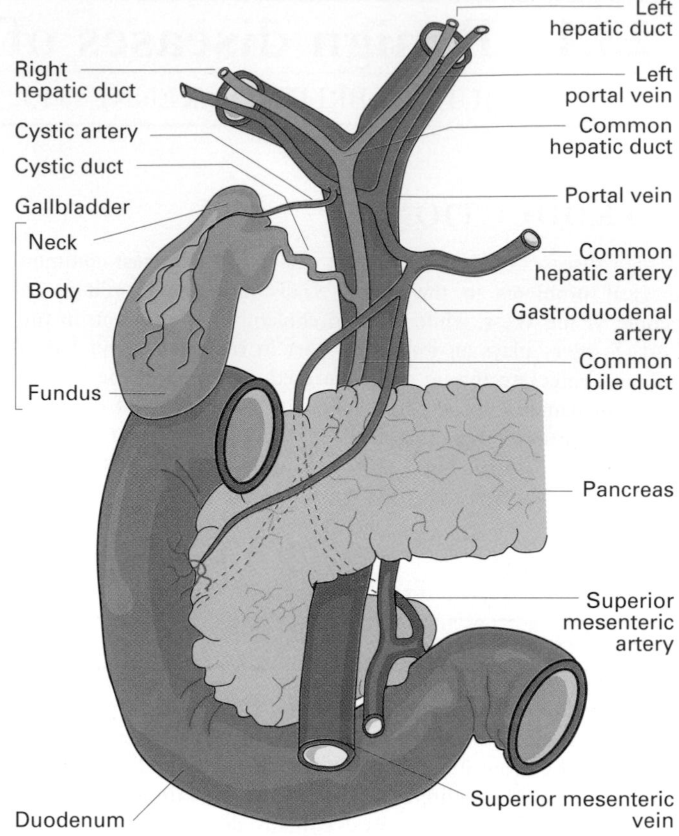

Fig. 3 Anatomy of the extrahepatic bile ducts and gallbladder.

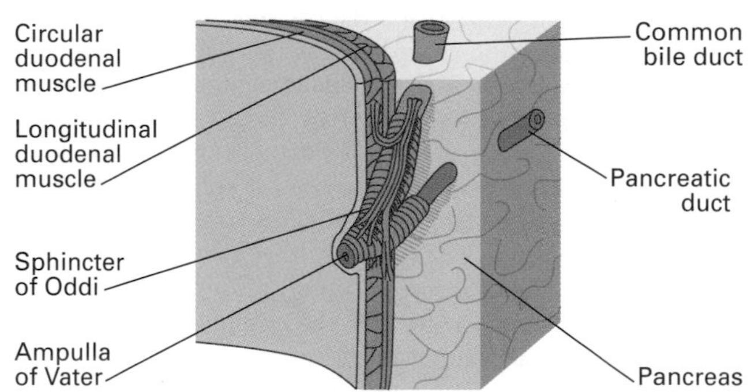

Fig. 4 Anatomy of the sphincter of Oddi.

Gallbladder and cystic duct

The gallbladder is a pear-shaped reservoir 5 to 12 cm in length and situated on the under surface of the liver along the junction between the right and the left liver. It is covered by peritoneum and separated from liver by the connective tissue of the cystic plate. Anatomically, the gallbladder is divided into the fundus, the body, and the neck. The fundus is the widest part of the gland and usually reaches to the free anterior edge of the liver. The neck leads to the cystic duct, and when distended by a stone has the appearance of a diverticulum known as Hartmann's pouch. This pouch occasionally lies very close to the common hepatic duct.

The gallbladder may lie more or less embedded within the liver, or it may be suspended on a mesentery formed from two layers of the peritoneum. The latter variation predisposes to torsion of the gallbladder. Other rare anomalies include agenesis of the gallbladder, in which the ventral pouch off the bile duct fails to form, and duplication or lobulation of the organ where the pouch itself divides to a variable extent.

The cystic duct runs from the neck of the gallbladder to the bile duct and is variable in length. The wall of the cystic duct contains muscle fibres which form the sphincter of Lutkens, while the mucosa is arranged in the spiral valves of Heister. The triangle bounded by the common hepatic duct medially, the cystic duct inferiorly, and the inferior surface of the liver superiorly is known as Calot's triangle. The fact that the cystic artery runs within the triangle makes this an important area of dissection during cholecystectomy. The cystic duct joins the supraduodenal portion of the bile duct either at an acute angle or after running parallel to the bile duct for a short distance. In 5 per cent of people the cystic duct spirals behind the common hepatic duct and enters the bile duct low down within the pancreas. Occasionally the cystic duct actually runs within the wall of the bile duct for a variable distance, and rarely it joins the right hepatic duct. These variations are important since the bile duct can easily be damaged if the precise anatomy is not recognized at operation.

Blood supply to the gallbladder and bile ducts

Within the liver the bile ducts are supplied by adjacent arteries. Outside the liver the supply to the bile duct is essentially axial and comes from two arteries that run along either side of the duct, known as the 3 o'clock and 9 o'clock arteries. About 60 per cent of blood flow to the duct arises inferiorly from the retroduodenal and gastroduodenal arteries whilst 38 per cent comes from the hepatic and cystic arteries superiorly (Fig. 5). The retropancreatic portion of the bile duct is supplied mainly from retroduodenal arteries.

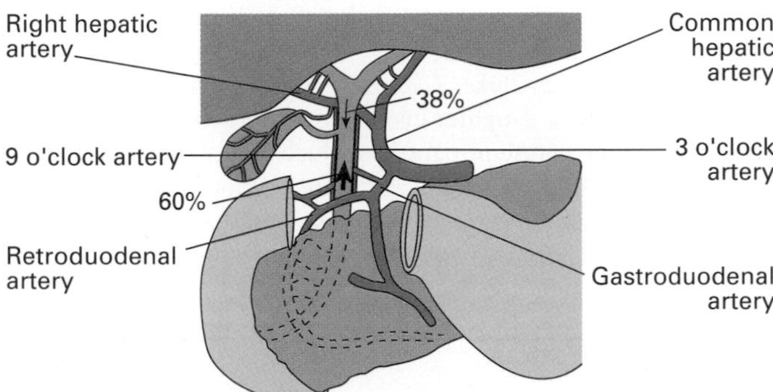

Fig. 5 Arterial supply of the extrahepatic bile ducts. The blood supply derives from two arteries, the 3 o'clock and the 9 o'clock arteries which run alongside the bile duct. Nearly two-thirds of the blood supply arises inferiorly and only two-fifths superiorly.

The principal blood supply to the gallbladder is derived from the cystic artery; a smaller component arises from vessels passing directly from the liver. The cystic artery runs above and behind the cystic duct and usually arises from the right hepatic artery after the latter has passed behind the bile duct. Variations in this anatomy are common. The cystic artery may arise from the common hepatic artery and pass in front of the bile duct. There may also be two separate cystic arteries supplying the anterior and posterior surfaces of the gallbladder. There are no discrete veins draining the gallbladder and bile duct, although all the arteries are normally accompanied by a small vein or venous plexus. Some veins drain directly from the gallbladder into the liver. Lymphatic drainage is first to the cystic lymph node which is usually seen adjacent to the cystic artery during a cholecystectomy and thence to the retroduodenal lymph nodes. Some lymphatic channels from the fundus drain to lymphatic channels in the liver capsule. Motor and sensory sympathetic nerves from the coeliac plexus reach the gallbladder along the hepatic artery and the parasympathetic motor supply comes from the right and left vagus nerves.

PHYSIOLOGY

Bile

The prime function of the biliary tract is to convey bile from the liver where it is formed to the duodenum. Along the way bile is stored and concentrated in the gallbladder until it is required. Bile helps in the digestion of certain foodstuffs and acts as a major excretory pathway.

Between 500 ml and 1000 ml of bile are secreted by human hepatocytes every day. The main constituent is water along with bile acids, bile pigments, cholesterol, phospholipids, and all the inorganic ions found in plasma (Table 1). The bile acids are the most important by weight. The precise concentrations of all these molecules are modified subsequently by the epithelium of both the bile ducts and the gallbladder. The pH of bile duct bile is generally above 7, and inorganic ions are normally present in concentrations slightly higher than in plasma with the exception of chloride which is usually lower (Table 2). This is important in clinical practice since patients with a significant bile fistula lose electrolytes rapidly.

Table 1 Composition of adult human hepatic bile

	g/l	Percentage
Water	—	98.0
Bile salts	6.5–14	0.7
Inorganic salts	—	0.7
Bile pigments	0.12–1.35	0.2
Fatty acids	1.6–4.1	0.15
Lecithin	—	0.1
Cholesterol	0.8–1.8	0.06

Between 250 and 1000 ml of hepatic bile is secreted in 24 h.

Table 2 Electrolyte content of adult human hepatic bile (mEq/l)

	Range	Mean
pH	6.2–8.5	7.5
Sodium	131–164	149
Potassium	2.6–12.0	5.0
Chloride	89–118	101
Bicarbonate	17–55	30
Calcium	3.3–4.1	—
Magnesium	1.4–3.0	—

The bile acids, cholic and chenodeoxycholic acid, are synthesized in the liver from cholesterol and are the major pathway of cholesterol excretion. In the colon they are metabolized by bacteria to deoxycholic and lithocholic acid, respectively; all except lithocholic acid are absorbed back into the portal circulation and are then re-excreted into the bile (Fig. 6). This enterohepatic circulation of bile salts takes place several times each day. Because of this continuous circulation there is always a pool of bile acids in the body. A small amount is lost from the pool each day in the stools and is made up by hepatic synthesis.

The main function of the bile acids in bile is to maintain cholesterol in solution, which they do by forming micelles. Hydrophobic cholesterol is encased in hydrophilic phospholipid and bile salts. Only when the concentration of cholesterol exceeds the capacity of the bile salts and phospholipid to maintain it in micellar solution does bile become lithogenic and liable to form stones. Clinically, increasing the concentration of bile salts in bile artificially makes it possible to render bile unsaturated in cholesterol and so enable dissolution of cholesterol gallstones (see Fig. 24 below). Ingestion

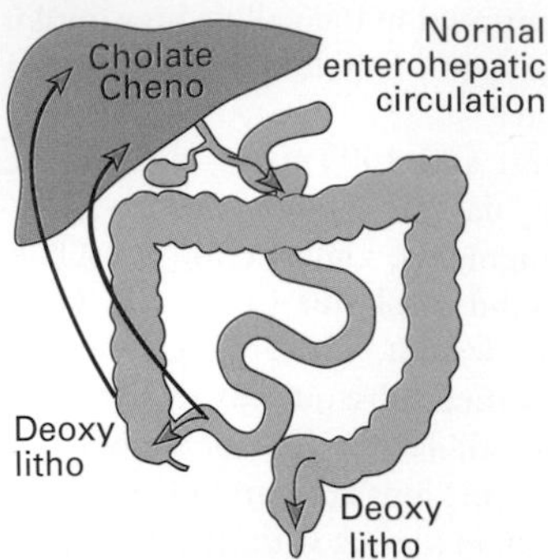

Fig. 6 Enterohepatic circulation of bile salts. Because of reabsorption of bile salts from the small and the large bowel only a small proportion of the bile salt pool is lost in the stool each day. This amount is replaced by synthesis of bile salts in the liver.

of food increases bile flow and this is probably mediated by vagal and hormonal stimuli, although bile salts themselves have a powerful choleretic effect.

Bilirubin, the major degradation product of haemoglobin, is conjugated with glucuronide by the hepatocyte and actively secreted into bile. Conjugated bilirubin is converted by the action of bacteria in the bowel into urobilinogen which is reabsorbed into the portal circulation and re-excreted. Some urobilinogen reaches the systemic circulation and is then excreted in the urine where it can be detected. The absence of urobilinogen from the urine implies complete obstruction of bile flow into the bowel.

The gallbladder acts as a store for bile in between meals and concentrates the bile by active reabsorption of water and electrolytes. About half the hepatic output of bile is stored in the gallbladder; the other half trickles into the duodenum continuously. Food, and especially fat, in the duodenum releases cholecystokinin, which is the most important stimulus for gallbladder contraction. Contraction of the gallbladder causes the sphincter of Oddi and the second part of the duodenum to relax. The bile duct acts purely as a conduit, for it does not show peristaltic activity. The sphincter of Oddi certainly plays an important part in bile duct function. The muscle of the sphincter is quite separate from duodenal wall muscle both embryologically and functionally, although the action of the two is usually co-ordinated. This coordination occasionally breaks down, but whether this is of clinical significance is not known. The role of the autonomic nerves to the gallbladder and the bile duct is also uncertain.

Biliary pain

At endoscopic retrograde cholangiopancreatography (ERCP), distension of the bile duct with contrast causes pain and it is probable that a similar effect occurs in normal life. While a rapid increase in intraductal pressure causes pain, slower increases lead to discomfort. Pain from stones in either the bile duct or the gallbladder probably results from acute obstruction to flow. Spasm of the sphincter of Oddi is probably painless, although it may also lead to a rapid rise in intraductal pressure. Pain nerve endings are widely distributed throughout the biliary tract. Most pain fibres return to the central nervous system via the splanchnic nerves, but a significant minority run with the vagus, right phrenic, and intercostal nerves. This wide distribution probably explains some of the clinical variations in the perception of biliary pain.

PATHOLOGY

Inflammation

Acute and chronic inflammation of the biliary tract are both common. Inflammation can be caused by chemicals, bacteria, or parasites; the aetiology of primary sclerosing cholangitis is unknown. Following obstruction of the gallbladder by a stone in the cystic duct, bile salts leak into the mucosa and cause inflammation. Bacterial infection soon follows. Bacteria are often present in normal bile, particularly if stones are present or if an anastomosis between the biliary tree and the bowel exists. The most common infecting bacteria are *Escherichia coli*, Klebsiella, and *Streptococcus faecalis*. Anaerobic bacteria are present in much smaller numbers. Most significant infections are due to multiple organisms. The frequent occurrence of bacteria in bile, even in the absence of acute inflammation, is the reason why prophylaxis with an appropriate antibiotic before any surgical or radiological procedure on the biliary tract is wise.

The Chinese liver fluke, *Clonorchis sinensis*, *Ascaris lumbricoides* and, occasionally, a daughter cyst from a ruptured hydatid cyst of the liver are the common parasites which infect the biliary tract, usually in the Middle East and Asia (see Section 41.17). Bacterial cholangitis is a common accompaniment, and malignant change in the biliary epithelium may follow chronic infection with *Clonorchis sinensis*.

Obstruction

Obstruction of the main bile duct leads to morphological changes in the liver with marked inflammatory infiltration of the portal tracts. Scarring and fibrosis around the bile ducts results in the eventual development, after weeks or months of obstruction, of secondary biliary cirrhosis. Hepatocyte function deteriorates progressively from the onset of obstruction and is slow to recover once the obstruction is relieved. Similar pathological changes can be seen in the gallbladder wall when chronic inflammation occurs secondary to gallstones. The gallbladder becomes shrunken, fibrotic, and non-functional (see Fig. 25 below).

Neoplasm

Neoplasia of the glandular biliary epithelium is unusual, and benign tumours are almost unknown. Occasionally adenomatous polyps are seen in the gallbladder or the bile duct.

INVESTIGATION OF THE BILIARY TRACT

Plain radiography

A plain abdominal radiograph may show radio-opaque gallstones (Fig. 7) or air in the biliary tree (Fig. 8). This is a useful investigation in patients who present acutely and is an essential preliminary to any contrast study of the biliary tract. Calcification in the right upper quadrant is not proof of biliary tract disease and neither does the presence of gallstones mean that they are the cause of the patients symptoms.

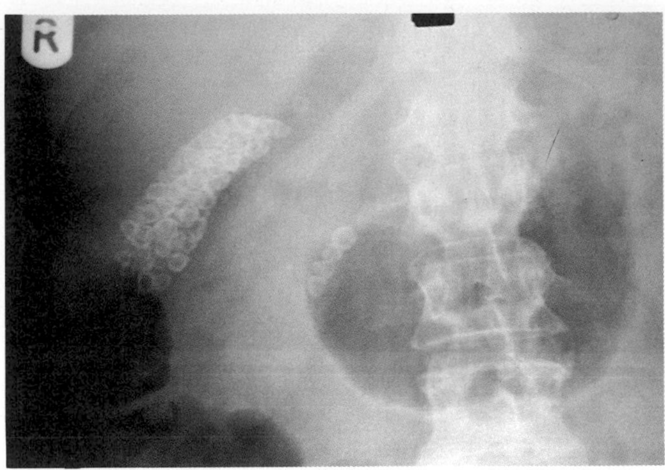

Fig. 7 Radio-opaque gallstones on a plain radiograph. The outline of the stones suggests that they are in the gallbladder and not the kidney.

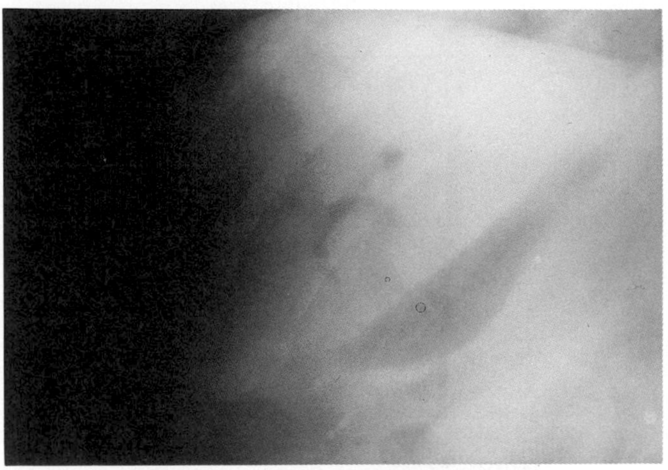

Fig. 8 Air in the biliary tree on a plain radiograph.

Two unusual appearances are diagnostic of biliary disease. Gas in the lumen or in the wall of the gallbladder is diagnostic of emphysematous cholecystitis, while the appearance of air in the biliary tree and distal small bowel obstruction suggests gallstone ileus. Another cause of biliary air is a biliary–enteric fistula, either created surgically (Fig. 8) or as a result of a stone ulcerating from the gallbladder into the bowel, usually the duodenum and very occasionally the colon.

Ultrasound

An ultrasound scan is the initial investigation in any patient suspected of biliary tract disease (see Section 6.5). It is non-invasive, painless, and can be easily performed on patients who are unwell. Adjacent organs can be examined simultaneously. Ultrasonography may provide unsatisfactory results in patients with obesity, ascites, and gaseous distension, and are dependent on the skill and experience of the operator.

Stones within the gallbladder can be detected with a sensitivity and specificity of over 90 per cent. They appear as reflective foci which cast an acoustic shadow (Fig. 9) and which move with changes in posture; they may form a layer in the gallbladder. The presence of local tenderness and the thickness of the gallbladder wall allow acute and chronic cholecystitis to be distinguished. A layer of oedema may also appear as a sonolucent zone between the gallbladder and the liver in patients with acute cholecystitis. Polyps within the lumen can be identified but ultrasound cannot, at present, assess gallbladder function accurately.

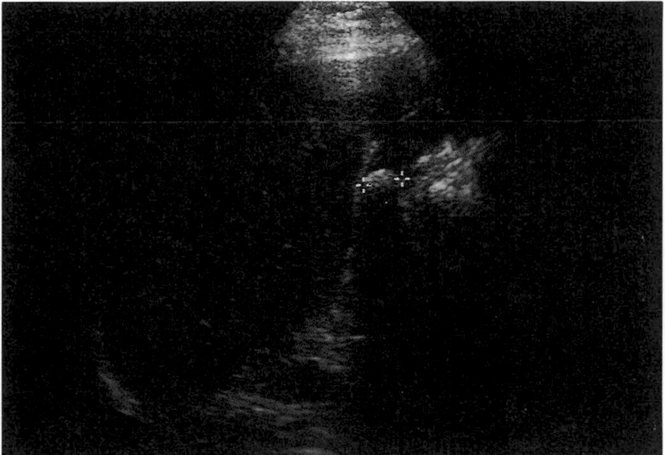

Fig. 9 Ultrasound picture showing gallstones in a contracted thick walled gallbladder.

Ultrasonograpy is always the first imaging technique used in a patient with jaundice or cholangitis. Dilatation of the ducts establishes an extrahepatic obstructive cause for the jaundice and may also identify stones in the ducts (Fig. 10). An expert can identify the site of the obstruction in three-quarters of patients and the cause in one-third. Ultrasound can also be used during surgery to detect bile duct stones.

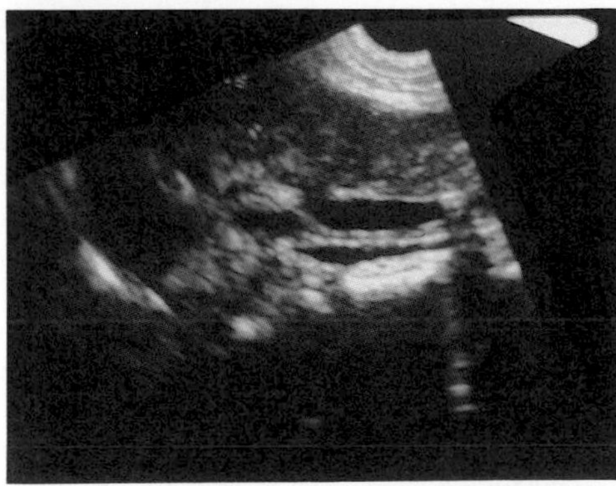

Fig. 10 Ultrasound picture showing a gallstone in a dilated common bile duct. There is a typical sonic shadow behind the stone.

Contrast radiology

Oral cholecystography

Although this was the standard method of investigating the gallbladder for many years, it is now been superseded by ultrasonography. A biliary contrast medium based on triiodobenzoic acid, which is primarily excreted by the liver, is taken by mouth. It is absorbed into the portal venous system, transported across liver cells into bile, and concentrated in the gallbladder, where it becomes visible on a radiograph (Fig. 11). Patients are then given a fatty meal: a normal gallbladder contracts. The examination is still useful in patients who present with gallbladder symptoms but in whom no abnormalities are detected on ultrasound examination. It is an essential examination when non-operative removal of gallstones is considered, since a functioning gallbladder is a prerequisite for effective treatment. Failure of the gallbladder to opacify is evidence of gallbladder disease, providing the contrast material has been absorbed and the patient is not jaundiced.

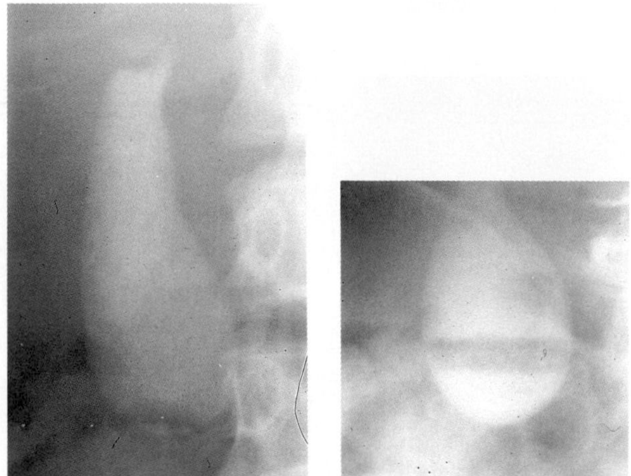

Fig. 11 Oral cholecystogram showing a layer of gallstones within the gallbladder. This is only seen when the patient stands erect (right hand picture).

Percutaneous transhepatic cholangiography

A 22-gauge flexible Chiba needle is advanced through the skin and well into the liver under local anaesthesia and antibiotic cover. Blood coagulation must be normal. Contrast medium is gently injected as the needle is slowly withdrawn. The procedure is watched on an image intensifier: when contrast medium enters a bile duct withdrawal is stopped. Contrast medium is then injected to fill the whole biliary tree (Fig. 12). In skilled hands this can always be achieved if the bile ducts are dilated, and is also possible in about two-thirds of patients in whom the ducts are normal in size. It may be necessary to puncture both the right and the left hepatic systems to outline all the ducts. Bile leakage into the peritoneum, cholangitis, and haemorrhage are the major complications, occuring in about 4 per cent of patients. For this reason it is still best to plan to relieve any obstruction, either surgically or by the percutaneous insertion of a drain or stent, during or fairly soon after the examination. The mortality rate associated with the procedure is about 0.5 per cent.

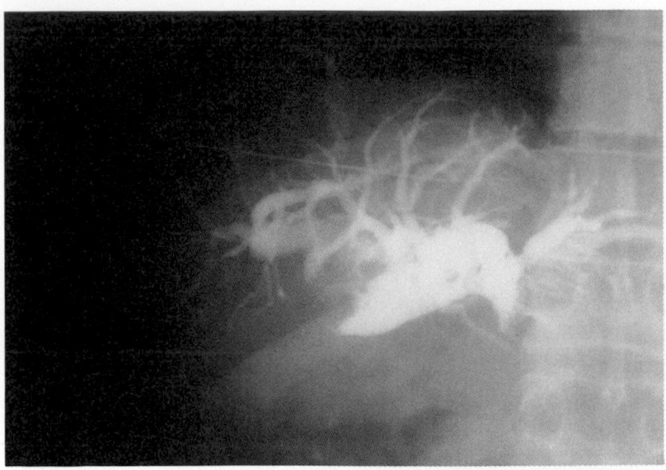

Fig. 12 Percutaneous transhepatic cholangiogram showing grossly dilated ducts. The stricture at the choledochojejunostomy developed 16 years after the original surgery which was performed to repair a damaged bile duct during a cholecystectomy. The Chiba needle can be seen at the top left of the picture.

Endoscopic retrograde cholangiopancreatography

A full description of this technique is given in Section 27.2. The ability to outline the biliary tree and the pancreatic duct as well as to inspect the ampulla of Vater has completely revolutionized the management of many benign biliary problems. Not only has diagnosis been improved (Fig. 13) but therapeutic techniques have been developed which have improved patient care significantly. Endoscopic retrograde cholangiopancreatography (ERCP) requires technical skill and sophisticated imaging, and is not as

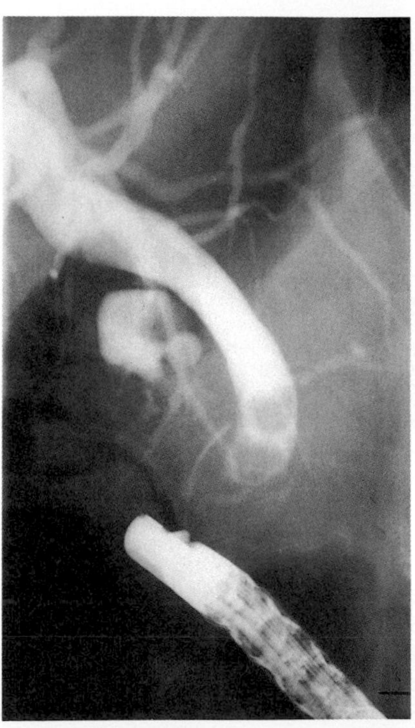

Fig. 13 Endoscopic retrograde cholangiogram showing stones in the common bile duct. This patient has had a previous Polya partial gastrectomy so that the endoscope approaches the ampulla backwards from the duodenojejunal flexure along the third part of the duodenum.

widely available as the percutaneous approach. The endoscopic route is preferred initially since it does not transgress the peritoneum, but there are occasions when it is essential to outline the bile ducts from above as well as from below.

Computed tomography

Computed tomography (CT) is useful in the diagnosis of biliary tract disease although the evidence is usually indirect. It is easier to identify pathology in the liver, the pancreas, and the gallbladder than the bile duct itself, although the ducts are easily seen when they are dilated (Fig. 14). CT is probably superior to ultrasonography in identifying the level and the cause of biliary obstruction, but the latter is cheaper, simpler, and safer.

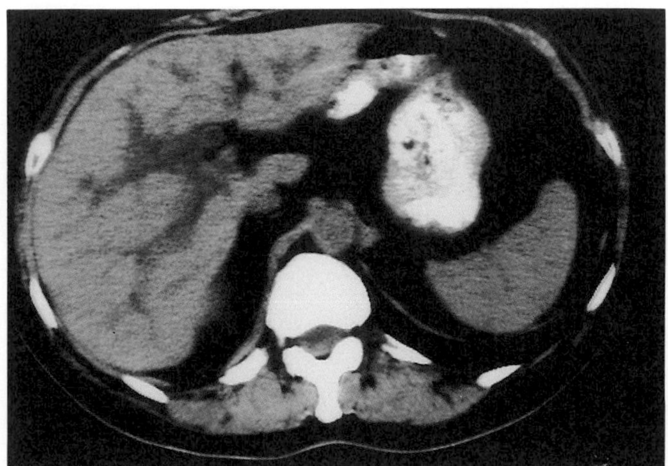

Fig. 14 Computed tomography scan of the liver showing grossly dilated bile ducts.

Malignant disease in or around the biliary tree can best be staged by CT; this may also be needed to allow a biopsy to be undertaken. It is not of great value in the management of the common inflammatory conditions, where ultrasound is of greater use. However ultrasound and CT should be regarded as complementary investigations and in difficult cases it is common to use both.

Other imaging techniques

A variety of other imaging techniques may be of value. Intravenous cholangiography, where the bile ducts are outlined directly following intravenous administration of contrast medium, has largely been superseded by ERCP and percutaneous transhepatic cholangiography, which provide better detail.

Isotopic scanning of the gallbladder may be useful in the diagnosis of acute cholecystitis. A technetium-labelled derivative of iminodiacetic acid (HIDA, PIPIDA) is administered intravenously and images are then recorded by a gamma-camera (Fig. 15). In acute cholecystitis the cystic duct is occluded and so the gallbladder will not opacify; opacification excludes acute cholecystitis. A HIDA scan is particularly useful in the diagnosis of acute acalculous cholecystitis. False positive results may occur in patients with alcoholic liver disease and in those maintained on total parenteral nutrition, in whom the gallbladder is atonic. The isotope may fail to enter the gallbladder despite a patent cystic duct.

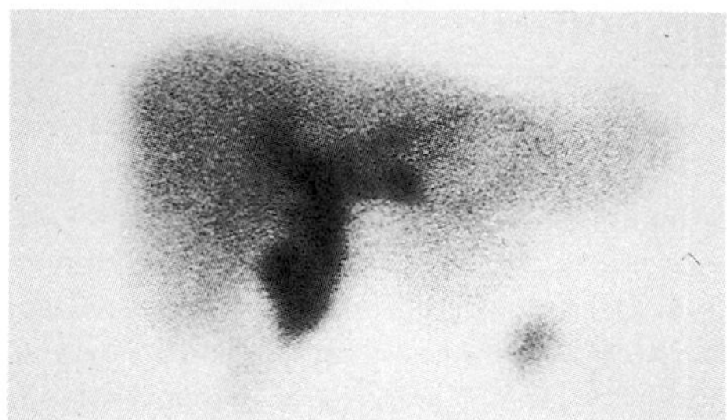

Fig. 15 HIDA scan of the liver and the bile ducts showing a normal excretion pattern. The gallbladder can just be seen as a small projection off the main bile duct.

Arteriography is essential before any major operation on the biliary system because of the wide variation in biliary arterial anatomy (Fig. 16). The liver, gallbladder, and pancreas can all be imaged by magnetic resonance (MRI), but the information currently provided is no better than that obtained from CT.

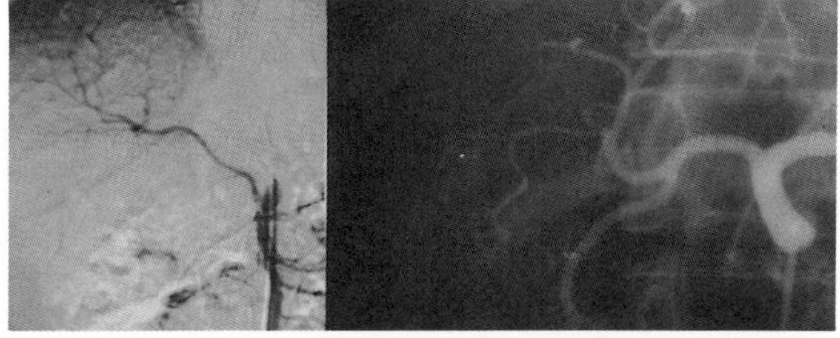

Fig. 16 Hepatic angiogram showing one of the common anomalies. The left hepatic artery arises from the coeliac plexus (the radiograph on the right) but the right hepatic artery comes from the superior mesenteric artery (the radiograph on the left). This arrangement is found in about 25 per cent of patients.

Liver function tests

Biochemical measures of liver function abound. In a surgical context interest has focused on bilirubin, alkaline phosphatase, which is excreted by liver cells, and transferase enzymes, which are predominantly located within liver cells. Changes in these three parameters have traditionally been used to differentiate between intra- and extrahepatic causes of jaundice. A rise in alkaline phosphatase signifies an extrahepatic obstruction while changes in enzyme levels indicate disease within the liver cells themselves. These changes are never totally reliable and they have been superseded by ultrasound and the demonstration of dilatation of the bile ducts. They are, however, useful indicators of disease severity, and their main use is to monitor the effects of treatment. Prothrombin time is also a useful measure of liver function, since it depends on the synthetic functions of the liver. Prolongation of the prothrombin time, which might lead to excessive haemorrhage, must be corrected by the administration of Vitamin K or fresh frozen plasma before embarking on any surgical procedure.

Biliary manometry

Biliary manometry is used to assess the function of the sphincter of Oddi. Pressure traces can be obtained either by placing a special perfusion catheter across the sphincter from below at ERCP or from above during surgical exploration of the common bile duct. The former is used to detect stenosis and dyskinesia of the sphincter of Oddi in patients with persistent pain following a cholecystectomy. Sphincter stenosis is diagnosed by an elevated basal sphincter pressure, and these patients are often cured of their symptoms by an endoscopic sphincterotomy. Other manometric abnormalities have been identified, such as rapid phasic contractions, excessive retrograde contractions, and a paradoxical response to cholecystokinin, but their clinical relevance is not yet clear. Manometry in conjunction with peroperative cholangiography can detect small stones in the bile duct, but the technique is time-consuming and difficult to perform accurately. It is not much used.

DISEASE OF THE BILIARY TRACT

Congenital abnormalities

Biliary atresia (see also Section 36.8)

Biliary atresia has an incidence of 1 in 12 000 live births and presents in the first week of life as cholestatic jaundice. Untreated it pursues a relentless course, with progressive liver failure and death before the age of 3 years. The cause of the atresia is unknown, but failure of vacuolation of the solid biliary bud in the early weeks of intrauterine life is one possible explanation. Inflammatory obliteration of previously patent ducts occurring about the time of birth is currently considered to be the cause. Viruses and metabolic disorders are two possible causes of such inflammation.

Classification

Three pathological types of atresia are recognized: Type 1, atresia of the common bile duct; Type 2, atresia of the common hepatic duct; and Type 3, atresia of the right and left hepatic ducts. Types 1 and 2 are relatively easy to correct surgically. In Type 3 disease there is often a conical area of fibrous tissue at the hilum of the liver which contains within it multiple small biliary radicals. The number of these ducts decreases with time and this adds to the urgency of diagnosis.

Diagnosis

Biliary atresia is notoriously difficult to diagnose. Jaundice in the newborn can be caused by hepatocellular disease, intrahepatic bile duct hypoplasia, or a choledochal cyst, as well as biliary atresia. Conventional methods of investigation which are useful in adults are less valuable in infants. For example there is rarely any intrahepatic duct dilatation, so that ultrasound is of limited help. Histological examination of a liver biopsy is the most reliable method of diagnosis, but in clinical practice a range of tests is usually needed.

Treatment

The discovery on microscopy of small biliary radicals in the fibrous tissue at the hilum of the liver has led to the development of portoenterostomy for the treatment of Type 3 biliary atresia. In this procedure all of the fibrous tissue and atretic ducts at the porta hepatis are resected *en bloc*. An open enterotomy in the antimesenteric border of a jejunal loop is then sutured to the edge of the fibrous tissue in the porta hepatis. Bile drains from the liver into the bowel through the tiny ducts at the liver hilum. This Kasai operation allows long-term survival of nearly half of the patients (Fig. 17). If atresia involves only the extrahepatic bile ducts, it is possible to anastomose the residual dilated hepatic ducts to a Roux-en-Y loop of small bowel. Unfortunately the results of hepaticojejunostomy are not much better than those of portoenterostomy. Various modifications of the Kasai procedure have been suggested, including bringing up the Roux loop to the skin surface in order to allow easy access to the hepatic anastomosis, but this appears to convey little advantage.

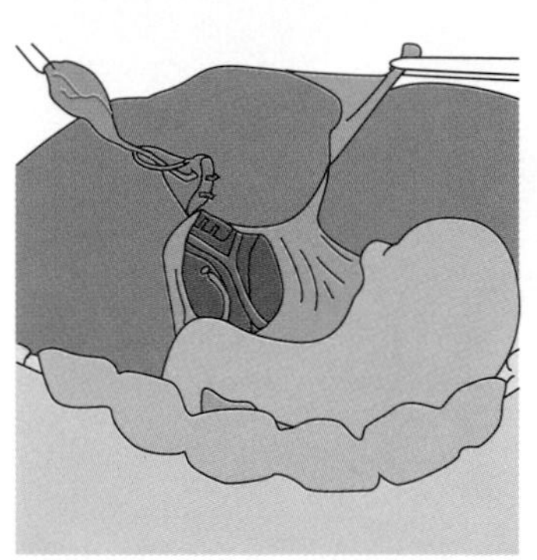
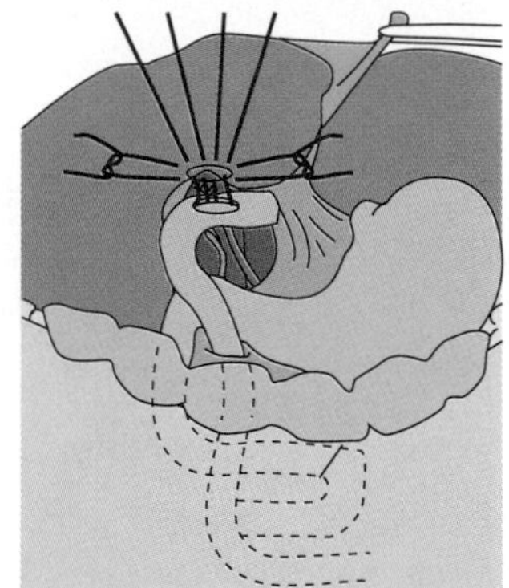

Fig. 17 The Kasai procedure. The abnormal tissue at the hilum of the liver is excised left and a Roux-en-Y loop of jejunum is sutured to the raw surface at the hilum of the liver right.

Bacterial cholangitis and portal hypertension are the two common complications of the Kasai operation. Cholangitis requires treatment with systemic antibiotics and the exclusion of a surgically correctable obstruction such as kinking of the Roux loop. Portal hypertension consequent upon hepatic fibrosis is a long-term problem: injection sclerotherapy is the treatment of choice for children who develop varices.

Even though the Kasai operation has markedly improved the management of biliary atresia the results are not completely satisfactory. However, the results of liver transplantation in children have improved so much that it is now the treatment of choice for children with end-stage liver failure (see Section 10.6). Since there are few paediatric liver donors it is necessary to reduce the size of an adult liver for transplantation into an infant, but the surgery and the immunosuppression is tolerated without difficulty. Portoenterostomy remains the first treatment for biliary atresia; liver transplantation is available when portoenterostomy is impossible or liver function fails.

Choledochal cyst

Choledochal cyst is an aneurysmal dilatation of the bile duct. It is a rare condition, with an incidence between 1 : 100 000 and 1 : 150 000 live births in the West, although it is probably more common in the East. Females are affected two to four times more often than are males. Most patients present in infancy, although a significant minority are diagnosed as adults.

Aetiology

The aetiology is unknown. Partial biliary obstruction and a weakness of the wall of the bile duct are the two basic defects required for the formation of a cyst: both these abnormalities may be congenital or acquired. Abnormal recanalization of the bile duct, which is complete by the fifth week of intrauterine development, may result in areas of stenosis and dilatation. This theory is supported by the occurrence of choledochal cysts in neonates and by the finding of multiple areas of stenosis and dilatation in some patients with a choledochal cyst. A cyst may also develop following trauma, or from fibrosis and stenosis of the distal common bile duct due to recurrent cholangitis associated with stones in the bile duct. Early changes of this type are sometimes seen at ERCP.

Classification

Cystic dilatation may affect any part of the biliary system: five patterns have been described. Type 1, a cystic or fusiform dilatation of the common bile duct, is the most common (82 per cent). Type 2 (3 per cent) is a supraduodenal diverticulum of the common bile duct, and Type 3 (5 per cent) is a diverticulum of the intraduodenal bile duct, or choledochocoele. Type 4 (9 per cent) consists of multiple cysts: Type 4A cysts affect both the intrahepatic and extrahepatic bile ducts, while Type 4B cysts affect the extrahepatic duct only. Type 5 (1 per cent) describes cysts of the intrahepatic bile ducts. These may be solitary or multiple, and this type includes Caroli's disease (Fig. 18). They can vary in size from 2 cm in diameter to giant cysts, and the wall is composed of fibrous tissue which may be up to 1 cm thick. The cyst is lined by cuboidal biliary epithelium, which is often ulcerated in adults.

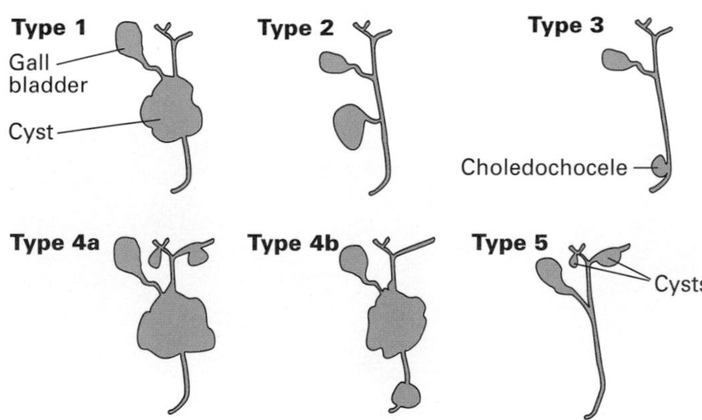

Fig. 18 Classification of choledochal cysts. Type 1 is commonest.

Diagnosis

Choledochal cysts present either as a mass or with biliary obstruction. The classic triad of abdominal pain, jaundice, and a mass occurs in less than one-half of patients. Most adults present with jaundice or cholangitis. Infants also present with jaundice, but may vomit due to duodenal compression and may also have a palpable mass in the abdomen.

Ultrasonography will usually confirm the diagnosis. Cholangiography is absolutely essential to delineate the biliary anatomy accurately and thus determine the best approach to surgical treatment. ERCP is the easiest method of obtaining a cholangiogram (Fig. 19), but percutaneous and operative cholangiography may also be needed. An arteriogram to delineate the relationship of the cyst to the hepatic artery and the portal vein may be very valuable before embarking on surgical treatment.

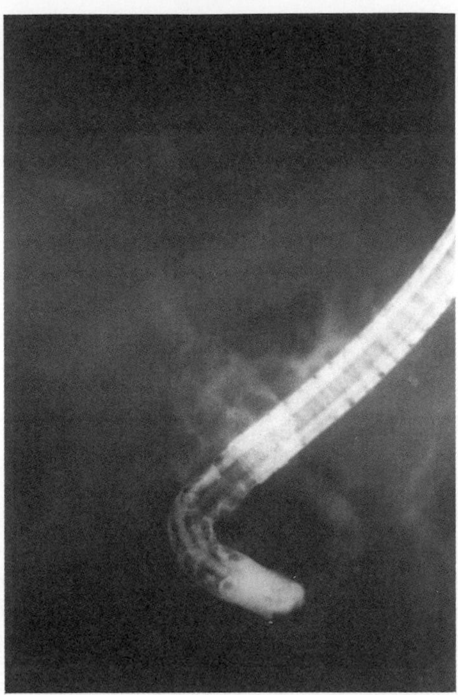

Fig. 19 Type I choledochal cyst packed with stones which presented in adult life. There is also a stricture of the common hepatic duct immediately at the junction with the cyst.

Treatment

Once diagnosed the treatment of a choledochal cyst is surgical. Although numerous operations have been described, a Type 1 cyst should ideally be excised completely. The distal bile duct is then anastomosed to the small bowel—usually the jejunum via a Roux-en-Y loop. In infants the structures may be sufficiently mobile to allow use of the duodenum. Anastomoses between the cyst wall and the bowel are usually unsatisfactory in the long term. The cyst wall is often devoid of mucosa and is lined only by granulation tissue, so that a stricture develops. This leads to recurrent cholangitis and the development of stones within the cyst. The high risk of carcinoma developing in a choledochal cyst is also a reason for complete excision. This is usually possible but if it is difficult it is acceptable simply to excise the lining of the cyst and thus protect the portal vein by a partial thickness of the cyst wall. Previous surgery, recurrent cholangitis, and portal hypertension all make treatment difficult.

Type 2 cysts can usually be excised, the defect in the common bile duct being repaired by primary suture over a T-tube brought out through a separate incision in the duct. Small choledochoceles (Type 3) may be treated by endoscopic sphincterotomy. Larger ones require a surgical sphincterotomy using the transduodenal approach. Type 4 cysts are treated by a combination of techniques, depending on the precise anatomy in each individual case. Segmental resection of the liver may be necessary, particularly if there are intrahepatic stones, strictures, or abscesses as well as an extra-hepatic cyst. Hepaticojejunostomy is then necessary to reconstitute biliary drainage.

Complications

Rupture may occur spontaneously in infants, and cholangitis develops in both adults and children. Gallstones can develop within the cyst, more commonly in adults (Fig. 19). Secondary biliary cirrhosis supervenes in 15 per cent of adults with chronic bile duct obstruction. Carcinoma develops within the cyst in 8 per cent of patients and is a fatal complication. The diagnosis is usually made at operation or at autopsy. Most patients are in their thirties, and 75 per cent of tumours are adenocarcinomas, although squamous carcinoma and cholangiocarcinoma also occur. The mean survival after diagnosis is 8.5 months.

Acquired disease

The most common acquired abnormality of the biliary system is gallstones. In most patients these remain dormant, but they may cause biliary colic simply by mechanical obstruction. More frequently, stones lead to acute or chronic inflammation within the biliary tree and causes symptoms. Inflammation without stones can occur in both the gallbladder and the bile duct, but is unusual, as are infarction of the gallbladder and benign neoplasms of the biliary tract. Damage to the bile duct occurs rarely at the time of cholecystectomy. It may lead to the development of a benign biliary stricture, which is one of the most serious complications of biliary tract surgery. Abnormalities of biliary function probably do occur but at the present time they are poorly understood.

Stones in the gallbladder

Prevalence

Gallstones are very common, with a prevalence at autopsy of 11 to 36 per cent. There are at least 5 million people in the United Kingdom and 25 million people in the United States of America with gallstones. Overall the prevalence has probably increased in Western societies over the last 50 years, and it certainly increases with age, from 4 per cent of people in the third decade to 27 per cent in the seventh. This may be related to changes in the biochemistry of bile with age. Women are three times more likely than men to develop stones, and first-degree relatives of patients with gallstones have a two-fold greater prevalence. There are geographical variations. The prevalence is very high in certain American Indian communities (Pima and Chippewa tribes), in Mexico, Sweden, Czechoslovakia, and Chile, and low in Greece, Japan, India, and China. Certain conditions predispose to the development of gallstones. Obesity is a risk factor for gallstones in women under the age of 50. Pregnancy, but not consumption of the oral contraceptive pill, probably predisposes to the development of gallstones (Fig. 20). Dietary factors which have been implicated include a high energy intake, increased consumption of unrefined carbohydrate, and diets low in fibre. Crohn's disease, terminal ileal resection, and jejunoileal bypass for obesity are associated with a four-fold increase in prevalence. Biliary infection and parasitic infestation of the biliary tree are important factors in the development of pigment stones in Asia but not in the West. Other diseases associated with the development of gallstones include diabetes mellitus, type IV hyperlipoproteinaemia, cirrhosis of the liver, gastric surgery, and total parenteral nutrition. Patients with haemolytic anaemia due to hereditary spherocytosis, sickle-cell disease, and thalassaemia also show an increased prevalence of pigment stones.

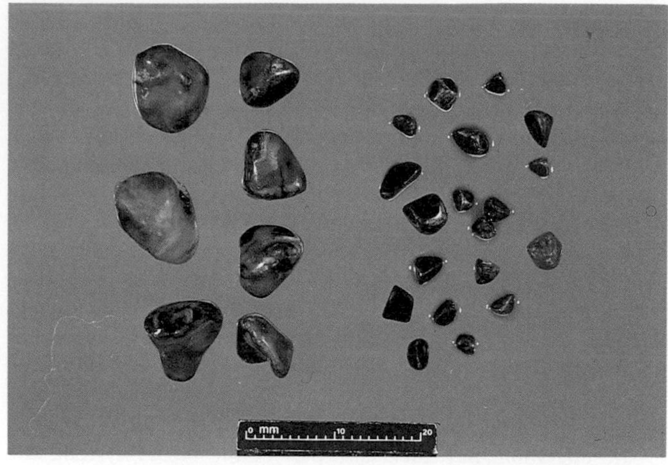

Fig. 20 Gallstones from a young woman with two children. The stones clearly divide into two groups of similar size and probably formed coincidentally with her two pregnancies.

Classification of stones

Cholesterol and bile pigments are the two principal constituents of gallstones. In addition, calcium carbonate, phosphate, and palmitate are present in variable amounts. Pure cholesterol and pure pigment stones do occur, but most stones are mixed (Fig. 21). Predominantly cholesterol stones account for 75 per cent of all gallstones in the West. They are single or multiple, hard, and usually layered on cross-section (Fig. 22). Pigment stones are most common in Asia. They are usually black or brown in colour; brown stones crumble when squashed (Fig. 23). About 10 per cent of stones contain enough calcium to be radio-opaque (Fig. 7).

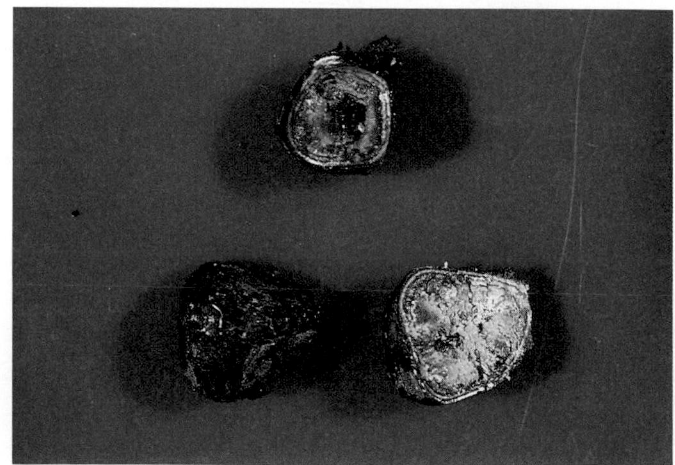

Fig. 21 Mixed stones. They are clearly faceted and consist of layers of pigment and cholesterol.

Formation of gallstones

Cholesterol stones

Cholesterol is insoluble in water, and is held in solution as micelles of cholesterol, phospholipids, and bile salts. Lecithin forms the

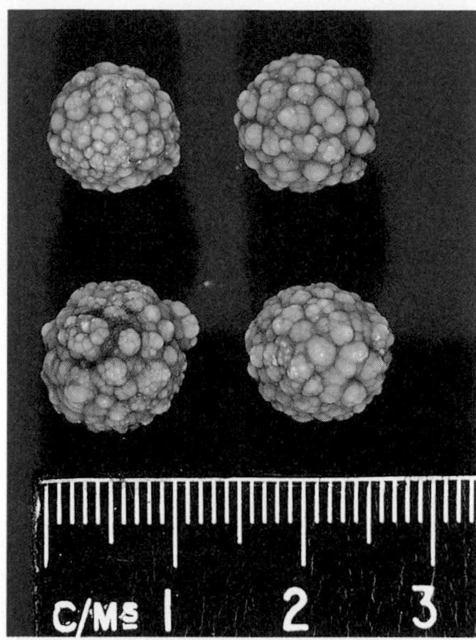

Fig. 22 Four pure cholesterol stones.

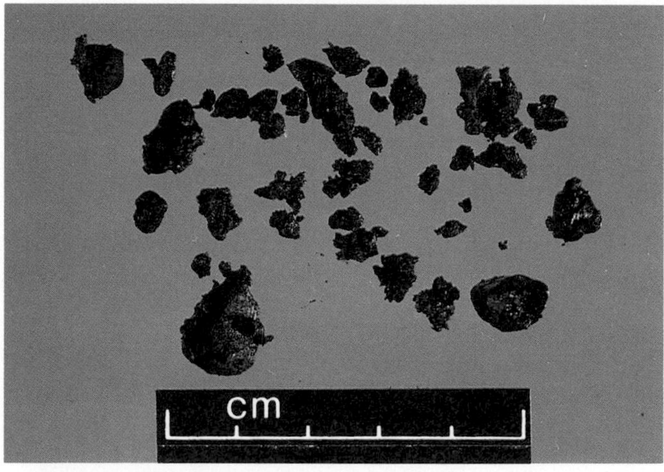

Fig. 23 Pigment gallstones. They are smaller and softer than mixed or cholesterol stones and they are classically associated with haemolysis.

major component of phospholipids while the bile salts are glycine or taurine conjugates. The physicochemical state of bile can be determined from a phase diagram (Fig. 24). The relative proportions of cholesterol, bile salts, and phospholipid are expressed as a percentage of the total lipid content and are plotted on triangular co-ordinates. An increase in the cholesterol concentration or a decrease in the bile salt concentration results in supersaturation of bile with cholesterol, and the formation of a liquid crystalline phase of cholesterol.

The biliary lipid composition of normal bile and gallstone bile is virtually identical, and since at least half of the Western population have supersaturated bile there must be another factor responsible for the formation of stones. Cholesterol will only crystallize from a supersaturated solution if there is a nidus on which the crystals can form. This process is called nucleation, and the time taken for supersaturated bile to form crystals of cholesterol is known as the nucleation time. Normal bile takes 15 days to form crystals, compared with 3 days for bile from patients with cholesterol gallstones. Mucus glycoproteins from the gallbladder wall and bilirubinate have both been proposed as nucleating factors, while a bile protein has been proposed as an inhibitor. The nucleation phenomenon also depends on gallbladder function: the motility of the wall determines the degree of stasis and mixing of the bile within the lumen. One other significant finding is that the size of the bile acid pool is reduced in many patients with gallstones, although the reason for this is unknown.

Pigment stones

Pigment gallstones are formed of calcium bilirubinate and contain less than 25 per cent cholesterol (Fig. 23). They are usually small and multiple, and about half are radio-opaque. As might be expected they are more prevalent in patients with haemolytic disorders such as hereditary spherocytosis or sickle-cell disease, and in patients with cirrhosis, who commonly have a mild degree of haemolysis. They are frequently found in oriental countries, where they are associated with parasitic infections. Bilirubin in bile is normally conjugated with glucuronide. The enzyme β-glucuronidase, which may be produced by bacteria such as *Escherichia coli*, splits the molecule and the unconjugated bilirubin precipitates as the calcium salt. Hydrolytic enzymes from gallbladder mucosa may act in the same way.

Clinical presentation of stones in the gallbladder

Since the sixteenth century it has been realized that most people who have gallstones remain asymptomatic throughout their lives. In a few patients stones are discovered by accident during the investigation of some other problem. In general these stones should be left alone. In a study of patients in whom gallbladder stones were discovered on screening, only 15 per cent developed biliary pain in the subsequent 15 years.

There may be a case for removing asymptomatic stones in diabetics because of their greater susceptibility to infection, and an incidental cholecystectomy for gallstones during a laparotomy for an unrelated condition may sometimes be appropriate because such patients are at greater risk of developing subsequent symptoms. There is no justification for removing the gallbladder with stones to prevent the later development of cancer.

Disease in the gallbladder affects only a small minority of people with gallstones. It presents with a variety of clinical syndromes, of which the most common are chronic cholecystitis, which appears slowly over time, biliary colic, and acute cholecystitis, both of which develop rapidly. Patients occasionally present with the complications of one of these three, either locally in the gallbladder or from stones in the bile duct, and very occasionally from a stone that has ulcerated through into the bowel.

Chronic cholecystitis

Pathology

About two-thirds of patients present with chronic cholecystitis. The pathological changes, which often do not correlate well with symptoms, vary from those of an apparently normal gallbladder with minor chronic inflammation in the mucosa to a shrunken organ with gross transmural fibrosis and organized adhesions

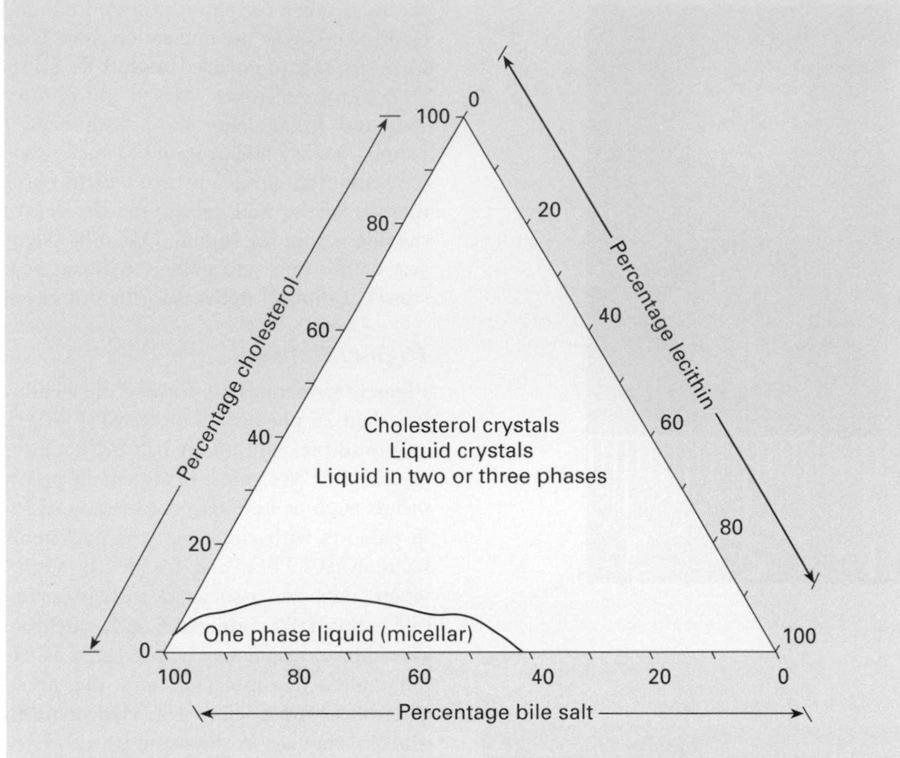

Fig. 24 Phase diagram of the solubility of cholesterol in bile. This diagram shows the physical state of all the possible combinations of bile salts in aqueous solutions. The area below the line in the bottom left represents the maximum amount of cholesterol solubilized by any mixture of lecithin and bile salt. Combinations above and to the right of this area means that cholesterol is present in bile in crystal or liquid crystal form (after Admirand and Small 1968).

(Fig. 25). The mucosa is initially hypertrophied but later becomes atrophied; the epithelium protrudes into the muscle coat, leading to the formation of Rokitansky-Aschoff sinuses. The most severe form is represented by cholecystitis glandularis proliferans in which there are buried areas of hyperproliferative epithelium within the wall of the gallbladder (see Fig. 28 below). Rarely, dystrophic calcification may occur, resulting in the formation of a porcelain gallbladder (Fig. 26).

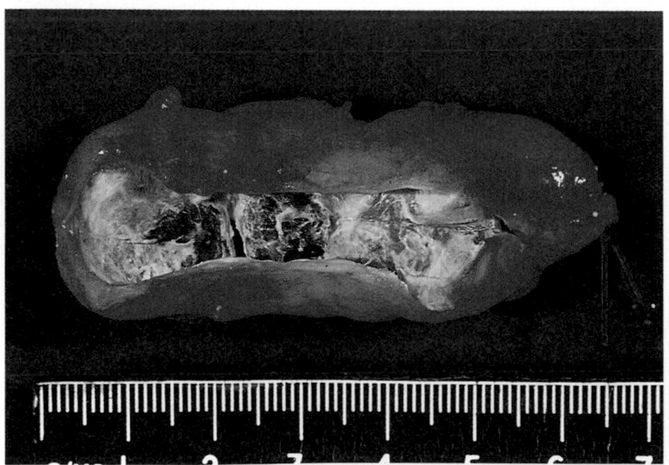

Fig. 25 Gallbladder removed at operation showing severe chronic cholecystitis.

Diagnosis

The typical patient complains of recurrent attacks of right hypochondrial or epigastric pain, usually after meals, and particularly after consumption of fatty foods. The pain, which often occurs at night, varies from mild indigestion after eating to persistent, moderately severe, right upper quadrant pain which may radiate round to the back and sometimes to the right shoulder or between the shoulder blades. The pain is often described as a tight band all the way round the upper abdomen; very occasionally the pain on the right hand side of the abdomen is suppressed and the patient presents only with left-sided pain.

Nausea usually accompanies the pain, sometimes associated with vomiting. There may be additional minor symptoms such as flatulence and abdominal distension, but these are equally common in patients who do not have gallstones. There may be mild right upper quadrant abdominal tenderness, but examination is usually unremarkable.

It is often possible to make a confident clinical diagnosis of chronic cholecystitis in a patient with classical symptoms, but the presence of gallstones should be confirmed by ultrasonography (Fig. 9). Occasionally an oral cholecystogram is also needed. When it is difficult to distinguish chronic cholecystitis from peptic ulceration, a hiatus hernia, or diverticular disease, further radiology and endoscopy may be required. The last two conditions often occur together with gallstones, a condition known as Saint's triad.

It is easy to ascribe the patient's symptoms to stones which are

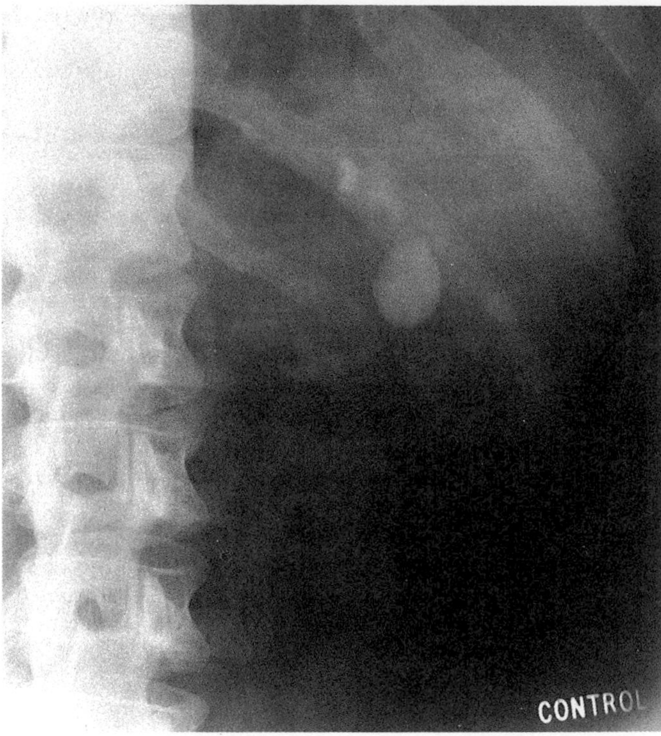

Fig. 26 A calcified gallbladder on a plain radiograph of porcelain gallbladder.

found on investigation when this is not the case: many patients with other conditions have gallstones. On the other hand patients with symptoms that show enough features related to proven gallstones are likely to improve on treatment.

Treatment

Once the diagnosis is established some form of active treatment is indicated since the symptoms will almost always continue. Some patients can control their symptoms by taking care over their diet. Others are only occasionally troubled and simply require mild analgesia. More commonly, some form of surgical treatment is needed to remove the stones, with or without the gallbladder. The risks of surgery must be balanced against the potential benefits, and the views of the informed patient are just as important as the opinion of the doctor. Most surgeons prefer the patient to request the operation.

Biliary colic

Biliary colic is due to impaction of a stone in the neck of the gallbladder. The severe pain starts abruptly in the epigastrium, often at night after a heavy meal, and lasts for several hours. It is usually continuous and is associated with restlessness, vomiting, and sweating. The pain may radiate through to the back but does not radiate to the shoulder, as in acute cholecystitis. General examination may disclose a patient in obvious severe pain with a mild tachycardia and normal temperature. Abdominal examination shows only mild tenderness in the epigastrium. In contrast to acute cholecystitis, tenderness over the gallbladder is absent. The gallbladder in patients with biliary colic is often normal in external appearance and shows only mild inflammatory changes on histological examination. Most patients need a strong analgesic given by injection, and after two attacks of severe biliary colic will want some form of definitive treatment.

Acute cholecystitis

Pathology

About one-fifth of patients first present with acute cholecystitis; in about one-third there is clinical or pathological evidence of previous chronic cholecystitis. It is usually due to persistent impaction of a stone in the neck of the gallbladder. The result is initially a chemical inflammation of the gallbladder wall perhaps due to the mucosal toxin lysolecithin, produced by the action of phospholipase on biliary lecithin. This is soon followed by bacterial infection. Because the cystic duct is occluded the inflammatory process is particularly aggressive and the gallbladder becomes acutely distended, with accompanying lymphatic and venous obstruction. The serosa may be covered by a fibrinous exudate and subserosal haemorrhage gives the appearance of patchy gangrene. The gallbladder wall itself is grossly thickened and oedematous and the underlying mucosa may show hyperaemia or patchy necrosis (Fig. 27). Histologically, three grades of inflammation are recognized: acute cholecystitis, acute suppurative cholecystitis, and acute gangrenous cholecystitis. Rarely an abscess or empyema develops within the gallbladder, while perforation of an ischaemic area leads to a pericholecystic abscess, bile peritonitis, or a cholecystoenteric fistula.

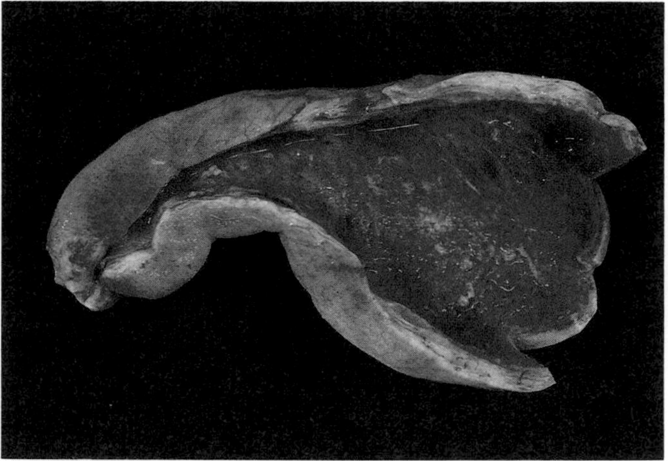

Fig. 27 A gallbladder removed at an emergency operation showing severe acute cholecystitis. Note the reddened mucosa and the thickening of the gallbladder wall.

Diagnosis

Patients present with acute upper abdominal pain that has often been present for 2 or 3 days. Because the inflammation extends to the parietal peritoneum the pain is well localized and it hurts the patient to move or to breathe. Patients feel generally unwell, may have been febrile, and are anorexic. Physical signs vary with the severity of the inflammation but there is usually some degree of fever and tachycardia. Mild jaundice is present in 10 to 15 per cent of patients. Right hypochondrial tenderness is invariable and there may also be guarding, rigidity, and rebound tenderness. If the latter physical signs are subdued it may be possible to feel the gallbladder itself. Murphy's sign (inspiratory arrest during subcostal palpation) is widely regarded as pathognomonic of cholecystitis. It is certainly present in patients with established acute cholecystitis, but it only reflects peritoneal inflammation in the right upper quadrant, other causes of which include chronic cholecystitis, acute hepatitis, and a localized abscess around a perforated duodenal ulcer. There is usually a clear distinction between acute cholecystitis and biliary colic: this is important since the management is different.

In elderly patients acute cholecystitis may present more insidiously and the frequent absence of typical physical signs results in a delay in diagnosis. In addition, the incidence of complications is higher and the prevalence of intercurrent illness combine to increase the mortality rate 10-fold. Acute cholecystitis is uncommon in children, most of whom have gallstones, sometimes as a complication of haemolytic disease. Acalculous cholecystitis occurs in children with severe sepsis.

Differential diagnosis

Clinically it can be difficult to distinguish acute cholecystitis from acute pancreatitis, acute appendicitis, acute pyelonephritis, perforation of a peptic ulcer, and, occasionally, biliary colic. A raised white cell count and serum amylase level may occur in several of these conditions, although patients with biliary colic rarely have a leucocytosis. Urine should always be examined under the microscope for pus cells and sent for culture if appropriate. One-quarter of patients have disturbed liver function tests, but not all will have stones in the bile duct. There are rarely any specific features of acute cholecystitis on plain radiology, but ultrasound may localize the tenderness to the gallbladder and may demonstrate stones. Free air under the diaphragm on a chest radiograph implies perforation of a viscus, usually a peptic ulcer. A normal HIDA scan excludes acute cholecystitis (Fig. 15).

Young women who present acutely with severe right upper quadrant pain and signs of peritonitis may have the Curtis–Fitz–Hugh syndrome. Clinically these patients appear to have acute cholecystitis but ultrasound examination fails to show gallstones or any signs of acute cholecystitis. At laparoscopy or laparotomy the gallbladder is normal but there are string-like adhesions between the liver and the peritoneum. This perihepatitis is caused by infection with *Chlamydia trachomatis*. There may also be evidence of genital tract infection with the same organism. The diagnosis can be confirmed by isolation of the organism from peritoneal fluid or by rising titres of chlamydial antibodies in serum. Treatment is with oxytetracycline 2 g daily for 10 days.

Acute viral hepatitis can sometimes present as acute cholecystitis. The acutely swollen liver is painful and tender but the systemic symptoms and the onset of jaundice soon make the true diagnosis clear.

Treatment

Acute cholecystitis resolves with conservative treatment in the majority of cases. If admission to hospital is necessary patients require intravenous fluids, analgesia, and suspension of oral intake. Vomiting is unusual, but if present nasogastric aspiration is helpful. If the patient fails to respond intravenous antibiotics are prescribed. Our present choice is cefuroxime 1.5 g three times a day.

Most patients should be offered cholecystectomy, which should normally be undertaken on the next convenient operating list. There is no advantage in letting the acute illness subside and removing the gallbladder 6 weeks later except in a patient who is unfit for surgery and whose condition could be improved by waiting.

Complications

An empyema of the gallbladder may be suspected clinically if the physical signs and symptoms fail to improve on conservative management. In particular, fever and right upper quadrant tenderness fail to abate, and there is a persistent or increasing leucocytosis. With time the gallbladder becomes necrotic and ruptures, resulting either in a localized abscess or in generalized peritonitis. An empyema is really an abscess within the gallbladder and it must therefore be drained. The best method is to insert a pigtail catheter into the gallbladder under ultrasound control, as the gallbladder is usually adherent to the peritoneum of the abdominal wall. If there is any doubt a transhepatic route for the catheter should be chosen. Percutaneous drainage is clearly less disturbing for the patient, who is usually quite ill and toxic. If it fails for any reason a conventional surgical approach must be adopted. Occasionally a safe cholecystectomy can be performed by an experienced surgeon. For everyone else a cholecystostomy is better.

Acute emphysematous cholecystitis

This is a severe and fulminant form of acute cholecystitis which accounts for less than 1 per cent of cases. Stones are absent in 30 to 50 per cent of patients, who are usually elderly men, and 40 per cent have diabetes mellitus. It is caused by a mixture of bacteria which includes gas-forming organisms, and the pathognomonic diagnostic sign is gas within the wall or the lumen of the gallbladder seen on a plain radiograph. The onset of the disease is abrupt and the condition of the patient deteriorates rapidly. There is a high incidence of gangrene and perforation, and emergency cholecystectomy is needed.

Xanthogranulomatous cholecystitis

This is a rare but severe form of chronic cholecystitis in which the gallbladder is thickened and irregular with extensions of yellow xanthogranulomatous inflammation to adjacent organs. Foamy macrophages and giant cells are seen within connective tissue in the wall of the gallbladder. The condition is thought to be due to bile penetrating deeply into the gallbladder wall. The appearances both on investigation and at operation resemble carcinoma of the gallbladder; frozen section histology at operation may be necessary because the two conditions are associated.

Acute acalculous cholecystitis

Acute cholecystitis can develop in the absence of gallbladder stones. It is most often seen in the intensive care unit and is associated with severe illness such as multiple trauma, extensive burns, major surgery, and sepsis, often in an elderly person. The aetiology is unknown, but is thought to be related to gallbladder distension and bile stasis. The normal contraction of the gallbladder is inhibited in patients with sepsis and those on total parenteral nutrition, especially if opiate analgesics are administered. This allows the development of biliary sludge, which may be demonstrated in the gallbladder of many patients with major illness, not all of whom develop acalculous cholecystitis.

Pathology

Pathological examination of the gallbladder reveals oedema of the serosa and muscular layers, with patchy thrombosis of arterioles and venules. Areas of necrosis develop and may affect the underlying mucosa. One possibility is that activation of factor VII by trauma may lead to thrombosis of blood vessels in the seromuscular layer of the gallbladder.

Diagnosis

In a severely ill patient, the development of acute acalculous cholecystitis is usually insidious. The clinical features are similar to those of acute calculous cholecystitis but they are often masked by the underlying condition. Ultrasound is the most useful investigation, and may show biliary sludge in a tender thickened gallbladder, but fails to demonstrate stones. All the indicators of liver function deteriorate, and a HIDA scan will fail to demonstrate the gallbladder.

Treatment

Once the diagnosis is made an immediate cholecystectomy is necessary because of the high incidence of gangrene of the gallbladder. The mortality rate varies with the nature of the underlying condition but is generally higher than that in patients with acute calculous cholecystitis.

Cholesterolosis

This is caused by the deposition of cholesterol in the mucosa and submucosa of the gallbladder wall and produces the classical 'strawberry gallbladder'. Microscopy shows macrophages loaded with cholesterol. Ultrasound identifies the cholesterol in the wall as bright shiny spots, and there may also be cholesterol stones within the lumen. Cholesterolosis may cause pancreatitis, perhaps as a result of small cholesterol crystals passing down the bile duct and briefly occluding the ampulla, so that symptomatic patients should be advised to undergo cholecystectomy.

Adenomyomatosis

Adenomyomatosis or cholecystitis glandularis proliferans is characterized by hypertrophic smooth muscle bundles and epithelial sinus formation. The gallbladder has a thickened wall which may be divided into two separate sections by a stricture of incomplete septum (Fig. 28). Granulomatous polyps develop in the lumen at the fundus. Inflammation develops later and gallstones are sometimes present. Symptomatic patients require a cholecystectomy. Others in whom the diagnosis is made but not treated require surveillance since adenomyomatosis may predispose to carcinoma.

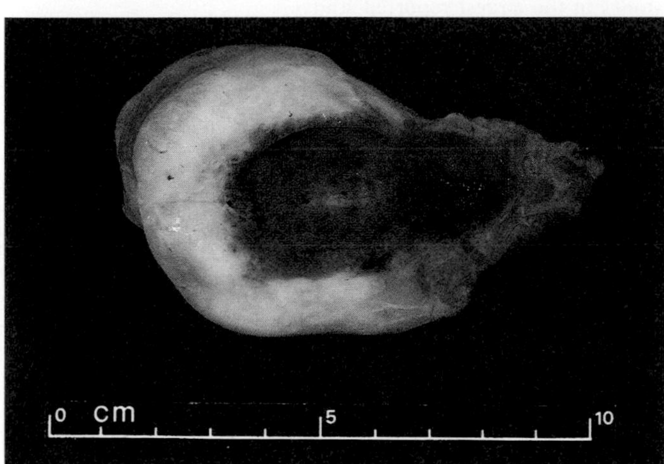

Fig. 28 Severe cholecystitis glandularis proliferans. The very thick wall of the gallbladder is white and rather mucoid in appearance when it is cut open.

Mucocele of the gallbladder

A mucocele of the gallbladder forms when a stone impacts in the cystic duct but bacterial infection does not occur. Bile is reabsorbed but the epithelium continues to secrete mucous, and the gallbladder becomes distended (Figs. 29, 30). It is easily palpable and may even be visible, but it is not tender. Such patients have somewhat subdued but nevertheless persistent symptoms, often including distressing nausea. If infection does occur an empyema may develop rapidly. In either circumstance a cholecystectomy is required. Rarely a mucocele of the gallbladder may perforate. Although pseudomyxoma peritonei has been reported to follow rupture of a mucocele it probably only follows rupture of a cystadenoma or cystadenocarcinoma of the gallbladder.

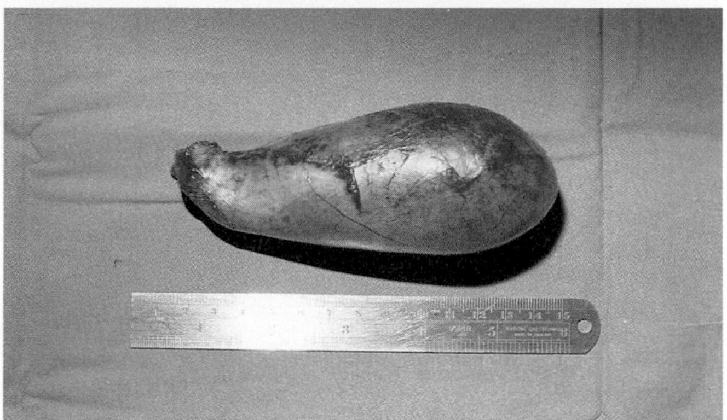

Fig. 29 A mucocele of the gallbladder—unopened.

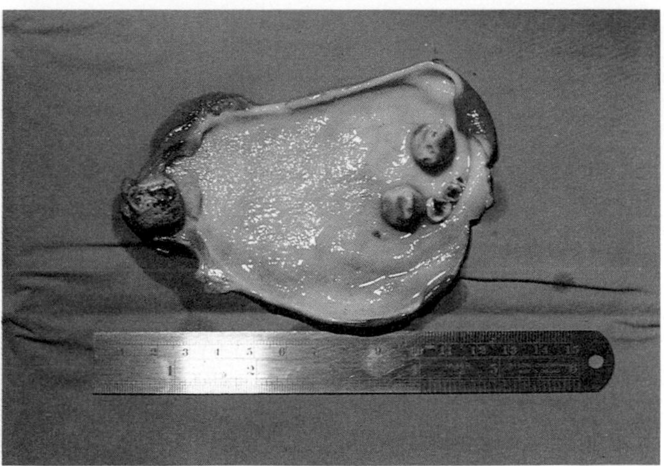

Fig. 30 The same specimen as Fig. 29 opened to show the white shiny mucosal surface and one stone stuck in Hartmann's pouch.

Torsion of the gallbladder

Infarction of the gallbladder due to torsion or volvulus is a rare event. Two anatomical anomalies permit torsion. Firstly the gallbladder may have no attachment to the liver, lying free in the peritoneal cavity suspended only by the cystic duct and artery. Secondly, and more commonly, the gallbladder is suspended from the liver by a narrow mesentery. Acute torsion causes right-sided abdominal pain and the tense, infarcted gallbladder may be palpable (Fig. 31). It is often misdiagnosed as acute appendicitis. Intermittent torsion can occur and produces periodic bouts of pain.

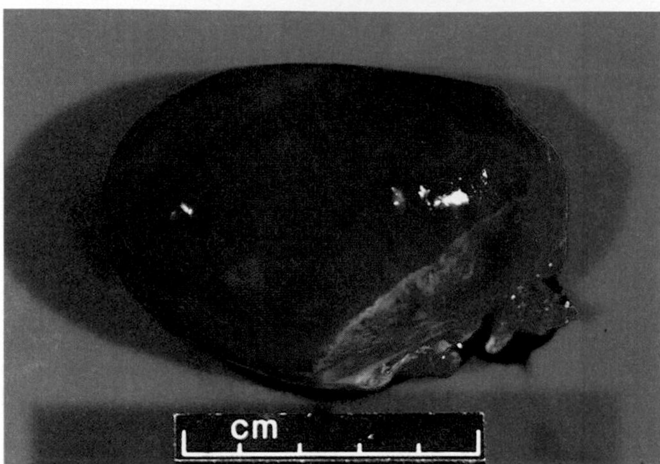

Fig. 31 Torsion of the gallbladder. The line across which the fundus of the gallbladder twisted can be clearly seen and the fundus is congested and gangrene is developing.

Biliary pain without stones

A small group of patients, usually young women, presents with pain in the right hypochondrium which, in the opinion of everyone who sees them, is typical biliary pain. However, all conventional biliary investigations, which may be repeated on several occasions, are normal. Furthermore a minority benefit from cholecystectomy even though no pathological abnormality is discovered in the gallbladder at operation.

Now that cholesterolosis and adenomyomatosis can be excluded by ultrasound studies before operation interest has centred on the possibility that these patients have a functional disorder of the biliary tract. This idea has received support from the discovery that some develop identical pain following an intravenous injection of cholecystokinin, and it was hoped that this would identify those who would benefit from a cholecystectomy. This test has not turned out to be so specific, but there are a number of other experimental tests of gallbladder and biliary function which may help us to understand these patients better in the future.

In practical terms, it is essential to exclude the irritable bowel syndrome which can produce symptoms very similar to those of biliary pain. After explaining the position very carefully to the patient it is reasonable to proceed to a cholecystectomy. Unfortunately the pain persists after operation in some patients; these form part of a group of patients with postcholecystectomy pain.

Management of gallbladder stones

The first successful cholecystectomy was performed by Langenbuch in 1882, and since then the operation has become the standard treatment for gallbladder stones. It is both safe and effective by modern surgical standards. However, there are deaths and complications following the operation and it takes 6 to 8 weeks to recover following a conventional open operation. An alternative to surgery would clearly be useful. Our understanding of the biochemistry of gallstone formation first led to the development of drugs which dissolve cholesterol gallstones. Further developments have produced a bewildering array of methods for removing or dissolving stones without the disadvantages of surgery.

Alternatives to cholecystectomy

Gallstone dissolution therapy

Cholesterol gallstones can be dissolved by decreasing the cholesterol saturation of bile. The naturally occurring bile salt chenodeoxycholic acid and the synthetic ursodeoxycholic acid when given by mouth achieve this. They probably have their effect by reducing the hepatic synthesis of cholesterol rather than by expanding the bile acid pool. Ursodeoxycholic acid is more efficient at reducing the cholesterol saturation of bile, but both drugs are equally good at dissolving gallstones *in vivo*. Because they work in slightly different ways there are advantages to giving them together. They are known to be safe, although chenodeoxycholic acid, which is by far the cheaper drug, causes diarrhoea and abnormalities of liver function tests in some patients. One interesting but unexplained benefit is that some patients experience relief of their symptoms whilst taking the drugs even though there is no effect on the size of their stones.

Dissolution therapy can only be used for non-calcified stones within a functioning gallbladder; as a consequence, less than 20 per cent of patients presenting to a doctor are suitable candidates. These drugs are obviously unsuitable for patients with acute symptoms and are less effective in obese patients and those with stones more than 15 mm in diameter.

The protocol for gallstone dissolution therapy is onerous. Prior to starting treatment the size of stones is measured. Either chenodeoxycholic acid (10–15 mg/kg.day) or ursodeoxycholic acid (8–12 mg/kg.day and up to 15 mg/kg.day in obese patients) is started. Liver function is carefully monitored and the stones are measured at 6 months. If there has been no reduction in size there is no point in continuing with treatment. Eighty per cent of small stones dissolve in 6 months, but larger stones require up to 2 years treatment. Even then only 14 per cent of patients were free of stones in the largest reported study.

Compliance may be a problem over such a long time, and female patients need to take adequate precautions against pregnancy. Better results are obtained in thin rather than obese patients, in women rather than men and in those patients with small lucent gallstones that 'float' as a layer on oral cholecystography (Fig. 11). Stones that are initially radiolucent occasionally calcify, in which case dissolution therapy is no longer effective. Gallstones recur within 5 years of treatment in 50 per cent of patients.

Overall, dissolution therapy provides a viable alternative to surgery in a small proportion of carefully selected patients. This mode of treatment may be particularly useful in patients who are poor anaesthetic risks or who refuse surgery.

Minimally invasive removal of gallstones

All of these techniques depend on the percutaneous puncture of the gallbladder and the removal of stones either mechanically or by dissolution. Some procedures can be performed under local anaesthesia, others require general anaesthesia, but none requires a conventional surgical incision. Mechanical removal of the stones, with or without crushing, can be achieved under direct vision after dilating the percutaneous track to the gallbladder, in a similar fashion to percutaneous nephrolithotomy. After removing all the stones attempts have been made to obliterate the gallbladder lumen by instilling drugs such as tetracycline.

Many chemicals have been tested for their ability to dissolve gallstones and a few of them are clinically useful. Methyl tert-butyl ether is an alkyl ether that rapidly dissolves cholesterol. It smells unpleasant and causes vomiting and sedation if it is absorbed; the catheter should take a transhepatic route to the gallbladder to minimize the possibility of intraperitoneal leakage. Small volumes of methyl tert-butyl ether, which will not overflow into the bile duct, are then instilled and aspirated cyclically until the stones have dissolved.

The stone recurrence rate following either procedure has not yet been assessed but there is no reason to think that it will be any different to the results following dissolution with oral therapy.

Extracorporeal shock wave lithotripsy (see Section 23.4 for detailed discussion)

Extracorporeal shock wave lithotripsy was first introduced for the management of renal calculi and has subsequently been adapted for fragmentation of both gallbladder and common bile duct stones. Once again the stones should be radiolucent and the gallbladder must function so that the tiny fragments of stone can pass spontaneously. Adjuvant oral dissolution therapy is required concurrently. The stones should be less than 30 mm in diameter and there should not be more than three (ideally only one). These criteria restrict the use of extracorporeal shock wave lithotripsy to between 5 per cent and 10 per cent of patients.

Shock waves are generated either by a spark gap system, a piezoelectric generator, or by the electromagnetic deflection of a metal membrane. They are then synchronized with the r wave of the electrocardiogram and focused on to the gallstone, which is imaged using either ultrasound or X-rays. With modern piezoelectric machines the treatment is virtually painless, even though more than one treatment and several thousand shocks may be required. Cutaneous petechiae, transient haematuria, and mild pancreatitis are recognized complications, and about one-third of patients experience biliary colic. Oral treatment with stone-dissolving drugs needs to continue, but in one reported series by the end of 2 years after extracorporeal shock wave lithotripsy the gallbladder was empty in all the patients who had solitary stones and in three-quarters of those with multiple stones.

Any fragments of stone which remain can act as a nidus for recurrent stones, but at the moment the recurrence rate after complete clearance of the gallbladder is not known.

Cholecystectomy

Cholecystectomy is the most common major abdominal operation in the Western world, and the rules for its safe execution are well established even though there are a number of different techniques. Elective operations, planned for the convenience of the patient and the surgeon, play an important role in training because a cholecystectomy teaches several important surgical principles. A routine operation requires careful dissection within a confined space in an important anatomical area and no major structure should be divided until the anatomy has been clearly identified. A certain degree of surgical skill is needed and successfully completing the operation is always a landmark in a young surgeon's career.

Patients who are admitted as emergencies may require an immediate operation by an experienced surgeon. More commonly they will respond to conservative treatment and should undergo operation on the next convenient list. There are no surgical advantages in waiting for 6 weeks while the inflammation subsides although there may, on occasion, be medical advantages. With the advent of ultrasound it is now easy to make the diagnosis acutely. A delayed operation is no easier and several trials have shown that the early operation is not associated with a greater risk of damage to the bile duct. Furthermore conservative treatment fails for one in seven patients, and a similar number are readmitted with a further acute attack before their planned admission date. From the economic point of view operation during the first admission saves money.

Preoperative preparation

Fluid depletion and electrolyte imbalance should be corrected in the acutely ill patient, and blood should be grouped and serum saved for crossmatching should blood transfusion be needed.

Routine preoperative antibiotic prophylaxis to prevent wound infection is always appropriate. Although the incidence of anaerobic bacteria in the biliary tract is low our present practice is to give everyone metronidazole 0.5 g and cefuroxime 1.5 g intravenously on induction of anaesthesia. This is probably sufficient, but some surgeons also give a second dose 12 h after operation.

Routine prophylaxis against deep venous thrombosis is also necessary. Patients undergoing elective operations should stop the contraceptive pill 1 month in advance and everyone should wear compression stockings on their legs. Patients as well as staff should appreciate the importance of mobility after the operation. Several drugs reduce the incidence of deep vein thrombosis, and some also reduce the incidence of pulmonary embolism. Our choice is to give 500 ml Dextran 70 during surgery and a further 500 ml during the first 24 h postoperatively. High-risk patients receive 6000 units heparin by subcutaneous injection 2 h before operation and every 12 h thereafter.

Operative technique

The principles of the operation are the same whichever surgical approach is used. They are to isolate, occlude, and divide the cystic artery and the cystic duct, and then to remove the gallbladder from the liver bed. A peroperative cholangiogram helps to delineate the biliary anatomy and to identify stones in the bile duct: the operation is best performed on an operating table suitably adapted for cholangiography. General anaesthesia with good relaxation provides the best exposure.

Open operation

Conventional incision

Four incisions can be used for cholecystectomy: midline, right paramedian, right subcostal, or right transverse. A midline incision is useful when the diagnosis is not definite, while a subcostal incision gives the best exposure when difficulties are expected. However, it does not provide good access to the rest of the abdomen. A transverse incision gives a good cosmetic result and less postoperative pain but provides more limited exposure. Choosing the most appropriate incision for any particular patient depends partly on the preference of the surgeon, partly on the build of the patient, and partly on the expected pathology. Improvements in preoperative diagnosis have reduced the need for a full diagnostic laparotomy. On the other hand it is easy and essential always to examine the gallbladder, the liver, the pancreas, the stomach, and the duodenum. In most operations it will be possible to assess the diameter of the bile duct.

Removal of the gallbladder

Calot's triangle

The operative field should be exposed by retraction of the liver upwards, with traction anteriorly and to the right on the neck of the gallbladder with a suitable forceps, while a damp pack held by the assistant retracts the colon and the duodenum inferiorly. Occasionally it is helpful to bring the whole liver down into the wound with a pack placed over the dome of the liver. If the gallbladder is tense and difficult to grasp the operation may be made easier by aspiration of the contents.

The peritoneum over the neck of the gallbladder is incised in front and behind and the contents of Calot's triangle displayed by a combination of blunt and sharp dissection (Fig. 32). Normally, the cystic duct lies in the inferior margin of the triangle with the common hepatic duct medially. The cystic artery crosses the triangle from left to right, running behind the bile duct and arising from the right hepatic artery, which may be visible. However the anatomy is very variable and the dissection must proceed until there is no doubt as to the identity of all the vascular and ductal structures which have been exposed. Once the cystic duct and artery have been definitely identified, the cystic artery is ligated in continuity and divided between ligatures. The cystic duct is dissected as far as is necessary to expose a sufficient length for easy cannulation for operative cholangiography. Any stones in the cystic duct are milked back into the gallbladder and the cystic duct is ligated close to the gallbladder. If cholangiography is to be performed it should be done at this stage. When satisfactory pictures have been obtained the cannula is removed and the cystic duct ligated or oversewn with an absorbable suture. The dissection of the gallbladder from the liver can begin either at the fundus or in the region of the cystic duct. Either way it is important to keep close to the gallbladder wall, and diathermy is needed to achieve haemostasis. Drainage after cholecystectomy is controversial, but we prefer to leave a vacuum drain in the gallbladder bed for 24 h after operation.

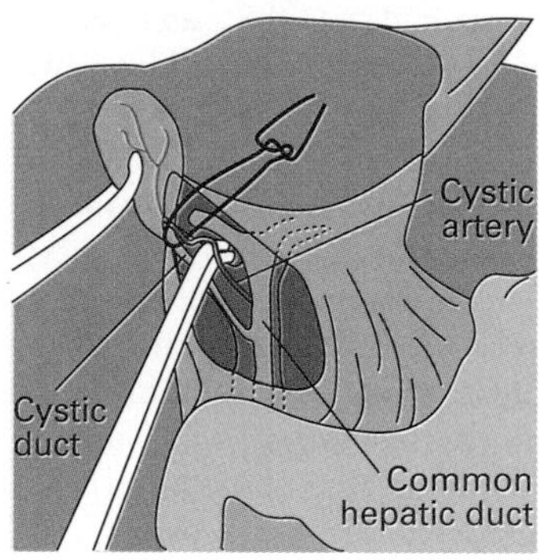

Fig. 32 Dissecting Calot's triangle as the first step in a cholecystectomy. The borders of Calot's triangle are the cystic duct laterally, the common hepatic medially, and the inferior margin of the liver superiorly.

Complications during cholecystectomy

Sudden arterial haemorrhage during a cholecystectomy usually arises from a torn cystic artery. The bleeding point should not be clipped; instead, the wound should be packed tightly with a small swab. It is then essential to wait while haemostasis develops. During this time the surgeon can ensure that the exposure and the illumination are optimal. The wound is then kept dry with a strong sucker while the bleeding point is sutured with a fine 4/0 or 5/0 Prolene stitch. Very occasionally the only way of controlling haemorrhage while the damage is repaired is by occluding the hepatic artery with the fingers and thumb of the left hand placed across the entrance of the lesser sac (Pringle's manoeuvre).

It is sometimes quite impossible to delineate the anatomy of the ductal system by dissection. In these circumstances a cholangiogram is absolutely vital. It is also invaluable when the anatomy is unclear and there is a leak of bile from an unidentified duct.

Peroperative cholangiography

There are good arguments for performing operative cholangiography routinely. From a practical viewpoint good cholangiograms are only obtained with regular practice but they also demonstrate the precise anatomy of the biliary tree (Fig. 33). On the other hand only a small proportion of cholangiograms disclose stones in the duct, some false positive results are obtained, and stones are actually removed from only two-thirds of ducts explored as a result of an abnormal peroperative cholangiogram. It is preferable, therefore, to select patients for operative cholangiography on the basis of a history of jaundice, abnormal preoperative liver function tests, small stones in the gallbladder, and dilatation of the bile duct on preoperative ultrasonography and at operation. A suitable cannula is tied into the cystic duct or a fine butterfly needle is introduced directly into the bile duct itself. After the careful elimination of any air bubbles from the syringe and cannula, dilute contrast material (25 per cent sodium diatrizoate) is then injected. Ideally this should be done during screening of the patient, but more commonly two radiographs are taken, the first

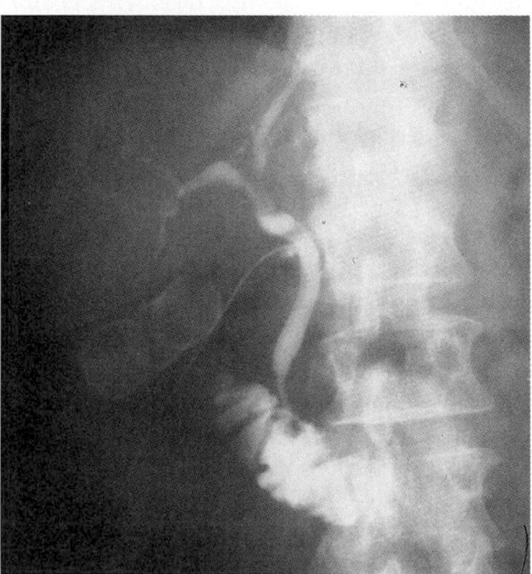

Fig. 33 An operative cholangiogram. Note the cannula inserted into the cystic duct stump (the same patient as in Fig. 25). The three large stones shown in the macroscopic specimen are clearly seen on the radiograph.

after injection of 3 to 5 ml and the second after a further 8 to 12 ml of contrast has been injected. On the first film the bile duct itself will be seen; the second film shows the intrahepatic biliary radicles and contrast in the duodenum. Filling defects in the contrast or the absence of flow into the duodenum are evidence of stones within the duct.

'Fundus first' cholecystectomy

Some surgeons feel that dissection of Calot's triangle first takes the surgeon too close to structures that should be avoided. They prefer to start the operation at the fundus and remove the gallbladder from the liver first. By keeping adjacent to the gallbladder wall the cystic artery and cystic duct are eventually exposed and can be tied well away from other important structures, which are often never seen. Operative cholangiography is performed towards the end of the operation if necessary. Bleeding from the gallbladder bed can be a nuisance and obscure the view of Calot's triangle, but this approach may be easier in a patient with an acutely inflamed gallbladder. It should certainly be adopted if the initial dissection of Calot's triangle in the conventional operation proves to be difficult.

Minicholecystectomy

Much of the morbidity associated with a conventional cholecystectomy arises from the abdominal wall wound which is needed to provide sufficient exposure. However, with modern imaging there is little need for either a laparotomy or an operative cholangiogram, which are the main reasons for a large wound. Minicholecystectomy is performed via a subcostal incision no more than 10 cm long placed right over the gallbladder, which is then dissected out fundus first. Metal clips are placed to occlude the cystic duct and the cystic artery. The incision is closed without drainage. There is little postoperative pain or systemic upset and patients can be discharged 2 or 3 days after surgery.

Laparoscopic cholecystectomy (described in detail in Chapter 13)

This is an extension of minicholecystectomy but it introduces a completely new concept into abdominal surgery. Laparoscopic cholecystectomy is rapidly replacing open cholecystectomy as the procedure of choice in developed countries.

The operation is performed through four laparoscopic ports inserted through the abdominal wall in the right upper quadrant (Fig. 34). The dissection is viewed on a television screen placed beside the operating table and the image is obtained from a television camera attached to a telescope inserted through the subumbilical port.

The cystic duct and the cystic artery are dissected out in exactly the same way as a conventional cholecystectomy, except that subtle alterations in manual dexterity and specialized instruments are required (Fig. 35). Clips are used to occlude the cystic duct and the cystic artery. It is perfectly possible to cannulate the cystic duct for cholangiography (Fig. 36). The gallbladder is dissected from the liver bed using diathermy or sharp dissection: this is often the most difficult part of the operation. The gallbladder is extracted from the abdominal cavity through the umbilical or epigastric incision which may need to be enlarged. A drain can be left to the gallbladder bed if desired. The procedure takes slightly longer than conventional cholecystectomy but postoperative recovery is faster. Pain and sepsis in the wounds are less of a problem (Fig. 37). It remains to be seen whether the mortality and morbidity associated with this procedure are better than those after conventional cholecystectomy.

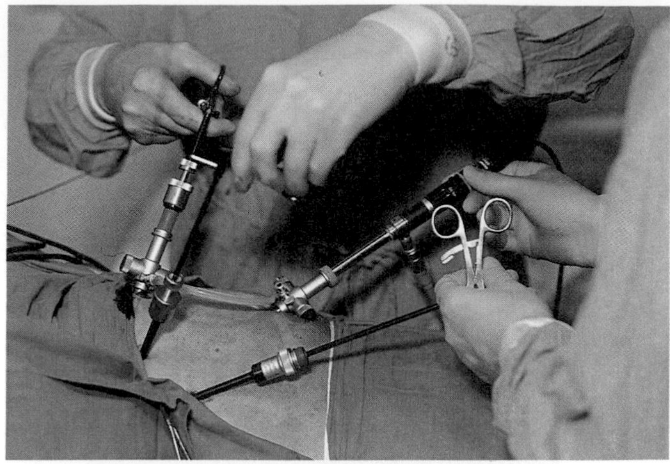

Fig. 34 A view of the abdomen to show the layout of the cannulae during a laparoscopic cholecystectomy.

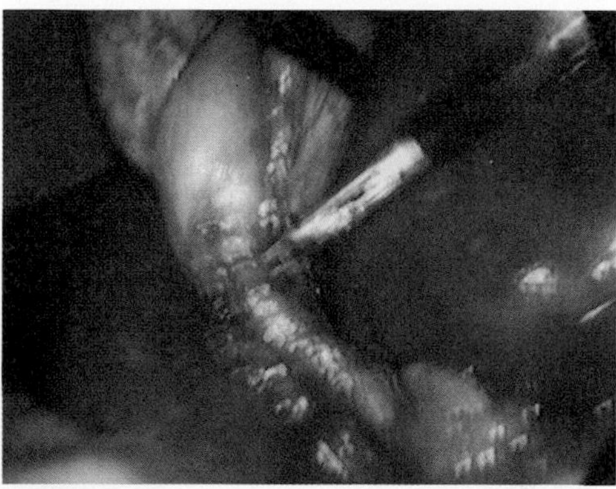

Fig. 35 View of Calot's triangle during a laparoscopic cholecystectomy.

Postoperative care

Most patients recover rapidly, irrespective of the method used for removing the gallbladder. Very few want anything to drink until the following day, except after a laparoscopic procedure when some patients will be able to eat and drink almost as soon as they return to the ward. Unless there is bile in the drain it can usually be removed after 24 h. Prolonged ileus is uncommon and most patients eat on the second postoperative day. After a conventional operation patients need to stay in hospital for 4 or 5 days, compared to 2 or 3 days after a laparoscopic or minicholecystectomy. Most patients need 6 to 8 weeks away from work after a conventional operation, whereas after a laparoscopic procedure 2 weeks is usually sufficient.

Cholecystostomy

Surgical drainage of the gallbladder is rarely necessary: percutaneous ultrasound-guided drainage can now achieve the same result with less disturbance to the patient. On the other hand the surgeon may embark on an urgent cholecystectomy only to realize that the pathology is too severe to allow a safe operation. In these circumstances it is much better simply to drain the gallbladder

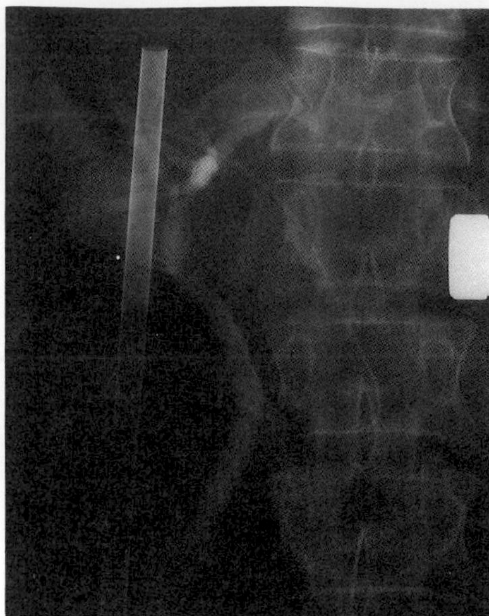

Fig. 36 Operative cholangiogram obtained during a laparoscopic cholecystectomy. The cystic duct is cannulated in the normal way and the cannula held in place either with a special instrument or with a removable metal clip. The laparoscopic cannulae need to be held out of the way during exposure of the radiographs. The 5 mm port at the neck of the gallbladder can be seen on the left of the picture.

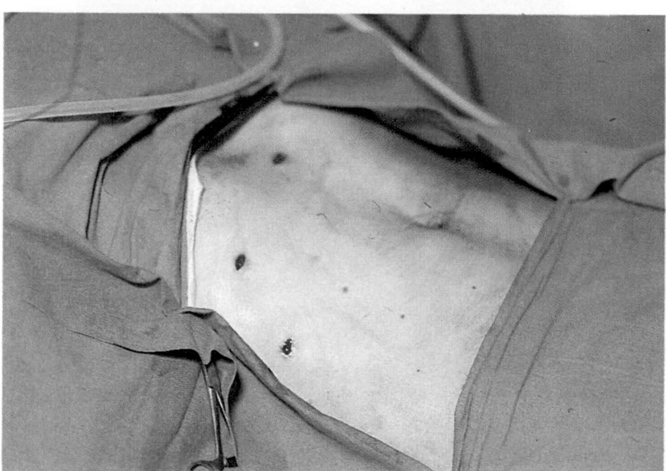

Fig. 37 Postoperative scars following a laparoscopic cholecystectomy.

with a large tube after removing all the stones, allow the inflammation to settle and to remove the gallbladder 6 weeks later.

Partial cholecystectomy

In the same circumstances an alternative to cholecystostomy is partial cholecystectomy. The gallbladder is evacuated of bile and stones and, starting at the fundus, it is dissected away from the liver as far as possible towards the neck of the gallbladder. Part of the wall of the gallbladder may be left in the gallbladder fossa if dissection of the gallbladder away from the liver bed proves difficult. Once the dissection has proceeded as close to the cystic duct and Calot's triangle as is safe, the remainder of the gallbladder is excised and its neck is oversewn. Operative cholangiography is not usually possible, but it is important to try and be sure that any stones in the cystic duct are removed and to leave a drain to the gallbladder bed.

Complications of cholecystectomy

Conventional cholecystectomy is a safe operation: although complications arise in about one to 10 patients they are rarely serious. Pulmonary complications are the most common; wound infection, deep vein thrombosis, and cardiovascular problems account for the remainder. Overall about 1 per cent of patients die. However, there is considerable variation in mortality rate with age. Cardiac and respiratory problems are more frequent in the elderly and it is more common to find complications from the stones themselves, such as an empyema or cholangitis: the mortality rate in patients over the age of 70 may reach 10 per cent.

Damage to the bile duct is a complication that everyone rightly fears (Fig. 38), and occurs roughly once in every 500 cholecystectomies. Damage is avoided by following every rule of the operation without fail on every occasion. If the duct is damaged it is important to recognize the injury and to repair it immediately. The results are then good. When the damage is only recognized some days after the operation, the patient is septic and a biliary fistula has developed.

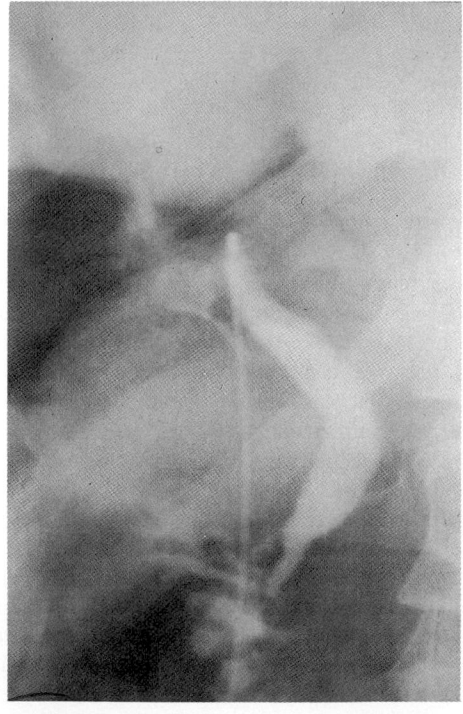

Fig. 38 Operative cholangiogram showing complete division of the bile duct with no contrast filling the intrahepatic ducts. The cannula is tied into the proximal common bile duct.

The postcholecystectomy syndrome

Persistent or recurrent symptoms, excluding early operative complications, are common after cholecystectomy and may be due to a number of conditions. In one prospective study 50 per cent of patients had symptoms 1 year after a cholecystectomy.

Fortunately the majority of patients have only mild complaints and often do not seek medical advice. Severe symptoms occur in 5 to 10 per cent of patients. They are more common in middle-aged patients with a long preoperative history and those who had a normal gallbladder removed. Upper abdominal pain and dyspepsia are common and may be acute and severe. Two-thirds of these patients experience symptoms similar or identical to those experienced before surgery.

When a patient presents with recurrent symptoms the first cause to exclude is a retained or recurrent stone in the bile duct. This accounts for about one-third of the patients. In a further one-third another cause, such as pancreatic or liver disease, peptic ulceration, or the irritable bowel syndrome, is found, and the original diagnosis of gallbladder disease was probably wrong.

Some patients, particularly those in whom the gallbladder was normal, have often had other intra-abdominal organs such as the appendix or the uterus removed. They may show symptoms of anxiety or depression, and they tend to focus a lot of attention on relatively mild symptoms. It is important to exclude the presence of objective organic disease in the biliary tract as far as possible, and then to offer these patients treatment for the underlying problem. Further surgery, including endoscopic sphincterotomy, should be avoided. Even after all the appropriate investigations have been done, no satisfactory cause for the symptoms is found in about one-quarter of such patients.

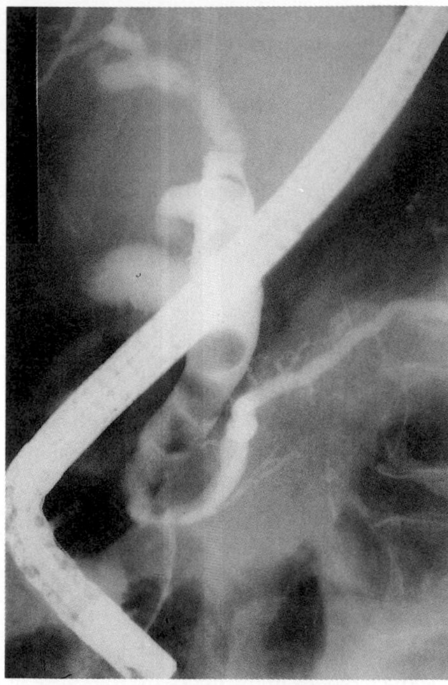

Fig. 39 Endoscopic cholangiogram of a patient admitted collapsed with septicaemia. *Escherichia coli* was grown from a blood culture.

Stones in the bile duct

Stones in the bile duct may lie dormant for many years and only come to light because of an episode of pain, jaundice, or cholangitis (Fig. 13). They may also be discovered by ultrasonography during investigation for stones in the gallbladder (Fig. 10) or by cholangiography during cholecystectomy (Fig. 33). Between 8 and 15 per cent of patients with stones in the gallbladder also have stones in the ducts (choledocholithiasis). The incidence increases with age: one-quarter of patients over 60 years of age have stones in both sites. In patients from the West, most stones are found in the common bile duct, whereas in the East hepatic duct stones are more usual.

Origin of common duct stones

Primary stones form within the bile duct. They are usually bilirubinate stones of the soft brown type, and they are associated with biliary stasis due to obstruction, infection, and the presence of foreign bodies such as food. In the Orient they are generally caused by infection, sometimes associated with parasites within the biliary tract. However, most common duct stones originate in the gallbladder and migrate through the cystic duct into the common bile duct. These secondary stones consist mostly of cholesterol and often grow in size within the duct.

Clinical presentation

Although stones in the bile duct may be silent, the development of symptoms is potentially serious; obstructive jaundice, ascending cholangitis, and acute pancreatitis are all associated with major morbidity and mortality.

Less seriously, stones in the ducts may cause bouts of abdominal pain or dyspepsia indistinguishable from symptoms of gallbladder disease or of intermittent biliary colic with transient jaundice. Elderly patients with bile duct stones sometimes present in apparently obscure ways with malaise, confusion, collapse, or septicaemia (Fig. 39). The cause is often only discovered when routine liver function tests are found to be abnormal. Until recently stones in the bile duct were most commonly discovered at operation. About one in every 10 patients undergoing cholecystectomy was discovered to have stones in the bile duct and required exploration of the duct, although stones were only recovered in perhaps two-thirds of the explorations. Nowadays most bile duct stones are diagnosed by ultrasound and removed endoscopically before cholecystectomy, although surgical exploration of the bile duct is still occasionally necessary.

Obstructive jaundice

Occasionally, a small stone passes into the bile duct and impacts at the ampulla, causing pain and jaundice. The severity of the jaundice depends on the duration of the obstruction, but as the stone passes on spontaneously the jaundice resolves. A solitary stone may disappear from the biliary tree in this way, but normally some stones remain in a thick walled gallbladder to support the diagnosis. Such patients need a cholecystectomy, and an operative cholangiogram is essential.

More commonly there is a larger stone or stones within a dilated bile duct. Sometimes a large number of stones in the duct leads to a significant impairment of bile flow. At other times a stone moves up and down within the duct and acts as a ball valve, causing pain and jaundice when it impacts but allowing the symptoms to resolve spontaneously when it moves away. The site of impaction is usually immediately above the ampulla, but it may be above a fibrotic narrowing in the bile duct caused by the stones themselves. Complete impaction of a stone causes severe progressive jaundice.

Stones in the bile duct usually cause pain. However, it is not easy to distinguish obstructive jaundice due to stones from that due to malignant disease on the basis of pain. Clinical examination normally discloses nothing except a jaundiced patient, and possibly some scratch marks from the intolerable itching. The gallbladder is not palpable since it is thick-walled and fibrotic, and it resists distension, although there is often mild tenderness in the right upper quadrant.

Many of these patients are elderly and require prompt endoscopic sphincterotomy and extraction of their stones. Cholecystectomy can be performed later when the jaundice has resolved. In practice only 10 per cent of such patients have continuing symptoms and need surgery. Patients under the age of 50 who are not profoundly jaundiced are best treated by cholecystectomy and exploration of the duct.

Ascending cholangitis

Ascending cholangitis is still a fatal disease and it must be treated as a medical emergency. Fortunately it is usually an easy diagnosis to make clinically, as most patients present with the classic symptoms of epigastric pain, rigors, and jaundice (Charcot's triad or Charcot's intermittent biliary fever). Elderly patients sometimes present simply with septicaemia or collapse with little or no jaundice, and rarely the origin of a Gram-negative septicaemia is eventually traced back to the bile duct.

Pathology

Cholangitis is always associated with some degree of obstruction within the bile duct: stones in the ducts are the cause in 80 per cent of cases. Many of the patients are elderly. Cholangitis is a rare presentation of malignant biliary obstruction, except in those with carcinoma of the ampulla. Patients with a benign biliary stricture commonly experience recurrent episodes of cholangitis and they always have bacteria in their bile, as do patients with an endoluminal prosthesis in place. Patients with stones nearly always have a positive bile culture, whereas this is only found in 10 per cent of patients with malignant jaundice.

Bacteriology

Most of the bacteria cultured from the bile in patients with cholangitis are also found in the bowel. *Escherichia coli*, *Streptococcus faecalis*, and *Klebsiella* species are the most common pathogens, but Staphylococcus, Pseudomonas, and Proteus may occasionally be present. Anaerobic bacteria such as *Clostridium perfringens* and *Bacteroides fragilis*, although rarely cultured from gallbladder bile, are an important feature in cholangitis. Bacteria reach the liver in the portal vein and are normally cleared there by the reticuloendothelial system. There is also evidence of cholangiovenous reflux of organisms into the circulation when the systemic symptoms of cholangitis become apparent. More than one organism is present in over half of all patients, and there is some evidence of synergy between the aerobic and anaerobic organisms. Antibiotic treatment, which should always be vigorous, must take account of the polymicrobial nature of most infections.

Treatment

The obstructed bile duct must be drained adequately, by the most effective route, and as quickly as possible. However, the patient must first be resuscitated with intravenous fluids and antibiotics. Antibiotic treatment of septicaemia will produce improvement in the patient for a short period, but it will not cure the patient unless the obstruction is relieved. Nowadays this can usually be achieved by an endoscopic sphincterotomy (Fig. 40), but occasionally conventional surgical drainage is still necessary.

Complications

Progression of the septic process within the bile ducts can occur in two separate ways. Sometimes pus develops within the ducts; intrahepatic abscesses may also appear. These abscesses may rupture through the hepatic capsule and give rise to intraperitoneal collections. Purulent cholangitis is often associated with a degree of tension within the biliary system, and there is a gush of purulent bile into the duodenum when the offending stone is released endoscopically.

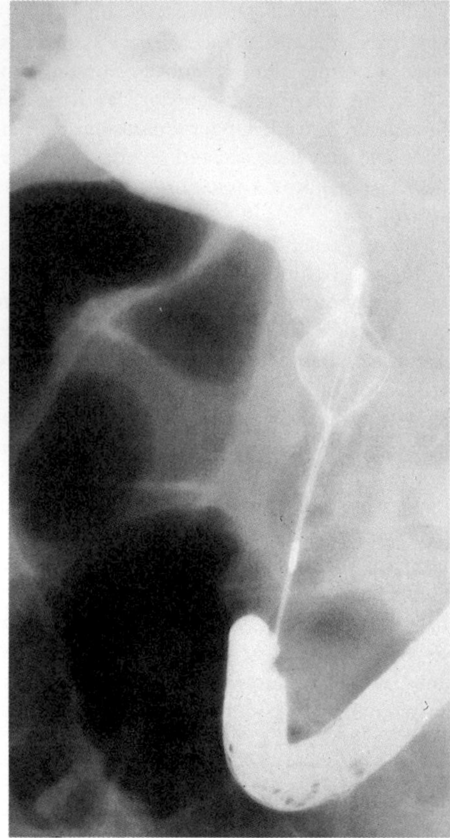

Fig. 40 Stone being extracted from the bile duct with a Dormier basket. This patient had also had a Polya gastrectomy performed some years previously. The endoscope approaches the ampulla along the afferent loop. This is always difficult and is only achieved in less than half the patients.

Alternatively the sepsis may become systemic. Progressive renal and cardiac impairment ensues, and patients develop septic shock. Dialysis or haemofiltration may be required. Occasionally, the presenting feature of cholangitis is complete renal failure or cardiovascular collapse; the mortality rate in these patients is very high.

Acute pancreatitis

Acute pancreatitis is associated with gallstones (see Section 25.1). Impaction of a small stone at the ampulla and occlusion of the pancreatic duct is a cause of pancreatitis in a minority of patients. An early ultrasound examination of the biliary tract is therefore essential in every patient who is admitted with acute pancreatitis, particularly if there is any change in the liver function tests. A few have evidence of stones in the bile duct and an immediate endoscopic sphincterotomy and extraction of the stone is well worthwhile in these patients, as it may abort the episode of pancreatitis immediately. There is no evidence that the pancreatitis is made worse by ERCP, although it is wise to avoid cannulating the pancreatic duct.

Mirizzi syndrome

This is an unusual and specific cause of obstruction of the common hepatic duct by a stone impacted in the cystic duct or Hartmann's pouch. The stone may simply press on the bile duct, but more commonly it ulcerates into the duct, creating a cholecysto-choledochal fistula. Patients present with obstructive jaundice, and cholangiography shows narrowing of the bile duct at the porta hepatis, which can have the appearance of a cholangiocarcinoma (Fig. 41, 42). The true pathology is eventually identified at surgery, but the operation is often extremely difficult because of severe inflammation and fibrosis. It is best to excise the gallbladder, and it is essential to remove the stone causing the obstruction. If this leaves a large gap in the wall of the bile duct, a biliary enteric bypass is needed. Reconstruction of the bile duct over a t-tube brought out through a separate stab incision is possible for smaller defects.

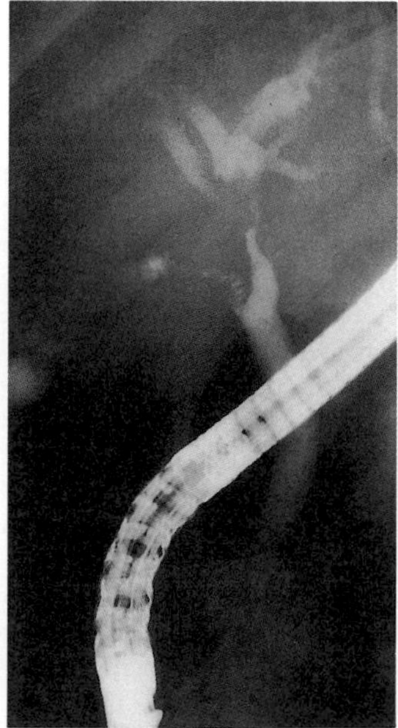

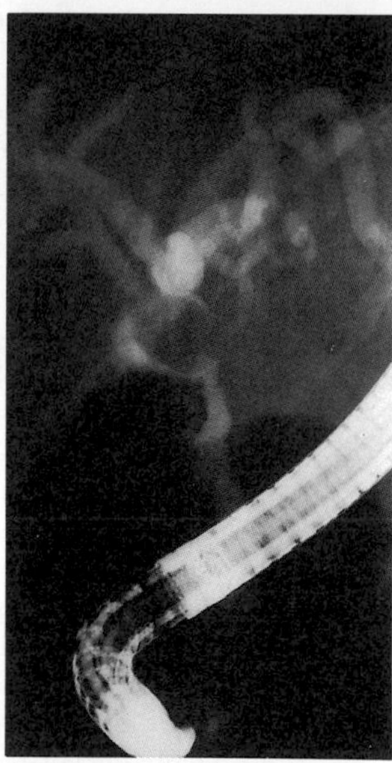

Fig. 41 and 42 Two cholangiograms of the same patient taken 6 weeks apart. The first picture was diagnosed as showing a typical cholangiocarcinoma and an attempt was made to place a stent across the tumour. Six weeks later, a second ERCP a large stone clearly shows in the common hepatic duct. It was easily removed at surgery. This is a classic example of Mirizzi's syndrome and an initial erroneous diagnosis of malignant biliary obstruction is not uncommon.

Investigation of common duct stones

The most important investigation is ultrasound examination of the liver, the bile duct, the gallbladder, and the pancreas. It should be undertaken on the least suspicion of stones or another obstructive lesion in the bile duct. The ultrasonographer need only decide whether or not the bile ducts are dilated. The normal common bile duct should not be greater than 7 mm in diameter when measured on ultrasound (Fig. 10). If the ducts are dilated, the patient has an extrahepatic obstructive cause for his or her symptoms. If the ducts are not dilated it is unlikely that there are stones in the bile duct, but there are two important exceptions to this rule. If the examination is done very soon after a stone has entered the bile duct there may have been insufficient time for dilatation to have developed. The examination should be repeated 1 week later. In patients with cirrhosis of the liver the intrahepatic bile ducts are simply not able to dilate. If there is clinical uncertainty about the presence of a stone within the ducts a cholangiogram is needed.

An experienced ultrasonographer can always detect dilation of the ducts, but the site of the obstruction will only be identified in two-thirds of patients, and the cause of the obstruction in one-third. Nevertheless stones and strictures can sometimes be identified on ultrasound.

Before the introduction of ultrasound, biochemical markers of liver function were important in differentiating surgical from medical jaundice. Their specificity and sensitivity were very poor and they are now only of historical interest. The main value of biochemistry nowadays is to quantify the severity and the duration of an obstruction and to monitor the effects of treatment.

Computed tomography (CT) has a limited place in the imaging of common duct stones. The ultrasound examination may raise the possibility of a malignant obstruction, and a CT scan may be obtained before ERCP. CT detects dilatation of the ducts very reliably (Fig. 14), and it is slightly better than ultrasound at identifying the site and the cause of an obstruction.

The prothrombin time is a marker of coagulation and should always be measured, even if the patient is not jaundiced. Patients with a prolonged prothrombin time should receive vitamin K and may also require fresh frozen plasma to correct a coagulation defect before embarking on an endoscopic sphincterotomy.

Any patient who has any degree of jaundice and a fever must have blood cultures taken before treatment with antibiotics. This may be the only opportunity to identify an organism.

It can still be very difficult to differentiate medical from surgical causes of jaundice and hepatitis occasionally develops in patients who also have stones in the ducts. As soon as this is suspected the immunological markers for hepatitis must be measured, and the laboratory must be warned.

Management of common duct stones

In a patient suspected of having stones in the bile duct and in whom dilatation of the ducts is seen on ultrasound, ERCP should be undertaken unless the patient is to proceed directly to surgery.

In most patients this will confirm the diagnosis and allow the stones to be removed through a sphincterotomy (Fig. 40). A detailed description of ERCP and sphincterotomy is given in Section 27.2. In certain circumstances percutaneous cholangiography is also helpful and other interventional techniques are sometimes needed. Once stones are discovered in the bile duct there should be little delay in removing them. The choice generally lies between an operation or an endoscopic sphincterotomy: the best approach primarily depends on whether or not the patient has undergone previous cholecystectomy.

Stones in the duct and the gallbladder present

Surgical removal is the most appropriate treatment for young or middle-aged patients without serious coexisting disease and with uncomplicated ductal stones. The morbidity and mortality associated with surgical exploration of the bile duct and endoscopic sphincterotomy are very similar in this group of patients, and most of them need their gallbladder removed anyway. Preoperative endoscopic clearance of the ducts may reduce the total time spent in hospital, but it has no other advantage and the risk of long-term complications from sphincterotomy is unknown.

Patients over the age of 60, poor-risk patients, and those with complicated ductal stones are best treated endoscopically. The morbidity and mortality associated with endoscopic treatment is much less in this group of patients, and only 1 in 10 elderly patients need subsequent cholecystectomy. Patients between the ages of 50 and 60 have to be treated on their individual merits.

Stones in the duct and the gallbladder absent

Patients with retained or recurrent stones following cholecystectomy should be treated endoscopically in the first instance, whatever their age. Retained stones are those detected soon after a choledochotomy. Residual stones come to light months or years later. ERCP and sphincterotomy are required as soon as retained stones are found, particularly if they have been deliberately left behind. They are occasionally difficult to remove, particularly if the ducts are small and if the stones lie above the t-tube. Some stones can only be removed once the t-tube has itself been removed, and time must pass to allow the t-tube track to mature before this is safe. Retained stones may pass spontaneously, and they can occasionally be flushed through the ampulla with saline, or dissolved by a solution with stone-dissolving properties; none of these techniques is totally reliable. Extracting retained stones along the mature t-tube track under radiological control (Burhenne technique) is very effective in skilled hands, but the patient has to keep his or her tube and its attendant bag for 6 weeks while the track matures. None of the methods is perfect, and a combination of a percutaneous and an endoscopic technique may be needed. Residual stones, which are often large, require a generous endoscopic sphincterotomy and removal of the stones with a basket or balloon (Fig. 40). Occasionally it is difficult to obtain a cholangiogram or to insert the sphincterotomy knife into the bile duct. Provided there is no doubt about the clinical diagnosis and the ultrasound findings, cutting into the ampulla with a needle knife is justified. This is a dangerous manoeuvre because of the risk of perforation, but once a small cut is made the proper knife will then enter the bile duct and the cut can be extended to a full sphincterotomy in order to extract the stones. Diverticula of the duodenum, which are more common in old age, can be a nuisance as they distort the anatomy of the ampulla and the distal bile duct.

The overall success in clearing the bile duct is about 85 per cent. Large stones are difficult to remove. The limitations of modern technology must be realized: conventional exploration of the common bile duct must be advised if appropriate. Alternatively, it may be possible to reduce the size of the stones with crushing baskets, stone-dissolving agents, or lithotripters. None of these methods work for everyone, all work sometimes. In very elderly and frail people insertion of a plastic stent into the bile duct is excellent palliation. The stent allows drainage of bile and prevents impaction of the stone.

Stones in the duct discovered at cholecystectomy

These stones may be suspected before operation or may appear unexpectedly on the operative cholangiogram (Fig. 33). It is normally appropriate to remove all the stones from the duct at one operation, but there are some exceptions. Small stones in small ducts, particularly if they are impacted at the ampulla, may be best left alone. The former may pass spontaneously whilst impacted stones should be extracted endoscopically after leaving a t-tube in the duct for safety. Similarly in poor risk patients it might be appropriate simply to close the wound, perhaps with a t-tube, and to arrange a prompt endoscopic extraction.

The action required when stones are discovered in the bile duct during a laparoscopic cholecystectomy is not yet clear. One option is simply to convert the operation to an open procedure and to remove the stones in the conventional way. Another is to complete the cholecystectomy, leave a drain in the abdomen, and perform an endoscopic sphincterotomy within a few days. Experts can clear the bile duct of stones laparoscopically, and in time this may well become the standard procedure.

Stones can be removed from the duct surgically, either from above (the supraduodenal approach) or from below (the transduodenal approach). Occasionally both approaches are needed together. The transduodenal operation has been largely superseded by the endoscopic approach which is safer and easier.

Supraduodenal exploration of the common bile duct

Following cholecystectomy and operative cholangiography the common bile duct is exposed above the duodenum. It is not necessary to expose the duct completely for fear of damaging the blood supply but it is helpful to mobilize the second part of the duodenum (Kocher's manoeuvre). The site of the choledochotomy should be as proximal as possible to allow choledochoduodenostomy if required and to leave the greatest length of bile duct above the choledochotomy against the unlikely possibility of the need for repair of a postoperative bile duct stricture.

Two stay sutures are placed on either side of the proposed choledochotomy and the duct is opened longitudinally along the anterior wall (Fig. 43). A sample of bile is sent for culture. Following careful removal of any obvious stones, the ducts are then flushed with an umbilical catheter. Choledochoscopy with either a rigid or a flexible instrument is then performed, first upwards into the intrahepatic ducts (Fig. 44) and then downwards to the ampulla. The saline infusion not only provides a view (Fig. 45) but also washes stones and debris out of the ducts. It is easier to see the intrahepatic ducts and much more difficult to be sure that the retroduodenal portion of the bile duct is clear of stones. Desjardin's forceps, a Fogarty balloon catheter, and a Dormia basket may all be helpful in extracting stones. The ampulla should never be dilated with metal bougies. They rarely dilate the ampulla but usually create a fistula into the duodenum immediately above the ampullary opening. Very narrow choledochoscopes with an outside diameter of 3 mm are now available. These pass down the

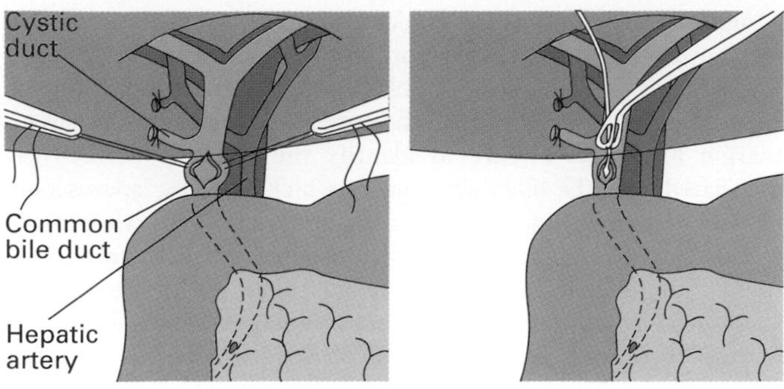

Fig. 43 The approach to supraduodenal exploration of the bile duct.

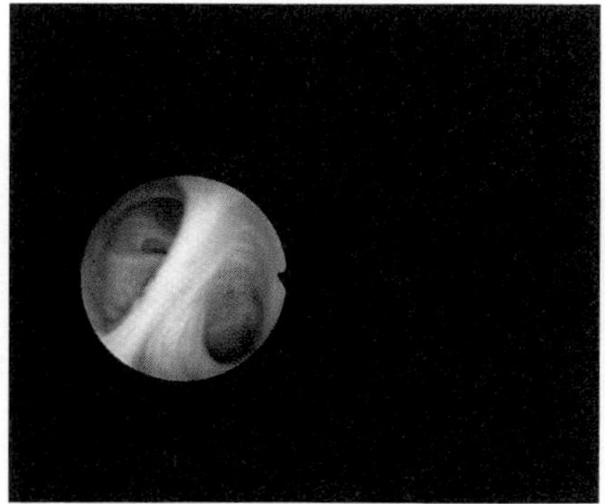

Fig. 44 The junction of the right and left hepatic ducts seen from within the bile duct at choledochoscopy. Second order bile ducts are seen beyond. This picture and the next were taken through a flexible choledochoscope.

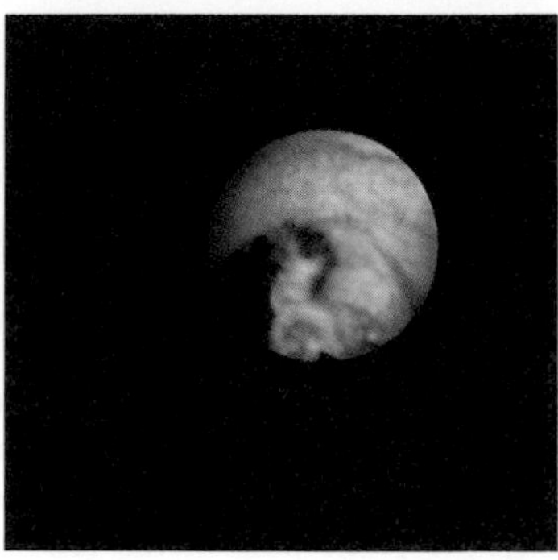

Fig. 45 A stone in the retroduodenal portion of the common bile duct seen at choledochoscopy.

cystic duct into the bile duct and they can be used through a laparoscope port.

Some surgeons like to repeat the cholangiogram to confirm that the duct has been cleared. However, it is difficult to obtain satisfactory pictures and the failure to remove all the stones at an exploration is not regarded as an error. It is sometimes safer and wiser to leave a difficult stone behind for later retrieval than to cause damage to the bile duct by prolonged attempts at its removal.

Once all the stones and debris have been removed a 16 Fg guttered latex t-tube is placed in the common bile duct. The free end is brought out laterally through the abdominal wall. This position keeps the radiologist's hands away from the X-ray beam during cholangiography, and the size of tube will allow percutaneous extraction of a retained stone if this becomes necessary. The choledochotomy is then closed with a fine absorbable suture and a drain is placed in the subhepatic space prior to closure of the wound.

Postoperatively the t-tube is allowed to drain freely into a sterile, closed, drainage bag. A t-tube cholangiogram is obtained 9 or 10 days after surgery (Fig. 46) and, if the duct is clear, the t-tube is clamped. Provided the patients does not develop any pain or discomfort the tube can be removed 24 h later. Drainage from the t-tube site usually ceases within 48 h.

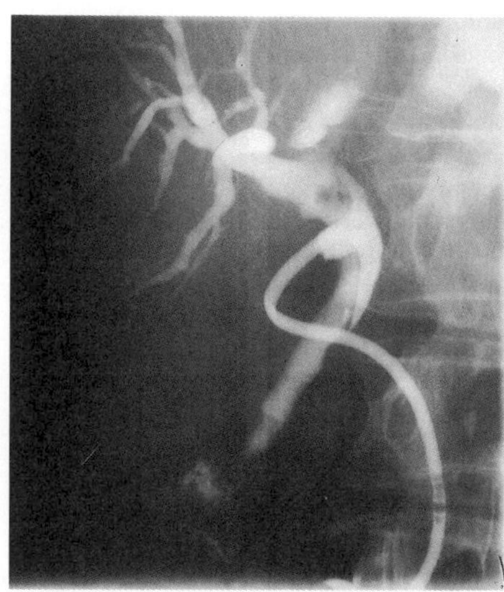

Fig. 46 T-tube cholangiogram showing a retained stone. The stone lies alongside the upper arm of the t-tube. It was removed at ERCP.

Transduodenal exploration of the bile duct

In this operation the bile duct is approached across the duodenum and through the ampulla. It is usually combined with a sphincteroplasty. The duodenum is fully mobilized and a longitudinal incision is made in the right lateral wall over the ampulla. A probe is then passed into the bile duct and the ampullary sphincter is divided with scissors. Fine catgut sutures are placed to appose the mucosa of the bile duct to the duodenum and the stones are then extracted with Desjardin forceps. The choledochoscope can be used to ensure that all the stones have been removed and the duodenum is then closed. The advantage of this approach is that any missed stone will pass spontaneously. The disadvantage is the risk of pancreatitis from interference with the ampulla. Most patients who need a transampullary approach to their bile ducts are better treated endoscopically.

Choledochoduodenostomy

Occasionally an alternative to closure of the common bile duct over a t-tube after a supraduodenal exploration is a choledochoduodenostomy. Provided the bile duct is more than 15 mm in diameter the operation is quick and easy to perform, and there are no worries about retained stones. The vertical incision in the common bile duct is sutured to a longitudinal incision in the duodenum with a single layer of stitches. Results in elderly patients are satisfactory, but in patients who have had the anastomosis for a number of years recurrent cholangitis may develop. This is known as the 'sump syndrome': infection arises from stones and vegetable matter which collect in the retroduodenal portion of the bile duct between the anastomosis and the ampulla. There may also be stenosis of the choledochoduodenostomy. Endoscopic sphincterotomy of the ampulla and balloon dilatation of the anastomosis may alleviate the symptoms, but treatment is not very satisfactory.

Biliary peritonitis

Percutaneous cholangiography is the most common cause of bile peritonitis, although there is usually blood present as well. Provided the signs are localized treatment can be conservative, although if there is a significant biliary obstruction it is likely that the leak will persist. It is still wise to perform percutaneous cholangiography only when it is also possible to relieve any obstruction, either radiologically or at an operation within 12 h.

Occasionally the acutely inflamed gallbladder perforates and fills the peritoneum with bile; this may also happen if a t-tube is removed too soon. Bile peritonitis can be difficult to diagnose clinically because uninfected bile is often not particularly irritant and the signs may be very subdued. Once the diagnosis is made laparotomy is usually needed, but for smaller more localized collections, as may occur after a percutaneous cholangiogram, ultrasound guided drainage may be sufficient.

Benign biliary structure

Postoperative stricture

Almost all injuries to the bile ducts occur during an easy cholecystectomy; the most common mistake is to confuse the common hepatic duct for the cystic duct. The 'duct' is tied and divided, thus excising a length of the common hepatic duct in the hilum of the liver (Fig. 38). A similar injury can occur during laparoscopic cholecystectomy. Very few patients have undergone operative cholangiography.

Aetiology and prevention

Poor surgical technique is the most common cause of a significant biliary injury. The precise individual anatomy has not been correctly identified, although various anatomical and pathological factors may have made this difficult. The surgeon thinks that narrow ducts are too narrow to be the bile duct. The cystic duct may run alongside the bile duct for a distance, which leads the surgeon into the wrong plane. Anatomical variations of the main ducts also predispose to damage. The cystic duct may enter the right hepatic duct; sometimes there is no right duct, and the right anterior hepatic duct runs very close to the cystic duct. Such anatomical variations are one of the justifications for performing operative cholangiography. During the operation excessive fibrosis and inflammation in the porta hepatis and sudden inadvertent haemorrhage are both dangerous and put the bile ducts at risk.

Inadequate exposure is the cause of most injuries. An adequate and correctly placed initial incision is essential Excessive traction is to be avoided and it is not necessary to trace the cystic duct right to the junction with the bile duct. Once any difficulty is encountered a cholangiogram is invaluable.

Two new operations have increased the risks of bile duct injury. Minicholecystectomy is undertaken through the smallest possible incision and exposure is therefore minimal. Dissection must stay immediately adjacent to the gallbladder wall until the cystic duct is reached. Correctly performed, the operation is safe, but there is no margin for error. Failure to identify the anatomy correctly is associated with the bile duct injuries which occur at laparoscopic cholecystectomy, but the causes are different. The two-dimensional television image causes difficulties in orientation and judgement of depth, and the necessary manual skills are strange to most surgeons. Exposure is not normally a problem and indeed the view of the anatomy, particularly in obese patients, is excellent (Fig. 35). If difficulty is encountered nothing must be divided until the anatomy is clear. A cholangiogram may help and an open operation must be undertaken if this would be a safer option.

Diagnosis

In about one-quarter of patients the injury is recognized at the time of operation and in a further third it comes to light within the next month. Most of these latter patients present with jaundice, sometimes with cholangitis and sometimes with a biliary fistula. The remaining patients present months or years later with recurrent cholangitis. In the early postoperative period ERCP is the most useful imaging technique for displaying the extent of the damage; this may provide an opportunity to place a stent if this is appropriate. Contrast medium injected along the track of a fistula may define the injury and the bile ducts adequately.

In patients who present later, both ERCP and percutaneous transhepatic cholangiography may be needed to display the superior and the inferior aspects of the stricture. It may also be possible to relieve the obstruction by placing a self expanding metal stent across the structure. These patients with long-standing incomplete obstruction and infection have a significant risk of liver damage and portal hypertension. The presence and the severity of these complications require investigations such as a liver biopsy and oesophagoscopy looking for varices.

Treatment

Many surgeons realize with horror during a cholecystectomy that they have just tied the bile duct. The tie should be removed and nothing further needs to be done. Strictures do not develop afterwards.

Immediate repair of a damaged duct

A serious injury may take one of three forms. First, there may be a short incision into the bile duct, perhaps with a ragged edge if tearing was a feature of the injury. This is commonly caused by inferior traction on the cystic duct at the junction with the bile duct. Second, the bile duct may be divided clean across, perhaps obliquely, but there is no loss of length. Third, a portion of the duct may be excised.

Most surgeons are able to deal with the first two injuries. In the first, the incision can be closed directly with fine absorbable sutures, over a t-tube if necessary. In the second case the bile duct should be repaired with interrupted fine absorbable sutures over a t-tube (Fig. 47). A t-tube should never be brought out through the damaged area of duct because the irritation, inflammation, and fibrosis is likely to increase the risk of subsequent stricture. It must always be placed through a separate stab incision above or below the repair.

The best results of treatment of the third type of injury are obtained if an experienced biliary surgeon is called to help. If a complete length of duct has been excised only a tiny stump of

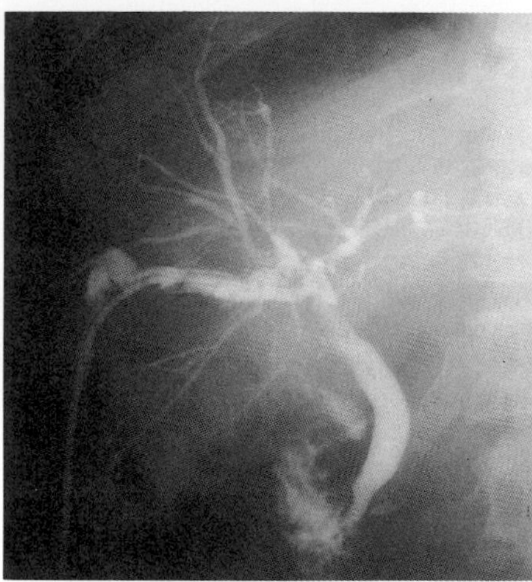

Fig. 47 Immediate end to end repair of a divided bile duct over a t-tube. The bile duct had been cut straight across and there was no loss of length. There is some leakage of contrast along the t-tube track but this was not clinically apparent. This is the same case as Fig. 38.

hepatic duct is likely to remain, and the wisest course is to reconstruct the biliary system at once with an hepaticojejunostomy to a Roux loop of jejunum. With experience a choledochoduodenostomy may be safe, but there is always the risk of excessive tension on the anastomosis and a subsequent stricture. Partial excision of one wall of the duct is the most dangerous injury of all. It is tempting to mobilize the duct above and below and to suture the defect transversely over a t-tube. Experience is required to judge whether the degree of tension is excessive. If there is any doubt an hepaticojejunostomy is safer.

Late repair of a damaged duct

Patients who present at any time after the original operation should be referred to a specialist unit. The first requirement is to control any sepsis by drainage of pus and appropriate antibiotics, and to ensure free drainage of bile so far as this is possible. It is then necessary to establish the precise nature and extent of the damage. The anatomy of all the bile ducts inside and outside the liver must be defined, and an arteriogram is essential if surgical reconstruction is planned. It is not uncommon to find concomitant damage to the hepatic artery or the portal vein. Many of these patients are malnourished and need parenteral nutrition. There should be no hurry to perform surgery.

The objective of treatment is to achieve long-term unobstructed drainage of bile to the bowel. Drainage can be achieved in several ways, but usually means a direct mucosa to mucosa anastomosis of the bile duct to a Roux loop of jejunum. There is a definite place for endoscopic or percutaneous balloon dilatation or stenting of a stricture, certainly as a temporary measure and occasionally as definitive treatment in high-risk patients. Inadequate treatment of a stricture is dangerous. The patient's symptoms may improve but there is nevertheless a slow and progressive deterioration in liver function, which ultimately proves fatal.

Complications and results

The best results are obtained when a bile duct injury is discovered immediately and when a suitable tension-free repair is performed, which heals with minimal scarring. The worst results arise in patients who have undergone multiple previous repairs and who have evidence of liver failure and portal hypertension. Injuries in the porta hepatis have a worse prognosis than more proximal damage probably because they are technically more difficult to repair.

The operative mortality is at least 5 per cent and uncontrollable haemorrhage and renal failure are common causes of death, often associated with infection and an external biliary fistula. Many patients experience one or more major complications. Bile duct repairs are notorious for the formation of a recurrent stricture. In the past about one in three patients could expect further trouble; recently this has fallen to one in 10 patients. Despite the difficulties they should be offered a further attempt at operation: previous failure does not preclude a successful outcome.

Postinflammatory stricture

Narrowing of the bile duct is often seen at ERCP in association with chronic inflammation in or around the duct usually from bile duct stones and sometimes from chronic pancreatitis. In patients with stones the stricture tends to be in the retroduodenal portion of the duct, and the important point from the endoscopist's point of view is to be sure that the stone will come through the narrow area if it is engaged in a basket. Failure to realize this problem is the most common cause of a trapped basket during attempted endoscopic removal of a bile duct stone (Fig. 48). Significant and short inflammatory strictures of the duct appear to respond well to balloon dilatation, although if dilatation fails surgery is needed. Rarely, chronic pancreatitis may cause narrowing of the proximal bile duct. Jaundice developing during an acute exacerbation

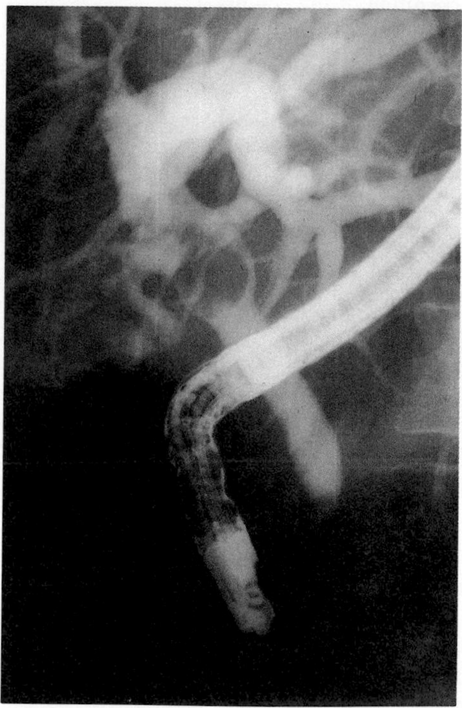

Fig. 48 The large stone in the common hepatic duct is wider than the proximal common bile duct. Unwisely the stone was trapped in a Dormier basket but it could not be retrieved through the narrow proximal common bile duct into the duodenum. The stone and the basket were both removed at an open operation performed the same day.

usually fades spontaneously. When there is evidence of long-term obstruction from severe fibrosis, an end-to-side choledochoduodenostomy is necessary.

Ampullary stenosis

The incidence of this condition is controversial. The main symptom that leads to investigation is episodic pain with features which strongly suggest a biliary origin. Most of these patients will have undergone previous cholecystectomy. There are no absolute diagnostic criteria, but the most useful are the combination of abnormal liver function tests, dilatation of the bile duct, delayed emptying of contrast, and difficulty in cannulating the ampulla at an ERCP performed by an experienced endoscopist. In specialist units manometric studies of ampullary function and special provocation tests may help to identify these patients and indicate those who will benefit from a sphincterotomy. The precise histological changes are uncertain, but in most cases there is excessive fibrosis and inflammation of both the mucosa and the muscle of the ampulla. If the diagnosis is well established before operation the results are good.

Sclerosing cholangitis

Sclerosing cholangitis is characterized by an obliterative inflammatory fibrosis of the biliary tract that leads to chronic liver disease. Sometimes the fibrosis is clearly secondary to stones in the bile duct or previous biliary surgery, but primary sclerosing cholangitis, in which these predisposing causes are absent, is a disease entity on its own. The appearance on cholangiography is diagnostic, although occasionally only time will exclude cholangiocarcinoma (Fig. 49). Primary sclerosing cholangitis was regarded as a rare disease but the advent of ERCP has resulted in greater recognition of the condition.

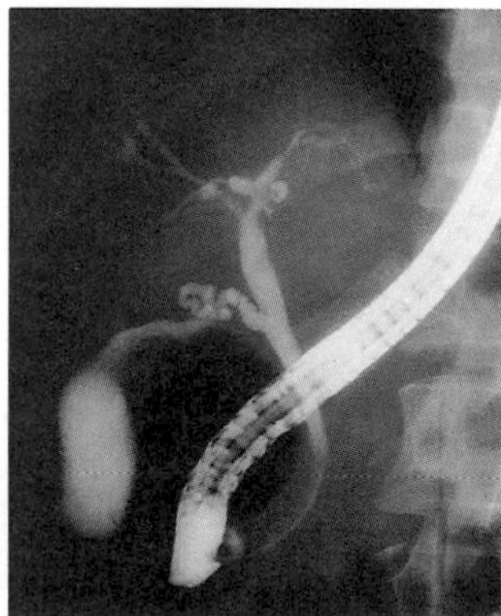

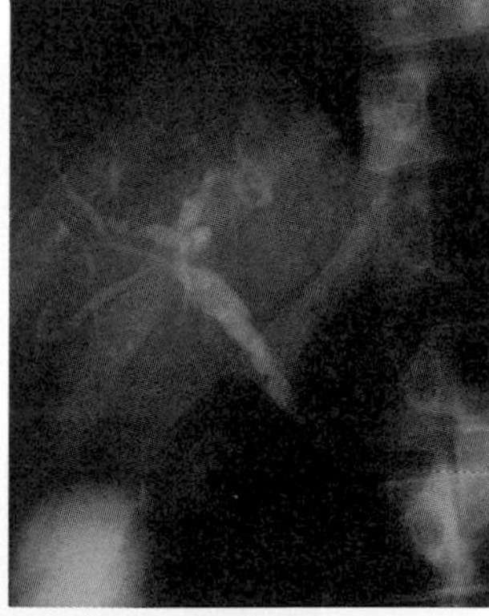

Fig. 49 Cholangiogram showing the typical appearances of primary sclerosing cholangitis with beading of both the intra- and the extrahepatic ducts. The cholangiogram on the right was obtained 2 years after the picture on the left and demonstrates the progression of the disease.

Aetiology

The cause of primary sclerosing cholangitis is unknown. The association with ulcerative colitis in two-thirds of patients suggests that chronic low-grade portal bacteraemia or the absorption of toxic bile acids from the diseased colon might be significant aetiological factors, but neither hypothesis has much experimental support. Recently, phenotyping studies have shown a much higher frequency of HLA-B8, DR3, DQ2, and DRw52A in patients with primary sclerosing cholangitis than in controls. These findings not only confirm the role of genetic factors but also suggest that the disease is immunologically mediated, as this phenotype is closely associated with a number of autoimmune diseases. Overall, current evidence suggests that primary sclerosing cholangitis is an immunologically mediated disease, perhaps triggered in genetically susceptible subjects by acquired toxic or infectious agents.

Diagnosis

Men are twice as commonly affected as are women and most patients present between the ages of 25 and 40. The usual symptoms are fatigue, intermittent jaundice, weight loss, upper abdominal pain, and pruritus. Attacks of acute cholangitis are surprisingly rare, unless there has been instrumental biliary intervention. Approximately half of all symptomatic patients have jaundice or hepatosplenomegaly. Many patients are discovered because of an abnormally high alkaline phosphatase on routine testing, usually during investigation of ulcerative colitis. Serum levels of bilirubin and alkaline phosphatase are usually elevated, the latter more than the former. These levels also fluctuate during the course of the disease. The cholangiogram is diagnostic, with typical beading from irregular stricturing and dilatation of both the intra- and extrahepatic ducts (Fig. 49). Occasionally only the intrahepatic ducts are involved; very rarely the disease affects only the extrahepatic system. Liver histology is not often diagnostic. The early features are periductal fibrosis, portal oedema, and bile ductular proliferation. Later fibrosis spreads into the liver parenchyma leading ultimately to biliary cirrhosis. Although primary sclerosing cholangitis and ulcerative colitis are closely linked the course of each disease is apparently independent. The colitis usually extends throughout the colon but causes few symptoms. Colectomy makes no difference to the course of the cholangitis.

Treatment

There is no curative treatment. Trials of corticosteroids, immunosuppressants, cholecystogogues, and antibiotics, either alone or in combination, have been universally disappointing. Management is directed towards minimizing symptoms and treating complications. Pruritus responds to cholestyramine; antibiotics are needed during episodes of cholangitis. Mechanical relief of a well-defined stricture is well worthwhile. In many patients the best approach is to place a stent across the obstruction either percutaneously or endoscopically. Balloon dilatation of the strictures may also be very effective.

Surgical treatment is controversial. Resection of extrahepatic strictures and reconstruction over Silastic stents produces good results in some series, but orthotopic liver transplantation is the only option available to young patients with primary sclerosing cholangitis and advanced liver disease. Recently, a 4-year survival rate of 70 per cent in 75 transplanted patients has been reported.

The average time between the onset of symptoms and death is about 7 years, and most patients die from hepatic failure. About one-quarter of patients with primary sclerosing cholangitis eventually develop a bile duct carcinoma, which frequently follows a very aggressive course.

Biliary fistula

Leakage of bile from the biliary tract can occur from the liver, the gallbladder, or the bile duct itself, and it may leak to the skin via the peritoneum or to the bowel. Some fistulae are created deliberately, such as a choledochoduodenostomy. Others develop from a pathological process, either from surgical complications, from ulceration of a stone, or from drainage of pus into an adjacent structure.

External biliary fistula

The most common external fistula develops following surgery. Even after a straightforward cholecystectomy there may be a little bile in the drain the following day. Larger volumes of bile occasionally drain, presumably because the tie on the cystic duct stump has slipped. Providing a stone has not been left in the bile duct and that there is no other cause of biliary obstruction the volume will decrease and the fistula will close spontaneously.

A t-tube in the common bile duct is technically a fistula. Normally a cholangiogram will be performed before the t-tube is removed to confirm that there is free flow into the duodenum; the fistula closes rapidly once the t-tube is removed. Any delay in closure implies some degree of obstruction, such as a residual stone, and an ERCP is necessary.

The late development of a fistula after an open cholecystectomy almost always signifies unrecognized damage to the bile duct and comes to light after the drainage of an abscess (Fig. 50). These patients are usually ill and septic. They need careful evaluation and investigation before any further surgical intervention. Biliary leaks from the cystic duct stump are a complication of laparascopic cholecystectomy. Placing a stent in the bile duct at ERCP normally stops these leaks at once.

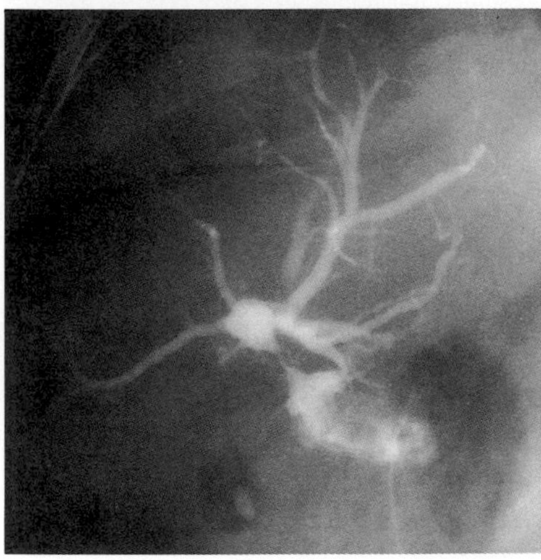

Fig. 50 External biliary fistula following a left hepatectomy for a chronic abscess in the left liver. The right posterior hepatic ductal system fills from a sinogram. The fistula was repaired with a loop of jejunum anastomosed to the right posterior hepatic duct.

Severe cholangitis occasionally leads to an intrahepatic abscess, which ruptures first into the perihepatic peritoneum. Biliary peritonitis rarely ensues because of surrounding adhesions, but when the abscess is drained externally a fistula results. Such a fistula will only close when the proximal obstruction that caused the cholangitis is removed or relieved. This may not be possible with a malignant obstruction.

Any significant bile loss externally is accompanied by rapid fluid and electrolyte depletion which must be vigorously replaced. If the patient will tolerate it bile can be returned to the bowel via a nasogastric tube.

Internal biliary fistula

Spontaneous internal fistulae are uncommon and are usually discovered at cholecystectomy when a communication between the gallbladder and the duodenum becomes apparent as Hartmann's pouch is dissected away from the bowel. This usually results when a stone has ulcerated into the duodenum and disappeared in the faeces. There are no specific symptoms to suggest that this has happened, except when a large stone escapes and impacts in the terminal ileum, giving rise to gallstone ileus. Rarely, the stone ulcerates into the stomach or the colon. In the latter instance patients have profuse diarrhoea as the bile is irritant to the colon.

The treatment is to remove the gallbladder and to close the hole in the bowel. It is very rarely necessary to resect the bowel, but it is wise to leave a drain in the wound.

Recurrent pyogenic cholangitis

A specific type of cholangitis occurs in patients of Asiatic or Oriental origin, affecting predominantly the intrahepatic bile ducts, which contain soft stones and strictures (see also Sections 41.5 and 41.6). The left hepatic system is more frequently affected than is the right, and liver abscesses are a common complication. Both sexes are affected equally, and the condition presents at a younger age than Western cholelithiasis. The gallbladder is only inflamed in about one-fifth of patients, and it rarely contains stones.

Pathology

Infection of small biliary radicles by bowel organisms, probably from an episode of gastroenteritis, is thought to be the cause. The disease is more common in malnourished people and in some populations there is an association with infection by *Clonorchis sinensis* and *Ascaris lumbricoides*. Bacterial enzymes split soluble conjugated bilirubin, forming bilirubinate sludge. Strictures of the ducts are also a constant feature, but it is uncertain whether the stones or the strictures appear first.

The primary pathology is in the bile ducts, and the liver is involved secondarily. In the acute stage the liver is oedematous and there is inflammation around the portal tracts and thrombophlebitis of the portal veins. After recurrent attacks the bile ducts become thickened and stenosed, surrounded by fibrous tissue and a chronic inflammatory infiltrate. Secondary changes develop in the liver.

Diagnosis

A clinical diagnosis is easy to make in the right context. There are typical symptoms of recurrent cholangitis in a young patient of Asian or Oriental origin and signs of chronic hepatic infection. Viral hepatitis is the principal differential diagnosis. Ultrasound and ERCP are the main diagnostic investigations required, but blood culture and examination of the stools for parasites are also important.

Treatment

Treatment of the acute stage is directed at controlling the infection with intravenous fluids and antibiotics. Surgery is avoided unless the patient's condition deteriorates because of septicaemia from severe obstruction or generalized peritonitis from pancreatitis, rupture, or an empyema of the gallbladder, or rupture of a distended hepatic duct on the surface of the liver. Acute operations are directed at draining the biliary tree with a t-tube through a choledochotomy after clearing the duct of as many stones as possible.

Elective surgery is intended to remove the stones from the biliary tract and to relieve any strictures that are present. This is difficult and tedious surgery, because the stones are very soft and do not wash away easily. On occasion some form of limited hepatic resection may be the best form of treatment; this is particularly useful if only the left hepatic system is diseased. Most surgeons also remove the gallbladder. As the name implies the disease tends to recur with time although the ultimate prognosis is very unpredictable. When complications develop the outlook is poor.

Biliary hydatid disease

The liver is the most common site for a hydatid cyst in man (see also Section 41.8). Such cysts grow slowly in size and about two-thirds of patients present with simple hepatomegaly. Of the remainder one in eight are found by accident and a similar number present with biliary colic and transient jaundice due to rupture of the cyst into the biliary tree. Attention is mostly directed towards treatment of the primary cyst, which includes treatment with drugs which kill the parasite. Imaging of the biliary system is important. If hydatid elements are present in the ducts they must be removed through a choledochotomy at the same time as removal of the main cyst. Choledochoscopy before closure is useful to ensure that the duct is clear, and the choledochotomy is then closed over a t-tube. Sometimes it is wise to perform a transduodenal sphincteroplasty to ensure free drainage of any residual hydatid material into the bowel. Nowadays it might be easier to do this endoscopically soon after removal of the cyst. Occasionally, a biliary fistula persists after removal of hydatid cyst: ERCP and sphincterotomy with removal of any daughter cysts or hydatid debris from the bile ducts should allow the fistula to close.

Benign tumours of the biliary tract

Neoplasia of the biliary tract is uncommon. Carcinoma of the gallbladder and bile duct appear infrequently, and benign tumours are decidedly rare.

Polyps in the gallbladder are sometimes seen on ultrasound or on a cholecystogram. The majority of these are cholesterol polyps or adenomyomas and are not, therefore, true tumours. If gallstones are also present and causing symptoms then the patient needs a cholecystectomy. If they are an isolated finding most surgeons believe that they sometimes cause symptoms; provided these are sufficiently severe surgery is justified. If surgery is not appropriate and the polyps are large they should be monitored radiologically, and removal is advised if they enlarge.

True adenomas do occur and they have a malignant potential. This is most likely to occur if they are larger than 10 mm in diameter and sessile. Such patients require cholecystectomy.

Papillomas of the bile duct occur most commonly at the ampulla and are usually small. They present with biliary tract obstruction or recurrent pancreatitis. ERCP reveals the lesion unfolding into the duodenum as the sphincterotomy is made. These lesions are usually regarded as premalignant, and they should be removed either surgically or endoscopically. Papillomas are sometimes multiple and when crowded together look like a villous adenoma (Fig. 51). These lesions tend to recur and to become malignant. It is obviously important to remove them; depending on their site in the biliary tract and their extent, this may require an hepatic resection.

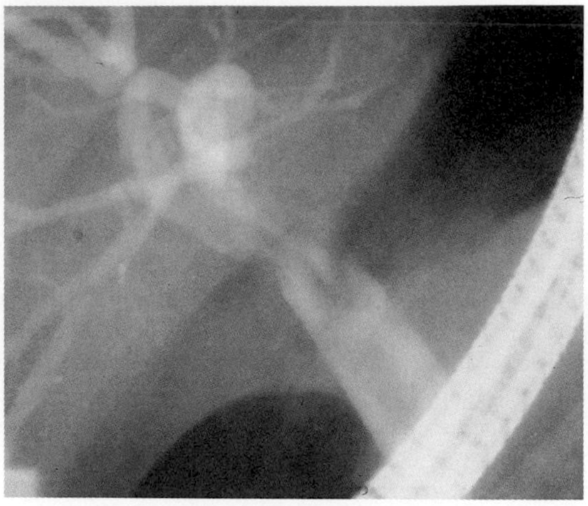

Fig. 51 Endoscopic retrograde cholangiogram of a patient with a villous adenoma of the left hepatic duct. The tumour can be seen extending out of the left hepatic duct and partially occluding the right hepatic duct. This was removed by a left hepatectomy.

FURTHER READING

Admirand WH, Small DM. The physicochemical basis of cholesterol gallstone formation in man. *J Clin Invest* 1968; **47**: 1043–52.

Aldridge MC, Bismuth H. Gallbladder cancer: the polyp-cancer sequence. *Br J Surg* 1990; **77**: 363–4.

Armstrong CP, Taylor TV, Jeacock J, Lucas S. The biliary tract in patients with acute gallstone pancreatitis. *Br J Surg* 1985; **72**: 551–5.

Ashby BS. Acute and recurrent torsion of the gallbladder. *Br J Surg* 1965; **52**: 182–4.

Baron RL, *et al.* A prospective comparison of the evaluation of biliary obstruction using computed tomography and ultrasonography. *Radiology* 1982; **145**: 91–8.

Belli L, Del Favero E, Marni A, Romani F. Resection versus pericystectomy in the treatment of hydatidosis of the liver. *Am J Surg* 1983; **145**: 239–42.

Benbow EW. Xanthogranulomatous cholecystitis. *Br J Surg* 1990; **77**: 255–6.

Blumgart LH, ed. *Surgery of the Liver and Biliary Tract*. Edinburgh: Churchill Livingstone, 1988.

Blumgart LH, Kelley CJ, Benjamin IS. Benign bile duct stricture following cholecystectomy: critical factors in management. *Br J Surg* 1984; **71**: 836–43.

Bodvall B. The postcholecystectomy syndromes. *Clin Gastroenterol* 1973; **2**: 103–26.

Bouchier IAD. Gall stones. *Br Med J* 1990; **300**: 592–7.

Boyden EA. The anatomy of the choledochoduodenal junction in man. *Surg Gynecol Obstet* 1957; **104**: 641–52.

Burhenne HJ. Percutaneous extraction of retained biliary tract stones: 661 patients. *Am J Roentgenol* 1980; **134**: 888–98.

Chapman RW, *et al.* Primary sclerosing cholangitis—a review of its clinical features, cholangiography and hepatic histology. *Gut* 1980; **21**: 870–7.

Chen HH, Zhang WH, Wang SS. Twenty-two year experience with the diagnosis and treatment of intrahepatic calculi. *Surg Gynecol Obstet* 1984; **159**: 519–24.

Chiverton SG, Inglis JA, Hudd C, Kellet MJ, Russell RCG, Wickham JEA. Percutaneous cholecystolithotomy: the first 60 patients. *Br Med J* 1990; **300**: 1310–2.

Cooperberg PL, Burhenne HJ. Real-time ultrasonography. Diagnostic technique of choice in calculous gallbladder disease. *N Engl J Med* 1980; **302**: 1277–9.

Cotton PB. Progress Report ERCP. *Gut* 1977; **18**: 316–41.

Couinaud C. *Le Foie: Études Anatomiques et Chirurgicales*. Paris: Masson & Cie, 1957: 9–12.

Csendes A, Carlos Diaz J, Burdiles P, Maluenda F, Nava O. Mirizzi syndrome and cholecystobiliary fistula: a unifing classification. *Br J Surg* 1989; **76**: 1139–43.

Degenshein GA. Choledochoduodenostomy, an 18 year study of 175 consecutive cases. *Surgery* 1974; **76**: 319–24.

DeMarco A, Nance FC, Cohn I. Chronic cholecystitis: experience in a large charity institution. *Surgery* 1968; **63**: 750–6.

Doyle PJ, Ward-McQuaid JN, McEwen-Smith A. The value of routine peroperative cholangiography: a report of 4000 cholecystectomies. *Br J Surg* 1982; **69**: 617–9.

Fox MS, Wilk PJ, Weissman HS, Freeman LM, Gliedman ML. Acute acalculous cholecystitis. *Surg Gynecol Obstet* 1984; **159**: 13–16.

Glenn F. A 26 year experience in the surgical treatment of 5037 patients with non-malignant biliary tract disease. *Surg Gynecol Obstet* 1959; **109**: 591–606.

Glenn F. Acute cholecystitis. *Surg Gynecol Obstet* 1976; **143**: 56–60.

Glenn F, Reed C, Grafe WR. Biliary enteric fistula. *Surg Gynecol Obstet* 1981; **153**: 527–31.

Gough MH. 'The cholecystogram is normal'—but—. *Br Med J* 1977; **274**: 960–2.

Gracie WA, Ransohoff DF. The natural history of silent gallstones. The innocent gallstone is not a myth. *N Engl J Med* 1982; **307**: 798–800.

Hand BH. An anatomical study of the choledochoduodenal area. *Br J Surg* 1963; **50**: 486–94.

Howard ER, Driver M, McClement JW, Mowat AP. Results of surgery in 88 consecutive cases of extrahepatic biliary atresia. *J R Soc Med* 1982; **75**: 408–13.

Kameda H, the Tokyo Co-operative Gallstone Study Group. Efficacy and indications of ursodeoxycholic acid treatment for dissolving gallstones. A multi-centre double-blind trial. *Gastroenterology* 1980; **78**: 542–8.

Keighley MRB. Micro-organisms in the bile. A preventable cause of sepsis after biliary surgery. *Ann R Coll Surg Engl* 1977; **59**: 328–34.

Kune GA, Sali A. *The Practice of Biliary Surgery*. 2nd edn. Oxford: Blackwell Scientific Publications, 1980.

Leow CK, Thompson MH. Endoscopic papillotomy without cholecystectomy for bile duct stones. *Ann R Coll Surg Engl* 1986; **68**: 300–1.

Le Quesne LP, Ranger I. Cholecystitis glandularis proliferans. *Br J Surg* 1957; **44**: 447–58.

Levine SB, Lerner HJ, Leifer ED, Lindheim SR. Intraoperative cholangiography: a review of indications and analysis of age-sex groups. *Ann Surg* 1983; **198**: 692–7.

Matolo NM, ed. Biliary Tract Disease. *Surg Clin N Am* 1981; **61**: 763–994.

May RE, Strong R. Acute emphysematous cholecystitis. *Br J Surg* 1971; **58**: 453–8.

McArthur P, Cuscheiri A, Sells RA, Shields R. Controlled clinical trial comparing early with interval cholecystectomy for acute cholecystitis. *Br J Surg* 1975; **62**: 850–2.

McClement JW, Howard ER, Mowat AP. Results of surgical treatment for extrahepatic biliary atresia in the United Kingdom 1980–1982. *Br Med J* 1985; **290**: 345–7.

Mentzer RM Jnr, Golden GT, Chandler JG. A comparative appraisal of emphysematous cholecystitis. *Am J Surg* 1975; **129**: 10–15.

Mirizzi PL. Operative cholangiography. *Surg Gynecol Obstet* 1937; **65**: 702–10.

Mitchell A, Morris PJ. Trends in the management of acute cholecystitis. *Br Med J* 1982; **284**: 27–30.

Motson RW, Wetter LA. Operative choledochoscopy: common bile duct exploration is incomplete without it. *Br J Surg* 1990; **77**: 975–82.

Mueller PR, Harbin WP, Ferrucci JT, Wittenberg J, Van Sonnenberg E. Fine needle transhepatic cholangiography: reflections after 450 cases. *Am J Roentgenol* 1981; **136**: 85–90.

Nardi GL, Michelassi F, Zannini P. Transduodenal sphincteroplasty 5–25 year follow-up of 89 patients. *Ann Surg* 1983; **198**: 453–61.

Neoptolemos JP, Carr-Lock DL, Fossard DP. Prospective randomised study of preoperative endoscopic sphincterotomy versus surgery alone for common bile duct stones. *Br Med J* 1987; **294**: 470–4.

Neoptolemos JP, Carr-Locke DL, London N, Bailey I, Fossard DP. ERCP findings and the role of endoscopic sphincterotomy in acute gallstone pancreatitis. *Br J Surg* 1988; **75**: 954–60.

Northover JMA, Terblanche J. A new look at the arterial supply of the bile duct in man and its surgical implications. *Br J Surg* 1979; **66**: 379–84.

O'Connor MJ, Schwartz ML, McQuarrie DG, Sumner HW. Acute bacterial cholangitis. An analysis of clinical manifestation. *Arch Surg* 1982; **117**: 437–41.

Porayko MK, *et al*. Patients with asymptomatic primary sclerosing cholangitis frequently have a progressive disease. *Gastroenterology* 1990; **98**: 1594–602.

Robertson HE. Silent gallstones. *Gastroenterology* 1945; **5**: 345–72.

Ruddell WSJ, Ashton MG, Lintott DJ, Axon ATR. Endoscopic retrograde cholangiography and pancreatography in investigation of post-cholecystectomy patients. *Lancet* 1980; **i**: 444–7.

Sackmann M, Delius M, Sauerbruch T. Shock-wave lithotripsy of gall bladder stones: the first 175 patients. *N Engl J Med* 1988; **318**: 393–7.

Safrany L, Cotton PB. A preliminary report: urgent duodenoscopic sphincterotomy for acute gallstone pancreatitis. *Surgery* 1981; **89**: 424–8.

Saharia PC, Zuidema GD, Cameron JL. Primary common duct stones. *Ann Surg* 1977; **185**: 598–604.

Sarles H, Sahel J. Cholestasis and lesions of the biliary tract in chronic pancreatitis. *Gut* 1978; **19**: 851–7.

Schein CJ, Gliedman ML. Choledochoduodenostomy as an adjunct to choledocholithotomy. *Surg Gynecol Obstet* 1981; **152**: 797–804.

Schoenfeld LJ, Lachin JM. Chenodiol (chenodeoxycholic acid) for dissolution of gallstones: the National Cooperative Gallstone Study. A controlled trial of efficacy and safety. *Ann Intern Med* 1981; **95**: 257–82.

Scragg RKR, McMichael AJ, Baghurst PA. Diet, alcohol, and relative weight in gall stone disease: a case-control study. *Br Med J* 1984; **288**: 1113–9.

Scragg RKR, McMichael AJ, Seamark RF. Oral contraceptives, pregnancy, and endogenous oestrogen in gall stone disease—a case-control study. *Br Med J* 1984; **288**: 1795–9.

Shanahan D, Lord PH, Grogono J, Wastell C. Clinical acute cholecystitis and the Curtis Fitz-Hugh syndrome. *Ann R Coll Surg Engl* 1988; **70**: 44–6.

Smith EEJ, Bowley N, Allison DJ, Blumgart LH. The management of post-traumatic intrahepatic cutaneous biliary fistulas. *Br J Surg* 1982; **69**: 317–8.

Smith L. Injuries of the liver, biliary tree and pancreas. *Br J Surg* 1978; **65**: 673–7.

Soloway RD, Trotman BW, Ostrow JD. Pigment stones. *Gastroenterology* 1977; **72**: 167–82.

Southern Surgeons Club. A prospective analysis of 1518 laparoscopic cholecystectomies. *N Engl J Med* 1991; **324**: 1073–8.

Spitz L. Choledochal cyst. *Surg Gynecol Obstet* 1978; **147**: 444–52.

Stanley RJ, Melson GL, Cubillo E, Hesker AE. A comparison of three cholecystographic agents. A double-blind study with and without a prior fatty meal. *Radiology* 1974; **112**: 513–7.

Stubbs RS. Wound infection after cholecystectomy: a case for routine prophylaxis. *Ann R Coll Surg Engl* 1983; **65**: 30–1.

Sykes D. The use of cholecystokinin in diagnosing biliary pain. *Ann R Coll Surg Engl* 1982; **64**: 114–16.

Taylor TV, Armstrong CP. Migration of gall stones. *Br Med J* 1987; **294**: 1320–2.

Thornton J, Heaton KW, Espiner HJ, Eltringham WK. Empyema of the gall bladder: reappraisal of a neglected disease. *Gut* 1983; **24**: 1183–5.

Todani T, Watanabe Y, Narusue M, Tabuchi K, Okajima K. Congenital bile duct cysts: classification, operative procedures, and review of thirty-seven cases including cancer arising from choledochal cyst. *Am J Surg* 1977; **134**: 263–8.

Toouli J. Sphincter of Oddi motility. *Br J Surg* 1984; **71**: 251–6.

Vellacott KD, Powell PH. Exploration of the common bile duct: a comparative study. *Br J Surg* 1979; **66**: 389–91.

Viceconte G, Viceconte GW, Pietropaolo V, Montori A. Endoscopic sphincterotomy: indications and results. *Br J Surg* 1981; **68**: 376–80.

Warshaw AL, Simeone J, Schapiro RH, Hedberg SE, Mueller PE, Ferrucci JT. Objective evaluation of ampullary stenosis with ultrasonography and pancreatic stimulation. *Am J Surg* 1985; **149**: 65–72.

Wenckert A, Robertson B. The natural course of gallstone disease. *Gastroenterology* 1966; **50**: 376–81.

23.2 Carcinoma of the gallbladder

DAVID L. BERGER AND RONALD A. MALT

Gallbladder cancer is the most frequent carcinoma of the biliary tract and the fifth most frequent carcinoma of the alimentary tract. The overall 5-year survival rate is less than 5 per cent, and the overall 1-year survival rate is less than 12 per cent. Gallbladder carcinoma is detected in about 2 per cent of patients undergoing gallbladder and biliary surgery. Because of the enhancing effect of female sex hormones on the formation of gallstones, women have more and larger stones than men, and there is a female : male ratio of 4 : 1 among patients with gallbladder carcinoma.

AETIOLOGY

A direct association exists between the presence of cholelithiasis and the pathogenesis of gallbladder cancer. In patients with gallbladder carcinoma, the incidence of cholelithiasis ranges from 54 to 97 per cent. The incidence of gallbladder cancer increases with age, especially in women with cholelithiasis. The incidence of gallbladder cancer is 0.03 per cent in women under the age of 50 with gallstones, 3.8 per cent those over the age of 50, and 8.8 per cent in those over the age of 65.

The risk of gallbladder cancer correlates with the increasing size of gallstones, and the epidemiology of cholelithiasis parallels that of gallbladder carcinoma. American Indians, Northeastern Europeans, Israelis, and Mexican Americans have a high incidence of gallbladder cancer. Black Americans and Africans have the lowest incidence. Although Americans in general have a 8 to 17 per cent incidence of cholelithiasis, gallstones are uncommon among black Americans. Patients may have cholelithiasis for 10 to 25 years without developing gallbladder cancer, and in autopsy studies only 1 to 2 per cent of patients with cholelithiasis harbour gallbladder carcinoma. Chronic cholecystitis is also associated with gallbladder carcinoma. End-stage chronic cholecystitis leads to a calcified or porcelain gallbladder. The incidence of gallbladder cancer in calcified (porcelain) gallbladders has been reported to range from 12 to 60 per cent, but the issue has not been subjected to epidemiological scrutiny.

Chemical carcinogens such as methylcholanthrene, dimethylnitrosamine, and α-aminoazotoluene induce gallbladder carcinoma in laboratory animals. The California Tumor Registry reported an increased incidence of gallbladder cancer in people who worked in rubber, automobile, wood-finishing, and metal-fabricating industries. However, despite 28 per cent of patients with gallbladder cancer in Akron, Ohio having worked in the rubber industry, the incidence of gallbladder carcinoma in the city was no higher than that reported across the United States.

An anomalous pancreaticobiliary ductal junction is associated with a 15 to 25 per cent incidence of gallbladder cancer. Such a junction allows bile and pancreatic juice to mix activating phospholipase A_2. This leads to increasing concentrations of lysophosphatidylcholine, which have cytotoxic effects, and cause mucosal hyperplasia and metaplasia, conditions that are almost obligatory substrates for carcinogenesis (Fig. 1). Endoscopic retrograde cholangiopancreatography revealed an anomalous pancreaticobiliary ductal union in 16.7 per cent of 95 patients with gallbladder cancer. An anomalous union was noted in only 2.8 per cent of 681 patients with hepatobiliary or pancreatic diseases excluding gallbladder carcinoma.

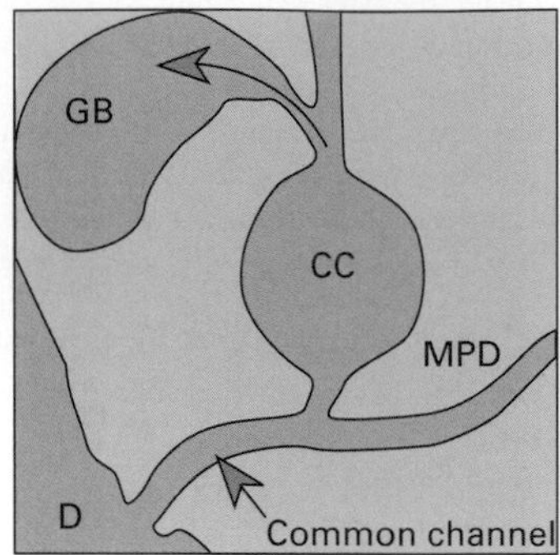

Fig. 1 Anomalous pancreaticobiliary duct function.

Adenomyomatosis, gallbladder adenomas, and epithelial dysplasia may be associated with gallbladder carcinoma. There are reports of gallbladder carcinoma arising in areas of adenomyomatosis. Epithelial dysplasia was found in 83 per cent of gallbladders resected for cholelithiasis, atypical hyperplasia was present in 13.5 per cent of the specimens, and carcinoma *in situ* in 3.5 per cent. One case of dysplasia occurred within an area of metaplasia in 277 cholecystectomy specimens, while dysplasia of metaplastic epithelium surrounded the neoplasm in 67 per cent of 15 carcinomatous specimens, suggesting that carcinoma may arise from the progression of metaplasia or hyperplasia to dysplasia and carcinoma. Since ultrasound examination has become widespread, the detection rate of gallbladder polyps has increased. In 1605 cholecystectomy specimens, 11 harboured benign adenomas, seven harboured adenomas with malignant change, and 79 harboured invasive carcinomas. A histological transition from benign adenoma to malignant carcinoma was recognized. All benign lesions were less than 12 mm in diameter.

PATHOLOGY

Gallbladder carcinoma manifests itself with thickening of the gallbladder wall, most often with the cancer originating in the gallbladder fundus. As the tumour progresses, the gallbladder may fill with tumour or may contain a mucinous exudate, with or without gallstones. Occasionally, the proteinaceous material within the lumen becomes infected and leads to cholangitis, either concomitantly or as a consequence.

Virtually all gallbladder cancer (80–95 per cent) is adenocarcinoma, the histological forms of which are papillary, tubular, mucinous, and signet-ring cell types. Undifferentiated or anaplastic carcinoma represents 2 to 7 per cent of cases, squamous cell cancer 2 to 5 per cent of cases, and adenoacanthoma or mixed adenosquamous tumour 1 to 3 per cent of cases. Carcinoid tumours, malignant melanoma, clear cell carcinoma, and spindle cell malignancies rarely occur.

Gallbladder cancer tends to spread locally, rather than by metastasis. The problem is that local spread can occur by lymphatic, vascular, intraneural, or intraductal invasion. Multiple channels of dissemination are responsible for the limited ability to restrain or cure the neoplasm. Direct invasion of the hepatic bed in the gallbladder fossa is seen in 45 to 90 per cent of patients with disseminated disease. The lymphatic drainage of the gallbladder begins in the intramural plexus, moves to the cystic nodes, into the hiatal nodes, to the superior and posterior pancreaticoduodenal nodes and, finally, to the periaortic chain. Lymphatic extension occurs in 20 to 70 per cent of cases. The venous drainage of the gallbladder is shown in Fig. 2. The number of cholecystic veins on the hepatic side of the gallbladder ranges from two to 20; these drain directly into segment IV of the liver. The venous drainage of the peritoneal side of the gallbladder consists of one or two veins that also drain into segment IV of the liver and rarely empty into the portal vein. Vascular extension is seen in 10 to 20 per cent of cases. Tumour spreads through the neural sheath in 24 per cent of patients and intraductally through the biliary system in 19 per cent.

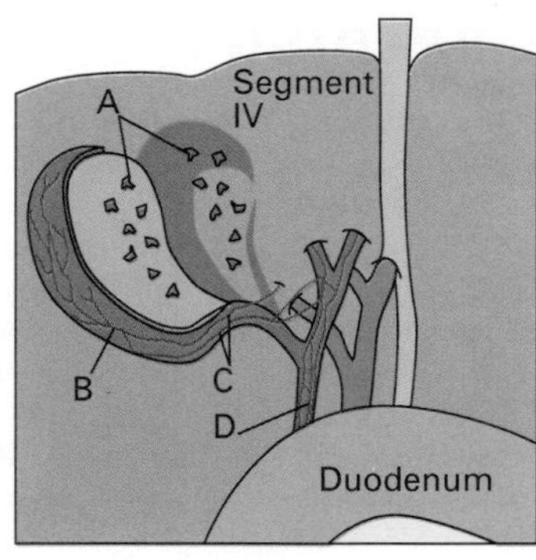

Fig. 2 Venous drainage of gallbladder: A, directly into segment IV of the liver; B, peritoneal veins; C, peritoneal veins draining into segment IV of the liver; D, venous drainage along cystic ducts.

DIAGNOSIS

Because the symptoms of gallbladder carcinoma are generally non-specific, the tumour is discovered either incidentally or at an advanced stage. Cancer is found in approximately 1 per cent of gallbladders removed for benign disease. Advanced disease commonly presents itself with multiple symptoms including abdominal pain, nausea and vomiting, weight loss, jaundice, anorexia, abdominal distension, and pruritus. Patients may have a palpable right upper quadrant mass. Eighty per cent of patients have symptoms for less than 6 months prior to their presentation. In only 10 to 25 per cent of patients is the correct diagnosis made before surgery. Laboratory tests, although abnormal, are non-specific. An arteriographic CT portogram, in which the superior mesenteric artery is injected with contrast material, is the best way to assess a gallbladder carcinoma for resectability. Neoplasms tend to be hypervascular and arteriographic CT portography delineates the extent of disease. Ultrasound findings of marked gallbladder wall thickening, of a complex mass filling the gallbladder, or of a polypoid or fungating tumour filling the gallbladder are indicative of carcinoma. Abdominal CT diagnoses gallbladder cancer with a 66 per cent accuracy.

STAGING

At least five staging systems for gallbladder carcinoma exist. Nevin devised a system from a review of 66 cases and a literature review of 399 cases that divided disease into five stages (Table 1). The Mayo Clinic proposed a modification of the Nevin system by placing contiguous extension of tumour into the liver into stage III rather than into stage V. The American Joint Commission on Cancer and the Union Internationale Centre de Cancer (UICC) established a staging system using the TNM classification with four stages (Table 2). Japanese surgeons stage gallbladder carcinoma according to the General Rules for Staging Carcinoma of the Biliary Tract into four stages. Another staging system was proposed in Japan which delineates patients into three stages. The lack of a definitive staging system for gallbladder carcinoma has made comparison of series of patients and analysis of results difficult to interpret.

Table 1 Nevin staging system for gallbladder cancer

Stage	Depth of invasion
I	Intramucosal only
II	Involvement of mucosa and muscularis
III	Transmural invasion
IV	Transmural invasion and cystic duct, lymph node metastasis
V	Metastasis

Table 2 American Joint Comission on Cancer staging system for gallbladder cancer

Stage	Depth of invasion
0	*In-situ* carcinoma
I	Involvement of the mucosa or muscularis
II	Transmural invasion
III	Transmural invasion and lymphatic invasion, or invasion of the liver <2 cm from the gallbladder fossa
IV	Involvement of two or more adjacent organs, invasion of the liver >2 cm from the gallbladder fossa, or distant metastasis

TREATMENT

Only surgery can cure gallbladder cancer: a universally accepted surgical treatment of gallbladder cancer does not exist. Only 10 to 30 per cent of patients have resectable disease on presentation.

Early experience failed to show a survival benefit following extensive resection: radical resection therefore fell out of favour. Modern delineation of the modes of spread of gallbladder cancer, however, has led to a resurgence of radical resection in an effort to remove microscopic tumour completely. The extent of radical surgery ranges from cholecystectomy with an accompanying hepatic wedge resection to an extensive resection including cholecystectomy, extended right hepatectomy, and pancreaticoduodenectomy with local and para-aortic lymphadenectomy. Anecdotal reports of long-term survival in patients with extensive disease following large extirpative procedures are common, but the morbidity rates associated with extensive resection reach 54 per cent, and mortality rates are around 5 per cent.

Direct comparisons between the results of radical and non-radical surgery do not show statistically significant differences in patient survival despite the attendant increases in morbidity and mortality. Both the Mayo Clinic and the Massachusetts General Hospital compared cholecystectomy with cholecystectomy and hepatic wedge resection and noted no statistically significant survival advantage. There is little evidence to support radical surgery for advanced disease.

Surgical treatment for incidentally discovered gallbladder carcinoma also remains controversial. In a Swedish study of 32 patients who underwent a cholecystectomy and were found to have microscopic gallbladder cancer, the 5-year survival rate was 64 per cent and the 10-year survival rate was 44 per cent when the tumour extended only to the gallbladder serosa. When tumour extended through the serosa, the 1-year survival rate was 30 per cent. Numerous reports cite a 100 per cent 5-year survival rate when tumour is limited to the gallbladder mucosa.

In a Japanese study of patients with inapparent carcinoma, 35 of 45 patients with tumour extending to the gallbladder serosa, but not through it, underwent cholecystectomy alone, with a 40 per cent 5-year survival. However, 10 patients who underwent cholecystectomy followed at a second operation by hepatic wedge resection, common bile duct resection and *en-bloc* dissection of regional lymph nodes had a 90 per cent 5-year survival rate. An increased survival rate was not seen in patients whose tumour extended through the gallbladder serosa. All patients with disease limited to the mucosa survived 5 years following cholecystectomy.

The effectiveness of adjuvant therapy in gallbladder cancer is unpredictable. The Eastern Cooperative Oncologic Group reported a randomized trial of 5-fluorouracil alone, 5-fluorouracil with streptozotocin, and 5-fluorouracil with methyl-CCNU. There was no difference in survival rates between regimens or compared with historical controls who received no chemotherapy. A non-significantly increased survival rate was found in a comparison of hepatic arterial infusion of mitomycin-C and 5-fluorouracil and controls.

Radiation therapy provides symptomatic relief. Eighty per cent of patients with end-stage gallbladder cancer reported palliation of pruritus and pain when treated with external beam radiation therapy with doses ranging from 3200 to 5000 cGy. Twenty patients who underwent postoperative radiation therapy (mean, 4200 cGy) showed no increase in survival rates over historical controls.

Intraoperative administration of radiation increases its specificity and intensity. Ten patients received such therapy for either gross residual disease or completely unresected disease with a median survival of 1 year. Seventeen patients who underwent radical resection combined with intraoperative radiation therapy were compared with nine patients who underwent radical resection alone. There was a small but statistically significant increase in ($p < 0.05$) 3-year survival among patients who received intraoperative radiation therapy. Intraoperative radiation therapy itself does not appear significantly to improve survival. Implantation of iridium-192 wire into the common bile duct is sometimes effective as palliative treatment, but rarely cures malignant biliary obstruction. Although cholangitis is a frequent complication of intraductal brachytherapy, its incidence can be decreased by endoscopically placing a 10 Fr biliary stent into the biliary duct 2 weeks before the iridium-192. As with other adjuvant therapeutic modalities the number of patients reported is small, patients so treated have usually had bile duct carcinoma, and the results are inconclusive.

CONCLUSION

Gallbladder cancer has a poor prognosis. The overall 5-year survival rate is approximately 5 per cent. Despite increasingly aggressive surgical resection, no improvement in survival has occurred in the last 30 years. Adjuvant therapy is ineffective. Simple cholecystectomy with postoperative radiation therapy is the treatment of choice for limited disease. Cholecystectomy and an accompanying biliary bypass procedure, when possible, are appropriate for extensive disease.

FURTHER READING

Albores-Saavedra J, Alcantra-Vazquez A, Cruz-Ortiz H. The precursor lesions of invasive gallbladder cancer: hyperplasia, atypical hyperplasia and carcinoma *in situ*. *Cancer*, 1980; **45**: 919–27.

Aldridge MC, Bismuth H. Gallbladder cancer: the polyp-cancer sequence. *Br J Surg*, 1990; **77**: 363–4.

Bergdahl L. Gallbladder carcinoma first diagnosed at microscopic examination of gallbladders removed for presumed benign disease. *Ann Surg*, 1980; **191**: 19–22.

Donohue JH, Nagorney DM, Grant CS, Tsushima K, Ilstrup DM, Adson MA. Carcinoma of the gallbladder: does radical resection improve outcome? *Arch Surg*, 1990; **125**: 237–41.

Fahim RB, McDonald JR, Richards JC, Ferris DO. Carcinoma of the gallbladder: a study of its mode of spread. *Ann Surg*, 1962; **156**: 114–24.

Falkson G, MacIntyre JM, Moertel CG. Eastern Cooperative Oncology Group experience with chemotherapy for inoperable gallbladder and bile duct cancer. *Cancer*, 1984; **54**: 965–9.

Houry S, *et al.* Gallbladder carcinoma: role of radiation therapy. *Br J Surg*, 1989; **76**: 448–50.

Kimura K, *et al.* Association of gallbladder carcinoma and anomalous pancreaticobiliary ductal union. *Gastroenterology* 1985; **89**: 1258–65.

Koga A, *et al.* Diagnosis and operative indications for polypoid lesions of the gallbladder. *Arch Surg*, 1988; **123**: 26–9.

Nevin JE, Moran TJ, Kay S, King R. Carcinoma of the gallbladder. *Cancer*, 1976; **37**: 141–8.

Ogura Y, *et al.* Radical operations for carcinoma of the gallbladder: present status in Japan. *World J Surg*, 1991; **15**: 337–43.

Piehler JM, Crichlow RW. Primary carcinoma of the gallbladder. *Surg Gynecol Obstet*, 1978; **146**: 929–42.

Shirai Y, Yoshida K, Tsukada K, Muto T. Inapparent carcinoma of the gallbladder: an appraisal of a radical second operation after simple cholecystectomy. *Ann Surg*, 1992; **215**: 326–31.

23.3 Carcinoma of the extrahepatic bile ducts

KIMBERLEY SAUNDERS KIRKWOOD AND RONALD A. MALT

Primary neoplasms of the extrahepatic biliary tract are found at postmortem examination at a rate less than 0.5 per cent. Discussions of bile duct tumours generally exclude carcinomas isolated to the intrahepatic ducts, gallbladder, pancreas, and ampulla of Vater. Bile duct cancer is more common in men (male : female ratio of approximately 1.5 : 1), with a peak incidence in the seventh decade of life.

PATHOLOGY

The site of the cancer is the most important prognostic factor in bile duct cancer. Fifty to 75 per cent of cancers are located in the upper third of the extrahepatic biliary tract at the level of the common hepatic duct or hepatic duct bifurcation. Cancers of the distal common bile duct or cystic duct–common duct junction are less common. An uncommon diffuse form of bile duct cancer carries a particularly poor prognosis.

Bile duct tumours are typically small, firm, well-circumscribed lesions involving the full thickness of the bile duct wall; they may occasionally have polypoid projections into the lumen of the duct. These tumours are adenocarcinomas with varying degrees of differentiation. The incidence of local metastases at operation approaches 50 per cent, spread to the liver and hepatoduodenal ligament being most common. Local spread does not necessarily represent a contraindication to resection. Metastases to distant organs are uncommon at the time the cancer is identified.

CLINICAL MANIFESTATIONS

Jaundice is the most common presenting symptom among patients with bile duct cancer, followed by weight loss, abdominal pain, and pruritus. Less frequently reported are signs and symptoms of cholangitis. Serum liver function tests typically reveal an obstructive pattern, often with marked elevations in total and conjugated bilirubin levels. As its clinical presentation is similar to that of benign biliary tract abnormalities, bile duct cancer is often unrecognized. Delays in diagnosis of several months are typical; many patients undergo several non-therapeutic procedures prior to the establishment of a definitive diagnosis.

Although radiographic imaging of bile duct tumours usually starts with ultrasonography or CT, detailed anatomical information regarding the site and the extent of the obstructive lesion is best obtained by endoscopic retrograde cholangiopancreatography or transhepatic cholangiography. When the diagnosis is made intraoperatively, operative cholangiography and choledochoscopy are helpful. Intraoperative choledochoscopy should be performed as a routine preliminary step to a planned curative procedure to exclude unsuspected multicentricity.

TREATMENT

The mainstay of treatment for patients with carcinoma of the extrahepatic bile ducts is surgery. The types of procedures performed fall into three categories: potentially curative resection, palliative surgical bypass, and operative intubation and drainage of ductal obstruction. Drainage can also be performed non-operatively.

Resection of the tumour generally entails anastomosis of the proximal ductal system to a loop of small intestine. The specific procedure selected depends upon the location and extent of the lesion. Approximately two-thirds of middle and distal common duct tumours are resectable, compared with less than one-third of proximal lesions. Recent advances in selection of patients and in perioperative care have led to marked reductions in operative mortality associated with tumour resection: operative mortality rates are now less than 5 per cent, even in elderly patients. The relative safety of these major biliary resections has led some authors to advocate radical vascular and hepatic resections for locally invasive proximal lesions. The impact of this aggressive approach on long-term survival is uncertain.

Palliative procedures aim to relieve biliary obstruction and its attendant sequelae. Most patients undergo operative palliation by either bilioenteric bypass of the obstructed segment(s) or ductal intubation. The advantages of operative versus non-operative palliation for the patient who is a candidate for surgery include accurate staging, pathological confirmation of the diagnosis, and possibly, improved biliary drainage and quality of life.

Both radiation and chemotherapy are employed as adjuvant treatments in patients with bile duct cancer. These treatments are generally delivered postoperatively for residual local disease. Prospective randomized studies evaluating the potential benefit of these adjuvant therapies are unavailable.

Overall survival figures for patients with bile duct cancer remain disappointing: less than half survive 1 year and less than 10 per cent are alive at 5 years. Patients with proximal cancers have a particularly poor prognosis. Most series report mean survival times of less than 1 year, and 5-year survival is extremely rare. Clearly, patients with neoplasms that are suitable for resection have the best prognosis.

FURTHER READING

Cameron JL, Pitt HA, Zinner MJ, Kaufman SL, Coleman J. Management of proximal cholangiocarcinomas by surgical resection and radiotherapy. *Am J Surg*, 1990; **159**: 91–8.

Gallinger S, Gluckman D, Langer B. Proximal bile duct cancer. *Adv Surg*, 1990; **23**: 89–118.

Hadjis NS, Blenkharn JI, Alexander N, Benjamin IS, Blumgart LH. Outcome of radical surgery in hilar cholangiocarcinoma. *Surgery*, 1990; **107**: 597–604.

Hall RI, Denyer ME, Chapman AH. Percutaneous endoscopic placement of endoprostheses for relief of jaundice caused by inoperable bile duct strictures. *Surgery*, 1990; **107**: 224–7.

Nimura Y, *et al.* Combined portal vein and liver resection for carcinoma of the biliary tract. *Br J Surg*, 1991; **78**: 727–31.

Reding R, Buard J, Lebeau G, Launois B. Surgical management of 552 carcinomas of the extrahepatic bile ducts (gallbladder and periampullary tumours excluded). *Ann Surg*, 1991; **213**: 236–41.

Sako S, Seitzinger GL, Garside E. Carcinoma of the extrahepatic bile ducts:

review of the literature and report of six cases. *Surgery*, 1957; **41**: 416–37.

Saunders KD, Longmire WP, Jr, Tompkins RK, Chavez M, Cates JA, Roslyn JJ. Diffuse bile duct tumours: guidelines for management. *Ann Surg*, 1991; **57**: 816–20.

Saunders KD, Tompkins RK, Longmire WP, Jr, Roslyn JJ. Bile duct carcinoma in the elderly. A rationale for surgical management. *Arch Surg*, 1991; **126**: 1186–90.

Tompkins RK, Thomas D, Wile A, Longmire WP, Jr. Prognostic factors in bile duct carcinoma. *Ann Surg*, 1981; **194**: 447–57.

Tompkins RK, Saunders K, Roslyn JJ, Longmire WP, Jr. Changing patterns in diagnosis and management of bile duct cancer. *Ann Surg*, 1990; **211**: 614–21.

Yeo CJ, Pitt HA, Cameron JL. Cholangiocarcinoma. *Surg Clin N Am*, 1990; **70**: 1429–47.

23.4 Lithotripsy of stones

RONALD A. MALT

Extracorporeal shock-wave lithotripsy (ESL) as a medical device was initiated by cocktail party speculation in Munich concerning the origin of small pits on the leading surfaces of airplane wings. When proof became available that the pits were the product of cavitating bubbles that imploded and released enormous energy in a tiny region, speculation turned to using the energy of cavitation for medical purposes.

CAVITATION

Cavitating bubbles arise at the surface of many objects subjected to intense, focused energy. Although every bubble is minute, the energy of each one as it implodes approximates the temperature at the surface of the sun: 5000°C. The collective energy can be transmitted to flaws in an appropriate target and reflected through it, just as a diamond cutter seeks cleavage planes along which to cut his stone (Fig. 1). A laser or other high-energy source can be used for this purpose: the shock waves specifically tailored for medical lithotripsy include electrohydraulic, acoustic, and piezoelectric waves.

ADVANTAGES AND DISADVANTAGES OF LITHOTRIPSY

The electrohydraulic lithotripter generates an intense underwater spark gap discharge at the F_1 focus of an ellipsoidal reflector. This energy is concentrated at the F_2 focus (Fig. 2).

Transmission of energy without loss obviously demands a medium for coupling. Since the body is largely water, a water bath provides a good coupling. This usually takes the form of a Silastic bag filled with water, applied to the patient's skin with ultrasound gel (Fig. 3).

The advantage of an electrohydraulic impulse is its intense energy. Its disadvantage is that the impact is of such high energy that it is uncomfortable for most patients unless they receive intravenous analgesia.

The acoustic generator works on the principle of the diaphragm of a home loudspeaker, but is many times more powerful. It can be focused, in the same way as a spark-gap device, but seems to be more endurable for patients than is the electrohydraulic generator.

Deformation of an array of piezoelectric crystals generates

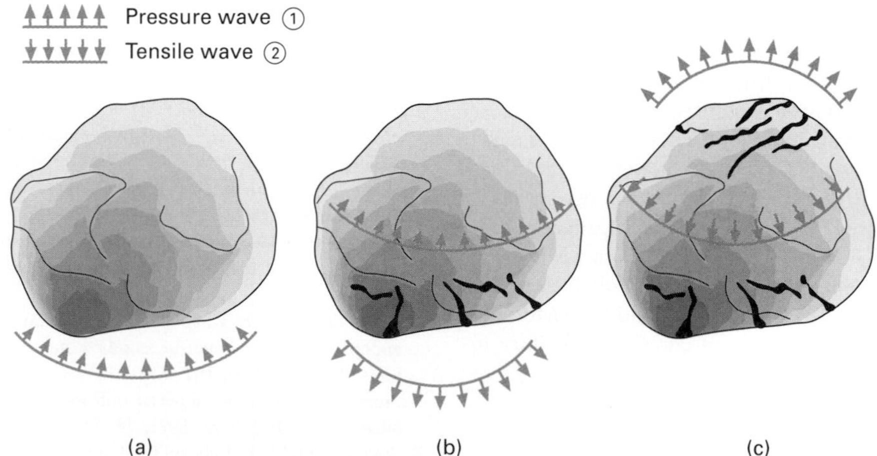

Fig. 1 Pressure and tensile waves cleaving faults in a stone. The pressure wave passes through the stone and is reflected from the back surface as a tensile wave.

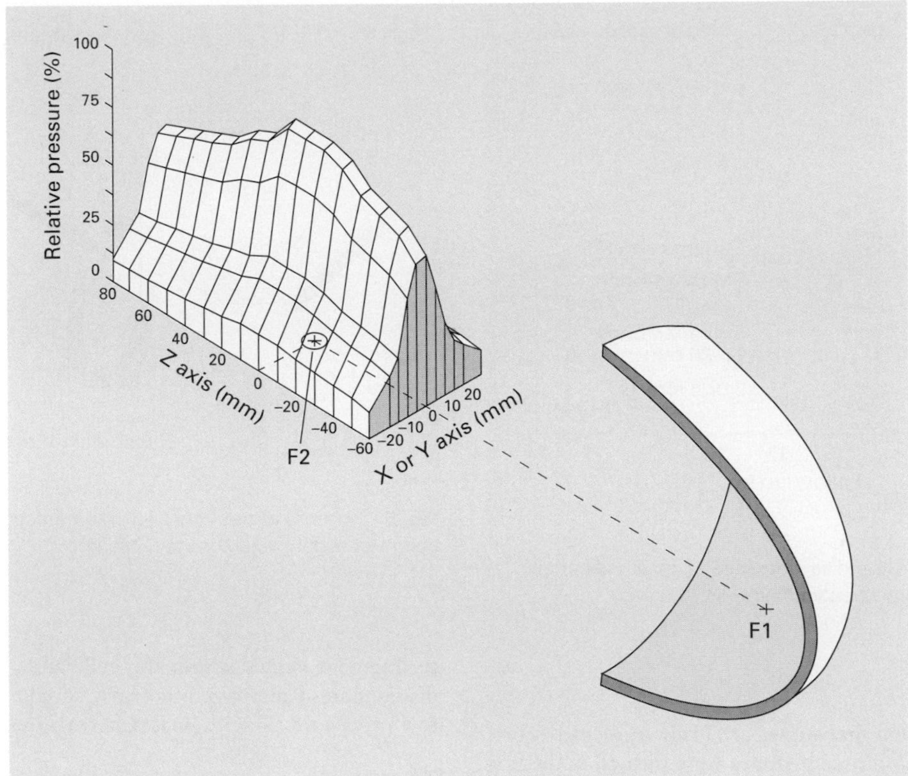

Fig. 2 Shock wave generated at F_1. Target at F_2 'focal point' is actually a complex geometric space.

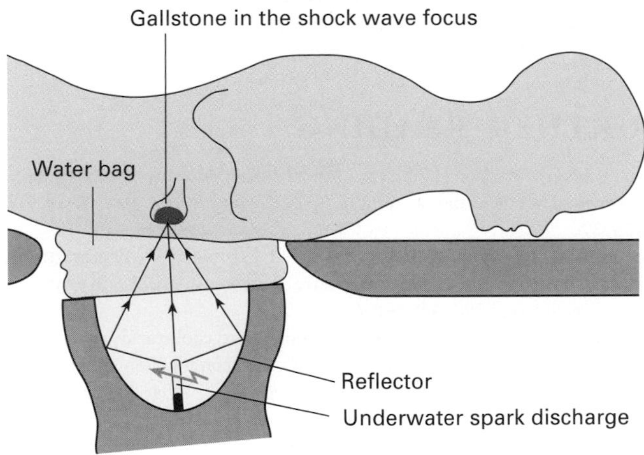

Fig. 3 Diagram of lithotripsy treatment.

shock waves proportional to the magnitude of incoming voltage. Like a dish for receiving electromagnetic waves from space, the piezoelectric array collects and distributes energy over a broad area. Discomfort during treatment is reduced, but multiple treatments are required to achieve good fragmentation of stones.

RENAL STONES (see Section 33.5)

Renal calculi are particularly attractive targets for lithotripsy. The physical nature of many is such that they can be pulverized easily and flushed through the ureters. Surgical removal of renal calculi formerly required a hospital stay of 10 to 12 days, and was associated with considerable morbidity. With lithotripsy, the hospital stay can be as short as 2 days.

GALLSTONE LITHOTRIPSY

Pure cholesterol gallstones or those containing only a nidus of non-cholesterol material are a good target for the lithotripter. In the hands of surgeons and physicians skilled in ultrasonic imaging excellent results can be achieved: 91 per cent disintegration of stones in 12 to 18 months. Nonetheless, elimination of the rubble produced is unpredictable unless the bile acid cholesterol solvent ursodeoxycholic acid is taken by mouth so that the gallstone dust becomes completely solubilized (Fig. 4). Except for a slightly increased frequency of bowel movement, there are no side-effects from use of this adjuvant. There are, however, hazards. For example, fragments of gallstones might drop from the gallbladder and into the pancreatic duct, inciting pancreatitis.

In the United States gallstone lithotripsy is not yet approved as a bona fide treatment. Only one of 10 American groups was able to duplicate the results of the German lithotripters. Thus, when laparoscopic cholecystectomy was introduced in 1988, lithotripsy for gallstones was largely abandoned. However, a single, large cholesterol gallstone precipitating recurrent biliary colic is suitable for lithotripsy as the primary form of treatment. Relief of pain is almost immediate, and the patient can return to work the next day without fear of a catastrophic event. The treatment can be repeated if required, or converted into a laparoscopic cholecyst-

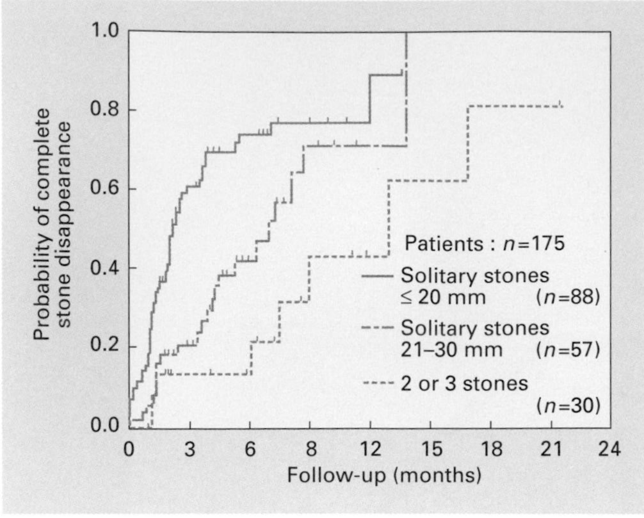

Fig. 4 Probability of complete disappearance of gallstones after lithotripsy with adjuvant oral chenodeoxycholic acid and ursodeoxycholic acid.

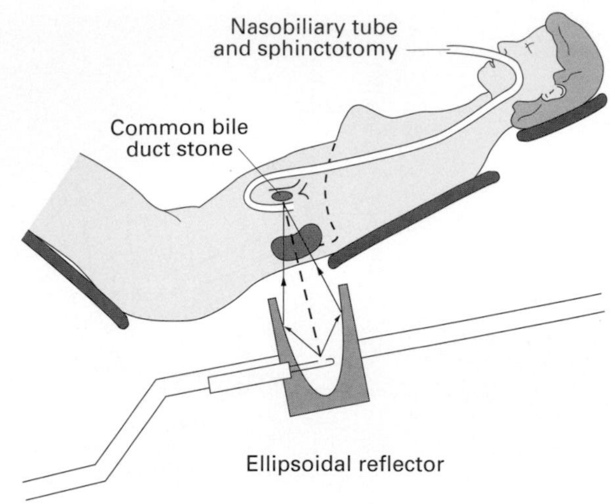

Fig. 5 Schema of treatment for fragmentation of gallstones in the common hepatic and common bile ducts.

ectomy. It could be argued that stones are likely to recur because the gallbladder itself is abnormal if stones were formed in the first place.

RETAINED COMMON BILE DUCT STONES

Stones in the common bile duct that cannot be removed by radiologically guided stone-crushing instruments in patients who still have a biliary T-tube are other appropriate targets for lithotripsy. The problems are that ductal stones can be up to 2 cm in diameter and multiple, patients are often old and weak, and a nasobiliary tube must be placed within the common duct to provide space for reverberation (Fig. 5). If all goes well, however, the fragments can be extracted following an endoscopic sphincterotomy of the bile duct, performed before or after the attempt at lithotripsy.

Although gallstone pancreatitis would seem to be a likely hazard of this form of treatment, pancreatitis is rare, but may eventuate long after anyone can remember that lithotripsy treatment was done. Bacteraemia is more common.

The alternative form of treatment if the patient has a T-tube still in place is laser lithotripsy. This involves passage of a fine fibreoptic bundle capable of transmitting laser energy through the T-tube into the area of the common bile duct where the stone is located. A coumarin green dye-tuned laser is used because its optical spectrum does not overlap that of haemoglobin, which is inevitably present in the lining of the bile duct: absorption of laser energy by haemoglobin would cause a ductal perforation. Provided that a choledochoenterostomy or an endoscopic sphincterotomy is in place, stone fragments normally pass into the gut without problems.

PANCREATIC STONES

Pancreatic stones are even more fragile than are common duct stones. Only 400 shockwaves, rather than the 2000 normally used to fragment stones within the gallbladder, cause these stones to disintegrate. Pancreatic lithotripsy should ideally precede a Puestow procedure (longitudinal pancreaticojejunostomy) routinely.

SALIVARY DUCT STONES

Stones in the submandibular duct may also be disintegrated by lithotripsy, but whether or not this effort is worthwhile awaits proof. Stones are normally easily extractable under local anaesthesia.

FURTHER READING

Barkun ANG, Ponchon T. Extracorporeal biliary lithotripsy: review of experimental studies and a clinical update. *Ann Intern Med*, 1990; **122:** 126–37.

Sackmann M, Ippisch E, Sauerbruch T, Holl J, Brendel W, Paumgartner G. Early gallstone recurrence rate after successful shock-wave therapy. *Gastroenterology*, 1990; **98:** 392–6.

Sackmann M, *et al.* Efficacy and safety of ursodeoxycholic acid for dissolution of gallstone fragments: comparison with the combination of ursodeoxycholic acid and chenodeoxycholic acid. *Hepatology*, 1991; **14:** 1136–41.

Sackmann M, Pauletzki J, Sauerbruch T, Holl J, Schelling G, Paumgartner G. The Munich gallbladder lithotripsy study: results of the first 5 years with 711 patients. *Ann Intern Med*, 1991; **114:** 290–6.

Sass W, Dreyer HP, Kettermann S, Seifert J. The role of cavitational activity in fragmentation processes by lithotripters. *J Stone Dis*, 1992; **4:** 193–207.

Sauerbruch T, Holl J, Sackmann M, Paumgartner G. Extracorporeal shock wave lithotripsy of pancreatic stones. *Gut*, 1989; **30:** 1406–11.

Sauerbruch T, Holl J, Sackmann M, Paumgartner G. Fragmentation of bile duct stones by extracorporeal shock-wave lithotripsy: a five-year experience. *Hepatology*, 1992; **15:** 208–14.

Schneider HT, *et al.* Pain in extracorporeal shock- wave lithotripsy: a comparison of different lithotripters in volunteers. *Gastroenterology*, 1992; **102:** 640–6.

Suslick KS. The chemical effects of ultrasound. *Sci Am*, 1989; **Feb:** 80–6.

Tint G, *et al.* Ursodeoxycholic acid: a safe and effective agent for dissolving cholesterol gallstones. *Ann Intern Med*, 1982; **97:** 351–6.

Portal hypertension 24

24.1 Aetiology, presentation, and investigation

GEORGE HAMILTON

AETIOLOGY

Many diseases of the liver or associated structures obstruct portal blood flow and result in portal hypertension. Such obstruction is accompanied by increased mesenteric blood flow, the so-called hyperaemia of portal hypertension. These phenomena are generally considered to be the two principal factors in the pathophysiology of portal hypertension.

Obstruction may occur in the hepatic veins, within the liver parenchyma, or in the portal vein itself. The most common cause of portal hypertension in Europe and North America is cirrhosis, which increases intrahepatic vascular resistance by fibrosis, thrombosis, and nodular regeneration. Portal vein obstruction by thrombosis or extrinsic compression is the second most common cause. Hepatic vein occlusion is the third most common, but much less frequent, cause.

A more precise classification of portal hypertension is by site of obstruction at the presinusoidal, sinusoidal, and postsinusoidal levels (Table 1). Intrinsic liver disease is usually absent in patients with presinusoidal obstruction: the natural history and prognosis of portal hypertension is therefore relatively good. Post-sinusoidal obstruction can result in hepatocellular damage as a secondary congestive phenomenon. In the acute phase of the illness this may result in death from liver failure rather than from variceal haemorrhage. In patients with sinusoidal block such as occurs in cirrhosis, the degree of hepatocellular damage is the most important factor in the natural history of the disease. Death may result not only from variceal haemorrhage but also from liver failure, malnutrition, or infection.

Irrespective of cause, portal hypertension results in the development of collateral channels between the portal and systemic venous circulations, of which the most important clinically are those that develop in the oesophagus. These varices are the source of spectacular haemorrhage and thus from a clinical viewpoint, the most important complication of portal hypertension.

Table 1 Classification of portal hypertension

Presinusoidal obstruction
- Portal vein thrombosis
  - Neonatal umbilical sepsis
  - Dehydration
  - Portal pyaemia
  - Hypercoagulable states (polycythaemia, oral contraceptives)
  - Periportal inflammation (pancreatitis)
  - Trauma (accidental, iatrogenic)
- Intrahepatic
  - Congenital hepatic fibrosis
  - Idiopathic portal hypertension, non-cirrhotic portal fibrosis
  - Schistosomiasis
  - Myeloproliferative disorders
  - Systemic mastocytosis
  - Primary biliary cirrhosis (early)
  - Toxic causes (arsenic, vitamin A intoxication, vinyl chloride, cytotoxics)
  - Sarcoidosis
  - Gaucher's disease
- Extrinsic compression (periportal lymphadenopathy tumours, pancreatitis)

Sinusoidal obstruction
- Cirrhosis
- Nodular regenerative hyperplasia
- Fatty liver
- Wilson's disease

Postsinusoidal obstruction
- Intrahepatic
  - Cirrhosis (alcoholic, postnecrotic, secondary biliary cirrhosis)
  - Alcoholic hepatitis
  - Viral hepatitis
  - Haemochromatosis
  - Budd–Chiari syndrome (hypercoagulable states, veno-occlusive disease)
- Extrahepatic
  - Budd–Chiari syndrome (hepatic vein and inferior vena cava thrombosis, congenital suprahepatic inferior vena cava webs)
  - Extrinsic inferior vena cava compression (hepatic, renal, and adrenal tumours)
- Chronic congestive cardiac failure
- Constrictive pericarditis

Increased flow portal hypertension
- Hepatic arterial-portal venous fistulae (congenital, traumatic, or malignant)
- Splenic or mesenteric arteriovenous fistulae
- Portal-hepatic venous shunts
- Massive splenomegaly (tropical splenomegaly syndrome)

Anatomical and physiological considerations

The liver has a dual supply from both the hepatic artery and the portal vein. The superior mesenteric and splenic veins drain the splanchnic and splenic beds and join to form the portal vein. Entering into the origin of the portal vein is the coronary or left gastric vein which drains the lesser curve of the stomach and the lower oesophagus. The inferior mesentric vein drains the left hemicolon and most of the rectum, and joins the splenic vein just before its confluence with the superior mesenteric vein (Fig. 1). After division into left and right branches, the hepatic artery parallels the portal system, and subsequently divides into branches corresponding to the segmental anatomy of the liver.

The portal venous system is entirely devoid of valves. Numerous small tributaries connect the portal and systemic venous systems, and these can evolve into major collateral channels when portal hypertension supervenes. Formation of such collaterals is triggered when portal pressure rises above the normal level of 5 to 10 mmHg. This absence of valves is a feature of practical importance, in that it allows portal venous pressure to be measured

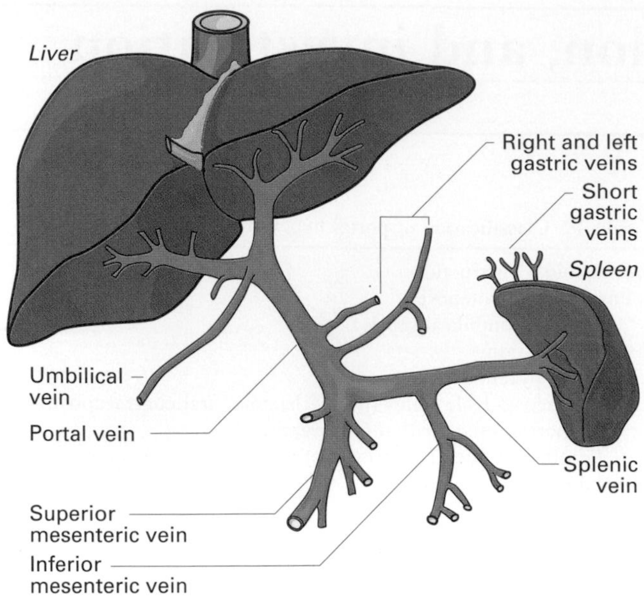

Fig. 1 Anatomy of the portal venous system.

during surgical procedures by cannulation of any small mesenteric or omental vein.

The most important of these portal-systemic channels is the left gastric or coronary vein, which connects the oesophagocardiac venous plexus with the splenic or portal vein; the short gastric and left gastroepiploic veins, which connect the oesophageal and gastric plexus with the splenic vein; numerous retroperitoneal portal radicles, which connect to the left renal vein via the left adrenal vein; the umbilical and periumbilical veins connecting to the left portal vein; and the inferior mesenteric vein connecting via the superior haemorrhoidal vein to the middle and inferior haemorrhoidal veins of the systemic circulation. The last are often responsible for the formation of large hypertensive haemorrhoids. Collaterals may also form across the diaphragm, within adhesions from previous abdominal surgery or from inflammatory bowel disease, or at mucocutaneous junctions, such as those that occur at ileostomies or colostomies (Fig. 2). In addition to these channels, intrahepatic shunts develop through which a significant proportion of portal venous flow can pass. These routes allow up to 80 per cent of the liver's blood supply to bypass the sinusoidal circulation.

The portal vein normally carries 75 per cent of the blood supply of the liver, with an average flow of 1200 ml/min. The hepatic artery supplies the remainder, at an average flow of 400 ml/min; it also provides 30 to 40 per cent of the liver's normal oxygen requirement since portal blood is already partly deoxygenated. When flow to the sinusoids is significantly reduced, a compensatory increase in hepatic arterial inflow takes place to provide the

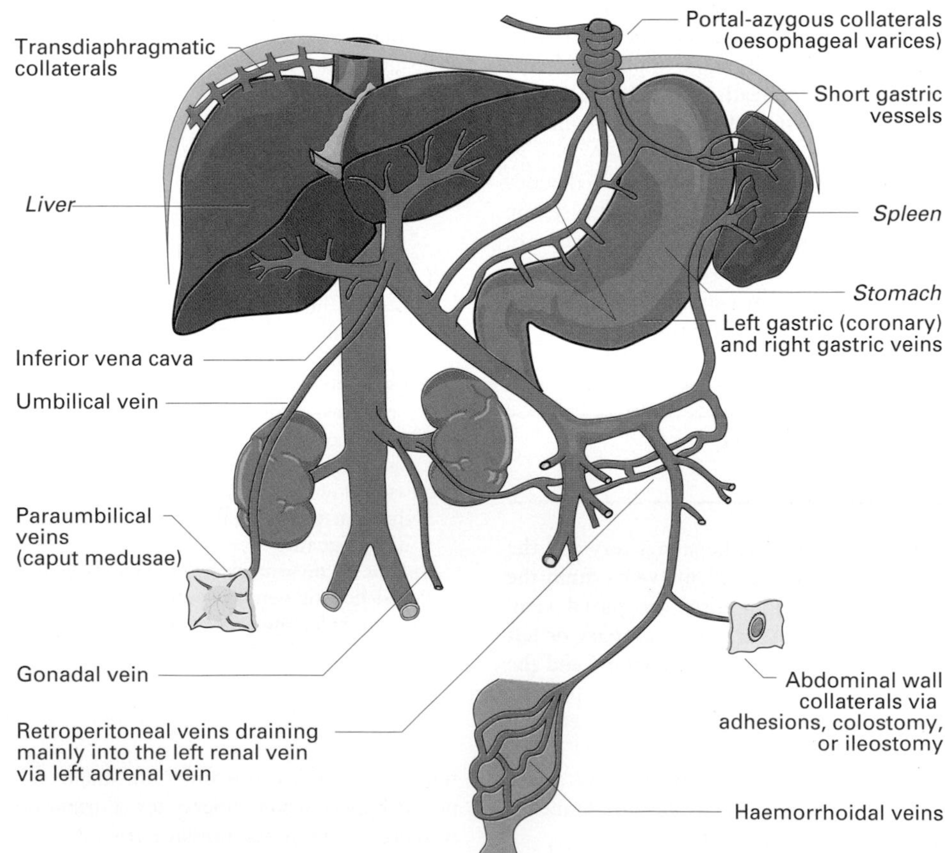

Fig. 2 Sites of portal-systemic collateral circulation in portal hypertension.

liver's oxygen requirements. However, intrahepatic shunting may cause up to 30 per cent of hepatic arterial flow to bypass the sinusoidal bed. Despite the compensatory increase in arterial flow, therefore, an overall significant reduction in hepatic tissue perfusion is highly likely to occur.

Haemodynamic considerations

An appreciation of the basic haemodynamic principles governing flow within blood vessels allows a better understanding of the pathophysiology of portal hypertension. As in all blood vessels, pressure within the portal system is determined by the interaction of flow and vascular resistance. As these parameters change, so does portal pressure. This relationship is expressed by Ohm's law,

$$D_p = Q \times R$$

where D_p is change in pressure, Q is flow, and R is resistance in a vessel.

Resistance is determined by several factors as expressed in Poiseuille's Law,

$$R = 8^n L / \pi r^4$$

where n is the coefficient of viscosity, L the vessel length, and r the vessel radius. Within the liver, viscosity and length of vessel are relatively constant and thus changes in vascular resistance are mainly due to changes in radius. Because the relationship is to the fourth power of the radius, small changes in portal vessel diameter will have profound effects on vascular resistance.

The normal liver has a very low resistance, but this increases dramatically in disease. As well as structural disturbances associated with cirrhosis, inflammatory changes in the hepatic venous tree and deposition of fibrous tissue around the terminal hepatic venules and adjacent sinusoids have been described. In cirrhotic livers, intrahepatic resistance may also be affected by proliferation of myofibroblasts around the sinusoids and terminal hepatic venules, resulting in increased contractility which may raise resistance and contribute to portal hypertension. Sinusoids may be compressed by hepatocyte enlargement in regenerating parts of the liver. This can occur as a result of several toxic, infectious, or metabolic insults to the parenchyma and may explain the portal hypertension seen in non-cirrhotic conditions such as alcoholic hepatitis.

The 'backward' and 'forward' theories of portal hypertension

Despite the decompressive effects of collaterals and intrahepatic shunts, with up to 80 per cent of the portal blood flow bypassing the liver, portal pressure remains elevated. Two major hypotheses have been advanced to explain this phenomenon.

The 'backward' theory postulates that portal hypertension is due to increased hepatic vascular resistance which develops as a specific response so that in the presence of normal flow, pressure must increase. Hypertrophy of myofibroblasts within the sinusoidal bed is one possible mechanism by which this could be achieved. Ohm's law suggests that portal hypertension would develop only if normal liver blood flow was maintained, but logically, in the presence of extensive low-resistance collaterals, blood flow should be diverted away and thus portal pressure should decrease. In reality, however, the portal and splanchnic circulation is not only markedly increased but hyperdynamic, thus negating the likelihood that this theory can explain portal hypertension.

The 'forward' theory was initially postulated by Banti in 1883. He suggested that splenomegaly, portal hypertension, and cirrhosis were the result of increased splenic arterial blood flow. The subsequent confirmation of increased splanchnic blood flow as a major feature of portal hypertension has led to further development of this theory. This now suggests that increased and hyperdynamic flow, together with decreased splanchnic precapillary resistance, maintain portal hypertension even in the face of extensive portal-systemic shunting. Since Banti first postulated his theory, opinions on the relative contribution of increased splanchnic blood flow to the development of portal hypertension have varied. More recently Groszmann and other workers have increasingly implicated both theories as being involved in the pathophysiology of this condition.

It is currently believed that the principal and initial abnormality is increased vascular resistance to portal flow and that portal hypertension is then maintained by increased blood flow into the portal circulation, a phenomenon which has been confirmed conclusively both experimentally and clinically. Blood flow to the stomach, spleen, and intestines is increased by 50 per cent in portal hypertension: this is achieved largely by splanchnic vasodilatation and raised cardiac output.

A hyperdynamic systemic circulation is frequently found in patients with portal hypertension. The intensity of this phenomenon was previously related to the degree of underlying hepatocellular dysfunction. However, this state is also seen in patients with extrahepatic causes of portal hypertension, in whom hepatic function is usually normal. It is, therefore, the extent of portal-systemic shunting which is the major determinant in the pathogenesis of this clinical feature. Various vasoactive substances produced locally in the splanchnic and portal circulations to modulate and increase blood flow are then transported via collaterals into the systemic side, where their vasoactive effects cause a generalized hyperdynamic circulation.

The role of vasoactive substances in portal hypertension

Several substances have been implicated as hormonal factors which act on both the splanchnic and systemic circulations to produce hyperaemia. The most important of these are bile acids, serotonin, glucagon, and prostaglandins, in particular prostacyclin.

Elevated levels of bile acids have been demonstrated in patients with liver disease and implicated as promoters of splanchnic hyperaemia. In the experimental situation however, lowering of serum bile acid levels to normal has no effect on the increased splanchnic blood flow, and their role remains uncertain.

Serotonin has a powerful vasoconstrictor effect on all vascular smooth muscle and is normally released into the portal circulation by the enterochromaffin cells of the gastrointestinal tract. In experimental portal hypertension, selective blockade of serotonin receptors reduces portal pressure, thus supporting the role of serotonergic mechanisms in the pathogenesis of portal hypertension.

Glucagon, a potent splanchnic vasodilator, is elevated in patients with portal hypertension, and probably accounts for 30 per cent of the increased splanchnic blood flow. The effect of somatostatin reducing portal pressure and blood flow may in part result from its inhibitory effect on the release of glucagon, in addition to its direct vasoactive properties.

Prostacyclin is another naturally occurring powerful vasodilator, production of which is elevated in the portal vein endothelium of rats with portal hypertension. Its production is directly related to the portal pressure. Prostacyclin production is also elevated in experimental arterial hypertension: this may represent a compensatory physiological response of endothelial cells to reduce hypertension. Cirrhotic patients have extremely high levels of urinary 6-ketoprostaglandin $F_{1\alpha}$, a stable metabolite of prostacyclin, and pharmacological inhibition of prostacyclin production reduces portal pressure in these patients.

Thus several important vasoactive substances are delivered directly into the systemic circulation via portal-systemic collaterals which carry 80 per cent of the portal blood flow. These substances will remain vasoactive since they have avoided deactivation by the hepatocytes. They provide a likely explanation for the systemic hyperaemia of portal hypertension.

EPIDEMIOLOGY AND NATURAL HISTORY OF PORTAL HYPERTENSION

Cirrhosis of the liver accounts for approximately 90 per cent of all cases of portal hypertension presenting in the West. In Eastern and tropical countries non-cirrhotic causes predominate. Distinct geographical distributions are found for non-cirrhotic portal fibrosis, schistosomiasis, and idiopathic portal hypertension.

In India, idiopathic portal fibrosis causes 20 to 30 per cent of all cases of portal hypertension; a further 20 to 30 per cent are due to portal vein thrombosis secondary to dehydration and portal infection in the neonatal period. In Japan approximately 10 per cent of cases of portal hypertension are idiopathic, as opposed to 1 to 6 per cent in the West. This condition remains most prevalent in the tropics.

Schistosomiasis affects more than 200 million people worldwide: *Schistosoma mansoni* is particularly prevalent in the Middle East, Africa, and South America, while *S. japonicum* is the causative agent in the Far East. Hepatic schistosomiasis is particularly common in Egypt, where oesophageal variceal bleeding secondary to this disease is the most common cause of upper gastrointestinal haemorrhage.

In children, extrahepatic portal vein obstruction is the main cause of upper gastrointestinal bleeding: this accounts for 40 to 50 per cent of all cases of portal hypertension in those under 17 years old. It is much more common in developing countries.

The natural history and prognosis of portal hypertension depends primarily on the underlying hepatic functional reserve. Conditions causing presinusoidal block but in which hepatocellular function remains good carry the best prognosis: the major lethal complication is haemorrhage from oesophageal varices. The mortality for each bleeding episode is about 5 per cent, and where facilities exist for prompt blood transfusion and injection sclerotherapy the long-term outlook is good. In postsinusoidal block (Budd–Chiari syndrome or veno-occlusive disease) severe secondary hepatocellular damage in the acute phase can result in death from liver failure and massive ascites rather than from haemorrhage.

In patients with cirrhosis the overall mortality rate from oesophageal variceal bleeding is about 40 per cent. If the patient recovers from the acute bleed the risk of recurrent haemorrhage during the same hospital admission is 60 per cent; this increases to more than 80 per cent at 2 years. The long-term survival of cirrhotics following variceal bleeding is poor, ranging from 6 to 35 per cent at 5 years. It is important to emphasize, however, that only about 30 per cent of cirrhotic patients will ever experience such bleeding. The remainder die of liver failure, cachexia, and infection.

The outlook in cirrhosis is generally determined by the severity of associated hepatocellular disease. In 1964 Child introduced a classification of severity of liver disease based on clinical findings and liver function tests. Classification into grades A, B, or C (Table 2) allows long-term survival and operative risk to be predicted for each patient. Groups A (good liver function) and B (moderate impairment of liver function) have a 70 to 80 per cent survival rate at 1 year while only 30 per cent of patients in group C (poor liver function) survive for 1 year. Child originally reported operative mortality rates of 5 per cent in groups A and B, and of 53 per cent in patients of group C undergoing portocaval shunting procedures. Using this classification, similar predictive patterns of mortality have been reported consistently throughout the literature. Patients with alcoholic liver disease or chronic active hepatitis also have particularly poor prognosis; patients with primary biliary cirrhosis generally have a better outlook.

Table 2 Child's classification of patients with chronic liver disease Clinical and laboratory data allow long-term prognosis and interventional or operative risk to be assessed. This also provides the best method of comparison of different forms of treatment in patients with portal hypertension.

Serum bilirubin			
(mmol/l)	<34	35–51	>68
(mg%)	<2	2–3	>3
Albumin (g/l)	35	28–35	<28
Prothrombin time			
(s prolonged)	1–4	4–6	>6
Ascites	Absent	Slight	Moderate
Encephalopathy	None	Minimal	Coma
Child's grade	A	B	C
points scored	5–6	7–9	10–15

Acute hepatic decompensation may occur during a bleeding episode. This may result in deterioration such that a patient initially in a good prognostic group enters a lower Child's grade. This phenomenon is of crucial importance in timing of intervention and most particularly, in analysis by Child's grading of the efficacy of specific interventional procedures.

OESOPHAGEAL VARICES

Rupture of oesophageal varices (and, less commonly, of gastric varices) is the most dramatic complication of portal hypertension and that which is most likely to require surgical management. Recent elegant anatomical studies have revealed in detail the complex and peculiar portal-systemic connection which occurs in the distal 2 to 5 cm of the oesophagus, precisely the zone where varices develop (Fig. 3). Four distinct layers of veins have been found

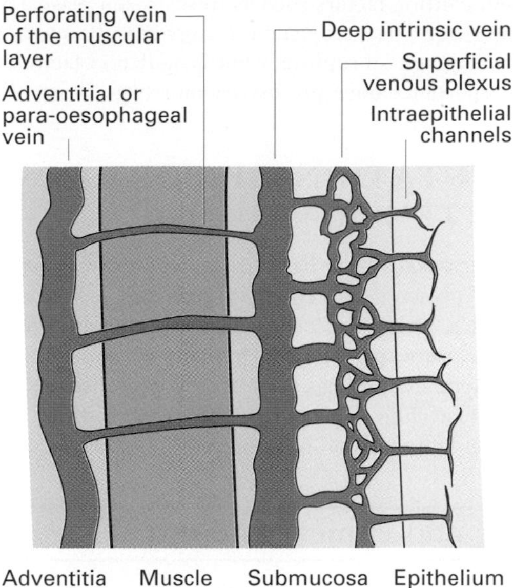

Fig. 3 Venous drainage of the distal oesophagus (after Kitano, 1986). Schematic, sectional representation of normal oesophageal wall displaying the venous anatomy.

in this zone, extending from the luminal surface to the adventitial layer. Intraepithelial veins or vascular epithelial channels drain into a superficial venous plexus, which lies just below the oesophageal epithelium. This plexus is in turn connected to a layer of deep intrinsic veins just outside the muscularis mucosae. The deep intrinsic veins connect with the outermost, external venous plexus coursing within the oesophageal adventitia via the perforating veins, which traverse the muscular layers of the oesophagus. Thus in this distal portion of the oesophagus, venous channels are concentrated largely in the mucosa and run in longitudinal pallisades. These connect with the more deeply located submucous plexus in the cephalad oesophagus and stomach respectively. This arrangement of veins probably underlies one of the intrinsic mechanisms of the physiological oesophageal sphincter, the so-called mucosal rosette, which is of importance in prevention of reflux.

In patients with portal hypertension this venous complex, situated at the watershed between the portal and systemic circulations, dilates dramatically and forms varices, classically running in three to five distinct trunks. The intraepithelial channels probably form the cherry red spots which can be seen endoscopically and are recognized as predictors of impending rupture. They are also found in histological specimens of oesophageal transection rings.

Studies using the oesophageal Doppler ultrasound probe have shown that blood flow and velocity within the palisade zone is complex and considerable. While flow is mainly cephalad, as would be expected, bidirectional flow has also been demonstrated, particularly where perforating veins from the deep adventitial plexus enter the varices. Turbulence of flow has also been demonstrated in these perforating veins. The palisade and perforating venous systems are therefore critical to the development of varices. Less severe variceal bleeds probably result from rupture of the intraepithelial channels, while torrential haemorrhage results from rupture of the deeper, high-flow intrinsic venous channels.

Gastric varices are a much less common source of haemorrhage, probably because of their deeper submucosal situation. These varices are mainly supplied by the short gastric veins and course into the deep intrinsic veins of the distal oesophagus. Congestive gastropathy, which is common in portal hypertension, is associated with mucosal congestion, resulting from increased submucosal arteriovenous communications which develop between the muscularis mucosae and dilated arterioles and venules. Such congested mucosa is particularly susceptible to gastritis and haemorrhage.

Rupture of oesophageal varices

Significant rupture occurs in only 30 per cent of patients, and the causes remain poorly understood. Two main theories for variceal rupture are commonly advanced. The erosive theory postulates that mucosal damage due to reflux oesophagitis causes erosion into the varix and thus haemorrhage. Reflux oesophagitis is not common, however, either at endoscopy or at operative inspection of the distal oesophagus. Inflammation is rarely found in specimens of oesophageal rings removed at transection, and controlled trials have found that cimetidine has no advantage over placebo in preventing recurrent variceal bleeding. Erosion of the oesophageal mucosa as a cause of rupture therefore seems unlikely.

The eruptive theory proposes that variceal rupture is related to pressure where the varix is in close proximity to the oesophageal lumen: thus it commonly occurs in the distal 2 to 5 cm of the oesophagus. Although increased portal pressure (>12 mmHg) is required for variceal development, a direct correlation between portal pressure and risk of variceal bleeding has not been found. There is more circumspect evidence to support a relationship between the severity of portal hypertension and risk of variceal haemorrhage. Portal pressure in alcoholic patients following a variceal bleed was higher in those who did not survive. In addition, angiography and blood volume expansion, both of which may increase portal pressure, occasionally precipitate haemorrhage. Variceal haemorrhage has also been reported to occur after deep inspiration, coughing, and following the Valsalva manoeuvre, all of which cause an increased pressure differential between oesophageal varix and lumen. Local factors such as variceal wall thickness and that of the overlying mucosa are obviously also of importance.

Variceal size has been reported to be a risk factor for haemorrhage, the larger varices being more likely to bleed. The lack of relationship between pressure and variceal size reinforces the importance of local factors in varix development, however.

Groszmann has proposed that variceal wall tension may be the unifying predictor of rupture. Tension in a variceal wall can be derived from a modification of Laplace's law

$$T = TP \times r/w$$

where T = tension, TP = transluminal pressure, r = vessel radius, w = wall thickness.

In oesophageal varices, transmural tension is the difference in pressure between the oesophageal lumen and that of the varix. Thus tension is directly related not only to this pressure difference, but also to the varix radius, and is inversely related to variceal wall thickness. These three variables correspond in the clinical situation to variceal size, thickness of epithelium overlying the varix, and degree of portal hypertension, all of which have been described as independent predictors of bleeding. When portal pressure is increased the more superficial protruding varix will have less supporting connective tissue and a larger radius than a deeper varix embedded in supporting tissue which is under identical pressure. Wall tension will therefore be higher in these superficial varices, and rupture will result when this tension is no longer in equilibrium with the outwardly directed expansile force of portal pressure. When the elastic limit of the vessel has been reached, small changes in volume or radius will result in large changes in wall tension and imminent rupture (Fig. 4).

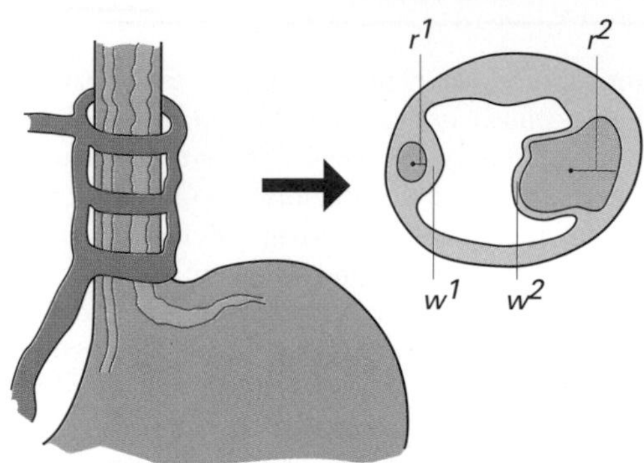

Fig. 4 Variceal wall tension (after Polio and Groszmann, 1986). Since $T = TP \times r/w$, variceal wall tension (T) is greater where radius (r) is larger and the wall (w) is thinner despite equal transmural pressure (TP); $T1$ is greater than $T2$.

The parameters considered in the above equation cannot be measured clinically. However endoscopic classification of varices according to size and presence of cherry red spots and red wall markings, both of which are related to thinness of the overlying epithelium, has markedly increased the clinician's ability to predict impending variceal haemorrhage.

Reduction of variceal pressure by shunting, disconnection, or by pharmacological means decreases transluminal pressure, vessel radius, and wall tension. Sclerotherapy, by causing dense perivariceal scarring, will increase the surrounding supporting tissue, strengthening the variceal wall and thus decreasing tension.

Once rupture has occurred the severity of haemorrhage will be affected by haemodynamic factors and by the disordered haemostasis that frequently accompanies liver disease. The relevant haemodynamic factors have been expressed by Groszmann in the following equation.

$$\text{severity of bleeding} = \frac{\text{area of rent}}{\text{blood viscosity}}$$

It follows that large holes under greater pressure will bleed more severely than small holes under lower pressure. Blood viscosity is directly related to the haematocrit: reduction of haematocrit after haemorrhage, in anaemia, and after volume replacement with crystalloids, may increase the severity of bleeding.

Patients with liver disease may show multiple disorders of haemostasis, including deficient production by the liver of the coagulation proteins, thrombocytopenia secondary to hypersplenism, impaired platelet function, and increased fibrinolytic activity. The relative importance of all these factors discussed in the clinical situation remains unclear. Haemorrhage generally responds most readily to transfusion of whole, preferably fresh, blood, and clotting factors such as fresh frozen plasma and platelets. Empirically, haemodynamic factors may be most important in the development of rupture, while coagulatory factors may be of greater importance once profuse haemorrhage is established.

PRESENTATION OF PORTAL HYPERTENSION

Portal hypertension *per se* has little in the way of clinical features, and usually presents with complications such as variceal haemorrhage, ascites, or hypersplenism. Haemorrhage occurs in only 30 per cent of these patients: the remainder may present with a clinical history and findings indicative of liver disease, particularly cirrhosis. The clinical history is therefore of major importance when portal hypertension is suspected.

History and clinical findings

Careful questioning of the patient about alcoholism, past jaundice or hepatitis, exposure to hepatotoxins, and a past history of blood transfusion or drug abuse should be routine. A history of neonatal or intra-abdominal sepsis, or of a myeloproliferative disorder is suggestive of an extrahepatic portal vein block. A history of myeloproliferative disorder may indicate the Budd–Chiari syndrome. The use of oral contraceptives or other sex hormone-containing medications is also significant.

The most common clinical presentation of portal hypertension is profuse gastrointestinal haemorrhage: the severity, frequency, and dates of these episodes must be determined. Elucidation of symptoms of hepatic decompensation, in particular ascites and portosystemic encephalopathy as manifested by intellectual dulling, confusion, or coma, is important. Haematemesis is the most common presentation, but episodes of melaena without haematemesis may also occur. A history of dyspepsia or past peptic ulceration suggests bleeding from one of these sources and the results of any previous barium studies or endoscopies may be informative.

Careful physical examination may reveal the stigmata of liver disease, but in the absence of hepatocellular decompensation the single most important finding is an enlarged spleen. If the spleen cannot be felt, or if splenomegaly is not confirmed on imaging, portal hypertension is unlikely to be present. Although enlargement of the spleen is progressive, the degree of hyperplenism is not related to the severity of portal hypertension. Abdominal wall veins from portal-systemic shunts may be visible, although this sign is uncommon. The caput medusae, in which several veins can be seen radiating out across the abdomen from the umbilicus is the most striking sign. In patients with obstruction of the inferior vena cava in the Budd–Chiari syndrome or as a result of severe ascites, abnormal veins course upwards across the abdomen from the iliac fossae to cross the costal margin and drain into superior vena cava territory.

Rarely, a murmur or venous hum may be heard in the region of the xiphoid process, arising from turbulent flow in a large umbilical collateral. A systolic murmur overlying the liver may indicate alcoholic hepatitis or a primary hepatocarcinoma. The liver may be enlarged, particularly in alcoholics, or shrunken: the latter can be confirmed by careful percussion. A shrunken liver is particularly common in portal hypertension and is reported to be associated with higher portal pressures. The consistency of the liver should also be assessed: a firm nodular liver indicates cirrhosis, while a smooth soft liver is suggestive of extrahepatic portal obstruction.

Ascites usually develops in hepatocellular decompensation and is rarely due to portal hypertension alone. Peripheral oedema is also frequently present. Further signs of liver failure include palmar erythema, spider naevi, white nails, jaundice, and portal-systemic encephalopathy. Rectal varices are common in portal hypertension but cannot be detected by digital examination alone. Bleeding from rectal varices is uncommon, rarely severe, and must obviously be distinguished from that associated with simple haemorrhoids.

Haemorrhage from oesophageal varices remains the most common presentation of portal hypertension: if these varices did not form, portal hypertension would be of virtually no clinical significance. Bleeding is typically dramatic and catastrophic, with massive haematemesis and circulatory collapse. Bleeding *per rectum* may also be profuse and fresh. A slow oozing of blood from varices may occasionally result in true melaena only. Variceal bleeding in patients with cirrhosis may cause marked deterioration of liver cell function. This, together with increased protein absorption from the blood-laden gut, may lead to portal-systemic encephalopathy and coma.

Non-variceal gastrointestinal bleeding is also common in alcoholic patients who may suffer from peptic ulceration, gastric erosions, and the Mallory–Weiss syndrome.

INVESTIGATION

Clinical evaluation of the patient is of utmost importance, particularly when surgical intervention is being contemplated. Operative procedures in patients with compromised liver function carry significantly increased risk. Evaluation of the patient's hepatocellular reserve is therefore of crucial importance when selecting treatment for bleeding varices. Such assessment may be best made in conjunction with a hepatologist or physician with a special interest in liver disease. Recommended laboratory investigations are listed in Table 3. Once the underlying liver disease has been diagnosed and liver function assessed, treatment should be selected on the basis of liver reserve, as classified by Child. The next stage in investigation is imaging of the varices and the portal circulation.

Table 3 General investigations of portal hypertension

1 Full blood count: anaemia, leucopenia, and thrombocytopenia in chronic liver disease and hypersplenism
2 Liver function tests: indicators of primary cause of liver disease
Serum albumin and prothrombin time are good measures of synthetic function
γ-Glutamyl transpeptidase is raised in patients with excess alcohol intake
3 Specific serum autoantibodies: markers of primary biliary cirrhosis and autoimmune chronic active hepatitis
4 Serological markers of hepatitis B and C
5 Tests for copper and iron metabolism (Wilson's disease and haemochromatosis)
6 Serum α_1-antitrypsin levels, any patient with cirrhosis, particularly with a past medical history of neonatal jaundice
7 Blood grouping

Endoscopy

Endoscopy allows rapid and safe confirmation of the source of bleeding from the upper gastrointestinal tract. It is of vital importance in the exclusion of other causes of bleeding, such as peptic ulceration, gastritis, duodenitis, or an oesophageal tear. During active haemorrhage the source of bleeding may be obscured, particularly if it is from gastric varices or gastritis. Repeat endoscopy after 3 to 4 h will often find the stomach emptied of clot or blood, allowing visualization of the source. Once the diagnosis of variceal haemorrhage is confirmed, a skilled endoscopist can undertake immediate treatment by injection sclerotherapy.

Endoscopy also allows the size, distribution, and colour of varices to be determined. Varices are normally white and opaque: red coloration and the presence of cherry red spots are accurate predictors of variceal bleeding. Larger varices are also more likely to bleed. Endoscopic assessment of scarring or ulceration following injection sclerotherapy is of major importance, particularly when bleeding continues or recurs and procedures such as oesophageal transection are being considered. Surgical intervention should be avoided in patients with injection site ulceration: this is a frequent cause of haemorrhage which usually responds to medical treatment.

IMAGING MODALITIES IN PORTAL HYPERTENSION

Plain radiographs of the abdomen and chest are of limited value in the management of portal hypertension, but they may yield useful information. In an abdominal radiograph liver and spleen size may be assessed and rarely, gas shadows in the portal circulation may be detected in patients with enterocolitis, intestinal infection, or disseminated intravascular coagulation syndromes (Figs. 5, 6).

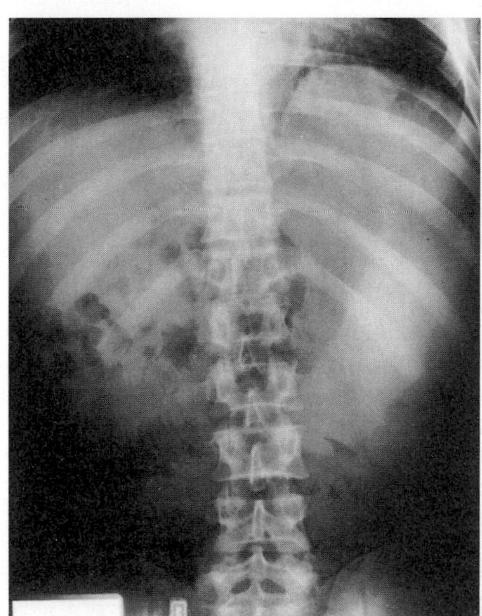

Fig. 5 Abdominal radiograph demonstrating gross splenomegaly secondary to portal hypertension.

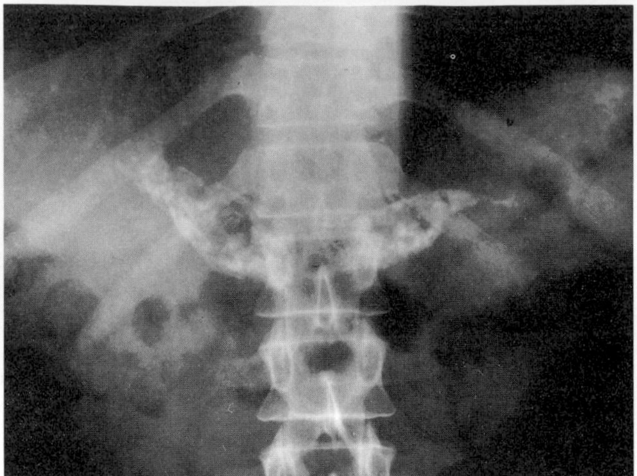

Fig. 6 Abdominal radiograph demonstrating calcified and thrombosed portal and splenic veins.

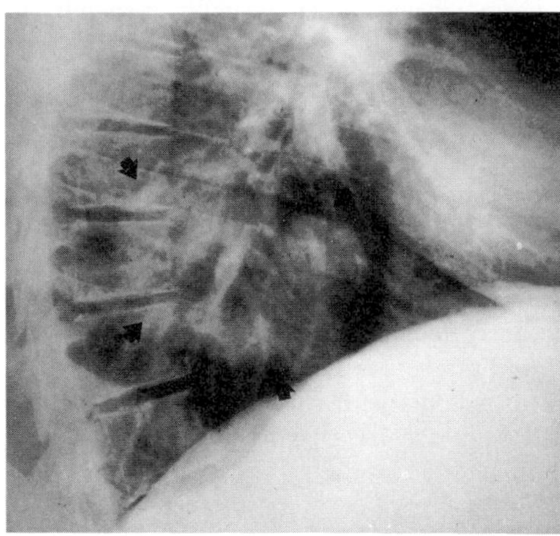

Fig. 7 Chest radiograph, lateral view: this shows a lobulated mass behind the heart due to para-oesophageal varices.

Widening of the left paravertebral shadow due to lateral displacement of the pleural reflection between aorta and vertebral column by a dilated hemiazygos vein may also be seen. Rarely, extensive para-oesophageal collaterals may appear as a posterior mediastinal mass (Fig. 7).

Where endoscopic facilities are not available, barium studies can be useful in demonstrating oesophageal and gastric varices (Fig. 8). The typical appearances are of a dilated oesophagus containing multiple irregular filling defects, usually in the distal third but occasionally running throughout the entire oesophagus. Barium studies are also useful in diagnosing other causes of bleeding, such as peptic ulceration. For this reason a full upper gastrointestinal barium study is preferable to a barium swallow alone.

Once the diagnosis is made and operative intervention is being considered, the anatomical details of the portal circulation are needed. Classically this is obtained by angiography, but less invasive techniques such as duplex ultrasonography, contrast-enhanced CT scanning, and magnetic resonance imaging are being increasingly employed.

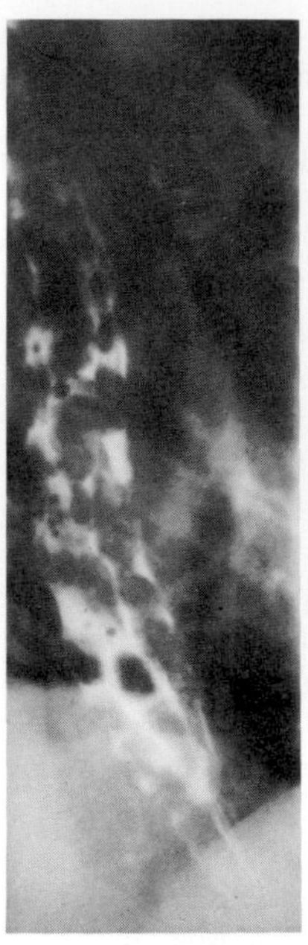

Fig. 8 Barium swallow. The characteristic sign of a string of beads in the oesophagus indicates oesophageal varices.

Diagnostic angiography

Angiography plays a major role in the investigation of portal hypertension. Hepatic blood flow, free and wedged hepatic pressures, and inferior vena cava pressures can all be measured during this procedure. The main indication, however, is visualization of the portal system, particularly for identification of major portosystemic collaterals and provision of a map to allow planning of surgical intervention. It is also particularly useful in the diagnosis and assessment of non-cirrhotic portal hypertension, such as that due to portal vein thrombosis, and when there is reason to suspect occlusion of a portal-systemic shunt. The portal circulation can be demonstrated by several angiographic techniques.

Coeliac and superior mesenteric angiography

Coeliac and superior mesenteric angiography is the safest, most commonly used, but indirect means of visualizing the portal venous circulation (Fig. 9). Using the Seldinger technique under local anaesthesia, the coeliac trunk and superior mesenteric artery are selectively and individually cannulated using a small bore arterial catheter (French 5) and 50 to 60 ml of contrast medium. The venous circulation is visualized awaiting the venous return of contrast after its arterial injection: this technique requires careful timing by the radiologist, and has been greatly simplified by the advent of digital subtraction angiography. Detailed imaging of the entire portal circulation with identification of major collaterals and shunts can be obtained routinely. Additional information such as the presence of hepatofugal flow, may influence the choice of surgical procedure.

Injection of contrast into the coeliac trunk allow the hepatic and splenic arterial circulation to be visualized. The intrahepatic circulation is frequently abnormal in cirrhosis, showing tortuosity or corkscrewing of the hepatic arterial branches. Haemangiomata, tumour circulation, hepatic artery-to-portal vein shunting, aneu-

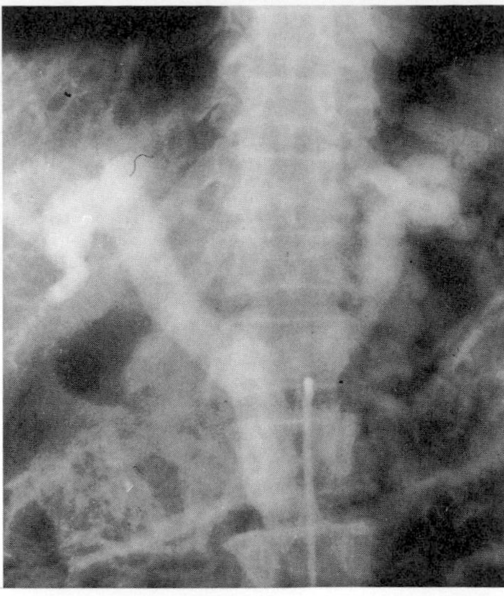

Fig. 9 Superior mesenteric angiogram. The venous phase shows a patent portal vein with a prominent left gastric vein and oesophageal varices.

rysms, or anatomical variations of the major arteries can be readily and accurately demonstrated. Injection of contrast into the splenic artery allows evaluation of the splenic vein and coronary vein, and demonstration of oesophagogastric varices. Superior mesenteric angiography is used to delineate the superior mesenteric and portal veins and their collaterals.

Indirect visualization of the portal tree suffers from a degree of loss of detail, but this is rarely severe enough to warrant direct venography. Digital subtraction angiography is being used increasingly often with good results, but resolution is often poorer than that of conventional angiography.

Splenic venography

The best imaging of the splenic and portal veins, and collaterals is obtained using this technique, but at the cost of increased risk. Splenic venography is of particular value in the investigation of extrahepatic portal vein obstruction or when cavernous transformation of a thrombosed portal vein is suspected (Figs. 10 and 11). After infiltration of local anaesthetic into tissues overlying the spleen, a fine bore catheter is passed into the spleen and splenic pulp pressure is measured. Venography is then performed by injection of contrast into the splenic pulp. Once imaging is completed, the catheter tract is sealed by injection of pledgets of gelatine foam. Providing any coagulopathy is corrected beforehand, this procedure is rarely complicated by significant haemorrhage, but extravasation of contrast around the spleen may cause pain, both local and referred to the left shoulder. The risk of complication remains higher than with angiography and splenic venography should therefore be reserved for patients in whom imaging by angiography is inadequate.

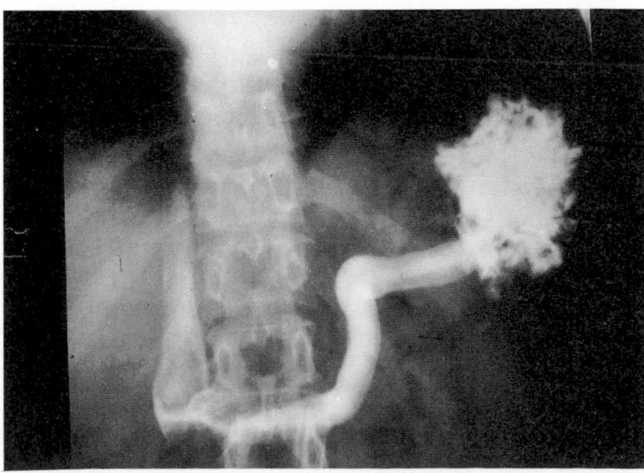

Fig. 10 Splenic venogram. The splenic injection gives the best definition of the portal venous circulation, here confirming the patency of a portacaval shunt.

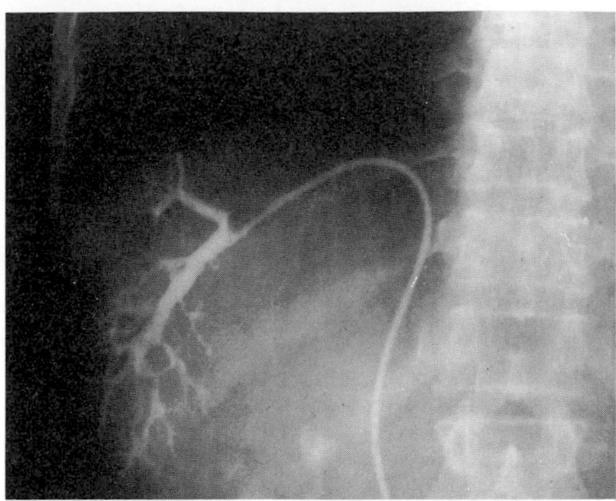

Fig. 11 Hepatic venogram, showing irregularity of the hepatic venous radicles indicating cirrhosis.

Transhepatic venography

This technique is performed by percutaneous puncture of the liver, introduction of a fine bore catheter into an intrahepatic radicle, and injection of contrast. Excellent imaging of the splenic and portal vein is obtained (Fig. 12) and varices can be embolized

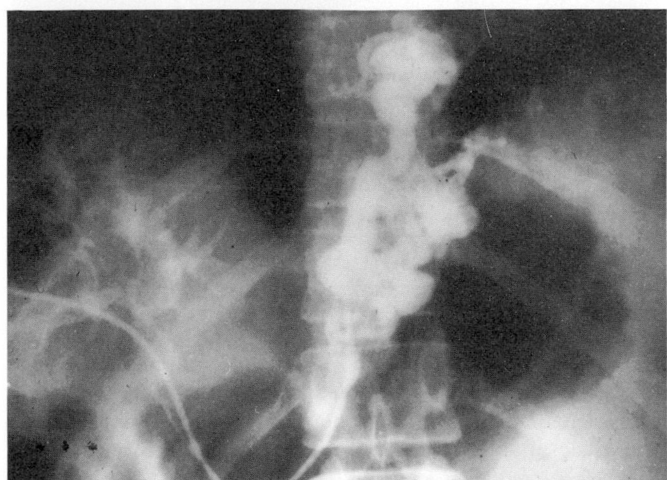

Fig. 12 Transhepatic portagram. Selective cannulation of the left gastric vein has been performed demonstrating oesophageal varices; embolization of bleeding varices is possible by this route but is now rarely employed because of technical difficulty and the high rebleeding rate.

via the coronary or larger collateral veins. Initial success in stopping variceal haemorrhage is high (80–90 per cent), but there is a 25 to 30 per cent rebleeding rate within a few days. This, together with a high complication rate and the technically demanding nature of the procedure, has led to its virtual abandonment.

Inferior vena cava and hepatic venography

In the Budd–Chiari syndrome the inferior vena cava is often severely stenosed or entirely occluded. The degree to which this vessel is compressed by the hypertrophied caudate lobe can be assesed both by visualization and measurement of the pressure gradient between the suprahepatic and infrahepatic inferior vena cavae (Fig. 13): a high gradient mitigates against treatment by portacaval shunt. Hepatic venography is of value in diagnosing hepatic vein thrombosis in patients with veno-occlusive disease associated with myeloproliferative disorders. Its most common use, however, is in measurement of free and wedged hepatic pressures in the assessment of cirrhosis and portal hypertension. These measurements are of particular value as a research tool in evaluation of the haemodynamic effects of drugs on the portal circulation.

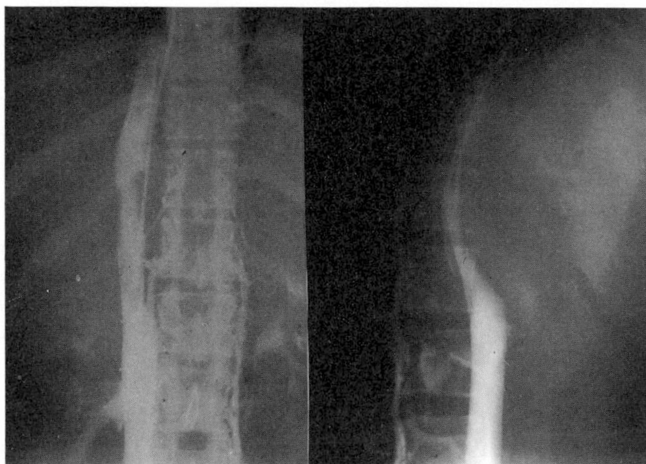

Fig. 13 Inferior vena cavogram. These anteroposterior and lateral views of the inferior vena cava confirm the diagnosis of Budd–Chiari syndrome with compression of the hepatic vena cava by the massively hypertrophied caudate lobe.

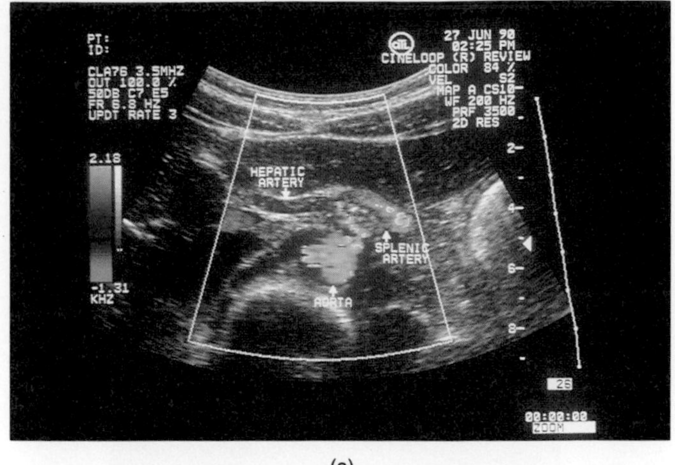

(a)

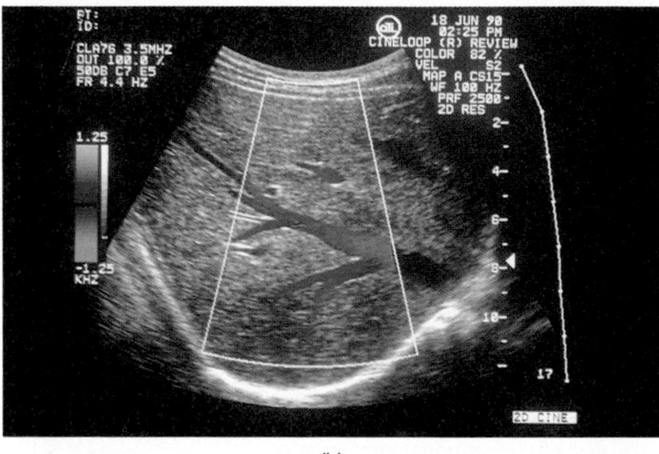

(b)

Fig. 14 Duplex scans of the portal and hepatic vessels. The portal, splenic and hepatic veins can be visualized by duplex scanning. Colour duplex, while not essential, facilitates imaging of deeper visceral vessels. Flow measurement and monitoring of blood flow direction can be routinely performed with this technique. Part (a) shows the structures at the coeliac axis; in (b) elegant images of a normal hepatic vein and its branches are shown.

Ultrasound and duplex scanning

Real-time ultrasound scanning can provide much detailed and accurate information by totally non-invasive means. It is of particular value for scanning the hepatic and splenic parenchyma for haemangioma, tumour, and cirrhosis. Thrombosis or occlusion of the portal, superior mesenteric, and splenic vein can be accurately detected. Large collaterals can be visualized, helping to confirm the diagnosis of portal hypertension. Although the results are often compromised by duodenal or intestinal gas, its absolute safety is making ultrasound scanning the first line of investigation in portal hypertension. Recent advances in duplex ultrasound technology, in particular colour-flow coding, allow faster and more accurate assessment of direction and flow in the portal circulation (Fig. 14). The accuracy is such that flow through portosystemic shunts can be measured, and duplex scanning is superseding angiography as the investigation of choice when graft occlusion is suspected. Duplex ultrasonography has become an important diagnostic and research tool with a promising future role in the investigation of portal hypertension.

Computerized axial tomography (CT scan)

The major advantage of CT scanning lies in the detection of focal liver disease and hepatosplenomegaly (Fig. 15). Used with contrast enhancement and dynamic scanning, portal vein patency and para-oesophageal and retroperitoneal portosystemic collaterals can be demonstrated readily. This is rarely the diagnostic pro-

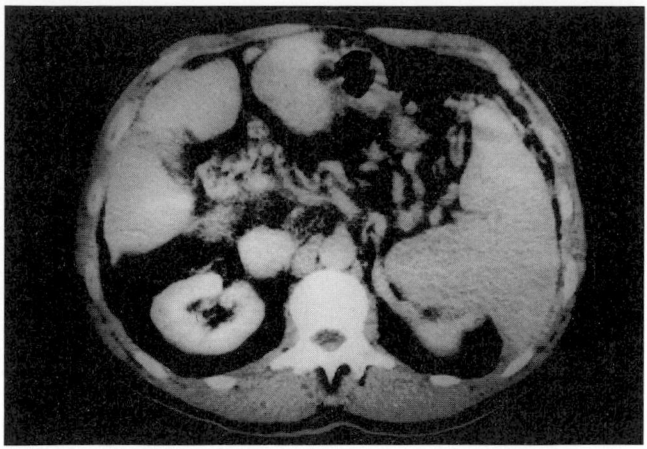

Fig. 15 Abdominal CT scan. Splenomegaly is clearly demonstrated with prominent retroperitoneal and hilar varices.

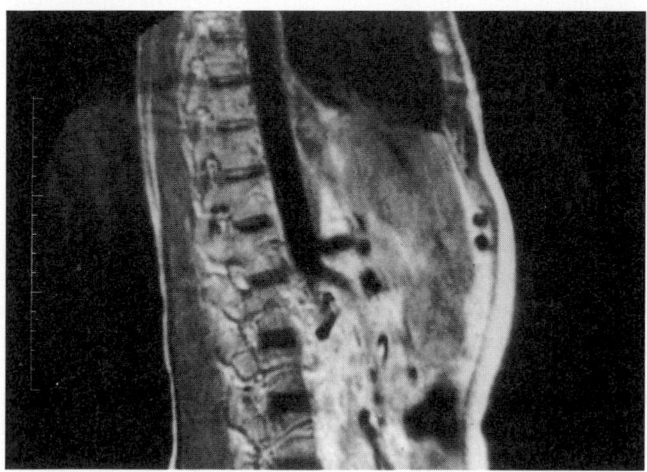

Fig. 16 Magnetic resonance imaging of the abdomen. The scan demonstrates the origins of the coeliac and superior mesenteric arteries. Note the large varices coursing along the anterior surface of the cirrhotic liver.

cedure of choice, however, since ultrasound, and increasingly magnetic resonance imaging, delineate these lesions more easily and accurately. CT assessment of liver parenchymal volume is used in some centres as part of the assessment and selection of candidates for liver transplantation.

Magnetic resonance imaging

This imaging modality allows excellent parenchymal visualization, imaging in any plane, and better blood vessel imaging than CT scanning. MRI angiography is currently limited by poor resolution and long imaging times. However development of this modality is progressing rapidly and it is very likely to supersede CT scanning and even conventional angiography in the future (Figs. 16 and 17).

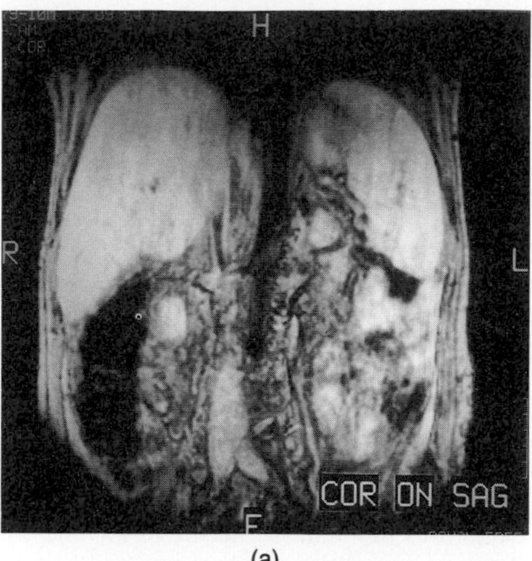

(a)

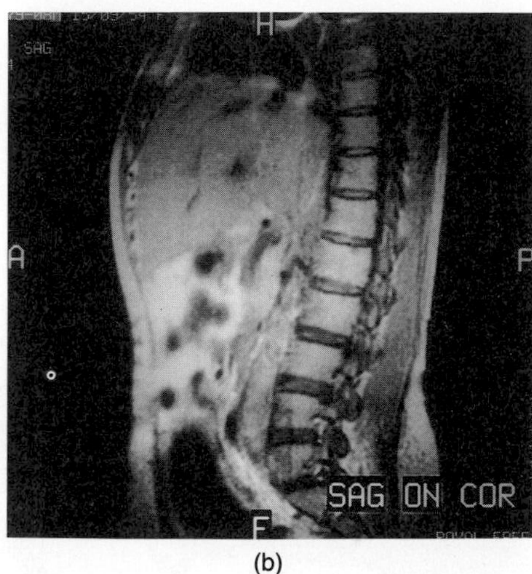

(b)

Fig. 17 (a and b) Magnetic resonance imaging, showing complete thrombosis of the hepatic and abdominal inferior vena cava of a patient with Budd–Chiari syndrome secondary to myeloproliferative disease. Note the collaterals in the anterior abdominal wall and running along the aorta.

FURTHER READING

Dick R. Angiography. In: Millward-Sadler GH, Wright R, Arthur MJP, eds. *Wright's Liver and Biliary Disease*. London: WB Saunders, 1992: 582–94.

Karin SK. Progress report. Non-cirrhotic portal fibrosis. *Gut* 1989; **30**: 406–15.

Kitano S, Terblanche J, Kahn D, Bornman PC. Venous anatomy of the lower oesophagus in portal hypertension: practical implications. *Br J Surg* 1986; **73**: 525–31.

Mahl TC, Groszmann RJ. Pathophysiology of portal hypertension and variceal bleeding. *Surg Clin N Am* 1990; **70**: 251–66.

Pilar Pizcueta M, Garcia-Pagan JC, Fernandez M, Casamitjana R, Bosch J, Rodès J. Glucagon hinders the effects of somatostatin on portal hypertension. A study in rats with portal vein ligation. *Gastroenterology* 1991; **101**: 1710–15.

Polio J, Groszmann RJ. Haemodynamic factors involved in the development and rupture of oesophageal varices: a pathophysiologic approach to treatment. *Semin Liver Dis* 1986; **6**: 318–31.

Sherlock S. *Disease of the Liver and Biliary System*, 8th edn. Oxford: Blackwell, 1991.

Sitzman JV, Bulkley GB, Mitchell MC, Campbell K. Role of prostacyclin in the splanchnic hyperaemia contributing to portal hypertension. *Ann Surg* 1989; **209**: 322–7.

Sitzman JV, Li S-S, Adkinson F. Evidence for role of prostacyclin as a systemic hormone in portal hypertension. *Surgery* 1991; **109**: 149–53.

Spence RAJ, Terblanche J. Venous anatomy of the lower oesophagus: a new perspective on varices. *Br J Surg* 1987; **74**: 659–60.

24.2 Emergency treatment of bleeding oesophageal varices

RONALD A. MALT

The most dangerous moment in the life of anyone with bleeding oesophageal varices caused by alcoholic cirrhosis is the instant of the first major haemorrhage (Fig. 1). The observed risk of death relative to baseline risk is increased 112-fold, and the overall mortality rate is increased by 35 to 70 per cent. More than 1 litre of blood can be lost in 1 h through a defect in the variceal wall only the size of a 22-gauge needle. Even though the chance of death decreases rapidly after the episode of bleeding subsides, rebleeding is common—perhaps even universal. In the evaluation of both clinical trials and the every day treatment of patients with variceal haemorrhage, control of the initial episode of bleeding and control of subsequent episodes of bleeding must be considered separately.

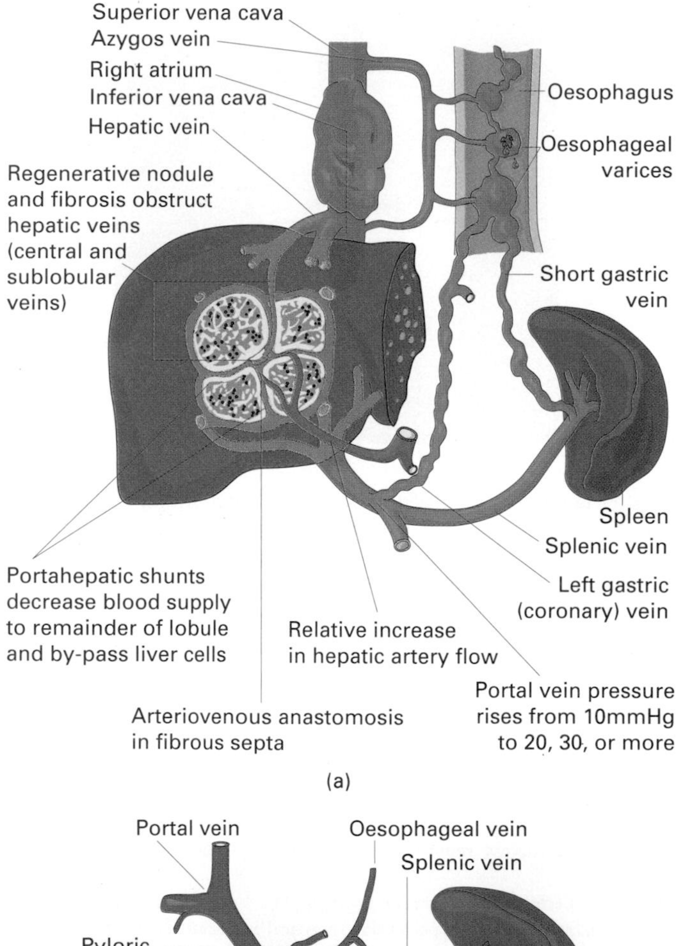

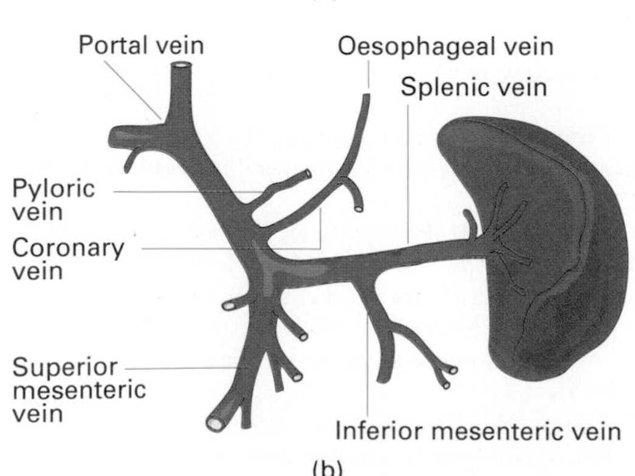

Fig. 1 (a) Bleeding oesophageal varices and the relevant splanchnic veins. (b) Schema of splanchnic veins (detailed).

FALLACIES OF RANDOMIZED TRIALS

Randomized trials to assess the value of surgery, of obliteration of varices by sclerotherapy, and of division of the variceal columns hinge not only on the variables known by the investigators, but also upon how they are presented. The choice of the zero timepoint of observation in reference to the entire clinical course may bias results. For example, a classic paper extolling the superiority of surgical treatment used as its zero point the time of death of all patients who died in hospital. Once the dead were eliminated, the survival rate of the remainder, who had proved their stamina by living through a major operation and its sequelae, was superb.

My opinion has not wavered from that expressed in 1976: the complexities of portal hypertension confound the best intentioned clinical trials. Studies on the therapeutic value of shunts require uniform and unequivocal diagnosis of bleeding varices, but this never has been achieved. Prospective stratification by age and by integrity of hepatic function of patients to be operated upon and of controls, even in a single hospital, is rarely feasible because the number of patients is too small except in multicentre trials. Cooperative trials are, however, beset by problems ranging from the differing selectivity of investigators to the criteria applied for interpreting findings. Violations of protocol because of the practicalities of clinical care introduce undetectable bias, making comparisons difficult. The several studies done in the 1970s showing that a prophylactic portacaval shunt merely changes the cause of death from variceal bleeding to liver failure are all flawed in light of modern knowledge about statistical power and β error.

A derivative of these arguments is that any patient whose liver function is so bad that blood clotting is impaired cannot do well. Although that observation is undeserving of a controlled trial, it persists in being substantiated by much investigative effort. Likewise, one would expect patients whose clinical status by Child's criteria for assessment of hepatic reserve (Table 1) puts them in

Table 1 Child's classification of cirrhotic patients in terms of 'hepatic functional reserve'

Variable	'A'	'B'	'C'
Serum bilirubin (mmol/l)	<35	35–51	>51
Serum albumin (g/dl)	>3.5	3.0–3.5	<3.0
Ascites	None	Easily controlled	Poorly controlled
Neurological disorder	None	Minimal	Advanced, 'coma'
Nutrition	Excellent	Good	Poor, 'wasting'

Modified from Child CG III, ed. The liver and portal hypertension. *Major Problems in Surgery*. Philadelphia: WB Saunders Co., 1964; **I**: 50.

Table 2 Massachusetts General Hospital scale for predicting the risk of postoperative death after portacaval or proximal splenorenal venous shunting. Calculation of a simple five-point predictive score

	Points assigned		
Predictor	0	1	2
Bilirubin (mg/dl) or [mmol/l]	(⩽0.99) [<35]	(1.00–1.99) [35–51]	(⩾2.0) [⩾51]
Ascites	None	Controlled (stable)	Uncontrollable
Operative urgency	Elective	Emergency	—

Score is the sum of points assigned for each predictor: minimum = 0, maximum = 5.

class A to do best, in class B, less well, and in class C, dismally, as they do. A valid means of predicting the likelihood of postoperative death, after either portacaval or proximal splenorenal shunting is shown in Table 2 and is depicted in Fig. 2.

The point of the foregoing paragraphs is to urge scepticism. Irrespective of what has been learned from clinical trials, treatment of bleeding varices is empirical. The fact that large varices are those most likely to bleed and that proper clotting is essential to survival are the unequivocal data to which one might repair.

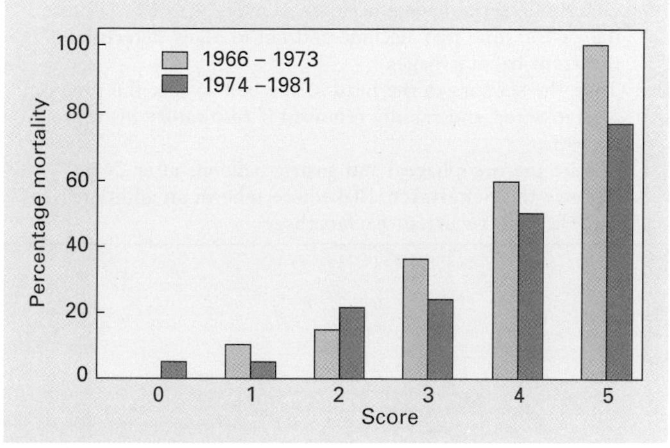

Fig. 2 Postoperative mortality rates predicted by Massachusetts General Hospital score after portacaval or splenorenal shunting in two eras.

EMERGENCY TREATMENT

No matter how much blood has been vomited by a patient with bleeding varices on admission to an emergency ward, the chances are better than even that bleeding will stop spontaneously. Letting the patient sit upright seems to help, but the patient who can tolerate sitting upright has to have a good intravascular volume and is thus a selected patient. Parenteral administration of vasopressin to constrict blood vessels, or of nitroprusside and other vasodilators is useless.

Tube tamponade

Insertion of a Sengstaken-Blakemore tube to tamponade oesophageal and gastric fundal varices is the first action. Table 3 outlines the criteria for safe use of the tube, as originally presented by Conn and as fitted to present-day criteria. The Minnesota modification of the tube refers to the presence of a fourth lumen, opening just above the inflated oesophageal balloon, which allows orotracheal secretions pooling above the balloon to be aspirated (Fig. 3). Formerly, a nasogastric tube for aspiration was tied to the Sengstaken tube above the oesophageal balloon. Since the Minnesota tube is now the only one being manufactured in the United States, there is no alternative. On the other hand, since the airway is protected by endotracheal or nasotracheal intubation with an inflated cuff on the tube to prevent aspiration of blood and secretion into the lungs, the fourth port of the Sengstaken tube is almost superfluous; the port seldom works as well as it should, anyway. The Idezuki tube, made of plastic components, rather than of rubber, is said to have more reliable and uniform characteristics of inflation.

Linton and Nachlas tubes, which have only a single large balloon, within the stomach, are used principally to tamponade gastric fundal varices (Fig. 4). Unlike the Sengstaken–Blakemore tube, traction must be applied to Linton and Nachlas tubes; hence, pressure necrosis of the oesophagogastric function can occur if they are left in place for more than 18 h.

Endoscopy

If bleeding is controlled upon removal of a tamponading balloon tube, upper gastrointestinal endoscopy is performed; extensive

Table 3 Protocol for use of the Sengstaken–Blakemore tube

Before insertion:
1. Establish nasotracheal intubation
2. Use a new tube and check the balloon for leaks
3. Attach a no. 18 F Salem sump tube above the oesophageal balloon if the Minnesota tube is not used, and sometimes when it is
4. Evacuate blood from stomach with a large tube. Insert the tube through the nose, rather than through the throat, if possible

After insertion:
1. Apply low, intermittent suction to the gastric tube
2. Apply constant suction to the Salem sump
3. Inflate the gastric balloon with 25-ml increments of air to 100 ml, observing whether the patient has pain, or not, and stopping if he does
4. By feel, snug the gastric balloon to the gastro-oesophageal junction
   Tape the tube to the nose under slight tension over a foam rubber pad
5. Add 150 ml of air to the gastric balloon
6. Place two clamps (one of which is then taped closed) on the tube to the gastric balloon
7. Inflate the oesophageal balloon to 25–45 mmHg. Clamp and check the balloon hourly
8. Perform a heavily penetrated upper abdomen–lower chest radiograph (portable) to confirm the position of the balloons
9. Determine serial haematocrit levels every 4 to 6 h, because the gastric tube may occlude and fail to allow detection of recurrent haemorrhages
10. Tape the scissors to the head of the bed so that the tube can be transected and rapidly removed if respiratory distress develops
11. Deflate the oesophageal and gastric balloons after 24 h
12. Remove the Sengstaken–Blakemore tube in an additional 24 h if there is no recurrent haemorrhage

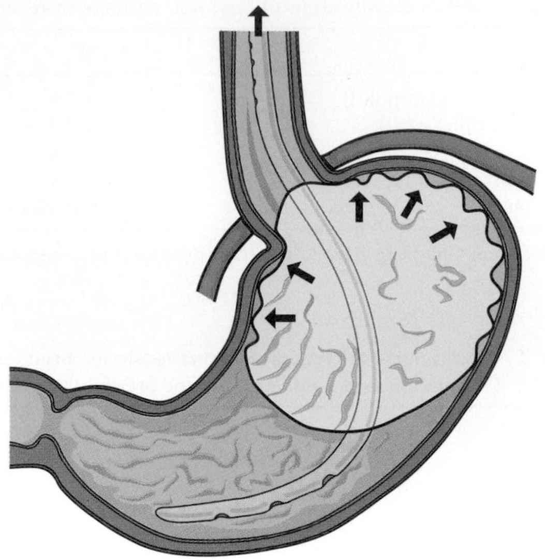

Fig. 4 Tamponade of gastro-oesophageal varices with Linton tube.

ice-water gavage is required to remove pooled blood in the stomach. The objectives thereafter are to identify non-variceal sources of bleeding that can be treated specifically, as well as confirming the diagnosis of bleeding oesophageal varices and to display bleeding gastric varices. Gastric varices require surgical control since they are generally endoscopically inaccessible to sclerotherapy. Although the statistic ingrained in reports is that 30 per cent of bleeding is caused by non-variceal disease, this seems an overestimate. The Sengstaken tube itself cannot be counted upon for long-term control: there is a 60 per cent chance of rebleeding after its removal.

If bleeding is uncontrollable by tube tamponade, by sclerotherapy, by oesophageal stapling, or by banding the varices with Neoprene rings, an emergency portasystemic shunt may be required.

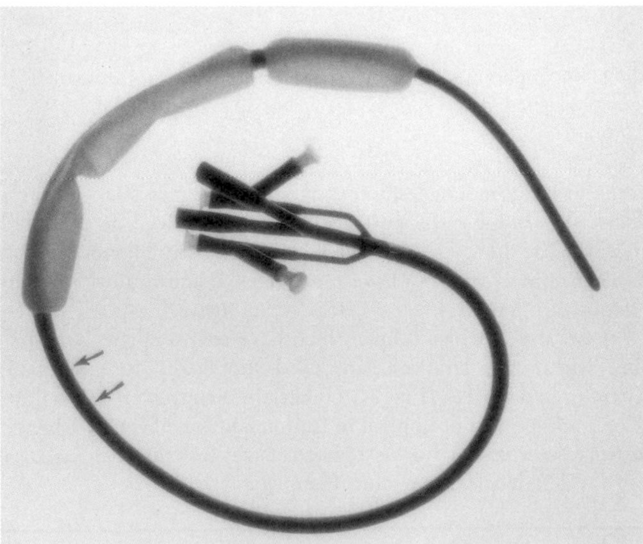

Fig. 3 Minnesota modification of Sengstaken–Blakemore tube with ports for aspiration of secretions dammed by inflated oesophageal balloon. Arrows indicate the suction ports.

Sclerotherapy and portacaval shunt

Child's class C patients are the most difficult to treat because of their poor liver function. Patients who need at least six blood transfusions have a mortality rate of about 50 per cent, irrespective of whether or not they are treated by sclerotherapy (Fig. 5) or by a portacaval shunt. The number of transfusions required is fewer after sclerotherapy, however. Costs of hospitalization are equal whether sclerotherapy or a portacaval shunt is used.

Sclerotherapy and stapling

Initially, oesophageal varices that are demonstrably or putatively the cause of haemorrhage are equally well controlled by sclerotherapy with any of a variety of sclerosants (usually ethanolamine oleate, ethanol, or sodium tetradecyl sulphate) or by oesophageal transection and reanastomosis with a stapling device (Figs. 6, 7). Neither sclerotherapy nor transection, however, prolongs life or prevents rebleeding. Sclerotherapy has the advantage of being a totally endoscopic technique. Its disadvantages are a rebleeding

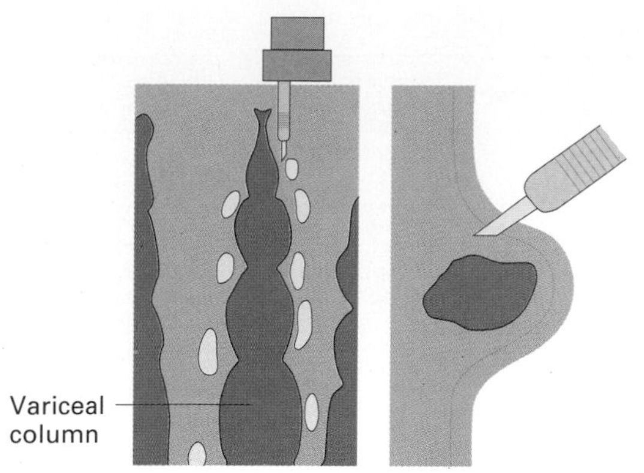

Fig. 5 Injection of sclerosant into variceal columns (far left) and paravariceal injections (B).

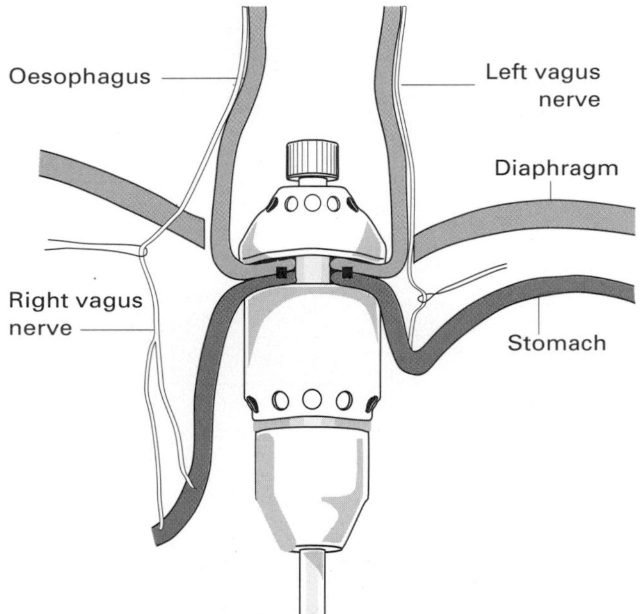

Fig. 6 Oesophageal transection and stapling to control bleeding varices. The vagus nerves are protected.

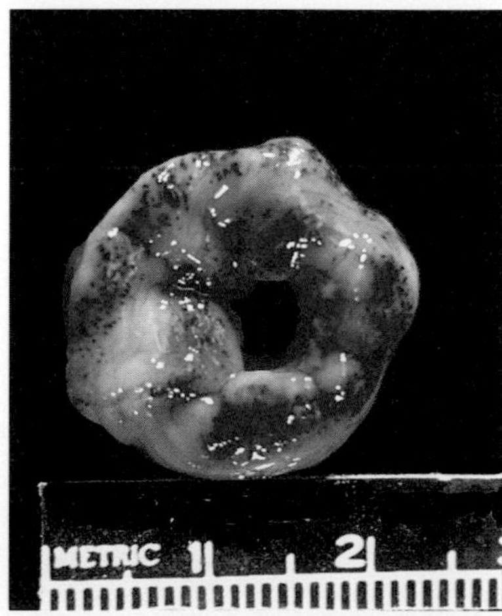

Fig. 7 Torus of oesophagus removed by stapling and anastomosis. Columns of varices are present.

rate of 62 per cent after one session of therapy and of 82 per cent after three sessions. There are myriad complications, some common and potentially severe—such as ulceration, and some rare, but potentially lethal, such as thrombosis of the splenic vein, perforation of the oesophagus, pneumomediastinum, pneumothorax, and pneumoperitoneum. Banding of varices with Neoprene rings, as in a haemorrhoidectomy, is currently thought to be safer.

Stapling has the disadvantage that it requires an intra-abdominal operation, with its attendent complications. Its advantage is that only a single treatment is required and that stapling is at least as good as sclerotherapy over the long term. In the short term, stapling is 88 per cent effective against rebleeding within 5 days of transection, as opposed to a 62 per cent rate of protection after a single sclerotherapy treatment.

Although vasoconstrictive therapy with a vasopressin analogue, β-adrenergic blockage with propanolol, and vasodilation with glyceryl trinitrate (nitroglycerine) or nitroprusside have all been employed, these modalities are useless in the treatment of acute, massive variceal bleeding. Propanolol in a dose sufficient to reduce the heart rate of cirrhotics by 25 per cent may delay or prevent the initial haemorrhage, but it has no effect on the mortality rate.

Recurrent massive variceal bleeding in a patient who has an open portal vein is better and more economically treated by an emergency portasystemic shunt than by sclerotherapy, if liver function and general health are adequate for surgery. Although one prospective, but uncontrolled trial detected little evidence of portasystemic encephalopathy after an emergency portasystemic shunt, encephalography occurs frequently. The best predictor of postoperative encephalopathy is the presence of preoperative encephalopathy.

Devascularization

In Japan, venous devascularization of the oesophagus and stomach from the level of the inferior pulmonary vein to the left phrenic and the short gastric veins, plus transection of the oesophageal mucosa and oversewing the mucosa, is a common form of treatment. In the West it has never been widely successful as a form of emergency therapy. A rate of recurrent bleeding after devascularization estimated as only 6.6 per cent by some authorities seems lower than that experienced by others.

Figure 8 shows an algorithm for the treatment of bleeding oesophageal varices.

FURTHER READING

Andreani T, *et al.* Preventive therapy of first gastrointestinal bleeding in patients with cirrhosis: results of a controlled trial comparing propanolol, endoscopic sclerotherapy and placebo. *Hepatology*, 1990; **12**: 1413–9.

Branicki FJ, *et al.* Emergency surgical treatment for nonvariceal bleeding of the upper part of the gastrointestinal tract. *Surg Gynecol Obstet*, 1991; **172**: 113–120.

Brooks, WS Jr. Sclerotherapy: analysis and review. *Endosc Rev* 1985; May/June; 11–53.

Burnett DA, Rikkers LF. Nonoperative emergency treatment of variceal hemorrhage. *Surg Clin N Am*, 1990; **70**: 291–306.

Burroughs AK, *et al.* A comparison of sclerotherapy with staple transection of the esophagus for the emergency control of bleeding from esophageal varices. *N Engl J Med*, 1989; **321**: 857–62.

Cello JP, *et al.* Endoscopic sclerotherapy versus portacaval shunt in patients with severe cirrhosis and acute variceal hemorrhage. *N Engl J Med*, 1987; **316**: 11–15.

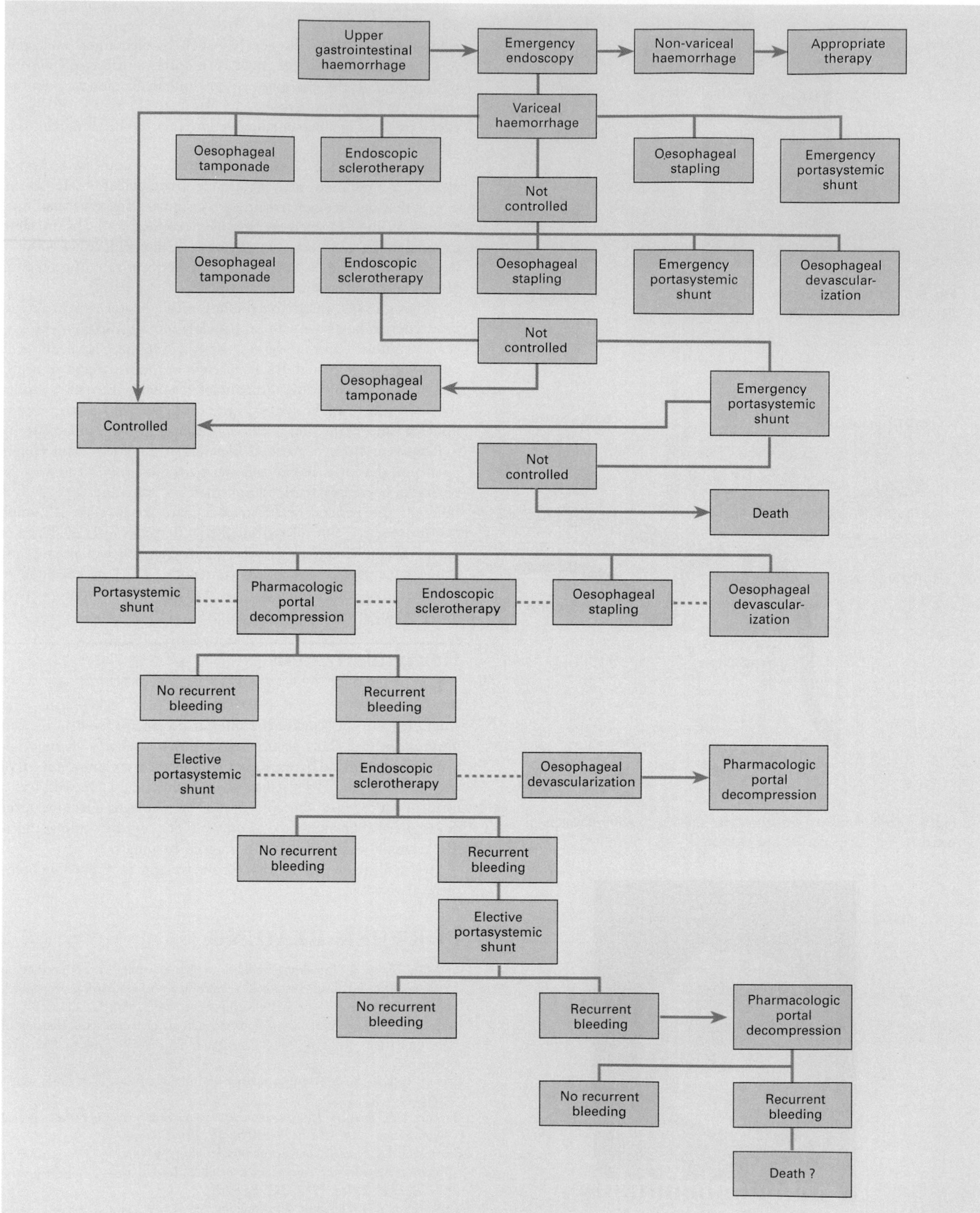

Fig. 8 Algorithm of treatment of bleeding varices.

Gitlin N. Treatment options in the management of varices. *Curr Opin Gastroenterol*, 1991; 7: 357–63.
Grace ND. Prevention of recurrent variceal bleeding—is surgical rescue the answer? *Ann Intern Med*, 1990; **112**: 242–4.
Henderson JM, *et al*. Endoscopic variceal sclerosis compared with distal splenorenal shunt to prevent recurrent variceal bleeding in cirrhosis. *Ann Intern Med*, 1989; **112**: 262–9.
Idezuki Y, *et al*. Current strategy for esophageal varices in Japan. *Am J Surg*, 1990; **160**: 98–104.
Jansen PLM. Current management of esophageal varices. *Curr Opin Gastroenterol*, 1990; **6**: 597–602.
Lacaine F, LaMuraglia GM, Malt RA. Prognostic factors in survival after portasystemic shunts: multivariate analysis. *Ann Surg*, 1985; **202**: 729–34.
Malt RA. Portasystemic venous shunts. *N Engl J Med*, 1976; **295**: 24–29, 80–86.
O'Connor KW, *et al*. Comparison of three nonsurgical treatments for bleeding esophageal varices. *Gastroenterology*, 1989; **96**: 899–906.
Orloff MJ, Bell RH. Long-term survival after emergency portacaval shunting for bleeding varices in patients with alcoholic cirrhosis. *Am J Surg*, 1986; **151**: 176–83.
Ottinger LW, Moncure AC. Transthoracic ligation of bleeding esophageal varices in patients with intrahepatic portal obstruction. *Ann Surg*, 1974; **179**: 35–8.
Planas R, *et al*. Portacaval shunt versus endoscopic sclerotherapy in the elective treatment of variceal hemorrhage. *Gastroenterology*, 1991; **100**: 1078–86.
Smith JL, Graham DY. The variceal hemorrhage: a critical evaluation of survival analysis. *Gastroenterology*, 1982; **82**: 968–73.
Sugiura M, Futagawa S. Esophageal transection with paraesophagogastric devascularizations (the Sugiura procedure) in the treatment of esophageal varices. *World J Surg*, 1984; **8**: 673–82.
Terblanche J, Burroughs AK, Hobbs KEF. Controversies in the management of bleeding esophageal varices. *N Engl J Med*, 1989; **320**: 1393–8, 1469–74.

24.3 Ascites and its complications

ROBERT M. STRAUSS AND JULES L. DIENSTAG

The term ascites is derived from the Greek word *askitos* (bladder, belly, bag) and denotes the presence of excessive fluid in the peritoneal cavity. It may present as an isolated clinical finding or be seen in the context of generalized oedema. Ascites is typically obvious: small amounts of fluid can be detected by diagnostic imaging.

CLASSIFICATION OF ASCITES AND DIFFERENTIAL DIAGNOSIS

Ascites may be caused by hepatic, renal, or cardiac decompensation; by hepatic venous outflow obstruction; and by malignant, inflammatory, or infectious processes in the peritoneum. Several different classification schemes have been proposed: one discriminating between transudative and exudative ascites has been adopted widely (Table 1).

Ascites is not the only cause of marked abdominal swelling. Gross obesity, gaseous distension, visceromegaly or abnormal masses can all be confused with fluid excess. A massive ovarian cyst, hydatid cyst, and, exceptionally, pregnancy with polyhydramnios or pregnancy alone may be confused with ascites.

PATHOGENESIS

Normally, there is just enough free fluid in the peritoneal cavity to lubricate the peritoneal surfaces.

Ascites occurs when there is an imbalance of factors that favour the flow of fluid from the vascular space or when there is exudation of fluid through infection or malignant implantation on the peritoneum, and represents a state of excess total body sodium.

Normally, the higher pressure at the arteriolar end of the capillary allows passage of fluid without protein into the pericapillary space, while reabsorption takes place at the venous end of the capillary where hydrostatic pressure is lower than oncotic pressure. In cirrhosis, portal venous hypertension increases the filtration pressure at the capillary level with transudation of fluid, while low albumin levels decrease vascular oncotic pressure. Two potential mechanisms have been proposed to explain the pathogenesis of ascites. The 'underfilling hypothesis' suggests that the primary abnormality is a sequestration of fluid within the splanchnic vascular bed secondary to portal hypertension and reduced oncotic pressure. These events cause a decrease in effective circulating blood volume, which leads to compensatory renal retention of sodium by increasing aldosterone production.

The 'overflow hypothesis' suggests that renal dysfunction (perhaps mediated by a hepatorenal reflex) is the primary event leading to sodium and water accumulation in the absence of intravascular volume depletion. This hypothesis is supported by the fact that acute constriction of the portal vein in dogs is associated with renal vasoconstriction, renal sodium and water retention, and renin stimulation. These effects can be abolished in the homolateral, denervated kidney, but not in the contralateral innervated kidney. Not all data, however, substantiate the 'overflow' hypothesis. For example, patients with decompensated cirrhosis show an activation of the sympathetic nervous and renin–angiotensin–aldosterone systems and non-osmotic release of vasopressin, which should be suppressed, not stimulated, by renal sodium and water retention with volume expansion.

A new hypothesis that integrates the underfill and overfill hypothesis into one is that of peripheral arterial vasodilation. The underlying assumption of this hypothesis is that patients have peripheral vasodilation as a consequence of arteriovenous shunts in the splanchnic, dermal, and pulmonary circulations. The peripheral vasodilation that accompanies arteriovenous shunts causes renal sodium retention. Because sodium retention may not be sufficient to fill the enlarged vascular compartment, renin, angiotensin, aldosterone, and vasopressin are not suppressed.

CLINICAL FEATURES

Patients may initially not be aware of the presence of fluid within the abdomen. As the amount increases, the patient may become

Table 1 Classification of ascites

I. *Transudative ascites*
  A. Hypoalbuminaemia
    1. Nephrotic syndrome
    2. Protein-losing enteropathy
  B. Venous hypertension
    1. Poor return of blood to the right side of the heart
      (a) Congestive heart failure
      (b) Tricuspid insufficiency (occasionally other valvular lesions)
      (c) Constrictive pericarditis
    2. Blockage of the hepatic veins and/or vena cava
      (a) Hepatic vein blocks (Budd–Chiari syndrome, webs, tumours)
      (b) Veno-occlusive disease
  C. Portal vein obstruction*
  D. Diffuse hepatic disease with portal hypertension
    1. Cirrhosis (all forms)
  E. Infiltrative processes of the liver
    1. Tumours, lymphomas, myeloid metaplasia†
    2. Granulomatous diseases

II. *Exudative ascites*
  A. Inflammatory diseases of the peritoneum
    1. Ruptured viscus with or without an intra-abdominal abscess: peptic ulcer, appendicitis, diverticulitis, cholecystitis, intestinal infarction
    2. Tuberculosis (peritoneal implants)
    3. Bacterial peritonitis
    4. Pancreatitis
    5. Bile peritonitis
  B. Malignant causes
    1. Metastasis to liver or peritoneum
    2. Primary hepatic tumours (hepatocellular carcinoma, cholangiocarcinoma)
    3. Primary mesothelioma

III. *Chylous ascites*
  A. Trauma to the thoracic duct
  B. Mediastinal tumours
  C. Filariasis
  D. Tuberculosis (occasionally)
  E. Cirrhosis (occasionally)

*Only when the process is chronic, leading to cirrhosis, or when there is primarily intrahepatic obstruction.
†Ascites may be exudative.

aware of distension, a sensation of fullness, or of tight-fitting clothes. Tense ascites may be associated with respiratory distress, anorexia, nausea, early satiety, pyrosis, ventral hernia, or abdominal pain. Body weight generally increases, but if the ascites is associated with alcoholism, poor nutrition, neoplasia or the wasting of end-stage chronic liver disease, weight may be stable or decreased. Some patients with tense ascites complain of numbness or paraesthesias with sensory loss in the distribution of the lateral cutaneous nerve of the thigh, presumably as a result of pressure where it emerges behind the inguinal ligament (meralgia paraesthetica).

Physical examination of patients with massive ascites reveals a tensely distended abdomen with tightly stretched skin, bulging flanks, and an everted umbilicus. Smaller amounts of fluid (in excess of 120 ml) may be detected by eliciting shifting abdominal dullness, a fluid wave, or periumbilical dullness with the patient on hands and knees; this last manoeuvre is known as a positive 'puddle sign'. When massive ascites is present, it is not uncommon to find presacral, scrotal, and pedal oedema, as well as pleural effusions, especially on the right side. Ascites is usually accompanied by other signs of chronic liver disease, such as jaundice, spider angiomata, hepatic or splenic enlargement, or prominent abdominal wall veins ('caput medusa'). Radiographic imaging examinations are helpful for confirming or extending impressions gained on physical examination. Ultrasonography and computed tomography can detect as little as 30 ml of ascitic fluid. Even routine plain radiographs of the abdomen may be helpful, demonstrating generalized haziness and loss of the psoas shadow, as well as centralization and separation of bowel loops by ascites.

Examination of the ascitic fluid

Diagnostic paracentesis is a simple, relatively safe procedure that should be done in every patient with new onset ascites and can help determine the cause of ascites. Points of entry into the peritoneal cavity with the patient in the supine position include the left or right lower quadrant and the avascular linea alba below the umbilicus. Previous scar sites should be avoided. Regardless of the point of entry patients should empty their bladders before paracentesis.

After selection of a needle insertion site, the area is disinfected with iodine solution, and skin and subcutaneous tissues can be infiltrated with a local anaesthetic. The operator's gloved hand retracts the skin caudad in relation to the abdominal wall while a needle is inserted (needle size is dependent on thickness of the panniculus). The direction of the needle is changed three times, in

'Z' fashion, to minimize the likelihood of post-tap ascites leak. The character of the fluid (clear, straw-coloured, thick, odorous, cloudy, milky, bloody) should be noted, and laboratory analysis should be performed. Traditionally, the concentration of protein in the ascitic fluid and the ascites: serum lactate dehydrogenase ratio are used to determine whether the ascites is exudative (protein > 2.5 g/100 ml, ascites serum lactate dehydrogenase ratio > 0.6) or transudative (protein < 2.5 g/100 ml, ascites serum lactate dehydrogenase ratio < 0.6). Unfortunately, the distinction between exudative and transudative ascites is not absolute. Some patients with infectious and malignant ascites have a transudate, while patients with cirrhotic ascites may have an exudate. The serum : ascites albumin concentration gradient (a difference rather than a ratio) is felt by some authorities to be more accurate than the exudate/transudate distinction in classifying ascites. This method is based on the concept of oncotic–hydrostatic balance; patients with portal hypertension have a large difference ($\geqslant$ 1.1 g/dl) between their serum and ascitic fluid albumin concentrations, while patients with ascites secondary to other processes have serum: ascites albumin gradients less than 1.1. For this method of classification to be accurate, however, the specimens must be obtained simultaneously (at least on the same day), the patient should be haemodynamically stable, and the specimens should be tested using the same assay system. The assay technique should also be accurate at low albumin ranges.

The serum: ascites albumin gradient provides information only about the presence or absence of portal hypertension, not about other causes of ascites. Patients with portal hypertension will have a high albumin gradient regardless of the presence of other superimposed conditions.

Ascitic fluid white blood and differential counts should be determined. An absolute count lower than 250 polymorphonuclear cells/mm^3 usually denotes uninfected ascites, while counts of above this suggest infection. Ascitic fluid lactic dehydrogenase (compared to serum level), albumin, total protein, glucose and triglyceride (if chylous ascites is suspected) concentrations should be measured; lactate levels may also be obtained when peritonitis is suspected. Cytology and bacteriological analysis should also be performed. Enough fluid should be obtained to perform Gram stains, routine cultures and staining for acid-fast bacilli. Mycotic and mycobacterial cultures should be performed if indicated, and amylase levels should also be determined.

An ascitic fluid polymorphonuclear count above 250/mm^3 has the accuracy for the diagnosis of spontaneous bacterial peritonitis. Although ascites pH and lactate levels have been proposed as helpful tests, they are not sufficiently discriminating to be of diagnostic value: ascitic pH values below 7.32 and lactate levels above 32 mg/dl are seen not only in spontaneous bacterial peritonitis, but also in malignant ascites, pancreatic ascites, and tuberculous peritonitis.

Chylous ascites refers to a milky or creamy appearance of peritoneal fluid resulting from the presence of thoracic or intestinal lymph. Chylous ascites contains Sudan-staining fat globules that can be detected microscopically and an increase in triglyceride level that can be documented by chemical examination.

MANAGEMENT

Some patients may respond to simple measures, while others may require a series of therapeutic approaches that will be only palliative. Generally speaking, the more advanced the liver disease, the worse the prognosis, and, therefore, the less effective therapy will be.

Medical management

General measures

As in any disease process, attention should be directed to treating the underlying cause. Attempts to improve liver function are worthwhile: patients should abstain from alcohol and receive optimal nutrition. Bedrest is usually recommended but is of little practical value, especially in patients whose urine sodium concentration is < 10 mEq/l. The theoretical benefit of bedrest derives from the fact that an upright posture activates the renin–angiotensin–aldosterone and α-adrenergic systems; however, the effect of bedrest is negligible compared with that of conventional therapy. Sodium intake should be restricted to 1.5 to 2 g day; lower limits are rarely practical in patients unless they are admitted to hospital. If renal function is normal and hyponatraemia is absent, fluid restriction is not indicated.

In cirrhotic patients with ascites, prostaglandins are felt to be helpful in preserving renal function by maintaining glomerular filtration rate and free water clearance. Administration of drugs that inhibit prostaglandin synthetase, such as non-steroidal anti-inflammatory drugs, should be avoided in such patients.

Diuretics

Most patients require diuretic therapy. Dye dilution studies have demonstrated that, in the absence of peripheral oedema, only 0.5 kg per day of ascitic fluid can be mobilized without compromising the intravascular compartment; however, many authorities advocate an approximate limit of 1 kg (1 litre) a day for medical diuresis. The presence of peripheral oedema with ascites permits a more liberal mobilization of fluid with diuretics. In the current climate which favours large volume paracentesis removing several litres of fluid, the applicability of these medical limits needs to be re-evaluated; however, excessive diuresis may result in azotaemia, hyponatraemia, encephalopathy, and hepatorenal syndrome.

Aldosterone antagonists

Spironolactone is an aldosterone antagonist that promotes natriuresis and potassium retention. The initial dose ranges from 50 to 200 mg/day given in two or four doses. A useful parameter to gauge the efficacy of natriuresis is the concentration of urinary sodium relative to potassium. It is practical to measure this in the first morning urine specimen, after the patient has abstained from sodium containing food for 8 to 12 h. If the sodium concentration of the urine remains lower than the potassium concentration, the diuresis is suboptimal and the dose of spironolactone should be increased by 50 to 100 mg every 2 to 3 days until urinary sodium exceeds urinary potassium. Theoretically, there is no absolute dose limit; however, hyperkalaemia and azotaemia usually prevent unlimited dose escalation. Most patients respond to a dose of less than 300 mg/day. Serum electrolytes should be monitored closely, depending on the responses to and duration of diuretic therapy. Gynaecomastia and galactorrhoea are recognized complications of spironolactone therapy and can be dose-limiting. If spironolactone causes hyperkalaemia, a potassium-wasting diuretic can be added.

Amiloride is another potassium sparing diuretic which, although not an aldosterone antagonist, has been used successfully to treat ascites. It increases renal excretion of sodium and chloride without significantly affecting the glomerular filtration rate.

Loop diuretics

These agents act by increasing the delivery of sodium to the distal tubule, where ability to reabsorb sodium is exceeded. The most common loop diuretic employed is frusemide and an initial dose of 20 mg/day may be sequentially increased, especially in patients with peripheral oedema. Loop diuretics should be used as supplements to spironolactone, not as the primary diuretic. Hypokalaemia may develop, despite administration of potassium-sparing diuretics, and hyponatraemia may also develop or worsen. Metabolic alkalosis and hepatic encephalopathy are other potential complications.

Thiazide diuretics

These are usually ineffective when given alone, and they may increase renal production of ammonia; they can, however, be used in conjunction with spironolactone either to reduce potassium retention or to provide a synergistic effect.

Large volume paracentesis

During the 1950s, before diuretics were available, large volume paracentesis was employed widely; this was, however, later implicated as a cause of hypotension, renal insufficiency, symptomatic hyponatraemia and encephalopathy, and the procedure was virtually abandoned for the next two decades. The procedure was resurrected in the 1980s by Rodés and his colleagues in Barcelona and by Kao and coworkers in the United States and was demonstrated to be safe and well tolerated, without haemodynamic, renal, or hepatic consequences. Numerous groups have since performed randomized studies comparing large volume paracentesis (with or without albumin infusion) with diuretic therapy and peritoneovenous shunting. Most studies have concluded that large volume paracentesis associated with intravenous albumin infusion is a fast, effective, and safe treatment for cirrhotic ascites. In general, patients undergoing paracentesis have a shorter hospital stay than those treated with diuretics. Recently, the Barcelona group has demonstrated the safety and clinical value of total volume paracentesis, performed over 1 to 2 h, with no effect on renal, hepatic, or hormonal features, provided that intravenous albumin is administered. Some groups have questioned the necessity for expensive salt-poor albumin infusion after paracentesis and have been treating patients quite successfully and safely without albumin infusions.

Paracentesis *per se* is quite simple. It should be performed in sterile conditions and under local anesthesia. The Barcelona group uses a needle (preferably a sharp metal needle within a 7-cm long, 17-gauge metal blunt-edged cannula with sideholes) that is inserted in the left lower abdominal quadrant. Once the needle has entered the peritoneal cavity, the inner part is removed and the fluid can be mobilized with the aid of a large volume capacity suction pump. After the procedure, patients remain recumbent for at least 2 h on the side opposite to the paracentesis to avoid leakage of fluid. Typically, after several days, diuretic therapy is resumed; paracentesis may be repeated when the clinical condition dictates—usually after several weeks but not uncommonly after a few days. In Barcelona, therapeutic paracentesis is 'first-line' therapy for patients with tense cirrhotic ascites; however, although quite widely used, large volume paracentesis has not been embraced by all centres. The need for rapid paracentesis is often not compelling, medical therapy is quite effective in most patients, the need to return for frequent procedures is difficult for many patients, and complications do occur. In addition, levels of opsonins have been shown to be reduced after paracentesis: this could theoretically predispose these patients to spontaneous bacterial peritonitis. Complications of paracentesis include infection, peritoneal dissection of fluid along fascial planes to the scrotum or pleural space, haemorrhage, perforation of the bowel with generalized peritonitis or abdominal abscess, and retention of catheter fragments in the abdominal cavity; however, these complications are rare in experienced hands.

Head out of water immersion

A few clinicians resort to this modality when conservative measures have failed. Head out of water immersion decreases plasma renin activity, aldosterone, vasopressin, and noradrenaline as well as increasing the percentage of water load and urinary sodium excretion. Obviously, encephalopathic patients cannot be subjected to this approach.

Surgical management

Peritoneovenous shunt

In 1974, LeVeen and colleagues developed a pressure activated one-way valve for uses as a peritoneovenous shunt. One limb of the shunt lies free in the peritoneal cavity, and the venous opening of the efferent limb inserts into the superior vena cava near its entrance into the right atrium. Flow in the shunt is maintained if there is a 3 to 5 cmH_2O pressure gradient between the valve and its venous end. If the gradient falls below this level, the valve closes, preventing blood from flowing back into the shunt tubing. Two additional shunts are available: the Denver Shunt and the Cordis-Hakim shunt, which incorporate a pumping mechanism at the abdominal end. Most patients, however, find 'manual pumping' of these shunts difficult, and they represent little improvement over the LeVeen shunt. Even with a peritoneovenous shunt, most patients require diuretics at a reduced dose. These shunts are also associated with concomitant improvement in renal blood flow.

A Veterans Administration Cooperative Study of LeVeen shunts diminished initial enthusiasm for this procedure. Over 3000 alcoholic patients with cirrhotic ascites were enrolled in this study; those refractory to diuretics were randomized to continued diuretic therapy plus therapeutic paracentesis versus LeVeen shunt placement. Patients randomized to LeVeen shunt therapy did not show improved survival, the number of infections increased, and the need for sodium restriction and diuretics continued, even in those with functioning shunts. Excessive shunt failure was also observed. A study published in 1989 compared medical treatment with peritoneovenous shunt therapy: the latter relieved the ascites promptly, reduced the length of hospital stay, and delayed recurrence of ascites. The duration of survival and number of complications in the medical and shunt groups were similar. This study suggests that peritoneovenous shunting is indicated in patients whose ascites is not treated satisfactorily by medical therapy, including those with recurrent ascites after multiple large volume paracentesis procedures and who have acceptable operative risk. If shunting is undertaken, current practice is to remove all or nearly all the ascitic fluid during the operation and to replace it with 5 l of isotonic sodium chloride solution.

Early complications of peritoneovenous shunts are valve malfunction, intravascular volume overload, pulmonary oedema, disseminated intravascular coagulation, hypokalaemia, air embolism, peritonitis, sepsis, and ascites leakage. Late complications are shunt occlusion (in about 30 per cent of patients), hepatic vein thrombosis, variceal haemorrhage, and peritoneal fibrosis with bowel obstruction. At least half of the patients will experience one or more complications. Mortality rates for these patients with end-stage cirrhosis and refractory ascites are quite high; about half succumb within the first postoperative year.

This procedure is contraindicated in patients with sepsis, heart failure, and active peritonitis. The best results are obtained in a limited subset of patients with diuretic-resistant ascites but relatively well preserved hepatic function.

Portasystemic shunts

Use of portasystemic shunts for treatment of cirrhotic ascites is warranted only in those patients in whom all other forms of therapy have failed. Many randomized trials have been done in the last 15 years comparing medical therapy with different types of portasystemic shunts, but most such studies were designed to evaluate shunts as therapy for bleeding oesophageal varices. The shunt operation that is most effective at relieving ascites has not been established; in fact, ascites is reduced after any type of portasystemic shunt as a consequence of decreased portal flow and decreased intrahepatic congestion. Among the most commonly performed shunts, splenorenal and portacaval shunts and their variants have been proven effective in relieving ascites. Ascites may actually increase transiently after distal splenorenal (Warren) shunt surgery, but, ultimately both distal and proximal (Linton) shunts lower the tendency to accumulate ascites. Between the two types of portacaval anastomosis, the end-to-side portacaval shunt decompresses the entire splanchnic bed but not hepatic sinusoids; after this shunt, ascites may persist. The side-to-side portacaval shunt, which decompresses both the splanchnic and hepatic sinusoidal beds, is very effective in relieving ascites; it is the decompressive shunt of choice for the treatment of ascites in the Budd–Chiari syndrome (when hepatic function is well-preserved).

The choice of portasystemic shunt should be individualized, taking into accounts factors such as the experience and preference of local surgeons.

Transjugular intrahepatic portasystemic shunt (TIPS)

Angiographically guided insertion of a metal stent between an intrahepatic hepatic vein and portal vein has been used to reduce portal hypertension in patients with bleeding oesophageal varices. Such transjugular intrahepatic portasystemic shunts (TIPS) have been shown to relieve intractable ascites as well. The role of TIPS in the management of refractory ascites—the object of current investigation—remains to be more full defined.

Liver transplantation

Although beyond the scope of this chapter, liver transplantation is the treatment of choice for patients with liver failure and otherwise intractable ascites, unless contraindications exist.

SPONTANEOUS BACTERIAL PERITONITIS

An important complication of ascites is spontaneous bacterial peritonitis, defined as an infection of ascites fluid in the absence of any obvious intraabdominal source.

Pathogenesis

Spontaneous bacterial peritonitis can occur in patients with ascites of any cause; the mechanisms underlying it remain unknown. Plausible contributing factors include transmural migration of bacteria secondary to increased permeability of the gut to enteric organisms, derangement in abdominal lymphatic circulation, haematogenous seeding from a distant source, decreased function of the reticuloendothelial system in patients with chronic liver disease, and impaired chemotaxis by blood monocytes and neutrophils in patients with cirrhosis.

Bacteriology

A single organism is the cause of over 90 per cent of cases. The most common organisms are *Escherichia coli* and *Streptococcus* species; other organisms may also be implicated (Table 2).

Table 2 Organisms causing spontaneous bacterial peritonitis

Causative organisms	Number of cases (%)
Gram-negative bacilli	69
Escherchia. coli	47
Klebsiella sp.	11
Other*	11
Gram-positive cocci	30
Streptococci–all species	26
S. pneumoniae	8
Enterococci	5
Other	12
Staphylococci	4
Anaerobes/microaerophils†	5
Miscellaneous‡	1
Polymicrobial	8

*Includes *Enterobacter* sp., *Citrobacter* sp., *Acinetobacter* sp., *Serratia liquefaciens, Proteus* sp., *Pseudomonas aeruginosa, Providencia* sp., *Aeromonas hydrophila*.

†Includes *Bacteroides fragilis, Bacteropides* sp., *Clostridia perfringens, Clostridia* sp., peptococci, lactobacilli, microaerophilic streptococci.

‡Includes diphtheroids, *Neisseria gonorrhoea, Candida albicans*.

Diagnosis

Prompt recognition of spontaneous bacterial peritonitis requires not only an awareness of the presenting symptoms and signs but also a high index of suspicion in any patient with ascites and clinical deterioration. Spontaneous bacterial peritonitis can vary in its presentation from being clinically dramatic to totally asymptomatic. Fever about 100°F is the most common presenting feature and occurs in 50 to 80 per cent of patients. Abdominal pain, usually diffuse, occurs in 25 to 72 per cent of patients; rebound tenderness is elicited in over 50 per cent of patients. None of these findings is specific for spontaneous bacterial peritonitis, however; abdominal complaints are common in cirrhotic patients with ascites in the absence of this complication, and spontaneous bacterial peritonitis can occur in the absence of fever or abdominal pain.

Other subtle indicators suggestive of spontaneous bacterial peritonitis include diarrhoea, worsening renal insufficiency, refractoriness to diuretics, hypothermia, and unexplained encephalopathy. Peripheral blood leucocytosis is common but may be masked by hypersplenism. Despite negative ascitic fluid cultures (which may occur in up to 50 per cent of patients), the presence of more than 250 polymorphonuclear cells per mm^2 in ascites suffices to establish a diagnosis and to mandate therapy.

Once the diagnosis is entertained, paracentesis is indicated. Ascitic fluid should be submitted promptly to the laboratory for aerobic and anaerobic cultures, cell count with differential, and Gram stain of centrifuged fluid, as well as other routine laboratory assessments. To increase the likelihood of a positive ascites fluid culture, the operator should inoculate 10 ml of ascitic fluid directly into blood culture bottles at the bedside. 'Bedside' inoculation increases the sensitivity of ascites culture and decreases the time between inoculation of the culture and appearance of bacterial growth.

The diagnosis of spontaneous bacterial peritonitis is based on a polymorphonuclear cell concentration of 250 cell/mm^2 or higher; ascitic pH below 7.3, a lactate level above 32 mg/100 ml. Glucose, specific gravity, and protein concentrations are not helpful. Most cases of peritonitis in cirrhotics are due to spontaneous bacterial peritonitis; therefore, the threshold for surgery, which can be fatal, should be very high. Conversely, peritonitis secondary to an intra-abdominal process such as a perforated ulcer or diverticulitis can occur in cirrhotics with ascites; failure to recognize such a source of infection and to intervene surgically and promptly is almost universally fatal. Hallmarks of 'surgical' peritonitis include polymorphonuclear cell counts above 10 000, polymicrobial peritonitis, low ascites glucose and high levels of lactate dehydrogenase and protein. A recent report suggested a diagnostic algorithm for patients with peritonitis: an ascitic fluid total protein above 1 g/dl, glucose below 50 mg/dl, and lactate dehydrogenase greater than the upper limit of normal for serum in the presence of polymorphonuclear cells provides evidence for non-spontaneous peritonitis (secondary to gut perforation).

Treatment

Once a presumptive diagnosis of spontaneous bacterial peritonitis has been made, prompt and appropriate intravenous antibiotic therapy should be instituted, long before culture results are known, and even if cultures are negative. Empirically, a third-generation cephalosporin should be used, unless a Gram stain suggests that a narrower-spectrum antibiotic will suffice. Aminoglycosides should be avoided; they are associated with a high risk of nephrotoxicity and have unpredictable distribution in cirrhotics. When antibiotic sensitivities of the organism are known, antibiotic coverage can be narrowed. Direct intraperitoneal instillation of antibiotics is not necessary. Treatment should continue for 10 to 14 days, although, shorter duration therapy with third-generation cephalosporins is effective. Response to antibiotics can be judged clinically; repeat paracentesis in 48 h may be helpful but is not usually necessary. Once an episode is treated, the frequency of recurrence is high, and the mortality is also high, a reflection of the underlying severity of the liver disease in these patients. Prophylaxis with daily quinolone therapy has been shown to reduce the frequency of recurrent spontaneous bacterial peritonitis.

HEPATORENAL SYNDROME

Progressive 'functional' renal failure occurs in patients with advanced liver disease, all of whom have decompensated cirrhosis, and most of whom have tense ascites. The kidneys are anatomically and histologically normal; if hepatic deterioration is reversed, for example by liver transplantation, the renal failure is also reversible.

Altered renal blood flow appears to be the primary abnormality. There is vasoconstriction of arterioles of the outer renal cortex with shunting of blood to the renal medulla, which results in decreased glomerular filtration rate and urine flow. These abnormalities are probably a result of decreased 'effective' blood volume and sympathetic overdrive. Accumulation of false neurotransmitters at nerve endings has also been proposed. Derangements in the renin–angiotensin and in the kallikrein–kinin system as well as altered synthesis of renal prostaglandins, vasoactive intestinal peptide, and endotoxins are also thought to be involved in the pathogenesis of the hepatorenal syndrome.

Diagnosis

Progressive azotaemia, oliguria (<500 ml/day), a concentrated urine with a urine: plasma osmolarity above 1.0, and a urinary sodium concentration below 10 mEq/l in the presence of a normal urinalysis are the typical features (Table 3). The urine may contain small amounts of protein, hyaline, and a few granular casts. Oliguria may occur spontaneously but usually follows diuretic therapy, diarrhoea, paracentesis, gastrointestinal haemorrhage, or sepsis. To establish this diagnosis, decreased intravascular volume must be excluded by fluid loading.

Table 3 Differential diagnosis of acute azotaemia in patients with advanced liver disease

Biochemical characteristic	Prerenal azotaemia	Hepatorenal syndrome	Acute renal failure
Urine sodium concentration (mEq/l)	<10	<10	>30
Urine to plasma creatinine ratio	<30:1	>30:1	<20:1
Urine osmolality	At least 100 mosmol > plasma osmolality	At least 100 mosmol > plasma osmolality	Equal to plasma osmolality
Urine sediment	Normal	Unremarkable	Casts, cellular debris

Treatment

There is no effective therapy for hepatorenal syndrome; however, precipitating factors should be eliminated. Diuretics should be withheld, blood volume replaced, serum electrolyte abnormalities corrected, infections treated promptly, and drugs known to inhibit prostaglandin synthesis as well as other nephrotoxic drugs discontinued.

A fluid challenge to increase effective plasma volume should be attempted; a combination of saline and salt-poor albumin should be administered while close monitoring, preferably including central venous pressure measurement, is undertaken. Numerous vasodilatory drugs (e.g. phentolamine, papaverine, metaraminol, phenoxybenzamine) have also been administered but have not been effective.

If the liver disease is reversible (for example, fulminant hepatitis), dialysis may be helpful, but dialysis is of no value in patients with end-stage chronic liver disease. Recovery from hepatorenal syndrome has been reported anecdotally following portasystemic shunts and liver transplantation. Nevertheless, most patients with this disorder are often too decompensated to be candidates for these surgical interventions. Occasionally peritoneovenous shunting reverses the hepatorenal syndrome.

FURTHER READING

Akriviadis EA, Runyon BA. Utility of an alogrithm in differentiating spontaneous from secondary peritonitis. *Gastroenterology* 1990; **98**: 127–33.

Bories P, *et al.* The treatment of refractory ascites by the LeVeen shunt; a multicenter controlled trial of 57 patients. *J. Hepatol* 1986; **3**: 212–18.

Conn HO. Transjugular intrahepatic portal-systemic shunts: the state of the art. *Hepatology* 1993; **17**: 148–58.

Epstein M. Derangements of renal water handling in liver disease. *Gastroenterology* 1985; **89**: 1415–25.

Epstein M. Hepatorenal syndrome. In: Epstein M, ed. *The Kidney in Liver Disease*. 3rd edn. Baltimore: Williams and Wilkins, 1988: 92.

Gines P, *et al.* Comparison of paracentesis and diuretics in the treatment of cirrhotics with tense ascites. *Gastroenterology* 1987; **93**: 234–41.

Gines P, *et al.* Randomized comparative study of therapeutic paracentesis with and without intravenous albumin in cirrhosis. *Gastroenterology* 1988; **94**: 1493–1502.

Kao HW, Rakov NE, Savage E, Reynolds TB. The effect of large volume paracentesis in plasma volume, a cause of hypovolemia? *Hepatology* 1985; **5**: 403–7.

Malt RA. Portasystemic shunts. *N Engl J Med* 1976; **295**: 24–8 and 80–5.

Nicholls KM, Shapiro MD, Kluge R, Hsaio-Min C, Bichet DG, Schrier RW. Sodium excretion in advanced cirrhosis: effect of expansion of central blood volume and suppression of plasma aldosterone. *Hepatology* 1986; **6**: 235–8.

Pinto PL, Amerian J, Reynolds TB. Large volume paracentesis in nonedematous patients with tense ascites: its effect in intravascular volume. *Hepatology* 1988; **8**: 207–10.

Quintero E, *et al.* Paracentesis versus diuretics in the treatment of cirrhotics with tense ascites. Lancet 1985; **i**: 611–2.

Ring-Larsen, Henricksen JM. Pathogenesis of ascites formation and hepatorenal syndrome: humoral and hemodynamic factors. *Semin Liver Dis* 1986; **6**: 341–52.

Runyon BA, Canawati HN, Akriviadis EA. Optimization of ascitic fluid culture technique. *Gastroenterology* 1988; **95**: 1351–5.

Runyon BA, Antillos RM, Montana AA. Effects of paracentesis on ascites fluid opsonic activity and serum complement. *Gastroenterology* 1989; **97**: 158–62.

Schrier RW. Pathogenesis of sodium and water retention in high-output and low-output cardiac failure, nephrotic syndrome, cirrhosis and pregnancy. *N Engl J Med* 1988; **319**: 1065–72 and 1127–33.

Shear L, Ching S, Gabuzda GI. Compartmentalization of ascites and edema in patients with hepatic cirrhosis. *N Engl J Med* 1970; **282**: 391–96.

Smajda C, Franco D. The LeVeen shunt in the elective treatment of intractable ascites in cirrhosis. *Ann Surg* 1985; **201**: 488–93.

Stanley MM, *et al.* Peritoneovenous shunting as compared with medical treatment in patients with alcoholic cirrhosis and massive ascites. *N Engl J Med* 1989; **321**: 1632–38.

Tito L, *et al.* Total paracentesis associated with intravenous albumin in management of patients with cirrhosis and ascites. *Gastroenterology* 1990; **98**: 146–51.

Wilcox CM, Dismukes WE. Spontaneous bacterial peritonitis. *Medicine* 1987; **66**: 447–56.

24.4 Portal hypertension and hypersplenism

Z. N. DEMIRJIAN

The common association between abnormal liver function, splenomegaly, and anaemia was recognized nearly a century ago, and was attributed to portal hypertension.

Long-standing elevated portal pressure, whether caused by intrahepatic or extrahepatic factors, invariably leads to congestive splenomegaly. Although the most common underlying factor is hepatic cirrhosis, portal hypertension also occurs in conditions associated with more or less normal hepatic morphology, such as malaria, and schistosomiasis. Whatever its cause, splenomegaly increases blood flow through the red pulp. This is especially evident in congestive splenomegaly, in which the increased volume of perfusing blood increases the filtering capacity of the spleen. When blood cells are sequestered and haematological parameters are altered, the condition is known as hypersplenism.

The term hypersplenism carries no aetiological implications, but merely signifies the presence of pancytopenia, with cellular elements affected in different degrees, accompanied by splenomegaly. Since bone marrow function is usually normal, splenectomy usually results in complete or partial correction of the pancytopenia.

The cytopenias which result from congestive splenomegaly are of variable severity. They are also influenced by the factors causing the portal hypertension. Anaemia is usually mild to moderate, the haematocrit rarely being below 25 per cent and stable in the absence of complications such as bleeding or nutritional deficiencies. The anaemia is due to several factors, including blood dilution secondary to increased plasma volume and splenic pooling of red cells, which can trap up to 25 per cent of the total circulating red cell mass, depending upon the size of the spleen. Red cell survival is also decreased, by up to 50 per cent, and this is also proportional to spleen size. This haemolysis is a result of repeated metabolic insults to red cells caused by splenic pooling. The consequent red cell changes become irreversible, and damaged cells are eventually phagocytosed by splenic reticuloendothelial cells. Depending upon the underlying aetiology of the portal hypertension, there may be an added element of inadequate bone marrow response to anaemia, as occurs in cirrhosis.

Splenic pooling of up to 35 per cent of circulating platelets occurs normally. Splenomegaly accentuates this phenomenon and leads to thrombocytopenia of variable severity. Commonly, there is a direct inverse correlation between spleen size and platelet count. Platelets in the spleen survive normally and some or most of them become available to the general circulation at times of stress. In hypersplenic patients, the total platelet mass is normal.

Finally, leucopenia is common, but is usually mild and mainly due to an absolute diminution of the granulocyte count. In one study, six patients with leucopenia and splenomegaly secondary to cirrhosis were studied with the DF ^{32}P lifespan technique. Five had shortened red cell survival, even though granulocyte production was normal. Although leucopenia may be due to the existence of a large splenic pool, there is normally no significant splenic pooling of granulocytes. This finding is further supported by a correlation between leucopenia and splenic size.

Splenectomy has long been advocated to correct the pancytopenias which result from the hypersplenism associated with portal hypertension. Even though this intervention may correct the haematological picture, it rarely changes the course of the underlying disease and it can give rise to serious septicaemia. A retrospective study of 563 patients concluded that splenectomy may be less satisfactory in correcting hypersplenism than is a distal splenorenal shunt, which often improves cytopenias and controls variceal bleeding. The efficacy of the distal splenorenal renal shunt has recently been challenged, however.

FURTHER READING

Aster RH. Platelet sequestration studies in man. *Br J Haematol* 1972; **22**: 259–63.

Bishop CR, *et al.* Leukocyte kinetics in neutropenia. *J Clin Invest* 1971; **50**: 1678–89.

Eichner ER. Splenic function: normal, too much and too little. *Am J Med* 1979; **66**: 311–20.

El-Kishen MA, Henderson JM, Millikan WJ, Kuter MH, Warren WD. Splenectomy is contraindicated for thrombocytopenia secondary to portal hypertension. *Surg Gynecol Obstet* 1985; **160**: 233–7.

Hess CE, *et al.* Mechanism of dilutional anemia in massive splenomegaly. *Blood* 1976; **47**: 629.

Iber FL. Portal hypertension in the presence of normal liver morphology. *Ann NY Acad Sci* 1970; **170**: 115–26.

Jacob HS. Hypersplenism: mechanisms and management. *Br J Haematol* 1974; **27**: 1–5.

Jandl JH. The anemia of liver disease: observations on its mechanism. *J Clin Invest* 1954; 390–402.

Reed IL, Barry P, Wong H, Greenberg MS. Granulocyte turnover in patients with cirrhosis. *Clin Res* 1966; **14**: 325.

24.5 Non-shunt procedures in management of variceal bleeding

GEORGE HAMILTON

INTRODUCTION

Most episodes of variceal haemorrhage will be successfully treated by resuscitation and injection sclerotherapy, and indeed the efficacy of this approach has now been confirmed by several well-controlled trials. Nevertheless, in a significant minority either acute bleeding will persist, or rebleeding will occur in the near or long term. In this situation there is little doubt that some form of portal–systemic decompression is the most successful treatment for bleeding.

However, this objective is achieved at a cost, because disabling portal–systemic encephalopathy and deterioration in liver function over subsequent years frequently develops in patients who have been treated by shunting. Also the operative mortality of emergency shunting procedures is high, even where hepatic reserve is good. Furthermore, in variceal bleeding from extrahepatic portal hypertension, 30 to 50 per cent of children and 40 to 50 per cent of adults will have extensive thrombosis of the splenic and mesenteric veins which makes decompressive procedures impossible. For all these reasons an alternative to portal decompression is required and clearly the repertoire of any surgeon involved in the treatment of variceal haemorrhage must include non-shunt procedures.

HISTORICAL BACKGROUND

Many different non-shunt approaches to the treatment of bleeding oesophageal varices have been developed ranging from the direct attack by oesophagogastrectomy to variations on the theme of portoazygous disconnection and these are listed in Table 1. Indeed this problem has taxed the ingenuity of surgeons since the late nineteenth century when splenectomy and omentopexy were originally performed. The wide range of procedures devised since then reflects the generally unsatisfactory results achieved, parti-

Table 1 Non-shunt procedures for variceal haemorrhage

Splenectomy	Total gastrectomy
Omentopexy, splenopneumopexy, etc.	Hepatic and splenic artery ligation
Coronary vein ligation	Splenectomy and coronary vein ligation
Transthoracic ligation of varices (Boerema, Crile, and Milnes Walker)	Tanner's procedure (subcardiac porta-azygos disconnection)
Boerema button	Hassab procedure
Stapled oesophageal transection	Sugiura procedure

cularly so in the presence of poor liver function. In recent years, the advent of stapling devices has reawakened interest in portoazygous disconnection as a suitable alternative to shunting. Currently, the importance of these procedures in comparison to injection sclerotherapy and portacaval shunting is under evaluation around the world.

INDICATIONS

In most centres the first line of management of variceal haemorrhage is by resuscitation, medical therapy with a variety of vasoactive agents, balloon tamponade as a holding procedure, and injection sclerotherapy of the varices. Operative treatment is generally reserved for continued bleeding, or where recurrent variceal haemorrhage is a problem (Table 2). For example, it is now clearly established that if bleeding is not controlled after two sets of variceal injection, high rebleeding and mortality rates result from further attempts at injection; in this group emergency operative intervention is the best option.

Table 2 Indications for non-shunt procedures

1. Failed sclerotherapy: mortality becomes very high after the second unsuccessful injection and emergency oesophageal transection is highly effective
2. Absence of suitable veins for shunting in extensive thrombosis of splenic and mesenteric veins causing extrahepatic portal hypertension
3. Mild liver dysfunction in the presence of splenomegaly and hypersplenism, e.g. mansonic schistosomiasis
4. High probability of portasystemic encephalopathy with a shunt, particularly where work demands a high level of skill or intellectual activity
5. Recurrent bleeding uncontrolled by injection in poor liver function, i.e. Child's grade C
6. Absence of expertise or facilities for emergency injection sclerotherapy: stapled oesophageal transection is as effective in controlling bleeding

Variceal bleeding in the presence of good hepatic function but a large spleen, for example in mansonic schistosomiasis, is a clinical scenario where a non-shunt procedure has many advantages over portal decompression. Usually massive splenomegaly and hypersplenism occur in a young patient with an excellent prospect of good life-long hepatocellular function. Shunting not only carries an immediate high incidence of portal–systemic encephalopathy but also in non-selective decompressive procedures an inexorable deterioration of liver function will take place over the years. This hepatocellular deterioration becomes highly relevant in patients with conditions such as schistosomiasis or extrahepatic portal hypertension where life expectancy and liver function are good. Oesophageal transection and oesophagogastric devascularization (Hassab and Sugiura procedures) offer low rates of rebleeding and advantages over shunting in terms of preserving liver function and avoiding portal–systemic encephalopathy. Unfortunately the dearth of properly constructed trials comparing shunt and non-shunt techniques makes it impossible to be more objective about these two surgical approaches. Obviously, when the splenic and superior mesenteric veins are thrombosed there is no alternative to using a non-shunt technique. Portosystemic encephalopathy is a devastating complication adversely affecting intellectual function.

Cirrhotic patients increasingly come to liver transplantation in the end-stages of their disease. Previous surgery, particularly portacaval shunting, will complicate the procedure but will also increase its morbidity and mortality, and adhesions around the left lobe of the liver and throughout the left upper quadrant from non-shunt procedures will undoubtedly increase the technical problems of the recipient hepatectomy. Arguably, however, dealing with these adhesions might be less difficult than the dissection around the portal structures with the added problems of sudden massive portal hypertension which occurs during the disconnection of patent portacaval shunt in a transplant. At present, where transplantation is not yet indicated, a mesocaval shunt is the operation most favoured by transplanters for control of variceal haemorrhage because of the minimal dissection around the liver. Simple oesophageal transection, however, will reliably control haemorrhage where injection sclerotherapy has failed, with much less adhesion development, and in this emergency situation must be the procedure of choice.

As in shunting, the more major devascularization procedures have a higher operative mortality in the emergency situation, particularly in the setting of poor hepatic reserve. Once again, an expeditiously performed simple oesophageal transection, using the stapler but without major devascularization, has been shown to be extremely effective in treatment of haemorrhage uncontrolled by medical therapy or injection.

PREOPERATIVE PREPARATION

Full investigation and assessment of liver disease and function is essential. Any clotting abnormality should be corrected, particularly in the presence of hypersplenism, and renal function assessed, monitored, and optimally maintained before, during and after the procedure. Preoperative angiography may be of value if devascularization is to be performed, providing a 'road map' of the collateral circulation around the oesophagogastric region. If splenectomy is to be performed, vaccination against pneumococcal infection is probably of value, as is maintenance low-dose penicillin cover for the perioperative period, and for at least 2 years afterwards.

CURRENT NON-SHUNT PROCEDURES

Techniques such as transthoracic ligation of oesophageal varices, Tanner's high gastric disconnection, and splenic artery and coronary vein ligation have little to offer over current medical and surgical treatment and have been largely abandoned. However, these methods find occasional use in the emergency situation, particularly where equipment and expertise may be lacking, and where transfer of a desperately ill patient across large distances to an experienced centre is not feasible. In the vast majority of centres, the currently favoured non-shunting procedures are simple stapled oesophageal transection, oesophagogastric devascularization, or a combination of the two.

Oesophageal transection

Interest in portoazygous disconnection was reawakened after Vanhemmel in 1974 first used a stapling device (the Russian

SPTU stapling gun) in transection of the oesophagus for bleeding varices. With the advent of simpler more effective stapling guns (Autosuture and Ethicon) came a worldwide upsurge of interest in oesophageal transection, particularly in the emergency situation.

The procedure is performed via a left subcostal or upper midline incision. The left lobe of the liver is retracted and the oesophagogastric junction identified; retraction may be difficult in a rigid cirrhotic liver and in this case, mobilization of the left lobe may be necessary. The overlying peritoneal reflection is incised using diathermy to coagulate the multiple small vessels which develop in this layer as a result of portal hypertension. The oesophagus is mobilized with its surrounding para-oesophageal tissues, from the oesophagocardiac junction to the upper margins of the diaphragmatic crus, a length of approximately 5 cm. Difficulty may be experienced with this mobilization in patients who have previously undergone injection sclerotherapy where thickening of the para-oesophageal tissues often develops. Despite this handicap it is always possible to mobilize the oesophagus without complication. Ideally the vagus nerves should be mobilized, although no postvagotomy complications were found in a recent large series from the Royal Free Hospital (London) where no specific attempt to mobilize the vagi was made. A strong linen thread is passed around the mobilized distal oesophagus and a short anterior gastrotomy is made. After assessing the lumen of the oesophagus with passage of calibrated obturators, the appropriate size of staple gun is passed into the oesophagus. The head is then separated from the anvil, and the linen thread tied tightly on to the shaft of the gun just above the oesophagogastric junction. After removal of any sling or tape around the oesophagus, the anvil and staple cartridge are approximated and the gun fired. In one manoeuvre, the oesophagus is transected with removal of a 1-cm ring of oesophagus, and the ends reanastomosed with a secure double layer of steel clips (Fig. 1).

The gun is opened and the doughnut inspected, a complete ring indicating a technically satisfactory transection. A nasogastric tube is carefully guided through the anastomosis and its tip placed in the body of the stomach before closure of the gastrotomy. The abdomen is closed without drainage, the patient allowed to take small sips of water, and the nasogastric tube usually removed after 2 days before allowing return to normal oral intake.

This technically straightforward procedure can be performed within 1 to 2 h and usually with little blood loss. Varying degrees of devascularization can be added to the procedure with most authors advocating ligation of peri-oesophageal collaterals and the left gastric or coronary veins.

Portoazygous disconnection

The principle behind this surgical approach is the disconnection of the venous circulation of the distal oesophagus and cardia from the hypertensive portal circulation by division of all the feeding vessels. The most frequently employed operations are the Hassab devascularization and Sugiura devascularization with oesophageal transection.

The Hassab procedure

The Hassab procedure consists of devascularization of the upper half of the stomach and oesophagus (Fig. 2). The first step is usually splenic artery ligation followed by careful mobilization of the spleen. This mobilization as in all dissections in portal hypertension, requires patient ligation and coagulation of multiple collaterals within the peritoneal reflections, and after individual ligation and division of the short gastric vessels, the spleen is removed. The whole proximal stomach is then devascularized from the terminal two branches of the left gastric artery at the incisura angularis upwards by ligation and division of the lesser and greater omentum, and of the posterior gastric adhesions. After division of the oesophagogastric reflection of peritoneum and mobilization of the vagi, the distal 7 to 8 cm of oesophagus is mobilized and all feeding vessels are ligated and divided. Exposure in this part of the procedure is much facilitated by the use of costal margin retractors. The distal 3 cm of oesophagus and proximal 5 cm of stomach may then be opened longitudinally thus displaying the varices and allowing obliteration of each variceal column by undersewing from as high as possible within the oesophagus with an absorbable suture. After positioning of a nasogastric tube the oesophagogastrotomy is carefully closed by suturing or stapling. Some authors recommend closure by swinging a flap of stomach wall into the oesophageal defect, thus minimizing oesophageal stricturing.

The Sugiura procedure

The Sugiura operation is a much more radical development of the above method, classically performed in two staged procedures. At the first operation, via a left thoracotomy, the distal intrathoracic oesophagus is devascularized and an oesophageal transection performed. Six weeks later, via an upper abdominal midline incision, the intra-abdominal oesophagus and proximal stomach are devascularized by lesser and greater curve division and splenectomy.

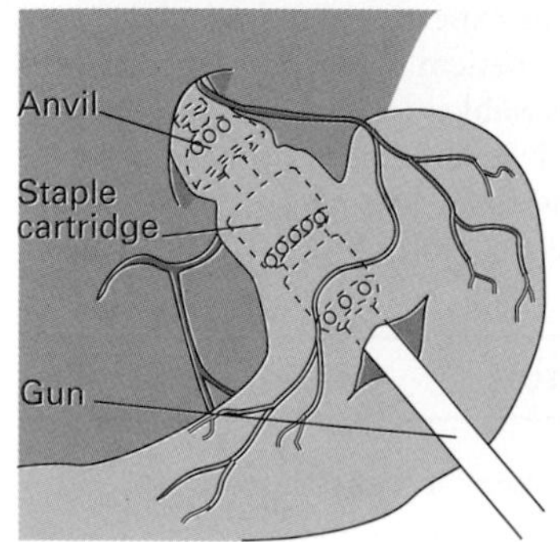

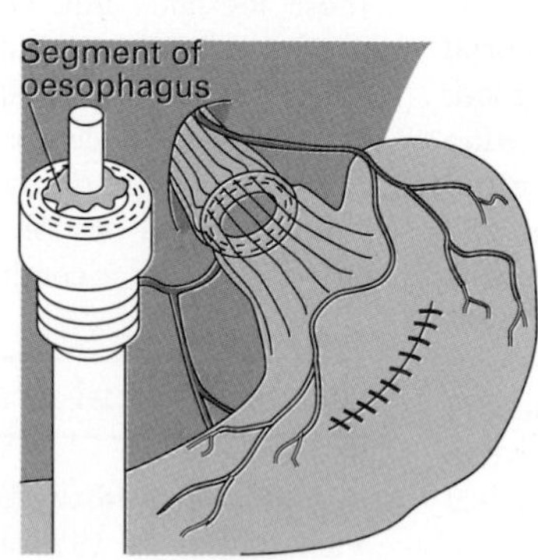

Fig. 1 Staple transection of the oesophagus. The head of the staple gun is introduced into the lower oesophagus via an anterior gastrotomy and a stout linen thread is tied firmly down on to the opened head of the gun about 1 cm above the oesophagocardiac junction. The head is closed on to the anvil and the gun fired, simultaneously transecting and removing a 1-cm ring of oesophagus and reanastomosing it with a double layer of staples. The 'doughnut' of resected oesophagus is inspected to ensure completeness of the transection.

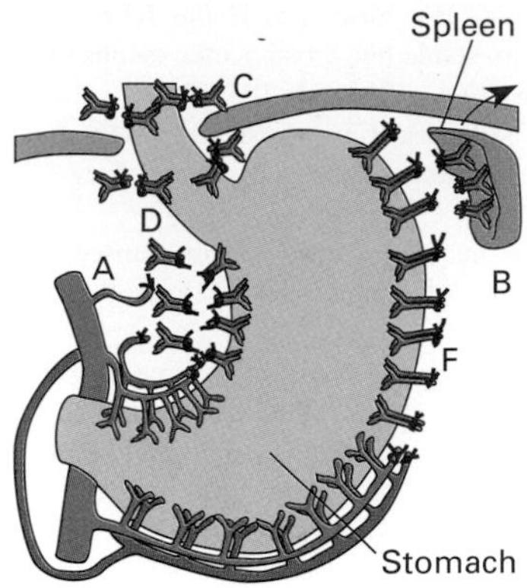

Fig. 2 The Hassab procedure. The distal oesophagus is mobilized by dissection via a midline or left transverse incision up to and including retraction or division of the diaphragmatic crura. A: the left gastric or coronary vein is divided. B: splenectomy is performed. C: the distal 8 to 10 cm of oesophagus is devascularized. D and F: the lesser and greater curves are devascularized. The oesophagus can be opened and the variceal trunks under-run with absorbable suture; a pyloroplasty is sometimes also performed.

Vagotomy and pyloroplasty are then performed (Fig. 3). This massive procedure has been modified into a one-stage operation using a transabdominal approach facilitated by the use of costal margin and sternal retractors. After division of the crura of the diaphragm, 10 cm of oesophagus can be devascularized, a staple transection performed via a gastrotomy and the rest of the abdominal part of the operation completed.

RESULTS OF NON-SHUNT PROCEDURES

Because of high long-term rebleeding rates of up to 50 per cent, simple oesophageal transection without some form of devascularization is rarely performed as a definitive, elective procedure. In the emergency situation however, transection alone has been shown to be highly effective at controlling variceal haemorrhage and in a randomized controlled trial from the Royal Free Hospital was found to have morbidity and mortality similar to injection sclerotherapy across all grades of liver disease. Rebleeding does not occur before 3 months but when it does develop, is frequently not from varices at all but from ulceration at the transection line which is readily controlled by omeprazole. The incidence of portal-systemic encephalopathy is very low and dysphagia, although frequent, is usually transient but when persistent, is cured by dilatation.

The major complications of devascularization procedures are those of the oesophageal transection, possibly compounded by devascularization ischaemia, namely dysphagia, ulceration, and stricture formation but with an extremely low rate of rebleeding and recurrence of varices when compared with simple transection alone. All of these procedures are characterized by little or no increase in portal-systemic encephalopathy.

The majority of series of devascularization procedures report a significantly high risk of rebleeding although there is considerable variability in reported results. The exception to this is Sugiura's results with his two-stage operation wherein he reported an overall mortality of 4.9 per cent with a mortality of 13.3 per cent for emergency procedures. In a different series from Kuwait, Abouna reported a similar overall mortality of 7.7 per cent for his one-stage modification of the Sugiura technique. Both series had extremely low rebleeding rates of 1.5 and 3.4 per cent respectively with no increase in portal-systemic encephalopathy. These results are the best reported for any treatment for oesophageal varices, but unfortunately no Western group has been able to reproduce them, largely it is claimed because of the higher preponderance of alcoholic cirrhosis and hepatitis in the West. Indeed the Western experience of the Sugiura technique is characterized by high morbidity and mortality. Excellent results however, have been reported in the management of variceal bleeding in schistosomal portal hypertension where long-term liver function is good. Devascularization procedures, in particular the modified Sugiura, provide the treatment of choice for this condition.

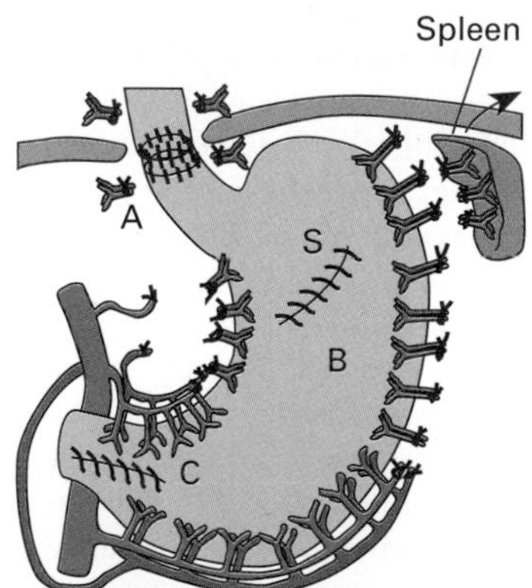

Fig. 3 The Sugiura procedure. This operation is performed either in two stages (thoracic then abdominal) or in one transabdominal procedure (modified Sugiura). A devascularization is performed as in the Hassab procedure, but with more extensive devascularization of the distal thoracic oesophagus; this can be achieved trans-hiatally without recourse to thoracotomy. A staple transection and usually pyloroplasty are then performed.

CONCLUSION

Despite the success of injection sclerotherapy there remains a place for surgical treatment of bleeding oesophageal varices which is being slowly defined. In general, non-shunt procedures offer advantages over portosystemic shunting mainly in terms of lower incidence of portosystemic encephalopathy and maintenance of portal perfusion of the liver. Simple oesophageal transection is a proven, effective means of controlling acute variceal haemorrhage, particularly where injection sclerotherapy has failed. In this emergency situation this simple approach has many advantages and is probably the treatment of choice. However, this method is less valuable in the elective situation because of its high rebleeding rate, and thus the modified Sugiura procedure has much to offer although Western experience has been disappointing. Because properly conducted comparison is not available, the choice of approach, shunt or non-shunt, is determined by the local disease patterns, local surgical expertise, and management bias.

FURTHER READING

Abouna GM, Baissony H, Al-Nakıb BM, Menkarios AT, Silva OSG. The place of Sugiura operation for portal hypertension and bleeding esophageal varices. *Surgery*, 1987; **101**: 91–8.

Bornman PC, Terblanche J, Kahn D, Jonker MA, Kirsch RE. Limitations of multiple injection sclerotherapy sessions for acute variceal bleeding. *S Afr Med J*, 1986; **70**: 34–6.

Burroughs AK, Hamilton G, Phillips A, Mezzanotte G, McIntyre N, Hobbs KEF. A comparison of sclerotherapy with staple transection of the esophagus for the emergency control of bleeding from oesophageal varices. *N Engl J Med*, 1989; **321**: 857–62.

Gouge TH, Ranson JH. Oesophageal transection and paraoesophagogastric devascularization for bleeding oesophageal varices. *Am J Surg*, 1986; **151**: 47–54.

Hassab MA. Gastro-oesophageal decongestion and splenectomy in the treatment of oesophageal varices in bilharzial cirrhosis: further studies with a report on 355 operations. *Surgery*, 1967; **61**: 169–76.

Hosking SW, Johnson AG. What happens to oesophageal varices after transection and devascularization. *Surgery*, 1987; **101**: 531–4.

Huizinga WK, Angorn PA, Baker LW. Esophageal transection versus injection sclerotherapy in the management of bleeding oesophageal varices in patients at high risk. *Surg Gynecol Obstet*, 1985; **160**: 539–46.

Kaye GL, McCormick PA, Siringo S, Hobbs KEF, McIntyre N, Burroughs AK. Bleeding from staple line erosion after esophageal transection: effect of omeprazole. *Hepatology*, 1992; **15**: 1031–5.

Matory WE Jr, Sedgwick CE, Rossi RL. Non-shunting procedures in management of bleeding esophageal varices. *Surg Clin N Am*, 1980; **60**: 281–95.

McCormick PA, *et al.* Esophageal staple transection as a salvage procedure after failure of acute injection sclerotherapy. *Hepatology*, 1992; **15**: 403–6.

Raia S, Mies S, Macedo AL. Surgical treatment of portal hypertension in schistosomiasis. *World J Surg*, 1984; **8**: 738–52.

Sherlock S. The portal venous system and portal hypertension. In: Sherlock S, ed. *Diseases of the liver and biliary system*. 8th edn. Oxford: Blackwell Scientific Publications, 1989: 151–207.

Sugiura M, Futagawa S. Results of six hundred and thirty-six oesophageal transections with paraoesophagogastric devascularization in the treatment of oesophageal varices. *J Vasc Surg*, 1984; **1**: 254–60.

24.6 Elective portasystemic shunts

RONALD A. MALT

INTRODUCTION

In the haemodynamic analysis of the splanchnic venous system, complex interplay among flow, resistance, shunting, and ignorance exceed the bounds of simple models and heuristic arguments prevail over logic. But one over-riding fact is that the principles of newtonian flow in rigid tubes do not hold when applied to the flexible, elastic veins. Moreover, the splanchnic venous system is not freely intercommunicating. Functional or anatomic blocks may isolate one part so that decompression of another part has no effect on it. For example, isolated splenic vein thrombosis causes left upper quandrant varices and is curable only by a splenectomy. To the contrary, the huge retroperitoneal collateral veins sometimes connecting the splenic vein to the renal vein in portal hypertension are ineffective decompression.

A 'total' shunt in a normal person deprives the hepatocytes of all splanchnic venous blood and leads to portasystemic encephalopathy. Modern research into the problems actually began with just such a preparation in a patient whose portal vein was purposely resected in 1952 during a pancreatectomy for cancer, followed by an end-to-side anastomosis of the superior mesenteric vein to the inferior vena cava. By and large, however, total shunts are infrequent nowadays, as compared with 1977, a decade ago, and patients with a normal liver rarely undergo a total shunt except in cases of portal-vein injury.

In patients with long-standing portal hypertension inferences that some shunts are total shunts because of apparent flow patterns of radiographic contrast media are heavily influenced by artefacts and are thus inexact. Doppler duplex ultrasonography seems more valid; it shows that in a 'total' side-to-side portacaval shunt total loss of splanchnic flow does not occur, an observation confirmed by other means. In almost every case, compensatory mechanisms increase hepatic arterial flow and collateral splanchnic venous flow so that perfusion of the hepatocytes continues—sometimes to a nearly normal level, sometimes very little; sometimes with considerable splanchnic venous blood, sometimes with almost none. Moreover, the relationship even between the classic Eck's fistula and 'meat intoxication' in dogs may have to be revised in light of studies showing that adequate nutrition prevents hepatic coma, but not hepatic atrophy.

By design, the end-to-side portacaval shunt removes residual direct splanchnic venous perfusion of the hepatocytes and should thus be 'total'. In addition, the side-to-side portacaval shunts, the proximal splenorenal shunts (with splenectomy), the mesocaval shunts, and the renoportal shunts also have the potentiality for being nominally total. Whether or not any one of them actually is depends on the balance among inflow pressures, intrahepatic and intravascular resistances, shunts between the hepatic arterial system and the portal venous system, and sites of decompression by collateral veins.

Only the selective distal splenorenal shunt is, indeed, selective in the sense of not depriving the liver of portal venous circulation in the early postoperative phase. But the choice of patients for a distal splenorenal shunt requires the preselection of those with 'prograde' (centripetal) flow of portal-vein blood, thus coincidentally selecting the best-risk patients—those whose cirrhosis is not so bad as to create a high resistance to splanchnic venous perfusion or to cause hepatic arterial shunting into the portal circulation. With time, even selective shunts become non-selective and act as functional side-to-side shunts. The pancreas may become overgrown with collateral veins, requiring a hazardous devascularization to correct it.

END-TO-SIDE PORTACAVAL SHUNTS

The end-to-side portacaval shunt is appropriate for both the emergency arrest of otherwise uncontrollable bleeding from oesophageal varices and the elective control of varices in patients who have bled. Results following its use may be as good as those following use of any of the more complicated shunts. The difficulty is in predicting which patients will do so well that their lives are almost normal, except for the limits imposed by the primary disease, and which will do badly from hepatic failure and portasystemic encephalopathy.

Prophylactic shunts should not be done for patients whose varices have never bled because they only change the mode of death from bleeding to hepatic encephalopathy and failure. For the patient whose varices have bled, conventional wisdom derived from results of randomized trials also says there is no value to shunting in prolonging life. Yet, analysis of the statistics from the studies on which this conclusion was reached indicates to the surgeon potential flaws in the arguments. Most patients entered into the trials were good risks, stratification was imprecise, the populations examined were usually small, varying skills of different surgeons and hospitals could not be controlled, and the β-error and power of negative observations was never calculated; the issue of statistical power was never calculated; the issue of power was considered only in studies done during the early 1980s. Thus, studies describing a 20 per cent increase in survival rate at 3 years after an end-to-side shunt may be more 'significant' than has been credited. An increase in the number of patients studied might have yielded generally accepted statistical significance.

Once it is granted that a shunt is appropriate treatment for a patient with varices that have bled—lesser measures having failed or being inappropriate—an end-to-side shunt is not only the easiest to do but the one most nearly certain to control variceal bleeding. An end-to-side shunt can even be done without preliminary imaging studies. It can be done with considerable confidence that the portal vein will be patent, otherwise suitable for use, and nearly certain to work. Doppler duplex ultrasonography promises to add certainty and reduce the need for preliminary angiography.

Although the techniques of end-to-side shunting are described elsewhere and will not be considered here, a few principles should be mentioned.

(a) The focus of dissection should be limited to the relevant portion of the inferior vena cava and the nearby portal vein.
(b) Initial exposure is facilitated by reflecting the duodenum with Kocher's manoeuvre, normally an easy dissection.
(c) Other structures in the portal triad should be retracted from the portal vein, not dissected individually.
(d) Only the exposure of the medial side of the portal vein entails a dangerous dissection.
(e) Clamping the hepatic end of the vein does not require good visualization of it, if an appropriate method is used.
(f) The vein must run in a good haemodynamic line to the medial aspect of the vena cava. The presence of a replaced hepatic artery running along the lateral aspect of the triad may require ingenious rerouting of portal vein; an impeding lip of pancreas or a wad of dense fat may require division.
(g) Caution should be exercised in using the vena cava as a conduit for decompression if there is angiographic or haemodynamic evidence of its compression by an engorged liver (as in Budd-Chiari syndrome) or a nodular caudate 'lobe'; nonetheless, most ostensible compression disappears when the patient is erect and any ascites present are drained. Actual anatomic obstructions in the vena cava (webs, for instance) are, of course, another story.

Failure of an end-to-side portacaval shunt to control oesophageal varices usually means that two walls of the vessels have been stitched together or that a clot has been allowed to form in the portal vein. The presence of postoperative ascites does not mean the shunt is thrombosed, internists' views to the contrary.

Aside from its utility in relieving portal hypertension, the end-to-side portacaval shunt can be used to correct metabolic disease by eliminating hepatic transformation of substances in the splanchnic venous circulation. It (and its modifications) can ameliorate hypoglycaemia and promote glycogenolysis in patients with some forms of glycogen storage disease, and can reduce synthesis of cholesterol and mobilize lipoprotein deposits in patients with homozygous familial hypercholesterolaemia.

SIDE-TO-SIDE PORTACAVAL SHUNT

Not only does the side-to-side portacaval shunt have the propensity for decompressing the distal portal vein and its tributaries, it can decompress the hepatic end of the portal vein, reducing intrahepatic portal venous pressure. While on the one hand this decompression may be desirable to remedy effects of a Budd-Chiari syndrome or to treat the now rare case of intractable ascites, it has the potential liability of depriving the liver of even more portal circulation than an end-to-side shunt, i.e., in cirrhotic patients the characteristic flow of hepatic arterial blood through arteriovenous shunts at the sinusoidal level could be diverted down the cephalic end of the side-to-side decompression, depriving the liver further of its vascular supply. As stated above, however, these arguments may not be valid. But because of this uncertainty and although it is widely used, the side-to-side shunt for emergency decompression of the splanchnic circulation is not considered appropriate by many authorities. It may, however, be useful in elective operations. Recent evidence suggests that a controlled 8-mm diameter side-to-side portacaval shunt has the potentiality for decompressing the portal circulation enough to prevent variceal bleeding, while permitting enough splanchnic hypertension to avoid the consequences of encephalopathy after total decompression.

The direct side-to-side shunt is more difficult to perform than the end-to-side portacaval shunt because the portal vein and the inferior vein may be too far apart to be joined easily or may have their potential route of connections blocked by an engorged caudate 'lobe' of the liver. Generalized engorgement of the liver may compress the intrahepatic vena cava, raising its pressure considerably and vitiating use of the vena cava as a low-pressure avenue for decompression. Narrowing of a side-to-side shunt from tension on the anastomosis caused by pulling two distant veins together predisposes to thrombosis. Indeed, the very disease for which this operation is best (Budd-Chiari syndrome) is the one most likely to give rise to all these problems. Thus, if division of several lumbar veins and dissection of the portal vein do not produce enough mobility for easy approximation of the portal vein and the inferior vena cava, an interposition ('H') graft of a vascular prosthesis or of autogenous vein is required. A double-barrel end-to-side portacaval shunt is particularly efficacious when circumstances allow its construction.

MESOCAVAL SHUNT (H-GRAFT)

The principle of a mesocaval shunt was originally proposed for decompression of portal hypertension in childhood, when the splenic vein and other peripheral splanchnic veins were considered too small for use.

Although one might anticipate this shunt would function like a mere side-arm tap off the portal vein—that is, like a side-to-side shunt—relationships of flow and resistance are such that it, too, can divert too much portal-vein blood into the systemic circulation. In terms of function, it has no advantage over a side-to-side portacaval shunt.

Nonetheless, the mesocaval shunt is undoubtedly valuable in decompressing the portal vein when the portal vein is occluded, but the superior mesenteric vein is open. It is an alternative to the side-to-side portacaval shunt for treatment of the Budd-Chiari syndrome. Extreme obesity and infrahepatic scarring may be relative indications for its use, as compared with a direct venovenous shunt. For glycogen storage disease and homozygous familial hypercholesterolaemia, the mesocaval shunt should work like the end-to-side portacaval shunt.

In terms of ease of use, those well-versed say it is a simpler operation than the portacaval shunt. Even if this assertion is correct, the H-graft mesocaval shunt must be considered less desirable than a portacaval shunt because it introduces problems of kinking and occlusion of the superior mesenteric vein, of clotting in the prosthesis, of infection, and of erosion into the duodenum. The international incidence of thrombosis and other complications is certainly 20 per cent and may actually be over 30 per cent. Use of autologous jugular vein as the H-graft offers no advantage in adult cirrhotics. In children with extrahepatic splanchnic venous occlusion or hypertension second to biliary atresia, cystic fibrosis, or congenital hepatic fibrosis, however, a high success rate may be possible, even if the vein has a diameter of only 5 mm.

For emergency shunting a small and imperfect randomized trial of the mesocaval shunt concluded it had no advantages over the end-to-side portacaval shunt for surgeons reared in the tradition of direct shunting. Instead, the facility of working with autogenous veins made the direct end-to-side portacaval shunt more appropriate.

MESOCAVAL SHUNT (END-TO-SIDE)

Haemodynamics of this shunt are doubtless the same as those of the H-graft, and its range of applications is the same. Its overwhelming utility is that it is unlikely either to erode into the duodenum or another structure, or to kink the superior mesenteric vein, because lines of stress on the vein wall are better. Too few operations have been done for the likelihood of thrombosis overall to be accurately assessed. In expert hands, a prevalence of patency over 90 per cent is possible.

MESOCAVAL SHUNT (SIDE-TO-SIDE)

Obliteration of the portal vein and of its intrahepatic branches from neonatal omphalitis and thrombophlebitis often spares the superior mesenteric vein. Until recently, the best shunt for children with portal hypertension from any extrahepatic block of this kind was a Marion–Clatworthy–Valdoni operation, which entails dividing the inferior vena cava, turning it up, and anastomosing it to the mesenteric vein for decompression. Nowadays the procedure is obsolescent because good results are possible by direct splenorenal anastomosis, even in small children, unless the splenic vein is also thrombosed (see below). The side-to-end shunt should never be used in adults because the frequent massive oedema of the lower extremities is too great a price to pay, as long as alternative forms of decompression exist.

PROXIMAL SPLENORENAL SHUNT WITH SPLENECTOMY

Because it is harder to perform than any of the shunts previously discussed, twice as liable to clot than the end-to-side portacaval shunt (29 versus 14 per cent worldwide), introduces the risk of overwhelming postsplenectomy sepsis in children, and is not suitable for emergency use because it decompresses the portal system too slowly, unique applications must be found if the proximal splenorenal shunt is to have a therapeutic role. The main acceptable indication is extrahepatic portal hypertension in children who have a patent splenic vein.

Figure 1 shows that decompression with the expectation of long-term patency is possible in young children. Results such as these and the 94 per cent patency rate in an earlier series are putting to rest the old saw that bleeding varices in childhood should be treated non-operatively, waiting until the child reaches his or her teens before attempting a shunt. While the traditional advice is true in the sense that children almost never die from variceal haemorrhage because their cardiovascular system is resilient, and some children stop bleeding as they age, the risks of hepatitis, cytomegalovirus infection, and acquired immune deficiency syndrome (AIDS) from blood transfusions may now be greater than those of surgery.

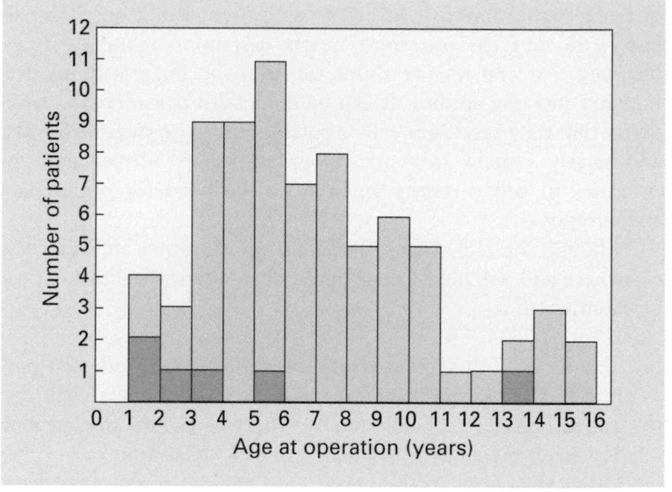

Fig. 1 Patency rates of splenorenal shunts in childhood. The hatched area represents the proportion of thrombosed shunts.

Relief of splanchnic venous hypertension and hypersplenism in patients with schistosomiasis and other forms of presinusoidal hypertension is also feasible with the proximal splenorenal shunt, but with the risk of a 31 per cent incidence of encephalopathy over the short term. However, the alternative operation, a selective distal splenorenal shunt, gives results at least as good in terms of control of varices and preservation of the spleen, and is associated with only a 13 per cent incidence of encephalopathy. (Oesophagogastric disconnection may in fact be superior to either.) The larger splenic vein in these diseases facilitates either type of anastomosis.

Considering the number of cirrhotic American patients only,

the great question is where the proximal splenorenal shunt with splenectomy stands in the priority list of operations for patients with bleeding varices. There is no question that some patients do superbly after this operation. Unfortunately, as with all portasystemic shunts, matching the type of shunt to the patient remains the dilemma.

As a result of an unpublished trial of 30 patients randomized between a proximal shunt and a distal shunt at our hospital, only two conclusions are justified: (a) It was impossible to predict from any preoperative study whether the proximal shunt or the distal shunt would be easier to do. Anatomic situations that looked difficult beforehand for one kind of operation turned out to be easy, and vice versa. (b) The patient with the worst encephalopathy had a selective distal splenorenal shunt.

PROXIMAL SPLENORENAL AND END-TO-SIDE PORTACAVAL SHUNTS: RESULTS COMPARED

Analysis of the results of shunting 120 patients in the 8 years from 1966 to 1973 (portacaval shunt, 57 per cent of total; proximal splenorenal shunt, 43 per cent) showed no differences in survival rates or encephalopathy rates between patients who underwent a portacaval shunt or a splenorenal shunt. These data were compared with those of 141 patients in the 8 years from 1974 to 1981 (portacaval shunt, 23 per cent of total; proximal splenorenal shunt, 58 per cent, mesocaval shunt, 12 per cent, distal splenorenal shunt, 6 per cent, coronary-caval shunt, 1 per cent).

Although the Child-Turcotte criteria (Table 1) were useful in predicting the mortality rate of operations, the criterion of 'encephalopathy' was not a specific one because it predicted the likelihood of future encephalopathy (83 per cent accuracy) rather than the probability of survival. Nutritional status was rarely assessed accurately.

Considering the 1974–1981 patients, the validity of a simple six-point scale to predict the likelihood of a postoperative death was confirmed (Table 2, Fig. 2) using the last data collected before an operation. An equation derived by logistic regression identified independent prognostic significance for an emergency operation, serum albumin and bilirubin concentrations, age, and sex (men, worse). With these data the cutpoint probability of 0.75 separated patients who had an 84 per cent chance of survival (above 0.75) from those below, who had at least a 77 per cent chance of death (Fig. 3).

Table 1 Child-Turcotte classification of cirrhotic patients according to functional reserve

Variable	Class A	Class B	Class C
Serum bilirubin (mg/dl)	<2.0	2.0–3.0	>3.0
Serum albumin (g/dl)	>3.5	3.0–3.5	<3.0
Ascites	None	Minimal	Poorly controlled
Neurological disorder	None	Minimal	Advanced, coma
Nutrition	Excellent	Good	Poor, 'wasting'

Table 2 Scale for predicting early postoperative mortality

	Points assigned*		
Variable	0	1	2
Bilirubin (mg/dl)	⩾0.99	1.00–1.99	2.0
Ascites	None	Stable	Uncontrollable
Operative urgency	Elective	Emergency	–

* Score is the sum of points established for all predictors: minimum = 0; maximum = 5.

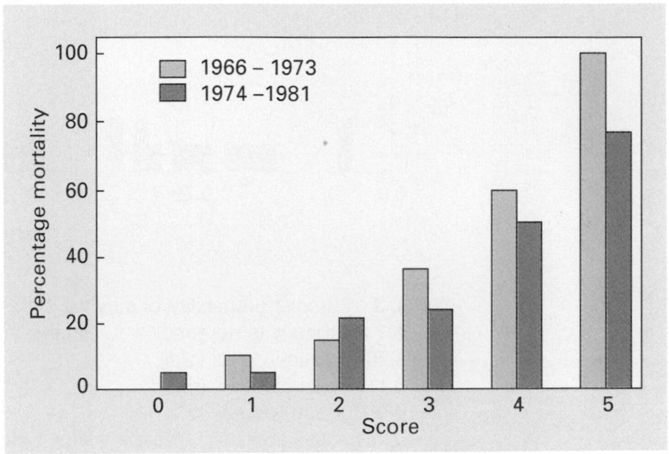

Fig. 2 Mortality rates of portacaval and splenorenal shunting by score (see Table 2): comparison of two intervals. S, predicted probability of survival for survivors. N, predicted probability of dying for non-survivors.

A Cox regression model for long-term survival after an emergency operation defined male sex and a prolonged partial thromboplastin time as poor prognostic factors, while after an elective operation only the serum albumin level was prognostic. Once a patient had survived the emergency operation (46 per cent mortality rate versus 9 per cent elective), his or her likelihood of 5-year survival (30 per cent) was as good as that of survivors of elective operations (37 per cent).

The rate of encephalopathy was 35 per cent among all patients and over all time, if encephalopathy was defined by the most sensitive criterion (any report of encephalopathy by any physician); the severity of encephalopathy was not assessable. The frequency of encephalopathy after end-to-side portacaval shunts in a randomized trial has been examined in only one study. That study showed an incidence in all of encephalopathy control (non-shunted) patients rising from 18 to 38 per cent during 4 years of observation, compared with 20 per cent, rising to 53 per cent, in shunted patients. The difference between 38 and 53 per cent was not statistically significant. The rate of severe encephalopathy, however, was 3 per cent in control subjects and 20 per cent after portacaval shunts. Contemporary repetition of such a study with all modern controls and means of estimating encephalopathy would be highly desirable, especially if extended to comparisons with proximal and the distal splenorenal shunts.

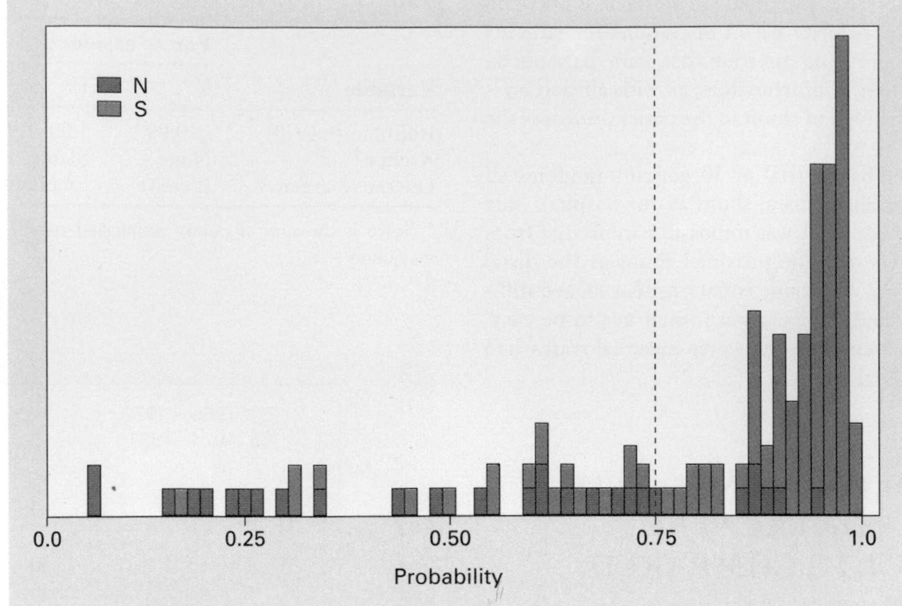

Fig. 3 Cutpoint probability of survival. Data were calculated from the equation:
0.907 × urgency (emergency = 1, elective = 2)
+ 1.26 × albumin level (g/dl)
− 0.11 × bilirubin level (mg/dl)
− 0.068 × age (years)
+ 0.561 × sex (male = 1, female = 2) + 1.45

FURTHER READING

Alvarez F, Bernard O, Brunelle, F, Hadchouel P, Odievre M, Alagille D. Portal obstruction in children. II. Results of surgical portasystemic shunts. *J Pediatr* 1983; **5**: 703–7.

Barsoum MS, Rizk-Allah MA, El-Said Khedr M, Khattar NY. A new posterior exposure of the splenic vein for an H-graft splenorenal shunt. *Br J Surg* 1982; **69**: 376–9.

Bismuth H. End-to-side splenorenal anastomosis. In: Malt RA, ed. *Surgical Techniques Illustrated.* Philadelphia: WB Saunders, 1985: 465–73.

Bismuth H, Franco D. Portal diversion for portal hypertension in early childhood. *Ann Surg* 1976; **183**: 439–46.

Callow, AD. Portacaval shunts. *World J Surg* 1984; **8**: 688–97.

Cello JP, *et al.* Factors influencing survival after therapeutic shunts: results of a discriminant function and linear logic regressions analysis. *Am J Surg* 1981; **141**: 257–65.

Child CG III, Turcotte JG. Surgery and portal hypertension. In: Child CG III, ed. *The Liver and Portal Hypertension*, Vol I. Dunphy JE, ed. *Major Problems in Clinical Surgery*. Philadelphia: WB Saunders, 1964:1–85.

Conn HO, Lindenmuth WW, May CJ, Ramsby GR. Prophylactic portacaval anastomosis. A tale of two studies. *Medicine* 1972; **51**: 27–40.

Donovan AJ. Surgical treatment of portal hypertension: a historical perspective. *World J Surg* 1984; **8**: 626–45.

Gliedman ML. Mesocaval shunt. In: Malt, RA, ed. *Surgical Techniques Illustrated.* Philadelphia: WB Saunders, 1985: 442–8.

Inokuchi K. Present status of surgical treatment of oesophageal varices in Japan: a nationwide survey of 3,588 patients. *World J Surg* 1985; **9**: 171–80.

Jackson FC, Perrin EB, Felix WR, Smith AG. A clinical investigation of the portacaval shunt: V. Survival analysis of the therapeutic operation. *Ann Surg* 1971; **174**: 672–701.

Lacaine F, LaMuraglia GM, Malt, RA. Prognostic factors in survival after portasystemic shunts: multivariate analysis. *Ann Surg* 1985; **202**: 729–34.

McDermott WV Jr. The treatment of cirrhotic ascites by combined hepatic and portal decompression. *N Engl J Med* 1958; **259**: 897–901.

McDermott WV Jr. *Surgery of the Liver and Portal Hypertension*. Philadelphia: Lea & Febiger, 1974: 117–23.

McDermott WV Jr, Adams RD. Episodic stupor associated with an Eck fistula in the human with particular reference to the metabolism of ammonia. *J Clin Invest* 1954; **33**: 1–9.

McNamara DJ, *et al.* Treatment of familial hypercholesterolemia by portacaval anastomosis: effect on cholesterol metabolism and pool sizes. *Proc Natl Acad Sci USA* 1983; **80**: 564–8.

Malt RA. Emergency and elective operations for bleeding oesophageal varices. *Surg Clin N Am* 1974; **54**: 561–71.

Malt RA. Portasystemic venous shunts. *N Engl J Med* 1976; **295**: 24–9, 80–6.

Malt RA. Proximal splenorenal venous shunts. In: Rutherford RB, ed. *Vascular Surgery*. 2nd edn. Philadelphia: WB Saunders, 1984: 1021–8.

Malt, RA, Abbott, WM, Warshaw AL, Vander Salm TJ, Smead WL. Randomized trial of emergency mesocaval and portacaval shunts for bleeding oesophageal varices. *Am J Surg* 1978; **135**: 584–8.

Mikkelsen WP. End-to-side portacaval anastomosis. In: Malt RA, ed. *Surgical Techniques Illustrated.* Philadelphia: WB Saunders, 1985: 436–41.

Ottinger LW. The Linton splenorenal shunt in the management of the bleeding complications of portal hypertension. *Ann Surg* 1982; **196**: 664–8.

Raia S, Mies S, Macedo AL. Surgical treatment of portal hypertension in schistosomiasis. *World J Surg* 1984; **8**: 738–52.

Resnick RH, Iber GL, Ishihara AM, Chalmers TC, Zimmerman H. A controlled study of the therapeutic portacaval shunt. *Gastroenterology* 1974; **67**: 843–57.

Reynolds TB, Donovan AJ, Mikkelsen WP, Redeker AG, Turrill FL, Weiner JM. Results of a 12-year randomized trial of portacaval shunt in patients with alcoholic liver disease and bleeding varices. *Gastroenterology* 1981; **80**: 1005–11.

Sanfey H, Cameron JL. Mesocaval shunts. In: Rutherford RB, ed. *Vascular Surgery*. 2nd edn. Philadelphia: WB Saunders, 1984: 1029–51.

Sarfeh IJ, Rypins EB, Mason GR. A systematic appraisal of portacaval H-graft diameters: clinical and haemodynamic perspectives. *Ann Surg* 1986; **204**: 356–63.

Sarr MG, Herlong HF, Cameron JL. Long-term patency of the mesocaval C shunt. *Am J Surg* 1986; **151**: 98–103.

Stipa S, Ziparo V. Mesentericocaval shunt (MCS) with autologous jugular vein. *World J Surg* 1984; **8**: 702–5.

Thompson JS, Schafer DF, Haun J, Schafer GJ. Adequate diet prevents hepatic coma in dogs with Eck fistulas. *Surg Gynecol Obstet* 1986; **162**: 126–30.

Turcotte JG, Erlandson EE. Portacaval shunts. In: Rutherford RB, ed. *Vascular Surgery*. 2nd edn. Philadelphia: WB Saunders, 1984: 1013–20.

Valayer J, Hay J-M, Gauthier F, Broto J. Shunt surgery for treatment of portal hypertension in children. *World J Surg* 1985; **9**: 258–58.

Voorhees AB Jr, Price JB. An update of portal systemic shunting and its complications. *World J Surg* 1984; **8**: 698–701.

Warren WD, *et al.* Splenopancreatic disconnection: Improved selectivity of distal splenorenal shunt. *Ann Surg* 1986; **204**: 346–55.

24.7 Splenorenal venous shunts

RONALD A. MALT

Normally intelligent and pragmatic surgeons spend too much time trying to decide which portasystemic shunt is best. They have done so for 40 years—a strange state of affairs given that only three impregnable concepts about surgical relief of portal hypertension have ever been enunciated. One of these concepts is that decompressing a high-pressure splanchnic venous circulation into a low-pressure systemic venous circulation reduces or eliminates the risk of bleeding from oesophagogastric varices, though at the risk of precipitating portasystemic encephalopathy. All other arguments are biased and in the absence of a unifying concept of the aetiology and treatment of bleeding varices, will continue to be.

THE IDEAL SHUNT

While there can be no doubt that the coronary–caval (Fig. 1) (left gastric) shunt is best, because it drains the specific venous compartment at risk immediately into the systemic circulation without diverting the flow of portal blood from the liver, this shunt is seldom feasible in Caucasian patients, as opposed to the frequency with which it can be usefully performed in Japanese patients. Although, over a period of 20 years we have found only five patients suitable for this operation, they have had no encephalopathy. The anatomy of the patient or the skill of the operator, or both, must be determinants of the result. In any event, the coronary–caval shunt is becoming increasingly feasible because of surgeons' ability to handle difficult venovenous anastomoses in patients with portal hypertension.

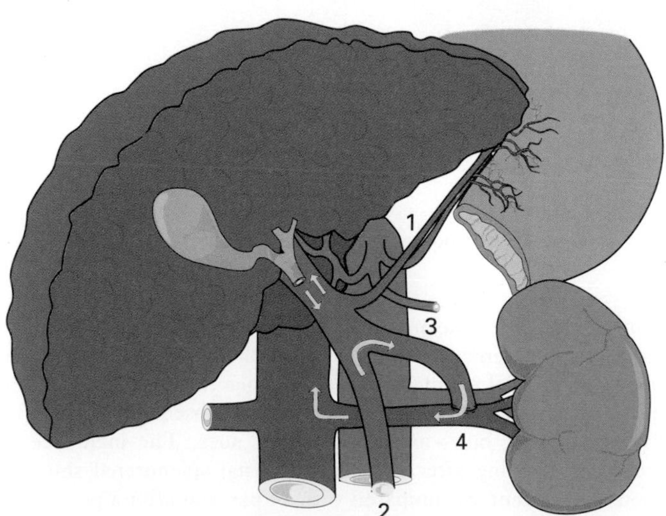

Fig. 1 Left gastric (coronary) vein anastomosis to inferior vena cava.

A key variable in almost every study of elective shunts is the extent to which the procedure being examined prevents or eliminates portasystemic encephalopathy. Divergent contentions about the incidence of portasystemic encephalopathy can be ignored, inasmuch as estimates of the incidence and prevalence of portasystemic encephalopathy are inaccurate. Despite hopes that computed electroencephalography would provide an objective assessment of the degree of encephalopathy, there is no unequivocal method of assessing the likelihood and the degree of portasystemic encephalopathy. Thus, stratification of patients and of results by the apparent degree of portasystemic encephalopathy is fraught with error and bias.

One should not be influenced by arguments masquerading as facts. The classical statement about the value of Warren's distal splenorenal shunt says that the incidence of encephalopathy after this procedure is about 5 per cent. Yet, in Grace's randomized prospective trial of the Warren shunt, as opposed to 'total' shunts, the chance of portasystemic encephalopathy was 51 per cent, granted that the skills of several operators in a multicentre trial might not equal the special talents of the originator of the procedure.

The surgeon should perform the kind of shunt he or she knows best how to do, without worrying about putative fine points of physiology.

One reason for inconstant results of any operation is that the splanchnic system itself is not freely interconnected. The flexible veins of the splanchnic circulation do not follow Poiseuille's law concerning the flow of liquids in rigid tubes. Each compartment is self-contained: the splanchnic, the splenic, the gastroduodenal, and the oesophageal (Fig. 2). Some compartments are freely interconnected; some are not. For example, when the splenic vein is clotted as a result of pancreatitis, variceal bleeding is cured by splenectomy, not by a shunt.

Conn once said, 'We must either learn to select better the patients we shunt or to shunt better the patients we select.'

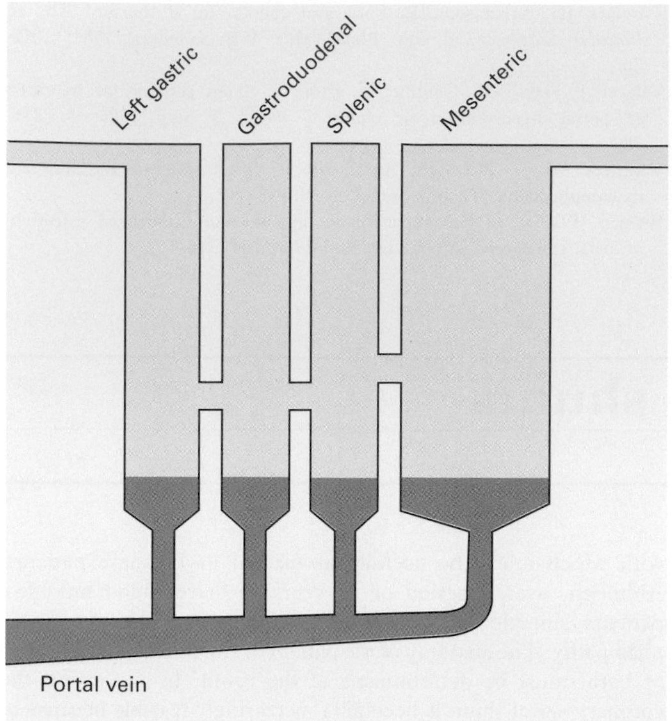

Fig. 2 Compartmentation of the splanchnic circulation. Some compartments are isolated, some flow into one another. The spillover levels are unpredictable.

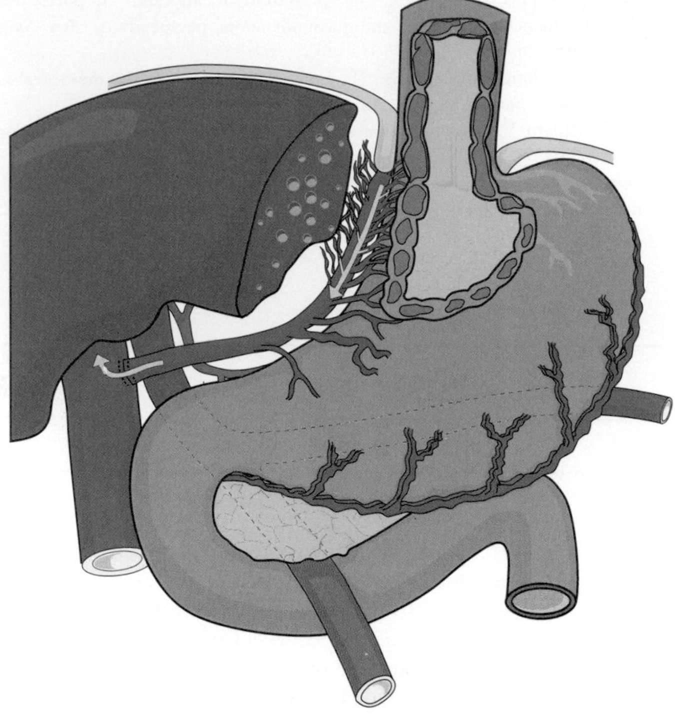

Fig. 3 Diagram of nominal venous flow patterns after a splenorenal shunt, designed to show that portal blood is not appreciably diverted, but which actually demonstrates the contrary.

SPLENORENAL SHUNT

Although the enthusiasts state that a central splenorenal shunt diverts less portal vein blood from the splanchnic circulation than does an end-to-side portacaval shunt, Fig. 3 shows what splenorenal shunting actually accomplishes. In fact, appreciable portal vein blood is diverted from the liver into the systemic circulation, and the functional anatomy is that of a side-to-side portacaval shunt. Nonetheless, the classical proximal (central) splenorenal shunt is as good as almost any other shunt, with the exception of a coronary–caval shunt. It is valuable for treating patients with severe hypersplenism and thrombocytopenia because the spleen is removed at the onset of the operation, facilitating thrombocytosis and coagulation. Extrahepatic portal hypertension in children, produced by neonatal thrombosis of the portal vein and causing oesophageal variceal haemorrhage at any age from birth to adolescence (Fig. 4), can be relieved by a central splenorenal venous anastomosis, sometimes as small as 4 mm in diameter, with only an 8 per cent chance of failure. The only issue is that children virtually never die from variceal bleeding, because their compensatory systems are so resilient. Today, they are mostly at risk from the consequences of infection by HIV and other contaminants in transfused blood.

Certain cases of schistosomiasis are also reasons to consider this procedure; however, the distal splenorenal shunt is probably superior for treatment of portal hypertension from bilharzial disease (schistosomiasis) because of its apparent lower incidence of portasystemic encephalopathy.

Despite the merits of a distal splenorenal shunt, it is not uniformly suitable for the emergency control of variceal bleeding, because it may decompress the splanchnic circulation too slowly to control bleeding. The proximal splenorenal shunt can often be used for emergency decompression, although it is less reliable than a portacaval shunt. However, neither the proximal nor the distal splenorenal shunt interferes with a subsequent orthotopic liver transplant, but a portacaval shunt does. The incidence of recurrent bleeding after a successful distal splenorenal shunt is about 29 per cent, as compared with 14 per cent after a portacaval shunt. Like a proximal splenorenal shunt, the distal splenorenal shunt is, or becomes, essentially a side-to-side portacaval shunt as collateral veins envelope the pancreas (Fig. 5).

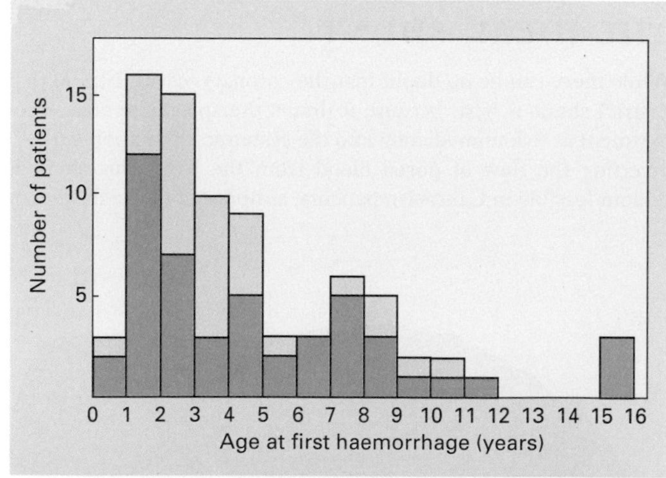

Fig. 4 Age of children at first haemorrhage from extrahepatic portal hypertension. The shaded areas indicate idiopathic causes.

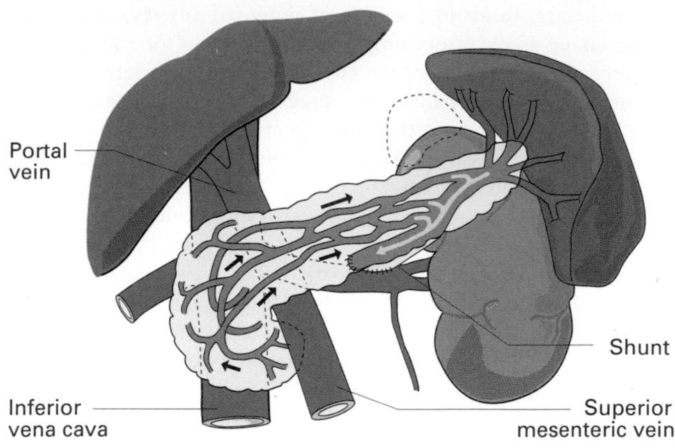

Fig. 5 Warren's schema of collateral veins surrounding the pancreas as alternative pathways continually form. The result is effectively that of a side-to-side portal caval shunt.

PROXIMAL SPLENORENAL VERSUS PORTACAVAL SHUNT

Over the years argument has raged about the merits of the proximal splenorenal shunt as opposed to those of the portacaval shunt. Although at one time the results of the proximal splenorenal shunt in terms of the incidence of portasystemic encephalopathy were clearly better than were those of the portacaval shunt, the reason for the seeming advantage was that the patients who had had a proximal splenorenal shunt were those who had survived a rigorous selection process. That is, a transthoracic transoesophageal ligation of bleeding varices was performed as a preliminary to a proximal splenorenal shunt. Obviously, anyone who had survived the first operation was preselected as an excellent candidate for any kind of surgery.

A postoperative mortality rate of about 20 per cent is common to both a proximal splenorenal shunt and a portacaval shunt. The 5-year survival rate of 42 ± 7.4 per cent (SE) for the proximal splenorenal shunt is not statistically different from the 29 ± 7.5 per cent survival rate after a portacaval shunt. Unlike the other portasystemic venous shunts, an end-to-side portacaval shunt, constructed with a patent inferior vena cava and a patent portal vein, almost never fails to cure bleeding oesophageal varices and to lower portal pressure, unless a neophyte surgeon puckers or occludes the anastomosis.

PREDICTORS

Table 1 shows a simple schema for predicting the likelihood of survival from data relating to the last blood samples drawn before either emergency or elective surgery. The bilirubin level is a parsimonious predictor of liver function and of the amount of blood products received. The presence of ascites reflects the serum albumin level (hence, the synthetic function of the liver) and the degree of portal hypertension. An emergency portasystemic shunt is an independent, ominous predictor. Obviously, if a patient's blood will not clot before surgery, it will be unable to clot afterwards. Overzealous administration of an electrolyte solution by the anaesthetist is a common cause of death from dilutional coagulopathy. In Fig. 2 of Section 24.5 the operative mortality after shunting based on the Massachusetts General Hospital score is shown during two eras of management.

TECHNIQUE

A transabdominal exposure is the easiest for the patient to tolerate (Fig 6). The need to use a transthoracic approach seldom arises, unless one can divine that the spleen is stuck tight to the diaphragm. Patients undergoing a splenorenal shunt for portal hypertension due to cystic fibrosis should always have an intra-abdominal operation, to avoid the added pulmonary hazards of a thoracoabdominal procedure.

The splenic vein is isolated from the splenic artery and surrounding structures (Fig. 7). It is hydrostatically dilated to increase its lumen (Fig. 8). The most difficult part of the operation is securing the small veins that drain from the pancreas to the splenic vein. These veins are fragile beyond belief, and they emit a torrent of blood out of proportion to their size.

The most common technical faults are:

1. Not freeing the splenic vein well enough from the pancreas;
2. Freeing the vein too well, so that the vein buckles when the organs shift;
3. Sewing the splenorenal union poorly. Very often, the anastomosis is done poorly as a result of lack of room to move, ordinarily as a result of having too many clamps in the field.

The only clamps required are three gentle bulldog clamps, which should be placed to occlude completely the medial and lateral aspects of the left renal vein and distal end of the splenic vein. Within broad limits, one does not need to be concerned about the effects of absent renal venous outflow from the left kidney, because the collateral veins (such as the adrenal, gonadal, and retroperitoneal veins) in a patient with portal hypertension divert enough blood to prevent venous infarction of the left kidney.

Table 1 Massachusetts General Hospital scale for predicting the risk of postoperative death after portacaval or proximal splenorenal venous shunting; calculation of a simple five-point predictive score

	Points assigned		
Predictor	**0**	**1**	**2**
Bilirubin (mg/dl) or [mmol/l]	(⩽0.99) [⩽35]	(1.00–1.99) [35–51]	⩾2.0) [⩾51]
Ascites	None	Controlled (stable)	Uncontrollable
Operative urgency	Elective	Emergency	–

Score is the sum of points assigned for each predictor: minimum = 0, maximum = 5.

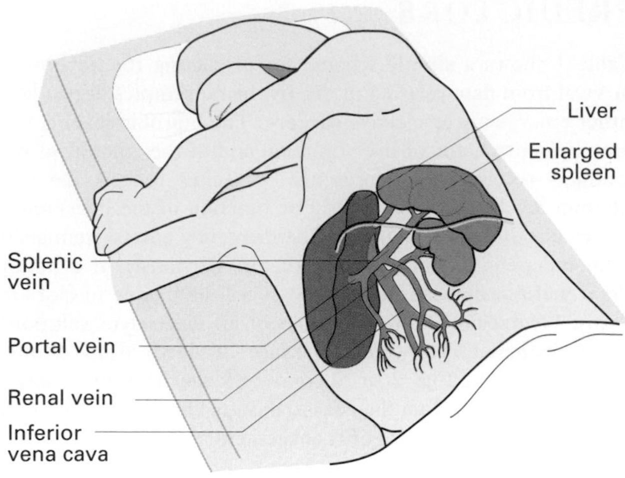

Fig. 6 Transabdominal approach for a splenorenal shunt. Although a thoracoabdominal incision is, in some senses, easier on the surgeon, it is fraught with more complications to the patient.

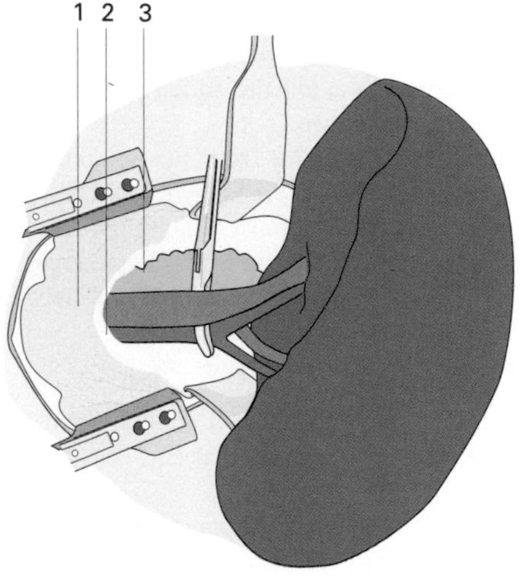

Fig. 7 Isolating the splenic vein. 1, Splenic vein; 2, splenic artery; 3, tail of pancreas.

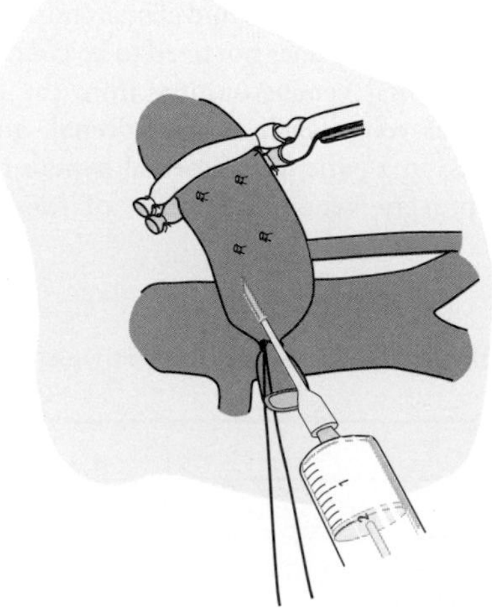

Fig. 8 Hydrostatic dilatation of the splenic vein increases its diameter.

Nevertheless, to avoid a source of potential anxiety, one should avoid taking an excretory urogram of the patient for a month after surgery. A recent study of the effects of ligating the left renal vein during aortic aneurysmectomy suggests that the consequences may be more important than have been supposed.

The freed splenic vein should be brought to the renal vein in as near a streamline as is possible. If the renal vein approaches the splenic vein from cephalad, the anastomosis ought to be constructed on the cephalad surface of the renal vein (Fig. 9). A small lenticular segment of the renal vein is cut from its surface. The anastomosis is carried out by stitching the veins together with fine polypropylene suture while the maximal circumference of the vein is maintained by the weight of fine haemostats at the end of stitches of diametrically opposite sutures. The stitches in the heel of the splenic vein, closest to the aorta, are continuous and encompass about 90° of the graft (Fig. 9). The rest are interrupted to permit the onlaid vein to billow. The veins are flushed free of clots (Fig. 10).

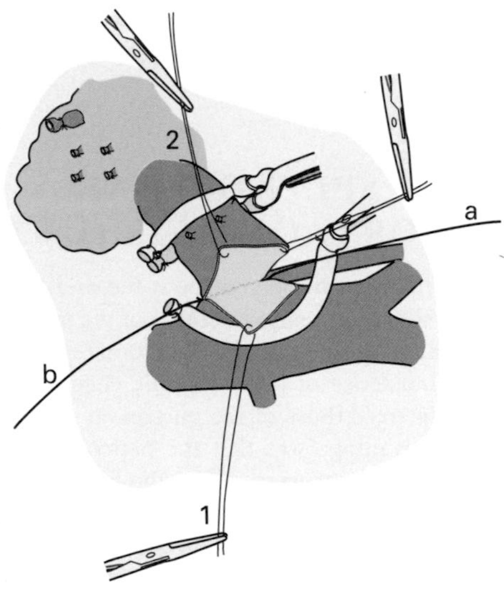

Fig. 9 Running stitch uniting the splenic and the renal veins. The cut and ligated ends of pancreatic veins that drained into the splenic vein are visible near the clamp with the number 2. Although a running, everting stitch is shown, a simple over-and-over stitch will do equally well. As specified in the text, vascular clamps are a nuisance. Bulldog clamps are better.

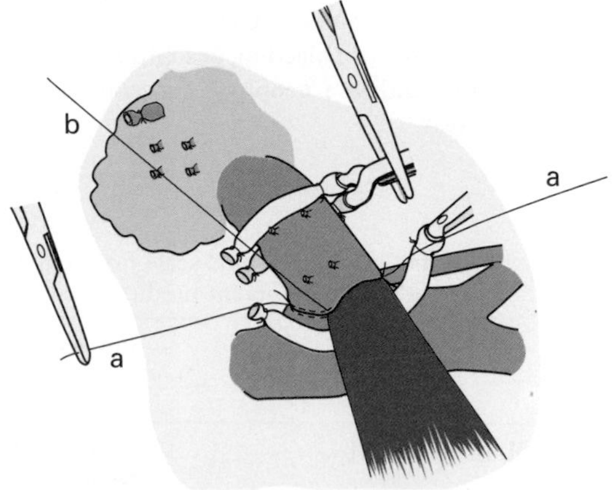

Fig. 10 Both veins are flushed to assure that they are not blocked by clot.

To guarantee patency of the anastomosis, both the renal vein and the splenic vein must be full of blood when the anastomosis is complete, and both must be capable of being emptied quickly by compressing them. Otherwise, splanchnic pressure should be measured, either by needle-puncture manometry within the veins or by Doppler scanning to ascertain flow. (Portacaval shunts do not require pressure measurements because the volume of blood is so great that one can easily feel and see the currents.) Persistent oozing of blood or lymph, or both, normally stops as soon as a patent shunt is opened.

FURTHER READING

Alvarez F, *et al.* Portal obstruction in children: II. Results of surgical portosystemic shunts. *J Pediatr* 1983; **103**: 703–7.

Bismuth H, Franco D, Alagille D. Portal diversion for portal hypertension in children: The first ninety patients. *Ann Surg* 1980; **192**: 18–24.

Calligaro KD, Savarese RP, McCombs P R, DeLauentis D A. Division of the left renal vein during aortic surgery. *Am J Surg* 1990; **160**: 192–6.

Collini FJ, Brener B. Portal hypertension. *Surg Gynecol Obset* 1990; **170**: 177–92.

Conn HO. To shunt or not to shunt. *Gastroenterology* 1974; **67**: 1065–71.

Ezzat FA, *et al.* Selective shunt versus nonshunt surgery for management of both schistosomal and nonschistosomal variceal bleeders. *Ann Surg* 1990; **21**: 97–108.

Fischer JE, *et al.* Comparison of distal and proximal splenorenal shunts: a randomized prospective trial. *Ann Surg* 1981; **194**: 531–44.

Grace ND. A hepatologist's view of variceal bleeding. *Am J Surg* 1990; **160**: 26–31.

Grace ND, Conn HO. Comparing nonselective and selective shunts (letter). *Hepatology* 1990; **12**: 377–8.

Grace ND, *et al.* Distal splenorenal vs. portal-systemic shunts after hemorrhage from varices: a randomized controlled trial. *Hepatology* 1988; **8**: 1475–81.

Lacaine F, LaMuraglia GM, Malt RA. Prognostic factors in survival after portasystemic shunts: Multivariate analysis. *Ann Surg* 1985; **202**: 729–34.

Langer B, Taylor BR, Greig PD. Selective or total shunts for variceal bleeding. *Am J Surg* 1990; **160**: 75–9.

Linton RR. *Atlas of vascular surgery*. Philadelphia: WB Saunders, 1973: 158–205.

Malt RA. Portasystemic venous shunts. *N Engl J Med* 1976; **296**: 24–9 & 80–6.

Malt RB, Malt RA. Tests and management affecting survival after portacaval and splenorenal shunts. *Surg Gynecol Obstet* 1979; **149**: 220–4.

Ottinger LW. The Linton splenorenal shunt in the management of the bleeding complications of portal hypertension. *Ann Surg* 1982; **196**: 664–8.

Rosemurgy AS, McAllister EW, Kearney RE. Prospective study of a prosthetic H-graft portacaval shunt. *Am J Surg* 1991; **161**: 159–64.

Rössle M, Gerok W. Comparing nonselective and selective shunts. (letter). *Hepatology* 1990; **2**: 377.

Salam AA, Ezzat FA, Abu-Elmagd KM. Selective shunt in schistosomiasis in Egypt. *Am J Surg* 1990; **160**: 90–2.

Sarfeh IJ, *et al.* Serial measurement of portal hemodynamics after partial portal decompression. *Surgery* 1986; **100**: 52–7.

Smith GW, Cameron JL, Malt RA, Turcotte JG. Total portosystemic shunts. In: Rutherford RB, ed. *Vascular surgery*. Philadelphia: W. B. Saunders, 1989: 1155–72.

Waddell WG, *et al.* Functional relations of the proximal components of the portal system: a preliminary report. *J Surg Res* 1972; **12**: 281–9.

Whipple AO. The problem of portal hypertension in relation to the hepatosplenopathies. *Ann Surg* 1945; **122**: 449–75.

25 The pancreas

25.1 Acute pancreatitis

DAVID W. RATTNER AND ANDREW L. WARSHAW

AETIOLOGY

A number of factors are capable of initiating acute pancreatitis although their mechanism of action is not known (Table 1). Alcoholism and biliary tract disease are the processes most commonly associated with pancreatitis: together they account for 80 per cent of acute cases. The number of patients with idiopathic pancreatitis depends on the extent to which rare causes are searched for.

Table 1 Factors capable of inciting acute pancreatitis

Ampullary block—gallstones, stenosis, duodenal diverticulum
Toxic and metabolic—alcohol, hypertriglyceridaemia, hypercalcaemia
Trauma
Endoscopic retrograde cholangiopancreatography
Infection—mycoplasma, mumps virus, Coxsackie virus, *Clonorchis* spp.
Ischaemia
Tumours
Drugs
Miscellaneous—scorpion sting, translumbar aortography, afferent loop obstruction, autoimmune disease

Acute pancreatitis may be the first manifestation of a tumour causing pancreatic duct obstruction: pancreatic carcinoma should be considered in non-alcoholic patients in whom no biliary disease is identified. Infectious agents which have been implicated as a course of pancreatitis include mumps virus, coxsackie virus, Mycoplasma, and parasites. Many drugs are capable of causing abdominal pain and hyperamylasaemia, though only a few have been implicated as clear causes of pancreatitis: these include thiazide diuretics, 6-mercaptopurine, L-asparaginase, azathioprine, oestrogens, frusemide, methyldopa, sulphonamides, tetracycline, pentamidine, DDI, enalapril, and procainamide. Patients with types I and V hypertriglyceridaemia frequently suffer from pancreatitis, usually associated with extremely high levels of serum triglycerides and lactescent serum. However, hypertriglyceridaemia can also be the result rather than the cause of pancreatitis. Postoperative pancreatitis can be fatal and is often due to iatrogenic pancreatic trauma. Pancreatitis following cardiopulmonary bypass is being recognized with increasing frequency; the majority of cases are mild or even subclinical, but evidence of severe pancreatitis is found in 25 per cent of patients who die following cardiac surgery.

PATHOGENESIS

The corrosive activity of pancreatic digestive enzymes is the driving force which differentiates acute pancreatitis from other abdominal inflammatory conditions. Although different agents may trigger acute pancreatitis by a variety of different mechanisms, they all ultimately result in intraparenchymal enzyme activation, tissue destruction, and ischaemic necrosis. The ultimate common finding in pancreatitis is the presence of activated proteolytic enzymes in the pancreatic parenchyma and retroperitoneum.

The pancreas is protected from autodigestion by several mechanisms. Pancreatic digestive enzymes are synthesized, transported, and secreted in the form of inactive precursors. From the time of their synthesis on the rough endoplasmic reticulum until their secretion by exocytosis, the potentially harmful digestive enzymes are sequestered from the cytosol in membrane bound organelles that contain potent inhibitors capable of inactivating prematurely activated trypsin. Other intracellular proteases that might be capable of activating trypsin are segregated from the zymogen granules in their respective organelles. Once discharged from the acinar cell, these proenzymes are transported to the gut through the pancreatic duct, which is not normally permeable to proteins of this size. When the zymogens reach the gut, enterokinase, an enzyme present in duodenal mucosa as well as in bile, cleaves trypsinogen to form activated trypsin. Trypsin then converts other inactive precursors to achieve forms in a cascade fashion.

The mechanism underlying the premature enzyme activation seen in acute pancreatitis, including the factors that inappropriately activate enzymes and the endogenous control mechanisms which combat the process, are poorly understood. α_1-Antitrypsin and α_2-macroglobulin, two potent protease inhibitors, are present in the pancreas, but their significance is unknown.

Once pancreatitis has been initiated, vascular events seem to play a major role in its propagation. Microinfarctions of the pancreas due to inflammation-induced microvascular thrombosis occur in most forms of severe acute pancreatitis. The severity of pancreatitis can be limited experimentally by preserving pancreatic blood flow with the use of dextran or isoproterenol. Conversely, factors which impair pancreatic blood flow are capable of converting mild pancreatitis to a severe form of the disease. It is not clear whether hypoxia or hypoperfusion alone can cause acute pancreatitis, but their role in the disease is supported by the small percentage of patients undergoing cardiopulmonary bypass and victims of accidental hypothermia who develop acute pancreatitis.

In mild pancreatitis the inflammatory response is well controlled. There may be oedema, usually confined to the pancreas, but tissue necrosis is uncommon. In severe pancreatitis the response is uncontrolled, leading to more widespread tissue injury and the many systemic manifestations of the disease. An inflammatory exudate rich in proteolytic enzymes, kinins, and vasoactive substances escapes from the pancreas into the lesser sac, retroperitoneum, and peritoneal cavity. It can then be absorbed into the systemic circulation leading to shock, respiratory failure, and renal failure.

The aetiology of shock in the early phase of acute pancreatitis is multifactorial. Sequestration of fluid in the interstitium, or third space, results in intravascular fluid depletion. However, restoration of a euvolaemic status, as indicated by central venous pressure and pulmonary capillary wedge pressure measurements may not restore normal blood pressure and haemodynamics. In addition, cross-circulation experiments have demonstrated the presence of humoral factors capable of causing hypotension in control animals without pancreatitis. Kinins, serotonin, and vasoactive amines have been implicated as mediators of diminished peripheral vascular resistance and increased vascular permeability. Although attempts to measure plasma levels of these compounds have not always correlated with the haemodynamic parameters, they are always present in high concentration in the peritoneal fluid during acute pancreatitis. Removal of this fluid by peritoneal lavage reverses the haemodynamic alterations.

In a study of 34 patients with severe acute pancreatitis, Cobo found that there was a failure of system vascular resistance to increase appropriately in the face of hypovolaemia. The difference between survivors and non-survivors in this series was the inability of the myocardium to compensate appropriately for this loss of peripheral resistance by increasing cardiac output. This was attributed to a myocardial depressant factor, although the circulating myocardial depressant factor which has been demonstrated in the plasma of hypotensive animals with severe pancreatitis has not been proved to exist in man. In most patients with acute pancreatitis the cardiac index is increased. Elevations in pulmonary vascular resistance have been documented, but these do not correlate with pulmonary capillary wedge pressure. When left ventricular stroke work was plotted as a function of wedge pressure (Sarnoff curve), the curve in patients with acute pancreatitis was shifted downward compared to that in normal patients. These data were interpreted to mean that myocardial performance was depressed even though the cardiac index was increased. The relationship between the Sarnoff curve and the elevated pulmonary vascular resistance is not clear, however, and the existence of a myocardial depressant factor in man remains in doubt.

The mechanism underlying the development of renal failure, a feared complication of acute pancreatitis, is also unclear. While hypotension and hypovolaemia may play some role, renal failure may also develop in patients who have had no preceding episode of shock and hypovolaemia.

In animal models of acute pancreatitis, significant reductions in glomerular filtration rate (GFR) occur prior to changes in peripheral circulation, and fluid resuscitation and restoration of normal cardiac output do not necessarily restore glomerular filtration rate to normal. These changes partially reflect an increase in renal vascular resistance. Most patients developing renal failure in association with acute pancreatitis are initially hypovolaemic with impaired renal perfusion and filtration. Progression to renal failure occurs even though systolic blood pressure is restored and is probably secondary to unidentified humoral factors that exert vasoconstrictive effects on the renal arterioles.

DIAGNOSIS OF PANCREATITIS

There is no foolproof diagnostic test for acute pancreatitis: the diagnosis rests on interpretation of clinical and laboratory information. In some cases the diagnosis is obvious, but the protean manifestations of this disease may make diagnosis difficult. The typical presentation includes upper abdominal pain, nausea, vomiting, and low grade fever. Tenderness is generally limited initially to the upper abdomen, although in severe cases diffuse peritoneal irritation may be present. In patients with severe peritoneal irritation laparotomy can be the safest means to establish a diagnosis and avoid missing a surgically correctable disease. When acute pancreatitis is found unexpectedly at laparotomy, it should not be a source of embarrassment but may provide the opportunity to treat any biliary pathology. Rarely, a patient has no pain, but presents with distension, ileus, fever, and tachycardia. This form of the disease is more often seen in patients with pancreatic infarction following cardiopulmonary bypass or accidental hypothermia.

Although the serum amylase level is the single most useful laboratory test, there is a significant incidence of false positive and false negative results. The serum amylase level in acute pancreatitis generally rises within 2 to 12 h of onset of symptoms and returns to normal over the next 3 to 5 days. Early resolution of hyperamylasaemia may indicate the early resolution of pancreatitis, but pancreatic necrosis may develop despite a normal serum amylase level, perhaps because of the extensive destruction of the gland. There is no correlation between serum amylase level and the aetiology, prognosis, or severity of the disease. The serum amylase is normal in up to 30 per cent of patients with acute pancreatitis, especially in alcoholics with underlying chronic pancreatitis or patients with hypertriglyceridaemia. Many non-pancreatic diseases may be associated with hyperamylasaemia (Table 2).

Table 2 Non-pancreatic causes of hyperamylasaemia

Acute and chronic renal failure
Salivary gland disease
Liver disease
Gastrointestinal disease
Common duct stones
Acute cholecystitis
Penetrating peptic ulcer
Intestinal obstruction
Crohn's disease
Mesenteric infarction
Diabetic ketoacidosis
Gynaecological disorders
Intracranial pathology
Macroamylasaemia

Hyperamylasaemia following abdominal surgery (most commonly biliary surgery and gastroduodenal surgery) is then due to genuine pancreatitis, presumably the result of operative trauma to the pancreas or trauma to the major or minor papilla. In many cases postoperative hyperamylasaemia is non-pancreatic in origin and reflects poorly understood metabolic changes. Isoamylase analysis can distinguish pancreatic from non-pancreatic sources of amylase, but this is not possible at most institutions.

Persistent unexplained hyperamylasaemia in a patient with normal renal function may be the result of macroamylasaemia, a term describing the presence of circulating amylase complexed with a macromolecule. This complex is too large to be filtered through the glomerulus and thus accumulates in the blood. The diagnosis is made by measuring amylase clearance, which is low. Macroamylasaemia occurs in 0.4 per cent of the general population and in 5.9 per cent of patients with hyperamylasaemia. Perhaps more common than macroamylasaemia is normal distribution hyperamylasaemia – a condition which the homeostatic balance between amylase production and breakdown is set at a high level. There is no predominant isoamylase type. This is the most likely explanation for persistent unexplained hyperamylasaemia in patients who are otherwise well, and it is important that this conditions is identified if unnecessary tests and treatment for non-existent pancreatitis are to be avoided.

The recent development of rapid accurate lipase assays has facilitated measurement of this enzyme as a marker for pancreatitis. Since the pancreas is the only known source of lipase this may represent a more specific marker for pancreatic disease than total serum amylase. The sensitivity and specificity of serum lipase determination may be equivalent to that of isoamylase measurement.

No radiographic technique is a sensitive index of acute pancreatitis, but some techniques can be important in confirming the clinical impression of pancreatitis, especially when the serum amylase level is normal. Radiography can assist in excluding other causes of acute abdominal pain and aid in the early detection of complications. Ultrasound yields abnormal findings in only 30 to 50 per cent of patients with acute pancreatitis. The major limitation of the tests is that the pancreas cannot be adequately seen in a large number of patients because intra-abdominal gas or excess body fat obscures tissue planes. Computerized tomography (CT) offers the advantages of better visualization of retroperitoneal structure and better overall visualization of the pancreas. The examination is more accurate regardless of the presence of abdominal gas, the patient's size, or clinical status. The changes detected by CT reflect pancreatic inflammation and oedema in approximately 70 per cent of proven cases. A normal CT scan or ultrasound does not exclude the diagnosis of pancreatitis; in fact these scans usually are normal in cases of mild pancreatitis. The CT scan is especially useful in diagnosing later complications of acute pancreatitis such as pancreatic necrosis, pseudocysts, abscess, or peripancreatic fluid collections. In severe pancreatitis, changes seen on early CT scans correlate with the subsequent development of pancreatic abscesses and pseudocysts, and early CT scans may therefore have some prognostic value, although similar information can also be discerned from Ranson's criteria (Table 3).

Table 3 Ranson's signs of severe acute pancreatitis

At admission:
Age > 55 years
Blood glucose > 200 mg/dl
Serum lactate dehydrogenase > 300 IU/l
SGOT > 250 units
White blood count > 16 000/mm^3
At 48 h after admission:
Haematocrit fall > 10%
Blood urea nitrogen rise > 5 mg/dl
Serum calcium < 8 mg/dl
Arterial $P\text{O}_2$ < 60 mmHg
Base deficit > 4 mEq/l
Estimated fluid

Diagnostic paracentesis has been used to demonstrate the presence of pancreatitis and predict the severity of the disease. Although the amylase concentration in the peritoneal fluid is of no diagnostic value, the physical properties of the fluid are of interest. A severe attack is heralded by the presence of dark peritoneal fluid and mild attacks by straw coloured fluid. The ability to aspirate more than 10 ml of free peritoneal fluid, regardless of colour may also be indicative of a severe attack. However, the Ranson criteria are at least as accurate as peritoneal aspiration and are less invasive, although it takes 48 h to gather the data.

MEDICAL TREATMENT OF ACUTE PANCREATITIS

Although many measures have been tried in an effort to modify the natural history of pancreatitis, no known agent arrests or reverses the inflammatory process. Most attacks of acute pancreatitis are self-limited and subside spontaneously. Existing treatment can only be supportive and directed at complications which may develop. Prevention of future attacks can be accomplished when a remediable cause is identified.

Fluid replacement

The most important requirement in the early treatment of pancreatitis is maintenance of adequate hydration. If the patient becomes hypovolaemic, and the splanchnic circulation is compromised, the pancreas may become ischaemic, with the potential for the development of complicated pancreatitis. In severe pancreatitis, where large fluid shifts occur, measurements of cardiac output and pulmonary capillary wedge pressure with Swan–Ganz catheters may be necessary, especially if cardiac or renal compromise complicate fluid management. Transfusion may be required if significant anaemia develops. When there is haemodynamic instability in spite of adequate fluid replacement, peritoneal lavage should be performed.

Treatment of hypoxaemia

Hypoxaemia is common in acute pancreatitis; 45 per cent of patients may have an arterial $P\text{O}_2$ level less than 50 mmHg. The four types of pulmonary disease associated with acute pancreatitis are early hypoxia without radiographic abnormality, respiratory insufficiency with non-specific radiological abnormalities (diaphragmatic elevation, atelectasis, pulmonary infiltrates, pleural effusions), pulmonary oedema occurring early in the illness, and late respiratory failure secondary to systemic sepsis. Respiratory failure is most likely to occur in the most severely ill patients and the need for intubation and ventilatory support indicates the likelihood of a fatal outcome.

Early hypoxaemia is usually associated with hypocarbia and is extremely common during the first 48 h of acute pancreatitis, whether clinically mild or severe. The only clues to the presence of hypoxaemia may be subtle tachypnoea and hyperventilation: the chest radiograph is usually normal. Impaired diffusion capacity, decreased compliance, increased airway resistance, and decreased vital capacity have all been demonstrated during this early phase, although the underlying cause or causes have eluded definitive documentation. Substances whose levels are known to be elevated in acute pancreatitis—amylase, lipase, elastase, insulin, fatty acids and triglycerides—increase oxyhaemoglobin affinity *in vitro*, and the hyperventilation and hypoxia observed without radiographic abnormality or sense of dyspnoea may relate to this altered affinity. Detection of early hypoxia depends less upon clinical observation than upon serial blood gas determinations. Since early hypoxaemia is both common and insidious, supplemental oxygen should be part of the routine treatment of older patients with acute pancreatitis. Although volume overload probably does not play a primary role in the aetiology, it is sensible to restrict intravenous fluids to a volume necessary to maintain adequate peripheral circulation and urine output rather than trying to achieve arbitrary central venous pressure or pulmonary capillary wedge pressure goals.

Between 30 per cent and 60 per cent of patients who survive beyond the first 48 h of illness develop radiographically demonstrable pulmonary complications. Unlike early occult hypoxaemia, these complications correlate directly with the severity of the underlying pancreatitis: they usually occur with continuing pancreatic injury and are associated with increased mortality. Atelectasis, bibasilar infiltrates, and diaphragmatic elevation are non-specific abnormalities common to any disease involving subdiaphragmatic inflammation, and are partly the result of splinting of the abdominal wall and restricted excursion of the diaphragm due to pain, localized peritonitis, and ascites. These phenomena usually resolve as the underlying pancreatitis subsides. Pneumonitis, commonly the result of aspiration of vomitus, may complicate recovery and its prevention remains a reason for using nasogastric suction in patients with acute pancreatitis. Pleural effusions that occur during the acute phase of the illness are sympathetic collections in response to subdiaphragmatic inflammation. They are usually sterile exudates with low amylase content and they are not generally large enough to compromise ventilation significantly and rarely require removal by thorocentesis.

Treatment of these forms of respiratory failure is supportive and directed primarily at the underlying pancreatitis. Humidification of the airways, supplemental tracheal suctioning, and ventilatory exercise to keep alveoli open are helpful. Antibiotics are not necessary unless radiographic evidence of pneumonia appears; choice of any should be based on the results of sputum Gram stain and culture. If the patient is already being treated with antibiotics for the pancreatitis, a resistant organism may have collected in the respiratory tract and a change of antibiotics is often necessary to treat the pulmonary infection effectively.

Non-cardiogenic pulmonary oedema occurs in 10 to 30 per cent of patients with acute pancreatitis, usually 2 to 4 days after the onset of the attack. The early circulatory dysfunction phase of pancreatitis is generally over by the time respiratory failure occurs; in fact, all of the other clinical features of the attack may be subsiding or may have resolved when respiratory failure first begins to evolve. The chest radiograph shows pulmonary vascular congestion, perihilar fluffy infiltrates, and finally full blown pulmonary oedema. The oedema fluid has a high protein content, unlike the situation in cardiogenic pulmonary oedema in which the fluid is a transudate. The clinical picture resembles that described as the adult respiratory distress syndrome but it evolves rapidly, without sepsis playing a part.

Attempts to understand the pathogenesis of this striking syndrome have focused on haemodynamic changes and on substances thought to affect endothelial permeability. Most patients have normal pulmonary capillary wedge and central venous pressures with normal or elevated cardiac output. Some studies have reported elevations of pulmonary vascular resistance, although the relationship of this to the pathogenesis of pulmonary oedema is not clear. The finding that pulmonary oedema fluid is exudative in the presence of relatively normal haemodynamics implies that pulmonary oedema is a consequence of abnormal permeability of alveolar capillaries. The mechanism of injury to the alveolar capillary membrane is unknown. Several possibilities exist: free fatty acids generated from serum triglycerides by lipase are directly toxic to this membrane and increased serum triglycerides are the best predictor of the likely development of pulmonary oedema. Another potential mechanism involves destruction of pulmonary surfactant. Phospholipase A_2 released from the pancreas is capable of splitting lecithin into lysolecithin and a fatty acid. There has not, however, been a consistent correlation between elevated serum phospholipase A_2 levels and the severity of pancreatitis or its respiratory complications. A third potential mechanism of endothelial injury involves vasoactive substances. Kinins, vasoactive amines, and other poorly characterized substances liberated in acute pancreatitis have been blamed for increased endothelial permeability, interstitial fluid leak, and hypotension. These substances might affect the permeability of the alveolar capillary membrane as well as that of other capillary beds. Finally, activated pancreatic proteolytic enzymes are capable of initiating intravascular coagulation, resulting in microthrombosis and microembolization in the pulmonary vascular system.

The treatment of pulmonary oedema secondary to pancreatitis is also primarily supportive. Diuresis can be beneficial if filling pressures are high but over diuresis should be avoided because of potential renal compromise. If severe pulmonary oedema and hypoxia supervene, endotracheal intubation, positive pressure ventilation, positive end-expiratory pressure are necessary. Ventilatory support may be required for several weeks, but the alveolar membrane injury usually heals within 7 to 10 days. It is important to be vigilant for the development of pneumonia in this setting: sputum should be obtained daily for Gram staining, and the development of purulent sputum with a predominant organism should be treated as evidence of bacterial pneumonia. The use of albumin and diuretics in this condition is controversial, but is likely to be ineffective when the alveolar capillary membrane is leaky. Likewise, there is no strong evidence that treatment with pharmacological doses of steroids or phospholipase A inhibitors is beneficial. If the hypothesis that lung injury is due to circulatory factors, whatever they may be, is correct, peritoneal lavage should be effective treatment for the pulmonary lesion as well as for the circulatory dysfunction which is its primary indication. However, since respiratory failure very rarely causes death in these patients, and since the current techniques of respiratory support are very effective, it is not an indication for either percutaneous or operative lavage.

Minimizing pancreatic secretion

'Putting the pancreas at rest' by fasting the patient has been a traditional part of medical treatment. Recent experimental and clinical studies have shown that pancreatic secretion is already below basal levels in acute pancreatitis and this finding may explain why somatostatin analogues, which inhibit pancreatic secretion, have little effect on the course of acute pancreatitis. Because studies of patients with mild pancreatitis do not show nasogastric suction to have any benefit it has been fashionable to decry it. Nonetheless, some patients suffer from clear recurrent inflammation when nasogastric suction is discontinued, and all patients with pancreatitis are at risk of vomiting and aspirating because of ileus. Therefore, when ileus or significant abdominal distension is present, a nasogastric tube is useful.

Although H_2-receptor blockers might theoretically confer the same benefits as nasogastric suction they have not been shown to have any effect on the course of pancreatitis. H_2-receptor blockers or antacids are still helpful in prophylaxis against haemorrhagic gastritis to which these patients are susceptible.

Nutritional support

Patients with severe pancreatitis often cannot be fed for several weeks or months. Once severe pancreatitis has developed total parenteral nutrition should be instituted. Intravenous fat emulsions do not exacerbate pancreatitis in patients with normal triglyceride levels. If triglyceride levels are raised, however, fat emulsion should not be used. Total parenteral nutrition should be continued until the patient appears clinically well. If there is a large inflammatory mass, residual abdominal tenderness, or hyperamylasaemia, total parenteral nutrition should be continued. When pancreatitis is fully resolved, oral feeding can begin cautiously. Since fat, protein, and solid food are strong stimulants of pancreatic secretion begin with a low fat liquid diet, rich in carbohydrates, and to advance the diet slowly. Rapid introduction of solid food may reactivate resolving pancreatitis.

Antibiotic therapy

Antibiotics are generally ineffective in preventing the late septic complications of acute pancreatitis, and their use may even promote selection of organisms that are more difficult to treat later on. It seems reasonable to withhold antibiotic therapy in alcoholic patients with mild to moderate pancreatitis. In severe pancreatitis, however, tissue necrosis is likely and there is a high risk of subsequent infection.

In a large German study 40 per cent of patients with severe pancreatitis requiring surgery had bacterial infection of the pancreas or peripancreatic tissue. The use of prophylactic broad spectrum antibiotics in this group of seventy ill patients has not been adequately studied. Bacteria can be recovered from the peripancreatic fluid in fulminant cases early in the course of the disease. Therefore, pre-emptive treatment with broad spectrum antibiotics might be justified in the hope of limiting bacteria invasion in this period of vulnerability. Since no clinical or biochemical parameter can reliably differentiate sterile pancreatic inflammation from early pancreatic infection, CT-directed percutaneous aspiration of inflammatory pancreatic masses should be used to guide therapy (Fig. 1). Pancreatic masses or fluid collections in patients with inflammatory signs should be sampled since some may be sterile and others infected. During the course of prolonged pancreatitis, repeated aspiration should be performed each time sepsis is suspected. The presence of infection requires either operative or percutaneous drainage as antibiotics alone have never been shown to cure a pancreatic abscess.

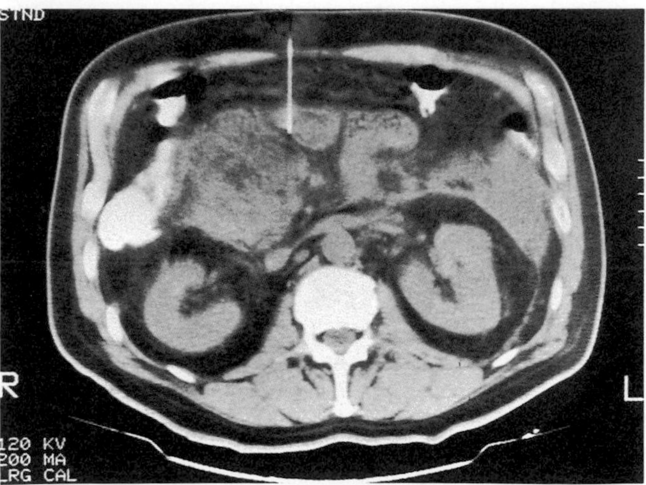

Fig. 1 CT scan of a patient with pancreatitis following cardiopulmonary bypass. This patient had a fever of unknown origin and ileus, but did not have abdominal tenderness or a palpable mass. Percutaneous CT guided aspiration of the phlegmon demonstrated bacterial infection and the patient subsequently underwent surgical debridement and drainage of the pancreatic abscess.

Antiprotease therapy

In spite of the central role of enzymatic digestion in its pathogenesis exogenous antiproteases are ineffective in limiting the progression of human acute pancreatitis.

Treatment of metabolic complications

Hypocalcaemia occurs in severe pancreatitis and a markedly reduced serum calcium is a poor prognostic sign. Only ionized calcium has physiological activity; any assessment of hypocalcaemia should therefore include either measurements of ionized calcium or a correction of the total calcium level on the basis of corresponding serum albumin level. Most cases of hypocalcaemia are due to reduction of serum albumin. Nonetheless hypoalbuminaemia does not account for all instances of hypocalcaemia in acute pancreatitis. Although extensive fat necrosis may be associated with deposition of large quantities of calcium in these areas, administration of exogenous calcium and the usual calcium homeostatic mechanism involving parathormone does not restore normocalcaemia. Studies of parathormone secretion have been contradictory, as have studies implicating calcitonin as a cause of hypocalcaemia. Hypomagnesaemia is common in alcoholic patients, and since this is necessary for both parathormone secretion and mobilization of calcium from bone, hypomagnesaemia may contribute to hypocalcaemia. In general, it is unnecessary to treat hypocalcaemia in these patients as they are rarely symptomatic. However, if neuromuscular irritability develops or the Q–T interval becomes prolonged intravenous calcium should be administered. Hypomagnesaemia and hypokalaemia, if present, must be corrected prior to administration of intravenous calcium.

Rigid control of blood glucose is unnecessary and unwise. Hyperglycaemia tends to be transient and is associated with high glucagon levels, which fall rapidly when the disease subsides. Therefore, insulin should be administered cautiously and blood glucose levels of 200 to 300 mg/dl should be tolerated.

SURGICAL TREATMENT OF PANCREATITIS

No single operative treatment and probably no operation cures pancreatitis. The role of surgery is reactive and responsive to particular complications as they evolve in a small minority of patients.

Attempts to modify the early course of pancreatitis

Gallstone pancreatitis

Gallstones can be recovered from the stools of most patients with gallstone pancreatitis, emphasizing the importance of gallstones passing into the common bile duct and then obstructing or injuring the pancreatic duct orifice. Over 60 per cent of patients have stones impacted at the ampulla during the first 48 h of gallstone-induced pancreatitis. This observation has led some to advocate early common duct exploration (within 48 h) to remove impacted stones, with the intention of aborting progression from oedematous to necrotizing pancreatitis. In one series, removal of the impacted stone during the first 48 h of the attack by common duct exploration and, if necessary, transduodenal sphincteroplasty seemed to reduce mortality from 16 per cent to 2 per cent.

The concept that early stone removal is beneficial has several flaws. First, the differentiation of gallstone-induced pancreatitis from other forms of the disease is often difficult. Biochemical criteria such as elevated transaminases are helpful, but direct cholangiography is needed to be sure. Secondly, transhepatic cholangiography in patients with gallstone pancreatitis easily demonstrates the presence of common duct stones, but these are rarely impacted. Thirdly, many of the patients studied have undoubtedly had only chemical hyperamylasaemia induced by the obstructing stone, not true pancreatic inflammation. Fourthly, many investigators have found higher complication and mortality rates among patients subjected to early biliary surgery. Ranson operated on 22 patients with gallstone pancreatitis during the first week after the attack with a 23 per cent mortality rate (three-quarters of the patients operated on within 48 h died), whereas there were no deaths among 58 patients treated non-operatively until the pancreatitis subsided, with subsequent cholecystectomy and common duct exploration. Similarly, in a study of 172 patients Kelley found impacted stones in 63 per cent of patients operated upon within 72 h, but had a 12 per cent operative mortality rate in these patients. In contrast, if operation was delayed by 5 to 7 days, only 5 per cent still had impacted stones and the operative mortality was nil. In 15 per cent of his patients the pancreatitis did not subside but progressed and forced earlier operative treatment.

Transduodenal sphincteroplasty in the presence of acute pancreatitis carries an appreciable risk of abscess or duodenal fistula formation. Because 95 per cent of cases of gallstone pancreatitis subside with medical management and without progression to a fulminant form, and 95 per cent of stones pass spontaneously in the first week, surgical intervention to remove the stone within 48 h does not seem justifiable at present. Cholecystectomy and, if still necessary, common duct exploration, may be safely and effectively delayed until pancreatitis subsides, generally during the same hospital admission.

Endoscopic retrograde cholangiopancreatography may be carried out safely by experienced endoscopists in up to 90 per cent of patients with gallstone pancreatitis. Prophylactic antibiotics should be administered and injections into the pancreatic duct should be avoided. The earlier endoscopic retrograde cholangiopancreatography is performed, the more frequently impacted stones are found, an observation confirming the studies of Kelley and Acosta. When an impacted stone is found and endoscopic sphincterotomy with stone removal is successful rapid improvement usually ensues. In patients with an impacted stone and complicating sepsis, a situation that is rare, urgent decompression is likely to be beneficial.

If gallstone pancreatitis is triggered by an initial insult from passage or impaction of a stone, removal of the stone after the insult may or may not alter the subsequent course of events. If early endoscopic sphincterotomy is to have an impact, however, it should be performed within 48 h. The challenge is to identify early in the presentation those patients who are likely to benefit from endoscopic sphincterotomy.

Pancreatic drainage and defunctionalization

The concept of an operation designed to drain the pancreatic bed and to reduce stimulation of the gland by placement of sump drains in the lesser sac, cholecystostomy tube or T-tube, gastrostomy, tube, and jejunostomy tube was popular in the 1970s. Review of the experience with this approach revealed that only patients who were judged to be dying in shock after 24 to 48 h of maximal supportive care seemed to benefit. The success of the operation in these patients was felt to be due to the removal of toxic ascites—a result which could also have been achieved with placement of percutaneous peritoneal lavage catheters.

Pancreatic resection

Major distal pancreatic resection can be accomplished in the face of acute pancreatitis with a mortality of approximately 40 per cent, while pancreaticoduodenectomy or total pancreatectomy carries a mortality rate of 60 per cent or more: the key question is how to select those patients likely to benefit. The surgeon must decide which part of the pancreas to resect, and how much to resect. This decision can be very difficult, because surface changes may not represent the degree of central pancreatic injury and because several days are required for the changes of pancreatic devitalization to become visible. In the first few days there is only massive swelling, with or without haemorrhagic staining. CT scanning following intravenous contrast administration may demonstrate which areas of the pancreas are being perfused and which are not. This has the potential to guide early surgical debridement, but there have been no reports demonstrating improved survival in patients with pre-emptive early resection compared with those treated by later debridement of clearly demarcated necrotic tissue. Since the operative mortality of early pancreatic resection is so high, it is preferable to delay surgery until areas of necrosis are clearly demarcated, or there is proven bacterial infection.

Recommended surgical responses to specific complications of acute pancreatitis

Early phase (first 4 days)

Peritoneal lavage

Many of the systemic effects of pancreatitis are believed to be mediated by kinins and other vasoactive amines such as kallikrein and bradykinin which can be found in the dark brown exudate which accompanies fulminant pancreatitis. The effects of these metabolic substances are manifested by capillary leak, low peripheral vascular resistance, and hyperdynamic shock. Peritoneal lavage to remove this toxic ascites frequently leads to a rapid improvement in haemodynamic and respiratory function, whereas haemodialysis does not.

The precise role of peritoneal lavage is controversial. Peritoneal lavage is not a treatment of pancreatitis itself, but only reverses some of the early phase systemic effects which are mediated by circulatory toxins. It is therefore of no benefit in mild to moderate degrees of pancreatitis and it does not alter the progression of pancreatic injury or prevent the intermediate or late phase developments of pancreatic necrosis and abscess. Likewise, there is no benefit in treating the signs and symptoms that develop after the first few days because the cause of late inflammation is more likely to be necrosis, abscess, or pseudocyst.

Attempts have been made to select patients in whom lavage would be helpful. Several carefully performed studies based on Ranson's signs or similar systems, which stratify for severity and risk of dying, have demonstrated no benefit in any objective parameter. However Ranson's signs are only overall predictors of mortality. No study has yet been performed which addresses the use of peritoneal lavage in the treatment of early phase shock or even identifies a subset of patients in early phase shock. These are precisely the patients in whom striking immediate improvement is commonly seen. Many still feel, therefore, that peritoneal lavage is beneficial when there is early evidence of major plasma volume loss, hypotension, pulse below 140 beats/min, or continued clinical deterioration. Lavage should be instituted within 24 h of the onset of illness.

Lavage is performed via a percutaneously placed dialysis catheter and 1 or 2 l of dialysate are used for each lavage. The fluid need not equilibrate, as is the case in peritoneal dialysis, but can be evacuated immediately. The purpose is to wash out the ascitic fluid and its toxins, and the process need be continued only until the systemic effects are reversed. The response to lavage should be quite rapid, within several hours. If not, there may have been an error in diagnosis, or the patient may be suffering from gallstone pancreatitis complicated by cholangitis, or inaccessible loculation of toxic ascites in the lesser sac. The latter may be reached by percutaneous catheter placed under ultrasound or CT guidance. Recent anecdotal reports suggest that lavage of the lesser sac is more effective than general peritoneal lavage.

Middle phase (4 days–2 weeks)

Irreversible tissue destruction becomes recognized after several days of acute pancreatitis. Phlegmon or swelling, due to oedema and inflammation, is apparent on ultrasound and CT in 30 to 50 per cent of patients and is palpable in 15 to 20 per cent. Intravenous contrast enhanced CT scans are sensitive for the early detection of ischaemic areas which subsequently become necrotic (Fig. 2). Several serum markers, including C-reactive protein and polymorphonuclear leucocyte-associated elastase, are associated with the development of necrosis and help determine which patients should undergo dynamic intravenous contrast enhanced CT scans. Serial CT scans remain the most accurate means for following the development of liquefaction necrosis. Liquefaction may occur in small well-defined patches or even in large segments such as the distal two-thirds of the gland, with extension of the necrotizing process into the retroperitoneum, perirenal spaces, and mesentery. This process is really regional necrosis, rather than just pancreatic necrosis. The combination of tissue ischaemia and release of activated enzyme into these areas can produce an ongoing necrotic process.

Three factors determine the ultimate outcome of necrosis: the amount, the extent of extrapancreatic necrosis, and, perhaps most important, bacterial contamination. Pancreatic necrosis is found to be infected in 40 per cent of patients. The incidence of infection is maximal during the third week of the disease process.

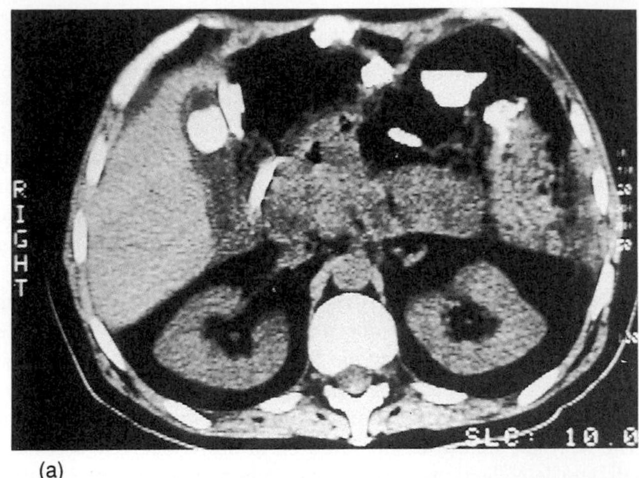

(a)

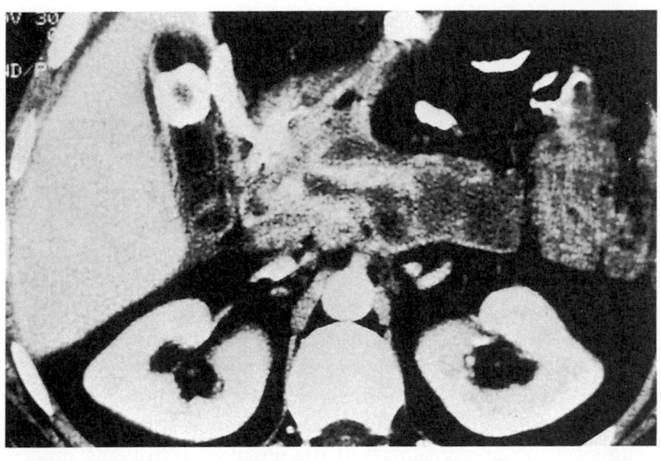

(b)

Fig. 2 (a) Abdominal CT scan of a patient in the middle phase of severe pancreatitis. A calcified gallstone is seen in the gallbladder and oral contrast lies within the gut lumen. Although there is a phlegmon in the pancreatic bed, one cannot discern from this image whether or not the tissue changes are merely reactive inflammation or necrosis. (b) Abdominal CT scan in the same patient with intravenous contrast demonstrating that much of the tissue in the pancreatic bed is non-perfused. At laparotomy, infected liquefaction and necrosis was debrided.

The appearance of infection, in general, correlates with higher mortality. In reports which differentiate between infected necrosis and pancreatic abscess, patients with infected necrosis require earlier surgery and have a higher mortality rate than those with pancreatic abscess. The combined effects of active pancreatitis and the infected necrosis force early surgical intervention in some of these patients. In contrast, patients whose active phase of pancreatitis is over, leaving them with necrotic tissue which was or would become infected, have a more indolent process which evolves over a longer period of time. When the indications for surgery finally become sufficient, the necrotic tissue has become fully liquefied—that is, an abscess has formed. Infected necrosis and pancreatic abscess are therefore not distinct entities, but are stages of a continuous spectrum of infectious complications.

Infection alone does not create the toxic state. Needle aspirations of pancreatic swellings show unexpectedly high rates of bacterial colonization, often with few or no clinical signs of infection. Furthermore, the haemodynamic consequences of pancreatic necrosis are virtually identical, whether it is infected or sterile. If infected necrosis can be indolent and sterile necrosis can produce severe haemodynamic consequences, the difference between the unstable patient with infected necrosis and the stable patient with a pancreatic abscess (and their correspondingly different mortality rates) must be due to another factor—probably the enzymatic and other biochemical events associated with ongoing acute pancreatitis.

Another area of controversy concerns how much necrosis can be safely observed. Operative mortality is rare in patients with sterile necrosis operated upon after the first week. However, postoperative complications such as fistula or abscess formation are frequent (13–24 per cent), leading some to question whether or not sterile necrosis should be operated on at all. If necrotic areas are small, sterile collections may resolve. When signs of inflammation are present, percutaneous aspiration should be undertaken to determine if infection is present: when bacteria are found in the aspirate, debridement and drainage are indicated. Larger necrotic areas are problematic because of concern that they will become infected before there is sufficient time for them to reabsorb and heal. The decision to operate on large collections is often made on the basis of clinical signs of inflammation; thus, the actual bacteriological status of the necrotic tissue does not necessarily alter the clinical decision. Sizeable collections which are not shown to be resolving on serial CT scans should be surgically debrided and drained irrespective of their bacteriological status (Fig. 3). Waiting for signs and proof of sepsis delays diagnosis and intervention, and may lower survival as complications increase.

Peripancreatic fluid collections occur in 10 to 20 per cent of patients with acute pancreatitis. Those persisting beyond the phase of acute inflammation become pancreatic pseudocysts. Pseudocysts occurring as part of the ongoing necrotizing process differ from those which are common in chronic pancreatitis. There is a 10 per cent death rate in patients with acute pseudocysts, due primarily to the severity of the underlying pancreatitis. Up to 15 per cent of patients with acute pseudocysts develop haemorrhage and sepsis while waiting for the cyst wall to become mature. Some acute pseudocysts may resolve spontaneously if the pancreatitis subsides, but those more than 6 cm in diameter which persist for 6 weeks after the onset of pancreatitis and those associated with ongoing pain and inflammation are unlikely to resolve and should be drained.

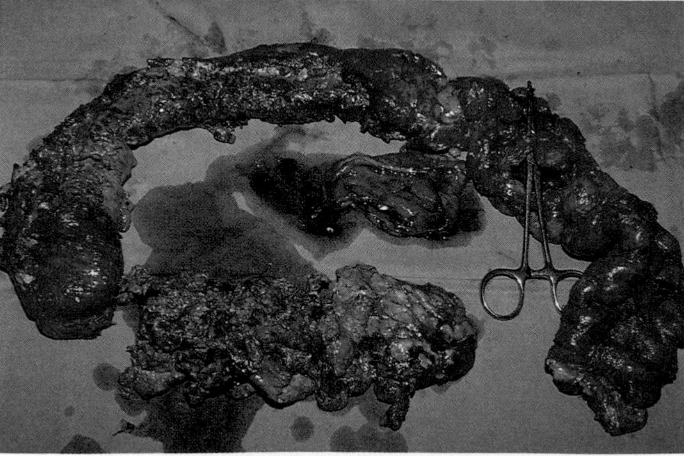

Fig. 3 Operative specimen from a patient with severe gallstone induced pancreatitis complicated by infarction of the left colon. This patient developed diarrhoea 1 week preoperatively and was found to have 'pseudomembranes' on sigmoidoscopy. The clamp traverses a site of transmural perforation. The gallbladder and necrotic peripancreatic tissue are also displayed.

Drainage by percutaneous aspiration is associated with a very high recurrence rate, and insertion of an indwelling catheter is necessary. Percutaneous drainage is generally not as effective as operative drainage since the cavity contains large amounts of necrotic material which cannot be adequately removed through small percutaneous catheters. Furthermore, if there is a persistent communication with the pancreatic duct in the presence of a proximal obstruction, an external fistula will ensue. The fistula may ultimately require a pancreatic resection for correction, whereas an internal drainage procedure performed in lieu of the initial percutaneous drainage would have been a safer and more definitive approach. There may be a subset of patients with pseudocysts who can be successfully treated with percutaneous catheters, but the criteria for identifying these patients are not yet well established. Pseudocysts may also be internally drained into the stomach or duodenum using endoscopic techniques. The safety of endoscopic cystgastrostomy for acute pseudocysts has yet to be established and for large cysts containing substantial amounts of necrotic material the procedure may be hazardous. Surgical internal drainage remains the standard therapy. Pseudocysts may be drained into the stomach, duodenum, or small bowel (Roux-en-Y limb with minimal morbidity and mortality. The choice of procedure depends on the topography of the pseudocyst and the experience and preference of the surgeon.

Cystgastrostomy is rarely utilized in Europe but is often the fastest and easiest procedure. Except in very large pseudocysts (> 15 cm diameter) cystgastrostomy is safe and effective. Giant pseudocysts and those that are not adherent to the stomach should be drained into a Roux-en-Y limb of jejunum. External drainage is necessary for 30 per cent of acute pseudocysts because the cyst wall is too friable to hold sutures. External drainage is frequently required when emergency pseudocyst drainage is performed for sepsis or haemorrhage.

Haemorrhage, a highly lethal complication, is caused by erosion of major blood vessels by elastase and other proteases. The initial lesion is a pseudoaneurysm in which infection is almost always present. If this ruptures, life threatening haemorrhage into a pseudocyst or retroperitoneum occurs. Angiography should be the management step: bleeding can often be fully controlled with angiographic techniques, allowing debridement and vessel ligation to take place under more favourable conditions. When bleeding originates from the main hepatic or splenic artery, angiographic control is difficult. Even if bleeding is not arrested, angiography provides a map that may assist the surgeon in planning the tactics of what is invariably a difficult operation. Although the effects on ultimate survival are difficult to establish without question, reduction in the rate of bleeding or complete cessation of bleeding saves blood, adds time for planning, and may reduce the expenditure of the patient's reserves. Surgery is inevitably required at some point for debridement of the associated regional necrosis and to control sepsis. If the affected area is inadequately drained or debrided, progression of sepsis, recurrence of bleeding, or both will inevitably follow, with fatal results.

Vascular thrombosis can involve the colic branches of the superior mesenteric artery, the splenic artery, or the gastro-

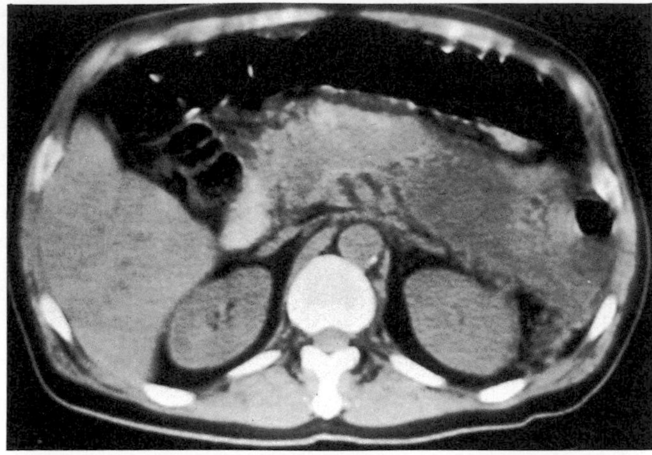

(a)

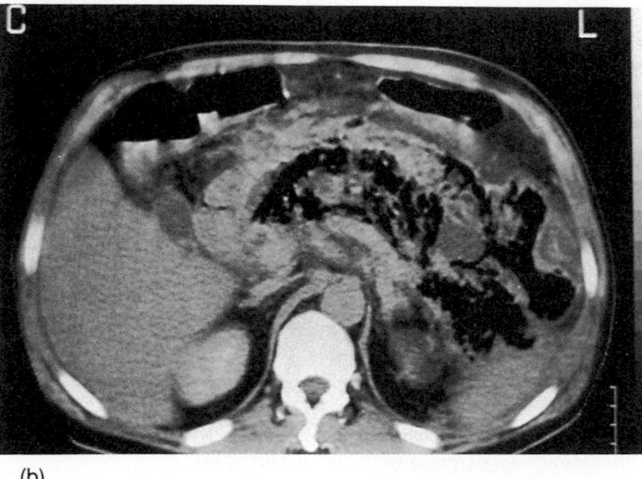

(b)

Fig. 4 The amount of necrosis that can be safely observed is unknown. (a) CT scan of a patient convalescing from a bout of severe pancreatitis. The patient was afebrile and had a normal white blood cell count. His physicians elected to discharge him from the hospital and observe the area of necrosis. (b) One week later the patient returned in septic shock. The CT scan obtained upon readmission demonstrates a large amount of retroperitoneal gas due to an extensive pancreatic abscess.

duodenal artery. Thrombosis manifests as gastrointestinal bleeding from sloughed mucosa, infarction with perforation, fistulae, or late stenosis and stricture. Colonic ischaemia may present with diarrhoea and endoscopic features of pseudomembranous colitis. If bowel infarction occurs it is necessary to exteriorize two stomas rather than risk breakdown of an anastomosis (Fig. 4). If the duodenum perforates, attempts at local repair are preferable to pancreaticoduodenectomy. Early channelling of any fistulae that develop is beneficial. When well drained, some fistulae close with healing of the underlying process. Gastric fistulae usually do not heal, and the rate of haemorrhage from the fistula tract is high. Biliary fistulae, particularly those developing after choledochotomy can be successfully treated by percutaneous or endoscopic placement of a biliary endoprosthesis.

Gastric outlet obstruction is generally due to duodenal compression and atony or localized ileus from the nearby phlegmon. Gastroenterostomy is occasionally necessary as gastric emptying may be impaired for long periods of time. A gastrostomy tube is helpful as one waits for resolution of the obstruction.

Partial common bile duct obstruction due to compression of the intrapancreatic portion of the common bile duct is common. The serum bilirubin may rise to 3 or 4 mg/dl. Operative decompression is almost never necessary unless common duct stones and cholangitis are present. The common bile duct always returns to its normal configuration when the pancreatitis subsides.

Late phase

Abscesses, which are the most common cause of death in acute pancreatitis, occur in approximately 2.5 per cent of all patients and are related to the severity of the attack. Abscesses are the most likely complication after the second week and arise from secondary infection of necrotic and liquefied pancreas. Abscesses usually contain enteric bacteria, but if broad spectrum antibiotics have been used, *Candida* species may become a major pathogen. Multiple organisms are cultured from nearly half of all pancreatic abscesses. Patients requiring peritoneal lavage in the early phase of their disease seem to have an increased incidence of abscess formation. However, it is probable that the need for early lavage is simply an indication of basic severity of the pancreatitis, rather than the portal by which infection entered.

The best method for diagnosing pancreatic abscesses is CT scanning. Although it is possible to predict which patients are statistically more likely to form abscesses by the use of early CT scan and a clinical severity score, patients must be evaluated individually. Early CT scan of the pancreas is recommend in patients with moderate or severe pancreatitis. Those with persistent clinical evidence of pancreatic inflammation should undergo CT evaluation every week to enable change in the retroperitoneal anatomy to be monitored. Fever and leucocytosis are not always present with infection and do not reliably differentiate infected from sterile collections. Unless extraintestinal gas is present, the CT scan often cannot distinguish sterile from infected collections, and needle aspiration may be quite helpful. Infections presenting early (in the first 2 to 3 weeks), especially in the patient who has never become free of inflammatory signs, are likely to be associated with ongoing pancreatitis. Abscesses manifesting late (3 weeks or later) in the disease tend to be more bland collections of pus and to behave similarly to other types of intra-abdominal abscesses. Adequate drainage is nonetheless essential; without it the mortality rate is 100 per cent. Antibiotics alone have never cured an abscess and, while limiting the bacteraemia, may select for late fungal superinfection.

Recently there has been guarded enthusiasm for percutaneous drainage of pancreatic abscesses with some authors claiming a success rate of up to 70 per cent. Others have not been as successful. The major shortcoming of percutaneous drainage is the inability to debride thick necrotic material and thus open all the extensions and loculations of what is usually a labyrinthine cavity. Abscesses presenting late in the course of pancreatitis and those developing after initial surgical drainage are most amenable to percutaneous catheter drainage. Most, however, require a combination of surgical and radiological drainage. Although the fluid component of the abscess is often adequately drained percutaneously, surgery is required to remove pieces of necrotic pancreatic debris (Fig. 5). Patients in whom the abscess can be successfully drained percutaneously often require multiple catheter insertions, multiple catheter manipulations, and long-term catheter drainage.

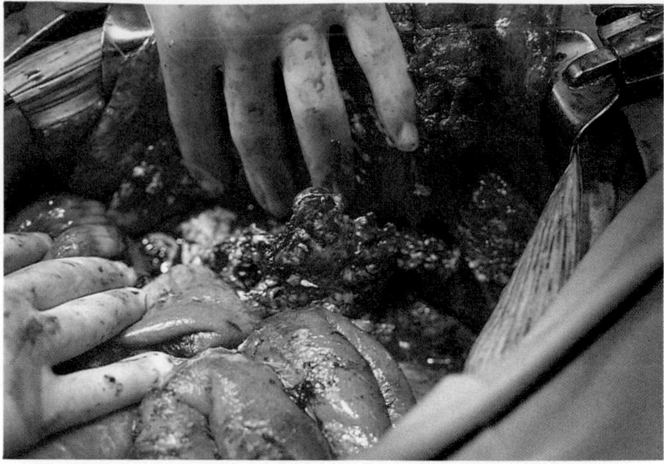

Fig. 5 Intraoperative photograph of infected necrosis. It is often easier to enter the lesser sac through the transverse mesocolon (held up by the assistant's hand) to the left of the ligament of Treitz than to try and dissect through the gastrocolic ligament.

In recent experience, with the use of aggressive surgical debridement, the mortality rate has been reduced to 5 per cent. Late endocrine and exocrine insufficiency are rare, probably because much of the tissue removed is peripancreatic tissue. Reoperation or subsequent percutaneous radiologically guided drainage is required by 20 per cent of patients. Complications occur frequently after abscess drainage and include fistulae, new abscesses, haemorrhage, renal failure, and wound infection; however most of the patients with these complications do not require further surgery.

Persisting pancreatitis

A few patients continue to have low grade signs of pancreatic inflammation for many weeks or even several months, without focal collections or areas of necrosis demonstrable by CT scan to target for debridement or drainage. Endoscopic retrograde cholangiopancreatography may identify irreversible injury to the pancreatic duct or underlying anomalies that do not allow the pancreatitis to subside. In other patients, there may be microabscesses or unrecognized duodenal wall injury. Resection of the pertinent area, even if it requires pancreaticoduodenectomy, however radical that may seem, may be the only option left. Distal pancreatectomy is indicated when the pancreatic duct becomes obstructed by the necrotizing process and its healing by scar.

FURTHER READING

Acosta JM, Pellegrini CA, Skinner DB. Etiology and pathogenesis of acute biliary pancreatitis. *Surgery* 1980; **88**: 118–25.

Beger HG, Bittner R, Block S, Buchler M. Bacterial contamination of pancreatic necrosis: prospective clinical study. *Gastroenterology* 1986; **91**: 433–8.

Cobo JC, Abraham E, Bland RD, Shoemaker WC. Sequential hemodynamic and oxygen transport abnormalities in patients with acute pancreatitis. *Surgery* 1984; **95**: 324–30.

Gerzof SG, *et al.* Early diagnosis of pancreatic infection by CT-guided aspiration. *Gastroenterology* 1987; **93**: 1315–20.

Ihse I, Evander A, Holmberg JT, Gustafson I. Influence of peritoneal lavage on objective prognostic signs in acute pancreatitis. *Ann Surg* 1986; **204**: 122–7.

Kelley TR. Gallstone pancreatitis: the timing of surgery. *Surgery* 1980; **88**: 345–50.

McMahon MJ, Playforth MJ, Pickford IR. A comparative study of methods for the prediction of severity of attacks of acute pancreatitis. *Br J Surg* 1980; **67**: 22–5.

Ranson JHC. The timing of biliary surgery in acute pancreatitis. *Ann Surg* 1979; **189**: 654–61.

Ranson JHC, *et al.* Prognostic signs and operative management in acute pancreatitis. *Surg Gynecol Obstet* 1974; **139**: 69–81.

Warshaw AL, Jin, G. Improved survival in 45 patients with pancreatic abscess. *Ann Surg* 1985; **202**: 408–15.

Warshaw AL, Rattner DW. The timing of surgical drainage for pancreatic pseudocysts: clinical and chemical criteria. *Ann Surg* 1985; **202**: 720–4.

25.2 Chronic pancreatitis

DAVID C. CARTER

INTRODUCTION

Controversy still surrounds the classification of acute and chronic pancreatitis. The most recent classifications define acute pancreatitis as a spectrum of inflammatory lesions in the pancreas and peripancreatic tissue with variable degrees of oedema, necrosis, and haemorrhage. Exocrine and endocrine function may be impaired to a variable extent and for a variable length of time. If the cause can be rectified and complications such as pseudocysts dealt with, then a clinical return to functional and morphological normality is usual. Acute pancreatitis rarely progresses to chronic pancreatitis.

Chronic pancreatitis is almost always associated with recurring or persisting pain. Chronic inflammation causes fibrosis with destruction of exocrine parenchyma leading to malabsorption and steatorrhoea. In the later stages, diabetes mellitus may follow destruction of the endocrine parenchyma.

INCIDENCE AND PREVALENCE

Chronic pancreatitis is relatively rare. Autopsy estimates of prevalence range from 0.03 to 0.4 per cent, but care has to be taken in the interpretation of postmortem findings. Pancreatic calculi are not uncommon after the age of 70 and are often associated with atrophy and fibrosis. However, these changes may be the result of squamous metaplasia of the ductal epithelium, are not associated with alcohol abuse, and do not produce the clinical picture of chronic pancreatitis.

In Europe and North America the incidence of chronic pancreatitis appears to be increasing, although this may reflect increased awareness and improved diagnosis. The prospective Copenhagen Pancreatitis Study found an annual incidence of 8.2 cases per 100 000 and a prevalence of 27.4 per 100 000. Extrapolation from these figures predicts a mean life expectancy of only 3.3 years from diagnosis, an estimate which is clearly too low, and it may be that the prevalence figure is an underestimate. In general, countries with a low alcohol intake have a low incidence of chronic pancreatitis, although there are many discrepancies. For example, Switzerland has a higher *per capita* alcohol consumption than Denmark and Sweden but a much lower incidence of chronic pancreatitis.

AETIOLOGY, PATHOGENESIS, AND PATHOLOGY

Two forms of chronic pancreatitis are generally recognized; a common 'calcific' form and a less common 'obstructive' form. Some accept the existence of a third 'inflammatory' form which can only be identified on histological examination and will not be considered further.

Chronic calcific pancreatitis

This type of pancreatitis is found in association with alcohol abuse (which now accounts for some 70 per cent of all cases in Western centres), hypercalcaemia, and malnutrition, and in hereditary and idiopathic chronic pancreatitis. The disease has a patchy lobular distribution, at least in its early stages, and inflammation leads to fibrosis, destruction of parenchyma, and eventual atrophy. Dilatation of the pancreatic duct system is often prominent. A common pathogenesis has been proposed in which the ductal system becomes occluded by protein precipitates or plugs which subsequently calcify. It is postulated that overstimulation of the acinar cells deranges intracellular transport of secretory proteins, resulting in an abnormal admixture of digestive enzymes and lysosomal hydrolases and/or storage of zymogens in acid compartments. Secretion of the iron binding protein, lactoferrin, is also increased; this molecule is known to associate strongly with acidic molecules to form complexes, a property that might facilitate formation of protein precipitates. In addition to secretory protein, pancreatic juice also contains a so-called pancreatic stone protein which can prevent nucleation and growth of calcium carbonate crystals.

Alcohol raises the viscosity of pancreatic juice by increasing secretory protein output and lactoferrin concentration, but it may also decrease biosynthesis of pancreatic stone protein (or increase its denaturation). Thus, the stage is set for the formation of protein plugs in the lumen of the acini and small ducts, and for their subsequent calcification. The calculi so formed consist of calcium carbonate, usually in the form of calcite (which constitutes approximately 95 per cent of their weight) and eosinophilic protein fibrils, which are thought to be a degraded form of pancreatic stone protein.

Although alcohol is heavily implicated in protein plug formation, less than 10 per cent of alcoholics develop chronic pancreatitis, and other factors must be involved. In addition, many patients with chronic pancreatitis have not abused alcohol and some are teetotal. Evidence suggesting that alcohol is more likely to cause chronic pancreatitis in individuals consuming a diet high in fat and protein is now contested: inadequate intake of antioxidant vitamins and trace elements may be more important. Induction of the detoxifying P450-I cytochromes occurs in the majority of patients with chronic pancreatitis regardless of cause. Such induction increases the production of oxygen free radicals and reactive toxic intermediates derived from ingested drugs and chemicals. If antioxidant intake is insufficient, failure of normal protective mechanisms could allow organelles within pancreatic acinar cells to become damaged. The trace elements zinc, copper, and manganese are required for activity of the free radical scavenger superoxide dismutase, while selenium is an essential component of glutathione peroxidase, an enzyme which controls endogenous peroxidase formation from unsaturated fatty acids in cell membranes. Alcoholics who smoke are at a higher risk of developing chronic pancreatitis than those who do not: cigarette smoking may increase free radical formation while at the same time diminishing antioxidant levels and the ability to scavenge free radicals.

A tropical form of chronic calcific pancreatitis is well recognized in underdeveloped areas of Africa and India, with a particularly high incidence in the Indian state of Kerala. Tropical pancreatitis characteristically presents with recurrent abdominal pain in childhood, development of diabetes at around puberty and death in early adulthood. The pancreatitis is associated with marked calcification and was once thought to result from the protein calorie malnutrition of kwashiorkor. However, it now seems more likely that pancreatic pain and insufficiency cause malnutrition rather than result from it. Dietary toxins, such as the cyanogenic glycosides found in cassava, a staple consumed in many areas affected by tropical pancreatitis, have also been implicated.

The incidence of chronic pancreatitis in patients with hyperparathyroidism has fallen from 5 to 10 per cent to around 1 to 2 per cent, probably as a result of earlier diagnosis and treatment of the parathyroid disorder. Hypercalcaemia stimulates the acinar cell and may also increase the concentration of calcium in pancreatic juice, thus favouring calculi formation.

Hereditary pancreatitis is a rare autosomal dominant disorder with incomplete penetrance. Pancreatitis is of early onset, calcification is marked, and there may be hyperlipidaemia and disorders of amino acid metabolism. The condition may increase the risk of pancreatic cancer, a risk reported to be as high as 25 per cent in some series. As in idiopathic pancreatitis (which is now thought to account for 10 to 30 per cent of cases of chronic pancreatitis) the mechanisms involved in the production of pancreatic inflammation are obscure but reduction in pancreatic stone protein levels may be involved.

Obstructive chronic pancreatitis

Obstruction of the duct due to papillary stenosis, scarring from acute pancreatitis or trauma, cysts or pseudocysts, or neoplasia may produce generalized diffuse inflammation and duct dilatation in the pancreas upstream of the point of blockage. Recurrent attacks of acute inflammation frequently precede chronic inflammation and more persistent pain. Characteristically, these acute attacks are less severe clinically than those which often develop in acute pancreatitis due to gallstones, and life threatening progression to necrosis and abscess formation is exceptional.

It is debatable whether pancreas divisum is a cause of obstructive pancreatitis. In pancreas divisum there is failure of fusion of the embryological dorsal and ventral pancreas so that most of the exocrine secretion has to pass through the smaller accessory papilla to gain the duodenum. The widespread use of endoscopic retrograde cholangiopancreatography (ERCP) indicates that pancreas divisum may be present in up to 10 per cent of the population, calling into question its role in pancreatitis. Nevertheless, pancreas divisum may be present in some patients with chronic pancreatitis and it may be such patients have superimposed papillary stenosis.

In contrast to chronic calcific pancreatitis, there may be considerable clinical and morphological improvement in obstructive pancreatitis once the obstructing lesion has been dealt with.

CLINICAL FEATURES

Pain

Only about 5 per cent of patients with chronic pancreatitis do not experience pain. In the remainder pain is usually the cardinal symptom, and it is by far the most common indication for surgery. The pain is recurrent or persistent, often incapacitating, and frequently requires administration of opiates for relief. It is usually experienced in the upper abdomen with radiation through to the back and is poorly localized, but may be lateralized to one or other hypochondrium and lower chest. The back pain can be particularly distressing. Some patients gain relief by leaning forwards while sitting, while some resort to kneeling on all fours. Lying flat in bed can be extremely painful and many patients sleep with the most painful side uppermost. Pain is often, but by no means invariably, exacerbated by food and alcohol intake and fatty foods may be particularly troublesome. Patients frequently apply heat to painful areas and permanent skin mottling (erythema ab igne) may result.

Attacks of acute inflammation may cause exacerbations of pain lasting for some days in the early stages of chronic pancreatitis. Although such exacerbations seldom produce a severe clinical illness, each attack should still be managed from the outset as a potentially life-threatening illness. With progression of chronic pancreatitis, acute exacerbations become less frequent and less severe, and serum amylase and lipase elevations become less marked as the gland loses its secretory capacity.

Obstruction of the pancreatic duct may cause attacks of pain which begin after eating and last for some hours. Pressure in the pancreatic duct is increased in most patients with chronic pancreatitis and it is tempting to assume that eating triggers exocrine secretion, increasing duct pressure and causing duct dilatation and pain. Pancreatic interstitial pressure is also raised and in general, operations designed to improve drainage reduce ductal and interstitial pressure. However, some patients with duct dilatation do not appear to suffer much pain, while others have pain in the absence of dilatation.

Pancreatic cysts and pseudocysts are common in patients with chronic pancreatitis and may cause pain as a consequence of the pressure within the fluid collection. While drainage often relieves pain, there is a variable relationship between pain, the presence of pseudocysts, and the magnitude of intracyst pressure.

Attention has centred recently on morphological changes in the nerves supplying the pancreas and their role in pain production. The mean diameter of the nerves is increased while the mean area served by each nerve is reduced. Oedema in nerve bundles is common and the perineurial sheath appears to serve as a less effective barrier between the surrounding connective tissue and its contents. Perineurial inflammation may be present, although its extent does not correlate with pain severity. Immunohistochemical studies suggest that there are increased amounts of neurotransmitters, such as substance P, in the nerve sheaths. Eosinophilic infiltration of the perineurial space has also been reported, particularly in those who have ingested alcohol recently, and the release of neurotoxins or pain mediators from eosinophils or mast cells has been suggested as a cause of pain.

Extrapancreatic causes of pain in chronic pancreatitis include stenosis or compression of the duodenum and common bile duct, and splenic vein thrombosis with splenic infarction. Duodenal and bile duct narrowing may result from fibrosis caused by long-standing pancreatic inflammation, from oedema in an acute exacerbation of pancreatitis, or from a pseudocyst. It is often difficult to determine the contribution of such extrapancreatic lesions to pain production but in general, pain is more often due to pancreatic causes. Duodenal ulceration is another potential cause of pain in chronic pancreatitis, the increased incidence of ulceration reflecting gastric hypersecretion and the diminished capacity of the pancreas to secrete bicarbonate and so neutralize acid in the duodenal bulb.

It is clear that there is no single cause of the pain of chronic pancreatitis and that there is great variation in its severity between individuals. Operations to relieve pain frequently have to be undertaken earlier in patients with alcohol-induced disease. Gross impairment of function with loss of secretory capacity and development of marked pancreatic calcification may be associated with increasing freedom from pain, but in many patients, an expectant approach is prevented by continuing severe pain and fears of opiate addiction.

Exocrine insufficiency

Development of steatorrhoea indicates that pancreatic exocrine secretory capacity has fallen to less than 10 per cent of normal. The stools are bulky, pale, difficult to flush and have a particularly offensive and pervasive smell which causes considerable embarrassment. Inadvertent passage of oily droplets with staining of underwear can also be a problem. Watery diarrhoea is unusual because fat is not hydrolysed to fatty acids until it has been exposed to bacterial lipase in the colon; thus fatty acids are not present in the small intestine to trigger a secretory diarrhoea. If watery diarrhoea does occur in chronic pancreatitis it may reflect failure of pancreatic bicarbonate secretion with lowering of intraduodenal pH, precipitation of bile salts, and failure to solubilize fatty acids for absorption.

Excessive loss of dietary protein from failure to secrete proteases is seldom as marked as steatorrhoea, but contributes to the weight loss and muscle wasting seen in patients with severe chronic pancreatitis.

Endocrine insufficiency

Failure of pancreatic endocrine function does not necessarily parallel the decline in exocrine function and occurs at a relatively late stage. When diabetes mellitus does develop it seldom responds to oral hypoglycaemic agents and exogenous insulin has to be prescribed. There is a real danger of insulin sensitivity as glucagon secretion is also reduced, with a resultant lowering of the capacity for gluconeogenesis. Insulin therapy must be monitored carefully and the patient made fully aware of the brittle nature of the diabetes. Diabetic ketoacidosis is rare in patients with chronic pancreatitis as there is usually enough residual insulin secretion to prevent release of fatty acids from adipose tissue and their subsequent metabolism in the liver to produce ketone bodies.

Miscellaneous features

Nausea, vomiting, and dyspepsia are common. Anorexia may be present but is often a reflection of the fact that the patient is afraid to eat rather than true loss of appetite. Weight loss and malnutrition with vitamin deficiencies are particularly common in alcohol-induced chronic pancreatitis. Gastrointestinal, retroperitoneal, and intraperitoneal bleeding may arise from erosion of pancreatic and peripancreatic vessels involved in inflammation. Bleeding from peptic ulceration, gastritis, and duodenitis is not rare and oesophageal varices may be present as a consequence of splenic vein thrombosis and segmental portal hypertension.

Pleural effusion and ascites are more often complications of acute pancreatitis but both can occur in chronic pancreatitis.

Associated disease

While evidence of biliary obstruction is commonly present on liver biopsy in patients with chronic pancreatitis, hepatic cirrhosis affects less than 5 per cent of patients. There may be a link between inflammatory bowel disease and chronic pancreatitis but pancreatitis may simply result from inflammation at the papilla of Vater. Primary sclerosing cholangitis is linked to exocrine pancreatic insufficiency but its relationship to chronic pancreatitis *per se* is uncertain. An association between chronic pancreatitis and pancreatic cancer remains speculative but the two can coexist and pose diagnostic difficulty. The increased incidence of non-pancreatic cancer in patients with chronic pancreatitis almost certainly reflects the smoking habits and alcohol consumption of this patient population.

DIAGNOSIS

Advanced chronic pancreatitis is seldom difficult to diagnose in the presence of calcification, malabsorption, and diabetes. The diagnosis of early disease is more difficult, and suspicions raised by the history are seldom accompanied by findings on physical examination. Tests of pancreatic function are of limited value given the functional reserve of the pancreas, and more reliance is now placed on imaging investigations which can detect changes in pancreatic morphology.

Tests of pancreatic exocrine function

An ideal test would detect pancreatic insufficiency before malabsorption became apparent, have a high specificity, and distinguish pancreatitis from pancreatic cancer. None of the tests available fulfils these criteria.

The secretin–cholecystokinin test

This is probably the best of the available tests of pancreatic function but it is now used rarely or not at all in many centres. Gastric contents are removed via a gastric tube and a duodenal tube is used to aspirate pancreatic secretions after stimulation by exogenous hormones. A marker such as ^{14}C-polyethylene glycol may be used to ensure that at least 85 per cent of duodenal juice is recovered. Output of bicarbonate, trypsin, and amylase can be measured, but lipase determination is difficult technically. The test has a sensitivity of 75 to 90 per cent but attempts to improve its specificity beyond 80 to 90 per cent simply lower sensitivity.

The Lundh test

This test used duodenal intubation to measure response to a test meal. It was even less sensitive than the secretin–cholecystokinin test and is now obsolete.

Tubeless indirect tests of pancreatic function

These remain in use although they are less sensitive and specific than the secretin–cholecystokinin test. In the bentiromide test, a synthetic tripeptide (*N*-benzoyl-L-tyrosyl-*p*-aminobenzoic acid) is given orally. In the presence of pancreatic chymotrypsin the tripeptide is cleaved to release *p*-aminobenzoic acid, which is absorbed from the small bowel, partially conjugated in the liver, and excreted in the urine. The pancreatolauryl test uses the same principle in that the ester fluorescein dilaurate is hydrolysed by pancreatic arylesterases to release fluorescein which is absorbed and excreted in the urine where it is detected spectrophotometrically. In patients with chronic pancreatitis judged to be severe on the basis of the secretin–cholecystokinin test, tubeless tests have a sensitivity of about 70 per cent; in mild to moderately severe disease this falls to below 50 per cent.

Other tests

Many have been described but not fully evaluated. The secretion of pancreatic lipase can be assessed by blood radioactivity levels after ingestion of ^{14}C-labelled triolein or by measuring breath $^{14}CO_2$. Lactoferrin concentration (and lactoferrin: lipase ratio) in pancreatic juice is increased in chronic pancreatitis, and plasma pancreatic polypeptide levels have been correlated with enzyme secretion during fasting and after pancreatic stimulation. Serum trypsin-like immunoreactivity and pancreatic isoamylase concentrations during fasting are also lower in chronic pancreatitis. None of these tests is used in routine clinical practice.

Tests of pancreatic endocrine function

Development of diabetes is assessed by testing for glycosuria, random blood glucose determinations, and an oral glucose tolerance test.

Imaging investigations

Ultrasonography

This is inexpensive, non-invasive and avoids ionizing radiation, and is the first investigation to be undertaken when chronic pancreatitis is suspected. Pancreatic size is assessed; in the early stages inflammation causes enlargement with an irregular outline, while in the advanced stages atrophy may ensue. There is often a heterogeneous pattern with increased echogenicity, and calculi charteristically produce very bright echoes. Pseudocysts and abscesses are readily detected. The pancreatic duct is frequently discernible and a diameter of more than 2 mm is regarded as abnormal. In normal individuals, injection of secretin produces an increase in duct diameter. In patients with chronic pancreatitis this may be prevented by surrounding fibrosis. Useful information may be obtained regarding primary disease in neighbouring organs, such as the liver and biliary system, which may be responsible for the patient's symptoms, and complications of pancreatitis affecting these organs, such as biliary obstruction and splenic infarction may be detected. Ultrasonography can also be used to guide percutaneous fine needle sampling for cytology or histology when the nature of a pancreatic mass lesion is uncertain, and can facilitate the aspiration or drainage of pseudocysts and abscesses. Percutaneous needle pancreatography can also be carried out under ultrasonographic control and Doppler ultrasonography can now be used to diagnose portal and splenic vein occlusion.

CT scanning

Since this investigation is more expensive than ultrasonography and requires exposure to ionizing radiation, it is not normally used as a first line investigation. It is, however, more sensitive than ultrasonography in the diagnosis of chronic pancreatitis (sensitivity 74 to 90 per cent as opposed to 60 to 70 per cent) and at least as specific (84 to 100 per cent versus 80 to 90 per cent respectively). Pancreatic size, density, and outline are readily assessed and CT scanning is the best method for detecting calculi. Pancreatic duct changes on CT scanning correlate well with those seen at endoscopic retrograde pancreatography, and duct size is best assessed after intravenous injection of contrast material. CT scanning also provides useful information about neighbouring organs and may distinguish between pancreatic cancer and chronic pancreatitis.

Endoscopic retrograde pancreatography

This is invasive, expensive, requires exposure to ionizing radiation and can give rise to complications which, on rare occasions, prove fatal. The Cambridge classification of radiological changes (Table 1) is generally accepted and this investigation is widely regarded as the most accurate means of diagnosing chronic pancreatitis and distinguishing it from pancreatic cancer. Endoscopic retrograde pancreatography helps to define the extent and distribution of chronic pancreatitis and outlines the duct system. This information may prove invaluable in the selection of operative procedure if surgery is to be undertaken. Useful information may also be provided about involvement of the biliary tree. However, technical reasons may prevent cannulation of the pancreatic duct and ductal narrowing or obstruction may prevent full visualization of the duct system when contrast is injected. In such cases, ultrasonography and CT scanning may provide some of the missing information, but ultrasonographically guided percutaneous pancreatography or operative pancreatography may be needed to provide a comprehensive picture of duct morphology.

Some patients with symptoms and other evidence of chronic pancreatitis have little or no abnormality visible on endoscopic retrograde pancreatography. This has given rise to the controversial concept of 'minimal change pancreatitis'.

Angiography and venography

Selective angiography and portal venography may be needed in selected patients, notably when portal or splenic vein thrombosis is suspected. Other imaging methods being evaluated at present include magnetic resonance imaging and endoscopic ultrasonography.

Table 1 Classification of pancreatograms in chronic pancreatitis (after Axon AT, *et al.*, *Gut*, 1984; **25**: 1107–12)

Terminology	Main duct	Abnormal side branches	Additional features
Normal	Normal	None	
Equivocal	Normal	Fewer than three	
Mild changes of chronic pancreatitis	Normal	Three or more	
Moderate changes of chronic pancreatitis	Abnormal	More than three	
Marked changes of chronic pancreatitis	Abnormal	More than three	One or more of: large cavity; obstruction; filling defects; severe dilatation; or irregularity

If pathological changes are limited to one-third or less of the gland they are said to be 'local' and designated as being in head, body, or tail; if more than one-third is affected, they are 'diffuse'.

Other investigations

Assessment of nutritional status, full blood count, and liver function should be performed periodically, and it is worth carrying out random blood alcohol samples when continuing alcohol abuse is suspected.

Recommendations in diagnosis

The value of a good history cannot be over emphasized. When there is overt steatorrhoea, pancreatic function tests are unnecessary and one should proceed to ultrasonography and/or CT scanning. Even in the absence of steatorrhoea, pancreatic function tests (such as the secretin–cholecystokinin test or tubeless tests) are of dubious value. They are certainly useless in distinguishing between chronic pancreatitis and pancreatic cancer, and guided fine needle aspiration or biopsy should be undertaken whenever cancer is suspected. The presence of pancreatic calcification does not exclude cancer and pancreatitis and cancer may coexist. Endoscopic retrograde cholangiopancreatography should be considered once the pancreas has been imaged by ultrasonography and/or CT scanning, particularly when the diagnosis remains in doubt, duct morphology has not been defined, and surgery is contemplated.

TREATMENT

The diagnosis of chronic pancreatitis is not in itself an indication for surgery. Some patients have little or no pain, while in others pain can be controlled without recourse to opiates. Surgery does not restore exocrine and endocrine function; indeed pancreatic resection may cause marked deterioration and precipitate the onset of diabetes. Chronic pancreatitis is often difficult to manage and when there are problems arising from alcoholism, social deprivation, and personality disorders it may be impossible to disentangle cause from effect. Good rapport and mutual trust are essential for successful long-term management and require frequent outpatient consultation with periods of inpatient assessment if appropriate.

Medical management

Pain

Effective pain relief is usually the most difficult aspect of management. Patients vary considerably in pain threshold and pain perception and many are already taking opiates when first referred for surgical consultation. They should be encouraged to abstain from alcohol, take frequent small meals rather than infrequent large ones, and avoid overtly fatty foods. Liquid meals and elemental diets are no longer prescribed in attempts to reduce pancreatic stimulation: liquids augment the gastric phase of pancreatic secretion while elemental diets stimulate cholecystokinin release. Pancreatic extracts are used to treat steatorrhoea and probably reduce pain by providing intraluminal trypsin which blocks release of cholecystokinin from the duodenal mucosa. Histamine H_2-receptor antagonists such as cimetidine or ranitidine may prevent or eradicate duodenitis and peptic ulceration, and theoretically reduce pancreatic stimulation by diminishing duodenal release of secretin.

Analgesics must be prescribed carefully, given the long-term nature of the problem and risk of opiate addiction. Unfortunately, non-opioid drugs such as aspirin and paracetamol are more effective at relieving musculoskeletal pain than visceral pain, and opiates are frequently essential. All opioid drugs may cause drowsiness, nausea and vomiting, and constipation (although this may be regarded as beneficial in patients with steatorrhoea). Sublingual bruprenorphine (200–400 μg every 6–8 h), and oral dihydrocodeine tartrate (30 mg every 4–6 h) or pentazocine (25–100 mg every 3–4 h after food) may give satisfactory pain control without recourse to injection. More severe exacerbations of pain may require injection of morphine (10–30 mg) or pethidine (50–100 mg) and long-lasting severe pain may need oral pethidine (50–150 mg every 4 h) or long-acting morphine preparations (such as morphine sulphate, MST Continus® 10–60 mg twice daily). Whenever such powerful opioid drugs are having to be prescribed frequently and/or continuously, serious consideration must be given to surgery.

The sensory sympathetic nerves which transmit pain impulses from the pancreas synapse in the coeliac ganglion on their way to the splanchnic nerves. Attempts to relieve the pain of chronic pancreatitis by CT guided injection of alcohol in and around the coeliac plexus have had extremely variable results and at best give pain relief for a few months. Coeliac blockade is no longer used in most centres.

Pancreatic exocrine insufficiency

In theory, provision of exogenous lipase supplements with every meal should readily eliminate steatorrhoea. In practice steatorrhoea may be difficult to abolish as gastric acid destroys up to 90 per cent of such enzyme activity by the time food reaches the distal duodenum. Antacids or H_2-receptor antagonists were once used to combat this problem. However, modern pancreatic exocrine supplements (e.g. Creon; one capsule of which contains 8000 units lipase, 9000 units amylase, and 210 units protease) consist of enteric coated granules of pancreatic extract contained in an outer gelatin capsule. The gelatin dissolves with a few minutes in the acidic stomach whereas the granules break down in the duodenum when luminal pH rises above pH 5.5. Microsphere preparations are more expensive than simpler preparations of pancreatic extracts but are well tolerated. The initial dose is 1 to 2 capsules with meals, rising to 5 to 15 capsules each day. If steatorrhoea persists, H_2-receptor antagonists should be prescribed. If steatorrhoea is still troublesome, alternative explanations (such as bacterial overgrowth in the small intestine or bile salt insufficiency) should be considered. If all else fails, fat intake should be reduced to below 40 g per day and the diet supplemented with medium chain triglyceride oil which requires less lipase for cleavage.

Diabetes mellitus

Insulin is needed if diabetes mellitus develops. As indicated earlier, the risk of hypoglycaemia is much greater than that of ketoacidosis.

Other measures

Nutritional status requires careful supervision. An adequate intake of calories and vitamins is essential, particular attention being paid to intake in alcoholic patients. Recent suggestions that antioxidant supplements may be of value in pain relief require further evaluation.

Surgical management

Pain is the most common indication for surgery. The decision to operate is only taken after full trial of medical therapy and comprehensive evaluation of the patient and his domestic situation. The patient must not be 'talked into' undergoing surgery and should be aware that many patients do not require surgery and that pain may gradually abate with time. He should have no illusions about the prospects following operation. Exocrine and endocrine function do not return to normal and arrest or slowing of functional deterioration is a realistic goal if a drainage operation is proposed. If resection is required, brittle lifelong diabetes may be precipitated and is inevitable after total pancreatectomy. Surgery does not always cure or improve pain and, even after total pancreatectomy, up to 20 per cent of patients still experience pain. A realistic guideline is that some 70 per cent of patients are still pain free or improved 5 years following operation. Many surgeons refuse to operate on alcoholics who are still drinking, and all agree that the prognosis after operation is much better in those who abstain.

Other factors which may indicate the need for surgery are the development of complications (see below) and uncertainty regarding the presence of pancreatic cancer.

Drainage operations

Longitudinal pancreaticojejunostomy

This is the standard operation when the pancreatic duct system is dilated to more than 7 to 8 mm in diameter. A complete pancreatogram is advisable and operative pancreatography (using needle puncture of the duct in the body or tail of the pancreas or transduodenal cannulation) may be needed if endoscopic retrograde pancreatography has been unsuccessful. The pancreas is exposed fully by division of the gastrocolic ligament and the pancreatic duct is opened fully along its length (Fig. 1). A minimum length of pancreatico-jejunal anastomosis of 10 cm is advised for

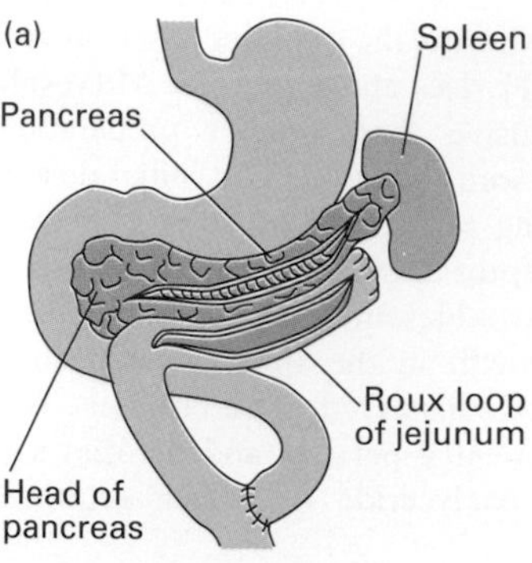

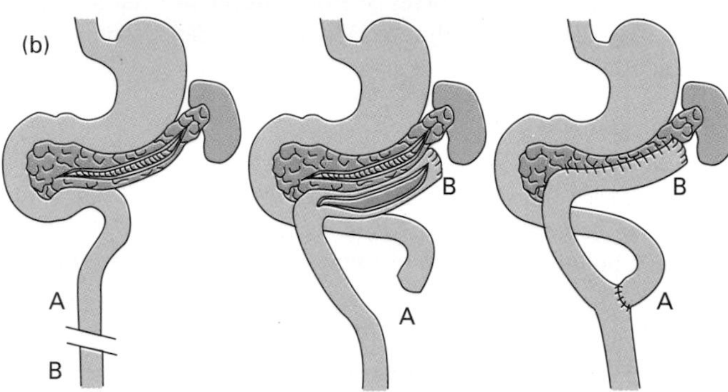

Fig. 1 Longitudinal pancreaticojejunostomy used in the treatment of chronic pancreatitis. Note that the blind end of the Roux loop is placed towards the tail of the pancreas. (a) Anastomosis about to be made between opened pancreatic duct and opened Roux loop of jejunum. (b) Schematic representation of steps.

long-term patency; the longer the anastomosis the better. Calculi are removed from the duct system and a Roux loop of proximal jejunum is brought through a window in the transverse mesocolon and anastomosed to the pancreatic duct in side-to-side manner. It is not necessary to remove the spleen during this operation. The Roux loop is orientated so that its end lies on the tail of the pancreas; this allows the same loop to be used for anastomosis to the biliary system should biliary obstruction develop. If biliary obstruction is already present, a side-to-side hepaticojejunostomy is undertaken at the time of pancreaticojejunostomy. Pseudocysts can also be drained into the Roux loop.

Alternatives to longitudinal pancreaticojejunostomy include caudal pancreaticojejunostomy and pancreaticogastrostomy. The former operation involves anastomosing a loop of jejunum to the cut surface of the pancreas after removing the tail; it is now obsolete. Pancreaticogastrostomy still has adherents but there is no objective evidence for its superiority over the conventional operation.

Transduodenal sphincteroplasty

This may be performed with or without removal of calculi from the pancreatic duct, and is of debatable value. Benefit has been claimed in small series of selected patients but for the vast majority it seems inherently unlikely that pancreatitis arises from obstruction of the terminal portion of the duct and that sphincteroplasty will give long-term success. This said, there is now a growing number of reports of treatment of chronic pancreatitis by endoscopic papillotomy or balloon dilatation, accompanied in some cases by insertion of a stent and destruction of calculi by extracorporeal shock wave lithotripsy. The long-term results are yet to be defined but the approach may defer or avoid operation in selected patients.

Accessory sphincteroplasty

Endoscopic and surgical means can be used in this manner to treat chronic pancreatitis associated with pancreas divisum. In the main, the results have been disappointing, calling into question the significance of pancreas divisum as an aetiological factor.

Resectional surgery

Distal pancreatectomy

Removal of 40 to 95 per cent of the pancreas was at one time popular, but its popularity waned with the realization that many patients still had pain after surgery and that marked exocrine and endocrine insufficiency often resulted. There is still a place for distal resection, conserving the spleen if possible, in patients in whom chronic inflammation appears to be confined to the distal pancreas.

The Whipple resection

This is regarded by many as the standard operation when the duct system is not sufficiently dilated for pancreaticojejunostomy. The head of the gland is often the most inflamed part, the operation conserves useful exocrine and endocrine function by retaining the body and tail, any biliary tract obstruction is dealt with, and the risk of leaving occult cancer in the head of the pancreas is avoided. The gallbladder should be removed to avoid subsequent gallstone formation and the jejunum is anastomosed to the common hepatic duct rather than common bile duct to reduce the risk of ischaemic breakdown of the anastomosis. Opinions vary as to whether antrectomy should be performed or whether the first part of the duodenum should be transected with preservation of the pylorus and entire stomach. One variant preserves the stomach and entire duodenum. The case for pylorus-preserving and duodenum-preserving pancreaticoduodenectomy rests on retention of more normal gastrointestinal physiology and function, but has yet to be accepted universally. Truncal vagotomy was once an integral part of the Whipple operation but the risk of marginal ulceration is now so small that few surgeons divide the vagi. Most surgeons attempt to retain exocrine function by anastomosing the cut surface of the remaining pancreas to the jejunum. Others attempt mucosa-to-mucosa apposition between the pancreatic duct and jejunum while some doubt the value of attempting to retain exocrine function and staple the transected pancreas or occlude its duct system.

Total pancreatectomy

This is a last resort given the inevitable diabetes and steatorrhoea which result. Most patients coming to total pancreatectomy have already failed to benefit from lesser surgical procedures and it must be re-emphasized that some 20 per cent of patients still complain of pain following total extirpation. Pylorus-preserving and duodenum-preserving forms of total pancreatectomy have been used. One advantage sometimes claimed for total pancreatectomy is that it avoids the need for anastomosis between residual pancreas and jejunum. However, this anastomosis is not as dangerous in chronic pancreatitis as it is in cancer surgery. In chronic pancreatitis the gland is fibrous and firm rather than friable, and the reduced exocrine secretory capacity lowers the risk of leakage and fistula formation.

Table 2 Results of surgery in chronic pancreatitis

Operation	*n*	Satisfactory pain control (%)	Insulin dependent diabetes (%) Preoperative	Postoperative	Late mortality (%)
Pancreatico-jejunostomy	228	74	26	50	39
80–95% distal pancreatectomy	108	72	11	62	36
Pancreatico-duodenectomy	276	68	28	64	30

Data taken from Eckhauser FE, *et al. Surgery*, 1984; **96**: 599–607.

Other operations

Attempts to relieve pain by excision of the coeliac ganglion and other forms of neurectomy have generally proved disappointing. Left transthoracic splanchnicectomy and bilateral truncal vagotomy has recently been advocated but requires further evaluation.

Comparison of surgical procedures (Table 2)

The ideal operation should have no operative mortality, provide permanent relief of pain, and conserve pancreatic exocrine and endocrine function. Additional aims would be minimal interference with normal digestive function and elimination of the risk of failing to remove occult pancreatic cancer. All operations should now carry a risk of operative mortality near to zero if performed in specialist hands. Pancreaticojejunostomy is safer than resection and offers a good prospect of pain relief with maximal conservation of pancreatic function. Unfortunately only some 20 to 30 per cent of patients have a duct system which is sufficiently dilated for this operation. It remains to be seen whether endoscopic procedures will retain a place in management as an alternative to surgical drainage.

Resection has become safer with improved operative and perioperative care but still carries a greater risk than drainage surgery. Tissue planes are frequently destroyed by inflammation, and operative damage to major vessels (particularly the portal and superior mesenteric vein) poses a real hazard. The greater the resection, the greater the risk of exocrine and endocrine insufficiency. Distal pancreatectomy is indicated when disease is confined to or is maximal in the body and tail and can be combined with drainage of the duct system of the remaining pancreas. The Whipple operation (or its variants) is now used in the majority of patients, while total pancreatectomy is reserved for patients in whom lesser procedures fail to relieve pain.

Management of complications

Pseudocysts

The availability of ultrasonography and CT scanning has improved our understanding of the natural history of pseudocysts in chronic pancreatitis. As a general rule pseudocysts which exceed 5 cm in diameter and which have been present for more than 6 weeks are unlikely to resolve spontaneously. When treatment is needed, internal drainage is safer and more effective than external drainage or resection. Biopsy of the pseudocyst wall is always advisable at surgery as cystic pancreatic neoplasms can cause confusion in diagnosis. A Roux loop of jejunum is usually recommended for internal drainage although on occasions the stomach or duodenum may be used. If a fluid collection proves to be an abscess, external drainage is advisable. False aneurysms can masquerade as pseudocysts and erosion of major vessels may cause bleeding into a pre-existing pseudocyst. It is always advisable to have a high index of suspicion, sample the cyst contents by needling before incision, and consider preoperative angiography when any doubt exists.

Biliary obstruction

Transient jaundice and elevation of serum alkaline phosphatase levels is common in chronic pancreatitis. Ultrasonography and, if necessary, endoscopic retrograde cholangiopancreatography can be used to define biliary morphology, and liver biopsy is indicated if there is long-standing derangement of liver function. However, alcoholic hepatitis and cirrhosis are surprisingly uncommon, even in patients with chronic alcohol-associated pancreatitis, secondary biliary cirrhosis is rare, and most patients merely have histopathological evidence of biliary obstruction with or without cholangitis. When the bile duct is narrowed a long segment of stenosis in the retropancreatic bile duct is usually found although hour-glass constriction or lateral displacement may occur (Fig. 2).

Bile duct obstruction in chronic pancreatitis is usually due to fibrosis of the surrounding pancreas rather than acute inflammation or pressure from a pseudocyst. Given the long-term risk of cholangitis and secondary biliary stenosis, fibrotic narrowing of the bile duct requires surgical treatment. Such surgery to relieve biliary obstruction is needed in 10 to 20 per cent of patients with chronic pancreatitis. Resection of the head of the pancreas may also be indicated because of pain, but if resection is not needed biliary drainage can be achieved by hepaticojejunostomy or choledochoduodenostomy. Cholecystojejunostomy is not recommended as it fails to ensure long-term bile flow and leaves the patients at risk of developing gallbladder disease. Temporary drainage can be obtained by endoscopic biliary stenting if there is a need to avoid operation.

Gastrointestinal obstruction

Transient duodenal obstruction may complicate an exacerbation of inflammation in the head of the pancreas. Chronic fibrotic obstruction is a relatively rare complication of chronic pancreatitis (<2 per cent of cases) and endoscopy is essential to exclude peptic ulceration, Crohn's disease, and pancreatic or periampullary cancer. Persisting fibrotic obstruction demands surgical relief. Gastroenterostomy is used if duodenal obstruction is the sole indication for surgery or when pancreaticojejunostomy is also needed. Where there is painful disease in the head of the pancreas and no duct dilatation, the Whipple operation is used.

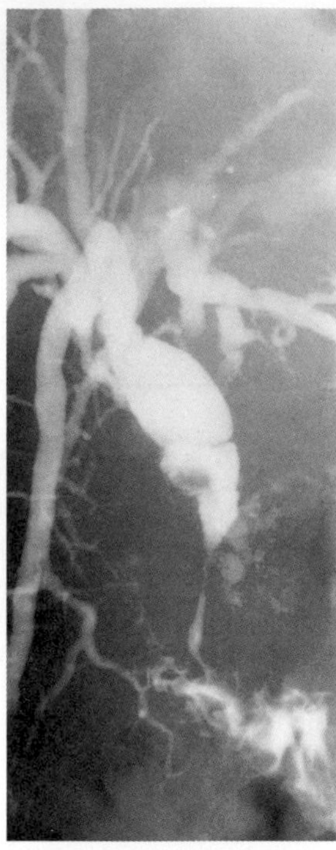

Fig. 2 Cholangiogram showing a long segment of stenosis in the retropancreatic common bile duct. The biliary system is distended and contains a calculus. Calcification is apparent in the head of the pancreas.

Colonic obstruction is rare; when it occurs it is usually transient, involving the distal colon or splenic flexure. Operation is only indicated if obstruction persists for more than a few weeks.

Haemorrhage

Arterial haemorrhage may result from necrosis of the vessel wall in areas of inflammation and pseudocyst formation. The splenic, gastroduodenal, pancreaticoduodenal, pancreatic, gastric, and hepatic arteries may be involved, in order of frequency. Rupture can result in pseudoaneurysm formation and bleeding can occur into the pancreatic duct, pseudocyst, retroperitoneal tissues, or peritoneal cavity. Endoscopy and selective angiography are useful investigations and although surgery is usually indicated, therapeutic embolization may be life saving in high risk patients.

Thrombosis

Thrombosis of the splenic vein, and less frequently of the portal and superior mesenteric vein, can be asymptomatic. Alternatively, the patient may bleed from gastric and oesophageal varices or present with a large spleen, leucocytopenia, and thrombocytopenia. Haemorrhage from colonic varices is exceptional. When variceal bleeding occurs after splenic vein occlusion, splenectomy is the treatment of choice. A preoperative arteriogram and venogram is advisable, partly to define the problem and partly to embolize the splenic artery to reduce collateral bleeding at operation.

Pleural effusion, fistula, and pancreatic ascites

Leakage of pancreatic juice from rupture of a pseudocyst or inflammation and necrosis of the pancreatic duct may result in rapid development of ascites and pleural effusions. The diagnosis is confirmed if the fluid protein content exceeds 25 g/l and if the amylase concentration of the fluid exceeds that of the serum. Conservative treatment with parenteral nutrition and the somatostatin analogue SMS201–905 (to reduce pancreatic secretion) may be employed initially but is seldom successful. Surgery should not be postponed beyond 2 to 3 weeks. Preliminary endoscopic retrograde pancreatography is invaluable to define the site of leakage. Leaks in the tail are usually treated by distal pancreatectomy, those elsewhere by pancreaticojejunostomy.

Internal pancreatic fistulae involving the gut may not require surgical intervention and are often discovered as incidental findings at endoscopic retrograde pancreatography. Pancreaticocutaneous fistulae frequently follow external drainage of pseudocysts or may complicate pancreatic surgery. They often respond to conservative measures but surgical resection of the involved pancreas may be needed.

Pancreatic cancer

Most workers accept that hereditary chronic pancreatitis predisposes to pancreatic cancer and there is now some epidemiological evidence suggesting that non-hereditary chronic pancreatitis may also be a premalignant condition. Definition of the relationship between chronic inflammation and cancer is difficult as the two conditions frequently coexist and an occluding cancer may give rise to inflammation.

PROGNOSIS

The prognosis in chronic pancreatitis depends on the frequency and severity of the attacks, need for surgery, and the development of complications, notably diabetes. Alcoholics who fail to stop drinking undoubtedly fare worse than non-alcoholics and alcoholics who abstain. Given the importance of alcohol as an aetiological factor and its associated personality and social upset, it is hardly surprising that patients with chronic pancreatitis have a lower life expectancy than the general population. The complications of the disease, drug addiction, depression, brittle diabetes, malnutrition, and increased risk of non-pancreatic cancer combine to reduce longevity. Reported survival rates vary greatly according to the nature of the series of patients studied. The cumulative survival rate based on life table analysis in alcoholics with or without surgery is about 50 per cent at 20 to 24 years from onset of the disease; non-alcoholic patients have survival rates which are some 20 per cent higher.

FURTHER READING

Ammann RW, Akovbiantz A, Largiader F, Schueler G. Course and outcome of chronic pancreatitis. Longitudinal study of a mixed medical-surgical series of 245 patients. *Gastroenterology* 1984; **86**: 820–8.

Axon AT, Classen M, Cotton PB, Cremer M, Freeny PC, Lees WR. Pancreatography in chronic pancreatitis: international definitions. *Gut* 1984; **25**: 1107–12.

Banks PA. Medical strategy in chronic pancreatitis. In: Carter DC, Warshaw AL, eds. *Pancreatitis*. Edinburgh: Churchill Livingstone, 1990; 133–47.

Bockman DE, Buchler M, Malfertheiner P, Beger HG. Analysis of nerves in chronic pancreatitis. *Gastroenterology* 1988; **94**: 1459–69.

Braasch JW, Vito L, Nugent W. Total pancreatectomy for end-stage chronic pancreatitis. *Ann Surg* 1978; **188**: 317–22.

Cooper MJ, *et al.* Total pancreatectomy for chronic pancreatitis. *Br J Surg* 1987; **74**: 912–15.

Copenhagen Pancreatitis Study. An interim report from a prospective epidemiological multicenter study. *Scand J Gastroenterol* 1981; **116**: 305–12.

Eckhauser FE, Strodel WE, Knol JA, Harper M, Turcotte JG. Near-total pancreatectomy for chronic pancreatitis. *Surgery* 1984; **96**: 599–607.

Grace PA, Pitt HA, Longmire WP. Pylorus preserving pancreatoduodenectomy: an overview. *Br J Surg* 1990; **77**: 968–74.

Greenlee HB, Prinz RA, Aranha GV. Long-term results of side-to-side pancreatico-jejunostomy. *World J Surg* 1990; **14**: 80–4.

Lambert MA, Linehan IP, Russell RCG. Duodenum preserving total pancreatectomy for end-stage chronic pancreatitis. *Br J Surg* 1987; **74**: 35–9.

Niederau C, Grendell JH. Diagnosis of chronic pancreatitis. *Gastroenterology* 1985; **88**: 1973–95.

Sarles H, Bernard JP, Gullo L. Pathogenesis of chronic pancreatitis. *Gut* 1990; **31**: 629–32.

Sauerbruch T, Holl J, Sackmann M, Paumgartner G. Extracorporeal shock wave lithotripsy of pancreatic stones. *Gut* 1989; **30**: 1406–11.

Singh SM, Reber HA. The pathology of chronic pancreatitis. *World J Surg* 1990; **14**: 2–10.

Stone HH, Chauvin EJ. Pancreatic denervation for pain relief in chronic alcohol associated pancreatitis. *Br J Surg* 1990; **77**: 303–5.

Wilson C, *et al.* Hepatobiliary complications in chronic pancreatitis. *Gut* 1989; **30**: 520–7.

Worning H. Incidence and prevalence of chronic pancreatitis. In: Beger H, Buchler M, Ditschuneit H, Malfertheiner P, eds. *Chronic Pancreatitis.* Berlin: Springer-Verlag, 1990: 8–14.

25.3 Trauma to the pancreas

ALAN R. BERRY

TRAUMA TO THE PANCREAS

Injury to the pancreas was first recognized and reported in 1827. Since that time the problem has become more familiar, though compared with the incidence of injury to other viscera, it is still uncommon, and therefore is frequently overlooked. If the injury is not diagnosed initially it usually becomes apparent subsequently, as complications occur up to 6 weeks after the event. At this time treatment is much more difficult, morbidity is high, and the mortality rate is about 20 per cent.

The trauma may be either blunt or penetrating in nature: the latter type is about three times more common and is associated with a higher mortality rate. Up to 90 per cent of patients also have other serious injuries: these contribute to the high mortality. Other viscera which are particularly liable to be damaged in patients with pancreatic trauma are the liver, spleen, and small intestine.

Pancreatic trauma occurs in between 1 and 3 per cent of patients who have suffered blunt or penetrating abdominal injuries. This figure is low, but is increasing with the increase in numbers of high-speed motor vehicle accidents and in civil violence. It is most commonly seen in young adults, and in men more frequently than women. At present, however, the experience of any one surgeon will be small and successful management will therefore be based on the accrued published experience of others. The possibility of pancreatic injury should always be considered in patients who have suffered abdominal trauma. If there is sufficient concern the pancreas should be examined thoroughly, either through a laparotomy, which may be being performed for other injuries, or by careful investigation. Ductal injury in particular must be identified early if complications are to be avoided.

INDICATORS OF PANCREATIC INJURY

Serum amylase levels are elevated in 50 to 90 per cent of patients with pancreatic trauma, but false-positive results are also common. Trauma is a common cause of acute pancreatitis in children, accounting for one-third of all such cases in the United States. The pancreas of a child is vulnerable and easily damaged during sledging or bicycle accidents or by physical abuse. Children often present late, the accident having been regarded as trivial; in these patients hyperamylasaemia is always present.

Ultrasound is a simple method by which patients suspected of having sustained pancreatic trauma can be assessed. It may demonstrate pseudocysts but it is unreliable in detecting ductal injury. Computed tomography, if available, is more reliable and will successfully detect pancreatic fractures and contusions, as well as post-traumatic pseudocysts. However, ductal integrity can best be assessed by endoscopic retrograde pancreatography: this is the investigation of choice, when pancreatic injury is suspected. The classification of pancreatic injuries is shown in Table 1.

Table 1 Classification of pancreatic injuries (Lucas 1977)

Grade I	Simple superficial contusions with minimal parenchymal damage (any portion of the pancreas can be affected but there is no question of disruption of the pancreatic head)
Grade II	Deep lacerations, perforations, or transection of the tail or the body of the pancreas with the possibility of pancreatic duct injury
Grade III	Severe transection, perforation, or crushing injuries to the head of the pancreas with or without ductal injury, but with an intact duodenum
Grade IV	Combined pancreaticoduodenal injuries. These are further classified as combined injuries with mild pancreatic injury or severe damage of the pancreas with ductal disruption

The majority of surgeons first encounter a pancreatic injury while performing a laparotomy for some more obvious coexisting injury. This is the best time to detect pancreatic injury, and correct treatment can avoid future complications and possible death. Examination of the pancreas in this situation is difficult however, particularly when other injuries seem more pressing and a planned approach is essential. Patients at risk are those who have received blunt trauma to the upper abdomen during a road traffic accident or who have an obvious penetrating injury to the upper abdomen. After other immediately life-threatening injuries have been dealt with, the pancreas should be examined. Clues to injury are the presence of blood in the lesser sac or, more commonly, a

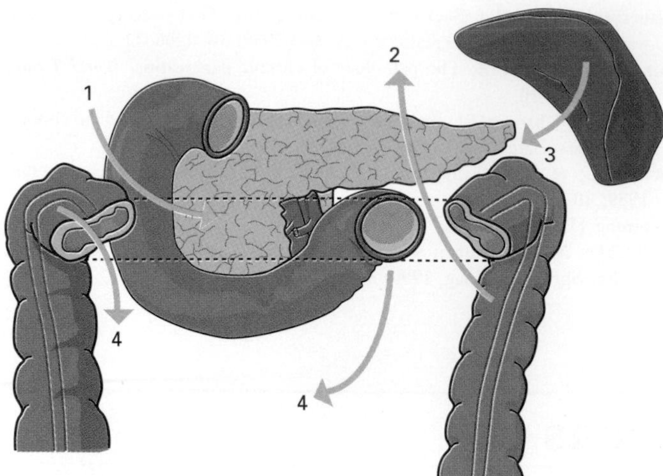

Fig. 1 Operative examination of the pancreas.

retroperitoneal haematoma in the upper abdomen that extends into the transverse mesocolon. There may be evidence of haematoma lateral to the second part of the duodenum. These findings demand thorough exploration and examination of the gland.

OPERATIVE EXAMINATION OF THE PANCREAS (Fig. 1)

Access to the head of the gland is gained by dividing the peritoneum lateral to the second part of the duodenum and lifting the head away from the posterior abdominal wall and to the left (Kocher's manoeuvre) (1). The body and tail of the gland are best examined from within the lesser sac. Access is gained by detaching the greater omentum from its avascular attachment to the transverse colon (2). This allows access deep to the omentum and superior to the transverse mesocolon. The tail of the gland can be approached by deflecting the spleen to the right (3). This is neither particularly easy nor quick, and in emergency situations the tail can be examined adequately without the need for this manoeuvre. Division of the ligament of Trietz and mobilization of the duodenojejunal flexure allows examination of the third and fourth parts of the duodenum (4). This may be made easier if the hepatic flexure of the colon is mobilized to the left.

Injury to the gland may be identified by the presence of a capsular tear, by obvious haemorrhage from the gland or, rarely, by complete gland disruption. Ductal injury, however, may be very difficult to confirm, with nothing more obvious than some bruising in the gland. If facilities allow, a pancreatic ductogram should be obtained at the initial laparotomy: this can be done by intraoperative endoscopic pancreatography or by performing a transduodenal cannulation of the pancreatic duct. In practice, however, such refined endoscopic techniques are only available in a few specialized centres, and even satisfactory transduodenal pancreatograms are extremely difficult to obtain and interpret when performed in an emergency situation.

MANAGEMENT

Grade I injuries can be safely managed by drainage of the pancreatic bed: this is best achieved by bringing large tube drains out posterolaterally through the loins. Unless there is definite evidence of ductal injury this is the treatment of choice.

If there is an obvious injury to the duct within the tail or body of the gland a distal pancreatectomy should be performed with ligation of the stump of the duct and drainage of the pancreatic bed. This approach in Grade II injuries carries fewer complications than drainage alone.

Grade III and IV injuries, in which the head of the gland is damaged, with or without trauma to the duodenum, may require a Whipple's pancreaticoduodenectomy to be performed. Fortunately this procedure is indicated only in 2 to 3 per cent of patients with pancreatic injuries. The operation is technically difficult, mainly because the very narrow calibre of the normal pancreatic and bile ducts makes reconstructions very difficult. In this situation the pancreatic anastomosis can be made by invaginating the stump of the gland into a loop of jejunum and the biliary anastomosis may be facilitated by ligating the distal common bile duct and anastomosing the gallbladder to an accessible loop of jejunum. Many authors have advocated drainage alone as the treatment for these severe injuries because of the technical difficulties of pancreaticoduodenectomy and the poor results of surgery. In critically ill patients with multiple trauma, it would seem prudent to institute drainage of the pancreas in the first instance. Appropriate investigations and secondary surgery can be performed at a later date in those patients who survive their other injuries. The results of surgical treatment of pancreatic trauma are disappointing: the overall mortality rate is about 20 per cent. The mortality associated with pancreaticoduodenectomy in these patients approaches 50 per cent, but the results of less radical treatment of these major injuries (Grades III and IV) are little better.

The prognosis of major pancreatic injuries (Grades III and IV) is unlikely to improve. However, with prompt diagnosis and early treatment, patients who have Grade I and II injuries should make a satisfactory recovery.

FURTHER READING

Lucas CE. Diagnosis and treatment of pancreatic and duodenal injury. *Surg Clin N Am*, 1977; **57**: 49–65.

Jones RC. Management of pancreatic trauma. *Am J Surg*, 1985; **150**: 698–704.

25.4 Pancreatic cancer

CARLOS FERNANDEZ-DEL CASTILLO AND ANDREW L. WARSHAW

AETIOLOGY AND EPIDEMIOLOGY

The incidence of pancreatic cancer in the United States was 9.2 per 100 000 in 1987: this represents a significant increase over that found in 1940, but has remained essentially unchanged for the last 15 years. Other developed countries have observed similar trends in the incidence of this disease. Pancreatic cancer is the second most common gastrointestinal malignancy after colorectal cancer, which affects five times more people. However, while colorectal cancer has a 5-year survival rate of over 50 per cent, that of pancreatic cancer is only 3.1 per cent: it is, in fact, the malignancy with the lowest 5-year survival.

Malignant neoplasms of the pancreas can occur at any age, but they are rare before the age of 40: the mean age of diagnosis is 64 years, after which the incidence increases rapidly.

The aetiology of pancreatic cancer is largely unknown; however, epidemiological studies have shown that several environmental factors are likely to be implicated. Cigarette smoking is the best established risk factor: smokers are two to three times more likely to develop pancreatic cancer than non-smokers, and they develop the disease at a median age 15 years younger. There is a direct relationship between the number of cigarettes smoked and the increase in risk.

The next most important risk factor is probably diet, which could also account in part for the wide variations in incidence found in different geographical regions, as well as for the altered risk that has been observed in certain migrant populations. A direct correlation between dietary fat intake and occurrence of pancreatic cancer has consistently been found in different populations, and the addition of unsaturated fats to the diet of azaserine-treated rats promotes development of pancreatic tumours. On the other hand, a high intake of fresh fruits and vegetables is associated with a significantly decreased incidence of pancreatic cancer in man. This protective effect has also been found with consumption of proteins of vegetable origin, such as beans and lentils, which contain high levels of protease inhibitors.

Exposure to several chemical agents, including naphthylamine, benzidine, and petrol has also been linked to pancreatic cancer. Workers from industries that produce or use these chemicals have been found to have up to a fivefold increase in mortality from this disease. Pancreatic cancer can be induced in rats with azaserine (*O*-diazoacetyl-L-serine) and in Syrian hamsters with nitrosamines.

Diabetes mellitus and chronic pancreatitis are both associated with pancreatic cancer, although the nature or even the direction of the cause–effect relationship has not been established. At least 15 per cent of patients with pancreatic cancer are discovered to have diabetes or have had diabetes diagnosed within the year prior to diagnosis of the cancer. It is unlikely that such new diabetes represents destruction of the pancreas by the tumour sufficient to cause endocrine insufficiency. A true association between pancreatic cancer and chronic pancreatitis is probably confined to familial and tropical forms of chronic pancreatitis.

Throughout the world, pancreatic cancer affects more men than women, with a male to female ratio of between 1.5 and 2. In experimental carcinogenesis, growth of azaserine-induced tumours is stimulated by androgens and is inhibited by antiandrogens or castration. Male patients with pancreatic cancer have low serum testosterone and high androstenedione levels and also show an altered testosterone:dihydrotestosterone ratio. These findings seem to be a consequence rather than the cause of the neoplastic disease: normal values are restored after resection of the tumour.

Much public and scientific controversy has been generated around the possible link between coffee consumption and pancreatic cancer. The first study to propose such an association appeared in 1981, and since then, more than 25 studies have attempted to answer this issue, with conflicting results. The majority of studies do not support a causal relationship between coffee and pancreatic cancer, but suggest rather that cigarette smoking, dietary habits, and other confounding factors were responsible for the association found in the earlier studies.

Prior surgery in the alimentary tract has also been implicated as a causative factor. Patients with a history of gastrectomy have at least a threefold greater risk of dying from pancreatic cancer. A relationship with cholecystectomy has also been proposed. The basis for these observations is not known.

The increased incidence of pancreatic cancer in certain populations such as Polynesians and the American black population suggests that genetic factors are also involved in its genesis.

PATHOLOGY

Malignant tumours of the pancreas can occur in either the exocrine parenchyma or in the endocrine cells of the islets of Langerhans (Table 1), but exocrine neoplasms are far more common. Adenocarcinoma accounts for around 80 per cent of pancreatic neoplasms, and is thought to be of ductal origin. It is twice as frequent in the head of the pancreas as in the body or tail, and at the time of diagnosis more than 85 per cent of these tumours have extended beyond the limits of the organ. Perineural invasion within and beyond the gland is particularly prominent in this type

Table 1 Classification of primary malignant tumours of the pancreas

Origin	Type of tumour
Ductal epithelium	Carcinoma: Adenocarcinoma, giant cell, adenosquamous, mucinous, microadenocarcinoma, cystadenocarcinoma, papillary cystic tumour, unclassified
Acinar cells	Acinar cell carcinoma
Islet cells	Malignant insulinoma, gastrinoma, VIPoma, glucagonoma, and others
Non-epithelial tissue	Fibrosarcoma, leiomyosarcoma, haemangiopericytoma, histiocytoma, lymphoma

of cancer, although lymphatic spread also leads to early metastasis to adjacent and distant lymph nodes. The most common sites of extralymphatic involvement are the liver and peritoneum. The lungs are the most frequently affected of the extra-abdominal organs. Rare carcinomas of the pancreas include giant cell, adenosquamous, and acinar cell varieties, all of which have a similar or worse prognosis than does ductal adenocarcinoma.

Malignant or potentially malignant cystic tumours of the exocrine pancreas, which include the mucinous cystadenoma–cystadenocarcinoma and the papillary–cystic tumour, behave quite differently. Most patients are women; in particular, papillary–cystic tumours almost exclusively affect young women. Both of these tumours tend to be large (>6 cm diameter on average) at the moment of diagnosis, and this fact, together with their cystic appearance on scan and at operation, usually allows them to be easily differentiated from ductal adenocarcinoma. The prognosis for these cystic neoplasms is very good if they are completely resected. The 5-year survival rate for all cystadenocarcinomas is 50 per cent, but reaches 75 per cent for the two-thirds of patients whose tumour is completely removed. The great majority of papillary–cystic tumours (up to 95 per cent) are cured.

Another pancreatic malignancy with a relatively favourable prognosis is lymphoma, which accounts for up to 5 per cent of all malignant pancreatic tumours in selected series and which is amenable to chemotherapy and irradiation.

The pancreas can also be the site of metastasis from malignant neoplasms of other organs. In autopsy studies, for every primary cancer of the pancreas there are three cases of metastatic carcinoma, breast and lung being the most common sites of origin.

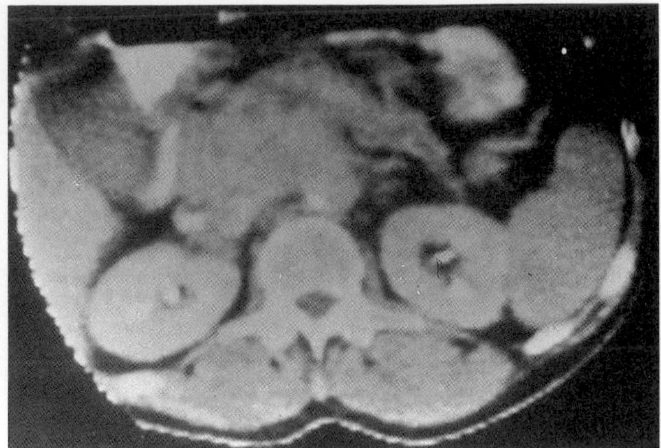

Fig. 1 CT scan showing a tumour in the pancreatic head with extension to retroperitoneal structures and obstruction of the pancreatic duct.

CLINICAL MANIFESTATIONS

At the time of presentation, most patients with pancreatic cancer have had symptoms for less than 4 months. Their principal complaints are pain, jaundice, and weight loss, usually developing insidiously. Pain is most commonly located in the epigastrium or left upper quadrant of the abdomen; it has a dull, aching nature and can radiate to the back. The patient may experience some relief when lying or sitting in a flexed or curled position. The pain becomes more severe as the disease advances and can become troublesome and difficult to control.

About 50 per cent of patients present with jaundice due to common bile duct obstruction. The jaundice is progressive and rarely regresses, is painless in up to one-third of cases, and is likely to be accompanied by pruritus.

Weight loss can be prominent; it is a result of decreased appetite, malabsorption, and other unknown factors which cause cancer cachexia. In advanced stages duodenal obstruction and perhaps disturbances of gastrointestinal motility from splanchnic nerve invasion can also be contributory.

Other symptoms include psychiatric disturbances, particularly depression, which are seen in up to 75 per cent of patients. Diabetes mellitus is present in 15 per cent, and is of recent onset in over 50 per cent of cases in which both entities are associated. An episode of acute pancreatitis is occasionally the first indication of the disease, but there is some sign of pancreatic inflammation in up to 14 per cent of cases. Gastrointestinal bleeding may also occur; this is most commonly secondary to gastric or duodenal invasion by the tumour, but may also originate from varices, which are the consequence of portal or splenic vein occlusion. Other rare manifestations include migratory thrombophlebitis and the appearance of tender subcutaneous nodules or polyarthritis secondary to metastatic fat necrosis. The last two have been particularly associated with acinar cell carcinomas.

In the early stages of pancreatic cancer, physical signs include jaundice, evidence of weight loss, and hepatomegaly, which reflects bile duct obstruction. A non-tender gallbladder can be palpated in 50 per cent of jaundiced patients (Courvoisier's sign). In advanced disease, ascites and a palpable mass are indicative of an unresectable tumour.

DIAGNOSIS AND DIFFERENTIAL DIAGNOSIS

The two methods most frequently used to confirm a clinical suspicion of pancreatic cancer are ultrasonography and computerized tomography (CT). Both of these can demonstrate pancreatic masses, dilation of the pancreatic duct as well as of the bile duct and gallbladder, hepatic metastasis, and extrapancreatic spread. An ultrasound scan usually shows pancreatic tumours to be less echogenic than the surrounding parenchyma, and accompanied by changes in the contour of the gland. Overall, the diagnostic sensitivity of this diagnostic method is about 70 per cent, and its specificity 95 per cent. Ultrasonography has the inconvenience that it relies heavily on the experience of the examiner and that a satisfactory scan cannot be obtained in about 20 per cent of patients because of obesity or the presence of intestinal gas.

Computerized tomography has a higher sensitivity than that of ultrasound, with a similar specificity; it should probably be used in all patients in whom a strong suspicion of pancreatic cancer exists. Diagnosis is also based on the presence of focal enlargement of the gland (Fig. 1). Additional signs, such as dilation of the pancreatic duct in the absence of intraductal or parenchymal calcification, can be highly suggestive of a pancreatic or ampullary malignancy. Neither CT nor ultrasonography are capable of identifying tumours less than 2 cm in diameter.

Magnetic resonance imaging has no advantage over CT. Recent reports have also described encouraging results with the use of endoscopic ultrasonography, especially for tumours located in the head of the pancreas.

Endoscopic retrograde cholangiopancreatography is a valuable tool in the differential diagnosis of the cause of obstructive jaundice when pancreatic or other periampullary cancer is suspected.

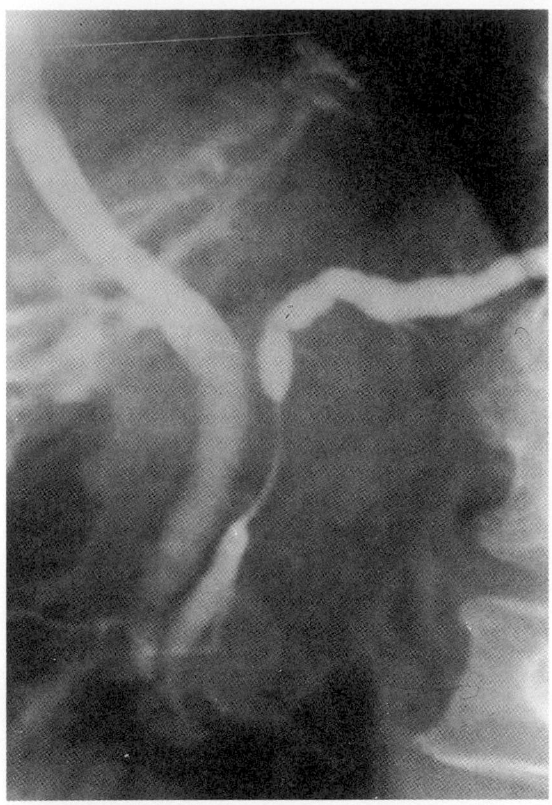

Fig. 2 Endoscopic retrograde cholangiopancreatography in pancreatic carcinoma, demonstrating encasement of the main pancreatic duct and retrograde dilation.

In certain cases, when the initial manifestation of the carcinoma is an episode of acute pancreatitis, this technique may demonstrate small tumours that could not otherwise be detected by CT. Virtually all pancreatic cancers show abnormalities in the pancreatogram, these consisting mainly of stenosis (Fig. 2) or obstruction of the pancreatic duct. In some patients, these findings may be difficult to differentiate from those of chronic pancreatitis. The study also permits visualization of the bile duct and placement of stents for the relief of jaundice. In selected cases, especially those in which the main suspicion is a proximal bile duct carcinoma, rather than a pancreatic or periampullary neoplasm, percutaneous transhepatic cholangiography may be preferred. This study is also used when endoscopic retrograde cholangiopancreatography fails or is not practicable due to the presence of anatomic barriers arising from prior gastric surgery.

The differential diagnosis of malignancies around the pancreatobiliary junction includes tumours of the head of the pancreas, ampulla, lower third of the bile duct, and duodenum. Pancreatic cancer is by far the most common of these, accounting for about 80 per cent of cases, followed by ampullary cancer (10 per cent). Certain clinical characteristics may aid in the differential diagnosis, such as the high frequency of intestinal bleeding in patients with ampullary and duodenal tumours, or the fluctuation of jaundice seen in some patients with ampullary carcinoma. Endoscopy and retrograde cholangiopancreatography are the mainstays in this differentiation, although in some patients definite diagnosis is not obtained until the tumour is resected.

Chronic pancreatitis can present a clinical and radiological picture indistinguishable from that of pancreatic cancer, and is the main benign condition from which this neoplasm has to be differentiated. Calcifications are uncommon in pancreatic carcinoma; their presence favours the diagnosis of chronic pancreatitis. However, more than 50 per cent of patients with chronic pancreatitis have no calcifications, and a diagnosis of malignancy cannot be definitely excluded. Although extremely rare, tuberculosis and sarcoidosis can also present as a pancreatic mass associated with pain or jaundice.

Several studies have been directed at the detection of serum markers to aid in this differential diagnosis of pancreatic cancer, as well as its diagnosis at subclinical stage. Such markers include tumour-associated antigens, enzymes and endocrine markers. The most extensively studied of these is the tumour-associated antigen CA19–9, the presence of which has a reported sensitivity for pancreatic cancer of over 90 per cent, but a relatively low specificity of about 75 per cent. Most of the false positive results occur in patients with other gastrointestinal malignancies, particularly ampullary and biliary carcinomas. One of the major drawbacks of this serum marker in common with most others, is that it is most likely to be positive in the advanced stages of the disease and most frequently negative in patients with the small tumours which are the easiest to cure. Two exceptions to this may be elevated levels of immunoreactive elastase and a testosterone: dihydrotestosterone ratio of 5 or less. These have been found to be positive in a high proportion (albeit or a small number) of stage I pancreatic cancers. A testosterone: dihydrotestosterone ratio of 5 or less is highly specific for pancreatic carcinoma and could therefore be useful in its differential diagnosis from chronic pancreatitis.

A definite diagnosis of pancreatic carcinoma can only be made following histological examination. Material obtained by percutaneous fine-needle aspiration of the tumour for cytological examination is invaluable, particularly for patients with advanced stage pancreatic cancer, who otherwise would require surgical exploration. The procedure is usually performed under direct guidance by ultrasonography or CT. A positive result reliably confirms the diagnosis of malignancy, but a negative one does not exclude it since there is a 10 to 20 per cent false negative rate. Percutaneous biopsy should not be used in patients with potentially resectable tumours since seeding of cancer cells along the needle track has been documented. There is also evidence that intraperitoneal spread may occur following this procedure.

STAGING

With few exceptions, only patients presenting with jaundice ever have a cancer which is potentially curable by resection; in fact, only 10 to 20 per cent of jaundiced patients have a resectable cancer. In the great majority of patients only a palliative procedure such as a biliary or duodenal bypass is feasible. Traditionally, most patients with pancreatic cancer underwent surgery to obtain tissue for diagnosis and to assess resectability. In the past few years this approach has been changing, as new techniques for percutaneous biopsy and preoperative evaluation have evolved, and preoperative staging is becoming one of the most important aspects in the management of patients with this neoplasm.

The goal of preoperative staging of pancreatic cancer is to ascertain the optimal treatment option for each patient. Specifically, the aim is to delineate which patients have tumours that are potentially resectable, which still have localized cancer, and which already have distant metastases. These facts in turn allow effective triage of patients, as well as a choice of therapeutic approach. Pancreatoduodenectomy in inexperienced hands can cause con-

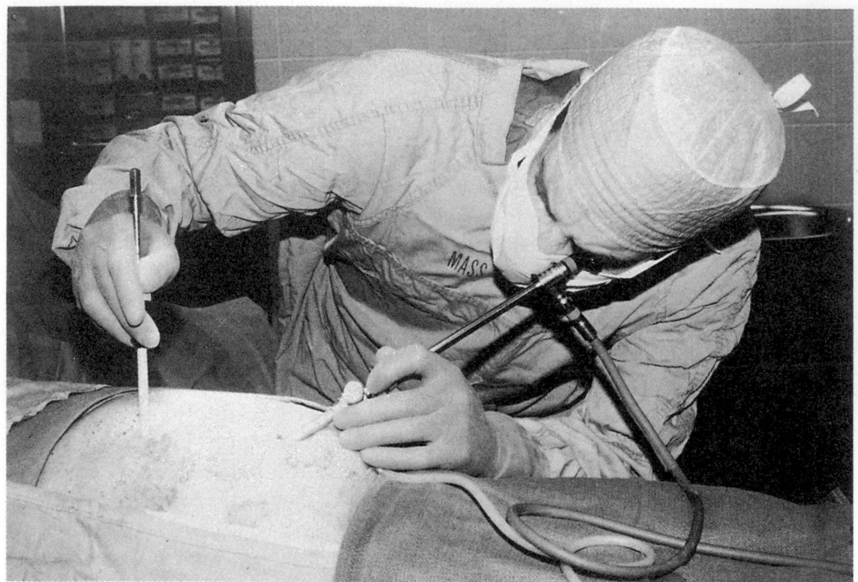

Fig. 3 Peritoneal and hepatic implants are present in 40 per cent of patients with pancreatic cancer, and can usually only be demonstrated preoperatively by laparoscopy.

Table 2 Staging of carcinoma of the pancreas

STAGE I	T 1–2, N 0, M 0. No direct extension and no regional nodal involvement
STAGE II	T 3, N 0, M 0. Direct extension into adjacent tissue but no lymph node involvement
STAGE III	T 1–3, N 1, M 0. Regional lymph node involvement with or without directed tumour extension
STAGE IV	T 1–3, N 0–1, M 1. Distant metastatic disease present

T 1: no direct extension of the primary tumour beyond the pancreas. Can be further subdivided into T 1a: tumour <2 cm, and T 1b: tumour >2 cm.
T 2: limited direct extension to duodenum, bile duct, or stomach.
T 3: advanced direct extension, incompatible with surgical resection.
N 0: regional lymph nodes not involved.
N 1: regional lymph nodes involved.
M 0: no distant metastasis.
M 1: distant metastasis present.

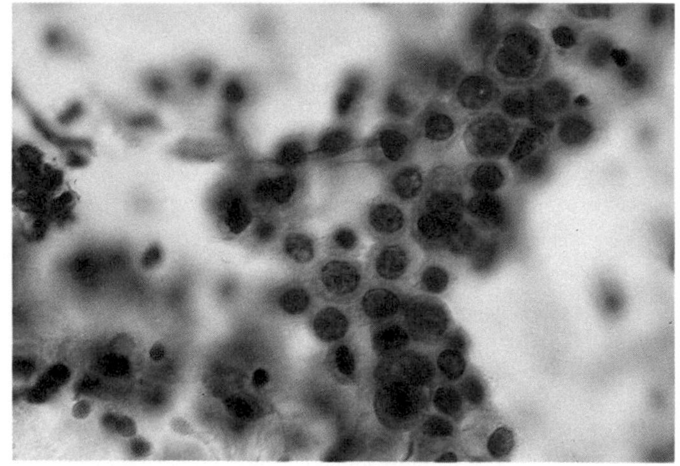

Fig. 4 Peritoneal lavage during laparoscopy or at laparotomy may demonstrate malignant cells, associated with a poor outcome.

siderable morbidity and up to 40 per cent mortality, although many specialized centres are currently reporting vastly improved results with less than 5 per cent mortality. It may therefore be appropriate to stage patients locally but to consider transfer to a regional centre if resection seems appropriate. On the other hand, patients who have a demonstrably unresectable cancer have a median survival of about 6 months. Many of these patients should be spared surgery. A tissue diagnosis can be obtained by percutaneous needle aspiration. Stents can be endoscopically or percutaneously placed to relieve biliary obstruction with efficacy equal to surgical bypass. Only patients with duodenal obstruction invariably require surgical intervention.

The staging classification for pancreatic cancer proposed by the American Joint Committee for Cancer is shown in Table 2. In some patients, the ultrasound or CT scan that was used to confirm the clinical diagnosis will already have demonstrated the presence of liver metastases or a large tumour with major vascular encasement or occlusion, thus effectively ending staging once tissue diagnosis is obtained percutaneously. If an initial ultrasound screening reveals no metastasis or major vascular invasion a CT scan should be performed: this gives a better outline of the pancreatic boundaries and is more sensitive in detecting liver and large nodal metastasis.

In our practice, the next step in staging is laparoscopy (Fig. 3). Laparoscopy will show evidence of hepatic or peritoneal spread in more than 40 per cent of patients, even when a CT scan is negative. Typically, the lesions seen at laparoscopy in these patients are 1- to 2-mm nodules on the surface of the liver, parietal peritoneum, or omentum—too small to be detected by any other means. Laparoscopy also allows for cytological examination of peritoneal washings, which, if positive (Fig. 4), indicates probable unresectability and a poor prognosis.

If laparoscopy is negative, the next study to be performed is angiography of the coeliac trunk and superior mesenteric artery, which will detect extrapancreatic arterial and especially venous encasement. Obstruction or narrowing of the portal (Fig. 5), splenic or mesenteric veins or of the coeliac, hepatic, or superior mesenteric arteries is usually an indication of unresectability, although some groups excise and reconstruct these vessels. Angio-

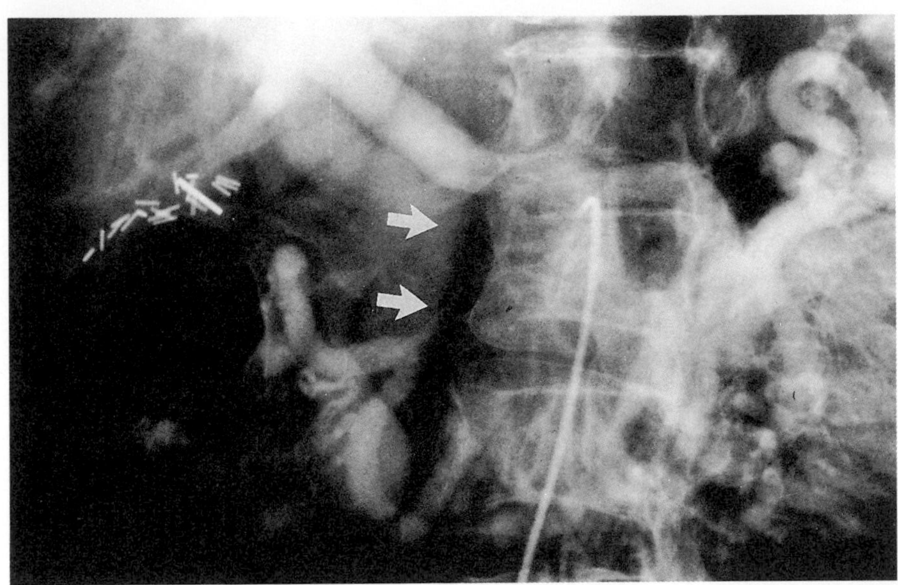

Fig. 5 Portal vein encasement and obstruction in a case of pancreatic carcinoma. Note tortuosity of the splenic vein, collateral circulation, and virtual absence of the portal vein (arrows).

graphy also gives valuable information on the vascular anatomy of the patient. An anomalous origin of the hepatic arteries is seen in about one-third of patients, and preoperative knowledge of this allows operative injury to these structures to be avoided.

CT scan, laparoscopy, and angiography give different indications of tumour resectability and are complementary. In our experience, 78 per cent of pancreatic head tumours can be resected in patients in whom all three tests are negative; if one or more of the three is positive, the resectability rate is only 5 per cent. In the future endoscopic ultrasonography may be refined enough to add another dimension to preoperative detection of lymph node metastases and extrapancreatic extension, thereby improving staging accuracy even further. It is also possible that future studies will establish the finding of a positive peritoneal cytology as a definite index of disseminated disease, even in the absence of obvious macroscopic metastasis, thereby precluding further consideration of resection.

TREATMENT

While the cure rate for pancreatic cancer is admittedly low, resection offers the only possibility of obtaining disease-free long-term survival. Radiotherapy, chemotherapy, and hormone therapy are sometimes used as adjuvants to resection, but they have practically no impact on survival when used alone. Pancreatoduodenectomy has been the standard operation for carcinoma of the pancreatic head since its demonstration by Whipple in 1935. Variations on this procedure include total, subtotal, and radical pancreatectomy, as well as the pylorus-preserving pancreatoduodenectomy. Carcinomas of the body and tail of the pancreas are somewhat less common; they are usually discovered at an advanced stage when they are not amenable to resection. Rarely, a small resectable tumour may be found in this location, usually by chance. Tumours to the left of the portal vein can theoretically be treated by distal pancreatectomy.

Histological proof of cancer

Many patients will undergo surgery before a histological diagnosis has been established. Traditionally, one of the first steps has been to establish the diagnosis of carcinoma, commonly by transduodenal needle biopsy of the tumour: this may be time consuming as well as a potential source of complications. Now that the morbidity and mortality of pancreatoduodenectomy are so low preoperative confirmation of malignancy is no longer mandatory. A biopsy is needed only if the surgical procedure is likely to differ significantly according to the diagnosis. However, the most commonly encountered diagnostic difficulty is differentiating between chronic pancreatitis and carcinoma, both of which will be well served by a pancreatoduodenectomy. Resection of the pancreatic head is therefore the procedure of choice both for cancer and for situations of diagnostic uncertainty.

If a diagnosis is required during surgery, tissue can be obtained by either incisional or needle biopsy of metastases or of the primary tumour mass. In some centres fine-needle aspiration has replaced needle-core biopsies for obtaining material for cytological examination because of the possibility of obtaining multiple samples with a lower complication rate. Whenever feasible, transduodenal needling is preferred to direct sampling.

Technique of pancreatoduodenectomy

The first step of the procedure is assessment of resectability. This entails a thorough exploration of all of the abdominal organs and peritoneal surfaces, extensive mobilization of the duodenum and head of the pancreas (Kocher's manoeuvre), and separation of the posterior neck of the pancreas from the superior mesenteric vein. Enlarged peripancreatic, periportal, and coeliac lymph nodes that might harbour metastases are biopsied. If there is no evidence of metastases, gross extrapancreatic invasion of the retroperitoneal structures or attachment of the cancer to mesenteric vessels, resection is started. The gallbladder is removed and the elements of the hepatic hilum are dissected. The common hepatic duct is divided above the cystic duct entry and its distal stump ligated. The fatty and lymphatic tissue anterior and lateral to the portal vein, as well as that surrounding the hepatic artery are dissected down towards the pancreas; both vessels are skeletonized. Care must be taken to preserve the right hepatic artery, which courses separately and to the right of the portal vein in 15 per cent of

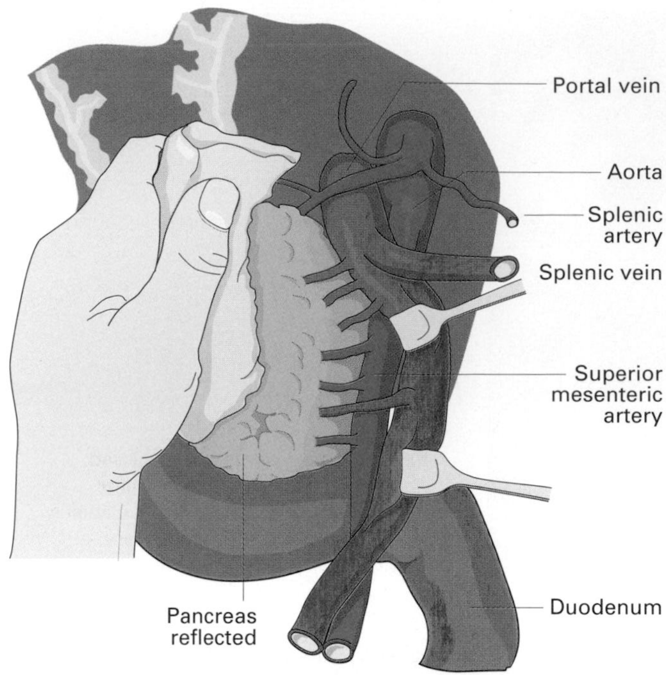

Fig. 6 One of the critical steps in pancreatoduodenectomy is dissection of the uncinate process from the posterior aspect of the mesenteric vessels. Adequate assessment of this area cannot be necessarily achieved by preoperative angiography or by palpation at the beginning of surgery. Sometimes a tumour that is thought to be resectable is found not to be so at this point in the operation.

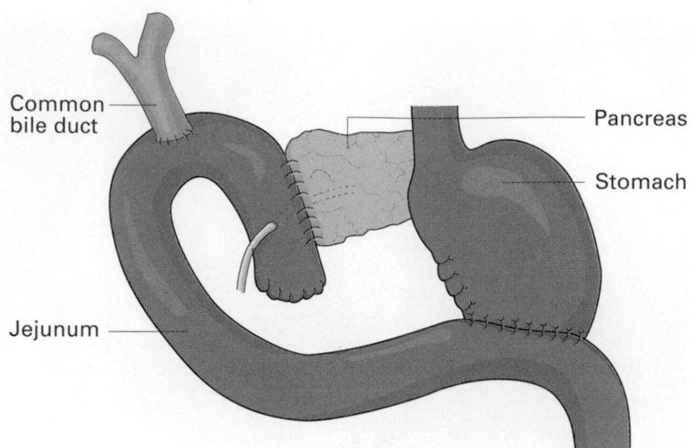

Fig. 7 Reconstruction after 'classical' pancreatoduodenectomy. We routinely stent the pancreatic anastomosis and leave the tube in place for at least seven days.

individuals. The gastroduodenal artery is then divided and ligated at its origin from the hepatic artery. This preparation allows further exposure of the portal vein to the point where it emerges above the pancreatic neck, thus completing the dissection behind the pancreatic neck to the superior mesenteric vein. Resection is continued by dividing the gastrohepatic omentum and reflecting this tissue down to the gastric antrum, dividing the right gastric and distal left gastric arteries. The gastrocolic omentum is opened and the lesser sac developed. After the gastroepiploic vessels have been ligated at the greater curvature the stomach is divided at the junction of the corpus and the antrum. The pancreas is then transected anteriorly or immediately to the left of the portal vein, and haemostasis of the distal stump carefully obtained with cautery and sutures. The proximal jejunum is divided, as is its mesentery down toward the ligament of Treitz, which is lysed. The proximal end of the jejunum is passed to the right under the mesenteric vessels, and the final steps of resection are then accomplished. The uncinate process of the pancreas must be dissected from the portal and mesenteric veins, carefully isolating and ligating the thin walled venous communications (Fig. 6). Finally, the retroperitoneal tissue and arterial branches to the uncinate from the superior mesenteric artery must be severed and ligated. After removal of the specimen, the peritoneum is closed at the ligament of Treitz.

Reconstruction of the alimentary tract is achieved by passing the distal jejunum through the right side of the transverse mesocolon and anastomosing the pancreas, bile duct, and stomach to the intestine, usually in that order (Fig. 7). It is thought that the alkaline pH of the pancreatic and biliary secretions are protective against marginal ulceration at the gastroenteric anastomosis, and also, if a troublesome leak develops from the pancreatojejunal anastomosis, the pancreatic remnant can be excised without disturbing the other connections. Pancreatojejunostomy can be carried out by invaginating the pancreatic remnant into the jejunum, or, as we prefer, by performing an end-to-side anastomosis approximating the mucosa of the pancreatic duct to that of the intestine. Interrupted fine polyglactin sutures are used for the mucosal anastomosis, which is routinely stented with a 5F paediatric feeding tube, brought out through the side wall of the jejunum and through the abdominal wall. An outer layer of interrupted silk sutures is also placed between the pancreas and the serosa of the jejunum. The biliary anastomosis is constructed in a similar fashion, but stents are generally unnecessary for the dilated bile duct. An antecolic gastrojejunostomy completes the reconstruction. Closed system soft silicone suction drains are left in the vicinity of the pancreatic and biliary anastomosis.

Complications of pancreatoduodenectomy are common: the most frequent are pancreatic (10–20 per cent) and biliary (5–10 per cent) fistulae, wound haemorrhage, cardiopulmonary events, and infection. Pancreatic fistulae are the principal source of postoperative morbidity and mortality, but the technique of stented mucosa–mucosa anastomosis has lowered our incidence of pancreatic fistula to 3 per cent (four of 140 cases), and has been innocuous in all but one case. Biliary fistulae are equally rare and will usually close spontaneously. Persistent fistulae may heal with the help of a percutaneous transhepatic stent bridging the anastomosis. Late postoperative haemorrhage is usually the consequence of vascular erosion associated with intrabdominal sepsis, most commonly related to a pancreatojejunal or other anastomotic leak. Other complications include wound abscess (which has become uncommon with routine use of antibiotic prophylaxis) and urinary and respiratory infections.

Mortality rates following the Whipple procedure have decreased markedly over the past 30 years. Prior to 1980 the average mortality in over 4000 patients from different sources was 17 per cent; however, in the last 5 years, at least six major institutions in the United States and Europe have reported substantial experiences with mortality rates of less than 5 per cent.

Survival rates 5 years after Whipple resection for pancreatic cancer have significantly improved: while such survival was rare 25 years ago, current reports quote figures between 5 and 18 per cent. In a series from Japan, the 5-year survival rate for patients

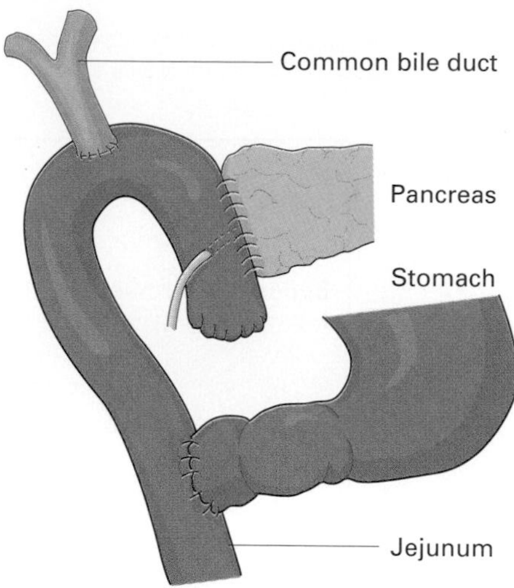

Fig. 8 Reconstruction after pylorus-preserving pancreatoduodenectomy.

with tumours less than 2 cm in diameter was 30 per cent, and 20 per cent of all those who underwent resection survived this long. The median survival of resected patients is about 18 months, which is significantly better than the figure of 6 months quoted for unresected patients, including those in whom the tumour was small and apparently confined locally. These observations suggest that resection of the tumour not only gives reasonable (and the only) hope of cure, but also the best palliation.

Pylorus-preserving pancreatoduodenectomy

This modification of the Whipple procedure was first proposed by Traverso and Longmire in 1978. The antrum, pylorus, and first 2 cm of duodenum are preserved (Fig. 8) with the intention of decreasing the frequency of marginal ulceration and improving postoperative nutritional status by avoiding postgastrectomy symptoms. The concern that this procedure might compromise the resection margins and the removal of potentially malignant lymph nodes, and therefore lessen the effectiveness of the resection, has not been borne out. Long-term survival has been equivalent to that of the conventional Whipple procedure. We currently use this operation in the treatment of carcinoma of the pancreatic head, provided that the first portion of the duodenum is not affected by the tumour and that the patient has no history of duodenal ulcer.

Total pancreatectomy

In an effort to improve the results of the Whipple procedure in the treatment of carcinoma of the pancreatic head, several groups started to perform total pancreatectomy in the 1970s. The arguments for this modification were that tumour was found either in the resection margin or distal to it in a multicentric fashion in up to one-third of patients, and that in extending the pancreatectomy a more complete lymphadenectomy could be achieved. It was also hoped that postoperative morbidity and mortality would be diminished by eliminating the pancreatic anastomosis. In a review of

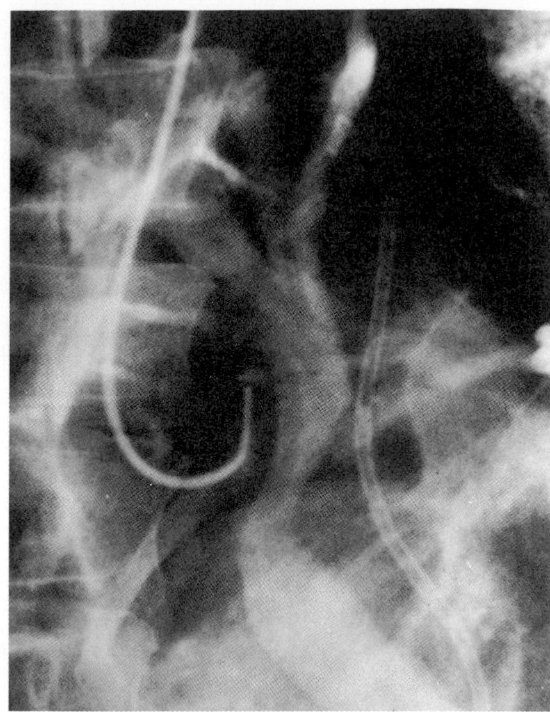

Fig. 9 Endoscopic stenting with large diameter tubes can provide long-term relief of jaundice. The catheter on the right was placed for angiography, and the image also shows partial obstruction of the portal vein.

more than 350 patients reported by different surgical groups, postoperative mortality was 17 per cent, mean survival 18 months, and 5-year survival 6.3 per cent. Thus, no advantage has been found to this approach, which also causes labile diabetes because of the absence of both insulin and glucagon. In hopes of avoiding this difficult diabetic state, some groups in Europe leave a small fragment of the pancreatic tail which is oversewn. The frequency of postoperative diabetes is less than that after total pancreatectomy and is easier to manage, but long-term results are not yet available. Total pancreatectomy should probably be reserved only for those resectable cases in which there is obvious involvement of the rest of the organ or in which tumour is found in the frozen section of the margin of the resected pancreas.

Regional pancreatectomy

In this operation, the pancreas and surrounding tissue are resected *en bloc*, along with a segment of the portal vein and, occasionally, segments of the hepatic or superior mesenteric arteries. The procedure entails either total or subtotal pancreatectomy. Its main advocate is Fortner, who described it in 1973. His operative mortality is now down to 8 per cent, but his long-term results are no different to those obtained with conventional pancreatoduodenectomy.

Palliative procedures

At the time of diagnosis curative surgical resection is already impossible for 90 per cent of patients with pancreatic cancer. Although this can usually be established by preoperative staging,

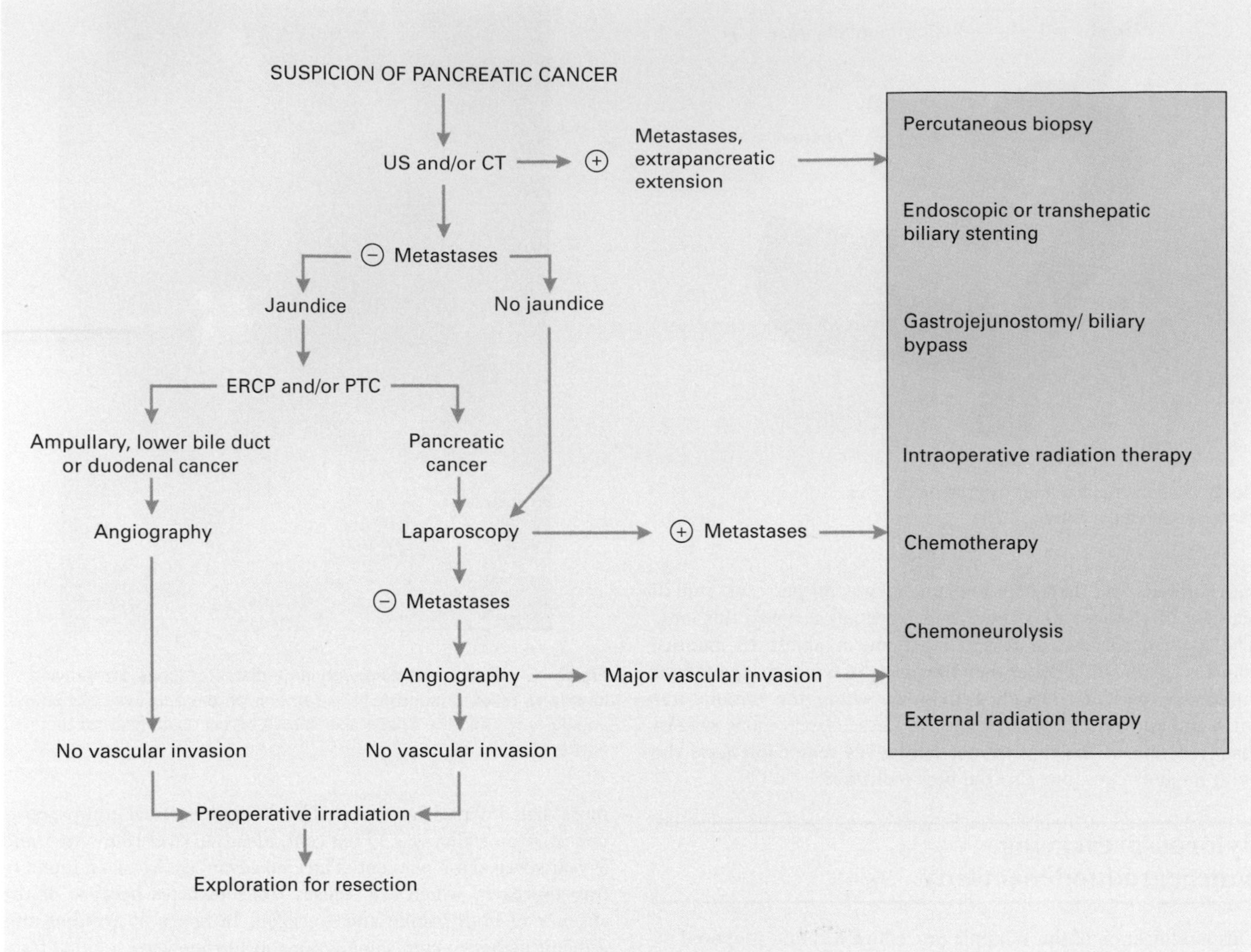

Fig. 10 Algorithm for the management of pancreatic cancer. ERCP = endoscopic retrograde cholangiopancreatography, PTC = percutaneous transluminal cholangiography.

unresectability may not be established before surgical exploration. Decompression of the biliary duct is indicated for relief of symptoms due to obstruction. Either cholecystojejunostomy or choledochojejunostomy may be suitable, but the latter is associated with a lower incidence of cholangitis and recurrent jaundice due to obstruction of the cystic duct by the tumour growing along the common duct. Anastomosis of the bile duct to the duodenum rather than the jejunum also works well; it is rarely prevented by cancer involving the proximal duodenum. For jaundiced patients in whom an unresectable or metastatic tumour is diagnosed preoperatively, and in those in whom tumour in the porta prevents access to the common duct, endoscopic stenting (Fig. 9) is the best option, especially now that large diameter tubes (10–12 Fr) can be used. Survival following stent compression is equal to that after surgical bypass, while cost and morbidity are reduced.

Biliary drainage achieved by a percutaneous stent is an option in patients for whom an endoprosthesis cannot be placed endoscopically. The time required to achieve placement of percutaneous endoprosthesis is greater than that for endoscopic placement, and complications are more common.

Obstruction of duodenal or gastric outlets can be another source of considerable distress for patients with inoperable pancreatic cancer and gastrojejunostomy is required. It has been stated that these patients have associated duodenal motility disorders which complicate the early postoperative course. For this reason, some surgeons insert a gastrostomy drainage tube at the time of gastrojejunostomy. Between 8 and 30 per cent of patients treated for biliary obstruction alone subsequently develop duodenal obstruction, perhaps justifying prophylactic gastrojejunostomy at the time of surgical biliary bypass.

In an effort to ameliorate pain from retroperitoneal nerve invasion, some surgeons perform chemical splanchnicectomy (chemoneurolysis) by infiltrating the coeliac plexus with phenol or 50 per cent ethyl alcohol at the time of palliative surgery. This may be of benefit for several months. Nerve blockade can also be achieved percutaneously, although the results may not be as durable.

Radiotherapy

External beam radiation therapy with 40 to 60 Gy may produce some palliation of pain for patients with unresectable pancreatic cancer, but survival is not significantly prolonged. The combination of radiotherapy with 5-fluorouracil was evaluated by the Gastrointestinal Tumor Study Group. The combined therapy produced a median survival of 10 months, patients who received only external beam radiation therapy survived 5.5 months. This combined modality was also tested in patients who underwent resective surgery with a curative intent, and the treated group had a significantly increased median survival of 21 months compared with 11 months in the untreated group. Although the number of patients treated was small, the findings suggest that combined adjuvant radiation and 5-fluorouracil can be of benefit after curative resection.

Radiation can be delivered to a pancreatic tumour in greater effective doses and with less injury to neighbouring viscera if it is performed during surgery. This objective has been accomplished with conventional orthovoltage, electron beams, and implantation of radioactive iodine. Only the electron beam therapy is said to prolong survival, and this treatment also appears to give substantial and lasting relief of pain in at least one-half of treated patients. Late duodenal ulceration and stenosis may result from radiation injury, and for this reason all patients treated with intraoperative electron beam also receive a gastrojejunostomy.

Chemotherapy

Several chemotherapeutic agents have been used in the treatment of pancreatic cancer, but only 5-fluorouracil, mitomycin C, streptozotocin, and ifosfamide have shown response rates above 20 per cent. The most extensively studied drug is 5-fluorouracil, which has a response rate of 28 per cent. However, the duration and value of the 'response' are minimal, and the end results of both single and combination drug treatment have been uniformly disappointing.

Endocrine therapy

Experimental pancreatic carcinoma is responsive to hormone manipulation, and human tumours bear sex steroid receptors. This, coupled with the androgen derangement (low testosterone, high androstenedione, and altered testosterone to dihydrotesterone ratio) seen in patients with this neoplasm, has prompted several groups to investigate endocrine treatment. Two phase II studies of tamoxifen treatment in patients with unresectable pancreatic cancer demonstrated an increase in median survival, as did a study with the use of an analogue of luteinizing hormone-releasing hormone. Phase III trials are currently in progress.

Figure 10 summarizes a suggested strategy for staging and treatment of pancreatic cancer.

FURTHER READING

Cameron JL, *et al.* Factors influencing survival following pancreaticoduodenectomy for pancreatic cancer. *Am J Surg* 1991; **161**: 120–25.

Grace PA, Pitt HA, Longmire WP. Pylorus preserving pancreatoduodenectomy: an overview. *Br J Surg*, 1990; **77**: 968–74.

Greenway BA. Carcinoma of the exocrine pancreas: a sex hormone responsive tumour? *Br J Surg* 1987; **74**: 441–2.

Gudjonsson B. Cancer of the pancreas; 50 years of surgery. *Cancer* 1987; **60**: 2284–303.

Fontham ETH, Correa P. Epidemiology of pancreatic cancer. *Surg Clin North Am* 1989; **69**: 551–67.

Warshaw AL. Implications of peritoneal cytology for staging of early pancreatic cancer. *Am J Surg* 1991; **161**: 26–30.

Warshaw AL, Swanson RS. Pancreatic cancer in 1988. Possibilities and probabilities. *Ann Surg* 1988; **208**: 541–53.

Warshaw AL, Zhuo-yun G, Wittenberg J, Waltman AC. Preoperative staging and assessment of resectability of pancreatic cancer. *Arch Surg* 1990; **125**: 230–3.

25.5 Insulinomas and other tumours

DAVID W. RATTNER

INTRODUCTION

Neuroendocrine tumours of the pancreas are being recognized with increasing frequency because of the development of radioimmunoassays for a growing number of circulating polypeptides. The clinical syndromes produced by excessive hormone secretion range from biochemical curiosities (PPoma) to life threatening derangements of homeostasis (insulinoma and VIPoma). Although characteristic groups of symptoms may trigger clinical suspicion, specific clinical diagnosis depends on measuring elevated levels of the circulating hormone. These tumours are generally slow growing and span the spectrum of behaviour from benign to malignant (Table 1).

Table 1 Spectrum of malignancy in islet cell tumours

Type	Malignancy (%)
Insulinoma	10–15
VIPoma	50
Somatostatinoma	50
PPoma	50
Non-functioning	60
Glucagonoma	60–70
Gastrinoma	60–70

The islets of Langerhans contain at least five cell types: β-cells, which produce insulin, were the first to be identified. Subsequent immunocytochemistry has identified α-cells, which produce glucagon, γ-cells, which produce somatostatin, and F cells which produce pancreatic polypeptide. The fifth islet cell type is the enterochromaffin cell, which produces serotonin. All islet cells are of neuroectodermal origin, contain neuron-specific enolase, and are capable of amine precursor uptake and decarboxylation. Individual islet cells can produce more than one hormone. They are also capable of producing hormones not usually found in the pancreas, such as gastrin, adrenocorticotrophin, vasoactive intestinal peptide, and growth hormone. Although many pancreatic islet cell tumours are multihormonal, one peptide generally predominates and is responsible for producing the clinical syndrome. Approximately 10 per cent of pancreatic islet cell tumours arise in association with multiple endocrine neoplasia type I. Conversely, 85 per cent of patients with this syndrome have pancreatic neuroendocrine tumours or hyperplasia. Pancreatic neuroendocrine tumours associated with multiple endocrine neoplasia type I are non-β-cell tumours, and tend to be multifocal. Non-functioning islet cell tumours comprise about 20 per cent of all pancreatic neuroendocrine tumours. They may produce as yet unidentified peptides with effects too vague to produce a clearly defined syndrome, or they may have defective release mechanisms of established peptides.

INSULINOMAS

Insulinomas are the most common pancreatic neuroendocrine tumours. The mean age of patients at presentation is 45 years, and the disease is rare in adolescence. Since the presentation may be insidious and the symptoms subtle, the diagnosis depends on carefully collected biochemical data, based on an understanding of normal insulin secretion and glucose homeostasis.

Physiology of insulin production

Since the measurement of insulin by radioimmunoassay is critical to the diagnosis of insulinoma, it is important to understand the mechanism of insulin synthesis, secretion, and release. Insulin is initially synthesized on the rough endoplasmic reticulum in a form known as pre-proinsulin. Following synthesis, a 24-amino acid peptide is cleaved to yield proinsulin, which is transported to the Golgi apparatus where it is packaged into secretory granules. Secretory granules contain proteases that cleave the C-peptide sequence of the molecule to yield biologically active insulin. Therefore, when insulin is secreted, equimolar amounts of C-peptide are also released; they can be detected in the plasma (Fig. 1).

Although some proinsulin is normally released from β-cells, it is usually less than 25 per cent of the amount of insulin. Serum levels of C-peptide and proinsulin are important in the differential diagnosis of hypoglycaemia (Fig. 2).

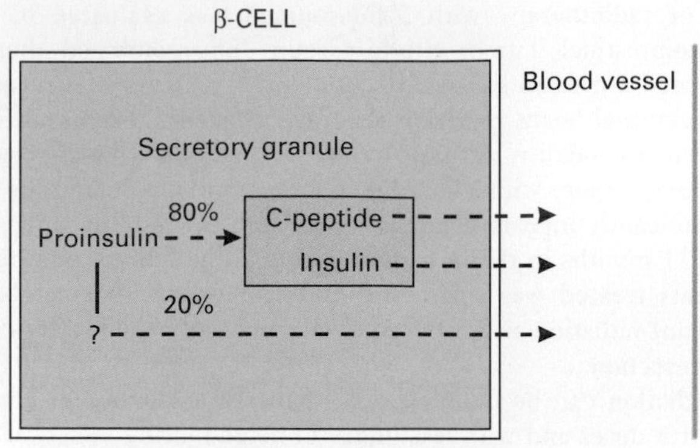

Fig. 1 Schematic drawing of a β-cell. Insulin is synthesized as an inactive precursor, proinsulin. Under normal conditions, most proinsulin is transported to secretory granules where it is cleaved into biologically active insulin and its cleavage fragment C-peptide. Insulin and C-peptide are secreted in equimolar quantities. Normally less than 20 per cent of proinsulin is released into the bloodstream.

Clinical presentation

The clinical presentation of insulinomas is hypoglycaemia in virtually all cases. Symptoms caused by local effects of the tumour mass are rare: most commonly, patients present with neurological effects of hypoglycaemia, such as visual disturbances, confusion, lethargy, weakness, or transient motor deficits. Erroneous psychiatric or neurological diagnoses are common and insulinomas may go undiagnosed for as long as 3 years. Hypoglycaemia also causes catecholamine release with consequent autonomic symptoms such as sweating, anxiety, and palpitations. Symptoms are due to reactive hypoglycaemia (i.e. postprandial) or induced by fasting or exercise; the distinction is important. Symptoms from insulinomas tend to be progressive over time and to occur while fasting. To avoid symptoms, many patients learn to eat frequent meals and thus are overweight. When hyperinsulinism is severe, symptoms may develop as early as 2 to 4 h after meals. This phenomenon can be demonstrated in oral glucose tolerance tests; reactive hypoglycaemia is followed by a rebound to normal plasma glucose levels if the hypoglycaemia is functional. In insulinoma, however, blood glucose levels remain depressed.

Diagnosis

In 1935, Whipple and Frantz proposed the diagnostic triad of symptoms of hypoglycaemia produced by fasting or exercise, blood glucose less than 45 (mmol/l), and symptoms relieved by administration of glucose. Advances in the ability to detect and measure insulin and its metabolites have allowed refinement of the diagnosis. The presence of hypoglycaemia in the face of inappropriately elevated levels of insulin is the key to diagnosis: this can be demonstrated by a prolonged fast in over 95 per cent of patients. Fifty-six per cent of patients with insulinomas will become hypoglycaemic within 14 h, 78 per cent by 18 h, and 87 per cent by 24 h. If the fast is extended to 72 h, over 95 per cent of patients will develop hypoglycaemia. If symptomatic or biochemical hypoglycaemia does not develop by 72 h, the patient should be exercised. This will provoke hypoglycaemia in virtually all insulinoma patients.

Absolute elevations of immunoreactive insulin concentrations are not found in all patients with insulinomas: the tumour may secrete in short bursts causing wide fluctuation in blood levels of immunoreactive insulin. While levels above 20 μu/ml are diagnostic, a normal level does not exclude the diagnosis. In normal subjects, blood immunoreactive insulin decreases with fasting to 3 to 7 μu/ml and changes in level parallel changes in glucose concentration. In insulinoma patients, the immunoreactive insulin levels may fluctuate, but they will not fall with fasting. The key in using measurements of immunoreactive insulin concentration for diagnosing insulinoma is the demonstration of inappropriate levels. After an overnight fast, the normal ratio of immunoreactive insulin (μu/ml)/glucose (mg/dl) is 0.3. States of insulin resistance such as obesity may cause an elevation of this ratio but these patients are not hypoglycaemic. In patients with organic

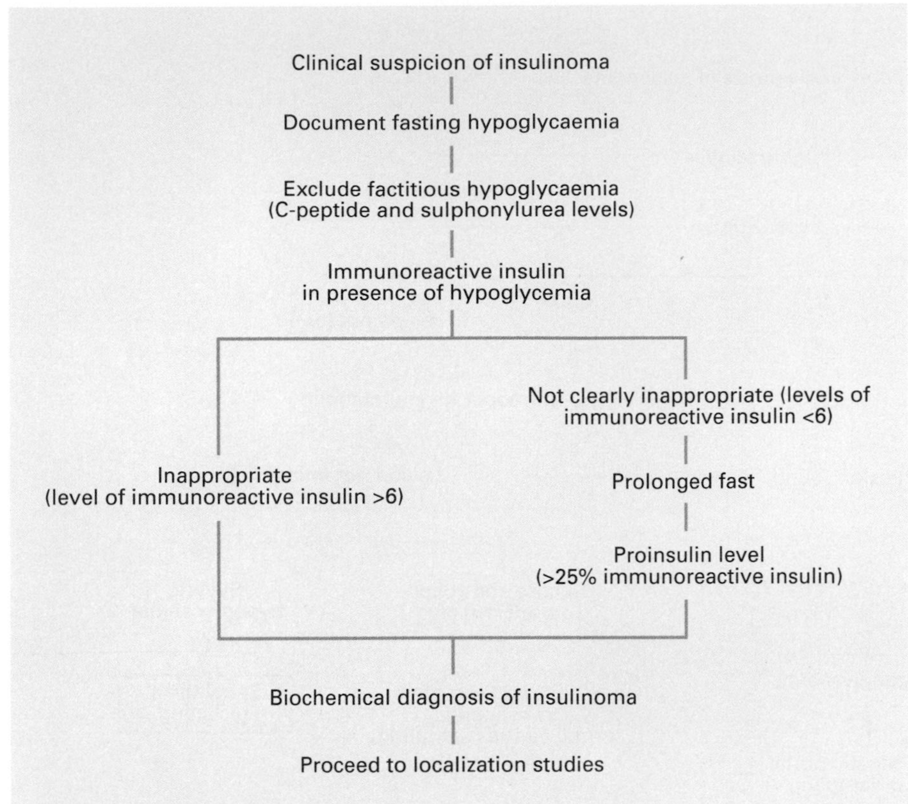

Fig. 2 Diagnostic algorithm for a suspected insulinoma.

hyperinsulinism, the ratio remains constant during fasting, but rises in the presence of insulinoma. This ratio should be studied with respect to its change over time during a fast, rather than as an absolute value. Another rule of thumb is that immunoreactive insulin levels above 6 μu/ml in the presence of a blood glucose concentration less than 40 mmol/l is diagnostic of insulinoma.

Proinsulin level is normally 10 to 20 per cent that of immunoreactive insulin but neoplastic tissue releases excess proinsulin. Up to 90 per cent of patients with insulinomas have proinsulin levels greater than 25 per cent that of immunoreactive insulin. Markedly elevated proinsulin levels serve as a marker for malignancy, although the overlap between benign and malignant disease is such that this finding is not an absolute discriminant. C-peptide levels should also be monitored: if factitious hypoglycaemia is produced by the administration of insulin appreciable amounts of this peptide will not be found. Sulphonylurea levels should also be measured. With the availability of radioimmunoassays, provocative tests such as the tolbutamide test are no longer employed.

Pathology

Between 75 and 80 per cent of insulinomas are solitary, benign lesions. Approximately 10 per cent occur as multiple adenomas associated with multiple endocrine neoplasia type I, and another 10 per cent are malignant. Five per cent represent diffuse microadenomatosis, in which multiple small non-encapsulated lesions are distributed throughout the pancreas (nesidioblastosis). Although common in childhood this is rare in adults.

Most benign insulinomas are between 0.5 and 2 cm in diameter and are distributed evenly throughout the pancreas. Pathological analysis alone cannot distinguish between benign and malignant insulinomas, although malignant lesions tend to be larger (average size 6.2 cm) and one-half of malignant lesions have metastasized at the time of diagnosis. Malignant spread is generally confined to the peripancreatic region and liver. When insulinomas arise in patients with multiple endocrine neoplasia type I, multiple adenomas or a combination of micro- and macroadenomatosis is common, yet surprisingly good results are obtained with resection, perhaps because multiple lesions do not all secrete at the same time.

Localization

Once the diagnosis of insulinoma is made, the location of the tumour should be sought. While some experienced surgeons are able to identify 75 to 90 per cent of these tumours, the literature is replete with examples of missed lesions. Since most insulinomas are less than 2 cm in diameter, CT scan and ultrasound examinations fail to detect at least half of them. Many of these lesions are hypervascular and can be visualized by arteriography, with success rates of 15 to 85 per cent. Subselective injections are more likely to demonstrate the lesion than coeliac trunk or superior mesenteric artery injections. The false positive rate is as high as 10 per cent, presumably because of accessory spleens or overlapping shadows.

If the arteriogram fails to localize the adenoma, some authorities recommend proceeding to laparotomy, while others perform transhepatic portal venous sampling. This requires a highly experienced team of angiographers, and the best results are reported by groups with the largest experience. Although success rates of

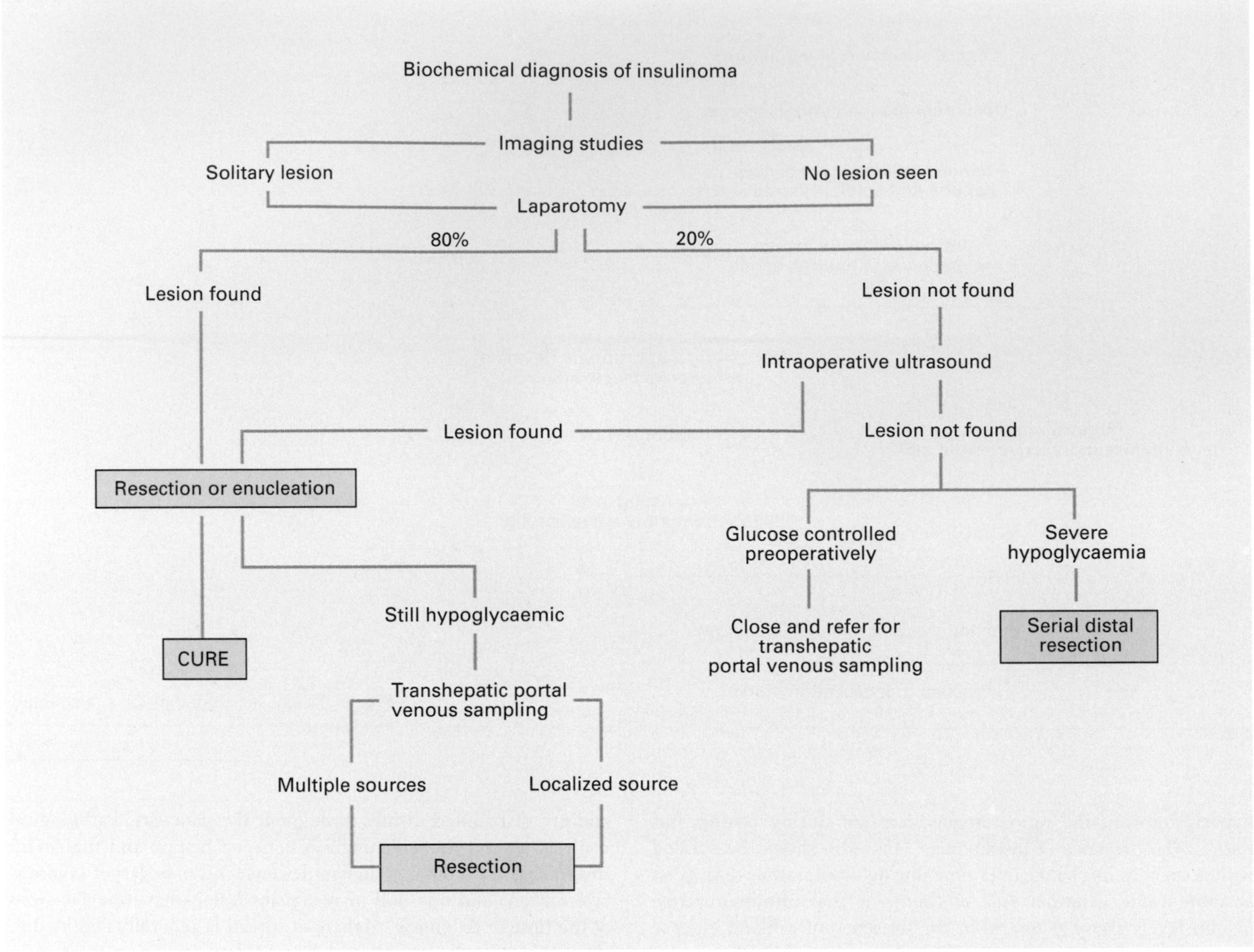

Fig. 3 Intraoperative decision making in insulinoma.

over 70 per cent are reported, the procedure is not without hazards, such as gallbladder perforation and haemobilia. Nonetheless, transhepatic portal venous sampling has theoretical attractions in being able to differentiate solitary adenomas from multiple lesions preoperatively, as well as directing the surgeon to one region of the pancreas if it is difficult to locate the lesion by palpation. At the time of surgery, intraoperative ultrasound may detect small lesions which are not readily palpable, particularly those in the head of the pancreas.

Treatment

Once the diagnosis of insulinoma is made, surgery need not be urgent. Symptoms can often be controlled medically: euglycaemia may be maintained by frequent small meals. Diazoxide, 200 to 600 mg/day, suppresses insulin release through unknown mechanisms. Approximately 60 per cent of insulinomas respond to diazoxide. The long-acting somatostatin analogue, SMS201–995 (octreotide) also suppresses insulin secretion to variable degrees. Non-surgical control of symptoms preoperatively allows time for localization studies and evaluation for multiple endocrine neoplasia type I. In patients with hypercalcaemia, parathyroidectomy should be performed before pancreatic surgery. Elevation of serum pancreatic polypeptide is suggestive of a polyendocrine adenopathy.

At the time of laparotomy, the pancreas should be fully exposed to allow complete bimanual palpation. After dividing the gastrocolic ligament, a wide Kocher manoeuvre should be performed. Reflection of the right colon after division of the attachments to the lateral abdominal wall facilitates exposure and examination of the uncinate process. The lateral peritoneal attachments of the spleen should be incised to elevate the tail of the pancreas. The peritoneum along the inferior surface of the gland may then be incised to allow bimanual palpation of the body and tail of the gland.

In general, adenomas should be enucleated to preserve remaining pancreatic endocrine parenchyma. Between 20 and 30 per cent of patients with insulinomas will develop diabetes postoperatively. Lesions in the tail of the gland may be either enucleated or encompassed by a spleen-preserving distal pancreatectomy: the incidence of fistula formation following enucleation is equivalent to the morbidity of distal resection. If multiple adenomas are found, all gross disease should be resected. In patients with multiple endocrine neoplasia type I, a subtotal pancreatectomy may be performed, but total pancreatectomy is not indicated as an initial procedure, even when diffuse disease is present. When the lesion cannot be located intraoperatively and the diagnosis of insulinoma is biochemically certain, the presence of an ectopic insulinoma is excluded, and preoperative diazoxide has not controlled symptoms, blind distal resection of up to 85 per cent of the gland should be performed in two steps, with serial sectioning of the pancreas as it is removed. If the patient's glucose level has been controlled with diazoxide, however, the operation should be terminated and the patient sent to a centre capable of performing transhepatic portal venous sampling so as to direct subsequent resection (Fig. 3).

When malignant insulinomas are discovered, aggressive attempts to remove all gross disease, including hepatic metastases, should be undertaken. Hepatic lesions should be excised by wedge excision. Formal anatomical hepatic resections probably should not be undertaken unless preoperative chemotherapy has been given and has failed. Ligation of the hepatic artery should be avoided because regional infusion chemotherapy may be necessary in future management. Malignant insulinomas tend to be slow growing with a disease-free interval of up to 5 years following radical resection. Collective opinions hold that long-term remission following resection of hepatic metastases is rare and must be compared with regression of 50 per cent of tumours and complete remission in 20 per cent of patients obtained with streptozotocin treatment. Nonetheless, in competent hands, wedge resection of hepatic metastases is simple, carries a low morbidity, and may provide a long period of effective palliation. Chemotherapy of malignant insulinomas, like all islet cell tumours, is based primarily on streptozotocin. This will reduce tumour mass in 50 per cent of all patients, and 60 per cent will have a reduction in plasma insulin levels. Streptozotocin is fairly toxic: virtually all patients experience nausea and vomiting while two-thirds develop some renal toxicity and hepatotoxicity. The addition of 5-fluorouracil to streptozotocin markedly improves the response rate, with 33 per cent of patients showing a complete response and median survival improving from 16 months in patients treated with streptozotocin alone to 26 months in patients receiving combination chemotherapy.

GASTRINOMA

The association of virulent peptic ulcer disease with a non-β pancreatic islet cell tumour was made in 1955 by Zollinger and Ellison. Subsequently the Zollinger–Ellison syndrome and gastrinoma have become synonymous. Gastrinomas are the second most common islet cell tumour and are found in patients of all ages without a significant predilection for sex, race, or socioeconomic status. Since the diagnosis rests on the radioimmunoassay of gastrin levels most reported cases are from cities with tertiary medical facilities.

Symptoms

Symptoms produced by gastrinomas are due to the effects of gastrin rather than to tumour mass. Gastric acid hypersecretion causes pain similar to typical peptic ulcer disease. One-third of patients, however, present with oesophagitis or diarrhoea due to hyperacidity. In the United States, 0.1 per cent of patients with duodenal ulcers have a gastrinoma. Patients diagnosed as having multiple peptic ulcers, ulcers in the postbulbar duodenum, ulcers resistant to medical therapy, or ulcers which relapse immediately upon cessation of medical therapy, should be suspected of having Zollinger–Ellison syndrome. Since 25 per cent of patients with gastrinomas have multiple endocrine neoplasia, a family history of endocrine disorders, hypercalcaemia, or ulcer diathesis should also raise suspicion that gastrinoma is present. Patients with multiple endocrine neoplasia type I generally present initially with hypercalcaemia.

Diagnosis

The *sine qua non* in the diagnosis of gastrinoma is the demonstration of an elevated fasting gastrin level in the presence of acid hypersecretion. Prior to embarking on an extensive evaluation for gastrinoma, achlorhydria must be excluded. A basal acid output above 15 mEq/hour is highly suggestive of gastrinoma and basal acid output greater than 25 mEq/h is virtually diagnostic. Prior to the proliferation of radioimmunoassays, extensive acid studies were performed. Nonetheless, studies of acid secretion have a 10 per cent false-positive rate and a 15 per cent false-negative rate. Their value is to exclude achlorhydria and to monitor the efficacy of medical therapy.

Although a gastrin level greater than 500 pg/ml in a patient with hyperacidity is diagnostic of Zollinger–Ellison syndrome, up to 60 per cent of patients have gastrin levels in the intermediate range (150–500 pg/ml). Earlier detection of patients has made this scenario more common. To differentiate gastrinoma from other causes of hypergastrinaemia, a secretin test is performed. Secretin is a potent stimulant of gastrin release from gastrinomas, but secretin has little effect on serum gastrin levels in all other causes of hypergastrinaemia. A secretin stimulation test is performed by injecting 2 U/kg of secretin as an intravenous bolus and collecting blood samples at zero, 2, 5, 10, 15, and 30 min from the time of infusion for gastrin assay. An immediate rise of over 200 pg/ml is considered a positive test and is diagnostic for gastrinoma. Rarely, patients with Zollinger–Ellison syndrome will have a non-diagnostic secretin test (i.e. less than two-fold or 200 pg/ml increase in gastrin). In these patients, a combined secretin–calcium test may detect gastrinomas: a 1-min infusion of calcium gluconate together with a bolus of secretin will evoke the expected 200 pg/ml increase in gastrin concentration. These tests also serve to distinguish patients with a retained gastric antrum and G-cell hyperplasia from those with gastrinomas. Patients with G-cell hyperplasia have an exaggerated response to test meals (>100 per cent increase in serum gastrin) whereas patients with gastrinoma have only a moderate response to meals (Table 2). Conversely, a test meal normally causes a two- to three-fold increase in plasma gastrin in normal patients, but there is only a minimal response in patients with gastrinoma because the high levels of circulating gastrin obscure the smaller physiologic response to the normal antral G-cells.

Pathology

Gastrinomas occur in both sporadic and familial forms: about 25 per cent occur in patients with multiple endocrine neoplasia type I; tumours are usually multiple but only 30 per cent prove to be

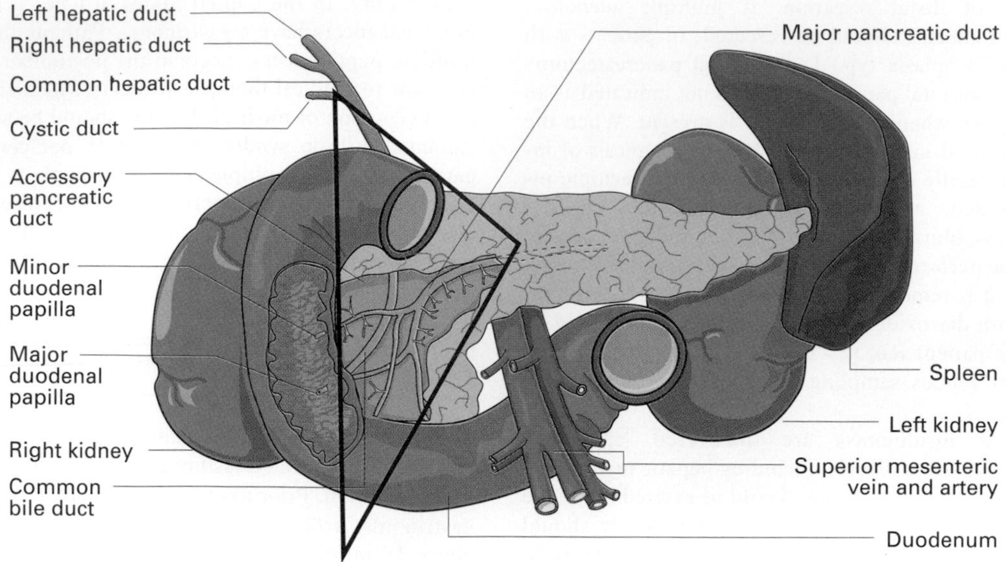

Fig. 4 Ninety per cent of gastrinomas lie within the gastrinoma triangle (outlined). Many of these are extrapancreatic, lying in lymph nodes or in the duodenal mucosa.

Table 2 The differential diagnosis of hypergastrinaemia

		Serum (gastrin) response to	
Cause of hypergastrinaemia	**BAO**	**Secretin test**	**Test meal**
Gastrinoma	+	++	+/−
Hypochlorhydic states	−	nc	nc
G-cell hyperplasia	+	nc	++
Retained antrum	+	nc	+
Short gut syndrome	+	nc	+
Gastric outlet obstruction	+	nc	+

nc = no appreciable change.
BAO = basal acid output.

malignant. Eighty-eight per cent of these patients are hypercalcaemic. Gastrin production in many of these patients occurs in duodenal microadenomas and not in other areas of pancreatic islet cell hyperplasia. If these findings are confirmed, many patients with Zollinger–Ellison syndrome and multiple endocrine neoplasia type I, previously felt to be inoperable, might be helped by duodenal tumour resection.

When Zollinger–Ellison syndrome occurs in sporadic form tumours are unifocal, but over 60 per cent are malignant. Historically, 50 per cent of these patients have metastases at the time of diagnosis, but with the current widespread use of radioimmunoassays, small solitary tumours are being found at an earlier stage. Neither size nor histological appearance is capable of differentiating benign from malignant gastrinomas: only the presence of metastases can attest to their malignant potential. In contrast to insulinomas, gastrinomas are not evenly distributed throughout the pancreas; they are frequently extrapancreatic, 90 per cent being contained in an area known as the gastrinoma triangle (Fig. 4). This area is bounded by the junction of the cystic and common ducts superiorly, the junction of the second and third portion of the duodenum inferiorly, and the junction of the neck and body of the pancreas medially. Solitary extrapancreatic tumours in the duodenal mucosa or lymph nodes are found in up to 25 per cent of patients. Patients whose gastrinomas are found in lymph nodes, with no apparent primary tumour, are presumed to have occult lesions in the duodenal mucosa. This subgroup of patients has an excellent prognosis and can be cured when rendered eugastrinaemic by removal of affected lymph nodes.

Localization

Once the diagnosis of gastrinoma is made, acid secretion should be controlled with H_2-receptor antagonists or omeprazole to allow time for localization studies. Localization should be undertaken in all patients, both to detect hepatic metastases and to aid the surgeon at laparotomy. Dynamic CT scanning is the single most accurate examination, detecting 75 to 80 per cent of all tumours. This result is comparable to those achieved using combined sonography, non-contrast enhanced CT, and selective arteriography. The sensitivity for detection of hepatic metastases is over 90 per cent. The success of dynamic CT scanning and selective arteriography is dependent to some extent on the experience of the radiological team.

In spite of these sophisticated imaging studies, a tumour will be found at laparotomy in nearly one-third of patients in whom all studies are negative. No preoperative test is superior to the ability of an experienced surgeon to find the offending gastrinoma. Intraoperative ultrasound may help to localize intrapancreatic tumours, but it is less helpful in identifying nodal gastrinomas and duodenal microadenomas. The value of transhepatic portal venous sampling is also debatable: it would seem to be of most use in patients in whom all of the localizing studies are negative. In such cases, the procedure should only be performed in centres with experience in the technique as the instance of false-positive results may be as high as 30 per cent.

Treatment

Prior to the introduction of potent antisecretory drugs, surgical therapy was directed at preventing complications of ulcer disease by the performance of a total gastrectomy. The introduction of H_2-receptor antagonists and, more recently, omeprazole initiated a wave of enthusiasm for non-surgical therapy in this disease. However, as patients have survived peptic complications only to succumb to metastatic disease, the importance of early tumour resection is now being re-emphasized. Zollinger reported a 76 per cent 5-year survival rate in patients with complete tumour resection, compared with a 21 per cent 5-year survival in those with incomplete resection. Since many tumours can now be detected earlier, curative resection may be possible in 40 per cent of patients, and all patients with apparent isolated gastrinomas and those in whom preoperative studies fail to demonstrate the site of a tumour should undergo surgical exploration. Extrapancreatic tumours, which frequently are not localized preoperatively, are the most curable; small intrapancreatic tumours may only be identified with careful surgical exploration and the use of intraoperative ultrasound. As with surgical exploration for insulinoma, the entire pancreas should be exposed and bimanually palpated. If no tumour is detected in the pancreas, all lymph nodes in the gastrinoma triangle should be examined and removed. If tumour is not detected by these manoeuvres, the duodenum should be opened and the mucosa everted and carefully inspected and palpated. Most microadenomas lie within 2 to 3 cm of the pylorus. Tumours in the body and head of the pancreas should be enucleated when possible. Distal pancreatectomy should be performed for lesions in the tail of the gland. Tumours located deep in the head or uncinate process may require a Whipple resection.

Occasionally no tumour is found at laparotomy: these patients may have either duodenal microadenomas, adenomatosis, or undiagnosed G-cell hyperplasia. The prognosis in these patients is excellent; indeed, they often outlive patients with resectable tumours. Patients with multiple endocrine neoplasia type I and no tumour demonstrable by preoperative studies often fall into this category; thus such patients should not undergo surgical exploration. However, patients with multiple endocrine neoplasia type I and a solitary lesion that can be localized preoperatively benefit from surgical excision of their gastrinomas.

Medical therapy

The goal of medical therapy is to prevent acid-mediated complications. Because symptoms are notoriously unreliable indicators of the efficacy of acid suppression, therapy should be monitored with acid studies or periodic endoscopic examinations. Drug dosages should be adjusted to maintain the basal acid output at 10 mEq/h or less; high daily doses, such as 3.5 g of cimetidine or 1.2 g of ranitidine, are frequently required. Antiandrogenic side-effects of these drugs are common at such high doses and contribute to the 40 per cent failure rate of medical therapy. Omeprazole is the most efficacious agent for control of acid secretion, but since the long-term effects of achlorhydria are unknown, the dosage should be adjusted to maintain basal acid output above 0 mEq/h but below 10 mEq/h. Long acting somatostatin analogues, often used in conjunction with omeprazole also show promise. Thus, the pharmacological tools to control acid secretion are now available but co-operation of the patient and meticulous attention to his or her clinical and endoscopic status are necessary for successful treatment.

Metastatic gastrinomas

Malignant gastrinomas tend to be more indolent than other islet cell carcinomas, and the presence of metastatic disease at the time of initial diagnosis does not necessarily imply rapidly advancing disease. Five-year survival for patients with metastases ranges from 20 to 60 per cent. Metastatic gastrinomas, like other islet cell carcinomas, can secrete multiple hormones, and the surveillance of these patients should include awareness of complications induced by these other peptides. Surgical resection of isolated metastases may be beneficial if all tumour is removed. Most patients with metastatic gastrinoma, however, are candidates for chemotherapy. The best response rate is seen after the use of a combination of streptozotocin and 5-fluorouracil (as with insulinomas). Total gastrectomy should be reserved for patients whose tumour cannot be removed and whose hyperacidity cannot be controlled with medical therapy. With the advent of omeprazole treatment, this group of patients can be expected to become smaller. Nonetheless, total gastrectomy is extremely well tolerated in patients with Zollinger–Ellison syndrome, and can be performed with 0 to 5 per cent mortality under elective circumstances. Total gastrectomy remains the most certain way to eliminate all acid-related complications in Zollinger–Ellison syndrome.

OTHER FUNCTIONING ISLET CELL TUMOURS

Glucagonoma

Hypersecretion of glucagon from α-cell neoplasms causes the 'diabetes–dermatitis' syndrome. While diabetes is mild, the rash, called necrotizing migratory erythema, is pathognomonic for glucagonoma. The rash involves the trunk, perineum, and thighs, and as the erythema spreads, central areas become necrotic and then heal. Other prominent features of this tumour, including weight loss, anaemia, and glossitis, are due to the catabolic effects of glucagon. Glucagon also has chronotropic activity; many patients manifest tachycardia, increased cardiac output, and constipation. The diagnosis, usually suspected on the basis of the rash, is confirmed by finding a plasma glucagon concentration greater than 50 pg/ml. Localization studies, as with insulinomas, are helpful in guiding surgical therapy and may be helpful in detecting metastases, as 50 per cent of tumours are malignant.

Preoperative correction of catabolism requires intravenous administration of amino acids, glucose, and supplemental insulin. Somatostatin analogues inhibit glucagon release and may palliate the rash. Prednisone is also beneficial. The surgical principles are similar to those described for insulinoma.

VIPoma

Vasoactive intestinal peptide is both an important neurotransmitter and hormone which is a potent stimulator of cAMP production by the gut, leading to massive secretion of water and electrolytes. The term 'pancreatic cholera' is an apt description of the full-blown effects of the tumour, with stool volumes sometimes being greater than 3 l a day. The diagnosis is made on the basis of watery diarrhoea, hypokalaemia, and achlorhydria in the presence of an elevated serum concentration of vasoactive intestinal peptide concentration. Flushing is also common because of the vasodilatory effects of the peptide. In the carcinoid syndrome, which has many similar symptoms, urinary levels of 5-hydroxyindole acetic acid are elevated and diarrhoea is less pronounced.

Ninety per cent of VIPomas lie within the pancreas; the remaining 10 per cent are found in neural tissue, including the adrenal medulla. Half of the tumours are malignant and 10 to 20 per cent are multifocal: localization studies are important to seek extrapancreatic tumours. Somatostatin analogues and indomethacin are useful in controlling diarrhoea, while dehydration and electrolyte abnormalities are corrected. Surgical principles are similar to those described for insulinomas.

Somatostatinomas

Somatostatinomas are rare, less than 50 having been reported. Symptoms are vague, including diabetes, cholelithiasis, indigestion, steatorrhoea, and hypochlorhydria. These tumours are often found coincidentally at the time of cholecystectomy. Half of the reported tumours have been found in extrapancreatic locations such as the duodenum, jejunum, and biliary tree.

NON-FUNCTIONING ISLET CELL TUMOURS

Non-functioning islet cell tumours present with symptoms caused by mass effect. If the tumour obstructs the pancreatic or bile duct, it may be detectable at a relatively early stage, but this is rare. The tumours are much larger than their functioning counterparts by the time they are diagnosed and thus they are more often malignant. In spite of their non-functional nature, immunoreactive cells are found in nearly 90 per cent of these tumours and 50 per cent contain multiple peptides. Their neuroendocrine origin is confirmed by finding neurone-specific enolase in the tumour, but there is little if any correlation between the immunohistochemical staining and clinical behaviour. All non-functioning islet cell tumours should be considered malignant because no gross or histological criteria, except the presence of metastases, can reliably establish the nature of the tumour. Aggressive surgical resection is indicated whenever this is feasible.

FURTHER READING

Delore R, Hermreck AS, Friesen SR. Selective surgical management of correctable hypergastrinema. *Surgery* 1989; **106**: 1094–102.

Fajans SS, Vinik AI. Insulin producing islet cell tumors. *Endocrinol Metab Clin N Am* 1989; **18**: 45–74.

Friesen SR. Update on the diagnosis and treatment of rare neuroendocrine tumors. *Surg Clin N Am* 1987; **67**: 379–93.

Howard TJ, Zinner MJ, Stabile BE, Passaro E. Gastrinoma excision for cure: a prospective analysis. *Ann Surg* 1990; **211**: 9–14.

Legaspi A, Brennan MF. Management of islet cell carcinoma. *Surgery* 1988; **104**: 1018–22.

Pipeleers-Marichal M, *et al.* Gastrinomas in the duodenum of patients with multiple endocrine neoplasia Type 1 and the Zollinger Ellison syndrome. *N Engl J Med* 1990; **322**: 723–7.

Proye C. Surgical strategy in insulinoma of adults. *Acta Chir Scand* 1987; **153**: 481–91.

Zollinger RM, Ellison EH. Primary peptic ulcerations of the jejunum associated with islet cell tumours of the pancreas. *Ann Surg* 1955; **142**: 709–28.

26 Abdominal wall, omentum, mesentery, and retroperitoneum

26.1 Abdominal wall trauma

CHARLES J. MCCABE

Abdominal trauma occurs frequently, and the presentation, evaluation, and treatment of damage to the intra-abdominal viscera are established. Isolated abdominal wall trauma is much less common and is rarely even considered in the initial assessment of the patient unless obvious signs are present. It is most commonly associated with musculoskeletal, head, or thoracoabdominal trauma, and its significance is, among other things, as a herald of underlying pathology.

EPIDEMIOLOGY

The aetiology depends on the demographics of the society and the environment, and includes blunt trauma (motor vehicle accident, pedestrian struck by a motor vehicle, motorcycle or bicycle accidents, falls), penetrating injuries (stab wounds, gunshot wounds), and blast injuries that have become common in some areas of the world.

Blunt forces that result from motor vehicle accidents vary depending upon the location of the accident, abuse of alcohol, and use of seatbelts. The incidence of penetrating injuries increase in an urban environment, and these are commonly associated with illicit drug use. The injuries that follow bombing or explosions caused by warfare or terrorist activity are rare, but such injuries may also occur in civilian locations such as mines, shipyards, and chemical plants. Flying glass, mortar, or other debris from the blast will have a penetrating force and the victim may become a projectile and suffer acceleration/deceleration forces when the abdomen strikes immobile objects.

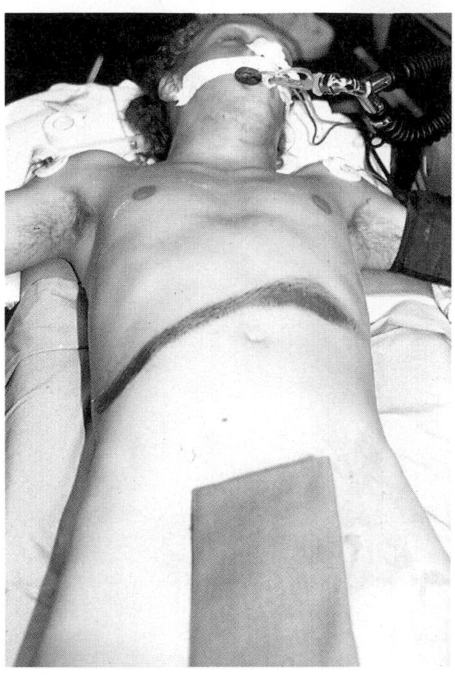

Fig. 1 Abdominal wall contusion resulting from a metal chain striking the abdomen as the patient rode a motorbike. This is a similar type of contusion that can occur as a result of the use of the lap belt (seatbelt sign).

MECHANISM AND VARIETY OF TRAUMA

The abdominal wall trauma that results from penetrating forces is usually obvious: stab wounds result in lacerations of the skin and subcutaneous tissue with deeper injuries causing lacerations of the muscle, fascia, and perhaps peritoneum. The effects of gunshot wounds vary, depending upon the calibre and velocity of the missile, but the kinetic energy generated causes major abdominal wall defects as the projectile passes through the tissue. In blunt trauma, the sudden application of a large force to the contracted abdominal wall musculature over a fulcrum is similar to the force that is responsible for diaphragmatic disruptions. The 'seatbelt syndrome' resulting from an improperly positioned lap belt is well recognized. The force can disrupt the body of the rectus abdominous muscle, as well as the external and internal oblique muscles, or cause an avulsion of the abdominal musculature from the costophrenic arch or pubis. Uniquely associated with the seatbelt syndrome is a fracture of the posterior process and/or the body of the lumbar spine. This was described by Chance in 1948 (and the fracture now bears his name) and results from hyperflexion of the spine about a fixed axis anterior to the vertebral column. These flexion/distraction fractures are often associated with the 'seatbelt sign' (Fig. 1). The injury is thought to arise from flexion over a fulcrum (the lap belt) causing distraction of the posterior elements of the spine.

CLINICAL PRESENTATION

Associated injuries to the head, thoracic, and extremity injuries often occupy the diagnostic and therapeutic attention. Clinical evidence of an abdominal wall injury may be obvious, with evisceration after a penetrating wound (Fig. 2) or a contusion from an improperly applied seatbelt ('seatbelt sign'). These should warn the physician of potential intra-abdominal injuries. The patient may complain of localized abdominal wall pain and a defect in the fascia may be palpated. There is often an abdominal wall mass.

The pathology seen depends on aetiology and includes lacerations of the abdominal wall skin, subcutaneous tissue, fascia, and muscles, following penetrating injuries, or contusions, haematoma formation, disruption of subcutaneous fat and abdominal wall muscle, and herniation from blunt forces. Traumatic hernia of the abdominal wall has a specific diagnostic triad: immediate appearance of a hernia with intact skin after blunt abdominal trauma, signs of injury at the time of the initial medical evaluation, and no identifiable hernial sac at exploration.

Intra-abdominal viscera are injured in 30 to 50 per cent of patients suffering abdominal wall trauma. The blunt forces involved cause a sudden increase in intra-abdominal and intraluminal pressure, with disruption of hollow viscuses; shearing forces may damage the mesentery (Fig. 3).

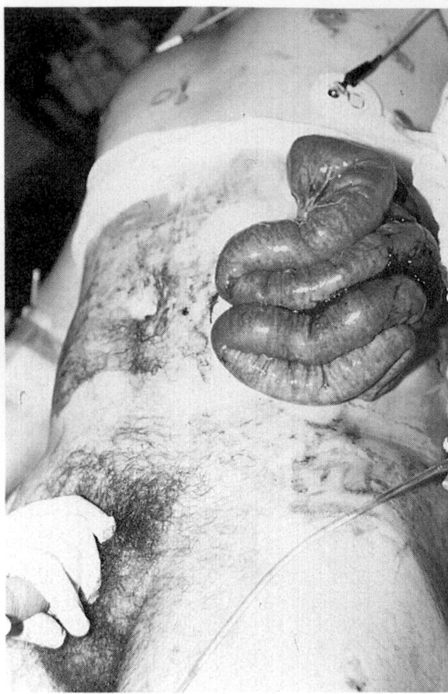

Fig. 2 The abdominal wall defect is obvious, resulting in the evisceration of several loops of small intestine. This occurred secondary to a stab wound of the abdomen.

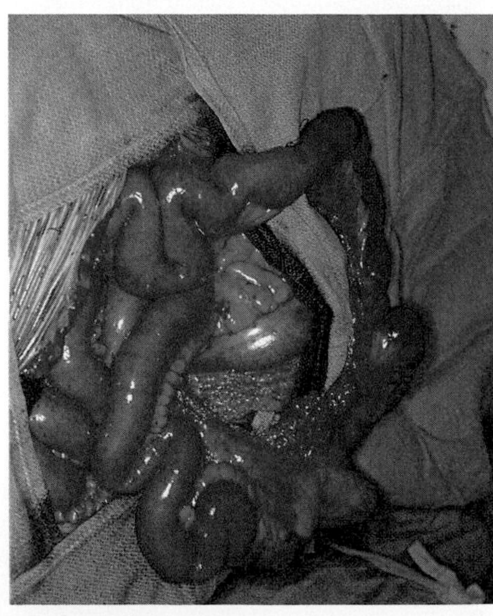

Fig. 3 Avulsion of the small bowel mesentery as the result of an acceleration/deceleration shearing force.

DIAGNOSIS

Diagnostic efforts are usually focused on the underlying intra-abdominal visceral injury. CT scan may reveal an abdominal wall defect with extrusion of small bowel. The hernia may present as an easily palpable anterior abdominal mass, but only become apparent during exploration of the abdomen.

THERAPY

The management of abdominal wall injuries should be a secondary consideration in the majority of patients. The evaluation and management of their associated and perhaps life-threatening injuries should be first priority.

Abdominal hernias should be repaired at the time of presentation, and this can normally be accomplished using non-absorbable suture (polypropylene, nylon). Rarely, the defect may be large and require a prosthetic graft to effect closure. The latter are normally hernias which have been neglected due to a delay in diagnosis. Injuries that result in tissue necrosis and significant contamination create enormous management problems and are fortunately rare. Contamination is a relative contraindication to the use of prosthetic material in closure of the abdominal wall, but this may be unavoidable.

Intra-abdominal visceral injuries are repaired, necrotic tissue is debrided, and the wound is vigorously irrigated. Appropriate antibiotics should be administered. If prosthetic grafts are required polytetrafluoroethylene has been successfully used and is reportedly resistant to infection.

Gunshot or shotgun wounds require local debridement, and large defects may be created as a result of tissue distribution. The defect should be required either primarily or as described for blunt trauma.

Sharp injuries to the abdominal wall are relatively simple to treat, with debridement of necrotic tissue and primary closure of the fascial edges. Polypropylene or nylon are an ideal closure material; drains are rarely indicated.

SUMMARY

Injuries to the abdominal wall are low on the list of priorities in the management of the patient with abdominal trauma. Local symptoms may make their presence more obvious, as will evisceration. Primary early repair is the ideal method of management. The presence of abdominal wall trauma should serve as a marker to alert the physician to the potential of injuries to the intra-abdominal viscera.

FURTHER READING

Appleby JP, Nagy AG. Abdominal injuries associated with the use of seatbelts. *Am J Surg* 1989; **157**: 457–8.

Asbun HJ, Irani H, Roe EJ, Bloch JH. Intraabdominal seatbelt injury. *J Trauma* 1990; **30**: 189–93.

Chance CQ. Note on a type of flexion fracture of the spine. *Br J Radiol* 1948; **21**: 452–3.

Dreyfuss DC, Flanchbaum L, Krasna IH, Tell B, Trooskin SZ. Acute transrectus traumatic hernia. *J Trauma* 1986; **26**: 1134–6.

Frykberg ER, Tepas JJ. Terrorist bombings: Lessons learned from Belfast to Beirut. *Ann Surg* 1988; **208**: 569–76.

Garrett JN, Braunstein PW. The seatbelt syndrome. *J Trauma* 1962; **2**: 220–38.

Guly HR, Stewart IP. Traumatic hernia. *J Trauma* 1983; **23**: 250–2.

Jones BV, Sanchez JA, Vinh D. Acute traumatic abdominal wall hernia. *Am J Emerg Med*, 1989; **7**: 667–8.

LeGay DA, Petrie DP, Alexander DI. Flexion distraction injuries of the lumbar spine and associated abdominal trauma. *J Trauma* 1990; **30**: 436–44.

Malangoni MA, Condon RF. Traumatic abdominal wall hernia. *J Trauma* 1983; **23**: 356–7.

Payne DD, Resnicoff SA, States JD. Seatbelt abdominal wall musculature avulsion. *J Trauma* 1973; **13**: 262–7.

Reid AB, Letts RM, Black GB. Pediatric chance fractures: association with intraabdominal injuries and seatbelt use. *J Trauma* 1990; **30**: 384–91.

26.2 Desmoid tumours

WILLIAM J. GALLAGHER

Desmoid tumours, also known as aggressive fibromatoses, are soft tissue neoplasms arising from musculoaponeurotic tissues. They belong to a family of fibroblastic proliferations that includes a variety of fibromatoses, as well as low-grade fibrosarcomas. These tumours are rare, a series of 44 patients treated for abdominal wall tumours being the largest reported. More than 75 per cent of these tumours arise in extra-abdominal sites, primarily the shoulder girdle, the inguinal area, and the lower extremities. Abdominal wall desmoids occur most commonly in women of child-bearing age during or shortly following pregnancy; they may be associated with scars from prior operations or trauma. The tumours are also seen in patients with familial polyposis coli (Gardner's syndrome), who may present with unresectable intra-abdominal tumours, as well as desmoid tumours at other sites. Desmoid tumours are often painless masses located deep in the abdominal wall, distinguishable in most situations from hernias or intra-abdominal masses by physical examination. They arise most commonly in the rectus abdominis muscles or the linea alba.

On microscopic examination, the tumours are composed of uniform, normal appearing fibroblasts distributed through dense collagenous stroma. Nuclei are thin and elongated; mitotic figures are seen typically in less than one per 50 high-power microscopic fields, and the fibroblastic component has neither the cellularity nor pleomorphism required for classification as low-grade fibrosarcoma. The lesions are never encapsulated. They insinuate themselves along fascial planes and muscle bundles in a fashion identical to that of sarcomas. The natural history of abdominal wall desmoid tumours is one of local progression with potential invasion of intra-abdominal structures, extremely rare pulmonary metastases, and multiple rapid local recurrences after excision: 80 per cent of recurrences develop within 2 years of excision. Because of the low incidence of dissemination, controversy regarding the inclusion of these lesions as bona fide sarcomas has existed for the last 50 years.

The diagnosis of desmoid tumour is confirmed by examination of a biopsy specimen. If the tumour is large or if there is a question of intra-abdominal extension or fixation to adjacent bony structures on physical examination, preoperative CT examination is useful. No search for distant metastases is necessary. If the lesion is less than 4 cm in diameter, excisional biopsy is appropriate. For larger lesions, incisional biopsy is preferred; evaluation of permanent sections of histological specimens to rule out sarcoma is then possible, and potential seeding of neoplastic cells along tissue planes for large distances as a result of a more extensive dissection is minimized. Haemostasis should be absolute. The biopsy incision should be placed so that it may be excised by a second, definitive excision.

Wide local excision of the tumour, which may require excision of the full thickness of the abdominal wall, is the operation of choice. Local recurrence rates are lower than for extra-abdominal tumours, ranging from 10 to 40 per cent. The rate increases with each recurrence. Although the presence of a pseudocapsule may give the surgeon a false sense of security when excising a presumably benign mass, tumour cells invariably extend beyond the grossly apparent tumour, making simple excisional biopsy a seemingly inadequate operation. There is, however, no clear correlation between margins of excision and local recurrence of these tumours: Posner found a highly significant correlation between the likelihood of local recurrence and the presence of inadequate or marginal excisions; on the other hand Reitamo *et al.* and Easter and Halasz found no such correlation. The lack of careful systematic evaluation of margins in most studies further confuses the issue. There is no correlation between tumour size and local recurrence rate. For tumours less than 5 cm in diameter, excision with a margin of 2 to 3 cm of grossly normal adjacent soft tissue is adequate, and primary closure of the abdominal wall is generally possible. The occult extension of larger tumours may be greater, and, if anatomically possible, a margin of excision approaching 5 cm should be considered. Synthetic materials or rotational flaps may be required to effect closure of the defect. Margins of excision should be carefully evaluated by the pathologist, and consideration given to additional therapy if excision of all gross tumour is not feasible. Recurrent tumours should be re-excised when the lesion can be resected grossly.

Radiation therapy to doses of 5000 to 6500 cGy is useful in controlling many unresectable tumours, producing complete responses, with long-term tumour control in 60 to 70 per cent of patients. Response to radiation is often slow and desmoid tumours may require 2 years to shrink. Since not all patients undergoing tumour excision with histologically positive margins suffer recurrence, postoperative radiation should be considered only when there is grossly evident residual tumour following an attempt at resection. For the postoperative patient with a small area of microscopically positive margin, careful follow-up and prompt treatment of recurrence with another excision or with radiation therapy is an effective alternative to adding radiation empirically.

A variety of hormonal, anti-inflammatory, and chemotherapeutic agents with acceptable toxicity have been evaluated on a very limited basis for therapy of desmoid tumours when surgery and radiotherapy are no longer options. Prolonged responses to therapy with vinblastine and methotrexate occurred in six of eight patients so treated; this regimen is currently the most active reported. Anecdotal responses have been seen to tamoxifen alone or in combination with indomethacin.

FURTHER READING

Easter DW, Halasz NA. Recent trends in the management of desmoid tumors: summary of 19 cases and review of the literature. *Ann Surg* 1989; **210**: 765 9.

Hardy JD. The ubiquitous fibroblast: multiple oncogenic potentials with illustrative cases. *Ann Surg* 1987; **205**: 445– 55.

Jones IT, Fazio VW, Weakley FL, Jagelman DG, Lavery IC, McGannon E. Desmoid tumors in familial polyposis coli. *Ann Surg* 1986; **204**: 94–7.

Kiel KD, Suit HD. Radiation therapy in the treatment of aggressive fibromatoses (desmoid tumors). *Cancer* 1984; **54**: 2051–5.

Leibel SA, Wara WM, Hill DR, *et al.* Desmoid tumors: local control and patterns of relapse following radiation therapy. *Int J Radiat Oncol Biol Phys* 1983; **9**: 1167–71.

Posner MC, Shiu MH, Newsome JL, Hajdu SI, Gaynor JJ, Brennan MF. The desmoid tumour: not a benign disease. *Arch Surg* 1989; **124**: 191–6.

Reitamo JJ, Scheinin TM, Hayry P. The desmoid syndrome; new aspects in the cause, pathogenesis, and treatment of desmoid tumors. *Am J Surg* 1986; **151**: 230–7.

Weiss AJ, Lackman. Low-dose chemotherapy of desmoid tumors. *Cancer* 1989; **64**: 1192–4.

26.3 The omentum

D. L. MCWHINNIE

TORSION OF THE OMENTUM

Torsion of the greater omentum is defined as a twist of the organ in its longitudinal axis around a narrow pedicle. It may be classified as primary or secondary.

Aetiology

In primary or idiopathic torsion, a redundant, mobile segment of omentum rotates around a proximal fixed point in the absence of any associated intra-abdominal pathology. This was first described by Eitel in 1899, but it remains a relatively rare condition, with fewer than 200 cases reported in the literature. Although the precise cause is unknown, both predisposing and precipitating factors in the pathogenesis of the condition can be identified.

Factors which predispose to torsion include anatomical abnormalities of the omentum itself, such as accessory omentum, bifid omentum, irregular accumulations of omental fat in the obese, and a narrowed omental pedicle. The normal anatomical arrangement of the omental vessels may also give rise to torsion. The omental veins are larger, longer, and more tortuous than the arteries and this redundancy allows venous kinking and obstruction, thereby providing a fixed point around which a self-perpetuating torsion may occur. The higher incidence of torsion on the right is related to the greater size and mobility of the right side of the omentum.

Factors that precipitate torsion are those which cause displacement of the omentum. These include blunt trauma to the abdomen, coughing and straining, heavy exertion, sudden change in body position, and hyperperistalsis from overeating.

Secondary torsion is more common than the primary type and is associated with pre-existing abdominal pathology. The omentum usually twists between two fixed points, with its distal edge attached directly or by adhesions to cysts, tumours, foci of intra-abdominal inflammation, postsurgical wounds or scarring, internal hernia, or external hernial sacs. The majority of cases occur in patients with inguinal herniae. The precipitating factors of primary torsion also initiate secondary torsion.

Pathology

The omentum twists a variable number of times around a pivotal point, usually in a clockwise direction. The venous return is compromised and the distal omentum becomes congested and oedematous. The resultant haemorrhagic extravasation stimulates an aseptic peritonitis with a characteristic accumulation of serosanguinous fluid in the peritoneal cavity. As the torsion proceeds, arterial occlusion leads to acute haemorrhagic infarction and eventual necrosis of the omental segment. If the mass is not excised it becomes atrophic and fibrotic and, on rare occasions, the pedicle may even auto-amputate.

Clinical features

Omental torsion usually occurs in the fourth or fifth decades of life. Men are affected twice as often as women and the majority of patients are overweight. The signs and symptoms reflect the underlying localized peritonitis. As the affected segment is usually on the right, the sudden onset of pain, with rebound tenderness and guarding is also usually right-sided, and is often mistaken for acute appendicitis or even acute cholecystitis or twisted ovarian cysts. The clinical features are not usually sufficient to allow an accurate preoperative diagnosis. This is of little consequence, as the clinical findings warrant laparotomy even in the absence of definitive diagnosis. The finding of free serosanguinous fluid in association with a normal appendix, gallbladder, pelvic organs, and bowel should alert the surgeon to the possibility of omental torsion.

Treatment

The condition only becomes clinically apparent once vascular thrombosis of the omental vessels has occurred and is irreversible even if the omentum is derotated. Treatment consists of resection of the affected portion of omentum. Any disease process associated with secondary torsion also requires correction. Although omental torsion is not life-threatening, segmental omentectomy reduces morbidity and removed inflammatory tissue which may later serve as a focus of intra-abdominal adhesions. Postoperative recovery is usually rapid and morbidity is minimal.

TUMOURS OF THE OMENTUM

Omental cysts

Pathology

Most cysts of the omentum are of lymphatic or mesothelial origin. All are rare.

Cystic lymphangioma

In childhood, omental cysts are usually caused by development abnormalities of lymphoid tissue, such as obstruction of lymphatic channels or by growth of congenitally misplaced lymphatic tissue. They are variously called chylous cysts, cystic hygromas, or cystic lymphangiomas, and are benign. They vary greatly in size, the smallest being only a few centimetres in diameter, and can be unilocular or multilocular. Histologically the cysts contain many foamy macrophages, giving the fluid a milky appearance, and each cyst has an endothelial lining similar to cystic hygroma of the neck.

Cystic mesothelioma

Omental cysts of mesothelial origin occur almost exclusively in adult life, usually in women under the age of 50 years. Although they are benign, local recurrence often occurs after surgical excision. They appear as large, multicystic masses similar to cystic lymphangiomas, but histologically they are lined by flattened or cuboidal mesothelial cells and the cyst fluid is clear, containing mucopolysaccharides. Although the aetiology is unknown there is no association with asbestos exposure.

Dermoid cysts

As with dermoid cysts elsewhere in the body, omental dermoid cysts are lined with squamous epithelium and may contain epithelial structures such as hair and teeth.

Pseudocysts

Omental pseudocysts are caused by fat necrosis or abdominal trauma with haematoma formation. They are lined with fibrous tissue and contain bloodstained fluid.

Clinical features and treatment

Many omental cysts are small and asymptomatic and may only be discovered incidentally at laparotomy or autopsy. Large cysts may present with diffuse abdominal distension or as a smooth, mobile, palpable mass in the lower midline. Characteristically they are non-tender unless complicated by torsion of the omentum or intestinal obstruction. Plain radiographs of the abdomen may demonstrate a soft tissue shadow and barium studies may show displacement of bowel. The differential diagnosis includes mesenteric, peritoneal, or retroperitoneal cysts and tumours, but the diagnosis is usually made at laparotomy. Treatment consists of surgical excision of the cyst.

Solid tumours of the omentum

Pathology

Secondary tumour

The vast majority of omental neoplasms are metastatic carcinomas arising from ovary, gastrointestinal tract, or pancreas, and these are often associated with abdominal ascites. The rare diffuse malignant mesothelioma of the peritoneum which is associated with exposure to fibrous minerals such as asbestos also consistently involves the omentum.

Primary tumour

Primary solid tumours of the omentum are exceptionally rare and may be benign or malignant. The majority are of smooth muscle origin and histologically may be of spindle-cell or epithelioid types. Malignant potential is difficult to predict from the histology but approximately one-third are frankly malignant. Before making a diagnosis of primary smooth muscle tumour of the omentum, leiomyosarcoma of the uterus or gastrointestinal tract giving rise to omental metastases must be carefully excluded. Other rare primary omental tumours include fibroma, fibrosarcoma, lipoma, and liposarcoma. Infantile myxoid hamartoma, found in infants under 1 year old, consists of multiple nodular lesions which show histological resemblance to myxoid liposarcoma; the clinical course is invariably benign.

Clinical features and treatment

Benign primary tumours of the omentum, when sufficiently large, present with a palpable abdominal mass or diffuse distension and require surgical excision. Malignant primary omental tumours are highly invasive and often present late with involvement of adjacent organs. Radical surgical excision of both the omentum and the involved organs may be required but often palliative surgery is the only treatment option.

FURTHER READING

Leitner MJ, Jordan CG, Spinner NH, Reese EC. Torsion, infarction and haemorrhage of the omentum as a cause of acute abdominal distress. *Ann Surg* 1952; **135**: 103–10.

Mainzer RA, Simoes A. Primary idiopathic torsion of the omentum. *Arch Surg* 1964; **88**: 974–83.

Morson BC, Dawson IMP, Day DW, Jass JR, Price AB, Williams GT. *Morson and Dawson's Gastrointestinal pathology*. 3rd edn. London: Blackwell, 1990.

Stout AP, Hendry J, Purdie FJ. Primary solid tumours of the great omentum. *Cancer* 1963; **16**: 231–43.

26.4 Mesenteric trauma

ALASDAIR K. T. CONN

INCIDENCE AND MECHANISM OF INJURY

Mesenteric injury occurs in 18 per cent of patients with penetrating abdominal injury and 5 per cent of those with blunt abdominal trauma. The latter figure has been substantiated by a recent review which reported 41 major mesenteric injuries in a population of 870 patients undergoing laparotomy for blunt abdominal trauma (4.7 per cent). Thirty-four patients had injury to the small bowel mesentery; 10 of these injuries involved the root, with disruption of either the superior mesenteric artery or vein. The colonic mesentery was damaged in seven patients and six of these injuries were in the right colon.

Mesenteric injury in blunt trauma arises from a shearing force (see Fig. 3, Section 26.1). In experimental animals the injury can be reproduced by compression between two opposing surfaces such as the abdominal wall and spine. In this animal model the site of injury cannot be related to the intraluminal pressure, the fixation of the bowel at the ligament of Treitz, or the presence or absence of air and fluid within the intestine. Such shearing forces can be generated not only by the traumatic incident itself but also by protective devices such as car safety belts during a sudden deceleration, especially if these are worn across the abdomen rather than across the bony pelvis. Experimentally, more severe intra-abdominal injuries are associated with higher abdominal compression loads.

DIAGNOSIS

Mesenteric injury is seldom diagnosed preoperatively: the injury tends to be found at exploratory laparotomy. The preoperative diagnosis of haemoperitoneum may be made from clinical findings, diagnostic peritoneal lavage, CT scan, or ultrasound and, in the adult population, this is an indication for surgical exploration. The patient with a bleeding mesenteric laceration has a clinical presentation of blood loss, hypotension, abdominal tenderness, a falling haematocrit, and abdominal distension. If pain is prominent, intestinal ischaemia should be suspected. It is the policy of the Massachusetts General Hospital that all penetrating gunshot wounds of the abdomen are explored; penetrating wounds from knives or similar objects entering the abdominal cavity are also explored, although some institutions advocate a selective approach.

All patients undergoing abdominal exploration for trauma require inspection of the entire length of the intestine as an integral part of operative management; a search should be made for mesenteric haematomas, tears in the mesentery and ischaemic bowel (Table 1).

MANAGEMENT

Mesenteric haematomas

Non-expanding haematomas and contusions of the mesentery should not be explored if the bowel is definitely viable. If a haematoma of the mesentery is expanding, proximal and distal control should be obtained and the haematoma explored. The management of injury to major intestinal vessels is out of the scope of this chapter.

If the haematoma appears to compromise intestinal viability, the surgeon needs to decide between resection and expectant observation; in the large bowel, exteriorization of the compromised section is an additional option. Intraoperative Doppler examination or intravascular injection of fluorescein may assist the surgeon in these difficult cases. A 'second look' should be considered, close re-examination of the bowel being performed within 24 h of the original laparotomy.

Mesenteric lacerations

If a laceration is actively bleeding, haemostasis should be obtained with artery forceps, after which sutures can be placed to preserve haemostasis, taking care not to compromise distal circulation and so avoiding intestinal ischaemia. Once haemostasis is obtained, the mesenteric defect should be closed using interrupted absorbable sutures. The defect may require both anterior and posterior surfaces to be closed, especially if the mesentery is thick, as in an obese patient. At the termination of the procedure, the viability of the bowel should be confirmed and noted in the operative record.

Mesenteric lacerations with devascularization

Following blunt trauma the mesenteric laceration may parallel the bowel and disrupt the arterial arcade, so that the surgeon at laparotomy will be presented with a bleeding mesentery and a section of ischaemic bowel, usually small intestine. In these patients there is no choice but to perform a bowel resection. After obtaining haemostasis, small bowel resection can be performed in one or two layers or with the use of a stapler. Once bowel continuity is restored, the surgeon should repair the mesenteric defect. The surgeon's options for treating ischaemic colon include resection with primary anastomosis, resection with colostomy (or ileostomy for an ischaemic right colon), mucus fistula, or Hartmann's pouch. If there is uncertainty, a segment of ischaemic colon can be exteriorized.

If there is a mesenteric injury and ischaemic bowel from a penetrating injury, the decision as to whether revascularization is to be attempted should be made soon after opening the abdomen. Issues such as the length of time that the bowel has been ischaemic, the mechanism of injury, the extent of other injuries, the length of bowel involved, and the likelihood of successful revascularization need to be considered.

COMPLICATIONS AND MISSED DIAGNOSIS

Complications following the repair of injured mesentery include bleeding, bowel ischaemia, and bowel obstruction. Bowel obstruction can arise from both adhesions or an internal hernia through a patent mesenteric defect. Continuing blood loss following laparotomy requires re-exploration to be performed. If there is concern over bowel viability, the patient should be re-explored within 24 h of initial surgery. A mesenteric defect that is either missed at laparotomy or inadequately repaired can serve as the site of an internal hernia with potentially fatal consequences; death may occur from septicaemia from a portion of gangrenous intestine.

SUMMARY

Mesenteric injury is common in both penetrating and blunt abdominal trauma. Although not often diagnosed preoperatively, surgeons should evaluate the mesentery as part of the trauma laparotomy; if appropriately managed, a cause of morbidity and even mortality may be avoided.

Table 1 Types of mesenteric injury

Types of injury	Abbreviated Injury Scale (1985 revision) rating
Haematoma within mesentery	2
Superficial tears of mesenteric peritoneum	2
Through and through lacerations of mesentery	3
Lacerations of mesentery; actively bleeding	3
Lacerations of mesentery with ischaemic bowel	4

FURTHER READING

American Association for Automotive Medicine. *The Abbreviated Injury Scale* (1985 revision). Illinois: American Association for Automotive Medicine, 1985.

Blaisdell FW. General assessment, resuscitation and exploration of penetrating and blunt abdominal trauma. In: *Trauma Management*, Vol. I, Abdominal trauma. New York: Thieme-Stratton Inc. 1982; 1–18.

Dauterive AH, Flancbaum L, Cox EF. Blunt intestinal trauma. *Ann Surg* 1985; **201**: 198–203.

McAlvanah MJ, Shaftan GW. Selective conservatism in penetrating abdominal wounds: A continuing reappraisal. *J Trauma* 1978; **18**: 206–12.

Miller MA. The biomechanical response of the lower abdomen to belt restraint loading. *J Trauma* 1989; **29**: 1571–84.

Williams RD, Sargent FT. The mechanism of intestinal injury in trauma. *J Trauma* 1963; **3**: 288–94.

Witte CL. Mesentery and bowel injury from automotive seat belts. *Ann Surg* 1968; **167**: 486–92.

26.5 Retroperitoneal fibrosis

DAVID CRANSTON

Retroperitoneal fibrosis was first clearly described by Albarran at the beginning of the century as 'stenosing periureteritis'. In 1902 he practised his operation of *libération externe*, designed to disengage the ureters from the scar tissue and fibrous masses that surrounded them. In 1948 Ormond described two patients with diffuse fibrosis of the retroperitoneal tissues, and established the clinical and pathological entity of idiopathic retroperitoneal fibrosis more clearly. An increasing number of causes of retroperitoneal fibrosis are now recognized and can be divided into benign and malignant.

BENIGN

Idiopathic retroperitoneal fibrosis, comprising two-thirds of the benign cases, is the best known of the group of fibrosing syndromes which include mediastinal fibrosis and sclerosing cholangitis. A dense plaque of fibrous tissue forms in the lower abdomen and extends laterally and downward from the renal arteries over the promontory of the sacrum, encasing, but not usually infiltrating, the hollow tubes, aorta, inferior vena cava, and ureters (Fig. 1). The central portion of the plaque consists of dense scar tissue, while the growing margins have the histological appearance of chronic inflammation, with a mixture of mononuclear cells interspersed with occasional giant cells and eosinophils. Idiopathic retroperitoneal fibrosis may occur in areas where the wall of the aorta or other arteries have severe atherosclerosis with damage of the media. When this occurs, insoluble lipid (ceroid) leaks into the periaortic tissue and induces an IgG-mediated immune response. Chronic periaortitis has been suggested as a more appropriate term for this condition (see Section 7.2).

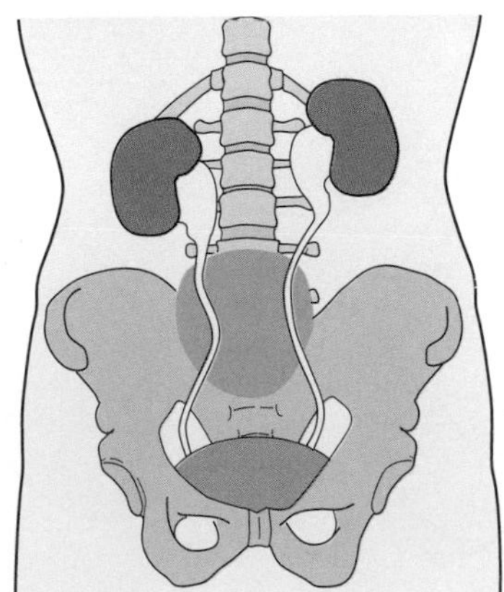

Fig. 1 The classical site of retroperitoneal fibrosis.

Idiopathic retroperitoneal fibrosis normally affects male patients in their fifth or sixth decade of life. One uncommon but well-recognized cause of this condition is the drug methysergide maleate which has been taken for migraine. Occasionally, long-standing urinary tract infections, especially with extravasation, can lead to retroperitoneal fibrosis, although extravasation in the absence of infection seldom leads to fibrosis. Haemorrhage into the retroperitoneal space from a leaking abdominal aortic aneurysm is said to be a cause of this condition, but this seems unlikely, and it is more probable that the association of abdominal aortic aneurysm with idiopathic fibrosis is due to an immune response to insoluble lipid.

MALIGNANT

The most common malignant tumour presenting as retroperitoneal is a lymphoma, and the diagnosis may be missed at laparotomy if a deep biopsy is not taken. Carcinoma of the breast, stomach, pancreas, colon, renal tract, and prostate, and carcinoid tumours may be associated with retroperitoneal fibrosis due to metastases. It may be difficult to identify the underlying metastatic tumour.

Radiotherapy in the treatment of cancer can also cause retroperitoneal fibrosis, although this is much less common today with more precise field localization before radiotherapy. Chemotherapy, especially following treatment of testicular tumours, may leave fibrous retroperitoneal masses which can involve the ureter. These may or may not contain residual tumour, and may require surgical removal.

CLINICAL PICTURE

The clinical picture may be associated with an underlying cause, such as an abdominal aortic aneurysm, or may be relatively nonspecific and include loss of appetite and weight, fever, sweating, and malaise. Hypertension may be present in up to 60 per cent of cases, and pyuria is a common finding. A girdle distribution of pain in the abdomen may be described. Classically the erythrocyte sedimentation rate is high. The major complication of retroperitoneal fibrosis is ureteric obstruction which, if bilateral, can lead to anuria and renal failure.

MANAGEMENT

If the patient is unwell due to renal failure, the obstruction can be relieved by double J stents, passed in either an antegrade or retrograde fashion, or nephrostomies if unsuccessful. In this situation it is important to watch for and correct the loss due to diuresis after relief of the obstruction. Once the immediate urgency of the situation has been resolved, there is time to find the underlying cause.

The classic appearance on the intravenous urogram or antegrade pyelogram is that of medical displacement of the ureters with dilatation of the ureter and pelvis above (Fig. 2). Ultrasound examination may demonstrate the fibrous plaque as an echo-free mass with smooth borders, thickest at the sacral promontory. Both computerized tomography scanning and magnetic resonance imaging can define the area of fibrosis precisely (Fig. 3). Fine-needle biopsy of the mass may be helpful in confirming the presence of malignant disease, but a negative result does not exclude malignancy.

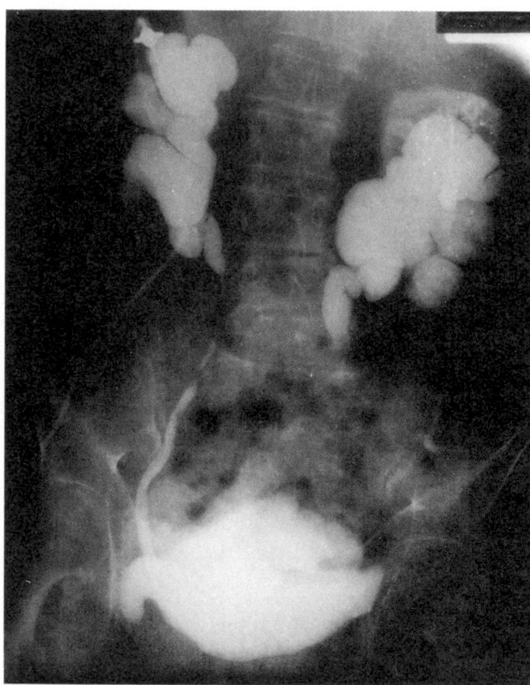

Fig. 2 Antegrade pyeolgram showing medial deviation of the ureter with obstruction.

The role of steroids remains a subject of debate. They may decrease the oedema often associated with retroperitoneal fibrosis and in this way help in resolution of the obstruction. If they are used, it is probably wise to terminate the steroids when the erythrocyte sedimentation rate returns to normal. Spontaneous resolution of retroperitoneal fibrosis in the absence of treatment is known to occur.

Laparotomy is often necessary to free the ureters from the encasing fibrous tissue. At the same time, biopsies should be taken to exclude an underlying malignant process. It is essential that large deep biopsies are taken for this purpose as it is very difficult to exclude malignancy with small, superficial biopsies. In patients who are unwell, or have one non-functioning kidney, it may be better to operate on only one side rather than both.

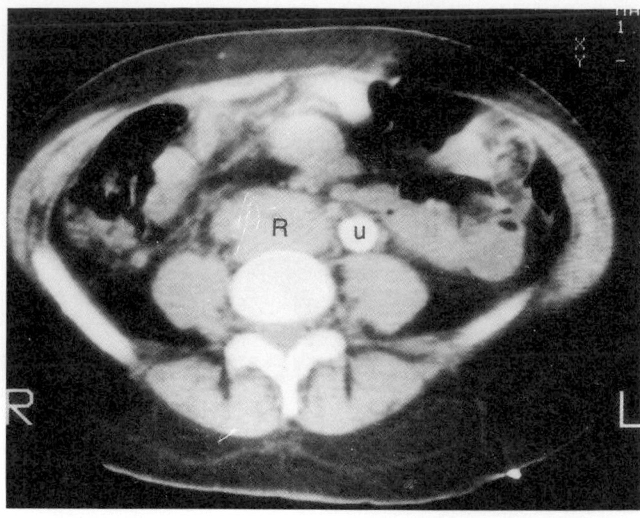

Fig. 3 Computerized tomography, showing retroperitoneal fibrosis (R) surrounding the aorta and inferior vena cava with ureteric obstruction (U).

In the presence of renal dysfunction, ureterolysis is performed. With care, a plane can usually be found between the ureters and fibrous tissue. It is often easier to begin just above the bladder, as the ureter is usually free at this point and, as the plaque is entered, a plane can be found between the ureter and the plaque. It is often helpful to place a sling around the ureter, and insert a right-angle

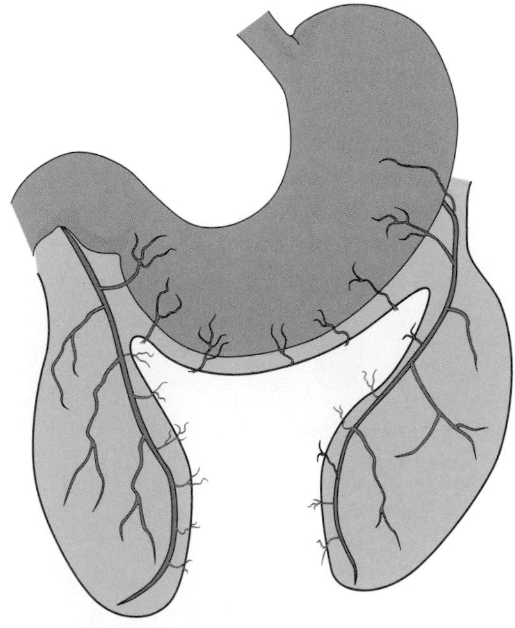

Fig. 4 Mobilization of the omentum before wrapping around the ureters.

forceps between the plaque and the ureter, and then cut down on to the forceps with a scalpel. The insertion of a stent or ureteric catheter up the ureter helps to identify it. Great care must be taken on the right-hand side to avoid damage to the inferior vena cava, which is often very difficult to identify in the inflammatory fibrotic mass of tissue.

After freeing the ureters from the fibrous sheath which surrounds them, omentum can be mobilized and used to wrap the ureters throughout their length, thus keeping them free of fibrous tissue (Fig. 4). In mobilizing the omentum, it must be remembered that the blood supply runs vertically down the gastroepiploic arch, and the majority of the blood to the arch comes from the right side. While wrapping the ureters in omentum does not guarantee freedom from recurrent obstruction, it seems to be better than other techniques.

Rarely, dense fibrosis is restricted to the lower ureters, and it is possible to reimplant a normal ureter into the bladder with a psoas hitch or Boari flap. Occasionally, long strictures form after the initial ureterolysis, and these may have to be treated by more specialized techniques, such as renal autotransplantation.

FURTHER READING

Albarran J. Retention renale par periureterité; libération externe de l'uretere. *Assoc France Urol* 1905; **9**: 511–17.

Baker LRI, *et al.* Idiopathic retroperitoneal fibrosis. A retrospective analysis of 60 cases. *Br J Urol* 1988; **60**: 497–503.

Charlton CAC. The use of steroids in a form of retroperitoneal fibrosis. *Proc Roy Soc Med* 1968; **61**: 875–6.

Degesys GE, Dunnick NR, Sivlerman PM, Cohan RH, Illescas FF, Castagno A. Retroperitoneal fibrosis: use of CT in distinguishing among possible causes. *Am J Roentgenol 1986;* **146**: 57–60.

Mikkelsen D, Lepor H. Innovative surgical management of idiopathic retroperitoneal fibrosis. *J Urol* 1989; **141**: 1192–6.

Mitchinson MJ. Retroperitoneal fibrosis revisited. *Arch Pathol Lab Med* 1986; **110**: 784–6.

O'Flynn D. Retroperitoneal fibrosis. In: McDougal WS, ed. *Rob and Smith's Operative Surgery (Urology)*. 4th edn. London: Butterworths, 1986: 243–54.

Ormond JK. Bilateral ureteral obstruction due to envelopment and compression by an inflammatory retroperitoneal process. *J Urol* 1948; **59**: 1072–9.

Suby HI, Kerr WS, Graham JR, Fraley E. Retroperitoneal fibrosis: a missing link in the chain of pathogenesis. *J Urol* 1965; **93**: 144–52.

Tresidder GC, Blandy JP, Singh M. Omental sleeve to prevent recurrent retroperitoneal fibrosis around the ureter. *Urol Int* 1972; **27**: 144–8.

Yuh WTC, Barloon TJ, Sickels WJ, Kramolowsky EV, Williams RD. Magnetic resonance imaging in the diagnosis and follow up of idiopathic retroperitoneal fibrosis. *J Urol* 1989; **141**: 602–5.

26.6 Retroperitoneal neoplasms

HERBERT C. HOOVER

INTRODUCTION

The retroperitoneum is a large potential space bounded anteriorly by the posterior peritoneum, posteriorly by the spine and back muscles, superiorly by the diaphragm, inferiorly by the levators, and laterally by the flank muscles at the level of the anterior superior spine of the iliac crest to the tip of the twelfth rib. In this vast potential space, retroperitoneal masses tend to become very large before producing signs or symptoms, thus accounting for the poor prognosis overall for malignant tumours arising there. Although the pancreas, kidneys, ureters, and adrenals are retroperitoneal structures, neoplasms of these organs are not generally included in the analysis of retroperitoneal neoplasms and will not be considered in this section. With rare exceptions, retroperitoneal neoplasms are sarcomas, lymphomas, or benign lesions. Lymphomas and benign tumours will be discussed only in terms of their differentiation from sarcomas, which will be the focus of our discussion. Retroperitoneal sarcomas are rare, representing only about 0.1 to 0.2 per cent of all malignancies overall and only about 10 to 15 per cent of all soft tissue sarcomas. They represent approximately 40 per cent of all retroperitoneal masses.

CLASSIFICATION OF RETROPERITONEAL NEOPLASMS

Most retroperitoneal tumours are of mesodermal origin and both benign and malignant tumours arising from every different tissue represented are seen, such as: adipose, lipoma and liposarcomas; smooth muscle, leiomyoma and leiomyosarcoma; connective tissue, fibroma and fibrosarcoma; striated muscle, rhabdomyoma and rhabdomyosarcoma; lymph vessels, lymphangioma and lymphangiosarcoma; lymph nodes, nodal hyperplasia and lymphoma; blood vessels, haemangiomas and haemangiosarcoma, or benign and malignant haemangiopericytoma. Benign and malignant tumours may also originate from the nervous system, including nerve sheath tumours such as non-encapsulated fibroma, encapsulated neurilemoma, or malignant schwannoma. Tumours arising from the sympathetic system include ganglioneuroma, sympathicoblastoma, or neuroblastoma. Rarely, tumours may arise from heterotopic adrenocortical and chromaffin tissue, such as carcinomas arising from adrenocortical tissue, malignant non-chromaffin paraganglioma, paraganglioma, and phaeochromocytoma. Urogenital ridge tumours are rare, as are tumours arising from embryonic remnants, such as benign and malignant teratomas and chordomas. At least eight cases of retroperitoneal synovial sarcomas have been reported. Primary tumours in virtually any organ can metastasize to the retroperitoneum, metastatic testicular carcinoma being common. Benign cysts also occur in the retroperitoneum, as they do in all other body cavities.

HISTOLOGY OF RETROPERITONEAL SARCOMAS

The histological types of retroperitoneal sarcomas seen most commonly in several major series are listed in Table 1. Malignant fibrous histiocytoma is being diagnosed with increasing

Table 1 Histological types of retroperitoneal sarcoma (composite of four major series—(294 cases)

Histological type	Number seen	Percentage of total
Liposarcoma	92	31
Leiomyosarcoma	70	24
Fibrosarcoma	33	11
Rhabdomyosarcoma	23	8
Neurofibrosarcoma	22	7
Miscellaneous	21	7
Malign fibrous histiocytosis	15	5
Spindle-cell carcinoma	7	2
Haemangiopericytoma	6	2
Synovial sarcoma	5	2

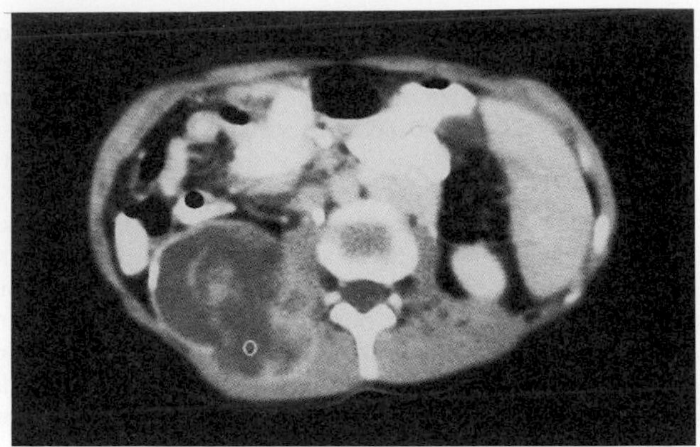

Fig. 1 CT scan of left retroperitoneal sarcoma with invasion into paraspinal muscles.

frequency, probably because of a better understanding of the histopathology of the tumour and the reclassification of many tumours previously diagnosed as pleomorphic variants of liposarcoma, fibrosarcoma, or rhabdomyosarcoma. Histological grade is of more prognostic significance than the cell of origin. Mesodermally derived tumours of different embryonic origin tend to behave in a similar biological fashion, but manifest increasingly aggressive behaviour clinically as they become less differentiated or assume a higher tumour grade. National Cancer Institute (USA) grading uses a composite of histopathological parameters that include necrosis, cellularity, pleomorphism, and mitosis. Each histological type has a spectrum of biological behaviour. Some tumours exhibit a narrow spectrum such as prolonged benign course (e.g. myxoid liposarcoma) but others such as synovial sarcomas are consistently aggressive and are always attributed a Grade 3 (highest grade). The degree of necrosis has the strongest predictive value for overall survival: prognosis is worse as the percentage of necrosis increases. All of these grading criteria are probably more applicable to soft tissue sarcomas in sites other than the retroperitoneum, where even low-grade lesions respond poorly to treatment, presumably because of their large size at presentation and the difficulty in achieving wide surgical margins on excision.

CLINICAL PRESENTATION

Unless found incidentally during a laparotomy or on a CT scan, retroperitoneal sarcomas are usually large at presentation. Physical signs are few, other than a palpable abdominal or pelvic mass, which is seen in 50 to 75 per cent of patients.

DIAGNOSTIC EVALUATION

CT scanning has revolutionized the investigation of patients with suspected retroperitoneal neoplasms and, if performed using radiographic contrast media may be the only study other than a chest radiograph that is needed preoperatively. Size and anatomical changes secondary to tumour growth are easily visualized and tumour invasion of adjacent organs can be demonstrated or suggested. CT scanning is, however, not useful in predicting the histological type or grade of soft tissue sarcomas. Most tumours in the retroperitoneum appear as soft tissue masses containing focal areas of necrosis (Fig. 1). If fatty elements are obvious, a diagnosis of liposarcoma is possible but differentiation from a benign lipoma is uncertain. CT scanning cannot reliably distinguish between retroperitoneal lymphomas and sarcomas: although lymphomas tend to be homogeneous on CT scanning and often envelope the inferior vena cava and aorta, while sarcomas are usually heterogeneous, these findings are unreliable.

The functional state of at least one kidney must be demonstrated by either an intravenous contrast CT scan or an excretory urogram because the *en bloc* resection of one kidney is often required for curative resections. Although upper gastrointestinal series and a barium enema study often demonstrate displacement or even invasion, these findings are easily demonstrated at laparotomy, and thus these imaging studies are usually unnecessary. It is not unreasonable to obtain a CT scan of the lungs, although pulmonary metastases are unusual at the time of presentation of retroperitoneal sarcomas. Arteriography is helpful in showing the extent of the lesion and the tumour's blood supply; it often reveals displacement of major vessels and should be performed in virtually all patients with extensive lesions. A 'flush' aortogram is usually obtained first, followed by selective arterial injections as indicated. Findings suggestive of neoplasia include neovascularity, venous lakes, tumour blush, and vessel encasement. Because malignant fibrous histiocytoma tends to occur in the renal area, the demonstration of an extrarenal arterial supply is helpful in deciding to save the kidney. A dominant lumbar or intercostal arterial supply adds to the likelihood that the tumour has a retroperitoneal origin. If the arterial supply is coeliac, or inferior or superior mesenteric, an intraperitoneal origin is likely, but retroperitoneal tumours are often supplied partially by the superior mesenteric artery or inferior mesenteric artery. Unfortunately, vascularity correlates poorly with the histological type and cannot reliably differentiate between benign and malignant tumours. Invasion and obstruction of arteries is rare, although veins, especially the vena cava, are more vulnerable. An inferior vena cavagram can be helpful in assessing tumour invasion of the vena cava and/or renal veins.

OPERATIVE CONSIDERATIONS

Percutaneous needle biopsies have little place in determining a histological diagnosis and may compromise a curative resection. All patients should undergo a full bowel preparation, because a limited resection of the colon or rectum is commonly required and an ample supply of banked blood should be on hand. Absence of metastatic disease must be assured.

A limited midline incision is usually best for the initial exploration; this should be placed directly over the centre of the mass so that it can be extended readily in either direction. If the tumour is in the upper retroperitoneum towards or invading the diaphragm, a thoracoabdominal approach may be indicated. The retroperitoneal or flank approach is less satisfactory than is an abdominal incision in allowing the surgeon to perform an *en bloc* resection of involved organs or to control the major arteries and veins supplying the tumour. The abdominal portion of the incision is opened first for the exploration to determine resectability and a careful search for hepatic or peritoneal metastases is performed. Assuming that biopsy of the tumour has not previously been performed, the surgeon has to decide whether or not a histological diagnosis is necessary. Incisional wedge biopsies should be obtained only from patients who have obviously technically inoperable disease or in patients in whom lymphoma is suspected. A retroperitoneal biopsy carries the risk of contaminating the entire peritoneal cavity and retroperitoneal space, potentially negating any chance for cure. Great care must be taken to isolate the area of biopsy and to obtain absolute haemostasis and a secure closure of the incision into the tumour.

Localized tumours, even those which are huge, should be completely removed to provide both biopsy material and ensure the most effective primary therapeutic approach. This should include an *en bloc* resection of involved organs, most commonly the kidney, tail of pancreas, or colon, the border of resection being well beyond the visible limits of the tumour whenever possible. The apparent encapsulation is usually a pseudocapsule containing normal as well as neoplastic cells. The surgeon must resist the temptation to remove the tumour from its pseudocapsule if a curative resection is the intent: although such dissection is often quite easy, recurrence is almost certain. Retroperitoneal sarcomas are often fixed as they invade muscles of the posterior parietal wall, which are themselves immobile. Fixation is not a sign of unresectability unless there is extensive involvement of irreplaceable or unremovable structures. The majority of these tumours become totally resectable with persistent dissection, though wide margins are usually not possible. Adequate drainage of the large space resulting from the resection using a closed drainage system is important.

Lymphomas tend to be more diffuse, in which case a limited biopsy specimen should be taken, and the margins of the tumour should be marked by clips. Rarely, localized lymphomas can be totally resected. It is more acceptable to resect totally what proves to be a lymphoma than to biopsy a potential sarcoma with the attendant risk of seeding. Surgical judgement is critical here. Unfortunately, the rarity of these tumours means that few surgeons have much experience in this evaluation.

RESULTS OF THERAPY

Resection rate

The resection rate varies considerably depending upon the outlook of the surgeon, but is usually about 50 per cent (Table 2). Liposarcomas and neurogenic sarcomas have the highest complete resection rate, and leiomyosarcomas are consistently the least resectable.

Table 2 Resectability and survival in retroperitoneal sarcoma

Series	Total no. of cases/no. resected (%)	Total 5-year survival (%)
UCLA (1981)	54/33 (61%)	
Memorial (1981)	158/77 (49%)	40
MCV (1984)	47/18 (38%)	50
Roswell Rark (1985)	68/27 (40%)	64
NCI (1985)	37/37 (100%)	38
Fort Sam Houston (1986)	20(7) (35%)	43
Sweden (1988)	32(16) (50%)	46
Minnesota (1989)	50(31) (62%)	48
Mean	(54%)	(47%)

Extent of resection

Resection of adjacent organs is commonly necessary for complete removal of retroperitoneal sarcomas and is required in up to 73 per cent of patients. Kidney and adrenal are the most commonly resected organs, followed by colon, pancreas, and small bowel.

Operative mortality

Several recent series report no deaths in the resection of retroperitoneal sarcomas. The mortality rate should be less than 5 per cent with modern anaesthesia and support.

Operative morbidity

Morbidity is obviously dependent upon the extent of resection and the adjacent organs resected. Common problems are related to small bowel and colonic ileus, small-bowel perforation, fistulae, and intra-abdominal abscess.

Survival

Interpretation of survival in the reported series (Table 2) is difficult. Scant data relative to histological grade and stage are usually given, the numbers of patients are generally small, and the follow-up period often short. However, some conclusions are obvious. Complete resection offers the only hope for long-term survival. Figure 2 shows the dramatic difference in survival between those patients with low and high grade sarcomas treated at Memorial Hospital in New York between 1971 and 1977.

Unfortunately, survival intervals even in patients whose sarcomas are totally resected continue to decline beyond 15 years, showing that retroperitoneal sarcomas are rarely totally cured. Recurrences are eventually seen in 70 to 80 per cent of patients: these are often in the original tumour bed and are often resectable. In the University of California, Los Angeles series, as in most, 85 per cent of the recurrences were local, and metastases occurred in only 15 per cent of patients—primarily to liver and/or lungs. Some series have reported up to seven re-excisions of the same tumour, producing long-term survival in spite of a very low eventual cure rate. Tumours often become less differentiated and more aggressive with each recurrence, with shorter tumour-free intervals.

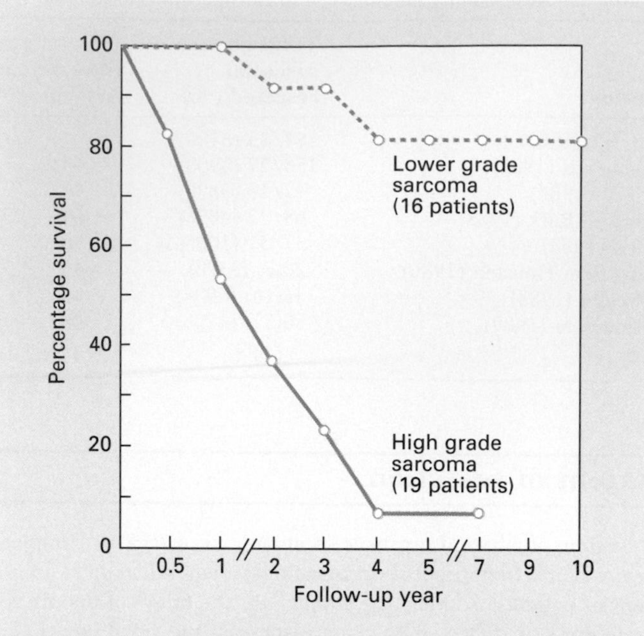

Fig. 2 Survival according to histological grade of 35 patients with retroperitoneal sarcoma (1971–77) following complete excision.

Role of chemotherapy

There is no evidence to suggest that chemotherapy used as an adjuvant to total surgical resection is of any benefit. It cannot be recommended outside of a clinical trial. Multiple drug chemotherapy (usually including Adriamycin) is usually recommended, but is of questionable benefit.

ROLE OF RADIATION THERAPY

The most important factor in obtaining long-term local control and disease-free survival is the complete resection of the tumour, although this produces a low likelihood of long-term tumour control. Essentially all series reporting good local control have employed high dose radiation following total resection. In the Massachusetts General Hospital series a dose of at least 6000 cGy was required for control. Adjuvant radiation therapy is recommended for all patients with Grade II or III sarcoma that is totally resectable. The role of intraoperative radiation therapy is being investigated. Combined radiotherapy and CT is more commonly used for patients with unresectable disease.

SUMMARY

Retroperitoneal neoplasms are rare but are most commonly sarcomas, lymphomas, or benign lesions. They usually reach a large size before presenting with a palpable abdominal or pelvic mass or with abdominal or back pain, often with weight loss and vague gastrointestinal symptoms. Of the sarcomas, liposarcomas are reported most often in the retroperitoneum, but malignant fibrous histiocytosis has been diagnosed with increasing frequency since its description. An abdominal and/or pelvic CT scan is the most important evaluation in planning resection, which is the only potentially curative therapy for retroperitoneal sarcomas. An arteriogram and inferior vena cavagram may also be helpful. An abdominal approach is usually advised for large retroperitoneal tumours to allow for the *en bloc* resection of involved adjacent organs and achieve optimum control of the major arterial and venous supply of the tumour. Potentially curable lesions should be radically resected and not removed from their pseudocapsule. Unfortunately, only about 50 per cent of tumours are resectable, and nearly 75 per cent require resection of adjacent organs. Operative mortality should be less than 5 per cent and morbidity rates should be low. Survival is dependent primarily upon the grade of malignancy and the stage with a 50 per cent 5-year survival overall. Unfortunately, nearly 80 per cent of patients eventually suffer a recurrence, but they may benefit from repeated resections. Adjuvant chemotherapy has no role outside of a controlled clinical trial. Adjuvant irradiation is probably of benefit but requires more definitive trials.

FURTHER READING

Bolin TE, Bolin SG, Wetterfors J. Retroperitoneal sarcomas. *Acta Chir Scand* 1988; **154**: 627–9.

Braasch JW, Mon AB. Primary retroperitoneal tumors. *Surg Clin N Am* 1967; **47**: 663–78.

Cody HS, Turnbull AD, Fortner JG, Hajdu SI. The continuing challenge of retroperitoneal sarcomas. *Cancer* 1981; **42**: 2147–52.

Costa J, Wesley RA, Glatstein E, Rosenberg SA. The grading of soft tissue sarcomas. Results of a clinicohistopathologic correlation in a series of 163 cases. *Cancer* 1984; **55**: 531–41.

Fortner JG, Martin S, Hajdu S, Turnbull A. Primary sarcoma of the retroperitoneum. *Semin Oncol* 1981; **8**: 180–4.

Glenn J, Sindelar WF, Kinsella T, *et al.* Results of multimodality therapy of resectable soft-tissue sarcomas of the retroperitoneum. *Surgery* 1985; **97**: 316–24.

Karakousis CP, Velez AF, Emrick LJ. Management of retroperitoneal sarcomas and patient survival. *Am J Surg* 1985; **150**: 376–80.

Karp W, Hafstrom LO, Jonsson PE. Retroperitoneal sarcoma: ultrasonographic and angiographic evaluation. *Br J Radiol* 1980; **53**: 525–31.

Kinsella TJ, Sindelar WF, Lack E, Glatstein E, Rosenberg SA. Preliminary results of a randomized study of adjuvant radiation therapy in resectable adult retroperitoneal soft tissue sarcomas. *J Clin Oncol* 1988; **6**: 618–25.

McGrath PC, *et al.* Improved survival following complete excision of retroperitoneal sarcomas. *Ann Surg* 1984; **200**: 200–4.

Neifeld JP, Walsh JW, Lawrence W. Computer tomography in the management of soft tissue tumors. *Surg Gynecol Obstet* 1982; **155**: 1–6.

Storm FK, Eilber FR, Mirra J, Morton DL. Retroperitoneal sarcomas: a reappraisal of treatment. *J Surg Oncol* 1981; **17**: 1–7.

Tepper JE, Suit HD., Wood WC, Proppe KH, Harmon D, McNulty P. Radiation therapy of retroperitoneal soft tissue sarcomas. *Int J Radiat Oncol Biol Phys* 1984; **10**: 825–9.

Solla JA, Reed K. Primary retroperitoneal sarcomas. *Am J Surg* 1986; **152**: 496–8.

Wist E, Solheim QP, Jacobsen AB, Blom P. Primary retroperitoneal sarcomas. *Acta Radiol* 1985; **24**: 305–10.

Zhang G, Chen KK, Manivel C, Fraley EE. Sarcomas of the retroperitoneum and genitourinary tract. *J Urol* 1989; **141**: 1107–10.

27 Endoscopy of the alimentary tract

27.1 Upper gastrointestinal endoscopy

PAUL C. SHELLITO

INTRODUCTION

Oesophagogastroduodenoscopy is useful for the diagnosis and treatment of upper gastrointestinal diseases. Endoscopy is more expeditious, sensitive, and specific than are barium radiographic studies, especially for superficial conditions such as oesophagitis and gastritis and for investigating gastrointestinal bleeding. Biopsy specimens may be obtained during endoscopy, further increasing its diagnostic value. In addition, therapeutic manoeuvres are possible with oesophagogastroduodenoscopy, especially staunching upper gastrointestinal bleeding, placing gastrostomy tubes, removing foreign bodies, and treating benign and malignant oesophageal strictures. Endoscopic retrograde cholangiopancreatography (ERCP) is a special type of upper gastrointestinal endoscopy specifically designed to assess the pancreaticobiliary system. In addition to the exquisite diagnostic power of ERCP, therapeutic manoeuvres such as removal of biliary stones and placement of tubular endoprostheses for palliation of malignant obstruction are possible. ERCP is considered in Section 16.2.1.

As discussed in Section 27.3, surgeons should perform endoscopy. Especially in cases of gastric ulcer or upper gastrointestinal bleeding, if surgery becomes necessary the plan for operation greatly depends upon the specific findings at oesophagogastroduodenoscopy. This information should preferably be first-hand.

Opportunities for therapeutic upper gastrointestinal endoscopy are growing. Surgeon endoscopists are most likely to make impartial choices between open surgery and endoscopic treatment. By temperament and training they are best equipped to perform endoscopic surgery and to deal with the possible complications.

EQUIPMENT AND PROCEDURE

An upper gastrointestinal endoscope is a thin flexible instrument, usually 100 cm long. An image is transmitted from the tip by either a fibreoptic bundle to the lens on the head of the scope or by a tiny video camera on the tip to a television screen. The end can be deflected in a wide arc by manipulating two steering knobs on the endoscopic head. There is a tiny air insufflation channel to produce stomach distension for inspection. Through this channel automatic water lavage of the scope tip may also be carried out to keep debris from obscuring the view. Another larger channel (and sometimes two) is available for suction or for passing instruments (biopsy forceps, grasping forceps, cytology brush, snare, injection needle, cauterizing probe, laser fibre).

The patient must have an empty stomach; nothing by mouth for 6 h beforehand is usually sufficient. Pharyngeal anaesthesia to blunt the gag reflex is achieved with benzocaine or lidocaine spray or gargle. Usually, the patient is also given intravenous sedation (narcotic and benzodiazepine) and is monitored during the procedure with blood pressure determinations, electrocardiography, and pulse oximetry.

To begin oesophagogastroduodenoscopy, most endoscopists place the patient on his or her left side, hold the instrument in the left hand, and alternately manipulate the scope controls and shaft with the right hand (or have an assistant manipulate the endoscope shaft). It is better to place the instrument in a bracket or chest harness, liberating the left hand to hold the shaft and the right hand to control the tip deflection knobs and instruments in the biopsy channel. The ability to control tip and shaft movements simultaneously gives facile and versatile operation, especially for endoscopic surgery. After placing a bite block between the patient's teeth, the endoscope is inserted into his or her mouth. The tongue is followed down to its base where the upper larynx can be seen (Fig. 1). The oesophagus is best entered under direct

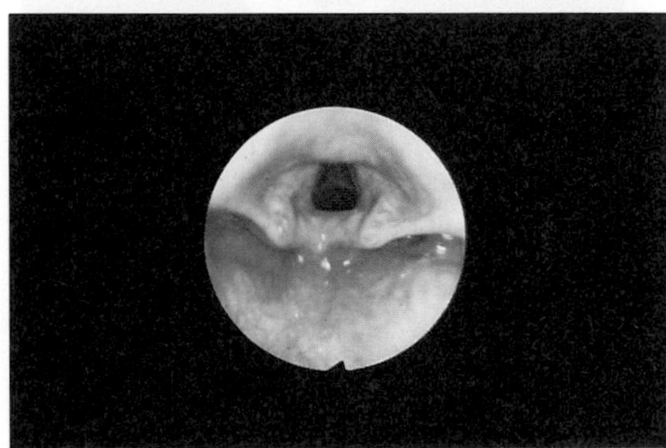

Fig. 1 Normal larynx seen at initial endoscope insertion.

vision; the scope is guided posterior to the arytenoid cartilages, where the view becomes obscured by the contracted cricopharyngeus muscle. While maintaining gentle pressure against the muscle with the scope, the patient is asked to swallow. This manoeuvre allows ready passage of the instrument into the upper oesophagus. If not, one should back up into the posterior pharynx, suction out any saliva with the scope, and try once more after the patient catches his breath. Keeping the gut lumen in the centre of the field of view (Fig. 2) the operator advances the scope distally with deflection of the tip and twisting of the shaft as necessary. Once in the stomach it is best to stay oriented by twisting the scope

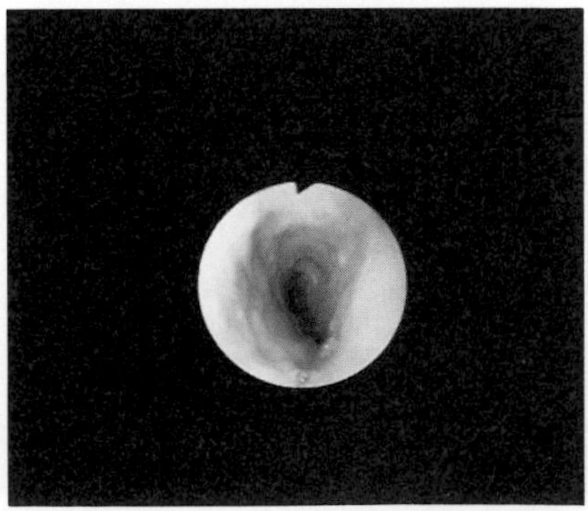

Fig. 2 Endoscopic view of the oesophagus.

(usually counter-clockwise at this point) so that the lesser gastric curvature lies at 12 o'clock with respect to the endoscopic view. Prominent rugae are visible in the gastric body (Fig. 3) and fundus, whereas the antral mucosa is rather flat (Fig. 4). The scope is then passed into the duodenum. Sometimes a moment of pressure with the instrument tip is required before the pylorus (Fig. 5) relaxes enough to permit the scope to traverse it. Care must be taken not to slip too quickly through the bulb (Fig. 6); a proximal lesion (just beyond the pylorus) can be missed.

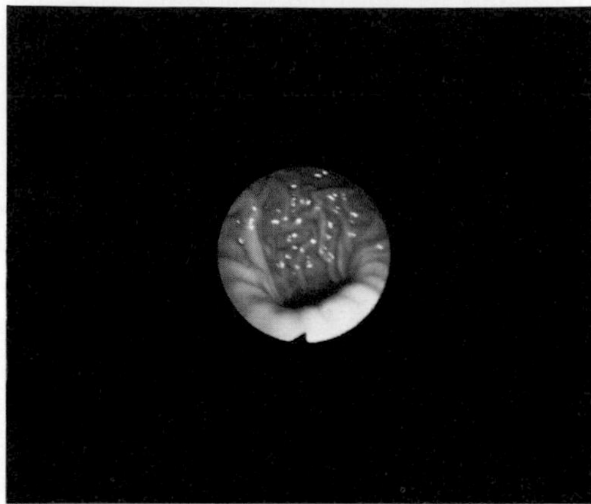

Fig. 3 Gastric body, with typical rugal folds.

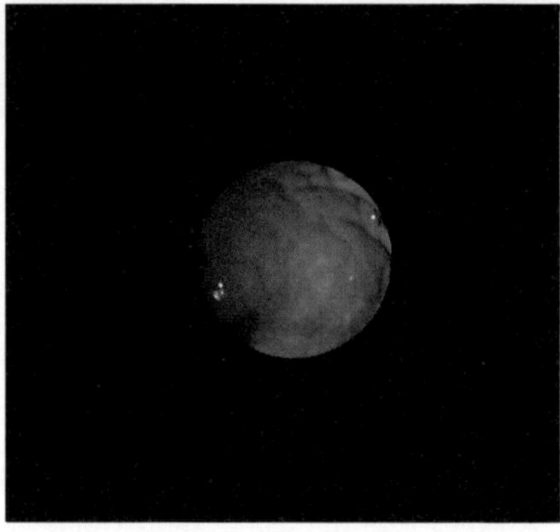

Fig. 4 Gastric antrum, which normally displays rather smooth mucosa.

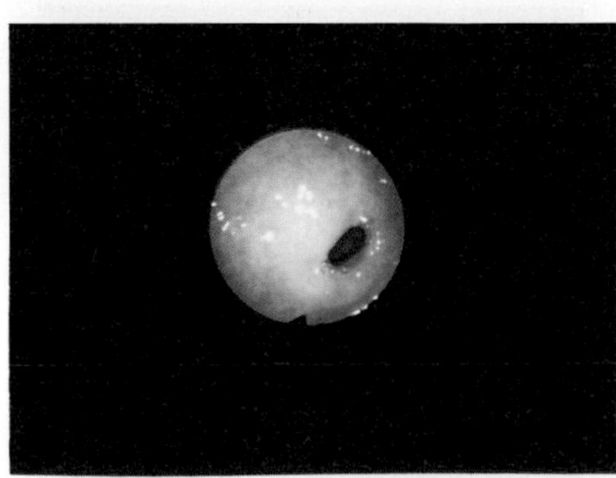

Fig. 5 Pylorus.

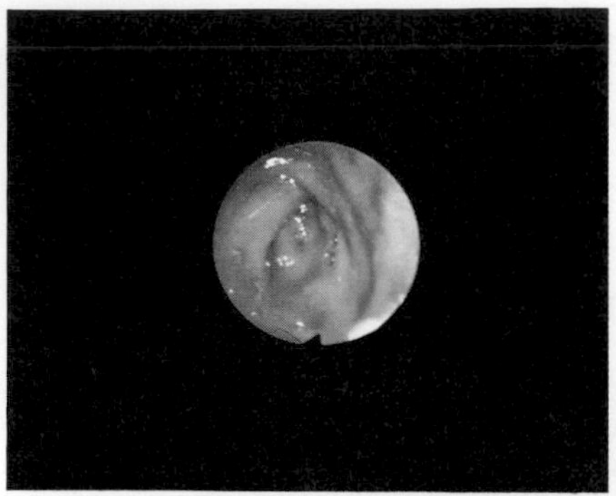

Fig. 6 Duodenal bulb.

The second portion of the duodenum is subsequently entered. Sometimes the angle between the first and second portions can be acute; if so, passage is easier if one remembers that the duodenum turns not only inferiorly, but also posteriorly. Circular mucosal folds differentiate the second portion of the duodenum from the smooth bulb (Fig. 7). Alternating insertion and withdrawal movements advance the endoscope into the second and third portions of the duodenum. The papilla of Vater is rarely seen without a side-viewing (ERCP) scope. Finally, the scope is withdrawn back into

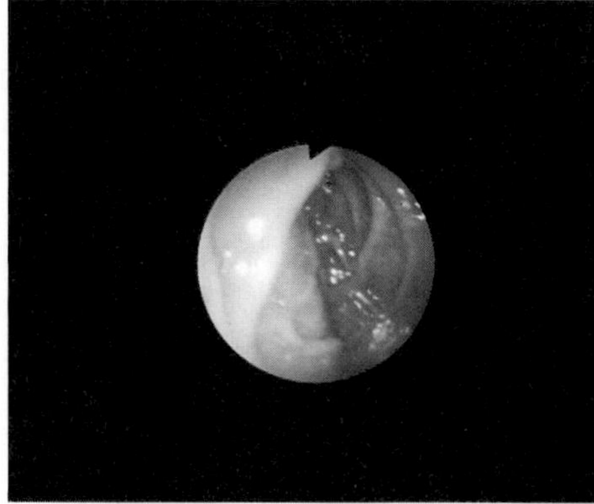

Fig. 7 Second portion of the duodenum. Bile staining and circular mucosal folds are usually prominent.

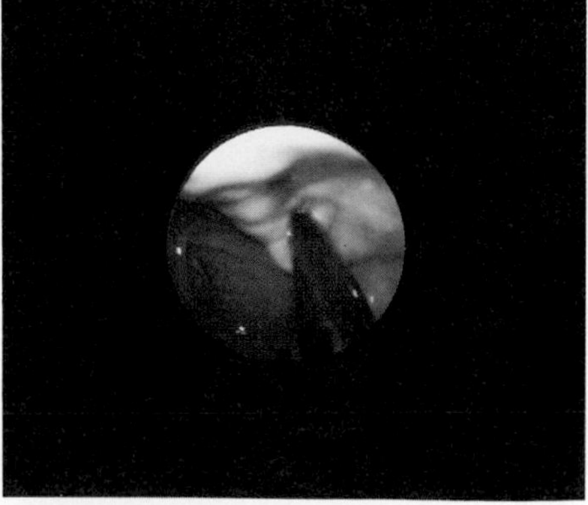

Fig. 8 'Retroflexed' endoscopic view of the gastro-oesophageal junction.

the stomach, and the tip is deflected 180° for 'retroflexed' inspection (Fig. 8). This gives the best view of the gastric incisura, the lesser curvature, and the fundus.

INDICATIONS, CONTRAINDICATIONS, AND COMPLICATIONS

Diagnostic osophagogastroduodenoscopy is especially valuable for evaluating upper gastrointestinal tumours, strictures, ulcers, varices, and mucosal changes such as oesophagitis and gastritis. It is less useful for judging functional or motility disorders or extraluminal lesions. Specifically, the major indications for diagnostic upper gastrointestinal endoscopy are:

(1) persistent upper abdominal pain or distress, especially if it is associated with symptoms or signs suggestive of serious disease (anorexia, weight loss, anaemia);
(2) persistent symptoms of gastro-oesophageal reflux despite treatment;
(3) swallowing difficulties;
(4) persistent vomiting of unknown cause;
(5) surveillance for upper gastrointestinal malignancy in high-risk patients;
(6) evaluation of upper gastrointestinal bleeding of unexplained iron deficiency anaemia;
(7) evaluation of ulcers, strictures, and tumours found by a barium meal examination.

The most important indications for therapeutic oesophagogastroduodenoscopy are:

(1) cauterization of injection of bleeding peptic ulcers (and occasionally vascular malformations);
(2) injection sclerosis of oesophageal varices that have bled;
(3) removal of foreign bodies or bezoars;
(4) removal of gastric polyps;
(5) dilatation of oesophageal strictures;
(6) palliative treatment of malignant upper gastrointestinal obstruction by dilatation, laser fulguration, or intubation;
(7) placement of gastrostomy tubes.

Percutaneous endoscopic gastrostomy is discussed in Section 27.5.

There are contraindications to oesophagogastroduodenoscopy. Endoscopy should be avoided if there is a possibility of a perforated viscus. If the stomach is not empty, little useful inspection is possible, and the risk of vomiting and aspiration pneumonia is great. A poor airway contraindicates upper gastrointestinal endoscopy. Respiratory arrest may result if there is a marginal passage (for example, pharyngeal tumour) combined with intravenous sedation, as well as partial occlusion and oedema induced by the endoscope. Endoscopy surgery should not be carried out if the patient is anticoagulated or has a coagulopathy.

Complications due to diagnostic oesophagogastroduodenoscopy are uncommon. Aspiration pneumonia may occur because of the combination of pharyngeal anaesthesia and instrumentation, especially in obtunded patients, or if there is active upper gastrointestinal bleeding. Although adverse cardiorespiratory events are rare, they may occur if the patient is frail or if sedation is excessive. Perforation and bleeding are infrequent unless endoscopic surgery is done. As is the case for colonoscopy, drug reactions, vasovagal reflex, bacteraemia, and superficial phlebitis are other less serious potential problems.

DIAGNOSTIC OESOPHAGOGASTRODUODENOSCOPY

Diagnostic upper gastrointestinal endoscopy is essential in the management of numerous lesions. It is the best way to evaluate the type and severity of oesophagitis (which may not appear on barium examination). A mass, a stricture, or an ulcer of the oesophagus or stomach require endoscopy and, usually removal of a biopsy specimen to determine whether malignancy is responsible. Cytological specimens obtained by brush or needle aspiration can augment simple biopsy. If gastric or oesophageal surgery becomes necessary, the type of incision as well as the extent of resection greatly depends upon the endoscopic assessment. Oesophagogastroduodenoscopy is the best first step in evaluating upper gastrointestinal bleeding. Contrast radiographic studies should be avoided in that situation because they often miss the lesion and because the barium hinders subsequent endoscopy or angiography. Endoscopy also reveals features of a lesion that predict the risk of rebleeding. Whenever small-bowel mucosal biopsies are needed, upper gastrointestinal endoscopy (perhaps with an extra-long scope) is the best way to obtain them. As discussed below, in a few specific circumstances oesophagogastroduodenoscopy is required for periodic surveillance for upper gastrointestinal cancers. Endoscopic ultrasound is a relatively new technique, which employs a small sonar instrument on the tip of a modified scope to provide a cross-sectional image of the oesophageal or stomach wall as well as adjacent viscera. It may be valuable for staging gastro-oesophageal tumours, assessing submucosal masses, and evaluating pancreatic lesions.

SURVEILLANCE FOR UPPER GASTROINTESTINAL NEOPLASMS

Oesophagogastroduodenoscopy is not appropriate for routine screening for upper gastrointestinal cancer, but it is worthwhile for patients at increased risk. Barrett's oesophagus and achalasia are premalignant conditions that warrant periodic (probably yearly) endoscopy. So is Plummer–Vinson syndrome, although it is rare. Gastric adenomatous polyps are unusual but, as in the colon, they may contain or transform to malignancy; they should be removed. Similarly, polyps are associated with a tendency to form metachronous lesions; periodic follow-up oesophagogastroduodenoscopy is indicated. Familial polyposis coli is associated with an excess risk of gastroduodenal neoplasms. After colectomy patients with familial polyposis coli require upper surveillance endoscopy. Atrophic gastritis, a postgastrectomy stomach remnant, oropharyngeal cancer, and lye-induced oesophageal stricture are other conditions that somewhat predispose to gastro-oesophageal cancer, but probably not enough to justify periodic oesophagogastroduodenoscopy.

Barrett's oesophagus is the most important upper gastrointestinal premalignant lesion. In this acquired condition, metaplastic columnar epithelium replaces the normal squamous epithelium in the distal oesophagus. It is strongly associated with gastro-oesophageal reflux, and there may be a concomitant hiatus hernia, oesophagitis, ulcer, or stricture. Nevertheless, reflux symptoms are sometimes mild. The typical endoscopic appearance is of velvety red mucosa extending circumferentially or in linear streaks proximally from the gastro-oesophageal junction. It may be difficult to differentiate a small hiatus hernia from Barrett's oesophagus, but there are usually longitudinal gastric folds in a hiatus hernia whereas the latter is a smooth, tubular structure above the most proximal gastric folds. Usually the metaplastic mucosa is readily discernible, but occasionally biopsy specimens are necessary for discrimination. Toluidine blue or Lugol's iodine sprayed on the mucosa enhances the detection of the columnar epithelium. Adenocarcinoma may arise in the Barrett's mucosa. The prevalence of cancer at initial diagnosis of Barrett's oesophagus is about 10 per cent. There is at least a forty-fold increased risk of developing distal oesophageal adenocarcinoma is patients with Barrett's oesophagus, about 1 to 2 per cent per year. These patients, including patients who have undergone successful antireflux surgery, should undergo yearly screening oesophagogastroduodenoscopy with random biopsies of the Barrett's mucosa. If persistent severe mucosal dysplasia is found, oesophagectomy should be considered.

Gastric polypectomy is different from colonic polypectomy. The stomach wall is thick and vascular. Removal of gastric polyps carries a greater risk of bleeding, but a lesser risk of perforation than in the large bowel. Therefore, more electrocoagulating energy must be applied when snaring gastric lesions. If the endoscope is withdrawn with the polyp suctioned on to its tip, care must be taken that the polyp is not pulled off by the cricopharyngeus muscle and aspirated into the trachea. An endoscope overtube obviates the problem. Because polypectomy leaves an iatrogenic stomach ulcer, a period of antacid therapy is advisable afterwards.

OESOPHAGOGASTRODUODENOSCOPY AND UPPER GASTROINTESTINAL BLEEDING

Endoscopy is an important early manoeuvre in the management of upper gastrointestinal bleeding. An experienced endoscopist can identify the bleeding source about 90 per cent of the time. A clear demonstration of the type and location of the responsible lesion helps guide subsequent treatment. This is especially important if urgent surgery becomes necessary; the surgeon must know where to focus the operation. The optimal arrangement is the surgeon and endoscopist as one person. Beyond diagnosis, however, treatment of a bleeding site is possible through the endoscope. In as much as upper gastrointestinal bleeding ceases spontaneously in about 80 per cent of cases, therapeutic endoscopy benefits primarily the small remaining group of 'high-risk' patients.

Both clinical and endoscopic features determine risk. Those most likely to die from bleeding are elderly patients, patients with other major medical problems, patients who begin bleeding while in hospital, and patients who bleed heavily (large transfusion requirement, haematemesis or haematochezia, hypotension, recurrent bleeding while in the hospital, need for emergency surgery).

Endoscopic findings also predict outcome. Varices or cancer correlate with a high mortality. For peptic ulcers, a visible vessel indicates up to a 50 per cent likelihood of rebleeding, whereas two other 'stigmata of recent haemorrhage' (adherent clot or active oozing) are associated with a 20 to 25 per cent risk of recurrent haemorrhage. Large ulcers are probably more likely to rebleed than are small ones, as are ulcers on the posterior wall of the duodenal bulb (overlying the gastroduodenal artery). Oesophageal varices, large vessels, or varices displaying overlying red spots are especially prone to bleed or rebleed. Therefore oesophagogastroduodenoscopy is worthwhile in all upper gastrointestinal bleeders, not only to identify the haemorrhage source, but also to help assess the danger of rebleeding and death. Endoscopic treatment can then be selected only for patients with high-risk features. In these candidates therapeutic endoscopy is of greatest benefit.

ENDOSCOPIC TREATMENT OF BLEEDING PEPTIC ULCERS

Numerous endoscopic techniques for haemostasis make use of instruments passed down the biopsy channel of the scope. The most common causes for upper gastrointestinal bleeding are peptic ulcers (Figs. 9–11) and oesophageal varices. For varices, injection sclerotherapy (as discussed below) is clearly the best choice. For ulcers, the available effective approaches are thermal coagulation with multipolar electrocautery ('BICAP'), a heater probe, or a neodymium: yttrium aluminium garnet (Nd: YAG) laser, as well as injection therapy with absolute ethanol (or perhaps adrenaline, hypertonic saline, or a mixture). Monopolar electrocoagulation and argon laser photocoagulation have largely been replaced by the other modalities. Topical agents, such as clotting factors, adrenaline, microcrystalline collagen, and cyanoacrylate glue, are

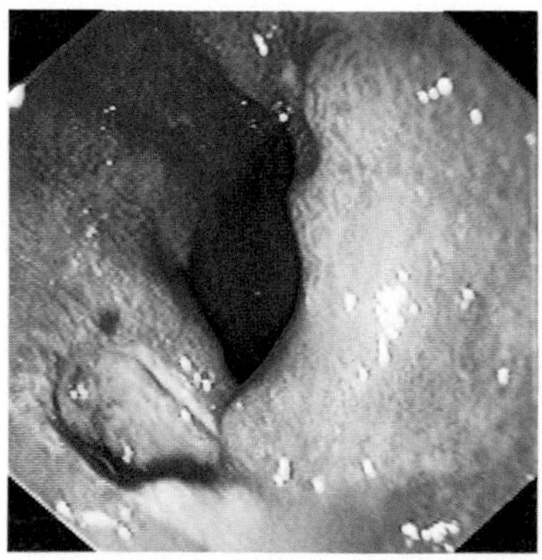

Fig. 9 A gastric ulcer.

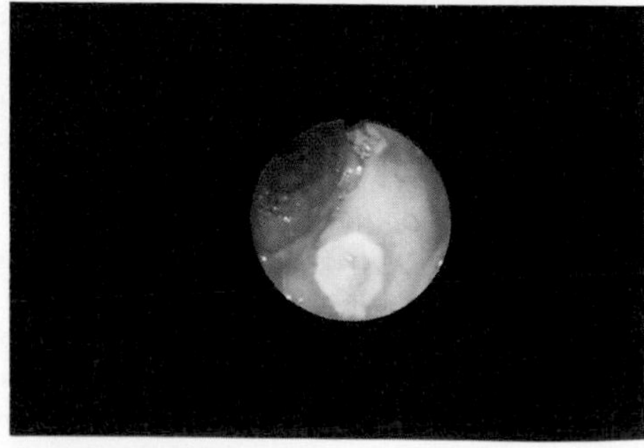

Fig. 10 A duodenal ulcer.

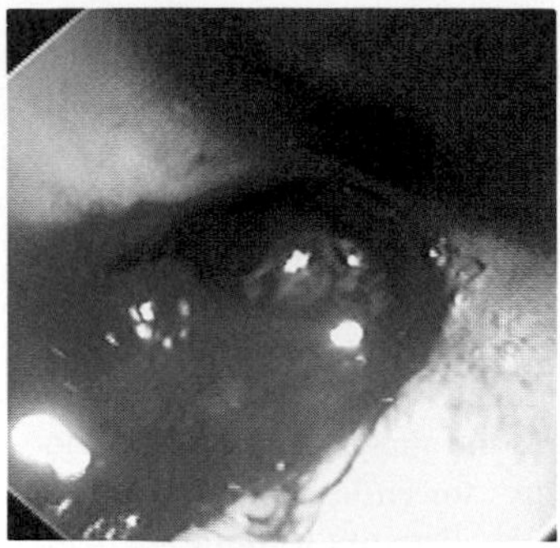

Fig. 11 A duodenal ulcer with an adherent clot and active oozing.

ineffective. No endoscopic method is free of problems. Massive haemorrhage and blood clots may obscure the view, ulcers in a deformed duodenum or elsewhere may be inaccessible, and much endoscopic skill is required. The patient must be able to co-operate with the examination, as well to remain haemodynamically stable enough to permit waiting, if necessary, for the examination and able to receive intravenous sedation. Bleeding may recur. Furthermore, the patient is at risk for aspiration pneumonia, gastrointestinal perforation, and even induction or exacerbation of bleeding due to the procedure.

The multipolar electrocoagulation probe is surrounded by three pairs of electrodes. Current is conducted between any pair of electrodes, and the depth of tissue injury is minimal. A bleeding vessel can be compressed with the probe before heat delivery (coaptive coagulation), which is superior to cauterization alone, especially for larger vessels (over 0.5 mm). Tamponade before coagulation also lets the operator know that the instrument tip is correctly placed. A built-in lavage channel is handy. Electrodes cover both the end and the sides of the probe tip so it can be applied tangentially when an *en face* approach to the vessel is impossible. The multipolar electrode delivers enough energy to coagulate, but not to vaporize tissue (which might induce bleeding). The equipment is portable and, compared to a laser, relatively cheap. Other attachments can be used with the unit to treat obstructing gastrointestinal tumours and haemorrhoids. Tissue adherence to the endoscope may be a problem, however; when the probe is withdrawn the coagulum may come also, with resumed bleeding.

The heater probe is a tiny Teflon-coated electrical resistance heater capable of delivering a precise amount of energy. It also incorporates an irrigating channel. Its advantages are the same as for the multipolar electrocoagulator, although it works a bit more slowly. Tissue adherence can also be a problem.

Laser photocoagulation takes advantage of the high power and precise control of laser light, which can be guided down a flexible quartz fibre in an endoscope channel. When the light is absorbed by tissue, it is converted to heat; no tissue contact is required. Adherence is therefore not a problem. A coaxial CO_2 jet clears the target area of blood and debris. The amount of energy delivered can be precisely determined but light (and heat) penetration is a little deeper than with the heater probe or multipolar unit. This effect can be an advantage when dealing with larger and deeper blood vessels, but might increase the perforation risk. Energy sufficient to vaporize tissue may be delivered, inducing bleeding. Lasers are perhaps the most technically difficult of the instruments to master and apply, and a direct *en face* approach to the lesion is required. Laser machines are not very portable, and are very expensive. The cost is somewhat mitigated by their versatility; Nd:YAG lasers can also be used for tissue ablation in the gastrointestinal tract and lung. They are ideal for the rapid treatment of multiple superficial mucosal vascular lesions (radiation telangiectasias (Figs. 12, 13), Osler–Weber–Rendu disease).

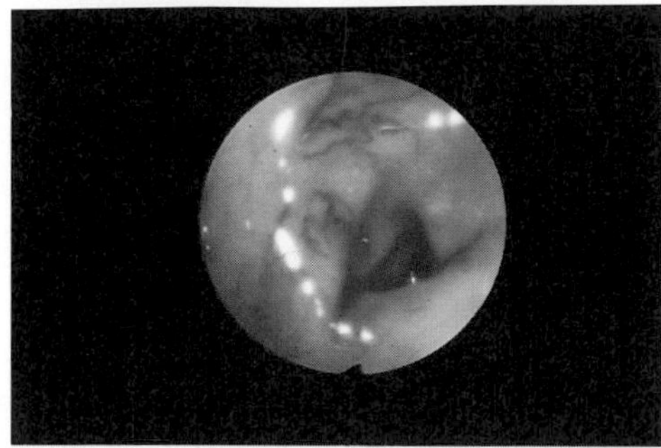

Fig. 12 Duodenal telangiectasis (which had caused bleeding) after pancreatic radiation therapy.

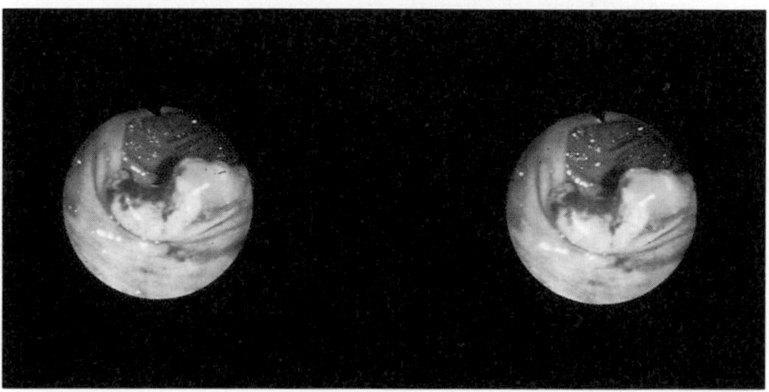

Fig. 13 Laser photocoagulation of duodenal telangiectasias.

Injection therapy (Figs. 14, 15) makes use of a thin flexible tube with a short retractable needle at its tip. This is the same item that is used for injection sclerosis of oesophageal varices (see Fig. 17)

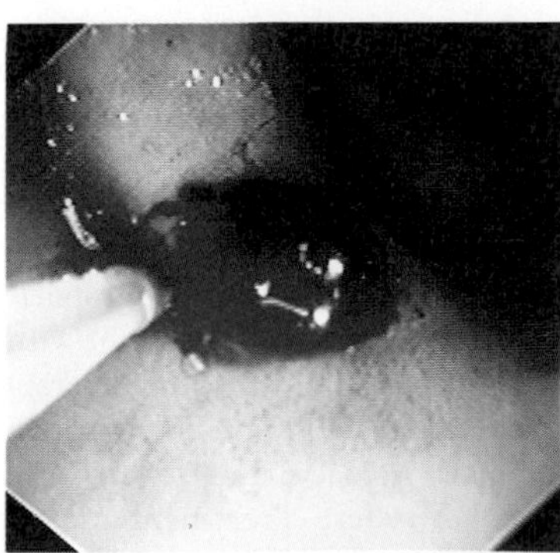

Fig. 14 Injection of absolute alcohol in and around the ulcer seen in Fig. 11.

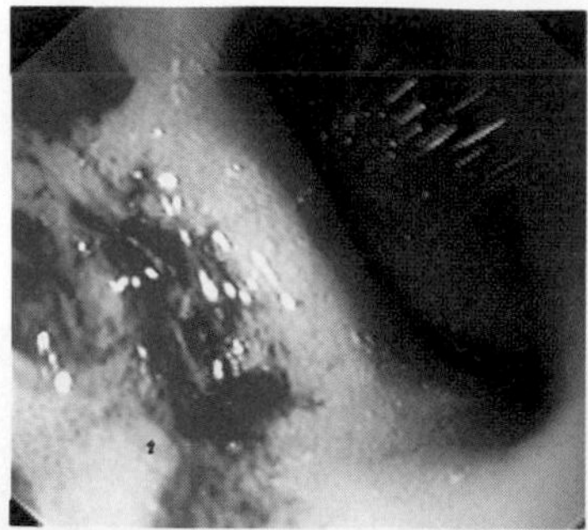

Fig. 15 Successful haemostasis after injection therapy.

but absolute alcohol, adrenaline, or hypertonic saline is usually employed for ulcer treatment. It is the simplest, cheapest, and most portable of all the treatment options. If precisely applied, it can bring about tissue coagulation with little necrosis, which may minimize the risk of perforation or induced bleeding. Nevertheless, it has no channel for simultaneous irrigation, and cannot easily be applied tangentially.

All four haemostatic techniques seem to be useful and effective. Nevertheless, results from clinical trials are often conflicting and inconclusive because of insufficient data or confounding variables. Few studies compare directly the various techniques, and the results from individual tests are roughly comparable. At present, a selection may be made based on the advantages and disadvantages enumerated above, and personal preference. In experienced centres, for patients with clinically severe bleeding from peptic ulcers displaying 'stigmata of recent haemorrhage', any one of these techniques will result in initial haemostasis in 80 to 100 per cent of patients, with rebleeding in 10 to 20 per cent. Reapplication produces an ultimate control rate of approximately 80 to 90 per cent, with the remainder of patients proceeding to emergency surgery (about 10 per cent) or death. Perforation occurs in 0 to 2 per cent, and uncontrollable bleeding is rarely induced. Trials comparing medical treatment alone to endoscopic treatment usually demonstrate superior haemostasis with the endoscopic method (a reduced proportion of patients with continued or recurrent bleeding, and a decreased number of transfusions). Often, but not always, the need for emergency surgery is decreased, and mortality improved. Even if surgery must eventually be performed, there is benefit from temporary haemostasis by endoscopic therapy; the patient can be resuscitated, stabilized, and operated upon electively rather than as an emergency.

A successful technique for endoscopic therapy begins with aggressive stomach lavage with a large orogastric tube to remove obscuring blood and clots. Changes in the patient's position can also shift blood out of the way. A double-channel endoscope is helpful because it allows simultaneous suction and use of the instrument. The likelihood of success is greatest when a clear and complete view (preferably *en face*) of the lesion is obtained before starting treatment. A heater probe or multipolar coagulator requires exact tamponade of the bleeding point with the instrument tip. Laser photocoagulation and injection therapy (0.2 ml increments of ethanol) begin in the immediately surrounding tissue to create a rim of oedema or coagulation to slow inflow, followed by targeting the actual bleeder. Treatment must be expeditious, before induced duodenal oedema obscures the view, and before the patient becomes excessively distended with air.

Endoscopic treatment of non-variceal upper gastrointestinal bleeding is feasible and safe, and reasonably (although not dramatically) effective. The most promising modalities are multipolar electrocoagulation, the heater probe, Nd:YAG laser photocoagulation, and injection therapy with absolute alcohol. Nevertheless, if the bleeding is truly torrential, endoscopic treatment is unlikely to be successful, and the patient should be taken directly to surgery. A posterior duodenal bulb bleeder or visible vessel may be the gastroduodenal artery and is also best treated surgically to avoid massive induced bleeding. Patients with active but not massive haemorrhage, and those with adherent clots or visible vessels, are ideal candidates for endoscopic therapy, especially if they are poor operative risks. Patients without stigmata of recent haemorrhage are not worth treating, since they rarely rebleed.

ENDOSCOPIC INJECTION SCLEROSIS OF OESOPHAGEAL VARICES

Bleeding oesophageal varices (Fig. 16) are difficult to treat and often fatal. Medical therapy, including transfusion, intravenous vasopressin, and balloon compression (Sengstaken–Blakemore tube) staunches the bleeding only some of the time. At least half the patients start bleeding again when the tube is deflated or when the infusion is stopped. Even without immediate rebleeding, there is a substantial likelihood of later recurrent haemorrhage and death, especially if liver function is poor. Urgent portasystemic shunting reliably cures the bleeding, but at the cost of a high morbidity and mortality.

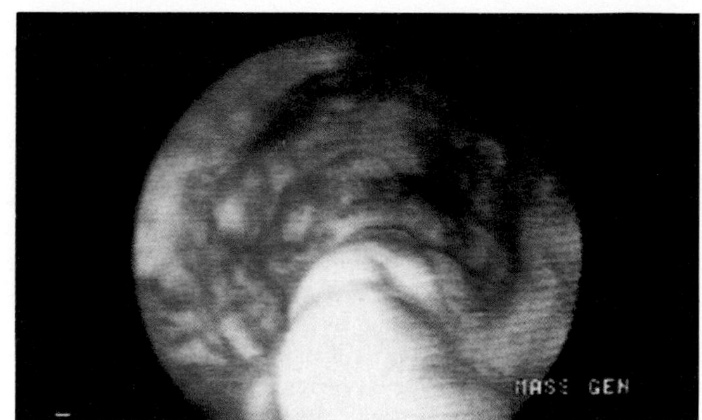

Fig. 16 Distal oesophageal varix.

Endoscopic injection sclerosis of varices is an attractive alternative. By means of a retractable needle inside a thin plastic tube (Fig. 17), which is passed down the biopsy channel of the scope, a small amount of sclerosing solution can be injected in and around the varices (Fig. 18). The injection causes thrombosis within the vein; inflammation and some necrosis of the endothelium, submucosa, and mucosa; and subsequent fibrosis and shrinkage of the varix. Large varices, and varices displaying overlying 'red spots' (red wales) are especially prone to bleed or to rebleed. Endoscopically determined variceal pressure (which correlates with vein wall tension) also predicts a tendency to bleed. Most important, the degree of cirrhosis or liver dysfunction correlates with variceal haemorrhage risk.

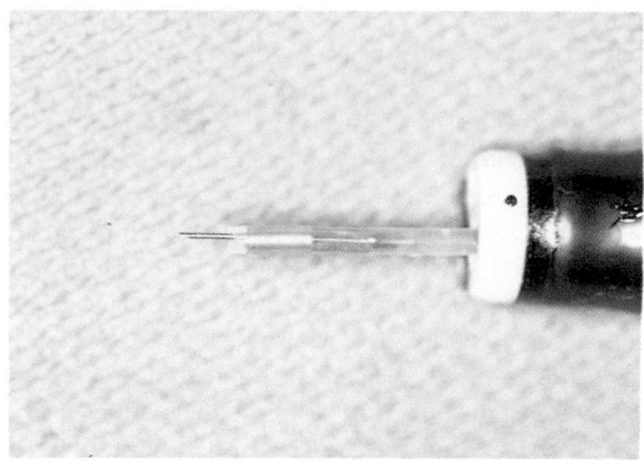

Fig. 17 Retractable endoscopic injection sclerosis needle.

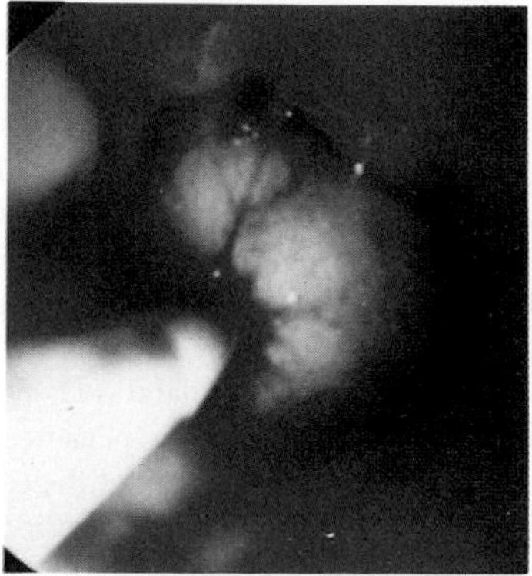

Fig. 18 Injection sclerosis of bleeding oesophageal varices.

Rates of survival, rebleeding, encephalopathy, and other complications are difficult to study in these heterogeneous and infirm patients. It has not been proved that survival after shunt surgery is prolonged compared to medical treatment; death from hepatic failure merely replaces death from haemorrhage. The stay in hospital for emergency surgery is typically long, complicated, and costly; encephalopathy is a considerable risk for survivors. In contrast, endoscopic injection sclerosis effectively reduces the frequency of rebleeding episodes and improves survival compared with medical therapy. Sclerotherapy also seems to result in improved survival and rebleeding rates compared with shunted historical controls. Nevertheless, little information is available to compare directly endoscopic therapy with surgery. The measure is made more difficult by the numerous variations in patient characteristics, as well as types and timing of surgical treatment. The few available comparisons of sclerosis with surgery do not clearly favour one over the other. Although acute and chronic control of bleeding is better with surgery, at least initial morbidity and mortality rates, as well as costs, are much lower with endoscopic therapy. With time, however, sclerosis patients probably catch up to their surgically treated partners, as rebleeding episodes gradually increase statistics for morbidity, mortality, and cost. In the final analysis, the outcome is determined more by liver function than by the type of treatment; the choice is whether to pay a price all at once or in instalments. It is reasonable to try the more benign endoscopic treatment first and to operate upon the failures. The primary disadvantage of injection sclerotherapy is that repeated treatments are required to obliterate the varices, and lifelong follow-up is necessary. A compliant patient is helpful. Until varices are eradicated, there is also the inconvenience of having occasionally to deal with recurrent bleeding episodes.

For active bleeders, management begins with resuscitation, and the sclerosis procedure is best done with the patient monitored in an intensive care unit or operating room. Administration of blood, clotting factors (fresh frozen plasma), and vitamin K may suffice to stem the haemorrhage. If bleeding persists, intravenous vasopressin or perhaps somatostatin and then balloon compression are appropriate manoeuvres to stabilize the patient's condition before gastroscopy (which can be done immediately or 6–24 h later). The rate of bleeding can at least be transiently checked in 80 to 90 per cent of patients, and the improved view greatly facilitates the endoscopic injection. Nevertheless, it is also reasonable, and perhaps more efficient, to skip medical manoeuvres and to carry out immediate endoscopic sclerosis, if equipment and personnel can be marshalled quickly. Encephalopathy, instrumentation, and iatrogenic sedation and pharyngeal anaesthesia predispose the patient to a disastrous aspiration of blood or vomitus; therefore, endotracheal intubation is wise. Gastric lavage with a large orogastric tube is necessary to clear the stomach of clots before the scope is passed. Flexible fibreoptic endoscopy has supplanted rigid oesophagoscopy for sclerotherapy, since it is easier, safer, and does not require general anaesthesia. Unless varices are clearly identified as the bleeding source, a brief oesophagogastroduodenoscopy before starting injection sclerosis is prudent. Cirrhotic patients sometimes bleed from peptic ulcers, gastritis, or from Mallory–Weiss tears. If non-bleeding varices are present, and there are no other important upper gastrointestinal lesions, the patient has probably bled from the varices and requires treatment accordingly. Gastric varices may also be seen. Often they are simply inferior extensions of oesophageal varices (being within 2–3 cm of the squamocolumnar junction). These usually disappear when the oesophageal varices are obliterated. More distant (fundal) gastric varices are unusual but problematic sources of gastrointestinal bleeding. Diagnosis can be difficult because they may resemble rugal folds or may flatten when the stomach is insufflated for endoscopy. Injection sclerosis of these 'true' gastric varices is usually fruitless; rebleeding often occurs, and there is probably an excess risk of perforation and ulceration.

The scope is with drawn into the distal oesophagus for injection. A small balloon placed around and just proximal to the endoscope tip is optional, but when inflated may produce relative stasis within the varices to hold the sclerosant in place until thrombosis occurs. Although blood flows in various directions within a varix, it most often moves cephalad. The balloon is also handy for tamponade to prevent back-bleeding from the injection needle hole. Injections are best aimed as low in the squamous mucosa over a varix as possible, since bleeding varices are always near the gastro-oesophageal junction. Sclerosant (1–3 ml) is injected into the lumen of three to five oesophageal varices. Intravariceal rather than submucosal paravariceal injections are the most widely advocated and probably minimize mucosal slough. Further injections at 3- to 4-cm intervals from distal to proximal oesophagus are optional. After withdrawing the injection needle, the needle hole is momentarily occluded with the needle sheath, the endoscope tip, or the balloon on the scope. Care must be taken not to overdistend the intestine with air during a long and difficult sclerosis procedure, especially in an unintubated patient; since it makes breathing more difficult. A nasogastric tube is preferably omitted after sclerosis to avoid mucosal erosion and rebleeding. Injection is repeated at 48 hours and at 1 week; the patient can then be discharged if stable.

Subsequent injection procedures can usually be done in an outpatient setting, unless active bleeding recurs. Since variceal size correlates positively with bleeding risk, the goal is to continue periodic injections until the varices are gone. After that, periodic surveillance endoscopy is wise, to check for recurrent varix formation. A reasonable schedule for follow-up sclerosis after an episode of acute bleeding is at 48 h, 1 week, every 4 to 8 weeks until the varices have shrunk, and then as necessary every 6 to 12 months for life. The sequence is restarted if the patient rebleeds.

Endoscopists differ about many technical details of injection sclerosis. Little objective information is available comparing the possible regimens, especially because so many variables can affect the outcome of sclerotherapy. The most common sclerosant solutions used in the United States are 5 per cent sodium morrhuate and 0.5 to 3.0 per cent sodium tetradecyl sulphate. Elsewhere, physicians also use 5 per cent ethanolamine oleate, 1 to 3 per cent polidocanol, and 50 to 95 per cent ethanol. Thrombin, a cephalosporin antibiotic, and 20 to 50 per cent dextrose are sometimes mixed in. Many endoscopists omit the balloon on the scope tip. Some workers use a flexible overtube with the fibreoptic endoscope; the tube has a distal slot to allow isolated prolapse of the target varix and compression of the remainder. Injections can be paravariceal, but most workers aim for an intravariceal location. The optimum number of injections and overall volume of sclerosant to administer per session is unknown. Similarly, the time interval between follow-up injections varies among sclerotherapists from a week to a few months. Numerous, frequent, and voluminous injections obliterate varices more rapidly, making rebleeding less likely. But intensive treatment is traded against an increased risk of local complications (ulceration, perforation, stricture) (Fig. 19). Laser photocoagulation of varices is of little benefit because of recurrent haemorrhage. Endoscopic elastic banding of varices has had reasonable early results (Fig. 20).

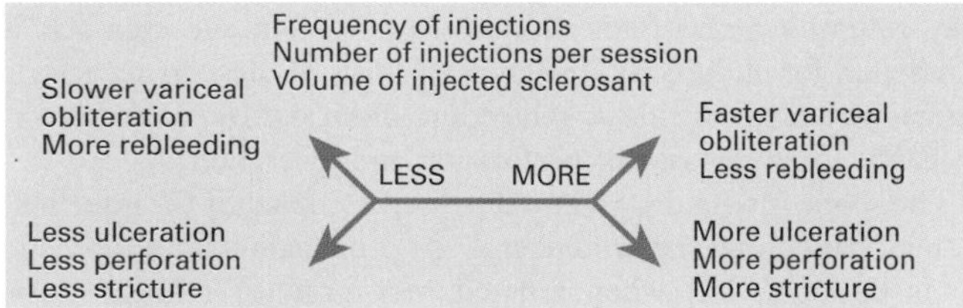

Fig. 19 Results of injection sclerosis.

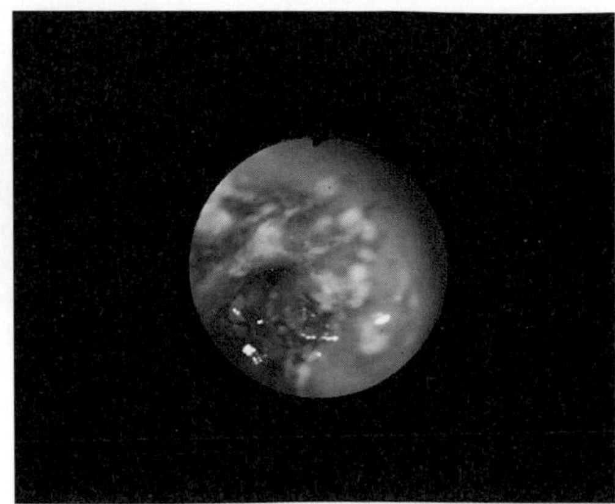

Fig. 20 Endoscopic rubber band ligation of oesophageal varix (the tiny black band visible in the lower portion of the photograph).

Although injection sclerosis is the safest non-medical treatment for bleeding varices, complications do occur. The sclerosis technique, the skill of the endoscopist, and the clinical state of the patient influence the morbidity rate. Transient substernal chest pain (probably from oesophageal spasm) odynophagia, fever, and pleural effusions are common in the first 24 to 72 h after injection, and are almost always inconsequential. Oesophageal mucosal ulceration due to tissue necrosis from the sclerosant is not uncommon, especially if follow-up endoscopies take place at short intervals. The ulcers usually heal spontaneously. Rarely, recurrent, bleeding issues from the ulcer. If an ulcer is seen at follow-up endoscopy, adjacent injections should be avoided. In a patient whose variceal bleeding has ceased, instrumentation can induce recurrent haemorrhage that might not be controllable endoscopically—fortunately an unusual problem. Instrumental acute oesophageal perforation does not occur, except when rigid oesophagoscopes are used; delayed necrosis and perforation with mediastinitis happens in 0 to 2 per cent. Aspiration pneumonia occurs in 2 to 10 per cent of patients, especially when sclerotherapy is undertaken during active bleeding. Although some sclerosant reaches the pulmonary circulation, respiratory function does not suffer. Even when thrombin is mixed with the sclerosant, no subclinical or overt systemic clotting abnormality results. Symptomatic distal oesophageal stricture develops in 2 to 20 per cent, especially when sclerotherapy is frequent and prolonged. Strictures usually respond well to dilatation.

Results of sclerotherapy are good in experienced centres. Active bleeding can be stopped 80 to 95 per cent of the time. About 20 per cent of patients rebleed during the initial period in hospital, but sclerotherapy can be repeated, giving a final acute control rate of 85 to 90 per cent. There is a 20 to 30 per cent short-term or 'hospital' mortality, usually from hepatic failure rather than bleeding. Endoscopic sclerotherapy is useful not only for acute haemostasis, but also for elective, long-term management of varices. Repeated injections, usually in an outpatient setting, gradually eradicate the lesions. Within the first 1 to 2 years of such a regimen, 20 to 30 per cent of patients rebleed; reinjection, however, ultimately controls the haemorrhage in 80 to 90 per cent of patients. Rebleeding most often appears during the first few months of treatment, before varices have become obliterated. Compliant patients do much better than average; those who faithfully attend follow-up endoscopy sessions rebleed less than 10 per cent of the time (these patients are also more likely to follow advice to stop drinking alcohol). Overall survival is about 50 per cent; again, death usually results from liver failure, not from bleeding. Hepatic function is the best predictor of death or rebleeding. Prophylactic endoscopic sclerosis of varices that have never bled is not worthwhile.

Endoscopic injection sclerosis is effective and safe, and is indicated for any patient with bleeding oesophageal varices. Once the haemorrhage has been staunched, the patient can recover, and decisions can be made about definitive elective treatment. Depending upon patient and physician preference, a shunt or continued sclerosis may be selected. Most cases can be nicely treated as outpatients with periodic injection sclerosis, but a non-compliant patient or the presence of gastric varices argues for surgery. Liver transplantation is now an alternative for selected cirrhotic patients. Episodes of repeat haemorrhage most often occur within the first few months of initiating sclerotherapy, before varices are obliterated. Occasionally, if rebleeding is frequent, or if the varices are not shrinking despite the injections, or if the patient is unco-operative, sclerosis should be abandoned in favour of surgery. Endoscopically uncontrollable bleeding (recurrent variceal haemorrhage despite two contiguous emergency injection treatments) leaves no alternative but shunt or oesophageal transection, but such patients usually have poor liver function and do poorly no matter what treatment is given them.

REMOVAL OF FOREIGN BODIES

Ingested foreign bodies usually occur in children. The remainder appear in adults who are most often edentulous, prisoners, or psychiatric patients. Fortunately, 80 per cent of foreign bodies pass spontaneously through the gastrointestinal tract. Nevertheless, if the object seems unlikely to pass, or fails to pass, or would be dangerous to allow to pass, it should be extracted. Fibreoptic endoscopy is effective and safe for this purpose; under most circumstances there is no longer any need for rigid oesophagoscopy and general anaesthesia. The success rate for foreign body extraction with a fibreoptic upper gastrointestinal scope is 90 to 95 per cent.

Decisions about management depend upon the type of foreign body, and its location in the body. Plain radiographs often provide the information. For oesophageal foreign bodies, lateral views are important, to be sure that the object is not in the trachea instead. In children, or anyone who cannot give an accurate history, radiographs encompassing the gut from mouth to anus are necessary to display the number and types of items present. Barium radiographic studies, however, should not be done, since the barium will later obscure the endoscopic view. If the object is in the cricopharyngeal area or oesophagus (foreign body or meat bolus), extraction should be carried out as soon as possible, to avoid possible aspiration or perforation. Removal is especially urgent if the object is sharp (such as a piece of bone) or if it is a miniature disc battery (serious corrosive damage can develop within hours). Attempted digestion of an impacted meat bolus with papain (meat tenderizer) is unwise because it can worsen oesophagitis (most of these patients have strictures), and it is dangerous if aspirated. An item in the stomach can often be left to pass spontaneously unless it is large or sharp. Passage usually occurs within 3 days, although the patient can be observed (with periodic radiographs) for up to 2 weeks. Surgery is required if the foreign body fails to progress through the gastrointestinal tract, or if signs of inflammation develop. If the object is thicker than about 2 cm or longer than about 5 cm, it often will not exit from the stomach; endoscopic removal is wise. Sharp, irregular, or pointed objects such as toothpicks, chicken bones, razor blades, or dental bridges should be extracted. If a sharp or pointed item has passed through the stomach into the small bowel, the patient should be admitted to the hospital for observation and daily radiographs. Laparotomy is necessary if the foreign body does not progress over a few days, or if signs of inflammation appear. If drugs in packets (cocaine, heroin) have been ingested for smuggling, they should not be endoscopically removed because packet rupture can cause rapid death from drug overdose. Laparotomy is necessary instead. Caustic (for example, lye or acid) ingestion should be promptly evaluated endoscopically. Removal is impossible of course, but it is helpful to assess the degree and extent of damage to the oesophagus and stomach. The scope should be advanced only to the most proximal level of major damage.

The technique of endoscopic removal begins with examination of an object similar to the one swallowed, if possible, in order to plan and practise the best way to grasp it. While making preparations for endoscopy, the patient should lie on his left side to discourage passage of the foreign body out of the stomach. The patient's airway is the most important consideration during the procedure. If during the process of removal the object is lost at the cricopharyngeus muscle, it may occlude the airway or be aspirated into the trachea. Concern is especially great in children, or any unco-operative patient. Items that are large (such as a coin in a child), irregular, or pointed, or smooth and difficult to grasp are also risky. Placing the patient in Trendelenburg position during withdrawal discourages aspiration. An overtube fitted on the outside of the endoscope is useful; once the endoscope is in place the tube can be slid down over the scope until its lower end is on the stomach or distal oesophagus. The endoscope and foreign body can be withdrawn (with or without simultaneous removal of the overtube) so that the cricopharyngeus cannot dislodge the object. The overtube also protects the oesophagus from laceration if the item is sharp, and can make multiple reinsertions easy (as for meat in the oesophagus, or multiple foreign bodies). If there is any doubt about maintaining an airway, the safest course is to do the endoscopy under general anaesthesia with orotracheal intubation.

If the object is at the level of the posterior pharynx or cricopharyngeus, removal is usually possible with an open rigid laryngoscope (anaesthesia type) and a plain forceps or clamp. For any other location, the flexible endoscope is needed. Extraction can be accomplished with an endoscopic snare, endoscopic forceps (alligator or rat-tooth), dormia basket, balloon catheter, or three-pronged polyp retriever. Hollow objects (such as rings) may be removed after passing a heavy thread through them with the scope instruments. A sharp or irregular object (such as an open safety pin) may need to be repositioned so that the pointed end is trailing when it is withdrawn, or so that it can be pulled into an overtube. Sometimes it is best to push an object from the oesophagus into the stomach, so that it can be turned. It is preferable to withdraw a pointed object and the endoscope through an overtube. If manipulation in that way is impossible, the next best manoeuvre is to at least pull the sharp end into the overtube, and remove the scope, overtube, and foreign body all together. Meat stuck in the oesophagus can usually be readily extracted with a snare. Sometimes it can simply be pushed into the stomach (gently). Most patients with impacted meat have an oesophageal stricture, which may not have been recognized previously. Gastric bezoars may be broken up with a snare, biopsy forceps, or irrigation. A lesion may be present that prevents normal gastric emptying.

DILATATION OF OESOPHAGEAL STRICTURES

Oesophagogastroduodenoscopy should be carried out on all patients with oesophageal strictures. Inspection and biopsy are necessary to be certain that cancer is not responsible. The oesophagus and stomach can be evaluated for associated lesions (such as oesophagitis, hiatus hernia, or peptic ulcer), which may not be apparent on upper gastrointestinal radiography. Beyond diagnosis, dilatation of oesophageal strictures is possible with the aid of endoscopy. Although fibrotic strictures from gastro-oesophageal reflux are the most common lesions treated, bougienage can also be applied for the dilatation of anastomotic strictures, malignant strictures, Schatzki rings, and, occasionally, caustic strictures.

Three types of dilating instruments are available: mercury-filled rubber bougies, guidewire dilators, and inflatable dilators that are passed through the biopsy channel of the endoscope.

Mercury-filled dilators (Maloney, Hurst) are passed blindly (or occasionally under fluoroscopy) and are simple to use. No simultaneous endoscopy is required. They are appropriate for mild to moderately narrow strictures that are relatively short, smooth, and straight. For tight, long, or irregular strictures, or strictures associated with a diverticulum, there is a greater risk of instrumental perforation, so wire-guided dilators are preferable. Eder–Puestow bougies are metal, 'olive tipped' graduated instruments. They are effective, but have largely been replaced by long, tapered, plastic dilators (Savary–Gillard; American). Inflatable 'through the scope' dilators are the latest addition to the array. These are passed down the endoscope channel and through the narrowed area under direct endoscopic view (no guidewire), and are expanded. Like guidewire bougies, they are appropriate for complex strictures, but are somewhat more troublesome to use. They are also expensive and have a limited lifespan. Their best application is in regions not accessible to other types of dilators, such as the pylorus, bile duct, or colon. Dilators are often sized in even-number increments of the French scale; each unit approximates 0.44 mm diameter (for example, 18 French = 6 mm diameter).

The procedure for dilatation begins with diagnostic upper gastrointestinal endoscopy. Rubber mercury-filled dilators are thereafter passed sequentially, with the patient sitting up so that gravity aids the process. For guidewire dilators, the wire is passed down the channel of the endoscope and through the stricture. The scope is then withdrawn, leaving the guidewire in place for the dilators to be passed over it. The goal is to position the wire completely through the stricture, with its end lying smoothly along the greater curve of the stomach (but not into the pylorus). Care must be taken that the wire does not perforate the oesophagus, curl above the stricture or in a hiatus hernia, or traverse only a portion of the stricture. The best assurance of proper placement is to first pass the endoscope (often the paediatric instrument) completely through the stricture. If that is not possible, fluoroscopic guidance is advisable (unless the stricture is short and straight). Indeed, whenever there is doubt about positioning a guidewire, or any difficulty with dilatation, fluoroscopy should be employed. Generally, in a single session only two or three dilator sizes (that is, 4–6 French units) should be passed beyond the first dilator that meets resistance. When passing wire-guided bougies, attention must be paid to the wire so that it does not become displaced.

Although many strictures recur, symptomatic relief after dilatation of benign strictures can be achieved in at least 80 per cent of patients. Dysphagia is usually relieved when dilatation to 40 to 45 French units is achieved (13–15 mm diameter). Symptomatic success is sometimes better than the objective change in stricture diameter. Perforation is the most important complication, and occurs in about 0.5 per cent of procedures. Strictures due to lye ingestion are especially fragile and prone to perforation during dilatation. Aspiration pneumonia, bleeding, and bacteraemia are other possible complications.

ENDOSCOPIC TREATMENT OF OESOPHAGEAL CANCER

Oesophageal carcinoma often has poor prognosis, and palliative treatment is sometime all that can be offered. The best palliation is an uncomplicated resection if possible. Radiation and chemotherapy or both, are also available. Another option is endoscopic treatment by dilatation, tumour ablation, or placement of an indwelling tubular stent. Some physicians resort to these measures only after failure of surgery or radiation, but endoscopic treatment may also be used initially, especially if the patient's life expectancy is short.

Numerous endoscopic options are available. Oesophageal dilatation, especially with a guidewire technique, is the simplest palliative treatment. Stenosis rapidly recurs, however, making frequent retreatment necessary. Tumour ablation with a laser (Nd:YAG) or bipolar electrocoagulator ('BICAP tumour probe') gives somewhat longer-lasting relief. The laser is applied under direct endoscopic view to vaporize intraluminal tumours. Boring a passageway sometimes requires several sessions, each a few days apart, especially if the tumour is treated from above down. Often, however, treatment may be completed in one or two sittings if the malignant stricture is first dilated, the scope passed through, and treatment applied from distal to proximal. This plan also makes it easier for the operator to stay properly oriented within the oesophageal lumen. The bipolar electrocoagulation instrument is passed through the tumour (usually after dilatation) under fluoroscopic guidance. As the probe traverses the tumour and power is applied, the cancer is circumferentially electrocoagulated; thus, it is appropriate only for circumferential lesions.

Tumour ablation is reasonably successful. It does have problems, however. Long or angled lesions are difficult to treat. Upper oesophageal tumours respond poorly even if a lumen is restored, probably because of dysmotility. Bothersome gastro-oesophageal reflux often results when a distal oesophageal or proximal gastric cancer is cored out. As tumours regrow, repeat treatments are required. Furthermore, therapy becomes increasingly difficult and ineffective as the extraluminal portion of the cancer enlarges. Fistulae and perforations occur, of course, especially if the tumour is large, or if radiation has been given previously. Enthusiasts report approximately 90 per cent technical success (restored lumen) with tumour ablation, but only 70 to 80 per cent functional success (improved dysphagia). Tracheo-oesophageal fistulae develop in 10 per cent, and perforations in 5 per cent. Bleeding is an occasional problem. Median survival is in the range of 3 to 12 months.

Oesophageal tube implantation is attractive because a single procedure can give immediate improvement in swallowing, which is more durable than tumour ablation. It is especially useful for the palliation of a malignant tracheo-oesophageal fistula. After initial dilatation or laser of the malignant stricture, a wire-guided introducer (like a dilator) is passed through the tumour. The prosthesis is then slid down over the introducer and positioned across the tumour under fluoroscopy. Alternatively, the endoscope is passed through the malignancy, and the implant is pushed down around the scope and positioned under endoscopic view. Although intubation is perhaps the best endoscopic palliation, the tubes can sometimes be difficult to place accurately. Oesophageal erosion or tube migration may occur, especially if the patient is subsequently radiated. Tumour overgrowth or food may obstruct the prosthesis (the patient should remain on a liquid diet indefinitely). As with tumour fulguration, intubation works poorly in the upper oesophagus, and promotes reflux in the lower oesophagus. In the limited available literature, 80 to 90 per cent of patients are reported to be improved.

FURTHER READING

American Society for gastrointestinal endoscopy. *Gastrointestinal endoscopy: diagnostic and therapeutic procedures: an information resource manual.* Manchester, MA.

Branicki FJ, *et al.* Bleeding duodenal ulcers: a prospective evaluation of risk factors for rebleeding and death. *Ann Surg* 1990; **211**: 411–18.

Dent TL, Kukora JS, Buinewicz BR. Endoscopic screening and surveillance for gastrointestinal malignancy. *Surg Clin N Am* 1989; **69**: 1205–25.

Fleischer D. Endoscopic therapy of upper gastrointestinal bleeding in humans. *Gastroenterology* 1986; **90**: 217–34.

Fleischer D, Sivak MV. Endoscopic ND:YAG laser therapy as palliation for esophagogastric cancer. *Gastroenterology* 1985; **89**: 827–31.

Hunter JG. Endoscopic laser application in the gastrointestinal tract. *Surg Clin N Am* 1989; **69**: 1147–66.

Infante-Rivard C, Esnaola S, Villeneuve JP. Role of endoscopic variceal sclerotherapy in the long term management of variceal bleeding: a meta-analysis. *Gastroenterology* 1989; **96**: 1087–92.

Overholt BF. Laser treatment of oesophageal cancer. *Am J Gastroenterol* 1985; **80**: 719–20.

Overholt BF. Laser treatment of upper gastrointestinal haemorrhage. *Am J Gastroenterol* 1985; **80**: 721–6.

Sacks HS, *et al.* Endoscopic hemostasis: and effective therapy for bleeding peptic ulcers. *JAMA* 1990; **264**: 494–9.

Schwesinger WH. Endoscopic diagnosis and treatment of mucosal lesions of the oesophagus. *Surg Clin N Am* 1989; **69**: 1185–1203.

Selivanov V, *et al.* Management of foreign body ingestion. *Ann Surg* 1984; **199**: 187–91.

Snady H. The role of sclerotherapy in the treatment of oesophageal varices: personal experience and a review of randomized trials. *Am J Gastroenterol* 1987; **82**: 813–22.

Snady H, Feinman L. Prediction of variceal haemorrhage: a prospective study. *Am J Gastroenterol* 1988; **83**: 519–25.

Steele RJC. Endoscopic haemostasis for nonvariceal upper gastrointestinal hemorrhage. *Br J Surg* 1989; **76**: 219–25.

Sugawa C. Endoscopic diagnosis and treatment of upper gastrointestinal bleeding. *Surg Clin N Am* 1989; **69**: 1167–83.

Terblanche J, Kahn D, Bornman PC. Long term injection sclerotherapy treatment for oesophageal varices. *Ann Surg* 1989; **210**: 725–31.

Terblanche J, Krige JEJ, Bornman PC. Endoscopic sclerotherapy. *Surg Clin N Am* 1990; **70**: 341–59.

Tytgat GNJ. Dilation therapy of benign oesophageal stenoses. *World J Surg* 1989; **13**: 142–8.

Webb WA. Oesophageal dilation: personal experience with current instruments and techniques. *Am J Gastroenterol* 1988; **83**: 471–5.

Webb WA. Management of foreign bodies of the upper gastrointestinal tract. *Gastroenterology* 1988; **94**: 204–16.

27.2 Biliary and pancreatic endoscopy

JULIAN BRITTON

INTRODUCTION

Endoscopic retrograde cholangiopancreatography (ERCP) is a combined endoscopic and radiological procedure which plays an essential role in the diagnosis and the management of diseases of the biliary tract and pancreas. The diagnostic technique was first described in 1968 and this was quickly followed by the development of therapeutic endoscopic procedures for the relief of obstructive jaundice and the extraction of stones from the bile duct. Although ERCP requires expensive equipment and technical skill, it is now widely available and it should be regarded as complementary to percutaneous transhepatic techniques.

INSTRUMENTS

Modern duodenoscopes are sophisticated side-viewing endoscopes, which are designed specifically for use within the duodenum. Older instruments produce an optical image from a congruent fibreoptic cable to which a television camera can be attached. In the future, video duodenoscopes, which incorporate the camera in the tip of the endoscope, will become the standard instrument. The television image is a real advantage as the endoscopy assistants are able to see what they are doing, and teaching the technique is made much easier. Endoscopes with instrument channels up to 4.2 mm in diameter are available. They are fully insulated and completely immersible, so that the whole instrument can be sterilized.

The basic diagnostic cannula is a plastic tube, 200 cm long, with an outside diameter of 1.6 mm, and a single terminal opening with a rounded tip marked at centimetre intervals for the last 5 cm (Fig. 1). The most important therapeutic instrument is the sphincterotomy knife (Fig. 2). This consists of a

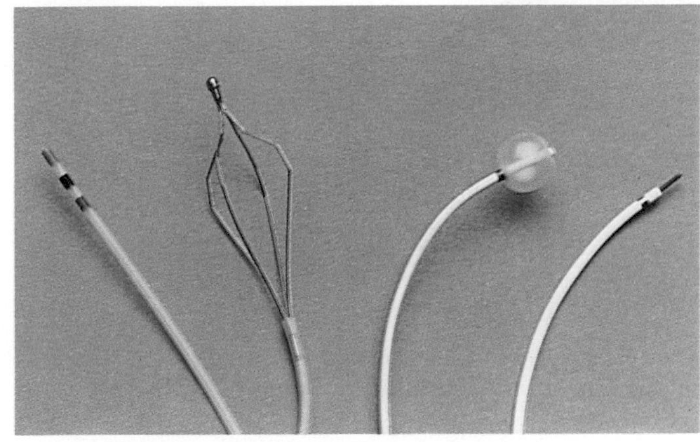

Fig. 1 A selection of endoscopic instruments. From the left they are: a diagnostic cannula, a Dormia basket, a balloon catheter, and a cannula and guidewire (note the metal collar on the cannula which enables easy visualization on the radiographic screen).

fine wire running down inside a plastic cannula and attached at the tip. For the final 3 cm the wire runs outside the plastic tubing. When the wire is shortened within the plastic tubing at the proximal end, the wire at the distal end 'bowstrings' across the tubing (Fig. 3). Other instruments are flexible guidewires, baskets, and balloons of a conventional design and suitable length and strength (Fig. 1).

A good-quality radiological screening unit with an image intensifier, which will also take still radiographs, is essential. A television screen should be placed behind the patient's head where the picture is comfortably visible to the endoscopist and the radiologist.

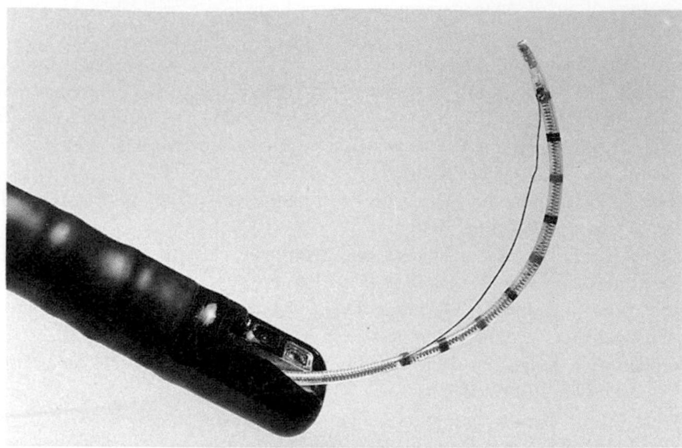

Fig. 2 A sphincterotomy knife in the relaxed position emerging from the instrument channel of a fibreoptic duodenoscope.

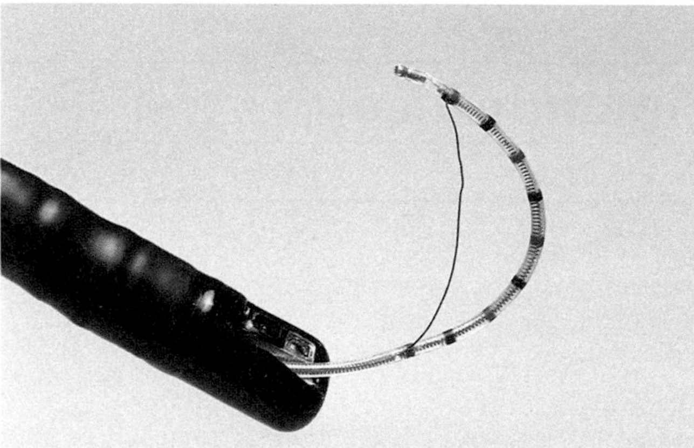

Fig. 3 A sphincterotomy knife in the tightened position.

INDICATIONS

The common indications for ERCP are extrahepatic obstructive jaundice and cholangitis. In most circumstances the endoscopist will attempt to relieve the obstruction or to remove the stones at the same examination. A diagnostic examination is appropriate in any patient in whom biliary or pancreatic disease is suspected, provided the same information cannot be obtained in a simpler or safer way. A preliminary ultrasound examination is always essential, and may, in expert hands, lead to a diagnosis. Even if diagnosis is not possible, the findings may influence management during the endoscopy.

There are no absolute contraindications. An ERCP cannot be performed if the patient has oesophageal, gastric, or duodenal obstruction. Patients with hepatitis or other infectious conditions should be examined at the end of the list, and the endoscopes should be cleaned and sterilized immediately afterwards.

PREPARATION

Most patients of any age and in any condition can tolerate an ERCP. Those with respiratory impairment require careful sedation, but patients who are severely ill, from cholangitis for example, are often better treated, after resuscitation, by this method rather than conventional surgery.

Blood coagulation must be normal. The prothrombin time should be less than 1.5 times the control value, and the platelet count must be within the normal range. Jaundiced patients receive vitamin K routinely, and fresh, frozen plasma is given immediately before the endoscopy if the prothrombin time remains abnormal. Patients are starved for at least 6 h beforehand and all of them receive intravenous fluids even though renal failure following an ERCP in a jaundiced patient is rare. When a therapeutic procedure is planned, the patient must receive an intravenous antibiotic 1 h beforehand, so as to minimize the risk of subsequent cholangitis. At the present time we use cefuroxime (1.5 g) or piperacillin (1 g).

Premedication is generally unnecessary. Children are best examined under general anaesthesia but adults are sedated with intravenous pethidine (50 mg) and midazolam (10 mg). One endoscopy assistant, equipped with a dedicated sucker, is solely responsible for looking after the patient throughout the procedure. Supplementary oxygen via nasal catheters is given to all the patients because respiratory depression can occur, and, since most of the procedure is conducted in semidarkness, physiological monitoring is essential. At the end of the examination the action of the sedative drugs is routinely reversed with naloxone (0.4 mg IV and 0.4 mg IM) and flumazenil (100 mcg IV).

Patients can eat and drink as soon as they have fully recovered from the sedation. They should stay in hospital for the night after the examination, since any complications usually develop within 12 h of the procedure.

TECHNIQUE

ERCP is technically the most difficult of all the common flexible endoscopic procedures. Patience, persistence, and perseverance are absolutely essential. Furthermore, a different endoscopist on a different occasion may succeed after an initial failure.

The patient lies on the X-ray table on his left side with his left arm behind him. The right arm lies up by the head with the intravenous cannula readily accessible to the endoscopist. The right knee and hip are fully flexed to begin with, while the left leg lies straight. The pelvis then lies more or less vertical and leaves the abdomen free. From this position it is easy to turn the patient on to his face when the endoscope is in the duodenum, simply by straightening the right leg. The weight of the patient on the abdomen then maintains the position of the endoscope across the stomach and within the duodenum. By good fortune, the X-ray beam then usually lies in exactly the correct plane for radiology of both the bile and the pancreatic ducts. A diathermy plate is placed around the left thigh when required.

Insertion of the duodenoscope requires practice. The endoscopist starts by facing the patient and passing the endoscope into the stomach. The easiest way to enter the duodenum is to push the endoscope around the greater curve of the stomach and obtain a face-on view of the pylorus. The tip of the instrument is then elevated and the endoscope advanced. The pylorus disappears from view, like the setting sun, and the endoscope enters the duodenum. The tip of the endoscope is then rotated and locked to the right, the endoscopist twists his body and thus the whole instrument to the right, and the excess length is withdrawn while maintaining a view of the duodenal lumen by manipulating the up–down control. During this manoeuvre the ampulla initially recedes from view, but then the tip of the endoscope advances and comes to lie immediately opposite the ampulla.

In this 'short' position, the endoscope lies in almost a straight line from the mouth to the duodenum, with the ampulla about 65 cm from the incisor teeth (Fig. 4). This is the easiest position in which to cannulate the ampulla. Occasionally, the 'long' position is better, particularly for cannulation of the bile duct. Here the original position of the endoscope around the greater curve of the stomach is maintained and virtually the full length of the endoscope may lie within the patient (Fig. 5).

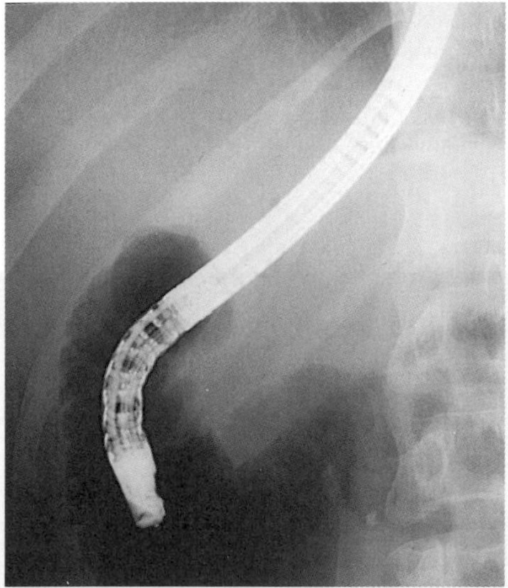

Fig. 4 Duodenoscope in the 'short' position, with the tip immediately opposite the ampulla and in the best position for cannulation.

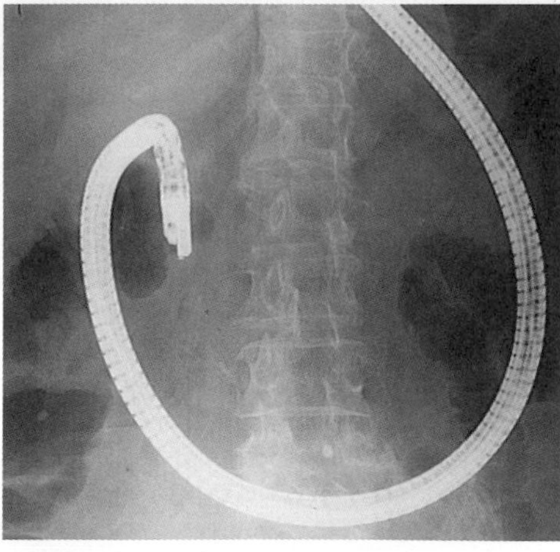

Fig. 5 Duodenoscope in the 'long' position. It is sometimes easier to cannulate the bile duct from here, although the instrument controls are always harder to work.

The key to successful cannulation is to position the endoscope correctly in relation to the ampulla. Until the endoscopist has a clear, face-on view of the ampulla (Fig. 6) attempts at cannulation are less likely to be successful. Duodenal peristalsis is a nuisance.

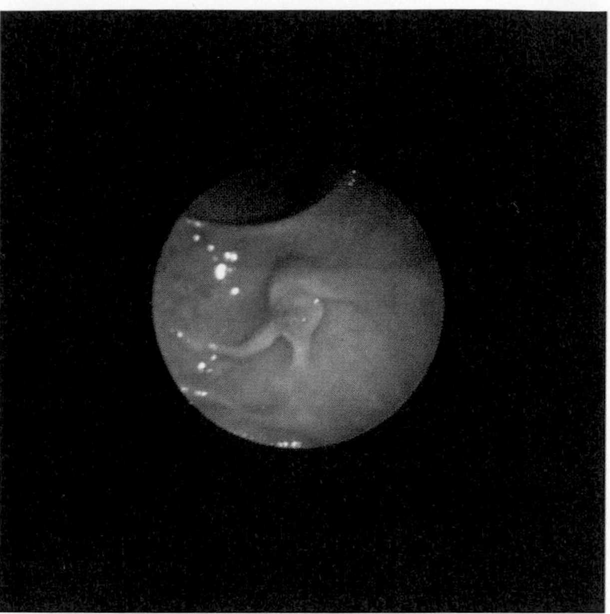

Fig. 6 A normal ampulla. This is a perfect position for cannulation of either duct.

Persistent insufflation of air may overcome the contractions, but the bowel can be paralysed with intravenous hyoscine-*N*-butylbromide (40 mg). Intravenous glucagon (1 mg) is an alternative.

Some manoeuvres may be helpful in achieving the correct position. Repeatedly pushing the endoscope further down the duodenum and then withdrawing, as described before, may help. Hooking the tip of the endoscope around the corner into the third part of the duodenum, at the same time as shortening the endoscope, is sometimes useful; and maintaining the patient on his left side occasionally helps. Patients who have had a previous Billroth II or Polya gastrectomy have to be intubated through the gastroenterostomy and backwards along the afferent loop. This may sometimes be easier with an end-viewing endoscope.

Orientation during endoscopy is always difficult. It is best not to try and orient oneself in relation to the position of the patient. It is helpful to imagine sitting in the second part of the duodenum facing the ampulla on the medial wall with your legs lying along the third part of the duodenum towards the duodenojejunal flexure. From this position the pancreatic duct runs almost horizontally away from the ampulla towards the spleen, while the bile duct passes vertically upwards behind the medial wall of the duodenum towards the liver which is above the endoscopist's head.

If the ampulla cannot be seen easily, the endoscopist should search the medial wall of the duodenum systematically, starting distally and working proximally. The endoscope is gently twisted from side to side and any suspicious mucosal folds should be elevated with a cannula. Diverticula require special attention and it may be necessary to place the tip of the endoscope actually within a diverticulum to find the ampulla. The papillary opening itself is usually obvious, except with ampullary tumours, when gentle probing with a cannula may help. The accessory ampulla can usually be seen 1 to 2 cm proximal and slightly to the right of the main ampulla. Once the main ampulla has been found, the tip of the cannula should be placed just within the orifice and a small bolus of contrast injected while screening the upper abdomen. If reflux of contrast into the duodenal lumen occurs, injection should stop immediately and the position of the cannula very gently adjusted, followed by a further injection of contrast. When a duct fills, suitable radiographic pictures are taken. The endoscopist should then withdraw the cannula a little, reposition the endoscope and the cannula, bearing in mind the comments in the paragraph above, and so fill the other duct (Figs. 7, 8). Sometimes it is immediately possible to advance the cannula some way into a duct. If this happens, it is wise to withdraw the cannula a little immediately prior to injecting contrast, in order to be sure that the tip of the cannula is not jammed into a side branch of the pancreatic duct.

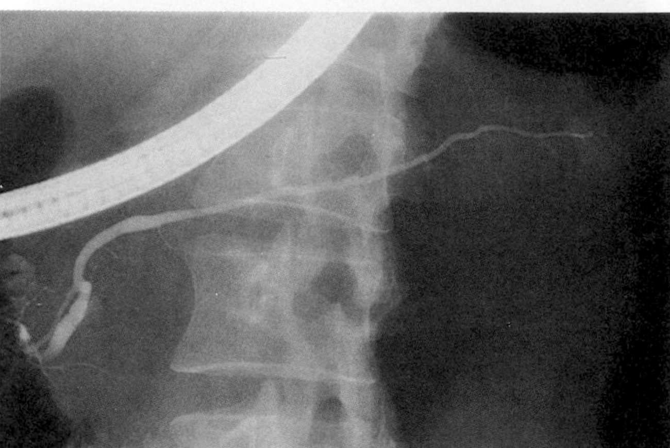

Fig. 7 A normal pancreatogram.

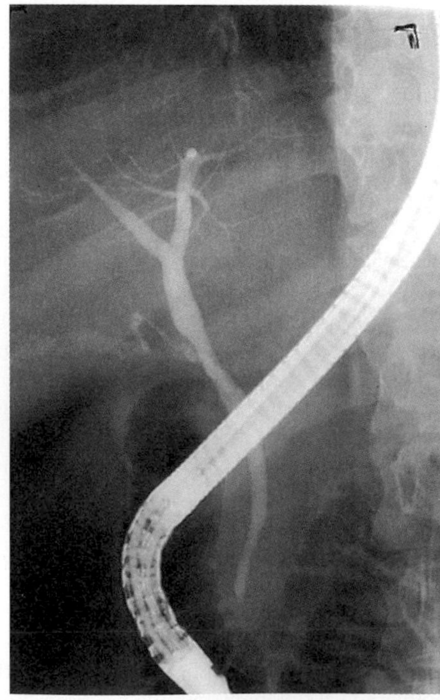

Fig. 8 A normal cholangiogram.

DIAGNOSIS

Endoscopy

Although the examination is primarily radiological, the endoscopic findings should not be ignored. A formal examination of the oesophagus and stomach is better done on a separate occasion, but the first and second parts of the duodenum are always seen clearly. Benign ulceration, malignant infiltration, and overt cancer may all be visible. Distortion of the duodenal anatomy and stenosis of the lumen may also be appreciated and may, on occasion, make it difficult to position the endoscope. Observation is particularly important in consideration of a carcinoma of the ampulla because, initially, histology and cytology may not make a definitive diagnosis (Fig. 9). All biopsy specimens should be taken just before removing the endoscope, when any bleeding will not interfere with cannulating

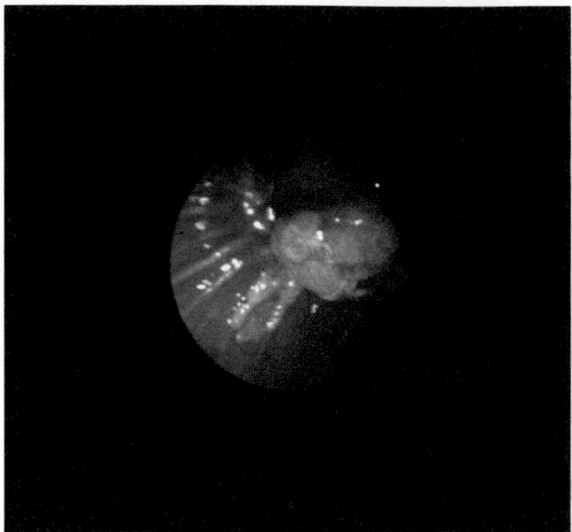

Fig. 9 A typical carcinoma of the ampulla.

the ampulla. The ampulla itself has a variable appearance. The most common appearance is shown in Fig. 6, where the ampulla appears as a nipple. Small mucosal fronds often pout out from the opening and there may be mild inflammation. Sometimes the ampulla is very flat and it is then often hard to find. A patulous, markedly inflamed, or oedematous appearance suggests either the recent passage of a stone or obstruction to lymphatic drainage by a tumour. Very rarely, there may be two separate orifices corresponding to the openings to the pancreatic and bile ducts.

Radiology

If chronic pancreatitis is suspected, a plain abdominal radiograph must be taken first, as calcification is rapidly obscured by contrast. During the procedure the assistance of a radiologist is invaluable so that the endoscopist can concentrate on the endoscopic appearance while the radiologist can position the patient and the X-ray beam to provide the best radiological image. Any of the standard contrast media can be used, but the concentration is important. If the contrast is too dense, stones in the bile duct may be obscured, and if it is too dilute, there is a risk of overfilling the pancreatic duct. We use 30 per cent and 60 per cent W/V meglumine iothalamate.

Attention to detail during the examination is essential and requires careful co-ordination between the endoscopy assistant, the endoscopist, and the radiologist. The pancreatic duct must be filled right to the tail of the gland, with some filling of the side branches but without filling the acini and producing a parenchymogram, which will almost always lead to pancreatitis.

During cholangiography early screening may be helpful but it may also be deceptive. If a stone is present in the bile duct it may rise up in the duct as the heavy contrast is injected, but the lucent whirlpool which is created when a fine jet of contrast is injected into a dilated duct may mimic a stone. Certainly, no therapeutic procedure should be performed until the diagnosis of choledocholithiasis has been definitely established on an radiographic film (Fig. 10).

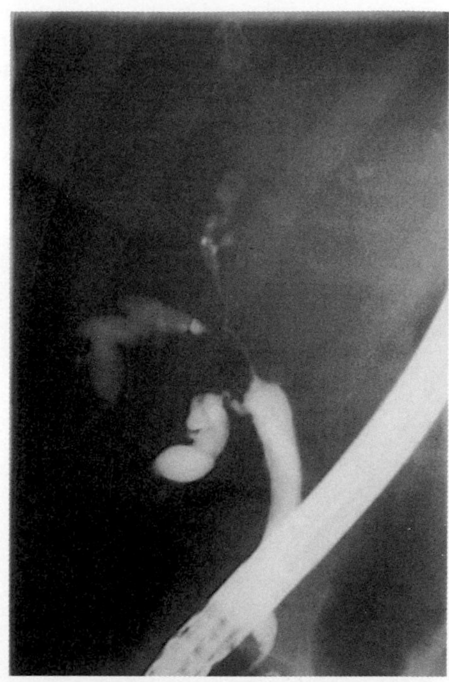

Fig. 11 A cholangiogram, showing a typical hilar stricture, probably due to cholangiocarcinoma.

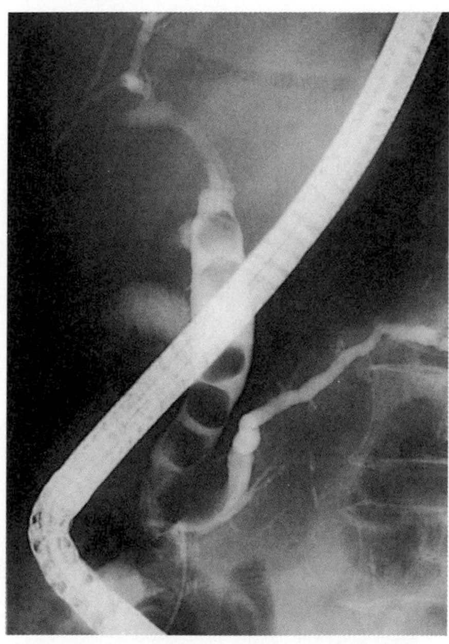

Fig. 10 A cholangiogram, showing multiple stones within the bile ducts.

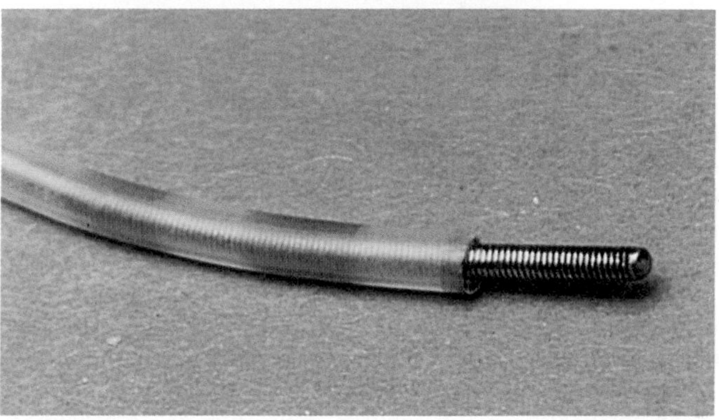

Fig. 12 A needle knife. A bare wire emerges from the end of the plastic cannula. Used for making a precut at the tip of the ampulla.

Ideally, contrast should outline both sides of a stricture because the diagnosis may rest almost entirely on the radiographic appearances. If this does not occur in the pancreatic duct, the proximal side-branches must be well filled, or even slightly overfilled, before an apparent narrowing or obstruction of the main duct can be accepted as significant. In the bile duct it may be necessary to jam the cannula deliberately into the bottom end of a stricture and then to inject contrast under a little pressure in order to obtain satisfactory pictures (Fig. 11).

Sometimes it is impossible to outline any duct. If there is a definite abnormality on ultrasound, it is usually justified to make a small precut in the tip of the ampulla, either with a needle knife (Fig. 12) or a sphincterotomy knife. Immediate cannulation of one or both ducts may then be possible, but it is often easier a few days later when there is some oedema of the ampulla. The use of this manoeuvre lessens with increasing experience.

TREATMENT

Endoscopic sphincterotomy

The basic therapeutic manoeuvre is to divide the ampullary sphincter and gain access to the bile duct. The relaxed sphincterotomy knife (Fig. 2) is inserted into the bile duct and the position confirmed on the television screen. The knife is slowly withdrawn until about half the wire is visible outside the ampulla. It is then gently tightened by the endoscopy assistant and the endoscopist divides the sphincter by using short bursts of cutting diathermy current. Three manoeuvres will extend the cut upwards through the sphincter—elevating the bridge, elevating the tip of the endoscope, and tightening the wire. Only one of these manoeuvres is used at a time so that the sphincter is divided slowly and in a controlled way (Fig. 13). If they are combined, there is a

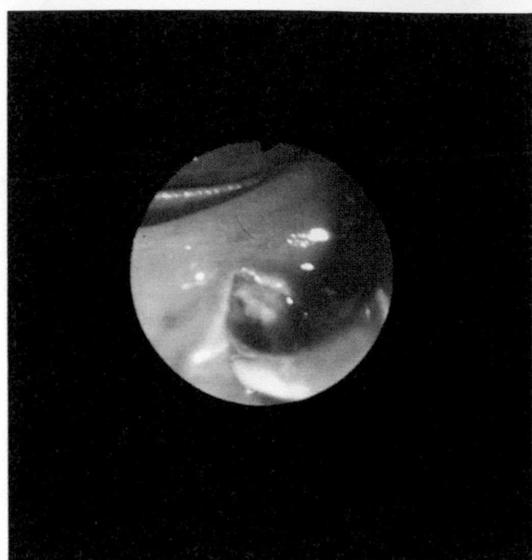

Fig. 13 The ampulla being divided with a sphincterotomy knife.

real risk that the wire will cut too far too fast, and the larger the cut the greater the risk of haemorrhage and perforation. It is rarely necessary to enlarge a sphincterotomy beyond the transverse mucosal fold, which lies immediately above the ampulla, and it is normally sufficient if the fully tightened knife will come through the opening easily. A sphincterotomy needs only to be big enough to allow removal of the largest stone.

Stones are removed from the duct with a balloon or a basket (Fig. 14). Very large stones and stones which are wider than the diameter of the proximal bile duct are not easy to remove. Such stones can sometimes be reduced in size by the use of dissolving agents instilled down a nasobiliary drain (Fig. 15), crushing baskets, laser light, ultrasound, and extracorporeal shock waves. None of these is particularly successful. If the duct cannot be completely cleared, it may be appropriate to leave a nasobiliary drain or a stent in place to allow adequate drainage while further management is considered.

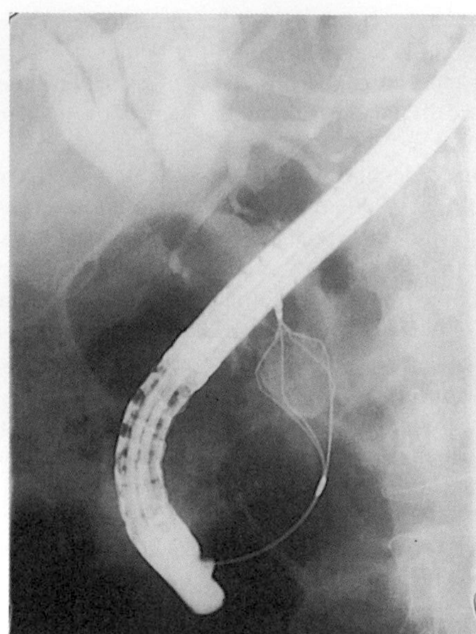

Fig. 14 A large stone being removed from the bile duct using a Dormia basket, following a sphincterotomy.

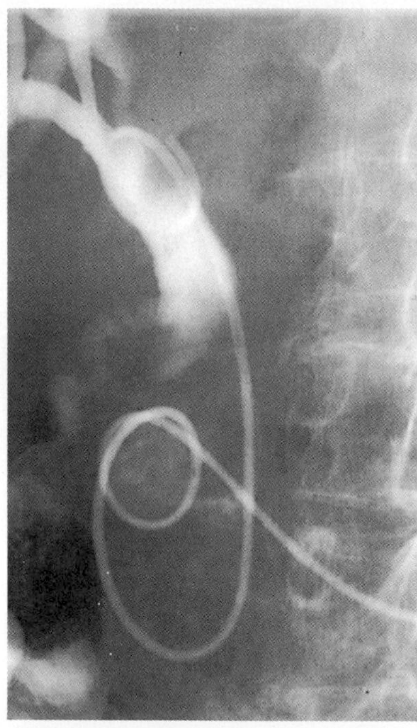

Fig. 15 A nasobiliary drain *in situ*. Mono-octonoin was infused down this tube, reducing the stone in size sufficiently for it to be removed endoscopically.

Biliary intubation

The other fundamental procedure is intubation of a duct with a flexible guidewire carried within a cannula. This is the basis for inserting any form of drainage into a duct, and is most often used to place a stent across an obstruction in the bile duct caused by a carcinoma of the pancreas (Fig. 16). The tip of the cannula is placed below the obstruction. The guide wire is manipulated across the stricture by careful co-ordination between the endoscopy assistant and the endoscopist, and is then followed by the cannula. The stent is 'railroaded' over the cannula and guidewire across the stricture. The proximal tip of the stent is placed well above the stricture, while the distal end lies just within the duodenum, so allowing bile to drain. Various diameters and lengths of stent are available, and the larger the diameter the longer they last. Our standard stent is 3.3 mm in outside diameter and 15 cm long. They last about 4 months. Recurrence of jaundice or cholangitis are signs that the stent needs changing, which is easy to do by removing the old stent with a basket or snare and inserting a new one using the original technique.

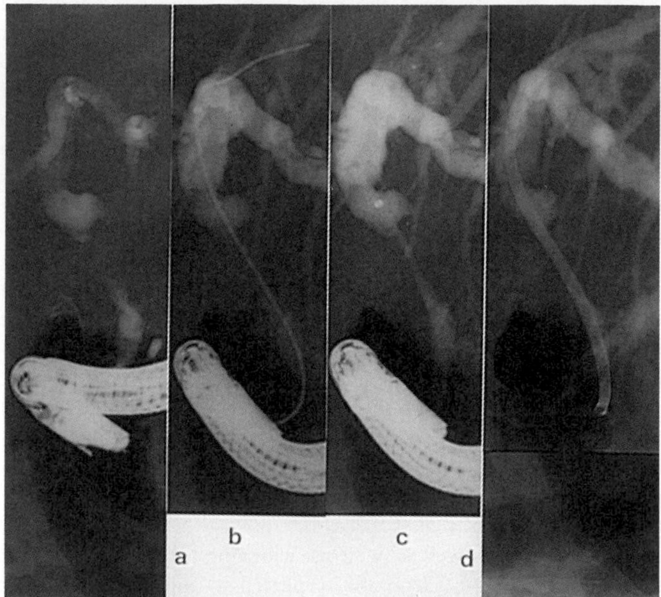

Fig. 16 Intubation of a biliary stricture. (a) Cholangiogram showing the obstruction; (b) cannula below the stricture and the guidewire across the stricture; (c) cannula and guidewire both across the stricture; and (d) stent 'railroaded' into place.

RESULTS

The ampulla can be found by experienced endoscopists in 98 to 99 per cent of patients. They will expect to cannulate both ducts in 90 per cent of patients, although the inexperienced find it slightly easier to cannulate the pancreatic duct. Most series report a 95 per cent success rate in performing a sphincterotomy and complete clearance of stones from the bile duct in nearly 9 out of 10 patients. Half the failures are because of large stones. Endoscopic intubation of the bile duct for malignant obstruction is rather less successful at present, with up to a quarter of attempts failing. Strictures high up and very low down in the bile duct are particularly difficult, but newer techniques, such as a combined percutaneous and endoscopic approach, may improve the results in the future.

COMPLICATIONS

The main complications are cholangitis, pancreatitis, and haemorrhage. The morbidity and mortality for a diagnostic ERCP are about 1 per cent and 0.1 per cent respectively, whereas after an endoscopic sphincterotomy the figures are 10 per cent and 1 per cent. There is a particular risk of haemorrhage after a sphincterotomy, and about half these patients will require a laparotomy. Less frequent problems are retroperitoneal perforation of the duodenal wall and impaction of a basket because a stone is trapped but is too large to remove.

Haemorrhage is usually apparent immediately, but pancreatitis becomes clinically obvious some hours later, and cholangitis can develop at any time. For these reasons we normally give any patient who has had a therapeutic procedure a second dose of antibiotics 12 h after treatment, and we also record the pulse and blood pressure half-hourly for 8 h afterwards.

FURTHER READING

Bickerstaff KI, Berry AR, Chapman RW, Britton BJ. Endoscopic sphincterotomy for bile duct stones. An institutional review. *Ann R Coll Surg* 1989; **71**: 384–6.

Carr-Lock DL, Cotton PB. Biliary tract and pancreas. In: Miller RA, Wickham JEA, eds. Endoscopic surgery. *Br Med Bull* 1986; **42**: 257–64.

Classen M, Demlin L. Endoskopische Sphinkterotomie der Papilla Vateri und Steinextraktion aus dem Ductus choledochus. *Deutsch Med Wochenschr* 1974; **99**: 496–7.

Cotton PB. Progress report ERCP. *Gut* 1977; **18**: 316–41.

Cotton PB, Williams CB. *Practical gastrointestinal endoscopy*. 3rd edn. Oxford: Blackwell Scientific Publications, 1990.

McCune WS, Shorb PE, Moscovitz H. Endoscopic cannulation of the ampulla of Vater: a preliminary report. *Ann Surg* 1968; **167**: 752–6.

Shepherd HA, Royle G, Ross APR, Diba A, Arthur M, Colin-Jones D. Endoscopic biliary endoprosthesis in the palliation of malignant obstruction of the distal common bile duct; a randomized trial. *Br J Surg* 1988; **75**: 1166–8.

Soehendra N, Reynders-Frederix V. Palliative bile duct drainage—a new method of introducing a transpapillary drain. *Endoscopy* 1980; **12**: 8–11.

27.3 Colonoscopy

PAUL C. SHELLITO

INTRODUCTION

Colonoscopy is an invaluable technique for the diagnosis and treatment of disorders of the large bowel. Impartial and direct comparisons to barium enema radiography are scarce, but endoscopy is appreciably more sensitive and specific than are radiographs. In particular, small lesions (especially under 1 cm) and mucosal changes (such as colitis) are much better evaluated by colonoscopy. The ability to do biopsies through the scope also enhances its value. Finally, while barium enema radiography is strictly diagnostic, various therapeutic manoeuvres are possible with colonoscopy, especially polyp removal and cauterization of some bleeding lesions. On the other hand, colonoscopy is probably somewhat more difficult to perform, although differences in patient comfort are arguable. Neither is endoscopy perfectly accurate; lesions can be missed if they are hidden by residual faeces, if located immediately behind flexures or mucosal folds, or if the caecum is not reached. The complication rate of colonoscopy is slightly higher than that for barium enema radiography. An isolated comparison of procedure cost favours radiography. Yet barium enema radiography is properly done in conjunction with a sigmoidoscopy, to avoid overlooking rectosigmoid lesions hidden by the enema tip balloon or by the rectosigmoid flexure. Also, barium enema radiography often leads to colonoscopy to verify, define, or remove a detected abnormality, or to be certain that a 'normal' radiograph is not falsely negative; however the reverse is rarely true. Thus the overall expense and expeditiousness of a colorectal evaluation beginning with colonoscopy by an experienced physician compares favourably with barium enema radiography.

It is particularly worthwhile for surgeons to practise colonoscopy. When colectomy is called for, it is preferable that the operating surgeon evaluate the nature and location of the lesion himself, rather than rely upon secondhand information from a medical physician. The issue is especially important when planning surgery for rectosigmoid carcinoma, because the precise location and size of the tumour greatly influence the type of resection. It is also vital when an endoscopically unresectable polyp is discovered or when a polyp is removed and found to contain invasive cancer. In these instances it may be impossible to palpate any lesion at laparotomy, and the surgeon must depend upon the previous endoscopic judgement to guide resection. Similarly, massive colonic bleeding, usually from diverticulosis or angiodysplasia, occasionally mandates difficult decisions about the segment of bowel that is responsible. An appropriate resection is more likely if the surgeon and the endoscopist are the same person. There is one final consideration. In many ways, modern surgery relies more and more upon less invasive techniques. The growing indications for therapeutic endoscopy reflect this trend. Surgeon endoscopists are most likely to make impartial choices between open surgery and endoscopy, and by temperament and training are best equipped to carry out the endoscopic surgery and deal with the possible complications.

EQUIPMENT AND PROCEDURE

A colonoscope is a thin flexible instrument, usually 160 cm long. An image is transmitted from the tip by either a fibreoptic bundle to a lens on the head of the scope, or by a tiny video camera on the tip to a television. The end can be deflected in a wide arc by manipulating two steering knobs on the endoscope head. Colonoscopes are equipped with a tiny air insufflation channel to permit bowel distension for inspection. Through this channel, automatic water lavage of the scope tip may also be carried out, to keep stool and debris from obscuring the view. Another, larger channel is available for suction or for passing instruments (biopsy forceps, electrocautery forceps, grasping forceps, cytology brush, polypectomy snare, injection needle, laser fibre). Mechanical bowel preparation is required before the procedure. Two or three days of a liquid diet, followed by laxatives and enemas gets the job done, but gut lavage by ingestion of a solution of polyethylene glycol and electrolytes (Golyteley, Colyte) is usually superior. Lavage requires only 4 to 6 h, clears the colon better, results in minimal fluid shifts, and is most often preferred by patients. The patient is usually given intravenous sedation (narcotic and benzodiazepine) and monitored during the procedure with blood pressure determinations, electrocardiography, and pulse oximetry. Fluoroscopy is dispensable.

To begin the procedure, most endoscopists place the patient on his or her left side, hold the instrument in the left hand, and alternately manipulate the scope controls and shaft with the right hand. It is better to place the patient on his or her right side, and to hold the instrument in a bracket or chest harness, thus liberating the left hand to hold the shaft and the right hand to control the tip deflection knobs and instruments in the biopsy channel. The ability to control tip and shaft movements simultaneously results in more facile and versatile instrument operation, especially for endoscopic surgery.

After digital rectal examination, the tip of the instrument is pressed sideways into the anal canal until the sphincter relaxes and the scope enters the rectum. Keeping the lumen in the centre of the field of view as much as possible, the scope is advanced proximally by deflecting the tip and twisting the shaft as necessary. When the view becomes obliterated by the scope tip lying against the bowel mucosa ('red out'), the scope must be partially withdrawn; advancing the shaft blindly invites perforation. Only a minimal amount of air should be insufflated during insertion. Colonic distension makes proximal passage more difficult by lengthening the bowel as well as widening it and making the flexures more acute. Generally, repeated to-and-fro movements with the scope are best, to progressively pleat the bowel over the shaft. Short withdrawal manoeuvre (which ought to be frequent) should usually be accompanied by clockwise rotation of the shaft to straighten the counter-clockwise sigmoid loop. When scope advancement becomes difficult, changing the patient's position (side, supine, even prone) or manually compressing the left lower quadrant of the abdomen often works. The goal is to reach the caecum with the shortest possible length of colonoscope. With a straight scope, the splenic flexure lies at 40 to 50 cm, the hepatic flexure at 60 to 70 cm, and the caecum at 80 to 100 cm. The instrument will then trace a smooth 'question mark' path to the caecum. Large loops or bows in the instrument stretch the bowel of mesentery and risk perforation, are painful to the patient, and, by placing the control cables on stretch, hamper the delicate tip manoeuvrability needed for thorough inspection and especially for therapeutic endoscopy. Residual stool and mucus should be meticulously suctioned out during instrument insertion, so that the obscuring fluid will not interfere with treatment of a lesion later, or make a detached polyp difficult to find. Experienced endoscopists reach the caecum 90 to 95 per cent of the time. Appearances of a 'blind end' can be misleading, however; the best assurance of traversing the entire colon is to see the appendiceal

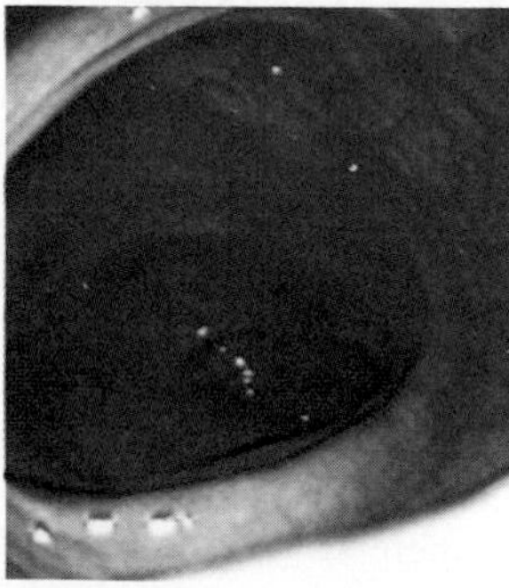

Fig. 1 An endoscopic view of a normal left colon. Typical mucosal folds are visible.

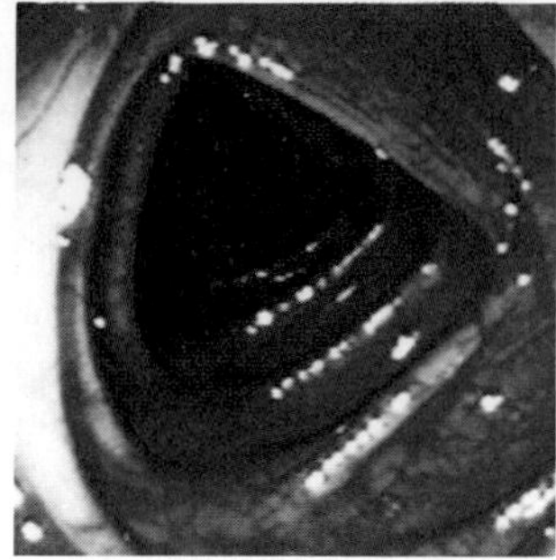

Fig. 2 The transverse colon; often it displays this triangular appearance.

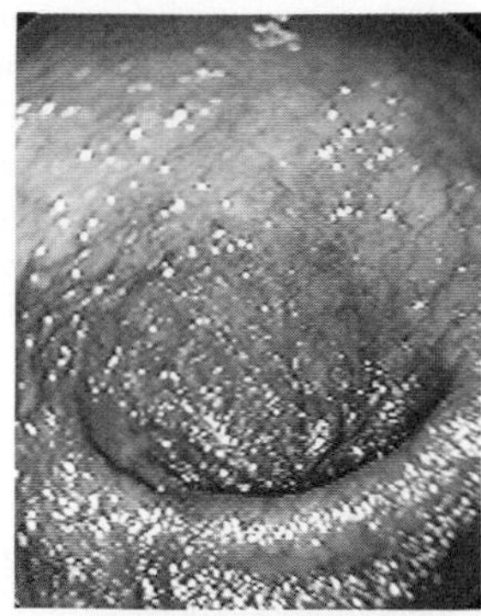

Fig. 4 Terminal ileum, with typical stippled appearance, due to villous mucosa and submucosal lymphoid follicles (colonic mucosa, in contrast, is smooth).

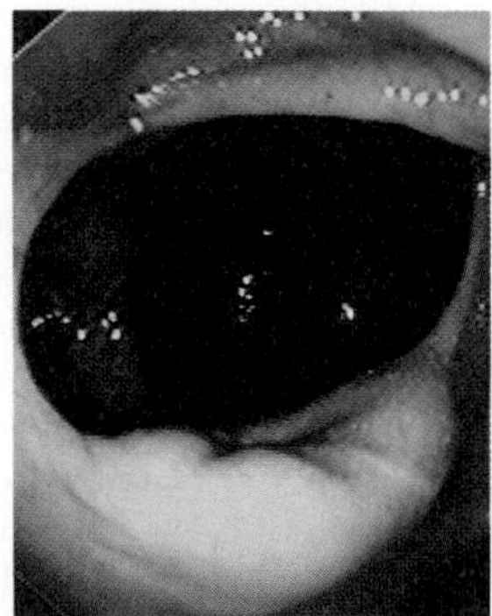

Fig. 3 Right colon, with ileocaecal valve visible inferiorly.

orifice and/or the ileocaecal valve (Fig. 3). Obstacles to reaching the caecum are a poor bowel clean-out, strictures or large tumours, fixed angulations in the bowel (usually from diverticular disease, previous pelvic surgery, or irradiation), or simply a long, tortuous colon. If a polyp is removed, its location within the colon or rectum should be judged carefully, and if multiple polyps are present, they should be submitted to pathology separately. Thus, if a lesion is later discovered to contain invasive cancer, the appropriate bowel resection can be performed.

INDICATIONS, CONTRAINDICATIONS, AND COMPLICATIONS

Diagnostic colonoscopy, including inspection and sometimes biopsy, is especially valuable for benign and malignant mucosal and submucosal tumours or strictures, as well as for mucosal changes caused by colitis (infection, infestation, radiation, ischaemia) or angiodysplasia. It is less satisfactory for judging functional or motility disorders, or extraluminal lesions (which may only cause extrinsic compression of the colon). Specifically, the major indications for diagnostic colonoscopy are:

(1) evaluation of a clinically important abnormality or possible abnormality seen on barium enema radiography;
(2) evaluation of lower gastrointestinal bleeding, faecal occult blood, or unexplained iron deficiency anaemia;
(3) surveillance for colon adenomas and carcinomas in high-risk patients;
(4) evaluation of persistent and important diarrhoea;
(5) evaluation of colitis.

The most important indications for therapeutic colonoscopy are:

(1) polyp removal;
(2) cauterization of some bleeding lesions;
(3) decompression of colonic ileus (Ogilvie's syndrome) or volvulus;
(4) possible treatment of obstruction by dilatation or incision of strictures, or laser fulguration of tumours.

On the other hand, colonoscopy is not ordinarily useful for:

(1) evaluation of abdominal pain (especially chronic pain) unless a category cited above is suspected;
(2) evaluation of acute limited diarrhoea;
(3) minor haematochezia in a patient with a convincing anorectal source after evaluation by anoscopy and flexible sigmoidoscopy.

There are also clear contraindications to colonoscopy. Any acute inflammatory process of the colon should deter the endoscopist. Endoscopy in the presence of acute diverticulitis will certainly be painful, and the associated manipulation and air insufflation may worsen the infection. Similarly, the suspicion of a perforated viscus contraindicates colonoscopy. So does fulminant colitis of any cause, because of perforation risks. Endoscopic surgery should not be carried out in an anticoagulated patient. Finally, a badly prepared bowel ought not to be colonoscoped. If a large amount of faeces is present, not only is diagnostic accuracy much decreased but also the risk of perforation is greater than usual because of the poor view.

The most important complications of colonoscopy are perforation and bleeding. Both are quite infrequent unless endoscopic surgery has been done. Perforation accompanies a diagnostic procedure in 0.1 to 0.5 per cent of cases. This may be a longitudinal antimesenteric tear from excessive pressure within a bowel loop (usually the sigmoid). In that event, the rent may not be immediately recognized since the side of the scope causes the tear while the tip remains in the lumen. Alternatively, the tip may directly poke through the bowel wall if the scope is not appropriately guided. This misfortunate is usually quickly apparent since small bowel or omentum can be seen. Diverticulosis (Fig. 5) predisposes

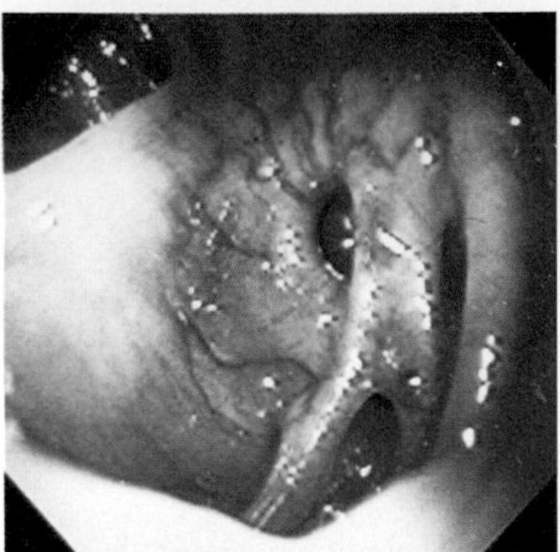

Fig. 5 Diverticulosis.

to perforation because of the thin diverticulum wall (mucosa only). The risk is also increased because of a frequently associated narrowed and tortuous sigmoid lumen, and possibly a fixed angulation from previous inflammation. Anything that weakens the bowel wall, such as colitis or pelvic radiation therapy, increases the danger. Also, radiation or simply adhesions from pelvic surgery add to the perforation risk by creating a relatively tortuous and immobile rectosigmoid. Bowel disruption by an antimesenteric tear or scope tip penetration requires prompt antibiotic administration and laparotomy for repair or (especially if there is associated diseased colon) resection. Nevertheless, colostomy is usually unnecessary because the colon has been mechanically prepared, and the injury is recognized immediately. Perforations after polypectomy, on the other hand, can often be treated conservatively (see below).

Appreciable bleeding is very rare after diagnostic colonoscopy even when biopsies have been done (0–0.1 per cent of cases). Haemoperitoneum from a splenic capsular tear has been reported. Other, usually less serious problems, are drug reactions (usually respiratory depression), vasovagal reflex, bacteraemia, and superficial phlebitis.

COLONOSCOPY AND GASTROINTESTINAL BLEEDING

Because of its superior sensitivity and specificity, colonoscopy should be the first choice for diagnosis of lower gastrointestinal bleeding whenever possible. The entire colon can be assessed in addition to the bleed site. Endoscopic treatment is sometimes feasible. Often, the terminal ileum, which may harbour angiodysplasia or Crohn's disease, can be inspected as well. The major disadvantage of endoscopy is that if the bowel is unprepared, or bleeding is rapid, the view is obscured. The diagnostic yield of colonoscopy in unselected patients with lower gastrointestinal bleeding is substantial, even if barium enema radiography is negative. An important lesion such as an adenoma, carcinoma, angiodysplasia, or inflammatory bowel disease will be found in 30 to 50 per cent of such patients. Thus even good-quality barium enema radiography which is normal (or shows only diverticulosis) should not terminate the search for a colonic lesion.

For patients with faecal occult blood, colonoscopy is the best initial test. Again, even when barium enema radiography is negative, colonoscopy is indicated because an important lesion will be found in about one-third of patients. If radiography shows an abnormality, endoscopy is still needed to confirm the presence and nature of the lesion, perhaps rule out synchronous neoplasms, and sometimes to treat the problem. If colonoscopy is unremarkable, oesophagogastroduodenoscopy may be considered, although the yield will be very low in patients with only guaiacum-positive faeces unless they have anaemia or upper gastrointestinal symptoms.

When melaena occurs, ordinarily oesophagogastroduodenoscopy is the appropriate initial manoeuvre. If that is normal, however, colonoscopy should follow, since in that setting a right colon lesion is often found. If both upper and lower endoscopy are negative, either a small lesion has been overlooked at endoscopy or a rare small bowel lesion is at fault (Meckel's diverticulum, leiomyoma, arteriovenous malformation, Crohn's disease).

Scanty intermittent haematochezia with bowel movement is a very common occurrence. An anal lesion is usually responsible, but up to 20 per cent of these patients have a proximal lesion (polyp, cancer, colitis), even if haemorrhoids or a fissure are seen. Small amounts of visible fresh blood, if not coming from the anus, usually come from the rectum or distal colon, so sigmoidoscopy (preferably flexible sigmoidoscopy) is always indicated. If the bleeding can be explained by an anal lesion, and the patient is under 40 years old without a prominent family history of colon neoplasms, ordinarily no further testing is necessary. For patients over 40, it is best to add barium enema radiography (or colonoscopy).

For patients presenting with active lower gastrointestinal bleeding, the fruits of colonoscopy are twice the yield in patients with only occult bleeding. Fortunately, frank haematochezia ceases spontaneously in at least 80 per cent of patients, so bowel preparation and endoscopy are usually possible. Barium enema radiography should not be done, not only because of its inferior accuracy, but also because barium in the bowel lumen would interfere with a later colonoscopy or angiogram. A meticulous bowel preparation is important (polyethylene glycol solution), to allow detailed inspection of the mucosa. Furthermore, if emergency colectomy becomes necessary, the mechanical bowel cleansing will have already been completed. Colonoscopy finds the source of active and substantial lower gastrointestinal haemorrhage in 80 to 90 per cent of patients. Bleeding diverticulosis and angiodysplasia are most often responsible, but the problem may also be due to inflammatory bowel disease, cancer, adenoma, ischaemic colon, or radiation telangiectasias. In massive unceasing bleeders, an option for initial diagnosis is laparotomy, intraoperative colonic lavage, and intraoperative colonoscopy, although mesenteric angiography is probably a better choice.

SURVEILLANCE FOR COLON NEOPLASMS

Colorectal cancer is decidedly appropriate for screening. It is common and frequently fatal. Adenocarcinoma develops slowly, most often beginning as a benign, precursory neoplastic polyp. After 5 to 15 years, a minority of adenomas degenerate into cancer. It is likely, although unproven, that removal of adenomas will decrease the incidence of colorectal cancer. The evidence is

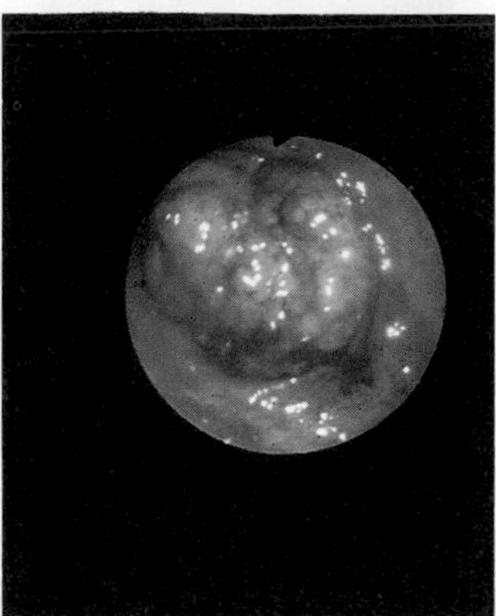

Fig. 6 Exophytic rectal carcinoma.

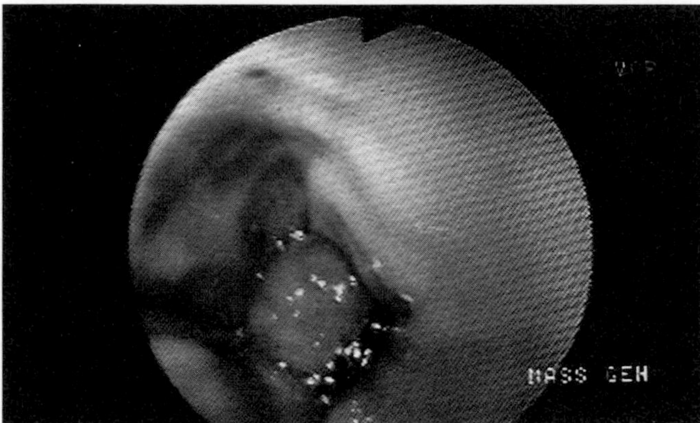

Fig. 7 Ulcerated right colon carcinoma.

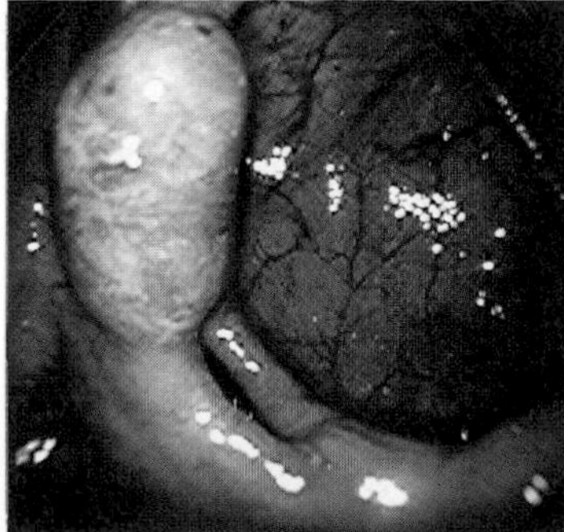

Fig. 8 Small carcinoma adjacent to the ileocaecal valve.

sufficient to justify strategies to detect and remove all colon adenomas. Since early stage cancers have a good prognosis, efficient identification of nascent carcinomas is also worthwhile. Because of risks and expense, aggressive screening is not appropriate for everyone. Colonoscopy is best offered to patients with a high risk for colorectal cancer. Characteristics denoting a high risk are:

(1) history of colorectal cancer;
(2) history of colorectal adenoma;
(3) strong family history of colorectal neoplasia;
(4) ulcerative colitis;
(5) familial polyposis or Gardner's syndrome;
(6) ureterosigmoidostomy;
(7) pelvic radiation;
(8) possibly a history of breast, endometrial, or ovarian cancer.

The first four are the most common and important. Familial polyposis is not an indication for screening, since colectomy should be done whenever the diagnosis is made. For other 'average-risk' patients, yearly faecal occult blood testing should be initiated at age 40, and flexible sigmoidoscopy every 2 to 3 years should start at age 50, as recommended by the American Cancer Society.

Whenever feasible, colon polyps should be removed. Adenomas may contain or transform to malignancy so excision is advisable, usually through a colonoscope. Tiny lesions (less than 5 mm in diameter) are often hyperplastic polyps, which are not premalignant. Nevertheless, histology cannot be inferred from gross appearance and so all polyps should be removed, since even small ones may be adenomas. In the rectum and left colon, 70 to 75 per cent of tiny polyps are hyperplastic and the remainder adenomas, but in the proximal colon the reverse is true—70 to 75 per cent are adenomas. Characteristics of an adenoma that correlate with increased likelihood of malignancy are large size (especially over 1.0 cm in diameter), villous histology (villous adenoma more than tubulovillous adenoma, more than tubular adenoma), and possibly sessile morphology. Simple biopsy of a polyp is often histologically misleading, so the whole lesion must be removed. Whenever a polyp is discovered by any means, the entire colon requires inspection, since 20 to 50 per cent of adenoma patients have at least one more adenoma, and 2 to 5 per cent have a synchronous cancer. Thus, sigmoidoscopy should be viewed as a sampling procedure; if a neoplasm is found, total colonoscopy is indicated. Periodic follow-up colonoscopy is also important because 20 to 50 per cent of patients will develop another adenoma. Multiple adenomas discovered on the initial examination correlate with an increased risk of metachronous lesions. Furthermore, 5 to 10 per cent of patients with adenomas produce a colorectal cancer later in life.

For persons who present with a colorectal cancer, the statistics for synchronous and metachronous neoplasms are virtually identical; this is consistent with the view that adenomas are precursor lesions to carcinomas. Of these patients, 2 to 5 per cent have synchronous colon cancers, 3 to 10 per cent develop metachronous malignancies (more if adenomas coexist with the initial tumour), 25 to 50 per cent have synchronous adenomas, and 20 to 40 per cent sprout adenomas later. Thus patients with colorectal cancer should have a perioperative, preferably a preoperative, colonoscopy. The synchronous lesions are not usually palpated at laparotomy, and often would have been excluded from the planned resection. Again, colonoscopy at regular intervals is useful after cancer resection, to detect metachronous neoplasms as well as to find the rare isolated anastomotic recurrence. Of all the possible tests available for follow-up of colorectal cancer patients (carcinoembryonic antigen, liver function tests, chest radiography, computerized scan, barium enema radiography, etc.), colonoscopy is probably the most worthwhile. For patients with either adenomas or cancers, the appropriate schedule for follow-up colonoscopy is unknown, but it is reasonable to carry out endoscopies yearly until no further polyps are found. The examination may then be repeated in 2 years and every 3 to 5 years thereafter (except in very elderly or frail patients).

The same colonoscopy schedule should apply to patients with strong family histories of colorectal cancer or adenoma. Inherited autosomal dominant colonic polyposis syndromes (familial polyposis and Gardner's syndrome), which always lead to cancer when untreated, aptly illustrate that there are powerful genetic determinants of at least some large bowel malignancies. Hereditary site-specific colon cancer, and cancer family syndrome (Lynch syndromes I and II), also autosomal dominant, markedly increase the risk of colorectal cancer, which arises at an uncharacteristically early age and proximal location (making sigmoidoscopy an ineffective screening tool), and with a high frequency of multiplicity. The latter condition is also associated with breast and endometrial cancer. When colon cancer and its precursor polyps are analysed together, inheritance patterns become even more recognizable. Inherited large bowel neoplasms may, in fact, be quite common. Even 'sporadic' colon neoplasms are genetic to some extent, inasmuch as first-degree relatives (parents, siblings, children) of colon cancer patients have three times the average risk for the disease. Thus periodic screening colonoscopy is appropriate possibly for individuals with one first-degree relative harbouring a colorectal cancer, and certainly for those with two afflicted first-degree relatives. Endoscopy should begin at approximately age 30.

Ulcerative colitis certainly predisposes to colon malignancy. The cancer may be multifocal, and is often flat and infiltrating, making recognition difficult, especially if severe mucosal inflammation coexists. Stage-specific survival is the same for ordinary colon malignancies, but diagnosis is often delayed until the cancer is deeply invasive. The cancer risk correlates chiefly with the amount of involved colon and the duration of the disease (not the activity of the disease). In patients with total colitis, the cancer danger becomes appreciable after 8 to 10 years. Thereafter, there is a risk of 0.5 to 1.0 per cent per year of disease duration. For left-sided colitis, the risk is diminished, and for proctitis only there is minimal danger. Colorectal cancer complicating ulcerative colitis is frequently associated with severe mucosal dysplasia. Thus, after 8 to 10 years, yearly screening colonoscopy with diffuse random biopsies should be initiated for those with extensive colitis. If persistent severe mucosal dysplasia is found, especially if a macroscopic abnormality is also present (such as a plaque, nodule, or stricture), the risk of a concomitant malignancy is high and prophylactic colectomy is indicated. Since mucosal changes are patchy, sigmoidoscopy and rectal biopsy alone are insufficient. Discontinuity is not the only problem with screening for mucosal dysplasia; 10 to 20 per cent of patients who develop carcinomas have no associated mucosal dysplasia, and only about one-third of patients with severe dysplasia get cancer. Accompanying severe mucosal inflammation makes recognition of dysplasia difficult. Furthermore, even under the best of circumstances the presence and degree of dysplasia is difficult to quantify, and pathological assessments may vary. Crohn's colitis also predisposes to cancer, although to a lesser extent, and screening colonoscopy may be helpful.

COLONIC POLYPECTOMY

Polyps are elevated growths of the colonic epithelium. Their shape may be sessile or pedunculated (Fig. 9). They are often adenomas, which are premalignant, but may also be hyperplastic polyps or, rarely, frank carcinomas. Since it is not possible to determine which polyps are adenomas until they are excised and studied microscopically, ordinarily all should be completely removed. Removal can usually be done endoscopically with low complication and recurrence rates. As discussed under the section on surveillance, the presence of any colon adenoma indicates the need for total colonoscopy, as well as periodic future examinations. Polyps 3 to 4 mm in diameter or smaller can be completely and easily removed with an enveloping biopsy cauterization forceps ('hot biopsy'). This tool preserves most or all of the lesion unharmed within its jaws for histological analysis, but electrocoagulates any residual polypoid tissue outside its grasp. Larger polyps are removed with an electrocautery snare. This is a retractable wire loop with a plastic sheath, which is passed through the endoscope and placed around the polyp base or stalk (Fig. 10).

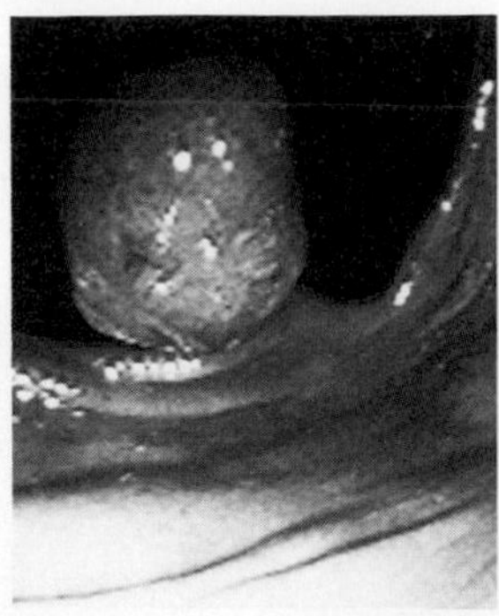

Fig. 9 A pedunculated colon polyp.

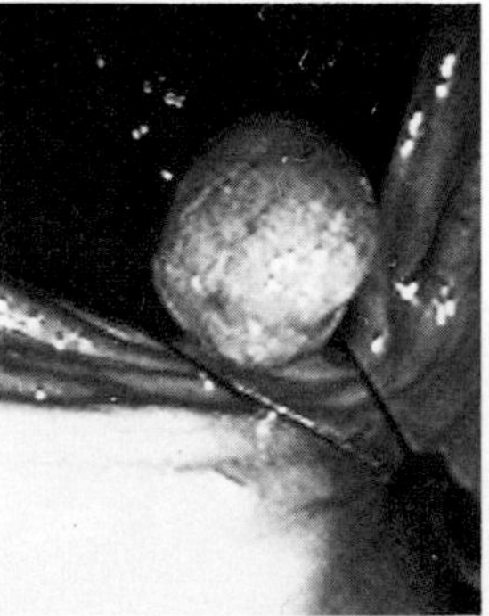

Fig. 10 A snare placed around the polyp.

The snare is tightened (Figs. 11, 12) as electrocoagulating current is passed through the wire, resulting in separation and haemostasis. Large polyps with a broad base may require multiple snare applications ('piecemeal resection'). Very large polyps are often best removed surgically, by either transanal excision under direct vision, or segmental colectomy.

The risks of colonoscopic polypectomy are somewhat greater than for simple diagnostic colonoscopy. Perforation occurs in 0.5 to 1.0 per cent. It is a bit more likely when the polyp lies in the right

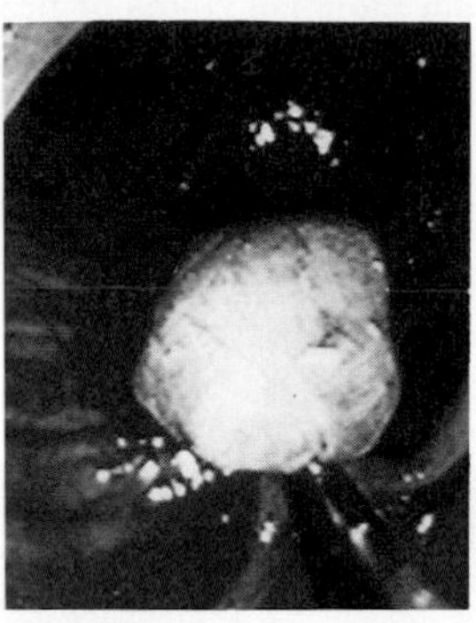

Fig. 11 The snare tightened around the base of the polyp.

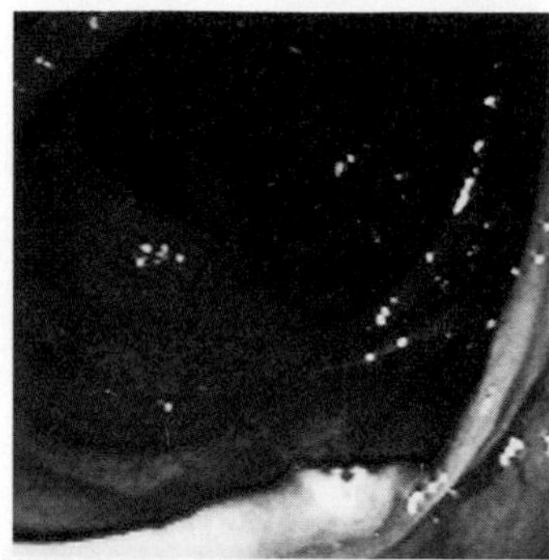

Fig. 12 The polyp neck transected by electrocautery snare.

colon, where the bowel wall is thin, or when the polyp is large and sessile. The risk of appreciable bleeding is 1 to 2 per cent, which may be delayed for days or even weeks. Large pedunculated polyps are probably the most likely to bleed after removal, since there may be a single large arteriole in the stalk. When bleeding or perforation is suspected after polypectomy, a frozen-section pathology report for the removed lesion will aid subsequent management. If the specimen contains invasive cancer, then colectomy can be carried out without delay. On the other hand, if the polyp is benign, then non-operative treatment may sometimes be attempted. When frank perforation occurs, marked by pneumoperitoneum and signs of spreading peritonitis, immediate laparotomy is needed, along with administration of broad-spectrum antibiotics. Since the colon has already been mechanically prepared, and since surgery quickly follows injury, repair without a colostomy is usually possible. If the patient develops only localized and non-progressive tenderness, often with a delayed presentation, the injury may simply be a small area of full-thickness coagulation. These patients will frequently recover without surgery if placed under careful hospital observation on broad-spectrum antibiotics and nothing by mouth. Even a small perforation with pneumoperitoneum may similarly resolve (especially if a water-soluble contrast enema radiograph shows no extravasation). Postpolypectomy bleeding can usually be treated conservatively. The patient should be kept in hospital for observation, and should be transfused as necessary. If the bleeding does not stop spontaneously, intravenous or intra-arterial vasopressin will usually succeed. Only a minority will continue to bleed and require surgery. If polyps from more than one segment of the colon have been removed, then angiography is a crucial guide for resection. Urgent repeat colonoscopy to recauterize a bleeding polyp stump is usually futile and unnecessary.

Malignancy within a polyp deserves special consideration. The appropriate treatment is difficult to study, but the important histological variables to consider are depth of invasion, polyp morphology, and margins or resection. A polyp should be considered 'malignant' if true invasive cancer is present, that is cancer penetrating the underlying muscularis mucosa. If the muscularis mucosa has not been broached (carcinoma *in situ*), then polypectomy alone is curative, and only routine follow-up endoscopy is required thereafter. Residual, recurrent, and metastatic disease have not occurred after local carcinoma *in situ*.

For snared sessile lesions containing invasive cancer, it is always difficult to be certain that the margins are free of tumour. Residual disease at the polypectomy site is found at colectomy or at follow-up endoscopy in 0 to 40 per cent. Furthermore, when colectomy is done after sessile polypectomy, positive lymph nodes are found in 10 to 40 per cent. Thus a formal colectomy is usually wise.

Cancer in pedunculated polyps metastasizes less often than does malignancy in sessile lesions. If the cancer extends down to the neck or stalk of a pedunculated polyp, the frequency of involved lymph nodes found by subsequent colectomy is 0 to 15 per cent, and the incidence of locally recurrent or residual disease is 0 to 10 per cent. On the other hand, if the cancer is limited to the head of a stalked polyp, the frequency of local disease and positive nodes approaches 0 per cent. Therefore, simple endoscopic polypectomy is usually sufficient treatment in the latter instance. Many authors recommend, however, that if the cancer in a pedunculated polyp is poorly differentiated, demonstrates invasion of lymphatics, or is present at the resection margin, colectomy should be done, even for a malignancy limited to the head, since residual or metastatic tumour will occasionally be found. In the absence of these special histological characteristics, however, the risk of colectomy probably outweighs the risk of recurrence for cancers only in the head of pedunculated polyps. A few investigators argue that endoscopic polypectomy is sufficient treatment for any malignant polyp as long as none of the above adverse microscopic features is present. Of course, the age and medical condition of the patient is an important consideration when judging the necessity for colectomy.

ENDOSCOPIC TREATMENT OF COLONIC BLEEDING

Not only is colonoscopy superior for diagnosis of lower gastrointestinal bleeding, but it can also be therapeutic. Angiodysplasia is an acquired submucosal and mucosal arteriovenous malformation which is one of the most frequent causes of lower gastrointestinal bleeding in elderly patients (Figs. 13, 15). As discussed in Section 18.7, the best treatment is endoscopic cauterization using a laser (Fig. 14) or electrocautery forceps. Rebleeding occurs in 10 to 30 per cent of cases, which compares favourably with the results of surgery. Perforation occurs in 0 to 7 per cent of cases.

For bleeding tumours, prompt laparotomy and radical resection is often best. Occasionally, however, non-operative therapy is preferable; the tumour may be inoperable, the patient may decline surgery, or, for an advanced malignancy, the physician may wish to delay laparotomy until preoperative adjuvant radiation therapy

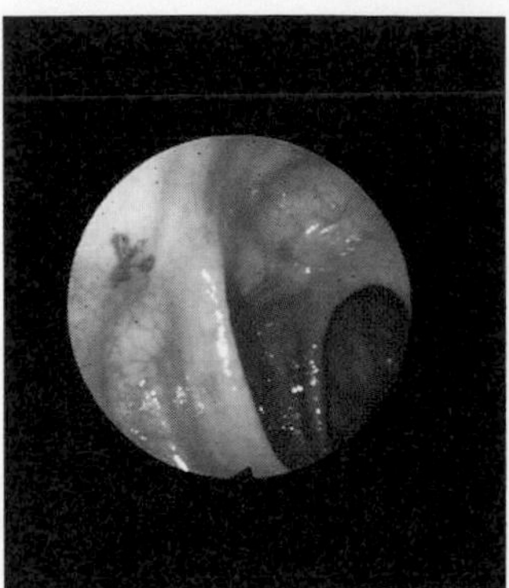

Fig. 13 Caecal angiodysplasia.

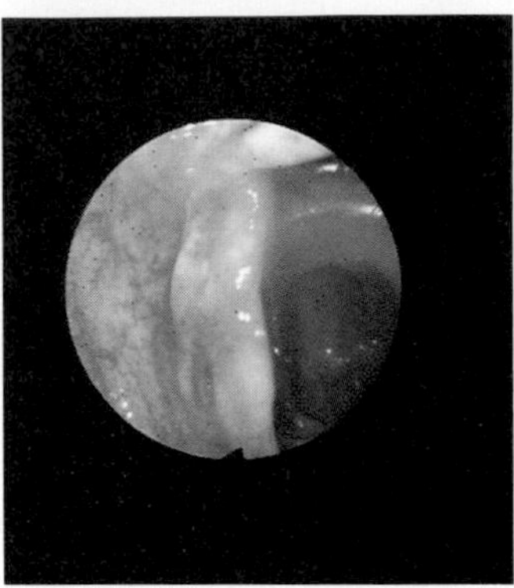

Fig. 14 Caecal angiodysplasia obliterated by laser photocoagulation.

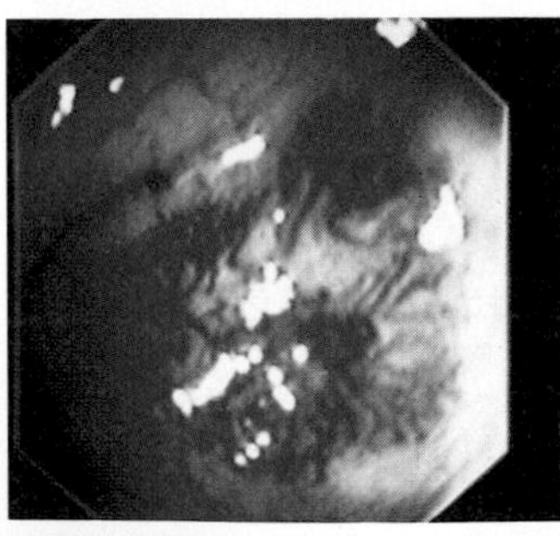

Fig. 15 Close-up view of caecal angiodysplasia, showing prominent mucosal and submucosal blood vessels.

can be given. Laser photocoagulation (usually a neodymium: yttrium aluminium garnet (Nd:YAG) laser) is attractive therapy for such cancers, since a larger surface area may be treated quickly, although two or three endoscopic treatment sessions may be required (see below). Polyps are unlikely to bleed heavily, but they are usually readily removable with snare electrocautery, as discussed above.

Haemorrhage from radiation colitis or proctitis is sometimes a chronic recurring problem. Mucosal telangiectasias superimposed upon a fibrotic and atrophic bowel wall are usually responsible (Fig. 16). Again, laser photocoagulation (Fig. 17) is attractive because a large surface area can be treated relatively easily, the

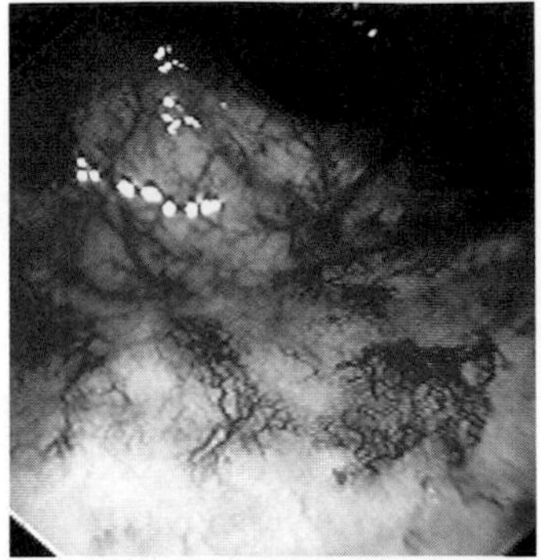

Fig. 16 Chronic radiation change in rectal mucosa (telangiectasias) after radiation therapy for cervical cancer.

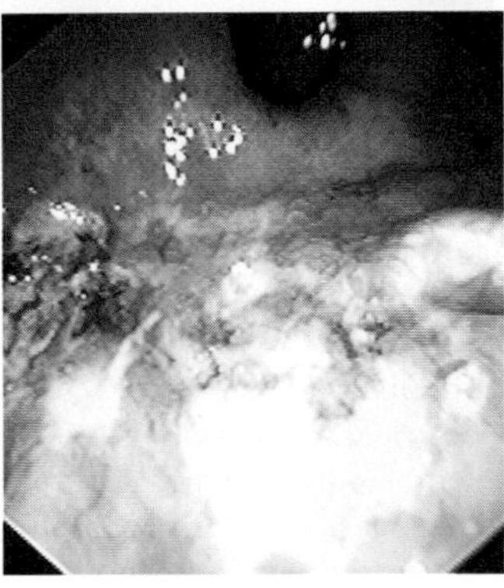

Fig. 17 Cauterization of rectal mucosal telangiectasias.

procedure can be done on outpatients, and the technique demonstrable reduces the number of bleeding episodes and the transfusion requirement. The risk and cost of laparotomy and resection is avoided, which is especially attractive since surgery for radiation-damaged colon has exceptional morbidity. Obliteration of the telangiectasias requires two or three sessions in the early phase. Also, periodic follow-up endoscopic coagulation is wise, since radiation damage is progressive, and the blood vessel malformations tend to recur and bleed again.

Rarely, diverticular bleeding may be treated endoscopically. Colonic diverticula occur at weak points in the muscularis, where blood vessels penetrate. This adjacent blood vessel may become eroded, perhaps by faecalith, and bleed. Although in practice it is rare to see a single diverticulum as a convincing bleeding point, if this is discovered or if there is a prominent blood vessel associated with a particular diverticulum and no other obvious bleeding source, endoscopic coagulation may be carried out. It is best to grasp the mucosa and the vessel with a hot biopsy forcep, lift the mucosa up off the underlying bowel wall (to minimize perforation risk), coagulate, and release (no actual biopsy taken). Because the wall of the diverticulum is very thin, coagulation should be performed adjacent to the orifice, not within it.

DECOMPRESSION OF COLONIC ILEUS AND VOLVULUS

When the colon is distended, there is a risk of perforation, especially when the caecal diameter reaches 10 to 12 cm. Thus, urgent manoeuvres to define the aetiology and decompress the colon are called for. Sometimes the diagnosis of volvulus or colonic ileus is fairly clear, just from the plain abdominal radiograph. (If a sigmoidoscopy is to be done, it should follow the abdominal film, so that insufflated air will not confuse the appearance of the site of obstruction.) If there is doubt about whether an obstruction colon tumour is present, an emergency contrast enema radiograph may be done. Water-soluble contrast rather than barium should be used in this circumstance, however, for two reasons. First, if colonoscopy is subsequently needed, barium obscures the view and obstructs the endoscope suction channel. Secondly, if urgent surgery becomes necessary, it is preferable not to have barium in the bowel lumen, because it potentiates faecal contamination. The water-soluble medium does not provide the same quality of radiographic detail as does barium, but in this situation detail is unimportant; one simply needs to know whether mechanical obstruction is present or not. In fact, it is often best to skip contrast radiography and go straight to colonoscopy.

The most important initial manoeuvre in a patient with sigmoid volvulus is non-operative decompression. An emergency sigmoid colectomy and anastomosis should ordinarily be avoided, since joining a colon distended and filled with faeces risks leakage. Usually, urgent sigmoidoscopy and possibly a long rectal tube will suffice for decompression. When that fails, however, a colonoscope will be long enough to do the job. Because volvulus has a high recurrence rate, bowel preparation and an elective sigmoid colectomy should soon follow. On the other hand, endoscopy is scarcely worthwhile for caecal volvulus. Colonoscopic decompression is much less successful than for sigmoid volvulus. An emergency right colectomy is usually safe, since the small bowel is anastomosed to non-dilated distal colon.

Colonic ileus (colonic pseudo-obstruction, Ogilvie's syndrome) is an idiopathic condition seen in association with many other medical problems, and can appear after surgery in a region unrelated to the colon. There may be massive colonic and caecal distension, although caecal perforation is probably unusual. If nasogastric suction and cessation of narcotics and anticholinergic agents, and correlation of electrolyte abnormalities, fails to resolve the situation, more direct decompression is required. Caecostomy is an option, but colonoscopy can often avert surgery. The endoscope is passed as far proximally as possible in the unprepared colon (a messy business) and the bowel is then suctioned out as the scope is withdrawn. Passage to the transverse colon is often sufficient. Frequently the procedure must be repeated every day or two for a total of two or three times. With this approach, the success rate is 50 to 80 per cent. The need for repeated colonoscopy can be avoided by endoscopically placing a long decompression tube (such as an overtube).

ENDOSCOPIC TREATMENT OF COLON STRICTURES AND TUMOURS

Symptomatic benign rectosigmoid strictures can sometimes be treated endoscopically. A guidewire may be passed via the colonoscope channel, and positioned across the narrowed area. The endoscope is then removed, leaving the guidewire in place. Dilators (for example, Savary) are then passed over the guidewire, perhaps under fluoroscopic view. Inflatable ('through the scope') dilators are also available for dilatation under endoscopic view. Finally, thin strictures, such as anastomotic strictures, may sometimes simply be endoscopically incised using a wire electrocautery papillotomy knife, or an Nd:YAG laser.

Rectosigmoid neoplasms have been treated by fulguration, usually with a laser. Although radical resection is usually the best primary treatment for potentially curable rectosigmoid cancer, local ablation may occasionally be employed for carefully selected patients with early low-rectal tumours. In general, however, transanal excision (full thickness for cancer, in the submucosal plane for adenomas) under direct vision is the best approach, rather than endoscopic fulguration. Meticulous excision gives the best chance that no neoplastic tissue remains and provides a complete specimen for pathological examination for the presence of invasive cancer, lateral margins, and depth of tumour invasion. Excision and closure also minimizes the likelihood of consequent fistula, abscess, or secondary bleeding.

Sometimes the goal is only palliation of a rectal cancer. A patient with a large tumour may refuse to accept a colostomy or be unable to manage one. Alternatively, because of advanced age or poor medical condition, an individual may be considered unfit for major surgery, although modern techniques of anaesthesia and perioperative care have nearly eliminated this category. And finally, incurable distant metastases may already be present by the time the rectal tumour is initially diagnosed. Electrocoagulation has been employed for palliation (and even potential cure), but endoscopic laser vaporization of tumours has recently supplanted this method. Most reports of laser fulguration have involved patients with rectosigmoid cancer rather than more proximal lesions, because access is easier, there is less risk of intraperitoneal perforation, a bigger operation would be required for resection, and there is a desire to avoid a stoma. Laser recanalization has also been occasionally used for obstructing yet potentially curable tumours, to permit a later one-stage resection. Nevertheless, most completely obstructing colorectal tumours lie near the splenic flexure, not the rectum, and the angulation of the flexure, as well as its intraperitoneal location, increase the perforation hazard. Fire near obstructed colon also invites explosion.

Even for rectal tumours, laser treatment has disadvantages. In coring out a large cancer, meticulous endoscopists will find spelunking amid smoke, blood, stool, and charred tissue unattractive. Repeated treatments are required, not only to initially carve away the lesion, but also to control tumour regrowth periodically thereafter. Surgery, on the other hand, would most likely fix the problem with a single stroke. As time passes, even with repeated laser applications, adequate palliation becomes more and more difficult to maintain.

Enthusiasts of laser fulguration report good initial results. Bleeding, obstruction (which may manifest itself as diarrhoea), and discharge are more amenable to laser treatment (especially the first) than are pain and tenesmus. Cancer cachexia and incontinence due to sphincter invasion by tumour are, of course, not improved at all. Relief of obstruction and/or bleeding sufficient to avoid surgery has been reported in 75 to 90 per cent of cases. Nevertheless, restoration of a lumen does not always abolish symptoms and restore function. Successful laser palliation of large circumferential tumours is difficult. Similarly, patients with locally recurrent cancers fare worse than do those with primary tumours, probably because there is a larger extraluminal mass responsible for most of the symptoms. Furthermore, time is the gremlin of the enterprise. Even with periodic treatments to destroy resurgent tissue, extraluminal tumour growth carries on unaffected by the laser. If the patient survives for long enough, the process leads to pain from nerve invasion, fistulization, or diffuse narrowing of the bowel, which is increasingly difficult to battle. Only about 40 per cent of surviving patients remain symptomatically well at 1 year, despite repeated laser fulgurations.

Complications compare favourably with major surgery. Bleeding requiring transfusion occurs in 1 to 5 per cent of cases, perforation in at least 1 to 3 per cent (especially if the tumour lies at or above the peritoneal reflection), symptomatic stenosis requiring dilatation or colostomy occurs in 0 to 5 per cent, rectovaginal fistula in 0 to 3 per cent (anterior low-rectal cancers in females), and perianal abscess in 0 to 1 per cent (presumably from a low microperforation).

Thus the best candidates for palliative laser therapy are those with severe local symptoms of obstruction or bleeding (more so bleeding) due to a relatively small cancer, but with a short life expectancy because of diffuse metastases (less than 6–12 months). Not many patients will fulfil these criteria.

FURTHER READING

Alexander TJ, Dwyer RM. Endoscopic Nd:YAG laser treatment of severe radiation injury of the lower gastrointestinal tract. *Gastrointest Endosc* 1988; **34**: 407–11.

American Society of Gastrointestinal Endoscopy. *Gastrointestinal endoscopy: diagnostic and therapeutic procedures: an information resource manual*. Manchester, MA.

Blackstone MO, Riddell RH, Rogers BHG, Levin, B. Dysplasia associated lesion or mass (DALM) detected by colonoscopy in long standing ulcerative colitis: an indication for colectomy. *Gastroenterology* 1981; **80**: 366–74.

Bown SG, Barr H, Matthewson K, *et al.* Endoscopic treatment of inoperable colorectal cancers with the Nd:YAG laser. *Br J Surg* 1986; **73**: 949–52.

Brunetaud JM, Maunoury V, Ducrotte P, Cochelard D, Cortot A, Paris JC. Palliative treatment of rectosigmoid carcinoma by laser endoscopic photoablation. *Gastroenterology* 1987; **92**: 663–8.

Cranley JP, Petras RE, Carey WD, Paradis K, Sivak MV. When is endoscopic polypectomy adequate therapy for colonic polyps containing invasive carcinoma? *Gastroenterology* 1986; **91**: 419–27.

Dent TL, Kukora JS, Buinewicz BR. Endoscopic screening and surveillance for gastrointestinal malignancy. *Surg Clin N Am* 1989; **69**: 1205–25.

Fitzgibbons RJ, *et al.* Recognition and treatment of patients with hereditary nonpolyposis colon cancer (Lynch Syndromes I and II). *Ann Surg* 1987; **206**: 289–94.

Fleischer DE, *et al.* Detection and surveillance of colorectal cancer. *JAMA* 1986; **261**: 580–5.

Fozard JBJ, Dixon MF. Colonoscopic surveillance in ulcerative colitis: dysplasia through the looking glass. *Gut* 1989; **30**: 285–92.

Guillem JG, Forde KA, Treat MR, Neuget AI, Bodian CA. The impact of colonoscopy on the early dètection of colonic neoplasms in patients with rectal bleeding. *Ann Surg* 1987; **206**: 606–11.

Lambert R, Sobin, LH, Waye JD, Stalder GA. The management of patients with colorectal adenomas. *CA* 1984; **34**: 167–76.

Manning AP, Bulgim OR, Dixon MF, Axon ATR. Screening by colonoscopy for colonic epithelial dysphasia in inflammatory bowel disease. *Gut* 1987; **28**: 1489–94.

Mathus-Vliegen EMH, Tytgat GNJ. Laser photocoagulation in the palliation of colorectal malignancies. *Cancer* 1986; **57**: 2212–16.

Nivatongs S, Vermeulen FD, Fang DT. Colonoscopic decompression of acute pseudoobstruction of the colon. *Ann Surg* 1982; **196**: 598–600.

O'Brien MJ, *et al.* The National Polyp Study: patient and polyp characteristics associated with high grade dysplasia in colorectal adenomas. *Gastroenterology* 1990; **98**: 371–9.

Olsen HW, Lawrence WA, Snook CW, Mutch WM. Review of current polyps and cancer in 500 patients with initial colonoscopy for polyps. *Dis Colon Rect* 1988; **31**: 222–7.

Overholt BF. Colonoscopy and colon cancer: current clinical practice. *CA* 1982; **32**: 180–6.

Panish JF. Management of patients with polypoid lesions of the colon: current concepts and controversies. *Am J Gastroenterol* 1979; **71**: 315–24.

Reasbeck PG. Colorectal cancer: the case for endoscopic screening. *Br J Surg* 1987; **74**: 12–17.

Richards WO, *et al.* Patient management after endoscopic removal of the cancerous colon adenoma. *Ann Surg* 1987; **205**: 665–70.

Rosenstock E, Farmer RG, Petras R, Sivak MV, Rankin GB, Sullivan BH. Surveillance for colonic carcinoma in ulcerative colitis. *Gastroenterology* 1985; **89**: 1342–6.

Schrock TR. Colonoscopic diagnosis and treatment of lower gastrointestinal bleeding. *Surg Clin N Am* 1989; **69**: 1309–25.

Strodel WE, Brothers T. Colonoscopic decompression of pseudoobstruction and volvulus. *Surg Clin N Am* 1989; **69**: 1327–35.

Van Cutsem E, *et al.* Risk factors which determine the long term outcome of neodymium YAG laser palliation of colorectal carcinoma. *Int J Colorect Dis* 1989; **4**: 9–11.

Wilcox GM, Anderson PB, Colacchio TA. Early invasive carcinoma in colonic polyps: a review of the literature with emphasis on the assessment of the risk of metastasis. *Cancer* 1986; **57**: 160–71.

27.4 Laparoscopy

P. JANE CLARKE

INTRODUCTION

The peritoneal cavity of a dog was examined in 1902 by Kelling, using air insufflation and the insertion of a cystoscope through the abdominal wall. The first clinical use was described in 1912 by Jacobaeus, although it was a further decade before a purpose-built scope was in use by Kalk (1929) and the era of modern-day laparoscopy (peritoneoscopy) began.

PROCEDURE (DIAGNOSTIC LAPAROSCOPY)

The patient is positioned supine on the operating table. A general anaesthetic with muscle relaxation is usually preferred, but it is possible to use local anaesthetic and sedation with intravenous benzodiazepines. The Verres needle is introduced via a stab incision. This is usually subumbilical in position, but the presence of scars may influence the precise location. The needle contains a spring-loaded blunt probe, and compression of the spring against the skin retracts the probe to expose the needle. Damage to intra-abdominal viscera can be minimized by holding up the anterior abdominal wall with one hand while inserting the needle with the other. When the needle has passed through the abdominal wall the resistance falls and the spring pushes forwards the probe covering the needle. Free flow of normal saline solution through the needle confirms that the linea alba and peritoneum have been punctured. The abdomen is then insufflated with carbon dioxide, using approximately 2 to 3 litres for an adult. During insufflation, the intra-abdominal pressure should not exceed 15 mmHg. The Veres needle is then withdrawn and the incision is enlarged to accommodate the laparoscope trocar, which is pushed down and back into the pelvis. The end- or side-view telescope is then inserted and laparoscopy commenced. Biopsy forceps and a palpating probe can be used in other, suitably placed stab incisions through the anterior abdominal wall. This allows the peritoneal contents to be inspected. Throughout the procedure, carbon dioxide is continually insufflated at low pressure.

CONTRAINDICATIONS

There are few absolute contraindications to the procedure, but certain conditions should alert the surgeon to potential problems. Multiple scars make introduction of the scope hazardous, and adhesions from repeated abdominal procedures may hinder the view within the peritoneum. Abdominal wall sepsis may introduce intraperitoneal infection. The procedure is not tolerated well in patients with severe pulmonary or cardiac problems, due to the intra-abdominal distension. Bleeding diatheses may result in body wall or intraperitoneal bleeding.

COMPLICATIONS

To minimize complications, laparoscopy is a procedure best performed by surgeons experienced in the technique, in an operating theatre equipped with the facilities to proceed to a laparotomy if necessary. Minor complications include abdominal wall bruising, subcutaneous emphysema, the development of a wound infection/hernia, and postoperative shoulder pain. Other complications are related to accidental visceral damage and bleeding from vessel injury. These problems should be noted at the time of laparoscopy and dealt with by prompt laparotomy if necessary. Mortality rates of 0.03 to 0.1 per cent are reported.

INDICATIONS (see Fig. 1)

Acute

In patients with localized peritonism, diagnostic laparoscopy is most commonly used in the management of patients with acute right iliac fossa pain, in an attempt to reduce the incidence of 'negative' surgical explorations for acute appendicitis, especially in young women. With the aid of a palpating probe inserted through the anterior abdominal wall of the right iliac fossa, the surrounding ileum and omentum may be manipulated away in order to see the appendix. In the case of a retrocaecal or retroileal appendix, it may be impossible to visualize the target organ, but other signs of acute inflammation may be noted. Alternatively, other causes of right iliac fossa pain may be apparent, and, if these require surgery, an appropriate incision can be made.

The role of diagnostic laparoscopy in the management of the patient with abdominal trauma is in conjunction with imaging techniques (CT and ultrasound scanning) and peritoneal lavage. The relative importance of each is not established clearly, although aggressive use of laparoscopy in this clinical situation may reduce the number of unnecessary laparotomies performed for minimal or moderate haemoperitoneum. The procedure can be performed in the accident and emergency department under local anaesthesia with intravenous sedation, and has been facilitated by the development of a 'mini' (5 mm) laparoscope.

Elective

In the management of patients with undiagnosed abdominal pain, opinion is divided as to the benefits of laparoscopy. The role of

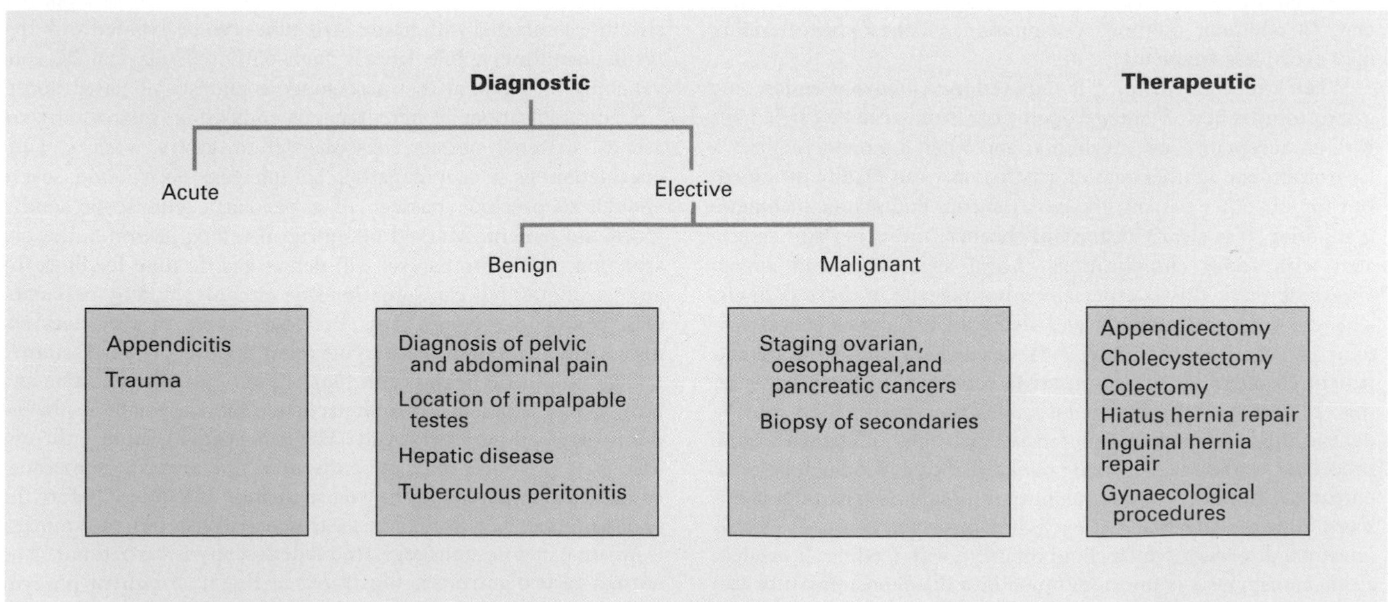

Fig. 1 Indications for laparoscopy.

laparoscopy is better established in the investigation of women with chronic pelvic pain, and is frequently performed by gynaecologists.

In children with impalpable testes, laparoscopy can be used to visualize the internal ring and the testicular vessels. These are followed to locate the testis, which may then be classified as being abdominal, pelvic, canalicular (the lower pole entering the orifice of the internal ring), or absent. The laparoscopic findings may then influence the site of a subsequent incision or obviate the need for an exploration.

Other indications for elective laparoscopy in benign disease include the diagnosis of various liver conditions (by direct visualization with or without biopsy), and tuberculous peritonitis.

Laparoscopy is commonly used in the management of intra-abdominal malignancy. As a staging investigation, laparoscopy is a more sensitive and accurate means of detecting small liver metastases and peritoneal seedlings compared with CT and ultrasound scanning. Biopsy may be performed using a Menghini needle under direct vision, which minimizes the risk of inadvertent visceral trauma, and increases the positive histological yield compared with a 'blind' percutaneous biopsy. Draining lymph nodes may also be seen and biopsied to exclude malignant involvement. The knowledge obtained by such procedures may avoid an unnecessary laparotomy if a palliative operation is not indicated.

Therapeutic

An increasing number of surgical operations are now feasible via the laparoscope (see Fig. 1). These are described, as appropriate, in the relevant chapters.

27.5 Percutaneous endoscopic gastrostomy

PAUL C. SHELLITO

When patients require nutritional support, the enteral route is always preferable if the gastrointestinal tract is functional. Tube feedings are no less effective than intravenous nutrition, and are also easier, safer, and much cheaper. Small, soft nasogastric feeding tubes work satisfactorily, especially if the need for nutritional support is expected to be short. Insertion of nasoenteric tubes can bring complications, however, such as pulmonary intubation leading to pneumothorax, hydrothorax, or pneumonia. Furthermore, nasogastric tubes are uncomfortable and certainly unsightly. With prolonged use, the tubes tend to clog, fall out, or get pulled out by the patient, who is often neurologically impaired. A tube gastrostomy, on the other hand, is more comfortable and easier to maintain. In addition, pulmonary aspiration and oesophageal reflux may occur less frequently.

When a tube gastrostomy is required, percutaneous endoscopic gastrostomy is best. Standard open gastrostomy can be carried out with an acceptably low morbidity, and when a patient requires a laparotomy for another reason, gastrostomy can readily be added. But for any other patient, the percutaneous endoscopic technique is superior. It is clearly faster and cheaper, and is perhaps associated with fewer complications. Local anaesthesia can almost always be used; this is especially advantageous in these patients, who are frequently elderly and debilitated. Open-tube gastrostomy can also be done under local anaesthesia, but exposure and patient co-operation are so unsatisfactory that surgeons rarely do this. If necessary, percutaneous endoscopic gastrostomy can be done at the bedside or in an intensive care unit, and pain after the procedure is minimal. In stable patients, it can even be done in an outpatient setting. The concomitant oesophagogastroduodenoscopy adds the advantage of excluding unsuspected upper gastrointestinal disorders, which could interfere with feeding. If needed, a thin transpyloric jejunostomy tube or a duodenostomy tube can also be placed by the percutaneous endoscopic gastrostomy route. Nevertheless, accurate placement of these tubes is tricky, and subsequent mechanical problems (occlusion, malposition) are common. They provide little extra protection against aspiration and pneumonia, since the problem in these patients is not often reflux of gastric contents, but rather inhalation of pharyngeal secretions.

Percutaneous endoscopic gastrostomy is indicated for any patient who cannot, or will not, eat and who therefore needs prolonged enteral tube feedings. Patients with neurological disorders, oropharyngeal dysfunction or tumours, or facial trauma often qualify. In addition, for anyone requiring prolonged gastric decompression, the discomfort, the difficulty in clearing pulmonary secretions, and the potential oesophagitis or even oesophageal stricture associated with nasogastric tubes can be avoided with this technique. Rarely, bile from a high-output fistula can be conveniently fed again after a percutaneous endoscopic gastrostomy.

Contraindications to percutaneous endoscopic gastrostomy are ascites, extreme obesity, oesophageal or gastric varices, anticoagulation or a coagulopathy, oesophageal obstruction severe enough to preclude passage of a paediatric endoscope, and a moribund patient. Marked oesophageal reflux, gastric outlet obstruction, and gastroparesis will defeat gastric tube feedings (by any technique) but can sometimes be circumvented by percutaneous endoscopic jejunostomy. Previous gastric surgery does not necessarily contraindicate percutaneous endoscopic gastrostomy.

The procedure begins with topical pharyngeal anaesthesia and intravenous sedation. A prophylactic antibiotic (usually cephalosporin) is given perioperatively. With the patient supine, the abdomen is swabbed with an antiseptic and draped. Sometimes oesophageal or posterior pharyngeal dilation is required before the endoscope can be passed. The gastroscope is inserted, the stomach is inflated, and oesophagogastroduodenoscopy is carried out. The normal gastric antrum is illustrated in Fig. 1. Frequent pharyngeal suctioning is helpful in a supine patient with an anaesthetized throat to minimize the risk of aspiration.

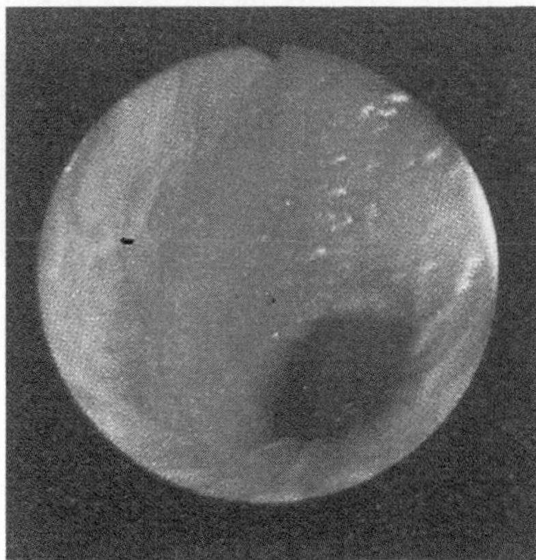

Fig. 1 Normal gastric antrum.

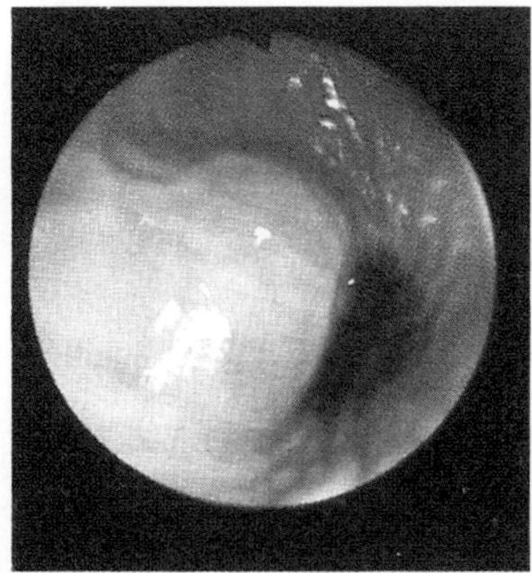

Fig. 2 The optimum gastrostomy site is selected by finger indentation.

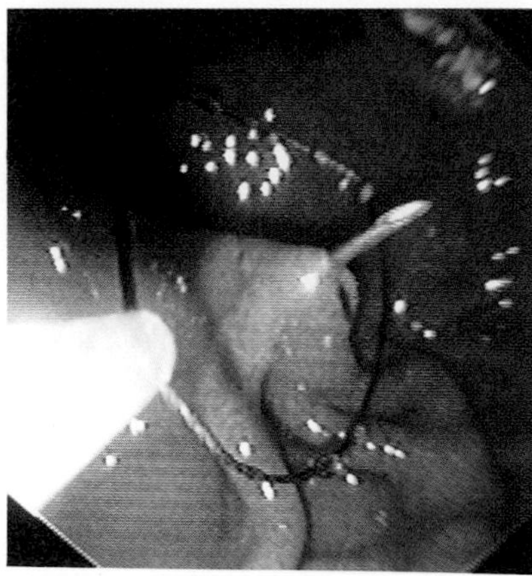

Fig. 3 A needle is inserted percutaneously into the stomach at the selected site. An endoscope snare is positioned around the needle tip.

The abdominal location for the gastrostomy is selected by transilluminating through the anterior stomach wall. A point in the left upper quadrant between the midline and the midclavicular line is often successful. Apposition of the stomach to the anterior abdominal wall is confirmed by finger indentation, which is readily visible through the endoscope (Fig. 2). If transillumination or finger indentation is equivocal, percutaneous gastrostomy should not proceed. After skin infiltration with local anaesthesia, a small stab incision is made at the selected site. The incision should be slightly larger than the diameter of the tube, to allow some later drainage of this inevitably contaminated wound. A needle is inserted through the incision, with simultaneous syringe suction (Fig. 3). Appearance of air in the syringe at the same time as the needle is seen entering the stomach ensures that the stomach, not the colon, is the first viscus entered. A heavy suture or a guidewire is then inserted through the needle (care must be taken not to allow the stomach to deflate through the needle) (Fig. 4). The suture or wire is snared by the endoscopist and is withdrawn through the mouth. A mushroom-tip gastrostomy tube (Fig. 5) is then drawn with the suture or guided over the wire back down through the mouth, stomach, and out through the abdominal wall (Fig. 6). The endoscope is reinserted to check the position of the tube (Fig. 7). An endoscopic technique using a peel-away introducer has also been described, which required only one insertion of the endoscope.

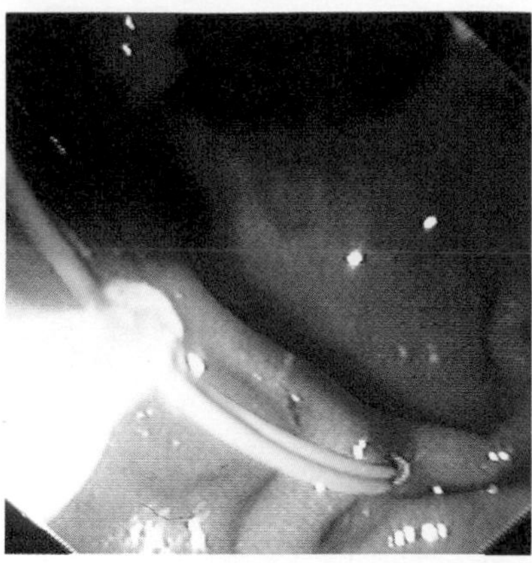

Fig. 4 A heavy suture or guidewire is passed through the needle, and snared by the endoscopist.

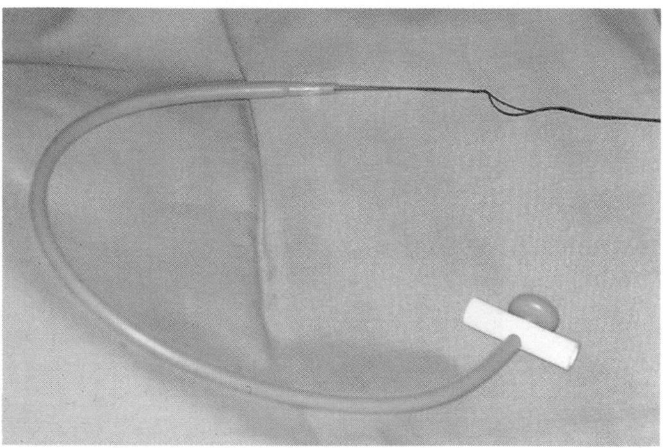

Fig. 5 The endoscope and the suture or guidewire are withdrawn back out through the mouth. The end of a gastrostomy tube is tied to the end of the suture or guidewire.

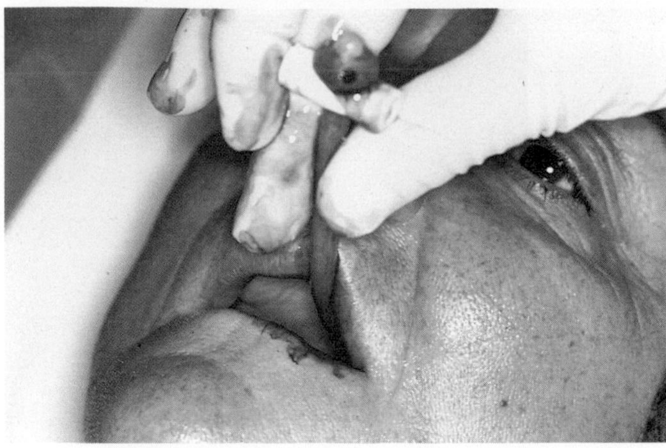

Fig. 6 The gastrostomy tube is then pulled down through the mouth, stomach, and out through the abdominal wall.

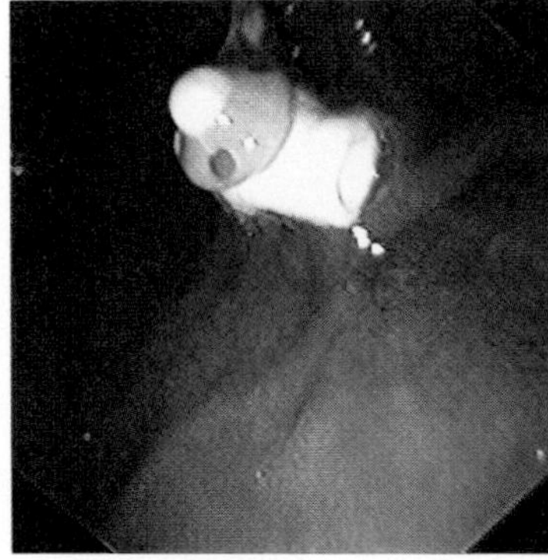

Fig. 7 The endoscope is reinserted and the gastrostomy tube is positioned properly.

An outer plastic cross-bar or disc is passed around the tube and positioned over the skin to hold the gastric and abdominal walls together. To avoid pressure necrosis of the skin or gastric wall, the tube should not be drawn up too tightly. Multiple heavy anchoring sutures at the skin insertion site minimize the likelihood that the tube will become displaced. Tube feedings may be started the next day. After about 2 weeks, a fibrous track will form, and the tube may be changed as needed. Tubes with soft tips that can be extracted through the skin are usually preferable to tubes that have non-deforming ends. In order to remove the non-deformable tube, the catheter must be cut at skin level, leaving the tip in the stomach. Since the plastic end may cause bowel perforation or obstruction, repeat endoscopy for extraction is required—an avoidable inconvenience. Percutaneous endoscopic gastrostomy is unsuccessful for technical reasons in 5 to 10 per cent of patients.

The complication rate for percutaneous endoscopic gastrostomy compares favourably with gastrostomy by laparotomy. Wound infection (cellulitis, abscess) occurs in no more than 1 to 5 per cent of patients if prophylactic antibiotics are administered. A few reports of severe necrotizing fasciitis have appeared, however. Aspiration pneumonia after percutaneous endoscopic gastrostomy is occasionally a problem, especially if the patient is neurologically impaired and has a previous history of aspiration. Of course, placing a gastrostomy tube will not alter a patient's tendency to inhale oropharyngeal secretions, and it is uncertain when aspiration pneumonia can be directly attributed to the procedure. It happens perhaps 1 to 5 per cent of the time. Haemorrhage requiring transfusion or surgery occurs in up to 2 per cent of patients, and an appreciable external leak around the tube appears in up to 1 per cent. None of the above complications is unique to the percutaneous endoscopic method. Since anterior gastropexy is not achieved with the endoscopic technique, however, an early inadvertent tube extrusion is particularly troublesome; a free intraperitoneal leak results. Up to 5 per cent of patients suffer tube dislodgement requiring surgery. An internal leak (without tube extrusion) or gastric perforation occurs in up to 2 per cent. Colon puncture or gastrocolic fistula is rare in adults. Asymptomatic pneumoperitoneum after percutaneous endoscopic gastrostomy is common and of no consequence. Respiratory arrest is a risk in patients with pharyngeal tumours, who might retain only a marginal airway. Further compromise comes from the presence of the scope, throat oedema from intubation, and sedation. If there is any question about airway adequacy, it is best to perform a tracheostomy first, or to postpone percutaneous endoscopic gastrostomy until after resection of the tumour.

FURTHER READING

Davis JB, Bowden TA, Rives DA. Percutaneous endoscopic gastrostomy: do surgeons and gastroenterologists get the same results? *Am Surg* 1990; **56**: 47–51.

DiSario JA, Foutch PG, Sanowski RA. Poor results with percutaneous endoscopic jejunostomy. *Gastrointest Endosc* 1990; **36**: 257–60.

Grant JP. Comparison of percutaneous endoscopic gastrostomy with stamm gastrostomy. *Ann Surg* 1988; **207**: 598– 603.

Hunter JG, Lauretano L, Shellito PC. Percutaneous endoscopic gastrostomy in head and neck cancer patients. *Ann Surg* 1989; **210**: 42–6.

Kaplan DS, Murphy UK, Linscheer WG. Percutaneous endoscopic jejunostomy: long term followup of 23 patients. *Gastrointest Endosc* 1989;**35**: 403–6.

Larson DE, Burton DD, Schroeder KW, MiMagno EP. Percutaneous endoscopic gastroscopy: indications, success, complications, and mortality in 314 consecutive patients. *Gastroenterology* 1987; **93**: 48–52.

Mamel JJ. Percutaneous endoscopic gastrostomy. *Am J Gastroenterol* 1989; **84**: 703–10.

Miller RE, Kummer BA, Kotler DP, Tiszenkel HI. Percutaneous endoscopic gastroscopy: procedure of choice. *Ann Surg* 1986; **204**: 543–5.

Ponsky JL. Percutaneous endoscopic stomas. *Surg Clin N Am* 1989; **69**: 1227–36.

Shellito PC, Malt RA. Tube gastrostomy: techniques and complications. *Ann Surg* 1985; **201**: 180–5.

Stern JS. Comparison of percutaneous endoscopic gastrostomy with surgical gastrostomy at a community hospital. *Am J Gastroenterol* 1986; **81**: 1171–3.

Stiegmann GV, Goff JS, Silas D, Pearlman N, Sun J, Norton L. Endoscopic versus operative gastrostomy: final results of a prospective randomized trial. *Gastrointest Endosc* 1990; **36**: 1–5.

Wolfsen HC, Kozarek RA, Ball TJ, Patterson DJ, Botoman VA. Tube dysfunction following percutaneous endoscopic gastrostomy and jejunostomy. *Gastrointest Endosc* 1990; **36**: 261–3.

27.6 Lasers in gastroenterological disease

HUGH BARR

PRINCIPLES OF LASER ACTION

The word laser is an acronym for 'Light Amplification by the Stimulated Emission of Radiation'. Some understanding of the nature of light is necessary to understand laser action. Light has a dual nature, behaving sometimes as a wave and at other times as a mechanical particle. The wave nature gives it wavelength; its particle side is manifested as the photon, which carries a discrete amount of energy. Both wave and particle viewpoints help towards an understanding of lasers but the particle theory is, in general, the more important.

Quantum mechanics limits atoms and molecules to certain discrete states of energy, the lowest of which is called the ground state. Atoms and molecules make instantaneous transitions between energy levels, which involve the absorption or release of energy. The transition energy is usually absorbed or released as a photon.

In order to understand the principle of a laser, consider a simple atom with orbiting electrons. The electrons orbiting the nucleus of the atom have specific energy levels; electrons away from the nucleus are in higher energy levels and electrons in the ground or lower energy states are closer to the nucleus. Now consider an incoming photon carrying a unit or quantum of energy that matches the difference between two energy levels of the atom. This photon can be absorbed, producing an excited atom in which an electron moves to a higher energy state; when this electron later spontaneously returns to the original lower energy state, the absorbed energy is released as another photon—'spontaneous emission'. There is another possibility, first predicted by Einstein in 1917: if the atom in the excited state is struck by another photon the energy is not absorbed, but it instead stimulates the atom to release a second photon of equal frequency and energy travelling in the same direction and in perfect spatial and temporal harmony with the stimulating photon (Fig. 1). This phenomenon is termed 'stimulated emission of radiation'. Thus a photon may be absorbed or stimulate emission of another photon.

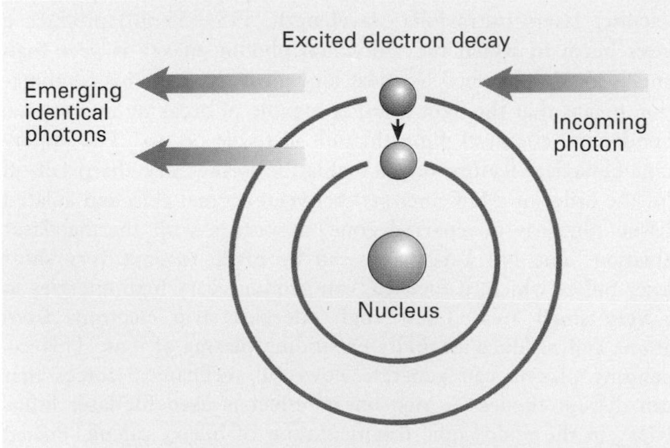

Fig. 1 Diagram to illustrate stimulated emission. An atom with orbiting electrons in an excited state is struck by a photon, causing the stimulated emission of two identical photons.

Left to themselves, atoms will always arrange themselves among their energy states in such a way that there are more in the lower energy states than in the higher states; in ordinary circumstances absorption always wins. Stimulated emission can, however, win over absorption, if for one pair of energy states there are more atoms in the higher than the lower state. Such a condition is called a population inversion, and is necessary for laser action.

Heating can increase the average energy of atoms or molecules, but heating alone cannot create a population inversion: heat moves all the atoms a little higher on the ladder, it does not increase the ratio of atoms in a higher state. Heat energy selectively excites atoms to certain high-energy states, where they keep their excess energy for an unusually long time. Atoms in a laser can be excited or pumped up to this state by light from other sources (even another laser), electrical currents passed through gases or semiconductors, by chemical reactions, or in other ways.

Stimulated emission produces light that travels in the same direction as the triggering light. In most lasers, however, stimulated emission is a weak effect that can build up to high power only after the light has travelled a long distance through the laser, interacting with other atoms. By placing a mirror at either end of the laser tube, the beam can be amplified to produce high powers. If one mirror is partially reflecting the laser beam can be allowed to emerge.

The light produced from lasers exhibits several special properties that differ in a number of respects from that of light from a domestic light bulb. Ordinary light is incoherent, whereas laser light is called coherent: the photons are travelling in the same direction and are identical, being in step with each other in both time and space. The coherence of laser light means that the divergence of a laser beam is very small (the beam is collimated). The full power of a laser beam can be focused on to a very small spot and it is this property of a laser that enables almost all of the power to be coupled into and transmitted through a small diameter fibreoptic guide which can in turn be passed through instrumentation channels of flexible endoscopes. Laser light consists of either one or just a few distinct colours. The beam of light from a laser is highly collimated, the irradiance (power per unit cross-sectional area) of the beam is very high, and can be focused to very tiny spots, producing enormous irradiance and localized power.

LASER LIGHT/TISSUE INTERACTION

An understanding of the interactions of laser light with tissue is fundamental to the rational use of lasers as instruments in surgery. Interactions are best considered by examining the fate of a laser beam externally irradiating a block of tissue (Fig. 2). On striking an air/tissue interface some of the photons are reflected from the tissue surface. On entering tissue a photon may be scattered; its energy is not significantly altered but the direction of travel is changed. Light that has penetrated deeper than a few hundredths

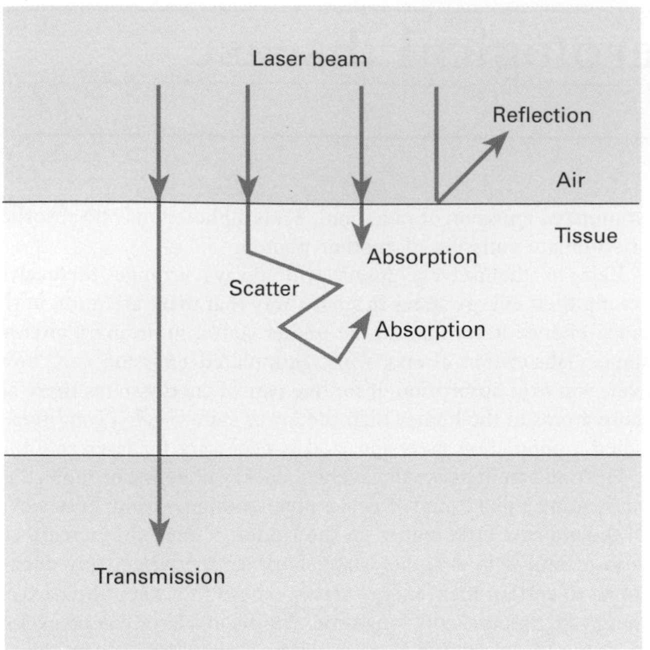

Fig. 2 The possible fate of laser light on penetrating tissue.

of a millimetre will have been subject to multiple scattering. It is important to note that scattered light does not produce any biological effect. Similarly, light that is transmitted through tissue exerts no biological effect: in order for a biological reaction to occur light must be absorbed by the tissue.

Non-specific absorption occurs when a variety of tissue agents absorb the light. In general absorption in tissue is determined by its constituents such as melanin, haemoglobin, myoglobin, and water. The absorption characteristics of individual tissues vary enormously and are also highly dependent on the wavelength of the light. The carbon dioxide laser beam (wavelength 10 600 nm, in the far infrared/invisible end of the spectrum) is strongly absorbed by water, whereas the argon ion laser beam (blue/green) is strongly absorbed by haemoglobin molecules and other pigments. In certain circumstances it may be desirable to administer an exogenous agent, to produce specific absorption of light in certain tissues such as malignant tumours. This allows photochemical reactions to be produced and is the basis of photodynamic therapy.

THERMAL EFFECTS

Absorption of a photon in a non-specific manner may produce thermal changes in the tissue. These are at present the most widely used and surgically useful biological effects produced by a laser beam. If the rate of delivery of the photons (laser power) is such that the energy is dissipated in the surrounding medium as quickly as it is delivered no significant rise in the tissue temperature will occur. However, if the light is delivered at high enough power the tissue temperature will rise. Initially, at low rates, the temperature rise may be great enough to cause thermal damage to biological reactions. Local heating of malignant tissue to temperatures in the region of 41 to 45°C may produce selective hyperthermic destruction of malignant cells, since they are more sensitive to such temperatures than is normal tissue. This differential killing ability is lost at temperatures above 45°C and all cells are rapidly killed above 50°C. Further heating of tissue causes thermal contraction and coagulation of proteins: as the tissue shrinks small vessels can be sealed, arresting haemorrhage, and thrombosis of the occluded vessel seems to occur as a secondary event. This haemostatic effect of laser light is best, when the volume of tissue heated is relatively large (>5 mm). The Nd YAG (neodymium yttrium aluminium garnet) laser (wavelength 1064 nm, in the near infrared) is able to seal vessels up to 1 mm in diameter. If more energy is used, tissue necrosis occurs, with vaporization, laser ablation, and burning. Vaporization occurs at 100°C, when cellular water boils. Three lasers are used for their thermal effects: carbon dioxide (CO_2), argon ion, and Nd YAG. The CO_2 laser beam is absorbed by water and so produces a very localized effect. The laser energy is rapidly absorbed by tissue, causing intracellular water to boil, disrupting cells, vaporizing, and cutting through the tissue. There is very little scattering of the CO_2 beam, and thus there is only a small area (0.1 mm) of coagulation beyond the vaporization crater.

The Nd YAG beam can produce coagulation at a depth of up to 6 mm into tissue, but superficial vaporization will occur if sufficient energy is used. At lower powers only coagulation will occur. This is very much in contrast to the CO_2 laser: a photon of light from the Nd YAG laser is 10 times more likely to be scattered than absorbed, and thus it will travel further into the tissue before it is absorbed.

NON-THERMAL EFFECTS

In certain circumstances the thermal effects of the laser beam are not required, but photons are required to drive photochemical reactions in tissue, similar to those which are the basis of photosynthesis in plants. Such reactions in tissue produce important biological effects at power and energy levels below those required to produce thermal damage. The most promising technique involves the administration of photosensitizing agents which are retained with some selectivity in malignant tissue. When activated by light of a wavelength that is absorbed mainly by the photosensitizer and less by non-specific tissue components, a cytotoxic substance (singlet oxygen) is produced and tissue destruction occurs. The higher concentration of photosensitizer in malignant tumours offers the possibility of selective tumour destruction.

Other non-thermal laser effects are the 'non-linear' reactions that occur when tissue is exposed to pulsed laser light. The excimer lasers (ultraviolet wavelength, 175–355 nm) produce a laser beam in which the individual photon energy is very high and is highly absorbed by most biological tissues. This combination means that the light beam is capable of breaking interatomic bonds, and chemical photoablation of tissue occurs. The important biological feature of photoablation is the very sharp cut-off (of the order of a few microns) between normal cells and ablated tissue: there is no charred zone, as occurs with thermal laser ablation. The Nd YAG laser can be made to emit very short laser pulses which, if focused, can produce very high energies in a very small area. These high energies strip electrons from atoms and produce a rapidly expanding plasma of ions. This expanding plasma can generate powerful mechanical forces that can disrupt tissues. A 'non-linear' effect is used for laser lithotripsy in the endoscopic fragmentation of biliary calculi. Pulsed Nd YAG and dye laser beams are transmitted down flexible optical fibres, the ends of which are placed just touching the stone. The laser pulses produce a localized shock wave that can pulverize stones.

LASER THERAPY FOR GASTROINTESTINAL HAEMORRHAGE

Upper gastrointestinal tract haemorrhage is responsible for up to 100 acute hospital admissions per 100 000 of the population per annum in the United Kingdom. Over 60 per cent of these are due to peptic ulcer haemorrhage. Although most stop spontaneously there is still significant mortality and morbidity associated with continued or repeated bleeding, and to arrest haemorrhage in frail patients is also a source of morbidity. Surgery may be avoided if the laser is used as a endoscopic haemostatic device to produce thermal contraction of the bleeding vessel.

The bleeding or visible vessel is identified, any clot washed off, and the lesion is ringed with several pulses of laser energy (50–80 W in 1-s pulses). The tissue turns white when it is coagulated and the feeding vessel has been occluded. Controlled trials have confirmed the efficacy of this treatment, with 1 per cent mortality in a laser-treated group compared with 12 per cent in control patients. It is now clear that the Nd YAG laser is the most appropriate laser to use. It is likely that cheaper methods, particularly endoscopic injection around the bleeding vessel, will ultimately prove to be as effective.

Endoscopic laser therapy has also proved useful for the treatment of angiodysplasias of the upper gastrointestinal tract and colon. The major problem is identifying the lesion that has bled, since multiple abnormalities may be present. The principles of treatment are similar to that for bleeding peptic ulcers. First a circumferential ring of tissue around the lesion is treated to produce thermal contraction of any feeding vessels. Finally the lesion itself is coagulated.

Lasers can be used to arrest repeated bleeding from inoperable or recurrent gastric carcinoma but conventional laser therapy can be difficult because of the large surface requiring treatment. Recently it has been possible to treat some of the lesions with interstitial laser therapy, slowly coagulating the tumour by inserting a laser fibre at several points into its centre and using low power (1–5 W) for 100 to 1000 s.

LASER THERAPY FOR GASTROINTESTINAL CANCER

Laser therapy is now widely used for the palliation of malignant dysphagia caused by oesophagogastric cancer and for the palliation of the symptoms produced by advanced, inoperable rectal cancer. Treatment is entirely local and the laser is used at high power (50–80 W in 1-s pulses) to coagulate and vaporize the tumour. Treatment starting at the distal extent of the tumour and working proximally (after dilatation if necessary) is safer than treatment starting at the upper end of the tumour, when the direction of the occluded segment is unclear. In the oesophagus there is a 5 per cent perforation rate but most of these can be managed conservatively (using intravenous fluids and antibiotics) without surgical intervention. The complication rate is lower than that of endoscopic intubation. This method is most suitable for the treatment of totally obstructing tumours and for tumours high in the oesophagus which are unsuitable for endoscopic prosthetic intubation. It is not useful if the tumour is extrinsic to the lumen or if a tracheo-oesophageal fistula is present: in these circumstances intubation is the preferred treatment. A further problem with laser therapy is that it must be repeated at monthly intervals in order to maintain the oesophageal lumen. The laser is also useful if there is obstruction by recurrent tumour growth following prosthetic tube insertion (Fig. 3).

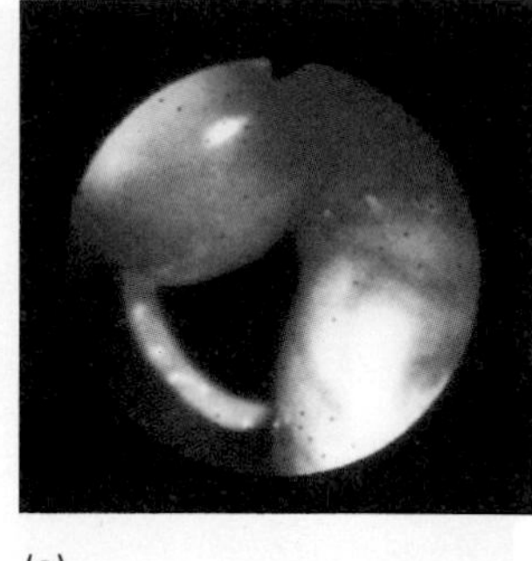
(a)

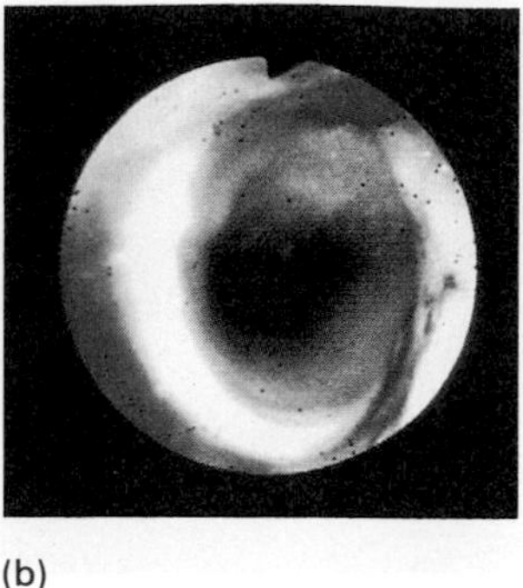
(b)

Fig. 3 (a) Tumour nodules occluding the lumen of an oesophageal tube. (b) Tumour nodules removed by endoscopic laser therapy.

Five per cent of patients with colorectal cancers have advanced metastatic spread or severe concomitant disease that render them unsuitable for surgery. Palliative colostomy will only bypass the obstruction and does little to relieve the local problems of discharge, bleeding, tenesmus, and incontinence. Local fulguration, cryotherapy, and transanal resection have provided some relief for these patients, but fulguration requires administration of a general anaesthetic and all techniques (except laser) are restricted to the management of low rectal cancers. Laser therapy aims to remove all of the exophytic tumour (Fig. 4), improving bleeding, discharge, and obstructive symptoms; incontinence is little improved and invasive pain is not helped at all. Occasionally laser therapy has been followed by prolonged survival. Measurement of quality of life in patients who have received palliative laser therapy has shown that little improvement occurs if the patient has pain as the predominant symptom or has only a short time to live (<10 weeks).

Colonoscopic Nd YAG laser therapy is also possible for benign colonic tumours. Although most polyps can be very effectively treated by snare diathermy, some large villous adenomas may be best treated with laser ablation. A large study reported complete eradication of 42 of 56 villous adenomas with the laser in patients monitored for up to 24 months.

Recently there has been an increasing interest in the use of interstitial laser hyperthermia for the treatment of solid tumours that are not resectable. Interstitial hyperthermia involves reducing the Nd YAG laser power from 50 to 80 W for 0.5 to 1 s to between 1 and 2 W delivered over a longer time (up to 1000 s) and inserting the fibre directly into tissue. Low power is used to avoid vaporization but produce hyperthermic destruction of the tissue. This technique has been investigated for the possible treatment of unresectable liver and pancreatic cancers. Multiple fibres are inserted into the tumour under ultrasound control. The progression of the damage can be monitored in real time by ultrasound or magnetic resonance, and the area of destruction can be matched to the size of the lesion.

PHOTODYNAMIC THERAPY

Photodynamic therapy is an interesting new technique with the potential for selective destruction of cancers, based on the systemic administration of certain photosensitizing agents that are

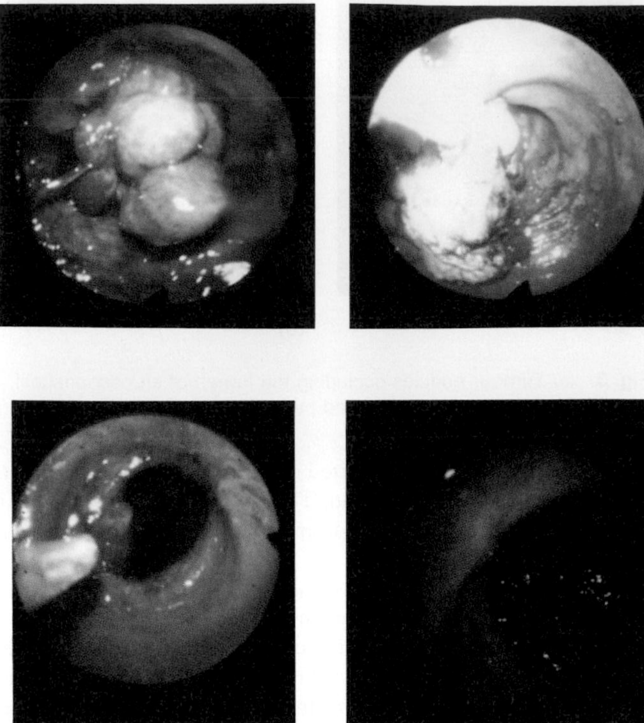

Fig. 4 Large obstructing exophytic tumour occluding the lumen of the descending colon. Treated with endoscopic laser therapy and completely removed.

retained with some selectivity in malignant tissue. When exposed to laser light of an appropriate wavelength, a cytotoxic reaction occurs, causing cellular destruction. The retention of these agents appears to be related to non-specific tumour factors rather than to the photosensitizer used. In extracranial tissues the maximum tumour:normal tissue ratio that can be obtained with a variety of photosensitizing agents is between 2 and 3:1. Investigation of photodynamic therapy in experimental colorectal neoplasms has demonstrated an important biological advantage over thermal laser destruction: full thickness colonic damage produced by photodynamic therapy, unlike thermal damage, does not reduce the mechanical strength of the bowel or cause perforation, because the submucosal collagen is preserved. However selective necrosis is limited to a small area. Initial clinical application in the gastrointestinal tract has demonstrated its potential.

LASER LITHOTRIPSY

Lasers may be used for the fragmentation of biliary calculi that are too large to be removed by endoscopic sphincterotomy. The biliary tree is approached either by percutaneous transhepatic cholangioscopy or retrogradely following endoscopic sphincterotomy. Treatment is performed under sedation with fluoroscopic control with a laser fibre passed up the duct. Treatment can also be performed under direct vision using a small endoscope (the laser fibre passed through the instrumentation channel) passed through the instrumentation channel of a large duodenoscope into the common bile duct. Successful fragmentation is possible with subsequent passage of the fragments from the bile duct. It is conceivable that gallstones could be similarly treated without the need for sphincterotomy. There is the potential for laser treatment in recanalizing malignant biliary strictures which are impassable by a guidewire to allow placement of an endoprosthesis.

FURTHER READING

Barr H, Krasner N, Boulos PB, Chatlani P, Bown SG. Photodynamic therapy for colorectal cancer: a quantitative pilot study, *Br J Surg*, 1990; **77**: 93–6.

Barr H, Krasner N. Interstitial laser photocoagulation for treating bleeding gastric cancer. *Br Med J*, 1990; **299**: 659–60.

Bown SG, *et al.* Endoscopic treatment of inoperable colorectal cancers with the Nd YAG laser. *Br J Surg*, 1986; **73**: 949–52.

Brunetaud JM, *et al.* Villous adenoma of the rectum. Results of endoscopic treatment with argon and Nd YAG lasers. *Gastroenterology*, 1985; **89**: 832–7.

Krasner N, Barr H, Skidmore C, Morris AI. Palliative laser therapy for malignant dysphagia. *Gut*, 1987; **28**: 792–8.

Lux G, *et al.* The first endoscopic retrograde laser lithotripsy of common bile duct stones in man using a pulsed Nd YAG laser. *Endoscopy*, 1986; **18**: 144.

Rutgeerts P, Broeckaert L, Janssens J, Vantrappen G, Coremans Hiele M. Comparison of endoscopic polidocanol injection and YAG laser therapy for bleeding peptic ulcers. *Lancet*, 1989; ii: 1164–6.

Steger AC, Lees WR, Walmsley K, Bown SG. Interstitial laser hyperthermia: a new approach to local destruction of tumours. *Br Med J*, 1989; **299**: 362–5.

Swain CP, Kirkham JS, Salmon PR, Bown SG, Northfield TC. Controlled trial of Nd YAG laser photocoagulation in bleeding peptic ulcers. *Lancet*, 1986; i: 1113–7.

The acute abdomen 28

28 The acute abdomen

JULIAN BRITTON

INTRODUCTION

Acute disease within the abdomen is common and many patients with abdominal symptoms present every day to doctors working in the community. Within a Western population of half a million people, between five and ten patients are admitted to a surgical ward each day with acute abdominal pain. One or two more will complain of acute abdominal symptoms after an accident. By definition the illness starts suddenly and most patients present to a hospital within 7 or 10 days of the onset of symptoms. In the majority of patients, symptoms arise from disease within the abdominal cavity itself, but occasionally they originate elsewhere in the body.

The range of disease, extends from the relatively trivial to the immediately life-threatening and attempts to reach a diagnosis must sometimes be curtailed in the interests of immediate treatment. More commonly there is time to take a history, to examine the patient, and to organize the investigations which will be helpful in establishing a diagnosis and planning treatment. Accurate recording of the relevant facts is vital and a clear understanding of the anatomy and pathophysiology of intra-abdominal disease is necessary for both diagnosis and treatment. These patients are therefore ideal for training junior members of a surgical team.

Some patients require early surgery. This itself varies from a simple straightforward procedure to a highly complex operation which stretches the ability and the skill of even the most experienced surgeon. The immediate feedback that an emergency operation provides on the accuracy and the adequacy of the preoperative assessment and preparation is another reason why the patient with an acute abdomen is an important part of surgical training.

ANATOMY

A good knowledge of normal and abnormal abdominal anatomy, and particularly surface anatomy, is essential. Variations within and between individuals are obvious, but normal anatomy also changes with age, posture, respiration, disease, and previous surgery. Nevertheless with experience most surgeons carry a remarkably accurate mental picture of the expected internal position of any particular organ in any particular patient.

The embryological development of the abdomen is relevant in two respects. The intestine and all its associated organs such as the liver and the pancreas develop initially as midline structures. Thus visceral pain is usually felt along the midline of the abdomen. The gut also has a segmental origin so that the division into foregut, midgut, and hindgut exactly correlates with the vascular supply and correspondingly pain is felt in the epigastrium, the umbilical area, and in the hypogastrium. Certain congenital abnormalities can predispose to acute abdominal complications.

In contrast to the visceral peritoneum, the parietal peritoneum is innervated by somatic nerves. Pain is therefore accurately localized to the site of irritation of the abdominal wall and is accompanied by a reflex contraction of the abdominal wall muscles. This applies both to the anterior and to the posterior abdominal wall. Psoas spasm from acute appendicitis and a scoliosis concave to the side of intra-abdominal inflammation are two good examples. Inflammation confined to the pelvis may not, however, be accompanied by anterior abdominal muscle spasm and this may cause clinical confusion. This is because the somatic nerves which supply the organs in the pelvis do not supply the anterior abdominal wall muscles.

When describing the findings of abdominal examination the surface is best divided into six areas by a transverse line going through the umbilicus and longitudinal lines running through the tip of the ninth rib on each side (Fig. 1). Thus there are epigastric and hypogastric areas in the middle and an iliac fossa and hypochondrium laterally. It is often also useful to describe a periumbilical area. However, it is important to realise that none of these divisions have a true anatomical basis.

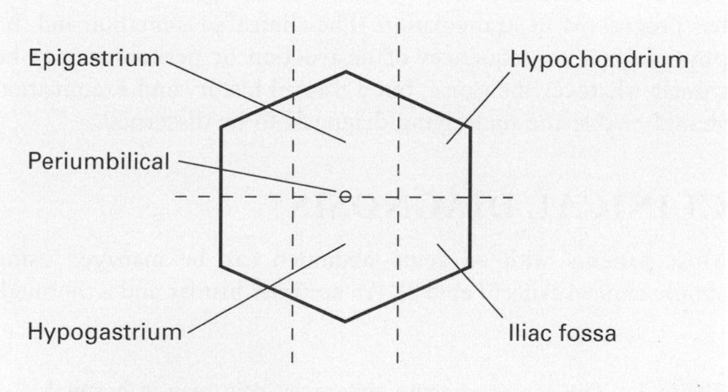

Fig. 1 The descriptive areas of the abdominal wall.

PHYSIOLOGY AND PATHOLOGY

Normal physiology is rapidly disrupted by the onset of acute intra-abdominal disease. Many patients vomit, and gastrointestinal secretion, absorption, and motility all change in the presence of obstruction, luminal infection, or peritonitis. Urine is reduced in volume and altered in content, usually secondary to redistribution of fluid in the body compartments but sometimes because of a direct toxic effect on the kidneys.

The mediation of abdominal pain is not well understood. It is perfectly possible to handle the intra-abdominal organs and even divide the bowel of a conscious patient without causing any pain. However, distension or stretching of the bowel wall is accompanied by reflex contraction of the smooth muscle in the wall, which is immediately painful. This may be due to transient ischaemia of the muscle. The pain fibres run with the splanchnic sympathetic nerves to the spinal column, where they are distributed segmentally. The pain is localized to the abdominal cavity but not to the precise segment of bowel which is being stretched. Other pathways within the spinal column are also stimulated and vomiting, which is a common accompaniment of severe pain, can also be centrally mediated.

The gastrointestinal tract is a significant source of a wide variety of hormones. These change in response to acute disturbances of function but whether this is a primary or a secondary effect is not yet clear. Inflammation is the most common cause of acute pathology within the abdomen, followed by obstruction, haemorrhage, trauma, and ischaemia.

Bacteria, viruses, fungi, parasites, and chemicals can all cause inflammation: bacteria from the bowel, such as *Escherichia coli*, *Streptococcus faecalis*, and various anaerobes are by far the most important. Other bacteria which cause acute abdominal pain are *Salmonella* and *Shigella* species, *Yersinia*, and *Campylobacter*. Acute inflammation normally develops into clinical significance over hours rather than minutes or days, and progression either to suppuration or resolution also takes time. Perforation and ischaemia develop in minutes and cause very acute symptoms. Resolution whatever the underlying pathology always takes longer than development. Neoplasia, neurogenic, and metabolic disorders occur less commonly but they are all well-recognized causes of acute abdominal pain.

Some of these pathological processes are closely interlinked. There are a number of causes of intestinal obstruction of which neoplasia is one. Peritonitis from perforation of the bowel into the potential peritoneal space usually arises from local ischaemia, but this may in turn be caused by inflammation or obstruction which has progressed to strangulation. The clinical presentation and the physiological consequences of obstruction or peritonitis may be similar whatever the cause, but a careful history and examination should enable the underlying diagnosis to be discerned.

CLINICAL DIAGNOSIS

Most patients with an acute abdomen can be managed using simple clinical skills (Table 1). An accurate history and a thorough examination are often sufficient to make a diagnosis and recommend treatment; modern investigations can help and may reassure the anaesthetist that the patient is fit for an operation. The primary objective, when the patient and the doctor first meet, is, therefore, to elicit the symptoms and the signs necessary to make a rapid and accurate diagnosis. It is sometimes obvious that the patient is in severe pain or seriously ill. The necessary immediate treatment must then take precedence over making a diagnosis.

Table 1 The causes of acute abdominal pain seen in hospitals in the developed world (after de Dombal 1991)

	Percentage of cases
Non-specific abdominal pain	34
Acute appendicitis	28
Acute cholecystitis	10
Small bowel obstruction	4
Acute gynaecological disease	4
Acute pancreatitis	3
Renal colic	3
Perforated peptic ulcer	2
Cancer	2
Diverticular disease	1
Miscellaneous	9

Unfortunately, even the most experienced clinicians only make a correct clinical diagnosis of acute abdominal pain on four occasions out of five; younger doctors and those who practise in the community are only right half the time. Many attempts have been made to improve on these results, and one method which has attracted much attention is computer-assisted diagnosis. By a curious coincidence this has simply taught us once again that taking an accurate history and examining the patient carefully are still the most important factors in making a correct diagnosis.

History

Many patients will make their own diagnosis as one listens to their story: the art of taking a history is to induce every patient to do so. Doctor and patient have not usually met before, and the style and the approach of the doctor really does matter. A relaxed confident manner and a smile always help and you must make it absolutely plain to the patient that they have your complete attention and that you have plenty of time to listen, even if this is not so. You should discourage interruptions by other members of staff or requests to answer the telephone.

Patients like to be treated as individuals. Go and sit by their bed knowing their name, and introduce yourself clearly with your own name. Some patients immediately start to describe their symptoms and must be left to continue. Others look for a cue from the doctor. Simple non-specific questions such as 'what has happened?' or 'why have you come to hospital?' are best. Some will then give their history spontaneously; others reply in only a few words and need prompting again. It is occasionally better initially to engage the patient in conversation about something entirely unrelated, such as their job or their family, and then when they are relaxed lead the discussion back to the acute problem. This is particularly useful with very anxious patients. The most difficult patient is the one who is garrulous about everything but the reason they have come for help. Often there is nothing for it but to stop the flow of words deliberately and redirect the patient to the current problem. It is difficult to do this without appearing rude or disinterested: beware of the temptation to assume that there is little wrong with these patients. They are sometimes simply frightened.

Most patients come to the end of their story spontaneously, and sometimes they have told you everything you need to know in perfect order. Never intervene to clarify a point of detail but do stop the patient when the information they offer becomes irrelevant: it is important not to overload the brain with too many facts. When the patient has finished there will usually be some points which need amplifying or some further information which is essential. This is best obtained by asking direct but not leading questions. It is very easy indeed to suggest the answer you want either by the words you use, your facial expression, or the manner in which you speak or behave. If you do this the answers will be unreliable. Asking questions is also an art which requires tact and skill. Short specific questions are best, and they must be phrased clearly without using jargon and in language the patient understands. Some patients, like most politicians, do not answer the question they are asked. You should insist, politely, on a specific answer if one is possible. No two doctors ever obtain exactly identical histories: a younger surgeon may be amazed to hear a patient give a totally contradictory reply to an apparently identical question from a senior colleague. It is also surprising how often the very last thing the patient says clinches the diagnosis.

Not everyone can give a history themselves. Most children are shy or frightened, although others, even the very young, sometimes tell a perfect story. The confused and the mentally handicapped are often unreliable as regards facts, while the memory of an elderly patient who is ill is often faulty. A relative or a friend must then relate the history, but the clinician should remember that his or her personality then intervenes. This is a particular problem if the patient is foreign and the history has to be taken through an interpreter.

Complete attention to the patient and absolute concentration on everything he or she says and how it is said it is essential. Observation of the patient is slightly different from inspection during the examination. It encompasses demeanour as well as an assessment of personality, mood, and reaction to the illness. Movement, particularly expressive movement of the hands, is always useful. Patients with peritonitis lie quite still and look ill, patients with colic really do roll around, and patients with cholelithiasis often describe the pain radiating round into the flanks with their hands for example. Obvious and significant physical signs such as gross abdominal distension with audible borborygmi, jaundice, or the smell of melaena should not be ignored: they all point to a specific pathology which may be confirmed by specific questions.

Allowing the patient to talk freely does not prevent recording the facts in a systematic fashion. In most hospitals this has to be done freehand but there are advantages in specially designed forms. The information is recorded systematically and omissions are obvious and can be corrected at once. Such forms also require the clinician to be specific about the features of certain symptoms.

Pain

Most patients admitted with an acute abdominal problem complain of abdominal pain. Cope in his classic book observed that acute pain lasting for more than 6 h in a previously fit patient usually has a surgical cause. It is also a most important symptom: detailed enquiry about the nature of the pain will often indicate the correct diagnosis.

Site

The first thing to establish is the precise site of the pain that the patient has now. Some patients are extraordinarily obtuse about this partly because they have difficulty in answering and partly because they often do not understand why you want to know. It is best to ask the patient to point with one finger to where the pain is worst and to record this site in the notes. Those who wave a hand vaguely everywhere probably do not have too much wrong with them. Pain often moves during the course of an illness and it is then worthwhile asking where the pain was situated at the beginning.

Radiation

Radiation of the pain to other parts of the body is often diagnostic. Radiation of the pain to the testicle in ureteric colic, to the shoulders in acute cholecystitis, and to the knee with an obstructed obturator hernia are specific and typical examples. Sometimes patients volunteer that a pain radiates elsewhere but more commonly it is necessary to ask directly.

Onset

Some patients can say exactly when the pain started. They may be able to give a time or say what they were doing. This always suggests a significant cause and an acute pathological process, such as perforation or strangulation. Pain which wakes the patient up at night is also significant, although it is not often possible to describe the acuteness of onset. Sometimes pain is not the first symptom the patient noticed and this may suggest a medical cause, as with the vomiting from gastroenteritis or the marked anorexia of hepatitis. The duration of the illness gives some idea how far any pathology may have progressed and this can be correlated with findings on clinical examination.

Some patients relate the onset of their pain to an injury. Apparently mild trauma is occasionally followed by serious intra-abdominal injury; on the other hand it is more common for patients, after the onset of the symptoms, to try and relate them to an injury. This can be dangerously misleading, with acute testicular torsion for example.

Frequency

There are two aspects to frequency. Alterations in the pain since this episode started are useful pointers to the immediate diagnosis, whereas pains which have come and gone in a similar way in the previous weeks or months suggest a longer-term and more chronic disease process. Variations in intensity in the short term can be classified into two types. Either the pain is constant or it comes and goes. If it comes and goes with some degree of regularity it is colic. Constant pain is associated with inflammatory conditions and colicky pain with distension of smooth muscle.

Aggravation and alleviation

Any movement makes the pain of peritonitis worse, while lying still makes it better. Acute exacerbation of the pain on walking, breathing, coughing, or going over a bump in the road on the ride to the hospital is equivalent to rebound tenderness on examination. Pain in the shoulder on lying down comes from diaphragmatic stimulation by an irritant fluid. The fluid is often blood from an intra-abdominal injury or an ectopic pregnancy. Analgesics usually make the pain better; this can be deceiving. Sometimes vomiting temporarily relieves the pain of obstruction.

Severity and type of pain

Pain is a very subjective symptom and people's reaction to it varies widely. Accompanying signs such as sweating and tachycardia give the observer some idea of severity, but this only establishes that there is something wrong with the patient which is often perfectly obvious anyway. Most patients find it very difficult to describe the nature of their pain and require prompting. No particular diagnoses are suggested by such descriptions as boring, dragging, sharp, or dull and they are best avoided.

Nausea and vomiting

These are two quite separate symptoms and both are useful in diagnosis. Nausea may precede vomiting but it need not do so and neither does vomiting always follow nausea. Nausea by itself is a less specific symptom, although it is a common accompaniment of gallstone disease. Anorexia is a separate and somewhat non-specific symptom since most people and particularly children lose their appetite when they are unwell. Pain normally precedes vomiting in surgical disease of the abdomen whereas the reverse is often the case in medical conditions.

Vomiting is a classic symptom of intestinal obstruction and it usually accompanies colic. Vomiting often occurs after a bout of pain in obstruction and the shorter the interval between the two the higher the obstruction. The vomit itself is initially green in colour but turns yellow and then frankly faecal as the obstruction persists. Retching without vomiting suggests acute torsion of an intra-abdominal structure.

Vomiting does not often accompany perforation of a peptic

ulcer nor intra-abdominal haemorrhage, and it is a late event in distal large bowel obstruction if it occurs at all. Nausea and anorexia are more common than vomiting in appendicitis.

Bowel function

Diarrhoea and constipation are two potentially confusing symptoms because they mean different things to different people. It is important first to establish the patient's normal bowel habit and the normal consistency of the stool and then to decide if there have been any recent changes. Diarrhoea to some people simply means frequent defecation of normal faecal material whereas repeated loose watery stools are of greater interest to the surgeon. When true diarrhoea is present it is important to establish whether other members of the household are afflicted. The presence of blood, slime, or the black tarry stools of melaena are all of obvious diagnostic value. If intestinal obstruction is suspected then failure to pass wind as well as stool is important.

Gynaecological symptoms

Symptoms arising from the uterus, fallopian tubes, and ovaries are a common reason for admission to hospital with acute abdominal pain. Furthermore the negative laparotomy rate is highest in young women. Questions about normal and abnormal menstrual function, vaginal discharge, and the risk of pregnancy are therefore essential. Tact and sensitivity are required but the answers really do matter: a ruptured ectopic pregnancy is a potentially lethal condition.

Urinary symptoms

Alterations in the pattern of micturition suggest urinary tract disease. Frequency is linked with inflammation, while anuria is most commonly caused by acute retention in elderly men. Pain on passing urine must be separated into two classes. Abdominal pain exacerbated by micturition suggests irritation of the peritoneal surface of the bladder, while stinging pain in the urethra on urination is characteristic of infection. Patients should also be asked about the colour of the urine and the presence of blood or pus. Dysuria is a symptom which means different things to different doctors, and the term should not be used without specifying what is meant.

Past history

Any previous medical problem may be relevant to the cause of an acute admission for abdominal pain and it will certainly be relevant to the management. Chronic indigestion can be a useful pointer to a possible cause of peritonitis. A past history of abdominal surgery is important because adhesions have now overtaken hernias as the commonest cause of intestinal obstruction. Patients often report previous episodes of abdominal pain and it is useful to establish whether this episode is identical. If it is chronic surgical diseases that flare intermittently must be considered. Recurrent acute pancreatitis would be a good example.

Drugs

Many people take therapeutic drugs. Most patients when asked think only of those prescribed by the doctor but in many countries in the world, including the United Kingdom, it is possible to buy drugs without a doctor's prescription and these may be relevant too. Diuretics and sympathomimetic drugs may be implicated in the onset of acute retention, digoxin overdose classically causes vomiting followed by abdominal pain, and many drugs cause cholestatic jaundice.

Not all patients know what drugs they are taking and pills may be transferred from bottle to bottle so that the labels are unreliable. Ultimately a direct enquiry to the doctor or the pharmacist who wrote or supplied the prescription may be necessary.

Examination

No experienced doctor completely separates examination from taking the history. Observation begins the moment the doctor meets the patient and does not end until they part company. Most clinicians rapidly assimilate, almost unconsciously, many features of a new patient and not all of them can easily be described in words. Attitude, alertness, mood, agitation, sweating, respiration, movement, the eyes, the colour, the facial expression, the pulse, the handshake, and many other factors are all put together to give an instant impression of the nature and severity of the illness the diagnosis. The restlessness of a patient with colic is in marked contrast to the immobility of peritonitis. The gaunt patient with sunken eyes, a weak thready pulse, and little respiratory or abdominal movement looks the same today as did patients two and a half thousand years ago when Hippocrates first described the facies of severe peritonitis.

First impressions may, of course, be false and they are not a substitute for a systematic examination. Some would say that examination does not add much to a well-taken history but more evidence to help unravel a diagnosis is usually welcome. As with the history, examination of the whole patient is relevant in the overall management, although here we are concerned with the signs which are important in the diagnosis of the acute abdomen.

Vital signs

Pulse rate, respiratory rate, temperature, and blood pressure are all essential observations. The initial values on admission may be misleading because of the hustle and bustle of the journey to hospital, but subsequent measurements are important in any patient whose condition is observed following admission. The charts may give a general clue as to the diagnosis. An increase in respiratory rate suggests pulmonary pathology rather than abdominal disease. An isolated rise in temperature certainly indicates disease but it does not specify where, nor does it necessarily signify infection. The height and the course of a fever in an adult may point to a diagnosis; in children fever is an unreliable guide as it is notoriously labile.

Consistent changes in these four vital signs over time are useful indicators of progressive pathology. A persistent rise in pulse with an accompanying fall in blood pressure is sure evidence that a peptic ulcer is still bleeding; increasing fever means that an empyema of the gallbladder needs draining. Changes in pulse and blood pressure following abdominal trauma are useful, although they usually indicate the need for active treatment rather than specifying the underlying diagnosis.

General features

There are many signs found elsewhere in the examination which indicate disease within the abdomen. General features of the patient such as anaemia, jaundice, and facial flushing all have a direct relevance to abdominal diagnosis. The pallor of fear must not be confused with the pallor of anaemia, and cyanosis often accompanies an acute intra-abdominal catastrophe. In children, acute inflammation of the upper respiratory tract can present with abdominal pain and examination is not complete until the tonsils and the ear drums have been inspected. Here, however, we are primarily concerned with the abdominal signs.

Examination of the abdomen

Physical examination of the abdomen follows the time-honoured sequence of inspection, palpation, percussion, and auscultation. Many signs can be seen and few patients, even young children, object to simple observation. Palpation may be painful and it is certainly unusual. Explaining what you are doing helps a patient to relax and so does distraction with conversation. Sometimes palpation with a stethoscope is useful. Percussion and auscultation are less useful in the abdomen than in examination of the chest.

Different doctors obtain different histories and variations in the interpretation of physical signs are even more marked. Natural variation is compounded by the lack of universal agreement on the definition of some physical signs. Despite this the basic findings should be recorded in the notes. Eponymous signs are best avoided. In practice they are rarely absolutely pathognomonic of one condition.

Inspection

Inspection of the abdomen is a subtle art. First and foremost both the patient and the examiner should be comfortable. The patient must lie as flat and as straight as possible with the head on a single pillow. The examiner should sit at the right hand side of the bed so that his arm and hand can lie parallel to the abdominal wall. Daylight and warmth are desirable and adequate exposure of the abdomen essential, although it is kind to keep the genitalia covered until they are actually examined.

Time should then be spent simply looking but looking in an intelligent and thoughtful way. Most important physical signs can often be seen (Fig. 2). The history will have given some clues as to possible diagnoses, and there will be specific signs to look for while remembering that negative findings are equally important. Previous abdominal operations will have been noted in the history and the scars can be examined. Their only importance now is that there may be an incisional hernia or underlying intraperitoneal adhesions. Obvious discoloration is always important. Bruising from a seat belt injury or the blue-grey discoloration in the flanks or around the umbilicus from haemorrhagic pancreatitis are both good examples.

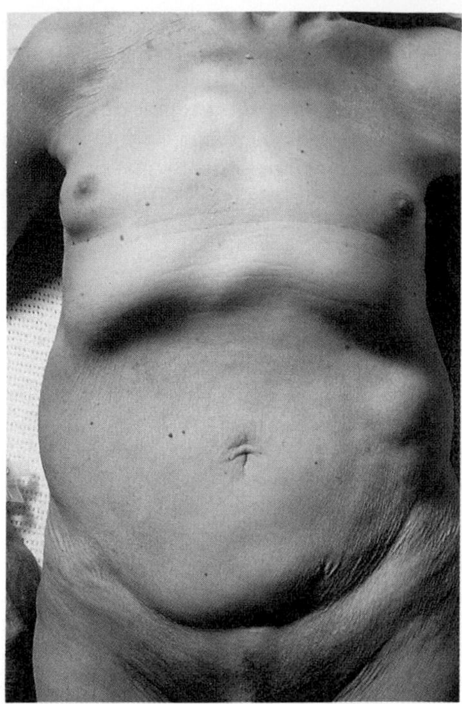

Fig. 2 All the necessary physical signs can be seen in this patient allowing a confident diagnosis of cancer of the pancreas. The patient is jaundiced, the skin is hanging loosely, indicating severe weight loss, and the distended gallbladder can be seen in the right hypochondrium.

Shape

The first thing to decide is whether the shape, symmetry, and contour of the abdominal wall are normal. Generalized distension is usually obvious except in obese patients, when it can be very difficult to decide whether the abdomen is simply fat. The most common cause of generalized distension in a woman is a fetus. Excess fluid and air in the gut and ascites are the common pathological causes of distension; this is usually symmetrical. Asymmetrical distension is best judged from the end of the bed and is caused either by a mass within the abdominal cavity or a lump in the abdominal wall. The two can be differentiated since the latter always moves with the abdominal wall whereas intraperitoneal lumps do not necessarily do so.

Movement

The abdominal wall normally moves with respiration. With the patient lying on his or her back the abdominal wall rises up on inspiration as the diaphragm descends and falls back on expiration. If this respiratory movement hurts then the patient will try to reduce or eliminate any movement by keeping the abdominal wall over the painful area still. This can often be seen and the effect can be enhanced by asking the patient to take a deep breath. Another common technique, but one that is less useful in the author's experience, is to ask the patient to blow his or her abdomen out and to suck it in. Patients with peritonitis find this painful, as they do when asked to cough. Sometimes in thin patients it is possible to see the abdominal wall muscles contract spontaneously in response to the painful stimulus. This is visible guarding.

Sometimes movement within the abdominal cavity can be seen on the surface. Aortic pulsation and fetal movements are both normal and so occasionally, in the elderly or those with gastroenteritis, is visible peristalsis. It is, however, a classic sign of intestinal obstruction. Distended loops of bowel can be seen through the abdominal wall and peristaltic contractions can often also be seen. These contractions are sometimes accompanied by borborygmi which are audible with or without a stethoscope. Patience is needed, and sometimes peristalsis can be stimulated by palpation of the abdomen.

Palpation

Palpation of the abdomen requires warm hands, short fingernails, and care. By convention the doctor sits on the patient's right with the right hand flat on the abdomen in a comfortable position. Students, however, should learn to be ambidextrous because sometimes only the left side of the patient is accessible and some organs, such as the gallbladder, are occasionally easier to feel from the left.

Superficial palpation should consist of gentle movements of the whole hand. Deep palpation is achieved by gentle pressure and by flexion of the metacarpophalangeal joints whilst keeping the fingers extended. It is best to begin by asking the patient where the abdomen hurts and then to start palpating in the opposite corner of the abdomen. Work towards the painful area but do take care. Once hurt few patients will relax. The signs then become difficult to interpret and are sometimes actually misleading.

The abnormalities of importance in the acute abdomen separate into three groups. There are the signs associated with peritonitis, those which accompany a mass or enlargement of one of the solid organs, and finally those that differentiate the causes of abdominal distension.

Signs of peritonitis

The four signs of peritonitis are tenderness, guarding, rigidity, and rebound tenderness. Eliciting these signs is painful and it is better to see than to hear the pain. A flicker of the eyelids or a facial grimace is quite sufficient to establish the presence of pain, although guarding and rigidity are usually felt.

Tenderness

This is present when any palpation of the abdominal wall causes pain. It is either present or absent, although it is also possible to establish the extent of the tenderness over the abdominal wall. It is not easy to assess severity because patients vary so much in their reaction to pain. It is useful to establish where in an individual patient the pain is worst. Pain arising from the parietal peritoneum is accurately localized and patients can often point to the site of most intense pain. The examiner can also ask the patient to compare the intensity of pain by direct pressure in the four quadrants of the abdomen.

Guarding

There are different opinions about the physical signs of guarding and rigidity, so the examiner must be specific about what he actually means. In the author's opinion guarding is present when there is reflex contraction of the abdominal wall muscles when the examining hand palpates the abdominal wall and thus causes slight pain. This may be seen but is more commonly felt.

Rigidity

Again there is no generally accepted definition of this sign but the most useful description is of an involuntary increase in the resting tone of the abdominal wall muscles. It may be localized or generalized. It is felt as an increased resistance of the abdominal wall to palpation. The intensity varies from minor increases in tension right up to the typical generalized board-like rigidity classically associated with perforation of a peptic ulcer.

Rebound tenderness

This is the most important physical sign of the four. It can be a difficult sign to elicit but when present it establishes the presence of peritonitis. It occurs when inflamed visceral peritoneum moves across and irritates the parietal peritoneum and is best detected by percussion. This produces small movements of the underlying tissues, causes least pain, and can even localize the sign to specific areas within the abdomen. The classical method of detecting rebound tenderness by gross depression of the abdominal wall with the hand and then sudden release (hence the term release tenderness) is both crude and unkind and while sometimes useful should generally be abandoned. Rebound tenderness is also a symptom. Movement such as walking or the jolting of a vehicle may exacerbate the abdominal pain, and it is always worth enquiring about this whilst taking the history.

Abdominal swellings

It is essential to establish the size of all the solid intra-abdominal organs during palpation and equally important to identify any abnormal masses. When the liver, spleen, and kidneys are enlarged there are certain specific signs that must be sought. When an abnormal mass is felt either within or separately from the solid organs then all the usual rules relating to the examination of lumps apply, although it may be impossible to assess swellings which lie deep within the abdominal cavity. Particular attention should be paid to the anatomical origin of the lump. Here mobility, and movement with respiration and pulsation are useful. It is always helpful to establish that a swelling is cystic. Sometimes tenderness and the other signs of peritonitis coexist with an abdominal swelling.

Abdominal distension

Abnormal abdominal distension may be caused by an abdominal swelling, but flatus, fluid, and faeces are more common. Pregnancy is generally obvious and faeces are easily discovered on rectal examination. Excess gas or fluid within the abdominal cavity is easy to demonstrate, but establishing the presence of free intraperitoneal air or ascites can be difficult.

Groins and genitalia

No abdominal examination is complete without examination of the groins and the genitalia, particularly in men. Hernias are common but not always obvious. A small femoral hernia in a large woman is easily missed. If the hernia is the cause of an obstruction it will also be tense, tender, and irreducible, but it may not be very large.

Scrotal abnormalities such as testicular torsion and epididymo-orchitis can present with abdominal pain, but there are always abnormal scrotal signs on examination.

Rectal and vaginal examination

No patient likes a rectal or a vaginal examination but they are essential. Again the examination needs to be conducted with thought. Consider all the anatomical structures in the pelvis including the prostate and the cervix and look at the glove for blood or pus when the examination is finished. Rectal tenderness on the patient's right side may be the only sign of pelvic appendicitis. A swelling in a fallopian tube on vaginal examination may be the only sign of an ectopic pregnancy.

Percussion

Percussion of the abdomen has three specific uses. First, it is the best method of eliciting rebound tenderness. Second, it is the most sensitive method for detecting enlargement of the bladder. Third, shifting dullness determines the presence or absence of ascites. It has a subsidiary role in confirming the size of the liver and spleen and may sometimes be useful in outlining an intra-abdominal mass.

Auscultation

Auscultation of the abdomen is not very helpful, but the presence or absence of bowel sounds is a useful physical sign. Qualitative observations are less reliable. Nevertheless an increase in the magnitude and the frequency of bowel sounds accompanies mechanical intestinal obstruction whilst a succussion splash, which can sometimes be heard without a stethoscope, is a sure sign of obstruction. Bowel sounds which definitely disappear during observation of a patient with abdominal pain and tenderness indicates the onset of peritonitis and the need for a laparotomy.

Investigation

Although investigations are more or less routinely requested in most patients with acute abdominal pain, very few of the tests are actually valuable in making a diagnosis. In a few patients no investigations are necessary because the diagnosis is clinically obvious. In the majority the cause of the pain is initially uncertain and it is hoped that tests will help. Older and more experienced surgeons maintain that it is preferable to wait and see in these circumstances. They argue that significant disease is usually progressive and when the patient is re-examined after an interval the physical signs are more marked and the diagnosis easier. Younger surgeons think that the delay gives time for complications to develop with a consequent increase in postoperative morbidity that diagnostic investigations might avoid. However, their enthusiasm for investigation can also delay a necessary operation if the tests take too long to perform. In a few patients an accurate diagnosis which is essential for correct treatment can only be made with the help of special investigations.

We are most concerned here with tests that will help in the diagnosis and the management of the patient within the first 24 h of admission. After that the number of tests that can sometimes be useful is vast and they are considered in the individual subject chapters. Analysis of venous blood and various radiographs are the most popular immediate investigations, with the recent addition of ultrasound examination. They can be divided into two groups—those tests that help in diagnosis and those that help in management.

Tests that are useful in diagnosis

Testing the urine

Simple clinical inspection of the urine should still be regarded as an essential part of examination of the abdomen. Urine containing tiny amounts of blood looks smoky. Infected urine smells unpleasant and may be cloudy or even contain frank blood. Sugar and ketone can also both be smelt and confirmation of all these findings using biochemical sticks is convenient and easy. Most clinicians should be able to identify pus cells in centrifuged urine using the ward microscope.

When a urinary tract infection is suspected a carefully collected urine specimen should also be sent immediately to the laboratory for analysis. It is not easy for any patient to provide a true midstream urine specimen, and they must be both helped and supervised. Even then contamination can be a problem and there are occasions, particularly in women and children, when a catheter specimen should be collected. Urethral catheterization is usually appropriate but suprapubic puncture of the bladder provides the least contaminated specimen and carries the least risk of introducing an infection. Even though the culture result will not be available for a few days the sample must be sent acutely otherwise the opportunity to identify the organism responsible may be lost, as most patients with a urinary tract infection presenting with acute abdominal pain will need immediate treatment with antibiotics.

Blood tests

White blood cell count

Many significant causes of acute abdominal pain are associated with some degree of inflammation. As a consequence an increase both in the absolute numbers of white cells and in the proportion of neutrophils might be expected. The reverse observation is also true: an increase in the white cell count indicates the existence of inflammation. It is always necessary to interpret the result in the clinical context, for the inflammation may not necessarily lie within the abdomen. A value within the normal range does not exclude intra-abdominal inflammation.

This very simple way of looking at the white cell count is not the most useful. It is more helpful to interpret the result in a statistical sense. In other words the probability of a patient with a normal white cell count having acute appendicitis, for example, is low whilst the chances of appendicitis in a patient with a raised count are higher (Table 2).

Table 2 The relationship between the total white blood cell count and the chance of appendicitis (after de Dombal 1991)

White cell count per mm^3	Chance of appendicitis (%)
1–8000	5
8001–10000	7
10001–12000	18
12001–15000	36
>15000	67

The same observations may be made about an excess of neutrophils in the differential white cell count. Indeed the results of all such tests used to establish a diagnosis should ideally be analysed in this way. In practice a normal white cell count is often used to reassure the surgeon who wants to wait and see while an increased count supports a decision to operate. The surgeon should realize, however, that the test is then being used to help in a management decision and not to make a diagnosis.

Serum amylase concentration

Acute pancreatitis usually presents with the symptoms and signs of peritonitis, and normally patients with peritonitis warrant an immediate laparotomy. Surgery is, however, best avoided in patients with acute pancreatitis. The rise in serum amylase concentration which usually accompanies pancreatitis allows the correct diagnosis to be made and a laparotomy is thus averted.

Because the result is so important for both diagnosis and treatment it is essential to appreciate the limitations of the test. Other intra-abdominal catastrophes such as a perforated peptic ulcer, a ruptured aortic aneurysm, or dead gut can cause a modest rise in the serum amylase level, while if the blood sample is taken too long after the onset of the pancreatitis the level may have reverted to normal and so give a false-negative result. Again a statistical approach can be adopted. A low level of serum amylase carries a low chance that the patient has acute pancreatitis whilst a high level implies a high chance (but not a certainty) that pancreatitis is indeed the diagnosis.

Radiological investigations

Plain abdominal radiographs

Controversy surrounds the use of plain abdominal radiology. Sometimes the films confirm the clinical diagnosis, add further detail, and modify the management of an individual patient. At other times the films are simply misleading, although occasionally they suggest a diagnosis which the clinician has not considered. One thing is certain. Not every patient with acute abdominal pain needs an abdominal radiograph. When it is requested the doctor should be clear what information he hopes to gain and he must have the skills to interpret the films if no radiologist is available.

Traditionally two films are taken, one with the patient lying supine and the other with the patient sitting or standing erect. Modern protagonists of a single supine film point out that little additional information is derived from the erect film and add that not every patient with acute abdominal pain can safely or comfortably sit or stand. Some radiologists prefer, as an alternative to the erect film, to lie the patient on their right side and then take a lateral radiograph (the lateral decubitus view). In the author's opinion an erect view does, on occasion, add useful information whereas the lateral decubitus view usually does not. It provides only a limited view of the abdominal cavity and free intraperitoneal gas is better seen on a chest radiograph.

Abdominal films are more use in some circumstances than in others. None of the radiological signs of acute appendicitis are truly helpful, but radiological examination should be performed in patients with suspected intestinal obstruction and those who have suffered abdominal trauma (Fig. 3). Stones in the kidney, the ureter, or the gallbladder are sometimes confirmed on a plain film, and calcification of the wall of an abdominal aortic aneurysm may be the only clue to its presence. Radiology of the abdomen is more useful in older patients, who tend to have more significant pathology and thus more abnormalities on such films. It is important to remember that the presence of abnormalities on any abdominal radiograph is valuable, but their absence is meaningless.

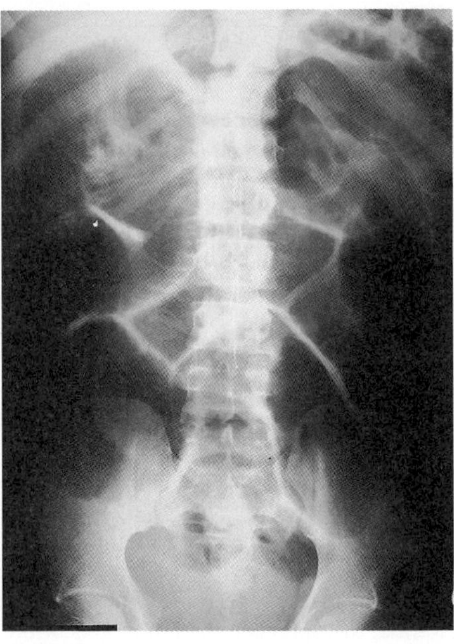

Fig. 3 A supine abdominal radiograph demonstrating grossly distended loops of small bowel typical of intestinal obstruction. (By courtesy of Dr D. Lindsell.)

Chest radiography

A good quality erect chest radiograph is the best film with which to confirm the presence of free intraperitoneal air (Fig. 4). This can be seen as a black crescent, sometimes with an air–fluid level, underneath one or both diaphragms. Proximal perforations of the bowel tend to lead to larger amounts of free air than distal perforations; if the perforation has occurred some time before presentation, as can happen in patients with diverticular disease, the margin of the pneumoperitoneum is often rather hazy and irregular. There may also be a small pleural reaction above the diaphragm.

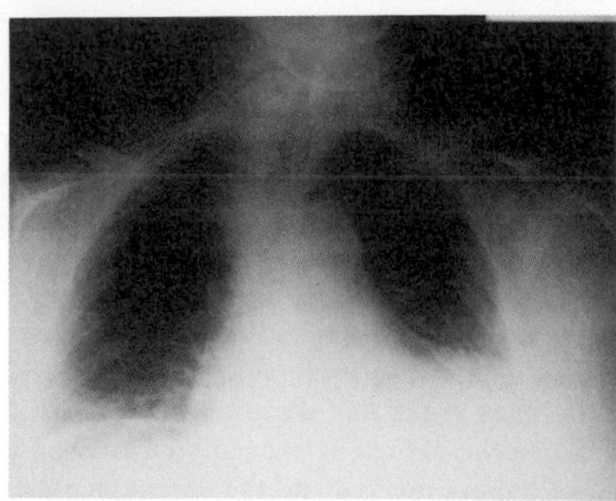

Fig. 4 An erect chest radiograph demonstrating free gas under the diaphragm.

In very old and very young patients pneumonia and pleurisy may present with referred abdominal pain. Lower rib fractures may indicate a ruptured spleen or lacerated liver.

Intravenous urography

Renal colic is usually an easy clinical diagnosis to make because of the characteristic distribution of the pain. When the diagnosis is in doubt an emergency intravenous urogram is frequently helpful: delayed excretion of contrast from the kidney on the side affected by pain confirms the diagnosis. A normal urogram effectively excludes the diagnosis, provided the examination is done during or within a short time of an episode of pain. Other causes of abdominal pain can then be considered. Although the film taken immediately after injection of contrast is sufficient for diagnosis, the examination is usually completed in order to determine the site of any obstruction, the size of an offending stone, and the degree of dilatation of the system.

Intravenous urography is also useful in patients who have suffered trauma to the urinary tract. Most such patients have haematuria. The degree and the site of any damage may be displayed, and the presence of a normally functioning kidney on the unaffected side can be confirmed.

Computed tomography

Clinical examination of the abdomen in the trauma victim is notoriously unreliable and computed tomography (CT) of the abdomen as a means of diagnosis is rapidly becoming routine in the seriously injured patient. Ultrasound is more readily available and should probably be the first investigation, but the examination is more limited.

Apart from trauma there are few indications for the use of CT in the immediate diagnosis of abdominal pain. It may be of occasional help in the diagnosis of an aortic aneurysm and acute pancreatitis, although in the latter case CT is of greater value in the identification of complications.

Ultrasound examination

Ultrasound is widely used in the diagnosis of acute abdominal pain. Its place in elective diagnosis of conditions affecting the upper abdomen, the pelvis, and the retroperitoneum is already established; it is also useful in the emergency patient. Gallstones and an aortic aneurysm are easily seen (Fig. 5), as are the oedematous gallbladder wall and a tear in an aneurysm. Hydronephrosis, and sometimes stones in the kidneys or ureter, can be seen, and ovarian cysts and swellings on the fallopian tubes can be identified in the pelvis. The ultrasound probe can also be used, like the examining hand, to identify the specific structure that hurts.

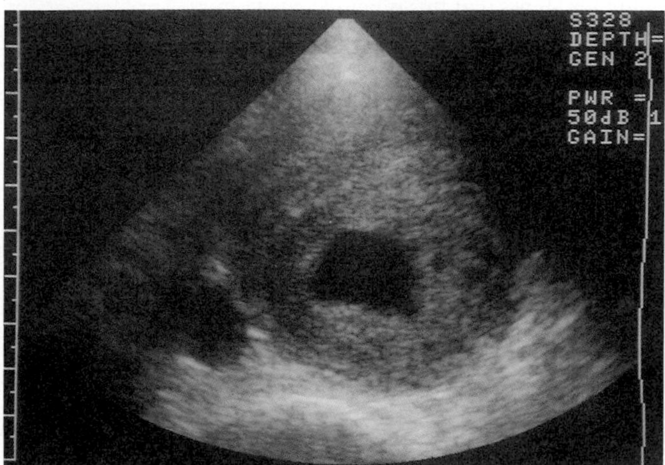

Fig. 5 A transverse ultrasound picture of the abdomen demonstrating a large aortic aneurysm filled with concentric rings of thrombus surrounding a residual lumen. (By courtesy of Dr D. Lindsell.)

Ultrasound is less useful in examining the bowel because of the presence of gas. However, the inflamed appendix often lies behind the caecum and contains little air. Certainly the ultrasound probe can localize the tenderness to this specific area and can sometimes demonstrate an oedematous tubular structure at the site where a retrocaecal appendix should lie.

Following trauma, ultrasound can demonstrate the presence of free intraperitoneal fluid and identify damage to the liver, spleen, kidneys, and pancreas. It cannot identify blood clot very well and it is of no practical use in looking for injury to the gut.

Doppler ultrasound, which demonstrates flow in vessels, can help decide the cause of acute testicular pain. The hyperaemia of epididymo-orchitis is in marked contrast to the ischaemia of torsion.

Tests useful in management

Many of the tests that are useful in diagnosis also have a role in management. A progressive reduction in the white cell count and improvement in the radiological signs of obstruction after treatment both indicate resolution of the pathology. A large number of other tests also help in the treatment of a patient, many of which are undertaken soon after the patient is admitted to hospital. Some of them also play a part in diagnosis.

Blood tests

Haemoglobin concentration and packed cell volume

The clinical diagnosis of anaemia is not always reliable, and in any patient who may possibly have an anaesthetic it is clearly important to know the oxygen-carrying capacity of the blood. The initial haemoglobin value does not indicate the volume of blood lost in patients with overt evidence of acute haemorrhage, but sequential measurements can give a rough guide, provided any blood transfused is taken into account. Occasionally the discovery of an unexpectedly low haemoglobin level can help in diagnosis: carcinoma of the caecum as a cause for intestinal obstruction with anaemia is a classic example. Packed cell volume accurately reflects the severity of fluid loss in a dehydrated patient and it is a good guide to the adequacy of rehydration.

Creatinine and electrolytes

Most patients with major intra-abdominal pathology should have serum creatinine and electrolyte concentrations measured on admission. The initial values must be interpreted in the clinical context, particularly if the patient is dehydrated; in most circumstances it is the serum potassium concentration which is the most important because of its role in cardiac function. Serial values are vital for proper postoperative fluid management.

Liver function tests

Most patients with an acute abdomen due to liver and biliary disease are jaundiced. The depth of the jaundice reflects the severity of the pathology, and it is rare to need to measure the liver function tests acutely. It is, however, essential to obtain a blood sample on admission for later analysis because subsequent deterioration in biochemical parameters, which may not be clinically obvious, will demand further action. This particularly applies to the elderly in whom the signs and symptoms of biliary disease are often obscure. The diagnosis is sometimes not even considered until abnormal liver function tests are discovered.

Calcium concentration

This is only of immediate value in patients with acute pancreatitis. Depleted values are an indirect guide to the diagnosis and are used in some severity scoring systems. When low calcium levels threaten to induce tetany, intravenous calcium supplements are needed. Calcium level is always measured in patients with renal colic, in whom evidence of hyperparathyroidism is sought, but hypercalcaemia is rarely found.

Blood gas analysis

Analysis of an arterial blood sample should be performed in a patient who is severely ill with an acute abdomen from whatever cause. Many such patients are covertly hypoxic, and the result of blood gas analysis may indicate the need for immediate ventilatory support. More commonly, patients will need ventilation after an emergency operation; preoperative values are then a useful indicator of the patient's progress.

Blood gas analysis is also a component of many scoring systems to assess the severity of acute pancreatitis.

Radiology

If a chest radiograph is not necessary for diagnosis it is unlikely that it will be needed in the management of the patient. Nevertheless there are times when, although a clinical diagnosis can be made, a chest radiograph should be obtained simply to provide a baseline. It is often useful to know that postoperative changes in a number of parameters, particularly the chest radiograph, were not present before surgery.

Contrast radiology

It is unusual for contrast radiology to be performed as an emergency although an urgent barium or air enema should be undertaken in a child with suspected intussusception. In adults with large bowel obstruction a limited barium enema examination is sometimes useful to establish the presence of a mechanical obstruction rather than pseudo-obstruction. In patients with small bowel obstruction where the cause is obscure or resolution is not occurring as fast as expected a small bowel enema is always useful.

Electrocardiography

Anyone over the age of 40 who presents with acute abdominal pain, particularly if the diagnosis is not straightforward, should undergo electrocardiography. Very occasionally a myocardial infarct will present with abdominal pain and recovery is unlikely to be helped by an unnecessary laparotomy.

Endoscopy and arteriography

Emergency gastroscopy and colonoscopy, occasionally performed on the operating table, are helpful in patients who present with acute gastrointestinal haemorrhage. Precise localization of the bleeding point is essential for effective treatment. Mesenteric angiography may also be needed. In both instances treatment as well as diagnosis may be possible.

Endoscopy has no part to play in the diagnosis of a perforated peptic ulcer, and may make matters worse by blowing air into the peritoneal cavity through the perforation.

Peritoneal lavage

This is a useful investigation in patients with abdominal trauma, particularly if they are unconscious or are otherwise unable to co-operate in an abdominal examination. The presence of significant amounts of blood or intestinal contents in the washout fluid is a clear indication for an urgent laparotomy.

In patients with acute abdominal pain the presence of excess neutrophils in fluid aspirated from or washed out of the peritoneum is a reliable indicator of peritonitis. The test is not widely used, probably because it does not indicate the underlying cause of the inflammation.

Laparoscopy

General surgeons have been slow to use the laparoscope, despite very good evidence that it can help in making a diagnosis. All that is set to change, partly because of the introduction of new video technology but also because of the development of laparoscopic surgery.

Many surgeons will consider that the opportunity to remove an appendix at the same time as confirming the diagnosis justifies the slight risks that laparoscopy entails. The current technique for laparoscopic appendicectomy is time-consuming and cumbersome, but McBurney's incision will undoubtedly become a relic of the past.

Laparoscopy also has a role in the management of the abdominal trauma victim. However, it is only used as a more sophisticated form of peritoneal lavage. If blood or intestinal contents are found in the peritoneum then the endoscopist must look for the source and also decide if the severity of the bleeding is sufficient to justify a laparotomy.

MAKING A DIAGNOSIS

No one really understands how a doctor makes a diagnosis, although the process has been analysed many times. In theory it is simply a matter of collecting all the relevant facts and analysing them correctly. The contrast between the junior clinician who takes time and trouble over the patient and yet makes the wrong diagnosis half the time and his senior colleague who asks a few questions, performs a limited examination, and is right eight times out of ten shows that this is not the whole story. Very few patients present with all the symptoms and signs of their disease and only experience can teach the clinician which few questions to ask, how to ask them, and how to interpret the answers correctly in the context of the individual patient. The last skill is particularly important when some of the facts conflict. Experience and constant practice are certainly essential for maximum accuracy.

In actual clinical practice, several methods are used to make a diagnosis. Some involve purely practical considerations whilst others look at the same data in different ways. Most clinicians use all the methods at one time or another, often together, and usually without giving the matter a second thought.

The classic case

In this unusual circumstance the patient gives the typical history of a classical cause of abdominal pain with every symptom in its correct place. Examination reveals all the expected signs and the diagnosis is obvious even to the least experienced clinician. There is really no place for a differential diagnosis nor are investigations necessary. All that is left to be done is to organize the correct treatment.

A question of elimination

More commonly a variety of diagnoses is suggested by the patient's initial complaint. Most doctors then ask further questions to support or exclude each individual diagnosis. The method reaches its peak with the most experienced clinician who makes a diagnosis on the basis of half a dozen questions and a very limited examination of the abdomen. This is the culmination of a natural development in most doctors. To begin with they are taught to obtain information in a systematic way and to record it all in a standard format. Later they learn that certain symptoms and signs are commonly associated with certain conditions and so they construct in their minds algorithms for each individual patient. With experience the method works well but it is dangerous for the beginner because of the risk of following the wrong pathway early in the decision tree.

Anatomy and pathology

Another approach is to consider which anatomical structure could be the cause of the symptoms and signs. Abdominal anatomy is broadly the same in everyone and most patients can localize their pain to one area of the abdomen. Each organ within that area is then considered in turn as the source of the symptoms. The most difficult area is the left upper quadrant where there are no structures which commonly cause acute abdominal pain. Anatomy can also be used to construct a list of all the other structures that could cause abdominal pain at any particular site.

A particular pathological process is suggested by certain symptoms and signs. This may, in turn, suggest a diagnosis. Acute intra-abdominal inflammation is usually accompanied by a fever and abdominal tenderness, while mechanical obstruction is characterized by colic and vomiting. Sometimes obstruction and inflammation coexist, but this in itself shortens the diagnostic list to only a few possibilities.

Age and sex

The importance of sex in relation to the possible causes of abdominal pain is obvious but age is an equally valuable discriminator. Cancer is more common in the old than the young, for example, whereas non-specific abdominal pain is a disease of the young.

Statistics

Acute appendicitis and non-specific abdominal pain account for approximately two-thirds of all the patients admitted to hospital with abdominal pain in Europe and North America (Table 1). This means that for two-thirds of the time the only important distinction the surgeon has to make is between these two conditions. Looked at another way this also means that if it was possible to separate these two diagnoses accurately from all the other possibilities then the clinician would make a correct diagnosis in two-thirds of the patients.

The pattern of disease

Common things occur commonly. The most common surgical cause of acute abdominal pain in a patient admitted to a hospital anywhere in the world is acute appendicitis. The next most common cause in Africa is small bowel obstruction; in the West it is acute cholecystitis. Knowledge of local epidemiology is therefore useful in the diagnosis of abdominal pain, although the patterns of disease will change over time.

Listing the possibilities

This is essential for the young clinician but a luxury for the surgeon in charge who has to decide on treatment. The latter keeps a list in his head but the former is wise to write the possibilities down, preferably in order of probability. There is truth in the saying that you will not make a diagnosis unless you think of it: making a list may jog the memory, as the rarities are easily forgotten. However, a list of possible diagnoses only provides a framework on which to base further enquiry. It is of no direct help in planning treatment.

A repeat visit

Most patients with abdominal pain will undergo some investigations on admission, particularly if the diagnosis is not obvious. The results usually support or refute a diagnosis that has already been considered, but they sometimes suggest another condition. This applies particularly to abdominal radiographs. It is then always worth repeating the clinical examination at once to test whether this possible diagnosis would fit with the findings. It is true that this is the reverse way to interpret information but it is, nevertheless, often a good way to make a correct diagnosis.

The return visit

Sometimes the initial symptoms and signs are insufficient to make a diagnosis. In these circumstances time is an invaluable ally. If spontaneous improvement occurs over the ensuing few hours then the need to make a prompt diagnosis lessens; if the disease process progresses the symptoms and particularly the signs will worsen. In practice the clinician returns to examine the patient again 3 or 4 h after admission. If the symptoms and signs are worse the diagnosis will usually be apparent. If there is improvement, no surgical treatment is needed, but it is also probable that no specific diagnosis will ever be made. If there has been no change, a further examination a few hours later is needed. Some people call this approach 'active observation'.

There are two risks attached to a 'wait and see' policy. The first is that the passage of time may allow a complication to develop with a consequent increase in morbidity. The second is a lack of intellectual rigour: the clinician waits until the patient has recovered or until it becomes obvious that a laparotomy is essential and never bothers to make a clinical diagnosis.

Computer assistance

Only a clinician can obtain the information that is needed from a patient with acute abdominal pain and decide on the best form of management. This information has first to be analysed in order to make a diagnosis before treatment can begin. It is here that computers can help, although this help does not derive entirely from sophisticated data analysis. In the Western world the diagnostic accuracy of the first doctor who sees a patient with acute abdominal pain in hospital is about 45 per cent. Improving the quality of the information obtained by the rigid definition of symptoms and signs and the amount of information collected with the use of special forms increases this initial accuracy to 60 per cent. This figure can be improved to about 70 per cent by giving feedback about their accuracy to individual doctors and by computer analysis of the data from individual patients in comparison with a large database of information from patients with abdominal pain of known cause. When the results of investigations are available, accuracy further improves to 75 per cent. Performance is improved at every level of surgical experience, and the very best clinicians can make an accurate diagnosis of the cause of acute abdominal pain 80 per cent of the time. This improvement in diagnostic accuracy is also reflected in an improved outcome for the patient, with a substantial reduction in the number of normal or perforated appendices removed at operation and fewer serious surgical errors.

The pragmatic approach

The pragmatists claim that the diagnosis lies between acute appendicitis and non-specific abdominal pain in two-thirds of the patients; the former need an operation whereas the latter do not.

They also claim that many of the remaining one-third of patients with another diagnosis will benefit from a laparotomy when the signs indicate that one is needed. The clinician faced with a patient with acute abdominal pain therefore has only one decision to make. Do the symptoms and signs justify a laparotomy? If the answer is yes then the diagnosis will become obvious at operation. If the answer is no then a period of active observation is all that is needed. The main disadvantages are a high negative laparotomy rate and the complications that ensue from inappropriate operations.

There are occasions when a practical approach has to be adopted. It may be obvious that a laparotomy is essential, but a diagnosis cannot be made because the patient is unconscious or is too ill to co-operate. Alternatively there may be no time to make a complete diagnosis. This will certainly be the case when the available surgical services are overwhelmed by multiple casualties. Absent bowel sounds as an indication of peritonitis would often be sufficient justification for a laparotomy in these circumstances.

The use of analgesia

It is a good rule that patients with acute abdominal pain are not given analgesia until a diagnosis has been made and treatment planned. However, common humanity often demands that pain is relieved before a surgical opinion is obtained. Provided that the time of administration and the dose of the drug is recorded, an experienced clinician should not be deceived. Analgesia does not eliminate all the physical signs but it does subdue them and due allowance must be made. Once a diagnosis has been made every patient must be given adequate analgesia at once, whatever other treatment is planned.

Some patients cannot be properly examined because of the severity of their pain. Adequate analgesia, perhaps given intravenously, may then make an examination, and a more accurate diagnosis, possible.

Spot diagnosis

This is included only to be condemned. Immediately visible symptoms and signs in the abdomen can often be interpreted in several ways. Furthermore, the doctor who jumps to conclusions tends to make subsequent observations fit his chosen diagnosis rather than to analyse them dispassionately. There are no circumstances where an instant diagnosis of the cause of an acute abdomen should be made. It is simply not safe.

LEARNING TO MAKE A DIAGNOSIS

How does the young clinician obtain the skills to match those of his seniors in the diagnosis of acute abdominal pain? A determination to make the correct diagnosis on every occasion and plenty of experience are the basic answers but there are a few techniques that will help.

Recording the facts

Computer analysis has shown the importance of obtaining all, but no more than all, the necessary information to make a diagnosis. Whilst it is usual for the house surgeon or intern to record a complete case history, residents or registrars should confine themselves to recording in their own writing the facts relevant to the diagnosis. This forces the clinician to decide which facts are important and starts the process of excluding more information than can be processed. This is easier if a special data collection form is used.

Always make a diagnosis

The surgical trainee must always decide upon and write down one diagnosis even if a list of other alternatives is appended. After all, a single diagnosis will become essential as soon as the trainee takes on the responsibility for deciding on treatment. To begin with the diagnosis will be wrong at least half the time, but as confidence and experience is gained this figure will improve.

Reporting to a senior

Asking a senior colleague for advice about the diagnosis and management of a patient is always good training. The discipline of putting the right facts together in a logical order and presenting them correctly is excellent practice at analysing the information.

Review the analysis

It is always worth comparing the findings on admission with the final diagnosis. It is often possible to identify where a sign or symptom was misinterpreted and also to appreciate that certain groups of findings correlate with certain diagnoses.

THE DIFFERENTIAL DIAGNOSIS

It is not the intention here to discuss in detail all the possible causes of acute abdominal pain. Rather it is to point out certain features which will help in the differentiation of the more common causes of pain and also to discuss a number of unusual problems which are not dealt with elsewhere.

There are various ways in which to classify the causes of acute abdominal pain. Bailey and Love compared the differential diagnosis of acute appendicitis to a house with two storeys corresponding to the upper and lower abdomen, the pelvis ('the basement'), the thorax ('the attic'), and the retroperitoneal structures ('the backyard') (Table 3). The underlying anatomical analysis is still useful, but in practice many experienced clinicians will first decide whether the features of the case suggest inflammation, obstruction, colic, a major catastrophe, or simply the presence of a mass. In many instances more than one pathology is involved. Inflammation can cause obstruction and unresolved obstruction will eventually lead to inflammation. Nevertheless the distinction is useful in practice because within each category there are then a number of possible causes for the findings.

Inflammation

Inflammation within the peritoneal cavity usually arises from one of the intra-abdominal organs although primary peritonitis does rarely occur in young girls. In most instances the inflammation is secondary to infection or ischaemia. Initially the inflammation is confined to the organ of origin and this makes the diagnosis easier as the physical signs will also be localized. Untreated and progressive inflammation will eventually lead to gangrene and necrosis, with consequent perforation of the viscus and the development of generalized peritonitis. Both the location of the initial signs and the speed of onset of generalized peritonitis will give a clue to the original site of the inflammation. The prognosis worsens with the progression of the pathology and so the clinician is always anxious to treat localized peritonitis before perforation occurs.

Localized peritonitis

Acute appendicitis

Many clinicians consider this to be a complete diagnosis in itself but in older textbooks acute catarrhal appendicitis, acute obstructive appendicitis, acute perforated appendicitis, and an appendix mass are all described as separate clinical entities. The last two certainly present a different clinical picture from the first two, and sometimes it is even possible to identify the colic and the vomiting which marks the start of an obstructed appendicitis. But with the exception of an appendix mass, where conservative management is usually preferred, the other three varieties all require an early operation so that differentiating between them is hardly worthwhile. Even so it is always wise to insist on adequate resuscitation of the patient with perforated appendicitis before surgery.

The other common error is to assume that all the patients with acute appendicitis present to a surgeon and, furthermore, that they all undergo appendicectomy. Acute inflammation sometimes resolves spontaneously, and acute appendicitis is no exception. A proportion of patients diagnosed as having non-specific abdominal pain probably have mild acute appendicitis, and a few such patients are readmitted a few days or weeks later with clear-cut appendicitis or an appendix mass.

Half the patients manifest all the classical symptoms and signs of appendicitis but the other half present in a variety of ways which varies from the misleading to the bizarre. The diagnosis is often difficult at the extremes of life and during pregnancy. The young may not be keen to reveal their symptoms and in the old there are often few physical signs. Stoical and muscular young men may have convincing symptoms but trivial tenderness. Pregnancy distorts the anatomy and the uterus can itself be the source of the pain. Diarrhoea and vomiting with abdominal pain will suggest gastroenteritis to most doctors, but they can be caused by appendicitis; appendicitis may also accompany gastroenteritis. The variable anatomical position of the appendix in normal people can also mislead the clinician. There may be few abdominal signs with pelvic appendicitis and the doctor who omits the rectal examination will miss the diagnosis. Retrocaecal appendicitis often causes microscopic haematuria due to inflammation of the adjacent ureter, and this can lead to an incorrect diagnosis of urinary tract infection or ureteric colic.

Bizarre presentations include a lumbar abscess from missed retrocaecal appendicitis, a perineal sinus from pelvic appendicitis, and appendicitis in the presence of an appendicectomy scar.

The list of differential diagnoses is very long: many conditions can mimic appendicitis, from right-sided pneumonia to salpingitis, and including a ruptured aortic aneurysm (Table 3).

At least one in five appendices removed at operation is normal on histology. This seldom matters, for another surgical cause for the pain is found at operation in about half these patients, although the complications that can ensue from an unnecessary operation should not be overlooked. A greater danger is to delay an operation until perforation has occurred, when the patient is worse, surgery is more difficult, and the complication rate is higher. The surgeon who never removes a normal appendix is undoubtedly exposing other patients to the risk of perforation.

Table 3 The differential diagnosis of acute appendicitis (after Bailey and Love 1962)

The attic
Pneumonia
Pleurisy
The upper storey
Perforated peptic ulcer
Acute cholecystitis
The ground floor
Gastroenteritis
Mesenteric adenitis
Intestinal obstruction
Crohn's disease
Meckel's diverticulitis
The basement
Salpingitis
Ectopic gestation
Ruptured luteal cyst
Twisted ovarian cyst
The backyard
Ureteric colic
Acute pyelonephritis
Ruptured abdominal aortic aneurysm
The electrical installation
Herpes zoster

Non-specific abdominal pain

Most patients with abdominal pain never discover the cause. Only about one patient in every 15 with pain is admitted to a hospital and of those who are admitted four out of every 10 leave without a diagnosis. Some patients find these statistics reassuring, but others find the doctor's inability to find a cause for their symptoms distressing. It is particularly important to reassure the latter group that a diagnosis of non-specific abdominal pain does not imply that there is no pain nor that there is no cause. The alternative title of non-surgical abdominal pain is more accurate in the sense that these patients do not need an operation, but it is inaccurate since there may still be an underlying surgical problem.

The predominant symptom is always pain, but there is usually abdominal tenderness as well, often in the right iliac fossa. This normally implies peritonitis but the signs are never sufficient to justify the diagnosis. Some people call this peritonism implying thereby irritation of the peritoneum without inflammation; this term is best avoided as it has no true pathological explanation.

Such patients are usually actively observed and the symptoms and the signs subside as mysteriously as they came. Up to a point, therefore, it is a diagnosis of exclusion and one that is only made in retrospect, but there are a few pointers towards a positive diagnosis. Most of the patients are young and two-thirds of them are women. The pain is rarely made worse by movement, it rarely moves its position in the abdomen, and about one-third of patients will keep their eyes closed during the abdominal examination (the 'closed eyes' sign).

Some of these patients do in fact have minor versions of recognized clinical conditions such as mesenteric adenitis, threadworm infestation, gynaecological pain from ovulation, or torsion of a colonic appendix epiploicae. Incomplete intestinal obstruction may not be clinically obvious and it may resolve before the diagnosis is made if the loop of bowel releases itself or the adhesion tears. Obscure abdominal pain in the elderly, which is uncommon, is often associated with cancer, particularly of the colon. Social and psychological factors play a very important role in some patients. This is usually because of anxiety about the minor abdominal pains which afflict everyone at some time or another rather than being a primary cause in themselves.

Acute cholecystitis

This is usually an easy diagnosis to make and even easier to confirm with the use of ultrasound. In the developed world it is the most common cause of acute abdominal pain in elderly people and the third most common cause in the younger age groups.

There are three important circumstances in which the diagnosis is difficult. In the elderly the symptoms are sometimes obscure and the signs minimal. There is often no fever and the white cell count is normal. Acute acalculous cholecystitis can develop insidiously in patients who are very ill for another reason. They are often being fed intravenously in intensive care. Ultrasound can confirm the diagnosis but only if it is considered. The third difficulty arises when a patient gives a classical history of acute gallstone disease but has no stones on ultrasound examination, even though the ultrasound probe may identify the gallbladder as the source of the pain. Sometimes the gallstones are too small to be seen, and occasionally the patient has passed their only stone. The diagnosis is then only made in retrospect when the stones have either reformed or grown in size. Alternative explanations for acute right upper quadrant abdominal pain in the absence of gallstones are exacerbation of a peptic ulcer, renal colic, and chlamydial perihepatitis (the Curtis-Fitzhugh syndrome).

Acute pancreatitis

Sometimes acute pancreatitis can be confidently diagnosed on the basis of the patient's symptoms and signs. A raised serum amylase merely confirms the clinical opinion. Constant epigastric pain radiating to the back and bruising in the flanks or around the umbilicus, which can be very difficult to see, are the key features. At other times it is difficult to distinguish pancreatitis from other causes of upper abdominal peritonitis, particularly a perforated peptic ulcer. The problem is compounded because a mild elevation of serum amylase is sometimes seen with a perforation and also in patients with ischaemic bowel or acute cholecystitis. Acute cholecystitis and acute pancreatitis can occur together. In the acute management of the patient with pancreatitis it is rarely helpful to decide whether gallstones or excess alcohol are the cause. Inflammation tends to be less severe in patients when the acute episode is superimposed on chronic pancreatitis.

Pancreatitis can also suddenly develop after any abdominal operation, and it is then almost impossible to diagnose clinically. It presents simply as an unexplained failure to recover from the surgery, perhaps accompanied by vomiting for no apparent cause. The diagnosis is only made when the serum amylase is measured as part of a biochemical screen.

This reinforces the general point that it is always wise to measure the serum amylase in any patient with predominantly upper abdominal peritonitis and then to re-evaluate the patient in the light of the result. High serum levels generally support the diagnosis of acute pancreatitis; modest elevations demand consideration of other possibilities.

Acute diverticular disease

This may present in a variety of ways, the most common of which is acute localized inflammation of a diverticulum. Less common presentations are generalized peritonitis from perforation of a diverticulum, a pericolic abscess, intestinal obstruction from adhesions, a faecal fistula, and acute rectal haemorrhage.

Acute pain and tenderness in the lower abdomen are the hallmarks of acute diverticulitis. Initially the symptoms and signs are fairly widely spread, even into the upper abdomen, but as the inflammation resolves the signs tend to localize to the left iliac fossa. There is usually an alteration in bowel habit and often frequency of micturition. A rectal examination is essential as tenderness or even a mass may be palpable; the most important differential diagnosis is carcinoma of the large bowel. A barium enema or a colonoscopy is best deferred until the acute episode has subsided because of the risk of perforating the inflamed diverticulum.

Acute ileitis

Some patients operated upon for appendicitis have acute inflammation of the terminal ileum. Crohn's disease can certainly present in this way, although there is usually a history of diarrhoea and weight loss as well as the recent pain. Infection with *Yersinia enterocolitica* can also cause a self-limiting ileitis. The diagnosis is made by sequential serological studies.

Acute caecal diverticulitis

This is a rare condition which presents in a similar fashion to acute appendicitis. At operation the appendix is normal and a large mass is felt in the caecum or ascending colon. Most surgeons mistake this mass for carcinoma and so perform a right hemicolectomy. If the correct diagnosis is made resection is unnecessary.

Acute gynaecological problems

Rupture of an ovarian follicle, ectopic pregnancy, salpingitis, ovarian cysts, and fibroids are common gynaecological causes of acute abdominal pain. Most of them present with other abdominal symptoms and signs which lead to confusion and a mistaken diagnosis of acute appendicitis, but all of them can be diagnosed clinically. A vaginal examination is essential. Reliable early pregnancy tests and pelvic ultrasound are also valuable aids to diagnosis, as is laparoscopy.

Salpingitis is the most common gynaecological cause of lower abdominal pain in women. It is often bilateral, is often accompanied by a fever and a vaginal discharge, may be associated with an intrauterine contraceptive device, and tends to be persistent and recurrent. The normal rupture of an ovarian follicle in the middle of the menstrual cycle (mittelschmerz) is sometimes accompanied by sufficient bleeding to cause significant lower abdominal pain. The diagnosis can often be made on ultrasound by the presence of a small amount of fluid in the pouch of Douglas. The bleeding is rarely of any magnitude and no treatment apart from rest and analgesia is usually needed. Haemorrhage from an ectopic pregnancy is often frightening and can be lethal. The difficulty is that many patients do not even realize that they are pregnant. Tactful but specific questions about the possibility of pregnancy are essential: never forget that previous sterilization does not mean that further pregnancy is impossible. Clips come adrift, ties come undone, and tubes recanalize. The residual damage to the fallopian tube means that an ectopic pregnancy is more likely than usual.

Benign ovarian cysts twist; malignant cysts can rupture, bleed, infiltrate surrounding structures, and cause small bowel obstruction. Twisted cysts are easy to diagnose as there is a tender central lower abdominal mass arising out of the pelvis, although they are not always easy to distinguish from a degenerating fibroid.

Urinary tract infection

This can mean anything from severe acute pyelonephritis to mild cystitis. The symptoms and the signs vary accordingly. Mild cystitis rarely presents to a hospital, but pyelonephritis certainly does and right-sided infection is easy to confuse with acute appendicitis. Normally the urine is obviously infected on testing but occasionally acute inflammation of the renal parenchyma can precede urinary symptoms and the appearance of pus in the urine by a day or two.

A perirenal abscess and a pyonephrosis both give rise to abdominal pain, but there are usually many other physical signs to suggest the true diagnosis.

Testicular pain

Occasionally patients with testicular torsion present with lower abdominal discomfort as the predominant symptom rather than severe scrotal pain. Confusion only arises when examination of the genitalia is omitted as part of the abdominal examination. The symptoms of acute epididymitis and torsion of a testicular appendage usually focus on the scrotum rather than any abdominal pain.

Meckel's diverticulitis

It is an exceptional diagnostician who can separate Meckel's diverticulitis from acute appendicitis. It can be done because the abdominal tenderness lies closer to the midline than with classical appendicitis but there are no other distinguishing features. The difference is of no practical importance since the true diagnosis is soon apparent at operation.

Generalized peritonitis

Generalized peritonitis is easy to diagnose, but the causes are legion. Up to a point identifying the precise cause is irrelevant, because a laparotomy is mandatory if the patient is to survive. The diagnosis is then immediately apparent. However, any surgeon knows the difficulty of oversewing a perforated duodenal ulcer in a fat patient from a lower left paramedian incision, and one incision is better than two for the patient, leaving aside the benefits to the surgeon's pride. Any abdominal organ can rupture as a result of inflammation, ischaemia, or trauma and flood the peritoneum with blood, bile, urine, or intestinal contents. It is always worth trying to decide which fluid is present and from whence it arises.

Perforation of the gut with leakage of intestinal contents is the most common problem. Bowel content is the most irritant substance and gives rise to all the classical symptoms and signs of peritonitis. The three common causes are a perforated peptic ulcer, perforated diverticular disease, and perforated appendicitis. Stercoral perforation of the colon due to severe constipation is a rare variant of perforated diverticulitis. Distinguishing between the various causes depends on taking a very careful history to try and decide the symptoms at the onset of the illness and an equally careful evaluation of the abdominal signs. Some patients are simply too ill to co-operate. Patients with a perforated ulcer may give a history of indigestion or the consumption of ulcerogenic drugs. Sometimes it is possible to decide that the signs are worst in one particular area of the abdomen.

Blood, bile, and urine are all rather less irritant to the peritoneum and give rise to less marked physical signs. Blood, which usually comes from a ruptured spleen, an ectopic pregnancy, or a ruptured aortic aneurysm characteristically gives rise to tenderness and rebound tenderness but very little guarding or rigidity. Uninfected urine and bile can both be present in the peritoneum in large amounts with very few signs at all, although once infection is present the signs are usually very marked.

Obstruction

Intestinal obstruction

Abdominal pain, vomiting, abdominal distension, and constipation are a quartet of very obvious symptoms and signs which make the diagnosis of intestinal obstruction easy. If the patient's presentation to the doctor is delayed the hyperactivity of the bowel which is so obvious at the onset of the obstruction may have been replaced by paralysis, with disappearance of the colicky pain and any visible peristalsis.

Not every patient with obstruction requires immediate surgery; it is important to try and decide on the cause. Uncomplicated obstruction due to adhesions, which is now the most common problem, is best treated conservatively to begin with, as many episodes will subside spontaneously. An obstructed hernia, which means occlusion of the lumen of the bowel within the hernia, requires a prompt operation. Strangulation implies impairment of the blood supply to the bowel and also demands an urgent operation. It is indicated by a shocked patient with peritonitis as well as the signs of obstruction, although these will not be present if only omentum or extraperitoneal fat are trapped in the hernia. An inguinal or incisional hernia should be obvious, but it is extraordinarily easy to overlook a small tense femoral hernia in a fat patient. The various rare intra-abdominal hernias are rarely diagnosed before surgery.

Both adhesions and hernias usually obstruct the small bowel. Large bowel obstruction is most commonly due to cancer, usually of the colon but sometimes of the ovary. Volvulus of the bowel, either large or small, initially causes obstruction but strangulation rapidly supervenes if the bowel is not untwisted.

If there is doubt about the reality or the severity of an obstruction contrast radiograph examination is always helpful. A small bowel enema is a useful way to decide whether small bowel obstruction needs surgical treatment. A conventional barium enema will help to plan an operation for large bowel obstruction and will identify patients with pseudo-obstruction.

Rare causes of obstruction such as gallstone ileus, bolus obstruction from worms or foodstuffs, an obturator hernia, and malrotation are usually diagnosed at laparotomy, although there is enormous satisfaction in making such a diagnosis in advance. This is sometimes possible if the diagnosis is considered and the relevant symptoms and signs are sought.

Acute retention of urine

Acute retention of urine also presents with abdominal distension and pain but the patient will volunteer that he or she has not passed urine for some time. Most patients are male and elderly. The tense distended bladder is easy to see and to feel and there is instant relief when a catheter is passed. The soft flaccid bladder associated with chronic retention, which sometimes presents acutely, is much more difficult to feel or to percuss, and ultrasound is often of help. Sympathomimetic drugs, sometimes in small doses in proprietary medicines, and constipation are two factors which can precipitate acute retention in susceptible people.

Patients with pelvic peritonitis are sometimes sent into hospital with a diagnosis of acute retention. The inflammation has led to dehydration and severe oliguria along with lower abdominal pain and distension. The true diagnosis is often not made until a catheter is passed and only a small amount of urine is retrieved.

Colic

Abnormal contraction of smooth muscle causes the regular and intermittent pain which is called colic. Within the abdomen only the gut, the renal tract, the uterus, and the biliary tract cause such a pain. The site and the distribution of the pain are different in each case and so they are easy to tell apart except, sometimes, for right-sided renal colic and biliary pain. The most severe intestinal colic accompanies gastroenteritis, although it is a classic sign of small bowel obstruction. Stones are the common cause of renal and biliary colic, although blood clot and pus can cause ureteric colic quite as severe as that due to a stone. Most, but not all, women know when they are pregnant and are about to deliver a baby, but uterine colic due to a miscarriage or even severe dysmenorrhoea sometimes presents as acute abdominal pain.

A major catastrophe

A ruptured abdominal aortic aneurysm, acute haemorrhagic pancreatitis, and acutely ischaemic bowel are the three common conditions causing a patient to present at hospital severely shocked immediately after the onset of acute abdominal pain. Shock is also seen in any patient with significant intra-abdominal pathology who presents some time after the onset of their symptoms, but the history will usually identify the delay and lead to the correct diagnosis.

A ruptured aneurysm is never easy to feel in a hypotensive patient and severe acute pancreatitis is sometimes only diagnosed at laparotomy. Patients with dead bowel inside the abdomen look and sometimes smell as though they are dying, which in one sense is correct. Those with strangulated gut usually show signs of obstruction, while a mesenteric embolus is easy to diagnose if the patient is fibrillating but very difficult if the thrombus lies on the endocardium after a silent myocardial infarct.

A mass

Occasional patients with abdominal pain who present acutely have a mass in the abdomen on palpation. The first rule is to try and define the organ from which the lump arises and then to describe all the physical characteristics of the lump, remembering particularly to test for pulsation. An ovarian cyst and an obstructed loop of bowel are common causes of a lump; apart from these, lumps are rare. They can arise from any intra-abdominal organ. Most obscure abdominal masses are subjected to intense preoperative investigation; in reality they all require exploration at laparotomy, when their nature and their origin will be revealed. Even then all the preoperative predictions are sometimes found to be wrong.

Specific diagnostic problems

Abdominal trauma

The injured patient with a rapidly distending abdomen and signs of exsanguination obviously requires an immediate laparotomy. However, it is often difficult to decide whether a trauma victim has significant intra-abdominal injury. Most such patients have other injuries, a few are unconscious, and alcohol is a factor in some. Complaints of abdominal pain should always be taken seriously, even though few patients can give a good history and abdominal examination is limited because the normal responses are impaired. Some abdominal injuries, particularly intestinal injuries, do not become apparent immediately: repeated reassessment is therefore essential.

It is always worth establishing the mechanism of injury as this can give some indication of the likely damage. Direct blunt trauma in a car crash or from the handlebars of a pedal cycle, kicks, punches, and falls from a height can all rupture the kidney, the spleen, or the liver. A lap and diagonal seat belt will tear the small bowel mesentery if the lap belt lies too tight across the abdomen. A fractured pelvis can perforate the bladder, and is often associated with rupture of the urethra.

The feasibility of a complete examination will vary but the abdominal surgeon should certainly pay attention to the general condition of the patient, the other injuries sustained and, in particular, to the chest. Unexplained and persistent tachycardia and hypotension despite active resuscitation implies continuing haemorrhage. If the site of bleeding is not visible the blood is either in the chest or in the abdomen. Fractured ribs can damage abdominal organs as well as the lungs.

Peritoneal lavage is a useful indicator of the need for a laparotomy. Frank blood, intestinal contents, or heavily bloodstained lavage fluid clearly indicates the need for a laparotomy. The kidney is the organ most frequently injured by blunt abdominal trauma, and intravenous urography is essential in the management of traumatic haematuria. Too many surgeons have removed an injured but solitary kidney. Computed tomography of the abdomen can identify retroperitoneal injuries which are not apparent on clinical examination and will also demonstrate the extent of an injury within a solid organ.

In civilian life penetrating abdominal wounds are less common than blunt injury, but most of the former will require surgical exploration. It is usually impossible to tell how far a wound has penetrated and no simple investigation, except perhaps laparoscopy, is helpful.

Common sense must always be applied: in the trauma victim it is almost always better to 'look and see' rather than to 'wait and see' if there is a continuing possibility of a significant intra-abdominal injury.

Acute abdominal pain in children

Nine of 10 children with abdominal pain either have acute appendicitis or non-specific abdominal pain (Table 4). The other child is likely to have either a urinary tract infection or intussusception. Urinary infection presents with the classical symptoms of fever, frequency, and stinging pain on micturition. The diag-

Table 4 The causes of acute abdominal pain in children seen in hospitals in the developed world (after de Dombal 1991).

	Percentage of cases
Non-specific abdominal pain	62
Acute appendicitis	32
Urinary tract infection	2
Intussusception	1
Miscellaneous	3

nosis is only confirmed when pus cells are found on microscopy of a correctly collected urine sample and a significant number of pathogenic bacteria grow on culture. In contrast, intussusception rarely presents with all the classical signs of colicky abdominal pain, a palpable abdominal mass, and redcurrant jelly stools. Any infant—most patients are under 5 years of age—who develops severe intermittent acute abdominal pain manifested as acute episodes of screaming should be suspected of harbouring an intussusception. An ultrasound examination will confirm the diagnosis and an enema either with barium, which can also make the diagnosis, or with air may also reduce the intussusception.

Two conditions which may cause non-specific abdominal pain in children deserve particular comment. Constipation is often said to be the most common cause of abdominal pain, although few such patients reach hospital. In young children, in whom a rectal examination is to be avoided, it is perhaps permissible to make the diagnosis on a plain abdominal radiograph, although even this is unnecessary if faecal masses can be felt in the abdomen. Secondly, examination of the ears and the throat are as essential as palpation of the abdomen in young children: both tonsillitis and otitis media can present with abdominal pain.

The acute abdomen in the tropics

Acute appendicitis and non-specific abdominal pain are the most common causes of abdominal pain all over the world. Disease patterns vary, however, and few patients with non-specific pain are admitted to hospital in the third world.

Of the specifically tropical diseases only two are of real concern. Firstly infestation with worms is a significant cause of abdominal colic, and sometimes of intestinal obstruction. Secondly, pain and tenderness in the right upper quadrant are more likely to be caused by amoebic hepatitis with a liver abscess rather than acute cholecystitis. Amoebic colitis can present with all the signs of peritonitis but the typical shallow shaggy ulcers seen on sigmoidoscopy should make the correct diagnosis clear, When the inflammation is confined to the caecum ('typhlitis') the signs mimic acute appendicitis.

Unusual problems

The abdominal wall

Rectus sheath haematoma

This rare condition can mimic intra-abdominal pathology. The haematoma develops from rupture of the inferior epigastric artery in the lower half of the abdomen. Pregnant women are particularly affected; there is sometimes a history of injury, and the right side is affected twice as often as the left.

The onset of the pain is acute and it is often accompanied by nausea and vomiting. There is marked tenderness in the iliac fossa, and it is easy to misdiagnose appendicitis. Two physical signs will reveal the true diagnosis. It may be possible to show that the tenderness, and the swelling if there is one, is confined to the abdominal wall. Secondly bruising of the skin may be visible. Sometimes this only appears a few days later and it is often at a distance from the site of maximum tenderness.

Once diagnosed the haematoma will slowly resolve with rest; in patients who undergo surgery the diagnosis becomes apparent as the abdominal incision is made. It is then worth tying off the bleeding vessel; this is also needed in the rare patient in whom the haemorrhage does not stop.

Similar bleeding sometimes arises from spontaneous rupture of an intercostal artery. The dramatic bruising of the abdominal wall spreading round from the lower thorax, often in a segmental distribution, is unmistakable. The haematoma will normally resolve with rest.

Abdominal wall hernia

Small epigastric, periumbilical, and tiny incisional hernias which usually contain only extraperitoneal fat can be very hard to find and are surprisingly painful, even without strangulation of the contents. Epigastric hernias often cause peculiar digestive symptoms, which can lead to diagnostic confusion.

Medical causes of abdominal pain

Many patients who need an operation for acute abdominal pain also have other medical problems, and some strictly medical conditions are treated by surgeons simply because they usually present as a surgical problem. Here we consider those patients who present with an acute abdomen but the underlying cause requires the care of a physician.

Pulmonary problems

Inflammation of the pleura at the base of the lungs can present as abdominal pain because of irritation of the lower intercostal nerves which supply the abdominal wall. Pneumonia in the very young and the very old, and pulmonary embolism at any age, can present in this way. Usually there are some symptoms and signs referrable to the chest, although in infants pneumonia may only be diagnosed on a chest radiograph.

Occasionally the chest abnormality is itself secondary to pathology below the diaphragm. Rarely, perforated diverticular disease produces minimal symptoms from the peritonitis but leads to some subphrenic infection. Pneumonia supervenes because of poor diaphragmatic movement and by the time the patient comes to the hospital the abdominal symptoms are long since forgotten. Conservative management of the abdominal problem is usually appropriate anyway, so the diagnostic error is rarely of serious consequence. Cholecystitis can sometimes present in the same way.

Cardiac causes

Occasionally pain from an acutely distended liver is the presenting feature of right-sided heart failure, although other physical signs are usually also present. Myocardial infarction is said, on occasion, to present with continuous epigastric pain. The main distinguishing feature is the complete lack of any epigastric tenderness.

Drugs

Warfarin and digoxin are the two common drugs that cause abdominal pain, although neither is as widely used as in the past. Digoxin toxicity presents with abdominal pain and vomiting. Warfarin anticoagulation can cause a spontaneous retroperitoneal haemorrhage with an associated paralytic ileus and severe abdominal pain radiating to the back. Haematuria is a clue to the diagnosis and the prothrombin time is usually excessively prolonged.

Diabetes

Very rarely diabetes mellitus first manifests itself with acute abdominal pain. The diagnosis is rarely difficult because the patient, who is usually an adolescent, is obviously severely ill with impairment of consciousness and marked dehydration. Sometimes the sweet ketotic smell typical of hyperglycaemic ketoacidosis pervades the whole examination room.

Hepatitis

Inflammation of the liver can sometimes cause intrahepatic cholestasis. If the acutely distended liver is also painful it is easy to think that the patient has extrahepatic obstructive jaundice. Both drugs and viral infections can produce this clinical picture, although the matter is resolved as soon as the bile ducts are of normal size on an ultrasound examination.

Blood

About half the children with Henoch-Schönlein purpura complain of abdominal pain. The pain is due to bleeding into the wall of the bowel and this can lead to an intussusception. The diagnosis will only be missed if the characteristic skin rash is absent. Spontaneous and painful intra-abdominal haemorrhage is also a feature of haemophilia.

Spurious abdominal pain

There are a few strange people in every society who enjoy being admitted to a hospital. Some of them are looking for a bed, some want drugs, some like attention, and a few need help. Most are well known to their own local medical services and some even achieve a wider notoriety.

Such patients usually present themselves in the accident and emergency department and give a dramatic history of some acute abdominal event. Renal colic, a potential rupture of the spleen, and a fall astride a bar are all popular. They can always simulate the necessary physical signs. They often appear in very severe pain. A tiny cut on the lip, a finger, or the genitalia is quite sufficient to produce haematuria. They will also claim to be allergic to intravenous contrast media so that it is impossible to confirm a diagnosis of renal colic. Many are admitted for observation and it may be some days before the true diagnosis is disclosed.

Many such patients are simply too good to be true. They fail to realize that it is exceptionally rare for any patient to have every recorded symptom of their chosen diagnosis. Most patients give an address which is a long way away and some describe themselves as lorry drivers. Other clues are early and repeated demands for opiate analgesia and many previous admissions to hospital. In the classical case of Munchausen's syndrome there are also multiple abdominal scars.

Even when the diagnosis is suspected it is difficult to confront the patient since doctors are naturally loath to accuse patients of lying. It is better to investigate the background by telephoning doctors who have treated the patient in the past, either in a hospital or in the community, and making it clear to the patient that this is taking place. Demands for pain relief should be met by the offer of non-opiate analgesics. Most patients simply leave the hospital, often without telling the staff, once this process of enquiry starts or when they fail to obtain the service which they were seeking.

CONCLUSION

The patient with acute abdominal pain always presents the surgeon with the challenge of making the correct diagnosis. Without that diagnosis the right treatment cannot be offered.

Making the correct diagnosis is never easy. It demands attention to detail in taking the history and examining the patient and clarity of thought in analysing the information that is obtained. Investigations may help but in many places in the world there are no facilities for further investigation. There the management of every patient depends entirely on the clinical skills of the doctor. Finally every surgeon should remember that for every five patients admitted to a hospital with abdominal pain at least one patient has his or her diagnosis changed during the course of the admission and two leave the hospital without being given a cause for their pain. This does not mean that there was no cause. It does mean that our skill in making a diagnosis needs to be improved.

FURTHER READING

Adams ID, *et al.* Computer aided diagnosis of acute abdominal pain: a multicentre study. *Br Med J* 1986: **293**: 800–4.

Bailey H, Love M. Vermiform appendix. In: *A Short Practice of Surgery.* 12th edn. London: Lewis, 1962: 978–1002.

Campbell JPM, Gunn AA. Plain abdominal radiographs and acute abdominal pain. *Br J Surg* 1988; **75**: 554–6.

Cope Z. *The Early Diagnosis of the Acute Abdomen.* 9th edn. London: Oxford University Press, 1948.

de Dombal FT. *Diagnosis of Acute Abdominal Pain.* 2nd edn. Edinburgh: Churchill Livingstone, 1991.

De Dombal FT, Leaper DJ, Horrocks JC, Staniland JR, McCann Ap. Human and computer-aided diagnosis of abdominal pain: further report with emphasis on performance of clinicians. *Br Med J* 1974: **1**: 376–80.

Editorial. Analgesia and the acute abdomen. *Br Med J* 1979; **279**: 1093.

Field S, Guy PJ, Upsdell SM, Scourfield AE. The erect abdominal radiograph in the acute abdomen: should its routine use be abandoned? *Br Med J* 1985; **290**: 1934–6.

Gallegos N, Hobsley M. Abdominal pain: parietal or visceral? *J R Soc Med* 1992; **85**: 379.

Gray DWR, Collin J. Non-specific abdominal pain as a cause of acute admission to hospital. *Br J Surg* 1987: **74**: 239–42.

Gray DWR, Dixon JM, Collin J. The closed eyes sign: an aid to diagnosing non-specific abdominal pain. *Br Med J* 1988; 297:837.

Hockerstedt K, Airo I, Karaharju E, Sundin A. Abdominal trauma and laparotomy in 158 patients. *Acta Chir Scand* 1982: **148**: 9–14.

Hoffman J, Rasmussen OO. Aids in the diagnosis of acute appendicitis. *Br J Surg* 1989; **76**: 774–9.

Jones DJ. Appendicitis. *Br Med J* 1992; **305**: 44–7.

Jones PF. Active observation in management of acute abdominal pain in childhood. *Br Med J* 1976; **274**: 551–3.

Jones PF. *Emergency Abdominal Surgery.* 2nd edn. Oxford: Blackwell Scientific Publications, 1987.

McAdam WAF, Brock BM, Armitage T, Davenport P, Chan M, de Dombal FT. Twelve years' experience of computer-aided diagnosis in a district general hospital. *Ann R Coll Surg* 1990; **72**: 140–6.

Macartney FJ. Diagnostic logic. *Br NMed J* 1987; **295**: 1325–31.

Masters K, Levine BA, Gaskill HV, Sirinek Kr. Diagnosing appendicitis during pregnancy. *Am J Surg* 1984; **148**: 768–71.

Mohammed R, Goy JA, Walpole BG, Brentnall EW, Miller T. Munchausen's syndrome. A study of the casualty 'Black books' of Melbourne. *Med J Aust* 1985; **143**: 561–3.

O'Shea B, McGennis A, Cahill M, Falvey J. Munchausen's syndrome. *Br J Hosp Med* 1984; **31**: 269–74.

Paterson-Brown S, Vipond MN, Simms K, Gatzen C, Thompson JN, Dudley HAF. Clinical decision making and laparoscopy versus computer prediction in the management of the acute abdomen. *Br J Surg* 1989; **76**: 1011–13.

Paterson-Brown S, Eckersley JRT, Sim AJW, Dudley HAF. Laparoscopy as an adjunct to decision making in the 'acute abdomen'. *Br J Surg* 1986: **73**: 1022–4.

Paterson-Brown S, Vipond MN. Modern aids to clinical decision making in the acute abdomen. *Br J Surg* 1990; **77**: 13–18.

Puylaert JBCM, *et al.* A prospective study of ultrasonography in the diagnosis of appendicitis. *N Engl J Med* 1987; **317**: 666–9.

Raheja SK, McDonald P, Taylor I. Non-specific abdominal pain—an expensive mystery. *J R Soc Med* 1990; **83**: 10–11.

Sawyers JL, Williams LF, eds. The acute abdomen. *Surg Clin N Am* 1988; **68**: 233–476.

Sherck JP, McCort JJ, Oakes DD. Computed tomography in thoraco-abdominal trauma. *J Trauma* 1984; **24**: 1015–21.

Siddiqui MN, Abid Q, Qaseem T, Hameed S, Ahmed M. 'Spontaneous' rectus sheath ahematoma: a rare cause of abdominal pain. *J R Soc Med* 1992; **85**: 420–1.

Stewart J, Finan PJ, Courtney DF, Brennan TG. Does a water soluble contrast enema assist in the management of acute large bowel obstruction: a prospective study of 117 cases. *Br J Surg* 1984; **71**: 799–801.

Thomson HJ, Jones PF. Active observation in acute abdominal pain. *Am J Surg* 1986; **152**: 522–5.

Williamson RCN, Cooper MJ, eds. *Clinical Surgery International*. Vol. 17. *Emergency Abdominal Surgery*. Edinburgh: Churchill Livingstone, 1990.

Winsey HS, Jones PF. Acute abdominal pain in children: analysis of a years admissions. *Br Med J* 1967: **1**: 653–5.

Wyatt GM, Spitz HB. Ultrasound in the diagnosis of rectus sheath haematoma. *JAMA* 1979; **241**: 1499–1500.

29 Hernias of the abdominal wall

29.1 Inguinal hernias

RICHARD COBB

INTRODUCTION

An inguinal hernia is defined as a protrusion of part of the contents of the abdomen through the inguinal region of the abdominal wall. Inguinal hernias are common throughout the world, but precise figures for prevalence and incidence are not available. Hernias in the inguinal region account for approximately 75 per cent of all forms of hernias and are more common in males than females.

Inguinal hernias are classified as indirect, direct, or recurrent, and may be reducible or irreducible. The possible contents of an inguinal hernial sac and their viability also allow further descriptive terms (Table 1).

Table 1 Some definitions relating to the contents of hernial sacs

Reducible: the contents of the hernia sac return to the abdominal cavity

Irreducible:
- Incarcerated: viable contents
- Strangulated: ischaemic or necrotic contents

Sliding (hernia-en-glissade): part of the wall of the sac may be colon on the left, caecum on the right, or bladder on either side

Richter's hernia: a hernia that has strangulated a part of the intestinal wall, without compromising the lumen. Thus the absence of intestinal obstruction does not exclude strangulation

Maydl's hernia: a hernia containing two adjacent loops of small intestine, with strangulation of the segment between the loops
Littre's hernia: a hernia containing a Meckel's diverticulum

Reduction-en-masse: reduction of the hernial sac into the abdominal cavity, without reduction of the contents of the sac. This may be associated with strangulation that is missed.

ANATOMY

Consideration of the anatomy of the inguinal region is fundamental to understanding both the development of inguinal hernias and the methods of surgical repair (Fig. 1 (a,b,c)).

Inguinal canal

The inguinal canal passes obliquely downwards and medially from the internal to external inguinal rings. In adults the inguinal canal is 3 to 4 cm long. The normal contents of the inguinal canal are, in the male, the spermatic cord and the ilioinguinal nerve; in the female they are the round ligament and the ilioinguinal nerve.

Anteriorly is skin, superficial fascia, and external oblique aponeurosis. Posteromedially is the conjoined 'tendon' (rarely tendinous) formed from the common insertion of the internal oblique and transversus abdominus muscles to the pubic crest. Posterolaterally, under the arching structures of the conjoined tendon, lies the transversalis fascia. Inferiorly is the inguinal ligament, formed from the inferior free border of external oblique aponeurosis. According to North American texts, immediately deep to the inguinal ligament is a structure named the iliopubic tract (an aponeurotic band formed from the inferior margin of the transversus abdominis muscle and aponeurosis). The iliopubic tract extends from the fascia of iliacus and psoas laterally to the pectineal ligament medially, and is described in the Cooper/McVay repair. However, the iliopubic tract is not referred to in English anatomy texts, and does not feature in the Shouldice method of repair.

Internal inguinal ring

The internal ring is the point at which the spermatic cord or round ligament passes through the transversalis fascia to enter the

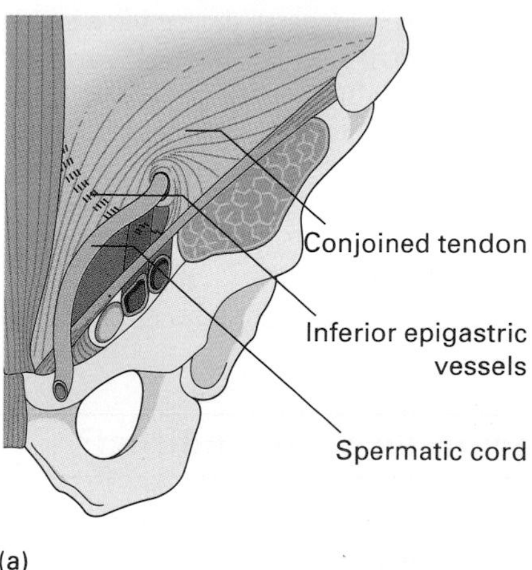

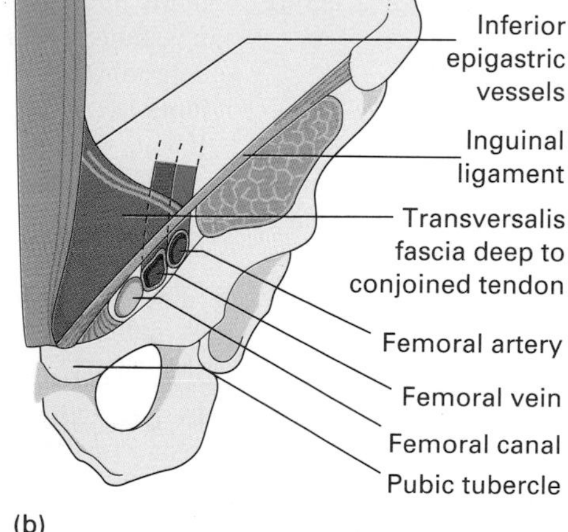

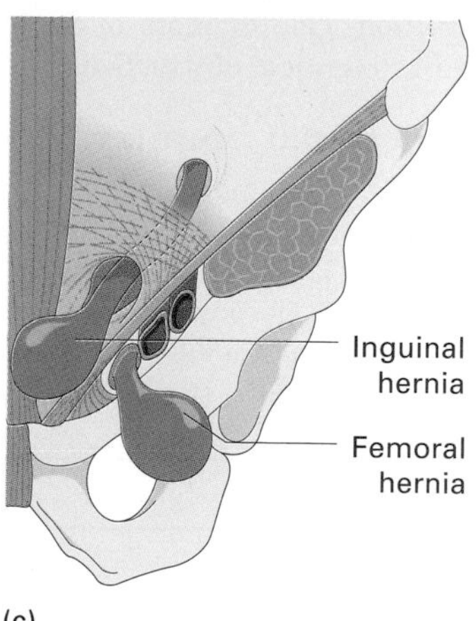

Fig. 1 The anatomy of the inguinal region.

inguinal canal. The transversalis fascia forms a U-shaped sling around the internal ring. This sling has two crura: the anterosuperior crus is in continuity with the transversus abdominis muscle and aponeurosis, and the posteroinferior crus is attached to the inguinal ligament/iliopubic tract. This U-shaped sling acts as a shutter when the transversus abdominis muscle contracts, preventing herniation in normal individuals.

The internal ring is bordered inferiorly by the inguinal ligament, medially by the inferior epigastric vessels, and superiorly and laterally by internal oblique and transversus abdominis. The surface marking of the internal ring, crucial in differentiating indirect from direct inguinal hernias, is 1.25 cm superior to the point midway between the anterior superior iliac spine and the pubic tubercle.

External inguinal ring

The external inguinal ring is a V-shaped defect immediately superior to the pubic tubercle, with the apex of the V superolaterally.

CLINICAL FEATURES

Symptoms

It is important to note the occupational history of the patient. Hernias often appear or become symptomatic in relation to strenuous physical activity. The symptoms of a hernia may limit ability to work: this is an indication for expeditious repair.

Local symptoms

Pain or discomfort may be present before a lump is noted by the patient. If pain develops in association with irreducibility of a previously reducible hernia, the contents must be assumed to be strangulated and emergency operation is indicated.

Many hernias are painless, and the patient notices a lump in the groin or scrotum. Some patients remark that the lump disappears after lying down or is largest at the end of the day.

Systemic symptoms

Colicky abdominal pain, vomiting, abdominal distension, and absolute constipation are the classical symptoms of intestinal obstruction. One or more of these symptoms is likely if a hernia causes intestinal obstruction.

Functional enquiry

Specific symptoms relevant to the development of hernias are any that indicate abdominal straining or raised intra-abdominal pressure. Thus, it is pertinent to enquire about persistent cough (commonly chronic bronchitis), difficulty with micturition (especially in middle-aged and elderly men) and constipation (more specifically, straining at defecation).

Signs

The diagnostic signs of a hernia are a lump that is reducible and has an expansile cough impulse. Accurate diagnosis that such a swelling is an inguinal hernia depends upon its position. Whether direct or indirect, inguinal hernias pass through the external

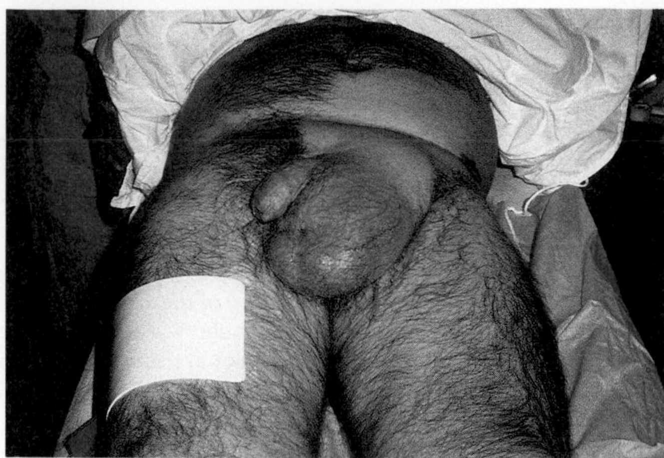

Fig. 2 A large inguinal hernia that has descended into the scrotum and is lying below and lateral to the pubic tubercle.

inguinal ring and are therefore always reduced through the abdominal wall above and medial to the pubic tubercle. However, large inguinal hernias often descend into the scrotum and may lie below and lateral to the pubic tubercle (Fig. 2).

A protocol for examination of an inguinal hernia

Both inguinal regions, and the scrotum must be examined with the patient standing and lying supine. If the former position is omitted small hernias, saphena varices, and varicoceles may be missed. The position, temperature, tenderness, shape, size, and consistency of groin and scrotal lumps must be determined during the course of clinical examination.

Inspection

Look for scars or any skin abnormalities as well as an obvious lump in either groin or the scrotum. Test whether a lump appears in the inguinal or femoral regions when the patient coughs.

Palpation

If a hernia is apparent on inspection, attempt to reduce it and decide whether it is inguinal or femoral by defining its relationship to the pubic tubercle. If the hernia is inguinal, determine whether it is indirect or direct (see Table 2). If a scrotal swelling is present, determine whether or not the lump has an upper border. If the lump has no upper edge, it is likely to be an inguinoscrotal hernia. If not, decide whether the lump is in the spermatic cord, the epididymis, the testis, or skin and fascial layers of the scrotum.

Percussion and auscultation

A hernia that contains gut may be resonant, and bowel sounds may be audible over it.

Is an inguinal hernia direct or indirect?

This question causes considerable anxiety, but is of little clinical significance. Not only does preoperative assessment of the type of inguinal hernia not affect management decisions, but even the most experienced clinicians reach the wrong diagnosis.

Table 2 Features distinguishing indirect from direct inguinal hernia

Indirect
1. Controlled at the internal ring
2. Often descends into the scrotum
3. Reduced upwards then laterally and posteriorly
4. The defect is not palpable
5. Appears at the mid-inguinal point, then expands medially and inferiorly

Direct
1. Not controlled at the internal ring
2. Rarely enters the scrotum
3. Reduced upwards then posteriorly
4. A defect may be palpable above the pubic tubercle
5. Appears medial to the mid-inguinal point, expanding anteriorly

An indirect inguinal hernia passes through the internal ring (i.e. lateral to the inferior epigastric vessels); direct inguinal hernias pass through defects in the transversalis fascia medial to the inferior epigastric vessels. Thus the cardinal distinguishing sign is whether or not the hernia is controlled at the internal ring. This is established by reducing the hernia fully, then applying pressure over the internal inguinal ring (1.25 cm above the midpoint between pubic tubercle and anterior superior iliac spine). If the hernia is controlled it is indirect; if not it is direct. Other features that distinguish indirect from direct inguinal hernias are summarized in Table 2.

DIFFERENTIAL DIAGNOSIS

Careful examination, with particular attention to anatomical relationships will distinguish inguinal hernia from most other lumps in the groin. A list of differential diagnoses, with distinguishing features is given in Table 3.

Table 3 Differential diagnoses of an inguinal hernia

Diagnosis	Distinguishing features
Femoral hernia	Below and lateral to pubic tubercle
Lymph node	No cough impulse Usually below inguinal ligament
Varicocele	Dilated veins in spermatic cord, visible with patient standing
Cyst of canal of Nuck (females only)	Able to get above lump
Hydrocele of cord (males only)	Not reducible
Undescended testis	Testis absent from scrotum May be associated with patent processus vaginalis

TREATMENT

Ideally all inguinal hernias should be repaired, but operation may be inappropriate for a few very unfit patients. In such cases the use of a truss may be considered. If prescribed, a truss must be properly fitted and maintained to avoid the potentially lethal application of a truss to a hernia that is not reduced. This may precipitate strangulation of the contents of the hernia.

Operations for inguinal hernia

There are many different techniques for the repair of inguinal hernias. Whatever method is used, meticulous technique is essential. The principles of repair are excision or reduction of the hernial sac, and repair of the posterior wall of the inguinal canal.

The hernial sac

Indirect hernias

For simple indirect hernias the sac is dissected out of the cord, transfixed at the internal ring, and excised. Sliding indirect hernias require dissection of the sac out of the cord so that the sac can be fully reduced, sometimes with excision of part of the sac distal to the sliding viscus. With large inguinoscrotal hernias it may be prudent to divide the sac at the internal ring, transfixing the proximal end and leaving the distal end open. Dissection of the sac of a large inguinoscrotal hernia out of the spermatic cord may result in a postoperative scrotal haematoma, and compromise of the blood supply to the testis.

Direct hernias

In all but very large direct hernias, the sac does not need to be excised. The hernia is reduced and the defect in the transversalis fascia closed either as part of the Shouldice technique, or prior to other methods of strengthening the posterior wall of the inguinal canal. If an obvious direct hernia is found, the spermatic cord must be opened and the cord carefully inspected at the internal ring. Even if there is no true indirect sac, there is usually a small crescentic peritoneal reflection (the remnant of the processus vaginalis). This reflection should be swept off the cord.

Repair of the posterior wall of the inguinal canal

The methods of repair may be classified in two broad groups: approximation or reinforcement of the structures of the posterior wall of the inguinal canal. The Shouldice technique combines elements of reinforcement with approximation, and is considered separately.

Approximation

The posterior wall of the inguinal canal may be repaired by approximation of the transversus abdominis aponeurotic arch either to the inguinal ligament (the Bassini technique, which has many variants) or to the iliopubic tract/Cooper's ligament (the McVay method). Both of these techniques were originally described using interrupted sutures. A relieving incision in the lateral aspect of the inferior part of the anterior rectus sheath is often required to prevent tension in the repair (Fig. 3).

Reinforcement

The posterior wall of the inguinal canal may be reinforced without tension (and therefore without requiring a relieving incision) by a loose but closely applied darn, the Shouldice method, or insertion of a prosthetic mesh. Prosthetic meshes are rarely used in primary hernia repairs, but are advocated by some surgeons for the repair of recurrent hernias.

Darns

Many variants of darn have evolved. Darns are between either Cooper's ligament or inguinal ligament and the conjoined tendon. It is important that the darn is secured superiorly to the tendinous

(a)

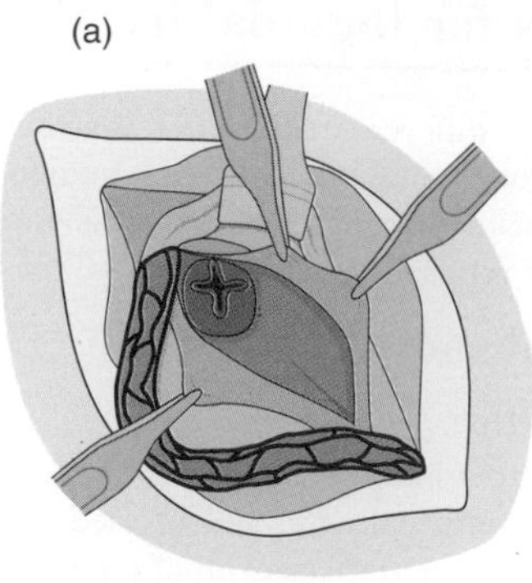

(b)

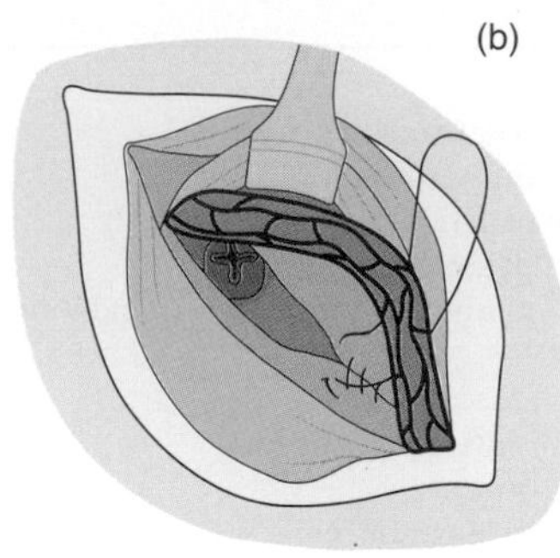

(c)

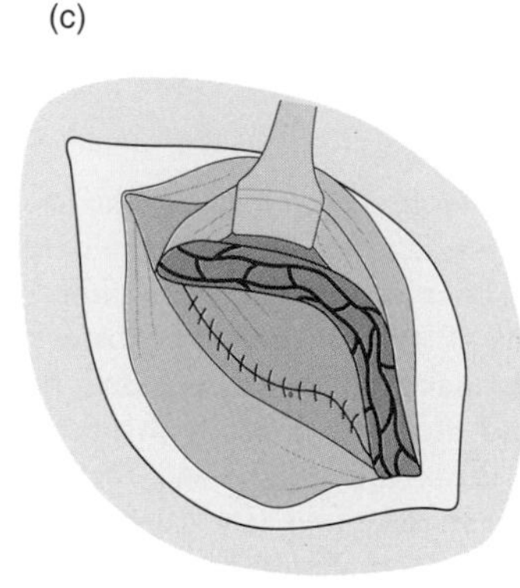

(d)

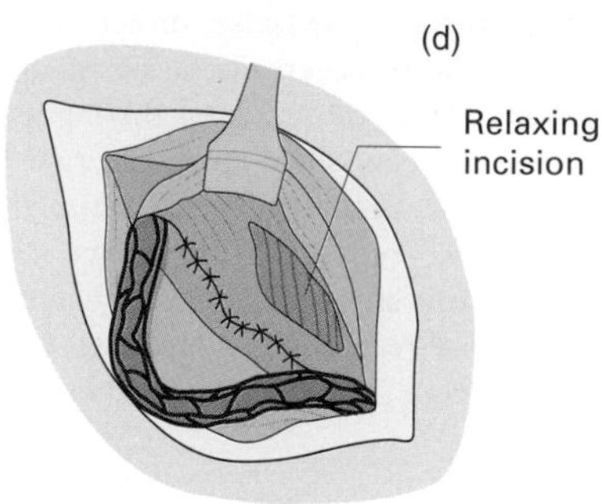

Fig. 3 The McVay Cooper's ligament operation: (a) clearing the anterior femoral sheath. (b) Suturing the transversus arch (fascia transversalis) to the iliopectineal line. (c) Continuing the repair by suturing the fascia transversalis to the anterior femoral sheath just proximal to the inguinal ligament. (d) The hernia repair opens the defect to the anterior rectus sheath (internal oblique and transversus tendons). The completion of the McVay Cooper's ligament repair with a rectus-relaxing incision.

aponeurosis of internal oblique/transversus abdominis rather than to the muscle. A variety of non-absorbable suture materials have been used. Initial strength is obtained by the darn itself. This strength is increased by fibrosis around the suture material used for the darn. Darns all share three features. First there must be no tension. This avoids the risks of either sutures tearing or development of a femoral hernia (if the inguinal ligament is used). Second, the suture should be continuous. This spreads the tension evenly. Finally, the lattice should have no defects (Fig. 4).

Shouldice technique

The method used at the Shouldice clinic differs from other repairs in two respects: the spermatic cord is freed at the internal ring by complete division of the cremaster muscle, and the posterior wall of the inguinal canal is repaired by dividing the transversalis fascia from the pubis to adjacent to the inferior epigastric vessels (which are preserved). The transversalis fascia is then 'double-breasted'. A continuous suture is employed starting at the pubic bone, attaching the free edge of the inferolateral flap to the undersurface of the superomedial flap of transversalis fascia. This extends to the internal ring, and the same suture is used to attach the free edge of the superomedial flap to the deep surface of the inguinal ligament working back to the pubic bone. A second suture runs from internal ring to the pubic bone and back again, bringing fibres of internal oblique and transversus abdominis to the deep aspect of the inguinal ligament (Fig. 5).

RECURRENT INGUINAL HERNIA

Incidence

The true incidence of recurrence following repair of inguinal hernias is difficult to determine: prolonged follow-up is necessary, and this is not feasible in most centres for logistic and financial reasons. In addition, there may be a bias towards reporting only good results. With these two caveats, the recurrence rates vary from 0.6 per cent reported in a personal series of 13 108 hernia repairs by Glassow to an estimate of 10 per cent of all hernia repairs performed in the United States of America.

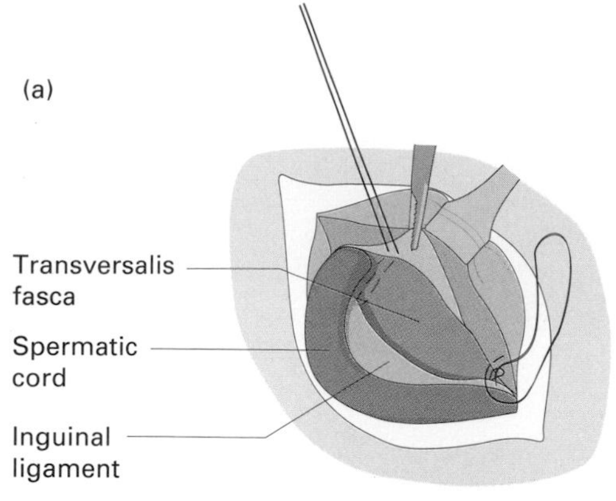

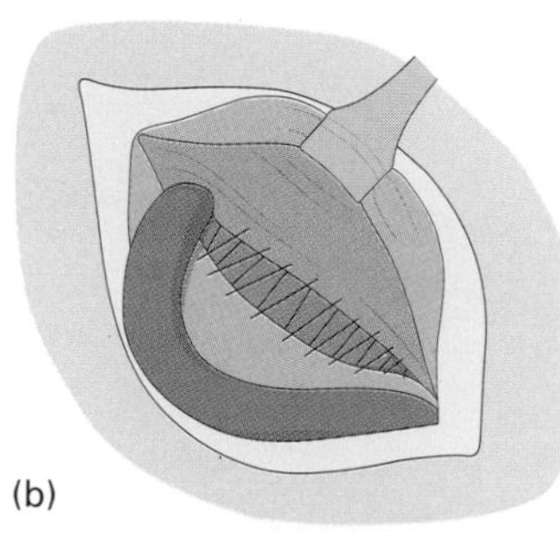

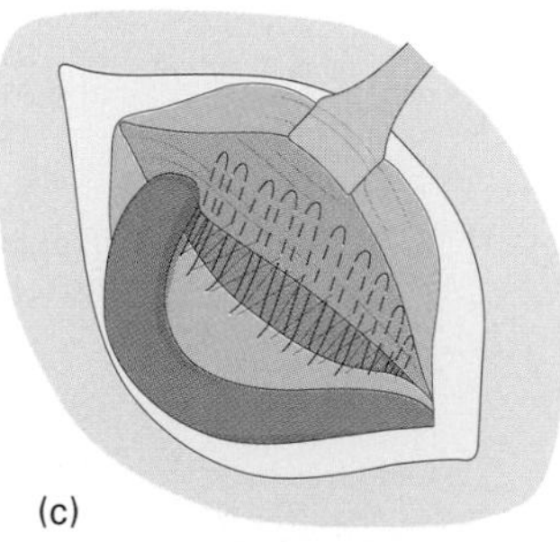

Fig. 4 Moloney's nylon darn repair of an inguinal hernia. (a) Initial suture reinforcing and tightening the internal ring. The start of the darn medially. (b) Loose continuous suture between the lower edge of the internal oblique muscle and the inguinal ligament. (c) Second layer of continuous suture, passing through the rectus sheath medially and the tendinous portion of the external oblique laterally.

Aetiology

Poor surgical technique is the most common cause of recurrence following primary repair of an inguinal hernia. The evidence for this is the wide variation in recurrence rate between reported series.

Wound infection following primary repair is associated with a high recurrence rate: meticulous asepsis is essential in hernia surgery. Persistent straining (cough, urinary outflow obstruction, or straining at defecation) is also a risk factor for the development of a recurrent hernia.

Surgical approaches to recurrent inguinal hernia

Direct repair after reopening the inguinal canal, except by the Shouldice method, is associated with a re-recurrence rate of greater than 2 per cent in all series. In contrast, insertion of a prosthetic mesh via a preperitoneal approach has a re-recurrence rate of less than 2 per cent in all series except one. However, no studies have compared these two methods directly.

Direct repair

The first step is to define the anatomy. This is often difficult because of the distortion and scarring caused by previous operations. Early identification of the external oblique aponeurosis well superior to the inguinal canal, and sharp dissection with a scalpel are useful techniques.

Small defects may be repaired by direct suture or onlay darn. For larger defects, the choice is between an onlay darn or insertion of a prosthetic mesh. Orchidectomy in the male (usually elderly) enables complete closure of the posterior wall of the inguinal canal.

The preperitoneal approach

The skin incision for the preperitoneal approach is placed superior to that used for primary repair of the hernia, and the preperitoneal space deep to the abdominal wall muscles is entered via an oblique incision in the rectus sheath with medial retraction of the rectus abdominis muscle (the McEvedy approach). This is an adaption of an earlier technique of lateral retraction of the rectus muscle (Cheatle/Henry). These approaches were originally described for the repair of femoral hernias, but access to the inguinal region is excellent, especially when the inguinal canal has been distorted by previous operations.

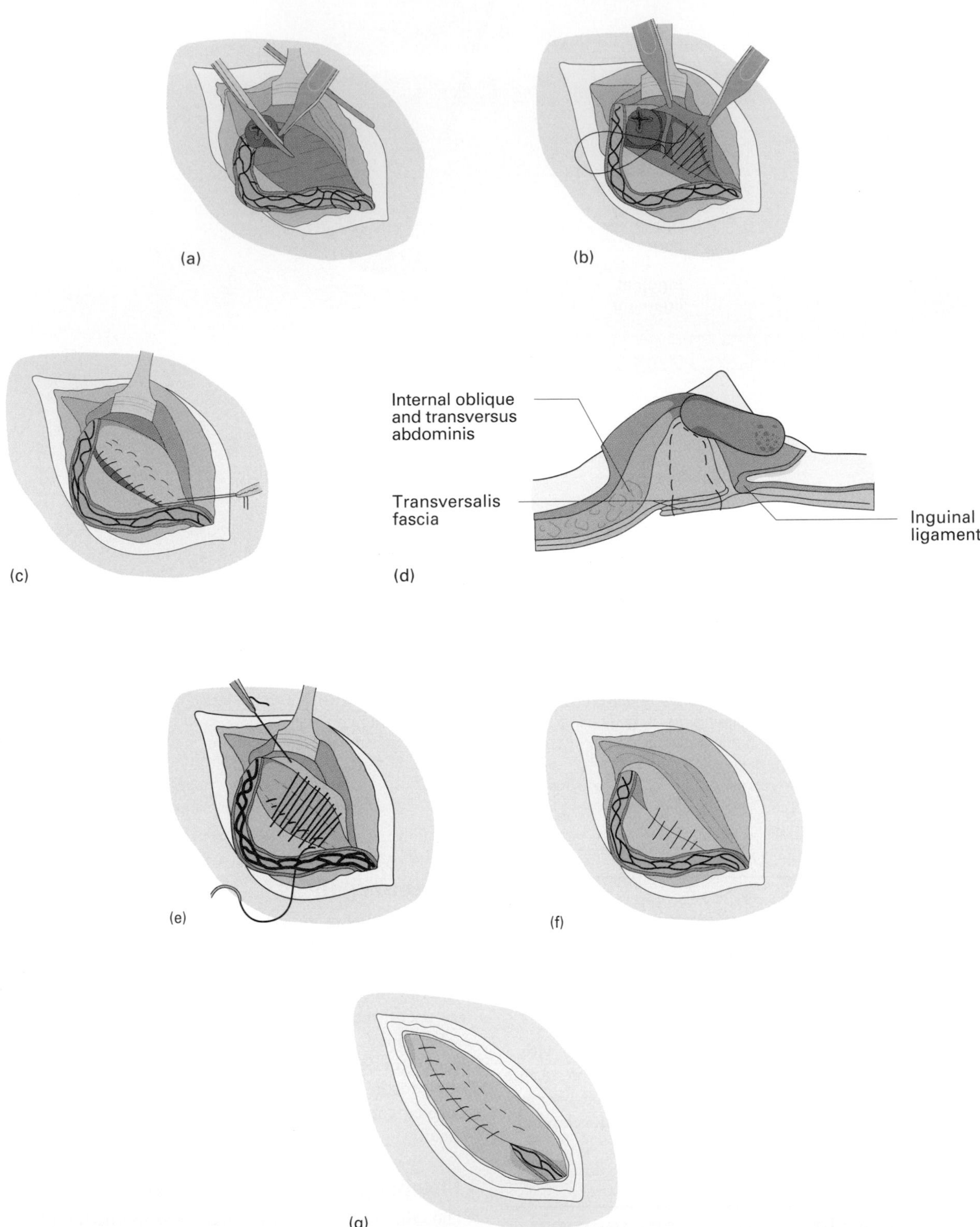

Fig. 5 The Shouldice repair. (a) Dissection of the fascia transversalis. (b) Suturing the lower lateral flap of fascia transversalis to the undersurface of the upper medial flap along the 'white line' or 'arch'. (c) and (d) Completing the overlap of the fascia transversalis repair. The margin of the upper medial flap is sutured to the anterior surface of the lower lateral flap. A neat closure up to the cord makes a new deep ring. (e) The aponeurotic, white part of the internal oblique tendon and the conjoint tendon are used to reinforce the repair. (f) The anterior aponeurotic surface of the internal oblique aponeurosis is loosely sutured to the aponeurosis of the external oblique. (g) The external oblique aponeurosis is closed, double breasted, anterior to the cord. Thus the inguinal canal is reconstituted with the cord obliquely traversing it.

The principle of the repair is to inlay a piece of prosthetic mesh (many types are available), securing the mesh to cover the inner aspect of the defect. This inlay technique has an obvious mechanical advantage over onlay meshes (placed in the inguinal canal) in that intra-abdominal pressure will plaster the former against the abdominal wall musculature and tend to push out the latter. Indeed some surgeons have placed prosthetic mesh via the preperitoneal approach without suturing, relying on intra-abdominal pressure to keep the mesh in place.

The main hazard of insertion of a large piece of mesh is infection. Scrupulous asepsis and prophylactic administration of broad-spectrum antibiotics are essential.

Laparoscopic repair of inguinal hernia

The recent rapid increase in laparoscopic access for surgical procedures has included use of this method in repair of inguinal hernias. A herniotomy equivalent is easily achieved, involving invagination, ligation, and excision of the hernia sac. This is only appropriate in indirect hernias with no muscular defect in the abdominal wall. Laparoscopic herniorrhaphy by insertion of synthetic mesh to eliminate the muscular defect associated with an inguinal hernia is now the procedure most widely used by surgeons who repair inguinal hernias laparoscopically.

However, all that has been proved to date is that the inguinal region can be operated on using laparoscopic methods. Proper evaluation must include comparison with standard methods in respect of early complications, hernia recurrence, and cost/benefit analysis. Such trials are in progress at this time.

FURTHER READING

Devlin HB. *Management of Abdominal Hernias*. London: Butterworth and Co., 1988.

Glassow F. Inguinal hernia repair using local anaesthesia. *Ann R Coll Surg Eng* 1984; **66**:381–7.

Inguinal Hernia. *Surg Clin N Am* 1984;**64**:

Nyhus LM, Condon RE, eds. *Hernia*. 3rd edn. Philadelphia: JB Lippincott Co., 1989.

Progress Symposium—Selected Topics in Hernia. *World J Surg* 1989;**13**: 489–596.

29.2 Femoral hernia

D. L. McWHINNIE

INTRODUCTION

A femoral hernia is a protrusion of peritoneum through the femoral canal. It may contain abdominal contents or extraperitoneal fat. Femoral hernias are the third most common type of groin hernia, after indirect and direct inguinal hernias and account for approximately 6 per cent of all abdominal wall hernias. They are twice as common on the right side as on the left. Although they are four times more common in women than in men, overall, the most common abdominal wall hernia in females remains the indirect inguinal hernia.

The aetiology of femoral hernias is unclear, although elevated intra-abdominal pressure and/or laxity of groin tissues is implicated. Femoral hernias are more common in parous than in nulliparous women and the incidence increases with advancing years, especially with those with weight loss, chronic cough, or constipation. Ten per cent of patients with femoral hernia have undergone previous groin surgery for inguinal hernia repair.

Femoral hernias may be described as reducible, irreducible, or strangulated. The higher incidence of irreducibility and strangulation in femoral hernias compared with inguinal hernias is related to the anatomy of the femoral canal.

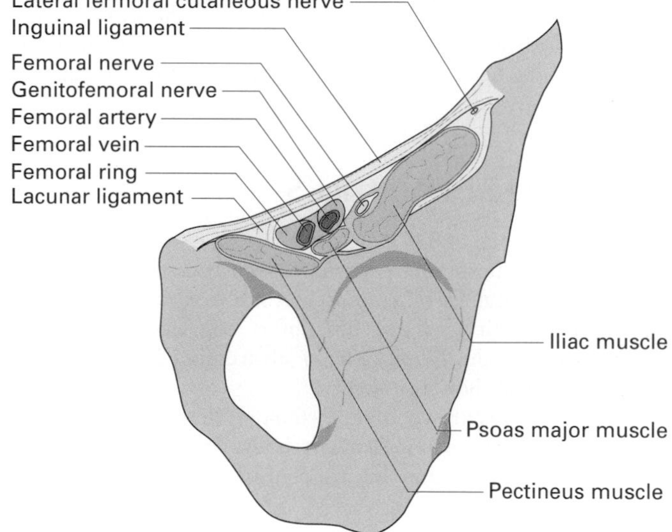

Fig. 1 Anatomical boundaries of the femoral canal.

ANATOMY

The femoral canal provides a conduit by which the femoral structures leave the abdomen and enter the upper thigh. The canal is bounded anteriorly by the inguinal ligament, posteriorly by the pectineal (Cooper's) ligament, medially by the unyielding lacunar ligament, and laterally by the iliopsoas muscle (Fig. 1). The contents of the canal consist of (from lateral to medial) the femoral nerve, the genitofemoral nerve, the femoral artery, and the femoral vein. Medial to the femoral vein lies the femoral ring, which contains loose areolar tissue, lymphatics, and the lymph node of Cloquet. The laxity of this tissue allows distension of the femoral vein during periods of increased venous return during exercise. The femoral vessels, but not the femoral nerve, are encased in the fibrous femoral sheath which is an extension of transversalis fascia. This forms a funnel extending down to the

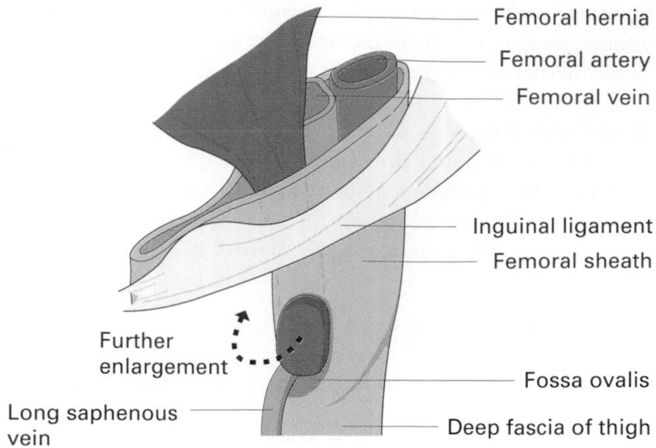

Fig. 2 Development of a femoral hernia. The hernia enlarges in the loose areolar tissue medial to the vein and emerges at the fossa ovalis. Fusion of the femoral sheath and the deep fascia of the thigh encourages the hernia to turn back on itself.

fossa ovalis where the long saphenous vein joins the deep femoral vein through the cribriform fascia.

The common site of a femoral hernia is through the femoral ring, in the loose areolar tissue medial to the vein. As the hernia enlarges within the femoral sheath, it emerges at the fossa ovalis (Fig. 2) and, by necessity, turns proximally into the loose subcutaneous tissue of the thigh. Distal progression is blocked by the fusion of the femoral sheath with the deep fascia of the thigh.

Although a femoral hernia may enlarge in the thigh, the femoral neck is bounded by the unyielding lacunar ligament medially. Any associated oedema of the hernial contents makes spontaneous reduction of the hernia unlikely, and progression to strangulation is common.

CLINICAL FEATURES

A reducible femoral hernia may present as an asymptomatic lump or as localized intermittent discomfort. If it becomes irreducible, the lump and localized discomfort become constant features. A mild pyrexia with localized discomfort suggests strangulated omentum within the hernial sac; if obstruction is also present strangulated small bowel is likely.

Richter's hernias are common in femoral hernias and result in strangulation of the antemesenteric intestinal wall without obstruction. Signs and symptoms are confusing and the diagnosing may be delayed.

Femoral hernias occasionally present with visible distension of the long saphenous vein. That indicates that the hernia has extended through the fossa ovalis and is compressing the saphenofemoral junction.

DIFFERENTIAL DIAGNOSIS

The differential diagnoses of a femoral hernia include inguinal hernia, groin lymph nodes, varicocele, maldescended testis, cyst of the canal of Nuck, or a hydrocele of the spermatic cord. The major feature distinguishing a femoral from an inguinal hernia is that the former lies below and lateral to the pubic tubercle.

TREATMENT

Conservative

Femoral hernias should not be treated conservatively: it is impossible to control the hernial neck with a truss and the incidence of strangulation is high, especially in elderly women. A non-tender femoral lump may be reduced by taxis in the shortterm but if any local tenderness suggesting strangulation is present, operative intervention is mandatory. Emergency repair of femoral hernias is ten times more common than elective operation. Elective repairs should not be delayed unduly.

Operative

The principles of femoral hernia repair, whether elective or emergency, are excision or reduction of the hernial sac, and narrowing of the stretched femoral opening.

Three approaches to femoral hernia repair are described, none of which is universally applicable.

The 'low' approach

This is suitable only for the uncomplicated small elective hernia in a thin patient. The incision is placed directly over the hernia, parallel to the inguinal ligament. The fundus of the sac often lies over the inguinal ligament, where it has turned proximally back on to itself. The various fascial layers are dissected and the neck freed circumferentially from the boundaries of the femoral canal. The fundus is opened and any contents of the sac inspected and returned to the abdomen. The sac is transfixed at its neck with an absorbable suture (Fig. 3) and redundant sac excised and allowed to recede into the abdomen.

The stretched femoral opening is narrowed by placing one or two non-absorbable sutures medial to the femoral ring, apposing the inguinal and pectineal ligaments (Fig. 4). A single figure-of-eight suture may also be used. This manoeuvre is most easily performed using a 'J'-shaped needle. The placement of these sutures is critical to the success of the procedure, as the femoral opening must be sufficiently narrowed to prevent hernial recur-

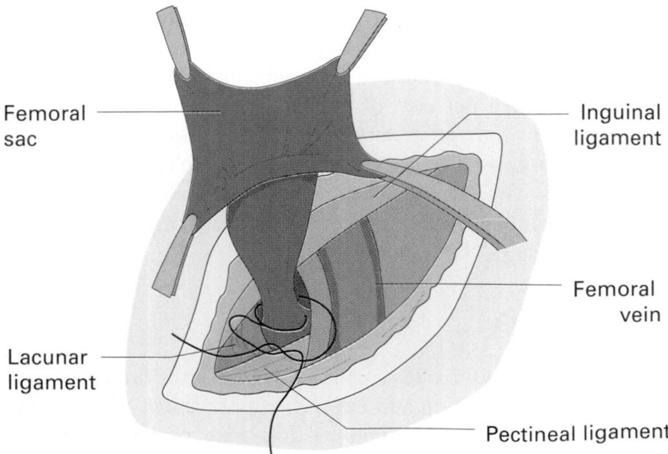

Fig. 3 The 'low' approach. The neck of the sac is transfixed and redundant sac is excised.

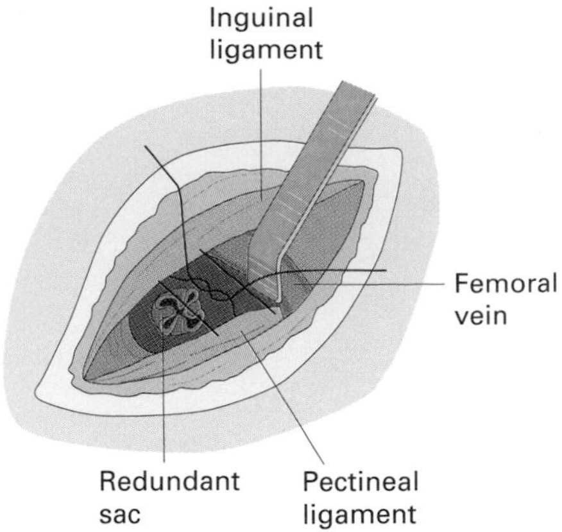

Fig. 4 The 'low' approach. Apposition of the inguinal and pectineal ligaments with a non-absorbable suture to narrow the stretched femoral opening.

rence, without compromising the femoral vein. On completion, the narrowed femoral opening should allow only the entry of the little finger of the hand. Further reinforcment of the apposed inguinal and pectineal ligaments has also been advocated, achieved by suturing an aponeurotic flap from the surface of pectineus muscle to the external oblique aponeurosis (Fig. 5).

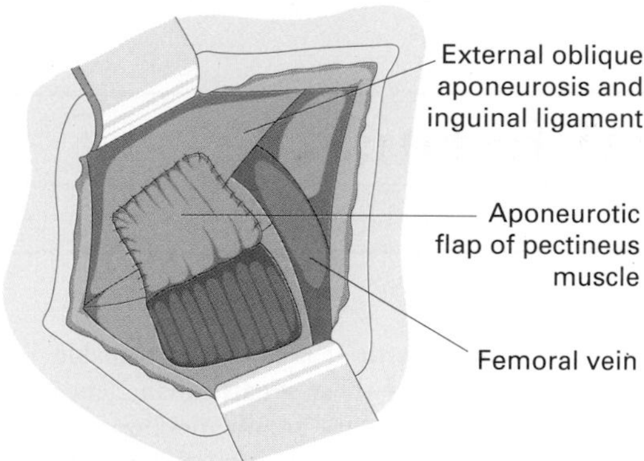

Fig. 5 The 'low' approach. Reinforcement of the repair with a flap of pectineus fascia.

The 'inguinal' approach

This is useful when a concomitant inguinal hernia needs to be repaired. It is obligatory when a femoral hernia is misdiagnosed as an inguinal hernia. The incision is the same as for an inguinal hernia. The femoral canal is approached through transversalis fascia on the back wall of the inguinal canal (Fig. 6). The femoral sac is delivered into the wound above the inguinal ligament and transfixed and excised (Fig. 7). The sutures to appose the inguinal and pectineal ligaments and narrow the canal are inserted on the pelvic aspect of the femoral opening. Closure of the tissue layers is then completed as for an inguinal hernia.

The 'preperitoneal' approach

This is mandatory for the emergency treatment of femoral hernia with obstruction or strangulation. It also allows better access for the elective repair of large or long-standing hernias, especially in obese patients. If, when using the low approach, a femoral hernia is found to be strangulated, an additional ipsilateral preperitoneal incision may facilitate inspection of the viscera or resection of the bowel. The rectus muscles are retracted through a pararectal or oblique incision (Fig. 8) to expose the extraperitoneal space. This is enlarged to identify the hernial sac entering the femoral canal.

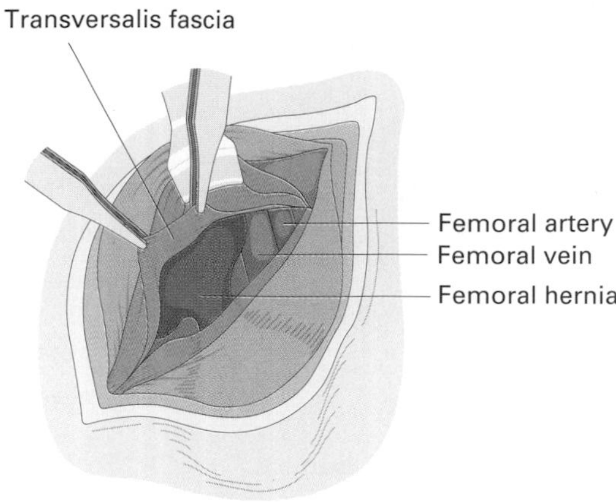

Fig. 6 The 'inguinal' approach. The femoral sac is mobilized through an incision in transversalis fascia.

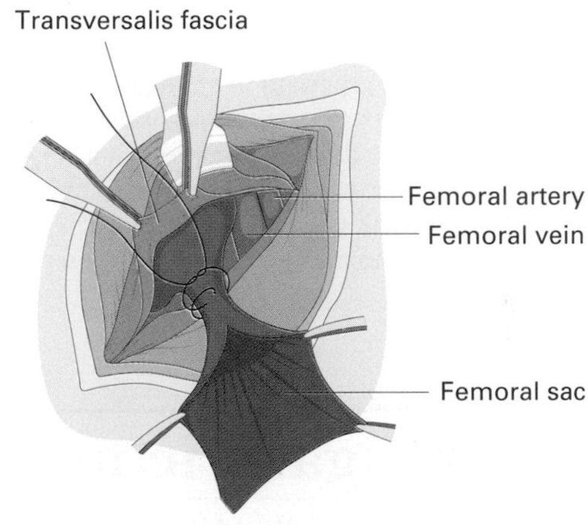

Fig. 7 The 'inguinal' approach. The femoral sac is transfixed at its neck and redundant sac is excised.

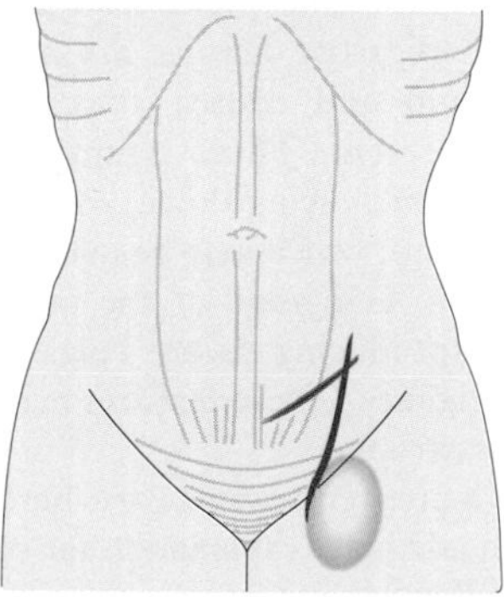

Fig. 8 The 'preperitoneal' approach. The hernia is approached through an oblique or pararectal incision.

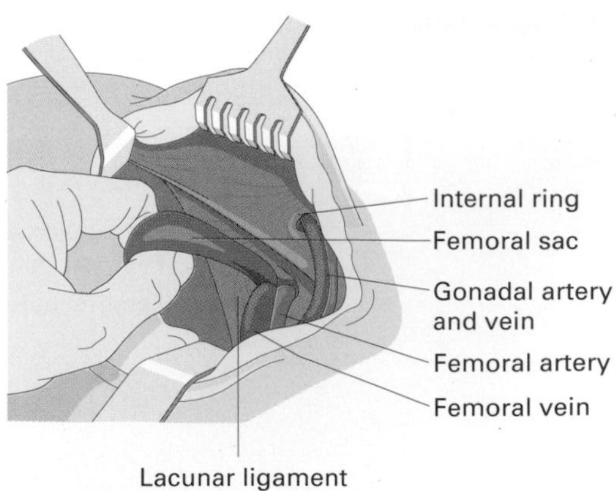

Fig. 9 The 'preperitoneal' approach. Viewed from within the pelvis, the hernial sac is delivered through the femoral opening.

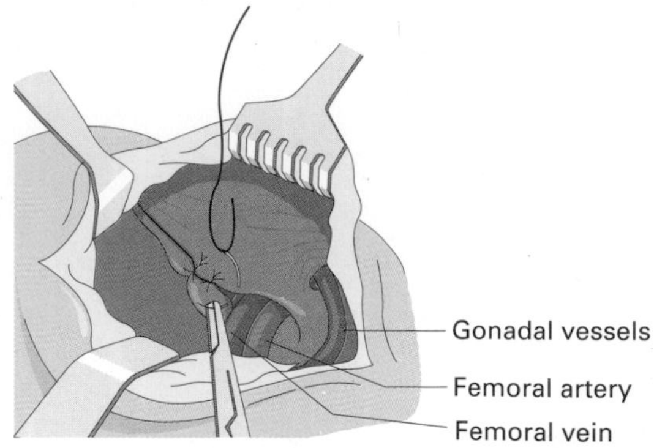

Fig. 10 The 'preperitoneal' approach. Apposition of the inguinal and pectineal ligaments to narrow the stretched femoral canal.

By sharp and blunt dissection, using external pressure on the hernial lump if necessary, the sac is returned to the pelvis (Fig. 9). The unyielding lacunar ligament often requires disruption to facilitate this manoeuvre, especially if strangulation is present.

The sac is opened and its contents are inspected. If bowel resection is necessary, exposure through this preperitoneal approach is more than adequate. The neck of the sac is transfixed and the redundant portion excised. As with the inguinal approach, the inguinal and pectineal ligaments are apposed by interrupted non-absorbable sutures on the pelvic aspect of the femoral canal (Fig. 10).

FURTHER READING

Devlin HB. *Management of Abdominal Hernias*. London: Butterworth and Co, 1988.

Nyhus LM, Condon RE, eds. *Hernia*. 3rd edn. Philadelphia: JB Lippincott Co, 1989.

29.3 Epigastric and umbilical hernia

HAMISH R. MICHIE AND ALAN R. BERRY

EPIGASTRIC HERNIA

An epigastric hernia is a protrusion of preperitoneal fat through a gap in the decussating fibres of the supraumbilical portion of the linea alba. The defect usually occurs where the linea alba is pierced by a blood vessel. A peritoneal sac may accompany fat through the defect and may contain omentum but only rarely bowel. This hernia may present at any age but is most common in adult males under the age of 40. An epigastric hernia is present in 5 per cent of individuals at autopsy; 25 per cent of individuals have multiple hernias.

The majority of epigastric hernias are asymptomatic. Vague upper abdominal pain and nausea associated with epigastric tenderness may be present. These symptoms tend to be more severe when the patient is lying down, owing to traction on the hernial contents. A lump, which may be tender, is usually palpable in non-obese subjects. Gangrene of the contents of the hernia occasionally occurs, producing severe epigastric tenderness and localized muscular rigidity. These features may mimic those of an intra-abdominal catastrophe.

The presence of a non-tender epigastric hernia should never be considered to be an adequate explanation for dyspepsia or epigastric pain except following extensive investigation of the upper gastrointestinal tract. Conversely, in obese patients with chronic upper abdominal symptoms an epigastric hernia may remain undiagnosed for years because it is often not palpable.

Symptomatic hernias and those greater than 2 cm in diameter are best repaired. The procedure entails mobilization and reduction of the protruding fat or peritoneal sac followed by closure of the defect in the linea alba with interrupted non-absorbable sutures.

UMBILICAL HERNIA

Three distinct types of hernia occur around the umbilicus: congenital (omphalocele or exomphalos), infantile umbilical hernia, and adult paraumbilical hernia.

Congenital (see also Chapter 36)

During intrauterine development the amniotic sac contains the embryological midgut. At 10 weeks of gestation the gut normally returns to the abdominal cavity. When this fails to occur normal rotation and fixation of the intestine is prevented. At birth the umbilicus is absent and a broad funnel-shaped defect in the abdominal wall is present through which viscera protrude into the umbilical cord. Peritoneum, but not skin, covers the protruding viscera. The peritoneal sac may rupture during, or shortly after birth. Defects less than 5 cm in diameter usually contain gut only (exomphalos minor) whereas defects greater than 5 cm usually contain liver and other viscera (exomphalos major). This condition occurs in 1 in 5000 births and is associated with other serious congenital abnormalities in 60 per cent of cases.

Urgent surgical repair should be performed before rupture of the sac occurs or infection supervenes. If the peritoneal sac has ruptured it is important to keep the bowel moist and protected with saline-soaked packs until prompt surgical repair can be performed. In exomphalos minor the viscera can usually be returned to the abdominal cavity with closure of the abdominal wall and skin defects. In exomphalos major the abdominal cavity is usually too small to allow return of the viscera and primary closure (attempts to achieve this usually resulting in respiratory embarrassment, obstruction of venous return, or intestinal obstruction). Initial treatment usually aims to cover the peritoneal sac with an artificial material such as a silastic bag which is sutured to the edges of the defect. This is followed by reduction of the contents as a staged procedure with eventual skin closure. Inevitably an incisional hernia results, which can be repaired in later childhood. Following such a staged closure it may be weeks or even months before normal intestinal function occurs and prolonged intravenous feeding may be necessary.

Infantile (see also Chapter 36)

At birth, following division of the umbilical cord the stump heals by granulation and scarring to fuse with the umbilical ring of the abdominal wall. Failure of fusion allows a peritoneal sac to protrude, usually at the superior margin of the ring. The infantile hernia, as opposed to the congenital type, is always covered with skin. This hernia is present in 10 per cent of caucasian infants (male:female ratio = 2:1) and 90 per cent of black infants. It is most common in premature babies.

This hernia is usually symptomless and presents as an easily reducible lump which becomes more prominent during crying and coughing. It rarely enlarges over time and will disappear in 93 per cent of children by the age of 2 years. The hernial contents usually remain virtually unchanged in size until just before final closure. Tapes, binders, and trusses to reduce the hernial contents are no longer generally advocated as they may lead to skin infection or necrosis.

Incarceration or strangulation of this hernia is extremely rare. Surgical repair is indicated if this occurs or if the hernia persists beyond the age of 2 years. Repair entails mobilization and reduction of the hernial sac followed by closure of the defect with one or two layers of interrupted non-absorbable sutures.

Adult paraumbilical hernia

This is an acquired hernia which occurs following disruption of the linea alba above, or much less commonly below, the umbilical cicatrix. Stretching of the abdominal wall due to obesity, multiple pregnancy, and ascites favour the development of this hernia. Deposition of fat in the abdominal wall in the obese may also be an aetiological factor. The condition usually occurs after the age of 35 and is five times more common in females.

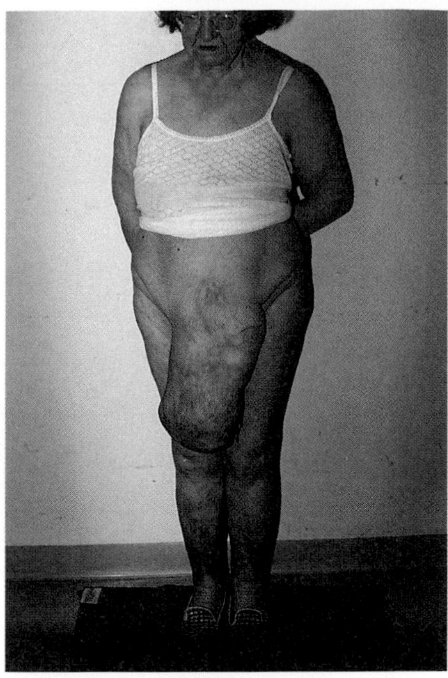

Fig. 1 A massive paraumbilical hernia.

This hernia tends to enlarge progressively over time and may produce localized dragging pain (Fig. 1). Gastrointestinal symptoms commonly occur due to traction between the hernial contents and the stomach and transverse colon. When the hernial sac contains bowel, colic due to intermittent intestinal obstruction is common. Intertrigo and necrosis of the skin may occur in patients with larger hernias.

The paraumbilical hernia usually has a small neck. Incarceration and strangulation are therefore common. Early operation is advisable. Repair comprises mobilization and excision of the sac following reduction of its contents. This is usually followed by the construction of flaps of rectus sheath and linea alba above and below the defect. The lower flap is then sutured under the upper flap. Finally, the upper flap is sutured anteriorly to produce a double-breasted repair (the Mayo repair).

FURTHER READING

Nyhus LM, Condon RE, eds. *Hernia*. 2nd edn. Philadelphia: JB Lippincott, 1978.

29.4 Rarer abdominal wall hernias

LINDA J. HANDS

OBTURATOR HERNIA

These hernias are uncommon: fewer than 600 were reported prior to 1980.

Anatomy

The hernia follows the obturator canal, a defect between the superior pubic ramus and the obturator membrane which normally transmits only the obturator nerve and vessels. The sac then spreads out deep to the adductor muscles in the groin, where it is difficult to detect clinically. The sac usually contains small bowel, often as a Richter's type hernia but occasionally including the complete circumference; less commonly omentum, colon, fallopian tube, ovary, or bladder are found. Strangulation is common because of the rigid neck to the sac.

Diagnosis

The majority of these hernias occur in elderly women who have recently lost weight. Sometimes straining because of constipation or other factors appears to be the immediate precipitating cause. The higher incidence in women is probably due to the wider pelvis, which changes the angle of the obturator canal.

Most patients present with acute groin pain; some also have abdominal symptoms, ranging from small bowel obstruction to mild and obscure discomfort. Approximately one-third report similar episodes in the past. The diagnosis is usually made during laparotomy for small bowel obstruction rather than preoperatively, mainly because the diagnosis is not entertained and the hernia itself difficult to palpate. Even if the correct diagnosis is suggested and the pathognomonic signs listed below are sought, they are positive in fewer than 50 per cent of cases.

1. Howship-Romberg sign—pain radiating to the medial thigh on extending, internally rotating, or adducting the hip.
2. Loss of the adductor reflex due to compression of the obturator nerve.
3. A hernial sac palpable as a tender mass on vaginal examination.
4. Bruising below the medial part of the inguinal ligament due to bloodstained exudate from a strangulated hernia.

In cases treated electively, usually with obscure groin pain as their only symptom, herniography may demonstrate the sac. Ultrasound is sometimes helpful.

Surgery

When the patient presents as an emergency with small bowel obstruction a laparotomy is advisable to allow bowel resection if necessary. Otherwise a preperitoneal approach is used. The hernia is found disappearing into the obturator canal and must be reduced by traction, the obturator canal being enlarged if necessary by incising posteromedial to the neck of the hernia, thereby avoiding damage to the obturator nerve. Bowel is resected if necessary, the sac inverted or excised, and its neck closed by suture. It may be possible to close the defect by direct suture but extra reinforcement is usually required. Bladder or non-absorbable Marlex mesh can be sutured across it.

There is a high mortality rate (13–40 per cent) in these patients because of their age, nutritional state, and coexistent diseases.

SPIGELIAN HERNIA

These are very uncommon.

Anatomy

The transversus abdominis muscle becomes aponeurotic at the semilunar line which stretches from the ninth rib to the pubic tubercle. Superficial to this muscle lies the internal oblique muscle, which splits lateral to the rectus muscle to run both anterior and posterior to it. The posterior layer is densely adherent to the transversus abdominis and forms the posterior rectus sheath. The lateral border of rectus muscle lies a variable distance medial to the semilunar line and the transversalis aponeurosis between the two, known as the Spigelian fascia, is an area of potential weakness. Furthermore it has bands of fibrous tissue running transversely; between these are well defined defects. It is through such a defect that a Spigelian hernia emerges, passing between the fibres of overlying internal oblique muscle and spreading out deep to the external oblique muscle. The hernia usually lies lateral to the rectus sheath and extends out towards the iliac fossa (Fig. 1); occasionally it lies within the sheath alongside the rectus muscle (Fig. 2). Only rarely does it penetrate the external oblique muscle to lie subcutaneously. The Spigelian fascia is only present in significant width below the umbilicus, and most Spigelian hernias occur in this region.

The sac may contain small bowel, colon, or omentum and may, like the obturator hernia, be a Richter's type hernia with only part

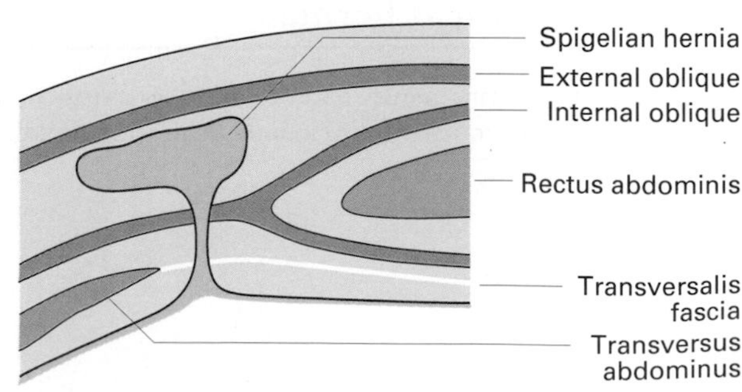

Fig. 1 A Spigelian hernia emerging lateral to the rectus sheath.

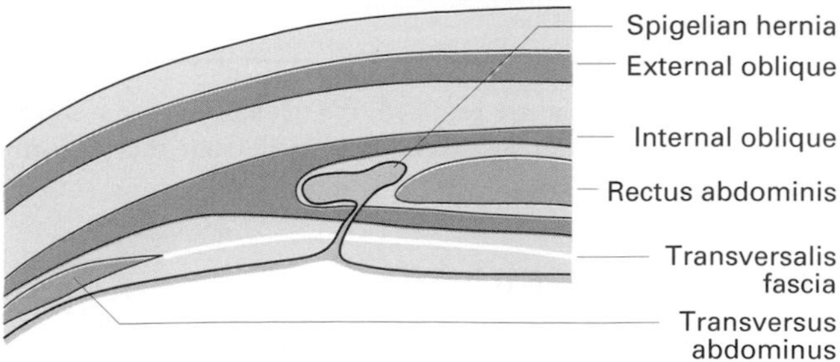

Fig. 2 A Spigelian hernia emerging within the rectus sheath.

of the bowel circumference involved. The rigid neck formed by the fibrous bands make strangulation common and repair is indicated wherever possible.

Diagnosis

The patient is usually over 50 years old and commonly female. The diagnosis is often difficult because the hernia is impalpable, especially in the plump patient, and the only symptoms are of obscure abdominal pain or small bowel obstruction. A mass with a cough impulse may be palpable in the iliac fossa when the patient is standing; this disappears on lying down. Twenty per cent of these hernias have strangulated at presentation and there is then a tender mass in the abdominal wall which may be difficult to differentiate from an abdominal wall haematoma, a muscle tear, or an intra-abdominal inflammatory mass, especially when associated with small bowel obstruction. However, in all cases there is localized tenderness over the neck of the hernia at the lateral margin on the rectus sheath.

Ultrasound and CT are equally useful in confirming the diagnosis. Herniography may give false-negative results and is of less use.

Surgery

This is a straightforward procedure when following confident preoperative diagnosis and localization. A transverse incision is made over the site, and external oblique fibres are split to expose the sac which is opened to check bowel viability. The defect can be enlarged laterally or medially to improve access if small bowel resection is required, or in order to reduce sac contents. The sac is excised and the defect closed by direct suture. If there is doubt over the diagnosis or location of the hernia then a vertical midline incision is made and an extraperitoneal approach made to the edge of the rectus sheath, where the hernia should be found disappearing through the Spigelian fascial defect. The contents are reduced, the sac excised, and the defect closed by direct suture from the inside.

LUMBAR HERNIAS

Massive incisional lumbar hernias often follow removal of an infected kidney with subsequent wound infection. These are the most common type of lumbar hernia; other forms occur infrequently.

Anatomy (Fig. 3)

In the area between the twelfth rib and the iliac crest a number of back and abdominal muscles come together and create an area of potential weakness. The likelihood of herniation depends on the extent of approximation or overlap of these muscles, and this is subject to individual variation. The area can be divided into the superior and inferior lumbar triangles. The inferior triangle (of Petit) is the usual site of congenital lumbar herniation, which accounts for 25 per cent of cases. The boundaries of this area are the iliac crest inferiorly, the latissimus dorsi muscle superomedially and the posterior boundary of the external oblique muscle superolaterally. Acquired hernias are rare in this area, except when both internal and external tables of iliac crest have been removed for bone grafting.

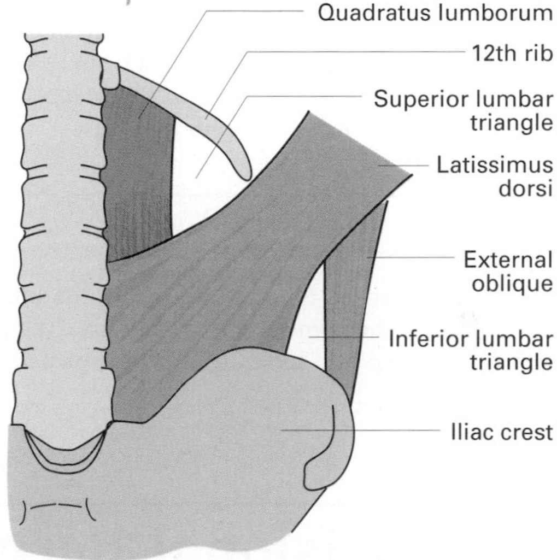

Fig. 3 The anatomy of the superior and inferior lumbar triangles.

The superior lumbar triangle is formed by quadratus lumborum, the twelfth rib, and the internal oblique muscle. It is the usual site of acquired hernias due to trauma (surgery, penetrating injury) or infection, or of those occurring spontaneously.

These hernias contain small or large bowel or omentum and have wide necks, so are at little risk of strangulation.

Diagnosis

Lumbar hernias usually occur in middle-aged men. They appear as a lumbar bulge that appears on standing and disappears on lying down, has a cough impulse, and over which bowel sounds may be heard. The only symptom is usually a dull ache.

Surgery

Surgery can be performed by a posterior approach with the patient in the lateral position, or through an anterior retroperitoneal approach. The sac is emptied, inverted, and can usually be closed off. Repairing the muscle defect is rather more difficult. If the hernia is small it may be possible to coapt adjacent muscles with non-absorbable sutures, but in most cases this is inadequate. Marlex mesh can be laid across the defect, preferably on its deeper aspect via the anterior, retroperitoneal approach. Alternatively a posterior approach is made with an additional vertical incision from the hernia down over the buttock, where a flap of fascia lata and gluteus maximus is mobilized and rotated up to close the defect.

SCIATIC HERNIAS

These are amongst the rarest of hernias.

Anatomy

The hernia sac finds its way out from the pelvis through either the greater sciatic foramen, above or below the piriformis muscle, or more commonly through the lesser sciatic foramen. The sac then lies deep to the gluteus maximus, where it is well hidden unless it is large enough to protrude below the buttock crease.

Diagnosis

This is usually made at the time of laparotomy for small bowel obstruction caused by the hernia. The bowel is seen disappearing out through a posterior pelvic defect, behind the broad ligament in women.

Surgery

The contents of the sac are reduced, the neck of the sac is ligated, and the defect covered by fascia mobilized from the piriformis muscle.

PERINEAL HERNIAS

Perineal hernias are uncommon. They occur through defects in the muscular pelvic floor and usually follow pelvic exenteration or abdominoperineal excision of the rectum. The hernial contents are usually small bowel or bladder and there are rarely associated symptoms.

Surgery

The usual approach is transabdominal. Once small bowel and bladder have been mobilized out of the way the defect is closed with Marlex mesh. If there is potential for infection synthetic implants are best avoided; gracilis muscle can be transposed from the thigh to form a sling across the defect via a perineal approach.

FURTHER READING

Beck DE, Fazio VW, Jagelman DG, Lavery IC, McGonagle BA. Postoperative perineal hernia. *Dis Colon Rect* 1987; **30**: 21–4.

Bjork KJ, Mucha P, Cahill DR. Obturator hernia. *Surg Gynecol Obstet* 1988; **167**: 217–22.

Devlin HB. *Management of Abdominal Hernias*. London: Butterworths, 1988.

Spangen L. Spigelian hernia. *Surg Clin N Am* 1984; **64**: 351–66.

29.5 Incisional hernia, including parastomal hernia

ADRIAN SAVAGE AND PETER M. LAMONT

INCISIONAL HERNIA

Wounds may fail in one of two ways. Wound dehiscence describes partial or complete disruption of an abdominal wound closure with protrusion or evisceration of the abdominal contents. Incisional hernia is defined as an abnormal protrusion of a viscus through the musculoaponeurotic layers of a surgical scar. Since the time at which a scar may be said to have formed is open to debate, the full healing of the skin incision is used to make a convenient distinction between wound dehiscence and incisional hernia. Dehiscence of the wound occurs prior to cutaneous healing, while incisional hernias lie under a well healed skin incision. A parastomal hernia is the result of an incisional hernia occurring adjacent to a surgically created stoma. In this section the epidemiology and management of abdominal wound disruption and incisional hernias, including parastomal hernias, will be discussed together. The factors contributing to these complications show similarities and wound dehiscence may be associated with the subsequent development of an incisional hernia.

Disruption of an abdominal wound occurs in less than 1 per cent of patients undergoing major abdominal surgery. Incisional hernia is more common, occurring in approximately 10 per cent of patients. The aetiology of wound failure is related to the preoperative condition of the patient, the technique of wound closure and postoperative complications.

Preoperative factors

The preoperative factors implicated in the aetiology of wound dehiscence and incisional hernia are age, male sex, previous irradiation, jaundice, uraemia, anaemia, diabetes, malnutrition, malignant disease, vitamin C depletion, obesity, and administration of steroids or cytotoxic drugs. Clinical studies of these variables in the aetiology of wound failure are sparse since they rarely occur in isolation. Experimental studies have, however, documented delayed healing of laparotomy wounds in uraemic and anaemic animals supporting a role for these factors in the aetiology of wound dehiscence. Some authors have reported malignant disease to be more common in patients with wound dehiscence (36 per cent) than in control patients (23 per cent), though others report no difference. There may also be an increased incidence of incisional hernia in patients with malignant disease. Jaundice is presumed to predispose to wound dehiscence because of its adverse effect on wound healing, but documentation of this is lacking. However, jaundice may be important in the subsequent development of incisional hernia. Malnutrition, as assessed by anaemia and protein depletion, increases the chance of wound dehiscence but probably not of incisional hernia. The role of obesity as a factor predisposing to wound dehiscence is supported by some but not others, in contrast to incisional hernia which is more common following laparotomy in the obese.

Operative factors

Norris wrote that 'the elimination of postoperative wound dehiscence is entirely within the jurisdiction of the operating surgeon'. The type of incision, the choice of suture material, and the method of wound closure are of major importance in the aetiology of wound dehiscence but less important in the development of incisional hernia. However, the exact role of each is obscure since the majority of studies have compared different suture techniques using different materials.

Type of incision

Wound dehiscence of appendicectomy incisions is less common than that of midline laparotomy incisions. There is a very low incidence of incisional hernia (0.37 per cent) and no wound dehiscence associated with the use of a lateral paramedian incision, but this approach is time-consuming to perform and not suitable for emergency situations. Midline, standard paramedian, and transverse incisions all have a similar incidence of incisional hernia. Upper abdominal incisions may be more prone to dehiscence than lower abdominal incisions. However, incisional hernia is considerably more common through incisions more than 18 cm in length and when a stoma is created through the wound.

Technique of closure

The theoretical advantages of a mass closure of abdominal incisions have found support in many clinical studies. For example, a 10.3 per cent wound dehiscence rate with layered closure with catgut has been reported and is to be compared with a rate of 0.93 per cent using a mass closure with interrupted steel sutures. The use of deep tension sutures to support a layered catgut closure was reported to prevent wound dehiscence but not subsequent incisional hernia. A reduction in the rate of wound dehiscence from 3.8 per cent to 0.8 per cent was reported on changing the technique of wound closure from layered catgut to mass closure with nylon or Dexon®. However, mass closure and layered closure of abdominal incisions are associated with similar rates of incisional hernia.

The technique of mass closure depends on the placement of sutures through all layers of the abdominal wall except the skin at a distance of more than 1 cm from the edge of the musculoaponeurotic layers of the anterior abdominal wall. Such sutures should not be placed more than 1 cm apart, and the total length of suture used in a continuous mass closure should be more than four times the length of the wound. The sutures should not be placed under tension, to allow for postoperative swelling of 30 per cent. Tension may be associated with ischaemia of the tissue enclosed within the mass closure and the development of incisional hernias.

Suture material

The use of catgut in the closure of all but appendicectomy wounds is now uncommon because of the high rate of wound dehiscence. Nylon suture is now most commonly used, since it is easier to handle than steel wire. The use of nylon sutures and a mass closure technique is associated with an incidence of wound dehiscence below 1 per cent. Jenkins reported only one dehiscence in 1505 abdominal wound closures. However, persistent wound sepsis and discharging sinuses have been associated with the use of non-absorbable sutures, and synthetic absorbable sutures that retain their strength far longer than catgut have certain theoretical advantages. Polyglycolic acid (Dexon®, polyglactin (Vicryl®) and polydioxanone (PDS®) have been used successfully for the closure of laparotomy wounds. The rate of wound dehiscence is comparable to that following mass closure with nylon, but there is no reduction in the rate of sinus formation and the incidence of incisional hernia is higher.

Postoperative factors

Increased intra-abdominal pressure due to inadequate postoperative analgesia, vomiting, the development of a postoperative chest infection resulting in coughing, and gross distension from paralytic ileus are important in the aetiology of both wound dehiscence and incisional hernia. Improvements in anaesthetic technique, postoperative care for the prevention of chest infection and good postoperative analgesia have contributed to the reduction in the incidence of wound disruption seen in recent years. Wound sepsis also predisposes to the development of wound dehiscence and incisional hernia.

Clinical features of wound disruption

Wound disruption may be occult or overt and partial or complete. Overt wound dehiscence follows removal of the skin sutures. The skin incision may partly or completely open to allow frank evisceration or show the presence of a herniation of bowel through a partial or complete defect in the musculoaponeurotic closure. Occult wound dehiscence occurs with disruption of the musculoaponeurotic layers beneath intact skin sutures.

Wound dehiscence is at least twice as common in men as in women and is more common in patients over the age of 60. Wound disruption occurs on the sixth to ninth postoperative day in over 55 per cent of patients. Twenty-one per cent of the dehiscences occur on removal of the sutures. The patient may show signs of gross dehydration, a rise in temperature and pulse rate, and a peripheral leucocytosis, especially if an occult dehiscence has been overlooked for more than 24 h. Signs of bronchopneumonia and meteorism may also be present. A copious serosanguinous discharge presages dehiscence in about one-third of patients. Alternatively, a boggy swelling or frank sepsis of the wound may be the only signs of dehiscence of the fascial layer.

Management of wound dehiscence

The first priority in the treatment of wound dehiscence is the correction of fluid depletion and electrolyte disturbance. Patients are often dehydrated, and cardiovascular collapse secondary to sepsis and shock from evisceration of the bowel must be treated prior to the administration of a general anaesthetic for repair of the dehiscence. If occult dehiscence is suspected, removal of skin sutures allows direct inspection of the fascial closure. While resuscitation is in progress, the dehiscence is covered by the liberal application of gauze swabs soaked in normal saline; a Velcro corset or many-tailed bandage may prevent further evisceration.

Confirmed dehiscence of an abdominal wound is best treated by resuture. At operation the skin sutures and the remnants of the previous fascial closure are removed. The edges of the wound are debrided of necrotic tissue and the wound resutured with a careful mass closure using No. 1 nylon. Gross abdominal distension may be due to an ileus or intestinal obstruction secondary to early formation of adhesions. Decompression of the bowel by retrograde milking of the intestinal contents into the stomach and nasogastric aspiration may considerably ease the process of closure of the wound; division of any obstructing adhesions is important.

Very rarely, the patient is unfit for surgery or the disrupted wound is too grossly contaminated to allow immediate surgery. Packing of the wound to return the bowel to the abdominal cavity followed by the application of strapping may allow the patient's condition to improve over a few days so that the wound may be closed as a secondary procedure. Wound dehiscence treated conservatively is inevitably followed by development of incisional hernia. Even after resuture, incisional hernia develops in almost 50 per cent of patients.

The prognosis of wound dehiscence is grave, and becomes worse with advancing age and with gross suppuration of the wound. Mortality rates of 24 and 15 per cent have been reported. The outcome is better if the wound disruption is recognized and treated early, in patients whose wounds are clean, and if prolapse of the intestine does not occur. Death is most commonly due to multisystem failure.

Clinical features of incisional hernia

Incisional hernias can develop at any age, although the mean age of patients developing this complication is 58 years, compared with 46 years for patients with intact wounds. Although clinical evidence of incisional hernia may be delayed for more than 10 years after laparotomy and less than 50 per cent of incisional hernias are apparent at 1 year, the use of radio-opaque markers has shown separation of the musculoaponeurotic layers as early as 1 month postoperatively in patients who subsequently develop incisional hernias.

The presentation of incisional hernia depends on the site of the original wound, the size of the neck of the hernia, the size of the hernia, and the presence of complications. Small defects in the scar may result in large hernias, and this may predispose to incarceration and strangulation. Large hernias are unsightly and may give rise to abdominal discomfort (Fig. 1). Pressure necrosis and ulceration may occur in the skin overlying a large hernia.

The majority of incisional hernias are asymptomatic, and the majority of symptomatic hernias may be managed by conservative measures. Obese patients benefit from weight reduction, since this reduces intra-abdominal pressure and may render a symptomatic hernia asymptomatic. Some patients find benefit from support by an elastic corset. In the fit patient, the indications for elective repair of incisional hernia are discomfort, enlargement, unacceptable appearance, or significant risk of strangulation. The presence of incarceration or strangulation is an indication for emergency surgery.

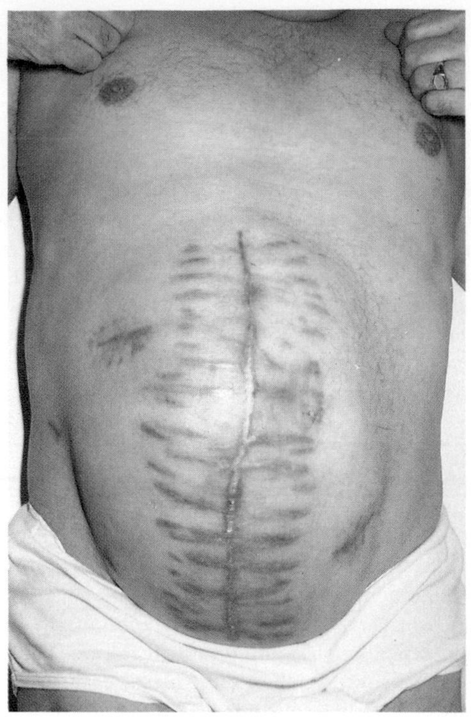

Fig. 1 Incisional hernia following laparotomy for peritonitis.

Factors which predispose to the development of incisional hernias are relative contraindications to repair. Weight reduction improves the chance of successful repair in obese patients. Cessation of smoking and optimization of respiratory function reduce the chances of postoperative cough. In patients with large incisional hernias, the contents of the hernia may have lost the right of domain in the abdomen: return of the contents of the hernia to the abdominal cavity may result in increased intra-abdominal pressure, splinting of the diaphragm, and a significant reduction in pulmonary reserve in patients with chronic respiratory disease. Recurrence of malignant disease, cachexia, ascites, renal failure, and hepatic failure are also contraindications to repair of an incisional hernia. The preoperative assessment of patients undergoing repair of incisional hernias is therefore important. Prophylactic administration of antibiotics is indicated to reduce the incidence of wound sepsis and the chance of failure of the repair.

Many different surgical approaches have been described for the repair of incisional hernias: no single technique is satisfactory for all hernias and surgical treatment has a high failure rate. The types of repair may be divided into five basic categories.

1. The defect may be repaired in the same way as a laparotomy wound is repaired, with a mass closure of No. 1 nylon.
2. The rectus sheath may be overlapped as in the 'Mayo' double-breasted 'vest over pants' repair.
3. The defect may be repaired by the use of a darn of nylon or fascia lata.
4. Lower midline incisions may be amenable to closure by swinging muscle over to close the defect.

5. Large defects may be repaired by implanting a non-absorbable mesh of tantalum, Marlex, Mersilene, or polytetrafluoroethylene (PTFE).

The initial steps in the repair of an incisional hernia are the same, irrespective of the technique used. Generally, the original incision is reopened, and it is often necessary to excise an ellipse of redundant skin. The skin and subcutaneous tissues are dissected from the hernia sac back to the defect in the musculoaponeurotic layers and 3 to 4 cm of the fascia around the hernia are exposed.

Mass closure of an incisional hernia may be appropriate if the defect can be approximated without undue tension. The peritoneum is opened, adhesions to the undersurface of the scar lysed to clear 3 to 4 cm on the peritoneal surface and the hernia sac, and its covering of weak scar tissue is excised. The hernia is then closed with a mass closure of interrupted or continuous non-absorbable suture such as No. 1 nylon. The sutures are placed according to the principles of mass closure of a primary wound. The repair may be reinforced by the addition of interrupted far-and-near sutures or with an onlay graft of Marlex mesh.

Opening of the peritoneum may result in postoperative ileus, and abdominal distension may compromise the security of the repair. In addition, dissection of the peritoneal and fibrous sac of the hernia may prove difficult and result in inadvertent enterotomy of underlying bowel. The 'keel operation' is an extraperitoneal repair for midline incisional hernias which avoids opening the peritoneum, minimizes postoperative ileus, and allows early mobilization. The hernial sac and the neck of the hernia are cleaned of fibrofatty tissue and the hernia is inverted by the placement of interrupted mattress nylon sutures to close the defect in the musculoaponeurotic layer. The use of relaxing incisions in the anterior rectus sheath should be avoided since the repair may fail through these incisions (Fig. 2).

The Mayo 'double-breasted' repair described for the repair of paraumbilical and epigastric hernias may be used to close small incisional hernias, especially if the direction of the original incision was transverse (for example, a hernia through an incision previously used for a transverse colostomy). After excising the hernial sac, the anterior rectus sheath is overlapped by a double layer of interrupted nylon mattress sutures so that the upper layer of the rectus sheath overlies the lower layer (Fig. 3).

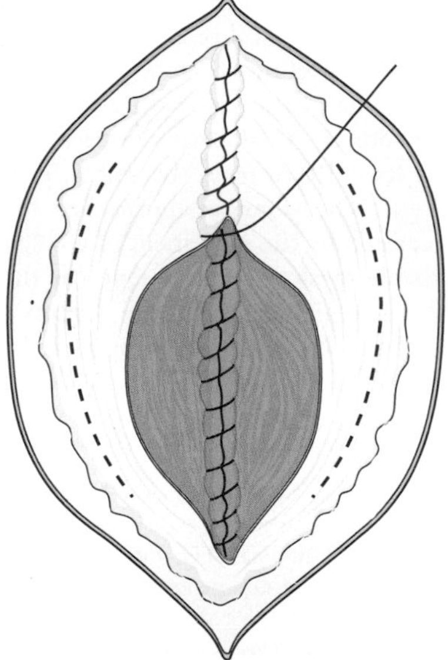

Fig. 2 The keel operation for extraperitoneal closure of an incisional hernia is performed by cleaning the edges of the hernia sac which is then inverted by two layers of interrupted mattress sutures. Relaxing incisions may be made as shown, but herniation through these incisions may occur.

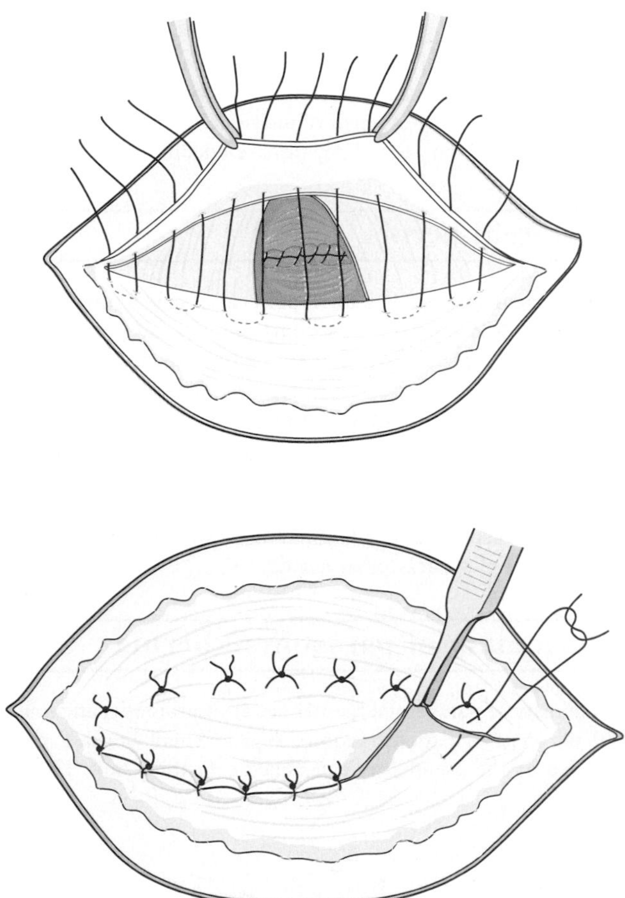

Fig. 3 The Mayo 'double-breasted' repair closes a defect by overlapping the upper part of the defect over the lower edge.

Fascia lata and nylon darn repairs have largely been replaced by the use of non-absorbable implants. However, midline incisional repairs may be repaired by incising the anterior rectus sheath 1 cm from the edge of the hernial defect on each side and suturing the medial edges of the anterior rectus sheath to invert the hernial sac. The repair is completed by placing a nylon darn between the lateral edges of the incision in the anterior rectus sheath.

Nuttall has described a repair of lower abdominal midline incisional hernias by overlapping the rectus abdominis muscle on each side. The anterior rectus sheath is incised on each side of the defect, and the rectus abdominis detached from its insertion as close as possible to the pubic symphysis. Each rectus abdominis muscle is then reattached to the opposite side of the pubic tubercle with nylon sutures, and the overlap of muscle loosely sutured together. The operation is completed by the closure of the anterior rectus sheath with non-absorbable sutures.

Large defects should be repaired by implanting a mesh of

non-absorbable material: the recurrence rate after mesh repair may be as low as 11 per cent, compared with 44 per cent after direct suture. Tantalum gauze has now been replaced with materials such as Marlex®, Mersilene®, and PTFE, though the last is expensive. The gauze is sutured to the edges of the defect in the musculoaponeurotic layers with a non-absorbable nylon suture. Both intraperitoneal and extraperitoneal placement have been described (Fig. 4).

A closed suction drain is placed deep to the skin closure and left until drainage has ceased. Postoperative care is as for any patient undergoing abdominal surgery, except that the patient is taught to sit up in ways which do not place tension on the repair. The recurrence rate following repair of incisional hernias is between 25 and 44 per cent, and second repairs are equally unsuccessful.

Parastomal hernia

Hernias develop alongside 5 to 10 per cent of colostomies and 3 to 10 per cent of ileostomies. Parastomal hernias are more common when the stoma is sited lateral to the rectus muscle than when the stoma is brought out through the rectus abdominis. The siting of a stoma in the incision used for laparotomy is associated with a very high incidence of incisional hernia. The extraperitoneal approach for the formation of a colostomy does not prevent the development of a parastomal hernia. A chronic cough, obesity, malnutrition, postoperative sepsis, and abdominal distension may predispose to the formation of a parastomal hernia.

Management of parastomal hernia

The majority of parastomal hernias are asymptomatic, and only 10 to 20 per cent of patients require repair. Small hernias may be controlled by the use of a well-designed colostomy belt. The indications for surgical intervention are mainly related to difficulties in maintaining the stoma appliance. If the hernia is large, it may be difficult to apply a bag. The patient may be unable to see the stoma because of a large hernia (Fig. 5). Reduction of the hernia on lying down and its prolapse on standing may cause the appliance to dislodge. The development of strangulation of a parastomal hernia is an absolute indication for repair. Some patients find large parastomal hernias cosmetically unacceptable. The contraindications to repair are the same as for repair of an incisional hernia.

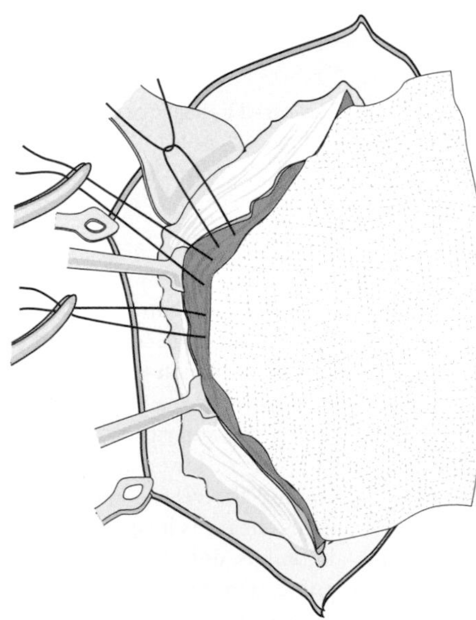

Fig. 4 Marlex or Mersilene mesh may be used to close a large defect. It is sewn in place with interrupted non-absorbable sutures. Usually, the mesh is placed outside the peritoneum but below the rectus abdominis.

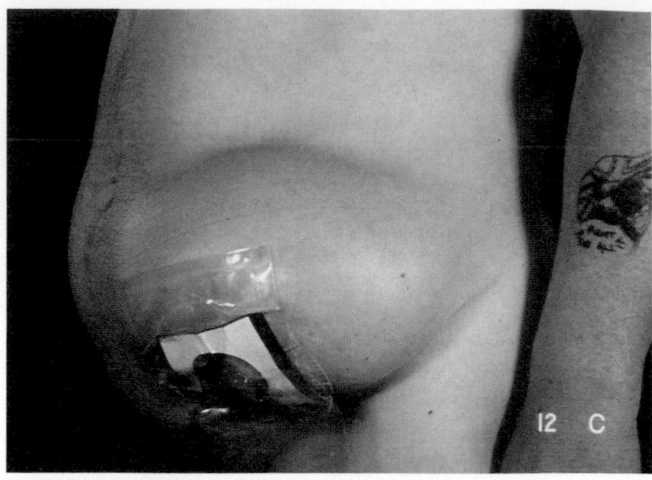

Fig. 5 A large parastomal hernia causing difficulty in the application of a colostomy bag.

Two surgical options are available for the repair of a parastomal hernia. The stoma may be resited elsewhere and the original stoma site closed, repairing the hernia at the same time: this is appropriate for patients in whom the original stoma site is unsatisfactory. In some patients who have had multiple abdominal incisions, however, the choice of sites for a stoma may be limited. Under these circumstances, local repair of the hernia is indicated.

Local repair may be performed via a peristomal incision. The defect in the abdominal wall musculature is then repaired with interrupted nylon sutures. An alternative is to approach the stoma via an incision at least 10 cm from the stoma, using the original laparotomy incision. The stoma is approached by subcutaneous dissection and repaired by the placement of a collar of Marlex or other non-absorbable mesh. The technique has the advantage of avoiding a fresh surgical incision in the vicinity of the stoma, which may cause problems with the fitting of an appliance.

FURTHER READING

Bucknall TE, Cox PJ, Ellis H. Burst abdomen and incisional hernia: a prospective study of 1129 major laparotomies. *Br Med J* 1982; **284**: 931–3

Donaldson DR, Hegarty JH, Brennan TG, Buillou PJ, Finan PJ, Hall TJ. The lateral paramedian incision-experience with 850 cases. *Br J Surg* 1982; **69**: 630–2

Dudley HAF. Layered and mass closure of the abdominal wall: a theoretical and experimental analysis. *Br J Surg* 1970; **57**: 664–7

Ellis H, Gajraj H, George CD. Incisional hernias: when do they occur? *Br J Surg* 1983; **70**: 290–1

Goligher JC, Irvin TT, Johnston D, de Dombal FT, Hill GL, Horrocks JC. A controlled clinical trial of three methods of closure of laparotomy wounds. *Br J Surg* 1975; **62**: 823–9

Grace RH, Cox S. Incidence of incisional hernia after dehiscence of the abdominal wound. *Am J Surg* 1976; **131**: 210–2

Greenall MJ, Evans M, Pollock AV. Midline or transverse laparotomy? A random controlled clinical trial. Part 1: Influence on healing. *Br J Surg* 1980; **67**: 188–90

Guiney EJ, Morris PJ, Donaldson GA. Wound dehiscence. *Arch Surg* 1966; **92**: 47–51

Lamont PM, Ellis H. Incisional hernia in re-opened abdominal incisions: an overlooked risk factor. *Br J Surg*; **75**: 374–6

Leaper DJ, Pollock AV, Evans M. Abdominal wound closure: a trial of nylon, polyglycolic acid and steel sutures. *Br J Surg* 1977; **64**: 603–6

Leslie D. The parastomal hernia. *Surg Clin N Am* 1984; **64**: 407–15

Maingot R. Umbilical and incisional hernia. In: Maingot R, ed. *Abdominal Operations*. New York: Appleton-Century-Crofts, 1980: 1618

Nuttall HCW. Rectus transplantation for midline incisional herniae. *Br J Surg* 1937; **25**: 344–50

Pearl RK. Parastomal hernias. *World J Surg* 1989; **13**: 569–72

Pollock AV, Evans M. Early prediction of late incisional hernias. *Br J Surg* 1989; **76**:953–4

Read RC, Yoder G. Recent trends in the management of incisional herniation. *Arch Surg* 1989; **124**: 485–8

Sjödahl R, Anderberg B, Bolin T. Parastomal hernia in relation to the site of the abdominal stoma. *Br J Surg* 1988; **75**: 339–41

Zrukowski ZH, Matheson NA. 'Button hole' incisional hernia: a late complication of abdominal wound closure with continuous non-absorbable sutures. *Br J Surg* 1987; **74**: 824–5

Index

Page numbers in **bold** refer to major discussions in the text and include major sections, subsections, and principal headings. Page numbers in *italics* refer to pages on which tables are to be found. 'vs' denotes differential diagnosis. This index is in letter-by-letter order, whereby hyphens and spaces within index headings are ignored in the alphabetization.

Abbreviations used in subentries (without explanation):

CT	Computed tomography
EBV	Epstein-Barr virus
ERCP	Endoscopic retrograde cholangiopancreatography
MRI	Magnetic resonance imaging
PDGF	Platelet-derived growth factor
PTCA	Percutaneous transluminal coronary angioplasty